D0845259

BROCKLEHURST'S
TEXTBOOK OF

Geriatric Medicine and Gerontology

fifth edition

BROCKLEHURST'S
TEXTBOOK OF

Geriatric Medicine and Gerontology

fifth edition

Edited by

Raymond Tallis, M.A., B.M., B.Ch., F.R.C.P., D.Litt.
Professor
Department of Geriatric Medicine
University of Manchester Medical School
Manchester, England
Honorary Consultant Physician
Department of Care of the Elderly
Hope Hospital
Salford, England

Howard Fillit, M.D.
Corporate Medical Director
Medicare NYLCare Healthplans, Inc.
Clinical Professor
Departments of Geriatrics and Medicine
Mount Sinai School of Medicine of the City University of New York
New York, New York

J.C. Brocklehurst, C.B.E., M.D., M.Sc., F.R.C.P. (Lond., Edin., Glas.)
Professor Emeritus
University of Manchester Medical School
Manchester, England

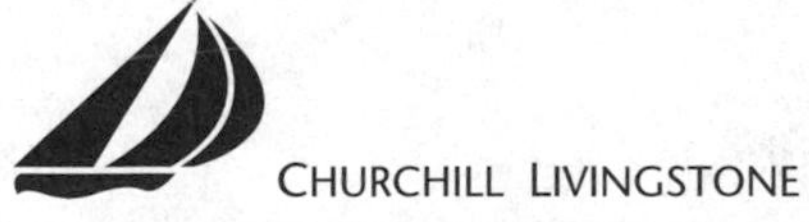

CHURCHILL LIVINGSTONE

Edinburgh, London, New York, Philadelphia, San Francisco, Sydney, Toronto

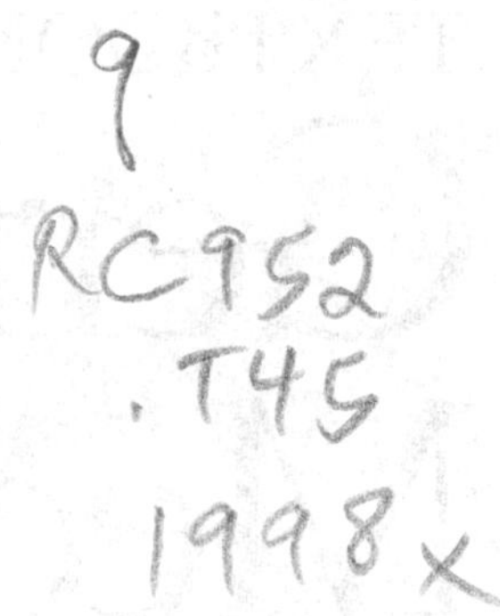

CHURCHILL LIVINGSTONE
A division of Harcourt Brace & Co. Ltd.

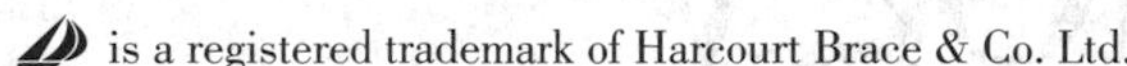

First published 1998

ISBN 0-443-05370-7

British Library Cataloguing in Publication Data
A catalogue record for this book is available from the British Library

Library of Congress Cataloging in Publication Data
A catalog record for this book is available from the Library of Congress

Medical knowledge is constantly changing. As new information becomes available, changes in treatment, procedures, equipment and the use of drugs become necessary. The editors/authors/contributors and the publishers have, as far as it is possible, taken care to ensure that the information given in this text is accurate and up to date. However, readers are strongly advised to confirm that the information, especially with regard to drug usage, complies with the latest legislation and standards of practice.

The Publishers have made every effort to trace the copyright holders for borrowed material. If they have inadvertently overlooked any, they will be pleased to make the necessary arrangements at the first opportunity.

Acquisitions Editor: *Sheila Khullar*
Production Editor: *Dave Terry*
Production Supervisor: *Sharon Tuder*
Cover Design: *Jeannette Jacobs*
Cover Illustration: Rembrandt: *An old man in an armchair*. Reproduced by courtesy of the Trustees, The National Gallery, London.

Printed in the United States of America

Contributors

Rebecca Allen-Burge, Ph.D.
Research Assistant Professor, Division of Gerontology/Geriatric Medicine, Department of Medicine, University of Alabama School of Medicine, Birmingham, Alabama

Tom Arie, C.B.E., M.A., B.M.(Oxon.), F.R.C.P.(Lond.), F.R.C.Psych., F.F.P.H.M.
Foundation Professor Emeritus of Health Care of the Elderly, University of Nottingham Medical School, Nottingham, England

Wilbert S. Aronow, M.D.
Adjunct Professor, Department of Geriatrics and Adult Development, Mount Sinai School of Medicine of the City University of New York; Medical Director, Department of Medicine, Hebrew Hospital Home, New York, New York

William H. Barker, M.D.
Associate Professor, Division of Preventive Medicine and Gerontology, Department of Community and Preventive Medicine, University of Rochester School of Medicine; Medical Attending Physician and Consultant in Health Services Research, Monroe Community Hospital, Rochester, New York

D. Barer, M.Sc., D.M., F.R.C.P
Professor of Clinical Geriatric Medicine, University of Newcastle, Queen Elizabeth Hospital, Gateshead, England

Craig Scott Bartlett III, M.D.
Fellow, Division of Trauma Service, Department of Orthopaedic Surgery, Hospital for Special Surgery, New York, New York

Paul E. Belchetz, M.A., M.D., M.Sc., F.R.C.P.
Consultant Endocrinologist, General Infirmary at Leeds, Leeds, England

Gerald C. J. Bennett, M.B., B.Ch., M.R.C.P.
Consultant Physician in Health Care for the Elderly, University of Nottingham Medical School, Nottingham, England

Steven L. Berk, M.D.
Professor and Chairman, Department of Internal Medicine, East Tennessee State University James H. Quillen College of Medicine, Johnson City, Tennessee

Gerald Blandford, M.B.B.S., F.R.C.P.(C.), F.A.C.P.
Clinical Professor, Division of Geriatrics, Department of Medicine, Albert Einstein College of Medicine of Yeshiva University; Medical Director, Loeb Center for Nursing and Rehabilitation, Montefiore Medical Center, Bronx, New York

Mary R. Bliss, M.B., B.S., M.R.C.P.(UK)
Consultant Physician, Department of Medicine for the Elderly, Hackney Hospital, London, England

Joan M. Braganza, M.B., B.S., M.Sc., F.R.C.P.
Consultant Senior Lecturer, Division of Gastroenterology, Department of Medicine, Royal Infirmary, Manchester, England

Lawrence J. Brandt, M.D., F.A.C.G., F.A.C.P.
Professor, Division of Gastroenterology, Department of Medicine, Albert Einstein College of Medicine of Yeshiva University; Director, Division of Gastroenterology, Department of Medicine, Montefiore Medical Center, New York, New York

J. C. Brocklehurst, C.B.E., M.D., M.Sc., F.R.C.P.(Lond., Edin., Glas.)
Professor Emeritus, University of Manchester Medical School, Manchester, England

Scott E. Brodie, M.D., Ph.D.
Assistant Professor, Department of Ophthalmology, Mount Sinai School of Medicine of the City University of New York; Associate Attending Opthalmologist, Department of Ophthalmology, Mount Sinai Hospital, New York, New York

Alan D. G. Brown, M.B., Ch.B., F.R.C.O.G., F.R.C.S. (Edin.)
Honorary Senior Lecturer, Department of Obstetrics and Gynaecology, University of Edinburgh Medical School; Consultant Obstetrician and Gynaecologist, Eastern General Hospital, Edinburgh, Scotland

Stuart Bruce, M.D., F.R.C.P.
Honorary Senior Clinical Lecturer, Institute of Human Performance, University College London, London; Consultant Physician, Department of Medicine for the Elderly, Conquest Hospital, St. Leonards on Sea, East Sussex, England

Alistair Burns, M.D., F.R.C.P., F.R.C.Psych.
Professor of Old Age Psychiatry and Honorary Consultant, University Hospital of South Manchester, Manchester, England

Robert N. Butler, M.D.
Professor, Department of Geriatrics and Adult Development, Mount Sinai School of Medicine of the City University of New York; Director, International Longevity Center, Mount Sinai Medical Center, New York, New York

Janet E. Carter, Ph.D., M.R.C.Psych.
Medical Research Council Clinician Scientist Fellow, Section of Old Age Psychiatry, Department of Neuroscience, Mandsley Hospital and Institute of Psychiatry, London, England

Andrew Casden, M.D.
Assistant Professor, Departments of Orthopaedics and Neurosurgery, Mount Sinai School of Medicine of the City University of New York; Chief, Spine Service, Department of Orthopaedics, Mount Sinai Medical Center, New York, New York

K. S. Channer, B.Sc., M.D., F.R.C.P.
Consultant Physician and Cardiologist, Department of Cardiology, Royal Hallamshire Hospital, Sheffield, England

John E. Clague, M.B., Ch.B., M.R.C.P., M.D.
Lecturer, Department of Geriatric Medicine, University of Manchester Medical School, Manchester, England; Honorary Consultant Physician, Department of Care of the Elderly, Hope Hospital, Salford, England

C. Clough, F.R.C.P.
Director, Department of Neurosciences, Kings College Hospital, London, England

Kenneth J. Collins, M.B., B.S., B.Sc., D.Phil., M.R.C.S.(Eng.), F.R.C.P.
Honorary Senior Clinical Lecturer and Staff Member, Medical Research Council, Department of Geriatric Medicine, University College and Hospitals, London, England

Martin J. Connolly, M.D., F.R.C.P.
Senior Lecturer, Department of Geriatric Medicine, University of Manchester Medical School, Manchester, England; Consultant Physician, Department of Geriatric Medicine, Barnes Hospital, Cheadle, England

Tara K. Cooper, M.B., B.Ch., B.A.O.(Hons.), M.R.C.O.G.
Consultant Obstetrician and Gynaecologist, St. John's Hospital, Livingston, England

Tim Cowen, B.Sc., Ph.D.
Senior Lecturer, Division of Basic Sciences, Department of Anatomy and Developmental Biology, Royal Free Hospital School of Medicine, London, England

R. A. Cowie, B.Sc., M.B., Ch.B., F.R.C.S.E., F.R.C.S.E.(S.N.)
Consultant Neurosurgeon, Hope Hospital and Salford and Royal Manchester Children's Hospital, Manchester, England

John Croker, F.R.C.P.
Honorary Senior Lecturer, Division of Medicine, Department of Care for the Elderly, University College London Hospitals; Consultant, Division of Geriatrics, Department of Medicine, Middlesex Hospital, London, England

Simon C. M. Croxson, B.M., M.R.C.P., M.D.
Consultant Physician, United Bristol Healthcare National Health Service Trust, Bristol General Hospital, Bristol, England

William J. K. Cumming, B.Sc., M.D., F.R.C.P., F.R.C.P.I., M.A.E., M.E.W.I.
Honorary Lecturer, Departments of Medicine and Cell and Structural Biology, University of Manchester Medical School, Manchester, England; Consultant Neurologist, Neuroscience Unit, Alexandra Hospital, Cheadle, England

J. L. Dall , M.D., F.R.C.P. (Glas. , Edin.), D.U. (Ottawa)
Consultant Physician and Honorary Senior Lecturer, Victoria Infirmary, Glasgow, Scotland; Visiting Professor, University of Ottawa Faculty of Medicine, Ottawa, Ontario, Canada

Ioan Davies, Ph.D.
Lecturer, Department of Geriatric Medicine, University of Manchester School of Biological Sciences, Manchester, England

Martin Dennis, M.D., F.R.C.P.(Ed.)
Reader in Stroke Medicine, Department of Clinical Neurosciences, University of Edinburgh Medical School; Honorary Consultant, Department of Medicine, Western General Hospital, Edinburgh, Scotland

Hugh Devlin, B.Sc., M.Sc., Ph.D., B.D.S.
Senior Lecturer, Division of Restorative Dentistry, Department of Dental Medicine and Surgery, University Dental Hospital of Manchester, Manchester, England

Aparjit Ballav Dey, M.D., M.B.B.S.
Associate Professor, Division of Geriatric Medicine, Department of Medicine, All India Institute of Medical Sciences; Consultant, Division of Geriatric Medicine, Department of Medicine, New Delhi Institute, New Delhi, India

T. Michael Dexter, Ph.D., D.Sc., F.R.C.Path., Hon.M.R.C.P., F.R.S.
Professor, Department of Experimental Haematology, University of Manchester Medical School; Director, Paterson Institute for Cancer Research, Manchester, England

Edward Dickinson, M.A., M.B.A., F.R.C.P.
Acting Director, Research Unit, Royal College of Physicians, London, England

Paul Dieppe, B.Sc., M.D., F.R.C.P.
Director, Medical Research Council Health Services Research Centre, University of Bristol Medical School, Bristol, England

Giuseppe DiGiovanni, M.D.
Resident, Division of Orthopaedics, Department of Orthopaedic Surgery, Mount Sinai Medical Center, New York, New York

Susie Dinan, Cert. Ed., P.G. Dip.
Clinical Exercise Practitioner, University Department of Geriatric Medicine, Royal Free Hospital School of Medicine; Clinical Exercise Practitions, Old Age Psychiatry Service Royal Free Hospital, London, England

Joanna H. Downton, M.D., F.R.C.P.
Consultant in Rehabilitation Medicine, Stockport Healthcare National Health Service Trust, St. Thomas's Hospital, Stockport, England

Shah Ebrahim, D.M., F.R.C.P., F.F.P.H.M., M.R.C.G.P.
Professor, Division of Clinical Epidemiology, Department of Primary Care and Population Sciences, Royal Free Hospital School of Medicine, London, England

William B. Ershler, M.D.
Visiting Scientist, Gerontology Research Center, National Institute on Aging, National Institutes of Health, Baltimore, Maryland

Marie Fallon, M.B.Ch.B., M.R.C.G.P.
Marie Curie Senior Lecturer, Department of Palliative Medicine, University of Glasgow Medical School; Consultant, Department of Palliative Medicine, Beatson Oncology Centre, Western Infirmary, Glasgow, Scotland

Mark W. J. Ferguson, Ph.D., B.Sc.(Hons.), B.D.S.(Hons.), F.F.D.
Professor, Department of Cell and Structural Biology, University of Manchester School of Biological Sciences, Manchester, England

Howard Fillit, M.D.
Corporate Medical Director, Medicare NYLCare Healthplans, Inc.; Clinical Professor, Departments of Geriatrics and Medicine, Mount Sinai School of Medicine of the City University of New York, New York, New York

R. M. Francis, M.B., Ch.B., F.R.C.P.
Senior Lecturer, Division of Geriatrics, Department of Medicine, University of Newcastle upon Tyne Medical School; Consultant Physician, Bone Clinic, Freeman Hospital, Newcastle upon Tyne, England

Michael L. Freedman, M.D.
Professor, Division of Geriatric Medicine, Department of Medicine, New York University School of Medicine; Director, The Diane and Arthur Belfer Geriatric Center, New York University Medical Center, New York, New York

A. J. Freemont, M.D., F.R.C.P., F.R.C.Path.
Professor of Osteo-articular Pathology, University of Manchester Medical School; Director, Division of Osteo-articular Pathology, Department of Pathological Sciences, Manchester Royal Infirmary, Manchester, England

Richard A. Frieden, M.D.
Assistant Professor, Department of Rehabilitation Medicine, Mount Sinai School of Medicine of the City University of New York; Assistant Attending Physician, Department of Rehabilitation Medicine, Mount Sinai Medical Center, New York, New York

George Fulop, M.D., M.S.C.M.
Assistant Clinical Professor, Division of Geriatrics, Departments of Community Medicine, Geriatric Medicine, and Psychiatry, Mount Sinai School of Medicine of the City University of New York, New York, New York; Director, Division of Medical Policy and Programs, Department of Medical Affairs, Merck-Medco Managed Care, L.L.C., Montvale, NJ

N. J. R. George, M.D., F.R.C.S., F.E.B.U.
Senior Lecturer and Consultant Physician, Department of Urology, University Hospital of South Manchester, Manchester, England

Gary Gerstenblith, M.D.
Professor, Division of Cardiology, Department of Medicine, Johns Hopkins University School of Medicine; Attending Physician, Division of Cardiology, Department of Medicine, Johns Hopkins Hospital, Baltimore, Maryland

Barbara A. Gilchrest, M.D.
Professor and Chairman, Department of Dermatology, Boston University School of Medicine; Chief, Department of Dermatology, and Director, Laser Center, Boston Medical Center, Boston, Massachusetts

Maria H. Gilleece, M.D., B.Sc.(Hons.), M.R.C.P., M.R.C.Path.
Research Fellow, Kay Kendall Leukemia Fund, Division of Hematological Malignancies, Dana Farber Cancer Institute, Boston, Massachusetts

Margot Gosney, M.D., M.R.C.P.
Senior Lecturer, Department of Geriatric Medicine, University of Liverpool School of Medicine, Liverpool, England

Stefan Gravenstein, M.D.
Associate Professor, The Glennan Center for Geriatrics and Gerontology, Eastern Virginia Medical School, Norfolk, Virginia

Christopher E. M. Griffiths, M.D., F.R.C.P.
Professor, Section of Dermatology, Department of Medicine, University of Manchester Medical School, Manchester, England; Honorary Consultant Dermatologist, Dermatology Centre, Hope Hospital, Salford, England

Emily Grundy, M.A., M.Sc., Ph.D.
Reader in Social Gerontology, Age Concern Institute of Gerontology, King's College, London, London, England

Michael Hahn, M.D.
Resident, Department of Orthopaedic Surgery, Mount Sinai Medical Center, New York, New York

Peter Hammond, M.A. M.D., M.R.C.P.
Consultant Physician, Harrogate District Hospital, Harrogate, England

R. N. L. Harland, M.D., F.R.C.S.
Consultant, Wigan Royal Albert Edward Infirmary, Wigan, England

John Harris, B.A., D.Phil.
Sir David Alliance Professor of Bioethics, University of Manchester Centre for Social Ethics and Policy, Manchester, England

Robert D. Helme, M.B.B.S., Ph.D., F.R.A.C.P.
Director, National Ageing Research Institute, Victoria, Australia

Michael A. Horan, M.A., Ph.D., F.R.C.P.
Professor, Department of Geriatric Medicine, University of Manchester Medical School, Manchester, England; Honorary Consultant Physician, Department of Care of the Elderly, Hope Hospital, Salford, England

Fraser G. Inglis, M.B.
Lecturer, Division of Ageing and Health, Department of Medicine for the Elderly, University of Dundee Medical School; Honorary Senior Registrar, Medicine for the Elderly, Dundee Healthcare National Health Service Trust, Dundee, Scotland

Sheldon Jacobson, M.D., F.A.C.E.P., F.A.C.P.
Professor and Chairman, Department of Emergency Medicine, Mount Sinai School of Medicine of the City University of New York; Chairman, Department of Emergency Medicine, Mount Sinai Medical Center, New York, New York

Oliver F. W. James, M.A., F.R.C.P.
Professor, Division of Geriatrics, Department of Medicine, University of Newcastle upon Tyne; Consultant, Department of Medicine, Freeman Hospital, Newcastle upon Tyne, England

Vanita Jassal, M.B., M.R.C.P.(UK), M.D.
Graduate Student, Division of Clinical Epidemiology, Department of Medicine, University of Toronto Faculty of Medicine; Clinical Fellow, Division of Nephrology, Department of Medicine, Toronto Hospital, Toronto, Ontario, Canada

Malcolm L. Johnson, B.A., D.S.A.S., F.R.S.A.
Professor, Department of Health and Social Policy, School for Policy Studies; Director, International Institute on Health and Ageing, University of Bristol, Bristol, England

David Jolley, M.Sc., F.R.C.Psych.
Medical Director, Wolverhampton Health Care National Health Service Trust, Wolverhampton, England

Rajendra Jutagir, Ph.D.
Clinical Assistant Professor, Department of Geriatrics and Adult Development, Mount Sinai School of Medicine of the City University of New York; Clinical Assistant Psychologist, Department of Geriatrics and Adult Development, Mount Sinai Hospital, New York, New York

Alexandre Kalache, H.Sc., M.D., Ph.D.
Chief, Ageing and Health Programme, World Health Organization, Geneva, Switzerland

Lalit Kalra, M.D., Ph.D., F.R.C.P.
Professor, Department of Health Care for the Elderly, and Honorary Consultant, Division of Medicine, King's College School of Medicine and Dentistry, London, England

Rosalie A. Kane, D.S.W.
Professor, Division of Health Services, and Director, National Long Term Care Research Center, University of Minnesota School of Public Health, Minneapolis, Minnesota

Evan Karas, M.D.
Attending Physician, Department of Orthopaedic Surgery, Westchester Hospital, Mt. Kisco, New York

Cornelius Katona, M.D., F.R.C.Psych.
Professor, Department of Psychiatry and Behavioral Sciences, University College London Medical School, London, England

Benny Katz, M.B.B.S., F.R.A.C.P.
Clinical Associate, National Ageing Research Institute and North West Hospital Pain Management for the Elderly, Victoria, Australia

Seymour Katz, M.D.
Clinical Professor, Department of Medicine, New York University School of Medicine, New York, New York; Attending Physician, Division of Gastroenterology, Department of Medicine, North Shore University Hospital, Manhasset, New York

Leslie I. Katzel, M.D., Ph.D.
Associate Professor, Division of Gerontology, Department of Medicine, University of Maryland School of Medicine; Clinical Director, Baltimore Veterans Affairs Medical Center, Baltimore, Maryland

Nicholas A. Kefalides, M.D., Ph.D.
Professor, Departments of Medicine and Biochemistry and Biophysics, University of Pennsylvania School of Medicine; Director, Connective Tissue Research Institute, University City Science Center, Philadelphia, Pennsylvania

David C. Kennie , M.B.Ch.B, F.R.C.P. (Glas., Edin.)
Honorary Senior Lecturer, Department of Medicine, University of Edinburgh Medical School, Edinburgh, Scotland; Consultant Physician in Geriatric Medicine, Department of Medicine, Royal Infirmary, Stirling, Scotland

Rose Ann Kenny, M.D., F.R.C.P.
Professor, Division of Geriatric Medicine, Department of Medicine, University of Newcastle upon Tyne Medical School; Consultant, Cardiovascular Investigation Unit, Royal Victoria Infirmary, Newcastle upon Tyne, England

U. J. Kirkpatrick, M.B., Ch.B., F.R.C.S.
Surgical Research Registrar, Department of Surgery, University Hospital of South Manchester, Manchester, England

T. B. L. Kirkwood, M.A., M.Sc., Ph.D.
Professor, Division of Biological Gerontology, Department of Geriatric Medicine, University of Manchester Medical School, Manchester, England

Mark Kosinski, D.P.M.
Associate Professor, Department of Medicine, New York College of Podiatric Medicine; Faculty Member, Mount Sinai Geriatric Education Center, New York, New York

Myrna I. Lewis, M.S.W.
Assistant Professor, Department of Community Medicine, Mount Sinai School of Medicine of the City University of New York, New York, New York

Michael Lye, M.D., F.R.C.P.
Professor, Department of Geriatric Medicine, University of Liverpool School of Medicine; Consultant Geriatrician, Department of Geriatric Medicine, Royal Liverpool and Broadgreen University Hospitals, National Health Service Trust, Liverpool, England

A. J. D. Macdonald, M.D., F.R.C.Psych.
Professor, Department of Psychiatry, United Medical and Dental Schools; Consultant, Department of Mental Health in the Elderly, Lewisham Hospital, London, England

James Malone-Lee, M.D., F.R.C.P.
Barlow Professor, Centre for Geriatric Medicine, Department of Medicine, University College London Medical School, London, England

David Michael Andrew Mann, Ph.D., F.R.C.Path.
Reader, Division of Molecular Pathology, Department of Pathological Sciences, University of Manchester Medical School, Manchester, England

R. E. Mansel, M.S., F.R.C.S.
Professor and Head, Department of Surgery, University of Wales College of Medicine, Cardiff, Wales

Kenneth G. Manton, Ph. D.
Director and Research Professor, Duke University Center of Demographic Studies, Durham, North Carolina

Anthony Martin, M.D., F.R.C.P.(Edin.), M.H.S.M.
Consultant Physician, Queen Victoria Hospital, East Grinstead, England: Chairman, Crawley Horsham Research Unit, Crawley Hospital, England; Chairman, Crawley Horsham National Health Service Trust, Crawley, England

E. J. Masoro, Ph.D.
Professor Emeritus, Department of Physiology, University of Texas Medical School at San Antonio, San Antonio, Texas

C. N. McCollum, M.D., F.R.C.S.
Professor, Department of Surgery, University of Manchester Medical School, Manchester, England

Declan M. McLoughlin, M.R.C.P.I., M.R.C.Pysch.
Alzeheimer's Disease Society Research Fellow, Section of Old Age Psychiatry, Department of Neurology, Mandsley Hospital and Institute of Psychiatry, London, England

Claudine McCreadie, M.A.
Research Associate, Age Concern Institute of Gerontology, King's College, London, London, England

Myron Miller, M.D.
Professor, Division of Geriatric Medicine and Gerontology, Department of Medicine, Johns Hopkins University School of Medicine; Director, Division of Geriatric Medicine, Department of Medicine, Sinai Hospital of Baltimore, Baltimore, Maryland

Richard A. Miller, M.D., Ph.D.
Professor, Department of Pathology and Associate Director for Research, Geriatrics Center, University of Michigan Medical School, Ann Arbor, Michigan

Kevin Morgan, B.Sc., Ph.D.
Director, Centre for Ageing and Rehabilitation Studies, School of Health and Related Research, Sheffield, England

William J. Mutch, M.B., F.R.C.P.(E.)
Consultant Physician in Medicine for the Elderly, Dundee Healthcare National Health Service Trust; Honorary Senior Lecturer, Department of Medicine, University of Dundee Medical School, Dundee, Scotland

James W. Myers, M.D.
Assistant Professor, Department of Internal Medicine, East Tennessee State University James H. Quillen College of Medicine, Johnson City, Tennessee

David Neary, M.D.
Professor and Consultant Neurologist, Department of Neurology, Manchester Royal Infirmary, Manchester, England

Mia Oberlink, M.A.
Director of Communications, International Longevity Center, Mount Sinai Medical Center, New York, New York

Shaun Timothy O'Keeffe, M.D., M.R.C.P.I.
Consultant Geriatrician, St. Michael's Hospital, Dublin, Ireland

Paul A. O'Neill, M.D., B.Sc.(Hons.), F.R.C.P.
Senior Lecturer, Department of Geriatric Medicine, University of Manchester Medical School; Consultant, Department of Geriatric Medicine, South Manchester University Hospitals National Health Service Trust, Manchester, England

Dimitrios G. Oreopoulos, M.D., Ph.D., F.R.C.P.(C.), F.A.C.P., F.R.C.P.S.(Glas.)
Professor, Division of Nephrology, Department of Medicine, University of Athens School of Medicine; Director, Peritoneal Dialysis Program, Division of Nephrology, Department of Medicine, Toronto Hospital, Toronto, Ontario, Canada

Joseph G. Ouslander, M.D.
Director, Division of Geriatric Medicine and Gerontology, Emory University School of Medicine; Chief of Medicine, Wesley Woods Geriatric Center at Emory University; Director, Atlanta Veterans Affairs Rehabilitation Research and Development Center, Atlanta, Georgia

M. S. J. Pathy, O.B.E., F.R.C.P., F.R.C.P.E.
Professor Emeritus, University of Wales College of Medicine; Research Director, Healthcare Research Unit, St. Woolos Hospital, Newport, England

Ann-Marie Plate, M.D.
Resident, Department of Orthopaedic Surgery, Mount Sinai Medical Center, New York, New York

P. Rabbit, M.A., M.Sc.
Professor, Age and Cognitive Research Center, University of Manchester Medical School, Manchester, England

Brion D. Reichler, M.D.
Assistant Professor, Department of Neurology, Mount Sinai School of Medicine of the City University of New York; Assistant Attending Physician, Division of Clinical Neurophysiology, Department of Neurology, Mount Sinai Medical Center, New York, New York

John F. Reinus, M.D., F.A.C.G.
Associate Professor, Division of Gastroenterology, Department of Medicine, Albert Einstein College of Medicine of Yeshiva University, New York, New York

Christopher Rodrigues, Ph.D., M.D., M.R.C.P.
Consultant Physician, Department of Medicine and Care for the Elderly, Kingston and Tolworth Hospitals, Kingston upon Thames, Surrey, England

David H. Rosenbaum, M.D.
Associate Professor, Departments of Neurology and Geriatrics and Adult Development, Mount Sinai School of Medicine of the City University of New York; Associate Attending Physician, Departments of Neurology and Geriatrics, Mount Sinai Medical Center; Consultant in Neurology, New York Medical Group, P.C., New York, New York

Laurence Z. Rubenstein, M.D., M.P.H., F.A.C.P.
Professor, Department of Medicine, University of California, Los Angeles, UCLA School of Medicine, Los Angeles, California; Director, Geriatric Research Education and Clinical Center, and Chief, Department of Geriatric Medicine, Sepulveda Veterans Affairs Medical Center, Sepulveda, California

Lisa V. Rubenstein, M.D., MSPH, FACP.
Professor, Department of Medicine, University of California, Los Angeles, UCLA School of Medicine, Los Angeles, California; Associate Chief of Staff, Department of Primary Care Medicine, and Chief, Department of General Internal Medicine, Sepulveda Veterans Affairs Medical Center, Sepulveda, California

Evelyn M. Russell, M.D., Ph.D., M.R.C.Psych.
Consultant in Old Age Psychiatry, Whittington Hospital, Manchester, England

G. Saldhana, B.A., M.B.B.S., M.R.C.P.
Clinical Fellow, Department of Neurology, Kings College Hospital, London, England

Laszlo Sarkozi, Ph.D.
Professor, Department of Pathology, Mount Sinai School of Medicine of the City University of New York; Director, Department of Chemistry, Mount Sinai Hospital, New York, New York

K. Warner Schaie, Ph.D.
Evan Pugh Professor of Human Development and Psychology, and Director, Gerontology Center, Pennsylvania State University, University Park, Pennsylvania; Affiliate Professor, Department of Behavioral Science and Psychiatry, University of Washington Medical School, Seattle, Washington

Malvin Schechter, M.A.
Assistant Professor (retired), Department of Geriatrics and Adult Development, Mount Sinai School of Medicine of the City University of New York, New York, New York

Edward L. Schneider, M.D.
Executive Director, Ethel Percy Andrus Gerontology Center; Professor and Dean, Leonard Davis School of Gerontology; Professor, Department of Medicine, and Adjunct Professor, Department of Biology, University of Southern California School of Medicine, Los Angeles, California

Andrew K. Scott, M.B., Ch.B., M.D., F.R.C.P.
Senior Lecturer, Department of Geriatric Medicine, University of Manchester Medical School; Honorary Consultant, Department of Care for the Elderly, Hope Hospital, Salford, England

David L. Scott, B.Sc., M.B., F.R.C.P.
Reader, Division of Medicine, Department of Clinical and Academic Rheumatology, King's College University of London; Consultant, Division of Rheumatology, Department of Medicine, King's College Hospital, London, England

D. Gwyn Seymour, B.Sc., M.D., F.R.C.P. (Lond.), F.R.C.P.(Edin.)
Professor, Division of Care of the Elderly, Department of Medicine and Therapeutics, University of Aberdeen Medical School; Consultant in Medicine for the Elderly, Woodend Hospital, Grampian Health Care Trust, Aberdeen, Scotland

N. M. Sharer, B.Sc., M.R.C.P.
Medical Coordinator, Department of Gastroenterology, Manchester Royal Infirmary, Manchester, England

David M. Simpson, M.D.
Associate Professor, Department of Neurology, Mount Sinai School of Medicine of the City University of New York; Director, Clinical Neurophysiology Laboratory, Department of Neurology, Mount Sinai Medical Center, New York, New York

Alan J. Sinclair, M.Sc., M.D., F.R.C.P.
Charles Hayward Professor of Geriatric Medicine and Gerontology, University of Birmingham Medical School; Consultant Physician in Diabetes, Birmingham Heartlands Hospital, Birmingham, England

Julie S. Snowden, Ph.D.
Clinical Scientist (Psychologist), Cerebral Function Unit, Department of Neurology, Manchester Royal Infirmary, Manchester, England

John D. Sorkin, M.D.
Assistant Professor, Division of Gerontology, Department of Medicine, University of Maryland School of Medicine; Epidermiologist, Gerontology Research Center, National Institute of Ageing, National Institutes of Health, Baltimore, Maryland

Robert W. Stout, M.D., D.Sc., F.R.C.P.
Professor, Department of Geriatric Medicine, and Provost of Medicine and Health Sciences, Queens University of Belfast Medical School, Belfast, Northern Ireland

Elton Strauss, M.D.
Clinical Assistant Professor, Division of Surgery, Department of Orthopaedics, Mount Sinai School of Medicine of the City University of New York; Chief, Division of Trauma and Reconstructive Surgery, Department of Orthopaedics, and Co-Chief, Orthogeriatric Service, Mount Sinai Medical Center, New York, New York

David G. Sutin, M.B.B.S.
Clinical Assistant Professor, Department of Medicine, New York University School of Medicine; Attending Physician, Geriatric Clinic, Bellevue Hospital, New York, New York

Stephanie Sweet, M.D.
Resident, Department of Orthopaedic Surgery, Mount Sinai Medical Center, New York, New York

C. G. Swift, Ph.D., F.R.C.P.
Professor, Department of Health Care of the Elderly, King's College (Dulwich) Hospital, London, England

Raymond Tallis, M.A., B.M., B.Ch. F.R.C.P., D.Litt.
Professor, Department of Geriatric Medicine, University of Manchester Medical School, Manchester, England; Honorary Consultant Physician, Department of Care of the Elderly, Hope Hospital, Salford, England

Robert E. Tepper, M.D.
Teaching Assistant, Department of Medicine, New York University School of Medicine, New York, New York; Assistant Attending Physician, Division of Gastroenterology, Department of Medicine, North Shore University Hospital, Manhasset, New York

Anita J. Thomas Ph.D., F.R.C.P.
Consultant Physician, Division of Health Care for the Elderly, Department of Medicine, Derriford Hospital, Plymouth, England

Rein Tideiksaar, Ph.D.
Director, Department of Geriatrics, Sierra Health Services, Inc., Las Vegas, Nevada

Anthea Tinker, B.Com., Ph.D.
Professor and Director, Age Concern Institute of Gerontology, King's College of London, London, England

Jonathan Tobias, M.D., Ph.D.
Senior Lecturer, Rheumatology Unit, Department of Medicine, University of Bristol Medical School; Consultant Rheumatologist, Bristol Royal Infirmary, Bristol, England

Arnold Wald, M.D.
Professor, Division of Gastroenterology and Hepatology, Department of Medicine, University of Pittsburgh School of Medicine; Associate Chief, Division of Gastroenterology and Hepatology, University of Pittsburgh Medical Center, Pittsburgh, Pennsylvania

Katherine Ward, D.P.M.
Instructor, Department of Medicine, New York College of Podiatric Medicine; Consultant in Podiatric Surgery, Veterans Affairs Medical Center, New York, New York; Captain, United States Army Reserves

Vivienne Watkin, M.R.C.Psych.
Senior Registrar, Department of Psychiatry, Whittington Hospital, London, England

Cyril Weinkove, B.Sc., M.B.Ch.B., Ph.D., F.C.P.(S.A.)
Senior Lecturer, Division of Clinical Biochemistry, Department of Medicine, University of Manchester Medical School, Manchester, England; Consultant Chemical Pathologist, Department of Clinical Pathology, Hope Hospital, Salford, England

Barbara E. Weinstein, Ph.D.
Professor and Program Director, Department of Speech and Theatre, Lehman College, City University of New York; Member, Doctoral Faculty, Ph.D. Program in Speech and Hearing Sciences, City University of New York, New York, New York

John Welsh, B.Sc., F.R.C.P.
Professor, Department of Palliative Medicine, University of Glasgow Medical School; Consultant, Division of Medicine, Department of Palliative Medicine, Hunters Hill Curie Centre, Glasgow, Scotland

Idris Williams, O.B.E., M.D., F.R.C.G.P.
Professor Emeritus, Department of General Practice, University of Nottingham Medical School, Nottingham, England

Sherry L. Willis, Ph.D.
Professor, Department of Human Development and Family Studies, Pennsylvania State University, University Park, Pennsylvania; Affiliate Professor, Department of Behavioral Sciences and Psychiatry, University of Washington School of Medicine, Seattle, Washington

Ken Woodhouse, M.D., F.R.C.P.
Professor, Department of Geriatric Medicine, and Vice Dean, Department of Medicine, University of Wales College of Medicine, Cardiff, Wales; Consultant Physician and Geriatrician, Department of Medicine, Llandough Hospital, Penarth, Wales

Archie Young, B.Sc., M.B.Ch.B., M.D., F.R.C.P. (Glas., Lond.)
Head, University Department of Geriatric Medicine, Roayl Free Hospital School of Medicine; Honorary Consultant Physicians in Geriatric Medicine, Royal Free Hospital, London, England

Preface

In advanced societies most people can now expect to live to old age. In developing societies, average life expectancy is less, but the massive populations of these societies mean that the old are numbered in millions. The impact of these demographic developments in the century now ending has been reflected in medicine and science by increasing research and knowledge, in society by improved services, and among elderly people themselves by increased expectations of health and social support. Gerontology and geriatric medicine are now firmly established disciplines throughout much of the world. In Great Britain, the specialty of geriatric medicine, officially recognized in 1948, is a major specialty, and the British Geriatrics Society has 1,600 members. General practitioners also have been stimulated to develop their knowledge of geriatric practice by the inauguration of the Diploma of Geriatric Medicine of the Royal College of Physicians. In commonwealth countries and much of Europe, the specialty is well founded and gaining official recognition through special qualifications and accreditation. In the United States, geriatric medicine has achieved recognition as an academic discipline, to be taught to medical students and to be researched, and the number of specialists practicing and researching has increased enormously. In recent years, family practitioners and internists in the United States have responded to the aging of their patients by developing a major interest in geriatric medicine and this has been acknowledged by a certification in geriatric medicine awarded by the American Boards of Internal Medicine and Family Practice. Eligibility for the certifying examination requires completion of fellowship training in an approved program in geriatric medicine.

Gerontology, the application of fundamental science to the process of aging, likewise continues to grow in stature, particularly in the United States. It is as important for clinicians dealing with elderly people to understand something of the physiology of aging as it is for pediatricians to understand the physiology of aging and development.

Advances in gerontology and in geriatric medicine are reflected by structural developments in care systems for the old—social, medical, and nursing. Practitioners in the medicine of old age must be aware of (and contribute toward) these developments.

This textbook, therefore, in its first edition in 1973, was presented in three main sections: gerontology, geriatric medicine, and services for the elderly. These sections have since been expanded to reflect the development of the subject. In this fifth edition, the second part has been subdivided, for ease of reference, into two major subsections covering systemic disease in the elderly and problem-based geriatric medicine. There is also a much expanded fourth section entitled "Provision of Care," which examines the problems posed to society by an aging population as well as the means of addressing these problems at all levels of health-care provision. As knowledge increases, so does specialism. An inevitable consequence is that subjects covered by one or two authors in the first edition are now divided among many more individuals, with special interests and knowledge generally based on their own research and scholarship. Whereas the first edition comprised 39 chapters written by a total of 44 authors, this fifth edition has 117 chapters contributed by 147 authors. Despite this, we have still kept the book a manageable size for the reader. To meet the increased editorial demands that these changes have brought about and also having in mind the burgeoning involvement of American physicians in geriatric medicine, the editorship was increased in the previous edition by the addition of Professor Raymond Tallis and Dr. Howard Fillit, both of whom are delighted to continue their association with this new edition.

The book, although extensively rewritten, broadly maintains the format of previous editions. Many of the authors are new and we have increased further the number of contributors from the United States. This increased American emphasis is reflected in the American spelling in the text. (Where measurements are given in SI units, the metric equivalent has been added in parentheses where appropriate.) It may be noted that where an individual patient is referred to in the text, the clumsy "him or her" or "them" have been eschewed and either "him" or "her" used (as may seem most appropriate) to imply both sexes.

In a work of this magnitude, acknowledgments and thanks are due to many people. Where illustrations have been taken from other publications, acknowledgment is made in the text. Thanks are due to medical illustration departments in many institutions in Great Britain and North America and likewise manuscript preparation to many secretaries. In particular, the hard task of editing has been lightened by the superb secretarial support of Penny Essex and Barbara Jones, whose excellent organizational skills have been crucial since the first stages of planning. Finally, grateful acknowledgment is made to the many authors involved, who have so excellently made their scholarship available to those who use this book.

As we approach the millennium, we hope that this textbook will continue to be a source of information, advice, and inspiration to the many practitioners and researchers who are at the sharp end of a demographic trend that is unlikely to change in the foreseeable future.

R. C. Tallis
H. M. Fillit
J. C. Brocklehurst

Contents

CHAPTER 1

The Epidemiology of Aging

EMILY GRUNDY

Epidemiology is commonly defined as "the study of the distribution of a disease or a physiological condition in human populations and of the factors that influence this distribution,"[1] and it is this emphasis on populations rather than individuals that most clearly distinguishes epidemiology from other health-related sciences. The study of the epidemiology of aging presents greater challenges than applying epidemiologic methods to the study of a particular disease and, as Greenhouse[2] noted, arriving at a satisfactory definition of what is meant by the epidemiology of aging is itself problematic. However, four elements that together constitute the core of the subject may be identified. These are

1. Studies concerned with the identification of risk factors that may elucidate the etiology of specific conditions primarily affecting elderly people
2. Studies in which epidemiologic methods are used in the evaluation of preventive or therapeutic interventions in elderly populations
3. Studies of the general health status of older populations, either descriptive or concerned with the identification of factors associated with variations in general indicators of health
4. Studies of age-related change in indicators of health status, both general and disease specific

In this chapter the chief focus will be on the more general studies included in the third and fourth categories listed above. The epidemiology of specific conditions, and the evaluation of therapeutic interventions, are of course important areas of activity, and references to these kinds of studies are included in other chapters in this volume. However, a more general inventory of the health status of older populations is essential for public health planning, and comparisons between populations and population subgroups may provide insight into factors associated with health problems in later life. Planning for the future requires an assessment of age-related changes in health status, which may also further our understanding of basic aging processes.

Major conceptual and methodologic problems make the compilation and interpretation of population-based statistics on aging and health particularly difficult. Health is an elusive concept, hard to measure or define at either the individual or population level. The World Health Organization (WHO) definition of health is "a complete state of physical mental and social well-being,"[3] which, while admirable in emphasizing the multifactorial nature of health, is hard to operationalize and, if applied rigorously, would probably consign most individuals in most populations to the ranks of the unhealthy. Research on "positive health" has recently attracted growing attention, but in practice, negative measures or morbidity—rather than health—predominate. Although perhaps simpler to conceptualize, morbidity is difficult to define. Should someone with occult or subclinical disease, for example, be considered healthy or unhealthy? Recent developments in genetics raise further complexities in this area. The consequences of particular pathologic processes for health more broadly defined may vary considerably as a result of psychosocial factors and host-environment interactions. The importance of the latter is recognized in the WHO distinction between impairments, disabilities, and handicaps.

For all these reasons it is now largely accepted that the distinction between health and ill health is a quantitative rather than a qualitative one, and that both the causes and consequences of particular pathologic processes may be multifactorial.[4]

Population Health

The measurement of health at the population level represents more than aggregation of individual level data and represents particular challenges. In some respects population level indicators should be simpler to devise than individual ones, if only because the degree of error associated with generalizing from large distributions is less than that associated with the prediction of particular observations. To take one example, chronologic age is an unreliable predictor of performance or health in an individual,[5] but at the population level is quite a sensitive discriminator between groups.[6] However, in many other respects, the measurement of health is more complex at the population level than for the individual. This is not simply a function of the problems associated with reliable ascertainment of health status in large groups, but also reflects the differing dynamics of health at the population and individual level. Health care interventions, environmental or behavioral changes that reduce the risk of disability from, for example, hypertension, may represent a health gain at the individual level but result in a higher prevalence of morbidity from this cause in the population. Selective survival effects may mean that the health trajectories of individuals differ from those in

Table 1-1 Deaths at ages 0–4 and 75+, England and Wales, 1901 and 1994

	% of All Deaths at Following Ages	
Year	**0–4**	**75+**
1901	37	12
1994	1	58

(Data from United Nations,[10] Office of Population and Census Surveys [OPCS].[11])

populations.[7] Cohort effects represent a further major factor complicating elucidation of trends over time or between age groups.

Possibly as a result of these methodologic problems, which will be referred to throughout this chapter, the epidemiology of aging is as yet an underdeveloped area[8] of a science itself in an early stage of development.[9]

These issues, and the basic questions of how to define and measure health, have become particularly pressing in contemporary developed populations with old age structures in which most deaths occur at advanced ages from degenerative diseases. As shown in Table 1-1, in England and Wales in 1994, over one-half of all deaths occurred among those aged 75 and over, and only a tiny proportion among infants and young children. In 1901, by contrast, well over one-third of all deaths occurred among infants under age 5. This enormous change reflects not just the welcome reduction in the risk of death early in life, but also age structure changes in the population.

Population Aging

The demographic determinants of a population's size and age structure are fertility, mortality, and migration. It has long been recognized that fertility is potentially the most important of these parameters in all but the highest of high mortality populations.[12–14]

Children, if they survive to maturity, will in most cases become the parents of children who themselves may reproduce. Each birth thus represents not just an addition to the current generation of children, but a potentially exponentially increasing contribution to the size of subsequent generations of children. Historically, and apparently paradoxically, improvements in mortality in the now developed world served to partially offset the trend toward population aging, as they chiefly benefited the young—and led to increases in the proportion surviving to have children themselves. Primary population aging—a once and for all shift to an older age structure—is a consequence of long-term downward trends in fertility. In much of the now developed Western World this shift, termed the "demographic transition," occurred in the late nineteenth or early twentieth century. As a consequence, as shown in the top panel of Figure 1-1, these countries today have 10 percent or more of the population aged 65 or more. In some, including the Nordic countries, the United Kingdom, Italy, and Germany (not all shown in the figure), more than 15 percent of the population are aged 65 or over. In the rest of the world, as illustrated in the bottom panel of Figure 1-1, the proportion of elderly people is much lower. However, a transition to lower, deliberately controlled fertility—the precursor of population aging—is now close to being a global phenomenon. In 1990, only 17 percent of the world's population lived in countries where no appreciable downturn in fertility was then evident[15] (and even in many of these countries there are now signs that this is occurring). In these populations, predominantly in sub-Saharan Africa, the proportion of elderly people aged 65 and over is very small and is not projected to increase significantly in the short-term future. It is important to remember, however, that these populations are rapidly growing and that this includes enormous growth in the *absolute* number of elderly people. In 1990, 60 percent of the world's population lived in countries where there had been significant and sustained downturns in fertility since 1950. In most of these populations the proportion aged 65 and over is currently below 10 percent (or even slightly below 5 percent in countries, such as Thailand, Turkey, and India, where the transition is relatively recent). These populations are, however, now aging rapidly.

Japan, with over 14 percent of its population aged 65 or more in 1995, was the first country outside the West to experience the demographic transition, and the speed of its decline in fertility was unprecedented. During the period from 1947 to 1957, the total fertility rate (average number of children that would be born to a woman experiencing the age-specific fertility rates of the period throughout the childbearing years) fell by more than one-half, from 4.5 to 2.0 children per woman.[16] Largely as a consequence of this, the pace of population aging in Japan has also been very fast, as illustrated in Figure 1-2, which compares the proportion aged 65 and over in England and Wales, the United States, and Japan over the course of the twentieth century, together with projections for the early decades of the next century.

In England and Wales the proportion aged 65 and over, which accounted for less than 5 percent of the total population at the start of the century, reached 10 percent by 1951 and 15 percent in 1981. In the United States the proportion aged 65 and over only reached 10 percent in 1971 and currently stands at 13 percent. The postwar "baby boom" in the United States (and Australia, Canada, and New Zealand) was sustained for a longer period, and at higher levels, than in England and Wales and other European countries. In the United States the total fertility rate in 1955 to 1960, for example, was 3.7, compared with 2.5 in England and Wales. This difference, and the rejuvenating effect of immigration on population age structure (as immigrants tend to be young) accounts for the slightly lower relative size of the elderly populations of the United States, Canada, Australia, and New Zealand in comparison with Northwest European countries such as England and

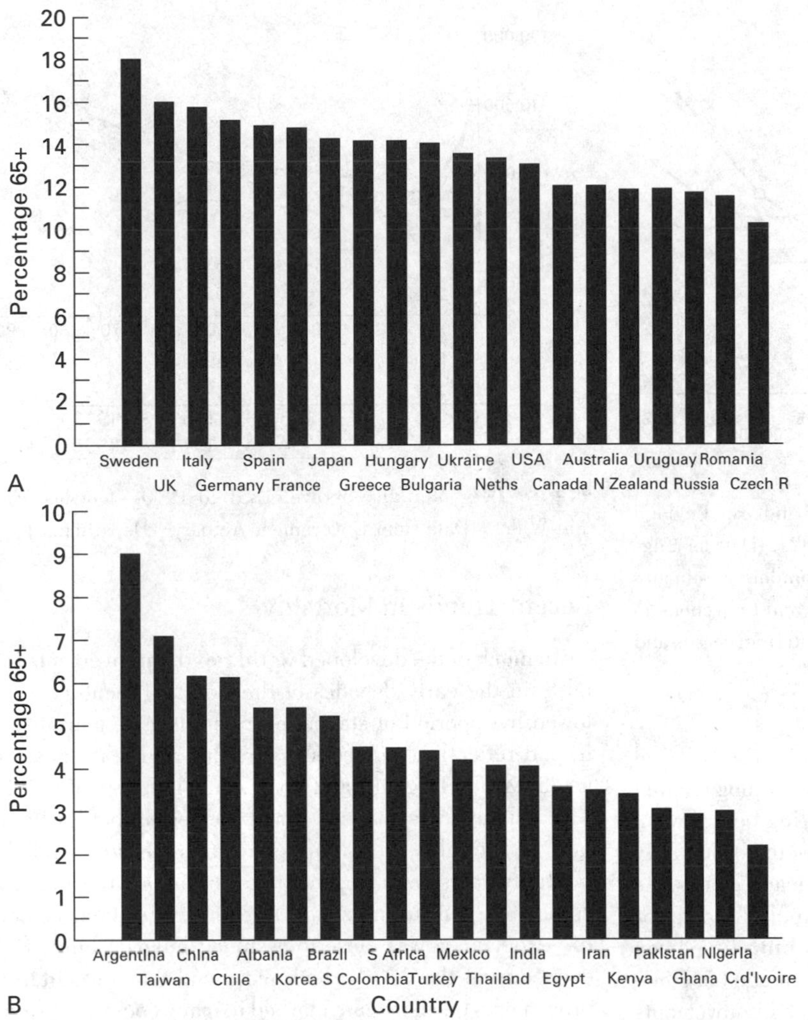

Figure 1-1 Percentage of the population aged 65 and over, 1995 (**A**) Selected countries in which this percentage >10% (**B**) Selected countries in which this percentage is <10%. (Data from Population Reference Bureau, 1990 World data sheet, Washington, DC.)

Wales, Sweden, and Germany. In Japan, the faster pace of fertility decline resulted in much more rapid population aging than in England and Wales or the United States. Recent trends in mortality have amplified this trend, as considered below.

Mortality, Morbidity and the Health Transition

As Preston[21] and others have documented, transitions from relatively high to low mortality have in all populations been associated with transformations in the age, sex and cause and structure of death. Omran[22] coined the term "epidemiologic transition" to describe this process; this concept has been expanded to include identification of separate phases of the transition.[23] There are two components to the epidemiologic transition: changes in the processes of health and disease that define the epidemiologic transition, and changes in the response of societies to these conditions.[24] The term "health transition" was posed as one that embraced both these phenomena. This transition, in all populations who have experienced it, involves substantial falls in death rates from infectious diseases (including respiratory tuberculosis, which was particularly important in England and Wales); bronchitis, pneumonia, and influenza; diarrheal diseases and maternal mortality (although in England and Wales declines in mortality from these causes occurred after the initial fall in infectious disease mortality). In England and Wales over one-half of the gain in life expectancy at birth between 1871 and 1911 was due to reduced infectious disease mortality. Declines in mortality from respiratory tuberculosis during this period led to an increase of nearly 2 years in life expectancy at birth among males and nearly 2.5 years for females—some 20 percent of the total gain.[25] The decline in these causes of death (from which the young benefited more than the old, and women more than men) meant that deaths at older ages accounted for a larger share of all deaths.

Long-term trends in mortality by age in England and Wales

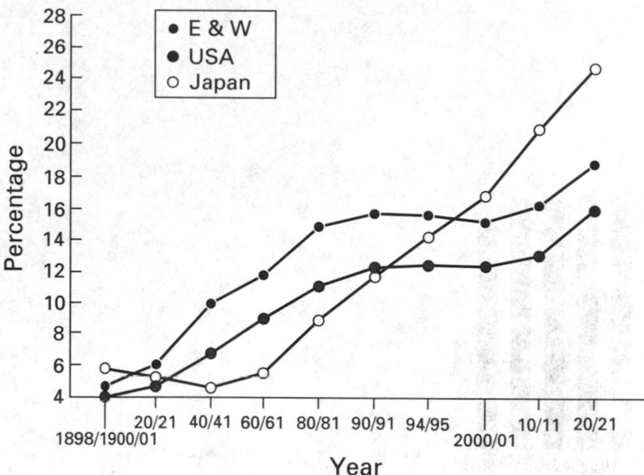

Figure 1-2 Proportion of the population aged 65 and over, England and Wales, the United States, and Japan 1900–2021. (Data for England and Wales from census reports and OPCS population estimates and projections; data for the US from census data and projections in Rosenwaike,[17] Tauber,[18] and Treas[19]; data for Japan from census and projections in Kono.[20])

are shown for men and women respectively in Figures 1-3 and 1-4. It can be seen that in all periods there is a strong relation between age and mortality, with the risk of dying being lowest prepuberty and then rising with age. Improvements in mortality over the whole have been greatest in younger age groups. As a result, as shown in Table 1-2, which also includes data for the United States, gains in life expectancy at birth have been more marked than gains in expectation of life at age 65. However, the table also reveals remarkable recent improvements in later life mortality. Male life expectancy at age 65 in both England and Wales and the United States increased more between 1970 and 1990 than in the whole period from 1900 to 1970.

Figure 1-3 Mortality by age, 1851 to 1990—males, England and Wales. (Data from Government Actuary's Department.)

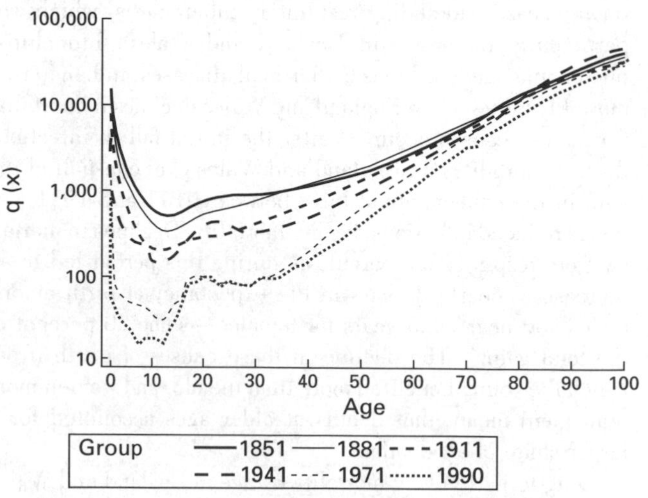

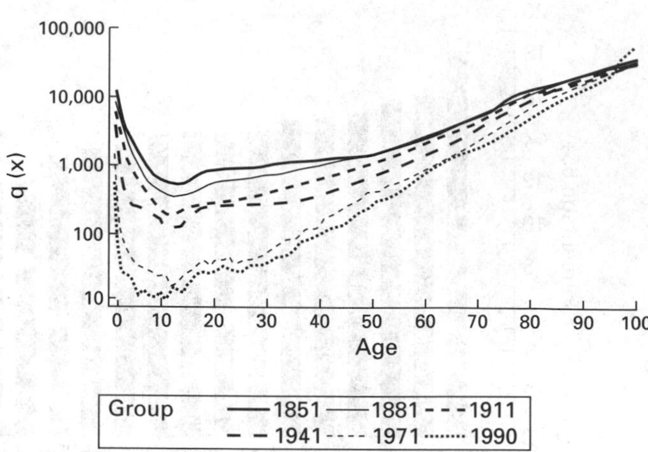

Figure 1-4 Mortality by age, 1851 to 1990—females, England and Wales. (Data from Government Actuary's Department.)

Recent Trends in Mortality

In much of the developed world rapid improvements in mortality in the early decades of the twentieth century were followed by a period of stagnation in adult male mortality rates, in part reflecting increases in circulatory disease death rates, as shown for England and Wales in Figures 1-5 and 1-6. It was assumed by some analysts of the period that further major falls in mortality were unlikely, either because endogenous mortality rates from degenerative diseases were inextricably associated with urbanization or industrialization, or because life expectancy was close to assumed biologic limits.[29] However, during the 1970s, both male and female mortality improvements became more marked in many countries (excluding Eastern Europe), in large part reflecting falls in circulatory disease mortality in North America and Australia and, slightly later, in Western Europe (Figs. 1-5 and 1-6).

Mortality Change at Older Ages and Further Population Aging

These more recent improvements in mortality have been greatest in absolute terms in adult (including elderly adult) age groups where the scope for further improvement was greatest. As a result, changes in death rates at older ages have come to play an increasingly important role in overall mortality change. Myers,[30] in a detailed examination of changes in six developed countries, found that in five of them the proportion of overall life expectancy increase in the 1980s due to gains among those aged 65 or more, was more than 40 percent for males and nearly 60 percent for females. In Japan, 48 percent of the female and 31 percent of the male gain in life expectancy at birth from 1985 to 1990 was due to falls in mortality among those aged 75 or over. In 1955 to 1960, by contrast, one-half of female and two-thirds of male gains were due to falls in mortality, while changes among those aged 65 or over had no or a negative effect on life expectancy.[31]

Not only have changes in late life mortality come to play a

Table 1-2 Trends in life expectancy at birth and at age 65, England and Wales and the United States

	England and Wales							United States						
	Life Expectancy (Years)							Life Expectancy (Years)						
	At Birth			At Age 65				At Birth			At Age 65			
Period	**M**	**F**	**Difference**	**M**	**F**	**Difference**	**Period**	**M**	**F**	**Difference**	**M**	**F**	**Difference**
1891–1900	44.1	47.8	3.7	10.3	11.3	1.0	1900[a]	46.3	48.2	2.0	11.5	12.2	0.7
1950–1952	66.5	71.5	5.0	11.7	14.3	2.6	1950	65.6	71.1	5.5	12.8	15.0	2.2
1970–1972	69.0	75.3	6.3	12.2	16.1	3.9	1970	67.1	74.7	7.6	13.1	17.0	3.9
1988–1990	73.0	78.5	5.5	14.0	17.8	3.8	1990	71.8	78.8	7.0	15.1	18.9	3.9

[a] *10 States and DC Colombia, age 65 data for 1900–1902 period.*
(Data from Treas,[20] *OPCS.*[26–28]*)*

much more dominant role in determining overall level and change in mortality, but in low fertility, low mortality populations with already relatively high proportions of elderly people, mortality changes are now the major determinant of further population aging. It has been estimated that 38 percent of the increase in the proportion of elderly people in the United Kingdom between 1951 and 1981 was due to mortality change,[32] and that in Sweden, Japan, and the United States, falls in mortality at older ages are now a major determinant of continued population aging.[33]

Sex Differentials in Mortality

Apart from age variations in the extent of mortality decline experienced during the transition period from relatively high to relatively low rates, a notable feature is the widening of sex differentials in death rates and so, life expectancy (Table 1-2), which is a general feature observed in populations experiencing mortality decline.[21] Waldron[34] has reviewed the literature on this subject and pointed to changes in the intrahousehold allocation of resources; declines in causes of mortality specifically or primarily affecting women (such as maternal mortality and tuberculosis); gender differences in health-related behavior and in exposure to occupational hazards; and the possibly greater susceptibility of males to stresses associated with socioeconomic change as causal factors. An important result of this sex differential in mortality is the high proportion of widows in elderly populations. As can be seen from Table 1-2, there are signs that the sex differential in mortality in England and Wales and the United States (and a number of other developed countries)[10] is beginning to narrow again. Changes in the relative propensity of men and women to smoke are undoubtedly an important factor in this. Figure 1-7 shows sex ratios in death rates from neoplasms from 1911 to 1991

Figure 1-5 Mortality from diseases of the circulatory system, 1911 to 1991 males, England and Wales. (Data from OPCS.)

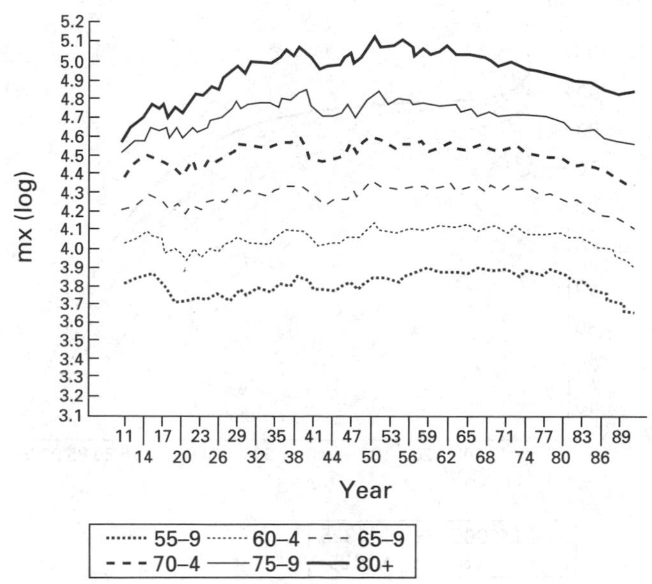

Figure 1-6 Mortality from diseases of the circulatory system, 1911 to 1991 females, England and Wales. (Data from OPCS.)

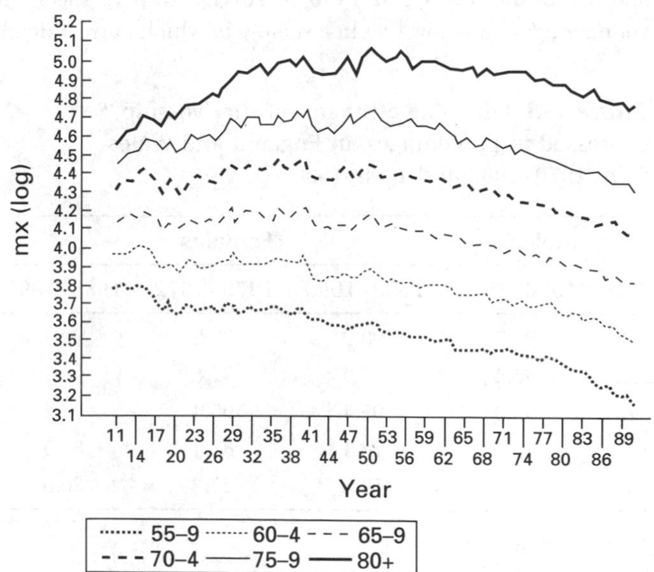

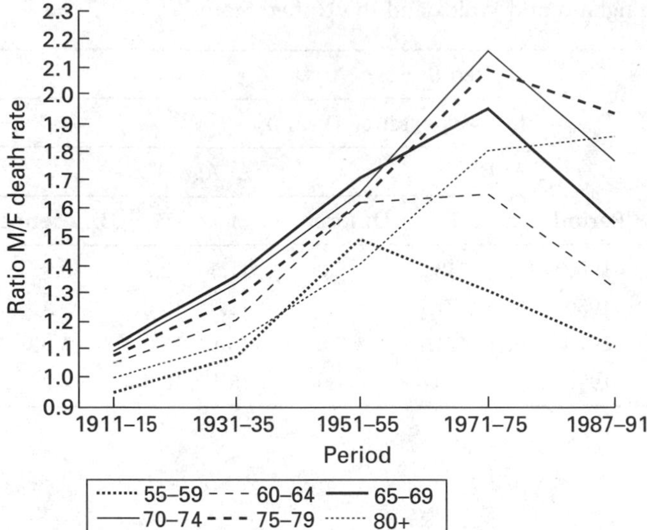

Figure 1-7 Sex ratios in death rates from neoplasms, England and Wales. (Data from OPCS.)

in England and Wales. Although these ratios rose substantially in the early and midcentury, since 1951 they have fallen again in younger age groups that comprise cohorts in which male and female exposures to smoking have been less divergent. This is an example of a cohort effect, a topic considered in more detail in Chapter 12.

The effect of recent changes in mortality on the chances of survival to high ages is illustrated in Table 1-3, which shows period life table estimates of survivorship based on the age-specific mortality schedules for England and Wales in 1970 to 1972 and 1989 to 1990. Already by 1970 to 1972, current mortality rates implied almost universal survival to age 45 and survival to age 65 for a substantial majority. By 1988 to 1990, the chance of survival to extreme old age had increased dramatically. Changes in survivorship from age 65 to age 85 were proportionately much greater than the changes between 1970 and 1972 and 1988 and 1990 in survivorship to specified younger ages. We now live in a society in which current death

Table 1-3 Life table estimates of survivorship,^{a} expressed in percentages, in England and Wales from 1970–1982 and 1988–1990

	Males		Females	
Age	1970–1972	1988–1990	1970–1972	1988–1990
5	97.7	98.9	98.2	99.1
25	96.4	97.9	97.6	98.7
45	93.3	95.4	95.4	97.2
65	70.4	78.4	82.4	86.5
85	11.4	18.5	27.2	36.6

^{a} *Based on period data.*
(Data from OPCS.[26–28]*)*

rates imply that over one-third of females can expect to celebrate their 85th birthday. Table 1-3, based as it is on mortality data for particular periods, can only give an indication of the implications of such mortality patterns if sustained for long periods. The hypothetical measures will diverge considerably from the actual experiences of particular cohorts if mortality ranges change.

Cohort Effects

The importance of cohort influences on health has long been recognized[35] and cohort differences in, for example, mortality from smoking-related diseases have been extensively documented.[36] Other causes of death, such as suicide, also show marked variations by birth cohort.[37] More recently there has been growing interest in the effects of wartime experiences on the subsequent health of the cohorts affected[38,39] and a renewed emphasis on early life influences on adult mortality.[40] Much of this research has focused on early (including in utero) nutritional influences on health in later life and the possible adverse consequences of early nutritional deprivation followed by relative affluence.[41,42] Although the methods employed in some of these studies, particularly those based on ecologic data, have been criticized,[43] clearly this issue is an important one, and a link between health in early and later life seems highly plausible. Figure 1-8 shows the survivorship of birth cohorts, which now comprise the elderly population in England and Wales. In each cohort the proportion surviving to specified ages has been greater. One result of this is that the oldest old, who comprise only a very small proportion of their original birth cohort, are more "selected" than their later born successors, and the extent of this selection varies by cohort. In England and Wales, for example, only 24 percent of men and 36

Figure 1-8 Survivorship of male and female 1905 and 1925 birth cohorts, England and Wales. (Data from Government Actuary's Department.)

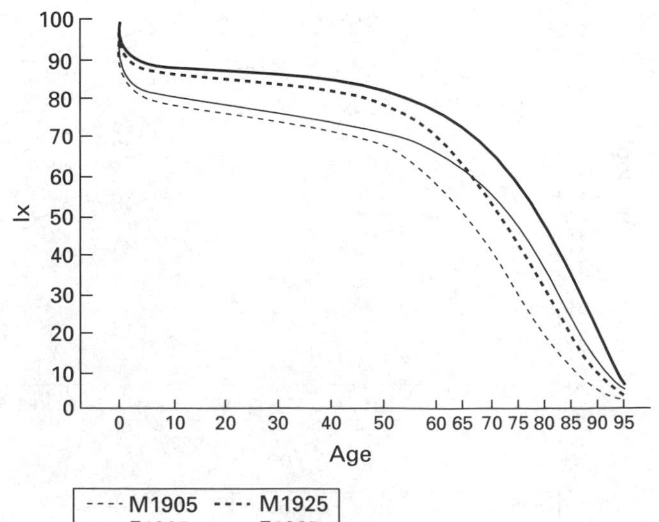

percent of women born in 1881 survived to celebrate their 75th birthday in 1956. Among those born 40 years later, the proportion surviving to age 75 (in 1996) were 41 percent and 58 percent respectively.[44]

Identifying and understanding trends in the relation between mortality and morbidity at older ages is complicated by the need to allow for these differences between cohorts and for the effects of selective survival.

Selective Survival and Health Status

Individuals are endowed at birth with different genetic and early environmental inheritances, and further differentiation occurs throughout the life span as a result of exposure to favorable and unfavorable environmental influences. Because weaker individuals tend to have a shorter survival, the older population includes a larger proportion of those with favorable health characteristics. The age trajectories of death rates for a population may differ substantially from the age pattern of risk for individual members of that population.[7] There is some evidence that the relation between mortality and age weakens in extreme old age,[45,46] which may reflect the status of centenarians as a healthy elite of survivors; although it is possible that this apparent pattern is artifactual.[47] Similarly, prospective studies often show a pattern of "unhealthy" groups becoming "healthier" with length of follow-up.[48] Manton and Stallard,[49] who have contributed extensively to the development and specifications of this thesis, have also suggested that selective survival may account for the apparent crossover in the mortality risks of blacks and whites in the United States, although again there is countervailing evidence that this may be an artifact.[50]

One problem in trying to assess the impact of increased survivorship on the health status of populations is that environmental changes or medical interventions are often likely to both increase survivorship among the frail (thus increasing population morbidity) and improve the health of those who would have survived even in the absence of any intervention (so decreasing ill health in the population, at least in the short term).

Mortality As an Indicator of Population Health

Mortality patterns in populations are of interest not just because of their effect on age structure, but also because of the inferences about health status, and about the process of aging itself, which may be drawn from them. Aging in the individual is associated with decrements in homeostatic mechanisms that bring about adaptive response to environmental challenges. The end result of this process is death, and increases in mortality with age are commonly used as an indicator of senescence.[4]

However, even the use of this most basic indicator poses a number of problems common to all areas of gerontologic research. First, there is the issue of measurement. Incomplete death registration, age misreporting, and numerator denominator biases in the registration and census data from which mortality rates are derived may all produce biases that distort the true pattern of mortality trends and differentials. While these problems are particularly serious in less developed countries, they may also influence the validity of mortality statistics in developed countries. Age misreporting by the very old is a problem in both the United States[51] and Britain[52] and numerator denominator biases mean that uncorrected mortality data for these age groups are unreliable. Comparisons of cause-specific mortality data may be further complicated by variations in coding practices.[53] These measurement problems aside, the usefulness of mortality data as an indicator of population health has been challenged.

Ruzicka and Kane[54] have argued that one important consequence of the epidemiologic or health transition has been a decline in the usefulness of conventional indicators of the health of a population, such as case fatality rates, cause-specific mortality, and life expectation. Although it is appropriate to calculate case fatality rates for many acute infectious diseases, this is not possible, or appropriate, for chronic degenerative diseases, given that the person affected may die, often after a long interval, from another cause. The usefulness of cause of death data (unless multiply coded) as an indicator of major health problems is also limited by the high, and apparently increasing, extent of comorbidity in older age groups.[55] Ruzicka and Kane's criticism of the unquestioning use of life expectancy as a measure of population health arises from the concerns expressed by some that recent reductions in mortality may be due partly to the prolongation of the process of dying rather than to an extension of healthy life.[56–59]

Adherents of this interpretation of recent trends in mortality and morbidity have argued that reductions in mortality at older ages have been achieved partly through medical interventions that postpone the lethal sequelae of chronic diseases, rather than by reducing the incidence or rate of progression of degenerative conditions. In short, the relationship between morbidity and mortality has changed, but with the unfavorable consequence of an increase in the prevalence of morbidity and disability. There is some evidence to support this view. The survival of old people with dementia, for example, seems to have increased.[60–62] However, this may reflect this group sharing the improvements in life expectancy experienced by the general population rather than any excess increase in survival.[63] Observed increases in the incidence of fractured neck of femur have also been associated with decreases in mortality,[64] possibly suggesting that the increased survival of more frail groups may be partly responsible. Finally, population surveys in Britain, France, Canada, and the United States show increases in the reported prevalence of chronic conditions.[65,66] As a result, calculations of disability-free life expectancy (which are discussed further below.) generally also show an unfavorable balance between years of "disabled" life gained to years of "active" life, at least if all degrees of disability, rather than just serious disability, are considered.

A diametrically opposed view of future morbidity trends has

been advanced by Fries[67] and rests on the concept of a fixed biologic limit to the life span. Fries argued that the limit to the life span was about 115 years and that in any population average life expectancy was unlikely to exceed 85. Improvements in health, brought about by the acceptance of personal responsibility for health and appropriate lifestyle changes, would result not in further mortality decline, but in a compression of morbidity at the end of the life span. Those who adopted the appropriate responsible behavior could hope to enjoy a vigorous life, followed by a short period of ill health, and then a natural death resulting from biological senescence rather than a specific disease process.

Fries' argument (largely unmodified in his more recent work) has been challenged on methodologic, theoretic, and empiric grounds.[68–70] Even if there is a fixed biologic limit to the life span—which many dispute[71]—far from reaching a mortality ceiling, many countries are experiencing continuing falls in mortality at advanced ages, and it has been argued that recent mortality data show a wider dispersion by age rather than signs of increasing concentration.[72] Recent analysis of data from Sweden, Japan, and the United States[73] indicates that mortality has been compressed and survival curves become more rectangular, but that this process has now slowed or been reversed.

Although the arguments of Fries on the one hand and Gruenberg on the other seem irreconcilable, adherents of both interpretations shared an assumption that the relation between morbidity and mortality was changing. A third hypothesis of "dynamic equilibrium" has been proposed by Manton.[74] He used United States multicause coded mortality data to examine the frequency with which certain chronic diseases were mentioned at all compared with the frequency with which they features as the underlying cause of death—in effect, a kind of chronic disease case fatality rate. This analysis led him to conclude that the prevalence of chronic diseases was increasing, but not as a result of the postponement of lethal sequelae. Rather, Manton suggested, the rate of progression of certain degenerative diseases had slowed down, partly as a result of medical interventions, resulting in a dynamic equilibrium between mortality and morbidity. This interpretation is consistent with a range of evidence suggesting that, even though overall levels of disability may have increased, there has been a decrease in the most serious forms of disability.[75–78] It should be noted that prospective studies of elderly people have shown that the best predictors of mortality are the markers of established disease or degree of functional capacity.[79–81] It is also clear that population subgroups with the highest mortality suffer more morbidity and the longest periods of disability.[75,82,83] This suggests a continuing strong link between morbidity and mortality.

Cause Specific Morbidity

Table 1-4 shows the prevalence per 1,000 of long-standing illness or disability by condition group for the population aged 65 and over in England in 1993. Among women, the most commonly reported cause of long-term illness or disability were disorders of the musculoskeletal system. These were also reported by more than one-quarter of elderly men, but among men, heart and circulatory system disorders were even more common.

Table 1-4 Rate per 1,000 of long standing illness or disability by condition group, England 1993, private household population aged 65+

Condition Group (ICD Chapter, 9th Revision)	Men		Women	
	Prevalence	Rank	Prevalence	Rank
Musculoskeletal	264	2	388	1
Heart and circulatory	342	1	262	2
Respiratory	135	3	92	4
Digestive	86	4	94	3
Endocrine and metabolic	75	5	79	5
Eye complaints	56	6	63	6

(Data from OPCS.[84])

Disorders such as arthritis may be indirectly associated with mortality (by, for example, increasing the risk of falls and other accidents) but they are rarely recorded as causes of death. Reliance on mortality data alone would tell us little about the problems arising from these common conditions. Heart and other circulatory diseases, by contrast, are associated with common causes of death among the elderly. Current age-and cause-specific mortality statistics imply that more than one-half of all older Americans (and a similar proportion of the United Kingdom population aged 65 and over) will eventually die from circulatory diseases.[85] Even so, morbidity as well as mortality data are needed in any assessment of the health impact of these diseases, as changes in case fatality rates,

Table 1-5 Percentage of population reporting ischemic heart disease, United States 1979–81 to 1985–87

Age and Sex	Period		
	1979–1981	1985–1987	Percent Change
Males			
55–64	7.8	9.9	+26.9
65–74	13.4	15.1	+11.3
75+	10.7	15.6	+14.6
Females			
55–64	4.2	4.5	+10.7
65–74	8.3	8.5	+10.2
75+	9.8	12.0	+12.2

(Data from Mermelstein et al.[86])

Table 1-6 Percentage change in death rates for diseases of the heart, United States 1980–1986

Age	Male	Female
55–59	−18.9	−13.8
60–64	−16.5	−10.7
65–69	−18.2	−13.3
70–74	−14.9	−12.7
75–79	−13.0	−12.8
80–84	−10.3	−11.4
85+	− 9.6	− 6.3

(Data from Furner et al.[87])

Table 1-8 Mean arterial blood pressure in three age cohorts of seventy year olds in Goteborg, Sweden

	Year of Birth		
	Cohort 1	Cohort 2	Cohort 3
Males	1901–1902	1906–1907	1911–1912
Systolic	159	160	157
Diastolic	96	92	84
Females			
Systolic	168	166	160
Diastolic	93	90	85
	Year of Measurement		
	1971–1972	1976–1977	1981–1982

(Data from Svanborg.[85])

rather than in incidence, may account for changes in mortality. As shown in Table 1-5, there have been marked increases in the reported prevalence of ischemic heart disease in the elderly population in the United States. However, as shown in Table 1-6, mortality from heart diseases fell substantially during the same period. It is possible that this increase in reported prevalence reflects increases in the survival of those with heart disease, partly as a result of medical interventions, which would lead to increases in prevalence even if incidence rates were unchanged, or even falling. An equally, if not more probable, explanation is that changes in the health awareness and expectations of both patients and doctors have led to increased reporting of heart disease. Certainly, increases in self-reported hypertension, in the absence of change in observed prevalence, were apparent in the United States in the 1970s, as shown in Table 1-7. In the early 1970s, the observed prevalence was much higher than the self-reported prevalence; by the late 1970s, this gap had narrowed due to increased self-reporting. Analysts of health trends with only this latter source of data available might conclude that hypertension rates were increasing alarmingly, whereas in fact, Table 1-7 suggests that is was awareness of the condition that increased.

Cohort differences also may distort cross-sectional relationships between age and measures such as blood pressure. Table 1-8 shows data taken from three successive cohorts of 70-year-

Table 1-7 Observed and self-reported hypertension in the United States, early and late 1970s

% Observed Hypertension (>160/95)[a] Measured by Nurse				% Self-Reported Hypertension			
	1971–1974	1976–1980	Change: Percentage Points		1972	1979–1981	Change: Percentage Points
Males—white				Males			
55–64	38	38	0	55–64	15	28	+13
65–74	41	44	+3	65–74	18	31	+13
Males—black							
55–64	54	54	0				
65–74	59	45	−6				
Females—white				Females			
55–64	39	39	0	55–64	22	30	+8
65–74	53	53	0	65–74	30	41	+11
Females—black							
55–64	64	62	+2				
65–74	69	77	+8				

[a] *And/or taking antihypertensive medication.*
(Data from Mermelstein et al.[86] and Havlik et al.[88])

olds included in the Gothenburg longitudinal studies.[89] It can be seen that mean diastolic pressure declined from cohort to cohort for both men and women; among women, statistically significant declines in mean systolic pressure were also found. This pattern of lower blood pressure in successive cohorts would tend to exaggerate the associations between age and blood pressure apparent in cross-sectional studies. Selective survival effects may also influence apparent relationships between age and blood pressure, as demonstrated by Kannel and Gordon's comparison of results from cross-sectional and longitudinal analyses of the Framingham study data.[90]

Data on morbidity from specific conditions are therefore subject to measurement biases, cohort, and selective survival effects, which may distort true relation between aging and disease processes. Changes in case fatality rates and in awareness and reporting of conditions further complicates the comparison of prevalence rates. For these reasons, incidence data are to be preferred to prevalence data in epidemiologic studies concerned with the etiology of particular diseases. However, such data are difficult and expensive to collect, and for service planning purposes both incidence and prevalence data are needed, particularly if changes in the duration or severity of the disease are suspected. For epidemiologists concerned with identifying possible risk factors, the incidence data are more revealing, but public health and other service planners also need to know about trends in prevalence. Even more importantly, information on the implications of morbidity for general health status, in the WHO sense of well-being, is needed. Elderly people vary enormously in the extent to which their activities are affected by disease processes; thus the same degree of arthritis may not result in the same level of disability. This is particularly true given the multiple pathology common at older ages. In the Alameda Country Study, for example, 41 percent of those aged 60 and over reported three or more diseases or health problems.[91] Social and environmental factors, as well as host differences, are also important influences on the general health implications of particular pathologic processes. For these reasons we need to consider general indicators of health, particularly functional health, and this is done in the following sections of this chapter.

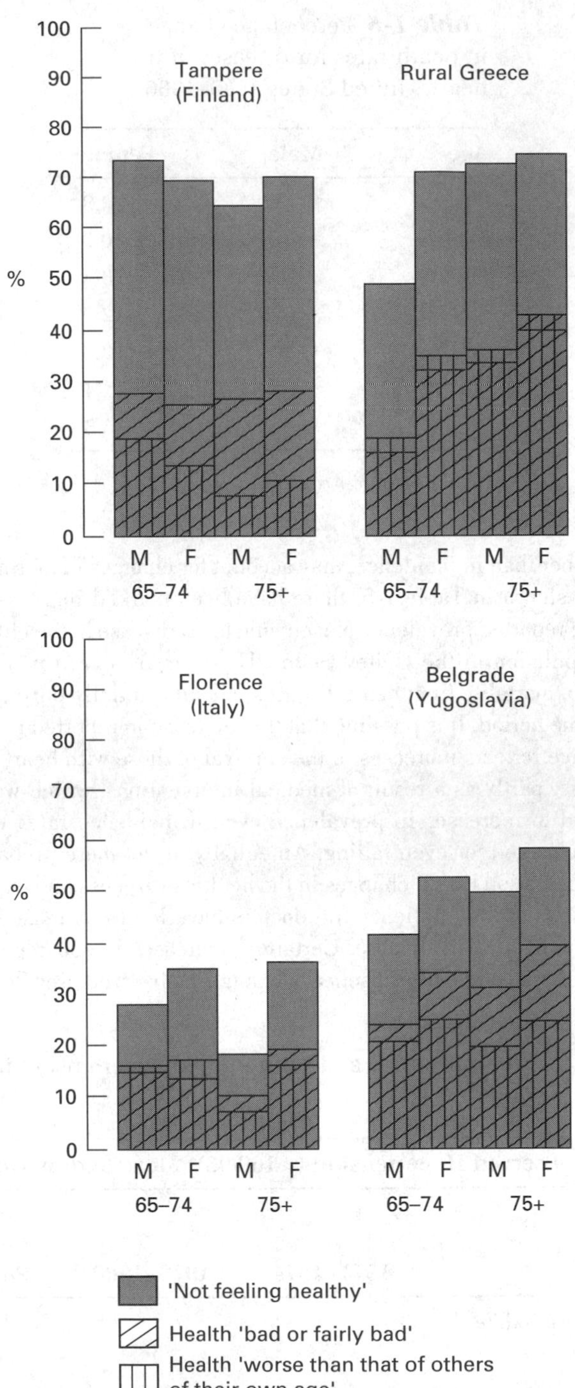

Figure 1-9 Self-reported health status among elderly people in four European countries, mid-1980s. (Data from Heikkinen et al.[94])

Self-reported Health Status

Two types of questions on self assessments of general health status are commonly included in population-based surveys and provide sources of international comparative data. The first asks respondents for a general assessment of their health, sometimes in relation to others of the same age. The second focuses on recent acute and chronic conditions, particularly those that affect usual activities.

Self perceptions of health have been shown in a number of studies to be fairly well correlated with other indicators, such as consultation rates and mortality.[92,93] Although this measure may therefore be useful for investigations into the health status of a defined population, unfortunately, it seems to be less helpful in making comparisons between populations that might throw light on factors influencing the health status of older people. The examination of trends over time, an extremely important issue, is also seriously complicated by possible changes in health expectations discussed above. Figure 1-9 shows data on self-reported health status collected in four of the European nations included in the WHO 11-country study.[94] The countries shown are all ones in which sample sizes were relatively large and included the institutional population. It can be seen that there are marked differences between the countries shown, not only in responses to the three questions on health status included in the (standardized) survey questionnaire, but also in the pattern of variation by age and sex. In rural Greece, for example, 75 percent of men aged 75 and over reported not feeling healthy compared with 50 percent of 65 to 74-year-old old men. In Belgrade, men in the older age group also reported not feeling healthy to a greater extent than younger men, although the differential was less marked. In Florence and Tampere, however, the proportions of 65- to 74-year-old men reporting not feeling healthy were greater than the proportions of men aged 75 or over. These data also show that elderly people in Florence consider themselves much healthier than in the other countries shown, particularly in comparison with Greece or Finland.

The WHO 11-country study also included questions on chronic conditions affecting activities. Respondents to the 11-country study were asked, "Have you had some accident, injury or chronic disease which affects activities of daily living, including work?" Respondents answering this in the affirmative were then asked, "Does this illness or disability limit your activities in any way?" Data gathered from these questions are shown in Figure 1-10. In Finland and Italy, the proportion reporting chronic conditions affecting their activities increases with age among both men and women. However, among Greek women, and both men and women in Belgrade, there is no clear relation to age. Greek levels of limiting chronic conditions are also noticeably higher than those in the other countries shown. These variations, not just in the level of reported health problems but also in the pattern of differentials by age and sex, suggest that the only safe conclusion to draw from the data shown in Figures 1-9 and 1-10, is that cultural differences in attitudes and in levels of customary activity strongly influence perceptions of health status.

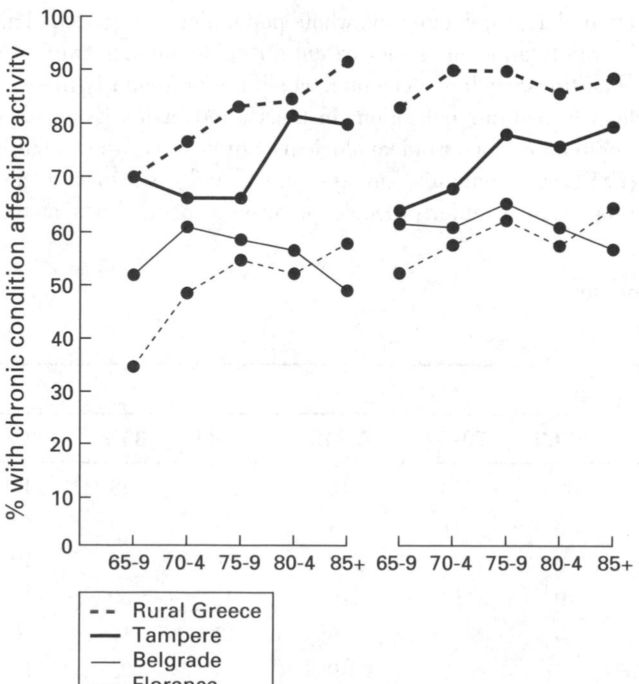

Figure 1-10 Elderly people reporting chronic conditions affecting their activities, four European countries, mid 1980s. (Data from Heikkiren et al.[94])

Functional Health Status

Measure based on indicators of functional ability such as Activities of Daily Living (ADL) and Instrumental Activities of Daily Living (IADL) scores are now very widely used both as an indicator of the health of elderly populations and population subgroups, and in clinical assessments. ADL scales usually include items on basic activities, such as eating and bathing, while IADL scales include questions about activities such as preparing food and shopping. Theoretically, these measures might appear preferable to self reports of perceived health; although influenced by environmental factors, a more standardized form of calibration may be possible. ADL and IADL measures have the advantage of being directly related to needs for services. Within populations, ADL measures also seem to correlate well with other indicators such as mortality and indeed self-assessed health. Data from the United States Longitudinal Study of Aging shown in Table 1-9, for example, illustrate clearly the strong relation between ADL status and survival over a 2-year follow-up period. The proportions surviving were highest for those who had no difficult with any of the ADLs considered, and lowest among those who had difficulty and were receiving assistance from another person. Those with some ADL difficulties were also more likely than those with no difficulties to be in a nursing home by time of follow-up. However, those who received help with ADLs in 1984 were, if anything, less likely to be in a nursing home than those not receiving help; presumably because although their functional disabilities were greater, the fact that they had a supporter able to provide help allowed them to remain in the community. This illustrates how closely health status and family or social circumstances may be linked, an association that severely constrains the inferences that may be drawn about health from data on proportions in institutions or use of community services.

Sensitivity and Specificity

As shown in Table 1-10, questions about mobility or ability to undertake tasks such as bathing certainly show much stronger associations with age than more general questions about perceived health status or limiting long-standing illness. This suggests greater specificity in questions relating to particular activities (as would be expected). On the other hand, questions about serious disabilities are obviously not designed to be sensitive to more prevalent mild or moderate limitations on health or activity.

Data on activities of daily living are widely used to derive indices of functional health.[97] These provide a useful summary measure well correlated with other health indicators. However, major differences between studies in estimates of functional disability have been reported,[98] suggesting that local environ-

Table 1-9 Outcome at 2 years follow-up by age and ADL[a] status in 1984, United States Longitudinal Study of Aging

Outcome		Difficulty with ADLs in 1984		
Age in 1984	Outcome in 1986[b]	No Difficulty	Some Difficulty: Help of Another Person Not Received	Some Difficulty: Help of Another Received
70–79				
Men	Deceased	5.1	20.6	37.5
	Nursing home	0.5	2.1	2.0
	Community	82.9	70.8	54.6
Women	Deceased	4.0	10.4	13.9
	Nursing home	0.7	1.6	9.0
	Community	87.0	75.3	69.1
80+				
Men	Deceased	19.1	27.0	45.5
	Nursing home	2.0	7.8	5.0
	Community	72.0	56.0	40.9
Women	Deceased	8.3	17.3	32.3
	Nursing home	3.4	10.4	7.1
	Community	78.4	61.2	54.8

[a] *Eating, toileting, dressing, bathing, walking, getting in and out of bed or chair, getting outside.*
[b] *9% were lost to follow-up, so these percentages sum to less than 100%.*
(Data from Miller et al.[95])

mental factors, methods of data collection, and other variables affect the results obtained.

Including the Institutional Population

The British GHS, United States NHIS, and several of the other sources referred to in this chapter, relate only to the population living in private households. As about one fifth of the oldest old aged 85 or over in Britain[99] and nearly one quarter in the United States[6] reside in institutions, this omission is important and for a comprehensive picture of age-related changes, data on the whole population are needed. This is true to an even greater extent for epidemiologic studies of conditions, such as dementia, which are particularly likely to lead to institutionalization. In the United States Established Population for Epidemiological Studies of the Elderly (ESPESE) community surveys, substantial differences in the proportion of elderly people performing poorly in a mental

Table 1-10 Indicators of health problems/disability by age and sex, Great Britain 1994 (private household population only)

		Age					
		65–69	70–74	75–79	80–84	85+	65+
Reported limiting long-standing illness	M	39	38	42	50	43	40
	F	35	41	43	46	54	42
Reported inability to manage one or more locomotion activities on their own	M	8	7	9	21	22	10
	F	10	13	19	27	50	19
Reported inability to usually manage bathing/showering/washing all over on their own	M	3	5	6	12	17	6
	F	5	7	9	15	23	10
Health in general in preceding year "not good"	M	21	20	22	31	17	22
	F	18	24	27	26	30	24

(Data from OPCS.[96])

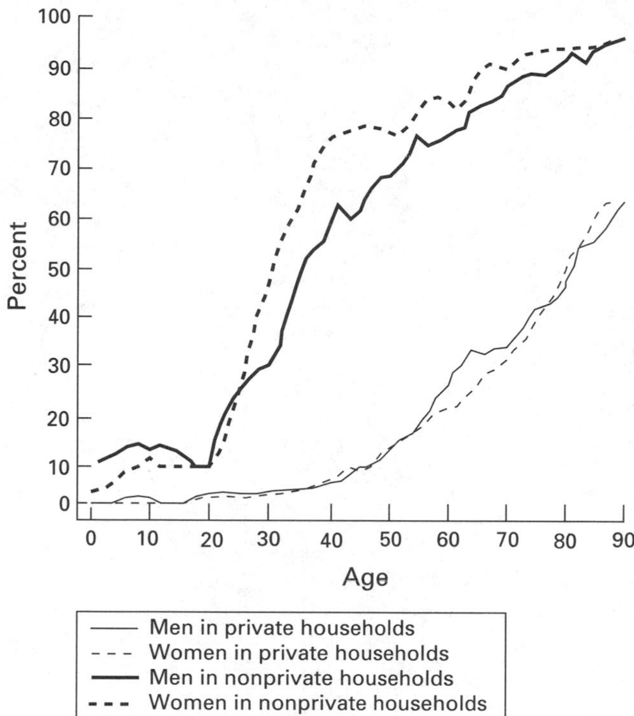

Figure 1-11 Long-term illness by age and type of residence, Great Britain 1991. (From Glaser et al.,[101] with permission.)

status questionnaire test were found between the three areas initially included in the project. These differences were found to reflect variations in the proportion of elderly people in institutions, who were not surveyed.[100]

Recent British data on the whole elderly population, including those in institutions, are available from the 1991 population census. Figure 1-11 shows the prevalence of self-reported long-term illness or serious disability, by age and sex for the private household (community) and nonprivate (institutional) populations.

The large differences, although not unexpected, caution against omitting those in institutions from epidemiologic studies. As residence in institutions is associated with a range of sociodemographic factors as well as health-related variables, such an omission will distort the relation between, for example, marital status and health, as well as resulting in an underestimation of health problems.[102]

Life Table Estimates of Active/Disabled Life Expectancy

A growing number of researchers have used life table methods to analyze data on mortality and on various estimates of disability to produce estimates of expectation of life divided into "active" or "disability-free" years and years with some form of impairment.[65,66,75,77,78,81] Health expectancy is the generic term used to described these and other conceptually similar indications, such as the World Bank's estimation of Disability Adjusted Life Years lost (DALYs).[103]

Health expectancy measures are useful summary indicators that may be readily interpreted. Largely under the auspices of the REVES group,[104] great advances have been made in standardizing terminology and methodology. Nevertheless, the estimates of health expectancy that have now been prepared for some 40 countries are not directly comparable because of the substantial differences in the methods and data used to derive them.[105]

Measures of health expectancy represent a major conceptual advance and a potentially valuable way for governments, health care providers, and individuals to asses health prospects and possibly the effects of interventions. However, the utility of any output measure depends crucially on the validity of the input data. In many cases, as discussed in preceding sections of this chapter, these are deficient. Despite these problems, some general conclusions can be drawn about differentials in health expectancy. In nearly all countries, for example, women have a longer life expectancy than men, but also spend proportionately longer in a state of impaired health.

For a few countries, estimates of health expectancy are available for different time periods, based on input measures that, at least in design, are consistent. Potentially, these results may hold the answer to the very important question of whether falls in mortality in older age groups are associated with reductions or increases in the extent of health limitations. At first sight the results of some of these studies suggest that much of the gain in life expectancy has been a gain in life with an impairment or disability. In the United States, for example, calculations based on NHIS data indicate that male life expec-

Figure 1-12 Percentage consulting general practitioner (family doctor) in preceeding 14 days; attending an outpatient or casualty department in preceeding 3 months; with inpatient stay in preceeding 12 months, Great Britain, 1994. (Data from General Household Survey.)

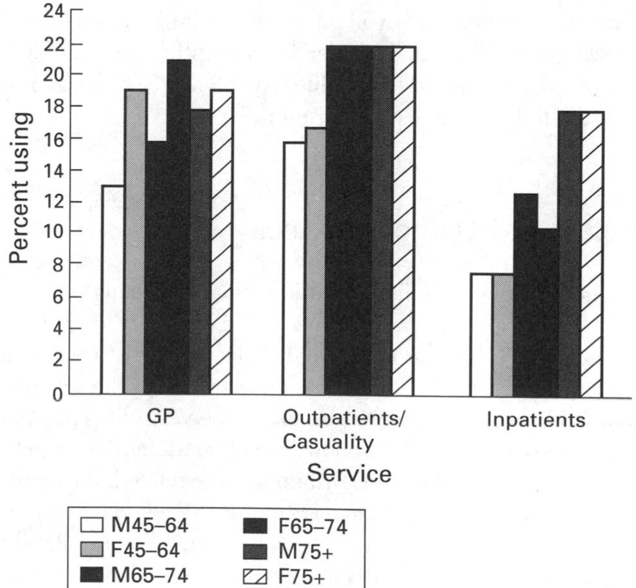

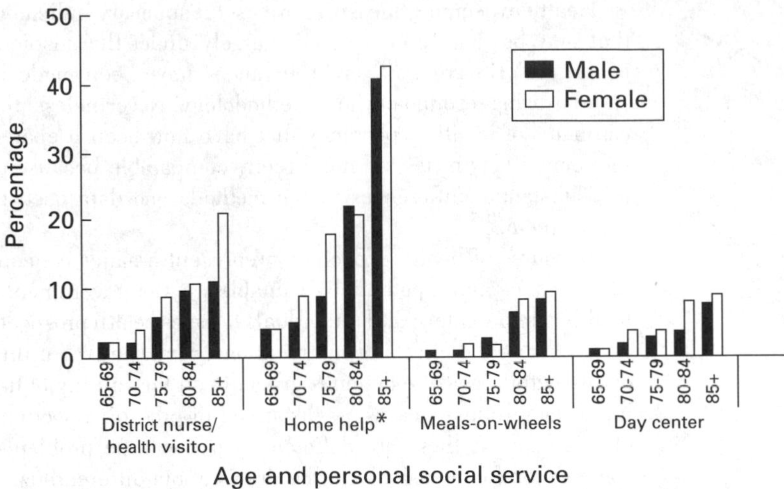

Figure 1-13 Percentage using specified social services in the month before interview, Great Britain 1991. (Data from OPCS, General Household Survey 1991, people aged 65 and over, London, HMSO, 1994.)

tancy in good health increased by only 0.3 years between 1962 and 1976, while life expectancy with an activity restriction increased by 1.5 years.[106] Results from Great Britain, similarly appear at first sight to suggest an unfavorable trend as far as life expectancy free of long-standing illness is concerned. Between 1976 and 1991, male life expectancy in long-term ill health increased by 1.6 years, while life expectancy free of long-term ill health increased by 1.4 years.[75] However, these results are based on responses to general questions in the General Household Survey that may well reflect changes in health *expectations* rather than health *expectancy*. Analyses based on the more detailed ADL questions suggest some reduction in at least the proportion of life lived with a more severe disability.[75] Recent data from the United States Long-Term Care surveys analyzed by Manton and Stallard suggest positive answer to the question of trends in health status. For very old people, the proportion of life expectancy free of disability appears to have increased during the 1980s.[107]

Aging and Use of Services

As the elderly are far more likely than the young to experience health problems, it is not surprising that their use of medical and other services is high. This of course is one of the reasons why policy makers are concerned about the economic implications of increases in the size of the very old population. As Figures 1.12 and 1.13 show, use of health and, even more so, social services in Great Britain are age related; the picture for other developed countries is similar. As noted earlier, service use depends on a range of factors, including availability of support at home and, of course, the extent of service provision, as well as health status.

Discussion

Aging is associated with biologic changes that increase the risk of morbidity, disability, and death. Later life is also marked by changes in economic status, family and household composition (resulting from, for example, widowhood), and in other relationships, all of which may be associated with changes in health status. Social aspects of aging are considered in detail in Chapter 2, but we should note here the evidence showing links between social networks and mortality[108]; the important role played by family and friends in supporting elderly people with disabilities,[109] and the likelihood that economic disadvantages may compound the effects of aging in some groups of the population.[110] Elderly populations are heterogeneous and their characteristics are influenced by historical events and the effects of selective survival. Health is an elusive concept, difficult to define and measure. It is not surprising, therefore, that studies of aging and health present major difficulties. Further methodologic work on overcoming these difficulties, and on collecting data that allows valid comparisons between and within populations at different points in time, is urgently needed to further our knowledge of the epidemiology of aging.

References

1. Lilienfeld DE: Definitions of epidemiology. Am J Epidemiol 1978;107:87–90
2. Greenhouse SW: Definitions of ageing. In Haynes SG, Feinleib M (eds): Proceedings of the Second Conference on the Epidemiology of Aging. Bethesda, Maryland: US, Department of Health and Human Services, Bethesda, Maryland, 1980
3. World Health Organization: Text of the Constitution of the

World Health Organization. Off Rec World Health Organ 1948;2:100

4. Evans JG: Ageing and disease. In: Evered D, Whelan J (eds): Research and the Ageing Population. Ciba Foundation Symposium 124 John Wiley, Chichester, 1988
5. Brouwer A: The nature of ageing. In: Horan MA and Brouwer A (eds): Gerontology: Approaches to Biomedical and Clnical Research. Edward Arnold, London, 1990
6. Seigel JS: A Generation of Change: A Profile of America's Older Population. Russell Sage Foundation, New York, 1992
7. Vaupel JW, Manton KG, Stallard E: The impact of heterogeneity in individual frailty on the dynamics of mortality. Demography 1979;16:439–454
8. Davies AM: Epidemiology and the challenge of aging. In Brody JA, Maddox GL (eds): Epidemiology and Aging. Springer, New York, 1988
9. Rothman KJ: Modern Epidemiology. Little Brown, Boston, 1986
10. United Nations: Population Bulletin No 25. United Nations, New York, 1988
11. Office of Population Censuses and Surveys (OPCS) Population Trends No. 83/1996; HMSO, London, 1996
12. Lotka A: Relation between birth rates and death rates. Science 1907;26:21–22
13. Notestein F: Some demographic aspects of aging. Proc Am Philosoph Soc 1954;98:229–233
14. Carrier N: Demographic aspects of the ageing of the population. In Welford AT, Argyle M, Glass DV, Morris JW, (eds): Society, Problems and Methods of Study. Routledge and Kegan Paul, London, 1962
15. United Nations Economic Commission for Europe/United Nations Fund for Population: Changing age Structures: Demographic and Economic Consequences and Implications. United Nations, Geneva, 1992
16. Kuroda T: Population ageing in Japan with reference to China. Asia-Pacific Population Journal 1987;2:3–22
17. Rosenwaike I: The Extreme Aged in America. Greenwood Press, Westport, Connecticut 1985
18. Taeuber C: Sixty-five plus in America. US Bureau of the Census Current Population Reports. Special Studies. US Government Printing Office, Washington DC, 1992
19. Kono S: Population ageing in Japan. Rev Clinical Geronto 1996;6:205–211
20. Treas J: Older Americans in the 1990s and beyond. Population Bulletin 50.2. Population Reference Bureau, Washington DC, 1995
21. Preston SH: Mortality Patterns in National Populations. Academic Press, New York, 1976
22. Omram A: The epidemiological transition: a theory of the epidemiology of population change. Millbank Mem Fund Quarterly 1971;64:355–391
23. Olshansky SJ, Ault AB: The fourth stage of the epidemiologic transition: the age of delayed degenerative diseases. Millbank Hem Fund Q 1986;64:355–391
24. Ruzicka L, Kane P: Health transition: the course of morbidity and mortality. pp. 1–26. In Caldwell J, Findley S, Caldwell C et al: What We Know About Health Transition: The Cultural, Social and Behavioural Determinants of Health. Vol. 2. Australian National University, Canberra, 1990
25. Casselli G: Health transition and cause specific mortality pp. 68–96. In: Schofield R, Reher D, Bideau A (eds). The decline of mortality in Europe. Clarendon Press, Oxford, 1991
26. OPCS: Mortality statistics serial tables 1841–1985 Series DHI No 19. HMSO, London, 1989
27. OPCS: Life tables 1970–72. Series DS No. 2. HMSO, London, 1979
28. OPCS: Mortality statistics, series DHI No. 24. HMSO, London; 1992
29. Bourgeois-Pichat J: Essai sur la mortalité "biologique" de l'homme. Population 1952;3:381–394
30. Myers G: Comparative study of mortality trends among older persons in developed countries. In Casselli G and Lopez A (eds): Health and Mortality Among Elderly Populations. Clarendon Press, Oxford, 1996
31. Kono S: Demography and population ageing in Japan. In: Ageing in Japan. JARC, Tokyo, 1994
32. Benjamin B: The demographic outlook. In: Benjamin B, Haberman S, Helowicz G, Kay G, Wilkie D (eds): Pensions: The Problems of Today and Tomorrow. Allen and Unwin, London, 1987
33. Preston SH, Himes C, Eggers M: Demographic conditions responsible for population aging. Demography 1989;26: 691–704
34. Waldron I: What do we know about sex differences in mortality? Population Bulletin No. 18. United Nations, New York, 1986
35. Kermack W, McKendrick A, McKinlay: Death rates in Great Britain and Sweden: some general regularities and their significance. Lancet 1934;226:698–703
36. Alderson MR, Ashwood F: Projection of mortality rates for the elderly. Pop Trends 1985;42:22–29
37. Murphy E, Lindesay J, Grundy E: Sixty years of suicide in England and Wales: a cohort study. Arch Gen Psych 1986; 43:969–976
38. Horiuchi S: The long term impact of war on mortality: old age mortality of First World War survivors in the Federal Republic of Germany. Population Bulletin No. 5 United Nations, New York, 1983
39. Caselli G: The influence of cohort effects on differentials and trends in mortality. In Vallin J, D'Souza S and Palloni A (eds): Measurement and Analysis of Mortality: New Approaches. Clarendon Press, Oxford, 1990
40. Barker DJP (ed): Fetal and infant origins of adult diseas. BMJ Publishing Group, London, 1992
41. Forsdahl A: Are poor living conditions in childhood and adolescence an important risk factor for arteriosclerotic heart disease? Br J Prevent So Med 1977;31:91–95
42. Forsdahl A: Living conditions in childhood and subsequent development of risk factors for arteriosclerotic heart disease. J Epidemiol Community Health 1978;32:34–37
43. Elo IT, Preston SH: Effects of early life conditions on adult mortality: a review. Population Index: 1992;58:186–212
44. Grundy E: The health and health care of older adults in England and Wales 1841–1991. In Charlton JC, Murphy M (eds): The health of Adult Britain 1841–1991. HMSO, London, 1997

45. Barrett JC: The mortality of centenarians. Arch Gerontol Geriat Medicine 1985;4:211–218
46. Barrett JC: The mortality of centenarians: a correction. Arch Gerontol Geriatr Medicine 1986;5:81
47. Coale A: Kisker EE: Defects in data on old age mortality in the United States: new procedures for calculating mortality schedules and life tables at the highest ages. Asian and Pacific Population Forum: 1990;4:1–31
48. Fox AJ, Goldblatt PO, Adelstein AM: Selection and mortality differentials. J Epidemiol Community Health 1982;36:69–79
49. Manton KG, Stallard E: Recent treands in mortality analysis. Academic Press New York, 1984
50. Preston SH, Elo IT, Rosenwaike I, Hill M: African-American Mortality at Older Ages: results of a matching study. Demography 1996;33:173–209
51. Kestenbaum B: A description of the extreme aged population based on improved Medicare enrollment data. Demography 1992;29:411–426
52. Thatcher AR: Trends and prospects at very high ages. In Charlton JC, Murphy M (eds): The Health of Adult Britain 1841–1991. London, HMSO, 1997
53. Alderson M: International Mortality Statistics. Macmillan Press, London, 1981
54. Ruzicka L, Kane P: Health transition: the course of morbidity and mortality. In Caldwell J, Findley S, Caldwell P et al (eds): What We Know About Health Transition: The Cultural, Social and Behavioural Determinants of Health Vol. 1. Canberra: Health Transition Centre, Australian National University, 1990
55. Israle Rosenberg Curtin, Am J Epidemiol 1986
56. Gruenberg EM: The failures of success. Millbank Mem Fund Q 1977;55:3–24
57. Kramer M. The rising pandemic of mental disorders and associated chronic diseases and disabilities. Acta Psych Scand 1980;62(suppl):285
58. Verbrugge L: Longer life but worsening health? Trends in health and mortality in middle-aged and older persons. Millbank Mem Fund Q, 1984;62:475–519
59. Rogers A, Rogers RG, Belanger A: Longer life but worse health? Measurement and dynamics. Gerontologist; 1990;30: 640–647
60. Blessed G, Wilson I: The contemporary natural history of mental disorder in old age. Br J Psychiat 1982;141:59–67
61. Christie A: Changing patterns in mental illness in the elderly. Br J Psychiat 1982;140:154–159
62. Gruenberg EM, Hagnell O: The rising prevalence of chronic brain syndrome in the elderly. In Levi L (ed): Society, Stress and Disease. Vol. 5, Old Age. Oxford: Oxford University Press, Oxford, 1987
63. Wood E, Whitfield E, Christie A: Changes in survival in demented hospital inpatients 1957–1987. Int J Geriat Israel Psychiatry 1991;6:523–528
64. Finsen V: Improvements in general health among the elderly: a factor in the rising incidence of hip fractures? J Epidemiol Comm Health 1988;42:200–203
65. Colvez A, Blanchet M: Disability trends in the United States population 1966–76: analysis of reported causes. Am J Public Health 1981;71:464–471
66. Robine JM, Blanchett M, Dowd JE: Health expectancy; 1st workshop of the International Health Life Expectancy Network (REVES). Studies on Medical and Population Subjects No. 54. HMSO, London, 1992
67. Fries J: Aging, natural death and the compression of morbidity. N Engl J Med 1980;303;130–135
68. Bromley D, Isaacs B, Bytheway B. Review symposium: ageing and the rectangular curve. Ageing and Society 1982;2: 383–392
69. Schneider E, Brody J. Aging, natural death and the compression of morbidity: another view. N Engl J Med 1983;309: 854–856
70. Grundy E: Mortality and morbidity among the old. BMJ 1984; 288:663–664
71. Gavrilov LA, Gavrilova NS: the biology of life span: a quantitative approach. Harwood Academic Publishers, London, 1991
72. Rothenberg R, Lentzner H, Parker R: Population aging patterns: the expansion of mortality. J Gerontol 1991;46:S66–70
73. Wilmoth JR, Curtsinger JW, Horiuchi S: Rectangularization revisited: survival curves for humans and fruit flies. Paper presented at the Annual Meeting of the Population Association of America, San Francisco, April 6–8, 1995
74. Manton KG: Changing concepts of morbidity and mortality in the elderly population. Millbank Mem Fund Q 1982;60: 183–224
75. Bone MR, Bebbington AC, Jagger C Morgan K, Nicolaas G Health expectancy and its uses. HMSO, London, 1996
76. Grundy E: Future patterns of morbidity in old age. In Caird FI, Evans JG (eds): Advanced Geriatric Medicine 6. John Wright, Bristol; 1987
77. Boshiuzen HC, Van de Water HPA: An international comparison of health expectancies. TNO Health Research, Leiden, 1994
78. Crimmins E, Saito Y, Ingegneri D: Changes in life expectancy and disability-free life expectancy in the United States. Population and Development Review 1989;15:235–267
79. Campbell J, Diep C, Reinken J, McCosh L: Factors predicting mortality in a total population sample of the elderly. J Epidemiol Community Health 1985;39:337–342
80. Warren MD, Knight R: Mortality in relation to the functional capacities' of people with disabilities living at home. J Epidemiol Community Health 1985;36:220–223
81. Ruigómez A, Alonso J, Auto JM: Functinal capacity and five year mortality in a sample of urban community elderly. Eur J Public Health 1993;3:165–171
82. Wilkins R, Adams O: Health expectancy in Canada, late 1970s: demographic, regional and social dimensions. Am J Public Health 1983;73:1073–1080
83. Preston SH, Taubman P: Socioeconomic differences in adult mortality and health status. pp. 279–318. In Martin LG, Preston JH (eds): Demography of Aging. National Academic Press, Washington DC, 1994
84. OPCS. Health Survey for England 1994. HMSO, London, 1995
85. WHO: World Health Statistics Annual 1988. WHO, Geneva, 1988
86. Mermelstein R, Miller B, Prohanska T et al: Measures of health In Van Nostrand JF, Furner DE, Suzman, R (eds): Health Data

on Older Americans: United States 1992. National Center for Health Statistics. Vital Health Stat (27) U.S. Department of Health and Human Services, Hyattsville, Maryland, 1993

87. Furner SE, Maurer J, Rosenberg H. Mortality. In Van Nostrand JF, Furner DE, Suzman, R (eds): Health Data on Older Americans: United States 1992. National Center for Health Statistics. Vital Health Stat (27) US Department of Health and Human Services, Hyattsville, Maryland, 1993
88. Havlik RJ, Lim BH, Kovar MG et al: Health statistics on older persons, United States 1986, Vital and Health Statistics. Series 3 No 23 DHHS Pub No (PHS) 87–1409. US Government Printing Office, Washington, D.C. 1987
89. Svanborg A: The health of the elderly population: results from longitudinal studies with age-cohort comparisons. In Evered D, Whelan J (eds): Research and the ageing population. Ciba Foundation Symposium 134. John Wiley Chichester, 1988
90. Kannel WB, Gordon T: Cardiovascular risk factors in the aged: the Framingham Study. In Haynes SG, Feinleib M (eds): Second conference on the epidemiology of ageing. U.S. Dept of Health and Human Services, Bethesda, Maryland, 1980
91. Seeman TE, Guralnik JM, Kaplan GA et al: The health consequences of multiple morbidity in the elderly. J Aging Health 1989;1:55–66
92. Blaxter M: Self definition of health status and consultation rates in primary care. Q J Soc Affairs 1985;1:131
93. Idler EL, Kasl S: Health perceptions and survival: do global evaluations of health status really predict mortality? J Gerontol 1991;46:S55–65
94. Heikkinen E, Waters WE, Brezezinski ZJ: The elderly in eleven countries, a sociomedical survey. WHO Regional Office for Europe Copenhagen, 1983
95. Miller B, Prohanska T, Mermelstein R, van Nostrand JF: Changes in functional status and risk of institutionalization and death. In Van Nostrand JF, Furner DE, Suzman, R (eds): Health Data on Older Americans: United States 1992. National Center for Health Statistics. Vital Health Stat (27) US Department of Health and Human Services, Hyattsville, Maryland, 1993
96. OPCS Living in Britain: results from the 1994 General Household Survey. HMSO, London 1996
97. Katz S, Branch LG, Branson MH et al: Active life expectancy. N Engl J Med 1983;309:1218–1224
98. Weiner JM, Hanley RJ, Clark R, Van Nostrand JF: Measuring the activities of daily living: comparisons across national surveys. J Gerontol 1990;45:S229–S237
99. Grundy E: Population Review: People aged 60 and over. Population Trends 1996; 83:14–20
100. White LR, Kohout F, Evans DA et al: Related health problems. In Coroni-Huntley J et al (eds): Established populations for epidemiological studies of the elderly. National Institute on Aging, US Dept. of Health and Human Services, Bethesda, Maryland; 1986
101. Glaser K, Murphy M, Grundy E: Limiting long-term illness and household structure among people aged 45 and over, Great Britain 1991. Ageing Soc 1996;17:3–20
102. Murphy M, Glaser K, Grundy E: Marital status and limiting long-term illness in Britain. Journal of Marriage and the Family 1997;59:156–164
103. World Bank: World Development Report 1993: Investing in Health, World Development Indicators. Oxford University Press Oxford; 1983
104. Robine JM, Romieu I, Cambois E et al: HPA, Boshuizen HC and Jagger C Contribution of the Network on Health Expectancy and the Disability Process. REVES Montpellier, 1995
105. Robine JM, Romieu I, Cambois E: Health expectancies in current research. Rev Clin Gerontol 1997:7;73–81
106. Serow WJ, Sly DF, Wrigley JM: Population Aging in the United States. Greenwood Press; New York, 1990
107. Manton K, Stallard E: Medical demography: interaction of disability dynamics and mortaly. p. 217–278. In Martin LG, Preston SH: Demography of Aging. National Academy Press, Washington DC 1994

C H A P T E R 2

Social Gerontology

MALCOLM L. JOHNSON

The processes of human aging involve individuals developing, changing, and adapting throughout their life-span. Their physical bodies grow and develop, then after a long plateau of change within adult maturity, decline in some degree and then more sharply in late old age. But the person is more than a body. Individuals exist in a social world of intimate and more formal relationships; live in a dwelling that is part of a neighborhood, in a community that is part of a nation state. Along with biologic growth, people change in their understanding of the social world, acquire knowledge and skills, and expand emotionally and spiritually. And in this journey along the life path, "life chances" are profoundly affected by experiences of childhood, family, education, and income.

Social gerontology concerns itself with the social and psychologic aspects of aging, with a particular focus on later life. Like many other areas of academic study, it is not easy to define with precision. *The International Glossary of Social Gerontology* says, it is "the sub-field of gerontology which studies the social and psychological aspects of ageing processes, societal attitudes to older persons, the place of older persons in society, and increasingly, how these relate to biological ageing."[1]

As a specialist area of study, social gerontology, like geriatrics, is a product of the second half of the twentieth century. Some important work was done before the Second World War, but it was only after it finished that knowledge began to accumulate in an identifiable way. The journal *Geriatrics* began in 1940 and the Gerontological Society of America was established in 1945—the same year as the first issue of the *Journal of Gerontology*. Physicians specializing in the medical treatment of old people were commencing work in British hospitals in the late 1940s with Lord Amulree and Marjory Warren emerging as early national standard bearers. Social scientists and psychologists began to publish important research-based books. Among the significant texts were Pollock's *Social Adjustment in Old Age*[2] and Havighurst and Albrecht's *Older People*[3] in America and Peter Townsend's two major books *The Family Life of Old People*.[4] and *The Last Refuge*.[5] in the United Kingdom. In the Netherlands, the psychologist Joep Munnichs was already in the field, as were Hans Thomae and Ursula Lehr in Germany and Leopold Rosenmayr in Austria.

This early work almost inevitably focused on the problems of old age. While geriatrics was preoccupied with strokes, falls, infections, and the biology of physical decline, social gerontologists studied social isolation, poverty, the apparent reduction in family support, inadequate housing, the poor quality of nursing and residential homes, impairments of cognitive functioning, mental illness, widowhood, loss and bereavement. Indeed, the pathology model has dominated the growth of the whole of gerontology, and only in the past decade has the literature taken "normal" and positive aging seriously. Baltes and Baltes' volume *Successful Aging: Perspectives from the Behavioural Sciences*[6] might be seen as a landmark that validated the holistic study of aging throughout the life span.

Like many of the new postsecond world war subdisciplines, gerontology was largely applied and empirical addressing what were seen as the major problems. The same was true in the parallel growth of criminology, the sociology of health and illness, urban studies, and the psychology of learning disabilities (mental handicap). In part this was the natural inclination of the researchers who were interested in conducting studies that would affect policy and practice to the benefit of older people. In part, it was because funding for research in these new areas was forthcoming only for the investigation of known and recognized social issues.

The treatment of aging and old age as the proper subject of serious research required scientists from each of the contributing disciplines to carry much of their prior academic baggage with them. This meant that the first and second generation of researchers did not neglect the theoretic and conceptual aspects of aging, but for the most part, they recycled theoretic notions that were already part of the wider discourse in their fields. For the sociologists, this meant a concern with role theory, family and generational relationships, class, status, power, and networks.

All of this can be observed in the remarkably visionary first edition of *Handbook of Aging and the Social Sciences*.[7] Its 25 chapters mapped social gerontology at a point when a distinct body of knowledge was emerging. Moreover, it astutely included contributions on emerging issues that have subsequently flourished as vital areas of the subdiscipline. Peter Laslett's chapter signalled an attention to the history of aging worldwide and carried within it formative statements about historic demography—the history of population structures.

This chapter draws upon material in Johnson ML: Dependency and Interdependency. In Bond J, Coleman P, Peace S (eds): Ageing in Society: An Introduction to Social Gerontology, Sage, London, 1993.

Vern Bengtson and Neal Cutler foreshadowed the major debate that ran throughout the 1980s and 1990s concerning the political economy of old age and the conflict between generations.

Harrold Sheppard's piece on work and retirement marked out a set of enduring and recurrently topical concerns about the importance of work, leisure, and income in later life. There were also sections on the economics of old age, death and dying, and legal aspects of life change and being old. Curiously, these three areas, important as they undoubtedly are, have not attracted the scholarly attention they deserve and remain underdeveloped. Economists have been very late to recognize the significance for world economic systems of the permanent shifts in age structures that Emily Grundy explains in her chapter in this volume. Similarly lawyers have shown little interest in gerontologic matters, despite the public interest in, for example, the depletion of personal capital to pay for nursing home care and its impact on inheritance. Nor are many attracted to the issues regarding citizenship for the increasing numbers of Alzheimer's disease sufferers. It is equally difficult to understand the modest size of the research literature on death, dying, and bereavement in old age when in this century, premature death has been so spectacularly reduced that death occurs almost exclusively (in developed economies) in old age.

Academic subjects are constantly changing and growing, so there cannot be a definitive statement that will permanently delineate their parameters. This is particularly so with social gerontology because its central dynamic themes, aging and changing, permeate every aspect of the human condition. There is no pre-existing area of knowledge that is unaffected by the consequences of the demographic revolution. Longer life for individuals all over the world has produced a structural shift of the first magnitude. It inevitably embraces all of the basic medical sciences and the practice of medicine, along with the established social and policy sciences. But it also intrudes into history, literature, art, philosophy, law, engineering, and even, apparently, disconnected fields like veterinary studies (companion animals and older people).

By now the reader will have become aware that one short chapter cannot possibly deal with the whole field of social gerontology. So it will be necessary to provide a slice through the ideas, concepts, and empirical evidence that reveal the nature of the subject. Mindful that this textbook is designed primarily for clinicians, I have selected the theme of *dependency* as the central focus of much of what follows. There are several reasons for this choice:

1. The medical literature itself is greatly preoccupied by the levels of functional capacity among older people, so it coincides with the perspectives adopted by other authors in this volume.
2. Although dependency is seen as a pathology, a sign of failing physical, social, or psychologic ability, it is also a concept that needs explanation. As is argued later, we are all dependent; so what does dependency mean and what are the desirable and undesirable components of it?
3. Dependency has probably been the major sociomedical field over the past 50 years.
4. It gathers in its wake a wide range of related issues, data, concepts, theories, and disciplines, and is thus representative of the true interdisciplinary character of social gerontology.

Again, it would be impossible to deal with the contexts and consequences of dependency in all societies. Therefore, the literature and data used here are principally from the United Kingdom, but set within the international body of knowledge. As the medical, social, and state systems vary from country to country, readers will need to make some translation to the settings in which they live or work. The references will provide a route to that information. But the issues are universal.

It would require considerable space to explain and illustrate for those readers who might need it, the use of concepts and theories in the social sciences and their application within social gerontology. Valuable sections can be found in the general texts by McPherson,[8] Fennell et al.,[9] and Hendricks and Hendricks.[10] However, the discerning reader will readily recognize in the remainder of this chapter the use of concepts such as reciprocity, social exchange, deviance, labelling, structured dependency, and political economy. Policy and practice implications are drawn out as a result of the combination of conceptual analysis and empirical research.

What is Dependency?

The implication of the term is that there is a majority of people who lead independent lives and a minority who do not, and that those in the latter group are in need of help. But is this a realistic set of assumptions? Who is independent in modern society? Whose lifestyle would remain unchanged if those who support them withdrew?

The Dutch psychologist Munnichs has highlighted the fallacy of the strict dichotomy between dependence and independence. He writes:[11]

> Dependency is always placed in contradiction to independency as if they exclude each other. In the opinion of many Western policy makers these concepts are even used to denote the object of policy aims and the means by which existing measures are tested. When these measures promote independency it is all right, if not, dependency is the root of the problem and then measures need to be changed.

Clark[12] has distinguished a range of sociopsychological and individual-psychological forms of dependency. She has identified (1) dependency of crisis (the loss of spouse or similar trauma), (2) neurotic dependency (where individuals develop a pathologic reliance on others), and (3) development or transitional dependency (arising from puberty, menopause, retirement, etc.), as afflictions that arise out of individuals. In further elaboration, Clark even begins to rank these conditions, nominating neurotic dependency as the worst form because "it persists throughout life as a dominant technique of adjustment and especially in stressful situations. The dependency is expressed in such attributes as self-effacement, dread of loneliness, ingratiation and indecision."[12]

The psychological conditions to which Clark draws attention would certainly reduce any individual's ability to manage their personal lives well. But so, too, would many other influences. Being grossly overweight or drinking too much alcohol would also inhibit social performance, as would the absence of educational qualifications or the inability to form worthwhile relationships. All of these elements would act as inhibitions to the achievement of personal potential. They can be seen as limits to our progress.

Equally they can be viewed as handicaps or disabilities, for these terms are often used loosely as synonyms for dependency. Yet there is a curious circumscription of the usage of these words, which confines their general application to particular categories of people. Wheelchair users who cannot do their own washing and ironing are "handicapped" and "dependent," but middle-aged bank managers who cannot do their own laundry are considered to be neither. Women who cannot change electric fuses and men who cannot cook are fundamentally dependent on others, but the term is never used. From these everyday examples it is evident that we live in an interdependent world. There is no one who in any proper sense is independent. In simpler societies than ours, individuals and families may be largely self-sufficient in food, clothing, and shelter. Apart from hermits and recluses who choose to lie outside of them, there is interdependence for all who exist in human societies. Indeed, the very notion of society, as a social system in which human beings live in community with each other, presupposes an agreed system of social rules and conventions that regulate our behavior and recognize the different contributions of others to the common good. These fundamental principles of social life require certain components to be present. Salient among these are mutual trust, a workable system of social exchange (of goods and services) and a willingness to involve every member of society in a way that provides them with recognized social roles and consequent livelihood.

In complex societies the extent of interdependence is greatly increased. We are all totally dependent on many strangers (who produce food, power, clothing, etc.) as well as on those with whom we live, work, and have other personal relations. These forms of universal dependence are acknowledged, but not encompassed in the usage of the word. The logic for this appears to be that we are all contributors as well as receivers and thus equal partners in a social contract. It is those who for some reason are unable to contribute, or are disbarred from contributing in economically recognized ways, who are prone to being labelled dependent. Thus, it is children, unemployed people, those who have physical and mental handicaps, the retired, and the old, who fall into this category.

Inclusion in the groupings of dependent people involves a process of *social* definition. Yet public and private reactions to those who have special need of the support of others to maintain their existence tends to be on an *individual* basis. While there is some recognition that illness is not their own fault, there remains a strong tendency to treat people who are handicapped in the performance of routine activities as personally responsible for their plight. Such victimization is not peculiar to any particular group of people, but is most strongly expressed in cases where incompetence can be observed, but the causes cannot.

People with hearing impairments or mental health problems are, in general, subject to less sympathetic and more controlling actions by others than wheelchair users or frail elderly people.[13,14]

David Wilkin[15] has helpfully refined these ideas in the process of applying them to the task of measuring dependency. He expresses reservations about the central use of helplessness and powerlessness as important dimensions, and dismisses them as too restrictive to be at the core of any definition or measure. Instead he argues that, "The key component is the reference to a social relationship," and goes on to offer his own definition, "a state in which an individual *is reliant* upon other(s) for assistance in meeting *recognized needs*." The analysis that led him to these conclusions was then applied to currently accepted causes and features of dependence. These were set alongside a summary list of recognized needs and presented in the form of a matrix (Fig. 2-1), with the intention of illustrating the complexity of dependency situations.

It is clear then that interdependency is a real phenomenon that is an integral component of citizenship. A special subset of this interdependency has been isolated and identified as dependency in modern societies. It is applied in the following circumstances:

- Where individuals, congenitally or by acquisition, are incapable, temporarily or permanently, of performing a range of actions that are assumed to be within the competence of full citizens of a given society.
- In particular, where there is an inability to carry out essential tasks related to personal maintenance, physical mobility, sensory functioning, mental stability, and communication (verbal or written).
- Where society by its laws, conventions, buildings, and social institutions places individuals in a dependent role or situation, such as children, or those who are unemployed, sick, financially insolvent, or otherwise deemed incompetent to live an independent and unsupervised life.

The interaction of personal factors and social mechanisms varies according to the characteristics of the person and the nature of the disability. For example, Cypriot or Pakistani women who come to Britain as non-English-speaking people are dependent and limited in their social participation in a similar way to a prelingually deaf person.[16,17] An unemployed person shares the same dependence on government agendas and the same restriction of consumer behavior as an elderly person on income support.

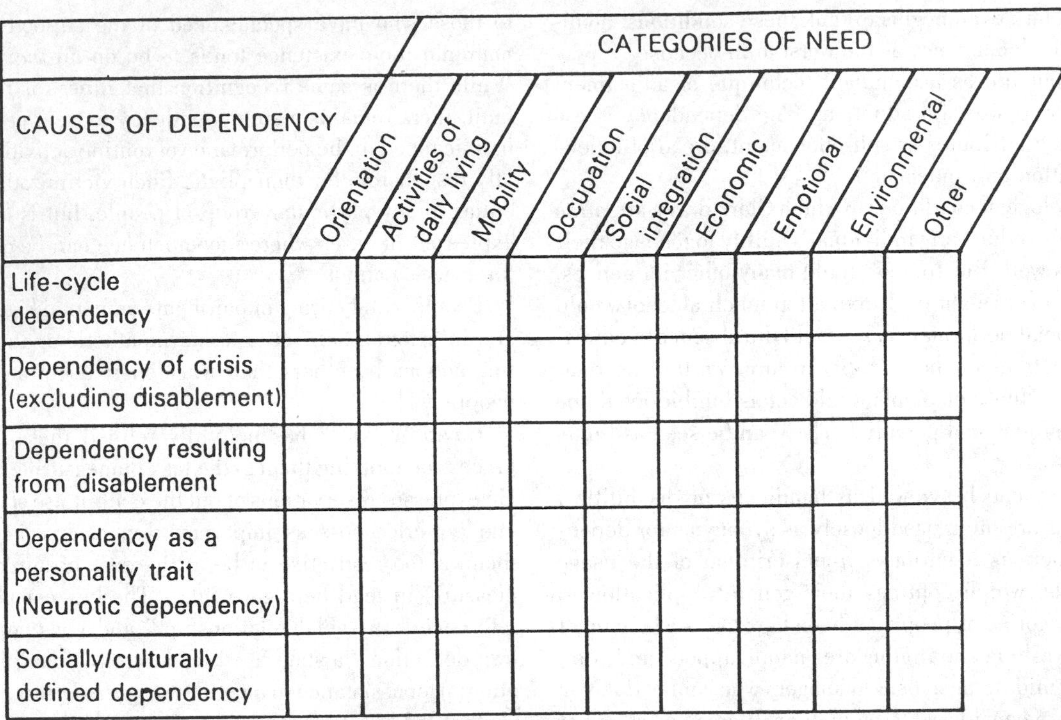

Figure 2-1 Classification matrix—dependency. (From Wilkin,[15] with permission.)

It will be necessary to look in more detail at the processes and circumstances that create dependent situations. However, it remains an inescapable fact that a significant minority of the population falls into this category. Millions of people can function as human beings only if others wash them, launder their clothes, clean their homes, cook their food, or transport them. Elderly people constitute the largest group within this pool. As evidenced by the Office of Population Censuses and Surveys (OPCS) survey,[18] the majority of people with hearing or visual impairments, mental health problems and mobility restriction are beyond the retirement ages. It is inevitable, therefore, that gerontologists have long been interested in the causes, consequences, and relief of dependency.

We have already encountered a set of definitional problems that need to be clarified if the notion of dependency is to be useful. More importantly, if ways are to be found of reducing dependency, it is essential that causation is understood. So, before examining the more practical problems that arise, some attention can usefully be given to a selection of key concepts that underpin both discourse and policy.

Reciprocity and Altruism

It is in the nature of dependency relationships that a person in profound need of help is given assistance, by one or more other people. They may do this as part of their paid occupation, and are therefore rewarded for the service they provide. But it is now well established that the overwhelming bulk of what is called caring is done by relatives, friends, and neighbors.[19–22] For them the help is given without direct payment. It is a gift. It may be a gift in return for gifts received in the past (children returning parental care) or in expectation of some return in the future (perhaps an inheritance). Equally, there may be no expectation of a reciprocal gift from the dependent person. The giver may give in the belief that if and when he or she needs help someone will be on hand. Or the aid may be provided with no expectation or hope of reward or exchange benefit—altruistic giving.

Since Mauss, in his classic essay *The Gift*,[23] and the anthropologist Malinowski, in his study of the Trobriand islanders,[24] formulated general propositions about the nature of social exchange, there has been much debate about its role in modern societies. These early studies postulated a set of powerfully stated social obligations to give to others both known and unknown. Accompanying sanctions reinforced the system, which ensured that there was a proper balance of reciprocity both direct and indirect. Not only is courtesy returned by courtesy, and favors by favors between people who know each other, but gifts are given to strangers in the expectation that yet other strangers will give to them.

Blau,[25] writing 40 years later, supported the notion of generalized exchange relationships, but drew attention to the highly developed sense of expected and observable reward that was generated by market transactions. Economic relations are fundamentally reciprocal exchanges, where all the parties involved are both givers and receivers. They involve trust; those who provide goods must trust that promises of payment will be honored. Blau also observed another distinct set of social exchanges characterized by unseeking generosity. In his important book *The Gift Relationship*, Titmuss[26] explored this quality of altruism through a study of blood donors. He believed that two forms of value have taken a grip on contemporary society—those of the marketplace and those of bureaucracy, where every action demanded a matching, measured, and inflexible response. His socialist conviction led him to conclude that a third and more moral force was essential to act as a counterbalance—that of gift values.

As a challenge to the rising view that altruism had no place in industrial societies, Titmuss set out to demonstrate that it was alive and well in such systems as blood donorship. Moreover, he argued that social exchanges that made people ask not, "Who is my neighbor?" but, "Who is my stranger?" were normally superior to market exchanges and should be fostered by governments. Subsequent empirical studies have provided less optimistic conclusions. The economist Hirsch[27] came to the view that the trend was for individuals to choose actions that were most likely to be to their personal benefit. Abrams'[28] research on informal care and neighboring was also broadly consistent with this view. He found that much neighboring activity was short-lived and highly instrumental. The mobile middle classes were seen to engage in neighborly activities as a way of gaining access to local social systems.

In Britain it is estimated that more than six million people are the primary, unpaid carers of dependent—mostly elderly—people.[19] In addition, unmeasured millions provide regular assistance to the older population. The motives and pressures which generate that help are still imperfectly understood. Yet governments in the western world are engaged in what is known as the interweaving of statutory services with informal care. Experiments like those in Thanet[29] and North Wales[30] consciously manipulated the willingness to give assistance by providing modest payments to family and other carers. They showed that financial inducements and sensitive organization can increase the quantity, quality, and cost effectiveness of care. But it could prove to be a further set of involvements to make informal care yet another saleable commodity.

It is frequently assumed that older people are the beneficiaries of giving relationships. For people who are very old, sick, or frail, there is certainly a marked shift in the balance, which would justify this view. However, as I show in detail later in this chapter, only about one in three of the retired population is placed in this "dependent" situation. Such people may require round-the-clock attention, which is very demanding indeed. But in considering their transfer into the receiver group, some countervailing factors must be taken into account.

Intergenerational giving

People who have lived to become old and sick have, by definition, lived through all the earlier stages of life in which they have been contributors to the social good—as workers, parents, friends, neighbors, supporters of their own elderly relatives, and contributors to wartime effort. They have usually given to the stock of social benefits more than they have received. It is by design that we ask the younger and more able-bodied to provide for their contemporaries who have neither of these characteristics, in return for similar aid when they too are in need. Old age is the classic example of the giver receiving back reciprocal gifts, presented and received over time.

Old age pensions are the most obvious example. To receive assistance in old age is an earned right, based upon an age-old social contract. When politicians and commentators speak of the "burden of the aged," they exhibit a lack of moral responsibility, a willingness to disregard time-honored arrangements or membership of that self-serving group that wants the well-to-do middle aged to further maximize their privileges and benefits. In the United States, this last set of motives has given rise to a movement that calls itself Americans for Generational Equity (AGE).

To argue that reciprocity between generations and over time is a necessary arrangement is not to say that any particular pattern or level of support is equally right. As the numbers of elders in need of help grow, it will be necessary to reassess constantly what is equitable and deliverable. AGE and bodies like it have a part in that debate. What would be regrettable and damaging is the substitution of accountancy and rationing solutions for ones based on the historic contributions of one generation to the welfare of its successors, and its reasonable expectations of reciprocity in the later stages of life. It should be remembered that the state assumed responsibility at the turn of the century for the support of elderly people, when other arrangements failed.[31]

The debate about intergenerational equity has become more vigorous during the past 10 years, drawing in economists, historians, philosophers, and lawyers. They have extended the discussion in three principal ways. The historians have enabled comparisons to be made over time that allow us to see how generous societies were in earlier time periods.[32] Philosophers have attempted to clarify what is meant by (1) the generational contract and (2) the nature of obligation.[33–36] Economic analysis has led to claims that the costs of supporting the growing population of retired people cannot be sustained under current conditions.[37]

As the discussion is still actively in process it is not possible to identify any outcome. But the existing consensual view of the intergenerational contract established in the welfare states of northern Europe in the early post-Second World War period is no longer unchallenged, even in those countries.[38,39] The reality of an upward trend in dependency and the demand for health and human services has produced strong attacks on the nature and extent of public and private support to the old and even on the existence of an obligation at all.[40]

Gift giving in old age

Another erroneous assumption is that retired people, because they are out of the remunerated work force, no longer make contributions to society. Once stated, this proposition becomes self-evidently inaccurate. The linkage between work and social value is an unreliable one, while the main weight of family caring falls on women aged 45 to 59.[20,41] Enid Levin and her colleagues[42] found that the average age of the supporters of confused old people was 61, and 30 percent were over age 70. This trend for the young old to care for the old old is projected to increase. At the same time, this group is known to provide financial and social support to their children and grandchildren. More specifically, as more women become economically active, the caring tasks they leave unfulfilled fall to the older generation.

The General Household Survey report *Informal Carers*[43] reports that there are more than 6 million carers in Britain, with 1.7 million caring for someone in their own home. Of these 6 million, 3.9 million are women and 2.9 million, men.[19] While there is no doubt that women are the principal contributors to "informal" care, it is worth noting that so many men are involved. Indeed, in the over-65 age group, male carers outnumber female carers.

There is also an observable rise in the involvement of the young old in voluntary bodies, self-help groups, and community activities. Within the older population itself there is a great deal of mutual aid. Keith[44] describes this graphically in *Old People, New Lives*. Her research in a new retirement community provides documentary accounts. Friends and neighbors check on each other daily; curtains not open by midmorning are a cue for a visit to make sure nothing is wrong. Meals are prepared, shopping done, and laundry washed and ironed for one blind resident.

> A look inside Merrill Court refrigerators also reveals an exchange network of food specialities. Except for the most extreme cases, such as the blind person, the exchanges are reciprocal. Of course, in a less tangible way, the blind man did offer a great deal in return to his caretakers. They enjoyed being the givers and carers, and they missed him bitterly when he died.[44]

Reciprocity and Receiving

Gift receiving need not be an ungracious act of taking what is offered. Qureshi's[45] study of carers in Sheffield indicates the wide variety of relationships that can exist. Some have always been one-sided. Others are based on mutual regard and long experience of mutual help. The following selection of quotations represents the range:

- Daughter: "I think she helps me more than I help her at the moment."
- Daughter: "Anytime I needed her she'd come at the drop of a hat, so I feel I owe it back, see, if she needs it. It works both ways doesn't it?"
- Son-in-law: "She's never been a mother as mothers should be. She was out every day of her life and she didn't want anyone . . . to upset her routine."
- Daughters: "He's never lifted a finger for anyone in his family."

Wright's[46] study of lone family carers confined itself to the debilitating effects of the caring task. It would be wrong to give the impression that the full-time care of sick elderly people is anything other than immensely demanding and exhausting. But it should be equally improper to presume that it is always unrewarding. The gift relationship that Titmuss[26] drew to our attention is an integral and durable part of intergenerational relations even when one of the parties did most of his or her giving in the past. The grateful and the thoughtful receiver is still a giver.

Finch and Mason's[22] major empirical study of family obligations in care giving concludes:

> However our main point is not so much that these experiences of giving and receiving help within families were common experience (though many of them were), but that they were treated as unremarkable experiences by many people who talked to us. They were seen as a characteristic part of family life.[22]

Labelling and Deviances

To carry the label "dependent" is to carry the burden of being a deviant, someone who no longer enjoys a place in the mainstream of society and whose behavior is abnormal. Others who share this status suffer a range of indignities and punishments that reinforce the deviance. Being excluded from social recognition and having no role in social relations is hurtful and damaging. Perhaps more importantly, it carries with it a set of attitudes, sanctions, and prohibitions that have the effect of dehumanizing the individual and engendering depression and reduction of self-esteem.

Social scientists have written extensively about the impact of labelling and the cluster of consequences that customarily accompany it. The literature encompasses criminals[47] drug users,[48] those who are deemed mentally ill,[49,50] and anyone—especially an elderly person—who becomes reliant on the services of others for their everyday existence.

What characterizes those who are subject to the labelling process is that the attribution of deviance results in negative stereotyping. Old age remains a deviant state in a society that celebrates youth and has not yet accustomed itself to the demographic revolution.[51] But it is the disabilities which accompany old age that attract the penalties. It is a response to perceptions of the abnormal, to the threatening and the unexpected. Such reactions are socially conditioned categories of action, rather than reflections on the individual.

Becker[46] summarized the construction of deviance when he wrote: Deviance is not a quality of the act the person commits but rather a consequence of the application by others of rules and sanctions to "an offender." The deviant is one to whom the label has been successfully applied; deviant behaviour that people so label.[48]

The existence of differences between older people and those of younger generations are well known, but exaggerated. There are, for example, few medical conditions exclusive to old age, so in that sense, they are sick in common with all ages. It is the association—often misinformed, or simply wrong—between aging and decline that provides the foundation for stereotypical treatment. Sadly, elderly people themselves and those who seek to represent their welfare frequently provide fuel for such misconceptions. Repetition of "Oh dear, it's my age," by elderly people or "What can you expect at your age?" by doctors only add to the conspiracy of ignorance against truth in the matter of aging. Even organizations that set out to promote the well-being of elderly people and know the scientific evidence, will amplify the negative features of later life in order to raise funds or make political points.

This "structural agism," which Scrutton[52] feels has such damaging consequences, especially for very old people, remains stubbornly persistent, despite the increasing reports of abuse and discrimination.[53]

It would not be proper, however, to make too much of the notion of old age as deviance, for it has too many flaws to be a worthwhile theory. What is valuable about the analysis of old age as a labelling phenomenon, is that it draws attention to the negative circumstance that the visible maladies attract.[54]

Measuring Dependency

With the definitional problems that remain unsolved, it is inevitable that statistical information about the nature and extent of dependency-creating disability and illness is subject to the same uncertainties. On the one hand, there are many research studies and population surveys that allow quantitative description of the retired population. On the other hand, much dispute exists about what these data mean. Before looking at the incidence of these conditions, we will look briefly at the technical definitions of dependency used by demographers, planners, and economists, who see old people as an economic burden.

Dependency Ratios

Economic analyses of population structure and change are preoccupied with the relative sizes of the economically active (i.e., in paid employment) segment of the population and those who are designated as dependent (all those not in paid employment, including children and retired people). The United Nations publication *The World Ageing Situation: Strategies and Policies*[55] summarizes the position well.

As the proportion of the population of working age increases, total dependency ratios (defined for the purposes of the present report as the number of young people, aged 0–14, plus the ageing, aged 60 and over, divided by the population of working age, aged 15–59) concurrently become lower. The total dependency ratio is often used as an indicator of economic potential, the principal argument being that a low dependency ratio implies relatively more workers and the need to divert fewer resources to dependent populations.[55]

As the total dependency ratio includes young and old, the two can be separated and their independent impact assessed and compared. Falkingham[56] has studied the United Kingdom figures that are used to measure the cost to the economy. She points out that as dependency is defined by age, the old age (gerontic) ratio will inevitably rise as the population ages. It has increased during this century from 12 old people (60/65+) per 100 in the working age ranges, to 34 in 1981, and this figure is projected to reach 38 by 2021. During the same period, the child dependency (neontic) ratio (aged 0–19) has fallen from 83 to 54. Projections indicate it will fall further by 2021, to 48. Figure 2.2 presents these trends graphically.

It is widely assumed that this shift in the balance of population is in itself bad and likely to damage the economy. As older

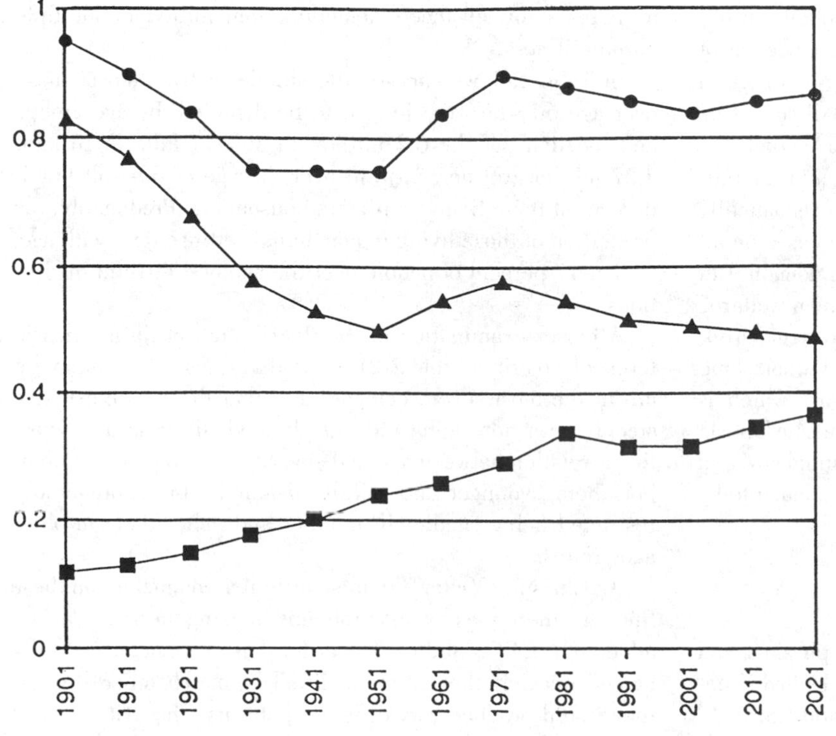

Figure 2-2 Dependency ratios, Great Britain, 1901–2021. ●, Gerontic ratio; ▲, neontic ratio; ■, total ratio. (From Falkingham,[56] with permission.)

people consume higher proportions of the national budget for health, social services, and social security, this has a somewhat self-evident aspect. Data such as that produced by Clark and Spengler[57] serve to encourage that view. For the United States, they estimate that the per capita costs for elderly persons are approximately three times those incurred by youth. Comparable figures for the developing world indicate that economic progress brings increased "dependency" costs. In Africa and East Asia, the costs of elderly people are only 1.5 times higher than for young people.[55] More recent studies[58] confirm these patterns.

The assumptions about relative costs and their damaging economic effects have come under attack from two separate quarters. First, from those who have adopted a political economy view of aging that sees old age as a period of dependency created by modern society. The other reaction comes from the ranks of demographers, economists, and historians, who have looked more closely at the real (as opposed to assumed) economic worth as well as the costs of old age. Falkingham[56] argues it is not necessarily the case that a change in the age structure will lead to a greater dependency cost. Demographic factors alone do not determine the ratio of workers to nonworkers. In addition, shifts in labor force participation involving many more women make dependency assumptions based on age and gender very suspect.[20]

Thane[59] sets out to quell the panic, first by drawing attention to the stability of the total dependency ratio throughout the twentieth century and the fact that this is scheduled to continue into the next. Within this framework she envisages a fall in per capita health and social services costs, as the increased healthiness of younger cohorts is transmitted into old age. This is a case also promoted by Bosanquet[60] and more recently using American data by Pifer and Bronte.[61] In a similar essay on the implications of greater activity in old age, Johnson[62] associated these arguments with evidence of considerable increases in the income and wealth of a portion of the elderly cohorts of the next century, who will constitute not an economic burden but a much sought after market.

In some ways, more fundamental than these technical arguments, is an ethical point about what counts as economically and socially worthwhile activity. Calculations are based on all income-generating activity recorded in the public domain. But is all of it worthy to count in the calculus of human welfare? Is the making and selling of hard drugs, pornography, or "stink bombs" to count equally with the production of wholesome food and nursing skill? And what about the work which is valued but not paid for (like informal care and domestic labor)? Not only are the dependency ratio calculations simplistic and inaccurate, they embody a set of values that leave much to be desired.

Disability and Dependence

The universal association of disability, both physical and mental, with increasing age is also present in the United Kingdom. There is some evidence to support Fries and Crapo's[63] claim that morbidity is being compressed into the later years of life, but there is no denying that incapacity increases significantly beyond the age of 70. Distinctions between those with different levels of impairment are therefore of importance, for both the self-perceptions and the reality experienced by most elderly people is that they are fit and able to lead their own lives.[64,65]

No national register of disability or disabled persons in Britain exists, despite the intentions set down in the Chronically Sick and Disabled Persons Act 1971. As a consequence, there is no census-based inventory from which reliable data can be drawn. Instead, we must look to a range of sample surveys and estimates shaped from a range of sources. Wicks and Henwood[66] calculated that 1.1 million people over the age of 65 are severely disabled constituting one in eight of the total age group. A further two million were estimated by Walker and Phillipson[67] to be moderately disabled.

As the result of a series of major surveys conducted by the OPCS during the late 1980s, we now have access to a more reliable data set. The studies, which are reported in two main publications,[18,68] draw on a large sample of the general population (100,000 addresses) including private households and communal establishments. Therefore they included people in hospitals, and residential and nursing homes, where the most frail elderly persons would be found. As part of the studies, those whom we deemed to be disabled were assessed on a range of dimensions to identify the nature and degree of disability. This allowed researchers to classify respondents on a scale of severity, from 1 (the lowest) to 10 (the highest). For example, someone in category 1 may have a hearing impairment in one ear; in category 6, a stroke or heart condition limits mobility and severely restricts self-care; while category 10 would include people who were totally dependent on others as a result of advanced dementia, immobility, or multiple chronic illness.

In Table 2-1 we can see the simple distribution of those over age 60 who were judged to be disabled, by age groups and location. Of the 6.2 million disabled adults in Britain, 4.27 million (69 percent) are over the age of 60—all but 7 percent of them living in private households. Predictably, the proportion of those living in communal settings rises with age, so that 17 percent of people over the age of 80 live in institutions.

A closer examination of the distribution of disabilities in terms of severity (Table 2-2) shows that the smallest numbers are in the most severe category and that those within it rise steeply with advancing old age. Indeed, there is an almost linear relation between age and severity, with the largest numbers being younger and mildly disabled—those profoundly restricted being smaller in number and more likely in older age groups.

As Christina Victor[69] points out in her commetary on these findings, there are obvious problems in using the kind of scale adopted by OPCS studies. The criteria used are not universally agreed ones. If they were modified to match other studies, they would produce very different patterns. She writes: For

Table 2-1 Estimates of disabled adults in Great Britain, 1988

Age	Numbers			Rate per 1,000	
	Private Households	Communal Establishments	Total	Private Households	Total
60–69	1,298	36	1,334	236	240
70–79	1,589	98	1,687	395	240
80+	1,037	217	1,254	674	714
All ages	5,780	422	6,202	135	142

(From Martin et al.,[18] with permission.)

example there were 1,186,000 adults in private households classified in severity category 1 compared to 102,000 in severity category 10. Changing the definition of disability so that severity category 1 was excluded would reduce the number of disabled people in the total population from 6,202,000 to 5,004,000 (a reduction of 1,198,000).[69]

A further anomaly is that older people are overrepresented in the more severe disability groups. Those over age 60 constitute 75 percent of the most severe disability group, but only 64 percent of the least severe category.

These methodologic points are important in alerting us to the uncertainties in national data about long-term illness, although there is every reason to be confident that the general patterns are correct. These problems beset information about mental illnesses, but are amplified by the greater difficulty in clinical diagnosis. Nonetheless, it is possible to say that two-thirds of all people with learning disabilities and physical impairments are over age 65. More than one-third of those over 65 (rising to one-half of those over 80) are estimated to have hearing impairment.[70] There are no wholly reliable figures for the numbers of people with significant visual handicap, but it is known that three-quarters of 100,000 people registered as blind are over 65. These conditions, along with other physical disabilities, mental frailty, incontinence, and limitations of poor housing, represent the range of handicap for older people.

Bond and Carstairs,[71] in their survey of elderly people in Scotland, identified heart conditions (15 percent), arthritis and related conditions affecting the back (10 to 15 percent), joints (15 to 35 percent), and sight defects (2 to 21 percent) as the most widely reported illnesses that restrict functional capacity. These in turn have consequences for the performance of activities of daily living (ADLs), where bending and stooping are ingredients in the process. The ability to cope with everyday tasks of personal hygiene and domestic tasks in the home is critical to the maintenance of an independent existence. These ADLs have received much attention in social surveys. Together they provide a picture of about one-half of the older population coping without assistance. As for the rest, there is again a steep rise with age.

McClone, commenting on the statistics shown in Table 2-

Table 2-2 Estimates of disabled adults by severity in Great Britain, 1988

Severity Category	Private Households				Communal Establishments			
	60–69	70–79	80+	Total, All Ages	65–69	70–79	80+	Total, All Ages
10	15	23	39	102	7	24	58	108
9	57	68	93	285	7	18	45	50
8	59	92	87	338	5	12	30	58
7	78	115	123	447	3	9	22	39
6	85	149	107	511	2	9	15	34
5	146	176	132	679	2	6	15	29
4	152	179	105	676	3	8	12	27
3	173	212	109	732	2	6	8	19
2	225	263	105	824	2	5	6	16
1	308	310	138	1,186	3	3	3	13
Total	1,298	1,589	1,037	5,780	36	98	217	422

(From Martin et al.,[18] with permission.)

Table 2-3 Inability to undertake mobility, self-care, and domestic tasks in the population over 65, 1985

	65–69	70–74	75–79	80–84	85+
Walk out of doors	5	7	14	24	47
Get up and down stairs and steps	4	5	10	17	31
Get around the house (on the level)	1	1	2	3	6
Get to the toilet	1	1	2	2	7
Get in and out of bed	1	1	3	2	7
Cut toenails	16	24	34	48	65
Bathe, shower, wash all over	4	5	10	16	31
Brush hair (females), shave (males)	1	1	1	3	7
Wash face and hands	0	1	1	1	2
Feed	0	1	0	1	2
Household shopping	7	10	16	29	56
Wash paintwork	8	13	24	34	62
Clean windows inside	9	13	21	34	63
Clean and sweep floors	5	7	13	20	45
Job involving climbing	17	25	36	52	76
Wash clothing by hand	4	5	9	12	32
Open screw-top jars	7	7	11	15	29
Cook a main meal	4	4	9	13	29
Use a frying pan	2	2	5	8	19
Make a cup of tea	1	1	3	3	8
N	1,062	1,025	788	395	240

(From Victor,[69] with permission.)

3, concludes that there is still only a minority of elderly people who are unable to cope.

Only 16 percent are unable to do their own shopping, 12 percent cannot sweep or clean floors, and 10 percent cannot open screw tops. Similarly, a very small percentage have problems with self care except for toenail cutting. Despite these small proportions, the numbers involved can be large. For example, there are an estimated 1.4 million people over 65 who cannot do their own shopping. Overall, at least 15 percent of the elderly population are likely to be dependent on others for the performance of some tasks they would previously have performed independently. This latter group is highly likely to contain those overage 65 who suffer strokes, and the 7 percent of males and 18 percent of females over 70 whom Vetter[72] reports as suffering from regular urinary incontinence.

Mental health problems are prevalent at all ages, but there is a cumulative effect that manifests itself in higher levels within postretirement populations. It is usual to separate organic syndromes (those with a physical cause) from affective disorders. Distinctions between the two are very difficult to sustain, with the result that both practical diagnosis and research leave large areas of doubt. Within the organic syndromes, dementia in its various forms and that of the Alzheimer's type in particular are both very disabling and relatively common in later life, although diagnostic uncertainty makes accurate estimates of prevalence difficult.

Moreover, as those with this condition are at high risk of institutionalization, community studies suffer from a number of well-known deficiencies both of sampling and methodology. Nonetheless, it is commonly accepted as Brayne and Ames[73] report that dementia occurs in about 5 percent of the population aged over 65 and up to 20 percent of those over 80. The rate of new cases is about 1 percent per year in those overage 65, rising with increasing age.

Of the functional mental illnesses, depression is the most prevalent. It is the most common psychiatric condition encountered in epidemiologic studies and routine medical practice alike. Again, because of the problems of definition as well as study methodology, research findings vary. Brayne and Ames's[73] tabulation of the most important British studies (Table 2-4) depicts a range from 6 to 26 percent of those over 65, greater than that of the much discussed forms of dementia.

It is essential to restate that the majority of elderly people in the United Kingdom lead lives as independent of the assistance of others as people in younger age groups. Media reports and even governmental statements about the "burden of dependency" serve only to reinforce unwarranted images.

Table 2-4 Depression in United Kingdom community samples

Study	Location and Age	n	Instrument	Findings
Kay et al., 1964	Newcastle	505	Psychiatrist interview	26% affective illness and neurosis
Parsons, 1965	Swansea 65+	228	Psychiatrist interview prevalence	0.9% endogenous depression (lifetime ED 6%)
Hare and Shaw, 1965	London 65+	211	Interview	11% depressive symptoms
Gurland et al., 1983	London 63+	396	Interview (CARE)	12.4% pervasive (inc. 1.3% manic depressive psychosis)
Maule et al., 1984	Edinburgh 62+	487	Psychiatrist interview	5.1% depression
Copeland et al., 1987	Liverpool 65+	1,070	Interview (GMSA/AGECAT)	11.3% depression (including 3.0% depressive psychosis)
Morgan et al., 1987	Nottingham 65+	1,042	Interview (SAD)	9.8% depression (4.9% met stricter clinical criteria)

(From Brayne and Ames,[73] with permission.)

Caring Services

It has already been established that family and informal carers provide the major part of the support given to dependent people. Nonetheless, the system of statutory and voluntary services—both health and personal social services—is an indispensable professional complement. Historically they have grown up in five unrelated organizational patterns: (1) local health authorities that provide hospital treatment, containing specialist geriatric provision, (2) primary health care teams providing general practitioner home nursing and health visitor services, (3) local authority social services departments offering a range of residential, day and domiciliary forms of care, (4) voluntary bodies, some of which offer residential accommodation and other community services including meals on wheels and day centers, and (5) private sector residential and nursing homes. To this range we must now add a variety of NHS and social services trusts that have taken over provision of some parts of the services previously supplied by health authorities and local government.

Following the full implementation of the United Kingdom NHS and Community Care Act on April 1, 1993, local social services departments became principally contractors or purchasers of services rather than direct providers as in the past.

The changes have been an accelerated version of those that have taken place since 1975 in the long-term care sector. At that stage there were 95,000 beds in LA old people's homes, with only 18,750 in private residential homes. There was a small voluntary sector. At the same time, there were 25,000 beds in private nursing homes. Today there are 328,000 beds in private long-term care (including nursing homes and other hospitals) and 140,000 in the public sector.[74,75] There are about 69,000 beds in private nursing homes.

Laing's[74] tabulation of the bed distributions and capital values in Table 2-5 provides an indication of the scale of what is now a major care industry.

Table 2-5 Market value of care of elderly, chronically ill, and physically disabled people, United Kingdom, annualized at March 1992

	Places	Million £
(A) Institutional Provision		
Private nursing homes	152,800	2,225
Private residential homes	162,400	1,572
Total Private Care Homes	315,200	3,797
Voluntary nursing homes	13,700	200
Voluntary residential homes	46,900	430
Total Voluntary Care Homes	60,600	630
NHS long-stay geriatric	41,300	942
NHS elderly mentally ill	24,300	554
NHS younger disabled	5,400	123
Local authority Part III	103,800	1,090
Total: Public Sector	174,800	2,709
Total: Institutional	550,600	7,136
(B) Nonresidential Care		
Private home care	—	422
Private aids and adaptations	—	146
Private Nonresidential	—	568
NHS district nursing	—	891
NHS day care	—	67
NHS chiropody	—	79
Local authority home care	—	815
Local authority day care	—	130
Local authority meals on wheels	—	90
Local authority other services	—	452
Public Nonresidential	—	2,524
Total Nonresidential	—	3,092
Grand Total	—	10,228
[Informal Care[a]]	—	[391,001]

[a] *Calculated following a method originally used by the Family Policy Studies Centre (1989), valuing each hour of informal care at £7.00 per hour (based on local authority pay rates).*
(From Laing,[98] with permission.)

The expansion has been driven largely by the dramatic growth in the numbers of very old dependent people (and in part by the failure of other support systems). To date, the public provider has borne the major task of supporting the largest proportion of very confused residents.

Long-stay care in geriatric hospitals or wards of general hospitals has become far less common than in the early 1980s and before. Extension of private provision has provided a ready discharge route for the chronically sick patient, leaving beds free for more acute care and rehabilitation. Evans[76] has reported that whereas consultants in general medicine had an average of 30 beds in their care, geriatricians had about 180, plus commitments to outpatients, day hospitals, and domiciliary visits. Even against these odds the length of hospital stay by elderly people has declined since 1970. Victor[77] reports that the mean length of stay for males aged 65 to 74 in 1974 was 18 days, but had fallen to 13 days by 1983 and continues to fall year to year.

For those who are sick at home or discharged from hospital, a variety of domiciliary services are supplied by the NHS and by local authority social services departments. Supplemented by home-based voluntary services, these inputs build upon family and other informal care. Linkages between hospital and community services have been notoriously poor, and the system's ability to coordinate services so that an elderly person returning home from hospital care gets home help, home nursing, or meals on wheels at the point of discharge is very limited. The Continuing Care Project's survey[78] showed that 14 days after discharge about one-half of all elderly patients could not cope with domestic tasks or personal care, of whom more than one-quarter had no one to help them. Of these two categories together, 84 percent either had a caring person who could not cope, or had no caring person at all. By 28 days after discharge, 39 percent of the principal caring persons were themselves found to be frail and at risk. Home visits from general practitioners (family doctors) are also delayed. The same survey showed that 63 percent of patients had not received a call by 14 days after discharge.

An increasingly impressive range of services exists for elderly people at home, but there is great geographic diversity in the extent and availability of them. Table 2-6 summarizes the domiciliary services available for elderly people in the United Kingdom. However, there are considerable variations in quantity and quality of these services across the country.

However, the identification of what individual clients need is determined by care managers (some of whom are social workers, but may also be nurses, health visitors, or other categories of staff). They arrange "packages" of care from different suppliers, and are responsible for coordinating and monitoring those services.

Up-to-date and reliable data on the delivery of these services are difficult to find, but Health and Personal Social Services Statistics 1985[79] reported findings for a 1-year period in 1982. It was found that, of those aged 65 or over, 605,462 received NHS chiropody services and 765,754 received the services of a home help. Such global figures tell only of relative magnitude and nothing of the effectiveness, match with needs, regularity, or duration. In general, research evidence indicates a shortfall of provision on all these principal services, adequacies in design to meet the needs of consumers, and failure to coordinate care packages for individuals.[80–84]

Table 2-6 Domiciliary services for elderly people

Service	Provider
Primary health care teams	NHS
Clubs	Local
Day centers	Local authority/voluntary
Meals on wheels	Local authority/voluntary
Luncheon clubs	Local authority/voluntary
Health visitors	NHS
Domiciliary physiotherapy	NHS
District nursing	NHS
Nursing auxiliaries	NHS
Aids for daily living/house adaptation	Local authority
Nail cutting services	Voluntary
Library service for housebound	Local authority/voluntary
Night sitting	Local authority/voluntary/private
Sheltered housing	Local authority/voluntary/private/trusts
Incontinence laundry	Local authority/NHS trusts
Community psychiatric nurse	NHS
Social worker	Local authority/voluntary/private
Respite care	Local authority/NHS/trusts
Geriatric day hospital	NHS/private
Good neighbor scheme	Voluntary
Community rehabilitation	NHS/trusts
Care managers	Local authority/NHS
Community physiotherapists	Local authority/NHS
Home care organizers	Local authority/private

Structured Dependency

Reference has already been made to the proposition that dependency among elderly people is amplified, if not created, by the manner in which modern societies are structured and organized. Such notions are not new, for it has been evident for some time that mandatory retirement that removes older people from the work force also reduces their income and social esteem. Similarly, it is well documented that the shortage of support services and the regimes in residential care establishments have created a reliance on others. Yet it was only in Townsend's article in *Ageing and Society*[85] that the concept of structured dependency was articulated. He drew upon his own extensive research, especially of residential care[4] to argue that the degree of dependency experienced by old people is unnecessary. He wrote:

I am arguing, then, that society creates the framework of institutions and rules within which the general problems of the elderly emerge and are indeed manufactured. Decisions are being taken every day in the management of the economy and in the maintenance and development of social institutions which govern the position which elderly people occupy in na-

tional life, and these also contribute powerfully to the public consciousness of different meanings of ageing and old age.[85]

The argument proceeds through a series of claims about the ways in which retired people are excluded from socially valued activities and status. Governments find it convenient to reduce unemployment figures by enforced retirement, while new technology makes their skills redundant or undervalued. Townsend adds: Less consideration tends to be given to sickness and disability at older than younger ages and, indeed, retirement is cavalierly associated with failing health and incapacity. Thus, the combined effects of industrial, economic and educational reorganisation are leading to more rigid stratification of the population by age.

This influential paper rapidly gave rise to a body of writings in the political economy of aging. Prior to its publication, the American gerontologist Estes[86] had produced her book *The Aging Enterprise*, which gave a critical edge to previous writings about old age and the state, by entering into a class analysis. Concurrently, Walker[87,88] was producing material that developed the same themes by examination of income and wealth in later life. His contention was:

. . . that poverty in old age is primarily a function of low economic and social status prior to retirement and the depressed social status of the retired, and secondarily, of the relatively low level of state benefits.[86]

Gaullier[89] analyzing postwar policies for retired people in France asserts that the government converted the positive aspects of the Third Age movement to create a new social ghetto. A similar process was described by Kohli et al,[90] based on their studies of prematurely retired tobacco workers in Germany. By the mid-1980s, volumes of collected papers began to emerge[91,92] to supplement monographs like Phillipson's,[93] which located the modern formula of retirement as a repressed social category in the development of western capitalism.

For one-half of a decade, the Townsend thesis had such a self-evident quality to it that no serious challenge was offered. But in more recent times, a number of criticisms have appeared. Johnson complains that the economic position of elderly people has been extensively examined by social policy analysts, yet virtually ignored by economists. In beginning to correct the imbalance he contends that:

Theories of "structured dependency" rest on the explicit or implicit argument that elderly people have experienced a constriction of economic liberty because of . . . the development of welfare and employment policies . . . [but] much of the detailed research that has made use of the concept of structured dependency has focused on the relatively small and exceptional group of elderly people living in institutions, for whom the concept of dependency seems more immediately relevant.[94]

Moreover, he suggests that the existence of old age pensions has given both a security of income and a range of choice, which sometimes exceeds what is available to younger people in employment.

Dant[95] takes issue even with the strongest part of the case as it relates to people in residential care. He points out that some may even prefer the "hotel" qualities of residential life, of not being bothered with cleaning and cooking. Townsend is further taken to task by claims that "He seems to regard both elderly people and all other people in society who do not have a functional role in the running of the state as 'cultural dopes' devoid of autonomy and self-determination."[96] In a more oblique way, Wilkin[96] also offers a critical refinement, by returning our attention to the detailed assessment of disability as a dependency-creating attribute. More sophisticated measures that place physical and mental impairments in the context of relationships and environment will produce the capacity to release elderly people from excessive dependence on others. His call for more focus on "dependency relationships" draws discussion back to individuals and their settings rather than the macroeconomic structure.

The structured dependency debate has a long way to go before it is concluded. What it has provided so far is a strongly presented alternative to the view that elderly people are not only the victims of old age, they are the unconscious perpetrators of its deprivations. Similarly, it has stimulated a more constructive view of the definitions, causes, and measurements of dependency. Whatever the outcome, it is inevitable that the political economy view of old age will have established itself as a permanent and proper vantage point for viewing problems in a more politically comprehensive way.

Conclusion

The seemingly simple notion of the dependency older people have on other people has proved to be both conceptually complex and methodologically difficult to measure. Earlier attempts to encapsulate the everyday requirements of people who have lost capacities to maintain themselves, by the use of check lists and rating scales now appear inadequate—even if still widely used. Exclusive attention to the shortcomings of the person in being able to carry out activities of everyday living is demonstrably incomplete, even if the measures are valid. If dependency is to gain a useful meaning—rather than being another negative label—it must be considered within both the local and national context. Much more attention is now being given to the specific identification of conditions that inhibit independent functioning and their matching with tested and effective social, medical, and financial support. Developments of this sort that individualize assessment and responses to it, while removing the individualization of the causes of pathology, appear to be fruitful lines of progress.

By using a much used and misued term—dependency—we have been able to explore a central arena of social gerontology and reveal its approaches and methods. In so doing we have confirmed Peter Berger's[98] dictum that the task of sociology is "to make the familiar, unfamiliar." At the same time, we have entered the common ground with medicine. The use of epidemiologic ideas and data, findings from clinical trials, and the discussion of the social meaning of illnesses, pathologies, and reductions in function have demonstrated the interdependent if not the symbiotic relation between social gerontology and the interests of geriatric medicine.

References

1. Gibson MJS, Nusberg C (eds): International Glossary of Social Gerontology. Van Nostrand Reinhold Co, New York, 1985
2. Pollock O: Social Adjustment in Old Age. Social Science Research Council Bulletin, 59, New York.
3. Havighurst R, Albrecht R: Older People. Longmans Green, New York, 1953
4. Townsend P: The Family Life of Old People. Routledge and Kegan Paul, London, 1957
5. Townsend P: The Last Refuge—A Survey of Residential Institutions and Homes for the Aged in England and Wales. Routledge and Kegan Paul, London, 1962
6. Baltes PB, Baltes MM (eds): Successful Ageing: Perspectives from the Behavioural Sciences. Cambridge University Press, Cambridge, 1990
7. Binstock R, Shanas E: Handbook of Aging and the Social Sciences. Van Nostrand Reinhold, London, 1976
8. McPherson BD: Aging as a Social Process. Butterworths, Toronto, 1990
9. Fennell G, Phillipson C, Evers H: The Sociology of Old Age. Open University Press, Buckingham, 1988
10. Hendricks J, Hendricks CD: Aging in Mass Society. 3rd Ed. Little and Brown, Boston, 1986
11. Munnichs JMA: Dependency, interdependency and autonomy: an introduction. pp. 3–8. In Munnichs JMA, and Van den Heuval WJA (eds): Dependency and Interdependency in Old Age. Martinus Nijhoff, The Hague, 1976
12. Clark M: Cultural values in later life. p. 263. In Cowgill DO, Holmes LD (eds): Aging and Modernisation. Appleton-Century-Crofts, New York, 1972
13. Herbst K: Communication problems of the elderly deaf. In: Deafness and the Elderly. Age Concern, London, 1976
14. Herbst K: Hearing. In Redfern S (ed): Nursing Elderly People. Churchill Livingstone, Edinburgh, 1991
15. Wilkin D: Dependency. In Peace SM (ed): Researching Social Gerontology. Sage, London, 1990
16. Blakemore K: Ageing in the inner city: a comparison of old blacks and whites. p.81 In Jerrome D (ed): Ageing in Modern Society. Croom Helm, London, 1983
17. Blakemore K: Ageing and ethnicity. In Johnson J, Slater R (eds): Ageing and Late Life. Sage, London, 1993
18. Martin J, Meltzer H, Elliot D: The Prevalence of Disability Among Adults. OPCS Surveys of Disability in Great Britain, Report No. 1. HMSO, London, 1988
19. Office of Population Censuses and Surveys: General Household Survey: Carers in 1990. HMSO, London, 1992
20. Arber S, Ginn J: Gender and Later Life. Sage, London, 1991
21. McGlone F: Disability and Dependency in Old Age: A Demographic Audit, Family Policy Studies Centre, London, 1992
22. Finch J, Mason J: Negotiating Family Responsibilities. Routledge, London, 1992
23. Mauss M: The Gift. Cohen, West, 1966 (English translation)
24. Malinowski B: Argonauts of the Western Pacific. Routledge & Kegan Paul, London, 1922
25. Blau P: Exchange and Power in Social Life. Wiley, New York, 1964
26. Titmuss RM: The Gift Relationship: From Human Blood to Social Policy. Allen and Unwin, London, 1970
27. Hirsch F: Social Limits to Growth. Routledge and Kegan Paul, London, 1977
28. Bulmer M: Neighbours: The Work of Philip Abrams. Cambridge University Press, Cambridge, 1986
29. Davies B, Knapp M: Matching Resources to Community Needs. Gower, Aldershot, 1987
30. Wenger GC: The Supportive Network. Allen and Unwin, London, 1984
31. Gunn PA: Legislating filial piety: the Australian experience. Ageing and Society 1986;6:135
32. Thomson D: The decline of social welfare: falling state support for the elderly since early Victorian times. Ageing and Society 1984;4:451
33. Laslett P, Fishkin JS (eds): Justice Between the Age Groups and Generations. Yale University Press, New Haven, 1992
34. Callahan D: Setting Limits: Medical Goals in An Aging Society. Simon and Schuster, New York, 1987
35. Daniels N: Am I My Parents' Keeper? An Essay on Justice Between the Young and the Old. Oxford University Press, Oxford, 1988
36. Selbourne D: The Principle of Duty. Sinclair Stevenson, London, 1994
37. Johnson P, Conrad C, Thomson D: Workers versus Pensioners. Manchester University Press in association with The Centre for Economic Policy Research, Manchester, 1989
38. Johnson ML: Generational relations under review. In Hobman D (ed): Intergenerational Solidarity: Fact or Fiction? Age Concern Publications, London, 1993
39. Johnson ML: Interdependency and the generational compact. Ageing and Society 1995;15:243
40. Epstein RA: Justice across the generations. p. 84 In Laslett P, Fishkin JS (eds): Justice Between Age Groups and Generations. Yale University Press, New Haven, 1992
41. Allen I: The elderly and their informal carers. p. 70. In DHSS (ed): Elderly People in the Community—Their Service Needs. HMSO, London, 1983
42. Levin E, Sinclair I, Gorbach P: Families, Services and Confusion in Old Age. Gower, Aldershot, 1988
43. Office of Population Censuses and Surveys: General Household Survey 1985. HMSO, London, 1988
44. Keith J: Old People, New Lives: Community Creation in a Resettlement Residence. University of Chicago Press, Chicago, 1977
45. Qureshi H: Responses to dependency: reciprocity and power in family relations. p. 167. In Phillipson C, Bernard M, Strang P (eds): Dependency and Interdependency in Old Age—Theoretical Perspectives and Policy Alternatives. Croom Helm, London, 1986
46. Wright F: Left to Care Alone. Gower, Aldershot, 1986
47. Matza D: Becoming Deviant. Prentice-Hall, Englewood Cliffs, 1969
48. Becker HS: Outsiders, Studies in the Sociology of Deviance. Free Press, New York, 1963
49. Scheff T: The Labelling Theory of Mental Illness. Am Soc Rev 1974;39:444

50. Skultans V: English Madness: Ideas on Insanity 1580–1890. Routledge and Kegan Paul, London, 1979
51. Laslett P: A Fresh Map of Life: The Emergence of the Third Age. Weidenfeld and Nicolson, London, 1989
52. Scrutton S: Ageism. In McEwan E (ed): Age: The Unrecognised Discrimination. Age Concern Publications, London, 1990
53. Eastman M: Old Age Abuse. Age Concern, London, 1985
54. Martin B: The cultural construction of ageing: or how long can the summer wine really last? In Bury M, MacNicol J (eds): Aspects of Ageing. Royal Holloway and Bedford New College, London, 1990
55. United Nations: The World Ageing Situation: Strategies and Policies. United Nations, New York, 1985
56. Falkingham J: Britain's Ageing Population: The Engine Behind Increased Dependency? Suntory Toyota International Centre for Economics and Related Disciplines, London School of Economics, London, 1987
57. Clark R, Spengler J: Dependency ratios: their use in economic analysis. p. 103. In Simon J, Devanzo J (eds): Research in Population Economics, Vol II. JAI Press, Greenwich, Connecticut, 1980
58. Johnson P, Falkingham J: Intergenerational transfers and public expenditure on the elderly in modern Britain. Ageing and Society 1988;8:129
59. Thane P: Economic Burden or Benefit? A Positive View of Old Age. Centre for Economic Policy Research, London, 1987
60. Bosanquet N: A Future for Old Age. Temple Smith/New Society, London, 1978
61. Pifer A, Bronte L (eds): Our Aging Society. W.W. Norton, New York, 1987
62. Johnson ML: Implications of greater activity in later life. In Fogarty M (ed): Retirement Policy—The Next Fifty Years. Heinemann, London, 1982
63. Fries JF, Crapo LM: Vitality and Aging: Implications of the Rectangular Curve. WH Freeman, San Francisco, 1981
64. Johnson ML: Self perception of need amongst the elderly: an analysis of illness behaviour. Sociol Rev 20:521–531, 1972
65. Office of Population Censuses and Surveys: General Household Survey 1989. HMSO, 1991
66. Wicks M, Henwood M: The Social and Demographic Circumstances of Elderly People. p.51. In: Gearing B, Johnson ML, Heller T (eds): Mental Health Problems in Old Age. Wiley, Chichester, 1988
67. Walker A, Phillipson C (eds): Ageing and Social Policy. Gower, Aldershot, 1986
68. Martin J, White A, Meltzer H: Disabled Adults: Services, Transport and Employment (OPCS). HMSO, London, 1988
69. Victor CR: Health and Health Care in Later Life. Open University Press, Buckingham, 1991
70. Coni N, Davidson W, Webster S: Ageing: The Facts. 2nd Ed. Oxford University Press, Oxford, 1992
71. Bond J, Carstairs V: Services for the Elderly: A Survey of the Characteristics and Needs of a Population of 5,000 Old People. Scottish Health Service Studies No. 42. Scottish Home and Health Department, Edinburgh, 1982
72. Vetter N: Urinary Incontinence in the Elderly at Home. The Lancet 1275, 1981
73. Brayne C, Ames D: The epidemiology of mental disorder in old age. p. 105. In Gearing B, Johnson ML, Heller T (eds): Mental Health Problems in Old Age. Wiley, Chichester, 1988
74. Laing W (ed): Laing's Review of Private Health Care. Laing and Buisson, London, 1990
75. Mitchell A: Community care act: implementation. This Caring Business. February 18, 1993
76. Evans JG: Hospital Care of the Elderly. p. 133. In Shegog R (ed): The Impending Crisis for Old Age. Oxford University Press, Oxford, 1981
77. Victor CR: Old Age in Modern Society. Croom Helm, London, 1987
78. Amos G (ed): Home from Hospital—To What? Community Care Project, Birmingham, 1980
79. DHSS: Health and Personal Social Services Statistics. HMSO, London, 1985
80. Johnson ML, di Gregorio S, Hughes B: Ageing, Needs and Nutrition. Policy Studies Institute, London, 1981
81. Midwinter E: Redefining Old Age. Centre for Policy on Ageing, London, 1987
82. Means R: Meals on Wheels. School for Advanced Urban Studies, Bristol, 1984
83. Clarke L: Domiciliary Services for the Elderly. Croom Helm, London, 1984
84. Allen I, Hogg D, Peace S: Elderly People: Choice, Participation and Satisfaction. Policy Studies Institute, London, 1992
85. Townsend P: The structured dependency of the elderly: creation of social policy in the twentieth century. Age Soc 1981;1:5
86. Estes C: The Aging Enterprise. Jossey-Bass, San Francisco, 1979
87. Walker A: The Social Creation of Poverty and Dependence in Old Age. J Soc Policy 1980;9:49
88. Walker A: Towards a Political Economy of Old Age. Ageing and Society 1981;1:73
89. Gaullier X: Economic crisis and old age: old age policies in France. Ageing and Society 1982;2:165
90. Kohli M, Rosenow J, Wolf J: The social construction of ageing through work: economic structure and life world. Ageing and Society 3:23, 1983
91. Guillemard AM (ed): Old Age and the Welfare State. Sage, London, 1983
92. Minkler M, Estes C (eds): Readings in the Political Economy of Aging. Baywood Publishing Co., Farmingdale, New York, 1984
93. Phillipson C: Capitalism and the Construction of Old Age. Macmillan, London, 1982
94. Johnson P: Structured Dependency of the Elderly: a critical note. Centre for Economic Policy Research, London, 1987
95. Dant T: Dependency and old age: theoretical accounts and practical understandings. Ageing and Society 1988;8:171
96. Wilkin D: Conceptual problems in dependency research. Soc Sci Med 1987;24:867
97. Berger P: Invitation to Sociology. Penguin, Harmondsworth, 1968
98. Laing W (ed): Laing's Review of Private Health Care. Laing and Buisson, London, 1993

CHAPTER 3

The Future of Old Age

KENNETH G. MANTON

The future of old age in the twenty-first century in the United States and other economically developed countries will be dynamic and will generate historically unprecedented demographic, social, and medical conditions. This is due to quantitative and qualitative population, social, and health factors. Some quantitative demographic factors are well known—although details of their operation are not fully appreciated.

First, in the United States, there were rapid declines in mortality at young ages from at least 1900 due to reductions in infectious disease risks and infant and maternal mortality. Responsible for these declines were improved nutrition, new antibiotic therapies, immunization and vaccination programs for childhood diseases, and improved public hygiene (e.g., improved sanitation, drinking water, and, recently, air quality). The likelihood of surviving to 65 for United States males in 1900 was 37.3 percent; for females 41.0 percent.[1] By 1950, this increased to 61.8 percent for males and 74.3 percent for females. From 1954 to 1968 United States mortality was viewed as static—male mortality rates increased 0.2 percent per year; female mortality rates, in contrast, declined 0.8 percent per year. Federal agencies began to plan, and operate, as if the upper limit to population life expectancy had been reached.[2] Projections of the Social Security beneficiary population in the mid-1970s assumed that mortality would decline no further.[3] This view was also expressed by epidemiologists who suggested that the third phase of the epidemiologic transition would have increased prevalence of chronic degenerative diseases[4] caused by adverse social[5] and public health conditions intrinsic to industrial society.[6]

Second, the size of birth cohorts increased. Post-WWII baby boom cohorts reached a maximum in 1963 in the United States. The first of those cohorts reaches age 65 in 2012, and age 85 in 2032. The largest cohorts reach age 65 in 2029 and 85 in 2049. The larger size of recent cohorts, and improved mortality up to age 65, will produce large future increases in the elderly population in the United States. Similar population dynamics operate in other developed, and some developing, countries. This will produce severe strains on economic and medical programs for elderly populations.

Third, after being static from 1954 to 1968, United States mortality above age 65 began to decline, in part due to the start of national research programs on chronic diseases. The National Heart Institute was created in 1949. The Framingham Heart Study began in 1950. Actually, although reductions in chronic disease mortality were identified as starting in 1968, a more comprehensive examination suggests that mortality declines for chronic diseases began earlier. From 1950 to 1992, age-standardized heart disease mortality rates declined 50.8 percent; stroke mortality declined 70.8 percent. Declines in stroke mortality can be traced back to at least 1925.[7] Declines in male heart disease prevalence became evident after examining data on US Civil War veterans age 65 and over who were assessed for pensions in 1910. A comparison of heart disease prevalence in Civil War veterans in 1910 with that in WWII veterans aged 65 and over in 1985 showed a decline of 66 percent in the intervening 75 years.[8]

Reductions in chronic disease mortality raised concern about society's "carrying" capacity for a growing elderly population, because it suggested that the number of years individuals live after age 65 would be significantly extended. Although Social Security finances benefit from an increasing number of persons living through their labor force years to age 65, living beyond 65 increases the financial burden on Social Security—and Medicare and Medicaid—programs. Recognition of the declines after 1968 in chronic disease mortality, and life expectancy increases above age 65, raised concerns about the long-term fiscal stability of the U.S. Social Security system. In 1982, in addition to payroll tax increases, increases in the Social Security normal retirement age from 65 to 67 were scheduled for early in the 21st century. Increases in the retirement age to age 70, or even 72, are currently being debated. Similar problems are faced in other developed countries. A Japanese study suggested that future economic growth could be compromised by population aging. That study anticipated that one-quarter of Japan's population will be over 65 by 2025—using estimates of life expectancy limits that were exceeded by 3 years by Japanese females in 1992.[9,10]

Policy and social responses to population aging depends upon a fourth dynamic—changes in the average health of the elderly. Was the health of a person age 70 in 1995 better, on average, than the health of a 70-year-old in 1970; will the health of an 80-year-old in 2020 be better than the health of an 80-year-old in 1995? U.S. data suggest that the answers to these questions are yes. Significant declines in the prevalence of chronic disability and morbidity in the elderly population were observed from 1982 to 1989—and continue to 1995 and beyond.[11–13]

Such health changes have profound effects on the social and economic institutions of a country—as well as on its health care delivery and financing system.[14] There are already popular responses in the perceived lower limit to "old age" in the United States. A recent survey suggested that persons age 50 thought a person has to reach age 80 before being "elderly." This was due to changing social perceptions, and economic realities due to the growing proportion of the total US population over age 65, and the effects on housing, insurance, and other private markets. Fundamental research issues involve determining parameters of the population health dynamics underlying changing social perceptions and economics. Whether or not improvements in health and functioning continue at late ages, and can be accelerated by judicious public health and medical innovations and investments, will affect how the United States' and other developed countries' social and economic institutions respond in the future to a growing elderly population.

A difficulty in anticipating future improvements in health at, for example, ages 85 and 95, is that changes depend upon both historical and future conditions. Historical factors are important because the individuals who will be the elderly and oldest-old cohorts in the next 65 years are already alive and have accumulated significant early exposures that partly determine the age trajectories of health parameters. Historical factors determine both the number of elderly persons (by reducing early mortality), and the mix of health problems they present (i.e., parameters of individual health changes with age vary due to differences in the prior experiences of birth cohorts). That is, depending both upon the cohort an elderly person is in, and the individual's life experiences, the principle health manifestations of aging may vary considerably. For example, very elderly cohorts may have little early smoking experience, and hence, little chronic pulmonary disease. Recent cohorts of postmenopausal females, due to the early use of exogenous estrogens, may have reduced osteoporosis and coronary heart disease (CHD) risks. An analysis of future conditions is necessary because we are in a historically unique period where many biomedical technologies, and their clinical application, are maturing so that many conditions once palliatively managed are now subject to disease-modifying treatments (e.g., rheumatoid arthritis[15]). Below we briefly review historical and future inputs to the health dynamics of the elderly population, and then forecast what "old age" will signify in the future.

Historical Determinants of the Future Health of the Elderly

The realized human life span is increasing. The first documented case of a centenarian was reported in 1800.[16] The first documented age of 110 years was achieved in 1932. The first documented age of 120 years (Jean Marie Calment; now age 122.3 years) was achieved in 1995. There are partly documented reports of ages of 125 years being achieved for a Brazilian female; 127 years for a US Hispanic female. Thus, the maximum documented human life span increased 10 years from 1800 to 1932, and over 12 years from 1932 to 1997, that is, at over twice the earlier rate. The number of centenarians in the United States increased 7 percent per year from 1960 to 1987—that growth continues with 54,000 centenarians estimated to be alive in 1995.[17] Similar rates of increase (7 percent) in the number of centenarians are found in other developed countries.[18] Thus, centenarians are no longer a rarity—although studies of their current, and past, health characteristics are.[19] The age range of new elderly and extreme elderly cohorts is now broad enough (e.g., 65 to 115 years of age) that the parameters of the health consequences of aging will differ significantly across the cohorts represented by that range (i.e., aging health changes are partly determined by historical processes).

Evidence suggests that the health of the extreme elderly is improving and that interventions can be successful at late ages. One factor in health improvements is the effect of early mortality on the health of very elderly populations; "high" early mortality in a cohort "selects out" its genetically less fit members between ages 50 to 85. In a Swedish study the relative risk of CHD mortality in monozygotic twin pairs was roughly 15 to 1 in middle age. Above age 85, the relative risk was 1.0.[20] Selection caused thyroid autoantibodies in Italian centenarians to be as only prevalent as they were at 50—even though their prevalence increased from ages 50 to 85.[21] Genetically determined lung cancer (due to defects in the cytochrome P-450 enzyme system) peak at 70 percent at age 50; by age 70 the genetic form of the disease is 20 percent of cases.[22] ApoE4, (apolipoprotein E4), associated with heart disease and dementia risk, declines with age from a prevalence of over 20 percent at age 80 to about 5 percent at age 100.[23] The null allele C4B*Q0 is associated with heart attack risk in middle-aged males, with such risks (and selection against the genotype) occurring at later ages for females.[24,25]

If mortality selection were the only factor determining the health of extreme elderly populations, their average health would decline as the percent surviving from birth to late ages in a cohort increased. However, many other factors affect the health of the extreme elderly.

A study of surgery performed on patients aged 90 to 103 showed that intraoperative mortality declined from 29 percent in the 1960s to 8 percent by 1985.[26] The study was performed because surgery rates over age 90 increased fivefold from 1979 to 1989. The 5-year survival of this group (mean age 93.5 years), was better than the general population (i.e., a 5-year survival of 21 percent versus 16 percent in regional life tables). A factor in the success of surgical interventions was the small number of "ever smokers" in the cohort and the low prevalence of chronic pulmonary disease.

Nutritional factors were thought to cause the reductions in chronic morbidity in Fogel's[8] study of Civil War veterans. One theory suggests that prenatal nutrition affects the risk of chronic disease at late ages[27–29] because the prenatal development of major organ systems is affected by maternal nutrition. In US Civil War veterans born 1825 to 1844, the high prevalence of chronic disease was thought to be due to poor maternal and early nutrition differentially affecting the development of major organ systems. Improvements 1910 to 1985 in physiological status at late ages was argued to be due to improved early nutrition between the experience of the 1825 to 1844, and 1900 to 1920, cohorts. This Fogel traced to temporal increases in stature and body mass index (BMI) on Waaler surfaces.[30]

Another theory suggests that improved food hygiene reduced exposures to viral and other chronic "slow" infections (e.g., cytomegalovirus [CMV], herpesvirus, *Chlamydia pneumoniae*[31,32]) in animal food sources causing latter reductions in atherosclerosis in adults.[33] They suggest that thermal food processing and tighter regulations on livestock production reduced the risk of chronic circulatory diseases and certain cancers[34] by reducing the risk of chronic viral and other infections.[33,35] That is, recent declines in heart disease mortality were traced to the ingestion of atherogenic viruses in pre-WWII, and postwar declines in infection rates as food hygiene improved. A number of events shaped these trends; vesicular exanthema, a viral disease of swine, was discovered in 1932. Controls for this and other livestock infections began in California in 1945 to 1949, a state showing early (1950) declines in heart disease. An outbreak of vesicular exanthema in 1952 mandated national regulations requiring thermal processing of livestock feed. Hog cholera eradication programs began in 1962. The Swine Health Protection Act was passed in 1980 to prevent another virus from entering the food chain. Thermal processing of prepared foods, although existing as a technology at the turn of the century, expanded rapidly after WWII. Some early models of atherosclerosis[36,37] suggested that infectious agents were involved—in addition to inflammatory processes, homeostatic factors, and blood lipids.[38] However, the technical ability (e.g., polymerase chain reaction [PCR] or fluorescence in-situ hybridization [FISH]) to detect the presence of agents, their genetic effects, or persistent immunologic responses is recent.[39]

Another model suggests that chronic circulatory disease change was, in part, due to changes in the dietary levels of micronutrients such as vitamins A, B, C, E, and D. A, C, and E are antioxidants and may reduce the rate of oxidation of low-density lipoprotein (LDL) cholesterol in macrophages (producing "foam cells")—a factor in atherogenesis.[38] Vitamins A and E are cellular redifferentiating agents reducing the risk of some cancers.[40] The dietary levels of vitamins A (and other retinoids) and C depends upon the availability of fresh fruits and vegetables—foodstuffs difficult to preserve before refrigeration and transportation technologies allowed persons in northern temperate climates to continue to consume such foodstuffs through the winter. This also could affect hypertension and stroke in that refrigeration reduced the use of salt as a food preservative. Increased consumption of fruits may have increased potassium intake and lowered hypertension.

Vitamin D has long been supplemented. Moon et al[41] noted that the curative effects of cod liver oil on rickets were documented in 1917. By 1923, the United States imported half a million gallons of fish liver oil, and nearly 3 million gallons in 1930. Ultraviolet radiation of milk began in the United States in 1924. Production of vitamin D rose from 35 pounds in 1948 to 14,000 pounds in 1972. Supplementation became problematic in that vitamin D is a potent hormonal agent with a narrow therapeutic trough. Thus, reductions in supplementation were mandated by the Food and Drug Administration (FDA) in 1972.

Vitamin D metabolism is complex, including effects on cellular calcium metabolism and parathyroid hormone production, possibly leading to hypertension.[42] Vitamin D interferes with the uptake of magnesium. Concomitant with increased vitamin D supplementation were declines in magnesium in the United States diet due to the use of nitrogen-based fertilizers. Vitamin D also increases the absorption of iron, so oversupplementation could affect heart disease by reducing magnesium (which could increase production of aldosterone[43]) and by increasing iron absorption-increasing LDL oxidation (also by causing increases in serum calcium and calcification of plaques), stroke (by affecting hypertension), and osteoporosis (by direct effects on osteoclasts and bone resorption).

A fourth model involves elevated homocysteine due to increased meat consumption and genetic or dietary deficiencies of vitamin B_6 and B_{12}. Decreasing renal function with age may adversely affect physiologic vitamin B levels, as may age changes in liver metabolism through the eighth decade of life. The homocysteine model suggests that atherosclerosis is, in part, a disease of protein toxicity whereby failure to detoxify certain sulfur-based amino acid products of protein metabolism leads to damage in arterial endothelium.[44] The homocysteine model may not only explain initiating events in circulatory disease,[45] but also possibly osteo- and rheumatoid arthritic changes (by affecting cartilage matrix formation) and increases in dementia.[46] Vitamin B_6 also has a wide range of physiologic effects (e.g., DNA binding and nuclear localization) on a super family of ligand activated transcription factors that exert biologic effects by regulating target gene expression.[47,48]

Current and Future Biomedical Inputs to Aging

The factors described above determined health parameters of persons now entering advanced age ranges. To respond to this heterogeneity of aging parameters, and recent changes in the physiologic manifestation of aging changes, are treatment modalities made possible by recent biomedical research. Research focused on aging per se, began in the United States with the creation of National Institute on Aging (NIA) in 1974. In the 1960s, biologic senescence was often viewed as a genetically determined cellular process operating universely in all tissue types, and chronic diseases were believed to be manifestations of its effects. Hayflick[49] suggested one model: under genetic control, human fibroblasts reproduced only 30 to 60 times. An experiment[50] challenging this view examined the number of cell replications remaining for fibroblasts drawn from persons aged 30 to 80 years. Cells lost one replication for every 5 years of life. Thus, if this is the basic mechanism of senescence, it would not limit life spans near current levels.

In the 1970s it became clear that many aging studies had

design flaws (i.e., the rate of loss of physiologic function was tracked in "representative" populations). This confounded the intrinsic physiologic rate of aging with the age-dependent prevalence of chronic disease determined by the history of environmental exposures. Studies of populations screened for existing chronic disease lowered estimates of the age rate of loss of physiologic functions, (e.g., the age rate of loss of cardiac function in an active elderly population was one-half that in earlier studies.[51]) Age-related disease processes were found to be physiologically more complex, with much wider variation in expression than previously thought.[52,53]

In the 1980s, medical science began to demonstrate potential for modifying chronic disease processes. Atherosclerosis was once thought to be a product of an aging circulatory system. Now it appears to be reversible by nutritional modification (e.g., cholesterol reduction) and other interventions,[54,55] with functional responses evident before anatomic changes[56,57] and facilitated by antioxidant therapy.[58] Left ventricular hypertrophy (LVH) was thought to be due to age-related remodeling of cardiomyocytes. However, angiotensin-converting enzyme (ACE)-II inhibitors, as well as controlling hypertension, can also cause regression of left ventricular hypertrophy,[59] possibly by blocking the effects of aldosterone in remodeling myocytes to fibrotic tissue.[60] Many classic signs of senescence, or old age, are now well-defined pathologic processes (e.g., frailty and osteoporosis, cognitive impairment and Alzheimer's disease). With the pathologic mechanisms identified, it is possible to develop disease-modifying interventions.

Some early chronic disease and aging interventions were initiated serendipitously. Exogenous estrogens were used by 3 million US women in 1985 for post menopausal symptoms. Now it appears that exogenous estrogens reduces the risk of osteoporosis and CHD[61] in postmenopausal women.[62] Aspirin has long been used as an analgesic and to control fever. Recently, its potential in secondary prevention of stroke and heart attack by affecting platelet adhesion has been realized.[63] An association of aspirin consumption with reduced risk of colorectal cancer was found, as has a speculative association with reductions in Alzheimer's disease risks. Nonsteroidal anti-inflammatory drugs (NSAIDs), by blocking inflammatory tissue responses, may affect other cancers by affecting the ability of tumor cells to metastasize and clonally organize.

Modeling senescence as the genetic control of the number of cell replications was given impetus by investigations of the end-segment of the human chromosome, the telomere, and an enzyme, telomerase, that induces its lengthening.[64] The evidence for the telomere controlling senescence is mixed. The telomere does decrease in length as the cell replicates. However, when a given length is reached, although the cell ceases to divide, it exhibits stable metabolism and function. Bone marrow and blood cells express low levels of telomerase, with that activity distributed across different cell types. Thus, there may not be an absolute shutoff of telomerase in somatic cells but continuing production at low levels. This is consistent with templates of telomerase ribonucleic acid (RNA) existing in somatic cells and the ability of tumor cells to express telomerase after a crisis phase.[65]

Evidence of the role of telomerase in neoplastic growth is clear. Normally, cells stop replicating while the telomere is still long. It may be that the p53 mediated pathway to apoptosis[66] is activated when the telomere drops below a functionally suboptimal length. Then, the cell enters a crisis phase that leads either to cell death or a reactivation of telomerase, a stabilized telomere length, and an immortal cell line.[67] Confirmation was found in that telomerase activity was present in 68 percent of stage I, and 95 percent of advanced stage breast tumors, but not in normal tissue. Telomerase was expressed in 45 percent of fibroadenomas, benign breast lesions.[68]

The search for universal mechanisms of senescence is difficult.[69] Many physiologic mechanisms associated with aging and cell growth prove to be more mutable by environmental factors, even at the genetic and molecular level, than once thought.[39,70,71] Some authors[72] argued that life expectancy is limited at 85 years, unless medical science developed interventions at the molecular level to modify parameters of aging. The problem with these arguments is defining molecular interventions; many existing interventions operate at a molecular level. Nutritional factors (e.g., vitamins A, B) may affect receptor structure in the cell membrane, the message to DNA, and the transcription of genetic code to specific proteins. Some interventions have been used for a long time, even though their mechanisms were initially not understood. The anthracycline, doxorubicin, is a potent chemotherapeutic agent disrupting cell replication by affecting nuclear proteins, Topoisomerase II α and β.[70] Early chemotherapeutic techniques were based on relatively simple principles where cell death was a function of drug concentration. Now the ways (e.g., interactions of c-*myc*, *bcl*-2 and *p53* genes[39]) in which apoptosis is induced, and interventions in ancillary processes such as angiogenesis, growth factor dependency, metastatic invasion, and cellular redifferention, are all therapeutic avenues being investigated at the molecular level.

To illustrate, an agent in use a long time, for which the mechanisms of molecular action are still being elaborated, is the antiestrogen, Tamoxifen. This compound was given to older women with advanced, estrogen receptor positive breast cancer, to control its growth.[73] At first, growth inhibition was attributed to competitive binding with estrogen in a tumor cell's estrogen receptors. This initially raised concern that Tamoxifen would exacerbate osteoporosis and heart disease. However, Tamoxifen's interaction with the receptor was more complex—sometimes being an agonist (i.e., it was protective against bone loss and circulatory disease). It appears that Tamoxifen affects the ability to induce transcriptional activity in the caboxy-terminal ligand binding domain.[74] Of further interest was that Tamoxifen affected estrogen receptor negative tumor cells, and in interaction with chemotherapeutic agents (e.g., cisplatin[75]), by synergistically interacting in inducing apoptosis with other agents (e.g., vitamin D[76]); possibly by increasing the expression of estrogen receptors; or by blocking the action of drug resistent genes by affecting the calcium channel membrane transport of the drug.[77,78] The effects on estrogen receptor negative breast cancer cells may be due to the induction of apoptosis by overexpression of *c-myc*, mRNA, and protein.[79] These effects may be enhanced by retinoic acid and vitamin D_3 analogs.[80,81] Interventions into the transcriptional expression of genotypes by known agents is interesting, given growing insights into the relation of carcinogenesis and senescence.[67,82,83]

The Future of Aging

The above suggest that (1) the physiologic expression of aging changes will vary in the future due to major changes in nutrition, infectious disease risks, and hygiene, some exposures inducing stable genetic abberations,[39,71] and (2) that we already have many agents and therapies affecting the molecular transcriptional expression of genotype, although our knowledge of the details of those mechanisms, and how to intervene, are not complete. It can be argued, however, that we have only recently developed the scientific tools (e.g., PCR, restriction fragment length polymorphism (RFLP); chromosome painting[39,71]) to accelerate our understanding of these mechanisms, and of the techniques and agents for intervening (e.g., rational drug design; nonimmunosuppressive cyclosporin, PSC833[84]).

Techniques intervening at a molecular level are not restricted to cancer treatments but also to many other disorders.[85] A promising area is the improved regulation of the aging immune system.[86] A promising recent development was the observation that interleukin-10 (IL-10) suppressed tumor growth and inhibited spontaneous metastasis.[87,88] This was a surprise because IL-10 suppressed macrophage and helper T-cell function, and delayed type hypersensitivity reactions. In suppressing macrophage activity, IL-10 suppressed release of proinflammatory cytokines, nitric oxide, and reactive oxygen intermediaries. It, however, stimulated natural killer (NK) cells, and chemoattraction of CD8+ cells and neutrophils. Inhibition of macrophage activity may have a tumor suppressive effect by reducing the local production of multiple growth or angiogenesis factors. Alterations of immune function (e.g., by vitamin A, C, or E supplementation[89,90]), and inflammatory responses and angiogenesis may be important in autoimmune disorders[91] and in certain stages of atherogenesis.[92,93] As in other cases, nutritional factors hold promise for modifying abnormal immunoresponse (e.g., the role of fish oil supplementation on MHC-II molecules and the membranes of human white blood cells affecting auto-immune disorders[94]). N-3 polyunsaturated fatty acids may protect against chronic obstructive lung disease in ever smokers.[95]

Thus, there is a matrix of interrelations of basic physiologic processes that underly the major chronic diseases expressed in old age. For example, the expression of Lp(a), a factor in circulatory disease risks, also has a strong association with breast cancer risk and its ability to metastasize.[96] The role of inflammatory response, and of the local production of growth factors, is likely crucial to both tumor growth and the development of atherosclerotic plaques.[88,92,93] There are likely associations of osteoporosis and atherosclerosis due to altered calcium metabolism.[97] Osteoporosis may be linked to hypertension and renal function by vitamin D metabolism.[85,98]

Because of this rapidly increasing understanding of disease processes and therapeutic interventions at the molecular level, it is reasonable to anticipate future and accelerating changes in disease and mortality risks at late ages. One of the crucial factors is to develop therapeutics with generally positive effect profiles. This is possible because of the above-mentioned matrix of physiologic functions that interrelate many age-dependent pathologies at the molecular level. For example, ACE-II inhibitors have positive effects on lipid and glucose metabolism, reduce LVH, and possibly increase β-receptor density as well as control hypertension.[99–101] Certain β-blockers may improve β-receptor activity in the myocardium by downregulating both response to norepinephrine and activity as an antioxidant.[102] The reason that IL-10 is promising is because it does not produce the serious side effects found with many other cytokines.[103]

One argument may be that this increased understanding of disease mechanisms may produce medical interventions too expensive to provide en masse to a rapidly growing elderly population. This may, however, be due to a misunderstanding of the economics of scientific innovation, in that the initial development of new technologies is expensive; the evolution of subsidiary production technologies reduce unit costs and more of the population is treated (i.e., development costs are amortized over larger numbers of patients and the full benefits for the population are realized). For example, ACE-II inhibitors reduce the number of days of hospitalization required for congestive heart failure (CHF).[104] As a result, the cost benefit ratio of ACE-II inhibitors, appropriately applied, can be quite high.[59] *Helicobacter pylori* was characterized in 1984. The role of *H. pylori* in the mechanism for most ulcers and gastric cancers[105] identified new treatment modalities that are very cost-effective. Antibiotic treatment for *H. pylori* costs about $200, compared to about $100 per month for the use of histamine blockers, which do not cure the disease. Given that there may be 4.5 million ulcer cases in the United States, the savings would be significant. Technologies also prove cost-effective, such as day surgery and plastic lens implants for cataracts;[106] newer forms of pacemakers more appropriate for cardiac functional decline at late ages, dual chamber pacemakers, can respond to the increasing role of arterial pulse in cardiac output with age.[107] Thus, the correct understanding of a disease mechanism and disease linkages may produce synergistic interventions that eventually prove economic, especially if disease control is also accompanied by functional increases at late ages. Estimates of the savings to Medicare of reductions in functional disability prevalence from 1982 to 1995 could be over 7 percent of costs; or $180 to $200 billion (in 1995 dollars[11]).

If costs are not a limiting factor to advancement of health at late ages, what might aging in the mid-twenty-first century look like? Projections for the United States suggest that control of major circulatory disease risk factors, over a long enough time for their regulation to affect existing disease, could significantly increase the mean age at which CHD and stroke deaths occur.[108] The predominant forms of CHD would involve interactions of hypertension, atherosclerotic change, and age-related declines in cardiac function (e.g., age-related loss of β-receptor binding efficiency) that would become further dominated by the age-related changes in cardiac function. Cancer mortality, especially for solid tumors, in the next 10 to 15 years will begin to show significant declines due to treatments now in clinical trials. Evidence suggests that significant breast cancer mortality reductions have occurred due to the use of Tamoxifen in estrogen receptor positive disease, and adjuvant therapy in early node negative disease.[109,110] Greenspan[111] suggests current chemotherapy, rigorously applied, could reduce the number of U.S. breast cancer deaths by one-third. The aging of the population could promote this trend, as recent studies indicate that very young women with breast cancer may respond less favorably than older women to chemotherapy.[112,113] This is due to the generally less aggressive nature of disease in older women and probably to better management of the adverse effects of more aggressive treatments at later ages (e.g., use of granulocyte-colony stimulating factor [G-CSF]). The mix of cancers affecting an older population will change significantly. This will be related to the nature of the host tissue in which the tumor arises. For example, cancer related to infectious processes (liver cancer, gastric cancer) or food spoilage may decline. Other neoplasia related to biologic aging processes (e.g., prostate cancer, multiple myeloma, certain types of lymphoma, late onset breast cancer) will increase in importance—although the mean age of death from those cancers will also increase. The effects of viral diseases on cancer risks and possibly on atherogenesis and general immunologic dysfunction (e.g., plasma cell dyscrias of unknown significance, which often progress to multiple myeloma[86]) will become more treatable as antiviral agents improve and as our understanding of the chronic effects of viruses on the immune system advances. Thus, there are a number of areas where therapeutic advances could occur, affecting multiple stages of very lengthy chronic disease processes. In addition, therapeutic advances could be supported by behavioral and lifestyle changes among middle aged and elderly persons. This can be anticipated in that (1) the proportion of elderly cohorts who are better educated is increasing, that is, better educated populations tend to be more amenable to public health messages,[114] and (2) physical activity has been shown to have benefits to extreme ages.[115–117]

These changes could increase life expectancy in the next 50 to 60 years (i.e., by 2050 to 2060) to 95 to 100 years.[118,119] This compares to U.S. Census Bureau high life expectancy projections for 2050 of 86.4 years for males and 92.3 years for females.[17] Census Bureau life expectancy estimates are based on extrapolations of mortality trends. Our higher estimates are based on using multiple risk factor data, their dynamics, and assumptions about the ability to jointly control those factors.[118,119] Our projections do not assume that heart disease, stroke, and cancer are eliminated. They do assume that the mean age at death for each is increased due to preventative and disease-modifying interventions. Those changes will also affect the proportion of deaths due to specific causes. Male cancer mortality would increase from about 20 to 40 percent of deaths at all ages. The largest changes would come from increased proportions of cancer deaths above age 85. For females, cancer mortality would increase relatively more (to about 60 percent of all deaths), because the adverse effects of menopausal changes in multiple cardiovascular disease (CVD) risk factors are assumed controlled in the projections. CVD risks would decline moderately (from 65 to 50 percent) for males as a proportion of all deaths, but those deaths would occur at later ages. For females, the projected declines in CVD deaths are much larger.

The two sets of projections imply different things for U.S. society's carrying capacity for the elderly. In census projections, the high life expectancy series project a U.S. population of 416 million by 2050. In this projection, 1 percent would be over age 100 (4.1 million), 7.2 percent would be over age 85 (30 million), and 23.3 percent would be over age 65 (97 million). The proportion of the population above a given age in the census projections is strongly affected by fertility assumptions. For example, Social Security Administration (SSA) cohort life tables for persons born in 1950 (which use less favorable mortality assumptions) imply that 5.6 percent of females and 1.5 percent of males live to age 100. Assuming a 3 to 1 survival advantage for females to age 100, this suggests that 4.6 percent of the 1950 cohort survives to age 100. For the 1990 cohort, survival to age 100 is 10.2 percent for females and 3.3 percent for males, or 8.4 percent combined. Thus, in a stable population, a large proportion of persons reach age 100 even in less optimistic SSA 1990 life tables. In our risk factor based projections, the US population is projected to be 456 million persons in 2050, with 14 percent over age 85, and 33 percent over age 65. Although these proportions are larger than in the census projections, they are not grossly different from the 25 percent of the Japanese population expected to be over age 65 in 2025. If fertility and immigration is lower than assumed in the census projections, then the proportion of the population over age 65 and over 85 would be higher. Even the extreme projections made from risk factor data do not take into account recent studies suggesting that human mortality never exceeds 50 percent at any age (i.e., 50 percent is the maximum mortality rate). This assumption has, for example, been built into the US Society of Actuaries 1994 group annuity tables.[120] Such estimates are consistent with estimates from multiple studies showing that the annual increase in mortality rates slows to very low values (2 to 3 percent) about age 100.[19] These slow increases in mortality are apparently due to the high mortality rates of very elderly persons with high levels of disability. Thus, the average level of disability about age 95 tends to stabilize due to the equilibrium with mortality rates at those ages.[108]

The question emerges of how a society can cope with a population with such a high proportion of elderly persons. This is a problem only if there is not a commensurate change in the age-specific health status of the population. The health-mortality factors discussed above suggest that their natural dynamics enforce this in part. There is also evidence of such changes in current health expenditures. Lubitz et al.[121] found that the average Medicare expenditure for those who died at age 70 was $35,511, compared to $65,633 for those who survived to age 101. Thus, the average Medicare expense per year for centenarians from ages 65 to 101 was $1,823, compared to $7,100 per year for those who died at age 70. Thus, the pattern of Medicare expenditures was in distinct contrast to the accumulated liability of increased life expectancy for Social Security.

If disability declines, as observed from 1982 to 1995, health costs will decrease even more rapidly at later ages. This pattern also seems consistent with the different patterns of medical problems that may be faced at late ages in the future. Thus, the primary response to the social costs of such large elderly populations would be increases in the normal retirement age for Social Security. Each year of increase in the normal retirement age for Social Security has a large fiscal impact. Thus, if the normal retirement age could be increased to age 70 or 72, because the physiologic status now at those ages is equivalent to the physiologic status at age 65 in, say, 1982—then a large portion of the fiscal burden of population aging could be addressed.

References

1. Social Security Administration: Life Tables for the United States Social Security Area 1900–2080 (Actuarial Study 107). Social Security Administration (SSA Pub No. 11–11536), Baltimore, 1992
2. National Center for Health Statistics: The change in mortality trends in the United States. Series 3, No. 1. Public Health Service, Washington, DC, 1964
3. Myers GC: Future age projections and society. In Gilmore AG (ed): Aging: A Challenge to Science and Social Policy. Oxford University Press, New York, 1981
4. Omran AR: The epidemiologic transition: A theory of the epidemiology of population change. Milbank Memorial Quarterly 1971;XLIX:509–538
5. Antonovsky A: Social class and the major cardiovascular diseases. J Chronic Dis 1968;21:65–106
6. Dubos R: Man adapting. Yale University Press, New Haven, 1965
7. Lanska DJ, Mi X: Decline in U.S. stroke mortality in the era before antihypertensive therapy. Stroke 1993;24:1382–1388
8. Fogel RW: Economic growth, population theory, and physiology: The bearing of long-term processes on the making of economic policy. American Economic Review 1994;84: 369–395
9. Nihon University: Population aging in Japan: problems and policy issues in the 21st Century. In Kuroda T (ed): International Conference on An Aging Society: Strategies for the 21st Century Japan. Nihon University Population Research Institute, Tokyo, 1982
10. World Health Organization: World health statistics annual. World Health Organization, Geneva, 1994
11. Manton KG: Future trends and perspectives in long term care. In Jolt H, Leibovici MM (eds): Health Care Management: State of the Art Review Series. Hanley & Befus, Philadelphia, 1997
12. Manton KG, Corder LS, Stallard E: Estimates of change in chronic disability and institutional incidence and prevalence rates in the U.S. elderly population from the 1982, 1984, and 1989 National Long Term Care Survey. J Gerontol: Soc Sci 1993;47:S153–S166
13. Manton KG, Stallard E, Corder LS: Changes in morbidity and chronic disability in the U.S. elderly population: evidence from the 1982, 1984, and 1989 National Long Term Care Surveys. J Gerontol 1995;50B:S194–S204
14. Ikegami N, Campbell J: Medical care in Japan. N Engl J Med 1995;333:1295–1299
15. Tugwell P, Pincus T, Yocum D et al: Combination therapy with cyclosporine and methotrexate in severe rheumatoid arthritis. N Engl J Med 1995;333:137–141
16. Thoms WS: Human longevity, its facts and its fictions. John Murray, London, 1873
17. Day JC: Population projections of the United States, by age, sex, race, and Hispanic origin: 1995 to 2050, Series P25–1130. U.S. Government Printing Office, Washington, DC, 1996
18. Vaupel JW, Jeune B: The emergence and proliferation of centenarians. Aging Research Unit, Odense University Medical School, Odense, Denmark, 1994
19. Manton KG, Stallard E: Longevity in the U.S.: age and sex specific evidence on life span limits from mortality patterns: 1962–1990. J Gerontol: Biol Sci 1996;B362–B375
20. Marenberg ME, Risch N, Berkman LF et al: Genetic susceptibility to death from coronary heart disease in a study of twins. N Engl J Med 1994;330:1041–1046
21. Marriotti S, Sansoni P, Barbesino G et al: Thyroid and other organ-specific auto-antibodies in healthy centenarians. Lancet 1992;339:1506–1508
22. Sellers TA, Bailey-Wilson JE, Elston RC et al: Evidence for Mendelian inheritance in the pathogenesis of lung cancer. J Natl Cancer Inst 1990;82:1272–1279
23. Louhija J, Miettinen HE, Kontula K et al: Aging and genetic variation of plasma apolipoproteins: relative loss of the apolipoprotein E4 phenotype in centenarians. Arterioscler Thromb 1994;14:1084–1089
24. Kramer J, Fulop T, Rajczy K et al: A marked drop in the incidence of the null allele of the B gene of the fourth component of complement (C4B*Q0) in elderly subjects: C4B*Q0 as a probable negative selection factor for survival. Hum Genet 1991;86:595–598
25. Kramer J, Rajczy K, Hegyi L et al: C4B*Q0 allotype as risk factor for myocardial infarction. Br Med J 1994;309:313–314
26. Hosking MP, Warner MA, Lodbell CM et al: Outcomes of surgery in patients 90 years of age and older. JAMA 1989; 261:1909–1915
27. Barker D, Meade T, Fall C et al: Relation of fetal and infant growth to plasma fibrinogen and factor VII concentrations in adult life. Br Med J 1992;304:148–152
28. Hale C, Barker D, Clark P et al: Fetal and infant growth

impaired glucose tolerances at age 64. BMJ 1991;303: 1019–1022

29. Barker DJP, Martyn CN: The maternal and fetal origins of cardiovascular disease. J Epidemiol Community Health 1992; 46:8–11
30. Waaler H: Height, weight, and mortality, the Norweigen experience. Acta Med Scand 1983;679(suppl. 1):1–56
31. Grayston JT: Chlamydia in atherosclerosis. Circulation 1993; 87:1408–1409
32. Linnanmäki E, Leinonen M, Mattila K et al: *Chlamydia pneumoniae*—specific circulating immune complexes in patients with chronic coronary heart disease. Circulation 1993;87: 1130–1134
33. Mozar HN, Bal DG, Farag SA: The natural history of atherosclerosis: an ecologic perspective. Atherosclerosis 1990;82: 157–164
34. Mozar HN, Bal DG, Farag SA: Human cancer and the food chain: an alternative etiologic perspective. Nutr Cancer 1989; 12:29
35. Melnick JL, Schattner A: Viruses and atherosclerosis. Isr J Med Sci 1992;28:463–465
36. Klotz O, Manning MF: Fatty streaks in the intima of arteries. J Pathol Bacteriol 1912;16:211
37. Frothingham C: The relation between acute infectious diseases and arterial lesions. Arch Intern Med 1911;8:153
38. Ross R: The pathogenesis of atherosclerosis—an update. N Engl J Med 1986;314:488–500
39. Sheer D, Squire J: Clinical applications of genetic rearrangements in cancer. Cancer Biol 1996;7:25–32
40. Prasad KN, Edwards-Prasad J: Vitamin E and cancer prevention: recent advances and future potentials. J Am Coll Nutr 1992;11:487–500
41. Moon RC, Rao KVN, Detrisac CJ, Kelloff GJ: Animal models for chemoprevention of respiratory cancer. J Natl Cancer Inst Monographs 1992;13:45–49
42. Eastell R, Yergery A, Vieira N et al: Interrelationship among vitamin D metabolism, true calcium absorption, parathyroid function, and age in women: evidence of an age-related intestinal resistance to 1, 25 dihydroxyvitamin A action. J Bone Mineral Res 1991;6:125
43. Ichihara A, Suzuki H, Saruta T: Effects of magnesium on the renin-angiotensin-aldosterone system in human subjects. J Lab Clin Med 1993;122:432–440
44. McCully KS: Homocystein theory of arteriosclerosis: development and current status. Arteriosclerosis 1983;2:157–246
45. von Eckardstein A, Malinow R, Upson B et al: Effects of age, lipoproteins, and hemostatic parameters on the role of homocyst(e)inemia as a cardiovascular risk factor in men. Arterioscler Thromb 1994;14:460–464
46. Riggs KM, Spiro A, Tucker K, Rush D: Relations of vitamin B-12, vitamin B-6, folate, and homocysteine to cognitive performance in the normative aging study. Am J Clin Nutr 1996; 63:306–314
47. Tully DB, Allgood VE, Cidlowski JA et al. The steroid hormone receptors and their mechanism of action. pp. 549–567. In: Nutrition and Gene Expression. CRC Press, Boca Raton, 1993
48. Allgood VE, Powell-Oliver FE, Cidlowski JA: Vitamin B_6 influences glucocorticoid receptor-mediated gene expression. J Biol Chem 1990;265:12424
49. Hayflick L: The limited in vitro lifetime of human diploid cell strains. Exp Cell Res 1965;37:614–636
50. Martin GM, Spaque CA, Epstein CJ: Replicative life-span of cultivated human cells: effects of donor's age, tissue and genotype. Lab Invest 1970;23:86–92
51. Kasch FW, Boyer JL, Van Camp SP et al: Effect of exercise on cardiovascular aging. Age Ageing 1993;22:5–10
52. Lakatta E: Health, disease, and cardiovascular aging. In: America's Aging: Health in an Older Society. National Academy Press, Washington, DC, 1985
53. Lakatta EG: Deficient neuroendocrine regulation of the cardiovascular system with advancing age in healthy humans. Circulation 1993;87:631–636
54. Ornish D, Brown SE, Scherwitz LW et al: Can lifestyle changes reverse coronary heart disease? The Lifestyle Heart Trial. Lancet 1990;336:129–133
55. Brown BG, Zhao XQ, Sacco DE, Alberts JJ: Lipid lowering and plaque disruption and clinical events in coronary disease. Circulation 1993;87:1781–1791
56. Treasure C, Klein J, Weintraub W et al: Beneficial effects of cholesterol-lowering therapy on the coronary endothelium in patients with coronary artery disease. N Engl J Med 1995; 332:481–487
57. Benzuly K, Padgett R, Kaul S et al: Functional improvement precedes structural regression of atherosclerosis. Circulation 1994;89:1810–1818
58. Anderson T, Meredith I, Yeung A et al: The effect of cholesterol-lowering and antioxidant therapy on endothelium-dependent coronary vasomotion. N Engl J Med 1995;332:488–493
59. Paul SD, Kuntz KM, Eagle KA, Weinstein MC: Costs and effectiveness of angiotensin converting enzyme inhibition in patients with congestive heart failure. Arch Intern Med 1994; 154:1143–1149
60. Weber K, Brilla C: Pathological hypertrophy and cardiac intersittium. Circulation 1991;83:1849–1865
61. Nabulsi A, Folsom A, White A et al: Association of hormone-replacement therapy with various cardiovascular risk factors in postmenopausal women. N Engl J Med 1993;328:1069–1075
62. Belchetz P: Hormonal treatment of postmenopausal women. N Engl J Med 1994;330:1062–1071
63. Antiplatelet Trialists' Collaboration: Collaborative overview of randomized trials of antiplatelet therapy–I: prevention of death, myocardial infarction, and stroke by prolonged antiplatelet therapy in various categories of patients. Br Med J 1994;308:81–106
64. Morin GB: The structure and properties of mammalian telomerase and their potential impact on human disease. Semin Cell Devel Biol 1996;7:5–13
65. Villeponteau B: The RNA components of human and mouse telomerases. Semin Cell Devel Biol 1996;7:15–21
66. Carson D, Ribeiro J: Apoptosis and disease. Lancet 1993;341: 1251–1254

67. Bacchetti S: Telomere dynamics and telomerase activity in cell senescence and cancer. Semin Cell Devel Biol 1996;7: 31–39

68. Hiyama E, Gollahon L, Kataoka T et al: Telomerase activity in human breast tumors. J Natl Cancer Inst 1996;88:116–122

69. Rowe J: Aging and geriatric medicine. In Wyngaarden W, Smith L (eds): Cecil, Textbook of Medicine. Harecourt, Brace Jovanovich, Philadelphia, 1988

70. Alton P, Harris A: Annotation: the role of DNA toppisomerases II in drug resistance. Br J Haematol 1993;85:241–245

71. Ramsey MJ, Moore DH, Briner JF et al: The effects of age and lifestyle factors on the accumulation of cytogenetic damage as measured by chromosome painting. Mutat Res 1995;338: 95–106

72. Olshansky SJ, Rudberg MA, Carnes BA et al: Trading off longer life for worsening health: expansion of morbidity hypotheses. J Aging Health 1991;3:194–216

73. McDonald C, Stewart H: Fatal myocardial infarction in the Scottish adjuvant tamoxifen trial. Br Med J 1991;303: 435–437

74. Wolf DM, Fuqua AW: Mechanisms of action of antiestrogens. Cancer Treat Rev 1995;21:247–271

75. McClay EF, McClay ME, Albright KD et al: Tamoxifen modulation of cisplatin resistance in patients with metastatic melanoma: a biologically important observation. Cancer 1993;72: 1914–1918

76. Welsh J: Induction of apoptosis in breast cancer cells in response to vitamin D and antiestrogens. Biochem Cell Biol 1994;82:537–545

77. Rowlands MG, Budworth J, Jarman M et al: Comparison between inhibitions of protein kinase C and antagonism of cal modulin by tamoxifen analogues. Biochem Pharmacol 1995; 50:723–726

78. Lam HY: Tamoxifen is a calmodulin antagonist in the activation of cAMP phosphodiesterase. Biochem Biophys Res Commun 1984;118:27–32

79. Kang Y, Cortina R, Perry RR: Role of c-*myc* in tamoxifen-induced apoptosis in estrogen-independent breast cancer cells. J Natl Cancer Inst 1996;88:279–284

80. Vink-van Wijngaarden T, Pols HA Buurman CJ et al: Inhibition of breast cancer cell growth by combined treatment with vitamin D_3 analogues and Tamoxifen treatment. Cancer Res 1994;54:5711–5717

81. Anzano MA, Byers SW, Smith JM et al: Prevention of breast cancer in the rat with 9-cis-retinoic acid as a single agent and in combination with Tamoxifen. Cancer Res 1994;54: 4614–4617

82. Cutler RG, Semsei I: Development, cancer and aging: possible common mechanisms of action and regulation. J Gerontol 1989;44:25–34

83. Warner HR, Fernandes G, Wange E: A unifying hypothesis to explain the retardation of aging and tumorigenesis by caloric restriction. J Gerontol: Biol Sci 1995;50:B107–B109

84. Sikic BI: Reversing multidrug resistance with the nonimmunosuppressive cyclosporin PSC 833. Cancer Invest: Abstracts 1996;14(suppl 1):55

85. Armbrecht H, Nemani R, Wongsurawat N: Protein phosphorylation: changes with age and age-related diseases. J Am Geriatr Soc 1993;41:873–879

86. Bowden M, Crawford J, Cohen H, Noyama O: A comparative study of monoclonal gammopathies and immunoglobulin levels in Japanese and United States elderly. J Am Geriatr Soc 1993; 41:11–14

87. Kundu N, Beaty TL, Jackson MJ, Fulton AM: Antimetastatic and antitumor activities of interleukin 10 in a murine model of breast cancer. J Natl Cancer Inst 1996;88:536–541

88. Allione A, Consalvo M, Nanni P et al: Immunizing and curative potential of replicating and non-replicating murine mammary adenocarcinoma cells engineered with interleukin (IL)-2, IL-4, IL-6, IL-7, IL-10, tumor necrosis factor α, granulocyte-macrophage colony- stimulating factor, and γ-interferon gene or admixed with conventional adjuvants. Cancer Res 1994; 54:6022–6026

89. Penn N, Purkins L, Kelleher J et al: The effect of dietary supplementation with vitamins A, C and E on cell-mediated immune function in elderly long- stay patients: a randomized controlled trial. Age Ageing 1991;20:169–174

90. Penn N, Purkins L, Kelleher J et al: Ageing and duodenal mucosal immunity. Age Ageing 1991;20:33–36

91. Carlquist J, Anderson J: HLA, autoimmunity, and rheumatic heart disease: apparent or real association. Circulation 1993; 87:2060–2062

92. Buja L, Willerson J: Role of inflammation in coronary plaque disruption. Circulation 1994;89:503–505

93. van der Wal A, Becker A, van der Loos C, Das P: Site of intimal rupture or erosion of thrombosed coronary atherosclerotic plaques is characterized by an inflammatory process irrespective of the dominant plaque morphology. Circulation 1994;89:36–44

94. Hughes DA, Pinder AC, Piper Z et al: Fish oil supplementation inhibits the expression of major histocompatiblity complex class II molecules and adhesion molecules on human monocytes. Am J Clin Nutr 1996;63:267–272

95. Shahar E, Folsom A, Melnick S et al: Dietary n-3 polyunsaturated fatty acids and smoking-related chronic obstructive pulmonary disease. N Engl J Med 1994;31:228–233

96. Kokoglu E, Karaarslan I, Karaarslan HM, Baloglu H: Elevated serum Lp(a) levels in the early and advanced stages of breast cancer. Cancer Biochem Biophys 1996;14:133–136

97. Moon J, Bandy B, Davison A: Hypothesis: etiology of atherosclerosis and osteoporosis: are imbalances in the calciferol endocrine system implicated. J Am Coll Nutr 1992;11: 567–583

98. MacGregor GA, Cappuccio FP: The kidney and essential hypertension: a link to osteoporosis? J Hypertens 1993;11: 781–785

99. Pollare T, Lithell H, Berne C: A comparison of the effects of hydroclorothiazide and captopril on glucose and lipid metabolism in patients with hypertension. N Engl J Med 1989;321: 868–873

100. Pouleur H, Rousseau M, van Eyll C et al: Effects of long-term enalapril therapy on left ventricular diastolic properties in patients with depressed ejection fraction. Circulation 1993; 88:481–491

101. Gilbert E, Sandoval A, Larrabee P et al: Lisinopril lowers cardiac adrenergic drive and increases b-receptor density in the failing heart. Circulation 1993;88:472–480

102. Packer M, Bristow MR, Cohn JN: The effect of carvedilol on morbidity and mortality in patients with chronic heart failure. N Engl J Med 1996;334:1349–1355

103. Nicolson GL: Bioregulators come of age in the control of tumor growth and metastasis. J Natl Cancer Inst 1996;88:479–480

104. SOLVD Investigators: Effect of enalapril on survival in patients with reduced left ventricular ejection fractions and congestive heart failure. N Engl J Med 1991;325:293–302

105. Fennerty M: *Helicobacter pylori*. Arch Intern Med 1994;154: 721–727

106. Taylor A: Cataract: relationships between nutrition and oxidation. J Am Coll Nutr 1993;12:138–146

107. Bush D, Finucane T: Permanent cardiac pacemakers in the elderly. J Am Geriatr Soc 1994;42:326–334

108. Manton KG, Stallard E, Woodbury MA, Dowd JE: Time-varying covariates in models of human mortality and aging: multidimensional generalization of the Gompertz. J Gerontol: Biol Sci 1994;49:B169–B190

109. Nab H, Hop W, Crommelin M et al: Changes in long term prognosis for breast cancer in a Dutch cancer registry. Br Med J 1994;309:83–86

110. Olivotto I, Bajdik C, Plenderleith I et al: Adjuvant systemic therapy and survival after breast cancer. N Engl J Med 1994; 330:805–810

111. Greenspan EM: The cure of breast cancer by combination chemotherapy. Cancer Invest 1996;14(suppl 1):70

112. Fowble BL: Section IV: Treatment. J Natl Cancer Inst Monographs 1994;16:67–68

113. Antman K, Ayash L, Elias A et al: High-dose cyclophosphamide, thiotepa, and carboplatin with autologous marrow support in women with measurable advanced breast cancer responding to standard-dose therapy: analysis by age. J Natl Cancer Inst Monographs 1994;16:91–94

114. Preston S: Demographic change in the United States, 1970–2050. In Manton K, Singer B, Suzman R (eds): Forecasting the health of elderly population. Springer-Verlag, New York, 1992

115. Fiatarone M, Marks E, Ryan N et al: High-intensity strength training in nonagenarians. JAMA 1990;263:3029–3034

116. Fiatarone M, O'Neill E, Doyle N et al: The Boston FICSIT study: the effects of resistance training and nutritional supplementation on physical frailty in the oldest old. J Am Geriatr Soc 1993;41:333–337

117. Fiatarone M, O'Neill E, Ryan N et al: Exercise training and nutritional supplementation for physical frailty in very elderly people. N Engl J Med 1994;330:1769–1775

118. Manton KG, Stallard E, Singer BH: Projecting the future size and health status of the U.S. elderly population. Int J Forecasting 1992;8:433–458

119. Manton KG, Stallard E, Singer BH: Methods for projecting the future size and health status of the U.S. elderly population. In Wise D (ed): Studies of the Economics of Aging. University of Chicago Press, Chicago, 1994

120. Society of Actuaries: 1994 group annuity mortality table and 1994 group annuity reserving table. Society of Actuaries, Exposure Draft, Schaumburg, IL, 1994

121. Lubitz J, Beebe J, Baker C. Longevity and medicare expenditures. N Engl J Med 1995;332:999–1003

CHAPTER 4

Evolution Theory and the Mechanisms of Aging

T. B. L. KIRKWOOD

The question "Why does aging occur?" calls for answers both at the level of proximate, physiologic mechanisms and also at the level of ultimate, evolutionary origins. This chapter provides an understanding of why aging has evolved and examines what evolution theory can tell us about the *kinds* of mechanisms we might regard as prime candidates to explain senescence.

Evolution theory is well recognized as a powerful tool with which to inquire about the genetic basis of the aging process.[1–3] Although human aging has its roots long ago in our past, the study of its evolution can throw important light on key present-day challenges. For example, recent analysis of longevity records for Danish twins born last century has established that there is a significant heritable component in human life spans.[4] Impelled in part by developments associated with the project to map and eventually sequence the human genome, there is interest in knowing how many and what kinds of genes are likely to be involved in this heritability.[5] There is also interest in human genetic disorders such as Werner syndrome that are characterized by acceleration of many aspects of the senescent phenotype. The recent identification by positional cloning of the gene responsible for Werner syndrome[6] raises interesting questions about its relation to other genes responsible for aging and age-associated diseases.

Before addressing these questions it is important to be precise about how the term "aging" is to be understood. In this chapter, aging is defined in the sense of a progressive, generalized impairment of function, resulting in a loss of adaptive response to stress and in a growing risk of age-related disease. The overall effect of these changes is summed up in the increase in the probability of dying, or age-specific death rate, in the population.

This definition of aging—in terms of a mortality pattern showing progressive increase in age-specific mortality—allows comparisons to be made even among species where the detailed features of the aging process may differ markedly. In phylogenetic terms, aging is widespread but by no means universal.[7–9] The fact that not all species show an increase in age-specific mortality indicates that aging is not an inevitable consequence of wear-and-tear. On the other hand, the fact that very many species do show such an increase is evidence that the evolution of aging has occurred under rather general circumstances.

Evolution of Aging

Theories on the evolution of aging seek to explain why aging occurs through the action of natural selection. The decline in survivorship, which is often also accompanied by a decline in fertility, means that there is an age-associated loss of Darwinian fitness that is clearly deleterious to the organism in which it occurs. Natural selection acts to increase fitness, so it is at once clear that selection should be expected, other things being equal, to oppose aging. The challenge to evolution theory is thus to explain why aging occurs in spite of its drawbacks.

Programmed or "Adaptive" Aging

It is sometimes suggested that in spite of its disadvantages to the individual, aging is beneficial and even necessary at the species level, for example, to prevent overcrowding.[10,11] In this case, genes that actively cause aging might have evolved specifically to program the end of life, in the same way as genes program development.

The difficulty with this view is that there is little evidence that aging serves as a major contributor to mortality in natural populations,[12] which means that aging apparently does not play the adaptive role suggested for it. The theory also embodies the questionable supposition that selection for advantage at the species level will be more effective than selection among individuals for the advantages of a longer life. Aging is clearly a disadvantage to the individual, so any mutation that inactivated the hypothetical adaptive aging genes would confer a fitness advantage, and therefore, the nonaging mutation should spread through the population unless countered by selection at the species or group level. Conditions under which "group selection" can work successfully are highly restrictive,[13] especially when there is selection in the opposite direction acting at the level of the individual. Briefly, it is necessary that the population be divided among fairly isolated groups, and that the introduction of a nonaging genotype into a group should rapidly lead to the group's extinction. The latter condition is necessary to provide the selection between groups that might, in principle, counter the tendency for selection at the level of individuals to favor the spread of nonaging mutants. It appears unlikely that these conditions will be met with sufficient generality to explain the evolution of aging.

Selection Weakens With Age

An observation of central importance to the evolution of aging is that the force of natural selection—that is, its ability to discriminate between alternative genotypes—weakens with age.[12,14–17] Because natural selection operates through the differential effects of genes on fitness, its discriminatory power must decline with age in proportion to the decline in the remaining fraction of the organism's lifetime expectation of reproduction. This is true whether or not the species exhibits aging.

The attenuation in the force of natural selection with age means inevitably that there is only loose genetic control over the later portions of the life span. For this reason it has been suggested that aging might be due to an accumulation in the germ-line of mutations, which potentially are deleterious but are not expressed, or which produce no phenotypic effect until late in life.[12]

The idea is that if deleterious mutations arc expressed so late that most individuals will already have died from some other cause, such as predation, even though the genes involved have the potential to cause harm they will be subject to very little selection against them. Over the generations a large number of such genes might accumulate. These would cause aging and death only when an individual is removed to a protected environment, away from the hazards of the wild, and so lives long enough to experience their negative effects.

A stronger version of this theory was by proposed by Williams,[15] who suggested that because of the declining force of natural selection with age, any gene that conferred an advantage early in life would be favored by selection even if the same gene had deleterious effects at older ages. Such pleiotropic genes could explain aging. The decline in the force of natural selection with age would ensure that even quite modest early benefits would outweigh severe harmful side effects, provided the latter occurred late enough.

Disposable Soma Theory

The disposable soma theory[1,18–20] explains aging through asking how best an organism should allocate its metabolic resources, primarily energy, between on the one hand, keeping itself going from one day to the next and on the other hand producing progeny to secure the continuance of its genes when it itself died. No species is immune to hazards such as predation, starvation, and disease. All that is necessary by way of maintenance is that the body remains in sound condition until an age after which most individuals will have died from accidental causes. In fact, a greater investment in maintenance is a disadvantage, because it eats into resources that, in terms of natural selection, are better used for reproduction. The theory concludes that the optimum course is to invest fewer resources in the maintenance of somatic tissues than are necessary for indefinite survival (Fig. 4-1). The result is that aging occurs through the gradual accumulation of unrepaired somatic defects, but the level of maintenance will be set so that the deleterious effects do not become apparent until an age when survivorship in the wild environment would be extremely unlikely.

Comparison of the Evolutionary Theories

The adaptive program theory is in a category of its own and support for this theory is weak; it will not be considered further in this chapter.

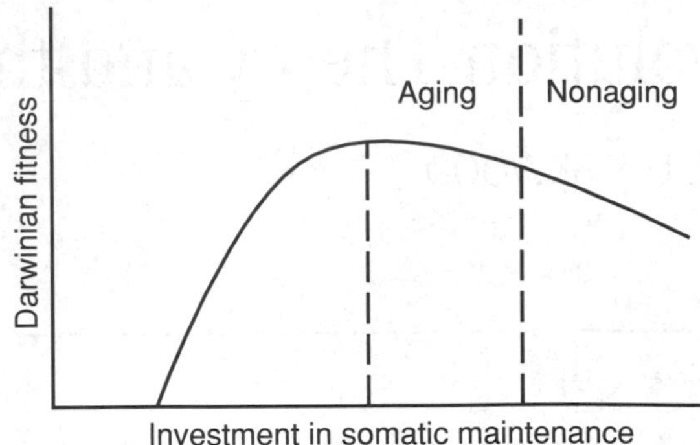

Figure 4-1 Relation between Darwinian fitness and investment in somatic maintenance predicted by the disposable soma theory of aging. Fitness is maximized at a level that is less than that which would be required for indefinite longevity (nonaging).

The disposable soma and pleiotropic genes theories are adaptive in the sense that aging is the result of positive selection for aspects of the organism's life history, but the essential difference is that aging itself is not adaptive but is a negative trait that arises only as a by-product or trade-off of some other benefit. The late-acting deleterious mutations theory assumes an essentially neutral evolutionary process, the accumulation of mutations reflecting the inability of natural selection to maintain tight control over the later portions of the life span.

Among the nonadaptive theories there is a common strand, namely that old organisms count less. This is not due to any implicit assumption of frailty or obsolescence (this would render the theories circular), but to the simple mathematics of mortality. Even if old organisms retain exactly the same vigor as young ones, to the extent that old and young are physiologically indistinguishable, the fact that each cohort becomes numerically attenuated with age means that the selection force weakens. The nonadaptive theories are not mutually exclusive. Thus, aging might in principle be due to a combination of any of them.

As regards the nature of gene action, the disposable soma theory is the most specific of the evolutionary theories, for it suggests not only why aging occurs but also predicts that the genetic basis of aging is to be found in the genes that regulate levels of somatic maintenance functions. Neither the pleiotropic genes theory nor the late-acting deleterious mutations theory is specific about the nature of the genes involved.

Genetics of Life Span

In this section we will look at the genetics of life span, first from the point of view of interspecies comparisons. That is we will ask the question why do species have the life spans they do? We will then look at intraspecies variation and heritability of life span. Finally, we will briefly discuss Werner's syndrome as a model of genetically accelerated senescence.

Species Differences in Longevity

In addition to explaining why aging occurs, evolution theory also must account for differences in species life spans. This raises basic questions about the genetic control of aging: specifically, how many genes are involved and how are these modified by selection to produce changes in life span?

For each of the nonadaptive theories, the generality of the selection forces that are involved suggests that multiple genes will be implicated. If there is a very large number of independent genes causing aging, however, the life span may be slow to change, because modifying a single gene may have little effect by itself and the probability of simultaneous independent modifications will be low. This suggests that either a reasonably small number of primary genes are responsible for aging, or that there exists some mechanism for coordinate regulation.

The evolution of increased life span is most readily explained if it is assumed that an adaptation occurs that results in a general lowering of the accidental (age-independent) death rate. In the late-acting deleterious mutations theory, this may result in new pressure to eliminate or postpone the deleterious gene effects. In the pleiotropic genes theory, the balance between early benefit and late cost may be shifted in favor of reducing the harmful effects on late survival. In the disposable soma theory, there may be selection to tune the optimum investment in maintenance to a higher level.

Variation Within Species

The variability in life span observed within a species or population clearly owes much to chance, but there is a significant heritable component as well.[4] Martin et al[3] have applied the terms "public" and "private" to denote genetic factors related to aging that may either be specific to individuals or shared across a population (perhaps even across species). Late-acting deleterious mutations are strong candidates for private genes, because the fate of such alleles is determined largely by random genetic drift. Public genes are more likely to be those that arise through trade-offs. In particular, the genes involved in regulating mechanisms of somatic maintenance are likely to be public genes of considerable importance. While these genes are "public" in the sense that all individuals have them, there may nevertheless be variations within a population in the precise levels at which these functions are set. These variations in setting may in turn be the cause of genetic variation in life expectancy.

As predicted by the disposable soma theory, the level of individual somatic maintenance systems should be set high enough so that the organism remains in sound condition through its natural expectation of life in the wild environment, but not much higher than this, or resources will be wasted. Numerous maintenance systems operate in parallel to preserve viability (Fig. 4-2). Depending on the levels at which they are set, each maintenance system can be thought of as "assuring" a given span of life (see also Cutler[21] and Sacher[22] for earlier discussion of the concept of "longevity assurance"). When any one of these critical mechanisms has exhausted its potential for assuring longevity, which happens because the accumulated defects threaten survival, the organism is liable to die.

If we now recall the shape of the fitness curve in Figure 4-1, we see that it is rounded instead of sharp, and so we can expect a fair amount of intrapopulation variance in the precise settings of maintenance processes; selection is expected to direct these settings toward the optimum, but once within the region of this optimum, the fitness differences on which selection can operate become quite small.

Putting these ideas together generates the prediction summarized in Figure 4-2. On the average, we expect the longevity assured by individual maintenance systems to be similar. This is because if the setting of any one mechanism is so low that it consistently fails before any of the others, then selection will tend to increase the level at which it is set. Conversely, if any mechanism tends always to fail after the others, then to the extent that this mechanism involves a metabolic cost, there will be selection to tune down the level at which it is set. In individuals, however, the genetic variance within the population is expected to result in variation in the extent to which the organism is predisposed to age from specific causes. For example, some individuals are likely to be less well protected against oxygen radicals than others, and these individuals will therefore experience greater oxidative damage.

Instances of extreme longevity, such as human centenarians, are of special interest for they are likely to be endowed

Figure 4-2 Polygenic control of longevity predicted by the disposable soma theory of aging. On average, the period of longevity ensured by individual somatic maintenance systems is predicted to be similar but some genetic variance about the average is also expected, as shown.

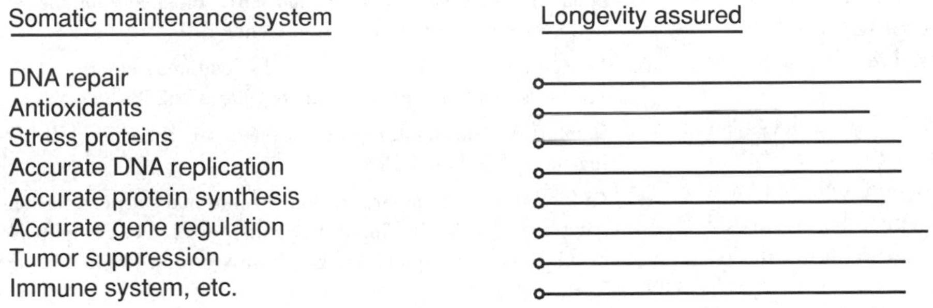

with unusually high levels of each of the important ingredients of the cellular defense network.[5] Such individuals may also be distinguished by their freedom from alleles that predispose toward diseases that otherwise might shorten life expectancy. Schächter et al[24] have performed a genetic study comparing centenarians with younger adult controls, which indicates the potential of this approach.

Werner Syndrome

Werner syndrome is a rare autosomal recessive disorder affecting around 10 in one million people, who prematurely develop a variety of major age-related diseases, including arteriosclerosis, ocular cataracts, osteoporosis, malignant neoplasms, and type II diabetes. Cells grown from Werner syndrome patients show reduced division potential and increased chromosomal instability compared to age-matched controls, and there is evidence that the pathology associated with Werner syndrome may be related rather generally to impaired cell proliferation.

Yu et al.[6] have recently identified the gene responsible for Werner syndrome and the predicted protein sequence shows significant homology to deoxyribonucleic acid (DNA) helicases, enzymes responsible for unwinding DNA for purposes of replication, repair, and expression of the genetic material. This discovery is interesting for it supports the general concept that accumulation of somatic defects is important in aging, while involving a gene that would not itself be regarded as a gene for maintenance. A defective helicase might, however, have the effects of both increasing the somatic mutation rate through interfering with replication and repair, and interfering with accuracy of gene expression. It is thus compatible with the scheme in Figure 4-2.

Tests of the Evolutionary Theories

For practical reasons, experimental tests of the evolutionary theories of aging have been mostly confined to short-lived species, in particular the fruit fly *Drosophila melanogaster*.

Evidence for trade-offs between early and late fitness components, as predicted by both the disposable soma and pleiotropic genes theories, comes from the success of indirect selection for increased longevity, based on a regimen in which females were selected for late reproductive ability.[25,26] An ingenious experimental regimen was recently used to select directly for longevity by Zwaan,[27] who reported results consistent with the disposable soma theory.

Work with the nematode *Caenorhabditis elegans* has also been instructive about the genetic basis of life span.[28,29] In this species a number of mutations have been found that have increased longevity. In general, these appear to be associated with increased resistance to stress, in accord with prediction from the evolutionary theory.[30]

Conclusions

Our answers to the question "Why does aging occur?" have broad implications for how we perceive the likely genetic basis of aging. Firstly, evolution theory can illuminate a long-running debate about whether programmed or stochastic events, such as DNA damage, drive the aging process. The weakness of evolutionary support for the adaptive aging genes hypothesis calls the program theory into question. Any notion of an aging "clock" needs to be qualified by recognition of this fact. The existence of temporal controls in development and in cyclic processes such as diurnal and reproductive cycles does not provide a sufficient basis to suggest the existence of a clock that regulates aging. Nor does the broad reproducibility of many features of aging provide any real evidence for an underlying active program. This is not to say, however, that the nature and rate of aging are not genetically determined. The issue that distinguishes programmed from stochastic theories of aging is not whether the factors that determine longevity are specified within the genome, but rather, how this is arranged.[31]

Secondly, evolution theory clearly indicates a polygenic basis for aging. Different mechanisms and even different kinds of genes may operate together. This presents a major challenge, and progress is likely to require a combination of approaches, including (1) transgenic animal models in which candidate genetic factors are altered by genetic manipulation, (2) comparative studies to identify factors that correlate positively or negatively with species' life spans, (3) studies of the extremely long-lived (e.g. human centenarians) to identify factors associated with above-average expectation of life, and (4) selection experiments to investigate the response of life span to artificial selection pressures.

References

1. Kirkwood TBL, Rose MR: Evolution of senescence: late survival sacrificed for reproduction. Phil Trans R Soc Lond B 1991; 332:15–24
2. Partridge L, Barton NH: Optimality, mutation and the evolution of ageing. Nature 1993;362:305–311
3. Martin GM, Austad SN, Johnson TE: Genetic analysis of ageing: role of oxidative damage and environmental stresses. Nature Genet 1996;13:25–34
4. McGue M, Vaupel JW, Holm N, Harvald B: Longevity is moderately heritable in a sample of Danish twins born 1870–1880. J Gerontol 1993;48:B237–244
5. Schächter F, Cohen D, Kirkwood TBL: Prospects for the genetics of human longevity. Hum Genet 1993;91:51
6. Yu C-E, Oshima J, Fu Y-H et al: Positional cloning of the Werner's syndrome gene. Science 1996;272:258–262
7. Comfort A: The Biology of Senescence. 3rd Ed. Churchill Livingstone, Edinburgh 1979
8. Kirkwood TBL: Comparative and evolutionary aspects of longevity. pp. 45–66. In Finch CE, Schneider EL (eds): Handbook of the Biology of Aging. 3rd Ed. Van Nostrand Reinhold, New York, 1985

9. Finch CE: Longevity, Senescence and the Genome. Chicago University Press, Chicago, 1990
10. Weismann A: Essays Upon Heredity and Kindred Biological Problems. Vol. 1. Clarendon Press, Oxford, 1891
11. Wynne-Edwards VC: Animal Dispersion in Relation to Social Behaviour. Oliver & Boyd, Edinburgh, 1962
12. Medawar PB: An Unsolved Problem of Biology. H.K. Lewis, London, 1952
13. Maynard Smith J: Group selection. Q Rev Biol 1976;51: 277–283
14. Haldane JBS: New Paths in Genetics. George Allen & Unwin, London, 1941
15. Williams GC: Pleiotropy, natural selection and the evolution of senescence. Evolution 1957;11:398–411
16. Hamilton WD: The moulding of senescence by natural selection. J Theor Biol 1966;12:12–45
17. Charlesworth B: Evolution in Age-structured Populations. Cambridge University Press, Cambridge 1980
18. Kirkwood TBL: Evolution of ageing. Nature 1977;270:301–304
19. Kirkwood TBL, Holliday R: The evolution of ageing and longevity. Proc R Soc Lond B, 1979;205:531–546
20. Kirkwood TBL: Repair and its evolution: survival versus reproduction. pp. 165–181. In Townsend CR, Calow P (eds): Physiological Ecology: An Evolutionary Approach to Resource Use. Blackwell Scientific Publications, Oxford, 1981
21. Cutler RG: Evaluating biology of senescence. pp. 311–360. In Behare JA, Finch CE, Moment GB (eds): The Biology of Aging. Plenum Press, New York, 1978
22. Sacher GA: Evolution of longevity and survival characteristics in mammals. pp. 151–167. In Schneider EZ (ed): The Genetics of Aging. Plenum Press, New York, 1978
23. Kirkwood TBL, Franceschi C: Is ageing as complex as it would appear? Ann New York Acad Sci 1992;663:412–417
24. Schachter et al
25. Rose MR: Laboratory evolution of postponed senescence in *Drosophila melanogaster*. Evolution 1984;38:1004–1010
26. Luckinbill LS, Arking R, Clare, MJ et al: Selection for delayed senescence in *Drosophila melanogaster*. Evolution 1984;38: 996–1003
27. Zwaan B, Bijlmstra R, Hoekstra RF: Direct selection on life span in *Drosophila melanogaster*. Evolution 1995;49:646–659
28. Johnson TE: Ageing can be genetically dissected into component processes using long-lived lines of *Caenorhabditis elegans*. Proc Natl Acad Sci U S A 1987;84:3777–3781
29. Kenyon C, Chang J, Gensch E et al: A *C. elegans* mutant that lives twice as long as wild type. Nature 1993;366:461–464
30. Lithgow GJ, Kirkwood TBL: Mechanisms and evolution of aging. Science 1997;273:80
31. Kirkwood TBL, Cremer T: Cytogerontology since 1881: a reappraisal of August Weismann and a review of modern progress. Hum Genet 1982;60:101–121

CHAPTER 5

Cellular Mechanisms of Aging

IOAN DAVIES

All multicellular organisms undergo changes with time. The progression of development, reproductive maturity, and aging is well recognized, although age-associated changes are not easily recognized until the postreproductive stages of the life span. The aging phenotype is progressively expressed over a long time-scale in the mammal, and attributing an accurate chronologic age is often difficult. Typical markers in humans include loss of height, a reduction in lean body mass, graying of hair, wrinkling of skin, changes in eyesight, and to some extent, less coordination of movement. Some or all of these changes may be present in elderly people. These alterations, along with others, have been described as "normal" aging.

In my view, aging is not satisfactorily defined, although the one commonly used is in Box 1.[1] Aging occurs at many different levels—social, psychological (behavioral), physiologic, morphologic, cellular, and molecular. A definition encompassing all of these strata does not exist, and may be impossible. It has been argued that aging changes should satisfy four criteria: they should be universal in the species, degenerative, progressive, and intrinsic.[2] These criteria were designed to separate aging from other time-related changes of development, maturation, and age-associated disease. However, no specific biologic event is featured in the definition, or the limiting criteria, and as such, they remain unsatisfactory. Most of the recognizable features of aging occur after the period of reproductive activity has ceased. The term "senescence" is often applied to this part of the life cycle and its usage has been considered more precise when referring to the degenerative effects associated with the passage of time.[1]

Extending our definition of aging of the whole organism to cellular aging is difficult. The fact that cells show age-associated changes is not questioned, but how aging is expressed in cellular terms is not obvious. We do not have the corollaries of aging of the whole organism—no gray hair, wrinkled skin, or altered gait. The other issue relating to cellular aging is how universal is the definition of aging: Is aging the same in mitotic and postmitotic cells? Biomedical gerontologists accept that an age-associated deterioration in cells leads to organ or tissue deficiencies and, ultimately, the expression of aging or disease. However, we need satisfactory biomarkers of aging at the cellular level; the most obvious change, the presence of the age-pigment, lipofuscin, is not a reliable indicator. This is an area of increasing interest,[3,4] although some disagree.[3,5]

Most gerontology textbooks show plots of physiologic function against time. These findings are usually derived from cross-sectional studies and show a decrease in physiologic effectiveness from about the age of 35 years onward. The graphs of nerve conduction velocity, cardiac index, maximum breathing capacity, and glomerular filtration rate show a considerable decline with age (Fig. 5-1). These data must be treated with caution, for reasons that are discussed in Chapter 14. However, data like these support part of our "definition" of aging, showing a potential increase in the vulnerability of multicellular organisms with time. Measuring complex physiologic functions shows the deterioration found in older animals and underscores the loss of integration of finely tuned regulatory mechanisms. Systems comprise subunits that act together to carry out a function that cannot be done by an individual component. The definition of aging refers to the failure of homeostasis by which the organism maintains a steady state in the face of environmental change. The subunits of a biologic system are easy to describe; organs, cells, and molecules are both the structure and the information needed to maintain that structure, so that it functions satisfactorily. An analysis of failure in homeostasis has to consider each of these factors. A simple system is described in Figure 5-2. All organisms, organs, and cells have systems for sampling the external and internal environments. Signals are transmitted from the sampling/receptor site to the central controlling system and then processed into suitable information for onward transmission. Some remote target site is then activated and transmits further information or acts to modify the organism's response to environmental change. Ultimately, when the sensory signals are no longer received, baseline activities are re-established in the system.

The central thesis of cellular and molecular gerontology is that breakdown of a complex organ system can be explained in cellular and molecular terms. Thus, a marked decline in liver function with age can probably be explained by alterations in the component cells and molecules. Laboratory rodents, frequently specific pathogen-free and of a carefully defined genetic background, form the backbone of material for researching tissue and cellular age changes in vivo.[6] The literature on aging also contains studies on invertebrates.[1,7] Many metazoan invertebrates are useful because of their mainly nonmitotic cell population, short life span, and ease of manipulation in strictly controlled environments. Studies on human cells are becoming increasingly important since changes seen here more likely pertain to alterations in patients. To many, this focus on human material is the "raison d'être" for aging research, and in vitro techniques offer the option of studying human mitotic cells directly.[8]

> ***Definition of aging***
>
> Aging is characterized by a failure to maintain homeostasis under conditions of physiologic stress, and this failure is associated with a decrease in viability, and an increase in vulnerability, of the individual.

Experimental studies of cellular and molecular mechanisms of aging are also subject to pathologic interference. The cells used in an investigation have to be derived from living animals. Cells must be derived from healthy humans or rodents; otherwise, significant errors can be made. Early research detected marked increases in albumin synthesis by the liver in rodents during the life span.[9] Explanations for this increase in protein synthesis included compensation for genomic damage from somatic mutations or other errors[10,11]; however, the reason was more commonplace, and related to the development of kidney pathology in old rodents. The result of age-associated kidney disease in aged rodents is proteinuria leading to a compensatory increase in plasma protein, particularly albumin, synthesis by the liver. This topic is discussed elsewhere,[12] but the study of changes in cellular function with age present many challenges.

Aging In Vitro

The historical background to the development of culture techniques for the study of individual cells is reviewed elsewhere.[13] Cells from a variety of normal human tissues proliferate in culture only for a defined period before degenerating and dying out.[14] These cultured cells are elongated and spindle-shaped, and are human diploid, fibroblast-like (HDF) cells. HDF cells only divide a certain number of times before they undergo replicative senescence (the "Hayflick" limit), and it

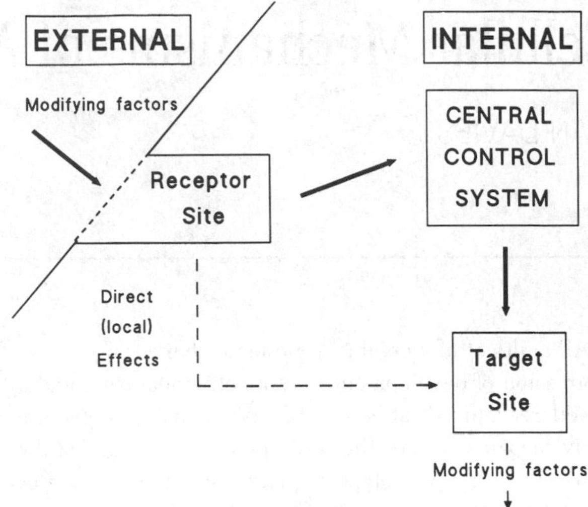

Figure 5-2 Simple biologic system indicating the connections between the external and internal environments. The simple model is applicable at different levels of organization.

is argued that this is the cellular expression of aging.[15] The in vitro model of cellular aging has been criticized. The limited survival of HDF may be due to deficiencies in the culture media.[16–18] However, a later study suggests that inadequacies in the culture medium may accelerate cell senescence by affecting the rate at which cells express their genetically predetermined replicative potential, but not replicative life span per se.[19] Perhaps more fundamental to the study of aging is the lack of interaction between different cells in this experimental system.[20] However, if these drawbacks are fully understood, then the in in vitro model is an extremely powerful tool in the study of aging mitotic cells.

Fibroblast-like cells from different species respond to culture conditions in different ways. Chick fibroblast-like cells

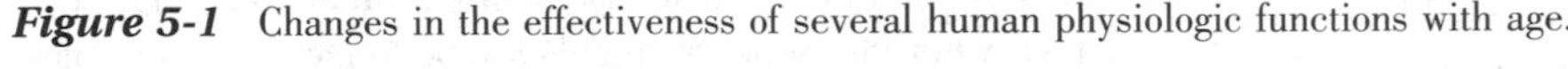

Figure 5-1 Changes in the effectiveness of several human physiologic functions with age.

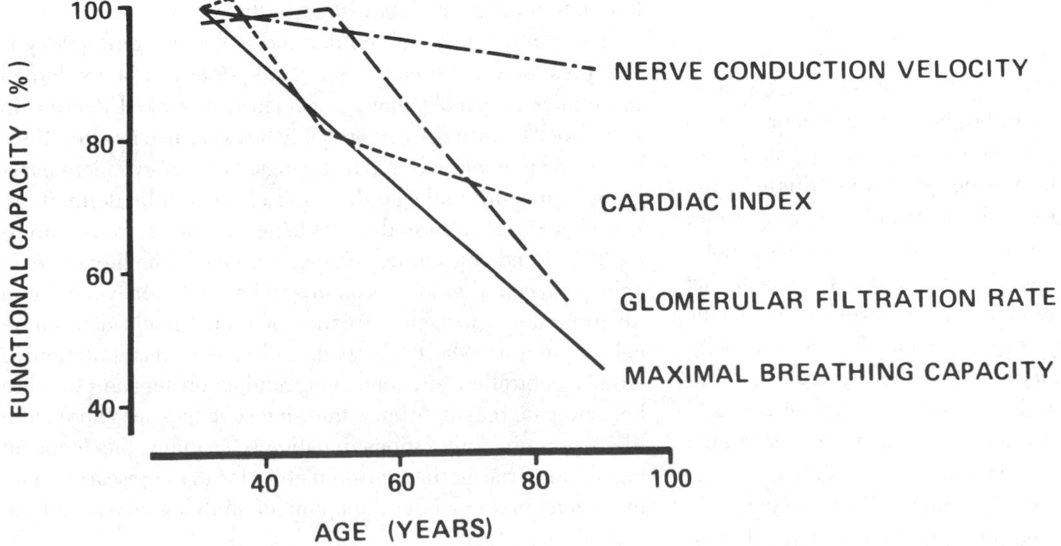

Factors affecting studies of cellular and molecular aging

- Age of donor
- Genetic background of the donor
- Pathologic status of the donor
- Composition of the diet and the effect it has on the expression of disease

have a stable, limited life span and never appear to produce "immortal" cell lines. Similar cells from mice and rats have a different growth pattern that comprises rapid proliferation of the cells followed by a decline, and then usually spontaneous transformation into an immortal cell line. Human cells on the other hand can be transformed to immortal cells by some treatment, such as exposure to the SV 40 virus.[21] The growth potential of cells in culture decreases with the age of the donor, and the outgrowth of cells from human skin explants takes longer with age. The delayed outgrowth increases linearly with age, although this phenomenon is subject to a great deal of individual variation that also depends on donor age.[22]

Accumulated population doublings are used as the measure of the age of a culture. The cells display different growth characteristics at different stages of the culture life cycle. In the early stages, the cells proliferate rapidly. The subcultivation intervals are short, but in the senescent phase of the culture the cells become larger and divide more slowly. The average number of population doublings of fetal lung and skin fibroblasts, before the senescent phase, are approximately 50, and the total number of doublings is 63 (Fig. 5-3).[13] Cells isolated from adult rather than fetal tissues show a reduction in the potential number of population doublings to 30 before the senescent phase.[23] It is frequently assumed that the end of cell division means cell death, although this is not so. Cultures can remain in the postreplicative state, if they remain sterile, for periods of more than 12 months, a situation more akin to cellular differentiation.[24,25] The cells continue to support many biosynthetic functions and only appear to differ from cells of earlier passage number in their ability to initiate deoxyribonucleic acid (DNA) synthesis before cell division.[26–28] The issue of differentiation, as opposed to senescence, has not been resolved. Critics of the in vitro model of aging cite Bayreuther,[25] while proponents refer to the huge catalogue of data generated by this approach. The field is discussed by Norwood et al[29] and Finch.[30]

The study of aging in vitro has led to the proposal of new theories to explain senescence in culture, such as the commitment theory[31] and the model of clonal attenuation.[32] Theoretic ideas on in vitro aging have developed rapidly and the reader is directed elsewhere for information on progress in this field.[13,33–39]

Genetic models of aging

Syndromes of accelerated aging in humans are primarily genetic conditions that have relevance to the pathobiology of human aging. Several so-called progeroid (accelerated aging) syndromes have been proposed as models of human aging.[40,41] Fibroblasts isolated from such individuals have been used to study age-associated changes in functional ability. The three classic progerias are Hutchinson-Gilford, Werner, and Cockayne syndromes,[40,41] which are characterized by young individuals having a senile appearance. Each of these conditions

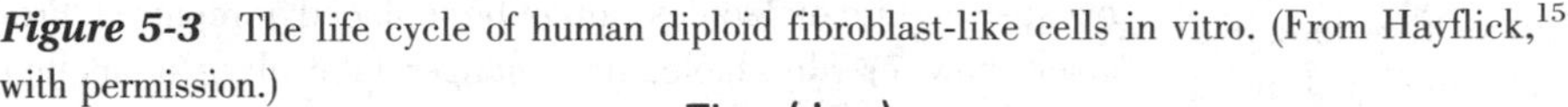

Figure 5-3 The life cycle of human diploid fibroblast-like cells in vitro. (From Hayflick,[15] with permission.)

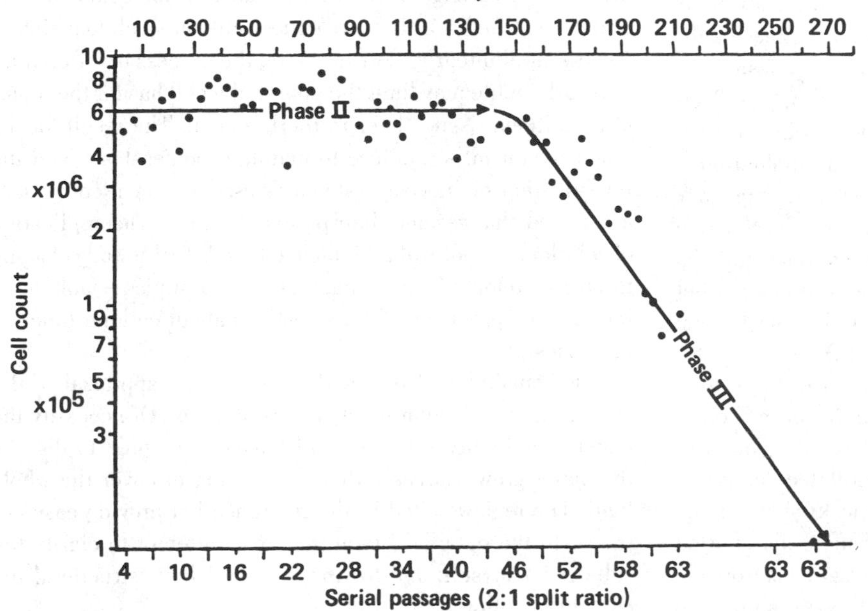

is autosomal recessive in its mode of inheritance.[41] HDF from individuals with these abnormalities have a shorter in vitro life span than cells from normal adults of the same age. The HDF from Hutchinson-Gilford and Werner patients undergo 10 doublings when compared with the average of 30 doublings in cells derived from normal adults. Decreases in mitotic activity, DNA synthesis, DNA repair efficiency, and cloning efficiency have been reported in cells isolated from people with progeria. The study of HDF from progeroid subjects could give valuable insights into both the genetic conditions themselves, and the genetic analysis of aging in humans.[41] Despite extensive study of the clinical and biochemical features of the disorder it was not until recently that a genetic linkage study identified proximity of the Werner syndrome mutation to a group of markers on chromosome 8.[42] One line of evidence implicated the structural gene for DNA polymerase β as a likely source of defective DNA metabolism in Werner syndrome cells. The structural gene for DNA polymerase β maps within the region of the Werner's syndrome mutation, on the short arm of chromosome 8, and is involved in both DNA repair and replication. However, the gene is just outside the main region of the mutation.[43] Subsequently, progress in the location and cloning of the gene has been rapid.[44,45] The gene responsible for Werner syndrome (now known as WRN) was identified by positional cloning. The predicted protein is 1,432 amino acids in length and is very similar to DNA helicases. Four mutations in Werner patients were identified. Two of the mutations are splice-junction mutations, with the predicted result being the exclusion of exons from the final messenger, ribonucleic acid RNA (mRNA). One of these mutations, which results in a frameshift and a predicted truncated protein, was found in the homozygous state in 60 percent of the Japanese Werner patients examined. The other two mutations are nonsense mutations.

The identification of a mutated putative helicase as the gene product of the Werner's syndrome gene suggests that defective DNA metabolism is involved in the complex process of aging in Werner patients.[45] An analysis of the replicative ability of HDF from Werner's syndrome patients shows that these cells exit, apparently irreversibly, from the cell cycle at a faster rate than do normal HDF cells. It has been proposed that the Werner syndrome gene is a gene that controls the number of times those human cells can divide before terminal differentiation.[46] A recent study of telomere length, telomeric DNA damage, and repair, in relation to the progression of aging, showed that telomeres are shorter in fibroblasts from old donors compared with those from young donors; shortest in cells from a patient with Werner syndrome; and relatively long in fibroblasts from a patient with Alzheimer's disease. Telomeric DNA repair efficiency was lower in cells from old donors than in those from young donors, normal in Alzheimer cells, and lower in Werner cells. It is possible that this decline in telomeric repair with aging is of functional significance to an age-related decline in genomic stability.[47] However, a study of the kinetics of the loss of telomeric repeats in Werner syndrome cells showed that the mean length of telomere restriction fragments from the earliest passages of Werner syndrome cells were similar to those of controls.[48] Thus, although accelerated loss of telomeric repeats may explain the rapid decline in proliferation of Werner's syndrome cells, it is possible that the cells exit the cell cycle through different mechanisms than those senescent cells from control subjects.

Down syndrome also shows certain features of accelerated aging.[41] Down syndrome is a condition of mental retardation with various associated abnormalities caused by the trisomy of chromosome 21. Brain autopsy specimens from old Down subjects have the neuropathologic signs associated with senile dementia. This very important finding has already generated interesting lines of research into possible genetic factors involved in Alzheimer's disease and its molecular pathology.[49]

Cell aging in vivo

The study of cells in vitro may be the accepted lore for cell biologic changes with age—but what about all those important postmitotic cells comprising the central nervous system or the skeletal muscles of the mammal? These cells do not grow readily in culture and have to be studied in vivo. The study of cells in vivo is more complicated. Although we can show changes in physiologic regulation with age, the identification of a cellular, or molecular, lesion as the cause of the disruption is not a simple matter. In physiologic systems we rarely know all of the steps in a chain of reactions. The difficulties of pinpointing defects in organs are not trivial due to the diverse cell populations involved. The deterioration of the vascular system (whether due to pathologic changes or what has been termed physiologic aging) is frequently a confounding factor in aging studies. Changes in circulation may produce effects that are incorrectly attributed to intrinsic alterations. The ultimate causes of aging will be due to molecular changes, probably because certain molecules cannot be replaced or repaired. Precisely how, or why, molecular changes take place is another matter. The passage of time may lead to a molecular defect, or defects, which will influence the ability of a cell to maintain its structural integrity. Furthermore, the process of differentiation early in life may limit the potential a cell has for the repair of constituent tissues later in the life span. The result for the intact organism is a failure to maintain homeostasis, and the investigation of in vivo systems is essential to identify age-associated changes and their precise location. The application of cellular and molecular biologic methods to the study of aging in vivo is fundamental because these techniques enable us to improve the precision of our questions about cellular function in tissues.

The remainder of this review will be an appraisal of the cellular and molecular mechanisms of aging. Of necessity the material is highly selected, and I have attempted to discuss the major growth areas rather than trying to cover the whole field. The reviews cited in the reference list provide easy entrance to the detailed literature. In an attempt to clarify the subject for myself, and for the reader, I have structured the content as follows:

- Changes in the principal components of the cell and their molecules
- Age-changes in processes
- Cellular homoeostasis

Changes in the Principal Components of the Cell and Their Molecules

The Nucleus, Genome, and DNA damage

No consistent structural alteration can be used to identify the nucleus of an aging cell, for example, as seen in cells undergoing programmed cell death.[50] On the other hand, declines in cell function imply some alteration in the DNA.

Chromosomes and chromatin

The DNA and chromatin of aging cells change (e.g, polyploidy leads to an increase in the DNA content of hepatocytes and some neurons from old animals). The thermal stability of chromatin increases, and chromatin template activity decreases, with age. However, these observations are not necessarily explained by changes in DNA, as the removal of proteins from the chromatin eliminates many age-associated differences. Overall, no change has been identified in the degradation of either histones or nucleotides with age in cell nuclei isolated from heart or brain. Nucleosome core size remains stable (approximately 140 base pairs) for all of the tissues investigated, and the nuclease, DNAse I, does not cleave DNA at different sites for the respective sets of young, mature, and old nuclei. No significant change was observed in the rate of attack on young or old chromatin after DNAase I treatment of brain and liver nuclei.

The use of reliable extraction techniques of whole organs suggests that neither nonhistone proteins (NHP), nor histones, show qualitative age-associated changes. Histones undergo chemical modifications during gene expression including phosphorylation, acetylation, and methylation. The NHP may also undergo similar chemical modifications. It has been reported that phosphorylation and acetylation of histones, and the acetylation of NHP, generally decrease with age. However, it is also claimed that the major drop in the acetylation of histone proteins is during the developmental period of the life span, rather than aging. Aging research frequently produces contradictory results and studies on chromatin structure are no exception. Some conclude that no age-associated, qualitative changes in histones have been reliably shown and that quantitative changes (if they exist) are small; others argue that detailed changes do take place. The differences between the various studies may have more to do with methodology. Without adequate tissue, or molecular fractionation, detecting age-associated alterations in chromatin structure and function will be difficult.

Chromosomal aberrations

Chromosomal aberrations are found with increasing frequency in aged cells.[51] The aberrations consist of chromosomal bridges and fragments seen in dividing cells, particularly the liver. In long-lived strains of mice the aberrations increase from an incidence of approximately 10 percent in 2-month-old animals to about 35 percent in 24-month-old mice. In short-lived mice they develop much more rapidly, from 20 percent at 2 months to 80 percent at 20 months (Fig. 5.4). Strains with intermediate life span have an intermediate rate of accumulation of aberrations. At first sight it seems that life span and the rate of development of chromosome aberrations are correlated.[51] However, some mice with very short life spans have a rate of accumulation of aberrations similar to that found in mice with long life spans.[51] These short-lived animals develop severe terminal pathology, such as leukemia or mammary carcinomas, and do not live to a life span achieved by other members of the species. Perhaps a more serious problem is that F_1 hybrids derived from parents with different life spans develop chromosomal aberrations at a rate intermediate between that of the parents, but live longer.

It is unclear whether or not changes in the incidence of chromosomal aberrations in adults are of physiologic significance. Aberration frequency does not change after 10 months of age in the CD1 mouse strain (median life expectancy of 16 months), but in the C57BL/6J strain it increases by 30 percent between 15 and 20 months of age. The data are difficult to interpret without statistical evaluation.[51] Recently, interest has renewed in chromosomal aberrations with old age.[52] Lymphocytes from aged individuals showed higher chromosomal aberration frequencies and longer G2 duration than cells from young individuals.[53] Chromosomal damage may be related to the action of reactive oxygen species, and some aberrations may be the result of errors in DNA replication as a function of use. Of particular interest is the peculiarly mammalian prop-

Figure 5-4 Incidence of chromosome aberrations in regenerating liver cells of two inbred strains of female mice plotted as function of age. The median life span of each strain is indicated by the arrows. (From Crowley and Curtis,[299] with permission.)

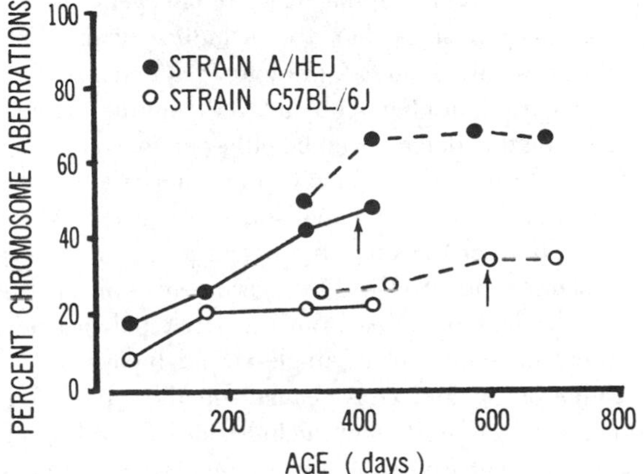

erty of the escape of cells from normal proliferative homeostasis into neoplasia[52] midway through the life span.

Telomeres

Research on cell replication in vitro has often been aimed at trying to identify the way that cultured cells count the number of cell divisions they undergo. It is now known that the telomeres, which are "tails" of nucleotide repeats at the ends of chromosomes, progressively shorten during aging of HDF. Immortalized tumor cells have stable telomeres that retain a constant length. In addition, the telomere length in stem cells is greater than that found in somatic cells, and the length of the telomeres in germ-line cells is constant, despite the age of the donor. Out of these observations came the telomere hypothesis of aging and immortalization.[54,55] Germ-line cells maintain the length of their chromosomes by the activity of an enzyme, telomerase, which extends one strand of the chromosome without a DNA template. At some stage during embryogenesis the telomerase becomes repressed, and in somatic cells telomere shortening takes place during cell division until the "Hayflick limit." When the Hayflick limit is reached, one or more telomeres will have lost most telomeric repeats, and the cells stop dividing. This hypothesis suggests a way in which the dividing cell may count its number of divisions, and may partially explain the loss of division potential in vitro. However, it probably has nothing to do with aging in cells that do not undergo cell division in the adult.

DNA damage

DNA is considered a prime target for age-changes. This macromolecule is unique; it has to replicate and maintain itself to preserve the primary genetic message of the cell through division and accidental events that may damage the DNA. In situations other than cell division, DNA has to be maintained so that its function as a template for other cellular molecules is preserved for the life span of the cell. However, in mammals, we know that the nuclear DNA of certain somatic cells undergoes a series of alterations that change it from the structure inherited through the germ line. Thus, the genome of certain cells in the immune system undergoes rearrangements and mutations of immunoglobulin genes during differentiation, and rearrangements and mutations occur in oncogenes in the later stages of oncogenesis. Other agents induce damage in DNA by either physical, chemical, or biologic actions. DNA can be broken, distorted, or chemically altered, and the source of the agent causing this damage can be either endogenous or exogenous.[56] Free radicals (see below) and other reactive metabolites of normal cellular metabolism, can cause cross-linkage of DNA to DNA, or DNA to intranuclear proteins. The fact that DNA molecules exist at a 37°C has been implicated as the cause of the loss of bases from the DNA polymer, and the subsequent development of single-strand breaks. Ultraviolet (UV) radiation, γ- and x-rays cause specific types of damage ranging from the distortion of the helix for UV, and either base removal or damage from free radicals generated by γ- or x-rays. Chemical mutagens and carcinogens also cause damage to DNA, as does viral DNA, which can be inserted into the genome of the host and alter the information content of the cell.

Mutations may also be a significant cause of age-associated dysfunction. They can arise from errors in DNA replication during the process of mitosis, by the mispairing of bases at the site of damage in the DNA molecule, or because of errors in the enzymic processes responsible for the synthesis of DNA. Mutations in somatic cells could cause changes in function, and two theories about aging were proposed incorporating this idea.[10,57] One theory assumed that dominant mutations were the cause of cell damage or death,[57] while the other considered that aging in diploid cells were due to recessive mutations.[10] If one of a pair of homologous genes was damaged or "hit," and subsequently inactivated, the other member of the pair would continue normal functioning; if both of the homologous genes were damaged, either through a previous hit or some hereditary fault, then both members of the pair would be inactive and cell damage would follow. Both versions of this theory have been discounted. The calculated rate of mutation in germ cells could not account for the life span of most species, so it was considered that recessive mutations could not affect the survival of somatic cells. One prediction of the theory is that inbred organisms should live longer than outbred ones. The inbred animal is homozygous at most loci, whereas outbred are heterozygous at many positions. Inbred organisms cannot be homozygous for genetic defects because this is often lethal, and since they will be heterozygous for very few "faults," it follows that they will express close to the species-specific life span. However, all the evidence obtained on inbreeding effects point to a reduction in life span.

Other observations are inconsistent with the notion of recessive mutations causing aging. Comparative studies on insects enabled the effect of different ploidy levels to be examined. Diploid organisms should have a longer life span than haploids, and haploids should be more susceptible to life-shortening effects such as ionizing radiation. Studies on the wasp *Habrobracon* have shown that such predictions are not true. The female wasps are diploid, but the males can be obtained with both haploid and diploid gene complements. The haploid males have the same life span as their diploid counterparts, which is inconsistent with the theory, but they are more susceptible to the effects of ionizing radiation.

Ionizing radiation is considered to accelerate aging because superficially, irradiated animals do show changes similar to those seen in old animals. Mice irradiated with a single dose of x-rays show a shortening of the life span proportional to dose. At postmortem it was shown that these rodents died of the acceleration of both malignant and nonmalignant causes of death. Although the types of pathologic changes observed are not identical to those seen in aging[58–60] (e.g., the onset of age-associated conditions), both benign and malignant neoplasms and senile cataracts are different between normal aging and radiation induced life-shortening.[58] Radiation causes mutations but does not clearly accelerate aging and furthermore, mutagenic chemicals (e.g., the bifunctional alkylating agents myleran and chlorambucil) shorten life but do not appear to hasten aging.[58]

A connection has been claimed between somatic mutations and chromosomal aberrations in aging cells.[51] Ionizing radiation also induces chromosomal aberrations, perhaps following somatic mutations. Aberrations increase in frequency up to 12 months of age in normal controls. In the same mice irradiated at 2 months of age, aberrations increase rapidly and then return slowly to normal levels. The decrease in chromosomal aberrations is due to repair activity, not to the removal of aberrant cells. However, this repair of x-ray-induced damage occurs over a period when chromosomal damage in control animals increases—events that are supposedly related to the somatic mutations causing aging. These data do not support the view that somatic mutations induce or precede chromosome aberrations. Furthermore, the evidence implies that artificial induction of somatic mutations, as reflected by the incidence of chromosome aberrations, is unimportant as far as the functional properties of cells containing them are concerned. This, in turn, throws doubt on the relevance of somatic mutations to aging, or alternatively, of the incidence of chromosome aberrations to somatic mutation frequency.

The effect of the various lesions described above depends on several factors (Fig. 5.5). Any alteration of the information content of the DNA can have substantial effects on cellular function. The various physiologic consequences following a mutation depend on whether the organism is a homo- or heterozygote, and whether or not the gene affected is dominant or recessive. Most mutations are probably not lethal, especially since, in a differentiated cell, much of the DNA is not expressed. Therefore, it is highly probable that a mutation would be in a nontranscribed (repressed) region rather than a transcribed one. A mutation in a repressed zone would be "silent." However, this could be changed if the cell had to either undergo division or respond to a hormone, and so utilize a previously unused region of the genome. Mutations in gene-control regions could cause gene repression or activation, which may then result in synthesis of the wrong molecules at the wrong time. If the mutation involves genes that control cell division, then abnormal cell proliferation may lead to tumor production or other diseases. A mutation in the transcribed region of the DNA would be expressed immediately in terms of altered RNA and hence protein (either structural proteins or enzymes).

Great efforts have been expended in trying to detect age-related changes in DNA. Increased numbers of strand breaks have been reported in DNA isolated from various sources including the thymus, neurons of the cerebellum, cardiac muscle, Küpffer cells, liver, and retinal photoreceptor cells.[61] Others were unable to demonstrate an age-associated increase in the digestion of mouse liver DNA by S1 nuclease (an enzyme specifically digesting single-stranded DNA).[62,63] In cultured HDF, qualitative changes in chromatin have been identified with alterations in circular dichroic properties,[64] and an accumulation of alkali-[65,66] and endonuclease-sensitive[67] sites. Quantitative studies have shown evidence for a loss of reiterated DNA sequences with age in culture.[68] The segregation of DNA at the time of cell division has been analyzed, and the range in values found for the 2C and 4C DNA contents differ. This is probably due to quantitative differences originating during semiconservative DNA synthesis, chromosome assembly, and segregation. Ultimately, this continuous rearrangement of the genome could lead to degeneration or a program of cellular differentiation.[69]

Certainly, in the literature up to 1990, chromosomal alterations, DNA cross-links, and strand breaks had been detected, but no clear, consistent pattern of increased damage in DNA had been reported.[70,71] Correlations between the ability to repair DNA and maximum longevity were identified but nonetheless, no general decline in DNA repair was found with increased age.[70] More recently, improved techniques for the detection of alterations in DNA have moved the field on, and advances have been made in the study of changes in both genomic and mitochondrial DNA.

DNA Oxidation

It has been claimed that oxidation of bases in DNA by intracellular oxidants is quantitatively the most important class of base alterations in mammalian cells.[72] The intracellular oxidants are free radicals and other reactive oxygen species. Free radicals are formed by the splitting of a covalent bond in a molecule so that each atom joined by the bond retains an electron from the shared pair. These reactions are common in normal cell physiology.[73,74] Uncontrolled free radical reactions may be an important source of pathologic cellular damage, and may initiate aging—the free radical theory of aging.[75] Free radical damage is thought to take place throughout the life span, causing a progressive deterioration of both nuclear and cytoplasmic components. The respiring organism faces a difficult dilemma; it respires and obtains energy from the metabolism of oxygen, but oxygen itself can be extremely toxic. To overcome these problems, several defense mechanisms have evolved to protect the cell. Most of the oxygen in an aerobic organism is reduced to water by the cytochrome oxidase enzyme complex of the inner mitochondrial membrane. However, some oxidases within the cell can generate hydrogen peroxide, which is extremely toxic, and in the presence of transition metal ions such as iron can decompose to form the hydroxyl radical ·OH.

$$Fe^{2+} + H_2O_2 = \cdot OH + Fe^{3+} + H_2O$$

Other enzymes catalyze oxidation reactions in which a single electron is transferred from a substrate onto each oxygen molecule; this produces the oxygen free radical known as superoxide $-O_2^{\cdot}$.

$$O_2 + e^- = O_2^{\cdot}$$

Superoxide is a by-product of various enzyme reactions (particularly in the mitochondrial and chloroplast electron

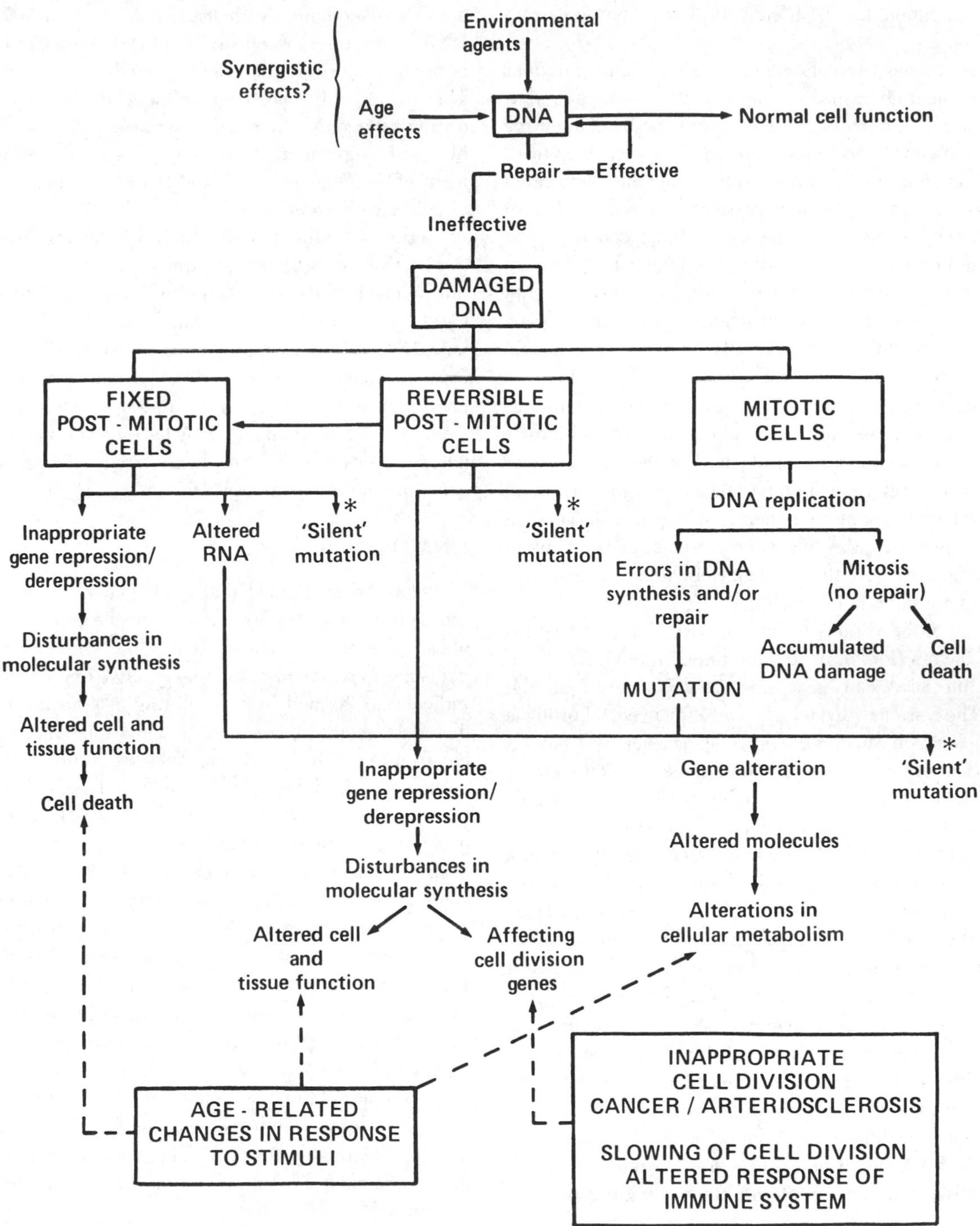

Figure 5-5 Diagrammatic view of the possible forms of damage to DNA and subsequent cellular responses. These changes are only of consequence during redifferentiation and/or stimulation of further mitoses.

transport systems), and can also be generated by environmental agents such as UV light, ultrasound, x-rays, gamma rays, toxic chemicals, and metal ions. Free radicals can also cause lipid peroxidation. Membrane lipids contain polyunsaturated fatty acid side chains that undergo lipid peroxidation involving the generation of carbon radicals and finally, lipid hydroperoxides. Lipid hydroperoxides decompose into cytotoxic aldehydes (e.g., malondialdehyde) and other products, causing damage to both enzymes and membranes. The various radicals react with, and damage, all molecules found within cells, but the lipid and protein components of membranes and mitochondrial DNA seem especially vulnerable.

Clearly cells do not continuously disintegrate because of free radical damage. Several protective, molecular mechanisms

Protection against reactive oxygen species

- Scavenging systems such as vitamin E (α-tocopherol)
- Peptides (e.g., glutathione—a tripeptide containing free sulfhydryl groups)
- Catalases and peroxidases—removal of hydrogen peroxide
- Superoxide dismutase (SOD)—removal of superoxide radical

have evolved to protect cells from free radical damage. Age-associated changes in glutathione, glutathione reductase, and superoxide dismutase (SOD) from blood cells,[76] liver,[77] and the eyes[78] have been reported. However, no correlation has been found between the maximum life span potential and levels of SOD in primates.[79] The fact that an increase in the oxygen: nitrogen ratio shortens the life span of *Drosophila* and leads to an increase in the concentration of lipofuscin has been used as evidence of the toxic effects of oxygen.[80] Experiments to extend animal survival by feeding antioxidants such as cysteine hydrochloride, ethoxyquin, 2-mercaptoethylamine hydrochloride, 2,2′-diaminodiethyldisulphide dihydroxide, and vitamin E through the life span are inconclusive.[81–83] Mean life span can increase by 10 to 15 percent depending on the strain of animal, but the maximum life span remains unaltered. The production of transgenic *Drosophila* overexpressing the gene for CuZn SOD led to small but statistically significant increases in the mean life span of several strains of this insect,[84] although maximum life span was not improved. Other transgenes, overexpressing both catalase and CuZn SOD showed significant extensions of life span in *Drosophila*.[85] Other attempts to genetically manipulate the enzymes involved in the metabolism of reactive oxygen species have been made, although they have not been successful in extending life span. Clearly, although the protective mechanisms against reactive oxygen species damage can be augmented with varying degrees of success, the developments in this field are unlikely to be rapid.

The dosing experiments are difficult to interpret. First, the studies have been conducted with too small numbers of animals to provide statistically reliable results. Second, no assessments have been made of the physiologic ages of the control and treated animals, to ensure that increased survival is in fact due to delayed aging and not to an effect on pathology. Third, most of these treatments result in a decrease in body weight,[81,82,86] so that these animals may be restricting their food intake, which can in itself lead to an extension of life. In spite of these reservations, the transgenic studies suggest that antioxidants do appear to influence the mean life span of some species. In addition, the feeding of antioxidants has been shown to reduce the levels of fluorescent pigments in animal tissues.[87,88] Conversely, diets inadequate in vitamin E are generally successful in accelerating the deposition of lipofuscin in both the nervous system and the adrenal glands of rats and mice.[89,90] Hence, the intracellular appearance of lipofuscin is highly likely to be associated with free radical damage within cells.

Estimates of the total number of oxidized bases formed in DNA on a daily basis range from 10^4 to 10^6 in each cell.[91] So-called small DNA oxidation products, thymine glycol, thymidine glycol, and hydroxymethyuracil, were first detected in the urine of rats and humans,[92] and were correlated with metabolic rate in mice, rats, and humans.[93] The concentration of 8-hydroxydeoxy-guanosine (8-OHdG) was found to increase with age in rat DNA.[94] In addition, DNA repair enzymes (glycosylases) that remove oxidized bases from DNA are positively correlated with life span in many mammals.[56] The mutagenic potential of oxidized bases in DNA is emphasized by the finding that the loss of the glycolase specific for the repair of 8-OHdG leads to an increase in the spontaneous mutation rate.[72]

Other modifications to genomic DNA by free radical intervention are postulated. The highly toxic carbonyl compound malondialdehyde is a major mutagenic and carcinogenic product of lipid peroxidation. The major compound produced by the reaction between malondialdehyde and DNA is the adduct *3 - β - D - 2′ - deoxyribofuranosylpyrimidol [1,2] - purin - 10(3H) - one*, but its relation to aging has yet to be established.[95] In addition, I-compounds, which are bulky covalent DNA modifications, can be detected as altered deoxyribonucleotides using extremely sensitive techniques.[95,96] These compounds accumulate with age in various tissues of laboratory rodents and have been termed indigenous compounds (hence, I-compounds).[97] The number and concentration of I-compounds are greatest in organs with high metabolic activity (e.g., liver and kidney). Studies of Fischer 344 rats show that, in a 2-year-old animal, the levels of these compounds is five times greater than at 1 month of age.[98] I-compounds are most likely derived from DNA-reactive intermediates generated during normal metabolism. These compounds have a wide range of chemical properties and appear to represent diverse molecular structures, suggesting they are derived from different precursors. The formation of I-compounds may be determined by genetics, environmental factors, and age, and their levels and type depend on species, strain, gender, diet, and exposure to potentially harmful chemicals. The argument for these compounds being indigenous in origin is the characteristic species- and tissue-dependent profiles that distinguish them from exogenous carcinogen-DNA adducts, which generally produce qualitatively identical patterns across tissues and species. In addition, a number of I-compounds in rodent liver exhibit diurnal changes that are not seen for carcinogen-DNA adducts. Thus, the indication is that these compounds are related to normal metabolic activity rather than exposure to environmental carcinogens. Two classes of I-compounds have been identified. The type 1 molecular modification is a consequence of normal metabolism and shows a positive, linear correlation, with median life span. The type 2 I-compounds are the result of oxidative damage and are bulky lesions that also increase with age. The role of type 1 I-compounds in carcinogenesis and neoplasia, and the effect of dietary restriction are discussed extensively by Randerath et al.[95] The data presented by these authors are very interesting and the relation between the formation of type 1 I-compounds and carcinogenesis suggests some intimate relation between their formation and malignant transformation. Evidence from dietary restriction studies indicates an increase in the occurrence of type 1 I-compounds with this treatment and may partially explain the reduction in malignancy observed in calorie-restricted rodents. However, the authors[95] primarily cite data for kidney and liver, and epithelial tumors are the least responsive malignancies to calorie restriction.[99] Oxidation of DNA in the test tube induces bulky DNA oxidation products that represent specific intrastrand cross-links, which can be increased several-fold after treating animals with carcinogens and pro-oxidant chemicals. These compounds are not derived from malondialdehyde, suggesting that these bulky, oxidative DNA lesions are due to endogenous mechanisms and are increased by carcinogens that induce oxidative stress in tissues. In addition, in rats, these type 2 I-compounds increase in the liver approximately twofold to threefold over the life span. The type 2 compounds are considered to be DNA lesions, whereas the type 1 are not.[95]

This field is in an early stage of development. The assays are extremely sensitive and the number of changes detected are extremely small.[100] The ability to measure this small level of DNA damage is a major advance in the field, but the low levels of damage, even though the percentage increase through the life span is quite large, suggest that genomic DNA damage may not be a major factor in aging without accompanying disease. The claim that the most likely source of these reactive oxygen species is leakage during oxidation in the mitochondria and the endoplasmic reticulum is reiterated frequently. That it is the source of oxidative damage to genomic DNA is, in my view, more questionable. These reactive oxygen species have a half-life of femtoseconds and are so highly reactive that whatever they meet in the way of lipid, or lipoprotein material, is highly likely to stop the moiety in its tracks. In that case, the damage must be local, and a far more likely recipient of the unwelcome attention of reactive oxygen species is the mitochondrial DNA.

Mitochondrial DNA

Mitochondrial DNA is a circular molecule and contains genes for two ribosomal RNAs (rRNAs), 22 transfer RNAs (tRNAs), and 13 peptides. These peptides are components of five multisubunit enzymes of the oxidative phosphorylation machinery of the inner mitochondrial membrane. Mitochondrial DNA is "naked" and attached to the inner mitochondrial membrane, and since about 2 percent of the oxygen reduced by the mitochondrion escapes as superoxide from the electron transport chain in the inner mitochondrial membrane, the DNA is very vulnerable to oxidative damage. Large deletions have been detected in mitochondrial DNA, and these increase markedly with increasing age in human, rats, mice, and nematodes.[95] The deletions detected usually involve large segments of the genome located between the origins of replication, and often involve directly repeated sequences that facilitate some form of intramolecular recombination. In addition, in some human myopathies and in diabetes, large sections of the mitochondrial genome have undergone rearrangements.[101]

Mitochondria are the most important intracellular source of reactive oxygen species. The DNA in mitochondria is subject to severe oxidative damage to a much higher degree than genomic DNA. The oxidative damage is detected by the presence of oxidized bases, particularly 8-OHdG. This base modification can lead to point mutations because of mispairing. The level of 8-OHdG in mitochondrial DNA increases with age in rat and human liver, muscle, and brain tissues. It also increases in the mitochondrial genome of the housefly.[95,102] The latter findings are interesting in that a decrease in the physical activity of the houseflies prolongs life span and reduces the level of 8OHdG in both nuclear and mitochondrial DNA.[102] These observations are discussed in greater detail elsewhere.[95] Mitochondrial DNA is also partially fragmented, possibly because of some of the deletions taking place. Recently, renewed interest has been expressed in the idea that defects in mitochondria are either contributing factors, or the cause of cellular aging.[103]

For many years it was considered that mitochondrial DNA did not have the facility to repair damage. However, this is now known to be incorrect and it seems that DNA repair processes in mitochondria resemble those seen in the nontranscribing DNA of the nucleus.[104] This finding must alter our view of how mitochondrial DNA may be affected by damage, but it does not preclude the possibility that mutations can accumulate in mitochondrial genomes, leading eventually to dysfunction of the cell. In addition, it is known that mitochondrial DNA can be inserted into nuclear DNA. This occurs continuously in yeast, and isolated sequences have been identified in human cells.[101,105] However, no evidence for the transfer of mitochondrial DNA sequences to the nucleus was found in aged human fibroblasts, suggesting that such transfers are rare in humans.[105] The whole issue of mitochondrial DNA damage in aging is discussed extensively in a recent review.[106] This is an exciting and growing field and is already proving extremely productive in the study of human disease. However, despite the very large increases in the alterations seen in mitochondrial DNA over the life span, particularly in postmitotic tissues, the overall level of mitochondrial genomes containing deletions is less than 0.1 percent of the total mitochondrial DNA in a given tissue. This rather general statement of damage may be misleading, because histochemical studies suggest that the mutant genomes are unevenly distributed and highly concentrated in cells where energy metabolism may be impaired. The photomicrographs of muscle tissue taken from human myopathies indicate that the changes in muscle fibers are extremely complicated. Much more work needs to be done in this area.[95]

DNA Repair

Under conditions of normal homeostasis, and particularly under conditions of physiologic stress, the integrity of the genome and consequently of gene expression depends on the

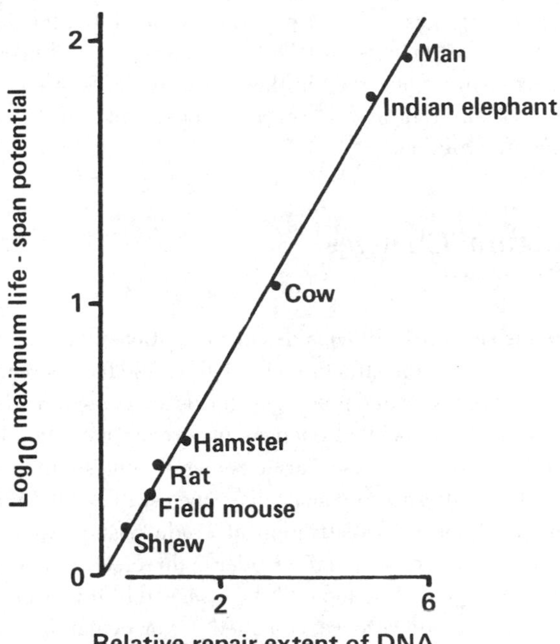

Figure 5-6 Diagrammatic representation of the correlation between the logarithm of the maximum life span potential of several species and the efficiency of repair of UV-damaged DNA in fibroblast cultures. (From Hart and Setlow,[109] with permission.)

ability to repair DNA damage; this mechanism is crucial to survival.[107] Alterations in DNA can be caused by UV radiation as an exogenous factor, and endogenous changes such as depurination or deamination of cytosine, or oxidative damage due to free radical attack.[107] In addition, the damage to DNA may or may not be random in nature, since the structure of the chromatin may make certain areas more susceptible to attack by outside agents. Repair of chromatin may also be restricted because of this limited accessibility.[56,108] Animals with long maximum life span potentials generally have a more efficient DNA repair system.[109] Evidence for this has been obtained from studies on fibroblast cultures exposed to high doses of UV radiation. Both the initial rate and maximum incorporation of radioactively labeled DNA precursors into DNA increases with the life span potential of the species as shown in Figure 5-6. Subsequent work has shown a strong correlation between DNA repair and longevity among mice[110,111] and primates.[112]

Endogenous changes in DNA are brought about as a result of living at 37°C.[107] It has been calculated that if such damage accumulated unchecked, 10 percent of the bases in the DNA of the average cell of an old human would be altered, and this is not compatible with life.[107] The repair of DNA damage is generally very effective, although the rate of damage caused by UV radiation in full sunlight is close to swamping the repair system.[107]

Few authors have examined the effect of age on the ability for DNA repair in nonmitotic tissues. Hamster lung and kidney shows little change in the ability to perform UV-induced, unscheduled DNA repair during the life span.[113] The cerebellar neurons from dogs up to 13 years of age were irradiated with x-rays and the resulting strand breaks repaired equally rapidly at all ages.[114] The results of the various studies of DNA repair and age are contradictory. An interesting investigation of several organs in rats of various ages highlights the confusion.[115] Four repair mechanisms were investigated: excision repair, single- and double-strand break repair, and Q-endonuclease susceptibility.[115] Repair capacity was highest in liver, spleen, kidney, and lung, and lowest in the brain, testes, and duodenum. An age-associated shift from excision repair to rejoining strands was noted in spleen, lung, heart, testes, skeletal muscle, and brain, with a complete loss of excision capacity at advanced age.[115] However, most investigations have centered on the ability of fibroblasts (i.e., mitotic cells) to repair damage under in vitro conditions.[38,108] Late passage cultures of HDF cells demonstrate less DNA repair activity than young cells after exposure to UV radiation.[116,117] These results indicate a decrease in the ability of senescent cells to integrate the various operations needed for DNA repair. However, the decline in UV-induced repair with culture age occurs only in the passage prior to cessation of cell division, prompting the conclusion that this deficiency in repair is not the basis of in vitro aging.[118] Recently, it has been suggested that the reduced capacity to repair double-strand breaks in human DNA appears to be more pronounced in older women than in older men (and may begin after age 65 years). Moreover, the reported age-related decline in double-strand break induction occurs more rapidly in women than in men. This analysis reveals a gender-specific pattern in the correlation between the percentage of double-strand breaks induced and the percentage of double-strand breaks rejoined. At comparable levels of double-strand break induction, cells from men rejoin a higher percentage than do cells from women.[119]

DNA polymerases

A reduction in the function of DNA in aging animals could depend on several factors besides alterations in chromatin structures that mediate the degree of gene activity, and changes in chromatin proteins. Reduced function may result from a decreased ability to synthesize new DNA, or more particularly, from a lowered fidelity of the process of replication or repair. Once again, variability is evident; a high molecular weight polymerase showed no age-associated changes in activity in the spleen of some mice.[120] However, a low molecular weight polymerase showed a marked reduction in activity in the spleen from the same old animals, but not in the liver or kidney, nor the spleen of another strain of mouse.[120] Recent studies on the activity and fidelity of chromatin-associated DNA polymerase β from aging mice of different life spans showed that the DNA synthetic activity of liver chromatin remained constant in both species throughout their life span.[121] Chromatin-directed and nonchromatin-directed copying of a dinucleotide polymer was similar in both *Mus musculus* (relatively short-lived), and *Peromyscus leucopus* (relatively long-lived), and was unaltered in older animals.[121] In addition, its fidelity using polydeoxycytidine as template was unchanged with age.[122] These studies suggest that the DNA polymerase from certain nonmitotic cells, aged in vivo, is mainly unchanged.

On the other hand, the fidelity of DNA polymerase enzymes are claimed to be reduced in extracts from aged HDF cells maintained in tissue culture, with error frequencies between 2 and 3.4 times greater than enzymes prepared from young cultures. The main mispairing that seems to take place is between guanine and thymine, but great care must be taken in the interpretation of these results, because the error frequency of DNA polymerase in vitro is much greater than when DNA is synthesized in vivo.[123] Recent studies of DNA excision repair in human cells showed a decline in efficiency as an apparent function of decreased DNA polymerase α-specific activity with increased age of the cell donor.[124] The data suggest that DNA polymerase α isolated from adult-derived human cells have low-activity and high-activity forms. The decreased specific activity of DNA polymerase α correlated with increased age of the donor appears to be a function of loss of an enzyme activator molecule resulting in diminished ability of the enzyme to bind DNA template-primer.

Ribosomes

The number of rRNA genes available for transcription varies at different stages of the life cycle, particularly during oogenesis.[125] However, estimations of the numbers of rRNA genes that can be transcribed late in the life span, when compared with early on, have been inconclusive. Age-dependent losses of rRNA genes have been described in mammals.[126,127] Others have noted that variation from the normal number of rRNA genes can affect the vigor of a species.[128] However, rRNA gene dosage was lower in the liver than in the brain of young mice, but after 12 months of age, the liver rRNA gene dosage increased to the levels found in the brain.[125] No difference in rRNA gene dosage for both the liver and brain, expressed as a function of either sex or age, could be detected in humans. The issue of organ complexity has been mentioned as a major problem in the interpretation of studies such as these, but a further source of confusion is differences between different tissues. Structural changes in the ribosomal populations of aging cells have been described,[129] and ribosomes isolated from old and young animals to investigate age-associated changes in protein synthesis. On balance, ribosomes do not appear to change markedly with age, and to our current knowledge they are not responsible for changes in the levels of protein synthesis that have been demonstrated in in vitro cell-free conditions.[108,130]

Changes in the complements of tRNAs have been recorded during developmental processes, cell differentiation, and hormone stimulation. Some claim to have shown age-associated changes in tRNA molecules in the rat, but the part of the life span investigated probably reflects maturational changes.[131] Others could not demonstrate changes in the nucleotide composition of tRNA from mature and old mice, nor from mature and old mosquitoes.[132] These experiments are difficult to interpret,[132,133] but changes in tRNA complements, and also the complex changes observed in the overall patterns of enzymes in cells of different ages,[134] may be consistent with the idea of codon restriction.[135,136]

Structural Changes in Proteins

In this section I will consider the alterations that may take place with age in the structure of proteins. The factors regulating gene expression and protein synthesis are considered later. Studies of age-associated changes in enzyme activities have shown increases, decreases, or no change—almost at random. The lack of pattern and consistency suggest that little can be concluded from an investigation of crude tissue extracts of enzyme activity per se and the reader is directed to two extensive reviews on this topic.[108,137] Research on structural changes in protein with age, so-called "error-containing" proteins, seemed more productive, in that here was an attempt to draw inferences about the molecular structure of proteins. Orgel[11,138] proposed a mechanism of aging whereby errors were made in protein synthesis, but withdrew his support for the idea at a later stage.[139] However, the original suggestion was that the incorporation of incorrect amino acids into proteins may take place with age, although the actual error frequency was uncertain. Preliminary estimates were a low value of 3 in 10^8 correct insertions, and a high one of 1 in 10^4 insertions. Incorrect amino acid insertions would have various effects, depending on where they were within a protein. If the "errors" were at the catalytically active site of an enzyme, for example, this could alter its activity, or specificity, for a substrate. An alteration at an allosteric site may result in a loosening of control over its activity, while a change at an amino acid residue involved in the maintenance of the three-dimensional structure of a protein might affect its biophysical characteristics.

In many proteins these changes may have little effect, such as in the case of proteins undergoing rapid turnover. However, errors in enzymes like the DNA and RNA polymerases could be potentially more damaging. These polymerases have long half-lives and catalyze a large number of reactions before they are degraded. Any alteration in their function could lead to the introduction of a large number of error-containing proteins that would accumulate within a cell. Orgel suggested that a critical level of such proteins may occur in a cell, and this would be followed by an "error catastrophe" and cell death. The theoretical argument concerning the possibilities and effectiveness of errors in protein synthesis on cellular function, particularly with respect to aging, continues,[140,141] although it is no longer considered a serious contender for the cause of aging in cells.[142]

Various experiments were conducted to test Orgel's hypothesis. Early studies used amino acid analogues, in place of the correct amino acids, to force cultured HDF to make errors, but no difference was found between the life spans of controls and treated cells, although the rate of cell division was slowed. It was also discovered that transformed, permanent cell lines that do not show in vitro senescence make larger numbers of errors than normal HDF. Clearly some mechanism must exist to enable the permanent cell lines to avoid an accumulation of altered proteins. Thus, permanent cell lines would be expected to show less sensitivity to the presence of amino acid analogues in the medium as compared to normal cells. However, the cell yield in the presence of analogues (as a percentage of the control culture) was reduced to a similar level in both transformed cell lines and HDF.[143] Other studies attempted to determine the ability of cells to discriminate between natural amino acids and their analogues. The ability of HDF cultures to discriminate between methionine and its analogue, ethionine, during protein synthesis, declines in senescence,[144] and in vivo experiments have shown that the ability to discriminate between methionine and ethionine during protein synthesis decreases with increasing age. There is also a failure to differentiate between the two analogues as donors of alkyl groups in the transmethylation of RNA bases.[145]

The accuracy of the translation mechanism has been examined in a cell-free protein-synthesizing system. Polyuridylic acid (an artificial mRNA) has been used to study the fidelity of polyphenylalanine synthesis in cell-free systems derived from animals of different ages. No decline could be detected in the accuracy or control of synthesis in cell-free systems derived from Fischer 344 rat brain, liver, or hippocampus.[146] However, although there was no significant age-associated change in the accuracy of this particular step in protein synthesis, the possibility remains that errors could occur with increasing frequency at other steps.

Abnormally heat-labile proteins

Much of the evidence for mutant proteins in aged cells comes from studies of the abnormal sensitivity of these macromolecules to heat denaturation. The thermal inactivation kinetics of proteins have been used to determine whether or not abnormal enzymes accumulate in cells during in vitro senescence. Glucose-6-phosphate dehydrogenase (G6PD) activity declines linearly when heated in crude extracts of young fibroblast cultures. On extrapolation of the regression line drawn through the data to zero time, an intercept value close to 100 percent activity is obtained (Fig. 5-7) suggesting negligible amounts of abnormally heat-labile enzyme in young HDF. On the other hand, the thermal denaturation characteristics of G6PD in senescent cells shows a biphasic decay in enzyme activity. The enzyme undergoes an initial, rapid inactivation, indicating the presence of abnormally heat-labile enzyme molecules, followed by a slower decay of activity, in which the rate of inactivation is the same as that observed for young cultures (Fig. 5-7). It was estimated that the error frequency was at least 1 in 10^3 in senescent HDF cultures, meaning that on average, about one-half of the G6PD molecules in senescent cells contained a misincorporated amino acid.[147]

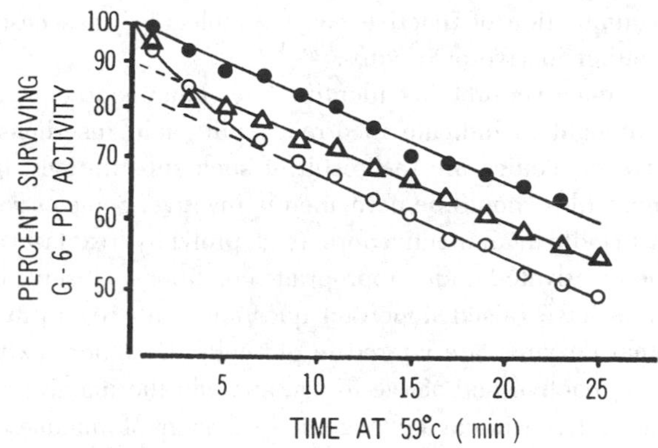

Figure 5-7 Thermal inactivation (59°C) of glucose-6-phosphate dehydrogenase from young, middle-aged, and senescent cultured MRC-5 fibroblasts. ●—young cells (passage 22); △—middle-aged cells (passage 48); O—old cells (passage 61). (From Holliday and Tarrant,[147] with permission.)

This study was followed by many others examining the thermal inactivation kinetics of enzyme proteins both in vitro and in vivo. The results have been contradictory.[142] One careful study showed an age-associated increase in the amount of abnormally heat-labile enzyme in the liver of the C57BL mouse.[148] The amount of heat-labile enzyme rose from about 2 percent at 3 months to a value of 12 percent at 12 months of age. However, no further significant increase in the levels of heat-labile protein were recorded. Thus, the levels of heat labile enzyme were 15 percent at 18 months, and 18 percent at 32 months of age. Similar results were reported for the enzyme glutathione reductase, where an abrupt increase was recorded in the amount of abnormally heat-labile material in the human lens at about 32 years of age, with no change thereafter.[149]

Immunoprecipitation techniques

Old nematodes have higher concentrations of inactive isocitrate lyase molecules.[150] Homogenates of *Turbatrix aceti* of different ages were prepared, and the activities of the extracts were adjusted to the same value with respect to the enzyme isocitrate lyase. An antiserum, which caused inactivation, or precipitation, of the enzyme, was then added to the extract and the activity of the isocitrate lyase determined. Homogenates from old worms required the addition of more antiserum to precipitate the same amount of enzyme activity as the homogenates of young nematodes. This was interpreted as showing a mixture of active and inactive molecules in old nematode cultures. This work has been confirmed for isocitrate lyase purified from 6- and 27-day old worms, but a more detailed study also showed that inactive forms of isoenzymes also occurred with increasing age.[151] Subsequent reports using this technique have described the occurrence and accumulation of inactive enzyme molecules in senescent organisms, but the results are contradictory. Inactive molecules of aldolase have been recorded in the muscle[152] and livers[153] of old mice, and in rabbit muscle.[154] However, other studies have not shown an accumulation of inactive enzyme molecules in senescent cells either in vivo or in vitro.[155–157]

The inactive proteins identified by immunoprecipitation were thought to indicate incorrect amino acid insertions. If inactive molecules are the result of such substitutions, then the molecules should be permanently inactive. Some enzymes occur in cells in an inactive form (e.g., prolyl hydroxylase) and can be reactivated under appropriate conditions. Observations like this have raised important questions with regard to the way that enzymes are altered in old cells. Do other enzymes exist as inactive and active forms, and can the inactive form become active without a change in the amount of immunoreactive protein? Changes in the molecular form of elongation factor 1 (EF1, an enzyme involved in protein synthesis) have been observed.[158] A decline in the specific activity of EF1, and an accumulation of inactive or partially active molecules during aging, has been reported in the nematode *T. aceti*. The molecular form of the enzyme also changed; in young animals most of the enzyme is present in aggregate form, whereas in old nematodes most of it is disaggregated. The decrease in the specific activity of EF1 with age may be related to the change in the degree of aggregation.

Viruses as probes of inaccurate protein synthesis

One ingenious, and elegant, investigation of protein synthetic function examined the ability of viruses to use the protein-synthesizing machinery of HDF cells grown in vitro to make new viral protein. If senescent cells contain a transcription and translation apparatus prone to errors, then this should result in either a reduction in the numbers of viruses produced, or abnormalities in the viral proteins. This in turn may make the assembly of the new viral particle less efficient, possibly altering the infectivity of new virus. Senescent cultures of HDF supported infections by three different viruses as well as young cultures, and the yields of new virus were equal in each case.[159] The infectivity of the viruses was also identical, and no increase in mutation rate was detected. These observations have been confirmed.[160,161]

The above discussion illustrates why there is doubt about whether errors in protein synthesis can be regarded as a primary mechanism in aging (although such a mechanism cannot be completely discounted).[142] Some predictions of the hypothesis have been confirmed. Some enzyme proteins do accumulate in the cells and tissues of aging organisms in forms that are enzymically inactive. This is not true for all enzymes, however, and although mechanisms have been suggested by which some proteins might accumulate in altered forms while others might not,[162] the fact that not all proteins are affected suggests that this is no universal phenomonenom in cells in vitro or in vivo.

Post-translational protein modifications

One factor consistently ignored by many of the investigators was the possibility of postsynthetic modifications in protein structure.[163–165] As human and rabbit erythrocytes age in vivo, several enzymes accumulate in inactive or abnormally heat-labile forms.[166] Since protein synthesis does not occur in erythrocytes at the time of this accumulation, the production of these abnormal proteins must be due to postsynthetic modifications. Altered proteins also accumulate in the fiber cells of the lens during aging, even though protein synthesis has ceased at this site also, again indicating that postsynthetic modifications must be occurring.[167] Various postsynthetic modifications to proteins have been recorded, including deamidation at asparagine or glutamine residues,[167] cleavage of peptide bonds,[167] acetylation of amino terminal residues,[168] and glycosylation of free amino groups.[169] Other reactions include phosphorylation at serine residues, sulfhydryl-disulphide bond interchange, changes involving cross-linking,[170] and oxidation.[171,172]

Detailed research has revealed clear conformational changes in certain enzymes from aged animals.[164,173–175] Studies on enolase in the free-living nematode *T. aceti* show that in old animals the enzyme has a lower specific activity and altered physical characteristics, including differences in secondary structure. These differences disappear when the respective proteins are "unfolded," suggesting an alteration in the conformation of the enzyme. Furthermore, this change is not a result of the oxidation or reduction of sulfhydryl groups as these are equal in number and they all exist in the reduced form. Nor do the altered properties appear to involve deamidation, phosphorylation, or partial proteolysis. "Old" enolase is relatively unstable to chromatography; during this treatment the enzyme is partly converted to a denatured "inactive" form, which can also be found in homogenates of old *T. aceti*. This inactive material cross-reacts with the antiserum prepared against "young" or "old" enzyme. Young enolase, although it is more stable than old, can be converted to a product similar to the latter by repeated chromatography. Studies on enolase turnover in the free-living nematode *T. aceti* show that the rate of synthesis and degradation of this enzyme, and the total soluble protein fraction slow with age.[173] A later paper shows that the young and old forms of the enzyme enolase are conformational isomers and that an in vivo transformation from young to old enzymes takes place by conformational changes without covalent modification.[165] This process may be related to the previously discussed reduction in turnover of enolase in *T. aceti*. Furthermore, such changes could not be due to errors in sequence. A similar mechanism applies to the enzyme phosphoglycerate kinase in the aging rat.[175]

The oxidation of amino acid residues in proteins can occur by direct or indirect mechanisms. Carbonyl groups are formed after putative free radical damage to amino acid side chains. The carbonyl content of proteins increases exponentially with age in cultured HDF.[176] It has been speculated that the oxidized protein in an aged animal may be as much as 30 to 50 percent of the total cellular protein, a value consistent with the reduced catalytic activity of many enzymes found in old animals.[177] If proteins are exposed to reactive oxygen species in vitro they undergo marked oxidative damage, although in my view this is hardly surprising. Carbonyl groups in proteins can also be generated by interacting with reducing sugars or reactive aldehydes in the cellular environment. Glycation of proteins involves the interaction of the carbonyl group of a reducing sugar with lysine residues of a protein to form Schiff base derivatives, which lead ultimately to fluorescent end products (Maillard products).[178] The contribution of glycation and other oxidative reactions to the total carbonyl content of tissues is not fully understood, but there are clearly a number of common pathways through the ubiquitous Schiff base reaction. It is interesting that when aged animals are fed compounds that prevent free radical damage, such as the spin-trap compound phenylbutylnitrone (PBN or N-*tert*-butyl-α-phenylnitrone), the carbonyl content of tissues decreases; when treatment is withdrawn the carbonyl groups reappear.[177]

Glycation, the process of nonenzymic addition of sugars to amino acid residues in proteins, is considered a major feature of aging in its own right.[179] These molecular changes are now considered a feature of the pathophysiology of aging. We know that adult onset diabetes with increased blood glucose raises the extent of the glycation of hemoglobin[180,181] and collagen.[182–184] The progressive glycation of collagen from human skin[182,183] and basement membranes[184] with age is well described, although the change is not universal in long-lived proteins (e.g., lens crystallins from normal human subjects).[185] The end products of the glycation process are now known as advanced glycation end products (AGE).[186] This area has been thoroughly reviewed elsewhere.[179,187]

Much of the early literature on aging included detailed analyses of the cross-linkage of macromolecules, particularly the connective tissue proteins collagen and elastin, although the cross-linkage of strands of DNA, and DNA protein within the chromosome, also fell into this general area. Collagen undergoes very low turnover rates in adult animals,[188] and is a very strong candidate for posttranslational changes. The formation of glycation products suggests that collagen can undergo modification unrelated to its normal maturation after synthesis. Recent research has examined some of the complex collagen cross-links, and this is reviewed by Finch.[30]

The presence of altered protein molecules in old cells may be a direct result of a decrease in the degradation of intracellular protein. It is now clear that several pathways exist for the removal of proteins within the cell. Short-lived proteins, in either normal or abnormal form, are degraded in a proteolytic pathway in the cytosol. One pathway involves ubiquitin as a marker, identifying proteins for rapid degradation. A substrate protein for degradation is "tagged" with ubiquitin in a covalent linkage that is ATP-dependent. The protease, which degrades the ubiquitin-labeled proteins, is also ATP-dependent, although it is thought that other proteases must exist. The cytosolic proteases, the calpains, which are calcium activated, also have a role in protein degradation.[189] The balance of evidence suggests that protein degradation in the intact animal decreases with age.[190] Some of the pitfalls involved in the study of intracellular proteolysis have been discussed above, but it is intriguing to speculate on the possible effects of age-associated changes in proteolysis,[191] and the effects they may have on cellular function and the process of cellular senescence.

Lysosomes and Lipofuscin

The most well-described change in the subcellular structure of nonmitotic cells is the presence of the so-called lipofuscin component, or aging-pigment granule (Fig. 5-8). This pigment

Figure 5-8 **(A)** Electron micrograph of lipofuscin from a neuron in the supraoptic nucleus of a 28-month-old mouse. Note the granular electron dense matrix with electron lucent inclusions. Scale bar = 1 μm. **(B)** Electron micrograph of lipofuscin from an adrenal cortical cell of a 28-month-old mouse. Note the differences in the appearance of the electron dense granules and the lack of electron lucent inclusions. Scale bar = 2 μm.

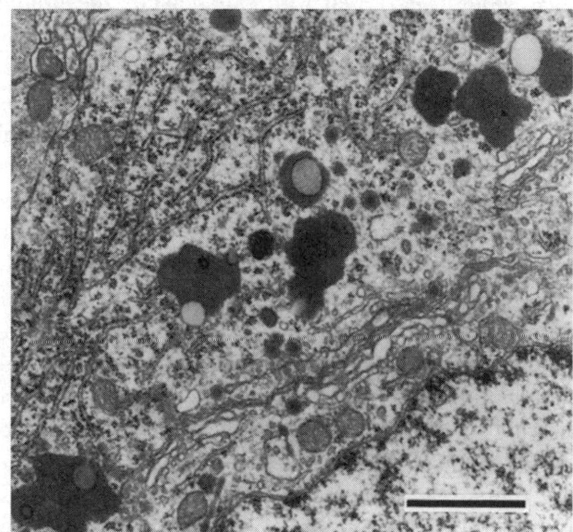

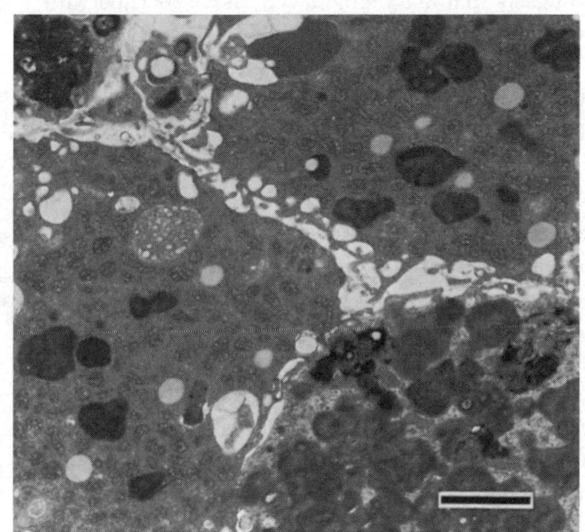

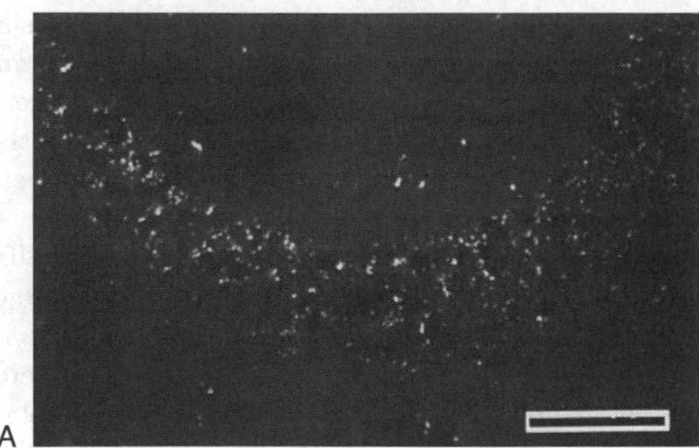

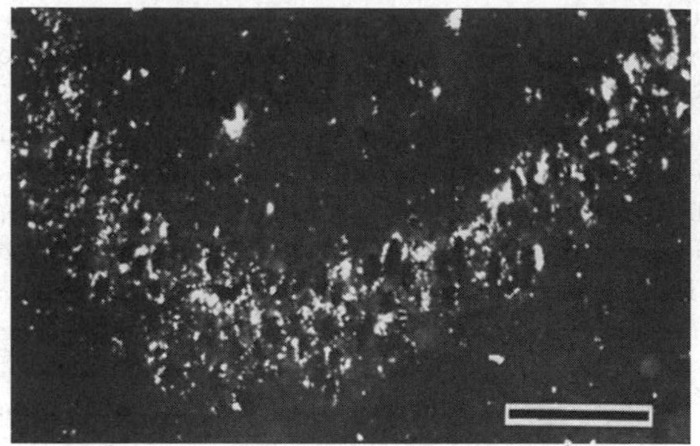

Figure 5-9 Photomicrographs showing the increase in the levels of the autofluorescent age-pigment, lipofuscin, in hippocampal neurons of mice. (**A**) Preparation from a 6-month-old animal (**B**) Preparation from a 28-month-old mouse. Scale bar = 100 μm.

emits a yellow-green to orange fluorescence when excited by UV light (Fig. 5-9). The lipofuscin granule is extremely heterogeneous; it contains proteins, carbohydrates, and lipids, and various enzymes associated with lysosomal activity and oxidative metabolism. In the electron microscope lipofuscin is highly irregular in shape, and the variation in structure is dependent on the cell type (Figure 5-8). Most reviews on this topic[192,193] have concentrated on how and why this material is generated in old cells, rather than addressing the question of what effects it has by being there. There are two schools of thought: first, that lipofuscin causes intracellular malfunction and second, that it is an indicator of age-associated cellular damage.

The first view is probably an over simplification based on obvious logic. Aging cells do not function as well as young cells, and lipofuscin is present to a greater extent in old cells. Therefore, lipofuscin causes a decline in function. The levels of lipofuscin and cytoplasmic RNA in tissue sections from autopsy samples of human central nervous system are negatively correlated.[194] However, there is little other quantitative evidence to support this viewpoint.

The high concentration of lipofuscin found in tissues from aging animals (and incidentally, from those with a vitamin E deficiency) suggests that age pigment may be associated with damage to subcellular components, possibly by way of free radical reactions and lipid peroxidation.[192,193] This view is supported by various studies. However, an investigation of the effects of age on the structure and function of neuroendocrine cells (the AVP- and oxytocin-producing cells) of the mouse hypothalamus has shown few changes with age. In spite of an age-associated increase in the concentration of lipofuscin, the volumes of other subcellular organelles measured in a quantitative morphologic study were not significantly different from those found in young mice.[195,196] In addition, an osmotic challenge, sufficient to cause the release of hormone from the neurohypophysis and stimulate hormone synthesis in the hypothalamic neurons, reduced the age-pigment concentration. On removal of the osmotic load and rehydration, the lipofuscin levels returned to control values. These data indicate that the lipofuscin compartment of the cell can be modified by physiologic stress, and suggests strongly that the material does not accumulate with age but increases in concentration, and may be dynamically controlled until late in the life span.[196]

The lysosome may contribute to cellular aging in a variety of ways. The leakage of lysosomal enzymes from damaged organelles could result in altered intracellular chemistry. Membranes may be damaged, cellular proteins lost or their conformation altered (see above, posttranslational modifications). RNA would be changed, so affecting the translation of protein, and DNA may become damaged, resulting in deletions and mutations. The major effects of such leakage would be centered mainly on nonmitotic cells, since the mitotic population would routinely remove damaged units and replace them with fresh daughter cells. However, there is little evidence for such disastrous alterations in nonmitotic cells.

It is clear that lysosomes are involved in the degradation of cellular organelles; they have also been implicated in the formation of lipofuscin. However, changes in the levels of lysosomal enzymes with age do not provide any consistent pattern with differences between tissues, or even between the diverse cells from the same tissue.

Early studies on lysosomal enzyme activities in crude homogenates should be viewed with skepticism. One problem may be the altered levels of protein encountered in old tissues, so that changes expressed per unit weight of protein may have little meaning. In addition, different levels of lysosomal enzymes are found in different cells, and if the proportion of cells of each type changes with age, the lysosomal enzyme levels would reflect this fact. This is a general drawback of crude biochemical investigations of organs. In the liver of 3-month-old rats, the activities of nine lysosomal enzymes differed between the hepatocyte (parenchymal), Küpffer, and endothelial (nonparenchymal) cell populations.[197] Approximately 66 percent of the liver consists of hepatocytes, the other 34 percent comprises mainly the Küpffer and endothelial cells. On a cell basis, hepatocytes show the highest enzyme activity, but because of their much greater protein content they have the lowest specific activity. The various cells show differential, age-associated changes in lysosomal enzymes. Parenchymal and nonparenchymal cells from rats of different ages were separated, and the activity of the lysosomal enzymes acid phosphatase, β-galactosidase, cathepsin D, and arylsulphatase β determined.[198] The most substantial change was a threefold increase of cathepsin D activity in hepatocytes between 12 and 30 to 35 months of age. In nonparenchymal cells no significant change was found during this period, but this was because there was a sharp fall in activity between 12 and 24 months, with a subsequent increase by 30 to 35 months. Overall, the changes in enzyme activities in the two cell populations did not correspond. Other authors have reported quite different results using unfractionated rat liver homogenates.[199] Acid phosphatase increases during maturation (between 1 and 16 months) and declines during senescence (between 16 and 27 months). β-Glucuronidase remains unchanged at first and then rises during senescence. In addition, levels of this enzyme were raised by phenobarbital administration, although less so in old than young rats. It is difficult to reconcile the findings from fractionated and unfractionated sources.

Age-associated alterations in lysosomal enzymes of rat and rabbit heart have also been recorded, with an increase in cathepsin D, no change in acid phosphatase, and a decrease in glucosaminidase in both species. The patterns of activity of a number of lysosomal enzymes were found to vary at different ages in the mouse heart, although acid phosphatase did not change significantly. No age-associated differences have been detected in the activities of a number of lysosomal enzymes in the frontal cortex of human brain, although the data show a considerable amount of scatter. Others have shown changes in β-glucuronidase and cathepsin D, but found a large increase in N-acetyl-β-glucosaminidase in 24-month-old compared with 2.5-month-old rat brain. Interestingly, acid phosphatase showed little change, in agreement with results for other tissues. There is little information regarding lysosomal turnover, although a significantly increased half-life of the lysosomal fraction in aged rats has been reported.[200]

Lysosomal enzyme activities show no consistent changes with age (they seem to be linked with several factors from sex to tissue of origin), and indeed, it is likely that they vary considerably in accord with the metabolic needs of tissue at a particular time.[201] The changes therefore are not necessarily a concomitant of age but more likely a reflection of an ongoing process of metabolic regulation.

Mitochondria

Mitochondria can undergo marked, age-associated changes in ultrastructure. Several reviews[202] have described the complex alterations seen in mitochondrial cristae, and there is evidence for the formation of myelin-like whorls of membrane in degenerating organelles (Fig. 5-10)

The respiratory activity of isolated mitochondria from both heart and skeletal muscles in the Fischer 344 rat has been studied at various ages.[203] Maximal respiratory capacity (state 3 respiration) was shown to decrease slowly up to 16 months of age and then more rapidly. Oxidative phosphorylation (state 4 respiration) in the presence of limiting concentrations of ADP was unchanged, and ADP:O ratios were close to the theoretical, suggesting that the integrity of mitochondria was maintained at advanced ages. Thus, there is a decrease in respiration in old mitochondria, and the defect is located before NAD reduction, implicating changes in dehydrogenase activity, anion transport, or other transport-associated systems.[203]

Matrix and inner-mitochondrial-membrane enzyme activities (malic dehydrogenase and cytochrome oxidase, respectively) were examined for a correlation between age-associated changes in mitochondrial morphology and enzyme activity in mice.[204] No age-associated effects were observed based on the concentration of protein in the mitochondria, and there was no cytochemical evidence for changes in location of the enzymes with age. There was no change in either state 4 or state 3 respiration, using succinate as substrate in agreement with previous investigators.[203] However, it was argued that enlarged and damaged mitochondria could be lost from the livers of old mice during the preparation procedure because of their putative "altered" properties.[205] The mitochondria from old animals were less stable on storage than those from young preparations, and the yield was lower. A loss of the most fragile organelles during preparation might explain the lack of an age-associated difference found in surviving mitochondria.

Since mitochondrial function is unaltered with age in a variety of tissues, it would seem unlikely that the organelles become damaged simply by surviving for extended periods in the cells from old animals. Either replacement components of mitochondria in old organisms are synthesized incorrectly, or they possess subtly altered membranes that are damaged rapidly by the microenvironment of old tissues. Thus, at any given time, and in spite of continuous turnover, a proportion of the mitochondria are in a damaged state. The observation that liver mitochondria in old mice show a range of forms from normal to enlarged does not tell us which of these two possibilities is correct.[205] Normal mitochondria may become altered if there was a decrease in turnover with age, although to my knowledge, no change in this variable has been detected.[206] In neuroendocrine cells subject to a physiologic challenge qualitative and quantitative changes are found in mitochondrial structure.[207,208] In young animals the number of mitochondria per unit area of cytoplasm drops temporarily and then increases to a stable level until the stress is withdrawn. No qualitative changes are observed during this period.[209] In old mice the number of mitochondria per unit area decreases and remains low throughout the stress. During this time qualitative changes could be seen in many of the mitochondria.[207] The relative volume of mitochondria within the cells of both age groups is similar, suggesting that the organelles in the neuroendocrine cells from old mice actually swell. In the control animals of both age groups no difference was found in the number of mitochondria per unit area of cytoplasm, or their volume. This suggests that the structural differences in the mitochondria of old, nonmitotic cells cannot be observed ultrastructurally until some stress is placed on the system.[208] Perhaps changes in

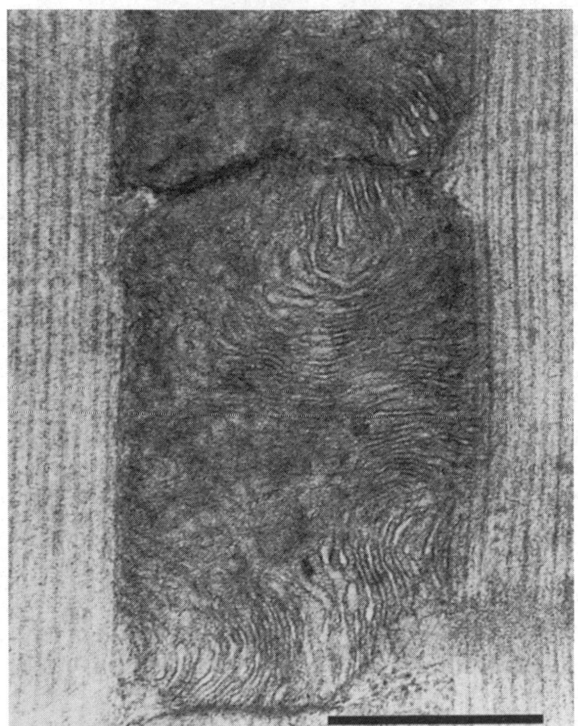

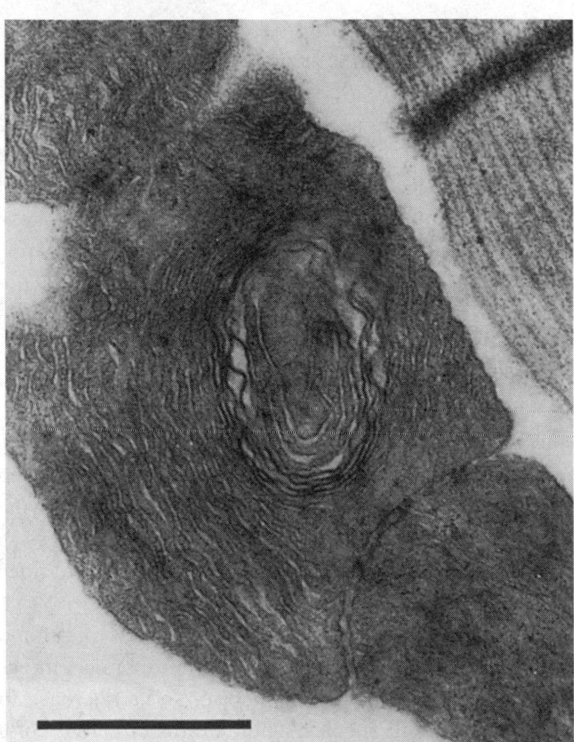

Figure 5-10 Electron micrographs of mitochondria from the flight muscle of the hymenopteran insect *Nasonia vitripennis*. (**A**) Mitochondrion is from a 3-day-old female. (**B**) Mitochondrion from a 19-day-old animal (maximum lifespan 21 days). Note the myelin-like change in the organelle from the old insect. Scale bar = 0.5 μm.

function have not been detected using biochemical techniques because the preparation procedures are too harsh, causing the loss of "damaged" mitochondria,[205] or because of a failure to separate different cell types in such investigations.

Mitochondria have been isolated from the brains of rats of various ages and differentiated into nonsynaptic and synaptic organelles.[210] State 3 oxidation of pyruvate and malate declined by 24 percent between 12 and 24 months of age in the nonsynaptic mitochondria. On the other hand, in synaptic mitochondria, a decrease occurred only between 3 and 12 months of age. Enzymes involved in fatty acid metabolism were also reduced; nonsynaptic mitochondria showed a drop in the state 3 respiration of glutamate-malate not observed in those from synapses.[211] These results may be due to a decrease in transport. Mitochondria from both sources showed age-associated changes in carbon dioxide production from glutamate or ketoglutarate. Others have failed to detect alterations in state 3 oxidation of pyruvate-malate-succinate, or glutamate-malate, in rat brain mitochondria from adult and old animals.[212]

Mitochondria appear to be substantially undamaged in both biochemical and morphologic terms, but they do show certain substrate-specific changes in function.[213] Such alterations may be attributed tentatively to the dehydrogenase involved, or to the carrier catalyzing transport across the mitochondrial membrane. Mitochondrial permeability also alters with age, and the composition of mitochondrial membranes change (see cell membranes below). However, while it may be possible to demonstrate age-changes in enzymes from mitochondria we must bear in mind the physiologic performance of the cell.[213] For example, energy transduction in the isolated, perfused heart from an old animal is very efficient, which raises doubts about some of the age-associated deterioration seen biochemically in isolated organelles. Another factor, frequently referred to in this review, relates to tissue complexity—in this case, metabolic heterogeneity within organs. This is often associated with differences in cell types, but in the liver can be extended to the location of the parenchymal cell within the liver lobule.[137]

Irrespective of the above considerations, the idea that mitochondria play a major role in aging and age-related illness has produced a burgeoning literature in the last 5 years. The damage to mitochondrial DNA described in an earlier section encourages the idea of reduced function in the bioenergetics of cells with advancing age. This topic is discussed in detail in a recent review.[106] However, it is clear that the small amount of damaged mitochondrial DNA, and the considerable reserve energy capacity in aged tissues, suggest that these organelles do not limit tissue function, although at the individual cell level damaged mitochondria may be critical. Wallace et al[106] argue that a system in bioenergetic decline could undergo severe failure if acutely stressed without prior conditioning. However, studies of old humans and rodents show considerable potential for improving aerobic capacity by training techniques,[214] and clearly, the mitochondrial populations of cardiac and skeletal muscle cells improve function under these conditions. This is an important area, since it is at the interface between changes in critical cell organelles and whole tissue metabolism. Clearly, if changes in diet, exercise, treatment with hormones, or compounds able to modify damage by reactive oxygen species can enable the reestablishment of cellular norms, this has great implications for the various cellular and molecular theories about aging.

Cell Membranes

Membranes are of primary importance in cellular function and age-associated changes in their structure and biochemistry have been investigated. Membranes regulate the passage of metabolites and ions in and out of the cell and the subcellular organelles; in addition, they are components of structural elements such as the respiratory assemblies of mitochondria and other membrane-bound enzymes and receptors.

Membrane composition

Studies of membrane composition have catalogued analyses of fatty acids, ratios of saturated to unsaturated fatty acids, the molar ratio of cholesterol to phospholipids, and the relative amounts of specific lipids. A consistent pattern of age-changes is found in the same type of membranes in different tissues, but no apparent relation between different membranes in the same tissue. In general, the cholesterol:phospholipid ratio seems to increase with age, and it has been postulated that this change would affect the fluidity of membranes. The reader is directed to major reviews that have tabulated the changes in membrane lipid composition with age,[108] and age-associated alterations in membrane composition of mitochondria.[213]

Membrane turnover

Using radioactive tracers it is possible to label lipids and obtain an estimate of the relative turnover rates of membranes. No age-associated change has been found in the turnover of phospholipid, neutral fractions or individual phospholipids (phosphatidyl ethanolamine and phosphatidyl choline), in either microsomes or mitochondria of rats. Others have shown no age-effect on mitochondrial membrane turnover.[206,215]

Membrane-associated proteins and enzymes

The ATPase required for calcium transport together with the steady-state concentration of membrane-lipid phosphorylated intermediates, and the rate of calcium transport, was measured at different ages in muscle membrane. In the steady state the phosphorylated intermediates were unchanged with age; however, ATPase activity fell between 2 and 12 months of age and rose between 24 and 28 months, ending at a higher level than younger animals. Calcium transport, although difficult to measure, was not reduced with age, but appeared to increase after 12 months. In fact, the efficiency of calcium uptake and Ca:Mg-ATPase activity may increase with age.

Alterations in membrane-bound enzymes have also been discovered in aging cells. It has been shown that ATPase activities decline in the sarcoplasmic reticulum of rat skeletal muscle between 2 and 12 months—and then rise to a high activity at 28 months of age. Others have shown that the Mg-ATPase and Na:K-ATPase activities in liver plasma membranes of old rats are decreased two fold when compared with young animals. These results are quite different from those described above for Ca:Mg-ATPase in rat sarcoplasmic reticulum membrane. One major difficulty in these studies is the use of animals under 3 months of age for comparison with old animals. It has been shown, for example, the Na:K-ATPase activity was constant in rat liver plasma membranes from about 5 to 22 months of age. However, a sharp reduction in activity occurred between 2.5 and 5 months of age. Thus, the examination of immature animals still undergoing active development could lead to erroneous conclusions about postreproductive aging. It is of interest that the activity of 5′-nucleotidase, a membrane-bound enzyme, drops between 6 and 22 to 29 months of age.

Qualitative evidence exists for age-changes in various membranes as shown by alterations in lipid composition, membrane-bound enzymes, and also hormone receptors. However, the lack of consistency in results from investigation to investigation leaves one uneasy about the quantitative aspects of these studies.[108]

Cellular Processes

Gene Expression

Early research focused on the ability of both exogenous (*E. coli*), and endogenous RNA polymerase to transcribe chromatin from rats and mice—chromatin template activity. The template activity of liver, kidney, and brain chromatin from young and old mice was reduced by 15 to 25 percent with age in all three tissues. The rate of radiolabeled uridine incorporation into RNA was greater per unit weight of DNA for chromatin from young liver. Since the length of the RNA chains formed from each age group were comparable, chromatin isolated from the young animal must have had more initiation sites to account for the increased incorporation of uridine. However, the use of homologous RNA polymerase extracted from the livers of young and old animals showed a surprising age-associated specificity; the polymerase prepared from the young liver was more active with the chromatin from young animals than that from old mice. The reverse was true when the polymerase extracted from the livers of old animals was used. In addition, if the polymerase and chromatin were age-matched they showed equal template activities.[216] Other investigators claimed that during neuronal aging the adaptive and regulatory mechanisms of chromatin template transcription are lost or become ineffective,[217,218] leading to a genetic restriction of neuronal chromatin. These changes suggest a severe age-associated restriction in the responsiveness of neurons from the cerebral cortex. More research is needed to clarify the situation, but it must be borne in mind that old cells may often react to stimuli, but only after a pronounced lag period. Studies of age-associated changes in neuronal plasticity *in vivo* suggest a continued ability to recover from damage at all ages, albeit at a slower rate with increasing age.[219]

Age-associated changes take place in the number and range of genes transcribed by cells. Age can be associated with a complete loss of function, an alteration in the rate of a particular process, or with some change in sensitivity to intra- and extracellular communication. Redundant (reiterated) DNA does not correlate with the maximum life span of several mammalian species,[220–222] but changes have been observed in the percentage of unique DNA sequences transcribed from brain tissue of young and old mice and humans. The number of rRNA genes expressed in liver, brain, kidney, and spleen of young and old mice decrease, but this variable undergoes constant modification during the life span. Preliminary studies of rRNA production in senescent HDF suggests some change in the kinetics of rRNA processing in these cells.[223]

The expression of genes, and the production of macromolecules late in the life span is of critical importance when trying to understand aging at the cellular level. The key question is to what extent somatic cells retain the ability to produce the correct synthetic responses to the demands of the body as a whole, and local functional demands. The sources of age-related changes in gene expression are therefore many and various. DNA sequences may be altered through a number of mechanisms: there may be epigenetic changes (e.g., DNA methylation, see below), altered rates of transcription, and splicing of macromolecules. The process of identifying age-associated changes in macromolecular synthesis, and of assessing the functionality of aged cells, is complicated by confounding factors relating to disease in either humans or rodents (see above).[12] It is naive to imagine that we will locate a universal alteration in gene expression with age. What is usually meant when we discuss age-associated changes in gene expression, is alterations in the stability of function in a particular tissue. For this reason, numbers of studies that examine whole organs, such as the brain or liver, without fractionating into specific cell types, are of little use.

The data available suggest that, qualitatively, there is very little difference in cell and tissue-specific gene expression with advancing age. Exceptions to this finding are the major involutions of organs like the thymus, and the ovary in the postreproductive stage of the life span.[224] Most cells appear to maintain function and differentiation throughout the life span, although once again, there are exceptions. The magnocellular nuclei of the hypothalamus produce the antidiuretic hormone, arginine vasopressin (AVP). The homozygous Brattleboro (*di/di*) rat cannot produce AVP because of a frameshift mutation, due to a single-base pair deletion in the AVP gene. This mutation prevents proper expression and secretion of AVP by the magnocellular neurones. However, in these animals, AVP immunoreactive neurones appear in a linear fashion from birth up to about 2 years of age, and then reduce slowly.[225] These solitary neurones are heterozygous, expressing both mutant protein and the normal, unprocessed neurophysin precursor protein. The most recent research suggests that this age-related reversion of the mutant phenotype is primarily due to a two-base pair, which restores the AVP coding sequence reading frame downstream of the deletion.[226] An additional feature of this work is that the same GA deletion is found in wild-type rats,[226] which suggests a much higher frequency of mutation in the AVP gene than for the overall somatic cell DNA mutation rate in these neurones. At present these are isolated observations, and they may be specific to the Long-Evans strain of rat.

Epigenetic Effects

Environmental and developmental factors can influence the expression of genes.[227] Changes in gene expression are essential components of aging, and there are detailed reviews of the range of age-associated alterations encountered.[30] The structure of chromatin at the site of a gene governs the way a gene is expressed. DNA methylation[228] has been strongly implicated as a factor in gene control. The expression of certain genes is correlated strongly with demethylation, particularly in embryonic and fetal tissues (e.g., globin genes in a variety of species, and genes from certain viruses).[229] This group of genes is demethylated in tissues where they are expressed, and methylated where they are not. In another group of genes, demethylation is not apparently correlated with expression in tissues, and in at least one case, methylation is associated with actual expression.[229]

DNA methylation may decrease with age, although this is not the case for all genes.[230] The level of 5′-methylcytosine in the DNA of human, mouse, and hamster diploid fibroblasts declines during serial subculture. The rate of decline is greatest in mouse fibroblasts and slowest in human cells, suggesting that the maintenance of methylation may be a prerequisite of long-term survival in vitro.[231] Since diploid fibroblasts are connective tissue cells, it is possible that demethylation may activate genes that are normally repressed, leading to their aging and death. This idea has some support from studies using the demethylating agents azacytidine, or azadeoxycytidine. A single treatment of young cells with a low dose of either of these compounds is followed by recovery, with a completely normal morphology and growth rate, but the cells die prematurely.[232] These studies are indirect evidence for the view that the maintenance of methylation is important for long-term survival of HDF.[233] There are other age-associated alterations in DNA methylation; for example, the genomes of certain endogenous viruses are demethylated in specific tissues with advancing age.[234] Thus, this epigenetic phenomenon may influence the aging of cells and tissues, and may prove to be a link between aging and cancer.[229]

The idea of aging being due to a loss of the differentiated state of cells has been discussed.[235] The early experiments, although interesting, were not conclusive. Certain genes are expressed in tissues from old animals that result in the production of proteins not considered appropriate for the tissue. There was a greater degree of expression of globin synthesis by the

DNA of old versus young brain, and the ratio of globin RNA to total RNA in the cytoplasm was increased with age for each age group.[236] However, no attempt was made to differentiate between the diverse cells found in brain tissue, thus negating the impact of the findings. Other observations were more persuasive. There is a random inactivation of one of the two X-chromosomes in each cell of female placental animals during early development. Apparently, this inactivation is stable through mitosis, so that all descendants have the same active X-chromosome and the same inactive one.[237] Each adult female is a mosaic with regard to X-chromosome activity.[237] An experiment conducted several years ago showed that the gene responsible for coat color in mice can be inactivated by inserting it into an X-chromosome. The gene involved is wild-type tyrosinase, which on inactivation, produces an albino coat. However, as these mice grew older, the animals became progressively more pigmented indicating that the tyrosinase gene was reactivated.[238] A similar observation was made on the expression of sex-linked ornithine carbamoyl transferase gene in the liver.[239] Methylation appears to play a role in maintaining the stability of the inactive X-chromosome, then the loss of methylation may be the cause of the reactivation process. Studies of another human, X-linked gene (hypoxanthine phosphoribosyltransferase), showed that heterozygous women with a severe deficiency of the enzyme, show rare, age-associated reactivation of the gene. However, demethylation with 5-azacytidine induced activity in white cells from old donors but not young ones.[240] These findings are not necessarily incompatible with the notion that imperfect inheritance of gene methylation patterns causes gene reactivation with increasing age.[241] Evolutionary reasons might mean that the control of X-inactivation is likely to be far tighter in long-lived, when compared with short-lived, species. The fact that the gene was reactivated more easily in white cells from old donors suggests that some demethylation had taken place, even though there was no detectable reactivation of the gene.

Control of gene expression

DNA methylation is one way of regulating gene expression, but there are many others. There are processes that mediate both gene activation and repression. The idea of differential gene expression goes with the process of cell differentiation. Transcription control involves the transfer of genetic information from DNA to RNA, with specific interaction of transcription regulatory proteins and specific regulatory DNA sequences. These processes occur in the promoter and enhancer regions of the gene. The regulatory DNA sequences are the cis-acting sequences, usually at the 5′ end of the coding region, although this is not always the case. The cis-acting sequences serve as recognition sites for the binding of specific trans-acting factors that serve to activate or repress gene expression. Recent research has focused on the signaling pathways associated with the expression of the so-called stress response genes that include the early immediate genes (*c-fos* and *c-jun*) and the heat shock proteins. Many of these genes undergo age-associated change, and the subject is reviewed extensively elsewhere.[242] The AP-1 cis-acting site binds fos-jun dimers that are members of a super family of trans-acting factors induced by polypeptide hormones, growth factors, cytokines, and neurotransmitters. These transcriptional factors undergo post-translational modifications that determine their level of activity. In rat hepatocytes there is a rise in constitutive levels of both c-fos and c-jun in the absence of known stress factors, suggesting chronic stress or constant stimulation of these genes.[243] In addition, AP-1 binding activity is more strongly induced in the hippocampus of aged rats.[244] Age-associated changes in heat shock protein have been detected in senescent HDF, hepatocytes, and hippocampus.[242] Induction of heat shock proteins (HSP70) by various stimuli in senescent HDF is significantly reduced, and is attributed to a reduction in the transcription of the HSP70.[245] The reduced transcription observed correlated with the loss of heat shock factor binding activity that activates the HSP70 gene.[246] Numbers of different lines of research are now converging with connections being made between heat shock gene expression, oxidative stress, and factors that may determine life span of animals. Mutant strains of the nematode *Caenorhabditis elegans* show a 70-percent increase in mean and maximum life span. The age mutations show an increased thermal tolerance to temperature stress and overexpression of a nematode heat shock protein—HSP16.[247]

This is a rapidly developing field and seems to be bringing together a number of different lines of research. However, what is not yet clear regarding the alterations in gene regulation of so-called stress response genes in vivo, is to what extent the changes are to do with the levels of stimulating factors at different ages.

RNA and Protein Synthesis

Changes in protein metabolism would be the major feature of age-associated differences in gene expression, and would have far-reaching effects on the physiology of cell, and ultimately organ homeostasis. Inadequate, or faulty replacement of protein components, particularly under conditions of maximum demand, could explain the lower physiologic capabilities of senescent animals. The obvious link between concentrations of RNA and protein synthesis has led to the study of the role of RNA in aging. Alterations in RNA levels may be brought about by a reduction in gene expression or changes in the activity of RNA polymerases. There is no experimental evidence to suggest that RNA synthesis is reduced to the extent that there is a damaging lack of protein synthesis, nor is there any undisputed evidence for loss of RNA polymerase activity with age. A careful study of specific mRNA species found in hepatocytes from animals of various ages showed that there was no general trend in the synthesis of mRNA with age.[248] Age did not seem to affect the size of the mRNA molecules, nor was there a change in the post-transcriptional processing of five mRNA species studied. The age-associated alterations in mRNA species were similar to the changes in the levels of the proteins coded for by these mRNAs. Thus, age-associated changes in the transcription of mRNA is the primary site of the regulation of protein concentrations at advanced ages.[248] Furthermore, the fidelity of transcription processes in nonmitotic cells is not affected by aging.[108,130]

The study of large-scale RNAs and protein synthesis with increased age shows little change with increasing age in rodents. Many of the early investigations of protein synthesis in old rodents examined enzyme activity, and no particular patterns emerged that could establish a general underlying cause of aging. Later studies looked at markers such as RNA sequence complexity, which gives a direct measure of the number of different active genes. These methods, although an improvement on the earlier approaches, do not give very precise measures of RNA concentrations, and would not detect quite large alterations in base mRNA species. However, most investigators agree that the overall mRNA levels do not change with age in either liver or brain.[249,250]

The fact that overall RNA and protein synthesis is maintained in old tissues and cells in rodents does not illuminate central issues of protein metabolism. There are a number of reviews that deal with this issue.[108,190,251,252] There are two viewpoints:

- Aging is accompanied by a reduction in overall RNA and protein synthesis.[108,251]
- The techniques used are not accurate enough to give unequivocal support for a decline in overall RNA and protein synthesis.[190,252]

Part of the reason for the disparate findings is the lack of information provided on the pool sizes of the constituents involved in protein synthesis, including the appropriate amino acid, tRNA and tRNA synthetase concentrations. In a review of this length it is difficult to present the arguments for and against these viewpoints. They are well covered elsewhere and the reader is directed to Finch's seminal work for a review of the issues.[30]

There are only a few definitive studies of protein metabolism that control appropriately for the same concentrations of precursor molecules. Studies of protein metabolism in intact animals show no significant change in the rate of incorporation of radiolabeled amino acids into the heart.[253] However, there is an increased uptake of leucine in the liver of old mice, and the hepatocytes from old animals show a decreased incorporation of Q-aminolevulinic acid (a precursor of the haem coenzymes) into the microsomal fraction. The decreased incorporation of amino acids involved in the synthesis of haem proteins may affect drug metabolism, and the increased leucine incorporation may reflect the increase in serum albumin synthesis with age.[253] On the other hand, there is a decrease in the incorporation of radiolabeled lysine in mitochondria-free cell supernatants from rat brain between 16 and 22 months of age.[254] Even though Finch's concerns about the techniques employed are valid, there is now a general acceptance that aging is accompanied by a reduction in RNA and protein synthesis. One relatively recent study examined protein synthesis in the liver of F344 rats using a perfusion technique that enabled the control of the specific activities of the amino acid valine and its tRNA. Both protein synthesis and degradation showed parallel changes at several ages,[255] with an overall reduction of 40 percent over 2 years of the life span.

Studies on humans show no age-changes of total protein synthesis in healthy, nonobese elderly men. Sophisticated techniques using radiolabeled glycine and leucine show that total body protein metabolism did not alter when normalized for body weight.[256–259]

These data suggest that in both humans and rodents the total body protein metabolism is probably unchanged. However, this is not particularly helpful when trying to assess the functional status of individual organs. The human material suggests that aging is associated with an alteration in tissue energy metabolism,[260] and this implies a change in protein metabolism. Elderly people are more likely to be affected by various biologic, environmental, and social factors that would generally increase protein needs above those for younger adults. The decline in energy intake in old people, together with its possible consequences for reducing the efficiency of dietary protein utilization, also will tend to increase the protein need for elderly subjects, relative to that for physically more active young adults. It has been advocated that an appropriate protein allowance would be 12 to 14 percent of the total energy intake.[261] Clearly, the consensus of opinion regarding protein metabolism in the rat is that there is a decline in protein synthesis in individual organs. This has clear implications for other aspects of protein structure dealt with previously.

The effect of age of the synthesis of specific proteins has also been investigated. One protein that has attracted particular attention is the liver protein α_{2u}-globulin. There are marked decreases with age in the production of mRNA, showing marked reduction of protein production at the transcription level. Both α_{2u}-globulin mRNA and its transcription decline in parallel after maturation.[262,263] The α_{2u}-globulin gene dissociates from the nuclear matrix when transcription decreases, whereas genes that continue to function throughout the life span do not.[264] Subsequent studies have shown that the subpopulation of hepatocytes that synthesize α_{2u}-globulin appear to disappear from the liver late in the life span.[265] Rats on a calorie-restricted diet show no age-associated change in α_{2u}-globulin transcription, and this has been related to hormone changes effected during this treatment.[263]

Tissue slices and short-term cell culture

There is considerable literature on this subject.[108] Some studies show an age-associated reduction in the uptake of labeled amino acids into tissue slices from the rat parotid gland,[266] but similar changes could not be found in the brain[267] or liver.[268] Intact rat hepatocytes show a marked increase in protein synthesis with age, although there are significant fluctuations throughout the life span.[108]

Cell-free preparations

Cell-free preparations of liver tissue have been used frequently for studies of age-associated changes in protein metabolism.[269] Other tissues have also been investigated, including rat testes, kidney, and brain, and mouse muscle. The overall conclusion is that in cell-free systems protein synthetic abilities appear to be reduced with age.[108] However, the actual rate of protein synthesis in these systems is approximately 1 percent of the activity found in vivo so the precise relation of these findings to the intact cell, organ, or organism is debatable.

Perhaps the major differences described in the literature are not necessarily associated with aging but, more likely, with methods of investigation and shortcomings in techniques.[146] This makes extrapolation from in vitro to in vivo situations more hazardous than usual. Thus, while the study of isolated cells and cell-free synthetic systems is of importance when trying to assess rate-limiting steps in cellular biochemistry, attention must always be paid to the physiologic changes seen in cells and organs when interprcting the changes.

Cellular Homeostasis

This brief, final, section is about the control of cell number with advancing age. Age-associated changes in cell proliferation are well described. Studies in vitro have established a limit to the number of cell divisions that normal HDF will go through before "replicative senescence" takes place.[15] One of the challenges that has faced in vitro researchers is in persuading those investigators who work on cells in vivo that their model means anything at the whole organism level. In vivo greatest concern is usually expressed over escape from the control of cell division with the prospect of neoplasia.[52] There are other issues regarding postmitotic cells: do they die throughout the life span, and if they do, how do they do it? And what happens in organisms that are essentially composed of postmitotic cells, except for germinal cells?

Cell Replication

Clearly, replicative senescence in vitro is well established. According to a number of investigators the process is controlled by multiple dominant-acting genes.[270] The idea that telomeres may control the number of cell divisions has been discussed above. We now know that senescent cells can begin the process of DNA synthesis by expanding nucleotide pools and inducing certain enzymes, but the genes needed for the progression of the cell cycle are repressed. The senescent cells survive for a prolonged period of time and there is now recognition that replicative senescence and differentiation may be one and the same thing,[25,270] although this is disputed territory (see above). The change in dermal fibroblasts after they have stopped dividing is quite marked, and it is argued that in their replicating state they are rapidly producing extracellular matrix, whereas, when they differentiate in vitro, they have a greater propensity for matrix degeneration.[271–273]

Campisi et al.[270] suggest two possible functions for replicative senescence:

- Senescent cells accumulate with age and contribute to age-related dysfunction.
- Replicative senescence is a tumor suppression mechanism.

The first is hardly a function, but more an indeterminate end to the replicative process. The assumption is that the observations made during the postreplicative differentiation process in vitro is similar to that seen in vivo. There is evidence for the apparent priming of certain proteases of fibroblast cells in aged skin,[274] although whether this can be construed as contributing to age-associated dysfunction is questionable. Observations made in vitro that are marshalled in support of this view include the age-associated reduction in proliferative ability of cells from old donors, the shorter life span of cells from short-lived species, the shorter replicative life span of progeriod subects, and altered control of gene regulation in senescent cells. The second idea relating to tumor suppression gains support from the following observations: many tumors contain cells that have passed the limits of replicative senescence; mutations that lead to neoplasia involve mechanisms that allow cells to escape replicative control; and activities of two well-known tumor suppressor genes are involved in the control of replicative senescence.[270]

A strong case has been made over the years for replicative senescence being under genetic control.[15] Hybridization experiments were carried out to investigate the role of cytoplasmic factors in in vitro senescence.[275] Hybrids between anucleate cytoplasms (cytoplasts) and inactivated normal HDF showed that the enzymes of untreated cytoplasts replaced inactivated enzymes of whole cells and permitted hybrid cell survival. The hybrids formed by old cytoplasts-old cells and young cytoplasts-old cells had a low doubling potential, whereas those hybrids involving young cells survived similar doubling to the controls.[275] Postmitotic, aged HDF may synthesize some specific repressor molecule(s) that inhibits the initiation of DNA synthesis.[276] Subsequent work showed that heterokaryons of old HDF, and either SV80-transformed HDF or HeLa cells, initiated DNA synthesis in the old nuclei.[277] These results strongly implicate positive control of DNA synthesis by the HeLa and SV80-transformed cells over that of the proposed repressor compound. If young HDF are in the S-phase of the cell cycle when they are fused to senescent cells, then DNA synthesis proceeds.[278] On the other hand, entry into the S-phase is inhibited because young HDF in the G1 phase of the cell cycle (when fused with senescent HDF), do not synthesize DNA.[278] These results are consistent with the hypothesis that senescence involves a block preventing cells in G1 entering the S phase.[279] It is possible to induce a superficial senescent phenotype in HDF cells using various manipulations, and it is possible to analyze and "dissect" cells from such treatments using hybridization procedures.[280,281] Fusions between different immortal human cells have led to the isolation of four distinct complementation groups.[282] Three of these complementation groups have been assigned to chromosomes 1, 4, and 7, although other chromosomes have induced a finite replicative life span in immortal cell lines.[283–285] Despite these findings with chromosomes, the genes involved have not been identified. There is some controversy over these findings. The number of chromosomes that induce senescence are greater than the number of complementation groups and, although explanations have been put forward to explain these observations, only the identity of the genes involved in the induction of senescence will suffice. It has been suggested that the complementation is due to delayed toxicity of the drugs used to select the hybrids,[286] but this has been refuted.[270]

The debate over replicative senescence rumbles on. However, in my view, the major question is not what occurs in culture (although considerable clarification is required on the role of genetic control over senescence) but what happens in vivo? There is not a great deal of evidence in support of replicative senescence in vivo. Postmitotic cell populations in skeletal muscle and the central nervous system appear to survive very much intact until late in the life span. There is debate about whether this is true in the cerebral cortex, but in the evolutionary older parts of the brain, the hypothalamus and the brain stem, neuronal populations stay intact.[287–289] The last 20 years of research into the morphology of the aged brain suggest that, in healthy individuals, atrophic change is more a feature of neuronal aging than cell death.[290,291] Are neurons, which presumably have undergone some form of replicative senescence, senescent cells that contribute to age-related dysfunction? Clearly, postmitotic cells do undergo senescent changes, but they occur late in the life span and are subject to complex alterations that take place in the environment of the body, whether this is related to levels of growth factors or even chronic stimulation with adrenal[292] or ovarian hormones.[293] Furthermore, although early transplantation studies of ovaries and skin between young and old animals suggested that young fertilized ovaries, or eggs, functioned less well in old compared with young recipients, the findings were generally equivocal.[294] In particular, the skin grafting results were difficult to interpret; in some cases the grafts from old animals grew as well as those from younger mice. During successive transplants the grafts became progressively smaller and many were lost, but this was common to samples from both young and old animals. A major problem was that cells from the host tissue migrated into the transplant during wound repair. Transplants of bone marrow stem cells were subsequently employed to reduce the problem of identifying the donor and host cells. The host was irradiated to kill all of its intrinsic stem cell population, and then was inoculated with donor cells. A chromosomal abnormality was used to identify donor tissue in an elegant study of the division capacity of marrow stem cells in mice.[295] Marrow cells were serially transplanted into recipients and this procedure was repeated annually. After four successive transplants, the stem cells had a reduced capacity to repopulate the host's marrow. It was concluded that the maximum life span of the mouse was very close to that of the functional division capacity of the marrow cells and that they were programmed in some way to age and die at the same time.

Subsequently, it was shown that successive transplantations caused nonspecific damage to stem cells; furthermore, the stem cell pool could be exhausted when constant division is stimulated.[296] The most definitive studies were carried out on mice with a genetic defect that causes hereditary anemia due to stem cell abnormalities.[297] In this case the mice do not require lethal irradiation and, if a transplant is successful, the anemia is cured. Red cell production was measured in the recipients after transplantation, so a direct measure of stem cell function was obtained. Since the cure of the hereditary anemia never occurs spontaneously, the donor cells are identified unambiguously, and the effects of cells from both young and old donor cells can be compared in the recipients. In these studies there was no evidence for intrinsic aging of the red-cell-producing stem cells.

Cell Death

One feature of aging cells that has only recently been addressed is the issue of cell death. A feature of senescent HDF in culture is they are resistant to apoptosis.[270,298] If HDF are resistant to programmed cell death in vivo, then there is the potential for the accumulation of nonfunctioning cells in tissues, (e.g., skin). Information on apoptosis in aged tissues in vivo is almost nonexistent. We have been examining the response of neurons to ischemic damage in aged mice and have evidence of apoptosis in the region of the infarct, although there is no qualitative difference between young and old animals up to 48 hours after the induction of ischemia (Davies et al, unpublished results). This is an area that requires further research.

Conclusion

The literature on aging has expanded dramatically during the past 20 years. Cell and molecular biologic studies are increasing our knowledge of the steps involved in cellular regulation and are posing new questions for us to ask. I am convinced that we have made real progress in our understanding of aging and age-associated changes, although I am concerned with our poor definition of what aging is. The challenge, as always, is to track down causes, and this, in my view, will be the difficult task. We are still relying too heavily on correlative data, and extrapolating too readily from factors that affect life span to effects on aging. Much of the genetic research is on survival of organisms and does not seem to have produced a mechanism for aging. The cellular mechanism that is considered the "hottest" area, the effect of reactive oxygen species, has been around for 40 years, and the evidence for it is still only correlative. In my view, we can expect little more. After all, we are dealing with the major frontier in biology.

References

1. Comfort A: The Biology of Senescence. 3rd Ed. Elsevier, New York, 1979
2. Strehler BL: Time, cells and ageing. Academic Press, New York, 1962
3. Harrison DE, Archer JR: Biomarkers of aging-tissue markers—future research needs, strategies, directions and priorities. Exp Gerontol 1988;23:309–321
4. Dean W, Morgan RF: In defense of the concept of biological aging measurement. Current status. Arch Geriatr Gerontol 1988;7:191–210
5. Costa PT, McCrae RR: Measures and markers of biological aging. A great clamoring of fleeting significance! Arch Geriatr Gerontol 1988;7:211–214
6. Gibson DC, Adelman RC, Finch C: Development of the Rodent as a Model System of Aging. U.S. Department of Health, Education and Welfare, Bethesda, 1978
7. Lints FA: Non-mammalian models for research on aging. S Karger, Basel, 1985
8. Schneider EL, Smith JR: The relationship of in vitro studies to in vivo human aging. Int Rev Cytol 1981;69:261–270
9. Beauchene RE, Roeder LM, Barrows Jr CH: The inter-relationships of age, tissue protein synthesis, and proteinuria. J Gerontol 1970;25:359–363
10. Szilard L: A theory of ageing. Nature 1959;184:957
11. Orgel LE: The maintenance of the accuracy of protein synthesis and its relevance to ageing. Proc Nat Acad Sci U S A 1963; 49:517–521
12. Finch CE: Longevity, Senescence and the Genome. University of Chicago Press, Chicago, 1990
13. Kirkwood TBL, Cremer T: Cytogerontology since 1891—a reappraisal of August Weismann and a review of modern progress. Hum Genet 1982;60:101–121
14. Hayflick L, Moorhead PS: The serial cultivation of human diploid cell strains. Exp Cell Res 1961;25:585–621
15. Hayflick L: The limited in vitro lifetime of human diploid cell strains. Exp Cell Res 1965;37:614–636
16. Hay RJ, Strehler BL: The limited growth span of cell strains isolated from the chick embryo. Exp Gerontol 1967;2: 123–135
17. Hay RJ, Menzies RA, Morgan HP, Strehler BL: The division potential of cells in continuous growth as compared to cells subcultivated after maintenance in stationary phase. Exp Gerontol 1968;3:35–44
18. Ryan JM, Sharf BB, Cristofalo VJ: The influence of culture medium volume on cell density and life-span of human diploid fibroblasts. Exp Cell Res 1975;91:389–393
19. Ryan JM, Nielsen PJ, Nelson LR: The effects of division rate-limiting amounts of fetal bovine serum on the proliferation and aging of cultured chick-cells. J Cell Physiol 1982;110: 175–182
20. Franks LM: Cellular aspects of ageing. Exp Gerontol 1970;5: 281–289
21. Cristofalo VJ, Stanulis BM: Cell aging: a model system. In Behnke JA, Finch CE, Moment GB (eds): The Biology of Aging. Plenum Press, New York, 1978
22. Waters H, Walford RL: Latent period for outgrowth of human skin explants as a function of age. J Gerontol 1970;25: 381–383
23. Martin GM, Sprague CA, Epstein CJ: Replicative lifespan of cultivated human cells. Effects of donor's age, tissue and genotype. Lab Invest 1970;23:86–92
24. Hornsby PJ, Gill GN, Bell E: Loss of division potential in culture; aging or differentiation. Science 1980;208:1482
25. Bayreuther K, Rodemann HP, Hommel R et al: Human skin fibroblasts in vitro differentiate along a terminal cell lineage. Proc Nat Acad Sci U S A 1988;85:5112–5116
26. Olashaw NE, Kress ED, Cristofalo VJ: Thymidine triphosphate synthesis in senescent WI- 38 cells: relationship to loss of replicative activity. Exp Cell Res 1983;149:547–554
27. Pendergrass WR, Saulewicz AC, Salk D, Norwood T: Induction of DNA polymerase alpha in senescent cultures of normal and Werner's syndrome cultured skin fibroblasts. J Cell Physiol 1985;124:331–336
28. Rittling SR, Brooks KM, Cristofalo VJ, Baserga R: Expression of cell cycle-dependent genes in young and senescent WI38 fibroblasts. Proc Nat Acad Sci U S A 1986;83:3316–3320
29. Norwood TH, Smith JR, Stein G: Aging at the cellular level: the human fibroblast like cell model. p. 131. In Schneider EL, Rowe JW (eds): Handbook of the Biology of Aging. Academic Press, San Diego, 1990
30. Finch CE: Longevity, Senescence and the Genome. University of Chicago Press, Chicago, 1990
31. Kirkwood TBL, Holliday R: Commitment to senescence: a model for the finite and infinite growth of diploid and transformed human fibroblasts in culture. J Theor Biol 1975;53: 481–497
32. Prothero J, Gallant JA: A model of clonal attenuation. Proc Nat Acad Sci U S A 1981;78:333–337
33. Holliday R, Huschtscha LI, Tarrant GM, Kirkwood TB: Testing the commitment theory of cellular aging. Science 1977;198: 366–372
34. Harley CB, Goldstein S: Retesting the commitment theory cellular aging. Science 1980;207:191–192
35. Holliday R, Kirkwood TB: Predictions of the somatic mutation and mortalization theories of cellular ageing are contrary to experimental observations. J Theor Biol 1981;93:627–642
36. Smith JR, Lincoln DW: Aging of cells in culture. Int Rev Cytol 1984;89:151–177
37. Stanulis-Praeger B: Cellular senescence revisited. A review. Mech Age Devel 1987;38:1–48
38. Macieira-Coelho A: Biology of normal proliferating cells in vitro. Relevance for in vivo aging. Karger, Basel, 1988
39. Angello JC, Prothero J: Independent evidence for a commitment model of clonal attenuation. Mech Age Devel 1989;49: 281–286
40. Epstein CJ, Martin GM, Schultz AL, Motulsky AG: Werner's syndrome. A review of its symptomatology, natural history, pathological features, genetics and relationship to the natural aging process. Medicine 1966;45:177–186

41. Martin GM: Genetic syndromes in man with potential relevance to the pathobiology of ageing. pp. 539. In Bergsma D, Harrison DE (eds): Genetic Effects of Ageing. Birth Defects. Vol. 14. Alan R Liss, New York, 1978
42. Goto M, Rubenstein M, Weber J et al: Genetic linkage of Werner's syndrome to five markers on chromosome 8. Nature 1992;355:735–738
43. Chang M, Burmer GC, Sweasy J et al: Evidence against DNA polymerase beta as a candidate gene for Werner syndrome. Hum Genet 1994;93:507–512
44. Goddard KA, Yu CE, Oshima J et al: Toward localization of the Werner syndrome gene by linkage disequilibrium and ancestral haplotyping: lessons learned from analysis of 35 chromosome 8p 11.1–21.1 markers. Am J Hum Genet 1996;58: 1286–1302
45. Yu CE, Oshima J, Fu YH et al: Positional cloning of the Werner's syndrome gene [see comments]. Science 1996;272: 258–262
46. Faragher RG, Kill IR, Hunter JA et al: The gene responsible for Werner syndrome may be a cell division "counting" gene. Proc Nat Acad Sci U S A 1993;90:12030–12034
47. Kruk PA, Rampino NJ, Bohr VA: DNA damage and repair in telomeres: relation to aging. Proc Nat Acad Sci U S A 1995; 92:258–262
48. Schulz VP, Zakian VA, Ogburn CE et al: Accelerated loss of telomeric repeats may not explain accelerated replicative decline of Werner syndrome cells. Hum Genet 1996;97: 750–754
49. Mann DMA: The pathological association between Down syndrome and Alzheimer disease. Mech Age Devel 1988;43: 99–136
50. Wyllie AH, Duvall E, Blow JJ: Intracellular mechanisms in cell death in normal and pathological tissues. p. 269. In Davies I, Sigee DC (eds): Cell Ageing and Cell Death. Cambridge University Press, Cambridge, 1984
51. Curtis HJ: Genetic factors in aging. Adv Genet 1971;16: 305–324
52. Martin GM, Fry M, Loeb LA: Somatic mutation and aging in mammalian cells. p. 7. In Sohal RS, Birnbaum LS, Cutler RG (eds): Molecular Biology of Aging: Gene Stability and Gene Expression. Aging. Vol. 29. Raven Press, New York, 1985
53. Pincheira J, Gallo C, Bravo M et al: G2 repair and aging: influence of donor age on chromosomal aberrations in human lymphocytes. Mutation Res 1993;295:55–62
54. Harley CA, Flutcher AB, Greider CW: Telomeres shorten during ageing of human fibroblasts. Nature 1990;345:458–460
55. Harley CB, Vaziri H, Counter CM, Allsopp RC: The telomere hypothesis of aging. Exp Gerontol 1992;27:375–382
56. Bernstein H, Gensler HL: DNA damage and aging. p. 89. In Yu BP (ed): Free Radicals in Aging. CRC Press, Boca Raton, 1993
57. Failla G: The ageing process and carcinogenesis. Ann NY Acad Sci 1958;71:1124–1135
58. Alexander P: The relationship between ageing and cancer; somatic mutations or breakdown of host defence mechanisms. Bull Schweiz Akad Med Wiss 1969;24:258–271
59. Yuhas JM: Age and susceptibility to reduction in life expectancy; an analysis of proposed mechanisms. Exp Gerontol 1971;6:335–344
60. Price GB, Makinodan T: Ageing: alteration of DNA-protein information. Gerontologia 1973;19:58–70
61. Bergtold DS, Lett JT: Alterations in chromosomal DNA and aging: an overview. p. 23. In Sohal RS, Birnbaum LS, Cutler RG (eds): Molecular Biology of Aging: Gene Stability and Gene Expression. Aging. Vol. 29: Raven Press, New York, 1985
62. Dean RG, Cutler RG: Absence of significant age-dependent increase of single-stranded DNA extracted from mouse liver nuclei. Exp Gerontol 1978;13:287–292
63. Finch CE: Susceptibility of mouse liver DNA to digestion by S1 nuclease: absence of age-related change. Age 1979;2:45–46
64. Maizel A, Nicolini C, Baserga R: Structural alterations in chromatin in phase III WI-38 human diploid fibroblasts. Exp Cell Res 1975;96:351–360
65. Icard C, Beaupain R, Diatloff C, Macieira-Coelho A: Effect of low dose irradiation on the division potential of cells in vitro. VI. Changes in DNA and in radiosensitivity during ageing of human fibroblasts. Mech Age Devel 1979;11:269–278
66. Suzuki F, Watanabe E, Horikawa M: Repair of x-ray induced DNA damage in ageing human diploid cells. Exp Cell Res 1980;127:299–308
67. Dell'Orco RT, Whittle WL: Evidence for an increased level of DNA change in high doubling level human diploid cells in culture. Mech Age Devel 1981;15:141–150
68. Shmookler Reiss RJ, Goldstein S: Loss of reiterated DNA sequences during serial passage of human diploid fibroblasts. Cell 1980;21:739–749
69. Macieira-Coelho A, Bengtsson A, Van der Ploeg M: Distribution of DNA between sister cells during serial subcultivation of human fibroblasts. Histochem 1982;75:11–24
70. Tice RR, Setlow RB: DNA repair and replication in aging organisms and cells. p. 173. In Finch CE, Schneider EL (eds): Handbook of the Biology of Aging. Van Nostrand Reinhold, New York, 1985
71. Rattan SIS: DNA damage and repair during cellular aging. Int Rev Cytol 1989;116:47–88
72. Marnett LJ, Burcham PC: Endogenous DNA adducts: potential and paradox. Chem Res Toxicol 1993;6:771–785
73. Halliwell B: Free radicals, oxygen toxicity and ageing. p. 1. In Sohal RS (ed): Age pigments. Elsevier/North Holland Biomedical Press, Amsterdam, 1981
74. Gutteridge JMC: Free radicals and aging. Rev Clin Geront 1994;4:279–288
75. Harman D: Ageing; a theory based on free radical and radiation chemistry. J Gerontol 1956;11:298–300
76. Glass GA, Gershon D: Enzymatic changes in rat erythrocytes with increasing cell and donor age—loss of superoxide-dismutase activity associated with increases in catalytically defective forms. Biochem Biophys Res Commun 1981;103:1245–1253
77. Stohs SJ, Al-Turk WA, Angle CR: Glutathione S-transferase and glutathione-reductase activities in hepatic and extra-

hepatic tissues of the female mice as a function of age. Bioch Pharm 1982;31:2113–2116

78. Dovart A, Gershon D: Rat lens superoxide-dismutase and glucose-6-phosphate-dehydrogenase—studies on the catalytic activity and the fate of enzyme antigen as a function of age. Exp Eye Res 1981;33:651–661

79. Tolmasoff JM, Ono T, Cutler RG: Superoxide dismutase—correlation with life-span and specific metabolic rate in primate species. Proc Nat Acad Sci U S A 1980;77:2777–2781

80. Miquel J, Lundgren PR, Bensch KG: Effects of oxygen-nitrogen (1:1) at 760 Torr on the life span and fine structure of *Drosophila melanogaster*. Mech Age Devel 1975;4:41–59

81. Harman D: Prolongation of the normal life-span and inhibition of spontaneous cancer by antioxidants. J Gerontol 1961;16: 247–255

82. Comfort A, Youhotsky-Gore I, Pathmanathan K: Effect of ethoxyquin on the longevity of C3H mice. Nature 1971;229: 254–255

83. Pryor WA: The free-radical theory of aging revisited: a critique and a suggested disease-specific theory. p. 89. In Warner HR, Butler RN, Sprott RL, Schneider EL (eds): Modern Biological Theories of Aging. Aging. Vol. 31. Raven Press, New York, 1987

84. Reveillaud J, Niedzwiecki A, Bensch KG, Fleming E: Expression of bovine superoxide dismutase in *Drosophila melanogaster* augments resistance to oxidative stress. Mol Cell Biol 1991; 11:632–640

85. Orr WC, Sohal RS: Extension of life-span by overexpression of superoxide dismutase and catalase in *Drosophila melanogaster*. Science 1994;263:1128–1130

86. Kohn RR: Effect of antioxidants on lifespan of C57BL mice. J Gerontol 1971;26:378–380

87. Epstein J, Gershon D: Studies on ageing in nematodes. IV. The effect of anti-oxidants on cellular damage and life-span. Mech Age Devel 1972;1:257–264

88. Freund G: Effects of chronic alcohol and vitamin E consumption on ageing pigments and learning performance in mice. Life Sci 1979;24:145–152

89. Tappel AL, Fletcher B, Deamer D: Effect of antioxidants and nutrients on lipid peroxidation fluorescent products and aging parameters in the mouse. J Gerontol 1973;28:415–424

90. Davies I, Davidson YS, Fotheringham AP: The effect of vitamin E deficiency on the induction of age pigment in various tissues of the mouse. Exp Gerontol 1987;22:127–137

91. Ames BN, Gold LS: Endogenous mutagens and the causes of aging and cancer. Mutation Res 1991;250:3–16

92. Ames BN, Saul RL, Schwiers E, Adelman R, Cathcart R: Oxidative DNA damage as related to cancer and aging: assay of thymine glycol, thymidine glycol and hydroxymethyuracil in human and rat urine. p. 137. In Sohal RS, Cutler RG (eds): Molecular Biology of Aging: Gene Stability and Gene Expression. Raven Press, New York, 1985

93. Adelman R, Saul RL, Ames BN: Oxidative damage to DNA: Relation to species metabolic rate and lifespan. Proc Nat Acad Sci 1988;85:2706–2707

94. Fraga CG, Shigenaga MK, Park JW et al: Oxidative damage to DNA during aging: 8-hydroxydeoxy-guanosine in rat organ DNA and urine. Proc Nat Acad Sci U S A 1990;87:4533–4537

95. Randerath K, Randerath E, Filburn C: Genomic and mitochondrial DNA alterations with aging. p. 198. In Schneider EL, Rowe JW (eds): Handbook of the Biology of Aging. Academic Press, San Diego, 1995

96. Randerath K, Reddy MV, Gupta RC: 32P-labeling test for DNA damage. Proc Nat Acad Sci U S A 1981;78:6126–6129

97. Randerath K, Li D, Nath R, Randerath E: Exogenous and endogenous DNA modifications as monitored by 32P-postlabeling: relationships to cancer and aging. Exp Gerontol 1992; 27:533–549

98. Randerath K, Hart RW, Zhou G-D et al: Enhancement of age-related increases in DNA I-compound levels by calorie restriction: comparison of male B-N and F-344 rats. Mutation Res 1993;295:31–46

99. Holehan AM, Merry BJ: The experimental manipulation of ageing by diet. Biol Rev 1986;61:329–368

100. Randerath K, Reddy MV, Disher RM: Age- and tissue-related modifications in untreated rats: detection by ^{32}P–postlabeling assay and possible significance for spontaneous tumour induction and aging. Carcinogenesis 7:1615–1617

101. Wallace DC: Mitochondrial DNA mutations in human disease and aging. p. 163. In Esser K, Martin GM (eds): Molecular Aspects of Aging. John Wiley and Sons, Chichester, 1995

102. Agarwal S, Sohal RS: DNA oxidative damage and life expectancy in house-flies. Proc Nat Acad Sci 1994;91: 12332–12335

103. Richter C: Oxidative damage to mitochondrial DNA and its relationship to ageing. p. 99. In Esser K, Martin GM (eds): Molecular Aspects of Aging. John Wiley and Sons, Chichester, 1995

104. Linn S: DNA repair in mitochondria: how is it limited? What is its function? p.191. In Esser K, Martin GM (eds): Molecular Aspects of Aging. John Wiley & Sons, Chichester, 1995

105. Shay JW, Werbin H, Piatyszek MA: Does aging favour translocation of mitochondrial DNA fragments to the nuclear genome? p. 179. In Esser K, Martin GM (eds): Molecular Aspects of Aging. John Wiley & Sons, Chichester, 1995 179–189

106. Wallace DC, Bohr VA, Cortopassi G et al: Group report: the role of bioenergetics and mitochondrial DNA mutations in aging and age-related diseases. p. 199. In Esser K, Martin GM (eds): Molecular Aspects of Aging. John Wiley & Sons, Chichester, 1995

107. Setlow RB: Theory presentation and background summary. p. 177. In Warner HR, Butler RN, Sprott RL, Schneider EL (eds): Modern biological theories of aging. Aging Vol. 31. Raven Press, New York, 1987

108. Rothstein M: Biochemical Approaches to Aging. Academic Press, New York, 1982

109. Hart RW, Setlow RB: Correlation between deoxyribonucleic acid excision repair and life-span in a number of mammalian species. Proc Nat Acad Sci U S A 1974;71:2169–2173

110. Hart RW, D'Ambrosio SM, Ng KG, Modak SP: Longevity, stability and DNA repair. Mech Age Devel 1979;9:203–224

111. Sacher GA, Hart RW: Longevity, aging and comparative cellular and molecular biology of the house mouse, *Mus musculus*, and the white-footed mouse, *Peromyscus leucopus*. p. 71. In Bergsma D, Harrison DE (eds): Genetic Effects on Aging. Birth Defects. Vol. 14 Alan R Liss, New York, 1978

112. Hart RW, Daniel FB: Genetic stability in vitro and in vivo. Adv Pathobiology 1980;7: 123–141

113. Gensler HL: The effect of hamster age on UV-induced unscheduled DNA synthesis in freshly isolated lung and kidney cells. Exp Gerontol 1981;16:59–68

114. Wheeler KT, Lett JT: On the possibility that DNA repair is related to age in non-dividing cells. Proc Nat Acad Sci 1974; 71:1862–1865

115. Niedermuller H: DNA repair during aging. p. 513. In Sohal RS, Birnbaum LS, Cutler RG (eds): Molecular Biology of Aging: Gene Stability and Gene Expression. Aging. Vol. 29. Raven Press, New York, 1985

116. Mattern MR, Cerutti PA: Age-dependent excision repair of damaged thymine from gamma-irradiated DNA by isolated nuclei from human fibroblasts. Nature 1975; 254:450–452

117. Hart RW, Setlow RB: DNA repair in late-passage human cells. Mech Age Devel 1976;5:67–77

118. Painter RB, Clarkson JM, Young BR: Ultra-violet induced repair replication in aging diploid human cells (WI-38). Rad Res 1973;56:560–564

119. Mayer PJ, Lange CS, Bradley MO, Nichols WW: Gender differences in age-related decline in DNA double-strand break damage and repair in lymphocytes. Ann Hum Biol 1991;18: 405–415

120. Barton RW, Wang WK: Low molecular weight DNA polymerase; decreased activity in spleens of old BALB/c mice. Mech Age Devel 1975;4:123–126

121. Fry M, Loeb LA, Martin GM: Nuclease digestion studies of mouse chromatin as a function of age. J Gerontol 1981;34: 672–679

122. Agarwal SS, Tufner M, Loeb LA: DNA replication in human lymphocytes during ageing. J Cell Physiol 1978;96:235–244

123. Murray V, Holliday R: Increased error frequency of DNA-polymerases from senescent human fibroblasts. J Mol Biol 1981;146:55–76

124. Busbee D, Sylvia V, Stec J et al: Lability of DNA polymerase alpha correlated with decreased DNA synthesis and increased age in human cells. J Natl Cancer Inst 1987;79: 1231–1239

125. Gaubatz JW, Prashad N, Cutler RG: Ribosomal RNA gene dosage as a function of tissue and age for mouse and human. Biochim Biophys Acta 1976;418:358–376

126. Johnson R, Strehler BL: Loss of genes coding for ribosomal RNA in ageing brain cells. Nature 1972;240:412–414

127. Johnson LK, Johnson RW, Strehler BL: Cardiac hypertrophy, ageing and changes in cardiac ribosomal RNA gene dosage in man. J Mol Cell Cardiol 1975;7:125–135

128. Medvedev ZA: Repetition of molecular-genetic information as a possible factor in evolutionary changes of life span. Exp Gerontol 1972;7:227–238

129. Miquel J, Johnson Jr JE: Senescent changes in the ribosomes of animal cells in vivo and in vitro. Mech Age Devel 1979;9: 247–266

130. Reff ME: RNA and protein metabolism. p. 225. In Finch CE, Schneider EL (eds): Handbook of the Biology of Aging. Van Nostrand Reinhold, New York, 1985

131. Wust CJ, Rosen L: Aminoacylation of methylation of rRNA as a function of age in the rat. Exp Gerontol 1972;7:331–343

132. Hoffman JL, McCoy MT: Stability of the nucleoside composition of tRNA during biological ageing of mice and mosquitoes. Nature 1974;249:558–559

133. Gusseck DJ: Anomalies of tRNA-aminoacylation reaction which could lead to misinterpretation of evidence for tRNA changes during development and ageing. Mech Age Devel 1974;3:301–311

134. Wilson PD: Enzyme changes in ageing mammals. Gerontologia 1973;19:79–125

135. Strehler BL, Hirsch G, Gusseck D et al: Codon restriction theory of ageing and development. J Theor Biol 1971;33: 429–474

136. Strehler BL, North D: Cell type specific codon usage and differentiation. Mech Age Devel 1982;18:285–313

137. Wilson PD: The histochemistry of ageing. Histochem J 1983; 15:393–410

138. Orgel LE: The maintenance of the accuracy of protein synthesis and its relevance to ageing. A correction. Proc Nat Acad Sci U S A 1970;67:1476

139. Orgel LE: Ageing of clones of mammalian cells. Nature 1973; 243:441

140. Goel NS, Islam S: Error catastrophe in and the evolution of the protein synthesising machinery. J Theor Biol 1977;68: 167–183

141. Kirkwood TBL: Error propagation in intracellular information transfer. J Theor Biol 1980;82:363–382

142. Rothstein M: Evidence for and against the error catastrophe hypothesis. p. 139. In Warner HR, Butler RN, Sprott RL, Schneider EL (eds): Modern biological theories of aging. Aging Vol. 31. Raven Press, New York, 1987

143. Ryan JM, Duda G, Cristofalo VJ: Error accumulation and aging in human diploid cells. J Gerontol 1974;29:616–622

144. Lewis CM, Tarrant GM: Error theory and ageing in human diploid fibroblasts. Nature 1972;239:316–318

145. Ogrodnik JP, Wulf JH, Cutler RG: Altered protein hypothesis of mammalian ageing processes. II. Discrimination ratio of methionine vs ethionine in the synthesis of ribosomal protein and RNA of C57BL/6J mouse liver. Exp Gerontol 1975;10: 119–137

146. Filion A-M, Laughrea M: Translation fidelity in the brain, liver, and hippocampus of the aging Fischer 344 rat. p. 257. In Sohal RS, Birnbaum LS, Cutler RG (eds): Molecular biology of aging: Gene stability and gene expression. Aging. Vol. 29. Raven Press, New York, 1985

147. Holliday R, Tarrant GM: Altered enzymes in ageing human fibroblasts. Nature 1972;238:26

148. Schofield JD, Hadfield JM: Age-related alterations in the heat-lability of mouse liver glucose-6-phosphate dehydrogenase. Exp Gerontol 1978;13:147–158

149. Harding JJ: Altered heat-lability of a fraction of glutathione reductase in aging human lens. Biochem J 1973;134: 995–1000

150. Gershon H, Gershon D: Detection of inactive enzyme molecules in ageing organisms. Nature 1970;227:1214–1217

151. Reiss U, Rothstein M: Age-related changes in isocitrate lyase from the free-living nematode *Turbatrix aceti*. J Biol Chem 1975;250:826–830

152. Gershon H, Gershon D: Altered enzyme molecules in senescent organisms; muscle aldolase. Mech Age Devel 1973;2: 33–41

153. Gershon H, Gershon D: Inactive enzyme molecules in ageing mice. Proc Nat Acad Sci U S A. 1973;70:909–913

154. Anderson PJ: Ageing effects on the liver aldolase of rabbits. Biochem J 1974;140:341–343

155. Rothstein M: Aging and the alteration of enzymes; a review. Mech Age Devel 1975;4:325–339

156. Oliveira RJ, Pfuderer P: Test for missynthesis of lactate dehydrogenase in ageing mice by use of a monospecific antibody. Exp Gerontol 1973;8:193–198

157. Pendergrass WR, Martin GM, Bornstein PM: Evidence contrary to the protein error hypothesis for in vitro senescence. J Cell Physiol 1975;87:3–14

158. Bolla R, Brot N: Age-dependent changes in enzymes involved in macromolecular synthesis in *Turbatrix aceti*. Biochem Biophys Acta 1975;169:227–324

159. Holland JJ, Kohne D, Doyle MV: Analysis of virus replication in ageing human fibroblast cultures. Nature 1973;245: 316–319

160. Tomkins GA, Stanbridge EJ, Hayflick L: Viral probes of ageing in the human diploid cell strain WI-38. Proc Soc Exp Biol Med 1974;146:385–390

161. Pitha J, Stork E, Wimmer EY: Protein synthesis during aging of human cells in culture. Direction by polio virus. Exp Cell Res 1975;94:310–315

162. Gershon D, Gershon H: An evaluation of the 'error catastrophe' theory of ageing in the light of recent experimental results. Gerontology 1976;22:212–219

163. Gershon D: Current status of age altered enzymes; alternative mechanisms. Mech Age Devel 1979;9:189–196

164. McKerrow JH: Non-enzymatic post-translational amino acid modifications in ageing. A brief review. Mech Age Devel 1979; 10:371–377

165. Sharma HK, Rothstein M: Altered enolase in aged *Turbatrix aceti* results from conformational changes in the enzyme. Proc Nat Acad Sci USA 1980;77:5865–5868

166. Fornaini G, Leoncini G, Segni P et al: Relationship between age and properties of human and rabbit glucose-6-phosphate dehydrogenase. Eur J Biochem 1969;7:214–232

167. VanKleef FSM, DeJong WW, Hoenders HJ: Stepwise degradations and deamidation of the eye lens protein crystallin in ageing. Nature 1975;258:264–267

168. Hoenders HJ, Schoenmakers JGG, Garding JJJ et al: The N-terminus of lens protein alpha-crystallin. Exp Eye Res 1968; 7:291–297

169. Bailey AJ, Robbins SP: Development and maturation of the crosslinks in the collagen fibres of the skin. Front Matrix Biol 1973;1:130–156

170. Zs-Nagy I, Nagy K: On the role of the cross-linking of cellular proteins in ageing. Mech Age Devel 1980;14:245–251

171. Kay MMB: Age effects on colony-forming human peripheral blood T and B cells. Gerontology 1985;31:278–284

172. Kay MMB, Bosman G, Notter M, Coleman P: Life and death of neurons: the senescent cell antigen. Ann NY Acad Sci 1988; 521:155–169

173. Sharma HK, Prasanna HR, Lane RS, Rothstein M: The effect of age on enolase turnover in the free-living nematode, *Turbatrix aceti*. Arch Biochem Biophys Acta 1979;194:275–291

174. Rothstein M: The formation of altered enzymes in ageing animals. Mech Age Devel 1979;9:197–202

175. Sharma HK, Prasanna HR, Rothstein MJ: Altered phosphoglycerate kinase in aging rats. J Biol Chem 1980;255: 5043–5050

176. Oliver CN, Ahn BW, Moerman EJ et al: Age-related changes in oxidised proteins. J Biol Chem 1987;262:5488–5491

177. Stadtman ER: Protein oxidation and aging. Science 1992;257: 1220–1224

178. Gutteridge JMC: Oxygen radicals, transition metals and aging. p. 1. In Aloj Totaro E, Glees P, Pisanti FA (eds): Advances in Age Pigments Research. Advances in the Biosciences. Vol. 64 Pergammon Press, Oxford, 1987

179. Harding JJ, Beswick HT, Ajiboye R et al: Non-enzymatic post-translational modification of proteins in aging. A review. Mech Age Devel 1989;50:7–16

180. Koenig RJ, Peterson CM, Jones RL et al: Correlation of glucose regulation and hemoglobin Alc in diabetes mellitus. Engl J Med 1976;295:417–420

181. Bunn HF: Nonenzymatic glycosylation of protein: Relevance to diabetes. Am J Med 1981;70:325–330

182. Schnider SL, Kohn RR: Glucosylation of human collagen in aging and diabetes mellitus. J Clin Invest 1980;66: 1179–1181

183. Schnider SL, Kohn RR: Effects of age and diabetes mellitus on the solubility and nonenzymatic glucosylation of human skin collagen. J Clin Invest 1981;67:1630–1635

184. Garlick RL, Bunn HF, Spiro RG: Nonenzymatic glycation of basement membranes from human glomeruli and bovine sources: effect of diabetes and age. Diabetes 1988;37: 1144–1155

185. Patrick JS, Thorpe SR, Baynes JW: Nonenzymatic glycosylation of protein does not increase with age in normal human lenses. J Gerontol 1990;45:B18–B23

186. Lee AT, Cerami A: Modifications of proteins and nucleic acids by reducing sugars: possible role in aging. p. 116. In Schneider EL, Rowe JW (eds): Handbook of the Biology of Aging. Academic Press, San Diego, 1990

187. Levine RL, Stadtman ER: Protein modifications with aging

p. 184. In Schneider EL, Rowe JW (eds): Handbook of the Biology of Aging. Academic Press, San Diego, 1996

188. Molnar JA, Alpert N, Burke JF, Young VR: Synthesis and degradation rates of collagens in vivo in whole skin of rats, studied with $^{18}O_2$ labelling. Biochem J 1986;240:431–435

189. Zeman R, Kameyama T, Matsumoto K et al: Regulation of protein degradation in muscle by calcium. Evidence for enhanced nonlysosomal proteolysis associated with elevated cytosolic calcium. J Biol Chem 1985;260:13619–13624

190. Makrides SC: Protein synthesis and degradation during ageing and senescence. Biol Rev 1983;58:343–422

191. Dice JF, Goff SA: Error catastrophe and aging: future directions of research p. 155. In Warner HR, Butler RN, Sprott RL, Schneider EL (eds): Modern biological theories of aging. Aging. Vol. 31. Raven Press, New York, 1987

192. Sohal RS: Age Pigments. Elsevier/North Holland Biomedical Press, Amsterdam, 1981

193. Aloj Totaro E, Glees P, Pisanti FA: Advances in Age Pigments Research. Pergammon Press, Oxford, 1987

194. Mann DMA, Yates PO: Lipoprotein pigments—their relationship to ageing in the human nervous system. I. The lipofusion content of nerve cells. Brain 1974;97:48–488

195. Davies I, Fotheringham AP: Lipofuscin—Does it affect cellular performance? Exp Gerontol 1981;16:119–125

196. Davies I, Fotheringham AP, Roberts C: The effect of lipofuscin on cellular function. Mech Age Devel 1983;23:347–356

197. Knook DL, Sleyster ECH: Isolated parenchymal, Küpffer and endothelial rat liver cells characterised by their lysosomal enzyme content. Biochem Biophys Res Comm 1980;96:250–257

198. Knook DL, Sleyster ECH: Lysosomal enzyme activities in parenchymal and nonparenchymal liver cells isolated from young, adult and old rats. Mech Age Devel 1976;5:389–397

199. Schmucker DL, Wang RK: Rat liver lysosomal enzymes: effects of animal age and phenobarbital. Age 1979;2:93–96

200. Comolli R, Ferioli ME, Azzola S: Protein turnover of the lysosomal and mitochondrial fractions of rat liver during ageing. Exp Gerontol 1972;7:369–376

201. DeMartino GN, Goldberg AL: Thyroid hormones control lysosomal enzyme activities in liver and skeletal muscle. Proc Nat Acad Sci U S A. 1978;75:1369–1373

202. Miquel J, Economos AC, Fleming J, Johnson Jr JE: Mitochondrial role in cell ageing. Exp Gerontol 1980;15:575–591

203. Chen JC, Warshaw JB, Sanadi DR: Regulation of mitochondrial respiration in senescence. J Cell Physiol 1972;80: 141–148

204. Wilson PD, Hill BT, Franks LM: The effect of age on mitochondrial ultrastructure. Gerontologia 1975;21:95–101

205. Wilson PD, Franks LM: The effect of age on mitochondrial enzymes and respiration. Gerontologia 1975;21:81–94

206. Menzies RA, Gold PH: The turnover of mitochondria in a variety of tissues of young adult and aged rats. J Biol Chem 1971;246:2425–2429

207. Davies I, Fotheringham AP: The influence of age on the response of the supraoptic nucleus of the hypothalamo-neurohypophyseal system to physiological stress. I. Ultrastructural aspects. Mech Age Devel 1981;15:355–366

208. Davies I, Fotheringham AP, Roberts C: The effect of osmotic challenge and subsequent rehydration on the aging hypothalamo-neurohypophyseal system. A quantitative morphological study of the supraoptic nucleus. Mech Age Devel 1984;26: 299–310

209. Davies I, Fotheringham AP: The influence of age on the response of the supraoptic nucleus of the hypothalamo-neurohypophyseal system to physiological stress. II. Quantitative morphology. Mech Age Devel 1981;15:367–378

210. Deshmukh DR, Owen OE, Patel MS: Effect of ageing on the metabolism of pyruvate and 3-hydroxybutyrate in mono-synaptic and non-synaptic mitochondria from rat brain. J Neurochem 1980;34:1219–1224

211. Deshmukh DR, Patel MS: Age-dependent changes in glutamate oxidation by non-synaptic mitochondria from rat brain. Mech Age Devel 1980;13:75–81

212. Chiu YJD, Richardson A: Effect of age on the function of mitochondria isolated from brain and heart tissue. Exp Gerontol 1980;15:511–517

213. Hansford RG: Bioenergetics in ageing. Biochim Biophys Acta 1983;726:41–80

214. Lakatta EG: Heart and circulation. p. 181. In Schneider EL, Rowe JW (eds): Handbook of the Biology of Aging. Academic Press, San Diego, 1990

215. Menzies RA, Gold PH: The apparent turnover of mitochondria, ribosomes and sRNA of the brain in young adult and aged rats. J Neurochem 1972;19:1671–1683

216. Hill BT: Influence of age on chromatin transcription in murine tissues using an heterologous and an homologous RNA polymerase. Gerontology 1976;22:111–124

217. Sarkander H-I: Age-dependent changes in the organization and regulation of transcriptionally active neuronal and nonastrocytic glial chromatin. p. 301. In Cervos-Navarro J, Sarkander H-I (eds): Brain Aging: Neuropathology and Neuropharmacology. Aging. Vol. 21. Plenum Press, New York, 1983

218. Lux RM, Cervos-Navarro J, Sarkander H-I: Modifications in the organization of neuronal nucleosomes in the course of aging. p. 329. In Cervos-Navarro J, Sarkander H-I (eds): Brain Aging: Neuropathology and Neuropharmacology. Aging. Vol. 21. Raven Press, New York, 1983

219. Cotman CW, Anderson KJ: Synaptic plasticity and functional stabilization in the hippocampal formation: possible role in Alzheimer's disease. p. 313. In Waxman S (ed): Physiological Basis for Functional Recovery in Neurological Disease. Raven Press, New York, 1988

220. Cutler RG: Redundancy of information content in the genome of mammalian species as a protective mechanism determining ageing rate. Mech Age Devel 1974;2:381–408

221. Cutler RG: Transcription of reiterated DNA sequence classes throughout the lifespan of the mouse. Adv Gerontol Res 1972; 4:219–321

222. Cutler RG: Evolution of human longevity and genetic complexity governing ageing rate. Proc Nat Acad Sci U S A 1975;72: 4664–4669

223. BeMiller PK, Pakar UA, Schmit JC: Cellular aging and ribosomal RNA. p. 223. In Sohal RS, Birnbaum LS, Cutler RG (eds): Molecular Biology of Aging: Gene Stability and Gene Expression. Aging. Vol. 29 Raven Press, New York, 1985

224. Bellamy D: Ageing: A Biometrial Perspective. John Wiley & Sons, Chichester, 1995

225. Van Leeuwen FW, Evans DA, Meloen R, Sonnemans MA: Differential neurophysin immunoreactivities in solitary magnocellular neurons of the homozygous Brattleboro rat indicate an altered neurophysin moiety. Brain Res 1994;635:328–330

226. Evans DAP, van der Kleij AAM, Sonnemans MAF et al: Frameshift mutations at two hotspots in vasopressin transcripts in post-mitotic neurons. Proc Nat Acad Sci U S A 1994;91: 6059–6063

227. Lamb MJ: Epigenetic inheritance and aging. Rev Clin Geront 1994;4:97–105

228. Holliday R, Pugh JE: DNA modification mechanisms and gene activity during development. Science 1975;187:226–232

229. Mays-Hoopes LL: DNA methylation: a possible correlation between aging and cancer. p. 49. In Sohal RS, Birnbaum LS, Cutler RG (eds): Molecular Biology of Aging: Gene Stability and Gene Expression. Aging. Vol. 29. Raven Press, New York, 1985

230. Vijg J, Uitterlinden AG, Mullaart E et al: Processing of DNA damage during aging: induction of genetic alteration. p. 155. In Sohal RS, Birnbaum LS, Cutler RG (eds): Molecular Biology of Aging: Gene Stability and Gene Expression. Aging. Vol. 29. Raven Press, New York, 1985

231. Wilson VL, Jones PA: DNA methylation decreases in aging but not in immortal cells. Science 1983;220:1054–1057

232. Holliday R: Strong effects of 5-azacytidine on the in vitro lifespan of human diploid fibroblasts. Exp Cell Res 1986;166: 543–552

233. Holliday R: Toward a biological understanding of the aging process. Pers Biol 1988;32:109–123

234. Ono T, Shinya K, Uehara Y, Okada S: Endogenous virus genomes become hypomethylated tissue-specifically during aging process of C57BL mice. Mech Age Devel 1989;50: 27–36

235. Cutler RG: Dysdifferentiative hypothesis of aging: a review. p. 307. In Sohal RS, Birnbaum LS, Cutler RG (eds): Molecular Biology of Aging: Gene Stability and Gene Expression. Raven Press, New York, 1985

236. Ono T, Cutler RG: Age-dependent relaxation of gene expression—increase of endogenous murine leukaemia virus-related and globin-related RNA in brain and liver of mice. Proc Nat Acad Sci U S A 1978;75:1431–1435

237. Holliday R: Ageing: X-chromosome reactivation. Nature 1987; 327:661–662

238. Deol MS, Truslove GM, McLaren A: Genetic activity at the albino locus in Cattanach's insertion in the mouse. J Embryol Exp Morphol 1986;96:295–302

239. Wareham KA, Lyon MF, Glenister PH, Williams ED: Age-related reactivation of an X-linked gene. Nature 1987;327: 725–727

240. Migeon BR, Axelman J, Beggs AH: Effect of ageing on reactivation of the human X-linked HRPT locus. Nature 1988;335: 93–96

241. Holliday R: X-chromosome reactivation and ageing. Nature 1989;337:311

242. Papaconstantinou J, Reisner PD, Liu L, Kuninger DT: Mechanisms of altered gene expression with aging. p. 150. In Schneider EL, Rowe JW (eds): Handbook of the Biology of Aging. Academic Press, San Diego, 1996

243. Fujita T, Maruyama N: Elevated levels of c-jun and c-fos transcripts in the aged rat liver. Biochem Biophys Res Comm 1991;178:1485–1491

244. Kaminska B, Kaczmarek L: Robust induction of AP-1 transcription factor DNA binding activity in the hippocampus of aged rats. Neurosci Lett 1993;153:189–191

245. Liu AY-C, Lin Z, Choi HS, Sorhage F, Li B: Attenuated induction of heat shock gene expression in aging diploid fibroblasts. J Biol Chem 1989;264:12037–12045

246. Liu AY-C, Choi HS, Lu Y-K, Chen KY: Molecular events involved in transcriptional activation of heat shock genes become progressively refractory to heat stimulation during aging of human diploid fibroblasts. J Cell Physiol 1991;149: 560–566

247. Lithgow GJ: Temperature, stress response and aging. Rev Clin Geront 1996;6:119–128

248. Richardson A, Rutherford MS, Birchenall-Sparks MC et al: Levels of specific messenger RNA species as a function of age. p. 229. In Sohal RS, Birnbaum LS, Cutler RG (eds): Molecular biology of aging. Gene stability and gene expression. Aging. Vol. 29. Raven Press, New York, 1985

249. Colman PC, Kaplan BB, Osterburg HH, Finch CE: Brain poly(A) RNA during aging: stability of yield and sequence complexity in two rat strains. J Neurochem 1980;34:335–345

250. Birchenall-Sparks MC, Roberts MS, Rutherford MS, Richardson A: The effect of aging on the structure and function of liver messenger RNA. Mech Age Devel 1985;32:99–111

251. Richardson A, Roberts MS, Rutherford MS: Aging and gene expression. Rev Biol Res Aging 1985;2:395–419

252. Finch CE: Longevity, Senescence and the Genome. University of Chicago Press, Chicago 1990

253. Du JT, Beyer TA, Lang CA: Protein biosynthesis in ageing mouse tissues. Exp Gerontol 1977;12:181–192

254. Dwyer BE, Fando JL, Wasterlain CG: Rat brain protein synthesis declines during postdevelopmental ageing. J Neurochem 1980;35:746–749

255. Ward WF: Enhancement by food restriction of liver protein synthesis in the aging Fischer 344 rat. J Gerontol 1988;43: B50–B53

256. Fukagawa NK, Minaker KL, Young VR et al: Glucose and amino acid metabolism in aging man: Differential effects of insulin. Metabolism 1988;37:371–377

257. Fukagawa NK, Minaker KL, Young VR et al: Leucine metabolism in aging humans: Effect of insulin and substrate availability. Am J Physiol 1989;256:E288–E294

258. Gersovitz M, Bier D, Matthews D et al: Dynamic aspects of whole body glycine metabolism: Influence of protein intake in young adult and elderly males. Metabolism 1980;29: 1087–1094

259. Gersovitz M, Munro HN, Udall J, Young VR: Albumin synthesis in young and elderly subjects using a new stable isotope

methodology: Response to level of protein intake. Metabolism 1980;29:1075–1086

260. Fukagawa NK, Bandini LG, Young JB: Effect of age on body composition and resting metabolic rate. Am J Physiol 1990; 259:E233–E238

261. Fukagawa NK, Young VR: Protein and amino acid metabolism and requirements in older persons. Clin Geriatr Med 1987;3: 329–341

262. Roy AK, Nath TS, Motwani NM, Chatterjee B: Age-dependent regulation of the polymorphic forms of α_{2u}-globulin. J Biol Chem 1983;258:10123–10127

263. Richardson A, Butler JA, Rutherford MS et al: Effect of age and dietary restriction on the expression of α_{2u}-globulin. J Biol Chem 1987;262:12821–12825

264. Murty CVR, Mancini MA, Chatterjee B, Roy AK: Changes in transcriptional activity and matrix association in alpha2u-globulin gene family in the rat liver during maturation and aging. Biochim Biophys Acta 1988;949:27–34

265. Motwani NM, Caron D, Demyan WF et al: Monoclonal antibodies to alpha$_{2u}$-globulin synthesizing hepatocytes during androgenic induction and aging. J Biol Chem 1984;259:3653–3657

266. Kim SK, Weinhold PA, Han SS, Wagner DJ: Age-related decline in protein synthesis in the rat parotid gland. Exp Gerontol 1980;15:77–85

267. McMartin DN, Schedlbauer LM: Incorporation of 14C-leucine into protein and tubulin by brain slices from young and old mice. J Gerontol 1975;30:132–137

268. Petell JK, Lebherz HG: Properties and metabolism of fructose diphosphate aldolase in livers of "old" and "young" mice. J Biol Chem 1979;254:8179–8184

269. Buetow DC, Moudgil PG, Eichholz RL, Cook JR: Protein synthesis in senescent liver. In Platt D (ed): Liver and Ageing. Schattauer Verlag, Stuttgart, 1977

270. Campisi J, Dimri G, Hara E: Control of replicative senescence. p. 121. In Schneider EL, Rowe JW, (eds): Handbook of the Biology of Aging. Academic Press, San Diego, 1996

271. West MD, Pereira-Smith OM, Smith JR: Replicative senescence of human skin fibroblasts correlates with a loss of regulation and overexpression of collagenase activity. Exp Cell Res 1989;184:138–147

272. Wick M, Burger C, Brusselbach S et al: A novel member of human tissue inhibitor of metalloproteinases (TIMP) gene family is regulated during G1 expression, mitogenic stimulation, differentiation and senescence. J Biol Chem 1994;269: 18953–18960

273. Millis AJ, Hoyle M, McCue HM, Martini H: Differential expression of metalloproteinase and tissue inhibitor of metalloproteinase genes in aged human fibroblasts. Exp Cell Res 1992;201:373–379

274. Ashcroft GS, Horan MA, Ferguson MWJ: The effects of ageing on cutaneous wound healing in mammals. J Anat 1995;187: 1–26

275. Wright WE, Hayflick L: Nuclear control of cellular ageing demonstrated by hybridization of anucleate and whole cultured normal human fibroblasts. Exp Cell Res 1975;96:113–122

276. Norwood TH, Pendergrass WR, Sprague CA, Martin GM: Dominance of the senescent phenotype in heterokaryons between replicative and post-replicative human fibroblast-like cells. Proc Nat Acad Sci 1974;71:2231–2234

277. Norwood TH, Pendergrass WR, Martin GM: Reinitiation of DNA synthesis in senescent human fibroblasts upon fusion with cells of unlimited growth potential. J Cell Biol 1975;64: 551–557

278. Yanishevsky RM, Stein GH: Ongoing DNA synthesis continues in young human diploid cells (HDC) fused to senescent HDC, but entry into S phase is inhibited. Exp Cell Res 1980;126: 469–472

279. Stein GH, Yanishevsky RM: Entry into S-phase is inhibited in two immortal cell lines fused to senescent human diploid cells. Exp Cell Res 1979;120:155–166

280. Norwood TH, Pendergrass W, Bornstein P, Martin GM: DNA synthesis of sublethally injured cells in heterokaryons and its relevance to clonal senescence. Exp Cell Res 1979;119: 15–22

281. Rabinovitch PS, Norwood TH: Comparative heterokaryon study of cellular senescence and the serum deprived state. Exp Cell Res 1980;130:101–109

282. Pereira-Smith OM, Smith JR: Genetic analysis of indefinite division in human cells: identification of four complementation groups. Proc Nat Acad Sci U S A 1988;85:6042–6046

283. Hensler P, Annab LA, Barrett JC, Pereira-Smith OM: A gene involved in control of human cellular senescence on human chromosome 1q. Mol Cell Biol 1994;14:2292–2297

284. Ning Y, Weber JL, Killary AM et al: Genetic analysis of indefinite division in human cells: evidence for a senescence-related gene(s) on human chromosome 4. Proc Nat Acad Sci U S A 1991;88:5635–5639

285. Ogata T, Ayusawa D, Namba M et al: Chromosome 7 suppresses indefinite division of nontumorogenic immortalized human fibroblast cell lines KMST-6 and SUSM-1. Mol Cell Biol 1993;13:6036–6043

286. Ryan PA, Maher VM, McCormick JJ: Failure of infinite lifespan human cells from different immortality complementation groups to yield finite life span hybrids. J Cell Physiol 1994; 159:151–160

287. Vijayashankar N, Brody H: A study of aging in the human abducens nucleus. J Comp Neurol 1977;173:433–439

288. Vijayashankar N, Brody H: Aging in the human brain stem. A study of the nucleus of the trochlear nerve. Acta Anat 1977; 99:169–173

289. Vijayashankar N, Brody H: Quantitative study of the pigmented neurons in the nuclei locus coeruleus and subcoeruleus in man as related to aging. J Neuropathol Exp Neurol 1979;38:490–497

290. Haug H, Barmwater U, Eggers R et al: Anatomical changes in aging brain; Morphometric analysis of the human prosencephalon. p. 1. In Cervos-Navarro J, Sarkander H-I (eds): Brain Aging: Neuropathology & Neuropharmacology. Aging. Raven Press, New York, 1983

291. Haug H: Macroscopic and microscopic morphometry of the human brain and cortex. A survey in the light of new results. Brain Pathol 1984;1:123–149

292. Landfield PW, Eldridge JC: Evolving aspects of the glucocorticoid hypothesis of brain aging: Hormonal modulation of neuronal calcium homeostasis. Neurobiol Aging 1994;15:579–588

293. Johnson SA, Finch CA: Changes in gene expression during brain aging: a survey. p. 300. In Schneider EL, Rowe JW (eds): Handbook of the Biology of Aging. Academic Press, San Diego 1996

294. Krohn PL: Review lectures on senescence. II. Heterochromic transplantation in the study of ageing. Proc Roy Soc Series B 1962;157:128–147

295. Ogden DA, Micklem HS: The fate of serially transplanted bone marrow cell populations from young and old donors. Transplantation 1976;22:287–298

296. Ross EAM, Anderson N, Micklem HS: Serial depletion and regeneration of the murine haematopoietic system: implications for haematopoietic organisation and the study of cellular aging. J Exp Med 1982;155:432–444

297. Harrison DE, Astle CM, Delaittre JA: Loss of proliferative capacity in immunohemopoietic stem cells caused by serial transplantation rather than aging. J Exp Med 1978;147:1526

298. Wang E, Lee MJ, Pandey S. Control of fibroblast senescence and activation of programmed cell death. J Cell Biochem 1994;54:432–439

299. Crowley C, Curtis MJ: Proc Natl Acad Sci U S A 49:626–628

CHAPTER 6

Physiology of Aging

E. J. MASORO

When broadly defined, aging refers to all time-associated events that occur during the life span of an organism. During this time, many changes occur in the physiologic processes. These changes may be beneficial, neutral, or deteriorative in nature. During the developmental period of life most changes are due to the maturation of the physiologic processes and tend to be beneficial. However, during the postmaturation period of life most of the changes are detrimental, although some may be neutral, such as the graying of the hair. Indeed, the term senescence is used to denote this postmaturation deterioration. Senescence is defined as the deteriorative changes with time during postmaturation life that underlie an increasing vulnerability to challenges, thereby decreasing the ability of the organism to survive. Although senescence is a subset of aging, in common usage, aging is often used to mean senescence. Unfortunately, this meaning is usually not explicitly stated. In this chapter, aging and senesence will be used as synonyms. This usage is particularly appropriate in a textbook of geriatric medicine.

This brief chapter can only cover concepts and provide a limited number of examples. Recently, the American Physiological Society has added a volume dedicated to aging[1] to its *Handbook of Physiology* series. That volume provides in-depth coverage of most age-changes in the physiologic systems and should be consulted by readers who desire further information in a particular subject area.

Physiologic Deterioration and the Aging Phenotype

A major characteristic of the aging phenotype is the difference in physiologic processes when the elderly are compared to the young adult. Age-specific mortality rate increases with increasing postmaturation age. The age-associated deterioration of the physiologic systems undoubtedly plays an important role in this increase in age-specific mortality rate. Therefore, it is of great value to have a knowledge of the age-changes in the physiologic systems and to understand the basis of this physiologic deterioration with advancing chronologic age.

Causes of Age-Associated Physiologic Deterioration

The progressive deterioration with age of the physiologic systems that starts during young adulthood is caused by the many damaging processes and agents that organisms encounter during life. Apparently, repair systems during postmaturational life are not able to fully eliminate the damage. The result is a progressive functional inadequacy of the physiologic systems due to the accumulation of damage. The extent of this functional inadequacy and its rate of occurrence varies among species and among individuals within a species, as well as among the physiologic systems of an individual. It is convenient to classify the damaging processes responsible for the age-associated physiologic deterioration in the following three categories: (1) Damage resulting from intrinsic living processes, (2) Damage caused by extrinsic factors, and (3) Damage resulting from age-associated diseases.

Category 1

Many of the processes essential to life also have damaging aspects. For example, aerobic metabolism, which enables organisms to readily generate metabolic energy from ingested nutrients, has the negative aspect of the generation of highly reactive compounds such as superoxide, hydroxyl radicals, and hydrogen peroxide due to the univalent reduction of oxygen. These oxygen-containing compounds are potentially highly damaging. Protection from and repair of damage from these substances has evolved, but these processes are not totally effective. Therefore, an accumulation of oxidative damage with increasing age occurs.[2] The extent of protection and the ability to repair the damage varies among species. Thus, it is not surprising that there is interspecies variation in the rate of accumulation of oxidatively damaged macromolecules. Another example involves glucose, a most important fuel for most organisms. However, in addition to serving as an energy source, glucose also participates in the glycoxidation of proteins and nucleic acids and, in this way, alters their biologic functions.[3] Again, there are protective mechanisms, as well as processes that eliminate the damaged macromolecules, which vary in efficacy among species. Probably there is no intrinsic living process that does not also have the ability to cause damage.

Category 2

There is general agreement that extrinsic factors contribute to the aging phenotype. However, many would not subscribe to the view that these extrinsic factors are part of the aging process. This view is based on long-held criteria for aging processes that were enumerated by Strehler[4] in 1977. One of the criteria is intrinsicality, the view that aging is entirely an intrinsic phenomenon. This criterion was considered necessary to distinguish aging from age-correlated changes, due to the effects of factors originating outside of the organism. In my opinion this criterion interferes with our thinking about aging processes and, in addition, is faulty for two reasons. First, if aging is the result of the progressive accumulation of unrepaired damage, it is irrelevant whether that damage originates from intrinsic living processes or is caused by extrinsic agents. Second, extrinsic agents cause damage only because of interactions with biologic materials and processes. Thus, all damage is intrinsic whether it originates as a result of basic living processes or from reactions to extrinsic factors. This issue has been addressed in a constructive way by Rowe and Kahn[5] in their concept of "usual" and "successful" aging. They classified the population without discernible disease into two groups. Those who exhibited the average amount of age-associated physiologic deterioration were classified as the usual aging group, while the smaller group who showed little deterioration with age in a constellation of physiologic functions was classified as the successful aging group. Rowe and Kahn suggested that the effects of the intrinsic aging processes have been exaggerated, and that the difference between the successful and the usual aging groups primarily relates to extrinsic factors. They considered that the major extrinsic factors responsible for usual aging are diet, lifestyle, personal habits, and psychosocial factors. It should be noted that if the concepts of Rowe and Kahn are correct, then much of the physiologic deterioration with advancing age is potentially quite modifiable. Moreover, based on their concepts, most of usual aging is the result of interactions between the organism and its environment.

That diet can markedly influence age-associated physiologic deterioration is clearly established by the many studies on the effects of restricting the intake of food by laboratory mice and rats to 50 to 60 percent of that eaten by ad libitum fed animals. This reduction of food intake maintains a broad array of physiologic processes in a youthful state until very advanced ages.[6] Examples of the scope include: the loss of gamma crystallins of the lens of the eye,[7] loss of dopamine receptors of the corpus striatum,[8] deterioration of immune function,[9] loss of ability to negotiate a maze,[9] loss of the ability of adipocytes to respond to lipolytic hormones,[10] loss of female reproductive function,[11] and attenuation of age-changes in gene expression.[12] Indeed, this reduction of food intake retards most, but not all age-associated changes in physiologic processes so far studied. For example, it was not found to attenuate the increase with age in the systolic blood pressure of rats.[13] It has been established that the reduction in energy (calorie) intake is the dietary factor responsible for this retardation of age changes in the physiologic systems.[14] There is no evidence that restricting energy intake of humans during adult life would globally retard age-associated physiologic deterioration, but there is also no evidence that it would not.

Indeed, there is evidence that diet can influence the occurrence or progression of age-associated human disease. For example, high fat, high calorie diets are believed to promote age-associated human pathology such as atherosclerosis,[15] hypertension,[15] and insulin resistance and impaired glucose tolerance.[16]

The lifestyle factor that has received the most attention relates to the fact that with increasing age many people become increasingly sedentary.[17] Studies on the effect of exercise training in old human subjects indicate that much of the decline in cardiovascular function with advancing age in sedentary people is due to the effects of exercise deficiency and, therefore, probably can at least in part be reversed by physical activity even at advanced ages.[18] Sketetal muscle mass and strength decrease with increasing age,[19] and both the mass and the strength of skeletal muscle can be increased by resistance training even at very advanced ages.[20] It is likely that the frequently occurring increase in body weight in people between the ages of 20 and 70 years is primarily the result of a sedentary lifestyle.[21] Exercise has also been found to attenuate the age-associated increase in body fat content.[22] Most importantly, exercise improves the distribution pattern of body fat in elderly men and women.[23] There is also evidence that exercise can prevent the increase in insulin resistance and the reduction in glucose tolerance that occurs in many people with advancing age.[24] There can be little doubt that the increasingly sedentary lifestyle with advancing age contributes greatly to the deterioration of physiologic functions of old people.

There is no clear demarcation between lifestyle factors and personal habits. For example, excessive exposure to the sun results in changes in skin structure and function that are generally considered to be part of the aging phenotype.[25] Such exposure may be an inevitable consequence of the occupation of individuals and/or the climatic conditions of the geographic region in which they reside. If so, excessive sun exposure probably should be in the lifestyle category. However, recreational choice leading to excessive exposure such as sunbathing can be viewed either as lifestyle or as personal habit. The personal habit that has received the most attention in regard to aging is cigarette smoking. It is established that wrinkling of the skin, a hallmark of aging, is promoted by smoking.[26] Also, many age-associated diseases that cause marked physiologic deterioration are promoted by smoking. Examples are chronic obstructive lung disease,[27] stroke,[28] and cataracts.[29]

Although yet to be intensively studied, there is suggestive evidence that psychosocial factors markedly influence age-changes in physiologic function.[30] For example, it has been established that autonomy and control (i.e., the extent to which an individual can determine his or her course of action), can significantly influence physiologic functioning.[5] Elderly people commonly encounter reductions in autonomy and control because of many factors, such as a reduction in economic resources and institutional living facilities,[31] which lead to the deterioration of physiologic functions. Also, both bereavement and residential relocation have been found to increase mortality and morbidity in the elderly and, therefore, it is likely that they negatively impact the physiologic systems. It has been proposed that a reduction in social support plays a causative role[5] in the physiologic deterioration of the elderly. The epidemiologic research[32] associating low educational level with an increased risk of a decline in mental function with increasing age focuses on another psychosocial factor capable of influencing age-changes in the physiologic systems. Clearly, the subject of the influence of psychosocial factors on human aging is in the very preliminary stages of study and requires much further investigation. In particular, the pathways linking the psychosocial factors to the physiologic systems must be delineated.

Category 3

There is general agreement that much of the physiologic deterioration of the elderly is secondary to age-associated disease. It is also recognized that the occurrence and progression of age-associated disease is strongly influenced by age-associated physiologic deterioration. However, there is disagreement as to whether age-associated disease is part of the normal aging process. Indeed, in order to study what many investigators call normal aging, great effort is made to exclude from the population to be studied subjects with age-associated disease.[33] Such studies are invaluable because such a reductionist approach is a powerful tool in dissecting the details of the aging processes. However, the view that normal aging does not involve the occurrence of age-associated disease is not conceptually sound in terms of basic biology. Evolutionary biologists propose that aging (senescence) occurs because of the decline in the force of natural selection with advancing age.[34] Because of this, biologic processes that result in detrimental effects expressed late in life cannot be selected against. It is for this reason that physiologic deterioration increases with increasing age, and it is for the same reason that age-associated disease increasingly expresses with advancing age. It is true that some people (a very small subset) can age without evidence of discernible age-associated disease, but this may relate to the ambiguity in the distinction between age-associated disease and age-associated physiologic deterioration. For example, loss of bone mass is a well-recognized age-associated physiologic deterioration and osteoporosis is a major age-associated disease; the boundary in this case separating physiologic change from disease is far from clear. For all of the above reasons, in this chapter, deterioration of physiologic systems secondary to age-associated disease will be considered to be an integral part of aging. Of course, it is always important to know the specific reason for the altered physiology, and when an age-associated disease is the major immediate cause, it should be identified.

Interspecies and Intraspecies Variation in Age-Associated Physiologic Deterioration

In general terms, mammalian species are remarkably similar in that a progressive, but usually not linear, deterioration in the physiologic systems occurs with advancing postmaturational age.[35] However, there is considerable interspecies variation in the details of these physiologic changes. For example, bone loss in humans occurs over much of postmaturational period of life,[36] while in rats it occurs only in the terminal period of life and is associated with renal failure.[37] Another example is a progressive fall in the hematocrit level with increasing postmaturational age in rats, while in humans a decrease in the hematocrit level occurs only late in the life span if it occurs at all.[38] A third example is the increase in basal plasma glucocorticoid levels in rats[39] with increasing age, which does not occur in humans.[40] Certainly, much of this difference is genetic in origin, but differences in environmental conditions among species may also be a factor.

There is also great intraspecies heterogeneity in age-changes in the physiologic systems, a phenomenon that has been well characterized for humans.[5] In the case of many physiologic processes, humans show substantial deterioration on average, but some individuals will exhibit little or no change. An excellent example of this heterogeneity are the findings on kidney function obtained in the Baltimore Longitudinal Study of Aging[41] summarized in Figure 6-1. The mean decrease in creatinine clearance in 446 male subjects followed over a 23-year period was 0.87 ml per minute per year. However, one-third of the subjects showed no decline in creatinine clearance, as illustrated by the data of six subjects plotted in the bottom panel of Figure 6-1. In contrast, the subjects recorded in the top panel exhibit a marked decline and those recorded in the middle panel, a small although statistically significant decline. Environmental factors are responsible for much of this intraspecies heterogeneity.[5] However, genetics also plays a role and this is well illustrated by the fact that almost all male F344 strain rats develop interstitial cell tumors of the testis[6] by middle age, while such tumors rarely occur in most other strains of rats.

Age-Changes in the Physiology of Specific Organs and Organ Systems

All organs and organ systems exhibit age-associated physiologic deterioration, if not in all individuals, at least in a significant fraction of the population. This subject area is so vast that it cannot begin to be covered in this brief chapter. The volume on aging[1] of the *Handbook of Physiology* series of the American Physiological Society provides a systematic and extensive coverage for those needing in-depth information about a particular organ or organ system. Also, the other chapters of this textbook provide a substantial discussion of age-changes on the physiology of specific organs and organ systems relevant to the subject matter of the chapter. In this chapter a few specific examples have been selected for discussion solely for the purpose of illustrating the general concepts presented above.

The age-changes in the physiology of the heart illustrate several of the concepts particularly well. The early studies on the effect of age on human cardiac function noted marked changes with advancing age. The results of recent studies have shown much less dramatic age changes. The major reason for the differences between the older and the more recent studies resides in the selection of the human subjects for study. The

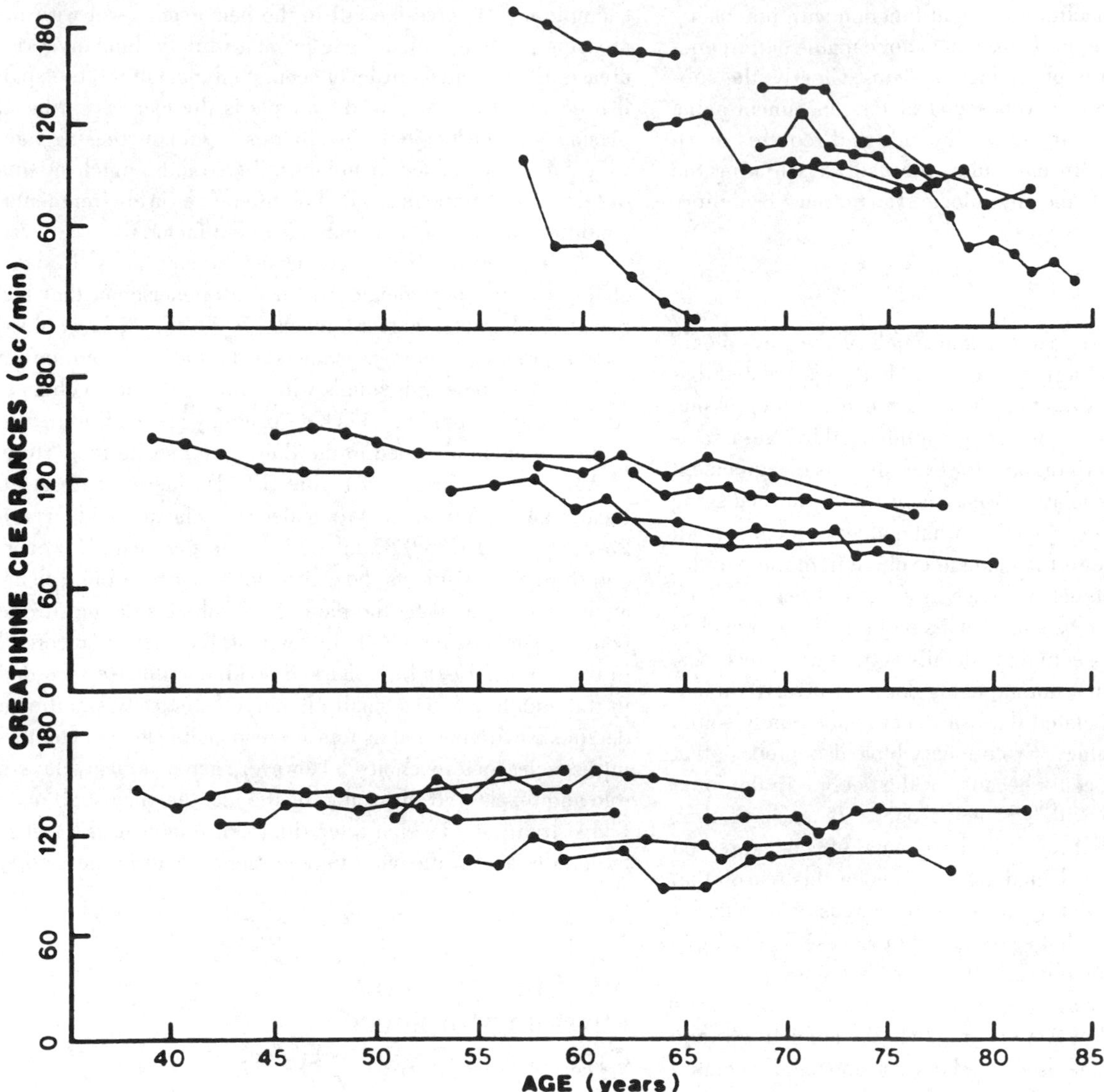

Figure 6-1 Age changes in creatinine clearance of male subjects studied serially in the Baltimore Longitudinal Study of Aging. Creatinine clearance is plotted on the x axis, and age in years of the subject on the y axis. The top panel presents the findings of six subjects from the group who exhibited marked decreases in creatinine clearance with increasing age; the middle panel presents the findings of six subjects from the group who exhibited a small but significant decrease in creatinine clearance with increasing age; the bottom panel presents the findings of six subjects from the group who exhibited no decrease in creatinine clearance with increasing age. (From Lindeman et al.,[41] with permission.)

investigators in the early studies did not recognize the need or often did not have the tools to carefully screen for physical fitness or age-associated disease, particularly occult coronary artery disease. For example, left ventricular wall thickness increases with increasing age in humans,[42] but in some individuals, the increase is moderate. Indeed, the extent of this age-change is markedly increased in individuals with coronary artery disease, those with hypertension, and in individuals with a sedentary lifestyle.[43] Resting cardiac output normalized to body surface area (i.e., cardiac index) has been reported to be markedly decreased with age,[44] mildy decreased,[45] and unchanged.[46] The reasons for these discrepancies in the literature is that resting cardiac index is influenced by hypertension, body composition, and undoubtedly other factors, and each of the populations studied probably differed in regard to these factors. In some studies, a reduced stroke volume index during vigorous exercise at advanced ages has been reported[47] while in other studies, either no change[48] or an increase[49] has been observed. The heterogeneity in these results is probably due to differences in the populations studied in regard to occult coronary artery disease, physical fitness, and body composition. However, not all changes in cardiac function with age have been related to age-associated disease, lifestyle, or body composition. For example, the reduced increase in heart rate in response to exercise has been observed in all subjects with advancing age, including those who are physically fit and free of occult coronary artery disease.[43] Another example is the decreased ability with advancing age of β-adrenergic agonists to increase heart rate;[50] it appears that aging blunts this response because of multiple changes in the molecular system coupling receptors and postreceptor mechanisms in all people with advancing age. Those age-changes in cardiac physiology that have not been related to disease, lifestyle, or environmental factors are felt to be due to intrinsic aging processes and inevitable. However, one cannot be certain that they do not arise from a yet to be recognized extrinsic factor or disease. Moreover, it is important to note that those age-changes in cardiac function that are secondary to lifestyle and other environmental factors are not inevitable and may be modifiable even at advanced ages, at least to some extent. Indeed, advances in medicine and public health have made modifiable some age-changes in cardiac function due to disease.

It has long been believed that a decrease in the glomerular filtration rate is an inevitable occurrence with advancing age.[51] This belief was based on cross-sectional studies. However, as discussed above, a longitudinal study has revealed that not all people exhibit a decline in glomerular filtration rate. Specifically, analysis of the findings of the Baltimore Longitudinal Study of Aging showed that a substantial fraction of that study population had little or no change in glomerular filtration rate with advancing age.[41] Unlike the heart, reasons for the differences among people in changes with age in kidney function have not been established. In a recent review article, Lindeman[52] has suggested that the decline in renal function noted in cross-sectional studies may be due to the fact that many in the population suffered from intervening pathology such as undetected glomerulonephritis or interstitial nephritis secondary to infections, immunologic insults, drugs and other toxic exposures, vascular occlusions resulting in ischemic injury, urinary tract obstruction, and infection. Indeed, it has been shown that hypertensive subjects have a more rapid age-associated decline in renal function than normotensive subjects.[53] It is also possible that lifetime dietary preferences play a role, since excessive dietary protein is believed to promote renal functional deterioration. Indeed, if the deterioration of renal function with age is primarily due to disease and environmental factors, then it is potentially modifiable by various public health measures.

The appearance of the skin is widely used as an indicator of the age of a person. The changes in skin underlying the altered appearance with increasing age are fine wrinkling, dryness, laxity, and proliferative lesions such as age spots, cherry angiomas, and seborrheic keratoses. However, most of these changes are not intrinsic but result from cumulative sun damage, since their extent is much reduced in skin areas protected from the sun.[54] Cigarette smoking is the other major factor that promotes skin wrinkling. Indeed, sun exposure and cigarette smoking appear to act synergistically to promote skin aging.[26] Thus, a commonly used marker of aging has little relation to intrinsic processes but primarily relates to environmental factors and can be readily modified by altering lifestyle. In addition to the change in appearance, many other skin functions deteriorate with age, including the barrier function, immune function, inflammatory response, wound healing, and Vitamin D production;[25] the extent to which the age-changes in these functions are secondary to sun exposure and cigarette smoking has yet to be carefully examined.

These three examples make clear that many age changes are not primarily due to intrinsic aging processes but, to varying degrees, are secondary to or at least promoted by age-associated disease or extrinsic factors or both. To view them as not part of the aging process removes from consideration major problems that confront individuals as they age, nor is there any biologic basis for such a view. It is true that deterioration due to disease or extrinsic factors may be preventable and, in some cases, reversible, but that hardly lessens their involvement in aging. Indeed, much of what we currently consider to be intrinsic may ultimately be found to be of extrinsic origin or at least influenced by extrinsic factors. And what is considered to be extrinsic has its actions by interacting with intrinsic processes. Indeed, what is considered to be lifestyle may have a strong intrinsic base. For example, the sedentary lifestyle adopted by many people as they age also occurs in laboratory rats,[55] which in the case of the rodent, is probably better viewed to be intrinsic rather than a lifestyle choice. Moreover, as discussed above, there are strong reasons to believe that most age-associated diseases are part of the aging process, making their separation from other aspects of aging arbitrary and of little value, other than providing detailed information about aging of some practical relevance and, in some instances, of theoretic importance.

Age-Changes in Organismic Function

Given the many deteriorative changes that occur in the physiology of organs and organ systems, it is to be expected that the functional competence of the organism is compromised with advancing age. Indeed, organismic functional deficits occur that can be classified in the following way: (1) reduced functional capacity, (2) compromised ability to cope with challenges, and (3) altered homeostasis. A few examples of these organismic functional deficits are presented below.

Ability to Cope with Challenges

The reduced ability to cope with challenges, or what are often referred to as stressors, is a hallmark of the aging phenotype.[56] It is well known that secretion of glucocorticoids by the hypothalmic-adenohypopyseal-adrenocortical system and an increase in the activity of the adrenal medullary-sympathetic nervous system are responses common to all stressors, and that they play an important role in enabling mammalian organisms to cope with all stressors.[40] Also, induction of the heat shock protein system is a common response, enabling organisms of almost all species to withstand many different cellular stressors.[57] Of course, in addition to these general responses, there are defenses that are specific for particular stressors or challenges. However, because the loss with advancing age in ability of organisms to cope appears to occur with all types of stressors, it might be expected that there is deterioration of one or more of the general mechanisms. The currently available evidence does not indicate that the ability of the hypothalmic-adenohypophyseal-adrenocortical system to respond to challenges by increasing the secretion of glucocorticoid hormone is compromised by aging.[58] Of course, that does not rule out the possibility of a reduced ability of the glucocorticoid target site to respond to the hormone, but studies designed to address this possibility have yet to be done. There is some indication that the response of the adrenal medullary-sympathetic nervous system to challenges may be attenuated with advancing age,[40] but these findings are hard to interpret because basal levels of catecholamines are elevated with increasing age. There is also evidence that there is a blunting with increasing age of at least some adrenergic responses in target tissues. Nevertheless, based on current information, it does not seem that an inadequate response of the adrenal medullary-sympathetic nervous system plays a major role in the reduced ability of the organism to meet challenges. In contrast to these neuroendocrine responses, the evidence is clear that the ability to induce heat shock proteins in response to cellular stressors markedly decreases with increasing age of mammals,[59] which may play a major role in the loss in ability to cope with stressors. However, because the deterioration in physiologic systems occurs with advancing age in most organs and organ systems, functional deficits in specific responses may underly the reduced ability of the aged to deal with a broad scope of challenges. A case in point is the decrease in the ability of the immune system to protect the organism from damage due to infectious agents.[60] Thus, although it has long been known that successfully meeting challenges is compromised with advancing age, the basis of this deficit remains to be fully elucidated.

Aerobic Capacity

The ability of the cardiopulmonary system to supply oxygen to exercising muscles and the ability of these muscles to use this oxygen in energy metabolism is referred to as the aerobic capacity. It is a measure of the maximum ability to carry out exercise and is determined by measuring the maximum rate of oxygen consumption attainable when performing an exercise test of increasing intensity that requires a large proportion of the total skeletal muscle mass. Aerobic capacity decreases in healthy sedentary men and women at the rate of about 10 percent per decade.[61] Since physical fitness markedly influences aerobic capacity, some of this decrease may be due to the fall in physical activity with advancing age. Of course, the decline in aerobic capacity is much greater in elderly suffering from chronic disease, particularly atherosclerotic disease. Well-trained endurance athletes at all ages have a higher aerobic capacity than untrained people of the same age. However, it is striking that the trained athlete also exhibits an age-associated decline in aerobic capacity, making it evident that a decrease in physical fitness is not the only factor underlying this age-related decline. Nevertheless, there is suggestive but not unequivocal evidence that the rate of decline in aerobic capacity with age is less in the trained athletes than in the untrained.[62] The aerobic capacity of sedentary men and women in the age range of 60 to 80 years can be increased by physical training,[63] but even if the training is maintained, the age-associated decline continues. Nevertheless, the elderly who continue the physical training maintain an aerobic capacity greater than that of their sedentary peers, which under certain circumstances, can significantly improve the quality of life. The decrease in aerobic capacity with advancing age is to a large extent due to alteration in cardiovascular function, but noncardiovascular factors such a reduction in skeletal muscle mass also play a role,[64] the extent of which varies among individuals.

Acid-Base Homeostasis

An analysis of data from many cross-sectional studies[65] has revealed that acid-base homeostasis is altered with advancing age. From age 20 to 80 years, the apparent steady-state plasma concentration of hydrogen ion was found to increase by 6 to 7 percent and that of bicarbonate ion to decrease by 12 to 16 percent. It has been suggested that this change in steady-state acid-base characteristics is due to a decline in renal function. If so, it would be expected that those subjects in the Baltimore Longitudinal Study of Aging—who did not have a change in renal function with age—would not exhibit this age-alteration in acid-base homeostasis. Such information has not been published and, if it is not available in the Baltimore Longitudinal Study of Aging data set, a longitudinal study should be carried out in which alterations with age in acid-base homeostasis and in renal function can be correlated. The low level metabolic acidosis that appears to occur in many people with advancing age may play a role in age-associated bone loss, a factor that has received little attention from those who study bone loss and aging.

Lean Body Mass

Lean body mass, or probably better called fat-free mass, is fairly stable in men and women through about 40 years of age, and then decreases with advancing age with the rate of loss accelerating with increasing age.[62] Clearly, the homeostatic system regulating fat-free mass is deranged at advanced age. Although an increasingly sedentary lifestyle is undoubtedly involved, physical fitness does not fully prevent the age-associated loss of fat-free mass, because it also occurs in trained athletes.[22] The principle component in this fall of fat-free mass is the loss of skeletal muscle mass with advancing age.[66] It is this loss of muscle mass that is the primary reason for the decrease in muscle strength with age.[67] Although muscle mass is lost with age in sedentary people and in athletes alike, exercise can improve the functional capacity of the elderly. High intensity resistance training has been found to increase muscle size and strength in the elderly,[68] which can be invaluable in enabling an elderly individual to maintain an independent existance of reasonable quality.

Fat Mass

Cross-sectional studies indicate that body fat mass increases with age in both men and women.[62] In women, a linear increase in percent body fat with age occurs through the eighth decade of life, with the average value being 25 percent and 41 percent at 25 and 75 years of age, respectively. In men the increase in body fat with age is similar to that of women through 50 years of age, but slows at more advanced ages. Even in those people whose body weight does not increase with age, body fat increases as lean body mass decreases. The homeostatic regulation of fat mass clearly becomes faulty with advancing age. Indeed, Pollack et al.[22] found that even in athletes that remain competitive there is a small increase in fat content with advancing age. Apparently, therefore, exercise can attenuate but not totally prevent the age-associated increase in body fat. In men, the increase in fat mass with age occurs primarily in the abdominal region, while such is not the case for women until after the age of 54 years.[69] Exercise not only decreases the age-associated increase in body fat but, most importantly, it also attenuates the disproportionate increase in abdominal fat.[70] The great concern about abdominal fat is due to the extensive evidence indicating that it is a risk factor for several age-associated pathologic problems including hypertension, type II diabetes, cardiovascular disease, as well as some types of cancer.[71] Thus, interventions aimed at preventing the abdominal accumulation of fat with advancing age are most important to develop.

Bone Mass

Every population that has been studied shows age-associated bone loss,[36] which suggests that it is an inevitable consequence of aging. Much progress is currently being made in regard to the molecular basis of this bone loss but, as of now, a clear understanding of the biologic basis has not emerged. Nearly all bones are affected to varying degrees. The age of onset of bone loss depends on gender and type of bone. Vertebral bone loss in women may start as early as the third decade of life, while the loss of appendicular bone occurs at a much older age.[72] Bone loss accelerates following menopause, with the inevitable occurence of estrogen deficiency being the major responsible factor.[73] Bone loss in men begins at an older age than in women and for some, the extent of loss is trivial. Although all people lose bone, the extent of bone loss and its clinical consequences vary among individuals. Black women have a higher bone mass as young adults and, as a consequence, are less prone to bone fractures with advancing age than white women.[74] There is evidence that exercise attenuates age-associated bone loss[75] and that an adequate intake of dietary calcium is needed to minimize loss.[76] Cigarette smoking and the consumption of alcohol and caffeine have been implicated as factors promoting age-associated bone loss.[77,78] Although the homeostatic ability to maintain bone mass becomes faulty in all people with advancing age, interventions are possible that will enable many to avoid much of the negative consequences during their lifetime. Estrogen replacement therapy markedly blunts the accelerated postmenopausal loss of bone, but its use must be evaluated in relation to the possible negative aspects of such therapy. Dietary supplements and exercise programs are also potential avenues of intervention. Moreover, giving up cigarette smoking, and moderation in other personal habits such as in the consumption of alcohol- and caffeine-containing beverages, should be helpful.

Body Temperature

The homeostatic regulation of body temperature and the ability to adapt to different thermal environments deteriorates with advancing age.[79] The extent of this deterioration varies among individuals and is influenced by health status, physical fitness, and personal habits such as cigarette smoking and alcohol consumption.[80] Part of the loss in ability to cope with extremes in environmental temperature stems from the reduction in the perception of the thermal environment. Because of this, individuals fail to make appropriate behavioral responses.[80] However, physiologic homeostatic failure also underlies the impaired ability to maintain body temperature. In response to a hot environment, the elderly are less able to increase cutaneous blood flow as effectively as young people.[81] Sweating is also impaired in the elderly[82] and this may be due to the decrease in physical fitness with increasing age.[83] The response to a cold environment is also compromised in the elderly,[84] with both the cutaneous vasoconstrictor response and the shivering response being less effective; in many cases, this can at least in part be traced to medications used to treat chronic age-associated diseases. To a great extent, the physiologic deficits can be compensated by appropriate conscious behavioral responses, but even this avenue becomes less trustworthy because of the perception deficit. The rise in body temperature in response to pyrogens is blunted with increasing age.[85] This deficit deprives the elderly of the possible benefits of fever in coping with infections.

Glucose Homeostasis

A diminished homeostatic regulation of plasma glucose concentration is a common characteristic of the aging phenotype.[16] When this regulatory ability declines sufficiently, a diagnosis of type II diabetes is made—a common age-associated disease in the elderly. The major tool for examining glucose homeostasis has been the oral glucose tolerance test. Typical findings are those of Chen et al.,[86] shown in Figure 6-2. They administered orally 100 g of glucose to groups of healthy old and young subjects; plasma glucose rose to higher levels and remained elevated longer in the old than in the young, while the rise in plasma insulin level was delayed in the old but with time

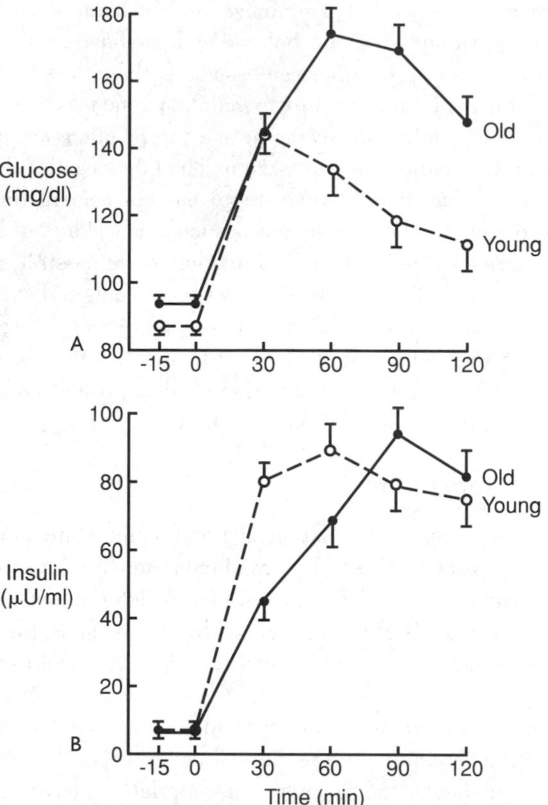

Figure 6-2 Influence of age on the response of plasma glucose and insulin concentration to an oral load of glucose. Young and old healthy human subjects were given orally 100 g of glucose. **(A)** Response of plasma glucose concentration; **(B)** response of plasma insulin. (From Chen et al.,[86] with permission.)

reached that of the young. A reduced ability to secrete insulin does not appear to be a major reason for this alteration in glucose homeostasis with age.[87] There is strong evidence that an increased resistance to insulin action is a major factor in the diminished homeostatic glucose regulation in old people.[88] With advancing age, people become increasingly sedentary and show an increase in body fat, particularly in the abdominal region—factors that are known to increase insulin resistance and to blunt the glucose homeostatic responses. Indeed, Zavaroni et al.[89] have reported that the effect of aging on glucose tolerance is essentially eliminated after correcting for the effects of physical inactivity and adiposity. This view is consistent with the finding that there are old people who are similar to young people in regard to glucose tolerance and insulin sensitivity.[90] However, there is evidence that indicates that a small component of glucose intolerance and insulin resistance with advancing age is independent of physical inactivity and adiposity.[91] Nevertheless, most people of middle-age and older can greatly improve their homeostatic regulation of glucose by modifying their lifestyle to reduce adiposity and increase physical fitness.

Summary and Conclusions

Physiologic deterioration is a hallmark of the aging phenotype. This deterioration is caused by (1) damage resulting from intrinsic living processes, (2) damage due to extrinsic factors such as diet, lifestyle, personal habits, and psychosocial factors, and (3) age-associated diseases. Although mammalian species are similar in that all show a progressive deterioration of physiologic processes with advancing age, the details of this deterioration varies among species. Thus, the detailed characteristics of the deterioration probably has a strong genetic component. There is also a considerable intraspecies variation in the rate and character of physiologic deterioration with advancing age. Much of the differences among individuals of the same species appears to relate to extrinsic factors. Age-associated deterioration occurs in all organs and organ systems. The extent to which extrinsic factors and age-associated disease play a role varies among organ systems and among individuals but, in most cases, they play a major role. These age-changes in the physiology of organs and organ systems compromise the functional abilities of the organism and underly the decreasing ability to survive with advancing age. The physiologic deficits of the aging organism can be summarized as (1) a reduced functional capacity, (2) a decreased ability to cope with challenges, and (3) an altered homeostasis. Because much of the physiologic deterioration with advancing age is caused by extrinsic factors, organismic aging can be modified by altering lifestyle and environmental factors. Also, the large role that age-associated disease plays in the physiologic deterioration can be modulated by presently available medical and public health measures and undoubtedly much more by those that will be developed in the future.

References

1. Masoro EJ (ed): Handbook of Physiology. Section 11. Aging. Oxford University Press, New York, 1995
2. Yu BP: Cellular defenses against damage from reactive oxygen species. Physiol Rev 1994;74:139–162
3. Sell DR, Lane MA, Johnson WA et al: Longevity and the genetic determination of collagen glycoxidation kinetics in mammalian senescence. Proc Natl Acad USA 1996;93:485–490
4. Strehler BL: Time, cells, and aging. 2nd Ed. Academic Press, New York, 1977
5. Rowe JW, Kahn RL: Human aging: usual and successful. Science 1987;237:143–149
6. Masoro EJ: Dietary restriction and aging. J Am Geriatr Soc 1993;41:994–999
7. Leveille PJ, Weindruch R, Walford RL et al: Dietary restriction retards age-related loss of gamma crystallins in the mouse lens. Science 1984;224:1247–1249
8. Roth GS, Ingram DK, Joseph JA: Delayed loss of striatial dopamine receptors during aging of dietarily restricted rats. Brain Res 1984;300:27–32
9. Ingram DK, Weindruch R, Spangler EL et al: Dietary restriction

benefits learning and motor performance of aged mice. J Gerontol 1987;42:78–81

10. Bertrand HA, Anderson WR, Masoro EJ, Yu BP: Action of food restriction on age-related changes in adipocyte lipolysis. J Gerontol 1987;42:591–595
11. Holehan AM, Merry BJ: Lifetime breeding studies in fully fed and dietary restricted female CFY Sprague-Dawley rats. I. Effects of age, housing conditions and diet on fecundity. Mech Aging Dev 1985;33:19–28
12. Yu BP: Putative interventions. p. 613. In Masoro EJ (ed): Handbook of Physiology. Section 11: Aging. Oxford University Press, New York, 1995
13. Yu BP, Masoro EJ, McMahan CA: Nutritional influences on aging of Fischer 344 rats. I. Physical, metabolic and longevity characteristics. J Gerontol 1985;40:657–670
14. Masoro EJ: Food restriction in rodents: an evaluation of its role in the study of aging. J Gerontol: Biol Sci 1988;43:B59–B64
15. Lipschitz DA: Nutrition and ageing. p. 119. In Evans JG, Williams TF (eds): Oxford Textbook of Geriatric Medicine. Oxford University Press, Oxford, 1992
16. Halter JB: Carbohydrate metabolism. p. 119. In Masoro EJ (ed): Handbook of Physiology. Section 11: Aging. Oxford University Press, New York, 1995
17. Cunningham D, Montoye H, Metzer H, Keller J: Active leisure time activities as related to age among males in a total population. J Gerontol 1968;23:551–559
18. Ehsani AA, Ogawa T, Miller TR et al: Exercise training improves left ventricular systolic function in older men. Circulation 1991;83:96–103
19. Lexell J, Taylor CC, Sjostrom M: What is the cause of the ageing atrophy? Total number, size and proportion of different fiber types studied in whole vastus lateralis muscles from 15 to 83 year-old men. J Neurol Sci 1988;84:275–294
20. Fiatarone MA, Marks EC, Ryan CN et al: High intensity strength training in nonagenarians. JAMA 1990;263:3029–3034
21. Hallfrisch J, Muller D, Drinkwater D et al: Continuing diet trends in men: the Baltimore Longitudinal Study of Aging (1961–1987). J Gerontol: Med Sci 1990;45:M186–191
22. Pollock ML, Foster C, Knapp D et al: Effect of age and training on aerobic capacity and body composition of master athletes. J Appl Physiol 1987;62:725–731
23. Kohrt WM, Obert KA, Holloszy JO: Exercise training improves fat distribution patterns in 60- and 70-year-old men and women. J Gerontol: Med Sci 1992;47:M99–M105
24. Rogers MA, King DS, Hagberg JM et al: Effect of 10 days of inactivity on glucose tolerance in master athletes. J Applied Physiol 1990;68:1833–1837
25. Chuttani A, Gilchrest BA: Skin. p. 309. In Masoro EJ (ed): Handbook of Physiology. Section 11: Aging. Oxford University Press, New York, 1995
26. Kadence DP, Burr R, Gress R et al: Cigarette smoking: a significant risk factor for premature facial wrinkling. Ann Intern Med 1991;114:840–844
27. Fletcher CM, Peto R, Tinker C, Speizer FE: The natural history of chronic bronchitis and emphysema. Oxford University Press, London, 1976
28. Hyman NM: Pathology of stroke. p. 297. In Evans JG, Williams TF (eds): Oxford Textbook of Geriatric Medicine. Oxford University Press, Oxford, 1992
29. Bron GA: The ageing eye. p. 557. In Evans JG, Williams TF (eds): Oxford Textbook of Geriatric Medicine, Oxford University Press, Oxford 1992
30. Berkman LF, Seeman TE, Albert M et al: High, usual, and impaired functioning in community-dwelling older men and women: findings from the Macarthur Foundation research network on successful aging. J Clin Epidemiol 1993;46: 1129–1140
31. Holmes TH, Rahe RH: The social readjustment rating scale. J Psychosom Res 1967;11:213–218
32. White L, Katzman R, Losonczy M et al: Association of education on the incidence of cognitive impairment in three established populations for epidemiological studies of the elderly. J Clin Epidemiol 1994;47:363–374
33. Rowe JW, Wang SY, Elahi D: Design, conduct, and analysis of human aging research. In Schneider EL, Rowe JW (eds): Handbook of the Biology of Aging. 3rd Ed. Academic Press, San Diego, 1990
34. Rose MR: Evolutionary Biology of Aging. Oxford University Press, New York, 1991
35. Finch CE: Longevity, senescence, and the genome. University of Chicago Press, Chicago, 1990
36. Kalu DN: Bone. p. 395. In Masoro EJ (ed): Handbook of Physiology. Section 11: Aging. Oxford University Press, New York, 1995
37. Kalu DN, Hardin RR, Cockerham R et al: Lifelong food restriction prevents senile osteopenia and hyperparathyroidism in F344 rats. Mech Aging Dev 1984;26:103–112
38. Masoro EJ, Mc Mahan CA, Shimokawa I et al: Longitudinal study of the hemocrit of *ad libitum* fed and dietary restricted male F344 rats. Aging: Clin Exper Res 1994;6:287–292
39. Sabatino F, Masoro EJ, Mc Mahan CA, Kuhn RW: Assessment of the role of the glucocorticoid system in the aging processes and in the action of food restriction. J Gerontol: Biol Sci 1991; 46:B171–B179
40. Mobbs CV: Neuroendocrinology of aging. p. 234. In Schnieder EL, Rowe JW (eds): Handbook of the Biology of Aging. 4th Ed. Academic Press, San Diego, 1996
41. Lindeman RD, Tobin JD, Shock NW: Longitudinal studies on the rate of decline in renal function with age. J Am Geriatr Soc 1985;33:278–285
42. Linzbach AJ, Akuamoa-Boateng E: Die alternsveranderungen des menschlichen herzens. Klin Wochenschr 1973;51: 156–163
43. Lakatta EG: Cardiovascular system. p. 413. In Masoro EJ (ed): Handbook of Physiology. Section 11: Aging. Oxford University Press, New York, 1995
44. Brandonfbrener M, Landowne M, Shock NW: Changes in cardiac output with age. Circulation 1955;12:557–566
45. Coggan AR, Spina RJ, Rogers MA et al: Histochemical and enzymatic characteristics of skeletal muscle in master athletes. J Applied Physiol 1990;68:1896–1901
46. Fleg JL, Gerstenblith G, Zonderman AB et al: Prevalence and

diagnostic significance of exercise-induced silent myocardial ischemia detected by thallium scintigraphy and electrocardiography in assymptomatic volunteers. Circulation 1990;81: 423–436

47. Kuickka JT, Lansimies E: Effect of age on cardiac index, stroke index and left ventricular ejection fraction at rest and during exercise as studied by radiocardiography. Acta Physiol Scand 1982;114:339–343
48. Fleg JL, Gerstenblith G, Schulman SP et al: Gender differences in exercise hemodynamics of older subjects: effects of conditioning status. Circulation 1990;82:III–239
49. Mann DL, Dennenberg BS, Gash AK et al: Effects of age on ventricular performance during graded supine exercise. Am Heart J 1986;111:108–115
50. Stratton JR, Cerquerira MD, Schwartz RS et al: Differences in cardiovascular responses to isoproterenol in relation to age and exercise training in healthy men. Circulation 1992;86:504–512
51. Rowe JW, Andres R, Tobin JD et al: The effect of age on creatinine clearance in men: a cross sectional and longitudinal study. J Gerontol 1976;31:155–163
52. Lindeman RD: Renal and urinary tract function. p. 485. In Masoro EJ (ed): Handbook of Physiology. Section 11: Aging. Oxford University Press, New York, 1995
53. Lindeman RD, Tobin JD, Shock NW: Association between blood pressure and the rate of decline in renal function with age. Kidney Int 1984;26:861–868
54. Gilchrest BA: Physiology and pathophysiology of aging skin. p. 1425. In Goldsmith L (ed): Physiology, Biochemistry and Molecular Biology of the Skin. 2nd Ed. Oxford University Press, New York, 1991
55. Yu BP, Masoro EJ, Mc Mahan CA: Nutritional influences on aging of Fischer 344 rats. I. Physical, metabolic and longevity characteristics. J Gerontol 1985;40:657–670
56. Masoro EJ: Aging: current concepts. p. 3. In Masoro EJ (ed): Handbook of Physiology. Section 11: Aging. Oxford University Press, New York, 1995
57. Lindquist S: The heat shock response. Ann Rev Biochem 1986; 55:1151–1191
58. Masoro EJ: Glucocorticoids and aging. Aging: Clin Exper Res 1995;7:407–413
59. Heydari AR, Gutsmann A, You S et al: Effect of dietary restriction on the genome function of cells: alterations in the transcriptional apparatus of cells. p. 213. In: Hart RW, Neumann DA, Robertson RT (eds): Dietary Restriction: Implications for the Interpretation of Toxicity and Carcinogenicity Studies. ILSI Press, Washington, DC, 1995
60. Miller RA: Aging and the immune response. p. 355. In Schneider EL, Rowe JL (eds): Handbook of the Biology of Aging. 4th Ed. Academic Press, San Diego, 1996
61. Buskirk ER, Hodgson JL: Age and aerobic power: the rate of change in men and women. Federation Proc 1987;46: 1824–1829
62. Holloszy JO, Kohrt WM: Exercise. p. 633. In Masoro EJ (ed): Handbook of Physiology. Section 11: Aging. Oxford University Press, New York, 1994
63. Kohrt WM, Malley MT, Coggan AR et al: Effects of gender, age, and fitness level on response of VO_{2max} to training in 60 to 71 year-olds. J Applied Physiol 1991;71:2004–2011
64. Spirduso WW: Physical Dimensions of Aging. Human Kinetics, Champaign, IL, 1995
65. Frassetto L, Sebastian A: Age and systemic acid-base equilibrium: analysis of published data. J Gerontol: Biol Sci 1996; 51A:B91–B99
66. Cohn SH, Vartsky D, Yasumura S et al: Compartmental body composition based on total-body potassium and calcium. Am J Physiol 1980;239:E524–E530
67. Evans WJ: What is sarcopenia? J Gerontol 1995;50A:5–8
68. Evans WJ: Effects of exercise on body composition and functional capacity of the elderly. J Gerontol 1995;50A:147–150
69. Shimokata H, Tobin JD, Muller DC et al: Studies in the distribution of body fat: I. Effects of age, sex, and obesity. J Gerontol: Med Sci 1989;44:M66–M73
70. Kohrt WM, Malley MT, Dalsky DP, Holloszy JO: Body composition of healthy sedentary and trained, young and older men and women. Med Sci Sports Exerc 1992;24:832–837
71. Elahi D, Dyke MM, Andres R: Aging, fat metabolism, and obesity. p. 147. In Masoro EJ (ed): Handbook of Physiology. Section, 11: Aging. Oxford University Press, New York, 1995
72. Riggs BL, Wahner HW, Dunn WL et al: Differential changes in bone mineral density of the appendicular and axial skeleton with aging. Relationship to spinal osteoporosis. J Clin Invest 1981;67:1487–1491
73. Slemenda C, Hui SL, Longcope C, Johnston CC: Sex steroids and bone mass: a study of changes about the time of menopause. J Clin Invest 1987;80:1261–1269
74. Garn SM: Bone loss and aging. p. 39. In Goldman R, Rockstein M (eds): Physiological and pathology of human aging. Academic Press, New York, 1975
75. Sandler RB, La Porte R, Sashin D et al: The epidemiology of physical activity and postmenopausal bone loss. First year of a clinical trial. p. 317. In Christiansen C, Arnaud CD, Nordin BEC et al (eds): Osteoporosis I. Aalborg Stiftsbogtrykkeri, Glostrup, 1984
76. Cuming RG: Calcium intake and bone mass: a quantitative review of the evidence. Calcif Tissue Int 1990;47:194–210
77. Heaney RP: Calcium intake, bone health and aging. p. 165. In Young EL (ed): Nutrition, Aging and Health. Alan R Liss, New York, 1986
78. Seeman E, Melton LJ, O'Fallon WM, Riggs BL: Risk factors of spinal osteoporosis in men. Am J Med 1983;75:977–983
79. Collins KJ, Exton-Smith AN: Thermal homeostasis in old age. J Am Geriatr Soc 1983;31:519–524
80. Lybarger JA, Kilbourne EH: Hyperthermia and hypothermia in the elderly: an epidemiologic view. p. 149. In Davis BB, Wood WC (eds): Homeostatic Function and Aging. Raven Press, New York, 1985
81. Kenney WL: Control of heat-induced cutaneous vasodilation in relation to age. Eur J Appl Physiol 1988;57:120–125
82. Inoue Y, Nakao M, Araki T, Murakami H: Regional differences in the sweating responses of older and younger men. J Applied Physiol 1991;71:2453–2459
83. Tankersly CG, Smolander J, Kenney WL, Fortney SM: Sweating

and skin blood flow during exercise: effects of age and maximum oxygen uptake. J Applied Physiol 1991;71:236–242

84. McCarter RJM: Energy utilization. p. 95. In Masoro EJ (ed): Handbook of Physiology. Section 11: Aging. Oxford University Press, New York, 1995

85. Norman DC, Grahn D, Yoshikawa TT: Fever and aging. J Am Geriatr Soc 1985;33:859–863

86. Chen M, Halter JB, Porte Jr, D: The role of dietary carbohydrate in the decreased glucose tolerance of the elderly. J Am Geriatr Soc 1987;35:417–424

87. Gumbiner B, Polonsky KS, Beltz WF et al: Effects of aging on insulin secretion. Diabetes 1989;38:1549–1556

88. Supiano MA, Hogikyan RV, Morrow LA et al: Aging and insulin resistance: role of blood pressure and sympathetic nervous system. J Gerontol: Med Sci 1993;48:M237–M243

89. Zavaroni I, Dall'Aglio E, Bruschi F et al: Effect of age and environmental factors on glucose tolerance and insulin secretion in a worker population. J Am Geriatr Soc 1986;34:271–275

90. Broughton DL, James OWF, Alberti KGMM, Taylor R: Peripheral and hepatic insulin sensitivity in healthy elderly human subjects. Eur J Clin Invest 1991;21:13–21

91. Shimokata H, Muller DC, Fleg JL et al: Age as an independent determinant of glucose tolerance. Diabetes 1991;40:44–51

CHAPTER 7

Connective Tissues and Aging

NICHOLAS A. KEFALIDES

The reciprocal role of aging and connective tissues is a complex issue, involving a variety of factors and interactions. One could inquire into the effects of aging on connective tissues and, conversely, one may ask how the components of connective tissue contribute to the aging process. To answer these questions, it becomes important to have some understanding of the structural biochemistry of connective tissues; the processes involved in their biosynthesis, modification, extracellular organization, and molecular genetics; as well as the factors affecting the properties of connective tissue cells and the extracellular matrix (ECM). Armed with this knowledge, it becomes apparent that there can be a huge number of events in the development of connective tissues that may be associated, directly or indirectly, in the processes or effects of aging. Over the past 25 years these have been and continue to be areas of intensive research.

This chapter presents an abbreviated discussion of the various components of the extracellular matrix, their structure, molecular organization, biosynthesis, modification, turnover, and molecular genetics. Some concepts on the effects of aging on the ECM and the effects of aging on the properties of various connective tissues, as well as the involvement of connective tissue physiology on diseases associated with aging will be discussed.

The Properties of Connective Tissues

The properties of connective tissues are derived primarily from the properties of the components of the ECM surrounding, and secreted by, the cells of those tissues. Some connective tissues such as cartilage or tendons may comprise primarily a single cell type (e.g., chondrocytes or fibroblasts) whose synthesis and secretion of ECM and other factors largely determines the properties of the tissue. Some tissues, such as bone and blood vessels, contain a number of different connective tissue cell types that contribute to both their structural and functional properties. Other tissues, such as cardiac muscle and kidney, may have properties dependent upon connective tissue components whose biologic roles are separate from the major physiologic function of the tissue and that may have influence over the properties of that tissue during the process of aging. Different cell types will exhibit different phenotypic patterns of ECM production that, in turn, will influence the structural properties of a given connective tissue.

The major components of the ECM fall into three general classes of molecules: the structural proteins, which include the collagens, of which there are now 19 types recognized; elastin, the proteoglycans, which contain several structurally distinct molecular classes; and the structural glycoproteins, whose contribution to the properties of connective tissues has been recognized only within the past 15 to 20 years. The interactions between these materials determines the development and properties of the connective tissues.

The Collagens

Structure

The collagens are a family of connective tissue proteins having a triple-stranded organization and containing molecular domains within which the strands are coiled around one another in a triple helix. The reader is referred to two recent reviews on collagen biochemistry.[1,2] At present, the genes of at least 19 distinct collagen types have been characterized.[1,2] The interstitial collagens—types I, II, III, and V—exist as large, extended molecules that tend to organize into fibrils.[2] There may be more than one collagen type within these fibrils.[3] Type IV collagen, also known as basement membrane collagen, does not exist in fibrillar form but rather, in a complex network of collagen molecules linked by disulfide and other cross-linkages, and associated with noncollagenous molecules such as laminin, entactin and proteoglycans, to form an amorphous matrix.[4,5] Although presently we recognize the existence of at least 19 genetically distinct collagen types, the protein of only the first 11 collagens has been isolated from tissues. Table 7-1 contains a summary of the collagen gene family. There are 33 genes corresponding to the α chains of 19 collagen types. The most abundant collagen and the most abundant protein in the body is collagen type I. The table classifies the various collagens into seven groups, depending on the nature of the fibrils they form. The basic unit of the type I collagen fibril is a triple helical heterotrimer, tropocollagen, consisting of two identical chains termed $\alpha 1(I)$ and a third chain, $\alpha 2(I)$.[2] The other collagen types have been given similar designations; however, some of the collagen types are homotrimers containing three identical chains, and some collagen types contain three genetically distinct α chains as indicated in Table 7-2. The collagen α chain has a unique amino acid composition, with glycine occupying every third position in the sequence. Thus the collagenous domains consist of a repeating peptide triplet, -Gly-X-Y-, in which X and Y are amino acids other than

Table 7-1 Collagen gene family

Fibrillar collagen genes	I, II, III, V, XI	9 genes
Fibril-associated collagens (FACIT)	IX, XII, XIV	5 genes
Network-forming collagen genes	IV	6 genes
Short chain collagen genes	VIII, X	3 genes
Collagens forming filamentous beads	VI	3 genes
Anchoring fibers	VII	1 gene
Multiple domain collagens	XIII, XV, XVI, XVII, XVIII, XIX	6 genes
Total		33 genes

glycine. A large percentage of amino acids in the Y position are occupied by proline. In addition, collagen contains two unique amino acids derived from posttranslational modifications of the protein, 4-hydroxyproline and hydroxylysine. The presence of hydroxyproline provides additional sites along the α chain capable of forming hydrogen bonds with adjacent α chains, which are important in stabilizing the triple helix so that it maintains its structure at body temperatures. If hydroxyproline formation is inhibited, the triple helix dissociates into its component α chains at 37°C. The presence of glycine in every third position, along with the extensive hydrogen bonding, provides the triple helix with a compact protected structure resistant to the action of most proteases. The structures of collagens can be stabilized further through the formation of covalent cross-linkages, derived from modification and condensation of certain lysine and hydroxylysine residues on adjacent α chains.[6] Cross-linkage formation is important in stabilizing collagen fibrils, and contributes to their high tensile strength.

Biosynthesis

Type I collagen α chains are synthesized as a larger precursor, procollagen, containing noncollagenous sequences at their C and N termini.[2,7] As each pro-α chain is synthesized, intracellular prolyl and lysyl hydroxylases act to form hydroxyproline and hydroxylysine. The triple helix is formed intracellularly and stabilized by the formation of interchain disulfide bonds near the carboxyl termini of the component pro-α chains. After secretion of the triple helical collagen, procollagen peptidases remove most of the noncollagenous portions at either end of the procollagen. Extracellular lysine and hydroxylysine oxidases oxidize the amino groups of lysine or hydroxylysine to form aldehyde derivatives, which can go on to form Schiff base adducts, the first cross-linkages. These can rearrange and become reduced to form the various other cross-linkages. The subject of collagen cross-linking is elegantly discussed in three reviews.[6,8,9] An increased number of collagen cross-links have been reported in a pathologic state known as scleroderma.

Collagenolysis

Extracellular degradation of collagen is accomplished by enzymes known as tissue collagenases. These enzymes cleave triple helical collagen at a site three-quarters from the amino terminus[10] resulting in the formation of two triple helical fragments, which denature at temperatures above 32°C to form nonhelical peptides, helical peptides that can now be degraded by tissue proteinases. Cleavage by tissue collagenase is considered to be the rate-limiting step in collagenolysis of triple helical collagen. Collagenolysis is the subject of a review by Harris et al.[10] Collagenolysis is an important physiologic process responsible, to a large extent, for the repair of wounds and processes of tissue remodeling in which undesired accumulations are removed as new connective tissue is laid down. However, in conditions such as rheumatoid arthritis and osteoporosis, as well as aging, the production of collagenases may be stimulated, resulting in an elevated degradation of synovial tissue or bone.

Table 7-2 Types of collagens

Type	Chain Composition	Tissue Distribution
I	$[\alpha 1(I)]_2\ \alpha_2(I)$	Skin, tendon, bone, cornea, blood vessels
II	$[\alpha 1(II)]_3$	Cartilage, intervertebral disc, vitreous body
III	$[\alpha 1(III)]_3$	Skin, blood vessels
IV	$[\alpha 1(IV)_2]\alpha 2(IV)$ $[\alpha 3\ (IV)_2]\alpha 5(IV)$ $[\alpha 4(IV)_2]\alpha 6(IV)$	Basement membranes
V	$[\alpha 1(V)]_2\alpha 2(V)$	Placenta, skin, cardiovascular system
VI	$\alpha 1(VI),\alpha 2(VI),\alpha 3(VI)$	Cornea, blood vessels
VII	$[\alpha 1(VII)]_3$	Skin, cornea, gastrointestinal tract
VIII	$[\alpha 1(VIII)]_2\ \alpha_2(VIII)$	Cardiovascular system, placenta, cornea
IX	$\alpha 1(IX),\alpha 2(IX),\alpha 3(IX)$	Cartilage, cornea
X	$[\alpha 1(X)]_3$	Cartilage
XI	$\alpha 1(XI,\alpha 2(XI),\alpha 3(XI)$	Cartilage
XII	$[\alpha 1(XII)]_3$	Tendons, periosteum
XIII	$[\alpha 1(XIII)]_3$	Many tissues
XIV	$[\alpha 1(XIV)]_3$	Skin, bone, cornea, blood vessels
XV	$[\alpha 1(XV)]_3$	Placenta, heart, colon
XVI	$[\alpha 1(XVI)]_3$	Placenta, heart, colon
XVII	$[\alpha 1(XVII)]_3$	Skin hemidesmosomes
XVIII	$[\alpha 1(XVIII)]_3$	Several tissues, particularly kidney and liver
XIX	$[\alpha 1(XIX)]_3$	Rhabdomyosarcoma cells

Tissue collagenases are secreted by connective tissue cells as a precursor, procollagenase, which must be activated to become enzymatically active. This can be achieved in vitro by the action of trypsin on the latent enzyme. Other proteinases—including lysosomal cathepsin B, plasmin, mast cell proteinase, and plasma kallikrein—also can activate latent collagenases.[10,11] Thus, inflammatory cells can secrete factors that lead to collagenase activation, accounting for the inflammatory sequelae of the arthritides. Eisen et al.[12] demonstrated that collagenases are also under the influence of plasma inhibitors, of which $\alpha 2$ macroglobulin accounts for most of the inhibitory process. In addition, inhibitors of plasminogen activation can indirectly prevent the activation of procollagenases by plasmin. Fibroblasts and other connective tissue cells also secrete inhibitors of collagenases, suggesting a complex system of extracellular control of collagenolysis.[10]

Elastin

The biochemistry and molecular biology of elastin have been subjects of some excellent reviews.[13,14] Like the interstitial collagens, glycine comprises about one-third of the amino acid content of elastin. Unlike collagen, however, glycine is not present in every third position. In addition, elastin is an exceedingly hydrophobic protein, with a large content of valine, leucine, and isoleucine. Elastin is synthesized as a precursor molecule, tropoelastin, with a molecular weight of about 70,000 kd. However, in tissues, elastin is found as an amorphous, macromolecular network. This is due to the condensation of tropoelastin molecules through the formation of covalent cross-linkages unique to elastin. These cross-linkages arise through the condensation of four lysine residues on different tropoelastin molecules to form the cross-linking amino acids, desmosine and isodesmosine, characteristic of tissue elastin. The reader is referred to the review by Eyre et al.[6] for a discussion of the details of collagen and elastin cross-linking.

The hydrophobicity, together with the formation of cross-linkages, endow elastin with its elastic properties as well as an extreme insolubility and amorphous structure. Elastin accounts for most of the elastic properties of skin, arteries, ligaments and the lungs. The presence of elastin has been demonstrated in other tissues such as the eye and the kidney. In most tissues, elastin is found in association with microfibrils, which contain several glycoproteins including fibrillin. Microfibrils have been identified in many tissues, and the importance of their assemblies as determinants of connective tissue architecture has been brought into focus by the identification of mutations in fibrillin in the heritable connective tissue disorder, Marfan syndrome.[15]

A recent elegant review summarizes the current knowledge of the structure of the elastin gene, including consideration of the heterogeneity observed in mature mRNA due to alternate splicing in the primary transcript.[16] Analysis of the bovine and human elastin genes revealed the separation of those exons coding for distinct hydrophobic and cross-linking domains. Comparison of the cDNA and genomic sequences, as well as S1 analyses, demonstrated that the primary transcript of both species is subject to considerable alternate splicing. It is likely that this accounts for the presence of multiple tropoelastins found in several species. It was suggested that the differences in alternate splicing may be correlated with aging.[16]

The Proteoglycans

Proteoglycans are characterized by the presence of highly negatively charged polymeric chains (glycosaminoglycans or "GAGs") of repeating disaccharide units covalently attached to a "core" protein. The disaccharide units comprise an N-conjugated amino sugar, either glucosamine or galactosamine, and a uronic acid, usually D-glucuronic acid or—in the instances of dermatan sulfate, heparan sulfate, and heparin—L-iduronic acid. In cartilage and in the cornea, another GAG, keratan sulfate, containing D-glucose instead of a uronic acid has been demonstrated. The amino group of the hexosamine component is usually acetylated, and the GAGs are usually O-sulfated in hexosamine residues (with some N-sulfation, instead of acetylation, in the instances of heparan sulfate and heparin). Depending upon the source and type of proteoglycan, the number of GAGs attached to the core protein can vary from three or four, all the way up into the twenties with each GAG having a molecular size in the tens of thousands. In addition, as in the case of the cartilage proteoglycans, there may be more than one type of GAG attached to the core protein. In cartilage several proteoglycan molecules may be associated with another very large GAG, hyaluronic acid, consisting of disaccharide units of glucuronyl N-acetylglucosamine. The compositional structure of the glycosaminoglycans is summarized in Table 7-3. The overall effect of these structures is the creation of huge, negatively charged, highly hydrophilic complexes. Some excellent reviews of proteoglycan biochemistry have been written.[17–19] The hydration and charge properties of these complexes causes them to become highly extended, occupying a hydrodynamic volume in the tissue much larger than would be predicted from their chemical composition. In the instance of synovial cartilage, it is suggested that the hydration endows the tissue with shock-absorbing properties in which applied pressure to the joint is counteracted by the extrusion of water from the complex, forcing a compression of the negative charges within the molecule. Upon the release of pressure, the electronegative repulsive forces drive the charges apart, with a concomitant influx of water to restore the initial hydrated state. The metachromatic staining properties of connective tissues are due mainly to their proteoglycan content.

In recent years, several proteoglycans have been identified in the pericellular environment, either associated with cell surfaces, or interacting with ECM components such as interstitial collagens, fibronectin, and TGF-β. In a recent review, Iozzo and Murdoch[20] described the structures of the protein cores, their gene organization, their functional characteristics and tissue distribution. Table 7-4, which is a modification of the one published by Iozzo and Murdoch,[20] lists the structure and biologic characteristics of pericellular proteoglycans. The first five on the list constitute a group of small leucine-rich proteoglycans (SLRP). They are multidomain assemblies of protein

Table 7-3 Properties and tissue distribution of glycosaminoglycans

Glycosaminoglycans	Composition	Distribution
Hyaluronic acid	N-acetylglucosamine D-glucuronic acid	Blood vessels, heart, synovial fluid, umbilical cord, vitreous
Chondroitin sulfates	N-acetylgalactosamine D-glucuronic acid 4- or 6- O-sulfate	Cartilages, cornea, tendon, heart valves, skin, etc.
Dermatan sulfate	N-acetylgalactosamine L-iduronic acid 4- or 6- O-sulfate	Skin, lungs, cartilage
Keratan sulfate	N-acetylglucosamine D-galactose O-sulfate	Cornea, cartilage, nucleus pulposus
Heparan sulfate	N-acetylglucosamine	Blood vessels, basement membranes, lung, spleen, kidneys
Heparin	N-sulfaminoglucosamine D-glucuronic acid L-iduronic acid O-sulfates	Mast cells, lung, Glisson's membranes

motifs with a relatively elongated and highly glycosylated structure having several protein domains shared with other proteins.

The presence of lumican (one of the leucine-rich proteoglycans) in articular cartilage was demonstrated in a study by Grover et al.[21] They showed that the relative abundance and size of lumican varied with age. Lumican was most abundant in adult cartilage extracts, where it exhibited a molecular size ranging from 55 to 80 k. Extracts from juvenile cartilage had a more restricted size variation, corresponding to the higher molecular size range present in the adult. In the neonate the sizes ranged from 70 to 80 kd.

The biosynthesis of proteoglycans begins with the synthesis of the core protein. The sugars of the GAG chain then are sequentially added to serine residues of the protein (in most instances), utilizing uridine diphosphate (UDP) conjugates of the component sugars, with sulfation following as the chain elongates. (The mechanism of sulfation is beyond the scope of

Table 7-4 Structure and properties of secreted pericellular proteoglycans

Designation (Gene Product)	Protein Core (kd)	Glycosaminoglycan Type	Chromosomal Location (Human)	Tissue Distribution
Decorin	36	CS/DS	12q21.3-q23	Ubiquitous, collagenous matrices, bone, teeth, mesothelia, floor plate
Biglycan	38	CS/DS	Xq28	Interstitium, cell surfaces
Fibromodulin	42	KS	1q32	Collagenous matrices
Lumican	38	KS	12q21.3-q22	Cornea, intestine, liver, muscle, cartilage
Epiphycan	36	CS/DS		Epiphyseal cartilage
Versican	265–370	CS/DS	5q13.2	Blood vessels, brain, skin, cartilage
Aggrecan	220	CS	15q26	Cartilage, brain, blood vessels
Neurocan	136	CS		Brain, cartilage
Brevican	100	CS		Brain
Perlecan	400–467	HS/CS	1p36	Basement membranes, cell surfaces, sinusoidal spaces, cartilage
Agrin	200	HS	1p32-pter	Synaptic sites of neuromuscular junctions, renal basement membranes
Testican	44	HS/CS	21	Seminal fluid

Abbreviations: CS, chondroitin sulfates; DS, dermatan sulfate; KS, keratan sulfate; HS, heparan sulfate.

this discussion). Most of the chain elongation and sulfation is associated with the golgi apparatus. The degradation of proteoglycans is mediated through the action of lysosomal glycosidases and sulfatases specific for the hydrolysis of the various structural sites within the GAG chain. Genetic abnormalities in the production or synthesis of these enzymes has been shown to be the main causes of the "mucopolysaccharidoses," whose victims may exhibit severe tissue deformities and a high incidence of mental retardation.

The Structural Glycoproteins

In addition to the collagen and elastin components of connective tissues, there are groups of glycoproteins, the structural glycoproteins, that have important roles in the physiology and structural properties of connective and other types of tissues. These proteins include fibronectin, laminin, entactin, thrombospondin, and others. These proteins are involved during development, in cell attachment and spreading, and in tissue growth and turnover.

Fibronectin

The best characterized of the structural glycoproteins is fibronectin. It originally was isolated from serum, where it was referred to as "cold-insoluble globulin" (CIG). As it became recognized that fibronectin was an important secretory product of fibroblasts and other types of cells, and was involved in cell adhesion, the term fibronectin replaced CIG. For more comprehensive reviews of fibronectin, see those by Yamada[22] and Ruoslahti.[23]

Fibronectin exists as a disulfide-linked dimer with a molecular weight of about 450 kd, each monomer having a molecular size of 250 kd. Fibronectin exists in at least two forms, a tissue form and plasma fibronectin. Plasma fibronectin is somewhat smaller, and is more soluble at physiologic pH than the cellular form. Spectrophotometric and ultracentrifugal studies indicate that both forms are elongated molecules composed of structured domains separated by flexible, extendible regions. Limited proteolytic digestion has revealed the presence of specific binding sites for a number of ligands including collagen, fibrin, cell surfaces, heparin (heparan sulfate proteoglycan), factor XIIIa, and actin. Fibronectin plays a role in blood clotting by becoming cross-linked to fibrin through the action of factor XIII transamidase which catalyzes the final step in the clotting cascade. Fibroblasts and other cell types involved in the repair of injury adhere to the clot by interacting with the cell-binding domain of fibronectin. Fibronectin also enables cells to migrate in developing embryos. Fibronectin contains a unique peptide sequence, arginylglycylaspartylserine (RGDS or RGD), which binds to specific cell surface proteins (integrins) that span the plasma membrane.[24] Purified RGD can inhibit fibronectin from binding the cells, and even can displace bound fibronectin. The integrins have a complex molecular organization and appear to interact with certain intracellular proteins, thereby providing a mechanism for the control of certain cellular events by components of the extracellular environment.

Fibronectin is encoded by a single gene, and its complete primary structure has been determined by the DNA sequencing of overlapping cDNA clones[25] From such studies, it became recognized that there are peptide segments derived from alternative splicing of fibronectin mRNA at three distinct regions termed extra domain A (ED-A), ED-B, and connecting segment (III CS). A middle region of the polypeptide containing homologous repeating segments of about 90 amino acids, called type III homologies, has been identified.[26] Using immunologic techniques with monoclonal antibodies, it was shown that the ED-A exon is omitted during splicing of fibronectin mRNA precursor in arterial medial cells, while the expression of fibronectin-containing ED-A is characteristic of modulated smooth muscle cells, such as those in culture or those involved in intimal thickening and atherosclerotic lesions. It would appear that this process of alternate splicing is used during embryonic development or tissue repair as a mechanism to generate different forms of fibronectin in the extracellular matrix by the inclusion or exclusion of specific segments.[27] This could be the source of differences between the plasma and cellular forms of fibronectin. This phenomenon of alternate splicing may also be involved in the synthesis of collagens and elastin and very well may be implicated in processes of aging.

Laminin

Laminin is the major structural glycoprotein of basement membranes. In addition to its association with the molecular components of basement membranes (e.g., type IV collagen, entactin, and heparan sulfate proteoglycan), it plays some important roles in cell attachment and neurite growth.[28–30] Laminin is difficult to isolate from whole tissues or from basement membranes due to its poor solubility, and most of our knowledge of it has been derived from extracts of tumor matrices.

Laminin is a very large complex composed of at least three protein chains associated by disulfide linkages. The largest of these, the $\alpha 1$ (formerly A chain), has a molecular weight of about 440 kd, whereas the smaller units, $\beta 1$ and $\gamma 1$ chains (formerly B_1 and B_2 chains), have molecular weights of about 200 to 250 kd. Several laminin isoforms have been described in recent years, necessitating a new nomenclature of its component chains.[31] The first new chain ($\alpha 2$ chain) has been found in preparations from normal tissues, but absent in those from neoplastic tissues.[32,33] Table 7-5 lists the various laminin isoforms and their tissue distribution. Laminin has been shown to have a twisted cruciform shape consisting of three short arms and a single long arm, with globular domains at the extremities of each arm. In several of the newer isoforms of laminin, the $\alpha 1$ chain has a smaller molecular size, lacking a portion of its amino terminus.

Laminin can influence processes of differentiation, cell growth, migration, morphology, adhesion, and agglutination, as well as being involved in the structural organization of basement membranes. It also has important roles in neurite outgrowth.[30] Many of these properties are related to specific interactions of laminin with connective tissue components and cell

Table 7-5 Isoforms of laminin

New Name	New Composition	Descriptive Name	Localization
Laminin 1	$\alpha1\beta1\gamma1$	EHS Laminin	All basement membrane except skeletal muscle
Laminin 2	$\alpha2\beta1\gamma1$	Merosin	Striated muscle, peripheral nerve, placenta
Laminin 3	$\alpha1\beta2\gamma1$	S-Laminin	Synapse, glomerus, arterial blood vessel walls
Laminin 4	$\alpha2\beta2\gamma1$	S-Merosin	Myotendinous junction, trophoblast
Laminin 5	$\alpha3\beta3\gamma2$	Kalinin/Nicein/Epiligrin	Dermal-epidermal junction, stromal-epidermal junction
Laminin 6	$\alpha3\beta1\gamma1$	K-Laminin	Dermal-epidermal junction, stromal-epidermal junction
Laminin 7	$\alpha3\beta2\gamma1$	KS-Laminin	Amnion, fetal skin
Laminin 8	$\alpha4\beta1\gamma1$		Lung, heart, blood vessels, smooth muscle, endothelial cells, placenta
Laminin 9	$\alpha4\beta2\gamma1$		Heart, blood vessels, placenta, lung
Laminin 10	$\alpha5\beta1\gamma1$	*Drosophila* Laminin	Heart, blood vessels, placenta, lung, kidney

surface receptors. It exhibits a preferential binding to type IV collagen as compared to other collagen types. Laminin contains domains similar to those of fibronectin, which bind to different proteins and cell surface components containing an RGD sequence on the $\alpha1$ chain and a YIGSR sequence on the $\beta1$ chain, both of which bind to different integrins on the cell surface and which are involved in cellular attachment and migratory behaviors.

Entactin

Entactin, a novel sulfated glycoprotein, is an intrinsic component of basement membranes. Entactin was first identified in the extracellular matrix synthesized by mouse endodermal cells in culture.[34] Subsequently, a degraded form, termed nidogen, was isolated from the Englebreth-Holm-Swarm sarcoma and mistakenly identified as a new basement membrane component.[35] Both terms, entactin and nidogen, are used interchangeably in the modern literature. Entactin forms a tight stoichiometric complex with laminin, and rotary shadowing electron microscopy revealed its association with the $\gamma1$ chain of laminin. Entactin recently has been shown to promote cell attachment via an RGD sequence, and calcium ions have been implicated in its properties.[36]

Thrombospondin

Thrombospondin is a large molecule (450 kd) composed of three identical disulfide-linked protein chains. It is one of the major peptide products secreted during platelet activation and also is secreted by a diversity of growing cells. Thrombospondin has 12 binding sites for calcium ion and depends upon it for its conformational stability. It binds to heparin (and heparan sulfate proteoglycan) and to cell surfaces, and appears to modulate a number of cell functions including platelet aggregation, progression through the cell cycle, and cell adhesion and migration. For a review of the properties of thrombospondin, see the paper by Mosher.[37]

Integrins

As indicated above, cell surfaces contain groups of proteins, the integrins that mediate cell-matrix interactions. The integrins behave as receptors for components of the extracellular matrix and interact, as well, with components of the cytoskeleton.[38] This provides a mechanism for the mediation by components of the ECM of intracellular processes, including control of cell shape and metabolic activity. The integrins exist as paired molecules containing an α and a β subunit. They appear to have a significant degree of specificity for ECM proteins that, apparently, is conferred by combinations of different α and β subunits. In addition to the integrins, cell attachment proteins (CAMs) are present on the cell surface. These confer specific cell-cell recognition properties. There are several reviews on integrins and CAMs.[38–40]

Aging and Factors Affecting the Properties of Connective Tissues

From the foregoing discussion, it becomes apparent that there can be a multitude of possible loci in the development, structural organization, metabolism, and molecular biology of connective tissues for the introduction of alterations in the properties of these tissues. For a given tissue, changes in the composition of the extracellular matrix, or changes in the factors that control the production of ECM can feed back through complex mechanisms to induce changes in the properties of the tissue. The process of aging may well involve some of these factors. It is probable that during the aging process, the phenotypic expression of ECM (i.e., the patterns of ECM composition) will change. It is also probable that many of the components of the ECM may evolve with time as a function of their long biologic half-lives and the enzymatic and nonenzymatic modifications that take place. These can include processes of maintenance and repair, responses to inflammation, nonenzymatic glycosylation, and cross-linkage formation. In a sense, it may be important to differentiate between those processes of senescence that are genetically programmed (i.e., innate senescence), and the contributions to aging induced by environmental factors. However, it becomes difficult to distinguish whether a given alteration is an effect or a cause of aging. In this section an attempt has been made to discuss some of the factors and conditions involving connective tissues that may be involved in the aging process. This will include aspects of senescence, inflammatory and growth factors, photoaging of the skin, diabetes mellitus, nonenzymatic glycosylation, the etiology of osteoporosis, osteoarthritis, collagen cross-linking, and the arthritides.

Cellular Senescence

A large body of research has established conclusively that normal diploid cells have a limited replicative life span and that cells from older animals have shorter life spans than those from younger animals.[41] Thus, the process of aging could be attributed to cellular senescence. A number of observations suggest that connective tissue proteins may be affected during cellular senescence. In an extensive study on the properties of murine skin fibroblasts, van Gansen and van Lerberghe[42] concluded that among the main effects of cellular mitotic age were a depression of chromatin plasticity, changes in the organization of cytoplasmic filaments, and changes in the organization of the ECM. They implicated an involvement of collagen fibers in the intracellular events both in vivo and in vitro. Although senescent fibroblasts may not be dividing, they are biosynthetically active, showing an increased synthesis of fibronectin[43] and increased levels of fibronectin mRNA.[44] However, both senescent and progeroid cells demonstrated a decreased chemotactic response to fibronectin and developed a much thicker extracellular fibronectin network than young fibroblasts.[43] There is some indication that, with increasing age, cells become less able to respond to mitogens[45] which may have a bearing on age-related differences in wound healing. It also was shown that senescent human skin fibroblasts in culture show a loss of collagenase regulation, with a twentyfold elevation in trypsin-activated collagenolytic activity.[46] Thus, it would appear that there is some correlation between cellular senescence and changes in the regulation of connective tissue metabolism and cellular interactions.

Inflammatory and Growth Factors

One of the active areas of contemporary connective tissue biology is the study of the influences of inflammatory and growth factors on the properties of connective tissues. It is well recognized that inflammatory cells accumulate in damaged and infected tissues as part of the inflammatory response. These cells secrete lymphokines, such as the interleukins, and other factors that may influence connective tissue metabolism. In addition, a number of growth factors, including epidermal growth factor (EGF), platelet- derived growth factor (PDGF), fibroblast growth factors (FGFs), and transforming growth factors (TGFs) can have extensive control over connective tissue metabolism. As indicated above, senescent cells may not respond to these factors as do young cells. In addition, it is possible that stimulation of cell replication by certain factors may accelerate the progression of cells towards senescence. To add to the complexity are the findings that many cells can synthesize certain of these factors—including interleukin 1, PDGF, FGFs, and TGFs—endowing the cellular components of tissues with autocrine and paracrine properties. In a recent review on the properties of TGF-β, Roberts and Sporn[47] emphasize this complexity. They indicate that this factor has profound effects upon all vascular cell types, including endothelial, smooth muscle, and adventitial cells. TGF-β plays a role in the vasculogenesis and angiogenesis characteristic of embryogenesis and inflammation, and also in the arterial thickening associated with hypertension. These actions of TGF-β are very complex, inhibiting vascular cell proliferation in vitro, but enhancing the organization of endothelial cells into tubular structures indicative of angiogenesis. TGF-β also increases fibronectin synthesis but decreases protease secretion by both endothelial cells and fibroblasts, both of which can influence the phenotypic patterns of extracellular matrix formation and structure, thereby contributing to the development of fibrosis. TGF-β also can regulate PDGF synthesis by these cells, adding another degree of complexity to these systems. In vivo, TGF-β is a chemoattractant for macrophages, and stimulates expression of mRNAs for several growth factors. PDGF, FGFs and EGF are powerful mitogens for smooth muscle cells, fibroblasts, and keratinocytes. The extent of involvement of these interacting factors in the aging process is not clear, but it is probable that these contribute to the process.

Photoaging of the Skin

It has begun to be realized that the alterations that take place in sun-exposed areas of the skin of aged individuals differ from those in protected areas of the same individuals.[48] It would appear, then, that two elements contribute to the aging of the skin: innate aging and the effects of solar exposure. The symptoms of photoaging are different from those of innate aging, and evidence suggests that these two processes have different mechanisms. In normal aging, despite a thinning of the epidermis, there is no indication that the protective function of skin is compromised either in the appearance or in the amounts of keratinization, and a well-formed stratum corneum is present.[49] However, there are some marked dermal-epidermal changes, the major change being a flat dermal-epidermal junction due to retraction of the epidermal papillae, resulting in a more fragile tissue that is less resistant to shearing forces. The major changes in the aged dermis concern the architecture of the collagen and elastin networks. The spaces between fibrous components are more compact, resulting from a loss of ground substance. Collagen bundles appear to unravel and there are signs of elastolysis. Imayama and Braverman,[50] in scanning electron microscopic studies of the three-dimensional arrangement of rat skin from animals ranging from 2 weeks to

24 months of age, showed that during postnatal growth, there was a dynamic rearrangement of the collagen and elastic fibers. An ordered arrangement of mature collagen bundles was attained by producing distortions of relatively straight elastic fibers. During adulthood, there was a tortuosity of these elastic fibers, coupled with an incomplete restructuring of the elastic network that was deposited to interlock with the collagen bundles. The authors imply that the tortuous elastic fibers become stretched beyond their capacity to recoil, thereby losing their elasticity and thus, tissue compliance. In the human this would lead to sags and wrinkles.

In recent reviews,[51,52] Kligman outlined the manifestations of the effects of photoaging. The dominant change in photoaging is hyperplasia of the elastic tissue, resulting in complete disorganization. Elastosis to this degree never occurs in normal protected skin, even of very old individuals. The main culprit appears to be the ultraviolet (UV)-B portion of the UV spectrum, although UV-A and infrared radiation also contribute to the damage. In UV-A-irradiated hairless mice, there appear to be alterations in the ratio of type III to type I collagen in addition to the elastosis. There also is an increase in the levels of the components of the ground substance in photoaged skin (predominantly dermatan sulfate, heparan sulfate, and hyaluronic acid). The fibroblasts in irradiated skin are more numerous, larger, with abundant cytoplasm, and appear to be highly metabolically active, but little is known about the molecular changes in these cells. In human aged skin, mast cells are numerous and appear to be degranulated. These cells are known to produce a variety of inflammatory mediators so that photoaged skin is chronically inflamed. In innate aging, the skin tends to be hypocellular. The microcirculation of the skin is also affected, becoming sparse, with the horizontal superficial plexus almost destroyed. Although atrophy may be presented in end-stage photoaging in the elderly, "ongoing photoaging is characterized by more, not less."[52]

The effects of photoaging could be totally prevented by broad spectrum sunscreens. Although severe photoaging in the human is considered to be irreversible, in hairless mice, it was found that repair could take place after the cessation of irradiation with the newly deposited collagen appearing totally normal. A similar repair was observed in biopsies of severely photodamaged human skin after several years of avoidance of exposure to the sun. It has been found that the administration of retinoic acid accelerated the repair in irradiated mice with the deposition of a repair zone of normal appearing collagen and with the appearance of numerous, metabolically active fibroblasts. This provides a potential opportunity for the development of a therapeutic approach to the connective tissue damage of photoaged skin.

Diabetes Mellitus

Diabetics often show signs of accelerated aging, primarily as a result of the complications of vascular disease and impaired wound healing so common in this disease. It is well documented that diabetics will exhibit a thickening of vascular basement membranes that, at least in part, is believed to be related to the observed susceptibilities.[53] The biologic basis for this thickening is as yet obscure but could well be related to abnormalities in cell attachment, or is the response to factors affecting basement membrane formation, to excessive nonenzymatic glycosylation of proteins, or to an abnormal turnover of basement membrane components. Fibroblasts from diabetic individuals exhibit a premature senescence in culture.[54] In a recent study, Sibbitt et al.[55] demonstrated—using normal fibroblasts—that mean population doubling times, population doublings to senescence, saturation density at confluence, tritiated thymidine incorporation, and response to PDGF were inhibited with increasing glucose concentrations in the media. They found that inhibitors of aldose reductase, sorbinil, and tolrestat, completely prevented these inhibitions. They also found that myoinositol had similar effects. However, no data were presented to indicate that aldose reductase inhibitors would reverse the premature senescence in fibroblasts from diabetic individuals. Thus, it is not clear if prevention of the formation of reduced sugars can have a therapeutic affect, nor is it clear that all of the aging effects of diabetes are mediated by reduced sugars.

Nonenzymatic Glycosylation and Collagen Cross-linking

When enzymes attach sugars to proteins, they usually do so at sites on the protein molecule dictated by the specificity of the enzyme for the regional sequence to be glycosylated. On the other hand, nonenzymatic glycosylation, a process long known to cause food discoloration and toughness, proceeds nonspecifically at any site sterically available.[56] The longer a protein is in contact with a reducing sugar, the greater the chance for nonenzymatic glycosylation to occur. In uncontrolled diabetics, elevated circulating levels of glucosylated hemoglobin and albumin are found. Since erythrocytes turn over every 120 days, the levels of hemoglobin A_{1c} are an index of the degree of control of hyperglycemia over a 120-day period. The same is true for glucosylated albumin over a shorter period. Proteins such as collagen, which is extremely long-lived, have also been shown to undergo nonenzymatic glucosylation. Sell and Monnier[57] demonstrated an accelerated age-related browning of human collagen in diabetes.

The nonenzymatic reactions between glucose and proteins are collectively known as the Maillard or browning reaction. The initial reaction is the formation of a Schiff base between glucose and an amino group on the protein. This is an unstable structure and can spontaneously undergo an Amadori rearrangement in which a new ketone group is generated on the adduct. This can condense with a similar product on another peptide sequence to produce a covalent cross-linkage.[56] The cross-linkages usually are fluorescent and, in a high enough content, can impart a brownish tinge to the protein. Bucala et al.[58] found that DNA incubated with glucose will also undergo this reaction, and it is possible that this reaction, although much slower than for proteins, may interfere with the genetic operation of the cell. In a recent review, Monnier[59] suggested that the fundamental aging process might be mediated by the Maillard reaction. In their *Scientific American* review, Cerami et al.[56] suggested that the irreversible advanced glycosylation end products (AGEs) of arterial collagen formed by exposure of arterial medial collagen to circulating glucose may trap cholesterol and lead to the initial development of atherosclerotic plaque. This could explain the greater susceptibility of the diabetic to cardiovascular disease. It is also possible, they propose, that the greater degree of collagen cross-linking associated with aging may be due not only to the accumulation of enzymatically derived cross-linking but perhaps to a greater extent, to nonenzymatic cross-linking.

The Arthritides

The development of rheumatoid diseases, particularly of osteoarthritis, is a common symptom in aging individuals. Older assertions that chondrocytes are terminally differentiated cells incapable of replication have come under challenge.[60] Studies have confirmed that articular chondrocytes from aged animals can proliferate both in vivo and in vitro and, furthermore, can synthesize macromolecules similarly to what is seen for younger animals. It has been reported that osteoarthritis is not the result of diminished metabolic activity, but rather that metabolic activity is elevated.[61] ECM synthesis and cell replication proceed at elevated rates in damaged tissue, but so do the levels of degradative lysosomal enzymes. Hollander et al.[62] have reported that in aging and osteoarthritis there is increased denaturation of type II collagen in cartilage. The damage starts at the articular surface and spreads into the deeper zones involving articular chondrocytes. Thus, proteoglycan content of articular cartilage decreases in proportion to the severity of the disease because of a greater rate of matrix degradation over synthesis.

In inflammatory arthritis, degradative enzymes including tissue collagenases are present in the rheumatoid lesion, leading to degradation of both cartilage and bone. It is believed that inflammatory factors stimulate abnormal levels of these enzymes.[63] Bunning et al[64] demonstrated that interleukin 1 (IL-1), originally believed to be produced by monocytes and macrophages, can also be produced by synovial cells. IL-1 is also mitogenic for synovial cells and can stimulate the production of collagenases, proteoglycanases, plasminogen activator, and prostaglandins. They suggest that IL-1 plays an important role in the pathogenesis of rheumatoid arthritis. It also has been shown that injections of type II collagen can lead to synovitis coupled to the appearance of antibodies against type II collagen. However, in spontaneously arthritic mice, synovitis appeared earlier than the peak levels of antibodies to type II collagen. It was suggested that in these mice, induction of antibodies to type II collagen is triggered by joint cartilage destruction with subsequent type II collagen release.

Osteoporosis

Bone mass loss associated with aging can lead to osteoporosis, which is associated with multiple bone fractures with impaired healing. Ferris et al.,[65] in a study of biopsy material from osteoporotic fractures of the iliac crest, demonstrated an altered orientation of the proteoglycan components of the noncollagenous bone matrix, although the amounts of the material seemed unchanged. This implied that the quality as well as the quantity of bone is affected in osteoporosis. In an experimental system using chronically (up to 7 months) immobilized monkeys as a model of osteoporosis, Yamauchi et al.[66] demonstrated a marked increase in the reducible (immature) cross-links of tibial type I collagen, which returned to control values after 40 months of ambulatory recovery. Mature, stable cross-link concentrations remained constant throughout immobilization and recovery. These studies strongly suggest that during the osteoporotic state, rapid new collagen synthesis took place. With long-term recovery, this returned to control values. Thus, it appears that progressive bone loss in osteoporosis may result from bone resorption in excess of bone deposition. Croucher et al.[67] have quantitatively assessed cancellous structure in 35 patients with primary osteoporosis. Their data demonstrate that for a given cancellous area, structural changes in primary osteoporosis are similar to those observed during age-related bone loss in normal subjects. Two recent studies have been reported on the use of a drug, etidronate, a diphosphonate compound that reduces bone resorption by inhibiting osteoclastic activity.[68,69] It was found that 2 or 3 years of therapy with the drug significantly elevated spinal bone mass and reduced the incidence of fractures, providing a new option for the treatment of osteoporosis. These findings strongly implicate an abnormal increase in the activity(ies) of osteoclast-derived resorption enzymes acting on the degradation of the extracellular matrix in the etiology of osteoporosis.

Werner Syndrome

Werner syndrome (WS) is a rare autosomal recessive condition with multiple progeroid features. WS may cause abnormalities in connective tissue metabolism that are rarely seen in normal aging, such as scleroderma-like skin.[70] Fibroblasts from WS patients grow poorly in culture. Recently, Arakawa et al.[70] reported increased collagen synthesis in fibroblasts from two WS patients. This was accompanied by a near doubling of the levels of procollagen mRNA over normal controls. Goldstein et al.[71] presented an interesting hypothesis to that the primary genetic abnormality in WS is a mutation of a trans-acting factor that normally represses a second genetic locus or its product, an inhibitor of DNA synthesis that is produced when cells reach the limit of their replicative life span. The result would be an early derepression of this locus, with resultant reduced DNA synthesis and premature replicative senescence.

Alzheimer's disease

In a recent review, Perlmutter and Chui[72] presented a summary of studies that implicated the vascular basement membrane in Alzheimer's disease. Ultrastructural analyses have revealed vascular basement membrane thickening, reduplication and vacuolization, with amyloid fibrils occasionally emanating from the abluminal basement membrane. Reduplication was observed as a folding or layering at the astrocytic surface. Immunocytochemical studies[72] using antibodies against type IV collagen, laminin, and heparan sulfate proteoglycan demonstrated in non-Alzheimer's patients that the capillary bed of the cerebral cortex existed as a highly interconnected network with smooth surfaces, consistent capillary diameters, and uniform distribution. However, in Alzheimer's patients, capillaries appeared ragged and irregular, with diameters of varying thickness and considerable variations from one region to another. In some areas, they were sparse while in others, they were tightly packed. All capillary beds stained with antibodies against type IV collagen, but heparan sulfate proteoglycans (HSGP) were disrupted at the endothelial surfaces with a significant colocalization of HSGP with amyloid deposits. It was suggested that the vascular basement membrane may serve as a nidus for senile plaque, playing a role in the development of both amyloid and neuritic elements in Alzheimer's disease.[73]

In a recent editorial, Fillit[74] reviewed the current knowledge concerning the role of amyloidogenesis and proteoglycans in the pathogenesis of Alzheimer's disease. It appears that with aging and senile dementia of the Alzheimer's type, morphologic changes of the synaptic terminal and presumably of the synaptic extracellular matrix occur. It is hypothesized that dysregulated synaptic plasticity or neuronal response to injury contributes to the evolution of amyloid deposition and senile plaque formation.

Summary

This chapter reviewed some of the aspects of connective tissue biochemistry and molecular biology, and discussed some aspects of the involvement of connective tissue in processes of aging. Discussion was made of the complexity inherent in the control of connective tissue structure, metabolism, and molecular biology, and how aging might contribute to alterations in these and vice versa. Among the phenomena that may prove central to the aging process are the processes of collagen crosslinking and nonenzymatic glycosylation, alternative gene splicing, effects of solar radiation, the interplay of cytokines, and growth factors on the control of connective tissue phenotype, production of degradative enzymes, factors that affect cell replication, connective tissue diseases, and intracellular factors that control senescence. The causes and effects of aging are an active area of contemporary research in which the involvement of connective tissue is an important segment.

References

1. Burgeson R, Mayne R: Biology of the extracellular matrix: function and structure of the collagen types. Academic Press, Orlando, 1987
2. Prockop DJ, Kivirikko, KI: Collagens: molecular biology, diseases and potentials for therapy. Annu Rev Biochem 1995;64: 403–430
3. Linsenmayer TF, Fitch JM, Birk DE: Heterotypic collagen fibrils and stabilizing collagens. Ann NY Acad Sci 1990; 580: 143–60
4. Yurchenko PD, O'Rear J: Supramolecular organization of basement membranes. p. 19. In Rohrbach DH, Timpl R (eds): Molecular and Cellular Aspects of Basement Membranes. Academic Press, San Jose, 1993
5. Kefalides NA, Alper R: Structure and organization of macromolecules in basement membranes. p. 73. In Nimni ME (ed): Collagen: Chemistry, Biology and Biotechnology. Vol. 2. CRC Press, Boca Raton, FL, 1988
6. Eyre DR, Paz MA, Gallop PM: Crosslinking in collagen and elastin. Annu Rev Biochem 1984;53:717–748
7. Mazzorana M, Gruffat H, Sergeant A, van der Rest M: Mechanisms of collagen trimer formation. Construction and expression of a recombinant mini gene in HeLa cells reveals a direct affect of prolyl hydroxylation on chain assembly of type XII collagen. J Biol Chem 1993;268:3029–3032
8. Richard-Blum S, Ville G: Collagen crosslinking. Cell Molec Biol 1989;34:581–90
9. Tanzer ML: Collagens and elastin: structure and interactions. Curr Opin Cell Biol 1989;1:968–73
10. Harris ED, Welgus GA, Krane SM: Regulation of mammalian collagenases. Collagen Rel Res 1984;4:493–512
11. Nagase H, Cawston TE, DeSilva M, Barrett AJ: Identification of plasma Kallikrein as an activator of latent collagenase in rheumatoid synovial fluid. Biochim Biophys Acta 1982;702: 133–42
12. Eisen AZ, Block KI, Sakai T: Inhibition of human skin collagenase by human serum. J Lab Clin Med 1970;75:258–63
13. Rosenbloom J, Abrams WR, Mecham R: Extracellular matrix 4: the elastic fiber. FASEB J 1993;7:1208–1218
14. Sandberg LB: Elastin structure in health and disease. Int Rev Connect Tissue Res 1976;7:159–210
15. Lee B, Godfrey, M, Vitale E et al: Linkage of Marfan syndrome and a phenotypically related disorder to two different fibrillin genes. Nature 1991;352:330–339
16. Bashir M, Indik Z, Yeh H et al: Elastin gene structure and mRNA alternate splicing. p. 48. In Davidson J, Tamburro A (eds): Elastin: Chemical and Biological Aspects. Galatina Congedo Editore, Italy, 1990
17. Carney SL, Muir H: The structure and function of cartilage proteoglycans. Physiol Rev 1988;68:858–910
18. Wight TN: Cell biology of arterial proteoglycans. Arteriosclerosis 1989;9:1–20
19. Bernfield M, Kokenyesi R, Kato M et al: Biology of the syndecans: a family of transmembrane heparan sulfate proteoglycans. Annu Rev Cell Biol 1992;8:365–393
20. Iozzo RV, Murdoch AD: Proteoglycans of the extracellular environment: clues from the gene and protein side offer novel perspectives in molecular diversity and function. FASEB J 1996; 10:598–614
21. Grover, J, Chen X-N, Korenberg JR, Roughley PJ: The human lumican gene. Organization, chromosomal location, and expression in articular cartilage. J Biol Chem 1995;270:21942–21949
22. Yamada KM. Fibronectins: Structure, functions and receptors. Curr Opin Cell Biol 1989;1:956–63

23. Ruoslahti E: Fibronectin and its receptors. Annu Rev Biochem 1988;57:375–413

24. Pierchbacher MB, Hayman EG, Ruoslahti E: Synthetic peptide with cell attachment activity of fibronectin. Proc Natl Acad Sci (USA) 1982;80:1224–27

25. Kornblihtt AR, Umezawa K, Vibe-Pedersen K, Baralle FE: Primary structure of human fibronectin: differential splicing may generate at lease 10 polypeptide from a single gene. EMBO J 1985;4:1755–59

26. Oldberg A, Ruoslahti E: Evolution of the fibronectin gene. Exon structure of the cell attachment domain. J Biol Chem 1986; 261:2113–16

27. French-Constant C, Hynes RO: Alternate splicing of fibronectin is temporally and spatially regulated in the chicken embryo. Development 1989;106:375

28. Kleinman HK, Sephel GC, Tashiro K-I et al: Laminin in neural development. Ann NY Acad Sci 1990;580:311–23

29. Timpl R, Aumailley A, Gerl M et al: Structure and function of the laminin-nidogen complex. Ann NY Acad Sci 1990;580: 311–23

30. Rao CN, Kefalides NA: Identification and characterization of a 43-kilodalton laminin fragment from the "A" chain (long arm) with high-affinity heparin binding and mammary epithelial cell adhesion-spreading activities. Biochemistry 1990;29: 6769–6777

31. Burgeson RE, Chiquet M, Deutzmann R et al: A new nomenclature for the laminins. Matrix Biol 1994;14:209–211

32. Ohno M, Martinez-Hernandez A, Ohno N, Kefalides NA: Laminin M is found in placental basement membranes but not in basement membranes of neoplastic origin. Connect Tiss Res 1986;15:199–207

33. Ohno M, Martinez-Hernandez A, Ohno N, Kefalides NA: Comparative study of laminin found in normal placental membranes with laminin of neoplastic origin. p. 3. In Shibata S (ed): Basement Membranes. Elsevier Science Publishers, Amsterdam, 1985

34. Chung AE, Freeman IL, Braginski JE: A novel extracellular membrane elaborated by a mouse embryonal carcinoma cell line. Biochem Biophys Res Commun 1977;79:859–68

35. Timpl R, Dziadek M. Fujiwara S et al: Nidogen: a new self-aggregating basement membrane protein. Eur J Biochem 1983; 137:455–65

36. Chakravarti S, Tam M, Chung AE: The basement membrane glycoprotein entactin promotes cell attachment and binds calcium ions. J Biol Chem 1990;265:10597–603

37. Mosher DF: Physiology of thrombospondin. Annu Rev Med 1990;41:85–97

38. Albelda SM, Buck CA: Integrins and other cell adhesion molecules. FASEB J 1990;4:2868–80

39. Buck CA, Horwitz AF: Integrin, a transmembrane glycoprotein complex mediating cell-substratum adhesion. J Cell Sci Suppl 1987;8:231–50

40. Ruoslahti E, Pierschbacher MD: New perspectives in cell adhesion: RGD and integrins. Science 1987;238:491–97

41. Cristofalo VJ, Stanulis-Paeger BM: Cellular senescence in vitro. Adv Cell Culture 1982;2:1–68

42. Van Gansen P, van Lerberghe N: Potential and limitations of cultivated fibroblasts in the study of senescence in animals. A review of the murine skin fibroblast system. Arch Gerontol Geriatr 1988;7:31–74

43. Shevitz J, Jenkins CS, Hatcher VB: Fibronectin synthesis and degradation in human fibroblasts with aging. Mech Aging Develop 1986;35:221–32

44. Smith JR, Pereira-Smith OM: Altered gene expression during cellular aging. Genome 1989;31:386–89

45. Albini A, Pontz B, Pulz M et al: Decline of fibroblast chemotaxis with age of donor and cell passage number. Collagen Rel Res 1988;8:23–37

46. West MD, Pereira-Smith OM, Smith JR: Replicative senescence of human skin fibroblasts correlates with a loss of regulation and overexpression of collagenase activity. Exp Cell Res 1989; 184:138–47

47. Roberts AB, Sporn MB: Regulation of endothelial cell growth architecture and matrix synthesis by TGF-beta. Am Rev Resp Dis 1989;140:1126–28

48. Uitto J: Connective tissue biochemistry of the aging dermis: age associated changes in collagen and elastin. Clin Geriatr Med 1989;5:127–47

49. Lavker RM, Zheng PS, Dong G: Aged skin: a study by light, transmission electron and scanning electron microscopy. J Invest Dermatol 1989;88 (suppl):44s–51s

50. Imayama S, Braverman IM: A hypothetical explanation for the aging of skin: three dimensional arrangement of collagen and elastic fibers. Am J Pathol 1989;134:1019–25

51. Kligman LH: Photoaging. Manifestations, prevention and treatment. Clin Geriatr Med 1989;5:235–51

52. Kligman LH: Skin changes in photoaging: characterization, prevention, and repair. In Balin AK, Kligman AM (eds): Aging and the Skin. Lippincott-Raven, Philadelphia, 1989

53. Reddi AS: Diabetic microangiopathy. I. Current concepts of the chemistry and metabolism of the glomular basement membrane. Metabolism 1978;27:107–24

54. Archer FJ, Kaye R: Aging of diabetic and non-diabetic skin fibroblasts in vitro: life span and sequential growth curves. J Gerontol 1989;44:M93–99

55. Sibbitt WL, Mills RG, Digler CF et al: Glucose inhibition of human fibroblast proliferation and response to growth factors is prevented by inhibitors of aldose reductase. Mech Aging Dev 1989;47:265–70

56. Cerami A, Vlassara H, Brownlee M: Glucose and aging. Scientific American 1987; 256:90–96

57. Sell DR, Monnier VM: Isolation, purification and partial characterization of novel fluorophores from aging human insoluble collagen-rich tissue. Connect Tiss Res 1989;19:77–92

58. Bucala R, Model P, Cerami A: Modification of DNA by reducing sugars: a possible mechanism for nucleic acid aging and age-related dysfunction in gene expression. Proc Natl Acad Sci U S A 1984;81:105–9

59. Monnier VM: Toward a Maillard reaction theory of aging. Prog Clin Biol Res 1989; 304:1–22

60. Hough AJ, Webber RJ: Aging phenomena and osteoarthritis: cause or coincidence? Ann Clin Lab Sci 1986;16:501–10

61. Bora FW, Miller G: Joint physiology, cartilage metabolism and the etiology of osteoarthritis. Hand Clin 1987;3:325–36

62. Hollander AP, Pidoux I, Reiner A et al: Damage to type II collagen in aging and osteoarthritis starts at the articular surface, originates around chondrocytes and extends into the cartilage with progressive degeneration. J Clin Invest 1995;96: 2859–2869

63. Mainardi CL: Biochemical mechanisms of articular destruction. Rheum Dis Clin North Am 1987;13:215–33

64. Bunning RA, Richardson HJ, Crawford A et al: The effects of interleukin-1 on connective tissue metabolism and its relevance to arthritis. Agents Actions 1986;18: (suppl) 131–52

65. Ferris BD, Klenerman L, Didds RA et al: Altered organization of non-collagenous bone matrix in osteoporosis. Bone 1987;8: 2285–88

66. Yamauchi M, Young DR, Chandler GS, Mechanic GL: Cross-linking and new bone collagen synthesis in immobilized and recovering primate osteoporosis. Bone 1988; 9:415–18

67. Coucher PI, Garrahan NJ, Compston JE: Structural mechanisms of trabecular bone loss in primary osteoporosis: specific disease mechanism or early aging? Bone and Mineral 1995;25: 111–121

68. Watts NB, Harris ST, Genant HK et al: Intermittent cyclical etidronate treatment of postmenopausal osteoporosis. N Engl J Med 1990;323:73–9

69. Storm T, Thamsborg G, Steinicke T et al: Effect of intermittent cyclic etidronate therapy on bone mass and fracture rate in women with post-menopausal osteoporosis. N Engl J Med 1990; 323:1265–71

70. Arakawa M, Hatamochi A, Takeda K, Ueki H: Increased collagen synthesis accompanying elevated mRNA levels in cultured Werner's syndrome fibroblasts. J Invest Dermatol 1990;94: 187–90

71. Goldstein S. Murano S, Shmookler-Reis RJ: Werner syndrome: a molecular genetic hypothesis. J Gerontol 1990;45:B3–8

72. Perlmutter LS, Chui HC: Microangiopathy, the vascular basement membrane and Alzheimer's diseasc: a review. Brain Res Bull 1990;23:677–86

73. Perlmutter LS, Chui HC, Saperia D, Athanikar J: Microangiopathy and the colocalization of heparan sulfate proteoglycan with amyloid in senile plaques of Alzheimer's disease. Brain Res 1990;508:13–19

74. Fillit H: Disorders of the extracellular matrix and pathogenesis of senile dementia of the Alzheimer's type. Lab Invest 1995; 72:249–253

CHAPTER 8

Clinical Immunology of Aging

STEFAN GRAVENSTEIN
HOWARD FILLIT
WILLIAM B. ERSHLER

As a fundamental organ necessary for the maintenance of life, the immune system first appeared in primitive organisms about 480 million years ago.[1] The intimate relation between acquired immunity and infection was apparent early in recorded history. Observing an epidemic of plague in 430 B.C., Thucydides reported that anyone who had recovered from the disease was never attacked again. The era of modern immunology was probably initiated by Jenner's report in 1798 on an effective vaccine employing cowpox pustules to prevent smallpox in humans. The linkage of advances in infectious disease and in immunology continued throughout the nineteenth and twentieth centuries. For example, identification of bacterial organisms ultimately resulted in the discovery of antibodies that could neutralize the toxins produced by these organisms, leading to modern methods for the development of vaccines. The discovery of antibody structure during the 1960s finally began the era of modern immunochemistry. With regard to cellular immunity, despite the early work of Metchnikoff and his followers, the role of cells in acquired immunity was not truly appreciated until the 1950s. Finally, although concepts of "recognition of self," and "autoimmunity" as a mechanism of disease appeared early in the twentieth century, the causes of autoimmune disease remain poorly understood.

Immunogerontology is a relatively new field, probably introduced by Walford in 1969.[2] Walford proposed that immune mechanisms play an important role in the pathogenesis, but not the etiology of the aging process. The immunologic theory of aging linked life span with the genetic repertoire of the individual via the major histocompatibility genes. Walford proposed that disorders in the immune system that occur with aging account for three major causes of disease in old age: increased autoimmunity causing organ-specific disease, including vascular disease; failing surveillance allowing the expression of cancers; and the increased susceptibility to infectious diseases. Current evidence supports the notion that the decline in immune function with aging may be viewed as a form of idiopathic acquired immunodeficiency in old age, which is generally mild in nature. More recent complexity has been added to our understanding of immune dysfunction in malignancies, including a component of immune dysregulation. The aged may also suffer secondary, potentially reversible causes of acquired immunodeficiency that may be clinically significant.[3]

Changes in the Human Immune System With Aging

Nonspecific Host Defense

Primary immunity is the first line of defense against invading pathogens. It differs from secondary immunity in that it does not require sensitization, or prior exposure, to offer protection. Examples of primary immunity include the mucocutaneous barriers, cellular barriers that perform the function of phagocytosis, and cellular (natural killer cells) and noncellular (complement) systems that mediate nonspecific lysis of foreign cells.

Phagocytosis

Phagocytosis involves the engulfment and usually lysis and/or digestion of foreign substances. The capacity of neutrophils, macrophages, and monocytes for phagocytosis is determined by their number and ability to reach the relevant site. Thus, absolute number, endothelial adherence and chemotaxis, and phagocytosis itself with subsequent digestion of the organism are critical factors determining the efficiency of this mechanism in primary immunity.[4] The study of alterations in phagocytosis with age must then involve examinations of each of these steps, and are inherently more difficult in human populations than in disease-free inbred animals.

Extrapolation of studies of senescent mice to humans would suggest that age itself does not attenuate response to bacterial capsular antigens in a well-vascularized area such as the lung; the pulmonary inflammatory reaction is similar between young adult and old animals.[5] Niwa and colleagues[6] reported a deterioration in neutrophil chemotaxis and increase in serum lipid peroxidase in the nonsurviving cohort of a 7-year longitudinal study, suggesting a preterminal but not necessarily "normal" aging alteration in these factors. However, age-related effectiveness in chemotaxis may be reduced in less vascular areas in vivo, such as in the skin, which also has a host of other changes that may impair the ability of cells in the vascular compartment to reach a site of infection.[7] Although in vitro neutrophil function, (including endothelial adherence, migration, granule secretory behavior, etc.) is insignificantly affected by age, significantly fewer neutrophils arrive at the skin abrasion sites studied in older people.[8] How this translates to immune response and immune-mediated repair in infected or otherwise physiologically stressed older people remains unknown.

Macrophage activation also appears to change with age; this may be partially attributable to a reduced gamma interferon signal from T lymphocytes.[9–11] Less signal at the site of infection could be a consequence of reduced numbers of activated T cells locally. Fewer T cells and the defective expression of homing markers to attract T cells from peripheral blood into inflamed tissues[12] suggests that increased susceptibility of old mice to, for example, tuberculosis, reflects an impaired capacity to focus mediator cells and the additional cytokine they may express at sites of infection[11] (more on T-cell changes with age, below). These observations may help explain why late-life tuberculosis, or, for that matter, reactivation tuberculosis occurs and remains clinically important.

Cell lysis

Cell lysis is mediated via a variety of pathways, including the complement system, natural killer (NK) cell activity, and neutrophil activity. Complement activity does not appear to decline significantly with age, and neutrophil function changes only arguably as noted above. However, kinetics of NK activity—lytic activity by cells that do not require prior exposure to the offending infected or malignant cells in order to lyse them—may be another factor that participates in infections such as tuberculosis. In longitudinal studies of nonhuman primates, NK activity does appear to be affected by age[13] and acute stressors such as illness.[14]

Specific Host Defense

Aging is accompanied by changes in the immune system, which are evidenced by alterations in both cellular and humoral immunity. Animal models have been used extensively to investigate these changes, but will not be discussed here in detail as more definitive reviews are available.[15–18]

Human aging is associated with decreased thymic function, an important factor for age-related changes in thymic dependent immunity.[19] Declines in serum thymic hormones precede the decline in thymic tissue. By the age of 60, few of the thymic peptides are measurable in human peripheral blood,[20] and most of the thymic epithelial tissue is replaced by fibrotic scar. Thymic hormone replacement may improve immune function in old age,[21,22] but there are no current clinical indications for the use of thymic hormones in practice.

In the cellular immune system, most studies show no significant changes with human aging in the total number of peripheral blood cells, including total lymphocytes, monocytes, NK cells, or polymorphonuclear leukocytes.[23–29] The appearance of lymphocytopenia is associated with mortality in the aged, but is not an age-related finding.[24,30,31] Most studies show no changes in the percentages of B- and T-lymphocyte populations in the peripheral blood,[23,26,28,32,33] although the chronically ill elderly may particularly have a decline in total T-cell numbers.[33] Equivocal changes in the ratio of helper cells to suppressor cells (T4/T8) occur in normal aging.[25,26,33–35] These findings are in contrast to human immunodeficiency virus (HIV)-induced acquired immunodeficiency syndrome (AIDS) associated with a decreased T4/T8 ratio.[36] Finally, there is a specific age-related increase in memory cells, cells that express the CD45 surface marker.[37–41]

The function of lymphocytes is altered with aging. There is a robust decline in the proliferative capacity of T lymphocytes to nonspecific mitogens.[29,32,35,42,43] In addition, antigen-specific declines in the proliferative potential of T cells to specific viruses have been demonstrated.[44,45] The number and the affinity of mitogen receptors on T lymphocytes do not change with age.[46] However, the number of T lymphocytes capable of dividing in response to mitogens is reduced, and the activated T cells do not undergo as many divisions.[47] The abnormality in T-cell proliferative capacity is not related to an abnormality in accessory cell function.[42] Changes in the fluidity of the cell membrane occur with aging in most cells, including lymphocytes,[48] which may impair the proliferative response by preventing cross-linking and capping of receptors, a process necessary for cell activation. Cell activation is also dependent on cellular shifts of calcium (Ca^{++}). Lymphocytes from old humans may have abnormalities in Ca^{++} signaling cascades that ultimately lead to deoxyribonucleic acid(DNA) synthesis.[49] There may be intrinsic T-cell defects in DNA mechanisms of proliferation that may be involved in this decline in proliferative capacity.[50] Fewer activated T cells from old humans progress through the cell cycle after activation, and fewer old human T cells re-enter the cell cycle and continue to proliferate.[51]

The decline in proliferation may also be caused by decreased T-cell lymphokine production and regulation, particularly interleukin 2 (IL-2), during the proliferative response to mitogens.[24,35,52,53] Decreases in the percentage of IL-2 receptor positive cells, IL-2 receptor density, and in the expression of IL-2 and IL-2 receptor specific mRNA in old humans have been reported.[35,54] IL-2 production in response to specific antigens also declines. Vaccination with influenza results in increased IL-2 secretion in response to viral antigen in vitro.[55,56] In addition, the number of influenza-specific cytotoxic T cells declines with age, with no increase after vaccination.[57] The sensitivity of T cells to prostaglandins is also altered in aging.[58,59] However, little decline has been noted in the serum levels or secretion of inflammatory cytokines; although chronically ill, frail patients may have elevated serum levels, which predict mortality,[60,61] and there is an age-related increase in IL-6 which is both age-related and appears to be inhibited by estrogen. IL-6 is of interest because it can be linked to other age-associated disorders (such as multiple myeloma and benign monoclonal gammopathy—see below) that are or have been suggested to be immune related (Alzheimer's disease[62,63] and osteoporosis[64]).[65]

There is a decline in delayed-type skin hypersensitivity

(DTH),[44] which may reflect the decline in in vitro lymphocyte proliferation.[44,45] Anergy, the lack of DTH to a battery of injected antigens, indicates incompetence of cell-mediated immunity.[66] Generally, a battery of skin test antigens (usually four to six antigens) is necessary to adequately assess DTH in the elderly. Anergy to both mitogens and specific antigens increases with age.[43,44,67,68] The number of skin test positive reactions declines with age from over 80 percent in young individuals to less than 20 percent in older individuals.[43] Variations in populations studied are important factors in determining rates of anergy in the elderly.[18] In one study,[68] 17.9 percent of subjects over age 66 years and living at home were anergic; 41 percent of subjects living in a nursing home but able to care for themselves were anergic; and 60 percent of subjects who were functionally impaired and living in a nursing home were anergic. In addition, a number of acute and chronic illnesses may impair the DTH response, suggesting the need for longitudinal studies of DTH to determine the nature of the defect in DTH present in an individual patient or in various populations.[66] Concomitant in vitro testing suggests that not all anergic patients have impaired in vitro measures of lymphocyte function such as proliferative capacity,[23,69] suggesting that both in vivo cutaneous DTH testing and in vitro lymphocyte testing may be necessary to identify individuals who are truly anergic and presumably immunodeficient.[70] Associations between anergy and mortality have been repeatedly demonstrated.[31,43,68,71–73] These changes in cellular immunity may be responsible for reactivation infections such as tuberculosis and varicella (shingles—more on this below) in aged individuals.

The issue of DTH testing in tuberculosis has also received particular interest because of the clinical implications of tuberculin skin reactivity for the diagnosis and treatment of tuberculosis in the elderly.[47,52,74–76] In this regard, the size of the skin test reaction appears to have some significance in the clinical interpretation of results. Positive skin tests are often found after repeated testing, suggesting the presence of a "booster" effect, requiring additional interpretation and analysis.[76]

In the humoral immune system, there are no changes in the number of peripheral blood B cells in old age.[77] Most studies indicate and increase in total serum immunoglobulin (IgG) and IgA levels, and no change in IgM.[78,79] Declines in antibody titers to specific foreign antigens have been noted, including naturally occurring antibodies to the isoagglutinins,[80] and titers of antibody to foreign antigens such as microbial antigens.[81–85] Both the primary[86] and secondary immune responses to vaccination are impaired. Elderly patients tend to have lower peak titers of antibody and more rapid declines in titers after immunization,[87,88] as well as the peak titer occurring slightly later (2 to 6 weeks rather than 2 to 3 weeks postvaccination) than in younger people.[89] In contrast, serum autoantibodies may have organ specificity, such as antiparietal cell, antithyroglobulin, and antineuronal antibodies.[90–97] Organ nonspecific autoantibodies, such as antibodies to DNA and rheumatoid factors, also increase with age. Circulating immune complexes may also increase with advancing age.[94,98] The reason why autoantibodies increase with age is not known. Several explanations are possible, including alterations in immune regulation and an increase in stimulation of B-cell clones due to recurrent or chronic infections or increased tissue degradation. Intrinsic B-cell abnormalities may be important in defective Ig production.[81,99–101] Changes in the human B-cell proliferative response, similar to the defect found in human T cells, have been investigated with varying findings.[29,102] Abnormalities in a specific B-cell subtype, the CD5+ B cell, may be responsible for the abnormal production of autoantibodies, particularly rheumatoid factors, and the occurrence of certain myeloproliferative disorders in old age.[103] Changes in T-cell function may contribute to the B-cell dysfunction with age.[82,100,101,104]

The Contribution of Immunosenescence to Disease in Old Age

Autoimmunity and Aging

Walford[2] speculated that autoimmunity plays an important role in the aging process. Kay[105] and others[106] have alternately proposed that autoimmunity may play an important physiologic role in the regenerative and reparative process that is ongoing during aging. Certain autoimmune diseases have their highest incidence in old age, such as pernicious anemia,[107] thyroiditis,[108–110] bullous pemphigoid,[111] rheumatoid arthritis,[112,113] and temporal arteritis,[114] suggesting that the age-related increase in autoantibodies may have clinical significance.

Autoimmunity may also play a role in vascular disease in old age.[115] Giant cell arteritis is a common disease in old age.[114,116] Of interest, giant cell arteritis is associated with degenerative vascular disease.[114] Indeed, immune mechanisms may result in atherosclerosis, a final common pathway of pathology secondary to a variety of vascular insults.[117,118] A number of antivascular antibodies have been described in man[119–122] that are associated with diseases of the vasculature. Antiphospholipid antibodies are associated with a variety of pathologic states of the vasculature, including stroke and vascular dementia,[123,124] temporal arteritis,[125] and ischemic heart disease.[126] However, the exact mechanism by which antiphospholipid antibodies cause vascular injury remains unknown.[127] The increased occurrence of antiphospholipid antibodies with age[128–130] and the association of these autoantibodies with vascular disease may represent a predisposing immunologic factor for immune-mediated vascular disease in the elderly. Autoantibodies to vascular heparan sulfate proteoglycans (vHSPG) may also be important in vascular injury in old age,[121] since vHSPG plays an important role in normal anticoagulation and cholesterol metabolism.[131]

Immunosenescence and Cancer in Old Age

Age is the single greatest risk for cancer.[132] Since immune mechanisms play an important role in the elimination of malignant clones via cytotoxic mechanisms, the decline of the im-

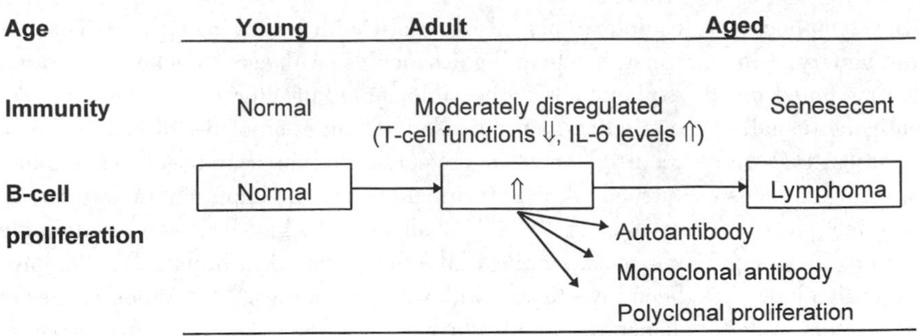

Figure 8-1 The relationship of immune changes with age and B-cell proliferation. A required second trigger such as *H ras* expression, is necessary for the development of lymphoma.

mune system in old age could be related to the increased rate of cancer in old age. Nevertheless, the exact relation between immunosenescence and the increased incidence of cancer is unknown. Among explanations of why tumors increase in frequency with age is the observation that tumors may go undetected for decades; thus, the reason for increased frequency in late life relates to easier detection when they finally achieve sufficient size, and the host has had sufficient time for the tumor to progress through each of the necessary promoting events. An alternative explanation suggests that the host and host factors change over time, favoring progression and expression in later life. These two hypotheses to explain the increase in late-life malignancy have aptly been described as "seed versus soil".[133]

From an immunologic and "soil" standpoint, there are two principle observations that relate to malignancies and age. There is both evidence of dysregulation of proliferation of cells directly controlled by the immune system, and evidence of increased malignancies in late life that could be hypothetically restrained by nonsenescent immunity. These will be discussed sequentially.

Proliferative disorders of the lymphocyte are common in old age. Although bimodal in incidence, the peak in late-life lymphoma includes a disproportionate incidence of nodular B-cell types.[134] Both old humans and mice have commonly exhibited a monoclonal gammopathy (paraprotein) in the last quartile of the life span.[135–139] Monoclonal gammopathies increase with age and may occur in 79 percent of sera from subjects over the age of 95 years.[140,141] Radl[139] has defined four categories of age-associated monoclonal gammopathy: (1) myeloma or related disorders; (2) benign B cell neoplasia; (3) immune deficiency, with T-cell greater than B-cell loss, and (4) chronic antigenic stimulation. He speculates that the third category is by far the most common, and that this is what occurs with immune senescence. It is possible that age-associated immune dysfunction is initially associated with markers of aberrant immune regulation such as paraproteinemia and/or autoantibody, and later contributes to the pathogenesis of lymphoma (Fig. 8-1).

Monoclonal gammopathies may cause morbidity, particularly renal disease in the absence of overt multiple myeloma.[142] In a minority of cases of monoclonal gammopathies, a malignant evolution may occur.[143–145] Multiple myeloma also has an age-related increase in incidence.[146] Although treatment is not generally indicated for monoclonal gammopathies,[145] treatment of myeloma is often useful. Another common malignant transformation of the lymphocyte in old age is chronic lymphocytic leukemia.[147] Non-Hodgkin's lymphoma increases in incidence with age, while Hodgkin's lymphoma has a bimodal distribution.[148] The increased prevalence of solid tumors[149] in old age may be related to defective immune surveillance, although this is now being disputed (more on immune surveillance below). An alternative theory holds that there is a natural balance where the immune system has both immune restraining as well as growth enhancing effects on the tumor, related in part to the cascade of cytokines released by the cells that infiltrate the tumor. With advancing age there may be an imbalance in these two factors that is more permissive or potentially can promote tumor growth (such as with multiple myeloma).[133]

Finally, a discussion of cancer development and aging would not be complete without considering the importance of the decline in immunity and associated failure of "immune surveillance." It has long been proposed that the decline in immune function contributes to the increased incidence of malignancy. However, despite the appeal of such an hypothesis, scientific support has been limited and the topic remains controversial.[150,151] Proponents of an immune explanation point to experiments in which outbred strains of mice with heterogeneous immune functions were followed for their life span.[152] Those who demonstrated better functions early in life (as determined by a limited panel of assays available at the time on a small sample of blood) were found to have fewer spontaneous malignancies and a longer life than those estimated to be less immunologically competent. Furthermore, it is difficult to deny that profoundly immunodeficient animals or humans are subject to a more frequent occurrence of malignant disease, and it would stand to reason that others with less severe immunodeficiency would also be subject to more malignancy, perhaps less dramatically so. However, the malignancies associated with profound immunodeficiency (e.g., with AIDS or after organ transplantation) are usually lymphomas, Kaposi's sarcoma, or leukemia and not the more common malignancies of geriatric populations (lung, breast, colon, and prostate cancers). Accordingly, it is fair to say that the question of the influence of age-acquired immunodeficiency on the incidence of cancer in the elderly is unresolved. However, there is much greater consensus on the importance of the immunodeficiency of aging in the clinical management of cancer, eluding the problems associated with infection and disease progression.

Immunosenescence and Infections in Old Age

Probably the most profound effect of immunosenescence in old age is to increase the morbidity and mortality from infections. Clearly, rates of a number of infections and their morbidity and mortality increase with age,[153] particularly influenza, pneumonia, urinary tract infections, skin infections, recrudescent latent infections (herpes zoster), and tetanus. There is also an increase in hospital-acquired and nursing home infections in the elderly. In addition to immunosenescence, impairments in primary host defenses also contribute to the increased rates of infection—such as a reduced cough reflex leading to aspiration pneumonia; urinary and fecal incontinence predisposing to urinary tract infections; and immobility predisposing to wound infections. Unusual organisms may also be due to previous antibiotic treatment, causing the expression of resistant organisms. Immunosenescence also results in the atypical presentation of infections in old age.[154] Infections are more frequent and prolonged in the elderly.[155]

Old individuals, particularly the old old, may fail to respond normally to therapy for infection, and may present with infections secondary to unusual organisms, recurrent infections with the same pathogen, or reactivation of quiescent diseases such as those caused by tuberculosis and herpes zoster virus. The impaired immune and inflammatory response in old age changes the clinical expression of infections. Typical signs of infection are often absent, and a high index of suspicion is necessary for infection in old age. Elderly patients may not present with typical hard signs of infections such as spiking fevers, leukocytosis, prominent inflammatory infiltrates on chest x-ray in patients with pneumonia, or rebound tenderness in patients with an acute abdomen. Lower baseline temperatures may require the need for monitoring the change in temperature, rather than the absolute temperature, in old age.[156]

Influenza

Most of the significant morbidity and excess mortality during influenza epidemics occurs in older adults.[157] Age itself, in addition to and separate from the many comorbid conditions of older people, is a significant risk factor for severe complications of influenza.[158] It is widely held that much of the increased susceptibility of elderly people to influenza and its complications is attributable to immunologic factors, including reduced antibody responsiveness and influenza-specific cell-mediated immunity. The role of humoral immunity, especially in the form of neutralizing antibody, is perhaps most important for preventing and limiting the initial infection[159] rather than promoting recovery. T-cell-mediated responses appear to be more important and primarily involved in postinfection viral clearance and recovery; influenza specific CTL activity correlates with rapid clearance of virus in infected human volunteers, even in the absence of detectable serum antibody,[160] and has been experimentally confirmed in adoptive transfer of influenza-specific CTL experiments using the mouse model.[161,162] No doubt influenza-specific antibody declines with age, whether due to natural infection or vaccination,[163–165] and this presumably translates to an increased risk of influenza infection. However, and perhaps equally importantly, CTL,[57,166] HLA restriction by influenza-specific T-cell clones, and lymphocyte proliferative responses[167] also decline with age. T-cell-mediated cytokine responses, such as IL-2, which mediate the humoral response to influenza may also decrease with age, although this has not been as clearly established for healthy elderly[56] as it has been for frail elderly people.[55] Together these observations can account for much of the age-related increase in influenza susceptibility and morbidity. It is important to note that, despite all of the changes occurring with age and comorbid conditions of age, that influenza vaccine still is highly cost-effective in reducing influenza-related infections and complications.[168,169]

Varicella zoster virus

Herpes zoster (shingles) is caused by varicella zoster virus (VZV) and is increasingly prevalent with advancing age, as are its severity and complications.[170–176] Incidence doubles to an annual attack rate of .8 percent from the age of 50 to 80 years,[172,173,176] and the majority of cases occurring after the age of 60.[170–176] Two major complications of herpes zoster, postherpetic neuralgia and cranial nerve zoster (often of the ophthalmic nerve, and not infrequently resulting in lower motor neuron paresis), are the most disabling. Postherpetic neuralgia occurs in over 25 percent of patients at least 60 years old and is strongly associated with sleep disturbance and depression.[170,171,175–182] Bell's palsy[183] and Menier's[184] disease, both conditions associated with advanced age, have also been linked to herpes zoster. VZV-specific cell-mediated immunity correlates closely with susceptibility to herpes zoster in large populations, such as patients with lymphomas, bone marrow transplant recipients, and immunocompetent elderly persons.[185–198] It is less clear whether boosting currently available measures of humoral or cellular immunity to VZV antigens will specifically reduce risk from developing herpes zoster,[190,194–201] but it is hoped that this will indeed be the case, making herpes zoster a vaccine preventable disease.

Secondary Causes of Acquired Immunodeficiency in Old Age

In contrast to the normative changes that may result in a mild idiopathic acquired immunodeficiency with aging, a variety of secondary causes of acquired immunodeficiency occur in the elderly that may be severe, yet reversible. The distinction between secondary causes of immunodeficiency from "normal" age-related changes represents an important clinical distinction. The clinician needs a high index of suspicion for acquired immunodeficiency in old age, since many of the causes are reversible and may be the primary reason for the susceptibility to infection, altered presentation of infection, or inadequate response to usual therapy.

The effects of malnutrition on the immune system may be profound, and clearly increase the risk of infection in the elderly.[202] Immune deficits in undernourished ambulatory elderly may be reversed by nutritional supplementation.[203] Malnutrition affects up to 50 percent of the hospitalized elderly and is highly associated with poor acute care outcomes, including death among the hospitalized elderly.[204–207] Severe protein, calorie, vitamin, and elemental deficiencies such as zinc (a cofactor for the function of thymic hormone) may cause immunodeficiency and poor outcomes in response to infection.[208] An absolute lymphocyte count below 1500 cells/mm^3 generally indicates some degree of malnutrition, and a count below 900 cells/mm^3 indicates severe malnutrition and immunodeficiency.[209] Chronic illnesses such as congestive heart failure[210] and Alzheimer's disease[211,212] may be associated with progressive cachexia despite adequate food intake, and may be mediated via tumor necrosis factor or other inflammatory mediators. In patients with dementia, despite adequate nutritional intake, malnutrition affected 50 percent of patients and was associated with a fourfold increase in infections.[212]

Since elderly people are frequently on several medications and often suffer polypharmacy, drug-induced acquired immunodeficiency is probably far more common than is generally clinically recognized. Numerous commonly used drugs cause neutropenia and lymphocytopenia.[213,214] Analgesics, nonsteroidal anti-inflammatory agents, steroids, antithyroids, antibiotics, antipsychotics, antidepressants, hypnotics/sedatives, anticonvulsants, antihypertensives, diuretics, (H_2) blockers, hypoglycemics, and other medications (such as allopurinol) commonly prescribed in old age may suppress the inflammatory immune responses. T lymphocytes also have calcium channels, and cholinergic, histaminic, and adrenergic receptors—all of which may have effects on immune function.[215] Hypogammaglobulinemia may also be induced by medications.[216] Recent studies have also demonstrated that medications may also be associated with an impaired[217] or enhanced response to vaccination.[218]

HIV infection may be a cause of acquired immunodeficiency in the elderly, and should always be considered part of the differential diagnosis of acquired immunodeficiency in elderly patients with lymphopenia and appropriate risk factors.[219–221] The most common source of AIDS in the elderly is from a transfusion.[222] Dementia is often a common presenting feature of AIDS,[223] and AIDS should be considered part of the differential diagnosis of dementia in aged patients with appropriate risk factors. The possibility that many cases of AIDS may go undetected in the elderly has considerable implications for geriatric health care workers.

Psychosocial isolation, depression, and stress are probable causes of immune dysfunction in old age.[224] There is an increased incidence of cancer during periods of psychosocial stress and depression related to bereavement.[225,226] Social isolation and marital discord may impair immune function.[227,228] Chronic stress in the form of caregiving for a demented spouse also reduces influenza vaccine response.[229] Interventions to enhance social contact improve immune function, as measured by a variety of laboratory measures.[230] Immobility may also cause immune dysfunction, and exercise may maintain function in old age in both animals and humans.[231,232] These aspects of psychoneuroimmunology obviously have particular relevance in the interdisciplinary practice of geriatrics, given the high prevalence of psychosocial problems in the elderly.

The tests necessary to perform an immunologic evaluation to establish the diagnosis of acquired immunodeficiency in old age are readily available to the clinician.[233] The humoral immune system is readily tested by measuring the serum protein electrophoresis, immunoelectrophoresis, and other methods for quantitation of Ig levels, as well as the measurement of specific antibody titers, such as isoagglutinins. The cellular immune system is tested by blood leukocyte counts, including absolute lymphocyte counts, delayed skin test hypersensitivity employing a panel of at least six antigens, and in vitro testing such as measurements of suppressor and helper lymphocyte ratios (T4/T8), and the ability of lymphocytes to proliferate in response to mitogens and specific antigens. The later tests are often performed in a standard clinical immunology laboratory. Other more sophisticated immune tests are also available from the clinical immunology consultant and laboratory.

Specific potentially reversible causes of acquired immunodeficiency, such as malnutrition or medications, should be sought in aged patients with recurrent or unusual infections, particularly those with lymphocytopenia and/or anergy. At a minimum, a medication review and a nutritional assessment should be performed, with monitoring of neutrophil or lymphocyte counts during nutritional supplementation or mediation withdrawal. HIV infections should always be considered in high risk patients, including the very old, particularly because of the risks for spread of HIV among health care workers and family members caring for frail elderly persons.[220,221]

Numerous interventions have been employed in an attempt to enhance immune function in old age. Thymic hormones, other hormones, mediations, and cytokines have been proposed as immunoenhancing agents, but none of these have gained clinical acceptance.[234,235] In animals, calorie restriction without undernutrition clearly prolongs life and is associated with immune competence into late life, but the benefits of calorie restriction in man remain unknown.[236] Zinc and other trace metals may have benefit in some older patients in restoring lymphocyte proliferation in vitro, and in enhancing delayed-type skin hypersensitivity reactions, but their effects in preventing or reducing the morbidity of infections or other problems potentially related to immunodeficiency in old age have not been demonstrated.[237] Vitamin C and other antioxidants may have beneficial effects on immune function.[235,238] Megadose dietary supplementation does not significantly improve immune function in the normal aged animal.[239]

Vaccinations are critically important in maintaining the health of the elderly in the face of declining immunity, and are effective in preventing pneumococcal and influenza pneumonia and tetanus and reduce mortality from these illnesses.[217,240–242] Although elderly people achieve lower peak titers and more rapid declines of serum antibody levels, the majority of healthy elderly achieve titers that are generally presumed protective.[87,88] However, chronically ill, frail elderly—particularly institutionalized, malnourished individuals—may not achieve adequate protective peak antibody titers against pneumococcal pneumonia or influenza when immunized with a single dose of vaccine, and supplemental doses may be required.[243–246] Older persons may require revaccination with tetanus toxoid more than every 10 years (as currently recommended) to maintain protective levels of antibodies in the serum.[82] The use of new protein conjugate[247] and immunoconjugate[248] vaccines may improve the response in older people.

Conclusions

Significant changes in the immune system occur with apparently normal aging. Impairments in immune function contribute to morbidity and mortality in old age by increased susceptibility to infection and other mechanisms. There are also reversible causes of acquired immunodeficiency in old age that result in morbidity and mortality, particularly in high risk, chronically ill elderly. Maintenance of adequate nutrition, the prevention of polypharmacy, the reduction of psychosocial stress, and other preventive measures such as the effective use of vaccines may minimize the morbid effects of immune dysfunction in old age. Newer therapeutic approaches may ultimately be useful in the treatment of acquired immunodeficiency in elderly people, particularly in high risk individuals who are substantially impaired by the effects of aging and diseases of old age on the immune system.

References

1. Silverstein AM: History of Immunology. p. 23. I Paul WE (ed): Fundamental Immunology. Raven Press, New York, 1984
2. Walford RL: The Immunologic Theory of Aging. Williams and Wilkins, Baltimore, 1969
3. Fillit H: Reversible acquired immunodeficiency in the elderly: a review. Age 1991;14:83–89
4. Lehrer RI, Ganz T, Selsted ME et al: Neutrophils and host defense. Ann Intern Med 1988;109:127–142
5. Esposito AL, Poirer WJ, Clark CA: In vitro assessment of chemotaxis by peripheral blood neutrophils from adult and senescent C57BL/6 mice: correlation with in vivo responses to pulmonary infection with Type 3 Streptococcus pneumoniae. Gerontology 1990;36:2–11
6. Niwa Y, Kasama T, Miyachi Y et al: Neutrophil chemotaxis, phagocytosis and parameters of reactive oxygen species in human aging: cross-sectional and longitudinal studies. Life Sci 1989;44:1655–1664
7. Branchet MC, Boisnic S, Frances C et al: Skin thickness changes in normal aging skin. Gerontology 1990;36:28–35
8. MacGregor RR, Shalit M: Neutrophil function in healthy elderly subjects. J Gerontol 1990;45:M55–M60
9. Orme IM, Miller ES, Roberts AD et al: T lymphocytes mediating protection and cellular cytolysis during the course of Mycobacterium tuberculosis infection. J Immunol 1992;148: 189–196
10. Murray HW: Interferon-gamma, the activated macrophage, and host defense against microbial challenge. Ann Intern Med 1988;108:595–608
11. Orme IM: Senescence of cellular immunity to tuberculosis infection in the mouse: some radical departures from previous thinking. pp. 27–40. In Powers DC, Morley JE, Coe RM (eds): Aging, Immunity and Infection. Springer Publishing, New York, 1994
12. Schimizu Y, Newman W, Tanaka Y, Shaw S: Lymphocyte interactions with endothelial cells. Immunology Today 1992;13: 106–112
13. Ershler WB, Coe CL, Gravenstein S et al: Aging and immunity in nonhuman primates: I. Effects of age and gender on cellular immune function in rhesus monkeys (Macacca mulatta). Am J Primatol 1988;15:181–188
14. Proust JJ, Bender BS, Nagel JE et al. Developmental biology and senescence. Natural Immun 1989;392–439
15. Goidl EA: Aging and the Immune Response. pp. 1–364. Marcel Dekker, New York, 1987
16. Doria G, Adorini L, Sabbadini E et al: Immunoregulation in aging. Ann N Y Acad Sci 1988;521:182–188
17. Miller RA: Aging and the immune response. pp. 157–180. In Schneider EL, Rowe JW (eds): Handbook of the Biology of Aging. Academic Press, San Diego, 1990
18. Fillit H, Mayer L, Bona C: Immunology of aging. pp. 71–90. In Brocklehurst JC, Tallis R, Fillit H (eds): Textbook of Geriatric Medicine and Gerontology. Churchill Livingstone, London, 1992
19. Boyd E: The weight of the thymus gland in health and disease. Am J Dis Child 1932;43:1162–1214
20. Lewis VM, Twomey JJ, Bealmear P et al: Age, thymic involution and circulating thymic hormone activity. J Clin Edocrinol Metab 1978;47:145–150
21. Weksler ME, Innes JB, Goldstein G: Immunological studies of aging. IV. The contribution of thymic involution to the immune deficiencies of aging mice and reversal with thymopoietin. J Exp Med 1978;148:996–1006
22. Gravenstein S, Duthie EH, Miller BA et al: Augmentation of influenza antibody response in elderly men by thymosin alpha one: a double-blind placebo-controlled study. J Am Geriatr Soc 1989;37:1–8
23. Barcellini W, Borghi MO, Sguotti C et al: Heterogeneity of immune responsiveness in healthy elderly subjects. Clin Immunol Immunopath 1988;47:142–151
24. Thompson JS, Wekstein DR, Rhoades JL et al: The immune status of healthy centenarians. J Am Geriatr Soc 1984;32: 274–281
25. Nagel JE, Chrest FJ, Adler WH: Enumeration of T lymphocyte subsets by monoclonal antibodies in young and aged humans. J Immunol 1981;127:2086–2088

26. Schwab R, Staiano-Coico L, Weksler ME: Immunological studies of aging. IX. Quantitative differences in T lymphocyte subsets in young and old individuals. Diagn Immunol 1983; 1:185–201
27. Weksler ME, Hutteroth TH: Impaired lymphocyte function in aged humans. J Clin Invest 1974;53:99
28. Gupta S, Good RA: Subpopulations of human T lymphocytes. X Alterations in T, B, third population cells, and T cells with receptors for immunoglobulin M or G in aging humans. J Immunol 1979;122:1214–1219
29. Murasko DM, Nelson BJ, Silver R et al: Immunologic response in an elderly population with a mean age of 85. Am J Med 1986;81:612–618
30. Bender BS, Nagel JE, Adler WH, Andres R: Absolute peripheral blood lymphocyte count and subsequent mortality of elderly men. J Am Geriatr Soc 1986;34:649–654
31. Proust J, Rosenzweig P, Debouzy C, Moulias R: Lymphopenia induced by acute bacterial infections in the elderly: a sign of age-related immune dysfunction of major prognostic significance. Gerontology 1985;31:178–185
32. Hallgren HM, Kersey JH, Dubey DP, Yunis EJ: Lymphocyte subsets and integrated immune function in aging humans. Cell Immunol 1978;10:65–78
33. Hallgren HM, Bergh N, Rodysill KJ, O'Leary JJ: Lymphocyte proliferative response to PHA and anti-CD3/Ti monoclonal antibodies, T cell surface marker expression, and serum IL-2 receptor levels as biomarkers of age and health. Mech Ageing Dev 1988;43:175–185
34. De Paoli P, Battistin S, Santini GF: Age-related changes in human lymphocyte subsets: progressive reduction of the CD4 CD45R (suppressor inducer) population. Cell Immunol 1988; 48:290–296
35. Nagel JE, Chopra RK, Chrest FJ et al: Decreased proliferation, interleukin-2 synthesis, and interleukin-2 receptor expression are accompanied by decreased mRNA expression in phytohemagglutinin-cells from elderly donors. J Clin Invest 1988;81: 1096–1102
36. Fauci AS, Masur H, Gelmann EP et al: The acquired immunodeficiency syndrome: an update. Ann Intern Med 1985;102: 800–823
37. Okumura M, Fujii Y, Takeuchi Y et al: Age-related accumulation of LFA-1^{high} cells in a $CD8^+CD45RA^{high}$ T cell population. Eur J Immunol 1993;23:1057–1063
38. Cossarizza A, Ortolani C, Paganelli R et al: CD45 isoforms expression on $CD4^+$ and $CD8^+$ T cells throughout life, from newborns to centenarians: implications for T cell memory. Mech Ageing Dev 1996;86:173–195
39. Utsuyama M, Hirokawa K, Kurashima C, et al: Differential age-change in the numbers of $CD4^+CD45RA^+$ and $CD4^+CD29^+$ T cell subsets in human peripheral blood. Mech Ageing Dev 1992;63:57–68
40. Miller RA: Short analytical review: accumulation of hyporesponsive, calcium extruding memory T cells as a key feature of age-dependent immune dysfunction. Clin Immunol Immunopathol 1991;58:305–317
41. Xu X, Beckman I, Ahern M, Bradley J: A comprehensive analysis of peripheral blood lymphocytes in healthy aged humans by flow cytometry. Immunol Cell Biol 1993;71:549–557
42. Schwab R, Hausman PB, Rinnooy-Kan E, Weksler ME: Immunological studies of aging. X. Impaired T lymphocytes and normal monocyte response from elderly humans to the mitogenic antibodies OKT3 and Leu 4. Immunology 1985;55: 677–684
43. Roberts-Thompson IC, Whittingham S, Youngchaiyud U, Mackay IR: Ageing, immune response, and mortality. Lancet 1974;ii:368–370
44. Burke BL, Steele RW, Beard OW et al: Immune response to varicella-zoster in the aged. Arch Intern Med 1982;142: 291–293
45. Miller AE: Selective decline in cellular immune response to varicella-zoster in the elderly. Neurology 1980;30:582–587
46. Antel J, Oger JJF, Dropcho E et al: Reduced T lymphocyte cell reactivity as a function of human aging. Cell Immunol 1980;54:184–192
47. Hefton JM, Darlington GJ, Casazza BA, Weksler ME: Immunologic studies of aging. V. Impaired proliferation of PHA-responsive human lymphocytes in culture. J Immunol 1980;125: 1007–1010
48. Rivnay B, Bergman S, Shinitzky M, Globerson A: Correlations between membrane viscosity, serum cholesterol, lymphocyte activation and aging in man. Mech Ageing Dev 1980;125: 1007–1010
49. Kennes B, Hubert C, Brohee D, Neve P: Early biochemical events associated with lymphocyte activation in aging. I. Evidence that Ca2+-dependent processes induced by PHA are impaired. Immunology 1981;42:119–126
50. Gutkowski JK, Innes J, Weksler ME, Cohen S: Induction of DNA synthesis in isolated nuclei by cytoplasmic factors. II. Normal generation of cytoplasmic stimulatory factors by lymphocytes from aged human with depressed proliferative responses: J Immunol 1984;132:559–562
51. Staiano-Coico L, Darsynkiewicz Z, Melamed MR, Weksler ME: Immunological studies of aging. IX. Impaired proliferation of T lymphocytes detected in elderly humans by flow cytometry. J Immunol 1984;132:1788–1792
52. Gillis S, Kozak R, Durante M, Weksler ME: Immunological studies of aging. Decreased production of and response to T cell growth factor by lymphocytes from aged humans. J Clin Invest 1981;67:937–942
53. Rabinowich H, Gosis Y, Reshef T, Klajman A: Interleukin-2 production and activity in aged humans. Mech Ageing Dev 1985;32:213–226
54. Orson FM, Saadeh CK, Lewis DE, Nelson DL: Interleukin-2 receptor expression by T cells in human aging. Cell Immunol 1989;124:278–291
55. McElhaney JE, Beattie BL, Devine R et al: Age-related decline in interleukin-2 production in response to influenza vaccine. J Am Geriatr Soc 1990;38:652–658
56. McElhaney JE, Meneilly GS, Beattie BL et al: The effect of influenza vaccination on IL2 production in healthy elderly: implications for current vaccination procedures. J Gerontol 1992;47:M3–M8
57. Powers DC: Influenza A virus-specific cytotoxic T lymphocyte activity declines with advancing age. J Am Geriatr Soc 1993; 41:1–5
58. Goodwin JS: Changes in lymphocyte sensitivity to prostaglan-

din E, histamine, hydrocortisone and x-irradation with age: studies in a healthy elderly population. Clin Immunol Immunopath 1982;25:243–251

59. Goodwin JS: Messner RP Sensitivity of lymphocytes to prostaglandin E2 increases in subjects over age 70. J Clin Invest 1979;64:434–439
60. Mooradian AD, Reed RL, Osterweil D, Scuderi P: Detectable serum levels of tumor necrosis factor alpha may predict early mortality in elderly institutionalized patients. J Am Geriatr Soc 1991;39:891–894
61. Mooradian AD, Reed RL, Scuderi P: Serum levels of tumor necrosis factor alpha, interleukin-1 alpha and beta in healthy elderly subjects. Age 1991;14:61–64
62. Huberman M, Sredni B, Stern L et al: IL-2 and IL-6 secretion in dementia: correlation with type and severity of disease. J Neurol Sci 1995;130:161–164
63. Hüll M, Berger M, Volk B, Bauer J: Occurrence of interleukin-6 in cortical plaques of Alzheimer's disease patients may precede transformation of diffuse into neuritic plaques. Ann NY Acad Sci 1996;777:205–212
64. Manolagas SC, Bellido T, Jilka RL: New insights into cellular, biochemical, and molecular basis of postmenopausal and senile osteoporosis: roles of IL-6 and gp 130. Int J Immunopharmacol 1995;17:109–116
65. Erhsler WB, Sun WH, Binkley N: The role of interleukin-6 in certain age-related diseases. Drugs Aging 1994;5:358–365
66. Zweiman B, Levinson AI: Cell-mediated immunity. p. 75. In Middleton E, Reed CE, Ellis EF (eds): Allergy: Principles and Practice. Mosby, St. Louis, 1983
67. Dorken E, Grzybowski S, Allen EA: Significance of the tuberculin test in the elderly. Chest 1987;92:237–240
68. Marrie TJ, Johnson S, Durant H: Cell-mediated immunity of healthy adult Nova Scotians in various age groups compared with nursing home and hospitalized senior citizens. J Allergy Clin Immunol 1988;81:836–844
69. Castle S, Peris T, Chang M et al: Correlation of delayed type hypersensitivity (DTH) with in vitro test of cell-mediated immunity in elderly nursing home patients. Gerontology 1989; 29:195A
70. Murasko DM, Wener P, Kaye D: Association of lack of mitogen-induced lymphocyte proliferation with increased mortality in the elderly. Aging: Immunol Infec Dis 1988;1:1–6
71. Cohn JR, Hohl CA, Buckley CE: The relationship between cutaneous cellular immune responsiveness and mortality in a nursing home population. J Am Geriatr Soc 1983;32:808–809
72. Stead WW, To T: The significance of the tuberculin skin test in elderly persons. Ann Intern Med 1987;107:837–842
73. Wayne SJ, Rhyne RL, Garry PJ, Goodwin JS: Cell-mediated immunity as a predictor of morbidity and mortality in subjects over 60. J Gerontol 1990;45:M45–48
74. Creditor MC, Smith EC, Gallai JB, Baumann M, Nelson KE: Tuberculosis, tuberculin reactivity, and delayed cutaneous hypersensitivity in nursing home residents. J Gerontol 1988;43: M97–M100
75. Barry MA, Regan AM, Kunches LM et al: Two-stage tuberculin testing with control antigens in patients residing in two chronic disease hospitals. J Am Geriatr Soc 1987;35:147–153
76. van den Brande P, Demedts M: Four-stage tuberculin testing in elderly subjects induces age-dependent progressive boosting. Chest 1992;101:447–450
77. Nagel JE, Adler WH: Immunology. pp. 299–309. In Kent B, Butler RN (eds): Human Aging Research: Concepts and Techniques. Lippincott-Raven, Philadelphia, 1988
78. Buckley CEI, Buckley EG, Dorsey FC: Longitudinal changes in serum immunoglobulin levels in older humans. Fed Proc 1974;33:2036–2039
79. Phair JP, Kauffman CA, Bjornson A et al: Host defenses in the aged: evaluation of components of the inflammatory and immune responses. J Infect Dis 1978;138:67–73
80. Makinodan T, Adler W: The effects of aging on the differentiation and proliferation potentials of cells of the immune system. Fed Proc 1975;34:153–158
81. Antel JP, Oger JJF, Wrabetz LG et al: Mechanisms responsible for reduced in vitro immunoglobulin secretion in aged humans. Mech Ageing Dev 1983;23:11–19
82. Kishimoto S, Tomino S, Mitsuya H et al: Age-related decline in the in vitro and in vivo synthesis of anti-tetanus toxoid antibody in humans. J Immunol 1980;125:2347–2352
83. Antonaci S, Jirillo E, Lucivero G et al: Humoral immune response in aged humans: suppressor effect of monocytes on spontaneous plaque forming cell generation. Clin Exp Immunol 1983;52:387–392
84. Pahwa SG, Pahwa RN, Good RA: Decreased in vitro humoral immune responses in aged humans. J Clin Invest 1981;67: 1094–1102
85. Kjeldsen K, Simonsen O, Heron I: Immunity against diphtheria and tetanus in the age group 30–70 years. Scand J Infect Dis 1988;20:177–185
86. Waldorf DS, Wilkens RF, Decker JL: Impaired delayed hypersensitivity in an aging population: association with antinuclear reactivity and rheumatoid factor. JAMA 1968;203:111–114
87. Shapiro ED, Berg AT, Austrian R et al: The protective effect of polyvalent pneumococcal polysaccharide vaccine. N Engl J Med 1991;325:1453–1460
88. Huang Y, Gauthey L, Martine M et al: The relationship between influenza vaccine-induced specific antibody responses and vaccine-induced nonspecific autoantibody responses in healthy older women. J Gerontol 1992;47:M50–M55
89. Levine M, Beattie BL, McLean DM, Corman D: Characterization of the immune response to trivalent influenza vaccine in elderly men. J Amer Geriatr Soc 1987;35:609–657
90. Hooper B, Whittingham S, Mathews JD et al: Autoimmunity in a rural community. Clin Exp Immunol 1972;12:79–87
91. Rosenthal M: Age and immunity: III. Circulating immune complexes in different age groups. Blut 1978;37:271–274
92. Hijmans W, Radl J, Bottazzo GF, Donlach D: Autoantibodies in highly aged humans. Mech Ageing Dev 1984;26:83–89
93. Pandey JP, Fudenberg JJ, Ainsworth SK, Loadholt CB: Autoantibodies in healthy subjects of different age groups. Mech Ageing Dev 1979;10:399–404
94. Goodwin JS, Searles RP, Tung KSK: Immunological responses of a healthy elderly population. Clin Exp Immunol 1982;48: 403–410
95. Hallgren HM, Buckley CE, Gilberstein VA, Yunis EJ: Lymphocyte phytohemagglutinin responsiveness, immunoglobu-

lins, and autoantibodies in aging humans. J Immunol 1973; 111:1101–1105

96. Manousskakis MN, Tziosfas AG, Sills MP et al: High prevalence of anti-cardiolipin and other autoantibodies in a healthy elderly population. Clin Exp Immunol 1987;69:557–565
97. Siskind GW, Weksler ME: The effect of aging on the immune response. Ann Rev Geriatr Geront 1982;3:3–26
98. Delespesse G, Gausset PH, Sarfati M et al: Circulating immune complexes in old people and in diabetics: correlation with autoantibodies. Clin Exp Immunol 198;40:96–101
99. Hollingsworth JW, Otte RG: B lymphocyte maturation in cultures from blood of elderly men: a comparison of plaque-forming cells, cells containing intracytoplasmic immunoglobulin and cell proliferation. Mech Ageing Dev 1981;15:9–18
100. Ceuppens JL, Goodwin JS: Regulation of immunoglobulin production in pokeweed mitogen-stimulated cultures of lymphocytes from young and old adults. J Immunol 1982;128: 2429–2434
101. Rodriquez MA, Ceuppens JL, Goodwin JS: Regulation of IgM rheumatoid factor production in lymphocyte cultures from young and old subjects. J Immunol 1982;128:2422–2428
102. Whisler RL, Williams JW Jr., Newhouse YG: Human B cell proliferative responses during aging. Reduced RNA synthesis and DNA replication after signal transduction by surface immunoglobulins compared to B cell antigenic determinants CD20 and CD40. Mech Ageing Dev 1991;61:209–222
103. Kipps TJ: The CD5 + B cell. Adv Immunol 1989;47:117–186
104. Delfraissy JF, Galanaud P, Dormont J, Wallon C: Age related impairment of the in vitro antibody response in the human. Clin Exp Immunol 1980;39:208–214
105. Kay MMB: Immunological aspects of aging. pp. 33–78. In Makinodan T (ed): Aging, immunity and arthritic disease. Raven Press, New York, 1980:33–78
106. Cohen IR: Autoimmunity: physiologic and pernicious. Adv Intern Med 1984;29:147–165
107. MacLennan WJ, Andrews GR, Macleod C, Caird FI: Anemia in the elderly. Quart J Med 1973;42:1–13
108. Blumenthal HT, Perlstein IB: The aging thyroid. II. An immuncytochemical analysis of the age-associated lesions. J Am Geriatr Soc 1987;35:855–863
109. Blumenthal HT, Perlstein IB: The aging thyroid. I. A description of lesions and an analysis of their age and sex distribution. J Am Geriatr Soc 1987;35:843–854
110. Tunbridge WMG, Evered DC, Hall R et al: The spectrum of thyroid disease in a community: the Whickham survey. Clin Endocrinol 1977;7:481–493
111. Rook AJ, Waddington E: Pemphigous and pemphigoid. Br J Dermatol 1953;65:425–431
112. Pope RM, Talal N: Autoimmunity in rheumatoid arthritis. Concepts Immunopathol 1985;1:219–250
113. Trentham DE, Dynesius RA, Rocklin RE, David JR: Cellular sensitivity to collagen in rheumatoid arthritis. N Engl J Med 1978;299:327–332
114. Machado EBV, Gabriel SE, Beard CM et al: A population-based case-control study of temporal arteritis: evidence for an association between temporal arteritis and degenerative vascular disease? Int J Epidemiol 1989;18:836–841
115. Mathews JD, Whittingham S, Mackay IR: Autoimmune mechanisms in human vascular disease. Lancet 1974;ii:1423–1427
116. Boesen P, Sorensen SF: Giant cell arteritis, temporal arteritis, and polymyalgia rheumatica in a Danish county. Arth Rheum 1987;30:294–299
117. Minick CR, Alonso DR, Rankin L: Role of immunologic arterial injury in atherogenesis. Thromb Haemostas 1978;39: 304–311
118. Beaumont JL: Immunologic factors in atherosclerosis. pp. 317–325. In Blumenthal HT (ed): Handbook of Diseases of Aging. Van Nostrand, New York, 1982
119. Fillit HM, Kemeny E, Luine V et al: Antivascular antibodies in the sera of patients with senile dementia-Alzheimer's type. J Geront 1987;42:180–184
120. Faaber P, Rijke TPM, van de Putte LBA et al: Cross-reactivity of human and murine anti-DNA antibodies with heparan sulfate. The major glycosoaminoglycan in glomerular basement membrane. J Clin Invest 1986;77:1824–1830
121. Fillit HM, Mulvihill M: Association of autoimmunity to vascular heparan sulfate proteoglycan and vascular disease in the aged. Gerontol 1993;39:177–182
122. Cines DB: Disorders associated with antibodies to endothelial cells. Rev Infect Dis 1989;11:s705–711
123. Briley DP, Coull BM, Goodnight SH: Neurological disease associated with antiphospholipid antibodies. Ann Neurol 1989;25:221–227
124. Asherson RA, Mercey D, Phillips G et al: Recurrent stroke and multi-infarct dementia in systemic lupus erythematous: association with antiphospholipid antibodies. Ann Rheum Dis 1987;46:605–611
125. McHugh NJ, James ID, Plant GT: Anticardiolipin and antineutrophil antibodies in giant cell arteritis. J Rheumatol 1990; 17:916–922
126. Klemp P, Cooper RC, Strauss FJ et al: Anticardiolipin antibodies in ischemic heart disease. Clin Exp Immunol 1988;74: 254–257
127. Lockshin MD: Antiphospholipid antibody and antiphospholipid syndrome. Curr Opin Rthem 1991;3:797–802
128. Mannoussakis MN, Tziousfas AG, Silis MP et al: High prevalence of anti-cardiolipin and other autoantibodies in a healthy elderly population. Clin Exp Immunol 1987;69:557–565
129. Ruffati A, Rossi L, Callgaro A et al: Autoantibodies of systemic rheumatic diseases in the elderly. Gerontol 1990;36:104–111
130. Alving CR: Antibodies to liposomes, phospholipids, and cholesterol: implications for autoimmunity, atherosclerosis, and aging. Prog Clin Biol Res 1990;343:41–51
131. Wight TN: Cell biology of arterial proteoglycans. Arteriosclerosis 1989;9:1–20
132. Newell GR, Boutwell WB, Morris DL: Epidemiology of cancer. pp. 3–32. In De Vita VTJ, Hellman S, Rosenberg SA (eds): Cancer: Principles and Practice of Oncology. Lippincott, Philadelphia, 1982
133. Ershler WB. Guest Editorial: Why tumors grow more slowly in old people. J Natl Ca Inst 1986;77:837–839
134. Cantor KP, Fraumeni JF Jr: Distribution of nonHodgkin's lymphoma in the United States between 1950 and 1975. Cancer Res 1980;40:2645–52

135. Radl J, Sepers JM, Skvaril F et al: Immunoglobulin patterns in humans over 95 years of age. Clin Exp Immunol 1975;22: 84–90
136. Radl J, Hollander CF, van den Berg P, de Glopper E: Idiopathic paraproteinaemia. I. Studies in an animal model—the ageing C57BL/KaLwRij mouse. Clin Exp Immunol 1978;33: 395–402
137. Radl J: Idiopathic paraproteinemia—a consequence of an age-related deficiency in the T immune system. Three-stage development—a hypothesis. Clin Immunol Immunopathol 1979; 14:251–5
138. Radl J, De Glopper ED, Schuit HR, Zurcher C: Idiopathic paraproteinemia. II. Transplantation of the paraprotein-producing clone from old to young C57BL/KaLwRij mice. J Immunol 1979;122:609–13
139. Ligthart GJ, Radl J, Corberand JX et al: Monoclonal gammopathies in human aging: increased occurrence with age and correlation with health status. Mech Ageing Dev 1990;52:235–43
140. Radl J, Weis J, Hoogeveen CM: Immunoblotting with (sub) class-specific antibodies reveals a high frequency of monoclonal gammopathies in persons thought to be immunodeficient. Clin Chem 1988;34:1839–1842
141. Kyle RA, Robinson RA, Katzmann JA: Clinical aspects of biclonal gammopathies. Am J Med 1981;71:999–1008
142. Buxbaum JN, Chuba JV, Hellman GC et al: Monoclonal immunoglobulin deposition disease: light chain and light and heavy chain deposition diseases and their relation to light chain amyloidosis. Ann Intern Med 1990;112:455–464
143. Fine JM, Lambin P, Muller JY: The evolution of asymptomatic monoclonal gammopathies. Acta Med Scand 1979;205: 339–341
144. Crawford J, Eye MK, Cohen HJ: Evaluation of monoclonal gammopathies in the "well" elderly. Am J Med 1987;82: 39–45
145. Kyle RA: Benign monoclonal gammopathy—after 20 to 35 years of follow-up. Mayo Clin Proc 1993;68:26–36
146. Cohen HJ: Multiple myeloma in the elderly. Clin Geriatr Med 1985;827–855
147. Stahl RL, Silber R: Chronic lymphocytic leukemia. Clin Geriatr Med 1985;1:857–867
148. Antin JH, Rosenthal DS: Acute leukemias, myelodysplasia and lymphomas. Clin Geriatr Med 1985;1:795–826
149. Dorn HF, Cutler SJ: Morbidity from cancer in the United States. Public Health Monographs 1956;56
150. Ershler WB: The influence of an aging immune system on cancer incidence and progression. J Gerontol 1993;48:B3–B7
151. Miller RA: Aging and cancer: another perspective. J Gerontol 1993;48:B8–B10
152. Covelli V, Mouton D, Mojo V et al: Inheritance of immune responsiveness, life span and disease incidence in interline crosses of mice selected for high or low multispecific antibody production. J Immunology 1989;142:1224–1234
153. Smith PW, Roccaforte JS, Caly PB: Infection and immune response in the elderly. Ann Epidemiol 1992;2:813–822
154. Berman P, Hogan DB, Fox RA: The atypical presentation of infection in old age. Age Aging 1987;16:201–207
155. Kohn P: Cause of death in very old people. JAMA 1982;247: 2793–2797
156. Castle SC, Norman DC, Yeh M et al: Fever response in elderly nursing home residents: are the older truly colder? J Am Geriatr Soc 1991;39:853–857
157. Glezen WP: Serious morbidity and mortality associated with influenza epidemics. Epidemiol Rev 1982;4:25–44
158. Barker WH, Mullooly JP: Impact of epidemic type A influenza in a defined adult population. Am J Epidemiol 1980;112: 798–813
159. Clements ML, Betts RF, Tierney EL et al: Serum and nasal wash antibodies associated with resistance to experimental challenge with influenza A wild-type virus. J Clin Microbiol 1986;24:157–160
160. McMichael AJ, Gotch FM, Noble GR et al: Cytotoxic T-cell immunity to influenza. N Engl J Med 1983;309:13–17
161. Taylor PM, Askonas BA: Influenza nucleoprotein specific cytotoxic T cell clones are protective in vivo. Immunol 1986;58: 417–420
162. Yap KL, Ada GL, McKenzie IFC: Transfer of specific cytotoxic T lymphocytes protects mice inoculated with influenza virus. Nature 1978;273:238–239
163. Davenport FM, Hennessey AV, Francis T Jr: Epidemiological and immunological significance of age distribution of antibody to antigenic variants of influenza virus. J Exp Med 1953;98: 641–656
164. Noble GR, Kaye HS, Kendal AP et al: Age-related heterologous antibody responses to influenza virus vaccination. J Infect Dis 1977;136:S686–692
165. Beyer WEP, Palache AM, Bljet M et al: Antibody induction by influenza vaccines in the elderly: a review of the literature. Vaccine 1989;7:385–394
166. Powers DC, Belshe RB: Effect of age on memory cytotoxic T lymphocyte responses to inactivated influenza virus vaccine. J Infect Dis 1993;167:584–592
167. Schwab R, Russo C, Weksler ME: Loss of MHC-restricted T cell recognition of influenza antigens in aging. Aging Immunol Infect Dis 1990;2:111–116
168. Nichol KL, Margolis KL, Wuorenma J, Von Sternberg T: The efficacy and cost effectiveness of vaccination against influenza among elderly persons living in the community. N Engl J Med 1994;331:778–784
169. Patriarca PA, Arden NH, Koplan JP, Goodman RA: Prevention and control of type A influenza in nursing homes: benefits and costs with four approaches using vaccination and amantadine. Ann Intern Med 1987;107:732–740
170. de Moragas JM, Kierland RR: The outcome of patients with herpes zoster. Am Arch Dermatol 1957;75:193–196
171. Burgoon CF Jr, Burgoon JS, Baldridge GD: The natural history of herpes zoster. JAMA 1957;164:265–270
172. McGregor RM: Herpes zoster, chicken-pox, and cancer in general practice. BMJ 1957;i:84–87
173. Hope-Simonson RE: The nature of herpes zoster: a long-term study and new hypothesis. Proc R Soc Med 1965;58:9
174. Molin L: Aspects of the natural history of herpes zoster. Acta Derm Venereol 1969;49:569–583
175. Rogers RS III, Tindall JP: Geriatric herpes zoster. J Am Geriatr Soc 1971;19:495–504
176. Ragozzino MW, Melton LJ III, Kurland LT et al: Population-

based study of herpes zoster and its sequelae. Medicine 1982; 61:310–316

177. Hope-Simpson RE: Posterpetic neuralgia. J Roy Coll Gen Pract 1975;25:571
178. Huff JC, Bean B, Balfour HH et al: Therapy of herpes zoster with oral acyclovir. Am J Med 1988;85:84–89
179. Wood MJ, Ogan PH, McKendrick MW et al: Efficacy of oral acyclovir treatment of acute herpes zoster. Am J Med 1988; 85:79–83
180. Harding SP, Lipton JR, Wells JCD: Natural History Of Herpes Zoster Ophthalmicus: predictors of postherpetic neuralgia and ocular involvement. Br J Ophthalmol 1987;71:353–358
181. Loeser JD: Herpes zoster and postherpetic neuralgia. Pain 1986;25:149–164
182. Watson CPN: Postherpetic neuralgia. Neurol Clin 1989;7: 231–248
183. Moffat MM, Ritchie L, Collacott I, Brown T: Is Bell's palsy a reactivation of varicella zoster virus? J Infect 1995;30:29–36
184. Welling DB, Daniels RL, Brainard J et al: Detection of viral DNA in endolymphatic sac tissue from Meniere's disease patients. Am J Otol 1996;15:639–643
185. Straus SE, Ostrove JE, Inchauspe G et al: Varicella-zoster virus infections; biology, natural history, treatment, and prevention. Ann Intern Med 1988;108:221–237
186. Arvin AM: Cell-mediated immunity to varicella-zoster virus. J Infect Dis 1992;166(suppl 1):S35–41
187. Dolin R, Reichman RC, Mazur MH, Whitley RJ: Herpes zoster-varicella infections in immunosuppressed patients. Ann Intern Med 1978;89:375–388
188. Goffinet DR, Glatstein EJ, Merigan TC: Herpes zoster-varicella infections and lymphoma. Ann Intern Med 1972;76: 235–240
189. Guinee VF, Guido JJ, Pfalzgraf KA et al: The incidence of herpes zoster in patients with Hodgkin's disease; an analysis of prognostic factors. Cancer 1985;56:642–648
190. Arvin AM, Pollard AM, Gamberg P et al: Cellular and humoral immunity in the pathogenesis of recurrent herpes viral infections in patients with lymphoma. J Clin Invest 1980;65:869
191. Meyers JD, Flournoy N, Thomas ED: Cell-mediated immunity to varicella-zoster infection after allogenic marrow transplant. J Infect Dis 1980;141:479
192. Schuchter LM, Wingard JR, Piantadosi S et al: Herpes zoster infection after autologous bone marrow transplantation. Blood 1989;74:1424–1427
193. Wilson A, Sharp M, Koropchak CM et al: Subclinical varicella-zoster virus viremia, herpes zoster, and T lymphocyte immunity to varicella-zoster viral antigens after bone marrow transplantation. J Infect Dis 1992;165:119–126
194. Miller AE: Selective decline in cellular immune response to varicella-zoster in the elderly. Neurology 1980;30:582–587
195. Berger R, Florent G, Just M: Decrease of the lymphoproliferative response to varicella-zoster virus antigen in the aged. Infect Immun 1981;32:24–27
196. Burke BL, Steele RW, Beard OW et al: Immune responses to varicella-zoster in the aged. Arch Int Med 1982;142:291–293
197. Hayward AR, Herberger M: Lymphocyte responses to varicella zoster virus in the elderly. J Clin Immunol 1987;7:174–178
198. Hayward A, Levin M, Wolf W et al: Varicella-zoster virus-specific immunity after herpes zoster. J Infect Dis 1991;163: 873–875
199. Brunell PA, Novelli VM, Keller PM, Ellis RW: Antibodies to the three major glycoproteins of varicella-zoster virus: search for the relevant host immune response. J Infect Dis 1987;156: 430–435
200. Giller RH, Winistorfer S, Grose C: Cellular and humoral immunity to varicella zoster virus glycoproteins in immune and susceptible human subjects. J Infect Dis 1989;160:919–928
201. Levin MJ, Murray M, Rotbart HA et al: Immune response of elderly individuals to a live attenuated varicella vaccine. J Infect Dis 1992;166:253–259
202. Chandra RK: Nutritional regulation of immunity and the risk of infection in old age. Immunology 1989;67:141–147
203. Chandra RK: The relation between immunology, nutrition and disease in elderly people. Age Aging 1990;19:s25–s31
204. Epstein AM, Leighton JR, Hoefer M: The relation of body weight to length of stay and charges for hospital services for patients undergoing elective surgery: a study of two procedures. Am J Public Health 1987;77:993–997
205. Agarwahl M, Acevedo F, Leighton LS et al: Predictive ability of various nutritional variables for mortality in elderly people. Am J Clin Nutr 1988;48:1173–1178
206. Weinsier RL, Hunker EM, Krumdieck CL, Butterworth CE: Hospital malnutrition: a prospective evaluation of general medical patients during the course of hospitalization. Am J Clin Nutr 1979;32:418–426
207. Lansey S, Waslien C, Mulvihill M, Fillit H: The role of anthropometry in the assessment of malnutrition in the hospitalized frail elderly. Gerontology 1993;39:346–353
208. Corman LC: The relationship between nutrition, infection and immunity. Med Clin North Am 1985;69:519–531
209. Lewis EF, Bell SJ: Nutritional assessment of the elderly. p. 73. In Morley JE, Glick Z, Rubinstein LZ (eds): Geriatric Nutrition. Raven Press, New York, 1990
210. Levine B, Kalman J, Mayer L et al: Elevated circulating levels of tumor necrosis factor in severe chronic heart failure. N Engl J Med 1990;323:236–241
211. Singh S, Mulley GP, Losowsky MS: Why are Alzheimer's patients thin? Age Aging 1988;17:21–28
212. Sandman P, Adolfsson R, Nygren C et al: Nutritional status and dietary intake in institutionalized patients with Alzheimer's disease and multiinfarct dementia. J Am Geriatr Soc 1987; 35:31–38
213. Dale DC: Neutropenia. pp. 807–816. In Williams WJ, Beutler E, Erslev AJ, Lichtman MA (eds): Hematology. McGraw-Hill, New York, 1989
214. Williams WJ: Lymphocytopenia. pp. 964–966. In Williams WJ, Beutler E, Erslev AJ, Lichtman MA (eds): Hematology. McGraw-Hill, New York, 1989
215. Plaut M: Lymphocyte hormone receptors. Ann Rev Immunol 1987;5:621–669
216. Travin M, Macris NT, Block HM, Schwimmer D: Reversible common variable immunodeficiency syndrome induced by phenytoin. Arch Int Med 1989;149:1421–1422
217. Gross PA, Quinnan GV, Weksler ME, et al: Relation of chronic

disease and immune response to influenza vaccine in the elderly. Vaccine 1989;7:303–308

218. Ershler WB, Hacker MP, Burroughs BJ et al: Cimetidine and the immune response: I. In vivo augmentation of nonspecific and specific immune response. Clin Immunol Immunopathol 1983;26:10–17

219. Moss RJ, Miles SH: AIDS and the geriatrician. J Am Ger Soc 1987;35:460–464

220. Fillit HM, Fruchtman S, Sell L, Rosen N: AIDS in the elderly: a case and its implications. Geriatrics 1989;44:65–70

221. Rosenzweig R, Fillit H: Probable heterosexual transmission of AIDS in an aged woman. J Am Geriatr Soc 1992;40: 1261–1264

222. Peterman TA, Jaffe HW, Feorino PM: Transfusion acquired immunodeficiency syndrome in the United States. JAMA 1985;254:2913–2917

223. Weiler PG, Mungas D, Pomerantz S: AIDS as a cause of dementia in the elderly. J Am Geriatr Soc 1988;36:139–141

224. Guidi L, Bartolini C, Frasca D et al: Impairment of lymphocyte activities in depressed aged subjects. Mech Ageing Dev 1991; 60:13–24

225. Bartrop RW, Lazarus L, Lockhurst E et al: Depressed lymphocyte function after bereavement. Lancet 1977:I:834–836

226. Schleifer SJ, Keller SE, Camerino M et al: Suppression of lymphocyte stimulation following bereavement. JAMA 1983; 250:374–377

227. Thomas RD, Goodwin JM, Goodwin JS: Effect of social support on stress-related changes in cholesterol level, uric acid level, and immune function in an elderly sample. Am J Psych 1985; 142:735–737

228. Kiecolt-Glaser JK, Fisher P, Ogrocki P et al: Marital quality, marital disruption and immune function. Psychosom Med 1987;49:13–34

229. Kiecolt-Glaser JK, Glaser R, Gravenstein S et al: Chronic stress alters the immune response to influenza virus vaccine in older adults. Proc Natl Acad Sci U S A 1996;93:3043–3047

230. Kiecolt-Glaser JK, Glaser R, Willinger D et al: Psychosocial enhancement of immunocompetence in a geriatric population. Health Psychol 1985;4:25–41

231. Pahlavani MA, Cheung TH, Chesky JA, Richardson A: Influence of exercise on the immune function of rats of various ages. J Appl Physiol 1988;64:2997–3001

232. Soppi E, Varijo P, Eskola J: Effect of strenuous physical stress on circulating lymphocyte number and function before and after training. J Clin Lab Immunol 1982;8:43–46

233. Grieco MH, Meriney DK: Immunodiagnosis for clinicans, Chicago, Year Book, 1983

234. Daynes RA, Araneo BA: Prevention and reversal of some age-associated changes in immunologic responses by supplemental dehydroepiandrosterone sulfate therapy. Aging Immunol Infect Dis 1992;3:135–155

235. Delafuente JC: Immunosenescence: clinical and pharmacologic considerations. Med Clin N A 1985;69:465–486

236. Masoro EJ: Dietary restriction and aging. J Am Geriatr Soc 1993;41:994–999

237. Gershwin ME, Beach R, Hurley L: Trace metals, aging and immunity. J Am Geriatr Soc 1983;31:374–378

238. Penn ND, Purkines L, Kelleher J et al: The effect of dietary supplementation with vitamins A, C and E on cell-mediated immune function in elderly long-stay patients: a randomized controlled trial. Age Ageing 1991;20:169–174

239. Goodwin JS, Garry PJ: Relationship between megadose vitamin supplementation and immunologic function in a healthy elderly population. Clin Exp Immunol 1983;51:647–653

240. Busby J, Caranasos GJ: Immune function, autoimmunity and selective immunoprophylaxis in the aged. Med Clin N A 1985; 69:465–474

241. Bentley DW: Pneumococcal vaccine in the institutionalized elderly: a review of past and recent studies. Rev Infect Dis 1981;3s:s61–70

242. Gross PA, Quinnan GV, Rodstein M et al: Association of influenza immunization with reduction in mortality in an elderly population. Arch Int Med 1988;148:562–565

243. Ammann AJ Schiffman G, Austrian R: The antibody responses to pneumococcal capsular polysaccharides in aged individuals. Proc Soc Exp Biol Med 1980;164:312–316

244. Forrester HL, Jahnigen DW, LaForce FM: Inefficancy of pneumococcal vaccine in a high-risk population. Am J Med 1987; 83:425–430

245. Peters NJ, Meiklejohn G, Jahnigen DW: Antibody response of an elderly population to a supplemental dose of influenza B vaccine. J Am Geratr Soc 1988;36:593–599

246. Simberkoff MS, Cross AP, Al-Ibrahim M et al: Efficacy of pneumococcal vaccine in high-risk patients. N Engl J Med 1986;315:1318–1327

247. Gravenstein S, Drinka P, Duthie EH et al: Efficacy of an influenza hemagglutinin-diphtherian toxoid conjugate vaccine in elderly nursing home subjects during an influenza outbreak. J Am Geriatr Soc 1994;42:245–251

248. Hibberd PL, Rubin RH: Immunization strategies for the immunocompromised host: the need for immunoadjuvants. Ann Intern Med 1989;110:955–956

CHAPTER 9

Aging of Memory

P. RABBITT

This review discusses changes in memory in normal, healthy old age. The effects of changes in memory efficiency that occur as a result of pathologies of the brain and central nervous system, which become increasingly common in old age, are described in another chapter. As healthy people grow old they invariably complain—citing convincing concrete instances—that their memories are becoming inconveniently unreliable. Large scale surveys in which older people have been asked to describe the difficulties that they experience confirm these anecdotal impressions. Guttman[1] found that after arthritis and rheumatism, memory loss was the second most frequent problem reported by elderly Canadians. et al[2] found that 70 percent of community-dwelling citizens of San Francisco reported that their memories had begun to fail. Hulicka[3] found that overall frequency of complaints of memory problems steadily increased from age 45 to 85. Given this striking consensus we might expect that the best way to learn about the prevalence, extent, and nature of changes in memory efficiency in old age, and to discover how these changes affect peoples' abilities to manage their everyday lives, must be to allow very large numbers of respondents to describe their problems while answering suitable questionnaires. Unfortunately, an extensive literature shows that individuals' subjective descriptions of their memory failures are poor indicators of their objective abilities. The reasons for this discrepancy between subjective impression and objective performance tells us much about the nature of memory and about the way in which we evaluate our own competence.

Self-Assessment of Memory by Young and Older Adults

Studies in which people are asked to assess their own mental competence have typically used questionnaires in which they rate, on a three- or five-point scale, their ability to cope with each of a variety of concretely specified everyday problems such as recalling names, telephone numbers, appointments, or shopping lists; to make and to carry through plans; and to recognize routes or faces. It was early apparent that young adults' ratings of their own competence in everyday tasks did not predict their objective performance on simple laboratory memory tasks, such as free recall of lists of words, or learning of paired associates that have been assumed to be useful tests of "general memory efficiency."[4] We may take this as evidence that we should not expect individual differences in performance of simple dull tasks to predict competence in the complex scenarios of everyday life, in which experience, interest, attention, and motivation may be decisive factors. A different conclusion might be that memory competence may be intensely task-specific, so that people who have developed remarkable memory skills in particular everyday situations may perform much less well in others. We must be wary of analogies between presumed levels of mental abilities, such as "memory" or "intelligence," and of physiologic indices such as "muscle tone" or "aerobic capacity." Memory is not strong or weak; its efficiency may markedly differ between situations. Thus, reliably excellent recall of paintings or visual images may be accompanied by relatively poor recall of verbal material or of past events. The idea that memory competence can be intensely situation-specific highlights the point that a suitable metaphor for memory is not an audiotape system, the accuracy of which is limited only by its fidelity, the interference it suffers, and the period over which its records degrade over time. Memory is, rather, a dynamically constructive and elaborative process that involves both selective and sustained attention, to encode and interpret new information in terms of knowledge that we accumulate about the world. This knowledge is organized into schemata or programs for dealing with particular classes of events, or some types of information and not others,[5] and for the retrieval of internally maintained information in response to externally perceived or internally generated demands. It is hard to think of any cognitive function that has been investigated by psychologists that does not, in some way, embody the functions that, in common language, we call "memory."

The diversity and complexity of mental abilities involved in memory may make it easier to understand why peoples' subjective, but global, impressions of their own competence are often not validated by the results of objective, but very limited experiments. It does not explain the further paradox that although nearly all elderly people complain in *general* terms about difficulties with memory, most studies have found that when asked to rate the relative frequency of their lapses in *particular* situations they usually report fewer lapses than do young adults.[6–10] Only a few studies have found no differences between old and young people,[11,12] and none have shown clear age-related increases in complaints.[13]

A sufficient explanation for this paradox is that people cannot make absolute judgments about their own mental capacities. They can only compare their own performance against some external, objective standard. Because common standards for comparison are only rarely available, the criteria that people use to make their subjective judgements tend to be personal, and so vary widely between individuals. An obvious criterion of mental competence is success in dealing with the demands of daily life. Very able middle-aged adults coping with demanding lives may have to remember and update information about many different appointments, telephone numbers, people, and events. They may often be distracted—by an unpredictable variety of urgent demands—from their attempts to follow the schedules of activity that they hold in mind. Because they inevitably make many lapses, and because they can only compare themselves against very able colleagues or partners, they may become convinced that they have unusually poor memories. In contrast, older people may cope extremely well with the lenient demands of their less demanding lives and so, quite accurately, report that they very rarely forget the few appointments, telephone numbers, or plans that see them through most of their days. An illuminating example of the relativity of self-assessment is peoples' appraisal of their own general health. Objectively, the incidence and prevalence of pathologies sharply increases in old age, but studies using self-assessment questionnaires have invariably found that people in their late seventies may give much more favorable ratings of their own health than do objectively healthier 50- or 60-year-olds. Mc Innes and Rabbitt[14] have shown that this is because older people tend to assess their health in relation to that of other members of their own age group. Fortunate individuals who have survived to answer health questionnaires late in their lives have also become increasingly conscious of their own relative well-being compared to that of most of their less fortunate peers.

The problem that people cannot rate themselves in absolute terms, and that they also usually cannot even make relative comparisons against any common standard, is compounded by the way in which most self-rating questionnaires have been designed and scored. For example, Reason[8,15] obtained descriptions of everyday mental lapses from a very large and representative sample of respondents, and derived from these paradigms of the most frequent categories of memory failures reported. He incorporated these as questions in his excellent self-rating questionnaire, the Short Inventory of Mental Lapses (SIML). Individuals' SIML scores are totals of the different types of lapses that they report, weighted by the frequency with which they have occurred. Within populations of people who all lead very similar lives and face similar levels of demands, it is possible that respondents' total tallies of lapses are useful indices of their relative proneness to memory failures. However, in gerontologic comparisons, a pervasive problem is that older adults may not only lead very different lives, with different levels of demands from those encountered by younger people, but that they may also experience problems in quite different kinds of situations.

Another issue is that in order to recognize their memory failures people need feedback from their lapses, or from their "near misses." As people age they tend to engage less often in cooperative activities and so have fewer opportunities to compare their own capabilities with those of others. They may also receive less pointed, but potentially useful criticism because, in their less demanding lives, the memory lapses that they inevitably make are, perhaps, also less often fraught with memorable consequences or are embarrassingly public. It is likely that peoples' ability to recognize and use their errors to monitor their own behavior diminishes with age, so that they recognize fewer of the errors that they make,[16] also, as they grow older, people tend to forget what they have forgotten.

Finally, peoples' responses to self-rating questionnaires are often as markedly influenced by their subjective feelings of depression and poor self-regard as by the objective reality of their everyday competence. It is pleasant to report that recent studies show that people do not necessarily experience higher levels of depression as they age,[17] and the more robust self-esteem of elite cohorts of older individuals who volunteer themselves for psychological investigations certainly contributes to their optimistic self-assessments. Rabbitt et al.[13] discussed these and other difficulties, and reviewed the literature on the on use of self-rating questionnaires to assess the elderly. For readers who may be tempted to agree with Reason[8] that responses to self-rating questionnaires are accurate reflections of objective reality and that the more favorable self-ratings given by older people on his SIML mean that everyday memory competence may not diminish but, in some cases, may even improve in old age, the following review of objective comparisons of older and younger adults on a variety of laboratory memory tasks may be provocative.

Population Studies of Changes in Memory With Increasing Age

The most convincing objective evidence that memory efficiency declines in old age is the great body of evidence from laboratory studies in which cumulatively, many thousands of elderly and young adults have been compared on many hundreds of different memory tasks. In almost all of these comparisons the elderly have performed much less well than the young participants. However, while these many comparisons confirm that older adults perform less well in a variety of tasks involving the encoding, retention, and retrieval of information, they give us little idea at what age competence first begins to decline, or how rapidly these declines then continue, or how to compare the rates of decline of memory efficiency with that of other cognitive functions. To answer these questions we must screen very large numbers of people, drawn from a wide range of ages on the same tasks. Of the many longitudinal studies that have been carried out few have included more than only one or two memory tasks. In the Manchester and Newcastle longitudinal study of over 6,000 individuals aged from 50 to 90 years,[18] seven different memory tests were used. Since all volunteers were also scored on the Mill Hill and

Wconsler Adult Intelligence Scale (WAIS) vocabulary tests, and since vocabulary test scores were found not to change within this age range and, in youth, are closely correlated with scores on tests of fluid general ability (intelligence tests), it is possible to match individuals of different ages in terms of their presumptive levels of general intellectual ability when they were young adults. When groups of participants of different ages are selected in this way, differences between average scores obtained from groups of individuals aged between 55 and 60 and those aged between 60 and 65 are small, but statistically reliable. Thereafter, declines in scores accelerate, and average scores markedly fall in the age range between 66 and 75, and even more so in the range between 76 and 85. However, variations in ability between individuals also markedly increase with group age, so that differences between the most and least able individuals in their seventies are very much greater than differences between the most and least able 50-year-olds. The implications of these increases in variability between individuals with group age becomes clearer when we consider overall correlations between memory test scores and age between 50 and 85 years. On all tests, correlations varied between $r = -0.25$ and $r = -0.46$. That is to say, if we consider all the sources of variance between individuals in scores on memory tests as 100 percent that proportion of this variance that was associated with their ages was only between 6.2 and 21 percent. Data from other recent large scale studies give very similar estimates (Dorly Deeg & Carolin Schmidt, personal communication, 1996 from the Amsterdam LASA study, Jellimer Jolles & Peter Houx, personal communication, 1996, from the Maastricht longitudinal study; Lars Goran Neilson, personal communication, 1996, from the Betula longitudinal study). As we shall see, these associations between test scores and chronologic age can be deceptive since, if we treat "years since birth" as a single, undifferentiated factor, we certainly confound the effects of very many other variables that are strongly associated with age: these include the reduction in level of complexity of everyday demands and so loss of daily practice at difficult everyday "memory tasks," and the greatly increased incidence of pathologies of all kinds and the consequently greater use of medication and of poorer states of general health in elderly samples.

Although these assessments are rough they are interesting, because they do confirm that there is a general, accelerating trend toward poorer memory performance in old age, they also show that the magnitude of changes in indices of memory competence in populations of healthy older people who volunteer for longitudinal studies may be very slight indeed. It seems that marked changes in ability do not occur until late in life. Longitudinal assessments of participants in the Manchester/Newcastle study now add to the finding that there are also very marked individual differences in rates of change in cognitive performance over time, such that some individuals have changed little or not at all, even between their mid-sixties and late seventies, while others have undergone substantial changes much earlier. It seems that these individual differences in rates of change are at least partly associated with individual differences in general health, and in the incidence of particular pathologies such as cardiovascular problems and late-onset diabetes. The possibility of discovering factors that make some individuals so much more fortunate than others in resisting age-related impairments is perhaps the most important practical goal of cognitive gerontology.

General Models of Change in Memory and Cognition With Age

It may be helpful to readers trained in other disciplines than psychology to recognize that, regrettably, we currently have models for changes in memory efficiency in old age that are derived either from behavioral or from neuropsychologic data, and that, at present, only weak and unsatisfactory links have been made between these two levels of description. Models that are entirely based on behavioral data are derived from comparisons between the performance of older and younger people on a great variety of experimental tasks. Models for the neurophysiology and neuropsychology of memory have been derived from the study of young and middle-aged adults with focal brain injuries. It is not a straightforward matter to relate these studies of focal and limited damage to interpret the behavioral results of normal brain aging, which produces global and diffuse rather than focal and limited changes.[19] Models derived from behavioural data have been regrettably limited in scope, because they have been developed to explain age-related changes in performance only in particular experimental tasks. One gallant exception has been the "information processing loss" model proposed by Salthouse.[20–22] It has long been recognized that aging is accompanied by slowing of mental performance.[23–24] Salthouse[20] has used this robust finding as the basis for a single factor theory of cognitive aging, proposing that changes in the rate at which humans processed information drive changes in their performance at all other cognitive skills, including memory. Thus functional models of cognitive aging may be very parsimoniously based on the idea that the entire gamut of all behavioral changes observed in human aging can be described as secondary consequences of this primary change in brain efficiency.

There is no doubt that older people do process information more slowly than the young, and there are good reasons why this should affect the efficiency with which they remember. For example, as Baddeley[25] and Baddeley and Hitch[26] have elegantly shown, the speed with which people can read or articulate words directly determines the number of different words that they can simultaneously hold in mind in order to understand complex sentences and to make correct inferences from temporally separated statements. In this sense, information-processing speed both determines the capacity of people's working memory for information presented to them, and also the efficiency with which they can bring many disparate kinds of information together in order to solve problems. Salthouse[27] and Salthouse and Babcock[28] have convincingly shown that working memory capacity diminishes with age and that this is, at least partly, because they have become slower at processing information. Speed of information processing also certainly affects the amount of information that people can remember over longer periods of time. Craik and Lockhart[29] and Craik and Tulving[30] have shown that people remember lists of words better when they are given the opportunity to encode them "deeply," by associating them as richly as possible to other words and information that they already hold in their long-term memories. It follows that individuals who process information faster will, as a consequence, be able to encode information more deeply, and to make more useful associations in unit time than those who are slower. Many studies, such as an exemplary experiment by Waugh and Barr,[31] have shown that older people may remember as much information as accurately as young adults if they are allowed longer study times to compensate for their slower uptake of information. However, the Salthouse, single factor model goes beyond these data, and is rigid in its insistence, not merely that slowing of information processing speed must reduce memory efficiency, but rather that it is entirely responsible for all of the changes in memory efficiency that occur in old age.

The single factor model does not survive closer inspection. One difficulty is evident from studies in which large numbers of healthy elderly people have been given batteries of many different tests, including intelligence tests, tests of information processing speed, a variety of different memory tests, and some neuropsychologic tests. Principal component analyses can be carried out on these results in order to discover which subsets of tests are most closely associated with each other, and which pick up most of the variance between individuals that is associated with their ages. A number of different studies of this kind carried out in our laboratory have found clear statistical separations between factors in which intelligence test scores and speed of information processing on the one hand, and memory tasks on the other, share common variance. Moreover, when individuals' ages are entered into these analyses as an additional variable, they are found to share common variance with memory test scores rather than with scores on tests of general intellectual ability, or of information processing speed.[32–34] In other words, such analyses do not support the ideas either that performance on memory tests is entirely accounted for by individual differences in information processing speed, or that people's scores on tests of information processing speed are more closely related to their ages than are their scores on all other tasks. On the contrary, they suggest that, if anything, changes in memory efficiency are more sensitive indices of cognitive aging than are changes in information processing speed.

This procedure makes the point that if we examine variance in performance across tests and between individuals, we find that differences in their information processing rates do not completely account for differences in their performance on memory tests. A different way to examine the relation between information processing speed and memory efficiency is to test whether, within individuals, relations between performance indices change with age. This was done by plotting individuals' scores on intelligence tests against their scores on memory tasks. This allowed us to determine which individuals showed the greatest disassociation between these measures, that is, which individuals had scores on memory tests that were much lower than would be predicted by their scores on intelligence tests. The numbers of such individuals located in large groups of volunteers increased with the age of the group sampled. Significantly more 70- and 80-year-olds than 50- and 60-year-olds showed marked dissociations between scores on intelligence and memory tests. In subsequent studies we compared correlations between scores on memory tests and on tests of information processing speed in individuals who did, and who did not, show disassociations between intelligence test scores and memory test scores. It emerged that identical, modest, but robust correlations between intelligence test scores and measures of information processing rate appeared in both groups. In the group whose better memories were predicted by their intelligence test scores, there were also modest correlations between measures of information processing speed and scores on memory tasks, just as Salthouse's[20,21] single factor theory would predict. However, within the group who had unusually poor memories relative to their intelligence test scores, there was no correlation between memory test scores and measures of information processing rate. It seemed that the changes in memory efficiency that these particular older individuals had suffered were not due either to a general decline in intellectual ability reflected in a decline in their performance on intelligence tests, nor to a decline in their information processing speed but, rather, to changes in some other factor that neither intelligence tests nor tests of information processing speed sensitively detect.[32] It seems that within, as well as between, individuals, memory efficiency and information processing speed are incompletely associated.[32,35] The failure of the parsimonious single factor model is regrettable because it is the only general account of cognitive changes in old age, and this means that we have to consider, piecemeal, evidence from comparisons between younger and older people on a great variety of different experimental tasks, without any overarching guiding framework of interpretation.

Laboratory Studies of Differences in Memory Competence Between Old and Young Adults

Preliminary Theoretical Orientation

As we have seen there are fundamental conceptual problems in discussing memory as a particular mental ability, or set of cognitive processes, which is distinct from others such as perception, attention, or problem-solving. Although this distinction is embodied in common language and so in everyday experience, it is not the most useful guide to our current functional models for cognitive processes or for the neurophysiologic architecture of the brain. We must recognize that our ability to recognize directly the nature and relevance of objects and relation in our visual, auditory, and haptic worlds are entirely dependent on information that we have processed and stored in the past. Insofar as "memory" is a common term for all of the information about the world that we maintain in our brains, our memories are a crucial component of our perceptual systems because, without access to information obtained from past experiences, we could not interpret and use the new input that our sense organs provide. In this sense, the efficiency of our selective attention also entirely depends on the integrity of information held in memory. Note that this information does not only include the results of previous experience that allow us to categorize the perceptual world into objects, and to recognize how some temporal sequences of changes reveal recurrent patterns from which we can infer causality and recognize events. The information we hold in our brains must also incorporate much more basic rules and procedures, learned rather than innate, that allow us to extract the maximum information from sensory input and impose structure on our sensory worlds. For example, we learn the rules of perspective and other cues that allow us immediately to judge which parts of the visual world can be related to each other to form "objects" and how far they are from each other and from us. The dynamic, interactive syntheses, which have been so illuminatingly described by Gregory[36] depend upon, and are guided by information held in memory.

In this context, an evolutionary insight by Sir Charles Sherrington is illuminating. He suggested that "distance receptors"—such as the primitive equivalents of eyes and ears—developed by ancestral organisms could not realize their full potential while, like the tactile receptors on their body surfaces, they could only provide information about things that have already happened. Sense organs must always operate at least a few milliseconds behind the temporal present. Organisms can overcome this crucial disadvantage of trying to survive on the basis of obsolete information about a rapidly changing environment if they can "grow" brains with sufficient computing power to use information about the past to predict the immediate future. These predictions can only be made on the basis of contingencies detected, and derived by recognizing and registering regular relations between events. At this point, Sherrington's insight cuts even deeper than his idea that memory has not been developed to archive the past but rather to predict the future: we could not use information about the past to predict the future if, like photograph albums, our memories were collections of discrete, detailed, representations of individual, separate, events. Past experience can only guide prediction if information about specific past events is collapsed and processed to reveal recurrent patterns, consistencies, or temporal regularities that define classes of "things" or patterns of recurrent relations between "things." In the battle for evolutionary survival it would have been a disaster to develop a memory that was, like a videotape, a faithful, unselective, temporally ordered record of the details of past sounds and sights. Information about the past guides us through the present only if we can discard incidental details that make particular events uninformatively unique, and can abstract and synthesize regularities, patterns of relations, and higher order organizing principles that allow us to interpret and predict our rapidly changing environments. An appropriate analogy for memory is not a computer database of detailed information that can be called up by inputting appropriate instructions; a better analogy is a dynamic computer program, which although it must be stored in the brain, runs constantly and constantly alters its logical structure as well as the representations of the past, present, and future that it embodies.

"Prospective Memory": A Reification of Sherrington's Insight

There has been a growing realization that people do not simply use their memories merely as archives of information about the past, but rather make active use of information stored in memory in order to plan and manage their lives. This has led to a distinction between "retrospective memory" for previously acquired information or experienced events, and "prospective memory" for what to do and when to do it. A review by Dobbs and Reeves[37] provides an excellent summary of work to date, and makes the point that progress in this interesting field has been slow because investigators have chosen to make the unhelpful assumption that prospective memory should be investigated as a distinct type of memory—a particular kind of cognitive activity by means of which people engage with the world, in contrast to the retrospective memory for information previously acquired, which has typically been studied in laboratory experiments. An equally helpful review by Maylor[38] shows that, so far, studies have been very limited, comparing young and older adults in their ability to remember to carry out single, simple actions at particular times. This is in marked contrast to the demands of everyday life, in which complex plans involving multiple contingencies have to be formulated and carried out in flexible ways, depending on changing environmental demands and opportunities.[39] As a discussion of the field by Craik[40] points out, most everyday activities require the use of information that has been previously learned, or the memory of plans that have previously been formulated, in order to direct our selective attention to pick up precisely the information that we need to guide us through purposive activities. The necessary continuous interactions between information and plans held in long-term memory, imminently received information held in short-term and working memory, rapid control of selective attention, and the ability to sustain attention over long periods of time illustrate the complexity of cognitive processes for which we as yet have no adequate models, and the impoverishment of experiments that have concentrated on the simple recall or recognition of previously encountered information.

Terminology and Categories of Experimental Paradigms

It is precisely because of the difficulties of dissociating memory from other cognitive processes that readers trained in other disciplines than cognitive psychology are likely to be exasperated and confused by our current models for memory, and by the limitations of the experiments that we have designed to test these models. Research on memory has progressed by attempting to base frameworks of description on dichotomies between hypothetical memory systems. These dichotomies usually reflect the variables that we can empirically manipulate when we design experiments to test how much, and what sorts of information people can retain over varying periods of time. For example, the time frame over which performance is analyzed has given us a distinction between short-term, intermediate-term, and long-term memory, or between primary and secondary memory. The period over which information must be retained turns out to produce qualitative as well as merely quantitative differences in what people can remember, and in the kinds of confusions that they tend to make. For example, although when disconnected pieces of information such as lists of words or digits are presented so rapidly that people do not have a chance to rehearse and learn them, they can retain only relatively few items. However, in this case, the temporal order in which this information was presented is automatically preserved and seems to offer a crucial structure for correct recall, since attempts to recall items in any other order than that in which they were presented result in increases in errors. Moreover, for spoken or written words, mistakes often occur because the temporal order of items that sound similar is transposed. In contrast, when people have the opportunity to consolidate information by repeated rehearsal, they can retain indefinitely large amounts of information over indefinitely long periods of time. However, in this case, although the temporal order in which information was encountered (e.g., the exact order in which a list of words was presented) can be preserved, this is generally possible only with some effort; it is not crucial to correct recall, and mistakes are often made by confusing the meanings, as well as the sounds or letter patterns of words presented for recall. We deduce that the systems involved in short-term and in long-term memory are functionally distinct, and that pieces of information, in this case words, held in these two systems are represented in characteristically different ways.

Another distinction that reflects the particular empiric manipulations in tests for retention of information sometimes are those between recognition and recall or between implicit and explicit memory. In this case, what is varied is the nature of the particular cues available to elicit memories; that is, participants may simply be given the instruction, "Recall the list of words," or be shown the words that they inspected once again, embedded among distracters that were not previously present, or be given tasks in which any information that they can remember about the words that they were given would be useful to them. Dichotomies between types of memory may also reflect distinctions between the kinds of information presented for later recall, implying the availability or lack of particular modes of representation of information (e.g., visual memory, phonological memory, auditory memory). Dichotomies may also reflect higher order logical distinctions between kinds of information about the world, or the particular uses to which this information is put in everyday life (e.g., the distinction between procedural, semantic, and episodic memory). They can reflect inferences about the nature of processes, such as the minimum number of temporally successive hypothetical mental operations necessary to register, maintain, and regain information (e.g., encoding versus storage versus retrieval). They may sometimes reflect inferences about the qualitative nature of one or more of these processes (e.g., deep versus shallow processing of information at encoding). They sometimes refer to hypothetical logical structures, in modern terminology, this is perhaps, the data base architecture in terms of which information is encoded, organized, and retrieved (e.g., schemata, scripts, scenarios, network structures). Experiments have typically been designed to explore these, and many other, putative dichotomies in order to discover whether the logical or empiric distinctions that they embody can be reified in terms of corresponding qualitative distinctions between hypothetical functional processes and, ultimately, be captured in terms of neuroanatomy and neurophysiology.

Readers who are unfamiliar with this literature, and also many cognitive psychologists, may be helped if they resolutely bear in mind that not all of these hypothetic dichotomies are of the same logical kind. It may also be helpful to bear in mind that those dichotomies that have survived as frameworks of description in the literature have done so because the experimental manipulations in which they are embodied reveal *qualitative*, rather than merely *quantitative* differences in performance. This is because it is hard to argue that manipulations that only reveal differences in the amount of information that can be remembered and retrieved tap functionally different processes. The case that a functional, as well as a logical, distinction is involved becomes very much better if comparisons between manipulations reveal qualitative distinctions in the kinds of information recalled, or in the kinds of errors or confusions made in recall.

The way this has worked out in practice is particularly clear in studies of aging memory. Comparisons between the abilities of older and younger people have invariably been made in terms of experimental paradigms that have been developed in work carried out with young adults to illustrate, or explore, one or other of these theoretical dichotomies. Because our knowledge about human memory is structured in terms of these frameworks of description, the existence of *quantitative* differences in performance between older and young adults has been considered uninteresting; that is, we can make little theoretic progress if we can only show that, under all the experimental tasks in which we compare them, older people perform less well than the young. When age differences have been found to be especially marked in some experimental conditions and minimal or absent in others, it has been argued that old age markedly affects some hypothetic functional processes or memory systems, but spares others. As we shall see, this is not a particularly strong argument, especially when—as is usually the case—older people perform relatively worse in just those experimental conditions that the young also find more difficult. We are then faced with the difficulty that the differences between younger and older groups only represent the failure of the old to cross a particular threshold of task difficulty. The case becomes much stronger if we not only discover that older people are more affected by differences between particular task conditions than the young, but also that task conditions not only determine how much they can remember, but also what they can remember, and the types of confusions that they make.

In summary, it is inevitable that all of the frameworks of description that have seemed successfully to differentiate memory processes, systems, and structures in young adults have been used in order to try to understand changes in memory competence in old age, or individual differences in memory competence associated with other measurable indices, such as general intellectual ability, which also decline in old age.[33] The resulting literature may be organized in terms of the distinctions between hypothetic memory systems that these various empiric comparisons have engendered.

Iconic, Primary, Secondary and Working Memory

There is good evidence both that the duration for which information is maintained in memory affects the way in which it is represented in memory, and also that different neurophysiologic processes and systems are involved in the maintenance of information over different periods of time.

Iconic memory

The type of memory with the briefest time-scale of operation, extending over only a few hundred milliseconds, is "iconic memory." Classic demonstrations by Averbach & Coriell[41] and Sperling[42] showed that when displays of visual information are briefly presented there is a finite time during which momentary changes, such as insertion of a symbol cueing one rather than others of a number of different letters, can be used to facilitate their subsequent identification and recall. This has been taken to mean that all of the information from very complex displays is potentially available at the moments at which they first appear, but that this rich sensory representation (iconic memory) very rapidly degrades over time. Because the speed at which information can be "read off" is limited, participants can only obtain some, but not all, of the information that is potentially available before the "iconic trace" degrades to an extent that makes it of no further use. The scanty evidence on age differences in maintenance of iconic traces appears paradoxic. Di Lollo et al.[43,44] report ingenious experiments in which they presented two regular 5 × 5 matrices of illuminated dots successively, side by side, on a computer screen. In one of these, one of the 25 possible dots was omitted. Although older observers were, on the whole, less accurate than young, there were suggestions that while the young could only locate the missing dot if the matrices were presented only between 40 msec and 90 msec apart, the old could sometimes make correct judgements when they were separated by longer intervals. These authors suggest that the duration of iconic traces is determined by the times taken to process them rather than by the rate at which they passively degrade. On this premise, Di Lollo and associates[44] infer that older people have longer lasting iconic traces because they process information much more slowly than the young.

Primary versus secondary memory

Once again the distinctions between these hypothetic systems is operational, in the sense that it implies that systems that hold information for different periods of time have different functional characteristics. The definition of primary memory stems from evidence that, for single unrelated items of any kind, such as words, digits, or letters, there is a fixed span of items that can be correctly reported, in the same order as they are presented, immediately after they have been heard or read. As Miller[45] pointed out, memory spans differ between different kinds of materials, being between seven and nine items for random digits, and somewhat less for words or letters. Miller also pointed out that a strong determinant of span is the relative efficiency with which items can be encoded or "chunked" for later retrieval. Individual subjects may have more practice, and hence expertise, at encoding some kinds of items than others. The equation of span with primary memory and its distinction from secondary memory arose from observations of the ways in which people immediately recall lists of items, such as words, which are so long that they cannot report all of them. In these cases people show marked "recency effects," usually correctly recalling a span of the last five to seven items in the list before they attempt less competent recall of other items. These final items are usually recalled in the same temporal order as they have been read or heard. In contrast, items from the middle of the list are usually recalled later, with less success, and usually not in the same order as that in which they were presented. Experimental manipulations such as delay of recall by additional tasks may reduce probability of correct recall of the final items but have less effect on the recall of earlier items. It has been concluded that this must be because the final items are held in a storage system with a rapid decay rate (primary memory) while earlier items have attained representation in a different storage system with a longer rate of decay (secondary memory).

In terms of this dichotomy it is natural to ask whether age affects primary more than secondary memory, or vice versa. The evidence is somewhat inconclusive. An obvious question is whether older individuals show greater decrements relative to the young in recall for early as against later items in supraspan word lists. Studies by Parkinson et al.[46] and Foos et al.[47] found no interactions between age and recall from different list positions. That is, there were equal age decrements in recall from the last few (primary memory) and from earlier (secondary memory) items in lists. In contrast, Delbecq-Derousne and Beauvoise[48] obtained a relatively pure measure of primary memory span in a well-planned experiment in which participants were instructed always to recall the final seven words in a list before attempting recall of any others. Under these conditions they found little age decrement in primary memory but a marked decrement in secondary memory.

If we equate primary memory with the maximum number of items that can be correctly recalled in the same order as they were presented, it seems clear that there are small but consistent reductions in span with increasing age.[28,49–51]

A difficulty in interpreting the results of studies that find that age reduces the number of items that can be recalled from primary more than from secondary memory or vice versa, is that the relative sizes of age differences obtained in these two systems appear to alter with the kind and familiarity of material to be remembered. For example, Wingfield et al.[52] found that groups of older and younger participants had identical spans for lists of digits but older participants had shorter spans for lists of words. Assuming that Wingfield et al.[52] were careful to equate the syllable lengths of the words and digits that they used, this suggests that elderly people can maintain spans for items such as lists of digits that they often have to encode and remember during their everyday lives, but are less successful at the task of remembering lists of random words, at which they have much less practice. Experiments have shown that when young adults are highly practiced, there appear to be no clear limits to the lengths of the spans of items that they can retain in primary memory. Ericcsen and his associates[53] have shown that, after modest amounts of practice, undergraduates can increase the numbers of digits that they immediately recall from the "normal" span of seven to nine, to 15 or more. They manage this by discovering, or inventing systems of encoding or grouping items. The systems that they use are specific to the particular materials for which they are designed. Individuals who have learned to greatly extend their digit spans show no benefits for letters, and *vice versa*. The fact that age differences in span may appear for unfamiliar, but not for familiar material means that although the bulk of evidence suggests that age does reduce the functional efficiency of the primary memory system, this conclusion is not logically secured until it has been shown that differences in spans between younger and older adults still exist after indefinitely lengthy periods of practice and, consequently, that span differences are not, simply, the results of disuse rather than of functional change. The fact that spans can almost indefinitely increase by improved encoding strategies means that we cannot regard them as measures of the maximum capacity of a static system such as a computer RAM, but rather as estimates of the current efficiency of a dynamic system that is constantly improving its techniques for encoding information.

However, there is other evidence that these two kinds of memory storage systems, primary and secondary memory, may be functionally distinct. It is possible to measure the speed with which people can retrieve information from these two systems by presenting them with lists of items and then asking them, as rapidly as possible, to make a decision whether a subsequently presented single probe was, or was not, one of the items presented. This allows us to measure how the time they take to decide whether or not a probe item was, or was not in the list presented to them varies as the length of the list of items that they have to remember is increased. Sternberg[54] found that the decision times for both positive (probe present in the memory list) and negative (probe not present in the memory list) decisions increased linearly with the number of items that had to be remembered. Significantly, the times taken for negative decisions increased more rapidly with list length than did times for positive decisions. Sternberg argued that this must be because people make a series of successive comparisons between the probe and memory representations of each item presented. Comparisons continue until a match is found, or no match can be detected. Because the search process terminates as soon as a match is found, decision times for "probe present" responses will increase, linearly as a function of (N + 1/2) where N is the number of items in the list. In contrast, "probe not present" decisions cannot be validated until all possible comparisons have been made. Thus, "probe not present" decision times will increase directly as a linear function of the number of items in a list. Results robustly fit these assumptions, so that Sternberg's[55] hypothesis of "serial self-terminating memory search" gains support. In contrast, for supraspan lists, which must at least partly be held in secondary rather than in primary memory, decision times increase much more slowly, or not at all with list length.[56] This operational distinction between a span-limited primary memory, in which serial self-terminating search is possible, and a span-unlimited primary memory, in which some other, presumably parallel search process is used, provides convincing evidence that these two types of memory storage systems may be functionally distinct, as well as different in the respect that they are supposed to hold material for shorter or longer periods of time.

These qualitative distinctions between the functional characteristics of primary and secondary memory offer a different way to ask whether old age affects them in different ways. Coyne et al.,[57] Craik & Rabinowitz,[58] and Lorsbach and Simpson,[59] report that older people take longer to retrieve information from both systems, but that age-related slowing of retrieval may be relatively longer from secondary than from primary memory. There is, however, a difficulty with all experiments that attempt to assess the effects of aging on hypothetically different functions or processes by comparing its effects on their relative speeds of operation. A masterly meta-analysis of age comparisons in reaction time tasks carried out by Cerella[60] showed that age has simple scalar effects on the rate of information processing such that, for all of a number of different types of tasks for which he could find published data, the average decision speeds for groups of older individuals could be accurately derived by multiplying the average decision speeds for groups of young adults by a simple constant, in the range 1.2 to 1.5. In other words, age slows difficult decisions more than easy decisions, but its proportionate effects are the same for decisions of all kinds and of all durations. There is no evidence that the effects of age on decision times vary with the qualitative nature of the functional processes involved. The relevance of Cerella's demonstration to experiments that compare the times that older and younger people take to retrieve matches to probes from primary and secondary memory is that people of all ages take longer to match secondary memory probes, so that age differences in decision times may increase in absolute terms, but still maintain the linearly scalar relations that Cerella uncovered. Many studies have shown that the effects of age on latencies for retrieval from long-term memory are also scalar.[61] The fact that age increases the absolute times required to retrieve information from one memory system more than it increases the absolute times taken to retrieve information from a supposedly different memory system is not, therefore, necessarily good evidence either that these systems must be functionally distinct, or that age reduces the efficiency of one system more than the efficiency of the other.

Working memory

The concept of "working memory" is both indispensable and vague. The term was coined by Baddeley and Hitch.[26] In their original formulation it referred to a particular model designed to explain quite limited data on memory for lists of words. Their elegant experiments showed that memory span for words was determined by their length, in the sense of the number of syllables that they contained. Moreover, increases in word span that occur as children grow up are directly and linearly related to the maximum rates at which they can repeatedly articulate the same list of three of four words. Repeated articulation of nonsense syllables interferes with immediate recall of word lists more than does concurrent listening to continuous speech or to lists of other random words. Similarly, spatial tracking or solution of problems involving imagery interferes less with retention of word lists than with retention of visual information—which is, also, less affected by concurrent articulation. These findings gave rise to an interesting model that assumes that information about lists of words that a person hears or reads is held in an "articulatory loop," where the articulatory representations of individual words rapidly decay unless they are refreshed by rehearsal in the order in which they were presented. Note that this provides a very tightly defined model in which the duration of survival of an articulatory representation of a word is determined by only two parameters: the rate at which it can be rehearsed (which can be inferred from maximum articulation rate for other material) and the rate at which an unrehearsed representation will decay and become unavailable. Representations of spatial or graphic information that cannot be encoded as words similarly are retained in a different store, the "visual scratch-pad." These sensory-based representation systems are under the active control of a device termed the "central executive." As Baddeley[25] has admitted, the central executive and its role are poorly defined. However, it is precisely this less well-developed aspect of the model that has gained it wide currency, since it captures Baddeley's important insight that we do not simply, passively, and involuntarily hold in mind information from the immediate present until it "decays" or becomes unavailable because of interference from later input. Rather, we combine information immediately gained from the world, and other information evoked from our long-term memories to solve particular problems. In this sense, working memory is, indeed, a work space in which new and old information can be selected, altered, and combined to derive necessary answers. Thus, while satisfactory descriptions of the central executive and what it does are not yet available, it seems an indispensable insight that there must exist a system that can dynamically initiate and control the "work" that working memory does.

Models for the subsystems that are envisaged as co-operatively constituting working memory offer clear opportunities for age comparisons. An initial question we may ask is whether the slight reductions in digit and word spans observed in older people are brought about by changes in one or both of the hypothetic system performance parameters of the articulatory loop system, whether fewer items can be held in the loop because decay is accelerated or rehearsal is slowed. Goward[62] tested this and found that declines in span were entirely attributable to age-related slowing of articulation rates and information processing rates, and that there was no evidence that age accelerates the rate at which representations of words in the articulatory store decay over time.

A second approach to age comparisons offered by the model derives from the assumption that working memory is involved whenever separate and independent decisions must be made about different aspects of the same information, and that the efficiency with which people can do this may change as they grow old. An ingenious paradigm developed by Just and Carpenter[63] has become the standard test. Participants read or hear statements one at a time, and have to make and announce a decision about each in turn, for example, whether it is true or false. They also have to try to remember the final word of each sentence. This involves simultaneous processing of information about each statement to determine its truth value, selection of the final word of each statement, and retention of as many of these words as possible. The maximum number of words that can be retained, while all sentences have been correctly evaluated, can be taken as an index of working memory capacity. On this criterion several studies report that declines in working memory capacity with advancing age are significantly greater than those observed in primary or secondary memory.[28,52,64–66]

Much of the interest in changes in working memory and, putatively, in the efficiency of the central executive with age stems from the idea that working memory is essential for the development and execution of plans and for the selective ordering of information, and that these functions are affected by damage to the frontal lobes. Although there are diffuse and widespread losses and degenerative changes in the tissue of the entire cortex in old age, postmortem and brain scan studies suggest that these may be especially marked in the frontal and temporal lobes. There has been increasing interest in exploring deficits of working memory in patients of all ages who have well-localized frontal lesions,[67] and in using working memory paradigms to seek for qualitative, rather than merely quantitative differences in the performance of normal elderly people and age-matched patients suffering from dementia of the Alzheimer's type. There is hope that work of this kind will eventually allow us to begin to relate functional to neurophysiologic changes in old age.

Some models of changes in working memory efficiency in old age seek parsimony by ascribing all changes to slowing of a single performance index; speed of information processing. This is captured in an attractive metaphor used by Salthouse,[27] who likens the capacity of working memory to the capacity of a restaurant, where the limitation is not merely set by the number of available tables but by the speed with which available staff can serve them. This seems logically parallel to the articulatory loop model proposed by Baddeley and Hitch[26] and Baddeley,[25] in which limitation to capacity is jointly set by information processing rate (rehearsal rate, the rate at which traces can be "served") and the rate at which unrehearsed memory traces are lost over time (decay rate). As we have seen, Goward[62] found no evidence that indices of trace decay rate changed with age, and concluded that age-related slowing of information processing rate provide a sufficient explanation for age changes in working memory capacity. Goward's findings have been replicated by several investigators and, in general terms, are consistent with studies by Salthouse et al.,[68,69] who show that working memory performance declines as a function of the complexity of the concurrent tasks that participants have to perform; that the rate of this decline with task complexity increases with age; and that a sufficient explanation for this is the well-documented global slowing of information processing rate (loss of processing resources) that occurs as age advances.

Although William of Occam would applaud explanations that postulate as few system performance characteristics as possible, it seems unlikely that such parsimony can do justice to the complexity of mental operations involved in selective attention, computation, and transformation of information held in memory. Other suggestions are emerging. For example, Hasher and Zacks[70] point to evidence that frontal lobe dysfunction is accompanied by a loss of selective attention and by increasing difficulties in suppressing irrelevant information. They suggest that, in addition to slowing of information processing rate, a different source of limitation to working memory capacity with age may be an increasing failure to suppress intrusion of unwanted information into working memory. Increasing evidence that both individuals with frontal lesions, and the elderly, do have increasing difficulty in tasks in which they have to discriminate between relevant and irrelevant information, or alternate types of decisions, makes this a promising line of speculation.

Information Retention for Long Durations

Readers unfamiliar with the psychological literature should once again patiently bear in mind that experiments testing longer term retention have been carried out in terms of dichotomies derived from many, different, and sometimes logically disparate frames of reference. Some of these dichotomies depend on distinctions between the kinds of information that are stored and retrieved (e.g., in procedural, semantic, and episodic memory), and attempt to derive from this categorization both an evolutionary chronology and functional distinctions between different memory systems.[71] Others depend on differences in the availability of information when elicited either directly or implicitly and, once again, argue that this implies functional, and possibly neurophysiologic distinctions between the processes or systems involved (implicit versus explicit memory systems). Others depend on distinctions between successive processes in a sequence that, it is assumed, must occur between the presentation of information and its later elicitation (encoding, storage, and retrieval processes; depth of processing and encoding specificity). Others contrast memory for higher and lower order structures in material, and for the ability to use previously acquired information and knowledge about the world to make correct inferences so as to interpret and organize material presented for later recall (e.g., distinctions between memory for the sense or logical structure of narratives, and specific details, incorporated in those narratives, which may be incidental or irrelevant to their main themes). A final distinction, which we shall argue is not dissimilar from that between the thematic structure and details of narratives, is that between memory for events or information, and memory for the source or context in which this information was acquired (source memory).

Inevitably, these dichotomies have become frameworks for comparisons between older and younger adults, so that the form of the questions that are invariably asked is, "Does old age affect episodic memory more than semantic memory? implicit memory more than explicit memory? encoding processes more or less than storage or retrieval processes? the ability to recognize and use principles of organization more than the ability to remember isolated details? memory for the sources or contexts in which information has been encountered more or less than memory for information without necessity for recall of source? It can be argued that questions framed in terms of these theoretic dichotomies do not necessarily provide the most informative means of discovering whether memory function in old age is *qualitatively* rather than merely *quantitatively* different from memory function in youth. This is because empiric answers to any and all of these questions can only be that age affects systems X and Y to the same extent, or that age affects system X more than system Y. However, since the distinctions made between systems X and Y or Z are usually cast in terms of the different kinds of material that they are supposed to maintain, or in terms of the different kinds of experimental manipulations that are made to elicit material from them, the only answers that such questions can provide (i.e., "more" or "less" or "the same") are unsatisfactory because they involve comparisons between logically incommensurable results. We shall return to this point at the end of this review, after we have considered the evidence that this process of enquiry has yielded.

Procedural, semantic, and episodic memory systems

This distinction between memory systems has been most explicitly developed by Tulving.[71,72] "Procedural memory" may be defined as memory for motor skills or other forms of acquired knowledge of how to do things, such as riding a bicycle, juggling, reading print, or adding up columns of figures. The idea that distinct neurophysiologic system maintain information about such acquired procedures came from early studies on amnesia following injury to the hippocampus and temporal lobes.[73,74] These found that even patients who are so profoundly amnesic that their ability to recall people or events and to acquire new information has been very severely impaired, may nevertheless retain previously acquired procedures, and may even be able to learn new procedures. Tulving has argued that these neuroanatomic and neurophysiologic dissociations are possible because procedural memory is the most evolutionarily ancient of all memory systems and so is physically distinct from later acquired systems. The second of these three hypothetic memory systems, semantic memory, is defined as "knowledge about the world," which is often, but not necessarily encapsulated in language. The third hypothetic system, "episodic memory," refers to events and objects that are dated and mapped in terms of the temporal or spatial episodes in which they occurred. So, for example, general knowledge about vases and the ability to recognize a particular vase would both be examples of semantic information. Recollection of the times and various contexts of different encounters with a particular vase would be an example of episodic recall. Similarly, in memory experiments, our knowledge of the meaning of a particular word would be classified as semantic memory, whereas our recollection that it was among other words that an experimenter presented to us on a specific occasion would be classified as episodic memory. Tulving[71] proposes that semantic memory is evolutionarily older than episodic memory, which is a comparatively recent development. As we have seen, there is good evidence that these different kinds of memory are unequally sensitive to brain damage, and also that procedural memory is least and episodic memory is most affected by the course of normal aging or of dementia.[75]

Although evidence for empiric dissociations between procedural, semantic, and episodic memory is convincing, there are some problems with this classification as a basis for assessing relative decrements in different kinds of memory with increasing age. It is difficult to assess the precise level of retention of a particular skill, such as juggling or reading mirror-image or upside-down print, in the same terms as retention of information about the world, precision of use of vocabulary, ability to remember the specific details of particular events, or the experimental contexts in which particular words were presented. For example, Kolers[76] has shown that there is some age decrement in the ability to remember how to read, or to learn to read transformed scripts; we would be surprised at the suggestion that, apart from anatomic and sensory problems, there is *no* loss of efficiency of acquired skills such as driving as age advances. Although there seems to be no decline between the ages of 50 and 86 years in the accuracy with which individuals can match words to the correct alternatives among lists of synonyms when given psychometric instruments such as the "Mill Hill A" or the WAIS vocabulary tests, the ability to produce exact definitions of words does show some decline over this period of the life-span.[32] Findings that all memory systems are, at least to some extent, affected by age, raise the problem of the baselines from which we are to calculate and compare these deficits, and the relative sensitivity of the very different kinds of experiments that we must carry out to assess deficits in these putatively different systems. A particular problem is that memory for an episode, an event recalled in unique detail and correctly assigned in terms of the location and time of its occurrence, demands availability of very much more information than does an undifferentiated outline, or schema, for a class of events that may have often been repeated. This point has been made by investigations of amnesiacs, who will often be able to correctly state a particular class of activity in which they often indulged during some periods of their lives (e.g., "I often went fishing with my father") but may also be unable to recall the specific details of any particular instance of this activity, in this case, any particular, unique fishing trip. The distinction between semantic and episodic memory, at least to some extent, reflects a distinction between an abstracted recollection of the general structure of a class of events (the class of vases, or fishing trips), and the availability of all of the considerable amount of additional information necessary to distinguish one unique event from another. In this respect, the distinction between semantic and episodic memory at least partly reflects distinction between the amount, as well as the kind of information that can be maintained and accessed. If we bear this in mind, the apparently greater effects of age on **semantic than on episodic memory** may be at least partly interpreted as the greater effects of age on the ability to cope with a more, rather than a less demanding memory task.

Implicit and explicit memory

The distinction between "explicit" and "implicit" memory is of philosophic as well as psychological interest, because it is a distinction between conscious recollection of information, and the possession of information which, although one is not consciously aware of its nature or provenance, nevertheless guides appropriate solutions for particular problems. As an example, people may be shown lists of words, and then are tested on their ability to recognize them when they are again presented among other distracter words that have not appeared during the course of the experiment. In a subsequent test, if words that they have failed consciously to recognize are presented in the form of anagrams for solution, these are solved faster than anagrams of other words that have not previously appeared during the course of the experiment. For complete reviews of analogous studies, see Jacobi and Witherspoon,[77] Schacter,[78] and Richardson-Klavehn & Bjork.[79] The striking conclusion is that information that is not consciously recalled can nevertheless affect behavior. The most important corollary finding has been that amnesic patients who are markedly impaired on conventional tests of conscious recall and recognition may nevertheless perform as well as normal controls on implicit memory tasks.[78] Parallel studies find that elderly people who perform worse than young adult controls on tests of conscious recall and recognition, nevertheless do as well on tests of implicit memory.[80,81] These dissociations in amnesic subjects and in the elderly have been taken as evidence that explicit and implicit memories are retained by functionally distinct systems, and that the former is much more sensitive than the latter to the effects of brain injury and normal aging.

Implicit memory has been tested in a variety of ingenious ways. For example, words that are pronounced in exactly the same way but nevertheless are spelled differently and have different meanings, (e.g. pear and pair) are said to be homophones of each other. Participants who are presented with one of a pair of homophones in a printed list, without being consciously aware of the reasons for their decision, tend subsequently to select that spelling and meaning for a spoken word for which either version might be appropriate. Howard[82] found that this effect was equally strong in old and young adults. Words that are presented in a list, but are not recognized when they are again presented on a later occasion, are nevertheless more easily identified than novel control words when presented at very brief exposures or obscured by random visual noise. This advantage from implicit memory of a word again seems to be as strong for old as for young adults.[83]

A recent variant of such studies is to compare individuals' ability specifically to remember having seen or heard a particular word in a list, and their feeling that although they have no specific memory of having seen or heard a word, a general feeling of familiarity leads them to be confident that it was, in fact, included. To test this, participants are given a list of words to remember and then asked to recognize these when they are presented among distracters, indicating, for each word that they recognize, whether they "remember" it being presented or, rather, only "know," because it is familiar, that it was one of those they earlier heard or saw. Parkin and Walter[84] report that, although these instructions may seem ambiguous and confusing, participants have little difficulty following them. Older individuals and patients with frontal lesions make fewer "remember" and more "know" responses than intact young adults. Some, but not all attempts to replicate these results have been successful. A persistent difficulty is whether or not "know" responses simply reflect less confident judgements than do "remember" responses. In this case, results from experiments that test the relative familiarity of words would not be evidence that implicit and explicit memory are served by functionally distinct systems, which are differentially sensitive to brain changes in old age and to frontal lobe pathology. They might, rather, simply reflect the fact that older people are less efficient at recall and recognition, and that their recognition of their poorer performance leads them to have less confidence in their judgement that they have seen or heard particular words.

Most comparisons that have been reported suggest that older people invariably perform less well than younger adults on explicit memory tasks but, in contrast, show no decrement on implicit memory tasks. However, this has not invariably been found to be the case.[85–87] Hultsch et al.[88] identify a methodologic problem with this, and with all other studies that have failed to find differences between old and young adults on some measures but not on others. They point out that since experiments have typically compared small groups of between 15 and 30 older and younger people, sample sizes have usually been too small to reassure us that the statistical comparisons made have been powerful enough for us to be confident of negative findings.

Recall and recognition

The distinction between implicit and explicit memory is based on empiric observation, as well as on logical distinctions between classes of experimental paradigms. Findings that older individuals and people with certain types of brain injuries perform less well on one class of paradigms than on the other have encouraged the hypothesis that these classes of paradigms involve functionally distinct and independent memory systems that are differently affected by age or injury. It must be stressed that this conclusion is plausible, but not logically obligatory. We must always consider the alternative possibility that differential age decrements on task performance reflect the fact that one class of task is easier than the other. Considered in this way, the demands made by implicit and explicit memory tasks are *quantitatively* as well as *qualitatively* different. That is, use of implicit knowledge to solve an anagram, or to recognize a briefly presented word may involve the retention and use of much less information than does explicit recognition or recall. This difference between the levels of demands that different classes of tasks make, and between the levels of information necessary to meet these demands, is clearly apparent in distinctions between recall and recognition.

In order to correctly recall a word, people have to encode, maintain, and reproduce all of the information that distinguishes it from other words in the lexicon that may look or sound similar, or that may have similar meanings. In a recognition task people are, in effect, cued by seeing the word itself among others. In this case, they may be able to identify correctly a word that they have seen or heard, even if they have been able to retain only fragmentary information about it. In order to recognize a word they only need to retain sufficient information to distinguish it from all of the other words in the particular list that they are inspecting. In order to recall a word, a person has to retain sufficient information to distinguish it from all other words in that language that they have previously encountered in other situations than the experiment in which they are engaged. The demands on information retention made by recognition tasks are, therefore, much smaller than those made by recall tasks. The general finding that older people perform relatively less well than the young on recall than on recognition tasks may, therefore, be explained by the assumption that any of the deficiencies from which they may suffer are more clearly revealed by the heavier demands of recall, rather than by the assumption that recall and recognition involve independent memory systems. However, a clever experiment by Craik and Mc Dowd[89] specifies and discounts an explanation in terms of one particular difference in terms of task demands. They point out that better performance in recognition tasks may simply reflect the fact that, in these situations, participants are able to guess among the alternatives provided. They convincingly show that age losses in performance on recognition are less than in recall, even when the probability of correct guessing has been taken into consideration. This classic experiment clearly defined the logical problem implicit in attempts to base arguments for the existence of functional distinctions on differences in performance on classes of tasks that make very different levels of informational demands. However, Craik and Mc Dowd's demonstration does not entirely settle the issue, because it still remains the case that people find recognition tasks easier because while they may retain insufficient information about words or events to completely describe them, the possession of even partial information will allow effective cueing on their reappearance in a recognition task. An illustration of this comes from a recent study by G. Smith in our laboratory (unpublished), who found that when some of the distracters presented in a recognition task are deliberately chosen to be similar in terms of their appearance, sound, or meaning to some of the target items that they have earlier experienced, older participants accept these lures significantly more often than do the young. A plausible explanation for this result is that while younger and more able individuals can retain sufficient information about the words that they saw to discriminate them even from closely similar lures, the attenuated information retained by the older and less able may often not be enough to discriminate lures from closely similar targets.

Note that Smiths' experiment raises several distinct issues. One is that the extent to which a word or other item is later confused with distracters may depend on the way in which it was initially encoded when it was first presented. For example, a word that is first encountered in a list that contains several other similar words may well deliberately be encoded in a way that emphasizes those of its features that most clearly distinguish it from them, and this may minimize the probability that it will later be confused with them. The nature of the context in which a word is first encoded may thus also determine the particular contexts in which it is most likely to be later recognized, and the particular distracters with which it is most likely to be confused. Another issue is that the probability with which words are recalled will also vary with the way in which they have initially been encoded. In particular, if the initial context in which words are presented obliges volunteers to encode them only in terms of their surface features, such as their sounds or orthographic structures, they are less likely to subsequently be recalled than if they have been encoded more elaborately, by the generation of meaningful associations.[29] A third issue is whether or not the cues and context that were available when the words were first presented and encoded recur again when they are to be recalled or recognized.[90,91] The general point is that this way of thinking about memory focuses on encoding and retrieval as dynamic processes that are, to a greater or less degree, under voluntary control, and that adaptively vary with the context in which words are first encountered or the context in which they are subsequently retrieved. In this framework of description, discussions of differences in memory efficiency between older and younger adults turn on issues such as whether older people can encode information as quickly as the young, so achieving the same level of depth or elaboration of processing within the limited study time allowed them; whether older people can achieve as deep or elaborate processing as the young only if their slower information processing speeds are compensated by allowing them extra study time, or whether, even if related slowing is compensated, the elderly cannot attain elaborative encoding or, perhaps, cannot use it to improve their retrieval; and whether older people can use all of the different kinds of cues, associations, structures, and context that may be implicitly or explicitly available in material to be remembered, or whether they cease to be able to use some cues that benefit the young.

Depth and elaboration of processing

A classic study by Craik and Lockhart[29] showed that if people were asked to "deeply" process a list of nouns presented for recall (e.g., by making semantic judgements by identifying each as a name of a living or nonliving entity), they correctly remembered more of them than if they were only asked to make surface judgements by saying whether each did or did not contain a particular letter for which they were asked to search. Craik and Tulving[30] replicated and extended these results, showing that recognition, as well as recall, was facilitated by deeper processing. It has long been recognized that age reduces the speed with which people can process information.[23,24] It was therefore a natural speculation that old age reduces the efficiency with which information can be encoded, and so impairs its maintenance in memory and its subsequent retrieval. Indeed, some experiments have directly shown that if older people are given enough time to study lists of words presented to them, their performance equalled that of their young adult controls.[36] This was seen as a very attractive line of investigation because it not only offers promise of practical remediation techniques for their memory difficulties but is theoretically a very economic way for accounting for all, or most, memory changes in old age. As Cohen[92] has pointed out, if we can show that older people suffer from encoding deficits, problems with maintenance or retrieval of information do not require any further explanation. It is not surprising that a very large number of studies have been carried out to investigate the extent to which age-related changes in recall and recognition are related to encoding difficulties.

Unfortunately, such comparisons are often difficult to interpret because of a methodologic problem that is common to nearly all studies in cognitive gerontology. If we compare the performance of older and younger people under conditions that do, and do not facilitate depth of encoding, we can expect one of only three outcomes: the encoding facilitation may benefit the young more than the old, may benefit the old more than the young, or may benefit both groups equally. The difficulty is to decide whether to assess relative gains in absolute terms, or in proportion to baseline. It is very likely that in the least favorable conditions, older individuals will remember fewer items than the young. As a result, if old and young show the same absolute gains from facilitation of encoding, the proportional, or percentage gains will be larger for the old. To decide whether or not encoding facilitation helps the old more than the young we need some theoretic rationale for deciding whether to use absolute or relative measures of improvement. The most straightforwardly interpretable finding would be that the experimental manipulation we have chosen to improve depth or elaboration of processing does not help the elderly at all, but markedly improves the performance of the young. In this case, it is safe to conclude that, for whatever reason, our older group cannot make use of the opportunities for improving encoding that we have provided. Another straightforward outcome would be one in which older participants show greater absolute improvement than the young. This is not ambiguous because, since they are almost certain to perform less well than the young, in absolute terms, on the less favorable condition, they will not only show a greater absolute, but an even greater proportional improvement. A finding that encoding facilitation helps older participants to recall some, but young participants many more items, is less easy to interpret. The absolute increase may be greater for the young than for the old, but the proportional increase over baseline performance may be equal for both groups or even, plausibly, less for the young. In the present state of theory this outcome is unhelpful, since available functional models provide no satisfactory rationale for deciding whether an absolute or a proportional change is the more sensible index.

Experiments on this issue can be categorized in two ways: first in terms of whether they show greater, less, or equal benefits for the old, and second in terms of whether they suggest that while older people can make use of some techniques, or opportunities for improving their encoding of information, they are less able to use others.

Most studies have found that young adults benefit more than the elderly when they are offered aids to study or encode the material that they have to remember. For example, Erber et al[93] asked older and younger volunteers to check for the presence or absence of letters in each of a list of target words and then to recall as many of these words as possible. They compared conditions in which their volunteers were told that they would have to recall the words, and so must try to learn them, and in which recall was unexpected. They found that instructions to intentionally learn the words benefited young more than older volunteers. Craik and Byrd[94] found that experimental conditions that increased depth of processing benefited people of all ages, but helped the young more than the old. Rabinowitz[95] compared older and young people under optimized study conditions, in which they could take as long as they felt necessary to learn the material presented to them, and were allowed to take notes to improve the way in which they structured material for later recall. All participants benefited, but the young improved more than the old. A number of studies have tested whether older or younger participants are differentially helped by the opportunity, or the instruction, to form mental images of material presented for recall. For example Treat and Reese[96] varied the rate at which participants inspected material presented to them, and their opportunities to use imagery, and Puglisi and Park[97] compared volunteers' memories for line drawing that they had inspected, and their memory for similar drawing that were presented to them unfinished and that they had to complete. Older participants were helped by beneficial encoding conditions, but the young improved even more.

However, in some studies, beneficial encoding conditions have helped older and younger participants to the same extent. For example, Goward[62] used a computerized task in which participants saw 30 words, one at a time, and made a timed decision about each. In a "deep processing" condition they pressed one of two keys to signal whether each word was, or was not, an animal name. In the other, "shallow processing," condition they decided whether or not the word contained the vowel "e." Immediately after each condition volunteers were shown, one at a time, a list of 60 words, among which the words they had just classified were randomly embedded. They made a timed decision about each word, identifying it either as one of the "old" words they had previously classified, or as a "new" word that had not previously appeared. Both young and old identified deeply classified words faster and more accurately than shallowly classified words, but these gains in speed and accuracy were equal for both groups.

There are also other experiments in which improved encoding has helped elderly more than young adults. Park et al.[98] showed volunteers pictures of pairs of objects that were either conceptually related, or unrelated to each other in terms of their previous experience. For example, a line-drawing of a spider and an ant, or of a spider eating a cherry. All participants, but especially the elderly, showed improved recognition for pictures in which the component items had been conceptually related. Rankin and Firnhofer[99] found that older improved more than younger people when they were asked to use distinctive rather than common adjectives as retrieval cues for nouns with which they had previously been paired. Hashtroudi, et al.[100] found that older individuals benefited more than younger from the provision of cues that facilitated their elaborative encoding of the items that they had to remember.

Given these inconsistencies between results, and given the problems of interpretation imposed by the question of whether absolute or proportional gains should be assessed, it is not surprising that the question whether the elderly benefit more or less from facilitation of encoding has been shelved as unprofitable. It has been replaced by the suggestion that the elderly are more likely than the young to suffer from difficulties in encoding that impair their later recall or recognition of material presented to them. Accordingly, attention has turned to improving explanations why older people come to suffer from encoding difficulties. The best articulated explanation to date has been the "transmission deficit" model of Macay and Burke,[101] who propose that the memory system can be modelled in terms of an associative network such as that described by Anderson.[102,103] They suggest that in such a network age damages the system so that the rate of transmission of information through the network is slowed, and the level of activation of the nodes in which information is encoded is reduced. New information will be better encoded if it activates nodes that, collectively, also act as representations of previously learned (old) information. This provides a formal explanation for the common observation that novel information can be learned more rapidly and is likely to be remembered for longer if it can be associated with previously learned information.

The practical implications that the Macay and Burke[101] model share with other thinking in this line of research are well illustrated in a paper by Craik[104] which suggests that, in old age, encoding is impoverished unless an enriched context is supplied. This can be done by manipulations carried out during a laboratory experiment, or in everyday life, by past experience of similar material or by the availability—at the moments of encoding and retrieval—of a variety of possible contextual or situational cues that may be collectively termed "environmental support." Craik suggests that, in general, older people may be less able than the young to generate, perceive, or use past experience or current environmental support to improve their performance. This disadvantage will be reduced to the extent that they can spontaneously learn or can be helped to do so and, most especially, to the extent to which environmental support is both available and optimal. In a similar vein, Craik[105] suggests that encoding of material for later recall involves interactions between processes that can be driven by external stimulation and those that require internal self-initiated processes. Because self-initiated processes tend to fail in old age, older people become increasingly dependent on environmental support from external stimulation.

A tacit assumption behind all these experiments has been that the cues incorporated in initial encoding, or the environmental support that is available when material is first encountered and encoded are again present when it is retrieved from memory. This opens the question whether deep or elaborative encoding of material facilitates later recall, even when the cues, associations, or contextual support that were present when the material was first encountered are absent, or are replaced by other cues and contexts when it is retrieved. In other words, does greater elaboration or depth of initial encoding facilitate later retrieval whether or not the same contexts or cues recur? This issue has been termed "encoding specificity."

Encoding specificity

Tulving and Thompson[91] reported an early and classic test of encoding specificity on young adults. They showed that the context in which material was first presented determined the way in which it was encoded, and that recall was much poorer if this context was altered, than if it was repeated when retrieval was required. Many experiments on young adults have replicated these findings, showing that advantages gained from elaborative encoding or from the provision of particular contexts—or in Craik's terms, of particular environmental support—are highly specific; that is, they are found only when the same cues or contexts present at encoding recur at recall. West and Boatwright[106] report that age differences are smallest when the specific cues provided at encoding are repeated, and are greatest when encoding and retrieval cues are different. In an exceptionally useful discussion of these effects, Craik and Jacoby[90] bring out the importance of encoding specificity for functional models of memory, suggesting that the processes of encoding and retrieval are, essentially, identical in as much as the same information processing structures or "network nodes" must be activated both when information is encoded and when it is retrieved. If all of the cues or contexts that are present at encoding recur, in identical form, at the moment when retrieval is required, the identical nodes or information processing networks will once again be activated, and recall or recognition will be maximally facilitated. If there is some, but not complete overlap in cues or contextual encoding and recall there will be some, but less facilitation. If contexts and cues entirely change, there will be no facilitation; there may even be interference, so that recall may be impaired.

An additional issue is whether people can passively and automatically obtain useful context or cues from the environment, or whether they must actively, and effortfully generate these cues and contexts for themselves. As we have seen, one explanation for some losses of memory efficiency in old age is that while older people may be able to use external or environmental cues to advantage, even to a point at which they equal the performance of the young, they are less able to generate their own encoding and retrieval cues. This raises the question of how far differences between older and younger people may be eliminated if, when they encode information, the old are forced to generate cues for the items that they must subsequently remember. Many investigators have explored such generation effects in relation to differences between old and young.

Elaborative encoding and generation effects

The "generation effect" has been used as a blanket term to acknowledge the facilitation in recall and recognition that occurs as a result of at least three different kinds of experimental manipulations. One manipulation is to compare peoples memory for material that they themselves have produced, relative to material that has been presented to them. A second is to compare their memory for material to which they have, deliberately generated associations, or that they have elaborated in various ways, against their memory for material for which they have not had the time, the opportunity, or the incentive to produce elaborative cues. A third is to test people's memory for the solutions of problems that they have solved by completing, or supplementing information given to them. An example of this last manipulation is reported by Jacobi,[107] who found that when young adults solved incomplete words given synonyms as guiding context (e.g., quick = F−ST?) they subsequently remembered them better than if they had been presented in entirety and only read aloud.

Age comparisons have concentrated on memory for self-generated items, and for items for which elaborative or associative encoding was encouraged. As in the case of experiments that have compared the benefits of depth of processing, results have been mixed.

Many studies have found that old and young benefit equally from elaborative encoding and from generation effects. Hashtroudi et al.[100] found equal cue-generation advantages for older and younger groups, as did Goward,[102] who asked her older and younger volunteers to produce either 0, 1, 2, or 3 different associates to each of a list of words presented one at a time. The speed and accuracy with which both older and younger participants subsequently recognized these target words when they were subsequently presented for recognition among distracters increased directly with the number of associations that they had produced to them. Older and younger volunteers benefited to the same extent. In the third category of tasks, in which participants generate the actual items that they later remembered and recalled, Johnson et al.,[108] Mc Daniel et al.,[109] Mitchell et al.,[110] Nilson and Craik,[111] (1990) and Rabinowitz,[112] also found equal gains for older and younger volunteers with respect to items that they had generated relative to those that they had only inspected. Mitchell et al.[110] made the interesting observation that older volunteers were less accurate than young at recalling whether they had previously seen or generated the items that they correctly recalled. This result is important because it makes a clear distinction between two possible sources for the generation advantage: one is that people encode and remember the act of generating, or of making an association to an item, and that it is this additional information that helps them to subsequently recall or recognize it. The second possibility is that facilitation of recall by memory for the deliberate act of generation or association may be unimportant relative to facilitation resulting from production of associations that are, again, generated at recall to act as retrieval cues. Mitchell et al.'s results suggest that memory for the act of generating associations may be less available to facilitate recall for the elderly than for the young. We shall review further evidence for this below.

We have seen that many studies report at least equal advantages for all age groups. Many others report relatively greater benefits for the old. Backman and Nilson[113] report that older people show as good recall as do the young for tasks that they themselves have performed. Backman[114] replicated this study, requiring participants either to learn verbal descriptions of series of actions or to perform them. Again, while older participants were less efficient at recalling descriptions of actions, they were equally good at recalling actions that they had, themselves, actually carried out. Kausler and Wiley[115] found that while age differences in efficiency of recall were not completely eliminated in recall of performed actions, older participants showed greater improvement than the young and these advantages persisted over long periods of time. Thus, in contrast with comparisons of the benefits of other forms of encoding enhancement, there seems to be evidence that generation effects benefit the elderly at least as much as, and possibly more than they benefit the young.

One explanation for the generation effect is that people may be, in effect, cued to remember items that they have produced, or to which they have actively generated associations, by their memory of these conscious and deliberate acts of generation. This possibility raises the more general question as to how well people can remember the sources of information that they have received, and use their memory for the source of information as a supplementary cue to aid its later retrieval.

Memory of sources

Rabbitt[116] carried out an early test of source memory in an experiment in which older and younger participants viewed television film of two or four different speakers who each made different comments on a related theme, for example, "ducks" or "weather." So long as the total number of comments presented did not exceed four, older participants were able to remember them as accurately as did the young. However, old people were much less accurate than the young at remembering which televised person had made each comment. Rabbitt interpreted these results as evidence that more information has to be encoded and retrieved in order to remember both the statements and their sources than to remember the statements alone. Because of their more limited information processing resources, older people are less able to encode and retrieve this additional information. McIntyre and Craik[117] replicated these results in a similar experiment in which they played their subjects lists of words that were read by two different speakers in random order. As usual, older participants recalled material presented to them less well than the young did, and, in addition, they were relatively worse at recalling the voice in which the words that they correctly remembered had been read. In an elegant extension of this line of research, Cohen & Faulkner[118] asked older and younger participants to listen to accounts of actions, perform actions themselves, or imagine performing actions. They found that older people have difficulty in remembering whether they have performed, imagined, or perceived actions that they can, nevertheless, accurately remember and describe. Later work by Hastroudi et al.[119] has confirmed this result.

Difficulties in remembering the sources of information recalled can have serious disadvantages in everyday life. In Cohen and Faulkner's[118] study, this was neatly demonstrated by a further experiment in which they tested their volunteers in an "eyewitness testimony" task in which, after a televised event that they were asked to remember had taken place, they were given further, deliberately misleading information about it before they were asked for their recall. Older volunteers were more often misled by this subsequently presented additional information than were the young. Cohen and Faulkner suggest that this is because they were less certain of the provenance of the different items of information that they were trying to recall and so were more likely to attribute the subsequently presented, deliberately misleading information to their original experience of an event. In our laboratory, Miranda Leslie has extended this line of research by asking volunteers to listen to short descriptions of events in which some details are overtly stated and others must be inferred from the context provided. She finds that although her older volunteers have no particular difficulty in making and recalling correct inferences, they are much less accurate than the young at reporting whether particular, correctly recalled items of information have been directly presented or had to be inferred from context. Memorial confusions between the possible sources of items of information and memorial confusions as to which elements of an account were inferred and which were overtly stated are evidently matters of practical concern not only in courts of law but also in everyday transactions between relatives, friends, and colleagues. Rabbitt's[120] finding that older people are less able than the young to remember who said what during a short exchange of remarks points to a further, everyday problem. The implicit content of a conversation can often only be properly understood if the different points of view expressed can be correctly attributed to the speakers involved. Loss of memory for this information disables the elderly in complex conversational interactions and may increasingly reduce their access to, and enjoyment of, conversations among groups of friends.

Encoding and retrieval: a summary

There is a consensus that many of the difficulties that older people experience with their memories occur because they can no longer encode information as efficiently as they once did. These difficulties can be reduced if they are given more time to study the material they have to remember, helped by environmental support from cues or context that recur at the point when they have to remember what they have learned and, in particular, asked actively to generate their own associations to material that they hope to recall. Unfortunately, it also seems that as people age they find it more difficult actively and consciously to generate new associations when encoding material that they encounter for the first time, or to generate appropriate associations to act as effective retrieval cues for material that they have encountered earlier. For this reason they may be helped, relatively more than the elderly, if environmental support for encoding or retrieval is available. This distinction between the relative efficiency with which older people can use externally provided, and the relative difficulty with which they can use self-generated encoding and retrieval cues parallels a distinction that forms the basis of a theory by Hasher and Zacks[121] that all conditions, including age, that reduce cognitive efficiency have little effect on automatic, unconscious, or effortless encoding but strikingly large effects on the ability to encode information in a controlled, conscious, or effortful way. This useful distinction has also been captured, in a slightly different way, by Craik and Jennings,[122] who summarize the literature with the comment that "if encoding offers advantages, but is only possible with expenditure of time and effort, then it is likely to benefit the young more than the old."

In any event, whether cues, associations, or context are self-generated or externally provided, in order to be maximally effective they should be as similar as possible at encoding and recall. Because the advantages of encoding are highly specific, once material has been encoded in terms of particular associations or contexts, attempts to use other cues, associations, or contexts as prompts will not improve, and may even impair subsequent recall. It is likely that the young are more able than the elderly to overcome the disadvantages of discrepancies in context and cues provided at encoding and retrieval. It may even be that the elderly show less generalization than the young, use a narrower range of retrieval cues, and so suffer even more from the disadvantages of encoding specificity.

The question of whether aids to encoding and retrieval help the elderly relatively more than the young has not, in general, been fruitful. This is partly because current models for human memory offer no guidance as to whether we should compare the benefits of encoding aids in terms of the absolute numbers of additional items remembered, or in terms of the proportional increases over baseline conditions in which aids are not provided. If we take as our index the absolute increase in the numbers of items recalled, a review of the literature suggests that older improve at least as much as younger adults in most, and substantially more than the young in some experimental paradigms. It follows that if we use proportional increases as our index we must conclude that older people, starting from a lower baseline, usually show markedly greater benefits than the young as the result of nearly all kinds of experimental assistance. In many experiments, older adults have achieved the same absolute levels of performance as the young, when given optimal help with encoding and retrieval, or tested on implicit rather than explicit memory. Such findings may be taken as evidence that particular memory systems or processes, such as the implicit memory system or automatic processing of information remain unaffected by old age, while others such as the explicit memory system or controlled information processing are vulnerable to age-related changes. We may take the further step of suggesting that the fact that brain changes due to increasing age affect these systems and processes to different extents is good evidence that they must be functionally, as well as logically, dissociable. Unfortunately, this still seems an unsafe conclusion, because to argue that age has *no* effect on a particular system or process, we must be certain that both younger and older adults have been tested at the upper limits of their possible ranges of performance. If tasks are made more difficult, young adults may begin to perform better than the old. Because we cannot be confident that any experiment available in the literature has actually tested age groups at their upper performance limits, it is prudent, for the moment, to adopt a more cautious provisional verdict on the literature. It is likely that age affects all memory processes and systems to some extent, but that the magnitude of age effects in undemanding tasks may be slight or imperceptible, expect by very sensitive experiments, but in demanding tasks, may become very marked indeed. This is, of course, just another way of raising the central unresolved question of whether age brings about *qualitative* changes in memory efficiency in the sense that it affects some systems or processes more than others, or simply brings about *quantitative* changes, in the sense that reduction of cognitive resources makes all tasks more difficult, but has proportionately greater effects on demanding than on undemanding tasks.

The question of how age affects memory can be approached in another way. Bartlett[5] carried out a classic series of studies that showed that people do not store information veridically—apart from gradual random losses over time—but rather dynamically interpret, encode and continuously adapt the information that they hold in memory using data structures or schemata that they have previously built up to interpret their knowledge about the world. Novel information, for which no existing schemata are available, is poorly remembered, or may be distorted to fit in with existing, inappropriate, schemata. In this latter case, the inferences in terms of which the novel information is comprehended are, of course, inappropriate or misleading. Within this framework of description, age can affect the encoding of complex information in a variety of different ways. As people age they may lose the patterns of organization or schemata that they have built up earlier during their lives. In this case because some principles of organization once available to them no longer exist, they will be at a disadvantage in making those types of inferences, and in encoding and recalling those types of information for which they no longer have bodies of organized data. This may be termed the "unavailability" model of principles of organization. Alternatively, the elderly may still retain the schemata and principles of organization that they built up in youth, but may no longer be able to use them, because in order to make the inferences necessary to understand relations and assimilate them into their mental data structures they need to hold substantial bodies of information in working memory. Progressive loss of working memory capacity and of information processing efficiency will result in progressively less effective use of schemata and data-encoding structures. This may be termed the "inaccessibility" model. A final possibility is that as people age they can still maintain schemata and higher order data structures, and can still use them to make inferences and to perceive relations within complex bodies of information that they process. However, as they age, the nature of these schemata, and so also the organization that they impose, gradually alters. In this case, organizational principles and modes of inference that are available to adults when they are young may gradually and idiosyncratically alter as they age. This may be termed the "altered schemata" model of aging memory. These three hypothetic possibilities can serve as a framework within which to review the evidence currently available.

Organization of Material in Memory

Schemata and organizational principles are, necessarily, very vague terms because they must encompass all possible systems of logical and associational relations that may be applied to all bodies of complex information about the world. Another difficulty with this line of research is that, in spite of the enormous ingenuity that investigators have shown, it has not been easy to find bodies of material for which there are generally agreed and clear-cut organizational principles. Consequent studies on age changes in the use of organizational principles have, almost without exception, been based on memory for main lines of argument and incidental and extraneous details in written or spoken series of propositions or brief stories and descriptions of events.

Age Differences in Memory for Direct Statements and Inferences

There is consensus that the elderly remember information that they have inferred less well than information that has been directly stated to them. In terms of the alternatives suggested above, the balance of evidence favors the inaccessibility hypothesis and, to a lesser extent, the unavailability hypothesis, but not the altered schemata hypothesis. That is, older people clearly can and do make inferences in the same way as do young adults, but their ability to do so seems to be reduced, probably because their working memory capacities and maximum information processing rates have declined.

A pioneering study by Cohen[123] showed that older people have relatively greater difficulty than the young in recalling information that they have inferred than information that has been directly presented to them. She found that these age-related deficits are particularly likely when, in order to make a correct inference, it is necessary to hold several separate premises simultaneously in mind. Deficits in making inferences are also especially marked when series of propositions are presented rapidly. Zacks et al.[124] also report that older people find it harder to recall implications than direct statements. There is also recent support for Cohen's[122] hypothesis that this change occurs partly because older people become unable to rapidly make and check inferences while reading text or listening to a conversation. Hamm and Hasher[125] found that their older volunteers were slower to detect and reject inappropriate interpolations in text comprehension tasks.

Reviews by Cohen[126] and by Zacks and Hasher[127] agree that the difficulties with comprehension that older people experience are due mainly to declines in the capacities of their working memories. Empiric studies, such as those by Spilich,[128] also conclude that the difficulties that older people experience with text comprehension are largely explained by progressive loss of information processing capacity. Studies such as that by Stine and Wingfield[129] make the additional point that while loss of information processing speed and working memory capacity may indeed account for age decrements in comprehension of simple sentences, older people also experience other sources of difficulty with complex sentences. Perhaps, as people age, they use or encounter complex constructions less often and so become less able to interpret or use them. There is support for this from Kemper,[130] who has been able to illustrate the reduction in use of complex sentences in old age in a particularly elegant way. She analyzed diaries that individuals had kept continuously from their youth into their old age and found that, as they grew older, they gradually altered their writing styles so as to reduce both the grammatic complexity and the length of the sentences that they used. This is consistent with the idea that people increasingly use short sentences and simple constructions to reduce demands on their failing working memories, but also with the idea that, as they age, increasing attenuation of communication may reduce the repertoire of grammatic constructions that people attempt.

In sum, the evidence on text comprehension and inference derivation suggests that older people continue to use the same organizational structures that they employed when they were young, but that the efficiency with which they can do so becomes increasingly restricted as their information processing rates decline, and their working memory capacities reduce. Age slows information processing rate and reduces the number of different elements of information that can simultaneously be held in mind, and this makes it increasingly difficult to use complex grammatic constructions or to correctly produce or interpret long sentences with many, multiply embedded, subordinate clauses. There are, however, suggestions from the literature that complex principles of organization may not only become inaccessible to older people, because they cannot use them, but that they may also gradually become unavailable, perhaps because of increasing disuse.

In order to understand speech or text, it is necessary not only to have sufficient information processing and working memory resources to use the syntactic rules required to make sense of patterns of words. It is also necessary to have background information about the world, and about the particular topics under discussion. Many studies have shown that age-related differences in text comprehension are greatest when the material presented is entirely novel, and are much less—or non existent—when it is familiar.[131] Such findings are often interpreted in terms of a distinction between the surface structure (the particular words or grammatical constructions in which information is presented), and the deep structure (the meaning that is to be conveyed). Cohen and Faulkner[132] read series of sentences to older and younger listeners and then asked them to recognize whether new versions of these sentences, later presented to them, had or had not been altered in terms of their deep and shallow structures. Older individuals found it relatively more difficult to recognize changes in deep structure than in surface structure. They argued that it must be because older people process information more slowly and so have time only to analyze and retain the surface structure but not the deep structure of propositions presented to them. In a subsequent review, Cohen[126] again concluded that her own work, and the bulk of the literature, suggest that age changes in efficiency of text comprehension are caused mainly by slowing of information processing rate and, consequently, also of working memory capacity. It should be noted that some apparently contradictory results on age differences in memory for surface and deep features do not contradict Cohen's conclusions, because they are explicable in terms of the particular nature of the tasks that volunteers have been asked to carry out. Holland and Rabbitt,[133] compared how well older and younger people, and those with relatively high and relatively low scores on intelligence quotient (IQ) tests were able to remember brief stories. Younger individuals, and those with high IQ test scores not only remembered the gist, or deep structure of the plots of stories, but could also correctly recall many details that were incidental or irrelevant to the plot. Older people, and lower test scorers showed equally good memory for plots or gist, but recalled fewer details. This difference in recall of plot and details was exaggerated when the difficulty of comprehending the deep structure of the stories was increased by including stories with two parallel subplots. In this case, both young and old people still recalled both plots equally well, but even the young began to show some loss of extraneous or irrelevant detail. Results of this kind are quite common in the literature, and can be reconciled with Cohen and Faulkner's[132] and Cohen's[126] findings if we consider that their studies investigated recall of single propositions rather than of passages of continuous narrative. In order to make any sense at all of a narrative, people of any age are obliged to process the deep structure of relations and events that constitute the plot. Failure to do this would result in retention of only disconnected fragments of information. When priority must be given to the plot, to process, register, and retain additional details that are extraneous or irrelevant, and so not necessarily logically cued by the plot, this requires the expenditure of additional processing capacity. The reduced processing capacities of older individuals, and of those of lower levels of general ability, make them less able to process and retain this additional, extraneous information.

Light and Anderson[134] found that their older were as able as their younger volunteers to use "scripts," that is, the logical structures of familiar classes of events such as visiting a restaurant, in order to understand and recall complex series of thematically related propositions. Hess et al[135] and Backman[136] also found that older adults can use knowledge structures, or schemata, scripts, and interpretation frameworks for events, in much the same way as the young do, but that on the whole, they may get less benefit from them. This conclusion is also endorsed by an ingenious experiment by Arbuckle et al[137] who showed that older volunteers were as able as young adults to use their general information about the conventional layout of rooms in domestic houses to understand and remember information about spatial relations given in the course of short prose passages. Collectively, all these results confirm the general conclusion that people can retain the knowledge structures that they have built up in their youth well into their old age, but that progressive losses of information processing efficiency make it increasingly difficult for them to use these structures to maximum advantage.

Summary

Our worlds and the languages that we use to describe them are very complex. In order to understand and encode events and discourse it is not enough to be able to recognize objects and words and to make simple associations between them. We must also have implicit or explicit knowledge of the logical relations and chains of causality that are expressed in terms of syntactic structures, and are embodied in terms of our implicit and explicit pragmatic knowledge about the world. Especially in the case of language, it is possible to categorize the bodies of information that we must hold in memory in terms of two different kinds of knowledge: semantic knowledge about the nature and properties of things, and actions and syntactic or grammatic knowledge, by means of which we put words in order to express relations between objects and concepts. It is clear that lack of either of these kinds of information impairs encoding and so reduces the amount of information that can subsequently be retrieved from memory by people of any age. The question of whether old age affects semantic more than syntactic memory is not particularly fruitful because the amount of semantic information and knowledge about the world and the rules that govern relations and contingencies within it are so varied and vast that estimates of relative losses are unobtainable. Instead of this it is possible to ask the question of whether older people are helped as much as the young by familiarity of semantic knowledge or by availability of syntactic structure and, if not, whether this is because they have lost knowledge of meaning, context, and structure, or because, although they retain this information, they can no longer make the best use of it. As is usual in psychological comparisons, the answer seems to be "both." It seems very likely that the total amount of semantic and syntactic knowledge declines with age. It is also the case that optimal use of syntactic and pragmatic structures, and probably also of semantics, meaning, and context, require the ability to process information rapidly, and the ability to hold as much as possible in working memory so that relations between different pieces of information can be made and appropriate inferences deduced.

These considerations partly answer the question of whether older people become less efficient than the young at remembering information over long periods of time. There is no known limit to the amount of information that humans can hold in long-term memory, nor any known limit, short of duration of survival, to the period for which it can be retained. Nevertheless, the amount, quality, and richness of the information that we remember will depend on the efficiency with which we can encode it and the adequacy of the structured schemata or systems of organization of information about the world that we have gradually built up in order to do so. If these organizational principles become unavailable as information processing efficiency and working memory capacity become increasingly inadequate to employ them to full advantage, the information encoded will both be impoverished and less well remembered, because appropriate structures of encoding and retrieval cues will cease to be available.

Long-term memory

Very many laboratory studies have compared older and younger adults at recalling lists of words or passages of text over periods of hours or weeks. As we have seen, the usual findings are that older people recall less than young, but that people of all ages benefit from any previous knowledge that they may have about the topics discussed, or from the opportunity to use the knowledge structures, the scripts as schemata that they may have previously acquired, which help them to interpret, encode, and subsequently retrieve the information that they have learned. However, when age changes in long-term memory are discussed, the questions asked are usually rather different because they relate to experiences in people's personal lives. That is, we may ask whether elderly people better recall public or private events that occurred during the last few days or months better or worse than those that occurred while they were children or young adults. In fact, as is notorious, elderly people so often report that, as they have aged, their recollections of their early lives have become progressively much sharper, clearer, and more detailed. Indeed, Ribot[138] suggested that as age progresses, more recently acquired memories are gradually lost or stripped away, improving access to previously buried memories of childhood and youth. This picturesque account fitted well with nineteenth century clinical experience that in disorders of memory, such as those associated with dementia of the Alzheimer's type, memories tend to be spared in direct proportion to their ages, so that some early memories may still be available while very few or no recent memories can be elicited. Descriptive ubiquity has gained this observation the status of Ribot's Law.

Although later evidence has called into question how far Ribot's Law is indeed an accurate description of changes in memory efficiency in old age, it still serves to generate useful questions to guide age comparisons. One such question is whether age-related difficulties in immediate memory for events or for connected discourse may not also be associated with some impairment in the quality of recall of early life events. Winthorpe and Rabbitt[139] and Holland and Rabbit[139] report experiments in which individuals aged between 60 and 85 years were tested for recall of brief stories. They found that greater age and lower scores on intelligence tests were associated with poorer recall, in the sense that incidental details in the stories were lost and only their narrative frameworks, or plots, were recalled. All volunteers were then asked to produce, in a relaxed conversational setting, accounts of any incidents from their early lives that they often spontaneously recalled, and that they felt to be particularly striking or important to them. Individuals who had been found to be relatively poor at immediate recall of stories also gave relatively impoverished accounts of their own life experiences, presenting the bare plots or scripts of events with little or nothing in the way of remembered detail. These results suggest that particular individuals may experience two nonexclusive changes in their ability to use their memories to recall both immediate and remote events. It seems likely that both their long-term and immediate memory were impaired in the sense that while some knowledge structures remained available, so that the rough outlines of events could be given, they had in fact lost the precise details of early events and could remember only very general scenarios or frameworks within which these events had occurred. The differential loss of memory for details and plot outlines seems as characteristic of attempts to recall complex, remote autobiographical events as to recall narrative information immediately. Further, and more specifically, reduced efficiency at recalling recent information predicts reduced efficiency at recalling remote autobiographical information, and vice versa. As our discussion has shown, there remains the residual question of whether old age and, perhaps, its associated pathologies degrade the schemata, and organizational structures themselves, or rather only compromise information processing ability and working memory capacity and so the extent to which even intact organizational structures can be used to encode and retrieve information. However, it must be stressed that even quite dated theoretic models for data storage and retrieval suggest that it may be entirely misleading to make any distinction between the structures within which data are stored and the details of the data themselves.[102,103] Thus, while the relative integrity of retention and access to details and structures remain very helpful guides for further empiric research, the premise that these two entities are functionally separated now seems a misleading guide for models of how human memory works, and how it changes in old age.

Memory for autobiographical events

Although elderly individuals' vehement assertions of the extreme subjective vividness of their recollections of their early lives must be accepted at face value, it is clearly necessary to distinguish between the subjective vividness and the objective accuracy of the information about their remote pasts that they can access. One issue is that the vividness or faintness of memories is an intensely personal quality that cannot be assessed by external observers and for which individuals themselves can have no absolute standards of comparison. Any person can judge only the vividness of one memory in relation to the vividness of others. In a case where all recent memories are uncertain and tenuous, distant memories may well subjectively appear to be much more exact and reliable but, in terms of objective accuracy, may not be so.

Fortunately for experimentalists, our lives and the public events that they span are now so overdocumented that it is possible to check the objective accuracy of peoples' memories of their early years against such objective criteria as school records or newspaper archives of descriptions of public events. This has allowed very laborious experiments by authors such as Williams and Santos Williams[140] and Williams and Holland,[141] who studied individuals' copious protocols of their verifiable early memories. Apart from deriving a descriptive model for the ways in which people go about searching for and retrieving information about distant events, they found clear evidence for considerable loss of crucial details and confabulation of information that apparently was no longer available. This provides good evidence, endorsed by other studies, that rather than improving, recall of distant events becomes increasingly unreliable as old age advances. Many other studies of individuals' recall of public events and personages bear out the idea that the more distant an event the less well it can be recalled by people of all ages, especially the old. For example, Stuart-Hamilton et al.[10] tested individuals aged from 50 through 85 on memory for information about public figures who had been intensely, but quite briefly, famous or notorious at various periods during their past lives. They found that people of all ages recognized fewer distantly than recently famous persons, and were also able to provide less information about the historically remote than about the relatively recent figures that they did recognize. Individuals with high current levels of intellectual ability, as assessed by their scores on intelligence tests, recalled more of, and more information about, both the recently and distantly famous. This suggests that in old age, recall of past people and events are compromised by two distinct deficits. Older people do, gradually, forget information about people and events in the distant past, and they probably also become increasingly less efficient at encoding and so retrieving information about current events and personages.

Other studies endorse the first, but not the second of these propositions. Howes and Katz[142] devised a questionnaire for public events that took place between 1920 and 1981 and administered it to people of all ages in the human life-span. The results suggested that memory for public events improves during adolescence and thereafter remains relatively constant. This study confirms that interest in public events, and possibly also the ability to effectively encode them improves during adolescence, but found no evidence that events experienced early in life are progressively forgotten. It is difficult to evaluate these discrepancies between investigations because studies of memory for public events and personages have many limitations. Most people first experience most public events as media reports. Not only has the intensity of media coverage of public events greatly increased over the last 50 years, but the particular mode through which they are experienced—such as newspapers, newsreels, radio, and television coverage—has greatly changed. Striking events continue to be topics of conversation for long periods after they occur, and both the amount of detail discussed and the level of interpretation of this detail are affected by the particular company in which these discussions take place and so also by the level of education and ability of the individuals involved. The numbers of times that public events are replayed in conversations, and in peoples' private rehearsals of their own recollections, is in direct in proportion to their significance. The durations of periods of replay also depend on a variety of factors. Especially significant events and people continue to have very extended life in historic works, media references, and carefully produced retrospectives. For example, it is now probably impossible for anyone who lived through the Kennedy assassination to disentangle media reports, images, and information gained at the time when it occurred from the overlay of those later encountered, and perhaps repeatedly re-encountered in media retrospectives during the last 30 years. Unless considerable trouble is taken to select those rare events and personages that were briefly prominent but have since received little or no exposure, as was the case for the Frith test used by Stuart-Hamilton et al.,[10] the frequent public rehearsal of significant events may be a sufficient explanation for their continued retention, even by older individuals.

The point that people become progressively less efficient at encoding new events as they grow old, has been elegantly made by a study by Cohen et al[143] Individuals sometimes report that their memories of particularly impressive events in their lives that may be personal or public (such as the Kennedy assassination) are remembered with exceptional vividness and accuracy. Such memories have become termed "flashbulb" memories. Cohen et al[144] compared the accuracy of older and younger adults' memories of a particularly striking public event, the resignation of Margaret Thatcher. Most individuals reported vivid memories for the details of precisely where they were, and what they were doing when they first heard that this event had taken place. However, when accounts given soon after this event were compared with accounts given some months later, older individuals showed strikingly more inaccuracy, confabulation, and loss of detail between the two recollections than did those given by young adults.

The variety of different factors that have to be taken into consideration in assessing the subjective quality and the objective accuracy of peoples' memories of life events have been explored by a technique developed by Francis Galton (1883), who asked them to recall and date as many incidents as possible from any and all parts of their lives, and compared the relative incidence of memories at different ages. Galton's original study, and its many subsequent replications,[144–146] have found that relatively few memories are recalled from early childhood and that the number of memories recalled increases steadily with age, except that there are clear signs of a reduction in the proportions of memories of recent events recalled by middle-aged and elderly adults.[147] More recently authors such as Fitzgerald[148] and Rabbitt & Winthorpe[149] have drawn attention to a "reminiscence bump" in memories reported by elderly people, such that the period of young adult life seems to be especially well documented in individuals' memories of their lives. Apart from asking older people to retrieve memories from different points of their life spans, Rabbitt and Winthorpe[149] persuaded them to rate these memories in terms of their levels of vividness, their dramatic or emotional impacts, and the relative frequencies with which they had been involuntarily rehearsed as they spontaneously came to mind or were triggered by other events. They found that rehearsal, or repeated reminiscence was the main factor predicting the relative subjective vividness of memories, and that memories from early adult life, during the period of the typical reminiscence bump, tended to be more dramatic, emotionally charged, more often rehearsed, and rated as more subjectively vivid than others from earlier or later periods. It seems likely that in most peoples' lives, this period of late adolescence and early adult life is most rich in significant, and memorable events. It may be a sad fact that the plots of individual's lives tend to contain increasingly fewer critical and memorable events as they pass into middle age. Recent studies have shown that these periods of intensely meaningful, or memorable events can be conditioned by external circumstances as well as by age. For instance, individuals of all ages who have lived through World War II tend to produce a high proportion of memories of events during its duration, irrespective of the particular periods of their lives during which it occurred. The factors that lead us to remember some events and not others are extremely complex, and include the nature of events and of their immediate and longer term significance in our lives, the efficiency with which we are capable of processing information at the moments when they occur and the number of times that we subsequently recall or discuss them, and the environmental support that we have when we do so. This complexity makes it difficult to interpret otherwise clear findings on individual differences in autobiographical memory. Rabbitt and McInnis[150] study of the earliest memories recalled by individuals aged between 50 and 86 years provides a good example of this situation. They found that individuals of all ages in this range who still had relatively high scores on a test of general intellectual ability, the Heim[151] AH 4, reported significantly earlier first memories than those with lower current scores. Many quite different factors might, individually or jointly, lead to this result. One is that individuals who still had relatively high scores had better recall of all events in their lives, including those in early childhood. Another is that individuals who were destined to have higher intelligence test scores throughout their lives had developed the ability to understand, interpret, and so remember events earlier than their less able coevals. A third is that individuals with relatively high levels of mental ability were also likely to be born into families with whom they were more likely to discuss events at an early age, and also perhaps more likely to reminisce, check, validate, date, and emend their earliest memories. Memory is not merely a biologic device for predicting the immediate future, but also the main repository of the social context in which we live our lives and of the data and structured narratives that allow us to impose such meaning and structure as we can on over lives. Perhaps it is now time to advance investigations of this rich social and existential aspect of memory independently of our theories of its functional and biologic substrate.

In sum, the quality, detail, and accuracy of individuals' memories of their lives tend to be conditioned by the uses that they make of their recollections of particular experiences. This is because the use to which particular memories are put, and the significance in the plot of an individual's life that they acquire, determines the frequency with which they are voluntarily or involuntarily recalled and rehearsed and the richness of the associational elaboration that they undergo. Rabbitt and Winthorpe[152] found that healthy and active individuals of all ages tend to produce a relatively high proportion of very recent memories, and that they report that these memories have been relatively often rehearsed. Rabbitt and Winthorpe suggest that this is because very recent events tend to provide the immediate bases and impetus for future plans, and so are often rehearsed while these plans are shaped. Memories of more distant archival events are usually not essential in day to day planning, but are nevertheless evoked, voluntarily or involuntarily, with a frequency determined by their relative degrees of significance, dramatic impact and emotional content or usefulness in conversational reference or as anecdotes. This leads us to consider the quality of memory for bodies of information and skills that are very often rehearsed because they are frequently practiced in everyday life, even into extreme old age.

Long-term retention of information cognitive skills

There is excellent evidence that even substantial bodies of information and complex skills can be excellently retained even in extreme old age, provided that they continue to be regularly practiced during everyday life. The classic evidence for this has been that verbal skills, information about the use of language, and social skills constitute a body of "crystallized intelligence" that robustly survives into old age in spite of other notable losses of "fluid" abilities such as speed of decision, working memory efficiency, and performance on tests of general intelligence.[153] Many studies of the extent to which people retain their vocabularies in old age have found that the number of words for which people can select exact synonyms among less precisely satisfactory alternatives remains constant, or may actually increase into the late 70s or early 80s.[154] These findings have often been replicated, even on very large populations of elderly volunteers.[32] However, as Salthouse[155] has pointed out, older people do perform less well than the young when they are compared on more demanding tests of lexical knowledge, such as the production, rather than recognition of precise definitions for words, or on tasks in which they are asked to generate as many words as possible within particular semantic categories such as "furniture", "fruits," or "animal names." It seems that although the continual use of language throughout life and into old age does substantially preserve the ability to understand and use words better than less practiced mental abilities there is, nevertheless, some loss.

Evidence for the reduced availability of even highly overlearned information in old age is the slowing of the rate at which it can be retrieved from memory. Perfect[61] questioned young adults and elderly volunteers to discover topics on which they were so exceptionally well informed that they might be regarded as "expert," and other topics about which they had only average information. He was then able to compare the times taken by older and younger adults to retrieve information on their expert and "novice" topics. Differences in retrieval times between young and elderly adults were much for their expert than for their novice topics. This implies that the frequent review and updating of information necessary to maintain expertise in particular areas does indeed reduce age differences in memory competence. However, even on their expert topics, on which they could correctly answer as many questions as their young controls, older people took longer to retrieve the necessary information from memory. Another difficulty with interpretation of this result is common to all comparisons between older and younger people that are based on the times that they take to do things. Cerella[60] found that across a variety of different tasks on which data have been published in the literature, the times taken by older people could be very precisely estimated by multiplying the times taken by younger adults by the same simple constant, between 1.2 and 1.5. The finding that slowing of decision times with age is proportionally the same for decisions of all levels of difficulty, and so of all durations applied also to Perfect's comparisons of the times that old and young people took to retrieve information about their expert and novice topics. That is, the proportionate slowing of retrieval times by age was the same in both cases.

The point that as people age they have increasing difficulty in retrieving from memory words that they have known and used for a lifetime is most evident in their reports of increasing incidence of "tip-of-the-tongue" states. That is, of failures, while speaking or writing, to find a particular word to continue what they want to say, in spite of the fact that they can recall very precisely the meaning that the word expresses, and often also enough information about it to reject less satisfactory alternatives and to correctly report surface rather than semantic information about it such as its syllabic length and its initial letter. These TOT states are, almost invariably, temporary and are eventually resolved because lost words can immediately be recognized in a thesaurus and words once mislaid may be spontaneously and easily retrieved and used hours or days later. However, the phenomenon may cause memorable social inconvenience and embarrassment because resolution often does not come about within a time frame acceptable during the course of a conversation. Experimenters have studied TOT states by asking volunteers to find appropriate words to precisely match careful definitions that they are given, noting the incidence of TOTs, the percentage of cases in which they are rapidly resolved, and the amount of partial information about the missing words that can be given before complete retrieval occurs. The general finding has been that TOTs do become increasingly frequent in older populations, that older people take significantly longer to resolve them and, at least in some studies, have been found to be able to generate significantly less partial information about missing words than young adults.[156,157] A related problem, that figures very prominently in older peoples' subjective reports of their memory lapses, is an extremely inconvenient increasing proneness to fail to remember proper names, even those that have been known and used for many years.[158,159] The evidence is slightly paradoxic. Older adults consistently perform much less well than the young at learning new information of all kinds,[101] and older adults also have relatively poorer delayed recall of newly learned names,[160] but the age-related deficit in learning names seems to be no larger than the age deficit in learning and immediately recalling other types of biographic information such as occupations or hobbies.[161] In studies of laboratory-induced TOT effects the age increases in the number of TOTs experienced was markedly greater for proper names than for other classes of words.[156] There is, therefore, objective evidence to support older peoples' subjective complaints that they have particular trouble in remembering proper names, but much less evidence that they have more trouble learning them in the first place.

Both of the two distinct explanations for the difficulty of remembering proper names inform our understanding of human memory and of the changes in its efficiency that occur in old age. The first explanation has been that proper names are unlike other items in the lexicon because they are arbitrary labels that have very specific referents, and in no way describe the properties of these referents or have useful associations with other words. There is no logical reason why the name "Dixon" should be assigned to one person rather than another and, like most other proper names, Dixon has no intrinsic meaning, use in the language, or semantic associations with other words in the language. Consequently, if we regard words as being represented in the brain as "nodes" in a "network," and suppose that they become available to consciousness when these nodes are activated by other nodes to which they are physically connected in the network because these represent other, semantically associated words, then it follows that the nodes representing proper names may well be less richly connected to other nodes than are the nodes for common nouns, which are embedded in more elaborate systems of semantic associations. If, further, we suppose that as brains age the neural networks of which they are composed increasingly lose components and connections, and perhaps acquire lower, overall levels of excitation, it is a plausible speculation that these changes more severely reduce the probability of excitation of sparsely than of richly connected nodes.[156,162] A second, different, but completely compatible explanation has been suggested by Jones and Rabbitt,[163] who compared age groups on their ability to learn and recall lists of pairs of proper names; that is, of first names and surnames. In different experimental conditions either the first name, or the surname, or both might be rare or common. The patterns of errors that occurred suggested that people of all ages, but especially the elderly, have difficulty both in initially learning and in subsequently retrieving proper names because these words are drawn from a fairly restricted set and so may be more easily confused with each other then members of very much larger sets such as common nouns, adjectives, or verbs. In a culture where many different people are called "John," "Peter," "Smith," or "Jones," it becomes difficult to assign correct pairings to particular people. This problem of confusion between names because of their multiple referents seems to become a particular problem in old age.

In sum, the evidence from studies of long-term retention of vocabulary and of the use of language is encouraging in the sense that it suggests that, on some criteria, people can retain, or even improve on their young adult competence until very late in their lives. However more detailed comparisons on more demanding tests of lexical competence reveal that there are increasing deficiencies in finding precise definitions for words, in rapidly generating lists of words, and in the speed with which information can be retrieved from memory, even if it has been well maintained by continued practice, and is, eventually, accurately available. The increase in old age of long, and embarrassingly unexpected, delays in finding the correct word with which to complete a sentence, and particular difficulties in remembering proper names, testify that although high levels of verbal competence can be maintained until very late in life, there is also some breakdown in the efficiency. The question of whether age affects long-term memory more or less than short-term, primary, secondary, or working memory seems to have no useful answer because of the incommensurability of the amounts of information with which these different systems deal. The limits to information that can be held in primary memory, short-term memory, or working memory are quite small and very clearly defined, so that it is easy to set at least approximate figures for their capacity, in terms of quantifiable units such as bits of information, and so to obtain what appear to be reassuringly very precise numeric estimates of the reduction in this capacity that occurs as people age. In contrast, there is no known limit to the amount of information that humans can retain in long-term memory, so that estimates of the proportionate reduction in this capacity that occurs with age or pathology are both unobtainable and, probably, uninformative. What is clear is that even when bodies of information held in long-term memory are continually rehearsed by their use throughout a lifetime, there is some decrement in the efficiency with which they can be maintained in, and retrieved from, long-term memory. It is also clear that these changes in the efficiency of both long-term and short-term retention of information have to be explained in terms of corresponding changes in qualitatively different functional processes. In the case of short-term memory, the critical factor seems to be change in the rate at which information can be encoded and handled. In the case of long-term memory, changes seem to refer to a gradual degradation of a complex representation system, which has the effect that information that is stored in terms of rich and varied patterns of associations is more robustly maintained and more rapidly and accurately retrieved than information that has been represented in terms of a more impoverished logical or associational structure. The question of relative impairment is not only uninteresting because it cannot be answered in any simple quantitative way, but because it may be less helpful to concentrate on the functional differences between these two systems than on the functional resemblances and, in particular, on the functional interactions between them. Most human activities require the application of information, procedures, and plans that have been learned and practiced over many years to the task of encoding of various different kinds of information that are immediately accessed from the environment and briefly retained for further analysis, management, and interpretation in working memory. Although we must accept the neuropsychologic evidence that long-term memory and working memory may be supported by distinct neurophysiologic systems, and that these systems may be differentially sensitive both to normal and to pathologic changes in the brain in old age, when we seek to describe the functional bases of the decisions that we continually make during our everyday lives it may be much more illuminating to consider how well these systems work together than what their separate characteristics may be. Information available from long-term memory is immediately and automatically available to recognize objects and interpret the dynamic relations between objects that we describe as "events." Immediately gathered information held in working memory cannot be encoded, or managed without the involvement of previously acquired information long resident in long-term memory. Rather than trying to describe these systems as discrete entities, and searching for evidence as to whether or not they have independent and asynchronous trajectories of aging, it seems more profitable to begin to consider how their mutual interactions are affected by aging of the brain.

These issues are most clearly brought out by a growing body of information on the long-term retention of cognitive skills that have been acquired over a lifetime and continue to be practiced into old age. Studies of maintenance of expertise at playing chess and bridge have been pioneered by Charness,[164,165] who found that expert players of bridge and chess, who continued to play frequently in old age, retained high levels of expertise. This allowed him to ask two important questions: The first was whether people who retain high levels of competence at these games do so because they also retained high levels of competence across a very wide range of other, different, cognitive skills, or whether maintenance of any skill is, rather, intensely "domain-specific" so that, for example, individuals who maintain high levels of performance at chess and bridge do not necessarily maintain competence even at other, quite closely related tasks. Charness's second question was possible because both of these complex games require players to hold, and continually to update and to use as much information as possible in working memory. In bridge this is necessary because it is important to remember, for instance, all of the cards that have been played, the order in which they have been played, and who played them. In chess it is crucial to hold in mind long sequences of moves and, in reviewing these, to recall which of them have, and which have not promising implications, and which have already been analyzed and rejected. Charness found that maintenance of high levels of competence at bridge by older adults does not necessarily generalize across other skills. For example, level of bridge expertise does not predict competence at other logical sequential problems such as solution of the "Tower of Hanoi" puzzle.

However, by the same token, it was clear that people could continue to maintain high levels of expertise at chess and bridge in spite of experiencing measurable losses in working memory capacity. It seems likely that, in ways that are not yet clearly understood, the acquisition of efficient schemata, programs, or scripts for playing bridge and chess reduce working memory load during play, and so allow older individuals to compensate, at least partially, for growing losses of the ability to simultaneously hold many different pieces of information in working memory, so that they can be effectively related to each other to execute complex plans. An effective theoretic rationale for this interaction between long-term and working memory is beginning to become available from work by Ericcsen and Polson[166] and Ericcsen et al.,[153] which develops earlier demonstrations by Ericcsen and associates. This is based on findings that even on very simple tasks such as immediate memory for lists of digits or letters, people who are practiced over very long periods of time can expand their immediate memory spans from the average young adult level of five to nine items to 20 items and over. They manage to do this by learning, and using, sometimes quite elaborate encoding rules and associated information held in working memory. For example, one volunteer encoded lists of digits as times for different running distances, a process that involved constant cross-referencing between information about distances, times, and athletic records held in his long-term memory while lists of 40 or more digits were being continuously inputted. A useful metaphor may be that by developing "expert" encoding systems, people can achieve "code compression," which allows them to very greatly increase the amount of information that they can process and then, later "play back." (See a classic account by Miller.[45])

Charness's conclusions have been confirmed and extended in our own laboratory by studies of the extent to which elderly people maintain expertise at crossword puzzle solving. Winder[167] selected volunteers aged between 50 and 83 for their ability to solve difficult cryptic crosswords within a severe time limit. She found, as expected, that all "experts" solved crossword cues much more rapidly and accurately than other volunteers, who were relative novices at crossword puzzle solving, but who had been carefully and individually matched to experts on the basis of their ages, genders, and scores on intelligence tests. Within both the expert and the novice groups, peoples' intelligence test scores declined with their ages in much the same way as in much larger populations of 6,500 or more screened by Rabbitt.[32] Within the control group, but not within the expert group, intelligence test scores modestly but robustly predicted crossword puzzle-solving skill. The experts preserved skill at crosswords although they had experienced identical declines in intelligence test performance to their controls. It follows that, as Charness found, highly practiced complex skills can be maintained at an expert level until very late in life, in Winders' experiment even into the early eighties. However, this maintenance by continual practice is intensely specific to the particular skill that is practiced, and does not generalize to other aspects of cognitive performance that are picked up by intelligence tests.

Forshaw[168] replicated and extended Winders[167] results, confirming that high expertise at crossword puzzle solving can be maintained into old age, and can be independent of maintenance of level of general intellectual ability as assessed by IQ test scores. Forshaw also found no evidence that maintenance of exceptional skill at crossword puzzle solving is necessarily dependent on maintenance of above average ability at working memory tasks, or of general speed of information processing. However, he also found clear evidence that maintenance of crossword solving skill did generalize to a variety of other tasks involving the use of language. Expert crossword solvers had higher scores on vocabulary tests than nonexperts. Further, although expert crossword solvers were no faster than nonexperts at tasks such as four choice reaction time, which did not involve the use of words, they were significantly faster and more accurate than their IQ test score-matched controls in tasks in which they had to make decisions about words; for example, when they had to decide whether horizontal strings of letter were or were not words, whether pairs of words were synonyms or homophones, and to solve anagrams. It seemed that maintenance of the overall skill of solving crossword puzzles also ensured maintenance of other, less complex, component skills in which decisions had to be made about words. Further, continued practice apparently cannot only maintain in memory the information, and procedures that are necessary to solve crossword puzzle clues, but also maintain the ability to make particular classes of less complex decisions very rapidly, as well as very accurately.

Another very useful, although extremely laborious, procedure for assessing learning and long-term retention of cognitive skills is to test peoples' recollection, at various points in their life spans, for systematic bodies of information that they acquired when they were adolescents or young adults. This line was pioneered by elegant studies in which respondents were asked for details about the previous layout of a city in which they had once lived, but had seldom or never visited since[169] or were assessed on their retention of a second language, Spanish, that they had learned at school. Bahrick found that, computing from the time when once well-learned knowledge was last practiced, recall declined exponentially over the first 3 to 5 years, changed very little over the next 20 years, and then showed further declines after 25 years. Bahrick concluded that after rapid initial loss, a body of knowledge enters a stable state, or "permastore," in which it remains available for a considerable period until, late in life, brain changes in old age make it increasingly inaccessible.

A necessary limitation of Bahrick's studies is that because he could probe only information acquired early in life, he could not simultaneously investigate changes in the stability of information acquired at different points during the life span. This has been rectified by a later, excellent pair of studies by Cohen et al.[170] who tested the recall of students of the Open University in the United Kingdom for material they had learned in psychology courses that they had completed at some time during a previous 12-year period. Because most students of the Open University are mature, and many are even elderly, Cohen et al. were able to assess the amount that they recalled both as a function of how old they were when they had initially taken the course, and of the time that had elapsed since.

Older students had generally obtained better grades than younger adults on their coursework, but had performed slightly less well on formal examinations, which they had taken under strict time constraints. Students of all ages lost information over a 12-year period. The resulting functions for loss of information over time closely resemble those obtained by Bahrick; there was an early rapid loss followed by only slight further declines. Losses were greatest for details, such as names of prominent individual scientists, but general concepts were relatively well remembered. This difference in accuracy of memory for concepts and for details was exaggerated by age. This study found no apparent differences in forgetting rates with age over a 12-year period. Thus, in contrast to other studies, this careful investigation finds no evidence that material learned late in life is more rapidly forgotten than material that has been encountered earlier. One distinction from previous studies is that, as we might infer from their advantages in the grades that they had earned for their coursework, older individuals, perhaps because they were relatively free of other commitments, had probably been able to give more time than the young to mastering the information they learned for their degrees. Once again, we encounter the methodologic problem that the rate at which material is forgotten may depend on the level at which it has been learned. Older people are evidently less able to extract and retain detailed information from complex events that are transient, and over whose time-course they have little control. In contrast, older individuals may assimilate complex information as well, and retain it as long as do the young, provided that they are allowed sufficient time to master it. Cognitive gerontology is, in many senses, a gray science, in which it is hard to find encouraging conclusions. Readers may be encouraged that this harrowing account of the increasing difficulties that people experience, as they age, in interpreting and remembering the world about them, can close on this relatively cheerful note.

References

1. Guttman JM: The elderly at home and in retirement housing: a comparative study of health problems, functional difficulties and support service needs. pp. 232–259. In Marshall VW (ed): Aging in Canada: Social Perspectives. Fitzhugh & Whiteside, Don Mills, Ontario; 1980
2. Buchler R, Pierce JT, Robinson P, Trier KS: Epidemiological Survey of Older Canadians. Government of Canada Report, Ottawa, HMSO, 1967
3. Hulicka IM: Memory function in late adulthood. In Craik FIM, Trehub, S (eds): Aging and Cognitive Processes, Plenum, New York, 1982
4. Herrmann D: Know thy memory: the use of questionnaires to assess and study memory. Psychol Bull 1982;92:434–452
5. Barlett FC: Remembering: A Study in Experimental and Social Psychology. Cambridge University Press Cambridge, 1932
6. Bennett-Levy J, Popwell GE: The subjective memory questionnaire (SMQ). An investigation into the self-reporting of "real-life" memory skills. Br J Soc Clin Psychol 1980;19:177–188
7. Bruce PR, Coyne AC, Botwinick J: Adult age differences in metamemory. J Gerontol 1982;37:354–357
8. Reason JT: Self-report questionnaires in cognitive psychology; have they delivered the goods? p. 406. In Baddeley AD, Weiskrantz LS (eds): Attention, Selection, Awareness and Control: A Tribute to Donald Broadbent. Oxford University Press Science Publications, Oxford, 1993
9. Rabbitt PMA, Abson V: "Lost and found" some logical and methodological limitations of self-report questionnaires as tools to study cognitive ageing. Br J Psychol 1990;82: 137–151

10. Stuart-Hamilton I, Perfect T, Rabbitt P: Remembering who was who. pp. 169–179. In Gruneberg MM, Morris PE, Sykes RN (eds): Practical Aspects of Memory Vol 2. John Wiley, Chichester, 1988

11. Devolder PA, Pressley M: Memory complaints in younger and older adults. Appl Cog Psychol 1991;5:443–454

12. Tenney YV: Aging and the misplacing of objects. Br J Psychol 1984;2:43–50

13. Rabbitt PMA, Maylor EM, Mc Innes L et al: What goods can self-assessment questionnaires deliver for cognitive gerontology? Appli Cog Psychol 1995;9:S127–S152

14. Mc Innes L, Rabbitt PMA: Subjective self-ratings as measures of health, J Gerontol (in press)

15. Reason JT: Lapses of attention in everyday life. pp. 515–549. In Underwood G, Stevens R (eds): Varieties of Attention. Academic Press, London, 1984

16. Rabbitt PMA: Age, IQ and awareness and recall of errors. Ergonomics 1990;33:1291–1305

17. Rabbitt PMA, Donlan C, Watson P, Mc Innes L, Bent N: Unique and interactive effects of depression, age, socio-economic advantage and gender on cognitive performance of normal healthy older people. Psychol Aging 1995;10:334–351

18. Rabbit PMA, Donlan C, Mc Innes L, et al: The University of Manchester Longitudinal Study of Cognitive Change in Normal Old Age. Zeitschrift fur Gerontologie 1993;26:176–183

19. Ivy GO, Mac Leod CM, Petit TL, Markus EJ: A physiological framework for perceptual and cognitive changes in aging. pp. 273–314. In Craik FIM, Salthouse TA (eds): The Handbook of Aging and Cognition. Erlbaums, Hillsdale, NJ, 1992

20. Salthouse TA: Speed of behaviour and its implications for cognition. pp. 400–426. In Birren JE, Schaie KW (eds): Handbook of the Psychology of Aging (2nd Edition). Van Nostrand Reinhold, New York, 1985

21. Salthouse TA: A theory of Cognitive Aging Elsevier, North Holland, 1985

22. Salthouse TA: Theoretical Perspectives in Cognitive Aging. Erlbaums, Hillsdale NJ, 1991

23. Birren JE: Psychophysiology and speed of response. Am Psychol 1972;29:808–815

24. Birren JE, Woods AM, Wiliams MV: Behavioural slowing with age: causes, organisation and consequences. pp. 293–308. In Poon LW (ed): Aging in the 1980s. American Psychological Association, Washington DC, 1980

25. Baddeley AD: Working Memory Oxford University Press, Oxford, 1986

26. Baddeley AD, Hitch G: Working memory. pp. 47–90. In GH. Bower (ed): The Psychology of Learning and Motivation. Vol 8.

27. Salthouse TA: Working memory as a processing resource in cognitive aging: limited resource model of cognitive development. Dev Rev 1990;10:101–124

28. Salthouse TA, Babcock RL: Decomposing adult age differences in working memory. Dev Psychol 1991;27:763–776

29. Craik FIM, Lockhart RS: Levels of processing: a framework for memory research. Journal of Verbal Learning and Verbal Behaviour 1972;11:671–684

30. Craik FIM, Tulving E: Depth of processing and retention of words in episodic memory. J Ex Psychol Gen 1975;104: 450–466

31. Waugh NC, Barr RA: Memory and mental tempo. In Poon LW, Fozard JL, Cermak LS, Arenberg D, Thompson LW (eds): New Directions in Memory and Aging. Erlbaums, Hillsdale, NJ, 1980

32. Rabbitt PMA: Does it all go together when it goes? O J Ex Psychol 1993;46A:385–434

33. Rabbitt PMA, Yang Q: Intelligence is not just mental speed. J Brosc Sci 1996;28:425–449

34. Robbins TW, James M, Owen AM et al: A neural systems approach to the cognitive psychology of ageing: studies with CANTAB or large samples of the normal elderly population. In Rabbitt PMA (ed): Methodology of Frontal and "Executive" Function. Hove Sussex, Erlbaums, 1997

35. Rabbitt PMA: Memory. pp. 463–478. In Grimley-Evans J, Franklin Wiliams T, (eds): Oxford Handbook of Geriatric Medicine. OUP Oxford, 1992

36. Gregory RL: The Intelligent eye. Mc Graw-Hill, New York, 1970

37. Dobbs AR, Reeves MB: Prospective memory: more than memory. pp. 199–226. In Brandimonte M, Einstein GO, Mc Daniel MA (eds): Prospective Memory: Theory and Applications. Erlbaums, Mahwah, NJ, 1996

38. Maylor EA: Does Prospective Memory Decline with Age? pp. 173–198. In Brandimonte M, Einstein GO, Mc Daniel MA (eds): Prospective Memory: Theory and Applications. Erlbaums, Mahwah, NJ, 1996

39. Rabbitt PMA: Commentary: why are studies of prospective memory planless? pp. 239–248. In Brandimonte M, Einstein GO, Mc Daniel MA (eds): Prospective Memory: Theory and Applications. Erlbaums, Mahwah, NJ, 1996

40. Craik FIM: Commentary: prospective memory: aging and lapses of attention. pp. 227–238. In Brandimonte M, Einstein GO, Mc Daniel MA (eds): Prospective Memory: Theory and Applications. Erlbaums, Mahwah, NJ, 1996

41. Averbach E, Coriell AS: Short-term memory in vision. Bell Systems Technical Journal 1961;40:309–328

42. Sperling G: The information available in brief visual presentations. Psychol Monographs, 1960;74:498

43. Di Lollo V: Temporal interaction in visual memory. J Exp Psychol Gen 1980;109:75–97

44. Di Lollo V, Arnett JL, Kruk RV: Age related changes in the rate of visual information processing. J Exp Psychol Hum Percept Perform 1982;8:225–237

45. Miller GA: The magical number seven, plus or minus two: some limits to our capacity for processing information. Psychol Rev 1956;63:81–97

46. Parkinson SR, Lindholm JM, Inman VW: An analysis of age differences in immediate recall. J of Gerontol 1982;37: 425–431

47. Foos PW, Sahal MA, Correl G, Mabley L: Age differences in primary and secondary memory. Bull Psychonomic Soc 1987; 25:159–160

48. Delbecq-Derousne J, Beauvoise MF: Memory processes and aging: a defect of automatic rather than control processes? Arch Gerontol Geriatr 1989;(suppl. 1):121–150

49. Botwinick J, Storandt M: Memory Related Functions and Age. C.C. Thomas, Springfield Ill, 1974

50. Johanssen B, Berg S: The robustness of the terminal decline phenomenon: longitudinal data for the digit-span memory test. J Gerontol Psychol Sci 1989;44:P184–P186

51. Parkinson SR: Performance deficits in short-term memory tasks: a comparsion of amnesic Korsakov patients and the aged. pp. 77–96. In Cermak LS (ed): Human Memory and Amnesia Erlbaums, Hillsdale NJ,

52. Wingfield A, Stine AL, Lahar CJ, Aberdeen JS: Does the capacity of working memory change with age? Exp Aging Res 1988;14:103–107

53. Ericcsen KA, Krampe R Th, Tesch-Romer C: The role of deliberate practice in the acquisition of expert performance. Psychol Rev 1993;100:363–406

54. Sternberg S: High speed scanning in human memory. Science 1966;153:652–654

55. Sternberg S: Memory scanning; new findings and current controversies. Q J Exp Psychol 1975;27:1–32

56. Ryan C: Decision and Control Processes in Recognition Memory. Ph.D. Thesis, University of Oxford, 1981

57. Coyne AC, Allen PA, Wickens DD: Influence of adult age on primary and secondary memory search. Psychol Aging 1986; 1:187–194

58. Craik FIM, Rabinowitz JC: The effects of presentation rate and encoding task on age-related memory deficits. J Gerontol 1985;46:309–315

59. Lorsbach TC, Simpson GB: Age differences in the rate of processing in short-term memory. J Gerontol 1984;39:315–321

60. Cerella J: Information processing rates in the elderly. Psychol Bull 1985;98:67–83

61. Perfect T: Age, Expertise and Long-Term memory Retrieval. PhD Thesis, University of Manchester, U.K., 1989

62. Goward LM: Am investigation of factors contributing to scores on intelligence tests. PhD Thesis, University of Manchester, Manchester U.K., 1987

63. Just MA, Carpenter PA: A capacity theory for comprehension: individual differences in working memory. Psychol Rev 1992; 99:122–149

64. Craik FIM, Rabinowitz JC: Age differences in the acquisition and use of verbal information. pp. 471–499. In Bouma H, Bouhuis DG (eds): Attention and Performance X. Erlbaum, Hillside, NJ, 1984

65. Dobbs AR, Rule BG: Adult age differences in working memory. Psychol Aging 1989;5:379–387

66. Wiegersma S, Meertse K: Subjective ordering, short-term memory and aging. Exp Aging Res 1990;16:73–77

67. Wiegersma S, Van der Scheer E, Hijman R: Subjective ordering, short term memory and the frontal lobes. Neuropsychologia 1990;28:95–98

68. Salthouse TA, Babcock RL, Shaw RJ: Effects of adult age on structural and operational capacities in working memory. Psychol Aging 1991;6:118–127

69. Salthouse TA, Mitchel DR, Skovronek E, Babcock RL: Effects of adult age and working memory on reasoning and spatial abilities. J Exp Psych Learning. Memory and Cognition. 1989; 15:507–516

70. Hasher L, Zacks RT: Working memory, comprehension and aging: a review and a new view. pp. 193–225. In Bower GH (ed): The Psychology of Learning and Motivation, Vol 22. Academic Press, New York, 1988

71. Tulving E: "How many memory systems are there?" Am Psychol 1985;40:385–398

72. Tulving E: Episodic and semantic memory. pp. 381–403. In Tulving E, Donaldson W (eds): Organisation of Memory. Academic Press, New York, 1972

73. Milner (1966)

74. Warrington EK, Weiskrantz LS: The effect of prior learning on subsequent retention in amnesic patients. Neuropsychologia 1974;12:419–428

75. Mitchell DB: How many memory systems? Evidence from aging. J Exp Psychol: Learning, Memory and Cognition 1985; 15:31–49

76. Kolers PA: Remembering operations. Memory and Cognition 1973;1:347–355

77. Jacobi LL, Witherspoon D: Remembering without awareness. Can J Psychol 1982;36:300–324

78. Schacter DL: Implicit memory: history and current status. J Exp Psychol: Learning, Memory and Cognition 1987;13: 368–379

79. Richardson-Klavehn A, Bjork RA: Measures of memory. Ann Rev Psychol 1988;39:475–543

80. Graf P: Lifespan changes in implicit and explicit memory. Bull Psychonom Soc 1990;28:353–358

81. Light LL, Burke DM: Patterns of language and memory in old age. pp. 244–271. In Light LL, Burke DM (eds): Language Memory and Aging, Cambridge University Press, New York, 1988

82. Howard DV: Aging and semantic activation: the priming of semantic and episodic memories pp. 77–100. In Light LL, Burke DM (eds): Language, Memory and Aging Cambridge University Press, New York, 1988

83. Light LL, Singh A: Implicit and explicit memory in young and older adults. J Exp Psychol: Learning, Memory and Cognition. 1987;13:531–541

84. Parkin AJ, Walter BM: Recollective experience, normal ageing and frontal dysfunction. Psychobiology, 1992;19:175–179

85. Rose TL, Yesavage JA, Hill RD, Bower GH: Priming effects and recognition memory in young and elderly adults. Exp Aging Res 1986;12:31–37

86. Howard DV, Shaw RJ, Heisey J: Aging and the time course of semantic activation. J Gerontol 1986;41:195–203

87. Chiarello C, Hoyer WJ: Adult age differences in implicit and explicit memory. Time course and encoding effects. Psychol Aging 1988;3:358–366

88. Hultsch DF, Masson MEJ, Snell BJ: Adult age differences in direct and indirect tests of memory. J Gerontol Psychological Sciences 1991;46:P22–P30

89. Craik FIM, McDowd JM: Age differences in recall and recognition. J Exp Psychol 1987;13:474–479

90. Craik FIM, Jacoby LL: Elaboration and distinctiveness in episodic memory. pp. 145–166. In Nilsson LG (ed): Perspectives in Memory Research. Erlbaums, Hillsdale, NJ, 1979

91. Tulving E, Thompson DM: Encoding specificity and retrieval processes in episodic memory. Psychol Rev 1973;80:352–373

92. Cohen G: Memory and learning in normal aging. pp. 43–58. In Handbook of the Clinical Psychology of Aging. In Woods RT (ed): Handbook of Clinical Psychology of Aging. John Wiley, Colchester, 1996

93. Erber JT, Herman TG, Botwinick J: Age differences in memory as a function of depth of processing. Exp Aging Res 1980;6: 341–348

94. Craik FIM, Byrd M: Aging and cognitive deficits: the role of informational resources. pp. 191–211. In Craik FIM, Trehub S. (eds): Aging and Cognitive Processes. New York, Plenum, 1982

95. Rabinowitz JC: Judgements of origin and generation effects: comparisons between young and elderly adults. Psychol and Aging 1989;4:259–268

96. Treat NJ, Reese HW: Age pacing and imagery in paired associate learning. Dev Psychol 1976;12:119–124

97. Puglisi JT, Park DC: Perceptual elaboration and memory in older adults. J Gerontol 1987;42:160–162

98. Park DC, Smith AD, Morrell RW et al: Effects of contextual integration on recall of pictures by older adults. J Gerontol Psychol Sci 1990;45:P52–P57

99. Rankin JL, Firnhofer S: Adult age differences in memory: effects of distinctive and common encodings. Exp Aging Res 1986;12:141–146

100. Hashtroudi S, Parker ES, Lewis JD, Reisen CA: Generation and elaboration in older adults. Exp Aging Res 1989;15: 73–78

101. Macay DG, Burke DM: Cognition and aging: a theory of new learning and the use of old connections. In Hess TM (ed): Aging and Cognition: A Theory of new learning and the Use of Old Connections. pp. 1–51. In Thomas M. Hess (Ed). Aging and Cognition: Organisation and Utilisation. Elsevier, Amsterdam, N. Holland, 1990

102. Anderson JA: A spreading activation theory of memory. J Verbal Learning and Verbal Behaviour 1983;22:261–295

103. Anderson JA: The Architecture of Cognition. Harvard University Press, Cambridge Mass, 1983

104. Craik FIM: On the transfer of information from temporary to permanent storage. Philosophical Transacitions of the Royal Society of London. Series B. 1983;302:341–349

105. Craik FIM: A functional account of age differences in memory. pp. 409–422. In Klix F, Hagendorf H, (eds): In Human Memory and Cognitive Capabilities. Mechanisms and Performances Elsevier, Amsterdam, N. Holland, 1986

106. West RL, Boatwright L: Age differences in cued recall under varying encoding and retrieval conditions. Exp Aging Res 1983;9:185–189

107. Jacobi LL: On interpreting the effects of repetition: solving a problem versus remembering a solution. Journal of Verbal Learning and Verbal Behaviour 1978;17:649–667

108. Johnson MM, Schmitt FA, Pietrukovitz M: The memory advantages of the generation effect: age and process differences. J Gerontol: Psychol Sci 1989;44:P91–P94

109. Mc Daniel MA, Ryan EB, Cummingham CJ: Encoding difficulty and memory enhancement for old and young readers. Psychol Aging 1989;4:333–338

110. Mitchell DB, Hunt RR, Schmitt FA: The generation effect and reality monitoring: evidence from dementia and normal aging. J Gerontol 1986;41:79–84

111. Nilson LG, Craik FIM: Additive and interactive effects in memory for subject-performed tasks. Eur J Psychol 2:305–324

112. Rabinowitz JC: Age deficits in recall under optimal study conditions. Psychol Aging 1989;4:378–380

113. Backman L, Nilson LG: Aging effects in free recall: an exception to the rule. Human Learning 1985;3:53–69

114. Backman L: Further evidence for the lack of adult age differences on free recall in subject performed tasks. Human Learning 1985;4:79–87

115. Kausler DH, Wiley JG: Effects of short-term retrieval on adult age differences in long-term recall of actions. Psychol Aging 1991;6:661–665

116. Rabbitt PMA: Talking to the Old. New Society, June 1980

117. Mc Intyre JS, Craik FIM: Age differences in memory for item and for source information. Can J Psychol 1987;41:175–192

118. Cohen G, Faulkner D: Age differences in source forgetting: effects on reality monitoring and eye-witness testimony. Psychol Aging 1989;4:10–17

119. Hastroudi S, Johnson MK, Chrosniak LD: Aging and qualitative characteristics of memories for perceived and imagined complex events. Psychol Aging 1990;5:119–126

120. Rabbitt PMA: Talking to the Old. New Society, 1980;212–214

121. Hasnner L, Zacks RT: Automatic and effortful processes in memory. J Exp Psychol Gen 1979;108:356–388

122. Craik FIM, Jennings JM: Human Memory. pp. 51–110. In Craik FIM, Salthouse TA (eds): The Handbook of Aging and Cognition. Erlbaums, Hillsdale NJ, 1992

123. Cohen G: Language comprehension in old age. Cog Psychol 1979;11:412–429

124. Zacks RT, Hasher L, Daren B et al: Encoding and memory of explicit and implicit information. J Gerontol 1987;42: 418–422

125. Hamm VP, Hasher L: Age and the availability of inferences. Psychol Aging 1992;7:56–64

126. Cohen G: Age differences in memory for text: production deficiency or word-processing limitations? pp. 171–190. In Light LL, Burke DM (eds): Language Memory and Aging. Cambridge University Press, New York, 1988

127. Zacks RT, Hasher L: Capacity theory and the processing of inferences. pp. 154–170. In Light LL, Burke DM (eds): Language, Memory and Aging. Cambridge University Press New York, 1988

128. Spilich GJ: Life-span components of text processing: structural and procedural differences. Journal of Verbal Learning and Verbal Behaviour 1983;22:231–244

129. Stine EAL, Wingfield A: The assessment of qualitative age differences in discourse processing. pp. 33–92. In Hess TM (ed): Aging and Cognition: Knowledge Organisation and Utilisation, Enevia Amsterdam, N. Holland, 1990

130. Kemper S: Geriatric psycholinguistics. pp. 58–76. In Light LL, Burke, DM (eds): Language Memory and Aging. Cambridge University Press, New York, 1988

131. Hultsch DF, Dixon RA: The role of pre-experimental knowledge in text processing in adulthood. Exp Aging Res 1985;9: 7–22

132. Cohen G, Faulkner D: Memory for discourse in old age. Discourse Processes 1981;4:253–265

133. Holland CA, Rabbitt PMA: Autobiographical memory and text recall in the elderly: an investigation of the processing resource deficit. O J Exp Psychol 1990;42A:441–470

134. Light LL, Anderson PA: Memory for scripts in older and younger adults. Memory and Cognition 1983;11:435–444

135. Hess JM, Vandermass MO, Donley J, Snyder SS: Memory for sex-role consistent and inconsistent actions in young and old adults. J Gerontol 42:505–511

136. Backman L: Recognition memory across the adult lifespan: the role of prior knowledge. Memory and Cognition 1991;19: 63–71

137. Arbuckle TY, Vanderleck VF, Harsony M, Lapidus S: Adult age differences in memory in relation to availability and accessibility of knowledge based schemata. J Exp Psychol Learning Memory and Cognition 1990;156:305–315

138. Ribot T: Diseases of Memory: An Essay on the Positive Psychology Smith WH trans. Appleton, New York, 1882

139. Winthorpe C, Rabbitt PM: "Working memory capacity, IQ, age and the ability to recount autobiographical events." pp. 175–179. In Gruneberg MM, Morris PE, Sykes RN (eds): Practical Aspects of Memory: Current Research and Issues. Vol 2. John Wiley, Chichester, 1988

140. Williams DM, Santos Williams SM: A method for exploring retrieval processes using verbal protocols. Attention and Performance, Vol. VIII. NJ, Erlbaums, Hillsdale, 1980

141. Williams DM, Hollan JD: The process of retrieval from very long-term memory. Cognitive Science, 1981;5:87–119

142. Howes JL, Katz AN: Assessing remote memory with an improved public events questionnaire. Psychol Aging 1988;3: 142–150

143. Cohen G, Conway MA, Maylor EA: Flashbulb memory in young and older adults. Psychol Aging 1994;9:454–463

144. Crovitz HF, Quina-Holland K: Proportion of episodic memories from early childhood by age. Bull Psychonom Soc 1976; 7:61–62

145. Crovitz HF, Schiffman H: Frequency of episodic memories as a function of their age. Bulle Psychonomic Soc 1974;4: 517–518

146. Rubin DC: On the retention function for autobiographical memory. J Verbal Learning and Verbal Behaviour 1982;21: 21–38

147. Cohen G, Faulkner D: Life-span changes in autobiographical memory. pp. 277–282. In Gruneberg MM, Morris PE, Sykes RN (eds): Practical aspects of memory: Current Research and Issues, Vol. 1. John Wiley, Chichester, 1987

148. Fitzgerald JM: Vivid memories and the reminiscence phenomenon: the role of self-narration. Human Development 1988; 31:261–273

149. Rabbitt P, Winthorpe C: What do old people remember? The Galton paradigm reconsidered. pp. 301–307. In Gruneberg MM, Morris PE, Sykes RN (eds): Practical Aspects of Memory. Vol. 1. John Wiley Chichester, 1988

150. Rabbitt PMA, McInnis L: Do clever old people have earlier and richer first memories? Psychol Aging. 1988;3:

151. Heim AW: AH 4 test. NFER/Nelson, Windsor, UK, 1968

152. Rabbitt P, Winthorpe C: What do old people remember? The Galton paradigm reconsidered. pp. 301–307. In Gruneberg MM, Morris PE, Sykes RN (eds): Practical Aspects of Memory. Vol. 1. John Wiley, Chichester, 1988

153. Horn JL: The theory of fluid and crystallised intelligence in relation to concepts of cognitive psychology and aging in adulthood. pp. 123–139. In Craik FIM, Trehubs (eds): Aging and Cognitive Processes. Plenum, Boston, 1982

154. Birren JE, Morrison DF: Analysis of the WAIS sub-tests in relation to age and education. J Gerontol 1961;16:363–369

155. Salthouse TA: Effects of aging on verbal abilities: examination of the psychometric literature. pp. 17–35. In Light LL, Burke DM (eds.) Language, Memory and Aging. Cambridge University Press, NY, 1988

156. Burke DM, Mackay DG, Worthley JS, Wade E: On the tip of the tongue: what causes word finding difficulties in young and older adults. J Memory and Language 1991;30:542–579

157. Maylor EA: Recognising and naming faces: aging, memory retrieval and the tip of the tongue state. J Gerontol Psychol Sci 1990;45:215–225

158. Cohen G, Faulkner D: Memory in old age: good in parts. New Scientist 1984;11:49–51

159. Sunderland A, Watts K, Baddeley AD, Harris JE: Subjective memory assessment and test performance in elderly adults. J Gerontol 1986;41:376–384.

160. Crook TH, West RL: Name recall performance across the adult lifespan. Br J Psychol 1990;81:335–349

161. Cohen G, Faulkner D: Memory for proper names. Age differences in retrieval. B J Psychol 1986;4:187–197

162. Cohen G: Recognition and retrieval of proper names. Age differences in the fan effect. Eur J Cog Psychol 1990;2:193–204

163. Jones SJ, Rabbitt PMA: (1994). Effects of age on the ability to remember common and rare proper names. Quarterly J Exp Psychol 1994;47A:1001–1014

164. Charness N: Component processes in bridge bidding and novel solving tasks. Can J Psychol 1987;41:223–247

165. Charness N: Age and expertise: responding to Talland's challenge. pp. 437–456. In Poon LW, Rubin DC Wilson B. (eds.) Everyday Cognition in Adulthood and Old Age. Cambridge University Press, NY, 1989

166. Ericcsen KA, Polson PG: (1987). An experimental analysis of memory skill for dinner orders. J Exp Psychol Learning, Memory & Cognition 1987;14:305–316

167. Winder B: The maintenance of skill in old age. Unpublished MSc thesis, University of Manchester, Manchester UK, 1993

168. Forshaw MJ: Expertise and ageing: the crossword puzzle paradigm. Unpublished PhD thesis, University of Manchester, 1994

169. Bahrick HP: Semantic memory content in permastore: 50 years of memory for Spanish learned in school. In Bower G (ed): The Psychology of Learning and Mortivation: Advances in Research and Theory, Vol. 17. Academic Press, New York, 1987

170. Cohen G, Conway M, Stanhope N: Age differences in the retention of knowledge by young and elderly students. Br J Devel Psychol 1992;10:153–164.

CHAPTER 10

The Aging Personality and Self

REBECCA ALLEN-BURGE
SHERRY L. WILLIS
K. WARNER SCHAIE

There is growing awareness that psychosocial issues in adulthood are intricately related to health outcomes, as well as to the treatment of chronic diseases associated with the aging process. The purpose of this chapter is to provide a broad overview of psychosocial development in adulthood and aging. Specifically, issues regarding personality, the interface of personality and cognition, motivation, and social/emotional support across the adult life span are included. In each section, current issues in the research literature are reviewed. Knowledge of stability and change within and among older adults regarding psychosocial issues may assist health care professionals in interpreting and treating health concerns and problems. This can be an exceptionally difficult task, given the myriad symptoms presented by many older adults.

First, theories and empirical work addressing stability and change in adult personality and conceptions of self are considered. Next, the field of social cognition, encompassing perceived control, self-efficacy, and metamemory is reviewed. The third section of the chapter deals with the interface of personality and cognition. Fourth, empirical findings regarding stability and change in motivation are examined. This is followed by a review of socioemotional selectivity, including a review of the relationship between social support and health. Throughout the chapter consideration is given to the implications of psychosocial issues for treatment and care of the elderly.

Personality and the Self

Overview

Personality has been defined as internal, dynamic biopsychosocial systems that shape an individual's interface with the world.[1,2] Two major issues in the study of personality development in adulthood concern the extent to which personality remains stable or changes in adulthood, and whether age differences, if observed, reflect change within an individual or merely differences between individuals born at different times (i.e., birth cohorts).[3] These issues have implications for attitudes toward aging that must be considered by health care professionals working with older adults. Theoretical paradigms that have been used to study personality across adulthood include stage theory, trait theory, and cognitive approaches to the self.

Each theoretical approach assumes a certain position regarding the possibility and likelihood of change in adult personality. For example, trait theories assume *stability*—the tendency for attitudes, behaviors, and perceptions of the self to be maintained across adulthood. In contrast, other approaches to personality such as stage theories assume an ordered sequence of *changes* in personality characteristics. Rather than assuming either stability or change, cognitive approaches focus on an individual's conceptualization of their personality (i.e., identity), and provide theoretical bases and mechanisms for when individual characteristics are likely to remain stable and when they are likely to change.

The implicit assumptions regarding stability and change underlying current theories of adult personality guide the research questions, methods, and interpretation of findings in specific ways that have an impact on their potential usefulness in medical practice. As health care professionals consider treatment recommendations, it is important to keep in mind relationships between personality and the presentation of symptoms. Consideration of psychosocial issues in adulthood involves not only an understanding of age-related changes in personality that occur as a person ages, but also recognition of differences among birth cohorts with regard to personality characteristics. Given rapid societal and technological change, health care professionals treating individuals across adulthood need to contemplate evidence from both kinds of investigations into adult personality in order to differentiate individual age-related change (i.e., maturation) from cohort-related differences.

Various birth cohorts can differ dramatically when studied at the same chronological age with regard to health and psychosocial factors. Consider the dramatic increase in average life expectancy for successive cohorts across this century, or the elimination of certain childhood diseases (e.g., smallpox, measles) in recent cohorts. Similar cohort differences are found for psychosocial variables, with studies showing increases across cohorts in need for abasement and sociability.[4] These behavioral characteristics may reflect cohort differences in a person's presentation of symptoms and/or manner of interacting with professionals. Therefore, health care professionals may need to spend a little more time with their older patients in order to ensure that the needs of the patient are clearly understood and that the patient clearly understands treatment recommendations. Without this extra effort, health care professionals may later find that older patients have not had their needs met or have not followed directions, because they simply agreed with the professionals' recommendations out of a sense that they need to defer to the experts without understanding the importance of their own input. Thus, consideration of stability and change within individuals and of cohort differences in personality characteristics will have direct impact on health care professionals' expectations regarding the cultural stereotype of the older adult hypochondriac, and are thus likely to impact health professional-patient communications.

In the following sections, we will review research from several theoretical approaches to adult personality. First we will review stage theories, emphasizing change in adult personality development. Second, we will discuss individual difference or trait approaches to the study of personality, with emphasis on the Five Factor model and stability. Finally, we will review cognitive conceptualizations of the self. These cognitive approaches to personality and identity emphasize the possibility of both stability and change. In each section, findings will be discussed in terms of their potential importance to health care professionals, and evidence of age changes will be differentiated from evidence of cohort differences.

Stage Models of Personality

Overview

The use of developmental stage models as a description of continuity and change within individuals across the life span has a long history in psychology.[2,5–7] Most of these models have their origins in the psychoanalytic tradition of Sigmund Freud, that identified stages of psychosexual development through adolescence.[8] Whereas Freud believed personality development to be essentially complete in adolescence, more recent stage theorists postulate that humans continue to seek ways to define the self throughout adulthood.[9]

Gender issues

Carl Jung[9,10] was one of the first theorists to propose that continued personality development was possible in adulthood. Jung focused attention on gender-role issues with his conceptualization of the anima, or feminine characteristics, and the animus, or masculine characteristics. He proposed that as individuals age, they achieve a balance between the expression of their masculine and feminine characteristics not previously observed. Using the Thematic Apperception Test (TAT), a projective personality test, Guttmann[11–13] found some support for Jung's hypothesis. Specifically, he found that men as they age are more likely to express feminine traits when asked to interpret ambiguous stimuli, and older women are more likely to express masculine traits.[9–13] Projective personality tests such as the TAT are based on the assumption that when individuals are presented with ambiguous stimuli and have open response options, they will impose order on the stimuli by projecting internal needs, motivations, and drives onto the stimulus material.[14] Thus, these studies provide evidence of changes in the expression of gender roles as assessed through interpretation of ambiguous stimuli, and may not be as readily observed when studied in a structured self-report format. Most research in the area of gender issues in personality change has been cross-sectional. Findings regarding increased balance of gender roles with age, however, have emerged in different cultures around the world.[2] This lends further support to Jung's proposition that there are age changes, not just age differences, in the presentation of gender role characteristics with age.[2]

Erikson's stages of psychosocial development

Extending Jung's proposition that there is personality development in adulthood, Erikson[2,5,9,15] proposed stages of psychosocial development that occur in midlife and in later adulthood. Erikson's theory incorporates both inner psychological and outer social influences. The sequence of Erikson's stages is based on the epigenetic principle that each psychosocial stage has its own special developmental period in which it becomes particularly salient. Erikson defined the psychosocial struggle of midlife as *generativity versus stagnation*. In this stage, individuals seek to give of their talents and experience to the next generation in order to ensure the perpetuation of society. If individuals succeed in focusing on generativity rather than becoming self absorbed (i.e., stagnation), trust in the ability of the next generation and a sense of care are obtained. Erikson's final stage of psychosocial development, typically reached after age 65, is *ego integrity versus despair*. In this stage, individuals become more aware of the nearness of death. Older adults engage in a process of life review, searching for a sense of meaning.[16] Older adults who have successfully completed earlier stages of psychosocial development are likely to look back on their life and find meaning. Those who examine their lives and find them meaningless experience despair.

Surprisingly little empirical research has investigated the Eriksonian model of developmental stages.[15] This is partially due to the lack of specification of how individuals reconcile crises and move from one stage to the next.[9,15] Some theorists have proposed that the themes of trust, achievement, and wholeness are dealt with repeatedly throughout life.[9] In one longitudinal empirical investigation of Erikson's stage theory, Whitbourne et al[17] assessed three cohorts over a period of 22 years using an inventory of psychosocial development. Results from this study showed significant age changes in terms of the resolution of developmental stages.[17] Middle-aged adults expressed emotions and cognition consistent with successful completion of more psychosocial developmental crises than did young adults.[17]

Loevinger's stages of ego development

Loevinger[6–7] extended Erikson's work by proposing a stage theory of ego development. Loevinger's theory relies heavily on findings from her validation of a scoring system for a projective sentence completion test. Using this approach, Loevinger's model identified six stages of adult personality development. These include: conformist, conscientious-conformist, conscientious, individualistic, autonomous, and integrated. Loevinger proposed that the progression of adults through these stages depended on their development in four areas: character (i.e., goals and values), interpersonal style, conscious preoccupations, and cognitive style.[9] We will briefly review the characteristics of these different stages.

The least developed stage of adult ego in Loevinger's theory is the *conformist* level.[7] Conformists obey external social rules to the letter and tend to relate to others in a superficial manner. Individuals at this stage tend to be ruled by a need for acceptance. The second stage of ego development, the *conscientious-conformist*, is the most common according to Loevinger.[7] At this stage, individuals differentiate societal norms from personal goals and recognize the impact of their actions on others. Although they are cognizant of their own needs, their cognitive style is to subjugate individual needs to group needs in the presence of conflict. Loevinger's third stage of ego development is the *conscientious* stage.[7] Individuals at this stage set their own ideals, goals, and standards and are self-monitoring of their progress. Their relationships are responsible, intense, and reciprocal.

Adults in the *individualistic* stage are differentiated from those at other stages by their respect for individual autonomy and their tolerance for self and others.[7] These individuals tend to resolve internal conflict by projecting discomfort externally. The fifth stage of ego development in Loevinger's model is the *autonomous* level, characterized by high tolerance for ambiguity and complexity in oneself and one's environment.[7] These individuals are able to balance dependence and interdependence in relationships with others and are comfortable with the idea that other people may hold different views. The final stage of ego development in Loevinger's model is the *integrated* stage.[7] This stage is marked by the resolution of inner conflicts.

Cross-sectional and longitudinal research shows that these stages are age related, albeit they show only modest correlations with chronological age.[2,9] Loevinger was most interested in explicating individual differences in personality stage. For example, her ego development score has been found to be associated with other measures of openness used in the study of personality aging, such as reasoning on social dilemma tasks and coping style.[9,18,19]

Stage of ego development may prove informative for health care professionals interacting with patients regarding health care decisions such as whether or not to have surgery or to execute a medical advance directive. For example, individuals at the conformist stage may be more likely than individuals at the individualistic or autonomous stages to base their decision on the recommendations of powerful others such as health care professionals or adult family members rather than on their own wishes. Thus, health care professionals wishing to preserve patient autonomy and to avoid surrogate decision making may want to adjust their presentation of treatment options according to an individual's stage of ego development. For example, health care professionals may wish to emphasize the personal importance of the impact of some decisions on quality of life with individuals in the conformist stage.

Summary of stage theories

In this section we have reviewed research findings from a stage approach to adult personality development, focusing on Erikson's and Loevinger's theories. Stage theories share specific perspectives regarding change in adult personality, the sequence of changes, and the role of the unconscious. In general, people are assumed to progress through stages chronologically in a prespecified order. Individuals move from one stage to the next as unconscious conflicts from the preceding stage are resolved. Stage theories allow for individual differences in the final stage of personality development reached, the rate of progression among stages, and the process by which movement among stages is experienced. Stage theories do not, however, take into consideration the possibility of cohort differences in proposed stages. Rather, stage theories assume that proposed stages hold true for each successive cohort and for all people.

The stage theories reviewed here each make significant contributions to our knowledge of adult personality. Jung introduced the idea that personality may continue to develop in adulthood, and focused on age changes in the expression of gender-related personality characteristics. Erikson was the first to specify adult stages of ego development, and to attempt to explain adult age differences in personality. Loevinger introduced the idea of the impact of individual differences in the final stage of ego development reached. In Loevinger's theory, only a small percentage of people reach the highest stage of ego development, and characteristics of these individuals can be identified. Like Loevinger, other researchers have focused on individual differences, but typically via trait approaches to life span personality development.

Trait Theories of Personality

In contrast to stage models that assume qualitative change over time, most trait theories assert that there is considerable stability in personality over time.[2,4,9,15] Traits are observable, characteristic patterns of behavior within an individual across time that differentiate the person from others.[20] Examples of traits include emotional stability, behavioral flexibility/rigidity, extraversion/introversion, warmth, and responsibility. The basic premises of a trait theory are that (1) traits are based on comparisons of individuals, (2) the qualities or behaviors making up a particular trait are distinctive from other traits, and (3) traits attributed to a person may be stable characteristics of the person.[21] Much of the recent research on personality in adulthood has used a trait approach. Studies have examined both the issue of stability versus change in personality traits within individuals across time, and the issue of cohort differences in personality. One prominent approach within trait theories is the Five Factor theory, proposed by Costa and McCrae.[3,4,20,21]

Five Factor theory

Costa and McCrae have conducted cross-sectional and longitudinal research that focused on identifying sets or groupings of traits that can explain individual differences in behavior and that can be helpful in examining the relationship between health and behavior in adulthood. Five broad dimensions of personality encompassing groups of related traits have been identified: neuroticism, extraversion, openness to experience, agreeableness, and conscientiousness.[2,4,9,20,21] *Neuroticism* encompasses such characteristics as anxiety, depression, emotional instability, self-consciousness, hostility, and impulsiveness. *Extraversion* deals with gregariousness, assertiveness, activity, and positive emotions. *Openness to experience* represents flexibility and a willingness to consider new ideas, to engage in new behaviors, and to dream. *Agreeableness* reflects attributes such as warmth and compassion that are considered pleasant and attractive to others. *Conscientiousness* encompasses responsibility, ambition, perseverance, and hard work.

Longitudinal stability and change

Results from longitudinal analyses suggest that maturational changes in personality continue through age 30, and then personality traits remain relatively stable for intervals of up to 30 years over the age range of 20 to 90.[2,20,22–23] Methodologies have included self-report and spousal ratings of personality traits, and the finding of stability remains.[3,4,15] The greatest instability is found for the period between late adolescence and early adulthood.[15,23]

In spite of the overwhelming evidence of stability in adult personality, small but consistent age changes have been found for some traits. For example, Schaie and colleagues[2,23] have investigated maturational and cohort differences in personality via the Seattle Longitudinal Study (SLS), a cohort-sequential study of adult intellectual development. Results from the SLS demonstrate that social responsibility increases with age through the mid-thirties and then remains stable. Level of social responsibility also varies greatly across age groups due to social and political events occurring during a particular historical period.[23]

Interestingly, although longitudinal studies suggest stability in personality traits, many individuals perceive that they have changed greatly over time.[4] Older adults are more likely to report that over the years they have become less extroverted, less open to experience, and less conscientious in comparison to younger adults.[22] The importance of an individual's perception of their own personality change will be explored further in the next section on cognitive approaches to identity.

Personality traits and health outcomes

Of particular interest to health care professionals are the findings regarding the relationship between personality traits and health outcomes. Prior studies have demonstrated relationships among stress (e.g., bereavement,[2,24,25] caregiving,[26] psychiatric illness[2,27]), behavior patterns (e.g., loneliness or driven behaviors[9,26–28]), and decrements in immune functioning. Additionally, discrepant findings regarding the relationship between personality characteristics and cardiovascular disease have been reported. For example, hostility and anger have been found to be related to risk factors for coronary heart disease (CHD), but a direct influence of hostility on CHD has not been established.[29] Cross-sectional and longitudinal analyses using the Five Factor approach to personality, however, have found no relationship between traits and certain health outcomes. Specifically, no association between hypertension and personality characteristics was found, controlling for the effects of age on hypertension.[3] Personality traits as measured within the Five Factor theory also do not predict later development of coronary disease, and coronary disease does not predict future personality traits.[3]

Some findings on the relationship between personality traits and health that should be of interest to health care professionals involve the influence of personality on symptom presentation. Personality traits, such as neuroticism, have been found to predict future complaints of angina in individuals with no electrocardiogram (ECG) signs of disease. Individuals who were less emotionally stable were more likely to report angina than individuals who did not report angina but who had abnormal or suspicious ECGs 20 years later.[3] Thus, findings regarding the association among specific personality characteristics and poor health outcomes (e.g., risk of CHD)[9,25–28] may be discrepant, but several personality traits have been shown to relate to symptom presentation.[3] The influence of personality variables on both actual health outcomes and symptom presentation are important for health care professionals in terms of the implications for consideration of long-term prognoses, relating these prognoses to patients, and medical decision making.

Cross-sectional age differences

Previous findings from cross-sectional studies showing age differences in personality traits can often be attributed to cohort effects. Schaie and colleagues[2,23] have found evidence of several positive and negative cohort differences in personality traits. For example, results from the SLS suggest that some age differences in gender roles may be due to a cohort effect. In other words, the current cohort of older adults had more traditional gender-role divisions of labor than current middle-aged or young adult cohorts. Additionally, there were negative cohort trends demonstrating that recent birth cohorts possess less social responsibility than earlier-born cohorts. In other words, individuals who were young adults in 1984 report lower feelings of responsibility toward others than individuals who were young adults in the 1940s. Successive cohorts since the turn of the century have scored lower at the same chronological age than earlier cohorts on other personality traits such as low self-sentiment, affectothymia (i.e., active extraversion), untroubled adequacy (i.e., self-assurance), and premsia (i.e., tender-mindedness). Beginning with the baby boomers, however, birth cohorts are now showing increases in affectothymia, untroubled adequacy, and premsia. Other traits show consistent increases across birth cohorts from the turn of the century through the baby boom generation, including threctia (i.e., threat reactivity), conservatism of temperament, group dependency, and superego strength. Downturns after the baby boomers (e.g., Generation X) have been observed for the latter three traits. Again, these cohort differences in personality traits are important for health care professionals due to their potential impact on the health care professional-patient relationship across time. For example, discussing treatment options with a 70-year-old in 1996 may involve different skills and organizational behaviors than discussing treatment options with a 70-year-old in 2016, due to cohort differences in the level of self-reported personality traits.

Identity and the Self: A Cognitive Approach

Rather than focusing on the components of adult personality such as traits, cognitive approaches to identity focus on the processes underlying stability and change in one's perception of the self. Identity is viewed as a dynamic construct influenced by internal and environmental factors. Thus, both age-related change and cohort differences in identity outcome are possible. The processes themselves, however, would not be expected to change significantly across time or different birth cohorts.

Whitbourne's theory of adult identity emphasizes a life span approach to one's core identity development, which is distinguished from observable manifestations of identity.[2,30–33] In Whitbourne's conceptualization, identity forms an internal organizing schema through which an individual's lifelong experiences are interpreted.[33] This model rests on two constructs, the scenario, representing an individual's expectations for their life path, and the life story, the personal history constructed after significant events have occurred. Individuals attempt to differentiate their scenario and life story from societal norms and expectations.[2]

The scenario and life story are the key concepts around which individuals assess the success of their lives in meeting their personal life goals. Evaluations of personal success in achieving goals are conducted through the processes of assimilation and accommodation.[2,33] Assimilation refers to the interpretation of life events via the cognitive and affective schemes of identity.[33] Individuals' reaction to medical illness, for example, will partially be determined by their interpretation of the illness and its meaning in regard to identity. Accommodation, in contrast, refers to the modification of cognitive and affective schemas of identity in light of life experiences.[33] One example of a life experience that can effect identity is insight-oriented psychotherapy.[34] For successful aging, identity must be a dynamic construct involving both assimilation and accommodation.[33] The lack of equilibrium, or rigid adherence to one process of identity development, may result in negative health outcomes.

Summary of Stage, Trait, and Cognitive Approaches

Stage, trait, and cognitive approaches have made unique contributions to the study of stability and change in personality and identity across adulthood. Stage theories attempt to characterize individual development in terms of resolution of conflicts or unconscious processes in cognitive, affective, and behavioral domains. Trait theories have demonstrated substantial stability in personality characteristics, in spite of significant events in the lives of individuals and changes in society as a whole. Cognitive approaches to identity, in contrast, have provided a means of looking at the process of identity development and maintenance across time. It is likely that all three approaches to personality in adulthood have some validity. For example, Schaie[23] proposed that personality characteristics could be differentiated into categories reflecting (1) stable traits, (2) characteristics consistent with a stage model that change with age and are mostly impervious to cohort or societal influences, and (3) characteristics that are readily modifiable by age, cohort, and time period influences. We will now turn our attention to personality concepts derived from the field of social cognition. These include control beliefs, self-efficacy, and metamemory.

Social Cognition: Control Beliefs, Efficacy, and Metamemory

Social-cognitive approaches to the study of the self have focused on the individual's beliefs regarding one's competence and whether control of life outcomes lies within the individual or is the result of chance, luck, or the actions of others. One dimension of control is efficacy, the belief that one can accomplish a task or goal.[35–37] Health care professionals familiar with older patients who complain about their memory will recognize the importance of the concepts of control and efficacy in individuals' evaluations of memory functioning. There is ample evidence that control beliefs and self-efficacy influence health outcomes and health behaviors, and growing evidence that beliefs about one's memory may do likewise.[37,38]

Perceived Control

Perceived control is the belief that one can regulate and influence one's own internal states and behavior, influence one's environment, and bring about desired outcomes.[39,40] Control beliefs involve internal and external orientations. Internal control focuses on beliefs regarding the individual's ability to affect personal outcomes, whereas external beliefs focus on chance and the influence of other people on individual outcomes. Having a more internal sense of control has been found to be associated with better memory and intellectual functioning, as well as higher educational attainment and socioeconomic status. It is a negative predictor of mortality and a positive predictor of psychological well-being (e.g., less depression, more openness and assertiveness).[2]

Research involving the relationship of control and health outcomes has demonstrated that individuals who have external control beliefs have poorer health habits and more illnesses, and are less likely to take active steps to treat their illness than are people with a greater sense of internal control.[37] Additionally, beliefs regarding the locus of control (e.g., internal, external) influence whether or not an event will be appraised as stressful, and the degree of one's reaction to stress. Research evidence is mounting that stress and perceptions of lack of control are strongly related to immunosuppression in older adults.[24–28,39] Specifically, undesirable and uncontrollable events precipitate stress and have been associated with negative health outcomes.[39] In contrast, interventions to enhance feelings of control in the elderly have had a positive impact on health.[39] Distinguishing situations in which it is beneficial to increase an older adult's feelings of control regarding health-related outcomes from those in which such an intervention could be detrimental (i.e., perceived control is unrealistic) needs further investigation.

Much prior research focused on the dimensionality of the control construct. The meaning and impact of global measures of control versus more domain-specific measurement is considered next. We provide an overview of these issues with specific examples of domain-specific control in the areas of intellectual functioning and health. Stability and change in control beliefs will also be considered.

Multidimensionality of control

Rotter's[41,42] original theory conceptualized personal control as a unidimensional trait with internal and external orientations as polar endpoints of the same phenomenon. This idea has since been refuted on conceptual and empiric grounds.[42] Conceptually, it seems perfectly logical that one could have an internal control orientation but still acknowledge the role of external, chance circumstances in a particular outcome (e.g., obtaining employment). Additionally, factor analyses of Rotter's original scale have demonstrated multiple factors with low intercorrelations, such as efficacy, control ideology, and political control.[42] Therefore, the multidimensionality of control beliefs has general acceptance in the current research literature, with the most common conceptualization of control encompassing "internal," "chance," and "powerful others" dimensions. Chance and powerful others are dimensions of external control, differing in whether fate or influential others are viewed as the locus of control.

Global and domain-specific control beliefs

A second issue involves global versus domain-specific specific control beliefs. Research has demonstrated that individuals have general conceptualizations about their degree of control over environmental outcomes in addition to ideas about their degree of control over specific domains of life.[40,41] For example, Lachman and colleagues[44] developed perceived control scales specific to intellectual functioning and compared them to global measures of control in terms of their relationships with primary mental abilities. The authors found that intellectual locus of control scales were more highly associated with ability domains. In a 5-year longitudinal study, Lachman and Leff[43] found no age changes in generalized control beliefs, a finding that has been replicated by others.[15,42–45]

Intellectual locus of control

In contrast to findings regarding generalized control beliefs, Lachman and Leff found age changes in control orientation involving the specific domains of intellectual functioning and health. Specifically, they found that participants reported increases over the 5-year period in reliance on powerful others in intellectual and health domains. Interestingly, those with higher education were more likely to show longitudinal decrements in internal intellectual control. Perhaps these individuals were more sensitive to age changes in ability level, and adjusted their control beliefs accordingly. They also found that individuals who maintained better health status were less likely to show decreases in internal control. Lachman and Leff suggest that generalized control may remain stable because it is not tied to specific domains such as intellectual functioning or health in which decrements are more likely to be perceived with advancing age.

Health locus of control

Investigations of health locus of control have focused on issues such as the extent to which individual differences in perceived control influence outcomes in persons with chronic disease, or on how control orientation influences compliance with a medical regimen.[37,45,46] For example, nursing home residents given control over their activities or responsibility for house plant care have been shown to demonstrate higher satisfaction, greater activity levels, better health, and one-half the mortality rate in comparison with residents without control.[47] Rodin[39] reported that healthy individuals higher in internal health control were more likely to engage in health promotive behavior such as exercise and good nutrition. According to Wallston,[48] however, internal health control beliefs may exert their influence through affecting the relationship between health status and health-promoting behavior rather than directly affecting health status itself. In other words, the tendency of individuals of a given health status to engage in health-promoting behavior varies with the individuals' locus of control. Comparing the tendency to engage in health-promoting behavior of people who differ in control beliefs regardless of health status, however, shows little direct influence of control beliefs on preventive health behavior.

Regarding stability and change, older individuals have been found to have lower internal control and less desire for control over health issues than younger adults.[47–49] Additionally, older adults held stronger beliefs in the importance of powerful others regarding health concerns than did young adults. These findings coincide with findings from Lachman and Leff's[43] longitudinal study, which showed that participants reported an increase in external control beliefs, specifically in terms of control of powerful others, over a 5-year time period. Interestingly, recent factor analytic studies of health locus of control have shown that the powerful others dimension may be separated into "doctors" and "other people."[50]

Summary

Older adults who are faced with declines in cognitive functioning and physical health have stronger external control beliefs in the domains of intellectual functioning and health. Specifically, the importance of powerful others increases significantly with age.[15,42,45] Older adults believe increasingly that others are better able to accomplish tasks than they are themselves, potentially leading to increased dependence on others to accomplish tasks in the intellectual and health domains. External control beliefs are more likely to be adopted initially by those with more medical problems and lower fluid intelligence.[2,42,43] In these individuals, external control orientations may be an adaptive coping response to their life circumstances. Likewise, increases in external control orientation with age may be an adaptive accommodation of beliefs in light of declining abilities. Alternatively, increases in external control orientation could represent a response to societal age bias within older individuals themselves.

These findings are particularly important for health care professionals, as they are likely to be perceived as powerful others by older adults in both the intellectual and health domains. This places health care professionals in a unique position of influence not only for medical, but also for psychological and social interventions with older adults. For example, it is a common occurrence in geriatric medical clinics to find that family members want physicians and other health care professionals to intervene in order to keep the older adult patient from driving.

Efficacy

Self-efficacy, or mastery, is the degree to which an individual believes that he or she has the knowledge and skills necessary to achieve a certain outcome.[2,36] Like control beliefs, efficacy measures are multidimensional and domain specific.[36] Domain-linked measures of personal efficacy typically predict changes in functioning better than do general measures. Self-percepts of efficacy activate the individual to pursue difficult goals more vigorously. For example, individuals with high efficacy beliefs regarding their cognitive functioning are likely to expend great effort in cognitive tasks and to persevere in the face of setbacks or failures. In contrast, individuals with low self-efficacy in the cognitive realm are likely to believe that failure experiences are the result of deficient aptitude and are prone to stress and depression. A resilient sense of efficacy enhances sociocognitive functioning in many ways. Of interest to health care professionals, feelings of self-efficacy enhance the older respiratory patient's effort to rehabilitate from health crises.[37]

Stability and change

Study findings differ on whether efficacy, measured as a sense of internal control, is maintained across the adult life span. It appears that some individuals are able to maintain a stable sense of self-efficacy even in the face of declining abilities and stable or increasing environmental demands.[42] This stability can be accomplished by evaluating one's performance in a valued skill in comparison with age peers, as opposed to comparisons with one's prior performance.[35,36] For example, an older man may maintain a stable sense of efficacy in relation to his golf game by maintaining social comparisons of his game relative to the performance of his age peers. Were such a man to compare his game at age 70 to his game at age 25, he may experience a decrease in efficacy beliefs. Alternatively, stability in efficacy beliefs can be accomplished via Whitbourne's process of accommodation. In other words, one's evaluation of the importance of a given skill domain may vary with one's ability to accomplish relevant tasks in that domain.

The issue of stability in self-efficacy is of interest to health care professionals involved in evaluating an older adult's capacity to live alone.[51] Such individuals must evaluate the accuracy of older individuals' self-efficacy beliefs in the context of their ability to perform tasks necessary for independent living such as maintenance of household and finances. It is important for professionals to keep in mind that, when people err in self-appraisal, they tend to overestimate their abilities.[35,36]

One area in which the study of internal control and self-efficacy beliefs has proven to be particularly useful is in self evaluations of memory performance.[52,53] Berry et al.[52,53] assessed the psychometric properties of a domain-specific memory self-efficacy questionnaire in young adult and elderly samples. They found age differences in memory self-efficacy level, but not in memory self-efficacy strength. In other words, younger adults endorsed their ability to perform more difficult memory tasks than did older adults, but individuals within both age groups were equally confident that they could perform the level of tasks they endorsed. Health care professionals are likely to be placed in positions requiring the evaluation of older adults' memory performance and as such are likely to consider older adults' evaluation of their own memory performance. Findings from longitudinal and cross-sectional investigations of metamemory will be reviewed in the next section.

Metamemory Assessments and Memory Complaints

In a broad sense, "metamemory" refers to an individual's knowledge and awareness of memory ability, knowledge of the mechanisms involved in storage and retrieval of information, and the ability to cope with declining memory skills.[54,55] Metamemory involves at least four major dimensions: memory self-efficacy, factual knowledge about how memory functions and the use of memory strategies, memory monitoring, and memory-related affect (e.g., depression, anxiety).[2] Several memory self-assessment inventories have been developed, but only two have been recommended for general use: (1) the Metamemory in Adulthood Questionnaire (MIA)[56–58] and (2) the Memory Functioning Questionnaire (MFQ).[59–62] Analyses of these instruments have shown that metamemory is a multidimensional concept.[57,60]

One dimension of metamemory involves memory complaints. Health care professionals with older patients are likely to encounter older individuals who present with memory complaints. Previous findings suggest that between 38 and 80 percent of older adults report subjective memory deficits.[61,63,64] Therefore, it is crucial that health care professionals understand the relationship between individuals' evaluation of their memory ability and actual memory performance. For example, memory complaints may not be specific indicators of concurrent cognitive decline.[62–66] Complaints vary with depressive symptoms, pessimism, or general psychopathology at the time of assessment.[67–69] In other words, individuals may rate their memory performance as worse than it really is as assessed by objective memory tests if they are depressed or have other psychopathology. Therefore, reliance on self-reports of memory functioning for insight into concurrent memory performance is problematic. Some investigators claim that one reason for the modest association between concurrent memory performance and metamemory is that the metamemorial abilities of older adults free of psychopathology do not keep pace with changes in actual memory skills.[70] They propose that older adults are likely to make predictions based on their past performance, and that their subjective evaluations of ability have not been adjusted for actual decline in ability over time. Therefore, assessment of memory complaints should include objective assessments of memory performance or reports from collateral sources.

Longitudinal investigations of metamemory evaluations and memory complaints

Until recently, there has been a paucity of research addressing the very question in which health care professionals are most likely to be interested: Do memory complaints predict subsequent memory decline?[38,64] Flicker and colleagues[64] conducted a longitudinal investigation of memory complaints and memory performance in 59 healthy (i.e., nondemented) individuals ranging from 60 to 84 years of age and having subjective memory complaints. At the 3-year follow-up, they found little evidence of progressive cognitive deterioration among the participants. There was evidence of decline in performance on only two of 12 tests in the assessment battery; these tests (vocabulary and category retrieval) assessed language ability. What is remarkable about these findings is that all participants were selected due to subjective complaints of memory loss, and thus should have demonstrated declines in performance if complaints were a reflection of early changes in memory ability. In contrast, Johansson et al. investigated the predictive utility of metamemorial judgments for subsequent decline in memory performance and subsequent diagnosis of dementia in a sample of individuals over 80 years of age.[38] They assessed metamemory evaluations, memory ability, and diagnosis of dementia across 6 years in a Swedish sample of the oldest old.[38] In contrast to the results of Flicker, these authors found that in cognitively intact individuals, metamemory evaluations at Time 1 predicted decline on specific tests of everyday memory and subsequent diagnosis of dementia at later testing occasions. Further research is needed to determine if this finding is due to the everyday nature of the memory tasks or the age of the participants.

Memory training

Health care professionals who see elderly patients with memory complaints may wish to refer these individuals to memory training programs, some of which have demonstrated modest ability to improve the memory performance of older adults.[67] For example, older adults with higher initial levels of internal intellectual control show the greatest training gains in intellectual functioning.[42] Lachman and Leff[43] suggest that individuals with higher internal control beliefs may profit most from training because they are most likely to persevere and are most motivated to improve performance. Research on memory training focuses on training older adults in the use of encoding strategies, affective components, and self-efficacy beliefs.[2,71–73] The effects of memory training may be more pronounced, however, in improving metamemory evaluations than in actually improving memory performance.

Several investigators have proposed that memory training in cognitive skills can produce more generalized and lasting effects if it raises self-efficacy beliefs as well as imparts skills.[35,36,74,75] For example, Dittmann-Kohli, et al.[74] examined the effects of different types of training on fluid abilities, everyday competence, and self-efficacy beliefs. The authors demonstrated that ability training and practice improved the cognitive performance of older adults, but only ability training resulted in increased self-efficacy for specific cognitive tasks.[74] Increases in efficacy were found only in regard to self-assessment of ability to perform the tests in which training occurred. There were no increases in general perceived efficacy or efficacy for nontrained cognitive measures.[74]

In a similar study examining the effects of different interventions on memory performance and memory self-efficacy, older adults' beliefs about the controllability of their memory were improved.[75] The most effective intervention consisted of cognitive restructuring plus self-generated memory strategy training, which was shown to increase favorable evaluations of memory in older adults. In contrast, memory self-efficacy was not improved by memory training that focused on self-generated memory skills. Certain interventions were effective in increasing the tendency of participants to report spontaneous use of memory strategies. Both the memory skills alone and the memory skills plus cognitive restructuring interventions were shown to increase spontaneous use of memory strategies in comparison with practice, cognitive restructuring only, and no-contact interventions. The authors concluded that older adults need direct intervention focused on beliefs about memory in order to develop awareness of the potential for improvement.[75]

Summary of Perceived Control Efficacy and Metamemory

Cognitive approaches to personality encompass control beliefs, self-efficacy beliefs, and metamemory. In general, individuals maintain their sense of efficacy into later adulthood, but develop increased belief in external control (e.g., powerful others) and evaluate their memory skills more poorly. As many as 80 percent of older adults complain that their memory skills have deteriorated.

Given recent findings that the powerful others dimension of control may be separated into doctors and other people,[50] health care professionals may represent a uniquely powerful force for intervention into the lives of older adults. Understanding the impact of internal control beliefs and self-efficacy can help health care professionals design treatments that fit the unique dispositions of adult patients. For example, individuals who assume primary responsibility for their own intellectual and health outcomes, and who believe they can accomplish a lifestyle change may respond to simple treatment recommendations to reduce stress, exercise, quit smoking, or improve nutrition. In contrast, those who believe their intellectual functioning and health are the result of fate and that nothing they as individuals can do will change their outcome, may not comply with such treatment recommendations and may need further intervention. Health care professionals need to consider the impact of personality variables on the decision-making abilities of patients across the adult life span. This interface will be explored in the next section.

Interface of Personality and Cognition

In this section, we review research concerning the relationship between control beliefs and primary mental abilities, wisdom, and the relationship between behavioral flexibility and cognition. We also present a stage model of adult intellectual development designed to encompass the impact of personality on the application of cognition to the pursuit of career and family. With knowledge of the impact of personality on cognitive competency across the adult life span, health care professionals and other professionals can effectively involve patients in treatment planning.

Cognitive Abilities and Control Beliefs

Intelligence has been defined as the capacity for learning or making wise choices, the ability to manipulate symbols, and proficiency in cognitive performance.[2] Currently, most researchers accept a multidimensional view of intelligence.[2,9,23] For example, Schaie's SLS conceptualizes intelligence as the aggregate of several unique primary mental abilities. These include verbal meaning, word fluency, number, spatial orientation, inductive reasoning, semantic memory, and perceptual speed.[2,23] Other researchers aggregate different abilities into higher-order dimensions. For instance, Baltes[76] differentiates between the mechanics (or basic processes) of intellectual functioning versus the pragmatics (or substantive content and life experience) of intelligence. Likewise, Horn and Cattell separate intelligence into fluid (e.g., inductive reasoning, spatial orientation) and crystallized (e.g., verbal meaning) dimensions.[2,23,77,78] In this review, we will use the concepts of fluid and crystallized intelligence in discussing the relation of control beliefs to primary mental abilities.

Stability and change in cognitive abilities

Schaie has shown that there is little longitudinal decline in the primary mental abilities until the mid-sixties.[2,23,77,78] In general, fluid abilities show earlier decrements with age, and crystallized abilities show stability in midlife and decline in the mid-seventies.[2,77–79] There are, however, vast individual differences in the rate of decline. For example, Schaie[79] demonstrated that at least 75 percent of those over age 53 maintained their ability level to age 60. Seventy percent of SLS participants at or beyond age 74 showed no change over the previous 7 years. Even by age 81, 60 percent of healthy, community-dwelling participants remained at a stable level of performance across the 7-year testing frame. Many of the differences in ability level between the current cohorts of young and old adults can be attributed to differences among generations in such attributes as education, health care, and health behavior.[2]

The relationship of control beliefs and abilities

Most studies have examined the relationship between control beliefs and cognitive ability at the same point in time. In contrast, relatively few research studies have explored the relationship of control beliefs and ability across time. The results of two longitudinal studies demonstrate that fluid intelligence and everyday task competence predict future intellectual control beliefs, but control beliefs do not predict future intellectual performance.[43,80] Specifically, individuals with lower fluid intelligence have shown greater increases in powerful-others-control beliefs over a subsequent 5-year period.[43] Additionally, better performance of everyday tasks has been shown to predict high self-efficacy beliefs 7 years later.[80] The finding that cognitive performance predicts future control beliefs is of interest due to its potential impact on medical practice. Just as training individuals' cognitive abilities can improve their performance now and reduce their risk of decline in the future,[2,81,82] educating older adults in coping with chronic illness before significant health problems occur may help individuals feel a greater sense of efficacy in the future when illnesses arise. Planning for future contingencies of life is part of wisdom.

Wisdom and Personality

Baltes and his colleagues[74] define wisdom as an expert knowledge system in the fundamental pragmatics of life (i.e., life experience), permitting individuals to exercise insight and to dispense advice on complex matters of the human condition. In their conceptualization, wisdom consists of the following criteria: (1) factual knowledge, (2) procedural knowledge, (3) life-span contextualism, (4) value relativism, and (5) ability to manage uncertainty. Procedural knowledge involves obtaining information, giving advice, and considering possible outcomes. Life-span contextualism deals with consideration of life stage, societal context, and individual priorities in the decision-making process. Value relativism is the ability to consider the values and opinions of others as well as one's own. Thus, in order to be considered wise, one must possess knowledge of one's own strengths and weaknesses, and plan to optimize the ratio between gains and losses in decision making and outcomes.

Using problem-solving tasks involving stage-appropriate life planning and existential crises, Baltes and colleagues have shown that younger and older adults do not differ in the ability to produce responses judged to be wise.[83,84] Older adults produce wiser responses, however, given problems to solve that are specific to their own age group.[2] Regarding the interface of wisdom and personality, studies suggest that longevity and greater openness to experience are necessary but not sufficient preconditions to the development of wisdom.[2,83] That is, individuals with more flexible lifestyles, beliefs, and attitudes may have greater exposure to and experience with dilemmas involving the fundamental matters of life. Thus, these individuals would be afforded greater opportunity to develop wisdom.

This hypothesis has received some support in studies showing that clinical psychologists and individuals nominated as wise (by prominent members of the press in Berlin, Germany) demonstrate higher levels of performance in wisdom-related tasks in comparison with professionals from disciplines outside the human service field.[83,84] Both clinical psychologists and prominent members of society considered by peers to exhibit wisdom would be expected to possess expertise, exposure to problems defining the human condition, and experience with the resolution of such problems.

Flexibility/Rigidity and Cognition

An important aspect of wisdom appears to be behavioral flexibility. One of the original premises of the SLS was that longitudinal changes in primary mental abilities might be related to an individual's degree of behavioral flexibility/rigidity.[23] Three cognitive style factors have been identified that represent unique domains of adult behavior separate from conceptions of intelligence or mental abilities: psychomotor speed, motor/cognitive flexibility, and attitudinal flexibility.[23,85]

Stability and change in flexibility/rigidity

Schaie and Willis[86] examined individual change and cohort differences in the observed measures constituting the Tests of Behavioral Rigidity for the first five waves of the SLS. In general, considerable stability across time was found within individuals regarding flexibility characteristics. In contrast, results showed substantial cohort differences in flexible personality styles and psychomotor speed tests. Regarding attitudinal, behavioral, and associational flexibility, substantial generational differences were found such that older adults (i.e., earlier-born cohorts) were shown to be less flexible as a result of their socialization.[86] Additionally, there were modest maturational changes in these measures, showing that attitudinal, behavioral, and associational flexibility increase through young adulthood and then decline from age 60.

Relationship of flexibility/rigidity and abilities

Significant concurrent relationships have been found between various mental abilities and different dimensions of flexibility. Longitudinal data indicate that flexible personality style at midlife reduces the risk of cognitive decline in later adulthood.[23] Specifically, cognitive style in midlife predicts the latent constructs of verbal and numeric ability in old age. Early cognitive abilities, however, do not predict later behavioral flexibility style. The predictive utility of flexibility measures for future cognitive performance may be of assistance to professionals in helping older adults plan for future health contingencies. Certain personality characteristics are associated with risk of future cognitive decline. Stated differently, personality can impact cognitive outcomes. This idea has been explored by Schaie in his stage model of adult intellectual development.

Stage of Intellectual Development

Historically, theories of intellectual development have focused on the acquisition of knowledge during childhood, adolescence, and young adulthood. In contrast, Schaie[2] proposed that Piaget's stages of intellectual development could be extended into adulthood, but that the focus must shift from the acquisition of knowledge to the application of knowledge. He proposed four stages of adult intellectual development. The *achieving* stage occurs in young adulthood and includes using one's knowledge in the establishment of career and family. Thus, the focus in this stage is the pursuit of individual long-term goals. Attending to the context and consequences of critical choices is necessary because the consequences of making a mistake are severe. In other words, mistakes can have detrimental effects in the success of establishing careers and families.

The second stage of adult intellectual development in Schaie's model is the *responsible* stage. This stage involves the application of cognitive skills to situations involving social responsibility and typically occurs in middle adulthood.[2] Individual goals must be considered and balanced with the needs of others in the family. An optional extension of the responsible stage experienced by a subset of adults is the *executive* stage, involving management of larger social groups and parts of organizations. Whether or not an individual will enter the executive stage depends on internal individual characteristics and motives, choice of career, and exposure to opportunities facilitating the rise.

Schaie's final stage of adult intellectual development is *reintegration*.[2] In this stage, the need to acquire new knowledge or to use existing knowledge in the realms of family and work has decreased. Thus, the acquisition and use of knowledge becomes more strongly tied to an individual's auxiliary interests, attitudes, and values. Individuals may begin to pursue hobbies or engage in activities for the first time as they identify new areas of interest for growth. Like other stage models, Schaie's model focuses on individual change rather than the possibility of intergenerational shifts in stage content or sequence.

Summary of the Personality and Cognition Interface

In this section, we examined research concerning the relationship between personality and cognition. Specifically, we reviewed research regarding the interface of control beliefs and mental abilities, wisdom, and flexibility. We also considered Schaie's stage model of adult intellectual development. The directionality of relationships between personality and cognition varies across dimensions. Several studies indicate prior cognitive ability influences subsequent control beliefs. The personality dimension of flexibility, however, has been shown to impact cognitive functioning in old age.

The interface of personality and cognition is of interest to professionals working with individuals across the adult life span due to the need for planning for future contingencies. Not only do personality variables influence the likelihood of individuals to plan for future needs, they can also influence future cognitive ability. Several investigators have suggested that motivation is also an important aspect of personality and cognition. We will now consider findings regarding motivation and its influence in adulthood.

Motivation

Although intuitively the concept of motivation has meaning, operational definitions of motivation vary and there is no comprehensive theory of motivational influence across the adult lifespan.[2,87] Instead, research interest has focused on the stability and change of specific types of motivation, such as anxiety and need for achievement. Maslow's[88] hierarchy of needs attempts to organize human motivations ranging from physiological needs necessary for the survival of the individual or the species to higher-order motives that are acquired through socialization.[2,88] We will review Maslow's conceptualization of human motivation, and then discuss findings regarding stability and change in anxiety, need for achievement, and emotion.

Overview of Maslow's Hierarchy of Needs

In Maslow's scheme, we are not pushed by drives, but pulled by needs to be fulfilled.[89] Lower needs must be met before the pursuit of higher-order needs begins. The most basic and paramount needs are *physiologic*, consisting of hunger, thirst, and sexual needs. *Safety and security needs* are next, and include the need for protection from danger, freedom from fear, and the need for stability, law, and order. Once safety and physiologic needs are met, individuals' need for *love and belongingness* emerges. In Maslow's next stage are those needs related to self-esteem. We need to respect ourselves, and we need the respect of others. At the top of Maslow's basic hierarchy is the need for *self-actualization*, the desire to become everything that one is capable of becoming. Once individuals reach self-actualization, even higher-order needs or "meta-needs" may emerge.[89] These include the pursuit of beauty, truth, or justice, which are expressed simultaneously in various degrees of intensity. Once experienced, the higher needs may become more compelling than lower needs.[2]

Basic Biologic Needs and the Influence of Socialization and Context

Maslow postulated that lower needs are basic processes determined by biology. Research has shown that physiologic changes affect eating and drinking behavior across the adult life span. As people age, they experience decrements in taste and olfaction, drops in basal metabolic rate due to slowing of the central nervous system, and changes in the hypothalamus leading to changes in the ability to regulate blood sugar levels.[2] All of these physiologic changes may lead to decreased food consumption in late adulthood.

It has been argued that even these basic needs reflect not only physiology but also cultural expectations, socialization, and learning.[2] For example, in this society, eating behavior is a reflection of cultural expectations of body image and the need for socialization. In young adulthood, eating disorders such as anorexia nervosa and bulimia flourish in young women.[90] In older adulthood, many social activities (i.e., at church or senior centers) revolve around meals. Older adults may therefore have difficulty with weight gain. In contrast, after bereavement, motivation to eat may decline because one must eat alone. Therefore, the study of such basic physiologic needs should take into account psychological processes and cognition.[2]

Anxiety

Needs for safety and security are threatened by the experience of anxiety. When faced with a situation perceived as threatening, individuals experience a set of autonomic symptoms and increased arousal, motivating a "fight or flight" response. Spielberger differentiates two types of anxiety: (1) trait anxiety and (2) state anxiety.[2] Individuals high in trait anxiety are likely to feel anxious in many situations. In contrast, state anxiety is a temporary experience specific to a certain situation. Costa and McCrae have shown that, as is characteristic of other traits, trait anxiety is a relatively stable characteristic of a person.[3,4,20,21] Research findings also suggest that state anxiety may decrease with age.[2,87]

Achievement Motivation

Achievement motivation is the desire to succeed in behaviors that will be evaluated by others or by oneself in terms of some standard of excellence.[2] Cross-sectional studies have found that the need for achievement was lower at older ages, except for single-career women.[2] One of the most frequently cited studies on achievement motivation is the AT&T study.[91] In this longitudinal study of employees of AT&T, achievement motivation is divided into the following components: (1) need for advancement and (2) inner work standards. Need for advancement is motivation to advance in one's career faster and further than one's peers. Inner work standards refers to having one's own high standards of work performance and motivation to perform to the best of one's ability. Howard and Bray[91] show that need for advancement declines across time, but internal work standards remain relatively stable, particularly for those individuals who achieve career success. Therefore, older workers who have been successful in their careers are likely to remain productive due to their personal commitment to quality work. Because careers and career success are partially individually defined, this stability in achievement motivation may be as applicable to homemakers as it is to executives.

In general, a domain-specific approach to the study of motivation may prove more fruitful than pursuing the elusive global concept. One area of interest to professionals working with older adults involves their motivation to engage in social relationships. It is toward a discussion of recent theories addressing this underlying need for affiliation to which we now turn.

Socioemotional Selectivity Theory

Selectivity theory proposes that purposeful selective reductions in social interaction begin in early adulthood, and that emotional closeness remains stable or increases within selected relationships as one ages.[92–94] In other words, adults select social relationships in which they want to invest their resources and in which they expect reciprocity, thereby optimizing their social contacts. Thus, older adults' social networks may shrink by choice, as individuals decrease contact with acquaintances but seek to maintain contact with certain relatives and close friends into their eighties and beyond.[92–94]

As one ages, there is greater emotional attachment invested in each chosen relationship. This idea is supported by the finding that older adults reduce the amount of social support they provide to others, while the amount of perceived support received from others does not change.[95] Thus, older adults with limited social contact may still perceive their social networks as supportive. Part of this perceived satisfaction may result from continuity in the quality of social interactions. Close social interactions that are evaluated positively are marked by reciprocity; that is, support is given and received by each member of the relationship.[96–102] This finding has important implications for professionals working with older adults in terms of judging the impact of social support networks on health status and health behavior. Specifically, it is important not to underestimate the beneficial health effects of relatively small social networks in which older adults still feel a sense of reciprocity.

A great body of research has shown that social support is related to health outcomes and behaviors, but the mechanisms by which social support influences health are less well understood. Social support during acute and chronic stressful events can attenuate decrements in immune functioning.[95,103] Additionally, previous research has shown that support and reciprocity can moderate the stressful effects of bereavement on depressive symptomatology.[101,102] Interestingly, bereaved individuals with high rates of reciprocity in their remaining support network may experience *greater* depressive symptoms.[102] This could be due to experiencing and utilizing the opportunity to grieve afforded by such a network, given the expectation that one's basic needs would be met. As would be expected following the resolution of grief, the relation between illness and bereavement was found to decrease over time.[104]

Additionally, previous research has shown that social support influences preventive health behaviors.[95,101–105] Previous findings illustrate that performance of preventive health behaviors that do not typically present imminent health benefits (e.g., seat belt usage, dental checkups, medical checkups) was related to feelings of personal control, higher socioeconomic status, and more frequent interactions with nonkin. In contrast, those preventive behaviors involving direct risk to health status (e.g., smoking, poor driving, poor personal hygiene) were only related to demographic variables such as older age and gender.[95] Specifically, older adults and women were *less* likely to smoke or demonstrate poor personal hygiene.

Synthesis of Findings and Future Directions

In this chapter, we reviewed the psychological literature concerning personality stability and change within and among individuals across the adult life span. We considered stage and trait theories and cognitive approaches to the study of personality in adulthood.

Consideration of cognitive approaches to personality lead to a review of research regarding stability and change in control beliefs, efficacy, and metamemory. The interface of personality and cognition was then considered in relation to control beliefs, primary mental abilities, the development of wisdom, and behavioral flexibility. Finally, we reviewed stability and change in motivation and socioemotionality across adulthood.

In general, personality characteristics, particularly when studied as traits, remain stable across the adult life span, but there is also evidence of plasticity and development. For example, aging brings with it the opportunity for the development of wisdom. Personality characteristics have been shown to influence current and future cognitive performance, such that individuals who are more open to experience and are more flexible are likely to maintain cognitive functioning.

There is also a great deal of evidence of generational or cohort differences in personality characteristics. This is important for professionals to bear in mind because older adults of tomorrow are not likely to interact with others or react to events in the same manner as older adults of today. Perhaps educational interventions undertaken with individuals in middle adulthood currently may help them to maintain a sense of individual efficacy in intellectual and health domains in later adulthood.

There is powerful evidence that personality dimensions can influence symptom presentation and thus interactions with medical professionals. There is also evidence that some aspects of personality can effect general health. For example, personality influences response to stress, choice of coping mechanisms, and motivation, which then influence health and health-related functioning. Personality traits per se, however, seem to have their greatest influence over health perceptions and complaints. Thus, even if personality characteristics do not exert direct influence on health outcomes, personality characteristics across the adult life span are likely to significantly impact the medical professional-patient relationship. Due to the perceived importance of doctors and possibly other health care professionals as sources of external control, these interactions may have significant impact on older adults' quality of life.

With the aging of society, questions regarding quality of life, the medical care of infirm older adults, and the allocation of limited medical resources have arisen. Questions such as at what point should the decision not to prolong life be made and who should make this decision have become not only the topic of research but also of legislation.[106] Therefore, the implications of the relation among the aging personality, cognition, motivation, and interactions with health care professionals are of great importance for society as a whole. Future development of knowledge of psychosocial issues across the adult life span is critical to ensuring an adequate quality of life for us all.

Acknowledgment

Preparatrion of this chapter was supported by funding from the National Institute on Aging to K. W. Schaie (R01AG08055) and to Sherry L. Willis (R01AG11032). R. Allen-Burge received postdoctoral funding by Training Grant MH 18904-07 from the National Institute of Mental Health.

References

1. Allport GW: Personality. Holt, Rinehart, and Winston, New York, 1937
2. Schaie KW, Willis SL: Adult Development and Aging, 4th Ed. Harper Collins, New York, 1996
3. Shock NW, Greulich RC, Andres R et al: Normal Human Aging: The Baltimore Longitudinal Study of Aging. National Institute of Health, Washington, DC, 1984
4. McCrae RR, Costa PT: Personality in Adulthood. Guilford Press, New York, 1990
5. Erikson EH: Childhood and Society. 2nd Ed. Norton, New York, 1960
6. Loevinger J, Wessler R: Measuring Ego Development 1. Construction and Use of a Sentence Completion Test. Jossey-Bass, San Francisco, 1970
7. Loevinger J: Ego Development: Conception and Theory. Jossey-Bass, San Francisco, 1976
8. Freud S: Three essays on the theory of sexuality. In Freud S (ed): The Standard Edition, Vol. VII. Hogarth, London, 1953
9. Cavanaugh JC: Adult Development and Aging. 2nd Ed. Brooks/Cole, Pacific Grove, CA, 1993
10. Jung CG: Analytical Psychology: Its Theory and Practice. Vintage, New York, 1968
11. Guttman DL: The cross-cultural perspective: notes toward a comparative psychology of aging. In Birren JE, Schaie KW (eds): Handbook of the Psychology of Aging. 1st Ed. Van Nostrand Reinhold, New York, 1977
12. Guttman DL: Reclaimed Powers: Toward a New Psychology of Men and Women in Later Life. Basic Books, New York, 1987
13. Guttman DL: Toward a dynamic geropsychology. pp. 284–295. In Barren J, Eagle M, Welitzky D (eds): Interface of Psychoanalysis and Psychology. American Psychological Association, Washington, DC, 1992
14. Walsh WB, Betz NE: Tests and Assessment. Prentice-Hall, Englewood Cliffs, New Jersey, 1985
15. Kogan N. Personality and aging. pp. 330–340. In Birren JE, Schaie KW (eds): Handbook of the Psychology of Aging. (3rd Ed) Academic Press, New York, 1990
16. Butler RN, Lewis MI: Aging and Mental Health. 3rd Ed. CV Mosby, St. Louis, MO, 1982
17. Whitbourne SK, Zuschlag MK, Elliot LB, Waterman AS: Psychosocial development in adulthood: a 22-year sequential study. J Personality Soc Psychol 1992;63:260–271
18. Blanchard-Fields F: Reasoning on social dilemmas varying in emotional saliency: an adult developmental study. Psychol Aging 1986;1:325–333
19. Labouvie-Vief G, Hakim-Larson J, Hobart CJ: Age, ego level, and the life-span development of coping and defense processes. Psychol Aging 1987;2:286–283
20. Costa PT, McCrae RR: Personality continuity and the changes of adult life. pp. 45–77. In Storandt M, VandenBos GR (eds): The Adult Years: Continuity and Change. American Psychological Association, Washington, DC, 1989
21. McCrae RR, Costa PT: Emerging Lives, Enduring Dispositions. Little, Brown and Co., Boston, 1984
22. Ryff CD, Heincke SG: Subjective organization of personality in adulthood and aging. J Personality Soc Psychol 1983;44: 807–816
23. Schaie KW: Intellectual Development in Adulthood: The Seattle Longitudinal Study. Cambridge, New York, 1996
24. Morley JE, Powers DC: Psychoneuroimmunology and aging. J Am Geriatr Soc 1993;41:572–573
25. Willis L, Thomas P, Garry PJ, Goodwin JS: A prospective study of response to stressful life events in initially healthy elders. J Gerontol 1987;42:627–630
26. Kiecolt-Glaser JK, Dura JR, Speicher CE et al: Spousal care-

givers of dementia victims: longitudinal changes in immunity and health. Psychosom Med 1991;53:345–362

27. Kiecolt-Glaser JK, Glaser R, Williger D et al. Psychosocial enhancement of immunocompetence in a geriatric population. Health Psychol 1985;4:25–41
28. Kiecolt-Glaser JK, Glaser R: Psychoneuroimmunology: can psychological interventions modulate immunity? J Consulting and Clinical Psychol 1992;60:569–575
29. Siegler IC: Hostility and risk: demographic and lifestyle variables. pp. 199–214. In Siegman AW, Smith TW (eds): Anger, Hostility, and the Heart. Lawrence Erlbaum Associates, Hillsdale, NJ, 1994
30. Whitbourne SK: The psychological construction of the life span. In Birren JE, Schaie KW (eds): Handbook of the Psychology of Aging (2nd Ed). Van Nostrand Reinhold New York, 1985
31. Whitbourne SK: The Me I Know: A Study of Adult Identify. Springer-Verlag, New York, 1986
32. Whitbourne SK: Openness to experience, identity flexibility, and life change in adults. J Personality Soc Psychol 1986;50: 163–168
33. Whitbourne SK, Angiullo LM: The developing self in midlife. In Willis SL, Reid JD (eds): Life in the Middle. Academic Press, San Diego (in press)
34. Garfield SL, Bergin AE: Handbook of Psychotherapy and Behavior Change. 3rd Ed. John Wiley & Sons, New York, 1986
35. Bandura A: Social Foundations of Thought and Action: A Social Cognitive Theory. Prentice-Hall, Englewood Cliffs, NJ, 1986
36. Bandura A: Regulation of cognitive processes through perceived self-efficacy. Develop Psychol 1989;25:729–735
37. Sarafino EP: Health Psychology: Biopsychosocial Interactions. 2nd Ed. John Wiley & Sons, New York, 1994
38. Johansson B, Allen-Burge R, Zarit SH: Self reports on memory functioning in a longitudinal study of the oldest old: relation to current, prospective, and retrospective performance. J Gerontol Psychol Sci 1997;52B:139–140
39. Rodin J: Health, control, and aging. pp. 139–165. In Baltes MM, Baltes PB (eds): The Psychology of Control and Aging. Erlbaum, Hillsdale, New Jersey, 1986
40. Wallston KA, Wallston BS, Smith S, Dobbins CJ: Perceived control and health. Curr Psychol Res Rev 1987;6:5–25
41. Rotter JB: Generalized expectancies for internal versus external control of reinforcement. Psychol Monogr 1966;80:609
42. Lachman ME: Personal control in later life: stability, change, and cognitive correlates. pp. 207–236. In Baltes MM, Baltes PB (eds): The Psychology of Control and Aging. Erlbaum, Hillsdale, New Jersey, 1986
43. Lachman ME, Leff R: Perceived control and intellectual functioning in the elderly: a 5-year longitudinal study. Develop Psychol 1989;25:722–728
44. Lachman ME, Baltes PB, Nesselroade JR, Willis SL: Examination of personality-ability relationships in the elderly: the role of the contextual (interface) assessment mode. J Res Personality 1982;16:485–501
45. Gatz M, Siegler IC, George LK, Tyler FB: Attributional components of locus of control: longitudinal, retrospective, and contemporaneous analyses. pp. 237–263. In Baltes MM, Baltes PB (eds): The Psychology of Control and Aging. Erlbaum, Hillsdale, New Jersey, 1986
46. Wallston BS, Wallston KA, Kaplan GD, Maides SA: Development and validation of the Health Locus of Control (HLC) scale. J Consult Clin Psychol 1976;44:580–585
47. Rodin J, Langer E: Long-term effect of a control-relevant intervention. J Personality Soc Psychol 1977;35:897–902
48. Wallston KA: Hocus-pocus, the focus isn't strictly on locus: Rotter's social learning theory modified for health. Cog Therapy Res 1992;16:183–199
49. Smith RP, Woodward NJ, Wallston BS et al: Health care implications of desire and expectancy for control in elderly adults. J Gerontol 1988;43:P1–P7
50. Wallston KA, Stein MJ, Smith CA: Form C of the MHLC scales: a condition-specific measure of locus of control. J Personality Assessment 1994;63:534–553
51. Willis SL: Assessing everyday competence in the cognitively challenged elderly. pp. 81–126. In Smyer MA, Schaie KW, Kapp M (eds): Older Adults' Decision-Making and the Law. Springer, New York, 1996
52. Berry JM, West RL, Dennehey DM: Reliability and validity of the memory self-efficacy questionnaire. Develop Psychol 1989;25:701–713
53. Lachman ME, Steinberg ES, Trotter SD: Effects of control beliefs and attributions on memory self-assessments and performance. Psychol Aging 1987;2:266–271
54. Devolder PA, Pressley M: Metamemory across the adult lifespan. Can Psychol 1989;30:578–587
55. Flavell JH: What is memory development the development of? Hum Develop 1971;14:272–278
56. Dixon RA, Hultsch DF, Hertzog C: The metamemory in adulthood (MIA) questionnaire. Psychopharmacol Bull 1988;24: 671–688
57. Hertzog C, Dixon RA, Hultsch DF: Relationships between metamemory, memory predictions, and memory task performance in adults. Psychol Aging 1990;5:215–227
58. Hultsch DF, Hertzog C, Dixon RA: Age differences in metamemory: resolving the inconsistencies. Can J Psychol 1987;41: 193–208
59. Gilewski MJ, Zelinski EM: Memory functioning questionnaire (MFQ). Psychopharmacol Bull 1988;24:665–670
60. Gilewski MJ, Zelinski EM, Schaie KW: The memory functioning questionnaire for assessment of memory complaints in adulthood and old age. Psychol Aging 1990;5:482–490
61. Zelinski EM, Gilewski MJ: Assessment of memory complaints by rating scales and questionnaires. Psychopharmacol Bull 1988;24:523–529
62. Zelinski EM, Gilewski MJ, Anthony-Bergstone CR: Memory functioning questionnaire: Concurrent validity with memory performance and self-reported memory failures. Psychol Aging 1990;5:388–399
63. Bolla KI, Lindgren KN, Bonaccorsy C, Bleecker ML: Memory

complaints in older adults: fact or fiction? Arch Neurol 1991; 48:61–64

64. Flicker C, Ferris SH, Reisberg B. A longitudinal study of cognitive function in elderly persons with subjective memory complaints. J Am Geriatr Soc 1993;41:1029–1032
65. Scogin F, Bienias JL: A three-year follow-up of older adult participants in a memory-skills training program. Psychol Aging 1988;3:334–337
66. Scogin F, Storandt M, Lott L: Memory skills training, memory complaints, and depression in older adults. J Gerontol 1985; 40:562–568
67. Scogin F, Prohaska M: Aiding Older Adults with Memory Complaints. Professional Resource Press, Sarasota, FL, 1993
68. Burt DB, Zembar MJ, Niederehe G: Depression and memory impairment: a meta-analysis of the association, its pattern, and specificity. Psychol Bull 1995;117:285–305
69. Kahn RL, Zarit SH, Hilbert NM, Niederehe G. Memory complaint and impairment in the aged. Arch Gen Psychiatry 1975; 32:1569–1573
70. Bruce PR, Coyne AC, Botwinick J: Adult age differences in metamemory. J Gerontol 1982;17:354–357
71. Yesavage J, Lapp D, Sheikh JA: Mnemonics as modified for use by the elderly. In Poon LW, Rubin D, Wilson B (eds). Everyday Cognition in Adulthood and Late Life. Cambridge University Press, Cambridge, England, 1989
72. Zarit SH, Cole KD, Guider RL: Memory training strategies and subjective complaints of memory in the aged. Gerontologist 1981;21:158–165
73. Zarit SH, Gallagher D, Kramer N: Memory training in the community aged: effects of depression, memory complaint, and memory performance. Educational Gerontol 1981;6:11–27
74. Dittmann-Kohli F, Lachman ME, Kliegl R, Baltes PB: Effects of cognitive training and testing on intellectual efficacy beliefs in elderly adults. J Gerontol Psychol Sci 1991;46: P162–P164
75. Lachman ME, Weaver SL, Bandura M et al: Improving memory and control beliefs through cognitive restructuring and self-generated strategies. J Gerontol Psychol Sci 1992;47: P293–P299
76. Baltes PB: The aging mind: potential and limits. Gerontologist 1993;33:580–594
77. Schaie KW: Intellectual development in adulthood. pp. 291–309. In Birren JE, Schaie KW (eds): Handbook of the Psychology of Aging. 3rd Ed. Academic Press, New York, 1990
78. Schaie KW: The course of adult intellectual development. Am Psychologist 1994;49:304–313
79. Schaie KW: Perceptual speed in adulthood: cross-sectional and longitudinal studies. Psychol Aging 1989;4:443–453
80. Willis SL, Jay GM, Diehl M, Marsiske M: Longitudinal change and prediction of everyday task competence in the elderly. Res Aging 1992;14:68–91
81. Willis SL, Schaie KW: Training the elderly on ability factors of spatial orientation and inductive reasoning. Psychol Aging 1986;1:239–247
82. Willis SL, Nesselroad CS: Long term effects of fluid ability training in old-old age. Develop Psychol 1990;26: 905–910
83. Baltes PB, Staudinger UM, Maercker A, Smith J: People nominated as wise: a comparative study of wisdom-related knowledge. Psychol Aging 1995;10:155–166
84. Smith J, Staudinger UM, Baltes PB: Occupational settings facilitating wisdom-related knowledge: the sample case of clinical psychologists. J Consult Clin Psychol 1994;66:989–999
85. Schaie KW, Dutta R, Willis SL: The relationship between rigidity-flexibility and cognitive abilities in adulthood. Psychol Aging 1991;6:371–383
86. Schaie KW, Willis SL: Adult personality and psychomotor performance: cross-sectional and longitudinal analyses. J Gerontol Psychol Sci 1991;46:P275–P284
87. Kausler DH: Motivation, human aging, and cognitive performance. pp. 171–182. In Birren JE, Schaie KW (eds): Handbook of the Psychology of Aging. 3rd Ed. Academic Press, New York, 1990;171–182
88. Maslow AH: Toward a Psychology of Being. 2nd Ed. Van Nostrand Reinhold, New York, 1968
89. Monte CF: Beneath the Mask: An Introduction to Theories of Personality. 3rd Ed. Holt, Rinehart, and Winston, New York, 1987
90. American Psychiatric Association: Diagnostic and Statistical Manual of Mental Disorders (DSM-IV). 4th Ed. American Psychiatric Association, Washington, DC, 1994
91. Howard A, Bray DW: Managerial Lives in Transition: Advancing Age and Changing Times. Guilford Press, New York, 1988
92. Carstensen LL: Age-related changes in social activity. pp. 222–237. In Carstensen LL, Edelstein BA (eds): Handbook of Clinical Gerontology. Pergamon, New York, 1987
93. Carstensen LL: Selectivity theory: social activity in life-span context. pp. 195–215. In Schaie KW, Lawton MP (eds): Annual Review of Gerontology and Geriatrics. Springer, New York, 1991
94. Carstensen LL: Social and emotional patterns in adulthood: support for socioemotional selectivity theory. Psychol Aging 1992;7:331–338
95. Krause N: Satisfaction with social support and self-rated health in older adults. Gerontologist 1987;27:301–308
96. Antonucci TC, Akiyama H: Social networks in adult life and a preliminary examination of the convoy model. J Gerontol 1987;42:519–527
97. Antonucci TC, Jackson JS: Social support, interpersonal efficacy, and health: a life course perspective. pp. 291–311. In Carstensen LL, Edelstein BA (eds): Handbook of Clinical Gerontology. Pergamon, New York, 1987
98. Krause N, Keith V: Gender differences in social support among older adults. Sex Roles 1989;21:609–628
99. Krause N, Markides K: Measuring social support among older adults. Int J Aging Human Develop 1990;30:37–53
100. McDaniel JS: Psychoimmunology: implications for future research. South Med J 1992;85:388–396

101. Kennedy S, Kiecolt-Glaser JK, Glaser R: Immunological consequences of acute and chronic stressors: mediating role of interpersonal relationships. Br J Med Psychol 1988;61: 77–85
102. Minkler M, Langhauser C: Assessing health differences in an elderly population: a five-year follow-up. J Am Geriat Soc 1988;36:113–118
103. Crawford CO, Preston DB: Differences in specific sources of social support for four healthy behaviors. pp. 215–228. In Rural Nursing. Sage, Newbury Park, CA, 1991
104. Langlie JK: Social networks, health beliefs, and preventive health behavior. J Health Soc Behav 1977;18:244–260
105. Potts MK, Hurwicz ML, Goldstein MS, Berkanovic E: Social support, health-promotive beliefs, and preventive health behaviors among the elderly. J Applied Gerontol 1992;11: 425–440
106. Omnibus Budget Reconciliation Act of 1990, P.L. 101–508, Section 4206 and 4751, codified at 42 U.S.C. Section 1395cc (a)(1)(Q), 1395 mm (c) (8), 1395cc (f), 1396a (57), (58), 1396a (w)

CHAPTER 11

The Pharmacology of Aging

KEN WOODHOUSE

Those who practice in the speciality of geriatric medicine pride themselves on their prescribing skills. The drug treatment of the older patient demands from the clinician an awareness of therapeutic goals, drug choice, dosage modification, and potential for adverse reactions that is considerably in excess of that required of the average prescriber. Physicians looking after elderly people make modifications to their prescribing that eventually become second nature. These include the following:

Avoidance of unnecessary drug therapy
Consideration of alternative treatments and quality of life
Consideration of compliance, information, and packaging
Appropriate drug choice and awareness of comorbidity
The use of a lower starting dose
Often the use of an extended dosing interval
Dose titration to achieve maximum therapeutic effect
Regular review of medication
An awareness of the potential for adverse reactions

This chapter examines the principles behind these changes and discusses some areas where theory and practice do not quite coincide.

Principles of Prescribing in the Elderly

Avoid Unnecessary Drug Therapy

The avoidance of unnecessary drug use would seem to be so obvious that it may hardly merit discussion. Indeed, most prescribers for the aged patient are particularly careful on this issue; geriatricians frequently comment that they stop more drugs than they start. Nonetheless, there is good evidence that older people are major consumers of prescribed and nonprescribed medication. This fact has been known for many years. As long ago as 1979, the Office of Health Economics in the United Kingdom[1] reported that one-third of National Health Service prescriptions were for the elderly, whereas they made up perhaps 15 to 18 percent of the population at that time. In addition, community-based studies have shown that older people may receive up to 13 prescriptions per annum, and consume a considerable number of nonprescription drugs.

Some of this drug use is clearly justified. With increasing age comes an increasing occurrence of the common, chronic, and disabling conditions that may require pharmacotherapy. Some examples are given in the accompanying boxed list. Nonetheless, when a breakdown of the *categories* of drugs prescribed is examined, cause for concern is evident. For example, diuretics are widely prescribed, but some studies have suggested that they may be safely withdrawn in up to half of recipients. Similarly, the overuse of nonsteroidal anti-inflammatory drugs (NSAIDs) is well recognized. Finally, one may question whether 24 percent of all drugs prescribed to the elderly need to be those acting on the central nervous system, often sedatives and hypnotics.[1–3]

Clearly, the aim of the astute prescriber should be to use drugs only when they are of proven benefit, and when the expected benefit will outweigh the risk and unpleasantness of possible adverse reactions. Examples of inappropriate drug use are familiar and include the following:

The use of potent diuretics for stasis edema
The use of neuroleptics such as prochlorperazine (Stemetil) for the treatment of "dizziness," when in fact the patient does not have vertigo, but simple age-related postural unsteadiness
The well-known use of NSAIDs where a simple analgesic would be more appropriate
The use of combination drugs where single agents are more appropriate, such as the use of cotrimoxazole for uncomplicated urinary tract infection rather than trimethoprim alone
One strategy for overcoming this excess drug usage is to consider other, nonpharmacologic approaches to treatment.

Treatment Alternatives and Quality of Life

Treatment strategies that rely on modalities other than drugs are probably not used enough in the older patient. The reasons for this are likely to be complex, but will include time constraints on the prescriber, the influence of the pharmaceutical companies, and the expectation of the patient. However, there is no doubt that under some circumstances it is appropriate to explore nondrug treatments before starting medication.[4] Possible examples include the following:

Dietary manipulations and exercise programs for noninsulin dependent diabetes
Low fat or low cholesterol diets for hyperlipidemias

Some chronic conditions in the elderly that necessitate increased drug usage

Cardiovascular
- Angina pectoris
- Heart failure
- Hypertension

Neurologic
- Stroke
- Parkinson's disease

Psychiatric
- Depression
- Confusion

Genitourinary
- Incontinence

Musculoskeletal
- Arthritis
- Osteoporosis

Reduction in alcohol and salt consumption, weight loss, and exercise for mild to moderate hypertension

Psychological approaches to the treatment of depression

Behavioral approaches to the management of insomnia

Therapy assessment and the provision of aids for postural instability

Physical therapy for arthritis

Transcutaneous electrical nerve stimulation, and possibly acupuncture, for a variety of pains, particularly neuropathic pain

These are but a few possible examples, all of which may be beneficial in some patients with some conditions. They may have the advantage not only of helping the target condition, but also of enhancing the patient's quality of life. Unfortunately, it is inevitable that in many people, for many diseases, drug treatment will be needed. It is in these patients that the art of bespoke prescribing comes into its own.

Compliance, Packaging, and Information

Compliance may be defined as the extent to which the patient's behavior coincides with that recommended by his or her attendants. Poor compliance does not simply relate to drug treatments; indeed, it can often be more difficult to persuade someone—particularly elderly patients with established habits—to modify their smoking, drinking, dietary, or exercise habits than to persuade them to take tablets.

Compliance is a graded phenomenon; a patient may take all, most, some, a little, or none of their treatment. How much this matters depends very much on the condition under treatment. For example, in some cases of simple urinary infections, taking only one or two doses of the prescribed regime may be effective. In some cases of difficult epilepsy, or Parkinson's disease, *missing* one or two doses can result in treatment failure.

It is commonly stated, and sometimes believed, that the elderly are very poor compliers. In fact, studies that have looked at the relatively fit, community-based, cognitively intact older person have shown, using digoxin compliance as a marker, that the elderly comply as well as if not better than, their younger compatriots.[5,6] Problems of compliance really only become apparent with complicated regimes of multiple drugs (a problem in the young too) or in patients who are cognitively impaired.[7,8]

Even if they are as good as the young—who are not particularly compliant themselves—attempts to improve compliance are worthwhile. Several strategies have been shown to be helpful,[9–11] and include the following:

In-hospital, predischarge training

Counselling by pharmacists

Information leaflets and written instructions

Drug diaries

Diary packaging

Pharmacy-filled, dated containers

Supervision

For some people, especially the confused and forgetful, it is only the last supervised treatment by carers or community nurses that really will ensure compliance with treatment. For all patients, though, compliance will be easier if they avoid side effects. The first stage in this process is choosing the right drug for that person.

Appropriate Drug Choice, Awareness of Comorbidity

The presence of multiple pathology in the older person makes the choice of drug particularly important. There is little point in treating one condition, only to make the patient feel worse because the prescribed drug has aggravated a coexisting disease. The potential number of such drug-disease interactions is enormous, but a few of the most important include the following:

β-Blockers, prescribed for angina or hypertension, worsening peripheral vascular disease

Thiazides, given for hypertension or heart failure, worsening glycemic control in diabetics

Calcium channel blockers, worsening ankle swelling in patients with stasis edema

NSAIDs, making hypertension or heart failure more difficult to control

Dopamine blockers, given as antiemetics or vestibular sedatives, precipitating or exacerbating parkinsonism

Drugs with anticholinergic effects, worsening confusion in cognitively impaired patients

Table 11-1 Some age-related physiologic changes that may influence pharmacokinetics

Change	Potentially Affecting	Ref.
Reduced gastric acid output	Absorption	12
Altered gastric emptying	Absorption	20
Reduced splanchnic blood flow	Presystemic elimination	13
Reduced body water	Distribution protein binding	14
Increased body fat	Distribution protein binding	15
Reduced lean body mass	Distribution protein binding	15
Reduced serum albumin	Distribution protein binding	10
Small liver	Hepatic clearance	17
Reduced liver blood flow	Hepatic clearance	17
Reduced glomerular filtration rate	Renal clearance	18
Reduced renal tubular function	Renal clearance	19

Sometimes it is not possible to choose an ideal drug, and one has to make do with the least risky. Even if it is possible to choose a fairly low risk agent, dosage modifications, at least at the start of treatment, are often prudent.

Lower Starting Dose

There are a variety of reasons why it is often prudent to reduce the dose of a drug given to an elderly person. These may relate to changes in systemic bioavailability; changes in distribution and protein binding; increased sensitivity because of receptor changes and homeostatic failure; and delayed elimination. For convenience, issues relating to drug elimination are dealt with in the next section.

The bioavailibility of a drug will depend on pharmaceutical factors, which are not related to the age of the patient, and to possible changes in absorption from the gastrointestinal tract or in presystemic metabolism, which may be age related.

Absorption from the gut

Some of the changes in physiology that are shown in Table 11-1 could, in theory, modify absorption of drugs; but in clinical practice, this is probably not too important. Furthermore, the literature is contradictory in relation to some of the minor changes that have been reported. For example, some authors have shown that drug absorption is just as complete in old as in young, although it may be rather slower.[21] By contrast, and using alternative methodologies, other groups have suggested that the early phases of gastric emptying may actually be more rapid in the elderly, resulting in more brisk absorption.[20] None of these changes, even if consistent, seem to have a major clinical impact.

First pass (presystemic) clearance

By contrast, age-related changes in presystemic elimination (Table 11-1) are very important. After absorption across the gut, drugs enter the portal circulation, and must pass through the liver before entering the systemic circulation. In the case of some drugs, especially those that are very lipid soluble, most of the drug is removed on this "first pass," resulting in a bioavailability of (in some cases) well under 10 percent. This can be very important, as relatively small changes in liver function, occuring with age, can have major effects. Thus, in the case of a drug that has a first pass elimination of 95 percent in the young (5 percent bioavailability), a small reduction with age, perhaps to 90 percent, would result in a bioavailability of 10 percent—an effective doubling. The literature is rather more consistent regarding the effect of age on first pass metabolism. Early studies by the Southampton group[22] showed that propranolol availability was much higher in geriatric patients than young volunteers, and later studies by the same group and others have shown that even in the case of fit old people, bioavailability of drugs such as nifedipine[23] is increased substantially. Clearly, if bioavailability increases, the oral dose given will have to be reduced to avoid excessive plasma levels and adverse drug reactions.

Distribution and protein binding

Body composition changes with age, and some of the most important alterations are shown in Table 11-1. With regard to drug distribution, the most important differences are an increase in body fat, and a relative decrease in body water. The decrease in body water is probably the most important change, which may necessitate a reduction in initial drug dosage. In the case of polar drugs, distributed to body water, a reduction in apparent volume of distribution will lead to higher plasma concentrations per unit dose. Examples include alcohol,[24] cimetidine,[25] and aminoglycosides.[26] Changes in body fat are more important in determining duration of action, and are dealt with later.

In addition, some plasma proteins alter with age. Even in "fit" elderly people, serum albumin tends to fall. This will result in higher free drug levels, with the potential for greater pharmacologic effect. In the short term, and with acute dosing, this may be important, and dosage reduction may be needed. In the longer term, with repeated dosing, free drug clearance will determine the free plasma drug level, rather than levels of plasma proteins. The other major drug binding protein, α-1-acid glycoprotein, shows no consistent age-related change in fit old people.[27–29]

Although it is important to be aware of these age-related differences in distribution and binding, it is unclear how crucial they are in determining the need for dose modification in the elderly.

Drug receptors and homeostasis

There can be little doubt that, on average, older people are more sensitive even to equivalent plasma drug concentrations. The potential explanation for these observations could theoretically relate to any of the ways in which most drugs exert their action, that is, via receptors. The intensity of a drug response will depend on receptor density, receptor affinity, postreceptor events and signal amplification, target tissue response, and effect of homeostatic mechanisms.

Receptors A lot of information is available in the literature regarding the relationship between age and drug receptors. The situation is very complex, and seems to vary between receptor types. Interestingly, with some few exceptions, receptors seem to become desensitized with age, which would result in a lowering of drug response, so it is unlikely that in most instances age-related drug sensitivity can be explained by these factors. Nonetheless, the findings are worthy of some consideration.

The most studied receptor type is the β-adrenoceptor. It has been known for some years that the cardiac chronotropic response to infused isoprenaline falls with age.[30] In simple terms, it is necessary to give a higher dose of isoprenaline to an old person to achieve the same increase in heart rate. Similarly, and perhaps surprisingly, the elderly seem to be relatively resistant to the effects of equivalent plasma concentrations of β-blockers.[30] The mechanisms behind these changes are still not entirely clear. Animal experiments show that β-receptor numbers on the surface of red cells,[31] adipocytes,[32] and brain cells[33] decline with age, a finding that has also been noted (admittedly rather inconsistently) in human lymphocytes.[34] Similarly, it has been suggested that the affinity of β-receptors may fall with age, and at least one study has shown this to be the case in human white blood cells.[35] The reasons for β-receptor changes with age are still under investigation, but some evidence suggests that it may be related to reduced levels of physical activity with aging.

Much less information is available about the interaction between aging and other receptors, partly because they are more difficult to study. As far as α-receptors are concerned, initial studies using rat models suggested that the effect of noradrenalin on myocardium and great vessels was reduced, but this finding has not been reproduced in humans.[36] One suggestion is that age-related changes depend on the α-receptor subtype, with α-2-receptors (which bind, for example, clonidine) exhibiting lowered responsiveness in the elderly, whereas α-1-receptors show little change.[37]

Cholinergic receptor function is again a matter of debate. Some experiments have suggested that atropine-induced tachycardia is diminished in the aged, and certainly some areas of geriatric rat brain show altered sensitivity to acetylcholine, but the clinical relevance of these findings remains unclear.[38]

Although not strictly speaking a receptor function, it is worth mentioning here the relationship between age and warfarin dynamics. It has long been known that the dose requirement for warfarin falls with age; furthermore, it has been shown that the degree of inhibition of clotting factor synthesis by a given plasma concentration of warfarin is greater in the elderly.

Benzodiazepines are widely used in old people, and it is well known that such patients are particularly prone to develop side effects from them. Part of the explanation for this is kinetic, but even for equivalent blood levels, the aged brain seems to be more sensitive—reflected in the occurrence of confusion, hangover, and increased body sway. One possible reason for this sensitivity may be increased penetration of the drug across the blood-brain barrier; certainly this has been shown in aged rats, using nitrazepam as a typical benzodiazepine. However, it is also possible that age-related changes in central nervous system benzodiazepine receptors occur, although animal experiments would not support this hypothesis.[39–41]

Homeostatic mechanisms likely to fail with aging

Postural blood pressure control
Posture control
Extrapyramidal system
Cognitive function
Thermoregulation

Homeostasis A variety of mechanisms have evolved to maintain the internal milieu of the human body, and to maintain its stability in the external environment. Those that are likely to fail with aging, and that are important in relation to drug therapy are shown in the accompanying boxed list.

Postural blood pressure control is one homeostatic mechanism that is often poor in the old; this failure is one important reason for the increased sensitivity of the elderly to the hypotensive effect of many drugs. Normally, on attaining the upright posture, a transient fall in blood pressure is sensed by baroreceptors in the carotid sinus and great vessels. The immediate response is a rise in heart rate, followed shortly thereafter by peripheral vasoconstriction to maintain blood pressure, and prevent syncope. Several studies are now available[42,43] that indicate that this series of reflexes is blunted in the aged person, even in those classified as relatively "fit." For example, when vasodilator drugs (e.g., nitrates or nifedipine) are given by infusion, the resulting positive chronotropic response is very much less in older people, resulting in a fall in blood pressure.[23] From a knowledge of these changes, it is apparent that old people are prone to postural hypotension; any drug with vasodilator or hypotensive actions will magnify this; and any compound that may prevent reflex tachycardia (e.g., β-blockers or some calcium channel blockers) may do the same.

Within the nervous system, the four most important homeostatic mechanisms with respect to aging pharmacology are postural control; extrapyramidal function; temperature regulation; and cognitive function.

Postural control is a most complex homeostatic process, involving many different neurologic reflexes. It can, however, be conveniently assessed by means of body sway measurements, which record the small corrective movements that are always occurring in order to maintain balance. Corrective movements become much more marked with aging, reflected in increased body sway.[44,45] Many drugs, especially those with sedative properties, will magnify these changes, leading to a greater risk of unsteadiness and falls. Indeed, epidemiologic studies show that the risk of falling and injury is much greater in the older person who takes such drugs.[46]

The extrapyramidal system is important not only in the maintenance of postural control, but also in many aspects of motor function. Various age-related changes in extrapyramidal function occur, principally related to a reduction in dopaminergic neuronal function. In some patients this may be regarded as subclinical Parkinson's disease. The main consequence of this change is that exposure of these people to dopaminergic blockade will result in the development of a clinically evident Parkinsonian syndrome, at a much lower drug dose than that which would be needed to produce extrapyramidal effects in younger people.[47–50]

The importance of thermoregulation cannot be overemphasized. Normally, a fall in core body temperature will result in shivering, a rise in metabolic rate, vasoconstriction, a perception of cold, and behavioral changes—all of which will serve to renormalize temperature. While it is probably safe to say that this series of reflexes is not universally impaired in the elderly, there is no doubt that a significant subset of older people do have blunted thermoregulatory reflexes, as evidenced by studies of survivors of accidental hypothermia.[51] Some drugs are known to have a negative effect on thermoregulation, and these will pose a particular risk for these people. Examples of potential problem agents include vasodilators (including ethanol), barbiturates, tricyclic antidepressants, and neuroleptics.

In humans, it is reasonable to classify higher mental function as, in part, a homeostatic process. Animal studies and studies in humans indicate that some age-related changes in neurotransmitters occur that are relevant to cognition,[52] even if this does not lead to overt clinical problems. For example, it seems that cholinergic function tends to fall off with age. The importance of this is that the administration of drugs such as the anticholinergics, which may further block these transmitters, may lead to the development of memory failure, or even florid acute confusion.

As can be seen from the above, a large number of factors are responsible for the necessary reduction in starting drug dose in the elderly. In addition to this change, however, it is often the case that the drug has to be given less frequently; the reasons for this are given in the next section.

Extended Dosing Interval

It is often the case that one can give a drug to an elderly person once or twice a day, whereas it would be necessary to give it to a younger person three times a day. The principal reasons for this are changes in distribution volumes, delayed renal elimination, and delayed hepatic clearance.

Distribution volumes

As discussed in the previous section, the changes in body composition that occur with age (Table 11-1), particularly the relative increase in body fat, may have important implications for drug elimination. Specifically, the apparent volume of distribution of lipid soluble drugs will increase. The net effect of this will be to increase the half-life of these drugs, *even if the clearance is maintained*. This will result in a prolonged duration of action. If clearance is reduced as well, as is often the case, this effect will be much greater.

These effects are particularly important for drugs such as the benzodiazepines, which are sedative, and where hangover effects may occur. Table 11-2 summarizes some of the kinetic data that are available for the benzodiazepines.

Renal clearance

It has been known for many years that there are important reductions in renal function with aging. Some of these are shown in Table 11-1. The net result of these changes is a reduction, on average, in the renal elimination of drugs. However, it is important to note that although *average* kidney function declines, this is by no means uniform between individuals, and some old people seem to maintain near normal levels of renal function even to quite an advanced age.

The clinical significance of these changes is very dependent upon the drug being given. In the case of some renally eliminated drugs, no modification in dose regime is required, as they have a very large therapeutic ratio, and toxicity is unlikely to occur. Many penicillins fall into this category.[56,57] By contrast, some drugs have a very narrow therapeutic ratio, and dose regimes have to be carefully monitored in order to avoid serious, and on occasion, life-threatening adverse events. Examples of drugs that may fall into this category are shown in Table 11-3.

Hepatic drug clearance

The liver is the most important site of drug metabolism in all mammalian species, and over the past few years, knowledge of the processes involved in hepatic drug metabolism, both in the young and in relation to age, has increased rapidly. Drug clearance by the liver is determined by a variety of parameters, the most important of which are shown in the boxed list; any of these could potentially be affected by age. Indeed, many studies are available in the literature that show that the hepatic clearance of drugs is reduced by up to 50 percent in the elderly, obviously necessitating dosage modification. Only recently have the mechanisms of these changes been clarified.

Liver size It has been suggested for many years that liver size decreased with age. Recent studies[13,17] have clearly shown that these changes are quite substantial; the liver may shrink by 25 to 35 percent between the third and tenth decade of life. Furthermore, we now know that this change is of sufficient magnitude to explain the reduced hepatic clearance of drugs

Table 11-2 The effect of age upon the pharmacokinetics of some benzodiazepines

Drug	Vd	Main Route of Elimination	Clearance t½	Total	Free Drug	Dose Modification	Ref.
Diazepam	↑	Oxidation	↑	↓			87
Nitrazepam	↑	Oxidation	↑	→		Yes	88
Chlordiazepoxide	↑	Oxidation	↑	↓			89
Midazolam	↑	Oxidation	↑	↓ males → females		Yes	90
Colabazepam (Clobazam)	↑	Oxidation	↑	↓ males → females	↓ males → females	Yes	91
Oxazepam		Glucuronidation	→	→	→	Yes	92, 93

seen in old age,[13,58–60] without invoking changes in any of the other parameters listed in the accompanying box.

Liver blood flow Because of its dual blood flow, techniques to measure hepatic perfusion have been quite difficult, and in practice, the clearance of highly extracted compounds has been used as a surrogate. The favorite such agent is indocyanine green. The clearance of this agent has been shown to fall substantially with age—in this case by up to 35 percent between third and tenth decades.[17]

Hepatic uptake Age-related changes in the uptake of drugs into the liver could, in theory, have an impact on hepatic clearance. This is another parameter that is difficult to measure, as it involves hepatic vein catheterization. The only study to have looked at uptake in relation to aging in a systematic way examined indocyanine green uptake in patients of a variety of ages who were undergoing right heart catheter for diagnostic purposes. This study showed that uptake was not reduced with aging.[61]

Enzyme activities The enzymes of drug metabolism are conventionally divided into two phases. Phase 1 reactions comprise oxidative, reductive, or hydrolytic reactions. Phase 2 reactions are conjugations. Conventional teaching was that the most important enzymes of phase 1 metabolism—the cytochrome P-450 dependent microsomal monooxygenases (MMO)—were reduced with aging, whereas conjugating enzymes were unaltered. We now know that the second statement is correct, and glucuronosyl transferases and sulphotransferases are similar in old and young liver tissue.[62,63] The decreased clearance of some conjugated drugs, seen in the elderly, is due to a reduction in liver size with age, as described above. By contrast, the first statement is true only of geriatric rodents. It has been well documented that there is a substantial fall in some MMO activities in aging male rats.[64,65] This is due to a progressive failure of the hypothalamic-pituitary-testicular axis in these aging animals, with a consequent loss of male sex-specific P-450 isoforms. Several studies have now indicated that such changes are not seen in primates, including humans, and P-450 levels do not fall with age in man.[65–70] As with conjugations, reduced clearance of phase 1 drugs is due to a smaller liver in the aged.[60]

Table 11-3 Examples of drugs cleared by the kidney that should be closely monitored in the elderly

Class	Drug	Ref.
Antibiotic	Gentamycin	26
	Streptomycin	26
	Kanamycin	26
β-Blocker	Atenolol	53
	Sotalol	53
Cardiac glycoside	Digoxin	54
Psychotropic	Lithium	55

Frailty, illness, and enzymes One set of circumstances where the enzymes of drug metabolism may begin to fail in old people is in relation to poor health. For example, plasma esterases, important in metabolizing some drugs, and probably reflecting hepatic enzyme activity, are markedly reduced in the chronically physically frail, after hip fracture and some forms of surgery, and in the sickest stroke patients. These changes will be additive to changes in liver size.[71,72]

Enzyme inhibition and induction Changes in these parameters could theoretically affect hepatic drug clearance in the older patient. In fact, there is no evidence that old people's enzymes are more sensitive to inhibitors than the young. The situation with regard to induction is rather more complex. Some in vivo kinetic studies have suggested that the induction of MMO enzymes in response to inducers such as cigarettes, rifampicin, and phenazone is less in the old, and that this may be partly responsible for reduced drug clearance.[73–80] However, it has to be noted that such changes have not been confirmed in isolated human cells.[81–84]

Hepatic clearance: summary The main factors behind reduced hepatic drug clearance in the elderly are a smaller

Determinants of hepatic drug clearance

Liver mass
Liver blood flow
Uptake of drugs and transport within hepatocyte
Enzyme affinity and activity
Enzyme induction and inhibition

liver and reduced blood flow. In some patients, physical frailty, injury, or disease may also be associated with a reduction in enzyme activities, but these are normal in most elderly people.

Dose Titration

Although it is common practice to use a lower starting dose in the elderly, and to extend the dosing interval, this can only be the start of the therapeutic process. One of the most important observations that has been made of aging populations is that the degree of heterogeneity increases markedly. This has already been alluded to in relation to renal function, where some elderly people have more or less normal renal function, and others suffer a dramatic decline.

The consequence of this observation is that it is necessary to titrate up the dose of a drug from the low starting level to achieve a therapeutic effect, but to avoid adverse reactions.

On current evidence, this process is not done particularly well. The emphasis on avoidance of adverse reactions has been so great that it is a common clinical observation that many old people are on homeopathic doses of drugs, which are, unsurprisingly, failing to have their desired effect. In this regard, a study performed in Irish nursing homes showed that, of those thought to have atrial fibrillation resistant to digoxin, about one-half had subtherapeutic blood levels.[85] This can happen even in the best units, as audit can reveal.[86]

Review of Medication and Awareness of Adverse Reactions

Medication review is vital, especially in the elderly. The aging process is a dynamic one, and the patient's status may change over the short or long term. For instance, new drugs may be added, the patient may become frail, new illnesses may develop, or occasionally, treatment may no longer be needed. Information technology has a major role to play in developing automatic medication review systems; many such systems are available for primary or secondary care settings.

Despite all of the changes in prescribing, described above, it is rather depressing to note that adverse drug reactions (ADR) are all too frequent in the elderly.[95] One of the largest studies of this issue was published in 1980. A review of all admissions to a number of geriatric units in the United Kingdom revealed that a drug side effect was the sole cause of admission in 1.8 percent of cases, and contributed to admission in a further 7.7 percent. Extrapolating these figures to the whole country would indicate that 4,000 admissions annually are due to an ADR alone, and in a further 11,000, an ADR is partly responsible.[96] The resource implications of this are obvious.

Table 11-4 Some underreported adverse reactions in elderly people

Drug Category	Side Effects
Anticholinergics (including some antidepressants)	Confusion, urinary problems, dry mouth, constipation, "off legs"
Antiemetics and neuroleptics	Parkinsonian syndrome, confusional states, orthostatic hypotension, tardive dyskinesia, drowsiness, susceptibility to hypothermia
Diuretics	Dehydration, electrolyte disturbance, hypotension
NSAIDs	Upper gastrointestinal upset, gastrointestinal hemorrhage, edema, heart failure
Sedatives and hypnotics	Hangover effect, "off legs," falls, confusional states

It is almost certain that such figures, bad as they are, represent only a small proportion of ADRs in the aged. Many such events mimic symptoms that are common in the elderly, as shown in Table 11-4, and it is known that only perhaps 10 percent of ADRs are ever reported to the authorities.

Finally, it should be remembered that, apart from all of the physiologic reasons for the increased rate of ADR in the old, the most important factor remains the fact that they take more drugs. Castleden and Pickles[96] have clearly shown that there is a close correllation between drug usage and ADR rate in the elderly.[96]

Conclusions

Prescribing for the elderly is a complex task, based on a wide variety of social, physiologic, and medical events. One would hope that an understanding of these changes, and an adherence to the guidelines given at the start of this chapter would minimize the risks of drugs in the elderly and maximize their benefits. Although it is probably inevitable that some older people will always have drug-related problems, it is important not to deny them the benefits of modern pharmacology because of overcaution or unrealistic fears of side effects.

References

1. Office of Health Economics (OHE) 1980 OHW Briefing No 13: Effect of prescription charges. OHE, London
2. Skoll SL, August RJ, Johnson GE: Drug prescribing for the

elderly in Saskatchewan during 1976. Can Med Assoc J 1979; 121:1074–81

3. Guttman D: Patterns of legal drug use by older Americans. Addict Dis Int J 1978;3:337–56
4. Woodhouse K, Pascual J: Hypertension in Elderly People. Martin Dunitz, London, 1996
5. Taggart AJ, Johnson GD, McDevitt DG: Does the frequency of daily dosage influence compliance with digoxin therapy? Br J Clin Pharmacol 1981;11:31–4
6. Hemminki E, Heikkila J: Elderly people's compliance with prescriptions and the quality of medication. Scand J Soc Med 1975; 3:87–92
7. Spriet A, Beiler D, Dechorgrat J, Simon P: Adherence of elderly patients to treatment with pentoxifylline. Clin Pharmacol Ther 1980;27:1–8
8. Baxendale C, Gourlay M, Gibson JM: A self medication retraining programme. BMJ 1978;2:1278–9
9. McDonald ET, McDonald JB, Phoenix M: Improving drug compliance after hospital discharge. BMJ 1977;2:618–21
10. Wandless I, Davie JW: Can drug compliance in the elderly be improved? BMJ 1977;1:359–61
11. Martin DC, Mead K: Reducing medication errors in a geriatric population. J Am Geriatr Soc 1982;20:258–60
12. Baron JH: Studies of basal and peak acid output with an augmented histamine test. Gut 1963;4:136
13. Woodhouse KW, Wynne HA: Age-related changes in liver size and hepatic blood flow. Clin Pharmacokinet 1988;15:287–94
14. Edelman IS, Leibman J: Anatomy of body water and electrolytes. Am J Med 1959;27:256
15. Forbes GB, Reina JC: Adult lean body mass declines with age: some longitudinal observations. Metabolism 1970;19:653–63
16. Hale WE, Stewart RB, Marks RG: Haematological and biochemical laboratory values in an ambulatory elderly population: an analysis of effects of age, sex, and drugs. Age Ageing 1983; 12:275–84
17. Wynne H, Cope L, Mutch E et al: The effects of age upon liver size and liver blood flow in man. Hepatology 1989;9:297–301
18. Davies DF, Shock NW: Age changes in glomerular filtration rate, effective renal plasma flow and tubular excretory capacity in adult males. J Clin Invest 1950;29:1950
19. Miller JH, McDonald RK, Shock NW: Age changes in the maximal rate of tubular reabsorption of glucose. J Gerontol 1952;7: 196
20. Rashid M: Some effects of drugs on gastrointestinal motility. M Phil Thesis, University of Newcastle-upon-Tyne, 1989
21. Castleden CM, Volan GN, Raymonds K: The effect of ageing on drug absorption from the gut. Age Ageing 1977;6:138–43
22. Castleden M, George C: The effect of ageing on hepatic clearance of propranalol. Br J Clin Pharmacol 1979;7:49–54
23. Robertson DRC, Waller DG, Renwick AG, George CF: Age-related changes in the pharmacokinetics and pharmacodynamics of nifedipine. Br J Clin Pharmacol 1988;25:297–305
24. Vestal RE, McGuire EA, Tobin JD et al: Ageing and ethanol metabolism. Clin Pharmacol 1977;21:343–54
25. Redolfi A, Borgogelli E, Lodola E: Blood level of cimetidine in relation to age. Eur J Clin Pharmacol 1979;15:257–61
26. Hansen J: Dose regimen of kanamycin and gentamycin. Acta Med Scan 1974;190: 521
27. Veering BTH, Burm AGL, Souverijn JHM et al: The effect of age on serum concentrations of albumin and α^1-acid glycoprotein. Br J Clin Pharmacol 1990;29:201–6
28. Hayes MJ, Langman MJS, Short AH: Changes in drug metabolism with increasing age. Warfarin binding and plasma proteins. Br J Clin Pharmacol 1975;2:69–72
29. Andreason F, Husted S: The binding of furosemide to serum proteins in elderly patients: displacing effect of phenoprocoumarin. Acta Pharmacol Toxicol 1980;47:202
30. Vestal RE, Wood AJJ, Shand DG: Reduced beta adrenoceptor sensitivity in the elderly. Clin Pharmacol Ther 1979;26:181–6
31. Bylund DM, Tellezi-Inon MH, Hollenberg MD: Age-related parallel decline in beta adrenergic receptors, adenylate cyclase and phosphodiesterase activity in rat erythrocyte membrane. Life Sci 1977;21:403–10
32. Giudicelli Y, Pecquery R: Beta adrenergic receptors and catecholamine sensitive adenylate cyclase in rat fat cell membranes: influence of growth, cell size, and ageing. Eur J Biochem 1978; 90:413–9
33. Greenberg LH, Dix RK, Weiss B: Age-related changes in the binding of 3H-dihydrooolprenolol in rat brain. p. 245. In Roberts J, Adelmann RC, Cristolfado VJ et al (eds): Pharmacological Intervention in the Ageing Process. Plenum Press, New York, 1978
34. Schocken D, Roth G: Reduced beta adrenergic receptor concentrations in ageing man. Nature 1977;276:856–8
35. Feldman RD, Limbird LE, Nadeau JL: Alterations in leukocyte beta receptor affinity with ageing. A potential explanation for altered beta adrenergic sensitivity in the elderly. N Engl J Med 1984;310:815–9
36. Scott PJW, Reid JL: The effect of age on the responses of human isolated arteries to noradrenaline. Br J Clin Pharmacol 1982; 13:237–9
37. Docherty JR: Ageing and the cardiovascular system. J Auton Pharmacol 1986;6:77–84
38. Dauchot P, Gravenstein JS: Effects of atropine on the electrocardiogram in different age groups. Clin Pharmacol Ther 1971;12: 274–80
39. Cook PJ, Flanagan R, James IM: Diazepam tolerance: effect of age, regular sedation and alcohol. BMJ 1984;289:351–3
40. Castleden CM, George CF, Marcer D et al: Increased sensitivity to nitrazepam in old age. BJ 1977;1:10–2
41. Swift CG, Ewan JM, Clarke P et al: Responsiveness to oral diazepam in the elderly: relationship to total and free plasma concentrations. Br J Clin Pharmacol 1985;20:111–8
42. Johnson RH, Smith AC, Spalding JMK: The effect of posture on blood pressure in elderly patients. Lancet 1965;1:731
43. Collins KJ, Exton-Smith AN, James MH: Functional changes in autonomic nervous responses with ageing. Age Ageing 1980; 9:17–24
44. Sheldon JH: The effect of age on the control of sway. Gerontology 1963;5:129

45. Swift CA: Postural instability as a measure of sedative drug response. Br J Clin Pharmacol 1984;18:87S–90S

46. Rae W, Griffin M, Schaffener W: Psychotropic drug use and the risk of hip fracture. N Engl J Med 1987;316:363

47. Cohen BM, Sommer BR: Metabolism of thioridazine in the elderly. J Clin Psychopharmacol 1988;8:336–9

48. Axelsson R, Martensson E: The concentration pattern of nonconjugated thioridazine metabolites in serum by thioridazine treatment and its relationship to psychological and clinical variables. Curr Ther Res 1977;20:561

49. Forsman A, Ohman R: Applied pharmacokinetics of haloperidol in man. Curr Ther Res 1977;21:396

50. Collins KJ, Dove C, Exton-Smith AN: Accidental hypothermia and impaired temperature homeostasis in the elderly. BMJ 1977;i:353–6

51. McGeer EJ: Ageing and neurotransmitter metabolism in human brain. p. 247. In Katzman R, Terry RD, Rick JR et al (eds): Alzheimers Disease: Senile Dementia and Related Disorders. Rover Press, New York, 1987

52. Barber HE, Hawksworth GM, Petrie JC et al: Pharmacokinetics of atenolol and propranolol in young and elderly subjects (abstract). Br J Clin Pharmacol 1981;12:118P

53. Cusack B, Kelley J, O'Malley K et al: Digoxin in the elderly: pharmacokinetic consequences of old age. Clin Pharm Ther 1979;25:772–6

54. Hewick DS, Newbury P, Hopwood S et al: Age as a factor affecting lithium therapy. Br J Clin Pharmacol 1977;4:201–5

55. Triggs EJ, Johnson JM, Learoyd B: Absorption and disposition of ampicillin in the elderly. Eur J Clin Pharmacol 1980;18: 195–8

56. Leikola E, Vartia KO: On penicillin levels in young and geriatric subjects. J Gerontol 1957;12:48

57. Woodhouse KW, James OFW: Hepatic drug metabolism and ageing. Br Med Bull 1990;46:22–35

58. Wynne HA, Cope LH, James OFW et al: The effect of age and frailty upon acetanilide clearance. Age Ageing 1989;18:415–8

59. Wynne HA, Cope LH, Herd B et al: The association of age and frailty with paracetamol conjugation in man. Age Ageing 1990; 19:419–24

60. Wynne H, Goudouvenous J, Adams P et al: Hepatic extraction of drugs: the effect of age using indocyanine green as a model substrate. Br J Clin Pharmacol 1990;30:634–7

61. Woodhouse KW, Herd B: The effect of age and gender on glucuronidation and sulphation in rat liver: a study using paracetamol as a model substrate. Arch Gerontol Geriatr 1993;16:111–5

62. Herd B, Wynne H, Wright P et al: The effect of age on glucuronidation and sulphation of paracetamol by human liver fractions. Br J Clin Pharmacol 1991;32:768–70

63. Kato R, Vassanelli P, Frontino G: Variation in the activity of liver microsomal drug metabolising enzymes in rats in relation to age. Biochem Pharmacol 1964;12:1037

64. Wynne H, Mutch E, James OFW et al: Effect of age on monooxygenase enzyme kinetics in rat liver microsomes. Age Ageing 1987;16:153–8

65. Sutter MA, Wood WG, Williamson LS et al: Comparison of the hepatic mixed function oxidase system of young adults and old non-human primates (Macca nemestrina). Biochem Pharmacol 1985;34:2983–7

66. Woodhouse KW, Mutch E, Williams FM et al: The effect of age on pathways of drug metabolism in human liver. Age Ageing 1984;113:328–34

67. Maloney AG, Schmucker DL, Vessey DS et al: The effects of ageing on the hepatic microsomal mixed-function oxidase system of male and female monkeys. Hepatology 1986;6:282–7

68. Wynne H, Mutch E, James OFW et al: The effect of age upon the affinity of microsomal monooxygenase enzymes for substrate in human liver. Age Ageing 1988;17:401–5

69. Schmucker DL, Woodhouse KW, Wang RK et al: Effect of age and gender on in vitro properties of human liver microsomal monooxygenases. Clin Pharm Ther 1990;48:365–74

70. O'Mahony MS, George G, Westlake H, Woodhouse K: Plasma aspirin esterase activity in elderly patients undergoing elective hip replacement and with fractured neck of femur. Age Ageing 1994;23:338–41

71. Emam SJ: A study of esterases in blood: the impact of influenza vaccination and acute stroke. PhD Thesis, University of Wales, 1996

72. Beckett AH, Triggs EJ: Enzyme induction in man caused by smoking. Nature 1967;216:587

73. Vestal RE, Norris AH, Tobin JD et al: Antipyrine metabolism in man: influence of age, alcohol, caffeine and smoking. Clin Pharmacol Ther 1975;18:425–32

74. Vestal RE, Wood AJJ, Branch RA et al: Effects of age and cigarette smoking on propranalol disposition. Clin Pharmacol Ther 1979;26:8–15

75. Mucklow JC, Fraser HS: The effects of age and smoking upon antipyrine metabolism. J Clin Pharmacol 1980;9:613–4

76. Crowley JJ, Cusack BJ, Jue SG et al: Ageing and drug interactions II. Effect of phenytoin and smoking on the oxidation of theophylline and cortisol in healthy man. J Pharmacol Exp Ther 1988;245:513–23

77. Bonde J, Pedersen LE, Bodtker S et al: The influence of age and smoking on the elimination of disopyramide. Br J Clin Pharmacol 1985;20:453–8

78. Salem SAM, Rajjayabun P, Shepherd AMM, Stevenson IH: Reduced induction of drug metabolism in the elderly. Age Ageing 1978;7:68–73

79. Twum-Barima Y, Finnigan T, Habbash AI et al: Impaired enzyme induction of rifampicin in the elderly. Br J Clin Pharmacol 1984;17:595–7

80. George G, Wynne HA, Woodhouse KW: The association of age with the induction of drug metabolising enzymes in human monocytes. Age Ageing 1990;19:364–7

81. George G, Wynne H, Woodhouse K: Age and the rate of induction in aryl hydrocarbon hydroxylase in isolated peripheral blood monocytes. Age Ageing 1991; 20:421–4

82. George G, Woodhouse K: Dose-dependent induction of the microsomal monooxygenase aryl hydrocarbon hydroxylase in isolated peripheral blood monocytes: the influence of age. Pharmacol Toxicol 1992;71:221–3

83. George G, O'Mahony S, Woodhouse K: Age, smoking and the activity of the monooxygenase aryl hydrocarbon hydroxylase in isolated human peripheral blood monocytes. Age Ageing 1994; 23:421–4
84. George G, O'Mahony MS, Woodhouse KW: Age, anticonvulsants, and benzo-α-pyrene hydroxylation in human monocytes. In Woodhouse KW, O'Mahony MS (eds): Topics in Ageing Research in Europe. Vol. 16. Eurage, Leiden, 1991
85. Shetty HGM, Woodhouse KW: Use of amiodarone for elderly patients. Age Ageing 1992;21:233–6
86. Kanto J, Maenpaa M, Mantyla R et al: Effect of age on the pharmacokinetics of diazepam given in conjunction with spinal anaesthesia. Anaesthesiology 1979;51:154–9
87. Kangas L, Iisalo E, Kento T et al: Human pharmacokinetics of nitrazepam. Effect of age and disease. Eur J Clin Pharmacol 1979;15:163–70
88. Roberts RK, Wilkinson GR, Branch RA, Shenker S: Effect of age and parenchymal liver disease on the disposition and elimination of chlordiazepoxide (Librium). Gastroenterology 1978; 75:479–85
89. Holazo AA, Winkler MD, Patel IH: Effects of age, gender and oral contraceptives on imtramuscular midazolam pharmacokinetics. J Clin Pharmacol 1988;28:1040–5
90. Greenblatt DJ, Divoll M, Puri S et al: Clobazepam kinetics and the elderly. Br J Clin Pharmacol 1981;12:631–6
91. Greenblatt DJ, Divoll M, Harmatz JS, Shader RI: Oxazepam kinetics: effects of age and sex. J Pharmacol Exp Ther 1980; 215:86–91
92. Murray TG, Chiang ST, Koepke HH, Walker BR: Renal disease, age and oxazepam kinetics. Clin Pharmacol Ther 1981;30: 805–9
93. Hurwitz N: Predisposing factors in adverse reaction to drugs. BMJ 1969;1:536–9
94. Seidl LS, Thornton GF, Smith JW, Cluff LE: Studies of the epidemiology of adverse drug reactions. Bull Johns Hopkins Hosp 1966;119:299
95. Williamson J, Chopin JM: Adverse reactions to prescribed drugs in the elderly. A multicentre investigation. Age Ageing 1980; 9:73–80
96. Castleden CM, Pickles H: Suspected adverse drug reactions in elderly patients reported to the Committee on Safety of Medicines. Br J Clin Pharmacol 1988;26:347–53

CHAPTER 12

Methodologic Problems in Research on Aging

JOHN D. SORKIN
LESLIE I. KATZEL

The principal aims of gerontology are to identify changes that occur during aging, to quantify the rate at which the changes occur, and to understand the mechanisms behind the changes. Aging is the result of (1) intrinsic biologic processes that are genetically determined (biologic aging), (2) age-associated lifestyle changes (e.g., decreased physical activity, increased obesity), and (3) age-associated increased incidence and prevalence of disease. This chapter will describe five study designs—cross-sectional, time-series, longitudinal, case-control, and cohort—that can be used to identify change, to quantify the rate at which change occurs at different ages, and to separate biologic aging from the effects of lifestyle and disease. Additionally, problems and limitations associated with the designs will be described.

Cross-sectional, Time-Series, and Longitudinal Designs

Cross-sectional Design

The cross-sectional design is the design most commonly used to study the relation between a variable of interest and age. A cross-sectional study is performed by assembling and studying a group of subjects of different ages at a fixed point in time, or over a short period of time. Each subject is examined only once (Fig. 12-1).

When a subject is examined, his or her age is recorded, and the variable of interest is measured. Subjects are placed into age groups, often decades of life, and the data are reported by presenting the mean value of the variable of interest for each age group. Alternatively, the data can be entered into a regression analysis that relates the parameter studied (the dependent variable Y) to the independent variable age (the X variable). If height were being studied, the equation obtained from the linear regression would be

$$\text{height} = \beta_0 + \beta_1 \text{ age}$$

The coefficient of the age term (β_1, the slope of age), gives the average difference in height between subjects who differ in age by 1 year. Cross-sectional studies are relatively easy, inexpensive, and quick. Unfortunately, inferences from cross-sectional studies are subject to two errors, either of which can lead to incorrect conclusions about the relation between age and the variable studied.

The first error, bias due to birth cohort effects, is a difference between subjects caused solely by the era in which the subjects were born (Fig. 12-2), not by any age difference between subjects. Progressive improvements in nutrition over the first half of this century, for example, may allow more recently-born subjects to achieve a greater adult height than subjects born years earlier. A cross-sectional study of height in a hypothetic population where there is no change in height with aging, will indicate that height decreases with age—not because height is lost as people get older, but because people born in the past did not grow to be as tall as people born recently.

The second error, bias due to selective mortality, occurs when the variable studied, Y, affects the survival of study subjects. If, for example, low values of Y are associated with an increased probability of survival to old age, and high values of Y with decreased probability of survival, the majority of old subjects will have low values of Y. Younger subjects, who are too young to have suffered significant mortality, will demonstrate the full range of values of Y. Even if Y does not change with age, a cross-sectional study of Y will lead to the conclusion that Y decreases with age (Fig. 12-3). Because of the problems inherent in the cross-sectional design (the potential for bias due to selective mortality and birth cohort effects), findings from cross-sectional studies should, whenever possible, be tested in longitudinal studies.

Because death is more common in older subjects, selective mortality can be a major confounder of studies of the oldest old.

Time-series Design

Gerontologists are often interested in examining differences that occur in a population over the course of time. For example, it may be of interest to know if the average cholesterol concentration in 45-year-old men in 1970 is the same as that seen in 45-year-old men in 1980 and 1990. A time-series design can answer this question. In a time-series study, a group of subjects of a given age (or a small age range) is assembled at a fixed point in time, and the group is examined once. Some time later, usually several years, a second group of subjects is assembled and examined. The second group is chosen so

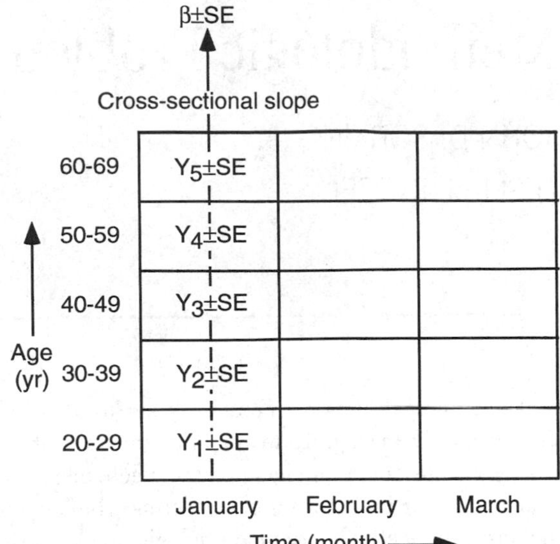

Figure 12-1 The design of a cross-sectional study. Over a short time period, 1 month in this example, a group of subjects 20 to 69 years of age is enrolled in a study. The subjects are divided into age decades. For each age decade, a mean and a standard error are calculated for the variable being studied ($Y_1 \pm$ SE through $Y_5 \pm$ SE). Additionally, a cross-sectional slope, $\beta \pm$ SE, is computed by entering all the data (ignoring the division into age decades) into a regression analysis in which the variable being studied, Y, is the dependent variable and age is the independent variable, X.

Figure 12-2 Differences related to a subject's birth cohort can bias the cross-sectional relation between a variable Y and age. There is no change in Y with age in any individual subject. Each subject's value of Y is determined solely by his date of birth. Subjects born in 1970 are 20 years old when examined in 1990. They were born with a Y value of 80, and maintain this value throughout their lives. This is indicated by the shortest horizontal line. (The next line is for subjects who are 30 years old when examined in 1990; they were born in 1960, and have a lifetime Y value of 70.) Recently-born subjects have higher Y values than subjects born years earlier. In 1990 40-year-old subjects have a Y value of 60, 60-year-old subjects 40, and 90-year-old subjects a Y value of 10. As a result of the birth cohort effect, a cross-sectional study performed in 1990 will lead to the incorrect conclusion that Y decreases with age.

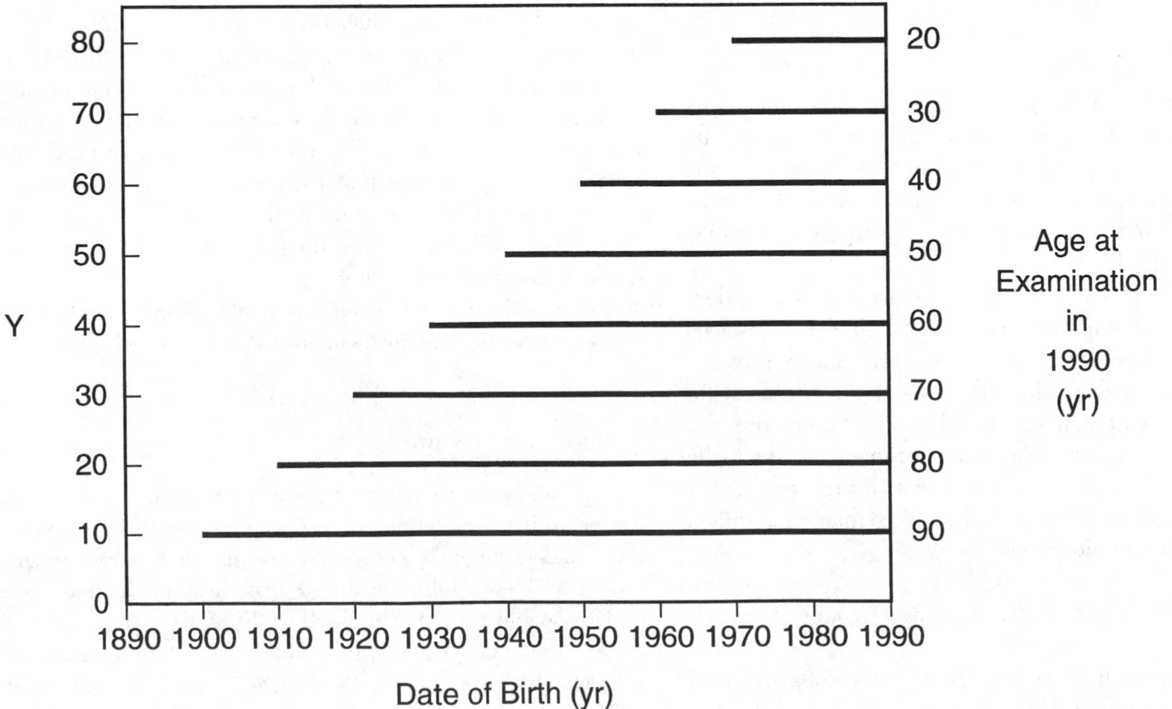

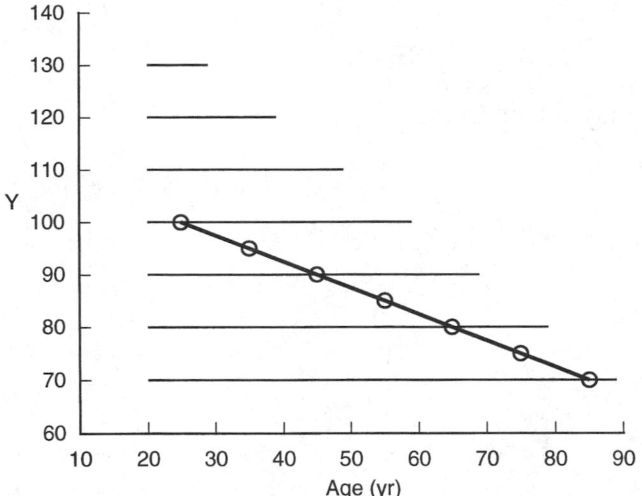

Figure 12-3 Selective mortality can bias cross-sectional studies. In this example, Y does not change with age in any individual subject (the horizontal lines), and high levels of Y are associated with early mortality. If a random cross-section of the population is recruited, all possible values of Y will be seen in young subjects. Thus, in subjects 20 to 29 years of age, the mean value of Y will be 100. Because all subjects with a Y value above 120 die before they reach 30 years of age, the mean value of Y in subjects 30 to 39 years of age is 95. Because only those subjects with the lowest value of Y survive beyond age 80, the only value of Y in subjects 80 to 89 years of age is 70. (The diagonal line in the figure indicates the cross-sectional mean values of Y seen at different ages.) Thus, although Y does not change with age in any subject, a cross-sectional study of Y would indicate that Y decreases with age.

that its age distribution, and mean age, are the same as were the age distribution and mean age of the first group when the first group was examined (Fig. 12-4). When a subject is examined, the age at which he or she is examined is noted as is the value of the parameter being studied.

Any difference between the groups can be ascribed to the time at which the groups were examined and not the age of the groups; the groups have the same mean age when they are examined. Data from a time-series study are reported by presenting the mean value of the parameter of interest by time period. Alternately, the data obtained from all subjects can be entered into a regression analysis, which relates the variable studied (the dependent variable Y) to the independent variable, X, the date of examination. The slope obtained from the regression gives the average difference in the variable of interest between two different subjects of the same age who were examined at two different periods of time.

Time-series studies are subject to two errors that can lead to incorrect conclusions about the association between the factor being studied and time. The first error occurs as a result of a biased selection of subjects in the time periods, a bias that affects the variable being studied. An example would be a

Figure 12-4 The design of a time-series study. At three distinct periods of time, 1970, 1980, and 1990, three distinct groups of subjects are recruited and studied once. The three groups are selected to have the same mean age at the time they are examined. For each of the three groups, a mean and a standard error are calculated for the variable being studied ($Y_1 \pm$ SE through $Y_3 \pm$ SE). Additionally a time-series slope, $\beta \pm$ SE, is computed by entering all the data (ignoring the division into time periods), into a regression analysis in which the variable being studied, Y, is the dependent variable and age is the independent variable, X.

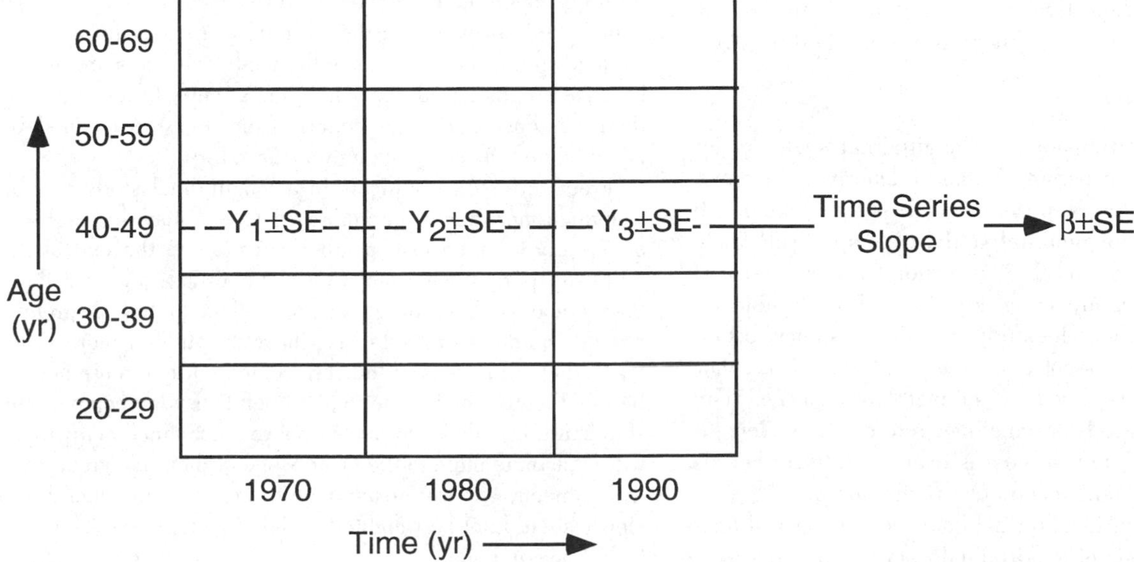

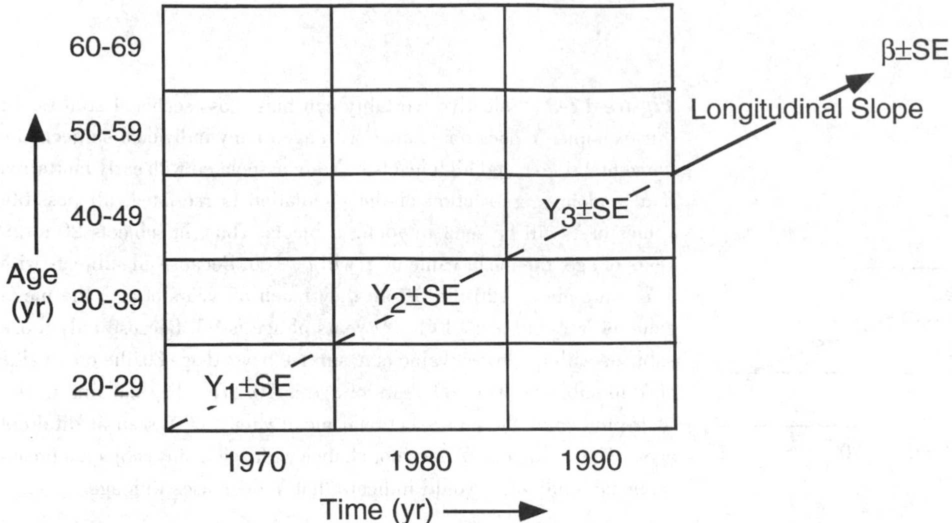

Figure 12-5 The design of a longitudinal study. In 1970, a group of subjects, 20-29 years old is recruited and studied. In 1980, the subjects who were 20 to 29 years old in 1970 are studied again. At this time they are 30 to 39 years old. In 1990, the subjects are 40 to 49 years old and they are studied one last time. For each of the three time periods, 1970, 1980 and 1990, a mean and a standard error are calculated for the variable being studied ($Y_1 \pm$ SE through $Y_3 \pm$ SE). A longitudinal slope, $\beta \pm$ SE, is computed using a two-stage random effects model. The slope characterizes the rate at which Y changes as subjects are aging from age 20 to 29 to age 40 to 49. See text for details.

study of height in which 40-year-old Lilliputians are studied in 1980 and 40-year-old giants are studied in 1990. The conclusion that 40-year-old people are taller in 1990 then were 40-year-old people in 1980 would be the result of studying subjects having different genetically determined heights, rather than a temporal change in height from 1980 to 1990. The second error occurs as a result of methodologic change or drift over time. For example, assume that cholesterol concentration is studied in 1980 and 1990. In 1980 one cholesterol assay is used and in 1990 a second assay that reads 5 mg/dl higher than the first. If the difference is not recognized, a time-series analysis of cholesterol concentration will suggest that cholesterol concentration has increased from 1980 to 1990.

Longitudinal Design

Subjects who participate in a longitudinal study are followed for an extended period of time to determine the rate at which a variable changes in the subjects as they get older. In order to conduct a longitudinal study, a group of subjects is assembled, examined, and then re-examined once, or several times, as the subjects are aging (Fig. 12-5). If each subject is examined exactly twice, the study is sometimes referred to as a cohort study. (This is not to be confused with birth cohort effects previously discussed.) If subjects are examined more than two times, the study is sometimes referred to as a longitudinal study. Each time a subject is examined, his or her age is noted and the variable of interest is measured.

Proper analysis of longitudinal data requires special techniques. If an analysis of longitudinal data is attempted using standard regression techniques (i.e., entering all the data into a single regression analysis), incorrect inferences may result (Fig. 12-6).

Several techniques have been used to analyze data obtained from a longitudinal study. The easiest to understand is the two-stage random effects model (Fig. 12-7). In the first stage of the model, a linear regression is performed for each subject. The regression relates the value obtained at each examination for the variable of interest (the dependent variable Y) to the age at which the datum was collected (the independent variable X). If 100 subjects were enrolled in the study, 100 slopes would be calculated. Each of the 100 slopes gives the average annual rate of change in the variable of interest for a single subject. In the second stage of the model, subjects are placed into age groups based upon their age at entry to the study (or their mean age during the course of the study). A mean slope is calculated for each age group (Fig. 12-8).

Frequently some subjects in a longitudinal study will be examined more times than others. Subjects may die, drop out of the study, or be lost to follow-up prior to the end of the follow-up period. This leads to an important question about the method used to compute the mean slope for the age groups. Should the slopes of subjects who were studied more times than other subjects (and thus are computed from more points) be weighted by the number of data points used to compute the slope? If this is done, subjects who were examined many times will contribute more to the mean slope of their age group than will subjects who were examined fewer times. In general, the slopes should not be weighted; weighting slopes can lead to a biased mean slope.

The problem produced by averaging weighted slopes is best understood by way of an example. Consider a longitudinal study of the change in serum cholesterol concentration. Each subject's cholesterol is measured annually for a maximum of 20 years. (Any subject can thus have his cholesterol measured up to 21 times.) High serum cholesterol concentrations are associated with early mortality. If two subjects of the same age have the same cholesterol concentration at entry to the study, the subject whose cholesterol concentration increases most rapidly will achieve higher levels at a younger age than will the subject whose concentration increases more slowly. Because high concentrations are associated with a high probability of death, the subject with the faster rate of increase will in all likelihood die at an earlier age than the subject whose rate of increase was slower. The subject with the faster rate of increase will therefore be less likely to remain in the study for 20 years than will the subject with the slower rate of increase. The slope for the subject with the faster rate of increase will be computed from fewer points than will the slope for the subject with the slower rate of increase. If the individual slopes are weighted by the number of points used to calculate the slope, the slope from subject with the faster rate of increase will have a smaller weight than the slope from the subject with the slower rate of increase. The average slope will thus be more heavily influenced by subjects with a slower rate of increase than by subjects with a faster rate of increase. The average slope will be biased; the longitudinal analyses will suffer from selective mortality. (The same bias occurs if the individual slopes are weighted by the inverse of their variance.) In general, if the rate of change of the variable studied is related to survival (i.e., the length of time a subject remains in the study), weighted slopes will result in a biased estimate of the rate at which the variable changes with aging.

Aside from the error that can result from the use of weighted slopes, unlike cross-sectional studies, two elements inherent in the design and execution of longitudinal studies keep the results of the study from being biased due to either selective mortality or birth cohort effects. The elements are (1) the requirement that the variable of interest be measured at least twice in each subject and (2) the fact that the slope for each age group is obtained by averaging the slopes calculated for each subject included in the age group, rather than by entering the data for all the subjects in the age group into a single regression analysis. If unweighted slopes are used, each subject will contribute equally to the average slope in his age group, regardless of the time at which the subject leaves the study, the number of points the subject contributes to the analysis, or the time at which the subject is lost to follow-up or dies. Thus longitudinal studies do not suffer from bias due to selective mortality. Birth cohort effects cause problems when subjects from different birth cohorts with different initial values of the variable studied are compared. In longitudinal analyses, individual subjects are not compared to each other. Slopes are computed for each individual, and the individual slopes

Figure 12-6 Standard regression techniques (i.e., entering all data into a single regression analysis) can result in an incorrect conclusion about the relation between a variable and age. In this example, data are plotted for five subjects (the five solid lines). For each subject Y decreases as the subject gets older. The regression line obtained by entering all the data into a single regression analysis is depicted by the dashed line. The dashed line incorrectly indicates that Y increases with age.

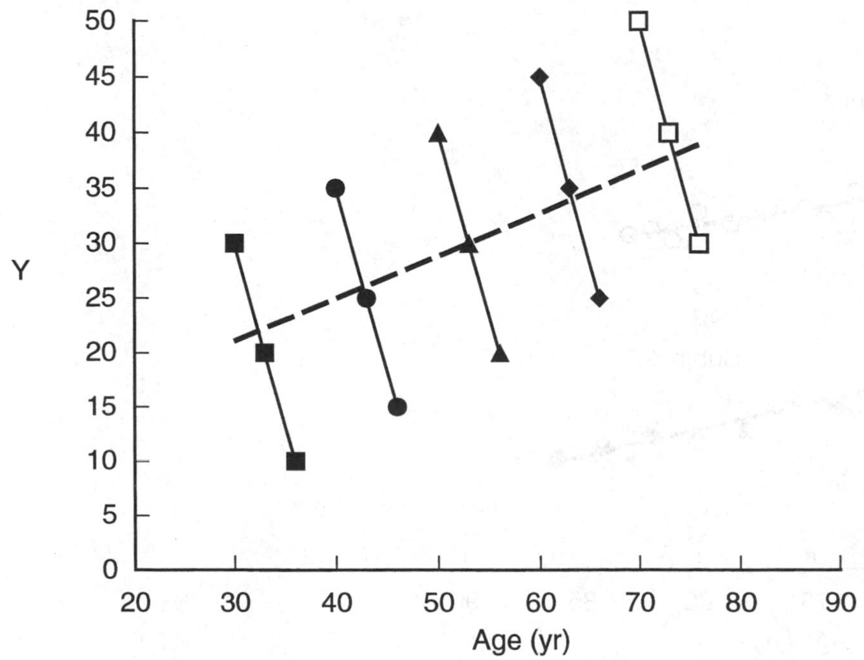

are averaged to get a mean slope for an age group. Because slopes are computed for each subject rather than for the entire group, individual subjects are not compared and thus, longitudinal studies are free from bias due to birth cohort effects.

Longitudinal studies can be very sensitive to small changes in assay methodology. These changes that can result from changing to a new instrument, a new reagent lot, or change in the personnel measuring the variable of interest. A small change in methodology can make a variable that does not change with age appear to change (Fig. 12-9).

Several steps can be taken to lessen the probability of methodologic change during the course of longitudinal study, including thorough training of study personnel (with periodic refresher courses), the use of a standard reference pool, and a crossover period when switching from an old to a new instrument. In the crossover period, duplicate samples are run on the new and old instruments, and a correction factor is generated that converts values from the new machine to values that would have been obtained on the old machine.

Even if great care has been taken to ensure assay stability, it remains important to look for methodologic error prior to data analysis. This is one of the most important steps in the analysis of longitudinal data; it is also one of the least frequently discussed. A review of techniques that can be used to test for methodologic error is beyond the scope of this chapter. A brief review of two techniques is presented in Elahi et al.[2]

The average life span of the subjects of longitudinal studies is usually longer than the period of time that any individual subject is studied. As a result, if the aim of a study is to understand the change in a variable that occurs over the course of adult life, the age range studied is generally broken into shorter intervals, often age decades. Each subject is placed into an age decade, based either upon his age at entry to the study, or his mean age during the period he participated in the study, and a mean slope is calculated for each age decade. If the average rate of change for each age decade is plotted (or tabulated) by the natural order of the age decades, a sense of the change of a variable over the entire adult life span will

Figure 12-7 An example of the first stage of a two-stage random effects model for the analysis of longitudinal data. In the first stage of the model, the rate at which a variable, in this case height, changes is calculated for each subject. This is accomplished by performing a separate linear regression for each subject in which the dependent variable, Y, is height and the independent variable is age, X. For subject 1, the regression is performed using data from 18 observations (the open circles), for subject 2, eight (the closed circles). In the second stage, each subject is placed into an age group (often an age decade) based upon age at entry to the study. In this example, subject 1 would be placed into the 60 to 69 year age decade, subject 2 into the 70 to 79 year age decade. (Alternately, each subject could be placed into an age decade based upon his mean age during the time he was studied. In this case, subject 1 would be placed into the 70 to 79 year age decade, subject 2 would also be placed into the 70 to 79 year age decade.) In the second stage of the model (Figure 12-8) each age group is characterized by the mean of the ages (either mean of the ages at entry or mean of each subject's mean age) and the mean of the slopes of the subjects assigned to the age group.

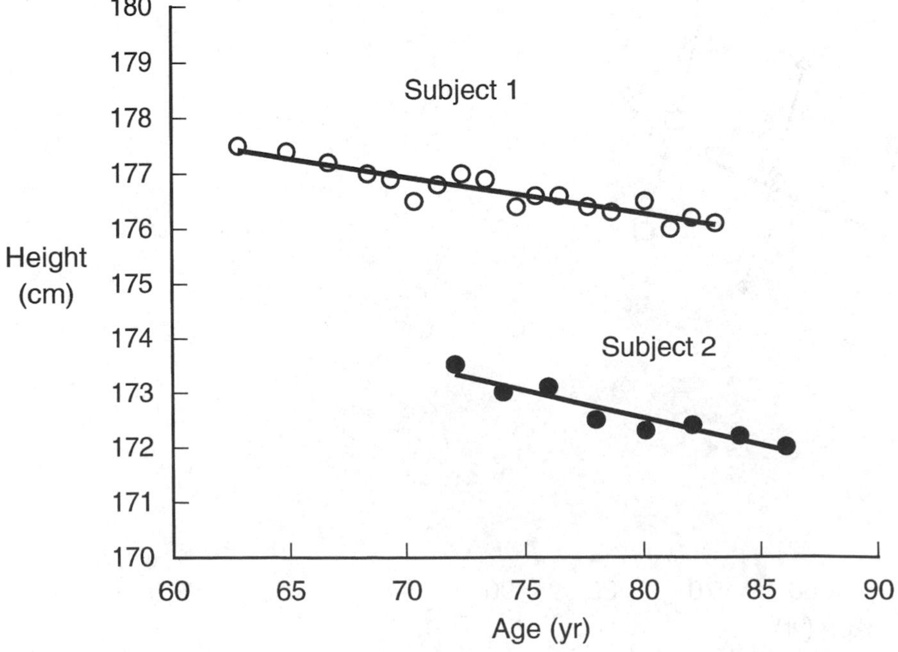

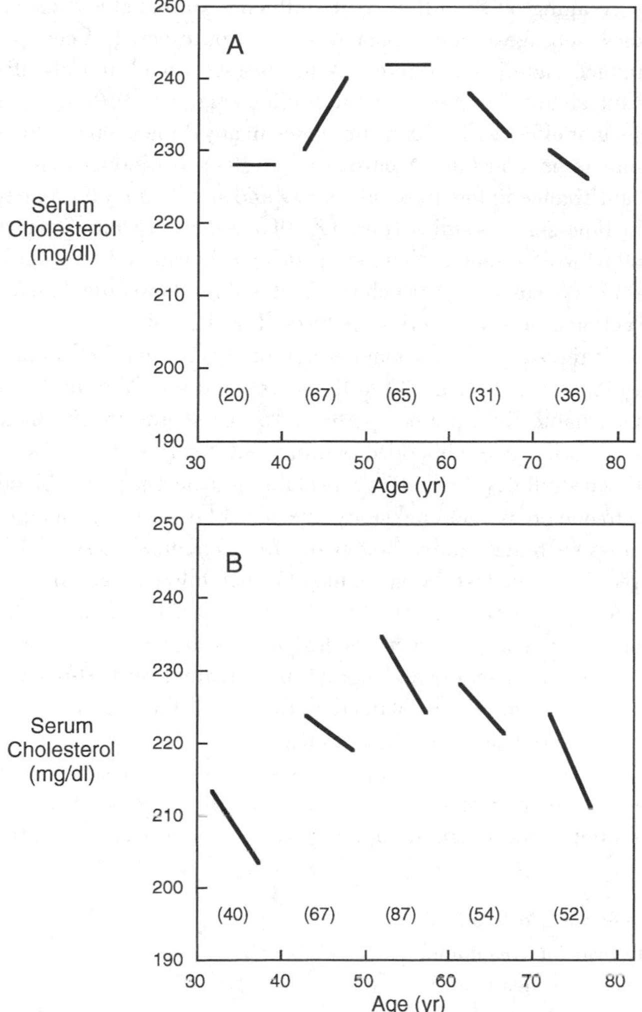

Figure 12-8 Longitudinal change in serum cholesterol in men from the Baltimore Longitudinal Study of Aging. The longitudinal change in each decade of life is represented by a line segment whose slope is the mean rate of change in cholesterol concentration for men whose mean age during longitudinal follow-up fell within the age decade. The midpoint of each line segment is plotted at the cross-sectional mean cholesterol concentration and cross-sectional mean age for the age decade. The horizontal length of each line (i.e., the difference between the age at the end and beginning of each line) represents the mean follow-up. The number of subjects included in each age decade is indicated by the numbers in parentheses. Fig. A depicts the change from 1963 through 1971. During this period cholesterol increased from young adulthood to middle age. Longitudinal analyses and cross-sectional analyses (represented by the midpoint of each line) show similar results. This pattern is consistent with a pure aging effect. Fig. B depicts the change from 1969 to 1977. In this period, cholesterol concentration drops in all five age decades; cross-sectional and longitudinal analyses disagree. In the youngest three age decades, the cross-sectional mean for each age decade, represented by the middle of each line segment, is at a progressively higher value as the mean age of the subjects increases; there is a cross-sectional increase in cholesterol with increasing age. ***Figure 12-8*** *(Continued)* During this period, the longitudinal slope in each of the age decades indicates that within each age decade cholesterol falls as subjects are aging. This pattern is consistent with a secular drop in cholesterol, which the authors felt was the result of "environmental factors." (From Hershcopf et al.[1] with permission.)

emerge. This methodology allows a pattern of nonlinear change to be seen (Fig. 12-8A). (Even if the lifetime trajectory of a variable is curvilinear, the change in most biologic variables over a short period of time, such as a decade, can be approximated as linear.)

A longitudinal study is more complex to design than a cross-sectional or time-series study. Important issues include the size of the group that must be studied, the number of measurements that should be obtained from each study participant, the frequency with which participants should be studied, and the length of time subjects should be followed. Factors that will influence the design include the rate at which the parameter of interest changes, the precision with which the parameter is measured, the day-to-day variability in the parameter, and the time and money available to perform the longitudinal study. An excellent discussion of the issues involved in planning a longitudinal study is contained in Schlesselman.[3,4]

Cautions About Inferences Derived From Cross-Sectional, Time-Series, and Longitudinal Studies

A statistically significant longitudinal change in a variable (a longitudinal slope that is significantly different from zero) does not ensure that the change is the result of aging. A secular trend in lifestyle could account for the change. A secular trend (sometimes referred to as a temporal trend) is a change occurring over a long time period, generally years or decades. Examples of secular trends include the decrease in cardiovascular disease mortality and infant mortality that has occurred in the United States over the last 45 years.[5] As an example of the effect of a secular trend, consider a longitudinal study of cholesterol concentration that finds a decrease in serum cholesterol with aging. The decrease might be due to biologic aging (i.e., the genetics of aging), but it might be due to a secular decrease in the consumption of fat over the course of the study, which in turn, leads to the decrease in serum cholesterol concentration.

Just as a significant change in a variable seen in a longitudinal study does not ensure that the change is due to aging, a significant difference in a cross-sectional study does not ensure that the difference is due to age. Consider a cross-sectional study that finds a cross-sectional decrease in height with age. Older subjects may be shorter than younger subjects because of biologic aging (e.g., an age-determined progressive loss of bone calcium leading to an increased incidence of compression fractures of the spinal vertebral bodies leading to loss of height), or the cross-sectional height differences may be due to birth cohort effects (Fig. 12-2).

As used above, a cohort effect (also known as a generation effect) is "a variation in health status that arises from the different factors to which each birth cohort in the population is exposed to as the environment and society changes."[6] A cohort effect that might affect height would be the progressively better nutrition in utero, infancy, and childhood that has occurred in the United States over the last century. The progressive improvement in nutrition during growth and development may allow more recently born subjects to achieve a greater fraction of their genetic height potential than was possible for subjects born earlier. Similarly, an apparent secular effect (often refered to as a temporal effect) seen in a time-series analyses may be confused with a birth cohort effect. Although a definitive determination of the etiology of a significant finding from a cross-sectional, time-series, or longitudinal study may be impossible from the usual study designs, an understanding of the effects of a pure aging, secular, or cohort effect is essential to understanding the possible etiologies of an observed effect.

Each of the three study designs—cross-sectional, time-series, and longitudinal—studies a single factor (time, date of birth, or age) while keeping one of the other two factors constant (Fig. 12-10A).

A longitudinal study explores the effect of aging, keeping date of birth constant (Fig. 12-10A). A cross-sectional study explores the effect of age, keeping time constant. A time-series study examines the effect of time, keeping age constant. A pure aging effect will exert its influence in any study design in which age is not constant. Thus, a pure aging effect will induce significant differences in cross-sectional and significant changes in longitudinal studies (Fig. 12-10B). A pure secular effect will exert its influence in any dimension in which time is not constant. A pure secular effect will induce significant change in longitudinal studies and significant differences in time-series studies (Fig. 12-10C). Finally, a pure cohort effect will be seen in those study designs in which date of birth is not constant. A pure cohort effect will therefore affect cross-sectional and time-series analyses (Fig. 12-10D).

If the subjects of a longitudinal study are recruited from a wide age range (e.g., 30 to 84 years), and are followed for a reasonable time period (perhaps 15 years), the longitudinal study will have embedded within itself a series of cross-sectional studies. (The first 5 years of the study might be combined into one cross-sectional study, the second 5 years into another cross-sectional study, etc.) If the first 5 years, the second 5 years, and the last 5 years of longitudinal follow-up are divided into age groups, perhaps by 5 years of age, the data can be analyzed using a time-series design. If all three analytic techniques (cross-sectional, longitudinal, and time-series) are used to analyze the data obtained during the follow-up period, a better understanding of the etiology of any observed effect will be possible than from an analysis of the data using only a longitudinal design. If significant effects are seen in cross-sectional and longitudinal analyses, and the effects are in the

Figure 12-9 A small change in assay methodology can have a profound effect on a longitudinal study. In this example, a new instrument is used to measure Y in the eighth year of a longitudinal study. The new instrument reads three units higher than the old instrument. Although there is no increase in Y with aging, the effect of the introduction of the new instrument is to change the slope for each subject from zero to a positive value. The average of the two slopes will be a positive number rather than the correct value of zero.

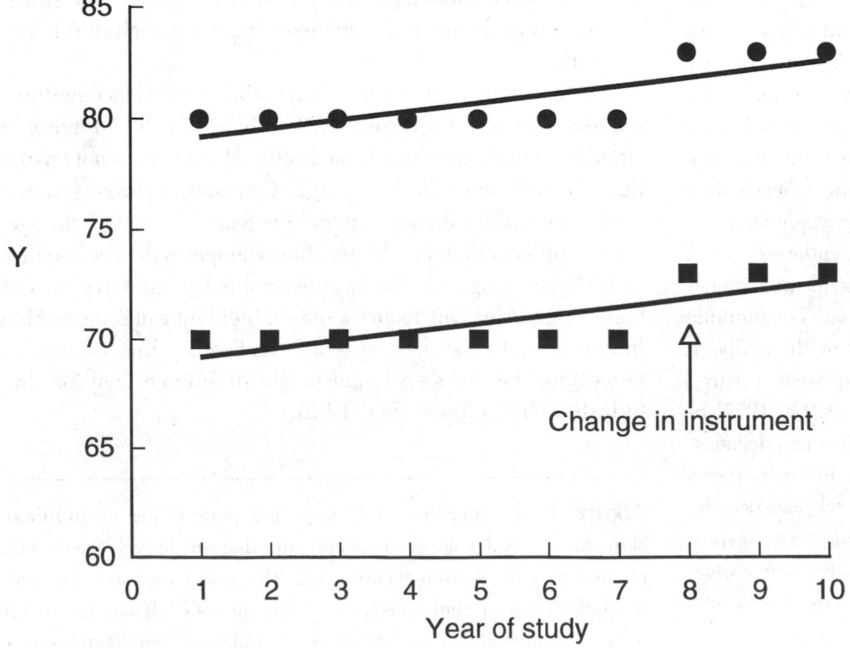

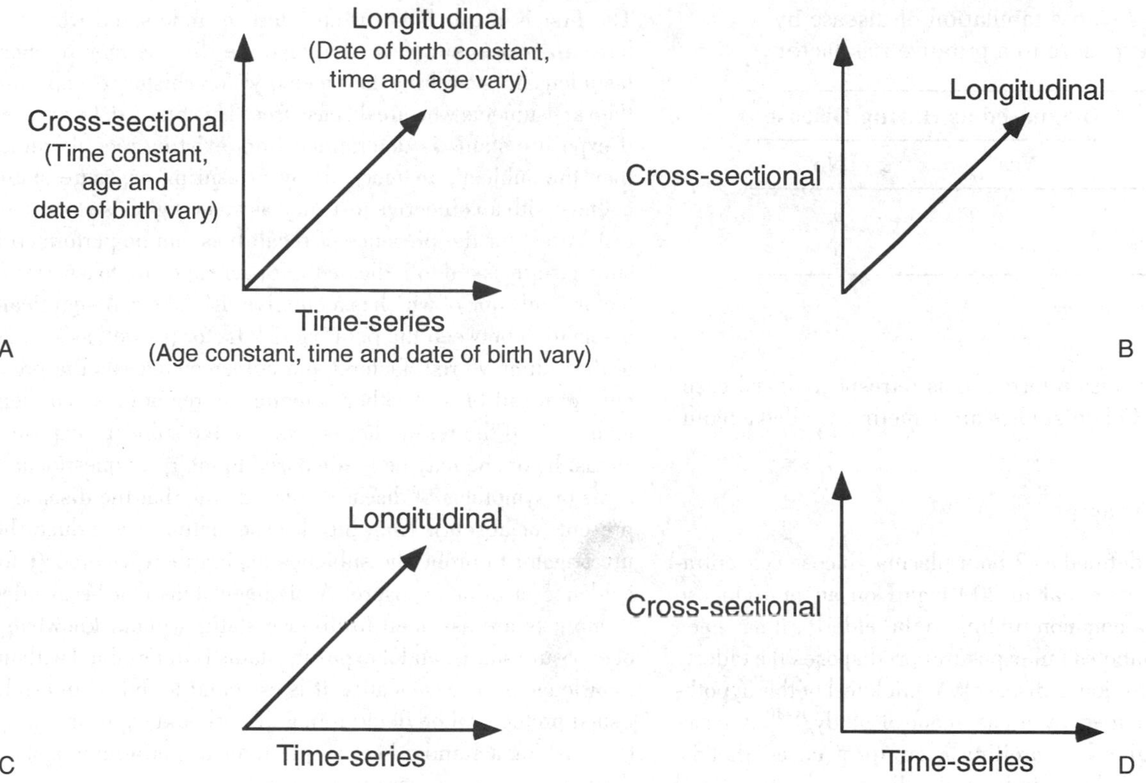

Figure 12-10 The effect of a pure aging, secular, and cohort effect on cross-sectional, time-series, and longitudinal studies. Fig. A identifies a unique axis for each of the three study designs (cross-sectional, longitudinal, and time-series) and indicates the effect that is held constant in each of the study designs. Fig. B indicates the study designs that are affected by a pure aging effect, Fig C by a pure secular effect, and Fig. D by a pure cohort effect.

same direction (both show an increase with age or both show a decrease with age) and are of similar magnitude, a pure aging effect can be postulated (Fig. 12-10B). If significant effects are seen in longitudinal and time-series analyses (and the effects are in the same direction and of similar magnitude) a pure secular etiology can be invoked (Fig. 12-10C). If cross-sectional and time-series analyses are significant (and are in the same direction and of similar magnitude), a pure cohort effect may be suspected (Fig. 12-10D). If significant effects are seen in all three analytic methodologies, a mixed effect is probably responsible. Conversely, a pure aging effect should be postulated only if consistent significant effects are seen in cross-sectional and longitudinal analyses and not in time-series analyses (Fig. 12-10B); a pure secular effect only if consistent significant effects are seen in longitudinal and time-series analyses but not in cross-sectional analyses; and a pure cohort effect only if consistent significant effects are seen in time-series and cross-sectional analyses but not in longitudinal analyses. An excellent description of a study in which longitudinal data were analyzed using longitudinal, cross-sectional, and time-series methodologies is presented in Elahi et al.[7]

Case-Control and Cohort Designs

The methodologies discussed up to this point for the analysis of data from cross-sectional, longitudinal, and time-series studies are applicable to continuous data that can take on a wide range of values (e.g., serum cholesterol concentration, or height). If the data can only have one of two values (i.e., the presence or absence of a characteristic such as being diabetic versus not being diabetic), other methods must be used. Two widely used methods for the analysis of data that can be classified as "0 versus 1" or "yes versus no" are the case-control and cohort designs.* A case-control study is related to a cross-sectional study in that each subject in a case-control study is examined only once. A cohort study is related to a longitudinal study in that every subject is examined at least twice. Case-

**The use of the term cohort in this context is unfortunate as it can be confused with a longitudinal study in which every subject is examined exactly twice. Hopefully, the context in which the word is used will make its intended meaning clear.*

Table 12-1 Cross tabulation of disease by history of exposure to a putative risk factor[a]

History of Exposure	Diagnosed as Having Disease	
	Yes	**No**
Yes	a	b
No	c	d

[a] *See text for explanation.*

control studies are also referred to as retrospective and case-referrent studies. Cohort studies are sometimes called longitudinal studies.

Case-Control Design

Type II diabetes, defined as 2-hour plasma glucose concentration greater than or equal to 200 mg/dl on an oral glucose tolerance test, is a common finding in the elderly. It has been postulated that diabetes (an exposure) predisposes the elderly to myocardial infarction (a disease). A quick test of this hypothesis could be provided by a case-control study.[8–10] A case-control study begins by enrolling a group of cases, that is, subjects tested and shown to have the disease of interest and a group of controls, subjects who are tested and shown not to have the disease of interest. At the time they are enrolled, cases and controls are examined for the presence of (or are asked to report if they were exposed to) a putative risk factor for the condition being studied. Although the history of exposure often comes from the subject's self-report or an examination of the subject, the history of exposure will at times be obtained from records (e.g., occupational, military, or medical). In the diabetes example, exposure status might be determined by a 2-hour glucose concentration greater than or equal to 200 mg/dl on an oral glucose tolerance test performed at the time subjects are enrolled in the study. On the basis of the presence or absence of the condition being studied and subjects' exposure history, a 2 × 2 table is produced that cross-tabulates disease status by exposure history (Table 12-1). The measure of the association between disease and exposure in a case-control study is the odds ratio. Using the symbols from Table 12-1, the odds ratio is defined as follows:

$$(a/c)/(b/d) = ad/bc$$

An odds ratio greater than one indicates that exposure is associated with disease. An odds ratio less than one indicates that exposure is associated with protection from disease. The rationale for using the odds ratio as the measure of association, its relation to the probability of disease in exposed subject compared to unexposed subjects, and the methods used to determine the statistical significance of an odds ratio are beyond the scope of this chapter. Interested readers are referred to Kahn and Sempos.[8]

Case-control studies are subject to several types of bias. The first is recall bias. In an effort to understand why they have a disease, subjects who have the disease may be more fastidious in "searching their memory" for a history of exposure then are subjects who are disease free. This bias can be avoided if exposure status is determined from existing records rather than the subject's memory, or by measuring exposure status at entry with an objective test such as an oral glucose tolerance test. A test for the presence of recall bias can be performed if subjects are asked to indicate their past exposure to a series of factors, only one of which is a putative risk factor. A significant association between the putative risk factor (as well as several of the "dummy" risk factors) and outcome suggests the presence of recall bias. Another potential source of bias is assignment bias. If the researcher is aware of the subject's exposure status, he or she may be predisposed to interpret questionable signs or symptoms of disease as indicating that the disease is present (or absent). Knowing disease status may induce the investigator to probe the subject's history more vigorously for evidence of prior exposure. Assignment bias can be avoided if subjects are assigned to disease status without knowledge of exposure status, and if exposure status is determined without knowledge of disease status. It is essential to follow an established protocol when determining disease and exposure status (e.g., asking a standard set of questions or performing a standard series of laboratory techniques).

Case-control studies have an important weakness; the inability to determine if there is a temporal association between exposure and the presence of disease. If the risk factor being studied causes disease, exposure to the risk factor must precede the appearance of disease. Because exposure and disease status are determined at the same time, at entry to the case-control study, it is not possible to determine if the putative risk factor resulted in the disease or if the disease process resulted in the observed status of the risk factor. A case-control study may indicate that elevated cholesterol concentration (defined as a serum cholesterol greater than or equal to 240 mg/dl) is associated with a history of myocardial infarction. Although this may be true, an alternate hypothesis would be that elevated cholesterol concentration promotes survival in those persons who suffer an infarction. If this hypothesis is true, people with low cholesterol concentrations will not survive their myocardial infarction. The pool of subjects who have had a myocardial infarction will be enriched with subjects whose cholesterol level is high (a from Table 12-1) and will have few subjects whose cholesterol is low (c from Table 12-1). The pool of subjects who did not have a heart attack will not be affected by this selection pressure. Increasing a and decreasing c without effecting b and d will bias the odds ratio ad : bc toward values greater than one. Thus case-control studies, much like cross-sectional studies, are subject to selective mortality. Case-control studies are often used to study rare diseases, diseases such as Binswanger's disease where it would not be practical to follow non affected subjects until they develop the disease. The problems inherent in the case-control design will often require a case-control study to be confirmed by a study conducted according to a cohort design.

Table 12-2 Cross tabulation of disease incidence during follow-up by exposure status at entry to a cohort study[a]

Exposure at Entry	Diagnosed as Having Disease During Follow-up: Yes	No	Total
Yes	a	b	a + b
No	c	d	c + d

[a] *See text for explanation.*

Cohort Design

Disability is an important problem for the elderly. It has been suggested that obesity in young adulthood (an exposure), defined as a BMI (body mass index, an index of weight adjusted for height) greater than 27 kg/m,[2] may lead to disability in old age (a disease). A cohort study could explore this question. A cohort study begins by screening a group of subjects to see if they have the condition being studied. The screening can be accomplished by examination, laboratory testing, or questioning the subject. Only those subjects who are free of the disease or condition of interest are enrolled into the study. At the time subjects are enrolled, a risk factor is measured and subjects are placed into an exposed or unexposed group. Some time in the future, at the time of follow-up, subjects are again screened to see if they have the disease or condition. On the bases of the results of the second screening, and the exposure status determined at entry to the study, a 2 × 2 table is created (Table 12-2).

The measure of the association between disease and exposure in a cohort study is the relative risk. The relative risk is defined (using the symbols from Table 12-2) as follows;

$$(a/(a + b))/(c/(c + d))$$

The relative risk, unlike the odds ratio, is a direct measure of the ratio of the rate of disease in exposed subjects to the rate of disease in unexposed subjects. A relative risk greater than one indicates that subjects who are exposed to the risk factor have a higher probability of developing the disease or condition than do subjects who are not exposed. Thus, a relative risk greater than one indicates that exposure is associated with disease. A relative risk less than one indicates that exposure is associated with protection from disease. The method used to determine the statistical significance of a relative risk is beyond the scope of this chapter. Interested readers are referred to Kahn and Sempos.[8] Because exposure status for each subject is determined at the time of enrollment into the study, before the disease or condition being studied develops, cohort studies, unlike case-control studies, are free from recall bias. Assignment bias can, however, occur if the person who evaluates subjects for the presence of disease at the end of the follow-up knows the subjects' exposure status. Cohort studies, as compared to case-control studies, can establish a temporal relation between exposure and disease incidence. Unfortunately, cohort studies take longer to complete and are more expensive than case-control studies.

Cohort studies can suffer from confounding as a consequence of loss to follow-up. If some subjects who were enrolled in the study never return for follow-up examination, they will not be included in the 2 × 2 table and hence will not be included in the computation of the relative risk. The computation of relative risk will be biased if the relation between exposure and disease is different in subjects lost to follow-up than it is in subjects who remain in the study. This survival bias is a form of selective mortality. As having no loss to follow-up is the only way to avoid survival bias, every attempt possible should be made to locate subjects who do not return for follow-up examination and convince them to return. Because some loss to follow-up is almost inevitable (subjects die, get sick, move, etc.), an important step in the analysis of a cohort study is to determine the potential effect of the loss to follow-up. Two methods have been used to accomplish this goal.

The first method is to assume that every subject who was lost to follow-up developed the condition being studied at the time they were lost to follow-up, and then reanalyze the data. This analysis is followed by one in which it is assumed that subjects who were lost to follow-up did not develop the condition being studied. If both analyses come to the same qualitative conclusion about the putative risk factor (i.e., both indicate that exposure increases risk, or both indicate that exposure is protective), and these results are qualitatively the same as those obtained from an analysis that excludes subjects who were lost to follow-up, then loss to follow-up might change the magnitude of the association between exposure and disease, but it will not change a protective factor into a risk factor for disease nor will it change a risk factor into a protective factor. If the two analyses come to different qualitative conclusions, the potential effect of loss to follow-up is uncertain, and any conclusion derived from the study is weakened.

The second method is to compare baseline characteristics of subjects lost to follow-up to baseline characteristics of subjects who were followed to the end of the study. A typical comparison might include age, sex, race, exposure status, and socioeconomic status. If there are no systematic differences between subjects who were lost to follow-up and those who were not, it is unlikely that subjects lost to follow-up had a different relation between exposure and outcome than did subjects who were not lost to follow-up. In this case, loss to follow-up is unlikely to have a substantial effect on the inferences derived from the study.

Extentions to the Case-Control and Cohort Designs

Case-control and cohort designs are important tools in the analysis of the relation between an outcome variable that can be in one of two states, diseased or not diseased, and a single independent variable, exposure status, which can take on two states, exposed or nonexposed. Rather straightforward modifications of the designs permit exposure status to have more than two discrete values.[8] These modifications, however, do not allow the exposure variable to be expressed as a continuous variable, and the modifications are limited in their ability to allow additional covariates to be added to the model. (In a study of the relation between diabetes and mortality, it might be of interest to include the subject's age as an additional covariate.) Logistic regression,[8] which is closely related to case-control methodology, and Cox proportional hazards regression,[11] which is closely related to cohort methodology, allow the exposure to be expressed as a continuous variable rather than as yes or no (e.g., actual cholesterol concentration rather than hypercholesterolemia versus a normal concentration). Although logistic regression and the Cox model are more "sophisticated" than are the case-control and cohort methodologies, they are subject to the same biases as are their respective simpler models.

Cautions About the Interpertation of Studies

A statistically significant relation between a risk factor and outcome, regardless of study design, does not guarantee that the association is "true." False associations can be produced by chance, bias, or confounding. A chance association is an association that is due to the random variation seen in a sample of a larger population. The paradigm followed in almost every study of the association between a risk factor and an outcome is to select a sample group of subjects from the total population and then perform a test to see if there is an association between the risk factor and outcome in the sample. Based upon the association (or lack of association) seen in the sample, an inference is made about the association of the risk factor and outcome in the entire population. The major problem with this paradigm is that the findings in the sample may not be generalizable to the total population. It is unlikely that the exact same relation between risk factor and outcome would be seen in two distinct samples of the population. There will always be some variation in the characteristics of the subjects that make up different samples (in the way in which the studies are performed in the samples, in the time of day the studies are performed, etc.), all of which will introduce variation in the relation between risk factor and outcome in different samples of the population. If the variation is large enough, it is possible that one sample will indicate that the risk factor is associated with disease and the second sample will indicate that the risk factor protects subjects from disease.

Chance variation between samples, or between a sample and the population, can be minimized by studying as large a random sample of the population as possible. Additionally, mathematic techniques are available to estimate the magnitude of the inter sample variation that might be expected due to chance alone. Statistical tests and the probability values (P values) obtained from the tests have been used to quantify the degree to which chance variability may account for the observed association. In medical research, a probability less than 5 percent ($P < 0.05$), is considered sufficient evidence to conclude that an association is unlikely to be due to chance variation (under the assumption of no association between exposure and outcome). A probability greater than or equal to 5 percent ($P > 0.05$), is considered insufficient evidence to exclude the possibility that chance variation is the source of the observed association. More recently, interest has focused on the computation of a confidence interval, which gives the range within which the true magnitude of an association lies with a certain degree of assurance. A discussion of the relative utility of P values versus confidence intervals is found in Rothman.[9]

Bias refers to any error in the planning, execution, or evaluation of a study that leads to a systematic error in the estimation of the association between a putative risk factor and outcome. Several, but not all, sources of bias, and techniques for dealing with them, have been discussed earlier in this chapter.

Confounding refers to a condition in which the association between a putative risk factor and outcome is distorted due to the effect of a third factor. Figure 12-11 depicts a hypothetic relation between a risk factor (BMI) and outcome—mortality in two groups of subjects, smokers and nonsmokers. The percentage of subjects who are smokers is inversely related to BMI throughout the range of BMIs seen in the population. At low BMI values, 90 percent of the subjects studied are smokers and the remaining 10 percent are nonsmokers. In the middle of the BMI range, 50 percent of all subjects are smokers and 50 percent are nonsmokers. At the highest BMIs seen, 10 percent of the subjects are smokers and 90 percent are nonsmokers.

The relation between BMI and mortality in smokers is shown by the upper dashed line; mortality increases with both high and low BMI. Minimal mortality occurs in the middle of the BMI range. The relation between BMI and mortality in nonsmokers (the lower dashed line) is the same as that seen in smokers; mortality increases with both high and low BMI. At any given BMI, however, the mortality rate is higher in smokers than it is in nonsmokers. If the relation between BMI and mortality is studied separately in smokers and nonsmokers (i.e, the analysis is "stratified by smoking status") the true "U"-shaped relation between BMI and mortality is seen. If, however, the relation between BMI and mortality is studied without regard to smoking status, (the subjects are analyzed as a single group), the relation between BMI and mortality seen is depicted by the solid line. At low BMI values, the mortality rate of the subjects will be close to that seen in smokers, since essentially all subjects are smokers. At high BMI values, the morality rate will be close to that of nonsmokers, since almost all subjects are nonsmokers. For subjects whose BMI is close to the middle of the BMI range, the overall morality rate will be close to midway between that seen in smokers and nonsmokers, because approximately one-half the subjects are smokers and the remaining one-half are nonsmokers. Thus, smoking confounds the relation between BMI and

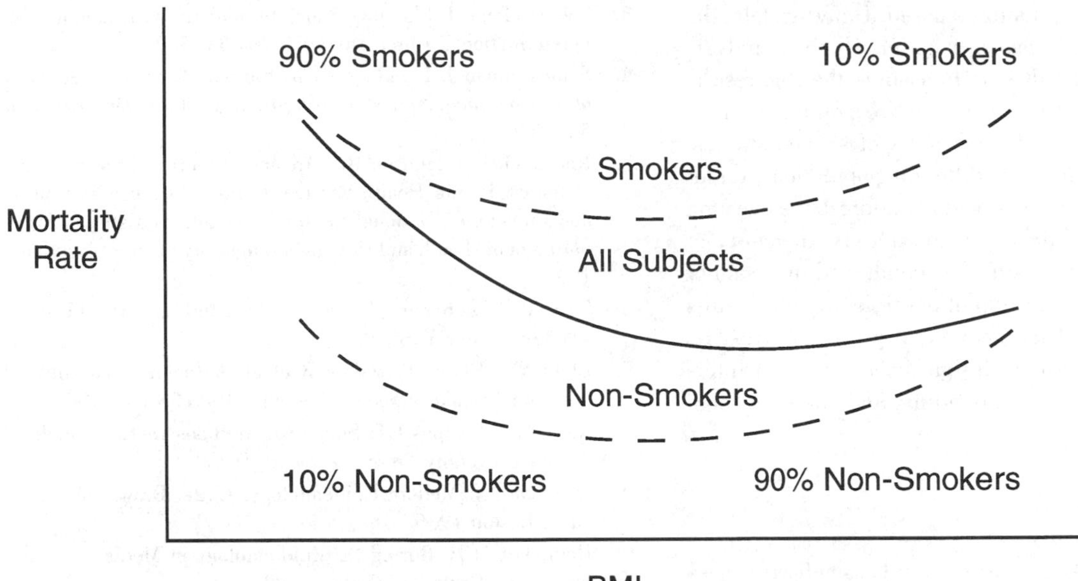

Figure 12-11 The hypothetical relation between a risk factor, BMI, is confounded by smoking status. See text for details.

mortality. If the confounding is not recognized and eliminated, the true "U"-shaped relation between smoking and mortality will not be seen.

Several steps can be taken to minimize the detrimental effects of confounding. (Attempting to eliminate the detrimental effects of confounding is often referred to as "adjusting" an analysis.) Stratification into groups based upon the value of a suspected confounder—for example, into smokers and non-smokers—will often allow the true relation between a risk factor and outcome to be seen if separate analyses are performed in each of the groups. A second method, restriction, is a technique in which analyses are performed in groups of subjects in which the potential confounder is restricted to a single, or in the case of a continuous confounder, to a small range of values. If age is believed to confound the relation between cholesterol and mortality, a study of the relation of cholesterol to mortality in the entire adult age range (i.e., 20 to 99 years) could be broken down into eight smaller analyses (20 to 29, 30 to 39 etc.). Within any age decade, the confounding due to age will be small because the subjects in any age decade are essentially the same age. A third method is the multvariate adjustment. This last technique is accomplished by adding the confounder as an additional independent variable to a model that includes the risk factor as an independent variable and the outcome as the dependent variable.

$$\text{Unadjusted model: mortality rate} = \beta_0 + \beta_1 BMI$$

$$\text{Adjusted model: mortality rate} = \beta_0 + \beta_1 BMI + \beta_2 \text{ smoking status}$$

where β_0 is the intercept; β_1 is the slope for BMI; and β_2 is the slope for smoking status.

A fourth technique is matching. In case-control analysis, subjects, at the time they are recruited, can be chosen so that cases and controls are "matched" on a potential confounder. If race is believed to be a confounder, for each of the cases selected, a control could be selected that is the same race as its respective control. Several races could participate in the study (as long as each case is matched with a control of the same race). Matching removes the racial difference between a case and its respective control. The case-control methodology previously described assumes that cases and controls were not matched. The analysis of a matched case-control study is slightly more complex than is the analysis of an unmatched case-control study.[8–10,12] Matching can also be performed in cohort studies.[9]

Regardless of the technique used to adjust for a potential confounder, if the relation between a putative risk factor and outcome is the same before and after adjustment, there is no confounding and the "confounder" can be ignored. If the results are different, the potential confounder is a true confounder, and the true relation between risk factor and outcome can only be determined after adjustment is performed. A complete discussion of chance, bias, and confounding, and the methods that can be used to avoid them is beyond the scope of this chapter. Interested readers are referred to any epidemiology text book including Rothman,[9] Hennekens et al,[10] and Kahn et al.[8]

The final methodologic problem in research on aging is determing the generalizability of the results of a study. Regardless of the care taken in the planning, execution, and evaluation of a study, unrecognized bias, confounding, and chance variation may be present. Thus, the results of a study may not be generalizable to the entire population. Many of the techniques used to lessen the probability of bias and the confounding result in restricting the population studied. Unfortunately, the more restrictive the conditions are under which a study is performed, the more difficult it is to assume that the results of a study can be generalized to the entire population. It is only through a comparison of the results of several studies, performed at different times, in different populations, under different conditions, that we can begin to address the question of the generalizability of an association. It is, therefore, of utmost importance that every study be conducted in a manner that will ensure, to as great an extent possible, that the results of the study are correct. This means that great care must be taken to assure that the study design, execution, and interpretation are as free of bias, confounding, and chance as possible.

References

1. Hershcopf RJ, Elahi D, Andres R et al: Longitudinal changes in serum cholesterol in man: an epidemiologic search for an etiology. J Chron Dis 1982;35:101–114
2. Elahi D, Muller DC, Rowe JW: Design, conduct, and analysis of human aging research. pp. 29–30. In Handbook of the Biology of Aging. Academic Press, San Diego 1995
3. Schlesselman J: Planning a longitudinal study. I. Sample size determination. J Chron Dis 1973;26:553–560
4. Schlesselman J: Planning a longitudinal study. II. Frequency of measurement and study duration. J Chron Dis 1973;26: 561–570
5. Kochanek KD, Hudson BL: Advance report of final mortality statistics. Public Health Service, Centers for Disease Control and Prevention, National Center for Health Statistics, US Department of Health and Human Services, Hyattsville, Maryland, 1995
6. Last JM: A Dictionary of Epidemiology. 2nd Ed. Oxford University Press, New York, 1988
7. Elahi VK, Elahi D, Andres R et al: A longitudinal study of nutritional intake in men. J Gerontol 1983;38:162–180
8. Kahn HA, Sempos CT: Statistical Methods in Epidemiology. Oxford University Press, New York, 1989
9. Rothman KJ: Modern Epidemiology. Little, Brown and Company, Boston 1986
10. Hennekens CH, Buring JE: Epidemiology in Medicine. Little, Brown and Company, Bostory, 1987
11. Lee ET: 10.2.2 Multivariate analysis: Cox proportional hazards model for survival data. pp. 250–263. In Statistical Methods for Survival Data Analysis. John Wiley & Sons, New York, 1992
12. Armitage P, Berry G: Statistical methods in medical research. Blackwell Scientific Publications, Oxford, 1971

CHAPTER 13

Anti-aging Interventions

EDWARD L. SCHNEIDER

RICHARD A. MILLER

For over five millennia, from the ancient Egyptians to Ponce de Leon, humans have sought ways to extend their life span. Today, many businesses flourish to serve the dreams of individuals to stay and look youthful. Few physicians are immune from the questions of patients who have heard through the media of the latest cure for aging or way to stay young. In this chapter, we review some of the more popular interventions that have been proposed to alter the basic mechanisms of aging and thus to prolong life span.

Before beginning this review, it is important to review some of the biologic aspects of aging that bear on some of the proposed interventions. First, what we see as normal human aging is the sum of many mechanisms operating at the molecular, cellular, tissue, and organ levels. Evolutionary studies also indicate that at least several hundred genes are involved in aging processes. Therefore, it is extremely unlikely, but admittedly not impossible, that a single intervention could reverse all aging processes, significantly alter the rate of aging, and substantially increase human life span. By contrast, we believe that it is likely that interventions may be developed that may have profound effects on certain specific aging changes. For example, there may be antioxidants developed that will inhibit, arrest, or reverse the oxidation of proteins that occurs with aging, or there may be immunomodulators introduced that slow down, arrest, or reverse the changes in the immune system that occur with aging.

Secondly, there are many interventions that have been reported to increase the life span of mice, and therefore are proposed to alter human longevity. However, these studies are flawed by a variety of factors: (1) the intervention produced significant weight loss, which, as described below, has a significant effect itself on the life span of rodents; (2) the intervention used animals that had shortened life spans and could therefore extend life span by treating one or more life-shortening diseases; (3) the intervention was a hormone correcting a deficiency in a hormone-deficient animal; and (4) poor research design, analyses, or interpretations.

Third, there may be changes with aging that are protective. Therefore, reversing these changes with anti-aging approaches could be dangerous. For example, with aging there is an increased prevalence of autoimmune disease. Thus, interventions that restored youthful levels of immune function in older persons might potentially increase the incidence of autoimmune disorders.

Finally, interventions that extend life span or reverse aging processes in rodents may not produce the same results in humans. For example, although dietary restriction, as described below, can extend the life span of rodents, it is not clear that this intervention will lengthen human life span.

The enormous volume of literature in this area precludes an exhaustive review of all interventions that have been proposed to have anti-aging effects. We focus on a few that have attracted great interest by the lay public and therefore, may be of interest to physicians responding to the questions of their patients in this area.

Immunomodulators: Agents That May Affect the Aging of the Immune System

With aging, there is a decline in a number of immune functions.[1] There is substantial, though not quite conclusive, evidence that poor immune function may be an independent risk factor for disease and death in elderly people. Several early studies documented an association between lower all-cause mortality and poor T-cell immunity, measured either as diminished in vitro mitogen responsiveness or as anergy to one or more recall antigens in tests of delayed-type hypersensitivity among nursing home or ambulatory elders.[2,3] These studies did not, however, either adjust for age, a likely confounder, or take special pains to identify and adjust for pre-existing illnesses that might have altered immune responsiveness and influenced survival. A more recent study,[4] including a 9-year follow-up period for 273 healthy individuals who were 60 years or older at the outset of the study, documented a 2.2-fold increased risk of all-cause mortality among the 74 anergic subjects. After adjustment for age, the risk ratio was still 1.9, with a 95 percent confidence interval of 0.94 to 3.79. There was also a trend toward increased cancer mortality among the anergic subset.

In a separate study[5] of 102 very old (range: 86 to 92) Swedish subjects, a cluster of immune phenotypes, including poor mitogenic responses, low B-cell numbers, and relatively low numbers of CD4 T cells, were associated with diminished 2-year survival.

Perhaps the strongest—albeit still indirect—evidence that assessments of immune function in early adulthood have prognostic value for longevity and disease comes from an analysis of hybrid mice produced from a mating between lines selected respectively for high immune responsiveness.[6] Among the progeny mice, those with the best antibody responses tended to have greatest life expectancy and the lowest age-adjusted incidence rates of several diseases, including neoplasia. A longitudinal analysis of another variety of genetically heterogeneous mice[7] has shown an association between rapid accumulation of T memory cells and relative early death.

These findings suggest that interventions aimed at improving immune function could have a significant effect on disease resistance and survival. Immune function in old mice can be restored to levels close to those of young mice by a combination of whole body irradiation, implantation of a thymus transplant from a genetically identical young donor, and injection of bone marrow cells from a young mouse. Mice reconstituted in this way do not exhibit improved longevity,[8] at least in a "specific pathogen-free" environment known to lack a defined set of viral and parasitic agents that can cause morbidity and mortality in less protected animal colonies. To guard against the possibility that damage induced by irradiation treatment, required for bone marrow transplantation, may have confounded detection of life span extension in these transplanted mice, the experiments were repeated in a congenitally anemic mouse strain that can accept bone marrow transplants without prior irradiation. In these recipients, the combination of bone marrow and thymus implantation led to a substantial restoration of immune competence, but no significant increase in longevity.[8]

A second group, using a F1 hybrid strain of long-lived mice, has also examined longevity after lethal irradiation combined with thymic implantation and transplant of young bone marrow.[9] Mice were treated at 17 months of age. Eleven months later the survivors exhibited immune function similar to that of 14-month-old animals and superior to that of 28-month-old untreated controls, but survival and tumor incidence in the treated and untreated groups was essentially identical (52 percent survival.) In a further series of experiments,[10] 18-month-old mice were given repeated implantations of thymic tissue from newborn animals at monthly intervals for 5 months. Treated animals had a subsequent mean life span (312 ± 38 days) that was somewhat above that of controls that had instead received repeated grafts of newborn splenic tissue, assumed to be inactive (214 ± 43 days; $P = 0.08$). Maximal life span, though much harder to measure with precision, was not altered by the treatment. Repeated transplants of thymic tissue (every 2 months from 3 through 21 months of age) also led to a marginal increase in mean life span (515 days versus 465 in control spleen-grafted mice; $P = 0.07$) of a mammary tumor-prone mouse strain, C3H/MTV[11]; a similar protocol did not extend significantly the life span of mice of the lymphoma-prone C57BL/6 strain. These protocols used specific pathogen-free mice; it is possible that immune restoration from this kind of cellular therapy might have led to prolonged survival in environments where infectious disease was a more serious threat.

Many groups have attempted to improve the immune function of elderly individuals by injection with purified or semi-purified proteins, or with synthetic peptides derived from the thymus, despite well-founded doubts about the evidence attributing endocrine effects to thymic products[12] and demonstrations that some of the best studied "thymic hormones" are, in fact, produced by a wide range of nonthymic tissues.[13] There have been isolated reports of dramatic effects of peptides whose sequences are derived from thymic materials. One group, for example, has reported[14] that a single injection of 16 ng of thymic humoral factor (THF)-g2 into 11-month-old mice led to a fourfold increase in T-cell help for antibody production in culture. A different peptide, thymopentin (TP5), was reported to increase mitogen-stimulated production of both interleukin-2 and interferon-γ in 120-week-old BALB/c mice when given at a dose of 1 mg/kg/day for 20 days; similar effects were seen in young control animals.[15] In this study, TP5 treatment was shown to protect old mice against the lethal effects of experimental *Leishmania* infection. Sporadic reports have also suggested effects of these substances in human subjects. Thus, for example, injection of TP5 (50 mg, 3 times/week for 4 weeks) into institutionalized elderly subjects selected for low baseline immune responsiveness was reported[16] to lead to improved delayed-type hypersensitivity, mitogen-induced proliferation, and in vitro IL-2 production; this report did not, however, include a group of placebo control subjects. In general, however, the results of studies on alleged thymic hormones have proven inconsistent and disappointing.[17,18]

Dehydroepiandrosterone

Dehydroepiandrosterone (DHEA) is a steroid present in human serum principally in its soluble sulfate form, DHEAS. DHEAS, produced largely by the zona reticularis of the adrenal gland,[19] is the most abundant adrenal steroid in human plasma. Levels of DHEA and DHEAS fall dramatically with age in adulthood, from mean levels of 3.5 mg/ml in men aged 20 to 24 years to mean levels of 0.7 mg/ml in men aged over 70 years; the corresponding values in women are 2.3 mg/ml and 0.5 mg/ml.[20] DHEA, thought to be the active moiety, is produced from DHEAS by specific DHEA sulfatases, and variation among tissues in sulfatase levels is thought to influence the amount of the active product available locally.[21] DHEA can exert either androgenic or estrogenic effects depending on other aspects of endocrine, and particularly sex hormone, status.[22] Despite its very high plasma level, there is as yet no clear consensus on the role played by DHEA in homeostasis, nor a consensus as to a biochemical basis for its effects on cells in target tissues.

The large differences among age groups in DHEAS concentration in humans are accompanied by large variations among people within any given age decade.[20] The interest in DHEA as a possible modulator of aging and late-life disease has been sparked by epidemiologic data suggesting a relationship between DHEAS concentration and risk of cardiovascular disease,[23] bladder cancer,[24] and breast cancer[25] and by arguments that the metabolic effects of DHEA should confer upon it antiatherogenic effects.[26] More recent work, however, has suggested that the relationship between serum DHEA levels and late-life illness does not simply represent a protective effect of DHEA against the ravages of age, but instead reflects a complex set of interactions among DHEA and other aspects of the hormonal environment. Thus, longer-term (i.e., 19 years) follow-up failed to document any statistically significant difference, among men with differing DHEAS levels, in death from ischemic heart disease or cardiovascular disease compared to men that did not die from these causes.[27] After multiple adjustments for age, cigarette and alcohol consumption, and other risk factors, high levels of DHEAS were associated in men with a modest reduction in relative risk of cardiovascular death when survivors were used as the comparison group. A similar study of 942 postmenopausal women, also with a 19-year follow-up period, found no evidence for any protective effect of DHEAS levels on cardiovascular mortality in women.[28] In a separate study,[29] low levels of DHEAS were associated with fatal coronary heart disease in men, but not with nonfatal myocardial infarction or with extent of atherosclerosis seen at autopsy, and the relative risk of fatal coronary disease was not statistically significant after adjustment for other risk factors. High levels of DHEAS also do not seem to protect men or women from cognitive decline,[30] or protect aging women from central obesity or glucose intolerance.[31] Levels of DHEAS were lower than control values among premenopausal women with mammary cancer, suggesting that high levels of DHEAS may protect against breast cancer in this age group, but in contrast postmenopausal breast cancer is associated with relatively high DHEAS levels[32,33]; the differences between men and women, and between pre- and postmenopausal women, suggest that the effects of DHEA are not "sex-neutral" but depend on interactions with other hormones or hormone-sensitive target tissues.

Several groups have demonstrated that oral administration of DHEA or DHEAS to rodents may protect against development of neoplasia. Almost all of these studies have used animals that are, for genetic reasons, unusually likely to develop tumors, or that have been treated with oncogenic agents to increase tumor yield. However, long-term exposure of rats to DHEA resulted in the production of hyperplastic nodules in their livers[34] as well as hepatocarcinomas.[35] Rodent work has also suggested that DHEA or DHEAS may repair many late-life abnormalities of immune function, although the most dramatic of these claims have not yet been replicated by other laboratories.[36–48]

Studies in which DHEA or DHEAS has been administered to human volunteers have focused on immunopotentiation or on fairly short-term (e.g., 6 to 12 months) analyses of metabolic variables. The results of these studies indicate little if any substantial changes in immune function in those individuals receiving DHEAS.[38,49]

To see if replacement therapy of DHEA might correct age-related changes in metabolic risk factors for late-life illness, Yen and his colleagues[50] administered DHEA to 13 men and 17 women aged 40 to 70 years at a dose of 50 mg/day for a 6-month period. They observed no significant changes in lipid profiles (except for a small decline in high density lipoproteins in women), no changes in insulin sensitivity, and no changes in body fat or growth hormone levels. Women experienced a twofold increase in androgen levels. The ratio of IGF-1 (insulin-like growth factor-1) to its binding protein increased by about 50 percent over placebo in both sexes. Remarkably, despite these relatively unimpressive changes in objective measures, 67 percent of the men and 84 percent of the women reported improved sense of well-being after the course of DHEA ingestion. A follow-up study[56] used a DHEA dose of 100 mg/day over a 1-year course for eight men and eight women aged 50 to 65 years, also using a double-blind, placebo-controlled protocol. These higher doses led to increased androgen levels in the females, which exceeded the upper limits of the normal distribution. This study replicated the observation of increased IGF-1 levels, and also showed a significant increase in lean body mass in the pooled group of subjects. Knee muscle strength increased by about 15 percent in the men, with the placebo effect accounting for about half of this change, and knee strength in DHEA-treated women was less than in the placebo group; lumbar muscle strength was unchanged in either sex. There was again no significant change in lipid or apolipoprotein profiles, insulin or glucose levels, nitrogen balance, or bone mineral density. Although interpretation is limited by the relatively brief period of DHEA administration, these data do not provide strong support for the idea that supplemental DHEA can greatly affect risk factors for late-life illness in humans.

Melatonin

Melatonin, *N*-acetyl-5-methoxytryptamine, is secreted by the pineal gland in response to light-dark cycles. Light reaching the retina produces a signal that is transmitted to the suprachiasmatic nucleus (SCN), which in turn sends the signal to the pineal gland, inhibiting melatonin synthesis. Blood levels of melatonin have a circadian rhythm, with peak levels of melatonin occurring during normal sleeping hours.

Melatonin is a potent antioxidant and appears to be effective in converting the highly reactive hydroxy radical into indolyl cation radical, which is relatively nonreactive.[44] It also appears to be protective against agents that cause oxidative damage to the lens of the eye and hippocampus.[44]

With aging there is a decline in production in both the daytime and the nocturnal blood melatonin levels.[45] But the variation between individuals is quite high, and some individuals at older ages fall into the younger age range and some younger individuals fall into the older age range. Melatonin synthesis commences in humans at 3 months of age. Peak melatonin levels are reached prior to puberty and the major decline in melatonin levels occurs between ages 5 and 15, and then declines slowly with aging and is very low at advanced ages. Peak melatonin levels and 24-hour levels decline from age 20 to 70,[46] with the major decline between age 30 and 40. Pineal melatonin levels also decline with aging. In a group of older insomniacs, one-half were low melatonin secretors and one-half had normal melatonin levels.[47] The 12-hour duration of peak melatonin nighttime blood levels was the same in these high and low melatonin secretors.[47] Therefore, with aging, there was no shortening of the duration of high melatonin secretion—just a decrease in the amplitude.

Much of the excitement about the proposed "anti-aging" properties of melatonin is derived from a series of experiments by Pierpaoli and his collaborators.[48] Mice who were fed melatonin at night in a water bottle lived significantly longer than control animals. Older mice (18 months) who received transplanted pineal glands from young mice (3 months) donors had significantly longer life spans than sham-operated animals. Old pineal glands implanted into young BALB/c mice resulted in a substantial decrease in life span.[49] The transplanted old animals with young pineal glands and the old animals given melatonin purportedly had restored reproductive gland functions.[49]

However, there has been considerable criticism of this work. Most inbred mice strains, such as the ones employed by Piepaoli and his colleagues, secrete very low levels of melatonin.[50] In a series of sophisticated genetic analyses, melatonin levels were found to be controlled by two genes that code for the key enzymes in melatonin synthesis, N-acetyl transferase, and hydroxy-indole-O-methyl transferase.

Furthermore, transplanting the pineal gland to another animal is extremely likely to sever sympathetic innervation and the signals for melatonin synthesis. Therefore, before one can accept any relationship between melatonin and life extension in the transplanted animals, it is critical to demonstrate that the transplanted pineal gland made melatonin. In the Pierpaoli studies, there was no evidence of melatonin production in the transplanted animals. Therefore, if there is a life-extending effect, it could be something else in the pineal gland, or perhaps some stimulation of the thymus where it is transplanted. In some of the transplant studies there was also a significant weight loss in the transplanted animals.[48] There is insufficient data to understand whether caloric restriction played a role in the increase in longevity of melatonin-treated or transplanted animals.

With aging there are significant alterations in sleep.[51,52] It takes longer to fall asleep, there are frequent awakenings, it is harder to return to sleep, and there is decreased rapid eye movement (REM) sleep.[52] Increase in sleep disorders with aging parallels use of hypnotics.[53] Since melatonin can induce sleep, decrease sleep latency, and increase total sleep time,[54–56] it has great potential to alter the decline in the quality and quantity of sleep obtained as we age. Furthermore, in older insomniacs, there are lower melatonin metabolites in the urine.[57] Older volunteers with insomnia were given 0.3 g of melatonin before their habitual sleep time, and were found to have decreased movement during sleep and better sleep patterns, decreased awakenings, and better self-reported restful sleep.[46]

However, a recent National Institutes of Health (NIH) workshop on "Sleep, Aging, and Melatonin" concluded that there was no clear evidence that taking melatonin improves sleep in a clinically significant fashion, and also no convincing evidence that decreasing melatonin levels with aging has anything to do with the sleep problems in the elderly. Clearly, further research is needed before one should routinely prescribe melatonin for the sleep problems associated with aging.

Antioxidants

As we age, we are continuously exposed to oxidative damage from free radicals from both our external environment and through the normal metabolic pathways necessary for sustaining life. For example, free radicals are continuously generated during normal mitochondrial oxidation, the synthesis of prostaglandins, and during macrophage phagocytosis. The body has several mechanisms for detoxifying free radicals including the enzymes superoxide dysmutase, catalase, and glutathionine peroxidase as well as vitamin E, vitamin C, uric acid, and β-carotene.[58] Although these mechanisms are highly efficient, it is clear that free radical damage does accumulate with aging.[58]

One of the best characterized results of age-related accumulation of free radical damage is seen in the increased concentration of oxidized proteins that occurs with aging.[59] There is also some evidence that these oxidized proteins are removed more slowly in aged cells.[59] As a result, certain enzyme activities may decline dramatically with aging.[60]

Another target of intracellular free radical damage is oxidative damage to deoxyribonucleic acid (DNA). Each day, our cells are faced with the challenge of removing thousands of altered DNA bases and replacing them without interfering with the fidelity of DNA replication and transcription.[61] The body has also evolved pathways that preferentially allow repair of DNA bases within expressed genes, thus providing a measure of additional safety to the process of transcription and replication.[62] However, it is likely that the frequency of damaged DNA bases does increase with aging.

Animals with shorter life spans produce increased levels of mitochondrial free radicals than longer-lived species,[63] suggesting that there may be a relationship between longevity and production of free radicals. Studies of two types of mice, the common laboratory mouse, *Mus musculus*, and the deer mouse, *Peromyscus leucopus*, reveal that *Peromyscus leucopus* produces less mitochondrial free radicals, and has lower levels of protein oxidation, higher levels of antioxidant enzymes, and a substantially longer life span.[64]

Furthermore, there is increasing evidence linking free radical damage to several age-related diseases and disorders such as Alzheimer's disease, Parkinson's disease, osteoarthritis, cataracts, arteriosclerosis, amyotrophic lateral sclerosis, and many cancers. We will leave it to the authors of the sections covering these diseases to discuss the role of oxidative damage in their pathogenesis.

As a result of the media's attention to the role of oxidative damage in aging and age-related disease, increasing numbers of persons are taking dietary supplements to augment their bodies' responses to free radical damage. Although many antioxidants can be obtained from dietary sources such as citrus fruits for vitamin C, it is difficult to take sufficient vitamin E with normal dietary intake. Thus, a rationale does exist to recommend augmentation of the diet with vitamins E and C. The recent results of studies with β-carotene certainly cloud recommending its use.

Dietary Restriction

Dietary restriction (DR)—limiting the amount of food calories available to a level 20 to 40 percent below that which a rodent would voluntarily consume, given free access—has been for many years the only well-documented method for extending mean and maximal longevity in mammals. Many excellent reviews have discussed the details of the method, the wide range of age-sensitive physiologic processes retarded by DR, and possible biochemical mechanisms by which DR delays the aging process.[65–67] Rather than recapitulate these overviews, we will here provide only a brief synopsis of the main points, and then emphasize a number of recent developments that merit additional attention.

Dozens of laboratories, following the lead of McCay,[68] have now demonstrated that rats and mice will live up to 50 percent longer if given only 60 percent of the amount of food consumed by controls fed ad libitum, provided that the diet is supplemented with sufficient levels of micronutrients to avoid malnutrition. Both mean and maximal life span are extended.[69] Although the largest effect is seen if the DR regime is imposed at weaning, substantial effects are still seen if DR is delayed until late middle-age.[70] DR not only delays most late-life diseases in rodents, including neoplastic and degenerative diseases.[71–73] but also retards most (though not all) age-dependent changes in biochemical, anatomic, and physiologic processes, including changes in gene expression, connective tissue cross-linking, immune function, exercise tolerance, and many others. Restriction can be accomplished in many ways—such as portion control or alternate-day feeding, natural-product or defined-component diets—and still be effective as long as caloric consumption is diminished.

Three groups have now begun to address the question of whether DR protocols will retard aging in nonhuman primates.[74–76] Although these studies have been under way for only a small percentage of the expected life span of the rhesus monkey, there are already preliminary indications that the DR protocol has led to effects reminiscent of those seen in restricted rodents, including reductions in core body temperature[77] and improvements in glucose tolerance and insulin sensitivity.[76,78,79] Some other age-sensitive measures, including measures of T-cell activation[80] seem not to be altered by DR during the initial 4 years, although it is possible that longer treatment will eventually reveal an effect. Attempts to estimate the biologic age of treated and control monkeys by factor analysis applied to a wide range of metabolic outcomes[81] has been less successful, in part because most of the tested animals were juveniles and adolescents, making it difficult to disentangle the putative effects of DR on aging from its effects on maturation and puberty. A clear answer to the key question—does DR retard disease and death in primates—will require many more years of observation.

References

1. Miller RA: Immune system. p. 555. In Masoro E (ed): Handbook of Physiology. Section 11: Physiology of Aging. Oxford University Press, New York, 1995
2. Murasko DM, Weiner P, Kaye D: Association of lack of mitogen-induced lymphocyte proliferation with increased mortality in the elderly. Aging: Immunol Infect Dis 1988;1:1
3. Roberts-Thomson IC, Whittingham S, Youngchaiyud U, Mackay IR: Ageing, immune response, and mortality. Lancet 1974;2: 368
4. Wayne SJ, Rhyne RL, Garry PJ, Goodwin JS: Cell-mediated immunity as a predictor of morbidity and mortality in subjects over 60. J Gerontol Med Sci 1990;45:M45
5. Ferguson FG, Wikby A, Maxson P et al: Immune parameters in a longitudinal study of a very old population of Swedish people: a comparison between survivors and nonsurvivors. J Gerontol A Biol Sci Med Sci 1995;50:B378
6. Covelli V, Mouton D, Di Majo V et al: Inheritance of immune responsiveness, life span, and disease incidence in interline crosses of mice selected for high or low multispecific antibody production. J Immunol 1989;142:1224
7. Miller RA, Turke P, Chrisp C et al: Age-sensitive T cell phenotypes covary in genetically heterogeneous mice and predict early death from lymphoma. J Gerontol 1994;49:B255
8. Astle CM, Harrison DE: Effects of marrow donor and recipient age on immune responses. J Immunol 1984;132:673
9. Hirokawa K, Sato K, Makinodan T: Restoration of impaired immune functions in aging animals. V. Long-term immunopotentiating effects of combined young bone marrow and newborn thymus grafts. Clin Immunol Immunopathol 1982;22:297
10. Hirokawa K, Utsuyama M: The effect of sequential multiple grafting of syngeneic newborn thymus on the immune functions and life expectancy of aging mice. Mech Ageing Dev 1984;28: 111
11. Hirokawa K, Utsuyama M: Combined grafting of bone marrow and thymus, and sequential multiple thymus graftings in various strains of mice. The effect on immune functions and life span. Mech Ageing Dev 1989;49:49
12. Stutman O: Role of thymic hormones in T cell differentiation. Clin Immunol Allergy 1983;3:9
13. Clinton M, Frangou-Lazaridis M, Panneerselvam C, Horecker BL: Prothymosin alpha and parathymosin: mRNA and polypeptide levels in rodent tissues. Arch Biochem Biophys 1989;269: 256
14. Goso C, Frasca D, Doria G: Effect of synthetic thymic humoral factor (THF-gamma 2) on T cell activities in immunodeficient ageing mice. Clin Exp Immunol 1992;87:346
15. Cillari E, Miland S, Dieli M et al: Thymopentin reduces the susceptibility of aged mice to cutaneous leishmaniasis by modulating CD4 T cell subsets. Immunology 1992;76:362
16. Meroni PL, Barcellini W, Frasca D et al: In vivo immunopotenti-

ating activity of thymopentin in aging humans: increase of IL-2 production. Clin Immunol Immunopath 1987;42:151

17. Hiramoto RN, Ghanta VK, Soong SJ: Effect of thymic hormones on immunity and lifespan. p. 177. In Goidl E (ed): Aging and the Immune Response. Marcel Dekker, Inc., New York, 1986
18. Ghanta VK, Hiramoto NS, Soong SJ, Hiramoto RN: Survey of thymic hormone effects on physical and immunological parameters in C57BL/6NNia mice of different ages. Ann NY Acad Sci 1991;621:239
19. Hornsby PJ: Biosynthesis of DHEAS by the human adrenal cortex and its age-related decline. Ann NY Acad Sci 1995;774: 29–46
20. Orentreich N, Brind JL, Rizer RL, Vogelman JH: Age changes and sex differences in serum dehydroepiandrosterone sulfate concentrations throughout adulthood. J Clin Endocrinol Metab 1984;59:551
21. Daynes RA, Araneo BA, Dowell TA et al: Regulation of murine lymphokine production in vivo. III. The lymphoid tissue microenvironment exerts regulatory influences over T helper cell function. J Exp Med 1990;171:979
22. Ebeling P, Koivisto VA: Physiological importance of dehydroepiandrosterone. Lancet 1994;343:1479
23. Bulbrook RD, Hayward JL, Spicer CC: Relation between urinary androgen and corticoid secretion and subsequent breast cancer. Lancet 1971;2:395
24. Nestler JE, Clore JN, Blackard WG: Dehydroepiandrosterone: the "missing link" between hyperinsulinemia and atherosclerosis? FASEB J 1992;6:3073
25. Barrett-Connor E, and Goodman-Gruen D: The epidemiology of DHEAS and cardiovascular disease. Ann NY Acad Sci 1995; 774:259–70
26. Barrett-Connor E, and Goodman-Gruen D: Dehydroepiandrosterone sulfate does not predict cardiovascular death in postmenopausal women. The Rancho Bernardo Study. Circulation
27. LaCroix AZ, Yano K, Reed DM: Dehydroepiandrosterone sulfate, incidence of myocardial infarction, and extent of atherosclerosis in men. Circulation 1992;86:1529
28. Barrett-Connor E, Edelstein SL: A prospective study of dehydroepiandrosterone sulfate and cognitive function in an older population: the Rancho Bernardo Study. J Am Geriatr Soc 1994; 42:420
29. Barrett-Connor E, Ferrara A: Dehydroepiandrosterone, dehydroepiandrosterone sulfate, obesity, waist-hip ratio, and noninsulin-dependent diabetes in postmenopausal women: the Rancho Bernardo Study. J Clin Endocrinol Metab 1996;81:59
30. Zumoff B, Levin J, Rosenfeld RS et al: Abnormal 24-hr mean plasma concentrations of dehydroisoandrosterone and dehydroisoandrosterone sulfate in women with primary operable breast cancer. Cancer Res 1981;41:3360
31. Gordon GB, Bush TL, Helzlsouer KJ et al: Relationship of serum levels of dehydroepiandrosterone and dehydroepiandrosterone sulfate to the risk of developing postmenopausal breast cancer. Cancer Res 1990;50:3859
32. Shibata M, Hasegawa R, Imaida K et al: Chemoprevention by dehydroepiandrosterone and indomethacin in a rat multiorgan carcinogenesis model. Cancer Res 1995;55:4870
33. Rao MS, Subbarao V, Yeldandi AV, Reddy JK: Hepatocarcinogenicity of dehydroepiandrosterone in the rat. Cancer Res 1992; 52:2977
34. Araneo B, Dowell T, Woods ML et al: DHEAS as an effective vaccine adjuvant in elderly humans. Proof-of-principle studies. Ann NY Acad Sci 1995;774:232–48
35. Araneo BA, Dowell T, Diegel M, Daynes RA: Dihydrotestosterone exertrs a depressive influence on the production of interleukin-4 (IL-4), IL-5, and γ-interferon, but not IL-2 by activated murine T cells. Blood 1991;78:688
36. Danenberg HD, Ben-Yehuda A, Zakay-Rones Z, Friedman G: Dehydroepiandrosterone enhances influenza immunization in aged mice. Ann NY Acad Sci 1995;774:297–9
37. Daynes RA, Araneo BA, Ershler WB et al: Altered regulation of interleukin-6 production with normal aging: possible linkage to the age-associated decline in dehydroepiandrosterone (DHEA) and its sulfated derivative. J Immunol 1993;150:5219
38. Caffrey RE, Kapasi ZF, Haley ST et al: DHEAS enhances germinal center responses in old mice. Adv Exp Med Biol 1994; 355:225–9
39. Risdon G, Cope J, Bennett M: Mechanisms of chemoprevention by dietary dehydrisoandrosterone. Inhibition of lymphopoiesis. Am J Pathol 1990;136:759
40. Garg M, Bondada S: Reversal of age-associated decline in immune response to Pnu-imune vaccine by supplementation with the steroid hormone dehydroepiandrosterone. Infect Immun 1993;61:2238
41. Pahlavani MA, Harris MD: Effect of dehydroepiandrosterone on mitogen-induced lymphocyte proliferation and cytokine production in young and old F344 rats. Immunol Lett 1995;47:9
42. Blauer KL, Poth M, Rogers WM, Bernton EW: Dehydroepiandrosterone antagonizes the suppressive effects of dexamethasone on lymphocyte proliferation. Endocrinology 1991;129: 3174
43. Padgett DA, Loria RM: In vitro potentiation of lymphocyte activation by dehydroepiandrosterone, androstenediol, and androstenetriol. J Immunol 1994;153:1544
44. Reiter RJ: The pineal gland and melatonin in relation to aging: a summary of the theories and of the data. Exp Gerontol 1995; 30:199–212
45. Waldhauser F, Weiszenbacher G, Tatzer E et al: Alterations in nocturnal serum melatonin levels in humans with growth and aging. J Clin Endocrinol Metab 1988;66:648–52
46. Wurtman RJ, and Zhdanova I: Improvement of sleep quality by melatonin [letter]. Lancet 1995;346:1491
47. Lewy AJ, Sack RL, Blood ML et al: Melatonin marks circadian phase position and resets the endogenous circadian pacemaker in humans. Ciba Found Symp 1995;183:303–21
48. Pierpaoli W, Regelson W: Pineal control of aging: effect of melatonin and pineal grafting on aging mice. Proc Natl Acad Sci USA 1994;91:787–91
49. Pierpaoli W: Exp Gerontology (in press)
50. Goto M, Oshima I, Tomita T, Ebihara S: Malatonin content of the pineal gland in different mouse strains. J Pineal Res 1989; 7:195–204
51. Foley DJ, Monjan AA, Brown SL, Simonsick EM, Wallace RB, and Blazer DG: Sleep complaints among elderly persons: An epidemiologic study of three communities. Sleep 1995;18: 425–32

52. Prinz PN, Vitiello MV, Raskind MA, Thorpy MJ: Geriatrics: sleep disorders and aging. N Engl J Med 1990;323:520–526
53. Wauquier A: Aging and changes in phasic events during sleep. Founding Congress of the World Federation of Sleep Research Societies Microstructure of Sleep Workshop (1991, Cannes, France). Physiol Behav 1993;54:803–806
54. Waldhauser F, Saletu B, Trinchard-Lugan I: Sleep laboratory investigations on hypnotic properties of melatonin. Psychopharmacology 1990;100:222–6
55. James SP, Sack DA, Rosenthal NE, Mendelson WB: Melatonin administration in insomnia. Neuropsychopharmacology 1990; 3:19–23
56. MacFarlane JG, Cleghorn JM, Brown GM, Streiner DL: The effects of exogenous melatonin on the total sleep time and daytime alertness of chronic insomniacs: a preliminary study. Biol Psychiatry 1991;30:371–6
57. Haimov I, Laudon M, Zisapel N et al: Sleep disorders and melatonin rhythms in elderly people. BMJ 1994;309:167
58. Pacifici RE, and Davies KJA: Protein, lipid and DNA repair systems in oxidative stress: the Free-Radical Theory of Aging revisited. Gerontology 1991;37:166–80
59. Stadtman E: Protein oxidation and aging. Science 1992;257: 1220–1224
60. Cabiscol E, Levine RL: Carbonic anhydrase III. Oxidative modification in vivo and loss of phosphatase activity during aging. J Biol Chem 1995;270:14742–14747
61. Ames BN, Shigenaga MK, Hagen TM: Oxidants, antioxidants and the degenerative diseases of aging. Proc Natl Acad Sci USA 1993;90:7915–22
62. Hanawalt PC: Transcription-coupled repair and human disease. Science 1994;266:1957–58
63. Ku HH, Brunk UT, Sohal RS: Relationship between mitochondrial superoxide and hydrogen peroxide production and longevity of mammalian species. Free Radical Biol and Med 1993; 15:621–27
64. Sohal RS, Ku HH, Agarwal S: Biochemical correlates of longevity in two closely related rodent species. Biochem Biophys Res Commun 1993;196:7–11
65. Masoro EJ: Food restriction in rodents: an evaluation of its role in the study of aging. J Gerontol 1988;43:B59
66. Weindruch R, Walford RL: The Retardation of Aging and Disease by Dietary Restriction. Charles C Thomas, Springfield, IL, 1988
67. Yu BP: Putative Interventions. p. 613. In Masoro EJ (ed): Handbook of Physiology. Section 11: Aging. Oxford University Press, New York, 1995
68. McCay CM, Crowell MF, Maynard LA: The effect of retarded growth upon the life span and upon ultimate body size. J Nutr 1935;10:63
69. Yu BP, Masoro EJ, McMahan CA: Nutritional influences on aging of Fischer 344 rats: I. Physical, metabolic, and longevity characteristics. J Gerontol 1985;40:657
70. Weindruch R, Walford RL: Dietary restriction in mice beginning at 1 year of age: effect on life span and spontaneous cancer incidence. Science 1982;215:1415
71. Sheldon WG, Bucci TJ, Hart RW, Turturro A: Age-related neoplasia in a lifetime study of ad libitum-fed and food-restricted B6C3F1 mice. Toxicol Pathol 1995;23:458
72. Maeda H, Gleiser CA, Masoro EJ et al: Nutritional influences on aging of Fischer 344 rats: II. Pathology. J Gerontol 1985; 40:671
73. Bronson RT, Lipman RD: Reduction in rate of occurrence of age related lesions in dietary restricted laboratory mice. Growth Dev Aging 1991;55:169
74. Kemnitz JW, Weindruch R, Roecker EB et al: Dietary restriction of adult male rhesus monkeys: design, methodology, and preliminary findings from the first year of study. J Gerontol 1993;48:B17
75. Cutler RG, Davis BJ, Ingram DK, Roth GS: Plasma concentrations of glucose, insulin, and percent glycosylated hemoglobin are unaltered by food restriction in rhesus and squirrel monkeys. J Gerontol Biol Sci 1992;47:B9
76. Bodkin NL, Ortmeyer HK, Hansen BC: Long-term dietary restriction in older-aged rhesus monkeys: effects on insulin resistance. J Gerontol A Biol Sci Med Sci 1995;50:B142
77. Lane MA, Baer DJ, Rumpler WV et al: Calorie restriction lowers body temperature in rhesus monkeys, consistent with a postulated anti-aging mechanism in rodents. Proc Natl Acad Sci USA 1996;93:4159
78. Lane MA, Ball SS, Ingram DK et al: Diet restriction in rhesus monkeys lowers fasting and glucose-stimulated glucoregulatory end points. Am J Physiol 1995;268:E941
79. Kemnitz JW, Roecker EB, Weindruch R et al: Dietary restriction increases insulin sensitivity and lowers blood glucose in rhesus monkeys. Am J Physiol 1994;266:E540
80. Grossmann A, Rabinovitch PS, Lane MA et al: Influence of age, sex, and dietary restriction on intracellular free calcium responses of CD4+ lymphocytes in rhesus monkeys (*Macaca mulatta*). J Cell Physiol 1995;162:298
81. Nakamura E, Lane MA, Roth GS et al: Evaluating measures of hematology and blood chemistry in male rhesus monkeys as biomarkers of aging. Exp Gerontol 1994;29:151

CHAPTER 14

Presentation of Disease in Old Age

MICHAEL A. HORAN

Aging, Disease, and Health

Distinguishing aging from disease would be of only philosophic interest were it not for the reactions that each concept can evoke. To the population at large, and for that matter many doctors, aging is simply a progressive deteriorative process that is the ultimate lot of all mankind. It is untreatable and does not seem to elicit any particular sympathy from others; nor is it regarded as a legitimate focus for medical attention. On the other hand, those with diseases often attract sympathy or even admiration at their fortitude and will usually have few problems in engaging medical interest.

In old age, a person may bear multiple pathologic lesions, not all of which will be symptomatic, and these will arise on a background of biologic aging. In this setting, any or all symptoms may be attributed to aging and it may be thought that nothing can be done about them, a conclusion that may well be shared by the doctor to whom any symptoms may be divulged. The emergence of geriatric medicine was largely an attempt to counteract such negative views, and with it came the much-quoted aphorism "aging is not disease and disease is not aging." Although this statement serves a practical purpose by counteracting the negative attitudes alluded to above, it does little to enhance the scientific foundations of the practice of geriatric medicine: quite simply, it does not stand up to scientific scrutiny. The issue revolves around the questions "What constitutes aging?" and "What constitutes a disease?" Unfortunately, the answer to neither question is entirely satisfactory.

Another important concept, intimately bound up with the concepts of aging and disease, is health. Like aging and disease, it defies adequate definition[1]: some view it in a narrow, biomedical perspective as the absence of disease, whereas others adopt the broad World Health Organization (WHO) definition of "a state of complete physical, mental and social well-being," which is so all-embracing as to be of little practical use. It has been reported that old people consistently rate their health as good in the presence of obvious, and often disabling, disease. In my own experience of recruiting "healthy" volunteers for research, only 20 to 25 percent of those who considered themselves to be healthy were considered to be so by the investigators. These older people obviously had rather different ideas about the meaning of "health" than did the clinical scientists. Interestingly, there has been quite a lot of research on how older people perceive health, but this has been conducted within a sociologic context rather than a biomedical one.[2,3]

The Nature of Aging

It is not my intention here to describe the various theories of aging, but rather to consider a framework in which they may be viewed, as well as some of the phenomena for which they must account. For the purposes of this discussion, aging is viewed as an accumulation of persistent changes that occur between conception and death, and it comprises two components: deleterious changes (senescence) and beneficial adaptive ones. Most research has concentrated on the former.

At a physiologic level, perhaps the most prominent characteristic of human (and animal) aging is its variability. Although increased age is associated with a gradual deterioration in average functional performances (Table 14-1), not all functions deteriorate at the same rate nor to the same extent, and this is the case both within individuals and between them.[4] In addition, there is considerable variation between individuals in the pattern of age-related pathology.[5,6] This interindividual variation may, in part, be due to genetic differences and one might envisage, for example, in an outbred population, that some individuals might have many more harmful, recessive traits than others. Longitudinal studies of aging twins revealed that intrapair differences in life span and the incidence of cancer were significantly smaller for monozygotic twins than for dizygotic ones.[7]

The functional declines alluded to above will proceed toward some threshold that, when exceeded, will result in decompensation in the relevant system. The gradual erosion of reserve capacity will limit the ability to respond to an increased demand. This is most likely to be clinically important for cardiopulmonary, renal, and cognitive functions. However, numerous studies of physiologic functions in relation to age confirm that senescence cannot be attributed to the failure of any single system, organ, tissue, or cell type. Instead, it has been suggested that the main manifestation of underlying aging processes in the intact organism is the disruption of the many regulatory processes that provide functional integration between cells, tissues, and organs.[8] The resulting impairment of the ability to coordinate the diverse functions necessary to defend homoeostasis (what Weksler calls *homeostenosis*) might also contribute to the vulnerability of the aged organism to both internal and external stresses.[8]

Thus, senescence may be understood in terms of reductions in reserve capacities together with alterations in the integration of the control mechanisms that regulate activities within and between cells, tissues, and organs, rather than simply as the

Table 14-1 The average decrease in some selected physiologic variables between the ages of 30 and 80 years

Variable	Percentage Reduction
Resting cardiac output	30
Vital capacity	50
Renal blood flow	50
Maximum breathing capacity	60
Maximum oxygen uptake	70

(From Shock et al,[59] with permission.)

failure of one or more organ systems. The various impairments may well interact in such a way that the overall effect is greater than their sum, though deterioration in a single system might well become the critical factor in a particular set of circumstances. This line of reasoning is consistent with the observation that although there is a gradual, linear decline in individual functions, the probability of dying increases approximately exponentially with time.[9]

All cell types undergo age-related deleterious changes (with the possible exception of hemopoietic stem cells and germ cells), and there is evidence that certain organ dysfunctions are the direct result of dysfunctions in their constituent cells.[10–12] In other words, organs probably senesce because their cells senesce. Cellular phenotypes must ultimately reflect what has come to be called the central dogma of molecular biology, that is, the flow of information encoded in genes (deoxyribonucleic acid [DNA] through ribonucleic acid (RNA) to protein, and it seems highly likely that cellular senescence has its origins in this information pathway.[13,14]

The Nature of Disease

Modern concepts of disease began with the systematic clinical descriptions that were related to the findings at postmortem examinations and, eventually, with changes at the microscopic level. Thus, the concept of disease became firmly rooted in pathology. With the great advances in microbiology, the notion of diseases in terms of specific etiology became more explicit and was enshrined in the postulates of Robert Koch. In this view, diseases are seen as attributable to a single, necessary, and sufficient cause (e.g., tuberculosis is caused by *Mycobacterium tuberculosis*), and those conditions not so characterized were of a fundamentally different nature. Within a few decades, this concept of disease had to be modified because of observations that not all individuals exposed to known "necessary causes" contracted the respective diseases, and the concept of differential susceptibility was born. As improved hygiene, immunization programs, and effective drugs brought about the decline of the great infectious diseases, the diseases of old age, many of which are chronic, acquired an increasing significance in the practice of medicine. Some of the diseases and disorders of old age are peculiar to this stage of life. This changing pattern of disease brought about changes in our concepts of the nature of disease, in particular an increasing emphasis on multiple predisposing factors. One concept of increasing importance is that the health of the mother and offspring during gestation and in the perinatal period can profoundly affect the susceptibility of the offspring to disease in later life,[15] particularly hypertension, heart disease, and chronic lung disease.

Koch's postulates for the diagnosis of infective diseases

The organism should be found in the lesion in a quantity adequate to account for its effects.

The organism should be cultivated in a pure state on an artificial medium.

The organism grown in artificial culture should be capable of producing a similar lesion in another member of the species.

Some diseases and conditions that are common only in old age

Polymyalgia rheumatica
Giant cell arteritis
Decubitus ulcers
Osteoarthritis
Paget's disease of bone
Multiple myeloma
Chronic lymphocytic leukemia
Prostatic cancer
Stroke syndromes
Dementia syndromes
Parkinson's disease
Accidental hypothermia
Urinary incontinence
Cataracts
Colonic angiodysplasia

Multiple Diseases and the Pathology of Advanced Age

Numerous studies have shown that multiple medical problems frequently coexist in aged individuals. For example, one study showed that those aged 65 to 74 suffered an average of 4.6 chronic conditions: 50 percent suffered from arthritis of some sort; 34 percent were forgetful; 33 percent reported persistent back pain; 32 percent had poor vision; 29 percent complained of indigestion; and 28 percent were breathless on only modest exertion.[16] For those over age 75, the mean number of ailments per person was 5.8, and only 10 percent reported no physical disabilities.

One never ceases to wonder at the abundance of pathologic lesions to be found at postmortem examination of old people.[17]

Indeed, Korenchevsky[18] wrote, "No human being has yet been identified whose old age, lifespan and death are physiologically normal. The aged individual is so subject to pathological defects that death as a natural biological phenomenon is yet beyond his reach." With such a variety of pathologic changes, it may be impossible to determine which, if any, was the actual cause of death. This problem led Kohn[19] to propose "that senescence be viewed as a disease and be accepted as a cause of death." It is not clear whether or not Kohn actually considered this multiplicity of lesions to be a manifestation of the aging process and that death came as a result of their accumulation. Loufbourrow[20] clearly separated these "secondary (or pathological) causes of aging" from some ill-defined primary process because they are not all systematically present in all individuals. He went on to say, "It is often difficult or impossible to determine the relative importance of physiological and pathological processes which contribute to aging. The best opportunity to study physiological aging is provided by animal colonies maintained in an environment which provides conditions as nearly ideal as possible."

Recent studies have shown that even specific pathogen-free rodents display as complicated a system of aging as man in the developed world. Regardless of whether such animals are allowed to live out their respective life span or members of a cohort (group of animals of the same age) are killed at intervals, multiple pathologic lesions are to be found.[21–23] Clearly, some lesions are genetically-determined artifacts of a particular inbred strain (e.g., retinal degeneration in WAG/Rij rats[23]) but, in the main, there is considerable heterogeneity between individuals in the nature of the pathologic lesions they acquire as they progress through their life span, even under near-optimal conditions. Indeed, the presence of such multiple and heterogeneous lesions has been incorporated into the definition of animals suitable for use in aging research.[23] It is likely that such individual variation in inbred animals is, to some extent, not present ab initio but emerges from continuous genetic and/or epigenetic alterations during aging in each individual. Thus, although the fundamental processes of senescence may well be universal, their manifestations need not be so. In other words, a specific pathologic lesion need not be present in every single individual to be regarded as a manifestation of aging.

Clinical Practice

The Atypical Presentation of Disease

The traditional model of medical practice derives predominantly from the presentation of disease in younger people, for whom it is often possible to account for all abnormal findings with a single diagnoses. A particular array of symptoms and signs is usually characteristic of a particular pathophysiologic state (e.g., heart failure) or disease. To the doctor who understands only this traditional model, deviations from it may lead to the erroneous conclusion that, because a characteristic pattern of symptoms and signs is absent, the patient could not have the disease so characterized. The most obvious way in which older people may deviate from the traditional model is that multiple diseases frequently coexist[16,17,22,24] so that the symptoms and signs that have been recorded may be attributable to several diseases. Furthermore, no single disease necessarily dominates the clinical picture. There may also be multiple complaints without a single major complaint, and even a major complaint that is not directly attributable to the most overt or most serious identifiable disease. Because of the age-related erosion of functional reserve in many systems and organs and because of impaired adaptive responses to challenge (e.g., waning immune response, blunted hypoxic and hypercapnic drives, reduced pain perception), and because of coincident pathology, a disease in one organ (e.g., respiratory infection) may precipitate decompensation in another (cardiac failure, acute confusion, falls), thus contributing to the atypical presentation of disease. Likewise, the nature of adverse drug reactions may be influenced by underlying senescent changes. In addition to age-related pharmacokinetic changes, there are also pharmacodynamic ones (see Ch. 11). These pharmacodynamic changes are particularly important in the brain;[25] many drugs may cause acute confusion, even digoxin,[26] whose primary site of action is in the heart. The presence of multiple diseases may also contribute to late or even silent presentations when disease at one site limits symptoms from another (e.g., stroke or arthritis limiting physical activity so that dyspnea does not appear until heart failure is very advanced).

The Giants of Geriatric Medicine

Several authors have rightly emphasized that certain patterns of disease presentation are peculiar to old people—immobility, instability (falls), incontinence, and intellectual impairment (confusion)[27–30] and that these have in common multiple causes, a chronic course, deprivation of independence, and no simple cure. They have been designated the "Giants of Geriatrics"[30] and are of immense importance in the practice of the medicine of old age, partly because they are very common[31] and partly because of the challenge they present to our diagnostic skills when we try to ascertain the precipitating cause(s) and identify treatable exacerbating factors. Almost any disease can present with these features and, conversely, any old person presenting in this way can have virtually any pathology. Indeed, one of the defining attributes of an effective geriatrician is the ability to assess and manage the Giants of Geriatric Medicine effectively.

The Late Presentation of Disease

The tendency for disease to present late and in an advanced form in old people is well established, and many factors associated with the patient and his/her doctor undoubtedly contribute to the failure to recognize that a potentially remediable problem is present. Of course, the disease may be particularly aggressive. Also, the patient may misinterpret the significance of symptoms, may have a low expectation of health, or may fear hospitalization due to the potential for loss of independence and self-determination, and deliberately conceal symptoms of illness.

There are certainly studies that show that older people tend to underconsult and that, when assessed, numerous ameliorable problems are to be found. For example, in a seminal study by Williamson,[32] diseases of the heart, lungs, and central nervous system were often well known to the family doctor, but locomotor disorders, dysfunctions of the bowels and bladder, depression, and confusion were often not recorded. Indeed, the latter two conditions (depression and confusion) very likely explain why comorbid conditions may present late in their course. More recent studies, however, do not confirm that old people are particularly prone to underconsultation.[33] There is even evidence that those old people not well known to their general practitioners may be an elite group enjoying unusually good health.[34,35]

There is reasonable evidence that older people may accept some symptoms as normal, particularly if mild and particularly if referable to the eyes, ears, or genitourinary system. More severe symptoms, particularly if referable to the cardiopulmonary system, abdomen, and locomotor system, are more readily attributable to disease.[36] Furthermore, beliefs about the significance of particular symptoms seem to be translated into actions in terms of the likelihood of consulting a doctor about them.[37] A recent study on out-of-hospital chest pain has shown that many older patients with a history of ischemic heart disease wait an alarmingly long time after the onset of severe pain before seeking medical help.[38]

The doctor may be unskilled at diagnosis in older people and wrongly interpret the significance of physical symptoms, some of which (e.g., nocturia) occur so commonly as to be of very little diagnostic significance.[39] Even worse, he may feel that strenuous diagnostic efforts are not worthwhile (agism). Even though most doctors would deny this latter assertion, there is clear evidence that seriously ill older people often fail to receive as vigorous diagnostic efforts and treatments as similarly ill younger patients, despite no age-effect on outcome between similarly managed patients.[40] Unskilled diagnosis and unwarranted assumptions may lead to inappropriate treatments (e.g., the use of diuretics for pedal edema in the absence of circulatory volume overload or the administration of anti-Parkinsonian drugs to people with essential tremor) or unnecessarily grave prognoses. Nieman and Holmes[41] have provided good evidence of the readiness to make clinical diagnoses of pancreatic cancer, unsupported by more dependable diagnostic tests. A wrong diagnosis of a terminal illness can have devastating effects on patient and family and seriously undermine quality of life.

Finally, patients may express themselves in terms a doctor cannot understand. The language of illness (like notions about aging, health, and disease) is determined by social as well as by regional and ethnic factors. For example, in old age the language of depression often focuses on somatic complaints, particularly those that are common in the old or are already problematic.[42] Other areas of particular difficulty include descriptions of pain, blackouts, and funny turns.

The Silent Presentation of Disease

The notion of the silent presentation of disease as a phenomenon peculiar to old age has almost achieved the status of holy writ. However, all diseases, regardless of the age of the patient, begin with a period of variable duration in which no symptoms are produced. There is no evidence that this period of silence is unusually prolonged in the aged.

What most people mean when referring to "silent presentations" is the absence or attenuation of typical features, such as painless myocardial infarction,[43–47] painless peritonitis,[48] painless perforation of abdominal viscera,[49] afebrile infections,[50–52] apathetic thyrotoxicosis.[53] Although it is undeniable that such phenomena exist, the evidence that they arise particularly commonly in the old is weak. Most studies have included no younger groups for comparison. In fact, recent studies on angina pectoris and myocardial infarction in people aged between 40 and 60 years demonstrate that silent episodes of myocardial ischemia (defined by objective evidence of ischemia in the absence of chest pain) may occur in 2 to 4 percent of healthy men and in 20 to 30 percent after myocardial infarction.[54] Furthermore, in patients with documented symptomatic coronary artery disease, 60 to 90 percent have additional periods of silent ischemia. However, there is recent evidence that older people with coronary heart disease have an increased perceptual threshold for chest pain, attributed by the authors to autonomic dysfunction,[55] but that may well have its origins in the brain.[56] These observations on silent myocardial ischemia in younger people raise serious questions about the silent presentation of other conditions, but equally rigorous studies have rarely been done. However, Gruber et al.[57] have shown that fever and leukocytosis are often absent in patients presenting to emergency departments and that this was no more likely in the old than in the young.

Frailty, Dependency, Social Crises, and the Pseudosilent Presentation of Disease

The ultimate measure of the impact of aging and disease on individuals is their functional capacity, degree of frailty, or ability to look after themselves. Aging takes place in a social context, and the ability to look after oneself is taken as a measure of *social fitness*. Significant impairments of this capacity must be compensated for in some way, usually by friends, family, voluntary organizations, and statutory social services provisions. In general, the greater the dependency, the greater the amount and complexity of the necessary support. Such people often have a precarious existence, and the appearance of a new problem (e.g., a urine infection with incontinence of urine) can lead to a sudden collapse of the support network, sometimes associated with anger, resentment, and recrimination. This is a *social crisis*. Regrettably, this presentation is the least likely to elicit sympathy from emergency medical services and the patient may simply be viewed as a potential "bed-blocker." Either through prejudice and/or ignorance, a proper assessment is not made and remediable factors are not identified. This presentation of the new problem has been termed *pseudosilent* because all the necessary information for diagnosis may well be present but go unrecognized.

Doctors must realize that most social crises have remediable (if not strictly medical) causes, and that a prompt and careful assessment will usually identify the underlying cause. When this is recognized and corrected, return home will generally be feasible. A tardy response deprives the patient of what is owed (in a moral sense) and is likely to severely test the good will of the carers who may then resist the patient's return home. As Williamson[58] has written: "Almost everything to do with the health of the elderly is a matter of urgency. If an old person is unwell on Monday, the chances are that he/she will be worse on Tuesday, and by the end of the week may be bedridden, dehydrated, confused and incontinent."

Conclusion

As we progress through our life span we undergo biologic aging, the deteriorative component of which (senescence) will become increasingly prominent. This intrinsic process will be modified by extrinsic, environmental factors during gestation and throughout life. This interaction may well produce overt disease. In practice, to try to distinguish between aging and disease is pointless; it is scientifically dubious and makes no difference to management. For clinicians, the major challenge is to formulate a patient's problems in such a way that they may be amenable to some sort of intervention, or at the least, be of some prognostic significance.

The classic disease-oriented model equips us poorly to address illness and disability in old age. What is needed, and what experienced geriatricians practice, is a problem-oriented model in which problems can be placed in hierarchies of functional importance. This done, attempts are made to determine how these problems arose so that management plans with specified goals can be constructed. The problems must be frequently re-evaluated to ensure that the goals are being met; if not, treatment must be changed or the goals modified.

In this chapter, I have attempted to address how old people fit poorly into the classic, disease-oriented model and I have tried to summarize the ways in which they do present their problems. These problems arise within a unique socioeconomic setting, which must always be taken into account when devising plans of management. Above all, this chapter should provide a framework within which to view the much more detailed discussions of health and disease in old age that constitute the rest of this book.

Acknowledgment

I wish to acknowledge my enormous debt of gratitude to Carel Hollander (former Director of the Institute for Experimental Gerontology, TNO, The Netherlands) for his guidance and inspiration. Without him, this chapter would have been impossible.

References

1. Lewis A: Health as a social concept. Br J Sociol 1953;4: 109–124
2. Victor C: Health and Health Care in Later life. Milton Keynes, Open University Press, 1991
3. Sidell M: Health in Old Age. Milton Keynes, Open University Press, 1995
4. Shock NW: Aging and physiological systems. J Chron Dis 1983; 36:137–142
5. McKeown EF: De Senectute. J R Coll Phys 1975;10:79–99
6. Tanaka Y: Pathology of the Extremely Aged. Vol. 1. Centenarians. Ishiyaku EuroAmerica, St. Louis, 1984
7. Bank L, Jarvik LF: A longitudinal study of aging human twins. p. 303–330. In Scheider EL (ed): The Genetics of Aging Plenum Press, New York, 1978
8. Shock NW: System integration. In CE Finch Handbook of the Biology of Aging. Hayflick L (eds): Von Nostrand Reinhold, New York, 1977
9. Timiras PS: Developmental Physiology and Aging. Macmillan, New York, 1972
10. Knook DL, Sleyster EC: Lysosomal enzyme activities in parenchymal and non-parenchymal liver cells isolated from young, adult and old rats. Mech Ageing Dev 1976;5:389–397
11. Knook DL: The isolated hepatocyte: a cellular model for aging studies. Proc Soc Exp Biol Med 1980;165:170–177
12. Wilson PD, Watson R, Knook DL: Effects of age on rat liver enzymes. Gerontology 1982;28:32–43
13. Sacher GA: Evolution of longevity and survival characteristics in mammals. pp. 151–165. In Schneider EL (ed): The Genetics of Aging. Plenum Press, New York, 1978
14. Kirkwood TBL: Repair and its evolution: survival versus reproduction. pp. 165–189. In Townsend CR, Callow P (eds): Physiological Ecology: An Evolutionary Approach to Resource Use. Blackwell Scientific Oxford, 1981
15. Barker DJP: Mothers, Babies and Disease in Later Life. London, BMJ Publishing Group
16. Abrams M: The health of the very elderly. In Isaacs B (ed): Recent Advances in Geriatric Medicine, 3. Churchill Livingstone Edinburgh, 1985
17. Howell TH: Fatal and contributory lesions in nonagenarians. J Clin Exp Gerontol 1985;7:155–162
18. Korenchevsky V: Physiological and Pathological Aging. Hafner, New York, 1961
19. Kohn RR: Causes of death in very old people. JAMA 1982; 247:2793–2797
20. Loofbourrow GN: Grow old along with me. J Kansas Med Soc 1969;LXX:109–116
21. Burek JD: Pathology of Aging Rats. CRC Press, West Palm Beach, California, 1978
22. Zurcher C, Hollander CF: Multiple pathological changes in aging rat and man. Exp Biol Med 1982;7:56–62
23. Hollander CF: Biological and clinical consequences of longitudinal studies in rodents: their possibilities and limitations. An overview. Mech Ageing Dev 1984;28:249–260
24. Wilson LA, Lawson IR, Bray W: Multiple disorders in the elderly: a clinical and statistical study. Lancet 1962;ii:841–843

25. Swift CG: Pharmacodynamics: changes in homeostatic mechanisms, receptor and target organ sensitivity in the elderly. Br Med Bull 1990;45:36–52
26. Portnoi VA: Digitalis delirium in elderly patients. J Clin Pharmacol 1979;19:747–750
27. Isaacs B: Current achievements in geriatrics: morbidity in elderly hospital patients. Cassel, London, 1964
28. Isaacs B: Is geriatrics a specialty? In Arie THD (ed): Health Care of the Elderly. Croom Helm, London, 1981
29. Cape RDT: Aging: Its Complex management. Harper & Rowe, Hagerstown, 1978
30. Isaacs B: The Challenge of Geriatric Medicine. Oxford Medical Publications, Oxford, 1992
31. Cape RDT: A geriatrics service. Midl Med Rev 1972;8:21–30
32. Williamson J, Stokoe IH, Gray S et al: Old people at home. Their unreported needs. Lancet 1964;i:1117–1120
33. Ford F, Taylor R: The elderly as under consulters: a critical reappraisal. J R Coll Gen Pract 1985;35:244–247
34. Ebrahim S, Hedley R, Shelldon M: Low levels of ill health among elderly non-consulters in general practice. BMJ 289: 1273–1275
35. Williams ES, Barley NH: Old people not known to the general practitioner: low risk group. BMJ 1985;291:251–254
36. Gjorup T, Hendriksen C, Lund E, Stromgard E: Is growing old a disease? A study of the attitudes of elderly people to physical symptoms. J Chron Dis 1987;40:1095–1098
37. Leventhal EA, Prohaska TR: Age, symptom interpretation, and health behaviour. J Am Geriatr Soc 1986;34:185–191
38. Tresch DD, Brady WJ, Aufderheide, TP et al: Comparison of elderly and younger patients with out-of-hospital chest pain. Arch Intern Med 1996;156:1089–1093
39. Hale WE, Perkins LL, May FE et al: Symptom prevalence in the elderly. An evaluation of age, sex, disease and medication use. J Am Geriatr Soc 1986;34:333–340
40. Hamel MB, Phillips RS, Teno JM et al: Seriously ill hospitalized adults: do we spend less on older patients? J Am Geriatr Soc 1996;44:1043–1048
41. Nieman JL, Holmes FF: Accuracy of diagnosis of pancreatic cancer decreases with increasing age. J Am Geriatr Soc 1989; 37:97–100
42. Blazer D, George L, Landerman R: The phenomenology of late life depression. pp. 143–152. In Bebbington PE, Jacoby R (eds): Psychiatric Disorders of the Elderly. Mental Health Foundation, London, 1986
43. Rodstein M: The characteristics of non-fatal myocardial infarction in the aged. Arch Intern Med 1956;98:84–90
44. Pathy MS: Clinical presentation of myocardial infarction in the elderly. Br Heart J 1967;29:190–199
45. Wrobleski M, Mikulowski P, Steen B: Symptoms of myocardial infarction in old age: clinical case, retrospective and prospective studies. Age Ageing 1986;15:99–104
46. Bayer AJ, Chadha JS, Farag RR, Pathy MSJ: Changing presentation of myocardial infarction with increasing old age. J Am Geriatr Soc 1986;34:263–266
47. Calle P, Jordaens L, De Buyzere M et al: Age-related differences in presentation, treatment and outcome of acute myocardial infarction. Cardiology 1994;85:111–120
48. Burston GR, Moore-Smith B: Occult surgical emergencies in the elderly. Br J Clin Pract 1970;24:239–243
49. Fulton JD, Peebles SE, Smith GD, Davie JW: Unrecognised viscus perforation in the elderly. Age Ageing 1989;18:403–406
50. Madden JW, Croker JR, Beynon GPJ: Septicaemia in the elderly. Postgrad Med J 1981;57:502–506
51. Chassagne P, Perol M-B, Doucet J et al: Is presentation of bacteraemia in the elderly the same as in younger patients? Am J Med 1996;100:65–70
52. Werner GS, Schulz R, Fuchs JB et al: Infective endocarditis in the elderly in the era of transoesophageal echocardiography: clinical features and prognosis compared with younger patients. Am J Med 1996;100:90–97
53. Trivalle C, Doucet J, Chassagne P et al: Differences in the signs and symptoms of hyperthyroidism in older and younger patients. J Am Geriatr Soc 1996;44:50–53
54. Droste K, Roskamm H: Silent myocardial ischaemia. Am Heart J 1989;118:1087–1092
55. Ambepitiya G, Roberts M, Ranjadayalan K, Tallis R: Silent exertional myocardial ischaemia in the elderly: a quantitative analysis of anginal perceptual threshold and the influence of autonomic function. J Am Geriatr Soc 1994;42:732–737
56. Rosen SD, Paulesu E, Frith CD et al: Central nervous pathways mediating angina pectoris. Lancet 344:147–150
57. Gruber PJ, Silverman RA, Gottesfeld S, Flaster E: Presence of fever and leukocytosis in acute cholecystitis. Ann Emergency Med 1996;28:273–277
58. Williamson J: Geriatric medicine: whose specialty? Ann Intern Med 1978;91:774–777
59. Shock NW, Greulich RC, Andres R et al: Normal Human Aging: The Baltimore Longitudinal Study of Aging. NIH Publication No. 84–2450. US Government Printing Office, Washington, DC

CHAPTER 15

Multidimensional Geriatric Assessment

LAURENCE Z. RUBENSTEIN
LISA V. RUBENSTEIN

Geriatric assessment is a multidimensional, often interdisciplinary, diagnostic process intended to determine a frail elderly person's medical, psychosocial, and functional capabilities and problems with the objective of developing an overall plan for treatment and long-term follow-up. It differs from the standard medical evaluation in its concentration on frail elderly people with their complex problems, its emphasis on functional status and quality of life, and its frequent use of interdisciplinary teams and quantitative assessment scales.

The process of geriatric assessment can be viewed as a continuum, ranging from a limited assessment by primary care physicians or community health workers focused on identifying an older person's functional problems and disabilities (screening assessment), to more thorough evaluation of these problems by a geriatrician or multidisciplinary team (comprehensive geriatric assessment), often coupled with initiation of a therapeutic plan. We shall discuss both limited geriatric assessment, such as can be performed by a single practitioner in an office setting, and comprehensive geriatric assessment, usually requiring a specialized geriatric setting.

Because the ultimate goal of geriatric assessment is to improve quality of life for elderly people, readers may find Figure 15-1 helpful.[1] As diagrammed, quality of life includes health status and socioeconomic and environmental factors. Health status can be quantified by both measures of disease, such as signs, symptoms, and laboratory tests, and measures of functional status. By functional status, we mean the individual's ability to participate fully in the physical, mental, and social activities of daily life. The ability to function fully in these arenas is strongly affected by an individual's physiologic health, and can often be used as a measure of the seriousness of a patient's multiple diseases. A comprehensive geriatric assessment should be able to evaluate and plan care for all these areas.

Brief History of Geriatric Assessment

The basic concepts of geriatric assessment have evolved over the past 65 years by merging elements of the traditional medical history and physical examination, the social worker assessment, functional evaluation and treatment methods derived from rehabilitation medicine, and psychometric methods derived from the social sciences. By incorporating the perspectives of many disciplines into a compact assessment format, geriatricians have attempted to create a practical means of viewing the "whole patient."

The first published reports of geriatric assessment programs came from the British geriatrician Marjory Warren, who initiated the concept of specialized geriatric assessment units during the late 1930s while in charge of a large London infirmary. This infirmary was filled primarily with chronically ill, bedfast, and largely neglected elderly patients who had not received proper medical diagnosis or rehabilitation and who were thought to be in need of lifelong institutionalization. Good nursing care kept the patients alive, but the lack of diagnostic assessment and rehabilitation kept them disabled. Warren systematically evaluated these patients, initiated active mobilization and selective rehabilitation, and was able to get most of the long bedfast patients out of bed and, in many cases, discharged home. As a result of her experiences, Warren advocated that every elderly patient receive comprehensive assessment and an attempt at rehabilitation before being admitted to a long-term care hospital or nursing home.[2]

Since Warren's work, the concepts of geriatric assessment have evolved. As geriatric care systems have been developed in countries throughout the world, geriatric assessment programs have been assigned central roles, usually as focal points for entry into the care systems.[3] Geared to differing local needs and populations, geriatric assessment programs vary in intensity and in many of their structural and functional components. They can be located in a number of different settings, including acute hospital inpatient units and consultation teams, chronic and rehabilitation hospital units, outpatient and office-based programs, and home visit outreach programs. Despite diversity, they share many common characteristics. Virtually all programs provide multidimensional assessment, utilizing one or more sets of measurement instruments to quantify functional, psychological, and social parameters. Most use interdisciplinary teams to pool expertise and enthusiasm in working toward common goals. Additionally, most programs attempt to couple their assessments with an intervention, such as rehabilitation, counseling, or placement.

In today's rapidly changing health care environment, geriatric assessment continues to evolve in response to increased pressures for cost-containment, avoidance of institutional

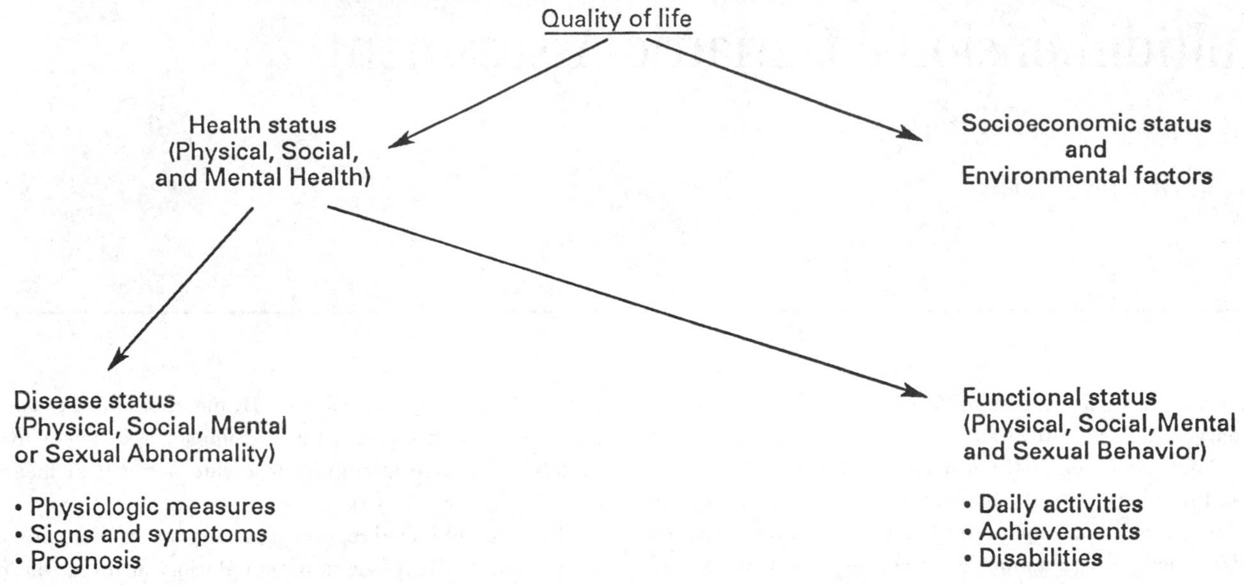

Figure 15-1 Conceptual components of quality of life—relationship to health and functional status. (Adapted from Rubenstein et al.,[1] with permission.)

stays, and active consumer demands for quality of care. In fact, the process of geriatric assessment can be extremely helpful both in achieving improved quality of care and in planning cost-effective care plans for individual patients. This has generally meant a greater emphasis on noninstitutional programs and shortened lengths of stay for hospital-based programs. Geriatric assessment teams are on the whole well positioned to develop creative responses to pressures for delivery of effective care for elderly persons within constrained resources. Geriatricians have long emphasized judicious use of technology, systematic preventive medicine activities, and minimization of institutionalization and hospitalization.

Structure and Process of Geriatric Assessment

Geriatric assessment begins with the identification of deteriorations in health status or the presence of risk factors for deterioration. These deteriorations include both worsening of disease and worsening of functional status. If disease alone has worsened, without affecting functioning, the patient should be able to be cared for in usual primary care settings. In addition, when functional status problems are mild and are not rapidly progressive, it is very appropriate for a primary care practitioner to proceed with the assessment. However, because families and patients identify functional status problems early, and because internists and family practitioners often are unfamiliar with the concept of "treating" functional status impairment as a problem in its own right, patients often self-refer to geriatric care settings for these functional status problems when such settings are available. Patients who have new severe or progressive deficits should ideally receive comprehensive multidisciplinary geriatric assessment. Figure 15-2 outlines an approach for evaluating elderly outpatients with health status deterioration and deciding who should be referred to multidimensional geriatric assessment settings.

Using this approach, an elderly patient presenting with a deterioration in health status of any kind, be it a markedly elevated blood glucose, a vertebral collapse, or a new inability to perform errands, should be evaluated briefly to determine the full extent of the functional disabilities present. Many experts believe that frail elderly people, defined generally as people over the age of 75, or over age 65 with chronic disease, should also be screened for functional disability or risk factors at regular intervals such as once a year, even when no known acute health insults have occurred.[1,4–7] When a new disability or high risk state is detected through screening, such patients may also be appropriate for a full geriatric assessment.

A typical geriatric assessment begins with a functional status "review of systems" that inventories the major domains of functioning. The major elements of this review of systems are captured in two commonly used functional status measures—basic activities of daily living (ADL) and instrumental activities of daily living (IADL). Several reliable and valid versions of these measures have been developed,[8–12] perhaps the most widely used being those by Katz,[13] Lawton,[14] and Barthel.[15,16] These scales are used by clinicians to detect whether the patient has problems performing activities that people must be able to accomplish to survive without help in the community. Basic ADL include self-care activities such as eating, dressing, bathing, transferring, and toileting. Patients unable to perform these activities will generally require 12- to 24-hour support by caregivers. Instrumental activities of daily living include heavier housework, going on errands, managing finances, and telephoning—activities that are required if the individual is to remain independent in a house or apartment.

To interpret the results of impairments in ADL and IADL, physicians will usually need additional information about the patient's environment and social situation. For example, the amount and type of caregiver support available, the strength of the patient's social network, and the level of social activities in which the patient participates will all influence the clinical approach taken in managing deficits detected. This information could be obtained by an experienced nurse or social worker. A screen for mobility and fall risk is also extremely helpful in quantifying function and disability, and several observational scales are available.[17,18] An assessment of nutritional status and risk for undernutrition is also important in understanding the extent of impairment and for planning care.[19] Likewise, a screening assessment of vision and hearing will often detect crucial deficits that need to be treated or compensated for.

Two other key pieces of information must always be gathered in the face of functional disability in an elderly person. These are a screen for mental status (cognitive) impairment and a screen for depression.[8,9,12] Of the several validated screening tests for cognitive function, the Folstein Mini-Mental State is one of the best because it efficiently tests the major aspects of cognitive functioning.[20] Of the various screening tests for geriatric depression, the Yesavage Geriatric Depression Scale,[21] and the Zung Self-Rating Depression Scale[22] are in wide use.

The major measurable dimensions of geriatric assessment, together with examples of commonly used health status screening scales, are listed in Table 15-1.[7–37] The instruments listed are short, have been carefully tested for reliability and validity, and can be easily administered by virtually any staff person involved with the assessment process. Both observational instruments (e.g., physical examination) and self-report (completed by patient or proxy) are available. Components of them—such as watching a patient walk, turn around, and sit down—are routine parts of the geriatric physical examination. Many other kinds of assessment measures exist and can be useful in certain situations. For example, there are several disease-specific measures for measuring stages and levels of dysfunction for patients with specific diseases such as arthritis,[31] dementia,[32] and parkinsonism.[33] There are also several brief global assessment instruments that attempt to quantify all dimensions of the assessment in a single form.[34–37] These latter instruments can be useful in community surveys and some research settings but are not detailed enough to be useful in most clinical settings. More comprehensive lists of available instruments can be found by consulting published reviews of health status assessment.[7–11,38]

A number of factors must be taken into account in deciding where an assessment should take place. These are outlined in Table 15-2. Mental and physical impairment make it difficult for patients to comply with recommendations and to navigate multiple appointments in multiple locations. Functionally impaired elders must depend on families and friends, who often must avoid job loss in the face of chronic and relentless demands on time and energy and in their roles as caregivers, and who may be elderly themselves. Each separate medical appointment or intervention has a high time-cost to these caregivers, which must be minimized if successful geriatric assessment is to occur. Patient fatigability during periods of increased illness may require the availability of a bed during the assessment process. Finally, enough physician time and expertise must be available to complete the assessment within the constraints of the setting.

Most geriatric assessments do not require the full range of technologic capacity nor the intensity of physician and nurse monitoring found in the acute care inpatient setting. Yet hospi-

Table 15-1 Measurable dimensions of geriatric assessment with examples of specific measures

Dimension	Basic Context	Specific Examples
Basic ADL[23,24]	Strengths and limitations in self-care, basic mobility, and incontinence	Katz (ADL)[15], Lawton Personal Self-Maintenance Scale,[14] Barthel Index[15,16]
IADL[23,24]	Strengths and limitations in shopping, cooking, household activities, and finances	Lawton (IADL)[14]; Older Americans Resources and Services, IADL Section[28]
Social activities and supports[25]	Strengths and limitations in social network and community activities	Lubben Social Network Scale[29]; Social Resources Section[28]
Mental health—affective[26,27]	The degree to which the person feels anxious, depressed, or generally happy	Yesavage Geriatric Depression Scale[21]; Zung Self-Rating Depression Scale[22]
Mental health—cognitive[27]	The degree to which the person is alert, oriented, and able to concentrate, and perform complex mental tasks	Folstein Mini-Mental State[20]; Kahn Mental Status Questionnaire[30]
Mobility—gait and balance[9]	Quantitative scale of gait, balance, and risk of falls	Tinetti Performance Oriented Mobility Assessment,[17] Get up and go test[18]
Nutritional adequacy[19]	Current nutritional status and risk of malnutrition	Nutrition Screening Initiative Checklist,[19] Mini-Nutritional Assessment[19]

Abbreviations: ADL, activities of daily living; IADL, instrumental activities of daily living.

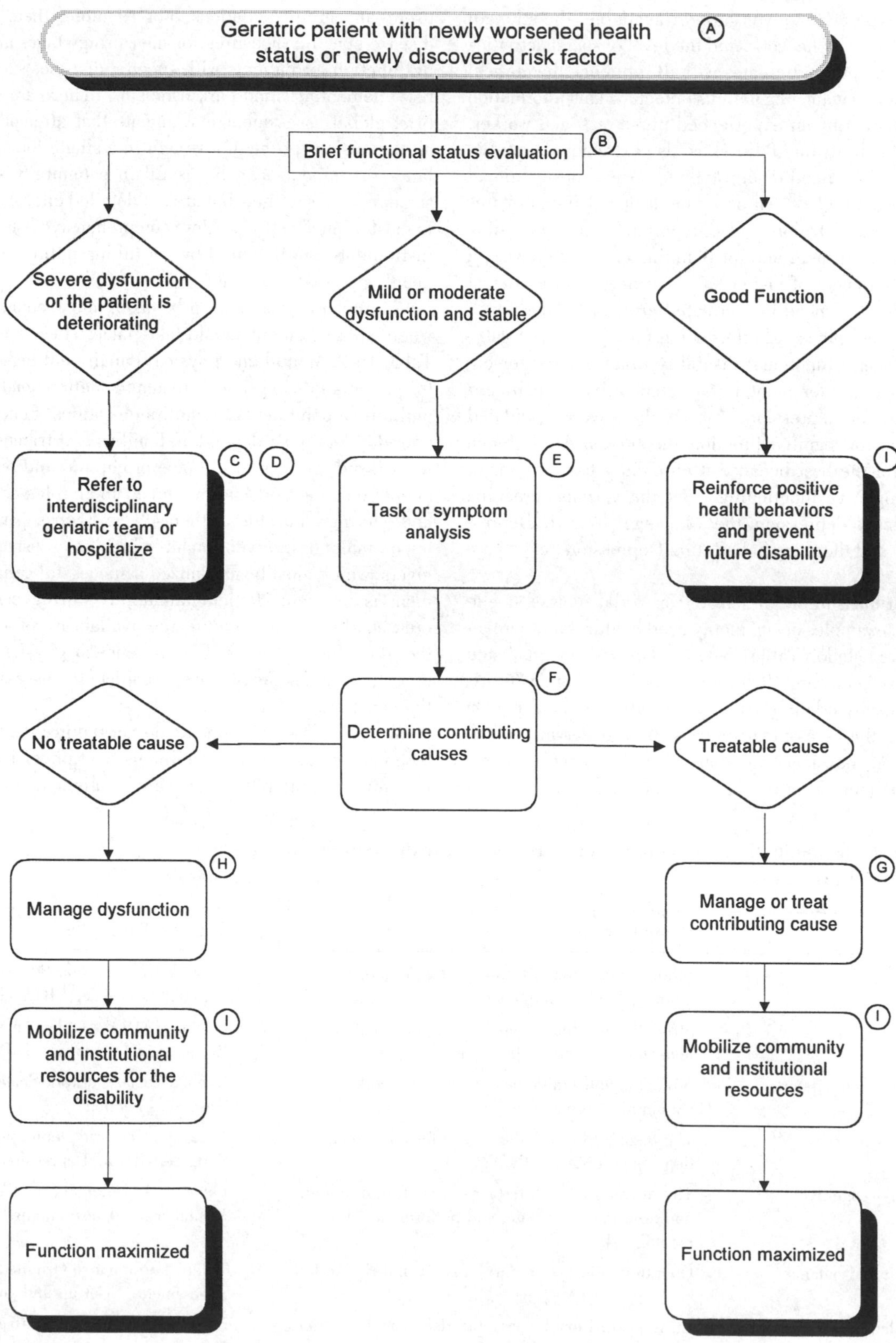
Geriatric patient with newly worsened health status or newly discovered risk factor
A
Brief functional status evaluation
B
Severe dysfunction or the patient is deteriorating
Mild or moderate dysfunction and stable
Good Function
Refer to interdisciplinary geriatric team or hospitalize
C
D
Task or symptom analysis
E
Reinforce positive health behaviors and prevent future disability
I
Determine contributing causes
F
No treatable cause
Treatable cause
Manage dysfunction
H
Manage or treat contributing cause
G
Mobilize community and institutional resources for the disability
I
Mobilize community and institutional resources
I
Function maximized
Function maximized

talization becomes unavoidable if no outpatient setting provides adequate intensity of resources to accomplish the assessment sufficiently fast. A specialized geriatric setting outside an acute hospital ward, such as a day hospital or subacute inpatient geriatric evaluation unit, will provide the easy availability of an interdisciplinary team with the time and expertise to provide needed services efficiently, an adequate level of monitoring, and beds for patients unable to sit or stand for prolonged periods. Inpatient and day hospital assessment programs have the advantages of intensity, rapidity, and ability to care for particularly frail or acutely ill patients. Outpatient programs are generally cheaper and avoid the necessity of an inpatient stay.

Assessment in the Office Practice Setting

A streamlined approach is usually necessary in the office setting. An important first step is setting priorities among problems for initial evaluation and treatment. The "best" problem to work on first might be the problem that bothers the patients the most or, alternatively, the problem upon which resolution of other problems depends (alcoholism or depression often fall into this category).

Figure 15-2 Evaluating and treating health status deterioration among geriatric outpatients.

A. Elderly patients with a new deterioration in health status or newly discovered risk factor(s) may need geriatric assessment. Examples of patients needing assessment include the following:
  1. Frail elderly people with a new functional disability or risk factor for deterioration detected on routine screening
  2. Elderly people with a new or worsened medical complaint or laboratory finding (e.g., "I fell last week" or the X-ray shows a new vertebral compression fracture)
  3. Elderly people with a new or worsened functional disability complaint ("I can't go to church because of my health")

B. Brief functional status evaluation should include the following:
  1. Activities of daily living (ADL)[13–16,23,24]
  2. Instrumental activities of daily living (IADL)[14,23,24]
  3. Mental status (e.g., Folstein Mini-Mental State)[20]
  4. Affective status (e.g., Yesavage Geriatric Depression Scale)[21]

C. Full multidimensional geriatric assessment and/or hospitalization is necessary for elderly patients with new severe or progressive functional disability

D. Targeted assessment for patients in office practice is appropriate for the following:
  1. Patients whose functional disabilities or medical problems are mild enough to make multiple appointment feasible
  2. Patients whose disability is stable enough to permit assessment over weeks to months

E. To perform task or symptom analysis, select the patient's major symptom or disability or chief complaint (the one that bothers him/her the most, the disability upon which resolution of other health problems depends, or the one that is the most treatable). Then, determine the exact maneuvers necessary to complete the task, or the exact components of the symptom (e.g., "difficulty getting dressed" due to difficulty putting on shoes because of inability to bend; or "difficulty with housework" because of failure to complete tasks despite adequate physical ability to perform them).

F. To determine contributing causes:
  1. Perform a targeted history, guided by the functional disabilities detected and by the known common occult causes of disability in the elderly (see text).
  2. Perform a targeted physical examination, always including postural blood pressure changes, vision and hearing screening, observations of gait (at least get up, walk 25 feet, turn around, sit down). Determine all specific physical disabilities such as hip flexor weakness, or poor hand mobility, that explain the observed functional disability.

G. Manage or treat contributing cause(s). Begin appropriate medical treatments and evaluations. Mobilize community and institutional resources as appropriate (low-vision resources for blindness; Alcoholics Anonymous for alcoholics, etc.). Identify key members of the multidisciplinary team and refer as needed (e.g., social worker for social isolation, physical therapist for gait disorder, or psychiatrist for depression).

H. When the disability cannot be reversed, maximize function using available services and behavioral or physical adaptation. For example, rearranging schedule to maximize activity, providing adaptive devices, or arranging for home support services might be indicated.

I. Always reinforce positive health behaviors.

Table 15-2 Determining the intensity and location of the geriatric assessment

	Office Setting	Outpatient Unit/Team	Inpatient Unit/Team
Level of disability	Low	Intermediate	High
Cognitive dysfunction	Mild	Mild to severe	Moderate to severe
Family support	Good	Good to fair	Good to poor
Acuity of illness	Mild	Mild to moderate	Moderate to severe
Complexity	Low	Intermediate	High
Transportation access	Good	Good	Good to poor

The second step in performing a geriatric assessment is to understand the exact nature of the disability through performing a task or symptom analysis. In a nonspecialized setting, or when the disability is mild or clear-cut, this may involve only taking a careful history. When the disability is more severe, more detailed assessments by a multidisciplinary or interdisciplinary team may be necessary. For example, a patient may present with difficulty dressing. There are multiple tasks associated with dressing, any one of which might be the stumbling block (e.g., buying clothes, choosing appropriate clothes to put on, remembering to complete the task, buttoning, stretching to put on shirts, or reaching downward to put on shoes). By identifying the exact areas of difficulty, further evaluation can be targeted toward solving the problem.

Once the history has revealed the nature of the disability, a systematic physical examination and ancillary laboratory tests are needed to clarify the type of physiologic abnormality responsible for the problem. For example, difficulty dressing could be caused by mental status impairment, poor finger mobility, or dysfunction of shoulders, back, or hips. Evaluation by a physical or occupational therapist may be necessary to pinpoint the problem adequately, and evaluation by a social worker may be required to determine the extent of family dysfunction engendered by or contributing to the dependency. Radiologic and other laboratory testing may be necessary.

Each of the types of abnormalities that could cause difficulty dressing suggests different treatments. By understanding the abnormalities that contribute most to the functional disability, the best treatment strategy can be undertaken. Often one disability leads to another—impaired gait may lead to depression or decreased social functioning; and immobility of any cause, even after the cause has been removed, can lead to secondary impairments in performance of daily activities due to deconditioning and loss of musculoskeletal flexibility.

Almost any acute or chronic disease can cause worsening of functioning. Common but easily overlooked causes of dysfunction in elderly people include impaired cognition, impaired special senses (vision, hearing, balance), unstable gait and mobility, poor health habits (alcohol, smoking, lack of exercise), poor nutrition, polypharmacy, incontinence, psychosocial stress, and depression. To identify contributing causes of the disability, the physician must thus look for worsening of the patient's chronic diseases, occurrence of a new acute disease, or appearance of one of the common occult diseases listed above. The physician does this through a refocused history guided by the functional disabilities detected and their differential diagnoses, and a focused physical examination. The physical examination always includes, in addition to usual evaluations of the heart, lungs, extremities, and neurologic function, postural blood pressure, vision and hearing screening, and careful observation of the patient's gait. The mini-mental state examination, already recommended as part of the initial functional status screen, may also determine what parts of the physical examination require particular attention as part of the evaluation of dementia or acute confusion. Finally, basic laboratory testing including a complete blood count and a blood chemistry panel, as well as tests indicated on the basis of specific findings from the history and physical examination, will generally be necessary.

Once the disability and its causes are understood, the best treatments or management strategies for it are often clear. When a reversible cause for the impairment is found, a simple treatment may eliminate or ameliorate the functional disability. When the disability is complex, the physician may need the support of a variety of community or hospital-based resources. In most cases, a strategy for long-term follow-up and often, formal case management should be developed to ensure that needs and services are appropriately matched up and followed through.

Multidimensional Geriatric Assessment

If referral to a specialized geriatric setting has been chosen, the process of assessment will probably be similar to that described above, except that the greater intensity of resources and the special training of all members of the multidisciplinary team in dealing with geriatric patients and their problems will facilitate carrying out the proposed assessment and plan more quickly, and in greater breadth and detail. In the usual geriatric assessment setting, key disciplines involved include, at a minimum, physicians, social workers, nurses, and physical and occupational therapists, and optimally may include other disciplines such as dieticians, pharmacists, ethicists, and home care specialists. Special geriatric expertise among the multidisciplinary team members is crucial.

The multidisciplinary (or interdisciplinary) team conference, which takes place after most team members have completed their individual assessments, has assumed a critical place in the assessment and treatment of functional disability. Most of the successful trials of geriatric assessment have included such a team conference. By bringing the perspectives of all disciplines together to develop a unified plan, the team conference generates new ideas, sets priorities, disseminates the full results of the assessment to all those involved in treating the patient, and avoids duplication or incongruity of therapies. Development of fully effective teams requires commitment, skill, and time as the interdisciplinary team evolves through the "forming, storming, and norming" phases to reach the fully developed "performing" stage.[39] Involvement of the patient (and carer if appropriate) at some stage is important in maintaining the principle of choice.[39,40]

Effectiveness of Geriatric Assessment Programs

A growing literature supports the effectiveness of geriatric assessment programs (GAPs) in a variety of settings. Early descriptive studies indicated a number of benefits from GAPs such as improved diagnostic accuracy, reduced discharges to nursing homes, increased functional status, and more appropriate medication prescribing. Because they were descriptive studies, without concurrent control patients, they were not able to distinguish the effects of the programs from simple improvement over time. Nor did these studies look at long-term, or many short-term, outcome benefits. Nonetheless, many of these early studies provided promising results.[41–45]

Improved diagnostic accuracy was the most widely described effect of geriatric assessment, most often indicated by substantial numbers of important problems uncovered. Frequencies of new diagnoses found ranged from almost one to more than four per patient. Factors contributing to the improvement of diagnosis in GAPs include the validity of the assessment itself (the capability of a structured search for "geriatric problems" to find them), the extra measure of time and care taken in the evaluation of the patient (independent of the formal elements of "the assessment"), and a probable lack of diagnostic attention on the part of referring professionals.

Improved living location on discharge from health care setting was demonstrated in several early studies, beginning with T. F. Williams' classic descriptive pre/poststudy of an outpatient assessment program in New York.[46] Of patients referred for nursing home placement in the country, the assessment program found that only 38 percent actually needed skilled nursing care, while 23 percent could return home, and 39 percent were appropriate for board and care or retirement facilities. Numerous subsequent studies have shown similar improvements in living location.[47–62] Several studies that examined mental or physical functional status of patients before and after comprehensive geriatric assessment coupled with treatment and rehabilitation showed patient improvement on measures of function.[47–51,55,59]

Beginning in the 1980s, controlled studies began to appear that corroborated some of the earlier studies and documented additional benefits such as improved survival, reduced hospital and nursing home utilization, and in some cases, reduced costs.[47–71] These studies were by no means uniform in their results. Some showed a whole series of dramatic positive effects on function, survival, living location, and costs, while others showed relatively few if any benefits. However, the GAPs being studied were also very different from each other in terms of process of care, and also accepted a wide variety of patient populations.

One of the more striking effects confirmed for GAPs was their positive impact on survival. Several controlled studies of different basic GAP models demonstrated significantly increased survival, reported in different ways and with varying periods of follow-up. Mortality was reduced for Sepulveda geriatric evaluation unit patients by 50 percent at 1 year, and the survival curves of the experimental and control groups still significantly favored the assessed group at 2 years.[47,63,64] Survival was improved by 21 percent at 1 year in a Scottish trial of geriatric rehabilitation consultation.[59] Two Canadian consultation trials demonstrated significantly improved 6-month survival.[55,56] Two Danish community-based trials of in-home geriatric assessment and follow-up demonstrated reduction in mortality,[48,61] and two Welsh studies of in-home GAPs had beneficial survival effects among patients assessed at home and followed for 2 years.[50,51] On the other hand, several other studies of geriatric assessment found no statistically significant survival benefits.[52,54,58,59]

Multiple studies followed patients longitudinally after the initial assessment and thus were able to examine the longer-term utilization and cost impacts of assessment and treatment. Some studies found an overall reduction in nursing home days.[47,59,65,66] Hospital utilization was examined in several reports. For hospital-based GAPs, the length of hospitalization was obviously affected by the length of the assessment itself. Thus, some programs appear to prolong initial length of stay[45,67,68] while others reduce initial stay.[53,59–61,69] However, studies following patients for at least 1 year have usually shown reduction in use of acute-care hospital services, even in those programs with initially prolonged hospital stays.[41,48,57]

Compensatory increases in use of community-based services or home care agencies might be expected with declines in nursing home placements and use of other institutional services. These increases have been detected in several studies[48,50,55,70] but not in others.[47,57,62] Although increased use of formal community services may not always be indicated, it usually is a desirable goal. The fact that several studies did not detect increases in use of home and community services probably reflects the unavailability of community service or referral networks rather than that more of such services were not needed.

The effects of these programs on costs and utilization parameters have rarely been examined comprehensively, due to methodologic difficulties in gathering comprehensive utilization and cost data, as well as statistical limitations in comparing highly skewed distributions. The Sepulveda study found that total first-year direct health care costs had been reduced due to overall reductions in nursing home and rehospitalization days, despite significantly longer initial hospital stays on the geriatric unit.[47] These savings continued through 3 years of follow-up.[63] Hendriksen's program[48] reduced the costs of medical care, apparently through successful early case-finding and referral for preventive intervention. Williams' outpatient GAP[57] detected reductions in medical care costs due primarily to reductions in hospitalization. Although it would be reasonable to worry that prolonged survival of frail patients would lead to increased service use and charges, or, of perhaps greater concern, to worry about the quality of the prolonged life, these concerns may be without substance. Indeed, the Sepulveda study demonstrated that a GAP could improve not only survival but prolong high-function survival,[47,63] while at the same time reducing use of institutional services and costs.

To resolve some of the discrepancies between study results, and to try to identify whether particular program elements were associated with particular benefits, a systematic meta-analysis was carried out in 1993.[72,73] This meta-analysis included published data from the 28 controlled trials completed as of that date, involving nearly 10,000 patients, and was also able to include substantial amounts of unpublished data systematically retrieved from many of the studies. The meta-analysis identified five GAP types: hospital units (six studies), hospital consultation teams (eight studies), in-home assessment services (seven studies), outpatient assessment services (four studies), and "hospital-home assessment services" (three studies) the latter of which performed in-home assessments on patients recently discharged from hospitals. The meta-analysis confirmed many of the major reported benefits for many of the individual program types. These statistically and clinically significant benefits included reduced risk of mortality (by 22 percent for hospital-based programs at 12 months, and by 14 percent for all programs combined at 12 months), improved likelihood of living at home (by 47 percent for hospital-based programs and by 26 percent for all programs combined at 12 months), reduced hospital (re)admissions (by 12 percent for all programs at study end), greater chance of cognitive improvement (by 47 percent for all programs at study end), and greater chance of physical function improvement for patients on hospital units (by 72 percent for hospital units).

Clearly not all studies showed equivalent effects, and the meta-analysis was able to indicate a number of variables at both the program and patient levels that tended to distinguish trials with large effects from ones with more limited ones. When examined on the program level, hospital units and home-visit assessment teams produced the most dramatic benefits, while no major significant benefits in office-based programs could be confirmed. Programs that provided hands-on clinical care and/or long-term follow-up were generally able to produce greater positive effects than purely consultative programs or ones that lacked follow-up. Another factor associated with greater demonstrated benefits, at least in hospital-based programs, was patient targeting; programs that selected patients who were at high risk for deterioration yet still had "rehabilitation potential" generally had stronger results than less selective programs.

The meta-analysis confirmed the importance of targeting criteria in producing beneficial outcomes. In particular, when use of explicit targeting criteria for patient selection was included as a covariate, increases in some program benefits were often found. For example, among the hospital-based GAPs studies, positive effects on physical function and likelihood of living at home at 12 months were associated with studies that excluded patients who were relatively "too healthy." A similar effect on physical function was seen in the institutional studies that excluded persons with relatively poor prognoses. The reason for this effect of targeting on effect size no doubt lies in the ability of careful targeting to concentrate the intervention on patients who can benefit, without diluting the effect with persons too ill or too well to show a measurable improvement.

Conclusion

Published studies of the effectiveness of comprehensive geriatric assessment have confirmed its efficacy in many settings. While there is no single optimal blueprint for geriatric assessment, the participation of the multidisciplinary team and the focus on functional status and quality of life as major clinical goals are common to all settings. Although the greatest benefits have been found in programs targeted to the frail subgroup of older persons, a strong case can be made for a continuum of GAPs—screening assessments performed periodically for all older persons and comprehensive assessment targeted to frail and high-risk patients. Clinicians interested in developing these services will do well to heed the experiences of the programs reviewed here in adapting the principles of geriatric assessment to local resources. Future research is still needed to determine the most effective and efficient methods for performing geriatric assessment and on developing strategies for best matching needs with services.

References

1. Rubenstein LV, Calkins DR, Greenfield S et al: Health status assessment for elderly patients: reports of the society of general internal medicine task force on health assessment. J Am Geriatr Soc 1989;37:562–569
2. Matthews DA: Dr. Marjory Warren and the origin of British geriatrics. J Am Geriatr Soc 1984;32:253–258
3. Brocklehurst JC: Geriatric care in advanced societies. MTP, Lancaster University Park Press, Baltimore, 1975
4. Canadian Task Force on the Periodic Health Examination: Can Med Assoc J 1979;121:1193–1254
5. Rubenstein LZ, Josephson KR, Nichol-Seamons M, Robbins AS: Comprehensive health screening of well elderly adults. J Gerontol 1986;41:343–352
6. US Congress, Office of Technology Assessment: Preventive health services for Medicare beneficiaries: policy and research issues (OTA-H-416). US Government Printing Office, Washington DC, 1990
7. Rubenstein LV: Using quality of life tests for patient diagnosis or screening. In Spilker B, (ed): Quality of Life and Pharmacoeconomics in Clinical Trials. 2nd Ed. JB Lippincott, Philadelphia, 1996
8. Rubenstein LZ, Campbell LJ, Kane RL: Geriatric Assessment. WB Saunders, Philadelphia, 1987
9. Rubenstein LZ, Wieland D, Bernabei R: Geriatric Assessment

Technology: The State of the Art. Kurtis Publishers, Milan, 1995

10. Kane RA, Kane RL: Assessing the elderly. Lexington Books, Lexington, Massachusetts, 1984
11. Feinstein AR, Josephy BR, Wells CK: Scientific and clinical problems in indexes of functional disability. Ann Intern Med 1986;105:413–420
12. Gallo JJ, Reichel W, Anderson L: Handbook of geriatric assessment. Aspen Publishers, Rockville, Maryland, 1988
13. Katz S, Ford AB, Moskowitz RW, et al: Studies of illness in the aged. The index of ADL: a standardized measure of biological psychosocial function. J Am Med Assoc 1963;185:914–919
14. Lawton MP, Brody EM: Assessment of older people: self-maintaining and instrumental activities of daily living. Gerontologist 1969;9:179–186
15. Mahoney FI, Barthel DW: Functional evaluation—the Barthel Index. Maryland State Med J 1965;14:61–65
16. Wade DT, Colin C: The Barthel ADL Index—a standard measure of physical disability. Int Disabil Studies 1988;10:64–67
17. Tinetti ME: Performance oriented assessment of mobility problems in elderly patients. J Am Geriatr Soc 1986;34:119–126
18. Mathias S, Nayak USL, Isaacs B: Balance in elderly patients: the "get up and go" test. Arch Phys Med Rehab 1986;67: 387–389
19. Vellas B, Guigoz Y: Nutritional assessment as part of the geriatric evaluation. In Geriatric Assessment Technology: The State of the Art. Kurtis Publishers, Milan, 1995
20. Folstein M, Folstein S, McHugh P: Mini-mental state: a practical method for grading the cognitive state of patients for the clinician. J Psychiatr Res 1975;12:189–198
21. Yesavage J, Brink T, Rose T et al: Development and validation of a geriatric screening scale: a preliminary report. J Psychiatr Res 1983;17:37–49
22. Zung WWK: A self rating depression scale. Arch Gen Psychiatr 1965;12:63–70
23. Branch LG, Meyers AR: Assessing physical function in the elderly. Clin Geriatr Med 1987;3:29–51
24. Hedrick SC: Assessment of functional status: activities of daily living. In Rubenstein LZ, Wieland D, Bernabei R (eds): Geriatric Assessment Technology: The State of the Art. Kurtis Publishers, Milan, 1995
25. Kane RA: Assessment of social function: recommendations for comprehensive geriatric assessment. In Rubenstein LZ, Wieland D, Bernabei R (eds): Geriatric Assessment Technology: The State of the Art. Kurtis Publishers, Milan, 1995
26. Gallagher D: Assessing affect in the elderly. Clin Geriatr Med 1987;3:65–85
27. Gurland BH, Wilder D: Detection and assessment of cognitive impairment and depressed mood in older adults. In Rubenstein LZ, Wieland D, Bernabei R (eds): Geriatric Assessment Technology: The State of the Art. Kurtis Publishers, Milan, 1995
28. Duke University Center for the Study of Aging and Human Development: The OARS Methodology. Duke University Press, Durham, North Carolina, 1978
29. Lubben JE: Assessing social networks among elderly populations. Family and Community Health 1988;8:42–52
30. Kahn R, Goldfarb A, Pollack M et al: Brief objective measures of mental status in the aged. Am J Psychiatr 1960;117:326–328
31. Chambers LW, MacDonald LA, Tugwell P et al: The McMaster Health Index Questionnaire as a measure of quality of life for patients with rheumatoid disease. J Rheumatol 1982;9: 780–784
32. Reisberg B, Ferris SH, DeLeon MJ et al: The global deterioration scale for assessment of primary degenerative dementia. Am J Psychiatr 1982;139:1136–1139
33. Hoehn MM, Yahr MD: Parkinsonism: onset, progression, and mortality. Neurology 1967;17:427–442
34. Stewart AL, Hays RD, Ware JE: Communication: the MOS short-form general health survey: reliability and validity in a patient population. Med Care 1988;26:724–735
35. Nelson E, Wasson J, Kirk J et al: Assessment of function in routine clinical practice: description of the Coop chart method and preliminary findings. J Chron Dis 1987;40:55S
36. Bergner M, Bobbit R, Carter WB: The sickness impact profile: validation of a health status measure. Med Care 1981;19: 787–805
37. Jette AM, Davies AR, Calkins DR, et al: The functional status questionnaire: reliability and validity when used in primary care. J Gen Intern Med 1986;1:143
38. Lohr KN, Ware JE: Advances in health assessment conference. J Chron Dis 1987;40:1S–5S
39. Campbell LJ, Cole KD: Geriatric assessment teams. Clin Geriatr Med 1987;3:99–110
40. Wieland D, Kramer BJ, Waite MS, Rubenstein LZ: The interdisciplinary team in geriatric care. Am Behav Sci 1996;39: 655–664
41. William J, Stokoe IH, Gray S et al: Old people at home: their unreported needs. Lancet 1964;i:1117–1120
42. Lowther CP, MacLeod RDM, Williamson J: Evaluation of early diagnostic services for the elderly BMJ 1970;3:275–277
43. Brocklehurst JC, Carty MH, Leeming JT, Robinson JH: Medical screening of old people accepted for residential care. Lancet 1978;ii:141–143
44. Applegate WB, Akins D, Vander Zwaag R et al: A geriatric rehabilitation and assessment unit in a community hospital. J Am Geriatr Soc 1983;31:206–210
45. Rubenstein LZ, Josephson KR, Wieland GD et al: Geriatric assessment on a subacute hospital ward. Clin Geriatr Med 1987; 3:131–143
46. Williams TF, Hill JH, Fairbank ME, Knox KG: Appropriate placement of the chronically ill and aged: a successful approach by evaluation. JAMA 1973;266:1332–1335
47. Rubenstein LZ, Josephson KR, Wieland GD et al: Effectiveness of a geriatric evaluation unit: a randomized clinical trial. N Engl J Med 1984;311:1664–1670
48. Hendriksen C, Lund E, Stromgard E: Consequences of assessment and intervention among elderly people: three-year randomized controlled trial. BMJ 1984;289:1522–1524
49. Thomas DR, Brahan R, Haywood BP: Inpatient community-based geriatric assessment reduces subsequent mortality. J Am Geriatr Soc 1993;41:101–104
50. Vetter NJ, Jones DA, Victor CR: Effects of health visitors working with elderly patients in general practice: a randomized controlled trial. BMJ 1984;288:369–372
51. Vetter NJ, Lewis PA, Ford D: Can health visitors prevent fractures in elderly people? BMJ 1992;304:888–890

52. Winograd CH, Gerety M, Lai N: A negative trial of inpatient geriatric consultation: lessons learned. Arch Intern Med 1993; 153:2017–2023
53. Collard AF, Bachman SS, Beatrice DF: Acute care delivery for the geriatric patient: an innovative approach. Qual Rev Bull 1985;(June):180–185
54. Allen CC, Becker PM, McVey LJ et al: A randomized controlled clinical trial of a geriatric consultation team: compliance with recommendations. J 1986;255:2617–2621
55. Hogan DB, Fox RA, Badley BWD, Mann OE: Effect of a geriatric consultation service on management of patients in an acute care hospital. Can Med Assoc J 1987;136:713–717
56. Hogan DB, Fox RA: A prospective controlled trial of a geriatric consultation team in an acute care hospital. Age Ageing 1990; 19:107–113
57. Williams ME, Williams TF, Zimmer JG et al: How does the team approach to outpatient geriatric evaluation compare with traditional care: a report of a randomized controlled trial. J Am Geriatr Soc 1987;35:1071–1078
58. Gilchrist WJ, Newman RH, Hamblen DL, Williams BO: Prospective randomized study of an orthopaedic geriatric inpatient service. BMJ 1988;297:1116–1118
59. Reid J, Kennie DC: Geriatric rehabilitative care after fractures of the proximal femur: one-year follow-up of a randomized clinical trial. BMJ 1989;299:25–26
60. Pathy MSJ, Bayer A, Harding K, Dibble A: Randomized trial of casefinding and surveillance of elderly people at home. Lancet 1992;340:890–893
61. Hansen FR, Spedtsberg K, Schroll M: Geriatric follow-up by home visits after discharge from hospital: a randomized controlled trial. Age Ageing 1992;21:445–450
62. Gayton D, Wood-Dauphine S, de Lorimer M et al: Trial of a geriatric consultation team in an acute care hospital. J Am Geriatr Soc 1987;35:726–736
63. Rubenstein LZ, Josephson KR, Harker JO, Wieland D: The Sepulveda GEU study revisited: long-term outcomes, use of services, and costs. Aging: Clin Exp Res 1995;7:212–217
64. Rubenstein LZ, Wieland D, Josephson KR et al: Improved survival for frail elderly inpatients on a geriatric evaluation unit (GEU): who benefits? J Clin Epidemiol 1988;41:441–449
65. Schuman JE, Beattie EJ, Steed DA et al: The impact of a new geriatric program in a hospital for the chronically ill. Can Med Assoc J 1978;118:639–645
66. Lefton E, Bonstelle S, Frengley JD: Success with an inpatient geriatric unit: a controlled study. J Am Geriatr Soc 1983;31: 149–155
67. Berkman B, Campion E, Swagerty E, Goldman M: Geriatric consultation teams: alternative approach to social work discharge planning. J Gerontol Soc Work 1983;5:77–88
68. Lichtenstein H, Winogard CH: Geriatric consultation: a functional approach. J Am Geriatr Soc 1984;32:356–361
69. Burley LE, Currie CT, Smith RG, Williamson J: Contribution from geriatric medicine within acute medical wards. BMJ 1979; 263:90–92
70. Tulloch AH, Moore V: A randomized controlled trial of geriatric screening and surveillance in general practice. J R Col General Pract 1979;29:733–742
71. Rubenstein LZ, Wieland D, Bernabei R: Geriatric assessment: international research prospective. Aging: Clin Exp Res 1995; 7:157–260
72. Stuck AE, Siu AL, Wieland GD et al: Comprehensive geriatric assessment: a meta-analysis of controlled trials. Lancet 1993; 342:1032–1036
73. Stuck AE, Wieland D, Rubenstein LZ et al: Comprehensive geriatric assessment: meta-analysis of main effects and elements enhancing effectiveness. In Rubenstein LZ, Wieland D, Bernabei R (eds): Geriatric Assessment Technology: The State of the Art. Kurtis Publishers, Milan, 1995

CHAPTER 16

Biochemical Tests

LASZLO SARKOZI

Biochemical tests are performed on various body fluids for several purposes. They are useful in physiologic assessment, diagnosis and treatment of diseases, and for monitoring therapeutic drug levels. A measured or observed laboratory test result from an individual is compared with a reference value.[1] Previously used terms, such as "normal value" and "normal range," are based on assumptions. Statistical distribution of biologic data most often does not fall into the gaussian symmetric "normal" bell-shaped distribution curve. In addition, by definition of the "95th percentile range," 5 percent of the healthy individuals would fall outside the normal range. Reference intervals (a range of values obtained from the reference value set) are based on the recommendations of the Expert Panel on Theory of Reference Values of the International Federation of Clinical Chemistry, and the published guidelines of the National Committee for Clinical Laboratory Standards, C28-P.[2]

Gradual physiologic changes that occur over time as part of the aging process affect several analytes. With the introduction of clinical laboratory automation and large scale multiphasic screening programs during the 1960s, it became possible to collect a sufficient database to document age and sex dependent changes and reference intervals for most biochemical diagnostic tests.[3–5]

Preanalytic and Analytic Variables

Biochemical test results are collected from reference populations under controlled preanalytic and analytic variables. Similarly, specimens from patient population must be obtained and processed under controlled circumstances. Several of the preanalytic variables to be considered are listed in Table 16-1.[2,6] Some of the variables might be more characteristic in the geriatric population.

Drug Regimen

The most commonly ignored preanalytic variable is the fact that elderly subjects are often on a drug regimen. Law and Chalmers[7] found in 1976 that in Great Britain, 87 percent of people over 75 years old living at home were on medication and 34 percent were on at least three different drugs daily. Drugs may have in vivo and/or in vitro effects on biochemical tests. Young[8] provides an updated list of these effects with very extensive references.

Multiple Disease and Severe Illness

Reference values are helpful in ruling out certain diagnoses. Values outside the reference may not be as valuable due to their lack of specificity. Several analytes, especially some elevated enzyme activities, may be the result of a chronic condition, eliminating their diagnostic utility.[9] Dehydration is a frequent condition in the elderly, with concurrent effect on renal function and homeostasis.

Recent Hospitalization, Prolonged Bed Rest

Calcium, sodium, potassium, and phosphate excretions are decreased, presumably due to decreased metabolism of skeletal muscle.[10] Fluid retention may result in decreased serum protein and albumin concentrations and, correspondingly, reduction of protein-bound constituents.

Geriatric Reference Values

A comprehensive book (86 contributors) on geriatric clinical chemistry presented data on 134 analytes.[11] Tietz et al.[12] determined 15,000 laboratory values in 236 individuals between the ages of 60 and 90 years, 22 individuals between 90 and 99 years, and 69 individuals at 100 years and above — an unprecedented wealth of information. They have avoided the use of the term "reference ranges" in the group of nonagenarians and centenarians. It is difficult to distinguish between symptoms of a disease and normal manifestation of aging. The selected individuals 90 years old or younger appeared to be mentally and physically fit and mobile; 72 of them had some health problems or some diseases that were controlled by medication. Although the number of observations in the groups aged over 90 years may not satisfy statistical requirements,[13] nevertheless, this is the first published data on these groups and presents valuable information. I have compiled these reports into a simplified format (Table 16-2) and will discuss only the tests whose mean values significantly differ from the young adult population.

Table 16-1 Selected preanalytic variables

Subject Preparation	Specimen Collection	Specimen Handling
Prior diet	Environmental conditions	Clotting
Fasting or nonfasting	Time	Transport
Drug regimen	Body posture	Centrifugation
Biologic rhythms	Specimen type	Storage
Physical activity	Collection site	Preparation for analysis
Stress	Technique	

(From National Committee for Clinical Laboratory Standards,[2] with permission.)

Selected Analytes

Albumin

In both males and females, serum albumin concentration decreases gradually with age but generally remains within the "normal" range.[14] This may not be the result of the aging process alone, but also of the decreased state of health of those individuals.[15] Significantly increased albumin concentration in urine was reported in one study[16] and correspondingly, there is a significantly increased urinary albumin/creatinine ratio in the oldest group.

Alkaline Phosphatase

The 60- to 90-year-old group of females has 20 to 25 percent elevated alkaline phosphatase activity, compared to young adults. This may be the result of postmenopause hormonal changes,[17] while in the same age group of males it remains constant. In the 90-years-and-older group, alkaline phosphate activities are equally elevated in both sexes. Elevated activities may not be only age related, they may be the result of subclinical osteomalacia associated with secondary hyperparathyroidism[18] or therapeutic drug administration.[19]

Cholesterol, Total

Total cholesterol levels are increased in the 60- to 90-year-old group, especially in the females. In the oldest group the cholesterol level decreased, more in the male group than in the female group.[20,21] The use of "desirable level," derived from prospective epidemiologic studies directly relating to coronary heart disease, is recommended instead of reference limits.

Insulin

In the 60- to 90-year-old group, insulin is sharply elevated, then it drops below the young adult mean. The increase has been attributed to progressively lessened sensitivity of muscular tissue to insulin,[22,23] insulin resistance,[24] and decreased number of insulin receptors in fat cells.[25] It has been suggested that obesity and glucose intolerance are more important determinants of insulin levels in the elderly than is age per se.[26]

Luteinizing Hormone

Mean values of luteinizing hormone (LH) increase six- to ten fold in the 90-years-and-older age group, as compared with values of young adults. In males it is probably due to the reduction of testosterone concentration.[27] The LH increase in females is attributed to the lack of negative feedback of ovarian steroids.[28]

Prostate-Specific Antigen

Prostate cancer occurs in 50 percent of the male population over the age of 70 years. As with other cancers, effective treatment of prostate cancer is more successful with early diagnosis.[29] Prostate-specific antigen (PSA) also is useful in monitoring treatment of patients with prostatic cancer. Elevated values may be seen in nonmalignant diseases of the prostate and other adjacent genitourinary tissues. Patients with confirmed prostatic carcinoma frequently have serum PSA concentrations within the range of those observed in healthy subjects. Serum PSA concentrations should be used only along with information from other diagnostic procedures and clinical evaluation of the patient.[30] PSA concentrations of 4 ng/ml or less are considered normal.

Triglycerides

Triglyceride levels in the 60- to 90-year-old age group are considerably higher than in the young adult group, followed by a decrease, especially in males.[31] Factors influencing the triglyceride levels in the elderly include adiposity, use of diuretics, weight loss, and genetic differences. Changes may relate to changes in lifestyle as individuals grow older.[32] Exercise levels tend to fall through adult life, and total energy expenditure falls appreciably as a consequence. Food consumption tends to fall[33] in parallel with the fall in energy expenditure, but body fat tends to increase with age up to a peak in late middle life, while muscle mass falls progressively in response to lower exercise level.

Urea Nitrogen

There is an age-related, steady increase of urea nitrogen, parallel with declining renal function.[34] The decrease in renal function is assumed to be due to the decrease in number of glomeruli, which are estimated to decrease by 33 to 50 percent in the population older than 70 years. Decreased renal function in this age group may also be due to decreased renal blood flow, as a result of decreased cardiac output, anatomic narrowing of blood vessels, and a persistent vasoconstriction.[35]

Therapeutic Drug Monitoring

When an elderly patient is being evaluated, a major part of that evaluation should be a thorough medication history. Elderly patients frequently have four to five simultaneous pre-

Table 16-2 Laboratory ranges (95th percentile) and mean values of young adults, 60- to 90-year-olds, and those 90 years old and older

			Young Adults		60–90		>90	
Analyte	**Method**	**Sex**	**Range**	**Mean**	**Range**	**Mean**	**Range**	**Mean**
Albumin, g/L	Rate nephelometry	M + F	34–48	41	32–46	40	29–45	36
Albumin, urine, mg/L	Rate nephelometry	M + F	2–24	6.7			1–100	21
Albumin/creatinine, urine, g/mol		M + F	0.22–1.48	0.57			0.3–12.2	3.0
α_1-Antitrypsin, g/L	Rate nephelometry	M	0.40–2.05	1.41			1.22–2.50	1.78
		F	0.64–2.53	1.53			1.30–2.36	1.80
ALP, U/L	PNPP substrate	M	53–128	85	56–119	81	56–155	97
	AMP buffer, 37°C	F	42–98	67	53–141	82	43–160	92
Amylase, U/L	Maltotetraose, 37°C	M + F	27–131	65	24–151	71		
	PNP-α-MP, PNP-α-MH, 37°C	M + F	20–104	55			25–147	73
ALT, U/L	Oxidation of	M	10–40	20			6–38	14
	NADH P-5′-P, 37°C	F	7–35	12			5–24	13
	Oxidation of	M	6–16	11	7–24	11.2		
	NADH 30°C	F	6–16	9	7–16	8.7		
Amylase P-type, U/L	PNP-α-MP, PNP-α-MH, and wheat germ inhibitor 37°C	M + F	27–70	48			<10–82	39
Andostenedione, ng/L	RIA after selective	M	750–2,050				270 1,160	681
	solvent extraction	F	850–2,750				30–2,250	566
nmol/L		M	2.6–7.2				0.9–4.1	2.4
		F	3.0–9.6				0.1–7.9	2.0
AST, U/L	Oxidation of	M	16–42	24.6			11–38	25
	NADH P-5′-P, 37°C	F	14–29	19			18–30	24
	Oxidation of	M	10–20	14	11–26	14.7		
	NADH 30°C	F	9–20	13	10–20	14.2		
Bilirubin, total mg/L	Modified Jendrassik-Grof	M + F	3–12	6	2–11	5	2–9	4.2
μmol/L			15–21	10	3–19	9	3–15	7
Bilirubin, conjugated mg/L	Jendrassik-Grof	M + F	1–3	2	<1–1	1	<1–2	1.1
μmol/L			2–5	3	<2	2	<2–3	2
C3 activator, mg/L	Rate nephelometry	M + F	200–470	320	220–440	330	220–480	325
Calcium, total mmol/L	o-Cresolphtalein complexone	M + F	2.15–2.50	2.30	2.20–2.55	2.35	2.05–2.40	2.25
Calcium, ionized, mmol/L	Ion-selective electrode	M + F	1.15–1.27	1.21	1.16–1.29	1.22	1.12–1.32	1.22
CEA, μg/L	Solid phase immunoenzymatic assay	M + F	Nonsmoker 0–3 Smoker 0–5				0.4–9.2	3.8
Ceruloplasmin, mg/L	Rate nephelometry	M	180–480	280			160–450	320
		F	200–560	340			240–460	350
Cholesterol, total, mg/L	Cholesterol oxidase	M	1,290–2,780 (recommended <2,000)	1,920	1,670–3,360	2,270	1,110–2,560	1,790
		F	1,260–2,800 (recommended <2,000)	1,750	1,680–3,480	2,460	1,480–2,690	2,010

(Continues)

Table 16-2 *(Continued)*

			Young Adults		60–90		>90	
Analyte	**Method**	**Sex**	**Range**	**Mean**	**Range**	**Mean**	**Range**	**Mean**
mmol/L		M	3.34–7.19 (recommended <5.17)	4.97	4.32–8.69	5.87	2.87–6.62	4.63
		F	3.26–6.83 (recommended <5.17)	4.53	4.34–9.00	6.36	3.83–6.96	5.20
Cl, mmol/L	Mercuric thiocyan.	M + F	98–107		98–107	103	98–111	104
CK, U/L	Reduction of NADP 37°C	M	52–200	112			21–203	50
		F	35–165	85			22–99	405
	Reduction of NADP 30°C	M	25–80	53	20–110			
		F	20–75	38	16–81			
CO_2, mmol/L	Cresol red	M + F	23–29	26	23–31	27		
	Enzymatic oxidation	M + F	20–29	25			20–29	26
Complement C_3, g/L	Rate nephelometry	M + F	0.78–1.75	1.16	0.82–1.70	1.19	0.82–1.58	1.05
Complement C_4, mg/L	Rate nephelometry	M	120–540	260			120–350	210
		F	110–340	220			140–420	240
Copper, μg/L	AAS	M	700–1,400		860–1,730	1,330	750–1,840	1,390
		F	800–1,550		1,070–1,890	1,500	1,000–1,970	1,490
μmol/L		M	11.0–22.0		13.5–27.2	20.9	11.8–29.0	21.9
		F	12.6–24.4		16.8–29.7	23.6	15.7–31.0	23.5
Corticobinding globulin (transcortin), μg/L	RIA in dilute serum	M + F	23–39				12–29	
Corticotropin ng/L	RIA	M + F	0–100				10–106	40
pmol/L			0–22				2–23	9
Cortisol, μg/L	RIA, competitive binding	M + F	50–230	150	78–225	140	56–230	140
nmol/L			138–635	414	215–621	386	154–635	386
C-peptide μg/L	RIA, competitive binding	M + F	1.4–4.3	2.3	1.5–4.9	2.7	0.6–4.4	2.1
Creatinine serum, mg/L	Jaffe, rate	M	9–13	11	8–13	10	10–17	12
		F	6–11	9	6–12	8	6–13	9
μmol/L		M	80–115	97	71–115	88	88–150	106
		F	53–97	80	53–106	71	53–115	80
DHEA, μg/L	RIA after column chromatography	M + F	1.60–8.00				0.17–1.69	0.79
nmol/L			5.5–27.8				0.6–5.9	2.7
DHEAS, μg/L	RIA in dilute serum after hydrolysis	M	1,800–4,500				40–750	287
		F	1,200–3,150				20–600	231
μmol/L		M	4.9–12.2				0.1–2.0	0.8
		F	3.3–8.5				0.1–1.6	0.6
Estradiol, ng/L	RIA after column chromatography	F	Follicular: 30–100 Luteal: 70–300				<5–20	6
pmol/L			Follicular: 110–367 Luteal: 257–1,101				<18–73	22
Estrone, ng/L	RIA after column chromatography	F	Follicular: 30–100 Luteal: 90–160				<5–58	29
pmol/L			Follicular: 110–370 Luteal: 333–592				<18–215	107

(Continues)

Table 16-2 *(Continued)*

Analyte	Method	Sex	Young Adults Range	Young Adults Mean	60–90 Range	60–90 Mean	>90 Range	>90 Mean
Folate, serum μg/L	RIA, competitive binding	M F	3.2–12.4 3.2–15.9	7.0 7.7	1.6–10.8 1.8–12.2	5.2 5.7	3.3–16.0 3.0–16.0	7.8 8.8
nmol/L		M F	7–28 7–36	16 17	4–24 4–28	12 13	8–36 7–36	18 20
FSH, milli-int. units/L	RIA	M F	2.2–14.0 (Midcycle: 12–33)	6.5			8–112 66–168	53 111
γ-Globulin, g/L	Electrophoresis	M + F	6.0–14	9	6.0–16.0	10.0	5.0–16.0	10.0
Gastrin, ng/L	RIA, competitive binding	M + F	0–100		85%: <100 15%: 100–800		40–150	80
GGT, U/L	g-Glutamyl p-nitroanilide and glycylglycerine 37°C	M F	10–34 7–30	19 13	11–42 9–55	25 23		
	g-Glutamyl p-nitroanilide and glycylglycerine 30°C	M F	7–47 4–25	17 11			3–47 4–44	15 15
Glucose, mg/L	Hexokinase	M + F	780–1,050	920	820–1,150	950		
mmol/L			4.3–5.8	5.1	4.6–6.4	5.3		
mg/L	Glucose oxidase	M + F	740–1,060	890			750 1,210	960
mmol/L			4.1–5.9	4.9			4.2–6.7	5.3
HDL cholesterol, mg/L	Cholesterol oxidase after PEG precipitation	M F	200–690 (recommended 280–700) 270–850 (recommended 370–910)	420 530	280–1,060 280–1,040	480 630	280–820 320–830	450 525
mmol/L		M F	0.52–1.78 (recommended 0.72–1.81) 0.70–2.20 (recommended 0.96–2.35)	1.09 1.37	0.72–2.53 0.72–2.69	1.24 1.63	0.72–2.12 0.83–2.15	1.16 1.36
HDL cholesterol, %	Calculated	M F	9–43 (Low risk: >37) 14–54 (Low risk: >40)	23 31	11–40 12–45	22 26	13–45 14–43	25.5 26
Hemoglobin, g/L	Coulter counter	M F	140–180 120–160				121–171 107–151	140 131
Hematocrit, %	Coulter counter	M F	0.40–0.54 0.37–0.47				0.36–0.51 0.32–0.46	0.42 0.39
Heptaglobulin, g/L	Rate nephelometry	M + F	0.28–1.78	0.94	0.36–1.73	1.08	0.22–1.97	1.15
Iron, μg/L	Colorimetric, ICSH method	M F	600–1,700 450–1,600	920 970			400–1,290 350–1,330	870 860
μmol/L		M F	11–30 8–29	16 17			7–23 6–30	16 15
IgA, g/L	Rate nephelometry	M F	0.76–5.46 0.74–4.20	2.31 1.99			0.94–9.56 0.98–8.18	3.28 2.95
IgD, mg/L	Radial immunodiffusion	M + F	0–80				0–60	10
IgE, Roto-int. units/L	Two-site sandwich immunoassay	M + F	0.7–463	71.5			1.2–352	69

(Continues)

Table 16-2 *(Continued)*

			Young Adults		60–90		>90	
Analyte	**Method**	**Sex**	**Range**	**Mean**	**Range**	**Mean**	**Range**	**Mean**
IgG, g/L	Rate nephelometry	M	7.36–13.86	10.32			1.56–17.50	12.06
		F	6.95–16.70	11.00			3.88–18.85	12.00
IgG, urine mg/L	Fixed-time nephelometry	M + F	<8.0				5.0–38	8.0
IgM, g/L	Rate nephelometry	M	0.52–2.99	1.48			0.28–1.98	0.91
		F	0.46–3.90	1.69			0.42–2.90	1.05
Insulin, mU/L	RIA, competitive binding	M + F	6–23	11.8	6.6–36.7	16.4	2.4–19.0	7.2
pmol/L		M + F	43–165	85	47–263	118	17–136	52
K, mmol/L	Flame emission	M + F	3.8–4.9	4.3	3.9–5.3	4.5		
	Ion select, electrode	M + F	3.7–4.8	4.3			3.6–5.5	4.4
LD, U/L	L → P, colorimetric (AM Blue 610), 37°C	M + F	93–184	138			99–284	163
	Reduction of NADP, 30°C	M + F	48–102	69	55–104	76		
Lead, μg/L	AAS	M + F	<250				<150	
μmol/L			<1.21				<0.72	
LH, milli-int, units/L	RIA	M	2.5–19.7	8.9			19–115	53
		F	3.5–31.0 (midcycle: 48–175)	8			35–154	82
Lipase U/L	Turbidimetric, 30°C	M + F	13–141	63	0–302			
	Modified turbidimetric 30°C	M + F	31–186	82			26–267	104
Magnesium mg/L	AAS	M + F	16–25		16–24	20	17–23	20
mmol/L			0.66–1.03		0.66–0.79	0.82	0.70–0.95	0.82
Microsomal antibodies	Hemagglutination	M + F	Negative				6.9% positive	
Na, mmol/L	Flame emission	M + F	137–143	140	137–144	140		
	Ion select, electrode	M + F	138–144	141			132–146	141
Osmolality, serum mOsm/kg	Freezing-point depression	M + F	278–299	286	280–301	290	277–301	290
pH	Potentiometric	M + F	7.35–7.45		7.31–7.42	7.37	7.26–7.43	7.35
Phosphorus, mmol/L	Molybdenum blue	M	0.87–1.32	1.07	0.74–1.20	0.97	0.71–1.26	0.97
		F	0.84–1.29	1.07	0.90–1.29	1.10	0.81–1.36	1.10
Prealbumin mg/L	Rate nephelometry	M	200–400	280			150–300	220
		F	150–290	220			140–360	230
Progesterone, ng/L	RIA after selective solvent extraction	M	130–970				<200–480	
		F	Follicular: 150–700 Luteal: 2,000–25,000				<200–540	
nmol/L		M	0.4–3.1				<0.6–1.5	
		F	Follicular: 0.5–2.2 Luteal: 6.4–79.5				<0.6–1.7	
Prolactin, μg/L	IRMA	M	3.9–22.1	9.5			8–25	15.5
		F	3.5–27.0	11.5			7–53	18
Prostatic acid phosphatase, mg/L	Solid phase enzyme immunoassay	M + F	<2.0				0–3.2	0.7

(Continues)

Table 16-2 (*Continued*)

			Young Adults		60–90		>90	
Analyte	**Method**	**Sex**	**Range**	**Mean**	**Range**	**Mean**	**Range**	**Mean**
PTH, pmol/ng midmolecule	RIA, competitive binding	M + F	36–86	54			49–118	71
RBP, mg/L	Radial immunodiffusion	M	34–88	58			26–96	56
		F	25–81	45			31–91	52
Sex hormone-binding globulin, μg/L	Competitive binding assay	M	9–19				11–45	23
		F	10–30				11–60	26
T_3, μg/L	RIA	M + F	1.12–2.12	1.56	1.00–2.00	1.43		
nmol/L			1.7–3.3	2.4	1.5–3.1	2.2		
μg/L		M + F	1.02–2.05	1.52			0.70–1.66	1.13
nmol/L			1.6–3.1	2.3		1.1–2.5	1.7	
T_4, μg/L	RIA	M + F	50–120	81	50–107	78		
nmol/L			64–154	104	64–138	100		
μg/L		M	46–105	74				
		F	55–110	78				
nmol/L		M	59–135	95			53–100	74
		F	71–142	100			68–129	95
TBG, mg/L	Two-site IRMA	M + F	16–34	22.6			18–29	22
Testosterone, free, ng/L	Equilibrium dialysis	M	52–280				11.8–74.6	26.7
pmol/L			180.3–971.8				40.9–258.8	92.6
Testosterone, % free	Calculated	M	1.5–3.2				0.4–1.3	0.8
Testosterone, bioactive μg/L	Competitive binding assay of non-SHBG bound fraction	M	1.28–4.30				0.27–1.76	0.67
nmol/L			4.4–14.9				0.9–6.1	2.3
Testosterone, % bioactive	Calculated	M	36.6–41.7				10.0–33.7	20.2
		F	11.0–26.0				8.2–28.2	16.5
Testosterone, total, μg/L	RIA after column chromatography	M	3.50–10.30				2.15–6.71	3.40
nmol/L			12.1–35.7				7.5–23.3	11.9
Thyroglobulin antibodies	Hemagglutination	M + F	Negative				17.2% positive	
Total protein g/L	Biuret	M + F	63–78	70	62–77		60–80	
Transferrin, g/L	Rate nephelometry	M + F	2.57–4.29	3.22	1.91–3.75	2.73	1.86–3.47	2.64
Triglycerides, mg/L	GPO Trinder	M	410–1,930	1010	310–3,500	1250	770–1,110	940
		F	(recommended		350–1,750		780–1,840	
			400–1,600)	820	440–2,910	1090	430–1,440	1,090
			300–1,850		350–1,500		430–2,370	
			(recommended 350–1,350)					
mmol/L		M	0.46–2.18	1.14	0.35–3.95	1.41	0.87–1.25	1.06
		F	(recommended		0.40–1.98		0.77–2.08	
			0.45–1.81)	0.93	0.50–3.29	1.23	0.49–1.63	1.23
			0.34–2.09		0.40–1.70		0.49–2.68	
			(recommended 0.40–1.52)					
Trypsin, μg/L	RIA	M + F	11–55	28	16–76	38		

(*Continues*)

Table 16-2 *(Continued)*

			Young Adults		60–90		>90	
Analyte	**Method**	**Sex**	**Range**	**Mean**	**Range**	**Mean**	**Range**	**Mean**
nmol/L		M + F	0.5–2.3	1.2	0.8–3.2	1.5		
TSH, milli-int. units/L	RIA	M + F	1.8–8.8	4.7	2.1–15.5	5.2		
	Two-site IRMA	M + F	0.7–7.0	2.8			0.4–7.2	2.8
Urea nitrogen, serum, mg/L	o-Phthalaldehyde reaction	M + F	60–200	122	80–230	150	100–310	197
nmol/L			2.1–7.1	4.4	2.9–8.2	5.4	3.6–11.1	7.0
Uric acid, mg/L	Reduction of phosphotungstate	M	44–76	62	42–80	61	35–83	60.5
		F	23–66	43	35–73	51	22–77	0
μmol/L		M	262–452	369	250–476	363	208–494	357
		F	137–393	256	208–434	303	131–458	297
Vitamin B_{12}, ng/L	RIA, competitive binding	M + F	128–701	399	110–769	380	58–872	318
pmol/L			94–517	294	81–567	280	43–644	235
Zinc, μg/L	AAS	M + F	700–1,500		630–1,070	850	520–990	750
μmol/L			10.7–23.0		9.6–16.4	13.0	8.0–15.1	11.5

Abbreviations: ALT, alanine transaminase; AST, aspartate transaminase; CEA, carcinoembryonic antigen; AMP, adenosine monophosphate; Cl, chloride; CK, creatine kinase; DHEA, dehydroepiandrosterone; NADP, nicotinamide adenine nucleotide phosphate; subluxation; RIA, radioimmunoassay; FSH, follicle-stimulating hormone; CGT, cortisol glucose tolerance; HDL, high-density lipoprotein; PEG, polyethylene glycol; ICSH, interstitial cell-stimulating hormone; PTH, parathyroid hormone; RBP, retinol-binding protein; TBG, thyrone-binding globulin; IRMA, immunoradiometric assay.
(From Tietz et al.,[12] with permission.)

scriptions, and they may also be self-medicating with over-the-counter drugs, or taking drugs offered by friends.[36] Pharmacodynamics (what a drug does to the body) and pharmacokinetics (what the body does to the drug) in the elderly have been explored, but no clear answers are available as yet.

The elderly have an increased sensitivity to some drugs and decreased or unchanged response to others. Because of decreased functioning of organs, the elderly are considered less able to maintain homeostasis than are younger patients. Pharmacokinetics (drug liberation, absorption, distribution, metabolism, excretion) in the elderly requires therapeutic drug monitoring more frequently than in younger adults.[37] Decisions to maintain, decrease, or increase dosage depend upon whether there is evidence of adequate response to therapy as well as evidence of possible toxic effects.

Decision Levels

Some people see things as they are, and say "Why?" I dream of things that never were, and say, "Why not?"...

R. F. Kennedy

Reference ranges are what they are, not what should be achieved by intervention. The Report of the National Cholesterol Education Program (NCEP) Expert Panel[38] of the National Heart, Lung and Blood Institute established the following criteria for interpreting serum total cholesterol values: Levels below 200 mg/dl are classified as "desirable," those 200 to 239 mg/dl as "borderline high," and those 240 mg/dl and above as "high blood cholesterol." The report of the NCEP noted that 240 mg/dl corresponds to the 75th percentile of the adult US population; but clearly, it was the change in risk of coronary heart disease (CHD), not the distribution of the cholesterol in the total population (nor the reference range derived from that distribution) that determined the selection of 240 mg/dl as a critical point. However, other factors also have to be considered, such as the selective effect of survival[31] (survival of the fittest). Characteristics that confer poorer prognosis may be eliminated by earlier death and so be seen less often in old age. An evaluation of the relationship between serum cholesterol level and all-cause CHD, and non-CHD mortality as a function of age, found that contrary to clinical expectations the 5-year survival rate of 73 percent for 80-year-old men in the highest two subgroups of cholesterol level (cholesterol level greater than 6.21 mmol/l greater than 240 mg/dl) was better than the 49 percent for those in the two lower subgroups (cholesterol level, 6.21 mmol/l).[39] They concluded that at the present time there is no definitive basis for recommending lipid-lowering treatment in men and women above 65 to 70 years of age. A decision level is a threshold value above which or below which a particular management action is recommended.[40] Reference intervals are insufficient for this task. One cannot necessarily deduce a clinical decision simply on the basis of whether a lab result is outside a particular reference interval.[41] Recent directions in laboratory medicine[42] such as patient-specific predictive values to guide in interpreting serial results, outcome-based reference end points (such as 200 mg/dl cholesterol level), and dynamic interpretation of biochemical laboratory results, will add greatly to the clinician's ability to make appropriate decisions.

References

1. Solberg HE: Establishment and use of reference values. pp. 182–191. In Burtis CA, Ashwood ER, (eds): Tietz Fundamentals of Clinical Chemistry. 4th Ed. Saunders, Philadelphia, 1996
2. National Committee for Clinical Laboratory Standards: NCCLS Document C28-P. How to define, determine, and utilize reference intervals in the clinical laboratory (ISBN 1-56238-143-1). NCCLS, Villanova, PA, 1992
3. Ratliff RR, Casey AE, Thrasher GS: Automatic instrumentation for mass screening procedures in metabolic profile studies. pp. 321–325. In Automation in Analytical Chemistry (Technicon Symposia 1966). Mediad, New York, 1967
4. Allerhand J, McCarrick L, Eisler L: The biochemical profile of blood-donors and healthy employees by AutoAnalyzer. pp. 61–65. In Automation in Analytical Chemistry (Technicon Symposia 1967). Mediad, New York, 1968
5. Tolls RE, Werner M, Hultin JV: Sex and age dependence of seven serum constituents in a large ambulatory population. pp. 9–14. In Advances in automated analysis (Technicon International Congress 1969). Vol 111. Mediad, New York, 1970
6. Statland BE, Winkel P: Selected preanalytical sources of variations in reference values. pp. 127–137. In Grasbeck R, Alstrom T (eds): Reference Values in Laboratory Medicine. John Wiley, New York, 1981
7. Law R, Chalmers C: Medicines and elderly people: A general practice survey. BMJ 1976;I:565–568
8. Young DS: Effects of Preanalytical Variables on Clinical Laboratory Tests. AACC Press, Washington, 1993
9. Friedman RB, Young DS: Effects of Disease on Clinical Laboratory Tests. 2nd Ed. AACC Press, Washington, 1993
10. Deitrick JE, Whedom GD, Shorr E: Effect of immobilization upon various metabolic and physiologic functions of normal men. Am J Med 1948;4:3–36
11. Faulkner WR, Meites S (eds): Geriatric Clinical Chemistry. AACC Press, Washington, 1994
12. Tietz NW, Shuey DF, Wekstein DR: Laboratory values in fit aging individuals—sexagenerians through centenarians. Clin Chem 1992;1167–1185
13. Lott JA, Mitchell LC, Moeschberger ML, Sutherland DE: Effects of reference ranges: how many subjects are needed? Clin Chem 1992;38:648–650
14. Greenblatt DJ: Reduced serum albumin concentration in the elderly. A report from the Boston collaborative drug surveillance program. J Am Geriatr Soc 1979;27:20–22
15. Campion EW, deLabry LO, Glynn RJ: The effect of age on serum albumin in healthy males: report from the normative aging study. J Gerontol 1988;43:M18–20
16. Rowe DJF, Dawnay A, Watts GGF: Microalbuminuria in diabetes mellitus: review and recommendation for the measurement of albumin in urine. Ann Clin Biochem 1990;27:297–312
17. Fülöp T Jr, Vórum I, Varga P et al: Blood laboratory parameters of carefully selected healthy elderly people. Arch Gerontol 1989;8:151–163
18. Kelly A, Munan L, PetitClerc C: Patterns of change in selected serum chemical parameters of middle and later years. J Gerontol 1979;34:37–40
19. Chen FWK, Millard PH: The effect of aging on certain biochemical values. Mod Geriatr 1972;March:92–106
20. Garry PJ, Hunt WC, VanderJagt DJ, Rhyne RL: Clinical chemistry referenve intervals for healthy elderly subjects. Am J Clin Nutr 1989;50:1219–1230
21. Garry PJ, Hunt WC, Koehler KM et al: Longitudinal study of dietary intakes and plasma lipids in healthy elderly men and women. Am J Clin Nutr 1992;55:682–688
22. Dilman VM: Age-associated elevation of hypothalmic threshold to feedback control, and its role in development, aging, and disease. Lancet 1971;I:1211–1219
23. Schrier RW, (ed): Clinical internal medicine in the aged. WB Saunders, Philadelphia, 1982
24. Barzilai N, Stessman J, Cohen P et al: Glucoregulatory hormone influence on hepatic glucose production in the elderly. Age 1989;12:13–17
25. Modan M, Karasik A, Halkin H et al: Effect of past and concurrent body mass on prevalence of glucose intolerance and type 2 (non-insulin-dependent) diabetes and on insulin response. Diabetologia 1986;29:82–89
26. Bjorntop P, Berchtold P, Tibblin G: Insulin secretion in relation to adipose tissue in man. Diabetes 1971;20:65–70
27. Harman SM, Tsitouras PD: Reproductive hormones in aging men. 1. Measurement of sex steroids, basal luteinizing hormone and Leydig cell response to human chorionicgonadotropin. J Clin Endocr Metab 1980;51:35–40
28. Sowers JR, Felicetta JV (eds): Endocrinology of aging. Raven Press, New York, 1988
29. Oesterling JE, Jacobsen SJ, Chute CG et al: Serum prostate-specific antigen in community-based population of healthy men. JAMA 1993;270:860–864
30. Catalona WJ, Smith DS, Ratliff TL et al: Measurement of prostate specific antigen in serum as a screening test for prostate cancer. N Engl J Med 1991;324:1156–1161
31. Alvarez C, Orejas A, Gonzales S et al: Reference intervals for serum lipids, lipoproteins, and apolipoproteins in the elderly. Clin Chem 1984;30:404–406
32. Hodkinson HM: Reference values for biological data in older persons. pp. 725–727. In Evans JG, Williams TF (eds): Oxford Textbook of Geriatric Medicine. Oxford University Press, Oxford, 1992
33. Garry PJ, Hunt WC, VanderJagt DJ, Rhyne RL: Clinical chemistry reference intervals for healthy elderly subjects. Am J Clin Nutr 1989;50:1219–1230
34. Landahl S, Aurell M, Jagenburg R: Glumerular filtration rate at the age of 70 and 75. J Clin Exp Gerontol 1981;3:29–45
35. Chen FWK, Millard PH: The effect of aging on certain biochemical values. Mod Geriatr 1972;March:92–106
36. Warner A: Therapeutic drug monitoring in the elderly. pp. 134–144. In Faulkner WR, Meites S (eds): Geriatric Clinical Chemistry. AACC Press, Washington, 1994
37. Cooper JW: Reviewing geriatric concerns with commonly used drugs. Geriatrics 1989;44:79–86

38. National Cholesterol Education Program, Report of the NCEP Expert Panel on Detection, Evaluation, and Treatment of High Blood Cholesterol in Adults. Arch Intern Med 1988;148:36–39
39. Kronmal RA, Cain KC, Zhan Y, Omenn GS: Total cholesterol levels and mortality risk as a function of age. Arch Intern Med 1993;153:1063–1073
40. Barnett R: Medical significance of laboratory results. Am J Clin Pathol 1968;50:671–676
41. Statland BE: Clinical decision levels for lab tests. Medical Economics, Oradell, NJ, 1983
42. Harris KE, Boyd JC: Statistical bases of reference values in laboratory medicine. Marcel Dekker, New York, 1995

CHAPTER 17

Social Assessment of Geriatric Patients

ROSALIE A. KANE

Social functioning is a broad concept, embracing all human relationships and activities. Social functioning, therefore, is multidimensional and cannot be measured meaningfully in a single scale. Physicians caring for older people will need routinely to assess at least some aspects of the social functioning of their patients. In some instances, physicians will also need to understand and use assessments done by the social worker on their own hospital teams, by local authority social workers (in the United Kingdom), or by case managers in community long-term care programs (in the United States). For these purposes, it is useful to consider the nature of available assessment technology, the particular aspects of social functioning that should be assessed, and the usefulness of the information derived for the actual planning of care.

Social Assessment as Part of Comprehensive Assessment

Particularly in the United States, but also in other developed countries, frail elderly persons often receive their first general, multidimensional assessment from a social worker or nurse who is defined as a case manager or care coordinator.[1–4] Such assessments are typically performed in the patient's own home, but they may also be performed in the hospital prior to the patient's discharge. The assessor uses a structured information-gathering schedule (often contained in a rather long booklet) to pose questions directly to the older person or (if the older person is incapable of participating) to a surrogate informant. Such assessments can take 1 hour or more to complete. They do not involve a physical examination or laboratory tests.

Multidimensional assessment used by case managers will typically include the following components:

Factual information about the older person's marital status, household composition, housing situation, and income

Assessment of physical health based on some combination of the following checklist: symptoms; diseases the respondent believes he or she has; reports of overall utilization of hospitals, physicians, and other health care; reports of days sick; reports of medications used; summary of deficits in hearing, vision, speech, and dentition; and self-reported estimate of one's own health

Assessment of the ability to perform basic activities of daily living using a standardized scale. Such scales, at a minimum, measure independence in bathing, dressing, toileting, transferring out of bed or chair, and feeding, but may also include information about mobility, hand control, continence, and endurance

Ability to perform more complex social skills associated with independent living, sometimes called IADL (instrumental activities of daily living). Items that may or may not be scored on such a scale include cooking, cleaning, doing laundry, shopping, using transportation, communicating by telephone, managing money, and taking medications

Direct screening for cognitive impairment (to determine whether the respondent is reliable)

Direct assessment of depressive affect and other possible psychological disturbances

Assessment of the social functioning of the older person in terms of the range of activities and relationships that the person pursues, the help available to or used by him or her, the presence of a confidante, and, perhaps, the subjective satisfaction of the older person with social interactions

Enumeration of the help the older person is receiving from family members and friends, from social programs, and from privately-paid helpers directly employed by the older person and family.

Such batteries of questions are common in the United States, where they are in wide use in public programs. Many are derived from an assessment protocol developed at the Older Americans Research and Service (OARS) program at Duke University and commonly called the OARS methodology,[5] which has had extensive work done on its psychometric properties[6] and which has been extensively adapted. Another multidimensional tool that has had substantial work is the CARE (Comprehensive Assessment and Referral Evaluation) interview, developed by Gurland and colleagues[7] for a collaborative study done in the United States and the United Kingdom and later refined by the development of scales.[8–11] But the protocols in actual use for case management programs vary enormously in the way they combine questions and scales.

Some general points can be made about these multidimensional assessment tools and their use by social workers and case managers with geriatric patients.

1. The batteries usually attempt a descriptive overview of physical and psychiatric functioning, but make no claims

to diagnostic capability. Rather, in the context of an overall social assessment, the questions on physical and psychological health are designed to point out when fuller geriatric or psychogeriatric assessments should be sought. Thus, the presence of questions about health status, health utilization, and medications are designed not to encroach on physicians' diagnostic prerogatives, but to identify persons needing medical attention as well as to take medical conditions into account in planning care.

2. Scores may be derived for various subsections of the assessment, but the assessments seldom can generate an overall well-being score that has clinical significance.
3. Comprehensive assessment protocols vary in the extent to which the information is based on queries made directly to the older person versus judgements of the assessor on the enumerated items. Unless careful instruction and training accompanies the assessment instrument, it is likely that the resultant information will not distinguish well between the older person's responses and the assessor's judgements.
4. Functional abilities are at the heart of the assessment, but are difficult to standardize and interpret. Although substantial agreement has been achieved on items for inclusion on ADL and IADL scales, variations occur in detail and approach to measurement. Sometimes, for example, the information about functioning is based on observation and sometimes on the older person's report. Sometimes the individuals are queried about what activities they are able to perform, and sometimes about activities they actually do perform. Sometimes the score is based on demonstration under test conditions, and sometimes professionals rate performance based on their observations. Widely varying time frames may be used (e.g., the last few weeks, the last few months, right now). There is also variation in the standard for adequate performance and the extent to which pain and discomfort of the older person, or elapsed time to complete a task are taken into account. Recent work has been done to combine ADL and IADL items in a general scale. Rather than using the conventional but arbitrary system of according equal points for each item, Finch et al.[12] did empiric work to develop a scale where items are weighted according to their overall importance in functional capacity.
5. When used by case managers or social workers, the assessment protocol is meant to inform decisions about the services that should be arranged and the priority the particular older person's needs should get. However, there is seldom a clear set of rules to guide the assessor in translating the information from the assessment into guidelines for a service plan. Work in progress by Glass shows the intimate relationship between social factors and ADL functioning. Taking advantage of a data set where respondents were asked about functiong in terms both of what they thought they could do and what they did do, he identified "underachievers" who failed to perform to their perceived capacity and, oddly enough, "overachievers" who claimed to do what they believed they were incapable of doing. Further inspection showed remarkable resourcefulness and creativity among the overachievers, and a variety of social and psychological factors (lack of wish to do the function, lack of transportation, lack of opportunity, lack of money, family factors) among the underachievers.[13]

Aspects of Social Functioning

The multidimensional, comprehensive batteries described above are composed of constituent parts, designed to measure various aspects of functioning. The groundwork for measuring those dimensions is often laid in earlier research with the particular set of questions or scales. Let us now consider what aspects of social functioning should be measured.

All behavior of human beings might be termed social. But many aspects of social functioning hardly need be measured in detail for geriatric care. In a multivolume review of measures pertaining to old people, Mangen and Peterson[14] devote chapters to measurement of dimensions such as religiosity, interspousal relationships, and filial relationships. Relevant social dimensions for geriatric care constitute a shorter list, which has been summarized in a number of review works.[15,16] Below we suggest the information on social functioning that is needed, excluding health utilization and basic performance of ADL, which are important components but are covered elsewhere in this volume. Note, however, that ADL and IADL performance will be enhanced or impeded by social factors, and, conversely, social factors can influence the repercussions of ADL or IADL impairment. To deal with the latter, Allen and Mor[17] elaborated on functional measures by incorporating follow-up questions designed to assess any deleterious consequences of insufficient help (e.g., "Have there been times in the past month when you were not able to bathe as often as you would have liked because no one was available to help you?" or "Have there been times in the past month when you were unable to eat when you were hungry because no one was available to help you?"). They refer to these as indices of unmet need.

First, the *ability to perform social roles*, sometimes called social skills, is relevant. For younger people, such measures usually encompass their performance as employees, family members, and citizens.[18] For older people, perhaps shortsightedly, the measurement of role performance is usually limited to ability to perform the so-called instrumental ADL (cooking, cleaning, laundry), which are, in turn, related to household management and independent living.

Second, information about *social relationships* (their frequency, context, and quality), *social activities* (again their frequency, nature, and quality), *social resources* (including income, housing, and environmental conditions) is useful to geriatric providers. Third, *social support* is a salient concept to examine; it may include the help the patient is receiving and can expect to continue to receive from others in the environment, and the degree to which this help is perceived as supportive. Fourth, *subjective social well-being* can be measured more generally.

A fifth area of social function—*family burden* or family stress—has come into prominence in the last decade. Although highly relevant to geriatric care, this measure pertains to family caregivers rather than to the older person receiving the care. The idea is that an understanding of the type and degree of burden that caregiving creates for the relative primarily responsible will help determine whether the arrangement is realistic, humane, and fair, and the extent to which relief for the family member is necessary.

A sixth emerging area concerns personal autonomy, values, and preferences. In recent years, there has been much interest in *personal autonomy and values* of older persons receiving long-term care.[19,20] This is fueled by growing social science literature that suggests that older people who perceive that they have lost control and choice over their lives experience adverse health outcomes, including depression, increased morbidity, and even increased mortality.[21–23] Some attempts have been made to approximate a measure of autonomy, although these measures are not ordinarily incorporated into everyday clinical practice. A related effort entails assessing the values and preferences that may be important to geriatric patients.[24]

Finally, since this textbook was last published, substantial work has been done to seek a satisfactory approach to assessing the older person's *satisfaction* with the care and help received. Before briefly discussing each of these areas, some general comments about the problems of measuring social functioning are warranted.

Problems in Assessing Social Functioning

First, social concepts such as social isolation, social support, or social well-being are value and abstract constructs, subject to interpretation. Thus, several scales containing different items may purport to measure the same thing, whereas scales that seem to be similar in content carry different labels.[14] It is important not to be deceived by the name of the scale, and to examine its contents.

Second, most social variables have both an objective and a subjective component. For example, one can measure social support by quantifying the support network and its activities, or by asking whether the older persons view themselves as supported in various ways. Similarly, one can examine the burden of caregivers by quantifying their objective tasks with the patient and their other obligations, or one can measure the extent to which they feel burdened. Both approaches may be important.

Third, adequate social functioning can be achieved through diverse patterns. One seldom finds clear norms for interpreting the results of social information. A person who states that he or she has 10 friends is not necessarily twice as well befriended as a person with five, nor can one say that a person who spends much time playing cards is better off than one who spends the same amount of time fishing. Growing out of this observation are two important points in interpreting social information: (1) a change in social functioning may be as important as the actual value on a scale; and (2) information about adequate thresholds of functioning is needed. Regarding the latter, the objective of social measurements for geriatric caregivers is not to achieve a perfectly scaled measure of a social property such as isolation or social support, rather, it is to determine whether these dimensions have fallen below some threshold that means that the patient is at risk.

Fourth, social role expectations for the elderly are unclear at best and vary according to ethnic groups as well as over time. Nobody seems to know what constitutes adequate role performance for a retiree, a grandparent, or an elderly widow or widower, and establishing these norms is more complicated because of their likely sensitivity to cultural differences. Finally, much social functioning involves people in interaction with others. They fill social roles, cope with stress, receive help from family members, and so on. How well a particular older person functions socially is, in part, dependent on the behavior of others, which complicates the assessment process. Glass and colleagues[25] have recently been pioneering in expanding the range of social functioning examined in older people. In studies underway at Yale and later at Harvard, the team has attempted to develop better measures of social functioning related to productive aging in social and economic roles, incorporating housework, yardwork, child care, and other family roles, paid work, and volunteer work.

Social Relationships, Activities, and Resources

The aggregated social relationships of a client, viewed descriptively, are sometimes called the social network. Social network refers to the web of social relationships and contacts that an individual may have. Although difficult because of the amount of data collection needed, objective properties of social networks can be described using terms such as size (i.e., how many people are in the network), density (i.e., the number of people who know each other in the network), homogeneity (i.e., similarity of network members on various characteristics), multiplexity (the number of different types of interactions exchanged), and reciprocity (the balance or imbalance between perception of giving and receiving support).[26] Researchers point out that social network is a static concept referring to relationships across the lifespan; the term "social convoy" has been suggested as a more dynamic concept.[27]

Though social networks have properties, such as size, density, frequency and intensity of contact, permeability, and directionality,[28–30] from the viewpoint of geriatric care, the large number of properties that can be elaborated upon for social research can be reduced to an interest in the frequency and nature of the patient's human contacts in the course of a day, week, or month. One approach, often incorporated into assessment, involves querying the patient about the frequency of contacts in person, by telephone, or by mail by categories of people (adult children, other relatives, friends, others), using a metric such as "frequently, occasionally, seldom, or never," or attempting more exact quantification (less than once a week, and so on). Such questions are sometimes followed up by asking the older person whether he or she has contact with these people more than desired, about the right amount, or less than desired. The OARS methodology, a multidimensional assessment tool described above,[7] contains an often-used measure of social contacts.

Some efforts have been made to combine social contacts and social activities in brief social network scales, designed to predict the individual's well-being and need for service. The Berkman Social Network Scale,[31,32] developed in a general population, and the Lubben Social Network Scale,[33] developed for the elderly, are examples. Typically, marital status, membership in formal groups, and religious participation are added to other brief measures of social contact.

To assess social resources, well-planned, consistently-asked questions are better than scales. Each assessment of social functioning does well to contain straightforward questions about household income and assets, and income and assets of the older person with the disability. It is also important to determine the composition of the household and the nature and adequacy of the housing. In some social contexts, access to a car and transportation is also an important social resource. Depending on the political context, information about insurance coverage, veteran status, and specific disability status may provide a key to resources that could be available for the person. Other information that is important in developing a plan and coming to know the individual includes information about the individual's occupation or former occupation, and interests; typically such items are overlooked.

Social Support

A description of the social network does not automatically translate into an understanding of how well the patient's needs are met by those around him, nor does it permit a prediction of how well the needs may continue to be met in the future. Being enmeshed in a large network of family and friends may, depending on the network, be reassuring or stressful, helpful or harmful, informative or misleading. Social support is the positive tangible and intangible assistance drawn from the social network.[34] A social network or convoy has multiple functions, which also can be measured.[35] These include giving informational support, such as facts and advice; affective support, such as comfort, encouragement, and love; social support and stimulation, such as companionship; and tangible help, such as money or physical assistance. It is obvious that the geriatric team has an interest in knowing whether a given patient has a network that can or does provide such support. The social network is the potential vehicle for social support, but may be associated with negative as well as positive effects. Social scientists have studied the complex stress process that involves interaction of life events, chronic life strains, self-concepts, coping skills, and social supporters.[36] If the geriatric patient already has tangible needs for physical help from others, one measure of social support is a straightforward tabulation of the kinds of help received and their frequency. Assessment tools usually attempt, however, to go beyond this simple count to an estimation of the likelihood that the help can continue into the future, and the prospects for a replacement, if the person giving most of the help cannot continue. Research suggests that often the patient's social support in terms of physical help depends on one person whose own health may be fragile, or who cannot continue indefinitely because of competing demands.[37] In such cases, planning can begin to broaden the base of social support. In other instances, additional relatives and friends are available to help, but the primary family caregiver assumes that nobody else is capable or willing. If the patient has not previously needed physical help, then an estimation of the likelihood of this help is needed. A few key questions can assist in making this prediction, for example, "If necessary, is there someone who could come and help you during the day?" or "Is there someone who could stay overnight with you if necessary?"

Subjective Well-Being

An overall measure of the patient's well-being is sometimes sought in a comprehensive assessment tool. Such measures are also often used to evaluate the worth of long-term care programs.[38,39] The two most frequently used measures in this regard are Lawton's Philadelphia Geriatric Center Morale Scale[40] and the Life Satisfaction Index (LSI-A) of Neugarten, Havighurst, and Tobin.[41,42] Both these scales are relatively brief and simple to administer, both have developed an extensive use history, and both measure elements of life satisfaction by asking clients to consider the extent to which their expectations in life were met. At the same time, both also measure aspects of existential well-being or happiness.

Although these two scales are often used for program evaluation, it is unclear how much these measures should change as a result of a worthwhile program. For example, a meal program may be performing an important and appreciated function, and yet the answer to the question "Overall, have I achieved most of my goals in life?" would remain the same. In general, it seems best to measure satisfaction with a program directly, through questions that specifically ask about satisfaction with various elements of the program, as described below.[14]

Caregiver Burden

On both sides of the Atlantic, social services authorities for the elderly recognize that their programs would be inadequate to meet the needs for care were it not for the volunteered efforts of family members. Indeed, unpaid family members give most of the personal care and housekeeping help that is received by community-dwelling older people. In the United States, almost 80 percent of in-home services for the elderly are given by family members. It has become a widespread program principle that social services should supplement and enhance family care, when appropriate, but should not replace it.

Given this situation, it becomes important to assess the well-being of family caregivers to estimate (1) how long such care may be expected to continue, and (2) legitimate needs for relief. Somewhat unfortunately because of its negative connotations, this area of measurement is often called measurement of "family burden." Many scales have developed in the last decade to assess family caregiver burden.[43–47] These scales are often themselves multidimensional (including, for example, physical burden, emotional burden, social burden, and financial burden), and they may concentrate on subjective burden or objective burden, or both. Other scales designed especially to examine the stress-engendering aspects of family care for persons with dementia specifically measure the presence and frequency of a range of troublesome behavior.

Many reviews compare and contrast burden scales.[48] Pearlin and colleagues[49] have contributed a careful conceptual model of the stress process related to family caregiving, complete with brief measures of the relevant aspects of the phenomenon (including problematic behavior, overload, relational deprivation, family conflict, job-caregiving conflict, economic strain, role captivity, loss of self, caregiving competence, personal gain, management of situation, management of meaning, and management of distress). This series of measures is designed for research rather than clinical practice, yet it reminds us that the concept of caregiver burden is by no means straightforward. In general, it has been well documented that objective needs of the older person and objectively defined tasks occasion varying degrees of burden. The Caregiving Hassles Scale[50] can be used to measure the extent to which care of an elderly relative causes small daily tribulations or, in the vernacular, "hassles." Some authorities believe that the daily hassles produce more stress than dramatic life crises. Less attention has been given to the positive aspects of caregiving, sometimes called "uplifts," though these, too, have been measured and studied.[51]

The stress or burden of family caregivers, balanced against positive aspects of the role, should be part of a comprehensive assessment of an older person. However, the social worker or case manager must then be prepared to interpret and use the information to decide when and how much relief should be offered to family members. It is important also to understand the information collected according to the relationship of the family caregiver to the patient (spouse, adult offspring, other relative) and the competing obligations of that family caregiver (which could include employment, care of younger children, care of another disabled or elderly relative, or even dealing with their own failing strength).

In addition to applying specific measures that generate scores, clinical teams can benefit by consulting a practical reference work by Lustbader and Hooyman,[52] which lists sets of assessment questions that are useful for specific caregiving situations. For example, when a spouse is a caregiver, they suggest that one ask about the length of the marriage prior to the illness; the health of the caregiving spouse; the predisability marital patterns; the timing of onset relative to the couple's retirement plans; the impact of the illness on the couple's financial resources; the impact on their sexual functioning; and the availability of backup help from other family and friends. If siblings are sharing caregiving, the assessment might include these questions: Is concern about a potential inheritance straining sibling relationships? Is there financial disparity among siblings? Is there a natural leader, a parental favorite? Is there a health care professional among them? Are there step-siblings among them? What have been the adult siblings relationships to each other? And what obligations must each sibling meet in addition to parental care?

Personal Autonomy, Preferences, and Values

In the last decade in the United States, there has been an attempt to record older people's preferences regarding life-sustaining medical treatment.[53–56] Such information is desired partly for legal reasons, to prevent liability, and partly to guide clinicians in giving good care. If taken seriously, however, assessment of such preferences is notoriously difficult. The validity of the data depends on whether accurate information has been adequately disclosed to the respondent and has been understood by the respondent. Some work has been undertaken to construct and study such measures, though in practice many assessment batteries merely contain a notation of the older person's preference for such services as cardiopulmonary resuscitation, artificial hydration, or respirators, and their preferences about who they want to act in their stead if they become temporarily or permanently unable to make decisions—without any assurance that the questions were asked or comprehended in any consistent way.

Others have sought to assess values of geriatric patients directly, a pursuit that is fraught with conceptual and methodologic difficulties.[57] Using a tool that is meant to be an exercise in self-discovery rather than precise measurement, Gibson, a philosopher, and her colleagues[58,59] developed a Values History, which they recommend for distribution to clients to complete at leisure and with discussion among families. At the other extreme, Doukas and McCullough[60] have developed an approach that uses a few true-false questions to tap into values about risk, life and death, and spirituality.

At the University of Minnesota, work has been done to assess systematically the ordinary values and preferences of older people that might be related to their care. Although not amenable to generating an overall scale, it is feasible to incorporate a list of topics that the patient rates in terms of importance, providing descriptive detail. Using a stem that relates the topic to care that they might need now or in the future, the instrument developed asks the person to rate the importance of the following: performing everyday routines in a particular way; participating in certain activities at home or away from home; personal privacy; specific events or milestones being anticipated or projects being completed; freedom from pain; taking risks as opposed to being protected but less free; involving or not involving family in their care; qualities desired in a helper; and qualities desired in a place to live. Older clients were willing to respond to such questions, revealing differences in the importance these issues hold and in the content of what they deemed important. However, clinicians were often somewhat reluctant to enter into such discussions, partly because of the time involved (about 20 minutes) and partly because of a sense of being intrusive or being unable to act on the preferences expressed.[61]

Although considerable hubris is involved in attempting to assess values and preferences, and assessors doing so must guard against believing that they have encapsulated the essence of another human being in a few simple items, it seems equally improper to ignore this arena. In fact, systematic efforts to assess the patient's values and preference are likely to restructure the encounter between social workers and geriatric patients in important ways. Moreover, insights into the values and preferences of the older persons served may be the best safeguard against inappropriate or paternalistic decision-making about their lives.

Satisfaction

Although the technical quality of care procedures may be assessed by professionals using objective criteria, increasing emphasis has been given to seeking a reliable way to elicit the patient's perspective, particularly with reference to home help and personal assistance. It is argued that the intimacy of care and its close connections to daily life requires that professionals have a way of determining how patients view that care. Indeed, evidence suggests that older people are often reluctant to accept the help suggested, and speculation has been that this reaction is related to dislike of the way services are offered. Geron[62,63] conducted focus groups with older home care clientele from varying ethnic backgrounds to identify the elements of quality important to consumers. With great consistency across ethnicity, older people identified the following elements of good care: humaneness (helpers who were likable, pleasant, courteous, caring), competence, dependability, continuity (i.e., if the previous two criteria were met, consumers preferred consistency rather than change, adequacy in terms of amount of help, and choice in the type and timing of help received). A tool to measure this multidimensional construct is being tested and should be available in 1997.

Other Areas of Social Assessment

Other areas of social assessment are amenable to measurement and may be important in specific situations. These include, for example, the following:

- Measures of social functioning for people with dementia: A large number of such scales have been developed for rating or assessing the social functioning of persons with dementia in terms of presence of appropriate behavior and absence of behaviors considered disruptive.[64,65]
- Measures of housing environments and housing satisfaction: This is an underdeveloped arena.
- Specific assessments of social functioning within the context of a nursing home or board and care home: This area of assessment is in its infancy in terms of scale development or systematic attention, although elaborate measures of environmental climates have been made for research purposes.
- Assessment of formal support in the form of help from personnel from health care and social service organizations: Such a measure of assistance may or may not be thought of as part of the social assessment, but, however classified, it is necessary. It is often helpful to divide "formal care" into types of tasks: nursing tasks, such as help with medicines or procedures; personal care, such as help with bathing, toileting, eating, and transferring; housekeeping tasks, such as laundry, cooking, cleaning; help with transportation; help with business matters; and help with arranging for services, such as case management. Assessments usually develop indicators of frequency (days/visits per month, week, or day) and intensity (total hours of help of each type in a given period).
- Assessment of the specific tasks performed by family carers: Some assessment tools develop parallel questions to use in inquiring about the type of tasks and the frequency and intensity provided by both formal and informal sources. It is only by comparing formal and informal help received with needs for assistance, that an estimation of unmet need is developed. Typically, care plans developed by social workers are designed to meet unmet needs.

Assembling the Assessment Protocol

As this chapter has suggested, assessment of social functioning can be as detailed as the geriatric team desires, touching on many of few dimensions of social functioning. The assessment may also vary in its mix of scales, single items, clinical ratings, and reliance on open-ended, unstructured approaches. This chapter recommends a consistent and standardized approach to assessing aspects of social functioning. Commitment to consistency and routine approaches is probably more important than which particular instrument is selected. Initial parsimony is also suggested, followed by more detailed assessment as necessary. It is highly likely that there will be an inverse relationship between the amount of information collected and the reliability and validity of the assessment interview.

A social worker is highly accepted as a member of a geriatric team. However, the importance of social information—whether collected specifically by a social worker or collected by a generalist who is gathering information to be used by all professionals on the team—has been insufficiently appreciated.

References

1. Davis D, Challis D: Matching Resources to Need in Community Care: An Evaluated Demonstration of a Long-Term Care Model. Gower Publishing Company, Aldershot, Hampshire, 1987

2. Kane RA: Case management and assessment of the elderly. In Kane RL, Grimley Evans J, Macfadyen D (eds): Improving the Health of Older People: A World View. Oxford University Press, Oxford, 1990
3. Kane RL, Kane RA: A Will and a Way: What the United States Can Learn From Canada About Caring for the Aging. Columbia University Press, New York, 1986
4. Pelham AO, Clark WF (eds): Managing Home Care For the Elderly: Lessons From Community Based Agencies. DC Health, Lexington, Massachusetts, 1986
5. Fillenbaum GL: Multidimensional Functional Assessment of Older Adults: The Duke Older Americans Resources and Services Procedures. Lawrence Erlbaum Associates, Hillsdale, NJ, 1988
6. George LK, Fillenbaum GG: OARS methodology: a decade of experience in geriatric assessment. Geriatr Soc 1985;33: 607–615
7. Gurland BJ, Kuriansky L, Sharpe L et al: The Comprehensive Assessment and Referral Evaluation (CARE): rationale, development and reliability. Int J Ageing Dev 1978;8:9–42
8. Gurland BJ, Wilder DE: The CARE interview revisited: development of an efficient, systematic, clinical assessment. J Gerontol 1984;29:129–137
9. Golden RR, Teresi JA, Gurland BJ: Development of indicator scales for the Comprehensive Assessment and Referral Evaluation (CARE) Interview Schedule. J Gerontol 1984;29:138–146
10. Teresi JA, Golden RR, Gurland BJ et al: Construct validity of indicator scales developed for the Comprehensive Assessment and Referral Evaluation Interview Schedule. J Gerontol 1984; 29:147–157
11. Teresi JA, Golden RR, Gurland BJ: Concurrent and predictor validity of indicator scales developed for the Comprehensive Assessment and Referral Evaluation Interview Schedule. J Gerontol 1984;29:158–167
12. Finch M, Kane RL, and Philp I: Developing a new metric for ADLs. Am Geriatr Soc 1995;43:877–884
13. Glass, TA: Hypothetical vs. Enacted: Conjugating the Tenses of Function. (in press)
14. Mangen D, Peterson W (eds): Research instruments in social gerontology. Yols. I–III. University of Minnesota Press, Minneapolis, 1982
15. Kane RA, Kane RL: Assessing the elderly: a practical guide to measurement. DC Heath, Lexington, Massachusetts, 1981
16. Kane RA: Assessment of social functioning. Recommendations for comprehensive geriatric assessment. In Rubenstein LZ, Wieland D, Bernebei R (eds): Geriatric Assessment Technology: The State of the Art. Editrice Kurtis, Milan, Italy, 1995
17. Allen SM, Mor V: The prevalence and consequences of unmet needs: contrast between older and younger adults with disability. Med Care (in press)
18. Kane R, Kane RL, Arnold S: Measuring social functioning in mental health studies: concepts and instruments. U.S. Department of Health and Human Services, National Institute of Mental Health, Rockville, Maryland, 1985
19. Kane RA: Personal autonomy for residents in long-term care: concepts and measurement. In Birren J, Lubben JE, Rowe JC, Deutchman DE (eds): The Concept and Measurement of Quality of Life in the Frail Elderly. Academic Press, Inc, San Diego, California, 1991
20. Hofland B (ed): The Gerontologist 1988;28(suppl)
21. Avorn J, Langer E: Induced disability in nursing home patients: a controlled trial. J Am Geriatr Soc 1982;30:797–400
22. Langer E, Avorn J: Impact of psychosocial environment of the elderly on behavior and health outcomes. In Hess B, Markson E (eds): Growing old in America, 3rd Ed. Transition Books, New Brunswick, New Jersey, 1985
23. Rodin J: Aging and health: effects of the sense of control. Science 233:1271–1275
24. Kane RA: Decision making, care plans, and life plans in long-term care; can case managers take account of clients' values and preferences. In McCullough LB, Wilson NL (eds): Long-Term Care Decisions: Ethical and Conceptual Dimensions. The Johns Hopkins University Press, Baltimore, Maryland, 1995
25. Glass TA, Seeman TE, Herzog AR et al: 1995 Change in productive activity in late adulthood: MacArthur studies of successful aging. J Gerontol: Soc Sci 1995;50B:S65–S76
26. Sauer W, Coward R (eds): Social Support Networks and the Care of the Elderly: Theory, Research, Practice, and Policy. Springer Publishing, New York, 1985
27. Antonucci TC: Social supports and social relationships. In Binstock RH, George LK (eds): Handbook of Social Science and Aging 3rd Edn. Academic Press, San Diego, 1990
28. Kahn R: Aging & social support. In Riley MW (ed): Aging From Birth to Death. Westview, Boulder, Colorado, 1979
29. Antonucci TC, Depner CE: Social support and informal helping relationships. In Wills T (ed): Basic processes in helping relationships. Academic Press, New York, 1982
30. Mitchell R, Trickett E: Task force reports: social networks as mediators of social support. J Community Mental Health 1980; 16:274
31. Berkman LF: The assessment of social networks and social supports in the elderly. J Am Geriatr Soc 1983;31:743–749
32. Berkman LF, Syme SL: Social network, host resistance, and mortality: a nine-year follow-up study of Alameda Country residents. Am J Epidemiol 1982;116:12–140
33. Lubben JE: Assessing social networks among elderly populations. Community Health 1988;11:42–52
34. Gottlieb GH: Social support strategies: guidelines for mental health practice. Sage, Beverly Hills, California, 1983
35. Hirsch BF: Psychological dimensions of social networks: a multimethod analysis. Am J Community Psychol 1979;7:263–277
36. Pearlin LI, Menaghan EG, Lieberman MA et al: The stress process. J Health Soc Behav 1981;22:337–356
37. Kulys R, Tobin S: Older people and their responsible others. Social Work 1980;25:130–145
38. Stock WA, Okun MA, Benin M: Structure of subjective well-being among the elderly. Psychol Aging 1986;1:91–102
39. Larsen RJ, Diener E, Emmons RA: An evaluation of subjective well-being measures. Soc Indicators Res 1985;17:1–17
40. Lawton MP: The Philadelphia Geriatric Center Morale Scale: a revision. J Gerontol 1975;30:85–89
41. Neugarten BL, Havighurst RJ, Tobin SS: The measurement of life satisfaction. J Gerontol 1961;16:141–43

42. Liang J: Dimensions of the Life Satisfaction Index A: a structural formulation. J Gerontol 1984;39:613–622
43. Kosberg JI, Cairl RE, Keller DM: Components of burden: interventive implications. Gerontologist 1990;30:236–242
44. Montgomery RV, Stull DE, Borgatta EF: Measurement and the analysis of burden. Res Aging 1985;7:137–152
45. Robinson B: Validation of a caregiver strain index. J Gerontol 1983;38:344–348
46. Zarit SH, Reever KE, Bach-Peterson J: Relatives of the impaired elderly: correlates of feelings of burden. Gerontologist 1980;20:649–655
47. Zarit SH, Zarit JM: The memory and behavior problem checklist and burden interview. Pennsylvania State University, Technical Report, 1983
48. Vitaliano PP, Young HM, Russo H: Burden: a review of measures used among caregivers of individuals with dementia. Gerontologist 1995;31:67–75
49. Pearlin LI, Mullan JT, Semple SJ et al: Caregiving and the stress process: an overview of concepts and their measures. Gerontologist 1990;30:583–584
50. Kinney J, Stephens MAAP: Caregiving Hassles Scale: assessing the daily hassles of caring for a family member with dementia. Gerontologist 1989;29:328–332
51. Brody EM, Hoffman C, Kleban MH et al: Caregiving daughters and their local siblings: perceptions, strains, and interactions. Gerontologist 1989;29:529–538
52. Lustbader W, Hooyman N: Taking care of aging family members. Free Press, New York, 1994
53. Diamond EL, Jemigan JA, Moseley RA et al: Decision-making ability and advance directive preferences in nursing home patients and proxies. Gerontologist 1989;29:622–626
54. Henderson M: Beyond the living will. Gerontologist 1990;30: 480–485
55. Wetle T, Levkoff S, Cwikel J et al: Nursing home resident participation in medical decisions: perceptions and preferences. Gerontologist 1988;28(suppl):53–58
56. Zweibel NR, Cassel CK: Treatment choices at the end of life: a comparison of decisions by older patients and their physician-selected proxies, Gerontologist 1989;29:615–621
57. Froberg D, Kane RL: Methodology for measuring health stale preferences, I-IV. J of Clin Epidemiol 1989;42:345–354, 459–471, 485–592, 675–685
58. Gibson JM: Values history focusses on life and death decisions. Medical Ethics 1990;5:1–2,17
59. Gibson JM: Continuity of care and ethics. Continuing Care 1990;11–32
60. Doukas DJ, McCullough LB: The values history: the evaluation of the patient's values and advance directives. J Family Practice 1991;32:145–153
61. Degenholtz H, Kane RA, Kivnick HQ: Preference and values of elderly community-based clients about their care: can case managers learn what's important to clients. (in press)
62. Geron SM: Using measures of subjective well-being and client satisfaction in health assessments of older persons. Health Care in Later Life (in press)
63. Geron. SM: The dimensionality of frail older consumers' satisfaction with home care and case management services. (in press)
64. Teresi JA, Lawton MP, Ory M, Holmes D: Measurement issues in chronic care populations: dementia special care. Alzheimer Disease and Associated Disorders 1994;8:S144–S183
65. Cohen-Mansfield J: Reflections on the assessment of behavior in nursing home residents. Alzheimer Disease and Associated Disorders 1994;8(suppl):S217–S222

CHAPTER 18

Surgery and Anesthesia in Old Age

D. GWYN SEYMOUR

This chapter provides a general overview of surgery and anesthesia in old age, but lays particular stress on those areas of the subject that are changing most rapidly and/or that are attracting most clinical and research interest. After a brief introduction dealing with epidemiologic trends, the older surgical patient is evaluated from a predominantly medical viewpoint. It is not possible to go into details of anesthetic or surgical technique here, but these have recently been considered at length elsewhere.[1–3] The rehabilitation of the elderly orthopaedic patient, important though it is, is also not dealt with here, as it is discussed elsewhere in this textbook.

Trends in Surgery and Anesthesia in Old Age

The surgical treatment of older patients is not a late twentieth century invention. Of 100 cases of strangulated hernia operated on by van Assen in Amsterdam between 1903 and 1906, 18 were between 50 and 70 years of age, 17 were between 70 and 80 years, and 3 were over 80.[4] Inhalational anesthesia was used in one-third of the cases, with local anesthesia in the others. There were only two deaths, but one of these was in a patient aged 81.

In the last 20 years, however, the increase in surgical activity in patients aged 65 and over has been much greater than would have been expected from demographic trends alone.[5,6] This increase has not just been in life-saving procedures, but has also been seen in procedures such as cataract surgery or total hip replacement, which are predominantly aimed at increasing quality of life. Figure 18-1 looks at Scottish trends in hospital admission rates to the specialties of general surgery and ophthalmology over the last 15 years. In both specialties, but particularly in ophthalmology, there has been a dramatic increase in admission rates in the older age groups, while admission rates in younger groups have been static or have increased much more slowly. Note that the rising admission rates in the old, and particularly the very old, in Figure 18-1 are not due to demographic changes, as these have already been allowed for by expressing referral rates relative to 100,000 patients of comparable age and gender in the general population.

Surgery for cataract and total hip replacements for osteoarthritis are two prime examples of high-technology approaches to a surgical problem that have had a major impact on the quality of life of older patients. They neatly refute the simplistic assumption that high technology "cures" are for the young, and low technology "care" is for the old. As Grimley Evans puts it, "curing is caring."[7] In recent years, some of the increased surgical activity in young and old alike has been due to technologic advances such as minimally invasive surgery. These techniques have had a major impact in urology, gynecology, and increasingly in general surgery,[1–3,8] and it is important to ensure that older people benefit from these techniques as least as much as the young.

Some of the changes in surgical activity in different age groups have followed naturally from changes in the incidence or prevalence of disease.[6] Thus, with the development of effective medical antiulcer therapy, surgery for peptic ulceration has become much less common in the last 20 years. On the other hand, there has been a marked increase in the number of hip fractures, partly due to demographic change but probably due to underlying changes in osteoporosis prevalence as well.[9] In the field of orthopaedic surgery, this "epidemic" of hip fractures threatens to limit the amount of elective orthopaedic surgery that can be carried out, particularly in those orthopaedic units where emergency and elective cases are competing for the same theater space.

In an ideal world, we would first assess medical and surgical needs in the community and then provide the appropriate services and resources to meet those needs. Those interested in trying to assess epidemiologic needs for surgical and medical services, as a stimulus to more rational planning, are recommended to read a series of reviews edited by Stephens and Raftery.[10] In the context of the elderly surgical patient, the chapters on colorectal cancer, total hip replacement, total knee replacement, cataract surgery, hernia repair, varicose vein treatment, and prostatectomy are particularly relevant.

Age, Surgery, and Outcome

The association between age, surgery, and postoperative outcome is a complicated one.

1. Many surgically treatable diseases become more common with age; for example, the incidence of colorectal cancer increases almost exponentially after the age of 40, so that 41 percent of affected people are aged 75 and over, while only 5 percent are under 50.[11]

2. Age may have an effect on surgical presentation; for instance, an acute abdomen in some older people may have less dramatic signs and symptoms, and may be harder to diagnose at an early stage.[12]
3. Ageist attitudes or misconceptions of the true risks of modern surgery and anesthesia may influence patients and professionals in decisions as to whether elective surgical referral is indicated.[13]
4. The incidence of nonelective presentation of surgical disease tends to rise sharply with age,[14] probably from a mixture of the above factors.
5. Nonelective surgical procedures have much higher rates of morbidity and mortality than elective procedures.[14–16]
6. Older surgical patients often have one or more coexisting medical conditions.[17] When these involve major organs such as the heart or lungs, then the risks of surgery and anesthesia tend to increase.[14,18]
7. Even in the absence of coexisting medical disease, gerontologic studies point to a diminution in homeostatic reserve with age. Under conditions of extreme stress it might be expected that the fit elderly patient would have less chances of survival than the fit young patient. This appears to be the case for multiple trauma or extensive burns,[19–22] but it is also true that vigorous intensive therapy in elderly patients with burns and multiple trauma has led to improved survival rates and quality of life over the last two decades.[21–23]

How can all these effects be disentangled? A fair summary of the available evidence is that it appears to be age-associated illness rather than the aging process itself that is the main reason for the increase in morbidity and mortality following surgery and anesthesia in old age.[24,25] Lines of evidence to support this assertion include:

- The APACHE III system, which looks at risk factors predicting mortality in intensive care unit patients, has indicated that almost 50 percent of the variability in mortality is due to the intensity of the acute illness, whereas only 3 percent is due to chronologic age.[26]
- In general surgical patients studied by the author in Dundee and Cardiff, the rate of postoperative complications for those aged 65 to 74 was almost the same as that for those aged 75 and over, provided that no preoperative medical problems were present (Fig. 18-2). Similar conclusions have been reached by Dunlop and colleagues[27] in a group of general surgical patients (where medical status was stratified using the Medisgroups system) and by Shabot and Johnson[23] in a group of trauma patients (stratified by the Simplified Acute Physiology Score and the Injury Severity Score).
- Multivariate analyses relating several preoperative risk factors to postoperative outcome in elderly general surgical patients have not usually shown age to be a major independent predictor of postoperative outcome. Once major clinical factors (such as cardiovascular function or the presence of malignancy or sepsis) are entered into multivariate analyses, the predictive effect of age becomes less or disappears altogether.[28] At first sight, the logistic regression analyses of Pedersen et al,[29,30] relating preoperative status to postoperative outcome appear to contradict this statement, as the variable "age 70 and over" is associated with an odds ratios of 7.1 for postoperative cardiovascular complications, 5.6 for respiratory complications, and 9.0 for in-hospital mortality. However, this variable is expressed relative to patients aged

Figure 18-1 General Surgery and Ophthalmology Admissions to Scottish Hospitals, 1978–1993. (Data courtesy of the Information and Statistics Division, Chief Scientist Office, Edinburgh, Scotland.)

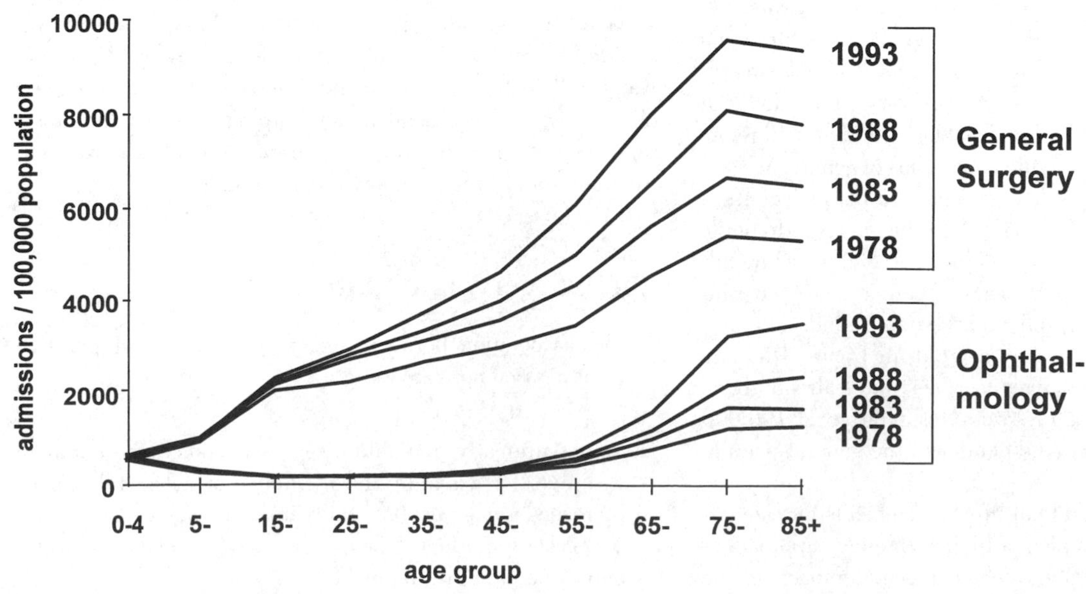

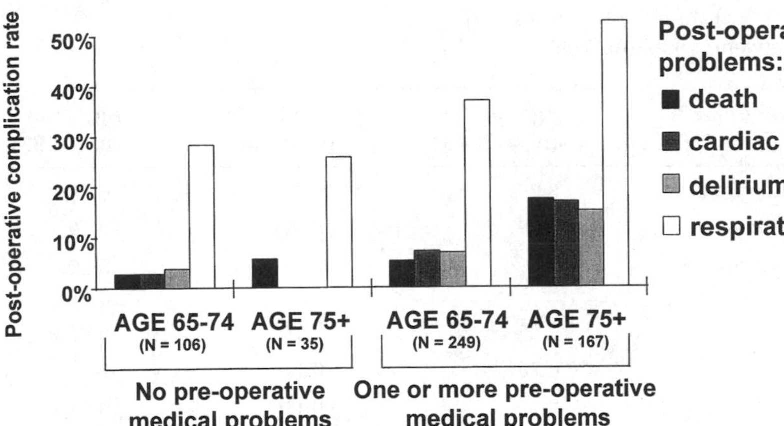

Figure 18-2 Age, preoperative medical status and postoperative outcome in general surgical patients aged 65 and over. (From Seymour,[13] with permission.)

between 20 and 49 years who are likely to have very little concomitant disease, and expressing the odds ratio relative to the age group 50 to 69 yields values of 2.0, 1.3, and 2.1. These are much lower than the odds ratios associated with major preoperative medical problems such as heart failure, ischemic heart disease, chronic lung disease, and renal failure.

Thus, attempts to set upper age limits for certain operations are suspect not simply from an ethical point of view, but are technically incompetent, because age by itself is such a poor predictor of adverse postoperative outcome in individual elderly people.[13,25,31] Each person with a surgical problem—whatever the age—needs and deserves an individual assessment. Moreover, it is important to realize that the aim of a preoperative assessment of an old person is identical to the aim of a preoperative assessment of a young person. In each case there is a need to estimate, on an individual basis, whether the potential benefits of operation outweigh the potential risks.

Anesthetic Factors

Morbidity and Mortality Following Anesthesia

In some elderly individuals, factors such as the extent and type of surgical pathology and the presence of serious coexistent medical disease may suggest that the potential risks of surgical intervention outweigh the potential benefits. Under such circumstances, in discussions with patient and relatives it is tempting to resort to the phrase that the patient is "not fit for an anesthetic." However, in fairness to our anesthetic colleagues and the published evidence, this temptation should be resisted, as postoperative deaths occurring solely because of anesthesia are very rare at any age. Reviewing a number of retrospective surveys, Pedersen[14] came up with an estimate of one death in 10,000 anesthetics. In his own prospective study of 7,306 consecutive anesthetics in patients of all ages studied between 1986 and 1987, one death in 2,500 was thought to be attributable to anesthesia, with about one-third of these being potentially preventable.[14]

The total in-hospital postoperative mortality in Pedersen's series was 1.2 percent (1:81), but it was difficult to judge whether or not anesthesia had contributed to individual deaths, many of which occurred in elderly patients having major surgery for malignant disease. Difficulties in attributing the relative contribution to postoperative mortality of multiple factors such as urgency of presentation, extent of medical and surgical pathology, age-changes, type of surgical procedure, and anesthetic technique is a constant problem in surgical audit, as the excellent and continuing series of reports from the National Confidential Enquiry into Post-Operative Deaths (NCEPOD)[32] has shown.

In Pedersen's[14] series of patients of all ages, complications directly attributable to anesthesia occurred in one patient in 170, whereas the overall rate of postoperative cardiopulmonary complications was as high as 1 in 11. Table 18-1 breaks down some of these data by age. Note that for complications directly attributable to anesthesia, there is no correlation with age. For problems not directly attributable to anesthesia, Table 18-1 indicates that in-hospital mortality and cardiorespiratory complications are rare below the age of 50, but that there is a steady increase in incidence of these postoperative problems for age groups 50 to 69, 70 to 79, and 80 and over.

Anesthetic Drugs in the Older Patient

Dodds[34] has described anesthesia as "applied clinical pharmacology with enough pathophysiology to confuse the picture." As both drug handling and pathophysiology are particularly variable in old age, the scope for "confusion of the picture" is greatly increased, particularly if pre-existing polypharmacy is present.

The recent review of anesthetic drugs in the elderly by Dodds[34] is recommended in its entirety as a concise guide to an enormous subject. However, nine key points from that review are highlighted here, with the permission of the author.

1. The minimum alveolar concentration (MAC) is that concentration of an anesthetic gas that suppresses movement in response to a surgical stimulus in 50 percent of subjects. MACs tend to fall with age: in one study, halothane had a

Table 18-1 Age and postoperative cardiopulmonary complications in a group of 7,306 Danish patients undergoing anesthesia between 1986 and 1987

	Age < 50 (n = 3965)	Age 50–69 (n = 2043)	Age 70–79 (n = 886)	Age ≥80 (n = 293)
All cardiovascular complications	2.6%	8.2%	14.3%	16.7%
All respiratory complications	2.3%	6.7%	8.9%	10.2%
Mortality in hospital	0.3%	1.8%	2.9%	5.8%
Complications attributable to anesthesia				
cardiovascular insufficiency	—	0.25%	0.45%	0.34%
cardiovascular problems after suxamethonium	0.03%	0.20%	0.11%	—
respiratory insufficiency	0.03%	—	0.11%	0.34%
regional anesthesia and brain dysfunction	0.10%	0.20%	0.11%	—
awareness under anesthesia	0.10%	0.20%	—	—
psychic decompensation after anesthesia	0.05%	—	—	—
miscellaneous (nerve palsy, oral trauma)	—	0.20%	0.11%	—
total	0.30%	1.03%	0.90%	0.68%

(Data from Pedersen[14] and Pedersen and Johansen.[33])

MAC of 1.08 percent in children but 0.64 percent at age 81.

2. With increasing age, there is a tendency to increased shunting in the lungs and decreased cardiac output. These pathophysiologic changes have complex effects on the uptake of volatile gases, as a low cardiac output favors rapid uptake, while a decreased lung function produces the opposite effect. Such effects are less with the more insoluble gases, which therefore tend to produce a more stable rate of induction.
3. Where there is pre-existing ischemic heart disease, the patient may be vulnerable to the cardiac depressant effects of some anesthetics. There is also a theoretic risk that isoflurane, enflurane, sevoflurane, and desflurane can "steal" blood from ischemic myocardium by increasing vasodilation in normal vessels.
4. Hepatic metabolism and/or clearance of drugs tends to be affected by age, but there is considerable variability. Insoluble anesthetic agents that require no hepatic metabolism should be safer than soluble agents. Some agents such as halothane also have potentially hepatoxic metabolites, and this agent may also produce a fall in protein synthesis.
5. Hepatic metabolism releases inorganic fluoride from some hydrocarbon anesthetics such as sevoflurane, and where blood fluoride levels exceed 50 μmol/L, nephrotoxicity can theoretically occur.
6. Because of reduced neuronal density and a reduced metabolic rate, the elderly may be more sensitive to a given amount of anesthetic drug. This raises the danger of overdosage. In patients with a delayed circulation time, there is increased potential for overdosage when intravenous agents are given too fast, as a delayed response may be mistaken for a lack of therapeutic effect, so that when the drug eventually reaches the brain, too much drug has been given. Smaller doses, slower rates of infusion, or repeated small boluses are recommended in the elderly.
7. Neuromuscular blocking agents can be classified into depolarizing types (of which suxamethonium is the only drug in common use), and nondepolarizing types. The nondepolarizing agents are usually favored in old age. Atracurium, vecuronium, and pancuronium are the nondepolarizing agents that have been most commonly used in general anesthetic practice, but atracurium has often been favored in the elderly because it is not dependent on renal and hepatic metabolism for its clearance.[35] Newer nondepolarizing agents such as mivacurium, rocuronium, and cisatracurium are now available, but there is less experience in the older patient.
8. The elderly appear to have an increased sensitivity to opiates, whether given as part of anesthesia or analgesia, and these agents may also predispose the patient to late postoperative hypoxemia, as is mentioned below.
9. Nonsteroidal anti-inflammatory agents (NSAIDs) are increasingly being used for analgesia in younger patients but may present increased hazards in the elderly because of nephotoxicity, fluid retention, and tendency to gastric irritation.

Respiratory Problems in the Older Surgical Patient

Incidence of Postoperative Respiratory Complications

Respiratory complications are common after surgery in elderly patients, and while the majority of such patients survive, deaths from respiratory causes still rank alongside cardiac and thromboembolic deaths as major potentially preventable causes of postoperative mortality.[14,18] The reported incidence of postoperative respiratory problems depends on the definitions used in individual research studies and on whether studies were prospective or retrospective.

In general surgical patients assessed prospectively in Cardiff using predefined clinical criteria, postoperative respiratory problems were found in 33 percent of those aged 65 to 74, and 50 percent of those aged 75 and over, but these percentages became 20 percent and 24 percent, respectively, when uncomplicated atelectasis was disregarded.[36] The risk of postoperative respiratory complications in these patients, all of whom were 65 years and over, was increased in the presence of clinical factors such as pre-existing lung disease, smoking, volume depletion, and incisions near the diaphragm.[37] In a logistic regression analysis of surgical patients of all ages, Pedersen et al.[38] found that age, major abdominal surgery, emergency operation, pre-existing chronic lung disease, prolonged anesthesia, and the presence of pancreatitis were all positively associated with an increased risk of postoperative respiratory problems.

Pathophysiology of Respiratory Problems in Older Surgical Patients

Lung abnormalities are common in older people even in the absence of smoking or known lung disease, although it is difficult to be sure how much of the abnormality of function is due to aging and how much to other factors such as recurrent respiratory infections or pollution.[39] Pulford and Connolly[39] have pointed to an increased closing volume (i.e., the lung volume at which basal airways begin to collapse) as one of the most consistent abnormal respiratory findings in old age. An increased closing volume appears to be important in the etiology of many postoperative respiratory complications, but the details of the pathophysiology are still being debated, not least because the accurate measurement of closing volume may be difficult in the anesthetized patient.[40]

Postoperative respiratory complications most commonly begin with basal atelectasis. Simple atelectasis may produce only minor signs and a low-grade hypoxemia but becomes clinically important when the lungs are already compromised and/or where the atelectasis develops into frank pneumonia. It should be noted that in the majority of postoperative patients, atelectasis is thought to be initiated not by retained secretions but by basal airway collapse.[18,40] A rise in closing volume or a fall in functional residual capacity favors airway collapse. Age is a risk factor for increased closing volume but in the surgical situation, incisions near the diaphragm, the supine posture, and postoperative sedation also play a part in causing the basal airways to collapse.[40] In addition, if anesthesia is given without periodic full inflation of the lungs (to mimic the spontaneous "sighs" that occur in the conscious patient about five to ten times an hour), atelectasis is more likely to occur.[40]

Implications of Research into Respiratory Pathophysiology

Classic methods of physiotherapy (which emphasize expiratory maneuvers and percussion) are unlikely to produce benefit in a patient in whom airway collapse rather than retained respiratory secretions is the initial event, and newer methods employ inspiratory maneuvers both before and after surgery. Devices such as incentive spirometers may be useful for encouraging deep inspiration,[41] and a systematic review of trials carried out between 1966 and 1992 concluded that incentive spirometry, intermittent positive pressure breathing, and deep breathing exercises were all more effective than no physical therapy in the prevention of pulmonary complications after upper abdominal surgery.[42] Classic "expiratory" methods of percussion and encouragement of coughing may have a role in those minority of cases where the retained secretions are the primary cause of respiratory complications, but if these techniques do not produce significant amounts of sputum, say 30 ml, then they may do more harm than good.[43]

Estimation of Respiratory Risk

In thoracic surgery, there is a large literature on the role of preoperative respiratory function testing as an aid to decision-making.[44–46] Research in thoracic surgery patients is continuing, but in recent years, researchers have also asked whether preoperative screening with respiratory function tests can help in the process of predicting postoperative complications in patients undergoing nonthoracic surgery.[47–51] The main conclusions so far have been that, in nonthoracic surgery, such tests must be interpreted along with clinical history and examination.[51] Future research reports will probably provide more precise guidelines, but in the meantime a pragmatic approach is suggested based on the current incomplete evidence (Table 18-2).

Late Postoperative Hypoxemia

In the early postoperative period, constant vigilance is needed to detect possible respiratory complications and/or hypoxemia, and the latter process has been greatly aided by the development of pulse oximeters (although the need for direct measurement of blood gases has not been removed entirely, as pulse oximeters indicate oxygen saturation rather than absolute oxygen tensions and give no indication as to carbon dioxide levels). Pulse oximeters have also had a major role in identifying a phenomenon, well known in anesthetic and surgical circles, for episodes of profound hypoxemia to develop 2, 3, 4, or even more days following surgery. The earliest research reports of prolonged hypoxia appeared over a decade ago,[53] and the basic underlying mechanisms are now reasonably well understood, although the conventional explanation offered here is probably an oversimplification.[40]

The classic clinical situation is that a patient who has had little or no hypoxemia for the first 1 or 2 postoperative days starts to develop episodes of profound hypoxemia (perhaps

Table 18-2 A pragmatic approach to perioperative pulmonary management

Several weeks before surgery:
Try to get patient to stop smoking (but 8 weeks abstinence is probably required).
Consider 2 weeks nutritional support in very malnourished patients (nutritional depletion may decrease respiratory muscle function).
In the very obese, weight reduction can improve arterial oxygen levels, but is of unproven clinical benefit to date.[52]
48 to 96 hours before elective surgery:
In patients with known lung disease consider drug therapy with bronchodilators, antibiotics if sputum is infected, and possibly corticosteroids.
Emphasize pre- and postoperative "inspiratory" physiotherapy techniques unless there is significant sputum (see text for details).
During anesthesia:
The use of warm humidified gases is logical as is the avoidance of very high oxygen concentrations.
The introduction of periodic full lung expansions should reduce atelectasis.
In the postoperative period:
In high-risk cases continue "inspiratory" physiotherapy into the postoperative period (but note that the most severe cases may require therapy every 1 to 2 hours while awake for 3 to 5 days).
Continuous positive airway pressure administered by mask may have a role.
Adequate analgesia, early removal of nasogastric tubes and early mobilization should be beneficial.
Be vigilant for signs of atelectasis or pneumonia. Pulse oximeters can be used to monitor for oxygen desaturations, but blood gases are required to monitor carbon dioxide levels and absolute arterial oxygen levels.
To reduce the risk of postoperative hypoxemia on the second to fourth postoperative night, consider giving prophylactic oxygen via nasal cannulae for 3 days and 5 nights postoperatively (see text for details).

(Adapted from Seymour et al.,[18] with permission.)

going below 60 percent saturation of oxygen), many times during the second, third, or fourth postoperative night. These desaturations often coincide with the presence of rapid eye movement (REM) sleep, which causes a disturbance of the respiratory mechanism similar to obstructive sleep apnea. The stress of surgery and, in particular, the use of opiates at the time of operation appear to suppress REM sleep for 2 or 3 days after major surgery, and it is when the REM sleep reappears that the episodes of desaturation occur.[54] Initially, the suppression of REM sleep was blamed entirely on opiates, but the phenomenon also occurs in patients who have not been given opiates.

Hypoxemia would be expected to cause arrhythmias and myocardial ischemia, particularly in patients with pre-existing heart disease, and it is tempting to conclude that some of the previously unexplained postoperative deaths around the third postoperative day were due to unrecognized hypoxemia.[55–58] However, it has been difficult to show a one-to-one relationship between episodes of hypoxemia and cardiac disturbance,[59] and other factors such as previous levels of hypoxemia and current carbon dioxide levels might be important as well. Hypoxemia might also have a detrimental effect on wound healing and cerebral function,[60,61] but again, there is need for further research in these areas.

The episodes of late hypoxemia can be prevented almost entirely by giving continuous oxygen by nasal cannulae for several days after surgery.[62] Common regimens are "three days and five nights." However, there are practical difficulties in identifying the patients who will be at risk from hypoxemia, and there is a balance to be struck between trying to monitor large numbers of patients with pulse oximeters and the alternative strategy of giving oxygen to a high proportion of patients even though some may not need it. Older patients, patients having major procedures, and those with respiratory disease would seem to be at increased risk of postoperative hypoxemia, but research is still continuing in this interesting area.

Cardiac Problems in the Elderly Surgical Patient

Incidence of Postoperative Cardiac Complications

Postoperative myocardial infarction has been reported after surgery in 1 to 4 percent of unselected general surgical patients aged 65 and over.[18] In unselected patients aged 75 and over, and in populations of patients with known ischemic heart disease, the incidence is at least twice as high. The association between increasing age and postoperative myocardial infarction is likely to be due in part to a secondary association between age and preoperative ischemic heart disease. Other risk factors that have been repeatedly reported to increase the chance of postoperative myocardial infarction include myocardial infarction within the last 6 months and active congestive cardiac failure.[63] A number of other factors have been highlighted by some studies including age, angina, hypertension, diabetes, arrhythmias, peripheral vascular disease, valvular heart disease, smoking, and previous cardiac surgery.[63]

Most surveys report that cardiac failure occurs more often than myocardial infarction, but that it is associated with similar preoperative risk factors.[63] More extensive electrocardiographic monitoring in the perioperative period has also revealed that many older patients have repeated episodes of subclinical myocardial ischemia that might be amenable to treatment. As mentioned above, some of these episodes might be precipitated by episodes of profound hypoxemia that are respiratory rather than cardiac in origin. This might help to explain why even the most sophisticated preoperative cardiac assessment cannot predict all adverse postoperative cardiac outcomes.

Diagnosis of myocardial infarction in the postoperative period may be difficult because the symptoms may be masked by analgesia or anesthesia, and the expected cardiac enzyme changes (such as a rise in creatine kinase) may be mimicked by surgical trauma to muscle. More specific enzyme tests are now becoming available, such as Troponin I and Troponin C, and these may have clinical as well as research value.[63,64] Once postoperative myocardial infarction has occurred, then the death rate has been reported to be as high as 50 percent.[14,18]

Cardiac Assessment of the Noncardiac Surgical Patient

It has been estimated that for every patient with known heart disease undergoing cardiac surgery, there are about 10 patients with (recognized or unrecognized) heart disease undergoing noncardiac surgery.[63] Many such patients are elderly. A large literature has therefore grown up on the "cardiac assessment of the noncardiac surgical patient."[65,66] Even though high-technology screening of cardiac and respiratory function might be able to predict many postoperative complications in such patients,[67,68] the large number of patients involved makes such a policy unfeasible. Apart from the practical and economic implications, there are also scientific objections to mass screening of patients with high-technology methods. Some of the cardiac tests are not without risk, and in addition, widespread preoperative cardiac screening in relatively low-risk patients would inevitably throw up large numbers of false positive results, which could result in the unnecessary postponement of much-needed surgery.

Are there strategies other than mass high-technology screening that would increase our chances of predicting postoperative cardiac complications? As Mangano[63] pointed out in his excellent review of the literature in 1990, the earliest research assessing cardiac risk in patients undergoing noncardiac surgery consisted of surveys in which risk factors were considered out one at a time (univariate analysis). Unfortunately, this type of data is difficult to use when more than one risk factor is present, and so Goldman and colleagues[69] in 1977 were pioneers in producing a multifactorial index of cardiac risk in general surgical patients aged 40 and over. This was refined by Detsky[70] in 1986.

The problem with any clinical risk index is that it tends to perform well on the data set from which it was constructed (i.e., the training data set) but usually performs less well on subsequent data sets (test data sets).[37] The original Goldman index was based on a training data set only, and subsequent attempts to validate it in other data sets have given rather variable results, particularly when more homogeneous subsets of patients such as those undergoing vascular surgery have been considered.[18] The modification of the index by Detsky in 1986 attempted to increase the predictive power of the index by taking into account the nature of the underlying surgical illness, but in a British context it is probably fair to say that indices of Goldman and Detsky are often quoted in reviews but as yet are rarely used in clinical practice.

The Goldman and Detsky indices are summarized in Table 18-3. This table gives an idea of the relative weights to be assigned to individual risk factors, but the type and extent of surgery being performed needs to be taken into account, and accuracy of prediction in individual patients (as opposed to groups of patients) may be disappointing. The potentials and limitations of cardiac risk predictors have recently been discussed by Goldman and Mangano,[65,66] and their two reviews are essential reading for those interested in risk prediction in general, and cardiac risk prediction in particular.

Table 18-3 Comparison of weightings in original cardiac risk index of Goldman and as subsequently modified by Detsky

	Points Allocated by Scoring System	
	Goldman[69]	**Detsky[70]**
Myocardial infarction within 6 months	10	10
Myocardial infarction more than 6 months		5
Canadian Cardiovascular Society angina		
class III		10
class IV		20
Unstable angina within 6 months		10
Alveolar pulmonary edema		
within one week		10
ever		5
S-3 or jugular venous distention	11	
Valvular disease		
suspected critical aortic stenosis		20
important aortic stenosis	3	
Arrhythmias		
rhythm other than sinus or sinus plus APBs on last preoperative ECG	7	5
more than five premature ventricular contractions at any time prior to surgery	7	5
Poor general medical status[a]	3	5
Age over 70	5	5
Emergency operation	4	10
Intraperitoneal, intrathoracic or aortic surgery	3	

Abbreviations: APB, atrial premature beat; ECG, electrocardiogram.

[a] *PaO_2 < 60 mmHg, $PaCO_2$ > 50 mmHg, K < 3.0 mEq/L; HCO_3 < 20 mEq/L, BUN > 50 mg/dl (18 mmol/L), creatinine > 3 mg/dl (260 mmol/L), abnormal SGOT, signs of chronic liver disease, bedridden from noncardiac causes.*

A Stepwise Approach to Cardiac Risk Prediction

The Goldman and Detsky indices might undergo a revival in interest because of modern tendencies to use them together with other more sophisticated methods of assessment. In the last 10 to 15 years, relatively noninvasive tests of cardiac function have become available in everyday medicine. These tests include include exercise stress testing, ambulatory electrocardiography, echocardiography (at rest, on exercise, and under influence of dobutamine), radionuclide ventriculography, and dipyridamole-thallium scanning. The role of these tests in predicting postoperative cardiac outcome has been extensively discussed, but the majority of the early investigations involved neither randomized controls nor observers who were blinded to the test results.

A consensus would now appear to be emerging[65,66] that the best strategy to employ when trying to predict cardiac risk in an individual patient is some sort of stepwise assessment. Thus, patients would initially be screened by simple clinical means, perhaps aided by one of the multifactorial indices. Patients judged to be at low risk would then proceed to surgery while higher risk patients would undergo further assessment by more sophisticated but noninvasive tests of cardiac function such as dipyridamole-thallium scanning, exercise testing, or ambulatory monitoring. These more sophisticated tests would give better delineation of cardiac risk and would suggest which patients could be operated on directly, which needed more invasive tests, and which would need prior intervention in the form of more intensive monitoring, or even surgical procedures on the coronary arteries.

Unfortunately, although the above stepwise strategy is theoretically sound, there is still considerable disagreement on the best sequence of testing and the optimal cutoff points of the various tests used to stratify patients. Mangano and Goldman[65] give some very useful interim recommendations, but the final recommendation of their authoritative review is that more randomized control trials are needed in this area.

Cardiac Surgery

Paradoxically, the prediction of risk in patients who are undergoing cardiac as opposed to noncardiac surgery is less of a problem, as most cardiac patients will have had sophisticated and invasive preoperative cardiac testing. Even more importantly, such patients are closely monitored postoperatively, usually in an intensive care unit. Under such circumstances, the mortality rate following cardiac surgery in patients aged 70 and over is of the order of 5 percent compared with a rate of about 2.5 percent in patients under 69.[71] Recent reports from Washington, D.C.[71] and from St. George's Hospital, London[72] have indicated that about one-quarter of cardiac surgical patients in both centers were currently over the age of 70. However, these are both teaching centers and there has been concern in Britain that referral practices and cardiac surgical rates in older patients are suboptimal.[73–75] Recent research has shown that the quality of life and functional improvement after cardiac surgery is at least as good for patients who are 70 or over as it is for those under 70.[76–78] Such studies add weight to the argument that cardiac procedures such as angioplasty, and operations such as coronary artery bypass grafting and aortic valve replacement should be more widely available in old people.

Nutrition

Undernutrition in middle-aged and elderly surgical patients is a subject of increasing research interest. Clinically, however, there remains concern in the United Kingdom that many medical students, doctors, and health workers are insufficiently trained in the field of nutritional assessment and therapy.[79]

Anthropometric methods of assessing nutrition that can be used in routine clinical practice are weight, height, body mass index (BMI) (weight in kilograms divided by the square of the height in meters), triceps skinfold thickness, mid-arm circumference, mid-arm muscle circumference, hand-grip strength, a history of weight loss, and measured weight change.[80] McWhirter and Pennington[80] point out that the BMI by itself is not a sensitive indicator of protein-energy malnutrition in adults, as it does not distinguish between depletion of fat or muscle. There are added problems in assessing BMI in older people, as some of them lose height as the result of osteoporosis. Some researchers substitute knee height or arm demispan for body height, but then, as for all the other anthropometric measurements, it is necessary to establish age- and sex-matched norms in a comparable general population.[80] Furthermore, in acutely ill surgical patients, even the measurement of body weight presents practical problems.

In addition to anthropometric measurements, clinicians may also measure serum proteins, and occasionally tests of immune function, but, as is discussed below, these can be affected by many surgical and medical problems in addition to protein depletion.

Prevalence of Malnutrition in Surgical Patients

Since the pioneering work of Bistrian and colleagues[81] in 1974, a popular study design in the field of surgical nutrition has been to take nutritional assessment methods that have been used in general population surveys and apply them to surgical patients in hospital.

Using this approach, Bistrian[81] concluded that one-half of all surgical patients were malnourished, and until recently, it was rare to find a publication in the field of surgical nutrition that did not begin with this statement. Although this statement had a stimulating effect on some clinicians, it caused a backlash among many practicing surgeons and physicians who simply could not believe that one-half of all their patients, of all ages and all surgical problems, were suffering from clinically important malnutrition.[82]

Recent reviews have tended to emphasize that severe (as opposed to moderate or mild) malnutrition is found in much less than 50 percent of the surgical population, and that it is on this severely malnourished group that our diagnostic and therapeutic efforts should be concentrated.[83,84] The evidence that led to this major re-evaluation of previous attitutes to surgical nutrition will now be briefly described.

Criticisms of Bistrian's 1974 estimates[81] of the prevalence of surgical malnutrition appeared as early as 1979. Gray and Gray[85] pointed out that the anthropometric norms used by Bistrian were not based on contemporaneous age- and sex-matched data from a comparable population. Even more importantly, the cutoff points were set as a simple percentage of the mean value rather than as a percentile or as a fixed number of standard deviations. This had bizarre effects, depending on the distribution and/or skewness of the parameter being considered. Thus, Gray and Gray calculated that over one-half of all young American women would be classified as malnourished on Bistrian's arm muscle circumference criteria, while one-half of all young American men would be classified as malnourished on the triceps skinfold criteria.[85]

Another criticism of Bistrian's nutritional criteria, albeit one that can be leveled at the majority of subsequent studies of surgical nutrition, is that the serum albumin was included as one of the nutritional parameters. In recent years, it has become clear that there are so many nonnutritional factors that can affect the serum albumin of an ill patient, that it should be regarded as a general index of illness severity rather than as an indicator of nutritional status.[82,86] For instance, in a surgical patient with a low serum albumin and an intra-abdominal abscess, it is more likely that the sepsis caused the low albumin than it is that malnutrition caused the sepsis.

However, the most fundamental criticism of the early surveys of malnutrition in hospitalized patients was made by McLaren.[86] He pointed out that much of the confusion in the literature on malnutrition in hospitals came about because concepts that had proved both informative and life-saving when applied to community surveys of malnourished children in developing countries, turned out to be misleading when applied to adult hospitalized patients in Europe and North America. One example offered by McLaren is that kwashiorkor is a very useful concept when assessing children in the Third World who have a protein deficiency in the presence of plentiful carbohydrate, but that this condition is very rare in adults in developed countries. In practice, almost all malnutrition seen in hospitalized adults is of the protein-energy-malnutrition (PEM) type.[86]

As many of the earlier nutritional assertions are now being questioned, what can be put in their place? From an evidence-based standpoint the main need is to move to properly control randomized studies whereby middle-aged and elderly surgical patients are (1) nutritionally assessed (taking into account the diagnostic difficulties noted above), (2) treatments are given, and (3) outcomes (in terms of morbidity, mortality, quality of life, and cost-effectiveness) are measured. The results of such studies are now starting to emerge.

Studies of Nutritional Supplementation in the Surgical Patient

To evaluate published research, however, it should be appreciated that performing nutrition studies in surgical patients is far from easy. Patients with the highest rates of preoperative malnutrition and postoperative morbidity tend to be elderly and/or emergency cases. The bedside nutritional evaluation of such patients is technically difficult. In addition, postoperative problems such as sepsis may have many causes, only some of which might be preventable by nutritional intervention. While in theory, a period of 2 weeks nutritional support might be advisable before surgery (see below), this is rarely practicable in emergency cases. An alternative experimental design has been to simplify data-gathering by excluding nonelective admissions, and by focusing on conditions such as gastrointestinal malignancy, where there is a strong likelihood of preoperative malnutrition.

The study of Bastow et al.[87] in 1983 is important both because of its findings, and because it addressed the difficult technical problem of nutritional assessment and therapy in patients with hip fractures. Almost all such patients are elderly, and so the study is of particular relevance here. Such patients present as emergencies and require urgent surgery, and so a prolonged period of preoperative nutritional therapy is not practicable. However, there is evidence that many such patients are malnourished and so Bastow and his colleagues set out to see if nasogastric feeding postoperatively had any benefits.

The study[87] had two key findings. First, postoperative nutritional support by the nasogastric route was shown to reduce postoperative morbidity rates and also appeared to reduce mortality rates (although the latter finding did not reach statistical significance). Second, the benefits of nutritional support were almost entirely confined to those with clear-cut malnutrition, (that is, those who were below the fifth percentile of nutritional status as judged by the primarily anthropometric methods used). A subsequent study by Delmi et al.[88] seemed to indicate that modern methods of oral feeding could be used to replace nasogastric feeding in hip fracture patients, but patient numbers were smaller, and the nutritional status of patients was not as clearly defined as it had been in the earlier Bastow study.[87]

The nutritional support of elective general surgical patients with proven or suspected nutritional deficiency has recently been explored by controlled trials.[84,89–94] The message from these studies is that when 10 to 14 days of preoperative therapy is possible in malnourished general surgical patients, then there are likely to be benefits in postoperative morbidity and possibly mortality. The benefits of shorter periods of nutritional support have been less easy to prove. Like the earlier work in hip fracture patients, the studies on general surgical patients also support the concept that it is the severely malnourished who need to be targeted—typically this has been the group of patients below the fifth percentile of whatever measurement technique was being used.[82–84,91]

The evidence that nutritional support is most likely to be of benefit when targeted on very malnourished patients is good news both for patients and health service managers. For instance, the recent study by McWhirter and Pennington,[80] indicated that 27 percent of general surgical patients, 39 percent of orthopaedic surgery patients, and 43 percent of medicine for the elderly patients were "undernourished." However, when only severe malnutrition was considered, the figures became 1 percent, 6 percent, and 19 percent, respectively, with moderate malnutrition being identified in 16 percent, 5 percent, and 20 percent.

Practical Treatment Strategies in the Malnourished Elderly Surgical Patient

From an academic standpoint, we might conclude that randomized control trials do not as yet permit the construction of detailed guidelines for nutritional assessment and support in elderly surgical patients. However, in the meantime, we need to do the best we can for our patients, and several lines of advice are available. A recent review by Rolandelli and Ullrich[95] has focused on the practical difficulties that can arise when assessing nutritional status in older surgical patients. Allison,[83] in a wide-ranging review of nutritional support in medical and surgical practice, points out that it is much easier to maintain physical and mental function by early feeding, that it is to regain function once it has been lost. His broad criteria for nutritional support are (1) weight loss of more than 10 percent and continuing, (2) continuing inadequate oral intake, and (3) the presence of disease whose known natural history is associated with likely accelerated weight loss and poor intake for 10 days or more. Guidelines from BAPEN and ASPEN (the British and American Societies for Parenteral and Enteral Nutrition) are published periodically and give detailed guidance on individual medical and surgical conditions.[79,96] On the organizational level, it is widely accepted that each major hospital needs a defined nutritional team to give advice and guidance on all aspects of nutritional support, but particularly where parenteral nutrition is contemplated.[79]

However, while further research evidence is awaited, a practical strategy for the bedside assessment of surgical patients has been devised by Windsor and Hill,[82,97,98] who are surgeons with an extensive experience in nutritional research. They have attempted to target nutritional therapy in surgical patients, by a structured clinical assessment together with basic anthropometric and laboratory tests. A summary of the methods that they advocate is shown in Table 18-4. The points to note from this table are that recent weight loss is probably of more importance than absolute body weight, and that where nutritional depletion appears to be affecting physiologic function (see Table 18-4 for definition), then there is more likely to be significant need for nutritional support than when physiologic function is not affected. The technique of Windsor and Hill is open to a degree of interobserver variation, and there may also be interpretational problems in older patients where physiologic impairment could well be due to coexistent disease rather than nutritional deficiences. However, until these questions are settled by further research, the practical benefits of the system far outweigh the disadvantages.

Table 18-4 Hill and Windsor's approach to nutritional assessment of surgical patients

The basic concepts
- Recent weight loss (in the last 3 months) is more important than earlier weight loss.
- Evidence of undernutrition together with significant impairment of function is more important than undernutrition alone.

The approach classifies patients into three groups
- Weight loss (in the last 3 months) less than 10% of body weight
- Weight loss of more than 10% of body weight, but no impairment of function
- Weight loss of more than 10% of body weight, and with impairment of function

A significant impairment in function is recorded when two or more of the following have coincided with the period of weight loss
- Reduction in activity level
- Reduction in skeletal muscle function (such as hand grip strength)
- Respiratory impairment (check respiratory effort and sound of coughing and dyspnea)
- Impaired wound healing (unhealed wounds, sores or scratches, and/or skin sepsis)
- Serum albumin less than 32 g/L
- Impaired psychological status (impaired mood, alertness, ability to concentrate, irritability)

Hill and Windsor found that only in group III patients were there statistically significant increases in postoperative pneumonia, septic complications, other major complications, and hospital stay. They recommend that nutritional support is concentrated on this group.

(Data from Windsor,[82] Hill,[97] and Windsor and Hill.[98])

Future Trends in Nutritional Support and Therapy

More fundamental laboratory-based research in the field of nutrition is also having an impact on clinical practice. At the cellular and molecular level, knowledge about the interactions of nutrition, immune function, stress response, and gene activation is growing rapidly.[99–103] This type of information has already led to clinical interest in the selective use of particular nutritional agents (such as glutamine, branched-chain amino acids, arginine, and omega-3 fatty acids) both as supplements and as pharmacologic agents to alter immune response.[83,100,101]

Obesity

The pathophysiology of obesity has been discussed by Bray,[104] who divides patients into five categories based on their BMI. Individuals who are not obese (class 0) have BMIs of 20 to 25 kg/m^2, while the BMIs of individuals in class I (low risk from obesity), II (moderate risk), III (high risk), and IV (very high risk) are 25 to 30, 30 to 35, 35 to 40 and greater than 40 kg/m^2 respectively. In reviewing the anesthetic risks of obesity, Wilson and Reilly[52] take 35 kg/m^2 or over as their definition, and have discussed the physiologic and anatomic changes that make the tasks of the anesthetist and surgeon more difficult. However, even in patients with severe obesity it has been difficult to demonstrate an increase in postoperative mortality; the main excess risk appears to be postoperative wound infections, with some studies also reporting an increase in thromboembolic complications.[52]

As Wilson and Reilly's review shows,[52] studies of postoperative outcome in mild or moderately obese patients are surprisingly uncommon in the literature. Garrow et al.[105] prospectively studied 469 patients undergoing abdominal surgery of whom 73 were classified as obese (taking a BMI of 27 or more in men and 30 or more in women so as to embrace the top 15 percent of BMIs in the population). The obese group had significantly more postoperative wound infections, but no differences were found in respect of deep venous thrombosis, pulmonary embolism, chest infections, urinary infections, and unexplained fever. Postoperative deaths (one in the obese group and six in the nonobese group) were too few for statistical analysis.

Garrow's series was not confined to the elderly, but in an earlier survey of general surgical patients aged 65 and over, patients above the 75th percentile of triceps thickness had twice the rate of postoperative wound infections, but no increase in postoperative chest infections or in-hospital mortality.[106] In a more recent study of elderly general surgical patients,[16] patients were classed as being underweight or overweight by simple visual inspection. It was the underweight patients who had the worst in-hospital mortality and 5-year mortality; patients classified as being overweight had a survival pattern that was identical with that of patients who were classified as normal (Seymour et al., unpublished observations). This is of interest, as there is evidence from a number of medical and population studies that, once a patient has achieved old age, it is being underweight rather than being overweight that is associated with the worse long-term survival.[107–109] There would seem to be a need for further research studies in older surgical patients, correlating both low and high body weight with postoperative outcome.

A retrospective study of perioperative morbidity following primary knee and hip replacement defined obesity as being 20 percent above ideal weight for height, based on life insurance tables. Of 154 patients 103 were classified as obese (joint replacement patients with osteoarthritis tend to be overweight, in contrast to hip fracture patients who tend to be underweight). While the obese patients had longer operative times, their stay in hospital, number of days with a fever, number of transfusions, and analgesic use were no different from the nonobese.[110]

Finally, in a retrospective study of 924 North American coronary artery bypass graft patients who were aged between 60 and 86, obesity was significantly related to a prolonged length of hospital stay, but was less important as a predictor than congestive cardiac failure, renal impairment, and being aged 75 years and over.[111]

Fluid and Electrolyte Imbalance In the Older Surgical Patient

The 1991–1992 National Confidential Enquiry Into Perioperative Deaths[32] stressed the critical importance of fluid balance in elderly surgical patients. However, the assessment and treatment of fluid and electrolyte disturbance in surgical patients is difficult, particularly in the case of emergency patients where the deficits are likely to be most severe. Guidelines are few and it may be simplistic to expect accurate guidelines ever to be produced in an area where there is inevitably so much variation in patient status. The sad news for the busy junior hospital doctor is that the best that can often be hoped for is to make an initial broad assessment of fluid and electrolyte needs, to start treatment on that basis, and to monitor progress constantly thereafter.

If guidelines are difficult to formulate for young surgical patients, then they are even more difficult to draw up for older patients; here, the increased prevalence of pre-existing renal disease and homeostatic impairment in the cardiovascular system and renal system[112] produces a need for tighter control, while at the same time the signs and symptoms of salt and/or water depletion are more difficult to interpret.[18,113]

Assessment of Fluid-Electrolyte Status

The standard surgical strategy when assessing perioperative fluid and electrolyte requirements in patients of any age is (1) to assess pre-existing deficits, (2) to estimate maintenance needs, and (3) to allow for continuing losses.[18,114]

The assessment of pre-existing fluid and electrolyte deficits is more difficult in older patients because many of the classical signs of water and salt depletion such as reduced skin turgor and postural hypotension are neither sensitive or specific in old age. For example, postural hypotension or lax skin tone may exist in elderly patients who are not volume-depleted, whereas a compensatory tachycardia may fail to develop in elderly people who are.[18,113,115] There is a need not just to examine the patient but to look at the whole clinical context over the previous few days. For instance, a patient who has been vomiting for 2 days is likely to be depleted both of salt and water even if the clinical signs are equivocal.

Water Depletion

Another of the basic principles of assessing electrolyte and fluid balance is to try to estimate the type of fluid that has been lost and to identify the main body compartment that has been affected. It is helpful to remember that losses predominantly of water have very different effects from losses of salt and water together.[18,114,115] When pure water depletion occurs, then the intracellular compartment is primarily affected, and the initial symptoms and signs are nonspecific, being drowsiness, irritability, and perhaps low grade fever.[18,113] In healthy younger patients, thirst is a reliable indicator of water depletion, but this may not be true in a proportion of healthy older patients,[112,115] and the symptom may in any case be impossible to elicit in acutely ill surgical patients. The main fact to remember about water depletion is that hypernatremia tends to develop, and Lye[116] has estimated that 90 percent of cases of hypernatremia in geriatric clinical practice are due to water depletion.

Salt and Saline Depletion

Loss of salt (or saline, as salt loss is usually associated with water loss as well) has its predominant effect on the extracellular compartment, which includes the vascular compartment.[8,114,115] Middle-aged patients with this type of depletion classically develop postural hypotension and tachycardia, but the presence or absence of these signs may be difficult to interpret in older patients where postural hypotension from other causes may occur in one-quarter of patients, and where autonomic reflexes are often blunted.[115]

The patient with severe salt (or saline) depletion will eventually develop circulatory collapse and poor peripheral circulation, but these are late signs. A low jugular venous pressure (obtained by lying the patient flat and observing the neck) is a test of volume depletion that is underused.[18] In severe cases, more invasive methods such as central venous pressure monitoring or the estimation of pulmonary artery pressure may be needed. Although noninvasive means of estimating pulmonary artery wedge pressure are being developed,[117,118] none have yet entered into routine medical practice. Whereas a high serum sodium can be used to diagnose water depletion, a low serum sodium is unfortunately not a good sign of salt depletion, as hyponatremia can occur in a variety of clinical conditions, including congestive cardiac failure, where total body stores of sodium tend to be high, and where intravenous administration of saline might lead to clinical disaster.

In a younger patient with salt and water depletion, the appropriate kidney response is to produce a urine that is concentrated and low in salt. If a young patient develops oliguria, and the urine has these features, then a "prerenal" deficit can be presumed and fluid challenge can be given. Where oliguria is not associated with such features, then permanent renal impairment is often inferred and caution is usually advised with fluids. In the older patient, where a degree of coincidental renal impairment is common, oliguria may develop primarily as a result of prerenal causes, but the urine may be misleading because the preexisting renal damage does not allow for salt and water conservation. Again, there is the need to take into account the whole clinical situation and not one set of biochemical results. If the clinical signs and history point to a likely volume depletion, then the correct course of action is to treat cautiously and monitor closely.

Defining Dehydration

In the discussion so far, the word "dehydration" has deliberately been avoided. Strictly this word should apply to water depletion on its own, and this is the way it is used by Levinsky.[119] However, in general usage, dehydration is often taken to mean a deficit of water or salt or both, and the classical signs of dehydration under this usage are actually signs of salt depletion such as postural hypotension. A recent useful review of salt and water depletion in elderly medical patients[115] appears to use the term dehydration in this more general sense. As has been argued above, the signs, symptoms, and treatment of salt depletion on the one hand, and water depletion on the other, are different. It is therefore unfortunate that the word dehydration is often used in a nonspecific sense to smudge both of these together. However, as the usage is so widespread, the best course of action is probably to avoid the word dehydration altogether and to try and specify the nature and amount of the fluid that has been lost, and which body compartment is primarily affected.

Practical Aspects of Fluid and Electrolyte Therapy

Some broad rules of thumb that may be useful in assessing and treating fluid/electrolyte disturbance in elderly surgical patients are as follows:

1. A water loss of 2 kg or more is probably significant in an older patient.[116]
2. In regard to younger adults, Shires and Canizaro[120] suggest that a saline loss of 4 percent of the body weight is "mild," 6 to 8 percent is "moderate," and 10 percent is "severe." Elderly patients are not specifically mentioned, but are probably at more risk from a given percentage of saline depletion, because of their more limited homeostatic reserve.
3. It has been estimated that, in the younger surgical patient, 4 L of saline are lost before signs of depletion appear, and 4 L of saline are gained before edema develops.[121] There appear to be no comparable estimates for older patients.
4. The recommended rate of fluid administration depends on the type of fluid that has been lost.
   a. In cases of water depletion, rapid replacement may be hazardous, as cerebral edema can result. Van Zee and Lowry[114] recommended that only one-half of the calculated water deficit should be administered over the first day, with the remainder being replaced over the next 1 to 2 days. Water repletion can be achieved by 5 percent dextrose infusions intravenously or subcutaneously. Water by oral or nasogastric route is an alternative.
   b. In cases of volume depletion, rapid replacement is usually desirable. In young patients with severe volume depletion, Shires and Canizaro[120] recommend an initial infusion rate of 2 L/hour, but state that this rate should be halved as soon as signs of improvement appear. Even then, when rates of infusion are above 1 L/hour, they recommend that a physician be in constant attendance. For older patients with severe volume depletion, Shires and Canizaro point out that the benefits of rapid repletion may be partly offset by the risks of fluid overload, and they state that monitoring by central venous line or a pulmonary artery catheter is desirable.

Central Nervous System

Postoperative Stroke

Postoperative stroke is a relatively rare complication following general surgery, although the incidence rises with age, being around 1 percent in the over-65 and 3 percent in the over-80 age group. However, as is discussed below, procedures on the carotid arteries and coronary artery bypass procedures, carry a higher risk than general surgical procedures. In the case of carotid endarterectomy for symptomatic stenosis, the balance of risks and benefits has been worked out in two recent controlled clinical trials, but the place of surgery in asymptomatic stenosis is still a matter for debate.[122–124]

The risk of stroke after open heart surgery appears to be falling but still remains higher than that for general surgery.[125] The improvement in outcome in cardiac bypass patients has usually been attributed to better techniques of extracorporeal circulation, but two recent studies of postoperative cardiac patients have claimed that the main risk of postoperative stroke is to be found in a small subset of patients with pre-existing cerebrovascular or carotid disease.[126,127] If these findings are confirmed, preventive strategies targeted on this subset of patients might show clinical benefit.

Postoperative Delirium

Postoperative mental impairment following surgery has been a topic of interest for many years. A proportion of patients develop postoperative delirium. This has an incidence of 10 to 40 percent depending on the type of operation, on the exact definition of delirium employed, and on whether the study was prospective or retrospective.[36,128] Many of the precipitants of delirium in the postoperative situation are the same as those causing delirium in the medical patient[129] and include acute illness (particularly infection), the effects of drugs, and withdrawal from alcohol or psychoactive drugs such as tranquilizers. However, delirium following surgery may also be due to premedication (especially with anticholinergics), anesthetic drugs, associated surgical complications, and episodes of late hypoxemia. Diagnosis of the cause of delirium may also be more difficult postoperatively. For instance, delirium tremens developing postoperatively in an emergency surgical patient who has been unwilling or unable to give a history of heavy alcohol intake prior to admission may be attributed to "surgical" causes.

A painstaking prospective study of the risk factors for postoperative delirium has recently been carried out[130] and has pointed to an age of 70 or over; self-reported alcohol abuse; poor cognitive status; poor functional status; markedly abnormal preoperative sodium, potassium or glucose; noncardiac thoracic surgery; and aortic aneurysm surgery as independent predictors of delirium. While it is sometimes stated that delirium is less common after regional as opposed to general anesthesia, in a large randomized controlled study of patients undergoing elective total knee replacement, Williams-Russo and colleagues[131] found no statistical difference between the incidence of postoperative delirium in patients following general anesthesia (12/128 or 9.4 percent) and that following epidural anesthesia (16/134 or 12 percent).

Although it is good practice to try to minimize risk factors that might cause delirium in older surgical patients, and minimal use of premedication in older surgical patients is one way of doing this, the main clinical requirement is probably to recognize delirium when it occurs and to treat the cause vigorously.

Postoperative Dementia

The more difficult question involving postoperative mental status is whether dementia ever occurs as a primary event following surgery and anesthesia. There has been argument about this in the literature for many years following two pioneering studies that attempted to identify patients who had "never been the same since their operation."[132,133] Since that time the search has been out for patients who had an apparently uneventful surgery and anesthesia but who suffered mental impairment thereafter. Many of the early studies in this area were uncontrolled and did not have a baseline mental assessment measurement.[134] Some were also associated with emergency surgical procedures where a number of factors such as hypotension or sepsis might have had a permanent effect on cerebral function that was not directly due to surgery or the anesthetic process.[134]

In recent years there have been attempts to carry out properly controlled trials, usually evaluating different techniques of anesthesia, with detailed psychological testing before and after surgery.[134] The problem with such trials is that the need to make precise preoperative psychological assessments tends to limit them to elective patients who are undergoing anesthesia under carefully controlled conditions and so the risk of postoperative complications of any type is likely to be small. Such formal trials have not demonstrated that anesthesia, whether general or regional, has a permanent effect on mental functioning. For instance, in the study of Jones et al.,[135] objective tests of cognitive function were not statistically significantly different before surgery and 3 months afterward, although there was a group of 21 out of the 129 patients who reported some subjective changes. It is not clear whether these patients had real but subtle changes in cognitive function that could not be picked up by the standard tests, or whether they had other conditions such as depression or postoperative fatigue that were not primary dementing processes. A subsequent prospective randomized study of local versus general anesthesia for cataract surgery in patients aged 65 to 98 years found no cognitive decline at 3 months after surgery, and no difference between the two anesthetic groups.[136]

Finally, in the largest study to date, Williams-Russo and colleagues found no long-term (6-month) difference in mental functioning between elderly patients undergoing elective orthopaedic surgery under regional anesthesia and those undergoing general anesthesia.[137] However, the cognitive function of 12 out of the 231 patients (7/114 of those having an epidural anesthetic and 5/117 having a general anesthetic) was worse at 6 months than it had been preoperatively. In the absence of long-term follow-up information of nonoperative patients using the same cognitive assessment protocols, it is difficult to assess whether or not a decline of this amount would have occured even in the absence of surgery.

This research area is still being explored but, at present, it is fair to advise elderly surgical patients that elective surgery under controlled conditions is unlikely to lead to a permanent memory problem, although a transient delirium is relatively common.

Postoperative sepsis

Wound sepsis is a common cause of postoperative morbidity, and large scale studies involving older patients have suggested that the incidence goes up with age. This might be due to subtle changes in immune function, but more prosaic explanations such as the tendency for older people to undergo more operations on the gastrointestinal tract and to present with more advanced surgical disease are probably more important. More serious sepsis such as intra-abdominal sepsis or widespread septicemia with multiorgan failure remains a major cause of postoperative mortality at all ages but particularly in the elderly. The pathophysiology of such states are complex[138] and mortality rates remain high despite intensive therapy.[139]

The concept of giving single doses of antibiotics to prevent postoperative sepsis has developed in recent years and is mentioned briefly here as it appears to run counter to normal antibiotic practice. Animal work over two decades ago[140,141] showed that sepsis in a wound or operative site was often initiated at the time of the first incision, and that this could be prevented if high levels of antibiotics were in the blood at that precise time. A single dose of an intravenous antibiotic given one-half hour before surgery is often sufficient to achieve this benefit, although subsequent doses are sometimes given during prolonged procedures. Antibiotic prophylaxis of this type is indicated where the risk of infection is high (such as in operations involving the gastrointestinal tract) or in situations where the risk of infection is low but the consequences of infection would be disastrous (such as in joint replacement surgery).[141] Where there is an established infection prior to surgery, such as in the case of a ruptured abscess, then full antibiotic courses need to be given and this should be distinguished from prophylactic antibiotic use. In practical terms, the administration of prophylactic antibiotics is usually in the hands of the surgical team, and there is a need to comply with local guidelines, particularly as antibiotic sensitivities can differ from place to place.

The area of antibiotic prophylaxis more familiar to the physician is that needed to prevent the development of bacterial endocarditis when a patient with a pre-existing heart valve lesion undergoes a procedure such as dental therapy, which might cause a transient bacteremia. The scope of this type of therapy has recently been extended to encompass surgical procedures on the urinary and biliary tract and also some procedures on the upper and lower bowel.[141] Again, there is a need to consult locally agreed guidelines.

Postoperative thromboembolism

Pulmonary embolism is difficult to diagnose clinically, particularly in the postoperative period, and its true incidence is almost certainly underestimated in older patients. In 1979, before prophylaxis was widely used, Palmberg and Hirsjarvi[142] reported that the postoperative death rate from pulmonary embolism in general patients aged 70 and over was 3 percent, accounting for one-third of the total postoperative mortality in their series.

The risk factors for thromboembolism in surgical patients are similar to those in medical patients and include presence of malignancy, age, and prolonged periods of immobility. The additional factor in surgical patients is that the surgical procedure itself may initiate the process of venous thrombosis.[18] For example, in general surgical patients, the period of calf flaccidity during general anesthesia may be enough to start off a process of thrombosis that can then spread proximally. In surgical operations involving the hip or pelvis there is danger of direct trauma to pelvic veins, which can cause thrombosis and subsequent pulmonary embolism. In the former situation, a dose of heparin, which would be insufficient to treat thrombosis once it develops, appears effective in preventing a large proportion of venous thrombosis.[18] This is the rationale for low-dose prophylactic subcutaneous heparin use prior to many general surgical procedures, the typical dose being 5,000 U twice a day until the patient is mobile.

More difficult decisions arise in the case of pelvic surgery or orthopaedic surgery. Here the risk of thrombosis is higher and may be more than subcutaneous heparin can deal with, but the risk of hemorrhage is also increased. Various regimens have attempted to either supplement low doses of heparin with other physical interventions, or to look at higher doses of anticoagulants, or to look at alternative antithrombotic methods.[143] As in the case of antibiotic prophylaxis, it is highly desirable to comply with local guidelines when prescribing prophylaxis for thromboembolism in surgical patients.

Surgical and Anesthetic Audit

Audit is a process that has been well established for many years among surgeons and anesthetists, and physicians have much to learn from their colleagues in these specialties. A major advance in Britain has been the establishment of a National Confidential Enquiry into Perioperative Deaths (NCEPOD) and the regular reports arising from this source are well worth reading.[32] These reports give illustrative case reports of situations where deaths of individual surgical patients might have been avoided, and as around two-thirds of all the deaths reported occur in patients over the age of 70, they are particularly relevant to the present discussion. Recurrent themes over the years have been the necessity for nonelective patients to be treated in units with appropriate facilities and by staff with the appropriate levels of experience. In some of the individual case reports, potentially preventable factors have included a lack of medical stabilization of patients prior to surgery. It must be acknowledged, however, that this is a difficult judgment to make, as excessive delay before surgery is also associated with increased complication rates in many conditions, including hip fractures.

As well as looking at the medical circumstances of individual cases, audits such as NCEPOD have also stressed the importance of having appropriate structures in place to deal with high risk groups such as the elderly emergency surgical patient. These structures involve the availability of adequate numbers of trained staff, the provision of high dependency units and intensive care beds, and the ready availability of operating theaters.[32] Less easy to define, but probably as important is the whole style and atmosphere of an individual surgical service. This is likely to involve its degree of cooperation with medical specialists including geriatricians in the preoperative period, the postoperative period, and during any rehabilitation that is necessary.

The establishment of audit, the general acceptance of well-designed guidelines for patient management, and thinking of an "evidence-based" type are all examples of general measures that are likely to improve postoperative outcome of all elderly surgical patients, but it may be difficult to prove the benefit of any individual intervention. This approach is complementary to the more usually discussed method of reducing risk in operative patients, which is to target high risk patients prior to surgery and to put in maximal effort at this point. It is becoming clear, however, that perfect targeting of patients is unlikely ever to be achieved and that a combined approach involving selective targeting, peri- and postoperative monitoring and close attention to the general environment, structure, and interprofessional links of the surgical service are all important.[25] A wider look at the subject might also consider the process of referral in the first place, and would also examine the attitudes of society to high-technology treatment in old age.[7,13,144] It is arguable, for instance, that if more older patients were referred at an earlier stage for surgery, then some emergencies could be avoided with a likely reduction in morbidity and mortality. While such approaches might have benefit, they need to be proven by controlled trials before they are introduced.

Quality of Life Measurement in the Elderly Surgical Patient

Surgeons and anesthetists have traditionally recorded deaths and surgical complications in the postoperative period as their only outcome measures. In so doing, they have given the lead to their physician colleagues, who have usually collected no outcome measures of any type. However, all groups of clinicians have realized in recent years that there is a need to look at the wider impact of treatment on a patient's ability to pursue those activities in life that are important to him or her. The exact definition of "health-related quality of life" is difficult, and, as McDowell and Newell[145] have pointed out, it is common for the terms "general health status measures" and "measures of health-related quality of life" to be used interchangeably. However, the aspects usually included in quality of life assessments are physical function and mobility, cognitive function, self-care, emotional status, sensory function, and pain.[146]

There is increasing interest in measuring health-related quality of life in surgical patients,[147,148] and studies are starting to have an impact on attitudes to surgery in old age. The measurement of quality of life after cardiac surgery[76–78] has supported the argument that more cardiac operations should be carried out in older people. Similarly, the decision whether or not to have a total hip replacement depends crucially on the ability of the surgery to reduce pain and increase activity, and thus to allow patients to pursue those activities in life that are most important to them.[149] Follow-up studies from intensive care units have started to consider qualititative aspects of outcome as well as simple survival.[146] Again, these studies seem to favor the more widespread use of intensive care for treatment of older people, as well as showing that age by itself has very little to do with the survival process.[146]

Questionnaires designed to measure health-related quality of life fall into three categories.

1. *Disease-specific measures*. These are designed to look at one particular surgical or medical problem. Thus, a questionnaire to look at patients following varicose vein surgery would be very different from that used to evaluate patients being treated for osteoarthritis.[150]
2. *Generic measures*. The second approach is to use more generic questionnaires such as the Sickness Impact Profile, the Short-Form-36 Health Survey, or the Nottingham Health Profile, which include questions about a wide range of physical, social, and mental function.[145] The advantages of generic questionnaires are that they allow different conditions to be compared in different populations, and that they are likely to have been well validated. The main disadvantage is that many of the questions may be of limited relevance for a specific clinical problem. For instance, questions on mobility are more relevant after hip replacement than after breast surgery. In practice, it is common for both disease-specific and generic scales to be used in individual surgical studies, as they tend to give complementary information.[149,151]
3. *Patient-specific measures*. A third approach to measuring Quality of Life in individual patients is to allow that individual to nominate those areas of life that are most important to him or her and then to devise a tailor-made scale to see how these areas change after therapy. These types of techniques are only in their infancy but include the MACTAR (The McMaster-Toronto Arthritis Patient Preference Disability Questionnaire),[152] the SEIQoL (schedule for the evaluation of individual quality of life),[153] and the PGI (Patient Generated Index).[154] To date, these scales have mainly been applied in the fields of orthopaedics and rheumatology, but they could easily be extended to other surgical situations.

Future Trends in Surgery and Anesthesia in Old Age

Factors Increasing the Number of Surgical Procedures in Old Age

It is highly likely that the technical developments in surgery and anesthesia that have occurred in the last two decades will continue in the future and will allow potentially beneficial surgery to be extended to ever older and frailer patients. Such developments are also likely to lead to more favorable attitudes to surgery in old age, so that more patients will be referred. Even if attitudes and techniques were not to change, demographic changes would lead to an increase in surgery in the old and the very old in the next two decades.

Factors Decreasing Surgical Procedures in Old Age

It is to be hoped that preventive medicine or novel forms of medical therapy will reduce the need for surgical intervention in some conditions in the future. This has already been seen in regard to modern medical therapy for peptic ulceration. An increase in minimally invasive techniques might also lead to a reduction in the number of major surgical operations being performed. For instance, gallbladder surgery is increasingly being performed by laparoscopic techniques rather than via a laparotomy.[8]

A reduction in surgical activity in some conditions because of better medical therapies or the substitution of less invasive procedures is obviously to be applauded. Much more sinister, however, is the tendency for politicians and health planners to contemplate that some forms of potentially beneficial surgery should be rationed on the basis of age, even though there is very poor evidence that age has any significant effect on the ability of a patient to benefit from a given surgical procedure.

If elderly patients are denied surgery simply on the basis of age, this is by definition ageist and such practices need to be challenged vigorously.[13,31] However, more subtle forms of discrimination may occur because of reduced equity of access of older people to medical and surgical services, and a Medical Research Council Review has concluded that "research is needed to examine the extent of differences in access to the NHS according to age group."[155] While detection of inequity of access is difficult for both medical and surgical conditions, the research is technically simpler in the surgical situation, as interventions and end points tend to be more clearly defined. Preliminary investigations by the author suggests that inequity of access for surgical patients on the basis of age does exist, but that this interacts with inequity based on patient deprivation.[13] Age-related inequity on the basis of age is probably decreasing with time, but inequity on the basis of deprivation category may be more resistant to change.[156]

References

1. Crosby DL, Rees GAD, Seymour DG (eds): The Ageing Surgical Patient: Anaesthetic, Operative and Medical Management. John Wiley & Sons, Chichester, 1992
2. Zenilman ME, Roslyn JJ (eds): Surgery in the elderly patient I. Surg Clin North Am 1994;74:1–221
3. Zenilman ME, Roslyn JJ (eds): Surgery in the elderly patient II. Surg Clin North Am 1994;74:223–495
4. Van Assen, quoted by Coley WB. Hernia. p.587. In Keen WW (ed): Surgery: Its Principles and Practice. WB Saunders, Philadelphia, 1913
5. Seymour DG: Surgery in the older patient. Geriatr Med 1994; 24:39–43
6. Seymour DG: Future trends. pp. 417–427. In Crosby DL, Rees GAD, Seymour DG (eds): The Ageing Surgical Patient: Anaesthetic, Operative and Medical Management. Wiley, London, 1992
7. Evans JG: Curing is caring. Age Ageing 1989;18:217–218
8. Fried GM, Clas D, Meakins JL. Minimally invasive surgery in the elderly patient. Surg Clin North Am 1994;74:375–387
9. Royal College of Physicians: Fractured neck of femur, prevention and management. J Roy Coll Phys Lond 1989;23:8–12
10. Stevens A, Raftery J (eds): Health Care Needs Assessment. The Epidemiologically Based Needs Assessment Reviews. Vols 1 and 2. Radcliffe Medical Press, Oxford, 1994
11. Mountney L, Sanderson H, Harris J: Colorectal cancer. pp. 379–410. In Stevens A, Raftery J (eds): Health care needs assessment. The epidemiologically based needs assessment review. Radcliffe Medical Press, Oxford, 1994
12. De Dombal FT: Acute abdominal pain in the elderly patient. pp. 161–171. In: Diagnosis of Acute Abdominal Pain, 2nd Ed. Churchill Livingstone, Edinburgh, 1991
13. Seymour DG: Ageing and ageism: a medical and surgical perspective. Aberdeen University Review 1996;195:344–359
14. Pedersen T: Complications and death following anaesthesia. A prospective study with special reference to the influence of patient-, anaesthesia-, and surgery-related risk factors. Danish Med Bull 1994;41:319–331
15. Le Néel J-C, Guiberteau B, Borde L et al: Prise en charge des patients âgés de plus de 75 ans presentant une pathologie digestive ou abdominale. A propos de 660 observations. Chirurgie 1993–1994;119:143–147
16. Edwards AE, Seymour DG, McCarthy JM, Crumplin MKH: A five year survival study of general surgical patients aged 65 years and over. Anaesthesia 1996;51:3–10
17. Arvidsson S, Ouchterlony J, Nilsson S et al: The Gothenburg study of perioperative risk. I. Pre-operative findings, post-operative complications. Acta Anaesth Scand 1994;38:679–690
18. Seymour DG, Rees GAD, Crosby DL: Introduction and general principles. pp. 1–90. In Crosby DL, Rees GAD, Seymour DG (eds): The Ageing Surgical Patient: Anaesthetic, Operative and Medical Management. John Wiley & Sons, Chichester, 1992
19. Day RJ, Vinen J, Hewitt-Falls E: Major trauma outcomes in the elderly. Med J Aust 1994;160:675–8
20. Smith DL, Cairns BA, Ramadan F et al: Effect of inhalation injury, burn size, and age on mortality: a study of 1447 consecutive burn patients. J Trauma 1994;37:655–9
21. Herruzo-Cabrera R, Fernandez-Arjona M, Garcia-Torres V et al: Mortality evolution study of burn patients in a critical care burn unit between 1971 and 1991. Burns 1995:21;106–9

22. Zoch G, Schemper M, Kyral E, Meissl G: Comparison of prognostic indices for burns and assessment of their accuracy. Burns 1992;18:109–12
23. Shabot MM, Johnson CL: Outcome from critical care in the "oldest old" trauma patients. J Trauma 1995;39:254–260
24. Lubin MF: Is age a risk factor for surgery? Med Clin North Am 1993;77:327–335
25. Seymour DG: The aging surgical patient—a selective review of areas of recent clinical and research interest. Rev Clin Gerontol 1993;3:231–244
26. Knaus WA, Wagner DP, Draper EA et al: The APACHE III prognostic system. Risk prediction of hospital mortality for critically ill hospitalized adults. Chest 1991;100:1619–36
27. Dunlop WE, Rosenblood L, Lawrason L et al: Effects of age and severity of illness on outcome and length of stay in geriatric surgical patients. Am J Surg 1993;165:577–80
28. Seymour DG: Prediction of Risk in the Elderly Surgical Patient. MD Thesis, University of Birmingham. Birmingham, England, 1988
29. Pedersen T, Eliasen K, Henriksen E: A prospective study of risk factors and cardiopulmonary complications associated with anaesthesia and surgery: risk indicators of cardiopulmonary morbidity. Acta Anaesthesiol Scand 1990;34:144–155
30. Pedersen T, Eliasen K, Henriksen E: A prospective study of mortality associated with anaesthesia and surgery: risk indicators of mortality in hospital. Acta Anaesthesiol Scand 1990; 34:176–182
31. Evans JG: This patient or that patient? pp. 118–124. In: Rationing in Action. BMJ Publishing Group, London, 1993
32. NCEPOD reports, available from The Administrator, National Confidential Enquiry into Peri-Operative Deaths, 35–43 Lincoln's Inn Fields, London WC2A 3PN
33. Pedersen T, Johansen SH: Serious morbidity attributable to anaesthesia. Considerations for prevention. Anaesthesia 1989; 44:504–8
34. Dodds C: Anaesthetic drugs in the elderly. Pharmacol Ther 1995;66:369–386
35. Slavov V, Khalil M, Merle JC et al: Comparison of duration of neuromuscular blocking effect of atracurium and vecuronium in young and elderly patients. Br J Anaesthesia 1995; 74:709–711
36. Seymour DG, Vaz FG: A prospective study of elderly general surgical patients II. Post-operative complications. Age Ageing 1989;18:315–26
37. Seymour DG, Green M, Vaz FG: Making better decisions: the construction of clinical scoring systems using the Spiegelhalter and Knill-Jones approach. BMJ 1990;300:223–6
38. Pedersen T, Viby-Mogensen J, Ringsted C: Anaesthetic practice and postoperative pulmonary complications. Acta Anaesthesiol Scand 1992;36:812–818
39. Pulford EC, Connolly MJ: Respiratory disease in old age. Rev Clin Gerontol 1996;6:21–39
40. Jones JC, Sapsford DJ, Wheatley RG: Postoperative hypoxaemia: mechanisms and time course. Anaesthesia 1990;45: 566–73
41. Hall JC, Tarala R, Harris J et al: Incentive spirometry versus routine chest physiotherapy for prevention of pulmonary complications after abdominal surgery. Lancet 1991;337:953–6
42. Thomas JA, McIntosh JM: Are incentive spirometry, intermittent positive pressure breathing, and deep breathing exercises effective in the prevention of pulmonary complications after upper abdominal surgery? A systematic overview and meta-analysis. Physical Therapy 1994;74:3–16
43. Murray JF: The ketchup bottle method. N Engl J Med 1979; 300:1155–7
44. Epstein SK, Faling LJ, Daly BD, Celli BR: Predicting complications after pulmonary resection. Preoperative exercise testing vs a multifactorial cardiopulmonary risk index. Chest 1993;104:694–700
45. Bolliger CT, Wyser C, Roser H et al: Lung scanning and exercise testing for the prediction of postoperative performance in lung resection candidates at increased risk from complications. Chest 1995;108:341–8
46. Ferguson MK, Reeder LB, Mick R: Optimizing selection of patients for major lung resection. J Thorac Cardiovasc Surg 1995;109:275–83
47. American College of Physicians: Preoperative pulmonary function testing. Ann Intern Med 1990;112:793–94
48. Zibrak JD, O'Donnell CR, Marton K: Indications for pulmonary function testing. Ann Intern Med 1990;112:763–771
49. Lawrence VA, Page CP, Harris GD: Preoperative spirometry before abdominal operations. A critical appraisal of its predictive value. Arch Intern Med 1989;149:280–5
50. Williams-Russo P, Charlson ME, MacKenzie R et al: Predicting postoperative pulmonary complications. Is it a real problem? Arch Intern Med 1992;152:1209–1213
51. Celli BR: What is the value of preoperative pulmonary function testing? Med Clin North Am 1993;77:309–326
52. Wilson AT, Reilly CS: Anaesthesia and the obese patient. Int J Obesity 1993;17:427–435
53. Catley DM, Thornton C, Jordan C et al: Pronounced, episodic oxygen desaturation in the postoperative period: its association with ventilatory pattern and analgesic regimen. Anesthesiology 1985;63:20–28
54. Knill RL, Moote CA, Skinner MI, Rose EA: Anesthesia with abdominal surgery lead to intense REM sleep during the first postoperative week. Anesthesiology 1990;73:52–61
55. Pateman JA, Hanning CD: Postoperative myocardial infarction and episodic hypoxaemia. Br J Anaesthesia 1989;63:648–50
56. Reeder MK, Muir AD, Foex P et al: Postoperative myocardial ischaemia: temporal association with nocturnal hypoxaemia. Br J Anaesthesia 1991;67:626–31
57. Gill NP, Wright B, Reilly CS: Relationship between hypoxaemic and cardiac ischaemic events in the perioperative period. Br J Anaesthesia 1992;68:471–3
58. Stausholm K, Kehlet H, Rosenberg J: Oxygen therapy reduces postoperative tachycardia. Anaesthesia 1995;50:737–739
59. Smith HL, Sapsford DJ, Delaney ME, Jones JG: The effect on the heart of hypoxaemia in patients with severe coronary artery disease. Anaesthesia 1996;51:211–218
60. Rosenberg J, Kehlet H: Postoperative mental confusion—association with postoperative hypoxemia. Surgery 1993;114: 76–81
61. Rosenberg J: Hypoxaemia in the general surgical ward—a potential risk factor? Eur J Surg 1994;160:657–61

62. McBrien ME, Sellers WFS: A comparison of three variable performance devices for postoperative oxygen therapy. Anaesthesia 1995;50:136–138
63. Mangano DT: Perioperative cardiac morbidity. Anesthesiology 1990;72:153–184
64. Adams JE, Sicard GA, Allen BT et al: Diagnosis of perioperative myocardial infarction with measurement of cardiac troponin I. N Engl J Med 1994;330:670–4
65. Mangano DT, Goldman L: Preoperative assessment of the patient with known or suspected coronary disease. New Engl J Med 1995;333:1750–1756
66. Mangano DT: Preoperative risk assessment many studies, few solutions. Is a cardiac risk assessment paradigm possible? Anaesthesiology 1995;83:897–901
67. Gerson MC, Hurst JM, Hertzberg VS et al: Prediction of cardiac and pulmonary complications related to elective abdominal and noncardiac thoracic surgery in geriatric patients. Am J Med 1990;88:101–7
68. Older P, Smith R, Courtney P et al: Preoperative evaluation of cardiac failure and ischaemia in elderly patients by cardiopulmonary exercise testing. Chest 1993;104:701–704
69. Goldman L, Caldera DL, Nussbaum SR et al: Multifactorial index of cardiac risk in noncardiac surgical procedures. N Engl J Med 1977;297:845–850
70. Detsky AS, Abrams HB, McLaughlin JR et al: Predicting cardiac complications in patients undergoing non-cardiac surgery. J Gen Intern Med 1986;1:211–219
71. Katz NM, Hannan RL, Hopkins RA, Wallace RB: Cardiac operations in patients aged 70 years and over: mortality, length of stay, and hospital charge. Ann Thorac Surg 1995;60: 96–101
72. Unsworth-White MJ, Holmes L, Treasure T: Cardiac surgery in older people. Br J Hosp Med 1993;49:457
73. Elder AT, Shaw TRD, Turnbull CM, Starkey IF: Elderly and younger patients selected to undergo coronary angiography. BMJ 1991;303:950–3
74. Lawson-Matthew PJ, Channer KS: Reporting on reports—cardiological interventions in elderly people. J Roy Coll Phys Lond 1995;29:11–14
75. Northridge D, Hall RC: Cardiological services for the elderly. Roy Coll Phys Lond 1995;29:9–10
76. Jaeger AA, Hlatky MA, Paul SM, Gortner SR: Functional capacity after surgery in elderly patients. JACC 1994;24:104–8
77. Walter PJ, Mohan R: Coronary bypass surgery in the elderly—a multi-disciplinary opinion. Summary of proceedings of an international symposium held at Antwerp, Belgium, March 9–11, 1994. Quality of Life Research 1995;4:279–287
78. Awad W, Cooper G, Blauth C: Cardiac surgery in the elderly. J Roy Coll Phys Lond 1995;29:252
79. Sizer T, Russell CA, Wood S et al: Standards and Guidelines for Nutritional Support of Patients in Hospital. A report by a Working Party of the British Association for Parenteral and Enteral Nutrition. Published by the British Association for Parenteral and Enteral Nutrition (BAPEN), Maidenhead, UK, 1996
80. McWhirter JP, Pennington CR: Incidence and recognition of malnutrition in hospital. BMJ 1994;308:945–8
81. Bistrian BR, Blackburn, Hallowell E, Heddle R: Protein status of general surgical patients. JAMA 1974;230:858–60
82. Windsor JA: Underweight patients and the risks of surgery. World J Surg 1993;17:165–172
83. Allison SP: The uses and limitations of nutritional support. Clin Nutr 1992;11:319–330
84. Campos ACL, Meguid MM: A critical appraisal of the usefulness of perioperative nutritional support. Am J Clin Nutr 1992; 55:117–130
85. Gray GE, Gray LK: Validity of anthropometric norms used in the assessment of hospitalized patients. J Paren Enteral Nutr 1979;3:366–8
86. McLaren DS: A fresh look at protein-energy malnutrition in the hospitalized patient. Nutrition 1988;4:1–6
87. Bastow MD, Rawlings J, Allison SP: Benefits of supplementary tube feeding after fractured neck of femur: a randomised controlled trial. BMJ 1983;287:1589–92
88. Delmi M, Rapin CH, Bemgoa JM et al: Dietary supplementation in elderly patients with fractured neck of the femur. Lancet 1990;335:1013–6
89. Meguid MM, Campos AC, Hammond WG: Nutritional support in surgical practice: Part I. Am J Surg 1990;159:345–58
90. Meguid MM, Campos AC, Hammond WG: Nutritional support in surgical practice: Part II. Am J Surg 1990;159:427–43
91. Veterans Affairs Total Parenteral Nutrition Cooperative Study Group: Perioperative total parenteral nutrition in surgical patients. N Engl J Med 1991;325:525–32
92. Von Meyenfeldt MF, Meijerink WJHJ, Rouflart MMJ et al: Perioperative nutritional support: a randomised clinical trial. Clin Nutr 1992;11:180–186
93. Rana SK, Bray J, Menzies-Gow N et al: Short term benefits of post-operative oral dietary supplements in surgical patients. Clin Nutr 1992;11:337–344
94. Hessov I: Impact of sip therapy on postoperative surgical outcome. Nutrition 1995;11(suppl 2):221–223
95. Rolandelli RH, Ullrich JR: Nutritional support in the frail elderly surgical patient. Surg Clin North Am 1994;74:79–92
96. American Society for Parenteral and Enteral Nutrition: Guidelines for the use of parenteral and enteral nutrition in adult and pediatric patients. J Paren Enteral Nutr 1993;17(suppl 4):1SA–52SA
97. Hill GL: Surgical nutrition: time for some clinical common sense. Br J Surg 1988;75:729–30
98. Windsor JA, Hill GL: Weight loss with physiological impairment. A basic indicator of surgical risk. Ann Surg 1988;207: 290–296
99. Gallagher HJ, Daly JM: Malnutrition, injury, and the host immune response: nutrient substitution. Curr Opin Gen Surg 1993:92–104
100. Saunders C, Nishiwaka R, Wolfe B: Surgical nutrition: a review. J Roy Coll Surg Edinb 1993;38:195–204
101. Mainous MR, Deitch EA: Nutrition and infection. Surg Clin North Am 1994;74:659–676
102. Udelsman R, Holbrook NJ: Endocrine and molecular responses to surgical stress. Curr Prob Surg 1994;31:653–720
103. Mainous MR, Deitch EA: Nutrition and infection. Surg Clin North Am 1994;74:659–676

104. Bray GA: Pathophysiology of obesity. Am J Clin Nutr 1992; 55:488S–494S

105. Garrow JS, Hastings EJ, Cox AG et al: Obesity and postoperative complications of abdominal operation. BMJ 1988;297: 181

106. Seymour DG: Medical Assessment of the Elderly Surgical Patient. Croom Helm, Beckenham, 1986

107. Campbell AJ, Spears GFS, Brown JS et al: Anthropometric measurements as predictors of mortality in a community population aged 70 years and over. Age Ageing 1990;19:131–135

108. Rajal SA, Haavisto HJ, Kaarela RH, Heikinheimo RJ: Body weight and the three year prognosis in very old people. Int J Obesity 1990;14:997–1003

109. Kushner RF: Body weight and mortality. Nutr Rev 1993;51: 127–136

110. Jiganti JJ, Goldstein WM, Williams CS: A comparison of the perioperative morbidity in total joint arthroplasty in the obese and nonobese patient. Clin Orthopaedics Related Res 1993; 289:175–179

111. Lahey SJ, Borlase BC, Lavin PT, Levitsky S: Preoperative risk factors that predict hospital length of stay in coronary artery bypass patients > 60 years old. Circulation 1992;86(suppl 5):II181–5

112. Phillips PA, Johnston CI, Gray L: Disturbed fluid and electrolyte homeostasis following dehydration in elderly people. Age Ageing 1993;22:S26–33

113. Gross CR, Lindquist RD, Woolley AC et al: Clinical indicators of dehydration severity in elderly patients. J Emergency Med 1992;10:267–274

114. Van Zee KJ, Lowry SF, American College of Surgeons: Emergency care. pp. 1–16. In: Surgery. Scientific American Inc, New York, 1995

115. Weinberg AD, Minaker KL, and the Council on Scientific Affairs, American Medical Association: Dehydration. Evaluation and management in older adults. JAMA 1995;274:1552–1555

116. Lye M: Electrolyte disorders in the elderly. Clin Endocrinol Metab 1984;13:377–98

117. McIntyre KM, Vita JA, Lambrew CT et al: A noninvasive method of predicting pulmonary-capillary wedge pressure. N Engl J Med 1992;327:1715–20

118. Vanoverschelde JL, Robert AR, Gerbaux A et al: Noninvasive estimation of pulmonary arterial wedge pressure with Doppler transmitral flow velocity pattern in patients with known heart disease. Am J Cardiol 1995;75:383–9

119. Levinsky NG: Fluids and electrolytes. pp. 242–253. In Isselbacher KJ, Braunwald E, Wilson JD et al. (eds): Harrison's Principles and Practice of Internal Medicine. 13th Ed. McGraw-Hill, New York, 1994

120. Shires GT, Canizaro PC: Fluid and electrolyte management of the surgical patient. pp. 64–86. In Sabiston DC et al: Textbook of Surgery. The Biological Basis of Modern Surgical Practice. 13th Ed. WB Saunders, Philadelphia, 1986

121. Tweedle DEF: Electrolyte disorders in the surgical patient. Clin Endocrinol Metab 1984;13:351–76

122. Rothwell PM, Slattery J, Warlow CP: A systematic review of the risks of stroke and death due to endarterectomy for symptomatic carotid stenosis. Stroke. 1996;27:260–5

123. Rothwell PM, Slattery J, Warlow CP: A systematic comparison of the risks of stroke and death due to carotid endarterectomy for symptomatic and asymptomatic stenosis. Stroke 1996;27: 266–9

124. Easton JD, Wilterdink JL: Carotid endarterectomy: trials and tribulations. Ann Neurol 1994;35:5–17

125. Sotaniemi KA: Long-term neurologic outcome after cardiac operation. Ann Thorac Surg 1995;59:1336–9

126. Ricotta JJ, Faggioli GL, Castilone A, Hassett JM: Risk factors for stroke after cardiac surgery: Buffalo Cardiac-Cerebral Study Group. J Vascular Surg 1995;21:359–64

127. Redmond JM, Greene PS, Goldsborough MA et al: Neurologic injury in cardiac surgical patients with a history of stroke. Ann Thorac Surg 1996;61:42–7

128. Dyer CB, Ashton CM, Teasdale TA: Post-operative delirium. a review of 80 primary data-collection studies. Arch Intern Med 1995;155:461–5

129. Schor JD, Levkoff SE, Lipsitz LA et al: Risk factors for delirium in hospitalized elderly. JAMA 1992;267:827–831

130. Marcantonio ER, Goldman L, Mangione CM et al: A clinical prediction rule for delirium after elective noncardiac surgery. JAMA 1994;271:134–139

131. Williams Russo P, Sharrock NE, Mattis S et al: Cognitive effects after epidural vs general anesthesia in older adults. A randomized trial. JAMA 1995;274:44–50

132. Bedford PD: Adverse cerebral effects of anaesthesia on old people. Lancet 1955;ii:256–263

133. Simpson BR, Williams M, Scott JF, Crampton Smith A: The effects of anaesthesia on old people. Lancet 1961;ii:887–893

134. Seymour DG: Anaesthetics and the mental state. pp. 995–1004. In Copeland JRM, Abou-Saleh MT, Balzer DG (eds). Principles and Practice of Geriatric Psychiatry. John Wiley & Sons, Chichester, 1994

135. Jones MJT, Piggott SE, Vaughan RS et al: Cognitive and functional competence after anaesthesia in patients aged over 60: controlled trial of general and regional anaesthesia for elective hip or knee replacement. BMJ 1990;300:1683–7

136. Campbell DNC, Lim M, Kerr Muir M et al: A prospective randomised study of local versus general anaesthesia for cataract surgery. Anaesthesia 1993;48:422–428

137. Williams Russo P, Sharrock NE, Mattis S et al: Cognitive effects after epidural vs general anesthesia in older adults. A randomized trial. JAMA 1995;274:44–50

138. Shaw JHF: Metabolic basis for management of the septic surgical patient. World J Surg 1993;17:154–164

139. Bender BS: Sepsis. Clin Geriat Med 1992;8:913–924

140. Condon RE, Wittman DH: Surgical Infections. pp. 27–44. In Morris PJ, Malt RA (eds): Oxford Textbook of Surgery. Oxford University Press, Oxford, 1994

141. Paluzzi RG: Antimicrobial prophylaxis for surgery. Med Clin North Am 1993;77:427–441

142. Palmberg GS, Hirsjarvi E: Mortality in geriatric surgery. Gerontology 1979;25:103–112

143. Merli GJ: Deep vein thrombosis and pulmonary embolism prophylaxis in orthopaedic surgery. Med Clin North Am 1993; 77:397–411

144. Evans JG: This patient or that patient? pp. 118–124. In: Rationing in Action. BMJ Publishing Group, London, 1993

145. Mc Dowell I, Newell C: Measuring Health. A Guide to Rating Scales and Questionnaires. 2nd Ed. Oxford University Press, New York, 1996
146. Chelluri L, Grenvik A, Silverman M: Intensive care for critically ill elderly: mortality, costs, and quality of life. Arch Intern Med 1995;155:1013–1022
147. Wood-Dauphinee SL, Troidl H: Assessing quality of life in surgical studies. Theoretical Surgery 1989;4:35–44
148. Fraser SCA: Quality-of-life measurement in surgical practice. Br J Surg 1993;80:163–169
149. Laupacis A, Bourne R, Rorabeck C et al: The effect of total hip replacement on health-related quality of life. J Bone Joint Surg 1993;75A:1619–1626
150. Bellamy N, Buchanan WW, Goldsmith CH et al: Validation study of WOMAC: a health status instrument for measuring clinically important patient relative outcomes to antirheumatic drug therapy in patients with osteoarthritis of the hip or knee. J Rheumatol 1988;15:1833–40
151. Bombardier C, Melfi CA, Paul J et al: Comparison of a generic and a disease-specific measure of pain and physical function after knee-replacement surgery. Medical Care 1995;33 (suppl):AS131–AS144
152. Tugwell P, Bombardier C, Buchanan WW et al: The MACTAR Patient Preference Disability Questionnaire—an individualized functional priority approach for assessing improvement in physical disability in clinical trials in rheumatoid arthritis. J Rheumatol 1987;14:446–51
153. O'Boyle CA, McGee H, Hickey A et al: Individual quality of life in patients undergoing hip replacement. Lancet 1992;339: 1088–91
154. Ruta DA, Garratt AM, Leng M et al: A new approach to the measurement of quality of life. The Patient-Generated Index. Medical Care 1994;32:1109–1126
155. Medical Research Council: The Health of the UK's Elderly People, MRC Topic Review. p. 42. Medical Research Council, London, 1994
156. Seymour DG, Garthwaite PH: Is there inequity of hospital referral on the grounds of age? An analysis of inguinal hernia surgery in men in Scotland. Poster presentation, British Geriatrics Society, Autumn Meeting, London, 1996

CHAPTER 19

Effects of Aging on the Heart

WILBERT S. ARONOW

Age-related changes in the cardiovascular system, overt and occult cardiovascular disease, and reduced physical activity affect cardiovascular function in elderly persons. With aging, there is a loss of myocytes in both the left and right ventricles, with a progressive increase in myocyte cell volume per nucleus in both ventricles.[1] With aging, there is also a progressive reduction in the number of pacemaker cells in the sinus node, with 10 percent of the number of cells present at age 20 remaining at age 75.[2]

Afterload

Afterload is the resistance to the ejection of blood by the left ventricle. Afterload is composed of two components: (1) peripheral vascular resistance, which is the steady-state component and the opposition to steady blood flow and (2) characteristic aortic impedance, which is the dynamic component and the opposition to pulsatile blood flow. Peripheral vascular resistance is calculated by dividing the mean arterial pressure by the cardiac output and is inversely proportional to the cross-sectional area of the peripheral vascular beds. Characteristic aortic impedance is measured as the time variation in mean arterial pressure/flow through the aorta and is inversely proportional to the arterial compliance (the distensibility of the arterial wall). An indirect measurement of afterload is the pulse wave velocity, which measures the propagation speed of pressure waves travelling from proximal to distal arterial segments and which increases as arteries become less compliant.

With aging, the large elastic arteries become dilated with a reduction in compliance.[3] Progressive thickening of the aortic media and intima are associated with aortic enlargement.[4] There is an age-associated increase in arterial stiffness resulting from changes in the arterial media such as thickening of the smooth muscle layers, increased fragmentation of elastin, an increase in the amount and characteristics of collagen, and increased calcification.[5] These structural changes are associated with a reduction in aortic distensibility due to increased aortic stiffness with an increase in pulse wave velocity.[6] These structural changes in the arterial wall are independent of coexisting atherosclerosis. Avolio et al.[6] demonstrated an increase in pulse wave velocity with age in farmers from Guanzhou Province in southern China despite a low prevalence of atherosclerosis in this population. The age-associated increase in stiffness and decrease in distensibility of large elastic arteries is not observed in distal arteries.[7]

Impedance spectral patterns have shown an age-related increase in characteristic aortic impedance and in peripheral vascular resistance.[8] The reduction in arterial compliance contributes more to the age-related increase in afterload than does the loss of peripheral vascular beds.[8] Peripheral vascular resistance was not age related in healthy Baltimore Longitudinal Study of Aging participants screened for occult coronary artery disease,[9] but was increased with age in persons not screened for occult coronary artery disease.[10] Arterial stiffening appearing as an increase in pulse wave velocity is associated with degeneration of the vascular media independent of atherosclerosis. Arterial stiffening causes earlier occurrence of wave reflection from peripheral sites to the ascending aorta during left ventricular ejection. Therefore, aortic and carotid phasic pressures increase to a greater magnitude at a later time during left ventricular ejection, causing an increase in systolic and pulse pressures and a delayed peak in the aortic pressure pulse contour.

Circulating levels of catecholamines increase with age, especially with stress. However, β-adrenergic vasodilation of vascular smooth muscle decreases with aging.[11] α-adrenergic vasoconstriction of vascular smooth muscle does not change with aging.[12] The impaired vasodilator response to β-adrenergic stimulation with age is most important during exercise and contributes to the increased afterload associated with aging.

Increased afterload causes an increase in blood pressure. With aging, there is an increase in systolic blood pressure and a widened pulse pressure. A slight reduction in diastolic blood pressure occurs after the sixth decade.[13] The increase in systolic blood pressure is due to interactions of aging, cardiovascular disease, and lifestyle factors such as dietary sodium intake, level of physical activity, and body weight. An age-associated increase in the index of aortic stiffening was not found in normotensive persons on a low sodium chloride diet.[14] The increase in carotid augmentation index (which is an index of aortic stiffening) in highly trained elderly men was one-half of that expected on the basis of age alone.[15]

As aortic compliance decreases with aging, the transfer of kinetic energy from the blood ejected during left ventricular systole to potential energy stored in the elasticity of the aortic wall is decreased. Consequently, the return of the potential energy stored in the elasticity of the aortic wall back to the kinetic energy of blood flow during diastole also is decreased. Therefore, the left ventricle must eject its stroke volume into a less compliant aorta with greater pressure and force to achieve an adequate cardiac output. The increased pulse wave velocity also causes the pressure in the aorta to increase and peak later in systole, contributing to the increased systolic blood pressure and widened pulse pressure.

Posterior left ventricular wall thickness increased with increasing age in normotensive men and women in the Baltimore Longitudinal Study of Aging participants screened for occult coronary artery disease.[3] Data from the Baltimore Longitudinal Study of Aging population suggested that the increase in left ventricular wall thickness associated with aging is mediated by an increase in systolic blood pressure.[16] Aging is also associated with an increase in the prevalence of hypertension and cardiovascular disease. Therefore, the prevalence of echocardiographic left ventricular hypertrophy increases with age.

Age-associated left ventricular hypertrophy is caused by an increase in the volume but not in the number of cardiac myocytes. Fibroblasts undergo hyperplasia, and collagen is deposited in the myocardial interstitium. Increased afterload causes an increase in left ventricular systolic stress and the addition of sarcomeres in parallel. This results in increased left ventricular wall thickness with a normal or decreased left ventricular chamber size and an increased relative wall thickness.

In the Framingham Heart Study, echocardiographic left ventricular hypertrophy was demonstrated in 33 percent of men and 49 percent of women older than 70 years.[17] In our elderly population, echocardiographic left ventricular hypertrophy was observed in 723 of 1,699 persons (43 percent, 70 percent women and 30 percent men) older than 60 years, mean age 81 years.[18] In our elderly population, hypertension was present in 108 of 215 blacks (50 percent), mean age 81 years; in 411 of 1,140 whites (36 percent), mean age 82 years; and in 19 of 54 Hispanics (35 percent), mean age 81 years.[19] Echocardiographic left ventricular hypertrophy was present in 66 of 92 hypertensive blacks (72 percent), in 194 of 346 hypertensive whites (56 percent), and in eight of 15 hypertensive Hispanics (53 percent).[19] However, echocardiographic left ventricular hypertrophy was present in only two of our 88 elderly persons (2 percent) without hypertension or overt cardiac disease.[20]

Preload

Preload is the filling volume of the left ventricle. Preload is determined by numerous factors that influence blood return to the heart and by the mechanical properties of the heart during diastolic filling of the left ventricle.

Resting left ventricular end-diastolic volume measured by echocardiography or by radionuclide ventriculography using multiple gated pool acquisition imaging is not age related in healthy persons, indicating that resting preload does not change with age.[3,9,21] However, although resting preload does not change with age, left ventricular early diastolic filling is reduced with aging.

Passive filling of the left ventricle occurs during the rapid filling and diastasis phases of early diastole. With aging, left ventricular stiffness is increased, left ventricular compliance is decreased, left ventricular wall thickness is increased, left ventricular relaxation is impaired, and left ventricular early diastolic filling is decreased. This may result in hypotension if preload is decreased. An age-related increase in systolic blood pressure also impairs left ventricular early diastolic filling, leading to hypotension if preload is reduced. Left ventricular filling during early diastole decreases 50 percent from age 20 years to 80 years.[3,22,23]

Despite the reduction in early diastolic filling of the left ventricle with aging, preload is maintained because left atrial contraction becomes more vigorous to increase late diastolic filling of the left ventricle.[3,21–27] Augmentation of late diastolic filling of the left ventricle prevents a decrease in left ventricular end-diastolic volume with aging. The ratio of late diastolic Doppler peak transmitral velocity (peak atrial or A-wave velocity) to early diastolic Doppler peak transmitral velocity (peak rapid filling or E-wave velocity) increases from approximately 0.6 at 30 years of age to 1.2 at 70 years of age.[28] A decrease in E/A-wave ratio with aging reflects a reduction in left ventricular compliance. An age-related increase in left atrial size resulting from increased wall stress due to increased left atrial pressure counteracts the effects of decreased left ventricular compliance with aging. In our elderly population, 579 of 1,699 elderly persons (34 percent) had echocardiographic left atrial enlargement.[18]

In the Framingham Heart Study, age was the most powerful independent variable for left ventricular filling in healthy persons.[29] Age was inversely associated with the E wave (peak early diastolic filling velocity) and was directly associated with the A wave (peak late diastolic filling velocity). Other independent variables contributing to a lesser degree of left ventricular filling were heart rate, PR interval measured from the electrocardiogram, gender, systolic blood pressure, and left ventricular systolic function. Increasing heart rate reduces peak early diastolic filling and increases peak late diastolic filling velocity. The PR interval on the electrocardiogram is inversely associated with peak early diastolic filling velocity. Women have slightly higher peak early diastolic filling velocities than men. Left ventricular systolic function is directly associated with peak early diastolic filling velocity. Increasing systolic blood pressure increases the peak late diastolic filling velocity.[29,30]

A reduction of preload is not well tolerated in older persons. Reduced intravascular volume, decreased venous return to the heart, vasodilation by drugs or disease states, and use of drugs such as nitrates or diuretics reduce preload and may cause a decreased cardiac output and hypotension in older persons. Decreased compliance of the left ventricle and reduced cardiac and vascular responsiveness to β-adrenergic stimulation[31] cause older persons to be greatly dependent on the Frank-Starling mechanism to increase cardiac output. Older persons are more susceptible to develop orthostatic hypotension.[32–34] Impaired baroreceptor reflex sensitivity,[35] decreased cardiac responsiveness to β-adrenergic stimulation,[31] loss of arterial compliance, decreased venous return due to increased venous distensibility, impaired compensatory mechanisms for maintenance of fluid volume and electrolyte balance, increased incidence of common precipitating diseases and disorders, and the use of multiple drugs contribute to orthostatic hypotension. Older persons are also more susceptible to develop postprandial hypotension.[36–38]

Since left atrial contraction can contribute up to 50 percent of left ventricular filling in a poorly compliant left ventricle, development of atrial fibrillation may cause a marked reduction in cardiac output because of the loss of left atrial contribution to left ventricular late diastolic filling. A rapid ventricular rate associated with atrial fibrillation will also reduce the time for diastolic filling of the left ventricle.

The incidence of chronic atrial fibrillation also increases with age.[39,40] In 2,101 elderly persons in a nursing home, the prevalence of chronic atrial fibrillation was 5 percent in persons aged 60 to 70 years, 13 to 14 percent in persons aged 71 to 90 years, and 22 percent in persons 91 years and older.[40]

Cardiac output is increased during exercise in healthy elderly persons by an increase in venous return to the heart, increasing diastolic filling of the left ventricle, and allowing an increased stroke volume to be ejected during exercise.[41] This is the Frank-Starling mechanism. In healthy persons in the Baltimore Longitudinal Study of Aging, the maximal heart rate response to exercise decreased with age.[9] However, exercise stroke volume increased with age to maintain the exercise cardiac output.[9] The increase in exercise stroke volume resulted from an increase in left ventricular end-diastolic volume (preload) by the Frank-Starling mechanism. In contrast, healthy nonelderly persons achieved an increase in exercise cardiac output primarily by an increase in heart rate. Exercise stroke volume increased in nonelderly healthy persons by a slight increase in left ventricular end-diastolic volume and by a large decrease in left ventricular end-systolic volume. The exercise-induced increase in heart rate and reduction in left ventricular end-systolic volume in nonelderly persons is probably mediated by β-adrenergic stimulation. The increase in left ventricular end-diastolic volume during exercise in healthy elderly persons suggests that the age-associated reduction in resting early diastolic filling of the left ventricle does not persist during exercise.

Contractility

The intrinsic ability of the heart to generate force does not change with age in healthy persons. However, the duration of contraction and relaxation is prolonged in senescent animals.[42,43] Prolongation of left ventricular ejection time[44] and of the pre-ejection period[45] with aging in healthy persons indicates that prolongation of contraction occurs with aging. Prolongation of the duration of contraction in senescent animals is associated with increased muscle stiffness and with prolongation of the action potential duration.[46] These age-related changes are associated with cellular changes in the excitation-contraction coupling mechanism,[47] and may be an adaptive response to preserve contractile function in response to an age-induced increase in afterload.

There is no reduction of resting left ventricular ejection fraction or circumferential fiber shortening in elderly persons with no evidence of heart disease.[3,9,21,48,49] Systolic function with exercise is impaired with aging. In the Baltimore Longitudinal Study of Aging, elderly persons showed less of an exercise-induced increase in left ventricular ejection fraction than did younger persons because of an age-related increase in left ventricular end-systolic volume.[9] However, absolute values of left ventricular ejection fraction at maximal exercise in healthy elderly persons rarely decreased from basal values.[9] Age-associated reductions in maximal heart rate and in left ventricular contractility during maximal exercise are manifestations of decreased β-adrenergic responsiveness with aging partially offset by exercise-induced dilation of the left ventricle.[50]

Diastolic Function

Aging is associated with prolongation of isovolumic relaxation time, a reduction in early diastolic filling of the left ventricle, and augmentation of late diastolic filling of the left ventricle.[22,25,28] Normal aging changes affecting left ventricular diastolic function include increase in systolic blood pressure, increase in left ventricular wall thickness, decrease in left ventricular early diastolic filling, prolongation of left ventricular diastolic relaxation, increase in left atrial size, and increase in left ventricular late diastolic filling.[51]

With aging occurs a slowing of the rate at which calcium is sequestered by the sarcoplasmic reticulum following myocardial excitation, which results in decreased relaxation of the left ventricle.[47,52,53] Accumulation of calcium at the onset of diastole may impair left ventricular diastolic relaxation and early diastolic filling.[52] Reduced oxidative phosphorylation and cumulative mitochondrial peroxidation occurring with aging may also impair left ventricular diastolic function.[54,55]

Increased left ventricular stiffness with aging due to increased interstitial fibrosis and cross-linking of collagen in the heart impairs left ventricular diastolic relaxation and filling.[1,56–58] Myocardial ischemia in the absence of coronary artery disease caused by reductions in capillary density and coronary reserve with aging may further impair left ventricular diastolic function in older persons.[1,59]

In addition to a reduction in left ventricular diastolic relaxation and early diastolic filling caused by aging, older persons are more likely to have left ventricular diastolic dysfunction because they have an increased prevalence of hypertension, myocardial ischemia due to coronary artery disease, and left ventricular hypertrophy due to hypertension, valvular aortic stenosis, coronary artery disease, hypertrophic cardiomyopathy, and other cardiac disorders. The increased stiffness of the left ventricle and prolonged left ventricular relaxation time impair left ventricular early diastolic filling and cause higher left ventricular end-diastolic pressures at rest and during exercise in elderly persons.[60,61]

Table 19-1 Prevalence of normal left ventricular ejection fraction in older patients with congestive heart failure

Study	Result
Wong et al.[63]	41% of 54 older patients, mean age 80 years, with CHF had normal LVEF
Aronow et al.[64]	47% of 247 older patients, mean age 82 years, with CHF had normal LVEF
Cardiovascular Health Study[65]	47% of 79 older patients with CHF had normal LVEF
Framingham Heart Study[66]	52% of 72 patients, mean age 73 years, with CHF had normal LVEF

Abbreviations: CHF, congestive heart failure; LVEF, left ventricular ejection fraction.

In congestive heart failure (CHF) associated with left ventricular systolic dysfunction, the left ventricular ejection fraction is less than 50 percent. There is a decreased amount of myocardial fiber shortening, the stroke volume is reduced, the left ventricle is dilated, and the patient is symptomatic.

In CHF due to left ventricular diastolic dysfunction with normal left ventricular systolic function, the left ventricular ejection fraction is normal. Kitzman et al.[62] demonstrated during exercise that persons with CHF and normal left ventricular systolic function but abnormal left ventricular diastolic function were unable to normally increase stroke volume, even in the presence of increased left ventricular filling pressure. Myocardial hypertrophy, ischemia, or fibrosis causes slow or incomplete left ventricular filling at normal left atrial pressures. Left atrial pressure increases to augment left ventricular filling, resulting in pulmonary and systemic venous congestion. The development of atrial fibrillation may also cause a reduction in cardiac output and the development of pulmonary and systemic venous congestion, because of the loss of left atrial contribution to left ventricular late diastolic filling and decreased diastolic filling time due to a rapid ventricular rate.

Elderly persons are more likely than nonelderly persons to develop CHF due to abnormal left ventricular diastolic dysfunction with normal left ventricular systolic function. Table 19-1 shows that the prevalence of normal left ventricular ejection fraction in older persons with CHF ranged from 41 to 52 percent.[63–66]

Left ventricular ejection fraction should be measured in all patients with CHF in order that appropriate therapy may be given.[67,68] For example, digoxin should not be used to treat patients with CHF and normal left ventricular ejection fraction if sinus rhythm is present.[51,69] By increasing contractility through increasing intracellular calcium ion concentration, digoxin may increase left ventricular stiffness, increasing left ventricular filling pressure, and adversely affecting CHF due to left ventricular diastolic dysfunction. Patients with CHF due to abnormal left ventricular ejection fraction tolerate higher doses of diuretics than do patients with CHF and normal left ventricular ejection fraction. Patients with CHF due to left ventricular diastolic dysfunction with normal left ventricular ejection fraction need high left ventricular filling pressures to maintain an adequate stroke volume and cardiac output and cannot tolerate intravascular depletion. These patients should be treated with a low salt diet with cautious use of diuretics, rather than with large doses of diuretics.

Cardiovascular Response to Exercise

The maximal oxygen consumption (VO_{2max}) is the best overall measurement of cardiovascular fitness.[70] VO_{2max} is the product of cardiac output and systemic arteriovenous oxygen difference at peak exercise. Maximal cardiac output is the heart rate multiplied by the stroke volume at peak exercise, and is a more direct measurement of cardiovascular reserve than is VO_{2max}.[70] VO_{2max} decreases with aging.[71,72] The degree of reduction of VO_{2max} with aging is affected by physical conditioning, subclinical coronary artery disease, smoking, and body weight. The boxed list summarizes the cardiovascular responses to exercise in healthy older persons.

In the Baltimore Longitudinal Study of Aging, older male athletes had a higher peak exercise VO_{2max} than older sedentary men.[73] The greater peak exercise VO_{2max} in older male athletes than in older sedentary men was achieved by a higher cardiac index and a greater systemic arteriovenous oxygen difference. The higher peak exercise cardiac index in older male athletes than in older sedentary men was due to a higher stroke volume index with similar maximal heart rates.

A decrease in maximal systemic arteriovenous oxygen difference occurs with aging.[74] The reduction in muscle mass

Cardiovascular responses to exercise in healthy older persons

Maximal heart rate decreases with aging.

Exercise stroke volume is increased with aging to maintain cardiac output.

Increased exercise stroke volume with aging results primarily from increase in left ventricular end-diastolic volume by Frank-Starling mechanism.

Decrease in muscle mass with aging plays role in age-associated reductions in systemic arteriovenous oxygen difference and in VO_{2max} at peak exercise.

Left ventricular end-diastolic and end-systolic volumes increase during peak exercise with aging.

Peak exercise left ventricular ejection fraction decreases with aging.

Exercise-induced reduction in left ventricular end-systolic volume index and increases in cardiac index, stroke volume index, and left ventricular ejection fraction from rest were greater in older men than in older women.

Table 19-2 Prevalence of some cardiovascular disorders in an elderly population in a long-term health care facility

Cardiovascular Disorder	Mean Age (Years)	Prevalence	
		Number	Percentage
Coronary artery disease[77]	81	774/1,793	43
Atherothrombotic brain infarction[78]	81	468/1,834	26
Peripheral arterial disease[78]	81	449/1,834	24
40% to 100% extracranial carotid arterial disease[79]	81	202/1,275	16
Congestive heart failure[64]	81	294/1,319	22
Hypertension[19]	81	538/1,409	38
Aortic stenosis[18]	81	287/1,699	17
Mitral annular calcium[18]	81	812/1,699	48
≥1 + mitral regurgitation[18]	81	554/1,699	33
≥1 + aortic regurgitation[18]	81	498/1,699	29
Rheumatic mitral stenosis[18]	81	20/1,699	1
Hypertrophic cardiomyopathy[80]	82	17/379	4
Atrial fibrillation[40]	81	283/2,101	13
Pacemaker rhythm[81]	82	50/1,153	4
Abnormal left ventricular ejection fraction[18]	81	399/1,699	23
Left ventricular hypertrophy[18]	81	723/1,699	43
Left atrial enlargement[18]	81	579/1,699	34

with aging may play a major role in the reduction in systemic arteriovenous oxygen difference at peak exercise and in VO_{2max} with aging.[75]

Fleg et al.[76] also investigated the effect of aging upon peak upright cycle exercise in healthy sedentary men and women aged 22 to 86 years in the Baltimore Longitudinal Study of Aging. Peak cycle work rate decreased with aging in both men and women but was greater in men than in women at any age. Both men and women had, at peak exercise, decreases in heart rate, cardiac index, and left ventricular ejection fraction and increases in left ventricular end-diastolic volume index and end-systolic volume index with aging. Peak exercise stroke volume index did not vary with age in either men or women. The exercise-induced reduction in left ventricular end-systolic volume index and increases in cardiac index, stroke volume index, and left ventricular ejection fraction from rest were greater in older men than in older women.

Cardiovascular Disease

In addition to age-related changes in cardiovascular function and deconditioning due to a sedentary lifestyle in many elderly persons, elderly persons also have a higher prevalence and incidence of cardiovascular disorders that impair cardiovascular performance than nonelderly persons. Table 19-2 lists the prevalence of some cardiovascular disorders in an elderly population in a long-term health care facility.[18,19,40,64,77–81]

Summary

The boxed list itemizes some age-related changes in cardiovascular function in healthy older persons. Decrease in arterial compliance contributes more to the age-related increase in afterload than does the loss of peripheral vascular beds. The impaired vasodilator response to β-adrenergic stimulation with aging is most important during exercise and contributes to the increased afterload associated with aging. Resting preload does not change with age. Left ventricular early diastolic filling is decreased with aging. Augmentation of late diastolic filling of the left ventricle prevents a decrease in left ventricular end-diastolic volume with aging. The maximal heart rate response to exercise decreases with age. Exercise stroke volume is increased with age to maintain the exercise cardiac output. The increase in exercise stroke volume with age results from an increase in preload by the Frank-Starling mechanism. Contractility at rest does not change with age. However, the duration of left ventricular contraction and relaxation is prolonged with aging. Age-associated decreases in maximal heart rate and in left ventricular contractility during maximal exercise are manifestations of decreased β-adrenergic responsiveness with aging partially offset by exercise-induced dilation of the left ventricle. VO_{2max} and systemic arteriovenous oxygen difference at peak exercise decrease with aging. In addition to age-related changes in cardiovascular function and deconditioning due to a sedentary lifestyle in many elderly persons, elderly persons also have a higher prevalence and incidence of cardio-

Some age-related changes in cardiovascular function in healthy older persons

Decrease in arterial compliance contributes more to age-related increase in afterload than does loss of peripheral vascular beds.

Resting preload does not change with age.

Left ventricular early diastolic filling is decreased with aging.

Augmentation of late diastolic filling of left ventricle prevents decrease in left ventricular end-diastolic volume with aging.

Contractility at rest does not change with aging.

Duration of left ventricular contraction and relaxation is prolonged with aging.

Cardiovascular responses to exercise with aging are listed in previous boxed list.

Age-associated decreases in maximal heart rate and in left ventricular contractility during maximal exercise are manifestations of decreased β-adrenergic responsiveness with aging partially offset by exercise-induced dilation of the left ventricle.

vascular disorders that impair cardiovascular performance than nonelderly persons. Elderly persons are more likely than nonelderly persons to develop CHF due to abnormal left ventricular diastolic dysfunction with normal left ventricular systolic function.

References

1. Olivetti G, Melissari M, Capasso JM, Anversa P: Cardiomyopathy of the aging human heart. Myocyte loss and reactive cellular hypertrophy. Circ Res 1991;68:1560–1568
2. Davies MJ: The pathological basis of arrhythmias. Geriatr Cardiovasc Med 1988;1:181–183
3. Gerstenblith G, Fredericksen J, Yin FCP et al: Echocardiographic assessment of a normal adult aging population. Circulation 1977;56:273–278
4. Safar M: Aging and its effects on the cardiovascular system. Drugs 1990;39(suppl 1):1–8
5. Yin FCP: The aging vasculature and its effects on the heart. pp. 137–214. In Weisfeldt ML (ed): The aging heart: its function and response to stress. Vol 12 Aging. Raven Press, New York, 1980
6. Avolio AP, Fa-Quan D, Wei-Qiang L, et al: Effects of aging on arterial distensibility in populations with high and low prevalence of hypertension: comparison between urban and rural communities in China. Circulation 1985;71:202–210
7. Boutouyrie P, Laurent S, Benetos A, et al: Opposing effects of ageing on distal and proximal large arteries in hypertensives. J Hypertens 1992;10:587–591
8. Nichols WW, O'Rourke MF, Avolio AP et al: Effects of age on ventricular-vascular coupling. Am J Cardiol 1985;55: 1179–1184
9. Rodeheffer RJ, Gerstenblith G, Becker LC et al: Exercise cardiac output is maintained with advancing age in healthy human subjects: cardiac dilatation and increased stroke volume compensate for a diminished heart rate. Circulation 1984;69: 203–213
10. Brandfonbrener M, Landowne M, Shock NW: Changes in cardiac output with age. Circulation 1955;12:557–566
11. Pan HY, Hoffman BB, Pershe RA, Blaschke TF: Decline in beta-adrenergic receptor-mediated vascular relaxation with aging in man. J Pharmacol Exp Ther 1986;239:802–807
12. Buhler F, Kowski W, Van Brumeler P: Plasma catecholamines and cardiac, renal and peripheral vascular adrenoceptor mediated response in different age groups in normal and hypertensive subjects. Clin Exp Hypertens 1980;2:409–426
13. Landahl S, Bengtsson C, Sigurdsson JA et al: Age-related change in blood pressure. Hypertension 1986;8:1044–1049
14. Avolio AP, Clyde KM, Beard TC et al: Improved arterial distensibility in normotensive subjects on a low salt diet. Arteriosclerosis 1986;6:166–169
15. Vaitkevicius PV, Fleg JL, Engel JH et al: Effects of age and aerobic capacity on arterial stiffness in healthy adults. Circulation 1993;88:1456–1462
16. Lima JAC, Gerstenblith G, Weiss JL et al: Systolic blood pressure, not age mediates the age-related increase in left ventricular wall thickness within a normotensive population (abstract). J Am Coll Cardiol 1988;11:81A
17. Levy D, Anderson KM, Savage DD et al: Echocardiographically detected left ventricular hypertrophy: prevalence and risk factors. The Framingham Heart Study. Ann Intern Med 1988;108: 7–13
18. Aronow WS, Ahn C, Kronzon I: Echocardiographic findings associated with atrial fibrillation in 1,699 patients >60 years old. Am J Cardiol 1995;76:1191–1192
19. Aronow WS, Kronzon I: Prevalence of coronary risk factors in elderly blacks and whites. J Am Geriatr Soc 1991;39:567–570
20. Aronow WS, Koenigsberg M, Schwartz KS: Usefulness of echocardiographic left ventricular hypertrophy in predicting new coronary events and atherothrombotic brain infarction in patients over 62 years of age. Am J Cardiol 1988;61:1130–1132
21. Gardin JM, Henry WL, Savage DD et al: Echocardiographic measurements in normal subjects: evaluation of an adult population without clinically apparent heart disease. J Clin Ultrasound 1979;7:439–447
22. Bryg RJ, Williams GA, Labovitz AJ: Effect of aging on left ventricular diastolic filling in normal subjects. Am J Cardiol 1987;59:971–974
23. Iskandrian AS, Aakki A: Age related changes in left ventricular diastolic performance. Am Heart J 1986;112:75–78
24. Spirito P, Maron BJ: Influence of aging on doppler echocardiographic indices of left ventricular diastolic function. Br Heart J 1988;59:672–679
25. Miyatake K, Okamoto J, Kinoshita N et al: Augmentation of atrial contribution to left ventricular flow with aging as assessed by intracardiac Doppler flowmetry. Am J Cardiol 1984;53: 587–589

26. Sartori MP, Quinones MA, Kuo LC: Relation of Doppler-derived left ventricular filling parameters to age and radius/thickness ratio in normal and pathologic states. Am J Cardiol 1987;59: 1179–1182
27. Fleg JL, Shapiro EP, O'Connor F et al: Left ventricular diastolic filling performance in older male athletes. JAMA 1995;273: 1371–1375
28. Gardin JM, Rohan MK, Davidson DM et al: Doppler transmitral flow velocity parameters: relationship between age, body surface area, blood pressure and gender in normal subjects. Am J Noninvas Cardiol 1987;1:3–10
29. Benjamin EG, Levy D, Anderson KM et al: Determination of Doppler indexes of left ventricular diastolic function in normal subjects (The Framingham Heart Study). Am J Cardiol 1992; 70:508–515
30. Villari B, Hess OM, Kaufmann P et al: Effect of aortic valve stenosis (pressure overload) and regurgitation (volume overload) on left ventricular systolic and diastolic function. Am J Cardiol 1992;69:927–934
31. Lakatta EG: Age-related alterations in the cardiovascular response to adrenergic mediated stress. Fed Proc 1980;39: 3173–3177
32. Robbins AS, Rubenstein LZ: Postural hypotension in the elderly. J Am Geriatr Soc 1984;32:769–774
33. Aronow WS, Lee NH, Sales FF, Etienne F: Prevalence of postural hypotension in elderly patients in a long-term health care facility. Am J Cardiol 1988;62:336
34. Lipsitz LA, Jonsson PV, Marks BL et al: Reduced supine cardiac volumes and diastolic filling rates in elderly patients with chronic medical conditions. Implications for postural blood pressure homeostasis. J Am Geriatric Soc 1990;38:103–107
35. Gribbin B, Pickering TG, Sleight P, Peto R: Effect of age and high blood pressure on baroreflex sensitivity in man. Circ Res 1971;29:424–431
36. Lipsitz LA, Nyquist RP Jr, Wei JY, Rowe JW: Postprandial reduction in blood pressure in the elderly. N Engl J Med 1983; 309:81–83
37. Vaitkevicius PV, Esserwein DM, Maynard AK et al: Frequency and importance of postprandial blood pressure reduction in elderly nursing-home patients. Ann Intern Med 1991;115: 865–870
38. Aronow WS, Ahn C: Postprandial hypotension in 499 elderly persons in a long-term health care facility. J Am Geriatr Soc 1994;42:930–932
39. Wolf PA, Abbott RD, Kannel WB: Atrial fibrillation as an independent risk factor for stroke: the Framingham Study. Stroke 1991;22:983–988
40. Aronow WS, Ahn C, Gutstein H: Prevalence of atrial fibrillation and association of atrial fibrillation with prior and new thromboembolic stroke in elderly patients. J Am Geriatr Soc 1996;44: 521–523
41. Poliner LR, Dehmer GJ, Lewis SE et al: Left ventricular performance in normal subjects: a comparison of the responses to exercise in the upright and supine positions. Circulation 1980; 62:528–534
42. Fraticelli A, Josephson R, Danziger R et al: Morphological and contractile characteristics of rat cardiac myocytes from maturation to senescence. Am J Physiol 1989;257:H259–H265
43. Capasso JM, Malhotra A, Remly RM: Effects of age on mechanical and electrical performance of rat myocardium. Am J Physiol 1983;245:H72–H81
44. Willems JL, Roelandt H, DeGeest H et al: The left ventricular ejection time in elderly subjects. Circulation 1970;42:37–42
45. Shaw DJ, Rothbaum DA, Angell CS, Shock NW: The effect of age and blood pressure upon the systolic time intervals in males aged 20–89 years. J Gerontol 1973;28:133–139
46. Lakatta EG: Do hypertension and aging have similar effects on the myocardium? Circulation 1987;75(suppl I):I69–I77
47. Lakatta EG, Yin FCP: Myocardial aging: functional alterations and related cellular mechanisms. Am J Physiol 1982;242: H927–H941
48. Port S, Cobb FR, Coleman RE, Jones RH: Effect of age on the response of the left ventricular ejection fraction to exercise. N Engl J Med 1980;303:1133–1137
49. Aronow WS, Stein PD, Sabbah HN, Koenigsberg M: Resting left ventricular ejection fraction in elderly patients without evidence of heart disease. Am J Cardiol 1989;63:368–369
50. Fleg JL, Schulman S, O'Connor F et al: Effect of acute β-adrenergic receptor blockade on age-associated changes in cardiovascular performance during dynamic exercise Circulation 1994;90:2333–2341
51. Tresch DD, McGough MF: Heart failure with normal systolic function: a common disorder in older people. J Am Geriatr Soc 1995;43:1035–1042
52. Wei JY, Spurgeon HA, Lakatta EG: Excitation-contraction in rat myocardium: alterations with adult aging. Am J Physiol 1984;246:H784–H791
53. Morgan JP, Morgan KG: Calcium and cardiovascular function: intracellular calcium levels during contraction and relaxation of mammalian cardiac and vascular smooth muscle as detected with aequorin. Am J Med 1984;77(suppl 5A):33–46
54. Bandy B, Davison AJ: Mitochondrial mutations may increase oxidative stress: implications for carcinogenesis and aging? Free Radic Biol Med 1990;8:523–539
55. Corral-Debrinski M, Stepien G, Shoffner JM et al: Hypoxemia is associated with mitochondrial DNA damage and gene induction: implications for cardiac disease. JAMA 1991;266:1812–1816
56. Lie JT, Hammond PI: Pathology of the senescent heart: anatomic observations on 237 autopsy studies of patients 90 to 105 years old. Mayo Clin Proc. 1988;63:552–564
57. Schaub MC: The aging of collagen in the heart muscle. Gerontologia 1964;10:38–41
58. Verzar F: The stages and consequences of aging collagen. Gerontologia 1969;15:233–239
59. Hachamovitch R, Wicker P, Capasso JM, Anversa P: Alterations of coronary blood flow and reserve with aging in Fischer 344 rats. Am J Physiol 1989;256:H66–H73
60. Ogawa T, Spina R, Martin III WH et al: Effects of aging, sex and physical training on cardiovascular responses to exercise. Circulation 1992;86:494–503
61. Manning WJ, Shannon RP, Santinga JA et al: Reversal of changes in left ventricular diastolic filling associated with normal aging using diltiazem. Am J Cardiol 1989;67:894–896
62. Kitzman DW, Higginbotham MB, Cobb FR et al: Exercise intolerance in patients with heart failure and preserved left ventricu-

lar systolic function: failure of the Frank-Starling mechanism. J Am Coll Cardiol 1991;17:1065–1072

63. Wong WF, Gold S, Fukuyama O, Blanchette PL: Diastolic dysfunction in elderly patients with congestive heart failure. Am J Cardiol 1989;63:1526–1528

64. Aronow WS, Ahn C, Kronzon I: Prognosis of congestive heart failure in elderly patients with normal versus abnormal left ventricular systolic function associated with coronary artery disease. Am J Cardiol 1990;66:1257–1259

65. Gardin JM, Arnold A, Kitzman D et al: Congestive heart failure with preserved systolic function in a large community-dwelling elderly cohort: the Cardiovascular Health Study (abstract). J Am Coll Cardiol 1995;25:423A

66. Vasan RS, Benjamin EJ, Evans JC et al: Prevalence and clinical correlates of diastolic heart failure: Framingham Heart Study (abstract). Circulation 1995;92(suppl I):I–666

67. Aronow WS: Echocardiography should be performed in all elderly patients with congestive heart failure. J Am Geriatr Soc 1994;42:1300–1302

68. Konstam MA, Dracup K, Baker DW et al: Heart Failure: Evaluation and Care of Patients With Left-Ventricular Systolic Dysfunction. No. 11 AHCPR Publication No. 94–0612. pp. 37–40. Agency for Health Care Policy and Research, Public Health Service, U.S. Department of Health and Human Services, Rockville, MD

69. Aronow WS: Digoxin or angiotensin converting enzyme inhibitors for congestive heart failure in geriatric patients. Which is the preferred treatment? Drugs Aging 1991;1:98–103

70. Fleg JL: Alterations in cardiovascular structure and function with advancing age. Am J Cardiol 1986;57:33C–44C

71. Dehn MM, Bruce RA: Longitudinal variations in maximal oxygen intake with age and activity. J Applied Physiol 1972;33: 805–807

72. Heath GW, Hagberg JM, Ehsani AA, Holloszy JO: A physiological comparison of young and older endurance athletes. J Applied Physiol 1981;51:634–640

73. Fleg JL, Schulman SP, O'Connor FC et al: Cardiovascular responses to exhaustive upright cycle exercise in highly trained older men. J Applied Physiol 1994;77:1500–1506

74. Julius S, Amery A, Whitlock LS, Conway J: Influence of age on the hemodynamic response to exercise. Circulation 1967; 36:222–230

75. Fleg JL, Lakatta EG: Role of muscle loss in the age-associated reduction in VO_{2max}. J Applied Physiol 1988;65:1147–1151

76. Fleg JL, O'Connor F, Gerstenblith G et al: Impact of age on the cardiovascular response to dynamic upright exercise in healthy men and women. J Applied Physiol 1995;78:890–900

77. Aronow WS, Ahn C: Correlation of serum lipids with the presence or absence of coronary artery disease in 1,793 men and women aged ≥62 years. Am J Cardiol 1994;73:702–703

78. Aronow WS, Ahn C: Correlation of serum lipids with the presence or absence of atherothrombotic brain infarction and peripheral arterial disease in 1,834 men and women aged ≳62 years. Am J Cardiol 1994;73:995–997

79. Aronow WS, Kronzon I, Schoenfeld M: Prevalence of extracranial carotid arterial disease and of valvular aortic stenosis and their association in the elderly. Am J Cardiol 1995;75:304–305

80. Aronow WS, Kronzon I: Prevalence of hypertrophic cardiomyopathy and its association with mitral anular calcium in elderly patients. Chest 1988;94:1295–1296

81. Aronow WS: Correlation of arrhythmias and conduction defects on the resting electrocardiogram with new cardiac events in 1,153 elderly patients. Am J Noninvas Cardiol 1991;5:88–90

CHAPTER 20

Atherosclerosis and Lipid Metabolism

ROBERT W. STOUT

Atherosclerosis is the most important disease in old age. It is responsible for the majority of deaths in old people and is the most common cause of disability and dependency in the later years of life. The principal organs affected by atherosclerosis are the coronary arteries, leading to myocardial infarction and chronic ischemic heart disease, cardiac failure, and cardiac arrhythmias; the cerebral circulation, leading to stroke, transient ischemic attacks, and multi-infarct dementia; the aorta, leading to aneurysm; and the peripheral arterial system, leading to intermittent claudication, chronic ischemia, gangrene, and amputation. Atherosclerosis has the characteristics of a chronic degenerative disease; it takes decades to develop, the underlying cause is unknown, and it is irreversible by the time it becomes clinically apparent.

Atherosclerosis is a disease of multiple causes with several mechanisms operating at different times in any individual. The advanced lesion with its cellular proliferation, connective tissue deposition, calcification, necrosis, and thrombosis is the final common pathway of a number of different mechanisms.

Pathogenesis

The Normal Artery

The arterial wall is divided into three layers: the adventitia, media, and intima.

The adventitia consists of fibrous and fatty connective tissue and is the means by which the artery is linked to the surrounding tissues. The adventitia appears to play no part in the development of atherosclerosis.

The media consists of smooth muscle cells and is separated from the intima by the fenestrated internal elastic lamina. Smooth muscle cells, by their contraction and relaxation, modify the size of the lumen of the artery and maintain blood pressure. They also are the major synthetic cells of the artery, manufacturing connective tissue, including collagen, fibrin, elastin, and proteoglycans, as well as cytokines and growth factors. Smooth muscle cells appear to exist in two phenotypic states—contractile or synthetic—and may change from one to the other depending on their environment.[1] In atheromatous lesions they appear to be in the synthetic state.

The intima consists of a single layer of epithelial-like cells, the endothelium, which is separated from the internal elastic lamina by connective tissue containing a variable number of smooth muscle cells. The number of smooth muscle cells in the intima increases with advancing age to form diffuse intimal thickening. The endothelium acts as a barrier that protects the inner part of the artery from injurious substances in the circulation and as a blood compatible container. It is selectively permeable and allows the passage of nutrients to the inner part of the artery. The endothelium, which in total is a very large organ, is metabolically active and secretes a number of important substances including prostacyclin; factor VIII antigen; endothelium-derived vasoactive factors such as nitric oxide, prostacyclin, and endothelin; and cytokines and growth factors.[1]

Atherosclerosis is a disease of the intima and inner part of the media of the artery.

Atherosclerosis

The term atherosclerosis or atheroma covers a number of lesions of which the most characteristic are the fatty streak and the fibrous plaque.[1,2] Fatty streaks are found in the lining of many arteries in children and younger adults. They are flat white or yellow longitudinal lesions on the intimal surface of the artery (Fig. 20-1) and consist of collections of lipid-engorged foam cells, overlain with an intact endothelium (Fig. 20-2). The foam cells originate from monocyte-macrophages and T lymphocytes. The fibrous plaque is the advanced atheromatous lesion (Fig. 20-3). It consists of a fibrous cap made up of connective tissue containing elastic fibers, collagen, proteoglycans, and basement membrane, in which are embedded smooth muscle cells, and beneath which are variable amounts of intracellular and extracellular lipids, smooth muscle cells, macrophages, T lymphocytes, connective tissue, and, in the depth of the lesion, necrotic debris, cholesterol crystals, and calcification (Fig. 20-4). The relative content of fibrous tissue and lipid within a plaque is variable, with lesions in the coronary arteries being largely fibrous. The surface of the fibrous plaque may be the site of thrombosis.

The relationship of fatty streaks to advanced lesions has been the subject of controversy. Although fatty streaks occur in sites that are prone to fibrous plaques, they also occur in areas that are not particularly susceptible to atherosclerosis and in populations that are relatively free from the disease. Evidence from both animals and humans supports the evolution of fatty streaks into fibrous plaques.[3,4] It appears that many fatty streaks, particularly those in the aorta, are harmless and disappear, but others, including at least some of those in the coronary arteries and in susceptible people, may develop into fibrous plaques. It is not known what determines whether a fatty streak evolves into a fibrous plaque, or what precipitates

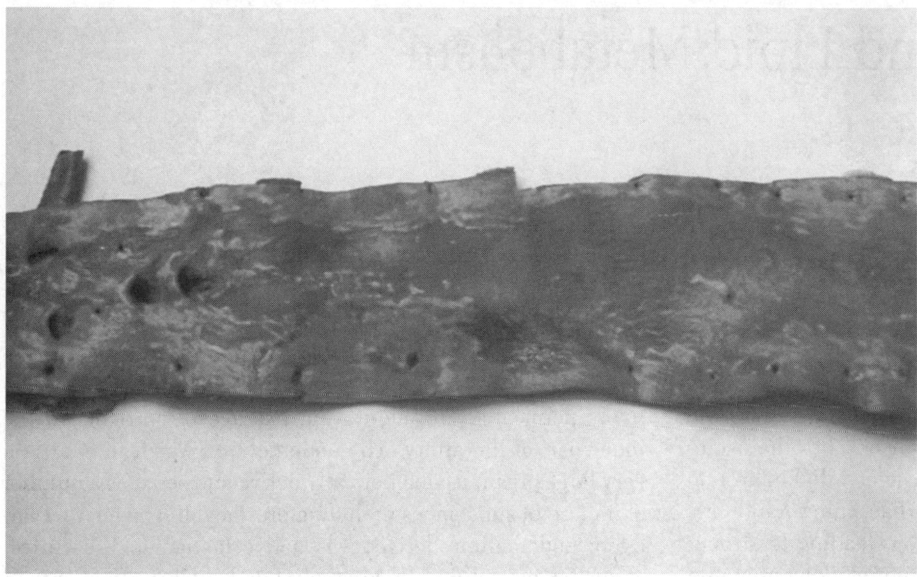

Figure 20-1 Surface of human aorta showing extensive involvement by fatty streaks. (Courtesy of Dr JD Biggart, Department of Pathology, The Queen's University of Belfast.)

thrombus formation on the plaque. The distribution of the lesion within the arterial system remains unexplained, although hemodynamic factors such as shear stress may account for the sites of some of the lesions.[5]

The cells of the lesions

Atherosclerosis results from the interaction of four cells—two arterial cells (endothelial and smooth muscle cells), and two circulating cells (platelets and monocyte-macrophages).[1] These interact with each other and with lipoproteins, hormones, hemodynamic factors, and connective tissue in the arterial wall. Each of the cells is able to synthesize and secrete a wide variety of cytokines, growth factors, coagulation factors, and vasoactive substances.[1] These can act locally on adjacent cells (paracrine function) and on the same cells (autocrine function). The interactions of these factors and circulating (endocrine) factors in the pathogenesis of atherosclerosis is complex and has not been completely elucidated.

Endothelial cells The endothelium consists of a single layer of epithelial cells whose growth and division is normally quiescent. Nevertheless, they are active in performing a number of essential functions. Endothelial cells regulate the transfer of metabolic substances between the plasma and the subendothelial space. They bind low density lipoprotein (LDL) and

Figure 20-2 Photomicrograph of fatty streak showing foam cells in subintimal tissues. (Courtesy of Dr J.D. Biggart, M.D., Department of Pathology, the Queen's University of Belfast.)

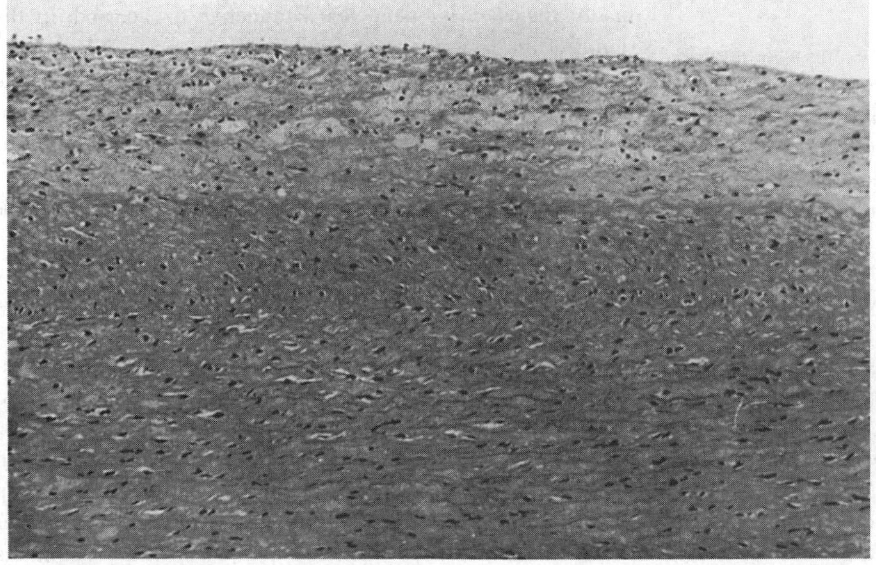

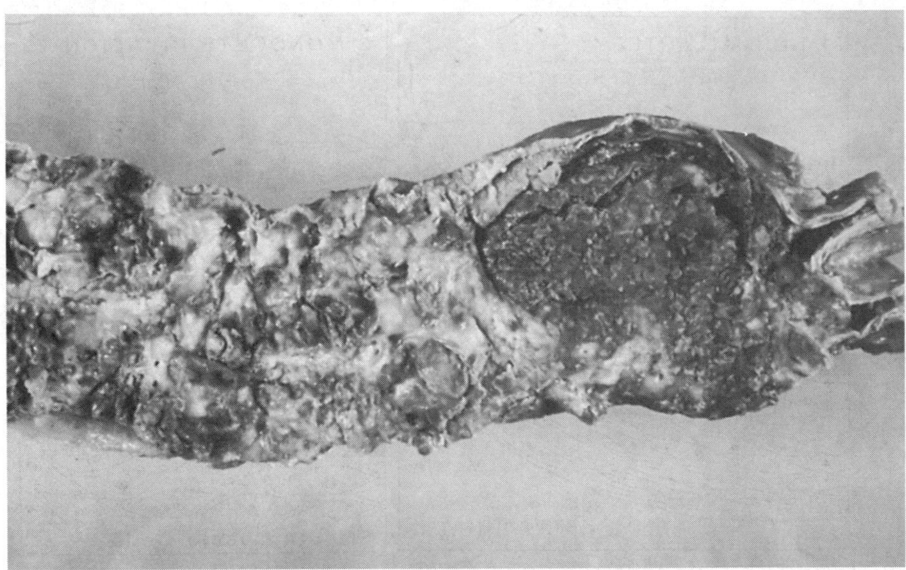

Figure 20-3 Surface of human aorta showing extensive involvement by fibrous plaques and a large thrombus. (Courtesy of Dr J.D. Biggart, M.D., Department of Pathology, The Queen's University of Belfast.)

"modify" it.[6,7] Modification by oxidation of LDL may be one of the most important early events in the development of atherosclerosis and may cause endothelial "injury."[1,7,8] The potential importance of this to atherogenesis is shown by the fact that experimental atherosclerosis can be prevented, without change in LDL levels, by the drug probucol, which has antioxidant properties.[9] They also bind insulin and other hormones, although they are resistant to the actions of these hormones.[10] They synthesize a number of biologically active molecules involved in hemostasis, in the regulation of vascular tone and in inflammation. Of particular relevance to atherosclerosis, endothelial cells synthesize a number of growth factors. In this way they may influence the growth and function of the other cells of the lesion and of themselves. Although the response to injury theory of atherogenesis presupposes an injury to the endothelial barrier, this "injury" may not result in loss of cells but may be a subtle alteration of endothelial function.[1]

Smooth muscle cells Proliferation of smooth muscle cells and their migration from the media to the intima is an

Figure 20-4 Photomicrograph of fibrous plaque showing fibrous cap with smooth muscle cells, foam cells and extracellular lipid, and necrotic debris. (Courtesy of Dr J.D. Biggart, M.D., Department of Pathology, The Queen's University of Belfast.)

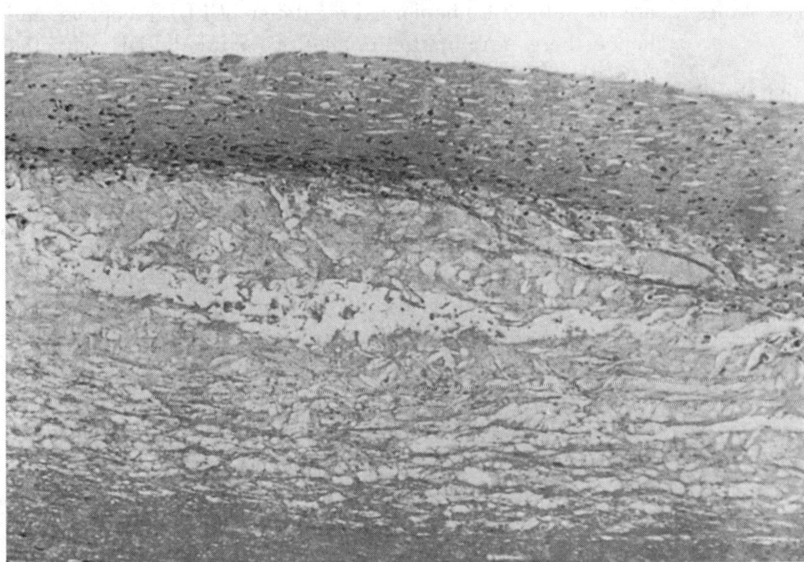

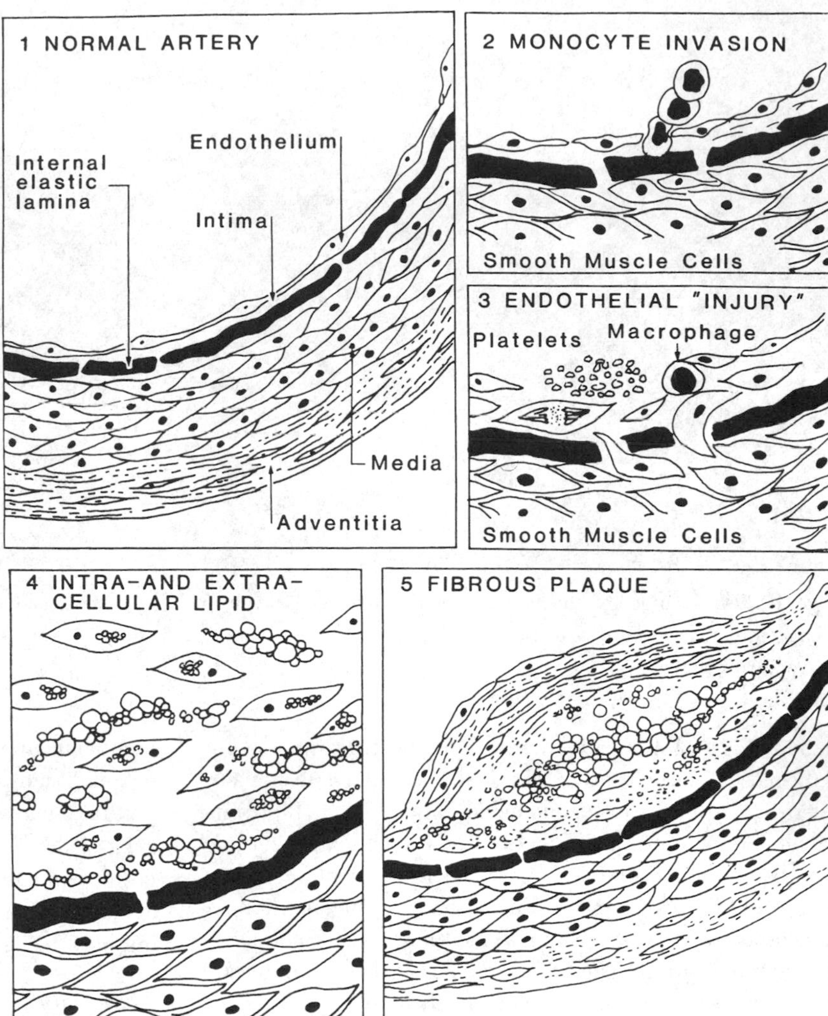

Figure 20-5 The pathogenesis of atherosclerosis. See text for details. (Adapted from Stout,[69] with permission.)

important event in the development of the fibrous plaque. Smooth muscle cells synthesize connective tissue, and are the major components of the fibroproliferative lesion of atherosclerosis. They synthesize and secrete growth factors and cytokines and factors that attract monocytes into the artery.[11]

Platelets These adhere to intimal surfaces that have been denuded of endothelium and release the contents of their granules, which include mitogens, platelet factor 4, β-thromboglobulin, and thromboxane A1. The platelet-derived growth factor (PDGF),[1] now known to be synthesized and secreted by many other cells as well as platelets, is particularly significant in atherogenesis, as it is a chemoattractant as well as a mitogen to smooth muscle cells and also stimulates the interaction of low density lipoproteins with their cell surface receptors.[11]

Monocytes/macrophages Circulating monocytes are the source of tissue macrophages and of many of the foam cells of the atheromatous lesion. In hypercholesterolemic animals, the earliest abnormality found in the arterial wall is attachment of monocytes to the surface of the endothelium. The monocytes then migrate between the endothelial cells into the subendothelium, where they accumulate lipid. Macrophages are considered to have a "scavenger" function in inflammatory reactions. They have scavenger receptors for modified LDLs that are not subject to the normal regulation of LDL receptors, and hence there is unlimited uptake of modified LDL, with the formation of foam cells.[6,12] Macrophages secrete many growth factors and cytokines, which act on the cells of the lesion. The mechanisms of the adherence and migration of monocytes in the artery wall are little understood.

Atherogenesis Current ideas on the development of atherosclerosis are based on the "response to injury" theory, a modern version of a hypothesis that is more than one century old.[1] This theory suggests that the early stages of the development of atherosclerosis involve the disruption or alteration of the endothelium's barrier function (the "injury") and infiltration of the artery by circulating monocytes, which become tissue macrophages (Fig. 20-5). Experimental evidence suggests that entry of monocytes may be the initial change and that this process further disrupts the endothelium.[12] Uptake of oxidized LDL appears to change the function of macrophages and leads to other events in atherogenesis.[7] Disruption of the integrity of the endothelium exposes the subendothelial connective tissue to which platelets adhere. The aggregating platelets release from their storage granules a number of active constituents, including the PDGF secreted from the α granules. PDGF and other growth factors, including hormones such as insulin,[13] and lipoproteins, act on the smooth muscle cells, causing them to proliferate and to migrate from the media to the intima through the pores in the internal elastic lamina.

This process is probably a repair and inflammatory process and normally leads to reconstitution of the integrity of the artery. The injury becomes covered by a continuous layer of endothelium, and the proliferating smooth muscle cells regress. However, in abnormal circumstances such as repeated injury or exposure to abnormal constituents of the circulation (e.g., hypercholesterolemia), the process changes from a repair to a proliferative process. This is characterized by an accumulation of smooth muscle cells in the arterial intima; the formation of extracellular connective tissue; the accumulation of foam cells, most of which are derived from monocyte macrophages that have engorged lipoproteins; calcification; ulceration; hemorrhage into the plaque; and superimposed thrombus formation. A small proportion of plaques are heavily engorged with lipid, both in foam cells and in the core of the lesion. These plaques appear to be unstable and at risk of fissuring, a process that predisposes to the formation of thrombus on the surface of the plaque.[2] It seems likely that there are a number of different stimuli that may be involved in the development of atherosclerosis, and that the advanced atherosclerotic lesion is the final common pathway of a number of pathogenic mechanisms.

Aging and atherosclerosis

Atherosclerosis and aging are intimately linked, and atherosclerosis is universally present in older humans. The exact relationship between atherosclerosis and aging is difficult to define. On the one hand, the pathogenesis of atherosclerosis may be related to a biologic aging process. On the other, the relationship between age and atherosclerosis may simply be the time required for its development.

Aging and atherosclerosis may be related by age changes in the artery, or by age changes in cardiovascular risk factors. Changes occur in the cells of the artery during senescence, which might contribute to the development of atherosclerosis[14] (Table 20-1). Endothelial cells lose their proliferative ability and hence their ability to repair an "injury" on the surface of the artery. The control of proliferation of smooth muscle cells and their interaction with lipoproteins is also altered with senescence. Hence, although atherosclerosis in old age is almost certainly the end point of a slow and prolonged process, it may be accelerated in older people because of changes in the cells that contribute to the development of the lesion.

Table 20-1 Changes in the biologic properties of arterial endothelial and smooth muscle cells in relation to in vivo or in vitro aging

Endothelial cells	Smooth muscle cells
Finite life span	Finite life span
Decreased population doublings	Decreased population doublings
Decreased binding and degradation of LDL	Longer latent period
No change in processing acetyl LDL	Reduced response to growth factors
Decreased angiotensin-converting enzyme activity	Decreased LDL degradation
	Decreased prostacyclin synthesis

Abbreviation: LDL, low density lipoprotein.
(Adapted from Stout,[14] with permission.)

Epidemiology of Atherosclerosis

Atherosclerosis is a universal condition that is present in all older people. It first appears in the late teens or early twenties; autopsy studies in young men killed as a result of war or accidents have revealed extensive atherosclerosis in these relatively young age groups.[15] However, atherosclerosis cannot be detected in life except by sophisticated imaging techniques, and hence epidemiologic studies measure other manifestations of cardiovascular disease, particularly coronary artery disease, either as sudden death, cardiovascular death, or as nonfatal myocardial infarction. Fewer epidemiologic studies have looked at stroke or peripheral vascular disease, which are less common than coronary artery disease and, therefore, more difficult to investigate.

Studies of the epidemiology of atherosclerosis have concentrated on the identification of risk factors for the disease. These are characteristics in asymptomatic people that predispose to cardiovascular disease, and are identified by prospective epidemiologic studies. Risk factors identify groups of people who are particularly susceptible to cardiovascular disease. They are not necessarily causal, but may be indirectly related to the disease or may even be early manifestations of the condition. As a result, alteration of a risk factor will not necessarily modify the course of the disease; intervention studies are required to test this. Risk factors that are associated with the clinical complications of atherosclerosis may or may not be related to the initiation of the disease in the vessel wall many years earlier, or to its progression to a stage where it causes clinical disease.

It is often assumed that risk factors for atherosclerosis are inoperative or less potent in old age. Recent data have cast doubt on this assumption, perhaps because there has been a change in risk factor distribution in recent years. Thus, increased survival may have reduced the selective mortality in populations where the levels of risk factors are high and hence, people with risk factors are now surviving into old age.[14]

The risk factors for atherosclerosis may be divided into intrinsic risk factors, which are currently not amenable to alteration, and extrinsic risk factors, which, to varying degrees, can be altered:

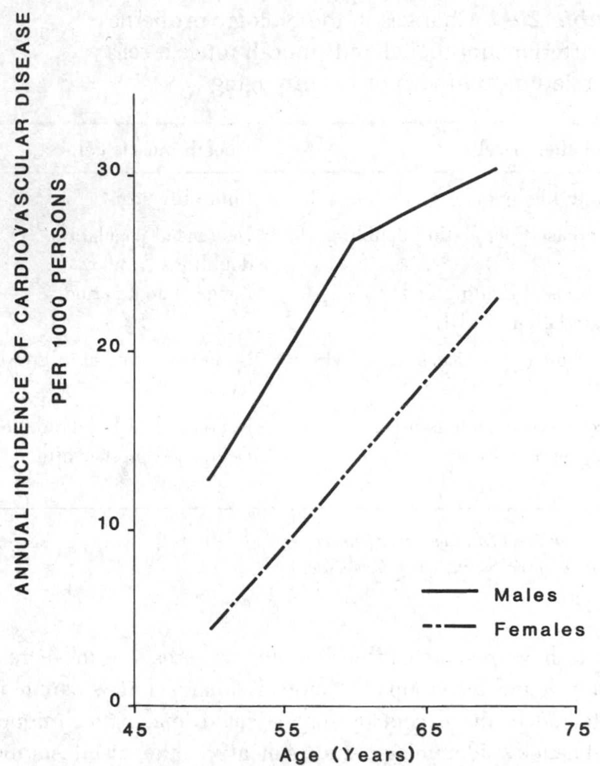

Figure 20-6 Incidence of cardiovascular disease by age and sex. (From Lerner and Kannel,[16] with permission.)

- Intrinsic
  - — Age
  - — Male sex
  - — Genetic and familial factors
- Reversible
  - — Cigarettes
  - — Hypertension
  - — Dyslipoproteinemia
  - — Hyperglycemia and diabetes mellitus
  - — Hyperfibrinogenemia
- Indirect
  - — Obesity
  - — Physical inactivity
- Others
  - — Hyperinsulinemia and insulin resistance
  - — Hemostatic factors
  - — Hyperuricemia
  - — Soft water

Intrinsic Risk Factors

Age is the most important risk factor for cardiovascular disease, which becomes progressively more common with advancing age in both men and women (Figs. 20-6 and 20-7). A reasonable hypothesis is that atherosclerosis is an age-related disease that is accelerated by the presence of other risk factors.

The male sex is another important risk factor for cardiovascular disease. Particularly in the younger age groups, men develop ischemic heart disease much more often than women.[16] Beyond the age of menopause the incidence tends to equalize, becoming similar at about the age of 70. This is because atherosclerosis increases in women after menopause.[17] The increased risk can be reduced by use of postmenopausal estrogens.[18] It is notable that the sex difference in incidence is less marked in stroke,[19] possibly because stroke tends to occur rather later in life than ischemic heart disease. The differences between the epidemiology of coronary heart disease and stroke, two complications of atherosclerosis, indicate the need for caution in extrapolating the results of studies of clinical end organ damage to disease of the arterial wall.

Genetic factors are important and may operate in two ways. Many cardiovascular risk factors are, to a greater or lesser extent, under genetic influence (e.g., hyperlipidemia).[20] However, after taking account of this, there still appears to be a genetic and familial susceptibility to premature cardiovascular disease. In the Framingham study, death due to coronary artery disease in parents was associated with a 30 percent increase in risk of coronary artery disease in siblings.[21] This association was found in men and women and was independent of the effect of other cardiovascular risk factors. Although present in those who developed coronary artery disease later than age 60 years, the effect was stronger with earlier onset of the disease.

Extrinsic Risk Factors

Cigarette smoking is totally extrinsic and the most completely preventable of all cardiovascular risk factors. Cigarette smoking is an important predisposing factor to premature cardiovascular disease, including ischemic heart disease[22] and stroke.[23] The risk increases with the number of cigarettes smoked. Cessation of smoking reduces the risk of myocardial infarction to that of those who never smoked in 2 or 3 years.[24] The mechanism by which cigarette smoking increases cardiovascular disease is not known, although some of the toxic products of cigarette smoke may act on the cells of the arterial wall, causing changes in their biological functions.[25] There is no doubt that elimination of cigarette smoking would result in a considerable increase in the health of the population.

Hypertension has a number of effects on the cardiovascular system. Hypertension itself may cause specific problems in the renal and retinal arteriolar circulation and also predisposes to Charcot-Bouchard aneurysms and intracranial hemorrhage. However, hypertension is an important risk factor for atherosclerotic cardiovascular disease, including ischemic heart disease[26] and stroke[27] (Fig. 20-8). Stroke is the most important cardiovascular complication of hypertension in terms of relative risk, although with respect to attributable risk, ischemic heart disease is numerically more important. Conversely, hypertension is the most important risk factor for stroke. Well-controlled therapeutic trials have shown that reduction of high blood pressure in people up to the age of 79 years prevents stroke but is less effective in preventing ischemic heart disease.[28]

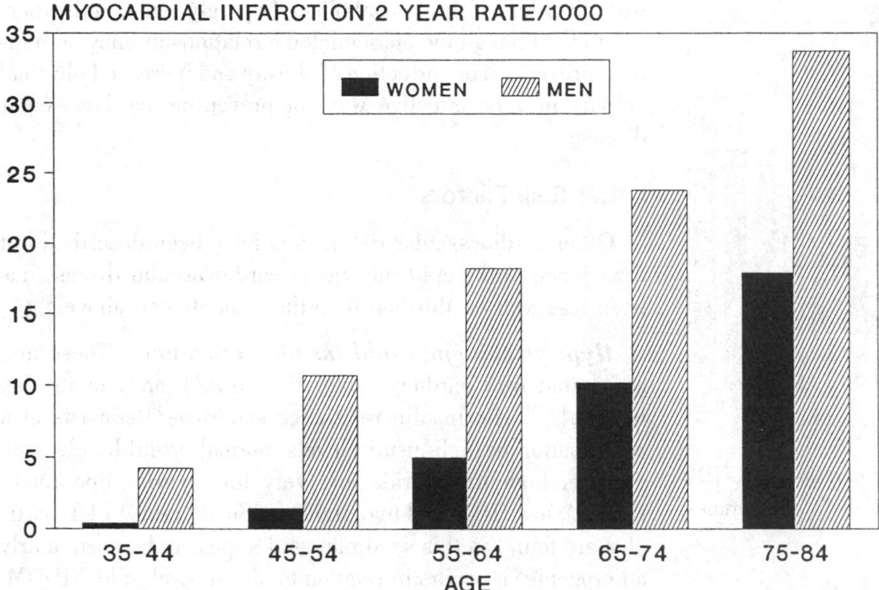

Figure 20-7 Incidence of myocardial infarction by age and sex. (From Lerner and Kannel,[16] with permission.)

Dyslipoproteinemia is a term that covers abnormal concentrations of plasma lipoproteins, including elevation of some lipoproteins (hyperlipoproteinemia) or decreased high density lipoproteins. The closest relation between lipids and cardiovascular disease is with plasma cholesterol[29,30] (Fig. 20-9). Cholesterol is carried in LDL and both cholesterol and LDL are positively correlated with the incidence of ischemic heart disease, even in old age,[31] and, to a somewhat lesser extent, with stroke[32] and peripheral vascular disease. There is an inverse relationship between the level of high density lipoprotein cholesterol (HDL) and cardiovascular disease.[33] Plasma triglyceride levels are also a risk factor for ischemic heart disease[34] and, although there has been controversy as to whether this relationship is independent of the effects of cholesterol,[35] evidence favors such a relationship.[36] Dyslipoproteinemia is related to both genetic[20] and dietary factors.[37] Lipid metabolism is discussed in more detail later in this chapter.

Diabetes mellitus is associated with an increase in the incidence of cardiovascular disease, which is present in both insulin-dependent diabetes mellitus (IDDM) and non insulin-dependent diabetes (NIDDM).[38] The atherosclerosis that occurs in diabetes is morphologically and biochemically indistinguishable from atherosclerosis in the general population and is not related to diabetic microangiopathy. Diabetes appears to confer a particularly high risk in women, so that in younger people with diabetes, the incidence of cardiovascular disease in women is equal to that in men (Fig. 20-10), while the excess risk associated with diabetes is present at least until age 75. Diabetes is the only condition in which the incidence of cardiovascular disease is the same in men and women at all ages. Diabetes is associated with other cardiovascular risk factors including dyslipoproteinemia and hypertension. However, even when these risk factors are taken into account, diabetes doubles the risk of cardiovascular disease. The risk is not

Figure 20-8 Cardiovascular mortality (per 10,000) in relation to hypertension in men and women. (From Kannel et al.,[29] with permission.)

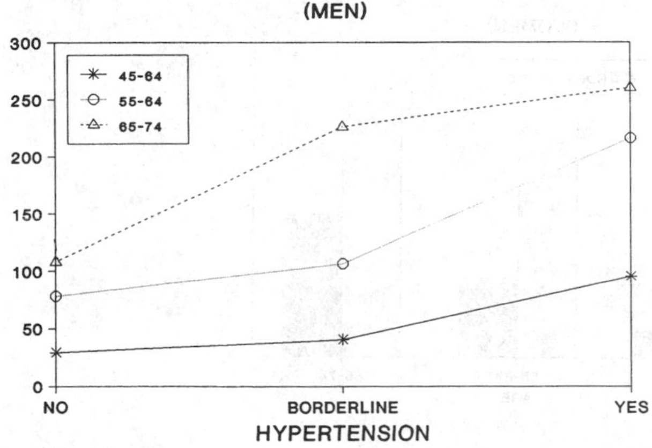

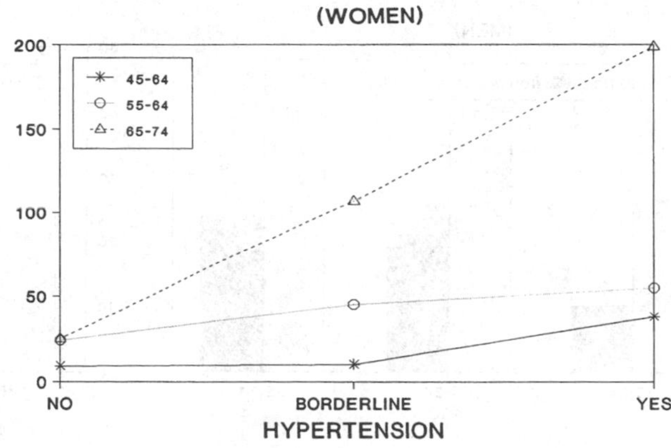

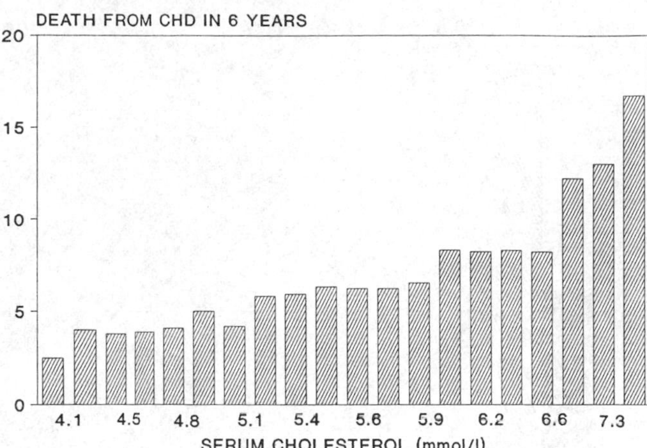

Figure 20-9 Six-year mortality from coronary heart disease (CHD) in relation to serum cholesterol. (From Martin et al.,[29] with permission.)

closely related to the blood sugar level, and currently available methods of treating diabetes do not prevent the excess frequency of cardiovascular disease.

Raised serum fibrinogen has been shown to be a risk factor for ischemic heart disease[40] and stroke.[41] Fibrinogen is involved in the coagulation process, and it seems likely that raised fibrinogen is related not only to the development of atherosclerosis but also to the thrombus, which often converts an atherosclerotic lesion into a complete occlusion of the artery.[2] Two longitudinal studies have shown that in older people, fibrinogen levels are higher in winter than in summer.[42,43] This parallels the seasonal variation in the prevalence of both fatal and nonfatal ischemic heart disease. Fibrinogen levels are influenced by a number of other factors including smoking, diet, and exercise; being an acute phase protein, fibrinogen is also influenced by inflammatory processes and other body stress.[44]

Indirect Risk Factors

There are a number of risk factors for cardiovascular disease that probably act indirectly. Prominent among these are obesity[45] and a sedentary lifestyle.[46] Both of these are associated with disorders of lipid metabolism, hyperglycemia, and hypertension. Although the epidemiologic relationship may be indirect, prevention or correction of obesity and increased physical activity may be effective ways of preventing cardiovascular disease.

Other Risk Factors

Other cardiovascular risk factors have been described but their place in the epidemiology of cardiovascular disease has been less well established than those mentioned above.[47]

Hyperinsulinemia and insulin resistance These are associated with cardiovascular disease and many of its risk factors.[48,49] The insulin resistance syndrome[49] consists of a combination of high insulin levels, normal or mildly elevated glucose, high triglyceride and very low density lipoprotein (VLDL), low HDL, and hypertension. Small, dense LDL particles are found in this syndrome and appear to be particularly atherogenic. It occurs in relation to obesity and mild NIDDM, but may be present in the absence of either. Although many people with cardiovascular disease have several or all of the components of the insulin resistance syndrome, prospective epidemiologic studies have shown that high insulin levels are independently associated with the development of ischemic heart disease.[48] As well as its effects on other risk factors, insulin has direct effects on the arterial wall, promoting smooth muscle cell proliferation and lipid accumulation. Hyperinsulinemia and insulin resistance may be corrected by avoiding obesity and by regular physical exercise.

Hemostatic factors As well as fibrinogen, a number of other factors that predispose to thrombosis have been associated with ischemic heart disease. Coagulation factor VII,[40] tissue plasminogen activator inhibitor (which inhibits fibrinolysis),[50] and activated protein C resistance (which promotes thrombosis)[51] have all been associated with coronary heart disease or other thrombotic disorders. Elevated white cell count has also been associated with coronary heart disease.[52] The exact role of these factors in atherosclerosis remains to be determined, as does their relation to aging.[53] They emphasize the fact that the classic risk factors for atheroscler-

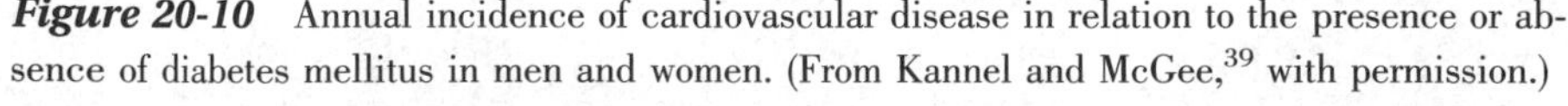
Figure 20-10 Annual incidence of cardiovascular disease in relation to the presence or absence of diabetes mellitus in men and women. (From Kannel and McGee,[39] with permission.)

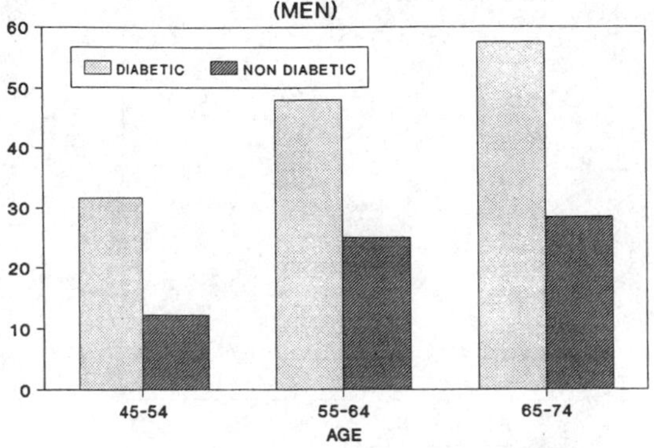

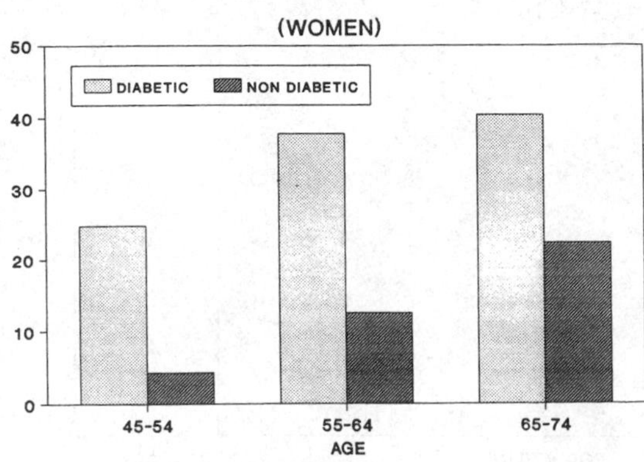

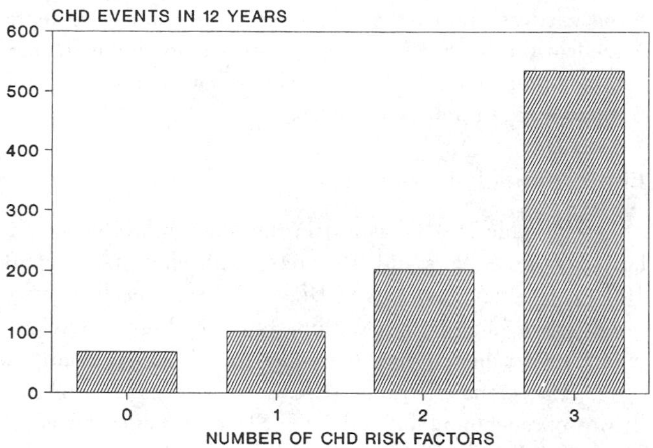

Figure 20-11 Annual incidence of coronary heart disease in relation to number of risk factors present. The risk factors are cigarette smoking, hypertension, and hypercholesterolemia. (From Kannel et al.,[54] with permission.)

sis—hypertension, smoking, and hypercholesterolemia—account for only a minority of cases of myocardial infarction and that the search for other factors must continue.

Hyperuricemia This may be related to ischemic heart disease simply as a by-product of lipid and carbohydrate metabolism, and there is no evidence that it is directly pathogenic.[47]

Soft water This has been suggested to be related to cardiovascular disease.[47] However, deficiency of trace elements in water may relate more to myocardial function than to atherosclerosis.

Multiple Risk Factors

Many patients have more than one risk factor for atherosclerosis. Often these are metabolically related—for example, obesity and diabetes, dyslipidemia and hypertension[49]—but some are unrelated, for example, cigarette smoking and other risk factors. Multiple risk factors act synergistically, the combined risk being greater than the sum of the individual risks[54] (Fig. 20-11). There have been several studies of intervention on multiple risk factors, including the Multiple Risk Factors Intervention Trial[55] in the United States and studies in Finland.[56,57] Unfortunately, these studies have not shown the expected beneficial results, apparently because the control group has also modified its behavior and hence, differences between study and control groups have not been apparent.

Evidence is accumulating that the predisposition to ischemic heart disease and stroke, and to many of their risk factors including changes in blood pressure and circulating lipids, diabetes, and insulin resistance, are determined in very early life—before, during or soon after birth.[58] Fetal and neonatal nutrition seem to 'programe' the individual for the future development of serious and life-threatening conditions. The possibility that health in old age is influenced by events around the time of birth is a new challenge to preventive gerontology.

Other Epidemiologic Findings

Geographic patterns of cardiovascular disease provide information on predisposing factors.[59] Migrant populations are very interesting to study in this respect. Coronary heart disease is particularly common in people who have originated from the Indian subcontinent and migrated to various parts of the world. The high rates cannot be explained by hypertension, smoking, or high serum cholesterol, but appear to be associated with low plasma HDL levels, high plasma triglyceride levels, and a high prevalence of NIDDM and hyperinsulinemia, suggesting a state of insulin resistance.[60]

One of the striking features of the epidemiology of atherosclerosis has been the decline in mortality rates from coronary heart disease that has occurred, particularly in the United States, since 1968.[61] Different countries have experienced different changes in coronary heart disease mortality over this time period.[62] It is not known whether the decline in mortality is due to a reduction in the case-fatality rate, resulting from better treatment of the patient with coronary heart disease, or whether there has been a reduction in the incidence of the disease. It seems likely that both mechanisms have contributed to the decline in mortality.[63] A decline in incidence may have resulted from modification of risk factors such as cigarette smoking, hypertension, and hypercholesterolemia. If so, it supports population-based strategies for health promotion. Mortality from stroke has also declined but the fall started earlier,[64] probably reflecting treatment of hypertension, or the decline in smoking.

Epidemiologic studies in which changes in plasma cholesterol levels or blood pressure have been related to changes in mortality from coronary heart disease have suggested that there is an 'incubation period' of at least 10 years between exposure to risk factors and the effects on mortality.[65] Studies in patients with diabetes have shown that atherosclerosis starts at the same time in patients with and without diabetes but progresses more rapidly in those with diabetes.[66] This suggests that the initiation and progression of atherosclerosis may be influenced by different factors.

Lipid Metabolism

Lipids

The major lipids of the circulation are cholesterol and fatty acids. Cholesterol is an essential structural component of cell membranes and a precursor of steroid hormones, bile acids, and other important molecules. Cholesterol is derived both from dietary animal fat, and from synthesis in the liver, although most tissues have the capacity to synthesize cholesterol. Fatty acids are the major energy source of the body and circulate either unesterified (free fatty acids), or as components of triglycerides, phospholipids, or cholesteryl esters. Fatty acids may be ingested in the diet or synthesized in the liver.

As lipids are insoluble in water, they circulate in lipid-protein complexes. Free fatty acids are loosely complexed with albumin, while cholesterol, cholesteryl esters, triglycerides, and phospholipids circulate in association with specific peptides (apolipoproteins) as macromolecular complexes, the lipoproteins. These systems transport cholesterol and fatty acids to the peripheral tissues and return cholesterol to the liver, where it is converted to bile acids and excreted, or repackaged into other lipoproteins.

Lipoproteins

The following lipoproteins occur in the circulation, in increasing order of density and decreasing order of size.

Chylomicrons are the largest lipoproteins and consist of triglyceride and cholesterol of dietary origin, and apolipoproteins (apo) B-48, E, and C-II. Normally, chylomicrons are cleared from the circulation within 4 hours of a meal by hydrolysis of triglyceride by the enzyme lipoprotein lipase; the resulting chylomicron remnants are present only transiently in the circulation and are taken up and metabolized by the liver.

Very low density lipoproteins are the main carriers of endogenously synthesized triglyceride. They also contain cholesterol, cholesteryl ester, phospholipids, and apolipoproteins B-100, C-II, and E. The triglyceride is hydrolyzed in capillaries by the enzyme lipoprotein lipase to create intermediate density lipoproteins (IDL), which are normally present only transiently in the circulation before being taken up by the liver.

Low density lipoproteins are the main carriers of cholesterol in the circulation. They also contain small amounts of triglyceride and phospholipids and apolipoprotein B-100.

High density lipoproteins contain nearly equal amounts of cholesterol and protein—apolipoproteins A-I and A-II. Two subclasses of HDL, HDL2 and HDL3, predominate in the circulation.

Lipid Metabolism

Lipid metabolism may be conveniently considered as occurring in three pathways: the exogenous lipid pathway, the endogenous lipid pathway, and reverse cholesterol transport.[67]

Exogenous fat transport

The majority of lipid that is ingested in the diet is triglyceride, although cholesterol is also taken in. Triglyceride is broken down in the gastrointestinal tract by lipases, reassembled in the intestinal epithelium, and absorbed into the lacteals, where it is complexed with cholesterol, also absorbed from the diet, and apoB-48, apoA-I, and apoA-IV to form chylomicrons.

In the circulation, chylomicrons acquire apoE and apoC-II, which is a cofactor for lipoprotein lipase. After a meal, particularly one containing fat, the triglyceride level in the blood greatly increases, and blood that is allowed to stand has a creamy layer representing the absorbed lipid. It is usually cleared in about 4 hours by the activity of the enzyme lipoprotein lipase, which is secreted from endothelial cells in adipose tissue capillaries and which hydrolyzes chylomicron triglyceride to fatty acids that are taken up by adipose cells and stored to be used as energy. The chylomicron remnants are reprocessed in the liver, which has specific chylomicron remnant cell membrane receptors. Hepatic lipase has an important role in remodelling remnant particles.

Endogenous Fat Transport

Triglyceride is synthesized in the liver from glucose and fatty acid precursors and is secreted with cholesterol, apoB-100, apoC-II, and apo-E as VLDL. VLDL triglyceride is hydrolyzed by the same lipoprotein lipase that hydrolyzes chylomicron triglyceride and the released fatty acids stored in adipose tissue. The remnant particles (IDL) are reprocessed in the liver by way of receptors that bind apoE. Some are cleared from the plasma while others are reformed into LDL. LDL is the main cholesterol-carrying lipoprotein and is cleared predominantly by the liver by way of the LDL receptor, which recognizes apoB-100.[68] LDL receptors are also present in most of the cells of the body. Interaction of LDL with its receptor results in internalization of the lipoprotein receptor complex (Fig. 20-12). This triggers a number of intracellular biochemical processes, which include catabolism of the lipoprotein in the lysosomes, inhibition of the activity of the enzyme hydroxymethyl glutyryl coenzyme A (HMG-CoA) reductase, the rate-limiting enzyme in the cholesterol synthetic pathway, and inhibition of further LDL interaction with cell membrane receptors. In this way, cellular cholesterol synthesis is finely regulated.

Reverse cholesterol transport

High density lipoprotein is responsible for reverse cholesterol transport, removing cholesterol from the tissues, and delivering it to the liver for reprocessing into other lipoproteins or for elimination by conversion to bile acids. Nascent HDL, secreted by the liver and the intestine, attracts material from the breakdown of chylomicrons and VLDL, and cholesterol from cells. The cholesterol is esterified by the enzyme lecithin cholesterol acyltransferase (LCAT), which uses apoA-I, present in nascent, HDL, as a cofactor. With incorporation of cholesteryl ester, HDL becomes larger and less dense, changing from HDL3 to HDL2. Some of the cholesterol of HDL2 is transferred to VLDL, IDL, and LDL by means of a cholesterol ester transfer protein (CETP). By this means, cholesterol is transported to the liver and can be eliminated from the body.

Control of lipid metabolism

Lipid metabolism is subject to many inherited and acquired disorders. Genetic disorders of most of the proteins involved in fat transport, the apolipoproteins, the cell membrane receptors, and the enzymes, have been described.[67] Many of the metabolic processes are influenced by hormones, particularly insulin but also thyroxine, corticosteroids, and catecholamines. Thus, conditions such as diabetes mellitus, obesity, hypothyroidism, and steroid therapy are associated with lipid abnormalities.[69]

Lipid and lipoprotein levels vary throughout the lifespan[70]

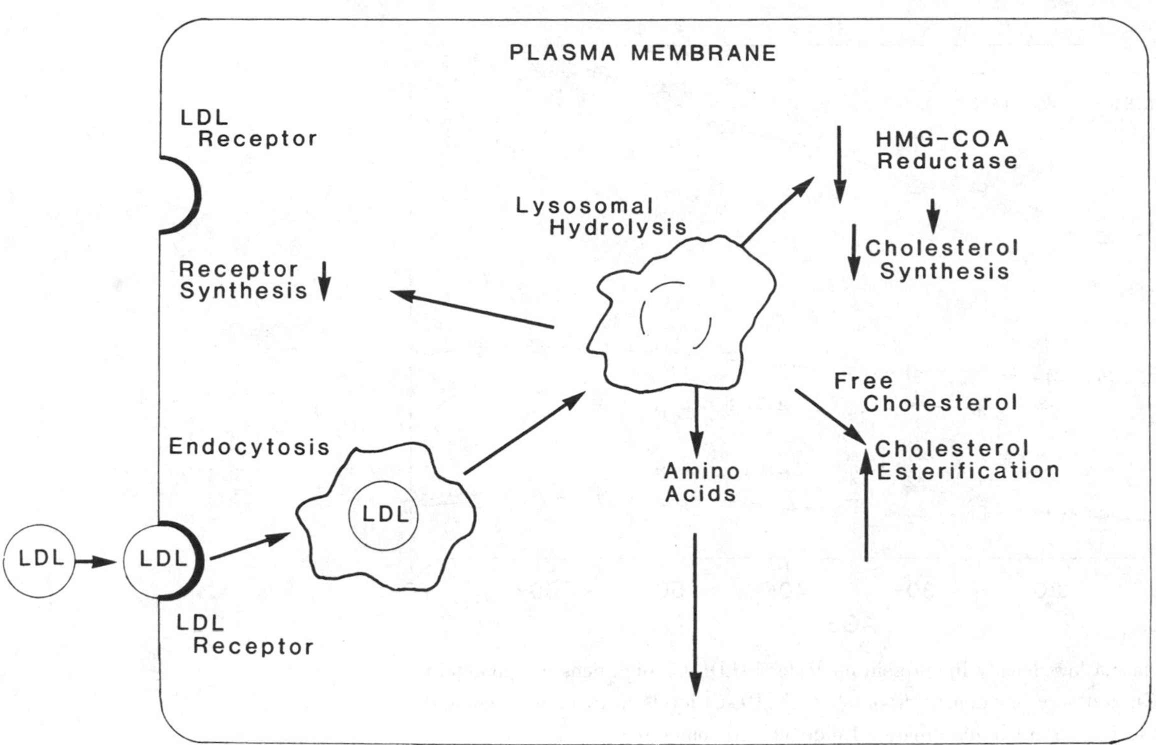

Figure 20-12 The low density lipoprotein receptor pathway. See text for details. (Adapted from Brown and Goldstein,[68] with permission.)

(Figs 20-13 and 20-14) in a way that parallels the incidence of atherosclerosis up to the age of about 50 years. The reduction in the rate of increase of lipids and lipoproteins after the age of 50 and the reduction in levels in old people[71] may be due to the phenomenon of exhaustion of susceptibles (i.e., those with high levels do not survive into old age), rather than a biologic age change. High HDL levels have been described in families with members of exceptional longevity,[72] although this has not been described in all studies.[73]

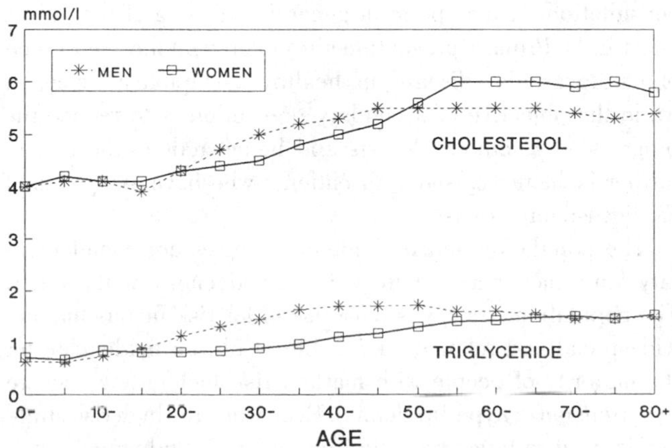

Figure 20-13 Plasma cholesterol and triglyceride levels in relation to age and sex. (Data from Lipid Research Clinics Program Epidemiology Committee.[70])

Lipids and Atherosclerosis

Cholesterol and low density lipoproteins

The combined weight of evidence from epidemiology, experimental pathology, cell biology, and intervention studies[74] leaves no doubt that cholesterol has a role in the development of coronary heart disease. There is inconsistent evidence that cholesterol is related to coronary heart disease in elderly people[75–77] The strength, consistency, and graded nature of the relation between serum cholesterol and coronary heart disease mortality makes a causal link very likely.[78] There is no association of total cholesterol levels with stroke[79]; it is possible, however, that studies of all strokes conceal different associations with ischemic strokes and hemorrhagic strokes. Cholesterol-lowering trials show that the prevention of coronary heart disease depends on the magnitude and duration of cholesterol reduction, not on the way it is achieved. Overviews of clinical trials on cholesterol lowering, by diet or drugs, have shown a consistent relationship between the reduction in plasma cholesterol and the reduction in coronary heart disease risk and the percent reduction in coronary risk is similar to that predicted from epidemiologic studies.

High density lipoproteins

Clinical and epidemiologic studies have shown an inverse relationship between HDL and coronary disease,[80,81] and it has been suggested that HDL has a protective role in atherogenesis.[82] The inverse relationship between HDL cholesterol

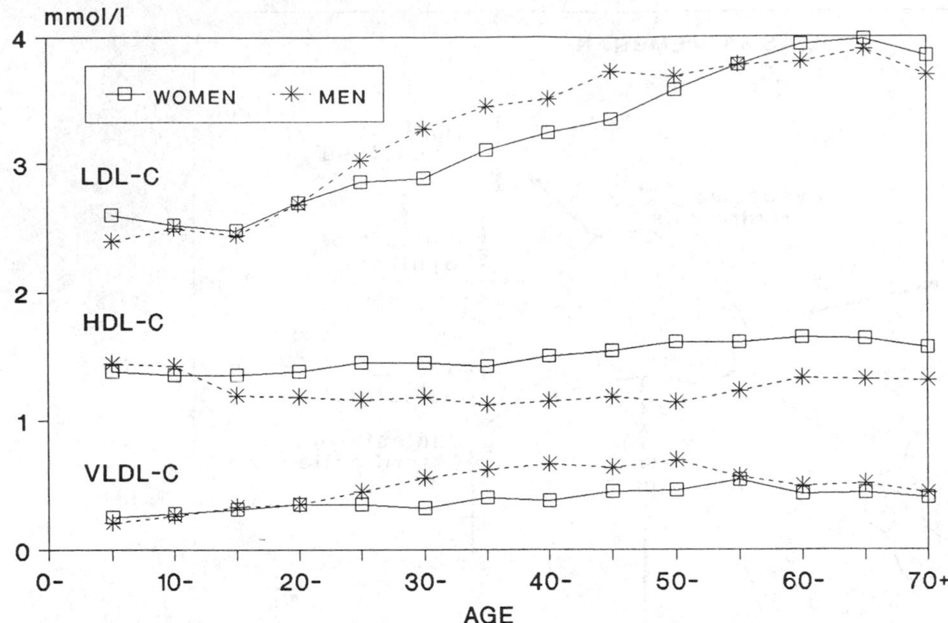

Figure 20-14 Plasma low density lipoprotein cholesterol (LDL-C), high density lipoprotein cholesterol (HDL-C), and very low density lipoprotein (VLDL-C) levels in relation to age and sex. (Data from Lipid Research Clinics Program Epidemiology Committee.[70])

and coronary heart disease mortality has been confirmed in elderly men[75,83] and women[83] but has also been refuted.[76] The mechanisms by which HDL levels are related to coronary heart disease remain unknown.

There is a decrement of 2 to 3 percent in coronary risk for each increment of 0.026 mmol/L in HDL cholesterol in men.[33] The ratio is slightly greater in women and does not decline with age. A reduction in the incidence of coronary heart disease and a simultaneous rise in HDL levels have been found in some clinical trials, but there has been no clinical trial designed specifically to test the effect of raising HDL levels, nor are there any drugs that increase HDL levels without affecting other lipoproteins.

Prevention of Atherosclerosis

Prevention of Cardiovascular Disease

Atherosclerosis is a universal condition closely related to aging and it is unlikely that it can be totally prevented. Slowing the progression of atherosclerosis with prevention or delay in its effects on the cardiovascular system is, therefore, the aim. Regression of atherosclerosis may also be possible. Regression has been described in experimental atherosclerosis in animals[84] and in wasting diseases in humans[85] and the results of angiographic studies in humans are consistent with regression of lesions in patients intensively treated with lipid lowering drugs.[86,87]

There are two possible strategies for prevention by risk factor reduction.[88,89] The *population strategy* is based on the realization that most cardiovascular disease results from the exposure of many people to moderately elevated levels of risk factors. This strategy, therefore, seeks to change people's behavior toward a healthier lifestyle by promoting, for example, healthy diets, exercise, and nonsmoking in the whole population. The *individual* or *`high risk' strategy* seeks to identify the relatively small number of people within the population who are at particularly high risk of cardiovascular disease. Those at high risk include people with a family history of cardiovascular disease occurring at an early age and those who have cardiovascular risk factors. The individual strategy may target risk factor assessment on people likely to have positive findings (selective screening); may use opportunistic screening by including an assessment of risk factors in the normal clinical consultation, or may perform general screening of the public (see Ch. 1). Primary prevention aims to prevent the occurrence of cardiovascular disease in healthy asymptomatic people, while the objective of secondary prevention is to reduce the progression of atherosclerosis and hence reduce the risk of further ischemic episodes in patients who have symptoms of cardiovascular disease.

The population and individual strategies are complementary, and each may enhance the effectiveness of the other. The population strategy is most useful for risk factors that are widespread and relatively mild, but would be inadequate for the minority of people with marked risk factors (e.g., severe hypertension or hyperlipidemia). Even when the high risk strategy is used to target specific risk factors in individuals, it is essential that the general burden of risk is addressed by changes in lifestyle.

One of the problems of assigning targets for risk-factor

modification is the fact that the relation between most of the risk factors and cardiovascular disease is continuous and linear or curvilinear. Thus, the definition of any target or 'normal' level is arbitrary. The synergistic effects of multiple risk factors must also be considered and any strategy must assess all risk factors, while assigning priority to the most important or the most readily modified. For example, in a cigarette smoker with diabetes, the importance of stopping smoking is overwhelming.

A number of trials have been carried out in order to try and prevent or delay the process of atherosclerosis. Those targeting lipids will be considered here; those involving other risk factors are described elsewhere in this book.

Lipid Metabolism

Two important prevention studies using the most effective means of reducing serum cholesterol levels, the HMG-CoA reductase inhibitors, have clarified the role of cholesterol lowering in the prevention of coronary heart disease. In the Scandinavian Simvastatin Survival Study (4S),[90] 4444 men and women aged 35 to 70 years with angina pectoris or previous myocardial infarction and serum cholesterol 5.5 to 8.0 mmol/L (212 to 309 mg/dl) on a lipid lowering diet were randomly allocated to double-blind treatment with simvastatin or placebo. The simvastatin group showed a marked reduction in death (relative risk 0.76), coronary death (relative risk 0.58), major coronary events (relative risk 0.66), and nonfatal myocardial infarction (relative risk 0.63). In the simvastatin group, total and LDL cholesterol were reduced by 25 percent and 35 percent respectively and HDL cholesterol increased by 8 percent. Side effects were few. The effect of simvastatin in reducing the risk of new coronary events was independent of the baseline total LDL and HDL cholesterol levels.[91] This study is important in showing an increase in survival without any suggestion of an increase in noncardiovascular deaths. It is also the first trial to show that cholesterol lowering reduces major coronary events in women and the first to show that it improves survival in older patients. The West of Scotland Coronary Prevention Study[92] looked at the effect of pravastatin, another HMG CoA reductase inhibitor, on coronary events and survival in 6,595 middle-aged men with mild hypercholesterolemia (cholesterol 7.0 ± 0.6 mmol/L) and no evidence of coronary disease. The treated group had a reduction in cholesterol levels of 20 percent and LDL cholesterol levels of 26 percent with a small reduction in triglycerides and a 5 percent increase in HDL cholesterol. Over a 5-year period, coronary events were reduced by one-third, as were coronary deaths, and there was a 22 percent reduction in overall mortality. There was no increase in noncardiovascular deaths and few adverse effects. These trials, together with earlier studies using other means of reducing cholesterol levels,[93–96] leave no doubt that reducing cholesterol levels reduces the incidence of coronary heart disease. They suggest that for every 1 percent reduction in cholesterol level, there is a 2 to 5 percent reduction in coronary heart disease incidence (the older the subjects, the lower the benefit), and the full effect of the reduction in risk is achieved by 5 years.[97] It seems likely that the reduction in clinical coronary heart disease associated with lipid lowering therapy results from depletion of cholesterol from the core of the atheromatous lesion and a decrease in the number of lipid-laden macrophage-derived foam cells.[87] In this way, the relatively small number of fatty lesions are stabilized, preventing fissuring and thrombosis.

The two most recent trials, together with evidence that cholesterol lowering slows the progression of atheromatous lesions or even results in their regression[86,87,98] provide convincing evidence in favor of attempting to reduce serum cholesterol levels. It is difficult to know how widely to extrapolate the results of trials, which use highly selected subjects, to the population as a whole and in particular to groups outside those studied. Women and elderly people tend to be excluded from trials on both treatment and prevention of heart disease.[99] There have been no published trials of primary prevention of cardiovascular disease in older people, and none of any prevention in people over 70 years old. Nevertheless, taking the results of all the studies, it would be difficult to argue that any age-sex group would not benefit from lowering elevated cholesterol levels. A concern that arose from some earlier studies, that a reduction in cardiovascular deaths was accompanied by an increase in deaths from noncardiovascular causes such as cancer[100] or violence, has not been a feature of more recent trials.[90,92,101]

A task force of the European Society of Cardiology, the European Atherosclerosis Society, and the European Society of Hypertension[89] and the United States National Cholesterol Education Program[102] suggest that the goal of lipid-lowering therapy should be to achieve plasma cholesterol concentrations of less than 5 mmol/L or 200 mg/dl. For those whose levels are between 5 and 6 mmol/L dietary advice and counseling on other risk factors should be given. Patients with levels between 6 and 7 mmol/L need more intensive dietary and general risk factor advice. If the cholesterol level is between 7 and 8 mmol/L, fasting lipids should be checked and secondary hyperlipidemia excluded. Intensive nutritional advice is indicated, and if this does not lead to a substantial reduction in plasma cholesterol over 3 to 6 months, drug treatment should be considered if the overall risk of cardiovascular disease is high. For those with cholesterol levels more than 8 mmol/L, full investigations of lipids, a search for causes of secondary hyperlipidemia, and consideration of familial hyperlipidemia are indicated. If intensive dietary advice does not reduce the plasma cholesterol to below 7 mmol/L (270 mg/dl) in 3 to 6 months, drug treatment should be considered. The most common causes of secondary hyperlipidemia are obesity, alcoholism, hypothyroidism, diabetes, and renal and hepatic disease. In considering the need for treatment, the presence of other risk factors, including existing cardiovascular disease, and the lipoprotein profile are taken into account. The diet should have less than 30 percent of daily food energy intake from fat with saturated fat contributing less than 10 percent of the total, less than 300 mg of cholesterol per day, and should contain foods rich in soluble fiber. Mild hypertriglyceridemia (3.0–6.0 mmol/L, 250–500 mg/dl) usually responds to weight reduction and decreased alcohol consumption; drugs may be used if this is not effective. Very high triglyceride levels (more than 6 mmol/L, 500 mg/dl) are associated with an increased risk of pancreatitis and should be vigorously treated with diet and drugs.

The choice of drug depends on the type of lipid disorder.[103] For hypercholesterolemia, the choice lies between the well-tested bile acid-sequestrating agents, such as cholestyramine, which may be difficult to take, or the HMG CoA reductase inhibitors, which are easy to take, effective, and to date, relatively free of adverse effects. Other drugs that may be used include nicotinic acid and fibric acid derivatives such as gemfribrozil, both of which have been shown to be effective in preventing coronary heart disease in long-term trials. Because of their relative freedom from adverse effects and proven effectiveness, the HMG CoA reductase inhibitors are the drugs of choice. The only reservation about this class of drugs is that they may not have been in use for long enough for long-term adverse effects to be apparent.

Another approach to the treatment of dyslipoproteinemia is to use long-chain polyunsaturated omega-3 fatty acids present in fish oil (e.g., Maxepa). These reduce serum triglycerides and raise HDL, and also inhibit the clotting process. However, they may raise cholesterol and LDL levels and increase blood glucose. There have been no reported studies of the effect of fish oils on cardiovascular disease, and their place in the management of lipid disorders remains to be decided.

Should hypercholesterolemia be sought and treated in elderly people?

It is not possible to give a definitive answer to this question, as the data on which a decision could be based are not available. There is some evidence, reviewed earlier, that cholesterol remains a risk factor for cardiovascular disease in old age. The potential for prevention is greatest in old age, since the incidence of cardiovascular disease increases with age, and postponement of a myocardial infarction, stroke, or amputation for even a few years would have major benefits on the lives of elderly people. However, it is possible that those who survive into old age with high cholesterol levels are protected in some way from their harmful effects. Although lipid-lowering treatment by diet or drugs seems to be as effective in older as in younger people,[104–106] none of the trials has studied people over the age of 70 years. A pragmatic approach should, therefore, be taken. After a full assessment of the patient's physical, mental, and functional states and measurement of cardiovascular risk factors, a decision on the benefits and risks of treatment can be taken. An independent healthy person with significant hypercholesterolemia may be offered treatment. This should first consist of advice on weight, exercise, diet, and smoking. There is no contraindication to a low fat, low cholesterol diet in older people. If, after adherence to this advice, cholesterol levels remain high, drug treatment may be instituted. If this approach is used, the need for drug treatment of hypercholesterolemia in old age will be rare.

Other Risk Factors

The beneficial effects of cessation of cigarette smoking are incontrovertible.

Hypertension is considered elsewhere in this book. Many studies, including one in elderly subjects,[28] have shown beneficial effects of treating hypertension on a number of fatal and nonfatal manifestations of cardiovascular disease.

There is no evidence that currently available methods of treating diabetes are effective in reducing the large vessel complications.[38] There are, of course, other benefits from controlling hyperglycemia. More attention is now being paid to control of other risk factors such as cigarette smoking, hypertension, and hyperlipidemia in diabetes in an attempt to reduce the cardiovascular complications.

Avoidance of obesity, and regular physical exercise have beneficial effects on several risk factors, and can be recommended as general health measures.

A different approach to prevention is to modify hemostatic function. Aspirin permanently inhibits cyclooxygenase-dependent platelet aggregation, and has been shown to be effective in the secondary prevention of cardiovascular disease.[107] Whether aspirin acts by reducing the progression of atheromatous lesions or by inhibiting thrombus formation on the lesions remains to be determined.

Conclusion

The burden of atherosclerosis in old age will increase as the aged population increases. Although there have been many advances in the treatment of cardiovascular disease, and many of these can be and are being used in elderly patients, they do not address the fundamental problem—atherosclerosis. Prevention of atherosclerosis requires a healthy lifestyle throughout the life span. Successful efforts at health promotion in younger people will not only result in increased survival but also a healthier old age.

References

1. Ross R: The pathogenesis of atherosclerosis: a perspective for the 1990s. Nature 1993;362:801–809
2. Fuster V, Badimon L, Badimon JJ, Chesebro JH: The pathogenesis of coronary artery disease and the acute coronary syndromes. N Engl J Med 1992;326:242–250:310–318
3. Pearson TA, Dillman JM, Solez K, Heptinstall RH: Clonal markers in the study of the origin and growth of human atherosclerotic lesions. Circulation Research 1978;43:10–18
4. Pearson TA, Dillman JM, Solez K, Heptinstall RH: Evidence for two populations of fatty streaks with different roles in the atherogenic process. Lancet 1980;ii:496–498
5. Schwartz CJ, Kelley JL, Nerem RM et al: Pathophysiology of the atherogenic process. Am J Cardiol 1989;64:23G–30G
6. Steinberg D, Parthasarathy S, Carew TE et al: Beyond choles-

terol: modifications of low-density lipoprotein that increase its atherogenicity. N Engl J Med 1989;320:915–924

7. Witztum JL: The oxidation hypothesis of atherosclerosis. Lancet 1994;344:793–795
8. Carew TE: Role of biologically modified low-density lipoprotein in atherosclerosis. Am J Cardiol 1989;64:18G–22G
9. Carew TE, Schwenke DC, Steinberg D: Antiatherogenic effect of probucol unrelated to its hypocholesterolemic effect: Evidence that antioxidants in vivo can selectively inhibit low density lipoprotein degradation in macrophage-rich fatty streaks and slow the progression of atherosclerosis in the Watanabe heritable hyperlipidemic rabbit. Proc Natl Acad Sci USA 1987;84:7725–7729
10. Stout RW: Hormone-endothelial interactions. pp. 301–312. In Cryer A (ed): Biochemical interactions at the endothelium. Elsevier Science Publishers, 1983
11. Mazzone T, Jensen M, Chait A: Human arterial wall cells secrete factors that are chemotactic for monocytes. Proc Natl Acad Sci USA 1983;80:5094–5097
12. Faggiotto A, Ross R: Studies of hypercholesterolemia in the nonhuman primate. II. Fatty streak conversion to fibrous plaque. Arteriosclerosis 1984;4:341–356
13. Stout RW, Bierman EL, Ross R: Effect of insulin on the proliferation of cultured primate arterial smooth muscle cells. Circulation Res 1975;36:319–327
14. Stout RW: Ageing and atherosclerosis. Age Ageing 1987;16: 65 72
15. Enos WF, Holmes RH, Beyer J: Coronary disease among United States soldiers killed in action in Korea. JAMA 1953; 152:1090–1093
16. Lerner DJ, Kannel WB: Patterns of coronary heart disease morbidity and mortality in the sexes: a 26-year follow-up of the Framingham population. Am Heart J 1986;111:383–390
17. Witteman JCM, Grobbee DE, Kok FJ et al: Increased risk of atherosclerosis in women after the menopause. BMJ 1989; 298:642–644
18. Sullivan JM, Vander Zwaag R, Lemp GF, et al: Postmenopausal estrogen use and coronary atherosclerosis. Ann Int Med 1988;108:358–363
19. Bamford J, Sandercock P, Dennis M et al: A prospective study of acute cerebrovascular disease in the community: the Oxfordshire Community Stroke Project 1981–86. I. Methodology, demography and incident cases of first-ever stroke. J Neurol Neurosurg Psychiatr 1988;51:1373–1380
20. Goldstein JL, Hazzard WR, Schrott HG, et al: Hyperlipidemia in coronary heart disease. 2. Genetic analysis of lipid levels in 176 families and delineation of a new inherited disorder, combined hyperlipidemia. J Clin Invest 1973;52:1544–1568
21. Schildkraut JM, Myers RH, Cupples LA, et al: Coronary risk associated with age and sex of parental heart disease in the Framingham Study. Am J Cardiol 1989;64:555–559
22. Fuller JH, Shipley MJ, Rose G et al: Mortality from coronary heart disease and stroke in relation to degree of glycaemia: the Whitehall study. BMJ 1983;287:867–870
23. Gill JS, Shipley MJ, Tsementzis SA et al: Cigarette smoking. A risk factor for hemorrhagic and nonhemorrhagic stroke. Arch Intern Med 1989;149:2053–2057
24. Rosenberg L, Palmer JR, Shapiro S: Decline in the risk of myocardial infarction among women who stop smoking. N Engl J Med 1990;322:213–217
25. Albers JJ, Bierman EL: The effect of hypoxia on uptake and degradation of low density lipoproteins by cultured human arterial smooth muscle cells. Biochem Biophys Acta 1976; 424:422–429
26. Kannel WB, Gordon T, Schwartz MJ: Systolic versus diastolic blood pressure and risk of coronary heart disease. The Framingham study. Am J Cardiol 1971;27:345–355
27. Kannel WB, Dawber TR, Sorlie P, Wolf PA: Components of blood pressure and risk of atherothrombotic brain infarction: The Framingham Study. Stroke 1976;7:327–331
28. Amery A, Birkenhager W, Brixko P et al: Mortality and morbidity results from the European Working Party on High Blood Pressure in the Elderly Trial. Lancet 1985;1:1349–1354
29. Martin MJ, Hulley SB, Browner WS et al: Serum cholesterol, blood pressure, and mortality: implications from a cohort of 361, 662 men. Lancet 1986;ii:933–936
30. Stamler J, Wentworth D, Neaton JD, for the MRFIT Research Group: Is the relationship between serum cholesterol and risk of premature death from coronary heart disease continuous and graded? Findings in 356,222 primary screenees of the Multiple Risk Factor Intervention Trial (MRFIT). JAMA 1986; 256:2823–2828
31. Castelli WP: Cholesterol and lipids in the risk of coronary artery disease—The Framingham Heart Study. Can J Cardiol 1988;4(suppl A):5A–10A
32. Iso H, Jacobs DR Jr, Wentworth D et al: Serum cholesterol levels and six-year mortality from stroke in 350,977 men screened for the multiple risk factors intervention trial. N Engl J Med 1989;320:904–910
33. Gordon DJ, Rifkind BM: High-density-lipoprotein—The clinical implications of recent studies. N Engl J Med 1989;321: 1311–1316
34. Carlson LA, Bottiger LE: Ischaemic heart-disease in relation to fasting values of plasma triglycerides and cholesterol. Stockholm prospective study 1972; Lancet i:865–868
35. Castelli WP: The triglyceride issue: A view from Framingham. Am Heart J 1986;112:432–437
36. Cambien F, Jacqueson A, Richard JL et al: Is the level of serum triglyceride a significant predictor of coronary death in 'normocholesterolemic' subjects? Am J Epidemiol 1986;124: 624–632
37. Kushi LH, Lew RA, Stare FJ et al: Diet and 20-year mortality from coronary heart disease. The Ireland-Boston-Diet-Heart-Study. N Engl J Med 1985;312:811–818
38. Stout RW (ed): Diabetes and Atheroslerosis. Kluwer, Dordrecht, 1992
39. Kannel WB, McGee DL: Diabetes and cardiovascular risk factors: The Framingham Study. Circulation 1979;59:8–13
40. Meade TW, Mellows S, Brozovic M et al: Haemostatic function and ischaemic heart disease: principal results of the Northwick Park Heart Study. 1986; Lancet ii:533–537
41. Kannel WB, Wolf PA, Castelli WP, D'Agostino RB: Fibrinogen and risk of cardiovascular disease. The Framingham Study. JAMA 1987;258:1183–1186
42. Stout RW, Crawford V: Seasonal variations in fibrinogen concentrations among elderly people. Lancet 1991;338:9–13

43. Woodhouse PR, Khaw KT, Plummer M et al: Seasonal variations of plasma fibrinogen and factor VII activity in the elderly: winter infections and death from cardiovascular disease. Lancet 1994;343:435–439
44. Ernst E, Resch KL: Fibrinogen as a cardiovascular risk factor: a meta-analysis and review of the literature. Ann Intern Med 1993;118:956–963
45. Hubert HB, Feinleib M, McNamara PM, Castelli WP: Obesity as an independent risk factor for cardiovascular disease: a 26 year follow-up of participants in the Framingham heart study. Circulation 1983;67:968–977
46. Morris JN, Chave SPW, Adam C et al: Vigorous exercise in leisure-time and the incidence of coronary heart-disease. Lancet 1973;i:333–339
47. Hopkins PN, Williams RR: A survey of 246 suggested coronary risk factors. Atherosclerosis 1980;40:1–52
48. Stout RW: Insulin and atheroma. 20-yr perspective. Diabetes Care 1990;13:631–655
49. Reaven GM: Role of insulin resistance in human disease. Diabetes 1988;37:1595–1607
50. Thompson SG, Kienast J, Pyke SDM et al. for the European Concerted Action on Thrombosis and Disabilities Angina Pectoris Study Group: Hemostatic factors and the risk of myocardial infarction or sudden death in patients with angina pectoris. N Engl J Med 1995;332:635–641
51. Ridker PM, Hennekens CH, Lindpaintner K et al: Mutation in the gene coding for coagulation factor V and the risk of myocardial infarction, stroke and venous thrombosis in apparently healthy men. N Engl J Med 1995;332:912–917
52. Kannel WB, Anderson K, Wilson PWF: White blood cell count and cardiovascular disease. Insights from the Framingham Study. JAMA 1992;267:1253–1256
53. Stout RW, Crawford VLS, McDermott MJ, et al: Seasonal changes in haemostatic factors in young and elderly subjects. Age Ageing 1996;25:256–258
54. Kannel WB, Doyle JT, Ostfeld AM et al: Optimal resources for primary prevention of atherosclerotic diseases. Atherosclerosis Study Group. Circulation 1984;70:(suppl)157A–205A
55. Multiple Risk Factor Intervention Trial Research Group: Multiple Risk Factor Intervention Trial. Risk factor changes and mortality results. JAMA 1982;248:1465–1477
56. Puska P, Tuomilehto J, Salonen J et al: Changes in coronary risk factors during comprehensive five-year community programme to control cardiovascular diseases (North Karelia project). BMJ 1979;2:1173–1178
57. Salonen JT, Puska P, Mustaniemi H: Changes in morbidity and mortality during comprehensive community programme to control cardiovascular disease during 1972–7 in North Karelia. BMJ 1979;2:1178–1183
58. Barker DJP (ed): Fetal and Infant Origins of Adult Disease. British Medical Association, London, 1992
59. Elford J, Phillips AN, Thomson AG, Shaper AG: Migration and geographic variations in ischaemic heart disease in Great Britain. Lancet 1989;i:343–346
60. McKeigue PM, Miller GJ, Marmot MG: Coronary heart disease in South Asians overseas: A review. J Clin Epidemiol 1989; 42:597–609
61. Levy RI: Declining mortality in coronary heart disease. Arteriosclerosis 1981;1:312–325
62. Marmot MG, Booth M, Beral M: Changes in heart disease mortality in England and Wales and other countries. Health Trends 1981;13:33–38
63. Gillum RF, Folsom AR, Blackburn H: Decline in coronary heart disease mortality. Old questions and new facts. Am J Med 1984;76:1055–1065
64. Haberman S, Capildeo R, Rose FC: Diverging trends in cerebrovascular disease and ischaemic heart disease mortality. Stroke 1982;13:582–589
65. Rose G: Incubation period of coronary heart disease. BMJ 1982;284:1600–1601
66. Krolewski AS, Kosinski EJ, Warram JH et al: Magnitude and determinants of coronary artery disease in juvenile-onset, insulin-dependent diabetes mellitus. Am J Cardiol 1987;59: 750–755
67. Breslow JL: Genetic basis of lipoprotein disorders. J Clin Invest 1989;84:373–380
68. Brown MS, Goldstein JL: A receptor-mediated pathway for cholesterol homeostasis. Science 1986;232:34–47
69. Stout RW: Hormones and atherosclerosis. MTP Press, Lancaster, 1982
70. Lipid Research Clinics Program Epidemiology Committee: Plasma lipid distributions in selected North American populations: The Lipid Research Clinics Program Prevalence Study. Circulation 1979;60:427–439
71. Ettinger WH, Wahi PW, Kuller LH et al: Lipoprotein lipids in older people. Results from the Cardiovascular Health Study. Circulation 1992;86:858–869
72. Glueck CJ, Gartside P, Fallat RW et al: Longevity syndromes: Familial hypobeta and familial hyperalpha lipoproteinemia. J Clin Lab Med 1976;88:941–957
73. Heckers H, Burkard W, Schmahy FW et al: Hyper-alpha-lipoproteinemia and hypo-beta-lipoproteinemia are not markers for a high life expectancy. Gerontology 1982;28:176–202
74. Steinberg D: The cholesterol controversy is over. Why did it take so long? Circulation 1989;80:1070–1078
75. Weijenberg MP, Feskens JM, Kromhout D: Total and high density lipoprotein cholesterol as risk factors for coronary heart disease in elderly men during 5 years of follow-up. The Zutphen Elderly Study. Am J Epidemiol 1996;143:151–158
76. Krumholz HM, Seeman TE, Merrill SS et al: Lack of association between cholesterol and coronary heart disease mortality and morbidity and all-cause mortality in persons older than 70 years. JAMA 1994;272:1335–1340
77. Jacobsen SJ, Freedman DS, Hoffmann RG et al: Cholesterol and coronary artery disease: age as an effect modifier. J Clin Epidemiol 1992;45:1053–1059
78. Marmot M: The cholesterol papers. Lowering population cholesterol concentrations probably isn't harmful. BMJ 1994;308: 351–352
79. Prospective Studies Collaboration: Cholesterol, diastolic blood pressure, and stroke: 13,000 stroke, in 450,000 people in 45 prospective cohorts. Lancet 1995;346:1647–1653
80. Gordon T, Castelli WP, Hjortland MC et al: High density lipoprotein as a protective factor against coronary heart disease. The Framingham Study. Am J Med 1977;62:707–714

81. Gordon DJ, Probstfield JL, Garrison RJ et al: High-density lipoprotein cholesterol and cardiovascular disease. Four prospective American studies. Circulation 1989;79:8–15

82. Miller GJ, Miller NE: Plasma-high-density-lipoprotein concentration and development of ischaemic heart-disease. Lancet 1975;i:16–19

83. Corti M-C, Guralnik JM, Salive ME et al: HDL cholesterol predicts coronary heart disease mortality in older persons. JAMA 1995;274:539–544

84. St Clair RW: Atherosclerosis regression in animal models: Current concepts of cellular and biochemical mechanisms. Progress in Cardiovascular Diseases 1983;26:109–132

85. Wilens SL: The experimental production of lipid depositions in excised arteries. Science 1954;114:389–393

86. MAAS Investigators: Effect of simvastatin on coronary atheroma: the Multicentre Anti-Atheroma Study (MAAS). Lancet 1994;344:633–638

87. Brown BG, Zhao X-Q, Sacco DE, Albers JJ: Lipid lowering and plaque regression. New insights into prevention of plaque disruption and clinical events in coronary disease. Circulation 1993;87:1781–1791

88. Oliver MF: Strategies for preventing and screening for coronary heart disease. Br Heart J 1985;54:1–5

89. Pyorala K, De Backer G, Graham I et al. on behalf of the Task Force of the European Society of Cardiology, European Atherosclerosis Society and European Society of Hypertension: Prevention of coronary heart disease in clinical practice. Eur Heart J 1994;15:1300–1331

90. Scandinavian Simvastatin Survival Study Group: Randomised trial of cholesterol lowering in 4444 patients with coronary heart disease: Scandinavian Simvastatin Survival Study (4S) Lancet 1994;344:1383 1389

91. Scandinavian Simvastatin Survival Study Group: Baseline serum cholesterol and treatment effect in the Scandinavian Simvastatin Survival Study (4S) Lancet 1995;345:1274–1275

92. Shepherd J, Cobbe SM, Ford I et al: Prevention of coronary heart disease with pravastatin in men with hypercholesterolaemia. N Engl J Med 1995;333:1301–1307

93. Lipid Research Clinics Program: The Lipid Research Clinics Coronary Primary Prevention Trial Results. 1. Reduction in incidence of coronary heart disease. JAMA 1984;251:351–364

94. Lipid Research Clinics Program: The Lipid Research Clinics Coronary Primary Prevention Trial Results. II. The relationship of reduction in incidence of coronary heart disease to cholesterol lowering. JAMA 1984;251:365–374

95. Frick MH, Elo O, Haapa K et al: Helsinki heart study: primary-prevention trial with gemfibrozil in middle-aged men with dyslipidemia. N Engl J Med 1987;317:1237–1245

96. Manninen V, Elo MO, Frick MH et al: Lipid alterations and decline in the incidence of coronary heart disease in the Helsinki Heart Study. JAMA 1988;260:641–651

97. Law MR, Wald NJ, Thompson SG: By how much and how quickly does reduction in serum cholesterol concentration lower risk of ischaemic heart disease? BMJ 1994;308:367–373

98. Furberg CD, Adams HP, Applegate WB et al: Effect of lovastatin on early carotid atherosclerosis and cardiovascular events. Circulation 1994;90:1679–1687

99. Gurwitz JH, Col NF, Avorn J: The exclusion of the elderly and women from clinical trials in acute myocardial infarction. JAMA 1992;268:1417–1422

100. Lackner KJ, Schettler G, Kubler W: Plasma Cholesterol, lipid lowering, and risk for cancer. An update of the results from epidemiologic studies and intervention trials. Klin Wochenschr 1989;67:957–962

101. Canner PL, Berge KG, Wenger NK et al: Fifteen year mortality in coronary drug project patients: long-term benefit with niacin. J Am Coll Cardiol 1986;8:1245–1255

102. Expert Panel on Detection, Evaluation and Treatment of Blood Cholesterol in Adults: Summary of the Second Report of the National Cholesterol Education Program (NCEP) Expert Panel on Detection, Evaluation and Treatment of High Blood Cholesterol in Adults (Adult Treatment Panel II) JAMA 1993;269:3015–3023

103. Havel RJ, Rapaport E: Management of primary hyperlipidemia. N Engl J Med 1993;332:1491–1498

104. Bach LA, Cooper ME, O'Brien RC, Jerums G: The use of simvastatin, an HMG CoA reductase inhibitor, in older patients with hypercholesterolemia and atherosclerosis. J Am Geriatr Soc 1990;38:10–14

105. Morisaki N, Mori S, Kobayashi J et al: Effects of long-term treatment with probucol on serum lipoproteins in cases of familial hypercholesterolemia in the elderly. J Am Geriatr Soc 1990;38:15–18

106. LaRosa JC, Applegate W, Crouse JR: Cholesterol lowering in the elderly. Results of the Cholesterol Reduction in Seniors Program (CRISP) Pilot Study. Arch Intern Med 1994;154:529–539

107. Hennekens CH, Buring JE, Sandercock P et al: Aspirin and other antiplatelet agents in the secondary and primary prevention of cardiovascular disease. Circulation 1989;80:749–756

CHAPTER 21

Cardiovascular Signs in Old Age

SHAUN TIMOTHY O'KEEFFE

MICHAEL LYE

In spite of the plethora of new investigative techniques, the physical examination remains an important part of the armamentarium of the modern physician. In a study conducted in a general medical clinic, Sandler[1] found that 56 percent of patients received a correct diagnosis by the end of a history and this figure increased to 73 percent after physical examination. Nevertheless, as with the findings of other diagnostic techniques, it is important to establish the reproducibility and diagnostic accuracy of physical signs. Disagreement over the performance and interpretation of physical examinations is common between different observers and even on reassessment by a single observer. Also, the diagnostic value of many time-honored physical signs has been found wanting in formal tests.

Of course, a single physical sign is rarely diagnostic; instead, clinical diagnosis usually depends on a comprehensive, chronologic history and the association of several physical findings. The ability to recognize patterns and derive meaningful diagnostic features often by employing subconscious fuzzy logic is a uniquely human facility. Computers using diagnostic algorithms may be helpful in some small focused areas, but are liable to blow a fuse when faced by the atypical 80-year-old. However, pattern recognition has its drawbacks; experienced physicians (and the more experienced, the greater the risk) will tend to find what they expect or hope to find on examination. Thus, it may become more apparent that the pulse is small in volume after auscultation has revealed the classical murmur of aortic stenosis. It has also been alleged that the "emperor's clothes syndrome" is particularly common in performance of the cardiovascular examination, and that the prestige and seniority of the carrier is a major factor in the spread of the disease[2]; classic signs include "I hear it," "It's very soft," and "It can only be heard in the sagittal decubitus."

Performance and interpretation of the physical examination in elderly people presents special difficulties.[3] The occurrence of age- and disease-related changes in the cardiovascular system and the frequent presence of noncardiac disease may reduce the sensitivity and, especially, the specificity of cardiovascular signs. Patients may be unable or unwilling to cooperate fully with the examination as a result of cognitive impairment or frailty. On the other hand, imaging procedures may be impossible for the same reasons. Also, cardiovascular and other disease may present atypically with one of the giants of geriatrics; physical findings can direct the choice of investigations in such patients.

Standard textbooks provide detailed descriptions of the techniques for eliciting and interpreting cardiovascular signs. This chapter will focus instead on the diagnostic value and reproducibility of these signs, with particular reference to the changes in these parameters wrought by the aging process. Sensitivity (true positive/[true positive + false negative]), specificity (true negative/[true negative + false positive]), and the κ statistic, which corrects interrater agreement for chance agreement, will be quoted wherever possible. As a rough guide, a κ score greater than 0.8 is excellent, 0.6 to 0.8 is good; 0.4 to 0.6 is moderate, and less than 0.4 is poor.

Hypertension

Blood pressure measurements in epidemiologic and treatment studies predict cardiovascular mortality and morbidity as effectively in elderly people as in young people. Nevertheless, because of the increased risk of side effects with antihypertensive treatment in elderly people, it is particularly important to ensure that the diagnosis of hypertension is accurate. This requires a meticulous technique for measuring cuff pressures. Also, because blood pressure variability is increased in old people, any single reading is less likely to be representative of blood pressure in general.[4] Hence, it is particularly important in this age group to carry out multiple readings before initiating therapy. Ambulatory blood pressure monitoring may be helpful in some patients; however, current diagnostic and therapeutic data in elderly patients are based on clinic readings. At the initial visit, blood pressure readings should be taken in both arms, since about 10 percent of elderly subjects have a between-arm difference of more than 10 mmHg. Blood pressure should subsequently be recorded in the arm with the highest pressure.[5]

The presence of atrial fibrillation greatly increases interobserver variability in the measurement of blood pressure.[6] There are as yet no clear guidelines for measuring blood pressure in patients with atrial fibrillation, but it seems prudent to take repeated recordings before making therapeutic decisions.

Pseudohypertension

Increased stiffness of the peripheral vessels with increasing age leads to increased systolic blood pressure in many elderly people. In some patients, it also leads to "pseudohypertension" due to overestimation of blood pressure using a mercury sphygmomanometer compared with intra-arterial readings. This may be suspected if patients with apparent hypertension exhibit no signs of end-organ damage. Messerli and colleagues[7] in 1985 reported that a maneuver described by Osler was an efficient way of identifying patients with pseudohypertension. Osler observed that sclerosed vessels remained palpable distal to a blood pressure cuff inflated above systolic pressure. Subsequent studies have found that interobserver reproducibility of this sign is poor (κ values of 0.26 to 0.38),[8] and that a positive Osler's maneuver is not predictive of pseudohypertension.[9,10] Fortunately, pseudohypertension is uncommon in the general elderly population.[10]

Fourth Heart Sound

The diagnostic value of an audible fourth heart sound (S4) is disputed but is probably poor in older people. Although an S4 is often heard in people with hypertension and left ventricular hypertrophy, it is also heard in about 60 percent of ostensibly normal people over the age of 50 years.[11] However, many patients in whom an S4 is heard do not actually have an S4 on phonocardiography[12]; it appears that even experienced cardiologists can mistake a split S1 for an S4–S1 sound in older patients.

Other Findings

Although fundoscopy is recommended on initial assessment of patients with hypertension, it should be recognized that, even in studies employing retinal pictures, interrater agreement for all but the most extreme changes is low.[13] A sustained "lift" on palpation of the apex of the heart is a reasonably specific, but insensitive sign of left ventricular hypertrophy.[14]

Congestive Heart Failure

Physical signs of heart failure can be difficult to interpret in elderly people.[15] Peripheral edema is common in immobile patients and those with hypoalbuminemia. It also occurs as a result of chronic venous insufficiency, which is present at about the same prevalence as heart failure in the community.[16] The presence or absence of peripheral edema is thus a poor guide to the diagnosis of heart failure or to the adequacy of treatment in patients with established heart failure. Basal pulmonary crackles frequently occur in the absence of significant cardiac or respiratory disease in immobile elderly people.[17] Hepatomegaly has many causes, and tachycardia is a very nonspecific sign.

Examination of Neck Veins

Elevated jugular venous pressure is a more useful test for the diagnosis of heart failure. Jugular venous pulsations are examined by inspecting the silhouette of the neck with the patient reclining at an angle of 45 degrees. The top level of the pulsations of the right internal jugular vein is taken as the venous pressure. The upper limit of normal is about 4.5 cm above the level of the sternal angle. The external jugulars are not in direct line with the superior cava and are relatively poor manometers. The right internal jugular is recommended because the left jugular pressure may be falsely elevated in some arteriosclerotic patients with unfolded aortic arch, causing compression of the innominate vein between the sternum and tortuous arterial branches.[18]

The abdominojugular test (originally the hepatojugular reflux test) is often used in conjunction with inspection of the jugular veins. The test is positive if there is a sustained rise in jugular venous pressure during 10 seconds of firm compression over the abdomen (not just over the liver) followed by an abrupt drop in venous pressure when compression ceases.[19] Even if the resting jugular venous pressure is within normal limits, a positive abdominojugular test suggests that venous pressure is high for that individual.

In patients with chronic heart failure, the presence of an elevated jugular venous pressure or positive abdominojugular test is a sensitive (65 to 81 percent) and specific (79 to 100 percent) indicator of elevated pulmonary capillary wedge pressure.[20–22] Thus, these signs can be used to determine optimal treatment with diuretics and vasodilators in such patients. Also, one or other of these tests is usually positive in patients with recent right ventricular infarction or isolated right ventricular failure.[23] However, a false rise in the height of the venous pulsations may occur in patients with severe lung disease who are unable to tolerate the resistance to downward movement of the diaphragm caused by abdominal compression. Interrater reliability for the assessment of the neck veins is good (κ score of 0.69 to 0.92).[22]

Apex Beat

Findings of cardiomegaly or a dyskinetic ventricular impulse on palpation of the precordium provide useful supporting evidence for heart failure. Cardiomegaly is usually diagnosed on the basis of a chest x-ray. However, clinical determination of heart size is useful for agitated patients or when patients are seen in the community. Many clinicians assess the position of the apex beat as a guide to heart size. Reasonable interrater reliability has been reported for palpability (κ score, 0.72) and displacement beyond the midclavicular line (κ score, 0.56) of the apex beat.[24] About 60 percent of unselected hospital patients with apex displacement have radiographic cardiomegaly, while 75 percent of patients without apex displacement have normal radiographic cardiac size.[25] Thus, this is a more useful test for excluding cardiomegaly than for confirming it. The apex beat is palpable in less than one-half of hospital patients; in particular, it is usually impalpable in obese patients or those with severe lung disease. However, the mere palpability of an apex beat in an older patient who is obese or has lung disease is suggestive of cardiomegaly. Palpation of the precordium is also less informative in patients with chest deformity.

Percussion of Cardiac Borders

Although percussion of the heart to detect cardiomegaly is rarely performed by physicians, recent studies suggest that it is more valuable than palpation of the apex beat. Heckerling and colleagues[26] reported in 100 hospital patients that dullness to percussion 10.5 cm lateral to the midsternal line was 94 percent sensitive and 67 percent specific for detection of radiographic cardiomegaly; interrater agreement was reasonable (κ score, 0.57).

Third Heart Sound

The presence of a third heart sound (S3) during systole is a classic feature of heart failure. In patients with established heart failure, an S3 is about 70 percent sensitive and 40 percent specific for detection of raised left ventricular filling pressure.[21] In people with acute myocardial infarction, presence of S3 is 70 percent sensitive and 70 percent specific for identification of reduced ejection fraction.[27] The presence of an S3 has also been reported to be useful as a guide to selecting heart failure patients in sinus rhythm who will benefit from digoxin therapy.[28] However, other data suggest that S3 is of little value in distinguishing heart failure with and without systolic dysfunction in the individual patient and that this sign is of least predictive value in elderly people.[29] Also, although agreement between cardiologists is good regarding the presence or absence of S3 (κ score, 0.60),[22] agreement is moderate or poor for noncardiologists (κ score, 0.1 to 0.5).[15,30]

Heart Failure With Normal Systolic Function

In recent years it has become apparent that a substantial proportion of people with clinical heart failure due to various etiologies have normal systolic function.[31] Data from hospital series suggest that heart failure with normal systolic function is more common in older patients. Some authors[32] have suggested that left ventricular S3 is suggestive of heart failure with systolic dysfunction and S4 suggestive of heart failure without systolic dysfunction. However, other reports[31,33] indicate that these findings are of little diagnostic value in individual patients.

Valvular Heart Disease

In general, accurate auscultation of the heart is more difficult in elderly people. One reason is that many elderly people have an increased anteroposterior chest diameter, especially at the base of the heart. Thick musculature or fat can reduce the audibility of heart sounds and murmurs. Conversely, many elderly patients with heart disease are poorly nourished, and it may be difficult to achieve a good air seal for the stethoscope in patients who are "skin and bone." The presence of coexisting lung disease such as emphysema can also reduce the audibility of cardiac sounds and murmurs. A variety of maneuvers, such as the Valsalva maneuver or squatting, may be helpful in the interpretation of auscultatory findings but are often not feasible in ill elderly people.[34]

At the onset of systole, the almost simultaneous closure of the mitral and tricuspid valves give rise to the first heart sound (S1). Closure of the aortic and pulmonary valves give rise to the two components of the second heart sound (S2). Aortic valve closure occurs first, giving rise to a splitting of S2, which is widest during inspiration. Although increased or decreased intensity of the sounds or abnormal splitting of S2 are described in a variety of conditions, these findings are rarely of diagnostic value in isolation from other cardiac signs. Also, there is remarkably little agreement, even between experienced physicians, regarding the normality or otherwise of S1 and S2.[35] Splitting of S2 is often inaudible in older patients, even during inspiration, due to a prolongation of the left ventricular ejection and isovolumic contraction times.[36–38] Conversely, splitting of S1 is often more marked in old age; this may lead to an erroneous diagnosis of an ejection click or a fourth heart sound.[12]

Aortic Stenosis Versus Sclerosis

Systolic murmurs are extremely common in older people and present major diagnostic difficulties. The most common murmur in this population is an aortic ejection murmur in the absence of aortic valvular stenosis; in one study,[39] such an "aortic sclerosis" murmur was present in about 50 percent of subjects over 50 years. The presence of hypertension further increases the incidence of this murmur, and it is twice as common in women as in men.[40] However, significant aortic stenosis is also increasingly common with advancing age, occurring in 13 percent of hospitalized patients over 80 years in one series.[41] Clinical distinction between sclerotic and stenotic murmurs is inaccurate in elderly people. Aortic sclerotic murmurs may radiate into the neck and may even be associated with a thrill.[40] Conversely, classic signs of aortic stenosis are often absent in elderly people.[42–45]

Palpation of peripheral pulses provides information regarding the rate of rise, the contour of the rise, and pulse volume. A slow rate of rise and low volume pulse are characteristic of significant aortic stenosis. There are few data regarding the predictive value of abnormal pulse quality for the diagnosis of aortic valvular disease. In a cardiology clinic, a slowly rising carotid pulse was reported to be a specific (95 percent) but insensitive (30 percent) indicator of significant aortic stenosis.[43] It is well recognized that elderly subjects with an aorta hardened by atherosclerosis may have a normal rate of rise in the peripheral pulses despite a significant aortic pressure gradient.[44] Thus, this sign is likely to be even more insensitive for the diagnosis of aortic stenosis in the elderly. More importantly, there is evidence that even experienced examiners cannot reliably distinguish normal from abnormal velocity of rise of carotid pulses. In a study of 20 consecutive patients with cardiac disease (seven of whom had aortic stenosis) by three cardiologists,[46] there was no significant interobserver agreement for designating pulse rise as slow, normal or rapid; also, there was no correlation between the ratings of any of the observers and independent measurement of the pulse rise velocity using a transducer.

As discussed earlier, the presence of an S4 is of little diagnostic value in older people. The quality of the murmur of aortic stenosis may also be altered in older people. In elderly people, high frequency components of the aortic murmur tend to radiate to the apex, where they may have a musical quality and be readily confused with a mitral regurgitant murmur; this is known as the Gallavardin phenomenon.[40] It is well recognized that the murmur may be very soft in patients with critical aortic stenosis and a reduced cardiac output. In elderly people, the murmur of aortic stenosis may be soft even in the absence of heart failure.[42]

Most importantly, clinical features do not accurately distinguish the severity of aortic stenosis. In a study by McKillop et al.,[47] 29 patients with aortic valve disease were examined by two physicians, one a cardiologist. Murmur intensity and the quality of the aortic closure sound did not correlate with the valve gradient on Doppler echocardiography, and clinical sensitivity for detecting a valve gradient greater than 30 mmHg was only 44 percent.

In conclusion, clinical examination is not an adequate substitute for echocardiography in symptomatic patients with aortic systolic murmurs.

Other Murmurs

In general, the typical features of other valvular diseases are similar in elderly and young patients, although the difficulties noted earlier in performing and interpreting findings on auscultation and on examination of the peripheral pulses in elderly patients still apply.

The murmur of mitral regurgitation is usually easily identified by its pansystolic quality, loudest intensity at the apex, and radiation toward the axilla. However, an aortic systolic murmur may occasionally mimic this pattern. Also, distinction of mitral and tricuspid regurgitant murmurs may be difficult if the heart is rotated.[40] In a study of 50 patients with systolic murmurs by two cardiologists,[34] the augmentation of intensity with inspiration and diminution with expiration differentiated right-sided systolic murmurs from all other murmurs with 100 percent sensitivity and 88 percent specificity. Increased intensity of the murmur after 1 minute of isometric handgrip exercise was 67 percent sensitive and 95 percent specific for distinguishing mitral regurgitation from aortic stenosis. In elderly patients, mitral valve prolapse frequently presents with a pansystolic murmur rather than the classic click and late systolic murmur.

Human hearing is relatively insensitive to low frequency sounds, and the diastolic murmur of mitral stenosis is easily missed even by experienced examiners.[48] This problem is of course compounded in patients presenting with fast atrial fibrillation or by using the diaphragm of the stethoscope. Clinically, silent mitral stenosis is also well recognized in elderly patients with apparent chronic pulmonary problems. The higher pitched diastolic murmur of aortic incompetence is more readily recognized, although clinical examination is less useful in determining the severity of the regurgitation. Also, mild and usually clinically insignificant aortic regurgitation is extremely common in patients with hypertension.[49]

Peripheral Vascular Disease

Carotid Bruits

Carotid bruits are best heard using the bell of the stethoscope over the area between the upper level of the thyroid cartilage and the angle of the jaw. In elderly people, the main cause of neck bruits to be distinguished from carotid bruits are systolic heart murmurs transmitted to the neck; the latter are usually louder over the precordium than over the neck. Agreement regarding the presence of a carotid bruit is good for experienced examiners (κ score 0.67). However, there is poor agreement regarding the intensity, pitch, or duration of a bruit (κ score of less than 0.4).[50] In a community study,[51] the frequency of asymptomatic carotid bruits increased from 2.3 percent in those aged 45 to 54 years to 8.2 percent in those aged 75 years or more; bruits were more common in women and in hypertensive people. In general, asymptomatic bruits are associated with an increased risk of both cardiovascular and cerebrovascular events. However, in patients older than 75 years, asymptomatic bruits may not be associated with increased risk of stroke.[52] Conversely, the absence of a bruit does not rule out severe carotid stenosis.[50]

Peripheral Pulses

Examination of the distal arterial pulses is important in the assessment of the patient with suspected peripheral arterial disease. The main difficulties arise in assessment of dorsalis pedis and the posterior tibial pulses in the foot. Anatomic variation in the location of these vessels is common, and leg edema may render an adequate examination impossible. Although one study[53] noted that interrater reliability for assessment of the foot pulses was very poor, two further studies,[54,55] one in a geriatric assessment unit,[54] have noted satisfactory reproducibility.

References

1. Sandler G: The importance of the history in the medical clinic and the cost of unnecessary tests. Am Heart J 1980;100: 928–1003
2. Gross F: The emperor's clothes syndrome. N Engl J Med 1971; 285:863
3. O'Keeffe ST, Smith T, Valacio R et al: Reproducibility of ankle jerk assessment in the elderly. Lancet 1994;344:1619–1620
4. Mancia G, Ferrari A, Gregorini L et al: Blood pressure variability in man: the relation to high blood pressure, age and baroreflex sensitivity. Clin Sci 1980;59:4015–4045

5. O'Brien E, O'Malley K: Blood pressure measurement. J Ir Coll Physic Surg 1990;19:281–294
6. Sykes D, Dewar R, Mohanuraban K et al: Measuring blood pressure in the elderly: does atrial fibrillation increase observer variability? BMJ 1990;300:162–163
7. Messerli FH, Ventura HO, Amodeo C: Osler's manoeuvre and pseudohypertension. N Engl J Med 1985;312:1548–1551
8. Tsapatsaris NP, Napolitano GT, Rothchild J: Osler's manoeuvre in an outpatient setting. Arch Intern Med 1991;151:2209–2211
9. Belmin J, Visintin J-M, Salvatore R et al: Osler's manoeuvre: absence of usefulness for the detection of pseudohypertension in an elderly population. Am J Med 1995;98:42–48
10. Kuwaijima I, Hoh E, Suzuki Y et al: Pseudohypertension in the elderly. J Hypertens 1990;8:429–432
11. Rectra EH, Khan AH, Pigott VM, Spodick DH: Audibility of the fourth heart sound. A prospective, "blind" auscultatory and polygraphic investigation. JAMA 1972;221:36–41
12. Jordan MD, Taylor CR, Nyhuis AW, Tavel ME: Audibility of the fourth heart sound. Relationship to presence of disease and examiner experience. Arch Intern Med 1987;147:721–726
13. Aoki N, Horibe H, Ohno Y et al: Observer variability and reproducibility for fundoscopic findings. Japan Circulat J 1977;41: 11–17
14. Roberts WC: Examining the praecordium and the heart. Chest 1970;57:567–573
15. The Task Force on Heart Failure of the European Society of Cardiology. Guidelines for the diagnosis of heart failure. Eur Heart J 1995;16:741–751
16. Belcaro G, Nicolaides AN, Veller M: Venous Disorders. WB Saunders, London, 1995
17. Krumpke PE, Knudson RJ, Parsons G, Reiser K: The ageing respiratory system. Clin Geriatr Med 1985;1:143–175
18. Sleight P: Unilateral elevation of the internal jugular pulse. Br Heart J 1962;24:726–728
19. Ewy GA: The abdominojugular test: technique and hemodynamic correlates. Ann Intern Med 1988;109:456–460
20. Stevenson LW, Perloff JK: The limited reliability of physical signs for estimating haemodynamics in chronic heart failure. JAMA 1989; 261:884–888
21. Chakko S, Woska D, Martinez H et al: Clinical, radiographic and haemodynamic correlations in clinical congestive heart failure: conflicting results may lead to inappropriate care. Am J Med 1991;90:353–359
22. Butman SM, Ewy GA, Standen JR et al: Bedside cardiovascular examination in patients with severe chronic heart failure. J Am Coll Cardiol 1993;22:968–974
23. Ducas J, Magder S, McGregor M: Validity of the hepatojugular reflux as a clinical test for congestive heart failure. Am J Cardiol 1983;52:1299–1303
24. O'Neill TW, Barry M, Smith M, Graham IM: Diagnostic value of the apex beat. Lancet 1989;1:410–411
25. Heckerling PS, Wiener SL, Wolfkiel CJ et al: Accuracy and reproducibility of precordial percussion and palpation for detecting increased left ventricular end-diastolic volume and mass. JAMA 1993;270:1943–1948
26. Heckerling PS, Wiener SL, Moses VK et al: Accuracy of precordial percussion in detecting cardiomegaly. Am J Med 1991; 91: 328–334
27. Gadsboll N, Hoilund-Carlsen PF, Nielson GG: Symptoms and signs of heart failure in patients with myocardial infarction. Eur Heart J 1989;10:1017–1028
28. Jaeschke R, Oxman AD, Guyatt GH: To what extent do congestive heart failure patients in sinus rhythm benefit from digoxin therapy? A systematic overview and meta-analysis. Am J Med 1990;88:279–285
29. Aronow WS, Starling L, Etienne F: Lack of efficacy of digoxin in treatment of compensated congestive heart failure with third heart sound and sinus rhythm in elderly patients receiving diuretic therapy. Am J Cardiol 1986;58:168–169
30. Ishmail AA, Wing S, Ferguson J et al: Interobserver agreement by auscultation in the presence of a third heart sound in patients with congestive heart failure. Chest 1987;91:870–873
31. O'Keeffe ST, Lye M: Heart failure in the elderly: the same syndrome as the clinical trials? pp. 41–71. In McMurray JJV, Cleland JGF (eds): Heart Failure in Clinical Practice. Martin Dunitz, London, 1996
32. Harizi RC, Bianco JA, Alpert JS: Diastolic function of the heart in clinical cardiology. Arch Intern Med 1988;148:99–108
33. Wong WF, Gold S, Fukuyama O, Blanchette PL: Diastolic dysfunction in elderly patients with congestive heart failure. Am J Cardiol 1989;63:1526–1528
34. Lembo NJ, Dell'Italia LJ, Crawford MH, O'Rourke RA: Bedside diagnosis of systolic murmurs. N Engl J Med 1988;318: 1572–1578
35. Raftery EB, Holland WW: Examination of the heart: an investigation into variation. Am J Epidemiol 1967;85:438–444
36. Aronow WS: Isovolumic contaction and left ventricular ejection times. Am J Cardiol 1970;26:328–331
37. Slodki SJ, Hussain AT, Luisada AA: The Q-2 interval. A study of the second heart sound in old age. J Am Geriatr Soc 1969; 17:673–678
38. Ehlers KH: Wide splitting of the second heart sound without demonstrable heart disease. Am J Cardiol 1969;23:690–695
39. Perez GL: Incidence of murmurs in the aged heart. J Am Geriatr Soc 1976;24:29–34
40. Constant J: Bedside Cardiology. 3rd Ed. Little, Brown, Boston, 1985
41. Aronow WS, Kronzon I: Prevalence and severity of valvular aortic stenosis determined by Doppler echocardiography and association with echocardiographic and electrocardiographic left ventricular hypertrophy and physical signs of aortic stenosis in elderly patients. Am J Cardiol 1991;67:776–777
42. Roberts WC, Perloff JK, Constantino T: Severe valvular stenosis in patients over 65 years of age. Am J Cardiol 1971;27:497–504
43. Forsell G, Jonasson R, Orinius E: Identifying severe aortic valvular stenosis by bedside examination. Acta Med Scand 1985; 218:397–400
44. Lombard JT, Selzer A: Valvular aortic stenosis: a clinical and haemodynamic profile of patients. Ann Intern Med 1987;106: 292–298
45. Stewart BF, Pearlman AS: Aortic stenosis or aortic sclerosis? Cardiol Elderly 1995;3:259–264

46. Spodick DH, Sugiura T, Doi Y et al: Rate of rise of the carotid pulse. An investigation of observer error in a common clinical measurement. Am J Cardiol 1982;49:159–162
47. McKillop GM, Stewart DA et al: Doppler echocardiography in elderly patients with ejection systolic murmurs. Postgrad Med J 1991;67:1059–1061
48. Wiener S, Nathanson M: Physical examination. Frequently observed errors. JAMA 1976;236:852–855
49. Cox N, McLenachan JM, Corrado OJ: Is an echocardiogram useful in heart failure in the elderly? Age Ageing 1994;23(suppl 4):4–5
50. Sauvé J-S, Laupacis A, Østbye T et al: Does this patient have a clinically important carotid bruit? JAMA 1993;270:2843–2845
51. Heyman A, Wilkinson WE, Heydon S et al: Risk of stroke in asymptomatic persons with cervical arterial bruits: a population study in Evans County, Georgia. N Engl J Med 1980;302: 838–841
52. Van Ruiswyk J, Noble H, Sigmann P: The natural history of carotid bruits in elderly persons. Ann Intern Med 1990;112: 340–343
53. Ludbrook J, Clarke AM, McKenzie JK: Significance of absent ankle pulse. BMJ 1962;1:1724–1727
54. Lawson IR, Ingman SR, Masih Y, Freeman B: Reliability of palpation of pedal pulses as ascertained by the kappa statistic. J Am Geriatr Soc 1980;28:300–303
55. Meade TW, Gardner MJ, Cannon P, Richardson PC: Observer variability in recording the peripheral pulses. Br Heart J 1968; 30:661–665

C H A P T E R 2 2

Chronic Cardiac Failure in the Elderly

MICHAEL LYE

Prevalence

The true prevalence of chronic cardiac failure in the elderly population is not accurately known. This is because of difficulties in definition and diagnosis compounded by the almost ubiquitous use of diuretics for any form of dependent edema in old people. Overall prevalence in general practice is estimated to be around 0.3 percent,[1] although the authors of this study comment that 83 percent of their patients were over the age of 65 years. Within a general practice population of diabetics of all ages the prevalence of cardiac failure was 12.2 percent.[2] In a rural population it was estimated that chronic cardiac failure had a prevalence of 6 percent in the over-65-year-olds and 10 percent in the over-75-year-olds.[3]

The longitudinal Framingham survey suggested that prevalence rates double every decade and reach approximately 10 percent for people in their eighties.[4] This study also emphasized a higher prevalence in men. Careful population studies from Sweden and Finland (Table 22-1) approximately confirm these studies but show a vast increase in prevalence of cardiac failure in the very old.[5,6] Webb and Impallomeni[7] calculated that there were at least 450,000 people over the age of 65 years with chronic cardiac failure in England and Wales. Estimates from prescribing data in the United Kingdom give lower prevalence of 0.1 percent in age groups 30 to 39 years and 5.45 percent in patients aged over 90 years.[8] Similar data from the United States based on nursing home admissions suggest that up to 1 in 5 elderly patients were being treated for chronic cardiac failure.[9] Whatever the true prevalence, there is no doubt that the brunt of this chronic disease in borne by the elderly and all who care for them must appreciate how common cardiac failure is. Equally, it is necessary that cardiologists treating patients with cardiac failure require "geriatric skills." The economic impact of chronic cardiac failure in an aging society is, and will continue to be, considerable.[10,11]

Pathophysiology

The ubiquitous nature of arteriosclerosis and coronary heart disease in the elderly of the developed world obscures to a large extent the effects of biologic aging upon the human cardiovascular system.[12] There are fortunately many so-called primitive populations who as yet do not have the "benefits" of modern lifestyles. These people, even when they become very old, do not show signs of arteriosclerosis.[13] The condition of their cardiovascular system is such that many of their elderly individuals regularly perform physical feats, especially endurance running, which cause Western anthropologists studying them to collapse with myocardial infarcts. The important age, as opposed to pathologic, changes are listed in the accompanying boxed list.

While resting heart rate changes little with increasing age,[14] the ability to accelerate the heart during exercise or other stress is attenuated.[15–17] The decrease in maximum heart rate starts at 40 years of age and proceeds linearly,[18] which is best described by the equation:

$$\text{Maximum fH} = 220 - \text{age (years)}$$

Ventricular weight increases without coronary artery disease or hypertension, not because of hyperplasia but due to accumulation of fat, fibrous tissue, lipofuscin, and amyloid.[19] The net result of these morphologic changes is to decrease ventricular compliance (i.e., the ventricles become stiffer).[20] Thus for unit cardiac output, the work as reflected by myocardial oxygen consumption increases disproportionately.

A stiffer myocardium affects both systolic and diastolic functions.[21] It is becoming increasingly apparent that the latter is affected much more than the former in the elderly.[21–23] This is probably not true in coronary artery disease or hypertension where systolic function is affected more than diastolic.[24] Impairment of diastolic function leads to underfilling of the ventricles, particularly the left ventricle, which even in otherwise healthy individuals may be improved by exercise training[25] or a calcium channel antagonist.[26] Earlier studies suggested a decrease in cardiac output of about 1 percent per annum beyond midlife.[27,28] It is now obvious that this was an overestimate and in healthy humans the rate is about half this amount.[22,29,30]

The reduction in cardiac output is, however, matched by a reduction in the body "demands" for a cardiac output as reflected by a reduced oxygen consumption.[31] The latter is caused by a reduction in lean body mass, especially muscle tissue, with increasing age.[32] Thus the alveolar-arterial oxygen difference (A-aO_2), a crude measure of the ratio oxygen supply: oxygen demand, is increased only slightly with increasing age.[17] The flattened Frank-Starling curve of the older patient[33–35] attenuates an important compensatory reflex by re-

Table 22-1 Prevalence (%) of chronic cardiac failure in the elderly based upon community surveys

Age (Years)	Males	Females
70–74	11	8
75–85	16	12
>85	53	48

(Data from Haavisto et al.[5] *and Landahl et al.*[6]*)*

ducing the increase in cardiac output caused by fluid retention and increased venous return (Fig. 22-1A).[22]

Paradoxically, the hormonal response to a reduced "effective" blood volume (Fig. 22-1B) is enhanced in the older cardiac failure patient. In particular, the higher rate of secretion of antidiuretic hormone,[36,37] the water-but not sodium-retaining hormone (arginine vasopressin, AVP), may explain why elderly patients seem more likely to develop hyponatremic cardiac failure than younger patients.[38,39] As assessed by plasma noradrenaline responses, sympathetic activity is higher in the elderly at rest,[40] during exercise,[41] and during chronic cardiac failure.[42] The significance of the increased output of atrial natiuretic peptide(s) by healthy old people[43,44] and further increases in cardiac failure[45,46] is not known.

The baroreflex arc (Fig. 22-1C) requires a greater fall in the effective blood volume to be triggered in older people, but still leads to marked peripheral arterial vasoconstriction.[47,48] This increases both aortic impedance and the damaging left ventricular wall tension. A further sympathetic mediated reduction in renal blood flow may well jeopardize an already precarious renal function. Adrenergic inotropic stimulation to the heart is also less effective[49] because of a down regulation of cardiac receptors, especially β-1-receptors.[50] There is an age-related inability of myofibrils to increase calcium uptake

Physiologic age-changes in cardiovascular function

Heart rate
- resting ±
- exercise ↓↓

Myocardial compliance ↓↓
Systolic function ±
Diastolic function ↓↓
Stroke volume ↓
Cardiac output ↓↓
Oxygen consumption ↓
A-aO_2 difference ↑

±, no change; ↓, slight decrease; ↑, slight increase; ↓↓, moderate decrease.

and thus increase their contractility.[51] The response of the renin-angiotensin-aldosterone axis (Fig. 22-1D) is not altered by aging,[52] though there is some increased peripheral vascular responsiveness to exogenous angiotensin II.[53,54]

Thus, homoeostatic mechanisms that counter the reduction in effective blood volume due to cardiac failure are much less efficient in the elderly patient.[55] They may be rendered even less efficient by pre-existing renal, venous, or neurologic disease. Equally, the addition of other pathologic conditions to pre-existing cardiac failure can cause the already precarious compensatory reflexes to fail. In the elderly cardiac failure patient this is often a respiratory infection; wet lungs provide an excellent nidus for infection.

Diagnosis

The diagnosis of chronic cardiac failure is not as simple as many of us believe. There is no agreed definition of cardiac failure and assessment is based primarily on the patient's description of symptoms and the physician's subjective evaluation of their importance.[56,57] Even in the research field there are no agreed-upon diagnostic criteria.[58,59] The much-used New York Heart Association functional classification system is arbitrary, imprecise, and subjective. The elderly patient with chronic cardiac failure presents even more difficulty in diagnosis and assessment (see Ch. 21).

The problem of late referral due to lack of symptoms is related to the hemodynamic consequences of the pathologic changes described previously. The classic Frank-Starling relationship describes the association of cardiac output (or cardiac work) to the distention of myofibrils during filling—left ventricular end-diastolic volume (Fig. 22-1A). The elderly patient with chronic cardiac failure has a curve that is depressed, moved to the right, and flattened. At rest the patient complains of nonspecific symptoms of a low cardiac output—weakness, tiredness, fatigue—and "takes to bed." Even quite limited exercise will increase end-diastolic volume sufficient to produce breathlessness but, because the patient has taken to bed, exertion is limited so there is little dyspnea. It is much more acceptable for old people to limit exercise than younger ones who would be demanding medical assistance urgently because of symptoms of breathlessness.[60,61]

Alternatively, chronic cardiac failure may be over diagnosed in elderly patients. Of particular concern is the practice of treating all old people who have dependent edema with diuretics, on the assumption that they have chronic cardiac failure and fluid overload. The most common cause in the elderly of dependent edema, which may be quite gross, is so-called postural or gravitational edema secondary to immobility.[62] The causes of immobility in the elderly are legion, with the main ones involving chronic neurologic, joint, and psychiatric diseases. Varicose venous insufficiency also increases the likelihood of postural edema.[63] Immobility may impair protein turnover, and the reduced albumin further

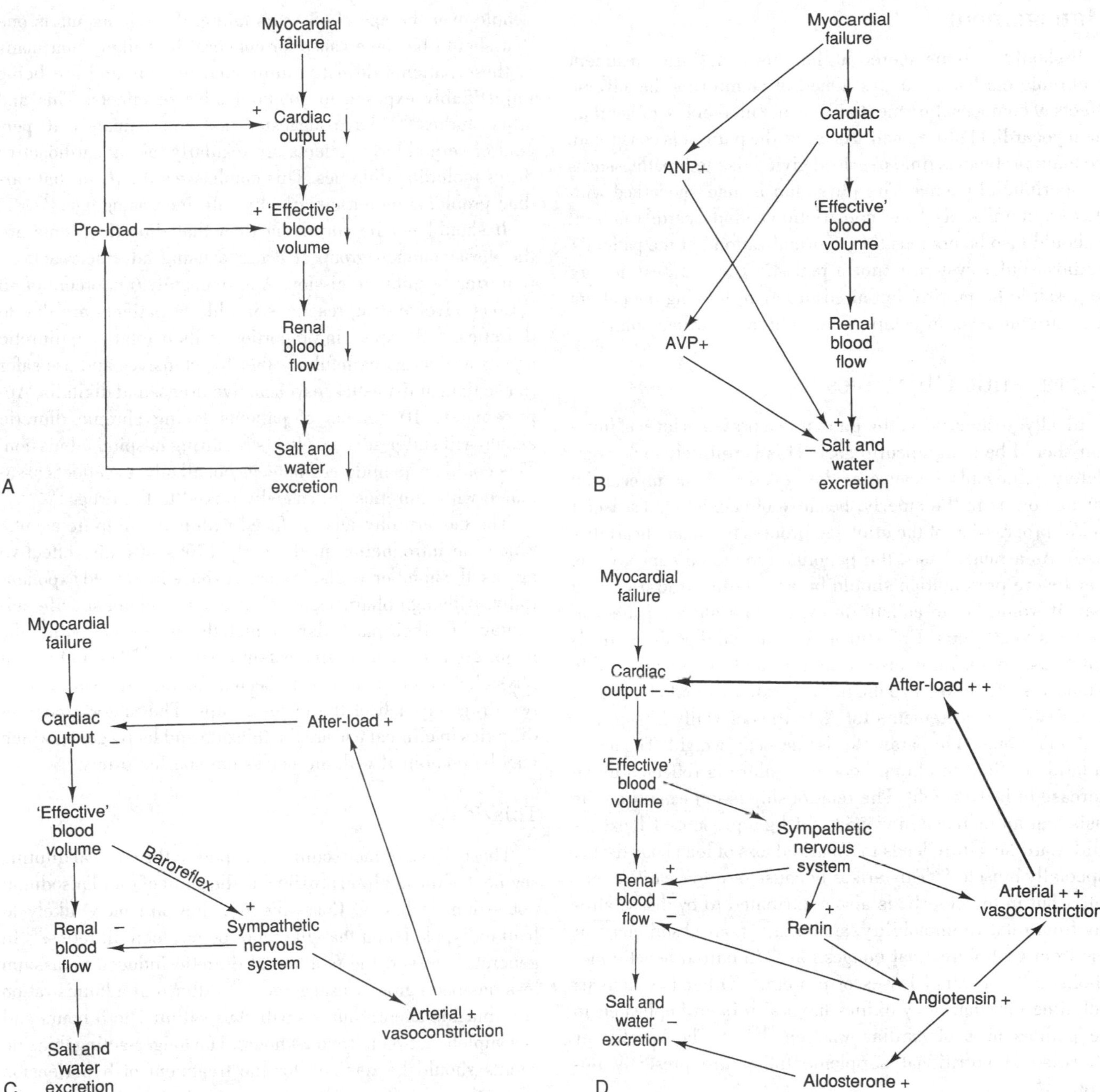

Figure 22-1 Hemodynamic and neurohumoral responses to reduced cardiac function. **(A)** Frank-Starling mechanism, **(B)** humoral response, **(C)** sympathetic neural response, **(D)** activation of R-A-A system. + and − compensatory (beneficial) increase or decrease. + + and − − overcompensatory increase or decrease.

increases edema.[64] Mobilization wherever possible is the cure, not diuretics.

The increasing availability of echocardiography represents a great step forward in diagnosis and management of chronic cardiac failure.[65] This relatively simple, noninvasive investigation not only helps etiologic diagnosis of cardiac failure,[66] but also differentiates between systolic and diastolic dysfunction.[67] The technique has already defined a form of cardiomyopathic cardiac failure confined to elderly patients.[68,69] Soon we probably could target specific therapy according to the cardiac dysfunction revealed by echocardiography.[70] All patients with cardiac failure, especially elderly ones, should undergo echocardiography at the time of initial diagnosis and assessment.[71–73]

Management

It should be remembered at the outset that drug treatment of chronic cardiac failure is aimed at countering the adverse effects of compensatory mechanisms detailed above rather than the myocardial failure itself. As far as the patient is concerned, the main problem is fluid overload giving rise to breathlessness and peripheral edema. The physician is also concerned with the peripheral arterial vasoconstriction and low cardiac output. It should also be obvious that "normalization" of the patient's cardiovascular system is not a realistic goal; at best, it may be possible to improve impaired function, leaving the patient at a variable level of compensated chronic cardiac failure.

Therapeutic Objectives

Ideally, restoration of the patient to a previous level of function should be a therapeutic goal. This is unlikely to be completely achievable because of the severity of the myocardial damage or, as in the elderly, because of coexisting disease(s) and/or progression of the etiologic process (coronary heart disease). As a rough basis, the patient's functional capacity one year before presentation should be ascertained and used as a goal. It would be unrealistic to expect to restore a patient of 80 years to 20 years. Unfortunately, functional goals are difficult to ascertain, imprecise in nature, and almost impossible to measure. Functional goals, to some extent, should be related to individual requirements for Activities of Daily Living.

A more objective parameter is the body weight. The accumulation of fluid in chronic cardiac failure is reflected by an increase in body weight. The relationship is not exactly on the basis that an increase in weight of 1 kg represents 1 L excess fluid. Cardiac failure leads to a marked loss of lean body tissue, especially muscle.[74] This arises because of a low cardiac output,[75] but in the elderly, is also contributed to by disuse atrophy from relative immobility, anorexia,[76] poor absorption[77] or loss from gastrointestinal congestion,[78] impaired hepatic metabolism,[76] and renal losses of protein.[79] Other mechanisms including circulating cytokines have also been implicated in the pathogenesis of cardiac wasting.[44,80,81] The benefits or otherwise of nutritional supplementation are presently unknown.[74]

Before starting treatment the patient's previous weight, 6 to 12 months earlier, should be determined. If it has increased, as it will usually have by the time of diagnosis, the increase represents excess salt and water. This body weight $\pm$ 0.5 kg should be the target to aim for, that when achieved, will represent neither gross over- nor undertreatment. Minimal peripheral edema that is not due to postural immobility suggests fluid overload of 4 L or more. Gross edema may represent up to 10 L excess.

Diuretic Agents

In a survey of nearly 2,000 patients admitted to departments of geriatric medicine across the United Kingdom, diuretic agents were being taken by 37 percent.[82] The figure of 1:3 people over the age of 65 years taking diuretic agents is one that should be some cause for concern. It is likely that many of these patients do not require such therapy and are being unjustifiably exposed to potential adverse effects. This and other studies[83,84] have suggested that approximately 40 percent of very elderly patients are regularly taking cardioactive drugs including diuretics. This emphasizes the point that cardiac problems increase markedly with increasing age.[85]

It should not be surprising then that diuretic agents are the most common group of drugs causing adverse reactions requiring hospital admission. Approximately 60 percent of all serious adverse drug reactions in elderly patients are due to diuretics.[82] However, in proportion to their total use, diuretic agents are not as harmful as other hypotensives and are safer in use than antispastics, psychoactive drugs, and digitalis. Approximately 10 percent of patients taking chronic diuretic agents will suffer adverse effects requiring hospital admission. This could be an underestimate, as not all adverse effects associated with diuretics are casually linked to the drugs.[86–88]

The modern physician is faced with many diuretic agents. Since the introduction in the early 1960s of orally effective agents, the number available seems to have increased exponentially. Although pharmaceutical companies claim specific advantages for their particular product, the differences within the major groups are to a large extent cosmetic.[89] The individual physician is recommended to become acquainted with one or two drugs of each of the major groups. The major groups of diuretics in clinical use are the thiazide and loop agents, which may be combined with the potassium-sparing drugs.

Thiazides

These drugs reduce sodium transport in the cortical diluting segment of the nephron proximal to the point of tubular sodium: potassium exchange. Consequently, they are more likely to lead to hypokalemia than the more potent loop diuretics.[90] In general, however, the problem of diuretic induced potassium loss has been grossly exaggerated.[91] After oral administration of a thiazide agent, diuresis will start within 1 to 3 hours and is complete between 8 and 24 hours. The longer-acting thiazide agents should be retained for the treatment of hypertension where they are effective hypotensives in low dose. Because the diuretic action of thiazides is reduced if the glomerular filtration rate is low, they are of little value on their own in chronic cardiac failure,[92,93] vide infra.

Loop Diuretics

These agents are much more powerful diuretics and exhibit a dose response curve.[94] When initiating therapy in elderly patients with fluid retention, low doses should be used initially to avoid the danger of excessive diuresis.[95] Loop diuretics act on the ascending loop of Henle by blocking movement of chloride ions and therefore sodium. They are less likely therefore to produce hypokalemia compared with thiazides and additionally, continue to be effective in patients with low glomerular filtration rates.[96,97]

Potassium-Sparing Agents

All three representatives of this group are by themselves weak diuretics and are therefore combined with either thiazides or loop agents. The structurally similar amiloride and triamterene act by blocking the exchange of sodium for potassium in the distal tubule. These agents unfortunately are widely used in treatment of cardiac failure and other forms of edema in old people.[91] The use of potassium-sparing agents is based on the hypothesis that the other more powerful diuretics produce potassium depletion and that by blocking the exchange of sodium for potassium in the distal tubule, potassium-sparing agents prevent hypokalemia and body potassium depletion. Unfortunately, these drugs are likely to produce serious hyperkalemia in some elderly patients.[98–100] In other patients they may produce hypokalemia.[99,101,102] Hyponatremia, which is often symptomatic and occasionally fatal, is associated with potassium-sparing diuretic usage in elderly patients with chronic cardiac failure.[103–106] Their use on a routine basis in the older patient cannot be supported.[91,107]

Choice of Diuretic Agent

For the elderly patient with chronic cardiac failure, the choice of diuretic agent should be based on consideration of the efficacy and adverse effects profile of the agent, and the social and medical circumstances of the individual patient. The range of diuretics available allows the physician to tailor the drug to meet individual patient's conditions. Rarely, in certain conditions—pre-existing urinary frequency or incontinence—a diuretic may not be first-line treatment; an angiotensin-converting enzyme (ACE) inhibitor may be a compromise solution.

The concept of stepped diuretic therapy is of value when planning treatment of the older patient. There is a tendency in clinical practice to commence treatment with too high a dose of a too powerful diuretic. The consequences of this in terms of adverse effects and patient compliance are not inconsiderable. Old people are not likely to continue taking a drug that confines them to a world within 5 m of the lavatory. Multiple pathology may mean a patient with chronic cardiac failure is immobile not from the failure but coexisting arthropathy or neurologic damage.[108] Physicians prescribing these drugs to relatively immobile old people should have personally experienced the effects of 80 mg of frusemide, preferably before setting out on a long car journey or attending the theater.

Efficacy

In the presence of normal renal function all diuretics are usually effective in most patients with chronic cardiac failure.[95] When initiating diuretic therapy for elderly patients with chronic cardiac failure, it is tempting to start with a low-dose thiazide agent.[109] However, it is important to remember that thiazides are ineffective diuretics if the glomerular filtration rate is reduced to below 30 to 40 ml/min.[66,110,111] In the elderly patient with chronic cardiac failure, renal function is impaired by virtue of increased age,[112,113] by the reduced cardiac output of cardiac failure itself,[114] and often, other coexistent pathologies.[115]

Metabolic adverse effects of diuretics in the elderly

Hyperkalemia
Hyponatremia
Uremia
Hyperglycemia
Hypercalciuria
Hypokalemia
Hyperuricemia

Therefore and considering different adverse effects profiles, vide infra, a loop diuretic is to be preferred to a thiazide for elderly patients with cardiac failure.[116,117] Where the condition is chronic, it is best to measure the plasma electrolytes first,[38,118] then introduce a low-dose loop agent such as frusemide 20 mg or bumetanide 0.5 mg daily. This dose can be titrated upwards at 48-hour intervals depending upon diuretic response. It may be necessary to rapidly increase oral doses of loop diuretics in some elderly patients because of the age-related increases in variability of pharmacokinetics and renal responsiveness.[119–121]

Without frank renal failure (blood urea greater than 30 mmol/L or creatinine clearance less than 15 ml/min), the vast majority of elderly patients will respond before reaching high oral doses of loop diuretics (e.g., less than 160 mg frusemide/4 mg bumetanide). Some elderly compliant patients without gross renal impairment may not respond to these doses. In these individuals changing to parenteral therapy for a few days may induce a diuresis.[66] The parenteral dose should be one-half the preceding oral dose and can be titrated upward if necessary. For patients living in the community, loop agents can be administered intramuscularly by a visiting nurse on a daily basis.[122] If patients do not respond to parenteral loop diuretics and are still grossly edematous, oral metolazone can be added after again halving the dose of loop agent.[123,124] Occasionally, this may result in a torrential diuresis with rapid and significant hypokalemia. This regimen should therefore be only started when the patient is in hospital, where close monitoring of urine output, blood pressure, and plasma electrolytes can be performed.[125] If necessary in refractory cases, a dopamine infusion may restore diuretic sensitivity, especially in elderly patients with gross renal impairment.[126,127]

Adverse Effects

It is not the purpose in this review to discuss all the adverse metabolic effects of diuretics, but to stress those problems that are pertinent to physicians treating elderly patients. For a general discussion of metabolic side effects the reader should consult some of the excellent reviews available.[84,128–130] Some of the main adverse metabolic effects of diuretics in elderly patients are listed in the accompanying boxed list.

Plasma Potassium

Plasma potassium levels do not decrease with increasing age in healthy individuals; indeed, on balance, there is a small but systematic increase.[131] Equally, while there is a decrease in body potassium content with increasing age, this does not represent body potassium depletion, as the reduction is proportional to a reduction in the body potassium capacity as represented by the lean body mass.[132,133] (For a full discussion of the effects of aging on potassium status, see Ch. 21).

The effects of chronic cardiac failure upon potassium status are becoming clear. Patients with untreated cardiac failure have on average higher plasma potassium levels than patients with untreated hypertension.[90] This is likely also to be the case in elderly patients.[91] Equally, cardiac failure seems to have little effect upon body potassium stores of both young[134–137] and elderly patients.[138,139] The conclusion, therefore, must be that neither aging, cardiac failure, nor their combination have significant or systematic effects on plasma potassium levels nor on body potassium content.[90,138]

Diuretics have been implicated in disturbances of potassium status of both young and old patients with chronic cardiac failure. It has been suggested that both thiazide and loop agents lead to hypokalemia and that this is especially likely in elderly patients.[83,140–143] In a population-based study Petri et al.[83] claimed that 28 percent of elderly patients taking thiazide agents were "hypokalemic." They also suggest that this proportion was halved in patients taking concomitant β-blocking drugs or captopril. Unfortunately, they do not state their lower limit of normal for plasma potassium, but the absolute range of their results in thiazide-treated patients—2.9 to 5.3 mmol/L (mmol/L = mEq/L)—suggests that very few had levels less than 3.0 mmol/L. It has been suggested that hypokalemia only below 3.0 mmol/L is significant in terms of adverse effects.[90,144–147] Some have claimed that levels below 3.5 mmol/L significantly affect cardiac conductivity.[148,149] The large Medical Research Council trial in mild to moderate hypertension found little relationship between plasma potassium levels and ventricular extrasystoles.[150] A recent well-controlled study showed that in elderly patients thiazide therapy did not affect the frequency of ventricular ectopics monitored over 24 hours.[151] This study also failed to find a relationship between hypokalemia and ectopic activity, and the addition of digoxin therapy did not increase ectopic activity. It is more likely that arrhythmic activity in elderly patients is related to increased age itself or to the degree of myocardial damage rather than any presumed metabolic effects of therapy.[151–153] It is likely that both the incidence and the significance of diuretic induced hypokalemia in elderly patients with cardiac failure have been grossly exaggerated.[91]

Alternatively, the problem of diuretic-induced hyperkalemia has not been sufficiently stressed. In a survey of nearly 5,000 patients taking diuretics with potassium supplements, Lawson[154] found that 3.6 percent of patients were hyperkalemic. In 16 percent of these hyperkalemic patients the level of potassium was life threatening; in 4 percent, the hyperkalemia was a contributory cause of death. There was a clear relationship between the incidence of hyperkalemia and increasing age. The danger of potassium supplements given to elderly patients with chronic cardiac failure was subsequently emphasized by Kassirer and Harrington.[155,156]

The propensity for elderly patients with cardiac failure to develop hyperkalemia is probably not completely attributable to increased age but, in addition, decreased renal function plays a part.[157–160] As discussed above, the combination of age-related decrease in renal blood flow and cardiac failure markedly decreases renal function. In addition, the elderly patient with cardiac failure may develop plasma volume depletion, usually secondary to dehydration, and thus a prerenal element is introduced (see Ch. 66).

Plasma Sodium

Hyponatremia (plasma sodium less than 130 mmol/L) on occasions is due to excessive dosage of thiazide[106,161] or loop diuretic agents.[140] The most frequent cause of hyponatremia in the elderly, however, is the use of potassium-sparing agents, in particular amiloride.[105,162–164] Hyponatremia is still a problem with other potassium-sparing agents such as triamterene.[165] Often the hyponatremia produced by these agents is symptomatic, leading to severe weakness, lethargy, and/or confusion,[166] or even death.[167] These symptoms may be mistakenly attributed to the underlying disease process rather than to the adverse effects of the drugs being administered. Uremia produced by potassium-sparing agents is especially likely in elderly patients with chronic cardiac failure.[86] Treatment of these metabolic consequences is the withdrawal of the potassium-sparing agent.[91]

Other Metabolic Adverse Effects

Diuretics lead to increases in serum cholesterol in patients of all ages including the elderly.[168,169] Whether this represents a risk factor for progression of coronary heart disease is debatable.[66,170] It is likely to be but a minimal danger in the face of the total mortality of established cardiac failure in the elderly patient.[171] Following the introduction of orally active diuretics there was anxiety that both thiazide[172] and loop diuretics[173] raise the serum uric acid and may therefore result in acute gout in elderly patients. In the event, however, it seems that the risk of gout is largely confined to elderly women in whom the gout is not acute but tophaceous.[174]

Following the introduction of orally active diuretics in the early 1960s, it was soon appreciated that both thiazide[175–177] and loop agents[178,179] could lead to impairment of glucose tolerance in diabetic and nondiabetic subjects. The impairment of glucose tolerance is usually reversible following withdrawal of the diuretic.[180] However, frank and nonreversible diabetes may be precipitated in patients who are presumed to be "prediabetic" or alternatively, have a strong family history for the disease.[181] In this situation, diabetes is nonreversible on withdrawing the diuretic. The elderly patient with pre-existing age-related carbohydrate intolerance is more likely to exhibit increases in blood sugar during diuretic therapy,[171,182] but the degree of carbohydrate intolerance in the elderly is no greater than in the young.[183] Loop agents are significantly less diabetogenic than thiazides in elderly subjects,[88] and bumetanide is probably less diabetogenic than frusemide.[184]

All loop diuretics are to a variable degree ototoxic.[185] Initially it was thought that ototoxicity only occurred following massive parenteral dosage with loop diuretics in patients with renal impairment.[186] This is not necessarily the case, as impaired hearing may follow standard dosage of loop diuretics in patients and experimental animals with normal renal function.[187,188] Bumetanide is the least likely to produce ototoxic problems.[189,190] Therefore, considering the lesser diabetogenic capacity of bumetanide, this agent is to be the preferred loop diuretic for elderly patients with chronic cardiac failure.[125]

Thiazide diuretics may affect calcium homeostasis by interfering with calcium absorption[191] or decreasing urinary calcium excretion.[83] They may even reduce the rate of recurrence of calcium urinary calculi.[192] However, loop agents have more significant effects upon calcium balance by markedly increasing distal tubular calcium excretion.[193] Sometimes the effect may be sufficient to compromise treatment of osteoporosis in elderly patients.[194] Changing to a thiazide agent may be necessary for patients with a combination of severe osteopenia and cardiac failure. The rate of hip fracture may be reduced by thiazide therapy in elderly patients.[195]

Physical Problems of Diuretics in the Elderly

By the very nature of their action, diuretic agents lead to an increased production of urine. Because the capacity of the bladder is finite, they increase both the frequency and volume of voiding. This response will seriously limit social activity of many patients. Patients often avoid taking their diuretic agents if they are leaving home for another activity such as shopping or visiting the outpatient clinic. A particular problem with the powerful loop diuretics in elderly patients is that they can produce or potentiate incontinence of urine.[108] Patients will be very unwilling to take drugs that produce this socially embarrassing situation. The prescriber must bear this in mind when choosing between the different agents. Thus, some patients may prefer a gentler prolonged diuresis, as will be produced by a thiazide or low-dose loop agent, whereas others would prefer a short duration brisk diuresis produced by high-dose loop agents. Discussion with the patient will lead to the best choice.

In elderly men with prostatic hypertrophy and bladder outflow obstruction, the sudden introduction of a high-dose loop diuretic may well result in acute retention of urine. This is obviously an extremely disturbing condition and may lead to the patient undergoing urgent urologic surgery. Acute retention of urine associated with a brisk diuresis also occurs in women with bladder neck outflow obstruction.[95] Patients with urinary leakage associated with an unstable bladder will find their symptoms worsened. To some extent, these problems of retention/incontinence can be avoided by the use of low-dose loop diuretics or the thiazide agents.

Physical problems of diuretics in the elderly

Incontinence
Retention
Hypotension
  supine
  postural
  postprandial
Urinary frequency/urgency
Hearing loss
Renal/bladder stones
Osteopenia

Hypotension and uremia are usually, although not always, a result of overdosage with diuretic agents.[88,155] On occasion, they may occur when diuretics have been inappropriately prescribed for immobility edema. A particular problem in elderly patients is the potentiation or precipitation of postural hypotension. This syndrome of many causes is a particular feature of the elderly[47] and diuretic agents used in excess[196] or, even in usual dosage,[197] may produce hypovolemia and aggravate the condition.[196] The treatment of these conditions is to reduce the dose of diuretic agent and, if necessary, add in other cardioactive drugs to maintain cardiovascular function.

Digoxin

William Withering[198] reported on the clinical efficacy in chronic cardiac failure of an infusion prepared from the purple foxglove. He also commented on the "narrow therapeutic window" and the toxicity of this preparation of digitalis. The positive inotropic action of digitalis as ouabain was demonstrated using papillary muscle preparations in 1938 by Cattell and Gold.[199] Since then, controversy has surrounded digitalis particularly as to its precise mode of action at cellular level.[200–203] This aspect need not concern us here. In this section, the use of digitalis preparations in the treatment of chronic cardiac failure in elderly patients will be considered from a purely clinical viewpoint.

There are more than 300 different cardioactive glycosides either naturally occurring, derived from various species of foxglove, or synthetic.[204] While some workers have laid stress on varying pharmacodynamic profiles of the different preparations of digitalis,[205,206] in clinical practice, the differences are largely irrelevant.[207] In the main, choice of digitalis preparation falls between digoxin, popular in Europe, and digitoxin, popular in North America. For a review of the important pharmacokinetic differences between different glycosides, the reader is referred to the review by Lye.[208] For clarity of discussion throughout the rest of this review, references to digoxin should be taken to include digitoxin and other available digitalis preparations unless stated otherwise.

Apart from being a positive inotrope, digoxin has many other actions. Effects on cardiac conduction and the autonomic nervous system are well known, but even within the therapeutic range, direct effects of digoxin are seen on the peripheral vasculature (venous and arterial constriction[209]), kidney (weak diuretic[210]), and gastrointestinal tract (gastric irritation[207]), and it also exhibits an estrogenic effect (gynaecomastia in men[211]). The noncardiac effects of digoxin become more obvious in overdosage and intoxication.

Inotropism

There are many trials and reviews showing that digoxin is a positive inotrope in patients with chronic sinus rhythm cardiac failure and, further, that digoxin-induced inotropism is clinically beneficial and well sustained.[94,212–218] Equally, there are many trials and reviews showing the opposite.[219–226] Several other studies have suggested that only some patients, usually the more disabled, respond to digoxin therapy.[227–231] Other reports extol the virtues of withdrawing digoxin from patients on long-term therapy for cardiac failure.[232–238] Although the designs and analyses of many of these studies have been criticized,[225,239–242] the general conclusion must be that there is some doubt about the effectiveness of digoxin as an inotropic agent in sinus rhythm chronic cardiac failure.[243]

The use of digoxin in patients with established atrial fibrillation and chronic cardiac failure is less controversial.[244,245] The therapeutic objective in this situation is to reduce ventricular response by enhancing atrioventricular block.[207] Slowing the heart rate in fast atrial fibrillation will improve ventricular filling and therefore, cardiac output.[246,247] The objective is to reduce resting heart rate to between 70 and 80 beats per minute.[248] Undue resistance of atrial fibrillation to adequate digoxin should lead to a consideration of other coexistent diseases. If the ventricular rate cannot be slowed in spite of plasma levels of digoxin being within the therapeutic range, verapamil[249] or diltiazem[250] should be carefully added.

Factors associated with "resistant" atrial fibrillation in the elderly

Compliance
Hyperthyroidism
Pulmonary emboli
Anemia
Endocarditis
Pericarditis
Amyloid
Myocarditis
Digoxin toxicity

Features of digoxin intoxication in the elderly

Weakness/lethargy
Depression
Confusion
Anorexia
Nausea/vomiting
Diarrhea
Xanthopsia/scotomata
Headache/dizziness
Any cardiac arrhythmia

Toxicity

Digoxin and all other preparations of digitalis have a narrow therapeutic window.[251] In the situation of the controlled clinical trial with strict inclusion and exclusion criteria associated with close monitoring, toxicity has not been reported to be a particular problem.[216,252] However, in the less strict environment of the clinical world, digoxin intoxication is a very frequent problem.[222,226,253–257] The incidence of digoxin toxicity may have decreased slightly in recent years following the introduction of serum measurements and increased awareness of the problem.[258–262]

If healthy, community-dwelling adult elephants can be killed by excess cardiac glycosides,[263] then we should not be surprised if frail elderly cardiac failure patients are equally at risk of digoxin poisoning. The elderly heart itself is probably more sensitive to the actions of digoxin.[262] Apart from this pharmacodynamic consideration, pharmacokinetic age differences are much more likely to lead to digoxin intoxication of the elderly patient. Digoxin clearance is directly related to renal function as measured by creatinine clearance.[226,264,265] As discussed previously, the elderly patient with chronic cardiac failure has reduced renal function by virtue of age and by virtue of cardiac failure. The addition of a prerenal element of dehydration, for example, due to respiratory infection, is likely to result in digoxin toxicity in an otherwise previously stable patient.[266] The symptoms of digoxin toxicity are then, attributed to the chest infection with dire consequences for the patient.

The age-related decrease in lean body mass[267–269] will lead to higher tissue levels of active digoxin as will the age-related decrease in plasma albumin binding capacity.[270,271] Polypharmacy is always a problem with elderly patients[82] and is likely to lead to potentially dangerous drug interactions, especially between digoxin and quinidine and amiodarone.[261,272] Finally, difficulties with compliance by elderly patients may increase the incidence of digoxin intoxication.[273,274]

The signs and symptoms of digoxin intoxication are well known. Unfortunately, for the poisoned patient, the vague symptoms of weakness, lethargy, and depression, which are the hallmarks of digoxin toxicity,[207] may be ascribed to the underlying condition of cardiac failure.[275] Anorexia, nausea, and diarrhea, which are early manifestations of toxicity in the young, are not so obvious in the elderly patient.[276] Central nervous system symptoms such as confusion and particularly, depression are common features of intoxication in the elderly.[208,277] Because of multiple pathology and/or polypharmacy, signs and symptoms of digoxin toxicity in elderly patients are easily unrecognized, with fatal consequences. Sometimes the first manifestation of digoxin toxicity—ventricular fibrillation—is the last.[278]

Other Inotropic Agents

Doubts about the efficacy of digitalis preparations in sinus rhythm cardiac failure have lead to the development of other inotropic agents. There are two main groups—the phosphodiesterase inhibitors and the sympathomimetic agents. After some initial enthusiasm,[279,280] it seems that despite the potential benefits (inotropism and vasodilation) all the phosphodiesterase inhibitors (amrinone, milrinone, and enoximone) have failed to produce benefits in clinical practice.[281–286] Their tendency to increase ventricular ectopy and induce life-threatening arrhythmias are likely to limit their use in all patients with chronic cardiac failure.[216,282,287] Additionally, overstimulation of the myocardium, by further damaging myocardial cells, may inevitably increase mortality in chronic cardiac failure.[288,289]

The sympathomimetic agents, dopamine[290] and dobutamine,[291] may benefit some elderly patients with chronic cardiac failure.[292] Unfortunately, both agents have to be given parenterally and should therefore be reserved for those resistant to diuretics or suffering severe cardiac failure; further, because of the development of tolerance, the drugs need to be given intermittently.[293] Using this regime, Van den Brande and colleagues[294] claim symptomatic and hemodynamic improvements in elderly patients with severe cardiac failure. Other workers have not been able to prove equal benefits.[295,296] Similarly, the adverse effects of the oral β-adrenergic agonists (isoprenaline, pirbuterol, zinternol) outweigh any benefits in hemodynamic function they may produce.[297,298] Thus, promising results from animal work have failed to translate into clinical practice.[299]

Conclusion

Digoxin is of value as a chronotropic antiarrhythmic agent in appropriate patients of all ages. This applies particularly to patients with fast atrial fibrillation with or without accompanying chronic cardiac failure. Unfortunately, the narrow therapeutic window for all digitalis preparations makes dangerous toxicity a likely event. Toxicity is both enhanced and more frequent in the elderly patient with chronic cardiac failure. Doubts about the beneficial inotropic activity of digitalis preparations have shifted the cost: benefit equation so much that now the conclusion must be that digitalis should no longer be used in the treatment of sinus rhythm cardiac failure of old people. Newer inotropic agents have yet to prove their value before entering clinical use in the treatment of cardiac failure in old people.[300–303] There are better and many safer alternative options, vide infra.

ACE Inhibitors

A major response to a reduction in effective plasma volume caused by cardiac failure is peripheral vasoconstriction brought about by angiotensin II (Fig. 22-1D). Angiotensin-converting enzyme inhibitors block the conversion of inactive angiotensin I to vasoconstricting angiotensin II.[304] Additionally, ACE inhibitors block aldosterone output and reduce, but do not abolish, sympathetic peripheral vasoconstriction.[305] Thus, these agents act as partial peripheral vasodilators, reducing cardiac afterload, while preserving some peripheral vasoactivity allowing maintenance of blood pressure regulation during, for example, change in posture. This is important in preventing postural hypotension in frail, at-risk elderly patients.[196]

Numerous well-conducted trials of ACE inhibitors have shown significant survival benefits as well as symptomatic improvement in patients with severe,[306] moderate,[307] and mild[308] cardiac failure. In addition, these agents have been shown to prevent or postpone the development of cardiac failure in patients at various degrees of risk with left ventricular dysfunction.[309–312] Finally, ACE inhibitors have been shown to increase well-being and reduce hospital admissions of cardiac failure patients with obvious and significant economic savings.[313–315] These otherwise laudable treatment trials have one major limitation: they mostly excluded those patients with the highest prevalence of cardiac failure—the elderly.[118,316] This omission has led some to question the role of ACE inhibitors in the management of elderly cardiac failure patients.[317]

Although extrapolation from ACE inhibitor trials in younger cardiac failure patients is potentially hazardous, there are sound theoretic reasons to support their use in the older patient. Angiotensin II selectively decreases renal blood flow[318] and ACE inhibitors can reverse this.[319–321] This should be of particular benefit to the older patient with age-related reduced renal blood flow combined with further reduction by virtue of cardiac failure and possibly other age-related pathology such as prerenal uremia associated with respiratory infection. All elderly cardiac failure patients with left ventricular dysfunction without specific contraindications (stenotic valve lesions) should be commenced on long-term ACE inhibitors.

They are best introduced using captopril at a dose of 6.25 mg given as the patient retires to bed at night. If there is no problem (fainting, dizziness, etc.) this is continued at 6.25 mg twice daily and after that, titrated upward until 50 mg twice daily is achieved. Then change to a once daily agent to aid compliance. The target dose should be the same as use in the various drug trials. The ATLAS (Assessment of Treatment with Lisinopril Survival) trial reports that lower maintenance doses may have been shown to be effective.[322] If problems do arise or the patient is high risk (hypotensive, dehydrated, uramic,

Table 22-2 Cardiovascular interaction of ACE inhibitors

NSAIDs	Fluid retention
Aspirin	Fluid retention De-unloading of LV
Antacids	Reduced bioavailability
Probenecid	Renal retention
Alcohol	Enhanced hypotension
SSRIs	Enhanced hypotension

Abbreviations: ACE, angiotensin-converting enzyme; NSAIDs, nonsteroidal anti-inflammatory drugs; LV, left ventricle; SSRIs, selective seratonin receptor inhibitors.

hyponatremic, hyperkalemic), the patient should be admitted to hospital for initiation of treatment.

Adverse Effects

For such powerful and effective drugs, the ACE inhibitors have proved to be remarkably safe in clinical use.[231,317,323] Not unexpectedly, the elderly cardiac failure patient is more likely to experience adverse reactions to ACE inhibitors than younger patients.[324] Initiating therapy in frail elderly patients who may be overtreated with diuretics is likely to cause severe symptomatic hypotension—first-dose hypotension.[325–327] This may be prevented by starting with a low dose[328] of a short-acting agent such as captopril[329] and excluding patients with a diastolic blood pressure less than 70 mmHg.[330] Reducing diuretic dose, or even withdrawing for 24 to 36 hours, may help to prevent first-dose hypotension.[331]

ACE inhibitors can worsen renal function or even result in renal failure in patients with renal artery atheroma.[329,332,333] Usually, any impairment in renal function rapidly resolves following withdrawal.[334] Paradoxically, ACE inhibitors may benefit renal function, especially proteinuria, in cardiac failure patients with diabetic nephropathy.[335,336] As diabetes is so common in elderly patients with cardiac failure, especially if treated with thiazide diuretics, this effect warrants further study. Potassium retention occurs with ACE inhibitors alone,[337,338] though is more likely when coprescribed with potassium supplements[339] or potassium-sparing diuretics.[340] In the first CONSENSUS trial,[306] hyperkalemia occurred only in those patients taking concurrent spironolactone.

Other adverse effects of ACE inhibitors are less frequent and/or less serious. Cough is a problem in some patients. Unfortunately, this is a class effect, and there is little value in changing to a different ACE inhibitor.[341] The use of disodium cromoglycate to suppress ACE inhibitor produced cough is not likely to be practical with elderly patients.[342] Table 22-2 lists some ACE inhibitor drug interactions that are of some consequence in patients with cardiac disease.

Conclusion

The introduction of ACE inhibitors has been a major advance in our management of elderly patients with chronic cardiac failure. ACE inhibitors cannot replace diuretics; they act synergistically with diuretics.[343,344] Differences between the different agents are marginal, and the clinician is advised to become familiar with perhaps just one short-acting and one long-acting agent. Used carefully and appropriately, the cost: benefit ratio of ACE inhibitors is very good and it is unlikely that the ratio is any less favorable in the elderly patient.[345–348] The evidence is now suggesting that ACE inhibitors on the basis of efficacy and safety should replace digoxin in the treatment of chronic cardiac failure in the elderly.

Vasodilators

Vasodilators were initially introduced for acute or intractable cardiac failure and especially cardiogenic shock.[349] Reduction in preload[350] and afterload[351] significantly improved survival in this critical condition.[352,353] The vasodilatory properties of morphine, especially within the pulmonary circulation, have been known and successfully used for many years.[354] Success of vasodilators in the acute phase of cardiac failure suggested they may have a role in chronic cardiac failure.

Initially, workers showed improvements in hemodynamic parameters associated with increased exercise capacity in patients with chronic cardiac failure given nitrates,[355,356] prazosin,[357] or hydralazine.[358,359] A particularly important study of vasodilators was the Veterans Administration Heart Failure Trial (V-HeFT). This study of 273 men with chronic cardiac failure compared prazosin with isorbide dinitrate plus hydralazine and concluded that the latter combination lowered mortality, whereas prazosin was ineffective.[360] This conclusion of the V-HeFT study has been widely accepted.[7,287,296,361] Unfortunately, the benefits claimed in the V-HeFT study were but marginal and the statistics have been severely criticized.[94] It should also be noted that the average age of participants in the V-HeFT study was only 58 years, and the results may not be extrapolated to elderly patients with chronic cardiac failure.

Other workers have found vasodilators, including nitrates,[362] prazosin,[363,364] hydralazine,[365–367] minoxidil,[368] and flosequinan,[369,370] to be variously ineffective, ill-sustained in benefit, or limited by unacceptable side effects. The conclusion is that both arterial and venous direct-acting vasodilators are of little use in the management of long-term chronic cardiac failure in the young[287,288,371] or elderly patient[296] and should be reserved for symptomatic patients unable to tolerate ACE inhibitors.[230]

Normal Systolic Function Cardiac Failure

The general availability of echocardiography has revealed that some people with chronic cardiac failure secondary to coronary artery disease have normal systolic function (i.e., contractility of the left ventricle is not impaired).[372–374] Prior to the introduction of widespread echocardiography, it had been assumed that cardiac failure with few exceptions was due to impaired left ventricular contractility (systolic dysfunction)—the classic picture.[375–377] Because of the effects of normal aging on left ventricular morphology, as detailed above, it is not surprising that a large proportion—probably up to 50 percent of elderly cardiac failure patients have normal systolic function.[316,378–381] It is important not to equate normal systolic function with diastolic dysfunction, as the latter can be only determined by invasive measures of ventricular filling pressures.[382,383] The phrase "diastolic cardiac failure" is often used as an unfortunate inexactitude.[384]

Symptomatically, cardiac failure patients with systolic dysfunction cannot be distinguished from those with normal systolic function.[316,385] For some reason as yet unknown, female cardiac failure patients are more likely than males to have normal systolic function.[386] The two conditions can be readily diagnosed by echocardiography or radionucleide scanning.[374,387] This is one reason why all elderly cardiac failure patients should undergo echocardiographic investigation.[57,388] While cardiac failure usually carries a very poor prognosis regardless of age and modern improvements in treatment,[317,389,390] patients with normal systolic function have improved survival compared with those showing even quite minimal systolic dysfunction in spite of the older age of the former.[391,392] Paradoxically, older patients with normal systolic function cardiac failure may sustain more symptomatic exacerbations of failure.[393]

Treatment

The management and treatment of classic cardiac failure with assumed systolic dysfunction have evolved since the use of scylla glycosides and opium, circa 50 A.D.,[394] via William Withering and digoxin[198] to using the results of the recent large and expensive drug trials.[395] No such sustained history guides our treatment of normal systolic function cardiac failure.[316] Treatment options are limited as there are no specifically lusitropic agents available for clinical use. Treatment recommendations therefore are based upon physiologic principles and anecdotal evidence. This approach underlines the urgent need for treatment trials in patients with normal systolic function failure, as well as including more older patients. Treatment of aggravating factors is obviously important, especially those causing hypertrophy or architectural deformation of the left ventricle.

Nonpharmacologic maneuvers have been shown to improve cardiac performance in subjects with normal systolic function cardiac failure.[316] They include weight reduction,[396,397] especially in diabetics,[397,398] and exercise training.[399] Restoration of synchronized atrial contraction in patients with atrial fibrillation will improve ventricular filling and therefore, cardiac output.[400–402] In elderly patients this is best accomplished by chemical conversion and maintenance using amiodarone.[403,404] Ultrafiltration, though effective in grossly fluid-overloaded patients, is not a realistic, routine proposal.[405] Lowering blood pressure in hypertensive cardiac failure patients is a very effective way of improving left ventricular architecture and diastolic function.[406–408] Finally, reducing uremia in renal failure leads to hemodynamic benefits, which are often maintained for some time.[409]

Specific drug treatments of normal systolic function cardiac failure include the use of diuretics mainly to improve symptoms.[410] However, it should be recalled that a high left ventricular filling pressure is important and should be maintained by avoiding overdiuresis.[411,412] Digoxin confers no hemodynamic benefit,[218] is arrhythmogenic, and therefore, dangerous in patients with normal systolic function.[226,413] Calcium channel antagonists improve left ventricular relaxation and filling but unfortunately, this is counterbalanced by their negative inotropic properties, especially a problem in older patients.[414–417] A further problem of calcium channel antagonists recently highlighted in elderly patients is increased danger of gastrointestinal bleeding[418] and possibly cancer.[419] The β-adrenergic antagonists suffer from the same drawback.[420,421] The ACE inhibitors, though underinvestigated, probably remain the best option after low to moderate dose diuretics.[316,410,422,423] In the future, large-scale drug trials in cardiac failure should select patients on the basis of ventricular dysfunction and if adequate numbers of old people are recruited, valid conclusions about diastolic dysfunction and its treatment could be drawn.[316]

"Resistant" Cardiac Failure

The most common cause for cardiac failure not to respond to drug treatment is the patient not taking the drugs.[274,424–426] There is little evidence that elderly patients are more or less conscientious in taking medication than young patients. A particular problem surrounds diuretic usage and the social inconvienience of urinary frequency or worse. Patients (of all ages) should be allowed to vary the time of day or frequency of taking diuretics in order to fit in with their activities such as shopping. If the patient is traveling, the diuretic can be omitted for a day; the patient will not have time to accumulate sufficient fluid to precipitate pulmonary edema.

Iatrogenic problems may underlie "resistance."[427] Nonsteroidal anti-inflammatory drugs (NSAIDs), so often prescribed to old people, cause fluid retention via prostaglandin synthetase inhibition and worsen cardiac failure.[428–430] Substitution with a paracetamol-like analgesic may restore diuresis. β-Adrenergic[431–433] and calcium channel[434–436] antagonists should be avoided because of their negative inotropic properties. In certain circumstances, such as normal systolic function cardiac failure, low dose or newer agents may be used on an experimental basis.[410,437–439] Topical β-adreneric antagonists used locally in the treatment of glaucoma probably do not worsen cardiac failure.[440]

Persistent or frequent transient arrhythmias may render cardiac failure difficult to treat.[61,247,441] Treatment of atrial fibrillation has already been discussed but bradycardias, although less common, are worth treating with a pacemaker if cardiac failure is proving resistant.[442] The routine use of antiarrhythmics to suppress ventricular ectopy and prevent sudden death cannot be recommended. Two recent trials of arrhythmia suppression have given conflicting results.[442–444] Hyperthyroidism is as relevant now[445] as it was 30 years ago.[446] Amyloid, though uncommon, should be suspected in very old patients with resistant failure, especially if associated with resistant atrial fibrillation.[447,448] Infections, including myocarditis, pericarditis, and endocarditis, are always worth seeking and treating in their own right.[449–452] Features of subacute bacterial endocarditis in elderly patients are often quite silent, apart from resistant cardiac failure.[453] Unsuspected valve lesions, especially aortic stenosis, are often overlooked but are easily revealed by echocardiography.[454] The results of surgery, even in the very old,[455] are very gratifying, and there is improvement in both resistant cardiac failure and quality of life.[456]

Future Perspectives

Until quite recently it was thought that angiotensin II was the main peripheral vasoconstricting hormone in chronic cardiac failure (Fig. 22-1D).[44,457–459] It is now apparent that activation of the endothelin-1 system is another component of the neurohormonal response to cardiac failure.[460–464] Levels of endothelin-1 in cardiac failure patients predict both exercise capacity[465–467] and survival.[468,469] Endothelin-1 receptor antagonists have markedly improved hemodynamics of rats with cardiac failure already on optimum treatment including ACE inhibitors.[470] If orally active antagonists and/or receptor blockers can be developed, it may provide a significant new approach to management.[471] As yet, there are no published studies in elderly patients (or elderly mammals), though if promise is fulfilled, the aged cardiovascular system is likely to benefit more than the younger system.[472] If this proves successful it may lead to a reappraisal of the value of low-dose peripheral vasodilators in cardiac failure.[230,473] An alternative approach to altered endothelial function in cardiac failure[474,475] would be by modification of nitric oxide in peripheral vessels,[81,476] or in the heart itself.[477,478]

Interest is growing in the use of β-adrenergic antagonists with α-1 vasodilatory properties both in hypertension[479,480] and cardiac failure. In particular, carvedilol has been shown to be effective in short-term[437] and longer term studies.[481] One problem, hypotension, may limit use in elderly cardiac failure patients.[482] It is possible that carvedilol will be of particular value in normal systolic function cardiac failure.[438] The future does not look bright for positive inotropes in cardiac failure, though trials of low-dose vesnarinone have been encouraging[302,483] and the drug has its advocates.[473,484] There is a suspicion that the drug in high dose may, like flosequinan,[370] increase mortality.[361]

One area that should receive more attention is prevention of thromboembolic complications in chronic cardiac failure.[485] Pulmonary embolism and infarction are particular problems in immobile elderly patients.[486,487] Treatment by full or low-dose oral anticoagulation reduces mortality of hospitalized elderly cardiac failure patients.[473,488,489] Certainly, patients with associated atrial fibrillation should be anticoagulated with warfarin.[490–492] A compromise using aspirin is probably not indicated, as the drug interacts with ACE inhibitors[493,494] and depresses myocardial function.[495] Unfortunately, it seems that cardiologists are more willing to use warfarin than geriatricians, who prefer aspirin.[496]

References

1. Parameshwar J, Shackell M, Richardson A et al: Prevalence of heart failure in two general practices. Br Heart J 1989;61: 114
2. Petri M, Gatling W, Hill LM et al: Cardiovascular disease and heart failure in a defined community based diabetic population. Clin Sci 1985;69:P1
3. Gibson TC, White KL, Klainer LM: The prevalence of congestive heart failure in two rural communities. J Chron Dis 1966; 19:141–52
4. Kannel WB, Belanger AJ: Epidemiology of heart failure. Am Heart J 1991;121:951–7
5. Haavisto M, Geiger U, Mattila K, Rajala S: A health survey of the very aged in Tampere, Finland. Age Ageing 1984;13: 266–72
6. Landahl S, Svanborg A, Astrand K: Heart volume and the prevalence of certain common cardiovascular disorders at 70 and 75 years of age. Eur Heart J 1984;5:326–31
7. Webb GC, Impallomeni MG: Heart failure in the elderly. Q J Med 1987;244:641–50
8. Clarke KW, Gray D, Hampton JR: How common is heart-failure—evidence from PACT (prescribing analysis and cost) data in Nottingham. J Pub Health Med 1995;17:459–64
9. Aronow WS: Prevalence of appropriate and inappropriate indications for use of digoxin in older patients at the time of admission to a nursing home. J Am Geriatr Soc 1996;44:588–90
10. McMurray J, Hart W, Rhodes G: An evaluation of the cost of heart failure to the National Health Service in the UK. Br J Health Econ 1993;6:99–110
11. McMurray J, Hart W: The economic impact of heart failure on the National Health Service. Br Heart J 1993;69:P19
12. Gerstenblith G, Fleg JL, Weiss J et al: Stress criteria redefines the prevalence of coronary artery disease in epidemiologic studies. Circulation 1980;62:304–8
13. Truswell AS, Hansen JDL: Medical research among the !Kung. In Lee RB, DeVore I, eds: Kalahari Hunter Gatherers. Harvard University Press, Harvard, 1976
14. Kostis JB, Moregra AE, Amendo MT et al: The effect of age on heart rate in subjects free of heart disease. Circulation 1982;65:141–5
15. Darr KC, Bassett DR, Morgan BJ, Thomas DP: Effects of age and training status on heart rate recovery after peak exercise. Am J Physiol 1988;254:H340–3
16. Rodeheffer RJ, Gerstenblith G, Becker LC et al: Exercise cardiac output is maintained with advancing age in healthy human subjects: cardiac dilatation and increased stroke volume com-

pensate for a diminished heart rate. Circulation 1984;69: 203–13

17. Gunnarsson L, Tokics L, Brismar B, Hedenstierna G: Influence of age on circulation and arterial blood gases in man. Acta Anaesthesiol Scand 1996;40:237–43
18. Kilbom A, Hartley LH, Saltin B et al: Physical training in sedentary middle-aged and older men. I. Medical evaluation. Scand J Clin Lab Invest 1969;24:315–22
19. Unverferth DV, Fetter JK, Unverferth BJ et al: Human myocardial histologic characteristics in congestive heart failure. Circulation 1983;68:1194–200
20. Weisfeldt ML, Loeven WA, Shock NW: Resting and active mechanical properties of trabeculae carnae from male rats. Am J Physiol 1971;220:1921–7
21. Aurigemma GP, Gaasch WH, McLaughin M et al: Reduced left-ventricular systolic pump performance and depressed myocardial contractile function in patients greater-than-65 years of age with normal ejection fraction and a high relative wall thickness. Am J Cardiol 1995;76:702–5
22. Wajngarten M, Negrao CE, Brandao MUP et al: Effects of aging on left-ventricular function during exercise. Cardiol Elderly 1995;3:125–31
23. Klein AL, Burstow DJ, Tajik AJ et al: Effects of age on left ventricular dimensions and filling dynamics in 117 normal persons. Mayo Clin Proc 1994;69:212–24
24. Linzbach AJ, Akuamoa-Boateng E: Die alternsveranderungen des menschlichen Herzens. 1. Das Herzgewight im Alter. Klin Wochenschr 1973;51:156–63
25. Levy WC, Cerqueira MD, Abrass IB et al: Endurance exercise training augments diastolic filling at rest and during exercise in healthy young and older men. Circulation 1993;88:116–26
26. Arrighi JA, Dilsizian V, Perronefilardi P et al: Improvement of the age-related impairment in left-ventricular diastolic filling with verapamil in the normal human heart. Circulation 1994;90:213–9
27. Brandfonbrenner M, Landowne M, Shock NW: Changes in cardiac output with ageing. Circulation 1955;12:557–66
28. Granath A, Jonsson B, Strandell T: Circulation in healthy old men studied by right heart catheterisation at rest and during exercise in supine and sitting position. Acta Med Scand 1964; 176:425–46
29. Sollott SJ, Lakatta EG: Normal aging changes in the cardiovascular system. Cardiol Elderly 1993;1:349–58
30. Folkow B, Svanborg A: Physiology of cardiovascular aging. Am J Physiol 1993;73:725–63
31. Owen OE: Resting metabolic requirements of men and women. Mayo Clin Proc 1988;53:503–10
32. Moore FD, Olsen KH, MacMurrey JD et al: The Body Cell Mass and its Supporting Environment. WB Saunders, London, 1963
33. Strandell T: Circulatory studies in healthy old men. Acta Med Scand 1964;414(suppl):1–44
34. Cleroux J, Giannattasio C, Bolla G et al: Decreased cardiopulmonary reflexes with aging in normotensive humans. Am J Physiol 1989;257:H961–8
35. Jacob R, Dierberger B, Kissling G: Functional significance of the Frank-Starling mechanism under physiological and pathophysiological conditions. Eur Heart J 1992;13(suppl E):7–14
36. Kirkland JL, Lye M, Goddard C et al: Plasma arginine vasopressin in dehydrated elderly patients. Clin Endocrinol 1984; 20:451–6
37. Johnson AG, Crawford GA, Kelly D et al: Arginine-vasopressin and osmolality in the elderly. J Am Geriatr Soc 1994;42: 399–404
38. Lye M: Electrolyte disorders in the elderly. Clinics Endocr Metab 1984;13:377–98
39. Elisaf M, Theodorou J, Pappas C, Siamopoulos K: Successful treatment of hyponatremia with angiotensin-converting enzyme inhibitors in patients with congestive heart failure. 1995;86: 477–80
40. Ziegler MG, Lake CR, Kopin IJ: Plasma noradrenaline increases with age. Nature 1976;261:333–5
41. Conway J, Wheeler R, Sannerstedt R: Sympathetic nervous activity during exercise in relation to age. Cardiovasc Res 1971;5:577
42. Vellodi C, Browne M, Vargas E, Lye M: Neurohumoral parameters in chronic heart failure in the elderly. Geriatr Cardiovasc Med 1988;1:151–4
43. Fenn WO, Noonan TR, Mullins LJ, Haege L: The exchange of radioactive potassium with body potassium. Am J Physiol 1941;135:149–63
44. Dutka DP, Olivotto I, Ward S et al: Plasma neuroendocrine activity in very elderly subjects and patients with and without heart-failure. Eur Heart J 1995;16:1223–30
45. Tissandier O, Nasr A, Rainfray M et al: Atrial natriuretic factor and brain natriuretic peptide—variations in elderly subjects with heart failure. Presse Med 1995;24:1837–41
46. Dutka DP, Olivotto I, Ward S et al: Effects of aging on neuroendocrine activation in subjects and patients in the presence and absence of heart failure with left ventricular systolic. Am J Cardiol 1996;77:1197–201
47. Lye M, Vargas E, Faragher EB et al: Haemodynamic and neurohumoral responses in elderly patients with postural hypotension. Eur J Clin Invest 1990;20:90–6
48. Watanabe T, Kobayashi F, Furui H et al: Assessment of sympathetic nerve activity controlling blood pressure in the elderly using head-up tilt. Environ Res 1993;62:251–5
49. Yin FCP, Spurgeon MA, Greene ML et al: Age-associated decrease in heart rate response to isoproterenol in dogs. Mech Ageing Dev 1979;10:17–25
50. Lye M: Autonomic dysfunction and abnormal vascular reflexes. pp. 191–211. In Tallis R (ed): The Clinical Neurology of Old Age. John Wiley & Sons, Chichester; 1989
51. Capasso JM, Remily RM, Sonnenblick EH: Age-related differences in excitation contraction coupling in rat papillary muscle. Basic Res Cardiol 1983;78:492–504
52. Vargas E, Lye M, Faragher EB et al: Cardiovascular haemodynamics and the response of vasopressin, aldosterone, plasma renin activity and plasma catecholamines to head-up tilt in young and old healthy subjects. Age Ageing 1986;15: 17–28
53. Duggan J, Nussberger J, Kilfeather S, O'Malley K: Aging and

human hormonal and pressor responsiveness to angiotensin II infusion with simultaneous measurement of exogenous and endogenous angiotensin II. 1993;6:641–7

54. Finn WL, Tunny TJ, Klemm SA et al: Ageing and blood pressure regulation: dose-response relationships for angiotensin, blood pressure, atrial natriuretic peptide and aldosterone in normal subjects of varying ages. Clin Exp Pharmacol Physiol 1993;20:392–4
55. Schrier RW: Pathogenesis of sodium and water retention in high-output and low-output cardiac failure, nephrotic syndrome, cirrhosis, and pregnancy. N Engl J Med 1988;319: 1127–34
56. Wilson JR, Rayos G, Yeoh TK et al: Dissociation between exertional symptoms and circulatory function in patients with heart-failure. Circulation 1995;92:47–53
57. Cleland JGF, Habib P: Assessment and diagnosis of heart failure. J Intern Med 1996;239:317–25
58. McKee PA, Castelli WP, McNamara M, Kannei WB: The natural history of congestive heart failure: the Framingham Study. N Engl J Med 1971;285:1441–6
59. Marantz PR, Alderman MH, Tobin JN: Diagnostic heterogeneity in clinical trials for congestive heart failure. Ann Intern Med 1988;109:55–61
60. Silvestri GA, Mahler DA: Evaluation of dyspnea in the elderly patient. Clin Chest Med 1993;14:393–404
61. Dargie HJ, McMurray JJV: Diagnosis and management of heart failure. BMJ 1994;308:321–8
62. De Jonge JW, Knottnerus JA, Van Zutphen WM et al: Short term effect of withdrawal of diuretic drugs prescribed for ankle oedema. BMJ 1994;308:511–3
63. McLachlin AD, McLachlin JA, Jory TA, Rawling EG: Venous stasis in the lower extremities. Ann Surg 1960;152:678–85
64. Lehmann AB, Johnston D, James OFW: The effects of old age and immobility on protein turnover in human subjects with some observations on the possible role of hormones. Age Ageing 1989;18:148–51
65. McDicken WN, Hoskins PR, Moran CM, Sutherland GR: New technology in echocardiography II: Doppler techniques. Heart 1996;75(suppl 2):2–8
66. Luchi RJ, Brown DL: Congestive heart failure. pp. 97–126. In Luchi RJ (ed): Clinical Geriatric Cardiology. Churchill Livingstone, Edinburgh, 1989
67. Topol EJ, Traill TA, Fortuin NJ: Hypertensive hypertrophic cardiomyopathy of the elderly. N Engl J Med 1985;312: 277–83
68. Lever HM, Karam RF, Currie PJ, Healy BP: Hypertrophic cardiomyopathy in the elderly: distinctions from the young based on cardiac shape. Circulation 1989;79:580–9
69. Lewis JF, Maron BJ: Elderly patients with hypertrophic cadiomyopathy: a subset with distinctive left ventricular morphology and progressive clinical course late in life. J Am Coll Cardiol 1989;13:36–45
70. Kitzman DW: Doppler assessment of diastolic function comes of age. J Am Geriatr Soc 1996;44:729–32
71. Clarke KW, Gray D, Hampton JR: Evidence of inadequate investigation and treatment of patients with heart failure. Br Heart J 1994;71:584–7
72. Aronow WS: Echocardiography should be performed in all elderly patients with congestive-heart-failure. J Am Geriatr Soc 1994;42:1300–2
73. Jennings M: Is echocardiography justified in the elderly. Cardiol Elderly 1995;3:265–8
74. King D: Cardiac cachexia in the elderly. Cardiol Elderly 1994; 2:102–6
75. Carr J, Stevenson LW, Walden JA, Harber D: Prevalence and hemodynamic correlates of malnutrition in severe congestive heart failure secondary to ischemic and dilated cardiomyopathy. Am J Cardiol 1989;63:709–13
76. Kubo SH, Walter BA, John DHA et al: Liver function abnormalities in chronic heart failure. Influence of systemic hemodynamics. Ann Intern Med 1987;147:1227–30
77. King D, Smith ML, Chapman TJ et al: Fat malabsorption in elderly patients with cardiac cachexia. Age Ageing 1996;25: 144–9
78. King D, Smith ML, Lye M: Gastrointestinal protein loss in elderly patients with cardiac cachexia. Age Ageing 1996;25: 221–3
79. Kark RH, Pirani CL, Pollack VE et al: Nephrotic syndrome in adults. Common disorder with many causes. Ann Intern Med 1958;49:751–74
80. Levine B, Kalman J, Mayer L et al: Elevated circulating levels of tumor necrosis factor in severe chronic heart failure. N Engl J Med 1990;323:236–41
81. Katz SD, Rao R, Berman JW et al: Pathophysiological correlates of increased serum tumor necrosis factor in patients with congestive heart failure: relation to nitric oxide-dependent vasodilation in the forearm circulation. Circulation 1994;90: 12–6
82. Williamson J, Chopin JM: Adverse reactions to precribed drugs in the elderly: a multicentre investigation. Age Ageing 1980;9:73–80
83. Petri M, Cumber P, Grimes L et al: The metabolic effects of thiazide therapy in the elderly: a population study. Age Ageing 1986;15:151–155
84. Nolan L, O'Malley K: Adverse drug reactions in the elderly. Br J Hosp Med 1989;41:446–57
85. Dewhurst G, Wood DA, Walker F et al: A population survey of cardiovascular disease in elderly people: design. Age Ageing 1991;20:353–61
86. Borland C, Amadi A, Murphy P, Shallcross T: Biochemical and clinical correlates of diuretic therapy in the elderly. Age Ageing 1986;15:357–63
87. MacLennan WJ: Diuretics in the elderly: how safe? BMJ 1988; 296:1551–2
88. Salive ME, Jones CA, Guralnik JM et al: Serum creatinine levels in older adults—relationship with health- status and medications. Age Ageing 1995;24:142–50
89. Beeley L: Errors and misconceptions in drug prescribing. J R Coll Phys Lond 1980;14:58–64
90. Morgan DB, Davidson C: Hypokalaemia and diuretics: an analysis of publications. BMJ 1980;1:905–8
91. Levy DW, Lye M: Diuretics and potassium in the elderly. J R Coll Phys Lond 1987;21:148–52
92. Brater DC: Pharmacodynamic considerations in the use of diuretics. Annu Rev Pharmacol Toxicol 1983;23:45–62

93. Taylor SH: Diuretics in heart failure. Br Heart J 1994; 72(suppl):S1–2

94. Rahimtoola SH: The pharmacologic treatment of chronic congestive heart failure. Circulation 1989;80:693–9

95. Lye M: Cardiovascular system—Diuretics. pp. 87–100. In Brocklehurst JC (ed): Geriatric Pharmacology and Therapeutics. Blackwell Scientific Publications Ltd., Oxford, 1984

96. Valacio R, Lye M: Diuretics and ACE inhibitors. Care Elderly 1994;6:294–6

97. Vanapruks C, Lye M: Loop diuretics and ACE inhibitors in heart failure patients. Geriatr Med (in press)

98. Shapiro S, Slone D, Lewis GP, Jick H: Fatal drug reactions among medical inpatients. JAMA 1971;216:467–72

99. Bender AD, Carter CL, Hansen KB: Use of a diuretic combination of triamterene and hydrochlorothiazide in elderly patients. J Am Geriatr Soc 1967;15:166–73

100. O'Connell JE, Colledge NR: Type-IV renal tubular acidosis and spironolactone therapy in the elderly. Postgrad Med J 1993;69:887–9

101. Adams KRH, Vargas E, Lye M: Electrolyte abnormalities and diuretics in the elderly. J Clin Exp Gerontol 1988;10:171–80

102. Sawyer N, Gabriel R: Progressive hypokalaemia in elderly patients taking three thiazide potassium-sparing diuretic combinations for thirty-six months. Postgrad Med J 1988;64: 434–7

103. Anderson RJ: Hospital-associated hyponatraemia. Kidney Int 1986;29:1237–47

104. Ashouri OS: Diuretic-induced hyponatremia in the elderly. A series of eight patients. Ann Intern Med 1986;146:1355–7

105. Sunderam SG, Mankikar GD: Hyponatraemia in the elderly. Age Ageing 1983;12:77–80

106. Ashraf N, Locksley R, Arieff AI: Thiazide-induced hyponatremia associated with death or neurologic patients. Am J Med 1981;70:1163–8

107. Saggarmalik AK, Cappuccio FP: Potassium supplements and potassium-sparing diuretics—a review and guide to appropriate use. Drugs 1993;46:986–1008

108. MacLennan WJ: Use and abuse of diuretics. pp. 127–133. In Evans JG, Caird FI (eds): Advanced Geriatric Medicine. 4th Ed. Pitman, London, 1984

109. Playfair AS: Picking a diuretic. BMJ 1975;3:42

110. Reubi FC, Cottier PT: Effects of reduced glomerular filtration rate on responsiveness to chlorothiazide and mercurial diuretics. Circulation 1961;23:200–10

111. Gerber JG: Antihypertensive agents and diuretics. p. 211. In Anders DJ, Schrier RW (eds): Clinical Use of Drugs in Patients with Kidney and Liver Disease. WB Saunders, Philadelphia, 1981

112. Epstein M: Effects of ageing on the kidney. Fed Proc 1979; 38:168–72

113. Lindeman RD, Tobin J, Shock NW: Longitudinal studies on the rate of decline in renal function with age. J Am Geriatr Soc 1985;33:278–85

114. Anand IS, Ferrari R, Kalra GS et al: Edema of cardiac origin studies of body water and sodium renal function hemodynamic indexes and plasma hormones in untreated congestive cardiac failure. Circulation 1989;80:299–305

115. Denham MJ, Hodkinson HM, Fisher M: Glomerular filtration rate in sick elderly inpatients. Age Ageing 1975;4:32–6

116. Smith SJ, Lye M: Cardiac failure in an elderly population. Rev Clin Gerontol 1994;4:199–211

117. Lye M: Heart disease in the elderly. pp. 1415–1429. In Julian DG, Camm AJ, Fox KM et al. (eds): Diseases of the Heart. 2nd Ed. WB Saunders, London, 1996

118. Valacio R, Lye M: Heart-failure in the elderly patient. Br J Clin Pract 1995;49:200–4

119. Andreasen F, Hansen U, Husted SE, Jansen JA: The pharmacokinetics of frusemide are influenced by age. Br J Clin Pharmacol 1983;16:391–7

120. Chaudhry AY, Bing RF, Castleden CM et al: The effect of aging on the response to frusemide in normal subjects. Eur J Clin Pharmacol 1984;27:303–6

121. Muhlberg W: Pharmacokinetics of diuretics in geriatric patients. Arch Gerontol Geriatr 1989;9:283–90

122. Lye M: Advances in cardiology. Geriatr Med 1983;13:71–4

123. Kiyingi A, Field MJ, Pawsey CC et al: Metolazone in treatment of severe refractory congestive cardiac failure. Lancet 1990; 335:29–31

124. Mulkerrin EC, Donovan K, Hampton D et al: Hormonal changes during combined metolazone and frusemide therapy in cardiac failure in the elderly. J Clin Exp Gerontol 1992; 14:269–82

125. Lye M: Diuretics for the patient with heart failure: select with care. Geriatr Med 1990;20:13–4

126. Seri I, Aperia A: Contribution of dopamine 2 receptors to dopamine-induced increase in glomerular filtration rate. Am J Physiol 1988;254:F196–210

127. Robinson T, Gariballa S, Fancourt G et al: The acute effects of a single dopamine infusion in elderly patients with congestive cardiac failure. Br J Clin Pharmacol 1994;37:261–3

128. Borst SE, Lowenthal DT: Cardiovascular drugs in the elderly. pp. 161–173. In Lowenthal DT (ed): Geriatric Cardiology. FA Davis Co., Philadelphia, 1992

129. McInnes GT, Yeo WW, Ramsay LE, Moser M: Cardiotoxicity and diuretics—much speculation—little substance. J Hypertens 1992;10:317–35

130. Bigger JT: Diuretic therapy, hypertension and cardiac arrest. N Engl J Med 1994;330:1899–900

131. Haavisto MV, Heikinheimo RJ, Mattila KJ, Rajala SA: Living conditions and health of a population aged 85 years or over: a five-year follow-up study. Age Ageing 1985;14:202–8

132. Lye M: Distribution of body potassium in healthy elderly subjects. Gerontology 1981;27:286–92

133. Mazariegos M, Wang ZM, Gallagher D et al: Differences between young and old females in the 5 levels of body composition and their relevance to the two-compartment chemical model. J Gerontol 1994;49:M201–8

134. Delwaide PA: Body potassium measurements by whole-body counting: screening of patient populations. J Nucl Med 1973; 14:40–8

135. Davidson C, Burkinshaw L, McLachlan MSF, Morgan DB: Effect of long-term diuretic treatment on body-potassium in heart-disease. Lancet 1976;2:1044–7
136. Lawson DH, Boddy K, Gray JMB et al: Potassium supplements in patients receiving long-term diuretics for oedema. QJ Med 1976;45:469–78
137. Cleland JGF, Dargie HJ, Robertson I et al: Total body electrolyte composition in patients with heart failure: a comparison with normal subjects and patients with untreated hypertension. Br Heart J 1987;58:230–8
138. Lye M: Body potassium content and capacity of elderly individuals with and without cardiac failure. Cardiovasc Res 1982; 16:22–5
139. Lye M: Body potassium content and severity of cardiac failure in old people. J Clin Exp Gerontol 1984;6:153–65
140. Greenblatt DJ, Duhme DW, Allen MD, Koch-Weser J: Clinical toxicity of furosemide in hospitalized patients. Am Heart J 1977;94:6–13
141. Lawson DH, Henry DA, Lowe JM et al: Severe hypokalaemia in hospitalized patients. Arch Intern Med 1979;139:978–80
142. Lowe J, Gray J, Henry DA, Lawson DH: Adverse reactions to frusemide in hospital inpatients. BMJ 1979;2:360–2
143. Kaplan NM, Carnegie A, Raskin P et al: Potassium supplementation in hypertensive patients with diuretic-induced hypokalemia. N Engl J Med 1985;312:746–9
144. Dargie HJ, Boddy K, Kennedy AC et al: Total body potassium in long-term frusemide therapy: is potassium supplementation necessary? BMJ 1974;4:316–9
145. Ramsey LE, Boyle P, Ramsey MH: Factors influencing serum potassium in treated hypertension. Q J Med 1977;46:401–10
146. Down PF, Polak A, Rao R, Mead JA: Fate of potassium supplements in six outpatients receiving long-term diuretics for oedematous disease. Lancet 1972;2:721–4
147. Ibrahim IK, Ritch AES, MacLennan WJ, May T: Are potassium supplements for the elderly necessary? Age Ageing 1978;7: 165–70
148. Poole-Wilson PA: Ventricular extrasystoles during thiazide treatment. BMJ 1983;287:1798–9
149. Steiness E, Olsen KH: Cardiac arrhythmias induced by hypokalaemia and potassium loss during maintenance digoxin therapy. Br Heart J 1976;38:167–72
150. Greenberg G: MRC trial of treatment of mild hypertension—principal results. BMJ 1985;291:97–104
151. Myers MG: Diuretic therapy and ventricular arrhythmias in persons 65 years of age and older. Am J Cardiol 1990;65: 599–603
152. Hoes AW, Grobbee DE, Peet TM, Lubsen J: Do non-potassium sparing diuretics increase the risk of sudden cardiac death in hypertensive patients. Recent evidence. Drugs 1994;47: 711–33
153. Papademetriou V: Effect of diuretics on cardiac arrhythmias and left ventricular hypertrophy in hypertension. Cardiol (Basel) 1994;84:43–7
154. Lawson DH: Adverse reactions to potassium chloride. Q J Med 1974;43:433–40
155. Kassirer JP, Harrington JT: Diuretics and potassium metabolism: a reassessment of the need, effectiveness and safety of potassium therapy. Kidney Int 1977;11:505–15
156. Kassirer JP, Harrington JT: Fending off the potassium pushers. N Engl J Med 1985;312:785–6
157. Hutcheon DE: Benefit-risk factors associated with supplemental potassium therapy. J Clin Pharmacol 1976;16:85–7
158. Beeley L, Brookes V: Drug prescribing in renal failure. Proc Br Pharmaceut Soc 1976;970P–1P
159. Wan HH, Lye M: Moduretic induced metabolic acidosis and hyperkalaemia. Postgrad Med J 1980;56:348–50
160. Allison SP: Fluid and electrolyte disorders. Potassium. Br J Hosp Med 1984;32:19–22
161. Cogan E, Abramow M: Diuretic-induced hyponatraemia in elderly hypertensive women. Lancet 1983;2:1249
162. Tarssanen L, Huikko M, Rossi M: Amiloride induced hyponatraemia. Acta Med Scand 1980;208:492–4
163. Clark BA, Shannon RP, Rosa RM, Epstein FH: Increased susceptibility to thiazideinduced hyponatremia in the elderly. J Am Soc Nephrol 1994;5:1106–11
164. Fidler HM, Goldman J, Bielawska CA et al: A study of plasma sodium-levels in elderly people taking amiloride or triamterene in combination with hydrochlorothiazide. Postgrad Med J 1993;69:797–9
165. Roberts CJC, Channer KS, Bungay D: Hyponatremia induced by a combination of hydrochlorothiazide and triamterene. BMJ 1984;288:1962
166. Booker JA: Severe symptomatic hyponatremia in elderly outpatients: the role of thiazide therapy and stress. J Am Geriatr Soc 1984;32:108–13
167. Tanneau RS, Bourbigot B, Richard P et al: Prognosis and neurologic outcome of severe hyponatremia in elderly patients. Eur J Intern Med 1993;4:311–8
168. Freis ED: The cardiovascular risks of thiazide diuretics. Clin Pharmacol Ther 1986;39:239–44
169. Pollare T, Lithell H, Berne C: A comparison of the effects of hydrochlorothiazide and captopril on glucose and lipid-metabolism in patients with hypertension. N Engl J Med 1989;321: 868–73
170. Wissler RW, Robert L: Aging and cardiovascular-disease—a summary of the 8th munster-international-arteriosclerosis-symposium. Circulation 1996;93:1608–12
171. Orme M: Thiazides in the 1990s. BMJ 1990;300:1668–9
172. Warshaw LJ: Acute attacks of gout precipitated by chlorothiazide-induced diuresis. JAMA 1960;172:802–6
173. Humphreys DM: Acute gout apparently precipitated by frusemide. BMJ 1966;1:1024–5
174. MacFarlane DG, Dieppe PA: Diuretic induced gout in elderly women. Br J Rheumatol 1985;24:155–7
175. Schwab RH, Perloff JK, Porus RL: Chlorothiazide-induced gout and diabetes. Arch Intern Med 1963;111:465–70
176. Goodman JM, Dornan J, Brown K, Plyley MJ: Exercise Training Following Coronary Artery Bypass Surgery in Older Patients. J Clin Exp Gerontol 1987;9:19–29
177. Wolff FW, Parmley WW, White K, Okeen R. Drug-induced

diabetes—Diabetogenic activity of long term administration of benzothiodiazides. JAMA 1963;185:568–71

178. Toivonen S, Mustala O: Diabetogenic action of frusemide. BMJ 1966;3:920–1

179. Breckenridge A, Welborn TA, Dollery CT, Fraser TR: Glucose tolerance in hypertensive patients on long term diuretic therapy. Lancet 1967;1:61–3

180. Lewis PJ, Kohner EM, Petrie A, Dollery CT: Deterioration of glucose tolerance in hypertensive patients on prolonged diuretic treatment. Lancet 1976;1:564–6

181. Shapiro AP, Benedek TG, Small JL: Effect of thiazides on carbohydrate metabolism in patients with hypertension. N Engl J Med 1960;265:1028–33

182. Amery A, DeSchaepdrijver A: Antihypertensive therapy in patients above age 60. Third interim report of the European Working Party on High Blood Pressure in Elderly (EWPHE). Acta Cardiol (Brux) 1978;33:113–34

183. Dall JLC: Diuretics in the elderly. BMJ 1978;1:1417

184. Chaudhuri MLD, Catania J: A comparison of the effects of bumetanide (Burinex) and frusemide on carbohydrate metabolism in the elderly. Br J Clin Pract 1988;42:427–9

185. Koegel L: Ototoxicity: a contemporary review of aminoglycosides, loop diuretics, acetylsalicylic acid, quinine, erythromycin and cisplatinum. Am J Otol 1985;6:190–9

186. Schwartz GH, David DS, Riggio RR et al: Ototoxicity induced by frusemide. N Engl J Med 1970;282:1413–4

187. David DS, Hitzig P: Diuretics and ototoxicity. N Engl J Med 1971;284:1328–9

188. Pillay VKG, Aimi K, Schwartz FD, Kark RM: Transient and permanent deafness following treatment with ethacrynic acid in renal failure. Lancet 1969;1:77–9

189. Tuzel IH: Comparison of adverse reactions to bumetanide and furosemide. J Clin Pharmacol 1981;21:615–9

190. Halstenson CE, Matzke GR: Bumetanide: a new loop diuretic. Drug Intell Clin Pharm 1983;17:786–97

191. Sakhaee K, Nicar MJ, Glass K et al: Reduction in intestinal calcium absorption by hydrochlorothiazide in postmenopausal osteoporosis. J Clin Endocrinol Metab 1984;59:1037–43

192. Churchill DN, Taylor DW: Thiazides for patients with recurrent calcium stones: still an open question. J Urol 1985;133: 749–51

193. Tambyah JA, Linn MKL: Effect of frusemide on calcium excretion. BMJ 1969;1:751–2

194. Drinka PJ, Nolten WE: Hazards of treating osteoporosis and hypertension concurrently with calcium vitamin D, and distal diuretics. J Am Geriatr Soc 1984;32:405–7

195. Ray WA, Griffin MR, Downey W, Melton LJ: Long-term use of thiazide diuretics and risk of hip fracture. Lancet 1989;1: 687–90

196. Lye M, Vargas E: Postural Hypotension. pp. 189–200. In Coodley EL (ed): Geriatric Heart Disease. PSG Publishing Company, Inc., Littleton, Massachusetts, 1985

197. Vardan S, Hill NE, Mehrotra KG et al: Hemodynamic response to orthostatic stress in the elderly with systolic systemic hypertension before and after long-term thiazide therapy. Am J Cardiol 1993;71:582–6

198. Withering W: An account of the Foxglove. In Willius FA, Keys TE (eds): Cardiac Classics. Dover Publications Inc, New York, 1985

199. Cattell M, Gold H: The influence of digitalis glycosides on the force of contraction of mammalian cardiac muscle. J Pharmacol Exp Ther 1938;62:116–22

200. Langer GA: Effects of digitalis on myocardial ionic exchange. Circulation 1972;46:180–6

201. Blood BE, Cohen I, Daut J, Noble D: Relation between ionic and inotropic actions of cardiac glycosides. 7th Eur Congr Cardiol 1976:551

202. Nayler WG: Ionic basis of contractility. pp. 154–165. In Oliver MF (ed): Modern Trends in Cardiology. Vol. 3. Butterworths, London, 1975

203. Weingart R, Kass RS, Tsien RW: Is digitalis inotropy associated with enhanced slow inward calcium current? Nature 1978;272:389–91

204. Smith TW, Haber E: Medical progress. Digitalis. N Engl J Med 1973;289:945–7

205. Runge TM: Clinical implications of differences in pharmacodynamic action of polar and non-polar cardiac glycosides. Am Heart J 1977;93:248–52

206. Caldwell KW, Nash CB: Comparison of a aminosugar cardiac glycoside with ouabain and digoxin on Na+. Am J Cardiol 1977;39:291–5

207. Hayward R, Hamer J: Digitalis. pp. 244–317. In Hamer J (ed): Drugs for Heart Disease. Chapman and Hall, London, 1979

208. Lye M: Cardiovascular system—Digitalis glycosides. pp. 71 to 86. In Brocklehurst JC (ed): Geriatric Pharmacology and Therapeutics. Blackwell Scientific Publications Ltd., Oxford, 1984

209. Demots H, Rahimtoola SH, Kremkau EL et al: Effect of ouabain on myocardial oxygen supply and demand in patients with chronic cronary artery disease. J Clin Invest 1978;58: 312–9

210. Torritti J, Hendler E, Weinstein L: Functional significance of Na-K-ATPase in the kidney: effects of ouabain in inhibition. Am J Physiol 1972;222:1398–401

211. Stoffer SS, Hynes KM, Jiang N-S, Ryan RJ: Digoxin and abnormal serum hormone levels. JAMA 1973;225:1643–5

212. Griffiths BE, Penny WJ, Lewis MJ, Henderson AH: Maintenance of the inotropic effect of dogoxin on long-term treatment. BMJ 1982;284:1819–22

213. Murray RG, Tweddel AC, Martin W et al: Evaluation of digitalis in cardiac failure. BMJ 1982;284:1526–8

214. Ware JA, Snow E, Luchi JM, Luchi RJ: Effect of digoxin on ejection fraction in elderly patients with congestive heart failure. J Am Geriatr Soc 1984;32:631–5

215. Hlatky MA, Fleg JL, Hinton PC et al: Physician practice in the management of congestive heart failure. J Am Coll Cardiol 1986;8:966–70

216. Dibianco R, Shabetai R, Kostuk W et al: A comparison of oral milrinone, digoxin, and their combination in the treatment of patients with chronic heart failure. N Engl J Med 1989;320: 677–83

217. Gheorghiade M, Hall VB, Jacobsen G et al: Effects of increasing maintenance dose of digoxin on left-ventricular function and neurohormones in patients with chronic heart-failure treated with diuretics and angiotensin-converting enzyme-inhibitors. Circulation 1995;92:1801–7
218. Vitarelli A, Fedele F, Dagianti A et al: A reexamination of the hemodynamic effects of digitalis relative to ventricular dysfunction. Cardiol (Basel) 1995;86:94–101
219. Braunwald E, Bloodwell RD, Goldberg LI, Morrow AG: Studies on digitalis. IV. Observations in man of the effects of digitalis preparations on the contractility of the nonfailing heart and on vascular resistance. J Clin Invest 1961;40:52–9
220. Fleg JL, Lakatta EG: How useful is digitalis in patients with congestive heart failure and sinus rhythm? Int J Cardiol 1984; 6:295–305
221. Bigger JT, Fleiss KR, Rolnitsky LM et al: Effect of digitalis treatment on survival after acute myocardial infarction. Am J Cardiol 1985;55:623–30
222. Anonymous: Needless digoxin. Lancet 1985;2:1048
223. Gheorghiade M, St Clair J, St Clair C, Beller GA: Hemodynamic effects of intravenous digoxin in patients with severe heart failure initially treated with diuretics and vasodilators. J Am Coll Cardiol 1987;9:849–57
224. Anonymous: Digoxin: new answers; new questions. Lancet 1989;2:79
225. Poole-Wilson PA: Positive inotropic agents in the management of heart failure in elderly patients. Cardiol Elderly 1994;2: 98–101
226. Eberhardt RT, Frishman WH, Landau A et al: Increased mortality in elderly individuals receiving digoxin therapy—results from the Bronx Longitudinal Aging Study. Cardiol Elderly 1995;3:177–82
227. Dobbs SM, Kenton WI, Dobbs RJ: Maintenance digoxin after an episode of heart failure: placebo-controlled trial in outpatients. BMJ 1977;1:749–52
228. Lee DC-S, Johnson RA, Bingham JB et al: Heart failure in outpatients. A randomized trial of digoxin versus placebo. N Engl J Med 1982;306:699–705
229. Guyatt GH, Sullivan MJJ, Fallen EL et al: A controlled trial of digoxin in congestive heart failure. Am J Cardiol 1988;61: 371–5
230. Baker DW, Konstam MA, Bottorff M, Pitt B: Management of heart failure. I. Pharmacologic treatment. JAMA 1994;272: 1361–6
231. Aumont MC, Agnola D, Juliard JM, Karrillon G: Classical treatment of chronic heart failure—what's new? Arch Mal Coeur Vaiss 1995;88:599–602
232. Starr I, Luchi J: Blind study on the action of digitoxin on elderly women. Am Heart J 1969;78:740–51
233. Dall JLC: Maintenance digoxin in elderly patients. BMJ 1970; 2:705–7
234. Hull SM, Mackintosh A: Discontinuation of maintenance digoxin therapy in general practice. Lancet 1977;2:1054–5
235. Johnston GD, McDevitt DG: Is maintenance digoxin necessary in patients with sinus rhythm? Lancet 1979;1:567–70
236. Gheorhiade M, Beller GA: Effects of discontinuing maintenance digoxin therapy in patients with ischemic heart disease and congestive failure in sinus rhythm. Am J Cardiol 1983; 51:1243–50
237. Mulrow CD, Feussner JR, Velez R: Reevaluation of digitalis efficacy. Ann Intern Med 1984;101:113–7
238. Carlson KJ, Lee DC, Goroll AH et al: An analysis of physicians' reasons for prescribing long-term digitalis therapy in outpatients. J Chron Dis 1985;38:733–9
239. Lye M, Faragher EB: Value of digitalis in heart failure. N Engl J Med 1982;307:625
240. Poole-Wilson PA: Digoxin in heart failure. Lancet 1989;2: 281–2
241. De Bono D: Digoxin in eurhythmic heart failure: PROVED or "not proven." Lancet 1994;343:128–9
242. Tauke J, Goldstein S, Gheorghiade M: Digoxin for chronic heart failure—a review of the randomized controlled trials with special attention to the PROVED and RADIANCE trials. Prog Cardiovasc Dis 1994;37:49
243. Lye M: Regional considerations in the use of digoxin in patients with eurhythmic heart failure. Drugs 1995;6:4
244. McCarthy DM, Hibbin J, Goldman JM: A role for 1,25-dihydroxyvitamin D3 in control of bone marrow collagen deposition. Lancet 1984;1:78–80
245. Channer KS: The drug treatment of atrial fibrillation. Br J Clin Pharmacol 1991;32:267–73
246. Lewis R, McClay J: Clinical pharmacology of chronic atrial fibrillation. J R Coll Physicians Lond 1988;22:252–7
247. McMurray J, Rankin A: Cardiology-II: treatment of heart failure and atrial fibrillation and arrhythmias. BMJ 1994;309: 1631–5
248. Williams P, Aronson J, Sleight P: Is a slow pulse-rate a reliable sign of digitalis toxicity? Lancet 1978;2:130–1
249. Cargnelli K, Domenghetti F, Ferrari M et al: Plasma digoxin concentrations in patients with atrial fibrillation and indications for association with other antiarrhythmic drugs. Int J Clin Pharmacol Ther Toxicol 1977;15:384–6
250. Theisen K, Haufe M, Peters J et al: Effect of the calcium antagonist diltiazem on atrioventricular conduction in chronic atrial fibrillation. Am J Cardiol 1985;55:98–102
251. George CF: Digitalis intoxication: a new approach to an old problem. BMJ 1983;286:1533–4
252. DiBianco R, Shabetai R, Kostuk W et al: Oral milrinone and digoxin in heart failure: results of a placebo-controlled trial. Circulation 1987;76:IV–256
253. Shapiro S, Slone D, Lewis GP, Jick H: The epidemiology of digoxin: a study in three Boston hospitals. J Chron Dis 1969; 22:361–71
254. Jorgensen AW, Sorensen OH: Digitalis intoxication: a comparative study on the incidence of digitalis intoxication during the periods 1950–52 and 1964–66. Acta Med Scand 1970; 188:179–83
255. Howard D, Smith CI, Stewart G et al: A prospective survey of the incidence of cardiac intoxication with digitalis in patients being admitted to hospital and correlation with serum digoxin levels. Aust N Z J Med 1973;3:279–84
256. Pahor M, Guralnik JM, Gambassi G et al: The impact of age

on risk of adverse drug-reactions to digoxin. J Clin Epidemiol 1993;46:1305–14

257. Woldow A, Wang RY, Rajagopal DE, Cohen JJ: The use of digoxin 0.125 mg versus 0.25 mg daily as maintenance dosage in patients older than 75 years of age. Cardiol Elderly 1993; 1:3–7

258. Vitti TG, Banes D, Byers TE: Bioavailability of digoxin. N Engl J Med 1971;285:1433–4

259. Duhm DW, Greenblatt DJ, Koch-Weser J: Reduction of digoxin toxicity associated with measurement of serum levels. Ann Intern Med 1974;80:516–9

260. Storstein O, Hansteen V, Hatie L et al: Studies on digitalis: XIII. A prospective study of 649 patients on maintenance treatment with digitoxin. Am Heart J 1977;93:434–43

261. Gheorghiade M, Rosman H, Mahdyoon H, Goldstein S: Incidence of digitalis intoxication. Primary Cardiol 1982;1:5–11

262. Smith TW, Antman EM, Friedman PL et al: Digitalis glycosides: mechanisms and manifestations of toxicity. (Part 1). Prog Cardiovasc Dis 1984;26:413–58

263. Brain C, Fox VEB: Suspected cardiac glycoside poisoning in elephants (Loxodonta africana). J South Afr Vet Assoc 1994; 65:173–4

264. Ewy GA, Kapadia GG, Yao L et al: Digoxin metabolism in the elderly. Circulation 1969;39:449–55

265. Nomura A, Kitabatake A, Kishino S et al: Digoxin dose adjusted according to estimated creatinine clearance in elderly patients with cardiac disease. Cardiol Elderly 1994;2:139–43

266. Mahowald JM, Himmelstein DU: Hypernatremia in the elderly: relation to infection and mortality. J Am Geriatr Soc 1981;29:177–80

267. Novak LP: Aging, total body potassium, fat free mass and cell mass in males and females between ages 18 and 85 years. J Gerontol 1972;27:438–43

268. Edmonds CJ, Jasani BM, Smith T: Total body potassium and body fat estimation in relationship to height, sex, age, malnutrition and obesity. Clin Sci Mol Med 1975;48:431–40

269. Womersley J, Durnin JVGA, Boddy K, Mahaffey M: Influence of muscular development, obesity and age on the fat free mass of adults. J Appl Physiol 1976;41:223–229

270. Friedman PJ, Campbell AJ, Caradoc-Davies TH: Hypoalbuminaemia in the elderly is due to disease not malnutrition. J Clin Exp Gerontol 1985;7:191–205

271. Keating FR, Jones JD, Elveback LR, Randall RV: The relation of age and sex to distribution of values in healthy adults of serum calcium, inorganic phosphorus, magnesium, alkaline phosphatase, total proteins, albumin and blood urea. J Lab Clin Med 1969;73:825–34

272. Mahdyoon H, Gheorghiade M: Digoxin therapy in elderly patients with heart failure. Geriatr Cardiovasc Med 1988;1: 243–6

273. Col N, Fanale JE, Kronholm P: The role of medication noncompliance and adverse drug reactions in hospitalization of the elderly. Arch Intern Med 1990;150:841–5

274. Monane M, Bohn RL, Gurwitz JH et al: Noncompliance with congestive heart failure therapy in the elderly. Arch Intern Med 1994;154:433–7

275. Lely AH, van Enter CHJ: Large scale digitoxin intoxication. BMJ 1970;3:737–8

276. Borison HC, Long TL: Physiology and pharmacology of vomiting. Pharmacol Res Commun 1953;5:193–202

277. Varriale P, Mossavi A: Rapid reversal of digitalis delirium using digoxin immune fab therapy. Clin Cardiol 1995;18: 351–2

278. Banka VG, Scherlag BJ, Helfant RH: Contractile and electrophysiological response to progressive digitalis toxicity. Cardiovasc Res 1975;9:65–72

279. Benotti JR, Grossman W, Braunwald E et al: Hemodynamic assessment of amrinone: a new inotropic agent. N Engl J Med 1978;229:1373–7

280. Klein NA, Siskird SJ, Frishman WH et al: Hemodynamic comparison of intravenous amrinone and dobutamine in patients with chronic congestive heart failure. Am J Cardiol 1981;48: 170–5

281. Wilmshurst PT, Walker JM, Fry CH et al: Inotropic and vasodilator effects of amrinone on isolated human tissue. Cardiovasc Res 1984;18:302–19

282. Massie B, Bourassa M, DiBianco R et al: Long-term oral amrinone for congestive heart failure: lack of efficacy in a multicenter controlled trial. Circulation 1985;71:963–71

283. DiBianco R: Acute positive inotropic intervention—the phosphodiesterase inhibitors. Am Heart J 1991;121:1871–5

284. Packer M, Carver JR, Rodeheffer RJ et al: Effect of oral milrinone on mortality in severe chronic heart failure. N Engl J Med 1991;325:1468–75

285. Wilmshurst P: Why inotropes continue to disappoint in heart failure. Br Heart J 1993;70:4

286. Cowley AJ, Skene AM: Treatment of severe heart failure: quantity or quality of life? A trial of enoximone. Br Heart J 1994; 72:226–30

287. Packer M: Therapeutic options in the management of chronic heart failure. Circulation 1989;79:198–204

288. Lipkin DP, Poole-Wilson PA: Treatment of chronic heart failure: a review of recent drug trials. BMJ 1985;291:993–6

289. Packer M: Do positive inotropic agents adversely affect the survival of patients with chronic congestive heart failure? J Am Coll Cardiol 1988;12:559–69

290. Rajfer SI, Goldberg LI: Dopamine in the treatment of heart failure. Eur Heart J 1982;3(suppl D):103–6

291. Leier C, Unverferth D: Diagnosis and treatment. Drugs five years later. Dobutamine. Ann Intern Med 1983;99:490–6

292. Robinson TG, Gariballa SE, Fancourt GJ et al: Acute effects of a single dopamine infusion in elderly patients with congestive cardiac failure. Age Ageing 1994;23(suppl 1):P8

293. Unverferth D, Blanford M, Kates R, Leier C: Tolerance to dobutamine after a 72 hour continuous infusion. Am J Med 1980;69:262–6

294. Van den Brande P, Van Meighem W, Demedts M: Intermittent dobutamine infusion in severe chronic heart failure in elderly patients. Gerontology 1990;36:49–54

295. Dies F, Krell MJ, Whitlow P et al: Intermittent dodutamine

in ambulatory outpatients with chronic cardiac failure. Circulation 1986;74(suppl II):1138

296. Jafri SM: Role of vasodilators and newer inotropic agents for treatment of heart failure. Geriatr Cardiovasc Med 1988;1: 247–50

297. Bing OHL, Brooks WW, Messer JV: Effect of isoproterenol on heart muscle performance during myocardial hypoxia. J Mol Cell Cardiol 1972;4:319–28

298. Weber KT, Andrews V, Janicki JS et al: Pirbuterol. Circulation 1982;66:1262–7

299. Altschuld RA, Starling RC, Hamlin RL et al: Response of failing canine and human heart cells to beta(2)-adrenergic stimulation. Circulation 1995;92:1612–8

300. Rector TS, Cohn JN, with the Pimobendan Multicenter Research Group: Assessment of patient outcome with the Minnesota living with heart failure questionnaire: reliability and validity during a randomized, double-blind, placebo-controlled trial of pimobendan. Am Heart J 1992;124:1017–25

301. Itoh H, Taniguchi K, Tsujibayashi T et al: Hemodynamic effects and pharmacokinetics of long-term therapy with ibopamine in patients with chronic heart failure. Cardiol (Basel) 1992; 80:356–66

302. Feldman AM, Bristow MR, Parmley WW et al: Effects of vesnarinone on morbidity and mortality in patients with heart failure. N Engl J Med 1993;329:149–55

303. Breall JA, Watanabe J, Grossman W: Effect of zatebradine on contractility, relaxation and coronary blood-flow. J Am Coll Cardiol 1993;21:471–7

304. Todd PA, Heel RC: Enalapril: a review of its pharmacodynamic and pharmackinetic properties and therapeutic use in hypertension and congestive heart failure. Drugs 1986;31: 198–248

305. Zimmerman BG: Adrenergic facilitation by angiotensin: does it serve a physiological function? Clin Sci 1980;60:343–8

306. The CONSENSUS Trial Study Group: Effects of enalapril on mortality in severe congestive heart failure. N Engl J Med 1987;316:1429–35

307. The SOLVD Investigators: Effect of enalapril on survival in patients with reduced left ventricular ejection fractions and congestive heart failure. N Engl J Med 1991;325:293–302

308. Cohn JN, Johnson G, Ziesche S et al: A comparison of enalapril with hydralazine-isosorbide dinitrate in the treatment of chronic congestive heart failure. N Engl J Med 1991;325: 303–10

309. Pfeffer MA, Braunwald E, Moye LA et al: Effect of Captopril on mortality and morbidity in patients with left ventricular dysfunction after myocardial infarction: results of the Survival and Ventricular Enlargement Trial. N Engl J Med 1992;327: 669–77

310. The Acute Infarction Rampril Efficacy (AIRE) Study Investigators: Effect of ramipril on mortality and morbidity of survivors of acute myocardial infarction with clinical evidence of heart failure. Lancet 1993;342:821–8

311. ISIS-4: ISIS-4: a randomised factorial trial assessing early oral captopril, oral mononitrate, and intravenous magnesium sulphate in 58 050 patients with suspected acute myocardial infarction. Lancet 1995;345:669–85

312. The SOLVD Investigators: Effect of enalapril on mortality and the development of heart failure in asymptomatic patients with reduced left ventricular ejection fractions. N Engl J Med 1992; 327:685–91

313. Cohn JN: The prevention of heart failure—a new agenda. N Engl J Med 1992;327:725–7

314. Riegger GAJ: ACE inhibitors in early stages of heart failure. Circulation 1993;87:IV—117—IV—119

315. Hart W, Rhodes G, McMurray J: The cost effectiveness of enalapril in the treatment of chronic heart failure. Br J Health Economics 1993;6:91–8

316. O'Keeffe ST, Lye M: Heart failure in the elderly: the same syndrome as the clinical trials? pp 47–71. In McMurray JJV, Cleland JGF (eds): Heart Failure in Clinical Practice. 1st Ed. Martin Dunitz Ltd, London, 1996

317. Garg R, Yusuf S, for the Collaborative Group on ACE Inhibitor Trials: Overview of randomized trials of angiotensin-converting enzyme inhibitors on mortality and morbidity in patients with heart failure. JAMA 1995;273:1450–6

318. Corcoran AC, Page IH: The effects of angiotonin on renal blood flow and glomerular filtration. Am J Physiol 1940;130:335–9

319. Dzau VJ, Hollenberg NK: Renal response to captopril in severe heart failure: role of furosemide in natriuresis and reversal of Hyponatremia. Ann Intern Med 1984;100:777–82

320. Cleland JGF, Dargie HJ, Ball SG et al: Effects of enalapril in heart failure: a double blind study of effects on exercise performance, renal function, hormones, and metabolic state. Br Heart J 1985;54:305–12

321. Van Hooft IMS, Grobbee DE, Derkx FHM et al: Renal hemodynamics and the renin-angiotensin-aldosterone system in normotensive subjects with hypertensive and normotensive parents. N Engl J Med 1991;324:1305–11

322. Komajda M, Wimart MC, Thibout E: The ATLAS study (Assessment of Treatment with Lisinopril Survival) justification and objectives. Arch Mal Coeur Vaiss 1994;87:45–50

323. Goodfriend TL, Elliott ME, Catt KJ: Drug-therapy—angiotensin receptors and their antagonists. N Engl J Med 1996;334: 1649–54

324. O'Neill CJ, Bowes SG, Sullens CM et al: Evaluation of the safety of enalapril in the treatment of heart failure in the very old. Eur J Clin Pharmacol 1989;35:143–50

325. Squire IB, Macfadyen RJ, Reid JL et al: Differing early blood pressure and renin angiotensin system responses to the first dose of angiotensin-converting enzyme inhibitors in congestive heart failure. J Cardiovasc Pharmacol 1996;27:657–66

326. Yodfat Y, Yodfat O: First-dose response and long-term effect of the ACE-inhibitor spirapril in hypertensive patients formerly treated with a diuretic. J Drug Develop Clin Pract 1995;7: 91–5

327. Squire IB, Macfadyen RJ, Lees KR et al: Hemodynamic response and pharmacokinetics after the first dose of quinapril in patients with congestive heart failure. Br J Clin Pharmacol 1994;38:117–23

328. Macfadyen RJ, Lees KR, Reid JL: Double-blind controlled study of low-dose intravenous perindoprilat or enalaprilat infu-

sion in elderly patients with heart failure. Br Heart J 1993; 69:293–7

329. Haffner CA, Kendall MJ, Struthers AD et al: Effects of captopril and enalapril on renal function in elderly patients with chronic heart failure. Postgrad Med J 1995;71:287–92

330. Hasford J, Ansari H, Lehmann K: Cart and logistic regression analyses of risk factors for first dose hypotension by an ACE inhibitor. Therapie 1993;48:479–82

331. Flapan AD, Davies E, Williams BC et al: The relationship between diuretic dose, and the haemodynamic response to captopril in patients with cardiac failure. Eur Heart J 1992; 13:971–5

332. Haffner CA, Kendall MJ, Struthers AD et al: Effects of captopril and enalapril on renal-function in elderly patients with chronic heart-failure. Postgrad Med J 1995;71:287–92

333. Schwartz D, Kornowski R, Schwartz IF et al: Prediction of renal impairment in elderly patients with congestive heart failure treated with captopril. Cardiovasc Drugs Ther 1996;10: 75–9

334. Mujais SK, Fouad FM, Textor SC et al: Transient renal dysfunction during initial inhibition of converting enzyme in congestive heart failure. Br Heart J 1984;52:63–71

335. Hallab M, Gallois Y, Chatellier G et al: Comparison of reduction in microalbuminuria by enalapril and hydrochlorothiazide in normotensive patients with insulin dependent diabetes. BMJ 1993;306:175–82

336. Mogensen CE, Keane WF, Bennett PH et al: Prevention of diabetic renal-disease with special reference to microalbuminuria. Lancet 1995;346:1080–4

337. Frost L, Bottcher M, Botker HE: Enalapril and exercise-induced hyperkalemia. A study of patients randomized to double-blind treatment with enalapril or placebo after acute myocardial infarction. Int J Cardiol 1992;37:401–5

338. Shionoiri H: Pharmacokinetic drug interactions with ACE inhibitors. Clin Pharmacokinetics 1993;25:20–58

339. Ponce SP, Jennings AE, Madias NE, Harrington JT: Drug induced hyperkalemia. Medicine 1985;64:357–70

340. Borra S, Shaker R, Kleinfeld M: Hyperkalemia in an adult hospitalized population. Mt Sinai J Med (NY) 1988;55:226–9

341. Parish RC, Miller LJ: Adverse-effects of angiotensin converting enzyme (ACE) inhibitors—an update. Drug Safety 1992; 7:14–31

342. Hargreaves MR, Benson MK: Inhaled sodium cromoglycate in angiotensin-converting enzyme-inhibitor cough. Lancet 1995; 345:13–6

343. Cody RJ, Covit AB, Schaer GL et al: Sodium and water balance in chronic congestive heart failure. J Clin Invest 1986;77: 1441–52

344. Richardson A, Bayliss J, Scriven A et al: Double-blind comparison of captopril alone against frusemide plus amiloride in mild heart failure. Lancet 1987;2:709–11

345. Romankiewicz JA, Brogden RN, Heel RC et al: Captopril: an update review of its pharmacological properties and therapeutic efficacy in congestive heart failure. Drugs 1983;25:6–40

346. Currie WJC, Cooper WD: Safety of angiotensin-converting-enzyme inhibitors. Lancet 1985;1:580–1

347. Edwards CRW, Padfield PL: Angiotensin-converting enzyme inhibitors: past, present and bright future. Lancet 1985;1: 29–34

348. O'Neill CJA, Bowes SG, Sullens CM: Evaluation of the safety of enalapril in the treatment of heart failure in the very old. Eur J Clin Pharmacol 1988;35:143–50

349. Northridge D: Frusemide or nitrates for acute heart-failure. Lancet 1996;347:667–8

350. Braunwald E: The control of ventricular function in man. Br Heart J 1965;27:1–8

351. DeLuz PL, Weil MH, Shubin H: Concepts on mechanism and treatment of cardiogenic shock. Am Heart J 1976;92:103–8

352. Hamer J: Fundemental aspects of myocardial performance. In Hamer J (ed): Recent Advances in Cardiology. Churchill Livingstone, Edinburgh 1973

353. Taylor SH: Heart failure. In Hamer J (ed): Recent Advances in Cardiology. Churchill Livingstone, Edinburgh, 1977

354. Anonymous: Vasodilators in heart failure. Lancet 1978;1: 972–3

355. Franciosa JA, Goldsmith SR, Cohn JN: Contrasting immediate and long-term effects of isorbide dinitrate on exercise capacity in congestive heart failure. Am J Cardiol 1980;69:559–66

356. Leier CV, Huss P, Magorien RD, Unverferth DV: Improved exercise capacity and differing arterial and venous tolerance during chronic isorbide dinitrate therapy in congestive heart failure. Circulation 1983;67:817–22

357. Aronow WS, Lurie M, Turbow M et al: Effect of prazosin vs. placebo on chronic left ventricular heart failure. Circulation 1979;59:344–50

358. Conradson TB, Ryden L, Ahlmark G et al: Clinical efficacy of oral hydralazine in chronic heart failure. One year double-blind placebo controlled study. Am Heart J 1984;108: 1001–6

359. Franciosa JA, Cohn JN: Sustained hemodynamic effects without tolerance during long-term isorbide dinitrate treatment of chronic left ventricular failure. Am J Cardiol 1980;45: 648–54

360. Cohn JN, Archibald DG, Ziesche S et al: Effect of vasodilator therapy on mortality in chronic congestive heart failure. N Engl J Med 1986;314:1547–52

361. Cohn JN: Drug therapy: the management of chronic heart failure. N Engl J Med 1996;335:490–8

362. Wieshammer S, Hetzel M, Hetzel J et al: Lack of effect of nitrates on exercise tolerance in patients with mild to moderate heart failure caused by coronary disease already treated with captopril. Br Heart J 1993;70:17–21

363. Colucci WS, Wynne J, Holman BL, Braunwald E: Long-term therapy of heart failure with prazosin: a randomized double blind trial. Am J Cardiol 1980;45:337–43

364. Markham RV, Corbett JR, Gilmore A et al: Efficacy of prazosin in the management of chronic congestive heart failure: a 6-month randomized double-blind placebo controlled study. Am J Cardiol 1983;51:1346–52

365. Franciosa JA, Weber KT, Levine B et al: Hydralazine in the

long-term treatment of chronic heart failure: lack of difference from placebo. Am Heart J 1982;104:587–94

366. Packer M, Meller J, Medina N et al: Hemodynamic characterization of tolerance to long-term hydralazine therapy in severe chronic congestive heart failure. N Engl J Med 1982;306: 57–62
367. Fonarow GC, Chelimsky-Fallick C, Stevenson LW: Effect of direct vasodilation with hydralazine versus angiotensin-converting enzyme inhibition with captopril on mortality in advanced heart failure: the Hy-C trial. J Am Coll Cardiol 1992; 19:842–50
368. Franciosa JA, Jordan RA, Wilen MM, Leddy CL: Minoxidil in patients with left heart failure: contrasting hemodynamic and clinical effects in a controlled trial. Circulation 1984;70: 63–9
369. Packer M, Rouleau J, Swedberg K et al: Effect of flosequinan on survival in chronic heart-failure—preliminary results of the PROFILE study. Circulation 1993;88:301
370. Barnett DB: Flosequinan. Lancet 1993;341:733–6
371. Anonymous: Flosequinan withdrawn. Lancet 1993;342:235
372. Soufer R, Wohlgelernter D, Vita NA et al: Intact systolic left-ventricular function in clinical congestive heart-failure. Am J Cardiol 1985;55:1032–6
373. Wheeldon NM, Clarkson P, MacDonald TM: Diastolic heart failure. Eur Heart J 1994;15:1689–97
374. Arrighi JA, Soufer R: Left ventricular diastolic function—physiology, methods of assessment, and clinical significance. J Nucl Cardiol 1995;2:525–43
375. Bedford PD, Caird FI: Congestive heart failure in the elderly. Q J Med 1956;25:407–26
376. Donald KW: Hemodynamics in chronic congestive heart failure. J Chron Dis 1959;9:476–97
377. Bing RJ, Bottcher D, Cowan C: What is heart failure? Am J Cardiol 1968;22:2–6
378. Stott DJ, Northridge D, Henderson E et al: Unexplained exertional dyspnea in elderly people is commonly associated with left-ventricular hypertrophy and diastolic dysfunction. J Clin Exp Gerontol 1992;14:33–44
379. Josephs W, Odenthal HJ, Lenga P et al: Diastolic left ventricular dysfunction—important differential diagnosis and therapy of cardiac insufficiency in old age. Z Gerontol 1992;25: 94–100
380. Cohn JN, Johnson G: Heart failure with normal ejection fraction: the V-HeFT Study. Circulation 1990;81(suppl III): III48–53
381. Zuccalà G, Sgadari A, Cocchi A et al: Effect of age and pathology on left-ventricular diastolic function—the diagnostic yield of Doppler echocardiography. J Gerontol Series A 1995;50: M78–82
382. Harizi RC, Bianco JA, Alpert JS: Diastolic function of the heart in clinical cardiology. Arch Intern Med 1988;148: 99–108
383. Aguirre FV, Pearson AC, Lewen MK et al: Usefulness of Doppler echocardiography in the diagnosis of congestive heart failure. Am J Cardiol 1989;63:1098–102
384. O'Keeffe ST: Diastolic dysfunction in elderly patients with dypnoea and normal left ventricular systolic function. Cardiol Elderly 1996;4:51–2
385. Cody RJ: Hypertensive heart disease and heart failure. Curr Opin Cardiol 1995;10:450–7
386. Aurigemma GP, Gaasch WH: Gender differences in older patients with pressure-overload hypertrophy of the left-ventricle. 1995;86:310–7
387. Goldsmith SR, Dick C: Differentiating systolic from diastolic heart-failure – pathophysiologic and therapeutic considerations. Am J Med 1993;95:645–55
388. Simpson IA: Echocardiography in the elderly—overview. Cardiol Elderly 1995;3:251–3
389. Acanfora D, Crisci C, Rengo C et al: Clinical determinants of long-term mortality in elderly patients with heart disease. Arch Gerontol Geriatr 1995;21:233–40
390. Kober L, Torppedersen C, Ottesen M et al: Influence of age on the prognostic importance of left-ventricular dysfunction and congestive heart failure on long term survival after acute myocardial infarction. Am J Cardiol 1996;78:158–62
391. Aronow WS, Ahn C, Kronzon I: Prognosis of congestive heart failure in elderly patients with normal versus abnormal left ventricular systolic function associated with coronary artery disease. Am J Cardiol 1990;66:1257–9
392. Gaasch WH: Diagnosis and treatment of heart-failure based on left-ventricular systolic or diastolic dysfunction. JAMA 1994; 271:1276–80
393. Lipsitz LA, Byrnes N, Hossain M et al: Restrictive left-ventricular filling patterns in very old patients with congestive heart failure—clinical correlates and prognostic significance. J Am Geriatr Soc 1996;44:634–7
394. Morley-Davies A, Nolan J: Heart failure: a historical context. pp. 1–13. In McMurray JJV, Cleland JGF (eds): Heart Failure in Clinical Practice. 1st Ed. Martin Dunitz, London, 1996
395. Katz AM: Scientific insights from clinical studies of converting-enzyme inhibitors in the failing heart. Trends Cardiovasc Med 1995;5:37–44
396. Dasgupta P, Ramhanmdany E, Brigden G et al: Improvement in left-ventricular function after rapid weight-loss in obesity. Eur Heart J 1992;13:1060–6
397. Jain A, Avendano G, Dharamsey S et al: Left-ventricular diastolic function in hypertension and role of plasma-glucose and insulin—comparison with diabetic heart. Circulation 1996; 93:1396–402
398. Vanninen E, Mustonen J, Vainio P et al: Left ventricular function and dimensions in newly diagnosed non-insulin-dependent diabetes mellitus. Am J Cardiol 1992;70:371–8
399. Belardinelli R, Georgiou D, Cianci G et al: Exercise training improves left-ventricular diastolic filling in patients with dilated cardiomyopathy—clinical and prognostic implications. Circulation 1995;91:2775–84
400. Takarada A, Kurogane H, Minamiji K et al: Congestive heart failure in the elderly—echocardiographic insights. Japan Circ J 1992;56:527–34
401. Wong WF, Gold S, Fukuyama O, Blanchette L: Diastolic dysfunction in elderly patients with congestive heart failure. Am J Cardiol 1989;63:1526–8

402. Frielingsdorf J, Gerber AE, Hess OM: Importance of maintained atrioventricular synchrony in patients with pacemakers. Eur Heart J 1994;15:1431–40

403. Lip GYH, Watson RDS, Singh SP: ABC of atrial-fibrillation—drugs for atrial-fibrillation. BMJ 1995;311:1631–4

404. Nolan J, Kearney MT: Heart-failure—an old problem. Br J Hosp Med 1995;54:43–6

405. Pepi M, Marenzi GC, Agostoni PG et al: Sustained cardiac diastolic changes elicited by ultrafiltration in patients with moderate congestive heart failure: pathophysiological correlates. Br Heart J 1993;70:135–40

406. Modena MG, Mattioli AV, Parato VM, Mattioli G: Effectiveness of the antihypertensive action of lisinopril on left ventricular mass and diastolic filling. Eur Heart J 1992;13:1540–4

407. Diez J, Laviades C, Mayor G: Diastolic dysfunction in elderly hypertensive patients. Cardiol Elderly 1993;1:9–14

408. Salcedo A, Lekuona I, Laraudogoitia E et al: Effect of antihypertensive therapy on left ventricular mass and diastolic filling in mild-to-moderate hypertension. Med Clin (Barc) 1993;100:646–50

409. Facchin L, Vescovo G, Levedianos G et al: Left-ventricular morphology and diastolic function in uremia—echocardiographic evidence of a specific cardiomyopathy. Br Heart J 1995;74:174–9

410. Tresch DD, McGough MF: Heart failure with normal systolic function: a common disorder in older people. J Am Geriatr Soc 1995;43:1035–42

411. Brutsaert DL, Sys SU, Gillebert TC: Diastolic failure—pathophysiology and therapeutic implications. J Am Coll Cardiol 1993;22:318–25

412. Kessler KM: Diastolic heart failure. Diagnosis and management. Hosp Pract 1989;24:137–48

413. Granger CB, Karimeddini MK, Smith VE et al: Rapid ventricular filling in left ventricular hypertrophy. I. Physiologic hypertrophy. J Am Coll Cardiol 1985;5:862–8

414. Visser CA, Reichert CLA, Hanrath P et al: Improved diastolic function with the calcium antagonist nisoldipine (Coat Core) in patients post myocardial infarction—results of the DEFIANT study. Eur Heart J 1992;13:1496–505

415. Parameshwar J, Poole-Wilson PA: The role of calcium antagonists in the treatment of chronic heart failure. Eur Heart J 1993;14(Sa):38–44

416. Pouleur H, Rousseau MF: Nisoldipine in severe ischemic left ventricular dysfunction. Eur Heart J 1993;14(Sa):45–7

417. Clavijo GA, de Clavigo IV, Weart CW: Amlodipine: a new calcium antagonist. Am J Hosp Pharmacy 1994;51:59–68

418. Pahor M, Guralnik JM, Furberg CD et al: Risk of gastrointestinal hemorrhage with calcium-antagonists in hypertensive persons over 67 years old. Lancet 1996;347:1061–5

419. Pahor M, Guralnik JM, Salive MF et al: Do calcium channel blockers increase the risk of cancer. Am J Hypertens 1996;9:695–9

420. Waagstein F, Bristow MR, Swedberg K et al: Beneficial effects of metoprolol in idiopathic dilated cardiomyopathy. Lancet 1993;342:1441–6

421. Waagstein F: The role of beta-blockers in dilated cardiomyopathy. Curr Opin Cardiol 1995;10:322–31

422. Dietz R, Waas W, Susselbeck T et al: Improvement of cardiac function by angiotensin converting enzyme inhibition—sites of action. Circulation 1993;87:108–16

423. Chapman D, Wang T, Gheorghiade M: Therapeutic approaches to heart failure in elderly patients. Cardiol Elderly 1994;2:89–97

424. Lowe CJ, Raynor DK, Courtney EA et al: Effects of self-medication program on knowledge of drugs and compliance with treatment in elderly patients. BMJ 1995;310:1229–31

425. Goodyer LI, Miskelly F, Milligan P: Does encouraging good compliance improve patients clinical condition in heart-failure. Br J Clin Pract 1995;49:173–6

426. Rich MW, Beckham V, Wittenberg C et al: A multidisciplinary intervention to prevent the readmission of elderly patients with congestive heart failure. N Engl J Med 1995;333:1190–5

427. Rich MW, Shah AS, Vinson JM et al: Iatrogenic congestive heart failure in older adults—clinical course and prognosis. J Am Geriatr Soc 1996;44:638–43

428. Marmot M, Ghodse AH, Jarvis S et al: Alcohol and the heart in perspective—sensible limits reaffirmed. J R Coll Physicians Lond 1995;29:266–71

429. Gurwitz JH, Avorn J, Ross-Degnan D, Lipsitz LA: Nonsteroidal anti-inflammatory drug-associated azotemia in the very old. JAMA 1990;264:471–5

430. Goorah R, Wynne H: The prescribing of nonsteroidal anti-inflammatory drugs in the elderly. Rev Clin Gerontol 1995;5:357–63

431. Walters EG, Horswill CE, Shelton JR, Akbar FA: Hazards of beta-blocker/diuretic tablets. Lancet 1985;2:220–1

432. Stott DJ, Ball SG: Treatment of essential hypertension. Br J Hosp Med 1986;36:261–9

433. Van Zyl A, Opie LH: Beta-blockade in the elderly. Lancet 1986;1:733

434. Wei JY: Use of calcium entry blockers in elderly patients. Special considerations. Circulation 1989;80:IV171–IV177

435. Anonymous: Calcium antagonist caution. Lancet 1991;337:885–6

436. Schwartz JB: Calcium antagonists in the elderly—a risk benefit analysis. Drugs Aging 1996;9:24–36

437. Krum H, Tonkin A, Trotter A et al: Effects of carvedilol, a vasodilator-beta blocker, in patients with congestive heart failure due to ischemic heart disease. Circulation 1995;92:212–8

438. Cleland JGF, Swedberg K: Carvedilol for heart-failure, with care. Lancet 1996;347:1199–201

439. de Vries RJM, Dunselman PHJM, Sung UGCK et al: Effects of lacidipine on peak oxygen-consumption, neurohormones and invasive hemodynamics in patients with mild-to-moderate chronic heart-failure. Heart 1996;75:159–64

440. Monane M, Bohn RL, Gurwitz JH et al: Topical glaucoma medications and cardiovascular risk in the elderly. Clin Pharmacol Ther 1994;55:76–83

441. Cecchi F, Montereggi A, Olivotto J: Symptoms of hypertrophic cardiomyopathy and their management in the elderly. Cardiol Elderly 1995;3:423–9

442. Stevenson WG: Mechanisms and management of arrhythmias in heart-failure. Curr Opin Cardiol 1995;10:274–81
443. Singh SN, Fletcher RD, Fisher SG et al: Amiodarone in patients with congestive-heart-failure and asymptomatic ventricular arrhythmia. N Engl J Med 1995;333:77–82
444. Hammill SC, Packer DL: Amiodarone in congestive heart failure—unraveling the GESICA and CHF-STAT differences. Heart 1996;75:6–7
445. Polikar R, Burger AG, Scherrer U, Nicod P: The thyroid and the heart. Circulation 1993;87:1435–41
446. Amidi M, Leon DF, deGroot WJ et al: Effect of the thyroid state on myocardial contractility and ventricular ejection rate in man. Circulation 1968;38:229–39
447. Hwang YT, Tseng CD, Hwang JJ et al: Cardiac amyloidosis presenting as sick sinus syndrome and intractable heart failure: report of a case. J Formosan Med Assoc 1993;92:283–7
448. Kyle RA: Amyloidosis. Circulation 1995;91:1269–71
449. Varma MPS, McCluskey DR, Khan MM et al: Heart-failure associated with infective endocarditis—a review of 40 cases. Br Heart J 1986;55:191–7
450. Gersh BJ: Infections: myocarditis, pericarditis, and endocarditis. Curr Opin Cardiol 1989;4:403–28
451. McKenna WJ, Beiras AC, Lado MP: The Cardiomyopathies. Br Heart J 1994;72 (suppl):S1–S56
452. Satoh M, Tamura G, Segawa I et al: Enteroviral RNA in dilated cardiomyopathy. Eur Heart J 1994;15:934–9
453. Burns JMA, Knight PV: Infective endocarditis in an elderly population: a five-year retrospective study. J Clin Exp Gerontol 1991;13:161–71
454. Roelandt JRTC, Meeter K: Diagnosis and management of valvular heart disease in the elderly. Cardiol Elderly 1993;1: 235–43
455. Sprigings DC, Forfar JC: How should we manage symptomatic aortic-stenosis in the patient who is 80 or older. Br Heart J 1995;74:481–4
456. Chocron S, Rude N, Dussaucy A et al: Quality-of-life after open-heart-surgery in patients over 75 years old. Age Ageing 1996;25:8–11
457. Samani NJ: The renin-angiotensin system in cardiovascular physiology and disease—new insights from molecular studies. Q J Med 1993;86:755–60
458. Francis GS, McDonald KM, Cohn JN: Neurohumoral activation in preclinical heart failure: remodeling and the potential for intervention. Circulation 1993;87:IV-90–IV-96
459. Sigurdsson A, Amtorp O, Gundersen T et al: Neurohormonal activation in patients with mild or moderately severe congestive heart failure and effects of ramipril. Br Heart J 1994;72: 422–7
460. Cody RJ, Haas GJ, Binkley PF et al: Plasma endothelin correlates with the extent of pulmonary-hypertension in patients with chronic congestive-heart-failure. Circulation 1992;85: 504–9
461. McMurray JJ, Ray SG, Abdullah I et al: Plasma endothelin in chronic heart-failure. Circulation 1992;85:1374–9
462. Benfante R, Reed D: Is elevated serum cholesterol level a risk factor for coronary heart disease in the elderly. JAMA 1990; 263:393–6
463. Kiowski W, Sutsch G, Hunziker P et al: Evidence for endothelin-1-mediated vasoconstriction in severe chronic heart-failure. Lancet 1995;346:732–6
464. Webb DJ: Evidence for endothelin-1-mediated vasoconstriction in severe chronic heart-failure—endothelin antagonism in heart-failure. Circulation 1995;92:3372
465. Krum H, Goldsmith R, Wilshireclement M et al: Role of endothelin in the exercise intolerance of chronic heart-failure. Am J Cardiol 1995;75:1282–3
466. Benians RG: Syncopal attacks in the elderly. Gerontol Clin 1970;12:229–34
467. Hornig B, Maier V, Drexler H: Physical-training improves endothelial function in patients with chronic heart-failure. Circulation 1996;93:210–4
468. Pacher R, Stanek B, Hulsmann M et al: Prognostic impact of big endothelin-1 plasma-concentrations compared with invasive hemodynamic evaluation in severe heart-failure. J Am Coll Cardiol 1996;27:633–41
469. Benjamin B: The span of life. J Inst Actuaries 1982;109: 319–57
470. Teerlink JR, Loffler BM, Hess P et al: Role of endothelin in the maintenance of blood-pressure in conscious rats with chronic heart-failure—acute effects of the endothelin receptor antagonist RO-47–0203 (bosentan). Circulation 1994;90:2510–8
471. Kaddoura S, Poole-Wilson PA: Endothelin-1 in heart failure: a new therapeutic target? Lancet 1996;348:418–9
472. Tschudi MR, Luscher TF: Age and hypertension differently affect coronary contractions to endothelin-1, serotonin, and angiotensins. Circulation 1995;91:2415–22
473. Gottlieb SS: New approaches to managing congestive heart failure. Curr Opin Cardiol 1995;10:282–7
474. Habib F, Dutka D, Crossman D et al: Enhanced basal nitric oxide production in heart failure: another failed counter-regulatory vasodilator mechanism. Lancet 1994;344:371–4
475. Lindsay DC, Holdright DR, Clarke D et al: Endothelial control of lower limb blood flow in chronic heart-failure. Heart 1996; 75:469–76
476. Winlaw DS, Smythe GA, Keogh AM et al: Increased nitric oxide production in heart failure. Lancet 1994;344:373–4
477. Susic D, Nunez E, Frohlich ED: Reversal of hypertrophy—an active biologic process. Curr Opin Cardiol 1995;10:466–72
478. Warren JB, Pons F, Brady AJB: Nitric oxide biology: implications for cardiovascular therapeutics. Cardiovasc Res 1994; 28:25–30
479. Lessem JN, Weber MA: Antihypertensive treatment with a dual acting beta-blocker in the elderly. J Hypertens 1993;11: S29–36
480. Rosendorff C: Beta-blocking agents with vasodilator activity. J Hypertens 1993;11:S37–40
481. Krum H, Sacknerbernstein JD, Goldsmith RL et al: Double-blind, placebo-controlled study of the long-term efficacy of carvedilol in patients with severe chronic heart-failure. Circulation 1995;92:1499–506
482. Krum H, Conway EL, Broadbear JH et al: Postural hypotension in elderly patients given carvedilol. BMJ 1994;309:775–6
483. Sasayama S: Current treatment for chronic heart failure—vesnarinone (OPC-8212). J Mol Cell Cardiol 1992;24: 36

484. Armstrong PW, Moe GW: Medical advances in the treatment of congestive heart failure. Circulation 1993;88:2941–52
485. Dunkman WB, Johnson GR, Ziesche S et al: Incidence of thromboembolic events in congestive heart failure. Circulation 1993;87:VI–94–VI–101
486. Ciuffetti G, Mercuri M, Rizzon MT et al: Age and blood cell rheology. Gerontology 1989;35:31–5
487. Stout RW, Crawford V: Seasonal variations in fibrinogen concentrations among elderly people. Lancet 1991;338:9–13
488. Weintraub NL, Chaitman BR: Newer concepts in the medical management of patients with congestive heart failure. Clin Cardiol 1993;16:380–90
489. Baker DW, Wright RF: Management of heart failure. IV. Anticoagulation for patients with heart failure due to left ventricular systolic dysfunction. JAMA 1994;272:1614–8
490. Raffaeli S, Paciaroni E: Stroke and atrial-fibrillation—risks, prevention and therapy in the elderly. Arch Gerontol Geriatr 1995;20:23–8
491. Barnett HJM, Eliasziw M, Meldrum HE: Drug therapy: drugs and surgery in the prevention of ischemic stroke. N Engl J Med 1995;332:238–48
492. Lip GYH, Lowe GDO: ABC of atrital fibrillation—antithrombotic treatment for atrial-fibrillation. BMJ 1996;312:45–9
493. Hall D, Zeitler H, Rudolph W: Counteraction of the vasodilator effects of enalapril by aspirin in severe heart failure. J Am Coll Cardiol 1992;20:1549–55
494. Schwartz D, Kornowski R, Lehrman H et al: Combined effect of captopril and aspirin in renal hemodynamics in elderly patients with congestive heart failure. Cardiol (Basel) 1992;81:334–9
495. Cleland JGF, Bulpitt CJ, Falk RH et al: Is aspirin safe for patients with heart-failure. Br Heart J 1995;74:215–9
496. King D, Davies KN, Slee A, Silas JH: Atrial-fibrillation in the elderly—physicians attitudes to anticoagulation. Br J Clin Pract 1995;49:123–5

CHAPTER 23

Diagnosis and Management of Ischemic Heart Disease in the Elderly

GARY GERSTENBLITH

The diagnosis and management of ischemic heart disease in the elderly is an increasingly frequent challenge. The elderly constitute the most rapidly growing segment of our society[1] and although they presently account for only approximately 10 to 16 percent of the total population, they represent a much larger proportion of patients with cardiac disease being treated in a hospital or in a physician's office. The increasing number of elderly is primarily accounted for by the more successful treatment of infectious diseases in the younger populations. Over the past 20 years, there has, in addition, been a significant decrease in cardiovascular mortality in middle-aged groups, primarily due to a decrease in stroke but also to a decline in cardiac mortality.[2] In the elderly, ischemic disease itself is responsible for over one-half of the deaths and the vast majority of patients with congestive heart failure and cardiac disability. This chapter will review whether, and if so, how the aging process itself alters the presentation and treatment of coronary disease.

Physiologic Changes Associated with Cardiac Aging

Age-related changes in cardiac function and structure are well described in normal man, and the mechanisms responsible for these are explored in animal models of aging.[3] Some of these alter the substrate upon which disease is superimposed and therefore, the presentation and diagnosis of ischemia. The most important of these are prolonged contraction and relaxation and a diminished response to β-adrenergic sympathetic stimulation.

Prolonged relaxation is evidenced by a decrease in the slope of early mitral valve closure on M-mode echocardiography,[4] a decrease in peak filling rate and an increase in the time to peak filling rate on radionuclide angiography studies,[5,6] and an increase in Doppler indices of atrial contribution to left ventricular filling.[7,8] In one study[8] of 69 individuals without overt evidence of cardiovascular disease, there was a significant linear increase in the ratio of the atrial contraction phase to the rapid filling phase (A/E) of left ventricular filling to age (A/E $=$ 0.14 [years in age] $+$ 0.153, r $=$ 0.82, $P < .001$).

Relaxation is prolonged in left ventricular trabeculae from senescent rat hearts,[9] and there is a constellation of changes on the subcellular level that manifest and/or are responsible for these findings. These include a prolonged aequorin light transient,[10] indicating a prolonged myoplasmic calcium transient, a decrease in the velocity of calcium accumulation by sarcoplasmic reticulum isolated from senescent cardiac muscle,[11] and a decrease in the percent of myosin isozyme that has the most rapid adenosine triphosphate (ATP) hydrolytic rate (the V_1 isomyosin) from over 50 percent in young adult rats to under 20 percent in muscle from senescent rat hearts.[12] It is possible that these changes are related to the mild increase in left ventricular wall thickness associated with aging,[4] which may result from increased stiffness of the central arteries and an increase in the force required for left ventricular ejection in late systole.[13] Prolonged contraction and delayed relaxation properties may also be related to changes in physical conditioning status and endocrine function, as exercise protocols and administration of thyroid hormone[12–14] reverse some of these age-related changes.

In addition to changes in relaxation parameters, both animal and human data indicate that aging decreases cardiovascular β-adrenergic responsiveness. This is true for the inotropic,[15–17] chronotropic,[18] as well as the vasodilating[19] effects of these agents. Diminished β-adrenergic responsiveness results in a decreased dependence on sympathetic-mediated increases in heart rate and contractility[20,21] during exercise stress, and a greater dependence on an increase in stroke volume mediated via an increase in end-diastolic volume—the Frank-Starling effect.

These changes may alter presenting symptoms in patients with ischemic disease. Ischemia, similar to aging, alters diastolic properties so as to increase end diastolic pressure for any given volume. Older individuals may therefore be more likely than younger patients to experience dyspneic symptoms for any given ischemic or tachycardic insult. Decreased dependence on sympathetic-induced cardiovascular changes to mediate an exercise response suggests that beta adrenergic blockers may be less effective anti-ischemic agents during exercise in an older population.

Importance of Risk Factors

Although the significance of risk factors for the development of coronary disease is well recognized in the younger and middle-aged groups, the importance of risk factor management in the elderly is sometimes debated. Epidemiologic data indicate that systolic blood pressure is an important discriminator of cardiovascular risk for middle-aged and older men and women.[22,23] In addition, several studies indicate that treating diastolic hypertension in individuals into the eighth decade of life reduces all cause mortality as well as cardiac and stroke mortality and morbidity.[23–25] In the Systolic Hypertension in the Elderly Program trial,[26] treatment of isolated systolic hypertension (systolic, 160 mmHg or more) in those 60 years of age or more resulted in a 36 percent decrease in fatal and nonfatal stroke, a 27 percent decrease in nonfatal myocardial infarction or coronary death, and a 32 percent reduction in all major cardiovascular events. Formulation of the treatment goals of antihypertensive therapy in patients with known ischemic disease should also consider a report indicating a "J"-shaped relationship between diastolic blood pressure reduction and cardiac outcomes in patients with known ischemic disease.[27] This study reported that in those with known coronary disease, cardiac outcomes were lowest if the treated diastolic pressure was in the 85 to 90 mmHg range and increased if diastolic pressures were lowered to below 85 mmHg.

The goals of antihypertensive therapy encompass lowering overall cardiovascular risk as well as decreasing blood pressure, per se. Since antihypertensive agents impact on other cardiovascular risk factors, as well as concomitant diseases that older individuals are more likely to have, the influence of agents on these variables should also be considered. Thus, potassium-sparing diuretics may have favorable effects on electrolyte balance; β-blockers and calcium blockers have anti-ischemic effects; β-blockers provide secondary prevention postinfarction; and angiotensin-converting enzyme (ACE) inhibitors slow the progression of renal disease in diabetic hypertensive patients, and improve outcomes in postinfarction patients with left ventricular dysfunction. Finally, it is recognized that left ventricular hypertrophy is an independent risk factor for the development of coronary disease in elderly men and women.[28] Regression of left ventricular mass is possible in older hypertensive patients and is associated with improved diastolic filling indices.[29] The diagnosis and appropriate treatment of hypertension is an important goal in the prevention of coronary outcomes in older patients.[30]

Another important remedial risk factor in the elderly is cigarette use. The effects of smoking cessation were evaluated in a subset of participants in the CASS Registry.[31] The relative risk (and confidence limits) of myocardial infarction or death over a 6-year period for those who continued to smoke, as compared to those who stopped, was 2.9 (1.4, 5.9) for those men and women 70 years of age and older and 1.5 (1.0, 2.3) for those aged 65 to 69 years. These were similar to or greater than the benefit in those under 65 years of age. Thus, there is strong suggestive evidence that even our older patients can reduce cardiac risk when they stop smoking.

A common risk factor in older individuals is elevated lipids. Although earlier data were conflicting, recent information indicates that lipids—in particular, the HDL (high-density lipoprotein) cholesterol level—are related to coronary mortality in older individuals. In the Established Populations for Epidemiologic Studies of the Elderly report,[32] there was a 17 percent increase in the risk for coronary heart disease (CHD) death for every 1 U increase in the total cholesterol/HDL cholesterol ratio in nearly 5,000 men and women aged 71 years or older. HDL cholesterol was also related to coronary outcomes in women and in those over 80 years of age. Although there are no data concerning the value of lipid lowering therapy for primary prevention in the older population, there are data regarding its effectiveness in older individuals with known coronary disease. In the Scandinavian study, HMG CoA reductase inhibitor therapy was associated with a 0.73 relative risk of all cause mortality and a 0.71 relative risk of a major coronary event, defined as coronary death, nonfatal myocardial infarction, or cardiac arrest in those 60 years of age or more.[33]

There are other risk factors that are associated with coronary disease and mortality, although no prospective, randomized trials yet indicate that changing these factors changes cardiovascular outcomes in the older population. Obesity is one; in a study of over 41,000 older women, body fat distribution indexed by the waist:hip ratio (but not body mass index [BMI]) was associated with a strong, monotonic increase in the risk of cardiovascular, cancer, and total mortality.[34] The waist:hip ratio is also the best marker for the metabolic hazards of obesity including insulin resistance, hypertension, and hyperlipidemia.[35] As age increases, the ratio of women to men in the patient population with ischemic heart disease also increases. Postmenopausal estrogen use is associated with a decrease in the development of coronary disease and cardiovascular mortality,[36] and of angiographic evidence of coronary atherosclerosis.[37] These benefits may be related to a rise in HDL levels, inhibition of endothelial proliferation, and a favorable influence on coronary vasoreactivity. In one study, the acute administration of estrogen attenuated acetylcholine-induced coronary vasoconstriction in postmenopausal women with coronary artery disease.[38] Other factors associated with decreased cardiovascular outcomes in older individuals are physical activity status,[39] dietary antioxidant flavonoid intake,[40] plasma fibrinogen and factor VII activity,[41] and dietary, although not supplemental vitamin E intake.[42]

Diagnosis and Evaluation of Severity

The diagnosis of coronary disease in an older individual should be considered with the realization that although silent ischemia is undoubtedly present in individuals of all age groups, it is particularly likely in the aged. In patients referred to a medical center for stress testing, the prevalence of exercise-induced silent ischemia increased from 7 percent in those less than 50 years of age to 36 percent in those 70 years of age or older.[43] In a report of 470 asymptomatic volunteers from the Baltimore Longitudinal Study of Aging population, the prevalence of exercise-induced silent ischemia, defined by both electrocardiographic and thallium scintigraphic criteria, increased from 2 percent in the fifth decade to 15 percent in the ninth decade of life.[44] The true, or autopsy, prevalence of significant stenoses is several-fold higher than the clinical prevalence if the latter is judged by symptoms of exertional chest discomfort or history of a myocardial infarction. In an autopsy study reported by investigators from the Mayo Clinic, 72 percent of men and 54 percent of women 70 years or older had 75 percent or greater stenoses of at least one major coronary artery.[45] The high prevalence of silent ischemia may be due to a diminished sensation of chest discomfort, the increased likelihood that ischemia will be manifest as dyspnea rather than more typical pain symptoms, and the fact that other, superimposed diseases may render the older individual less likely to exercise to the point at which anginal symptoms occur.

It is important, therefore, to go beyond just a negative history if a degree of certainty is required regarding the absence of ischemic disease in the elderly. Often the most useful objective test is the exercise electrocardiogram. Although the specificity is somewhat less in the older age group,[46] it is generally useful with some known caveats. The first is that the predictive accuracy of a positive test is low in the setting of an abnormal baseline electrocardiogram. This is more likely in older individuals because of the increased prevalence of left bundle branch block, left ventricular hypertrophy, and digitalis ingestion. In these circumstances, an exercise isotope exam would be useful. It should also be noted that the predictive accuracy of a negative test is low in a population with a high prevalence of disease. Thus, a negative test in an older man with risk factors and some symptoms, who may have a 80 percent pretest likelihood of disease, may still be associated with a 50 percent post-test likelihood of significant disease. A third concern in the older population is an inability, because of other medical problems such as arthritis or pulmonary insufficiency, to exercise to 85 to 90 percent of the predicted maximum heart rate. In this setting, the predictive accuracy of a negative test is low, and pharmacologic testing with dipyridamole, adenosine, or dobutamine in conjunction with electrocardiographic, isotope, or echocardiographic monitoring is useful.[47,48] For patients in whom good quality echocardiograms can be obtained, this tool provides additional information that may be particularly useful in the older individual. These include the significance of aortic stenosis (at times associated with angina symptoms in the elderly), the presence of left ventricular hypertrophy, and global and regional assessment of left ventricular function.

Prognosis in patients with stable coronary disease is dependent upon coronary anatomy and left ventricular function. Although the severity of symptoms is one means of evaluating the severity of atherosclerosis, the absence or the presence of only minimal symptoms, particularly in the older age groups, cannot be relied upon to indicate the presence of only minimal disease. In this situation as well, the noninvasive stress electrocardiogram is useful, not only in diagnosing disease, but also in assessing the likelihood of triple vessel or left main coronary stenoses. Indicators of severe disease, even in asymptomatic or minimally symptomatic patients,[49] include an early positive test, one that remains positive for more than 8 minutes after the termination of exercise; more than 2 mm of ST-segment shift (in the presence of a normal baseline); changes in the anterior *and* inferior leads with stress; a systolic fall in pressure of more than 10 to 20 mmHg; and exercise-induced malignant ventricular arrhythmias.

Treatment

It is often useful to consider whether noncardiac factors are present in an older individual who presents with new onset angina or a change in anginal pattern. Anemia, for example, frequently presents with ischemic symptoms in this age group. Hyperthyroidism in the elderly often presents with cardiac manifestations, including arrhythmias and ischemia, rather than noncardiac symptoms, which are more common in the young. Supraventricular arrhythmias, hypertension, and congestive heart failure are all more common in the elderly and increase myocardial oxygen demand requirements as well as decrease supply. Identification and reversal of these precipitating factors, therefore, may return the older individual to the symptomatic status enjoyed previously.

Medical Therapy

If medical therapy is needed, sublingual nitrates are the most effective agents for the relief of an acute ischemic episode. Continuous nitrates alone, however, are not capable of providing continuous prophylaxis because of tolerance, which is present for oral, topical, as well as continuous intravenous use. Tolerance is not present for β-blockers and calcium antagonists, and both classes are effective anti-ischemic agents. The choice of an anti-ischemic β-blocker can be based on associated medical conditions and patient convenience. These can be used to decide whether to use a hydrophilic or lipophilic agent, as well as whether to use a relatively cardioselective agent. The latter, however, are cardioselective in only low doses and may lose their relative selectivity when moderate and high doses are employed. An additional consideration in the postinfarction patient is whether the β-blocker provides secondary prevention (vide infra). Calcium antagonists may provide additional benefit in patients who continue to experience angina despite β-blocker therapy. Some calcium antagonists have antihypertensive, as well as anti-ischemic, properties and are therefore especially useful in those angina patients with associated hypertension.

Coronary Angioplasty

Angioplasty is an increasingly attractive option in elderly individuals with continued symptoms despite medical therapy. This is particularly true in those who are at increased risk with bypass surgery (vide infra) because it avoids the thoracotomy, general anesthesia, and prolonged convalescence associated with surgery. Although the National Heart Lung Blood Institute (NHLBI) Percutaneous Transluminal Coronary Angioplasty

(PTCA) registry initially reported a lower success rate and a higher complication rate, including death and need for subsequent bypass surgery, in patients over 65 years of age,[50] more recent data indicate that age itself is not associated with a higher failure rate.[51–53] The development of newer techniques and increased experience in the treatment of multivessel disease has increased the number of elderly who are likely to experience significantly improved symptoms with angioplasty. In a recent report of 768 patients 65 years of age or more undergoing angioplasty, the technical success rate was 93.5 percent, in-hospital death rate was 1.4 percent; and 6-month death or myocardial infarction rate was 7.1 percent.[51] Longer-term follow-up of 1 year or greater also indicates that the proportion of patients experiencing sustained benefit, 65 to 75 percent, is also similar to that of the younger population.[52] The International Society and Federation of Cardiology and the World Health Organization Task Force on Coronary Angioplasty lists angina in patients 75 years of age or older as a "Class Two," or "evolving" indication for coronary angioplasty.[53]

Coronary Bypass Surgery

Perioperative survival and long-term follow-up following bypass surgery in elderly individuals are reported by several centers.[54–57] In view of the fact that surgery is often reserved for older patients who have few other options, it is not surprising that perioperative survival is lower, and complications—including cognitive dysfunction[58]—higher in older age groups. This can be related to increased prevalences of left main disease, left ventricular dysfunction, and advanced coronary disease in older patients undergoing revascularization. It is also related to other associated diseases, most importantly, pulmonary and renal dysfunction. Despite a higher perioperative mortality, postdischarge survival is comparable to that in younger patients,[54] and in the CASS Registry report, surgical survival in patients over 65 years of age actually trended higher than survival in those treated with medical therapy over a 6-year follow-up period.[56] In a study of 100 octogenarians undergoing open heart surgery, however, 24 percent of patients undergoing bypass alone died in the perioperative period or within 3 months of surgery.[57] When other options are limited, surgery can be successful in a high proportion of patients. Successful results with bypass surgery are reported in patients in their eighth and ninth decades, for example, who present with ischemia-induced recurrent pulmonary edema despite an intensive medical regimen.[59] A retrospective, case-control analysis of 195 patients over 70 years of age undergoing angioplasty, and 195 patients undergoing surgical revascularization matched for left ventricular function, age, and gender, found that hospital stay, death, Q-wave infarction, and stroke were less in the angioplasty group, but that the surgical group experienced less recurrent angina, required fewer repeat revascularization procedures, and experienced fewer Q-wave infarctions during follow-up.[60] Five-year survival in the two groups was the same. However, it should be noted that although data from the prospective, randomized Bypass Angioplasty Revascularization Investigation (BARI) trial of patients with stable angina undergoing revascularization also indicate no survival difference in the general population of patients, the subset of patients with diabetes on medical therapy experienced significantly worse survival with angioplasty than with bypass surgery.[61]

Acute Myocardial Infarction

Symptoms of infarction in the elderly are more likely to include dyspnea and those related to decreased cardiac output, including mental status changes, rather than typical chest pain.[62] Older individuals are also more likely to have an enzyme pattern consisting of an elevated MB fraction in the presence of a normal total creatinine kinase (CK). In one report, this pattern was present in 20 percent of those over 70 years of age but in only 10 percent of those under 70 years who met other criteria for acute infarction.[63] Treatment of acute myocardial infarction in the elderly should be tempered by the knowledge that older individuals are several-fold more likely to suffer serious complications of the infarct, including death, congestive heart failure, recurrent infarction, and rupture than are their younger counterparts.[64–66] In the prethrombolytic era, the Multicenter Investigation of the Limitation of Infarct Size (MILIS) Study Group reported that 65- to 74-year-old patients with acute infarction have a higher frequency of congestive heart failure (44 versus 28 percent) in hospital death (14 versus 7 percent) and 1-year mortality for hospital survivors (19 versus 5 percent) than those less than 65 years of age.[64] The influence of age on mortality in patients with first myocardial infarction was reported by the Gruppo Italiano per lo Studio della Sopravvivenza nell'Infarto Miocardio (GISSI)-2 investigators.[65] In over 9,700 patients receiving thrombolytic therapy for acute infarcts, mortality, congestive heart failure, and echocardiographic evidence of left ventricular dysfunction increased with age. There was no increase, however, in the investigators' measures of infarct size, including CK elevation and number of electrocardiographic leads involved with the infarct. The most striking finding on autopsy was a marked age-related increased finding of rupture. Rupture was present in over 80 percent of those older than 70 years of age who died and had autopsy examination. It is not clear why this was so high, particularly since there was no age-related increase in the extent of fixed coronary disease in these patients with first myocardial infarction. The rupture finding may relate to impaired healing in older individuals; to increased load on the infarcted regions because the noninfarcted territory cannot compensate as well for the myocardium, which has been lost as a result of the infarct; or to the fact that all of the patients received thrombolytic therapy.

The Thrombolysis in Myocardial Infarction (TIMI)-2 investigators also studied the impact of age on outcomes and the influence of postlytic management strategies in older infarct patients.[66] They reported an increase in mortality, complications, and recurrent infarctions. This may have been related to an age-related increase in delay to administration of the thrombolytic, perhaps due to the increased likelihood of atypical presentations in the older population, and to the fact that fewer older individuals were eligible to receive concomitant β-blocker therapy. There was no difference in clinical outcomes between those 65 to 74 years of age who were randomized to an early intervention strategy with catheterization and revascularization, and patients who underwent an early conservative strategy in which revascularization was performed only if they had evidence of recurrent ischemia during the early postinfarction period.

There are several limitations of thrombolytic therapy, and some of these are particularly relevant in the older population. Older individuals are less likely to be eligible to receive thrombolytic therapy because of hypertension and/or a history of central nervous system or other major bleeding. Best results are probably achieved with TIMI-3 flow; this is present in only about 60 percent of patients who undergo lysis. In addition, the risks of thrombolytic therapy may be increased in the older population. For these and other reasons, investigators compared primary angioplasty with thrombolytic therapy for patients with acute infarctions. In the large PAMI trial, separate results were not reported for those over 70 years of age.[67] However, in a meta analysis combining the Primary Angioplasty in Myocardial Infarction (PAMI) results with a Netherlands trial,[68] primary angioplasty was associated with a significant survival advantage and a decrease in stroke risk, as compared to thrombolytic therapy in those 70 years of age or older.

Postinfarction risk stratification is based on the same factors as those in the younger patient, that is, left ventricular function, the frequency and complexity of ventricular arrhythmias, and subjective or objective evidence of recurrent ischemia. Of several factors assessed in a prognostic study, Killip Class was the most powerful predictor of survival in those aged 65 years or more.[69] The low-level treadmill test may be particularly useful in older patients who may not have initially presented with chest pain symptoms. Those who are at increased risk because of poor left ventricular function may benefit from revascularization procedures with angioplasty or bypass surgery, if viable myocardium is dysfunctional due to low flow. Alternatively, if poor function is due to extensive scar, ACE inhibitor therapy improves survival, decreases left ventricular filling pressures and cavity size, and improves exercise tolerance.[70] The reduction in fatal and nonfatal events following infarction in patients with ejection fractions of 40 percent or less in the Survival and Ventricular Enlargement (SAVE) trial, was the same in those older and younger than 65 years of age.[70] There is less to offer those judged to be at increased risk on the basis of postinfarction arrhythmias. The inability of antiarrhythmics to decrease mortality in these individuals is highlighted by the data from the Cardiac Arrhythmia Suppression Trial, which indicated that the class 1C agents encainide and flecainide were actually associated with an increase in cardiac mortality in patients over 60 years of age, in whom the risk ratio was four- to fivefold higher in the treated, as compared with the placebo groups.[71] Some reports indicate amiodarone may improve survival.[72]

Those who have recurrent ischemic symptoms, or who have a positive electrocardiogram on stress testing, are at increased risk of recurrent infarction or death over the ensuing year and are generally considered for more aggressive diagnostic evaluation, including cardiac catheterization, in order to assess the suitability for revascularization procedures. If individuals are judged to be at low risk, one aspirin a day may be effective prophylaxis. Older patients also benefit from the routine use of β-blockers. Both the Norwegian Timolol study and the Beta-Blocker Heart Attack (BHAT) propranolol study demonstrated a significant improvement in survival for those over 60 to 65 years of age in the β-blocker as compared with the placebo groups.[73,74] Finally, an extensive trial of continuing versus discontinuing anticoagulation following myocardial infarction in 878 patients over 60 years of age indicated that anticoagulation reduced the 2-year incidence of recurrent infarction (from 15.9 percent in the placebo group to 5.7 percent in the treated group) and of total mortality (from 13.4 percent in the placebo group to 7.6 percent in the treated group) over a 2-year follow-up period.[75] This benefit was not outweighed by significant intracranial or extracranial bleeding events.[76]

References

1. Bureau of the Census: Current population reports. Special studies. Sixty-five plus in America. Government Printing Office, Washington, D.C., 1993
2. Thom TJ, Epstein FH: Heart disease, cancer, and stroke mortality trends and their interactions: an international perspective. Circulation 1994;90:574–582
3. Lakatta EG: Cardiovascular regulatory mechanisms in advanced age. Physiol Rev 1993;73:413–467
4. Gerstenblith G, Fredericksen J, Yin FCP et al: Echocardiographic assessment of a normal adult aging population. Circulation 1977;56:273–278
5. Bonow RO, Vitale DF, Bacharach SL et al: Effects of aging on asynchronous left ventricular regional function and global ventricular filling in normal human subjects. J Am Coll Cardiol 1988;11:50–58
6. Schulman SP, Lakatta EG, Fleg JL et al: Age-related decline in left ventricular filling at rest and exercise. Am J Physiol 1992;263(32):H1838–H1932
7. Kuecherer H, Ruffmann K, Kuebler W: Effect of aging on Doppler echocardiographic filling parameters in normal subjects and in patients with coronary artery disease. Clin Cardiol 1988;11:303–306
8. Miyatake K, Okamoto M, Kinoshita N et al: Augmentation of atrial contribution to left ventricular inflow with aging as assessed by intracardiac doppler flowmetry. Am J Cardiol 1984;53:586–589
9. Lakatta EG, Gerstenblith G, Angell CS et al: Prolonged contraction duration in aged myocardium. J Clin Invest 1975;55:61–68
10. Orchard CH, Lakatta EG: Intracellular calcium transients and developed tensions in rat heart muscle. A mechanism for the negative interval-strength relationship. J Gen Physiol 1985;86:637–651

11. Froehlich JP, Lakatta EG, Beard E et al: Studies of sarcoplasmic reticulum function and contraction duration in young and aged rat myocardium. J Mol Cell Cardiol 1978;10:427–438
12. Effron MB, Bhatnagar GM, Spurgeon HA et al: Changes in myosin isoenzymes, ATP-ase activity, and contraction duration in rat cardiac muscle with aging can be modulated by thyroxine. Circ Res 1987;60:238–245
13. Avolio AP, Fa-Quan D, Wei-Qiang L et al: Effects of aging on arterial distensibility in populations with high and low prevalence of hypertension: comparison between urban and rural communities in China. Circulation 1985;71:202–210
14. Spurgeon HA, Steinbach MF, Lakatta EG: Chronic exercise prevents characteristic age-related changes in rat cardiac contraction. Am J Physiol 1983;244:H513–H518
15. Lakatta EG, Gerstenblith G, Angell CS et al: Diminished inotropic response of aged myocardium to catecholamines. Circ Res 1975;36:262–269
16. Guarnieri T, Filburn CR, Zitnik G et al: Contractile and biochemical correlates of β-adrenergic stimulation of the aged heart. Am J Physiol 1980;239:H501–H508
17. Jiang MT, Moffat MP, Narayanaan N: Age-related alterations in the phosphorylation of sarcoplasmic reticulum and myofibrillator proteins and diminished contractile response to isoproterenol in intact rat ventricle. Circ Res 1993;72:102–111
18. Yin FCP, Spurgeon HA, Greene HL et al: Age-associated decrease in heart rate response to isoproterenol in dogs. Mech Ageing Dev 1979;10:17–25
19. Pam HY, Hoffman RR, Perskin RA et al: Decline in beta adrenergic receptor-mediated vascular relaxation with aging in man. J Pharmacol Exp Ther 1986;239:802–807
20. Rodeheffer RJ, Gerstenblith G, Becker LC et al: Exercise cardiac output is maintained with advancing age in healthy human subjects: cardiac dilatation and increased stroke volume compensate for a diminished heart rate. Circulation 1984;69: 203–213
21. Port S, Cobb FR, Coleman E, Jones RH: Effect of age on the response of the left ventricular ejection fraction to exercise. N Engl J Med 1980;303:1133–1137
22. Kannel WB, Dawber TR: Hypertension as an ingredient of a cardiovascular risk profile. Br J Hosp Med 1974;2:508–516
23. Glynn RJ, Field TS, Rosner B et al: Evidence for a positive linear relation between blood pressure and mortality in elderly people. Lancet 1995;345:825–829
24. Amery A, Birkenhager W, Brixko P et al: Mortality and morbidity results from the European Working Party on high blood pressure in the elderly trial. Lancet 1985;1:1349–1354
25. Insua JT, Sacks HS, Lau T-S et al: Drug treatment of hypertension in the elderly: a meta-analysis. Ann Intern Med 1994;121: 355–362
26. SHEP Cooperative Research Group: Prevention of stroke by antihypertensive drug treatment in older persons with isolated systolic hypertension. JAMA 1991;265:3255–3264
27. Cruickshank JM, Thorp JM, Zacharias FJ: Benefits and potential harm of lowering high blood pressure. Lancet 1987; 581–584
28. Levy D, Garrison RJ, Savage DD et al: Left ventricular mass and incidence of coronary heart disease in an elderly cohort. Ann Intern Med 1989;62:707–714
29. Schulman SP, Weiss JL, Becker LC et al: The effects of antihypertensive therapy on left ventricular mass in elderly patients. N Engl J Med 1990;322:1350–1356
30. National High Blood Pressure Education Program Working Group Report on Hypertension in the Elderly: NIH Publication No. 94–3527. National Institutes of Health, Washington D.C., 1994
31. Hermanson B, Omenn GS, Kronmal RA, Gersh BJ: Beneficial six-year outcome of smoking cessation in older men and women with coronary artery disease: results from the CASS registry. N Engl J Med 1988;319:1365–1369
32. Corti M-C, Guralnik JM, Salive ME et al: HDL cholesterol predicts coronary heart disease mortality in older persons. JAMA 1995;274:539–544
33. Scandinavian Simvastatin Survival Study Group: Randomized trial of cholesterol lowering in 4444 patients with coronary heart disease: the Scandinavian Simvastatin Survival Study (4S). Lancet 1994;344:1383–1389
34. Folson AR, Kaye SA, Sellers TA et al: Body fat distribution and 5-year risk of death in older women. JAMA 1993;269: 483–487
35. Bjorntorp: The associations between obesity, adipose tissue distribution and disease. Acta Med Scand 1988;723(suppl): 121–134
36. Stampfer MJ, Colditz GA, Willett WC et al: Postmenopausal estrogen therapy and cardiovascular disease: ten-year follow-up from the Nurses' Health Study. N Engl J Med 1991;325: 756–762
37. Sullivan JM, Vander Swaag R, Lemp GF et al: Postmenopausal estrogen use and coronary atherosclerosis. Ann Intern Med 1988;108:358–363
38. Reis SE, Gloth ST, Blumenthal RS et al: Ethinyl estradiol acutely attenuates vasomotor responses to acetylcholine in postmenopausal women. Circulation 1994;89:52–60
39. Paffenbarger RS, Hyde RT, Wing AL, Hsieh C: Physical activity, all-cause mortality, and longevity of college alumni. N Engl J Med 1986;314:605–613
40. Hertog MGL, Feskens EJM, Hollman PCH et al: Dietary antioxidant flavonoids and risk of coronary heart disease: the Zutphen Elderly Study. Lancet 1993;342:1007–1011
41. Woodhouse PR, Khaw KT, Plumer M et al: Seasonal variations of plasma fibrinogen and factor VII activity in the elderly: winter infections and death from cardiovascular disease. Lancet 1994; 343:435–439
42. Kushi LH, Folsom AR, Prineas RJ et al: Dietary antioxidant vitamins and death from coronary heart disease in postmenopausal women. N Engl J Med 1996;334:1156–1162
43. Callaham PR, Froelicher VF, Klein J et al: Exercise-induced silent ischemia: age, diabetes mellitus, previous myocardial infarction and prognosis. J Am Coll Cardiol 1989;14:1175–1180
44. Fleg JL, Gerstenblith G, Zonderman AB et al: Prevalence and prognostic significance of exercise-induced silent myocardial ischemia detected by thallium scintigraphy and electrocardiography in asymptomatic volunteers. Circulation 1990;81: 428–436

45. Elveback L, Lie JT: Continued high incidence of coronary artery disease at autopsy in Olmstead County, Minnesota. Circulation 1950 to 1979;70:345–349

46. Hlatky MA et al: Factors affecting sensitivity and specificity of exercise electrocardiography. Multivariable analysis. Am J Med 1984;77:64–71

47. Bateman TM, O'Keefe JH Jr: Pharmacological (stress) perfusion scintigraphy: methods, advantages, and applications. Am J Cardiac Imaging 1992;6:3–15

48. Beleslin BD, Ostojic M, Stepanovic J et al: Stress echocardiography in the detection of myocardial ischemia: head-to-head comparison of exercise, dobutamine, and dipyridamole tests. Circulation 1994;90:1168–1176

49. Blumenthal DS, Weiss JL, Mellits ED, Gerstenblith G: The predictive value of a strongly positive stress test in patients with minimal symptoms. Am J Med 1981;70:1005–1010

50. Mock MB, Holmes DR, Vlietstra RE et al: Percutaneous transluminal coronary angioplasty (PTCA) in the elderly patient: experience in the National Heart, Lung, and Blood Institute PTCA registry. Am J Cardiol 1984;53:89C–91C

51. Thompson RC, Holmes DR, Grill DE et al: Changing outcome of angioplasty in the elderly. J Am Coll Cardiol 1996;27:8–14

52. Dorros G, Janke L: Percutaneous transluminal coronary angioplasty in patients over the age of 70 years. Cathet Cardiovasc Diagn 1986;12:223–229

53. Bourassa MG, Alderman EL, Bertrand M et al: Report of the joint ISFC/WHO task force on coronary angioplasty. Circulation 1988;78:780–789

54. Horneffer PJ, Gardner TJ, Manolio TA et al: The effect of age on outcome after coronary bypass surgery. Circulation 1987; 76(suppl V):V-6–V-12

55. Peterson ED, Jollis JG, Bebchuk JD et al: Changes in mortality after myocardial revascularization in the elderly: the national Medicare experience. Ann Intern Med 1994;121:919–927

56. Gersh BJ, Kronmal RA, Schaff HV et al: Comparison of coronary artery bypass surgery and medical therapy in patients 65 years of age or older. N Engl J Med 1985;313:217–224

57. Edmunds LH, Stephenson LW, Edie RN, Ratcliffe MB: Open-heart surgery in octogenarians. N Engl J Med 1988;319: 131–136

58. Newman MF, Croughwell ND, Blumenthal JA et al: Effect of aging on cerebral autoregulation during cardiopulmonary bypass: association with postoperative cognitive dysfunction. Circulation 1994;90:II-243–II-249

59. Kunis R, Greenberg H, Yeoh CB et al: Coronary revascularization for recurrent pulmonary edema in elderly patients with ischemic heart disease and preserved ventricular function. N Engl J Med 1985;313:1207–1210

60. O'Keefe JH, Sutton MB, McCallister BD et al: Coronary angioplasty versus bypass surgery in patients >70 years old matched for ventricular function. J Am Coll Cardiol 1994;24:425–430

61. Ferguson JJ: NHLBI BARI clinical alert on diabetics treated with angioplasty. Circulation 1995;92:3371

62. Solomon CG, Lee TH, Cook EF et al: Comparison of clinical presentation of acute myocardial infarction in patients older than 65 years of age to younger patients: the multicenter chest pain study experience. Am J Cardiol 1989;63:772–776

63. Heller GV, Blaustein AS, Wei JY: Implications of increased myocardial isoenzyme level in the presence of normal serum creatine kinase activity. Am J Cardiol 1983;51:24–27

64. Tofler GH, Muller JE, Stone PH et al: Factors leading to shorter survival after acute myocardial infarction in patients ages 65 to 75 years compared with younger patients. Am J Cardiol 1988; 62:860–867

65. Maggioni AP, Maseri A, Fresco C et al: Age-related increase in mortality among patients with first myocardial infarction treated with thrombolysis. N Engl J Med 1993;329:1442–1448

66. Aguirre FV, McMahon RP, Hueller H et al: Impact of age on clinical outcomes and postlytic management strategies in patients treated with intravenous thrombolytic therapy: results from the TIMI II study. Circulation 1994;90:78–86

67. Grines CL, Browne KF, Marco J et al: A comparison of immediate angioplasty with thrombolytic therapy for acute myocardial infarction. N Engl J Med 1993;328:673–679

68. O'Neill WW, Zijlstra F, Suryapranata H et al: Meta-analysis of the PAMI and Netherlands randomized trials of primary angioplasty versus thrombolytic therapy of acute myocardial infarction. Circulation 1993;88:I–106

69. Olmsted WL, Groden DL, Silverman ME: Prognosis in survivors of acute myocardial infarction occurring at age 70 years or older. Am J Cardiol 1987;60:971–975

70. Pfeffer MA, Braunwald E, Moye LA et al: Effect of captopril on mortality and morbidity in patients with left ventricular dysfunction after myocardial infarction: results of the Survival and Ventricular Enlargement Trial. N Engl J Med 1992;327: 669–677

71. The Cardiac Arrhythmia Suppression Trial (CAST) Investigators: Preliminary report: effect of encainide and flecainide on mortality in a randomized trial of arrhythmia suppression after myocardial infarction. N Engl J Med 1989;321:406–412

72. Pfisterer ME, Kiowski W, Brunner H et al: Long-term benefit of 1-year amiodarone treatment for persistent complex ventricular arrhythmias after myocardial infarction. Circulation 1993;87: 309–311

73. The Norwegian Multicenter Study Group: Timolol-induced reduction in mortality and reinfarction in patients surviving acute myocardial infarction. N Engl J Med 1981;304:801–807

74. Beta Blocker Heart Attack Study Group: The Beta-Blocker Heart Attack Trial. JAMA 1981;246:2073

75. Report of the Sixty Plus Reinfarction Study Research Group: A double-blind trial to assess long-term oral anticoagulant therapy in elderly patients after myocardial infarction. Lancet 1980; ii:989–994

76. Second Report of the Sixty Plus Reinfarction Study Research Group: Risks of long-term oral anticoagulant therapy in elderly patients after myocardial infarction. Lancet 1982;i:64–68

CHAPTER 24

Hypertension

ANDREW K. SCOTT

Hypertension is a common problem in older adults. It is a major risk factor for two of the most important causes of death in elderly patients—ischemic heart disease and cerebrovascular disease. Despite this and attention given to hypertension research in younger adults, it has received relatively little attention until the last 10 to 15 years, though happily this situation is changing.

Management of such a common and important condition should be second nature to all medical practitioners. However, the reality is that all aspects of care of patients with hypertension are less than satisfactory both in hospital and general practice. Measurement of blood pressure is poor; application of basic guidelines in establishing a diagnosis of sustained hypertension is inadequate; choice of medication is guided more by marketing than evidence-based medicine; and long-term follow-up has too many accidental escapees.

Although more research is necessary into hypertension in elderly patients, management could be greatly improved by applying the knowledge we already have. Undertreatment and overtreatment need to be replaced by appropriate treatment of patients likely to benefit from intervention. This chapter aims to cover all aspects of the management of hypertension in older patients, and to highlight areas where our practice needs to improve.

Epidemiology

The relationship between blood pressure and age has been assessed in many cross-sectional studies[1,2] but also in a small number of longitudinal studies, notably the Framingham study.[3] For example, in the Health Survey for England[2] systolic blood pressure increased with age in both men and women, whereas diastolic blood pressure increased until age 50 to 60 and then tended to plateau in both sexes but with a suggestion of a fall in very elderly men. Although the average blood pressure values differ between populations (developed and developing) the trend with age is similar.[4]

How prevalent is hypertension in elderly people? The figure obtained depends partly on the definition or cutoff point for hypertension, but also on how many measurements are made and the procedure for measuring blood pressure. The most widely accepted pressures are a systolic above 160 mmHg or a diastolic over 95 mmHg. Most studies use only a single measurement or two or three measurements at a single visit. This will give a higher prevalence than multiple measurements over a series of visits but the latter is usually impractical in a large scale epidemiologic study. The influence of who measures blood pressure, and how it is measured, on the figure obtained is discussed in the section on blood pressure measurement.

In the Health Survey for England, systolic blood pressure over 160 mmHg was observed in 35 percent of men and 37 percent of women aged 65 to 74, increasing to 41 percent of men and 49 percent of women aged 75 and above. Overall, 50 percent of the population aged 65 to 74 was classified as having high blood pressure, comprising 13 percent treated hypertensives, 12 percent treated but still with elevated blood pressure, and 26 percent untreated high blood pressure. In the older age group (over age 75) the figures were higher, with 56 percent of men and 70 percent of women labelled as having high blood pressure.

Clearly, this is an overestimate of sustained hypertension, but the results emphasize the need to take great care in making an accurate diagnosis before starting treatment. The actual level of sustained hypertension over several measurements is about one-third of that for casual recordings.[5,6] This large difference is accounted for by several factors, including increased variability of blood pressure in old age,[7] "white coat" hypertension, and regression to the mean. Care also needs to be taken with the timing of measurement, as postprandial falls in blood pressure are well documented. Seasonal variation is important, with higher pressures in winter.[8]

Isolated systolic hypertension (ISH) is almost entirely a disorder of elderly people with a prevalence of only 0.8 percent at age 50 compared with 12.6 percent at 70 and 23.6 percent at 80 years,[9] although again these figures are based on casual recordings. ISH is more common in women and tends to be more difficult to treat, although in the past there has been a tendency to concentrate on treating diastolic pressure.

Several "environmental" factors affect blood pressure and may differ in elderly people. The relationship between sodium intake and blood pressure is well known. There is an increased effect in older patients at least up to the age of 60 to 69 years. An increase in sodium of 100 mmol/day is associated with a 10- to 15-mmHg rise in systolic pressure compared with a 4- to 5-mmHg rise in younger adults.[10] Obesity results in an increased blood pressure with a 10-kg difference in body weight, giving a 3-mmHg difference in blood pressure.[11] This appears to continue in old age, and significant obesity in older people is not uncommon.

Physical exercise is known to reduce blood pressure but many older people are unable to exercise on a regular basis. Excessive alcohol elevates blood pressure, although consumption tends to fall in older age. With these and other factors it is not clear how much is due to tracking of blood pressure due to exposure in earlier life, and how much is because of an enhanced effect in older people.

Target Blood Pressure

Although an arbitrary definition of hypertension, such as blood pressure greater than 160/95 mmHg, is used, there is no sharp cutoff in cardiovascular risk between normotension and hypertension. Both stroke and coronary heart disease show a continuous relationship between diastolic blood pressure in the range 70 to 110 mmHg and the risk of a cardiovascular event.[12] In population terms, the majority might benefit from a reduction in blood pressure. For individual patients, a decision to treat, especially drug treatment, depends on the degree of risk from the level of blood pressure set against the expected benefit and adverse effects of treatment. Much of the available data come from middle-aged and young elderly people. In the very elderly (over 85 years) some studies have shown that survival is improved with high blood pressure, although overall the evidence is conflicting.

When dealing with an individual patient, the blood pressure level should not be considered in isolation. The patient's overall risk of a cardiovascular event should be assessed, taking other known risk factors into consideration—smoking, excessive alcohol, diabetes mellitus, obesity, cholesterol concentration, and age—as well as the blood presure. Treatment of hypertension is more likely to produce a worthwhile level of benefit in higher risk patients, that is, patients with multiple risk factors or very high blood pressure. Elderly patients are a high risk group and blood pressure above 160/100 mmHg is worth treating even in the absence of other risk factors. A decision needs to be made as to the size of risk that is worth treating, and this is related to the number of patient years of treatment necessary to prevent one cardiovascular event. For comparison, 850 patients were required to be treated for 1 year to prevent one event in younger adults with mild hypertension,[13] but only about 30 patient years of treatment are necessary for the same benefit in elderly people.[14,15] Some bodies are now advocating clearer guidelines as to when treatment should be started; for example, the National Advisory Committee on Core Health and Disability Support Services in New Zealand has suggested a 20 percent chance of a major event in the next 10 years.[16]

The optimum target blood pressure on treatment remains to be established. There has been considerable debate about the existence of a "J"- or "U"-shaped curve with higher death rates in patients with lower blood pressures. Some studies have shown such a relationship initially, but this has disappeared when corrected for concurrent illness.

Pathogenesis

Hypertension in most elderly patients is primary, or "essential." Secondary hypertension is responsible for less than 10 percent of cases, although the exact figure is uncertain. Treatable underlying causes are very rare.

Blood pressure depends on peripheral resistance and cardiac output. In hypertension it is clear that the problem is one of increased peripheral resistance.[17] The vessels that make the major contribution to peripheral resistance are at the arteriolar level. The primary underlying cause of the increased peripheral resistance is uncertain, although several factors have been suggested. Research in this area is difficult. Many experimental models involve relatively acute rises in blood pressure rather than the more usual clinical scenario of development over months or years.

It has been suggested that the chronic increase in peripheral resistance in patients with hypertension occurs through structural narrowing of resistance vessels.[18] This concept explains why it takes a long time for these structural changes to be reversed and permit blood pressure to fall to acceptable values in patients with long-standing hypertension. Any attempt to establish the cause of hypertension must look at the mechanisms responsible for these structural changes.

Detailed consideration of the responsible factors is beyond the scope of this book. In brief, genetic influences are polygenic; renal factors such as the renin-angiotensin system are undoubtedly of considerable importance; local endothelial factors such as endothelin probably play a role; and central autonomic factors are also important. Individual substances implicated include nitric oxide, acetylcholine, kinins, atrial natriuretic peptide, and catecholamines.

More specifically in elderly patients, the loss of elastic tissue function results in a loss in arterial compliance, higher systolic pressures, and left ventricular hypertrophy. Renal function as measured by creatinine clearance declines with age, but it is uncertain whether or not this is responsible for more hypertension in elderly patients.

At a different level, but one at which we can have an effect, are environmental factors known to raise blood pressure. Blood pressure tends to respond fairly quickly to changes in these lifestyle influences. The effect of salt has been extensively debated, and it now seems clear that salt has a major influence on blood pressure. Since about 75 percent of our salt intake is in processed foods, there is clear scope for intervention at government level. Action can also be taken against excessive alcohol consumption and obesity, although both of these tend to be resistant to change.

Secondary hypertension is most often due to renal or renovascular problems. Renal failure is a well-known cause of hypertension, although the degree of impairment necessary to result in a rise in blood pressure is variable. Renal artery stenosis is relatively common in older adults along with other vascular disease. It should be seriously considered where there is worsening control of blood pressure after a period of stability. Endocrine causes are rare.

Complications of hypertension

Cardiac
- Myocardial infarction
- Angina
- Cardiac failure
- Left ventricular hypertrophy

Stroke
- Ischemic
- Hemorrhagic

Renal failure

Accelerated/malignant hypertension

Hypertensive encephalopathy

Complications

Hypertension is best considered not as a disease but as a risk factor for the complications it causes. This is important for two reasons when it comes to choosing treatment. Firstly, we have as yet no drugs that cure the problem by acting on the primary cause. Secondly, it needs to be remembered that we are not lowering the blood pressure for its own sake but to reduce the risk of complications. Cardiovascular mortality has been shown in the Framingham study to be about three times as high in hypertensive elderly people compared with those with normal blood pressure. The complications of untreated hypertension are shown in the accompanying boxed list.

The most important complications are cardiac disease and stroke. Cardiac disease is the most frequent problem in terms of absolute numbers, but the relative risk of stroke is greater when compared to the normotensive population.

Both cardiac disease (Chs. 22 and 23) and stroke are covered in detail elsewhere (Ch. 34). The high level of cardiac morbidity and mortality in patients with hypertension is due to two mechanisms. Firstly, there is accelerated development of atheroma of the coronary arteries, resulting in ischemic heart disease. Secondly, left ventricular hypertrophy occurs due to the increase in left ventricular workload. Left ventricular hypertrophy is related to the severity and duration of the hypertension and serves as a prognostic marker. These two factors may work together, such that the left ventricular hypertrophy makes the myocardium more susceptible to ischemic injury in association with coronary atheroma. Left ventricular oxygen consumption per unit weight is increased.

Both thromboembolic and hemorrhagic strokes are more common in hypertensive patients. Renal disease is a less common problem with adequate treatment of blood pressure, and it is often difficult to determine whether the hypertension is due to or the cause of the renal impairment. Accelerated phase or malignant hypertension is much less common now. The classification of retinal changes in terms of their prognostic value requires revision, and a scheme for this has been published recently.[19]

Measuring Blood Pressure

Blood pressure measurement is one of the most frequent observations made on patients both in hospital and general practice. Reliable performance of this technique should be second nature to all doctors and nurses. Regrettably, however, the evidence is that blood pressure measurement is far from satisfactory. Accurate measurement of blood pressure requires reliable, well-maintained equipment, a properly trained observer, and a knowledge of factors known to affect the blood pressure. There are problems in all of these areas.

Equipment

The gold standard for routine blood pressure measurement is a standard mercury column sphygmomanometer. Surveys have shown that a significant proportion of sphygmomanometers have defects even in major hospitals. Common faults are perished rubber tubing, bad connections, sticking valves, and the mercury level not being at zero. These are easily spotted and avoidable with regular servicing. Electronic machines also develop faults and require regular servicing. Faults are less likely to be noticed by the user than with the mercury column sphygmomanometer.

Whichever type of machine is used, it is important to use a suitable sized cuff. The standard bladder size is 23 × 12 cm. This is too small for many arms, and it has been recommended that the larger 35 × 12 cm cuff is more suitable for most patients, though debate continues. The optimum cuff size for older patients has not been adequately evaluated. The average arm circumference is less in older patients and thus, overcuffing may be a significant problem. In one study in older adults it has been shown that there is little difference in measured blood pressure with different cuff sizes (23 × 12, 30 × 13, 35 × 15), providing that the center of the cuff is carefully placed over the brachial artery.[20] In a small number of patients, however, there were larger and clinically more important discrepancies between cuff sizes. The standard 23 × 12 cm cuff is suitable for most elderly patients, but a larger cuff should be used for larger arms.

Trained Observer

Good technique in blood pressure measurement needs to be taught from the start, yet many medical schools devote little time to it. In the United Kingdom, experience and published data on doctors in training suggest that many are unaware how to measure blood pressure according to British Hypertension Society guidelines. Common errors are failure to check the sphygmomanometer before use; too rapid deflation rate; reinflation without full deflation to check an uncertain value; use of a too short cuff in patients with obese arms; and digit preference (most often to the nearest 10 mmHg).

Observers should be trained to measure blood pressure ac-

British Hypertension Society Guidelines for Blood Pressure Measurement

Patient seated

Conventional mercury column sphygmomanometer with cuff bladder size appropriate for patient arm circumference

Diastolic reading—phase 5—disappearance of sound

Record to nearest 2 mmHg

At least two blood pressure measurements at each visit

At least four visits to establish sustained hypertension (over 3 to 6 months in mild cases; shorter time if severe hypertension or end-organ damage)

Standing blood pressure measurement if orthostatic hypotension is likely (e.g., elderly)

cording to national guidelines, for example as shown in the boxed list for the United Kingdom.

Factors Affecting Blood Pressure

It is important to measure blood pressure in an environment as stress free as possible. A relaxed clinic atmosphere with a friendly staff and a firm commitment to run to time are important. This is easier to provide in a session dedicated to hypertension than in a general clinic where other matters take priority. It is essential that the patient is allowed time to settle before the measurement is made—at least 3 minutes for sitting or lying and 1 minute for standing recordings. Arm position is important, with a requirement for the cuff to be at heart level with the arm gently supported. Excessive talking to the patient also raises blood pressure and any discussion should be kept until after the pressure has been measured. In elderly patients, it is best to avoid measuring blood pressure too soon after meals, as postprandial hypotension is not uncommon. Blood pressure lability (especially systolic) is greater in elderly adults, more so in females.

Determining Whether Hypertension Is Sustained

A single raised blood pressure reading does not necessarily mean sustained hypertension and does not require immediate treatment. All national guidelines suggest that at least three blood pressure measurements should be made over a period of time. If the initial blood pressure is very high, measurements should be made over weekly intervals (unless there is evidence of accelerated phase hypertension or a clinical picture that requires more urgent action). For mild elevations in blood pressure the recordings should be spread over 3 to 6 months. Overtreatment is common. Local audit has shown a high percentage of elderly patients are started on treatment without adequate evidence of need. Even in the large, multicenter trials, 20 to 50 percent of patients in the placebo arm had normal blood pressure throughout the study. Also, trials of stopping treatment (by patient or doctor) show that about one-half remain normotensive off treatment. It is essential to establish that hypertension is sustained before starting treatment so that resources are aimed at those most likely to benefit. We do not know whether patients with a high initial blood pressure but who subsequently remain normotensive have a cardiovascular event risk similar to the rest of the population. If this group is at increased risk, then the level of risk is likely to be lower than for sustained hypertension, and any benefit of treatment may be too small to be worthwhile.

Waiting 6 months to see if the hypertension is sustained may be wasting valuable time in elderly patients. Ambulatory blood pressure recording allows most patients with "white coat" hypertension to be detected and is a more accurate reflection of the patient's blood pressure load. Ambulatory blood pressure has been shown to correlate better than clinic measurements with left ventricular hypertrophy. As yet there are no published data looking at ambulatory blood pressure recording and cardiovascular event rates, but such studies (e.g., SYSTEUR, Systolic Hypertension in the Elderly in Europe) are ongoing. Elderly patients have potentially much to gain from an early diagnosis of sustained hypertension, and further studies with ambulatory blood pressure measurement in this age group are required.

Clinical Features

Uncomplicated hypertension is not in itself associated with symptoms. Raised blood pressure is often an incidental finding when the patient presents with other illness or undergoes routine screening (as in those over 75 in the United Kingdom). Headache is not a specific feature of hypertension but any pain will increase blood pressure. Inquiry should be made as to the symptoms of possible complications of hypertension, such as chest pain due to myocardial infarction or angina; breathlessness due to cardiac failure; limb weakness or dysphasia due to stroke. The clinical signs of these complications should be sought.

Clinical assessment also requires consideration of possible underlying causes though, apart from renal disease, these are rare (e.g., Cushing's disease, Conn syndrome, pheochromocytoma). Fundal examination is essential to exclude accelerated phase hypertension. More severe grades of retinopathy point to a poorer prognosis.

Full clinical assessment of past and present problems will detect existing complications and point to diseases that are relative contraindications to therapy with some antihypertensive agents. Examples are obstructive airway disease and β-blockers; gout or diabetes mellitus and diuretics; peripheral vascular disease, renal artery stenosis, and angiotensin-converting enzyme (ACE) inhibitors. In the past, peripheral vascular disease has been seen as a contraindication to β-blockers but this has been questioned.[21] A social and drug history will note past or present smoking, alcohol intake, and drugs likely to raise blood pressure (e.g., steroids) or interfere with treatment (e.g., NSAIDs, nonsteroidal anti-inflammatory drugs).

Investigation

Fashions change, and fortunately, the era of intravenous urography for everyone has disappeared. Investigations are required for three reasons—to identify an underlying cause, to look for evidence of end-organ damage, and to detect risk factors for cardiovascular disease or drug therapy.

Underlying Cause

Measurement of plasma urea and creatinine and urinalysis for protein are of value, as renal disease is the only common underlying cause. Plasma electrolytes are done as a routine with urea, and low potassium suggests the possibility of Conn syndrome. Other investigations should be considered only if there are specific clinical indications.

End-Organ Damage

A standard 12-lead electrocardiogram (ECG) should be performed on all patients, though it is not the best measure of left ventricular hypertrophy. Echocardiography would be better, but it is not a feasible investigation for all patients in most centers and should be reserved for those in whom there are clear additional indications such as cardiac failure or doubt as to whether treatment should be initiated. Chest x-ray is worthwhile if there are signs or symptoms of cardiac failure or chest disease, but it is not a useful guide to the presence of left ventricular hypertrophy.

Risk Factors

Serum lipid profile should be considered, although there is debate as to which elderly patients should be treated. Blood glucose should be measured to exclude diabetes mellitus. It is a safe policy to check a full blood count, liver function tests, and urate before drugs are given.

Other tests need to be considered if clinically indicated. Common requirements are thyroid function tests and serum calcium. If the patient has peripheral or general vascular disease then renal artery stenosis should be considered before starting an ACE inhibitor. Renal ultrasound will show a difference in renal size and isotope renogram (+/− captopril) is a relatively noninvasive method of looking at renal blood flow. If these tests are suggestive, patients require renal artery angiography. Detailed endocrine assessment for Cushing's, Conn's, or acromegaly is occasionally necessary.

General measures in the management of hypertension

Blood pressure reduction
- reduced salt intake
- increased potassium intake
- weight reduction
- reduce alcohol intake
- exercise

Reduce other risk factors
- stop smoking
- reduce saturated fat intake
- weight reduction
- optimize alcohol intake
- exercise

Management

As with any disorder, it is worth thinking of the following four general steps: (1) establish diagnosis, as discussed above (2) remove underlying cause (rarely possible, as already noted) (3) general measures and (4) specific drug treatment.

General Measures

General nondrug treatments should be thought of in two parts—measures to reduce blood pressure and measures to reduce other cardiovascular risk factors.

Blood pressure reduction

Salt The influence of salt on blood pressure and the value of reducing salt intake in lowering blood pressure have been debated fiercely. Many interpopulation studies have shown a relationship between sodium intake and blood pressure. However, the relationship has been less clear cut within population studies. In the Intersalt studies[22] there was a positive correlation between salt intake and blood pressure in most populations, and when the regression coefficients were combined this was highly significant, though weak. Of added interest for geriatricians was the observation that the increase in blood pressure with age was accentuated in those populations with a high sodium intake. There is also evidence from intervention studies to show that increasing salt intake in hypertensive patients on a low salt diet does raise blood pressure. An overview of such trials confirmed the value of reducing salt in lowering blood pressure and showed that older patients were more responsive to the effects of salt restriction.[23] This has been confirmed in more recent studies such as one which found a fall of 8/0 mmHg in clinic pressures and 3/1 mmHg in 24-hour ambulatory blood pressure with an 80 mmol/24-hour reduction in sodium intake in elderly patients (mean age 73 years).[24] The enhanced effect of sodium restriction in elderly patients is to be expected because they tend to have low renin, volume-dependent hypertension.

There are thus clear benefits from reducing salt intake for overall population blood pressure and thus, population risk of stroke. For individual patients in routine practice, however, there are difficulties. Firstly, about 75 percent of our sodium intake is due to the presence of salt in processed foods. Major dietary changes may therefore be necessary to achieve a significant salt reduction. Reduction of blood pressure in most patients will be small compared to the effects of drug treatment. In patients with a high salt intake due to addition of excessive salt in cooking and at table, there is more to be gained because of the potential for a greater reduction in intake. It is at least worth persuading patients to add no salt at table, little during cooking, and to consider use of reduced sodium "salts" that replace about 70 percent of the sodium with potassium (if renal function is satisfactory). If patients also consume much salt laden processed foods, then a more drastic change in diet should be considered—but is very difficult in practice.

In summary, major success can be achieved in a few patients with very high salt intake who can be persuaded to change their habits. For most patients, the effect on blood pressure will be small but could be worthwhile as part of an overall management package.

Potassium There is a weak negative correlation between potassium intake and blood pressure. Randomized trials have shown a significant fall in blood pressure with a roughly twofold increase in potassium intake, though results have been variable. As with sodium, there is a relationship between the size of the blood pressure reduction and the starting blood pressure.[25] Sodium-restricted patients fail to respond to increasing potassium,[26] and it has been suggested that these interventions work via a common final pathway. In a group of elderly patients (mean age 75) with high initial blood pressure (181/97 mmHg), potassium supplements of 60 mmol/day resulted in a 10/6 mmHg fall in clinic blood pressure and 5/2 mmHg fall in daytime ambulatory blood pressure.

These results support the use of replacing sodium with potassium in table salt as a general strategy. Care must be taken to avoid hyperkalemia in patients with impaired renal function.

Obesity There is a strong relationship between body weight and blood pressure, independent of possible confounding factors, in younger adults. However, in older adults, the effect of body weight on blood pressure may be less or even nonexistent. Blood pressure is more difficult to measure in obese arms and a suitable sized cuff must be used. The relationship between body weight and blood pressure has been shown to be independent of measurement artifact due to large arm circumference.

Weight loss in younger adults shows a clear fall in blood pressure of the order of 3/2 mmHg for each kilogram lost. An overview of eight intervention studies found that substantial weight loss results in a 15 percent reduction in blood pressure.[27] This effect is much greater and more consistent than other nonpharmacologic methods and is similar to the expected response from a single antihypertensive drug.

There are only limited data in elderly patients and a reluctance to encourage dieting because of a belief that elderly patients will find it impossible to lose weight. However, such pessimism may be unjustified. A comparison of doctor's advice, doctor's advice plus a written diet sheet, and referral to a dietician in obese hypertensive patients yielded favorable results[28] (see Ch. 63). Patients referred to the dietician fared best with a mean weight loss of 5.1 kg at 1 year. The other groups also achieved a useful reduction of 2.3 kg in that time. In terms of compliance with weight-reducing diets, older females achieved greater weight reductions than older males or younger adults of either sex.[29]

Although there is inadequate firm evidence in terms of blood pressure reduction in elderly patients, it seems reasonable to encourage weight loss, preferably with referral to a dietician. This may result in a fall in blood pressure, and other health benefits more than justify the effort.

Alcohol Recent evidence strongly supports the beneficial effects of regular intake of moderate amounts of alcohol in reducing cardiovascular risk. Initial studies supported the value of red wine, and interest concentrated on other factors, such as flavanoids, in the wine. Further research seems to suggest that most forms of alcoholic drinks are beneficial. However, regular consumption of excessive amounts of alcohol raises blood pressure. The gap between a beneficial amount and an adverse intake may be small. Two to three units of alcohol per day reduce risk, but subjects taking three or more drinks each day have significantly higher blood pressure than those drinking less.[30] The effect of age and gender on this relationship is unclear. One study found a stronger association between alcohol intake and blood pressure in older males[31] while another found a stronger relationship in younger adults and in females.[32]

Alcohol intake tends to decrease after retirement, perhaps due to reduced income and removal from the social aspects of employment. There is a problem in identifying excessive drinkers as most patients understate or underestimate their intake. It is also difficult to persuade patients to reduce their alcohol intake, especially the most at risk heavy drinkers. This does not appear to have been studied as a way of reducing blood pressure in elderly hypertensive patients. Excessive alcohol consumption should be suspected if there is an unexplained elevation in mean corpuscular volume or γ-glutamyl transpeptidase concentration or if the patient smells of alcohol when seen. General advice should be to restrict alcohol intake to 1 to 2 drinks per day rather than complete abstinence.

Exercise Regular exercise has been known to reduce blood pressure for many years, though not all studies have found a beneficial relationship. The effect of exercise on blood pressure is seen soon after starting training but also disappears in about 2 weeks if sedentary habits are resumed. Exercise has received less attention than other nonpharmacologic methods but again, most of the evidence comes from younger adults.

The prevalence of both systolic and diastolic hypertension in women up to the age of 89 years is lower in those who exercise compared to sedentary individuals.[33] The biggest difference in blood pressure (20 mmHg) occurred in those undertaking vigorous exercise. In another study, in 60- to 69-year-olds vigorous exercise reduced blood pressure and peripheral vascular resistance and increased cardiac output.[34]

The amount and type of exercise required to obtain optimum benefit is not clear. A common suggestion is for 20 minutes of vigorous (e.g., running) exercise or 40 minutes moderate (e.g., brisk walking) exercise three times per week. It is essential to give advice on exercise that is appropriate for the individual patient. Cycling and swimming are good forms of exercise but it is unreasonable (and probably dangerous) for a 75-year-old man to take to the roads if he has not cycled for 50 years. Lack of availability of swimming pools is a problem in many areas. An exercise bicycle is one option but may be too expensive for many patients, and such exercise tends to be boring unless attempted while watching a favourite soap opera. Regular brisk walking is cheap and convenient for most elderly patients and can be built into the daily routine. Exercise is beneficial for health in all elderly people, and specialized classes have been developed for residents of nursing homes and those unable to walk.[35]

Other risk factors

Smoking The excess risk of cardiovascular disease in smokers is well known and stopping smoking has been shown to reduce the risk of myocardial infarction.[36] Hypertensive patients who smoke are at greater risk of cardiovascular events than hypertensive nonsmokers, although most of the evidence is from younger adults. In the Medical Research Council (MRC) trial in younger adults, the reduction in stroke in the propranolol treated group was found only in nonsmokers.[13] Both smokers and nonsmokers benefitted from bendrofluazide. The relationship of outcome to smoking was not evaluated in the Systolic Hypertension in the Elderly Program (SHEP)[37] or Swedish Trial of Old Patients (STOP) with hypertension[14] trials. However, in the MRC study in elderly patients, the benefit in terms of stroke reduction was seen mainly in nonsmokers treated with diuretics.[38] Specific studies to evaluate the additional benefits of stopping smoking at the time of diagnosis on cardiovascular events in elderly hypertensive patients have not been done. A randomized trial would not be possible because of the clear overall health benefits from stopping smoking. Smoking is by far the most important preventable risk factor, and it is sensible to encourage cessation as part of the holistic approach to the management of hypertension.

Plasma lipids Lipid metabolism and atheroma is covered in more detail elsewhere (Ch. 20). Elevated plasma cholesterol is clearly a risk factor for cardiovascular disease. However, there has been considerable debate as to the value of treatment in terms of overall mortality and the level of cholesterol at which to intervene. In younger adults, reduction of cholesterol concentration by diet and drug therapy reduced the risk of ischemic heart disease but not overall mortality because of an increase in deaths due to trauma and suicide.[39] More recent studies have confirmed the clear benefits of reduction in ischemic heart disease and have shown a reduction in overall mortality. In the 4S study, simvastatin was used to treat postmyocardial infarction survivors aged 35 to 70 with a plasma cholesterol of greater than 5.4 mmol/L (208 mg/dl).[40] This required 16 patients to be treated for 5 years to prevent one major coronary event. There was no increase in noncoronary mortality. Further evidence comes from the West of Scotland study, which showed benefit from treating middle-aged men without coronary heart disease and a cholesterol greater than 6.4 mmol/L (247 mg/dl) using pravastatin.[41]

It is thus clear that in the patients included in these studies there is benefit from treating cholesterol concentrations over 5.4 if there is pre-existing coronary heart disease and 6.4 if not. However, patients over age 70 were not included and we do not have a clear answer to the problem of elevated cholesterol in elderly patients. In population terms it is reasonable to aim for a reduction in plasma cholesterol concentrations by dietary changes. When dealing with an individual elderly patient we need to consider all aspects of the patient's care. Aggressive management with major dietary changes and drug treatment is reasonable for very high cholesterol concentrations if the patient agrees. Less drastic dietary change is a reasonable target in all other patients, though the likely reduction in cholesterol will be small. Drug treatment for primary prevention in patients over the age of 70 with a cholesterol of 5.5 to 8.0 requires more evidence before it can be justified. Interestingly, recent guidelines from the American College of Physicians recommend a more selective approach to screening for cholesterol than has been usual for that country. They make no recommendation one way or the other for 65- to 75-year-olds. For those over 75 they suggest that routine screening is not required, since there is no evidence that high cholesterol is a risk factor for heart disease in this age group.[42]

When treating hypertension we are trying to alter several aspects of the patient's behavior, and it is important not to overburden the patient with too many changes at once. For most patients, it is reasonable to treat the other risk factors and only consider measuring cholesterol and treating elevated levels in selected individuals.

Obesity This is an independent risk factor for sudden cardiac death and coronary disease.[43] Weight reduction is justified for this reason, as well as the blood pressure-lowering effects discussed above.

Exercise Exercise may protect against stroke independently of the effect on blood pressure. Vigorous exercise in early adulthood, as well as recent vigorous exercise and regular walking, protects against stroke in later life.[44] Clearly, it is too late to influence our elderly patients' past lifestyle but we can encourage regular walking or other suitable exercise. Though the evidence of specific benefit in reducing stroke risk is not strong, the effect on blood pressure and general well-being justifies this approach.

Left ventricular hypertrophy (LVH) LVH is an independent risk factor for cardiovascular events. We hope that treating the blood pressure will cause this to regress. At present, specific treatment to achieve regression is not generally used. ACE inhibitors are more effective than thiazide diuretics at reversing LVH. Outcome studies using ACE inhibitors are awaited to see if this will be translated into more effective reduction in the risk of cardiovascular events.

Diabetes mellitus Diabetes should be treated in the usual way with diet, oral hypoglycemics, and insulin as necessary. Should this influence our choice of antihypertensive agent? Although higher doses of thiazide diuretics have an effect on blood sugar, this is rarely a problem at low doses such as 2.5 mg of bendrofluazide. This seems a reasonable first choice agent. However, ACE inhibitors have been shown to reduce albumin excretion and preserve renal function in diabetes and may be considered where diabetic nephropathy is suspected or if blood glucose is difficult to control.

Overview

Nonpharmacologic measures should not be thought of as replacing drug treatment, but as supporting and enhancing it. General measures are useful to improve the health of most patients but the individual drop in blood pressure is relatively small for most patients with sustained hypertension. Initial benefits may appear greater if measures are introduced at first presentation because of the tendency for higher blood pressures to decrease with time. Drug treatment alone reduces the risk of stroke by only 30 to 40 percent and heart disease by less. Greater benefits can be achieved only by tackling multiple risk factors where appropriate. The above discussions have centered on individual factors, though the reality is that all should be considered together. Such a strategy has not been formally studied in elderly patients. In middle-aged hypertensive patients, long-term studies have shown that it is feasible to implement and maintain an assault on multiple factors—in this case weight, salt, and alcohol reduction.[45,46] The interventions did lower blood pressure and had a treatment-sparing effect when compared to control groups not given this advice. This is considered further in comparison with drug treatment below.

Specific Drug Treatment

The main drug groups for treating hypertension are diuretics, β-blockers, ACE inhibitors, calcium channel blockers, α-blockers and others, such as methyldopa, hydralazine, and minoxidil.

Older, more toxic agents such as reserpine, adrenergic neurone blockers, and ganglion blockers are very rarely used now. Important features of the main drug groups are considered before looking at the proven benefits of treatment.

Diuretics

Diuretics include bendrofluazide, hydrochlorothiazide, chlorthalidone, and frusemide. Thiazide diuretics are first choice agents for treating hypertension in elderly patients. Loop diuretics such as frusemide have little long-term effect on blood pressure when used alone, but are valuable in combination with an ACE inhibitor. Thiazides have been available for over 30 years, but their exact mechanism of action remains uncertain. Although there is an initial response due to natriuresis, the long-term effect is to reduce peripheral vascular resistance.

Most thiazides are well absorbed from the gastrointestinal tract and elimination is by a combination of liver metabolism and renal excretion of unchanged drug. Plasma half-life varies from 3 hours for bendrofluazide to 90 hours for chlorthalidone. Despite this, all thiazides have a prolonged effect on blood pressure and can be given once daily. No specific data are available for older adults. As with many antihypertensive drugs, initial doses were high. It is now clear that low doses (e.g., bendrofluazide 2.5 mg) are as effective as higher doses in controlling blood pressure and have been used in the later stages in some outcome studies. Even lower doses (1.25 mg bendrofluazide) have a similar effect on blood pressure without metabolic adverse effects, but are not available for routine use. There are few absolute contraindications to thiazide use, which are best avoided if there is pre-existing hyponatremia, hypokalemia, or hyperuricemia. Higher doses should be avoided in patients with diabetes. Thiazides are not effective in patients with renal failure when the glomerular filtration rate falls below 30 ml/hour.

Serious adverse effects are rare with low doses. A small fall in plasma potassium occurs but rarely requires intervention. Routine coprescription of a potassium-sparing agent is not necessary. In a few patients there is a more significant degree of hypokalemia or hyponatremia, which requires attention. Gout may be precipitated but is rare with the low doses now used. Idiosyncratic reactions such as skin rashes, acute pancreatitis and blood dyscrasias also occur rarely. Higher doses cause impotence but it is unclear whether this occurs with low dose treatment.

β-Blockers

β-Blockers include atenolol, bisoprolol, and propranolol. Like the thiazides, β-blockers have been used for many years and remain one of the main drug groups in younger adults. They are effective in elderly patients, but widespread use is limited by more frequent contraindications in the elderly. The exact mechanism of action is uncertain but seems to be more than just antagonism at the peripheral β-receptor.

There are marked differences in the kinetics of different drugs. Lipid soluble agents such as propranolol are well absorbed after oral administration but undergo extensive presystemic metabolism such that bioavailability is low and variable. Propranolol has an elimination half-life of about 6 hours, and there is reduced clearance in elderly patients. Water soluble drugs such as atenolol are poorly absorbed and excreted predominantly unchanged by the kidney. The half-life is longer than for propranolol and it is suitable for once daily dosing without formulation in a slow release preparation. Atenolol clearance declines in proportion to the reduced renal function in elderly people.

Dose should be kept as low as possible. In most elderly patients the starting dose of atenolol should be 25 mg once daily with an increase to 50 mg if necessary. Although an occasional older patient may require 100 mg, there is no benefit in exceeding this dose. Doses of lipid soluble drugs are more variable but again, low doses should be used to begin treatment.

As already noted, the main problem with this group of drugs in elderly patients is the presence of contraindications such as cardiac failure, asthma/obstructive airways disease, cardiac conduction defects, and severe peripheral vascular disease. Care also needs to be taken in patients with diabetes mellitus.

Adverse effects are more common than with thiazides and are mainly those expected from antagonism of the β-receptor in different tissues. All of these drugs may precipitate asthma, which may be fatal. Selective drugs such as atenolol are less likely to do so but are not completely safe. All may precipitate heart failure—often in a patient with pre-existing cardiac dilatation. General weakness and tired legs are common, though many patients adapt to these with time. Cold extremities are a particular problem in winter. Central side effects such as depression, sleep disturbance, and nightmares are more common with the lipid soluble drugs, which readily cross the blood-brain barrier. Sudden withdrawal is best avoided, especially in patients with underlying coronary artery disease. This may result in angina and progress to myocardial infarction in some patients.

ACE inhibitors

ACE-inhibitors include captopril, enalapril, and lisinopril. Although these drugs were initially introduced for patients with refractory or renovascular hypertension, they now have a licence for treating all grades of hypertension. Unfortunately, there is as yet no evidence that they reduce cardiovascular events when used to treat hypertension, although studies are ongoing. On the positive side, several drugs have been shown to be of benefit in reducing morbidity and mortality in patients with cardiac failure and after myocardial infarction. It is thus difficult to justify these drugs as first-line agents in elderly hypertensive patients, but they are a reasonable choice in the many patients who also have cardiac failure—in which case combination with a thiazide may be appropriate.

As the name implies, ACE inhibitors are competitive inhibitors of ACE and thus reduce the conversion of angiotensin I to angiotensin II. This results in a fall in the level of the pressor hormone, angiotensin II, and a resultant reduction in aldosterone secretion. Blood pressure is thus lowered by a fall in peripheral resistance. ACE inhibitors are effective in the pressence of both high and low renin levels.

The ACE inhibitors are generally well absorbed after oral administration, but most are given as the prodrug (e.g., enalapril), which requires de-esterification in the liver to release the active moiety (enalaprilat). Elimination is mainly by renal excretion of the unchanged drug with a small amount of hepatic metabolism. Fosinopril has balanced 50:50 hepatic:renal elimination, which is claimed to be safer in elderly patients who have a degree of renal impairment. It is debatable whether this property is of any real clinical advantage. Plasma half-life varies from around 8 hours for captopril to 30 hours for lisinopril and 110 hours for ramipril. Most can be given once daily for control of blood pressure, but captopril must be given two to three times daily, and there is debate as to whether enalapril has a true 24-hour effect when smaller doses are used.

There is a wide dose range, though clearly the lowest effective dose should be used. There are no robust data in elderly patients as to the equipotent doses of the different agents in this group.

ACE inhibitors should be avoided in patients with known hypersensitivity and used with extra caution in collagen vascular disorders. However, the most common contraindication to their use is renal impairment and renovascular disease. It is difficult to give a clear cutoff as to the safe level of renal function at which to prescribe these drugs. Cautious use with regular monitoring of renal function is required. Severe deterioration may occur in patients with renal artery stenosis. This is a particular problem in elderly patients, as many have atheromatous disease affecting the aorta and renal arteries. There is a greater risk if patients are known to have other evidence of vascular problems such as peripheral vascular or coronary artery disease. It is impractical to test all elderly patients for renal artery stenosis. However, it is essential to monitor the serum creatinine on a regular basis and stop treatment if there is a significant rise while the condition is reversible. Such changes may occur early in the course of treatment or be delayed for months or years.

The most frequent adverse reaction is cough, which occurs in up to 15 percent of patients and may necessitate drug withdrawal. This is a class effect and rarely benefits from a change to another ACE inhibitor. First dose hypotension may occur, particularly in patients who are volume depleted due to diuretic therapy. It is sensible to withhold diuretics for 24 hours before the first dose is given. Renal failure is not infrequent, as discussed above.

Calcium channel blockers

Calcium channel blockers include amlodipine, nifedipine, and verapamil. There are three categories of calcium channel antagonist—dihydropyridines (e.g., nifedipine, amlodipine), phenylalkylamines (e.g., verapamil), and benzothiazepines (e.g., diltiazem). All can be used to treat hypertension but differ in their other properties. Like the ACE inhibitors, there is as yet no evidence that they reduce the risk of cardiovascular events in mild-moderate hypertension. There has been a suggestion that shorter-acting dihydropyridines like nifedipine actually increase the total mortality. This has been fiercely debated but definitive outcome study results are required. At present, these drugs should be third-line treatment when other agents have failed or are contraindicated.

There are marked kinetic differences between the drugs. Nifedipine is well absorbed at a rapid rate after oral administration but like propranolol, undergoes extensive first-pass metabolism. Elimination is by hepatic metabolism with a half-life of about 4 hours. Amlodipine, on the other hand, is more slowly absorbed and without significant first-pass metabolism. Plasma half-life is about 30 hours. The difference in kinetics between these drugs may explain the difference in vascular side effects. Nifedipine has a high incidence of headache and flushing, and slower release forms have been developed to try to reduce these effects. Although in different categories, verapamil and diltiazem resemble nifedipine in their pharmacokinetic properties.

The dose of nifedipine is variable because of the extensive first pass metabolism and variation in bioavailability. Amlodipine, in contrast, has a relatively narrow dose range. As always, the lowest effective dose should be used.

The most important relative contraindication is cardiac failure. Diltiazem and verapamil should be avoided in second- and third-degree heart block and in sick sinus syndrome. All these agents are best avoided in patients with aortic stenosis, as severe hypotension may occur due to a rapid reduction in peripheral resistance.

Side effects are particularly common with the dihydropyridines. Vasodilator effects such as headache, flushing, and reflex tachycardia have resulted in about one-third of patients stopping treatment in some series. With longer term administration, leg edema becomes a problem, especially in females. The edema is due to local vascular effects rather than fluid retention or heart failure. Although vasodilator side effects are less of a problem with diltiazem and verapamil, constipation can be a limitation to their use in elderly patients. A recent study has found an almost twofold increase in risk of gastrointestinal hemorrhage with these drugs.[47]

α-Blockers

α-Blockers include doxazosin, prazosin, and indoramin. Problems with early drugs in this group have resulted in few centers using them other than as second- or third-line agents. There is evidence of a beneficial effect on the lipid profile, but as with other newer drugs, there are no published outcome trials to show whether or not this results in real clinical benefit.

All these drugs are well absorbed. Prazosin undergoes extensive first-pass metabolism in the gut and liver, but this does not occur to a significant extent with doxazosin. All are metabolized in the liver. Plasma elimination half-life is short at 3 hours for prazosin and longer at 22 hours for doxazosin.

The biggest problem with prazosin is first-dose hypotension. This tends to occur when patients have forgotten to take their medication then restart. Orthostatic hypotension occurs even with regular dosing. Such problems are particularly serious in elderly patients. Urinary incontinence may occur, though the bladder effects are beneficial in patients with prostatism. Intolerance is more common than with most other antihypertensive agents.

Others

Methyldopa is used rarely now because of its tendency to cause tiredness and depression. However, much of the problem was due to excessive dosing and it still has a place when other agents fail. Initial dose should be low at 125 mg twice daily and not increased above a total of 750 mg daily.

Hydralazine use declined as newer drugs became available and because of concern over problems with drug-induced lupus. To obtain maximum benefit from it in long-term use, patients should be on a *β*-blocker. The place for hydralazine in elderly patients is thus limited.

Minoxidil is a potent vasodilator but requires to be given in combination with a diuretic and a *β*-blocker to counteract its tendency to cause edema and reflex tachycardia. It is thus rarely used in elderly patients.

Nonpharmacologic Versus Drug Therapy

In reality, we normally adopt both approaches at the same time, but do need to consider the relative merits of the two approaches for patients who wish to discuss the possibility of avoiding drugs. There are two main studies that have looked at this, but not specifically in older adults.

One study[45] compared obese men aged 40 to 69 years with previously untreated hypertension and randomized to diet (weight reducing, sodium restricted, reduced alcohol) or drugs (stepped care, atenolol first) for 1 year.

Weight was reduced by 7.8 kg in the diet group, but increased by 1.0 kg in the drug group. Sodium excretion fell by 42 mmol/day on diet and by 10 mmol/day on drug treatment. There was no difference in alcohol intake or potassium excretion.

Blood pressure was 7/6 mmHg higher in the diet compared to the drug-treated group. Diastolic blood pressure was below 90 mmHg in 73 percent of the drug-treated group but only 29 percent of the diet-treated group. Lipid profile was more favorable in the diet group.

In the second study,[46] less severe hypertensive patients were randomized to three groups: (1) stop drugs and reduce weight, salt and alcohol (2) stop drugs but no nutrition program and (3) continue drugs with no nutrition program. Patients of both sexes with a mean age of 56 were followed for 4 years.

Weight was reduced by 1.8 kg in the nutrition group but increased by 2 kg in the other groups. Sodium excretion was reduced by 60 mmol/day in the nutrition group but increased by 20 mmol/day in group 2.

Of those given dietary treatment, 39 percent remained normotensive and off treatment, compared with only 5 percent in group 2. Blood pressure was 11/5 mmHg higher in the group randomized to dietary advice whether or not they had to restart drug treatment. The diet group who stayed off drug treatment had lower serum cholesterol and fasting glucose concentrations.

Patients avoiding drug treatment had higher blood pressure and, overall, there is a clear advantage for drug treatment. Nonpharmacologic measures should therefore be used to sup-

Table 24-1 Summary of main outcome studies of drug treatment for hypertension in older adults

	C & W[50]	EWPHE[15]	STOP[14]	MRC[38]	SHEP[37]
No. of patients	884	840	1627	4396	4736
Age	60–79	60–97	70–84	65–74	>60
BP entry					
systolic	>170	160–239	180–230	160–209	160–219
diastolic	>105	90–119	90–120	<115	<90
BP obtained					
active	162/78	149/85	167/87	152/79	144/68
placebo	180/89	172/94	186/96	167/85	155/71
Events (% reduction in event rates)					
Nonfatal					
stroke	27	35	38[a]	30	37[a]
all cardiac	26	9	—	13	40[a]
all CVS	26	36[a]	—	25[a]	36[a]
Fatal					
stroke	70[a]	32	73[a]	12	29
all cardiac	+1	38[a]	25	22	20
all CVS	22	27[a]	43[a]	9	20
All events					
stroke	42[a]	36[a]	47[a]	25[a]	36[a]
all cardiac	15	20	13	19	27[a]
all CVS	23[a]	34[a]	40[a]	17[a]	32[a]

Abbreviations: C & W, Coope and Warrender; EWPHE, European working party on high blood pressure in the elderly; STOP, Swedish trial in old patients with hypertension; MRC, Medical Research Council; SHEP, Systolic hypertension in the elderly program; BP, blood pressure; CVS, cardiovascular.
[a] $P < 0.05$.

plement the benefits of drug treatment and not replace or postpone it, unless the patient has strong views about avoiding drugs.

Benefits of Treatment

Benefits of treating hypertension must be assessed in terms of reduction in the risk of the major complications—cardiovascular and cerebrovascular disease. These conditions are common and the incidence varies depending on the presence of risk factors in a population. Large multicenter trials are necessary to show whether or not there is benefit from treating hypertension. Since such trials are very expensive, it is not surprising that there are no published outcome studies using nondrug treatments, and manufacturers of newer agents have been slow to finance evaluation of their products. The risk of both stroke and heart disease is greater for elderly than for younger patients with the same level of blood pressure. Although bad for the individual, this has the advantage that a study to evaluate the treatment of hypertension in elderly patients requires fewer patients and can be carried out more quickly and at lower cost than a study with the same power in younger adults. Details of the five main studies that have included patients over 70 years of age are shown in Table 24-1.

Most of the studies had an upper age limit of 84 or less. The two studies with no upper age limit recruited few patients above the age of 80. There are thus few data on the benefits or otherwise of treating hypertension in the very elderly population. Drugs used were various thiazide diuretics alone or in combination with a potassium-sparing agent and β-blockers (mainly atenolol). The EWPHE study used methyldopa as add on therapy if diuretics were insufficient. Mean diastolic blood pressure at entry was around 100 mmHg except for the MRC study (91 mmHg) and SHEP, which excluded patients with a diastolic greater than 90. Systolic pressures were higher in the studies of mixed hypertension than in SHEP, which was confined to patients with isolated systolic hypertension. All studies showed a fall in the placebo group compared to entry blood pressure after placebo run-in; indeed, the mean placebo blood pressures were not "hypertensive" in several of the studies. However, there was a significant drug effect in all of the studies. These figures emphasize how the significant drug effects observed are occurring in a mildly hypertensive population.

There is clear evidence of benefit from thiazide diuretic-based treatment in the reduction of stroke (nonfatal and fatal) and all cardiovascular events. The size of the reduction ranged from 25 to 47 percent in all strokes and 17 to 40 percent for all cardiovascular events. Overall, the reduction in stroke is about one-third, but the biggest benefit was seen in the study with the highest entry blood pressure and highest blood pressure on placebo (STOP-hypertension). This population was at greater risk and thus had more potential for benefit. In most of the studies, the reduction in cardiac risk did not reach statistical significance. There is an overall pattern of benefit, though less than for stroke, at about 25 percent. Where there were sufficient numbers of patients to compare thiazide with β-blockers, the benefits were almost entirely due to the thiazide diuretics.

The drugs were well tolerated by most patients, with thiazides again being better than β-blockers. The low doses of thiazide used in some of the studies confirmed the safety of this treatment. The side effects reported in the trials were those expected. Thiazides caused problems such as muscle cramps, nausea, gout, and skin rashes. The risk of significant hypokalemia was small and in SHEP, the mean serum potassium fell from 4.4 to 4.1 mmol/L on thiazide alone. The reported incidence of impotence was also low at 4.8 percent compared with 3.2 percent on placebo. β-blocker effects were also those expected such as cold hands, breathlessness, and lethargy.

The figures quoted above are for reduction in stroke risk, but percentage figures may be misleading. It is better to think in terms of absolute risk when deciding if treatment is worthwhile. In the MRC study in younger adults (as noted above), it was necessary to treat 850 patients for 1 year to prevent one stroke.[13] The higher risk of a cardiovascular event in elderly adults means that the benefits of effective treatment are greater. For example, in the STOP-hypertension trial, only 70 patient years of treatment were required to prevent one stroke and one death[14]; in SHEP, 165 patient years were required to prevent one cardiovascular event[37]; and in the MRC study in older adults, overall about 150 patient years prevented one cardiovascular event, but only 60 patient years were necessary in the higher risk patients.[38]

Treatment Based on Overall Cardiovascular Risk

Although the overall figures are convincing and justify treatment of hypertension in elderly patients at least up to the age of 80 to 84 years, we need to consider individual patients. For each hypertensive patient we try to assess the cardiovascular risk by looking for other risk factors and dealing with these as discussed above. At present, such an approach is based on an overall impression rather than hard facts to calculate the true risk of an event over the next few years. Papers are now beginning to appear that tackle this problem.

Haq and colleagues[48] consider age-related risk for a range of serum cholesterol concentrations in the presence or absence of four other risk factors—hypertension, smoking, diabetes, and left ventricular hypertrophy (LVH). They have produced a table to be used to determine if an individual patient's coronary risk is greater than 1.5 percent per year. The table is intended to be used in decision-making for primary prevention, which may be worthwhile above this level of risk. The table clearly highlights the effect of age and the gender difference in risk. As an example, a 70-year-old hypertensive male smoker with LVH should be treated for a cholesterol of above 5.5 mmol/L, but a similar female would not require lipid-lowering treatment.

A report from New Zealand suggests that "decisions to treat raised blood pressure should be based primarily on the estimated absolute risk of cardiovascular disease rather than on blood pressure alone."[16] They suggest that treatment should be given only if there is a 20 percent or greater chance of a major cardiovascular event over the next 10 years. This is equivalent to treating 150 people to prevent one cardiovascular event per year (i.e., similar to the proven benefit in several of the outcome studies). The authors of the report feel that this approach is better than standard guidelines. As an example, a 60-year-old woman with a diastolic pressure of 100 mmHg and no other risk factors would be treated, whereas a 70-year-old man with a diastolic pressure of 95 mmHg and multiple risk factors would not be treated by most guidelines—despite the fact that the 60-year-old woman has only a 10 percent risk of a cardiovascular event in the next 10 years and the 70-year-old man's risk is 50 percent. Treatment of blood pressure would reduce the risk to 7 percent for the 60-year-old woman and 33 percent for the 70-year-old man. Using their criteria, all men over the age of 70 with mild hypertension (more than 150/90 mmHg) should be treated, whereas elderly women should be treated only if blood pressure is greater than 170/100 mmHg or greater than 150/90 mmHg with one or more other risk factors.

Further research is required, but this approach clarifies the rationale for treating elderly hypertensive patients. More complex calculations are required for younger adults.

Quality of Life

Benefits from treatment need to be set against any effects on the patient's well-being. Overall quality of life depends on many factors, including drug adverse effects. The literature on quality of life is confusing, with some conflicting results. The main drugs used in the outcome studies—thiazides and atenolol—have no significant effect on global quality of life. Similarly, the newer drugs such as the ACE inhibitors and the calcium channel antagonists show no important overall effect although some studies with ACE inhibitors claim extra benefit. At present, it is better to compare drugs in terms of their adverse effect profile rather than quality-of-life scores. Future research may develop such scores, which are more appropriate for elderly patients and which show clear differences between treatments.

Economics

Detailed economic assessment is beyond the scope of this chapter, although this is a rapidly developing field. Such studies need to consider all aspects of the management of hypertension, rather than just drug costs. If newer drugs such as the ACE inhibitors are shown to produce benefits that are similar to or slightly greater than thiazide diuretics in outcome studies, then economic arguments will become more important.

For drug costs alone, thiazides are by far the cheapest option. Low dose bendrofluazide in the United Kingdom costs around £2 per year. It is therefore an effective, safe, and cheap form of treatment. If ACE inhibitors are also found to be effective, then thiazides would still be the clear first-choice drug if efficacy was similar. However, if ACE inhibitors produced a reduction of 30 percent in risk of cardiac disease, compared to the 25 percent for thiazides, would this be worth the extra cost (£100 to 200 per year)? A good quality study taking all costs into consideration is required. A decision can then be made as to whether it is worth spending this money on hypertension or if it would be better spent elsewhere.

Delivering a Service

Effective reduction of the complications of hypertension within a population requires detection of those at risk, adequate treatment, and regular monitoring to ensure good control of the blood pressure and well-being. The "rule of halves" states that about one-half of hypertension in a population is undetected; one-half of that detected is untreated; and one-half of that treated is not well controlled. In other words, only one-eighth (12.5 percent) of those with hypertension are well controlled. Until recently, this finding, which was first noted over 30 years ago, still seemed to hold true. However, there is some recent hope that detection and treatment rates are higher, though the degree of good control of those treated is still about 50 percent.[49]

Consideration needs to be given to the most cost-effective way of delivering a service to treat hypertension. For a common problem such as hypertension, the emphasis must be on community services with a lesser role for hospital specialists. The ideal services should provide prompt, accurate diagnosis followed by effective treatment where indicated and a safe follow-up procedure. Some general practitioners run their own specialized hypertension clinic and refer only the troublesome problems to hospitals. Others have a higher referral rate. Success depends on both general practitioner and hospital specialist having an interest in hypertension. Some centers have established shared-care schemes so that both hospital and general practitioner services provide seamless care. Hypertension is well suited to such an approach.

Detection of all hypertension requires whole population screening on a regular basis. This approach is expensive and causes problems in false-positive cases. Most patients in the United Kingdom visit their general practitioner within a 5-year period. This allows opportunistic screening at little extra cost if the individual practitioner is motivated to measure the blood pressure during a routine visit for another problem. Initiation of treatment in patients with sustained hypertension requires commitment to see the patient several times, consider other risk factors and nonpharmacologic measures, and use an effective drug where indicated. The longer-term follow-up is more difficult, as patients may default for many reasons. Noone should be lost because of an inadequate follow-up system. Computers can be used to indicate those patients who are overdue, and send a reminder.

Summary

Many treatments used in elderly patients have not been evaluated properly in this age group. Although much more research is necessary in hypertension, there is at least clear evidence of benefit from using thiazide diuretics and, to a lesser extent, β-blockers. Management of most hypertension is not difficult but does require close attention to detail and procedure. Most of the current problems of management are due to ignorance and lack of commitment to the required level of follow-up.

Successful management of hypertension in an elderly patient requires the following:

- Good blood pressure measurement technique
- Establishing a diagnosis of sustained hypertension
- Evaluation of overall cardiovascular risk
- Encouragement to the patient to make appropriate lifestyle changes
- Selection of sensible drug treatment—usually starting with low dose thiazide
- Adequate follow-up and supervision of blood pressure control and any drug-related problems

References

1. Stamler J, Stamler R, Riedlinger WF et al: Hypertension screening of 1 million Americans: Community Hypertension Evaluation Clinic (CHEC) Program, 1973–75. JAMA 1976;235: 2299–2306
2. OPCS Social Survey Division: Health survey for England 1993. HMSO, London, 1994
3. Kannel WB, Gordon T: Evaluation of cardiovascular risk in the elderly: the Framingham Study. Bull N Y Acad Med 1978;54: 573–591
4. Whelton PK, He Jiang, Klag MJ: Blood pressure in Westernised populations. pp. 11–21. In Swales JD (ed): Textbook of Hypertension. Blackwell Scientific Publications, Oxford, 1994
5. Miall WE, Greenberg G: Mild hypertension—is there pressure to treat? Cambridge University Press, Cambridge, 1987
6. Colandrea MA, Friedman GD, Nichaman MZ, Lynd CD: Systolic hypertension in the elderly: an epidemiologic assessment. Circulation 1970;41:239–245
7. Veerman DP, Imholz BP, Wieling W et al: Effects of aging on blood pressure variability in resting conditions. Hypertension 1994;24:120–130

8. Woodhouse PR, Khaw Kay-Tee, Plummer M: Seasonal variation of blood pressure and its relationship to ambient temperature in an elderly population. J Hypertens 1993;11: 1267–1274
9. Staessen J, Amery A, Fagard R: Isolated systolic hypertension in the elderly. J Hypertens 1990;8:393–405
10. Law MR, Frost CD, Wald NJ: By how much does dietary salt reduction lower blood pressure. I—Analysis of observational data among populations. BMJ 1991;312:811–815
11. Dyer AR, Elliot P: The INTERSALT study: relations of body mass index to blood pressure. J Hum Hypertens 1989;3: 299–308
12. McMahon S, Peto R, Cutler J et al: Blood pressure, stroke and coronary heart disease. Part I, prolonged differences in blood pressure: prospective observational studies corrected for the regression dilution bias. Lancet 1990;335: 765–774
13. Medical Research Council Working Party: MRC trial of treatment of hypertension: principal results. BMJ 1985;291: 97–104
14. Dahlof B, Lindholm LH, Hansson L et al: Morbidity and mortality in the Swedish trial in old patients with hypertension (STOP-Hypertension). Lancet 1991;338:1281–1285
15. Amery A, Birkenhager WH, Brixho P et al: Mortality and morbidity results from the European working party on high blood pressure in the elderly. Lancet 1985;i: 1349–1354
16. Jackson R, Barham P, Bills J et al: Management of raised blood pressure in New Zealand: a discussion document. BMJ 1993; 307:107–110
17. Heagerty AM, Aalkjaer C, Bund SJ et al: Small artery structure in hypertension. Dual processes of remodelling and growth. Hypertension 1993;21:391–397
18. Folkow B: Hypertension—pathophysiology, diagnosis and management. Lippincott-Raven, Philadelphia, 1990
19. Dodson PM, Lip GYH, Eames SM et al: Hypertensive retinopathy: a review of existing classification systems and a suggestion for a simplified grading system. J Hum Hypertens 1996:10: 93–98
20. Oates A, Scott AK: Arm size and blood pressure measurement in elderly patients. Age Ageing 1995;24(suppl 1):39
21. Solomon SA, Ramsay LE, Yeo WW et al: Beta-blockade and intermittent claudication: placebo controlled trial of atenolol and nifedipine and their combination. BMJ 1991;303: 1100–1104
22. Intersalt Cooperative Research Group: The Intersalt study. J Hum Hypertens 1989;3:279–320
23. Grobbee DE, Hofman A: Does sodium restriction lower blood pressure? BMJ 1986;293:27–29
24. Fotherby MD, Potter JF: Effects of moderate sodium restriction on clinic and 24 hour ambulatory blood pressure in elderly hypertensive subjects. J Hypertens 1993;11:657–663
25. Swales JD: Non-pharmacological antihypertensive therapy. Eur Heart J 1988;9(suppl G):45–52
26. Smith SJ, Markandu ND, Sagnella GA, MacGregor GA: Moderate potassium chloride supplementation in essential hypertension: is it additive to moderate sodium restriction? BMJ 1985; 291:110–113
27. Andrews G, MacMahon SW, Austin A, Byrne DG: Hypertension: comparison of drug and non drug treatments. BMJ 1982; 284:1523–1526
28. Ramsay LE, Ramsay MH, Hettiarachchi J et al: Weight reduction in a blood pressure clinic. BMJ 1978;ii:244–245
29. Ramsay LE: Compliance with weight reduction in hypertensive patients. J Hypertens 1985;3(suppl 1):81–85
30. Klatsky AL, Freidman DG, Siegelaub AB, Gerard MJ: Alcohol consumption and blood pressure: Kaiser-Permanente multiphasic health examination data. N Engl J Med 1977;296: 1194–1200
31. Klatsky AL, Freidman DG, Armstrong MA: The relationships between alcoholic beverage use and other traits to blood pressure: a new Kaiser-Permanente study. Circulation 1986;73: 628–636
32. Weissfeld JL, Johnson EH, Brock BM, Hawthorne VM: Sex and age interactions in the association between alcohol and blood pressure. Am J Epidemiol 1988;128:559–569
33. Reaven PD, Barret-Connor E, Edelstein S: Relation between leisure time physical activity and blood pressure in older women. Circulation 1991;8:559–565
34. Hagberg JM, Mountain SJ, Wade H et al: Effect of exercise training in 60–69 year old persons with essential hypertension. Am J Cardiol 1989;64:348–353
35. McMurdo MET, Burnett L: A trial of exercise in the elderly. Age Ageing 1992;21(suppl 2):18
36. Perkins J, Dick TBS: Smoking and myocardial infarction: secondary prevention. Postgrad Med J 1985;61:295–300
37. SHEP Co-operative Research Group: Prevention of stroke by antihypertensive drug treatment in older persons with isolated systolic hypertension. Final results of the systolic hypertension in the elderly program (SHEP). JAMA 1991; 265:3255–3264
38. Medical Research Council Working Party: MRC trial of treatment of hypertension in older adults: principal results. BMJ 1992;304:405–412
39. Anonymous: Secondary prevention of coronary disease with lipid-lowering drugs. Lancet 1989;i:473–474
40. Scandinavian Simvastatin Survival Study Group: Randomised trial of cholesterol lowering in 4444 patients with coronary heart disease: the Scandinavian simvastatin survival study. Lancet 1994;344:1383–1389
41. Shepherd J, Cobbe SM, Ford I et al: Prevention of coronary heart disease with pravastatin in men with hypercholesterolaemia. N Engl J Med 1995;333:1301–1307
42. Garber AM, Browner WS, Hulley SB: Cholesterol screening in asymptomatic adults, revisited. Ann Intern Med 1996;124: 518–531
43. Anonymous: Sudden cardiac death in obesity and hypertension. Lancet 1988;i:628–629
44. Shinton R, Sagar G: Lifelong exercise and stroke. BMJ 1993; 307:231–234
45. Berglund A, Andersson OK, Berglund G, Fagerberg B: Antihy-

pertensive effect of diet compared with drug treatment in obese men with mild hypertension. BMJ 1989;299:480–485

46. Stamler R, Stamler J, Grimm R et al: Nutritional therapy for high blood pressure: final report of a four year randomized controlled trial—the Hypertension Control Program. JAMA 1987;257:1484–1491

47. Pahor M, Guralnik JM, Furberg CD et al: Risk of gastrointestinal haemorrhage with calcium antagonists in hypertensive persons over 67 years old. Lancet 1996;347:1061–1065

48. Haq IU, Jackson PR, Yeo WW, Ramsay LE: Sheffield risk and treatment table for cholesterol lowering for primary prevention of coronary heart disease. Lancet 1995;346:1467–1471

49. Ford GA, Duggan S, Aylett M, Eccles M: Validation of primary care notes based hypertension audit tool. Age Ageing 1996; 25(suppl 2):66

50. Coope J, Warrender TS: Randomised trial of treatment of hypertension in the elderly in primary care. BMJ 1986;293: 1145–1151

C H A P T E R 25

Valvular Heart Disease in Old Age

K. S. CHANNER

If the human heart beats on average 70 times per minute, then after 65 years the aortic, mitral, pulmonary, and tricuspid valves have opened and closed 2,391.5 million times. It is hardly surprising, therefore, that they begin to show signs of wear and tear. Most of the causes of valvular heart disease in the young also affect the old, but the majority of valvular heart disease in the elderly is degenerative. All the valves may be affected, but the mitral and aortic valves are more commonly affected[1] because they are subjected to greater pressure and trauma. Aortic and mitral valve dysfunction is more important clinically because of the consequences for the systemic circulation. Valvular dysfunction in the aging heart is not as well tolerated as in youth. The compensatory physiologic mechanisms of ventricular hypertrophy and dilatation still occur, but these functional adaptations are limited by age-related degeneration in the cardiac muscle (senile amyloid deposition and fibrosis) and the high frequency of associated disease, especially coronary artery disease. Other changes occur in the physiology of the heart and circulation in aging.[2] The left ventricle hypertrophies with age and increases in weight. This is associated with a decrease in compliance. Left ventricular diastolic filling changes as a consequence, and Doppler studies[3,4] have shown that atrial systole becomes increasingly important with advancing age and may contribute up to 50 percent of cardiac output at age 80 years compared with 10 percent at age 20 years. Ventricular myocardium is less responsive to catecholamines, and exercise-induced changes in heart rate are often blunted. The cardiac conduction tissue also degenerates, and as a consequence, bradyarrhythmias associated either with sinus or atrioventricular node dysfunction increase with age. Atrial and ventricular extrasystoles and tachycardias are much more common in the elderly, making interpretation of 24-hour ambulatory electrocardiographs more difficult. Arterial compliance also decreases, causing a rapid upstroke in the carotid pulse and higher peak systolic pressures. These changes and interactions are important since they influence the presentation, history, and prognosis of valvular heart disease. For example, atrial fibrillation occurs more frequently in the elderly in association with valvular heart disease than it does in the young, and it is of more significance because atrial systole is more important in the aging heart.[5] Another important clinical interaction is the association with other organ dysfunctions. For example, degenerative valvular heart disease is commonly associated with renal dysfunction. This has important implications for drug and surgical treatment.

Investigations

In recent years the investigation and assessment of valvular heart disease has become easier. Electrocardiography and chest X-ray changes assist in the diagnosis of valvular heart disease, but Doppler echocardiography has brought major advances. This technique is simple, quick, noninvasive, reproducible, and repeatable. It carries no risk for the patient, operator, or environment. With modern echocardiographic equipment it is possible not only to make a qualitative accurate diagnosis but also to quantify the severity of stenotic valve lesions. The cardiac adaptations that occur as a consequence of severe aortic and mitral valve disease, namely left ventricular hypertrophy and dilatation, can be accurately measured by echocardiography, and serial measurements provide an insight into the natural history of the lesion in the individual patient. Pulmonary hypertension complicates serious mitral valve disease, and this causes pulmonary arterial and right ventricular and right atrial dilatation—all of which are discernible on echocardiography. More accurate assessments of pulmonary artery pressures can be made with Doppler. In pulmonary hypertension, right ventricular dilatation stretches the tricuspid annulus, and the valve therefore becomes incompetent. The peak velocity measured by Doppler of the tricuspid regurgitant jet of blood can be used to derive the pressure gradient between the right atrium and right ventricle. If the right atrial pressure is known (from the jugular venous pressure wave) and is added to the gradient, an estimate of right ventricular pressure is made. Assuming that there is no pulmonary stenosis, the right ventricular and pulmonary artery pressures are equal.

Doppler echocardiography is undoubtedly the technique of choice in the elderly because of its noninvasive nature. It can be performed at the bedside and interferes little with the patient and as a consequence, is very well tolerated. The alternative technique of cardiac catheterization involving right and left heart cannulation is invasive and carries a considerable morbidity, a definite mortality, and is much more expensive.

Echocardiography relies on ultrasound reflected back from interfaces within the chest, for example, the heart muscle. Unfortunately, air absorbs ultrasound; in patients with emphysema or other chest deformities, transthoracic echocardiographic images may be obscured by overlying lung tissue. In perhaps 10 percent of patients, suboptimal transthoracic echocardiographic images are obtained. In order to obtain clearer cardiac images, transesophageal echocardiography has been

Indications for transesophageal echocardiography

Failure of transthoracic echocardiography
Location of cardiac source of embolism
Assessment of prosthetic valves
Diagnosis of infective endocarditis
Diagnosis of intra-atrial thrombus prior to cardioversion
Assessment of inter-atrial septal integrity
Diagnosis and assessment of atrial disease
Perioperative assessment during mitral valve repair
Diagnosis of aortic dissection
Assessment of congenital heart disease before and after corrective surgery in adolescents and adults

developed.[6] In this technique the ultrasound probe is mounted on a fiberoptic endoscope and passed into the esophagus through the mouth. The heart is then imaged from the esophagus. Images derived by this technique are of high quality. Antibiotic prophylaxis is not necessary, since the risk of endocarditis following esophageal intubation is very low. Some structures that lie posteriorly are visible only by the transesophageal route (e.g., the left atrial appendage). Prosthetic valves reflect and scatter ultrasound because of their metal parts, and better images are obtained from the esophagus. The aorta can only be easily imaged for its first few centimeters by transthoracic echocardiography, but with transesophageal echocardiography, virtually the whole of the ascending arch and proximal descending aorta can be seen. Transesophageal echo is therefore particularly valuable for the diagnosis of aortic dissection.[7] Indications for transesophageal echo are shown in the accompanying boxed list.

Other noninvasive techniques for the investigation of cardiac conditions have been developed. None of these has a great part to play in the investigation of valvular heart disease, but they are helpful in the assessment of left ventricular function, which may influence management. The most useful is isotope blood pool imaging or multiple gated acquisition scanning (MUGA). In the technique, red cells are labeled by technetium-99m (^{99m}Tc) and changes in the ventricular isotope activity in systole and diastole can be used to derive the ejection fraction. It is possible to estimate the ejection fraction for the right ventricle and left ventricle separately.

The prevalence of valvular heart disease in the elderly is considerable, but its severity is variable. Routine echocardiography in patients over 70 years of age will often demonstrate mitral and aortic valve thickening, and sensitive Doppler techniques routinely show these valves to be incompetent. Minor degrees of incompetence are so frequently found as to be considered a normal finding in the elderly patient. Hemodynamically significant valve disease is still relatively rare in old age. On the other hand, aortic flow murmurs are common. These are caused by turbulence of blood in the ascending aorta and are usually labeled as aortic sclerosis.

The pattern of valve disease—stenosis or incompetence—is the same in old age as in youth, but the causes are often different.

Aortic Stenosis

Aortic stenosis is the most common lesion requiring valve replacement in the elderly.[8] Although postinflammatory stenosis due to commissural fusion may present in the elderly, most patients with rheumatic valve disease present by the fifth decade. Aortic stenosis presenting for the first time in the sixth decade is usually due to calcific degeneration of a congenitally abnormal valve, and aortic stenosis presenting in the seventh decade may be due to calcific degeneration of a previously normal aortic valve.[9]

"Bicuspid" aortic valves are present in 1.5 to 2 percent of live births and represent the most common congenital cardiac abnormality.[10] The anatomic abnormality is associated with premature calcific degeneration, which causes stenosis and rarely, primary incompetence, unless there has been concomitant endocarditis. Virtually all stenosed valves will be shown to be incompetent at Doppler echocardiography, but this is frequently not of hemodynamic significance. There is an age-related increase in the degree of stenosis, with a 46 percent prevalence at age 50 years compared with a 73 percent prevalence at age 70 years.[11]

Calcific degeneration of the aortic valve may involve the ventricular septum and damage to the atrioventricular node and bundles of His.[10] There is, thus, an increased incidence of complete heart block in association with calcific stenosis. There is an estimated nine-fold increase in aortic dissection in patients with bicuspid aortic valves, and presentation occurs earlier at an average age of 55 years in patients with bicuspid valves, compared with an average age of 63 years in patients with tricuspid valves.[12]

Senile calcific aortic stenosis of a tricuspid valve has been found in 10 to 31 percent of cases at postmortem.[9] The valve leaflets are thickened and large nodules of calcium prevent their full excursion. The condition is associated with calcification in the mitral annulus and is more common in females.[13]

Whatever the pathology, the natural history of aortic stenosis is such that by the time symptoms develop, the stenosis is severe. Without surgery, untreated symptomatic aortic stenosis carries a life expectancy of between 2 and 3 years.[14] The classic triad of exertional syncope, exertional dyspnea, and angina pectoris may not always occur in the elderly. About 20 percent of elderly patients will present with heart failure.[8] Fatigue and lethargy are common. On examination, the pulse is characteristic, with a slow upstroke and prolonged plateau phase. However, because of the loss of arterial compliance in aging, many elderly patients have a rapidly rising pulse. The systemic blood pressure is usually low, but about 20 percent of elderly patients have significant systemic hypertension.[8] The left ventricle is

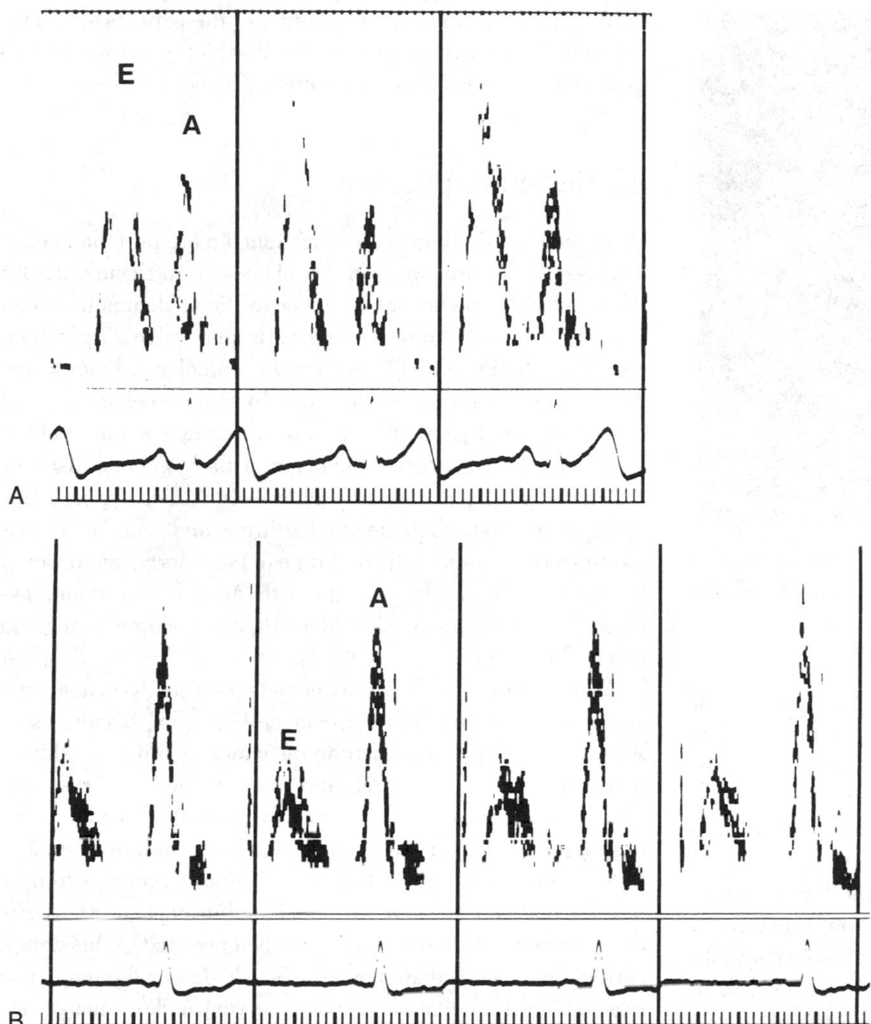

Figure 25-1 **(A)** Normal transmitral Doppler flow pattern. The early flow velocity (E) is greater than the flow velocity generated by atrial systole (A). **(B)** Reversal of flow pattern as seen in left ventricular hypertrophy. (From Channer,[46] with permission.)

hypertrophied, and this is clinically recognizable by a thrusting or heaving apical impulse. The apex beat is not displaced unless there is associated left ventricular dilatation. The murmur of aortic stenosis is of ejection type and maximal in the aortic area radiating into the neck over the carotid arteries. However, it is often atypical in the elderly. It can be high pitched and musical and is often heard all over the precordium. Ejection clicks are classically associated with compliant aortic stenosis, which occurs in young people, and they are virtually never audible in the elderly. The second heart sound is usually soft but distinct, and a fourth heart sound may be heard. This is caused by left atrial systole. When the left ventricle is hypertrophied its compliance is reduced and early diastolic filling is less. Atrial systole occurring toward the end of diastole compensates by causing an increased contribution to filling. This is readily demonstrated with pulsed Doppler traces of transmitral diastolic blood flow (Fig. 25-1). This physiologic compensation explains why left ventricular hypertrophy is so often associated with left atrial hypertrophy and also why patients may decompensate and develop left ventricular failure when atrial fibrillation occurs.

Investigations

Significant aortic stenosis is associated with left ventricular hypertrophy, which can be seen on electrocardiography. It should be remembered that precordial voltage criteria for the diagnosis of left ventricular hypertrophy are neither sensitive nor specific. The criteria of Sokolow and Lyon[15] have a sensitivity of about 55 percent and a false-positive rate of at least 10 percent. More strict criteria of Romhilt and Estes[16] are more specific but lose sensitivity to only about 30 percent. Echocardiography is, however, more sensitive and specific[17] and is the method of choice for assessing the presence of left ventricular hypertrophy. Left bundle branch block is a common consequence of left ventricular hypertrophy and especially of severe calcific aortic stenosis. As mentioned earlier, higher degrees of atrioventricular block may also occur.

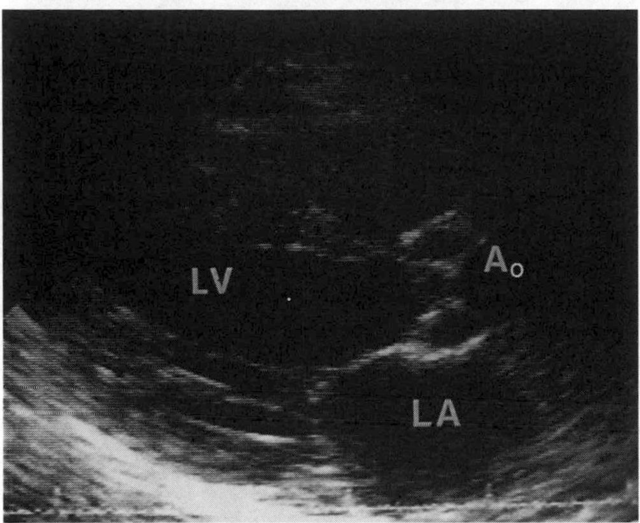

Figure 25-2 Long axis view of the left ventricle (LV), mitral valve (closed), and left atrium (LA). The aortic valve is thickened and restricted in its opening as in aortic stenosis.

The chest x-ray may not show cardiomegaly in severe aortic stenosis until left ventricular dilatation, a sign of left ventricular decompensation, occurs. The ascending aorta is unfolded because of poststenotic dilatation, but aortic unfolding is common in the elderly. Penetrated posteroanterior and lateral views usually show calcium in the region of the aortic valve.

Echocardiography shows a hypertrophied left ventricle, often with normal systolic function. Only about one-third of patients with severe aortic stenosis will have abnormal systolic function.[18] The aortic valve is thickened and restricted in its opening (Fig. 25-2). Echogenic masses around the valve ring often obscure leaflet detail but scans can be made from three or four different planes. The left atrial dimension is usually increased. Doppler echocardiography will show a significant stenotic jet, and gradients of more than 50 mmHg are associated with severe stenosis. It is important, however, to recognize the limitations of Doppler assessment of gradients. Aortic incompetence accompanying stenosis causes higher Doppler gradients when compared with those measured during cardiac catheterization. More importantly, if the Doppler beam is not positioned in the center of the aortic jet, lower gradients will be obtained. Abnormal valves typically generate eccentric jets, and as a consequence, it is important to estimate gradients from as many angles and different Doppler windows as possible. The valve leaflet excursion can also be measured and aortic orifice planimetered. An effective valve area of less than 1 cm^2 is associated with severe stenosis (normal is 2 to 4 cm^2).

Management

If the patient has symptomatic aortic stenosis and the preceding noninvasive evaluation has shown left ventricular hypertrophy and a significant Doppler gradient, the only effective treatment is aortic valve replacement. Cardiac catheterization and coronary angiography will usually be necessary in the elderly patient because about one-half of the patients will have associated coronary artery disease. Many surgeons would also graft significant coincidental coronary stenotic lesions.

Aortic Incompetence

Isolated aortic incompetence is much more rare than aortic stenosis. There are two basic mechanisms: intrinsic valvular damage as a consequence of endocarditis or rheumatic fever, and dilatation of the ascending aorta and valve ring, which causes stretching of the leaflets and eventually incompetence. Aortic ring dilatation is the more common mechanism, and causes include hypertension, myxomatous degeneration of the aortic wall, and dissecting aneurysm. Other systemic diseases associated with aortic incompetence—including syphilis, ankylosing spondylitis, rheumatoid arthritis, and giant cell arteritis—rarely present for the first time in the elderly, and it would be most unusual for patients with Marfan syndrome, osteogenesis imperfecta, or Ehlers-Danlos syndrome even to reach old age.

Minor degrees of aortic incompetence usually accompany aortic stenosis, and Doppler echocardiography, because it is so sensitive, would demonstrate incompetence in most elderly hypertensive patients. Patients with clinically significant chronic aortic incompetence usually present with increasing dyspnea. This is caused by left ventricular failure and so is initially exercise related, but will eventually progress to dyspnea at rest and nocturnal dyspnea and orthopnea. Many patients present late with severe incompetence, and in this group, corrective surgery does not always alleviate symptoms. The reason for this is that permanent left ventricular damage has already occurred by the time symptoms have developed. The ventricle is able to tolerate chronic volume overload much better than pressure overload, and moderate-to-severe aortic incompetence can be asymptomatic for years.

Examination will reveal a collapsing pulse with wide pulse pressure. However, this is a normal consequence of aging, because of a loss of compliance of the arterial tree. The carotid arteries may visibly pulsate (Corrigan sign) and the head may bob with systole (deMusset sign). Capillary pulsation in the fingertips may be visible (Quincke sign). The heart is enlarged and the apex beat is displaced laterally and inferiorly. The left ventricle is usually easily felt. The early diastolic decrescendo murmur of aortic incompetence is best heard down the left sternal edge and may be associated with a mitral middiastolic rumble (the Austin-Flint murmur). This is caused by the aortic incompetent jet interfering with mitral inflow. Color flow Doppler frequently shows the aortic jet streaming over the anterior leaflet of the mitral valve. The murmur of aortic incompetence is high pitched and sighing and may be well localized. It is best heard by leaning the patient forward and listening in held expiration.

Acute aortic regurgitation, which develops in endocarditis or aortic dissection, will be associated with less obvious peripheral signs. The clinical picture is usually dominated by severe left ventricular failure with tachycardia, vasoconstriction, and pulmonary edema.

Investigations

Significant aortic incompetence will cause an increase in heart size, which is readily seen on chest x-ray. The aortic root may appear dilated with unfolding of the ascending aorta. Calcification of the aortic valve is uncommon in pure aortic incompetence, but often present when it accompanies aortic stenosis. The electrocardiograph will usually show signs of left ventricular hypertrophy. The echocardiogram shows a dilated left ventricle with good systolic function usually. When the left ventricular end systolic diameter exceeds 5.5 cm, then the ventricle is said to be overdilated, requiring valve replacement. The interventricular septum and free wall of the left ventricle may not be thickened, although overall left ventricular muscle mass is increased because of the large volume ventricle. The echocardiogram will help to distinguish intrinsic aortic valve disease from aortic root disease. The anterior mitral leaflet shows fluttering or shattering as the aortic incompetent jet causes it to vibrate as it opens. This shatter is also sometimes seen on the interventricular septum. Doppler traces will demonstrate the presence of aortic incompetence, but are not accurate at predicting its severity. Color flow Doppler provides a visual demonstration of the jet; a wide jet that descends deep into the ventricle usually represents severe incompetence. The incompetence can also be visualized by aortic angiography and the severity of the lesion assessed by the amount of contrast medium visible in the left ventricle. This technique also has a high interobserver variability.

Management

One of the most difficult clinical decisions in cardiology is to predict the timing of valve replacement in aortic incompetence. Because the lesion is tolerated so well for so long, reliance should be placed on more objective changes. These include increasing cardiac dimensions on chest x-ray—remembering that the volume overload of aortic incompetence will be associated with about 1 cm difference in transverse cardiac dimension between systole and diastole, so that serial changes in transverse diameter must be progressive. Left ventricular dimensions and function can be more accurately measured by echocardiography. A serial increase in left ventricular diastolic and systolic dimensions may herald left ventricular decompensation. Some authors suggest that objective assessment of left ventricular function should be monitored by repeated measurement of exercise capacity on a treadmill in asymptomatic subjects.[8]

Mitral Stenosis

Mitral stenosis is usually caused by rheumatic fever and sometimes presents for the first time in the elderly. Calcification of the mitral annulus, which is associated with aging, may rarely interfere with mitral leaflet excursion, causing functional stenosis. The lesion causes a progressive increase in left atrial dimensions and pulmonary venous hypertension, with a consequent compensatory increase in pulmonary artery pressure and right-sided filling pressure. Left ventricular filling is reduced, and this is associated with low cardiac output.

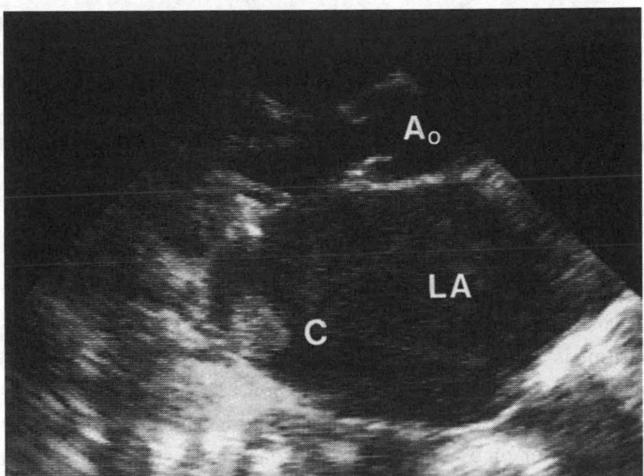

Figure 25-3 Long axis view showing severe mitral stenosis with markedly dilated left atrium (LA). There is a thrombus (C) attached to the posterior wall of the left atrium. Note the different echogenic appearance of blood in the LA compared with that in the aorta (A). This is caused by marked turbulence and red cell aggregation.

The natural history of mitral stenosis is long, and patients may not notice a progressive deterioration in effort tolerance. Eventually, however, dyspnea impinges on daily activities like dressing and washing. Nocturnal dyspnea and orthopnea are characteristic. Acute decompensation occurs when the left atrial dilatation is associated with atrial fibrillation, since the loss of atrial systole causes a sudden severe decrease in left ventricular filling. Under these circumstances, the patient may present with severe, even fatal, pulmonary edema. All patients who present with recent onset of atrial fibrillation and heart failure should have mitral stenosis excluded by echocardiography. Other symptoms include hemoptysis from pulmonary venous hypertension, and palpitation from paroxysmal or persistent atrial fibrillation. Atrial fibrillation, especially when it is combined with mitral stenosis, is commonly associated with systemic embolism from thrombus formation within the left atrium and its appendage[19,20] (Fig. 25-3). Patients presenting with systemic embolism should always have echocardiography to exclude mitral stenosis or myxoma.

Clinical signs of mitral stenosis include atrial fibrillation, a low volume pulse, and characteristic malar flush on the cheeks. The right-sided pressures are usually elevated, causing a raised jugular venous pulse (JVP) and right ventricular dilatation and palpable parasternal impulse. The apex beat is not displaced, as the left ventricle is small, but is tapping in quality. The first heart sound is loud, and in diastole an opening snap is followed by a low pitched rumbling diastolic murmur. This is usually localized to the apex and is best heard with the bell of the stethoscope lightly applied with the patient in the left lateral position. The opening snap can often be heard more widely and may be mistaken for a split second sound or a third heart sound. In the presence of pulmonary hypertension the pulmonary component of the second heart sound is loud and is best appreciated in the left second interspace. Hepatomegaly may be present as may ankle or sacral edema.

Investigations

Electrocardiography usually shows atrial fibrillation. If the patient is in sinus rhythm, left atrial hypertrophy is seen as a bifid P wave in V1 or P mitrale in lead II. Chest X-ray shows an enlarged left atrium seen as a double shadow to the right heart border or by splaying of the carina. Posteriorly, the left atrium indents the esophagus, and this can clearly be seen on a lateral barium swallow. The mitral valve may have calcium within it and be visible on a penetrated posteroanterior or lateral film. The pulmonary arteries may be dilated, and the lung fields are congested with prominent upper lobe veins and Kerley B lines. Echocardiography is the diagnostic test. The mitral valve is thickened and restricted and shows a characteristic plateau. The posterior leaflet is tethered and moves forward with the anterior leaflet instead of away from it during valve opening. The left ventricle fills more slowly than usual and the free wall and interventricular septum show a characteristic diastolic slope. Doppler traces of transmitral blood flow are also characteristic, with a high turbulent velocity and prolonged flow. An estimate of the severity of the valve stenosis can be derived from the pressure half time, from which the effective valve area can be calculated. Valve areas of less than 1 cm^2 are considered to be severe stenosis. Estimates of pulmonary arterial hypertension can be derived from the tricuspid regurgitation jet as previously described. Thus, the severity of the stenosis can be assessed noninvasively and surgery can be recommended on this basis. There is frequently no need to embark on further invasive cardiologic assessment by cardiac catheterization unless coincidental coronary artery disease is suspected and thought likely to influence surgical management.

Management

Mitral valve replacement is required in symptomatic patients with pulmonary hypertension and effective valve areas of less than 1 to 1.5 cm^2. Patients in atrial fibrillation should have long-term anticoagulation to prevent atrial thrombus formation and systemic embolism.

Mitral Incompetence

Mitral incompetence is probably the most common valvular lesion in the elderly. As in aortic incompetence it can be caused by intrinsic mitral valve disease following endocarditis and rheumatic fever or by damage to its supporting structures. Papillary muscle dysfunction following ischemic damage or myxomatous degeneration of the chordae tendineae cause mitral valve prolapse. This is now the most common indication for mitral valve replacement in elderly men. Alteration in the geometry of the mitral annulus, which occurs in left ventricular dilatation and heart failure, inevitably causes mitral incompetence. Similarly, calcification of the mitral annulus, which occurs with advancing age causes the valve to leak. Mitral ring calcification occurs in about 3.2 percent of women aged less than 70 years but rises to 44 percent of women over 90 years.[21] The incidence in males is approximately one-half of this, but there is an increased incidence of rupture of the chordae tendineae in males because of their higher systolic blood pressure and greater hemodynamic load.[22] Mitral annulus calcification is increased in patients with chronic renal failure, hypercalcemia, diabetes mellitus, systemic hypertension, and aortic stenosis.

Most patients with clinically significant mitral incompetence present with dyspnea. Initially this is on exertion but will gradually progress and be associated with paroxysmal nocturnal dyspnea and orthopnea. Increasing pulmonary venous congestion will be associated with pulmonary hypertension and right-sided heart failure, characterized by ankle swelling and anorexia and right upper abdominal tenderness from hepatic congestion. Left atrial dilatation secondary to mitral incompetence will cause atrial fibrillation and a feeling of palpitation. In some patients, the left atrium enlarges so much as to cause dysphagia by pressure on the esophagus.[23]

In severe mitral incompetence the examination will reveal atrial fibrillation in some patients and often a rather bounding pulse. The central venous pressure will usually be raised. The apex beat is displaced and forceful and the right ventricle is palpable. The pansystolic murmur is best heard at the apex and often radiates widely into the back and up into the neck and over the carotid arteries. The murmur encroaches onto the second heart sound, which is usually soft except in pulmonary hypertension when the loud pulmonary component is best heard in the pulmonary area. The liver is enlarged and tender, and ankle or sacral edema is present.

Mild mitral incompetence may only be associated with a soft midsystolic murmur localized at the apex and no evidence of left ventricular or right ventricular enlargement. Mitral valve prolapse will often be accompanied by a systolic click preceding the murmur.

Investigations

Electrocardiography shows atrial fibrillation, or if the patient remains in sinus rhythm, left atrial enlargement will be seen (see mitral stenosis above). Severe mitral incompetence is associated with left ventricular hypertrophy in about 50 percent of cases. About 15 percent of patients will also show signs of right ventricular hypertrophy[24] (right axis deviation, prominent R wave in V1, or partial or complete right bundle branch block). The chest x-rays shows cardiomegaly with left atrial enlargement. The lung fields are congested, and in pulmonary hypertension the proximal pulmonary arteries are di-

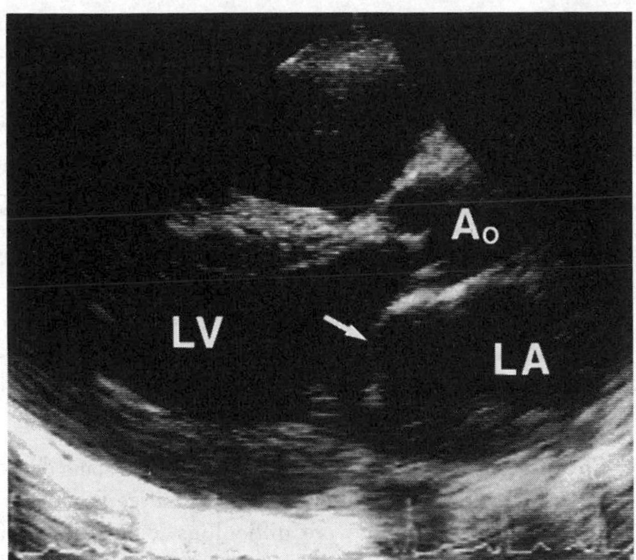

Figure 25-4 Long axis view showing severe prolapse of the anterior mitral leaflet (arrow).

lated, making the hila prominent. Calcification may be seen in the valve or more commonly in the annulus. Echocardiography shows a dilated volume-overloaded left ventricle with increased septal and free wall thickness. The mitral valve apparatus is clearly visible on two-dimensional imaging, and prolapse of either mitral valve leaflet can often be seen. The mitral apparatus, including papillary muscles, chordae, and ring, may show thickening or calcification. Two-dimensional scans may also show mitral leaflet prolapse during systole (Fig. 25-4). Left atrial dimension is increased, and in the presence of pulmonary hypertension the pulmonary artery, right ventricle, and right atrium will also be dilated. Doppler examination confirms systolic turbulence behind the mitral valve in systole. Accurate assessment of the degree of mitral regurgitation cannot be made by Doppler, although techniques aimed at measuring the regurgitant fraction are being developed. Nevertheless, as in mitral stenosis, the secondary complications of mitral incompetence, including left ventricular dilatation and failure and the development of pulmonary hypertension, can be detected by echocardiography.

In view of the fact that mitral incompetence is often associated with left ventricular dysfunction, which may be caused by coronary artery disease, most patients will require coronary angiography prior to mitral valve replacement so that simultaneous coronary artery bypass grafting can be done.

Management

As in aortic incompetence, the left ventricle can tolerate the volume overload of mitral incompetence for some time. Symptoms usually develop after the left ventricle has failed, and surgery should then be actively considered. Some authors suggest that objective assessments of effort tolerance should be used to help the physician judge the time of the operation.[8] Patients in atrial fibrillation should have life-long anticoagulation unless there are contraindications.

Infectious Endocarditis

Infectious endocarditis remains a rare but important cause of morbidity and mortality in patients with valvular heart disease. The condition is more common in the elderly, with more than 50 percent of patients having their first episode of endocarditis after the age of 60 years.[25] The elderly are more at risk of endocarditis, probably because valvular endocardial disruption is more common, immunity is impaired, and nutrition may be poor. Infection risk is also related to the size of the inoculum and the virulence of the organism. Bacteremia complicating dental treatment remains an important etiologic factor, and the severity of the bacteremia is increased by the presence of peridontal disease.[26]

Presentation in the elderly is, however, often atypical. Patients may be asymptomatic or have vague and nonspecific complaints like anorexia or nausea and vomiting. Fever occurs only in 50 to 70 percent of cases, and neurologic symptoms and signs may be predominant (in about one-third). Confusion or focal neurologic signs may be dismissed as features of cerebrovascular diseases.[27–29]

The aortic valve is most frequently infected (20 to 40 percent of cases), with the mitral valve next in frequency (25 to 35 percent of cases), and both valves are infected in about one-quarter of the cases.[30] The infecting organisms are most often streptococci and enterococci associated with bowel and urinary tract disease. Staphylococcal endocarditis, particularly *Staphylococcus epidermidis*, is most commonly associated with prosthetic valve endocarditis and is probably introduced at the time of surgery.[31] Males are at greater risk if they have mitral incompetence. Mortality is higher and this is probably because of late or missed diagnosis.

The diagnosis of infectious endocarditis is made by a combination of fever, embolic phenomena, and evidence of cardiac involvement[32] (changing murmurs or heart failure). Any elderly patient with a heart murmur and malaise, especially if there is associated fever, must be considered to have endocarditis. Blood cultures must be taken with care before any antibiotics are given. Unfortunately, they may be negative in the elderly. A high index of suspicion should be maintained and a low threshold for blood cultures. Other useful diagnostic hints include a high erythrocyte sedimentation rate (ESR), normochromic normocytic anemia, and proteinuria and hematuria. Echocardiography has been heralded as a useful diagnostic tool for endocarditis. This is not so. The sensitivity and specificity of echocardiography is low.[33] It is common to find echogenic areas around and on degenerative valves in the elderly, and it is not possible to distinguish these from infected vegetations especially early on in the disease process. As mentioned earlier, valve thickening and incompetence detected by Doppler are almost universal findings in the elderly. However, large

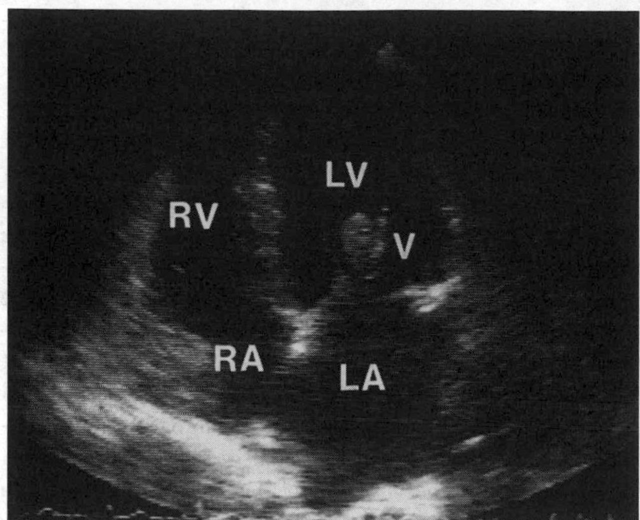

Figure 25-5 Apical four chamber view showing a large vegetation (2 cm × 1 cm) on the mitral valve leaflets. (RV, right ventricle; RA, right atrium; LV, left ventricle; LA, left atrium; LV, left ventricle.)

masses on valves are unlikely to be anything other than vegetations (Fig. 25-5).

Management

Intravenous antibiotics appropriate for the infecting organism should be given for 2 weeks and then oral antibiotics given for a further 4 weeks. The indications for surgery include (1) hemodynamic deterioration, (2) evidence of persisting uncontrolled sepsis, and (3) large vegetations seen on echocardiography or abscess cavities in the septum or aorta.[34]

All patients with heart murmurs must be reminded to maintain good dental hygiene by regular visits to the dentist and to report the fact of their murmur to their medical and dental attendants so that prophylactic antibiotic therapy can be given when appropriate.[35]

Surgery of Valve Disease in the Elderly

Establishing that a patient has significant valve disease that may be helped by valve replacement is only the first step in deciding whether this is in the patient's best interest. Before recommending surgery it is necessary to determine the natural history of the disease that is present and to balance that against the risks in the short and long term of any intervention. Surgery for prognostic reasons will be influenced by the age of the patient, since this will affect life expectancy and operative risks. The overall risk of surgery when the indication is for symptomatic reasons is less influenced by age and more by comorbidity, since the ability of patients to withstand major surgery decreases with impaired visceral function and concomitant coronary artery disease and impaired left ventricular function. Biologic aging is not always related to chronologic age, and some patients have little to gain by any intervention because of advanced degenerative disease of the body in general.

Certain associated diseases will lead to an increased risk of surgery and, if severe, may prohibit it.

Cerebral disease Patients who have had cerebrovascular accidents tend to deteriorate after open heart surgery; sometimes this is only temporary. Patients with intra- or extracerebral vascular disease are at risk from the neurologic complications that can follow cardiac surgery in any age group. Very careful assessment of neurologic function and identifying possible risk factors such as carotid artery disease is important in selecting patients for surgery.

Chronic pulmonary disease There is always some deterioration of lung function after open heart surgery and this extra insult may lead to severe difficulties if no reserve of function is available. The pulmonary route is a major portal of infection after cardiac surgery.

Gastrointestinal disease Peptic ulceration after surgery can be life-threatening and will need appropriate treatment before and after surgery.

Investigation Before Surgery

The same diagnostic cardiac investigations are required in young and old alike. Echocardiography remains the prime investigation. Depending on the skills and experience of the echocardiography department it may be possible to dispense with invasive cardiac catheterization in the assessment of the nature and severity of the valve disease per se.

Risk Diagnosis

Investigation is necessary not only to elicit a diagnosis but also to provide information on those features that may increase the risks of operative surgery.

Coronary arteriography

One of the major risk factors in the treatment of valvular heart disease in the adult population is the presence of coronary heart disease. Older patients are especially prone to this. Coronary arteriography, therefore, is indicated in every patient except in exceptional circumstances. This investigation is at present the only way to detect concomitant coronary heart disease. Whether or not coronary artery surgery is also performed when concurrent coronary disease has been detected will depend on its pattern of distribution, the nature of the valve disease, and the condition and age of the patient.

Combined valve surgery and coronary artery surgery is performed if the pattern of disease and the nature of the valvular lesion make the chances of myocardial infarction—either immediately or later—a likely event. For instance, a patient with mitral valve disease and angina due to coronary artery lesions is greatly at risk from this complication. A patient with aortic stenosis and no angina but angiographically proven coronary artery lesions is at low immediate risk of infarction, although the risk of this is higher in the medium to long term. Thus, in those elderly patients without angina, the surgeon may conclude that the extra risks of concomitant coronary artery surgery are unjustified and settle for a quick operative procedure. Although some reports suggest that the mortality of the combined operation is identical to that of simple valve replacement,[36] others suggest significant extra risk.[37,38] Craver et al.[37] showed that the risk of aortic valve replacement in patients of 70 years and more was 7.3 percent for the simple operation and 11.6 percent for the combined procedure. The additional risk of neurologic damage caused by a longer bypass time in the elderly patient was 8.4 percent as opposed to 3.0 percent in younger patients.

Carotid Doppler studies

Carotid Doppler studies are indicated if there is any evidence of a carotid bruit, in order to assess the severity of carotid artery disease. There is not complete agreement that carotid artery disease should be treated surgically at the same time as the cardiac surgery is performed, nor about the staging of the operations if the two procedures are judged to be necessary to avoid cerebral damage during the period of cardiopulmonary bypass. Most surgeons at present would regard carotid artery disease only as significant if there was a history of transient ischemic attacks or other manifestations of the cerebral effects of the lesions.

Gastrointestinal endoscopy

A history of dyspepsia should lead to a suspicion of peptic ulceration. Definitive diagnosis is provided by endoscopy. Cardiac surgery should be delayed until any peptic ulceration is controlled, in view of the risks of gastrointestinal hemorrhage.

Operative Strategies

All procedures on diseased valves should be regarded as palliative. Several choices are available for the treatment of valve disease: (1) surgical valve repair, (2) surgical valve replacement, and (3) percutaneous valvuloplasty.

Surgical repair and replacement must be done under vision with an arrested heart and artificial circulation to preserve the tissues of the body (extracorporeal circulation, ECC). ECC is relatively nonphysiologic and there is always a degree of visceral dysfunction after its use, which is mainly due to hypoxic damage of the tissues. In the elderly patient with fewer reserves, there is a risk of organ failure as a result of ECC. In addition, the surgical procedure involves emptying the heart of its blood and then refilling it at the end of the operation in an effort to remove all the air. In virtually every case this process is incomplete to a lesser or greater degree and air embolism results. This is a particularly common cause of cerebral damage.

Surgical Valve Repair

These procedures are most successful in mitral and tricuspid valve disease. By means of a series of plasty procedures the valves may be repaired. These operations are particularly suitable for degenerative disease of the mitral and tricuspid valves and less successful with the cicatrized valves following inflammatory reactions as in rheumatic fever. Degenerative disease of the mitral valve is a common finding in echocardiographic studies and increases in incidence with advancing age. The pathologic process is characterized by progressive weakness and stretching of the fibrous stroma of the valves, leading to elongation of the ring, cusps, and suspensory chordae of the valve. This process may be detected echocardiographically before regurgitation occurs. When the valve does leak, the patient will complain of progressive symptoms. Carpentier[39] has developed a rational scheme of analysis of the causes of degenerative valvular regurgitation and the subsequent corrective procedures and has applied this philosophy to the treatment of many patients. Long-term follow-up of such patients reveals good functional results and a low reoperation rate. The good functional results are in large part due to the preservation of the suspensory apparatus of the valves, which appear to be important in the efficient functioning of the ventricles. Another benefit of valve repair is the fact that the native valve is capable of self repair under the stresses of normal functioning. These two features of repair are particularly advantageous to the elderly patient. The possibility of avoiding anticoagulant therapy is also a benefit. Carpentier's techniques have been applied widely by other centers with equally good results. It is now generally accepted that a policy of trying to repair rather than replace diseased valves is beneficial to all patients, but the type of valve disease most suitable for repair, usually degenerative disease of the mitral valve, is particularly found in the elderly.

Valve Replacement

Replacement of the diseased valve is necessary for nearly all aortic valve disease and atrioventricular valve disease, which is too extensive for repair. All valvular prostheses are imperfect and differ only in the type of imperfection, which is usually a consequence of the method of manufacture and the materials used.

Hazards associated with valvular prostheses

Hazards of valvular prostheses include thromboembolism, durability, infection, and unphysiologic function.

Thromboembolism and durability are particularly difficult problems. Valvular prostheses are constructed of two different materials. First, there are the bioprostheses, usually made from animal aortic valve or pericardium and mounted on a cloth-covered frame. Second, there are the mechanical prostheses made from a synthetic material, nowadays usually pyrolytic carbon. Bioprostheses tend to work well, and often there is no need for anticoagulation because of their low thrombogenic properties. However, their durability is less than the mechanical type and most will fail in a 10- to 12-year period. Mechanical valves are much more durable than this but are highly thrombogenic and therefore, lifelong anticoagulation is required, with all the possible complications of this therapy. There is no uniformity of view as to the best prosthesis to use at all times, but there is widespread consensus that the biologic valve is the best choice for the elderly patient if there is a reasonable certainty that the durability of the valve exceeds the life expectancy of the patient who is to receive it.

Percutaneous Valvuloplasty

These procedures were introduced by Cribier in 1986[40] as a simple and relatively noninvasive method for the relief of stenosis of the mitral aortic and tricuspid valves. The procedure consists of inserting a catheter by the femoral route into the heart. The catheter has at its tip an inflatable balloon that can be passed through a stenotic valve. With inflation of the balloon the valve is stretched and the obstruction reduced. This technique has been mostly used for the relief of aortic and mitral stenosis, and those experienced in its use claim good results as judged by patient survival and abolition or reduction of stenotic gradients. The use of the technique has been advocated for the elderly frail patient in particular.[41]

In general terms, balloon valvuloplasty for calcific aortic stenosis is of no value.[42] Although good initial results were obtained, the medium-term results are poor with no appreciable reduction in the degree of stenosis and no improvement in prognosis. The degenerative nature of calcific aortic stenosis make commisural splitting by the valvuloplasty balloon impossible. Where successful valvuloplasty has been achieved it is nearly always associated with leaflet damage, tearing, and moderate or even severe aortic incompetence. Occasionally, the technique may buy time for valve replacement in patients who are shocked and in heart failure in order to improve their operative risk. Mitral balloon valvuloplasty by comparison has been more successful. There are many reasons for this. First, the disease process responsible for mitral stenosis is much more commonly rheumatic rather than degenerative. The rheumatic process causes scarring and commisural fusion of the valve leaflets, which themselves remain pliable for many years. It is possible to split the commisures by balloon valvuloplasty, which has replaced closed valvotomy in this group of patients. The key to the success of balloon valvuloplasty for mitral stenosis has been the careful selection of patients. Suitable patients are younger, have pliable valve leaflets without appreciable calcification, and no significant mitral incompetence, or intra-atrial clot. Nowadays, there is only a small group of patients in the United Kingdom for which valvuloplasty would appear to give as good results as closed valvotomy. A large proportion of suitable patients would be found in Third World countries, where rheumatic fever is still common.[43] Most elderly patients with rheumatic mitral stenosis have secondary degenerative changes, including annular calcification and chordal calcification, which disqualifies them for valvuloplasty. Most also have concomitant incompetence. Occasionally, however, elderly patients with less than optimal anatomy may benefit from mitral valvuloplasty if surgery is considered of too high a risk because of other serious associated disease. The risk of increasing the degree of mitral incompetence must be balanced against the advantage of significantly reducing the transmitral pressure gradient, and improving forward flow through into the ventricle.

Valve Replacement

Aortic Stenosis

Untreated, severe calcific aortic stenosis carries a bad prognosis, with a 3-year survival after the development of symptoms of 20 percent. The operative risk (30 day mortality) of aortic valve replacement in the elderly ranges from 5.3 to 8.3 percent, and in octogenarians is about 10 percent.[44] These figures can be considered to be the most optimistic; when it is necessary to combine aortic valve replacement with coronary artery surgery the mortality doubles to about 20 percent. The best predictor of outcome is the degree of left ventricular dysfunction. Complications are more common in the elderly, but the most serious morbidity is associated with postoperative stroke, which occurs in up to 11 percent of patients.

Despite these daunting figures, aortic valve replacement undoubtedly improves prognosis and, if successful, returns 80-year-olds to the survival pattern of their peers without aortic valve disease. Symptoms and quality of life also improve, since most patients are in functional class III or IV prior to surgery, and afterward are in a lower functional class.

Mitral valve disease

The operative mortality for mitral valve replacement is around 5 percent, although this may be lower following repair rather than replacement. Mortality is higher in patients 70 years and older, and in those with poor left ventricular function, severe symptoms (functional class IV), and concomitant ischemic heart disease. Eleven-year survival is about 65 percent[45]; the main complications of mitral valve replacement are bleeding and thromboembolism, which occur in up to 50 percent of patients over this period.

References

1. Pomerance A: Cardiac pathology in the elderly. In Noble RJ, Rothbaum DA (eds): Geriatric Cardiology. Cardiovascular Clinics. FA Davies, Philadelphia, 1981
2. Wenger NK, O'Rourke RA, Marcus FI: The care of elderly patients with cardiovascular disease. Ann Intern Med 1988; 109:425–428
3. Kuo LC, Quinones MA, Rokey R et al: Quantification of atrial contribution to left ventricular filling by pulsed Doppler echo-

cardiography and the effect of age in normal and diseased hearts. Am J Cardiol 1987;59:1174–1178

4. Spirito P, Maron BJ: Influence of ageing on Doppler echocardiographic indices of left ventricular diastolic function. Br Heart J 1988;59:672–679
5. Kannel WB, Abbott RD, Savage DD, McNamara PM: Epidemiological features of chronic atrial fibrillation: the Framingham Study. N Engl J Med 1982;306:1018–1022
6. Daniel WG, Mugge A: Transoesophageal echocardiography. N Eng J Med 1995;332:1268–1279
7. Cigarroa JE, Isselbacher EM, DeSanctis RW, Eagle KA: Diagnostic imaging in the evaluation of suspected aortic dissection. N Engl J Med 1993;328:35–43
8. Rahimtoola SH, Cheitlin MD, Hutter AM: Valvular and congenital heart disease. J Am Coll Cardiol 1987;10:60A–62A
9. Cohle SD, Graham MA, Dowling G, Pounder DJ: Sudden death and left ventricular outflow disease. Pathology Annual 1988; 23:97–124
10. Roberts WC: Congenital cardiovascular abnormalities usually "silent" until adulthood: morphological features of the floppy mitral valve, valvular aortic stenosis, discrete subvalvular aortic stenosis, hypertrophic cardiomyopathy, sinus of valsalva aneurysm and the Marfan syndrome. Cardiovas Clin 1979;10: 407–453
11. Fenoglio JJ, McAllister HA, DeCastro CM et al: Congenital biscupid aortic valve after age 20. Am J Cardiol 1977;39: 164–169
12. Larson EW, Edwards WD: Risk factors for aortic dissection: a necropsy study of 161 cases. Am J Cardiol 1984;53:849–855
13. Roberts WC, Perloff JK, Constantino T: Severe valvular aortic stenosis in patients over 65 years of age. A clinicopathological study. Am J Cardiol 1987;27:497–506
14. Frank S, Johnson A, Ross J Jr: Natural history of valvular aortic stenosis. Br Heart J 1973;35:41–46
15. Sokolow M, Lyon TP: The ventricular complex in left ventricular hypertrophy as obtained by unipolar, precordial and limb leads. Am Heart J 1949;37:161–186
16. Romhilt DW, Estes EH: Point score system for the ECG diagnosis of left ventricular hypertrophy. Am Heart J 1968;75: 752–758
17. Reichek N, Devereaux RB: Left ventricular hypertrophy: Relationship of anatomic, echocardiographic and electrocardiographic findings. Circulation 1981;63:1391–1398
18. Murphy ES, Lawson RM, Starr A, Rahimtoola SH: Severe aortic stenosis in patients 60 years of age or older: left ventricular function and 10 year survival after valve replacement. Circulation 1981;64(suppl 11):184–188
19. Coulshed N, Epstein EJ, McKendrick CS et al: Systemic embolism in mitral valve disease. Br Heart J 1970;32:26–34
20. Fleming HA, Bailey SM: Mitral valve disease, systemic embolism and anticoagulants. Postgrad Med J 1971;47:599–604
21. Pomerance A Pathological and clinical study of calcification of the mitral valve ring. J Clin Pathol 1970;23:354–361
22. Rowland ML, Fulwood R: Coronary heart disease risk factor trends in blacks between the first and second nations. Health and Nutritional Examination Surveys 1971–1980. Am Heart J 1984;108:771–779
23. Chesshyre MH, Braimbridge MV: Dysphagia due to left atrial enlargement after mitral Starr valve replacement. Br Heart J 1971;33:799–802
24. Braunwald E: Valvular heart disease. In Braunwald E (ed): Heart Disease: A Textbook of Cardiovascular Medicine. WB Saunders, Philadelphia, 1984
25. Von Reyn CF, Levy BS, Arbeit RD et al: Infective endocarditis: an analysis based on strict case definitions. Ann Intern Med 1981;94:505–518
26. Silver JG, Martin AW, McBride BC: Experimental transient bacteraemias in human subjects with varying degrees of plaque accumulation and gingival inflammation. J Clin Peridontol 1977;4:92–99
27. Bayles TB, Lewis WH Jr: Subacute bacterial endocarditis in older people. Ann Intern Med 1940;13:2154–2163
28. Gleckman R, Hibert D: Afebrile bacteraemia: a phenomenon in geriatric patients. JAMA 1982;248:1478–1481
29. Thell R, Martin FH, Edwards JE: Bacterial endocarditis in subjects 60 years of age and older. Circulation 1975;51:174–182
30. Applefeld MM, Hornick RB: Infective endocarditis in patients over 60. Am Heart J 1974;88:90–94
31. Bayliss R, Clarke C, Oakley C et al: The teeth and infective endocarditis. Br Heart J 1983;50:506–512
32. Channer KS, Bukis E, Rees JR: Overdiagnosis of infectious endocarditis. Lancet 1988;i:1395–1396
33. Lintas EM, Roberts RB, Devereaux RB, Prieto LM: Relationships between the presence of echocardiographic vegetations and the complication rate in infective endocarditis. Am Heart J 1986;112:107–113
34. Anonymous: Fever in infective endocarditis. Lancet 1986;ii: 202
35. Friedlander AH, Yoshikawa TT: Pathogenesis, management and prevention of infective endocarditis in the elderly dental patient. Oral Surg, Oral Med, Oral Pathol 1990;69:177–181
36. Tsai TP, Matloff JM, Chaux A et al: Combined valve and coronary artery bypass procedures in septuagenarians and octogenarians: results in 120 patients. Ann Thorac Surg 1986;42: 681
37. Craver JB, Weintraub WS, Jones EL et al: Predictors of mortality complications and length of stay in aortic valve replacement for aortic stenosis. Circulation 1988;78 (suppl 1):85–90
38. McGovern JA, Pennock JL, Campbell DB et al: Aortic valve replacement and combined aortic valve replacement and coronary artery bypass grafting: predicting high risk groups. J Am Coll Cardiol 1987;9:38
39. Carpentier A: Cardiac valve surgery—the "French Correction". J Thorac Cardiovasc Surg 1983;86:323–337
40. Cribier A, Savin T, Saoudi N et al: Percutaneous transluminal valvuloplasty of acquired aortic stenosis in elderly patients: an alternative to valve replacement? Lancet 1986;i:63–67
41. Letac B, Cribier A, Konig R, Lefebvre E: Aortic stenosis in elderly patients aged 80 or older. Treatment by percutaneous

valvuloplasty in a series of 92 cases. Circulation 1989;80: 1514–1520

42. Hall R, Kirk R: Balloon dilatation of heart valves. BMJ 1992; 305:487–8
43. Reyes VP, Raju BS, Wynne J et al: Percutaneous balloon valvuloplasty compared with open surgical commisurotomy for mitral stenosis. N Engl J Med 1994;331:961–967
44. Sprigings DC, Forfar JC: How should we manage symptomatic aortic stenosis in the patient who is 80 or older? Br Heart J 1995;74:481–84
45. Hammermeister KE, Sethi GK, Henderson WG et al: A comparison of outcomes in men 11 years after heart-valve replacement with a mechanical valve or bioprosthesis. N Engl J Med 1993; 328:1289–96
46. Channer KS: Doppler Insights into atrial systole. Cardiol Pract 1990;8:26–28

CHAPTER 26

Cardiac Arrhythmias

ANTHONY MARTIN

Cardiac arrhythmias occur with increasing frequency with advancing age both in apparently healthy individuals and in those with cardiopulmonary disease. Rhythm disturbances produce many challenges to the physician. The diagnosis may be complex, because the presentation in older people may be related to organ systems other than the heart. The effect of an arrhythmia on the individual may be out of proportion to the severity of the arrhythmia because the circulation may be impaired by other forms of heart disease and the effects of aging on the cardiovascular system.

In general, the management of an arrhythmia does not differ with the age of the patient. However, because of the more sinister symptomatology in elderly people, the aggressiveness of treatment may need to be increased. A summary of the more important arrhythmias is shown in Table 26-1.

The Mechanisms of Arrhythmias

There are two principal mechanisms in the generation of arrhythmias. Increased automaticity in cardiac cellular tissue leads to an increased likelihood of many cardiac tissues to generate an inherent and independent rhythm. This may result in an ectopic focus of accelerated activity actually displacing the sinus node as the cardiac pacemaker. This is the mechanism thought to be responsible for atrial tachycardias.

The other mechanism that may produce an arrhythmia is the re-entry phenomenon. This probably accounts for the great majority of arrhythmias in old age. Re-entry consists of a wave of electrical excitation repeatedly circulating around a fixed anatomical obstacle, such as an area of infarction. The Lown-Ganong-Levine and the Wolf-Parkinson-White syndromes present the most well-known examples of true reentry due to electrical circulation around bypass tracts between the atria and ventricles, thus bypassing the atrioventricular node.

Re-entry may also occur around an area of functional block maintained in a refractory state by the circulation itself and probably accounts for the generation of atrial flutter. The mechanism giving rise the most common arrhythmia in old age, atrial fibrillation, is the appearance of multiple small wavelets occurring irregularly in the myocardium and invading adjacent excitable cardiac tissue.

Symptomatology of Arrhythmias

Arrhythmias may give rise to a wide variation of symptoms, usually related to the heart, the lungs, or the nervous system. As a general rule, tachycardias give rise to shortness of breath, angina, palpitations, and dizziness or fainting. Bradycardias most commonly present as dizziness or fainting, but may also present as shortness of breath or angina on exertion. Atrial fibrillation may also be complicated by thromboembolism and give rise to strokes or peripheral emboli.

The mechanism for this common symptomatology is cardiac failure and hypoperfusion of the brain. Hypoperfusion of other organs may also occur, such as the kidney and gut, but interference with the circulation in these organs does not usually give rise to presenting symptoms. The presenting symptoms may be exacerbated by other underlying pathology, such as chronic lung disease, anemia, or carotid and cerebral artery disease. There may also be concurrent cardiac disease such as senile cardiac amyloidosis and valvular disease. Thyroid disease may also precipitate cardiac arrhythmias; for example thyrotoxicosis is almost invariably associated with atrial fibrillation in the elderly and myxoedema is associated with myocardial infiltration.

Syncope (see Ch. 32) is a good example of the complex problems that face physicians. Syncope is a common and highly morbid syndrome. It accounts for up to 2 to 3 percent of all medical emergency admissions to hospital each year.[1] Approximately 25 percent of frail institutionalized elderly people have a history of syncope over a preceding 10-year period and 6 percent of nursing home residents experience syncope each year.[2]

One of the characteristic features of advancing age is the accumulation of degenerative and multiple disease processes. Some or many of these may interact to impair cerebral oxygenation and increase the risk of syncope. When cerebral oxygenation falls below a critical threshold, syncope occurs. Cardiovascular disease may cause between 21 to 34 percent of syncopal episodes in elderly people[1]—most commonly myocardial infarction, aortic stenosis, sick sinus syndrome, ventricular tachycardia, and heart block. Carotid sinus sensitivity and vagal hypersensitivity are also important contributors to syncope and are discussed in detail in Chapter 32.

Because syncopal episodes are often isolated or infrequent and the occurrence of cardiac arrhythmias very high,[3] it is often

Table 26-1 Types of cardiac arrhythmias

Bradycardias and conduction defects	
Sinus node	Sinus bradycardia Sinoatrial block Sinus arrest Sick sinus syndrome
Atrioventricular block	1st degree 2nd degree 3rd degree (complete heart block)
Bundle branch block	Left Right
Tachycardias	
Atrial	Atrial premature beats Atrial tachycardia Atrial flutter Atrial fibrillation
Nodal	AV Nodal re-entrant tachycardia AV re-entrant tachycardia
Ventricular	Ventricular premature beats Ventricular tachycardia Ventricular fibrillation

very difficult to relate the symptoms directly to demonstrable arrhythmias. The finding of atrial premature beats or repetitive ventricular premature beats in a patient being investigated for syncope is not an indication for pharmacological intervention because the treatment is likely to cause a more adverse outcome than the arrhythmia itself. Indeed, these common arrhythmias have not been shown to be associated with subsequent coronary events.[4] However, documented episodes of cardiac standstill, as in the sick sinus syndrome or heart block, or substantial periods of tachycardia, as in atrial fibrillation or ventricular tachycardia, do require treatment.

The Diagnosis

Arrhythmias must always be documented by electrocardiographic evidence. Even experts can confuse atrial fibrillation with frequent ventricular premature beats on clinical examination. A resting 12-lead electrocardiogram (ECG) will only demonstrate a small proportion of arrhythmias. Ambulatory electrocardiography or dynamic electrocardiography (DCG) will demonstrate about five times as many arrhythmias as a resting ECG, but is really only applicable to patients who have frequent episodes of arrhythmias because it is rarely practicable to record DCGs for more than 24 to 48 hours. For more infrequent arrhythmias an "events" recorder which is patient-activated is the investigation of choice. Modern events recorders have a loop facility which records the ECG tracing for some 20 seconds before the "event". Many of these devices have the ability to transmit telephonically and can enable instant diagnosis. For more complex arrhythmias, electrophysiological investigation may be required.

For dynamic ECG investigation it is important to try and correlate the event with a rhythm abnormality, but in practice this is difficult in older people. However, an absence of rhythym abnormalities in a patient with many and frequent symptoms can be a useful way of excluding an arrhythmia as the cause of the symptomatology. Table 26-2 presents electrocardiographic techniques used in the diagnosis of rhythm abnormalities.

Bradycardias and Heart Block

Sinus node function

The decline in the sinus node discharge rate with advancing years is hardly significant.[5] Sinus bradycardia does not appear to be a normal response to aging[6] and the finding of 4 percent in our series of ambulant elderly individuals was most probably due to the concurrence of underlying heart disease.[3]

Sinus arrhythmia is known to decrease with age.[3,7] Similarly, there may be a marked reduction in the dynamic range of heart rate.[3] These findings are probably due to latent myocardial disease, age-related partial autonomic paresis or degenerative sinus node disease—a variety of the sick sinus syndrome. The following table shows sinus node function in three reported studies in apparently healthy ambulant elderly individuals (Table 26-3).

Sinus pauses are one of the features of the sick sinus syndrome (Fig. 26-1). This syndrome is a result of muscle cell degeneration in the sinus node and their replacement with fibrous tissue.[9] Sinus pauses may be prolonged and lead to

Table 26-2 Electrocardiographic techniques used in the diagnosis of arrhythmias

Passive techniques	
Resting electrocardiography	12-lead surface ECG Esophageal electrogram
Ambulatory monitoring	Telemetry Holter monitoring Holter/statistical features in implanted pacemakers
Events monitoring	Transtelephonic devices "Memory loop" recorders
Provocative techniques	
Exercise testing	Treadmill Bicycle ergometer
Drug bolus injection	Adenosine Isoprenaline Atropine
Autonomic maneuvres	Valsalva maneuvre Diving reflex Carotid sinus massage
Electrophysiological study	Programmed electrical stimulation

Table 26-3 Sinus node function in three reported studies in apparently healthy ambulant elderly individuals

Author	No.	Age	Definition of Study Group	Sinus Bradycardia (%)	Sinus Pauses (%) (<40 beats/min) (>2 s)
Camm et al.[3]	106	75–95	Ambulatory, elderly subjects living at home	4	0
Fleg and Kennedy[4]	98	60–85	Normal physical, ECG, chest X-ray, exercise test. No cardiovascular medications	2	0
Manyari et al.[8]		60–96	Normal physical, ECG, chest X-ray, biochemistry, M-mode echo, spirometry. No cardiovascular medication	0	0

syncopal attacks. Occasionally, they may be associated with alternating periods of atrial fibrillation and sinus bradycardia—the "Tachycardia-bradycardia" syndrome (Fig. 26-2). This syndrome produces a very challenging hemodynamic situation and nearly always leads to major symptoms.

Atrioventricular block

First degree atrioventricular (AV) block, with a P-R interval greater than 0.22 seconds increases with age and does not appear to be related to clinical heart disease.[10] First degree AV block occurs in between 5 to 10 percent of apparently healthy old people. It is usually an incidental finding, unless associated with digitalis toxicity, and is not associated with an adverse prognosis.[11]

Higher degrees of AV block are rarely found in the healthy older person and intermittent incomplete heart block has been reported as occurring in only 1 to 4 percent in studies of ambulant elderly people.[3,6,12] Incomplete heart block may cause symptoms and, if so, should be treated with permanent cardiac pacing. If asymptomatic, no specific treatment is required. Complete, or third degree, AV block is almost always associated with symptoms, usually syncope, and is an indication for permanent cardiac pacing (Fig. 26-3).

Cardiac Pacing

A comprehensive review of cardiac pacing would be inappropriate in this chapter. However, the increasing need to pace more and more elderly people with the sick sinus syndrome or complete AV block has raised several issues about the specific considerations that pertain in people of this age group. The indications for pacing in sinus node disease are shown in Table 26-4 and the indications for pacing in atrioventricular block are shown in Table 26-5.

The first cardiac pacemaker was implanted in Sweden in 1958. Since that time remarkable progress has occurred. The development of lithium battery technology has allowed greatly increased longevity and diminished size of the pulse generator. Microprocessor-based circuitry has made pacemaker programmability and telemetric functions possible. Advances in lead technology and transvenous implantation techniques has led to single and dual chamber rate-adaptive pacing.

The complexity of modern pacing systems has led to the development of a generic pacemaker code by a joint working party of the North American Society of Pacing and Electrophysiology (NASPE) and the British Pacing and Electrophysiology Group (BPEG).[13] Table 26-6 shows the generic pacemaker code.

Pacing systems can be characterized as single lead ventricular, such as VVI or ventricular sensing and pacing and inhibited, or atrial based, such as AAI or atrial demand. Dual chamber pacing is becoming increasingly used and DDD refers to atrial and ventricular units that sense and pace both atrium and ventricle and the response to pacing may be triggered and inhibited.

Rate-responsive, or rate-adaptive, systems utilize nonatrial sensors to control the pacing rate on exercise. In the pacemaker code rate-responsive pacemakers are designated with a fourth letter, R, so that a VVI unit that is rate-responsive becomes VVIR.

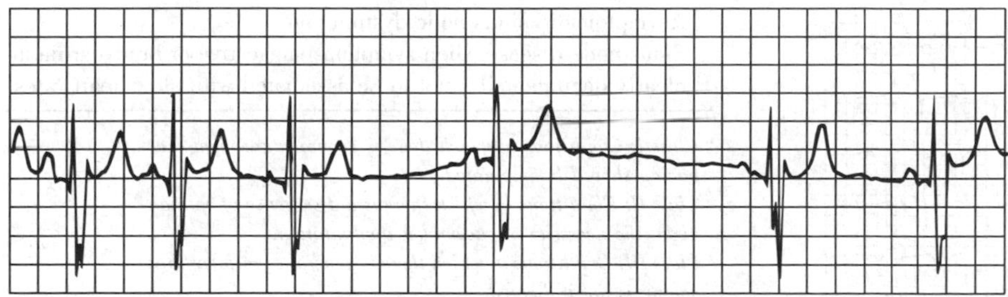

Figure 26-1 Sinus pause interrupted by an atrial escape beat.

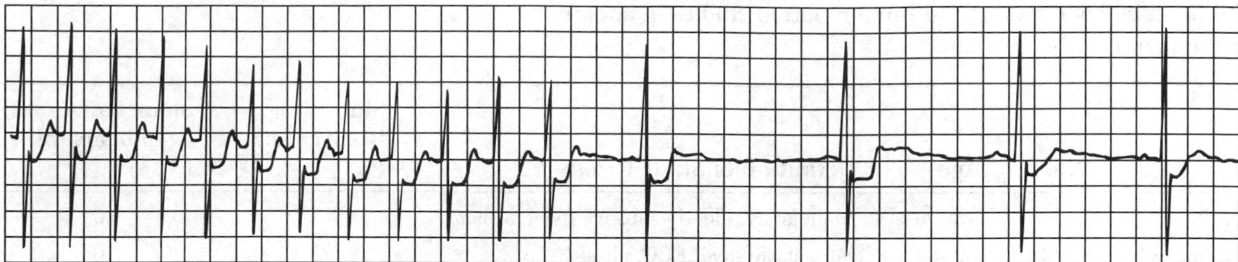

Figure 26-2 Tachycardia-bradycardia syndrome. A run of supreventricular tachycardia followed by sinus bradycardia.

Most pacemaker recipients are elderly, so age alone should never be a contraindication to pacing, or indeed, the use of complex and expensive units. No longer should pacing be regarded as simply a way to prevent Stokes-Adams attacks or life-threatening bradyarrhythmias. Recently, the advantage of maintaining atrial function and atrioventricular synchrony in elderly people has been recognized and dual chamber pacing produces much greater exercise tolerance and higher quality-of-life measures. Single ventricular pacemakers, even if rate-responsive (VVIR), are functionally far inferior to atrial-based systems in those with the sick sinus syndrome.

The mechanism for the increased contribution of atrioventricular synchrony to cardiac output is that elderly hearts have both reduction and delay in passive diastolic left ventricular filling, due to reduced left ventricular compliance. In older patients there is a twofold increase in the atrial contribution to resting cardiac output compared with younger patients.[14]

Another important factor in elderly people is the "pacemaker syndrome". This may be defined as "the signs and symptoms related to the adverse haemodynamic and electrophysiological consequences of ventricular pacing".[15] This syndrome occurs in the presence of a normally functioning ventricular pacemaker. It may more rarely occur in dual chamber pacing and then it is due to inadequate timing of atrial and ventricular contractions.

Many patients with the sick sinus syndrome have preserved ventriculoatrial conduction and about 30 to 40 percent of patients with partial or complete AV block may also exhibit ventriculoatrial conduction. It is this reverse conduction, especially seen with VVIR pacemakers, that is principally responsible for the pacemaker syndrome. The loss of atrioventricular synchrony is not the only direct mechanism for the pacemaker syndrome, because reversed ventriculoatrial conduction may produce a "negative" atrial kick. Thus atrial fibrillation with ventricular pacing cannot produce the pacemaker syndrome.

Not all patients with the pacemaker syndrome have symptoms, which are generally caused by sudden falls in cardiac output. This situation may be manifested by a myriad of symptoms, which include syncope, cardiovascular collapse, heart failure, dyspnoea, and reduction in exercise tolerance. The syndrome may occur some time after the pacemaker has been implanted. Many patients are more comfortable and energetic when changed from a VVI to DDD pacing, even if they do not have significant prior symptoms.[16] The pacemaker syndrome is an iatrogenic condition[17] and can simply be cured by restoring atrioventricular synchrony, usually with a dual chamber pacemaker.

Pacing in the sick sinus syndrome should be with an atrial-based dual chamber system, unless there is chronic atrial fibrillation. This method will reduce the incidence of the pacemaker syndrome because ventricular-atrial conduction is more common in the sick sinus syndrome. Atrial pacing will also reduce the occurrence of supraventricular arrhythmias, especially atrial fibrillation. Atrial-based pacing is not only more

Figure 26-3 Complete atrioventricular block.

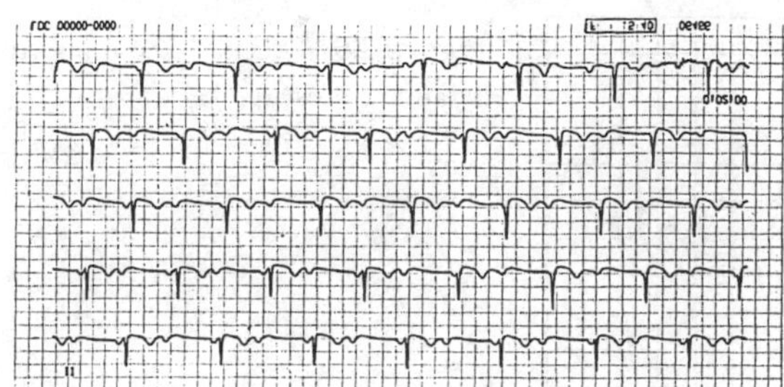

Table 26-4 Indications for pacing in sinus node disease

Class I[a]
Sinus node disease with documented symtomatic bradycardia
Class II[b]
Sinus node disease with heart rates below 40 bpm with no clear association of bradycardia and symptoms
Class III[c]
Asymptomatic sinus node dysfunction
Sinus node disease when symptoms suggestive of bradycardia are clearly documented—not to be associated with slow heart rates

[a] *Class I: Conditions in which there is general agreement that pacing should be implanted.*
[b] *Class II: Conditions in which there is a divergence of opinion about the necessity of pacemaker implantation.*
[c] *Class III: Conditions in which there is general agreement that pacing is not indicated.*

Table 26-5 Indications for pacing in atrioventricular block

Class I
- Complete heart block (intermittent or persistent) with
  - Symptomatic bradycardia
  - Congestive heart failure
  - Asystole of more than 3 sec
  - Heart rates less than 40 bpm
  - Confusional states that clear with temporary pacing
- Second degree heart block with symptomatic bradycardia
- Atrial fibrillation or flutter with any of the above conditions

Class II
- Asymptomatic complete heart block with heart rates greater than 40 bpm
- Asymptomatic Type 11 second degree heart block

Class III
- First degree heart block
- Asymptomatic type 1 (Wenckebach) second degree heart block

effective than VVI pacing, but will reduce the mortality as well as increasing quality-of-life measures.[16] Many feel that VVI pacing in the sick sinus syndrome is contraindicated, even if there are paroxysmal supraventricular arrhythmias, and that the only indication for VVI or VVIR pacing modes is chronic atrial fibrillation or atrial flutter with atrioventricular block or a slow ventricular response.[18]

Tachyarrhythmias

Atrial

Atrial premature beats (APBs) occur with great frequency in elderly people.[3] Frequently occurring APBs may be difficult to distinguish from atrial fibrillation clinically. APBs increase in frequency with advancing years and in those with known heart disease. Although APBs may trigger a paroxysm of atrial fibrillation or supraventricular tachycardia they are of no clinical significance when found as an incidental finding.

Multifocal atrial tachycardia

This condition is characterized by an atrial rate greater than 100 beats per minute (bpm) and usually less than 150 bpm. P waves of varying morphology and variable P-P, P-R, and R-R intervals. It is an uncommon condition and is frequently misdiagnosed.[19] It usually occurs in acutely ill old people, especially those with chronic pulmonary disease. It is often precipitated by β-agonists, digoxin, and toxic levels of tricyclic antidepressants. It may be associated with a high mortality unless properly treated with a β-blocking agent, such as metoprolol or sotalol. Chronic multifocal atrial tachycardia may degenerate into atrial fibrillation.

Atrial tachycardia with AV block

If the atrial rate exceeds 150 bpm, second degree heart block usually occurs. Atrial tachycardia with AV block is another manifestation of digoxin toxicity and is usually seen in patients with organic heart disease. Merely stopping the digoxin and maintaining the serum potassium level at the upper range of normal may be sufficient treatment. Other antiarrhythmic therapy may not be necessary and may, indeed, complicate the management. Phenytoin is the drug of choice if such therapy is deemed necessary.

Atrial fibrillation

Atrial fibrillation (AF) is the most common and important clinically significant arrhythmia in elderly people. In our own series of 106 apparently healthy ambulant subjects over the age of 75 years we found that 11 percent had either established (chronic) or paroxysmal AF.[3] Manyari et al.[8] found that only 3 percent of their subjects had AF, but their age spectrum was broader (60 to 96 years). It appears that the incidence of AF rises with age.[20] The underlying pathology is degenerative or ischemic disease in the sinoatrial node leading to the sick sinus syndrome. Atrial fibrillation is one characteristic of this syndrome.

Atrial fibrillation may also be associated with hypertension

Table 26-6 The NASPE/BPEG generic pacemaker code

Position: Category:	I Chamber(s) Paced	II Chamber(s) Sensed	III Response to Sensing	IV Programmability, Rate Modulation	V Anti-tachyarrhythmia Function(s)
	0 = none	0 = none	0 = none	0 = none	0 = none
	A = atrium	A = atrium	T = triggered	R = Simple programmable	P = Pacing (anti-tachyarrhythmia)
	V = ventricle	V = ventricle	I = inhibited	M = Multiprogrammable	S = Shock
	D = Dual (A + V)	D = Dual (A + V)	D = Dual (T + I)	C = communication R = rate modulation	D = Dual (P + S)
Manufacturers' designation only	S = single (A or V)	S = Single (A or V)			

and this mechanism accounted for about one half of the cases of AF in the Framingham study. However, the age range in this study did not extend to the very old and it is likely that hypertension is only a minor cause in elderly people.

Rheumatic heart disease, especially mitral valve disease, is associated with AF. The mechanism is probably left atrial dilatation. These patients are greatly at risk of thromboembolism. However, although patients with minor degrees of rheumatic heart disease may graduate into old age or even appear clinically for the first time in later life, their number is relatively small compared to the more usual cases of nonrheumatic AF.

Hyperthyroidism has long been recognized to contribute to the incidence of AF.[20] Indeed, the occurrence of AF with thyrotoxicosis rises with age and it is rare not to find this arrhythmia in patients with hyperthyroidism over the age of 75 years. In elderly people the arrhythmia may not disappear with treatment of the thyroid condition.

Atrial fibrillation is important for a number of reasons. It is a manifestation of significant heart disease, because apart from signifying sinus node disease, due either to ischemia or degeneration, it frequently co-exists with rheumatic mitral valve disease, which may appear clinically for the first time in elderly people. In the majority of patients AF is associated with a rapid ventricular response and this produces symptoms of heart failure and angina and requires treatment to increase the AV block and control the ventricular rate. Finally, the existence of AF, from whatever cause, is associated with an increased incidence of thromboembolic disease. The prognostic significance of AF in the elderly has been the subject of much dispute, but the studies of Martin et al.[21] and Kulbertus et al.[22] have suggested that there is a significant increased risk of mortality.

Fleg and Kennedy[6] and Manyari et al.[8] have demonstrated the existence of slow atrial tachycardia in up to 30 percent of their subjects. This is likely to be a benign variant of AF.

The hemodynamic consequences of AF are considerable. The two principle effects are first the loss of the atrial "kick" with the fibrillating atria, which may account for as much as a 10 percent loss of cardiac output. The second is the rapid ventricular rate, which prevents adequate diastolic filling and ineffective ventricular contraction. The combination of poor ventricular contraction and the loss of atrioventricular synchrony result in a catastrophic fall in cardiac output, which can be reversed by the cessation of AF or the control of the ventricular rate.

The clinical features of AF very much depend on whether it is paroxysmal or chronic and how fast is the ventricular rate. Paroxysmal AF may present as palpitations, angina, dizziness, or acute left ventricular failure since the ventricular rate tends to be fast during paroxysms of AF. Established or chronic AF is more likely to present as reduced exercise tolerance and heart failure, although patients also complain of palpitations due to recognition of an irregular rhythm. Acute left ventricular failure in elderly people is probably most commonly due to AF, although acute myocardial infarction is also an important cause of acute left ventricular failure and may itself be associated with AF in the acute phase.

Atrial fibrillation may also present with the effects of thromboembolism. The risk of a patient with AF having a stroke is about 5 percent per year. About 15 percent of all stroke cases present with AF and even non-rheumatic AF increases the risk of stroke fivefold compared with controls in sinus rhythm.[23] Other thromboembolic manifestations of AF are systemic emboli, usually in the legs.

Atrial fibrillation and stroke

The risk of embolization in patients with AF due to rheumatic heart disease is extremely high and at least 17 times those in sinus rhythm. Therefore, full anticoagulation is mandatory unless there are major contraindications. In patients with nonrheumatic atrial fibrillation the picture has, in recent times, become clear. Evidence from the Framingham Study[24] and the Oxford Community Stroke Project[25] has suggested that there is a significant increase risk of stroke in those patients with nonrheumatic AF compared to those in sinus rhythm. Furthermore, the greatest danger of death from thrombo-embolism is in the first 30 days after the stroke event.[25]

In recent years there have been five major trials that have examined the role of antithrombotics and anticoagulants in this situation. The Copenhagen AFASAK study[26] examined patients with non-rheumatic AF with a mean age of 74 years. They reported a significant reduction (59 percent) in strokes and transient ischemic attacks in those fully warfarinized, but a reduction of only 14 percent in those given aspirin. The Stroke Prevention in Atrial Fibrillation (SPAF) trial[27a] reported a 67 percent reduction in stroke in those given low dose warfarin (INR = 1.5 to 3.0), but patients over 75 years were excluded from warfarin treatment in the first phase of this study and the mean age of patients given warfarin was 65 years. The second SPAF trial[27b] included 385 patients over 75 years and they were followed up for 2 years. Warfarin reduced the incidence of stroke more than aspirin in these subjects, but the absolute benefit was offset by a higher incidence of bleeding than seen in other primary prevention trials (4.2 percent per annum compared with 1.6 percent with aspirin). These results may, in part, be due to the level of anticoagulation (INR = 2.0 to 4.5). Interestingly, those under 75 years with no other risk factors for stroke other than AF treated with aspirin had a very low rate of thromboembolism (0.5 percent annually). The Boston Area Anticoagulation Trial for Atrial Fibrillation (BAATAF) study[28] also showed a significant reduction in both stroke occurrence and mortality on low-dose warfarin and 10 percent of their patients were over 80 years. The Canadian Trial[29] using low-dose warfarin was concluded early because of the positive results shown in other trials at the time but the relative risk reduction of stroke was 37 percent in the 378 patients recruited. The Veterans Affairs Study[30] also showed a significant reduction in stroke incidence on low-dose warfarin.

The risk of bleeding in these trials of warfarin was surprisingly low and ranged from 0.5 to 1.5 percent per annum. The risks of intracranial hemorrhage increased from 0.1 to 0.3 percent per annum. There are certain measures that should be taken to minimize the risk of bleeding with warfarin. These include controlling hypertension, avoiding alcohol excess, excluding liver disease, avoiding treatment in those whom have had a cerebral hemorrhage, and avoiding concomitant aspirin or other nonsteroidal therapy. Warfarin treatment should not be started after a stroke unless cerebral hemorrhage has been excluded by computed tomography (CT) of the brain.

Aspirin has an important antiplatelet action and has been shown to decrease the risk of stroke, but is only half as effective as warfarin.[27a] Aspirin is clearly easier to monitor than warfarin and may have a place in patients with a low risk of stroke or in whom there are contraindications to warfarin treatment[31, 32] Patients with a high risk of stroke include those who have previous strokes or transient ischemic attacks, long-standing AF, large left atria, and diabetes.

Rhythm control of atrial fibrillation

Paroxysmal AF It is generally assumed that paroxysmal AF ultimately develops into established AF. The management of paroxysmal AF, therefore, should be aimed at preventing the paroxysms which will remove unwanted symptoms and, theoretically, prevent or delay the onset of established AF. The alternatives are using either Vaughan Williams Class 1 or 111 drugs. Of the Class 1c drugs, flecainide and propafenone are effective.[33,34] Despite the fears generated by the CAST study when Class lc drugs were used in the suppression of ventricular arrhythmias following myocardial infarction,[35] flecainide and propafenone have a good safety record for the management of paroxysmal AF.[36] They should probably be avoided in patients with known ischemic heart disease and heart failure. It should be remembered that all antiarrhythmic agents have some proarrhythmic effect.

Class III agents are also effective in controlling paroxysmal AF. Sotalol is useful and can be of especial benefit in those with exercise-induced AF.[34] Amiodarone is highly effective in controlling paroxysmal AF, but should be reserved for refractory cases since its unwanted effects are very extensive. The main side effects in elderly people involve the skin and thyroid. On long-term treatment with amiodarone, biochemical hypothyroidism is common and hyperthyroidism may also occur. Amiodarone is an iodinated compound and although it frequently affects the thyroid biochemistry it does not always cause clinical signs of thyroid disease. If this does occur, however, the dose of amiodarone should be reduced or stopped. The maintenance dose in elderly people can be as low as 200 mg twice a week. It is also important to remember that it interacts with both digoxin and warfarin, so care should be taken when using these combinations.

The risk of stroke in paroxysmal AF is a matter of dispute. Most authors agree that the risks are much less than in established AF, but are still greater than those in sinus rhythm. It is essential, therefore, to control the paroxysms.

Digoxin is still used by some physicians for the control of paroxysmal AF. A study examining the effects of digoxin in paroxysmal AF retrospectively showed that the paroxysms of AF were longer and the heart rate in these paroxysms was not reduced.[37] However, a later randomised, placebo-controlled trial showed that digoxin reduced both the frequency of symptomatic attacks and the heart rate during the attacks.[38] However, digoxin in not particularly useful in the management of paroxysmal AF.

Established AF Established AF may be persistent—in that sinus rhythm may be possible—or permanent, when it is impossible to produce sinus rhythm. In elderly people the permanent variety is very much more common and there are few people who can benefit from attempted cardioversion, whether electrically or by drug treatment. At the onset of AF it is not always possible to be sure whether AF is persistent or permanent. In this situation a conservative approach is reasonable. The majority of people with persistent AF will tend to return to sinus rhythm whether treatment is instituted or not. Clearly, if the heart rate is high and cardiac decompensation results, then treatment with digoxin or a calcium-channel blocker, such as dilitiazem, or a β-blocker, such as esmelol, (pindolol), is indicated.

The mainstay of rate control in established permanent AF in the resting state remains digoxin. It is effective in controlling the heart rate in the majority of people, but in those with AF due to accessory pathway re-entry AF, digoxin may worsen the arrhythmia. Digoxin is not be very effective in controlling the heart rate during exercise since its mechanism of action is vagotonic. If this is the case the addition of a β-blocking drug with intrinsic sympathomimetic properties, such as pindolol 5 mg b.d. may be very useful.[39] It is usually possible to reduce the dose of digoxin to at least 0.0625 mg using this combination. If this regimen is not effective, the addition of diltiazem or amiodarone to a small dose of digoxin may prove effective.

Digoxin has a very narrow therapeutic ratio and in elderly patients is likely to induce toxic effects. This is especially likely in patients with renal impairment, and is is worth remembering that elderly people often have impaired renal function even in the presence of normal serum urea and creatinine levels. Potassium reduction in the serum may also induce toxic effects of digoxin and it is important to supplement loop diuretics with oral potassium. Digoxin also interacts with amiodarone and quinidine and extreme care should be taken with these combinations. The first signs of digoxin toxicity in the elderly are likely to be serious arrhythmias because nausea and vomiting are usually absent.

In North America there is a tendency to use Class la drugs, such as quinidine and disopyramide, for the control of AF, especially after cardioversion. However, these agents are prone to cause serious proarrhythmic effects and in particular, *torsades des pointes*. Cardioversion for elderly patients with permanent AF due to degenerative or ischemic causes is very unlikely to lead to sustained sinus rhythm and is not generally recommended. If it proves impossible to control the ventricular rate in AF, His bundle ablation can be performed and permanent ventricular or dual chamber pacing instituted under local anesthetic.

Atrial Flutter

Atrial flutter is a much less common arrhythmia. The atrial rate is usually about 300 bpm. The flutter waves are positive in lead VI and usually associated with a 2:1 AV block. It is probably caused by a single re-entrant circuit, usually in the right atrium and may be associated with cor pulmonale.

Atrial flutter is often difficult to treat in old people. Digoxin may control the ventricular rate by increasing the AV block. Amiodarone or one of the Class 1c antiarrhythmics may convert atrial flutter to sinus rhythm, but generally the only way to effectively restore sinus rhythm is by DC cardioversion followed by oral antiarrhythmic therapy. Over time, atrial flutter usually degenerates into atrial fibrillation.

Ventricular Arrhythmias

Ventricular ectopic activity is very high in those over 65 years. Studies have shown that ventricular premature beats may occur in up 80 percent of apparently healthy old people.[3,6] This is probably a reflection of ischemic and degenerative heart disease, but may also be influenced by drugs often used in the elderly, such as digoxin and β-agonists, and electrolyte disturbances that are due to the injudicious use of diuretics. A number of studies have shown that simple ventricular premature beats when associated with apparently normal hearts have no prognostic significance.[21,40]

The most common significant ventricular arrhythmia that occurs in clinical practice is monomorphic ventricular tachycardia (VT) (Fig. 26-4). The symptoms depend on the degree of hemodynamic change and this is related to the rate of the tachycardia, the length of the episode, and the association of underlying heart disease. It may present as palpitations, dizziness, syncope, or even sudden death.

Ventricular tachycardia causes a broad complex tachycardia on the electrocardiogram. In the past, many cases of VT were misdiagnosed as supraventricular tachycardia with bundle branch block. Algorithms, such as the one suggested by Dancy and Ward,[41] have been developed to enable accurate diagnosis using the 12-lead ECG. Ventriculoatrial dissociation is diagnostic of VT but only occurs in about a quarter of cases. Structural heart disease, such as myocardial infarction or ischemia, is a very strong pointer to VT. An important development in verifying the diagnosis of broad complex tachycardia has been the introduction of the very short-acting drug adenosine given intravenously.[42] Adenosine induces temporary AV block and slows the ventricular response in atrial flutter, atrial fibrillation, and supraventricular tachycardias. It will abolish junctional tachycardias but has no effect on VT.

Partly because it is usually associated with structural heart disease, VT has an adverse prognosis and may be a precursor of sudden cardiac death, especially if there is depressed ventricular function.[43]

The management of VT is difficult. Emergency treatment is best with intravenous lignocaine, which has a short half life. If this is ineffective intravenous flecainide or disopyramide can be used. If these fail DC cardioversion should be used. The long-term management of VT can also be with drugs, and amiodarone is probably the most effective, despite its high side effect profile (see above). Because of the importance of of controlling VT it is important to monitor treatment with Holter ambulatory monitoring and use signal averaged electrocardiography to detect late potentials. Programmed electrical stimulation is also useful because it can empirically test the efficacy if different drugs.

The management of asymptomatic ventricular premature beats is not to give drug therapy. This advice is based on evidence from the CAST study, where there was an increased mortality on treatment with encainide and flecainide.[35]

β-blocking drugs are known to have a protective effect after myocardial infarction and are just as effective in the elderly as they are in the young. The specific mechanism by which β-blocking drugs reduce sudden cardiac death is unknown but, unless contraindicated, should be used in the elderly.

The management of serious ventricular arrhythmias associated with structural heart disease and a low ejection fraction may require aggressive interventional procedures. These include cardiac surgery, including coronary artery bypass grafting, ventricular resection, and ablation. It has been shown that despite a higher operative mortality, the benefits may be as great in the old as in the young.[44] Implantation of automatic implantable cardioverter defibrillators may also have a place in older people if it is difficult to control the ventricular arrhythmia by simpler means.[45]

Figure 26-4 Ventricular tachycardia.

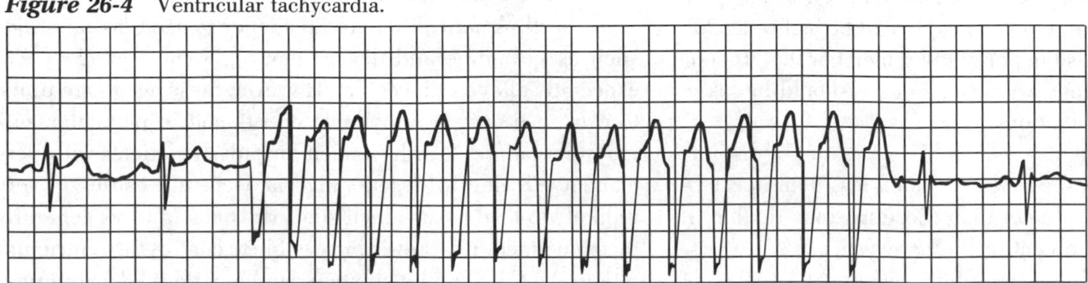

References

1. Lipsitz LA: What's different about syncope in the aged. Am J Ger Cardiol 1993;2:37–41
2. Lipsitz LA, Wei JY, Rowe JW: Syncope in an elderly, institutionalised population: prevalence, incidence and associated risk. Q J Med 1985;216:45–54
3. Camm AJ, Evans KE, Ward DE, Martin A: The rhythm of the heart in active elderly subjects. Am Heart J 1980;99:598–603
4. Fleg JL, Kennedy HL: Longterm prognostic significance of ambulatory electrocardiographic findings in apparently healthy subjects over 60 years of age. Am J Cardiol 1992;70:748–751
5. Landowne M, Brandfonbrener M, Shock NW: The relation of age to certain measures of performance of the heart and circulation. Circulation 1955;11:567
6. Fleg JL, Kennedy HL: Cardiac arrhythmias in a healthy elderly population: detection by 24-hour ambulatory electrocardiography. Chest 1982;81:302–307
7. Faulkner JM: The significance of sinus arrhythmias in old people. Am J Med Sci 1980;180:42–47
8. Manyari DE, Peterson C, Johnson D et al: Atrial and ventricular arrhythmias in asymptomatic active elderly subjects: correlation with left atrial size and left ventricular mass. Am Heart J 1990; 119:1069–1076
9. Davies MJ, Pomerance A: Quantitative study of ageing changes in the human sinoatrial node and internodal tracts. Br Heart J 1972;34:150–152
10. Fisch C, Genovese PK, Dyke RW et al: The electrocardiogram in persons over 70. Geriatrics 1957;12:616–620
11. Rodstein M, Brown M, Wolloch L: First degree atrioventricular heart block in the aged. Geriatrics 1968;23:159–165
12. Glasser SP, Clark PI, Appelbaum HJ: Occurrence of frequent complex arrhythmias detected by ambulatory monitoring: findings in an apparently healthy asymptomatic elderly population. Chest 1979;75:565–568
13. Bernstein AD, Camm AJ, Fletcher RD et al: The NASPE/BPEG generic pacemaker code for antibradyarrhythmia and adaptive-rate pacing and antitachyarrhythmia devices. PACE 1987;10: 794–799
14. Barold SS: Permanent cardiac pacing in the elderly patient: is selection of the pacing mode important? Am J Geriatr Cardiol 1993;2:12–29
15. Ausubel K Furman S The pacemaker syndrome. Ann Intern Med 1985;103:420–429
16. Hesselson AB, Parsonnet V, Bernstein AD et al: Deleterious effect of long-term single-chamber ventricular pacing in patients with sick sinus syndrome. The hidden benefits of dual chamber pacing. J Am Coll Cardiol 1992;19:1542–1549
17. Travill CM, Sutton R: Pacemaker syndrome: an iatrogenic condition. Br Heart J 1992;68:163–166
18. Clarke M, Sutton R, Ward D et al: Recommendations for pacemaker prescription for symptomatic bradycardia. Report of a working party of the British Pacing and Electrophysiology Group. Br Heart J 1991;66:185–191
19. Kupfer YY, Arsura EL, Ismail YA, Tessler S: Multifocal atrial tachycardia: a commonly misdiagnosed rhythm in the elderly. Cardiol Elderly 1993;3:191–194
20. Sandler G, Wilson GM: The nature and prognosis of heart disease in thyrotoxicosis. QJ Med 1959;111:347–352
21. Martin A, Benbow LJ, Butrous G et al: Five year follow-up of 106 elderly subjects by means of long-term ambulatory monitoring. Eur Heart J 1984;5:592–595
22. Kulbertus H, De Laval-Rutten F, Barsch P, Pettit JM: is lone atrial fibrillation benign in the elderly? J Am Coll Cardiol 1983; 1:583
23. Lip GYH, Beavers DG, Singh SP, Watson RDS: ABC of atrial fibrillation: aetiology, pathophysiology and clinical features. Br Med J 1995;311:1425–1428
24. Wolf PA, Abbott RD, Kannel WB: Atrial fibrillation: a major contribution to stroke in the elderly. Arch Intern Med 1987; 147:1561–1564
25. Sandercock P, Warlow C, Bamford J et al: Is a controlled trial of long-term oral anticoagulants in patients with stroke and non-rheumatic atrial fibrillation worthwhile? Lancet 1986;1: 788–792
26. Petersen P, Boysen G, Gotdfresen J, Andcrsen ED: Placebo controlled, randomised trial of warfarin and aspirin for prevention of thromboembolic complications in chronic atrial fibrillation Lancet 1989;1:175–179
27. Stroke Prevention in Atrial Fibrillation Study Investigators: The stroke prevention in atrial fibrillation study: patient characteristics and final results of placebo comparisons. Circulation 1991; 84:527–539
28. The Boston Area Atrial Fibrillation Investigators: The effect of low-dose warfarin on the risk of stroke in patients with non-rheumatic atrial fibrillation. N Engl J Med 1990;323: 1505–1511
29. Connolly SJ, Laupacis A, Gent M et al: Canadian atrial fibrillation anticoagulant (CAFA) study. J Am Coll Cardiol 1991;18: 349–355
30. The Veterans Affairs Stroke Prevention in Nonrheumatic Atrial fibrillation investigators: N Engl J Med 1992;327:1406–1412
31. Atrial Fibrillation Investigators: Risk factors for stroke and efficacy of antithrombotic therapy in atrial fibrillation. Arch Intern Med 1994;154:1449–1452
32. Laupacis A, Albers GW, Dalen JE et al: Antithrombotic therapy in atrial fibrillation. Chest 1995;108(suppl):352–359S
33. Anderson JL, Gilbert EM, Alpert BL et al: Prevention of symptomatic recurrence of paroxysmal atrial fibrillation in patients initially tolerating antiarrhythmic therapy: a multicentre, double-blind crossover study of flecainide and placebo with trans-telephonic monitoring. Circulation 1989;80:1557–1570
34. Antman EM, Beamer AD, Cantillon C, et al: Therapy of refractory symptomatic atrial fibrillation and atrial flutter: a staged care approach with new antiarrhythmic drugs. J Am Coll Cardiol. 1990;15:698–707
35. The Cardiac Arrhythmia Suppression Trial (CAST) Investigators: Preliminary report: effect of encainide and flecainide on mortality in a randomised trial of arrhythmia suppression after myocardial infarction. N Engl J Med 1989;321:406–412
36. Pritchett EL, Wilkinson WE: Mortality in patients treated with flecainide and encainide for supraventricular arrhythmias. Am J Cardiol 1991;67:976–980

37. Rawles JM, Metcalfe MJ, Jennings K: Time of occurrence, duration and ventricular rate of paroxysmal atrial fibrillation: the effect of digoxin. Br Heart J 1990;63:225–227
38. Murgatroyd FD, O'Nunain S, Gibson SM et al: The results of the CRAFT-1: a multicenter, double-blind, placebo-controlled crossover study of digoxin in paroxysmal atrial fibrillation. J Am Coll Cardiol 1993;21(abstr):478
39. Wang R, Camm AJ, Ward D et al: Treatment of chronic atrial fibrillation in the elderly. J Am Ger Soc 1980;28:529–534
40. Cruz-Jentoft AJ, Zamorano JL, Perez-Casar F, Ribera JM: Holter monitoring in healthy elderly subjects: a five year follow-up study. Cardiol Elderly 1993;2:97–101
41. Dancy M, Ward DE: Diagnosis of ventricular tachycardia: a clinical algorithm. Br Med J 1985;291:1036–1038
42. DiMarco JP, Miles W, Akhtar M: Adenosine for paroxysmal supraventricular tachycardia: dose ranging and comparison with verapamil. Assessment in placebo-controlled, multicenter trials. The Adenosine for PSVT Study Group. Ann Intern Med 1990; 113:104–110
43. Mukharji J, Rude RE, Poole W et al: Risk factors for sudden death after acute myocardial infarction: two year follow-up. Am J Cardiol 1984;54:31–36
44. Tresch DD, Platia EV, Guarnieri T et al: Refractory symptomatic ventricular tachycardia and ventricular fibrillation in elderly patients. Am J Med 1987;83:399–404
45. Tresch DD, Troup PJ, Thakur RK et al: Comparison of efficacy of automatic implantable cardioverter-defibrillator in patients older and younger than 65 years of age. Am J Med 1991;90: 717–724

CHAPTER 27

Vascular Surgery

U. J. KIRKPATRICK
C. N. McCOLLUM

Atherosclerosis affects the entire arterial system with consequent effects on different organ systems. The prevalence increases with advancing age, and therefore it is hardly surprising that the majority of a vascular surgeon's patients are elderly and have a full range of concomitant diseases typical of such patients. Equally, specialists in medicine for the elderly frequently find vascular disease in the patients they treat. Decisions regarding treatment need to be balanced against cardiac and respiratory risk factors, and in many patients neither invasive investigation by arteriography nor vascular surgery will be indicated. Vascular surgery is now being performed with increasing safety and patients now have longer life expectancies. These principles of balancing benefit against risk of treatment will be emphasized throughout this chapter.

We have concentrated on those subjects particularly relevant to the practice of geriatric medicine. The elderly suffer a range of vascular conditions, but we will cover the three most common problems presenting to vascular surgeons: (1) abdominal aortic aneurysm; (2) carotid disease; and (3) vascular disease of the limb—either acute or chronic. New techniques are rapidly changing the approach to the management of vascular conditions; for example, the use of percutaneous transluminal angioplasty as the sole treatment for lower-limb critical ischemia[1] and the introduction of endovascular stent-grafts for the treatment of abdominal aortic aneurysms.[2]

Abdominal Aortic Aneurysms

Prevalence and Definition

Abdominal aortic aneurysms are common. Mortality statistics from the Office of Population Censuses and Surveys show that each year approximately 10,000 deaths are due to aortic aneurysm in England and Wales. However, quoted statistics may vastly underestimate the number of deaths related to aortic aneurysms as most aneurysms remain undiagnosed and may be certified as myocardial infarction following sudden unexplained death in the elderly. Deaths from rupture are rare below the age of 50 years; deaths from rupture peak in men aged 75 to 79 years.[3]

The prevalence of true aortic aneurysms is increasing, though some would argue that this finding merely reflects improved diagnosis, changing patterns of referral, and an increased awareness of the disease.[4,5] Difficulties arise in estimating the prevalence and mortality of aneurysms because of varying definitions of aneurysm and operative mortality, especially as aneurysm is still most frequently diagnosed on postmortem examination.

The Vascular Surgery Society proposed that an aneurysm was by definition 50 percent dilated above normal, normal being an estimate taken from the literature and adjusted for gender and radiologic modality.[6] Collin suggested that an abdominal aortic aneurysm was present by definition when the infrarenal aorta was at least 4 cm in diameter or exceeded the maximum diameter of the aorta between the origin of the superior mesenteric and left renal arteries by at least 0.5 cm.[7] Sterpetti has suggested that an abdominal aneurysm is present when the ratio of infrarenal to suprarenal measurements is 1.5 or greater.[8] Screening of 4,237 men and women aged 65 to 80 years around Chichester, U.K. yielded aneurysms of 3 cm or more in 4.3 percent of cases and *aneurysmal changes* can be detected in 10.7 percent of men in the eighth decade of life.[9,10] The prevalence rates of aneurysms are higher in certain subgroups such as male hypertensives over the age of 50, first-degree male relatives of patients with proven aneurysms, and patients with peripheral vascular disease.[11–13]

Clinical Presentation

Although most aneurysms are asymptomatic or present with rupture, they may cause back or abdominal pain. This is not always classic lumbar back pain, and all vague abdominal pains in patients with an abdominal aortic aneurysm should be attributed to the aneurysm until proved otherwise. Alternatively, first presentation may be that of acute leg ischemia due to distal emboli from the aneurysm, although this is surprisingly rare.

When an aortic aneurysm ruptures, the patient presents with severe back or abdominal pain and hemorrhagic shock. Patients with retroperitoneal rupture, where the bleed is contained by the pressure of surrounding tissues, are more likely to reach hospital alive, but still the vast majority of patients die before arrival at the hospital.[14] Less common presentations include rupture of the aneurysm into the vena cava (leading to a massive arteriovenous fistula and high-output cardiac failure) or gastrointestinal tract (hematemesis and melena) due to an aortoduodenal fistula.

Natural History

Aneurysms less than 5 cm seldom rupture, but the outlook for larger aneurysms is grim; the 2-year mortality for aneurysms greater than 6 cm may be as high as 72 percent, though this high mortality does reflect a bias against operating on patients who are unfit at diagnosis. However, the majority of deaths in patients with large aneurysms are due to aneurysm rupture.[15,16] The expansion rate of abdominal aortic aneurysms depends on aneurysm size and in small aneurysms is approximately 2 mm/year, but growth is neither consistent, steady, or predictable.[17] Growth rates tend to accelerate as the aneurysm size increases and the only reliable predictor of aneurysm rupture is aneurysm size.[8,15,18] Irrespective of size, aneurysms that are giving rise to symptoms, or that are tender, should be investigated with a view to surgery as soon as possible.

Diagnosis

Most aneurysms are detected as asymptomatic findings, usually either on physical examination or on abdominal ultrasound (Fig. 27-1). Physical examination tends to overestimate aneurysm size by about 20 percent owing to overlying retroperitoneal tissue and the thickness of the abdominal wall.[19] Although ultrasound is the most cost-effective imaging method for diagnosis and follow-up, further information should be obtained prior to elective repair. The relationship to the origin of the renal arteries should be defined, and patency and diameter of the iliac arteries confirmed. Most aortic aneurysms are infrarenal. If there is suprarenal extension of the aneurysm, the operative difficulty increases, as does the operative mortality due to the need to cross-clamp above the renal arteries with subsequent increased risk of renal embolization and renal failure. Specialist centers favor either computed tomography (CT) (Fig. 27-2) or nuclear magnetic resonance imaging (MRI) for this assessment. Both are noninvasive and are sensitive to the level of the renal arteries.[20] Neither provides adequate information on occlusive arterial disease, either viscerally or peripherally, although MRI angiography is an option. Arteriography has been found to be unhelpful as it underestimates the extent of the aneurysm due to luminal thrombus.

Mortality From Rupture

The operative mortality for a ruptured aneurysm varies between centers from 31 to 64 percent.[21,22] However, this represents only the tip of the iceberg, as the overall mortality is greater than 85 percent with only a minority of patients reaching hospital alive.[14] Mortality rates for emergency surgery have improved very little over the years, with an overall mortality rate in the UK of around 70 percent but with lower mortality rates in specialized vascular centers.[23]

Operative Mortality

The 30-day mortality for elective aneurysm surgery ranges from 1.9 to 7.5 percent depending on the series of patients and the center.[24,25] Generally, in the U.K. mortality rates for elective surgery should be around 5 percent.

Operative mortality is increased by symptomatic occlusive atherosclerotic disease, chronic pulmonary disease, hypertension, and impaired renal function.[26] Intraoperative hypotension, left renal vein ligation, and blood loss greater than 4

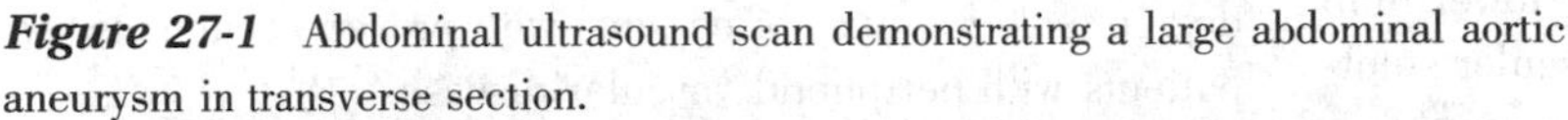

Figure 27-1 Abdominal ultrasound scan demonstrating a large abdominal aortic aneurysm in transverse section.

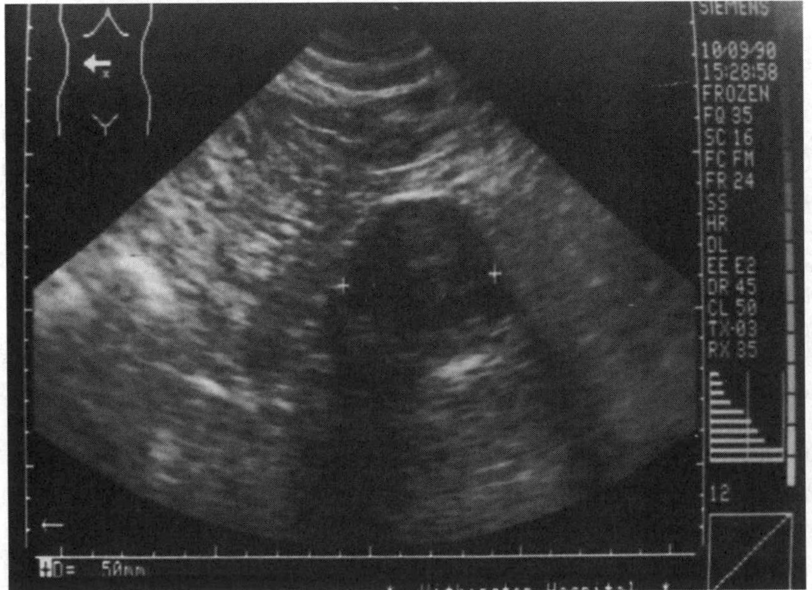

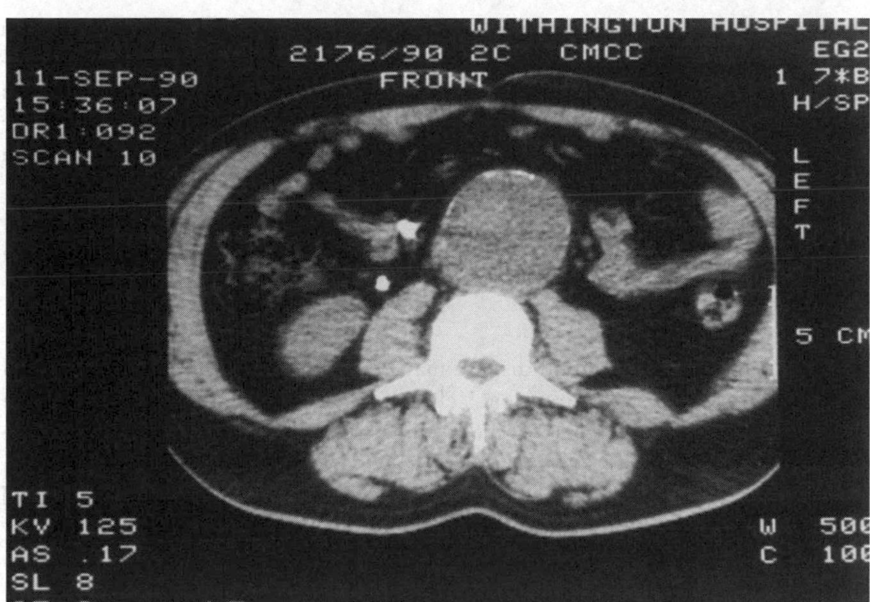

Figure 27-2 CT scan showing a large (8-cm diameter) abdominal aortic aneurysm. Note the heavily calcified wall.

units are associated with increased mortality.[27,28] Postoperative renal failure is the strongest predictor of death.[22] Following successful aneurysm repair, prognosis is excellent, with a life expectancy comparable to an age- and sex-matched population.[26]

Cardiac Complications

Aneurysm patients tend to have increased operative risk due to concomitant cardiac and pulmonary disease. Just under half of these patients have a prior history of cardiac symptoms.[29,30] Myocardial infarction is the most frequent cause of death in patients undergoing elective aneurysm repair. If there is a history of significant angina, coronary angiography should be considered to define the extent of coronary artery disease prior to elective surgery. An echocardiogram may be of some value in identifying segmental wall motion abnormalities indicative of underlying ventricular dysfunction and in providing an estimate of the left ventricular ejection fraction. Patients with an ejection fraction greater than 60 percent are unlikely to run into significant cardiac problems postoperatively, but a low ejection fraction is not necessarily a good predictor of complications.

Respiratory Complications

Severe pulmonary insufficiency with dyspnea at rest is a contraindication to surgery. A simple clinical assessment based on ability to walk or climb a flight of stairs without a rest identifies most "problem" patients, but arterial blood gases and pulmonary function tests may be useful in defining the extent of pulmonary insufficiency. Those patients with less severe obstructive lung disease require careful preoperative physiotherapy and bronchodilators to increase pulmonary capacity, thereby reducing postoperative morbidity and mortality.

Surgical approach may also influence outcome; abdominal aortic aneurysm repair has traditionally been performed via a transperitoneal approach, but an extended retroperitoneal approach may be less stressful for the elderly and those with limited pulmonary reserve.[31]

Renal Complications

After cardiac causes, renal insufficiency is the next most frequent cause of death following aortic aneurysm repair. Approximately 5 to 10 percent of patients undergoing elective abdominal aortic aneurysm repair have an elevated serum creatinine preoperatively.[29] The worse the preoperative renal function, the greater the risk of postoperative renal failure. This pre-existing renal insufficiency may be caused by repeated embolization from an atheromatous aorta, coexisting atheroma of the renal arteries, or concomitant disease such as hypertension or diabetes. It is especially important to avoid perioperative hypovolemia in these patients.

Cerebrovascular Complications

Stroke is an infrequent complication of aneurysm repair.[26] Noninvasive duplex Doppler investigation reliably identifies potentially treatable carotid artery stenosis, but carotid surgery is only of proven benefit in patients with appropriate symptoms in the relevant carotid territory.

Decreasing Operative Mortality

There are many ways to improve the outcome for patients undergoing elective abdominal aortic surgery. Patients undergoing aortic surgery should have the benefit of standard intensive monitoring including electrocardiogram (ECG), arterial pressure monitoring, and pulse oximetry, but intensive or high-dependency facilities must be available for ventilation and postoperative monitoring as required. This type of monitoring has led to a progressive decrease in morbidity and mortality, as well as a decrease in the incidence of renal complications, by minimizing periods of hypotension.[32]

Modern vascular surgery should also include a strategy for managing blood transfusion. Techniques such as preoperative donation, perioperative hemodilution, and the use of salvage autotransfusion result in an appreciable saving of bank blood transfusion, and the many risks inherent in blood transfusions are obviated.[33]

The osmotic diuretic mannitol has been used sporadically in aortic surgery for the last 30 years to maintain urine output during aortic cross-clamping.[34] More recently, mannitol has been shown to be an effective scavenger of oxygen free radicals that are produced upon the restoration of blood flow to ischemic tissues, and these are important in the development of ischemia-reperfusion injury. A prospective randomized clinical trial in elective aortic aneurysm repair has shown a significant benefit in postoperative pulmonary function in those patients who received mannitol prior to cross-clamping.[35]

Aortic Aneurysm Repair in the Elderly

Aneurysm surgery is well-tolerated in octogenarians and mortality for repair of a ruptured aneurysm is unrelated to age.[21,22] Regrettably, in a recent British survey nearly half of general practitioners would not refer an 80-year-old with a palpable aneurysm.[36] Clearly, we should take advantage of the current enthusiasm for continued medical education to ensure that appropriately selected patients are offered elective repair before rupture occurs.

New Techniques

Endovascular prosthetic stents have now been used successfully to bypass abdominal aortic aneurysms in selected patients.[37] The stent is inserted into the aorta via the femoral artery at operation; this avoids a laparotomy with its associated cardiac and respiratory morbidity in this group of high-risk patients. However, only a minority of patients are suitable for this technique as a widely patent and not too tortuous iliac system through which the graft can reach its destination is required. A suitable length of nonaneurysmal aorta below the renal arteries is essential, as is a normal aorta above the bifurcation or acceptable iliac arteries for stent attachment.[2] These measurements are all taken during spiral CT or MRI imaging.

Management of Small Aneurysms

The management of small abdominal aortic aneurysms (less than 5 cm in diameter) is controversial. Most prospective studies generally support an observational policy for aortic aneurysms less than 5 cm in maximum diameter.[38] The conservative management of patients with aneurysms less than 5 cm does not mean that the patients are discharged to await their fate, but rather involves regular ultrasound follow-up at 6- or 12-month intervals. The results of the MRC-funded UK Aneurysm Study and Small Aneurysm Trial should help resolve this controversy. This is a controlled trial that randomizes patients with abdominal aortic aneurysms between 4 and 5.5 cm to either early elective surgery or to management by close observation with regular ultrasound scanning.

Carotid Disease

Diagnosis

Carotid disease may be asymptomatic or may present with stroke, transient ischemic attacks (TIA), or possibly with vague symptoms such as dizziness. Carotid artery stenosis may cause stroke by hypoperfusion or by emboli; indeed many strokes are preceded by TIA that are often ignored by the patient and their doctor.

Carotid bruits can occur in the absence of significant internal carotid artery disease and severe carotid disease may not produce a bruit. Thus, a bruit is not a reliable indicator of underlying carotid disease.[39,40] In a study examining the predisposing factors for acute cerebral infarction, only 14 percent had cervical bruits.[41] All patients presenting with either stroke with good recovery or a TIA, who would be fit for carotid surgery, should have some form of carotid imaging; significant carotid artery disease is found in just over 30 percent of those with anterior circulation infarcts as classified by the Oxford Community Stroke Project Classification.[42,43]

Investigation of Carotid Artery Disease

Noninvasive techniques to assess the carotid arteries include color duplex Doppler, which incorporates continuous wave Doppler to estimate blood velocity and B-mode ultrasound to image the whole vessel. High-resolution B-mode scanning has also been shown to give prognostic information: echolucent (soft) plaques may have a greater propensity for embolization than echo-dense (hard) plaques.[44]

Portable continuous-wave Doppler (Fig. 27-3) can be used to assess the blood flow at the bifurcation and both the internal and external carotid arteries as far as the mandible. An experienced vascular technologist can readily distinguish the wave forms from each of these three vessels. Those from the internal carotid artery have a high diastolic component caused by low peripheral resistance from the cerebral circulation. In comparison, the external signal is more pulsatile with a sharp initial peak and usually a characteristic small second peak resembling the flow signals from the peripheral arteries. Increased blood velocity through a stenotic area is detected by increased frequency in the Doppler shift so that the grade of stenoses over 50 percent may be determined. As stenoses less than 50 percent have little or no hemodynamic significance, diagnostic accuracy and the value of the investigation improves as the degree of stenoses increases.

Although this method is simple, quick, and accurate for detecting stenoses of greater than 50 percent, mistakes may be made in heavily calcified vessels that may appear occluded

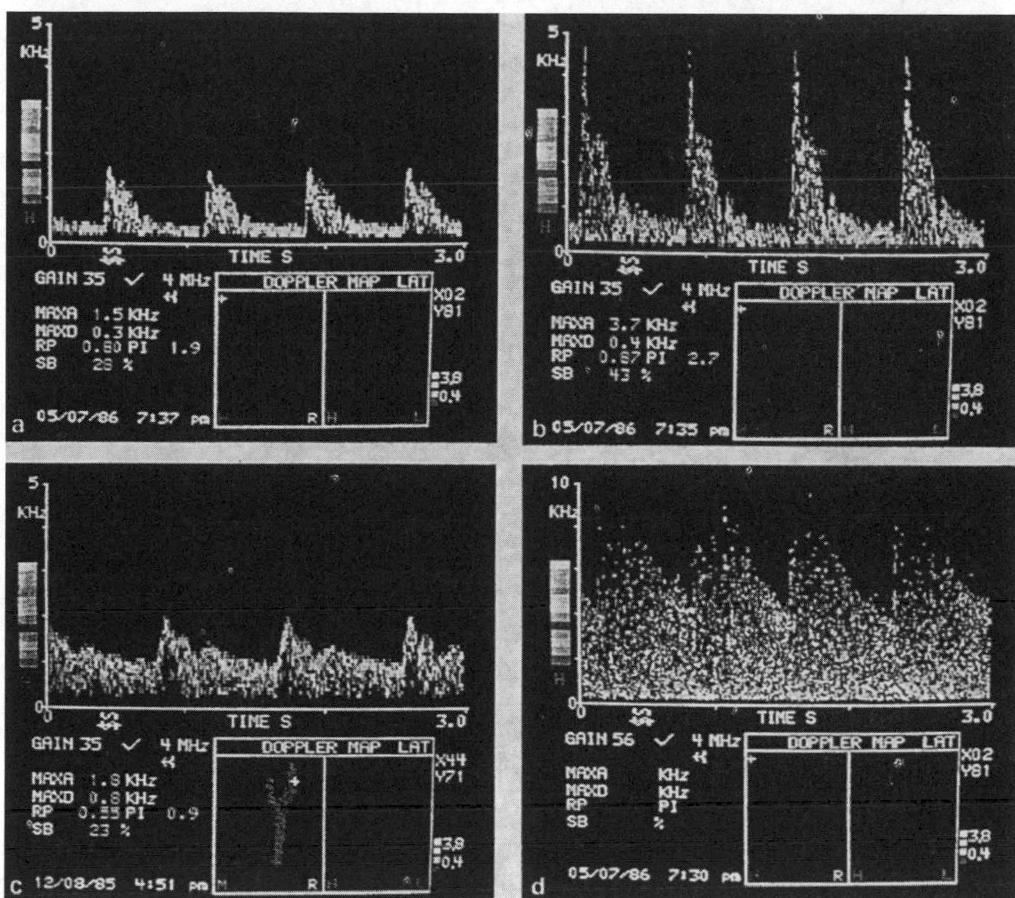

Figure 27-3 Spectrum analysis of Doppler flow signals in **(A)** normal common carotid artery; **(B)** normal external carotid artery; **(C)** normal internal carotid artery, with flow map of the common, internal, and external carotid arteries; **(D)** a stenosed internal carotid artery where there is an increase in the frequency on the vertical axis.

because the calcification may prevent ultrasound from penetrating the vessel. In these circumstances, and where there are clinical symptoms relevant to carotid artery disease, duplex Doppler (Fig. 27-4) should be used to guide therapy. Occasionally, even a duplex scan may be difficult to interpret and, in particular, the diagnosis of total occlusion may be inaccurate due to a failure to detect trickles of blood flow through a very tight stenosis. In these cases digital subtraction angiography is indicated.

The most important risk of angiography is transient or permanent neurologic deficits, with estimates ranging from 0.5 to 4 percent and 0.09 and 1.3 percent, respectively. Local complications include hematoma, dissection of the femoral artery, and embolism. Systemic complications such as allergic reactions and renal failure also occur. The overall complication rate varies from 0.9 to 10 percent.[45–48]

In contrast, color duplex ultrasound is noninvasive and essentially risk free. The issue of whether ultrasound alone is adequate as the definitive investigation prior to surgery is controversial. Advocates of angiography argue that angiography is the "gold standard" of assessment. However, atherosclerotic plaques often form on one side of the carotid artery and expand asymmetrically.[49] Angiography may well under- or overestimate the degree of carotid stenosis if a large plaque is situated asymmetrically within the vessel lumen. It is also argued that angiography is necessary to exclude additional stenotic lesions elsewhere in the cerebral circulation, typically in the carotid siphon, or coincidental cerebral aneurysms, but the relevance of these so-called tandem lesions is uncertain.[50] A recent large study suggested that carotid siphon stenosis did not alter either short- or long-term morbidity following carotid surgery.[51] If a decision is made to consider carotid surgery in patients with a recent acute stroke and significant carotid artery stenosis, a cerebral CT scan (Fig. 27-5) should be performed to exclude intracerebral hemorrhage.

In our practice, we feel that the risks and cost of angiography do not justify its routine use prior to carotid surgery. The exceptions to this policy are if the Duplex imaging is inconclusive or if the artery appears to be occluded on ultrasound when it is important to exclude the possibility of "trickle flow" through a very tight stenosis. However, there is no consensus on the use of angiography prior to carotid surgery.

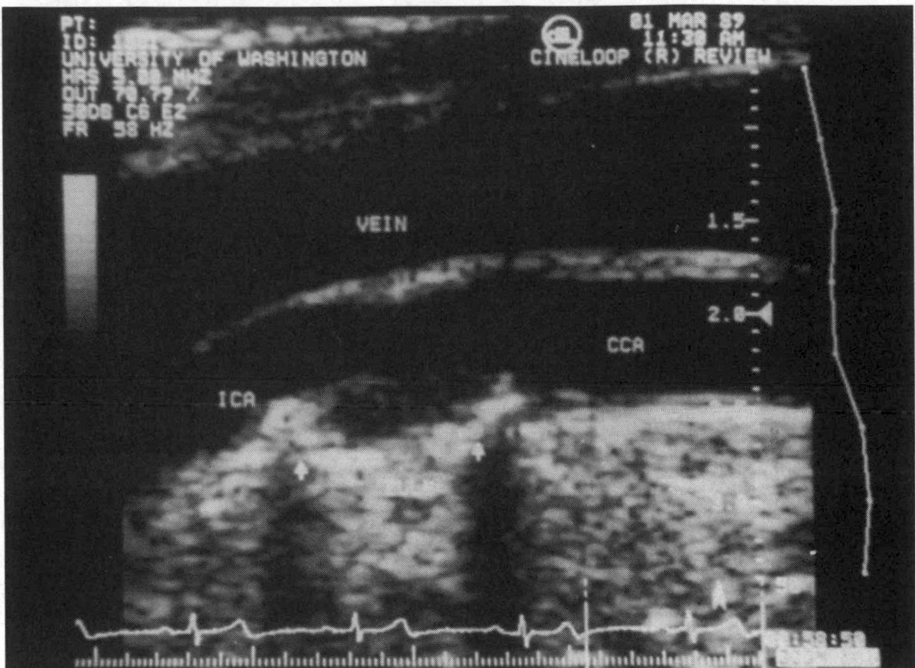

Figure 27-4 B-mode image of the carotid bulb region, demonstrating the jugular vein, common carotid (CCA), and internal carotid arteries (ICA). An ulcerated, calcified plaque is demonstrated at the origin of the internal carotid (between arrows).

Benefits of Carotid Surgery

The role of carotid surgery in the prevention of stroke in symptomatic patients with severe stenosis (70 to 99 percent) of the internal carotid artery is now well-established.[52,53] The North American Carotid Surgery Trial randomized patients from 50 clinical centers with internal carotid stenosis and a history of a hemispheric or retinal transient ischemic attack or nondisabling stroke within 120 days of onset. In patients with 70 to 99 percent stenosis (diameter reduction on angiography) of the symptomatic artery[53]: the cumulative estimated risk of an ipsilateral stroke was 26 percent in the 331 medical patients at 2 years and 9 percent in the 328 surgical patients. For a major or fatal ipsilateral stroke, the corresponding rates were 13.1 and 2 percent. The perioperative stroke and death rate was 5.8 percent, but only 2.1 percent for major stroke and death. The European Carotid Surgery Trial randomized patients who after a carotid territory nondisabling ischemic stroke, a transient ischemic attack, or amaurosis fugax were found to have a stenosis of the relevant carotid artery[52]: In 374 patients with mild carotid stenosis (less than 40 percent) there was low 3-year risk of ipsilateral stroke, so any 3-year benefit in surgery was outweighed by the risk of surgery. In patients with severe carotid stenosis (greater than 70 percent), there was a 7.5 percent risk of stroke or death within 30 days of surgery. However, during the next 3 years the risks of ipsilateral stroke were only 2.8 percent for surgery patients and 16.8 percent for control patients. At 3 years, the total risk of death or any stroke was 12.3 percent for surgery and 21.9 percent for control patients.

Figure 27-5 CT brain scan demonstrating a large cerebral infarct in the right parietal region.

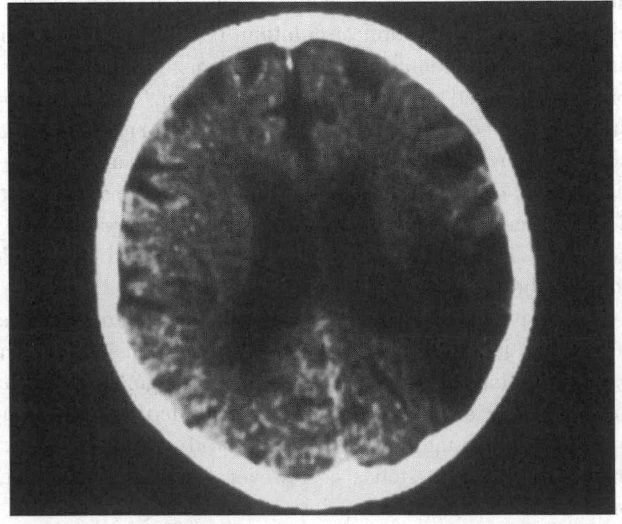

Recent data from the European Carotid Surgery Trial on 1,590 patients with symptomatic carotid stenosis of 30 to 69 percent has not supported the use of carotid endarterectomy in the management of those patients with only moderate stenosis.[54]

Asymptomatic Carotid Artery Stenosis

The question of whether to offer carotid endarterectomy to patients with asymptomatic carotid artery disease remains unanswered. The Asymptomatic Carotid Atherosclerosis Study

(USA) results suggested that endarterectomy holds a slight benefit for asymptomatic patients with 60 percent internal carotid artery stenosis.[55] However, there were methodologic anomalies and this is the first large randomized study to reach this conclusion. This finding would also have massive cost implications as it would be necessary to undertake approximately 40 carotid endarterectomies for each stroke saved. The European equivalent, the asymptomatic Carotid Surgery Trial is still ongoing and we recommend a conservative approach until the results of this study are known.

Mortality for Carotid Surgery

Current mortality and complication rates for carotid endarterectomy in the UK and Ireland are low: there is a 1.3 percent mortality and 2.1 percent stroke rate by 30 days postoperatively.[56] A combined stroke/death rate of 1.8 percent at 30 days for a small group of elderly patients aged 76 years or greater is lower, but not significantly so.[57] Other studies have also confirmed that carotid endarterectomy can be performed safely in the elderly, including nonagenarians, but outcome is dependent on the individual surgeon.[58–61] Clearly, the key issues in the decision to offer carotid surgery are the risk of stroke and the quality of life enjoyed by the patient.

Timing of Carotid Surgery After Stroke

Traditionally, surgery is delayed for 2 months in patients with acute stroke. In the 1960s several studies of the role of urgent carotid surgery were published. The results were poor, and postmortem studies often demonstrated intracerebral hemorrhage.[62,63] It was concluded that urgent surgery precipitated hemorrhage within the infarct. However, CT was not available then to exclude a primary intracerebral hemorrhage, where surgery would be clearly inappropriate. Furthermore, many of the patients in these early studies had dense neurologic deficits and were in "coma, semicoma or stupor."[64]

Interest in the role of urgent carotid surgery following acute stroke was renewed by reports of improvement in neurologic deficits in patients with progressing stroke and limited deficit.[65] The rationale for carotid surgery in such patients is twofold: first to restore cerebral perfusion and limit neuronal death, and second, to reduce early recurrence or progression of stroke due to further emboli from the diseased carotid. Urgent surgery in patients with progressing strokes and acute stable strokes have shown better results than the natural history of acute stroke in small studies, but there has been no adequate trial on carotid surgery in acute stroke since CT scans were introduced.[66–68]

Arterial Disease of the Limb

Most patients with peripheral vascular disease present with symptoms of chronic ischemia; this may range from intermittent claudication with a benign prognosis to critical ischemia presenting with rest pain, gangrene, ischemic ulceration, and the threat of amputation.

Acute ischemia of a limb may be due to emboli, but is now more usually secondary to thrombosis in diseased arteries. The majority of emboli lodge at the bifurcation of a main vessel, giving rise to distal dysfunction. Acute ischemia may present with some or all of the classical symptoms such as pain, pallor, paresthesia, paralysis, and pulseless.

Prevalence of Chronic Peripheral Vascular Disease

Atherosclerosis is the most common disease affecting peripheral arteries in the elderly and may severely limit mobility and quality of life.[69] Amputation for peripheral vascular disease or gangrene is the second most common operation in patients aged over 90 years.[70] At least one-third of patients with arterial stenosis or arterial occlusion, particularly involving the superficial femoral artery at the adductor canal, are asymptomatic.[71] However, approximately 50 percent of patients presenting with intermittent claudication have a superficial femoral artery occlusion.[72] The prevalence of claudication has been shown to be 1.0 to 1.5 percent in men aged under 50 years but rises substantially in the elderly with quoted prevalence up to 20 to 25 percent in those over 85.[73,74]

Prognosis in Chronic Vascular Disease

Only 10 percent of individuals with intermittent claudication consult a doctor and only a minority of these will ever come to surgery.[75] The outlook for the legs in patients with claudication is good, but peripheral vascular disease is a strong predictor of subsequent mortality, which more than doubles that of nonclaudicants.[76–78] The majority of claudicants die from associated cardiovascular events, in particular stroke and myocardial infarction, and this high mortality risk is only partly explained by the expected association of peripheral vascular disease with coronary artery disease due to the generalized nature of atherosclerosis.[79–81] The Speedwell prospective heart disease study has shown that men with intermittent claudication have a 30 percent 5-year mortality compared with 6 percent in men without intermittent claudication.[81]

Investigation of Chronic Vascular Disease

Investigation of patients with intermittent claudication should concentrate on identifying risk factors for cardiac and cerebrovascular events. Smoking is strongly associated with intermittent claudication and there are higher incidences of peripheral arterial disease in patients with diabetes, hypertension, and those with a high total triglyceride level.[76,81,82] In diabetic patients there is an increased frequency of involvement of small vessels with distal artery occlusion, which carries a poor prognosis.[77]

The ankle-brachial pressure index (ABPI) may be helpful in quantifying the severity of peripheral vascular disease, but only a minority of patients with abnormal APBIs are symptomatic.[83] As a general rule, patients with a mean ABPI of less than 0.6 who have symptoms or low leg ulcers need vascular surgical assessment.[84]

Rest pain, ischemic ulceration, or gangrene is an absolute indication for investigation with a view to treatment. Duplex scanning or angiography may be used to identify the sites of stenotic or occlusive lesions, but are only indicated if surgery or angioplasty is being considered. Duplex scanning has become increasingly important in the diagnosis and follow-up of arterial lesions. This is a noninvasive technique and can be repeated on many occasions to monitor the progress of the disease, graft patency, and the need for intervention. It identifies arterial occlusions and hemodynamically significant stenoses with a sensitivity and specificity of 92 and 97 percent respectively, and has the potential to replace angiography. The presence of multiple stenoses is the main limitation on diagnostic accuracy.[85–87] Duplex scanning alone can predict the indication for percutaneous transluminal angioplasty in 84 percent of cases.[88]

Treatment for Chronic Vascular Disease

The best advice for patients with claudication is to stop smoking, lose weight if appropriate, and keep walking. Exercise training can improve claudication distances by over 100 percent in 12 weeks.[89] Treatment is directed at control of risk factors for cardiovascular and cerebrovascular mortality, such as the control of hypertension, hyperlipidemia, and diabetes. Surgery or angioplasty for peripheral vascular disease is rarely indicated for intermittent claudication, but may be offered to those whose symptoms are intolerable for their lifestyle despite a period of conservative care.

The treatment for rest pain, ischemic ulceration, or gangrene depends on the state of the peripheral circulation. Development of new treatment modalities has revolutionized the revascularization of lower-limb ischemia. Percutaneous transluminal angioplasty is becoming the most frequent option in the treatment of both claudication and revascularization for critical ischemia.

Figure 27-6 A sequence of arteriograms from a patient presenting with acute on chronic right lower limb ischemia. **(A)** Demonstrates the limitations of standard preoperative angiography in this setting. There is no visualization of "run-off" below the recent occlusion in the proximal popliteal artery. **(B)** An on-table angiogram via the distal popliteal artery revealed a possible patent anterior tibial artery. This film taken on completion of the bypass (with reversed saphenous vein) demonstrates the patent run-off vessel.

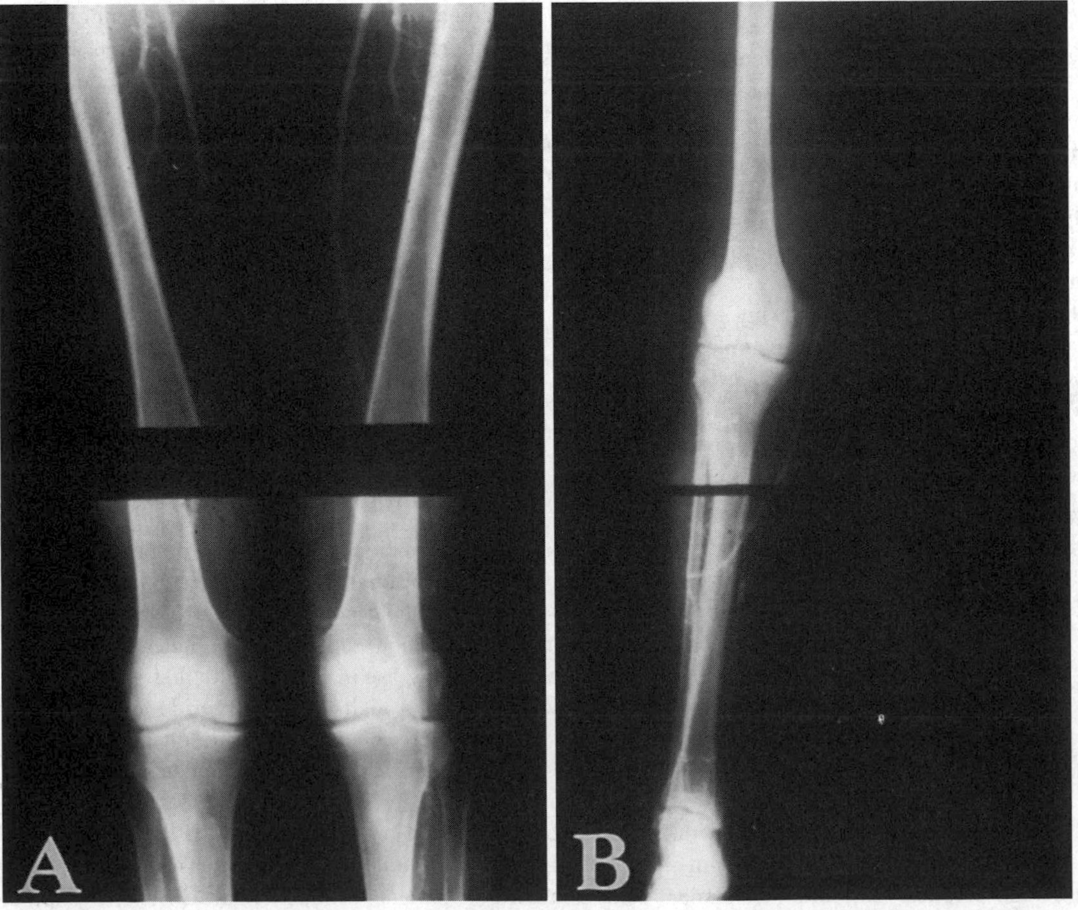

If there is a lesion amenable to angioplasty, then this should be treated. Alternatively, reconstructive surgery is indicated dependent on the level and length of arterial occlusions and the multiplicity of stenoses.

Acute Limb Ischemia

The clinical distinction between thrombosis or embolism can be difficult, but errors in diagnosis lead to a higher surgical failure rate and higher hospital mortality.[90,91] Acute ischemia of the lower limb may occur due to embolization into a previously normal arterial tree but is now more likely to be due to thrombosis in diseased arteries. The most frequent site of origin for an acute arterial embolus is from the heart, either due to poor atrial emptying in atrial fibrillation or from a mural thrombus following myocardial infarction. Alternatively, an embolus may originate from a previously undiscovered ventricular or aortic aneurysm.

Arterial emboli to the arm are usually seen only in the elderly. Approximately two-thirds of emboli are of cardiac origin, though peripheral aneurysm may account for over 20 percent of cases.[92,93] Conservative management is appropriate for many of these patients if the hand is viable and the pressure index (relative to the opposite normal arm) is greater than 0.6.[94,95] Surgical embolectomy can be performed under local anesthesia and achieves excellent results. However, there is an associated mortality of greater than 10 percent related predominantly to the underlying cardiac condition.[92]

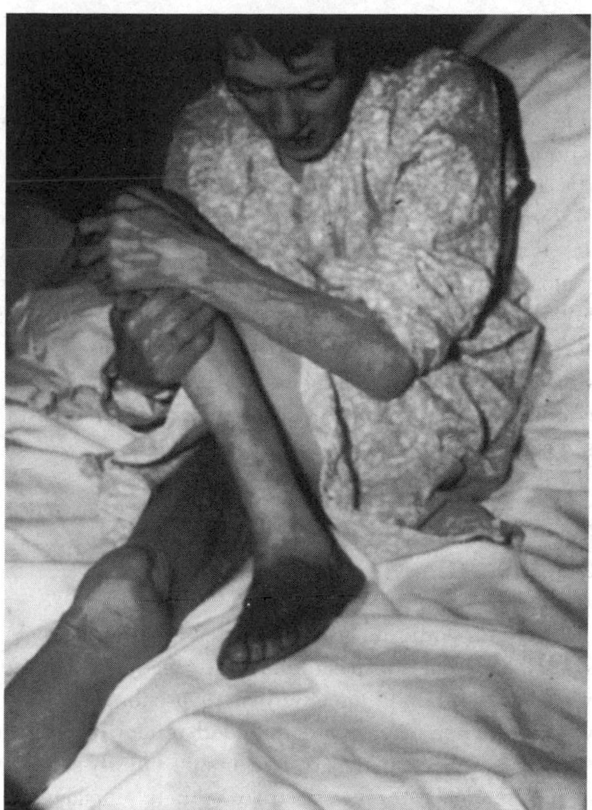

Figure 27-7 This picture demonstrates the distress, malaise, and general disability resulting from prolonged rest ischemia, often treated by opiates. Physiotherapy should be started immediately to try and release the flexion contracture of the knee.

Management of Acute Ischemia of the Leg Due to Embolism

Most surgeons in the past proceeded directly to femoral embolectomy in those patients with a strong clinical suspicion of an embolus, such as those with a short history of ischemia (less than 72 hours), a risk factor such as atrial fibrillation suggesting an embolic source, and no past history of intermittent claudication.[96] Acute embolism may be successfully treated surgically via embolectomy with a Fogarty catheter, but is associated with a 16 to 26 percent mortality due predominantly to coexisting cardiac disease.[96–98] Following embolectomy, the patient should be given long-term anticoagulant therapy, initially by heparin infusion and then with oral anticoagulants. Patients who develop an acute embolus should be investigated at least with echocardiography and possibly abdominal aortic ultrasound.

Management of Acute Ischemia Due to Thrombosis

In contrast, the management of acute or chronic ischemia is one of the more demanding surgical emergencies and should only be dealt with by an experienced vascular team. There is usually a little more time to make the diagnosis and arrange treatment as a collateral circulation may offer some protection. The patient with acute or chronic ischemia should be heparinized as soon as possible to reduce extension of the thrombus. If the limb is not completely anesthetic or paralyzed there should be sufficient time for adequate preoperative investigations by urgent duplex Doppler and angiography if indicated to assess the distal arterial tree.

Intra-arterial thrombolysis achieves lysis of such thrombi (or emboli) in approximately two-thirds of cases.[99] Accelerated techniques of lysis such as the pulse-spray method may be undertaken in as little as 30 minutes, but the higher doses of thrombolytic agents tend to increase the risk of hemorrhagic complications.[100] Following lysis the underlying arterial disease should be treated either by transluminal angioplasty or by arterial reconstruction. If percutaneous techniques are unavailable or there is little chance of success with these techniques, then surgical reconstruction is imperative. If there is insufficient time for these investigations, then "on table" operative angiography may be performed (Fig. 27-6) to assess what needs to be done, and then repeated on completion to check the adequacy of surgery and give intimation of prognosis.

Outcome of Limb Salvage for Severe Ischemia

With an aggressive policy of revascularization, limb and patient survival rates of approximately 75 percent each at 1 year may be obtained even in the elderly.[101] Almost all patients with severe leg ischemia should therefore undergo some form of limb salvage procedure as this is associated with a better quality of life (Fig. 27-7).[102] The availability of specialist vascular surgeons has been shown to reduce the frequency of major lower limb amputations with a concomitant increase in the number of distal reconstructions.[103] Even in the very elderly, arterial reconstruction to save the leg and alleviate pain is preferable to an amputation; few elderly patients regain long-term mobility with artificial limbs after lower limb amputation and most require a wheelchair from the outset with their homes adapted for wheelchair use.[97] Although the initial operative costs of reconstructive surgery are higher than those of amputation, this cost is more than offset by the duration of inpatient stay and the high community costs of amputation even in the first year.[98]

Conclusion

Surgery for aortic aneurysm enables a patient to look forward to the normal life span of his or her age-matched contemporaries. Carotid endarterectomy or revascularization for peripheral vascular disease are intended primarily to enhance quality of life. Without such treatments the elderly patient may lose independence through a stroke or limb amputation. The loss of independence and long-term care costs required by the elderly patient after limb amputation or stroke argue for the cost-effectiveness of an aggressive policy of early revascularization for limb salvage or carotid disease.

Informed consent for surgery in the elderly is especially important because of concomitant risks, but surgical intervention in appropriately selected patients is beneficial and well-tolerated. The aim of surgeons is to enhance the quality of life of the elderly patient and vascular surgery makes a particularly important contribution to this aim.

References

1. London NJM, Varty K, Sayers RD et al: Percutaneous transluminal angioplasty for lower-limb critical ischaemia. Br J Surg 1995;82:1232–1235
2. Andrews SM, Cuming R, MacSweeney ST et al: Assessment of feasibility for endovascular prosthetic tube correction of aortic aneurysm. Br J Surg 1995;82:917–919
3. Office of Population Censuses and Surveys (ed): Mortality Statistics Cause Series DH2 Ed. Vol. 19. England and Wales: HMSO, 1992
4. Fowkes FGR, Macintyre CCA, Ruckley CV: Increasing incidence of aortic aneurysms in England and Wales. Br Med J 1989;298:33–35
5. Collin J: The increasing incidence of aortic aneurysms. Br Med J 1989;298:387–388
6. Johnston KW, Rutherford RB, Tilson MD et al: Suggested standards for reporting on arterial aneurysms. J Vasc Surg 1991;13:444–450
7. Collin J: A proposal for a precise definition of abdominal aortic aneurysm: a personal view. J Cardiovasc Surg 1990;31: 168–169
8. Sterpetti AV, Schultz RD, Feldhaus RJ et al: Factors influencing enlargement rate of small abdominal aortic aneurysms. J Surg Res 1987;43:211–219
9. Scott RAP, Ashton HA, Kay DN: Abdominal aortic aneurysm in 4237 screened patients: prevalence, development and management over 6 years. Br J Surg 1991;78:1122–1125
10. Bengtsson H, Bergqvist D, Ekberg O et al: A population based screening of abdominal aortic aneurysms (AAA). Eur J Vasc Surg 1991;5:53–57
11. Twomey A, Twomey E, Wilkins RA, Lewis JD: Unrecognised aneurysmal disease in male hypertensive patients. Int Angio 1986;5:269–273
12. Collin J, Walton J: Is abdominal aortic aneurysm familial? Br Med J 1989;299:49
13. Galland RB, Simmons MJ, Torrie EPH: Prevalence of abdominal aortic aneurysm in patients with occlusive peripheral vascular disease. Br J Surg 1991;78:1259–1260
14. Drott C, Arfvidsson B, Örtenwall P, Lundholm K: Age-standardized incidence of ruptured aortic aneurysm in a defined Swedish population between 1952 and 1988: mortality rate and operative results. Br J Surg 1992;79:175–179
15. Glimaker H, Holmberg L, Elvin A et al: Natural history of patients with abdominal aortic aneurysm. Eur J Vasc Surg 1991;5:125–130
16. Szilagyi DE, Elliott JP, Smith RF: Clinical fate of the patient with asymptomatic abdominal aortic aneurysm and unfit for surgical treatment. Arch Surg 1972;104:600–606
17. Cronenwett JL, Sargent SK, Wall MH et al: Variables that affect the expansion rate and outcome of small abdominal aortic aneurysms. J Vasc Surg 1990;11:260–269
18. Collin J, Heather B, Walton J: Growth rates of subclinical abdominal aortic aneurysms—implications for review and resceening programmes. Eur J Vasc Surg 1991;5:141–144
19. Brewster DC, Darling RC, Raines JK et al: Assessment of abdominal aortic aneurysm size. Circulation 1972;56(suppl 2):164
20. Salaman RA, Shandall A, Morgan RH et al: Intravenous digital subtraction angiography versus computed tomography in the assessment of abdominal aortic aneurysm. Br J Surg 1994;81: 661–663
21. Robson AK, Currie IC, Poskitt KR et al: Abdominal aortic aneurysm repair in the over eighties. Br J Surg 1989;76: 1018–1020
22. Harris LM, Faggioli GL, Fiedler R et al: Ruptured abdominal aortic aneurysms: factors affecting mortality rates. J Vasc Surg 1991;14:812–820
23. Berridge DC, Chamberlain J, Guy AJ, Lambert D: Prospective audit of abdominal aortic aneurysm surgery in the northern region from 1988 to 1992. Br J Surg 1995;82:906–910
24. Mutirangura P, Stonebridge PA, Clason AE et al: Ten-year review of non-ruptured aortic aneurysms. Br J Surg 1989;76: 1252–1254
25. Johansson G, Nydahl S, Olofsson P, Swedenborg J: Survival

in patients with abdominal aortic aneurysms. Comparison between operative and nonoperative management. Eur J Vasc Surg 1990;4:497–502

26. Olsen PS, Schroeder T, Agerskov K et al: Surgery for abdominal aortic aneurysms. J Cardiovasc Surg 1991;32:636–642
27. Amundsen S, Skjaerven R, Trippestad A, Sfreide O: Members of the Norwegian Aortic Aneurysm Trial. Abdominal aortic aneurysms—a study of factors influencing postoperative mortality. Eur J Vasc Surg 1989;3:405–409
28. AbuRahma AF, Robinson PA, Boland JP et al: Elective resection of 332 abdominal aortic aneurysms in a southern West Virginia community during a recent five-year period. Surgery 1991;109:244–251
29. Johnston KW, Scobie JK: Multicentre prospective study of non-ruptured abdominal aortic aneurysms. I. Population and operative management. J Vasc Surg 1988;7:69–81
30. Johnston KW: Multicenter prospective study of nonruptured abdominal aortic aneurysm. Part II. Variables predicting morbidity and mortality. J Vasc Surg 1989;9:437–447
31. Leather RP, Shah DM, Kaufman JL et al: Comparative analysis of retroperitoneal and transperitoneal aortic replacement for aneurysm. Surg Gynecol Obstet 1989;168:387–393
32. Cohen JR, Mannick JA, Couch NP, Whittemore AD: Abdominal aortic aneurysm repair in patients with peri-operative renal failure. J Vasc Surg 1986;3:867
33. Clifford PC, Kruger AR, Smith A et al: Salvage autotransfusion in aortic surgery: initial studies using a disposable reservoir. Br J Surg 1987;74:755–757
34. Barry KG, Cohen A, Kuchel JP et al: Mannitol infusion: the prevention of acute functional renal failure during resection of an aneurysm of the abdominal aorta. N Engl J Med 1961; 264:967–971
35. Paterson IS, Klausner JM, Mannick JA et al: Pulmonary oedema after aneurysm surgery is modified by mannitol. Ann Surg 1990;210:796–801
36. Michaels JA, Galland RB: General practitioner referral of patients with symptoms of peripheral vascular disease. J R Coll Surg Edinb 1994;39:103–105
37. Parodi JC, Palmaz JC, Clem MF et al: Intraluminal bypass of abdominal aortic aneurysm: feasibility study. Radiology 1992; 184:185–190
38. Brown PM, Pattenden R, Gutelius JR: The selective management of small abdominal aortic aneurysms: the Kingston study. J Vasc Surg 1992;15:21–27
39. Chambers BR, Norris JW: Clinical significance of asymptomatic neck bruits. Neurology 1985;35:742–745
40. Crevasse LE, Logue RB: Carotid artery murmurs. Continuous murmur over carotid bulb—a new sign of carotid artery insufficiency. JAMA 1958;167:2177–2182
41. Sandercock PAG, Warlow CP, Jones LN, Starkey IR: Predisposing factors for cerebral infarction: the Oxfordshire Community Stroke Project. Br Med J 1989;298:75–80
42. Bamford J, Sandercock P, Dennis M et al: Classification and natural history of clinically identifiable subtypes of cerebral infarction. Lancet 1991;337:1521–1526
43. Mead GE, Murray H, Farrell A et al: The potential role of carotid surgery in acute stroke. Br J Surg 1995;82:A1558
44. Feeley TM, Leen EJ, Colgan MP et al: Histologic characteristics of carotid artery plaque. J Vasc Surg 1991;13:719–724
45. Grzyska U, Freitag J, Zeumer H: Selective cerebral intraarterial DSA. Complication rate and control of risk factors. Neuroradiology 1990;32:296–299
46. Waugh JR, Sacharias N: Arteriographic complications in the DSA era. Radiology 1992;182:243–246
47. Hankey GJ, Warlow CP, Molyneux AJ: Complications of cerebral angiography for patients with mild carotid territory ischaemia being considered for carotid endarterectomy. J Neurol Neurosurg Psych 1990;53:542–548
48. Mani RL, Eisenberg RL, McDonald EJ et al: Complications of catheter cerebral arteriography: analysis of 5,000 procedures 1. Criteria and incidence. Am J Roentgenol 1978;131: 861–865
49. Spencer MP, Reid JM: Quantitation of carotid stenosis with continuous-wave (C-W) doppler ultrasound. Stroke 1979;10: 326–330
50. Schuler JJ, Flanigan DP, Lim LT et al: The effect of carotid siphon stenosis on stroke rate, death and relief of symptoms following elective carotid endarterectomy. Surgery 1982;92: 1058–1067
51. Mattos MA, van Bemmelen PS, Hodgson KJ et al: The influence of carotid siphon stenosis on short- and long-term outcome after carotid endarterectomy. J Vasc Surg 1993;17: 902–911
52. European Carotid Surgery Trialists' Collaborative Group: MRC European Carotid Surgery Trial: interim results for symptomatic patients with severe (70–99%) or with mild (0–29%) carotid stenosis. Lancet 1991;337:1235–1243
53. North American Symptomatic Carotid Endarterectomy Trial Collaborators: Beneficial effects of carotid endarterectomy in symptomatic patients with high grade carotid stenosis. N Engl J Med 1991;325:445–453
54. Rothwell PM, Warlow CP: The efficacy of carotid endarterectomy for 30–69% symptomatic carotid stenosis in the ECST, abstracted. Br J Surg 1996 (in press)
55. Executive Committee for the Asymptomatic Carotid Atherosclerosis Study: Endarterectomy for asymptomatic carotid artery stenosis. JAMA 1995;273:1421–1428
56. McCollum PT, Da Silver A, De Cossart L: Carotid endarterectomy in the UK and Ireland, abstracted. Br J Surg 1996 (in press)
57. McCollum PT, Da Silver A, De Cossart L: Carotid endarterectomy in the elderly patient abstracted. Br J Surg 1996 (in press)
58. Perler BA, Williams GM. Carotid endarterectomy in the very elderly: Is it worthwhile? Surgery 1994;116:479–483
59. Ouriel K, Penn TE, Ricotta JJ et al: Carotid endarterectomy in the elderly patient. Surg Gynecol Obstet 1986;162:334–336
60. Schultz RD, Sterpetti AV, Feldhaus RJ: Carotid endarterctomy in octogenarians and nonagenarians. Surg Gynecol Obstet 1988;166:245–251

61. Brook RH, Park RE, Chassin MR et al: Carotid endarterectomy for elderly patients: predicting complications. Ann Intern Med 1990;113:747–753

62. Wylie EJ, Hein MF, Adams JE: Intracranial haemorrhage following surgical revascularisation for treatment of acute strokes. J Neurosurg 1964;21:212–215

63. Hunter JA, Julian OC, Dye WS, Javid H: Emergency operation for acute cerebral ischemia due to carotid artery obstruction. Review of 26 cases. Ann Surg 1965;162:901–904

64. Bauer RB, Meyer JS, Fields WS et al: Joint study of extracranial arterial occlusion: 3. Progress reports of controlled study of long term survival in patients with and without operation. JAMA 1969;208:509–518

65. Goldstone J, Moore WS, Moncure AC et al: Emergency carotid artery surgery in neurologically unstable patients. Arch Surg 1976;111:1284–1291

66. Gertler JP, Blankensteijn JD, Brewster DC et al: Carotid endarterectomy for unstable and compelling neurologic conditions: do the results justify an aggressive approach? J Vasc Surg 1994;19:32–40

67. Khanna HL, Garg AG: 774 carotid endarterectomies for strokes and transient ischaemic attacks: comparison of results of early vs. late surgery. Acta Neurochir, suppl. 1988;42: 103–106

68. Greenhalgh RM, Cuming R, Perkin GD, McCollum CN: Urgent carotid surgery for high risk patients. Eur J Vasc Surg 1993; 7(suppl):25–32

69. Pell JP, Scottish Vascular Audit Group: Impact of intermittent claudication on quality of life. Eur J Vasc Surg 1995;9: 469–472

70. Adkins RB, Scott HW. Surgical procedures in patients aged ninety years and older. S Med J 1984;77:1357–1364

71. Widmer LK, Greensher A, Kannel WB. Occlusion of peripheral arteries—a study of 6400 working subjects. Circulation 1964;30:836–842

72. Wilson SE, Schwartz I, Williams RA, Owens ML: Occlusion of the superficial femoral artery. What happens without operation? Am J Surg 1980;140:112–117

73. Dormandy J, Mahir M, Ascady G et al: Fate of the patient with chronic leg ischaemia. J Cardiovasc Surg 1989;30:50–57

74. Hale WE, Marks RG, May FE et al: Epidemiology of intermittent claudication: evaluation of risk factors. Age Ageing 1988; 17:57–60

75. Reid DD, Brett GZ, Hamilton PJ et al: Cardiorespiratory disease and diabetes among middle aged male civil servants. Lancet 1974;1:469–473

76. Kannel WB, McGee DL: Update on some epidemiologic features of intermittent claudication: the Framingham study. J Am Geriatr Soc 1985;33:13–18

77. Jonason T, Ringqvist I: Mortality and morbidity in patients with intermittent claudication in relation to the location of the occlusive atherosclerosis in the leg. Angiology 1985;36: 310–314

78. Jelnes R, Gaardsting O, Hougard Jensen K: Fate in intermittent claudication: outcome and risk factors. Br Med J 1986; 293:1137–1140

79. O'Riordain DS, O'Donnell JA: Realistic expectations for the patient with intermittent claudication. Br J Surg 1991;78: 861–863

80. Reunanen A, Takkunen H, Aromaa A: Prevalence of intermittent claudication and its effect on mortality. Acta Med Scand 1982;211:249–256

81. Bainton D, Sweetnam P, Baker I, Elwood P: Peripheral vascular disease: consequence for survival and association with risk factors in the Speedwell prospective heart disease study. Br Heart J 1994;72:128–132

82. Fowkes FGR: Aetiology of peripheral atherosclerosis. Br Med J 1989;298:405–406

83. Paris BE, Libow LS, Halperin JL, Mulvihill MN: The prevalence and one-year outcome of limb arterial obstructive disease in a nursing home population. J Am Geriatr Soc 1988;36: 607–612

84. Yao ST: Haemodynamic studies in peripheral arterial disease. Br J Surg 1970;56:676–679

85. Whelan JF, Barry MH, Moir JD: Color flow doppler ultrasonography: comparison with peripheral arteriography for the investigation of peripheral vascular disease. J Clin Ultrasound 1992;20:369–374

86. Legemate DA, Teeuwen C, Hoeneveld H et al: The potential of duplex scanning to replace aorto-iliac and femoro-popliteal angiography. Eur J Vasc Surg 1989;3:49–54

87. Allard L, Cloutier G, Durand L-G et al: Limitations of ultrasonic duplex scanning for diagnosing lower limb arterial stenoses in the presence of adjacent segment disease. J Vasc Surg 1994;19:650–657

88. van der Heijden FHWM, Legemate DA, van Leeuwen MS et al: Value of duplex scanning in the selection of patients for percutaneous transluminal angioplasty. Eur J Vasc Surg 1993; 7:71–76

89. Hiatt WR, Regensteiner JG, Hargarten ME et al: Benefit of exercise conditioning for patients with peripheral arterial disease. Circulation 1990;81:602–609

90. Jivegard L, Holm J, Schersten T: The outcome in arterial thrombosis misdiagnosed as arterial embolism. Acta Chir Scand 1986;152:251–256

91. Fogarty TJ: Management of arterial emboli. Surg Clin North Am 1979;59:749–753

92. Vohra R, Lieberman DP: Arterial emboli to the arm. J R Coll Surg Edinb 1991;36:83–85

93. Davies MG, O'Malley K, Feeley M et al: Upper limb embolus: a timely diagnosis. Ann Vasc Surg 1991;5:85–87

94. Abbott WM, Maloney RD, McCabe CC et al: Arterial embolism: a 44 year perspective. Am J Surg 1982;143:460–464

95. Baird RJ, Lajos TZ: Emboli to the arm. Ann Surg 1964;160: 905–909

96. Scott DJA, Davies AH, Horrocks M: Risk factors in selected patients undergoing femoral embolectomy. Ann R Coll Surg Engl 1989;71:229–232

97. Collin C, Collin J: Mobility after lower-limb amputation. Br J Surg 1995;82:1010–1011

98. Humphreys WV, Evans F, Watkin G, Williams T: Critical limb ischaemia in patients over 80 years of age: options in a district general hospital. Br J Surg 1995;82:1361–1363

99. Earnshaw JJ: Thrombolytic therapy in the management of acute limb ischaemia. Br J Surg 1991;78:261–269

100. Braithwaite B, Birch P, Davies C et al: Accelerated high-dose bolus tissue plasminogen activator extends the role of peripheral thrombolysis but may increase risk. Br J Surg 1994; 81:A619

101. Sayers RD, Thompson MM, Hartshorne T et al: Treatment and outcome of severe lower-limb ischaemia. Br J Surg 1994;81: 521–523

102. Shearman CP, Ashley EMC, Gwynn BR, Simms MH: Rehabilitation of patients after vascular reconstruction for critical limb ischaemia. Br J Surg 1990;77:A346

103. Lindholt JS, Bøvling S, Fasting H, Henneberg EW: Vascular surgery reduces the frequency of lower limb major amputations. Eur J Vasc Surg 1994;8:31–35

CHAPTER 28

Venous Thrombotic Disease and Varicose Ulcers

PAUL A. O'NEILL

Deep vein thrombosis and pulmonary embolus are the main manifestations of venous thrombotic disease. Thromboembolism occurs with increasing frequency with age[1] and is potentially treatable, yet all surveys indicate that it is underrecognized and often misdiagnosed. As many as two-thirds of patients with a deep vein thrombosis may remain symptom-free[2] and symptoms suggestive of a deep vein thrombosis may be due to another condition in approximately 50 percent of patients.[2,3] Pulmonary embolus is discussed in detail in Chapter 77, but it has been estimated to be the cause of death in 3 to 6 percent of the general population in both the United Kingdom and the United States[4,5] and postmortem studies show an incidence as high as 69 percent.[1] Antemortem diagnosis is low: 90 percent of fatal pulmonary emboli may not be recognized in life[6] and often the condition is not even considered.

Venous-thrombotic disease is treatable. Intravenous heparin and subsequent oral anticoagulation have been the cornerstones of treatment for many years. A study by Largerstedt et al.[7] showed that the recurrence rate at 3 months for deep vein thrombosis was reduced from 29 percent when treated with compression stockings alone, to 0 percent after anticoagulation. If the development of the condition is thought likely, prophylaxis is available. In an overview of the rates of venous thrombosis after general surgery, Colditz et al.[8] found that the rate on no prophylaxis was 29 percent compared with 9.6 percent when subcutaneous heparin was used.

Epidemiology

The reported prevalence of deep vein thrombosis not only depends on what etiological factors are operating, but how the diagnosis is made. A clinical diagnosis will be confirmed in less than half of all patients.[9] The relative merits of the different diagnostic techniques are discussed below. The minimum incidence of the condition can be gauged by the statistics from the Office of Population Censuses and Surveys (OPCS)[10] in the UK, which reported that there were 1,700 female deaths and 750 male deaths in 1986 from venous embolus and thrombosis (ICD code 451–453) and 480 deaths from pulmonary emboli (ICD code 415.1). This compares with over 100,000 deaths from acute myocardial infarction alone. The figures relate to a single cause of death and are a gross underestimate of the true incidence of fatal pulmonary emboli.

The gold standard for determining the true prevalence of deep vein thrombosis might be expected to be postmortem examination. However, the majority of the published surveys were carried out over 25 years ago and the rates vary from between 27 and 83 percent. The most recent study by Havig[1] in patients over the age of 30 years reported a prevalence of 62 percent. The difference in figures is due to the variation in the medical and surgical causes of death, the ages of the patients studied and whether the postmortem included all, or just selected, patients. The final factor relates to the completeness of the examination of the venous system by an experienced pathologist.

General Factors

In thrombus formation, the interactions between the vessel wall and the cellular and noncellular constituents of blood are crucial. The coagulation system is stimulated by "tissue factors" released at sites of endothelial damage via factor VII (extrinsic) and factor VIII (intrinsic) leading to thromboplastin formation. The end product is activated factor X which acts in conjunction with factor V, calcium, and phospholipids to convert prothrombin to thrombin. Very low concentrations of thrombin can activate platelets causing expression of the anionic phospholipid membrane. This stimulates the components of the hemostatic system to produce a clot at the site of the tissue damage. Both heparin and the oral anticoagulants interfere with these cascade reactions (see below).

Thrombin production is limited by the surrounding healthy endothelium. Normally, the vascular endothelium provides a non thrombogenic surface. Antithrombin molecules are concentrated on the endothelial surface together with thrombomodulin molecules. If thrombin is generated, the healthy endothelium quickly neutralizes it through binding to thrombomodulin and activating the anticoagulant protein C system. There are other inhibitory systems, particularly antithrombin III (heparin cofactor). If generated, thrombus can be dissolved through the fibrinolytic system.

Stasis is a major factor in the development of deep vein thrombosis as it inhibits the removal of activated clotting elements and prevents mixing with natural inhibitors. Interestingly, although severe varicose veins have been cited as a risk factor for DVT,[11] there is no evidence of an association in the absence of other risks.[12]

The immobility that often occurs with advancing years reduces the efficiency of the muscle pump, particularly if other factors are also in operation, such as deep vein valvular incompetence (because of previous thrombosis).[11] The promotion of mobility, especially postsurgery, may prevent the development of thrombosis, though studies in other areas do not always bear this out.[11] An alternative means of prevention is compression of the leg to increase venous return (see below).

Etiologic Factors

Age

The risk of developing a deep vein thrombosis rises with increasing age[1,13,14] (Fig. 28-1). Havig[1] reported that the percentage of patients with a thrombosis diagnosed at postmortem rose from less than 20 percent in those under 40 years to approximately 100 percent in those over 90 years, but the number of very old patients studied was small. In life, the annual incidence for DVT increased from 1.8/1,000 population at age 65 to 69 years to 3.1/1,000 at age 85 to 89 years.[15]

Most studies have not considered age as a factor independent from the presence of conditions such as stroke, which are also common with advancing years and which predispose to thrombosis.[11] Immobility is also a confounding variable (see above). Both Havig[1] and Beckering and Titus[16] reported a correlation between the incidence of deep vein thrombosis and the duration of bed rest, the effect being more apparent in those over the age of 70 years.

Sex and Obesity

The majority of studies have shown a slightly increased risk of developing a deep vein thrombosis in females compared to males,[1,17] though Kniffen et al.[15] did not find an association using Medicare data. There is also an association between venous thrombosis and obesity.[1]

Figure 28-1 The rising incidence of deep vein thrombosis with increasing age in two surveys. (Data from Havig[1] and Sevitt and Gallagher.[14])

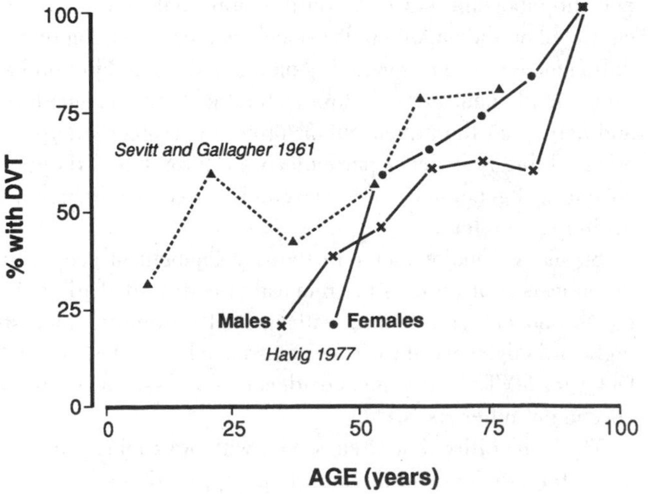

Surgery (Including Trauma)

Thrombosis is a common complication following hip replacement, regardless of whether it is carried out because of arthritis or fracture of the neck of femur. One study[18] reported an incidence of 54 percent. Yet, Campbell[19] found only 4 percent who were anticoagulated; however no diagnostic investigation was carried out, illustrating the gross underestimation by clinical diagnosis alone. At postmortem, 40 to 60 percent of patients who had died following a fractured femur or tibia had a deep vein thrombosis.[14]

There is an increased risk of venous thrombosis in patients who have had general surgery. A mean incidence of 27 percent was found, using fibrinogen uptake, in 31 trials of prophylaxis.[8] The relationship to the magnitude of the operation is not clear. Neither Havig[1] nor Allgood et al.[20] found any correlation, but Hills et al.[21] reported that, in the absence of malignancy, age and the severity of the operation were the most important etiological factors.

The type of anesthesia employed during surgery is important. Epidural[22] and spinal[23] anesthesia reduced the risk of deep vein thrombosis during total hip replacement.

Heart Disease

Heart failure predisposes a patient to the development of a deep vein thrombosis[24,25] with reported incidences varying from 30 to 60 percent. A similar relationship exists in acute myocardial infarction. A working party on anticoagulant therapy in coronary thrombosis[26] found that over 8 percent of those dying from a myocardial infarct had had a pulmonary embolus. In life, the reported incidence of deep vein thrombosis using fibrinogen scanning varied from 19 to 37 percent.[27,28] The high incidence was not simply due to prolonged immobility as the rate was much higher for the same duration of bed rest in those who had had a myocardial infarction compared with those with chest pain who subsequently did not infarct.[27,28]

Stroke

It was believed that the risk of thromboembolism in cerebrovascular disease was linked to bed rest and the age of the patient.[29] However, venous thrombosis occurs in the majority of patients following a stroke. Warlow et al.[30] reported that, using fibrinogen scanning, 60 percent of patients had a venous thrombosis. This was confirmed in a subsequent paper[11] and, again, the vast majority occurred in the paralyzed leg. No effect of age was found and the incidence was the same whether or not the patient was mobilized early. Other workers[31,32] have confirmed the association between deep vein thrombosis and acute stroke. As with myocardial infarction, the development of a deep vein thrombosis is related to changes in the coagulation system.

Malignancy

There is an association between malignancy and thromboembolic disease,[1,33] classically seen as thrombophlebitis migrans. Armand Trousseau (Physician, 1801–1867) stated that it, ". . . foretells with an almost mathematical precision that a capital (i.e. visceral malignancy) condition is lurking in the background."[34] It has been suggested that this may be a fortuitous relationship due to the increasing frequency of neoplasia with age.[29] However, Hills et al.[21] found that although the risk of a deep vein thrombosis rose with age in patients without malignancy, this association was lost in those with a tumor. Over 50 percent of patients with cancer had evidence of a venous thrombosis as demonstrated by fibrinogen scanning.[21]

Adenocarcinoma is a common cause. The causal relationship is complex and part of the spectrum of disseminated intravascular coagulopathy.[35,36] It can be caused by direct invasion of the tissues and release of tissue factor, activation of leucocytes and secretion of tissue factor (leukemic cells) or direct activation of the clotting cascade by mucin or a specific cancer procoagulant. Typically, the venous thrombosis associated with maligancy can be treated and prevented by heparin, but not by warfarin.[37]

Seasonal and Circadian Variation

There is a seasonal variation in thromboembolic disease[38] with peak fatal episodes occurring between January and April. There is no difference for males and females. It has been postulated that the risks may be due to changes in the blood including flow and clotting[39] and that the reduction in mobility and increase in morbidity of elderly people in the winter may be contributing factors.[38] A circadian rhythm has been described[40] with a peak risk of pulmonary embolus in the morning.

Diagnosis

Clinical

The clinical diagnosis of a deep vein thrombosis is based on the classical symptoms of pain and swelling of the calf together with increased calf circumference, local warmth, induration of the soleus and gastrocnemius muscle bed, tenderness on palpation and a positive Homans' sign (Surgeon, 1877–1954), which is pain in the calf on dorsiflexing the foot. However, two-thirds of patients with venous thrombosis may not have any symptoms or signs[2] and, if the signs are present, these may be due to another condition in at least half of patients (e.g., ruptured Baker's cyst or cellulitis).[2,3] In one study,[21] signs were detected in only 9 of the 53 legs with thrombosis, and these developed at least 2 days after a positive fibrinogen scan.

Recently, the view that clinical signs are unreliable[41] has been challenged. Landfield et al.[42] found that swelling above or below the knee, recent immobility, cancer and fever were independent predictors of acute proximal deep vein thrombosis. If venography had been carried out only in patients with one or more of these factors, it would have diagnosed 97 percent of cases and would have been avoided in 26 percent of patients with normal test results. By combining clinical findings with venous ultrasonography, Wells et al.[43] confirmed that it is posible to stratify patients into high, moderate, and low pretest probabilities, limiting the need for invasive venography.

Venography

Other than detailed postmortem studies, the visualization of the venous drainage of the lower limb by injection of radio-opaque contrast media (venography) remains the gold standard with which other imaging procedures are compared. The impact of venography on patient management can be marked. Ramsey[41] found that among general medical patients with an initial diagnosis of deep vein thombosis, the final diagnosis remained the same in only 25 percent after the introduction of venography compared to 83 percent before and hospital stay was shortened from 14 to 7 days.

It has been estimated that venography identifies at least 95 percent of clinically reported thromboses[44] (Fig. 28-2), but it may have a 5 to 10 percent false positive rate. Interobserver variation also reduces the accuracy.[45] Venography is limited by the technical difficulty in cannulating a small foot vein in the presence of edema or with a noncooperative patient. The problems of a high osmotic media have largely been solved by improved techniques and the use of low osmotic media, but venography cannot be used for serial monitoring because of the changes induced in the venous system.[46,47]

Fibrinogen Scanning

The ^{125}I fibrinogen uptake test is the standard method for screening at risk patients. The technique depends on the developing thrombus taking up and incorporating radiolabeled fibrinogen as it is converted into fibrin. Sodium iodide is given orally to block uptake of the isotope into the thyroid and then the radiolabeled compound is injected. With the legs slightly elevated to reduce venous pooling, a scintillation counter records the activity at a series of set points over the thigh and calf. The counts are related to the activity over the precordium. A deep vein thrombosis is diagnosed if the count is 15 or 20 percent (depending on the collimator[46]) greater than the adjacent point on the same leg or the corresponding point on the opposite leg and the difference is sustained for at least 24 hours (Fig. 28-3).

The overall accuracy of the technique compared to venography ranges from 70 to 90 percent[46] with particular problems with false positives (specificity). It also lacks sensitivity when screening the upper thigh; Harris et al.[48] showed that only 50 percent of venographically proven thrombosis were detected in elective hip surgery patients postoperatively. Labeled fibrinogen uptake also occurs in any incisions, cellulitis, trauma, or ruptured Baker's cyst. Hence, it is not of great value in assessing patients with clinical signs of a possible thrombosis. Its major role is in screening asymptomatic patients.

Impedence Plethysmography

Ohm's law states that $R = V/I$ where R is the electrical resistance, V the voltage drop, and I the current. As blood is a very good conductor of electricity, any pooling causes a drop

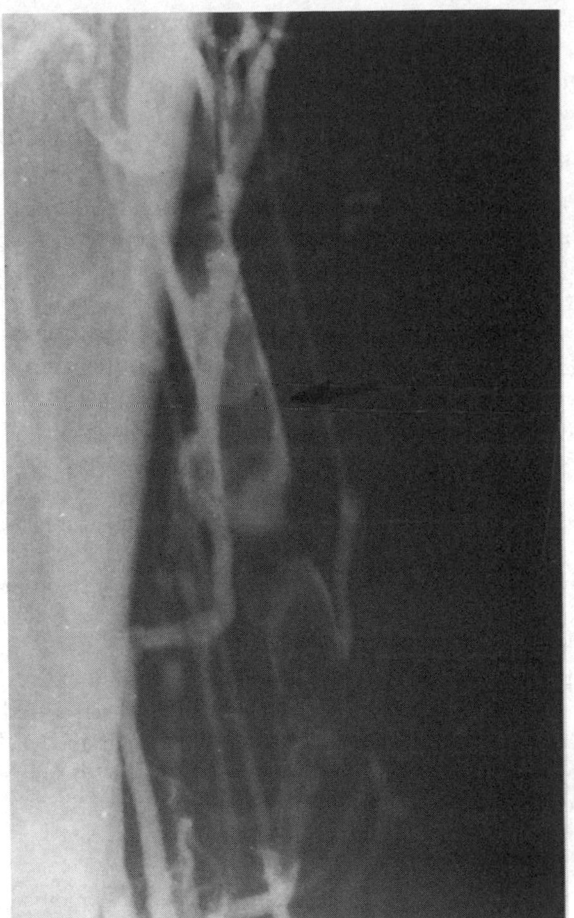

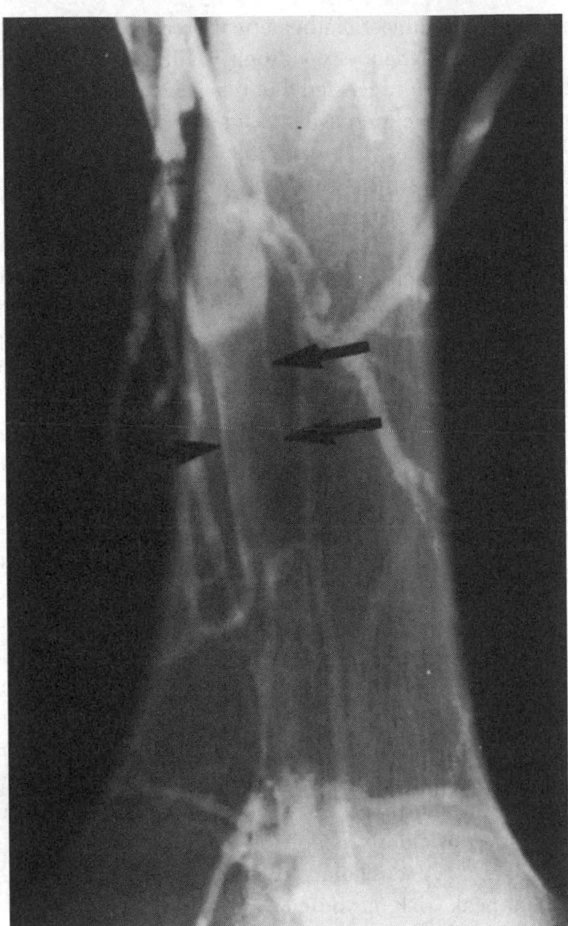

Figure 28-2 **(A&B)** Appearances of a major thrombus in the popliteal and femoral veins, with the characteristic tramlines (arrows).

in resistance. Thus, during respiration, current at a constant voltage will rise with inspiration and any blockage of venous drainage will abolish this (Fig. 28-4). A refinement of this technique is to measure changes in current when a pressure cuff is applied to the leg (see Fig. 28-4).

Figure 28-3 The typical results from fibrinogen scanning in a patient with an extensive left deep vein thrombosis. The difference has been maintained for 24 hours.

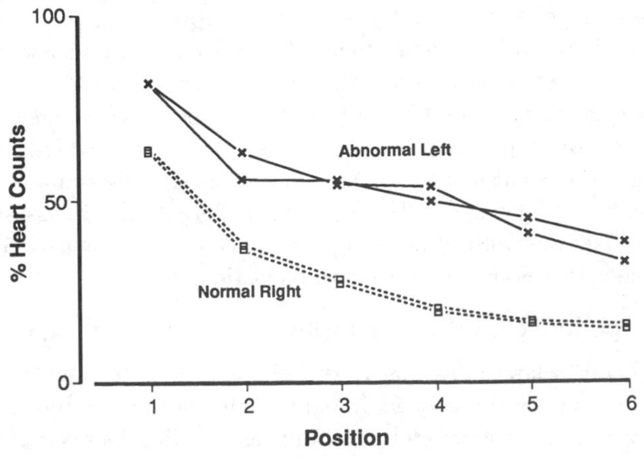

The major drawback, apart from noncooperation in a confused elderly patient, is the lack of change in impedence with calf thrombi or nonobstructing thigh vein thrombi. False positives may occur in other conditions interfering with venous return, for example, congestive cardiac failure, marked peripheral edema or chronic venous insufficiency.

The technique has an accuracy of 85 to 90 percent in patients with popliteal or thigh vein thrombi.[49,50] Consequently, its use depends on the costs in terms of morbidity and mortality if small calf vein thrombi are missed (see below).

Doppler Ultrasound

In 1842 Christian Doppler first described the effect of motion (either the source, the medium, or observer) on the observed frequency of a waveform. Clinically, the effect depends on the relative movement of a column of blood. In the detection of thrombosis a transducer emitting a 5 to 10 mHz beam is used. Typical normal waveforms recorded over the femoral artery and vein are shown in Figure 28-5. Doppler ultrasound is useful in bedside screening. A number of designated points are scanned with the patient supine. The results are interpreted using changes in the waveform with respiration and with distal and proximal compression.

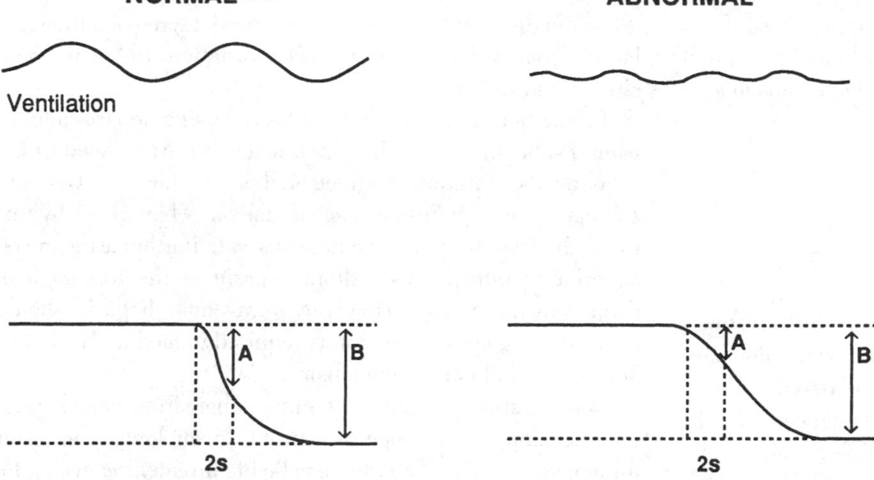

Figure 28-4 The variation in current recorded by impedence plethysmography during respiration (top) and during application of a pressure cuff (bottom). The abnormal trace shows the loss of respiratory pattern, and once the cuff is released the decline in current is slow (A/B is reduced).

The sensitivity of Doppler ultrasound is limited by nonocclusive thrombi (particularly distal). Meadway[51] reported an overall accuracy of only 27 percent. With improved techniques, Dosick et al.[52] claimed a 94 percent accuracy compared to venography. Combined with impedence plethysmography, an accuracy of 95 percent has been obtained with a 10 percent false positive and a 0 percent false negative rate.[53]

Doppler ultrasound combined with duplex B-mode scanning allows visualization of the thrombosis. It is valuable in symptomatic patients.[54,55] In a study of 220 patients with clinically suspected deep vein thrombosis, 100 percent of thigh vein thrombi were detected, but 66 percent of calf ones were not.[56] False positive results can occur with heart failure, venous insufficiency, or external venous compression.[57] As discussed above, ultrasound combined with clinical findings can avoid the need for venography,[43] though it cannot yet supplant it.[58]

Other Methods

Many other methods have been used to diagnose deep vein thrombosis including: thermography, blood screening (plasma fibrinogen chromatography and fibrinogen degradation products), and other isotope techniques (e.g., ^{99m}Tc, ^{111m}In label-

Figure 28-5 Doppler ultrasound recording over the femoral artery and vein with the typical phasic pattern during the respiratory cycle over the vein.

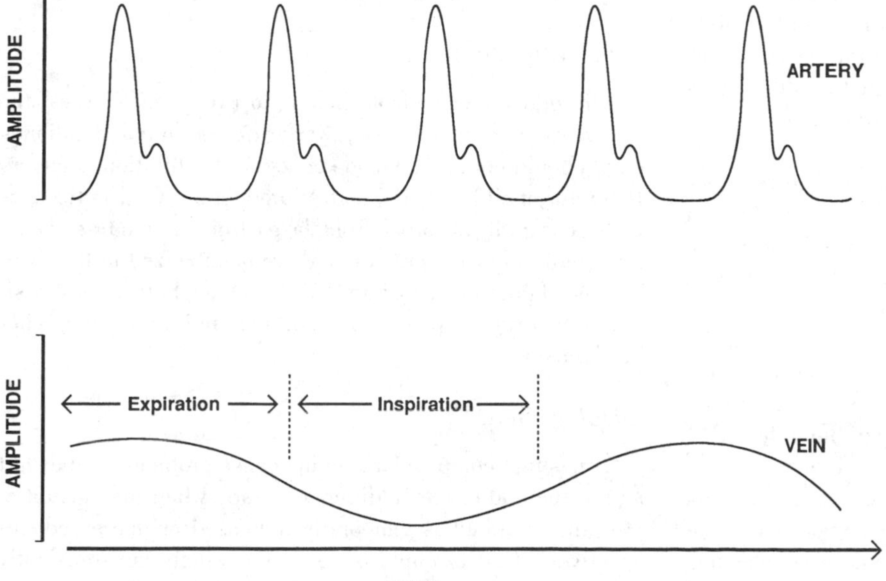

ing). None have any proven value. More recently, the measurement of D-dimer has shown promise as a simple blood test[59] It is a specific degradation product of cross-linked fibrin that is released when fibrinolyis occurs in fresh venous thromboemboli.

Treatment

Risk of Pulmonary Embolus

The sequelae of a deep vein thrombosis include postphebitic syndrome and venous ulceration (see below). Pulmonary embolus is the most feared complication. The associated mortality from this has continued to rise and may account for 12 percent of all deaths in elderly people.[60] Kniffen et al.[15] found that the in-hospital mortality associated with pulmonary embolism was 21 percent compared to only 3 percent with deep vein thrombosis. Most cases of major embolism are not diagnosed during life[61] and, in the majority of the fatal cases, death occurs within 30 minutes of the event.[62] The emphasis should therefore be on prevention. If thromboembolism does occur, it should be promptly treated.

Major emboli originate from the large proximal iliac and femoral veins. However, most thrombi that embolize begin in the deep veins of the calf muscular bed.[63] It is rare for these to embolize without first propagating to the major veins, although it can occur[66] and propagation may take place in 12 hours or less. The need for treatment is supported by the high incidence (51 percent) of silent pulmonary emboli in patients with a proven deep vein thrombosis[65]; these may herald a major, possibly fatal, event.

Heparin

Heparin is the prime treatment in the immediate management of thromboembolism. It acts mainly by augmenting the natural inhibitors of the clotting mechanism, particularly by increasing the activity of antithrombin III; this in turn inhibits the formation of IXa, Xa, and XIa. The cascade reaction has a large amplification factor, which means that small amounts of heparin can prevent thrombosis being initiated, but once in progress, larger amounts are required.

The half-life of heparin is between 1.5 and 2 hours. Constant intravenous infusion is the optimum method of delivery; a lower total dose is required and gives rise to fewer hemorrhagic complications when compared to bolus doses.[66] The drug is metabolized in the liver and excreted as uroheparin.

The aim is to achieve and maintain the activated partial thromboplastin time (APTT) or kaolin cephalin clotting time at 1.5 to 2.5 times the control value. At this level, the production and extension of thrombosis is abolished, but if the APTT drops below 1.5 for only 24 hours, thrombosis may recur.[67] Hemorrhage is the most serious and common complication of heparin therapy; in one series, it was the most common cause of drug-related death in hospital.[68] The incidence of bleeding is related to the degree of anticoagulation, rising eightfold if the APTT is over three times the control value.[69] Unfortunately, it is often difficult to achieve the required degree of anticoagulation,[70] partly due to the day-to-day variations in heparin sensitivity and delivery.[71]

Full anticoagulation can be achieved using heparin administered subcutaneously. Therapeutic levels are achieved within 2 hours; the duration of effect is about 10 hours.[72] Calcium salt causes less pain than the sodium salt when given by this route. In one study,[73] subcutaneous calcium heparin proved superior to intravenous sodium heparin in the treatment of deep vein thrombosis. However, intravenous heparin should be used when anticoagulation is required immediately, that is, after major pulmonary embolism.

Complications of heparin therapy, apart from hemorrhage, include alopecia, osteoporosis (when given long term), and thrombocytopenia. The latter may be life threatening even after as little as 7 days treatment.[74]

Low molecular weight (LMW) heparins are smaller fragments of standard heparin produced by chemical or enzymatic breakdown of the heparin molecule. As they are too small to inhibit factor IIa effectively, their antithrombotic effect is mainly due to factor Xa inhibition. The low molecular weight heparins have a longer half-life and greater bioavailability when given subcutaneously. In a meta-analysis, Leizorovicz et al.[75] found that in the initial treatment of deep vein thrombosis, LMW heparins, compared to unfractionated heparin, was associated with less thrombus extension. However, there were no differences in the other outcome measures (recurrence, major hemorrhage, mortality). Simplified therapy using LMW heparin may allow the treatment of uncomplicated proximal deep vein thrombosis as an outpatient.[76]

Oral anticoagulants are usually started immediately once a diagnosis of deep vein thrombosis is made. In one study there was no difference in the recurrence rate whether warfarin was started on day 1 or 7 of treatment.[77] In massive iliofemoral thrombosis or pulumonary embolus, oral anticoagulants are often delayed until after day 3.[72]

Oral Anticoagulants

The oral anticoagulants belong to two major classes, the courmarin derivatives (e.g., warfarin) and the indandiones (e.g., phenindione). The mode of action is inhibition of factors II (prothrombin) VII, IX, and X production. Oral anticoagulants are rapidly absorbed from the gastrointestinal tract, heavily bound to plasma protein, and are metabolized in the liver. The list of possible drug interactions is long, but can be classified into drug displacement, enzyme inhibition, and other mechanisms.

Displacement

Drugs that compete for binding cause problems at the start and at the end of any additional therapy when the amount of free anticoagulant is temporally increased or decreased, respectively. One example is naproxen, which can transiently increase the amount of unbound warfarin by 10 percent,[78] though there is no difference in the degree of anticoagulation while the drug is being taken. Consequently, this interaction is of less importance than enzyme inhibition.

Enzyme inhibition

Drugs that cause enzyme inhibition (e.g., cimetidine)[79] increase free anticoagulant so long as the inhibitor is being taken. Consequently, the warfarin dose needs to be reduced.

Other mechanisms

Other mechanisms influencing anticoagulant control include: enzyme induction; a reduction in vitamin K_1 availability; alterations in receptor sensitivity; changes in hemostasis; and a decrease in absorption. These mechanisms have been reviewed by Serlin and Breckenridge.[80]

Elderly people have increased sensitivity to oral anticoagulants, which is partly due to increased receptor affinity.[81] However, there is limited evidence that age, per se, increases the risks of bleeding from anticoagulation. The risk of recurrence of thrombosis is reduced by achieving an international normalized ratio (INR) between 2:3 increasing the ratio simply heightens the risk of hemorrhage, which is related to the prothrombin time in a log linear fashion.[82]

The criteria for adequate control have changed,[84] especially since the introduction of the INR.[84] Consequently, the results from older studies, particularly from North America where high-intensity treatment has been used,[85] are difficult to compare with current UK practice. Unless there are other factors to consider, the INR should be maintained at 2 to 3.[72] For patients with recurrent thromboembolism, an INR of 3 to 4.5 is recommended.[72] The degree of control obtained can be monitored using computer systems.[86]

In order to assess the risk of bleeding, Levine et al.[87] reviewed the published studies using elderly patients. In the majority of studies, there were insufficient data in crucial areas such as the duration of therapy and quality of control for analysis to be attempted. Pooled bleeding rates ranged from 6 to 29 percent of patients treated; for major hemorrhage the rate was 2 to 8 percent. Levine et al. attempted to look at age as an independent factor, but found that the data were inadequate for analysis. Another study concluded that there was no relationship between age and the risk of bleeding complications.[88] Wickramasinghe et al.[89] reported that in patients attending a geriatric medical clinic, age did not influence the bleeding rate nor the degree of control. In contrast, an inverse relationship was found between the control obtained and the number of drugs prescribed. In patients who bled, poor control had been observed from the outset. Generally, many would feel that the risk:benefit ratio for the use of oral anticoagulants has not been established at any age.[90,91] However, in a prospective study, Landfield et al.[92] reported that age (>65 years), along with a history of stroke, gastrointestinal bleeding, or a serious comorbid condition, was associated with a risk of major bleeding, particularly during the first month of therapy.

There is lack of agreement about the duration of therapy. It was originally proposed that warfarin therapy should continue for a minimum of 4 months.[93] Subsequently, it was suggested that 4 weeks' therapy may achieve the optimum risk: benefit ratio when treating the first episode of thrombosis.[82] More recently, Schuman et al.[94] compared 6 weeks with 6 months of therapy. In patients with a first occurence of deep venous thrombosis, fewer recurrences occured in patients treated for the longer period. This reduction was seen during treatment, after cessation the recurrence rate was similar. There was no increase in hemorrhage rate with 6 months of therapy. The inference is that patients should be treated for 6 months. However, the evidence from other studies suggest that anticoagulants can be stopped after 4 to 6 weeks in patients with transient risk factors such as surgery or temporary immobilization.[95,96] In those patients with idiopathic thrombosis, therapy should be for at least 6 months[96] and for those with continuing risk factors, such as malignancy or antithrombin III deficiency[97] therapy may need to be lifelong.[82,95,96]

Thrombolytic Therapy

Although thrombolytic therapy has been used to treat deep vein thrombosis, its use is generally restricted to life-threatening pulmonary emboli (see Ch. 77). It has no proven value in the treatment of proximal deep vein thrombosis.[98]

Prevention

Low Dose Heparin

The need for prophylaxis has been considered above. Ideally, any agent used should be well tolerated, can be given infrequently, requires no special monitoring, and should have a low incidence of side effects, particularly bleeding. Calcium heparin is currently widely used, though it does not fulfill all of the foregoing requirements, needing repeated subcutaneous injections that can be painful (though less than with the sodium salt) and can cause local bruising. The main mode of action is to promote the activity of antithrombin III. Its use has been reviewed by Kakkar.[99]

Low molecular weight heparins prevent venous thrombosis more effectively than standard heparins and the once daily dosage is an advantage, though the risk of major bleeding is probably the same.[100]

Prophylaxis is of value in some medical conditions. Four out of five studies showed a significant reduction in the incidence of deep vein thrombosis[99] after myocardial infarction. McCarthy et al.[101,102] reported a large reduction in venous thrombosis following a stroke, as demonstrated by fibrinogen scanning.

There are clear benefits for patients undergoing general surgery. Colditz,[8] in an overview analysis, found a reduction in thrombosis from 27 to 10 percent with the use of subcutaneous heparin. For patients following hip surgery, the rate was reduced from 50 to 20 percent.[99] The final end point in prophylaxis must be to lower the incidence of fatal pulmonary

Table 28-1 Stratification of risk of thromboembolism and strategies for prevention

Low Risk	Moderate Risk	High Risk
Minor surgery	Major surgery, age >40 yr, or other risk factors	Major orthopedic surgery—pelvis, lower limb
Major surgery, age <40 yr	Minor surgery, but previous history of thrombosis/thrombophilia	Major pelvic surgery for cancer
Medical illness	Cancer	Lower limb paresis (e.g., stroke)
	Major medical illness	Major surgery/trauma with previous history of thrombosis/thrombophilia
Strategies for prevention		
Graduated compression stockings	Graduated compression stockings	Graduated compression stockings
	Low dose heparin	Intermittent pneumatic compression
		Adjusted dose heparin

(Data from Refs. 104 and 105.)

embolus. In a large multicenter trial of over 4,000 patients[103] only 2 of those treated with heparin died from a pulmonary embolus compared with 16 in the control group. In any strategy for prevention, patients should be stratified and treated according to the estimated risk of thromboembolism (Table 28-1).[104,105]

Other Methods

There are other methods for prophylaxis. Low dose warfarin reduced the risk of deep vein thrombosis in gynecology patients postoperatively.[106] Hills et al.[21] reported that intermittent pneumatic calf compression was of value in general surgical patients, which was confirmed by Colditz et al.[8] They found that a combination of compression stockings and intermittent pneumatic compression was even more effective than heparin. Graduated elastic stockings alone were of less use.

The current evidence does not support the use of aspirin or other antiplatelet treatment for venous thromboprophylaxis, particularly as there are effective alternatives (see above).[107]

Varicose Ulcers

Epidemiology and Etiology

Leg ulcers are common and their care consumes large amounts of resources. The point prevalence of active ulceration has been estimated at 0.62 to 1.48/1,000 total population.[108,109] Women are more frequently affected. The vast majority of ulcers are in older people; in one survey, 90 percent of patients were over the age of 60 years.[108] This means that 75,000 to 90,000 patients have a leg ulcer at any point in time in the UK, and 2 percent of all females over 80 years of age are affected.[108,110] Given this high prevalence, it is not suprising that over £39 million per year are spent on dressing materials alone, and the total cost of care is over £236 million per year for the UK.[111]

There have been several series examining the frequency of different etiological factors in leg ulceration (Table 28-2). Most cases are associated with venous disease, either varicose veins, a history of deep venous thrombosis, or episodes during which venous thrombosis was likely to have occurred. The consequent incompetence of the valves within the deep veins or superficial peforators leads to chronic venous congestion. In turn, there are fibrotic changes within the capillary network and dermis.

Most ulcers (90 percent) are in the "gaiter" area around the malleoli[109] and are long-standing. In one survey, the median duration of current ulceration was 26 weeks (range 4 weeks to 30 years).[109] Due to the chronic venous hypertension and skin changes, venous ulceration is a chronic relapsing and remitting condition with over three-quarters of patients having recurrence over many years.[109]

Table 28-2 Etiologic factors in leg ulcers

Cause	Proportion (%)
Varicose veins	43–68
History of venous thrombosis	17–25
Diabetes	10
Obesity	48
Immobility	32–38
Peripheral arterial disease	21–31
Long-standing hypertension	17
Previous fracture	10–25
Rheumatoid arthritis	9–11
Generalized skin disorders	8
Neurologic disease	5

(Data from Baker et al.,[109] Cornwall et al.,[110] and Ruckley et al.[112])

Management

Although the majority of leg ulcers are due to venous disease, it is important that a positive diagnosis is made. Consideration should be given to the conditions highlighted in Table 28-2. An unusual site for the ulcer should raise suspicions. Similarly, features such as a raised edge make biopsy mandatory to exclude malignancy.

As the mainstay of treatment of venous ulceration is compression bandaging, peripheral vascular disease must be excluded. Many patients can be identified from clinical assessment, but this may miss more than 40 percent of patients.[110] It is mandatory to measure ankle brachial pressure indices using ultrasound and exclude patients for compression bandaging with values less than 0.8.[113] Failure to do this will result in limb ischemia.

Using multiple layer high compression bandaging, over 80 percent of ulcers can be healed within 6 months.[114] A number of groups have examined the factors which predict slow or nonhealing. Franks et al.[113] found that ulcer size, fixed limb joints, ulcer duration, and general mobility were independent predictors of a poor outcome. Skene et al.[115] also identified older age and deep vein involvement as additional factors.[115]

Despite good evidence for the use of high compression bandaging,[114] many patients are still managed ineffectively[111] due to inadequate training of staff, lack of simple Doppler ultrasound equipment to exclude arterial ischemia, Drug tarrif limitations on appropriate bandaging, and failure to transfer resources appropriately. Yet Bosanquet et al.[116] showed that community leg ulcer clinics are cost effective with vastly improved healing (80 vs. 22 percent) at a 61 percent cost reduction. As with many potential advances in health care, the way forward is to put into practice what is already known.

References

1. Havig O: Deep vein thrombosis and pulmonary embolus. Acta Churg Scand 1977;478(suppl):1–93
2. Salzman EW: Venous thrombosis made easy. N Engl J Med 1986;314:847–848
3. Cranlley JJ: Diagnosis of deep vein thrombosis: fallability of clinical symptoms and signs. Arch Surg 1976;111:34–36
4. Dalen JE, Alpert JS: Natural history of pulmonary embolus. Prog Cardiovasc Dis 1975;17:259–270
5. Dismulie SE: Pulmonary embolus as a cause of death. JAMA 1986;255:2039–2042
6. Horrowitz PE, Tatter D: Lethal pulmonary embolism. In Sherry S, Brinkhouse KM, Stengle JM (eds): Thrombosis. National Academy of Science, Washington D.C., 1969
7. Lagerstedt CI, Olson C, Fagher BO et al: Need for longterm anticoagulant treatment in symptomatic deep vein thrombosis. Lancet 1985;2:515–518
8. Colditz GA, Tuden RL, Oster G: Rates of venous thrombosis after general surgery: combined results of randomised clinical trials. Lancet 1986;2:143–146
9. Hull R, Hirsch J, Sackett DL, Stoddart G: Cost effectiveness of clinical diagnosis, venography, and non-invasive testing in patients with symptomatic deep vein thrombosis. N Engl J Med 1981;304:1561–1567
10. OPCS: Death by cause. 1986–1987 registrations OPCS monitor Ref. DH2 87/4. 1987
11. Warlow C, Ogston D, Douglas AS: Deep vein thrombosis of the legs after strokes. Part I: Incidence and predisposing factors. Part II: Natural history. Br Med J 1976;1:1178–1183
12. Campbell B: Thrombosis, phlebitis and varicose veins. Br Med J 1996;312:198–199
13. Morrell M: The post mortem incidence of pulmonary embolism in a hospital population. Br J Surg 1968;55:347–352
14. Sevitt S, Gallagher NG: Venous thrombosis and pulmonary embolism. A clinico-pathological study in injured and burned patients. Br J Surg 1961;48:475–488
15. Kniffen JR, Baron J, Barrett J et al: The epidemiology of diagnosed pulmonary embolism and deep vein thrombosis in the elderly. Arch Intern Med 1994;154:861–866
16. Beckering RE, Titus JL: Femero-popliteal venous thrombosis and pulmonary embolus. Am J Clin Pathol 1969;52:530–537
17. Kemble JVH: The incidence of deep vein thrombosis. Br J Hosp Med 1971;6:721–726
18. Louden JR, Thorburn J, Graham J, Vallance R: Deep vein thrombosis after hip replacement. Br Med J 1978;1: 1550–1551
19. Campbell AJ: Femoral neck fracture in elderly women: a prospective study. Age Ageing 1976;5:102–109
20. Allgood RJ, Cook JH, Weedon BJ et al: Prospective analysis of pulmonary embolism in post-operative patients. Surgery 1970; 68:116–122
21. Hills NH, Pflug JJ, Jeyasingh K et al: Prevention of deep vein thrombosis by intermittent pneumatic compression of calf. Br Med J 1972;1:131–135
22. Modig J, Maripuu E, Sahlstedt B: Thromboembolism following total hip replacement. A prospective investigation of 94 patients with emphasis on efficacy of lumbar epidural anaesthesia in prophylaxis. Reg Anaesthiol 1986;11:72–79
23. Thorburn J, Lauden JR, Vallance R: Spinal and general anaesthesia in total hip replacement: frequency of deep vein thrombosis. Br J Anaesthiol 1980;52:1117–1121
24. Consensus Conference: Prevention of venous thrombosis and pulmonary embolus. JAMA 1986;256:744–749
25. Forbes CD, Lowe GD: Low dose heparin for prevention of deep vein thrombosis and pulmonary embolus in medical patients. Scot Med J 1987;32:67–68
26. Report of a working party on anticoagulant therapy in coronary thrombosis. Br Med J 1969;1:335–342
27. Murray TS, Lorimer AR, Cox FC, Lawrie TDV: Leg vein thrombosis following a myocardial infarction. Lancet 1970;2: 792–793
28. Maurer BJ, Wray R, Shillingford JP: Frequency of venous thrombosis after a myocardial infarction. Lancet 1971;2: 1385–1387
29. Denham MJ: The incidence of deep vein thrombosis and pulmonary embolus. pp. 93–106. In McCarthy ST (ed): Peripheral

Vascular Disease in the Elderly. Churchill Livingstone, Edinburgh, 1983

30. Warlow C, Ogston D, Douglas AS: Venous thrombosis following strokes. Lancet 1972;1:1305–1306
31. Prasad BK, Banerjee AK, Howard H: Incidence of deep vein thrombosis and the effect of pneumatic compression of the calf in elderly hemiplegics. Age Ageing 1982;11:42–44
32. Denham MJ, Farran H, James G: The value of 125I-fibrinogen in the diagnosis of deep vein thrombosis in hemiplegia. Age Ageing 1973;2:207–210
33. Coon WW: Risk factors in pulmonary embolism. Surg Gynaecol Obst 1976;143:385–390
34. Clain A: Hamilton Bailey's Demonstration of Physical Signs in Clinical Surgery. 15th Ed. John Wright, Bristol, 1973
35. Williams E: Disseminated invascular coagulation. pp. 921–944. In Loscalzo J, Schafer A (eds): Thrombosis and Hemorrhage. Blackwell Scientific Publications, Boston, 1994
36. Marder V, Felstein D, Francis C, Coleman R: Consumptive thrombohemorrhagic disorders. pp. 1023–1063. In Colman R, Hirsch J, Marder V, Salzman E (eds): Hemostasis and Thrombosis. 3rd Ed. Lippincott-Raven, Philadelphia, 1994
37. Bell W, Starksen N, Tong S, Porterfield J: Trousseau's syndrome: devasating coagulopathy in the absence of heparin. Am J Med 1985;79:423–430
38. Colantonio D, Casale R, Natali G, Pisqualetti P: Seasonal periodicity in fatal pulmonary embolism after hip arthroplasty. Lancet 1990;1:56–57
39. Bell RB, Simon TL: Current status of pulmonary thromboembolic disease: pathophysiology, diagnosis, prevention and treatment. Am Heart J 1982;103:239–262
40. Colantonio D, Casale R, Abruzzo BP et al: Circadian distribution of fatal pulmonary thromboembolism. Am J Cardiol 1989; 64:403–404
41. Ramsey LE: Impact of venography on the diagnosis and management of deep vein thrombosis. Br Med J 1983;286: 698–699
42. Landfeld CS, McGuire E, Cohen AM: Clinical findings associated with acute proximal deep vein thrombosis: a basis for quantifying clinical judgement. Am J Med 1990;88:382–388
43. Wells PS, Hirsch J, Anderson DR et al: Accuracy of clinical assessment of deep-vein thrombosis. Lancet 1995;345: 1326–1330
44. Browse N: Diagnosis of deep vein thrombosis. Br Med Bull 1978;34:163–167
45. McLachlan MSF, Thomson JG, Taylor DW et al: Observer variation in the interpretation of lower limb venograms. Am J Roentol 1979;132:227–229
46. Bettman MA, Salzman EW: Recent advances in the diagnosis of deep vein thrombosis and pulmonary embolus. pp. 287–317. In Poller L (ed): Recent Advances in Blood Coagulation. 3rd Ed. Churchill Livingstone, Edinburgh, 1981; 287–317
47. Schmitt HE: Phlebography in deep vein thrombosis. pp. 126–149 In McCarthy ST (ed): Peripheral Vascular Disease in the Elderly. Churchill Livingstone, Edinburgh, 1983
48. Harris WH, Salzman EW, Atlansoulis CA et al: Comparison of 125I fibrinogen count scanning with phlebography for detection of venous thrombi after elective hip surgery. N Engl J Med 1975;292:665–667
49. Sasahara AA, Sharma GURK, Parisi AF: New developments in the detection and prevention of venous thromboembolism. Am J Cardiol 1979;43:1214–1224
50. Hirsch JB, Hull R: Comparative value of tests for the diagnosis of venous thrombosis. World J Surg 1978;2:27–38
51. Meadway J, Nicolaides AW, Walker CJ, O'Connell JD: Value of Doppler ultrasound in the daignosis of clinically suspected deep vein thrombosis. Br Med J 1975;4:552–554
52. Dosick SM, Blakemore WS: The role of Doppler ultrasound in acute deep vein thrombosis. Am J Surg 1978;136:265–268
53. Lepore TJ, Savron J, Van de Water J et al: Screening for extremity of deep vein thrombosis. Am J Surg 1978;135: 529–534
54. Langsfield M, Hersbey FB, Thorpe L et al: Duplex B-mode imaging for the diagnosis of deep vein thrombosis. Arch Surg 1987;122:587–591
55. Aitken AGF, Gadden DJ: Real time ultrasound diagnosis of deep vein thrombosis: a comparison with venography. Clin Radiol 1987;38:309–313
56. Lensing AWA, Pradoni P, Brandjes D et al: Detection of deep vein thrombosis by real time B-mode ultrasonography. N Engl J Med 1989;320:342–345
57. The diagnosis of deep vein thrombosis. Leader Lancet 1989; 2:23–24
58. Becker DM: Clinical assessment plus ultrasonography accurately predicted deep vein thrombosis. ACP Journal Club 1996;124:19
59. Moser KM: Diagnosing pulmonary embolism. Br Med J 1994; 309:1525–1526
60. Taubman LB, Silverstone FA: Autopsy proven pulmonary embolism amongst the institutionalised elderly. J Am Geriatr Soc 1986;34:752–756
61. Freiman DG, Suyemoto J, Wessler S: Frequency of pulmonary thromboembolism in man. N Engl J Med 1965;272: 1278–1280
62. Donaldson GA, Williams C, Scannell JG, Shaw R: A reappraisal of the Trendelenburg operation to massive fatal embolism. N Engl J Med 1963;268:171–174
63. Kakkar VV, Howe CT, Flanc C, Clarke MB: Natural history of post-operative deep vein thrombosis. Lancet 1969;2:230–232
64. Salzman EW, Davies GC: Prophylaxis of venous thromboembolism: analysis of cost effectiveness. Ann Surg 1980;191: 207–218
65. Huisman MV, Buller HR, Ten Cote JW et al: Unexpected high prevalence of silent pulmonary embolism in patients with deep vein thrombosis. Chest 1989;95:499–502
66. Wilson JE, Bynum LJ, Parkey RW: Heparin therapy in venous thromboembolism. Am J Med 1981;70:808–816
67. Hull RD, Raskab GE, Hirsch J et al: Continuous intravenous heparin compared with intermittent subcutaneous heparin in the initial treatment of proximal vein thrombosis. N Engl J Med 1986;315:1109–1114

68. Porter J, Hershel J: Drug related death among medical inpatients. JAMA 1977;237:879–881

69. Landefield CS, Cook EF, Flatley M et al: Identification and preliminary validation of prediction of major bleeding in hospitalised patients starting anticoagulant therapy. Am J Med 1987;82:703–713

70. Fennerty AG, Thomas P, Backhouse G et al: Audit of heparin control. Br Med J 1985;290:27–28

71. Fennerty AG, Levine MN: Non-biological factors in day to day variation of heparin requirements Br Med J 1989;299: 1012–1013

72. Anonymous: How to anticoagulate. Drugs Therapeut Bull 1992;30:77–80

73. Walker MG, Shaw JW, Thomson GJL et al: Subcutaneous calcium heparin versus intravenous sodium heparin in treatment of established acute deep vein thrombosis of the legs: a multicentre prospective randomised trial. Br Med J 1987;294: 1189–1192

74. Bell WR, Tamaswo PA, Alving BM, Duffy TP: Thrombocytopenia occuring during the administration of heparin. A prospective study in 52 patients. Ann Int Med 1976;85:155–160

75. Leizorovicz A, Simonneau G, Decousus H, Boissel JP: Comparison of efficacy and safety of low molecular weight heparins and unfractionated heparin in initial treatment of deep vein thrombosis: a meta-analysis. Br Med J 1994;309:299–304

76. Hull RD, Raskob GE, Pineo GF et al. Subcutaneous low molecular weight heparin compared with continuous intravenous heparin in the treatment of proximal-vein throbosis. N Engl J Med 1992;326:975–982

77. Gallus A, Jackman J, Tillet J et al: Safety and efficacy of warfarin started early after submassive venous thrombosis or pulmonary embolism. Lancet 1986;2:1293–1296

78. Jain A, McMahon GF, Slattery JT, Levy G: Effect of naproxen on the steady state serum concentration and anticoagulant activity of warfarin. Clin Pharm Ther 1979;25:61–66

79. Serlin MJ, Mossman S, Sibean RG et al: Cimetidine interaction with oral anticoagulants in man. Lancet 1979;2:317–319

80. Serlin MJ, Breckenridge AM: Drug interactions with warfarin. Drugs 1983;25:610–620

81. O'Malley K, Stevenson IH, Ward CA et al: Determinants of anticoagulant control in patients receiving warfarin. Br J Clin Pharm 1977;4:309–314

82. Fennerty A, Campbell IA, Routledge PA: Anticoagulants in venous thromboembolism. Br Med J 1988;297:1285–1288

83. Poller L: The operative range in anticoagulant administration. Br Med J 1985;290:1683–1686

84. Poller L: INR and the therapeutic range. Biol Clin Haematol 1987;9:203–213

85. Poller L, Taberner DA: Dosage and control of oral anticoagulants. An international survey. Br J Haematol 1982;51: 479–485

86. Ryan PJ, Gilbert M, Rose PE: Computer control of anticoagulant dose for therapeutic management. Br Med J 1989;299: 1207–1209

87. Levine MN, Raskob G, Hirsch J: Haemorrhagic complications of long-term anticoagulant therapy. Chest 1986;89(suppl 2): 16S–25S

88. Forfar JC: A 7-year analysis of haemorrhage in patients on long-term anticoagulant treatment. Br Heart J 1979;42: 128–132

89. Wickramasinghe LSP, Basu SK, Bansal SK: Long-term anticoagulant therapy in elderly patients. Age Ageing 1988;17: 388–396

90. Lowe GDO: Anticoagulants in the elderly: valuable in selective patients. Br Med J 1988;297:1260

91. Scott PJW: Anticoagulants in the elderly: the risks usually outweight the benefits. Br Med J 1988;297:1261

92. Landfeld CS, Goldman L: Major bleeding in outpatients treated with warfarin: incidence and prediction by factors known at the start of outpatient therapy. Am J Med 1989;87:144–152

93. Coon WW, Willis PD: Recurrence of venous thromboembolism. Surgery 1973;73:823–827

94. Schuman S, Rhedin AS, Lindmarker P et al: A comparison of six weeks with six months of oral anticoagulant therapy after a first episode of venous thromboembolism. N Engl J Med 1995;332:1661–1665

95. Chesterman CN: After a first episode of venous thromboembolism. Br Med J 1995;311:700–701

96. Hirsch J: The optimal duration of anticoagulant therapy for venous thrombosis. N Engl J Med 1995;332:1710–1711

97. Familial antithrombin III deficiency. Leader Lancet 1983;1: 1021–1022

98. Verstraete M: Thrombolytic treatment. Br Med J 1995;311: 582–583

99. Kakkar VV: The prevention of venous thromboembolism. pp. 150–164. In McCarthy ST (ed): Peripheral vascular disease in the elderly. Churchill Livingstone, Edinburgh, 1983

100. Anonymous: Low molecular-weight heparins in orthopaedic surgery. Drugs Ther Bull 1993;31:39–40

101. McCarthy ST, Turner JJ, Robertson D, Hawkey CJ: Low dose heparin as a prophylaxis against deep-vein thrombosis after acute stroke. Lancet 1977;2:800–801

102. McCarthy ST, Turner JJ: Low dose subcutaneous heparin in the prevention of deep vein thrombosis and pulmonary embolus following acute stroke. Age Ageing 1986;15:84–88

103. International Multicentre Trial: Prevention of post-operative pulmonary embolus by low doses of heparin. Lancet 1975;2: 45–51

104. Thromboembolic Risk Factors (THRIFT) Consensus Group: Risk and prophylaxis for venous thromboembolism in hospital patients. Br Med J 1992;305:567–574

105. Anonymous: Preventing and treating deep vein thrombosis. Drugs Ther Bull 1992;30:9–12

106. Poller L, McKernan A, Thompson JM et al: Fixed minidose warfarin: a new approach to prophylaxis against venous thrombosis after major surgery. Br Med J 1987;295:1309–1312

107. Cohen AT, Skinner JA, Kakkar VV: Antiplatelet treatment for thromboprophylaxis: a step forward or backwards? Br Med J 1994;309:1213–1217

108. Callum MJ, Ruckley CV, Harper DR, Dale JJ: Chronic ulceration of the leg: extent of the problem and provision of care. Br Med J 1985;290:1855–1856
109. Baker SR, Stacey MC, Jopp-Mckay AG et al: Epidemiology of chronic venous ulcers. Br J Surg 1991;78:864–867
110. Cornwall JV, Dore CJ, Lewis JD: Leg ulcers: epidemiology and aetiology. Br J Surg 1986;73:693–696
111. Freak L, Simon D, Kinsella A et al: Leg ulcer care: an audit of cost-effectiveness. Health Trends 1995;27:133–136
112. Ruckley CV, Dale JJ, Callum MJ, Harper DR: Causes of chronic leg ulcer. Lancet 1982;ii:615–616
113. Franks PJ, Moffatt CJ, Connolly M et al: Factors associated with healing leg ulceration with high compression. Age Ageing 1995;24:407–410
114. Moffatt CJ, Franks PJ, Oldroyd M et al: Community leg ulcer clinics and impact on ulcer healing. Br Med J 1992;305: 1389–1392
115. Skene AI, Smith JM, Doré CJ et al: Venous leg ulcers: a prognostic index to predict time to healing. Br Med J 1992;305: 1119–1121
116. Bosanquet N, Franks P, Moffatt C et al: Community leg ulcer clinics: cost-effectiveness. Health Trends 1993;25:146–148

CHAPTER 29

Neurobiology of Aging

DAVID MICHAEL ANDREW MANN

Age-associated deficiencies in the musculoskeletal, cardiovascular, and endocrine systems producing arthritis, hypertension, stroke, and diabetes are all too apparent in our elderly population, yet internally caused failures in the function of the nervous system provide the extremely common, and mostly intractable, problems of memory and intellect or locomotion in old age that face and frustrate clinicians.

Neurologic and neuropsychological complaints are widespread even in otherwise physically healthy old people. Forgetfulness is common, and while this could be equated with what has popularly been termed "benign senescent forgetfulness" it might represent an insidious forerunner of neurodegenerative disease. Mental status investigations show that although vocabulary, attention, and concentration are often well preserved into later life, semantic knowledge (object naming) and verbal fluency (word generation) decline. The ability to retain information over a brief period of time (short-term memory) is compromised, while the recall of past events may be less affected. Visuospatial abilities diminish, as does the capability to conceptualize ideas and think in abstract terms. Dizziness, poor posture, and impaired balance are frequent complaints, even in the absence of musculoskeletal deficiencies. These may represent disturbances of visual, vestibular, and sensory inputs. Impairment of smell, hearing, sight, and taste are commonplace. Elderly individuals show a decrease in muscle strength and sometimes display minor degrees of clumsiness, especially for finicky locomotor tasks, and a slowing of movement. Sleep difficulty is frequent, with nocturnal leg cramps or spasms being common. Whether such clinical changes are pathologic or form part of "normal aging" is difficult to ascertain; a (variable) contribution by both processes is perhaps likely with the balance between each differing much among individuals.

While such functional changes may in part reflect the "efficiency" with which brain cells operate in later life, and the extent to which their interconnections (pathways) are used, it is nonetheless an expectation that actual alterations in tissue organization or structure should occur in the elderly brain and that these will underlie many of the clinical signs of a failing system. In this chapter the structural and chemical characteristics of many of the pathologic changes taking place in the elderly brain are presented. It is well known that those features usually associated with the common neurologic and psychiatric disorders of old age (i.e., Alzheimer's disease or Parkinson's disease) are also frequently seen, albeit usually to a lesser extent, in the brains of old persons apparently clinically free from such disorders. In this review no useful purpose is served by attempting to draw anatomic distinctions between such clinical diagnostic groups. In broad terms, a plaque is a plaque or a tangle is a tangle whether these be in a 60-year-old patient with clinical Alzheimer's disease or in an apparently mentally healthy centenarian. Hence, the following pathologic descriptions are given without deference to the clinical setting in which the changes occur and apply to any particular pathologic structure equally well regardless of the state of health of the person bearing that change. Nevertheless, it has to be emphasized that the far greater mass of knowledge regarding the structure and chemistry of such pathologic changes has been gained from studies of the diseased, rather than the "normal," state, though this in no way detracts from its applicability to all situations where that change might be present. Distinctions between clinical settings are based more upon the amount or distribution of a particular pathology rather than its presence per se. Such quantitative differences may relate principally to etiological variations, such as genetic or environmental factors, that determine whether or not this pathology occurs and, if so, to what extent it is manifest.

Brain Imaging Studies

Over the past decade noninvasive neuroimaging techniques such as computed tomography (CT), magnetic resonance imaging (MRI), and positron emission tomography (PET), have all been extensively employed to investigate the structure and function of the brain in living patients, especially elderly people, and particularly those with neurodegenerative disease.

Computer tomography scans of healthy elderly persons[1–4] show that the volume of cerebrospinal fluid within and surrounding the brain increases with age, the ventricles enlarge and the gaps (sulci) between certain major gyri widen. Yet, within this generality perhaps as many as 50 percent of individuals have a CT scan not dissimilar to that seen in young persons. When cerebral atrophy is present, however, it is usually slight and diffusely distributed and ventricular enlargement is uniform, though sometimes focal emphasis in frontal or parasagittal parietal sulci can occur. Furthermore, between one-third and one-half of all normal elderly persons show some degree of white matter change, this being seen as periventricular translucencies (leukoaraiosis), which refer to local cerebrovascular insufficiencies affecting the deep white matter, usually that of the centrum semiovale. Magnetic resonance imaging (MRI)[5–9] reveals similar findings to those seen on CT scanning,[1–4] though recent quantitative studies have suggested a preferential atrophy of the medial temporal lobe[10] and hippocampus[11–14] in old age. In PET, decreases in brain energy metabolism, as measured by fluorodeoxyglucose uptake, have been reported in some studies,[15–19] but not in others.[20–21] Similarly, studies of basal ganglia function, using fluorodopa uptake, have been contradictory.[22,23] Such discrepancies remain unresolved, but they may be due to patient recruitment criteria because in those studies where no changes were noted on PET[20,21,23] only high performers on mental test examinations were used; in other studies[15–19,22] patients were not so rigorously screened.

Hence, neuroimaging reveals a number of inconstant, though generally mild, changes in gray and white matter structure and function, which may affect as many as half of all elderly persons. What is obvious though, is that there is no clear and universally applicable definition of brain change in later life and many individuals appear to be completely spared of (observable) tissue alterations, even in advanced old age.

Gross Changes in the Brain at Autopsy

At autopsy, the brains of elderly persons again frequently show a number of inconstant macroscopic changes, these reflecting the variances seen on neuroimaging. The arachnoid is often thickened by fibrosis, especially over the parasagittal cortex and the arachnoid granulations may be increased in size. External inspection of the brain surface often shows that some shrinkage of the overlying gyri may have occurred, either focally or more diffusely. The fresh weight of the brain may be reduced. The brain attains maximum weight at about 20 years of age and remains at this weight until 40 to 50 years of age after which it decreases in weight at a rate of 2 to 3 percent per decade, eventually reaching a value some 10 percent below maximum by 80 years of age.[24–27] As the brain is reduced in size, the fluid-containing space surrounding it is increased and there is a gradual fall with aging in the ratio between brain size and intracranial capacity (skull volume), the latter remaining constant throughout life.[26] As the subarachnoid space increases, so the meninges may become lax. The lateral ventricles may increase in size, particularly at the centrum semiovale where a rounding of the angles can be apparent, as do their extensions into the temporal lobe; the III and IV ventricles and aqueduct may also become enlarged.[28–31]

Simplistic correlations involving a falling brain weight or volume with age at death have popularized the concept that the human brain loses one million nerve cells every day of its life. This, however, may be an overestimation of the true extent of change. Secular analyses[32–34] have shown that the brain, like the rest of the body, has in fact undergone a real increase in size over the past century, this presumably being due to better diet, health care, etc. A lower brain weight in elderly persons may therefore, in part, simply reflect an initially smaller brain and when this is corrected for it is seen that brain weight, on average, remains fairly constant up until 60 years of age, after which a gradual decline sets in leading to an eventual loss of only some 5 percent of the original weight (60 to 70 g) by the nineth decade.[34] Studies[26] relating brain volume to cranial capacity, a measure not influenced by secular changes, confirm these data.

How this actual loss of tissue is distributed through the brain is not clear. While the amounts of both gray and white matter decrease with age, the ratio between these follows an unusual course such that it decreases from 20 to 50 years of age, then progressively increases thereafter.[32,35] Such data suggest that during the first half of life a preferential loss or shrinkage of gray matter components occurs whereas thereafter white matter changes predominate, these perhaps involving a loss of myelin and axons. The white matter hyperintensities observed on MRI,[6–9] and the periventricular translucencies seen on CT,[1–4] indicative of cerebrovascular damage common in old age would concur with such a preferential fallout of white matter elements in later life.

Changes in Nerve Cell Number with Aging

It is a natural assumption that the loss of brain tissue in later life should be represented by a fallout of the brain's principal cells, the neurones. Yet, it is possible that shrinkage of the nerve cell body or its processes (axons and dendrites) or both, could achieve this same net tissue loss without any actual change in cell number having occurred. Indeed, some combination of both processes might take place. Furthermore, a loss of tissue elements other than neurones (e.g., blood vessels) might influence brain weight, and it is also possible that age related *increases* in glial cells could, in part, counterbalance any change due to neuronal atrophy and loss. Hence, microscopic investigations are needed to clarify the cellular counterpart of these gross tissue changes. However, despite more than half a century of scientific effort, it is still far from clear as to what extent, and in what areas of the brain, any age-related attrition in neuronal number might take place.

Cerebral Cortex

Accurate quantification of nerve cell numbers in the cerebral cortex presents great difficulty, partly because out of necessity only a small proportion of the total tissue can be sampled, but also because of the cytoarchitectonic variations that occur within and between cortical regions. Nonetheless, most early studies,[36–42] based on total nerve cell counts or counts of specific cell populations, like pyramidal cells, within single tissue sections, generally demonstrated a progressive decline in nerve cell number with aging in areas such as the temporal cortex (middle and inferior temporal gyri), the pre- and postcentral gyrus, the striate cortex, and the inferior and superior frontal cortex, leading to average overall losses in old age ranging from about 10 to 50 percent with the greatest changes occurring in the frontal and temporal cortex. No consensus regarding what nerve cell types might be affected, however, has been reached. In some studies[39,40,42] emphasis was placed on the larger, presumably pyramidal, cell population, but in others[36,37] involvement of small cells (interneurones) was stressed; in the remainder[38,41] no preferential cellular involvement was detected, or at least mentioned. Furthermore, in (most of) these studies, little or no attempt was made to correct these "raw" cell density measurements for any overall or local changes in tissue volume taking place in later life[27,32,42,43] that might lead to a compacting down of surviving tissue elements and produce an artifactually high numerical density value. Hence, the actual cell loss, correcting for this cortical atrophy, will in all likelihood be somewhat in excess of figures quoted. A density value indicating no change in cell number with age will probably mean that an actual loss of cells will have taken place, but only up to a level that matches the overall degree of tissue shrinkage. This may explain later findings[27] in which no overall change in nerve cell density was found in several cortical regions with age, because here no compensation for this cortical atrophy was made. In this same study,[27] however, it was noted that the density of "large" cells in the tissue did in fact decrease with age, though this was counterbalanced by an increase in density of "small" cells, and it was concluded that while some cell loss was likely in old age, most tissue change related to a shrinkage, rather than an actual loss of, the large pyramidal cells. Haug and colleagues[33,34,44,45] and Braak and Braak[46] have likewise concluded that nerve cell loss is slight in old age and cell shrinkage may be more important than actual perikaryal loss in producing local or overall decreases in cerebral cortical volume[32,44] and brain weight[34] in later life.

Hence, while most early studies point toward a substantial decrease in the number of nerve cells, and perhaps particularly the larger pyramidal cells, in old age later studies have stressed that only a shrinkage of neurones occurs with little actual numerical change. Clearly, methodologic problems arising from the examination of small amounts of tissue in relatively few individuals and using an assortment of counting techniques are likely to account for much of these discrepancies; at present a definitive answer to the question of cell loss from the cerebral cortex in aging is still awaited. Nonetheless, on balance, it does seem that some nerve cell loss is likely in many elderly people, but this may be much less than was formerly thought to be the case. The extent of neuronal shrinkage (atrophy) may be a more important factor in dictating the functional efficiency of brain tissue in old age.

Hippocampus

Possible changes in the nerve cell complement of the hippocampus have been studied on many occasions, and while in some instances the entire structure has been sampled, in others only specific subregions, usually areas CA1 or subiculum, have been investigated. In many studies[41,42,47–51] a loss of pyramidal cells, ranging from 20 to 50 percent, from areas CA1 or subiculum or both, have been recorded though in others[52–54] little or no (significant) change was found in these or other parts of the hippocampus. While, as with the cerebral cortex, the problems of wide interindividual variation and small sample sizes will militate against detecting a significant decline (even if this does actually occur) in some studies[52,54] it is also notable that in others[42,48–50] a statistically significant decrease in neurone number was achieved only when a correction for the *overall* atrophy of the hippocampus was made. However, because Davies et al.[54] have found that the width of the pyramidal cell band itself remains unchanged in later life, such corrections of raw cell counts for atrophy based on *overall* hippocampal size may actually be erroneous and basic cell counts may be sufficient. Hence, at present, it is strongly suspected that some loss of nerve cells from one or other part of the hippocampus may occur in old age, though again a definitive study that encompasses sufficient individuals of wide enough age range and addresses the possible affects of *local* atrophy is still awaited.

Amygdala

Only a single study[55] has investigated changes in nerve cell number in the amygdala and in this only small, though significant, decreases ranging from 3 to 9 percent were found in cortical, medial, and central nuclei, with no losses being detected in other areas of this brain region.

Cerebellum

A clear loss of Purkinje cells from the cerebellar cortex with aging has been detected in all of those studies[56–59] that have addressed this issue, this amounting to about 20 to 35 percent of the original cell number by 90 years of age. No change in cell number, however, has been found among the nerve cells of the dentate nucleus.[60]

Subcortical Regions

The relative ease of defining anatomical boundaries and discriminating nerve cell types has made it possible to investigate age-related changes in many subcortical regions with a greater degree of accuracy than has been possible so far for most cortical structures. Hence, a higher degree of unaniminity has been achieved among the various studies that have examined these.

Many of the cranial nerve nuclei of the brain stem such as those of the cochlear,[61] trochlear,[62] abducens,[63] and facial[64] nerves show no reduction in nerve cell number with aging. However, among the catecholaminergic cell groups a substantial loss of cells with aging has been consistently shown for the locus ceruleus complex,[65–73] the substantia nigra,[74–78] and the dorsal motor vagus,[79] though no change was seen in the dorsal raphe.[67,68] While one study[80] found a 20 percent reduction in the number of nerve cells in the inferior olivary nucleus, two others[81,82] have reported no changes. Tomlinson and Irving[83] found no change in the number of anterior horn cells in the spinal cord before 60 years of age, though 30 percent of these were eventually lost by 90 years of age.

In the basal ganglia, one study[84] has reported a decrease

in neuronal density in the putamen whereas two others[45,85] have found no change in cell number. There have been three reports[86–88] showing an age-related decline in nerve cell number in the nucleus basalis of Meynert complex though other studies[89–91] have claimed this not to occur. Finally, in the hypothalamic region, Wilkinson and Davies[92] detected no cell loss from the mammillary bodies with age and the density of nerve cells in the supraoptic and paraventricular nucleus remains unchanged.[93,94] While vasopressin-containing cells of the suprachiasmatic nucleus and the sexually dimorphic nucleus[95] are decreased in number with aging, there are no changes in the vasoactive intestinal peptide (VIP)-containing cells of these regions.[96]

Regressive Changes in Neurones with Aging

As has already been argued, an actual loss of nerve cells may not necessarily be the only route whereby the function of any particular brain region might become compromised in later life. A fall in the number, or a reduction in the size of, synapses or dendrites without overt perikaryal loss may impair function just as drastically as if a loss of the entire nerve cell had taken place.

Dendritic Changes

Dendrites comprise some 95 percent of the total receptive cell surface area that neurones offer for contact with other neurones.[97] Hence, maintenance of the dendritic tree is paramount in ensuring the integrative capacity of an individual nerve cell, or the region in which such cells are contained. Failure to maintain dendrites may lead to a deterioration in function should this fall below a critical threshold.

Early studies using the rapid Golgi technique,[98–100] suggested a reduction in the size of the dendritic tree with ageing in pyramidal cells of the hippocampus and cerebral cortex, this being associated with morphological changes involving a loss of dendritic spines and a swelling and distortion of the dendrites themselves. However, Golgi procedures of this kind are notoriously capricious to perform and highly selective in the cells they impregnate. Later work,[101,102] using a more reliable Golgi-Cox procedure,[103] failed to replicate these earlier studies and, moreover, demonstrated a net *increase* in the dendritic tree of pyramidal cells of the entorhinal cortex in later life suggestive of a compensatory response on the part of surviving cells to loss of their neighbors. Other studies by these same workers[104,105] likewise detected an increase in the dendritic extent of hippocampal granule cells between 52 and 73 years of age, though this response was lost in extreme old age (90 years) where a net reduction of dendrites, compared to the 73-year-old group, was seen. Nevertheless, pyramidal cells in the frontal[106] and motor[107] cortex have been shown to regress continually throughout life. Hence, it is still unclear whether, and to what extent, the dendritic system of nerve cells might regress in old age. Much local variation seems to occur especially in terms of cell type with some cells (e.g., those in the hippocampal formation) apparently possessing capacity for adaptive change, but others (as in the neocortex), not. Perhaps local events, such as deafferentation, glial cell changes, or vascular insufficiencies, might impact upon the microenvironment of nerve cells and help to dictate these regionally variable changes in dendritic plasticity during aging.

Axonal Changes

The difficulties in obtaining suitably preserved tissue for ultrastructural analysis and the problems of accurately and representatively determining synaptic density in minute portions of tissue have led to a paucity of information concerning synaptic changes with aging. An age-related decrease in synaptic density has been demonstrated in some cortical areas, such as the precentral gyrus[108,109] and frontal cortex,[110,111] but not in others, like the postcentral gyrus[108,109] and temporal cortex.[110,111] However, any effect of an actual loss of synapses may be (at least partially) offset by compensatory changes involving a lengthening of the contact zone of remaining synapses,[108,112] which increase the presynaptic contact area. In this way even a substantial numerical loss of synapses may be tolerated without (appreciable) tissue dysfunction.

Perikaryal Changes

The overall reduction in nerve cell size with aging[27,34,41,46] has already been commented upon, though the structural and molecular causes of this perikaryal atrophy are not known. These may involve a reduction in the amount of internal membrane (e.g., rough endoplasmic reticulum) since several studies[67,68,113,114] have shown a progressive loss of cytoplasmic RNA with aging from nerve cells of a variety of types. Whether such nucleic acid changes are primary and relate to genomic defects is not known; they may "simply" reflect adaptive responses to an anatomically reduced dendritic tree or axonal plexus or represent a physiologic "underactivity" of neurotransmission. Other perikaryal changes with aging, involving a formation and accumulation of inclusion bodies, such as neurofibrillary tangles, Lewy bodies, granulovacuoles, or pigment granules will be discussed later.

Amyloid Plaques

The Prevalence of Plaques in the Elderly

A deposition of amyloid β protein (Aβ) in the form of plaques, principally within the gray matter of the cerebral cortex, but also elsewhere in the brain, occurs in many old people with perhaps as many as 70 percent or more of those over 80 years of age showing some degree of plaque formation.[115–126] However, not *all* elderly people seem to accumulate such plaques in their brains no matter how long they live; an absence of amyloid deposits in many octogenarians and even in some centenarians is documented[122,126,127] though others[124] have shown a universal involvement in subjects 100 years of age and older. Such observations imply that the potential to deposit Aβ in later life is commonplace and only small or subtle differences in biological factors that promote this deposition may be required to ensure that this strong inherent, and possibly inherited, tendency takes place.

The Distribution of Amyloid Plaques in the Brain

When present, amyloid plaques occur most commonly, and at greatest densities, within the association areas of the neocortex, particularly the frontal, temporal, cingulate, insular, and occipital regions. Plaques are less likely in the primary motor and sensory cortices. However, archicortical regions such as the hippocampus (especially areas CA1 and subiculum), amygdala (cortical and medial nuclei particularly), and hypothalamus can be affected, as can subcortical structures such as the caudate nucleus and putamen, the medial thalamus, and sometimes the cerebellar cortex and periaqueductal gray matter.[115–126] Plaques do not occur in the deep gray nuclei of the cerebellum and brain stem, nor are they seen in the gray matter of the spinal cord; white matter regions likewise contain no amyloid deposits.[115–126]

The Morphology of Plaques

The Size of Plaques

Plaques can measure any size from 5 to 200 μm in cross section. Size frequency distributions show a positive skewed distribution with few deposits being less than 10 μm in diameter, and most having a diameter between 20 to 40 μm; the frequency of larger deposits progressively decreases with increasing plaque diameter.[128,129] This size frequency profile approximates to a negative exponential distribution and does not reflect sectioning artifacts of objects of fairly even size. Plaque size may be related to the size or frequency of those cells responsible for its production with the greater the number (density) of cells present, or the larger such cells might be, producing a bigger plaque. Nonetheless, in the later stages of plaque evolution some compacting of its constituents may result in a decrease in overall size.

The Appearance of Plaques

The principal component of plaques is Aβ. When tissue sections are immunostained using antibodies against this protein, most plaques in the cerebral cortex, and indeed virtually all of those (when present) in the caudate nucleus, putamen, thalamus, hypothalamus, and cerebellum, appear as areas where the stained Aβ is finely and evenly distributed.[119–126] Such plaques are known as "diffuse plaques." However, other plaques, particularly in the cerebral cortex, hippocampus, and amygdala adopt a form where the Aβ is compacted, these sometimes appearing to have a dense central core of material surrounded by a paler staining "halo" of Aβ. These latter plaques have been variously termed "cored" plaques, "mature" plaques, "classical" plaques or more historically, "senile plaques." Not only is this kind of plaque less common in the cerebral cortex, but it may be absent in some instances even when (many) diffuse plaques are regularly seen. The Aβ within these cored plaques (this of the above terms is preferred and will be used subsequently) is present in a β-pleated sheet structure and as such can be easily detected by dyes like Congo red, where it appears as a red-green birefringence when viewed under polarized light, or thioflavine S as a bright yellow fluorescence. In diffuse plaques the Aβ is poorly organized, if at all, into this β-pleated structure and accordingly such plaques are not detectable using these latter techniques. This may explain why the diffuse plaque went unrecognized for so long, since early methodologies commonly employed to detect plaques used only one or other of these two stains. Normal appearing axons often cross diffuse plaques and the Aβ may enclose nerve cell bodies or blood vessels, particularly when present as large conglomerates.[130–135]

There are other important distinctions, apart from the density and distribution of Aβ, between cored and diffuse plaques. Cored plaques, when stained using "classic" silver impregnation techniques like the Bielschowsky, Bodian, or Palmgren methods, but not diffuse plaques, contain swollen, densely staining filamentous structures called "neurites"; these relate to damaged nerve terminals, both axonal and dendritic in origin. Such plaques have been called, for obvious reasons, "neuritic plaques" though because this was the first type of plaque originally observed in Alzheimer's disease (senile dementia) early this century, using these same kinds of silver staining methods, the name "senile plaque" was applied. Neuritic (senile) plaques are much less common than diffuse, non-neuritic plaques and may be seen, even in the cerebral cortex, in only about 10 to 15 percent of elderly but nondemented individuals.[30,119,121,136–138] Other differences exist: glial cells, both microglial and astrocytic, are common within cored plaques but are sparse, and often absent, in diffuse plaques. These glial cell changes may represent differences in the maturation state (evolution) of plaques. However, despite these differences, both diffuse and cored plaques show a common presence of a wide variety of so-called amyloid-associated proteins or "chaperone" proteins, like the apolipoproteins (Apo) A1, E, and J, heparan sulfate proteoglycan (HSPG), amyloid P component, α-1 antichymotrypsin (α-ACT), and complement factors, all of which may play a role(s) in favoring the deposition of Aβ within the tissue or in its "organization" into the fibrillary β-pleated structure.

Hence, amyloid plaques represent complex foci of damage to, and destruction of, brain tissue. Given the multiplicity of cellular and noncellular elements they contain, it is understandable that under the light microscope they will present, in any one person or even in any given region of tissue, with a wide spectrum of morphologies, and often also with wide-ranging densities according to the particular component being sought and the staining procedure being used.

The Ultrastructural Appearance of Plaques

Although early ultrastructural studies[139–142] claimed that the Aβ within diffuse plaques existed as an amorphous nonfibrillary material, termed "preamyloid", later work,[143,144] using well-preserved biopsy or autopsy tissues, showed that Aβ is always in fibrillary form, such plaques being composed of bundles of amyloid, or single fibrils, loosely interwoven between neuronal and neuritic elements and the cell bodies and processes of glial cells. Each single, unbranched amyloid fibril is 5 to 10 nm in thickness and longitudinally narrows every 30 to 40 nm through a helical winding of the pair of filaments from which it is composed. All amyloid is present extracellularly and the fibrils run haphazardly, though sometimes they originate (especially in cored plaques) from an obvious central mass of a similar substance. The neuritic elements with which they intermingle contain numerous dense lamellar and multivesicular bodies, these probably originating from degenerate mitochondria. Many neurites also contain variable numbers of structures called paired helical filaments (PHF) which are also present, as neurofibrillary tangles (NFT) in the perikaryon of nerve cells, and neuropil threads in the proximal dendrites or dendritic sprouts of affected neurones.[145] The structure and origin of these will be described later.

The Evolution of Plaques

It is now accepted that plaques are dynamic structures that can exist in the tissue for many years over which period of time they may undergo a substantial modification and reorganization of their component parts. It has been widely assumed that because diffuse plaques far outweigh numerically the cored and neuritic plaques, the former may represent the morphological forerunner of the latter. Studies in Down syndrome,[116,134,146–152] where the development of the pathologic changes of Alzheimer's disease by middle age is entirely predictable,[146] substantiate this view. In most younger persons with Down syndrome, diffuse plaques will have appeared in the cerebral cortex by 30 years of age. These quickly acquire many of the extra-cellular protein (ApoE, HSPG, complement factors, α-ACT) and cellular (microglia) characteristics of the cored plaques, though the latter are not regularly present until after 40 years of age. The presence of neuritic and astrocytic changes in cored plaques and NFT in nerve cell bodies is not seen until at least 10 to 15 years after the onset of Aβ deposition.

These data have challenged the original postulates[153] that (1) the abnormal neurite is the initial structural manifestation of plaque formation with the earliest (so-called primitive) plaques being composed of a cluster of distended neurites with few or no amyloid fibrils and, (2) that amyloid deposition increases according to the spread of the neuritic changes. Instead, it is now widely believed that plaque formation starts with the extracellular deposition of Aβ as a diffuse plaque and that (at least a proportion of) these evolve with time into the cored, neuritic plaques. However, because the diffuse amyloid plaques of the cerebellum and corpus striatum never evolve into cored plaques nor acquire neurites,[148,154] neither do the diffuse-type plaques in the cerebral cortex of aged animals,[155–157] it remains possible, though perhaps unlikely, that each plaque type originates separately and evolves independently. Nevertheless, because the earliest, and possibly the most critical, changes associated with plaque formation seem to involve Aβ deposition, much effort has been made recently toward characterizing the biochemical and molecular features of Aβ, identifying its cellular source and investigating factors which might influence its deposition within the tissue.

The Composition of Aβ

Chemical Studies

About 25 percent of the dry weight of the plaque core is protein. Much of the rest may contain inorganic elements like aluminium and silicon, these perhaps being present as an aluminosilicate,[158–161] though this is disputed.[162,163] Some 70 percent of the protein part is Aβ.[164] Initial studies[161] showed that the Aβ extractable from plaque cores is composed of a peptide of molecular mass around 4.2 kd, but its actual length varies from 39 to 43 amino acids. Later analyses[164–171] have substantiated this and confirmed that the extractable amyloid is indeed of variable length and occurs mostly as $A\beta_{x-42}$, where x is mainly asp-1 or leu-17, though numerous other start points are also possible, especially at glu3 or glu11, with both of these being converted into pyroglutamate. Isomerization or racemization of asp-1 may also take place. Analysis of tissue regions rich only in *diffuse* plaques again shows some Aβ to be composed of $A\beta_{x-42}$ though here $A\beta_{17-42}$ appears a major peptide species.[155,168] Interestingly, there appears to be little carboxy-terminal heterogeneity and only minor quantities of peptide terminating at val39, val40, or thr43 are detected.

Immunohistochemical Analyses

Immunohistochemical studies using antibodies end-specific for val40 or ala42 (thr43) of the Aβ sequence[150,151,154,172–179] show that the major Aβ peptide species within cored plaques terminate at ala42 (i.e., $A\beta_{42}$) with only minor and varying amounts terminating at val40 (i.e., $A\beta_{40}$). Furthermore, the diffuse type of plaque contains *only* $A\beta_{42}$, irrespective of whether this is located in the cerebral cortex, the cerebellum, or the corpus striatum. Indeed, these observations hold firm for diffuse and cored plaques whether they occur in the nondemented elderly, in Alzheimer's disease, or in Down syndrome. Hence, it is likely that $A\beta_{42}$ represents the predominant, and also the initial, Aβ peptide species that is deposited in plaques of all morphologic forms. $A\beta_{40}$ becomes present only in a subset of plaques, relating chiefly to those of a cored variety. The amino-terminal heterogeneity in plaque amyloid, apparent in protein chemistry, is also seen by immunohistochemistry.[151,180,181] Both diffuse and cored plaques show strong immunoreactivity for Aβ species commencing at asp-1, with or without racemization or isomerization, and pyroglutamate-3, again irrespective of anatomical location or clinical setting. However, apparently very little $A\beta_{17-42}$ can be detected immunohistochemically[181] even though chemical analyses[155,168] suggest otherwise.

Hence, taken together, chemical and immunohistochemical analyses suggest that $A\beta$ might deposit within the tissue initially as unmodified $A\beta_{1-42}$, then undergo amino-terminal modifications, involving racemization, isomerization, or proteolysis and pyroglutamation of the initial two amino acids to give $A\beta_{3-42}$. Alternatively, $A\beta_{3-42}$ might also be an initial product that again undergoes modification. Whether these amino-terminal modifications precede tissue deposition, or occur following the deposition of $A\beta$ as plaques is not known, though their effect in either case will be to hamper the proteolysis of $A\beta$ by aminopeptidases and contribute to its stability once deposited within the tissue.

The Source of $A\beta$

$A\beta$ deposits vary much in size and shape. Diffuse plaques are often large, irregular in outline, and frequently merge into conglomerate deposits. Cored plaques are usually smaller, fairly constant in size, and are often rounded in shape (they may even be spherical in three dimensions). The factors that determine these appearances are not known but they may relate to the actual cellular source of the $A\beta$. Diffuse plaques are topographically associated with neuronal cell bodies[130–135] whereas cored plaques contain many microglial cells and their processes[134,149,182,183] and sometimes also blood vessels.[135,184,185] Whether these relationships represent more than chance associations between geographically common structures is not clear. It is possible that the initial deposition of $A\beta$ in diffuse plaques relates to a release of this from nerve cells while subsequent development into what are considered to be more mature, cored plaques rests with the presence of associated glial cells. A hematogenous source for $A\beta$, although a popular concept at one time, is unlikely.

The Amyloid Precursor Protein

$A\beta$ is not a native genomic product but is derived from the proteolytic breakdown of a larger precursor, known as amyloid precursor protein (APP). The APP gene is located on the long arm of chromosome 21 and contains 19 coding regions (exons), extending over 400 kb.[186–188] Alternative splicing of the single mRNA transcript of this gene produces multiple isoforms of which APP_{695}, APP_{751} and APP_{770} are the predominant ones expressed in brain tissue.[189–191] Because the gene sequence transcribing $A\beta$ lies across two neighboring exons (exons 16 and 17), $A\beta$ cannot be produced by any aberrant or minor splicing mechanism. In the brain, APP mRNA is abundant in neurones and endothelial cells[191–194] mostly as APP_{695}, whereas APP_{751} and APP_{770} are transcribed fairly uniformly across the brain and are the species principally produced by glial cells,[195–198] especially microglial cells and particularly upon their activation. All translated proteins are modified through N- and O-glycosylation, tyrosine sulfation, or phosphorylation[199,200] within the Golgi apparatus to produce a family of gene products, Mr110 to 135 kd.[201,202] These are transported by axonal flow[203] to the nerve cell terminals where some are proteolytically cleaved along the way and secreted into the extracellular space (as secreted APP), and some are inserted, in full length form, into the cell membrane, probably at the synapse.[204] Changes in APP expression with aging, favoring a relative increase in APP_{751} and APP_{770} species[205,206] may represent an increased glial cell activity in later life, rather than a shift in the pattern of neuronal expression toward old age. The absence of $A\beta$ deposits in any tissue other than the brain, except for perhaps the skin,[207,208] despite the almost universal tissue expression of the APP gene, implies either a particular idiosyncracy in the manner whereby APP is catabolized in the brain, or how $A\beta$ is cleared from the brain tissue once formed.

The biological function(s) of APP currently remain unknown, though the secreted forms of $APP_{751/770}$, derived from platelets, are identical to protease nexin II, a protease inhibitor secreted by fibroblasts, and the inhibitor of coagulation factor XIa.[209–212] These may function in terms of wound repair or in the regulation of the coagulation cascade. Cells in peripheral tissues showing high APP expression are characterized by their high membrane fusion capacity, suggesting that APP might function in relationship to tissue maintenance and repair, affecting cell-cell and cell-matrix interactions.[213–215] Membrane-bound forms might act as a G-protein receptor[216] or a signal transductor.[217,218]

The expression of APP increases in times of trauma,[219] hypoxia/ischemia,[220,221] or intoxication[222,223] and this may follow upregulation of the APP gene by glial cell released interleukin-1.[224–227] Hence, increased APP expression may form part of an acute cell or tissue response to "stresses" of diverse kinds and APP may play a vital role in mediating or modulating reactive or adaptive changes to this in terms of maintenance of tissue integrity.

The Processing of APP into $A\beta$

$A\beta$ is a proteolytic fragment of APP comprising the first 28 amino acids immediately amino-terminal to the membrane surface (when inserted therein) plus the first 12 to 15 residues of the putative transmembrane domain. Hence, $A\beta$ must be formed as a result of two separate proteolytic events occurring at both the amino- and the carboxyl-sides of the $A\beta$ sequence. However, most full-length APP produced by the cell follows a secretory processing route involving the enzyme α-secretase, which cuts the full-length APP molecule around, though usually between, residues 16 and 17 of the $A\beta$ sequence.[199,228,229] As a result of this a large amino-terminal secreted portion (Mr = 105 to 124 kd) is produced and released into the extracellular space[201,202] and a small carboxy-terminal fragment of ~8 kd, consisting of the last 82 amino acids of the APP sequence is retained intracellularly.[230] This is cut by a further enzyme,

γ-secretase, acting at or around residues 40 or 42/43 of the Aβ sequence to produce fragments of 3 kd (i.e., Aβ_{17-40}, Aβ_{17-42}), collectively known as P3 peptide,[231] which are then released from the cell, presumably as a waste product. Hence, processing of APP along this route will preclude the formation of full-length Aβ and thereby avoid the possibility of Aβ depositing in plaque form.

α-Secretase mediated secretion of APP is regulated by the phosphorylative action of phosphokinase C[232] this in turn being driven by acetylcholine through its action on muscarinic receptors on the neuronal cell surface[233] or via interleukin-1.[224–227] Inhibitors of phosphokinase C have the opposite effect, reducing APP secretion and importantly, *increasing* the release of Aβ. These presumably cause a diversion of APP along pathways that involve a degradation by enzymes other than α-secretase. Hence, the degradation products Aβ and P3 occur in opposing balance; when APP secretion is high, Aβ levels are low, but P3 levels are high. Reductions in APP secretion lower P3 levels and increase Aβ production. Such observations imply the existence of competing routes for APP catabolism.

This competing mechanism involves a further enzyme, β-secretase, which cuts APP close to the amino-terminus of Aβ, at or around amino acid 672 of the APP_{770} sequence, and acts mainly on the APP_{695} isoform principally produced by neurones.[234,235] This again produces a secreted APP molecule of about 93 kd, but retains a carboxyl terminal fragment of 11 kd that starts with, and contains the whole of, the Aβ sequence. This fragment can likewise act as a substrate for γ-secretase, which again removes the carboxyl-terminus to produce Aβ molecules between 39 and 43 amino acids long. These are released in soluble form into the extracellular tissue fluid[231,235,237–240] or the cerebrospinal fluid.[236,241,242]

Analysis of the APP carboxyl domain structure shows a consensus sequence for endocytosis via clathrin-coated pits. Hence, presumably, full-length APP molecules can be reinternalized from the cell surface or the extracellular space into the endosomal-lysosomal compartment of the cell. Degradation, again via secretase activity, produces a range of carboxyl-terminal fragments containing both Aβ and P3 peptide sequences[232,239,243,244]; these could be released into the extracellular space as Aβ or P3 following further catabolism.

Most of the Aβ formed via these various routes appears to be secreted as Aβ_{1-40}, with lesser (~ 17 percent) amounts of Aβ_{1-42} and other minor species being produced. The intracellular sites of APP processing are not known, though much of the newly formed APP is likely to be processed within the late Golgi apparatus, on its way to the cell surface for secretion.[245] At this site both α- and β-secretases can compete for the same APP molecules, according to the state of "activation" of the nerve cell and local requirements for secreted APP; the relative amounts of Aβ and P3 produced will reflect the balance of these enzyme activities. Any "spare" full-length APP molecules, destined for insertion as such into the cell membrane, can be subsequently broken down in endosomal compartments following their reinternalization.

Thus, although the actual deposition of Aβ within brain tissue is widely thought of as a pathologic event, the mechanisms whereby it is produced occur as part of the normal metabolic profile of the nerve cell. Nonetheless, once secreted from cells, Aβ molecules, because of their high hydrophobicity, have a great propensity to aggregate into fibrils, and in so doing are capable of forming tissue deposits of amyloid.

Plaque Formation

When first secreted into the extracellular space, Aβ molecules are present in soluble form[246,247] and must therefore be brought "out of solution" for fibrillization and subsequent aggregation into plaques to take place. The conversion of soluble Aβ molecules into insoluble Aβ fibrils proceeds via a nucleation type process[248,249] whereby soluble molecules form dimers and higher aggregates, eventually producing a nucleus that "seeds" fibril formation. Fibrillization can occur once the Aβ peptide concentration has reached a critical threshold with the prevailing local concentration of Aβ depending upon the rate at which soluble Aβ peptides are produced (as opposed to P3 peptides) and the rate at which they are removed from the extracellular fluid, either passively into the cerebrospinal fluid, or actively via extracellular proteolysis or internal catabolism following uptake by other (glial) cells. Also, the amino-acid, and particularly the carboxyl-terminal, characteristics of the secreted Aβ peptides influence the rate of fibrillization, because forms of Aβ terminating at residues 42 and 43 have a much higher propensity to fibrillize than those terminating at residue 40.[248,250,251] Similarly, the rate of accumulation of fibrils (plaque formation) will depend upon the balance drawn between rates of production and removal. Changes in particular local factors like the concentration of ApoE E4 protein,[249,252] zinc,[253,254] aluminium or iron,[254] HSPG,[255] or α-ACT[252] can all promote the conversion of Aβ peptides into fibrils either by reducing the lag time to nucleation or by favoring the rate of seeding once the process has begun.

It will not have gone unnoticed that the principal Aβ peptide species secreted by cells is Aβ_{1-40} while that eventually deposited as plaques in the brain is Aβ_{x-42} where x = 1, 3, 10, 17 among other start points. Thus, while Aβ species terminating at residue 42 are a minor constituent of secreted Aβ they form (because of their higher tendency to fibrillize[248]) the major, and indeed the initial, components of deposited Aβ. Analysis of readily solubilized Aβ from early diffuse plaques[246,247] shows this to be exclusively Aβ_{42} (see also immunohistochemistry[150,151,154,174–179]) and probably Aβ_{1-42}. Furthermore, this peptide species exists in the extracellular fluid even before Aβ fibrils become detectable by immunohistochemistry.[247] Following deposition of Aβ as diffuse amyloid plaques, amino-terminal modifications may take place. Aβ_{40} appears later in the course of plaque evolution, this perhaps "seeding" upon pre-existing Aβ_{42}-containing plaques, these enhancing the fibrillization of this former species which when present "normally" within the extracellular fluid is relatively resistant to aggregation. The region of Aβ critical for fibrillization appears to reside between residues 25 to 35, this being the part of the molecule with greatest hydrophobicity and that also confers the β-pleating characteristics of the peptide.[250,256]

The Neurotoxicity of Aβ

As in the primary and secondary amyloidoses affecting other tissues and organs of the body, it has been argued that the large amounts of Aβ deposited as plaques might similarly and adversely affect brain function. The presence of damaged nerve endings (dystrophic neurites) surrounding at least some of the amyloid plaques in the cerebral cortex further suggests that Aβ might actually take part in inducing this neurofibrillary pathology. Despite much experimental work, however, it still remains uncertain whether Aβ is neurotoxic in vivo, and if so by what mechanism toxicity might be invoked, though it does seem that neurotoxicity depends upon the aggregation state of Aβ.[257–260] Possible neurotoxic mechanisms might involve apoptosis[259–262] or necrosis[263] following oxidative stress,[258,264] or an increased vulnerability to Ca^{2+} mediated excitotoxic damage,[217] an interference with K^+ channels,[265] a predisposition towards hypoglycemia,[266] or an induction of microglial cell activation with production of neurotoxic substances.[267]

It is possible, however, that only certain Aβ peptide species possess (significant) neurotoxic properties. The diffuse plaques of the cerebellum and corpus striatum, which contain only Aβ_{42},[154] never acquire PHF-containing dystrophic neurites no matter how long they are present in the tissue.[134] Such data imply either that (unaggregated) Aβ_{42} is not neurotoxic, or that these latter brain regions are "insensitive" to its deposition. Further, the early diffuse plaques in the cerebral cortex, which again contain only Aβ_{42},[150,151] are apparently free from neuritic pathology and many seemingly remain so during their lifetime. On the other hand, neuritic plaques, in which neuronal damage is presumed to occur, always contain Aβ_{40}.[150,151] Hence, although a minor and late component of plaques, Aβ_{40}, and not Aβ_{42}, may be the peptide responsible in vivo for neurotoxicity when this is deposited in a suitably aggregated state upon pre-existing Aβ_{42}-containing plaques. The cellular source of Aβ_{40} in plaques is uncertain, but it may be produced by microglial cells.[149,183,197,198]

Amyloid-Associated Molecules

Most amyloid plaques, whether they be diffuse or cored (neuritic) or occur in the cerebral cortex or elsewhere, contain certain other proteins known as amyloid-associated proteins or "chaperone" proteins, which are tightly bound to, or are closely associated with, the Aβ fibrils. Principal among these are the apolipoproteins A1, E, and J, HSPG, α-ACT, complement factors, and amyloid P component, though many others such as fibronectin, laminin, collagen type IV, basic fibroblast growth factor, interleukins, transthyretin, α2-macroglobulin, lactoferrin, and complex oligosaccharides can also be present. The significance of many of these latter molecules particularly, in terms of amyloid deposition or plaque formation, remains unknown; some may simply bind passively to the Aβ protein because they happen to be present in the vicinity of the plaque in the extracellular fluid. Nonetheless, others may play important roles either by helping to bring Aβ molecules out of solution and into fibrillar form or by modifying the physicochemical state of the fibril once formed thereby influencing its stability in the tissue and determining the rate of build up of the amyloid deposit. They may also affect the course of evolution (maturation) of plaques over the many years that they are present within the tissue.

Apolipoprotein E

Apolipoprotein E (ApoE) is a polymorphic protein that facilitates the movement of cholesterol in and out of cells. Two common polymorphisms, at residues 112 and 158 of the ApoE gene, determine the three major allelic forms, E2, E3, and E4, and produce the six genotypes E2/E2, E2/E3, E2/E4, E3/E3, E3/E4, and E4/E4 of which the latter three are the most common. Two observations implicate ApoE in the pathogenesis of plaque formation. Firstly, numerous immunohistochemical studies[151,268–273] show that, as in systemic amyloids, ApoE can bind to Aβ in plaques. Secondly, possession of the E4 allelic variant of the ApoE gene is a major genetic determinant of some cases of early onset, and many cases of late onset, Alzheimer's disease,[274–280] this disorder being characterized by a widespread brain deposition of amyloid plaques.

How ApoE protein might influence the course of Aβ deposition is not clear though, because not all early diffuse plaques contain this,[151,281] binding may occur *after* Aβ has been deposited within the tissue in fibrillar form, rather than *while* Aβ is still in a soluble nondepositable form. Hence, ApoE may influence how much or in what form Aβ is deposited in the tissue, rather than determining whether deposition will occur or not. In this context, the E4 isoform may have a greater effect than the other isoforms, E2 and E3, and accordingly many studies[270,271,282–291] have compared the amount of Aβ deposited in the brain, mostly in cases of Alzheimer's disease, in the presence or otherwise of the E4 allelic form. While some reports[270,271,282–285] have suggested an increased Aβ deposition in cases possessing an E4 allele, and particularly in those homozygous in this respect, others[286–291] have not found this to be so. Much of these variations in findings may be due to the wide range in extent of Aβ deposition that can often occur between cases of AD of any given ApoE genotype or the small numbers of cases examined in each group, differing plaque load assessment methodologies, different staining techniques employed, or varying antibody specifications. Despite this, recent work[287,289] has shown that while the total amount of Aβ deposited as Aβ_{42} does not vary between genotype groups, the amount of Aβ_{40} does in fact increase with ApoE E4 allele copy number; possessors of one E4 allele have about twice as much Aβ_{40} in their brains as those with no E4 alleles, and those with two E4 alleles have more than three times as much. Because $A\beta_{40}$ is present in cored, rather than diffuse, plaques,[151,172] it is possible that the ApoE E4 protein facilitates, relative to the E2 and E3 isoforms, the subsequent aggregation of $A\beta$ into such cored masses. Alternatively, when bound to $A\beta$, the E4 isoform may increase its "attractiveness" to microglial cells compared to E2 or E3 proteins. In this context, it is notable that the diffuse plaques of the cerebellum and corpus striatum contain less ApoE protein than those of the cerebral cortex[273,281] and that these plaques also lack microglial cells[134] and do not contain $A\beta_{40}$.[154] Hence, ApoE, and particularly ApoE E4, protein may play a role in determining the subsequent maturation of plaques, though it does not seemingly influence the amount of $A\beta$ that is initially deposited in the tissue as $A\beta_{42}$.

Heparan Sulfate Proteoglycan

As in other systemic amyloids, heparan sulfate proteoglycan (HSPG) is present in both the diffuse and the cored plaques of the cerebral cortex,[292–297] but is absent from the diffuse plaques of the cerebellum.[297] The role of HSPG in plaque formation is unknown, though it may promote the aggregation of $A\beta$ fibrils into the β-pleated configuration characteristic of all amyloids. The absence of HSPG in the non-congophilic, thioflavine-negative diffuse plaques of the cerebellum[297] would be consistent with this role, but many diffuse plaques in the cerebral cortex remain non-congophilic yet these still contain HSPG[293]; presumably, in these the level of β-pleating is low and insufficient for visualization by these methods. The source of HSPG within plaques is not known, though this may originate from microglial cells[298–299]; again the lack of HSPG in cerebellar diffuse plaques,[297] which are also deficient in microglial cells,[134] would accord with this.

Complement Factors

Most of the complement factors and complement inhibitors characteristic of the activation cycle of the classic, but not the alternative, pathway are present in all amyloid plaques in the cerebral cortex, and are particularly rich in those of the cored variety with the diffuse cerebellar and striatal plaques containing little, if any, complement.[300–304] Complement factor Clq binds directly to $A\beta$ and in this way may signal engagement of the activation cycle without the need for immunoglobulin to be present.[304,305] Binding of Clq, however, depends upon the aggregation state of $A\beta$[306] and this may explain the relative absence of complement factors in cerebellar and striatal plaques where the $A\beta$ exists in a noncongophilic form.

Microglial cells express complement (Fc) receptors, especially when activated,[307,308] and because the presence of complement in plaques predates that of microglial cells binding of Cl to $A\beta$ may be the trigger to migration and activation of microglial cells, rather than the presence of $A\beta$ itself. The paucity of microglial cells in cerebellar plaques[134] lacking Cl[300–302] would accord with this. Immunoreactivity for the terminal membrane attack complex (MAC), C5b-9, is also seen, but only in neuritic plaques[304,308,309] suggesting that only in these plaques has the full classic pathway been activated; in diffuse plaques complement activity terminates at C3.

The complement inhibitors, vitronectin, clusterin (apolipoprotein J), and protectin (CD59) are also present in diffuse and neuritic plaques of the cerebral cortex.[310–313] While these might represent an attempt to minimize bystander lysis via MAC, they may also play a part in amyloidosis. Indeed, specific ionic reactions between ApoJ and $A\beta$[314] may maintain the solubility of the latter in extracellular fluids. This molecule, together with ApoA1 and ApoE, may act in concert to regulate the solubility of $A\beta$ and changes in the relative balance of these may favor the subsequent deposition of $A\beta$ in fibrillary form.[314–317]

Other Proteins

The diffuse and cored plaques of the cerebral cortex, and the diffuse plaques of the cerebellum, all contain α-ACT.[318–320] The purpose of this is uncertain, but it may, in conjunction with the apolipoproteins, promote the assembly of $A\beta$ peptides into amyloid fibrils.[252] Like the systemic amyloids, all amyloid plaques in the brain, irrespective of their morphologic type or topographic location, contain amyloid P component.[301,309,321–323] P component is highly resistant to proteolysis and its binding to $A\beta$ may be an important factor in maintaining the persistence of $A\beta$ deposits in brain tissue.[324]

While these amyloid-associated proteins may all play some part in fibrillogenesis, it is unlikely that one single protein is wholly responsible for this. The "balance" between the various proteins in plaques may exert a "net effect" deciding between $A\beta$ solubility and insolubility. Indeed, specific interactions between the amyloid-associated molecules themselves seem to occur[252,325] and particular regional variations in their distribution may determine the topography of plaques throughout the brain or their morphological characteristics.

Neuritic Changes

Although dystrophic neurites are characteristically seen in the cored amyloid plaques of the cerebral cortex, it has been suggested[326] that many of the diffuse plaques of this region may also contain such neurites, though to a much lesser extent. Diffuse plaques in the cerebellum and corpus striatum, however, do not contain neurites no matter how long they might persist in the tissue.[154] The actual origin of these altered nerve endings is not clear and it is likely that both axons and dendrites contribute. Under the electron microscope neurites contain many dense lamellar and multivesicular bodies, these probably being the remains of degenerate mitochondria, and the PHF typically present in NFT. While many neurites may indeed derive from axons, no one single nerve type is involved with neurites displaying a wide range of immunoreactivities for (markers of) neurotransmitters like acetylcholine,[327,328] noradrenalin,[329] somatostatin,[330–333] substance P,[334] and neuropeptide Y.[333,335] Damage to nerve endings in plaques may thus occur unselectively with most, or even all, types of terminal being affected irrespective of its morphological characteristics or neurotransmitter type; the actual mix of transmitters involved in the plaque may depend solely on the local relative proportions of each at the site of damage.

In accordance with the neuritic dystrophy, there is also axonal damage and loss of synapses and axons from tissue regions containing such plaques.[336–339] Synaptic loss, however, does not occur in areas of diffuse amyloid deposition.[339] Hence, neuritic plaques can be considered as "malignant" plaques whose presence damages brain tissue and (presumably) interferes with brain function. On the other hand, no obvious destructive changes are associated with diffuse plaques, even in those of the cerebral cortex, and these may be thought of as "benign" deposits.

Neurites also contain much APP[340–346] and while this might signal the neurite as a site of catabolism of APP and a potential source of Aβ deposition, it may simply reflect the damming up of newly delivered, but unused, APP to these damaged nerve endings. Some neurites also contain the growth associated protein, GAP-43[347,348] suggesting these may be regenerating, rather than degenerating, nerve endings.

Glial Cells in Plaques

Apart from the extracellular Aβ and the neuritic changes, plaques also contain glial cells, both astrocytic and microglial in nature, this being particularly so in the case of the cored, neuritic plaque types with much less or no glial reaction being seen in the diffuse amyloid deposits.[134] Within cored plaques the microglial cells are large and plump, being known as ameboid or activated microglial cells, whereas in diffuse plaques the microglial cells are smaller and have long thin processes—ramified microglia. The microglial cells and processes are closely associated with the amyloid deposits, particularly in cored plaques where they lie in between the clumps and bundles of fibrils; indeed at electron microscope level, microglial cell processes appear to come into direct contact with Aβ fibrils that in some instances seem to be streaming into, or away from, the microglial cell body.[349–351] Diffuse plaques are not so closely associated with microglial cells or their processes,[352] especially the diffuse plaques of the cerebellum and corpus striatum which are usually devoid of such cells.[134]

Astrocytes are also frequent within cored plaques[134, 353–357] but are much less common in diffuse plaques, again especially those of the cerebellum.[134] In contrast to microglial cells, astrocyte cell bodies are typically present around the margins of the plaque though they may direct their processes inwards toward the plaque core.

The Chronology of Glial Cell Involvement

Early diffuse Aβ deposits do not contain glial cells of any kind. Presently, these come to contain microglial cells, the numbers of which increase as the plaques adopt a cored appearance.[134] Immunohistochemistry[149,183] shows that the presence of microglial cells is correlated with the appearance of Aβ_{40} in plaques and as long as plaques remain solely Aβ_{42}-reactive, the microglial presence stays low. Likewise, astrocytes are absent from early diffuse plaques and may remain so throughout their lifetime.[134] Astrocytes only become widely present in cored plaques, and then only after many microglial cells have infiltrated the plaque and neuritic changes are well established.[134]

The factors that stimulate these glial reactions are not known. Because microglial cells express Fc receptors,[307,308] it is possible that Aβ becomes chemotactic for these once it has received a coating of complement Clq, or perhaps apolipoprotein E, particularly the E4 isoform. Microglial cells produce interleukin-1[358]; release of this may engage the migration and activation of astrocytes within plaques, though this could also be directly triggered by damage to nerve endings.

The Role of Glial Cells in Plaques

The appearance of glial cells after the deposition of Aβ in plaques suggests a "reactive" role for both microglial cells and astrocytes; these cells may be responsible for many of the evolutionary changes in morphology that occur in plaques over the numerous years they exist.

Glial Cells and Amyloidosis

The close anatomic proximity of microglial cells to Aβ fibrils suggests a role in amyloidosis. However, it is clear that the tissue deposition of Aβ, as diffuse deposits, predates the presence of microglial cells[134,149,182,183,358] implying that, even though they are capable of expressing APP message[197,198,359–361] and may also contain APP protein, these cells are unlikely to be the primary or initial producers of Aβ. The reciprocal relationship between Aβ_{42} and Aβ_{40} staining of plaques[150,151] and the concurrence of Aβ_{40} and microglia[149,183] suggest that microglial cells may be the source of the Aβ_{40} in cored plaques. They may produce this from their own endogenous APP following activation[197,198,359–361] or it may result from a proteolytic trimming by them of the last two amino acids from pre-existing Aβ_{42}. Release of interleukin-1 from microglia[358,362] may cause upregulation of APP production in nearby neurones[224–227] which, following processing, may increase neuronal release of Aβ_{40} and Aβ_{42} with incorporation of this into the amyloid deposits. The absence of Aβ_{40} in the microglial-free diffuse plaques of the cerebellum[134,154] would accord with this scenario.

Because of their phagocytotic capabilities, microglial cells may participate in the proteolytic degradation and removal of Aβ.[363] However, Aβ deposits in elderly stroke victims seem to be cleared by circulating macrophages rather than by resident microglial cells.[364] This may occur because of the breach of the blood brain barrier in this latter condition, this usually remaining intact in old age and in neurodegeneration.

Microglial cells can secrete HSPG[298,299] and might thus encourage the adoption by Aβ of the β-pleated configuration typical of cored plaques, this perhaps being facilitated by removal of the final two amino acids from Aβ_{42}. Again, the lack of HSPG in diffuse cerebellar deposits,[297] where the Aβ is not β-pleated and microglial cells are absent,[134] would be in keeping with this role.

Although astrocytes can also express APP message and contain APP protein when activated,[195,196,365] it is uncertain whether they play any direct part in the production of the Aβ in plaques. Remodeling of the Aβ might, however, be achieved through release of α-ACT or ApoE, for which astrocytes appear to be the main cellular source within the CNS.

Glial Cells and Neurotoxicity

Microglial cells also possess high peroxidative capacity and might therefore produce excessive amounts of free radicals or nitric oxide,[267,366,367] which could damage nerve cell membranes and even induce neuritic or neurofibrillary changes if unscavenged. Again, the lack of PHF-containing neurites in diffuse cerebellar plaques and NFT in nearby Purkinje and other cells of the cerebellum[134] would accord with this. Astrocytes too produce potentially neurotoxic cytokines and nitric oxide and could also contribute to tissue damage through the release of these. Furthermore, expression of S-100 protein in astrocytes is increased in neuritic plaques[357,368–370] and this may play a part in stimulating the neuritic response; the lack of increased S-100 expression in the astrocyte-free diffuse cerebellar plaques[357] could again help to explain the absence of neuritic changes in this region.

Glial Cells and Inflammation

Microglial cells, particularly those of the cored and neuritic plaques, strongly express the major histocompatibility Class II antigen,[371,372] the usual purpose of which is to bind and present antigen to T-helper/inducer lymphocytes. They also express, at lower level, Class I antigen which interacts with T-cytotoxic/suppressor lymphocytes.[373] Because only few, and usually no, lymphocytes occur in plaques, these changes may simply reflect a change in activation state and need not necessarily imply an increased potential for T-lymphocytic interactions. The increase in reactive astrocytic processes in and around plaques[134,353–357] may serve as a physical barrier restricting the amount of tissue damage caused by plaque formation. However, the presence of much glial scar tissue, and the secretion of inhibitory factors by astrocytes, may limit the potential for regeneration of damaged tissue.

Hence, glial cells may play several important and complementary roles in plaque formation and evolution in line with their wide ranging capabilities. They could influence amyloidosis, induce neurotoxic changes, mediate acute phase responses, and engage in phagocytotic or "healing" reactions. Because glial cell changes concur with the neuritic alterations, clarification of the roles that these cells play in plaque pathogenesis may lead to therapies which could suppress many of the seemingly malignant changes taking place in plaques of these kinds, leaving perhaps only the relatively benign accumulation of diffuse amyloid, as Aβ_{42}, to bear testament to the site of tissue damage.

Neurofibrillary Tangles

The Prevalence and Distribution of Tangles

A few, widely scattered NFT occur in the brains of many (and perhaps most) nondemented elderly people.[30,47,120,121,126,137,374–377] In general, the number of NFT, particularly in the hippocampus and temporal cortex, increases with age though nonagenarians and centenarians may actually suffer less from NFT formation than those individuals between 70 and 90 years of age.[126] When present in such elderly subjects, NFT are most likely to occur, and to be most numerous, in the large stellate cells of layer II of the entorhinal cortex[376] which, for reasons still not understood, appear exquisitely sensitive to this change. Nonetheless, they can also commonly occur in the pyramidal cells of areas CA1 and subiculum, especially of the hippocampus and in the cells of the cortical and medial nuclei of the amygdala. Outside these regions NFT are usually rare, but can sometimes be seen in the pyramidal cells of layers III and V of the cerebral neocortex (inferior and middle temporal gyri) and in cells of subcortical regions like the nucleus basalis of Meynert, the locus ceruleus, and the raphe nuclei. Some nerve cell types apparently never form NFT, the Purkinje cells of the cerebellum and the large motor nerve cells of the cranial nerve nuclei, spinal cord, and precentral gyrus being notable examples.

The Morphologic Appearance of NFT

The morphologic appearance of NFT varies greatly according to the cell type in which it is contained. In smaller neurones of the cerebral cortex, NFT may appear as a single band of material looping around the nucleus and extending from the basal, toward the apical, dendrite. In larger pyramidal cells the NFT resembles a skein or tangle of wool, and in the hippocampus, and particularly in CA1 cells, it adopts the archetypical "flame" or "torch" shape. In subcortical regions NFT look like a ball of wool and are termed "globose." NFT are not easily seen in routinely stained sections, but are intensely argyrophilic, irrespective of their anatomical location, and are best demonstrated using silver impregnation methods like Bielschowsky, Palmgren, or Bodian techniques. Because the neurofibrillary material exists in a β-pleated configuration, NFT can also be visualized using Congo red and thioflavine S methods.

Although in most instances the cell outline and nucleus can still be seen in affected neurones, where the thick fibrils may weave tortuously throughout the cell body, on other occasions the NFT seems to be devoid of cytoplasmic material, apparently lying freely within the neuropil. These NFT have been called extracellular tangles or "ghost" (skeleton) tangles and represent an end-stage pathology where the affected nerve cell has died and the cell membranes have degenerated, liberating the residual tangle into the extracellular space.

Similar appearing neurofibrillary material can be seen extending into the dendrites of affected cells where, on sectioning, it appears as thread-like profiles, aptly called "neuropil threads."[145] These may also occur as dystrophic neurites within plaques.

The Ultrastructure of NFT

Ultrastructurally, NFT consist of numerous long, unbranched, but aligned filaments each being made up of a pair of filaments 15 nm in diameter wound around each other in a left-handed, α-helical manner.[378,379] Such an appearance led to the term "paired helical filaments" (PHF) as a descriptor of their morphology. Hence, because of this helical winding, each PHF is of maximum width of 24 nm and minimum width of 15 nm, with a periodicity of about 150 nm. Mixed in with, and sometimes forming a distinct segment of, the PHF are "straight filaments" of 15 nm in diameter.[380–384] When assembled, each strand of the PHF resembles a long stack of C-shaped subunits which in PHF are organized in a "base to base" manner whereas in the straight filament the same subunits are organized "back to back"; the latter produces a rounded cross-section instead of the helical alignment of PHF.[384] The straight filament is therefore a structural variant of the PHF and is not a separate anatomical or molecular entity. Individual PHF may be cross-linked, holding the bundles of filaments tightly together, and this in part accounts for their high insolubility and proteolytic resistance, enabling them to remain virtually unchanged in the tissue over a period of many years.

Molecular Characteristics of PHF

The intense insolubility characteristics of PHF have much hindered their analysis and it was not until about 10 years ago that immunohistochemistry first revealed them to be strongly reactive to antibodies against the microtubule associated protein, tau.[385–389] These findings were quickly confirmed by protein chemistry,[390–393] which further showed the tau to be incorporated into the PHF structure by its carboxyl third, this part of the molecule containing the microtubule binding domain. Nonetheless, immunohistochemistry shows PHF also to be reactive to many other cytoskeletal and noncytoskeletal proteins such as neurofilament protein,[394–399] MAP2,[400] vimentin,[401] and ubiquitin.[402,403] Of these, only the presence of ubiquitin has been directly confirmed by protein chemical analysis.[403] In some instances, the apparent immunoreactivity for neurofilament protein was due to a cross-reactivity between epitopes shared with tau.

This apparent mix of proteins within PHF seems at odds with their ordered structure. However, ultrastructural analysis of *isolated* PHF shows these to consist of an inner protease resistant "core" and an outer protease labile "fuzzy coat".[404] Following protease digestion, analysis of the core region shows it to be composed solely of tau.[393] Hence, it seems that the inner core of PHF is pure tau, to which a fuzzy coat containing more tau, but also including other proteins like ubiquitin and neurofilament protein, is more loosely adherent. It is not clear how much of the tau sequence is actually present in PHF and some amino- and carboxyl-truncation of the tau molecule seems to occur before its incorporation into the PHF structure.[404–406]

Tau protein normally exists in one of six isoforms, these being derived by the alternative splicing of a single transcript encoded on chromosome 17.[407] The isoforms differ according to the number (3 or 4) of tandem repeats containing the microtubule binding domain at the carboxy-terminus and the number (0, 1, or 2) of inserts toward the amino-terminus.[407] The tandem repeat section is rich in basic amino acids and binds to the acidic domain of tubulin, thereby maintaining the integrity of the microtubule system and its capacity for intracellular transport of proteins. In cells affected by NFT, there is a redistribution of tau proteins, from where they are normally present in the axonal compartment into the somatodendritic compartment, this being associated with a decrease in solubility into a form capable of self-assembly into PHF.[408,409]

When tau proteins are extracted from tissues rich in NFT, as in Alzheimer's disease affected brain, and "run" on polyacrylamide gels (with Western blotting) they show a reduced mobility, compared to tau from NFT-free tissues, appearing as characteristic bands at Mr55, 64, and 69 kd[410–412]; tau normally has Mr45 to 62 kd. This shift in mobility appears to be due solely to an increase (compared to normal tau) in the phosphorylation state of the pathologic tau, this incidently also increasing its resistance to proteolysis and favoring its assembly into PHF. All six isoforms of tau seem equally implicated in the formation of PHF. Hence, whereas normal tau has 2.5 to 3.5 moles of phosphate per mole of protein, pathologic tau has 10 to 12 moles of phosphate. How much of the abnormal tau exists in this hyperphosphorylated state is uncertain, though this may actually be as little as 10 percent[405] with half of this being present within the core structure and half in the fuzzy coat.[413]

It is still unclear whether the hyperphosphorylation of tau precedes the amino- and carboxyl truncation of the molecule prior to assembly into PHF, or whether truncation of some tau occurs as a separate and initiating event leading to the self-formation of the core structure upon which other, hyperphosphorylated, full-length tau molecules are deposited within the fuzzy coat region. Both concepts have been argued fiercely[405,414–416] and the relevance of phosphorylation as a key or critical stage in the process of PHF formation is still debated.

Phosphorylation of tau occurs mainly at Serine-Proline or Threonine-Proline motifs, of which there are 17 distributed across the tau molecule, 14 being shared by all 6 isoforms. It has long been uncertain whether the overphosphorylation of tau is due to the presence of extra phosphate at all 17 sites, or whether certain specific sites are involved while others retain a normal phosphorylation state. Early autopsy comparisons[417–419] of tau from normal and PHF-containing tissues (artifactually) suggested a preferential phosphorylation of certain sites in PHF tau, for example at Ser,[202] Ser,[396] and Ser.[404] However, more recent work[420–422] has shown that normal tau, when extracted promptly from biopsy tissue, is phosphorylated, but to a lesser extent, at nearly all the same sites as tau from PHF-rich tissues and that while all such phosphates long remain associated with PHF in autopsy tissues many quickly dissociate from normal tau at certain sites after death. Hence, overall differences in phosphate binding between normal tau and tau associated with PHF may be solely quantitative with the extent of phosphorylation at every site being consistently greater in PHF-tau. Nonetheless, it is not clear whether the hyperphosphorylation at *all* sites in PHF-tau is of *functional importance* and in this context phosphorylation at Ser[262] may be critical.[423] The major *functional* difference between PHF-tau and normal tau lies in its inability to bind to tubulin and therefore to stabilize microtubules. Of all the phosphorylation sites lying within the microtubule binding domain of tau only Ser[262] has been shown in autopsy tissues to be (over) phosphorylated in PHF-tau.[424,425] Phosphorylation at this particular site strongly inhibits the binding of tau to microtubules.[426] On the other hand, many of the sites phosphorylated in PHF-tau, including Ser,[262] are also phosphorylated in *a proportion of* fetal tau molecules and tau molecules derived from biopsy tissues,[421,427] yet the tau extracted from these tissues can bind to tubulin normally and promote correct microtubule assembly. Hence, phosphorylation of tau, particularly at Ser,[262] may form part of the normal phosphorylation/dephosphorylation, inactivation/activation cycle that regulates microtubule assembly/disassembly. (Over) phosphorylation of an excessive proportion of tau molecules at critical sites like Ser[262] may be sufficient to precipitate the abnormal accumulation of phosphorylated tau and the formation of PHF.

An increase in the phosphorylation state of tau might be due to an increase in protein kinase activity or a reduction in protein phosphatase activity, or some combination of both. The enzymes mitogen activated protein kinase (MAP kinase)[428,429] glycogen synthetase kinase (GSK) 3α and 3β,[430] and others such as casein kinase II,[431] proline directed protein kinase,[432] cyclin dependent kinases CDK2 and CDK5[433,434] and cyclic AMP-dependent protein kinase (CAMP-PK) and calcium/calmodulin dependent protein kinase II (CaMkII)[423] can all phosphorylate tau in vitro at those sites known to be phosphorylated in PHF-tau. Which of these enzymes is actually responsible, in situ, for increasing the net phosphorylation state of tau is uncertain though GSK 3β, CAMP-PK, and CaMkII are the only ones so far shown to be capable of in vitro phosphorylation of tau *within cells*.[423,435] Importantly, CAMP-PK and CaMkII can phosphorylate tau at Ser[262] (and Ser[356])—sites critical for the efficient binding of tau to tubulin when nonphosphorylated[423]—whereas GSK 3β operates mostly at Ser[235] and Ser.[404,430]

Of the many possible phosphate-removing enzymes that could play a role, it is known that phosphatases 1, 2A, and 2B can remove phosphates from Serine-Proline and Threonine-Proline tau motifs[436–439] though of these only phosphatase 1 and 2A can remove phosphates from Ser[262] (and Ser[356]) motifs.[427]

NFT and Cell Function

While the relevance of phosphorylation of tau to the pathogenesis of PHF formation remains contentious, the effect of this change in respect of microtubule assembly and intracellular protein transport is abundantly clear. Hyperphosphorylation of tau, particularly in the microtubule binding domain, will impair its binding to tubulin[426] and destabilize microtubules. This, plus a shift in cellular distribution of tau away from axonal and into somatodendritic compartments,[408,409] will have the effect of disrupting axonal transport and preventing the dispatch of macromolecules from the sites of production in the cell body to the points of utilization at the cell terminals. Derangement of cell metabolism and function will occur, continued damage undoubtedly causing the nerve cell to dysfunction and ultimately die.

Even a cursory microscopic inspection of nerve cells containing NFT suggests them to be incapable of normal function, at least during the later stages of PHF accumulation when the cell becomes densely packed. Indeed, indices of protein synthesis like nucleolar size or cytoplasmic RNA content show these to be lowered in NFT-bearing cells compared with their nontangled counterparts.[113,440,441] Ultrastructurally,[442] reductions in the number of ribosomes, extent of endoplasmic reticulum, and the density of mitochondria all correlate with increases in the amount of PHF in cortical pyramidal cells. NFT-containing cells are thus unlikely to be healthy cells, though they may retain (partial) function during the early stages of PHF accumulation.[443] Eventually, however, metabolism will fail and the affected cell will die. When this occurs the outer cell membrane is lost, and the perikaryal remains are liberated into the extracellular space. Such extracellular tangles (and neurites) progressively lose their tau and ubiquitin immunoreactivity[444–448] due to the proteolytic removal of amino-terminal fragments of tau and other molecules in the fuzzy coat region, though changes involving epitope accessibility may also occur. Proteolysis may be due to microglial cell action, these being common in the vicinity of extracellular NFT,[445,448,449,450] though actual phagocytosis of tangle remains by microglia seems unlikely.[352] Eventually, when much of the fuzzy coat components have been lost, the remaining core structure becomes immunoreactive to carboxyl-terminal tau antibodies[405,414,415,447] and, following further crosslinking of filaments,[451–454] remains long in the tissue, resistant to further degradation. The PHF skeleton may become infiltrated by astrocytes which may degrade, disperse, or phagocytose some of the residuum.[455–457] However, because counts of tangled (intracellular and extracellular) and nontangled cells in the hippocampus in some cases of Alzheimer's disease remain similar to counts of unaffected cells in normal persons,[458] it seems the capacity to remove such extracellular debris by glial cells is limited.

NFT and Other Proteins

Apart from tau, NFT contain various other principal proteins among which are ubiquitin and HSPG. It is well known from immunohistochemistry[402,403,459] and protein chemistry[403] that NFT contain ubiquitin protein. Ubiquitination of proteins serves to identify those effete or redundant proteins for intracellular proteolysis. Because NFT are so labeled, it is believed that the cell "recognizes" PHF (or phosphorylated tau) as unwanted protein and attempts to degrade it along recognized routes. Failure to achieve this leads to the progressive accumulation of PHF. Following cell death, extracellular NFT also lose their ubiquitin immunoreactivity[444–448] as the fuzzy coat proteins (of which ubiquitin is one) are removed by microglial cells or astrocytes.[445,448–450,455–457] Ubiquitination may be part of a wider "stress" response in NFT-containing cells since there are also increases in other "stress" proteins like HSP27,[460] HSP70,[461] and heme oxygenase-1 (HSP32)[462,463] and these may indicate an ongoing oxidative stress within tangle-bearing cells.

NFT-containing nerve cells stain strongly for the proteoglycans, HSPG[292–295] and chondroitin sulfate proteoglycan (CSPG),[464] these molecules again being located in the fuzzy coat region. The role of proteoglycan in NFT formation is unknown, though because HSPG also binds to Aβ[292–296] and probably helps to favor the adoption of a β-pleated configuration by this latter molecule it may similarly facilitate the β-pleating of PHF.

NFT, and particularly extracellular tangles, stain for apolipoprotein E[268,271,465,466] and Aβ[446,467–471] though these changes may only represent a secondary (passive) deposition and play no significant part in the formation or structural organization of PHF within NFT.

NFT persist in the tissue for many years and changes occur over time that increase their stability. These involve a binding with reducing sugars, such as glucose, and a participation in Maillard condensation reactions, involving glycation and oxidation steps, to produce end products like pyrraline and pentosidine.[451–454,472] Such reactions work especially strongly with lysine-rich proteins like tau[472] and may be invoked because of the delayed turnover of tau, following its phosphorylation, in the presence of reducing sugars. Reactions like these produce much cross-linking of proteins and this explains why NFT (and Aβ, which can also participate in similar condensation reactions) are difficult to remove from the tissue either by extracellular proteolysis or phagocytotic degradation. Moreover, such glycated end-products can impart oxidative stress upon cells[453,454] and these might be responsible, at least partially, for the induction of heme oxygenase-1 and other "stress" proteins in NFT-containing cells[460–463] and could thereby contribute to the ultimate demise of the affected neurone.

Lewy Bodies

The Prevalence of Lewy Bodies

Lewy bodies are typically, and most commonly, seen in the pigmented neurones of the substantia nigra, locus ceruleus, and dorsal motor nucleus of the vagus nerve, though they also occur in many other of the monoaminergic neurones of the midbrain and brain stem.[66,473–476] However, nonaminergic cells like those of the cholinergic nucleus basalis of Meynert and cerebral cortical pyramidal cells can be affected as can nerve cells in the peripheral parasympathetic and sympathetic ganglia[477,478]; even neurones in the nerve plexi of the gastrointestinal tract occasionally contain Lewy bodies.[479]

Although the widespread presence of Lewy bodies in neurones of these regions is considered to be pathognomonic for the idiopathic form of Parkinson's disease, about 3 to 10 percent of apparently healthy elderly persons in the general population also show occasional Lewy bodies, particularly in cells of the substantia nigra and locus ceruleus,[66,474,475,480,481] with the proportion of cells so affected increasing with each decade. Such cases have been termed[481] "incidental Lewy body disease" and may represent instances of preclinical Parkinson's disease. When cortical Lewy bodies are present along with those in brain stem regions the disorder cortical Lewy body disease (CLBD) is said to be present[482–484] and this may coexist with variable degrees of Alzheimer-type pathology (amyloid plaques, NFT) in about 75 percent of cases.

The Morphology of Lewy Bodies

Lewy bodies, particularly those in brain stem and midbrain structures, can be easily seen in routine hematoxylin-eosin stained sections where they appear as roughly circular structures, 5 to 30 μm in diameter, typically possessing a dense core, a body with or without concentric lamellae, and a clear surrounding halo.[481] They can occur singly or multiply within cells at any given level of section and although they usually appear rounded when cut in cross-section, tracing of such structures in consecutive sections shows them to be more elongate or serpentine in shape. Following the death of affected neurones, Lewy bodies may be seen lying extracellularly in the neuropil; they may eventually be removed from the tissue, though how this is achieved is not known. Electron microscopy[485,486] shows them to consist of a dense central mass of filaments and granular material with a periphery of looser radiating fibrils, each measuring 7 to 20 nm in diameter.

Along with well-formed Lewy bodies, cells of the substantia nigra, particularly locus ceruleus and nucleus basalis, may contain "pale bodies".[487] These are larger, rounded, homogeneously eosinophilic structures whose relationship to Lewy bodies is unknown, though they may represent morphologic forerunners of the latter. Indeed, the Lewy bodies in the cerebral cortex closely resemble these brain stem pale bodies in morphology and typical Lewy bodies are only occasionally seen here. In the cerebral cortex the larger pyramidal cells in layers V and VI are most often affected with temporal, frontal, cingulate, insular, and parahippocampal gyri being the usual sites of involvement.[481–483,488]

The Composition of Lewy Bodies

Given their relative scarcity in the tissue, it has not yet been possible to purify Lewy bodies sufficiently for biochemical investigation, though immunohistochemistry and other in situ analytical techniques have provided insight into their composition. Immunohistochemistry shows both brain stem and cortical Lewy bodies to stain strongly with antibodies against ubiquitin protein[459,484,489,490] and enzymes associated with ubiquitin-mediated proteolysis.[491] All three members of the neurofilament protein triplet are present,[489,492,493] as is MAP2[489] but *not* tau protein or actin. Some Lewy bodies are also immunoreactive to αB crystallin.[489,493,494]

Hence, present data suggest Lewy bodies are derived from neurofilament protein and, like NFT and Hirano bodies, may represent a disordering of the cytoskeleton. In common with NFT, Lewy bodies also contain proteoglycan, both as HSPG[295] and CSPG[495]; these again may facilitate the interlinking of filaments in Lewy bodies conferring resistance to proteolysis and their persistence within the cell.

Brain stem Lewy bodies may differ slightly in CLBD from those in Parkinson's disease with some containing tau[496] or tropomyosin.[497] HSPG may be absent in brain stem Lewy bodies in CLBD even though CSPG is present in both disorders.[495] Neurofilaments in Lewy bodies in CLBD can be solubilized[498] whereas those in Parkinson's disease cannot.[499] Whether these variations represent disease-specific differences in the basic mechanism underlying Lewy body formation is not known; they may simply represent local differences in the internal microenvironment of nerve cells related to the particular functional disturbance ongoing in each disorder.

The Effects of Lewy Bodies

Whether the presence of Lewy bodies within nerve cells, or the processes leading to their formation, exert any deterimental effect upon cell function is not known. However, a disordering of the neurofilament axis causing, or resulting from, their formation might precipitate a dying back of the axon thereby disconnecting the affected nerve cell from its afferent target. The presence of ubiquitin[459,484,489–491] and ubiquitin-associated enzymes[491] in Lewy bodies suggests they might represent cellular attempts to remove abnormal or defunct cytoskeletal proteins. On the other hand, their formation may be just one facet of a wider spectrum of degenerative changes going on in affected cells. The presence of iron within Lewy bodies[500,501] raises their potential participation in free-radical mediated reactions, though they could simply act as an inert "sink" for this potentially neurotoxic element.

Hirano Bodies

The Prevalence of Hirano Bodies

Hirano bodies are pathologic structures that occur most commonly, but not exclusively, within the pyramidal cell layer of the hippocampus, and especially in area CA1 of this brain region. Although seen here in greatest numbers in persons suffering from Alzheimer's disease[42,502] and other dementias like Pick's disease[503] and the amyotrophic lateral sclerosis-Parkinsonism dementia complex of Guam[504] and in alcoholic encephalopathies[505] they are also widely present, though fewer in number, in many nondemented elderly individuals.[42,502,506] Hirano bodies are occasionally seen in these clinical conditions in areas other than the hippocampus, especially the cerebellum,[507,508] and they may also occur in tissues outside of the CNS.[509–512]

The Morphology of Hirano Bodies

Hirano bodies are easily seen in routine hematoxylin-eosin stained sections, appearing as brightly eosinophilic, slightly hyaline, and often elongate structures, measuring up to 15 μm in short axis and sometimes more than 30 μm in long axis. They usually appear to be lying freely within the neuropil, often close or adjacent to the pyramidal cells, and may actually occur within the dendrites of such cells[513]; a glial location is, however, also possible.[514,515] Electron microscopy[513,515–519] demonstrates a paracrystalline structure composed of a lattice of crossing filaments, each measuring 6 to 10 nm in diameter and 60 to 100 nm in length.

Immunohistochemistry indicates the protein lattices to be composed of actin, especially F-actin[520–522] though other proteins like α-actinin, vinculin, and tropomyosin,[520] tau,[523] MAP-2,[524] or neurofilament[525] may also be present. Interestingly, they do not appear to be reactive against ubiquitin antibodies.[526]

The Significance of Hirano Bodies

The precise molecular composition and mode of formation of Hirano bodies is still unclear and their preferential location in the CA1 region of the hippocampus remains unexplained. Nonetheless, as NFT represent a disordering of the neuronal microtubule network, and Lewy bodies a disordering of the neurofilament axis, Hirano bodies might reflect a cytoskeletal change of actin filaments. Whether the structures contribute to the dementia of Alzheimer's disease, or that of other conditions where they are found is not known though their location within the dendrites of CA1 pyramidal cells, which make contact with branches of the incoming perforant pathway and the Schaffer collaterals of areas CA3/4, make them ideally placed either to impair directly, or to reflect an impairment of, pathways critical to the proper functioning of this brain region.

Granulovacuolar Degeneration

Prevalence of Granulovacuolar Degeneration

Granulovacuolar degeneration (GVD) is a pathologic change principally affecting the pyramidal nerve cells of area CA1 of the hippocampus, though cells in other regions of the hippocampus may also be involved, but to a lesser extent, as occasionally can cells in the nucleus basalis of Meynert, the amygdala, the olfactory bulb, the frontal, temporal, and cingulate cortices, and certain brain stem nuclei. The number of hippocampal cells affected by this change increases with age, but generally remains low in nondemented persons with less than 10 percent of cells being involved.[527–529] However, in Alzheimer's disease[527–529] the proportion of cells so affected increases greatly, though, as with Hirano bodies, GVD is severe and common in other neurodegenerative disorders like Pick's disease and the parkinsonism dementia-amyotrophic lateral sclerosis complex on Guam.[503,515]

The Morphological Appearance of Granulovacuolar Degeneration

Affected cells can contain up to as many as 20 clear, rounded vacuoles each measuring 3 to 5 μm in diameter and containing a single hematoxylinophilic, argyrophilic granule 0.5 to 1.5 μm in width.[527,528] When present in large numbers the vacuoles may cause the cell to bulge and displace the nucleus towards the margin of the cell.

Preservation of GVD at autopsy is usually poor, and electron microscopy contributes little further information; in this GVD appears simply as an electron-dense amorphous core within an electron-lucent, membrane-bound sphere.[516] Histochemistry is likewise uninformative, the granules being negative in stains for carbohydrates, nucleic acids, or glycosaminoglycans. Immunohistochemistry has shown reactivity of the granular part for neurofilament protein,[530] tubulin,[531] and tau[387,532–534] suggesting that GVD, like NFT, Lewy and Hirano bodies may represent or reflect a cytoskeletal abnormality. Indeed, GVD and NFT may coexist in the same cell, though this is exceptional. Although some studies[459,533,535] have shown ubiquitin immunoreactivity of the granule,[526] not all workers[526] have found this to be so.

The Significance of Granulovacuolar Degeneration

GVD might represent an autophagic abnormality in which (ubiquitinated) cytoskeletal elements are degraded. Clearly, the presence of such granulovacuoles is detrimental to cell function, or is at least indicative of an unhealthy cell; affected cells are much deficient in cytoplasmic RNA.[536] However, it is not known how they might cause neuronal dysfunction, or stem from the same, nor is it again clear why these particular hippocampal nerve cells should be so vulnerable. Nonetheless, as with Hirano bodies, their location in many cells in the CA1 region of the hippocampus may help to disrupt connections within the hippocampus and its output to other cortical regions and by so doing, GVD could also contribute to the catastrophic disturbances in memory that occur in dementia.

Neuropigments

Many nerve cells of diverse types come to contain, and progressively accumulate, pigment granules as they get older. In most cells the pigment is known as lipofuscin, though in the pigmented cells of the substantia nigra, locus ceruleus, ventral tegmentum, and dorsal motor vagus nucleus, this is known as neuromelanin. The two pigment types share many properties; indeed, it is widely believed that neuromelanin is actually a "melanized" form of lipofuscin, its preferred presence in the aforementioned cell types being related to their use, and catabolism of, catecholamines as neurotransmitter.

Lipofuscin

Lipofuscin has a native yellow-brown color and is strongly autofluorescent yellow when subjected to illumination by near ultraviolet light. It appears to be a heterogeneous mix of carbohydrate, lipid, and protein and contains many hydrolytic enzymes, particularly acid phosphatases and acid esterases.[537] Ultrastructurally, lipofuscin appears as membrane-bound material with a dense granular matrix and a homogeneously pale lipid globular component.[485,486,538]

Lipofuscin is generally thought to arise from the gradual transformation of active lysosomes into residual bodies,[539] though it may also arise from autophagic vacuoles containing acid phosphatases.[540] Its chemical composition does not suggest a functional role and most workers believe that it represents an accumulation of metabolically inactive residues. Nonetheless, it could act as a "trap" for substances that might damage the cytoplasm.

There is characteristic topography to the distribution of lipofuscin in the brain. It is particularly prominent in cells of the inferior olives and the dentate nucleus of the cerebellum,[541–543] but also occurs substantially in anterior horn cells[83] and other motor neurone types, in dorsal root ganglion cells, and in cells of the lateral geniculate bodies.[544] By contrast, Purkinje cells of the cerebellum are almost free from pigment, even at extreme old age,[542] and while pyramidal cells of the cerebral cortex and hippocampus and neurones of the thalamus and globus pallidus are usually intermediate in terms of lipofuscin accumulation, occasional cells can become densely packed.[542,543]

Lipofuscin can appear in some cells, such as those of the inferior olives, as early as the perinatal period[541] and accumulates with age in almost a linear fashion.[541,542,544,545] Nevertheless, any effects its accumulation might have on cellular metabolism or function are unknown. Accumulation of pigment within cells of the inferior olives has been linked to a gradual loss of ribosomal RNA and a decrease in the size of the nucleolus,[541,542] suggesting an associated decline in protein synthetic capability and possible dysfunction; Barden[546] noted a reduction in the Golgi apparatus enzyme within these same cells. Yet, even in such cell types where accumulation of pigment and RNA losses are maximal,[541,542] the actual number of nerve cells may remain unchanged in later life.[81,82] It is possible, however, that cellular metabolism or its efficiency might be mechanically disrupted by an expanding pigment bulk, though not to such an extent as to lead to overt cell death. Nonetheless, other age-related processes occurring in parallel could be responsible for these perikaryal changes. In nerve cell types where pigment accumulation is low (e.g., Purkinje cells and pyramidal cells of the hippocampus) protein synthetic capacity is reduced by less than 10 percent in old age[542] and the Golgi apparatus is unaltered.[546] Nevertheless, the number of Purkinje cells is reduced in old age by 25 percent[58] and those in the hippocampus by about 20 percent[41,42,47–50] (See also References 53 and 54). Cerebral cortical neurones also accumulate only modest amounts of lipofuscin,[543] yet they too may be much reduced in number.[36–42] Clearly, in all these latter cell types, factors other than lipofuscin accumulation alone must be responsible for their downfall in later life.

Hence, it is still uncertain whether lipofuscin accumulates in cells simply as an innocent bystander, solely marking the passage of time, or whether in some insidious way it contributes to, or even hastens, a deterioration in function in old age in certain vulnerable cell types.

Neuromelanin

The neuromelanin-containing cells of the brain form two continuous columns extending along either side of the brain stem from a position central to the motor nucleus of the oculomotor nerve to the caudal end of the medulla.[547] Of all the cell groups within these columns, the substantia nigra, locus ceruleus, and dorsal motor vagus nucleus are the most pigmented and probably the best known. Neuromelanin, like lipofuscin, contains acid phosphatases and acid esterases[537] and at ultrastructural level has the same granular matrix and lipid components, though other coarse electron dense particles are also present on the matrix.[485,486,538,548] Neuromelanin and lipofuscin are thus probably related—neuromelanin being a "melanized" form of lipofuscin—with their slightly differing structure resulting from interactions between lipofuscin and the products (quinones) of catecholamine auto-oxidation.[549] Neuromelanin granules are rich in iron,[550] which could play a role in free radical mediated cell death in later life.

Neuromelanin first appears in cells of the locus ceruleus around birth,[551,552] but cells of the substantia nigra are not regularly pigmented until around 18 months of postnatal life,[552] this possibly reflecting the onset of sustained physiologic function in such cells. Nonetheless, pigment accumulates steadily in both cell types up to about 60 years of age,[552,553] after which average cell levels of pigment gradually decrease. This fall in pigmentation may be due to a preferential fallout in later life of the more heavily pigmented cells,[554] leaving the lesser pigmented cells to survive further into old age. Such observations suggest that neuromelanin may have direct cytotoxic potential or that its presence in excess amounts exerts a metabolic "weakening" of cells predisposing to cell damage and death.

Indeed, age-related increases in neuromelanin in the substantia nigra are associated with reductions in nerve cell cytoplasmic RNA content and nucleolar volume[76] and decreases in the content of dopamine synthetic enzymes[75,555] and dopamine production[556–559] in the corpus striatum. In cells of the substantia nigra there is a 25 percent decrease in protein synthetic capacity in old age, though the actual loss of nerve cells (50 percent) far exceeds this.[74–77] However, in the locus ceruleus there is less cell loss[66–73] and protein synthetic capacity is better maintained[66]; levels of the noradrenalin-synthesizing enzyme, dopamine β-hydroxylase[560] as well as noradrenaline itself[557,559] within projection areas of the cerebral cortex are not reduced. This less severe change in cells of the locus ceruleus may partly reflect their lower pigment concentration[76] though the degradative products of noradrenaline are much less cytotoxic than those of dopamine.[549]

Therefore, as with lipofuscin, it is uncertain whether the accumulation of neuromelanin within these cell types carries with it any metabolic or cytotoxic (free radical) repercussions; again it may simply accumulate as a marker of the passage of time upon cells of these types.

Other Neuronal Changes

Intranuclear Inclusions

The frequency of certain intranuclear inclusions, such as paracrystalline rodlets[561] or spherical bodies[562] may increase with age.[563,564] The composition of these inclusions is uncertain but they may consist of microfilaments. Any relevance they might have to cell function is unknown, but they could be important reflecting changes in DNA transcription and protein synthesis since their presence may increase in situations of metabolic disturbance associated with, for example, viral infections like subacute sclerosing panencephalitis (SSPE)[565–567] or Creutzfeldt-Jakob disease.[568]

Eosinophilic inclusions have been reported in the nucleus of pigmented neurones of the substantia nigra and locus ceruleus.[569–571] Such structures, called Marinesco bodies,[571] are round or oval in shape and stain pink with eosin or Masson trichrome. Up to four inclusions, each measuring 2 to 10 μm in diameter, may be seen within a single nucleus. They consist of nonmembrane-bound, aggregated, osmiophilic granular material occasionally associated with filamentous structures.[572] While their origin and significance remains unknown, and their presence may be age-related,[571] they are particularly increased in number in encephalopathies associated with liver[569] or lung[573] disease.

Intracytoplasmic Inclusions

In most normal people, especially in the elderly, clusters of eosinophilic granules can be seen lying among the pigment granules in the cytoplasm of cells of the substantia nigra and locus ceruleus. Ultrastructurally,[574] these consist of groups of parallel filaments, about 8 nm in diameter, connected by finer filaments. They are present within the distended cisternae of the rough endoplasmic reticulum. These same sort of granules have also been seen within altered mitochondria of these cell types[575] and similar structures have been reported in neurones of the dorsal root ganglia[576] and thalamus.[577,578] Although their origin is uncertain and their significance unknown, they are considered to represent some kind of age-related process occurring within affected cells.

Polyglucosan Bodies

Polyglucosan bodies consist mostly of glycogen-like material (glucose polymers) mixed with a small amount of protein and glycosaminoglycan.[579–585] The best known of these are corpora amylacea, these being rounded (5 to 20 μm in diameter) structures, bluish or grey in color in hematoxylin-eosin stained sections, frequently having a denser core. Corpora amylacea occur mostly in subpial, perivascular, or subependymal areas of gray and white (especially) matter and their numbers increase with age or in the presence of neurodegenerative disease.[586, 587] Ultrastructurally, they usually occur in astrocytic processes[588] but sometimes are present in those of neurones too.[587,589–591] They consist of randomly arranged 6.5 nm filaments, which form whorls, and are not bounded by a limiting membrane. The filaments often become more compact within the center and may contain electron-dense floccular material.

The low quantities of protein within corpora amylacea are, however, strongly immunoreactive for markers of oligodendroglial cells or axonal (myelin) elements.[592] They are also ubiquitinated[579,580,592,593] and contain low molecular weight heat shock proteins[593,594] and complement factors.[595] The cellular source of corpora amylacea remains unknown, though the presence within them of mitochondrial proteins and DNA suggests[586] they might represent the autophagic remains of organelles that have undergone an oxidative stress-mediated degeneration leading to their accumulation within the processes of astrocytes, or other cells. Following the death of affected cells they build up extracellularly in white matter (especially periventricular) regions. X-ray microprobe analysis[587,596] shows corpora amylacea to contain much sodium, phosphorus, sulfur, and chloride with minor amounts of aluminium, silicon, copper, iron, potassium, and calcium; they may therefore contain inorganic ions or compounds such as sodium chloride or calcium phosphate. Although usually regarded as being of no pathologic significance, it has been suggested[595] that they could usefully act as "traps" for the end-products of myelin damage or neuronal degeneration brought about by complement activation. In this context, they might prevent a recognition of such immunogenic proteins by lymphocytes or microglial cells and by doing so limit tissue damage. Others[596] have suggested that they may firstly adsorb, then absorb, inorganic material extravasated from the blood and cerebrospinal fluid that has been taken up by astrocytes following failures in blood-brain, or blood-cerebrospinal fluid, barriers during aging or neurodegeneration.

Tissue Mineralization

Basal Ganglia Calcification

While a severe calcification of the basal ganglia, thalamus, and dentate nucleus is frequent in persons suffering from parathyroid hormone deficiency,[597] a much milder calcification is commonplace in the brains of apparently mentally normal old people and other persons of all ages with a wide variety of neurological illnesses.[598–604] The calcification involves either the walls of the large arteries of the globus pallidus, which lose their muscle and elastic coats and become thickly fibrosed and calcified, or is seen as "strings" of calcospherites lying alongside capillaries or occurring freely in the neuropil of this region.[604] Occasionally, the dentate nucleus of the cerebellum or the fascia dentata of the hippocampus can be similarly affected. The significance of this pathology is unknown, though it may be related to an aging process fairly specific to blood vessels of the globus pallidus, but one that is not obviously related to co-existing cerebrovascular disease.[604] Chemical analysis shows the calcospherites to contain variable amounts of polysaccharide and protein enriched with calcium, iron, manganese, and aluminium[597] though the particular presence of these elements is probably not indicative of any homeostatic disorder of metals.

Iron Deposition

In and around areas of old tissue infarction, surviving nerve cells may become coated with iron and calcium, this conferring a positive Prussian Blue reaction for iron and a positive von Kossa reaction for calcium. This is known as ferrugination or mineralization of nerve cells. Hemosiderin deposition following subarachnoid hemorrhage gives an orange-yellow discoloration to the meninges. A similar pigmentation over the surface of, or within, brain tissue marks the site of a prior contusion. Both these changes can be seen as incidental findings in the brains of some old persons, particularly those prone to cerebrovascular insults or ones who may have suffered minor head trauma in the past.

Axonal Changes

Axonal torpedoes are argyrophilic swellings that are typically seen in the cerebellum and occur most often on the proximal part of the axon of the Purkinje cell before the origin of collateral branches. They are frequently seen in old age, but are particularly common in neurodegenerative disorders involving the cerebellum such as multisystem atrophy and Creutzfeldt-Jakob disease.[605,606] The axon torpedo is characterized by a dense central accumulation of haphazardly arranged 10 nm neurofilaments that displace the usual mitochondria and endoplasmic reticulum to the periphery.[607] Axon torpedoes are distinct from the retraction bulbs that typically form at the ends of damaged or severed axons following traumatic head injury and which contain many lamellar, multivesicular, and dense bodies. Axon torpedoes may, therefore, represent a regenerating, rather than a degenerating, state within the nerve cell. Similar, but more rounded, structures measuring over 20 μm in diameter have been seen in the axons of motor neurones, particularly in amyotrophic lateral sclerosis.[608]

Granular glycogen bodies, measuring 5 to 50 μm in diameter and consisting of densely packed accumulations of α or β (but not both) glycogen granules, can sometimes be seen in both myelinated and unmyelinated axons.[609,610] In Alzheimer's disease they often lie close to the dystrophic neurites in plaques. Although so far only reported in this particular disorder[609,610] glycogen bodies like these may be more commonplace, their limited descriptions reflecting the difficulty in obtaining suitable (biopsy) tissues for their demonstration. Their formation may relate to disturbances in the transport of carbohydrate within nerve processes, possibly because of interruptions in axonal flow.

References

1. LeMay M: Radiologic changes of the aging brain and skull. Am J Radiol 1984;143:383–389
2. Schwartz M, Creasey H, Grady CL et al: Computed tomographic analysis of brain morphometrics in 30 healthy men, aged 21 to 81 years. Ann Neurol 1985;17:146–157
3. Pfefferbaum A, Zatz LM, Jernigan TL: Computer-interactive method for quantifying cerebrospinal fluid and tissue in brain CT scans: effects of aging. J Comput Assist Tomogr 1986;10: 571–578
4. Drayer BP: Imaging of the aging brain. Radiology 1988;166: 785–796
5. Creasey H, Rapoport SI: The aging human brain. Ann Neurol 1985;17:2–10
6. Bradley WG, Waluch V, Brant-Zawadzki M et al: Patchy, periventricular white matter lesions in the elderly: a common observation during NMR imaging. Noninvas Med Image 1984; 1:35–41
7. Brant-Zawadski M, Fein G, Van Dyke C et al: MR imaging of the aging brain: patchy white-matter lesions and dementia. Am J Neuroradiol 1985;6:675–682
8. George AE, de Leon MJ, Kalnin A et al: Leukoencephalopathy in normal and pathologic aging. II. MRI of brain lucencies. Am J Neuroradiol 1986;7:561–570
9. Fazekas F, Chawluk JB, Alavi A et al: MR signal abnormalities at 1.5 T in Alzheimer's dementia and normal aging. Am J Neuroradiol 1987;8:421–426
10. Sullivan EV, Marsh L, Mathalon DH et al: Age-related decline in MRI volumes of temporal lobe gray matter but not hippocampus. Neurobiol Aging 1995;16:591–606
11. Coffey CE, Wilkinson WE, Parashos IA et al. Quantitative cerebral anatomy of the aging human brain: a cross-sectional study using magnetic resonance imaging. Neurology 1992;42: 527–536
12. Bhatia S, Bookheimer SY, Gaillard WD, Theodore WH: Measurement of whole temporal lobe and hippocampus for MR volumetry: normative data. Neurology 1993;43:2006–2010
13. Jack CR, Petersen RC, O'Brien PC, Tangalos EG: MR-based hippocampal volumetry in the diagnosis of Alzheimer's disease. Neurology 1992;42:183–188
14. Golomb J, De Leon MJ, Kluger A et al: Hippocampal atrophy in normal aging: an association with recent memory impairment. Arch Neurol 1993;50:967–973
15. Kuhl DE, Metter EJ, Riege WH, Phelps ME: Effects of human ageing on patterns of local cerebral glucose utilization determined by the (18 F) flurodeoxyglucose method. J Cereb Blood Flow Metab 1982;2:163–171
16. Stoessl AJ, Tuokko H, Martin WRW et al: Cerebral glucose metabolism in normal aging. Neurology 1986;36:104
17. Chawluk JB, Alavi A, Dann R et al: Positron emission tomography in aging and dementia: effect of cerebral atrophy. J Nucl Med 1987;28:431–437
18. Yoshii F, Barker WW, Chang JY et al: Sensitivity of cerebral glucose metabolism to age, gender, brain volume, brain atrophy and cerebrovascular risk factors. J Cereb Blood Flow Metab 1988;8:654–661
19. DeCarli C, Atack JR, Ball MJ et al: Post-mortem regional neurofibrillary tangle densities but not senile plaque densities are related to regional cerebral metabolic rates for glucose during life in Alzheimer's disease patients. Neurodegeneration 1992;1:113–121
20. De Leon MJ, Ferris SH, George AE et al: Positron emission tomographic studies of aging and Alzheimer disease. Am J Neuroradiol 1983;4:568–571
21. Duara R, Margolin RA, Robertson-Tschabo EA et al: Cerebral glucose utilization as measured with positron emission tomography in 21 resting healthy men between the ages of 21 and 83 years. Brain 1983;106:761–775
22. Martin WRW, Palmer MR, Patlak CS, Calne DB: Nigrostriatal function in humans studied with positron emission topography. Ann Neurol 1989;26:535–542
23. Sawle GV, Colebatch JG, Shah A et al: Striatal function in normal ageing: implications for Parkinson's disease. Ann Neurol 1990;28:799–804
24. Blinkov SM, Glezer II: The human brain in figures and tables. Plenum, New York, 1968
25. Dekaban AS, Sadowsky D: Changes in brain weights during the span of human life: relation of brain weights to body heights and body weights. Ann Neurol 1978;4:345–356
26. Davis PJM, Wright EA: A new method for measuring cranial cavity volume and its application to the assessment of cerebral atrophy at autopsy. Neuropathol Appl Neurobiol 1977;3: 341–358
27. Terry RD, De Teresa R, Hansen LA: Neocortical cell counts in normal human adult ageing. Ann Neurol 1987;21:530–539
28. Last RJ, Tompsett DH: Casts of the cerebral ventricles. Br J Surg 1953;40:525–543
29. Barron SA, Jacobs L, Kinkel WR: Changes in size of normal lateral ventricles during ageing determined by computerized tomography. Neurology 1976;26:1011–1013
30. Tomlinson BE, Blessed G, Roth M: Observations on the brains of non-demented elderly people. J Neurol Sci 1968;7: 331–356
31. Hubbard BM, Anderson JM: Age, senile dementia and ventricular enlargement. J Neurol Neurosurg Psych 1981;44: 631–635
32. Miller AKH, Alston RL, Corsellis JAN: Variation with age in the volumes of grey and white matter in the cerebral hemispheres of man: measurements with an image analyser. Neuropathol Appl Neurobiol 1980;6:119–132
33. Haug H: Macroscopic and microscopic morphometry of the

human brain and cortex. A survey in the light of new results. Brain Pathol 1984;1:123–149

34. Haug H: Are neurones of the human cerebral cortex really lost during aging? A morphometric examination. pp. 150–163 In Traber J, Gispern WH (eds): Senile Dementia of the Alzheimer Type. Early Diagnosis, Neuropathology and Animal Models. Springer-Verlag, Berlin, 1985

35. Harris GJ, Schlaepfer TE, Peng LW et al: Magnetic resonance imaging evaluation of the effects of ageing on grey-white ratio in the human brain. Neuropathol Appl Neurobiol 1994;20: 290–293

36. Brody H: Organization of the cerebral cortex. III. A study of ageing in the human cerebral cortex. J Comp Neurol 1955; 102:511–556

37. Brody H: Structural changes in the ageing nervous system. Interdiscip Top Gerontol 1970;7:9–21

38. Colon EJ: The elderly brain. A quantitative analysis in the cerebral cortex of two cases. Psych Neurol Neurochir 1972; 75:261–270

39. Shefer VF: Absolute numbers of neurones and thickness of the cerebral cortex during ageing, senile and vascular dementia, and Pick's and Alzheimer's diseases. Neurosci Behav Physiol 1973;6:319–324

40. Henderson G, Tomlinson BE, Gibson P: Cell counts in human cerebral cortex in normal adults throughout life using an image analysing computer. J Neurol Sci 1980;46:113–136

41. Anderson JM, Hubbard BM, Coghill GR, Slidders W: The effect of advanced old age on the neurone content of the cerebral cortex. Observations with an automatic image analyser point counting method. J Neurol Sci 1983;58:233–244

42. Mann DMA, Yates PO, Marcyniuk B: Some morphometric observations on the cerebral cortex and hippocampus in presenile Alzheimer's disease, senile dementia of Alzheimer type and Down's syndrome in middle age. J Neurol Sci 1985;69: 139–159

43. Hubbard BM, Anderson JM: A quantitative study of cerebral atrophy in old age and senile dementia. J Neurol Sci 1981; 50:135–145

44. Haug H, Kuhl S, Mecke E, Sass N-L, Wasner K: The significance of morphometric procedures in the investigation of age changes in cytoarchitectonic structures of human brain. J Hirnforsch 1984;25:353–374

45. Haug H, Eggers R: Morphometry of the human cortex cerebri and corpus striatum during aging. Neurobiol Aging 1991;12: 336–338

46. Braak H, Braak E: Ratio of pyramidal cells versus non-pyramidal cells in the human frontal isocortex and changes in ratio with ageing and Alzheimer's disease. pp. 185–212. In Swaab DF, Fliers E, Mirmiran M et al (eds): Progress in Brain Research. Elsevier Biomedical, 1986

47. Ball MJ: Neuronal loss, neurofibrillary tangles and granulovacuolar degeneration in the hippocampus with ageing and dementia. A quantitative study. Acta Neuropathol 1977;37: 111–118

48. Shefer VF: Hippocampal pathology as a possible factor in the pathogenesis of senile dementias. Neurosci Behav Physiol 1977;8:236–239

49. Mouritzen Dam A: The density of neurones in the human hippocampus. Neuropathol Appl Neurobiol 1979;5:249–263

50. Miller AKH, Alston RL, Mountjoy CQ, Corellis JAN: Automatic differential cell counting on a sector of the normal human hippocampus. The influence of age. Neuropathol Appl Neurobiol 1984;10:123–141

51. West MJ: Regionally specific loss of neurons in the ageing human hippocampus. Neurobiol Aging 1993;14:287–293

52. Brown MW, Cassell MD: Estimates of the number of neurones in the human hippocampus. J Physiol 1980;301:58–59P

53. Mani RB, Lohr JB, Jeste DV: Hippocampal pyramidal cells and ageing in the human; a quantitative study of neuronal loss in sectors CA1 to CA4. Exp Neurol 1986;94:29–40

54. Davies DC, Horwood N, Isaacs SL, Mann DMA: The effect of age and Alzheimer's disease in pyramidal neurone density in the individual fields of the hippocampal formation. Acta Neuropathol 1992;83:510–517

55. Herzog AG, Kemper TL: Amygdaloid changes in ageing and dementia. Arch Neurol 1980;37:625–629

56. Ellis RS: A preliminary quantitative study of Purkinje cells in normal, subnormal and senescent human cerebella with some notes on functional organization. J Comp Neurol 1919; 30:229–252

57. Ellis RS: Norms for some structural changes in the human cerebellum from both to old age. J Comp Neurol 1920;32: 1–33

58. Hall TC, Miller AKH, Corsellis JAN: Variations in the human Purkinje cell population according to age and sex. Neuropathol Appl Neurobiol 1975;1:267–292

59. Torvik A, Torp S, Lindboe CF: Atrophy of the cerebellar vermis in ageing. A morphometric and histologic study. J Neurol Sci 1986;76:283–294

60. Hopker von W: Das altern des nucleus dentate. Z Altersforsch 1951;5:256–261

61. Konigsmark BW, Murphy EA: Neuronal populations in the human brain. Nature 1970;228:1335–1336

62. Vijayashankar N, Brody H: Ageing in the human brain stem. A study of the nucleus of the trochlear nerve. Acta Anat 1977; 99:169–172

63. Vijayashankar N, Brody H: A study of ageing in the human abducens nucleus. J Comp Neurol 1977;173:433–438

64. Van Buskirk C: The seventh nerve complex. J Comp Neurol 1945;171:501–516

65. Vijayashankar N, Brody H: A quantitative study of the pigmented neurones in the nuclei locus caeruleus and subcaeruleus in man as related to ageing. J Neuropathol Exp Neurol 1979;38:490–497

66. Mann DMA, Yates PO, Hawkes J: The pathology of the human locus caeruleus. Clin Neuropathol 1983;2:1–7

67. Mann DMA, Yates PO, Marcyniuk B: Monoaminergic neurotransmitter systems in presenile Alzheimer's disease and in senile dementia of Alzheimer type. Clin Neuropathol 1984;3: 199–205

68. Mann DMA, Yates PO, Marcyniuk B: Alzheimer's presenile dementia, senile dementia of Alzheimer type and Down's syndrome in middle age form an age-related continuum of patho-

logical changes. Neuropathol Appl Neurobiol 1984;10: 185–207

69. Tomlinson BE, Irving D, Blessed G: Cell loss in the locus caeruleus in senile dementia of Alzheimer type. J Neurol Sci 1981;49:419–428
70. Marcyniuk B, Mann DMA: The topography of nerve cell loss from the locus caeruleus in elderly persons. Neurobiol Aging 1989;10:5–9
71. German DC, Manaye KF, White CL et al: Disease specific patterns of locus caeruleus cell loss: Parkinson disease, Alzheimer's disease and Down's syndrome. Ann Neurol 1992;32: 667–676
72. Wree A, Braak H, Schleicher A, Zilles K: Biomathematical analysis of the neuronal loss in the ageing human brain of both sexes, demonstrated in pigment preparations of the pars cerebellaris loci caerulei. Anat Embryol 1980;160:105–119
73. Chan-Palay V, Asan E: Quantitation of catecholamine neurons in the locus coeruleus in human brains of normal young and older adults and in depression. J Comp Neurol 1989;287: 357–372
74. Hirai S: Ageing of the substantia nigra. Adv Neurol Sci 1968; 12:845–849
75. McGeer PL, McGeer EG, Suzuki JS: Ageing and extrapyramidal function. Arch Neurol 1977;34:33–35
76. Mann DMA, Yates PO: The effects of ageing on the pigmented nerve cells of the human locus caeruleus and substantia nigra. Acta Neuropathol Berlin 1979;47:93–97
77. Fearnley JM, Lees AJ. Aging and Parkinson's disease: substantia nigra regional selectivity. Brain 1991;114:2283–2301
78. German DC, Manaye KF, Smith WK et al: Mid brain dopaminergic cell loss in Parkinson's disease: computer visualization. Ann Neurol 1989;26:607–614
79. Mann DMA, Yates PO, Hawkes J: The noradrenergic system in Alzheimer and multi-infarct dementias. J Neurol Neurosurg Psych 1982;45:113–119
80. Sandoz P, Meier-Ruge W: Age related loss of nerve cells from the human inferior olives and unchanged volume of its grey matter. IRCS Med Sci 1977;5:376
81. Monagle RD, Brody H: Effects of age upon the main nucleus of the inferior olive in the human. J Comp Neurol 1974;155: 61–66
82. Moatamed F: Cell frequencies in the human inferior olivary nuclear complex. J Comp Neurol 1966;128:109–116
83. Tomlinson BE, Irving D: The number of limb motor neurones in the human lumbosacral cord throughout life. J Neurol Sci 1977;34:213–219
84. Bugiani O, Salvarani S, Perdelli F et al: Nerve cell loss with ageing in the putamen. Eur Neurol 1980;17:286–291
85. Bottcher J: Morphology of the basal ganglia in Parkinson's disease. Acta Neurol Scand 1975;52 (suppl 62):1–87
86. McGeer PL, McGeer EG, Suzuki JS et al: Ageing, Alzheimer's disease and the cholinergic system of the basal forebrain. Neurology 1984;34:741–745
87. Mann DMA, Yates PO, Marcyniuk B: Changes in nerve cells of the nucleus basalis of Meynert in Alzheimer's disease and their relationship to ageing and the accumulation of lipofuscin pigment. Mech Ageing Dev 1984;25:189–204
88. De Lacalle S, Iraizoz I, Ma Gonzalo L: Differential changes in cell size and number in topographic subdivisions of human basal nucleus in normal aging. Neuroscience 1991;43: 445–456
89. Whitehouse PJ, Parhad IM, Hedreen JC et al: Integrity of the nucleus basalis of Meynert in normal ageing. Neurology 1983; 33(suppl 2):159
90. Clark AW, Parhad IM, Folstein SE et al: The nucleus basalis in Huntington's disease. Neurology 1983;33:1262–1267
91. Chui HC, Bondareff W, Zarow C, Slager U: Stability of neuronal number in the human nucleus basalis of Meynert with age. Neurobiol Aging 1984;5:83–88
92. Wilkinson A, Davies I: The influence of age and dementia on the neurone population of the mammillary bodies. Age Ageing 1978;7:151–160
93. Goudsmit E, Hopman MA, Fliers E, Swaab DF: The supraoptic and paraventricular nuclei of the human hypothalamus in relation to sex, age and Alzheimer's disease. Neurobiol Aging 1990;11:529–536
94. Fliers E, Swaab DF, Pool CW, Verwer RWH: The vasopressin and oxytocin neurons in the human supraoptic and paraventricular nucleus; changes with aging and in senile dementia. Brain Res 1985;342:45–53
95. Swaab DF, Fliers E, Partiman TS: The suprachiasmatic nucleus of the human brain in relation to sex, age and senile dementia. Brain Res 1985;342:37–44
96. Zhou J-N, Hofman MA, Swaab DF: VIP neurons in the human SCN in relation to sex, age, and Alzheimer's disease. Neurobiol Aging 1995;16:571–576
97. Schade JP, Baxter CF: Changes during growth in the volume and surface area of cortical neurones in the rabbit. Exp Neurol 1960;2:158–178
98. Scheibel ME, Lindsay RD, Tomiyasu U, Scheibel AB: Progressive dendritic changes in the ageing human cortex. Exp Neurol 1975;47:392–403
99. Scheibel ME, Lindsay RD, Tomiyasu U, Scheibel AB: Progressive dendritic changes in the ageing human limbic system. Exp Neurol 1976;53:420–430
100. Scheibel ME, Tomiyasu U, Scheibel AB: The ageing human Betz cell. Exp Neurol 1977;56:598–609
101. Buell SJ, Coleman PD: Dendritic growth in the aged human brain and failure of growth in senile dementia. Science 1979; 206:854–856
102. Buell SJ, Coleman PD: Quantitative evidence for selective dendritic growth in normal human ageing but not in senile dementia. Brain Res 1981;214:23–41
103. Buell SJ: Golgi-cox and rapid Golgi methods as applied to autopsied human brain tissue: widely disparate results. J Neuropathol Exp Neurol 1982;41:500–507
104. Flood DG, Buell SJ, De Fiore CH et al: Age related dendritic growth in the dentate gyrus of human brain is followed by regression in the "oldest old". Brain Res 1985;345:366–368
105. Flood DG, Buell SJ, Horwitz GJ, Coleman PD: Dendritic extent

in human dentate gyrus granule cells in normal ageing and senile dementia. Brain Res 1987;402:205–216

106. Coleman PD, Flood DG: Neurone numbers and dendritic extent in normal ageing and Alzheimer's disease. Neurobiol Aging 1987;8:521–545

107. Nakamura S, Akiguchi M, Kameyama M, Mizuno N: Age-related changes of pyramidal cell basal dendrites in layers III and V of human motor cortex: a quantitative Golgi study. Acta Neuropathol 1985;65:281–284

108. Cragg BG: The density of synapses in neurons in normal, mentally defective and aging human brains. Brain 1975;98:81–90

109. Adams I: Plasticity of the synaptic contact zone following loss of synapses in the cerebral cortex of aging humans. Brain Res 1987;424:343–351

110. Huttenlocher PR. Synaptic density in human frontal cortex: developmental changes and effects of aging. Brain Res 1979; 163:195–205

111. Gibson PH: EM study of the numbers of cortical synapses in the brains of ageing people and people with Alzheimer-type dementia. Acta Neuropathol 1983;62:127–133

112. Scheff SW, Price DA: Synapse loss in the temporal lobe in Alzheimer's disease. Ann Neurol 1993;33:190–199

113. Doebler JA, Markesbery WR, Anthony A, Rhoads RE: Neuronal RNA in relation to neuronal loss and neurofibrillary pathology in the hippocampus in Alzheimer's disease. J Neuropathol Exp Neurol 1987;46:28–39

114. Mann DMA, Sinclair KGA: The quantitative assessment of lipofuscin pigment, cytoplasmic RNA and nucleolar volume in senile dementia. Neuropathol Appl Neurobiol 1978;4: 129–135

115. Davies L, Wolska B, Hilbich C et al: A4 amyloid protein deposition and the diagnosis of Alzheimer's disease: prevalence in aged brains determined by immunocytochemistry compared with conventional neuropathologic techniques. Neurology 1988;38:1688–1693

116. Rumble B, Retallack R, Hilbich C et al: Amyloid (A4) protein and its precursor in Down's syndrome and Alzheimer's disease. N Engl J Med 1989;320:1446–1452

117. Ogomori K, Kitamoto T, Tateishi J et al: β amyloid protein is widely distributed in the central nervous system of patients with Alzheimer's disease. Am J Pathol 1989;134:243–251

118. Ikeda S-I, Allsop D, Glenner GG: The morphology and distribution of plaque and related deposits in the brains of Alzheimer's disease and control cases: an immunohistochemical study using amyloid β protein antibody. Lab Invest 1989;60: 113–122

119. Mann DMA, Brown AMT, Prinja D et al: A morphological analysis of senile plaques in the brains of non-demented persons of different ages using silver, immunocytochemical and lectin histochemical staining techniques. Neuropathol Appl Neurobiol 1990;16:17–25

120. Price JL, Davis PB, Morris JC, White DL: The distribution of plaques, tangles and related immunohistochemical markers in healthy ageing and Alzheimer's disease. Neurobiol Ageing 1991;12:295–312

121. Arriagada PV, Marzloff K, Hyman BT: Distribution of Alzheimer-type pathologic changes in non-demented elderly individuals matches the pattern in Alzheimer's disease. Neurology 1992;42:1681–1688

122. McKee AC, Kosik KS, Kowall NW: Neuritic pathology and dementia in Alzheimer's disease. Ann Neurol 1991;30: 156–165

123. Mackenzie IRA: Senile plaques do not progressively accumulate with normal ageing. Acta Neuropathol 1994;87:520–525

124. Delaere P, He Y, Fayet G et al: βA4 deposits are constant in the brain of the oldest old: an immunocytochemical study of 20 French centenarians. Neurobiol Aging 1993; 14:191–194

125. Coria F, Moreno A, Rubio I et al: The cellular pathology associated with Alzheimer β-amyloid deposits in non-demented aged individuals. Neuropathol Appl Neurobiol 1993; 19:261–268

126. Giannakopoulos P, Hof PR, Mottier S et al: Neuropathological changes in the cerebral cortex of 1258 cases from a geriatric hospital: retrospective clinicopathological evaluation of a 10-year autopsy population. Acta Neuropathol 1994; 87:456–468

127. Morris JC, McKeel JDW, Storandt M et al: Very mild Alzheimer's disease: informant-based clinical, psychometric, and pathologic distinction from normal aging. Neurology 1991;41: 469–478

128. Hyman BT, West HL, Rebeck GW et al: Quantitative analysis of senile plaques in Alzheimer disease: Observation of log-normal size distribution and molecular epidemiology of differences associated with apolipoprotein E genotype and trisomy 21 (Down syndrome). Proc Natl Acad Sci (USA) 1995;92: 3586–3590

129. Armstrong RA, Myers D, Smith CUM: What determines the size frequency distribution of β-amyloid (Aβ) deposits in Alzheimer's disease patients? Neurosci Lett 1995;187:13–16

130. Allsop D, Haga S-I, Haga C et al: Early senile plaques in Down's syndrome brains show a clear relationship with cell bodies of neurones. Neuropathol Appl Neurobiol 1989;15: 531–542

131. Cras P, Kawai M, Siedlak S et al: Neuronal and microglial involvement in β-amyloid protein deposition in Alzheimer's disease. Am J Pathol 1990;137:241–246

132. Pappolla MA, Omar RA, Sambamurti K et al: The genesis of the senile plaque. Further evidence in support of its neuronal origin. Am J Pathol 1992;141:1151–1159

133. Probst A, Langui D, Ipsen S et al: Deposition of β/A4 protein along neuronal plasma membranes in diffuse senile plaques. Acta Neuropathol 1991;83:21–29

134. Mann DMA, Younis N, Jones D, Stoddart RW: The time course of pathological events concerned with plaque formation in Down's syndrome with particular reference to the involvement of microglial cells. Neurodegeneration 1992;1:201–215

135. Armstrong RA: Factors determining the morphology of β-amyloid (Aβ) deposits in Down's syndrome. Neurodegeneration 1995;4:179–186

136. Dayan AD: Quantitative histological studies on the aged human brain. I. Senile plaques and neurofibrillary tangles in "normal" patients. Acta Neuropathol 1970;16:85–94

137. Mann DMA, Tucker CM, Yates PO: The topographic distribution of senile plaques and neurofibrillary tangles in the brains of non-demented persons of different ages. Neuropathol Appl Neurobiol 1987;13:123–139
138. Ulrich J: Alzheimer changes in nondemented patients younger than sixty-five: possible early stages of Alzheimer's disease and senile dementia of Alzheimer type. Ann Neurol 1984;17: 273–277
139. Tagliavini F, Giaccone G, Frangione B, Bugiani O: Preamyloid deposits in the cerebral cortex of patients with Alzheimer's disease and non demented individuals. Neurosci Lett 1988; 93:191–196
140. Verga L, Frangione B, Tagliavini F et al: Alzheimer patients and Down patients: cerebral preamyloid deposits differ ultrastructurally and histochemically from the amyloid of senile plaques. Neurosci Lett 1989;105:294–299
141. Yamaguchi H, Nakazato Y, Hirai S et al: Electron micrograph of diffuse plaques. Am J Pathol 1989;135:593–597
142. Hachimi KH, Verga G, Giaccone G et al: Relationship between non-fibrillary amyloid precursors and cell processes in the cortical neuropil of Alzheimer patients. Neurosci Lett 1991; 129:119–122
143. Davies CA, Mann DMA: Is the "preamyloid" of diffuse plaques in Alzheimer's disease really non-fibrillar? Am J Pathol 1993; 143:1594–1605
144. Yamaguchi H, Nakazato Y, Shoji M et al: Ultrastructure of diffuse plaques in senile dementia of the Alzheimer-type: comparison with primitive plaques. Acta Neuropathol 1991;82: 13–20
145. Braak H, Braak E, Grundke-Iqbal I, Iqbal K: Occurrence of neuropil threads in the senile human brain and in Alzheimer's disease: a third location of paired helical filaments outside of neurofibrillary tangles and neuritic plaques. Neurosci Lett 1986;65:351–355
146. Mann DMA: The pathological association between Down syndrome and Alzheimer disease. Mech Ageing Dev 1988;43: 99–136
147. Mann DMA, Brown AMT, Prinja D et al: An analysis of the morphology of senile plaques in Down's syndrome patients of different ages using immunocytochemical and lectin histochemical methods. Neuropathol Appl Neurobiol 1989;15: 317–329
148. Mann DMA, Jones D, Prinja D, Purkiss MS: The prevalence of amyloid (A4) protein deposits within the cerebral and cerebellar cortex in Down's syndrome and Alzheimer's disease. Acta Neuropathol 1990;80:318–327
149. Mann DMA, Iwatsubo T, Fukumoto H et al: Microglial cells and amyloid β protein (Aβ) deposition; association with Aβ40 containing plaques. Acta Neuropathol 1995;90:472–477
150. Iwatsubo T, Mann DMA, Odaka A et al: Amyloid β protein (Aβ) deposition: Aβ42(43) precedes Aβ40 in Down syndrome. Ann Neurol 1995;37:294–299
151. Lemere CA, Blusztajn JK, Yamaguchi H et al: Sequence of deposition of heterogeneous amyloid β-peptides and APO E in Down syndrome: implications for initial events in amyloid plaque formation. Neurobiol Dis 1996;3:16–32
152. Wisniewski HM, Wegiel J, Kotula L: Some neuropathological aspects of Alzheimer's disease and its relevance to other disciplines. Neuropathol Appl Neurobiol 1996;22:3–11
153. Wisniewski HM, Terry RD: Re-examination of the pathogenesis of the senile plaque. Prog Neuropathol 1973;2:1–26
154. Mann DMA, Iwatsubo T: Diffuse plaques in the cerebellum and corpus striatum in Down's syndrome contain amyloid β protein (Aβ) only in the form of Aβ42(43). Neurodegeneration 1996;5:115–120
155. Wisniewski T, Lalowski M, Bobik M et al: Amyloid β1–42 deposits do not lead to Alzheimer's neuritic plaques in aged dogs. Biochem J 1996;313:575–580
156. Wegiel J, Wisniewski HM, Dziewiatkowski J et al: Fibrillar and non-fibrillary amyloid in the brain of aged dogs. pp. 703–707. In Iqbal K, Mortimer JA, Winblad B, Wisniewski HM (eds): Research Advances in Alzheimer's disease and Related Disorders. John Wiley & Sons, 1995
157. Cork LC, Masters C, Beyreuther K, Price DL: Development of senile plaques. Relationship of neuronal abnormalities and amyloid deposits. Am J Pathol 1990;137:1383–1392
158. Candy JM, Oakley AE, Klinowski J et al: Aluminosilicates and senile plaque formation in Alzheimer's disease. Lancet 1986;1:354–357
159. Duckett S, Galle P: Mise en evidence de l'aluminium dans les plaques seniles de la maladie d'Alzheimer, etude la microsonde de lastaing. CR Academy of Science 1976;282: 393–395
160. Nikaido T, Austin JH, Trueb L, Rinehart R: Studies in ageing of the brain. II. Microchemical analyses of the nervous system in Alzheimer patients. Arch Neurol 1972;27:549–554
161. Masters CL, Simms G, Weinman NA et al: Amyloid plaque core protein in Alzheimer disease and Down syndrome. Proc Natl Acad Sci (USA) 1985;82:4245–4249
162. Chafi AH, Hauw J-J, Rancurel G et al: Absence of aluminium in Alzheimer's disease brain tissue: electron microprobe and ion microprobe studies. Neurosci Lett 1991;123:61–64
163. Landsberg JP, McDonald B, Watt JF: Absence of aluminium in neuritic plaque cores in Alzheimer's disease. Nature 1992; 360:65–68
164. Miller DL, Papayannopoulos IA, Styles J et al: Peptide compositions of the cerebrovascular and senile plaque core amyloid deposits of Alzheimer's disease. Arch Biochem Biophys 1993; 301:41–52
165. Selkoe DJ, Abraham CR, Podlisny MB, Duffy LK: Isolation of low-molecular-weight proteins from amyloid plaque fibres in Alzheimer's disease. J Neurochem 1986;46:1820–1834
166. Roher AE, Lowenson JD, Clarke S et al: Structural alterations in the peptide backbone of β-amyloid core protein may account for its deposition and stability in Alzheimer's disease. J Biol Chem 1993;268:3072–3083
167. Mori H, Takio K, Ogawara M, Selkoe DJ: Mass spectrometry of purified amyloid β protein in Alzheimer's disease. J Biol Chem 1992;267:17082–17086

168. Gowing E, Roher AE, Woods AS et al: Chemical characterization of Aβ17-42 peptide, a component of diffuse amyloid deposits of Alzheimer disease. J Biol Chem 1994;269:10987–10990

169. Naslund J, Schierhorn A, Hellman U et al: Relative abundance of Alzheimer Aβ amyloid peptide variants in Alzheimer disease and normal aging. Proc Natl Acad Sci (USA) 1994;91:8378–8382

170. Tamaoka A, Odaka A, Ishibashi Y et al: APP717 mis-sense mutation affects the ratio of amyloid β protein species (Aβ1-42/43 and Aβ1-40) in familial Alzheimer's disease brain. J Biol Chem 1994;269:32721–32724

171. Gravina SA, Ho L, Eckman CB et al: Amyloid β protein (Aβ) in Alzheimer's disease brain. J Biol Chem 1995;270:7013–7016

172. Iwatsubo T, Odaka N, Suzuki N et al: Visualization of Aβ42(43)-positive and Aβ40-positive senile plaques with end-specific Aβ monclonal antibodies: evidence that an initially deposited species is Aβ1–42(43). Neuron 1994;13:45–53

173. Mann DMA, Iwatsubo T, Ihara Y et al: Predominant deposition of Aβ42(43) in plaques in cases of Alzheimer's disease and hereditary cerebral haemorrhage associated with mutations in the amyloid precursor protein gene. Am J Pathol 1996;148:1257–1266

174. Mann DMA, Iwatsubo T, Cairns NJ et al: Amyloid (Aβ) deposition in chromosome 14-linked Alzheimer's disease: predominance of Aβ42(43). Ann Neurol 1996;40:149–156

175. Murphy GM, Forno LS, Higgins L et al: Development of a monoclonal antibody specific for the COOH-terminal of β-amyloid 1-42 and its immunohistochemical reactivity in Alzheimer's disease and related disorders. Am J Pathol 1994;144:1082–1088

176. Mak K, Yang F, Vinters HV et al: Polyclonals to β-amyloid (1–42) identify most plaque and vascular deposits in Alzheimer cortex, but not striatum. Brain Res 1994;667:138–142

177. Fukumoto H, Asami-Odaka A, Suzuki N et al: Amyloid β protein (Aβ) deposition in normal aging has the same characteristics as that in Alzheimer's disease: predominance of Aβ42(43) and association of Aβ40 with cored plaques. Am J Pathol 1996;148:259–265

178. Yamaguchi H, Sugiahra S, Ishiguro K et al: Immunohistochemical analysis of COOH-termini of amyloid beta protein (Aβ) using end-specific antisera for Aβ40 and Aβ42 in Alzheimer's disease and normal aging. Amyloid: Int J Clin Invest 1995;2:7–16

179. Kida E, Wisniewski KE, Wisniewski HM: Early amyloid-β deposits show different immunoreactivity to the amino- and carboxy-terminal regions of β-peptide in both Alzheimer's disease and Down's syndrome brain. Neurosci Lett 1995;193:1–4

180. Saido TC, Iwatsubo T, Ihara Y et al: Dominant and differential deposition of distinct β-amyloid peptide species, AβN3(PE) in senile plaques. Neuron 1995;14:457–466

181. Iwatsubo T, Saido TC, Mann DMA et al: Full-length Aβ(1–42(43)) as well as amino-terminally modified and truncated Aβ42(43) deposit in diffuse plaques. Am J Pathol 1996;149:1823–1830

182. Ohgami T, Kitamoto T, Shin R-W et al: Increased senile plaques without microglia in Alzheimer's disease. Acta Neuropathol 1991;81:242–247

183. Fukumoto H, Asami-Odaka A, Suzuki N, Iwatsubo T: Association of Aβ40 positive senile plaques with microglia cells in the brains of patients with Alzheimer's disease and non-demented aged individuals. Neurodegeneration 1996;5:13–17

184. Luthert PJ, Williams JA: A quantitative study of the coincidence of blood vessels and A4 protein deposits in Alzheimer's disease. Neurosci Lett 1991;126:110–112

185. Kawai M, Kalaria RN, Harik SI, Perry G: The relationship of amyloid plaques to cerebral capillaries in Alzheimer's disease. Am J Pathol 1990;137:1435–1446

186. Kang J, Lemaire H-G, Unterbeck A et al: The precursor of Alzheimer's disease amyloid A4 protein resembles a cell surface receptor. Nature 1987;325:733–736

187. Goldgaber D, Lerman MI, MacBride OW et al: Characterization and chromosomal localization of a cDNA encoding brain amyloid of Alzheimer's disease. Science 1987;235:877–880

188. Tanzi RE, St. George-Hyslop PH, Haines JH et al: The genetic defect in familial Alzheimer's disease is not tightly linked to the amyloid precursor protein gene. Nature 1987;329:156–157

189. Ponte P, Gonzalez DeWhitt P, Schilling J et al: A new A4 amyloid mRNA contains a domain homologous to serine proteinase inhibitors. Nature 1988;331:331–525

190. Tanzi RE, McClatchey AI, Lamperti ED et al: Protease inhibitor domain encoded by an amyloid protein precursor mRNA associated with Alzheimer's disease. Nature 1988;331:528–530

191. Kitaguchi N, Takahashi Y, Tokushima Y et al: Novel precursor of Alzheimer's disease amyloid protein shows protease inhibitory activity. Nature 1988;331:530–532

192. Goedert M: Neuronal localization of amyloid β protein precursor mRNA in normal human brains and in Alzheimer's disease. EMBO J 1987;6:3627–3632

193. Bahmanyar S, Higgins GA, Goldgaber D et al: Localization of amyloid β protein messenger RNA in brains from patients with Alzheimer's disease. Science 1988;237:77–80

194. Neve RL, Finch EA, Dawes LR: Expression of the Alzheimer amyloid precursor gene transcripts in the human brain. Neuron 1988;1:669–677

195. Stern RA, Otvos L, Trojanowski JQ, Lee VM-Y: Monoclonal antibodies to a synthetic peptide homologous with the first 28 amino acids of Alzheimer's disease: β protein recognize amyloid and diverse glial and neuronal cell types in the central nervous system. Am J Pathol 1989;134:973–978

196. Siman RL, Card JP, Welson RB, Davis LG: Expression of β-amyloid precursor protein in reactive astrocytes following neuronal damage. Neuron 1989;3:275–285

197. Haass C, Hung AY, Selkoe DJ: Processing of β-amyloid precursor protein in microglia and astrocytes favours an internal

localization over constitutive secretion. J Neurosci 1991;11: 3783–3793

198. Banati RB, Gehrmann J, Czech C et al: Early and rapid de novo synthesis of Alzheimer βA4-amyloid precursor protein (APP) in activated microglia. Glia 1993;9:199–210

199. Weidmann A, Konig G, Bunke D et al: Identification biogenesis and localization of precursors of Alzheimer's disease A4 amyloid protein. Cell 1989;57:115–126

200. Oltersdorf F, Ward PJ, Beattie EC et al: In vitro mutagenesis of the β-amyloid precursor protein. Neurobiol Aging 1990;11: 219

201. Podlisny MB, Mammen AL, Schlossmacher MG et al: Detection of soluble forms of the β-amyloid precursor protein in human plasma. Biochem Biophys Res Commun 1990;167: 1094–1101

202. Palmert MR, Podlisny MB, Witker DS et al: The beta-amyloid protein precursor of Alzheimer's disease has soluble derivatives found in human brain and cerebrospinal fluid. Proc Natl Acad Sci (USA) 1989;86:6338–6342

203. Koo EH, Sisodia SS, Archer DR et al: Precursor of amyloid protein in Alzheimer's disease undergoes fast anterograde axonal transport. Proc Natl Acad Sci (USA) 1990;87: 1561–1565

204. Schubert W, Prior R, Weidmann A et al: Localization of Alzheimer β/A4 amyloid precursor protein at central and peripheral sites. Brain Res 1991;563:184–194

205. Oyama F, Shimada H, Oyama R: Differential expression of β amyloid precursor protein (APP) and tau m-RNA in the aged human brain: individual variability and correlation between APP-751 and four repeat tau. J Neuropathol Exp Neurol 1991; 50:560–578

206. Konig G, Beyreuther K, Masters CL et al: Pre-A4 RNA distribution in brain areas. Prog Clin Biol Res 1989;317: 1027–1036

207. Joachim CL, Mori H, Selkoe DJ: Amyloid β-protein deposition in tissues other than brain in Alzheimer's disease. Nature 1989;341:226–230

208. Soininen H, Syrjanen S, Heinonen O et al: Amyloid β-protein deposition in skin of patients with dementia. Lancet 1992; 339:245

209. Bush AI, Martins RN, Rumble B et al: The amyloid precursor protein of Alzheimer's disease is released by human platelets. J Biol Chem 1990;265:15977–15983

210. Van Nostrand WE, Wagner SL, Suzuki M et al: Protease nexin-II, a potent antichymotrypsin, shows identity to amyloid β precursor. Nature 1989;341:545–549

211. Smith RP, Higuchi DA, Broze GJ: Platelet coagulation factor X1a-inhibitor, a form of Alzheimer's amyloid precursor protein. Science 1990;248:1126–1128

212. Oltersdorf T, Fritz LC, Schenk DB et al: The secreted form of the Alzheimer's amyloid precursor protein with the Kunitz domain is protease nexin II. Nature 1989;341:144–147

213. Schubert D, LaCorbiere M, Saitoh T, Cole G: Characterization of an amyloid β precursor protein that binds heparin and contains tyrosine sulfate. Proc Natl Acad Sci (USA) 1989;86: 2066–2069

214. Breen KC, Bruce M, Anderton BH: Beta amyloid precursor protein mediates neuronal cell-cell and cell-surface adhesion. J Neurosci Res 1991;28:90–100

215. Beer J, Masters CL, Beyreuther K: Cells from peripheral tissues that exhibit high APP expression are characterized by their high membrane fusion activity. Neurodegeneration 1995; 4:51–59

216. Nishimoto I, Okamoto T, Matsuura Y et al: Alzheimer amyloid protein precursor complexes with brain GTP-binding protein Go. Nature 1993;362:75–79

217. Mattson MP, Rydel RE: β amyloid precursor protein and Alzheimer's disease: the peptide plot thickens. Neurobiol Aging 1992;13:617–621

218. Furukawa K, Barger SW, Blalock ER, Mattson MP: Activation of K+ channels and suppression of neuronal activity by secreted β-amyloid precursor protein. Nature 1996;379: 74–78

219. Gentleman SM, Nash MJ, Sweeting CJ et al: β-amyloid precursor protein (β-APP) as a marker for axonal injury after head injury. Neurosci Lett 1993;160:139–144

220. Kawarabayashi T, Shoji M, Harigaya Y et al: Expression of APP in early stages of brain damage. Brain Res 1991;563: 334–338

221. Kalaria RN, Bhatti SU, Palatinsky EA et al: Accumulation of β-amyloid precursor protein at sites of ischemic injury in rat brain. NeuroReport 1993;4:211–214

222. Shigematsu K, McGeer PL: Accumulation of amyloid precursor protein in damaged neuronal processes and microglia following intracerebral administration of aluminium salts. Brain Res 1992;593:117–123

223. Shigematsu K, McGeer PL: Accumulation of amyloid precursor protein in neurones after intraventricular injection of colchicine. Am J Pathol 1992;140:787–794

224. Goldgaber D, Harris HW, Hla T et al: Interleukin-1 regulates synthesis of amyloid β-protein precursor mRNA in human endothelial cells. Proc Natl Acad Sci (USA) 1989;86: 7606–7610

225. Donnelly RJ, Friedhoff AJ, Beer B et al: Interleukin-1 stimulates the beta-amyloid precursor protein promoter. Cell Mol Neurobiol 1990;10:485–491

226. Buxbaum JD, Oishi M, Chen HI et al: Cholinergic agonists and interleukin-1 regulate processing and secretion of the Alzheimer β/A4 amyloid protein precursor. Proc Natl Acad Sci (USA) 1992;89:10075–10078

227. Sheng JG, Boop FA, Mrak RE, Griffin ST: Increased neuronal β-amyloid precursor protein expression in human temporal lobe epilepsy: association with interleukin-1α immunoreactivity. J Neurochem 1994;63:1872–1879

228. Esch ES, Keim P, Beattie EC, Blancher RW et al: Cleavage of amyloid β peptide during constitutive processing of its precursor. Science 1990;248:1122–1124

229. Zhong Z, Higaki J, Murakami K, Wang Y et al: Secretion of

β-amyloid precursor protein involves multiple cleavage sites. J Biol Chem 1994;269:627–632

230. Estus S, Golde TE, Kunishita T et al. Potentially amyloidogenic carboxy-terminal derivatives of the amyloid protein precursor. Science 1992;255:726–728

231. Busciglio J, Gabuzda DH, Matsudaira P, Yankner BA: Generation of β-amyloid in the secretory pathway in neuronal and non-neuronal cells. Proc Natl Acad Sci (USA) 1993;90:2092–2096

232. Buxbaum JD, Gandy SE, Cicchetti P et al: Processing of Alzheimer β/A4 amyloid precursor protein: modulation by agents that regulate protein phosphorylation. Proc Natl Acad Sci (USA) 1990;87:6003–6006

233. Nitsch RM, Slack BE, Wurtman RJ, Growdon JH: Release of Alzheimer amyloid precursor derivatives stimulated by activation of muscarinic acetylcholine receptors. Science 1992;258:304–307

234. Kennedy H, Kamctani K, Allsop D: Only Kunitz inhibitor-containing isoforms of secreted Alzheimer amyloid precursor protein show amyloid immunoreactivity in normal cerebrospinal fluid. Neurodegeneration 1992;1:59–64

235. Seubert P, Vigo-Pelfrey C, Esch F et al: Isolation and quantification of soluble Alzheimer's β-peptide from biological fluids. Nature 1993;359:325–327

236. Seubert P, Oltersdorf T, Lee MG et al: Secretion of β-amyloid precursor protein cleaved at the aminoterminus of the β-amyloid peptide. Nature 1992;361:260–263

237. Davis D, Sinha S, Schlossmacher MG et al: Isolation and quantification of soluble Alzheimer's β-peptide from biological fluids. Nature 1992;359:325–327

238. Haass C, Schlossmacher MG, Hung AY et al: Amyloid β-peptide is produced by cultured cells during normal metabolism. Nature 1992;359:322–325

239. Haass C, Koo EH, Mellon A et al: Targeting of cell-surface β-amyloid precursor protein to lysosomes: alternative processing into amyloid bearing fragments. Nature 1992;357:500–502

240. Shoji M, Golde TE, Ghiso J et al: Production of the Alzheimer amyloid β protein by normal proteolytic processing. Science 1992;258:126–129

241. Dovey HF, Suomesaari-Chrysler S, Lieberburg I et al: Cells with a familial Alzheimer's disease mutation produce authentic β-peptide. Neuro Report 1993;4:1039–1042

242. Vigo-Pelfrey C, Lee D, Keim P et al: Characterization of β-amyloid peptide from human cerebrospinal fluid. J Neurochem 1993;61:1965–1968

243. Golde TE, Estus S, Younkin LH et al: Processing of the amyloid protein precursor to potentially amyloidogenic derivatives. Science 1992;255:728–730

244. Knops J, Lieberburg I, Sinha S: Evidence for a nonsecretory, acidic degradation pathway for amyloid precursor protein in 293 cells. J Biol Chem 1992;267:16022–16024

245. Haass C, Lemere CA, Capell A et al: The Swedish mutation causes early-onset Alzheimer's disease by β-secretase cleavage within the secretory pathway. Nature Med 1995;1:1291–1296

246. Tabaton M, Nunzi MG, Xue R et al: Soluble amyloid β-protein is a marker of Alzheimer amyloid in brain but not in cerebrospinal fluid. Biochem Biophys Res Commun 1994;200:1598–1603

247. Teller JK, Russo C, de Busk LM et al: Presence of soluble amyloid β peptide precedes amyloid plaque formation in Down's syndrome. Nature Med 1996;2:93–95

248. Jarrett JT, Berger EP, Lansbury PT: The carboxy terminus of the β-amyloid protein is critical for the seeding of amyloid formation. Implications for the pathogenesis of Alzheimer's disease. Biochemistry 1993;32:4693–4697

249. Evans KC, Berger EP, Cho GG et al: Apolipoprotein E is a kinetic but not thermodynamic inhibitor of amyloid formation; implications for the pathogenesis and treatment of Alzheimer's disease. Proc Natl Acad Sci (USA) 1995;92:763–767

250. Hilbich C, Kisters-Woike B, Reed J et al: Aggregation and secondary structure of synthetic amyloid βA4 peptides of Alzheimer's disease. J Molec Biol 1991;218:149–163

251. Burdick D, Soreghan B, Kwon M et al: Assembly and aggregation properties of synthetic Alzheimer's A4/β amyloid peptide analogies. J Biol Chem 1982;267:546–554

252. Ma J, Yee A, Brewer B, Das S, Potter H: Amyloid-associated proteins of α-1 antichymotrypsin and apolipoprotein E promote assembly of Alzheimer β protein into filaments. Nature 1994;372:92–94

253. Bush AI, Pettingell WH, Multhaup G et al: Rapid induction of Alzheimer Aβ amyloid formation by zinc. Science 1994;265:1464–1467

254. Mantyh PW, Ghilardi JR, Rogers S et al: Aluminium, iron, and zinc ions promote aggregation of physiological concentrations of β-amyloid peptide. J Neurochem 1993;61:1171–1174

255. Snow AD, Sekiguchi R, Nochlin D et al: An important role of heparan sulphate proteoglycan (Perlecan) in a model system for the deposition and persistence of fibrillar Aβ amyloid in rat brain. Neuron 1994;12:219–234

256. Halverson K, Fraser PE, Kirschner DA, Lansbury PT: Molecular determinants of amyloid deposits in Alzheimer's disease: conformational studies of synthetic β-protein fragments. Biochemistry 1990;29:2639–2644

257. Pike CJ, Walencewicz-Wasserman AJ, Kosmoski J et al: Structure-activity analyses of β-amyloid peptides: contributions of the β25–35 region to aggregation and neurotoxicity. J Neurochem 1995;64:253–265

258. Schubert D, Behl C, Lesley R, Brack A et al: Amyloid peptides are toxic via a common oxidative mechanism. Proc Natl Acad Sci (USA) 1995;92:1989–1993

259. Shearman MS, Ragan CI, Iversen LL: Inhibition of PC12 cell redox activity is a specific, early indicator of the mechanism of β-amyloid-mediated cell death. Proc Natl Acad Sci (USA) 1994;91:1470–1471

260. Shearman MS, Hawtin SR, Tailor VJ: The intracellular component of cellular 3-(4,5-dimethylthiazol-2-yl)-2,5-diphenyltet-

razolium bromide (MTT) reduction is specifically inhibited by β-amyloid peptides. J Neurochem 1995;65:218–227

261. Loo DT, Copani A, Pike CJ et al: Apoptosis is induced by β-amyloid in cultured central nervous system neurons. Proc Natl Acad Sci (USA) 1993;90:7951–7955
262. Forloni G, Chiesa R, Smiroldo S et al: Apoptosis-mediated neurotoxicity induced by chronic application of beta amyloid fragment. NeuroReport 1993;4:523–526
263. Behl C, Davis B, Klier FG, Schubert H: Amyloid beta peptide induces necrosis rather than apoptosis. Brain Res 1994;645: 253–264
264. Behl C, Davis JB, Lesley R, Schubert D: Hydrogen peroxide mediates amyloid β protein toxicity. Cell 1994;77:1–20
265. Etcheberrigaray R, Ito E, Kim CS, Alkon DL: Soluble β-amyloid induction of Alzheimer's phenotype for human fibroblast K+ channels. Science 1994;264:276–279
266. Copani A, Koh J, Cotman CW: β-amyloid increases neuronal susceptibility to injury by glucose deprivation. NeuroReport 1991;2:763–765
267. Meda L, Cassatella MA, Szendrei GI et al: Activation of microglial cells by β-amyloid protein and interferon-γ. Nature 1995;374:647–650
268. Namba Y, Tomonaga M, Kawasaki H et al: Apolipoprotein E immunoreactivity in cerebral amyloid deposits and neurofibrillary tangles in Alzheimer's disease and Kuru plaque amyloid in Creutzfeldt-Jakob disease. Brain Res 1991;541:163–166
269. Wisniewski T, Frangione B: Apolipoprotein E: a pathological chaperone protein in patients with cerebral and systemic amyloid. Neurosci Lett 1992;135:235–238
270. Schmechel D, Saunders AM, Strittmatter WJ et al: Increased amyloid β peptide deposition in cerebral cortex as a consequence of apolipoprotein E genotype in late-onset Alzheimer disease. Proc Natl Acad Sci (USA) 1993;90:9649–9653
271. Rebeck GW, Reiter JS, Strickland DK, Hyman BT: Apolipoprotein E in sporadic Alzheimer's disease: allelic variation and receptor interactions. Neuron 1993;11:575–580
272. Yamaguchi H, Ishiguro K, Sugihara S et al: Presence of apolipoprotein E on extracellular tangles and on meningeal blood vessels precedes the Alzheimer β-amyloid deposition. Acta Neuropathol 1994;88:413–419
273. Kida E, Golabek AA, Wisniewski T, Wisniewski KE: Regional differences in apolipoprotein E immunoreactivity in diffuse plaques in Alzheimer's disease brain. Neurosci Lett 1994; 167:73–76
274. Saunders AM, Strittmatter WJ, Schmechel D et al: Association of Apolipoprotein E4 with late-onset familial and sporadic Alzheimer's disease. Neurology 1993;43:1467–1472
275. Strittmatter WJ, Saunders AM, Schmechel D et al: Apolipoprotein E: high-avidity binding to β-amyloid and increased frequency of type 4 allelle in late-onset familial Alzheimer's disease. Proc Natl Acad Sci (USA) 1993;90:1977–1981
276. Corder EH, Saunders AM, Strittmatter WJ et al: Gene dose of apolipoprotein E Type 4 allele and the risk of Alzheimer's disease in late onset families. Science 1993;261:921–923
277. Houlden H, Crook R, Duff K et al: Confirmation that the apolipoprotein E4 allele is associated with late onset familial Alzheimer's disease. Neurodegeneration 1993;2:283–288
278. Mayeux R, Stern Y, Ottman R et al: The apolipoprotein E4 allele in patients with Alzheimer's disease. Ann Neurol 1993; 34:752–754
279. Pickering-Brown SM, Roberts D, Owen F, Neary D: Apolipoprotein E4 alleles and non-Alzheimer forms of dementia. Neurodegeneration 1994;3:95–96
280. Saunders AM, Schmader K, Breitner JCS et al: Apolipoprotein E4 allele distribution in late onset Alzheimer's disease and in other amyloid forming diseases. Lancet 1993;342:710–711
281. Davies CA, Mann DMA: Co-localization of apolipoprotein E and amyloid β protein in Down's syndrome. Ann Neurol 1997; (in press)
282. Berr C, Hauw J-J, Delaere P et al: Apolipoprotein E allele E4 is linked to increased deposition of the amyloid β-peptide (A-β) in cases with or without Alzheimer's disease. Neurosci Lett 1994;178:221–224
283. Hyman B, West HL, Rebeck GW et al: Neuropathological changes in Down's syndrome, hippocampal formation: effect of age and apolipoprotein E genotype. Arch Neurol 1995;52: 373–378
284. Ohm TG, Kirca M, Bohl J et al: Apolipoprotein E polymorphism influences not only cerebral senile plaque load but also Alzheimer-type neurofibrillary tangle formation. Neuroscience 1995;66:585–587
285. Polvikoski T, Sulkava R, Haltia M et al: Apolipoprotein E, dementia, and cortical deposition of β-amyloid protein. N Engl J Med 1995;333:1242–1247
286. Harrington CR, Louwagie J, Rossau R et al: Influence of apolipoprotein E genotype on senile dementia of the Alzheimer and Lewy body types. Am J Pathol 1994;145:1472–1484
287. Mann DMA, Iwatsubo T, Pickering-Brown SM, Saido TC: Preferential deposition of amyloid β protein (Aβ) in the form Aβ_{40} in Alzheimer's disease is associated with a gene dosage effect of the apolipoprotein E E4 allele Neurosci Lett 1997;221: 81–84
288. Benjamin R, Leake A, Ince PG et al: Effects of apolipoprotein E genotype on cortical neuropathology in senile dementia of the Lewy body type and Alzheimer's disease. Neurodegeneration 1995;4:443–448
289. Gearing M, Mori H, Mirra SS: Aβ peptide length and apolipoprotein E genotype in Alzheimer's disease. Ann Neurol 1996; 39:393–399
290. Heinonen O, Lehtovirta M, Soininen H et al: Alzheimer pathology of patients carrying apolipoprotein E E4 allele. Neurobiol Aging 1995;16:505–513
291. Itoh Y, Yamada M: Apolipoprotein E and the neuropathology of dementia. N Engl J Med 1996;334:599–600
292. Snow AD, Mar H, Nochlin D et al: The presence of heparan sulphate proteoglycans in the neuritic plaques and congophilic angiopathy in Alzheimer's disease. Am J Pathol 1988;133: 456–463
293. Snow AD, Mar H, Nochlin D et al: Early accumulation of heparan sulphate in neurones and in the β amyloid protein

containing lesions of Alzheimer's disease and Down's syndrome. Am J Pathol 1990;137:1253–1270

294. Su JH, Cummings BJ, Cotman CW: Localization of heparan sulfate glycosaminoglycan and proteoglycan core protein in aged brain and Alzheimer's disease. Neuroscience 1992;51: 801–813

295. Perry G, Siedlak SL, Richey P et al: Association of heparan sulphate proteoglycan with the neurofibrillary tangles of Alzheimer's disease. J Neurosci 1991;11:3679–3683

296. Buee L, Ding W, Anderson JP et al: Binding of vascular heparan sulfate proteoglycan to Alzheimer's amyloid precursor protein is mediated in part by the N-terminal region of A4 peptide. Brain Res 1993;627:199–204

297. Snow AD, Seikiguchi RT, Nochlin D et al: Heparan sulphate proteoglycan in diffuse plaques of hippocampus but not of cerebellum in Alzheimer's disease brain. Am J Pathol 1994; 144:337–347

298. Threlkeld A, Adler R, Hewitt AT: Proteoglycan biosynthesis by chick embryo retina glial-like cells. Dev Biol 1989;132: 559–568

299. Fluharty AL, Davis LD, Trammell JL et al: Mucopolysaccharides synthesized by cultured glial cells derived from a patient with Sanfilippo A syndrome. J Neurochem 1975;25:429–435

300. Lue L-F, Rogers J: Full complement activation fails in diffuse plaques of the Alzheimer's disease cerebellum. Dementia 1992;3:308–313

301. Kalaria RN, Perry G: Amyloid P component and other acute phase proteins associated with cerebellar Aβ deposits in Alzheimer's disease. Brain Res 1993;631:151–155

302. Rozemuller JM, Eikelenboom P, Stam FC et al: A4 protein in Alzheimer's disease: primary and secondary cellular events in extracellular amyloid deposition. J Neuropathol Exp Neurol 1989;48:674–691

303. Eikelenboom P, Hack CE, Kamphorst W et al: The sequence of neuroimmunological events in cerebral amyloid plaque formation in Alzheimer's disease. pp. 165–170. In Corain B, Iqbal K, Nicolini M, Wisniewski H, Zatta P (eds): Alzheimer Disease: Advances in Clinical and Basic Research. John Wiley & Sons, Chichester, 1993

304. Rogers J, Cooper NR, Webster S et al: Complement activation by β-amyloid in Alzheimer disease. Proc Natl Acad Sci 1992; 89:10016–10020

305. Jiang H, Burdick D, Glabe CG et al: β-Amyloid activates complement by binding to a specific region of the collagen-like domain of the C1q A chain. J Immunol 1994;152:5050–5059

306. Snyder SW, Wang GT, Barrett L et al: Complement C1q does not bind monomeric β-amyloid. Exp Neurol 1994;128: 136–142

307. Akiyama H, McGeer PL: Brain microglia constitutively express β2 integrins. J Neuroimmunol 1990;30:81–93

308. McGeer PL, Akiyama H, Itagaki S, McGeer EG: Activation of the classical complement pathway in brain tissue of Alzheimer's patients. Neurosci Lett 1989;107:341–346

309. Zhan S-S, Veerhuis R, Kamphorst W, Eikelenboom P: Distribution of beta amyloid associated proteins in plaques in Alzheimer's disease and in the non-demented elderly. Neurodegeneration 1995;4:291–297

310. Zhan SS, Veerhuis R, Janssen I et al: Immunohistochemical distribution of the inhibitors of the terminal complement complex in Alzheimer's disease. Neurodegeneration 1994;3: 111–117

311. McGeer PL, Walker DG, Akiyama H et al: Detection of the membrane inhibitor of reactive lysis (CD59) in deceased neurons of Alzheimer brain. Brain Res 1991;544:315–319

312. Choi-Miura NH, Ihara Y, Fukuchi K et al: SP-40,40 is a constituent of Alzheimer's amyloid. Acta Neuropathol 1992;83: 260–264

313. Akiyama H, Kawamata T, Dedhar S, McGeer PL: Immunohistochemical localization of vitronectin, its receptor and beta-3 integrin in Alzheimer brain tissue. J Neuroimmunol 1991;32: 19–28

314. Wisniewski T, Golabek A, Matsubara E et al: Apolipoprotein E: binding to soluble Alzheimer's β-amyloid. Biochem Biophys Res Commun 1993;192:359–365

315. Matsubara E, Soto C, Governale S et al: Apolipoprotein J and Alzheimer's amyloid β solubility. Biochem J 1996;316: 671–679

316. Golabek A, Marques M, Lalowski M, Wisniewski T: Amyloid β binding proteins *in vitro* and in normal human cerebrospinal fluid. Neurosci Lett 1995;191:79–82

317. Koudinov A, Matsubara E, Frangione B, Ghiso J: The soluble form of Alzheimer's amyloid β protein is complexed to high density lipoprotein 3 and very high density lipoprotein in normal human plasma. Biochem Biophys Res Commun 1994; 205:1164–1171

318. Abraham CR, Selkoe DJ, Potter H: Immunochemical identification of the serine protease inhibitor α1-antichymotrypsin in the brain amyloid deposits of Alzheimer's disease. Cell 1988; 52:487–501

319. Shoji M, Hirai S, Yamaguchi H et al: Alpha 1-antichymotrypsin is present in diffuse senile plaques. A comparative study of β-protein and α-1-antichymotrypsin immunostaining in the Alzheimer brain. Am J Pathol 1991;138:247–257

320. Rozemuller JM, Abbink JJ, Kamp AM et al: Distribution pattern and functional state of α1-antichymotrypsin in plaques and vascular amyloid in Alzheimer's disease. Acta Neuropathol 1991;82:200–207

321. Kalaria RN, Galloway PG, Perry G: Widespread serum amyloid P immunoreactivity in cortical amyloid deposits and the neurofibrillary pathology of Alzheimer's disease and other degenerative disorders. Neuropathol Appl Neurobiol 1991;17: 189–201

322. Duong T, Pommier EC, Scheibel AB: Immunodetection of the amyloid P component in Alzheimer's disease. Acta Neuropathol 1989;78:429–437

323. Coria F, Castrano E, Prelli F et al: Isolation and characterization of amyloid P component from Alzheimer's disease and other types of cerebral amyloidosis. Lab Invest 1988;58: 454–458

324. Tennent GA, Lovat LB, Pepys MB: Serum amyloid P component prevents proteolysis of amyloid fibrils of Alzheimer's dis-

ease and systemic amyloidosis. Proc Natl Acad Sci (USA) 1995;92:4299–4303

325. Ji Z-S, Fazio S, Lee Y-L, Mahley RW: Secretion-capture role for apolipoprotein E in remnant lipoprotein metabolism involving cell surface heparan sulfate proteoglycans. J Biol Chem 1994;269:2764–2772

326. Rifenburg RP, Perry G: Dystrophic neurites define diffuse as well as core-containing senile plaques in Alzheimer's disease. Neurodegeneration 1995;4:235–237

327. Struble RG, Cork LC, Whitehouse PJ, Price DL: Cholinergic innervation in neuritic plaques. Science 1982;213:413–415

328. Armstrong DM, Bruce G, Hersh LB, Terry RD: Choline acetyltransferase immunoreactivity in neuritic plaques of Alzheimer brain. Neurosci Lett 1986;71:229–234

329. Kitt CA, Struble RG, Cork LC et al: Catecholaminergic neurites in senile plaques in prefrontal cortex of aged nonhuman primates. Neuroscience 1985;16:691–699

330. Struble RG, Kitt CA, Walker LC et al: Somatostatinergic neurites in senile plaques of aged non-human primates. Brain Res 1984;324:394–396

331. Armstrong DM, LeRoy S, Shields D, Terry RD: Somatostatin-like immunoreactivity within neuritic plaques. Brain Res 1985;338:71–79

332. Morrison JH, Rogers J, Scherr S et al: Somatostatin immunoreactivity in neuritic plaques of Alzheimer's patients. Nature 1985;314:90–94

333. Nakamura S, Vincent SR: Somatostatin- and neuropeptide Y-Immunoreactive neurons in the neocortex in senile dementia of Alzheimer's type. Brain Res 1986;370:11–20

334. Armstrong DM, Terry RD: Substance P immunoreactivity within neuritic plaques. Neurosci Lett 1985;58:139–144

335. Dawbarn D, Emson PC: Neuropeptide Y like immunoreactivity in neuritic plaques of Alzheimer's disease. Biochem Biophys Res Commun 1985;126:289–294

336. Benes FM, Farol PA, Majocha RE et al: Evidence for axonal loss in regions occupied by senile plaques in Alzheimer cortex. Neuroscience 1991;42:651–660

337. Masliah E, Honer WG, Mallory M et al: Topographical distribution of synaptic-associated proteins in the neuritic plaques of Alzheimer's disease hippocampus. Acta Neuropathol 1994; 87:135–142

338. Masliah E, Terry RD, Mallory M et al: Diffuse plaques do not accentuate synapse loss in Alzheimer's disease. Am J Pathol 1990;137:1293–1297

339. Masliah E, Mallory M, Deerinck T et al: Re-evaluation of the structural organization of neuritic plaques in Alzheimer's disease. J Neuropathol Exp Neurol 1993;52:619–632

340. Cummings BJ, Su JM, Geddes JW et al: Aggregation of the amyloid precursor protein within degenerating neurons and dystrophic neurites in Alzheimer's disease. Neuroscience 1992;48:763–777

341. Cras P, Kawai M, Lowery DE et al: Senile plaque neurites in Alzheimer's disease accumulate amyloid precursor protein. Proc Natl Acad Sci (USA) 1991;88:7552–7556

342. Shoji M, Hirai S, Yamaguchi H et al: Amyloid β-protein precursor accumulates in dystrophic neurites of senile plaques in Alzheimer's disease. Brain Res 1990;512:164–168

343. Tate-Ostroff B, Majocha RE, Marotta CA: Identification of cellular and extracellular sites of amyloid precursor protein extracytoplasmic domain in normal and Alzheimer's disease brains. Proc Natl Acad Sci (USA) 1989;86:745–749

344. Joachim CL, Games D, Morris J et al: Antibodies to non-Beta regions of the beta-amyloid precursor protein detect a subset of plaques. Am J Pathol 1991;138:373–384

345. Kawai M, Cras P, Richey P et al: Subcellular localization of amyloid precursor protein in senile plaques of Alzheimer's disease. Am J Pathol 1992;140:947–958

346. Masliah E, Honer WG, Mallory M et al: Topographical distribution of synaptic-associated proteins in the neuritic plaques of Alzheimer's disease hippocampus. Acta Neuropathol 1994; 87:135–142

347. Masliah E, Mallory M, Hansen L et al: Localization of amyloid precursor protein in GAP43-immunoreactive aberrant sprouting neurites in Alzheimer's disease. Brain Res 1992;574: 312–316

348. Six J, Lubke U, Lenders M-B et al: Neurite sprouting and cytoskeletal pathology in Alzheimer's disease: a comparative study with monoclonal antibodies to growth-associated protein B-50 (GAP43) and paired helical filaments. Neurodegeneration 1992;1:247–255

349. Wisniewski HM, Wegiel J, Wang KC et al: Ultrastructural studies of the cells forming amyloid fibres in classical plaques. Can J Neurol Sci 1989;16:535–542

350. Wisniewski HM, Vorbrodt AW, Epstein MH: Nucleoside diphosphatase (NDPase) activity associated with human β-protein amyloid fibres. Acta Neuropathol 1991;81:366–370

351. Perlmutter LS, Barron E, Chui HC: Morphologic association between microglia and senile plaque amyloid in Alzheimer's disease. Neurosci Lett 1990;119:32–36

352. Wegiel J, Wisniewski HM: The complex of microglial cells and amyloid star in three-dimensional reconstruction. Acta Neuropathol 1990;81:116–124

353. Mancardi GL, Liwnicz BH, Mandybur TI: Fibrous astrocytes in Alzheimer's disease and senile dementia of Alzheimer's type. Acta Neuropathol 1983;61:76–80

354. Mandybur TI, Chuirazzi BA: Astrocytes and the plaques of Alzheimer's disease. Neurology 1990;40:635–639

355. Schechter R, Yen S-HC, Terry RD: Fibrous astrocytes in senile dementia of the Alzheimer type. J Neuropathol Exp Neurol 1981;40:95–101

356. Frederickson RCA: Astroglia in Alzheimer's disease. Neurobiol Ageing 1992;13:239–253

357. Van Eldik LJ, Griffin WST: S100β in Alzheimer's disease: relation to neuropathology in brain regions. Biochim Biophys Acta 1994;1223:398–403

358. Sheng JG, Mrak RE, Griffin WST: Microglial interleukin-1α expression in brain regions in Alzheimer's disease: correlation with neuritic plaque distribution. Neuropathol Appl Neurobiol 1995;21:290–301

359. Konig G, Monning U, Czech C et al: Identification and differential expression of a novel alternative splice form of the βA4 amyloid precursor protein (APP) mRNA in leucocytes and brain microglial cells. J Biol Chem 1992;267: 10804–10809

360. Sandbrink R, Masters CL, Beyreuther K: βA4-amyloid protein precursor mRNA isoforms without exon 15 are ubiquitously expressed in rat tissues including brain, but not in neurons. J Biol Chem 1994;269:15510–15517

361. Monning U, Sandbrink R, Weidemann A et al: Extracellular matrix influences the biogenesis of amyloid precursor protein in microglial cells. J Biol Chem 1995;270:7104–7110

362. Griffin WST, Sheng JG, Roberts GW, Mrak RE: Interleukin-1 expression in different plaque types in Alzheimer's disease: Significance in plaque evolution. J Neuropathol Exp Neurol 1995;54:276–281

363. Naidu A, Quon D, Cordell B: β-Amyloid peptide produced *in vitro* is degraded by proteinases released by cultured cells. J Biol Chem 1995;270:1369–1374

364. Wisniewski HM, Barcikowska M, Kida E: Phagocytosis of β/A4 amyloid fibrils of the neuritic neocortical plaques. Acta Neuropathol 1991;81:588–590

365. Card JP, Meade RP, Davis LG: Immunocytochemical localization of the precursor protein for β amyloid in the rat central nervous system. Neuron 1988;1:835–846

366. Boje KM, Arora PK: Microglial-produced nitric oxide and reactive nitrogen oxides mediate neuronal death. Brain Res 1992;587:250–256

367. Chao CC, Molitor TW, Hu S: Neuroprotective role of IL-4 against reactive microglia. J Immunol 1993;151:1473–1481

368. Griffin WST, Stanley LC, Ling C et al: Brain interleukin 1 and S-100 immunoreactivity are elevated in Down syndrome and Alzheimer disease. Proc Natl Acad Sci (USA) 1989;86: 7611–7615

369. Marshak DR, Pesce SA, Stanley LC, Griffin WST: Increased S100β neurotrophic activity in Alzheimer's disease temporal lobe. Neurobiol Aging 1991;13:1–7

370. Sheng JG, Mrak RE, Griffin WST: S100β protein expressed in Alzheimer disease: potential role in the pathogenesis of neuritic plaques. J Neurosci Res 1994;39:398–404

371. Mattiace LA, Davies P, Yen S-H, Dickson DW: Microglia in cerebellar plaques in Alzheimer's disease. Acta Neuropathol 1990;80:493–498

372. Styren CD, Civin WH, Rogers J: Molecular, cellular, and pathologic characterization of HLA-DR immunoreactivity in normal elderly and Alzheimer disease brain. Exp Neurol 1990; 110:93–104

373. Jamada M, Mehraein P: Distribution of senile changes in the brain: the part of the limbic system in Alzheimer's disease and senile dementia. Neurologie 1968;211:308–324

374. Itagaki S, McGeer PL, Akiyama H: Presence of T-cytotoxic suppressor and leukocyte common antigen positive cells in Alzheimer's disease brain tissue. Neurosci Lett 1988;91: 259–264

375. Morimatsu M, Hirai S, Muramatsu A, Yoshikawa M: Senile degenerative brain lesions and dementia. J Amer Geriat Soc 1975;23:390–406

376. Braak H, Braak E: Neuropathological staging of Alzheimer-related changes. Acta Neuropathol 1991;82:239–259

377. Bouras C, Hof PR, Morrison JH: Neurofibrillary tangle densities in the hippocampal formation in a non-demented population define subgroups of patients with differential early pathologic changes. Neurosci Lett 1993;153:131–135

378. Kidd M: Paired helical filaments in electron microscopy of Alzheimer's disease. Nature 1963;97:192–193

379. Terry RD: The fine structure of neurofibrillary tangles in Alzheimer's disease. J Neuropathol Exp Neurol 1963;22: 629–642

380. Shibayama H, Kitoh J: Electron microscopic structure of the Alzheimer's neurofibrillary changes in case of atypical senile dementia. Acta Neuropathol 1978;41:229–234

381. Yagishita S, Itoh Y, Wang N, Amano N: Reappraisal of the fine structure of Alzheimer's neurofibrillary tangles. Acta Neuropathol 1981;54:239–246

382. Metuzals J, Montpetit V, Clapin DF: Organization of the neurofilamentous network. Cell Tissue Res 1981;214:455–482

383. Crowther RA, Wischik CM: Image reconstruction of the Alzheimer paired helical filament. EMBO J 1985;4:3661–3665

384. Crowther RA: Straight and paired helical filaments in Alzheimer's disease have a common structural unit. Proc Natl Acad Sci (USA) 1991;88:2292–2298

385. Delacourte A, Defossez A: Alzheimer's disease tau proteins, the promoting factors of microtubule assembly, are major components of paired helical filaments. J Neurol Sci 1986;76: 173–186

386. Ihara Y, Nukina N, Miura R, Ogawara M: Phosphorylated tau protein is integrated into paired helical filaments in Alzheimer's disease. J Biochem Japan 1986;99:1807–1810

387. Grundke-Iqbal I, Iqbal K, Tung Y-C et al: Abnormal phosphorylation of the microtubule-associated protein (tau) in Alzheimer cytoskeletal pathology. Proc Natl Acad Sci (USA) 1986; 83:4913–4917

388. Kosik KS, Joachim CL, Selkoe DJ: Microtubule associated protein tau is a major antigenic component of paired helical filaments in Alzheimer's disease. Proc Natl Acad Sci (USA) 1986;83:4044–4048

389. Wood JG, Mirra SS, Pollock NJ, Binder LI: Neurofibrillary tangles of Alzheimer's disease share antigenic determinants with the axonal microtubule associated protein tau. Proc Natl Acad Sci (USA) 1986;83:4040–4043

390. Kondo J, Honda T, Mori H et al: The carboxyl third of tau is tightly bound to paired helical filaments. Neuron 1988;1: 827–834

391. Kosik KS, Orecchio LD, Binder L et al: Epitopes that span the tau molecule are shared with paired helical filaments. Neuron 1988;1:817–825

392. Goedert M, Wischik C, Crowther RA et al: Cloning and sequencing of the cDNA encoding a core protein of the paired

helical filament of Alzheimer's disease: identification as the microtubule associated protein tau. Proc Natl Acad Sci (USA) 1988;85:4051–4055

393. Wischik C, Novak M, Thagersen HC et al: Isolation of a fragment of tau derived from the core of the paired helical filament of Alzheimer's disease. Proc Natl Acad Sci (USA) 1988;85: 4506–4510

394. Anderton BH, Breinburg D, Downs MJ et al: Monoclonal antibodies show that neurofibrillary tangles and neurofilaments share antigenic determinants. Nature 1982;298:87–96

395. Sternberger NH, Sternberger LA, Ulrich J: Aberrant neurofilament phosphorylation in Alzheimer disease. Proc Natl Acad Sci (USA) 1985;82:4274–4276

396. Perry G, Rizzuto N, Autilio-Gambetti L, Gambetti P: Alzheimer's paired helical filaments contain cytoskeletal components. Proc Natl Acad Sci (USA) 1985;82:3916–3920

397. Ulrich J, Haugh M, Anderton BH et al: Alzheimer dementia and Pick's disease: neurofibrillary tangles and Pick bodies are associated with identical phosphorylated neurofilament epitopes. Acta Neuropathol 1987;73:240–246

398. Gambetti P, Shecket G, Ghetti B et al: Neurofibrillary changes in the human brain. An immunohistochemical study with a neurofilament antiserum. J Neuropathol Exp Neurol 1983;42: 69–79

399. Miller CCJ, Brion J-P, Calvert R et al: Alzheimer's paired helical filaments share epitopes with neurofilament side arms. EMBO J 1986;5:269–276

400. Yen S-HC, Gaskin F, Terry RD: Immunocytochemical studies of neurofibrillary tangles. Am J Pathol 1981;104:77–89

401. Yen S-H, Gaskin F, Fu SM: Neurofibrillary tangles in senile dementia of the Alzheimer type share an antigenic determinant with intermediate filaments of the vimentin class. Am J Pathol 1983;113:373–381

402. Perry G, Friedman R, Shaw G, Chau V: Ubiquitin is detected in neurofibrillary tangles and senile plaque neurites of Alzheimer's disease brains. Proc Natl Acad Sci (USA) 1987;84: 3033–3036

403. Mori H, Kondo J, Ihara Y: Ubiquitin is a component of paired helical filament in Alzheimer's disease. Science 1987;235: 1641–1644

404. Wischik CM, Novak M, Edwards PC et al: Structural characterization of the core of the paired helical filament of Alzheimer's disease. Proc Natl Acad Sci (USA) 1988;85:4884–4888

405. Wischik CM, Lai R, Harrington CR et al: Structure, Biochemistry and molecular pathogenesis of paired helical filaments in Alzheimer's disease. pp. 9–39. In Goate A, Ashall F (eds): Pathobiology of Alzheimer's Disease. Academic Press, London, 1995

406. Poulter L, Barratt D, Scott CW, Caputo CB: Locations and immunoreactions of phosphorylation sites on bovine and porcine tau proteins and a PMF-tau fragment. J Biol Chem 1993; 268:9636–9644

407. Goedert M, Spillantini MG, Jakes R et al: Multiple isoforms of human microtubule-associated protein tau: sequences and localization in neurofibrillary tangles of Alzheimer's disease. Neuron 1989;3:519–526

408. Mukaetova-Ladinska EB, Harrington CR, Hills R et al: Regional distribution of paired helical filaments and normal tau proteins in aging and in Alzheimer's disease, with and without occipital lobe involvement. Dementia 1993;3:61–69

409. Mukaetova-Ladinska EB, Harrington CR, Roth M, Wischik CM: Biochemical and anatomical redistribution of tau protein in Alzheimer's disease. Am J Pathol 1993;143:565–578

410. Lee VM-Y, Balin BJ, Otvos LJ, Trojanowski JQ: A major subunit of paired helical filaments and derivatized forms of normal tau. Science 1991;251:675–678

411. Goedert M, Spillantini MG, Cairns NJ, Crowther RA: Tau proteins of Alzheimer paired helical filaments: abnormal phosphorylation of all six brain isoforms. Neuron 1992;8:159–168

412. Flament S, Delacourte A, Mann DMA: Phosphorylation of tau proteins: a major event during the process of neurofibrillary degeneration. Comparisons between Alzheimer's disease and Down's syndrome. Brain Res 1990;516:15–19

413. Lai RYK, Gertz HJ, Wischik DJ et al: Examination of phosphorylated tau protein as a PHF-precursor at early stage Alzheimer's disease. Neurobiol Aging 1995;16:433–445

414. Mena R, Edwards P, Perez-Olvera O, Wischik CM: Monitoring pathological assembly of tau and β-amyloid proteins in Alzheimer's disease. Acta Neuropathol 1995;89:50–56

415. Mena R, Edwards PC, Harrington CR et al: Staging the pathological assembly of truncated tau protein into paired helical filaments in Alzheimer's disease. Acta Neuropathol 1996;91: 633–641

416. Lee VM-Y, Trojanowski JQ: Tau proteins and their significance in the pathobiology of Alzheimer's disease. pp. 41–58. In Goate A, Ashall F (eds): Pathobiology of Alzheimer's Disease. Academic Press, London, 1995

417. Goedert M, Jakes R, Crowther RA et al: The abnormal phosphorylation of tau protein at Ser-202 in Alzheimer's disease recapitulates phosphorylation during development. Proc Natl Acad Sci (USA) 1993;90:5066–5070

418. Biernat J, Mandlekow E-M, Schroter C et al: The switch of tau protein to an Alzheimer-like state includes phosphorylation of two serine-proline motifs upstream of the microtubule binding region. EMBO J 1992;11:1593–1597

419. Bramblett GT, Goedert M, Jakes R et al: Abnormal tau phosphorylation at Ser^{396} in Alzheimer's disease recapitulates development and contributes to reduced microtubule binding. Neuron 1993;10:1089–1099

420. Garver TD, Lehman RAW, Lee VM-Y et al: Tau phosphorylation in human, primate and rat brain: evidence that a pool of tau is highly phosphorylated in vivo and is rapidly dephosphorylated in vitro. J Neurochem 1994;63:2279–2287

421. Matsuo ES, Shin RW, Billingsley ML et al: Biopsy-derived adult human brain tau is phosphorylated at the same sites as Alzheimer's disease paired helical filaments. Neuron 1994; 13:989–1002

422. Sergeant N, Bussiere T, Vermersch P et al: Isoelectric point differentiates PHF-tau from biopsy-derived human brain tau proteins. NeuroReport 1995;6:2217–2220

423. Litersky JM, Johnson GVW, Jakes R et al: Tau protein is phosphorylated by cyclic AMP-dependent protein kinase and calcium/calmodulin-dependent protein kinase II within its mi-

crotubule-binding domains at Ser262 and Ser356. Biochem J 1996;316:655–660

424. Hasegawa M, Morishima-Kawashima M, Takio K et al: Protein sequence and mass spectrometric analyses of tau in the Alzheimer's disease brain. J Biol Chem 1992;267:17047–17054

425. Morishima-Kawashima M, Hasegawa M, Takio K et al: Ubiquitin is conjugated with amino-terminally processed tau in paired helical filaments. Neuron 1993;10:1151–1160

426. Biernat J, Gustke N, Drewes G et al: Phosphorylation of serine^{262} strongly reduces the binding of tau protein to microtubules: distrinction between PHF-like immunoreactivity and microtubule binding. Neuron 1993;11:153–163

427. Watanabe A, Hasegawa M, Suzuki M et al: In vivo phosphorylation sites in fetal and adult rat tau. J Biol Chem 1993;268: 25712–25717

428. Drewes G, Lichtenberg-Kraag B, Doring F et al: Mitogen activated protein (MAP) kinase transforms tau protein into an Alzheimer-like state. EMBO J 1992;11:2131–2138

429. Gustke N, Steiner B, Mandelkow E-M et al: The Alzheimer-like phosphorylation of tau proteins reduces microtubule binding and involves Ser-Pro and Thr-Pro motifs. FEBS Lett 1992; 307:199–205

430. Hanger DP, Hughes K, Woodgett JR et al: Glycogen synthase kinase-3 induces Alzheimer's disease-like phosphorylation of tau: generation of paired helical filament epitopes and neuronal localization of the kinase. Neurosci Lett 1992;147: 58–62

431. Greenberg SM, Koo EH, Selkoe DJ et al: Secreted β-amyloid precursor protein stimulates mitogen-activated protein kinase and enhances tau phosphorylation. Proc Natl Acad Sci (USA) 1994;91:7104–7108

432. Vulliet R, Halbran SM, Braun RK et al: Proline directed phosphorylation of human tau protein. J Biol Chem 1992;267: 22570–22574

433. Baumann K, Mandelkow E-M, Biernat J et al: Abnormal Alzheimer-like phosphorylation of tau protein by cyclin dependent kinases cdk2 and cdk5. FEBS Lett 1993;336:417–424

434. Paudel HK, Lew J, Ali Z, Wang JH: Brain proline-directed protein kinase phosphorylates tau on sites that are abnormally phosphorylated in tau associated with Alzheimer's paired helical filaments. J Biol Chem 1993;268:23512–23518

435. Lovestone S, Reynolds CH, Latimer D et al: Alzheimer's disease-like phosphorylation of the microtubule-associated protein tau by glycogen synthase kinase-3 in transfected mammalian cells. Current Biol 1994;4:1077–1085

436. Gong C-X, Singh TJ, Grundke-Iqbal I, Iqbal K: Phosphoprotein phosphatase activities in Alzheimer disease brain. J Neurochem 1993;61:921–927

437. Gong CX, Singh TJ, Grundke-Iqbal I, Iqbal K: Alzheimer disease abnormally phosphorylated tau is dephosphorylated by protein phosphatase-2B (calcineurin). J Neurochem 1994;62: 803–806

438. Harris KA, Oyler GA, Doolittle GM et al: Okadaic acid induces hyperphosphorylated forms of tau protein in human brain slices. Ann Neurol 1993;33:77–87

439. Billingsley ML, Ellis C, Kincaid RL et al: Calcineurin immunoreactivity in Alzheimer's disease. Exp Neurol 1994;126: 178–184

440. Dayan AD, Ball MJ: Histometric observations on the metabolism of tangle-bearing neurons. J Neurol Sci 1973;19: 433–436

441. Mann DMA, Yates PO: The relationship between formation of senile plaques and neurofibrillary tangles and changes in nerve cell metabolism in Alzheimer-type dementia. Mech Ageing Dev 1981;17:395–401

442. Sumpter PQ, Mann DMA, Davies CA et al: An ultrastructural analysis of the effects of accumulation of neurofibrillary tangle in pyramidal cells of the cerebral cortex in Alzheimer's disease. Neuropathol Appl Neurobiol 1986;12:305–319

443. Salehi A, Ravid R, Gonatas NK, Swaab DF: Decreased activity of the hippocampal neurons in Alzheimer's disease is not related to the presence of the neurofibrillary tangles. J Neuropathol Exp Neurol 1995;54:704–709

444. Endoh R, Ogawara M, Iwatsubo T et al: Lack of the carboxyl terminal sequence of tau in ghost tangles of Alzheimer's disease. Brain Res 1993;601:164–172

445. Ikeda K, Haga C, Oyanagi S et al: Ultrastructural and immunohistochemical study of degenerate-neurite bearing ghost tangles. J Neurol 1992;239:191–194

446. Bondareff W, Wischik CM, Novak M et al: Molecular analysis of neurofibrillary degeneration in Alzheimer's disease: an immunohistochemical study. Am J Pathol 1990;137:711–723

447. Su JH, Cummings BJ, Cotman CW: Subpopulations of dystrophic neurites in Alzheimer brain with distinct immunocytochemical and argentophilic characteristics. Brain Res 1994; 637:37–44

448. Mann DMA, Prinja D, Davies CA et al: Immunocytochemical profile of neurofibrillary tangles in Down's syndrome patients of different ages. J Neurol Sci 1989;92:247–260

449. Cras P, Kawai M, Siedlak S et al: Neuronal and microglial involvement in β-amyloid protein deposition in Alzheimer's disease. Am J Pathol 1990;137:241–246

450. Ikeda K, Akiyama H, Haga C, Haga S: Evidence that neurofibrillary tangles undergo glial modification. Acta Neuropathol 1992;85:101–104

451. Smith MA, Taneda S, Richey PL et al: Advanced Maillard reaction end products are associated with Alzheimer disease pathology. Proc Natl Acad Sci (USA) 1994;91:5710–5714

452. Smith MA, Rudnicka-Nawrot M, Richey PL et al: Carbonyl-related posttranslational modification of neurofilament protein in the neurofibrillary pathology of Alzheimer's disease. J Neurochem 1995;64:2660–2666

453. Yan S-D, Chen X, Schmidt A-M et al: Glycated tau protein in Alzheimer disease: a mechanism for induction of oxidant stress. Proc Natl Acad Sci (USA) 1994;91:7787–7791

454. Yan SD, Yan SF, Chen X et al. Non-enzymatically glycated tau in Alzheimer's disease induces neuronal oxidant stress resulting in cytokine gene expression and release of amyloid β-peptide. Nature Med 1995;1:693–699

455. Nakano I, Iwatsubo T, Otsuka N et al: Paired helical filaments in astrocytes: electron microscopy and immunohistochemistry in a case of atypical Alzheimer's disease. Acta Neuropathol 1992;83:228–232

456. Ikeda K, Haga C, Akiyama H, Kase K, Iritani S: Coexistence of paired helical filaments and glial filaments in astrocytic processes within ghost tangles. Neurosci Lett 1992;148: 126–128

457. Probst A, Ulrich J, Heitz PU: Senile dementia of Alzheimer type: astroglial reaction to extracellular neurofibrillary tangles in the hippocampus. Acta Neuropathol 1982;57:75–79

458. Cras P, Smith MA, Richey PL et al: Extracellular neurofibrillary tangles reflect neuronal loss and provide further evidence of extensive protein cross-linking in Alzheimer disease. Acta Neuropathol 1995;89:291–295

459. Lowe J, Blanchard A, Morrell K et al: Ubiquitin is a common factor in intermediate filament inclusion bodies of diverse type in man, including those of Parkinson's disease, Pick's disease, and Alzheimer's disease, as well as Rosenthal fibres in cerebellar astrocytomas, cytoplasmic bodies in muscle, and Mallory bodies in alcoholic liver disease. J Pathol 1988;155:9–15

460. Renkawek K, Basman GJCGM, de Jong WW: Expression of small heat-shock protein hsp27 in reactive gliosis in Alzheimer disease and other types of dementia. Acta Neuropathol 1994; 87:511–519

461. Hamos JE, Oblas B, Pulaski-Salo D et al: Expression of heat shock proteins in Alzheimer's disease. Neurology 1991;41: 345–350

462. Smith MA, Kutty RK, Richey PL et al: Heme oxygenase-1 associated with the neurofibrillary pathology of Alzheimer's disease. Am J Pathol 1994;145:42–47

463. Smith MA, Richey PL, Kutty RK et al: Ultrastructural localization of heme oxygenase-1 to the neurofibrillary pathology of Alzheimer disease. Molec Chem Neuropathol 1995;24: 227–230

464. DeWitt DA, Silver J, Canning DR, Perry G: Chondroitin sulfate proteoglycans are associated with the lesions of Alzheimer's disease. Exp Neurol 1993;121:149–152

465. Buee L, Perez-Tur J, Leveugle B et al: Apolipoprotein E in Guamanian amyotrophic lateral sclerosis/parkinsonism-dementia complex: genotype analysis and relationships to neuropathological changes. Acta Neuropathol 1996;91:247–253

466. Yamaguchi H, Ishiguro K, Sugihara S et al: Presence of apolipoprotein E on extracellular tangles and on meningeal blood vessels precedes the Alzheimer β-amyloid deposition. Acta Neuropathol 1994;88:413–419

467. Perry G, Cras P, Siedlak SL et al: β Protein immunoreactivity is found in the majority of neurofibrillary tangles of Alzheimer's disease. Am J Pathol 1992;140:283–290

468. Tabaton M, Cammarata S, Mancardi G et al: Ultrastructural localization of β-amyloid, tau and ubiquitin epitopes in extracellular neurofibrillary tangles. Proc Natl Acad Sci (USA) 1991;88:2098–2102

469. Hyman BT, Van Hoesen GW, Beyreuther K, Masters CL: A4 amyloid protein immunoreactivity is present in Alzheimer's disease neurofibrillary tangles. Neurosci Lett 1989;101: 352–355

470. Yamaguchi H, Nakazato Y, Shoji M et al: Secondary deposition of beta amyloid within extracellular neurofibrillary tangles in Alzheimer-type dementia. Am J Pathol 1991;138:699–705

471. Allsop D, Haga S-I, Bruton C, Ishii T, Roberts GW: Neurofibrillary tangles in some cases of dementia pugilistica share antigens with amyloid β-protein of Alzheimer's disease. Am J Pathol 1990;136:255–260

472. Ledesma MD, Bonay P, Colaco C, Avila J: Analysis of microtubule-associated protein tau glycation in paired helical filaments. J Biol Chem 1994;269:21614–21619

473. Greenfield JG, Bosanquet FD: The brain stem lesions in Parkinsonism. J Neurol Neurosurg Psych 1953;16:213–226

474. Forno LS: Concentric hyaline intraneuronal inclusions of Lewy type in the brains of elderly persons (50 incidental cases); relationship to Parkinsonism. J Am Geriat Soc 1969;17: 557–575

475. Forno LS, Alvord EC: The pathology of Parkinsonism. pp. 120–161. In Recent Advances in Parkinson's disease. Blackwell Scientific Publications, Oxford, 1971

476. Ohama E, Ikuta F: Parkinson's disease: distribution of Lewy bodies and monoamine neuron system. Acta Neuropathol 1976;34:311

477. Forno LS, Murphy GM, Eng LF: Immunocytochemical study of Lewy bodies in sympathetic ganglia. Neurodegeneration 1992;1:135–144

478. Oyanagi K, Wakabayashi K, Ohama E et al: Lewy bodies in the lower sacral parasympathetic neurons of a patient with Parkinson's disease. Acta Neuropathol Berlin 1990;80: 558–559

479. Wakabayashi K, Takahashi H, Takeda S et al: Parkinson's disease: the presence of Lewy bodies in Auerbach's and Meissner's plexuses. Acta Neuropathol 1988;76:217–221

480. Forno LS, Langston JW: Lewy bodies and aging: relation to Alzheimer's and Parkinson's diseases. Neurodegeneration 1993;2:19–24

481. Gibb WRG: Idiopathic Parkinson's disease and the Lewy body disorders. Neuropathol Appl Neurobiol 1986;12:223–234

482. Perry RH, Irving D, Blessed G et al: Senile dementia of Lewy body type. A clinically and neuropathologically distinct form of Lewy body dementia in the elderly. J Neurol Sci 1990;95: 119–139

483. Hansen L, Salmon D, Galasko D et al: The Lewy body variant of Alzheimer's disease: a clinical and pathological entity. Neurology 1990;40:1–8

484. Dickson DW, Crystal H, Mattiace LA et al: Diffuse Lewy body disease: light and electron microscopic immunocytochemistry of senile plaques. Acta Neuropathol 1989;78:572–584

485. Roy S, Wolman L: Ultrastructural observations in Parkinsonism. J Pathol 1969;99:39–44

486. Duffy PO, Tennyson VM: Phase and electron microscopic observations of Lewy bodies and melanin granules in the substantia nigra and locus ceruleus in Parkinson's disease. J Neuropathol Exp Neurol 1965;24:398–414

487. Dale GE, Probst A, Luthert P et al: Relationships between Lewy bodies and pale bodies in Parkinson's disease. Acta Neuropathol 1992;83:525–529

488. Ince P, Irving D, MacArthur F, Perry RH: Quantitative neuropathological study of Alzheimer-type pathology in the hippocampus: comparison of senile dementia of Alzheimer type, senile dementia of Lewy body type, Parkinson's disease and non-demented elderly control patients. J Neurol Sci 1991;106: 142–152

489. Galloway PG, Grundke-Iqbal I, Iqbal K, Perry G: Lewy bodies contain epitopes both shared and distinct from Alzheimer neurofibrillary tangles. J Neuropathol Exp Neurol 1988;47: 654–663

490. Lennox G, Lowe J, Morrell K et al: Anti-ubiquitin immunocytochemistry is more sensitive than conventional techniques in the detection of diffuse Lewy body disease. J Neurol Neurosurg Psych 1989;52:67–71

491. Lowe J, McDermott H, Landon M et al: Ubiquitin carboxylterminal hydrolase (PGP 9.5) is selectively present in ubiquitinated inclusion bodies characteristic of human neurodegenerative diseases. J Pathol 1990;161:153–160

492. Goldman J, Yen S-H, Chiu F, Peress N: Lewy bodies of Parkinson's disease contain neurofilament antigens. Science 1983; 221:1082–1084

493. Bancher C, Lassmann H, Budka H et al: An antigenic profile of Lewy bodies: immunocytochemical indication for protein phosphorylation and ubiquitination. J Neuropathol Exp Neurol 1989;48:81–93

494. Lowe J, McDermott H, Pike I et al: αB crystallin expression in non-lenticular tissues and selective presence in ubiquitinated inclusion bodies in human disease. J Pathol 1992;166:61–68

495. DeWitt DA, Richey PL, Praprotnik D et al: Chondroitin sulfate proteoglycans are a common component of neuronal inclusions and astrocytic reaction in neurodegenerative diseases. Brain Res 1994;656:205–209

496. Galloway PG, Bergeron C, Perry G: The presence of tau distinguishes Lewy bodies of diffuse Lewy body disease from those of idiopathic Parkinson disease. Neurosci Lett 1989;100:6–10

497. Galloway PG, Perry G: Tropomyosin distinguishes Lewy bodies of Parkinsons's disease from other neurofibrillary pathology. Brain Res 1991;541:347–349

498. Pollanen MS, Bergeron C, Weyer L: Detergent-insoluble cortical Lewy body fibrils share epitopes with neurofilament and tau. J Neurochem 1992;58:1953–1956

499. Galloway PG, Mulvihill P, Perry G: Filaments of Lewy bodies contain insoluble cytoskeletal elements. Am J Pathol 1992; 140:1–14

500. Jellinger K, Paulus W, Grundke-Iqbal I et al: Brain iron and ferritin in Parkinson's and Alzheimer's diseases. J Neural Transm Park Dis Dement Sect 1990;2:327–340

501. Hirsch EC, Brandel JP, Galle P et al: Iron and aluminium increase in the substantia nigra of patients with Parkinson's disease: an x-ray microanalysis. J Neurochem 1991;56: 446–451

502. Gibson PH, Tomlinson BE: Numbers of Hirano bodies in the hippocampus of normal and demented people with Alzheimer's disease. J Neurol Sci 1977;33:199–206

503. Schochet SS, Lampert PW, Lindenberg R: Fine structure of the Pick and Hirano bodies in a case of Pick's disease. Acta Neuropathol 1968;11:330–337

504. Hirano A, Malamud N, Elizan TS, Kurland LT: Amyotrophic lateral sclerosis and parkinsonism-dementia complex on Guam. Arch Neurol 1966;2:225–232

505. Laas R, Hagel C: Hirano bodies and chronic alcoholism. Neuropathol Appl Neurobiol 1994;20:12–21

506. Ogata J, Budzilovitch GN, Cravioto H: A study of rod-like structures (Hirano bodies) in 240 normal and pathological brains. Acta Neuropathol 1972;21:61–67

507. Yamamoto T, Hirano A: Hirano bodies in the perikaryon of the Purkinje cell in a case of Alzheimer's disease. Acta Neuropathol 1985;67:167–169

508. Nagara H, Yajima K, Suzuki K: An ultrastructural study on the cerebellum of the brindle mouse. Acta Neuropathol 1980; 52:41–50

509. Tomanaga M: Hirano bodies in extraocular muscle. Acta Neuropathol 1983;60:309–313

510. Atsumi T, Yamamura Y, Sato T, Ikuta F: Hirano bodies in the axon of peripheral nerves in a case with progressive external ophthalmoplegia with multisystem involvement. Acta Neuropathol 1980;49:95–100

511. Fu Y-S, Ward J, Young HF: Unusual, rod-shaped cytoplasmic inclusions (Hirano bodies) in a cerebellar hemangioblastoma. Acta Neuropathol 1975;31:129–135

512. Ho K-L, Allevato PA: Hirano body in an inflammatory cell of leptomeningeal vessel infected by fungus Paecilomyces. Acta Neuropathol 1986;71:159–162

513. Schochet SSJ, McCormick EF: Ultrastructure of Hirano bodies. Acta Neuropathol 1972;21:50–60

514. Gibson PH: Light and electron microscopic observations on the relationship between Hirano bodies, neuron and glial perikarya in the human hippocampus. Acta Neuropathol 1978;42: 165–171

515. Okamoto K, Hirai S, Hirano A: Hirano bodies in myelinated fibers of hepatic encephalopathy. Acta Neuropathol 1982;58: 308–310

516. Hirano A, Dembitzer HM, Kurland LT, Zimmerman HM: The fine structure of some intraganglionic alterations. Neurofibrillary tangles, granulovacuolar bodies and "rod-like" structures as seen in Guam amyotrophic lateral sclerosis and parkinsonism-dementia complex. J Neuropathol Exp Neurol 1968;27: 169–182

517. Tomonaga M: Ultrastructure of Hirano bodies. Acta Neuropathol 1974;28:365–366

518. O'Brien L, Shelley K, Towfighi J, McPherson A: Crystalline ribosomes are present in brains from senile humans. Proc Natl Acad Sci (USA) 1980;77:2260–2264

519. Mori H, Tomonaga M, Baba N, Kanaya K: The structure analysis of Hirano bodies by digital processing on electron micrographs. Acta Neuropathol 1986;71:32–37

520. Galloway PG, Perry G, Gambetti P: Hirano body filaments contain actin and actin-associated proteins. J Neuropathol Exp Neurol 1987;46:185–199

521. Goldman HE: The association of actin with Hirano bodies. J Neuropathol Exp Neurol 1983;42:146–152

522. Goldman JE, Horoupian DS: An immunocytochemical study of intraneuronal inclusions of the caudate and substantia nigra.

Reaction with anti-actin antiserum. Acta Neuropathol 1982; 58:300–302

523. Galloway PG, Perry G, Kosik KS, Gambetti P: Hirano bodies contain tau protein. Brain Res 1987;403:337–340

524. Peterson C, Kress Y, Vallee R, Goldman JE: High molecular weight microtubule-associated proteins bind to actin lattices (Hirano bodies). Acta Neuropathol 1988;77:168–174

525. Schmidt ML, Lee VM-Y, Trojanowski JQ: Analysis of epitopes shared by Hirano bodies and neurofilament proteins in normal and Alzheimer's disease hippocampus. Lab Invest 1989;60: 513–522

526. Manetto V, Abdul-Karim FW, Perry G et al: Selective presence of ubiquitin in intracellular inclusions. Am J Pathol 1989; 134:505–513

527. Tomlinson BE, Kitchener D: Granulovacuolar degeneration of hippocampal pyramidal cells. J Pathol 1971;106:165–185

528. Ball MJ, Lo P: Granulovacuolar degeneration in the ageing brain and in dementia. J Neuropathol Exp Neurol 1977;36: 474–487

529. Xu M, Shibayama H, Kobayashi H et al: Granuolovacuolar degeneration in the hippocampal cortex of aging and demented patients: a quantitative study. Acta Neuropathol 1992;85:1–9

530. Kahn J, Anderton BH, Probst A et al: Immunohistological study of granulovacuolar degeneration using monoclonal antibodies to neurofilaments. J Neurol Neurosurg Psych 1985;48: 924–926

531. Price DL, Altschuler RJ, Struble RG et al: Sequestration of tubulin in neurons in Alzheimer's disease. Brain Res 1986; 385:305–310

532. Dickson DW, Ksiezak-Reding H, Davies P, Yen S-H: A monoclonal antibody that recognizes a phosphorylated epitope in Alzheimer neurofibrillary tangles, neurofilaments and tau proteins immunostains granulovacuolar degeneration. Acta Neuropathol 1987;73:254–258

533. Dickson DW, Liu W-K, Kress Y et al: Phosphorylated tau immunoreactivity of granulovacuolar bodies (GVB) of Alzheimer's disease: localization of two amino terminal tau epitopes in GVB. Acta Neuropathol 1993;85:463–470

534. Bondareff W, Wischik CM, Novak M, Roth M: Sequestration of tau by granulovacuolar degeneration in Alzheimer's disease. Am J Pathol 1991;139:641–647

535. Okamoto K, Hirai S, Iizuka T et al: Reexamination of granulovacuolar degeneration. Acta Neuropathol 1991;82:340–345

536. Mann DMA: Granulovacuolar degeneration in pyramidal cells of the hippocampus. Acta Neuropathol 1978;42:149–151

537. Barden H: The histochemical relationship of neuromelanin and lipofuscin. J Neuropathol Exp Neurol 1969;28:419–441

538. Hirosawa K: Electron microscopic studies on pigment granules in the substantia nigra and locus caeruleus of the Japanese monkey. Zeitschri Zellforsch 1968;88:187–203

539. Sekhon SS, Maxwell DS: Ultrastructural changes in neurones of spinal anterior horns of ageing mice with particular reference to accumulation of lipofuscin pigment. J Neurocytol 1974;3:59–72

540. Brunk U, Ericsson JLE: Electron microscopical studies on rat brain neurons. Localization of acid phosphatase and mode of formation of lipofuscin bodies. J Ultrastruc Res 1972;38:1–15

541. Mann DMA, Yates PO: Lipoprotein pigments: their relationship to ageing in the human nervous system. I. The lipofuscin content of nerve cells. Brain 1974;97:481–488

542. Mann DMA, Yates PO, Stamp JE: Relationship of lipofuscin pigment to ageing in the human nervous system. J Neurol Sci 1978;35:83–93

543. Brody H: The deposition of aging pigment in the human cerebral cortex. J Gerontol 1960;15:258–261

544. Scholtz CL, Brown A: Lipofuscin and trans-synaptic degeneration. Virchows Arch Anat Histol 1978;381:35–40

545. Samorajski T, Keefe JR, Ordy JM: Intracellular localization of lipofuscin age pigments in the nervous system. J Gerontol 1964;19:262–272

546. Barden H: Relationship of Golgi thiamine pyrophosphatase and lysosomal acid phosphatase to neuromelanin and lipofuscin in cerebral neurones of ageing rhesus monkey. J Neuropathol Exp Neurol 1970;29:225–240

547. Bazelon M, Fenichel GM, Randall J: Studies on neuromelanin. I. A melanin system in the human adult brain stem. Neurology 1969;17:512–519

548. Moses HL, Ganote CE, Beaver DL, Schuffman SS: Light and electron microscope studies of pigment in human and rhesus monkey substantia nigra and locus caeruleus. Anatom Rec 1966;155:167–184

549. Graham DG, Tiffany SM, Bell WR: Auto-oxidation versus covalent binding of quinones as the mechanism of toxicity of dopamine, 6-hydroxydopamine and related compounds towards C1300 neuroblastoma cells in vitro. Molec Pharmacol 1978;14:644–653

550. Jellinger K, Kienzl E, Paulus W et al: Presence of iron in melanized dopamine neurons in Parkinson's disease. J Neurochem 1992;59:1168–1171

551. Foley JM, Baxter D: On the nature of pigment granules in the cells of the locus caeruleus and substantia nigra. J Neuropathol Exp Neurol 1958;17:586–598

552. Mann DMA, Yates PO: Lipoprotein pigments: their relationship to ageing in the human nervous system. II. The melanin content of pigmented nerve cells. Brain 1974;97:489–498

553. Graham DG: On the origin and significance of neuromelanin. Arch Path Lab Med 1979;103:359–362

554. Mann DMA, Yates PO, Barton CM: Variations in melanin content with age in the human substantia nigra. Biochem Exp Biol 1977;13:137–139

555. McGeer PL, McGeer EG: Enzymes associated with the metabolism of catecholamines, acetylcholine and GABA in human controls and patients with Parkinson's disease and Huntington's Chorea. J Neurochem 1976;26:65–76

556. Carlsson A, Winblad B: Influence of age and time interval between death and autopsy on dopamine and 3-methoxytyramine levels in human basal ganglia. J Neural Transm Park Dis Dement Sect 1976;38:271–276

557. Winblad B, Adolfsson R, Gottfries CG et al: p. 253. In: Frigerio A (ed): Recent Advances in Mass Spectrometry in Biochemistry and Medicine. Academic Press, New York, 1978

558. Barden H, Barret R: Localization of catecholamine fluores-

cence to dog hypothalamic neuromelanin bearing neurones. J Histochem Cytochem 1973;21:175–183

559. Spokes EGS: An analysis of factors influencing measurements of dopamine, noradrenaline, glutamic acid decarboxylase and choline acetyl transferase in human post mortem brain tissue. Brain 1979;102:333–346

560. Cross AJ, Crow TJ, Perry EK et al: Reduced dopamine-β-hydroxylase activity in Alzheimer's disease. BMJ 1981;1: 93–94

561. Bouteille M, Kalifat SR, Delarue J: Ultrastructural variations of nuclear bodies in human disease. J Ultrastruc Res 1967; 19:474–486

562. Seite R, Leonetti J, Luciani-Vuillet JL, Vio M: Cyclic AMP and ultrastructural organization of the nerve cell nucleus: stimulation of nuclear microtubules and microfilaments assembly in sympathetic neurons. Brain Res 1977;124:41–51

563. Field EJ, Peat A: Intranuclear inclusions in neurones and glia. A study in the ageing mouse. Gerontologia 1971;17:129–138

564. Toper S, Bannister CM, Lincoln J et al: Nuclear inclusion bodies in Alzheimer's disease. Neuropathol Appl Neurobiol 1980;6:245–253

565. Zurhein GM, Chou SM: Subacute sclerosing panencephalitis. Neurology 1968;18:146–160

566. Oyangi S, Rorke LB, Katz M, Koprowski H: Histopathology and electronmicroscopy of 3 cases of SSPE. Acta Neuropathol 1971;18:58–73

567. Martinez AJ, Oya T, Jabbour JT et al: Subacute sclerosing panencephalitis (SSPE). Reappraisal of nuclear, cytoplasmic and axonal inclusions. Ultrastructure of 8 cases. Acta Neuropathol 1974;28:1–13

568. Grunnet ML: Nuclear bodies in Creutzfeldt-Jakob and Alzheimer's disease. Neurology 1975;25:1091–1093

569. Shiraki H, Yamamoto T: Histochemical aspects of hepatocerebral diseases. Adv Neurol Sci 1960;5:73–80

570. Ishii T, Hamada S: Histological and histochemical studies on the eosinophilic intranuclear inclusions of the pigmented cells of the substantia nigra. Adv Neurol Sci 1960;5:111–116

571. Yuen P, Baxter DW: The morphology of Marinesco bodies (paranucleolar corpuscles) in the melanin pigmented nuclei in the brainstem. J Neurol Neurosurg Psych 1963;26:178–184

572. Leestma JE, Andrews JM: The fine structure of the Marinesco body. Arch Pathol 1969;88:431–437

573. Hirai S, Okamoto K: Marinesco body. Neurol Med (Tokyo) 1986;24:457–462

574. Schochet SSJ, Wyatt RB, McCormick WF: Intracytoplasmic acidophilic granules in the substantia nigra. Arch Neurol 1970;22:550–559

575. Sekiya S, Tanaka M, Hayashi S, Oyanagi S: Light- and electron-microscopic studies of intracytoplasmic acidophilic granules in the human locus coeruleus and substantia nigra. Acta Neuropathol 1982;56:78–80

576. Sasaki S, Hirano A: Study of intracytoplasmic acidophilic granules in the human dorsal root ganglia. Neurol Med (Tokyo) 1983;19:263–268

577. Culebras A, Feldman GR, Merk F: Cytoplasmic inclusion bodies within neurons of the thalamus in myotonic dystrophy. J Neurol Sci 1973;19:319–329

578. Pena CE: Intracytoplasmic neuronal inclusions in the human thalamus. Acta Neuropathol 1980;52:157–159

579. Cisse S, Lacoste-Royal G, Laperriere J et al: Ubiquitin is a component of polypeptides purified from corpora amylacea of aged human brain. Neurochem Res 1991;16:429–433

580. Cisse S, Perry G, Lacoste-Royal G et al: Immunocytochemical identification of ubiquitin and heat-shock proteins in corpora amylacea from normal aged and Alzheimer's disease brains. Acta Neuropathol 1993;85:233–240

581. Austin JH, Sakai M: Corpora amylacea. pp. 29–61. In Minckler J (ed): Pathology of the Nervous System. McGraw-Hill, New York, 1972

582. Sakai M, Austin J, Witmer F, Trueb L: Studies of corpora amylacea. I. Isolation and preliminary characterization by chemical and histochemical techniques. Arch Neurol 1969; 21:526–544

583. Liu HM, Anderson K, Caterson B: Demonstration of a keratan sulfate proteoglycan and a mannose-rich glycoconjugate in corpora amylacea of the brain by immunocytochemical and lectin-binding methods. J Neuroimmunol 1987;14:49–60

584. Steyaert A, Cisse S, Merhi Y et al: Purification and polypeptide composition of corpora amylacea from aged human brain. J Neurosci Methods 1990;31:59–64

585. Stam FC, Roukema PA: Histochemical and biochemical aspects of corpora amylacea. Acta Neuropathol 1973;25:95–102

586. Cisse S, Schipper HM: Experimental induction of corpora amylacea-like inclusions in rat astroglia. Neuropathol Appl Neurobiol 1995;21:423–431

587. Singhrao SK, Neal JW, Newman GR: Corpora amylacea could be an indicator of neurodegeneration. Neuropathol Appl Neurobiol 1993;19:269–276

588. Ramsey HJ: Ultrastructure of corpora amylacea. J Neuropathol Exp Neurol 1965;24:29–39

589. Takahashi K, Agari M, Nakamura H: Intra-axonal corpora amylacea in ventral and lateral horns of the spinal cord. Acta Neuropathol 1975;31:151–158

590. Anzil AP, Herrlinger H, Blinzinger J, Kronski D: Intraneuritic corpora amylacea. Virchows Archives 1974;364:297–301

591. Yagashita S, Itoh Y: Corpora amylacea in the peripheral nerve axon. Acta Neuropathol 1977;37:73–76

592. Singhrao SK, Neal JW, Piddlesden SJ, Newman GR: New immunocytochemical evidence for a neuronal/oligodendroglial origin for corpora amylacea. Neuropathol Appl Neurobiol 1994;20:66–73

593. Martin JE, Mather K, Swash M et al: Heat shock protein expression in corpora amylacea in the central nervous system: clues to their origin. Neuropathol Appl Neurobiol 1991;17: 113–119

594. Prabhakar S, Kurien E, Gupta RS et al: Heat shock protein immunoreactivity in CSF: correlation with oligoclonal banding and demyelinating disease. Neurology 1994;44:1644–1648

595. Singhrao SK, Morgan BP, Neal JW, Newman GR: A functional role for corpora amylacea based on evidence from complement studies. Neurodegeneration 1995;4:335–345

596. Tokutake S, Nagase H, Morisaki S, Oyanagi S: X-ray microprobe analysis of corpora amylacea. Neuropathol Appl Neurobiol 1995;21:269–273
597. Lowenthal A, Bruyn GW: Calcification of the striopallidodentate system. pp. 703–729. In Vinken PJ, Bruyn GW (eds): Handbook of Clinical Neurology. North-Holland, Amsterdam 1968
598. Hurst EW: On the so-called calcification in the basal ganglia of the brain. J Pathol 1926;24:65–84
599. Neumann MA: Iron and calcium dysmetabolism in the brain. J Neuropathol Exp Neurol 1963;22:148–163
600. Strassman G: Iron and calcium deposits in the brain. J Neuropathol Exp Neurol 1949;8:428–435
601. Slager UT, Wagner JA: The incidence, composition, and pathological significance of intracerebral vascular deposits in the basal ganglia. J Neuropathol Exp Neurol 1956;15:417–431
602. Takashima S, Becker LE: Basal ganglia calcification in Down's syndrome. J Neurol Neurosurg Psych 1985;48:61–64
603. Wisniewski KE, French JH, Rosen JF et al: Basal ganglia calcification (BGC) in Down's syndrome (DS): another manifestation of premature aging. Ann NY Acad Sci 1982;396: 179–189
604. Mann DMA: Calcification of the basal ganglia in Down's syndrome and Alzheimer's disease. Acta Neuropathol 1988;76: 595–598
605. Escourolle R, Poirer J: Manual of Basic Neuropathology. WB Saunders, Philadelphia, 1973
606. Beck E, Matthews WB, Stevens DL et al: Creutzfeldt-Jakob disease. The neuropathology of a transmission experiment. Brain 1969;92:699–716
607. Mann DMA, Stamp JE, Yates PO, Bannister CM: The fine structure of the axonal torpedo in Purkinje cells of the human cerebellum. Neurol Res 1980;1:369–378
608. Carpenter S: Proximal axonal enlargement in motor neuron disease. Neurology 1968;18:841–851
609. Gertz HJ, Cervos-Navarro J, Frydl V, Schultz F: Glycogen accumulation of the aging human brain. Mech Ageing Dev 1985;31:25–35
610. Mann DMA, Sumpter PQ, Davies CA, Yates PO: Glycogen accumulations in the cerebral cortex in Alzheimer's disease. Acta Neuropathol 1987;73:181–184

CHAPTER 30

Neurologic Signs in Old Age

M. S. J. PATHY

Time-related changes characterize all multicellular organisms. Viewed from afar, old people are readily distinguished from the young by their stance, gait, or morphologic configuration. Close up, subtle physiognomic changes or more obvious wrinkled or blemished skin, graying hair, and changes in voice quality are common hallmarks of aging.

In the Central nervous system (CNS), accumulation of age-associated cellular changes and molecular and neurochemical deficits may lead to altered function. New synapse formation may compensate to a greater or lesser extent for age-associated neuronal loss.[1] This adaptation is limited. Neurologic reserves, though generous, are finite. Changes due to disease, occult or overt, may be superimposed upon, or masquerade as, senescence. Non-neurologic disease or disability or adverse effects of drugs may coexist with neurologic signs, and the distinction between the features of nonpathologic aging and disease may be at times indefinite.

The essence of neurologic assessment in old age is to distinguish signs, positive or negative, of CNS disease from age-related phenomena or non-neurologic disorders. Clinical presentations in old age are often colored or modified by a complex amalgam of disease and nondisease and psychological, nutritional, and multi-drug therapy effects. An apparently absent neurologic sign in an apprehensive, tense, or bewildered old person is too easily dismissed as an age-related change. Tendon reflexes are particularly difficult to elicit in this setting or when joint pain is prominent. Interpretation of neurologic signs at any age require a detailed history, including past illness or trauma, drug usage, and alcohol intake.

Critchley,[2] in his *Goulstonian Lectures*, played a pivotal role in drawing attention to the influence of age on neurological signs. Since that time the literature has been awash with a bewildering array of conflicting reports on the putative effects of age on clinical signs in the nervous system. Much of this lack of unanimity is due to studies on widely differing populations and to considerable variations in examination methodology.

Motor Signs

Muscle strength appears well preserved until age 50[3] but it progressively declines after this age in the leg muscles[4] and in the arm muscles.[5] Maximum muscle strength diminishes with advancing age[6] and a 30 percent decline in cross-sectional area of muscles may occur between ages 50 and 80 years.[7] Age-related reduction in muscle mass is associated with loss of both Type I and Type II fibers, but particularly type II (fast twitch) fibers.[5,8] In a cross-sectional study of healthy elderly subjects age 65 to 89, Skelton[9] and her colleagues reported a progressive decline of leg extension power and isometric knee extension strength. The men in this study were substantially stronger than the women in muscle strength tests standardized for body weight. (See also Ch. 79.)

Both in the aged experimental animal and in human aging, motor unit numbers decrease, but information on motor unit population for individual muscles has been limited as earlier findings relied on laborious manual counting methods. The introduction of automated techniques has greatly facilated motor unit counting and reduced the subjectivity inherent in the older methods. Advancing old age is associated with the progressive loss of motor units for the small muscles of the hand or foot, but probably not for the biceps brachii.[10]

The denervation–reinnervation cycle is associated with re-innervation of variable numbers of surviving motor units. The maintenance of muscle strength depends to a considerable extent on the degree of successful reinnervation.

The presence of ragged red fibers[11] in aged muscles has no known effect on function, but they are also found in some myopathic conditions.

Paratonia (Gegenhalten)

Gegenhalten is a condition characterized by excessive muscle tone during passive manipulation of the limbs, often suggestive of deliberate resistance, and may be accentuated by rapid passive flexing and extending of the limbs. The resistance may not be apparent if the movements are performed slowly. The rigidity of Gegenhalten is inconstant in contrast to the persistent plastic rigidity in parkinsonism.

Increased muscle tone has been noted in old age,[2,12,13] but community-based studies in clinically healthy subjects have shown no significant increase in tone in the upper limbs.[14,15] Odenheimer and her colleagues,[15] however, found increased tone and rigidity in the lower limbs in old age. Critchley[2] noted the tendency to a flexed posture with age may progress to marked general curvature. In advanced dementia, this postural state may develop through a phase of paratonic rigidity to episodic flexion of the arms and legs and finally, sustained curving of the trunk and permanent flexion of the upper and lower limbs[16]—fortunately, an uncommon findings these days. Although paratonia may occur in normal old age, advanced Alzheimer's disease is the predominant cause of severe paratonia.[17]

Sensory Changes

Subjective sensory complaints are common, particularly formication and paresthesiae and intractable symptoms of tic douloureux and postherpetic neuralgia are more likely to occur in older people.[2] However, aging does not appear to effect heat-induced pain.[18] Thresholds to some kinds of painful stimuli are increased in elderly subjects.[19] Decreased density of receptors subserving cutaneous sensibility may contribute to age-associated sensory changes.[20] Sensitivity to light touch diminishes in older individuals.[21–24] When spatial acuity for the sense of touch is represented by the four dimensions of skin site; area or length of skin surface stimulated; orientation along or across the skin; and awareness of surface discontinuity, the threshold for each of these domains has been shown to increase with age at approximately 1 percent per year between the ages of 20 and 80 years.[25] Pressure perception for one- or two-point discrimination alters with age[26] as does the temporal discrimination of repeated brief cutaneous or lingual stimuli.[27] Using a forced choice adaptive method,[28] Stevens confirmed a progressive age-related decline in two-point discrimination and emphasized the important impact of these changes on activities such as the use of Braille and Optacon. (See also Ch. 35).

Tactile vibratory threshold, particularly for higher frequencies,[29] progressively increases with age probably due to changes in Pacinian corpuscle receptor sensitivity.[30,31] The vibratory threshold for elderly women is lower than that for older men,[20,32] but when body height, which has a positive correlation with vibration threshold, is taken into account, older women have a higher threshold than age-equivalent men.[33] In old age the ability to detect vibration sense decreases more rapidly in the fingers than in the toes, but the differential threshold is maintained with a higher threshold in the toes.

As vibratory and thermal sensitivity tests are used as modes for the quantitative assessment of large and small nerve fiber function, respectively, in diabetic neuropathy it is crucial that the test methods are reproducible.[33] Studies to evaluate the influence of age on thermal perception have given conflicting findings. Substantial evidence points to a decrease in cutaneous temperature perception with age.[18,34–37] However, other investigators[38–40] have not confirmed these age-associated changes. Thermal perception thresholds increase more in older men than in women, but body height appears to influence temperature perception, and when this variable is included no gender difference has been found in some studies.[33] Nevertheless, the influence of height on temperature sensitivity is not a consistent finding.[18] Regional (body) and interindividual variation in cutaneous thermal sensitivities are considerable and may explain some of the conflicting findings. Warm-cold difference threshold increases with age.

Face-Hand Test

This test of perceptual ability to appreciate and localize two simultaneously administered tactile stimuli to widely spaced areas of the body was first described by Bender[41] and has been used as a measure of cognitive status in old age. The examiner, seated in front of the subject, simultaneously touches the side of the face and the dorsum of the contralateral hand of the examinee. An error is a failure (on two attempts) to perceive the two stimuli (extinction) or accurately to localize the site of the stimulus (displacement). Extinction errors are substantially more common in healthy aged persons than in healthy young adults.[42] Displacement errors are more likely to be found in Alzheimer's disease.[42] Simple modification of the face-hand test allows assessment of an order of dominance in perceptual responses over the body and the detection of interaction between visual and tactile stimuli.[43–45]

Color Perception

In subjects over age 60 who are not color blind, Bender[46] found that 48 percent had defects in color perception. Color discrimination deteriorates with age,[47–49] particularly for short wavelength colors.[50] Cataracts cause substantial loss of appreciation of short wavelength colors. Critical flicker fusion frequency—the frequency at which a flashing light source appears as a continuous light—decreases with age at all levels of brightness.[51]

Taste and Smell

The sense of taste and smell decline with age[52] and the taste threshold for many substances is elevated. The decreased gustatory ability spans the four primary tastes of sweet, sour, bitter, and salt. Though the salt taste threshold is elevated in normal elderly subjects, it is higher in smokers than nonsmokers. In addition to smoking habits, alcohol consumption, wearing of dentures and medication, and long-term avoidance or use of salt or sour tasting foods may modify the sense of taste.[53] The demonstration of discrete areas of taste loss in the aging tongue with preservation of whole mouth taste sensitivity[54] suggests that much of the reported change in taste appreciation with advancing age is related to the methodology of taste testing. However, substantial age-related dysfunction has been demonstrated by applying brief stimuli to well-defined localized areas of the tongue.[55] As Doty and Zadra[56] note the large array of reputed tastes is due to olfactory nerve stimulation; the foods include banana, chocolate, strawberry, pizza sauce, vanilla, root beer, cola, licorice, steak sauce, steak, fried chicken, apple, and lemon. As implied, the appreciation of taste is closely related to the sense of smell. Using threshold tests, olfactory function shows a decrease in normal persons after the age of 65 and in an ear, nose, and throat, setting anosmia or hyposmia is found in most patients with olfactory symptoms.[57] Olfactory function is influenced both by age and by disease. Symptomatic smell impairment is usually due to disease and the most common causes include inflammatory changes of the mucosa of the nasal cavity and sinuses,[58] viral or bacterial upper respiratory infections,[59] head trauma,[60] Parkinson's disease,[61] and Alzheimer's disease.[62]

In old age, discrimination of both quality of odor and distinction between different odors is diminished.[63] Peak smell identification performance is between the third and fifth decade with considerable decline after the seventh decade.[64] Nonsmokers retain a more effective sense of smell than smokers, and women outperform men at all ages with gender difference becoming more pronounced in old age.[64] This may be at least in part due to the smaller number of female smokers.

Auditory Perception

A progressive decline in hearing ability from the third decade onward is well documented and this bilateral age-related sensorineural impairment is evident initially for higher sound frequencies, particularly in men. Women are less sensitive than men to low sound frequencies. Impairment of speech understanding is largely due to a decline in peripheral sensorineural ability. However, in a proportion of elderly people there is a discrepancy between the degree of hearing loss due to peripheral presbyacusis and the level of speech understanding.[65–68] Central presbyacusis is ascribed to changes in auditory structures and in the auditory pathways in the brain stem and cortex. It occurs in 23[69] to 35 percent[70] of clinically fit elderly subjects. Low-frequency hearing loss appears to be due to central factors[71] and may explain the age-related gender difference in peripheral/central dysfunction.[72] The impact of central auditory system dysfunction on speech understanding was first reported by Gaeth[73] and it was later shown that sentence recognition as well as word understanding was impaired due to these central changes.[66–74] Cognitive impairment has not been established as the basis of impaired speech understanding associated with central auditory dysfunction.[68–75] (See Ch. 47.)

Tendon Reflexes

Tendon reflexes may be difficult to elicit in old people either because of their apprehension or because of musculoskeletal changes. The ankle jerk has been reported to be the first and most frequent tendon reflex to be lost in old age,[2,21,76,77] but a community survey by Hobson and Pemberton[78] noted knee and ankle jerks to be absent with equal frequency. The achilles tendon reflex time increases with age[79] and more so in elderly women.[80] Several recent well-conducted community studies of clinically healthy and independently living elderly subjects have confirmed an increased prevalence of tendon reflex loss in old age,[14,15,81] but significant differences between the very old (aged 85 and over) and the young old (65 to 74) have not been demonstrated in functionally active old people.[81]

Primitive Reflexes

These reflexes are normally found in early infancy, but disappear as the child matures. Their reappearance in old age has been ascribed to the presence of diffuse irreversible brain disease,[82] but considerable controversy exists as to the association with aging or neuropathologic changes. Even in carefully conducted community studies of ostensibly healthy elderly subjects substantial differences in the prevalence of primitive reflexes are reported: thus Odenheimer et al.[15] found subjects age 84 and over to be significantly more likely to have snout and grasp reflexes (vide infra) compared to the young old whereas Nichols et al.[81] found primitive reflexes to be only exceptionally present in healthy centenarians. Undoubtedly, the inconsistencies between studies are due to multiple factors. Earlier studies were often hospital-based with neurologists, psychiatrists, and general physicians (internists) dealing with different patient populations with different age structures but all labeled "old". Dissimilar groups of primitive reflexes have been reported and as Vreeling and his colleagues[83] have emphasised, techniques for the eliciting of these reflexes vary, with consequent poor inter- and intraobserver consistency. In a series of papers[83–85] Vreeling and colleagues have demonstrated that marked improvement in clinical consistency can be obtained by using standard methodologic protocols. In general, single primitive reflexes can be demonstrated in a proportion of healthy adult subjects and the prevalence of these reflexes increases with advancing age. There is agreement that multiple primitive reflexes are rare in healthy old age and are normally associated with advanced brain disease, especially chronic dementing states. Most reports have recorded an association between the severity of dementia and the prevalence and multiplicity of these reflexes.[85] However, Molloy et al.[86] found no correlation with the degree of cognitive impairment in Alzheimer's disease, but a significant association with the level of functional impairment.

The glabella tap, snout, and palmomental reflexes have been considered nocioceptive as it is believed that facial muscle contraction is a reponse to a perceived noxious stimulus.[17] As grasp and suck reflexes have an obvious grasping character, these have been termed prehensile.[17,87] In a large Canadian study of health and aging,[88] primitive reflexes were commonly found in association with dementia and the presence of prehensile primitive reflexes in demented subjects was associated with significantly more functional and cognitive impairment.

The Palmomental Reflex

Momentary contraction of the mentalis muscle elicited by stroking the thenar eminence of the ipsilateral hand was first demonstrated by Marinesco and Radovici.[89] It has a latent period of 50 ms.[90] Otomo[91] found a positive reflex in 2.3 percent of students aged 15 to 64, 27.1 percent of persons in the fifth decade, and 53.5 percent of subjects aged 60 and over, but the frequency of this reflex in reputedly healthy adults has varied in different reports.[92–95] An increasing prevalence with increasing age has not been universally reported.[96] These conflicting findings may be related to differences in examination technique because sufficiently strong stimuli produced electromyographic evidence of mentalis contraction in all subjects.[97] The palmomental reflex is normally bilateral when present in healthy old age. The presence of a unilateral response is suggestive of focal neurologic impairment.[42,98] The palmomental reflex is commonly present in Parkinson's disease.[84,94,96,99,100] It has been suggested that this association may be an age-related phenomenon.[101] However, although the palmomental reflex increases in frequency with age, it does not reach the prevalence found in Parkinson's disease.[84]

Snout (Pouting) Reflex

Pouting or sucking movements of the lips on gently pressing the middle phalanx of the flexed index finger against the lips is a positive sign. The reflex may also be elicited by pressure over the philtrum of the upper lip or tapping the same area with the forefinger or patella hammer. The presence of a snout reflex correlates with advanced age.[13,15,17,92] A correlation between the snout reflex and impairment of cognition on psychomotor testing[102] is in keeping with evidence of diffuse brain damage reported in earlier observations.[82] The reflex is present twice as often in Alzheimer's disease as in age-matched clinically healthy controls[103] and is a common finding in Parkinson's disease.[84,99,104]

Nuchocephalic Reflex

Rapid turning of the shoulders to the right or left with the eyes closed is followed by turning of the head in the same direction. In infants and children up to 4 years of age the head remains central on rapidly rotating the shoulders. The reflex is present in normal old age,[13] but it may be elicited more frequently in Parkinson's disease[105] and dementia.[106]

Glabellar Tap Reflex

First described by Myerson,[107] this sign is a blink response to lightly tapping the glabellar prominence. The blink reflex following the tap has two components: an initial shorter and a subsequent longer latency component.[108] Reflex closure of the eyelids is dependent on the harmonious relaxation of the levator palpebrae and contraction of the orbicularis oculi assisted by the elastic properties of the eyelid.[109] By comparing normal subjects with patients with facial neuropathy, Snow and Frith[110] were able to separate the two main muscle components. They showed that early lid movement following the glabellar tap was initiated by the levator palpebrae relaxation and full closure resulted from the elastic action of the eyelid. Blinking in response to the first few taps is common in normal subjects, but in Parkinson's syndrome the blink continues with repeated taps[107,111,112] and has been considered the most reliable sign for monitoring the severity of Parkinson's disease.[99] However, the reflex is often present in nonbasal ganglia brain disease.[96] A positive blink reflex has been found in 60 percent of patients over age 60 in the absence of clinical parkinsonism,[113] but the correlation with age[114] has not been invariably found.[96] However, a positive glabellar tap reflex occurs more often in Parkinson's disease than normal adults[96] and in this disorder repeated taps result in positive eye blinks despite habituation of the second longer latency component of the reflex. Antiparkinsonian medication may abolish the reflex,[115–117] but there are contrary findings.[118]

The glabellar tap is one of the more prominent release signs[119,120] with an early occurrence. It is found more frequently in vascular dementia than in Alzheimer's disease.[85] As already noted Franssen et al.[17] considered the glabellar tap with the snout and palmomental reflexes as nocioceptive. They found that although they were present in the intact CNS they have a greater prevalence in cognitively impaired individuals.

Corneomandibular Reflex

This reflex was first described by von Solder[121] in 1902. Short and long latency components of the reflex have been described.[122] There are several methods for testing the reflex. The most commonly used technique is to touch the lateral margin of the cornea with a wad of cotton wool while holding the upper lid to prevent corneal reflex blinking. A positive response is a brief contralateral deviation of the jaw due to the action of the lateral pterygoid muscle of the stimulated side. Grossman and Jacobs[101] maintain that touching the cornea with the surgically gloved forefinger elicits the reflex most consistently. This reflex is present in 50 percent of newborn infants[123] and in approximately 6 percent of young adults[122] and older persons.[92] A substantially higher prevalence has been reported in the very old[93] and may be partly due to methodologic factors that may have a considerable impact on response rate[92] or population sampling. It is generally agreed that the corneomandibular reflex is uncommon in health[124] and a combination of corneomandibular, snout, and palmomental reflex is present only with CNS disease.[95]

Grasp Reflex

The reflex is a flexion of the fingers with adduction of the thumb in response to stroking across the palm of the hand or placing two fingers across the palm of the hand with the patient's attention distracted. If the patient grasps the examiner's fingers he or she is asked to desist and the test is repeated. If a flexion response is again elicited the test is positive. A closely related phenomenon of forced groping may be demonstrated when the eyes are closed and the palmar surface of the fingers lightly touched. The fingers close on the object and the hand and an arm move towards the stimulus. This reflex response is almost invariably found in the newborn, but may reemerge in senescence. However, the grasp reflex is uncommon in healthy old age and its presence correlates with cognitive scores[102] and it is clear that the reflex is increasingly likely to occur with progressive dementia.[104,120,125] No correlation between a positive reflex and CT evidence of brain atrophy has been demonstrated.[126]

However, cortical atrophy on CT scanning is common in healthy old age. The frequency of the grasp reflex in Alzheimer's disease may correlate more closely with the severity of daily living functional impairment than with cognitive function.[86]

A unilateral grasp reflex may be present in frontal lobe cerebrovascular lesions and tumors. However, this finding may be on the same side or contralateral side of a large frontal lobe lesion.[127] Analogous with the palmar grasp reflex is flexion and adduction of the toes, often associated with inversion and incurving of the foot, when the sole is stimulated—foot grasp reflex. As direct pressure on the sole of the foot may evoke the reflex, gait may be affected. The prevalence of this reflex closely parallels the palmar grasp reflex. It is similarly uncommon in healthy old age and more common in advanced stages of dementia.[17]

Suck Reflex

This reflex is elicited by gently placing the index finger between the lips or stroking the lips and a positive response is closure of the lips around the fingers associated with sucking movements of the lips, tongue, and jaw. The reflex is invariably present in infancy and is of survival import at this phase of life. This reflex occurs only infrequently with normal aging[85] and is usually inconsistent. It occurs more often in dementia[103]—though even with this disorder it remains an uncommon finding—and correlates with the severity of cognitive impairment.[128] In some patients the head may move toward the stimulus as in infancy.

Root Reflex

This is closely allied to the suck reflex and is elicited by lightly stroking the corner of the mouth with the tip of the finger. A positive response is movement of the corner of the mouth toward the examiner's finger. The root reflex is rarely present with normal aging and is largely a late phenomenon of advanced dementia.[17,129]

Head Retraction Reflex

This reflex was first described in essence by Nemlicher and colleagues[130] and the term "head retraction reflex" was coined by Wartenberg.[131] Though several methods of eliciting the reflex have been used, Wartenberg himself considered the best method is to encourage the patient to relax the neck muscles with the head slightly bent forward and to apply a tap to the upper lip and a brief head retraction jerk is a positive response. This reflex occurs in approximately 5 percent of healthy elderly individuals, but it is much more frequently found in Parkinson's disease and the strength of the neck extension is more marked in this disorder than in fit elderly subjects.[132] Anti-Parkinsonian medication does not influence the reflex response.[132] The reflex occurs no more frequently in the presence of dementia than in normal elderly control subjects.[132]

Eyelids

Ptosis of the upper eyelid (blepharoptosis) is a common feature of old age and is largely due to changes in the levator palpebrae aponeurosis. In a community study[133] 11.5 percent of subjects aged 50 and over had evidence of ptosis of the eyelids and the frequency of this finding increases substantially after the age of 80. Upper eyelid position decreases by 0.4 mm per decade over the age range 20 to 80 years.[134] Of central importance is the distinction of age-related ptosis from that due to neurologic disease. In the study by Sridharan et al.[133] ptosis was bilateral in 57 percent and unilateral in 39 percent of subjects. In this study ptosis was considered acquired in 92 percent and congenital in 8 percent of subjects and primary aponeurotic disinsertion was the principle causal factor. Previous ophthalmic surgery and occular inflammation and trauma[133,135] are important causes of secondary aponeurotic disinsertion. Blepharoptosis may be accentuated in downgaze[136–138] and the degree of downgaze blepharoptosis increases with age.[134] This may be of clinical importance if it gives rise to symptomatic visual field restriction during downgaze activities such as reading. Minor levator aponeurotic resection resolves the field restriction.[137] In acquired unilateral ptosis the interpalpebral fissure remains narrower on downgaze on the ptotic side, but in congenital unilateral ptosis the fissure is wider on the ptotic side during downgaze.[139]

Pupils

The aging pupil is characteristically small and minor differences in the size of the two pupils is not uncommon. Pupil size diminishes progressively from the second decade.[140] A pupil diameter of 1 mm or less becomes increasingly common with advancing age and is most frequently seen with age-related bilateral ptosis.[133] In the aging eye, the speed of pupillary constriction is slower, latency is prolonged,[141] and the reaction to light is diminished.[142] Visual acuity declines substantially between the ages of 60 and 80.[142] Central acuity is tested by standard Snellen chart. The use of spatial contrast sensitivity gratings provides a more balanced estimate of functional visual performance.[143] The age-related impairment of high-spatial frequencies of contrast sensitivity is probably due to a combination of optic and neural causes.[144,145]

Dark Adaptation

The ability to adapt from bright to dark surroundings is progressively diminished with age and is most likely due to a combination of optical and retinal changes. Photopigmentation regeneration slows with age[146] and this supports the likelihood of a retinal contribution to age-associated reduction in dark adaptation.

Visual Fields

Despite the methodologic weaknesses of many earlier reports, more stringent studies using automated perimetry have confirmed an age-related contraction of visual fields[147] due to neural changes,[148] but optical factors may also play a role.

The range of eye movements, particularly, elevation[149] and the velocity of saccadic movements diminish with age.[150] The age-related decline in accommodation becomes all too obvious when the printed word has to be held ever further from the eyes to keep it in focus.

Tremor

Physiologic tremor is present in the limbs of all ages and though difficult to see with the naked eye can be readily identified by simple linear accelerometers. Accurate characterization of tremors can be determined by the application of spectral analyses. Physiologic tremor is polyrhythmic with frequencies in the range of 8 to 12 Hz, which appears to be inherent in the mechanical properties of a jointed bone system[151] subjected to the irregular subtetanic recruitment of motor units leading to unfused contraction of muscle fibers and to the ballistic forces (recoil and impact) of left ventricular activities.[152] Population studies have not substantiated the reputed age-related increased prevalence of physiologic action tremor.[153] The distinction between tremulousness and tremor is ill-defined and often semantic.

Enhanced physiologic tremor is visible, may be symptomatic, and has the frequency of physiologic tremor. Enhanced physiologic tremor is characteristically seen with fear, anxiety, or other causes of increased β-adrenergic stimulation. Old people are particularly sensitive to increased β-2 adrenoreceptor stimulation from bronchodilator drugs and may exhibit marked tremor. Excess thyroid hormone production or administration, hypoglycemia, drug/alcohol withdrawal states, and excessive intake or sensitivity to caffeine may be responsible for this overt form of physiologic tremor. Physiologic tremor or enhanced physiologic tremor represents a spectrum in which there is no evidence of segmental stretch reflex at one extreme and EMG evidence of repetitive stretch reflexes at the other end.[152] The additive nature of tremors is commonly observed when enhanced physiologic tremor due to anxiousness exaggerates essential tremor or Parkinsonian tremor.

Essential Tremor

The term "senile tremor" is misleading in that it refers to essential tremor recognized for the first time in old age—careful enquiry will often establish the involuntary shaking as an exaggeration of a mild tremor extant for many years. Essential tremor occurs at a frequency of 8 to 12 Hz. Aging may reduce tremor frequency and increase the amplitude of the oscillations.[155] The possible mechanisms of these age-related changes have been authoritatively reviewed by Elble.[156] It has been postulated that an 8 to 12 Hz component of physiologic action tremor is a forme fruste of essential tremor[157] or this may be regarded as a subtype of essential tremor.[158]

Essential tremor is the most common form of tremor and may occur at any age, with a positive family history in about half of the patients. It is a postural tremor which is absent at rest and is not substantially enhanced by exercise. It may be associated with tremor of the head (titubation) in 50 percent of patients.[159] The tremor has often surprisingly little impact on function, but when pronounced it may make activities such as writing, doing up buttons and zips, and drinking difficult or impossible. Three percent of those afflicted may be severely disabled.[160] Alcohol often decreases the tremor,[160,161] but β-adrenergic anatgonists, particularly propanolol, are the most effective agents.[162]

Orthostatic Tremor

This benign form of tremor occurring in the lower limbs and trunk was first described by Heilman[163] and termed orthostatic tremor, but more recently Walker[164] referred to it as isometric tremor. It is possibly a variant of essential tremor.[165] It occurs in late middle to old age and typically has a frequency of 14 to 16 Hz. Characteristically, the tremor occurs in the legs and trunk on standing following a brief latent period, but to a lesser extent it may occurs in the arms of 60 percent of sufferers.[164] The cause is unknown with no defined pathology and a benign course. The tremor responds to valproate and primidone.

Posture

Normal postural control requires maintenance of the body's center of gravity over the support base, both during stance and active movement, to secure effective balance in the face of potential external or voluntary destabilization forces. This control, predominantly integrated through the CNS, depends on complex systems with central processing, motor, sensory, vestibular, and biomechanical components. In healthy old age effective posture is retained and much of the reputed age-related change is due to concomitant neurologic or musculoskeletal disorders.[166]

Normal erect posture becomes less common in late old age.[167] A tendency to stand with slightly flexed hips and knees is common in the very elderly and is probably largely due to altered neuromuscular control, diminished muscle power, and degenerative joints disease. Vestibular function plays little role in static posture or in righting reactions,[168] but when the individual is sitting or standing on an unstable base, balance may be seriously compromised if vestibular function is impaired.[169]

Posture is dependent on proprioceptive feedback where vision cannot be used as in blindness or darkness. Ability to cope in the dark progressively deteriorates with age and closely parallels the incidence of falls. In both blindness and darkness women are considerably more affected than men. Defective stance control increases the risk of falls[170] and age-associated changes in the central and peripheral nervous system may contribute to declining balance in aging individuals.[171] Movement of the standing surface during stance induces stretch reflexes, which can be readily measured by surface electromyography over the anterior tibial and soleus muscles. The latency of these stretch-induced reflexes increases with age[172] and may increase the risk of falls when, for example, attempting to compensate for a stumble.

Postural Sway

Sway is a normal phenomenon and is determined by oscillations of two distinct frequencies. Fast oscillations are consequent on information from the ankle joints[173] and feet. Slow oscillations appear to depend, at least in part, on vestibular influences. Looking at the feet influences normal postural sway probably due to reduced peripheral visual information.[173] Postural sway is substantially greater in elderly female[174] and male[175] volunteers than in young adults. Sheldon[175] showed that control of stance as judged by static sway was poor in early childhood but reaches an optimum in early adulthood and progressively deteriorates from the 50s onward. Among the subjects of all ages studied by Sheldon, one-third of those over the age of 60 were unable to minimize the amplitude of static sway by visual endeavor. This subgroup consisted predominantly of women, and all had sustained one or more falls. Increased sway is most evident in old people with a history of falls, loss of balance, and giddiness.[176,177] Proprioceptive impairment, particularly of vibration sense, may be associated with increased sway.[178–180]

Early studies of sway were concerned with recording the overall area of sway around the vertical in relation to global balance ability and were not able to distinguish relevant age-related components. It is now appreciated that the integration of visual, vestibular, musculoskeletal, and somatosensory systems is central to postural control and to understanding the effect of age on sway.[181–184] Sensory organization testing permits the standing surface to be static and stable or unstable to evaluate proprioceptive input; eyes open or closed or unexpected movements of visual reference point to assess visual contribution. Sway shows no age-related increase when tested on a stable surface with intact visual input,[182,183,185,186] but it increases in both young and elderly subjects when they are deprived of proprioceptive or visual information. The effect of isolated proprioceptive impairment on age-associated sway remains debatable. Increased sway has been found in elderly subjects when proprioception and/or visual feedback is restricted, albeit the effects are greater when the combined modes of information are curtailed.[186] However, in clinically healthy subjects, increased sway following reduction of proprioceptive information when the eyes are open has been reported to occur only in the very elderly (over age 85).[184] Sway compensation is mainly through the ankle joint (so-called ankle strategy), but older people tend to use muscle responses at the hip joint (hip strategy)[187] possibly due to lack of ability to produce adequate ankle torque.

Many earlier studies on age-related changes in sway did not specifically exclude overt disease. Sway has been shown to be substantially greater in elderly in-patients and day-patients than in healthy old people at home.[180]

Gait

In the course of normal gait cycle there is a stance phase (60 percent of the cycle) in which part of the foot is in contact with the ground and a swing phase (40 percent of the cycle) in which no part of the foot is in contact with the ground. During the initiation of limb or trunk perturbations posture is modulated to maintain the centre of gravity within the support base.[188,189] In old age walking speed diminishes by 15 to 20 percent[190–192] largely due to shorter stride length. Step width (distance between the feet) and double support time (gait phase in which at least part of each foot is in contact with the ground) increases in individuals over 80 years of age by 20 percent when compared to young adults.[190]

Gait in old age is influenced by a multiplicity of factors—musculoskeletal, neurologic, metabolic, and drugs, including alcohol. Cross-sectional data suggests that about one third of people from age 75 have gait impairment.[193]

Conclusion

There is no clear concensus as to what we mean by healthy old age. Commonly, it is regarded as the absence of symptoms and clinical signs of disease, but these features may be dismissed by the patient and physician as the product of old age.[194] Clinicians have more ready access to patients than to elderly healthy subjects and many studies of age-related neurologic changes have failed to exclude the effects of disorders on either the CNS or musculoskeletal system. A recent large community study by Waite et al.[195] demonstrated that with the exception of impaired vibration sense and upward gaze and bradykinesia, all neurologic signs are associated with neurodegenerative disorders and stroke, and is a salutory reminder to us to be critically circumspect in ascribing neurologic changes to age per se.

References

1. Cotman CW: Synaptic plasticity neurotropic factors and transplantation in the aged brain. pp. 255–274 In Schneider EL, Rowe JW (eds): Handbook of Biology of Ageing. Academic Press, San Diego, 1990
2. Critchley M: Neurology of old age. Lancet 1931;i:1119–1127; 1331–1336
3. Rodgers MA and Evans WJ: Changes in skeletal muscle with aging: effects of exercise training. Exerc Sports Sci 1993; RPV.21:65–102
4. Danneskiold-Samsoe BV, Kofod V, Munter J et al: Muscle strength and functional capacity in 78–81 year old men and women. Eur J Appl Physiol 1984;52:310–314

5. Grimby G, Saltin B: The ageing muscle. Clin Physiol 1983; 3:209–218
6. Young A: Muscle function in old age. In Peripheral nerve change in the elderly. New Issues in Neurosciences 1988;1: 141–156
7. Booth FW, Weeden SH, Tseng BS: Effect of ageing on human skeletal muscle and motor function. Med Sci Sports Exerc 1994;26:556–560
8. Lexell JC, Taylor C, Sjostrom M: What is the cause of the ageing atrophy? Total number, size, and proportion of different fiber types studied in whole vastus lateralis muscle from 15 to 83 year old men. J Neurol Sci 1988;84:275–294
9. Skelton DA, Greig CA, Davies JM, Young A: Strength, power and related functional ability of health people aged 65–89 years. Age Ageing 1994;23:371–337
10. McCosmas AJ, Galea V, de Bruin H: Motor unit populations in healthy and diseased muscles. Physical Ther 1993;73: 868–878
11. Tomonaga M: Histo-chemical and ultra-structural changes in senile human skeletal muscle. JAGS 1977;25:125–131
12. Prakash C, Stern G: Neurological signs in the elderly. Age Ageing. 1973;2:24–27
13. Jenkyn LR, Reeves AG, Warren T et al: Neurological signs in senescence. Arch Neurol 1985;42:1154–1157
14. Kaye JA, Oken BS, Howieson DB et al: Neurological evaluation in the optimally healthy oldest old. Arch Neurol 1994; 51:1205–1211
15. Odenheimer G, Funkenstein HH, Beckett L et al: Comparison of neurologic changes in successfully aging persons vs the total aging population. Arch Neurol 1994;51:573–580
16. Yakolev PI: Paraplegia in flexion of cerebral origin. J Neuropathol Exp Neurol 1954;13:267–196
17. Franssen EH, Reisberg B, Kluger A et al: Cognition-independent neurologic symptoms in normal aging and probable Alzheimer's disease. Arch Neurol 1991;48:148–154
18. Meh D, Denislic: Quantitative assessment of thermal and pain sensitivity. J Neurol Sci 1994;127:164–169
19. Procacci P, Bozza G, Buzzelli G, Della Corte M: The cutaneous pricking pain sensation in old age. Gerontol Clin 1970;12: 213–218
20. Gescheider GA, Bolanowski SJ, Hall KL et al: The effects of ageing on information-processing channels in the sense of touch: I. Absolute sensitivity. Somatosens Mot Res 1994;11: 345–357
21. Howell T: Senile deterioration of the central nervous system: Clinical study. Br Med J 1949;i:56–58
22. Axelrod S, Cohen LD: Senescence and embedded-figure performance in vision and touch. Percept Psychophysiol 1961; 12:283–288
23. Dyck PJ, Schultz PW, O'Brien PC: Quantitation of touch-pressure sensation. Arch Neurol 1972;26:465–473
24. Thornbury JM, Mistretta: Tactile sensitivity as a function of age. J Gerontol 1981;86:34–39
25. Stevens JC, Patterson MQ: Dimensions of spatial acuity in the touch sense: changes over the life span. Somatosens Mot Res 1995;12:29–47
26. Dellon ES, Mourey R, Dellon AL: Human pressure perception values for constant and moving one and two point discrimination. Plast Reconstr Surg 1992;90:112–117
27. Petrosino L, Fucci D: Temporal resolution of the ageing tactile memory systems. Percept Motor Skills 1989;68:288–290
28. Stevens JC: Aging and spatial acuity of touch. J Geront (Psych Sci) 1992;47:35–40
29. Goff GD, Rosner BS, Detre T, Kennard D: Vibration perception in normal man and medical patients. J Neurol Neurosurg Psych 1965;28:503–509
30. Verrillo RT: Age related changes in sensitivity to vibration. J Gerontol 1980;35:185–193
31. Frisina RD, Gescheider GA: Comparison of child and adult vibrotactile thresholds as a function of frequency and duration. Percept Psychophys, 1977;22:100–103
32. Steiness I: Vibratory thresholds in normal adults. A biothesiometer study. Acta Med Scand 1957;158:315–325
33. Nico J, de Neeling D, Beks PJ et al: Sensory thresholds in older adults: reproducibility and references values. Muscle Nerve 1994;17:454–461
34. Bertelsmann FW, Heimans JJ, Weber EJM et al: Thermal discrimination thresholds in normal subjects and in patients with diabetic neuropathy. J Neurol Neurosurg-Psych 1985;48: 686–690
35. Bravenboer B, van Dam PS, Hop J et al: Thermal threshold testing for the assessment of small fibre dysfunction: normal values and reproducibility. Diabetic Med 1992;9:546–549
36. Claus D, Hilz MJ, Neundörfer B: Thermal discrimination thresholds: a comparison of different methods. Acta. Neurol. Scand. 1990;81:533–540
37. Doeland HJ, Nauta JJP, van Zandbergen JB et al: The relationship of cold and warmth cutaneous sensation to age and gender. Muscle Nerve 1989;12:217–715
38. Arezzo JC, Schaumburg HH, Lavdadio C: Thermal sensitivity tester. Device for quantitative assessment of thermal sense in diabetic neuropathy. Diabetes 1986;35:590–592
39. Armstrong FM, Bradbury JE, Ellis SH et al: A study of peripheral diabetic neuropathy. The application of age-related reference values. Diabetic Med 1991;8:594–599
40. Merchut MP, Toleikis C: Aging and quantitative sensory thresholds. Electromyogr Clin Neurophysiol 1990;30: 293–297
41. Bender MB, Fink M, Green M: Patterns in perception on simultaneous tests of face and hand. Arch Neurol Psych (Chicago). 1951;66:355–362
42. Basavaraju NG, Silverstone FA, Libow LS, Paraskevas R: Primitive reflexes and perceptual sensory tests in the elderly: their usefulness in dementia. J Chron Dis 1981;34:367–377
43. Bender MB: Perceptual interaction. In William D (ed) Modern Trends in Neurology, Butterworth, London, 1970
44. Bender MB, Feldman M: The so called "visual agnosia". Brain 1972;95:173–186
45. Green M, Fink M: Simultaneous tactile perception in patients with conversion sensory deficits. M Sinai J Med 1974;41: 141–143

46. Bender M: The incidence and type of perceptual deficiencies in the aged. pp. 18–33. In Fields WS (ed): Neurological and Sensory Disorders in the Elderly. Medical Book Corporation, Stratton International, New York, 1975

47. Verriest G: Further studies on acquired deficiency of color discrimination. J Op Soc Am 1963;53:185–195

48. Cooper BA, Ward M, Gowlands C, Mclntosh JM: The use of the Lanthony New Color Test in determining the effects of aging on color vision. J Gerontol 1991;46:320–324

49. Roy MS, Podgor MJ, Collier B, Gunkel RD: Vision and age in normal North American population. Graefes Arch Clin Exp Ophthalmol 1991;229:139–144

50. Pitts DG: The effects of aging on selected visual function: dark adaptation, visual acuity, stereopsis and brightness contrast. pp. 131–159. In Seculer R, Kline D, Dismukes K (eds): Aging and Human Visual Function. Alan R Liss, New York, 1982

51. Kline DW, Schieber FJ: Visual persistence and temporal resolution. pp. 231–244. In Secular R, Kline D, Dismukes K (eds): Aging and Human Visual Function. Alan R Liss, New York, 1982

52. Grzegeorczyk PB, Jones SW, Mistretta CM: Age related differences in salt-taste acuity. J Gerontol 1979;34:834–840

53. Chauhan J: Relationship between sour and salt taste perception and selected subject attributes. J Am Diet Assoc 1989; 89:652–658

54. Bartoshuk LM: Taste. Robust across the age span? Ann NY Acad Sci 1989;561:65–75

55. Matsuda T, Doty RL: Regional taste sensitivity to NaCl: relationship to subject age, tongue locus and areas of stimulation. Chem Senses 1995;20:283–290

56. Doty RL, Zrada Smell and taste in the elderly. In Pathy MSJ (ed): Principles and Practice of Geriatric Medicine, 3 ed. John Wiley & Sons, Chichester, (in press)

57. Cairn WS: Testing olfaction in a clinical setting. Ear, Nose Throat J 1989;68:322–328

58. Duncan HJ, Smith DV: Clinical disorders of olfaction. pp. 345–365. In Doty RL (ed.) Handbook of Olfaction and Gustation. Macel Dekker New York, 1995

59. Deems DA, Doty RL, Settle RG et al: Smell and taste disorders: a study of 750 patients from the University of Pennsylvania Smell and Taste Center. Arch Otolaryngol Head Neck Surg 1991;117:519–528

60. Costanzo RM, Zasler ND: Head trauma. pp. 711–730. In Getchell TV, Doty RL, Bartoshok LM, Snow JB Jr. (eds): The Chemical Senses in Health and Disease. Raven, New York, 1991

61. Doty RL, Deems DA, Stellar S: Olfactory dysfunction in Parkinson's disease: a general deficit unrelated to neurologic signs, disease state or disease duration. Neurology. 1988;38: 1237–1244

62. Doty RL: Olfactory dysfunction in neurodegenerative disorders. pp. 735–751. In Getchell TV, Doty RL, Bartoshuk LM, Snow JB, Jr. (eds): The Chemical Senses in Health and Disease. Raven, New York, 1991

63. Stevens JC, Cairn WS, Schiet FT, Oatley MW: Olfactory adaptation and recovery in old age. Perception 1989;18:265–276

64. Doty RL, Shamon P, Applebaum SL et al: Smell identification ability: changes with age. Science 1984;226:1441–1443

65. Jerger J: Audiological findings in aging. Adv Otolaryngol 1973;20:115–124

66. Jerger J, Hayes D: Diagnostic speech audiometry. Arch Otolaryngol 1977;103:216–222

67. Dubno JR, Dirks DD, Morgan DE: Effects of age and mild hearing loss on speech recognition in noise. Acoust Soc Am 1984;76:87–97

68. Jerger J, Jerger S, Oliver T, Pirrozolo F: Speech understanding in the elderly. Ear Hear 1989a;10:79–89

69. Cooper JC, Gates GA: Hearing in the elderly. The Framingham Cohort: 1983–1985. Part III. Prevalence of central auditory processing disorders. Ear Hear 1991;12:304–311

70. Stach BA, Spretnjak ML, Jerger JF: The prevalence of central presbyacusis in a clinical population. J Am Acad Audiol 1990; 1:109–145

71. Hansen CG, Reske-Nielsen E: Pathological studies in presbyacusis. Arch Otolaryngol 1965;82:115–132

72. Jerger J: Can age-related decline in speech understanding be explained by peripheral hearing loss? J Am Acad Audiol 1992; 3:33–38

73. Gaeth J: A study of phonemic regression in relation to hearing loss. Unpublished disseration, Northwestern University. Cited by Wallace E, Hayes D, and Jerger J. 1994. Neurology of ageing: the auditory system. pp. 448–464. In Martin LA, Knoeffel JE (eds) Clinical Neurology of Ageing. 2nd Ed. Oxford University Press, New York, 1948

74. Shirinian M, Arnst D: Patterns in performance-intensity functions for phonetically balanced word lists and synthetic sentences in aged listeners. Arch Otolaryngol 1982;108:15–20

75. Jerger J, Stach B, Pruitt J et al: Comments on speech understanding and aging. J Acoust Soc Am 1989b;85:1352–1354

76. Bryndum B, Marquarsden J: The tendon reflexes in old age. Gerontol Clin 1964;6:257–265

77. Klawans HL, Tufo HM, Ostifield AN et al: Neurologic examinations in an elderly population. Dis Nerv Syst 1971;32: 274–279

78. Hobson W, Pemberton J: The health of the elderly at home. Br Med J 1958;I:587–593

79. Bhattia SP, Irvine RE: Electrical recording of the ankle jerk in old age. Gerontol Clin 1973;15:357–360

80. Carel RS, Korczyn AD, Hochberg Y: Age and sex dependency of Achilles tendon reflex. Am J Med Sci 1979;278:57–63

81. Nichols ME, Meadors KJ, Loring DW et al: Age related changes in the neurologic examination of healthy sexagenarians, octogenarians and centenarians. J Geriat Psych Neurol 1994;7:1–7

82. Paulson G, Gottlieb G: The appearance of foetal and neonatal reflexes in aged patients. Brain 1968;91:37–52

83. Vreeling FW, Jolles J, Verhey FRJ, Houx PJ: Primitive reflexes in healthy adult volunteers and neurological patients: methodological issues. J Neurol 1993;240:495–504

84. Vreeling FW, Verhey FRJ, Houx PJ, Jolles J: Primitive reflexes

in Parkinson's disease. J Neurol Neurosurg Psych 1993;56: 1232–1326

85. Vreeling FW, Houx PJ, Jolles J, Verhey FRJ: Primitive reflexes in Alzheimer's disease and vascular dementla. J Geriatr Psych Neurol 1995;8:111–117
86. Molloy DW, Clarnette RM, Mcllroy WE et al: Clinical significance of primitive reflexes in Alzheimer's Disease. J Am Geriatr Soc 39:1160–1163
87. Franssen EH: Neurologic signs in ageing and dementia. pp. 144–174. In Burns A (ed) Ageing and Dementia: A Methodological Approach. Edward Arnold, London, 1993;144–174
88. Hogan DB, Ebly EM: Primitive reflexes and dementia: results from the Canadian Study of Health and Aging. Age Ageing. 1995;24:275–381
89. Marinesco G, Radovici A: Sur un réflexe cutane nouveau: réflexe palmomentonnier. Rev Neurol 1920;27:237–240
90. Moldaver A: Etude de la courbe de sommation central du réflexe palmomentonnier de l'homme. CR Soc Biol 1932;109: 1143–1148
91. Otomo E: The palmomental reflex in the aged. Geriatrics 1965; 20:901–905
92. Jacobs L, Grossman MD: Three primitive reflexes in normal adults. Neurology 1980;30:184–188
93. Orefice G, Modafferi N, Selvaggio M et al: Archaic reflexes in normal elderly people. Acta Neurol 1991;13:19–24
94. Maertens de Noordhout A, Delwaide PJ: The palmomental reflex in Parkinson's disease. Neurology, 1988;4:425–427
95. Isakov E, Sazbon L, Costeff H et al: The diagnostic value of three common primitive reflexes. Eur Neurol 1984;23:17–21
96. Jensen JPA, Gron U, Parkenberg H: Comaprison of three primitive reflexes in neurological patients and in normal individuals. J Neurol Neurosurg Psych 1983;46:162–167
97. Reis DJ: The palmomental reflex. A fragment of a general nocioceptive reflex: a physiological study in normal man. Arch Neurol 1961;4:486–498
98. Marx P, Reschop J: The clinical value of the palmomental reflex. Neurosurg Rev 1980;3:173–177
99. Klawens HL, Paulson GW: Primitive reflexes in Parkinsonism. Confinia Neurol 1971;33:32–52
100. Jimenez-Roldan S, Esterban A, Abad YJ. Reflejo palmomentoniano en infermedad de Parkinson. Archr Neurbiol (Madrid) 1976;39:233–248
101. Grossman MD, Jacobs L: Three primitive reflexes in Parkinsonian patients. Neurology 1980;30:189–192
102. Tweedy J, Reding M, Garcia C et al: Significance of cortical disinhibition signs. Neurology 1982;32:169–173
103. Galasko D, Kwo-on-Yuen PF, Klauber M, Thal L: Neurological findings in Alzheimer's disease and normal aging. Arch Neurol 1990;47:625–627
104. Girling DM, Berrios GE: Extra-pyramidal signs, primitive reflexes and frontal lobe function in senile dementia of the Alzheimer type. Br J Psych 1990;157:888–893
105. Pearce J, Aziz H, Gallagher JC: Primitive reflex activity in primary and symptomatic Parkinsonism. J Neurol Neurosurg Psych 1968;31:501–508
106. Jenkyn LR, Walsh D, Culver C, Reeves AG: The nuchocephalic reflex in diffuse cerebral disease. Neurology (Minneapolis) 1974;24:358–363
107. Myerson A: Tap and blink responses in Parkinson's disease. Arch Neurol Psych (Chicago) 1944;51:480–484
108. Kimura J, Belisa J, Hallett M: An AAEE workshop. pp. 1–11. American Association of Electromyography and Electrodiagnosis, Rochester, 1984
109. Evinger C, Shaw M, Peck CK et al: Blinking and associated eye movement in humans, guinea-pigs and rabbits. Neurophysiol 1984;52:323–339
110. Snow BJ, Frith RW: The relationship of eye movement to the blink reflex. J Neurol Sci 1989;91:179–189
111. Garland HG: Parkinsonism. Br Med J 1952;2:153–155.
112. Schwab RS, England AC: Parkinson's disease. J Chron Dis 1958;8:488–509
113. Wright WB, Boyd RV: The glabellar tap sign in the elderly patient. Gerontol Clin 1964;6:124–128
114. Koller WC, Glatt S, Wilson R, Fox JH: Primitive reflexes and cognitive function in the elderly. Ann Neurol 1982;12: 302–304
115. Mesina C, Di Rosa AE, Tomasello F: Habituation of blink reflexes in Parkinsonian patients under levodopa and amantadine treatment. J Neurol Sci 1972;17:141–148
116. Sandrini G, Alfonsi E, Martignoui E et al: Effects of lisuride on blink reflex habituation in Parkinson's disease. Eur Neurol 1985;24:374–379
117. Penders CA, Delwaide PJ: Blink reflex studies in patients with Parkinsonism before and during therapy. J Neurol Neurosurg Psych 1971;34:674–678
118. Bronisch FW: Dierflexe. Thieme Verlag, Stuttgart, 1979
119. Huff FJ, Growdond JH: Neurological abnormalities associated with severity of dementia in Alzheimer's disease. Can J Neurol Sci 1986;13:403–405
120. Huff FJ, Boller F, Luchelli F et al: The neurological examination in patients with probable Alzheimer's disease. Arch Neurol 1987;44:929–932
121. von Solder F: Der corneomandibular reflex. Neurol Centralbl 1902;31:111–113
122. Ansink BJJ: Physiologic and clinical investigations into 4 brainstem reflexes. Neurology 1962;12:320–328
123. Paulson GW, Bird NT: The corneo-mandibular reflex. Confinia Neurol 1971;33:116–119
124. Gordon RM, Bender MB: The corneomandibular reflex. J Neurol Neurosurg Psych 1971;34:236–242
125. Förstl H, Burns A, Levy R et al: Neurologic signs in Alzheimer's disease: results of a prospective clinical and neuropathologic study. Arch Neurol 1992;49:1038–1042
126. Moylan JJ, Saldias CH: Developmental reflexes and cortical atrophy. Ann Neurol 1979;5:499–500
127. De Jong RN: The Neurological Examination. Hoeber, New York, 1967
128. Bakchine S, Lacomblez L, Palisson E et al: Relationship between primitive reflexes, extrapyramidal signs, reflective

apraxia and severity of cognitive impairment in dementia of the Alzheimer type. Acta Neurol Scand 1989;79:38–46

129. Delwaide PJ, Dijeux L: Réflexes néonataux et dykinésies bucco-linguo-faciales dans la démence sénile. Actualité Gérontol 1980;6:126–133.

130. Nemlicher L, Schetzer M, Schmelkin D: Über ein neues symptom bei doppelseitgen affectionen des hirnstammes. Dtsch Z Nervenheilkd 1931;120:184–190

131. Wartenberg R. Head retraction reflex. Am J Med Sci 1941; 201:553–561

132. Sandyk R, Fleming J, Brennan MJW: The head retraction reflex: its specificity in Parkinson's disease. Clin Neurol Neurosurg 1982;84:159–162

133. Sridharan GV, Tallis RC, Leatherbarrow B, Forman WM. A community survey of ptosis of the eyelid and pupil size of elderly people. Age Ageing. 1995;24:21–24

134. Stoller SH, Meyer DR: Quantitating the change in upper eyelid position during downgaze. Ophthalmology 1994;101: 1604–1607

135. Millay DJ, Larrabee WF: Ptosis and blepharoplasty surgery. Arch Otolaryngol Head Neck Surg, 1989;115:198–201

136. Patipa M: Visual field loss in primary gaze and reading gaze due to acquired blepharoptosis and visual field improvements following ptosis surgery. Arch Opthalmol 1992;110:63–67

137. Wojno TH: Downgaze ptosis. Ophthal Plast Reconstr Surg 1993;9:83–89

138. Dryden RM, Kahanic DA: Worsening of blepharoptosis in downgaze. Ophthalmol Plast Reconstr Surg 1992;8:126–129

139. Waller RR, McCord CD. Jr, Tanebaum M: Evaluation and management of the ptosis patient. pp. 331–333. In McCord CD, Tanebaum M (eds) 2nd Ed. Raven Press, New York, 1987

140. Loewenfeld IE: Pupillary changes related to age. pp. 124–150. In HS Thompson (ed) Topics in Neuro-ophthalmology. Williams & Wilkins, Baltimore, 1979

141. Bourne PR, Smith SA, Smith SE: Dynamics of the light reflex and the influence of age on the human pupil measured by television pupillometry. J Physiol (London) 1979;293:1–10

142. Pitts DG: Effects of aging on selected visual functions: dark adaptation, visual acuity stereopsis and brightness contrast. pp. 131–159. In Sekuler R, Kline D, Dismukes K (eds) Aging and Human Visual Function. Alan R Liss, New York, 1982

143. Ippolit CA, Katz M, Katz B: Neuro-ophthalmology of aging. pp. 421–447. In Albert ML, Knoefel JE (eds) Clinical Neurology of Aging. 2nd Ed. Oxford University Press, New York, 1994

144. Celesia GC, Kaufman D, Core S: Effects of age and sex on pattern electroretinograms and visual evoked potentials. Electroencephalgr Clin Neurophysiol 1987;68:161–171

145. Adachi-Usami E: Senescence of visual function as studied by visual evoked cortical potentials. Jpn Ophthalmol 1990;38: 81–94

146. Coile DC, Baker HD: Foveal dark adaptation, photopigment regeneration and aging. Vis Neurosci 1991;9:27–39

147. Jaffe GJ, Alvarado JA, Juster RP: Age-related changes of the normal visual field. Arch Ophthalmol 1986;104:1021–1025

148. Frisen L High-pass resolution perimetry and age-related loss of visual pathway neurons. Acta Ophthalmol (Copenhagen) 1991;69:511–515

149. Chamberlain W. Restriction in upward gaze with advancing age. Trans Am Ophthalmol Soc 1970;68:235–244

150. Pitts MC, Rawles JM: The effect of age on saccadic latency and velocity. Neuro-ophthalmology. 1988;8:123–129

151. Freund HJ, Dietz V. The relationship between physiological and pathological tremor, Vol 5. pp. 66–89. In Desmedt JE (ed) Progress in Clinical Neurophysiology. Karger, Basel, 1978

152. Elble RJ, Koller WC: Tremor. John Hopkins University Press, Baltimore, 1990

153. Mortimer JA: Human motor behaviour and aging. Ann NY Acad Sci 1988;515:54–66

154. Young RR, Hagbarth KE: Physiological tremor enhanced by manoevres affecting the segmental stretch reflex. J Neurol Neurosurg Psych 1980;43:248–256

155. Elble RJ, Higgins C, Leffler K, Hughes L: Factors influencing the amplitude and frequency of essential tremor. Mov Disord 1994;9:589–596

156. Elble RJ: The role of aging in the clinical expression of essential tremor. Exp. Gerontol 1995;30:337–347

157. Elble RJ: Physiologic and essential tremor. Neurology 1986; 36:225–231

158. Marsden CD: Origins of normal and pathological tremor. pp. 37–84. In Findley LJ, Capildeo R (eds) Movement Disorders: Tremor. Macmillan, London, 1984

159. Marsden CD: The mechanism of physiological tremor and their significance for pathological tremor. Vol 3, pp. 1–77. In Desmedt JE (ed) Physiological tremor, Pathological Tremor and Clonus. Karger, Basel, 1978

160. Koller W, Biary N, Cone S: Disability in essential tremor: effects of treatment. Neurology 1986;36:1001–1004

161. Lou JS, Javonic J: Essential tremor: clinical correlates in 350 patients. Neurology 1991;41:234–238

162. Koller W, Vetere-Overfield: Acute and chronic effects of propanolol and primidone in essential tremor. Neurology. 1988; 35:1587–1588

163. Heilman KM: Orthostatic tremor. Arch Neurol 1984;41: 880–881

164. Walker FD, McCormick GM, Hunt VP: Isometric features of orthostatic tremor: an electromyographic analysis. Muscle Nerve 1990;13:918–922

165. Fitzgerald PM, Janovik J: Orthostatic tremor: an association with essential tremor. Mov Disord 1991;6:60–64

166. Gabell A, Nyak VSC: The effect of age on variability in gait. J Gerontol 1984;39:662–666

167. Horenstein S: Managing gait disorders. Geriatrics 1974;29: 86–94

168. Martin JP: Myotatic kinesthetic and vestibular mechanisms. p. 92. In de Reuck AVA and Kim J (eds): Ciba Foundation Symposium, Churchill, London, 1967

169. Martin JP: Tilting reactions and disorders of the basal ganglion. Brain 1965;874–885

170. Horak FB, Shupert CL, Mirka A: Components of postural dyscontrol in the elderly: a review. Neruobiol Aging 1988;10: 727–738
171. Stelmach GE, Philips J, Di Fabio RP, Teasdale N: Age, functional postural reflexes, and voluntary sway. J Gerontol 1989; 44:B100–106
172. Nardone A, Siliotto R, Grasso M, Schiepatti M. Influence of ageing on leg muscle reflex responses to stance perturbation. Arch Phys Med Rehab 1995;76:158–165
173. Begbie GH. Myotatic, kinesthetic and vestibular mechanisms. pp. 80–92. In de Reuck AVS and Knight J (eds.) Ciba Foundation Symposium. JA Churchill, London, 1967
174. Hasselkus BR, Shambes GM: Aging and postural sway in women. J Gerontol 1975;30:661–667
175. Sheldon JH: The effect of age on the control of sway. Gerontol Clin 1963;5:129–138
176. Overstall PW, Exton-Smith AN, Imms FJ, Johnson AL: Falls in the elderly related to postural imbalance. Br Med J 1977; 1:261–264
177. Lichtenstein MJ, Shields SL, Shiavi RG, Burger MC: Clinical determinants of biomechanics of platform measures of balance in aged women. JAGS 1988;36:996–1002
178. Era P, Keikkinen E: Postural sway during standing: an unexpected disturbance of balance in random samples of men of different ages. J Gerontol 1985;4:287–295
179. Brocklehurst JC, Robertson D, James-Groom P: Clinical correlates of sway in old age: sensory modalities. Age Ageing 1982; 11:1–10
180. Duncan G, Wilson JA, MacLennan WJ, Lewis S: Clinical correlates of sway in old people living at home. Gerontology 1992; 38:160–166
181. Black FO, Nashner LM: Postural control in four classes of vestibular abnormalities. pp. 271–281. In Ingarashi M, Black FO (eds) Vestibular and Visual Control on Posture and Locomotor Equilibrium. Karger, Basel, 1985
182. Woolacott MH, Shumway-Cook A, Nashner LM: Age and posture control changes in sensory organisation and muscular coordination. Int J Aging Human Dev 1986;23:97–114
183. Peterka RJ, Black FO: Age-related changes in human posture control: sensory organisation tests. J Vest Res 1990;1:73–85
184. Panzer V, Kaye J, Edner A, Holme L: Standing postural control in the elderly and very elderly pp. 220–231. In Woolacott M, Horak F (eds) Posture and gait: control Mechanisms. University of Oregon Books, Eugene, 1992
185. Ledin T, Kronhed AC, Moller M et al: Effects of balance training in elderly evaluated by dynamic posturography. J Vest Res 1990;1:129–138
186. Whipple R, Wolfson L, Derby C et al: Altered sensory function and balance in older persons. J Gerontol 1993;48:71–76
187. Manchester D, Woolacott M, Zederbauer-Hylton N Marin O: Vestibular and somatosensory contributions to balance control in the older adult. J Gerontol 1989;44:M118–127
188. Cordo PJ, Nashner LM. Properties of postural adjustment associated with rapid arm movement. J Neurophysiol 1982;47: 287–302
189. Basalgette D, Zattara M, Bathien M et al: Postural adjustments associated with rapid voluntary arm movements in patients with Parkinson's disease. pp. 371–374. In Yarr MD, Bergman KJ (eds) Advances in Neurology. Vol. 45. Raven Press, New York, 1986
190. Murray MP, Kory RC, Klarkson BH: Walking patterns in healthy old men. J Gerontol 1969;24:169–174
191. Imms FJ, Edholm OG: Studies of gait and mobility in the elderly. Age Ageing. 1981;10:147–156
192. Elble RJ, Thomas SS, Higgins C, Colliver J: Stride dependent changes in gait in older people. J Neurol 1991;238:1–5
193. Akhtar AJ, Broe GA, Crombie A et al: Disability and dependence in the elderly at home. Age and Ageing. 1973;2: 102–110
194. Path MSJ, Bayer A, Harding K, Dibble A: Randomised trial of case finding and surveillance of elderly people at home. Lancet 1992;340:890–893
195. Waite LM, Broe GA, Creasey H et al: Neurological signs, aging and the neurodegenerative syndromes. Arch Neurol 1996;53: 498–503

CHAPTER 31

Epilepsy

RAYMOND TALLIS

There has been increasing interest in epilepsy in older adults over the last decade. Until quite recently, only a tiny proportion of the huge epilepsy literature was specifically devoted to elderly patients. The growing awareness among epileptologists in geriatric patients is reflected in designated sessions at international meetings and in the publication of at least two textbooks[1,2] on epilepsy of old age in the the last couple of years.

The paucity of literature on seizures in old age might be due to several misconceptions: that epilepsy is rare in old age; that it matters less in an elderly person than in a younger one; and that it is the same as epilepsy in younger adults, so that whatever is learned about the latter can be applied directly to the former. The importance of seizures in old age should not need to be spelled out. Even though epilepsy no longer carries the stigma it once did, the psychological impact of an epileptic fit may be profound. Elderly patients, in particular, may have childhood memories that go back to a time when epilepsy was poorly controlled, was often associated with serious brain damage, and was stigmatized.

In many respects, the problem of epilepsy is comparable to that of recurrent falls: although the condition is episodic, the anxiety it causes may be constant. An elderly person may worry, and not without reason, that future fits may lead to injury—to road traffic accidents, fractures, burns, etc. The prolonged postictal states seen in old age[3] may add further hazards. Moreover, discontinuity of consciousness undermines self-confidence at the deepest level; to an elderly person, a fit may seem a harbinger of death. For these reasons, as will be discussed, reassurance—based upon information and education—is a crucial aspect of management.

Definition

Seizures are defined pathophysiologically as being due to paroxysmal discharges of cerebral activity, in which a critical mass of neurones fires synchronously.

"Epilepsy" should not be used to refer to a *single* seizure, but to a continuing *tendency* to epileptic seizures. In epidemiologic studies, the term is usually used when a patient has suffered from more than one nonfebrile seizure of any type. It follows that a diagnosis of epilepsy cannot strictly be made on the basis of a single seizure, especially if the seizure has an external provocation. The distinction, however, is not as sharp as is sometimes implied; in old age at least, the majority of individuals who present with a single seizure will go on to have further seizures.[4–6]

Epidemiology

Many doctors have the impression that seizures are comparatively rare in elderly people and that elderly-onset epilepsy is uncommon. Twenty-five percent of general practitioners[7] in one postal survey thought they had never seen epilepsy presenting for the first time in old age.

The belief that elderly-onset seizures are uncommon has no foundation in the recent literature. Twenty years ago, Hauser and Kurland[8] reported a rise in the prevalence of epilepsy above the age of 50 and an even steeper rise in incidence—from 12 per 100,000 in the 40 to 59 age range to 82 per 100,000 in those over 60.

This rise has been confirmed in their more recent studies[9–10] and Luhdorf[11] reported a similar incidence of 77 per 100,000. This has also been confirmed by studies based in primary care. The United Kingdom National General Practice Survey of Epilepsy and Epileptic Seizures,[4] a prospective-based, community-based study found that 24 percent of new cases of definite epilepsy were in subjects over the age of 60. A study of a primary care database covering 82 practices and nearly 370,000 subjects, 62,000 of whom were over the age of 60, revealed a continuing rise in the incidence of seizures in old age[12]: whereas the incidence for the overall population was 69 per 100,000, the incidence in the 65 to 69 age group was 87, in the 70s 147 per 100,000, and in the 80s 159 per 100,000. Over one-third of all incident cases placed on antiepileptic drugs (AEDs) were individuals over the age of 60. Analysis of an expanded primary care database of over 3,000,000 subjects has generated very similar findings (Tallis et al. in preparation). Finally, a recent literature review[13] incorporating additional data from detailed studies in Switzerland has further underlined the dramatic increase in the incidence of seizures in old age. Jallon and colleagues[13] found that, in a population with an overall incidence of initial seizures of 73 per 100,000, the rate increased from 65 for patients in their 50s to just under 200 for those in their 80s.

The high incidence is observed for both definite epilepsy and single seizures. Loiseau[14] found an annual incidence for all seizures (single and recurrent) of 127 in subjects over age 60 and that those over age 60 accounted for 28 percent of cases of confirmed epilepsy (two or more unprovoked seizures)

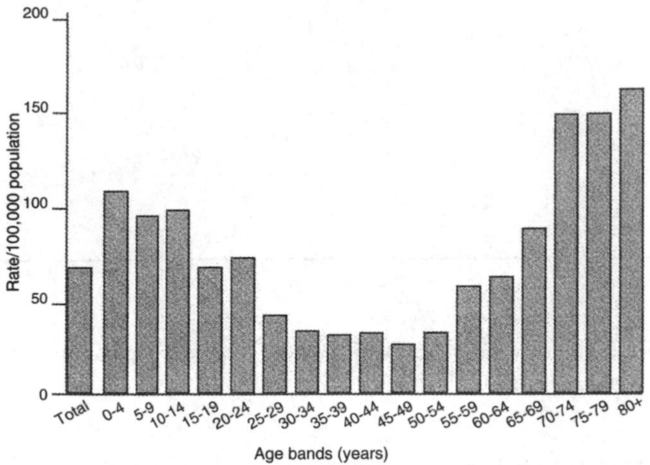

Figure 31-1 The age-related incidence of seizures (From Tallis et al.,[14] with permission.)

and 52 percent of acute symptomatic seizures. The Rochester Minnesota survey[10] also found that both single unprovoked seizures and definite epilepsy increased sharply with age.

The dramatic rise of the incidence of seizures with age is shown in Figure 31-1. In view of the predicted rise in the elderly population we may anticipate a parallel rise in the number of cases of elderly-onset seizures.

Prevalence studies in epilepsy are less straightforward than studies of incidence because of the difficulty of arriving at an agreed definition of definite, active epilepsy. Nevertheless, the recent literature, in contrast with earlier reports, shows a striking upsurge in prevalence of epilepsy in the older population compared with younger people. This is particularly true of the older elderly population, namely the over 75s. For example, in the Rochester study, Hauser[15] found a prevalence of 14.8 per 1,000 in subjects over 75, compared with an overall population average of 6.8 per 1,000. In the Rotterdam study[16] there was a rise in prevalence from 7 per 1,000 in those aged 55 to 64 to 12 per 1,000 in people aged between 85 and 94, with an overall prevalence in elderly people of 9. Hauser[15] noted a dramatic increase in the prevalence in elderly people between the years 1940 and 1980—1.9 to 14.8 per 1,000 in the over 75s.

This secular trend will have been in part due to improved case ascertainment, but this is clearly not the whole story. Because cerebrovascular disease is the main cause of seizures in old age (see below) and there has been a decline in overt stroke during this period, the trend may seem paradoxical. However, it is possible that the increase in the prevalence of seizures may reflect an increase in the burden of "minor" or occult cerebrovascular disease that is sufficiently advanced to predispose to seizures, but not expressed as overt stroke or, where it is expressed in stroke, carries a lower mortality.

Whatever the explanation, these data show that epilepsy is the third most common serious neurologic disease of old age, following dementia and stroke. Why should its incidence and prevalence be so underestimated? Minor seizures may not be reported; they may not be recognized for what they are, getting lost in the pathologically rather busy situation of the biologically aged person; or, even if recognized, not referred to the hospital and included in hospital-based or hospital-biased series. In the NGPSE,[4] 20 percent of elderly patients with seizures were not referred to a hospital, compared with only 4 percent of younger patients. This is despite the fact that elderly people contributed a disproportionate number of additional cases of "possible" or "probable" epilepsy, confirming the increased diagnostic uncertainty in the aged.

Types of Seizures

The manifestations of epilepsy are complex and varied and the methods of classifying seizures correspondingly complex. The revised 1981 International League against Epilepsy classification[17] correlates clinical seizure types with ictal and interictal electroencephalographic features. Table 31-1 gives those parts of the classification relevant to elderly patients.

Primary generalized seizures are those in which the first clinical events suggest involvement of both hemispheres from the outset. This is confirmed by electroencephalogram (EEG) discharges during a fit that are bilateral from the outset. Such seizures may be convulsive or nonconvulsive. In the former case, motor manifestations are bilateral from the outset. In nonconvulsive seizures, there is impairment or interruption of consciousness without motor manifestations. Impairment of consciousness also may be the first event in a convulsive seizure. In partial seizures, the *first* changes suggest activation of neurones limited to part of one cerebral hemisphere. A partial seizure is classified as "simple" if consciousness is *not* impaired and as "complex" if it *is* impaired. Impairment of consciousness in a partial seizure usually implies bilateral spread of seizure activity. The clinical correlate of such generalized electrical activity may also include tonic-clonic features supervening on initially focal symptoms.

It may be useful to map the current, more precise terminology onto the older terminology with which some readers may be more familiar. (For obvious reasons, the mapping cannot be exact and the older, more imprecise terminology should no longer be used.) Primary generalized convulsive seizures roughly correspond to the classical "grand mal" attack without a preceding aura. A grand mal attack preceded by an aura or other focal features corresponds to "partial seizures evolving to secondary generalised seizures". "Minor" or "focal" epilepsy covers simple and complex partial seizures. Most of the latter were previously classified as "temporal lobe epilepsy" as, among the focal seizures, it is those originating in the temporal lobes that are most likely to be associated with disturbances of consciousness. Some temporal lobe attacks may take the form of simple partial seizures with autonomic or psychic symptoms.

The *classification* of seizures in old age in epidemiologic studies is rarely satisfactory. Large, population-based studies do not have full electrophysiologic evaluation—this is a seri-

Table 31-1 Partial seizures: focal onset

Simple: consciousness unimpaired throughout
- With motor symptoms:
  - Focal motor with or without march
  - Versive
  - Postural
  - Vocalization
- With somatosensory or special-sensory symptoms:
  - Somatosensory
  - Visual
  - Auditory
  - Olfactory
  - Gustatory
  - Vertiginous
- With autonomic symptoms or signs:
  - Epigastric sensations
  - Pallor
  - Sweating
  - Flushing
  - Piloerection
  - Pupillary dilation
- With disturbances of higher cerebral function:
  - Dysphasic
  - Dysmnestic
  - Cognitive
  - Affective
- Illusions (e.g., macropsia)
- Structured hallucinations (e.g., music, scenes)

Partial seizures: focal onset
- Complex: Consciousness Impaired at Some Point[a]
  - Beginning as simple partial seizures and progressing to complex seizures
  - Consciousness impaired from the outset:
    - Impairment of consciousness only
    - Impairment of consciousness with automatism
- Partial Seizures becoming secondarily generalized (with convulsive manifestations)

Generalized Seizures: Onset is Generalized
- Myoclonic seizures
- Clonic seizures
- Tonic seizures
- Tonic-clonic seizures
- Atonic seizures

[a] *Brief absences occurring in older people are most often due to complex partial seizures (they used to be called ``temporal lobe absences" rather than ``petit mal".) Primary generalised absences in older people are rare.*

(Modified from Commission on Classification and Terminology of the International League Against Epilepsy,[17] with permission.)

ous omission because seizures that appear clinically to be primarily generalized may actually be focal in origin (and symptomatic) though generalization occurs too rapidly to be noted by an observer. Studies in which investigation has been adequate enough to ensure accurate classification are often derived from atypical populations attending neuromedical centers. The literature on the respective frequencies of different types of seizures has been usefully reviewed in Jallon and Loiseau.[13]

Current evidence suggests that at least 75 percent of elderly-onset seizures are focal or focal in origin.[4,11,13] The actual figure may be higher as it seems unlikely that primary generalized seizures occur spontaneously for the first time in old age. An individual with an idiopathic-lowered seizure threshold would have expressed this earlier in life. This said, a recent study has suggested that idiopathic generalized epilepsy may, after all, occur for the first time in late middle or old age—the author[18] even suggested a second peak in the incidence of these epilepsies (which typically present in childhood and adolescence) in older subjects.[18] Interictal EEGs showed generalized spike-wave or polyspike abnormalities at about 3 Hz with no consistent asymmetrical discharges. Neuroimaging ruled out focal lesions. Jallon et al.[13] also discuss elderly-onset idiopathic primary generalized epilepsies.

Simple partial seizures have been reported as being more frequent than complex seizures.[13] This, however, may be because brief loss or impairment of consciousness may not be observed or reported. Moreover, Hauser[15] found that complex partial seizures accounted for nearly 50 percent of seizures in old age, while simple partial seizures accounted for only 13 percent. Among generalized seizures, over 90 percent are tonic-clonic, myoclonic seizures being exceptionally rare (about 2 percent of cases). Epileptologists have increasingly drawn attention to absence status in elderly patients (see below). Finally, and not surprisingly, there is a high proportion of unclassifiable seizures in older people—in roughly 10 percent of cases.[4] The proportion of *misclassified*—as opposed to *unclassified*—seizures is probably even higher. Much remains to be done in this area.

Etiology

An epileptic fit may be regarded as the result of an interaction between an individual predisposition, which is constitutional or hereditary, and a provoking cause that may be either an epileptogenic lesion in the brain or a systemic disturbance lowering the convulsive threshold. In elderly patients presenting with fits for the first time, it may be reasonably assumed that the contribution of the provoking cause usually outweighs that of the individual predisposition, because the latter would have already expressed itself earlier in life.

Cerebrovascular Disease

It is becoming increasingly clear that cerebrovascular disease is the main cause of epilepsy in older adults, accounting for between 30 and 50 percent of cases in different series.[4,11,14,19,20] It accounts for an even higher proportion—up to 75 percent[4]—of cases in which a cause is found.

Cerebrovascular disease and seizures may be linked in different ways: (1) in association with overt stroke, early (peristroke, onset) seizures and late (post-stroke) seizures; and (2) in association with otherwise occult stroke disease, as evidenced by concurrent CT scan finding and/or subsequent development of stroke. There have been recent important studies investigating the relationship between overt stroke and early and late seizures. Kilpatrick et al.[21] found that about 4 percent of patients had early seizures. Seizures occurred within 5 years of an ischemic stroke in about 10 percent of cases in the Oxford Community Stroke Project (Sandercock, personal communication). The Oxford study found a much higher incidence of poststroke seizures in hemorrhagic stroke and this was also observed by Lancman.[22]

The recently published population-based study of over 500 patients with ischemic stroke by So et al.[23] must be regarded as definitive. They divided seizures into early (within 1 week of the stroke) and late (after 1 week). Six percent of subjects developed early seizures, 78 percent of these within 24 hours. Late seizures developed in 5.5 percent of subjects. The cumulative probabilities of developing an initial late seizure were 3 percent at 1 year, nearly 5 percent at 2 years, and 7.5 percent at 5 years. Early seizure occurrence was a strong predictive factor for initial late seizures. Overall, ischemic stroke increased the chances of an individual developing epilepsy 17-fold.

The relationship between otherwise occult cerebrovascular disease and seizures is more problematic. It is true that the more carefully cerebrovascular disease is sought in epileptic patients, the more frequently it is found. One series[24] compared the computed tomography (CT) scan appearances of patients with elderly-onset epilepsy and no evidence of cerebral tumor with those of age- and sex-matched controls. There was an excess of ischemic lesions in epileptic patients. In half of the epileptic patients who were found to have CT evidence of vascular disease, clinical examination was normal. This observation, however, may have to be treated with caution: the presence of areas of ischemia on a CT scan may not mean that they are the primary or even a contributory cause of the seizures. Studies have also shown an excess of previous seizures in patients admitted to the hospital with acute stroke compared with controls, suggesting that in a proportion of elderly patients seizures may be the earliest manifestation of cerebrovascular disease.[25] The practical significance of this is that any elderly patient with unexplained seizures should be fully screened for cardiovascular risk factors and treatment with low-dose aspirin or other preventative measures should be instituted where appropriate.

The strong relationship between age and the incidence and prevalence of cerebrovascular disease—as reflected in the almost exponential relationship between age and first-ever stroke—underlines the growing importance of this cause of elderly-onset seizures, particularly as the elderly population is itself aging.

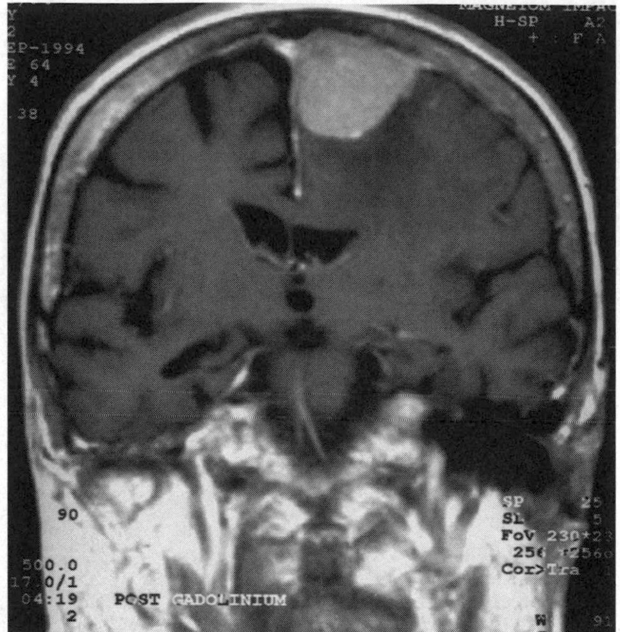

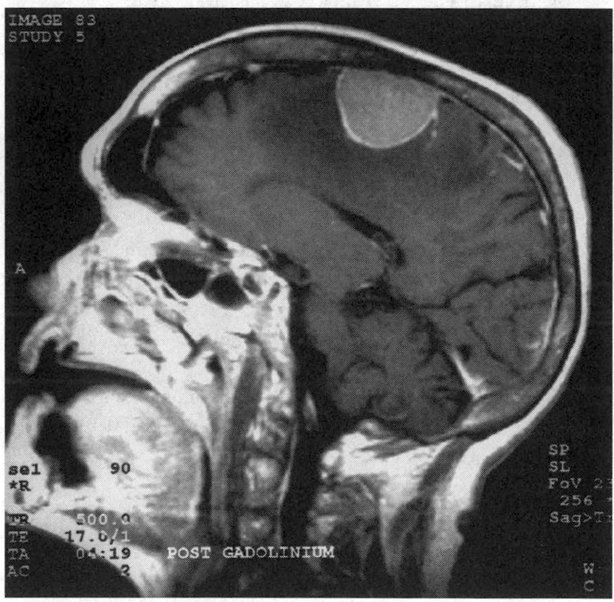

Figure 31-2 **(A and B)** MRI scans showing a meningioma in an 82-year-old woman who presented with seizures commencing 2 years earlier. (Courtesy of the Department of Magnetic Resonance Imaging, Salford Royal Hospitals Trust.)

Other Cerebral Disorders

Cerebral tumors

Clinicians are often concerned that elderly-onset epilepsy may indicate a cerebral tumor. Most series indicate that this applies only to a minority of cases.[4,11,19,20] There is a large variation, presumably due to the different populations being studied (itself a reflection of different referral patterns), to the different extent of which patients are investigated and, related to this, the different proportion of cases in which no cause is found. The most reliable figures so far suggest that about 10 to 15 percent of elderly-onset epilepsy may be due to neoplasm. In most cases, tumors are either metastatic or (inoperable) gliomas, though a few meningiomas are found. Until there is information on adequately documented, investigated, and sufficiently large population-based series, one cannot be certain what proportion of cases of very late-onset epilepsy are due to treatable and nontreatable tumors. Even less is known regarding the proportion of patients with seizures due to tumors in which there are no other pointers on history or examination to a space-occupying lesion. In my own experience, these are fairly rare but do occur from time to time (Fig. 31-2).

Nonvascular Cerebral Disease

A variable proportion of seizures is attributed to non-vascular cerebral degeneration. Again, the data are insufficient and will remain so until large series with uniform access to CT scanning facilities are reported. Mcareavy et al.[26] have suggested that Alzheimer dementia may cause seizures and this has been reiterated by Hesdorffer et al.[27] who reported a sixfold increased risk of unprovoked seizures. However, in neither study were "gold standard" criteria used for diagnosing Alzheimer's dementia and differentiating Alzheimer's from multi-infarct dementia or mixed Alzheimer's and multi-infarct dementia.

Subdural hematoma is an important but remediable cause, especially as very elderly patients are prone to this condition because of cerebral atrophy. Because it may occur after a relatively trivial injury, the diagnosis may be missed.[28] Direct brain damage due to head injury is itself a relatively uncommon cause of elderly-onset epilepsy, except in one series,[20] where it accounted for over 20 percent of cases over the age of 60. This unusually high figure, however, derived from a tertiary referral hospital responsible for head injury.

Seizures may occur during the course of severe cerebral infections (meningitis, encephalitis, or cerebral abscess), but under such circumstances should not strictly be called "epilepsy". Following recovery from such infections, however, epilepsy may arise due to scarring. This is a rare cause of epilepsy in the elderly.

Metabolic and Toxic Causes

Recent series[14] have underlined the importance of toxic and metabolic causes of seizures in old age. Alcohol is an important factor at any age.[29–30] Pyrexia and other acute conditions may precipitate seizures in older people[14] and pneumonia, which in the biologically aged may be more likely to cause hypoxia,[31] may predispose to seizures, or precipitate them in an individual who has otherwise well-controlled epilepsy. The accompanying box shows toxic and metabolic causes of seizures in elderly patients.

A wide range of drugs has been suspected of causing convulsions.[32–33] It is often difficult to prove that a given drug caused convulsions in a particular case, but in certain drugs the probability of a causal relationship seems to be high. Drug-induced seizures are particularly likely to occur when the drug is given in high dosage, parenterally, or to patients with impaired drug handling. Aminophylline, which has a narrow therapeutic index, and whose disposition may be altered by cigarette smoking, is especially prone to cause generalized seizures. Psychotrophic drugs, including trycyclic antidepressants and phenothiazines, are also particularly important. Benzodiazepines may cause withdrawal fits. Repeated hypoglycemic episodes due to excessive insulin or oral hypoglycemics may precipitate recurrent seizures. Drugs suspected of being epileptogenic are listed in Table 31-2. Strictly, epileptic seizures provoked by metabolic and toxic causes, even if they are recurrent, should not be called "epilepsy".

Occasionally, one encounters a patient whose seizures are apparently idiopathic, presenting for medical help for the first time in old age. Such patients may have had a lifetime of

- Pyrexia
- Hypoglycaemia
- Electrolyte disturbances (including water overload)
- Hypoxia with or without respiratory failure
- Severe myxoedema
- Hepatic failure
- Renal failure
- Drugs and drug withdrawal
- Alcohol and alcohol withdrawal

Table 31-2 Drugs that may cause seizures

Antibiotics
Benzylpenicillin
Oxacillin
Carbenicillin
Isoniazid
Cycloserine
Hormones
Insulin
Oral hypoglycemics
Prednisone
Local anesthetics/antiarrhythmics
Lignocaine
Procaine
Disopyramide
Anticholinergics in overdose
Psychotropic drugs
Chlorpromazine
Other phenothiazines
Tricyclic antidepressants
Lithium
Analeptic drugs
Aminophylline
Doxapram
Anaesthetic agents
Ether
Methohexitone
Ketamine
Halothane
Althesin
Radiographic contrast media
Meglumine
Metrizamide (very rare)
Withdrawal fits
Benzodiazepines
Alcohol

(Modified from Chadwick,[32] with permission.)

untreated epilepsy. Without such a long history, it is difficult to sustain a diagnosis of idiopathic epilepsy, though the possibility of elderly-onset idiopathic primary generalized seizures has already been discussed.[18]

Diagnosis and Investigation

The diagnostic task when a patient presents with suspected seizures is complex. These are the questions that should be addressed:

- Are the events seizures?
- What sort of seizures are they?
- Why did they occur?
  (a) Was there some unusual precipitant? (e.g., a prescribed drug)
  (b) Is there some continuing underlying cause (e.g., cerebrovascular disease)?
- Are there other concurrent illnesses?

The most powerful tool for answering these questions is a detailed history. In the context of a well-defined aura; clear progression from a tonic to a clonic phase; tongue-biting; incontinence or focal neurologic features during an attack; and stupor or prolonged confusion, headache, and transient neurologic signs after the attack, diagnosis is straightforward. Post-event confusion and headache are particularly useful pointers to a fit. For obvious reasons, the history from the patient may be unsatisfactory and eyewitness reports must be sought. This may be difficult in a patient who lives alone and who has simply been "found on the floor". Even evidence from individuals who did not see the event itself but observed the patient's postevent state—neighbours, ambulance drivers, casualty staff—may be helpful. In the case of an elderly person living alone, this may be the only source of useful history. The next most powerful tool is a wide-ranging, open-minded, physical examination. The third most powerful tool is time. It is better to wait and see than to initiate inappropriate treatment. Specialist investigations such as the EEG are only occasionally helpful in either positively diagnosing epilepsy or ruling it out. More useful, as we shall see, are tests of cardiovascular function that may positively diagnose syncope as a cause of transient loss of consciousness.

Are the Events Seizures?

The most common feature of epilepsy in elderly people, as at any other age, is transient impairment or loss of consciousness. Sometimes disturbances of consciousness may be forgotten and the patient will report only a fall. The differential diagnosis will then encompass the numerous other causes of falls in elderly people. A fall occurring in the absence of any obvious environmental cause and which cannot be confidently attributed to orthopedic, cardiovascular, or nonepileptic neurologic factors, should raise the suspicion of a fit.

- Syncope
- Hypoglycemia
- Transient ischemic attacks
- Recurrent paroxysmal behavioral disturbances secondary to organic brain disease
- Drop attacks and other nonepileptic causes of falls
- Transient global amnesia
- Psychogenic attacks
  - Panic attacks
  - Hyperventilation
  - Pseudoseizures

In the case of a classic generalized or partial seizure, the diagnosis can be readily made on the basis of the history. Unfortunately, fits may be difficult to differentiate from a variety of nonepileptic paroxysmal events that also occur in old people. Some of these latter may, however, be relatively easily ruled out. The accompanying box lists nonepileptic events that may be confused with epileptic fits.

Hypoglycemia is rare in a patient not on hypoglycemic medication. Where it does occur, however, it may not be associated in an old person with characteristic autonomic features.[34] Nocturnal hypoglycemia due to longer-acting oral hypoglycemics such as chlorpropamide and glibenclamide may occasionally cause fits and present as early morning confusion and postictal headache. (Such oral hypoglycemics should be avoided in elderly people).

Transient ischemic attacks do not typically cause disturbance of consciousness. They tend to have negative features, such as weakness and numbness, whereas focal seizures have positive features such as twitching and tingling or lancinating sensations.[35]

Recurrent paroxysmal behavioral disturbances are seen in dementias, in particular multi-infarct states. They may be confused with complex partial seizures (or vice versa, see below). Unlike the latter, they tend to have a predictable diurnal pattern, occurring as darkness falls—the so-called "sundowner effect"—or in the latter half of the day.[36]

Drop attacks[37] are associated with immediate (rather embarrassed) recovery, and do not cause loss of consciousness. A patient might say, "my legs just gave way, doctor." They tend to occur in a cluster and spontaneously remit. Other causes of recurrent falls may be inappropriately attributed to seizures. However, the reverse error is equally likely: fits may not be considered when the only available history is that of the patient repeatedly being found on the floor.

Transient global amnesia may be confused with complex partial seizures causing temporal lobe dysfunction and consequent memory disturbance. However, it is less common, and has characteristic features (anguished disorientation and repeated asking of the same questions), typically lasts for 24 hours, and usually does not recur.[38]

Psychogenic attacks (Appleton et al.[39]) do not usually occur for the first time in old age and there are typically other features of functional psychiatric illness and precipitating factors such as bereavement.

The most difficult differential diagnosis is *syncope*—transient loss of consciousness due to acute cerebral anoxia secondary to a fall in cerebral perfusion. Even when there is a reasonably good history, the features that characteristically differentiate fits from faints may not be as decisive as in younger adults, as is set out in Table 31-3. The diagnosis and management of syncope is covered in Chapter 32 and comprehensively reviewed in Kenny's[40] recent definitive textbook. It will therefore be only briefly touched on here.

Differentiating fits from faints may be even more difficult when there are coexistent conditions predisposing to both syncope and seizures. It is well-known that transient cerebral anoxia, as for example in carotid sinus syncope—now recognized to be much more more common than before realized[41]—may itself cause convulsions. Recurrent cardiac arrhythmias are particularly important: in one series of patients referred to a neurologic department with a diagnosis of epilepsy, 20 percent were found to have cardiac arrhythmias that caused or significantly contributed to their symptoms.[42] The situation may be particularly confusing, as complex partial seizures affecting the temporal lobes may present with autonomic features and recent attention has been drawn to the ictal bradycardia syndrome, in which episodic bradycardia or even asystole leading to syncope may itself be an ictal event.[43]

It may, therefore, prove impossible to determine whether transient cerebral symptoms are cardiac or cerebral in origin. Even ambulatory 24-hour ECG, with or without other cardiovascular tests, and prolonged EEG monitoring may not permit a confident diagnosis. Nonspecific abnormalities on an EEG, or cardiac arrythmias recorded on a 24-hour tape unrelated to the symptoms, may add to the confusion. Head-up tilt for up to 45 minutes with or without carotid sinus massage may induce bradycardia and/or hypotension and thus help differentiate convulsive syncope from epilepsy.[40] The golden rule is to avoid, as much as possible, approaching the patient with preconceptions—"as ye seek, so shall ye find". (The correlative of this is that, presumably, one should not establish isolated epilepsy clinics or syncope clinics for older people but, perhaps, "paroxysmal disorder clinics".)

Some genuinely epileptic events may not be appreciated for what they are (Table 31-4). The temporal lobe is the terminus of the vestibular pathways; consequently, seizures originating in this area may present with episodic vertigo, often associated with nausea.[44] Sometimes these fits may evolve to full-blown tonic-clonic seizures, but until this happens they may be dismissed as nonspecific dizziness, especially in an elderly person. Complex partial seizures with or without automatisms, may be labeled as nonspecific confusional states or even, where there are affective[45] or cognitive features or hallucinations, as manifestations of functional psychiatric illnesses. Patients with nonconvulsive epileptic status may present with acute, behavioral changes—withdrawal, mutism, delusional ideas, paranoia, vivid hallucinations, and fugue states.[46] Fluctuating mental impairment may easily be attributed to other

Table 31-3 The differences between faints and fits: problems in older patients

	Usual Distinction		
Features	**Faints**	**Fits**	**Modification in Older Patients**
Posture	Usually occur in the upright position	Not position-dependent	Faints in older people are not always position-dependent because they are often due to significant, position-independent, pathology
Onset	Gradual	Sudden	Loss of consciousness may be quite abrupt in syncope in an older person; complex partial seizures may have a gradual onset
Injury	Rare	More common	A syncopal attack may be associated with significant soft tissue or bony injury in an older person
Incontinence	Rare	Common	An individual prone to incontinence may be wet during a faint; partial seizures will not usually be associated with incontinence
Recovery	Rapid	Slow	A fit may take the form of a brief (temporal lobe) absence; a faint associated with a serious arrhythmia may be prolonged
Postevent confusion	Little	Marked	A prolonged hypoxic episode due to a faint may be associated with prolonged postevent confusion
Frequency	Usually infrequent with a clear precipitating cause	May be frequent and usually without precipitating cause	Faints associated with cardiac arrythmias, low cardiac output, postural hypotension or carotid sinus sensitivity may be very frequent

Table 31-4 Seizures that may be confused with other conditions

Epileptic Event	Possible Misdiagnosis
Epilepsia partialis continua (partial motor status)	Extrapyramidal movement disorder
Sensory epilepsy	Transient ischemic attack
Complex partial seizures	Organic or functional psychosis
Atonic seizures	Drop attacks/hysteria
Epileptic vertigo (due to temporal lobe attacks)	Brain stem/vestibular disease/nonspecific dizziness
Todd's palsy	Stroke/transient ischaemic attack
Any kind of seizures	"Falls"

causes of recurrent confusional states or even misread as part of a dementing process.[47–48] Thomas[49] has recently reviewed epileptic confusional states in elderly people due to either absence status or partial complex status and noted how often they are triggered by psychotropic medication (usually in excessive doses), though there are often metabolic causes. The role of antiepileptic drugs—as opposed to the removal of the underlying cause—is very limited. Occasionally, patients present with abrupt loss of consciousness without tonic/clonic movements—so-called atonic seizures.[50] Perhaps because of age-related changes in the brain, but more likely because epilepsy in the elderly usually takes place against the background of cerebral damage, postictal states may be very prolonged, and this may be another source of diagnostic confusion. At least 14 percent of patients in one series suffered a confusional state lasting 24 hours or more and in some cases it could persist as long as a week.[3] A focal postictal paresis (Todd's Palsy) is also more frequent in elderly patients. Todd's paresis after a fit may be misdiagnosed as stroke; in one series this was the most common nonstroke cause of referral to a stroke unit.[51] This is particularly likely where fits occur against a background of known cerebrovascular disease, and a recurrence of stroke may be incorrectly diagnosed.[52]

In the face of such difficulties, the clinician's primary duty is to acknowledge uncertainty where it exists and, if uncertainty remains after a careful history, examination, and appropriate investigations, simply to wait and see. A "therapeutic trial" of anticonvulsants as a diagnostic test is not recommended: it will rarely produce a clear answer and will add the burden of possibly unnecessary drug treatment to the patient's troubles.

Investigations

Investigations will be directed toward confirming the clinical diagnosis of epileptic seizures (and so differentiating this from other causes of "funny turns" and other transient impairments), defining the type of epilepsy (although it can be safely assumed that the vast majority of cases of epilepsy in old age are focal in origin), and identifying remediable underlying causes.

General Investigations

The choice of investigations will, of course, be determined by the history and by the findings on examination as well as by consideration of likely causes. Routine tests should include a full blood count, erythrocyte sedimentation rate, biochemical investigations (including urea, electrolytes, glucose, and liver function tests), electrocardiograph and chest X-ray. It is important to rule out metabolic causes (see the section, Metabolic and Toxic Causes, above) as they will usually be amenable to treatment. An estimate of γ-glutamyl transferase may be a useful marker of recent alcohol consumption. The threshold for carrying out thyroid function tests should be low, as myxoedema (which is occasionally associated with seizures) is common in older people and may present atypically. Diabetic control should be reviewed, especially where the presenting problem is that of nocturnal seizures in a patient on oral hypoglycemic agents. The choice of other investigations, such as serum tests for syphilis, will be influenced by history and findings on examination.

Specialist Investigations

The hardest diagnostic challenge is often, as already indicated, to differentiate between fits and faints. If it decided that there is strong chance that the episodes are syncopal, then the patient should be carefully investigated along the lines suggested in Chapter 32.

In the absence of features suggesting acute infection of the nervous system, there is no indication for lumbar puncture which may, anyway, be dangerous if a space-occupying lesion has not been ruled out by neuroimaging. The remote possibility of neurosyphilis will be even more remote if blood testing does not show abnormal serology. A chest X-ray may reveal a relevant primary neoplasm. While a skull X-ray may show evidence of raised intracranial pressure, intracranial calcification, or other evidence of an intracerebral neoplasm, it is rarely helpful.

A recent survey[53] of American neurologists' management of a single, unprovoked seizure showed a wide variation in the use of electroencephalography and neuroimaging. Some neurologists routinely ordered both investigations, some one, but not the other, and some neither. There is clearly scope here for studies evaluating these different approaches to investigation.

Electroencephalography

Excessive reliance upon an EEG to make or to refute a diagnosis of epilepsy is potentially dangerous. A routine EEG may support the diagnosis of epilepsy, especially if clear-cut paroxysmal discharges are observed. The absence of such activity on a routine recording does not, however, rule out the diagnosis; after all, most recordings last for only 20 minutes and ictal or diagnostic interictal activity occurs only intermittently. The range of "normal" increases with age so that discriminating normal from abnormal is more difficult in an elderly patient. Nonspecific abnormalities are more common in old age. In summary, while the EEG may provide useful supporting evidence for the diagnosis of epilepsy, it should not overrule the clinical diagnosis nor, with rare exceptions such as nonconvulsive status, provide its sole basis. It should also be added that an EEG, in this age group as in any other, cannot alone determine the need for a treatment in a newly diagnosed case, establish the adequacy of treatment, or predict the safety of discontinuing therapy.

A focal abnormality on an EEG may support the clinical diagnosis of a focal origin for fits and suggest a local neurologic cause. In those fits where there is an inadequate history or where the focal phase is too brief to be observed clinically, its observation may suggest a focal origin for the first time and guide further investigation. Persistent gross localized abnormalities on an EEG would strongly support a focal structural lesion. The EEG may be particularly useful in diagnosing nonconvulsive status or epilepsy presenting with recurrent behavioral disturbance or other neuropsychiatric manifestations (see above).

Neuroradiology

The older the age of presentation with epilepsy the greater the chance of a positive CT scan: as many as 60 percent of very late onset epilepsy patients may show a structural lesion.[54] This, however, would be an argument for routine scanning only if identification of such lesions influenced management[55]—as in the case of a space-occupying lesion amenable to neurosurgical removal (see Fig. 31-2). However, in only a minority of patients with elderly-onset epilepsy is a neoplasm or subdural hematoma the cause and in only a small proportion of tumor cases would neurosurgical intervention be appropriate. As already noted, in most series tumors are more likely to be gliomas or metastases than meningiomas. Even where a meningioma is diagnosed, neurosurgical treatment may not be indicated.[56] There is an impression that some meningiomas in old age may be relatively inert and there is no doubt that craniotomy is often tolerated poorly by elderly patients. The discovery of an otherwise inert meningioma, especially if it is nonoperable because of its site or the patient's general condition, may not be of benefit to the patient. Even so, it is sometimes useful to have a definitive diagnosis, though treatment for the underlying condition may not be available or considered inappropriate. Arguable indications for CT scanning are given in the accompanying box.

Magnetic resonance imaging (MRI) has been assessed in patients with seizures in whom there was no clear cause and CT scans have been normal. In some such cases, MRI has given diagnostically helpful information, confirming that it is a powerful and sensitive diagnostic tool; however, how often the information obtained using it would alter management in elderly-onset epilepsy remains to be seen.[57]

Indications for computerized tomography in elderly-onset seizures.

Strong
- Unexplained focal neurologic signs
- Progressive or new neurological symptoms, especially those of raised intracranial pressure
- Progressive or new neurologic signs
- Poor control of fits not attributable to poor compliance with anti-epileptic drugs or continued exposure to precipitants such as alcohol

Less strong
- Clear cut, stereotyped focal fits
- Persistent marked slow-wave abnormality on the EEG

Management

Doctors tend to think of the care of patients with epilepsy predominantly in terms of drug treatment. Management, however, extends far beyond drug treatment.

General Measures

Reassurance

Reassurance is of paramount importance: that, in the vast majority of cases, fits do not indicate serious brain damage; that they are unrelated to psychiatric disturbance; and that they can be controlled by medication. Patients should be told that anyone's brain is capable of having seizures if the circumstances are right and that fits are the most common neurologic problem after headache.

Patients may want to know whether fits are brought on by any particular activity and whether, for this reason, they should lead restricted lives. The advice in this age group is the same as that given to any patients: avoid only those activities that would mean immediate danger if a fit occurred.

The regulations relating to driving vary from country to country and even, as in the US, from state to state. In the UK, anyone holding a driving licence diagnosed as having epilepsy must notify the Driver and Vehicle Licensing Authority and stop driving until further directed by the Authority. The onus of responsibility to inform the Authority lies with the patient and not with the doctor. The regulations in the UK have recently been revised. They have been usefully summarized by Shorvon[58] and the essence of his summary is contained in Appendix 31-1.

As so often in old age medicine, management is multidisciplinary. A fit may cause severe loss of confidence and, in individuals who already have locomotor or other disability, this may lead not only to voluntary restriction of activities and a shrinkage of "life space", but may be also the beginning of a progressive descent into a vicious spiral of reduced mobility.

In such patients, encouragement of mobility, assessment for walking or other aids, and a review of the home circumstances and need for social support services will require input from remedial therapists and social workers. A home visit by an occupational therapist to look for potential sources of dangers—unguarded fires, etc.—may be helpful. Where fits are frequent, especially when there is a warning aura, a personal alarm may be useful.

Factors that are known to precipitate fits, such as inadequate sleep or excess alcohol, should be avoided. The patient should be warned that alcohol will increase the side effects of medication and that other drugs may trigger seizures or interact with AEDs. Patients should be encouraged to remind their doctors that they have epilepsy when they are seen about other conditions for which they may receive prescriptions. In any patient presenting with seizures, existing medication should be reviewed and drugs with a known epileptogenic potential or liable to interfere with AEDs withdrawn if possible.

Contact numbers for local branches of the national Epilepsy Associations may be useful, though older patients may find the rest of the membership rather young. With the patient's permission, spouses, relatives, neighbors, and other caretakers should be advised as to how to manage seizures if they occur.

Drug Treatment

Though the literature on anticonvulsant drug therapy is enormous, it contains relatively little specific reference to elderly patients. In those few drug trials from which elderly patients are not actually excluded, they are seriously under-represented. Most of what we think we know about anticonvulsant therapy in the aging brain has therefore been extrapolated from studies on younger patients, many of whom do not have the focal lesions that are typical in elderly epileptic patients and all of whom lack the age-related changes seen in older people. The advice that follows, therefore, falls rather short of the ideals of evidence-based medicine.

When Should Antiepileptic Drugs Be Started?

Epilepsy is defined as a tendency to recurring seizures and implicit in treatment with AEDs is the assumption that a patient does have such a tendency. A single seizure—especially if it has an obvious precipitating cause such as fever or alcohol—does not count as epilepsy, the assumption being that it does not imply an underlying tendency to recurrence. Here the correct approach is not AEDs, but removal of the cause. Where there is a single apparently unprovoked seizure, the decision whether or not to treat with AEDs is more difficult. It will be influenced by several considerations: the severity of the index seizure; the clinician's view as to the likelihood of recurrence (estimates range from 27 to 80 percent[59–60]; the estimate of the risks such as injury associated with a recurrent seizure; the conjectured hazards of AEDs; and the credibility one gives to the notion that "fits breed fits" so that early treatment may prevent epilepsy becoming chronic or intractable. At present, we have inadequate information upon which to base rational decisions as to whether a single unprovoked major seizure in an older person should be treated. Age itself is not a consistent predictor of recurrence although the presence of a clear cut etiological factor, such as a focal cerebral lesion, is. The relative dangers of non-treatment (injury due to recurrence) and of treatment (adverse effects of medication) have never been assessed in a systematic population-based, prospective manner. Until this has been done—and we have the results of the long-term outcome of trials such as the First[61–62] and MESS[63] studies—the decision whether or not a single unprovoked fit should be treated is partly personal prejudice.[64]

At present, it seems reasonable to treat a single unprovoked major seizure only if it is prolonged or if it has a clear cut underlying cause such as a previous stroke or a cerebral tumor. Where there is no such cause, and the fit has not been prolonged, the decision is more difficult. In the case of a short-duration generalized convulsive seizure or a partial or nonconvulsive seizure, it is probably best to wait. In a patient who has had a single fit, it is important to emphasize prompt treatment of conditions such as chest infections that might lead to hypoxia and so precipitate further fits. Two or more unprovoked major seizures warrant AED treatment, for then the risk of recurrence is about 70 percent in the general adult population[39] and it will probably be higher in the older adult population, where there is more often a continuing underlying cause.

There is even less information regarding the prognosis of untreated minor seizures. Treatment of a single minor episode is probably overzealous and it would seem to be reasonable to wait and see how frequent and how upsetting the episodes are before embarking on drug therapy.

Which AED Should Be Prescribed?

The majority of adult patients with either primary or secondary generalized seizures or partial seizures can be controlled with a single drug.[65] Nearly 70 percent of patients can expect a 5-year remission. Phenytoin, carbamazepine, and sodium valproate are equally effective as first-line, broad-spectrum AEDs.[65] Monotherapy should, therefore, be preferred to polytherapy. In younger subjects, where monotherapy is unsuccessful, this is very often due to poor compliance or sometimes associated with a serious underlying cerebral condition. Adding a second drug frequently contributes only additional side effects. It has been shown that in patients who are on more than one drug, withdrawal of the second or third drug may actually improve control. The idea that epilepsy is better controlled with smaller doses of more than one drug makes even less sense in older people who may already be on other medication. If monotherapy with one anticonvulsant gives unsatisfactory control, it is worthwhile trying monotherapy with another.[66] Although monotherapy should be the aim, there will be a proportion of patients who will require two AEDs—so-called "rational polypharmacy"—but before embarking on this course, the advice of an expert should be sought. In future, when we have "cleaner" drugs whose actions are both more precise and better understood, it may be possible to tailor-make a "cocktail" of drugs with complementary actions, each given in relatively low doses. However, this approach lies in the future.

Few trials have recruited enough elderly people to be able to compare the efficacy and side-effect profiles of different drugs in this age group. What little information there is, suggests that there is no overall advantage of one drug compared with another. In a recent multicenter comparative trial of efficacy in over 150 patients,[67] both sodium valproate and phenytoin proved to be useful first-line, broad-spectrum AEDs in elderly-onset seizures. Although there there was marginally better seizure control and there were fewer side effects on sodium valproate, the differences were not statistically significant. Interestingly, actuarial analysis suggested that a 6-month remission by 12 months follow-up would be enjoyed by 78 percent of the patients on valproate and 76 percent of patients on phenytoin—very similar to the findings from monotherapy studies in the general adult population.[65]

Because phenytoin, carbamazepine, and sodium valproate will have approximately equal efficacy in both generalized tonic-clonic and in partial seizures, the choice of drug will be greatly influenced by considerations of toxicity and, to a lesser extent, cost. The toxicity of AEDs has been investigated intensively, although relatively few studies have included significant numbers of elderly patients.

AEDs may cause acute dose-related, acute idiosyncratic, and chronic toxic effects. These adverse effects are usefully summarized in Appleton et al.[39] and the reader is strongly advised to be familiar with them when an AED is prescribed.

The gross *neurologic* side effects include ataxia, dysarthria, nystagmus, dizziness, unsteadiness, blurring and doubling of vision, reversible dyskinesias, and asterixis. Again, reviews of the literature indicate that although some neurotoxic effects may occur more frequently with certain drugs, there is so much overlap that most cannot be regarded as specific to any one drug.[65] The effects are generally dose related, and in the general adult population can usually be avoided or minimized by careful dosage titration.

Effects on cognitive function are of particular relevance. Earlier studies suggested that, of the commonly used broad spectrum AEDs, maximum adverse impact was seen with phenytoin and lesser effects with sodium valproate and carbamazepine.[68] Interestingly, this difference has not been found in elderly patients in a recent detailed study comparing the impact of sodium valproate and phenytoin on various aspects of cognitive function, including attention, concentration, psychomotor speed, and memory. There was little difference between phenytoin and sodium valproate in terms of impact on cognitive function.[69] Indeed, phenytoin seemed to have slightly *less* adverse impact on cognitive function than sodium valproate and neither drug had a major adverse impact. This failure to show a major difference between the two drugs is in keeping with more recent literature comparing effects of anticonvulsants on cognitive function in the general adult population, which also has failed to demonstrate significant difference.[70] Craig and Tallis[69] concluded that, if the dose of AEDs is kept low, adverse cognitive effects are probably not important; and where there are no gross adverse effects, subtle ones are not seen either. Other neurologic or neuropsychiatric side effects—for example, subjective feelings of unsteadiness and tiredness—may, however, still be significant and there may be important differences in the frequency and severity of these. A recent survey of the general population of patients with seizures found that over 80 percent experienced feelings of tiredness.[71] These aspects still need systematic study in patients with elderly-onset seizures.

Of the many non-neurological side effects, osteomalacia[72,73] may be especially relevant since this is more likely to occur in patients whose poor dietary intake of vitamin D and reduced exposure to sunlight already puts them at risk. Phenytoin, in particular, induces metabolizing enzymes in the liver, and so accelerates metabolism of vitamin D. There may, therefore, be a case for routine vitamin supplementation in patients on this AED. Sodium valproate, unlike phenytoin or carbamazepine, does not cause hypocalcemia or reduced vitamin D levels. Carbamazepine-induced hyponatremia increases significantly with age[74] and may occur at very low doses. The risk of hyponatremia may be even greater with oxcarbazepine.[75] This will be important in patients on diuretics—especially potassium sparing ones—or who have cardiac failure.

Other considerations may influence the choice of anticonvulsants. Unlike conventional formulation sodium valproate and carbamazepine, phenytoin may be taken in a single daily dose[76]—an advantage in those patients who depend on others to help with their medication. Sustained release sodium valproate, which may also be taken once a day, is available. Phenytoin also has the advantage of a predictable relationship between blood levels and efficacy and between blood levels and side effects, though physicians should be aware of the implications for dosage increments of the saturation kinetics it exhibits in the therapeutic range. Dosage adjustments should be in *small* increments—as little as 25 mg—to prevent a swing from subtherapuetic to toxic blood levels. If this is not recognized, then there is serious danger of causing significant adverse effects.

In summary, so far as conventional AEDs are concerned, there is no blanket recommendation for "the elderly". There may be individual drugs that are more suited to individual patients. Whatever drug is chosen, the prescribing physician should be familiar with its effects, kinetics, and its side effects.

New Antiepileptic Drugs

The multicenter comparative study of AEDs in elderly-onset seizures referred to earlier[67] indicated a high rate of adverse effects (20 percent). Most of these were minor, but it might be anticipated that "minor" adverse effects in older patients who are often near to the threshold of failure, may translate into a significant difference of function. Moreover, just over 20 percent of patients were not satisfactorily controlled. Herein lies the potential attraction of the new generation of AEDs: to obtain the same, or better, levels of efficacy with fewer adverse effects. Two other important considerations seem relevant to the new AEDs: lack of drug interactions and relatively simple kinetics associated with a wide therapeutic window.

The drugs that have been most extensively evaluated at present are lamotrigine, gabapentin, topiramate, and vigabatrin. I shall give a brief account of these and then make some general comments about the new generation AEDs. The reader is referred three excellent recent reviews for further information.[77–79]

Lamotrigine,[80] like phenytoin, acts by blockage of sodium-dependent channels. It exhibits linear kinetics and is not bound to plasma protein. It has been shown to be effective as add-on treatment in refractory partial seizures. Recent studies of monotherapy with lamotrigine in patients with newly diagnosed partial or generalized tonic-clonic seizures did not demonstrate the superior efficacy of lamotrigine over phenytoin[81] or carbamazepine.[82]

Gabapentin[83] acts via both sodium-channel blocking effects and potentiation of GABA responses. Although it does not have linear kinetics (exhibiting saturability of gastrointestinal absorption), it is a relatively easy drug to use because it is excreted unchanged in the kidney, is unbound to protein, and has a wide therapeutic window. It has no interactions with other drugs; a potentially important benefit in a patient population exposed to polypharmacy. Gabapentin has been shown to be effective as add-on therapy in refractory seizures, but again there is little evidence available from head-to-head comparisons with the conventional AEDs in the general patient population.

Vigabatrin[79] was the first tailor-made AED, being designed to slow the breakdown of γ-aminobutric acid (GABA) by inhibiting GABA-transaminase. It, too, exhibits linear kinetics, is not protein-bound, and is renally excreted. Moreover, because the inhibition of GABA-transaminase is irreversible, its effect outlasts its presence in the blood and it is feasible to use it once daily. There were anxieties initially that it might have marked adverse neuropsychiatric effects, especially in patients with cerebral injury, but recent studies have not shown a higher rate of withdrawal from treatment due to this cause than with other new AEDs. A recent monotherapy trial, however, has not shown a superior efficacy of vigabatrin over carbamazepine.[84]

Topiramate, the most recent of the new AEDs to be licensed in the UK, acts in at least four different ways and its use could be justifiably described as "single drug polypharmacy". Again, the kinetics are simple, with nonsaturability, mostly renal excretion, and lack of protein binding. There is little evidence that it has any significant interactions. It is effective as an add-on therapy in refractive seizures, but there are no data for monotherapy or in the generality of patients with seizures.

What most of these new drugs have in common are: the promise of enhanced efficacy, either alone or in combination with other drugs, in cases of intractable seizures; simpler kinetics; fewer or (as in the case of gabapentin) no drug interactions; and the possibility of less frequent or less marked adverse effects. However, they also have other features in common: they are much more expensive than the conventional drugs; they are less well-tried and tested; and none has been specifically evaluated in an elderly population, although trials of lamotrigine and gabapentin are ongoing. The physician who is looking for an alternative first-line monotherapy for the broad range of seizures in old age must, therefore, wait a while. To quote a recent authoritative review:[78] "At present, the main use of the new agents is in patients refractory to first-line drugs . . . and further studies are required to characterize their activity spectrum as well as their potential value in monotherapy. In most patients, new drugs cannot be recommended for first-line use until evidence is obtained that potential advantages in tolerability or ease of use outweigh the drawback of their high cost."

On the basis of the present data, Marson and colleagues[79] suggest that, if add-on treatment is required with the drugs discussed above, gabapentin and lamotrigine offer the best option for patients with drug intolerance but adequate seizure control, while in patients with poor seizure control in whom potency is the main issue, topiramate and vigabatrin might be the optimal choice. In either case, for the practicing geriatrician, these drugs should be used only in patients with seizures unresponsive to the conventional therapy and, hence, on the advice of a specialist. If at present they are to be used as first-line monotherapy in older patients, this should usually be in the context of an ongoing drug trial in older people. More generally, it is important that when the new drugs have demonstrated their efficacy in the younger adult population, they should be separately evaluated in older people; until such studies have been done, they should not be routinely recommended for people with elderly-onset seizures.

For the present, a sensible strategy is to use a conventional drug with which one is familiar, unless the considerations set out above dictate the choice of one of the other AEDs. If this works, well and good; if, despite adequate dosage and good compliance, there is poor control, then one of the other first line broad-spectrum AEDs should be tried. In a small minority of patients it may be necessary to use more than one AED at a time; such patients should be referred to a physician with a special interest in seizures.

Some patients may not be fully controlled even with optimal AED treatment. This should not prompt ever increasing, toxic doses of multiple drugs, but a more modest goal: to achieve a reduction in fit frequency to tolerable levels without unacceptable drug side effects. Feeling continually wretched from the adverse effects of AEDs may be even worse than suffering the intermittent unpleasantness of a fit.

Dosages

The dosages recommended for the general adult population may be inappropriate for elderly patients. There is considerable evidence to support an age-related increase in pharmacodynamic sensitivity to certain anticonvulsants.[85] For example, a study of carbamazepine found a greater effect on body sway with one 400 mg dose, despite the absence of pharmacokinetic differences. Even more important than age-related changes in pharmacodynamic sensitivity, are the altered pharmacokinetics of anticonvulsants in older patients.

The concentration of anticonvulsants in the nervous system reflects the free or unbound concentration in the plasma rather than that bound to protein. Since albumin concentrations tend to be lower in the elderly—especially the ill elderly—higher free concentrations of certain drugs are to be expected. This has been demonstrated in the case of phenytoin, sodium valproate, and certain benzodiazepines. The differences are particularly marked with valproate. There is also reduced clearance of certain anticonvulsants. Single-dose studies have shown reduced clearance of valproate and in multiple-dose studies the maximum rate of phenytoin clearance and the clearance of unbound valproate are both reduced. In the case of phenytoin, there is an increased plasma half-time. This is due in part to reduced clearance, but also to the fact that the volume of distribution for lipid soluble drugs is increased in elderly people because of the increase of fatty tissue as a proportion of the total body mass. There is, therefore, a longer interval between initiation of a drug dosage and the attainment of a steady state. This does not appear to apply to valproate.

The information just given should not lead to an exaggerated estimate of present knowledge of age-related changes in pharmacodynamics or pharmacokinetics or its applicability to an individual patient. Such changes are often derived by comparing mean values for young and old groups. Differences within these groups may be at least as important as differences between them. In the case of phenytoin, for example, only 20 percent of the inter-individual variation noted in one series was attributable to age alone.[86] In this context, as so often in clinical geriatrics, age is more important as a source of unpredictable variability than of predictable change.

Other sources of unpredictability arise from concurrent diseases, particularly those that affect hepatic metabolism or that, for a variety of reasons, lead to a further reduction in albumin, and hence, protein binding. Renal impairment appears to be less important for most anticonvulsants. The multiple pathology associated with old age will often mean multiple medication; many drugs interact with anticonvulsants and they interact with one another. Interactions affecting anticonvulsants occupy over 10 percent of the Drug Interaction Appendix of the British National Formulary.[87] Predicting plasma levels in a patient who is on more than two interacting drugs is even more difficult.

Finally, there is the problem of compliance. People of all age groups with epilepsy tend to comply poorly with their medication—which is not surprising in view of the chronicity of treatment, the purely prophylactic nature of the benefit, and the frequency of side effects. There is little evidence that most elderly patients are much less compliant than younger people; nevertheless, poor or variable compliance will be another reason for the lack of predictable relationship between prescribed dose and plasma level and between the doctor's action and the patient's response.

All of this should make clear that to suggest specific doses "for the elderly" is misconceived. All that can be recommended is a general strategy: "start low and go slow" and be prepared to find that the response, either in terms of adverse effects or efficacy is not precisely what one had expected or hoped for. There is now sufficient evidence to suggest that the initial dose of phenytoin in an elderly person should not be more than 200 mg, possibly lower. Most patients will be controlled on 150 to 250 mg daily. It would seem reasonable to commence carbamazepine at 100 to 200 mg total daily dose, with a maintenance dose of about 0.6 to 1.2 g daily. Sodium valproate should be started at 400 mg total daily dose increasing to about 1 to 1.2 g total daily dose. Except where fits are frequent and control is a matter of urgency, dosage increases should be gradual. This is particularly applicable to phenytoin where, as already noted, near the therapeutic range, an increment of as little as 25 mg may cause a marked rise in blood levels.

Anticonvulsant Monitoring

The long-term management of epileptic patients has been enormously improved by the introduction of anticonvulsant monitoring.[88] This is particularly useful where fits are not controlled by average doses of drugs, there are doubts about compliance, signs of intoxication, or odd neuropsychiatric syndromes, there is a sudden loss of control of fits, new interacting drugs are introduced, or where there are other diseases that may complicate treatment. The increased unpredictability between prescribed dose and blood levels in the patient make anticonvulsant monitoring particularly appropriate in the elderly.

It must be appreciated, however, that the most important part of *patient* monitoring is not measurement of anticonvulsant levels, but the use of information derived from history and examination. The patient or relative should keep a record of seizures; moreover, the patient should always be accompanied by a well-informed relative, neighbor, or caretaker to ensure that an accurate as possible account of events is obtained. Independent witnesses may also help the physician to pick up adverse effects that may be subtle in elderly people, and if not actively looked for, missed. Some attempt should be made to assess compliance and this should always be discussed with the patient. Increasing the dose because poor control due to variable compliance has been misinterpreted as implying insufficient dosage may lead to disaster. It is vital to emphasize the need to take medication consistently and indefinitely; some patients may have the impression that anticonvulsants need to be taken only when fits occur or as a "course". Finally, doctors should be aware that generic substitution may be associated with alteration in control and/or an increase in side effects. This is particularly important with phenytoin, where different preparations have markedly different bioavailability.

Anticonvulsant levels are most useful when they are used to answer a particular question or to resolve a particular uncertainty. Phenytoin is especially suitable for monitoring. First, its saturation kinetics mean a nonlinear relationship between dose and blood level: near the therapeutic range there will be a very steep dose-blood level curve. Second, it has a propensity to produce adverse neuropsychiatric effects that may present nonspecifically or be lost in the noise of other neurologic and other non-neurologic pathology. Third, interindividual variation in kinetics is more marked than with the other two broad spectrum anticonvulsants. Fourth, there is a close correlation, at least at the population level, between blood values of this drug and, on the one hand, efficacy and, on the other, side effects. Finally, because of the long half-life of phenytoin, single samples taken at random give a good approximation of the steady state level.

The place of anticonvulsant monitoring is less well-defined for carbamazepine[90] and valproate.[91] The dosage of carbamazepine is a poor predictor of serum concentration (though after the initial period of enzyme induction the relationship between dose and plasma concentration in an individual is relatively linear) and many of the side effects do appear concentration dependent. The relationship between carbamazepine concentration and clinical response is complicated by varying degrees of metabolism to its active metabolite and individual pharmacodynamic variability. The values given for the therapeutic range should be interpreted with caution: seizure control may be achieved throughout a very wide range of concentrations. Moreover, a single measurement may be meaningless because of great variations of concentration during a dosage interval. Both peak (3 to 4 hours after a dose) and trough (just after the next dose) levels need to be measured. In the case of sodium valproate, there is little correlation between blood levels and pharmacologic effect and, because there may be diurnal variation in drug clearance, repeated levels on the same dose may show wide variation. Only a few of the side effects, such as tremor, are concentration-dependent. Monitoring, however, may help to rationalize treatment in patients on polypharmacy and to identify the cause for treatment failure when a patient is on an apparently adequate dose. Samples should be taken at a standard time in relation to doses.

Overdoing or overinterpreting anticonvulsant levels may lead to mismanagement.[89] As already indicated, levels are only a small part of the clinical assessment and the results obtained from the laboratory must be interpreted in the light of the larger picture. Therapeutic ranges defined on general adult populations may not apply to the elderly population and certainly will not necessarily apply to any individual elderly patient. Doses should not be adjusted in fit-free nontoxic patients simply to bring the levels into the "therapeutic range". A patient with symptoms suggestive of intoxication should not be required to continue on the same dose of an anticonvulsant simply because the values from the laboratory fall within the notional therapeutic range. It must be remembered that laboratory results may be incorrect for all sorts of technical reasons, ranging from the time the specimen was taken, through the labeling of the specimen, to the method used in the measurement.

In a recent extermely helpful review, Richens[92] has set out the situations in which monitoring might be used: when seizure control is being established; if seizure control is lost; if adverse events occur; if the patient develops concomitant illnesses; if the patient's psychological state changes; and before withdrawing therapy. Limiting therapeutic monitoring to these patients, Richens suggests, will strike the best cost-effective balance.

Improving Compliance

As already noted, there is little evidence that elderly patients are any worse at compliance than younger adults.[93] However, there are special problems for an older patient who may be be on several drugs in addition to AEDs. These are some of the ways in which compliance may be assisted:

- Simplifying regimes
- Giving clear instructions, both orally and written
- Making sure that medication is clearly labeled
- Making sure that medication is accessible (childproof bottles and blister packs may defeat the patient)
- Co-opting the help of caretakers, relatives, and others where appropriate
- Using compliance aids, such as dosette containers
- Adopting a nonadversarial approach to compliance
- Trying to determine the reason for noncompliance if it is detected

Prognosis

Prognosis for Control of Fits

There is little information on the proportion of elderly-onset patients who are satisfactorily controlled on AEDs. A retrospective study[94] of admissions to a geriatric unit found that readmission due to poor control was very uncommon. In a recent comparison of phenytoin with sodium valproate,[67] failure due to poor control was found in only 2 percent of patients on valproate and 4 percent of subjects on phenytoin (this difference was not significant), though 10 and 14 percent, respectively, had withdrawn due to adverse effects. We need larger numbers of subjects followed over a longer period of time to get a reliable picture.

Can Drugs Be Withdrawn?

When should AEDs be withdrawn in patients with elderly-onset seizures? The literature (e.g., the Medical Research Council AED withdrawal study[95]) addresses much younger populations. Because, however, late-onset epilepsy, partial and secondarily generalized seizures (which are, of course, more common in the elderly), and the presence of known cerebral pathology (also more common in elderly epileptic patients) are associated with an increased rate of relapse, one may have to reluctantly concede that withdrawal of therapy should not be attempted in most elderly patients who have had a good reason to be placed on anticonvulsants in the first place.

Prognosis: Mortality

Mortality is increased in epileptic patients. However, the relative increase—the standard mortality ratio—may be less marked in those diagnosed over 60 years of age than in those diagnosed in youth or middle age. Hauser et al.[96] found that the death rate from cardiac disease was increased in patients with elderly-onset epilepsy, but that the incidence of sudden cardiac death was increased only in patients with symptomatic epilepsy in whom cerebrovascular disease was the attributed cause. Luhdorf[97] followed 251 patients for a minimum period of 2 years. Survival at 6 years was 60 percent of what was expected. Most deaths were related to cerebrovascular disease or tumors and when patients with tumors or overt cerebrovascular disease were excluded, mortality was no higher than that of the age-matched population. It would appear that epilepsy per se does not load mortality.

In summary, what little evidence we have suggests that, in the absence of serious progressive disease, the prognosis both for control of seizures and for survival is good in elderly-onset cases. However, more prospective long-term studies are required, particularly because a recent report from Alabama[98] suggested a high death rate (4 percent) in elderly patients discharged from hospital with a primary diagnosis of convulsions.

Services for Patients with Epilepsy

The challenge presented by a patient whose complaint suggests seizures is formidable. There is the diagnostic challenge: are these events seizures and what is there underlying cause? Answering this question may require a good deal of clinical acumen and, sometimes, access to sophisticated investigative tools. Beyond this, there is the task of ensuring that patients are fully informed about their condition and its implications and that the necessary reassurance, education, and counseling is given. Finally, there is the challenge of ensuring that the appropriate medication is prescribed, and taken, in the appropriate amounts over many years of a fluctuating condition affecting a patient who may have other illnesses that may influence the effects and adverse effects of the medication.

The nature of these challenges clearly argues for the development of specialist services. Perhaps these should not be addressed specifically to patients with epilepsy but should be open to patients who suffer from paroxysmal disorders of all kinds. Diagnosis specific clinics—such as separate epilepsy clinics and separate syncope clinics—tend to prejudge diagnoses. Enthusiasts for the former may have a bias towards the diagnosis of epilepsy and for the latter towards syncope. We tend to find what we seek. If such specialist services were developed, a crucial element would be specific diagnostic facilities because the most difficult phase in management is confirming the diagnosis of seizures.

At present, there is little experience of such specialist services for older people. Elderly people with seizures may fall between two stools—between specialist geriatrics services and specialist epilepsy services. The clinic should be supported by, and reach out to, the wider geriatric medical services and to community services. There should be clear definition of the roles of general practitioners and specialists in what will, inevitably in a chronic disease, be "shared care". Crucial to such services will be the specialist epilepsy nurse who has proved to be very effective[99] and cost-effective[100] in supporting patients with epilepsy in the long term, meeting their needs for information, education, counseling, and monitoring.

Areas for Research

For the reasons given at the outset of this chapter, geriatric epileptology is a relatively underdeveloped and under-researched field.

Causes of Seizures

Although it now seems clear that cerebrovascular disease is the most common cause of seizures in old age, the connection may be exaggerated because of the frequency of CT scan evidence of vascular disease in the general elderly population. More studies are needed to determine the frequency and type of cerebral tumors as a cause.

The Physical Impact of Seizures

Seizures might be expected to have more adverse physical effects in old people. Is this the case? How frequent are fractures and other significant injuries?

The Psychosocial Impact of Seizures

Jacoby and colleagues[101] have emphasised how "impact of a chronic illness is experienced not only through its physical symptoms, but also as a result of its effect on psychosocial functioning. In the case of an illness such as epilepsy, where the physical manifestations are transient, the psychosocial consequences may, with time, come to be of greater concern." We know little or nothing about this in older people. What do they think about seizures? What misconceptions and/or fears do they have and how much do they contribute to inducing dependency and shrinking lifespace? What are their information needs? How should those needs be best met?

When to Use AEDs?

Should one treat a single unprovoked tonic-clonic seizure in old age or wait for two or more seizures? What are the chances of recurrence where there is no overt cause? Prospective studies are needed to answer related questions: how easy are seizures to control in old age; could elderly people be more controlled with lower blood levels of anticonvulsants than younger people?

The Role of the Newer Generation of AEDs

What is the place of monotherapy using the new generation of anticonvulsants in the de novo treatment of elderly onset seizures? Studies addressing these questions should focus not simply on the traditional endpoints such as seizure control. The importance of newer AEDs may lie more in reducing subtle adverse effects on gait and mobility than in improved seizure control, especially as "minor" effects of this sort may, in a frail elderly person, translate into significant dysfunction.

The Organization of Epilepsy Services

How best should we provide a service for elderly people with seizures? What are the elements of an optimal overall comprehensive service? Who should provide it? How should we evaluate it? If we had answers to these questions our management of seizures in old age would be considerably better than it is now.

References

1. Tallis RC: Epilepsy in Elderly People. Martin Dunitz, London, 1995
2. Rowan AJ, Ramsay GR: Seizures and Epilepsy in The Elderly. Butterworth-Heineman, Boston, 1997
3. Godfrey JW, Roberts MA, Caird FI: Epileptic seizures in the elderly: 2. Diagnostic problems. Age Ageing 1982;11:29–34
4. Sander JWAS, Hart YM, Johnson AL, Shorvon SD: National General Practice Study of Epilepsy: newly diagnosed epileptic seizures in general population. Lancet 1990;336:1267–1270
5. Chadwick D: Epilepsy after first seizures: risks and implications. J Neurol Neurosurg Psych 1991;54:385–387
6. Beghi E, Ciccione A: The First Seizure Trial Group: Recurrence after a first unprovoked seizure. Is it still a controversial issue? Seizure 1992;2:5–10
7. Craig I, Tallis RC: General practitioner knowledge and management of elderly-onset epilepsy. Care of the Elderly 1991; 3:69–72
8. Hauser WA, Kurland LT: The epidemiology of epilepsy in Rochester, Minnesota, 1935 through 1967. Epilepsia 1975; 16:1–66
9. Hauser WA et al: Prevalence of epilepsy in Rochester, Minnesota: 1940–1980. Epilepsia 1991;32:429–445
10. Hauser WA, Annegers JF, Kurland LT: Incidence of epilepsy and unprovoked seizures in Rochester, Minnesota: 1935–1984. Epilepsia 1993;34:453–468
11. Luhdorf K, Jensen LK, Plesner AM: Epilepsy in the elderly: incidence, social function, and disability. Epilepsia 1986;27: 135–141
12. Tallis RC, Craig I, Hall G, Dean A: How common are epileptic seizures in old age? Age Ageing 1991;20:442–448
13. Jallon P, Loiseau P: Epileptic Seizures and Epilepsies in the Elderly. Sanofi Winthrop, Scipp Vincennes, 1995
14. Loiseau J, Loiseau P, Duche B et al: A survey of epileptic disorders in Southwest France: seizures in elderly patients. Ann Neurol 1990;27:232–237
15. Hauser WA: Seizure disorders: the changes with age. Epilepsia 1992;33:S6–S14
16. de la Count A, Brezeler M, Meinardi H, et al: A prevalence of epilepsy in the elderly: the Rotterdam study. Epilepsia 1996;37:141–147
17. Commission on Classification and Terminology of the International League Against Epilepsy: Proposal for revised clinical and electroencephalographic classification of epileptic seizures. Epilepsia 1981;22:489–501
18. Luef G, Schauer R, Bauer G: Idiopathic generalised epilepsy of late onset: a new epileptic syndrome? Epilepsia 1996; 37(suppl 4; abstr):4
19. Luhdorf K, Jensen LK, Plesner A: Etiology of seizures in the elderly. Epilepsia, 1986;27:458–463
20. Sung C-Y, Chu N-S: Epileptic seizures in elderly people: aetiology and seizure type. Age Ageing, 1990;19:25–30
21. Kilpatrick CJ, Davis SM, Tress BM, et al: Epileptic seizures in acute stroke. Arch Neurol 1990;47:157–160
22. Lancman ME, Golimstok A, Norscini J, Granillo R: Risk factors for developing seizures after stroke. Epilepsia 1993;34: 141–143
23. So EL, Annegers JF, Hauser WA et al: Population-based study of seizure disorders after cerebral infarction. Neurology 1996; 46:350–355
24. Shorvon SD, Gilliatt RW, Cox TC, Yu YL: Evidence of vascular disease from CT scanning in late onset epilepsy. J Neurol Neurosurg Psych 1984;47:225–230
25. Shinton RA, Gill JS, Zezulk AV, Beevers DJ: The frequency of epilepsy preceding stroke. Lancet 1987;i:11–13
26. Mcareavey BJ, Ballinger BR, Fenton GW: Epileptic seizures in elderly patients with dementia. Epilepsia 1992;33:657–660
27. Hesdorffer DC, Hauser WA, Annegers JF et al: Dementia and adult-onset unprovoked seizures. Neurology 1996;46: 727–730
28. Jones SC, Bamford JM, Heath J, Heatley RV: Multiple forms of epileptic seizures secondary to a small chronic subdural haematoma. Br Med J 1989;299:439–441
29. Heckmatt JA: Seizure induction by alcohol in patients with epilepsy. Experience in two hospitals. J R Soc Med 1990;83: 6–9
30. Lechtenberg R, Worner TM: Total ethanol consumption as a seizure risk factor in alcoholics. Acta Neurol Scand 1992;85: 90–94
31. Tallis RC: Biological ageing, illness in old age, and geriatric medicine J Hong Kong Geriatr Soc 1993;4:4–11
32. Chadwick DW: Convulsions associated with drug therapy. Adverse Drug React Bull 1981;87:316–319
33. Swift C: Drug-induced neurological disease pp. 391–406 In Tallis RC (ed): The Clinical Neurology of Old Age. John Wiley & Sons, Chichester 1988
34. Puxtey J: The neurological complications of metabolic nutritional and endocrine disorders pp. 309–322. In Tallis RC

(ed) The Clinical Neurology of Old Age. John Wiley & Sons, Chichester,1988

35. Hankey GJ: Cerebrovascular disease: a clinical approach. Rev Clin Gerontol 1994;4:289–310
36. Jarvik LF, Lavretsky EP, Neshkes RE: Dementia and delirium in old age pp. 326–349. In Brocklehurst JC, Tallis RC, Fillit HM (eds); Textbook of Geriatric Medicine and Gerontology. Churchill Livingstone, Edinburgh, 1992
37. Overstall P: Drop attacks, In Kenny RA (ed): Syncope in the Older Patient. Causes, Investigations and Consequences of Syncope and Falls. Chapman & Hall, London, 1996
38. Miller JW, Peterson RC, Metter EJ et al: Transient global amnesia: clinical characteristics and prognosis. Neurology 1987;37:733–737
39. Appleton R, Baker G, Chadwick D: Epilepsy. 3rd Ed. Martin Dunitz, London, 1993
40. Kenny RA (ed): Syncope in the Older Patient. Causes, Investigations and Consequences of Syncope and Falls Chapman & Hall, London, 1996
41. McIntosh S, DaCosta D, Kenny RA: Outcome of an integrated approach to the investigation of dizziness, falls and syncope in elderly patients referred to a "syncope" clinic. Age Ageing 1993;22:53–58
42. Schott GD, Macleod AA, Jewitt ED: Cardiac arrhythmias that masquerade as epilepsy Br Med J 1977;i:1454–1457
43. Reeves AL, Nollet KE, Klass DW, Sharbrough FW: The ictal bradycardia syndrome. Epilepsia 1996;37 (suppl 5; abstr):82
44. Kogeorgos J, Scott DF, Swash M: Epileptic dizziness Br Med J 1981;282:687–689
45. Blumer D: Epilepsy and disorders of mood. Adv Neurol 1991; 55:185–195
46. Rowan AJ: Ictal amnesia and fugue states. Adv Neurol 1991; 55:357–367
47. Ellis JM, Lee SI: Acute prolonged confusion in later life as an ictal state. Epilepsia 1978;19:119–128
48. Jamal GA, Fowler CJ, Leslie K et al: Non-convulsive status epilepticus as a cause of acute confusional state in the over-60 age group. J Neurol Neurosurg Psych 1988;51:738
49. Thomas P: Epileptic confusional states in the elderly. Epilepsia 1996;37 (suppl 4):36
50. Godfrey JW: Misleading presentation of epilepsy in elderly people. Age Ageing 1989;18:17–20
51. Norris JW, Hachinski VC: Mis-diagnosis of stroke. Lancet 1982;i:328–331
52. Fine W: Post hemiplegic epilepsy in the elderly. Br Med J 1967;1:199–201
53. Gifford DR, Vickrey BG: Neurologists vary in their test ordering and treatment decisions for a single, unprovoked seizure. Epilepsia 1995;36 (suppl 4; abstr):95
54. Ramirez-Lassepas M, Cipolle RJ, Morillo LR, Gumnit RJ: Value of computed tomography scan in the evaluation of adult patients after their first seizure. Ann Neurol 1984;15:436–443
55. Young AC, Costanzi JB, Mohr PD, Forbes WS: Is routine computerised axial tomography in epilepsy worthwhile? Lancet 1982;ii:1446–1447
56. Chadwick D: How far to investigate the elderly patient with epilepsy. pp. 21–30 In Tallis RC (ed) Epilepsy and the Elderly. Royal Society of Medicine Services, London, 1988
57. Kilpatrick CJ, Tress BM, O'Donnell C et al: Magnetic resonance imaging and late-onset epilepsy. Epilepsia 1991;32: 358–364
58. Shorvon S: Epilepsy and driving. Br Med J 1995;310:885–886
59. Chadwick D: Epilepsy after first seizures: risks and implications. J Neurol Neurosurg Psych 1991;54:385–387
60. Berg AT, Shinnar S: The risk of seizure recurrence following a first unprovoked seizure: A quantitative review. Neurology 1991;41:965–972
61. Beghi E, Ciccione A The First Seizure Trial Group: Recurrence after a first unprovoked seizure. Is it still a controversial issue? Seizure 1992;2:5–10
62. Beghi E: First Seizure Trial Group. A randomised clinical trial of the efficacy and safety of the treatment of the first unprovoked epileptic seizure. Neuroepidemiology 1992;11:50–51
63. Medical Research Council Multi-centre study of early epilepsy and single seizures (MESS).
64. Reynolds EH, Chadwick D: Controversies in treatment and management. Do anticonvulsants alter the natural course of epilepsy? Br Med J 1995;310:176–167
65. Treiman DM: Efficacy and safety of antiepileptic drugs: a review of controlled trials. Epilepsia 1987;28 (suppl 3):S1–S8
66. Schmidt D, Richter K: Alternative single anticonvulsant therapy for refractory epilepsy. Ann Neurol 1986;19:85–87
67. Tallis RC, Easter D, Craig I: Multicentre trial of sodium valproate and phenytoin in elderly patients with newly diagnosed epilepsy. Age Ageing 1994; 23(suppl 2, abstr):5
68. Trimble MR: Anticonvulsant drugs and cognitive function: a review of the literature. Epilepsia 1987;28 (suppl 3):37–S45
69. Craig I, Tallis R: The impact of sodium valproate and phenytoin on cognitive function in elderly patients: results of a single-blind randomised comparative study. Epilepsia 1994;35: 381–390
70. Meador KM, Loring DW, Huh K et al: Comparative cognitive effects of anticonvulsants. Neurology 1990;40:391–394
71. Brown SW: The Treatment of Epilepsy. A Patient's Viewpoint. British Epilepsy Association, London, 1996
72. Ashworth B, Horn DB: Evidence of osteomalacia in an outpatient group of adult epileptics. Epilepsia 1977;18:37–43
73. Gough H, Goggin T, Bissessar A et al: A comparative study of the relative influence of different anticonvulsants, UV exposure and diet on vitamin D and calcium metabolism in outpatients with epilepsy Q J Med 1986;59:569–577
74. Lahr MB: Hyponatraemia during carbamazepine therapy. Clin Pharmacol Ther 1985;37:693–696
75. Houtkooper MA, Lammertsma A, Meyer JWA: Oxcarbazepine: a possible alternative to carbamazepine. Epilepsia 1987;28: 693–698
76. O'Driscoll K, Ghadiali E, Crawford P, Chadwick D: A comparison of single daily dose and divided dose of phenytoin in epileptic outpatients Acta Therap 1985;11:375–385
77. Wyllie E (ed): New developments in antiepileptic drug ther-

apy. Special edition of Epilepsia. Epilepsia 1995;36: (suppl 2)

78. Perucca E: The new generation of antiepileptic drugs: advantages and disadvantages. Br J Clin Pharmacol 1996;42: 531–543
79. Marson AG, Kadir ZA, Chadwick DW: New antiepileptic drugs: a systematic review of their efficacy and tolerability. Br Med J 1996;313:1169–1174
80. Richens A: Overview of the clinical efficacy of lamotrigine. Epilepsia 1991;32(suppl 2):S13–16
81. Steiner TJ, Silveira C, Yuen AWC North Thames Lamictal Study Group: Double-blind comparison of lamotrigine (Lamictal) and phenytion in newly-diagnosed epilepsy. Epilepsia 1994;35(suppl 7; abstr):61
82. Brodie MJ, Richens A, Yuen AW: Double-blind comparison of lamotrigine and carbamazepine in newly diagnosed epilepsy. Lancet 1995;345:476–479
83. Chadwick D: The role of gabapentin in epilepsy management. pp. 59–65 In Chadwick D (ed): New Trends in Epilepsy Management: the Role of Gabapentin. RSM Services Ltd London, 1993
84. Kalviainen R, Aikia M, Saukkonen AM et al: Vigabatria versus carbamazepine monotherapy in patients with newly diagnosed epilepsy: a randomised controlled study. Arch Neurol 1995; 52:989–996
85. Mawer G: Specific pharmacokinetic and pharmacodynamic problems of anticonvulsant drugs in the elderly. pp. 21–30 In Tallis RC (ed): Epilepsy and the Elderly. Royal Society of Medicine Services, London, 1988
86. Bauer LA, Blouin RA: Age and phenytoin kinetics in adult epileptics. Clin Pharmacol Ther 1982;31:301–304
87. British National Formulary 19 (March 1990): British Medical Association and the Royal Pharmaceutical Society of Great Britain. London.
88. Rimmer EM, Richens A: Clinical pharmacology and medical treatment. In Laidlaw J, Richens A, Oxley J (eds): A Textbook of Epilepsy, 3rd Ed. Churchill Livingstone, Edinburgh, 1988
89. Chadwick DW: Overuse of monitoring of blood concentrations of anti-epileptic drugs. Br Med J, 1987;294:723–724
90. Brodie MJ Hallworth MJ: Therapeutic monitoring of carbamazepine. Hosp Update 1987:57–63
91. Leading article. Sodium valproate. Lancet 1988;ii:1229–1231
92. Richens A: How valuable is therapeutic drug monitoring? Epidata Bull No. 8. British Epilepsy Association London 1996
93. Weintraub M: Compliance in the elderly. Clinics in Geriatric Medicine WB Saunders, Philadelphia, 1990
94. Ghose K: Incidence and presentation of epilepsy in an acute geriatric unit. Proc 4th Br, Dan, Dutch Epilepsy Congress 7–10th Sept 1988 Amsterdam. (abstr) p. 61.
95. Medical Research Council Antiepileptic Withdrawal Study Group: A randomised study of antiepileptic drug withdrawal in patients in remission of epilepsy. Eng J Med 1991;337: 1175–1180
96. Hauser WA, Annegers JF, Elveback LR: Mortality in patients with epilepsy. Epilepsia 1980;21:399–412
97. Luhdorf K, Jensen LK, Plessner AM: Epilepsy in the elderly: life expectancy and causes of death. Acta Neurol Scand 1987; 76:183–90
98. Geyer J, Kuzniecky R, Faught E: Admission and mortality rates for convulsive seizures in patients aged 65 years and older. Epilepsia 1995;36(suppl 4):148
99. Brown SW et al: An epilepsy needs document. Seizure 1993; 2:91–103
100. Hartshorn JC: A nurse-managed clinic for individuals with epilepsy. Epilepsia 1995;36(suppl 4; abstr)99
101. Jacoby A, Baker G, Smith D et al: Measuring the impact of epilepsy: the development of a novel scale. Epilepsy Res 1993; 16:83–88

Driving and Epilepsy: New U.K. Regulations for Ordinary Licence Holders—August 1994

- A patient may drive only if he or she is free of epileptic attacks during the year before the date when the licence is granted
- If epileptic attacks occur only during sleep, the patient must have had a sleep-only pattern for 3 years or more
- His or her driving must be unlikely to endanger the public where driving is compromised by drug treatment or associated neurologic or neuropsychiatric disturbances

Seizures

Single Seizures

Single seizures are not regarded as epilepsy by the DVLA unless a continuing liability can be shown (usually by EEG or imaging). However, the DVLA usually prohibits driving for 12 months after a single seizure.

Provoked Seizures

Provoked seizures are defined as seizures precipitated by exceptional nonrecurring circumstances in nonepileptic subjects. Driving is usually allowed once the provoking factor has been successfully treated or removed. The precipitating factor must be truly exceptional. Alcohol and illicit drugs do not qualify.

Mild Seizures

Mild seizures are defined as, for example, myoclonic jerks and seizures not associated with loss of conciousness. These are treated the same as other attacks.

Attacks Occurring During Changes in Drug Treatment

Regulations apply to these attacks. Licence will be barred regardless of whether deliberate or accidental. Driving should be suspended during changes in drug treatment (advisory not regulatory). When drugs are being totally withdrawn, driving should be suspended from the time withdrawal begins until 6 months after completion.

EEG Changes

Without overt seizures, these are not usually a bar to driving. The exception is unequivocal 3 Hz spike/wave in primary generalized seizures.

(From Shorvon S: Epilepsy and driving. Br Med J 1995;310: 885 ± 886 with permission.)

C H A P T E R 32

Syncope

ROSE ANN KENNY
APARJIT BALLAV DEY

Syncope is a term used to describe transient loss of consciousness lasting for usually a few seconds to a few minutes resulting from temporary cessation of cerebral function. Loss of postural control, and spontaneous and complete recovery without resuscitation are typical features of syncope. Usually there are no residual symptoms such as confusion, drowsiness, or headache after recovery, but some elderly subjects may occasionally experience these symptoms. Presyncope or near syncope is a sensation of impending unconsciousness that may or may not precede syncope.

Epidemiology of Syncope

The epidemiology of syncope in old age has not been well studied. The greatest difficulty in assessing the magnitude of this problem is the overlap between syncope and falls. A substantial number of elderly subjects with syncope present with unexplained and recurrent falls. For example, nearly two-thirds of elderly patients with orthostatic hypotension,[1] and one-third of patients with carotid sinus syndrome,[2] present with falls and deny loss of consciousness, possibly because of amnesia for loss of consciousness.[1,2] An accurate witness account of falls and syncope is not available in up to half of elderly patients.[3] A history from the patient may be unreliable, particularly if cognitive function is impaired or if the patient has amnesia for loss of consciousness. The problem is further complicated by the presence of multiple disorders that may synergistically cause syncope and by methodologic difficulties in determining a relationship between circumstances, medications, and symptoms.

Accurate estimates of the prevalence and incidence of syncope are not available. From available data, syncope accounts for 3 percent of emergency room attendances and 1 percent of medical admissions to a general hospital.[4] In addition, unexplained and recurrent falls (a frequent presentation for syncope) were responsible for 7 percent of attendances to an accident and emergency department of an inner-city university hospital among 12,480 elderly patients (age >65 years) in an ongoing study.[5] In a study of 711 elderly subjects (mean age 87 years) living in a chronic care facility, the prevalence of syncope was reported to be 23 percent over a 10-year period with an annual incidence of 6 percent and recurrence rate of 30 percent, over a 2-year prospective follow-up.[6] This is undoubtedly an underestimate because falls were excluded. A cause of syncope could not be determined in 40 percent of patients among 210 community-dwelling elderly subjects (mean age 71 years).[7] Syncope due to a cardiac cause is associated with higher mortality rates irrespective of age.[7] In patients with a non-cardiac or unknown cause of syncope, older age, a history of congestive cardiac failure, and male sex were important prognostic factors of mortality.[7] This study predated establishment of standardized tests for baroreflex sensitivity and did not specifically investigate all patients for baroreflex abnormalities, namely carotid sinus syndrome (CSS), orthostatic hypotension, and vasovagal syncope. These conditions are likely to be responsible for a substantial proportion of unexplained syncope in the elderly.

Pathophysiology of Syncope in the Elderly

The temporary cessation of cerebral function that causes syncope results from transient and sudden reduction of blood flow to parts of the brain (brain stem reticular activating system) responsible for consciousness. Age-related physiologic impairments in heart rate, blood pressure, cerebral blood flow, in combination with comorbid conditions and concurrent medications account for the increased prevalence of syncope in the elderly. Baroreflex sensitivity is blunted with aging, manifesting as a reduction in the heart rate response to hypotensive stimuli.[8,9] The elderly are prone to reduced blood volume due to excessive salt wasting by the kidneys as a result of a decline in plasma renin and aldosterone,[10] a rise in atrial natriuretic peptide,[11] and concurrent diuretic therapy. Low-blood volume together with age-related diastolic dysfunction can lead to a low cardiac output, which increases susceptibility to orthostatic hypotension and vasovagal syncope. Cerebral autoregulation, which maintains a constant cerebral circulation over a wide range of blood pressure changes, is altered in the presence of hypertension and possibly by aging.[8,9,12] As a result, sudden mild to moderate declines in blood pressure can affect cerebral blood flow markedly and render an older person particularly vulnerable to presyncope and syncope. Multiple age-related diseases and medications influencing circulation, together with these physiologic alterations predispose as well as influence the outcome of syncope in the elderly.

Etiology

Syncope is a common symptom experienced by up to 30 percent of healthy adults at least once in their lifetimes.[13,14] A wide variety of conditions, benign as well as life-threatening, are causally related to syncope. An attributable cause of syncope can be identified by detailed history, examination, and specific laboratory investigations in most patients.[15–17] A subset of patients, however, will remain undiagnosed with recurrent syncope despite extensive investigations, particularly older patients who have marginal cognitive impairment and for whom a witnessed account of events is only available in 40 percent.[2] The common causes of syncope are enumerated in Table 32-1. Strict diagnostic criteria are essential for accurate diagnosis and management. In some reports, syncope of cardiac origin has been distinguished from that due to noncardiac causes by higher mortality rates.[7] However, it is not clear whether the higher mortality is related to underlying heart disease or to syncope.

Overlap Between Syncope and Falls

Syncope and falls are often considered as two separate entities with different etiologies. Though controversial, an overlap between syncope and falls has become increasingly evident from published literature.[1–4,18–21] In the elderly, determining the cause of a fall may be difficult. Approximately 30 percent of cognitively normal elderly subjects fail to recall documented falls 3 months later,[22] and up to one-half of syncopal episodes go unwitnessed.[3] Nearly 40 percent of patients with carotid sinus syndrome (CSS) present with unexplained falls and deny loss of consciouness.[2] Amnesia for loss of consciousness has been observed in one-half of patients with CSS who present with falls[20] and one-fourth of all patients with CSS irrespective of presentation[21] have amnesia for loss of consciousness. Amnesia for loss of consciousness has also been observed in syncope induced through a sequence of hyperventilation, orthostasis, and Valsalva maneuver.[23] In addition, similar hemodynamic changes have been observed in elderly patients complaining of falls or syncope in association with postprandial hypotension[24] and orthostatic hypotension,[1,3] suggesting that the phenomenon is generalized for cardiovascular syncope. Amnesia for loss of consciousness combined with loss of postural stability (due to hypoperfusion of those parts of the brain responsible for posture) result from hemodynamic changes associated with syncope. Thus, syncope and falls are often indistinguishable and in fact are manifestations of similar pathophysiologic processes.

Table 32-1 Etiology of syncope in elderly patients

Cardiac arrhythmia
Bradyarrhythmia: sick sinus syndrome, high atrioventricular block
Tachyarrhythmia: supraventricular, ventricular
Neurocardiogenic syncope including
Vasovagal syncope
Situational syncope
Micturition syncope
Defecation syncope
Tussis syncope
Orthostatic hypotension
Carotid sinus syndrome
Drug-induced syncope
Postprandial syncope
Syncope associated with low cardiac output
Myocardial infarction
Pulmonary embolism
Aortic stenosis, mitral stenosis
Hypertrophic cardiomyopathy
Pulmonary hypertension
Hyperventilation syncope
Swallow syncope
Glossopharyngeal syncope
Subclavian steal syndrome
Transient ischemic attack
Epilepsy

Diagnostic Evaluation of Syncope in Elderly Subjects

Diagnostic evaluation of syncope in the elderly requires: (1) clarification of the presenting symptom by differentiation from other similar entities such as falls, drop attacks, seizures, dizziness, and vertigo, and (2) a detailed noninvasive cardiovascular investigation to determine the attributable cause(s) of loss of consciousness. Multiple illnesses are very common in the elderly: subjects over 65 years have on average 3.5 illnesses.[25] It is thus important to carefully attribute a diagnosis, rather than assume that the presence of an abnormality known to produce syncope or hypotensive symptoms is the cause. In order to attribute a diagnosis, patients must have symptom reproduction during investigation and preferably alleviation of symptoms with specific intervention during follow up. In addition, various hypotensive disorders coexist[21] in the same patient, often rendering a precise diagnosis for the symptom difficult.

History and Physical Examination

A detailed history and physical examination can result in a diagnosis in up to 40 percent of cases.[7] An accurate witnessed account can help to differentiate syncope from an accidental fall. Witnessed features of prodrome (e.g., pallor, sweating, presence or absence of loss of consciousness, presence or absence of involuntary movements) and clinical events after the episode (e.g., confusion, vomiting) are crucial in constructing a diagnostic picture. Nonetheless, a witnessed account is often not available. The majority of episodes of syncope or falls, even in institutional care, occur in the bedroom or bathroom and are unwitnessed.[26] A witnessed account was available in only 40 percent of older patients attending a dedicated syncope outpatient facility.[3] Clincial features suggestive of specific causes of syncope are detailed in Table 32-2.

Table 32-2 Clinical features suggestive of a specific cause of syncope

Symptoms	Diagnostic consideration
After sudden unexpected pain, unpleasant sight, sound or smell, prolonged standing	Vasovagal syncope, carotid sinus syndrome
During micturition, defecation, cough	Situational syncope Carotid sinus syndrome
With neuralgia	Neuralgic syncope (glossopharyngeal, trigeminal)
Upon standing	Orthostatic hypotension
Taking antihypertensive medication	Drug-induced (vasovagal syncope, orthostatic hypotension)
After meals	Postprandial, carotid sinus syndrome
Changing position	Atrial myxoma, LA thrombus
With exertion	Aortic stenosis, mitral stenosis, pulmonary hypertension
With head rotation	Carotid sinus syndrome
Associated with vertigo, diplopia, dysarthria, other motor and sensory symptoms of brain stem ischaemia	Vertebrobasilar insufficiency, steal
With arm exercise	Subclavian steal

Patients frequently complain of dizziness alone or as a prodrome to syncope and unexplained falls. The clinical features of dizziness can further help to identify an underlying cause of symptoms. Four categories of dizzy symptoms—vertigo, disequilibrium, light-headedness, and others—have been recognized.[27] Light-headedness is often associated with an underlying cardiovascular cause of symptoms, vertigo with peripheral or central lesions, and unsteadiness with an underlying central lesion.[28] In addition, dizziness is most likely attributable to a cardiovascular diagnosis if associated with pallor, syncope, prolonged standing, or the need to lie down or sit down when symptoms occur.[28]

Physical examination should include morning orthostatic blood pressure measurement, observation of carotid and cardiac bruits, heart rate and rhythm, and the presence of atherosclerotic disease: for example peripheral vascular disease, hypertensive retinal changes, etc. Assessment of gait, mobility, muscle strength, and use of walking aids are important in patients complaining of unexplained falls and possible syncope. Assessment of vision, hearing, and signs of Parkinson's disease are also important.

Orthostatic Blood Pressure Measurement

Supine blood pressure measurements should be taken after a minimum of 10 minutes of rest. Blood pressure should then be recorded for up to 2 minutes while standing unaided. In 90 percent of patients who have orthostatic hypotension, a significant reduction in standing blood pressure will have occurred by 1 minute during standing. Some studies have recorded blood pressure for up to 20 minutes.[29] However, prolonged standing may lead to overlap of orthostatic symptoms and vasovagal symptoms.[30] A sustained 20 mmHg fall of systolic blood pressure, a 10 mmHg fall in diastolic blood pressure, or a fall of systolic blood pressure to 90 mmHg or less is considered diagnostic for orthostatic hypotension. However, in practice, patients can have symptom reproduction (dizziness) during transient falls in orthostatic blood pressure that are not sustained or which changes do not meet the standard criteria for orthostatic hypotension. This is particularly so in frailer elderly persons in whom cerebral autoregulation is compromised. Digital photoplethysmography (Finapres) is a useful noninvasive technique for beat-to-beat blood pressure measurement during orthostasis. Alternatively, other systems for automated recording of blood pressure or repeated manual sphygmomanometry can be used but will miss transient hypotension. Reproducibility of orthostatic hypotension depends on the time of day of measurement and on autonomic nervous system function.[1] Where possible, the procedure should be carried out in the morning. In patients with unexplained syncope an attributable diagnosis of orthostatic hypotension depends on reproduction of symptoms.

12-Lead Electrocardiogram

Causes of syncope such as acute myocardial infarction, bradyarrhythmias, or tachyarrhythmias can be diagnosed from surface ECG. However, an abnormal ECG is not necessarily the cause of symptoms—up to 32 percent of normal healthy unselected elderly have an abnormal surface ECG.[31] Ischemic changes in the ECG together with a history of palpitation may indicate an underlying arrhythmogenic cause of syncope.[32]

Ambulatory Cardiac Monitoring

Ambulatory cardiac monitoring is usually performed for 24 hours or for its multiples and the diagnostic yield increases with the duration of monitoring. In a study of 95 patients (median age 66 years) in whom the etiology of syncope was not apparent from history, physical examination, and routine ECG, major ECG abnormalities in ambulatory cardiac monitoring were detected in 15 percent of patients on day 1, an additional 11 percent on day 2, and a further 4 percent on day 3.[33] The complement to these findings is the observation that among patients who had episodes of dizziness or syncope without concurrent arrhythmias, 14 percent were evident on day 1, 12 percent on day 2, and 4 percent on day 3. Considering the yield of usefulness in this group of patients by the duration of monitoring, 28 percent benefited diagnostically from 1 day of ambulatory cardiac monitoring, an additional 12 percent from 2 days, and a further 7 percent from 3 days. Most episodic supraventricular and ventricular arrhythmias and atrioventricular blocks can be diagnosed by ambulatory cardiac monitoring.[34,35] Other ambulatory diagnostic interventions such as memory loop recorder, real-time cardiac monitors, and signal average ECG have not been studied in detail in older patients with syncope.[36–38]

Ambulatory Blood Pressure Monitoring

Ambulatory blood pressure monitoring is predominantly used in the management of hypertensive disorders. It can, however, play a major role in the diagnosis and management of hypotensive disorders. Information such as the pattern of diurnal blood pressure behavior, postprandial dips in blood pressure, and blood pressure changes after medication are useful in patients suffering from syncope and dizziness. A reversal of the diurnal blood pressure pattern is observed frequently in symptomatic orthostatic hypotension.[39]

Carotid Sinus Massage

Carotid sinus massage comprises measurement of heart rate and blood pressure responses during and after longitudinal massage over the point of maximum carotid impulse, usually located at the level of the upper border of the thyroid cartilage (Fig. 32-1). Heart rate responses are recorded using a continuous surface electrocardiogram. Blood pressure is best measured by noninvasive phasic blood pressure monitoring equipment that allows accurate assessment of the blood pressure nadir (around 18 seconds after the onset of massage).[21,40] Massage should be carried out initially supine and then tilted head-up to 70°. This is because up to 10 percent of patients with carotid sinus syndrome have a normal response to massage while supine, but an abnormal response only when upright.

Head-Up Tilt Testing

Prolonged head-up tilting tests the baroreflex response to prolonged standing. The optimal protocol for the test is as yet undefined. Thus, a variety of methods are recommended concerning the angle of tilt, duration of tilt, and use of additional provocation to induce syncope. A tilting angle within the range of 60 and 80 degrees provides the necessary orthostatic stress.[41] Duration of tilting in various studies has varied from 30 to 60 minutes. Concurrent administration of intravenous isoprenaline reduces duration of the test to about 10 minutes with improved sensitivity.[42] The test should be carried out during morning hours after an overnight fast and after withdrawal of all cardioactive drugs for at least 5 half-lives. The subject should be rested supine for periods of 15 to 30 minutes after which baseline blood pressure and heart rate is recorded. Blood pressure is ideally recorded by digital photoplethysmography (Finapres), which records beat-to-beat changes. Alternatively, other systems for automated blood pressure recording or repeated manual sphygmomanometer blood pressure recording and continuous surface ECG can be used for monitoring. The authors consider a tilting angle of 70° and duration of 45 minutes as adequate in most patients. The test is positive if the patient develops syncope and or presyncope together with hypotension and/or bradycardia during the upright period. The patient should be immediately lowered to supine position and the study terminated. Symptom reproduction during hemodynamic changes is preferable in order to attribute cause.

Figure 32-1 Technique for carotid sinus massage.

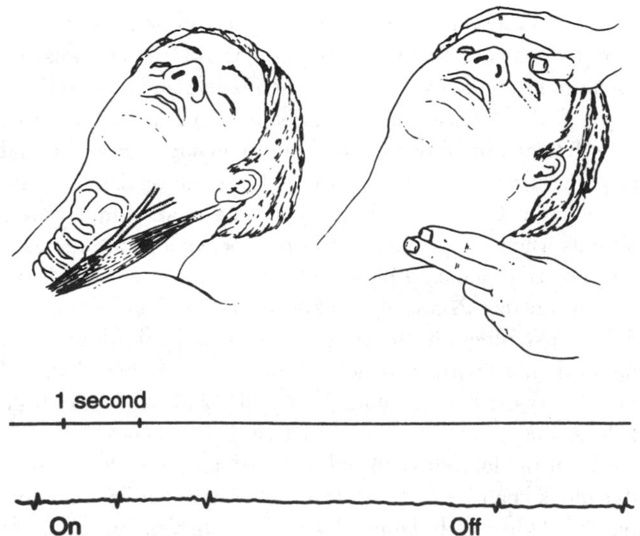

Head-up tilting is a very useful investigation in the following instances:

1. The diagnosis of neurocardiogenic syncope. Additional provocative tests include intravenous isoprenaline,[43,44] sublingual or intravenous glyceryl trinitrate,[45,46] and intravenous cannaultion.[47]
2. The diagnosis of orthostatic hypotension.[1]
3. The diagnosis of cardioinhibitory carotid sinus syndrome (up to 10 percent of patients have a hypersensitive response only when tilted upright[21]).
4. It is a useful procedure (reproducing "syncope") in patients with psychiatric disorders without any change in blood pressure and heart rate.[3]
5. The diagnosis of hyperventilation syncope, where patients hyperventilate with reproduction of symptoms, but without developing hypotension or bradyarrhythmia.[48]
6. The diagnosis of central dizziness. Movement of tilt bed can reproduce symptoms of dizziness without accompanying hemodynamic changes.[3]

Electrophysiologic Studies

In a study of 400 patients with syncope, 1 percent of 190 younger patients and 2 percent of 210 elderly subjects were diagnosed by electrophysiologic study.[7] However, abnormal electrophysiologic studies in a majority of patients with syncope have been reported by several investigators.[49–51] Most of the patients studied in these reports had structural heart disease and multiple electrophysiologic abnormalities. Thus, in the absence of symptom reproduction during electrophysiologic abnormalities, it is difficult to attribute a diagnostic value to abnormal findings.

Investigation Protocol

In most early reports, the cause of syncope in older subjects could not be established in between one-third and one-half of patients studied.[52] However, in a recent report from a dedicated outpatient "syncope and falls" facility for older patients, using an integrated approach to unexplained syncope, dizziness and falls, over 70 percent had an attributable diagnosis (Table 32-3).[3] This approach comprised of:(1) full clinical evaluation including a detailed history and pursuance of witnessed account, (2) baseline laboratory investigations, (3) 12-lead surface ECG, (4) repeated morning orthostatic blood pressure measurements, (5) supine and upright carotid sinus massage, (6) 24-hour ambulatory ECG and blood pressure monitoring, and (7) passive head-up tilt studies with or without additional provocative tests during head-up tilt with isoprenaline or glyceryl trintrate. Abnormal historical and physical findings should be further investigated with echocardiography, carotid Doppler ultrasound study, treadmill stress testing, intracardiac electrophysiological study, EEG, and head CT scan, as appropriate. Certain clinical variables have predictive value on test outcomes; for example, male sex is commonly associated with a diagnosis of CSS, orthostatic hypotension is more frequent in patients who have cognitive impairment, arrhythmias during ambulatory monitoring are common if syncope is accompanied by palpitations or if the patient is taking diuretics, and falls are a more likely presentation of syncope in older patients and in those with cognitive impairment.[32] Carotid sinus massage and orthostatic blood pressure measurements together with an accurate history, physical examination, and surface ECG can diagnose up to 60 percent of cases. Inclusion of other tests increases diagnostic yield to 80 percent.[32] An algorithm for the diagnostic approach to older patients with syncope is presented in Figure 32-2.

Table 32-3 Final diagnosis after integrated investigation program in elderly patients with syncope referred to a dedicated outpatient facility

Diagnosis	(%)
Carotid sinus syndrome	45
Orthostatic hypotension	32
Vasodepressor syndrome	11
Cardiac arrhythmia	21
Epilepsy	9
Cerebrovascular accident	8
Benign positional vertigo	8
Cough syncope	2
Drop attacks	2
Conversion reaction	2
Unexplained	6

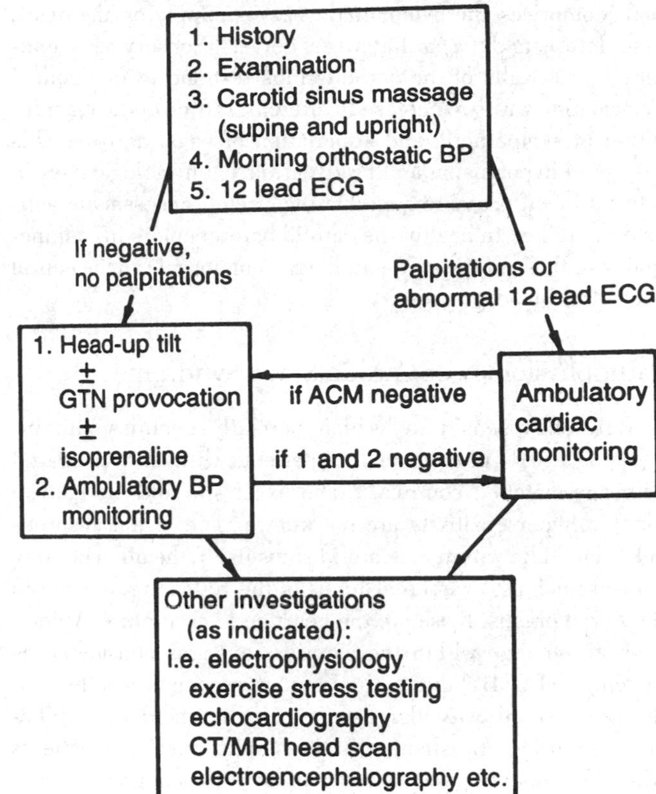

Figure 32-2 Protocol for investigation of older patients with syncope.

Carotid Sinus Syndrome

Carotid sinus syndrome is an important but frequently overlooked cause of syncope and presyncope in the elderly.[53] Episodic bradycardia and/or hypotension resulting from exaggerated baroreceptor-mediated reflexes or carotid sinus hypersensitivity (CSH) characterize the syndrome. The syndrome is diagnosed in subjects with unexplained symptoms, when 5 seconds of carotid sinus massage produces asystole exceeding 3 seconds (cardioinhibitory), or a fall in systolic blood pressure exceeding 50 mmHg in the absence of cardioinhibition (vasodepressor) or a combination of the two (mixed).[54,55] The first recognized case of CSS was reported in 1930,[56] though slowing of the heart rate in response to carotid pressure was first published in 1799.[57] However, it was only in the 1920s that the anatomy and physiology of the carotid baroreflex were described in detail.[58]

Anatomy and Physiology

The carotid sinus is the dilated portion of the internal carotid artery at the level of the carotid bifurcation.[59] The sinus wall is rich with elastic tissue. Sensory nerve endings emerge from the sinus as the carotid sinus nerve of Hering, before joining the glossopharyngeal nerve. Some of the fibers also join the vagus, hypoglossal, and cervical sympathetic nerves.[55] The afferent limb of the carotid sinus reflex terminates at the nucleus of the tractus solitarius in the medulla.[60] The efferent limb comprises the sympathetic nerves supplying the heart, vasculature, and the cardiac vagus nerve.[61] Sensory nerve endings in the walls of the carotid sinus respond to mechanical deformation with an increase in afferent traffic-producing inhibition of sympathetic and stimulation of vagal activity. This results in hypotension and bradycardia.[61] Physiologic rises in arterial blood pressure generate the stretch necessary to activate the reflex. In health, the carotid baroreceptors in conjunction with those of the aortic arch play a major role in the neural control of blood pressure.

Pathophysiology of Carotid Sinus Syndrome

Baroreflex sensitivity, which normally declines with increasing age,[62] is enhanced in patients with CSS compared with age-matched controls.[63] The exact site and mechanism for this hypersensitivity are not known. The lesion, theoretically, could lie within the carotid sinus itself, the afferent limb, central nucleus, or efferent limbs of the reflex arc, or even in the target organs, those are the heart and vasculature. Atherosclerotic change within the carotid sinus was considered as the cause of CSH[64] due to the frequent association of the syndrome with cardiovascular disease. A higher incidence of bilateral atherosclerotic changes in the carotid arteries of patients with CSS was observed using Doppler ultrasonography, compared with controls matched for atherosclerotic risk factors.[65] The frequent occurrence of CSH in the presence of neck pathology supported this theory. However, the occurrence of symptoms that are not triggered by head movement,[21] the frequent overlap with vasovagal syncope, dissociation of cardioinhibition, and vasodepression in many patients and the normal release of arginine vasopressin during hypotension (for which intact afferent connections to the hypothalamus are essential) in patients with the syndrome[66] argue against this hypothesis. The efferent limb of the reflex arc; that is the vagus nerve, is responsible for the heart rate slowing response during carotid sinus massage.[67] Vagally mediated depression of sinoatrial automaticity and sinoatrial block lead to sinoatrial arrest and asystole.[68] Atropine in a dose of 400 mcg can abolish bradycardia in 80 percent of subjects whereas 700 mcg will abolish the response in all patients.[69] Complete atrioventricular block may also occur and is reported to coexist with sinus arrest in up to 70 percent of patients.[53]

Carotid sinus syndrome and sick sinus syndrome are two separate diagnostic entities, although up to 5 percent of patients with CSS can have abnormal intrinsic sinus node function.[70] Conversely, a proportion of patients with sick sinus syndrome have altered autonomic tone.[71] It is possible that CSS results from a central abnormality of baroreflex gain.[72] The frequent association of CSS with atherosclerotic comorbidities has led to speculation that ischemia may play an important role in its pathogenesis.[73] Myocardial ischemia causing activation of vagal afferents capable of influencing central baroreflex pathways or ischemia at brain stem level may result in abnormalities of neurotransmitter function.[74] A recent hypothesis[75] suggests upregulation of central postsynaptic α_2-adrenoceptors as the primary abnormality in CSH. This upregulation may represent denervation supersensitivity of dominant postsynaptic α_2-receptors subsequent to relatively reduced afferent impulse traffic from an atherosclerosed carotid sinus.[75] Carotid sinus stimulation, during carotid sinus massage, can cause an exaggerated baroreflex-mediated efferent response, leading to hypotension (stimulation of central α_2-adrenoceptor leads to a sympatholytic effect) and (vagally mediated) bradycardia.[76]

Prevalence of Carotid Sinus Hypersensitivity and Carotid Sinus Syndrome

The prevalence of carotid sinus reflex hypersensitivity in asymptomatic individuals is not known. However, it definitely increases with age and is rare in patients with syncope who are aged less than 50 years.[77] Early reports suggested that 10 percent of the healthy aged population had carotid sinus reflex hypersensitivity and that the prevalence was even higher in the presence of coronary artery disease or hypertension.[78–81] Such studies predated the standardization of diagnostic criteria for reflex hypersensitivity and involved long periods of carotid sinus massage, leading to scepticism regarding the existence of CSS as a disease entity rather than an epiphenomenon for atherosclerotic vascular disease. However, recent studies suggest that it is not a feature of normal aging.[82] In a study of 25 healthy elderly subjects, none developed diagnostic or symptomatic cardioinhibition or vasodepression during carotid sinus massage.[82] In another series, abnormal cardioinhibition was reported in 2 percent of 288 healthy subjects (age range 17 to 84 years).[83] Carotid sinus hypersensitivity was demonstrated in 19 percent of 538 patients (age >50 years) who presented to an accident and emergency department of an inner-city university hospital with unexplained falls, the prevalence increased to 21 percent among fallers aged more than 65 years.[5] Abnormal responses to carotid sinus massage are more likely to be observed in asymptomatic individuals with coronary artery disease[73] and those on vasoactive drugs known to influence reflex sensitivity (digoxin, β-blockers, and α-methyldopa).[84–86] The prevalence of drug-induced CSH among elderly fallers was 11 percent.[5] Though it is still generally considered as a very rare condition (only 1 in a series of 204 syncopal patients[52]), referral centers that routinely perform carotid sinus massage in all older patients presenting with syncope diagnose CSS in up to 45 percent of them.[3]

Carotid Sinus Massage

Carotid sinus reflex sensitivity is assessed by measuring heart rate and blood pressure responses to carotid sinus massage. In normal subjects, carotid sinus massage induces both cardioinhibition as well as vasodepression. In a study of 25 healthy elderly subjects cardioinhibition of 1,038 (± 195) ms and vasodepression of 21 (±14) mmHg was observed following 5 seconds of carotid sinus massage.[82] No subject developed diagnostic cardioinhibition or vasodepression when supine though 12 percent of subjects had asymptomatic vasodepression of more than 50 mmHg during upright carotid sinus massage. Cardioinhibition and vasodepression were more marked on right-sided carotid sinus massage and there was no fixed relationship between rate of heart rate slowing and fall in blood pressure. In patients with cardioinhibitory CSS, over 70 percent have a positive response to right-sided carotid sinus massage either alone or in combination with left-sided carotid sinus massage.[21]

Carotid sinus massage is a crude and unquantifiable technique and is prone to intra- as well as interobserver variation. More scientific diagnostic methods using neck chamber suction[63] or drug-induced changes in blood pressure[62] can be used for carotid baroreceptor activation, but neither of these methods is suitable for routine use. The duration of carotid sinus massage was previously controversial and varied widely between investigators, with some applying this stimulus for 30 seconds.[78] However, a standardized 5 to 10 second stimulus has been accepted by most current investigators as safe and effective (maximum fall in heart rate usually occurs within 5 seconds of the onset of massage).[55,72]

Complications resulting from carotid sinus massage include cardiac arrhythmias and neurologic sequelae.[87–89] Fatal arrhythmias, both asystolic and ventricular, are extremely uncommon and have generally occurred in patients with underlying heart disease undergoing therapeutic rather than diagnostic massage.[87,90] Digoxin toxicity has been implicated in most cases of ventricular fibrillation.[53] Neurologic complications are thought to result from either occlusion of or embolization from the carotid artery. Several authors have reported cases of hemiplegia following carotid sinus stimulation, often in the absence of hemodynamic changes.[89] Complications from carotid sinus massage, however, are extremely uncommon (0.14 percent).[91] Only 12 patients, in a retrospective analysis[92] of 16,000 instances of carotid sinus massage, developed neurologic complications, which resolved within 24 hours in 8 patients and within 1 week in 2 patients. Neurologic deficits persisted in two patients. Serious ventricular arrhythmias were never encountered. Complications were immediate and in two-thirds of occasions followed a vasodepressor response to carotid sinus massage. Carotid Doppler studies in these cases did not reveal significant carotid obstruction compared to age-matched controls. It was not possible to predict either from clinical characteristics or from Doppler findings those who developed neurologic sequelae.

It has been suggested that carotid sinus massage should not be performed in patients with known cerebrovascular disease or carotid bruits unless there is a strong indication.[55] It should also be avoided immediately following myocardial infarction when reflex sensitivity may be increased.[72] It is prudent to rest patients for at least 10 minutes if there is a significant hypotensive response during the stimulus before standing them up for other tests.

Diagnostic Criteria for Carotid Sinus Syndrome

Carotid sinus syndrome should be diagnosed when CSH is documented in a patient with otherwise unexplained dizziness or syncope and in whom carotid sinus massage reproduces symptoms.[55] Three subtypes of CSH or of CSS are currently recognized. The cardioinhibitory subtype is diagnosed if carotid sinus massage produces asystole exceeding 3 seconds, the vasodepressor subtype if there is a fall in systolic blood pressure exceeding 50 mmHg in the absence of significant cardioinhibition (or 30 mmHg in the presence of symptoms), and a mixed subtype if both responses are present.[54,55,67] The independent vasodepressor response can be confirmed by repeating carotid sinus massage after abolishing significant cardioinhibition using either A-V sequential pacing or intravenous atropine.[67,93] Asystole exceeding 1.5 seconds should be regarded as "significant" in this regard. The frequency of each of the subtypes is similar. In a series of 64 consecutive cases with CSS, a third each had cardioinhibitory, vasodepressor, and mixed responses.[21] A cerebral subtype has been described in which facial pallor and symptoms of cerebral hypoperfusion occurred during massage in the absence of any hemodynamic change.[94] These changes were attributed to reflex cerebral vasoconstriction. More recently, it has been shown that such symptoms develop as a result of carotid occlusion in the presence of contralateral carotid disease and the existence of the cerebral subtype has largely been discredited.[90]

Symptom reproduction during carotid sinus massage was regarded by early investigators as essential in the diagnosis of CSS,[55] but is not always justified in patients with reproducibly abnormal responses.[53,72] Spontaneous symptoms usually occur in the upright position.[55] So it is still worth repeating the procedure, with the patient upright, even after demonstrating a positive response when supine. This aids in attributing a diagnosis with reproduction of symptoms especially in patients with unexplained falls who deny loss of consciousness and have CSH.

Clinical Characteristics

Carotid sinus syndrome is virtually unknown before the age of 50 and its incidence increases with age thereafter.[53] Males are more commonly affected and the majority have either coronary artery disease or hypertension.[95] The symptoms are usually precipitated by mechanical stimulation of the carotid sinus; that is by head turning, tight neckwear, neck pathology, and by vagal stimuli such as prolonged standing.[21,55] Other recognized triggers for symptoms are postprandial state, straining, looking or stretching upwards, exertion, defecation, and micturition. In a significant number of patients no triggering event can be identified.[95] Abnormal response to carotid sinus massage may not always be reproducible, necessitating repetition of the procedure if the diagnosis is strongly suspected.

Carotid sinus hypersensitivity is frequently associated with other hypotensive disorders such as vasovagal syncope and orthostatic hypotension,[21] indicating a common pathogenetic process. Overlap of hypotensive disorders can make attributable diagnosis more difficult. However, every attempt must be made to arrive at an attributable diagnosis as interventions may vary and methods for assessment of response depend on the initial diagnosis. Carotid sinus syndrome is associated with appreciable morbidity. Approximately one-half of patients may sustain an injury during symptomatic episodes while fractures (especially of femoral neck) were sustained by 25 percent.[21] In a prospective study of falls in nursing home residents, a threefold increase in the fracture rate in those with CSH was observed.[96] Indeed, CSH can be considered as a modifiable risk factor for fractures of the femoral neck.[97] Carotid sinus syndrome is not associated with an increased risk of death. The mortality rate in patients with the syndrome is similar to that of patients with unexplained syncope and the general population matched for age and sex.[98] Mortality rates are similar for the three subtypes of the syndrome.[98]

Natural History

The natural history of asymptomatic subjects with CSH or patients with CSS has not been well investigated. In one study, the majority (90 percent) of asymptomatic subjects remained symptom free during a mean follow-up period of 19 months while half of those who present with syncope got symptom recurrence.[99] Similar observations were made in another study where 57 percent of patients with CSS were randomized to a nontreatment protocol during an average follow-up of 36 months.[100]

Treatment

No treatment is necessary in subjects with asymptomatic CSH. However, there is no consensus on the timing of therapeutic intervention in the presence of symptoms. Considering the high rate of injury in symptomatic episodes as well as low recurrence rate of symptoms, it is prudent to treat all patients with a history of two or more symptomatic episodes. The need for intervention in those with a solitary event should be assessed on an individual basis, taking into consideration the severity of the event and the patient's lifestyle.[53]

Treatment strategies in the past included carotid sinus denervation achieved either surgically or by radioablation.[101,102] Success rates with radioablation were variable and the procedure has largely been abandoned. Surgical denervation has been reported to relieve symptoms in approximately two-thirds of patients,[55] but is not without risk of post-operative orthostatic hypotension and hypertensive crises.[101,103] Denervation surgery is still occasionally considered in patients with coexisting neck pathology[104] or with vasodepression resistant to drug therapy.[105]

The treatment of patients with cardioinhibition has largely been superseded by newer treatment modalities. Cardioinhibition can be treated with anticholinergic agents such as atropine and propantheline bromide; and some benefit has been reported.[106] However, frequent cholinergic adverse effects, particularly in the elderly, limit this treatment option.

Cardiac pacing, first used nearly a quarter of a century ago, is currently the treatment of choice in patients with symptomatic cardioinhibitory CSS. Atrial pacing is contraindicated in view of the high incidence of both sinoatrial and atrioventricular block in patients with CSH.[72] Ventricular pacing abolishes cardioinhibition but fails to alleviate symptoms in a significant number of patients. Such symptoms result from either aggravation of a coexisting vasodepressor response or the development of pacemaker-induced hypotension (pacemaker syndrome).[107] The latter occurs when ventriculoatrial conduction is intact and this is so for up to 80 percent of patients with the syndrome.[72] Atrioventricular sequential pacing is the treatment of choice for patients with symptomatic cardioinhibition. Dual-chamber pacing has been shown to result in significantly less vasodepression than ventricular pacing during both supine and upright carotid sinus massage.[108] Moreover, with maintenance of atrioventricular synchrony, there is no risk of pacemaker syndrome. Randomized double-blind studies have demonstrated that a substantial number of patients prefer atrioventricular pacing.[109,110] Both DDI and DDD pacing modes have been widely used; DDD pacing carries a theoretical risk of inducing endless loop tachycardia but this has rarely been encountered.[53] With appropriate pacing, syncope is abolished in 85 to 90 percent of patients with cardioinhibition.[72,98]

In a recent report 67 (mean age 73 years) patients with cardioinhibitory CSS were assessed for their response to treatment with modifiable rate drop response pacemaker.[111] There was a significant improvement in syncope (prepacing, 82 percent,[111] postpacing 12 percent), falls (prepacing, 31 percent; post-pacing, 11 percent) and need for hospitalization (prepacing, 43 percent, post pacing, 0), whereas 41 out of 43 patients continued to experience dizziness though the intensity of symptoms was reduced in 20 patients.

Treatment of vasodepressor CSS is less successful due to poor understanding of its pathophysiology. Ephedrine has been reported to be useful,[76] but long-term use is limited by side effects. Dihydroergotamine is effective, but poorly tolerated.[112] Fludrocortisone, a mineralocorticoid widely used in the treatment of orthostatic hypotension, is used in the treatment of vasodepressor CSS with good results, but its use is limited in the longer term by adverse effects.[113] The medical treatment of vasodepressor CSS remains unsatisfactory.

Orthostatic Hypotension

Orthostatic or postural hypotension is arbitrarily defined as either a 20 mmHg fall in systolic blood pressure or a 10 mmHg fall in diastolic blood pressure on assuming an upright posture from a supine position.[114] Orthostatic hypotension implies abnormal blood pressure homeostasis and is a frequent observation with advancing age. Prevalence of postural hypotension varies between 4[6] and 33 percent[115] among community living elderly persons depending on the methodology used. Higher prevalence and larger falls in systolic blood pressure have been reported with increasing age[116] and often signifies general physical frailty. Orthostatic hypotension is reported to be associated with excessive mortality.[117]

Physiology of Orthostasis

Orthostasis is a physiologic stress related to upright posture. On standing, the force of gravity in the vertical axis causes venous pooling in the lower limbs, a sharp decline in venous return, and reduction in filling pressure of the heart, which increase further on prolonged standing due to shifting of water to interstitial spaces and hemoconcentration.[118] These mechanical events can cause a marked reduction in cardiac output and consequent fall in arterial blood pressure. However, in normal people, cardiac output and blood pressure are maintained by powerful compensatory mechanisms involving a rise in heart rate.[119] Consequently, the fall in stroke volume is compensated for and cardiac output declines only slightly. Blood pressure is maintained by a rise in peripheral resistance. These compensatory phenomena are initiated by the baroreceptors located at the aortic arch and carotid bifurcation. The baroreceptor input to brain stem centers leads to inhibition of cardiac vagal control, stimulation of sympathetic ganglia, and release of noradrenaline from sympathetic nerve endings. Noradrenaline has a positive chronotropic and inotropic effect on the heart and also causes venous and arteriolar vasoconstriction.[120] Thus, the compensatory response to orthostasis involves stimulation of the sympathetic nervous system and inhibition of the parasympathetic nervous system, and reflects the integrity of the total arterial baroreflex arc. Orthostatic hypotension results from failure of the arterial baroreflex, most commonly due to disorders of the autonomic nervous system.[121]

Aging and Orthostasis

The heart rate and blood pressure responses to orthostasis occur in three phases: (1) an initial heart rate and blood pressure response, (2) an early phase of stabilization, and (3) a phase of prolonged standing—all are influenced by aging.[122–125] The maximum rise in heart rate and the ratio between the maximum and the minimum heart rate in the initial phase decline with age, implying a relatively fixed heart rate irrespective of posture.[123–125] Despite a blunted heart rate response, blood pressure and cardiac output are adequately maintained on standing in active, healthy, well-hydrated, and normotensive elderly subjects.[124] The underlying mechanism involves decreased vasodilatation and reduced venous pooling during the initial phases and increased peripheral vascular resistance after prolonged standing. However, in elderly subjects with hypertension and cardiovascular disease receiving vasoactive drugs, these circulatory adjustments to orthostatic stress are disturbed, rendering them vulnerable to postural hypotension.[126]

Hypertension and Orthostatic Hypotension

Aging is associated with an increased risk for hypertension as well as hypotension. Hypertension itself increases the risk of hypotension by impairing baroreflex sensitivity and reducing ventricular compliance.[127,128] A strong relationship between supine hypertension and orthostatic hypotension has been reported among unmedicated institutionalized elderly subjects.[129] Hypertension increases the risk of cerebral ischemia from sudden declines in blood pressure. Elderly hypertensives are more vulnerable to cerebral ischemic symptoms even with modest and short-term postural hypotension as their threshold of cerebral autoregulation is set at a higher level by prolonged elevation of blood pressure.[130] In addition, antihypertensive agents impair cardiovascular reflexes and further increase the risk of orthostatic hypotension.

Table 32-4 Commonly used drugs causing orthostatic hypotension

Class of Drug	Mechanism of Orthostatic Hypotension
Antihypertensives	
Calcium channel blocking agents	Vasodilatation
ACE inhibitors	Inhibition of angiotensin II production
Adrenergic nerve blocking agents	α-Adrenergic blockade
α-Adrenoceptor antagonists	α-Adrenergic blockade
Coronary vasodilators	
Nitrates	Vasodilatation
Diuretics	
Thiazide, other loop diuretics	Volume depletion
Psychotropic drugs	
Phenothiazines	α-Adrenergic blockade
Tricyclic antidepressants	α-Adrenergic blockade
Anti-Parkinsonian drugs	
Levodopa	Not clearly understood
Bromocriptine	Activation of vascular dopaminergic receptors
CNS depressants	
Ethanol	Vasodilatation

Etiology of Orthostatic Hypotension

Several pathologic conditions are associated with orthostatic hypotension. Autonomic failure[131] and drugs[132] (Table 32-4) are important causes of orthostatic hypotension. Establishing a causal relationship between a drug and orthostatic hypotension requires identification of the culprit medicine, abolition of symptoms by withdrawal of the drug, and rechallenge of the drug to reproduce symptoms.[133] Rechallenge is an important step in the diagnosis, but often omitted in clinical practice in view of the potential serious consequences. In the presence of polypharmacy, which is so common in the elderly, it becomes difficult to identify the culprit drug because of the synergistic effect of different drugs and drug interactions.[132] A number of non-neurogenic conditions are also associated with postural hypotension. They include myocarditis, atrial myxoma, aortic stenosis, constrictive pericarditis, hemorrhage, diarrhea, vomiting, ileostomy, burns, hemodialysis, salt-loosing nephropathy, diabetes insipidus, adrenal insufficiency, fever, and extensive varicose veins.

Primary Autonomic Failure Syndromes

These are three distinct clinical entities, namely: pure autonomic failure (PAF), multiple system atrophy (MSA), or Shy Drager syndrome (SDS), and autonomic failure associated with idiopathic Parkinson's disease (IPD). PAF, the least common and a relatively benign entity was previously known as idiopathic orthostatic hypotension. This condition presents with orthostatic hypotension, defective sweating, impotence, and bowel disturbances. No other neurologic deficits are found and resting plasma noradrenaline levels are low. MSA is the most common of all and carries the poorest prognosis. Clinical manifestations include features of dysautonomia and motor disturbances due to striatonigral degeneration, cerebellar atrophy, or pyramidal lesions. Additional neurologic deficits include muscle atrophy, distal sensorimotor neuropathy, pupillary abnormalities, restriction of ocular movements, disturbances in rhythm and control of breathing, life-threatening laryngeal stridor, and bladder disturbances. Psychiatric manifestations and cognitive defects are usually absent. Resting plasma noradrenaline levels are usually within the normal range but fail to rise on standing or tilting. The prevalence of autonomic failure in Parkinson's disease is not precisely known. Cerebellar and pyramidal signs are not seen. Orthostatic hypotension in Parkinson's disease can be due to factors other than dysautonomia, for example, side effects of antiparkinsonian drugs (levodopa, bromocriptine), accompanying effects of aging, autonomic neuropathy complicating coexisting diabetes mellitus, side effects of drug therapy for other coexisting diseases (vasodilators for hypertension, α-adrenergic antagonists for benign prostatic hypertrophy), and confusion with early MSA with predominant parkinsonian features.[131] Clinical manifestations of primary autonomic failure syndromes are summarized in Table 32-5.

Secondary Autonomic Dysfunction

Availability of sensitive tests of autonomic function has led to the identification of autonomic nervous system involvement in several systemic diseases. A large number of neurologic disorders are also complicated by autonomic dysfunction, which may involve several organs leading to a variety of symptoms in addition to orthostatic hypotension, namely: anhidrosis, constipation, diarrhea, impotence, retention of urine, urinary incontinence, stridor, apneic episodes, and Horner syndrome. Important among them are multiple sclerosis, brain stem lesions, compressive and noncompressive spinal cord lesions, demyelinating polyneuropathies (Guillain-Barré syndrome), diabetic polyneuropathy, chronic renal failure, chronic liver disease, and connective tissue disorders.[131] In the absence of well-recognized conditions causing primary and secondary autonomic failure, aging can also be considered as a cause of autonomic failure.

Manifestations of Orthostatic Hypotension

The clinical manifestations of orthostatic hypotension are due to hypoperfusion of the brain and other organs. Depending on the degree of fall in blood pressure and cerebral hypoperfusion, symptoms can vary from dizziness to syncope associated with a variety of visual defects, from blurred vision to blackout.[134] Other reported ischemic symptoms of orthostatic hypotension are nonspecific lethargy and weakness, suboccipital and paravertebral muscle pain, low backache, calf claudication, and angina.[134,135] Several precipitating factors for orthostatic hypotension have been identified; namely, speed of positional change, prolonged recumbency, warm environment, raised intrathoracic pressure (coughing, defecation, micturition), physical exertion, and vasoactive drugs.

Orthostatic hypotension is an important cause of syncope accounting for 14 percent of all diagnosed cases in a large series on syncope.[7] In a tertiary referral clinic dealing with unexplained syncope, dizziness and falls, 32 percent patients (age >65 years) had orthostatic hypotension.[3] Irrespective of symptoms, orthostatic hypotension increases the risk of falls in elderly patients. Nineteen percent of elderly fallers attending an accident and emergency department had a diagnosis of orthostatic hypotension.[20] Orthostatic hypotension was the cause of "drop attacks" in 15 percent of 35 elderly patients (age >50 years) and probably contributed to unexplained falls in a similar proportion of patients.[136]

The diagnosis of orthostatic hypotension involves a demonstration of a postural fall in blood pressure after active standing. Reproducibility of orthostatic hypotension depends on the time of measurement and on autonomic function.[1] The diagnosis may be missed on casual measurement during the afternoon. The procedure should be repeated during the morning after maintaining supine posture for an adequate period (10 minutes). Sphygmomanometer measurement is as sensitive as sophisticated phasic blood pressure measurements and active standing is as diagnostic as head-up tilting.[1] In patients with unexplained syncope or falls, an attributable diagnosis of orthostatic hypotension depends on reproduction of symptoms.

Table 32-5 Clinical manifestations of primary autonomic failure syndromes

	Autonomic Dysfunction	Extra-Pyramidal Signs	Pyramidal Signs	Olivoponto-cerebellar Signs
Pure autonomic failure	+++	−	−	−
Idiopathic Parkinson's disease	−	+++	−	−
Parkinson's disease plus autonomic failure	++	+++	−	−
Multiple system atrophy	+++	++	+	+
Dementia of Lewy body type	++	++	+	−

Management of Orthostatic Hypotension

The goal of therapy for symptomatic orthostatic hypotension is to improve cerebral perfusion. There are several nonpharmacologic interventions for orthostatic hypotension that include avoidance of precipitating factors for low blood pressure, elevation of the head of the bed at night,[137] and application of graduated pressure from a support garment to the lower limbs to reduce venous pooling. There are reports to suggest benefit from implantation of cardiac pacemakers, in a small number of patients, by increasing heart rate during postural change.[138] However, the effects of tachypacing on improving cardiac output in patients with maximal vasodilatation remains conjectural. A large number of drugs have been used to raise blood pressure in orthostatic hypotension. Of all of these agents three drugs are commonly used. They include fludrocortisone, midodrine, and desmopressin (DDAVP). Fludrocortisone (9-α-fluhydrocortisone) in a dose of 0.1 to 0.2 mg, causes volume expansion, reduces natriuresis, and sensitizes α-adrenoceptors to noradrenaline. The drug is poorly tolerated in larger doses and for long periods. Reported adverse effects in the elderly include hypertension, cardiac failure, depression, edema, and hypokalemia.[139] Midodrine is a directly acting sympathomimetic vasoconstrictor of resistance vessels. Treatment is started at a dose of 2.5 mg three times daily and requires gradual titration to a maximum dose of 45 mg per day. The adverse effects include pilomotor erection, gastrointestinal symptoms, and cardiovascular and central nervous system toxicity. Side effects are usually controlled by dose reduction. Midodrine is comparable in its efficacy with other sympathomimetic agents, but better tolerated. In a recent double-blind placebo controlled trial, midodrine was found to be an effective and well-tolerated treatment for moderate to severe orthostatic hypotension.[140] It significantly increased standing blood pressure and improved symptoms of orthostatic hypotension. Side effects were mostly mild and only 7 percent of patients discontinued treatment due to supine hypertension. DDAVP has potent antidiuretic and mild pressor effects. Intranasal doses of 5 to 40 μ at bedtime are useful. One side effect is water retention. This agent can be combined with fludrocortisone with synergistic effect. The drug treatment for orthostatic hypotension requires frequent monitoring for supine hypertension, electrolyte imbalance, and congestive heart failure.

Neurocardiogenic Syncope

Clinical Characteristics

The hallmark of neurocardiogenic or vasovagal syncope is hypotension and/or bradycardia sufficiently profound to produce cerebral ischemia and loss of neural function. Vasovagal syncope has been classified into cardioinhibitory (bradycardia), vasodepressor (hypotension), and mixed (both) subtypes depending on the blood pressure and heart rate response.[141] In most patients, the manifestations occur in three distinct phases: a prodrome or aura, loss of consciousness, and postsyncopal phase.[142] A precipitating factor or situation is identifiable in most patients which include extreme emotional stress, anxiety, mental anguish, trauma, physical pain or anticipation of physical pain (e.g., anticipation of venesection), sight of blood, accident, warm environment, air travel, and prolonged standing. The most common triggers in older individuals are prolonged standing and vasodilator medication.[3] In the authors' experience, drug-induced syncope is more often due to vasovagal syncope than orthostatic hypotension. Some patients experience symptoms in specific situations, namely: micturition, defecation, and coughing. Prodromal symptoms include extreme fatigue, weakness, diaphoresis, nausea, visual defects, visual and auditory hallucinations, dizziness, vertigo, headache, abdominal discomfort, dysarthria, and paresthesias. The duration of prodrome varies greatly from seconds to several minutes, during which patients take actions such as lying down to avoid an episode. The syncopal period is usually brief, during which patients may develop involuntary movements from tonic-clonic movements to myoclonic jerks. Recovery is usually rapid, but patients can experience protracted symptoms such as confusion, disorientation, nausea, headache, dizziness, and a general sense of ill health.

Pathophysiology of Neurocardiogenic Syncope

The normal physiologic responses to orthostasis, as described earlier, are an increase in heart rate, rise in peripheral vascular resistance (increase in diastolic blood pressure), and minimal decline in systolic blood pressure, to maintain an adequate cardiac output. In patients with neurocardiogenic syncope, these responses to prolonged orthostasis are paradoxical. The precise sequence of events leading to neurocardiogenic syncope are not fully understood. The possible mechanism involves a sudden fall in venous return to the heart, rapid fall in ventricular volume, and virtual collapse of the ventricle due to vigorous ventricular contraction.[30,143] The net result of these events is stimulation of ventricular mechanoreceptors and activation of the Bezold-Jarisch reflex leading to peripheral vasodilatation (hypotension) and bradycardia.[143] Negative inotropic agents (β-blockers, disopyramide) can avert or diminish these responses in spontaneous or head-up tilt-induced neurocardiogenic syncope.[144] Several neurotransmitters, namely serotonin, endorphins, and arginine vasopressin, play an important role in the pathogenesis of neurocardiogenic syncope, possibly by central sympathetic inhibition, although their exact role is not yet well understood.

Healthy elderly subjects are not particularly prone to neurocardiogenic syncope compared to younger adults. Due to an age-related decline in baroreceptor sensitivity, the paradoxical responses to orthostasis (as in neurocardiogenic syncope) are possibly less marked in elderly subjects. Thus, situational syncope is less common in old age. However, in the presence of hypertension and atherosclerotic cerebrovascular disease, excessive loss of baroreflex sensitivity leads to dysautonomic responses to prolonged orthostasis (in which blood pressure and heart decline steadily over time) and patients become susceptible to neurocardiogenic syncope. Diuretic or age related contraction of blood volume further increases the risk of syncope.

Diagnosis

Several methods have evolved over the years to determine an individual's susceptibility to vasovagal syncope such as the Valsalva maneuvers, hyperventilation, and ocular compression. However, these methods are poorly reproducible and lack correlation with clinical events. Using the strong orthostatic stimulus of head-up tilting and maximal venous pooling, reflex neurocardiogenic syncope can be reproduced in a susceptible individual in the laboratory. Head-up tilting as a diagnostic tool was first reported in 1986[145] and since then validity of this technique to identify susceptibility to neurocardiogenic syncope has been established.[146–150] Syncope induced by head-up tilting has several similarities with neurocardiogenic syncope, namely: the basic sequence of blood pressure and heart rate changes, changes in plasma catecholamine levels prior to syncope and prodromal symptoms. A classification of vasovagal responses to head-up tilting has been suggested by some investigators as outlined in the following sections.[141]

Type 1—mixed

Heart rate rises on head-up tilting and later falls at the time of syncope with ventricular rate 40 bpm or less for less than 10 seconds with or without asystole for 3 seconds. Blood pressure may rise initially with tilting, but then falls before the heart rate falls.

Type 2a—cardioinhibitory

Heart rate rises on head-up tilting, but then falls at the time of syncope with ventricular rate less than 40 bpm for more than 10 seconds or asystole occurs for more than 3 seconds. Blood pressure may rise initially with tilting but then falls before the heart rate falls.

Type 2b—cardioinhibitory

Heart rate rises on head-up tilting and then falls at the time of syncope with ventricular rate less than 40 bpm for more than 10 seconds or asystole occurs for more than 3 seconds. Blood pressure may rise initially with tilting but only falls to hypotensive levels (less than 80 mmHg systolic) at or after the onset of rapid and severe heart rate fall as defined above.

Type 3—pure vasodepressor

Heart rate rises progressively after adoption of the head-up position and does not fall more than 10 percent from its peak at the time of syncope. Blood pressure falls during tilt to cause syncope. There are a few exception to these criteria: (1) chronotropic incompetence: no heart rate rise during head-up tilting possibly due to underlying sinoatrial disease; (2) excessive heart rate rise: excessive heart rate rise both at the onset and through out the head-up tilt (> 130 bpm), can be associated with types 1 to 3 due to different pathophysiology; and (3) association of carotid sinus hypersensitivity with any of the subtypes.

The sensitivity of head-up tilting can be further improved by provocative agents that accentuate the physiologic events leading to vasovagal syncope. The most widely used agent is intravenous isoprenaline, which enhances myocardial contractility by stimulating β-adrenoreceptors. Isoprenaline is infused, prior to head-up tilting, at a dose of 1 mcg per minute and gradually increased to a maximum dose of 5 mcg per minute to achieve a heart rate increase of 25 percent.[42] Though the sensitivity of head-up tilt testing improves by about 15 percent,[151] the specificity is reduced.[42,43] In addition as a result of the decline in β-receptor sensitivity with age isoprenaline may be less useful as a provocative agent in elderly patients with a higher incidence of adverse effects.[152] The other agent which can be used as a provocation is nitroglycerin which, by reducing venous return due to vasodilatation, can enhance the vasovagal reaction in susceptible individuals. The drug can be administered by intravenous infusion,[46] but more conveniently sublingually[45,153] with improved sensitivity and reduced period of tilting. The positivity of head-up tilting can also be improved by intravenous cannulation,[47] providing a useful provocative stimulus without any adverse effects.

The precise sensitivity of head-up tilting is difficult to determine as no gold standard is available for comparison. However, the estimated sensitivity of head-up tilting in various reports is between 30 percent and 80 percent.[41,143,154] Vasovagal syncope can be produced by head-up tilting in less than 10 percent of healthy elderly subjects.[155–157] Healthy young subjects are more likely to experience syncope compared to elderly controls reflecting declining baroreflex sensitivity in old age.[154] Specificity of head-up tilting must be considered with the fact that neurocardiogenic syncope results from a normal (though exaggerated) reflex response, which can be induced in most individuals with proper conditioning. Therefore, it must be recognized that in the absence of recurrent and unexplained syncopal symptoms, the value of positive head-up tilt is limited. Head-up tilt testing has a symptomatic reproducibility of 80 to 90 percent in patients with recurrent syncope.[157–160] Thus, in symptomatic patients this test has great value in assessing the efficacy of intervention.

Treatment

Patient education involving avoidance of precipitating factors, vasodilator drugs, and taking evasive action for example, lying down, during prodromal symptoms has great value in avoiding many episodes of vasovagal syncope. However, many patients experience symptoms without warning, and these require drug therapy. A number of drugs are reported to be useful in alleviating symptoms. β-Blockers (atenolol 50 mg/day) by their negative inotropic actions decrease the force of ventricular contraction, and thereby reduce the degree of mechanoreceptor discharge, and are useful in vasovagal syncope.[42] Disopyramide (200 mg twice daily) by its negative inotropic and anticholinergic effects,[161] transdermal scopolamine (1 patch every 3 days) by its anticholinergic effects,[150] and fludrocortisone (100 to 200 mcg/day) by its volume expanding effect,[143] are of value in neurocardiogenic syncope. Recent reports suggest that serotonin antagonists such as fluoxetine (20 mg/day) and sertraline hydrochloride (25 mg/day) are effective in symptom relief.[162] The efficacy of midodrine in the management of vasovagal syncope has been recently observed in a double-blind randomized controlled trial.[163] More than 50 percent of patients experienced significant symptomatic improvement, delayed response to head-up tilting, and improvement in quality of life. Midodrine presumably acts by reducing peripheral venous pooling and thereby improving cardiac output. Elastic support hose and relaxation techniques (biofeedback) are useful adjuvant therapy in neurocardiogenic syncope. Permanent cardiac pacing has been used in some patients,[164] dual chamber pacing being the preferred mode of pacing.[165] However, pacing influences the bradycardia component of the response and not vasodilatation and hypotension, which frequently dominate. Its utility is limited in some instances to prolongation of the prodrome in order to allow other evasive action.[166]

Postprandial Hypotension

The effect of meals on the cardiovascular system was appreciated from post-prandial exaggeration of angina which was demonstrated objectively by deterioration of exercise tolerance following food.[167] Postprandial reductions in blood pressure manifesting as syncope and dizziness were subsequently reported[168,169] leading to extensive investigation of this phenomenon. In healthy elderly subjects, systolic blood pressure falls by 11 to 16 mmHg,[170–172] and heart rate rises by 5 to 7 bpm[170,171] 60 minutes after variously composed meals of varying energy content. However, the change in diastolic blood pressure is not as consistent. In elderly subjects with hypertension, orthostatic hypotension, and autonomic failure, the postprandial blood pressure fall is much greater with no corresponding rise in heart rate.[173] These responses are marked if the energy and simple carbohydrate content of the meal is high.[174] However, in the majority of fit as well as frail elderly subjects, most of these hypotensive episodes go unnoticed. Postprandial physiologic changes include increased splanchnic and superior mesenteric artery blood flow at the expense of peripheral circulation[175] and a rise in plasma insulin levels[174,176,177] without corresponding rises in sympathetic nervous system activity. Vasodilator effects of insulin[178] and other gut peptides, namely, neurotensin and VIP, are thought to be responsible for postprandial hypotension although the precise mechanism remains uncertain. The clinical significance of a fall in blood pressure after meals is difficult to quantitate. However, postprandial hypotension is causally related to recurrent syncope and falls in elderly subjects.[8,179,180] In this authors' experience postprandial hypotension occurs in at best 20 percent of patients with orthostatic hypotension. A reduction in simple carbohydrate content of food, its replacement with complex carbohydrates, and frequent small meals are effective interventions for postprandial hypotension. Drugs useful in the treatment are indomethacin,[181] octreotide,[182] and caffeine.[183,184] Given orally along with food, caffeine prevents hypotensive symptoms in fit as well as frail elderly subjects.[185,186]

Consequences of Syncope

Adverse consequences of syncope can be summarized as: (1) hazards related to the underlying cause, (2) hazards related to the trauma of fall, and (3) risk borne by others from a syncopal episode.

The Underlying Cause

The risk of death in an elderly individual who had at least one syncopal episode is approximately 27 percent over the ensuing 2 years (compared to 8 percent in younger subjects).[7] The risk of death increases to 38 percent if the underlying cause is cardiovascular, whereas it is 11.6 percent in the case of a non cardiovascular cause and 20.4 percent if no specific cause is established. The expected mortality, for comparison, from all causes for a cohort drawn from the general population between the ages 70 to 72 is 4.1 percent (for the original cohort) and 5.9 percent for those who reach the age of 70 years.[187]

The Trauma of Fall

Information on trauma brought on by syncope is very scant. The rate of injury per episode of fall may be as high as 35 percent. Of these, one-sixth of injuries are serious—namely, fracture, subdural hematoma, and injury to internal organs.[4,188] Other obvious consequences of syncope are hospitalization, anxiety, depression, institutionalization, and automobile accidents. The psychological impact of syncope has not been well evaluated. The functional disability is comparable to that seen in arthritis, emphysema, or diabetes mellitus in its effect on employment, driving and interpersonal relationships.[189] Fear of falling can lead to a debilitating spiral of loss of confidence, limitation of mobility, and restriction of social activities and loss of independence.[190]

Risk Borne by Others From a Syncopal Episode

The risk of hazards to others in the vicinity of the patients are sometimes very serious. This is best exemplified by the threat of automobile accidents if the driver suffers from an episode of syncope.

References

1. Ward C, Kenny RA: Reproducibility of orthostatic hypotension in symptomatic elderly. Am J Med 1996;100:418–422

2. Kenny RA, Traynor G: Carotid sinus syndrome: clinical characteristics in elderly patients. Age Ageing 1991;20: 449–454
3. McIntosh SJ, DaCosta D, Kenny RA: Outcome of an integrated approach to the investigation of dizziness, falls and syncope in elderly patients referred to a syncope clinic. Age Ageing 1993;22:53–58
4. Day SC, Cook EF, Funkenstein H, Goldman L: Evaluation and outcome of emergency room patients with transient loss of consciousness. Am J Med 1982;72:15–23
5. Richardson DA, Shaw FE, Bond J, Kenny RA: Prevalence of carotid sinus hypersensitivity among unexplained fallers presenting to an accident and emergency department. PACE 1997;20:820–823
6. Lipsitz LA, Wei JY, Rowe JW: Syncope in an elderly, institutionalised population: prevalence, incidence and associated risk. Q J Med 1985;55:45–55
7. Kapoor W, Snustad D, Peterson J et al: Syncope in elderly. Am J Med 1986;80:419–428
8. Lipsitz LA, Pluchino FC, Wei JY, Rowe JW: Syncope in institutionalised elderly: the impact of multiple pathological conditions and situational stress. J Chron Dis 1986;39: 619–630
9. Lipsitz LA: Altered blood pressure homeostasis in advanced age: clinical and research implications. J Gerentol 1989;44: 179–183
10. Crane MG, Harris JJ: Effect of ageing on renin activity and aldosterone secretion. J Lab Clin Med 1976;87:947–959
11. Epstein M, Hollenberg MK: Age a determinant of renal sodium conservation in normal man. J Lab Clin Med 1976;87: 411–417
12. Strandggard S, Oleseng J, Skinhoj E, Sassenn A: Altered regulation of brain circulation in severe arterial hypertension. Br Med J 1973;1:507–510
13. Dermksian G, Lamb LE: Syncope in a population of healthy young adults: incidence mechanism and significance. J Am Coll Cardiol 1958;168:122–127
14. Murdoch BD: Loss of consciousness in healthy South African men: incidence, causes and relationship to ECG abnormality. S Afr Med J 1980;57:771–774
15. Schilinford JP: Syncope. Am J Cardiol 1970;26:609–612
16. Friedberg CK: Syncope: pathologic physiology, differential diagnosis and treatment. Mod Concepts Cardiovasc Dis 1971; 40:54–63
17. Wright KE Jr, McIntosh HD: Syncope: a review of pathophysiologic mechanisms. Prog Cardiovasc Dis 1971;13:580–594
18. Rubenstein LZ, Robbins AS, Josephson KR et al: The value of assessing falls in an elderly population. Ann Int Med 1990; 113:308–316
19. Lipsitz LA: Abnormalities in blood pressure homeostasis that contribute to falls in the elderly. Clin Geriatr Med 1985;91: 637–648
20. Davies AJ, Kenny RA: Falls presenting to the accident and emergency department: types of presentation and risk factor profile. Age Ageing 1996;25:362–366
21. McIntosh SJ, Lawson J, Kenny RA: Clinical characteristics of vasodepressor, cardioinhibitory and mixed carotid sinus syndrome in the elderly. Am J Med 1993;95:203–208
22. Cummings SR, Nevitt MC, Kidd S: Forgetting falls: the limited accuracy of recall of falls in the elderly. J Am Geriatr Soc 1988;36:613–616
23. Lempert T, Bauer M, Schmidt D: Syncope: a videometric analysis of 56 episodes of transient cerebral hypoxia. Ann Neurol 1994;36:233–237
24. Aronow WS, Ahn C: Postprandial hypotension in 499 elderly persons in a long term health care facility. J Am Geriatr Soc 1994;42:930–932
25. Besdine RW: Geriatric medicine: an over view. Ann Rev Gerontology 1980;1:135–153
26. Dimant T: Accidents in the skilled nursing facility. NY State J Med 1985;85:202
27. Drachman DA, Hart CW: An approach to the dizzy patient. Neurology 1972;22:323–324
28. Lawson J, Birchall JP, Fitzgerald J, Kenny RA: Benefits of an integrated diagnostic approach to the investigation of dizziness in the community. Age Ageing 1994;23:19
29. Patel A, Maloney A, Damato AN: On the frequency and reproducibility of orthostatic blood pressure changes in healthy community dwelling elderly during 60 degrees head-up tilt. Am Heart J 1993;126:184–188
30. Streeten DP, Andersen GH Jr, Richardson R, Deaver TF: Abnormal orthostatic changes in blood pressure and heart rate in subjects with intact sympathetic nervous function: evidence for excessive venous pooling. J Lab Clin Med 1988;111: 326–335
31. Camn AJ, Evans KE, Ward DE, Martin A: The rhythm of the heart in active elderly subjects. Am Heart J 1980;99:598–603
32. McIntosh SJ, Lawson J, Reeve P, Kenny RA: Clinical variables which predict the outcome of cardiovascular tests in the elderly: A modified investigation profile for older syncopal patients. Age Ageing 1994;23:19
33. Bass EB, Curtis EI, Arena VC et al: The duration of Holter monitoring in patients with syncope: is 24 hours enough? Arch Intern Med 1990;150:1073–1078
34. Kapoor WN: Diagnostic evaluation of syncope. Am J Med 1991;90:91–106
35. Gibson TC, Heitzman MR: Diagnostic efficiency of 24 hour electrocardiographic monitoring for syncope. Am J Cardiol 1984;53:1013–1017
36. Cumbe SR, Pryor RE, Linzer M: Cardiac loop ECG recording a new non-invasive diagnostic test in recurrent syncope. South Med J 1990;80:39–43
37. Frazier HW: The diagnosis of syncope in the elderly. Int J Tech Assess Health Care 1993;9:102–111
38. Strasberg B, Sagie A, Rechavie E et al: The non-invasive evaluation of syncope of suspected cardiovascular origin. Am Heart J 1989;117:160–163
39. Senard JM, Charmontin B, Rascol A, Montastruc JL: Ambulatory blood pressure in patients with Parkinson's disease without and with orthostatic hypotension. Clin Autonomic Res 1992;2:99–104
40. Mathias CJ, Armstrong E, Browse N et al: Value of non-

invasive continuous blood pressure monitoring in the detection of carotid sinus hypersensitivity. Clin Auton Res 1991;1: 157–159

41. Benditt D, Remole S, Bailin S et al: Tilt table testing for evaluation of neurally mediated syncope: rationale and proposed protocols. PACE 1991;14:1528–1537
42. Almquist A, Goldenberg I, Milstein S et al: Provocation of bradycardia and hypotension by isoproterenol and upright posture in patients with unexplained syncope. N Engl J Med 1989; 320:346–351
43. Kapoor WN, Brant N: Evaluation of syncope by upright tilt testing with isoproterenol. A nonspecific test. Ann Int Med 1992;116:358–368
44. Kapoor WN, Smith MA, Miller NL: Upright tilt testing in evaluating syncope: A comprehensive literature review. Am J Med 1994;97:78–88
45. McIntosh SJ, Lawson J, Kenny RA: Use of sublingual GTN as a provocative test for vasovagal syncope. Cardiol Elderly 1996; 4:33–37
46. Raviele A, Gasparini G, diPede F et al: Usefulness nitroglycerin infusion during head-up tilt for the diagnosis of vasivagal syncope. J Am Coll Cardiol 1993;21:111A
47. McIntosh SJ, Lawson J, Kenny RA: Intravenous cannulation alters the specificity of head-up tilt testing for vasovagal syncope in elderly patients. Age Ageing 1994;23:317–319
48. Taylor R: Metabolic and endocrine causes of syncope. In Chapman and Hall (eds): Syncope in the older patient. 1996
49. Doherty JU, Pembrook-Rogers D, Grogan EW et al: Electrophysiologic evaluation and follow-up characteristics of patients with recurrent unexplained syncope and presyncope. Am J Cardiol 1985;55:703–708
50. Surgue DD, Holmes DR, Gresh BJ et al: Impact of intracardiac electrophysiologic testing on the management of elderly patients with syncope or near syncope. J Am Geriatr Soc 1987; 35:1079–1083
51. Denes P, Uretz E, Ezri MD, Borbola J: Clinical predictor of electrophysiologic findings in patients with syncope of unknown origin. Arch Int Med 1988;146:1922–1928
52. Kapoor W, Karp FM, Wieand S et al: A prospective evaluation and follow up of patients with syncope. N Engl J Med 1983; 309:197–204
53. Strasberg B, Sagie A, Erdman S et al: Carotid sinus hypersensitivity and the carotid sinus syndrome. Prog Cardiovasc Dis 1989;31:379–391
54. Franke H: Uber das Karotissinus-Syndrome und den Sogenannten Hyperaktiven Karotissinus-Reflex. Friedrich-Karl Schattauer-Verlag, Stuttgart, 1963
55. Thomas JE: Disease of the carotid sinus—syncope. pp. 532–551. In Vinken PJ, Bruyn GW, (ed) Handbook of Clinical Neurology, Vol 11. North-Holland, Amsterdam, 1972
56. Roskam J: Un syndrome nouveau. Syncopes cardiaques graves et syncopes repetees par hyperreflectivite sinocarotidienne. Presse Med 1930;38:590–591
57. Parry CH: An Enquiry into Symptoms and Causes of Syncope Anginosa, Commonly Called Angina Pectoris. R Cruttwell, Bath, 1799
58. Hering HE: Der Sinus caroticus an der ursprungsstelle der carotis interna als ausgangsort eines hemmenden herzreflexes und eines depressorischen gefassreflexes. Munch Med Wschr 1924;71:701–704
59. Binswanger O: Anatomische untersuchungen uber die ursprungsstelle und den anfongstheil der carotis interna. Arch Psych Nervenkr 1879;9:351–368
60. Crill WE, Reis DJ: Distribution of carotid sinus and depressor nerves in cat brainstem. Am J Physiol 1968;214:269–276
61. Thomas JE: Hyperactive carotid sinus reflex and carotid sinus syncope. Mayo Clin Proc 1969;44:127–139
62. Bristow D, Honour J, Pickering GW et al: Diminished baroreflex sensitivity in high blood pressure. Circulation 1969;39: 48–54
63. Dehn TCB, Morley CA, Sutton R: A scientific evaluation of the carotid sinus syndrome. Cardiovasc Res 1984;18:746–751
64. Salomon S: The carotid sinus syndrome. Am J Cardiol 1958; 2:342–350
65. Wiedermann G, Grotz J, Bewermeyer H et al: High-resolution real-time ultrasound of the carotid bifurcation in patients with hyperactive carotid sinus syndrome. J Neurol 1985;232: 318–325
66. Kenny RA, Lyon CC, Ingram AM et al: Enhanced vagal activity and normal arginine vasopressin response in carotid sinus syndrome: implications for a central abnormality in carotid sinus hypersensitivity. Cardiovasc Res 1987;21:545–550
67. Walter PF, Crawley IS, Dorney ER: Carotid sinus hypersensitivity and syncope. Am J Cardiol 1978;42:396–403
68. Gang ES, Oseran DS, Mandel WJ, Peter T: Sinus node electrogram in patients with the hypersensitive carotid sinus syndrome. J Am Coll Cardiol 1985;5:1484–1490
69. Kenny RA, McIntosh SJ, Wynne H: Pattern of inhibition of parasympathetic activity in response to incremental bolus doses of atropine in the carotid sinus syndrome. Clin Autonom Res 1994;4:63–66
70. Morley CA, Hudson WM, Kwok HT et al: Is there a difference between carotid sinus syndrome and sick sinus syndrome? Br Heart J 1983;49:620–621
71. Brignole M, Menozzi C, Gianfranchi L et al: Naturally mediated syncope detected by carotid sinus massage and head-up tilt test in sick sinus syndrome. Am J Cardiol 1991;68: 1032–1061
72. Morley CA, Sutton R: Carotid sinus syncope [editorial]. Int J Cardiol 1984;6:287–293
73. Brown KA, Maloney JA, Smith HC et al: Carotid sinus reflex in patients undergoing coronary angiography: relationship of degree and location of coronary artery disease to response to carotid sinus massage. Circulation 1980;62:697–703
74. Wentink JRM, Jansen RWMM, Hoefnagels WHL: The influence of age on the response of blood pressure and heart rate to carotid sinus massage in healthy volunteers. Cardiol Elderly 1993;1:453–459
75. O'Mahony D: Pathophysiology of carotid sinus hypersensitivity in elderly patients. Lancet 1995;346:950–952
76. Almquist A, Gornick C, Benson DW et al: Carotid sinus hyper-

sensitivity: evaluation of the vasodepressor component. Circulation 1985;71:927–936

77. Nathanson MH: Hyperactive cardioinhibitory carotid sinus reflex. Arch Intern Med 1946;77:491–502
78. Heidorn GH, McNamara AP: Effect of carotid sinus stimulation on the electrocardiograms of clinically normal individuals. Circulation 1956;14:1104–1113
79. Sigler LH: The hyperactive cardioinhibitory carotid sinus reflex as an aid in the diagnosis of coronary disease. N Engl J Med 1942;226:46–51
80. Smiddy J, Lewis D, Dunn M: The effect of carotid sinus massage in older men. J Gerontol 1972;27:209–211
81. Sigler LH: Hyperactive vasodepressor carotid sinus reflex. Arch Intern Med 1942;70:983–1001
82. McIntosh SJ, da Costa D, Lawson J, Kenny RA: Heart rate and blood pressure responses to carotid sinus massage in healthy elderly subjects. Age Ageing 1994;23:57–61
83. Brignole M, Gigli G, Altomonte F et al: Cardioinhibitory reflex provoked by stimulation of carotid sinus in normal subjects and those with cardiovascular disease. G Ital Cardiol 1985; 15:514–519
84. Quest JA, Gillis RA: Effect of digitalis on carotid sinus baroreceptor activity. Circ Res 1974;35:247–255
85. Reyes AJ: Propanolol and the hyperactive carotid sinus reflex syndrome. Br Med J 1973;2:662
86. Bauerfeind Hall C, Denes P, Rosen KM: Carotid sinus hypersensitivity with alpha methyldopa. Ann Int Med 1978;88: 214–215
87. Hilal H, Massumi R: Fatal ventricular fibrillation after carotid sinus stimulation. N Engl J Med 1966;275:157–158
88. Askey J: Hemiplegia following carotid sinus stimulation. Am Heart J 1946;31:131–137
89. Calverley JR, Millikan CH: Complications of carotid manipulation. Neurology 1961;11:185–189
90. Lown B, Levine SA: The carotid sinus: clinical value of its stimulation. Circulation 1961;23:766–789
91. Munro NC, McIntosh SJ, Lawson J et al: Incidence of complications after carotid sinus massage in older patients with syncope. J Am Geriatr Soc 1994;42:1248–1251
92. Davies AJ, Haslam P, Richardson DA, Kenny RA: Complications of carotid sinus massage: a review of patient characteristics. Age Ageing; 1997;26:60
93. Stryjer D, Friedensohn A, Schlesinger Z: Carotid sinus hypersensitivity: diagnosis of vasodepressor type in the presence of cardioinhibitory type. PACE 1982;5:793–800
94. Weiss S, Baker JP: The carotid sinus reflex in health and disease: its role in the causation of fainting and convulsions. Medicine (Baltimore) 1933;12:297–354
95. Draper AJ: The cardioinhibitory carotid sinus syndrome. Ann Int Med 1950;32:700–716
96. Murphy AL, Rowbotham BJ, Boyle RS et al: Carotid sinus hypersensitivity in elderly nursing home patients. Aust N Z Med 1986;16:24–27
97. Ward C, McIntosh S, Kenny RA: The prevalence of carotid sinus syndrome in elderly patients with fractured neck of femur (abst). Age Ageing 1993;23(suppl 1):A16
98. Brignole M, Oddone D, Cogorno S et al: Long-term outcome in symptomatic carotid sinus hypersensitivity. Am Heart J 1992; 123:687–692
99. Blanc JJ, Boshat J, Penther P: Hypersensibilite sino-carotidienne. Evolution a moyen terme en fonction du traitement et des symptomes. Arch Mal Coeur 1984;77:330–336
100. Brignole M, Menozzi C, Lolli G et al: Long-term outcome of paced and nonpaced patients with severe carotid sinus syndrome. Am J Cardiol 1992;69:1039–1043
101. Trout HH, Brown LL, Thompson JE: Carotid sinus syndrome treatment by carotid sinus denervation. Ann Surg 1979;189: 575–580
102. Greeley HP, Smedal MI, Morset W: The treatment of the carotid sinus syndrome by irradiation. N Engl J Med 1955;252: 91–94
103. Ford FR: Fatal hypertensive crisis following denervation of the carotid sinus for the relief of repeated attacks of syncope. Case history. Bull Johns Hopkins Hosp 1957;100:14–16
104. Frank JI, Ropper AH, Zuniga G: Vasodepressor carotid sinus syncope associated with a neck mass. Neurology 1992;42: 1194–1197
105. Wenger TL, Dohrmann ML, Strauss HC: Hypersensitive carotid sinus syndrome manifested as cough syncope. PACE 1980;3:332–339
106. Sugrue DD, Gersh BJ, Holmes DR et al: Symptomatic "isolated" carotid sinus hypersensitivity: natural history and results of treatment with anticholinergic drugs or pacemaker. J Am Coll Cardiol 1986;7:158–162
107. Morley CA, Perrins EJ, Grant P et al: Carotid sinus syncope treated by pacing. Analysis of persistant symptoms and role of atrioventricular sequential pacing. Br Heart J 1982;47: 411–418
108. Madigan NP, Flaker GC, Curtis JJ et al: Carotid sinus hypersensitivity: beneficial effects of dual-chamber pacing. Am J Cardiol 1984;53:1034–1040
109. McIntosh SJ, Lawson J, Bexton RS et al: A study comparing UVI and DDI pacing in elderly patients. Heart 1997;77: 553–557
110. Morley CA, Perrins EJ, Chan SL, Sutton R: Longterm comparison of DDI and VVI pacing in carotid sinus syndrome. pp. 929–935. In Steinbach K, Gloggar D, Laszkowicz A et al. (eds): Proceedings of the VIIth World Symposium on Cardiac Pacing. Steinkopff-Verlag, Darmstadt, 1983
111. Davies AJ, Bexton RS, Kenny RA: Retrospective analysis of RDR pacing in carotid sinus syndrome. (Submitted to PACE)
112. Morley CA, Perrins EJ, Sutton R: Pharmacological intervention in the carotid sinus syndrome. PACE 1983;6:A16
113. da Costa D, McIntosh S, Kenny RA: Benefits of fludrocortisone in the treatment of symptomatic vasodepressor carotid sinus syndrome. Br Heart J 1993;69:308–310
114. Mathias CJ, Bannister R: Investigation of autonomic disorders. pp. 255–290. In Bannister R, Mathias CJ (eds): Autonomic Failure: A Textbook of Clinical Disorders of the Autonomic Nervous System. Oxford Medical Publications, Oxford, 1992
115. Palmer KT: Studies into postural hypotension in elderly patients. N Z Med J 1983;96:43–45

116. Caird FI, Andrews GR, Kennedy RD: Effect of posture on blood pressure in the elderly. Br Heart J 1973;35:527–530

117. Schatz IJ, Masaki KH, Burchfiel CM et al: Orthostatic hypotension (OH) as a predictor of two year mortality in elderly men; the Honolulu heart program. Clin Autonomic Res 1995;5:321

118. Sjostrand T: Regulation of the blood distribution in man. Acta Physiol Scand 1952;26:312

119. Ziegler MG: Postural hypotension. Ann Rev Med 1980;31: 239–245

120. Rowe JW, Troen BR: Sympathetic nervous system and ageing in man. Endocrinol Rev 1980;1:167–179

121. Bannister R, Mathias CJ: Clinical features and manifestations and investigation of primary autonomic failure syndromes. pp. 531–547. In Autonomic Failure: A Textbook of Clinical Disorders of the Autonomic Nervous System. Bannister R, Mathias CJ (eds): Oxford Medical Publications, Oxford, 1992

122. Wieling W, van Brederode JFM, deRijk LG et al: Reflex control of heart rate in normal subjects in relation to age: a data base for cardiac vagal neuropathy. Diabetologia 1982;22: 163–166

123. Wieling W: Laboratory assessment of disturbances in cardio vascular control. pp. 47–71. In Kenny RA (ed): Syncope in the Older Patient: Causes, Investigations and Consequences of Syncope and Falls. Chapman & Hall, London, 1996

124. Imholz BPM, Dambrink JHA, Karemaker JM, Wieling W: Orthostatic circulatory control in the elderly evaluated by non-invasive continuous blood pressure measurement. Clin Sci 1990;79:73–79

125. Wieling W, Veerman DP, Dambrink JHA, Imholz BPM: Disparieties in circulatory adjustment to standing between young and elderly subjects explained by pulse contour analysis. Clin Sci 1992;83:149–155

126. Van Dijk JG, Tjon-A-Tsien AML, Kamjoul BA et al: Effect of supine blood on interpretation of standing up test in 500 patients with diabetes mellitus. J Autonom Nerv Syst 1994;47: 23–31

127. Gribbin B, Pickering TG, Sleight P, Peto R: Effect of age and blood pressure on baroreflex sensitivity in man. Circ Res 1971; 29:424–431

128. Lakatta EG: Do hypertension and aging have a similar effect on myocardium. Circulation 1987;75:169–177

129. Lipsitz LA, Storch HA, Minaker KL, Rowe JW: Intra-individual variability in postural blood pressure in the elderly. Clin Sci 1985;69:337–341

130. Strandgaard S: Autoregulation of cerebral blood flow in hypertensive patients: the modifying influence of prolonged antihypertensive treatment on the tolerance to acute drug induced hypotension. Circulation 1976;53:720–727

131. Mathias CJ: The classification and nomenclature of autonomic disorders: ending chaos, resolving conflict and hopefully achieving clarity. Clin Autonom Res 1995;5:307–310

132. Wynne HA, Schofield S: Drug induced orthostatic hypotension. pp. 137–154. In Syncope in the Older Patient: Causes, Investigations and Consequences of Syncope and Falls. Kenny RA (ed): Chapman & Hall, London, 1996

133. Naranjo CA, Busto U, Sellers EM et al: A method of estimating the probability of adverse drug reactions. Clin Pharmacol Ther 1981;30:239–245

134. Mathias CJ: Primary autonomic failure in association with other neurological features: the syndromes of Shy-Drager and multiple system atrophy. pp. 237–248. In Kenny RA (ed): Syncope in the Older Patient: Causes, Investigations and Consequences of Syncope and Falls. Chapman & Hall, London, 1996

135. Bleasdale-Barr K, Mathias CJ: Suboccipital (coat hanger) and other muscular pains: frequency in autonomic failure and other neurological problems, and association with postural hypotension. Clin Autonom Res 1994;4:82

136. Dey AB, Stout NR, Kenny RA: Cardiovascular syncope is the commonest cause of drop attacks in the older patient. Eur JCPE 1996;2:84–88

137. Bannister R, Ardill L, Fentem P: An assessment of various methods of treatment of idiopathic orthostatic hypotension. Q J Med 1969;38:377–395

138. Moss AJ, Glaser W, Topol E: Atrial tachypacing in the treatment of a patient with primary orthostatic hypotension. N Engl J Med 1980;302:1456–1457

139. Hussain RM, McIntosh S, Lawson J, Kenny RA: Fludrocortisone in the treatment of hypotensive disorders in the elderly. Heart 1996;76:507–509

140. Jankovic J, Gilden JL, Hiner BC et al: Neurogenic orthostatic hypotension: a double blind placebo controlled study with midodrine. Am J Med 1993;95:38–48

141. Sutton R, Petersen M, Brignole M et al: Proposed classification for tilt induced vasovagal syncope. Eur J Cardiac Pacing Elelctrophysiol 1992;2:180–183

142. Wayne HH: Syncope: physiologic considerations and an analysis of the clinical characteristics in 510 patients. Am J Med 1961;30:418–438

143. Samoil D, Grubb BP: Vasovagal (neurally mediated) syncope: pathophysiology, diagnosis, and therapeutic approach. Eur J Cardiac Pacing Electrophysiol 1992;2:234–241

144. Rea R: Neurally mediated hypotension and bradycardia: which nerves? How mediated. J Am Coll Cardiol 1989;14: 1663–1664

145. Kenny RA, Ingram A, Bayliss J, Sutton R: Head-up tilt is a usefull tool for investigating unexplained syncope. Lancet 1986;2:1352–1354

146. Fitzpatric A, Sutton R: Tilting towards a diagnosis in unexplained recurrent syncope. Lancet 1989;1:658–660

147. Grubb BP, Temesy -Armos P, Hahn H, Elliot L: Utility of head upright tilt table testing in the evaluation and management of syncope of unknown origin. Am J Med 1991;90:6–10

148. Strasburg B, Rechavia E, Sagie A et al: Usefulness of head-up tilt table test in evaluating patients with syncope of unknown origin. Am Heart J 1989;118:923–927

149. Raviele A, Gasparini G, DePede F et al: Usefulness of head-up tilt table test in evaluating syncope syncope of unknown origin and negative electrophysiologic study. Am J Cardiol 1989;65:1322–1327

150. Abi-Samara F, Maloney J, Fouad FM, Castle L: The usefulness

of head-up tilt table testing and hemodynamic investigations in the workup of syncope of unknown origin. PACE 1987;10: 406–410

151. Grubb BP, Samoil D: Neurocardiogenic syncope. pp. 91–106. In Kenny, RA (ed): Syncope in the Older Patient: Causes, Investigations and Consequences of Syncope and Falls. Chapman & Hall, London, 1996
152. Brignole M, Menozzi C, Gianfranchi L et al: Carotid sinus massage eyeball compression and head-up tilt test in patients with syncope of uncertain origin and in healthy control subjects. Am Heart J 1991;122:1651–1664
153. Raviele A, Menozzi C, Brignole M et al: Value of head-up tilt testing with sublingual nitroglycerin to assess the origin of unexplained syncope. Am J Cardiol 1995;76:267–272
154. Fish F, Benson DW: Tilt testing for unexplained syncope. Primary Cardiol 1992;18:87–97
155. Shvartz E: Relaibility of quantifiable tilt table data. Aerospace Med 1968;39:1094–1096
156. Shvartz E, Meyerstein N: Tilt tolerance of young men and women. Aerospace Med 1970;41:253–255
157. Fitzpatrick AP, Theodorakis G, Vardas P, Sutton R: Methodology of head upright tilt table testing in patients with unexplained syncope. J Am Coll Cardiol 1991;17:125–130
158. Chen XC, Chen MY, Remole S et al: Reproducibility of head upright tilt table testing for elliciting susceptibility to neurally mediated syncope in patients without structural heart disease. Am J Cardiol 1992;69:755–760
159. Sheldon R, Spelaniski J, Koestner J et al: Reproducibility of isoproterenol tilt table testtests in patients with syncope. Am J Cardiol 1992;69:1300–1305
160. Grubb BP, Wolfe D, Temesy Amos P et al: Reproducibility of tilt table test results in patients with syncope. PACE 1992; 15:1477–1481
161. Milistein S, Buetikofer J, Lesser J et al: Usefulness of disopyramide for prevention of upright tilt induced hypotension and bradycardia. Am J Cardiol 1990;65:1339–1344
162. Grubb BP, Wolfe DA, Samoil D et al: Usefulness of fluoxetine hydrochloride for prevention of resistant upright tilt induced syncope. PACE 1993;16:458–464
163. Ward C, Gilroy J, Bishop J, Kenny RA: Midodrine in vasovagal syncope: a randomised controlled trial. Heart 1997 (in press)
164. Fitzpatrick A, Theodorakis R, Ahmed T et al: Dual chamber pacing aborts vasovagal syncope induced by head-up 60 degree tilt. PACE 1991;14:13–19
165. Samoil D, Grubb BP. Brewster P et al: Comparison of single and dual chamber pacing techniques in prevention of head upright tilt induced vasovagal syncope. Eur J Pacing Electrophysiol 1993;1:36–41
166. Grubb BP, Wolfe D, Samoil D et al: Adaptive rate pacing controlled by right ventricular pre-ejection interval for severe refractory orthostatic hypotension. PACE 1993;16:801–805
167. Goldstein RE, Redwood DR, Rosing DR et al: Alterations in the circulatory response to exercise following a meal and their relationship to post prandial angina pectoris. Circulation 1971; 44:90–100
168. Seyer-Hansen K: Postprandial hypotension. Br Med J 1977; 2:1262
169. Lipsitz LA, Nyquist RP, Wei JY, Rowe JW: Postprandial reduction in blood pressure in the elderly. N Engl J Med 1983; 309:81–83
170. Lipsitz LA, Fullerton KJ: Postprandial blood pressure reduction in healthy elderly. J Am Geriatr Soc 1986;34:267–270
171. Westenend M, Lenders JWM, Thein T: The course of blood pressure after a meal: a difference between young and elderly subjects. J Hypertens 1985;3:S417–419
172. Peitzman SJ, Berger SR: Postprandial blood pressure decrease in well elderly persons. Arch Int Med 1989;149:286–288
173. Jansen RWMM, Penterman BJM, vanLier HJJ, Hoefnagels WHL: Blood pressure reduction after oral glucose loading and its relation to age, blood pressure and insulin. Am J Cardiol 1987;60:1087–1091
174. Potter JF, Heseltine D, Hartley G et al: Effects of meal composition on the postprandial blood pressure, catecholamine and insulin changes in eldely subjects. Clin Sci 1989;77:265–272
175. Sidery MB, Cowley AJ, Macdonald IA: Cardiovascular responses toa high fat and high carbohydrate meal in healthy elderly subjects. Clin Sci 1993;84:263–270
176. Jansen RWMM, Peeters TL, vanLier HJJ, Hoefnagles WHL: The effect of oral glucose, protein, fat and water loading on blood pressure and the gastrointestinal peptides VIP and somatostatin in hypertensive elderly subjects. Eur J Clin Invest 1990;20:192–198
177. Heseltine D, Dakak M, Macdonald IA et al: Effects of carbohydrate type on postprandial blood pressure, neroendocrine and gastrointestinal hormone changes in the elderly. Clin Autonom Res 1991;1:219–224
178. Mathias CJ, daCosta DF, Fosbraey P et al: Hypotensive and sedative effects of insulin in autonomic failure. Br Med J 1987; 295:161–163
179. Jonsson PV, Lipsitz LA, Kelly M, Koestner J: Hypotensive responses to common daily activities in institutionalized elderly. Arch Int Med 1990;150:1518–1524
180. Vaitkevicius PV, Esserwein DM, Maynard AK et al: Frequency and importance of postprandial blood pressure reduction in elderly nursing-home patients. Ann Int Med 1991;115: 865–870
181. Robertson D, Wade D, Robertson RM: Postprandial alterations in cardiovascular hemodynamics in autonomic dysfunctional states. Am J Cardiol 1981;48:1048–1052
182. Raimbach SJ, Cortelli P, Kooner JS et al: Prevention of glucose induced hypotension by the somatostatin analogue octreotide (SMS 201–995) in chronic autonomic failure, hemodynamic and hormonal changes. Clin Sci 1989;77:623–628
183. Haigh R, Fotherby M, Harper G et al: Duration of caffeine abstention influences the acute blood pressure response to caffeine in elderly normotensives. Eur J Clin Pharmacol 1993; 44:549–553
184. Potter JF, Haigh R, Harper G et al: Blood pressure, plasma catecholamine and renin response to caffeine in elderly hypertensives. J Hum Hypertens 1993;7:273–278

185. Lenders JWM, Morre HLC, Smits P, Thien TH: The effect of caffeine on the postprandial fall in blood pressure in the elderly. Age Ageing 1988;17:236–240

186. Heseltine D, Dakak M, Woodhouse K et al: The effect of caffeine on postprandial hypotension in the elderly. J Am Geriatr Soc 1991;39:160–164

187. National Center for Health Statistics: Vital Statistics of the US vol 2. Public Health Service, Washington DC, 1990

188. Kapoor WN: Evaluation and outcome of patients with syncope. Medicine 1990;69:160–175

189. Linzer M, Pontinen M, Gold DT et al: Impairment of physical and psychological function in recurrent syncope. J Clin Epidemiol 1991;44:1037–1043

190. Vellas B, Cayla F, Bocquet H et al: Prospective study of restriction of activity in old people after falls. Age Ageing 1987;16:189–193

CHAPTER 33

Headache and Facial Pain

C. CLOUGH
G. SALDHANA

Wolff prefaced the first edition of his now famous handbook with the pertinent observation that, "Headache may be equally intense whether its implications are malignant or benign, and though there are few instances in human experience where so much pain may mean so little in terms of tissue injury, failure to separate the ominous from the trivial may cost life or create paralysing fear."

The extent of the headache problem is difficult to evaluate as few epidemiologic studies have been carried out. In 1 year in the US, 70 percent of the general population had a headache, 5 percent of whom sought medical attention.[1] Less is known about the frequency of headache in the elderly, although in a large population based study carried out in East Boston, Massachusetts.[2] some 17 percent of patients over 65 years of age reported frequent headache with 53 percent of women and 36 percent of men reporting headache in the previous year. There is thus a preponderance of females over males.[2] The prevalence in the elderly age group ranged from 5 to 50 percent.[3,4] Overall, headache appears to be less frequently reported in the elderly population[5] and shows a decline with age.[2] Most studies agree that the prevalence of primary headache syndromes declines with increasing age.[6–9] One obvious limitation of these studies is that none is longitudinal and so may not differentiate an effect of aging from cohort or period effects. In addition, elderly patients may complain less or the emergence of other more serious problems may have suppressed the reporting of a benign symptom such as headache.

In elderly people headache is more likely to represent organic pathology.[10] This was confirmed by a clinic-based retrospective case record study[11] that concluded that while it was less likely that the elderly would attend a hospital as outpatients for diagnosis of headache, there was a tenfold increase in the likelihood of finding organic pathology. Recruitment bias is a problem in these studies. Nevertheless, it is likely that headache is a more serious complaint from the elderly.

A large lifetime prevalence study[12] utilizing a population-based questionnaire found that while migraine and tension-type headache appeared to decrease with increasing age, chronic tension headache has significantly higher prevalence rates in the elderly.

The authors conclude that headache remains an extremely common condition of the elderly, much of it has benign origin, but more care needs to be taken with older patients to rule out underlying pathology especially when they present for the first time.

Migraine

Migraine is an episodic disorder that is diagnosed from the history. Epidemiologic studies are difficult to carry out and dogged by numerous problems.[13] There has been much controversy whether migraine headache and tension headache are separate entities or different points on a continuum of headache disorder.[14] Only 5 percent of migraine sufferers consult specialists[15] and so clinic-based studies will suffer from referral bias. Despite this limitation, a number of population-based studies have been carried out.[16–18] Criteria for the diagnosis of headache have been developed by the International Headache Society[19] and there has been evaluation of these criteria.[20]

Rasmussen[16] did not find a decrease in migraine prevalence with increasing age in contrast to the findings of Stewart et al.[17] who also showed that it is uncommon for migraine to start in the elderly.[9] The female preponderance of migraine persists in this age group.[15]

Diagnosis and Treatment

The diagnosis of migraine has improved since the adoption of the criteria of the International Headache Society.[19] Migraine is now classified into two main forms, migraine with aura (formerly "classical migraine") and migraine without aura (formerly "common migraine"). Other varieties of migraine include ophthalmoplegic migraine, retinal migraine, and complications of migraine such as migrainous infarction (a neurologic deficit not reversible in 7 days) and status migrainosis (an attack of headache or aura lasting >72 hours). Migraine aura can exist without headache and the same patient may at different times experience headache with aura, headache without aura, and aura without headache.[21,22]

To diagnose certain migraine without aura five attacks are needed, each lasting 4 to 72 hours and having two of the following four characteristics: unilateral location, pulsating quality, moderate or severe intensity, and aggravation by routine physical activity. In addition, the attacks must have at least one of the following: nausea and/or vomiting and/or photophobia and phonophobia.

Migraine with aura is diagnosed when there have been at least two attacks with any three of the following features: one or more fully reversible aura symptoms; aura developing over more than 4 minutes; aura lasting less than 60 minutes; and headache following aura with a free interval of less than 60 minutes.

A simpler working definition for the clinical diagnosis of migraine was proposed by Solomon and Lipton.[23] A positive diagnosis could be made on any two of the following four symptoms: unilateral headache, pulsating quality, nausea, photophobia, and phonophobia. A similar headache must have occurred in the past and structural disease excluded.

Migraine attacks may generally be divided into five phases: the prodrome (hours or days before the headache); the aura (migraine with aura); the headache; the headache termination; and the postdrome phase.[24] Symptoms of the prodrome may include mental, neurologic and/or general (constitutional, autonomic) symptoms. The patients may experience depression, euphoria, irritability, restlessness, mental slowness, hyperactivity, and drowsiness. General symptoms may include a feeling of coldness, sluggishness, thirst, anorexia, diarrhea, constipation, fluid retention, and food cravings. Photophobia and phonophobia may also occur.

The aura is a group of neurologic symptoms that precede or accompany the attack. They may be visual, sensory, or motor and may also cause language or brain stem disturbance. Headache usually occurs within 60 minutes of the end of the aura,[19] but may begin with the aura. Most patients may have more than one type of aura and progress from one type to another.

Common visual symptoms are the positive phenomena such as hemianopic photopsia (flashes of light) and teichopsia or fortification spectra. Scotomota may follow. Complex visual distortions and hallucinations are reported, but are more common in younger patients.[21]

Sensory phenomena, typically paresthesia with anatomical march of symptoms may occur and motor disturbance may result in hemiparesis. Aphasia has also been reported.[7,25]

Acephalgic migraine is an entity characterized by the neurologic dysfunction of the aura but without headache. This is strictly a diagnosis of exclusion especially in the elderly. These so-called migraine accompaniments may occur for the first time in the older age group[26] and can be easily confused with transient ischemic attacks (TIAs) except in the most classic of cases. Migraine with aura and acephalgic migraine can both be confused with TIAs and vice versa. Headache occurred with 36 percent of TIAs in one series.[65] Migrainous aura in the elderly presents a particularly difficult diagnostic dilemma. Transient hemiparetic or hemisensory symptoms occurring in the elderly for the first time should be assumed to be vascular (i.e. TIA) in etiology until proved otherwise. Alternating hemisensory/paretic symptoms are more likely to be migrainous, but still could have an embolic cause. Investigation including carotid Doppler studies and echocardiography will be necessary to manage potentially treatable embolic sources. Visual disturbance is more likely to be helpful as fortification spectra and colored zigzag lines are unlikely to occur in straightforward TIAs and are almost always migrainous in origin. Migraine with aura can occur for the first time in the elderly and may reflect the development of vascular change. It is often helpful in these cases to elicit a previous history of common migraine earlier in life.

The headache of migraine is typically throbbing in nature and exacerbated by exercise.[27] The pain may be unilateral in 60 percent of cases, but bilateral at the outset in up to 40 percent.[7] Unilateral headache may later become bilateral during the attack. The intensity is moderate to severe and pain may radiate down the neck to the shoulder. Some 40 percent of migraine sufferers report short-lived jabs of pain lasting seconds and having a "needle"-like quality, the so called "ice pick" pains.[28]

The common accompanying symptoms of nausea and vomiting may make it difficult for the patient to take oral medication. There is usually photophobia and phonophobia; many patients retire to a dark room for rest. Constitutional, mood, and mental changes are universal[7] and the patient is usually left feeling tired and washed out for a variable period of time after the attack.

Basilar migraine is a variant characterized by brain stem dysfunction such as ataxia, dysarthria, diplopia, vertigo, nausea and vomiting, and alteration in cognition and consciousness. Headache is invariable. In the elderly these symptoms should be assumed to be of vascular origin until proven otherwise.

Ophthalmoplegic migraine is rare and can be confused with the presentation of berry aneurysm. Attacks of migraine-like pain occur around the eye with oculomotor nerve dysfunction and dilatation of the pupil. The ophthalmoplegia may last from hours to months and the differential diagnosis includes orbital inflammatory disease and diabetic mononeuropathy.

Migraine attacks may vary in frequency from a few a year to one or more a week. Trigger factors include foods such as chocolates, red wine, cheese, lack of sleep, and stress. Environmental triggers include flickering lights, noise, and even certain types of weather. Head injury may lead to migraine attacks.

Once the diagnosis has been established, reassuring the patient may suffice. Any obvious precipitating cause such as diet, lack of sleep or environmental factors should be discussed. Relaxation therapy may be helpful but special diets have little place in management.

Pharmacotherapy includes treatment of the acute attack and consideration of prophylactic therapy. Acute treatment should be started by the patient at the outset of an attack, and is best limited to simple soluble analgesics such as paracetamol or aspirin. Combination analgesics such as coproxamol should be avoided, if possible, because of side effects and risk of addiction. For more severe headache, nonsteroidal anti-inflammatory drugs are used.[29] Ibuprofen (200 mg tds) may be obtained without prescription or naproxen (250 mg tds) by prescription or diclofenac 75 mg twice daily. This group of drugs should

Table 33-1 Drugs of use in the treatment of migraine[a]

Migraine Attack Treatments	Migraine Prophylaxsis
Soluble aspirin	Propranolol
Soluble paracetamol	Pizotifen
Antiemetics such as domperidone suppositories	Calcium antagonists
Nonsteroidal anti-inflammatory drugs	Methysergide
Sumatriptan (subcutaneous or oral)	Sodium valproate
Medihaler ergotamine and other ergotamine preparations	
Combination analgesia	

[a] *Care must be taken with possible interactions with pre-existent treatments and conditions such as asthma (if β-blockers are to be prescribed). The table lists medication in order of preference.*

be administered with caution in the elderly because of the increased risk of serious gastrointestinal hemorrhage especially when there is a past history of peptic ulceration[30,31] or renal insufficiency. Table 33-1 lists drugs used to treat migraine.

For moderate to severe migraine not responding to simple analgesia sumatriptan can be tried. The initial dose is 50 mg orally and can be increased to 100 mg if there is no response. Subcutaneous self administration is the preferred route when there is significant nausea or vomiting. Sumatriptan is a $5HT_1$ agonist and is thought to act as a selective cerebral vasoconstrictor. Up to 80 percent of patients obtain relief from headache within 2 hours after an injection[32] and up to 65 percent after a tablet dose.[33] The advantage is that the drug may be administered at any point during an attack and repeated if necessary. Flushing, tingling in the neck and head, and chest tightness can occur in up to 5 percent of patients.[34] Because it may cause coronary vasoconstriction it is contraindicated in patients with ischemic heart disease, Prinz-metal's variant angina, and uncontrolled hypertension. Special care in the elderly is required because the loss of subcutaneous fat may lead to intramuscular injection and more rapid absorption. In addition to pharmacotherapy most patients derive benefit from rest and sleep.

Ergotamine preparations are best reserved for occasional (>1 month interval) severe headaches. It is a potent vasoconstrictor and is best avoided in patients with a history of vaso-occlusive disease, peripheral vascular disease, hypertension, and those on β-blockers or with a history of Raynaud's phenomenon. Patients should be encouraged strongly to avoid overuse of these drugs, because it can lead to resistant headaches and perpetuate a vicious cycle of increasing ergot use and increasing headache. Admission for drug withdrawl is required when this occurs.

The accompanying symptoms of nausea and vomiting are often as disabling as the headache and require treatment in their own right. Metoclopramide is the most commonly used antiemetic and by promoting gastric emptying aids absorption of coadministered medication. It can cause extrapyramidal side effects especially in the elderly. Domperidone is less likely to cause this problem as it does not cross the blood brain barrier but does not aid gastric emptying.

Prophylactic therapy is indicated when there is severe recurrent headache causing disruption to daily life; as a guide, more than two severe headaches per month. Various drugs are used including β-blockers, antidepressants, serotonin antagonists, calcium-channel blockers, and occasionally anticonvulsants. Treatment is started at a low dose and built to maintenance. Possible side effects should be discussed and the regimen kept as simple as possible as many patients in this age group are likely to have coexistent medication. Patients should be weaned from therapy every 4 to 6 months.

Of the β-blockers, propranolol, metoprolol, timolol, nadolol, and atenolol have all been shown to be effective in up to 60 to 80 percent of patients producing a greater than 50 percent reduction in attack frequency.[35] The starting dose of propranolol is usually 20 mg bd and the top dose 160 mg daily. Patients may complain of fatigue, dizziness, nightmares, and cold extremities and care should be taken when there is peripheral vascular disease and combination with ergotamine.

The tricyclic antidepressants have been used in migraine prophylaxis although the evidence for their efficacy is largely based on anecdotal reports or uncontrolled trials. Their effect in headache may be independent of their antidepressant effect.[36,37] Amitriptyline is most commonly used although fluoxetine, a newer atypical tricyclic, has fewer anticholinergic side effects and causes less weight gain.[38] Because of their common side effect of drowsiness, the tricyclics are administered at the lowest effective dose at bedtime and slowly increased as necessary. The elderly are more vulnerable to the muscarinic side effects. The typical starting dose for amitriptyline should be 10 mg increasing to 150 mg if needed.

Calcium-channel antagonists are not licensed for migraine prophylaxis in the UK, but have been shown to be of benefit.[35] The mechanism of action of these compounds in migraine is uncertain and side effects are common including edema, flushing, dizziness, and not infrequently an initial increase in headache frequency. Improvement of headache may require several weeks of treatment.[39]

Of the serotonin antagonists the two mostly commonly prescribed drugs are pizotifen and methysergide. Pizotifen is a $5HT_2$ antagonist that is usually commenced in a dose of 0.5 mg at night and increased in stepwise manner to a dose of 4.5 mg. It has mild antidepressant activity, but unfortunately stimulates appetite and leads to weight gain if diet is not controlled. It can produce beneficial effects in 40 to 79 percent of patients.[40] Methysergide is also a $5HT_2$ antagonist with some affinity for the $5HT_1$ receptor. It is effective prophylaxis in up to 60 percent of migraine, possibly with better results in those with migraine with aura.[41] Side effects are common and include myalgia, weight gain, nausea, and hallucinations (especially after the first dose). The complication of retroperitoneal, endocardial, and pulmonary fibrosis is rare and prevented by stopping treatment for 3 to 4 weeks every 4 to 6 months that the patient is being treated. The starting dose is 1 mg at night but may be increased to 6 mg daily in divided dose.

Feverfew (*Tenacetum parthenium*) is a herbal remedy long used for headache treatment. It has limited effect and the side effects include mouth ulceration and loss of taste.[42,43]

Tension Headache

The Classification Committee of the International Headache Society, 1988, define episodic tension headache as recurrent headaches lasting for 30 minutes to 7 days with fewer than 15 headache days per month and at least two of the following pain characteristics:

1. Pressing/tightening (non pulsating) quality
2. Mild or moderate intensity
3. Bilateral location
4. Nonaggravation by walking stairs or similar routine physical activity

There should not be photophobia and phonophobia, although either alone is permitted within the definition. Patients should not experience nausea or vomiting (although the IHS criteria allow for nausea but not vomiting in the diagnosis of chronic tension type headache). Chronic tension headache has similar characteristics to the episodic form, but with a frequency of more than 15 headache days per month for more than 6 months. In both types of headache there may be pericranial muscle tenderness with or without increased electromyographic activity, although this does not imply that muscle tension is the cause of the headache.[44] In all age groups tension-type headache is the most common form of headache. However, only 5 percent of patients with chronic tension-type headache report onset after the age of 60 years.[45] Within all age groups tension headache remains more common in females.[16]

The pain of tension-type headache is usually described as a constant ache that is infrequently pulsatile. Patients may describe a tight band about the head or a sensation of wearing a tight cap. There may be associated stiffness of the neck and upper back; in contrast to migraine the pain is usually of lesser intensity. Scalp tenderness may lead to avoidance of hair brushing. This symptom is also recorded in migraine sufferers and it may persist for some days after the headache has subsided.[46] The headache may be unilateral or bilateral, commonly occipital or frontal, but may involve any site. It can be relieved by changing position.

Patients with episodic tension headache may experience pericranial muscle tenderness with palpable nodules.[47] Depression, anxiety, and other psychological factors are important in the pathogenesis of tension headache though not infrequently patients may initially deny any role.

Depression is common in the community at large, and in an average family practice in the UK is the fourth most commonly diagnosed disorder.[48] The headache associated with depression can have features described for tension-type headache and the headaches are often present for years or even through out the patient's life. The headache is typically diurnal, usually worse in the morning and in the evening. There may be identifiable emotional, physical, and psychic complaints. These problems merit attention in their own right especially in the elderly when organic pathology is more likely anyway. The presence of severe depression in the elderly may be easily overlooked. Other headache associated with depression can be described more bizarrely with almost a delusional tone. Such headaches may indicate serious psychiatric disorder and should lead to urgent psychiatric referral.

Treatment of tension headache includes reassurance, simple analgesia as abortive treatment for the acute attack, and treatment of any psychopathology that may be present. Paracetamol is the drug of choice and amitryptyline may be added as appropriate. The latter is especially useful when sleep disturbance is a prominent symptom. Fluoxetine in a dose of 20 mg daily is less sedating. Monoamine amine oxidase inhibitors should be avoided if possible. Psychiatric help may be appropriate though its need is often initially rejected by patients. Relaxation therapy and biofeedback may also have a role.

The mixed headache syndrome, that is, migraine and tension-type headache in the same patient, usually responds to treatment with tricyclic antidepressants with the addition of analgesia for acute episodes.

Headache Arising From the Neck

Cervical spondylosis, affecting the neck vertebrae, has a strong association with age.[49] Degenerative changes lead to a loss of intervertebral height with narrowing of the central canal and the intervertebral foramina. Spondylotic changes may compress cervical nerves and or spinal cord and lead to symptoms and signs. Symptomatic cervical spondylosis is more common in men than women and produces symptoms typically in the fifth and sixth decades. Neck pain and headache may result and although most of the population over the age of 40 years has radiologic changes consistent with cervical spondylosis without symptoms, in those with symptomatic disease (brachalgia or myelopathy) 40 percent reported headache as a chief symptom and 25 percent reported it as a major symptom.[50] Overall cervical spondylosis is an uncommon cause of headache.

The head pain resulting from cervical degenerative disease is frequently occipital in distribution, but may radiate to the vertex or even the frontal area. The greater occipital nerve (C2) provides much of the sensory input from the back of the head and irritation of this nerve typically causes occipital headache. The pain is usually described as constant, nonthrobbing, and of moderate intensity. Associated muscle tenderness, perhaps secondary to spasm, may be present and this may make differentiation from tension headache difficult. It is disputed whether the cervical spine itself gives rise to headache per se, but headache may arise as a secondary phenomenon due to muscle spasm in the neck.[49] Movements of the cervical spine may aggravate the headache and examination will reveal reduced range of movement and suboccipital tenderness with muscle spasm.

Treatment is usually conservative with the use of a cervical collar and analgesia. Collars should be used only for weeks and combined with referral to a physiotherapist for neck exercises. Surgery is considered when there is myelopathy or radiculopathy especially when progressive.

Lesion of the bones of the upper cervical spine and base of skull can give rise to occipital ache by pressure on the cervical nerves. Myeloma, osteomyelitis, metastatic tumor, and erosive inflammatory disease, such as rheumatoid arthritis, may all cause headache and neurologic deficit. Paget's disease can cause basilar invagination with traction on the upper cervical nerves and or hydrocephalus, both of which may result in headache.[50]

Sinus Disease and Dental Disease

Head and facial pain may be referred from the cranial sinuses. Experiments have shown that inflammation of the sinus lining is rarely painful, but that pain arises from inflammation of the ducts and ostia of the sinuses or inflammation of the nasal turbinates.[51] Disease of the frontal sinuses causes ache localized over these sinuses; that of the antrum is usually referred to the maxillary region and into the zygomatic or temporal areas. Headache associated with sphenoidal and ethmoidal disease is mainly felt behind the eyes and over the vertex of the skull.

The pain of sinus disease is usually deep-seated and dull, aching, and nonpulsatile. Adopting a recumbent position may relieve the headache of sinus disease and so these headaches are less prominent at night than during the day. Pain may be exacerbated by shaking the head or adopting a head down position. Coughing or straining also exacerbates the pain by raising intracranial venous pressure. The treatment of sinusitis is symptomatic with decongestants and analgesia, but unremitting pain may indicate a more sinister cause and merits further investigation.

Dental disease is referred to the distribution of the trigeminal nerve. In general upper jaw disease is referred to the maxillary division and lower jaw disease to the mandibular division. The etiology of such pain is usually obvious, but continued facial pain may merit referral to a maxillofacial surgeon. Examination of the patient with facial pain includes assessment of the teeth and a search for tooth sensitivity with percussion.

Facial Neuralgias and Atypical Facial Pain

Trigeminal Neuralgia

Trigeminal neuralgia is diagnosed clinically. It rarely begins before the age of thirty.[52,53] The symptoms are pathognomonic. The pain is periodic, of high intensity, and lancinating in nature, lasting from 20 to 30 seconds followed by a period of relief lasting a few seconds to a minute, which may be followed by further paroxysms of pain. The pain usually commences in the maxillary and mandibular divisions of the trigeminal nerve and in less than 5 percent of cases begins in the ophthalmic division. In some 10 to 15 percent of cases all the divisions are involved and the symptoms may be bilateral in 3 to 5 percent.[54] Apart from the quality and characteristic site of pain the patient usually can identify trigger factors such as brushing the teeth, washing the face, shaving, biting, chewing, or even a gust of cold wind on the face. Avoidance behavior is common. Slightly more females than males are affected.

The pain may occur daily for weeks or months followed by remission of varying periods; unfortunately, there is a tendency for the disorder to deteriorate, with increased frequency of attacks increasingly resistant to treatment. Clinical examination should be normal, and any loss of facial sensation prompt investigation, preferably MRI of the skull, to rule out a compressive lesion of the trigeminal nerve.

The etiology of this condition is unexplained. The presence of chronic irritation of the roots of the trigeminal nerve has been demonstrated to cause neuralgia. This may also with more peripheral lesions. Animal laboratory data, however, are more consistent with a central mechanism mediated by the loss of segmental inhibition within the spinal trigeminal sensory nucleus. To reconcile these observations, Fromm and Colleagues[55] proposed that spontaneous peripheral activity from the irritated nerve, in the presence of the failure of the normal central inhibitory mechanisms, may cause paroxysmal bursts of neuronal activity within the trigeminal nucleus and in thalamic relays perceived as neuralgia by the patient. This has been likened to a form of "sensory reflex epilepsy."[56] Some evidence for the peripheral component of this hypothesis comes from the common finding of vascular loops in association with the nerve root in a majority of symptomatic patients.[57] Because vessels tend to become more ectactic with age this may explain why the condition is "more" common with increasing age.

The treatment of this condition is firstly medical.[58–60] Occasionally, the symptoms are so severe that hospital admission is required to control symptoms and prevent a downward spiral of increasing pain and depression.

The drugs of choice are anticonvulsants and it is usual to begin with carbamazepine. Pain relief is usually obtained within 4 to 24 hours. Carbamazepine is commenced at 100 mg three times daily and increased every 48 hours in a stepwise manner until symptom relief or side effects occur. Patients should be warned of the potential for drowsiness, rash, and unsteadiness. A baseline full blood count is recommended because leucopenia does occur commonly and agranulocytosis rarely. Treatment is stopped immediately if the latter occurs. Although carbamazepine is usually effective at blood levels of 25 to 50 μL, the dose can be titrated to the maximum tolerated in resistant cases. Therapy should be maintained until the patient has been free of pain for at least 4 weeks after which slow reduction of dose by decrements of 100 mg of carbamazepine each week may allow for complete withdrawal of the drug.

If adequate pain relief is not obtained with standard doses of carbamazepine, then a second drug such as baclofen 10 mg three times daily up to 1.03 mg/kg daily can be administered. This may aggravate drowsiness. Alternatively, phenytoin, clonazepam, or sodium valproate can be added. However, polypharmacy should be avoided if possible because of additional side effects and problems with compliance.

Surgical intervention should be considered if medical treatment fails. Up to 50 percent of patients may eventually require some form of surgical treatment. There are two main options, rhizotomy or microvascular decompression.

Radiofrequency rhizotomy or alternatively glycerol rhizolysis is relatively safe and simple. Patients require only light anesthesia and the procedure is carried out under radiographic screening control. Selective root lesioning is achieved if a stimulating electrode is employed and this reduces the side effects (see below). Glycerol injection into Meckel's cave acts as a neurotoxin.

The main side effect is sensory loss (usually less with glycerol injection). Corneal hypoesthesia is a problem which may result in ulceration. Rarely there may be masseter weakness. Both forms of treatment have about 90 percent success and the patient can be discharged home within 24 hours. Unfortunately, the reported recurrence rates are about 25 percent.

Microvascular decompression involves major neurosurgery with a posterior fossa approach. This procedure was pioneered by Janetta.[61] If a blood vessel is found in close association with the trigeminal root or deforming it, it is mobilized and a small sponge of polyvinylchloride interposed between the nerve and the vessel. The nerve root can also be surgically compressed. In the elderly this is a procedure of last resort because of a 1 percent mortality rate, additional morbidity, and the length of hospital admission.

Glossopharyngeal Neuralgia

This syndrome has the same symptom characteristics as trigeminal neuralgia, but the pain is felt in the region of the tonsil and ear. Trigger factors include swallowing, coughing, and talking and the distribution of the pain is in the sensory territory of the glossopharyngeal nerve and the auricular and pharyngeal branches of the vagus nerve. Rarely the patient may become unconscious during an attack due to asystole.[62] Neurologic examination is normal unless the syndrome is secondary to pathology such as neoplasia, infection, or inflammatory disease.

Treatment is the same as for trigeminal neuralgia with carbamazepine and other drugs; failing this microvascular dissection of the intracranial section of the glossopharyngeal nerve and upper two rootlets of the vagus can be undertaken.

Postherpetic Neuralgia

Postherpetic neuralgia occurs following 10 percent of attacks of shingles but this figure rises to 50 percent in the over 60s. The most common site is the ophthalmic division of the trigeminal nerve. The virus has a predilection for the trigeminal and upper cervical ganglia and in the acute stages the herpetic eruption is seen in the appropriate distribution. The Ramsay Hunt syndrome is due to herpetic infection of the facial nerve. Excruciating pain may precede the eruption of vesicles by 1 to 3 days. The latter are seen over the external auditory meatus and mastoid process and may occur with edema and redness of the ear, making examination difficult. Occasionally, other cranial nerves may be affected with involvement of the trigeminal nerve leading to loss of sensation on the face and numbness of the palate occurring when the ninth nerve is affected. A careful search for vesicles around the ear and in the mouth will make the diagnosis clear. Involvement of the fourth, sixth, and oculomotor nerves may also occur,[63] with the possibility of long-term paralysis.

The syndrome of postherpetic neuralgia is characterized by a constant burning or aching pain with occasional stabbing components and occurs following healing of the rash. It may take several weeks or months to emerge. There is sensory loss over the affected area and invariably allodynia develops.

Treatment is symptomatic. Acyclovir oral and topical can be used for the acute eruption, but it is unclear whether this or the use of corticosteroids during the acute phase reduces the likelihood of developing the postherpetic syndrome. Opiate analgesia may be required. For chronic cases, amitriptyline is of proven benefit[64] and carbamazepine may help to control the stabbing component of the pain. Transcutaneous electrical nerve stimulation (TENS) may sometimes be useful. The condition is notoriously difficult to treat and presently there is no role for surgery.

Atypical Facial Pain

This syndrome is rare in the elderly. It is characterized by a continuous, chronic head or facial pain that does not follow dermatomal boundaries nor conform to any of the known patterns of headache or cranial neuralgia. The diagnosis can be made only after the exclusion of organic pathology, including dental and sinus disease. Many patients are believed to be depressed[65] and receive tricyclic antidepressants, generally with a good result. Lance[54] has proposed an organic basis to this syndrome. However, tricyclics remain the treatment of choice together with the judicious use of baclofen. Occasionally, the pain may have a throbbing vascular nature, and when intermittent it is worth considering a diagnosis of facial or "lower half" migraine. In this case, a trial of β-blockers or sumatriptan may be useful.

Vascular Disorders and Headache

Giant Cell Arteritis

This condition is rare below the age of 50 years, with incidence rising tenfold between the sixth and ninth decades. The female:male ratio is approximately 4:1 and the overall prevelance was found to be 133 per 100,000.[66] Headache is the most common symptom (85 percent at some point in the disease). It is usually a severe, persistent ache with an additional throbbing component. Many patients also report an additional burning quality to the headache. The pain is usually bitemporal, but may be unilateral, frontal, or generalized. Scalp tenderness is a common symptom and patients may avoid grooming the hair. The rare symptom of jaw claudication (facial pain when chewing) is virtually pathognomonic of this condition. Infarction of the tongue can follow this symptom. Although primarily a condition pathologically affecting the extracranial arteries, any vascular bed may be involved. Thus, a plethora of symptoms can occur and there is an association with polymyalgia rheumatica. Patients may report a number of constitutional symptoms such as fatigue and malaise, lethargy, anorexia, and a low-grade fever. Weight loss and sweating are common.

Transient ischemic attacks can occur and sudden visual loss may affect up to 7 percent of cases.[66] This is a result of ischemia of the posterior ciliary arteries and secondary ischemic optic neuropathy, or infarction of the choroid.

The affected vessels become nodular, tortuous, and swollen. The superficial temporal artery may become palpable, tender, and pulseless. There is medial necrosis with formation of granulomatous tissue and invasion of lymphocytes and giant cells. Often there is thrombosis of the lumen. Unfortunately, the pathology is not continuous and "skip lesions" mean that there is a good chance that a temporal artery biopsy will be negative.

The sedimentation rate is a vital diagnostic test, but can be normal in up to 10 percent of cases.[67] Nonspecific abnormalities include a mild normochromic normocytic anemia, and leucocytosis. Plasma fibrinogen levels are elevated and other acute phase proteins. Liver function tests are often abnormal with an elevated alkaline phosphatase and elevated transaminases. An elevated creatine phosphokinase does not occur and should lead to a search for an alternative diagnosis.

If clinical suspicion is high the patient should be commenced on high-dose corticosteroids immediately because failure to act may cost the patient loss of vision. Prednisolone between 60 to 80 mg is given usually with rapid clinical effect. Failure of the symptoms to respond within 24 to 48 hours should lead one to review the diagnosis. This high dose is maintained for 1 to 2 weeks and then tapered gradually depending on the sedimentation rate and the patients symptoms. Patients will be on treatment for many months and most for several years. After stopping treatment the patient's sedimentation rate and symptoms should be monitored for at least 6 months to a year in case of relapse.

Temporal artery biopsy should be undertaken in all suspected cases to confirm the diagnosis, but this is not essential. It should not delay treatment if clinical suspicion is high. Biopsy can be undertaken after a few days of treatment and still be positive. Unfortunately, this is a disorder that can be easily overlooked with potential disastrous consequences. Any elderly person with malaise, arthralgia, depression, and vague headache should be considered a possible case until proven otherwise.

Cerebrovascular Disease and Hypertension

Headache is a common accompaniment to cerebrovascular disease[68,69] and may occur before, during, or after transient ischemic attack or stroke. The pain is often throbbing in nature and exacerbated with effort. Usually it is lateralized to the side of ischemia. It occurs most frequently when there is parenchymal hemorrhage (57 percent), but also with TIA (36 percent), thromboembolic infarct (29 percent) and lacunar infarction (17 percent).

Headache does not occur more frequently in the hypertensive than in the nonhypertensive general population unless it is of extreme degree or associated with rapid rises of blood pressure as in pheochromocytoma.[70] Occasionally, however, one meets cases where migraine has undoubtedly been aggravated by the occurrence of hypertension.

Carotid and Vertebral Artery Dissection

Carotid artery dissection and occlusion gives rise to ipsilateral pain involving the face and forehead and occasionally the neck. The pain is described as burning or throbbing but can be sudden and stabbing. A Horner's syndrome may be present ipsilateral to the involved artery with contralateral neurologic signs.[67] Occasionally there are no associated neurologic signs.

Vertebral artery dissection is associated with neck and occipital pain[71] and may occur more commonly than is thought in patients diagnosed with vertebrobasilar insufficiency. The occipital headache associated with this form of dissection is almost always associated with neurologic deficits from the brain stem.

Cluster Headache

This condition, although more common in young adults, may have its onset in the seventh decade.[72,73] The International Headache Society classification divides the condition into episodic and chronic cluster headache, the latter being more common in the elderly.

It is characterized by bouts of severe pain often described as "boring" in nature. The pain is constant for several hours during which patients walk around trying to find relief in contrast to those with migraine who lie quietly. The pain is often centered on one eye and there may be ipsilateral watering of the eye with nasal stuffiness and a runny discharge. There is usually conjunctival injection and there may be an associated ptosis and miosis. The pain may spread to the whole side of the face. Bouts of pain occur 1 to 3 times per day with alarm clock regularity and last from 45 minutes to a few hours. The cluster period typically lasts for 1 to 2 months and then subsides. During the cluster attacks alcohol is a potent precipitant as are vasodilatory drugs such as nitrates. The chronic form continues without remission often for many years.

Treatment is symptomatic. Oxygen at 100 percent is useful in the casualty department and can be given at home. More practically, sumatriptan by subcutaneous injection is the drug of choice for acute attacks. Nocturnal ergotamine may prevent nightly attacks but should be avoided as a long-term solution. Steroids (prednisolone 40 mg daily for a week and reducing by 10 mg a week) may abbreviate cluster attacks. No one thing works for everybody and other drugs such as methysergide, verapamil, and sodium valproate[74] may need a trial in resistant cases. Lithium carbonate given in standard psychiatric doses and monitored accordingly is useful in chronic cluster.

Rarely, surgical intervention is necessary; percutaneous radiofrequency trigeminal gangliorhizolysis or posterior fossa trigeminal sensory rhizolysis have been performed but are of unproven benefit. Operation can cause a reduction in facial sensation and corneal hypoesthesia with increased risk of corneal ulceration.[75]

Cluster headache is an underdiagnosed cause of recurrent paroxysmal cranial pain in the elderly. It may not have the usual classic features in this age group. Treatment may need to be given empirically when there is doubt.

Subarachnoid Hemorrhage

Intracerebral aneurysms are usually silent except when aneurysms cause compression of neural structures to produce focal signs and headache or when they rupture. The sudden, severe catastrophic headache of subarachnoid hemorrhage is easily diagnosed and in the elderly the prognosis is usually poor.[76] Warning leaks are a concern and may presage fatal hemorrhage. Patients with sudden, severe headache may need screening urgently for the possibility of aneurysmal bleed.

Chronic Subdural Hemorrhage

This condition usually presents in an insidious manner and a history of head trauma may be absent or forgotten. Coagulopathy, particularly with a background of excessive alcohol consumption, is a well recognized predisposing factor. Headache with fluctuating neurologic signs, cognitive impairment, and a suggestive history should be investigated by means of a CT brain scan. Large symptomatic hematomas are usually evacuated, but smaller hematomas may be left and the patient's neurologic state monitored clinically. The resolution of the hematoma is reviewed by serial CT scans.

Intracranial Tumors

As in most age groups, the most common intracranial mass lesions in the elderly are secondary tumors. Some tumors may grow to a large size in the elderly before symptoms and signs are evident. This is attributed to the increased space within the cranium secondary to cerebral atrophy.

The typical features of raised intracranial pressure are the same in the elderly as in all age groups; morning headache, vomiting, and gradual visual loss. The headache is exacerbated by coughing, straining, or bending forward. There may be incontinence, gait disturbance, and mental deterioration. Papilloedema is often absent. Mass lesions may cause less easily recognized types of headache. Stretching of dural structures by tumors may cause persistent focal headache. Occasionally, tension headache and migraine may be mimicked. Thus, further investigation including brain scan may be indicated in the elderly whenever there is recent onset of head pain syndrome. Headache persisting for more than 6 months is unlikely to have a structural cause. However, rarely, pituitary tumors that distort the sella turcica can cause long-term headache that is often deep seated, and retro-orbital.

The most common benign primary brain tumors are meningiomas, which are usually operable with good result in the otherwise fit elderly patient where there is headache. Asymptomatic meningiomas can be managed conservatively if monitored regularly.

Drugs Causing Headache

There are a large number of drugs prescribed for the elderly that cause headache, (Table 33-2). The pain is usually described as involving the whole head, but may be occipital or frontal.

Chronic Analgesic Abuse Syndrome

The overuse of analgesics and ergotamine can lead to the development of chronic refractory headache and this leads to increasing dependence on medication. Patients with initially intermittent migraine or tension-type headache may develop chronic daily headache because of analgesic abuse. These patients have higher depression scores and attempted discontinuation leads to withdrawal symptoms and a refractoriness to prophylactic treatments.[77] Side effects of the medication are also more likely such as ergotism, analgesic nephropathy, and gastrointestinal problems.

The only option is to stop the analgesics although this almost inevitably precipitates a temporary worsening of the head-

Table 33-2 Drugs that can cause headache

Calcium-channel blockers	Nitrates
Indomethacin	Dipyridamole
Lithium	Corticosteroids
Hydralazine	Sympathomimetics
MAO inhibitors	Cimetidine
Ranitidine	Theophyllines

aches. Patients with severe headache should be admitted for drug withdrawal, and given temporary cover with opiates and steroids along with instigation of antidepressant therapy and consideration of migraine prophylaxis.[78]

Headache and the Eye

The eye and orbit derives a rich innervation from the first division of the trigeminal nerve and these structures are common causes of pain around the eye and of headache. In the elderly population, glaucoma can be an important cause of eye pain and headache. Although the condition may be acute or chronic, it is the acute closed angle glaucoma that causes sudden onset of severe constant pain centered on the affected eye. This may spread to give a generalized headache and there are visual symptoms such as colored haloes in the visual field and misting of vision. There is photophobia and nausea or vomiting. Patients may be diagnosed as suffering from subarachnoid hemorrhage unless the history or signs of eye disease are discovered. Clinically there is limbic injection, corneal edema (hazy appearance), and the globe will be hard and tender to palpation. This condition represents an ophthalmologic emergency that requires immediate referral to an ophthalmic casualty department for further treatment. Opiate analgesia will be necessary.

Proptosis, ophthalmoplegia, and pain can be caused by orbital pseudotumor. Often there is an elevated sedimentation rate and a rapid response to high-dose corticisteroids. The differential diagnosis includes dysthyroid eye disease, orbital neoplasia (secondary spread from e.g., melanoma). Superior orbital fissuritis (Tolosa-Hunt syndrome) is one end of the spectrum of orbital inflammatory disease. MRI of the skull and/or CT of the skull should differentiate between these conditions, but often the response to steroids aids the diagnosis.

Painful oculomotor paresis with retro-orbital pain is usually due to two main pathologies. If the pupil is fixed and dilated then a surgical cause is likely, with aneurysm of the posterior communicating artery being the most common cause. If the pupil reacts to light then the cause is likely to be non-surgical and diabetes is the most common cause. Angiography may still be necessary to rule out aneurysm even if the blood sugar is elevated.

Anterior and posterior uveitis are also causes of eye pain and visual disturbance. There may be evidence of coexistent systemic pathology to aid diagnosis. Refractive disorders (so called "eye strain") rarely cause headache. Orbital pain may arise from entrapment of the greater occipital nerve as it emerges from between the occiput and first cervical vertebra. Pain usually starts in the occipital region and radiates forward to the eye although it may be isolated to the orbit. Treatment is symptomatic and a soft collar can be tried for a short period.

Miscellaneous Causes of Head Pain

The hypnic headache syndrome was first described by Raskin[79] and reviewed by Newman, Lipton, and Solomon.[80] It is an uncommon form of headache occuring only in the elderly. Headaches wake the patient from sleep at a regular time each night. They are generalized and usually pulsating in quality. They may last up to 30 minutes and recur the same night. There are no associated autonomic symptoms. This disorder is believed to be related to a disturbance of REM sleep. It is difficult to treat; lithium carbonate may produce a remission but the limiting factor is side effects, particularly tremor and gastrointestinal symptoms.

The exploding head syndrome[81] is another benign cause of disturbance experienced more commonly by the elderly. It is not a pain or headache, but a loud noise occurring in the twilight of sleep and waking the patient. It may occur for a short period of weeks or months on an infrequent basis or recur irregularly but more frequently. The noise is deep in the center or back of the head and causes fear in the patient. Some may describe momentary difficulty in breathing, tachycardia, or sweating. There are no sequelae and usually patients do not have a preceeding illness or history of neurologic disease. The etiology of the condition is unknown and it is almost certainly underreported. Reassurance is usually all that is required.

About one-third of patients with Parkinson's disease report occipital headache, usually dull in nature. The cause of this is not clear and it is not associated with nuchal rigidity.[82] Amitriptyline may be effective.

Diagnostic Approach to Headache

As in any branch of medicine, the diagnosis rests heavily on the history of the complaint and use of appropriate investigations after a thorough physical examination. The duration of symptoms and their mode of onset together with the tempo of their development provide valuable diagnostic clues. Quality of headache is a less useful feature, but position and intensity together with radiation of the pain and the presence of exacerbating and relieving factors should be asked for. A complete drug history should be obtained and appraisal of the patient's mood, sleep, and vegetative functions are helpful in discerning the impact of the illness and possible psychological background.

Although the vast majority of headaches in all age groups are benign, in the elderly the risk of organic pathology is increased. The diversity of symptoms of temporal arteritis can often lead to a delay in diagnosis. Chronic malaise, myalgia, and arthralgia are not infrequently seen in giant cell arteritis but easily dismissed as nonspecific symptoms and resulting from the aging process. Severe pain of sudden onset, pain that is persistent and progressively worsening with time, early morning headache with vomiting, and exacerbation by coughing, straining, and bending forward all suggest underlying organic disease. Migraine can be identified when there is a long history or classic symptoms, but complicated migraine may be difficult to differentiate from TIAs[26] and complete investigation is warranted. The presence of other symptoms such as drowsiness, confusion, and memory loss will raise the index of suspicion. Other worrying symptoms include progressive visual disturbance, weakness, clumsiness, and loss of balance. It is important to realize that the cranial neuralgias are not associated in their simple form with neurologic deficits and have a strict definition for a positive diagnosis. The description of bands of pain or tight caps on the head is more likely to result from muscle tension as seen in tension-type headache or disease of the neck, but can be a symptom of a more serious disease. Injury to the head may precede the formation of subdural hematoma, which is more likely with coagulopathy or chronic alcohol abuse. Brachalgia together with myelopathy should point to the neck as the source of headache. A normal neurologic examination will often help rule out serious underlying disease and prevent unnecessary investigation.

References

1. Siberstein SD, Silberstein MM: New concepts in the pathogenesis of migraine headache. Pain Manage 1990;3:297–302
2. Cook NR, Evans DA, Funkenstein HH et al: Correlates of headache in a population-based cohort of elderly. Arch Neurol 1989; 46:1338–1344.
3. Newland CA, Illis LS, Robinson PK et al: A survey of headache in an English city. Res Clin Stud Headache 1978;5:1–20
4. Serratrice G, Serbanesco F, Sambuc R: Epidemiology of headache in elderly: correlations with life conditions and socio-professional environment. Headache 1985;25:85–89
5. Waters WE, O'Connor PJ: Epidemiology of headache and migraine in women. J Neurol Neurosurg Psych 1971;34:148–153
6. Nikiforow R: Headache in a random sample of 200 persons: a clinical study of a population in northern Finland. Cephalalgia 1981;1:99–107
7. Selby G, Lance JW: Observations on 500 cases of migraine and allied vascular headache. J Neurol Neurosurg Psych 1960;23: 23–32
8. Rasmussen BK, Olesen J: Migraine epidemiology [letter; comment]. Cephalalgia 1993;13:216–217
9. Stewart WF, Linet MS, Celentano DD et al: Age- and sex-specific incidence rates of migraine with and without visual aura. Am J Epidemiol 1991;134:1111–1120
10. Hale WE, May FE, Marks RG et al: Headache in the elderly: an evaluation of risk factors. Headache 1987;27:272–276
11. Pascual J, Berciano J: Experience in the diagnosis of headaches that start in elderly people. J Neurol Neurosurg Psych 1994; 57:1255–1257
12. Gobel H, Petersen-Braun M, Soyka D: The epidemiology of headache in Germany: a nationwide survey of a representative sample on the basis of the headache classification of the International Headache Society [see comments]. Cephalalgia 1994;14: 97–106
13. Linet MS, Stewart WF: Migraine headache: epidemiologic perspectives. [Review]. Epidemiol Rev 1984;6:107–139
14. Featherstone HJ: Migraine and muscle contraction headaches: a continuum. Headache 1985;25:194–198
15. Silberstein SD, Lipton RB: Epidemiology of migraine. [Review]. Neuroepidemiology 1993;12:179–194
16. Rasmussen BK, Jensen R, Schroll M, Olesen J: Epidemiology of headache in a general population: a prevalence study. J Clin Epidemiol 1991;44:1147–1157
17. Stewart WF, Lipton RB, Celentano DD, Reed ML: Prevalence of migraine headache in the United States. Relation to age, income, race, and other sociodemographic factors. JAMA 1992; 267:64–69
18. Henry P, Michel P, Brochet B et al: A nationwide survey of migraine in France: prevalence and clinical features in adults. GRIM [see comments]. Cephalagia 1992;12:229–237
19. Headache Classification Committee of the International Headache Society (1988): Classification and diagnostic criteria for headache disorders, cranial neuralgia, and facial pain. Cephalgia 1988;8(suppl 7):1–96
20. Rasmussen BK, Jensen R, Olesen J: A population-based analysis of the diagnostic criteria of the International Headache Society. Cephalalgia 1991;11:129–134
21. Silberstein SD: Saper JR: Wolff's Headache and other Head Pain. 6th Ed. Oxford University Press, 1996
22. Ziegler DK, Hassanein RS: Specific headache phenomena: their frequency and coincidence. Headache 1990;30:152–156
23. Solomon S, Lipton RB: Criteria for the diagnosis of migraine in clinical practice. [Review] Headache 1991;31:384–387
24. Blau JN: Migraine prodromes separated from the aura: complete migraine. Br Med J 1980;281:658–660
25. Jensen K, Tfelt-Hansen P, Lauritzen M, Olesen J: Classic migraine. A prospective recording of symptoms. Acta Neurol Scand 1986;73:359–362
26. Fisher CM: Late-life migraine accompaniments-further experience. [Review]. Stroke 1986;17:1033–1042
27. Iversen HK, Langemark M, Andersson PG et al: Clinical characteristics of migraine and episodic tension-type headache in relation to old and new diagnostic criteria. Headache 1990;30: 514–519
28. Raskin NH, Schwartz RK: Icepick-like pain. Neurology 1980; 30:203–205
29. Pradalier A, Clapin A, Dry J: Treatment review: non-steroid anti-inflammatory drugs in the treatment and long-term prevention of migraine attacks. [Review]. Headache 1988;28: 550–557
30. Johnson AG, Day RO: The problems and pitfalls of NSAID therapy in the elderly (Part I). [Review]. Drugs Aging 1991;1: 130–143
31. Garcia Rodriguez LA, Jick H: Risk of upper gastrointestinal bleeding and perforation associated with individual non-steroidal anti-inflammatory drugs [published erratum appears in Lancet 1994;343:1048]. Lancet 1994;343:769–772
32. The Subcutaneous Sumatriptan International Study Group (1991): Treatment of migraine attacks with sumatriptan. N Engl J Med 1991;325:316–321
33. The Oral Sumatriptan and Aspirin plus Metaclopramide Comparative Study Group: A study to compare oral sumatriptan with oral aspirin plus oral metaclopramide in the acute treatment of migraine. Eur Neurol 1992;32:177–184

34. Brown EG, Endersby CA, Smith RN, Talbot JC: The safety and tolerability of sumatriptan: an overview. Eur Neurol 1991;31: 339–344

35. Andersson K, Vinge E: Beta-adrenoceptor blockers and calcium antagonists in the prophylaxis and treatment of migraine. Drugs 1990;39:355–373

36. Couch JR, Ziegler DK, Hassanein R: Amitriptyline in the prophylaxis of migraine. Effectiveness and relationship of antimigraine and antidepressant effects. Neurology 1976;26:121–127

37. Ziegler DK, Hurwitz A, Hassanein RS et al: Migraine prophylaxis. A comparison of propranolol and amitriptyline. Arch Neurol 1987;44:486–489

38. Adly C, Straumanis J, Chesson A: Fluoxetine prophylaxis of migraine [see comments]. Headache 1992;32:101–104

39. Meyer JS, Hardenberg J: Clinical effectiveness of calcium entry blockers in prophylactic treatment of migraine and cluster headaches. Headache 1983;23:266–277

40. Peatfield R: Headache. Springer-Verlag, Berlin, 1986

41. Drummond PD: Effectiveness of methysergide in relation to clinical features of migraine. Headache 1985;25:145–146

42. Johnson ES, Kadam NP, Hylands DM, Hylands PJ: Efficacy of feverfew as prophylactic treatment of migraine. Br Med J (Clin Res Ed) 1985;291:569–573

43. Murphy JJ, Heptinstall S, Mitchell JR: Randomised double-blind placebo-controlled trial of feverfew in migraine prevention. Lancet 1988;2:189–192

44. Silberstein SD: Tension-type and chronic daily headache. [Review]. Neurology 1993;43:(9):1644–1649

45. Langemark M, Olesen J, Poulsen DL, Bech P: Clinical characterization of patients with chronic tension headache. Headache 1988;28:590–596

46. Drummond PD: Scalp tenderness and sensitivity to pain in migraine and tension headache. Headache 1987;27:45–50

47. Hatch JP, Moore PJ, Cyr-Provost M et al: The use of electromyography and muscle palpation in the diagnosis of tension-type headache with and without pericranial muscle involvement. Pain 1992;49:175–178

48. Marsland DW, Wood M, Mayo F: Content of family practice. Part I. Rank order of diagnoses by frequency. Part II. Diagnoses by disease category and age/sex distribution. J Fam Pract 1976; 3:37–68

49. Iansek R, Heywood J, Kamaghan J, Balla JI: Cervical spondylosis and headaches. Clin Exp Neurol 1996;175–178

50. Edmeads J: The cervical spine and headache [see comments]. Neurology 1988;38:1874–1878

51. Stevenson DD, Delassio DJ, Silberstein SD (eds): Allergy, atopy, nasal disease, and headache. pp. 291–333. In Wolff's Headache and Other Head Pain. 6th Ed. Oxford University Press, 1993

52. Rothman KJ, Monson RR: Epidemiology of trigeminal neuralgia. J Chronic Dis 1973;26:3–12

53. Katusic S, Beard CM, Bergstralh E, Kurland LT: Incidence and clinical features of trigeminal neuralgia, Rochester, Minnesota, 1945–1984. Ann Neurol 1990;27:89–95

54. Lance JW: Mechanism and Management of Headache. 5th Ed. Butterworth-Heinemann Ltd, Oxford, 1993

55. Fromm GH, Terrence CF, Maroon JC: Trigeminal neuralgia. Current concepts regarding etiology and pathogenesis. Arch Neurol 1984;41:1204–1207

56. Pagni CA: The origin of tic douloureux: a unified view. J Neurosurg Sci 1993;37:185–194

57. Tash RR, Sze G, Leslie DR: Trigeminal neuralgia: MR imaging features. Radiology 1989;172:767–770

58. Zakrzewska JM, Patsalos PN: Drugs used in the management of trigeminal neuralgia. [Review]. Oral Surg Oral Med Oral Pathol 1992;74:439–450

59. Sidebottom A, Maxwell S: The medical and surgical management of trigeminal neuralgia. [Review]. J Clin Pharm Ther 1995;20:31–35

60. Green MW, Selman JE: Review article: the medical management of trigeminal neuralgia. [Review]. Headache 1991;31: 588–592

61. Jannetta PJ: Treatment of trigeminal neuralgia by suboccipital and transtentorial cranial operations. Clin Neurosurg 1977;24: 538–549

62. Dalessio D, Delassio DJ, Silberstein SD (eds): The major neuralgias, postinfectious neuritis, and atypical facial pain. pp. 345–364. In Wolff's Headache and Other Head Pain. 6th Ed. Oxford University Press, Oxford: 1993

63. Ragozzino MW, Melton LJ, III, Kurland LT et al: Population-based study of herpes zoster and its sequelae. Medicine (Baltimore) 1982;61:310–316

64. Watson CP, Evans RJ, Reed K et al: Amitriptyline versus placebo in postherpetic neuralgia. Neurology 1982;32: 671–673

65. Lascelles RG: Atypical facial pain and depression. Br J Psych 1966;112:651–659

66. Huston KA, Hunder GG, Lie JT et al: Temporal arteritis: a 25-year epidemiologic, clinical, and pathologic study. Ann Intern Med 1978;88:162–167

67. Kansu T, Corbett JJ, Savino P, Schatz NJ: Giant cell arteritis with normal sedimentation rate. Arch Neurol 1977;34: 624–625

68. Edmeads J: The headache of ischemic cerebrovascular disease. Headache 1979;19:345–349

69. Portenoy RK, Abissi CJ, Lipton RB et al: Headache in cerebrovascular disease. Stroke 1984;15:1009–1012

70. Waters WE: Headache and blood pressure in the community. Br Med J 1971;1:142–143

71. Caplan LR, Zarins CK, Hemmati M: Spontaneous dissection of the extracranial vertebral arteries. Stroke 1985;16:1030–1038

72. Ekbom K: Patterns of cluster headache with a note on the relations to angina pectoris and peptic ulcer. Acta Neurol Scand 1970;46:225–237

73. Ekbom K: A clinical comparison of cluster headache and migraine. Acta Neurol Scand 1970;(suppl):41:1

74. Hering R, Kuritzky A: Sodium valproate in the treatment of cluster headache: an open clinical trial. Cephalalgia 1989;9: 195–198

75. Mathew NT, Hurt W: Percutaneous radiofrequency trigeminal gangliorhizolysis in intractable cluster headache. Headache 1988;28:328–331

76. O'Sullivan MG, Dorward N, Whittle IR et al: Management and long-term outcome following subarachnoid haemorrhage and intracranial aneurysm surgery in elderly patients: an audit of 199 consecutive cases. Br J Neurosurg 1994;8: 23–30
77. Mathew NT: Drug-induced headache. Neurol Clin 1990;8: 903–912
78. Clough C: Treating migraine [see comments]. [Review]. Br Med J 1989;299:141–142
79. Raskin NH: The hypnic headache syndrome. Headache 1988; 88:534–563
80. Newman LC, Lipton RB, Solomon S: The hypnic headache syndrome: a benign headache disorder of the elderly. Neurology 1990;40:1904–1905
81. Pearce JM: Clinical features of the exploding head syndrome. J Neurol Neurosurg Psych 1989;89:907–910
82. Indo T, Naito A, Sobue I: Clinical characteristics of headache in Parkinson's disease. Headache 1983;83:211–212

CHAPTER 34

Stroke: Pathology and Epidemiology

SHAH EBRAHIM

Definitions and Criteria

Stroke is defined clinically rather than pathologically as "rapidly developing clinical signs of focal (or global) disturbance of cerebral function, with symptoms lasting 24 hours or longer or leading to death, with no apparent cause other than of vascular origin."[1] Events lasting less than 24 hours are classified as transient ischemic attacks (TIAs) and are excluded by the definition, whereas subarachnoid hemorrhages are included. In population surveys of stroke prevalence, which are of value in the development and evaluation of health services, the simple question "Have you ever had a stroke?" performs well.[2]

The underlying vascular origins of stroke may be divided into two broad categories: occlusion (i.e., thrombosis or embolism) and hemorrhage. For decades, this approach has provided clinicians with a practical means of grouping patients with similar problems and management needs. Alternative classifications such as reversible ischemic neurologic deficit (RIND)[3] and major and minor stroke are widely used terms but lack agreed-on operational criteria.[4] However, a fuller understanding of the pathologic processes is essential if attempts are to be made to reduce the amount of brain damage in acute stroke, avoid recurrence, make an accurate prognosis, and examine risk factors without misclassification bias.

Clinical diagnostic scales,[5,6] relying largely on symptoms and signs associated with raised intracranial pressure and meningism, can distinguish between large hemorrhagic and thrombotic stroke but are not sufficiently accurate for clinical management of patients. Computed tomography (CT) scanning is helpful in diagnosis, but in one-third to one-half of patients no CT abnormality is found despite clinical evidence of stroke.[7,8]

An appraisal of stroke subtype requires information about the underlying pathogenesis or mechanism (i.e., thrombosis, embolus, hemorrhage, hemodynamic); the arterial site affected (i.e., internal carotid artery, middle cerebral artery, small perforating arteries, and so on); and the clinical picture (i.e., sudden death, associated cardiac disease, and so on). A classification based on clinical criteria of the region and extent of arterial circulation affected (Table 34-1) may have value in improving prognostic information[9,10] and may be helpful in describing more homogeneous groups of stroke patients for inclusion in clinical trials.

The clinical value of classifications based on complex criteria is limited, and the accuracy of categorization of patients depends to a large extent on the intensity of investigation. A simple scheme is shown in Figure 34-1. For older people, the most important purpose of defining stroke subtypes is to distinguish between hemorrhagic and occlusive stroke: in the former prophylaxis with antiplatelet agents may be hazardous, but in the latter this treatment reduces the risk of recurrent stroke.

A practical advantage of considering the pathologic mechanism of stroke is a raised index of suspicion of rare underlying causes of stroke[11] (Table 34-2) that are important to exclude clinically as they often require different management and usually have a different natural history. Unfortunately, the assessment of older stroke patients is often poor,[12] and not only are rare causes of stroke missed but conditions (such as subdural hematoma and hypoglycemia) that masquerade as stroke go unrecognized as well, with potentially devastating consequences for the patient.

Pathologic Mechanisms

Hemorrhage

Cerebral hemorrhage is caused by bleeding from small microaneurysms (Charcot-Bouchard aneurysms) associated with changes in the arterial walls (lipohyalinosis) due to long-term hypertension.[13] In older patients amyloid angiopathy is the most common cause of hemorrhagic stroke[14] and results from weakness in arterial walls infiltrated with amyloid. Binswanger's disease may cause stroke and is diagnosed from the appearance on a CT scan of diffuse white matter changes around the lateral ventricles.[15] In Binswanger's disease the underlying pathology may be related to amyloid angiopathy, and small white matter lacunae are found in association with lipohyalinosis.[16] Subarachnoid hemorrhage is uncommon in older patients and is associated with berry aneurysms occurring largely in the anterior cerebral circulation.

Bleeding into the brain parenchyma results in hematoma formation with raised intracranial volume, reduction in cerebral compliance, and a potential for raised intracranial pressure and reduced cerebral perfusion.[17] Sometimes decompression occurs by extension of the hematoma into the ventricular system. Many large hemorrhages are rapidly fatal because of these direct effects, but in the case of smaller hemorrhages, resolution occurs through invasion of the hematoma by phagocytic glial cells, new blood vessel formation, and breakdown of hemoglobin by macrophages over several weeks.

Table 34-1 A clinical classification of ischemic stroke subtypes and associated mortality

Stroke Subtype	**Proportion in Community Series (%)**	**Mortality at 6 Months (%)**
Anterior circulation infarct (ACI)		
Total anterior circulation infarct (TACI) (i.e., cortical and subcortical impairment)	17	56
Partial anterior circulation infarct (PACI) (i.e., only cortical impairment)	34	10
Lacunar anterior circulation infarct (LACI) (i.e., pure motor, pure sensory, motor-sensory, ataxic syndromes	25	7
Posterior circulation infarct (POCI) verterbrobasilar circulation impairment	24	14

(Data from Oxford Community Stroke Study, Bamford et al.[10]*)*

Table 34-2 Rare causes of stroke

Occlusive
- Arteritis
  - Collagen-vascular diseases (PAN, SLE)
  - Takayasu's disease
  - Granulomatous intracranial arteritis
- Hyperviscosity syndromes
  - Polycythemia (primary and secondary)
  - Myeloma
  - Waldenstrom's macroglobulinemia
- Infections
  - Subacute bacterial endocarditis
  - Endarteritis obliterans associated with tuberculosis, syphilis
- Atrial myxoma
- Arterial dissection
- Inherited collagen disorders
  - Ehlers-Danlos syndrome
  - Marfan's syndrome
  - Pseudoxanthoma elasticum
  - Homocysteinuria

Hemorrhagic
- Bleeding diatheses
- Ateriovenous malformations
- Warfarin treatment
- Head injury
- Cerebral tumors
- Amphetamine abuse

Occlusion

Occlusion of arteries often occurs at sites of atheroma where the endothelium has been damaged,[18] leading to the activation of platelets which become sticky and leak adenosine diphosphate (ADP) and thromboxane A_2, both of which cause more platelets to clump together. Activated platelets also switch on the coagulation cascade, and the conversion of prothrombin to thrombin results in the formation of a platelet thrombus. Endothelial cells also have a counterbalancing role, converting arachidonic acid to prostacyclin via the cyclo-oxygenase pathway, which leads to platelet disaggregation and vasodilatation.[16]

Following occlusion of the cerebral circulation, a series of complex inter-related mechanisms come into play, initially in an attempt to maintain delivery of oxygen and glucose to neurons and subsequently to reduce the metabolic demands of neurons by a reversible reduction in electrophysiologic activity. Finally, an irreversible phase associated with failure of calcium homeostasis follows, and cell death occurs.[19] The speed with which cell death takes place depends on the sever-

Figure 34-1 A simple scheme of pathologic mechanisms in stroke.

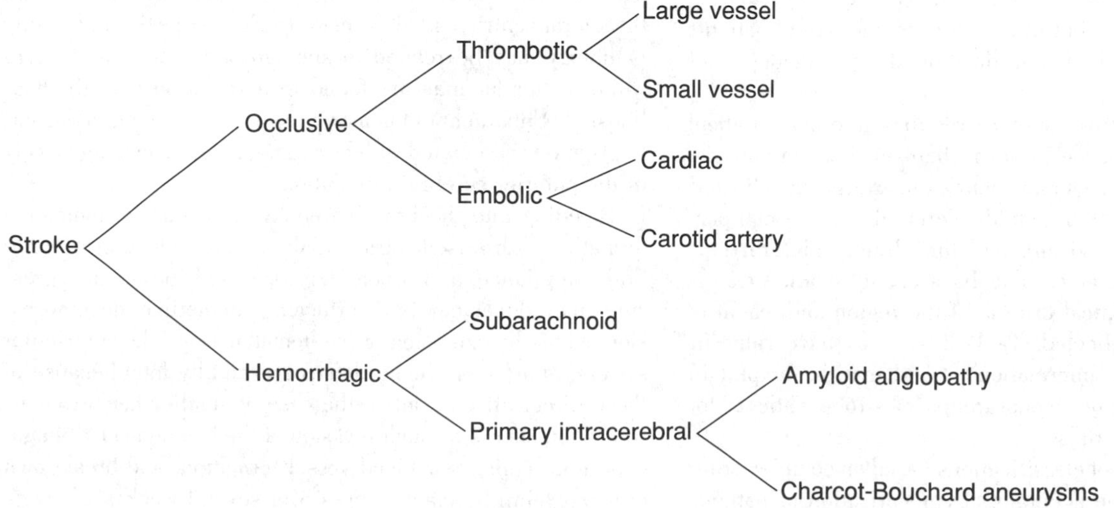

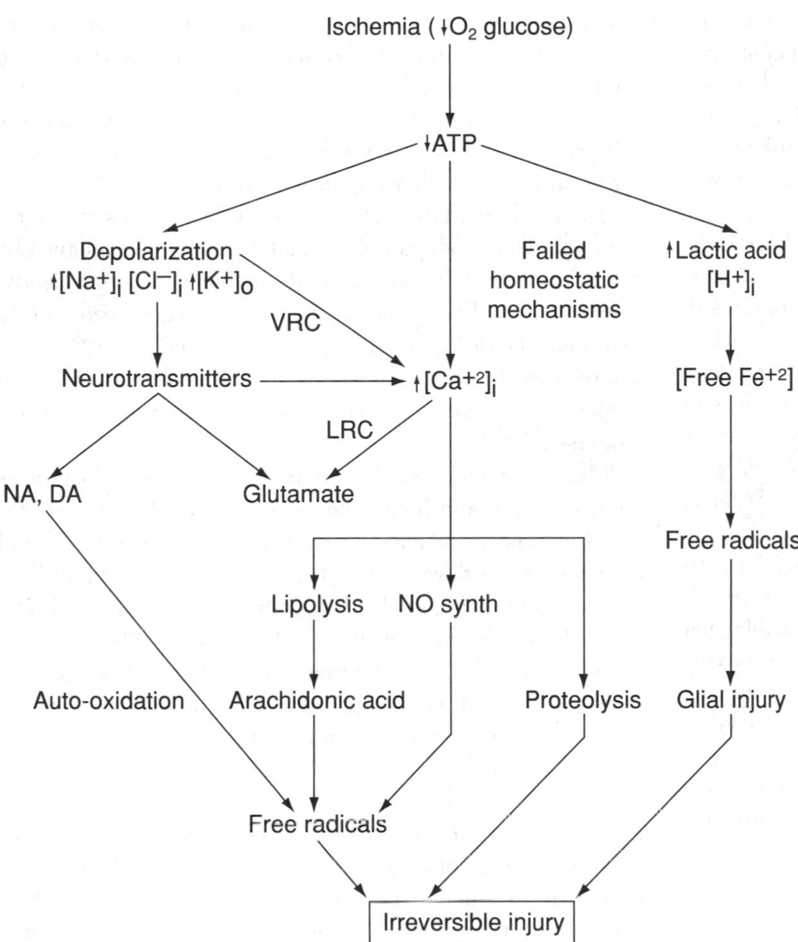

Figure 34-2 Potential mechanisms of ischemic brain damage. VRC, Voltage-regulated calcium channels; LRC, ligand-regulated calcium channels; NA, noradrenaline (norepinehrine); DA, dopamine; NO synth, nitric oxide synthase. (From Pulsinelli,[19] with permission.)

ity of occlusion; typically the process evolves over a period of a few hours. The area of brain immediately around the occluded artery is the first to undergo cell death, and areas more distant from the center form an ischemic "penumbra"[20] in which reversible infarction has occurred, creating the possibility of salvage of neurons by maintaining cerebral blood flow or drugs preventing extension of infarction to the penumbra.[21]

Cellular processes of lactic acidosis, free radical damage, excitatory neurotransmitter release, and calcium influx into neurons are of particular importance in the "ischemic cascade."[22] The steps in this cascade have generated substantial research interest as they offer the possibility of new therapeutic approaches to reducing acute cellular damage[19] (Fig. 34-2).

Epidemiology

An understanding of the distribution and determinants of stroke in populations is essential for health services planning and evaluation and for rational approaches to stroke prevention through risk factor reduction.

Since stroke comprises two major pathologic mechanisms—hemorrhage and occlusion—it is logical to examine the epidemiology of each type of stroke separately. However, it is not possible to accurately distinguish hemorrhagic from occlusive stroke subtypes clinically or from routine sources of information,[5,23–25] although clinical diagnosis of specific subtypes of cerebral infarction may be reliable.[26] Consequently, most of the epidemiologic information on stroke combines both hemorrhagic and occlusive stroke, although the picture is dominated by occlusive stroke which predominates in most western countries. With increased use of CT scanning in population-based stroke studies, it is becoming feasible to examine the distribution, risk factors, and natural history of subtypes of stroke.

Burden of Stroke

Stroke is the third most common cause of death and the leading cause of severe disability in most of the developed world.[27] In China there are about 1 million deaths per year attributed to stroke,[28] and worldwide each year approximately 44 million disability-adjusted life-years (DALYs) are lost because of stroke, of which only 5 million DALYs occur in countries with established market economies.[29] Given the rapid aging profile that is affecting most of the developing world, stroke will become an increasingly important cause of mortality and disability, and a high priority must be given to its prevention.[30]

In England and Wales, each year over 130,000 people suffer a first or recurrent stroke, and about 70,000 deaths are attributed to stroke, with the majority occurring in people over the age of 65. Although many people die rapidly from the stroke, there are about 300,000 stroke survivors living in the community, of whom one-half are unable to use public transport, one-quarter need help from a district nurse, and one-twentieth require long-term institutional care.[31]

Stroke is an expensive disease in terms of health services. In the United States is estimated that $30 billion is spent each year,[32] and about 4 to 5 percent of total British National Health Service spending is on stroke.[33] However, direct health service costs (bed-days, investigations, treatments) account for only about half of total costs when loss of earnings and costs of family caregiving are considered.[34,35] Total lifetime costs are dominated by long-term care rather than acute hospital care costs,[36] although economic appraisals have tended to focus on the costs of acute care.

Projections of the future burden of stroke disability are difficult to make. While demographic trends will inevitably result in an increase in the number of strokes, it is possible that selective mortality of the most disabled and elderly survivors will lead to only modest increases in the number requiring institutional care.[37] However, secular trends in case fatality are falling,[38–41] and possible increases in incidence, changes in the balance of care provided by public and private sources, and number of available family caregivers may make estimates of the future burden unreliable.

Variation in Time, Place, and Person

Time Trends

Stroke mortality rates have fallen over the twentieth century (Fig. 34-3), and the decline has been more rapid since the 1970s, with falls of 20 to 70 percent over two decades in many countries.[27] However, the situation in central and eastern Europe and the former USSR shows an opposite trend, with mortality rates rising by 1 to 50 percent over the same time period.[27] The reason for the declining mortality trend in more affluent countries is not entirely clear,[42] and the study of secular variation in incidence is beset with problems.[43]

The fall in mortality rates mirrors a decline in stroke incidence,[44,45] although part of the pattern might be explained by a fall in case fatality and a stable incidence. More recently, the rate of decline in mortality and incidence seems to be slowing, but case fatality still appears to be declining.[38–41,46,47] Interestingly, hemorrhagic and occlusive stroke have followed similar declining trends in studies capable of examining stroke subtypes.[40,48,49]

Changes in major cardiovascular risk factors—blood pressure, smoking, and blood cholesterol—over the last few decades have occurred and may explain between one-third[50] and as much as two-thirds of the decline in stroke mortality.[51] In Japan, despite a rise in blood cholesterol levels from the 1960s to the 1980s, stroke rates have fallen dramatically.[52]

Better detection and treatment of high blood pressure is often put forward as an explanation for the declining risk of stroke.[53,54] However, in Australia and New Zealand, only marginal reductions in blood pressure have occurred,[55] and it is estimated that only 10 percent of the decline in mortality among people younger than 70 years old can be attributed to treatment of high blood pressure.[56] In the United States better treatment does not seem to be the explanation.[45,57,58] Older people have also enjoyed a reduction in stroke mortality, which suggests that better detection and treatment of high blood pressure is an unlikely explanation as these individuals are less likely to be treated than younger people.

The divergent secular trends in western and eastern European countries indicate that stroke risk is modifiable and therefore preventable. Furthermore, the era of declining rates is

Figure 34-3 Stroke death rates, England and Wales, 1901–1991.

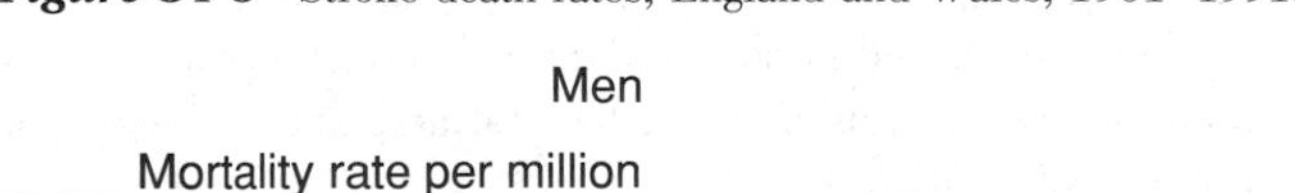

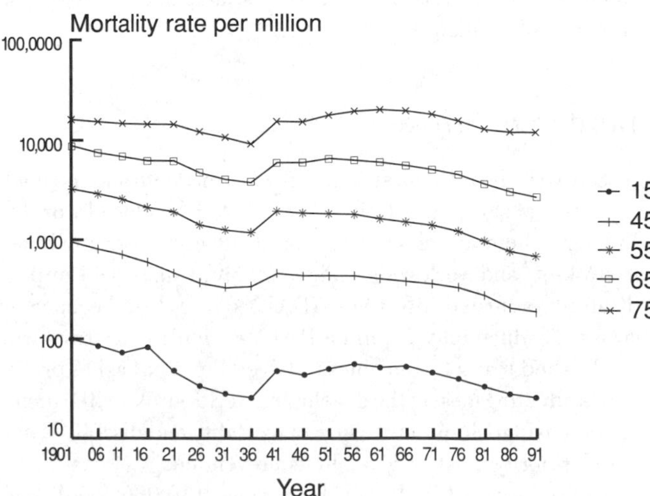

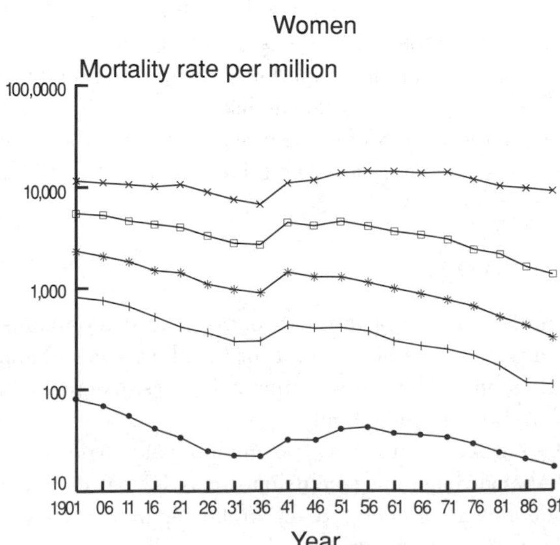

probably coming to an end in affluent countries,[41,46,47,59] which suggests that some of the factors responsible may change in an adverse direction despite apparent progress. These trends are probably due in part to changes in cardiovascular risk factors and in part to social and economic differentials among and within populations.

Geographic Trends

Stroke mortality varies by fivefold among countries, with the highest rates in Bulgaria and China and the lowest rates in North America[27] (Fig. 34-4). Stroke incidence also shows considerable variation among countries, but there are major methodologic problems in obtaining comparable data.[60] Mortality rates also vary within countries, with rates twice as high in the north of England as in the south,[61,62] and higher in the north than the south of China.[63] Interestingly, people who migrate from areas of high mortality to low mortality acquire the low risk of the area to which they migrate,[64,65] suggesting that current environmental factors are more important determinants of risk than genetic or early-life factors.[66,67]

The differences among and within countries are a source of the optimistic view that stroke is preventable. Possible reasons for variation among populations include differences in the major risk factors (e.g., blood pressure, smoking), the underlying determinants of these risk factors or other unknown risk factors. One likely explanation involves salt intake, which shows a large variation among countries[68,69] and accounts for some of the variation in population blood pressure distributions[70] and may also contribute to secular trends in stroke risk.[71–74]

Vitamin C and potassium intake derived from fresh fruit and vegetables, which also varies between rich and poor countries and has changed over time, may provide an explanation for differences in stroke risk both over time and from place to place.[75–81]

Individual Risk Factors

Variation among people is of major importance in guiding prevention policy and strategy. Risk factors can be classified[82] as inherent biologic traits such as genes, age, and gender, physiologic characteristics such as blood pressure, behaviors such as smoking, social characteristics such as social class, and environmental factors such as temperature. Prevention policy and practice vary depending on the strength of evidence implicating risk factors, their position in the causal chain, and the ease and cost with which they can be modified.

Inherent biologic traits

Age is the most important, but immutable, stroke risk factor, with an exponential increase in mortality risk of 100-fold between the ages of 30 to 40 years and 80 to 90 years.[83–85] By the age of 85 years, one in four men and one in five women currently aged 45 can expect to suffer a stroke.[86] With increasing age the strength of association between some risk factors and stroke tends to weaken, but because the absolute risk of stroke increases with age, the contribution of such risk factors remains important.[12,87]

People from different ethnic groups show variations in stroke mortality risk, with the highest rates in those born in

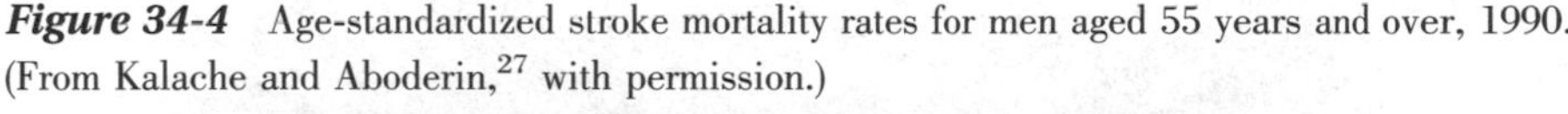

Figure 34-4 Age-standardized stroke mortality rates for men aged 55 years and over, 1990. (From Kalache and Aboderin,[27] with permission.)

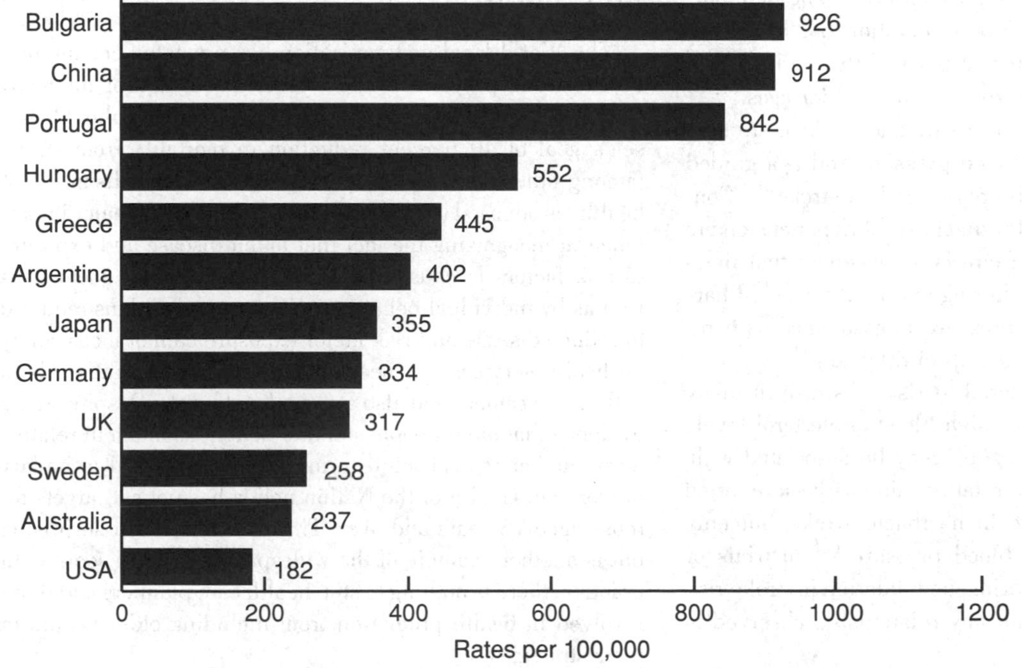

the Caribbean.[88,89] The explanation for ethnic variation is not clear, and several of the factors listed above may be implicated. In the United States, the excess risk of stroke among blacks compared with whites is associated with higher blood pressure levels, raised blood cholesterol, and diabetes mellitus.[90,91]

Stroke tends to run in families,[12,92,93] but the genetic contribution to stroke as determined by studies on twins is unclear: in a well-conducted Swedish twin registry trial with high levels of follow-up, similar concordance rates for stroke mortality in both monozygotic and dizygotic twins were found.[94] However, in an American study on twins with 60 percent follow-up and analysis of prevalent rather than fatal or incident stroke, a fourfold increase in concordance among monozygotic compared with dizygotic twins was found.[95] Thus there is continued uncertainty about the relative contributions of genetic and environmental factors in stroke.

Homocysteinemia is an interesting example of the way in which genetic inheritance can be modified by environmental factors. Homocysteinuria is an autosomal recessive inborn error of metabolism which, in addition to causing skeletal defects similar to those of Marfan's syndrome, is associated with increased risk of venous and arterial thrombosis. Heterozygous states are relatively common and may be associated with homocysteinemia, which is associated with increased risk of stroke.[96–100] As one of the common metabolic pathways affected in this condition is pyridoxine and folate dependent, dietary deficiency may lead to increased stroke risk, possibly explaining the increased risk with age. It is not known whether treatment with pyridoxine or folate reduces homocysteinemia in heterozygotes or decreases the risk of stroke.

Physiologic characteristics

Raised blood pressure has long been known to be an important stroke risk factor.[101,102] This observation has been confirmed in many studies in different parts of the world,[103–108] and the association remains strong even at older ages.[87,109] The relationship between blood pressure and stroke is stronger for systolic than for diastolic blood pressure and is a graded response with no threshold of increased risk of stroke.[103] Consequently, clinical thresholds for diagnosis of hypertension are somewhat arbitrary, although there is a consensus that pressures over 160/95 require monitoring and treatment.[110] Pharmacologic reduction of blood pressure is associated with reduced risk of stroke even at ages up to 80 years.[111]

Blood cholesterol is not related to risk of stroke in many populations,[87,112] although very high blood cholesterol levels [greater than 8 mmol/L (309 mg/dl)] may be associated with occlusive stroke.[113] An inverse relationship has been reported between blood cholesterol and hemorrhagic stroke, but only in men with raised diastolic blood pressure.[114] In trials of pharmacologic cholesterol lowering, no reduction in stroke risk has been found, suggesting that any relationship observed is not causal.[115]

Behaviors

Smoking is of much greater importance than was initially thought,[116] and several studies have confirmed its adverse consequences for stroke risk.[103,105,117–121] Cessation of smoking is associated with a rapid reduction in stroke risk.[117] The interaction of smoking with high blood pressure is of great importance, with a 12-fold increased stroke risk among people who are both hypertensive and smoke.[103]

Other factors

Past history of ischemic heart disease and heart failure,[122] atrial fibrillation,[123–125] diabetes mellitus,[126–128] and intermittent claudication[129] are all associated with increased risk of stroke.

A very wide range of risk factors have been described from large-scale prospective studies[103,104,106–108] which have confirmed the importance of age, raised blood pressure, smoking, past cardiovascular disease, and diabetes mellitus as major determinants of stroke risk. Other factors associated with risk of stroke are shown in Table 34-3.

Risk factors for stroke subtypes

Several studies have examined the etiology of hemorrhagic and occlusive stroke subtypes. In general, raised blood pressure,[107,177–182] smoking,[121,155,181–184] and alcohol consumption[152,154,178,181,182] are associated with both hemorrhagic and occlusive stroke. Diabetes mellitus is not associated with hemorrhagic stroke.[128,129] Atrial fibrillation is associated with risk of cortical but not lacunar[185] or primary hemorrhagic stroke.[124] Minor ischemic stroke, lacunar stroke, and TIA have many risk factors in common.[185,186]

Prevention

The World Health Organization has promoted community-based stroke prevention and hypertension control for many years.[187] In England, the Health of the Nation policy[188] has set a goal of 40 percent reduction in mortality from stroke (among other diseases) over 10 years. The establishment of health, as opposed to health service, policies is of major importance in recognizing the fact that much disease and exposure to risk factors is caused by social and economic factors, as well as by individual behaviors. Consequently, plans required to reduce disease and risk factor exposure cannot focus solely on health services but need much wider collaboration, both within government and also at more local levels. Despite strong evidence that older people stand to benefit as much in relative terms, and more in absolute terms, from primary and secondary prevention, Health of the Nation policy has not set targets for those aged 75 years and over. This omission is not surprising but is another example of the widespread agism in society. In practice, there is nothing to stop health care planners and those involved in health promotion from including older people in their strategies.

Table 34-3 Stroke risk factors

Factor	Relative Risk[a]
Inherent traits	
Genetic	
Homocysteinemia	1–3[96–100]
Family history	2–3[92,93,104,105,130,131]
Monozygotic twin	1–5[94,95]
Age (55–64 versus 75+)	5[103,109,132]
Race	—[88,89,133–135]
Physiological characteristics	
High blood pressure	3[102,103,136,137]
Low forced expiratory volume	2[104,138]
Blood cholesterol	—[87,113,114]
Lp (a)	—[139,140]
Raised fibrinogen	—[104,141,142]
Raised hematocrit	—[143]
Endogenous tissue plasminogen activator	3.5[144]
Obesity	1–2[145–148]
Snoring	2[149–151]
Behaviors	
Alcohol consumption (30+ units/wk)	2.5–4[103,121,152–154]
Smoking	2[105,118,120,155,156]
Low dietary vitamin C	1.5[79,80]
Low dietary potassium	2–5[81]
Exercise	0.3–0.5[157–161]
Life events (e.g., bereavement, loss of job)	2[162]
Hormone replacement therapy	0.5–2[161,163–165]
Environmental factors	
Low temperature	—[166]
Air pollution	—[167,168]
Social characteristics	
Lower social class	1.6[62,169,170]
Other factors	
Early-life environment and maternal nutrition	—[66,67,171]
Comorbid conditions	
Heart failure	5[122]
Atrial fibrillation	5–7[123–125]
Carotid bruit	1–2[172,173]
TIA	7[174]
Diabetes mellitus	2–3[126–128]
Acute infection	5[175]
Warfarin treatment	7–10[176]

[a] *Relative risk estimates for continuous variables are generally lowest compared with the highest quintiles of distributions. No estimate is given when the publication did not calculate a relative risk.*

High-Risk Approach

Identification of people at high risk of stroke is an essential step in primary prevention. An efficient stroke risk score has been developed[189] comprising age, systolic blood pressure, smoking, and presence of anginal symptoms. The score derived from these risk factors can be used to identify individuals who will subsequently suffer a stroke. Those in the highest quintile (fifth) of the score distribution suffer 80 percent of strokes occurring over a period of 5 years. Use of such a scoring system in primary care would reduce the amount of work required in identifying and targeting preventive strategies such as antihypertensive treatment, use of antiplatelet agents, and antismoking advice. The costs of primary prevention must also be considered, and in the case of blood pressure detection and treatment may range widely from £1000 to £30,000 per DALY gained.[190]

Population Approach

Lowering population distribution risk factors will also result in a reduction in the proportion of high-risk individuals.[191] It has been suggested that the high-risk approach is inefficient because only a third of excess stroke deaths would be avoided if those with a systolic blood pressure over 170 mmHg were detected and treated.[82] Such calculations ignore the increased risk of stroke in individuals with multiple risk factors and therefore underestimate the value of high-risk approaches to prevention.

However, public health measures for lowering the dietary consumption of salt and alcohol might be expected to result in lower blood pressure distributions,[68,69] although there is doubt about the size of the reduction that could be achieved[192] and whether such changes can be achieved in practice.

Reduction in smoking and increase in physical activity are both measures that are of general importance in the control of other diseases as well as stroke.

It is worth emphasizing that these preventive measures are of benefit in people already suffering from clinical evidence of cardiovascular disease.[193] A more vigorous approach to preventing recurrent disease is required in these circumstances.

References

1. World Health Organization: Cerebrovascular disease: a clinical and research classification. WHO Offset Publ 43, 1978.
2. O'Mahony PG, Dobson R, Rodgers H et al: Validation of a population screening questionnaire to assess prevalence of stroke. Stroke 1995;26:1334–1337
3. National Institute of Neurological Disorders and Stroke: Classification of cerebrovascular diseases III. Stroke 1990;21: 637–676
4. Bamford J: Clinical examination in diagnosis and subclassification of stroke. Lancet 1992;339:400–402
5. Celani MG, Righetti E, Migliacci R et al: Comparability and validity of two clinical scores in the early differential diagnosis of acute stroke. BMJ 1994;308:1674–1676
6. Poungvarin N, Viriyavejakul A, Komontri C: Siriraj stroke score and validation study to distinguish supratentorial intracerebral haemorrhage from infarction. BMJ 1991;302: 1565–1567
7. Sandercock P, Molyneux A, Warlow C: Value of computed

tomography in patients with stroke: Oxfordshire Community Stroke Project. BMJ 1985;290:193–197

8. Foulkes MA, Wolf PA, Price TR et al: The Stroke Data Bank: design, methods and baseline characteristics. Stroke 1988;19: 547–554
9. Bamford J, Sandercock P, Jones L, Warlow C: The natural history of lacunar infarction: the Oxfordshire Community Stroke Project. Stroke 1987;18:545–551
10. Bamford J, Sandercock P, Dennis M et al: Classification and natural history of clinically identifiable subtypes of cerebral infarction. Lancet 1991;337:1521–1526
11. Anonymous: Uncommon causes of stroke. Lancet 1989;1:26
12. Ebrahim S: Clinical Epidemiology of Stroke. Oxford University Press, Oxford, 1990
13. Russell RW. How does blood-pressure cause stroke? Lancet 1975;2:1283–1285
14. Shuaib A, Hachinski VC: Mechanisms and management of stroke in the elderly. Can Med Assoc J 1991;145:433–443
15. Caplan LR: Binswanger's disease—revisited. Neurology 1995;45:626–633
16. Allen CMC, Harrison MJG, Wade DT: The management of acute stroke. Castle House Publications, Tunbridge Wells, United Kingdom, 1988
17. Diringer MN: Intracerebral hemorrhage: pathophysiology and management. Crit Care Med 1993;21:1591–1603
18. Davies MJ, Woolf N: Atherosclerosis: what is it and why does it occur? Br Heart J 1993;69(suppl):s3–s11
19. Pulsinelli W: Pathophysiology of acute ischaemic stroke. Lancet 1992;339:533–536
20. Heiss WD, Graf R: The ischemic penumbra. Curr Opin Neurol 1994;7:11–19
21. Siesjo BK: Pathophysiology and treatment of focal cerebral ischemia. I. pathophysiology. J Neurosurg 1992;77:169–184
22. Collins RC, Dobkin BH, Choi DW: Selective vulnerability of the brain: new insights into the pathophysiology of stroke. Ann Intern Med 1989;110:992–1000
23. Hawkins GC, Bonita R, Broad JB, Anderson NE: Inadequacy of clinical scoring systems to differentiate stroke subtypes in population-based studies. Stroke 1995;26:1338–1342
24. Sandercock PA, Allen CM, Corston RN et al: Clinical diagnosis of intracranial haemorrhage using Guy's Hospital score. BMJ 1985;291:1675–1677
25. Weir CJ, Murray GD, Adams FG et al: Poor accuracy of stroke scoring systems for differential clinical diagnosis of intracranial haemorrhage and infarction. Lancet 1994;344:999–1002
26. Lindley RI, Warlow CP, Wardlaw JM et al: Interobserver reliability of a clinical classification of acute cerebral infarction. Stroke 1993;24:1801–1804
27. Kalache A, Aboderin I: Stroke: the global burden. Health Policy Plan 1995;10:1–21
28. Bonita R, Beaglehole R, Asplund K: The worldwide problem of stroke. Curr Opin Neurol 1994;7:5–10
29. World Bank: World Development Report 1993: Investing in Health. Oxford University Press, Oxford, 1993
30. Pearson TA, Jamison DT, Trejo-Gutierrez J: Cardiovascular disease. In Jamison DT, Mosley WH, Measham AR, Bobadilla JL (eds): Disease Control Priorities in Developing Countries. Oxford University Press, Oxford, 1993 p. 577–594
31. Wade DT: Stroke (Acute Cerebrovascular Disease). In J (eds): Health Care Needs Assessment. Vol. 1. Stevens A, Raftery J, (eds): Ratcliffe Medical Press, Oxford, 1994
32. Gorelick PB: Stroke prevention. Arch Neurol 1995;52: 347–355
33. Isard PA, Forbes JF: Cost of stroke to the National Health Service in Scotland. Cerebrovasc Dis 1992;2:47–50
34. Mills E, Thompson M: The economic cost of stroke in Massachusetts. N Engl J Med 1978;299:415–418
35. Adelman SM: National Survey of Stroke: economic impact. Stroke 1981;12(suppl 1): I-69–I-87
36. Bergman L, van der Meulen JH, Limberg M, Habbema JD: Costs of medical care after first-ever stroke in the Netherlands. Stroke 1995;26:1830–1836
37. Malmgren R, Bamford J, Warlow C et al: Projecting the number of patients with first ever strokes and patients newly handicapped by stroke in England and Wales. BMJ 1989;298: 656–660
38. Bonita R, Broad JB, Beaglehole R: Changes in stroke incidence and case-fatality in Auckland, New Zealand, 1981–91. Lancet 1993;342:1470–1473
39. McGovern PG, Burke GL, Sprafka JM et al: Trends in mortality, morbidity, and risk factor levels for stroke from 1960 through 1990: the Minnesota Heart Survey. JAMA 1992;268: 753–759
40. Sarti C, Tuomilehto J, Sivenius J et al: Declining trends in incidence, case-fatality and mortality of stroke in three geographic areas of Finland during 1983–1989: Results from the FINMONICA stroke register. J Clin Epidemiol 1994;47: 1259–1269
41. Harmsen P, Tsipogianni A, Wilhelmsen L: Stroke incidence rates were unchanged, while fatality rates declined, during 1971–1987 in Göteborg, Sweden. Stroke 1992;23:1410–1415
42. Bonita R, Beaglehole R: Explaining stroke mortality trends. Lancet 1993;341:1510–1511
43. Malmgren R, Warlow C, Bamford J, Sandercock P: Geographical and secular trends in stroke incidence. Lancet 1987;2: 1196–1200
44. Garraway WM, Whisnant JP, Furlan AJ et al: The declining incidence of stroke. N Engl J Med 1979;300:449–452
45. Ostfeld AM: A review of stroke epidemiology. Epidemiol Rev 1980;2:136–152
46. Alfredsson L, von Arbin M, de Faire U: Mortality from and incidence of stroke in Stockholm. BMJ 1986;292:1299–1303
47. Broderick JP, Phillips SJ, Whisnant JP et al: Incidence of stroke in the eighties: the end of the decline in stroke? Stroke 1989;20:577–582
48. Kagan A, Popper J, Reed DM et al: Trends in stroke incidence and mortality in Hawaiian Japanese men. Stroke 1994;25: 1170–1175
49. Chang CC, Chen CJ: Secular trend of mortality from cerebral-

infarction and cerebral hemorrhage in Taiwan, 1974–1988. Stroke 1993;24:212–218

50. Tuomilehto J, Bonita R, Stewart A et al: Hypertension, cigarette smoking, and the decline in stroke incidence in eastern Finland. Stroke 1991;22:7–11
51. Vartiainen E, Sarti C, Tuomilehto J, Kuulasmaa K: Do changes in cardiovascular risk factors explain changes in mortality from stroke in Finland? BMJ 1995;310:901–904
52. Shimamoto T, Komachi Y, Inada H et al: Trends for coronary heart disease and stroke and their risk factors in Japan. Circulation 1989;79:503–515
53. Garraway WM, Whisnant JP: The changing pattern of hypertension and the declining incidence of stroke. JAMA 1987; 258:214–217
54. Whisnant JP: The decline of stroke. Stroke 1984;15:160–168
55. Bonita R: Stroke trends in Australia and New Zealand: mortality, morbidity, and risk factors. Ann Epidemiol 1993;3: 529–533
56. Bonita R, Beaglehole R: Does treatment of hypertension explain the decline in mortality from stroke? BMJ 1986;292: 191–192
57. Casper M, Wing S, Strogatz D et al: HA Antihypertensive treatment and U.S. trends in stroke mortality, 1962 to 1980. Am J Public Health 1992;82:1600–1606
58. Jacobs DR Jr, McGovern PG, Blackburn H: The U.S. decline in stroke mortality: what does ecological analysis tell us? Am J Public Health 1992;82:1596–1599
59. Terent A: Increasing incidence of stroke among Swedish women. Stroke 1988;19:598–603
60. Asplund K, Bonita R, Kuulasmaa K et al: Multinational comparisons of stroke epidemiology: evaluation of case ascertainment in the WHO MONICA Stroke Study: World Health Organization monitoring trends and determinants in cardiovascular disease. Stroke 1995;26:355–360
61. Office of Population Censuses & Surveys OPCS. Mortality: Area. HMSO, London, 1993
62. Acheson RM, Sanderson C: Strokes: social class and geography. Popul Trends 1978;12:13–17
63. Li SC, Schoenberg BS, Wang CC et al: Cerebrovascular disease in the People's Republic of China: epidemiologic and clinical features. Neurology 1985;35:1708–1713
64. Strachan DP, Leon DA, Dodgeon B: Mortality from cardiovascular disease among interregional migrants in England and Wales. BMJ 1995;310:423–427
65. Syme SL, Marmot MG, Kagan A, Rhoads G: Epidemiological studies of coronary heart disease and stroke in Japanese men living in Japan, Hawaii, and California: introduction. Am J Epidemiol 1975;102:477–480
66. Barker DJ, Osmond C, Pannett B: Why Londoners have low death rates from ischaemic heart disease and stroke. BMJ 1992;305:1551–1554
67. Barker DJ, Osmond C: Death rates from stroke in England and Wales predicted from past maternal mortality. BMJ 1987; 295:83–86
68. Intersalt Cooperative Research Group: Intersalt: an international study of electrolyte excretion and blood pressure: results for 24 hour urinary sodium and potassium excretion. BMJ 1988;297:319–328
69. Elliott P, Stamler J, Nichols R et al: Intersalt revisited: further analyses of 24 hour sodium excretion and blood pressure within and across populations. BMJ 1996;321: 1249–1253
70. Law MR, Frost CD, Wald NJ: By how much does salt restriction lower blood pressure? I. analysis of observational data among populations. II. analysis of observational data within populations. III. analysis of data from trials of salt reduction. BMJ 1991;302:811–824
71. Joosens JV, Kestelloot H, Amery A: Salt intake and mortality from stroke. N Engl J Med 1979;300:1396
72. Walker JW: Changing U.S. life style and declining vascular mortality: cause or coincidence? N Engl J Med 1977;297: 163–165
73. Simpson FO: Salt and hypertension: a sceptical review of the evidence. Clin Sci 1979;57:463s–480s
74. Cummins RO: Recent changes in salt use and stroke mortality in England and Wales: any help for the salt hypertension debate? J Epidemiol Commun Health 1983;37:25–28
75. Bulpitt CJ: Vitamin C and vascular disease. BMJ 1995;310: 1548–1549
76. Khaw KT, Woodhouse P: Interrelation of vitamin C, infection, haemostatic factors, and cardiovascular disease. BMJ 1995; 310:1559–1563
77. Gale CR, Martyn CN, Winter PD, Cooper C: Vitamin C and risk of death from stroke and coronary heart disease in cohort of elderly people. BMJ 1995;310:1563–1566
78. Barer DH, Ebrahim S, Pengally D: Vitamin C and stroke: case control study. J Clin Epidemiol 1989;42:625–631
79. Gillman MW, Cupples LA, Gagnon D et al: Protective effect of fruits and vegetables on development of stroke in men. JAMA 1995;273:1113–1117
80. Acheson RM, Williams DR: Does consumption of fruit and vegetables protect against stroke? Lancet 1983;1:1191–1193
81. Khaw KT, Barrett-Connor E: Dietary potassium and stroke-associated mortality: a 12-year prospective population study. N Engl J Med 1987;316:235–240
82. Marmot MG, Poulter NR: Primary prevention of stroke Lancet 1992;339:344–347
83. Bamford J, Sandercock P, Dennis M et al: A prospective study of acute cerebrovascular disease in the community: the Oxfordshire Community Stroke Project—1981–86. 2. incidence, case fatality rates and overall outcome at one year of cerebral infarction, primary intracerebral and subarachnoid haemorrhage. J Neurol Neurosurg Psychiatry 1990;53:16–22
84. Bamford J, Sandercock P, Dennis M et al: A prospective study of acute cerebrovascular disease in the community: the Oxfordshire Community Stroke Project 1981–86. 1. methodology, demography and incident cases of first-ever stroke. J Neurol Neurosurg Psychiatry 1988;51:1373–1380
85. Bonita R, Beaglehole R, North JDK: Event, incidence, and case-fatality rates of cerebrovascular disease in Auckland, New Zealand. Am J Epidemiol 1984;120:236–243

86. Bonita R: Epidemiology of stroke. Lancet 1992;339:342–344

87. Prospective Studies Collaboration: Cholesterol, diastolic blood pressure, and stroke: 13,000 strokes in 450,000 people in 45 prospective cohorts. Lancet 1995;346:1647–1653

88. Balarajan R: Ethnic differences in mortality from ischaemic heart disease and cerebrovascualr disease in England and Wales. BMJ 1991;302:560–564

89. Marmot MG, Adelstein AM, Bulusu L: Lessons from the study of immigrant mortality. Lancet 1984;1:1455–1458

90. Kittner SJ, White LR, Losonczy KG et al: Black-white differences in stroke incidence in a national sample. The contribution of hypertension and diabetes mellitus. JAMA 1990;264: 1267–1270

91. Sacco RL, Kargman DE, GU Q, Zamanillo MC: Race-ethnicity and determinants of intracranial atherosclerotic cerebral infarction: the Northern Manhattan Stroke Study. Stroke 1995; 26:14–20

92. Khaw KT, Barrett-Connor E: Family history of stroke as an independent predictor of ischaemic heart disease in men and stroke in women. Am J Epidemiol 1986;123:59–66

93. Wannamethee G, Shaper AG, Ebrahim S: Family history and stroke. Stroke 1996;27:1492–1498

94. de Faire U, Friberg L, Lundman T: Concordance for mortality with special reference to ischaemic heart disease and cerebrovascular disease. Prev Med 1975;4:509–517

95. Brass LM, Isaacsohn JL, Merikangas KR, Robinette CD: A study of twins and stroke. Stroke 1992;23:221–223

96. Clarke R, Daly L, Robinson K et al: Hyperhomocysteinemia: an independent risk factor for vascular disease N Engl J Med 1991;324:1149–1155

97. Boers GH, Smals AG, Trijbels FJ et al: Heterozygosity for homocystinuria in premature peripheral and cerebral occlusive arterial disease. N Engl J Med 1985;313:709–715

98. Verhoef P, Hennekens CH, Malinow MR et al: A prospective study of plasma homocyst (e)ine and risk of ischemic stroke. Stroke 1994;25:1924–1930

99. Berwanger CS, Jeremy JY, Stansby G: Homocysteine and vascular disease. Br J Surg 1995;82:726–731

100. Perry IJ, Refsum H, Morris RW et al: Prospective study of serum total homocysteine concentration and risk of stroke in middle-aged British men. Lancet 1995;346:1395–1398

101. Colandrea MA, Friedman GD, Nichaman MZ, Lynd CN: Systolic hypertension in the elderly: an epidemiologic assessment. Circulation 1970;41:239–245

102. Kannel WB, Wolf PA, Verter J, McNamara PM: Epidemilogic assessment of the role of blood pressure in stroke: the Framingham Study. JAMA 1970;214:301–310

103. Shaper AG, Phillips AN, Pocock SJ et al: Risk factors for stroke in middle aged British men. BMJ 1991;302:1111–1115

104. Welin L, Svardsudd K, Wilhelmsen L et al: Analysis of risk factors for stroke in a cohort of men born in 1913. N Engl J Med 1987;317:521–526

105. Thompson SG, Greenberg G, Meade TW: Risk factors for stroke and myocardial infarction in women in the United Kingdom as assessed in general practice: a case-control study. Br Heart 1989;61:403–409

106. Wolf PA, D'Agostino RB, Belanger AJ, Kannel WB: Probability of stroke: a risk profile from the Framingham Study. Stroke 1991;22:312–318

107. Harmsen P, Rosengren A, Tsipogianni A, Wilhelmsen L: Risk factors for stroke in middle-aged men in Goteborg, Sweden. Stroke 1990;21:223–229

108. Boysen G, Nyboe J, Appleyard M et al: Stroke incidence and risk factors for stroke in Copenhagen, Denmark. Stroke 1988; 19:1345–1353

109. Khaw KT, Barrett-Connor E, Suarez L, Criqui MH: Predictors of stroke-associated mortality in the elderly. Stroke 1984;15: 244–248

110. Starr JM, Bulpitt C: Hypertension. pp. 245–252. In Ebrahim S, Kalache A (eds): Epidemiology in Old age. British Medical Journal Publications, London, 1996

111. Mulrow CD, Cornell JA, Herrera CR et al: Hypertension in the elderly: implications and generalisability of randomized trials. JAMA 1995;272:1932–1938

112. Chen Z, Peto R, Collins R et al: Serum cholesterol concentration and coronary heart disease in population with low cholesterol concentrations. BMJ 1991;303:276–282

113. Lindenstrom E, Boysen G, Nyboe J: Influence of total cholesterol, high density lipoprotein cholesterol, and triglycerides on risk of cerebrovascular disease: the Copenhagen City Heart Study. BMJ 1994;309:11–15

114. Iso H, Jacobs DR Jr, Wentworth D et al: Serum cholesterol levels and six-year mortality from stroke in 350,977 men screened for the multiple risk factor intervention trial. N Engl J Med 1989;320:904–910

115. Hebert PR, Gaziano JM, Hennekens CH: An overview of trials of cholesterol lowering and risk of stroke. Arch Intern Med 1995;155:50–55

116. Dawber TR: The Framingham Study. Harvard University Press, London, 1980

117. Wannamethee SG, Shaper AG, Whincup PH, Walker M: Smoking cessation and the risk of stroke in middle-aged men. JAMA 1995;274:155–160

118. Shinton R, Beevers G: Meta-analysis of relation between cigarette smoking and stroke. BMJ 1989;298:789–794

119. Wolf PA, D'Agostino RB, Kannel WB et al: Cigarette smoking as a risk factor for stroke: the Framingham Study. JAMA 1988; 259:1025–1029

120. Kawachi I, Colditz GA, Stampfer MJ et al: Smoking cessation and decreased risk of stroke in women. JAMA 1993;269: 232–236

121. Lee TK, Huang ZS, Ng SK et al: Impact of alcohol consumption and cigarette smoking on stroke among the elderly in Taiwan. Stroke 1995;26:790–794

122. Kannel WB, Wolf PA, Verter J: Manifestations of coronary disease predisposing to stroke: the Framingham Study. JAMA 1983;250:2942–2946

123. Flegel KM, Shipley MJ, Rose G: Risk of stroke in non-rheumatic atrial fibrillation. Lancet 1987;1:526–529

124. van Merwijk G, Lodder J, Bamford J, Kester AD: How often

is non-valvular atrial fibrillation the cause of brain infarction? J Neurol 1990;237:205–207

125. Wolf PA, Abbott RD, Kannel WB: Atrial fibrillation: a major contributor to stroke in the elderly: the Framingham Study. Arch Inter Med 1987;147:1561–1564

126. Abbott RD, Donahue RP, MacMahon SW et al: Diabetes and the risk of stroke: the Honolulu Heart Program. JAMA 1987; 257:949–952

127. Manson JE, Colditz GA, Stampfer MJ et al: A prospective study of maturity-onset diabetes mellitus and risk of coronary heart disease and stroke in women. Arch Intern Med 1991;151: 1141–1147

128. Burchfiel CM, Curb JD, Rodriguez BL et al: Glucose intolerance and 22-year stroke incidence: the Honolulu Heart Program. Stroke 1994;25:951–957

129. Jamrozik K, Broadhurst RJ, Anderson CS, Stewart-Wynne EG: The role of lifestyle factors in the etiology of stroke: a population-based case-control study in Perth, Western Australia. Stroke 1994;25:51–59

130. Graffagnino C, Gasecki AP, Doig GS, Hachinski VC: The importance of family history in cerebrovascular disease. Stroke 1994;25:1599–1604

131. Kiely DK, Wolf PA, Cupples LA et al: Familial aggregation of stroke: the Framingham Study. Stroke 1993;24:1366–1371

132. Oxfordshire Community Stroke Project: Incidence of stroke in Oxfordshire: first year's experience of a community stroke register. BMJ 1985;287:713–717

133. Broderick JP, Brott T, Tomsick T et al: The risk of subarachnoid and intracerebral hemorrhages in blacks as compared with whites. N Engl J Med 1992;326:733–736

134. Caplan LR: Strokes in African-Americans. Circulation 1991; 83:1469–1471

135. Yatsu FM: Strokes in Asians and Pacific-Islanders, Hispanics, and Native Americans. Circulation 1991;83:1471–1472

136. MacMahon S, Peto R, Cutler J et al: Blood pressure, stroke, and coronary heart disease. 1. prolonged differences in blood pressure: prospective observational studies corrected for the regression dilution bias. Lancet 1990;335:765–774

137. Kannel WB, Dawber TR, McGee DL: Perspectives on systolic hypertension: the Framingham Study. Circulation 1980;61: 1179–1182

138. Strachan DP: Ventilatory function as a predictor of fatal stroke. BMJ 1991;302:84–87

139. Shintani S, Kikuchi S, Hamaguchi H, Shiigai T: High serum lipoprotein (a) levels are an independent risk factor for cerebral infarction. Stroke 1993;24:965–969

140. Woo J, Lau E, Lam CW et al: Hypertension, lipoprotein (a), and apolipoprotein A-I as risk factors for stroke in the Chinese. Stroke 1991;22:203–208

141. Kannel WB, Wolf PA, Castelli WP, D'Agostino RB: Fibrinogen and risk of cardiovascular disease: the Framingham Study. JAMA 1987;258:1183–1186

142. Wilhelmsen L, Svardsudd K, Korsan-Bengtsen K et al: Fibrinogen as a risk factor for stroke and myocardial infarction. N Engl J Med 1984;311:501–505

143. Gagnon DR, Zhang TJ, Brand FN, Kannel WB: Hematocrit and the risk of cardiovascular disease—the Framingham Study: a 34-year follow-up. Am Heart J 1994;127:674–682

144. Ridker PM, Hennekens CH, Stampfer MJ et al: Prospective study of endogenous tissue plasminogen activator and risk of stroke. Lancet 1994;343:940–943

145. DiPietro L, Ostfeld AM, Rosner GL: Adiposity and stroke among older adults of low socioeconomic status: the Chicago Stroke Study. Am J Public Health 1994;84:14–19

146. Abbott RD, Behrens GR, Sharp DS et al: Body mass index and thromboembolic stroke in nonsmoking men in older middle age: the Honolulu Heart Program. Stroke 1994;25: 2370–2376

147. Folsom AR, Prineas RJ, Kaye SA, Munger RG: Incidence of hypertension and stroke in relation to body fat distribution and other risk factors in older women. Stroke 1990;21:701–706

148. Larsson B, Svardsudd K, Welin L et al: Abdominal adipose tissue distribution, obesity, and risk of cardiovascular disease and death: 13 year follow up of participants in the study of men born in 1913. BMJ 1984;288:1401–1404

149. Koskenvuo M, Kaprio J, Telakivi T et al: Snoring as a risk factor for ischaemic heart disease and stroke in men. BMJ 1987;294:16–19

150. Palomaki H: Snoring and the risk of ischemic brain infarction. Stroke 1991;22:1021–1025

151. Palomaki H, Partinen M, Juvela S, Kaste M: Snoring as a risk factor for sleep-related brain infarction. Stroke 1989;20: 1311–1315

152. Gill JS, Shipley MJ, Tsementzis SA et al: Alcohol consumption—a risk factor for hemorrhagic and non-hemorrhagic stroke. Am J Med 1991;90:489–497

153. Gill JS, Zezulka AV, Shipley MJ et al: Stroke and alcohol consumption. N Engl J Med 1986;315:1041–1046

154. Kiyohara Y, Kato I, Iwamoto H et al: The impact of alcohol and hypertension on stroke incidence in a general Japanese population: the Hisayama Study. Stroke 1995;26:368–372

155. Robbins AS, Manson JE, Lee IM et al: Cigarette smoking and stroke in a cohort of U.S. male physicians. Ann Intern Med 1994;120:458–462

156. Bonita R, Scragg R, Stewart A et al: Cigarette smoking and risk of premature stroke in men and women. Br Med J 1986; 293:6–8

157. Shinton R, Sagar G: Lifelong exercise and stroke. BMJ 1993; 307:231–234

158. Wannamethee G, Shaper AG: Physical activity and stroke in British middle aged men. BMJ 1992;304:597–601

159. Paffenbarger RS Jr, Laughlin ME, Gima AS, Black RA: Work activity of longshoremen as related to death from coronary heart disease and stroke. N Engl J Med 1970;282:1109–1114

160. Lapidus L, Bengtsson C: Socioeconomic factors and physical activity in relation to cardiovascular disease and death: a 12 year follow up of participants in a population study of women in Gothenburg, Sweden. Br Heart J 1986;55:295–301

161. Lindenstrom E, Boysen G, Nyboe J: Lifestyle factors and risk of cerebrovascular disease in women: the Copenhagen City Heart Study. Stroke 1993;24:1468–1472

162. House A, Dennis M, Mogridge L et al: Life events and difficulties preceding stroke. J Neurol Neurosurg Psychiatry 1990; 53:1024–1028

163. Falkeborn M, Persson I, Terent A et al: Hormone replacement therapy and the risk of stroke: follow-up of a population-based cohort in Sweden. Arch Intern Med 1993;153:1201–1209

164. Paganini-Hill A, Ross RK, Henderson BE: Postmenopausal oestrogen treatment and stroke: a prospective study. BMJ 1988;297:519–522

165. Wilson PW, Garrison RJ, Castelli WP: Postmenopausal estrogen use, cigarette smoking, and cardiovascular morbidity in women over 50: the Framingham Study. N Engl J Med 1985; 313:1038–1043

166. Pan WH, Li LA, Tsai MJ: Temperature extremes and mortality from coronary heart disease and cerebral infarction in elderly Chinese. Lancet 1995;345:353–355

167. Zhang ZF, Yu SZ, Zhou GD: Indoor air pollution of coal fumes as a risk factor of stroke, Shanghai. Am J Public Health 1988; 78:975–977

168. Knox EG: Meterological associations of cerebrovascular disease mortality in England and Wales. J Epidemiol Commun Health 1981;35:220–223

169. Marmot MG, McDowall ME: Mortality decline and widening social inequalities. Lancet 1986;2:274–276

170. Howard G, Russell GB, Anderson R et al: Role of social class in excess black stroke mortality. Stroke 1995;26:1759–1763

171. Barker DJ, Osmond C: Infant mortality, childhood nutrition, and ischaemic heart disease in England and Wales. Lancet 1986;1:1077–1081

172. Wolf PA, Kannel WB, Sorlie P, McNamara P: Asymptomatic carotid bruit and risk of stroke: the Framingham Study. JAMA 1981;245:1442–1445

173. Van Ruiswyk J, Noble H, Sigmann P: The natural history of carotid bruits in elderly persons. Ann Intern Med 1990;112: 340–343174. Dennis M, Bamford J, Sandercock P, Warlow C: Prognosis of transient ischemic attacks in the Oxfordshire Community Stroke Project. Stroke 1990;21:848–853

175. Grau AJ, Buggle F, Heindl S et al: Recent infection as a risk factor for cerebrovascular ischemia. Stroke 1995;26:373–379

176. Hart RG, Boop BS, Anderson DC: Oral anticoagulants and intracranial hemorrhage: facts and hypotheses. Stroke 1995; 26:1471–1477

177. Juvela S, Hillbom M, Palomaki H: Risk factors for spontaneous intracerebral hemorrhage. Stroke 1995;26:1558–1564

178. Calandre L, Arnal C, Ortega JF et al: Risk factors for spontaneous cerebral hematomas: case-control study. Stroke 1986; 17:1126–1128

179. Brott T, Thalinger K, Hertzberg V: Hypertension as a risk factor for spontaneous intracerebral hemorrhage. Stroke 1986; 17:1078–1083

180. Lin CH, Shimizu Y, Kato H et al: Cerebrovascular diseases in a fixed population of Hiroshima and Nagasaki, with special reference to relationship between type and risk factors. Stroke 1984;15:653–660

181. Stemmermann GN, Hayashi T, Resch JA et al: Risk factors related to ischemic and hemorrhagic cerebrovascular disease at autopsy: the Honolulu Heart Study. Stroke 1984;15:23–28

182. Tanaka H, Ueda Y, Hayashi M et al: Risk factors for cerebral haemorrhage and cerebral infarction in a Japanese rural community. Stroke 1982;13:62–73

183. Abbott RD, Yin Y, Reed DM, Yano K: Risk of stroke in male cigarette smokers. N Engl J Med 1986;315:717–720

184. Gill JS, Shipley MJ, Tsementzis SA et al: Cigarette smoking: a risk factor for hemorrhagic and nonhemorrhagic stroke. Arch Intern Med 1989;149:2053–2057

185. Lodder J, Bamford JM, Sandercock PA et al: Are hypertension or cardiac embolism likely causes of lacunar infarction? Stroke 1990;21:375–381

186. Dennis MS, Bamford JM, Sandercock PA, Warlow CP: A comparison of risk factors and prognosis for transient ischemic attacks and minor ischemic strokes: the Oxfordshire Community Stroke Project. Stroke 1989;20:1494–1499

187. Hatano S, Shigematsu I, Strasser T: Hypertension and Stroke Control in the Community. World Health Organization, Geneva 1976

188. Secretary of State for Health: Health of the Nation. HMSO, London, 1992

189. Coppola WG, Whincup PH, Papacosta O et al: Scoring system to identify men at high risk of stroke: a strategy for general practice. Br J Gen Pract 1995;45:185–189

190. Ebrahim S: Stroke. pp. 262–269. In Ebrahim, S, Kalache A (eds): Epidemiology in Old Age. British Medical Journal Publications, London, 1996

191. Rose G: The Strategy of Preventive Medicine. Oxford University Press, Oxford 1993

192. Davey Smith G, Phillips AN: Inflation in epidemiology: "the proof and measurement of association between two things" revisited. BMJ 1996;312:1659–1661

193. Ebrahim S, Davey Smith G: Health Promotion for Coronary Heart Disease and Stroke in Older People. Health Education Authority, London, 1996

CHAPTER 35

Stroke: Clinical Presentation and Management

LALIT KALRA

The term *cerebrovascular disease* refers to a broad group of disorders and includes any abnormality of the brain resulting from pathologic processes involving blood vessels that leads to ischemia, infarction, or hemorrhage (Fig. 35-1). These disorders are classified into three main clinical categories: transient ischemic attacks (TIAs), stroke (occlusive or hemorrhagic), and cerebral multi-infarct states (cortical, subcortical, or diffuse).

Stroke is the cardinal manifestation of cerebrovascular disease and is defined as the acute onset of a neurologic deficit lasting more than 24 hours or leading to death with no apparent cause other than vascular disease.[1] The neurologic deficit is generally focal and is representative of the site and size of the anatomic lesion. Global presentations, associated with loss of consciousness, are occasionally seen. The abruptness of onset of the neurologic deficit (minutes, hours, or days) is the characteristic feature of stroke. Another important characteristic is its clinical course: there is arrest of the neurologic deficit followed by regression—depending on pathology to a greater or lesser extent—in all but fatal strokes.

Stroke ranks first in frequency, and probably urgency, among serious neurologic disorders and accounts for nearly half of all neurologic admissions seen in general hospitals.[2] It is a leading cause of death and disability in the western world. Nearly one-half of stroke patients die within 1 year of the acute episode,[3] with another 10 percent of survivors dying every year thereafter. Only a third of survivors make good recovery, and stroke is estimated to be responsible for 14 to 25 percent of cases of severe disability in the community.[4] The human cost of stroke to the individual, family, and society cannot be overestimated. The financial costs of managing stroke patients are high, irrespective of whether treatment takes place in a hospital or in the community. Overall, about 20 percent of the medical beds in a general hospital are occupied by stroke patients, and in western countries half of the survivors spend at least 4 weeks in the hospital.[5] There are concerns that these costs are likely to escalate as a consequence of demographic changes and the changing epidemiology of stroke.

In the past, stroke management has been dominated by negative and nihilistic attitudes, not only among physicians but also among patients and their families. Much of this pessimism has reflected the absence of effective medical treatment for acute stroke, ignorance about the benefits of nonpharmacologic interventions, and a perception of universally poor outcome in this patient group. Fortunately, attitudes are changing, in part because of developments in therapeutics (which offer hope for the future) and also because of changes in the philosophy of stroke management. The transition from a disease/organ-centerd approach to a holistic patient-centerd approach in recent years has been shown to be associated with a better outcome for patients at reduced service costs because of better organization of care.[6] Awareness of the true costs of poor management of stroke patients and fears of spiraling costs in the future have provided further impetus to adopting a more positive attitude, with stroke prevention and treatment receiving high priority in most national health programs.

Stroke is primarily a disorder of the aging population and, in the United Kingdom at least, much of the care of stroke patients is undertaken by professionals with a special interest in geriatrics. The association with aging has several important implications. Acute and late mortality are higher in this age group compared with that for younger stroke patients.[7,8] Older patients are more likely to be hospitalized because of severe loss of function and lack of adequate support mechanisms at home.[9] They are also more likely to have other pathology—notably ischemic heart disease, chronic heart failure, chronic pulmonary disease, arthritis, and visual or auditory impairment—which must addressed as a part of overall stroke management. Background levels of chronic cognitive impairment increase with age and are likely to affect outcome, especially because much of rehabilitation involves learning and retention of new skills. Despite these considerations, there is no evidence suggesting that age per se affects neurologic recovery or the duration of hospital stay in stroke patients.[10]

It is important to emphasize that stroke affects several domains of human performance and behavior, many of which lie outside traditional medical models of assessment and management. The whole philosophy of stroke assessment and management is based on multidisciplinary practice requiring the skills of many people including doctors, nurses, therapists, social workers, and other professionals who may be called on to help in the care of patients. Although this chapter will concentrate mainly on the medical aspects of stroke presentation and management in an elderly population, emphasis will also be placed on a holistic approach to assessment and treatment based on multidisciplinary practice.

Clinical Aspects

Terminology

TIAs are arbitrarily distinguished from completed stroke by the duration of neurologic dysfunction, which is stipulated as being less than 24 hours. If symptoms (not necessarily signs)

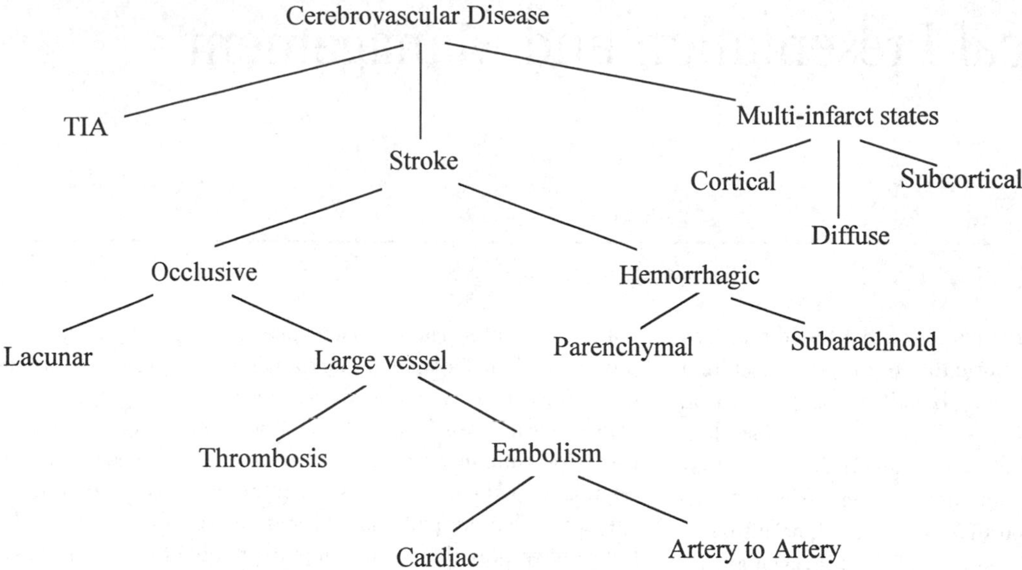

Figure 35-1 Classification of cerebrovascular diseases.

resolve within 1 week (3 weeks in North America)[11] the term *reversible ischemic neurologic deficit* (RIND) is often used. It is important to remember that there are no differences in pathogenesis, epidemiology, risk factors, management, or long-term prognosis between a TIA and a nondisabling ischemic stroke. The increasing use of computed tomography (CT) has led to the identification of asymptomatic areas of cerebral ischemia in patients with first stroke as well as infarcts in relevant cerebral areas in patients who have had a TIA. The term *cerebral infarction with transient symptoms* (CITS) has been suggested for these presentations but is not universally accepted.[12]

Classification

Stroke is a syndrome resulting from a range of heterogeneous conditions that affect cerebral vasculature or blood flow but have a common clinical presentation. Strokes may be divided into those due to arterial occlusion and those due to hemorrhage (Fig. 35-1). Approximately 85 percent of strokes are occlusive[3]: the occlusion may affect large vessels (thrombosis or embolism), small vessels (lacunar stroke) associated with hypertension, or, possibly, embolism. Some experts prefer to classify lacunar stroke (seen in about a one-fourth of occlusive stroke patients) separately because of differences in pathology, prognosis, and management compared with large vessel disease. Hemorrhagic stroke occurs in 15 percent of stroke patients. It may be primary, due to microaneurysms (11 to 12 percent), or secondary, due to extracerebral rupture of intracranial vessels (3 to 4 percent).[3]

Thrombotic stroke

The most commonly cause of thrombotic stroke is atherosclerosis in the arteries of the brain which parallels, but is somewhat less severe than, atherosclerosis of the aorta, coronary, or renal arteries. The common sites of involvement are the internal carotid artery at the carotid sinus in the neck, the junction of the vertebral and basilar arteries, the main bifurcation of the middle cerebral artery, the posterior cerebral artery around the cerebral peduncle, and the anterior cerebral artery over the corpus callosum.[2] It is rare for cerebral arteries to be affected significantly beyond their first bifurcation.[2] Degeneration, hemorrhage into atheroma, or rupture of atheromatous plaques damage the vascular endothelium and exposes subendothelial collagen. This, in association with other stimuli, activates platelets, leading to aggregation, adhesion, and thrombus formation. The thrombus may occlude the vessel at the site of formation or be carried downstream to lodge in a vessel with a smaller lumen (artery-to-artery embolism).

Thrombotic strokes are classically described as having "stuttering" intermittent progression over several hours or days after commencement. However, this intermittency is not seen in the majority (60 percent) of patients, in whom there is but a single progressive episode.[2] Thrombotic stroke is said to be particularly common during sleep or shortly after waking. Headache is uncommon but may be seen in 15 percent of thrombotic stroke patients and can antedate the stroke by several days. TIA may precede thrombotic stroke, and it is estimated that half of all TIAs are due to thromboembolic complications of atherosclerosis of the arteries leading to the brain. Carotid bruits are an unreliable sign of carotid obstruction in thrombotic stroke. An ipsilateral carotid bruit is present in only 64 percent of patients with 50 percent or greater stenosis of the internal carotid artery, while 11 percent of patients with less than 50 percent stenosis have a bruit.[13]

Thrombotic strokes are dynamic and may progress after the initial episode. This can be the result of increasing stenosis of the involved artery, growth of the mural thrombus, and/or propagation of the thrombus into other branches, hindering anastomotic flow. Retrograde thrombosis in the middle cerebral artery can extend back to the mouth of the anterior cerebral artery with the possibility of causing secondary infarction in the territory of that vessel. In addition, embolic particles traveling from the site of thrombosis to other vessels may precipitate abrupt changes in the neurologic deficit after the main event.

Embolic stroke

The heart is the source of emboli in most cases of cerebral embolism, but artery-to-artery embolism may occur as mentioned previously. Although any region of the brain can be affected, the territory of the middle cerebral artery is most frequently involved. Cerebral embolization from the heart can be caused by atrial fibrillation; damaged, infected, or prosthetic valves; or damaged or dyskinetic myocardial segments. Cerebral emboli can be associated with severe neurologic deficits because the rapidity of onset of complete occlusion prevents collateral perfusion from becoming established. Embolic stroke does not have any prodromal features and has been classically described as "a bolt out of the blue"; the full-blown neurological deficit develops within a few minutes of onset. Occasionally, in its passage along an artery, an embolus may produce significant neurologic deficits which are transitory and resolve as the embolus breaks up or passes into a small branch supplying a relatively silent area of the brain. The clinical picture is then that of a TIA. Cardiogenic emboli are responsible for TIAs in 20 percent of patients presenting with transient weakness.[14] TIAs due to cardiogenic emboli are characterized by episodes in different vascular territories with differing patterns of neurologic deficit since it is unlikely that successive emboli will lodge at identical sites.

Hemorrhagic transformation

In many cases, the embolic clot subsequently breaks up into fragments which then enter smaller vessels before disappearing completely. Recanalization of the previously occluded vessel may then lead to bleeding in the necrotic area. Hemorrhagic transformation is estimated to occur in 30 percent of embolic infarcts.[15] Although hemorrhagic transformation is particularly linked to embolic stroke, this is not always the case. The extent of hemorrhagic transformation is dependent on the depth and duration of ischemia as well as on the intensity of reperfusion. Serial CT studies have shown that this is a dynamic process and can occur at any time during the first 2 weeks after stroke.[15] Although hemorrhagic transformation is being more frequently recognized because of widespread use of CT scans in stroke, little is known about its clinical or therapeutic implications.

Hemorrhagic transformation is of particular significance in relation to early use of drugs that affect hemostatic mechanisms and is more likely to occur in patients already on such drugs at the time of their stroke.[15] The relationship with antithrombotic or antiplatelet drugs given after a cerebral infarct is less clear. There is some evidence suggesting that the use of thrombolytic agents in established infarcts is associated with a higher risk of intraparenchymal bleeding and increased mortality.[16,17] The benefits of preventing clot propagation and early recurrence must be balanced against the risks of hemorrhagic transformation in the development of thrombolytic interventions for management of acute stroke.

Lacunar stroke

Lacunar lesions of the brain are a pathologic diagnosis obtained at autopsy and include the residua of small infarcts, small hemorrhages, or dilatation of the perivascular spaces. The term is conventionally used to describe an area of infarction within the territory of a single perforating artery.[18] Patients with such lesions may or may not present with clinical features of stroke, and recent CT evidence suggests that as many as 80 percent of lacunar infarcts may be clinically silent.[19] Approximately 21 percent of occlusive strokes are lacunar, and their frequency increases with age.[20]

Lacunar strokes result from the occlusion of small perforating arteries which branch off from the major cerebral arteries and have few anastomotic branches. The areas most commonly affected are the caudate and lenticular nuclei, thalami, basis pontis, and cerebral or cerebellar white matter. The arteries are blocked not by platelet or fibrin thrombi (as would be expected in large vessel disease) but by a poorly understood process known as lipohyalinosis. In some instances, lipohyalinosis results in false aneurysm formation resembling Charcot-Bouchard aneurysms of intracerebral hemorrhage. As lacunar strokes can affect any fibers descending from the cortex, they can cause a host of clinical syndromes. A small number of clinical syndromes appear to occur more commonly and have been correlated with relevant lacunae observed during subsequent autopsy. These are regarded as "classic" lacunar syndromes and include pure motor stroke, pure sensory stroke, dysarthria-clumsy hand syndrome, ataxic hemiparesis, and sensorimotor stroke.[21] The term *extended lacunar stroke* is used to describe cases in which lacunar strokes have been associated with additional features such as psychological disturbances or eye movement abnormalities. Little is known about this condition, which may have different pathophysiology and clinical implications compared with lacunar infarcts. A "corona radiata lacune," more commonly seen in the elderly, is not a true lacunar infarct but a partial watershed infarct between the area of supply of the medullary branches of the cortical middle cerebral artery and the lenticulostriate penetrating branches of the middle cerebral artery. It is usually larger, less distinct, and more superficial than a lacunar infarct.[22]

Pure motor stroke is the most common presentation of lacunar infarcts. The deficit is likely to evolve over hours and does not have any cortical features such as language problems, visual field defects, inattention, or visuospatial difficulties. Significant headaches, seizures, or impairment of consciousness are all uncommon in lacunar strokes. TIAs in 20 percent of patients may be due to the involvement of small perforating arteries and are a result of incipient occlusion rather than cardiogenic or artery-to-artery emboli (as in the case of large vessel disease). Incipient occlusion may also explain the crescendo of attacks (frequency and duration) sometimes seen immediately before the completion of deficit (capsular warning syndrome).[21]

Although lacunar strokes are more common in patients with hypertension, atherosclerosis, and diabetes, the underlying pathophysiology appears—as already described—to be different from that of large-vessel occlusion. Significant ipsilateral carotid stenosis (resulting in artery-to-artery embolism) or potential cardiac sources of embolism (in particular atrial fibrillation) are less prevalent in lacunar stroke patients[23] and, where they are seen, their contribution to the disease process remains to be proven. Consequently, there is debate about the choice of special investigations, antiplatelet therapy, and anticoagulation for these patients. A diagnosis of lacunar stroke should not preclude further investigation in elderly patients because these strokes develop in an atherogenic milieu similar to that of large vessel infarcts. The possibility that any proximal vascular lesions may be coincidental to the presenting stroke, however, should be borne in mind.[21]

Anatomic Classification of Cerebral Infarcts

In almost all patients classification of infarcts according to site and size can be achieved with considerable accuracy on the basis of clinical signs and symptoms alone. This approach has been favored by epidemiologists and clinical trialists because of its simplicity, lack of dependence on extensive investigations, and correlation with outcome and the uniformity of pathophysiologic mechanisms within individual groups. A currently popular version, used in several clinical trials in Britain, classifies ischemic stroke into total anterior circulation infarction (TACI) partial anterior circulation infarction (PACI), posterior circulation infarction (POCI), and lacunar infarction.[25]

TACI is a result of occlusion of either the internal carotid artery or the proximal stem of the middle cerebral artery and involves almost all of the carotid territory. The grouping includes, but does not distinguish, patients who may have added anterior cerebral artery infarction. The proportion of TACIs caused by in situ thrombosis, cardiogenic embolism, or artery-to-artery embolism from the internal carotid artery to the middle cerebral artery is not known. TACI is associated with high levels of mortality (more than 50 percent dead at 1 year) and dependence, suggesting that acute thrombolysis may be most worthwhile in this group of patients.[25] PACI is generally due to involvement of smaller branches of the middle cerebral artery and is most frequently embolic in origin. There is a high risk of recurrence of stroke in these patients, especially within the first 3 months.[25] This suggests that patients with PACI need early investigation and institution of secondary preventive measures even—or especially—when there is relatively minor neurologic deficit. Infarction in the border zones between two main arterial territories may occasionally present as PACI. This is usually caused by hemodynamic disturbance and if unilateral may indicate a tight stenosis of the ipsilateral internal carotid artery. The ratio of thrombotic to embolic events in POCI is 4:1. It is usually difficult to determine exact vascular involvement in this area because of the rich anastomoses in the posterior fossa. Lacunar anterior circulation infarction (LACI) is associated with less mortality and morbidity than other infarcts and does not have cortical features. Recurrence occurs at a steady rate subsequent to the initial event, suggesting that another perforating artery needs to be involved before further symptoms arise. Data from the Oxford Community Stroke Project suggest that 17 percent of cerebral infarcts are TACI, 34 percent are PACI, 24 percent are POCI, and 25 percent are LACI.

Stroke subtyes according to site and size

Total anterior circulation infarction (TACI)
- Motor and sensory deficit
- Ipsilateral hemianopia
- Evidence of cortical dysfunction (dysphasia, visuospatial problems, and so on)

Partial anterior circulation infarction (PACI)
- Any two of the above, or
- Isolated disturbance of higher cerebral function

Posterior circulation infarction (POCI)
- Unequivocal signs of brain stem involvement, or
- Isolated hemianopia

Lacunar infarction (LACI)
Any one of the following:
- Pure motor stroke
- Pure sensory stroke
- Pure sensorimotor stroke
- Ataxic hemiparesis

Hemorrhagic stroke

The most common type of hemorrhagic stroke is primary intracerebral hemorrhage (PICH) and is associated with hypertension and increasing age. The nature of the vascular lesion that leads to arterial rupture is not fully known, but it is thought to be due to arterial wall changes secondary to hypertension and aging, leading to segmental lipohyalinosis or formation of microaneurysms from which bleeding occurs. These microaneurysms are usually located on small arteries, especially the lenticulostriate branches of the middle cerebral artery and the cerebellar and pontine branches of the basilar artery. The extravasation forms a roughly oval or circular mass which disrupts the surrounding tissue and depending on the size of the bleed, may cause a mass effect. The most common sites for PICH, in order of frequency, appear to be the putamen and the adjacent internal capsule (50 percent of cases), various parts of the central white matter (frontal lobe, corona radiata, extension from the putamen), thalamus, cerebellar hemisphere, and pons.

Hemorrhagic stroke is said to have an abrupt onset, usually associated with activity, and a relentlessly progressive course dependent on the speed of bleeding. Hypertension is common, but there are no recognizable warning or prodromal symptoms. Moderate to large intracerebral bleeds (depending on hemorrhage volume and ventricular extension) are associated with a persistent and often severe neurologic deficit from which rapid improvement is not to be expected. There is, however, increasing awareness that smaller bleeds, which are confined to cerebral parenchyma, may have a clinical course similar to that of cerebral infarction.[26] Severe headache occurs in only 50 percent of patients, and vomiting once or twice at the onset of hemorrhage may be an important feature. Epileptic fits occur in 10 percent of patients during the first few days of a stroke, especially in those with subcortical "slit hemorrhages" at the junction of white and gray matter. Once bleeding has stopped, early rebleeding is uncommon.

Diagnostic Issues

The clinical features of stroke are so distinctive that diagnosis is self-evident. Despite this, uncertaininty about the clinical diagnosis was the main or a contributory reason for admission in half of patients entering the hospital with stroke.[9] The three major criteria underpining a diagnosis of stroke are clinical setting, temporal profile, and evidence of focal brain damage. If this information is lacking, a diagnosis can still be established by undertaking CT scans of the brain. It should be remembered that a significantly large proportion of acute CT scans in patients with clinically definite stroke do not show any relevant abnormality. In such circumstances, confirmation of diagnosis can be made by extending the period of observation and resorting to the golden rule that a physician's best diagnostic tool is the second and third examinations.[2] Factors that may contribute to difficulties in diagnosis in elderly patients include nonavailability of a reliable history because of the absence of a witness, dysphasia, dementia or confusion, unusual symptoms or signs due to preexisting cerebrovascular disease, and multiple pathology which may mask or confound the clinical diagnosis of stroke.

The diagnosis of TIA depends almost entirely on clinical history, as signs are seldom present during examination and there are no objective investigations that can confirm or exclude the diagnosis. Approximately 15 percent of patients having their first stroke have a history of TIA, although in only half has this event been correctly identified.[14] Accuracy of diagnosis of TIA in the elderly is compromised by problems of obtaining a reliable history in some patients and nonspecificity of symptoms (especially if they involve the vertebrobasilar territory), as well as a multiplicity of other conditions that may have a similar presentation (syncope, hypoglycemia, epilepsy).[27] In addition, there is considerable interobserver variability in the diagnosis of TIA between general physicians and neurologists and even between experienced neurologists.[28] The difficulties in the diagnosis of TIA are due to lack of detail in the widely used definition and the absence of any precise, valid, reliable, generally acceptable criteria for diagnosis.[27] There have been attempts to develop and evaluate computer-assisted programs and clinical algorithms for evaluating patients with TIA. These programs take into account variables such as setting of symptoms (presence of risk factors), rapidity of onset and temporal profile (arrest and rapid resolution) of neurologic symptoms, focal nature of the deficit, and the presence or absence of associated symptoms.[29] In patients with vague or uncharacteristic symptoms or in whom symptoms occur under unusual circumstances, a diagnosis of "possible TIA" should be made pending confirmation by witness accounts or reassessment over a period of time.[30] The annual risk of stroke following a TIA is increased sevenfold over the first 5 years. It is hence imperative that patients with TIA or possible TIA be investigated as a matter of urgency, especially as the risk of stroke is highest during the first few weeks after the TIA.[14]

The clinical presentation of thrombotic and arterial occlusion depends on the occluded artery and varies according to the availability of collateral blood flow. There are countless variations in the size, shape, and completeness of infarcts, depending on the speed of occlusion, cerebral autoregulation, and oxygenation variables. Focal ischemic lesions have traditionally provided one of the most instructive approaches in localizing function in the brain, with doctors learning neurology "stroke by stroke."[2] Although specific impairments may vary in different patients and according to the location and size of the infarct, there is sufficient uniformity to permit diagnosis within major vascular territories. In general, unilateral signs predominate in carotid system involvement (hemiplegia, hemianesthesia, hemianopia, dysphasia, and agnosia), whereas bilateral motor or sensory signs with cranial nerve or cerebellar involvement are more commonly found in vertebrobasilar disease. In general, hemorrhage within these vascular territories gives rise to effects similar to those observed with occlusive stroke. The overall clinical picture, however, is apt to differ from that for infarcts because of deep extension of the hemorrhage into other vascular territories and because of a mass effect giving rise to midline shift and raised intracranial pressure. Determination of the arterial territory involved in TIA is important because carotid endarterectomy may be a possible intervention for carotid circulation syndromes. It is usually possible to distinguish between carotid territory (80 percent) and vertebrobasilar territory (20 percent) involvement on the basis of clinical presentation and symptoms, especially if they are related to cortical function or include transient monocular blindness. The difficulty arises when the neurologic symptoms are limited to pathways that receive their blood supply from the carotid or basilar circulation at different levels (e.g., corticospinal tracts, spinothalamic tracts, optic radiation). In such instances, interobserver reliability is even worse than for diagnosis of TIA,[28] and ancillary investigations provide little help in resolving diagnostic problems.

Differences Between Hemorrhage and Infarction

The distinction between cerebral hemorrhage and infarction has become extremely important because of recent advances in the acute management and secondary prevention of stroke.

It is particularly important to make this distinction before considering treatment with thrombolytics and in patients who may already be on drugs that modify hemostatic function. Accuracy of pathologic diagnosis is also required in patients who may be candidates for invasive interventions aimed at secondary stroke prevention (anticoagulation, carotid angiography, carotid endarterectomy). It has been traditional to differentiate between hemorrhagic and ischemic strokes using clinical features derived retrospectively from autopsy series. These distinctions have been made on the basis of time of onset, temporal profile of symptoms, progression of deficit, and associated features of headache and vomiting. This method of clinical distinction, even when clinical scoring systems are used, is neither sensitive nor reliable because nearly 60 percent of stroke patients have a similar presentation regardless of pathology.[2] Differentiation based on clinical features alone is also not supported by CT scan data, which show considerable overlap in clinical presentation between primary intracerebral hemorrhage and cerebral infarction, especially in patients with smaller peripheral hemorrhages that have not ruptured into the ventricular system.[31] CT scanning soon after the initial episode is the only reliable way of distinguishing between an infarct and a hemorrhage as a cause of stroke. The radiologic density of a hemorrhage changes with time, and delays beyond 2 weeks may necessitate magnetic resonance imaging (MRI) to distinguish reliably between hemorrhage and infarction (see below).

Investigations in Stroke

The diagnosis of stroke and TIA are mainly clinical, and there are few situations where investigations are needed solely for this purpose.[20] Investigations, however, play a major role in determining the pathology and etiology of stroke, which is essential for management and secondary stroke prevention. All stroke patients need basic investigations to detect treatable vascular risk factors and other disorders that would alter management. Investigations may also be needed to identify a possible treatable complication of stroke. The issue of appropriateness is important in determining the level of investigation in stroke patients. Although age in itself should never be a contraindication to undertaking further investigations, investigative zeal must be tempered by the clinical state of the patient and the potential for functional recovery, comorbidity (which may preclude aggressive management), risk-benefit appraisal of management options (some of which may actually favor elderly people), and suitability (as well as willingness) to undergo further investigation or intervention.

Baseline investigations in all stroke patients should include a full blood count (polycythemia, thrombocyte disorders), erythrocyte sedimentation rate (hyperviscosity, vasculitis), blood glucose (glycemic status), urea and electrolytes (diuretics, renal function), serum cholesterol, electrocardiogram (atrial fibrillation, myocardial infarct), and a chest radiograph (metastatic disease, cardiomegaly, aspiration). Serum cholesterol levels are representative only if a fasting specimen has been taken within 24 hours of stroke, otherwise they should be measured at least 6 weeks after the acute episode. Further investigations should be dictated by age of the patient (atherosclerosis being uncommon in the young), presence or absence of vascular risk factors, and atypical features in presentation. Investigations may involve echocardiography, hemostatic profile, screening for dyslipoproteinemias, hemoglobinopathies, abnormal proteins (antithrombin III, proteins C and S), immunologic profile, plasma electrophoresis, syphilis serology, and anticardiolipin antibodies. Angiography, tests for inherited metabolic disorders, and tests for rare granulomatous diseases tend to be reserved for young patients who have no vascular risk factors.

CT Scanning

CT scan studies are the cornerstone investigation in stroke. Although seldom needed to diagnose stroke per se, there are some situations in which an adequate diagnosis cannot be established on the basis of clinical features alone and a CT scan becomes imperative. Indications for CT scanning for diagnostic purposes include nonavailability of a clear history (unconscious or acutely confused patient) or presentation with atypical symptoms or signs. Patients suspected of having cerebellar stroke or subarachnoid hemorrhage or known to be on anticoagulants (hemorrhage versus subdural hematoma) also need to be scanned urgently because definitive treatment may be delayed or denied in the absence of a scan. CT scanning may also be necessary to establish vascular pathology in stroke patients with underlying malignant disorders in whom metastases may be an alternative explanation for focal neurologic deficits.

The most important indication for undertaking CT scanning in stroke patients is the need to distinguish between hemorrhagic and ischemic stroke. CT is extremely sensitive in detecting intracerebral bleeding soon after the onset of stroke, which is seen as an area of high attenuation within the cerebral parenchyma. The sensitivity of CT scanning in detecting hemorrhages decreases with time because areas of high attenuation may become isodense or even hypodense with respect to surrounding brain tissue after 2 weeks of onset, making differentiation between hemorrhage and infarction difficult. CT scanning is less sensitive in detecting infarction in the acute phase and is negative in 33 to 50 percent of patients presenting with clinically established stroke.[32] This may be because the scan has been performed too early (CT scan infarction changes may take 1 to 2 days to appear) or because of the transitory "fogging effect" due to which infarcts may not be visible (infarcted areas become isodense within 1 to 3 weeks in 50 percent of cases).[33] Other reasons are that infarcts are too small to be seen on CT scans or are located in the posterior fossa, which is not well visualized by this technique. Although the number of infarcts seen increases with repeated scanning, there is no justification for this in mainstream practice. In situ thrombosis may be seen occasionally as a diffuse area of high density in an artery on an ordinary CT scan, and follow-up scans may show a decrease in vessel density due to thrombus resolution.[34] CT scanning has a sensitivity of 80 percent in detecting hemorrhagic infarcts, which are seen as areas of patchy high density, often in the territory of the middle cerebral artery.[35] It can, however, be difficult to distinguish between a hemorrhagic infarct and PICH on a CT scan. Although this may not present significant problems in medical management (antihemostatic treatment being contraindicated in both conditions), it may make surgical decisions regarding possible endarterectomy (which may be required in some patients with hemorrhagic infarcts secondary to artery-to-artery embolization) more difficult.

Contrast-enhanced CT scanning is of limited value in stroke patients. There are fears that large amounts of contrast given in the acute phase may be toxic to ischemic neurons and may increase the severity of neurologic deficit. Enhanced scans are not necessary in most stroke patients because excluding hemorrhage (which is hyperdense) is usually the main indication for the procedure. Contrast-enhanced scans may be helpful in the diagnosis of cerebral infarction in patients with isodense lesions on CT scans (fogging effect)[33] in whom the study shows contrast enhancement around an area of isodensity. These appearances may be difficult to differentiate from that of a cerebral tumor and a repeat scan may be needed after an interval of 4 to 6 weeks.

As already noted, lack of sensitivity in detecting ischemic lesions does not limit the benefits of CT scanning significantly because it is more important to exclude hemorrhage than to demonstrate infarction in acute stroke. The widespread availability of CT scanning and its ability to reliably demonstrate bleeding in the first 2 weeks of onset makes it the most practical initial imaging technique for patients with acute stroke. In the United Kingdom, there has been considerable controversy about the level of investigation, especially CT scanning, needed in stroke patients. In many cases, they have been considered superfluous because of their perceived inability to affect management decisions.[20] Fortunately, this perception is changing rapidly, and the strong case for undertaking CT scanning in nearly all stroke patients to establish the nature and pathology of the lesion is now being accepted.[36] Accuracy in diagnosis is important for prognosis, acute intervention (hemorrhage versus infarction), determining the need and nature of secondary prevention (large versus small vessel disease), and establishing specific rehabilitation needs (site and size of lesion), although the latter is influenced more by the overall clinical picture.

MRI Scanning

MRI is more sensitive than CT scanning in detecting infarcts, particularly if undertaken early or if the infarcts are small or occur in the posterior fossa.[37] The sensitivity of MRI in detecting hemorrhages or hemorrhagic infarcts in the acute phase is less than that of CT scanning, although its performance can be increased by undertaking special studies.[38] In contrast to that of CT scanning, the sensitivity of MRI in detecting hemorrhage increases with time. This is because of the formation of methemoglobin in 3 to 5 days, which results in an increased signal on T_1 and T_2 images and hemosiderin at the edge of the bleed in about 2 weeks which shortens the T_2 image, resulting in a low-intensity rim around the edge of the hematoma. MRI does not have any significant advantages over CT scanning in differentiating between primary intracerebral hemorrhages and hemorrhagic transformation of infarcts.[39]

MRI is a second-level investigation in stroke patients and should be undertaken only in situations where CT scanning does not provide relevant answers. MRI is expensive, not universally available, and contributes little toward resolving diagnostic issues important in acute stroke management over and above CT scanning. It is important to remember that nearly a fifth of patients with acute stroke are unable to undergo an MRI examination because of claustrophobia or contraindications, such as pacemakers.[40]

Other Imaging Techniques

In the past the emphasis of imaging in stroke has been on delineation of the anatomy and pathology of the lesion. In recent years, there has been considerable interest and developments in imaging techniques for studying the physiologic aspects of stroke. Significant developments in this area include positron emission tomography (PET), single photon emission computed tomography (SPECT), xenon CT, and magnetic resonance spectroscopy (MRS). Most of these techniques are research tools and are being used to study the pathophysiology (vascular and neurologic) of acute stroke, the effect of acute interventions, and the changes associated with recovery, reactivation, and rehabilitation. Although these techniques have not been introduced in clinical practice, an overview is essential to facilitate better understanding of current research and its future implications.

Xenon CT and SPECT have been used primarily to study cerebral blood flow in the acute phases of stroke. Xenon CT can demonstrate the site and size of cerebral ischemic injury before any changes are seen on ordinary CT scans.[27] Xenon CT scanning can be performed immediately after conventional CT scanning and may have the potential of selecting patients for thrombolysis because of its ability to distinguish between patients with low cerebral blood flow (who are likely to benefit) and those with high cerebral blood flow (who are unlikely to benefit).[41] Xenon CT scanning may be of limited value in the evaluation of treatments for acute thrombotic stroke because xenon per se increases cerebral blood flow.[42] SPECT is essentially a research tool which provides high-resolution images of cerebral blood flow changes associated with acute stroke within 20 to 30 minutes of injection of a tracer isotope. The technique needs further refining because perfusion data are semiquantitative and uptake of commonly used tracer isotopes does not appear to relate specifically or linearly to changes in cerebral blood flow.[42] SPECT has been used for studying temporal changes in cerebral blood flow after acute stroke and in monitoring the effects of acute treatment.[43]

PET and MRS have been employed in the study of cerebral perfusion, oxygen consumption, and metabolic changes following stroke and their relationship to recovery. It is now possible to examine the metabolic consequences of ischemia, the threshold between reversible and irreversible ischemia, and metabolic factors involved in neurologic recovery.[44] It may be possible to predict which patients are most likely to benefit from acute stroke intervention on the basis of perfusion and oxygen consumption patterns observed on PET scanning.[45] Studies using PET have suggested that there are changes in the metabolic activity of both the affected and the unaffected sides of the brain during recovery, with reactivation of previously silent areas.[46] This has considerable implications in the evaluation of recovery and therapy inputs in stroke. It may also be possible to identify biochemical markers of prognosis and response to therapy in acute stroke using PET or MRS techniques.[27]

Vascular Studies

Vascular studies are necessary in patients with recent carotid territory TIA or nondisabling stroke. They are most urgent in patients with PACI because of the high risk of recurrence. There continues to be controversy about the relevance of these investigations in patients with lacunar syndromes, as discussed previously. Investigations include noninvasive procedures, such as carotid ultrasound and magnetic resonance angiography, and invasive tests such as conventional angiography, intra-arterial digital subtraction angiography (IA-DSA), and intravenous digital subtraction angiography (IV-DSA).

Carotid Ultrasound

Extracranial

Duplex carotid ultrasound, which combines the high reliability of Doppler studies in detecting hemodynamically significant internal carotid artery stenosis (more than 50 percent of diameter) with the high reliability of B-mode imaging in detecting mild to moderate lesions (25 to 50 percent diameter), is the most effective noninvasive method of detecting extracranial carotid disease.[47] Doppler flow studies have high sensitivity (90 to 100 percent) and moderate specificity (55 to 90 percent in detecting moderate to severe stenosis but are less reliable in detecting milder disease that produces normal flow patterns. In contrast, B-mode imaging readily detects mild to moderate lesions with a high sensitivity (70 to 100 percent) but cannot reliably detect more advanced stenosis because of scattering of sound waves due to fibrosis or calcification. As advanced stenosis is usually accompanied by flow velocity changes, this limitation of B-mode echo is overcome by the Doppler flow element of the investigation.

Carotid duplex studies are fast gaining acceptance as a screening procedure for carotid artery disease but may be limited by high carotid bifurcation, difficulty in distinguishing the internal from the external carotid artery in some patients, incomplete plaque characterization, inability of sound waves to penetrate calcified atherosclerotic plaques, and persisting difficult in distinguishing tight stenosis from occlusion. The reliability of carotid duplex studies is also dependent on the expertise of the examiner. In trained hands, this procedure can detect mild atherosclerotic disease in an extracranial artery with a sensitivity of 90 percent and a specificity of 85 to 95 percent.[47] The sensitivity of carotid duplex studies in detecting hemodynamically significant disease (more than 50 percent stenosis) is even higher (greater than 95 percent).[47] The major problem encountered in such studies in mainstream practice is difficulty in differentiating between a tight but patent stenosis and complete occlusion. The positive predictive value of duplex in detecting occlusion is low (53 to 86 percent), suggesting that 14 to 37 percent of patients in whom a duplex study suggests an occlusion actually have a tight but patent internal cranial artery stenosis.[48] This has important implications because occlusion of the internal carotid artery precludes patients from carotid endarterectomy, whereas a tight symptomatic stenosis in the same territory is a definite indication for the procedure. It is hence appropriate that angiography be undertaken in all patients potentially suitable for endarterectomy suspected of having internal carotid artery occlusion on duplex studies because a significant proportion of them will be found to have treatable tight stenosis.[48]

Transcranial

Intracranial components of the cerebral circulation are difficult to investigate ultrasonically because they are surrounded by bone. The acoustic barrier of the brain has been overcome by using lower than conventional ultrasound frequencies and directing the beam through the natural foramina (foramen magnum) or the thinnest regions of the skull (temporal bone). Despite this, it is not possible to penetrate the acoustic barrier of the skull in 10 percent of patients, particularly elderly females and those of Afro-Caribbean or Asian origin (failure rate 30 percent).[49]

Transcranial Doppler is a noninvasive procedure for measuring blood flow in the major intracranial arteries using a small, portable unit. This method has been used to evaluate cerebral collateral flow in patients with extracranial carotid disease, monitor middle cerebral artery blood flow velocity during carotid endarterectomy, detect cerebral embolism during surgical procedures or in acute stroke, assess acute cerebral infarction and vessel recanalization, and detect posterior circulation flow disturbances in vertebrobasilar insufficiency.[49] Transcranial Doppler is also used to evaluate the presence of hemodynamically significant intracranial stenosis of the major arteries. The procedure is highly operator dependent (more so than duplex scanning) and is limited by the accessibility of cranial windows in some patients, patient cooperation, anatomic anomalies of the circle of Willis, inaccuracies in vessel identification, effect of pathologic structural abnormalities, and abnormal collateral flow states. The data provided by the procedure reflect blood velocity and not volume flow, which may be a more relevant measure.[50]

Future developments

Carotid ultrasound is also being used in studying plaque morphology, early changes in the carotid arterial wall, and longitudinal progression of carotid disease. These applications are still being developed and are not a part of mainstream clinical practice. Technologic advances include the development of color duplex sonography which combines real-time ultrasound imaging with semiquantitative color encoding of Doppler information, which allows turbulent flow to be more easily detected. This development has the potential of overcoming the most important current limitation of carotid duplex sonography because tight stenoses are likely to be associated with greatest turbulence in flow, whereas there should be no turbulence in cases of occlusion. Similar advances have been made in sonographic intracranial imaging with the development of low-frequency duplex color probes (transcranial color-coded sonography) for transcranial use. Although color-coded sonography requires a better acoustic window than conventional intracranial Doppler studies, it has the advantage of allowing more precise identification of vessels and structural abnormalities and more accurate measurement of blood flow velocities. It is likely that these developments in extra- and intracranial ultrasound imaging techniques will provide a noninvasive, safe, reliable alternative to angiography in stroke patients.

Angiography

Selective intra-arterial angiography, whether conventional or digitally subtracted, continues to be the gold standard for diagnosing vascular abnormality in stroke. An angiogram is indicated in stroke patients who are potential candidates for carotid endarterectomy. It may also be indicated in other patients with ischemic infarcts in whom carotid duplex studies have failed to demonstrate significant atheromatous disease. These patients include young individuals with no risk factors, suspected subclavian steal syndrome, or arteritis, and patients with neck trauma or pain before stroke suggestive of carotid artery dissection. In addition, it may be necessary to undertake angiography in nondisabled survivors of cerebral hemorrhage, depending on the site of bleeding (e.g., lobar hematoma) and the lack of any obvious underlying cause (hypertension or bleeding diathesis). The objective is to exclude significant aneurysms or arteriovenous malformations which may be a treatable cause of the hemorrhage.

Eligibility for carotid endarterectomy is by far the most common indication for angiography in acute stroke. Carotid angiography should be undertaken if duplex studies show significant levels of stenosis (70 to 99 percent) in the extracranial section of the relevant internal carotid artery. The carotid artery on the symptomatic side is studied first, and if a potentially operable lesion is demonstrated (70 to 99 percent stenosis), the contralateral carotid is studied unless already well shown by duplex scanning. As the risk of recurrence or stroke after TIA is highest during the first few weeks after the initial event, it is logical that angiography and possibly carotid endarterctomy be performed as soon as the patient has recovered and is fit enough to undergo the procedure. In practice, this usually means surgery 4 to 6 weeks after the stroke although it is being undertaken earlier at some facilities. Carotid angiography is a major procedure and has its own risks. The neurologic complication rate of conventional angiography in patients suffering TIA or minor strokes is about 4 percent, with 1 percent of patients suffering disabling stroke resulting in permanent neurologic deficit.[51] The risks are greatest for patients with tight stenosis of the external internal cerebral artery.[52] Arch angiography is probably less risky than selective studies but of inferior resolution. It is likely that IA-DSA may be associated with less severe complications (being a shorter procedure), but there have been no prospective studies on complications associated with this procedure.[27] The risks of angiography must be balanced by the potential benefit of endarterectomy for the patient. There is no indication for undertaking angiography in stroke patients in whom carotid duplex studies have demonstrated mild to moderate stenosis. Even in those shown to have significant disease, it is important to ascertain that they are willing to proceed with carotid endarterctomy, if indicated, before being offered angiography. All patients should be told of the relative risk of stroke before and after endarterectomy, as well as the possibility of neurologic complications caused by angiography and carotid endarterectomy, to help in the decision making process. Although age in itself is not a criterion, there is no justification for proceeding with angiography in elderly patients who may not wish to undergo carotid endarterectomy for personal or cultural reasons or for fear of disabling consequences.

IV-DSA has been superseded by carotid duplex studies in investigating extracranial internal carotid artery disease in stroke. IV-DSA is nonselective and has poor spatial resolution. Large amounts of contrast are required, and the patient must have good cardiac function and be cooperative. The procedure lacks accuracy: only 80 percent of the studies are interpretable, and the rate of systemic complications, estimated at 19 percent, is unacceptably high.[51] MRA has a limited role in the evaluation of stroke patients. The procedure is not widely available, and its value appears to be limited to patients with technically inadequate duplex studies (because of a high carotid junction) or in whom it is important to distinguish internal carotid artery occlusion from tight stenosis accurately and noninvasively.[53] MRA lacks the spatial resolution, selectivity, and dynamic character of conventional intra-arterial angiography, which remains essential for a more detailed assessment of cerebral circulation abnormalities.[53]

Echocardiography

The role of routine echocardiography in the evaluation of stroke patients is controversial. Large series on echocardiography in stroke have shown low yields of clinically relevant lesions.[54] There is little evidence that management decisions, such as those regarding anticoagulation, are influenced by echocardiographic findings. An abnormal echo does not prove that the ischemic lesion was caused by embolism or that the heart was the source of this embolism. Similarly, a normal echo does not exclude a cardiac source of embolism because the whole clot may have embolized, leaving no trace, or the clot may be less than 2 mm in diameter, too small to be detected by conventional echocardiography but not too small to lodge in a branch of the middle cerebral artery. The type of echocardiographic scan used is also important. The conventional two-dimensional transthoracic echo may occasionally detect intraventricular thrombi as small as 5 mm in diameter but cannot visualize the left atrium and appendage reliably. It is also of limited value in obese patients and those with emphysema, chest deformity, or prosthetic valves.[55] Some of these limitations can be overcome by using transesophageal echocardiography, but it is expensive, has limited availability, and does not visualize the cardiac apex as well as the transthoracic procedure.[56]

The clinical value of echocardiography depends on appropriate patient selection and awareness of the relevance of the information it provides. It is now accepted that unrestricted use of echocardiography in stroke patients is unjustified and unnecessary.[20] Echocardiography should be restricted to stroke or TIA patients with no significant evidence of atheromatous disease or risk factors; those with evidence of relevant cardiac disease on clinical examination, chest radiograph, and electrocardiography (atrial fibrillation, aortic or mitral valve disease, vegetations, myocardial dyskinesia); and those with a family history of atrial myxoma or cardiomyopathy. Symptomatic patients with a high probability of atrial thrombus should be referred for transesophageal echocardiography if the two-dimensional echo is normal. Other cardiac techniques important from a stroke management point of view include contrast echocardiography, ultrafast (cine) cardiac CT, and wide-field transesophageal ultrasonic echocardiographic tomography.[57,58] These techniques are still being evaluated but hold promise for the future.

Management of Stroke Patients

Management of stroke patients is a complex process ranging from acute medical intervention to treatment of long-term disability and involves several specialities, disciplines, and settings. There is no single measure which in itself can overcome the burden of stroke to the patient, to health services, and to society. Management of stroke patients is based on a pragmatic strategy involving intervention at several levels. Effective management of stroke also requires true integration of services across different areas of interest (e.g., medical, rehabilitation, and social services) to ensure mechanisms for timely mobilization of appropriate resources and to achieve a seamless service from the onset of stroke to long-term care.[59]

Acute Management

Most patients with acute stroke are admitted to a hospital despite there being no widely accepted specific treatment for this disorder. Although there may be good medical reasons to admit these patients (confirmation of diagnosis and investigation, assessment of vascular risk, prevention or management of complications) in most cases this is done to meet nursing, rehabilitation, and social needs.[9] The proportion of stroke patients who are admitted to hospitals also varies from area to area and is as low as 50 percent and as high as 90 percent in some districts.[60,61] There is a view that a significant proportion of admissions to hospitals are unnecessary and that this leads to inappropriate use of resources.[62] Several observational studies have suggested that outcome in terms of physical independence is equally good in patients treated at home compared with that of those treated with conventional hospital services.[20] However, a nonrandomized controlled trial showed that acute at-home care for stroke patients involving additional care and rehabilitation was neither feasible nor effective because there were no reductions in hospital admission rate, length of hospital stay, functional or social disability, or care giver stress.[63] Preliminary results from ongoing research at our institution suggest that more than half of stroke admissions to hospitals are from emergency services with little input from family doctors, limiting their ability to prevent these admissions. An overwhelming proportion of admissions appear to be appropriate based on predefined criteria of medical need (e.g., unconscious patient, swallowing problems, atypical clinical features, and so on). In addition, a significant proportion of patients (10 to 15 percent) sustained their stroke while in the hospital for other reasons, which is in keeping with results from other studies.[5] Developments in community services may make it feasible to provide effective at-home acute care to a well-defined group of stroke patients in the future and are currently being investigated. Until such time, most acute stroke patients will continue to be managed in hospital settings.

Once a stroke has occurred, the predominant aim of management is to restore function. This can be achieved by reducing the size of the lesion (acute interventions aimed at the

Management of stroke patients

Effective treatment
- Medical intervention to minimize impairment
- Prevention and early treatment of acute complications
- Rehabilitation to minimize disability
- Adaptations to minimize handicap

Effective prevention (strokes and TIAs)
- *Modification of risk factors*: e.g., hypertension, smoking, lifestyle
- *Medical treatment*: antiplatelets, anticoagulants
- *Surgical treatment*: carotid endarterectomy

Effective support
- *Patient and family*: Counseling, education, training
- *Health services*: community nursing, domiciliary rehabilitation
- *Statutory services*: personal care, respite care
- *Voluntary agencies*: clubs, information, day centers

pathology of stroke), thereby reducing the severity of impairment, or alternately, by treating impairment to prevent or reduce disability (acute rehabilitation). Acute medical treatment of stroke can be divided into three parts: (1) general medical management in the acute phase, (2) measures to restore circulation and arrest the pathologic process, and (3) measures to prevent further strokes and progression of vascular disease.

General medical measures

The management of patients with acute stroke requires the skills of a well-coordinated multidisciplinary team because of the number of problems associated with stroke (e.g., impaired consciousness, dysphagia), the high risk of stroke-related complications (e.g., aspiration pneumonia, venous thrombosis) that may affect outcome,[64] and the specialized needs (e.g., communication problems, visuospatial impairment) of this patient group. Most of the treatment in acute stroke is supportive, allowing time for neurologic injury to settle with minimization of further direct risk to the area of damage and indirect risk from complications that may arise.[65] This includes maintaining stable respiratory and cardiovascular function, with particular attention to oxygenation and appropriate blood pressure; correction of fluid electrolyte imbalance and monitoring blood glucose levels; ensuring adequate nutrition; preventing hypo- or hyperthermia and complications such as aspiration pneumonitis, urinary retention or infection, venous thromboembolism, seizures, pressure sores, contractures, and dislocated or frozen shoulder. Despite the lack of direct evidence from controlled prospective studies, it is likely that interactive general management of stroke patients in the acute phase results in lower mortality and morbidity.[66, 67] Areas that need special attention include the following.

1. *Maintenance of airways and oxygenation:* Despite its obvious importance in restricting the damage associated with stroke, this aspect of care is frequently poorly managed in clinical settings. It is particularly important in elderly patients, in whom alterations in consciousness level following stroke are common and who are more likely to suffer from chronic pulmonary disease or desensitization of central ventilatory mechanisms. Interventions include proper positioning, adequate nasopharyngeal suction, and oxygen administration. Aminophylline may be used in patients with Cheyne-Stokes breathing. Assisted ventilation and hyperbaric oxygen have been used in patients with acute stroke but their effectiveness remains to be demonstrated.
2. *Management of hypertension:* High blood pressure is commonly seen in patients with acute stroke.[68,69] There is considerable controversy regarding optimal blood pressure control in acute hypertensive intracerebral hemorrhage. Persistent marked elevation of blood pressure can promote further bleeding, increase cerebral blood flow, and raise intracranial pressure.[70] Markedly elevated blood pressure (higher than 125 mmHg diastolic) on admission and persistent inadequate blood pressure control have been shown to adversely affect the prognosis in intracerebral hemorrhage.[70] There appears to be a case for controlling high blood pressure in patients with cerebral hemorrhage, although persistent hypotension (which may lead to secondary ischemia) should be avoided.

   It is generally accepted that hypertension should not be treated soon after ischemic stroke.[71] Cerebral autoregulation is lost in the area around cerebral infarction, and perfusion is dependent on systemic blood pressure.[72] Observational studies have shown that in the acute phase of ischemic stroke, elevation of blood pressure in the first few days helps to restore cerebral perfusion and activates collateral arterial supply.[73] SPECT has shown that reducing blood pressure carries the risk of reducing the blood flow to the penumbra and increasing the area of infarct.[74] The effects of iatrogenic hypotension may be more significant in elderly hypertensives in whom age and hypertension may already have impaired cerebral autoregulatory mechanisms.[72] Studies have shown a marked fall in systolic and diastolic blood pressure levels during the first 7 days after acute stroke in most patients,[75] and a wait-and-see policy is recommended. Antihypertensive treatment may be indicated in patients who continue to be hypertensive beyond the first week of stroke.[75] The aim should then be to reduce blood pressure gradually into the high normal range.[72] There may be benefits in using angiotensin-converting enzyme inhibitors, α-adrenergic blockers, or β-adrenergic blockers, which preserve cerebral blood flow, in preference to cerebral vasodilators such as nitroprusside and certain calcium channel blockers, which may result in cerebral edema or vascular steal from the ischemic area.[74,76]

   Early antihypertensive treatment may be necessary for stroke patients presenting with persistent high diastolic blood pressure levels greater than 145 mmHg or features of malignant hypertension.[76] A recent report suggests that systolic hypertension in acute stroke may be associated with early progression, but the causal relationship between systolic hypertension and early progression was not established.[77] Confirmation of this relationship has the potential of altering future antihypertensive management in acute stroke, especially if shown to be amenable to therapeutic interventions.
3. *Hydration and biochemical imbalance:* Stroke is frequently associated with disturbances of water, glucose, and salt mechanisms. These conditions may be due to impaired consciousness, inability to perceive or respond to hunger and thirst, or hypothalamic disturbances causing salt losing or retaining syndromes. Hydration should be maintained with care to reduce the risk of cerebral or pulmonary edema (chronic heart failure being common in the elderly) and hyponatremia. In the absence of diabetes mellitus, hyperglycemia has been associated with poor outcome in stroke

patients, although this is not universally accepted.[78] In most patients, hyperglycemia resolves spontaneously within the first few days. Care should be taken in patients who require antihyperglycemic treatment because of the dangers of hypoglycemia.

4. *Nutrition:* Malnutrition is common in acute stroke patients, especially if they have swallowing problems. Elderly patients are at greater risk than their younger counterparts because of the increased prevalence of background malnutrition in this age group.[79] Research has shown that the nutritional status of stroke patients (regardless of the presence of dysphagia) tends to decrease in the first few months after stroke.[80] This is compounded by low mood, anorexia, and starvation-induced weakness of the pharyngeal and respiratory muscles, leading to further malnutrition.[81] It is not known whether nutritional supplementation, over and above daily requirements, can influence recovery or outcome in stroke patients. Despite the awareness of nutritional depletion in such individuals, there are no universally accepted guidelines for feeding acute stroke patients. The decision to maintain nutrition depends on the clinical state of the patient, expected prognosis, and clinical practice at individual centers. In general, assisted nutrition (nasogastric or via a gastrostomy) may not be appropriate in deeply unconscious patients with poor prognosis. Swallowing problems in most other patients resolve rapidly in the first 2 weeks after stroke, and persistent problems are seen in only 10 to 15 percent of stroke survivors after this time. Adequate nutrition in these patients can be achieved through a nasogastric tube (with its inherent problems) or by undertaking a percutaneous endoscopic gastrostomy (PEG), which is a relatively simple and safe (although not widely available) procedure for establishing nutrition in stroke patients. Although PEG has theoretical advantages over nasogastric feeding, there is no agreement on the timing of the procedure or its benefits over nasogastric feeding in patients who may recover rapidly in a few days.[82] Early PEG may be indicated in patients for whom clinical assessment by a speech and language therapist suggests that swallowing problems are unlikely to resolve in the near future.[83] The assessment and management of dysphagia is discussed in greater detail in a later section.

Specific therapies

Rationale for acute intervention Specific therapies have been developed mainly for acute ischemic stroke due to large vessel disease and are aimed at re-establishing blood flow or limiting the neuronal consequences of hypoxia. Complete occlusion of the blood supply due to thrombosis or embolism leads to neuronal death within 5 to 10 minutes because of the high oxygen requirement of these cells. The effects of occlusion, however, are modified by the presence of collateral perfusion, leading to a small central area of infarct surrounded by an oligemic region between the infarcted area and healthy tissue. This area, called the ischemic penumbra is defined as "the area of brain where blood flow is sufficient to prevent neuronal death, but not sufficient to sustain normal electrical activity."[84] It is characterized by impaired synaptic transmission but preserved ionic gradients and cell morphology. A flow rate just below the threshold necessary for electrical activity can be tolerated for several hours (Fig. 35-2). If the insult is sustained, cell death invariably occurs.

Neuronal death is a result of impaired energy metabolism in a cell due to disruption of oxidative phosphorylation and reduced adenosine triphosphate (ATP) production. This results in a loss of control over the transport of ions (particularly calcium) and neurotransmitters (particularly glutamate and aspartate) across the cell membrane. The flux of these neurotransmitters overstimulates the *N*-methyl-D-aspartate (NMDA) receptor, a subtype of glutamate receptor present on a large number of neurons, which initiates a massive influx of calcium ions in toxic doses through the NMDA-gated ionic channels

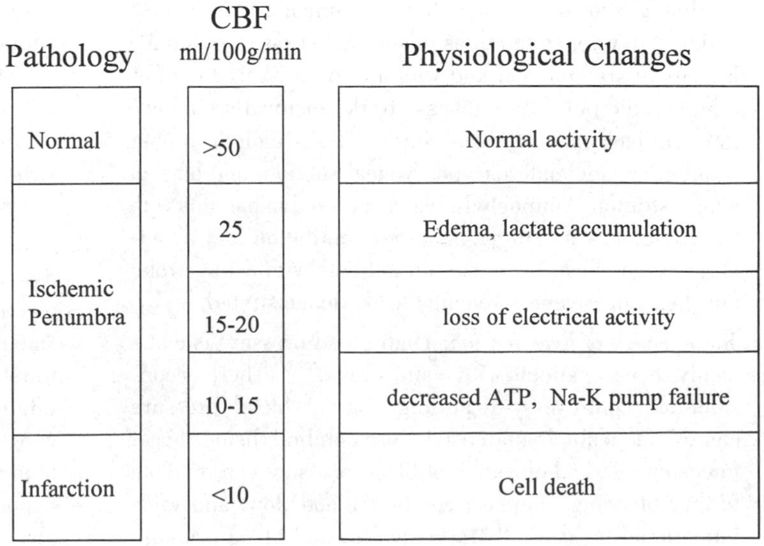

Figure 35-2 Pathophysiology of stroke.

Pathology	CBF ml/100g/min	Physiological Changes
Normal	>50	Normal activity
Ischemic Penumbra	25	Edema, lactate accumulation
	15-20	loss of electrical activity
	10-15	decreased ATP, Na-K pump failure
Infarction	<10	Cell death

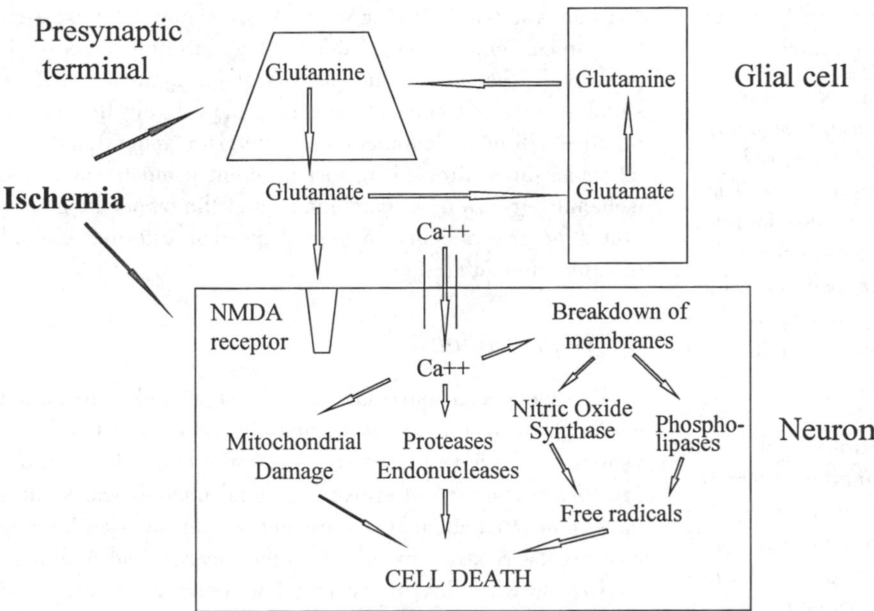

Figure 35-3 Simplified diagram of the ischemic cascade.

into neurons and their mitochondria (Fig. 35-3). The massive influx of calcium against a background of homeostatic failure activates lipases, proteases, and endonucleases, resulting in cell destruction (ischemic cascade). Calcium-activated phospholipases and intracellular metabolites also contribute to cell injury by stimulating nitric oxide synthase and the generation of highly reactive free radicals. These metabolites further compromise membrane and cellular processes, cause vascular vasospasm, increase local thrombogenesis, and release glutamate in huge quantities, fueling further calcium influx. The structural consequences of the ischemic cascade are swelling of the cells, which takes place between 24 and 48 hours after the acute injury and is followed by extracellular edema which occurs 3 to 5 days after stroke.[85] This may be seen clinically in association with large infarcts and causes deterioration after initial clinical improvement.

Therapeutic interventions have been targeted at these mechanisms and are specifically directed toward rescuing the ischemic penumbra. The possible strategies include the following.

- Early restoration of blood flow to ischemic tissue to prevent infarction or improve the ischemic penumbra to reduce the size of the infarct
- Protection of ischemic neurons from consequences of the ischemic cascade by blocking excitatory pathways, inhibiting calcium influx, or scavenging free radicals
- Management of cerebral edema to improve capillary circulation and prevent herniation
- Reduction of energy requirements of neurons and other cells in the brain.

Treatments aimed at restoration of blood flow and oxygenation include thrombolysis using streptokinase or tissue plasminogen activator (tPA), anticoagulation with heparin or warfarin, and inhibition of platelet aggregation using aspirin or prostacyclin. Other studies have investigated the role of improving cerebral perfusion using vasodilators, vasopressors, or hemodilution.[65] The effects of improved oxygenation have been examined using continuous oxygen therapy and hyperbaric oxygen. Interventions aimed at reducing the oxygen requirement of the brain include treatment with naftidrofuryl (an agent claimed to modify oxygen utilization)[86] and selective hypothermia of the injured cortex.[87] Other strategies that have been investigated include the use of steroids and osmotic agents such as glycerol to reduce cerebral edema[88, 89] and, alternately, craniectomy to allow the brain to expand in the case of large infarcts with midline shift.[90] Free radical scavengers, such as 21-aminosteroids and vitamins E and C, which block peroxidization and lipoxygenase activity, may decrease ischemic and postischemic brain swelling.[91] Initial results using free radical scavengers have been encouraging, and further studies are currently in progress.[92] In general, most of these interventions have failed to live up to expectations and are currently thought to have little role in the management of patients with acute stroke. The developing areas of interest, which may have a potential for the future, include thrombolysis, neuroprotection with NMDA receptor antagonists, and the use of aspirin and/or heparin. In long-term secondary prevention trials for stroke and TIA, aspirin has been shown to prevent arterial occlusion and reocclusion.[93] Antiplatelet therapy, alone or in combination with anticoagulation, may have potential benefits in patients with acute stroke and have lesser risk than thrombolysis. The roles of aspirin and heparin in acute stroke are being investigated in the International Stroke Trial. Preliminary results suggest that in acute stroke aspirin reduces mortality and recurrence but that high-dose heparin may be associated with a higher risk of early mortality. Data are currently being analyzed, and the final results of the study are awaited.

Thrombolysis Experimental models of cerebral infarction have shown that, when given intra-arterially or intravenously, thrombolytic agents such as streptokinase, tPA, and urokinase may lyse acute clots and reduce infarct size. These studies also showed that there was a narrow window for intervention, requiring that the drugs be given within 6 hours of the acute episode. Initial studies on stroke patients, which were mostly isolated and poorly controlled, showed mixed results but suggested potential benefits.[94] Several multicenter randomized controlled trials are currently underway, and results are available for the European Cooperative Acute Stroke Study (ECASS) and the Multicentre Acute Stroke Trial—Italy (MAST-I).[16,17] The ECASS study showed significant benefits in neurologic and functional recovery in the treated group, but there was no difference in mortality between the two groups.[16] The occurrence of large parenchymal hemorrhages was significantly more frequent in patients receiving thrombolysis. In contrast, the MAST-I study showed a highly significant increase in early mortality in patients treated with streptokinase.[17] Although combined-case fatality and disability were reduced at 6 months in the treated group, this result was not of statistical significance. The difference between the MAST-I and ECASS may due to differences in patient selection criteria or differences between the interventions used (streptokinase versus tPA).

At present thrombolysis seems to have limited application in future practice. Potential benefits of thrombolytic treatments need to be weighed against the risk of early death or intracerebral bleed. Evidence suggests that thrombolysis should be limited to carefully selected stroke patients because treating unselected populations is associated with an unacceptable increase in hemorrhagic complications and death. The limited therapeutic window presents a challenge because very few patients in Britain present within 6 hours of stroke.[95] It is also estimated that only 5 to 10 percent of patients presenting with acute stroke would be eligible for any such intervention.[96] In addition, most settings lack the facilities for undertaking CT scanning within 4 to 6 hours after stroke or for the intensive monitoring required in patients receiving thrombolytic therapy.

Neuroprotection Cytoprotective therapies in acute stroke are directed toward limiting the abnormal biochemical events (the ischemic cascade) associated with acute ischemia and thereby salvaging the peri-infarct penumbra. Experimental work has shown that NMDA receptor antagonists effectively attenuate ischemic brain injury in animal models, with dramatic reductions in infarct size both in the cortex and subcortical areas.[97] Unfortunately, as in the case of thrombolysis, the therapeutic window is limited to 6 to 8 hours after stroke. Unlike thrombolysis, CT scanning is not mandatory prior to commencing treatment, and special monitoring facilities may not be needed. A large number of drugs are currently undergoing phase III clinical trials, and the few results available to date have been disappointing.[98] The results of other ongoing trials are awaited, following which it will be important to assess the clinical implications of this strategy in future practice. It is unlikely that any single pharmacologic approach will be suitable for all stroke patients. It is more likely that future practice will be a combination of synergistic general and specific measures directed against different components of the ischemic process (e.g., combinations of thrombolysis, neuroprotection, free radical scavenging) aimed at restoring cerebral function after infarction.

Stroke prevention

The role of aggressive strategies aimed at stroke prevention cannot be overestimated. It is generally accepted that no intervention would have a greater impact on quality of life in old age than prevention of stroke.[99] Several unequivocal studies have shown that adequate control of hypertension significantly reduces the risk of stroke.[100,101] Identification and treatment of patients with TIA in the first few weeks after the initial episode is another important intervention that significantly reduces, if not prevents, the possibility of a stroke.[14]

Antiplatelet drugs (e.g., aspirin 75 to 300 mg/day) in patients with atherosclerosis, TIA, or minor stroke reduce the risk of recurrence by 25 percent.[93,102] There is also evidence that aspirin may decrease the risk of first-ever stroke and possibly recurrent stroke in patients with atrial fibrillation.[103] Despite the widespread use of aspirin in vascular disease, there are several questions that remain unanswered. It is not known whether inadvertent aspirin administration can worsen the condition of patients with primary intracerebral hemorrhage or whether patients on stroke prophylaxis with aspirin are more likely to have hemorrhagic infarcts. There is also considerable debate about when aspirin should be started after an ischemic stroke (risk of hemorrhagic transformation), what the effective dose should be (higher doses may not offer a greater benefit: risk ratio), and for what period of time it should be continued. It is also possible that the benefits of aspirin are limited to large vessel occlusive disease and may not extend to patients with lacunar infarcts because of the difference in pathophysiology. It is hoped that some of these questions will be answered when the final results of the International Stroke Trial become available.

Atrial fibrillation, common in elderly patients, is an important cause of thromboembolic stroke. Trials of anticoagulation in stroke have consistently shown a two-thirds reduction in risk compared with a 25 percent reduction in risk seen with aspirin.[104–107] The risks of stroke, and hence the benefits of anticoagulation, are greatest in patients with structural valve disease involving the mitral and aortic valves, prosthetic or infected valves, cardiomyopathy, and chronic heart failure. The risks are also higher in patients with a previous history of stroke and other vascular risk factors. The benefits of anticoagulation need to be counterbalanced by the risks involved, especially in elderly patients who may be prone to falls, suffer from cognitive impairment compromising compliance and ability to monitor adverse events, take a large number of drugs (some of which may interfere with anticoagulation), or have significant comorbidity (recent bleed, peptic ulcer disease, malignancy, or alcoholism). In general, elderly patients with atrial fibrillation who have moderate to high risk of stroke should be considered for anticoagulation if there are no other contraindications.[108] Low-dose anticoagulation [International ratio (INR) 2.0 to 3.0] with or without aspirin may be preferable in elderly patients because of a lower incidence of adverse effects. The relative effectiveness of such measures in preventing strokes is not known and is currently under investigation. In patients with atrial fibrillation for whom the risks of anticoagulation outweigh its benefits, treatment with aspirin may be a safe, although not as effective, alternative.

Lifestyle changes are an important aspect of stroke prevention.[109–111] There is evidence that lifestyle changes such as cessation of smoking,[112,113] lowering cholesterol levels,[114] and exercising[115] may reduce the risk of stroke. Moderate alcohol consumption has been found to be protective, and the benefits are not limited to any particular type of alcoholic beverage.[116] The success of any preventative program based on lifestyle changes is dependent on adequate resources, targeting (individual risk approach), acceptance rate, and ability to provide effective continued intervention and follow-up.[111,117]

The increasing availability and proven efficacy of carotid endarterectomies (CEAs) has been another important development in prevention of stroke.[118–120] CEA is indicated in patients with a recent TIA or nondisabling stroke in whom the CT scan is compatible with a diagnosis of cerebral ischemia and duplex scanning has demonstrated a hemodynamically significant stenosis of the relevant extracranial internal carotid artery. Selective angiography is needed to demonstrate that the stenosis is amenable to surgery and that there are no other distal lesions that may preclude surgical intervention. The risks of surgery include minor neurologic deficits which may be seen in 10 to 20 percent of patients and are usually transitory. Major neurologic sequelae leading to permanent disability or death are seen in 1 to 5 percent of patients depending on the expertise available in the operating room and the skill of the surgeon.[118] CEA is of proven effectiveness in patients with 70 to 99 percent extracranial internal carotid artery stenosis where the benefit for stroke reduction outweighs the risks of the procedure and angiography. Age per se should not be a contraindication to CEA because the risk of stroke increases with age and elderly people with significant stenoses are likely to accrue greater health benefit than younger patients, provided that they are medically fit and willing to undergo the operation. CEA is of little benefit in patients with mild carotid stenosis (0 to 29 percent reduction in diameter), for whom the risks of the procedure are greater than the risk of stroke. The risk/benefit ratio in patients with moderate stenosis remains unclear. Progression in degree of stenosis occurs in about one-fourth of these patients, half of whom will develop a severe stenosis within 10 years.[121] The cumulative risk of stroke in these cases has been estimated at 11 percent after 7 years.[121] At present it is conventional not to offer surgery to patients with moderate stenosis except under specific circumstances.[122] Recent advances in interventional neurovascular radiology have led to the development of cerebral percutaneous transluminal angioplasty as an alternative to surgical endarterectomy.[123] This procedure is undergoing further evaluation, but preliminary data suggest a success rate of 90 percent with less than 10 percent morbidity.[123] Despite their ability to prevent strokes in selected patients with tight carotid stenosis, carotid endarterectomy and angioplasty may not have a significant impact on stroke incidence. It is estimated that even if the availability of CEA were unrestricted, only one stroke per year would be prevented for every 20 procedures performed (estimated reduction in stroke incidence less than 1 percent), limiting its impact as a major stroke prevention strategy.[14]

Conclusions

Based on evidence from randomized trials and statistical overviews, the current accepted view on acute interventions is that there is little that medical treatment and nothing that vascular surgery can do to alter the immediate outcome after cerebral infarction.[124,125] The lack of convincing evidence may not be because there are no potentially useful treatments in acute stroke but because of the inadequacies of studies to date. This view may change in the near future as currently ongoing trials with thrombolytics and neuroprotective agents near conclusion. The availability of potentially effective treatments for acute stroke will revolutionize clinical practice and have a significant impact on stroke management strategies. However, it may be a few years before these advances result in changes in mainstream clinical practice. Until such time, early and planned multidisciplinary rehabilitation will remain the cornerstone of stroke management.

Recovery and Rehabilitation

Recovery

Most patients who survive a stroke make significant functional recovery. Recovery is of two types; intrinsic, which involves a degree of return of neural control, and adaptive, in which alternative strategies are used to overcome disability. The majority of patients show some degree of both intrinsic and adaptive recovery. In general, older patients and those who have had previous strokes are less likely to do well and are more likely to have higher mortality and poor functional outcome. Other significant factors associated with poor recovery in elderly patients include prestroke disability (and dependence), urinary incontinence, and inability to feed themselves or maintain posture. Patient motivation, especially in the very elderly, may be another factor that can influence functional recovery in stroke patients.[126]

Recovery is the fastest in the first few weeks after stroke, with a further 5 to 10 percent occurring between 6 months and 1 year. About 30 percent of survivors are independent within

3 weeks, and by 6 months this proportion rise to 50 percent.[127] Measurable recovery seldom occurs after 12 months, although every clinician is aware of at least one patient who is an exception to this rule. Later neurophysiologic recovery can continue for several years but is rarely significant in terms of improvement in overall functional ability.[128] Completeness of recovery depends largely on the severity of the initial deficit. The more severe the initial deficit, the less likely is it that complete recovery will occur. The pattern of recovery is not uniform and shows considerable variation between individuals and also between different deficits in the same individual. There is currently no validated method for predicting the precise mode or degree of recovery for a given individual. In addition, there can be considerable variation in day-to-day progress of individual patients, which may mask overall recovery or at times give rise to false optimism. This problem can be overcome by monitoring patients over time, as overall trends are more important than "one-off" assessments. Recovery may be affected adversely by the development of stroke-related complications. Although intensive and appropriate therapy may hasten recovery, it is debatable whether the ultimate overall extent of recovery is affected. Comorbidity in elderly patients is another variable that affects overall recovery and rehabilitation.

Rate of recovery varies for different impairments and disabilities. Some problems such as homonymous hemianopia, dysphagia, and sitting balance resolve very quickly in stroke survivors, whereas arm paralysis and language impairment recover more slowly and less completely. Perceptual problems may persist or take a very long time to recover.

Homonymous hemianopia Improves within 4 weeks, usually within 10 days. Hemianopia present after 4 weeks usually persists.[129]

Urinary incontinence Urinary incontinence has been suggested as a prognostic measure in stroke,[130] although its clinical relevance may be limited by other variables such as conciousness, mobility, and nursing practices in different settings. About 60 percent of elderly stroke survivors are incontinent at 1 week, 42 percent at 4 weeks, 25 percent at 3 months, and 15 percent at 1 year. Persistence of urinary incontinence is associated with poor functional outcome, but it is not clear at what point in time this should be measured.

Dysphagia Swallowing problems are common in stroke and occur in up to 60 percent of patients within the first 24 hours of an acute episode.[81] Most swallowing difficulties in acute stroke, however, are transient and resolve in most patients within 2 weeks (mean 8.5 days) of the acute episode. Less than 15 percent of patients are symptomatic beyond 2 weeks,[131] less than 2 percent beyond 3 months.[132]

Dysphasia Dysphasia is normally slow to recover, maximum recovery occurring by 3 months. Some patients continue to recover up to 6 months.[128] The variability between the speed and degree of recovery among patients, compounded by lack of knowledge about predictors of recovery, has made prognostication difficult in this area. Spontaneous recovery is not influenced by the type of dysphasia or the age of the patient, which in turn does not influence functional recovery.[133, 134]

Sitting balance Nearly 60 percent of stroke survivors recover sitting balance by 10 days, and 90 percent by 4 weeks.[135] Inability to maintain sitting balance at 3 months is associated with poor prognosis and is usually due to further strokes.[132]

Arm weakness Improvement in arm function is independent of overall stroke severity: 40 percent of patients gain full voluntary movement, and another 40 percent make partial recovery.[136] In general, if there is no recovery by 4 weeks, the prospects of full recovery are poor, although some patients may still show nonfunctional gains. The rate of arm recovery varies in different muscle groups. Wrist and finger flexors recover better than extensors, and shoulder movement is twice as likely to recover as hand movement.[136]

Walking Leg function recovers quickly in patients who will finally walk: 45 percent of patients walk independently indoors by 4 weeks.[137] Walking outdoors presents greater problems, with only 25 percent of patients achieving this by 6 months. Improvement in walking is not usually seen past the first 6 months.

Perceptual disorders The natural history of perceptual disorders is difficult to determine because of problems involving definition and measurement. Some perceptual problems, such as unilateral visual neglect and anosagnosia, tend to recover more quickly than other problems such as sensory inattention and sensory neglect. The presence of perceptual problems adversely influences speed of functional recovery, length of hospital stay, and destination of discharge even in the presence of good recovery in terms of other impairment.[138]

Functional recovery Functional recovery depends the level of initial impairment and disability.[139] Mild to moderately disabled patients make measurable improvements up to 3 months following stroke, after which the recovery curve flattens.[140] There is evidence showing that the rate of functional recovery can be influenced by coordinated rehabilitation (Fig. 35-4). Patients with severe stroke may continue to show further functional improvement between 3 and 6 months.[141] The pattern of functional recovery often predicts the pattern of discharge from the hospital and the length of hospital stay (Fig. 35-4). If all stroke survivors are considered, 62 percent are independent in self-care at 3 months and 66 percent at the end of 1 year, despite persistence of neurologic deficit in some patients.[142]

Rehabilitation

Rehabilitation in stroke is not simply a matter of being treated by a therapist or a group of therapists but involves a whole range of approaches to managing disability provided by a coordinated multidisciplinary team and tailored to restore patients to their fullest possible physical, mental, and social capability.[143, 144] The goals of rehabilitation are not always

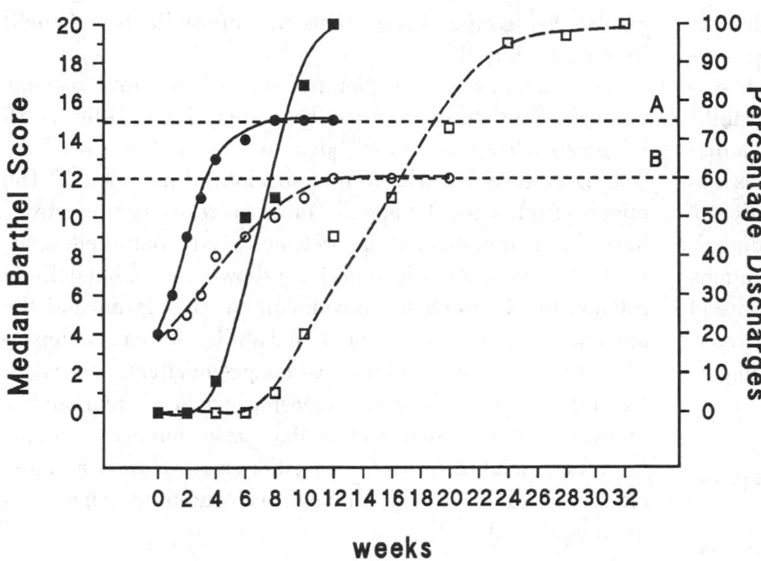

Figure 35-4 Weekly median Barthel scores and discharge rates of stroke survivors on stroke unit ($n = 73$) and general wards ($n = 69$) ●, median Barthel score (stroke unit); ■, percentage discharges (stroke unit); ○, median Barthel score (general ward); □, percentage discharge (general ward).

easy to define because it deals with many aspects of human performance. In general, rehabilitation should aim to maximize patients' role fulfillment and independence in their environment within the limitations imposed by underlying impairment and availability of resources.[145] It should help them to make the best adaptation possible to any difference between the roles desired and the roles achieved following stroke. Another important objective of the rehabilitation process is to monitor regularly the services provided to ensure that the best possible value is being obtained for the money and effort being expended.[143]

Progress in the development of rehabilitation techniques in stroke has been slow because of the absence of an agreed-on framework or model for rehabilitation. Recent consensus on the pathology-impairment-disability-handicap model[146–148] provides the basic framework for defining and evaluating appropriate assessments and interventions in stroke rehabilitation. It is accepted that the focus of attention should pass from pathology to handicap and from patient to environment during the course of rehabilitation. The major areas of concern in rehabilitation are disability and handicap. Disability is defined as "restriction, or lack of ability, to perform an activity in the manner or within the range considered to be normal."[146] Disability relates to function, and the ability to undertake basic activities of self-care is fundamental to any physical rehabilitation program. Handicap, the social consequence of disability, is defined as "limitations faced by stroke patients in fulfilling their normal role in the society."[146] It is not always possible to differentiate handicap from disability, and most pragmatic approaches tend to combine these two dimensions, referring to them as social disability.[149]

Process of rehabilitation

Rehabilitation in stroke is essentially a multidisciplinary activity which has been described as a problem-solving educational process focusing on disability and intended to reduce handicap.[145] The basic principles that should be applied throughout rehabilitation of stroke patients are the following.

- Documentation of impairments, disabilities, and handicaps and, where possible, measuring them using simple, valid scales
- Maximization of independence and minimization of learned dependency
- Holistic approach to patients, taking into account their physical and psychosocial background as well as their environment

The process of rehabilitation has four important components: assessment, planning, intervention, and evaluation.

Assessment Assessment includes measurement of deficits, identification of problems, and analysis of underlying causes. Assessment is necessary to ascertain the precise nature and severity of deficits prior to commencement of a rehabilitation program. It provides a logical basis for treatment and management and enables monitoring of patients' progress.[143] As rehabilitation deals with the ill-defined concept of human performance, there are many areas for potential assessment, but it may be pragmatic and productive to select a small group of scales relevant to the objectives of intervention rather than to use comprehensive assessments to evaluate the overall outcome of rehabilitation.[150] As all other processes of rehabilitation and the quality of overall management of stroke patients are dependent on performing appropriate, adequate assessments, this aspect of stroke management will be discussed in detail in a later section.

Planning Planning is the process of goal setting based on identification of aims, objectives, and targets. Many difficulties arise in stroke rehabilitation because the goals of intervention are not set in advance or because these goals have not been discussed and agreed on by all relevant parties.[145] The two major problems that arise in goal setting include failure to use a common language in communication between various professionals or between professionals and patients and, second, failure to agree on a time frame within which the rehabilitation process must be accomplished.[151] There is often a discrepancy between the goals of patients and their families and those of professional staff members. An essential function of the whole rehabilitation team is to identify and modify unrealistically high (and sometimes unjustifiably low) expectations of patients and their families by making them more aware of the nature of residual deficit and expected prognosis as soon as these are reasonably clear.[145] The areas of practical importance in goal setting are as follows.

- *Accommodation*: Where will the patient live and what physical adaptations will be needed?
- *Personal support*: What help will be essential for the patient?
- *Life satisfaction*: What roles will the patient be fulfilling within his or her social setting and how will they be occupying their time?

Intervention The minimum requirement of any stroke intervention is to provide care necessary to maintain the status quo and prevent deterioration of the patient's condition or functional ability due to poor management or complications. Further intervention should be aimed at facilitating recovery and improving outcome by minimizing disability and preventing handicap. Traditional therapy input lacks a proper physiologic basis because little is known about the processes underlying the return of neurologic function.[144] A recent study using PET suggested that "new" cerebral areas, usually in the frontal cortex and not normally used, are activated during the recovery process.[46] In addition, activation of the unaffected side is altered, suggesting considerable changes in brain activity following stroke. These preliminary observations need wider confirmation, and further research is required in conjunction with therapy disciplines to provide a scientific basis for rehabilitation in stroke.

Literature on therapeutic intervention in stroke is limited and deals largely with poorly designed studies undertaken with small groups of patients.[20,143] An overview of these studies suggests that, because of ethical considerations, it is virtually impossible to design trials comparing therapy with no therapy, despite the absence of proof of effectiveness. Of the few trials that compared different therapeutic techniques, none showed conclusively that one technique was superior to any other in the major areas of physical therapy[152–155] or in speech and language function.[156–160] Randomized studies on social services intervention[161] and on counseling and education of caregivers[162,163] have also failed to show any significant differences between study and control groups. There appears to be a direct relationship between severity of stroke and amount of therapy actually given. More severely disabled patients tend to receive more therapy,[164,165] and there are concerns that intensive treatment is being offered to patients who are unlikely to benefit from such input.[164]

The amount of formal therapy received by stroke patients is small. One study suggests that it may be as little as 46 minutes each working day[165] or 3 to 4 percent of a patient's waking time each week, even at specialized facilities.[166] The effects of intensive therapeutic input on recovery from stroke have been investigated in well-designed controlled studies.[167,168] These investigations have shown a small but definite relationship between the amount of therapy given and the amount of improvement in functional ability, which is independent of the nonspecific effects of changes in attention or adaptive mechanisms. There is increasing evidence from studies at stroke rehabilitation centers that early, intensive therapy has a beneficial effect on the speed of early recovery and discharge from the hospital, although the long-term benefits remain equivocal.[6, 140]

Evaluation Evaluation is the process of monitoring a patient's progress (or lack of it) and assessing the effectiveness of the rehabilitation process itself. Objective assessment of effectiveness of stroke rehabilitation has proved difficult for several reasons. These include the confounding effect of spontaneous recovery from stroke, difficulty in defining the extent of need, and perceptions of good outcome, which may vary with the perspective of different observers. Most patients who survive stroke exhibit varying degrees of spontaneous recovery due either to return of neural control mechanisms or to adaptive processes involving the use of alternative strategies. As recovery is fastest during the first 3 months[61,128,141] and coincides with the period during which patients are likely to receive maximum rehabilitation input, it is difficult to disentangle the effects of rehabilitation from those of spontaneous recovery.

The extent of need is also difficult to define. Although most patients have some disabilities and problems related to the stroke, it is unlikely that the level of disability will always correlate with the scale of problems encountered by stroke patients. A severely disabled person who needs nursing home care seemingly has a lesser need for formal rehabilitation and does not seem to pose as serious a management problem. The rehabilitation needs of a moderately disabled person who chooses to live alone in inappropriate accommodations, on the other hand, are great and require an inordinately high level of resource input.

Similarly, differences in expectations and, consequently, perceptions of what is considered good outcome, have resulted in considerable variability in evaluating the effectiveness of stroke rehabilitation programs. It is accepted that goals of rehabilitation vary according to the expectations of the parties involved.[144] The goal of hospitals may be to discharge patients as soon as possible, whereas the goal of patients may be to return to their previous functional status even if this is unattainable. The goal of caregivers may be to minimize the level of input they need to provide even at the cost of institutionalization. Many of the difficulties ultimately faced in managing patients and in evaluating the effectiveness of interventions can be traced back to conflicts between the goals and objectives of different parties.[145]

Conclusions There is consensus that well-organized well-planned rehabilitation guided by well-defined goals based on adequate assessment and sensitive negotiation with patients and caregivers reduces disability and long-term institutionalization. There is, however, no evidence supporting any specific treatment technique for stroke patients. A pragmatic functional approach individualized for each patient's needs is recommended, and strict adherence to theories with little scientific basis or clinical evidence of effectiveness should be discouraged. There is also evidence suggesting that early, intensive intervention by therapists may speed recovery and hasten discharge from the hospital without increasing the total amount of therapeutic input.

Assessments in Stroke Rehabilitation

In rehabilitation assessment is acquisition of the information needed to define rehabilitation goals. A large number of neurologic, physical, and functional assessments are currently available and can be divided into global assessments (which determine the overall impact of stroke) and specific assessments (which deal with a single level or domain of impairment or disability). There are numerous scales for measuring global disease severity, which often use composite scoring systems.[169] Composite scores for global disease severity are unreliable because of the dominance of speech and language function over other indexes and because, when quite different disabilities are combined into one score, much specific information is lost.[170] Most scores also mix a variety of impairments and disabilities without considering their interactions.[169] A considerable amount of work has been undertaken in developing and validating simpler and more specific measures of stroke disability that are more appropriate in assessing and comparing stroke patients and their treatment. It may well be that these more specific measures will make global measures of disease severity redundant.

Ideally all component items of an assessment at a given time should relate to the level being measured.[169] Some overlap between assessments for different levels, however, is likely to occur in clinical settings because these levels are not discrete but form a continuum. The importance of knowing what information is wanted and why, that is, the purpose of a measure, is central to choosing any measure in rehabilitation.[171] It is also important to decide on the least amount of information necessary to achieve this purpose. The temptation to collect large amounts of data should be resisted because this practice is expensive in time and effort and often results in reduced accuracy and completeness of the data collected. Assessment protocols based on a small selection of easy-to-use relevant measures have been recommended for wider use.[150] The necessary characteristics of suitable measures are validity, reliability, sensitivity, simplicity, and communicability. It is best to use existing measures wherever possible provided that they are valid for the purpose in mind, reliable in the circumstances proposed, and appropriate to the needs and resources. Moreover, the use of established measures makes communication and interpretation of data easier.

The major reasons for undertaking assessments in stroke patients are (1) to define the type of patient and the potential for recovery and/or responding to intervention (prognostication); (2) to identify the main areas of difficulty and their underlying causes, the extent of disability, and the aims of the patient and the family; (3) to monitor the process of rehabilitation (evaluation); and (4) to assess the degree of recovery and residual disability at the end of the rehabilitation process (outcome).

Prognostication in Stroke

Nature of stroke

PICH has traditionally been associated with high mortality and severe disability. Over two-thirds of patients with PICH die within 3 weeks of onset.[172] However, the increasing use of CT scanning has shown that some minor strokes are due to small hemorrhages deep within the parenchyma of the brain and are associated with good functional outcome. The functional outcome of patients with severe stroke who survive cerebral hemorrhage has also been improved considerably by the development of rehabilitation techniques, especially stroke rehabilitation units, in recent years.[173] The anatomic classification of stroke[25] is of prognostic significance in patients with cerebral infarction, as described earlier. The prognosis of patients with hemorrhagic transformation remains unknown. In general, CT scan appearances of severe edema, midline shift, or herniation in association with a vascular lesion are indicative of poor outcome.

Stroke severity

Prognosis after stroke is directly related to the severity of initial impairments and disabilities, and there are several ways of predicting outcome. These may utilize simple specific indicators or more complex assessment approaches including weighted formulas based on multivariate analysis. Simple indicators include urinary incontinence,[130,174] changes in conciousness levels,[175] and severity of individual motor, speech, or perceptual impairment.[169] The more complex methods of determining prognosis include assessments of aggregated motor deficit,[176,177] functional impairment scores,[178,179] or a combination of motor and functional impairment scores incorporated into multivariate scores.[180–183]

There has been considerable controversy over the relative merits of these different prognostic indicators and their applicability to stroke practice. Various studies have shown that prognostic indicators based on neurologic examination can predict mortality or severe handicap but are of limited use in predicting functional outcome, destination of discharge, or care needs following discharge from the hospital.[180,184,185] Scores that include functional assessments are more predictive of functional outcome but often involve the use of multivariate formulas.[178–80,183,186] There are some reservations about the use of multivariate formulas in predicting stroke outcome because of their perceived complexity and their lack of validity in data sets other than those from which they were derived.[187] There is a trend toward promoting the use of simple single indicators, such as urinary incontinence, as predictors of outcome in clinical practice[144,187] despite concerns about the sensitivity and reliability of any single indicator in predicting outcome.[188,189] Although urinary continence has been demonstrated to be superior to five multivariate scales in predicting outcome,[130] It may not always be easy to assess incontinence in intensive care units.[183] In addition, urinary continence may continue to improve over several weeks, limiting its predictive value in the early phase of stroke management. Early in the course of their treatment, it is possible and clinically more relevant to group stroke survivors for expected outcome and resource use (health benefit grouping) using a simple validated beside scoring system based on clinical assessment of power, balance, proprioception, and cognition.[182,183] Grouping of patients according to outcome and resource use has applications in monitoring the appropriateness of care for individual patients and in undertaking comparisons of the effectiveness of various therapy interventions or models of stroke care. It is important to remember that no prognostic criteria are applicable to all patients in all settings. These criteria must be used as part of overall clinical evaluation of individual patients when determining management strategies.

Monitoring Rehabilitation

The wide variety of impairments and disabilities associated with stroke, as well as the large number of instruments available to measure each impairment and disability, have contributed significantly to the lack of a common assessment data set for stroke management. This problem has been addressed by the British Stroke Research Group, which has recommended a battery of assessments that are well-validated and reliable and pertain to key areas in stroke rehabilitation.[144,145,169] Core assessments include Motoricity Index and Trunk Control Test for motor loss, Star Cancellation Test for neglect, Frenchay Aphasia Screening Test for aphasia, Abbreviated Mental Test for orientation and memory, Barthel Activities of Daily Living Index (ADL) for functional abilities, Rivermead Mobility Index, and a Timed Walking Test. Other assessments may be used in specific circumstances. Despite some agreement on what should be assessed and how it should be measured, the number of assessments recommended remains large and it may not always be possible or necessary to undertake all of them, especially if repeated measurements are needed. A sensible approach is to use simpler assessments more frequently during the rehabilitation process to monitor and adjust the treatment program.

A review of studies on stroke rehabilitation has shown the predominance of ADL scales in monitoring the rehabilitation process.[190] This may be because ADL scales measure independence (and, by implication, dependence on others) in undertaking basic daily activities, which is a fundamental goal of the rehabilitation process. The level of independence in ADL is not only the basis for more complete recovery but is also important in determining the care needs of, and resource use by, patients who continue to be dependent. Widespread use of ADL scales is further supported by the general agreement on the core ADL components (bladder and bowel function, feeding, cleanliness, dressing, and mobility),[191–193] high interrater reliability in clinical settings which is not influenced by the method of data collection,[194] and communicability within multidisciplinary teams. Hence, although the development of ADL scales has followed observed practice rather than being developed from a consistent theory or framework, they appear to be a suitable measure of rehabilitation outcome.[195]

The limitations of ADL scales should be acknowledged. The distinction between impairment and disability is often blurred, and ADL scales include items that could be considered impairments. Items on these scales may not be independent of each other or may be influenced by other aspects of disability (e.g., communication or orientation) that are not measured.[169] ADL scales have a low ceiling effect and cannot identify the reasons why patients fail to achieve goals (e.g., incontinence may be due to immobility or bladder dysfunction) or how patients achieve independence (the quality of functional recovery).

Measurement of Outcome

Successful outcome means different things to different people (e.g., patients, caregivers, professionals), evaluation of outcome after stroke rehabilitation is complex, and it has been consistently difficult to identify a single outcome measure that satisfies all needs. Measures such as mortality and handicap have long been used in epidemiologic research. Judging the outcome of rehabilitation, in contrast, depends on assessment of a broad range of ill-defined functions and requires the use of more complex, sensitive measures.

The recommended minimum outcome information required in normal clinical practice is the Barthel ADL index.[169] It is an important surrogate indicator of quality of life because most quality-of-life measures are primarily concerned with ADL functions. Barthel scores were also shown to have a good correlation with the Rankin Handicap Scale.[196]

Three additional outcome measures are important in hospital settings. Mortality continues to be important because of its inclusion in several epidemiologic and stroke outcome studies. Mortality in stroke can be divided into three phases: (1) early mortality due to brain damage, which is unlikely to be influenced by rehabilitation but may be affected by acute interventions; (2) delayed hospital mortality due to stroke-related complications, which is an indicator of quality of care; and (3) late mortality, which is multifactorial depending on the severity of stroke, rehabilitation, care requirements, community intervention, and comorbidity.

The setting into which an individual is discharged after rehabilitation, when premorbid accommodation has been taken into account, has long been one of the most frequently used outcome indicators.[150] Institutionalization implies unsuccessful rehabilitation, loss of freedom to live at home, and high costs to society. Destination of discharge, however, not only is dependent on the level of residual disability or success of rehabilitation but is also influenced by comorbidity, family support, and social variables which may be outside the control of the rehabilitation process.[110] Despite these limitations, institutionalization has been used in several previous studies and is accepted as useful outcome measure in stroke research.[150]

Length of hospital stay is a fashionable outcome measure in the current climate of health care provision. However, this measure is often policy-driven and influenced by several factors such as availability of beds, pressure on services, and financial constraints in insurance-driven systems. Nevertheless, it is still regarded as a proxy measure for the efficiency of the rehabilitation process, especially for organizational aspects aimed at expediting discharge from the hospital once rehabilitation goals have been achieved. In the British system, average length of hospital stay remains an important determinant of the overall hospital cost of stroke and is an important consideration in planning the delivery of health services in the future.

Sequelae of Stroke

Stroke patients may suffer a range of problems associated with primary pathology or due to secondary medical or neurologic complications. Stroke-related disorders that are significant in patient management include visual problems (hemianopia or inattention), dysphagia with the risk of aspiration and infection, communication problems, venous thrombotic disease, urinary and bowel problems, spasticity and contractures, pressure sores, shoulder pain, associated reactions, cold hemiplegic arm, and edema of the limbs. The main neurologic complications include depression, seizures, behavioral changes and, rarely, thalamic pain. Stroke patients are also at a higher risk of falls which, in association with osteoporotic bone changes in the hemiplegic limb, often result in fractures on the stroke side.[197] Various studies have shown that complications occur in about 60 percent of stroke patients undergoing rehabilitation and are more frequent in patients with severe disability.[64] The clinical aspects of some of the more important problems are discussed in the following sections.

Dysphagia

Swallowing problems are common after stroke and have been attributed in the past to brain stem or bilateral cerebral lesions. New research, however, suggests that this condition is also seen in a significant number of patients with unilateral hemispheric lesions.[198,199] Swallowing problems are associated with increased incidence of aspiration, chest infection, dehydration, and malnutrition.[81] The presence of dysphagia, in itself and in association with its complications, is linked with poor outcome following stroke.[200] Despite this, dysphagia is poorly recognized and poorly managed in most acute settings.

The diagnosis of dysphagia is conventionally dependent on clinical examination and a demonstrated absence of the gag reflex in stroke patients. There is considerable evidence suggesting that this reflex is not a reliable sign of dysphagia, being present in some patients with significant swallowing problems and absent in others who may have no swallowing problems.[201] Dependence on this sign may result in inappropriate management, especially as a speech therapy assessment may not be available on an on-call basis in most hospitals. Bedside swallowing assessment may be a simple, feasible, reliable alternative method for screening patients for swallowing problems.[81] This assessment should be undertaken in patients with relevant neurologic deficits (facial weakness, dysarthria, dysphonia), reasonable sitting balance, and ability to cooperate with the examination (appropriate sensorium). The patient is given a teaspoonful of water and observed for dribbling, cough, altered respiration, breathing problems, or wet dysphonia before being given more liquid and then a solid. Oral intake should be restricted in patients with definite or probable swallowing problems pending full assessment by a speech and language therapist.

The development of videofluoroscopic techniques has greatly facilitated objective assessment of swallowing problems.[202] Videofluoroscopy allows analysis of various phases of deglutition in great detail and can measure transit times for the bolus to complete the pharyngeal swallow accurately.[203] It can demonstrate problems with initiating swallow (e.g., poor tongue control, inability to form bolus or move bolus to the pharynx), with swallowing itself (e.g., poor swallow reflex, inadequate laryngeal elevation, pooling, aspiration), or in the postpharyngeal pharyngeal phase of swallow (e.g., esophageal spasm). It also shows the presence of aspiration (entry of food or barium below the level of the true vocal cords) even when there are no clinical signs of a compromised airway or aspiration.[204] Videofluoroscopy has made it possible to assess objectively and reliably the effectiveness of various interventions aimed at improving swallowing in stroke patients. It is important to remember that this procedure is not necessary in most stroke patients (who recover rapidly and spontaneously) and should be reserved for patients with atypical or persistent dysphagia or those with unexplained or recurrent pneumonia.

Most swallowing difficulties in acute stroke are transient and resolve in most patients within 2 weeks of the acute episode. The remainder respond well to compensatory techniques and dietary modifications under the supervision of speech and language therapists and dieticians, which remain the mainstay of treatment of dysphagia in stroke patients.[205–207] Treatment of patients with persistent dysphagia, however, presents problems. Most current strategies are directed toward establishing alternative means of nutrition (e.g., nasogastric tubes, PEG) until normal feeding can be established using conventional speech and language therapy. There are no accepted interventions aimed directly at improving the swallowing process. The identification of cortical center involved in swallowing presents the exciting possibility of using measures such as cortical stimulation with magnetic fields to stimulate the swallowing reflex.[199,208] Insertion of artificial electrical pacemakers to trigger laryngeal elevation is also being investigated.[209] Intervention studies to date have been limited to animal models and have methodologic problems, but they provide the basis for further research in this area.[208,209]

Dysphasia

Dysphasia is a defect in language function manifesting as impairment in speech production, comprehension, reading, or writing in the absence of motor disturbances of voice production or writing, visual or auditory deficits, and intellectual or cognitive impairment. Although the left hemisphere is traditionally associated with speech in most people, there is evidence suggesting that the right hemisphere has some capacity for language even in right-handed people.[210] In left-handed people, lesions of the left hemisphere can still result in speech problems because this is the dominant hemisphere in 70 percent of these individuals. In the remaining 30 percent, language functions are situated in the right hemisphere in 20 percent and equally distributed between the two hemispheres in 10 percent. Consequently, left-handed people are more likely to suffer from dysphasia as a group, regardless of which hemisphere is damaged. Dysphasia in left-handed patients, however, tends to be less severe and to recover more rapidly than that in right-handed patients, probably because of bilateral representation.[210] Evidence suggests that damage to subcortical nuclei may also result in dysphasia.[210] Structures mainly involved are the thalamus and the basal ganglia. Language deficits associated with lesions in these areas include alterations in fluency, nominal aphasia, hesitancy, word blocking, and impairment in reading and comprehension.[210]

Patients may present with nonfluent dysphasia, which at its most severe consists of complete loss of speech and phonation. This is nearly always associated with an inability to comprehend anything but the most simple commands. Often there is buccofacial apraxia. Recovery is associated with the ability to phonate simple yes or no responses (or similar monosyllablic utterances) which are usually out of context and inappropriate. Less severe, and more common, forms present as agrammatic speech, although the information content may be adequate to convey appropriate meaning to a patient listener despite the hesitancy and distorted articulation. Fluent dysphasia is characterized by spontaneous speech which is abnormal and often incomprehensible because of the use of nonexistent words, wrong words (paraphasia), or inappropriately arranged words, which lose their meaning.

Impaired ability to understand speech is common in dysphasic patients. The difficulty in comprehension increases with increasing linguistic complexity of the speech presented and length of sentences used. The extent to which a dysphasic patient can understand what is being said is frequently overestimated, which can result in misunderstandings between patients and their families or professionals involved in patient care. It is important that speech and language problems be identified early in stroke patients because many therapy interventions are dependent on this function.

The more severe forms of dysphasia are often easy to diagnose on clinical examination in most stroke patients. The diagnosis of mild dysphasia may be more difficult, especially if the patient has a high-level language deficit. It is also important to differentiate dysphasia from confusion secondary to cognitive impairment. Enquiries about the patient's language background (native language, profession, social and educational status), previous speech problems (e.g., stuttering) and hand dominance should be part of the examination. Problems in comprehension are particularly difficult to assess. A bedside measure can be obtained by assessing the patient's ability to respond to commands of increasing complexity, either in content or in linguistic structure. It should be remembered that in some patients errors may occur because of dyspraxia or memory problems. Problems with expression usually present as difficulty in finding words, problems with naming objects, or inability to read or write during a bedside assessment. All patients suspected of having dysphasia should be assessed by speech and language therapists regardless of the severity of the impairment. Appropriate treatment of dysphasic patients consists of individualized therapy programs supervised by speech and language therapists, development of simple communication strategies to enable multidisciplinary rehabilitation, and educating caregivers in communication techniques appropriate to the patient's level of impairment.

Perception

Perception is an important but sadly neglected aspect of stroke management. The outcome of rehabilitation frequently depends on effective management of perceptual problems rather than on motor recovery alone. Despite this, perceptual problems are poorly understood and difficult to assess objectively because of the paucity of valid assessment instruments. Their management is equally difficult and a subject of great controversy.[155]

Perceptual problems after stroke can be divided into (1) neglect, which is the disregard of, and failure to attend to, one half of external space; (2) agnosias, which comprise problems with interpreting sensory data from the environment or the body (visual, tactile, autotopagnosia); and (3) apraxias, the collection of problems involving formulating, initiating, or sequencing motor activity. Although it is traditional to consider perceptual problems a consequence of nondominant (right) hemisphere lesions, there is increasing evidence that these difficulties may be equally common in both hemispheres but are hard to assess in patients with left hemisphere lesions because of dysphasia.[211]

Total neglect of one side of the body is a result of extensive hemisphere damage and is usually combined with dense hemiplegia. Patients with visuospatial neglect tend to ignore objects on the affected side and classically leave food on one side of the plate or bump into objects on the affected side despite no obvious hemianopia. Common agnosias seen in stroke patients include visual agnosia (failure to recognize objects by sight alone) and problems with depth and movement perception. Visual problems are common and are present in about 25 percent of stroke survivors in the acute phase. Visuospatial dysfunction may significantly affect visual depth and movement perception and can be particularly disabling in stroke patients, as it affects their ability to judge distances and relationships between objects or between self and objects in a three-dimensional setting, causing severe restrictions in daily living activities.[138] Some patients with perceptual difficulties lose left-right discrimination, leading to inappropriate action, whereas others may suffer impairment of topographic awareness of the environment, causing them to become lost even in familiar surroundings. Some patients may be aware of their deficit but are unable to overcome it without paying extra attention to affected functional abilities.[210]

The simplest and perhaps most sensitive test for visuospatial impairments involves asking the patient to draw a clock face. Affected individuals fail to put numbers on the affected side.[212] More formal tests include star or number cancellation tests and the Rivermead Perceptual Test Battery. It is not known whether these deficits respond to general stimulation or to specific remedial measures. Recent research suggests that neglect may be amenable to therapeutic interventions.[213,214] Electrical stimulation may also be of benefit in patients with neglect, but further studies are required to confirm this benefit.[215] Although visuospatial problems delay or compromise functional recovery in most patients, some individuals eventually make full recovery.[216]

Other major agnosias affecting functional recovery are loss of body image, resulting in failure to identify parts of the body (autotopagnosia) and denial of the stroke or underestimation of its severity (anosoagnosia). Autotopagnosia is usually revealed when patients try to dress themselves and fail to dress completely, ignoring the affected part of the body. Some patients with right parietal lobe lesions complain about "phantom limbs" or other bizarre phenomenon (e.g., having "withered" or "demonic" limbs), which can be very frightening for them. The clinical presentation of body agnosia is very characteristic, but further confirmation can be made by asking the patient to name body parts or draw a picture of a human body. More formal confirmation can be made by one of the many perceptual test batteries available (e.g., Rivermead Perceptual Assessment Battery). In patients with anosognosia the lack of awareness of any problem makes their rehabilitation difficult. Despite this, improvement is possible with specialist input provided by therapists trained in stroke management.

Apraxia is difficulty in performing purposive movements at will in the absence of sensation, comprehension, motor, or coordination deficits adequate to explain this inability. Learned skilled movements are performed incorrectly but may be performed spontaneously in response to subconscious stimuli. Several types of apraxia affect different activities (e.g., orofacial, gait, dress) and occur singly or in combination. In some patients apraxia is seen on the unaffected side (sympathetic apraxia). There is no effective treatment for apraxia. Management currently focuses on increasing the patient's awareness of the condition and its effects in the stroke setting, early recognition of the problem and its impact on the patient, education, and teaching of adaptive skills and coping strategies to patients and their relatives.

Tone and Spasticity

Doctors and therapists have differing perceptions and definitions of tone and spasticity and different views regarding its clinical significance. Spasticity is a consequence of increased tone and is defined as the resistance to passive stretch of muscles. Tone is often reduced in the early days after a stroke, and return of tone is usually associated with good outcome. Physiotherapists emphasize that tone is a more dynamic, complex process that is part of an overall pattern of posture and movement. Appropriate management of tone is one of the fundamental principles of the Bobath method of facilitative physiotherapy in stroke patients, which gives priority to normalization of tone and improving symmetry even at the cost of postponing standing or walking.[217]

The management of abnormal tone and spasticity is difficult, as it depends on achieving the right balance between hypo- and hypertonia between different muscle groups. The problem is compounded by the fact that spasticity varies between different groups of muscles and times of day and with the emotional state of the patient, activity being undertaken, and posture of the limb. Inappropriate exercise can result in inappropriate tone patterns to the ultimate detriment of the patient. If not managed correctly, spasticity leads to bad gait patterns, contractures, and loss of function. Management of spasticity should be undertaken jointly by doctors and physiotherapists. Treatment of abnormal tone is usually initiated by physiotherapists, who can offer a range of interventions (posture, exercises, splints) to reduce spasticity and its complications. Drug therapy should be initiated in consultation with therapists and adjusted to achieve optimal effects. Its main drawback is its lack of selectivity; since all muscle groups are affected equally, there may be undesirable hypotonia in some muscle groups (e.g., drugs for reducing spasticity in arm muscles may affect walking). In certain patients with severe spasticity, tenotomy, localized phenol or botulin toxin injection may be helpful.[218, 219]

The Hemiplegic Shoulder

Shoulder pain, restriction of movement, and subluxation of the shoulder joint are common problems in stroke patients. In hypotonic patients, the loss of muscle strength around the shoulder joint and the weight of the paralyzed arm may result in malalignment of the humeral head in the shallow glenoid cavity, predisposing to inferior subluxation of the shoulder. This can easily be detected clinically in the sitting or standing patient and confirmed on radiographs in the erect position.

There is considerable variation in the reported incidence of subluxation in stroke patients, but it is estimated that one in every five patients is affected.[220,221] The clinical implications of subluxation and its effects on eventual recovery of function are not known.

Shoulder pain is more common and inconsistently related to subluxation,[222] although its exact prevalence remains unknown.[223] It is encountered in rehabilitation settings with disconcerting frequency and may be a result of spasticity in the shoulder muscles, glenohumeral subluxation, reflex sympathetic dystrophy (the shoulder-hand syndrome), or orthopedic causes such as rotator cuff injury, arthritis, or adhesive capsulitis made worse by immobility. Contributory factors include careless handling of patients and incorrect position of the hemiplegic arm. Management is empirical with no agreed-on guidelines. It should be undertaken in collaboration with physiotherapists and includes measures such as proper positioning of the arm during periods of inactivity, avoidance of abnormal arm movements causing excessive strain on the shoulder joint or inappropriate pulling of the hemiplegic arm during transfers, and early passive exercise to prevent joint stiffness and contractures. Patients should be advised to avoid overzealous, self-assisted arm movements. Treatment with analgesics and nonsteroidal anti-infammatory drugs may help in some patients. Steroid injections in the shoulder may be helpful, but data on their effectiveness and safety in treating shoulder pain are inadequate.[224]

Edematous Limbs

Swelling of the limbs on the affected side is common after stroke. It causes considerable discomfort and concern to stroke survivors, especially because it may never resolve in some patients. Swelling of the leg is seen in about 25 percent of stroke survivors and in most cases is caused by underlying phlebothrombosis.[225] This swelling is more common in elderly patients, increases with stroke severity, and predisposes to venous thrombosis. Management is conservative and includes measures such as early mobilization, avoidance of trauma, and leg elevation at rest. The role of stockings and long-term heparin prophylaxis remains to be determined. Anticoagulation may be necessary if there is proven deep vein thrombosis.

The precise etiology of edema of the hand of the paralyzed arm is not known, but it is thought to be due to reflex sympathetic dystrophy, posture, and lack of muscle activity. It is often unsightly and painful, especially on flexion of the fingers. Edema fluid has a high protein content and is unlikely to respond to diuretics. Treatment modalities include elevation of the hand, massage, and application of elastic bandages. Immersion of the hand in a tank of water cooled to 10°C has been shown to reduce the swelling considerably.[226]

Seizures

Cerebrovascular disease is the most common cause of elderly onset seizures (see also Ch. 31). Fits occurring at the onset of stroke are seen in about 2 to 6 percent of patients and are associated with lesions in carotid artery distribution.[227,228] These fits are most likely the result of acute local brain metabolic alteration induced by ischemia, and once these derangements are reversed, the seizures disappear.[229] Treatment with anticonvulsants hence may not be appropriate in these patients until further fits occur.[227] In acute stroke seizures do not correlate with the size of the lesion, functional outcome, or mortality. In clinical practice, it is not always easy to distinguish between a stroke causing a seizure (anticonvulsants not indicated) or a seizure with a strokelike presentation (possible treatment indicated), and it may be appropriate to undertake further investigations (including imaging) before making therapeutic decisions. It is important to remember that the risk of subsequent late seizures and poststroke epilepsy is increased in patients with early seizures.[229]

Late-onset seizures (those appearing more than a week after the stroke is completed) can occur months to years after the stroke and are probably due to structural brain abnormalities leading to development of an epileptic focus. A longitudinal study has shown that the risk of developing epilepsy is 3 ± 2 percent at 1 year and 5 ± 4 percent at 5 years after stroke.[230] The risk of seizures is greatest with cortical lesions and least with subcortical or infratentorial lesions. The pathology of stroke is important: about 10 percent of patients with cerebral infarction, 25 percent of patients with primary intracranial hemorrhage, and over 30 percent of patients with subarachnoid hemorrhage developed epilepsy within 5 years of the original event in the Oxford Community Stroke Project. Late-onset seizures need to be treated and respond well to anticonvulsant treatment.

Depression

It is estimated that between 30 and 60 percent of stroke patients have clinically significant depression, the highest prevalence and severity occurring in the first 2 years.[231] Three different types of mood disorders have been recognized in stroke patients: (1) severe depression that meets the diagnostic criteria for major depression, (2) minor depressive illness fulfilling most of the criteria for a dysthymic disorder except the time frame, and (3) an indifferent, apathetic mental state often associated with false cheerfulness.[232] Diagnosis of mood disorders in patients with acute stroke is difficult because changes in appetite, sleep, or interest (all indicative of depression) may be a normal adjustment response to physical disability and changed roles.[233] The diagnosis of depression in stroke is further hampered by the presence of dysphasia and impairments in attention and concentration which make assessment difficult. The presence of autonomic and psychological depressive symptoms (e.g., palpitations, anxiety, excessive sweating, loss of energy, concentration difficulties, pessimistic thoughts including suicide), however, strongly favors depression in the acute stroke period.[233]

It is commonly accepted that depression in stroke is frequently associated with left hemisphere lesions despite some studies suggesting no laterality.[234,235] The frequency and severity of depression appears to be related to the proximity of the anterior boundary of the lesion to the left frontal pole. Anatomic work suggests that the deep nuclei of the forebrain and associated structures (mainly the head of the caudate and the anterior limb of the internal capsule) may play a special role in the pathogenesis of depression in stroke. There is no convincing evidence that the size of the lesion correlates with the severity of the depression observed. Depression is less frequent following right hemisphere lesions and is associated with posterior or retrorolandic pathology. Poststroke depression appears to be more common in patients with a family or personal premorbid history of depression.[234]

Poststroke depression may last for 7 to 8 months or more without treatment and is highly correlated with failure to resume premorbid social and physical activities.[236] Depression also has a negative effect on functional and cognitive recovery, integration into the family environment, and caregiver stress in stroke patients.[237] There is growing evidence suggesting that early recognition of depression in stroke and early treatment with appropriate antidepressants can facilitate recovery, although most series are small.[236,238,239] Antidepressant therapy, however, needs to be used with caution and monitored carefully because of potential toxicity. It is also important to remember that the expectation of benefits from antidepressant therapy is based on extrapolation of existing data on depression in the general population to stroke patients. The role of antidepressant drugs in stroke patients has not been demonstrated equivocally in well-designed prospective intervention studies. Equally importantly, the role of nonpharmacologic interventions has not been properly evaluated. There is little information on which types of antidepressants are most effective in stroke patients, the time when antidepressants should be started, and the duration for which they should be continued. There is a prima facie case for preferring serotonin-specific reuptake inhibitor (SSRI)-type drugs over tricyclics because of the latter's side effects, but this as well and their effectiveness has yet to be supported in a satisfactory clinical trial.

Apathy

Apathy is a frequent sequela of stroke and is associated with older age, cognitive impairment, and premorbid deficits in activities of daily living.[240] Although it frequently coexists with depression, apathy can also present without marked depressive features. It appears to be more common in patients with lesions in the posterior limb of the internal capsule. The presence of this condition significantly affects functional recovery in stroke patients. It is not known whether apathy responds to drug intervention. It may be possible to improve motivation in these patients by adopting an enthusiastic approach, setting achievable goals, and praising achievements regardless of their magnitude.

Psychosocial Aspects and Support

Stroke is a major life event which few, if any, are prepared for and presents major difficulties for patients, their spouses, and their families. It not only may result in physical dependency but also requires a wide range of emotional and social adjustments within families, often leading to role reversals and establishment of new hierarchies. The poststroke phase is a period of considerable turmoil during which patients and their families need to be supported in order to achieve good outcomes. The major areas of relevance are the following.

Bereavement The reaction to stroke is akin to bereavement.[241] Initially, there is a phase of shock during which patients and caregivers have so much to cope with that they may not assimilate much of what is told to them about the illness. This is followed by a phase of realization of the enormity of the event and is usually associated with despondency. Then a period of positive thinking and optimism sets in as patients focus on the activities of the rehabilitation team, and many harbor unrealistic hopes of sudden recovery. It is important for the clinician to introduce the notion of gradual and perhaps incomplete recovery at this phase to prevent unrealistic expectations of outcome. This reduces the chances of ultimate disappointment, and it may pave the way to more successful adaptation to the reality of residual disability. As the recovery curve begins to reach a plateau, there may be a second phase of depression which may be aggravated when the patient leaves the hospital or is discharged from outpatient care. Stroke patients understandably feel rejected: they had expected to be cured yet remain disabled. They need counseling as well as practical support because they feel uncertain or gloomy about the future.[242]

Fear: Another significant psychological problem faced by stroke patients is fear. They may be frightened of disfigurement, loss of physical function, falls, insanity, leaving the hospital, poverty, and even death.[243,244] They worry about sexual impairment and wonder whether it will be safe to try to resume sexual activity. Fear of further stroke can be eased to some extent by explaining that 90 percent of survivors do not have a stroke in any given year, that drugs such as aspirin reduce the chances of further occlusive vascular disease, and that strokes are not caused by stress or exertion.

Personality changes Alterations in personality may commonly occur after stroke and are a source of great distress to spouses and caregivers of stroke patients. One of the saddest comments made by spouses of stroke patients is "He (or she) is not the person I married." The changes noted are irritability, aggression, and anxiety[241]; the patient may be described as "difficult." Some disabled stroke victims are models of good behavior in the hospital but become demanding tyrants after they go home.[245] They may revert to childish behavior, eat messily, and be reluctant to cooperate.

Loss of self-esteem People who were very active and independent feel distressed when they must rely on others to wash and shave them, cut their food, dress and bathe them, or wipe their bottom. The loss of esteem may lead to apathy and even depression if not addressed early during a patient's treatment. This is more likely to happen in the paternalistic environment of hospitals, and the attitude and approach of the medical team are crucial in enabling the patient to maintain dignity. Esteem plummets when patients are not given much attention on hospital rounds or are depersonalized by staff who refer to them as "CVAs" or "hemis" rather than considering them unique individuals.

Guilt: Even in secular societies, stroke may be seen as punishment for real or imaginary sins of omission or commission. The doctor must explain to the patient and family that no one is responsible for this illness; it was not caused by stress or overwork or nagging or anything else done by the victim or his or her relatives.[246] The knowledge that a stroke is a reflection of the state of one's cardiovascular system and not of one's soul can be reassuring.

Care at Home

Most stroke patients return home. Of these, a quarter are dependent on someone for feeding, dressing, and toileting.[247] In one survey, 65 percent of those relying on caregivers needed help with bathing, 54 percent with dressing, 38 percent with toileting, and 21 percent with feeding; 18 percent required attention every night.[248] Most stroke patients are cared for by their families with little outside support.[249] These informal caregivers who often shoulder a heavy burden,[250] are mostly women and are often elderly themselves.

Caregivers, especially elderly people, may have their own health problems and suffer further physical ill health because of lifting (backache, hernias, injury) or accidents. Depression is common (50 percent of caregivers are depressed at 3 years) and is frequently unrecognized.[251] Depression is also common in caregivers of minimally disabled patients. In addition, they may have made significant changes in their lifestyle,[252] such as giving up work (resulting in loss of income and self-esteem) or social pursuits. Being tied to the home is one of the most burdensome aspects of caregiving. There may be marital stress, especially if the patient is dysphasic, demanding, depressed, or irritable.[253]

It is not uncommon for caregivers to feel exhausted, isolated, and depressed from time to time and to require support in their own right. Despite the heavy burden of care, most relatives who provide support have little respite: only one-third leave the patient unattended for all or part of the day. Those who provide the most care (because the patient is more severely disabled) are less likely to have frequent contact with neighbors. There is an increasing awareness that stroke families need continuing care and support which may be required for many years. Support for stroke victims and their families is high on the agenda of many health and social service organizations. A large number of services supporting stroke patients and their caregivers are also being developed within the voluntary sector.

There continues to be a medical role in the long-term management of stroke. This input should consist of monitoring of secondary preventive measures (e.g., lifestyle changes, cessation of smoking, and control of hypertension, hyperlipidemia, or diabetes); monitoring of disease progression (especially in patients with known moderate internal carotid artery stenosis); assessment of changes in disability or handicap and their potential for reversibility using therapy or environmental interventions; and identification of psychological and social support needs of patients and caregivers that may require referral to appropriate social or community care agencies. Long-term medical management goals can be achieved by regular review of stroke patients by their general practitioners, backed up with review by a specialist once or twice a year. Many disabled stroke patients survive for many years, and it is important that we ensure that their quality of life is as good as possible.[254]

Cerebral Multi-infarct States

There is considerable heterogeneity of multi-infarct states associated with cerebrovascular disease. In general, cortical multi-infarct disease is characterized by clear-cut repeated atherothrombotic or cardioembolic strokes, obvious sensorimotor deficits, more severe aphasic disturbances, and abrupt onset of cognitive failure.[255] Subcortical multi-infarct states, on the other hand, are associated with pseudobulbar signs, isolated pyramidal deficits and depression or emotional lability, mildly impaired memory, disorientation, apathy, lack of concentration, preseveration, and other behavioral problems attributable to frontal lobe dysfunction.[256] Cerebral multi-infarct states are classified into five major clinicoanatomic subtypes, although there is debate about classification and overlap between different subgroups.

Cortical multi-infarct disease Cortical multi-infarct disease appears to be a result of multiple thromboembolic infarcts too small individually to produce a major clinical incident but synergistically causing impairment of cortical function. It is more common in the elderly, and the diagnosis is straightforward when a patient has repeated thromboembolic episodes (TIAs or physically nondisabling strokes) and brain imaging shows more than one cortical infarct. Depending on the location of infarcts, the clinical picture shows a combination of deficits in higher function (e.g., dysphasia, apraxia, neglect) with a significant memory disorder.[255] Not infrequently, apraxic gait disturbance becomes clinically significant before the onset of cognitive impairment.[257]

Distal field infarction Distal field infarction usually involves the anterior circulation and is thought to be due to disturbances of the frontal border zone perfusion secondary to internal carotid artery disease. The areas affected are distant from the centroslyvian structures with widespread or multifocal infarction (often bilateral) which includes the association areas of the anterior and posterior cerebrum.[258] A frontal syndrome predominates and is associated with aphasia, dyspraxia, or neglect rather then hemiparesis or hemianesthesia. Because the syndrome is related to a tight carotid artery stenosis, carotid endarterectomy theoretically may prove effective in slowing the progression of this form of dementia.

Lacunar multi-infarct disease Lacunar dementia is due to multiple deep infarcts and exhibits the classic features of subcortical multi-infarct disease—gait, continence, and emotional problems—which may be early markers for this syndrome.[259] Frontal lobe features often predominate and overshadow cognitive decline, which is usually subtle or mild. In some patients, however, infarcts in the thalamus, caudate nucleus, or genu may have a disproportionate effect on cognitive function. These cases may be wrongly diagnosed as cortical multi-infarct disease.

Binswanger's disease Binswanger's disease shares several of the features of, and is often clinically indistinguishable from, lacunar multi-infarct states. These features include pseudobulbar speech and abulic delay, prominent mood and behavior changes, bilateral pyramidal signs, and a mild memory disorder.[260] The clinical course features slow but relentless mental deterioration punctuated by transient focal symptoms. The most prominent pathologic finding is severe white matter atrophy with sparing of the cortex. Imaging shows a high frequency of white matter lesions, although these may be seen in elderly patients not suffering from Binswanger's disease. The diagnosis is dependent on the demonstration of extensive deep white matter rarefaction with multiple deep infarcts on brain imaging in the clinical setting of dementia with frontal lobe and focal signs and evidence of cerebrovascular disease or risk factors.[261]

Amyloid angiopathy Two presentations of this rare condition are recognized: multiple lobar hemorrhages in an elderly nonhypertensive patient with preceding or supervening dementia, and diffuse white matter or focal cortical ischemic lesions with or without concomitant Alzheimer's disease.[259] A third, more recently described presentation is a syndrome of recurrent transient neurologic symptoms, responding to anticonvulsants and suggestive of seizures provoked by microhemorrhages.[262] In all types, there is deposition of amyloid β protein in the cortical arterioles, replacing normal smooth muscles.

Cerebral multi-infarct disease is often associated with significant cognitive impairment and is the second most common cause of dementia after Alzheimer's disease. The true incidence of dementia due to multi-infarct states is not known and, as stroke and Alzheimer's disease frequently coexist, it is often difficult to determine whether vascular disease is a cause of or is coincidental with the dementia.[258] Despite this limitation, it is estimated that dementia secondary to multi-infarct states occurs in about 25 percent of stroke patients and in about 3 percent of patients without a history of stroke.[258,263] The diagnosis of dementia due to cerebral multi-infarct states requires that a patient have (1) evidence of cerebrovascular disease (history, examination, brain imaging); (2) memory impairment with at least two other cognitive deficits that interfere with ADL and are not explained by stroke-related physical deficits (e.g., dysphasia, agnosia, apraxia); (3) evidence of causality that includes a temporal relationship between dementia and stroke, stepwise deterioration with a fluctuating course, or specific brain image findings in relevant areas.[264] Supportive evidence includes a history of cerebrovascular risk factors, early appearance of gait disturbances[257] or frequent falls, urinary incontinence not explained by urological disease, frontal lobe or extrapyramidal features, and pseudobulbar features with or without emotional liability. Cortical infarcts are seen in about 38 percent of patients with vascular dementia, subcortical in 46 percent, and combined lesions in the remaining 16 percent.[259] Multiple lesions predominate, although a small number of patients may have single lesions (strategic infarct dementia). These focal forms of dementia are due to damage to the temporal lobe and hippocampus (posterior type), basal ganglia or thalamus (basal type), or frontal lobes (frontal type).[259] The clinical features depend on the specific location but are associated with confusion and significant memory loss.

Management of Cerebral Multi-infarct States

Interest in cerebral multi-infarct states has increased in recent years, not only because of the realization that they are more common than previously supposed but also because they may be more amenable to prevention and treatment at present than other forms of dementia. Generally speaking, the risk factors for most cerebral multi-infarct states are the same as those for stroke and include hypertension, diabetes mellitus, advanced age, male gender smoking, and cardiac disease.[265] In addition to the established association between hypertension and stroke, hypertension is an independent risk factor for Binswanger's disease.[266] Other rarer causes include lipohyalinosis, cerebral amyloid angiopathy, disruption of the blood-brain barrier, and altered regulation of cerebral blood flow.[267] Extracerebral causes include ischemic hypoxic dementia, vasculitis, hyperviscosity, and hemostasis abnormalities.[267] This heterogeneity of causes of cerebral multi-infarct diesease should be taken into account in developing a management approach for this group of disorders.

The evolving clinical approach to multi-infarct disease consists of several options aimed at preventing further cerebrovascular damage and managing related symptoms.[268] These include lifestyle changes (e.g., cessation of smoking, starting an exercise program, dietary changes) and treatment of hypertension, elevated cholesterol, and atrial fibrillation. In the presence of early signs of cerebrovascular disease, such as TIAs or subtle cognitive deficits supported by changes on brain imaging, a more aggressive approach may be warranted. This may include aspirin, anticoagulants, or even carotid endarterectomy. Most of the current management of cerebral multi-infarct disease is empirical and based on extrapolation of stroke data to this group of disorders. The effectiveness of any of the possible interventions in either preventing or slowing the progression of this condition has yet to be supported by appropriately designed prospective clinical trials.

References

1. World Health Organisation Special Report Stroke: Recommendations on stroke prevention, diagnosis, and therapy. Stroke 1989;20:1407–1431

2. Adams RD, Victor M: Cerebrovascular diseases. pp. 777–874. In Adams RD, Victor M: Principles of Neurology, McGraw-Hill, New York, 1977
3. Bamford J, Sandercock P, Dennis M, Warlow C: A prospective study of acute cerebrovascular disease in the community: the Oxfordshire Community Stroke Project. II. incidence, case fatality rates and overall outcome at one year of cerebral infarction, primary intracerebral and subarachnoid haemorrhage. J Neurol Neurosurg Psychiatry 1990;53:16–22
4. Gresham GE, Phillips TF, Wolf PA et al: Epidemiological profile of long-term stroke disability: the Framingham study. Arch Phys Med Rehabil 1979;60:489–495
5. Aho K, Harmsen P, Hatano S et al: Cerebrovascular disease in the community: results of a WHO collaborative study. Bull WHO 1980;58:113–130
6. Stroke Unit Trialists Collaboration: A systemic overview of specialist multidisciplinary team (stroke rehabilitation unit) care for stroke inpatients. In Warlow C, Van Gijn J, Sandercock P (eds): Stroke Module of Cochrane Database of Systematic Reviews. BMJ Publishing, London, Disk issue 1, 1995
7. Posner JD, Gorman KM, Woldow A: Stroke in the elderly: 1. epidemiology. J Am Geriatr Soc 1984;32:95–102
8. Sheikh K, Bretinan PJ, Meade TW et al: Predictors of mortality and disability in stroke. J Epidemiol Community Health 1983; 357:70–74
9. Bamford J, Sandercock P, Warlow C, Gray M: Why are patients with acute stroke admitted to hospital? Br Med J 1986;1: 1369–1372
10. Kalra L: Does age affect benefits of stroke unit rehabilitation? Stroke 1994;25:346–351
11. National Institute of Neurological Disorders and Stroke: Classification of cerebrovascular diseases III. Stroke 1990;21: 637–676
12. Bogousslavsky J, Regii F: Cerebral infarction with transient signs (CITS): do TIAs correspond to small deep infarcts in internal carotid artery occlusion? Stroke 1984;15:536–539
13. Hankey GJ, Warlow CP: Symptomatic carotid ischaemic events: safest and most cost-effective way of selecting patients for angiography, before carotid endarterectomy. Br Med J 1990;300:1485–1491
14. Warlow CP, Davenport RJ: The management of transient ischaemic attacks. Prescriber's J 1996;36:1–8
15. Laureno R, Shields RW, Narayan T: The diagnosis and management of cerebral embolism and haemorrhagic infarction with sequential computerised cranial tomography. Brain 1987; 110:93–105
16. Hacke W, Kaste M, Fieschi C et al: Intravenous thrombolysis with recombinant tissue plasminogen activator for acute hemispheric stroke: the European Cooperative Acute Stroke Study (ECASS). JAMA 1995;274:1017–1025
17. Multicentre Acute Stroke Trial—Italy: Randomised controlled trial of streptokinase, aspirin and combination of both in treatment of acute ischaemic stroke. Lancet 1995; 346:1509–1514
18. Poirier J, Derouesne C: Cerebral lacune: a proposed new classification. Clin Neuropathol 1984;3:266
19. Tuszynski MH, Petito CK, Levy DE: Risk factors and clinical manifestations of pathologically verifiable lacunar infarctions. Stroke 1989;20:990–999
20. Wade DT: Epidemiologically Based Needs Assessment: Stroke. District Health Authorities: Research Programme, National Health Service Management Executive, London, 1992
21. Bamford J: Classic lacunar syndromes. pp. 366–372. In Bogousslavsky J, Caplan L (eds): Stroke Syndromes. Cambridge University Press, Cambridge, 1995
22. Angeloni U, Bozzao L, Fantozzi L et al: Internal border zone infarction following acute middle cerebral artery occlusion. Neurology 1990;40:1196–1198
23. Lodder J, Bamford JM, Sandercock PAG et al: Are hypertension or cardiac embolism likely causes of lacunar infarction? Stroke 1990;21:375–381
24. Bamford J: Is it a stroke and what sort of stroke is it? Hosp Update 1991;17:890–899
25. Bamford J, Sandercock P, Dennis M et al: Classification and natural history of clincally identifiable subtypes of cerebral infarction. Lancet 1991;337:1521–1526
26. Jorgensen HS, Nakayama H, Raaschou HO, Olsen TS: Intracerebral haemorrhage versus infarction: stroke severity, risk factors and prognosis. Ann Neurol 1995;38:45–50
27. Hankey GJ: Recent advances in cerebrovascular disease. Rev Clin Gerontol 1992;2:187–206
28. Kraaijeveld CL, van Gijn J, Schouten HJA, Staal A: Observer agreement for the diagnosis of transient ischaemic attacks. Stroke 1984;15:723–725
29. Sandercock PAG: Recent developments in the diagnosis and management of patients with transient ischaemic attacks and minor ischaemic stroke. Q J Med 1991;286:101–112
30. Whisnant JP: Classification of cerebrovascular diseases III. Stroke 1990;21:637–676
31. Weir CJ, Murray GD, Adams FG et al: Poor accuracy of stroke scoring systems for differential clinical diagnosis of intracranial haemorrhage and infarction. Lancet 1994;344:999–1002
32. Foulkes MA, Wolf RA, Price TR et al: The Stroke Data Bank: design, methods and baseline characteristics. Stroke 1988;19: 547–554
33. Skriver EB, Olsen TS: Transient disappearance of cerebral infarcts on CT scan, the so-called fogging effect. Neuroradiology 1981;22:61–65
34. Hankey GJ, Khangure MS, Stewart-Wynne EG: Detection of basilar artery thrombosis by computed tomography. Clin Radiol 1988;39:140–143
35. Ladurner G, Sager WD, Hoefier H et al: Computerised tomography (CT) correlated with anatomic pathology in stroke. pp. 75–80. In JS Meyer, H Lechner, Reivich M (eds): Cerebral Vascular Disease 2. Excerpta Medica, Amsterdam, 1979
36. Wardlaw JM: Is routine CT in strokes unnecessary? Br Med J 1994;309:1498–1500
37. Bryan RN, Levy LM, Whitlow WD et al: Diagnosis of acute cerebral infarction: comparison of CT and MR imaging. AJR Am J Roentgenol 1991;157:585–594

38. Ramadan NM, Deveshwar R, Levine SR: Magnetic resonance and clinical cerebrovascular disease: an update. Stroke 1989; 20:1279–1283

39. Moseley I: Acute disturbances of cerebral function: stroke and cerebrovascular disease. pp. 20–34. In Magnetic Resonance Imaging in Diseases of the Nervous System: an introduction. Blackwell, Oxford, 1988

40. Hommel M, Besson G, Le Bas JF et al: Prospective study of lacunar infarction using magnetic resonance imaging. Stroke 1990;21:546–554

41. Hughes RL, Yonas H, Gur D, Latchaw R. Cerebral blood flow determination within the first 8 hours of cerebral infarction using stable xenon-enhanced computed tomography. Stroke 1989;20:754–760

42. Hankey GJ, Warlow CP: The role of imaging in the management of cerebral and ocular ischaemia. Neuroradiology 1991; 33:381–390

43. Baird AE, Donnan GA, Austin MC et al: Reperfusion after thrombolytic therapy in ischaemic stroke measured by single-photon emission computed tomography. Stroke 1994;25: 79–85

44. Brooks DJ: PET: its clinical role in neurology. J Neurol Neurosurg Psychiatry 1991;54:1–5

45. Marchal G, Serrati C, Rioux P et al: PET imaging of cerebral perfusion and oxygen consumption in acute ischaemic stroke: relation to outcome. Lancet 1993;341:925–927

46. Weiller C, Chollet F, Friston KJ et al: Functional reorganisation of brain in recovery from striatocapsular infarction in man. Ann Neurol 1992;31:463–472

47. Carroll BA: Carotid sonography. Radiology 1991;178: 303–313

48. Humphrey P, Sandercock P, Siattery J: A simple method to improve the accuracy of non- invasive ultrasound in selecting TIA patients for cerebral angiography. J Neurol Neurosurg Psychiatry 1990;53:966–971

49. Martin PJ, Naylor AR: Transcranial sonography and its clinical applications. Hosp Update 1994;20:479–488

50. Petty GW, Wiebers DO, Meissner I: Transcranial Doppler ultrasonography: clinical applications in cerebrovascular disease. Mayo Clin Proc 1990;65:1350–1364

51. Hankey GJ, Warlow CP, Sellar RJ: Cerebral angiographic risk in mild cerebrovascular disease. Stroke 1990;21:209–222

52. Hankey GJ, Warlow CP, Molyneux AJ: Complications of cerebral angiography for patients with mild carotid territory ischaemia being considered for carotid endarterectomy. J Neurol Neurosurg Psychiatry 1990;53:542–548

53. Caplan LR, Wolpert SM: Angiography in patients with occlusive cerebrovascular disease: views of a stroke neurologist and neuroradiologist. Am J Neurolog Radiol 1991;12:593–601

54. Come PC, Riley MF, Bivas NK: Roles of echocardiography and arrhythmia monitoring in the evaluation of patients with suspected systemic embolism. Ann Neurol 1983;113: 527–531

55. Popp RL: Echocardiograpy. N Engl J Med 1990;323: 101–109, 165–172

56. Pop G, Sutherland GR, Koudstaal PJ et al: Transesophageal echocardiography in the detection of intracardiac embolic sources in patients with transient ischaemic attacks. Stroke 1990;21:560–565

57. Love BB, Struck LK, Stanford W et al: Comparison of two-dimensional echocardiography and ultrafast cardiac computed tomography for evaluating intracardiac thrombi in cerebral ischaemia. Stroke 1990;21:1033–1038

58. Seward JB, Khandheria BK, Tajik AJ: Wide-field transoesophageal echocardiographic tomography: feasibility study. Mayo Clin Proc 1990;65:31–37

59. Wade DT: Evaluating outcome in stroke rehabilitation. Scand J Rehabil Med 1992;(suppl 26):97–104

60. Wandless I: Hospital referral in acute stroke. Public Health 1983;97:197–203

61. Marquardsen J: The Natural History of Acute Cerebrovascular Disease: A Retrospective Study of 769 Patients. Munksgaard, Copenhagen, 1969

62. Wade DT, Langton Hewer R: Hospital admission for acute stroke: who, for how long and to what effect? J Epidemiol Community Health 1985;39:347–352

63. Wade DT, Langton Hewer R, Skilbeck CE et al: Controlled trial of home care service for acute stroke patients. Lancet 1985;1:323–326

64. Kalra L, Yu G, Wilson K, Roots P: Medical complications during stroke rehabilitation. Stroke 1995;26:990–994

65. Harper G: Treatment of stroke in older patients: a state of the art review. Drugs Aging 1995;6:29–44

66. Wade DT, Rivermead Speciality Team: Services for people with stroke. Qual Health Care 1993;2:263–266

67. Bath P, Butterworth RJ, Soo J, Kerr J: The King's College Hospital Acute Stroke Unit. J Roy Coll Physicians 1996;30: 13–17

68. Wallace JD, Levy LL: Blood pressure after stroke. JAMA 1981;246:2177–2180

69. Britton M, Carlsson A, de Faire U: Blood pressure course in patients with acute stroke and matched controls. Stroke 1986; 17:861–864

70. Dandapani BK, Suzuki S, Kelley RE et al: Relation between blood pressure and outcome in intracerebral haemorrhage. Stroke 1995;26:21–24

71. Lees KR, Dykes AG: Diagnosis and therapeutic aspects of stroke. Netherlands J Med 1995;47:195–198

72. Strandgaard S: Autoregulation of cerebral blood flow in hypertensive patients. Circulation 1976;53:720–727

73. Brainin M: Antihypertensive therapy in stroke: acute therapy, primary and secondary prevention. Acta Med Austriaca 1995; 22:54–57

74. Lisk DR, Grotta JC, Lamki LM et al: Should hypertension be treated after acute stroke? a randomised controlled trial using SPECT. Arch Neurology 1993;50:855–862

75. Harper G, Castleden CM, Potter JF: Factors affecting changes in blood pressure after acute stroke. Stroke 1994;25: 1726–1729

76. Powers WJ: Acute hypertension after stroke. Neurology 1993; 43:461–467

77. Jorgensen HS, Nakayama H, Raaschou HO, Olsen TS: Effect

of blood pressure and diabetes on stroke progression. Lancet 1994;344:156–159

78. Matchar DB, Divine GW, Heyman A, Feussner JR: The influence of hyperglycemia on outcome of cerebral infarction. Ann Intern Med 1992;117:449–456
79. Ek AC, Larsson J, von Schenck et al: The correlation between anergy, malnutrition and clinical outcome in an elderly population. Clin Nutr 1990;9:185–189
80. Axelsson K, Apslund K, Norberg A, Eriksson S: Eating problems and nutritional status during hospital stay of patients with severe stroke. J Am Diet Assoc 1989;89:1092–1096
81. Smithard DG, O'Neill MD, Park C et al: Complications and outcome following acute stroke: does dysphagia matter? Stroke 1996;27:1200–1204
82. Wanklyn P, Cox N, Belfield P: Outcome in patients who require a gastrostomy after stroke. Age Ageing 1995;24: 510–514
83. Norton B, Homer-Ward M, Donnelly MT et al: A randomised prospective comparison of percutaneous endoscopic gastrostomy and nasogastric tube feeding after acute dysphagic stroke. Br Med J 1996;312:13–16
84. Astrup J, Symon L, Siejbo BK: Thresholds in cerebral ischaemia—the ischaemic penumbra. Stroke 1981;12:723–725
85. Randall JB, Hoff JT: In Weinstein PR, Faden AI (eds) Protection of the brain from ischaemia. Williams and Wilkins, Baltimore, 1990
86. Harper GD, Castleden CM: Drug therapy in patients with recent stroke. Br Med Bull 1990;46:181–201
87. Kakuda W, Naritomi H, Shimizu T et al: Cerebral blood flow and metabolic outcome in stroke patients undergoing hypothermia therapy in the acute phase. Cerebrovasc Dis 1996; 6(suppl 2):4
88. Mulley GP, Wllcox RG, Mitchell JRA: Dexamethasone in acute stroke. Br Med J 1978;2:994–996
89. Steiner TJ, Rose FC: Trials in acute stroke. Lancet 1987;1: 1032
90. Schabitz WR, Dorfler A, Forsting M et al: Decompressive craniotomy in experimental "malignant" hemispheric stroke. Support for an aggresive therapeutic approach. Cerebrovasc Dis 1996;6(suppl 2):24
91. Goldstein LB, Davis JN: Restorative neurology: drugs and recovery following stroke. Stroke 1990;21:1636–1639
92. Hall ED, Pazara KE, Braugler JM: The 21-aminosteroid lipid peroxidation inhibitor protects against cerebral ischaemia in gerbils. Stroke 1988;19:997–1002
93. Antiplatelet Trialists Collaboration Group: Collaborative overview of randomised trials of antiplatelet therapy. I. prevention of death, myocardial infarction and stroke by prolonged antiplatelet therapy in various categories of patients. Br Med J 1994;308:81–106
94. Levine SR, Brott TG: Thrombolytic therapy in cerebrovascular disorders. Prog Cardiovas Dis 1992;34:235–262
95. Harper GD, Haigh RA, Potter JF, Castleden CM: Factors delaying admission to hospital after stroke in Leicestershire. Stroke 1992;23:835–838
96. Panayiotou BN, Fotherby MD, Potter JF et al: Eligibility of acute stroke patients for pharmacological therapy. Age Ageing 1994;23:384–387
97. Scatton B, Carter C, Benavides J, Giroux C: *N*-Methyl-D-aspartate receptor antagonists: a novel therapeutic perspective for the treatment of ischaemic brain injury. Cerebrovasc Dis 1991; 1:121–135
98. Heros RC: Stroke: early pathophysiology and treatment—summary of the Fifth Annual Decade of the Brain Symposium. Stroke 1994;25:1877–1881
99. World Health Organisation: Cerebrovascular diseases: prevention, treatment and rehabilitation. World Health Organisation Technical Report Series, 469. World Health Organisation, Geneva, 1971
100. MacMahon S, Peto R, Cutler J et al: Blood pressure, stroke and coronary heart disease. I. prolonged differences in blood pressure: prospective observational studies corrected for regression dilution bias. Lancet 1990;335:765–774
101. Collins R, Peto R, MacMahon S et al: Blood pressure, stroke and coronary heart disease. 2. short-term reductions in blood pressure: overview of randomised drug trials in their epidemiological context. Lancet 1990;335:827–838
102. Antiplatelet Trialists Collaboration Group: Secondary prevention of vascular disease by prolonged antiplatelet treatment. Br Med J 1988;296:320–331
103. European Atrial Fibrillation Trial Study Group: Secondary prevention in non-rheumatic atrial fibrillation after transient ischaemic attack or minor stroke. Lancet 1993;342: 1255–1262
104. Stroke Prevention in Atrial Fibrillation Study Group: Preliminary report of the Stroke Prevention in Atrial Fibrillation Study. N Engl J Med 1990;322:863–868
105. Stroke Prevention in Atrial Fibrillation Study Group: the Stroke Prevention in Atrial Fibrillation Study: final results. Circulation 1991;84:527–539
106. Petersen P, Boysen G, Godtfredsen J et al: Placebo-controlled, randomised trial of warfarin and aspirin for prevention of thromboembolic complications in chronic atrial fibrillation: the Copenhagen AFASAK study. Lancet 1989;i:175–179
107. Albers GW, Sherman DG, Gress DR et al: Stroke prevention in non-valvular atrial fibrillation: a review of prospective randomised trials. Ann Neurol 1991;30:511–518
108. Lip GY, Lowe GD: ABC of atrial fibrillation: antithrombotic treatment for atrial fibrillation. Br Med J 1996;312:45–49
109. Rose G: Strategy for prevention: lessons from cardiovascular disease. Br Med J 1981;282:1847–1850
110. Ebrahim S: Clinical Epidemiology of Stroke. Oxford University Press, Oxford, 1990
111. OXCHECK Study Group of the Imperial Cancer Research Fund: Prevalence of risk factors for heart disease in OXCHECK trial: implications for screening in primary care. Br Med J 1991;302:1057–1060
112. Shinton R, Beevers G: Meta-analysis of relation between cigarette smoking and stroke. Br Med J 1989;298:789–794
113. Shaper AG, Phillips AN, Pocock SJ et al: Risk factors for stroke in middle aged British men. B M J 1991;302: 1111–1115

114. Scandinavian Simvastatin Survival Study Group: Randomised trial of cholesterol lowering in 4444 patients with coronary heart disease. Lancet 1994;344:1383–1389

115. Shinton R, Sagar G: Lifelong exercise and stroke. Br Med J 1993;307:231–234

116. Hendriks HFJ, Veenstra J, Velthius-te Wierik et al: Effect of moderate dose of alcohol with evening meal on fibrinolytic factors. Br Med J 1994;308:1003–1006

117. OXCHECK Study Group of the Imperial Cancer Research Fund: Effectiveness of health checks conducted by nurses in primary care: results of the OXCHECK study after one year. Br Med J 1994;308:308–312

118. European Carotid Surgery Trialists Collaborative Group: MRC European Carotid Surgery Trial: interim results for symptomatic patients with severe (70–99%) or with mild (0–29%) carotid stenosis. Lancet 1991;337:1235–1243

119. North American Symptomatic Carotid Endarterectomy Trial (NASCET): Beneficial effect of carotid endarterectomy in symptomatic patients with high-grade carotid stenosis. N Eng J Med 1991;325:445–453

120. Brown MM, Humphrey PRD: Carotid endarterectomy: recommendations for management of transient ischaemic attack and ischaemic stroke. Br Med J 1992;305:1071–1074

121. Johnson BF, Verlato F, Bergelin RO et al: Clinical outcome in patients with mild and moderate carotid artery stenosis. J Vasc Surg 1995;21:120–126

122. Moore WS, Barnett HJ, Beebe HG et al: Guidelines for carotid endarterectomy: a multidisciplinary consensus statement from the ad hoc committee, American Heart Association. Stroke 1995;26:188–201

123. Higashida RT, Halbach VV, Tsai FY et al: Interventional neurovascular techniques for cerebral revascularisation in the treatment of stroke. AJR Am J Roentgenol 1994;163:793–800

124. Rothrock JF, Hart RG: Antithrombotic therapy in cerebrovascular disease. Ann Intern Med 1991;115:885–895

125. Sandercock P, Willems H: Medical treatment of acute ischaemic stroke. Lancet 1992;339:537–539

126. Henley S, Pettit S, Todd-Polwopek A, Tupper A: Who goes home? Predictive factors in stroke recovery. J Neurol Neurosurg Psychiatry 1985;48:1–6

127. Wade DT, Langton Hewer R: Functional abilities after stroke: measurement, natural history and prognosis. J Neurol Neurosurg Psychiatry 1987;50:177–182

128. Skilbeck CE, Wade DT, Hewer RL, Wood VA. Recovery after stroke. J Neurol Neurosurg Psychiatry 1983;46:5–8

129. Gray CS, French JM, Bates D et al: Recovery of visual fields in acute stroke: homonymous hemianopia associated with adverse prognosis. Age Ageing 1989;18:419–421

130. Gladman JR, Harwood DM, Barer DH: Predicting the outcome of acute stroke: prospective evaluation of five multivariate models and comparison with simple methods. J Neurolo Neurosurg Psychiatry 1992;55:347–351

131. Gordon C, Hewer RL, Wade DT: Dysphagia in acute stroke. Br Med J 1987;295:411–414

132. Wade DT, Hewer RL: Motor loss and swallowing difficulty after stroke: frequency, recovery and prognosis. Acta Neurol Scand 1987;76:50–54

133. Undrum W, Lincoln NB: Spontaneous recovery of language in patients with aphasia between 4 and 34 weeks after stroke. J Neurol Neurosurg Psychiatry 1985;48:743–748

134. Oder W, Binder H, Baumgartner CH: Is aphasia an additional prognostic factor in ischemic stroke with regard to the severity of hemiparesis in the subacute phase? Acta Ncurol Scand 1988;78:85–89

135. Partridge CJ, Johnston M, Edwards S: Recovery from physical disability after stroke: normal patterns as a basis for evaluation. Lancet 1987;1:373–375

136. Bard G, Hirschberg GG: Recovery of voluntary motion in upper extremity following hemiplegia. Arch Phys Med Rehabil 1965; 46:567–572

137. Christie D: Aftermath of stroke: an epidemiological study in Melbourne, Australia. J Epidemiol Community Health 1982; 36:123–126

138. Edmans JA, Lincoln NB. The relationship between perceptual deficits after stroke and independence in ADL. Br J Occup Ther 1990;53:139–142

139. Kalra L, Smith D, Crome P: Stroke in patients aged over 75 years: outcome and predictors. Postgrad Med J 1993;69: 33–36

140. Kalra L: The influence of stroke unit rehabilitation on functional recovery from stroke. Stroke 1994;25:821–825

141. Andrews K, Brocklehurst JC, Richards B, Laycock PJ: The rate of recovery from stroke and its measurement. Int Rehabil Med 1981;3:155–161

142. Kotila M, Waltimo O, Niemi ML et al: The profile of recovery from stroke and factors influencing outcome. Stroke 1984;15: 1039–1044

143. Langton-Hewer R: Rehabilitation after stroke. Q J Med 1990; 279:659–674

144. Wade DT: Is stroke rehabilitation worthwhile? Curr Opin Neurol Neurosurg 1993;6:78–82

145. Wade DT: Stroke: rehabilitation and long-term care. Lancet 1992;339:791–793

146. World Health Organisation: The international Classification of Impairments, Disabilities and Handicaps. World Health Organisation, Geneva, 1980

147. Duckworth D: The need for a standard terminology and classification of disablement. pp. 1–113. In Granger CV, Gresham GE (eds): Functional Assessment in Rehabilitation Medicine. Williams & Wilkins, Baltimore, 1984

148. Granger CV: A conceptual model for functional assessment. pp. 14–25. In Granger CV, Gresham GE (eds): Functional Assessment in Rehabilitation Medicine. Williams & Wilkins, Baltimore, 1984

149. Grimby G, Finnstam J, Jette A: On the application of the WHO handicap classification in rehabilitation. Scand J Rehab Med 1988;20:93–98

150. Keith RA: Status of measurement in stroke rehabilitation outcomes. Stroke 1990;21(suppl III):30–31

151. Davis AM, Davis S, Moss N et al: First steps towards an interdisciplinary approach to rehabilitation. Clin Rehabil 1992;6: 237–244

152. Logigian MK, Samuels MA, Falconer J, Zagar R: Clinical exercise trial for stroke patients. Arch Phys Med Rehabil 1983; 64:364–367

153. Dickstein R, Hocherman S, Pillar T, Shaham R: Stroke rehabilitation: three exercise therapy approaches. Phys Ther 1986; 66:1233–1238

154. Lord JP, Hall K: Neuromuscular re-education versus traditional programmes for stroke rehabilitation. Arch Phys Med Rehabil 1986;67:88–91

155. Edmans JA, Lincoln NB: Treatment of visual perceptual deficits after stroke: single case studies on four patients with right hemiplegia. Br J Occup Ther 1991;54(4):139–144

156. David RM, Enderby P, Bainton D: Treatment of acquired aphasias: speech therapists and volunteers comapared. J Neurol Neurosurg Psychiatr 1982;45:957–961

157. Howard D, Patterson K, Franklin S, Orchard-Lisle MJ: Treatment of word retrieval deficits in aphasia: a comparison of two therapy methods. Brain 1985;108:817–829

158. Lincoln NB, Pikersgill MJ, Hankey AI, Hilton CR: An evaluation of operant training and speech therapy in the language rehabilitation of moderate aphasics. Behav Psychother 1982; 10:162–178

159. Lincoln NB, Pickersgill MJ: The effectiveness of programmed instruction with operant training in the language rrehabilitation of severely aphasic patients. Behav Psychother 1984;12: 237–248

160. Lincoln NB, McGuirk E, Mulley GP et al: Effectiveness of speech therapy for aphasic stroke patients: a randomised controlled trial. Lancet 1984;i:1197–1200

161. Towle D, Lincoln NB, Mayfield LM: Service provision and functional independence in depressed stroke patients and the effects of social work intervention on these. J Neurol Neurosurg Psychiatry 1989;52:519–522

162. Lincoln NB, Jones AC, Mulley JP: Psychological effects of speech therapy. J Psychosom Res 1985;29:467–474

163. Evans RL, Matlock AL, Bishop DS et al: Family intervention after stroke: does counselling or education help? Stroke 1988; 19:1243–1249

164. Brocklehurst JC, Andrews K, Richards B, Laycock PJ: How much physical therapy for patients with stroke? Br Med J 1978;i:1307–1310

165. Wade DT, Skilbeck CE, Langton-Hewer R, Wood VA. Therapy after stroke: amounts determinants and effects. Int Rehabil Med 1984;6:105–110

166. Tinson DJ: How do stroke patients spend their day: an observational study of the treatment regime offered to patients in hospital with movement disorders following stroke. Int Disabil Stud 1989;11:45–49

167. Smith DS, Goldenberg E, Ashburn A: Remedial therapy after stroke: a randomised controlled trial. Br Med J 1981;282: 517–520

168. Sunderland A, Tinson DJ, Bradley EL et al: Enhanced physical therapy improves recovery of arm function after stroke: a randomised controlled trial. J Neurol Neurosurg Psychiatry 1992; 55:530–535

169. Wade DT: Measurement in Neurological Rehabilitation. Oxford University Press, Oxford, 1992

170. Capildeo R, Clifford-Rose F: The assessment of neurological disability. pp. 106–116. In Greenhalgh RM, Clifford-Rose F (eds): Progress in Stroke Research 1. Pitman Press, Tunbridge Wells, 1979

171. Feinstein AR, Josephy BR, Wells CK: Scientific and clinical problems in indexes of functional disability. Ann Intern Med 1986;105:413–420

172. Abu-Zeid HAH, Won Choi N, Hsu PH, Maini KK: 1978 Prognostic factors in the survival of 1484 stroke cases observed for 30 to 48 months. 1. diagnostic types and descriptive variables. Arch Neurol 35:121–125

173. Kalra L, Eade J: The role of stroke rehabilitation units in managing severe disability after stroke. Stroke 1995;26: 2031–2034

174. Wade DT, Skilbeck CE, Langton Hewer R: Predicting Barthel ADL score at 6 months after an acute stroke. Arch Phys Med Rehabil 1983;64:24–28

175. Teasdale G, Jennett B: Assessment of coma and impaired conciousness: a practical scale. Lancet 1974;2:81–83

176. Allen CMC: Predicting recovery after acute stroke. Br J Hosp Med 1984;31:428–434

177. Allen CMC: Predicting the outcome of acute stroke: a prognostic score. J Neurol Neurosurg Psychiatry 1984;47:475–480

178. Shah S, Vanclay F, Cooper B: Stroke rehabilitation: Australian patient profile and functional outcome. J Clin Epidemiol 1991; 44:21–28

179. Asberg KH, Nydevik I: Early prognosis of stroke outcome by means of Katz Index of activities of daily living. Scand J Rehabil Med 199;23:187–191

180. Prescott RJ, Garraway WM, Akhtar AJ: Predicting functional outcome following acute stroke using a standard clinical examination. Stroke 1982;13:641–647

181. Stone SP, Patel P, Greenwood RJ: Selection of acute stroke patients for treatment of visual neglect. J Neurol Neurosurg Psychiatry 1993;56:463–466

182. Kalra L, Crome P: The role of prognostic scores in targeting stroke rehabilitation in elderly patients. J Am Geriatr Soc 1993;41:396–400

183. Kalra L, Dale P, Crome P: Evaluation of a clinical score for prognostic stratification of elderly stroke patients. Age Ageing 1994;23:492–499

184. Feigenson J, McDowell F, Meese P et al: Factors influencing outcome and length of stay in a stroke rehabilitation unit. I. analysis of 248 unscreened patients: medical and functional prognostic indicators. Stroke 1977;8:651–656

185. Young A: Assessment for rehabilitation after stroke. Ann Acad Med Singapore 1988;17:267–274

186. Newman M: The process of recovery after hemiplegia. Stroke 1972;3:702–710

187. Barer DH, Mitchell JRA: Predicting the outcome of acute stroke: do multivariate models help? Q J Med 1989;261: 27–39

188. Anderson TP: Studies up to 1980 on stroke rehabilitation outcomes. Stroke 1990;21:1143–1145

189. Granger CV, Hamilton BB, Fiedler RC: Discharge outcome after stroke rehabilitation. Stroke 1992;23:978–982

190. Seale C, Davies P: Outcome measurement in stroke rehabilitation research. Int Disabil Stud 1986;17:358–360

191. Law M, Letts L: A critical review of scales of activities of daily living. Am J Occup Ther 1989;43:522–528

192. Eakin P: Assessments of activities of daily living: a critical review. Br J Occup Ther 1989;52:11–15

193. Barer DH, Nouri F: Measurements of activities of daily living. Clin Rehabil 1990;3:179–187

194. Collin C, Wade DT, Davis S, Horne V: The Barthel ADL index: a reliability study. Int Disabil Stud 1988;10:61–63

195. Norstrom T, Thorslund M: The structure of IADL and ADL measures. Age Ageing 1991;20:23–28

196. Wolfe CDA, Taub NA, Woodrow EJ, Burney PGJ: Assessment of scales for disability and handicap for stroke patients. Stroke 1991;22:1242–1244

197. Askham J, Glucksman E, Owens O et al: A Review of Research on Falls Among Elderly People. Age Concern Institute of Gerontology, London, 1990

198. Robbins J, Levine RL, Master A et al: Swallowing after unilateral stroke of the cerebral cortex. Arch Phys Med Rehabil 1993;74:1295–1300

199. Hamdy S, Aziz Q, Rothwell JC et al: The cortical topography of swallowing motor function in man. Nature Medicine, 1996; 2:1217–1224

200. Kidd D, Lawson J, Nesbitt R, MacMahon J: The natural history and clinical consequences of aspiration following acute stroke. Q J Med 1995;88:409–413

201. Davies AE, Kidd D, Stone SP, MacMahon J: Pharyngeal sensation and gag reflex in healthy subjects. Lancet 1995;345: 487–488

202. Logemann J: Evaluation and Treatment of Swallowing Disorders. College Hill Press, San Diego, 1983

203. Jones B, Donner MW (eds): Normal and Abnormal Swallowing: Imaging in Diagnosis and Therapy. Springer-Verlag, New York, 1991

204. Dantas RO, Kern MK, Massey BT et al: Effect of swallowed bolus variables on oral and pharyngeal phases of swallowing. Am J Physiol. 1990;258:G675–G681

205. Gresham SL: Clinical assessment and management of swallowing difficulties after stroke. Med J Aust 1990;48:397–399

206. Logemann JA: Non invasive approaches to deglutitive aspiration. Dysphagia 1993;8:331–333

207. Logemann JA, Kahrilas P, Kobara M Vakil N: The benefit of head rotation on pharyngoesophageal dysphagia. Arch Phys Med Rehabil 1989;70:767–771

208. Valdez DT, Salapatek A, Niznik G et al: Swallowing and upper oesophageal sphincter contraction with transcranial magnetic-induced electrical stimulation. Am J Physiol 1993;264: 213–219

209. Broniatowski M: Dynamic control of the larynx and future prospects in the management of deglutitive aspiration. Dysphagia 1993;8:334–335

210. Oxbury J, Wyke MA: Disturbances of higher cerebral function. pp. 21.33–21.39. In Weatherall DJ, Leddingham JGG, Warrell DA (eds): Oxford Textbook of Medicine. 2nd Ed. 1989

211. Edmans JA, Lincoln NB: The frequency of perceptual deficits after stroke. Clini Rehab 1987;1:273–281

212. Andrews K, Brocklehurst JC, Richards H, Laycock PJ: The prognostic value of picture drawings by stroke patients. Rheum Rehabil 1980;19:180–188

213. Robertson IH, Tegner R, Tham K et al: Sustained attention training for neglect: theoretical and rehabilitation implications. J Clin Exp Neuropsychol 1995;17:416–430

214. Antonucci G, Gauriglia C, Judica A et al: Effectiveness of neglect rehabilitation in a randomised group study. J Clin Exp Neuropsychol 1995;17:383–389

215. Prada G, Tallis RC: Treatment of the neglect syndrome in stroke patients using a contingency electric stimulator. Clin Rehabil 1995;9:77–86

216. Wade ST, Wood VA, Hewer RL: Recovery of cognitive function soon after stroke: a study of visual neglect, attention span and verbal recall. J Neurol Neurosurg Psychiatry 1988;51:10–13

217. Bobath B: Adult Hemiplegia: Evaluation and Treatment. Heinemann, London, 1978

218. Koyama H, Murakami K, Suzuki T, Suzaki K. Phenol block for hip flexor muscle spasticity under ultrasonic monitoring. Arch Phys Med Rehabil 1992;73:1040–1043

219. Hesse S, Lucke D, Malezic M et al: Botulinum toxin treatment for lower limb extensor spasticity in chronic hemiparetic patients. J Neurol Neurosurg Psychiatry 1994;57:1321–1324

220. Smith RG, Cruikshank JG, Dunbar S, Akhtar AJ: Malalignment of the shoulder after stroke. Br Med J 1982;284: 1224–1226

221. Fitzgerald-Finch OP, Gibson IIJM: Subluxation of the shoulder in hemiplegia. Age Ageing 1975;4:16–18

222. Van Langenberghe HVK, Hogan BM: Degree of pain and grade of subluxation in the painful hemiplegic shoulder. Scand J Rehabil Med 1988;20:161–166

223. Roy CW: Shoulder pain in hemiplegia: a literature review. Clin Rehabil 1988;2:35–44

224. Dacre J, Beeney N, Scoot D: Injections and physiotherapy for the painful stiff shoulder. Ann Rheum Dis 1989;48:322–325

225. Cope C, Reyes TM, Skversky NH: Phlebographic analysis of the incidence of thrombosis in hemiplegia. Radiology 1973; 109:581–584

226. Moon AH, Gragnani JA: Cold water immersion for the oedematous hand in stroke patients. Clin Rehabil 1989;3:97–101

227. Shinton RA, Gill JS, Melnick SC et al: The frequency, characteristics and prognosis of epileptic seizures at the onset of stroke. J Neurol Neurosurg Psychiatry 1988;51:273–276

228. So EL, Annegers JF, Hauser WA et al: Population-based study of seizure disorders after cerebral infarction. Neurology 1996; 46:350–355

229. Asconape JJ, Penry JK. Post stroke seizures in the elderly. Clin Geriatr Med 1991;7:483–492

230. Viitanen M, Eriksson S, Asplund K: Risk of recurrent stroke,

myocardial infarction and epilepsy during long-term follow up after stroke. Eur Neurol 1988;28:227–231

231. Sharpe M, Hawton K, House A et al: Mood disturbances in long-term survivors of stroke: associations with brain lesion location and volume. Psychol Med 1990;20:815–828
232. Robinson RG, Lipsey JR, Pearlson CD: The occurrence and treatment of post-stroke mood disorder. Compr Ther 1984;10: 19–24
233. Fedoroff JP, Starkstein SE, Parikh RM et al: Are depressive symptoms non-specific in patients with acute stroke? Am J Psychiatry 1991;148:1172–1176
234. Hermrmann M, Wallesch CW: Depressive changes in stroke patients. Disabil Rehabil 1993;15:55–66
235. Agrell B, Dehlin O: Depression in stroke patients with left and right hemisphere lesions: a study in geriatric rehabilitation in-patients. Aging Clin Exp Res 1994;6:49–56
236. Tiller JW: Post stroke depression. Psychopharmacology 1992; 106(suppl):S130–133
237. Angeleri F, Angeleri VA, Foschi N et al: The influence of depression, social activity and family stress on functional outcome after stroke. Stroke 1993;24:1478–1483
238. Anderson G, Vestergaard K, Lauritzen L: Effective treatment of post-stroke depression with the selective serotonin reuptake inhibitor citalopram. Stroke 1994;25:1099–1104
239. Morris PL, Raphael B, Robinson RG: Clinical depression is associated with impaired recovery from stroke. Med J of Aust 1992;157:239–242
240. Starkstein SE, Fedoroff JP, Price TR: Apathy following cerebrovascular lesions. Stroke 1993;24:1625–1630
241. Jarman CMB: Psychiatric aspects of strokes. Br J Clin Pract 1978;(suppl 2):32–35
242. Lawrence L, Christie D: Quality of life after stroke: a three year follow up. Age Ageing 1979;8:167–172
243. Charatan FB, Fisk A: Mental and emotional results of strokes. NY State J Med 1978;78:1403–1405
244. Goodstein RK: Overview: CVA and the hospitalized elderly—a multidimensional clinical problem. Am J Psychiatry 1983;140:141–147
245. Issacs B, Neville Y, Rushford I: The stricken: the social consequences of stroke. Age Ageing 1976;5:188–192
246. Mykyta LJ, Bowling JH, Nelson DA, Lloyd EJ: Caring for relatives of stroke patients. Age Ageing 1976;5:87–90
247. Brocklehurst JC, Morris P, Andrews K et al: Social effects of stroke. Soc Sci Med 1981;15:35–39
248. Ebrahim S, Nouri F: Caring for stroke patients at home. Int Rehabil Med 1987;8:171–173
249. Legh-Smith J, Wade DT, Hewer RL: Services for stroke patients one year after stroke. J Epidemiol Community Health 1986;40:161–165
250. Anderson R: The unremitting burden on carers. Br Med J 1987;294:73–74
251. Camworth TCM, Johnson DAW: Psychiatry morbidity among spouses of patients with stroke. Br Med J 1987;294:409–411
252. Holbrook M: Stroke: social and emotional outcome. J R Coll Physicians Lond 1982;16:100–104
253. Kinsella GJ, Duffy FD: Psychosocial readjustment in the spouses of aphasic patients. Scand J Rehabil Med 1979;11: 129–132
254. A Report of the Royal College of Physicians Stroke: Towards Better Management. Royal College of Physicians, London, 1989
255. Erkinjuntti T: Types of multi-infarct dementia. Acta Neurol Scand 1987;75:391–393
256. Stuss DT, Cummings JL: Subcortical vascular dementia. In Cummings JL (ed): Subcortical Dementia. Oxford University Press, Oxford, 1990
257. Wilkieson C, Stott DJ, Wardlaw JM, Caird FI: Cerebral multi-infarct states: Rev Clin Gerontol 1994;4:29–42
258. Tatemichi TK: How acute brain failure becomes chronic: a view of the mechanisms and syndromes of dementia related to stroke. Neurology 1990;40:1652–1659
259. Tatemichi TK: Dementia. In Bogousslavsky J, Caplan L (eds): Stroke Syndromes, Cambridge University Press, Cambridge, 1995
260. Caplan L, Schoene WC: Clinical features of subcortical arteriosclerotic encephalopathy (Binswanger's disease). Neurology 1978;28:1206–1215
261. Bennett DA, Wilson RS, Gilley DW, Fox JH: Clinical diagnosis of Binswanger's disease. J Neurol Neurosurg Psychiatry 1990;53:961–965
262. Greenberg SM, Vonsattel JPG, Stakes JW et al: The clinical spectrum of cerebral amyloid angiopathy: presentations without lobar haemorrhage. Neurology 1993;43:2073–2079
263. Suzuki K, Kutsuzawa T, Nakajima K, Hatano S: Epidemiology of vascular dementia and stroke in Akita, Japan. pp. 16–24. In Hartmann A, Kuchinski W, Hoyer S (eds): Cerebral Ischaemia and Dementia, Springer-Verlag, Berlin, 1991
264. Roman CG, Tatemichi TK, Erkinjuntti T et al: Vascular dementia: diagnostic criteria for research studies—report of the NINDS-AIREN International Workshop. Neurology 1993;43: 250–260
265. Skoog I: Risk factor for vascular dementia: a review. Dementia 1994;5:137–144
266. Johansson BB: Pathogenesis of vascular dementia: the possible role of hypertension. Dementia 1994;5:174–176
267. Parnetti L, Mari D, Mecocci P, Senin U: Pathogenetic mechanisms in vascular dementia. Int J Clin Lab Res 1994;24: 15–22
268. Anonymous: Vascular dementia: an updated approach to patient management: a roundtable discussion 3. Geriatrics 1994; 49:39–46

CHAPTER 36

Stroke: Organization of Services

MARTIN DENNIS

A few years ago no editor of a textbook on geriatric, general, or neurologic medicine would have considered including a chapter on the organization of stroke services. However, things have changed, and after years of being largely ignored by doctors and health services managers, as well as by editors, the organization of stroke care has become an important issue. The frequency of stroke and its impact on patients' survival and function have led governments in many countries to identify stroke as a key area for improving health care.[1] Several reports have suggested that stroke care is too often poorly organized and not tailored to the individual.[2] Perhaps this is not surprising since in many countries no specialist group has taken stroke on as, for example, cardiologists have taken on myocardial infarction.

Until recently there was little reliable evidence that it mattered how services for stroke patients were organized. Since the 1960s, several randomized controlled trials (RCTs) had individually provided little to justify setting up stroke units. In 1991 a small RCT evaluating a stroke unit in Trondheim demonstrated that patients managed in the unit had reduced mortality and a better functional outcome than patients managed in a general medical setting.[3] This stimulated Langhorne and colleagues[4] to perform a systematic review of all RCTs, comparing the outcome of stroke unit care with that in a general medical setting. Despite the methodologic problems associated with performing a meta-analysis of RCTs of relatively heterogeneous interventions and that measured different outcomes, this study provided fairly robust evidence that care in a stroke unit is associated with a significant reduction in mortality.[4] These data have focused attention on how stroke services should be organized, although it provides little direct evidence about the optimum type of general care and rehabilitation.

When considering the organization of stroke services, it is useful to list the components of care to ensure that each is adequately addressed to provide a comprehensive service so that particular groups of patients are not disadvantaged (see accompanying box). There has been little formal evaluation to establish the optimum method for delivering those components of stroke care not included within the functions of a stroke unit. However, one can make some commonsense recommendations based on what we know about patients' problems and needs and the clinical epidemiology of stroke. In this chapter I will address some of the choices offered at different stages in a patient's treatment and discuss the rationale, or the evidence if any exists, for competing models of stroke service. I will conclude by outlining some of the issues surrounding the monitoring and integration of stroke services.

Immediate Management

Patients who recognize the initial symptoms of a stroke should be advised to (1) contact their family doctor, or (2) call an ambulance or go straight to the nearest hospital.

The rationale for immediate self-referral to a hospital is that it reduces the delay in getting medical attention[5] and that if acute medical treatment for stroke is going to be successful it is likely to be most effective if initiated early. There is evidence supporting this. RCTs of thrombolytic therapy in acute ischemic stroke suggest that the benefits of treatment may be greater (and the risk of treatment, i.e., hemorrhagic transformation, less) if administered within the first 3 hours.[6] If these findings are confirmed, we will have to modify the preadmission care of stroke patients, perhaps including the kinds of arrangements currently made to ensure minimum delay between onset of myocardial infarction and thrombolysis therapy which have been used to facilitate the evaluation of early thrombolysis in acute stroke.[7] Currently, few medical centers use routine thrombolytic therapy, and therefore emergency admission of all patients is not easily justified and patients probably lose little by contacting their family doctor. Of course if acute medical treatments that can be safely administered in the community without prior imaging are identified, the need for hospitalization will be reduced. However, it seems likely that the initial evaluation of such treatments would be hospital-based.

Hospital Referral

Family doctors seeing patients with a stroke or transient ischemic attack (TIA) have two choices regarding referral to a hospital: (1) Managing patients themselves in the community or refering them to a hospital, and (2) referring patients for outpatient (ambulatory) or inpatient care.

The proportion of stroke patients admitted to hospitals varies widely from place to place.[8,9] This must reflect factors including the quality and confidence of family doctors; the population's perception of stroke and their expectations concerning acute treatment, general care, and rehabilitation; and the access to facilities in the community and in a hospital. Social factors, such as whether the patient lives alone, are often decisive.[8] There have been no completed RCTs to compare inpatient and outpatient management.

There is an increasing consensus that all, or at least almost all, patients with stroke and TIA should be referred to a hospi-

Aspects of Stroke Management

Initial diagnosis (how can the patient access the appropriate services?)

Full assessment to identify the type, cause, and consequences of the stroke (crucial to the planning of all other aspects of care)

Specific acute medical and/or surgical treatment (of relatively little importance at present because of the lack of evidence regarding the effectiveness of these interventions but this is likely to change)

General care in the acute period (although there may be little evidence supporting the use of specific acute treatments, a lot can be done to prevent and treat the complications and coexistent pathology in stroke patients)

Terminal care (an area bristling with ethical dilemmas)

Rehabilitation (often thought of as comprising simply physical therapies but should probably be thought of as a wider process which merges seamlessly with general care, i.e., rehabilitation should start immediately)

Long-term placement

Secondary prevention (an area where there are several interventions of proven effectiveness)

Management of long-term disability and handicap (some argue that stroke-specific services are most relevant in the first few months of a patient's stroke and that generic services for the disabled should become involved at this stage because of the complex interrelationship of disabilities due to different pathologies)

tal for a detailed assessment.[10,11] Referral is usually justified on the basis that a specialist with hospital-based facilities can offer a more accurate and thorough assessment than a family doctor. Although, the clinical diagnosis of stroke is usually reliable, the diagnosis of TIAs is prone to considerable interobserver variation.[12,13] However, a complete assessment includes a search for the underlying cause, which involves investigations to define the pathologic type of stroke and in some patients with ischemic stroke to identify cardiac and extracranial vascular disease, and so the clinician needs ready access to appropriate imaging facilities.

Timing of Referral

The history of an event and its neurologic signs are most easily interpreted as soon as possible after the event. Computerized tomagraphy (CT) scanning can reliably distinguish cerebral infarction from primary intracerebral hemorrhage only if it is performed within 2 weeks of onset.[14] This means that patients should see a specialist as soon as possible and has prompted the development of stroke or neurovascular clinics that provide early clinical assessment and fast track investigation for patients who do not require hospital admission. The situation in many institutions where only inpatients have access to early investigation reflects a lack of organization and is bound to increase the service costs by encouraging unnecessary admissions to hospitals. Family doctors sometimes delay admission to see how the patient progresses, but this strategy has some inherent dangers. It can put undue pressure on the family who may later, even after a period of inpatient rehabilitation, be reticent about further involvement in the patient's long-term care. Also, inexpert handling at home may lead to injury to the patient or the caregiver.

Accessing the Multidisciplinary Team

Even after the diagnosis of stroke has been confirmed, the likely cause identified, and treatable underlying causes excluded, patients often require further detailed assessment. Thus, in all but the mildest or most transient cases, the patient should have prompt access to a team comprising at least a nurse, physiotherapist, speech and language therapist, and occupational therapist. In most places this usually requires referral to a hospital.

Stroke Units

Initial Placement

Once the decision has been made to admit the patient to a hospital, the next choice is whether the patient should be admitted to (1) a general medical, geriatric, or neurologic unit, or (2) a specialized acute stroke unit, that is, a unit that accepts direct, unselected admissions with stroke from the community.

There are few data from RCTs that help inform this choice. Acute stroke units make some sense since they facilitate

- The introduction of guidelines and protocols to ensure consistently high standards of assessment and early treatment, perhaps including an assessment proforma[15,16]
- Research, especially to test the effectiveness of medical treatments for acute stroke
- Early involvement of specialists and members of a multidisciplinary team
- Monitoring of the performance of the unit since all cases are more easily identified at an early admission stage

Stroke Intensive Care Units

Some have suggested that acute stroke patients should initially be managed in high-tech stroke intensive care units where a range of physiologic parameters, for example, intracranial pressure, can be monitored and attempts made to optimize them.[17] However, little is known about the benefits, or indeed the risks, of manipulating these parameters. It seems unlikely that any improvement in outcome from such interventions would be dramatic, and thus we need to look for evidence of effectiveness from RCTs. Unfortunately little such evidence is available, and that from nonrandomized studies has not been particularly encouraging.[18–20] These factors, taken in combination with the likely increased cost of such units, means that we should not set up stroke intensive care units unless it is to evaluate them or unless some acute intervention is shown to be effective and requires such close monitoring of patients.

The Post Acute Period—Triage

Once the diagnosis has been made, investigations completed, and any early medical or surgical treatment given, patients can usually be divided into three groups depending on their condition. For each of these three groups of patients one must provide facilities that match their individual needs. Noted that about 10 percent of patients do not survive more than a few days.

Mild Strokes

Some patients, perhaps 20 to 30 percent, have minimal functional sequelae and are able to be discharged home within a few days. Their further treatment should primarily be directed at secondary prevention, although we should not underestimate their psychologic needs. After all they may perceive their stroke as a major threat to their survival and independence. These patients should probably remain in the acute admission area or stroke unit until an early discharge. The period of inpatient care can be usefully employed in educating and informing the patient and relatives about stroke, although this process may need to be carried through into the postdischarge period. Once a strategy for secondary prevention has been developed, it should probably most sensibly be monitored in primary care, where this is well organized but, alternatively, the neurovascular clinic could fulfill this role.

The Severest Strokes

Some patients have been so badly damaged by the stroke itself or have coexistent pathologies, for example, dementia, that they are unable to participate actively in rehabilitation. Such patients may die, may remain in a severely dependent state, or may require time to improve to a level where they might benefit from a rehabilitation environment. For instance, those who remain in a coma or medically unwell might remain in the acute area where they can receive good nursing care and appropriate medical treatment. Obviously issues such as prevention of pressure sores, aspiration, deep venous thrombosis, dehydration, and malnutrition are important during this period. Where patients are likely to survive with an acceptable quality of life, they require active medical management of such problems. Such individuals often raise difficult ethical dilemmas, which makes good communication between professionals and with relatives particularly important. This may be an important reason for managing such patients in a designated area.

Strokes of Intermediate Severity

Many patients fall into an intermediate group who have neurologic impairments and disabilities that make immediate discharge impossible. Such individuals need rehabilitation, and this can be provided in several different environments including (1) acute general medical, geriatric, or neurologic units, (2) specialized stroke rehabilitation units, and (3) generic rehabilitation units.

The systematic review of all RCTs of stroke units referred to in the introduction provides compelling evidence that patients, particularly those in the intermediate category, are better managed in a stroke rehabilitation unit. The care provided in a stroke unit compared with that offered in a general medical setting has been associated with a 20 percent reduction in the odds of death within the first year and a 34 percent reduction in the odds of death or long-term institutionalization.[21,22] Several characteristics may account for their effectiveness,[23] including

- Involvement of a multidisciplinary team whose members are interested in and have specialized in stroke care
- Regular (at least weekly) meetings of the multidisciplinary team to discuss progress and to plan treatment of patients
- In-service training for the staff
- Involvement and education of caregivers in the management of patients

Of course there are many different ways of delivering these services, and unfortunately there is little evidence supporting one particular model. There are, however, practical arguments for pursuing certain models of stroke unit care.

Combining or Separating Acute Care and Rehabilitation

Some of the more successful hospital units have combined both acute and rehabilitation functions.[3] The danger of this is that less acute patients compete unsuccessfully for nursing time, as occurs in an acute hospital setting where the needs of the acute patient (e.g., treatment of ischemic chest pain) may be perceived as more urgent and perhaps more important than those of the rehabilitating patient (e.g., regular toileting to maintain continence). Some splitting of the functions seems logical, but if this can be achieved in one unit, continuity of care and thus consistency of approach will be improved.

Stroke Units Versus Mobile Stroke Teams

Most of the evidence from RCTs supported the concept of a geographically defined unit rather than one based in several locations that relies on the input from a roving multidisciplinary team. One of the main advantages of a geographically defined unit is that it facilitates full participation of the nurses in the multidisciplinary team. After all, the aim is for patients to receive consistent help toward regaining independence around the clock and not just during therapy sessions. Only one of the RCTs included in the overview evaluated a roving stroke team.[24]

Maintaining Flexibility

One of the major disadvantages of a geographically defined unit is that unless one has extremely flexible staffing arrangements and use of beds, the number of patients who can be accommodated is limited. In most hospitals there are likely to be substantial fluctuations in the number of patients who might benefit from stroke unit care. Many of these fluctuations are due to random effects, although seasonal variation in stroke incidence and admission may play a part.[25] When the number of stroke admissions rises or the proportion of patients with severe stroke increases (so increasing mean length of stay), some patients cannot get into the unit. One partial solution is to operate a mobile stroke team which manages patients wherever they are as well as those in the stroke unit. An ideal solution is to have an expandable unit sized to match changing demands.

Generic Rehabilitation Centers

In many countries patients are moved from acute care facilities, which may be stroke-specific or not, to generic rehabilitation facilities. The latter are often in separate departments of or even at a different site than the acute facility. Such rehabilitation facilities may provide excellent multidisciplinary care but can lead to a loss of continuity of care. Also, if rehabilitation locations are scarce, patients may have to wait at an acute facility. Patients who are waiting for rehabilitation may become frustrated and may not receive the sort of care that will ensure their continued progress. There needs to be close integration of acute and rehabilitation facilities where these are geographically separated. It is still unclear whether generic rehabilitation services, which might include geriatric services, are as effective as stroke-specific ones.

Many other issues will need to be addressed in future RCTs, including questions regarding the optimum type of stroke unit and which features contribute most to its effectiveness.

Duration of Hospitalization

Once a patient has been admitted to a hospital, it must be decided how long they should remain there. The length of stay varies greatly from place to place and depends on how much emphasis is placed on rehabilitation and what community facilities are available to provide care. For instance, in many developing countries the length of stay may be short because rehabilitation facilities are limited, and the extended family can provide a home environment in which a disabled patient can receive at least basic care. In some countries prolonged hospital care may be an option only for those who can afford to pay. In many countries there are considerable pressures to reduce length of hospital stay to limit the spiraling costs of medical care. Stroke accounts for a significant proportion of available bed days because of its high frequency and prolonged length of stay.[26] There is evidence that stroke unit care is associated with reduced length of hospital stay.[21] Patients with disabling stroke require enough care to be able to live at home as well as to continue therapy to ensure that they reach their optimum outcome as regards function. "Early supported discharge" or "hospital at home" schemes that combine these two elements of care in the patient's own home are models that might reduce length of hospital stay. Several randomized trials are currently addressing the important question whether such care can provide better, or at least equivalent, outcomes at less cost than conventional care.

Outpatient Rehabilitation

Once patients have been discharged from an inpatient facility, whether the stay was prolonged or shortened by an early supported discharge scheme, some may benefit from further input from members of the team. Those responsible for organizing services may choose whether this input is provided (1) in the hospital, either in an outpatient or a day hospital environment, or (2) in the patient's own home.

In two randomized trials comparing the cost-effectiveness of hospital- and home-based continued therapy for stroke patients,[27–30] there were no convincing differences in patient outcome or in the cost of care.

Long-term Care

For patients with continuing disability one can choose to (1) provide enough continuing support in the community to allow them to return home, or (2) provide care in institutions (e.g., long-term hospital care or nursing home care).

Some patients may be so badly disabled by their stroke that a return to their previous accommodation is not possible given the resources in the community (family or social services). Of course, given unlimited resources it is possible to maintain anyone, whatever their functional status and care needs, at home. Those responsible for funding long-term care have to determine the balance between providing community and institutional care, a decision that should take account of patients' needs and wishes as well as the comparative costs.

After a stroke the timing of the decision to move a patient into long-term care is often difficult. Institutions may not provide the facilities or environment to ensure that the patient continues to improve or even maintain their level of independence. The patient may need to stay in the rehabilitation facility until everyone involved in their care, including the family and sometimes even the patient, is convinced that further rehabilitation is unlikely to make a long-term difference in their quality of life.

There is considerable uncertainty about the value of long-term maintenance therapy. One frequently sees patients who deteriorate after discharge from rehabilitation, perhaps because of an overly protective family and lack of practice, which can partly be avoided by properly instructing the caregiver. However, some patients seem to require long-term input, or at least intermittent input, from therapists to maintain their functional level. In such cases, this interaction may be essential to allow them to remain at home.

Monitoring Stroke Services

A system of monitoring stroke services might demonstrate good or poor performance and identify particular problems that need to be addressed. Any system may depend on monitoring various aspects of care: (1) structure, (2) process, and (3) outcome.

There are few recommendations we can make about the structure of a service that are based on reliable evidence, but these include the recommendation that patients be managed in stroke units rather than in a general medical setting. Monitoring the process of care is more promising since several specific interventions have been shown to improve the outcome after stroke, most in the area of secondary prevention.[31–34] Therefore it seems sensible to monitor the use and appropriateness of well-defined interventions such as antiplatelet drugs, anticoagulants, and carotid surgery. The value of monitoring other aspects of process, such as use of imaging, quality of assessment, and access to a multidisciplinary team, is less certain since their effectiveness has not been demonstrated in RCTs. Also, it may be difficult to measure these aspects of care reliably.[35] The patient's survival and physical, social, or psychological outcome are perhaps the most relevant indications of the quality and effectiveness of stroke services. However, the outcome of patients managed by a particular service depends not only on the quality and effectiveness of care but also on the "case mix," the method of measuring outcome, and luck. The case mix is probably the most important determinant of outcome, its effect swamping any differences attributable to the treatment provided.[36–39] Also, most stroke services do not manage sufficiently large numbers of patients to provide a precise enough estimate of, for example, the case fatality rate, to allow comparisons to be made between units or within the same unit in different periods. Of course if a service has consistently poor outcomes, possible causes should be sought. Any differences or changes in the patients' outcomes must be interpreted in the light of detailed information about the case mix and with the utmost caution.

Providing Integrated Stroke Services

In the preceding sections we have discussed some of the choices available to those planning stroke services. It is often not a matter of choosing one model or another but rather of finding a balance between them. For instance, how far does one strive to maintain disabled patients in their own home? In many areas there is little reliable evidence about how services are best organized. Thus choices often have to be based on local decisions taking into account existing resources, local geography, and funding arrangements. However, it seems clear that stroke services should be well organized and their structure based on some knowledge of patients' needs. Facilities need to ensure that all aspects of management can be provided, from acute care through long-term support for severely disabled survivors. Also, with rapid advances in our knowledge and treatment of patients with stroke, it is vital that services be flexible enough to incorporate changes dictated by developments. One example is the introduction of an acute drug treatment for stroke which might have dramatic a effect on the structure of stroke services. However, the precise structure of a stroke service is probably less important than having an individual or small group of people who are willing to take on the responsibility of organizing services for stroke patients. The latter should ensure that services are constructed to meet local needs and conditions.

References

1. Secretary of State for Health: The Health of the Nation. HMSO, London, 1992
2. King's Fund Consensus Conference: Treatment of stroke. Br Med J 1988;297:126–128
3. Indredavik B, Bakke F, Solberg R et al: Benefit of a stroke unit: a randomised controlled trial. Stroke 1991;22:1026–1031
4. Langhorne P, Williams BO, Gilchrist W, Howie K: Do stroke units save lives? Lancet 1993;342:395–398
5. Fogelholm R, Murros K, Rissanen A, Ilmavirta M: Factors delaying hospital admission after acute stroke. Stroke 1996;27:398–400
6. Wardlaw J, Yamaguchi T, del Zoppo G, Hacke W: Thrombolysis in acute ischaemic stroke. In Warlow C, Van Gijn J, Sandercock P (eds): Stroke Module of the Cochrane Database of Systematic Reviews. BMJ Publishing Group, London, 1996
7. Alberts MJ, Perry A, Dawson DV, Bertels C: Effects of public and professional education on reducing the delay in presentation and referral of stroke patients. Stroke 1992;23:352–356
8. Bamford J, Sandercock P, Warlow C, Gray M: Why are patients with acute stroke admitted to hospital? BMJ 1986;292:1369–1372
9. Asplund K, Bonita R, Kuulasmaa K et al: Multinational comparisons of stroke epidemiology: evaluation of case ascertainment in the WHO MONICA Stroke Study. Stroke 1995;25:355–360
10. Adams HP, Brott TG, Crowell RM et al: Guidelines for the management of patients with acute ischemic stroke: a statement for health care professionals from a special writing group of the Stroke Council, American Heart Association. Stroke 1994;25:1320–1335
11. Adams HP Jr: The importance of the Helsingburg declaration on stroke management in Europe. J Intern Med 1996;240:169–180
12. Koudstaal PJ, Van Gijn J, Staal A et al: Diagnosis of transient ischemic attacks: improvement of interobserver agreement by a check-list in ordinary language. Stroke; 1986;17:723–728
13. Quik-van Milligen MLT, Kuyvenhoven MM, de Melker RA et al: Transient ischemic attacks and the general practitioner: diagnosis and management. Cerebrovas Dis 1992;2:102–106

14. Dennis MS, Bamford JM, Molyneux AJ, Warlow CP: Rapid resolution of signs of primary intracerebral haemorrhage in computed tomograms of the brain. BMJ 1987;295:379–381
15. Davenport RJ, Dennis MS, Warlow CP: Improving the recording of the clinical assessment of stroke patients using a clerking proforma. Age Ageing 1995;24:43–48
16. Royal College of Physicians Research Unit and UK Stroke Audit Group: Stroke Audit Package. Royal College of Physicians, London, 1994
17. Hacke W, Schwab S, De Georgia M: Intensive care of acute ischaemic stroke. Cerebrovasc Dis 1994;4:385–392
18. Drake WE, Hamilton MJ, Carlsson M et al: Acute stroke management and patient outcome: the value of neurovascular care units (NCU). Stroke 1973;4:933–945
19. Pitner SE, Mance CJ: An evaluation of stroke intensive care: results of a municipal hospital. Stroke 1973;4:737–741
20. Kennedy FB, Pozen TJ, Gabelman EH et al: Stroke intensive care—an appraisal. Am Health J 1970;80:188–196
21. Stroke Unit Trialists Collaboration 1996: A systematic review of specialist multidisciplinary team (stroke unit) care for stroke patients. In Warlow C, Van Gijn J, Sandercock P (eds): Stroke Module of the Cochrane Database of Systematic Review. BMJ Publishing, London, 1996
22. Dennis MS, Langhorne P: So stroke units save lives: where do we go from here? BMJ 1994;309:1273–1277
23. Langhorne P: What is a stroke unit? A survey of the randomised trials, abstracted. Proceedings of the 4th European Stroke Conference, Bordeaux, France. Cerebrovasc Dis 1995;5:288
24. Wood-Dauphinee S, Shapiro S, Bass E et al: A randomized trial of team care following stroke. Stroke 1984;15:864–872
25. Rothwell PM, Wroe SJ, Slattery J, Warlow CP: Is stroke incidence related to season or temperature? Lancet 1996;347: 934–936
26. Isard PA, Forbes JF: The cost of stroke to the National Health Service in Scotland. Cerebrovasc Dis 1992;2:47–50
27. Young JB, Forster A: The Bradford Community Stroke Trial: results at six months. BMJ 1992;304:1085–1089
28. Young J, Forster A: Day hospital and home physiotherapy for stroke patients: a comparative cost-effectiveness study. J Roy Coll Phys Lond 1993;27:252–257
29. Gladman JRF, Lincoln NB: Follow-up of a controlled trial of domiciliary stroke rehabilitation (DOMINO Study). Age Ageing 1994;23:9–13
30. Gladman J, Forster A, Young J: Hospital- and home-based rehabilitation after discharge from hospital for stroke patients: analysis of two trials. Age Ageing 1995;24:49–53
31. Antiplatelet Trialists' Collaboration: Collaborative overview of randomised trials of antiplatelet therapy. I. prevention of death, myocardial infarction, and stroke by prolonged antiplatelet therapy in various categories of patients. BMJ 1994;308:81–106
32. EAFT (European Atrial Fibrillation Trial) Study Group: Secondary prevention in non-rheumatic atrial fibrillation after transient ischaemic attack or minor stroke. Lancet 1993;342:1255–1262
33. North American Symptomatic Carotid Endarterectomy Trial Collaborators: Beneficial effect of carotid endarterectomy in symptomatic patients with high-grade carotid stenosis. N Engl J Med 1991;325:445–453
34. European Carotid Surgery Trialists' Collaborative Group: MRC European Carotid Surgery Trial: interim results for symptomatic patients with severe (70–99%) or with mild (0–29%) carotid stenosis. Lancet 1991;337:1236–1243
35. Gompertz P, Dennis M, Hopkins A, Ebrahim S: Development and reliability of the Royal College of Physicians stroke audit form. Age Ageing 1994;22:378–383
36. Daley J, Jencks S, Draper D et al: Predicting hospital-associated mortality for Medicare patients: a method for patients with stroke, pneumonia, acute myocardial infarction and congestive heart failure. JAMA 1988;260:3617–3624
37. Jencks SF, Daley J, Draper D et al: Interpreting hospital mortality data: the role of clinical risk adjustment. JAMA 1988;260: 3611–3616
38. Gompertz P, Pound P, Briffa J, Ebrahim S: How useful are non-random comparisons of outcomes and quality of care in purchasing hospital stroke services? Age Ageing 1995;24: 137–141
39. Davenport RJ, Dennis MS, Warlow CP: Effect of correcting outcome data for case mix following stroke. BMJ 1996;312: 1503–1505

C H A P T E R 37

Disorders of the Autonomic Nervous System

KENNETH J. COLLINS

TIM COWEN

This chapter describes recent advances in the neurobiology of aging in the autonomic nervous system (ANS) and attempts, as far as possible, to interpret the etiology of some familiar syndromes of autonomic dysfunction in the elderly. The ANS embodies four principal nerve groups: the sympathetic, parasympathetic, and enteric divisions, together with autonomic centers in the brain. Brain stem and peripheral autonomic centers have afferent inputs which also form part of the autonomic system. All autonomic nerves exhibit marked plasticity affecting many features of their organization and requiring dynamic regulation; their neurons have multiple neurotransmitters and receptors. It is believed that the idea of aging as a continuous, generalized loss of neurons, including those of the ANS, is not tenable based on present evidence. The plasticity of autonomic neurons involves interactions with target organs and with other neurons, and it is as vital to mature and aging autonomic neurons as it is to developing neurons. Thus, trophic factors released from the target organ, for example, nerve growth factor (NGF), can influence the plasticity of the innervating neuron, and conversely, neurons may be capable of influencing the trophic status of the target organ. What are perceived as autonomic disorders in old age may arise from many sources, of which alteration in trophic interactions between nerve and effector appears to be a major contributor. Pathologic changes in specific components of an autonomic reflex arc are difficult to identify, and in tests of autonomic function it may be helpful first to assess the function of the target organ, as much as possible independently of its innervation. When effector function is impaired, then clearly, abnormal responses to tests of reflex integrity might occur. If normal autonomic reflex responses were obtained under conditions in which effector function was impaired, it would indicate adaptive changes in the system. Influences on aging processes are more easily characterized in animals. However, even in animal investigations, it is rare that specific pathogen-free, barrier-protected animals are used to differentiate cellular aging from the accumulated effects of a lifetime of undocumented disease. Clinical investigations of autonomic function in the elderly suffer to an even greater degree from this lack of precision.

Neurobiology of the Aging Autonomic Nervous System

Nature of Aging

Autonomic dysfunction is common in the elderly and affects a number of different systems. Autonomic control is impaired in the vasculature, heart, thermoregulatory system, gut, bladder, and iris,[1–3] with evidence of sympathetic involvement in the majority of instances. The popular concept that aging involves the widespread degeneration and death of many neurons, including those of the ANS, is probably misleading (see reviews[4,5]). Extensive cell death has been reliably demonstrated only in the enteric nervous system of aged animals,[6] while earlier studies have indicated cell loss in the intermediolateral column of elderly subjects, estimated at 5 to 8 percent per decade.[7] Other areas of the ANS appear to be relatively well maintained, with no evidence of dramatic cell loss in humans or laboratory animals. The extensive functional deficits in the ANS therefore do not appear to be the result of large-scale death of autonomic neurons.

Quantitative microscopic methods have been used to characterize and assess peripheral autonomic motor and sensory nerve fibers and their associated neurotransmitters (Fig. 37-1). Age-related changes in these features are often local in nature, and even in the affected areas not all the nerves supplying a particular tissue are involved. In many cases, no changes are observed. Where they do occur, changes are frequently species-specific and may involve increases, for example, in nerve fiber density or transmitter expression, as well as decreases. The changes seen are frequently sufficiently subtle to require measurement.[5] An area that has been relatively extensively studied because of its possible relevance for the blood supply to the aging brain, is the autonomic nerve supply to the major cerebral arteries of the circle of Willis.[8] In humans (seventh and eighth decades) and rats (24 to 36 months) these nerves decline with increasing age.[9–11] However, in humans the loss of nerve fibers affects mainly the anterior choroidal, posterior communicating, and internal carotid arteries, while in rats the changes affect middle and posterior cerebral and basilar arteries of the circle of Willis.[8,9] In rats, where the changes can be studied in more detail, sympathetic vasoconstrictor nerves decline significantly in density between 18 and

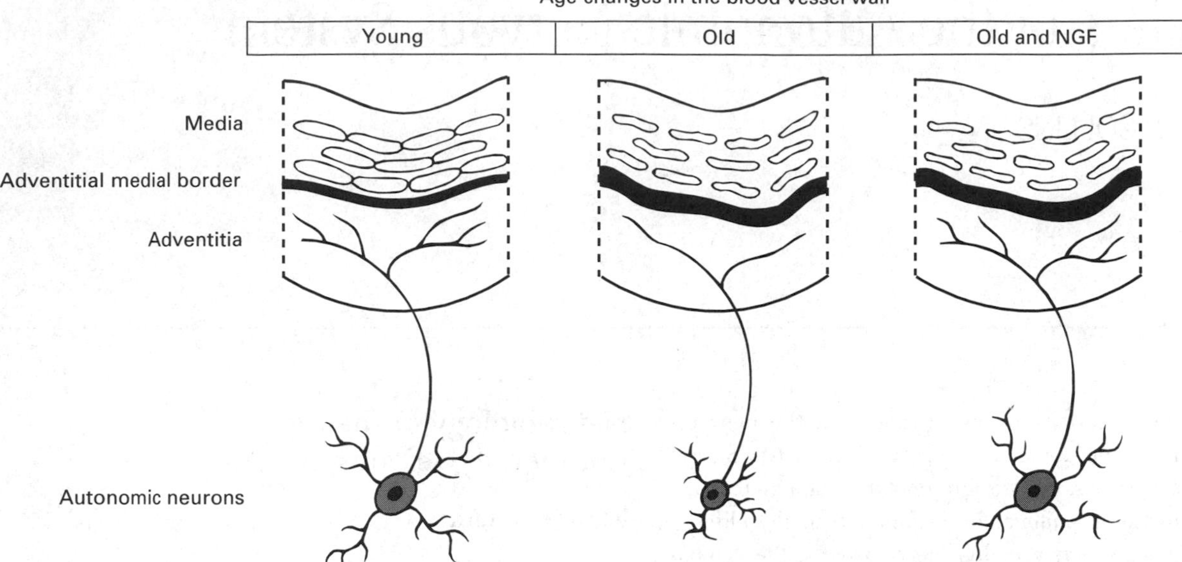

Figure 37-1 Diagrams showing changes in nerve and smooth muscle in the aging blood vessel wall. With aging there is atrophy of autonomic neurons, including loss of axon collaterals and shrinkage of dendrites and nerve cell body, and also shrinkage of muscle cells and thickening of basal lamina at the adventitial medial border (AMB). Following NGF treatment there is regrowth of neurons, including axon collaterals, cell body, and dendrites. (Modified from Gavazzi and Cowen,[28] with permission.)

24 months,[11] while vasodilator nerves, including sensory and parasympathetic fibers, may increase. Although sympathetic nerves in the rat cerebral vasculature decline in density with age, it appears that levels of the noradrenaline-synthesizing enzyme tyrosine hydroxylase may increase within these nerve fibers.[10] Tracing studies using retrogradely transported dyes[12] have shown that the soma and dendrites of neurons projecting to different targets, including cerebral arteries, tend to be reduced in size and length, respectively, in parallel with the age changes in their peripheral axons.

In support of the evidence for impaired thermoregulation in the elderly, local deficits have been demonstrated in the structure and function of sympathetic (cholinergic) nerves around the sweat glands of elderly subjects. Sweat output, which is known to be a vital part of thermoregulation, declines after the seventh decade, in parallel with reduced size of glandular acini and reduced density of the periacinar sympathetic nerves.[13] Similar changes were found in the eccrine sweat glands of the rat footpad.[14]

Other tissues have been investigated but only in laboratory animals. Sympathetic nerve fibers from the coeliac-superior mesenteric ganglion complex of aged rats, supplying the enteric nervous system, were much reduced,[15] as was the sympathetic nerve supply to the renal vasculature at the level of the renal artery in rabbits[16] and around intrarenal arterioles in rats.[17] In the iris of the aged rat, sensory and parasympathetic nerves were reduced in density by 20 to 30 percent, while sympathetic nerves increased in density.[18] From these immunohistochemical studies it seems likely that combinations of growth changes (lengthening, retraction, or atrophy) of axons and dendrites and alterations in soma size and neurotransmitter expression occur in different situations. Because neurotransmitter markers are generally used to identify the peripheral fibers of particular nerve groups in tissues with multiple innervation, it is not always possible to know whether a change in staining pattern indicates altered levels of neurotransmitter, altered growth of nerve fibers, or both.

Dystrophic changes in neurites have been identified in sympathetic ganglia of aged human subjects and rodents.[19,20] Not very much is known about the changes with increasing age in central neurons of the ANS. There is some evidence of selective neuron loss in the hypothalamus[21] and brain stem regions[22] controlling autonomic activity, while earlier studies on the human spinal cord showed cell losses in the lateral horn of preganglionic sympathetic neurons[7] amounting to 5–8 percent per decade.

The divergent changes in peripheral autonomic neurons with age (growth as well as atrophy of axons and dendrites, and neurotransmitter changes) suggest that compensatory changes occur in neurons and groups of neurons as they attempt to respond to the altered demands of old age. These extra demands may include the loss of neighboring neurons. Alteration of the autonomic centers of the brain and spinal cord (see above) and in the dendrites of postganglionic sympathetic neurons in aging suggests altered patterns of central connectivity. The overall picture is of relatively small quantitative changes which, perhaps because of accumulated effects at several levels of neural organization, lead to the rather more widespread deficits in autonomic function that have been observed clinically.

Plasticity in Mature and Aging ANS

Plasticity in mature autonomic neurons includes changes associated with growth (or retraction) of axons and dendrites to expand their territory, regeneration of nerves after injury, growth or shrinkage of cell soma, and changes in expression of neurotransmitters and other markers of dynamic behavior. While plasticity is generally associated with the developing nervous system, it has become increasingly clear that it continues to be an important feature of the mature, and even aged, nervous system (see above) as it attempts to respond to altered demand. Plastic changes in the aging nervous system use mechanisms "inherited" from earlier stages of development. The peripheral processes of mature autonomic and sensory neurons continually grow and retract over periods of a few days.[23,24] The mechanism proposed to control this form of plasticity is the synthesis and release by target tissues (the end organs of autonomic control such as smooth muscles and glands) of limiting amounts of neurotrophic factors (see below). Developing autonomic neurons are thus intimately related to their targets, providing them with appropriate signals for activation and receiving in return trophic messages required for neuronal growth.

Trophic interactions with target tissues are important elements of plasticity at all stages of life, but the nature of these interactions may change with age. During early development, it is well known that targets control survival of autonomic and other neurons,[25] and, in addition, the establishment of appropriate patterns of growth, connectivity, and neurotransmitter phenotype.[26,27] In later periods of life, the survival of autonomic neurons becomes largely independent of target support. However, interactions between autonomic neurons and their targets remain important for the regulation of growth of axons, soma, and dendrites and of neurotransmitter expression.[28] Studies on experimentally induced hypertrophy of smooth muscle in gut and bladder have shown that associated autonomic neurons undergo a parallel hypertrophy,[29] providing strong evidence of the influence that target tissues can have on their innervating neurons. Trophic interactions between nerves and end organs are therefore a vital feature of maintenance and plasticity in the mature ANS, and alterations in this relationship are likely to be critical determinants in the aging process.

Studies on the cells and molecules involved in plasticity of mature autonomic neurons generally require the use of animal models (see below). Denervation studies show that collateral sprouting (the capacity of axons to expand their territory) is impaired in sympathetic neurons of the aged rat.[30] However, it is not clear from these studies whether the defect lies in the neurons themselves, in the target tissues, or more generally in the "old" environment in which nerve growth takes place.

Transplantation studies have explored this issue by placing target tissues from young and old donor rats, with known age changes in their autonomic innervation, in contact with the axons of autonomic neurons of young host rats.[28] The donor tissues are denervated on removal, providing new territory over which host nerves can grow. Transplants of old middle cerebral or basilar arteries, in which the density of autonomic nerve fibers is reduced by about 50 percent with age, become reinnervated by strikingly fewer host nerves than similar transplants of young arteries. This result holds for the overall (sensory, sympathetic, and parasympathetic) nerve supply, as indicated by nonspecific neuron markers, as well as for the sympathetic population of nerve fibers, as indicated by specific markers. Similar studies have attempted to find out whether target tissues can influence age changes in neurotransmitter expression as well as peripheral nerve fiber density. Eccrine sweat glands are innervated by sympathetic neurons, which are unusual in using acetylcholine as their peripheral neurotransmitter. Evidence from early development shows that these neurons switch their neurotransmitter phenotype from catecholaminergic to cholinergic at the time when their peripheral axons first contact their target sweat glands.[31] Again using transplantation, it has been shown that sweat glands from aged rats, in which density of innervation is normally reduced, were, like rat cerebral arteries, less attractive to host nerves. However, they remained competent to invoke cholinergic characteristics in the reinnervating host neurons,[32] suggesting that different target-associated factors regulate nerve growth and transmitter expression.

Transplantation has also been used to study the other side of the plasticity equation—the autonomic neuron.[33,34] Aged sympathetic neurons from the superior cervical ganglion transplanted into different environments in young hosts have generally shown unimpaired plasticity in terms of survival as well as extent of neurite outgrowth. However, in the few studies in which transplants were made into old host rats, both young and old[35] neurons were impaired in their capacity for neurite outgrowth, suggesting that changes in the environment as well as changes in the neurons themselves in old age, could contribute to altered plasticity.

These observations demonstrate that target tissues retain a considerable, dynamic influence over the pattern and density of their innervating autonomic neurons and over their patterns of neurotransmitter expression, and that this ongoing influence extends throughout maturity into old age. In addition, intrinsic changes in neurons and alterations in their environment contribute to age-related changes in plasticity. These mechanisms allow constant adjustment of autonomic neurons to altered functional demands.

Neurotrophic Mechanisms

Soluble factors

Target tissues achieve their influence over innervating neurons through the production of neurotrophic factors. The first of these, NGF, was discovered during investigations of a mouse sarcoma that induced extravagant growth of sympathetic nerve fibers.[25] It took 35 more years to discover that NGF was a member of a larger family—the neurotrophins—which has trophic effects on many different neurons in the central and peripheral nervous systems. In addition to NGF, neurotrophins now include brain-derived neurotrophic factor (BDNF), NT3, NT4–5, and NT6.[36] Their effects on particular neurons are specified by receptors of two main types: tyrosine kinase (trk) receptors, which are relatively specific as to which neurotrophin they bind, and nonspecific glycoprotein p75 receptors,[37] which bind all neurotrophins with varying affinities but whose role remains controversial. Although trk receptors can transduce most of the known effects of neurotrophins, p75 NGF receptors are probably important in modulating some of these effects, particularly in later stages of development.[38] For example, recent evidence implicates a mutation of p75 receptors in the induction of hypertension.[39] In addition to neurotrophins, there are a number of other cytokines—such as ciliary neuronotrophic factor (CNTF), fibroblast growth factors (FGFs), and retinoic acid—with important neurotrophic effects on developing sympathetic and other neurons.[40]

The neurotrophic theory[26,41] states that during early development neurons compete with their neighbors for a share of limited quantities of target-derived trophic factors such as NGF. Success results in the survival and connectivity of an appropriate number of neurons. Similar relationships and factors are thought to govern the survival of other autonomic neurons. The small, unmyelinated sensory afferent neurons, including those that provide afferent input to the ANS, also depend on NGF for survival. A survival factor for parasympathetic neurons remains to be discovered.

Trophic support from targets continues to be important for the maintenance and plasticity of the mature ANS. Mature neurons inherit dependence on particular factors from earlier stages of life but, through changes in receptors and intracellular signaling, respond in a different way. Thus, mature autonomic neurons remain dependent on NGF for growth,[42] for collateral sprouting,[43] and for neurotransmitter expression (see above). However, unlike developing neurons, they are probably not dependent on neurotrophic factors for survival, and regeneration of sympathetic and sensory nerves in mature animals is also not NGF-dependent.[43]

The continued influence of trophic factors such as NGF on plasticity in autonomic neurons raises the possibility that these factors can be used therapeutically to rescue neurons from age-related neurodegeneration, and preliminary experiments on animals have been moderately encouraging. Because of the wide range of effects of NGF on immune and other systems[25] and its ability to encourage inappropriate nerve growth (e.g., in an animal model of causalgia,[44] these experiments have required the use of local infusion techniques with miniosmotic pumps. Infusion of NGF into the third ventricle or subdural space of aged rats at relatively high concentrations induces the recovery of atrophic cerebrovascular nerve fibers around the internal carotid artery[45] or middle cerebral artery[77] (and see above) to levels similar to those in young rats. Sprouting of fibers mainly involved the sympathetic nerves, while sensory nerves responded to NGF infusion with elevated calcitonin gene-related peptide (CGRP) levels.[46] Dendrites of the sympathetic neurons projecting to cerebral blood vessels were also found to be capable of regrowth following local treatment of their peripheral axons with NGF.[47] Withdrawal of treatment predictably resulted in atrophy, indicating the need for continuous therapy to replace an ongoing, probably increasing deficit. Trials using systemic treatment with neurotrophic factors for diseases such as motoneuron disease have resulted in some cases in significant side effects including weight loss and pain, indicating that additional research will be required before the use of neurotrophic factors as therapeutic agents becomes feasible.

It is not clear at present whether the effects of treatment with NGF on growth of mature autonomic nerves are evidence of a pharmacologic effect or whether it supplements target-derived endogenous NGF in the regulation of neuronal plasticity. Whereas in early postnatal life target levels of either the NGF protein or its mRNA tend to correlate with the density of sympathetic innervation,[48,49] as would be expected from the limiting relationship previously described, this correlation seems to be lost in tissues from aged rats.[50] This implies either that other factors, or combinations of factors, become more important influences on plasticity in aged neurons or that neuronal responsiveness to neurotrophins is altered in old age.

Bound insoluble neurotrophic factors in the extracellular matrix

While studies on NGF have yielded important information about plasticity in mature and aged autonomic neurons, it is probable that we are only beginning to identify the different trophic factors that affect aging neurons. The extracellular matrix (ECM) contains a number of insoluble bound factors with important neurotrophic activities to which autonomic (and other) neurons respond. Indeed, recent work on Hirschsprung's disease implicates inappropriate expression of the ECM glycoprotein laminin in the failure of enteric neurons to differentiate and migrate to the distal bowel.[51] ECM element's are found in basal laminae at sites of neuroeffector junctions of somatic and autonomic neurons and are therefore ideally positioned to influence dynamic growth processes of the kind described above through contact with terminal nerve fibers. In this context, it is interesting to note the involvement of ECM in neural changes associated with the muscular dystrophies. Dystrophin-glycoprotein complexes are expressed in muscle and brain where they link cytoskeletal elements to ECM and provide receptors for laminin and other molecules. Dystrophin deficiency in Duchenne muscular dystrophy results in mental retardation as well as muscle degeneration, while laminin deficiency in congenital muscular dystrophy (CMD) results in peripheral neuropathy, cognitive deficits, and muscle degeneration.[52] Although the role of ECM molecules in aging has not been extensively investigated, recent studies implicate laminin and ECM in autonomic (including sensory) nerve fiber atrophy in aged rats,[53] and it is possible that, like other neurotrophic factors, laminin and NGF act synergistically on plasticity in autonomic neurons.

A likely scenario is that combinations of factors will be identified with trophic influences on particular groups of autonomic neurons and that the particular factor(s) identified will have roles that are specific for particular stages of development.

Neuronal Responsiveness to Trophic Factors

Recent evidence indicates developmental shifts in the responsiveness of sympathetic neurons to NGF, some of which have been described (see above). Later in life, further changes occur that may require a revision of our understanding of the role of NGF in the mature ANS. Aged sympathetic neurons become less able to scavenge and utilize available NGF,[18,50] making them vulnerable to trophic factor deprivation and providing an explanation for the reduced capacity for collateral sprouting previously described.[30,35] In vitro studies also indicate reduced responsiveness of aging sympathetic neurons to NGF.[54] While NGF binding is reduced in aged sympathetic ganglia,[55] it is not yet known for certain which NGF receptors are involved in these changes, although some lines of evidence point to the p75 receptor. In the absence of changes in irideal NGF levels, reduced NGF responsiveness of aging sympathetic neurons projecting to the iris suggests that NGF receptor expression is no longer as tightly coupled to levels of NGF at the target (see above) as it was during early development. The search for alternative influences on the responsiveness of aged autonomic neurons to trophic factors forms an important area for further study and may have implications for future therapy.

By virtue of their large size and surface area and high metabolic requirements, neurons are exposed to a number of local and systemic changes during the aging process, which may influence plasticity. In addition to the target-associated factors already described, growth hormone (GH) levels decline substantially with age, resulting in undetectable serum levels of GH in 50 percent of all subjects by their seventh decade.[56] Declining GH levels have been proposed as a major influence on aging and perhaps on the nervous system.[57] The most likely pathway for neural effects is that mediated by the insulin-like growth factors (IGF-1 and IGF-2), which have been shown to influence development and outgrowth of cultured peripheral neurons.[58] Altered levels of sex hormones may affect targets of autonomic neurons such as sweat glands[59] and thereby influence their autonomic innervation (see above). In addition, aging autonomic neurons are increasingly likely to encounter the damaging effects of partial ischemia or raised levels of free radicals. These changes are relatively specific to old age and introduce a negative influence on neuronal plasticity not present at earlier stages of development. In regard to the role of free radicals in aging, it is interesting to note that enteric autonomic neurons that synthesize nitric oxide (itself a free radical) appear to be relatively well protected from the cell death that affects their neighbors,[60] although how they achieve this apparent invulnerability is not understood.

Neurotransmission

Experimental studies on the effects of age on neurotransmission are beyond the scope of this chapter and have been reviewed extensively elsewhere.[61,62] In humans, aging is accompanied by increases as well as decreases in different aspects of sympathetic function; for example, sympathetic nerve activity and plasma noradrenaline levels are generally increased in the elderly,[63–65] perhaps as a result of increased noradrenaline release[66] (see section on cardiovascular system). However, there is controversy over the possible explanation for these phenomena, in particular whether reduced reuptake of noradrenaline also contributes to elevated levels in plasma.[67] Cholinergic mechanisms in parasympathetic nerves are also affected by aging.[68]

Techniques and Models

Because of its multifactorial nature, aging poses numerous problems for research. Its study requires the combination of a wide range of methods. In the ANS, these include epidemiologic studies and investigations of altered function in humans to identify the key areas, and the establishment and use of animal models for the elucidation of mechanisms at tissue, cellular, and molecular levels. A new area, which has only begun to be developed because of technical difficulties, concerns the use of tissue culture techniques for the isolation and experimental manipulation of molecular influences in aging.

Human studies

Investigations of autonomic function in elderly people have been made in cross-sectional and, more rarely, longitudinal studies in normal volunteer subjects and in clinical tests of autonomic function in patients. These studies are discussed according to different physiologic systems in the following sections.

Animal models

A wide range of animals have been used in aging studies, including guinea pigs, rabbits, and chickens.[6,16,68] However, laboratory rodents, in particular rats and mice, have been most extensively used.[17,42] Because there are interspecies and interstrain differences, each area of study requires independent verification of a model system. However, in areas where direct comparisons have been possible, aged rats and humans have exhibited some similarities. Thus, in both species plasma noradrenaline levels are elevated with age. Atrophy has been demonstrated in the autonomic nerve supply to cerebral arteries[10] and to the eccrine sweat glands[13,14] in 24-month-old Sprague-Dawley rats and in humans from the seventh or eighth decade, although there are fundamental differences between the sweating apparatus in humans and in rats. Bladder dysfunction is seen in patients with Parkinsonism, who are often elderly,[69] while deficits in the noradrenergic innervation of the bladder have been observed in aged rats.[70–72]

Experimental studies on mechanisms involved in neuronal aging have continued to use rat or mouse models for a number of reasons, including the need for species-specific baseline data and the relative tolerance of rats and mice for infusion, transplantation, selective denervation, and other experimental manipulations. The development of transgenic models involving gene deletion or insertion seems likely to increase the use of mice in aging studies. Neurons from both species are generally preferred for tissue culture studies.

One aspect of aging that has had a major impact on technique concerns its gradual, relatively subtle nature. Aging rarely if ever is accompanied by all-or-nothing changes, whatever the aspect under investigation. Biochemical, electrical, functional, and morphologic changes are almost invariably quantitative, generally in the range of 10 to 50 percent. A further problem affecting aging studies is that individual variation tends to increase with age, in animals as well as humans, making it necessary to sample increasing numbers or to carry out longitudinal studies on identified individuals. A recent study on sympathetic nerve activity changes with age[65] showed that only a longitudinal experimental design could demonstrate a significant effect of age on nerve activity because of the large, increasing, interindividual variation with age.

These features of aging have driven the search for appropriate techniques in a number of areas, for example, in human research involving measurement of altered function, power spectrum analysis of autonomic control of the heart, and intraneural recording (see "The Cardiovascular System," below). Biochemical changes have been measured using, for example, highly sensitive enzyme-linked immunoabsorbant assay (ELISA) for trophic factors[73] and high-pressure liquid chromatography (HPLC) combined with electrochemical detection for catecholamines.[74] Receptor changes can be measured using ligand-binding studies with biochemical or morphologic methods of assessment, the latter generally using radioisotope labeling. Morphologic changes in neurons have been quantified by cell counting techniques that take account of cell size and changes in tissue volume and shape,[6] while changes in peripheral nerve fibers and dendrites have been quantified using computerized image analysis in combination with light and, more recently, confocal laser-scanning microsopy.[75,76]

Autonomic Dysfunction and the Nervous System

In recent years, advances in neuroanatomic techniques involving immunohistochemistry and axoplasmic transport tracing have provided abundant new information on the regions of the brain and spinal cord that control the ANS.[78] New ideas have been developed to justify revision of classic concepts of anatomic and neurochemical organization and are gradually being applied to the study of aging and the ANS. Some progressive decline in autonomic control is thought to result from aging processes, and there is a wide range of pathologic conditions known to affect central and peripheral autonomic function, the most important of which appear in the accompanying list. Widespread involvement of the ANS is seen in multiple system atrophy which, although a comparatively rare disease, presents with obvious manifestations of autonomic failure including orthostatic hypotension, defective sweating, visual disturbances, and bladder, bowel, and sexual dysfunction. There is a spectrum of autonomic involvement in extrapyramidal and cerebellar disorders, and autonomic studies can be helpful in distinguishing these disorders.[79] Autonomic pathways may also be damaged in central cerebral lesions involving the hypothalamus and midbrain and in spinal cord lesions.[80] Psychotropic drugs and other centrally acting drugs have a profound global effect on autonomic responses, particularly in the elderly. The peripheral components of the ANS show neuropathy in many diseases affecting the nervous system,[81] and in both younger

Autonomic dysfunction associated with diseases affecting the nervous system

- Central disturbances
  - Primary autonomic failure
  - Multiple system atrophy (Shy-Drager syndrome)
  - Cerebrovascular disease
  - Trigeminal zoster
  - Parkinsonism
  - Wernicke's encephalopathy
  - Brain tumors
  - Alzheimer's disease
  - Hypothalamic degeneration
  - Traumatic cord lesions
  - Traumatic brain lesions
  - Multiple sclerosis
  - Transverse myelitis
  - Syringomyelia
  - Tabes dorsalis
  - Holmes-Adie syndrome
- Peripheral neuropathy
  - Diabetes mellitus
  - Guillain-Barré syndrome
  - Acute inflammatory and acute autonomic neuropathies
  - Amyloidosis
  - Alcoholism
  - Vitamin B complex deficiency
  - Vitamin B_{12} deficiency
  - Rheumatoid arthritis
  - Chronic renal failure
  - Chronic liver disease
  - Malignancy
  - Chemical toxicity

and elderly patients this is overwhelmingly more common in diabetes mellitus.

Primary Autonomic Failure

Primary autonomic failure may occur in pure form without any other neurologic signs or in association with quite different degenerations of the nervous system such as multiple system atrophy and Parkinsonism. Virtually all patients with primary autonomic failure are found at postmortem to have severe loss of intermediolateral column cells. A clinical classification of primary autonomic failure identifies three disorders[82]: (1) pure autonomic failure, formerly called idiopathic orthostatic hypotension, (2) autonomic failure with multiple system atrophy, and (3) autonomic failure with Parkinson's disease. Cytoplasmic neuronal inclusions (Lewy bodies) characteristic (but not pathognomic) of Parkinson's disease, are also found in brains of patients with pure autonomic failure without Parkinsonian features, but very rarely in patients with multiple system atrophy. The above three classes of disorder are chronic in nature, but acute and subacute types of primary autonomic failure, termed pandysautonomia or cholinergic dysautonomia, have also been described.[82]

Multiple system atrophy

Autonomic failure as part of multiple system atrophy was originally described by Shy and Drager.[83] Multiple system atrophy in the form of striatonigral degeneration may occasionally occur, however, without the symptoms of autonomic failure.[84] In primary autonomic failure, patients are usually middle-aged or elderly, and in multiple system atrophy, males are affected more often than females. Commonly, the presenting feature is orthostatic hypotension, and the onset of somatoneurologic manifestations is usually insidious, following the orthostatic hypotension by 6 months to 2 years. The neurologic changes are accompanied by marked depletion of dopamine, noradrenaline, and tyrosine hydroxylase in brain regions normally rich in catecholamines. In the substantia nigra, there is depletion of tyrosine hydroxylase-containing dopaminergic neurons, these neurons projecting primarily to the putamen. The reciprocal relationship between the substantia nigra and the putamen, which forms part of the nigrostriatal loop, appears to be damaged. These findings contrast with Parkinson's disease, where nigral dopaminergic neurons are depleted but the striatonigral projection fibers are preserved.[85] Magnetic resonance imaging (MRI) may show abnormalities in the cerebellum and brain stem, the putamen, or both.[86] The amount of diagnostic help gained from MRI depends on the clinical picture.[87] If it includes obvious cerebellar ataxia, finding cerebellar atrophy on MRI will not help much. If Parkinsonism dominates the clinical picture and clinically masks cerebellar involvement, obvious cerebellar atrophy on MRI might contribute toward diagnosis.

In elderly patients with multiple system atrophy, dementia is no more common than might be expected on the basis of chance. It is surprising to observe preserved intellectual function in a patient who is almost completely incapacitated in terms of motor control, orthostatic blood pressure regulation, and bladder disturbance. This is in striking contrast to the neuronal degeneration of Alzheimer's disease in which there is degeneration of cholinergic ascending projections from the reticular system. It also contrasts with the intellectual impairment that is a feature of many cases of Parkinson's disease.[88]

Parkinson's disease

In the original description of the disease named after him, James Parkinson included several dysautonomic symptoms, and over the years autonomic disturbances such as orthostatic hypotension, sweating abnormalities, and sexual dysfunction have received comment.[89,90] Many patients with classical Parkinson's disease have mild orthostatic hypotension when compared with controls, and there are reports that resting levels of plasma noradrenaline are in a lower than normal range in these individuals.[91] However, patients with classic Parkinson's disease do not have abnormalities of cardiovascular reflex control linked with baroreceptor defects and intermediolateral column cell loss characteristic of the autonomic failure syndrome. Mild symptoms of autonomic dysfunction occurring with aging, together with the need to evaluate autonomic function in an objective manner, make it difficult to assess the significance of minor autonomic disturbances in elderly Parkinsonian patients. The influence of dopaminergic therapy in Parkinson's disease needs particular consideration, as demonstrated by the changes in autonomic function tests induced by L-dopa and bromocriptine in treated and untreated patients.[92] In an analysis of patients with idiopathic Parkinson's disease, it was found that older age, medication, and higher Hoehn and Yahr disability scores were each associated with poor autonomic responsiveness.[93] Multiple stepwise regression analysis showed that older age explained most of the heart rate variability, and the only significant Parkinson's disease-related factor was the use of medication. Unmedicated Parkinson's disease patients with mild disease of short duration showed no evidence of autonomic dysfunction. It is apparent that the vast majority of patients with Parkinson's disease do not show evidence of autonomic failure if strict criteria in autonomic testing are applied. Involvement of the ANS is best defined by a series of tests using changes in specific measurable physiologic and biochemical criteria.

Alzheimer's disease

The cholinergic pathways in the brain are important in learning and memory, and their function declines with normal aging. This transmitter system is severely impaired in Alzheimer's disease. Current research is attempting to understand the molecular mechanism of the functional decline in the disease and to develop therapies for reversing it.[94] Accompanying autonomic dysfunction in Alzheimer's disease, there is reported to be a reduction in the cholinergic ascending projections from the substantia innominata of the reticular formation, together with loss of noradrenergic projections from cells in the locus coeruleus.[95] To assess whether Alzheimer's disease affects the sympathetic or parasympathetic influences on heart rate, power spectrum analysis of heart rate variability has been used.[96] Compared with normal controls, patients with Alzheimer's disease exhibited a relative hypersympathetic and hypoparasympathetic state. It must be said, however, that age-matching of elderly patients and controls investigated (71 ± 8 years versus 65 ± 2 years) was not precise. It was concluded from this study that although Alzheimer's disease is a dementing illness, organs and tissues remote from the central nervous system (CNS) may be involved as well. Similar changes in cardiovascular autonomic function have also been reported by other investigators.[97]

Stroke

Autonomic failure is known to manifest commonly in stroke, but little attention has been given to various features of sympathetic dysfunction in cerebrovascular disease. Impaired sympathetic skin responses reflecting suppression of reflex activity of the sympathetic nervous system have been recorded in patients with brain infarction.[98] Researchers have also tested sympathetic skin responses between 1 and 72 months after cerebrovascular accident on normal and hemiplegic sides and found no differences.[99] It is probable that the divergence of findings reflects differences in the timing of the studies.

Secondary Autonomic Failure

Autonomic fibers are damaged secondarily in a variety of disorders, most commonly in diabetes mellitus and alcoholism but also in a wide range of acute and chronic peripheral neuropathies. Secondary autonomic failure can be a complication of various autoimmune, collagen, or connective tissue diseases such as rheumatoid disease and may also occur in renal failure and severe liver disease.[100] Impairment of autonomic function is common in patients with terminal uremia, and disturbances of sympathetic and parasympathetic function have been demonstrated by many investigators. It is suggested that chronic renal failure with hypertension may be accompanied by an afferent signal arising in the failing kidneys. The rate of sympathetic nerve discharge does not, however, appear to be correlated with either plasma noradrenaline levels or plasma renin activity.[101]

Dysfunction of the ANS is well-recognized in some cases of Guillain-Barré syndrome[102] and in complications of infections such as syphilis and botulism. Several varieties of acute and subacute autonomic neuropathy have been reported in patients with no other evidence of systemic disease or sensorimotor neuropathy. It is possible that they represent a selective form of Guillain-Barré syndrome.[80] A study on 50 cases of rheumatoid arthritis investigated by heart rate variability during deep breathing and postural change showed no neurologic or autonomic signs, although there was an inflammatory syndrome.[103] There was a significant difference between rheumatoid patients and the controls only for the Valsalva maneuver, but there was no obvious correlation between autonomic dysfunction in rheumatoid arthritis and markers of inflammation or presence of rheumatoid factor. ANS dysfunction in rheumatoid arthritis appears to be subclinical and probably isolated from other peripheral or CNS damage.

Alcoholism

In cases of Wernicke's encephalopathy showing characteristic ophthalmoparesis, ataxia, and Korsakoff's psychosis, orthostatic hypotension and peripheral neuropathy may be present. The condition is due to thiamine deficiency, and there is a "dying back" neuropathy identical to that of beri-beri. The most distal parts of the longest fibers in the vagus nerve appear to be affected earliest, and the shorter, more proximal, fibers of the sympathetic system are affected later, when the peripheral neuropathy is severe. Peripheral sympathetic vasomotor control is relatively well-preserved in alcoholics until the peripheral neuropathy reaches an advanced stage. Definite evidence of vagal damage in chronic alcoholics has been demonstrated by impaired heart rate responses to Valsalva maneuver, deep breathing, change in posture, neck suction, and atropine.[104] Alcoholics with vagal neuropathy have an increased mortality rate.[105] A significant reduction in the density of myelinated fibers in distal parts of the vagus and carotid sinus nerves has been demonstrated in chronic alcoholic patients,[106,107] although the splanchnic nerves are relatively spared. Orthostatic hypotension is more likely to occur if the splanchnic outflow is involved, and the lack of pathology in splanchnic nerves is consistent with the relatively normal response to postural change in these cases.

Diabetic autonomic neuropathy

Significant clinical symptoms occur in relatively few diabetic patients even though evidence of diffuse autonomic dysfunction is often detected. Autonomic neuropathy is probably the direct result of inadequate metabolic control, and it can manifest itself in a number of ways. Autonomic damage often begins with loss of sweating in the extremities, impotence, and bladder dysfunction, and then progresses through abnormalities in cardiovascular reflexes to a final stage of symptomatic postural hypotension, gastroparesis, diarrhea, and bladder atony. Disorders of potency and orthostatic hypotension are usually the main problems. Autonomic neuropathy carries a poor prognosis, with mortality over 2 years in diabetic patients being twice as great when symptomatic autonomic neuropathy is present.[108] The cause of diabetic neuropathy affecting the small fibers is not known, but there is evidence that immunologically mediated damage can contribute to the pathologic changes in autonomic nerves.[109] Immune complexes appear to be increased. The idea has also been advanced that antibodies to exogenous insulin might interfere with the action of NGF. This factor is required for the growth and survival of sympathetic nerves, and it can be shown to accumulate in denervated effector organs such as the iris.[110]

The prevalence of peripheral and autonomic neuropathy in insulin-dependent diabetics appears to have different age distributions as shown in a study[111] where peripheral neuropathy was defined as the absence or impairment of ankle reflexes and a vibration threshold greater than the 95th percentile for age-matched controls without diabetes. The presence of peripheral neuropathy increased progressively with age, whereas that of autonomic neuropathy peaked in the fifth decade and then declined. Both were related to the duration of diabetes, but the prevalence of autonomic neuropathy apparently declined after 25 years' duration. Interpretation of these data on prevalence (as opposed to incidence) is complicated, but the differences are probably due to different patterns of mortality.

Severe secondary autonomic dysfunction is most likely to result from conditions such as diabetes mellitus that affect small myelinated and unmyelinated fibers in the baroreceptor afferents, vagal innervation of the heart, and sympathetic efferent fibers in the mesenteric vascular bed, or from Guillain-Barré syndrome in which there is acute segmental demyelination in the sympathetic and parasympathetic nerves. In Friedrich's ataxia, in which the large-diameter fibers in peripheral nerves are predominantly affected, there appears to be no accompanying disturbance of autonomic function.[112]

Investigation of autonomic function in peripheral nerve disease can involve (1) tests of reflex responses mediated through autonomic pathways, (2) microelectrode recordings of sympathetic nerve activity, (3) measurement of altered pharmacologic responses of denervated tissues, (4) detection of immunocytochemical changes, and (5) biopsy, which is not widely used but can provide useful information in some conditions, for example, findings on sural nerve biopsy which generally reflect the changes in the ANS in peripheral autonomic failure due to diabetes mellitus, amyloidosis, chronic alcoholism, and inflammatory neuropathies.[113]

The Cardiovascular System

Autonomic control of cardiovascular responses to postural, pressor, and exercise stress in older individuals is of considerable importance in helping to assess the cardiovascular potential in elderly patients and in diagnosis and management of primary cardiovascular disease. Hypotensive events such as orthostatic and postprandial hypotension are found more frequently in elderly than in young or middle-aged patients,[114] and this has led to the hypothesis that reflexes involved in blood pressure homeostasis become impaired with age, failing to compensate with adequate vasoconstriction and cardiac stimulation and leading to a reduction in cardiac output.[115] In addition, resting heart rate is generally slightly elevated and heart rate variability is diminished with advancing age.

Cardiovascular Reflexes and Aging

A number of cardiovascular reflexes have been shown to change with aging, including respiratory sinus arrhythmia, vagal baroreflex responses, cardiopulmonary reflexes, tachycardia caused by chemoreflex action, facial cooling bradycardia, and cold pressor reflexes.[116,117] The control of heart rate during changes in arterial pressure, which primarily provides an index of vagal activity, is reduced with age. In both young and elderly, cholinergic blockade virtually eliminates the relationship between heart rate and arterial blood pressure.[118] In animal studies, arterial baroreflex control of heart rate, renal sympathetic activity, and arterial blood pressure are all significantly diminished in older animals, and this is shown to represent a defect in control of both parasympathetic and sympathetic limbs of the baroreflex.[119] An area that is likely to receive attention in the future is the effect of endothelial cell function on cardiovascular regulation. Endothelial cells produce a variety of relaxing and contracting substances, some of which (e.g., endothelin) are known to influence afferent signaling and central baroreflex modulation.[120] Activation of the baroreflex is thought to release endothelin into plasma, possibly from the neurohypophysis.[121] Whether endothelin levels change with age is at present controversial.

Reactions of the cardiovascular system to physiologic stimuli such as meals or standing upright differ in the elderly compared to young people partly because age modifies the balance between the parasympathetic and sympathetic control systems.[122] In the elderly, there appears to be a progressive decline in parasympathetic function, which controls the initial heart rate response to standing. Splanchnic blood pooling and endocrine reactions after meals appear to produce hypotension because of cardiovascular modifications in old people. The main factors contributing to these different response patterns in arterial baroreflexes include reduced compliance of the vascular tree, impaired vagal activity, and decreased sympathetic nerve response to orthostatic stress.

Cardiopulmonary reflexes

Deformation of the cardiac chambers and pulmonary arteries and veins is sensed by mechanoreceptors in the walls, and together with arterial baroreceptors contributes to autonomic cardiovascular control. Like baroreflexes, cardiopulmonary reflexes provide a tonic inhibitory influence on the sympathetic control of the peripheral circulation.[123] They are also involved in restraint of sympathetic tone in the kidney and in release of renin, thereby contributing to both blood pressure and blood volume homeostasis.[124] Cardiopulmonary reflexes are found to be impaired in studies on aged humans[114] and animals.[125] The impaired ability of cardiopulmonary receptors to alter plasma renin activity in elderly subjects might be explained by the reduced responsiveness of juxtaglomerular cells to neural stimuli. Aging may affect the central nervous integration of cardiopulmonary reflexes, and signals originating from the cardiopulmonary volume receptors may be affected as the result of receptor degeneration. Elderly subjects show less change in left ventricular diastolic volume when central venous pressure is increased or decreased,[126] and so a reduction in cardiac distensibility may also be involved.

Investigation of Cardiovascular Autonomic Function

Few clinical tests of the integrity of the ANS can distinguish between pure sympathetic and parasympathetic abnormalities nor can the site of dysfunction in the afferent, central, or efferent pathways be clearly identified. Before reflex tests are undertaken, it is logical to identify whether there have been any alterations in the ability of the target organ(s) to react. There are nearly always age-related decrements in effector function that influence the interpretation of autonomic tests. In human studies, the normal interplay between different cardiovascular and cardiopulmonary reflexes makes it difficult to interpret reflex tests of autonomic function. A critical approach is essential and, if possible, the investigative technique should ensure that the reflex stimulus is as physiologic as possible; the stimulus-response relation should be defined completely, stimuli should be applied repeatedly and averaged, and the interventions should be brief and selective.[116] The outcome of proper assessments is important, for it has been suggested that the association of variables such as the increase in blood pressure and decrease in baroreflex function in the elderly may lead to greater cardiovascular morbidity and mortality.[127] Moderate cardiac vagal tone is regarded as protective, and high sympathetic tone tends to reduce ventricular stability. Sudden death has been reported in patients who have low baroreflex vagal activity.[128]

Sinus arrhythmia

During quiet respiration there is generally a shortening of the R-R interval of the electrocardiogram (ECG) with inspiration (increased heart rate) and a lengthening during expiration (decreased heart rate). The sinus arrhythmia is due to neural activity, the efferent limb being vagal. Two principal factors have been identified that are responsible for the generation of sinus arrhythmia: (1) central nervous interactions, for example, an overflow or irradiation of impulses from the respiratory center to the cardioinhibitory center, thereby diminishing vagal tone, and (2) cardiorespiratory reflexes evoked during respiratory movements.[129] The occurrence of sinus arrhythmia decreases with age,[118] as it does in patients with diabetic neuropathy. It does not follow, however, that this decrease is necessarily due to efferent vagal neuropathy. Many other factors can influence sinus arrhythmia, including reduced thoracic compliance, sinoatrial dysfunction, afferent neuropathy, cerebral damage, or even circulating antibodies to muscarinic receptors.

Heart rate response to standing or head-up tilt

In normal subjects, head-up tilt or standing results in minimal changes in blood pressure. In autonomic disorders, blood pressure often falls, and the degree and rapidity of fall and extent of recovery can vary considerably even within the same individual. A lack of increase in heart rate during postural change in the presence of a substantial fall in blood pressure is indicative of baroreflex abnormality, as in parasympathetic and sympathetic failure. Heart rate responsiveness to standing is diminished with age.[118,130] In young adults the increase may be nearly 20 beats per minute, and in middle and old age, 15 to 10 beats per minute. At least 10 minutes lying supine is necessary for baseline measurements. After standing, readings should be taken at 30 seconds if possible, and then at 2-minute intervals after standing for the next 10 minutes.[131] The short-term circulatory adaptation to the upright position has been arbitrarily divided into an initial phase (first 30 seconds), with marked changes in heart rate and blood pressure, and an early steady-state response (after 1 to 2 minutes standing). Prolonged standing is defined as at least 5 minutes upright.[132] (See also below discussion of orthostatic hypotension.)

Lower-body negative pressure

The application of lower-body negative pressure (LBNP) has been used to study reflexes from the heart and lungs. By pulling blood from the central circulation to the periphery, cardiac filling pressure is reduced and mechanoreceptors on the low-pressure side of the central circulation are stimulated. Physiologic responses include tachycardia, reduction in peripheral blood flow, and decreased cardiac output. A progressive LBNP test is generally well-tolerated by elderly people using suction of −20, −30, −40, and −50 mmHg, each applied for 2 minutes with intervening 3-minute control periods.[117,118] When small negative pressures are used, the central venous pressure can be reduced without a change in mean arterial pressure or pulse pressure. Thus, it is assumed that the activity of the arterial baroreceptors is unchanged.[133] Even small negative pressures (less than −10 mmHg) unload and thus stimulate cardiopulmonary baroreceptor afferents. This increases sympathetic neural activity in normal subjects but not in those with sympathetic vasoconstrictor failure, in whom blood pressure then rapidly falls.

Neck suction

The technique of neck suction to stimulate carotid baroreceptors is based on the principle that afferent baroreceptor traffic can be increased by either positive pressure inside or negative pressure outside a baroreceptor artery. Positive or negative pressure applied to a chamber fixed over or around the neck is transmitted to the carotid arteries in human subjects and provokes nearly linear reductions or increases in carotid artery diameter. Responses to baroreflex forcings are assessed with ECG R-R intervals, muscle sympathetic nerve activity, ventricular stroke volumes, and plasma neurotransmitter concentrations. The method has been used in studies on aging in subjects up to 60 years old.[114] A detailed critique of the method is given by Eckberg and Sleight.[116]

Valsalva maneuver

The Valsalva maneuver is commonly used to provide information about both the sympathetic and vagal baroreflex systems. The subject blows with an open glottis to maintain a

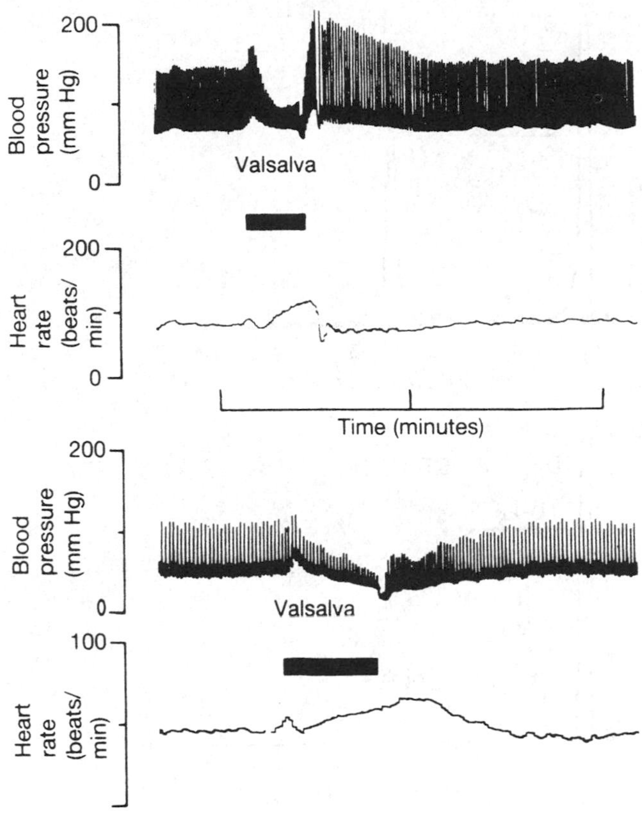

Figure 37-2 The effect of a Valsalva maneuver on intra-arterial blood pressure and heart rate in a normal subject (upper traces) and in a patient with autonomic dysfunction (lower traces). (From Mathias and Bannister,[134] with permission.)

forced expiratory pressure of 20 to 40 mmHg for 10 seconds. With the rise in intrathoracic pressure, the venous return to the heart falls, along with the blood pressure (Fig. 37-2). When intrathoracic pressure is released in a normal subject, there is a blood pressure overshoot because of the persistence of sympathetic activity. Baroreflex activation produces a secondary fall in heart rate to below baseline levels.[134] When there is autonomic dysfunction, the Valsalva maneuver results in a continual fall in blood pressure with no stabilization, and after release there is no blood pressure overshoot or compensatory bradycardia. Although often used as a standard test of autonomic function, the Valsalva maneuver is an extremely complex test dependent on the mechanical status of the circulation, the integrity of several populations of autonomic receptors, central autonomic interactions, and efferent sympathetic and parasympathetic effectors.[116]

Pressor tests

A number of techniques are employed to stimulate sympathetic efferent pathways and raise blood pressure. These include isometric exercise and the application of a cold stimulus to a hand (cold pressor test). There is often an important cerebral component, and the use of stimuli such as a sudden noise or mental arithmetic is dependent predominantly on cerebral stimulation. The cold pressor test requires the hand to be immersed in cold water at 4°C for up to 10 minutes,[135] which is unlikely to be suitable for most elderly patients. Muscle sympathetic activity is influenced by the cold pressor test, and there is a positive correlation between the frequency of sympathetic bursts in muscle nerves and plasma concentrations of noradrenaline in forearm venous blood.[136]

Facial cooling

Facial cooling induced by immersion of the face in cold water, facial contact with an ice bag or gel pack, or convective cooling with cold air initiates the cardiovascular changes seen in the "diving response."[137] Receptors in the nasal mucosa and face innervated by the trigeminal nerve initiate a bradycardia and an increase in total peripheral resistance. Convective cooling of the face by a cold air stream has been found to be an acceptable test in healthy elderly people.[117] With facial cooling, cardiac vagal efferents and sympathetic vascular responses can be tested while avoiding the cardiopulmonary reflexes involved in breath-holding diving responses.

Sympathetic microneurography

The function of the efferent limb of an autonomic reflex may be measured directly by microneurography. Recordings of cardiac vagal traffic in humans have not been made, but it has been possible to obtain direct measurements of previously inaccessible postganglionic muscle and skin sympathetic nerve activity with safety.[138,139] Cutaneous sympathetic activity is affected principally by thermal stimuli, in contrast to muscle sympathetic activity which responds to maneuvers activating baroreceptors and is time-locked to blood pressure changes within the cardiac cycle.

Power spectral analysis

The phenomenon of rhythmic fluctuations in cardiovascular variables such as heart rate and blood pressure has led to computer techniques for quantifying the oscillations based on Fourier transformations. In humans, assessment of autonomic function by spectral analysis provides a quantitative, noninvasive means of analyzing short-term cardiovascular autonomic control mechanisms. Heart rate variability due to rhythmic fluctuations is mainly the result of autonomic nervous influences, and this can be measured in a frequency-specific way. By using specific blocking agents, fluctuations in heart rate occurring at about 0.25 Hz high frequency [HF]) appear to be related to vagal-cardiac activity, while fluctuations at about 0.10 Hz (low frequency [LF]) seem to be determined by both vagal and sympathetic outflows. Relative LF power and the LF/HF ratio take account of sympathovagal interactions, while absolute LF power is considered to be mainly a marker of sympathetic function. LF fluctuations in supine subjects appear to be mediated entirely by the parasympathetic nervous system. On standing, the LF fluctuations increase and are jointly mediated by both autonomic divisions (Fig. 37-3).

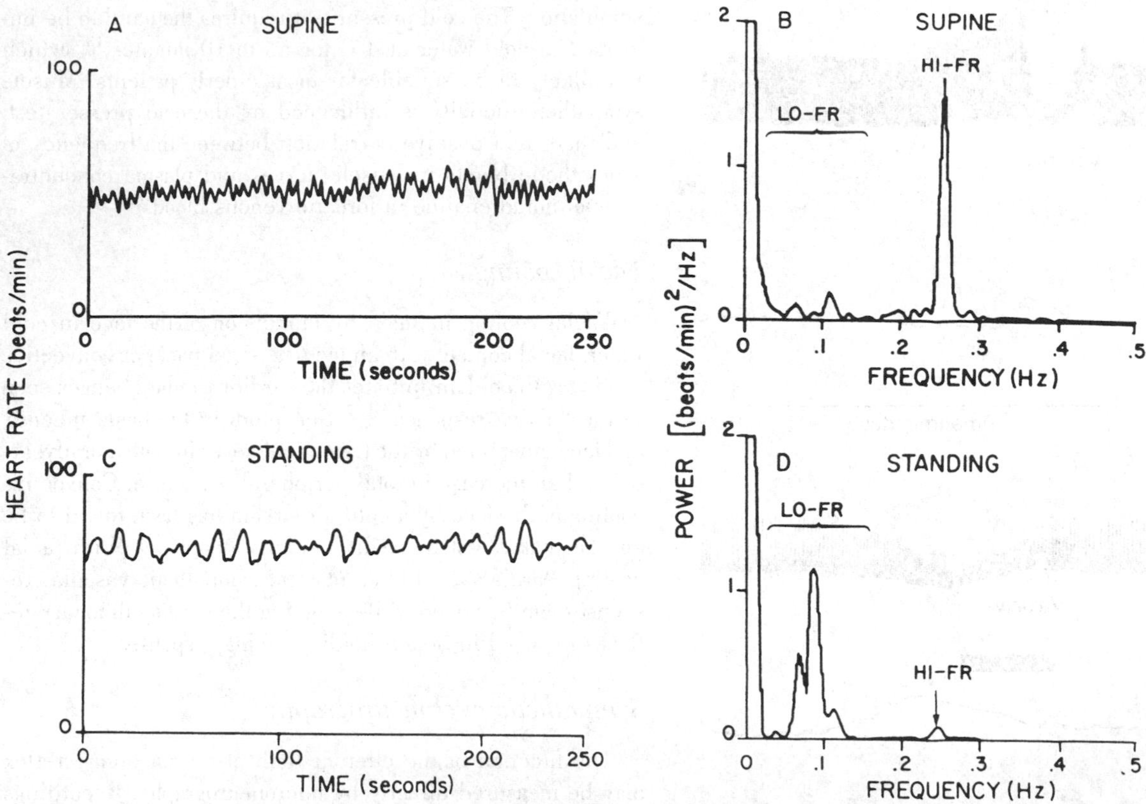

Figure 37-3 Assessment of autonomic function by heart rate spectral analysis in a young adult. (**A**) Heart rate in supine position showing high-frequency oscillations (respiratory sinus arrhythmia). (**B**) Power spectrum of A, with a small low-frequency (LO-FR) peak and large high-frequency (HI-FR) peak. (**C**) Heart rate on standing showing low-frequency oscillations. (**D**) Power spectrum of B, with prominent LO-FR peak and small HI-FR peak. (From Pomeranz et al.,[140] with permission.)

Comparison of heart rate variability in supine and upright positions in healthy young and elderly subjects has shown that spectral power in the LF and HF components is significantly lower in diabetic patients and healthy elderly subjects.[141] An important potential advantage of spectral analysis of R-R interval power lies in the possibility that this approach can be used to estimate the levels of sympathetic-cardiac nerve traffic, and this has been applied in studies on elderly subjects.[142] It may be that power spectral analysis is a more sensitive indicator of baroreflex control, particularly of vagal control, than the direct evidence of autonomic imbalance.[143] A disadvantage is that the technique may not have been validated adequately. Direct comparisons need to be made between recordings of sympathetic and vagal-cardiac traffic with measurements derived from spectral analysis.

Orthostatic Hypotension

Orthostatic (postural) hypotension occurs frequently in elderly people. It is recognized as a cardinal feature of autonomic nervous dysfunction, although there are also other nonneurogenic etiologies. Arterial blood pressure is strongly dependent on cardiac filling, and body fluid volume expansion is therefore a primary measure in alleviating orthostatic hypotension. The syndrome is often linked to recurrent falls and resultant injury. It is arbitrarily defined as a decrease of more than 20 mmHg systolic blood pressure, and sometimes the definition also includes a decrease of more than 10 mmHg diastolic blood pressure. Orthostatic hypotension can be asymptomatic when cerebral autoregulation maintains normal cerebral blood flow.[144] The prevalence has been reported to range from 5 to 30 percent in elderly people,[145] with the higher proportion in those over 75 years and in old people in institutional care. An overall prevalence of 10 percent is more likely in elderly people living in the community. In an analysis of 50 cases of orthostatic hypotension, only 14 percent had overtly postural symptoms,[146] and it is therefore a condition that can easily be overlooked. A 10-year follow-up to determine prognostic importance in the elderly showed that diastolic, but not systolic, blood pressure predicted excess cardiovascular mortality.[147] However, this relationship disappeared in the multivariate analysis, suggesting that the association was apparently related to background factors such as cardiovascular disease. Very old people with multiple pathology are at high risk of orthostatic hypotension, falls, and associated morbidity and mortality.

Pathophysiology

Maintenance of blood pressure depends on a number of factors including (1) structural factors of the heart and blood vessels involved in maintaining cardiac output and peripheral resistance, (2) circulating hormones such as the renin-angiotensin-aldosterone system, (3) intravascular volume, and (4) activity of autonomic reflexes. Impairment of any one or more of these components during a head-up postural change may threaten blood pressure homeostasis. In elderly patients with chronic cardiovascular medical conditions reduced cardiac volume and impaired early diastolic filling contribute.[148] Since some patients have marked reduction in pulse pressure on standing, venous pooling is likely to be involved,[149] and consideration should be given to possible functional deficiencies in the skeletal muscle pump in the lower limbs.

On standing, about 700 mL of blood normally leaves the thorax and is rapidly pooled in the venous reservoirs of the abdomen and legs. The pressure in the right atrium falls to or below the mean intrathoracic pressure, and there is diminished return of blood to the right side of the heart. Cardiopulmonary and arterial baroreflexes are thus activated to normalize blood pressure. It is likely that arterial (primarily diastolic) hypotension mediates increases in sympathetic nerve activity during standing.[116] In maintaining blood pressure during orthostasis, increases in sympathetic vasoconstrictor activity to the splanchnic and skeletal muscle vessels is arguably the most crucial.[150] There are age-related changes in muscle sympathetic nerve activity (MSA). In the supine position, MSA increases with age, but on standing there is less of an increase in MSA bursts compared to that in young subjects. Supine hypertension, however, is apparently not related to the development or degree of orthostatic hypotension in the elderly.[151]

Nonneurogenic causes of orthostatic hypotension (other than the effects of drugs) may fall into three categories: the effects of cardiac impairment (e.g., from aortic stenosis or cardiomyopathy), low intravascular volume (e.g., from fluid loss or from renal or endocrine causes such as Addison's disease), and excessive vasodilatation (e.g., from the effects of heat or alcohol). It has been postulated that a change in vascular distensibility is sufficient to explain the postural fall in blood pressure.[152] This theory has received some support from the finding that changes in plasma noradrenaline levels, as a marker of sympathetic nerve activity, were normal in a sample of elderly people with orthostatic hypotension.[153] Loss of elasticity of arterial walls with aging has been well-documented, and a loss of baroreflex sensitivity could be explained by changes in arterial distensibility. Although diminished sensitivity of baroreceptors has been suggested,[154] experiments on humans and animals have provided little evidence of selective degeneration of the baroreceptor organs in arterial walls.

Autonomic responses to standing have been related to changes in plasma noradrenaline level.[155] Standing evokes a diffuse increase in sympathetic nervous activity with enhanced release of noradrenaline. However, an increase in the level of plasma noradrenaline on standing is not found in some patients with orthostatic hypotension.[156] The similarity in neurohumoral responses during tilt tests on normal elderly and on those with orthostatic hypotension suggested that there was target organ failure rather than autonomic failure. In patients who had orthostatic hypotension and supine hypertension, it was found that measures of cardiopulmonary volume and systemic vascular resistance differentiated between venous pooling and autonomic insufficiency but that head-up tilt tests and plasma catecholamine measurements did not.[157]

Drugs are a major cause of orthostatic hypotension in the elderly. Many have effects on the ANS, both centrally and peripherally, and on fluid balance. Important among drugs with hypotensive effects are diuretics, calcium channel blockers, nitrates, L-dopa, phenothiazines, and antidepressants (even in low dosage).[158] Alcohol and drugs such as vincristine can cause autonomic neuropathy.

Clinical features and diagnosis

Orthostatic hypotension occurs in many elderly people, even when they are not taking medication or have no obvious disease in which hypotension is a complication. When cerebral autoregulation fails, possibly as the result of cerebrovascular disease, or if the fall in blood pressure on standing is excessive, the patient complains of weakness, faintness, dizziness, loss of balance, or blacking out. Symptoms are brought on by common activities of daily life such as rapid standing or standing after prolonged recumbency especially in a warm environment, raised intrathoracic pressure during swallowing or coughing, straining during micturition or defecation, and physical exertion. A common clinical picture is that of a patient whose legs give way when an attempt is made to stand. This is associated with clouding of consciousness, confusion, pallor, cyanosis, tremor, unsteadiness, and finally loss of consciousness. Symptoms are usually worse in the morning and on rising. Impairment in other systems under autonomic control such as defective sweating, impotence, and urinary bladder disturbance favors a neurogenic cause.[159] Orthostatic hypotension can also rarely induce transient ischemic attacks with focal signs.[160] Nocturnal polyuria and natriuresis can cause a substantial overnight fluid loss, and this contributes to low blood pressure in the morning. Some patients experience the symptoms of orthostatic hypotension for a considerable time after getting up.

There are three main modes of presentation in the elderly: falls or mobility problems, acute or chronic mental confusion, and predominantly cardiac symptoms. Medication was found to be responsible for orthostatic hypotension in 66 percent of patients in one study, and striking examples of polypharmacy were encountered in many patients.[146] However, there is probably an overestimation of the prevalence of orthostatic hypotension, defined as a decline in systolic blood pressure of 20 mmHg, because of variations in standardization of procedures in standing or tilt-table tests.[131,161] Many of the problems of blood pressure recording, including observer bias, may be resolved by using an automatic recording device. A Finapres system, which measures finger arterial pressure (with good agreement with intra-arterial pressure) is suitable for elderly patients.[162]

Management

There are several general and specific approaches to the management of orthostatic hypotension, most of which have their limitations. Treatment is first directed toward rectifying the underlying cause, and if drugs are responsible, they should be withdrawn or the dose reduced. Nonneurogenic causes such as diminished intravascular volume should be dealt with specifically. In orthostatic hypotension due to autonomic failure, there are considerable difficulties in attempting to re-establish the role of sympathetic or parasympathetic efferent activity.[163]

General measures Initially, the patient should be instructed to avoid situations that may worsen the condition; for example, small frequent meals can reduce postprandial hypotension, and hot baths or bathing when alone at home should be avoided. Pooling of blood in the lower extremities when standing can be limited by mechanical means such as wearing an antigravity suit or elastic stocking.[164] Stockings should not be taken off at night, lest patients fall when getting out of bed. Simple maneuvers such as crossing the legs, tensing the calf muscles, and abdominal compression are also useful as a temporary means of overcoming symptoms[165] but are not possible for all elderly patients. Head-up tilt at night (by as much as 10 degrees or as much as can be tolerated) is a useful procedure, particularly in combination with fludrocortisone therapy.[166] Orthostatic tolerance can sometimes be developed by "training" baroreflexes by frequent changes of posture. Cardiac pacing designed to sense a patient's fall in blood pressure when sitting and augmenting the heart rate accordingly has been used to prevent syncope on standing.[167] Pacing does not normally have a place in management except for severe refractory orthostatic hypotension of neural origin.

Drug treatment The wide range of drugs employed in treatment of the condition, in spite of known serious drug side effects, implies that orthostatic hypotension is difficult to treat successfully. A difficult therapeutic dilemma occurs, for example, in patients who suffer from supine hypertension in addition to orthostatic hypotension.[168] Ambulatory monitoring may be a useful technique for assessing a therapeutic effect.[169] A number of different therapeutic approaches have been used, of which the following are most commonly employed.

1. *Expansion of blood volume*: The expansion of circulatory volume by mineralocorticoids such as fludrocortisone is often used, although this drug (along with many others) is not specifically licensed for treatment of orthostatic hypotension.[163] Fludrocortisone is nevertheless a first-line drug, starting with 100 to 200 μg/day and preferably given at night. The high doses often required to be effective may lead to supine hypertension, ankle edema, and hypokalemia and may even precipitate cardiac failure. In patients with nocturnal polyuria, especially that associated with bladder dysfunction, nocturnal use of the vasopressin-V2 receptor agonist desmopressin (5 to 40 μg intranasally) can be of value in reducing orthostatic hypotension.[170]
2. *Increased vasoconstriction*: Sympathomimetics such as ephedrine, initially 15 mg tds, with the first dose being given before getting up in the morning, produce an increase in vascular resistance and in venous tone. With higher doses, adverse effects include CNS stimulation, tachycardia, and tremor. In the elderly it can give rise to acute retention of urine even in small doses and is, therefore best avoided. Because of these indirect effects, ephedrine is more useful in central autonomic disorders.[171] In peripheral autonomic dysfunction, mididrone, an α agonist with selective vasoconstrictor properties, is more likely to be effective.[172] It can, however, produce supine hypertension. Dihydroergotamine, an α-adrenergic agonist, has been shown to produce significant improvement in orthostatic hypotension when given as 2 mg tds. The effects are due to a powerful, relatively selective constrictor action on venous capacity reservoirs in the peripheral circulation.[173] The low, erratic bioavailability of oral preparations has, however, hindered its use. After excluding patients with coronary or peripheral artery disease, successful treatment of orthostatic hypotension has been reported with the use of inhaled dihydroergotamine,[174] and no side effects were recorded.
3. *Increased cardiac output*: Drugs that block β-adrenoreceptors but also have partial sympathomimetic activity, such as pindolol[175] and xamoterol,[176] may improve orthostatic hypotension by increasing cardiac output. Early reported benefits of these drugs have not been confirmed, and there are potential dangers in using them, particularly with elderly patients.
4. *Reduced vasodilatation*: Drugs that inhibit the vasodilator activity of prostaglandins have been helpful in improving orthostatic hypotension and raising systemic vascular resistance. Prostaglandin synthetase inhibitors such as indomethacin[177] and flurbiprofen[178] have been used, but they have side effects including gastrointestinal intolerance and hemorrhage, which may exclude them from use in many elderly patients. Somatostatin analogs (e.g., octreotide), which act by blocking vasodilator peptides including those released following food ingestion, and caffeine, have been advocated for the treatment of postprandial hypotension.
5. *Other more recent treatments*: Dopamine receptor blocking agents such as domperidone have been used to help patients in whom hypotension has been enhanced by L-dopa or bromocriptine. The value of erythropoietin in increasing red cell mass has been described in patients with mild to moderate anemia associated with orthostatic hypotension.[179] Orthostatic dizziness improved during treatment, and mean

systolic and diastolic blood pressure did not increase significantly in the supine position. Possible long-term effects, however, are not known. There is a possibility that the increase in red cell mass may increase vulnerability to stroke and myocardial infarction.

Postprandial Hypotension

Postprandial reduction in systolic blood pressure may predispose some elderly people to symptomatic hypotension and produce syncope and falls.[180] There is a large increase in splanchnic blood flow after eating a meal, as has been demonstrated by noninvasive measurements of superior mesenteric artery blood flow.[181] Insulin can lower blood pressure substantially in autonomic failure, and it seems likely that it causes the splanchnic vasodilatation. A decrease in total systemic vascular resistance, a reduction in venous return to the heart, a reduction in stroke volume and cardiac output, and postprandial hypotension may result, especially in the elderly and in patients with ANS dysfunction who have impaired sympathetic reflex activity.[182] An effective drug in preventing postprandial hypotension is the somatostatin analog octreotide, a synthetic, long-acting, peptide release inhibitor.[183] It reduces postprandial hypotension even in low dosages (25 to 50 μg twice a day subcutaneously). Abdominal colic and diarrhea are adverse side effects. Octreotide prevents the rise in insulin, neurotensin, and a range of other hormones in response to food, but it has no effect on cardiac output or muscle or skin blood flow, suggesting that it prevents postprandial hypotension largely by exerting its effect on the splanchnic vasculature.

Temperature Regulation

The ANS fulfills three principal roles in thermoregulation: control of thermoregulatory neuroeffector systems, contributing to the neural control of metabolic heat production, and central hypothalamic control of body temperature.

Neuroeffector Systems

Physiologic regulation of heat loss or gain from the skin surface depends largely on sympathetic vasomotor and sudomotor activity. A reduced capacity to vasoconstrict in the cold[2,184] and reduced vasodilatation in the heat[185] are key factors in reducing the efficiency of thermoregulation in elderly people. However, diminished vasomotor responses do not necessarily signify that there is dysfunctional autonomic neural control. It has been shown, for example, that the sensitivity of peripheral blood vessels to vasoconstrictor and vasodilator substances is reduced with advancing age.[186] It has also been found that, in cold environments, peripheral blood flow decreases less in elderly people who demonstrate reduced blood vessel compliance, and these changes are exaggerated in elderly patients with arteriosclerosis and peripheral vascular disease.[187] Similarly, reduced sweating responses in elderly people can be explained by effector organ dysfunction accompanying senile atrophy of the skin and peripheral detraining of sweat glands as well as regressive changes in peripheral sympathetic nerves.[13]

Metabolic Heat Production

As the proportion of body mass made up of functionally active cells is reduced with age, a decline in basal metabolic rate and total heat production follow. Shivering, an important component in thermogenesis under cold conditions, is, however, under the control of somatic rather than autonomic nerves. Shivering ability is not lost with age, but changes occur in the efficiency and intensity of shivering, probably as the result of reduction in muscle bulk and changes in fast and slow muscle motor units. The sympathetic and sympathoadrenal systems, on the other hand, provide control of nonshivering thermogenesis. Sympathetic nerves can directly affect metabolic activity by increasing hepatic glycogenolysis (e.g., in hypoglycemia) and by regulating blood flow in adipose tissue.[188] The thermogenic effect of food is a relatively small but potentially important component of total daily energy turnover. It varies with factors such as obesity, anaerobic fitness, insulin resistance, and meal composition, and it has been shown to be significantly lower in elderly people.[189] In particular, the facultative component of the thermogenic reaction is associated with the sympathetic nervous response to a meal, and this may be reduced as part of a decrease in autonomic function attributable to old age.

Central Nervous Control

Little is known about possible changes in the threshold of response or sensitivity of the hypothalamic control system in the elderly, although indirect evidence from studies on thermal comfort, behavioral thermoregulation, circadian temperature rhythms, and effects of changes in sleep-wake cycles indicate alterations in the integrative function of the CNS.[190] Desynchronization of circadian rhythms occurs more frequently in old age,[191] and some studies have concluded that temperature rhythm variables such as phase and amplitude are altered in elderly patients with Alzheimer's disease.[192,193] It is known that serotonin (5-hydroxytryptamine) is a key modulator of thermoregulation in the preoptic region of the hypothalamus and that deficits in serotoninergic neurons occur in Alzheimer's disease.[194] There are decreases in other neuropeptides in the brain that participate in central thermoregulatory control. It may, therefore, be expected that widespread disruption of circadian rhythms, including body temperature, will occur in advanced Alzheimer's disease. However, elderly patients with mild Alzheimer's disease studied in a carefully health screened community showed that entrainment of temperature rhythm was little affected.[195]

Hypothermia in the Elderly

Reduced efficiency of autonomic thermoregulatory responses in elderly people leads to greater sensitivity to cold environments[196] and sometimes to hypothermia. Recent experience suggests that the prevalence of hypothermia in the United Kingdom is much less than that predicted in the 1960s. Present statistics on hypothermia as a cause of mortality in England and Wales, mostly among elderly patients, imply that hypothermic deaths amount to only about 1 percent of excess winter mortality.[197] The registration of deaths from hypothermia, however, presents difficulties because of the uncertainty as to whether hypothermia is a primary or a secondary event.[196] Hypothermia includes all conditions associated with a deep body temperature of less than 35°C (95°F). Primary hypothermia arising from inherent impairment of the central nervous control of thermoregulation is rare in elderly people; secondary hypothermia associated with central or peripheral pathology or other medical conditions, and accidental hypothermia from the effects of cold exposure are the more common forms of presentation. Many elderly individuals display an unresponsive attitude toward cold, partly because of blunted thermal perception, and this is aggravated by reduced mobility and mild confusional states affecting behavioral thermoregulation. Centrally acting drugs most commonly associated with hypothermia in old people include psychotropics (notably phenothiazines), hypnotics, anxiolytics, and antidepressants.[198] Alcohol predisposes to hypothermia by virtue of its properties as a vasodilator, a CNS depressant, an anesthetic, a cause of hypoglycemia, and a risk factor for trauma and environmental exposure.

Pathophysiology

Low deep body temperature can develop because of extrinsic (environmental) and intrinsic (physiologic) factors which act to increase heat loss from the body surface and/or reduce production and conservation of heat. Many elderly hypothermic patients are found in their own homes after an accidental fall. Thinness or undernutrition is thought to impair thermoregulation and predispose to injury, especially fracture, due to accidental falls.[199] Secondary hypothermia may accompany autonomic dysfunction in metabolic disorders such as diabetes mellitus and neurologic disorders, for example, Parkinsonism, Wernicke's encephalopathy, and cerebrovascular disease. There is often a marked deterioration in vital functions, especially in association with malnutrition or existing illness or infection. It is something of a paradox that infection can be linked with hypothermia. Infections were thought to be the immediate cause of hypothermia in a large proportion of elderly cases reviewed in a Jerusalem hospital.[200] Mortality was high (74 percent), and the hypothermic patients were often critically ill, cachectic, and poorly nourished. A third of these patients developed hypothermia during the warm season. A similar high incidence of hypothermia in elderly patients with infections has been observed in a U.K. hospital.[201] A spontaneous fall in deep body temperature can occur during the course of overwhelming general infection, and hypothalamic dysfunction may be the common link between various infectious disorders and hypothermia. It may also be seen in vascular or degenerative lesions of the hypothalamus or in primary hypothyroidism or hypopituitarism.

Clinical features and diagnosis

Clinical presentation of hypothermia depends on the rate of decline and extent of the lowering of body temperature. At first a confusional state is usually a salient feature. Drowsiness is also apparent, and when body temperature drops below 32°C (90°F), there is a gradual loss of consciousness. With a slow progression of the condition, the patient develops a grey color due to pallor and cyanosis, a distinct doughy consistency of subcutaneous tissues, and a "myxoedematous" appearance. Normally warm regions of the body such as the abdomen, axillae, and groin feel cold. The heart rate slows as a result of the direct effect of low core temperature, and there is sinus bradycardia or slow atrial fibrillation. Shivering is replaced by generalized muscular rigidity, and vital signs become unrecordable. Acute pancreatitis is commonly found at postmortem, though few typical signs are evident in the hypothermic patient.

The diagnosis can be established by measuring the rectal temperature using a low-reading clinical thermometer. Examination usually reveals bradycardia, hypotension, slow and shallow respiration, diminished tendon reflexes, and absent or reduced bowel sounds. The ECG may show some degree of heart block with an increase in PR interval in patients in sinus rhythm, and there is a delay in intraventricular conduction. The appearance of a J-wave (Osborn wave), a characteristic deflection at the junction of the QRS and ST segments, is typical but not pathognomic since it has been reported in normothermic patients.[202] Gastric dilatation is frequently present, and there is a risk of aspiration of gastric contents. Renal blood flow, glomerular filtration, and tubular function are impaired, and acute tubular necrosis may occur. Hemoglobin and hematocrit values may be raised because of a decrease in plasma volume. Body temperature has a marked effect on the partial pressure of blood gases. A 1°C (2°F) drop in the temperature of blood sealed in an anaerobic environment lowers the $PaCO_2$ by 4.4 percent, and the PaO_2 by 6 percent.

Management

Slow surface rewarming using blankets in a warm room at about 25°C (77°F) is the method usually employed in treating elderly patients. The patient is warmed gradually at the rate of a 0.5°C (1°F) rise in core temperature per hour. The rectal temperature is monitored continuously, together with ECG and blood pressure taken at 30-minute intervals. Other general measures include protection of the airway, correction of fluid and electrolyte balance, and intravenous broad-spectrum antibiotics which should be given routinely as bronchopneumonia is difficult to diagnose in these cases. Thyroid hormone replacement is given when there is definite evidence of hypothyroidism. If the blood pressure falls as the core temperature rises, the patient is immediately cooled by fans and rewarmed again after the blood pressure is stabilized.[203] Although rapid, active warming of the body surface and internal warming by intravenous and irrigation fluids can be practized in young adults with accidental hypothermia, such procedures are hazardous in the elderly and can lead to circulatory collapse. The initial "after-drop" in core temperature with rapid warming may precipitate hypotension and cardiac dysrhythmias. At some centers, however, active warming of even elderly patients in an intensive care unit has been successful.[204] During rewarming, arrhythmias are the most dangerous complication, ventricular fibrillation occurring most frequently at and below deep body temperatures of 28°C (83°F). Extracorporeal blood rewarming using a heat exchanger has been effectively used in such severe cases. Mortality in hypothermia is often due to associated illnesses, but recovery is possible even in advanced old age.

Hyperthermia in the elderly

Heat-related illnesses can occur in urbanized communities during heat waves in temperate areas, as well as in tropical and subtropical regions.[205] In the United States about 4,000 deaths a year are attributed to heat-related illnesses, and 80 percent of these deaths are in persons over 50 years of age, especially the elderly. In one study in St. Louis and Kansas City during the 1980 summer heat wave, the heat stroke rate in persons aged 65 years or more was 12 to 13 times that in the remainder of the population. Consequently, urban risk factors for heat-related illness in the elderly have been the subject of special study.[206] For the United Kingdom annual total death rates registered as due to excessive heat are usually in single figures. Thermoregulatory impairment due to diminished sweating and peripheral vasodilatation in older people is thought to be one of the factors responsible for heatstroke under hot conditions. In addition to autonomic dysfunction, physiologic factors controlling water balance, the secretion of and renal response to vasopressin, and the control of sodium balance and osmolality, all crucial in the response to heat stress, may be altered by age. There are dangers in prescribing psychotropic drugs under hot conditions, particularly phenothiazines which interfere with central and peripheral thermoregulation, and anticholinergic drugs which decrease sweating.[198] Elderly patients are often treated with diuretics, which is a risk factor for dehydration and electrolyte disturbances under hot conditions. Active management to reduce core temperature includes placing the patient in a cool room, removing clothing, tepid water sponging, and creating air movement. Excess heat wave deaths in the aged population are usually due to the effects of increased cardiovascular strain in patients with ischemic heart or cerebrovascular disease.[207]

Blunted or absent fever responses to infections have been reported in approximately 30 percent of geriatric patients with bacteremia.[208] Experimental evidence from animals suggests age-related impairments in fever induced by exogenous pyrogens and an attenuated response to leukocyte-derived endogenous pyrogen.[209] Tumor necrosis factor α, a powerful endogenous pyrogen thought capable of causing fever by acting on the hypothalamus and by stimulating the synthesis of interleukin-1, causes a significantly greater rate of increase and a higher peak temperature in young than in old animals.[210]

The Gastrointestinal System

There is general agreement that the parasympathetic innervation of the digestive tract is primarily excitatory, and that of the sympathetic system, inhibitory. It has become apparent that a third division of the ANS, the enteric nervous system, provides the important autonomous control of the entire gut from esophagus to anorectum. The enteric nervous system consists of the intrinsic nerve plexuses, the myenteric plexus (Auerbach's plexus), and the submucous plexus (Meissner's plexus). This intrinsic system supplies all the motor innervation of the smooth muscle of the gut, but sensory information is transmitted not only to the enteric nervous system but also from it via the sympathetic and parasympathetic divisions to the CNS. Experimental evidence points to the conclusion that the enteric nervous system provides not only the motor neurons for the smooth muscle but control circuitry containing the program of motor activity.[211] Periodic gastrointestinal motor activity is an expression of the activity of the enteric nervous system.

Autonomic Dysfunction

Although autonomic control is important in terms of gut motility, there is good evidence for autonomic control of secretion, absorption, and blood flow in the gastrointestinal tract. However, changes in motor activity have been demonstrated most often.[211] Motility disturbances are seen in Parkinsonism[212] and with autonomic neuropathy in alcoholism. The presence of Lewy bodies in the myenteric plexus of the esophagus and colon in Parkinson's disease suggests that the disease may also affect the enteric nervous system. Diffuse esophageal spasm (presbyesophagus) has been described as an abnormality associated with aging.

In general, autonomic dysfunction results in delay or arrest of transit through the bowel. Since this resembles intestinal obstruction due to mechanical obstruction as occurs with tumors or volvulus, the condition is often referred to as pseudo-obstruction. The clinical presentation of complete or relative pseudo-obstruction varies according to the region(s) affected.[211]

- *Esophagus*: dysphagia, regurgitation, retention of food in the esophagus, aspiration pneumonia
- *Stomach*: epigastric fullness, vomiting
- *Small bowel*: distension, colic, constipation, diarrhea secondary to bacterial overgrowth, malnutrition due to bacterial overgrowth
- *Large intestine*: distension, colic, constipation, diarrhea.

It is difficult to determine whether the enteric nervous system or the parasympathetic and sympathetic system is responsible for the functional deficit. Primary pseudo-obstruction refers to disease confined to the bowel wall that is not associated with disease elsewhere, that is, involving only the enteric nervous system. The presence of normal periodic activity provides evidence of the relative integrity of the enteric nervous system, and its absence strongly suggests dysfunction of the enteric nervous system.

Diarrhea due to autonomic neuropathy may be suspected when other common causes of diarrhea and fecal incontinence have been excluded. Nocturnal or early morning diarrhea occurs in some patients with autonomic dysfunction. Diabetic diarrhea is associated with bacterial overgrowth, and abnormalities of small bowel motility have been reported.[213]

Delayed colonic transit time through the cecum and large intestine has been associated with aging in animal studies.[214] Reduced responsiveness to neurotransmitters and a deficit in gut innervation suggest a possible basis for delayed transit. In other investigations on aged guinea pigs, a marked reduction in myenteric neuron number has also been observed.[6]

Irritable bowel syndrome is a disorder associated with young and middle-aged patients. Its existence as a disease entity remains a matter of debate, and it is diagnosed only reluctantly in the elderly. The syndrome is characterized by irregular defecation, abdominal pain, bloating, and stool mucus. There are no good studies relating age to colonic motility; in the young the symptoms are ascribed to irritable colon syndrome and in the elderly to diverticular disease. It is probably premature to characterize irritable bowel syndrome as an autonomic dysfunction, but it does seem that autonomic dysfunction is at least a component of this syndrome. The role of the ANS has been supported by findings that associate cholinergic abnormality with a constipation-predominant subgroup, and adrenergic abnormality with diarrhea predominance.[215]

The Urogenital System

Renal Sympathetic Nerve Activity

Under physiologic conditions, basal efferent sympathetic nerve activity appears to be too low to influence renal hemodynamics. When renal sympathetic activity is elevated above baseline, however, its effect on renal hemodynamics can be profound. Nerves within the cortical microcirculation have been localized to both the afferent and efferent glomerular arterioles. Renal nerve stimulation decreases single-nephron glomerular filtration rate and single-nephron plasma flow.[216] In investigations of renal sympathetic nerve activity with aging, a more marked increase in activity has been recorded in older animals than is expected from impairment of arterial and cardiopulmonary baroreflexes.[119,125] It is known that activation of left atrial mechanoreceptors (cardiopulmonary volume receptors) decreases renal sympathetic nerve traffic[216] so that impairment of cardiopulmonary reflexes with age might have caused the greater renal sympathetic nerve outflow. The increase in baseline renal sympathetic nerve activity, however, appears to represent a true increase in central sympathetic drive, probably of central origin, and it is consistent with increased muscle sympathetic nerve activity which is related to age in humans.[217] The finding of an elevated renal sympathetic outflow to the kidney may partly account for the diminished glomerular filtration rate and renal blood flow observed with advancing age.[218]

Renal sympathetic nerve activity also stimulates juxtaglomerular β-adrenergic receptors to release renin. However, it is also found that levels of plasma renin fall with age, and the response of elderly subjects to orthostasis or salt depletion is less than in younger subjects. Basal renin levels in plasma are estimated to be diminished by 30 to 50 percent in older persons,[219] and changes in renin activity accompanying cardiopulmonary reflex stimulation are reduced.[114] The impaired ability of increased renal sympathetic nerve activity to alter plasma renin that characterizes older individuals might be explained by reduced responsiveness of juxtaglomerular cells to neural stimuli.[144]

Lower Urinary Tract Dysfunction

Disturbances of micturition occur commonly in patients with autonomic dysfunction which may be due to aging processes and/or to neuropathology. Patients suffering from progressive autonomic failure with primary degeneration of autonomic neurons show a characteristic inability to contract the distal urethral sphincter.[220] Detrusor instability can be due to abnormalities of detrusor muscle activity and/or neural control.[221] Elderly patients with atonic bladder were found to have marked autonomic impairment.[222] A general reduction in the number of autonomic nerves in detrusor smooth muscle has also been observed.[223] Since there is no treatment to restore autonomic innervation to the bladder, the management of urinary dysfunction arising from autonomic failure is essentially symptomatic. The autonomic nervous supply to the lower urinary tract illustrates some of the most remarkable examples of plasticity.[224] For example, the number of autonomic axon profiles per square millimeter of detrusor muscle decreases with age in humans and is matched by a linear decrease in the density of acetylcholinesterase-positive fibers in the bladder.[3] These changes may involve nerve redistribution or transmitter and receptor expression leading to rearrangement of nerve pathways and altered function in pathologic or normal physiologic conditions such as aging. In disease states involving lower motor spinal cord lesions, the expression of these transmitters changes, and there appears to be some form of reorganization of the innervation of the bladder.[225]

Drug therapy for detrusor instability and hyperreflexia has focused largely on muscarinic receptor antagonists, particularly those that have greater specificity and fewer side effects. The muscarinic subtype responsible for contracting the bladder has been identified by using pharmacologic antagonist studies combined with immunoprecipitation and ligand binding techniques.[226]

Erectile Dysfunction

Impotence is principally a disorder of older men; a substantial level of impotence has been reported in association with medical disorders such as diabetes mellitus and neurologic diseases affecting the ANS.[227] Penile erection is a complex behavioral response dependent on the integration of vascular, endocrine, and neurologic mechanisms. Details of many aspects of the neurohumoral control of erection are still uncertain, but three types of peripheral nerves—lumbar sympathetic, sacral parasympathetic, and somatic—together with various populations of neurons in the CNS appear to be involved. The central and peripheral neural pathways are sensitive to the hormonal environment and depend on a variety of transmitters including monoamines, amino acids, acetylcholine, and neuropeptides. Neurologic disease and pelvic surgery may affect potency by interrupting autonomic fibers of the nervi erigentes. In recent years these pathways have been traced in humans so that even radical prostatectomy can be carried out with preservation of potency.[228] Diabetes mellitus is one of the most common causes of erectile failure. The prevalence of erectile impotence is about 50 percent in unselected diabetics, increasing with age to reach 98 percent in patients attending a geriatric diabetic clinic.[229] Several processes may contribute, including large vessel disease, microangiopathy and autonomic neuropathy, as well as psychogenic factors. There is no direct means of testing the autonomic innervation of the corpora. Prolongation of the bulbocavernosus reflex, however, is sometimes cited as evidence of peripheral neuropathy in diabetic patients with impotence. Impaired relaxation of corporeal smooth muscle from diabetic men with impotence has been shown to occur in in vitro studies with autonomic nerve stimulation or after acetylcholine administration.[230]

Acknowledgment

We thank Dr. Leo Wollner for his contributions to the literature search and final preparation of this chapter.

References

1. Benetos A, Huguet F, Albaladejo P et al: Role of adrenergic tone in mechanical and functional properties of carotid artery during aging. Am J Physiol 1993;265:H1132–H1138
2. Collins KJ, Exton-Smith AN: Thermal homeostasis in old age. J Am Geriatr Soc 1983;31:519–524
3. Gilpin SA, Gilpin CJ, Dixon JS et al: The effect of age on the autonomic innervation of the urinary bladder. Br J Urol 1986; 58:378–381
4. Finch CE: Neuron atrophy during aging: programmed or sporadic? Trends Neurosci 1993;16:104–110
5. Cowen T: Ageing in the autonomic nervous system: a result of nerve-target interactions? a review. Mech Ageing Dev 1993; 68:163–173
6. Gabella G: Fall in the number of myenteric neurons in aging guinea pigs. Gastroenterology 1989;96:1487–1493
7. Low PA, Okazaki H, Dyck PJ: Splanchnic preganglionic neurons in man. I. morphometry of preganglionic cytons. Acta Neuropathol 1977;40:55–61
8. Cowen T: Regulation of the autonomic innervation of blood vessels during development and ageing. pp. 25–40. In Edvinnson L, Uddman R (eds): Vascular innervation and receptor mechanisms: new perspectives. Academic Press, London, 1993
9. Bleys RLAW, Cowen T, Groen GJ, Hillen B: Perivascular nerves of the human basal cerebral arteries. II. changes in ageing and Alzheimer's disease. J Cereb Blood Flow Metab 1996;16:1048–1057
10. Thrasivoulou C, Cowen T: Regulation of rat sympathetic nerve density by target tissues and NGF in maturity and old age. Eur J Neurosci 1995;7:381–387
11. Mione MC, Dhital KK, Amenta F, Burnstock G: An increase in the expression of neuropeptidergic vasodilator, but not vasoconstrictor, cerebrovascular nerves in aging rats. Brain Res 1988;460:103–113
12. Andrews TJ, Thrasivoulou C, Nesbit W, Cowen T: Target-specific differences in the dendritic morphology and neuropeptide content of neurons in the rat SCG during development and aging. J Comp Neurol 1996;368:33–44
13. Abdel-Rahman TA, Collins KJ, Cowen T, Rustin M: Immunohistochemical, morphological and functional changes in the peripheral sudomotor neuro-effector system in elderly people. J Aut Nerv Syst 1992;37:187–198
14. Abdel-Rahman TA, Cowen T: Neurodegeneration in sweat glands and skin of aged rats. J Aut Nerv Syst 1993;46:55–63
15. Baker DM, Santer RM: A quantitative study of the effects of age on the noradrenergic innervation of Auerbach's plexus in the rat. Mech Ageing Dev 1988;42:147–158
16. Cowen T, Haven AJ, Wen Qin C et al: Development and ageing of perivascular adrenergic nerves in the rabbit: a quantitative fluorescence histochemical study using image analysis. J Aut Nerv Syst 1982;5:317–336
17. Vega JA, Ricci A, Amenta F: Age-dependent changes in the sympathetic innervation of the rat kidney. Mech Ageing Dev 1990;54:185
18. Gavazzi I, Canavan REM, Cowen T: Influence of age and anti-NGF treatment on the sympathetic and sensory innervation of the rat iris. Neuroscience 1996;73:1069–1079
19. Schmidt RE, Beaudet L, Plurad SB et al: Pathologic alterations in pre- and postsynaptic elements in aged mouse sympathetic ganglia. J Neurocytol 1995;24:189–206
20. Schmidt RE, Plurad SB, Parvin CA, Roth KA: Effect of diabetes and aging on human sympathetic autonomic ganglia. Am J Pathol 1993;143:143–153
21. Miller MM, Joshi D, Billiar RB, Nelson JF: Loss of LH-RH neurons in the rostral forebrain of old female C57BL/6J mice. Neurobiol Aging 1990;11:217–221
22. Sturrock RR: A comparison of age-related changes in neuron number in the dorsal motor nucleus of the vagus and nucleus ambiguus of the mouse. J Anat 1990;173:169–176
23. Purves D, Voyvodic JT, Magrassi L, Yawo H: Nerve terminal remodelling visualized in living mice by repeated examination of the same neuron. J Neurosci 1987;238:1122–1126

24. Harris LW, Purves D: Rapid remodelling of sensory endings in the corneas of living mice. J Neurosci 1989;9:2210–2214
25. Levi-Montalcini R: The nerve growth factor: 35 years later. Science 1987;237:1154–1162
26. Purves D, Snider WD, Voyvodic JT: Trophic regulation of nerve cell morphology and innervation in the autonomic nervous system. Nature 1988;336:123–128
27. Landis SC: Target regulation of neurotransmitter phenotype. Trends Neurosci 1990;13:344
28. Gavazzi I, Cowen T: Can the neurotrophic hypothesis explain degeneration and loss of plasticity in mature and ageing autonomic nerves? J Aut Nerv Syst 1996;58:1–10
29. Gabella G: Hypertrophy of visceral smooth muscle. Anat Embryol. 1990;182:409–424
30. Kuchel GA: Alterations in target innervation and collateral sprouting in the aging sympathetic nervous system. Exp Neurol 1993;124:381–386
31. Schotzinger RJ, Landis SC: Acquisition of cholinergic and peptidergic properties by sympathetic innervation of rat sweat glands requires interaction with normal target. Neuron 1990; 5:91–100
32. Cowen T, Thrasivoulou C, Shaw SA, Abdel-Rahman TA: Transplanted sweat glands from mature and aged donors determine cholinergic phenotype and altered density of host sympathetic nerves. J Aut Nerv Syst 1996;60:215–224
33. Stieg P, Stromberg I, Olson L: Effects of donor age on superior cervical ganglion transplants—evaluation by Falck-Hillarp histochemistry and immunocytochemistry. Exp Brain Res 1991;85:55–65
34. Gavazzi I, Cowen T: Axonal regeneration from transplanted sympathetic ganglia is not imparied by age. Exp Neurol 1993; 122:57–64
35. Gavazzi I: Collateral sprouting and responsiveness to nerve growth factor of ageing neurons. Neurosci Lett 1995;189: 47–50
36. Jelsma TN, Aguayo AJ: Trophic factors. Curr Opin Neurobiol 1994;4:717–725
37. Bothwell M: Functional interactions of neurotrophins and neurotrophin receptors. Ann Rev Neurosci 1995;18:223–255
38. Miller FD, Speelman A, Mathew TC et al: Nerve growth factor derived from terminals selectively increases the ratio of p75 to trka NGF receptors on mature sympathetic neurons. Dev Biol 1994;161:206–217
39. Nemoto K, Kageyama H, Hagiwara T et al: Mutation of low affinity nerve growth factor receptor gene in spontaneously hypertensive and stroke-prone spontaneously hypertensive rats: one of the promising candidate genes for hypertension. Brain Res 1994;655:267–270
40. Patterson PH: Cytokines and the function of the mature nervous system. C R Acad Sci Paris 1993;316:1150–1157
41. Purves D: Body and Brain: A Trophic Theory of Neural Connections. Harvard University Press, Cambridge, MA, 1988
42. Ruit KG, Osborne PA, Schmidt RE et al: Nerve growth factor regulates sympathetic ganglion cell morphology and survival in the adult mouse. J Neurosci 1990;10:2412–2419
43. Gloster A, Diamond J: Sympathetic nerves in adult rats regenerate normally and restore pilomotor function during an anti-NGF treatment that prevents their collateral sprouting. J Comp Neurol 1992;326:363–374
44. McLachlan EM, Jang W, Devor M, Michaelis M: Peripheral nerve injury triggers noradrenergic sprouting within dorsal root ganglia. Nature 1993;363:543–546
45. Isaacson LG, Saffran BN, Crutcher KA: Nerve growth factor-induced sprouting of mature, uninjured sympathetic axons. J Comp Neurol 1992;326:327–336
46. Isaacson LG, Ondris D, Crutcher KA: Plasticity of mature sensory cerebrovascular axons following intracranial infusion of nerve growth factor. J Comp Neurol 1995;361:451–460
47. Andrews TJ, Cowen T: Nerve growth factor enhances the dendritic arborization of sympathetic ganglion cells undergoing atrophy in aged rats. J Neurocytol 1994;23:234–241
48. Shelton DL, Reichard LF: Expression of the B-nerve growth factor gene correlates with the density of sympathetic innervation in effector organs. Proc Nat Acad Sci USA 1984;81: 7951–7955
49. Ebendal T, Olson L, Seiger A: The level of nerve growth factor (NGF) as a function of innervation. Exp Cell Res 1983;148: 311–317
50. Cowen T, Gavazzi I, Weingartner J, Crutcher KA: Levels of NGF protein do not correlate with changes in innervation of the rat iris in old age. Neuroreport 1996;7:2216–2220
51. Parikh DH, Tam PK, van Velzen D, Edgar D: Abnormalities in the distribution of laminin and collagen type IV in Hirschsprung's disease. Gastroenterology 1992;102:1236–1241
52. Leyten QH, Gabreels FJ, Renier WO et al: White matter abnormalities in congenital muscular dystrophy. J Neurol Sci 1995; 129:162–169
53. Gavazzi I, Boyle KS, Edgar D, Cowen T: Reduced laminin immunoreactivity in the blood vessel wall of ageing rats correlates with reduced innervation in vivo and following transplantation. Cell Tiss Res 1995;281:23–32
54. Uchida Y, Tomonaga M: Effects of nerve growth factor and heart cell conditioned medium on neurite regeneration of aged sympathetic neurones in culture. Brain Res 1985;348: 100–106
55. Uchida Y, Tomonaga M: Loss of nerve growth factor receptors in sympathetic ganglia from aged mice. Biochem Biophys Res Commun 1987;146:797–801
56. Shetty KR, Duthie EH: Anterior pituitary function and growth hormone use in the elderly. pp. 213–231. In Gambert SR, Gupta KL (eds): Endocrinology and Metabolism Clinics of North America. WB Saunders, Philadelphia, 1995
57. D'Costa AP, Ingram RL, Lenham JE, Sonntag WE: The regulation and mechanisms of action of growth hormone and insulin-like growth factor I during normal ageing. J Reprod Fertil Suppl 1993;46:87–98
58. Recio-Pinto E, Rechler MM, Ishii DN: Effects of insulin, insulin-like growth factor-II, and nerve growth factor on neurite formation and survival in cultured sympathetic and sensory neurons. J Neurosci 1986;6:1211–1219
59. Rees J, Shuster S: Pubertal induction of sweat gland activity. Clin Sci 1981;60:689–692
60. Belai A, Cooper S, Burnstock G: Effect of age on NADPH-diaphorase-containing myenteric neurones of rat ileum and proximal colon. Cell Tiss Res 1995;279:379–383

61. Burnstock G: Integration of factors controlling vascular tone: overview. Anesthesiology 1993;79:1368–1380

62. Burnstock G: Plasticity in expression of co-transmitters and autonomic nerves in aging and disease. Adv Exp Med Biol 1991;296:291–301

63. Kelly J, O'Malley K: Adrenoceptor function and ageing. Rev Clin Gerontol 1984;66:509–515

64. Ng AV, Callister R, Johnson DG, Seals DR: Endurance exercise training is associated with elevated basal sympathetic nerve activity in healthy older humans. J Appl Physiol 1994; 77:1366–1374

65. Fagius J, Wallin BG: Long-term variability and reproducibility of resting human muscle nerve sympathetic activity at rest, as reassessed after a decade. Clin Aut Res 1993;3:201–205

66. Duckles SP, Tsai H, Bucholz JN: Evidence for decline in intracellular calcium buffering in adrenergic nerves of aged rats. Life Sci 1996;58:2029–2035

67. Duckles SP: Effect of norepinephrine uptake blockade on contractile responses to adrenergic nerve stimulation of isolated rat blood vessels: influence of age. J Pharm Exp Ther 1987; 243:521–526

68. Giacobini E: The cholinergic system in ageing. pp. 665–692. In Whittaker VP (ed): The Cholinergic Synapse. Springer-Verlag, New York, 1988

69. Betts DC, Fowler CJ: Investigation and treatment of bladder and sexual dysfunction in diseases affecting the autonomic nervous system. pp. 462–478. In Bannister R, Mathias CJ (eds): Autonomic Failure: A Textbook of Clinical Disorders of the Autonomic Nervous System. 3rd ed. Oxford University Press, Oxford, 1992

70. Nishimoto T, Latifpour J, Wheeler MA et al: Age-dependent alterations in beta-adrenergic responsiveness of rat detrusor smooth muscle. J Urol 1995;153:1701–1705

71. Warburton AL, Santer RM: Sympathetic and sensory innervation of the urinary tract in young adult and aged rats: a semiquantitative histochemical and immunohistochemical study. Histochem J 1994;26:127–133

72. Saito M, Kondo A, Gotoh M et al: Age-related changes in the response of the rat urinary bladder to neurotransmitters. Neurourol Urodyn 1993;12:191–200

73. Crutcher KA, Weingartner J: Hippocampal NGF levels are not reduced in the aged Fischer-344 rat. Neurobiol Aging 1991; 12:449–454

74. Jackowski A, Crockard A, Burnstock G, Lincoln J: Alterations in serotonin and neuropeptide Y content of cerebrovascular sympathetic nerves following experimental subarachnoid hemorrhage. J Cerebr Blood Flow Metab 1989;9:271

75. Cowen T: Quantification of nerves and neurotransmitters using image analysis. pp. 335–380. In Springall DR, Polak JM, Wooton R (eds): Image Analysis in Histology: Conventional and Confocal Microscopy. Cambridge University Press, Cambridge, 1995

76. Cowen T, Thrasivoulou C: A microscopical assay using a densitometric application of image analysis to quantify neurotransmitter dynamics. J Neurosci Meth 1992;45:107–116

77. Andrews TJ, Cowen T: In vivo infusion of NGF induces the organotypic regrowth of perivascular nerves following their atrophy in aged rats. J Neurosci 1994;14:3048–3058

78. Loewy AD, Spyer KM: Central Regulation of Autonomic Functions. Oxford University Press, Oxford, 1990

79. Sandroni P, Ahlskog JE, Fealey RD, Low PA: Autonomic involvement in extrapyramidal and cerebellar disorders. Clin Aut Res 1991;1:147–155

80. Walton J: Disorders of the autonomic nervous system and hypothalamus. pp. 677–689. In Walton J (ed): Brain's Diseases of the Nervous System. 10th ed. Oxford University Press, Oxford, 1993

81. McLeod JG: Autonomic dysfunction in peripheral nerve disorders. Curr Opin Neurol Neurosurg 1992;5:476–481

82. Bannister R, Mathias CJ: Clinical features and investigation of the primary autonomic failure syndromes. pp. 531–547. In Bannister R, Mathias CJ (eds): Autonomic Failure: A Textbook of Clinical Disorders of the Autonomic Nervous System. 3rd ed. Oxford University Press, Oxford, 1992

83. Shy GM, Drager GA: A neurological syndrome associated with orthostatic hypotension. Arch Neurol 1960;3:511–527

84. Fearnley JM, Lees AJ: Striatonigral degeneration: a clinicopathological study. Brain 1990;113:1823–1842

85. Goto S, Hirano A, Matsumoto S: Subdivisional involvement of nigrostriatal loop in idiopathic Parkinson's disease and striatonigral degeneration. Ann Neurol 1989;26:766–770

86. Fulham MJ, Dubinsky RM, Polinsky RJ et al: Computed tomography, magnetic resonance imaging and positron emission tomography with [^{18}F]fluorodeoxyglucose in multiple system atrophy and pure autonomic failure. Clin Aut Res 1991;1: 27–36

87. Quinn N, Wenning G: Multiple system atrophy. Curr Opin Neurol 1995;8:323–326

88. Brown RG, Marsden CD: How common is dementia in Parkinson's disease? Lancet 1984;ii:1262–1265

89. Aminoff MJ: Autonomic dysfunction in central nervous system disorders. Curr Opin Neurol 1992;5:482–486

90. Koller WC, Vetere-Overfield B, Williamson A et al: Sexual dysfunction in Parkinson's disease. Clin Neuropharm 1990; 13:461–463

91. Turkka J: Autonomic dysfunction in Parkinson's disease. Acta Univ Ouluensis 1986;D142:14–66

92. Durrien G, Senard JM, Tran MA et al: Effects of levodopa and bromocriptine on blood pressure and plasma catecholamines in parkinsonians. Clin Neuropharm 1991;14:84–90

93. van Dijk JG, Haan J, Zwinderman K et al: Autonomic nervous system dysfunction in Parkinson's disease: relationships with age, medication, duration and severity. J Neurol Neurosurg Psychiatry 1993;56:1090–1095

94. Goldman JE, Calingasan NY, Gibson GE: Aging and the brain. Curr Opin Neurol 1994;7:287–293

95. Rosser MN: Parkinson's disease and Alzheimer's disease as disorders of the isodendritic core. Br Med J 1981;283: 1588–1590

96. Aharon-Peretz J, Harel T, Revach M, Ben-Haim SA: Increased sympathetic and decreased parasympathetic cardiac innervation in patients with Alzheimer's disease. Arch Neurol 1992; 49:919–922

97. Algotsson A, Vitonen M, Winbled B, Solders G: Autonomic dysfunction in Alzheimer's disease. Acta Neurol Scand 1995; 91:14–18

98. Korpelainen JT, Tolonen U, Sotaniemi KA, Myllyla VV: Suppressed sympathetic skin response in brain infarction. Stroke 1993;24:1389–1392
99. Zimmermann KP, Monga TN, Darouiche RO, Lawrence SA: Post-stroke autonomic nervous function: palmar sympathetic skin responses thirty or more days after cerebrovascular accident. Arch Phys Med Rehab 1995;76:250–256
100. Lenz K, Hortnagl H, Magometschnigg D et al: Function of the autonomic nervous system in patients with hepatic encephalopathy. Hepatology 1985;5:831–836
101. Converse RL, Jacobsen TN, Toto RD et al: Sympathetic overactivity in patients with chronic renal failure. N Engl J Med 1992;327:1912–1918
102. Zochodne DW: Autonomic involvement in Guillain Barré syndrome. Muscle Nerve 1994;17:1145–1155
103. Toussirot E, Serratrice G, Valentin P: Autonomic nervous system involvement in rheumatoid arthritis. J Rheumatol 1993; 20:1508–1514
104. Duncan G, Johnson RH, Lambie DG, Whiteside EA: Evidence of vagal neuropathy in chronic alcoholics. Lancet 1980;ii: 1053–1056
105. Johnson RH, Robinson BJ: Mortality in alcoholics with autonomic neuropathy. J Neurol Neurosurg Psychiatry 1988;51: 476–480
106. Guo YP, McLeod JG, Baverstock J: Pathological changes in the vagus nerve in diabetics and chronic alcoholics. J Neurol Neurosurg Psychiatry 1987;50:1449–1453
107. Tamura N, Baverstock J, McLeod JG: A morphometric study of the carotid sinus nerve in patients with diabetes mellitus and chronic alcoholism. J Aut Nerv Syst 1988;23:9–15
108. Ewing DJ, Campbell IW, Clarke BF: The natural history of diabetic autonomic neuropathy. Q J Med 1980;49:95–108
109. Sundqvist G, Lind P, Bergstrom B et al: Autonomic nerve antibodies and autonomic nerve function in type I and type II diabetic patients. J Intern Med 1991;229:505–510
110. Edmonds ME, Watkins PJ: Clinical presentation of diabetic autonomic failure. pp. 698–720. In Bannister R, Mathias CJ (eds): Autonomic Failure: A Textbook of Clinical Disorders of the Autonomic Nervous System. 3rd ed. Oxford University Press, Oxford, 1992
111. O'Brien IAD, Corrall RJM: Epidemiology of diabetes and its complications. N Engl J Med 1988;318:1619–1620
112. Ingall TJ, McLeod JG: Autonomic function in Friedrich's ataxia. J Neurol Neurosurg Psychiatry 1991;54:162–164
113. Galassi G, Nemni R, Baraldi A et al: Peripheral neuropathy in multiple system atrophy with autonomic failure. Neurology 1982;32:1116–1120
114. Mancia G, Cleroux J, Daffonchio A et al: Reflex control of circulation in the elderly. Cardiovasc Drugs Ther 1990;4: 1223–1228
115. Ferrari AU, Grassi G, Mancia G: Alterations in reflex control of circulation associated with ageing. pp. 39–50. In Anvery A, Staesson J (eds): Handbook of Hypertension. Vol. 12. Elsevier Science Publishing, Amsterdam, 1989
116. Eckberg DL, Sleight P: Human Baroreflexes in Health and Disease. pp. 153–215. Oxford University Press, Oxford, 1992
117. Collins KJ, Abdel-Rahman TA, Easton JC et al: Effects of facial cooling on elderly and young subjects: interactions with breath-holding and lower body negative pressure. Clin Sci 1996;90:485–492
118. Collins KJ: Autonomic failure and the elderly. pp. 489–507. In Bannister R (ed): Autonomic Failure: A Textbook of Clinical Disorders of the Autonomic Nervous system. 1st ed. Oxford University Press, Oxford, 1983
119. Hajduczok G, Chapleau MW, Johnson SL, Abboud FM: Increase in sympathetic activity with age. I. Role of impairment of arterial baroreflexes. Am J Physiol 1991;260: H1113–H1120
120. Chapleau MW, Hajduczok G, Abboud FM: Paracrine modulation of baroreceptor activity by vascular endothelium. News Physiol Sci 1991;6:210–214
121. Kaufmann H, Oribe E, Oliver JA: Plasma endothelin during upright tilt: relevance for orthostatic hypotension? Lancet 1991;338:1542–1545
122. de-Biase L, Amorosi C, Sulpizii L et al: Cardiovascular reactions to physiological stimuli in the elderly and the relationship with the autonomic nervous system. J Hypertens Suppl 1988; 6:63–67
123. Mark AL, Mancia G: Cardiopulmonary baroreflexes in humans. pp. 795–813. In Shepherd JT, Abboud FM (eds): Handbook of Physiology. Sec. 2: The Cardiovascular System. Vol. III. American Physiology Society, Washington, DC, 1982
124. Grassi G, Giannattasio C, Saino A et al: Cardiopulmonary receptor modulation of plasma renin activity in normotensive and hypertensive subjects. Hypertension 1988;11:92–99
125. Hajduczok G, Chapleau MW, Abboud FM: Increase in sympathetic activity with age. II. role of impairment of cardiopulmonary baroreflexes. Am J Physiol 1991;260:H1121–H1127
126. Cleroux J, Giannattasio C, Bolla G et al: Decreased cardiopulmonary reflexes with aging in normotensive humans. Am J Physiol 1989;257:H961–H968
127. Lipsitz LA: Orthostatic hypotension in the elderly. N Engl J Med 1989;321:952–957
128. Schwartz PJ, La Rovere MT, Vanoli E: Autonomic nervous system and sudden cardiac death: experimental basis and clinical observations for post-myocardial infarction risk stratification. Circulation 1992;85(suppl 1):1–77
129. Daly M de B: Interactions between respiration and circulation. pp. 529–594. In Handbook of Physiology: The Respiratory System II. American Physiology Society, Bethesda, MD, 1985
130. Dambrink JHA, Wieling W: Circulatory response to postural change in healthy male subjects in relation to age. Clin Sci 1987;72:335–341
131. Macrae AD, Bulpitt CJ: Assessment of postural hypotension in elderly patients. Age Ageing 1989;18:110–112
132. Wieling W: Non-invasive continuous recording of heart rate and blood pressure in the evaluation of neurocardiovascular control. pp. 291–311. In Bannister R, Mathias CJ (eds): Autonomic Failure: A Textbook of Clinical Disorders of the Autonomic Nervous System. 3rd ed. Oxford University Press, Oxford, 1992
133. Shepherd JT, Mancia G: Reflex control of the human cardiovascular system. Rev Physiol Biochem Pharmacol 1986;105: 1–99

134. Mathias CJ, Bannister R: Investigation of autonomic disorders. pp. 255–290. In Bannister R, Mathias CJ (eds): Autonomic Failure: A Textbook of Clinical Disorders of the Autonomic Nervous System. 3rd ed. Oxford University Press, Oxford, 1992

135. Le Blanc J, Dulac S, Cote J, Girard B: Autonomic nervous system and adaptation to cold in man. J Appl Physiol 1975; 39:181–186

136. Victor RG, Leimbach WN, Seals DR et al: Effects of the cold pressor test on muscle sympathetic nerve activity in humans. Hypertension 1987;9:429–436

137. Heath ME, Downey JA: The cold face test (diving reflex) in clinical autonomic assessment: methodological considerations and repeatablity of responses. Clin Sci 1990;79:139–147

138. Wallin BG: Intramural recording of normal and abnormal sympathetic activity in man. pp. 359–377. In Bannister R, Mathias CJ (eds): Autonomic Failure: A Textbook of Clinical Disorders of the Autonomic Nervous System. 3rd ed. Oxford University Press, Oxford, 1992

139. Eckberg DL, Wallin BG, Fagius J et al: Prospective study of symptoms after human microneurography. Acta Physiol Scand 1989;137:567–569

140. Pomeranz B, Macaulay RJB, Candill MA et al: Assessment of autonomic function in humans by heart rate spectral analysis. Am J Physiol 1985;248:H151–H153

141. Korkushko OU, Shatilo VB, Plachinda Y, Shatilo TV: Autonomic control of cardiac chronotropic function in man as a function of age: assessment by power spectral analysis of heart rate variability. J Aut Nerv Syst 1991;32:191–198

142. Luutonen S, Antila K, Neuvonen P et al: Spectral analysis of heart rate variability in evaluation of sympathetic function in elderly subjects. Age Ageing 1994;23:473–477

143. Sleight P, La Rovere MT, Mortarn A et al: Physiology and pathophysiology of heart rate and blood pressure variability in humans: is power spectrum analysis largely an index of baroreflex gain? Clin Sci 1995;88:103–109

144. Wollner L, McCarthy ST, Soper NDW, Macy DJ: Failure of cerebral autoregulation as a cause of brain dysfunction in the elderly. Br Med J 1979;i:1117–1118

145. Alli C, Avanzini F, Betelli G et al: Prevalence and variability of orthostatic hypotension in the elderly: results of the Italian study of blood pressure in the elderly. Eur Heart J 1992;13: 178–182

146. Craig GM: Clinical presentation of orthostatic hypotension in the elderly. Postgrad Med J 1994;70:95–117

147. Raiha I, Luutonen S, Piha J et al: Prevalence, predisposing factors, and prognostic importance of postural hypotension. Arch Intern Med 1995;155:930–935

148. Lipsitz LA, Jonsson PV, Marks BL et al: Reduced supine cardiac volumes and diastolic filling rates in elderly patients with chronic medical conditions: implications for postural blood pressure homeostasis. J Am Geriatr Soc 1990;38:103–107

149. Streeten DHP, Scullard TF: Excessive gravitational blood pooling caused by impaired venous tone is the predominant non-cardiac mechanism of orthostatic intolerance. Clin Sci 1996;90:277–285

150. Rowell LB: Human Cardiovascular Control. Oxford University Press, New York, 1993

151. Vargas E, Lye M: Is there a relationship between supine systemic blood pressure and orthostatic hypotension in the elderly? Clin Auton Res 1993;3:345–349

152. Lye M: Autonomic dysfunction and abnormal vascular reflexes. pp. 191–211. In Tallis R (ed): The Clinical Neurology of Old Age. Wiley, Chichester, 1988

153. Robinson BJ, Johnson RH, Lambie DG, Palmer KT: Do elderly patients with an excessive fall in blood pressure on standing have evidence of autonomic failure? Clin Sci 1983;64: 587–591

154. Pfeiffer MA, Weinberg CR, Cook D et al: Differential changes of autonomic nervous function with age in man. Am J Med 1983;75:249–258

155. Ziegler MG. Postural hypotension. Ann Rev Med 1980;31: 239–245

156. Lye M, Vargas E, Faragher EB et al: Haemodynamic and neurohumoral responses in elderly patients with postural hypotension. Eur J Clin Invest 1990;20:90–96

157. Masuo K, Mikami H, Ogihara T: The frequency of orthostatic hypotension in elderly patients with essential hypertension, isolated systolic hypertension and borderline hypertension. J Hypertens 1993;11(suppl 5):S306–S307

158. Robertson D, Robertson RM: Causes of chronic orthostatic hypotension. Arch Intern Med 1994;154:1620–1624

159. Mathias CJ. Autonomic neuropathies—aspects of diagnosis and management. pp. 95–117. In Ashbury AK, Thomas PK (eds): Peripheral Nerve Disorders II. Butterworth Heinemann, Oxford, 1995

160. Riley TL, Friedman JM: Stroke, orthostatic hypotension and focal epilepsy. JAMA 1981;245:1243–1244

161. Mo R, Omvik P, Lund-Johansen P: The Bergen blood pressure study: estimated prevalence of postural hypotension is influenced by the alerting reaction to blood pressure measurement. J Hum Hypertens 1994;8:171–176

162. Imholz BPM, Dambrink JHA, Karemaker JM, Wieling W: Orthostatic circulatory control in the elderly evaluated by non-invasive continuous blood pressure measurement. Clin Sci 1990;79:73–79

163. Mathias CJ: Orthostatic hypotension. Prescribers J 1995;35: 124–132

164. Palmer K: Graduated compression stockings. Br Med J 1980; 28:389–390

165. Wieling W, van-Lieshout JJ, van-Leeuwen AM: Physical manoeuvres that reduce postural hypotension in autonomic failure. Clin Auton Res 1993;3:57–65

166. Ten-Harkel AD, van Lieshout JJ, Wieling W: Treatment of orthostatic hypotension with sleeping in the head-up-tilt position alone and in combination with fludrocortisone. J Intern Med 1992;232:139–145

167. Grubb BP, Wolfe DA, Samoil D et al: Adaptive rate pacing controlled by right ventricular pre-ejection interval for severe refractory orthostatic hypotension. Pacing Clin Electrophysiol 1993;16:801–805

168. Schutzman J, Jaeger F, Maloney J, Fouad-Tarazi F: Head-up tilt and hemodynamic changes during orthostatic hypotension in patients with supine hypertension. J Am Coll Cardiol 1994; 24:454–461
169. Breuetti G, Chiariello M, Bonaduce D et al: 24-hour blood pressure recording in patients with orthostatic hypotension. Clin Cardiol 1985;8:406–412
170. Mathias CJ, Fosbraey P, da Costa DF et al: The effect of desmopressin on nocturnal polyuria, overnight weight loss and morning postural hypotension in patients with autonomic failure. Br Med J 1986;293:353–354
171. Brooke DJ, Redmond S, Mathias CJ et al: The effects of orthostatic hypotension on cerebral blood flow and middle cerebral artery velocity in autonomic failure, with observations on the action of ephedrine. J Neurol Neurosurg Psychiatry 1989;52: 962–966
172. Jankovic J, Gilden JL, Hiner BC et al: Neurogenic orthostatic hypotension: a double blind, placebo controlled study with midodrone. Am J Med 1993;95:38–48
173. Said G: Action of dihydroergotamine in severe orthostatic hypotension: 16 cases. Presse Med 1987;16:800–803
174. Biaggioni I, Zygmunt D, Haile V, Robertson D: Pressor effect of inhaled ergotamine in orthostatic hypotension. Am J Cardiol 1990;65:89–92
175. Davies IB, Bannister R, Mathias CJ, Sever P: Pindolol in postural hypotension. Lancet 1981;ii:982–983
176. Mehlsen J, Trap-Jensen J: Xamoterol, a new selective B-1-adrenoceptor partial agonist in the treatment of postural hypotension. Acta Med Scand 1986;219:173–177
177. Imaizumi T, Taleshito A, Ashihara T et al: Increase in reflex vasoconstriction with indomethacin in patients with orthostatic hypotension and central nervous system involvement. Br Med J 1984;52:501–504
178. Watt ST, Tooki JE, Perkins CM, Lee MR: The treatment of idiopathic orthostatic hypotension: a combination of fludrocortisone and flurbiprofen. Q J Med 1981;198:205–212
179. Hoeldtke RD, Streeten DH: Treatment of orthostatic hypotension with erythropoietin. N Engl J Med 1993;329:611–615
180. Lipsitz LA, Fullerton KJ: Postprandial blood pressure reduction in healthy elderly. J Am Geriatr Soc 1986;34:267–270
181. Kooner JS, Armstrong E, Bannister R et al: Octreotide (SMS 201–995) prevents superior mesenteric artery vasodilatation and post-prandial hypotension in human autonomic failure. Br J Pharmacol 1990;29:154P
182. Mathias CJ: Postprandial hypotension: pathophysiological mechanisms and clinical implications in different disorders. Hypertension 1991;18:694–704
183. Hoeldtke RD, O'Dorisio TM, Boden G: Treatment of autonomic neuropathy with a somatostatin analogue, SMS 201–995. Lancet 1986;ii:602–605
184. Richardson D, Tyra J, McCray A: Attenuation of the cutaneous vasoconstrictor response to cold in elderly men. J Gerontol 1992;6:M211–M214
185. Rooke GA, Savage MV, Brengelmann GL: Maximal skin blood flow is decreased in elderly men. J Appl Physiol 1994;77: 11–14
186. Fleisch JH: Age-related changes in the sensitivity of blood vessels to drugs. Pharmacol Ther 1980;8:477–487
187. Collins KJ: Effects of cold on old people. Br J Hosp Med 1987; 38:506–514
188. Collins KJ: The autonomic nervous system and the regulation of body temperature pp.212–230. In Bannister R, Mathias CJ (eds): Autonomic Failure: A Textbook of Clinical Disorders of the Autonomic Nervous System. 3rd ed. Oxford University Press, Oxford, 1992
189. Schwartz RS, Jaeger LF, Veith RC: The thermic effect of feeding in older men: the importance of the sympathetic nervous system. Metabolism 1990;39:733–737
190. Collins KJ, Abdel-Rahman TA, Goodwin J, McTiffin L: Circadian body temperatures and the effects of a cold stress in elderly and young subjects. Age Ageing 1995;24:485–489
191. Brock MA: Chronobiology and aging. J Am Geriatr Soc 1991; 39:74–91
192. Touitou Y, Reinberg A, Bogdan A et al: Age-related changes in both circadian and seasonal rhythms of rectal temperature with special reference to senile dementia of Alzheimer type. Gerontology 1986;32:110–118
193. Diamond PT, Diamond MT: Thermoregulatory behaviour in Alzheimer's disease. J Am Geriatr Soc 1991;39:532
194. Hussain MM, Nemeroff CB: Neuropeptides in Alzheimer's disease. J Am Geriatr Soc 1990;38:918–925
195. Prinz PL, Moe KE, Vitello MV et al: Entrained body temperature rhythms are similar in mild Alzheimer's disease, geriatric onset depression, and normal aging. J Geriatr Psychiatry Neurol 1992;5:65–71
196. Collins KJ: Hypothermia—The Facts. Oxford University Press, Oxford, 1983
197. Curwen M: Excess winter mortality: a British phenomenon? Health Trends 1990;22:169–175
198. Lomax P, Schonbaum E: Environment, Drugs and Thermoregulation. Karger, Basel, 1983
199. Bastow MD, Rawlings J, Allison SP: Undernutrition, hypothermia, and injury in elderly women with fractured femur: an injury response to altered metabolism? Lancet 1983;i: 143–146
200. Kramer MR, van Dijk J, Rosin AJ: Mortality in elderly patients with thermoregulatory failure. Arch Intern Med 1989;149: 1521–1523
201. Darowski A, Najim Z, Weinberg JR et al: Hypothermia and infection in elderly patients admitted to hospital. Age Ageing 1991;20:100–106
202. Patel A, Getsos JP, Moussa G, Damato AN: The Osborn wave of hypothermia in normothermic patients. Clin Cardiol 1994; 17:273–276
203. Golden FStC: Rewarming. pp. 194–208. In Pozos RS, Wittmers LE (eds): The Nature and Treatment of Hypothermia. University of Minnesota Press, Minneapolis, 1983
204. Ledingham IMcA, Mone JG: Treatment of accidental hypothermia: a prospective clinical study. Br Med J 1980;280: 1102–1105
205. Hope W, Donnell HD, McKinley TW, Sikes RK: Illness and death due to environmental heat—Georgia and St. Louis 1983. JAMA 1984;252:20–23
206. Martinez BF, Annest JL, Kilbourne EM et al: Geographic distribution of heat-related deaths among elderly persons: use of

county-level dot maps for injury surveillance and epidemiological research. JAMA 1989;262:2246–2250

207. Fish PD, Bennett GC, Millard PH: Heatwave morbidity and mortality in old age. Age Ageing 1985;14:243–245

208. Gleckman R, Hibert D: Afebrile bacteremia: a phenomenon in geriatric patients. JAMA 1982;248:1478–1481

209. Norman DC, Yamamura RH, Yoshikawa T: Fever response in old and young mice after injection of interleukin-1. J Gerontol 1988;43:M80–M85

210. Miller D, Yoshikawa T, Castle SC et al: Effects of age on fever responses to recombinant tumor necrosis factor alpha in a murine model. J Gerontol 1991;46:M176–M179

211. Wingate DL: Autonomic dysfunction and the gut. pp. 510–528. In Bannister R, Mathias CJ (eds): Autonomic Failure. 3rd ed. Oxford University Press, Oxford, 1992

212. Edwards LL, Quigley EMM, Pfeiffer RF: Gastro-intestinal dysfunction in Parkinson's disease. Neurology 1992;42:726–732

213. Dooley CP, el Newihi HM, Zeidler A, Valenzuela JE: Abnormalities of the migrating motor complex in diabetics with autonomic neuropathy and diarrhoea. Scand J Gastroenterol 1988; 23:217–223

214. McDougal JN, Miller MS, Burks TF, Kreulen DL: Age-related changes in colonic function in rats. Am J Physiol 1984;247: G542–G546

215. Aggarwal A, Cutts TF, Abell TL et al: Predominant symptoms in irritable bowel syndrome correlate with specific autonomic nervous system abnormalities. Gastroenterology 1994;106: 945–950

216. Kopp VG, Di Bona GF: The neural control of renal function. pp. 1157–1204. In Seldin DW, Giebisch G (eds): The kidney: physiology and pathophysiology. Lippincott-Raven, New York, 1991

217. Yamada YE, Miyajima E, Tochikubo O et al: Age-related changes in muscle sympathetic nerve activity in essential hypertension. Hypertension 1989;13:870–877

218. Brown WW, Davis BB, Spry LA et al: Aging and the kidney. Arch Intern Med 1986;146:1790–1796

219. Tsunoda K, Abe K, Goto T et al: Effect of age on the renin-angiotensin-aldosterone system in normal subjects: simultaneous measurement of active and inactive renin, renin substrate, and aldosterone in plasma. J Clin Endocrin Metab 1986;62: 384–389

220. Kirby RS, Fowler CJ, Gosling JA, Bannister R: Vesico-urethral dysfunction in progressive autonomic failure with multiple system atrophy. J Neurol Neurosurg Psychiatry 1986;49:554–562

221. Malone-Lee J: A clinical approach to urinary incontinence in the elderly. pp. 93–102. In Andreucci VE, Fine LG (eds): International Yearbook of Nephrology, Dialysis, Transplantation. Vol. 10. Oxford University Press, Oxford, 1995

222. Collins KJ, Exton-Smith AN, James MH, Oliver DJ: Functional changes in autonomic nervous responses with ageing. Age Ageing 1980;9:17–24

223. Gilpin SA, Gilpin CJ, Dixon JS et al: The effect of age on the autonomic innervation of the urinary bladder. Br J Urol 1986; 58:378–381

224. Lincoln J, Burnstock G: Autonomic innervation of the urinary bladder and urethra. pp. 33–68. In Maggi CA (ed): Nervous Control of the Urogenital System. Harwood Academic, Chur, Switzerland 1993

225. Crowe R, Burnstock G, Light JK: Adrenergic innervation of the striated muscle of the intrinsic external urethral sphincter from patients with lower motor spinal cord lesions. J Urol 1989; 141:17–49

226. Dorje F, Levey AI, Braun MR: Immunological detection of muscarinic receptor subtype proteins (ml–m5) in rabbit peripheral tissues. Mol Pharmacol 1991;40:459–526

227. Newman HF, Marcus H: Erectile dysfunction in diabetes and hypertension. Urology 1985;26:135–137

228. Walsh PC, Mostwin JL: Radical prostatectomy and cystoprostatectomy with preservation of potency. Br J Urol 1984;56: 694–697

229. Korenman SG. Impotence. pp. 1146–1154. In Hazzard WR, Andres R, Bierman EL, Blass JP (eds): Principles of Geriatric Medicine and Gerontology. 2nd ed. McGraw Hill, New York, 1990

230. Saenz de Tejada I, Goldstein I, Azadzoi K et al: Impaired neurogenic and endothelium-mediated relaxation of penile smooth muscle from diabetic men with impotence. N Engl J Med 1989;320:1025–1034

CHAPTER 38

Parkinsonism and Other Movement Disorders

WILLIAM J. MUTCH
FRASER G. INGLIS

Movement disorders can be divided into those with lack of movement in the absence of weakness or spasticity (rigid-akinetic or Parkinsonian states) and those with excess movement (hyperkinetic or dyskinetic states). Most arise from dysfunction in the basal ganglia and their connections.

Basal Ganglia

Terminology in this area can be confusing, with structures often having more than one name. The term *basal ganglia* is generally applied to five structures on each side of the brain: the caudate nucleus, the putamen (which is structurally and functionally linked to the caudate nucleus), the globus pallidus, the functionally related subthalamic nucleus (body of Luys), and the substantia nigra (Fig. 38-1).

A substantial body of knowledge has now accumulated about the structure and connections of the striatum,[1–6] pallidum,[6] substantia nigra,[7–12] and subthalamic nucleus.[6]

The main afferents to the basal ganglia terminate in the striatum. The entire neocortex sends topographically specific glutaminergic axons to the ipsilateral striatum. Its gross appearance is largely formed by Wilsons pencils—bundles of nerve fibers radiating through its substance—converging on or radiating from the globus pallidus. Within the striatum there are neurochemically defined areas (striosomes and matrix) which have different cortical inputs, varying neurochemical features, and distinct outputs. Acetylcholine and α-aminobenzoic acid (GABA) act as neurotransmitters,[13] and various neuropeptides such as substance P and somatostatin may modulate the activity of transmitters.[14,15]

The substantia nigra can first be defined at the end of the third month of fetal life. It is derived from the intermediate primary cerebral vesicle and is probably comprised of neuroblasts of both basal and alar plates.

The substantia nigra is composed of a deep, cell-rich pars compacta and a superficial, larger but less cellular pars reticularis. The pars compacta, together with the smaller pars lateralis, forms the cell group A9 of Dahlstrom and Fuxe,[16,17] and together with the retrorubral nucleus (A8) it comprises most of the dopaminergic neuron population of the midbrain and is the source of the mesostriatal dopamine system. All these neurons are thought to contain acetylcholine in addition to dopamine, and there is evidence that up to 25 percent of them are in fact cholinergic.

The principal output from the basal ganglia is from the internal segment of the globus pallidus to the thalamus. From the thalamic nuclei fibers project to the prefrontal and motor cortex. The main feature of the connections of the basal ganglia is the formation of feedback loops.[18] Five loops have been described, a motor loop, an oculomotor loop, two prefrontal loops, and a limbic loop.[19] The formation of these loops permits specific regions of the striatum to enable the decisions of the cerebral cortex to be translated into overt (motor) behavior and allows midaction adjustments to be made when necessary. For example, the head of the caudate nucleus is essential for overt performance of a response involving planning, strategy, and working memory, and the inferior putamen for responses dependent on detailed visual analysis.

The Striatum and Its Connections

Thus, we have a system of nuclei in which the striatum has a pivotal role and receives inputs from all parts of the brain, those from the cortex being highly organized. Reciprocal innervations between basal ganglia structures and cortical inputs to separate nuclei allow a sophisticated system of modulation and cross-checks. The concept of independent pyramidal and extrapyramidal systems projecting down to the spinal cord is no longer tenable. Rather, the extrapyramidal (basal ganglia) system exerts its influence on cortically led movement via feedback loops as described above. The substantia nigra, however, is also recognized to project to the brain stem reticular formation and the spinal cord. The function of the basal ganglia in movement may be to act as a repository of basic patterns important in the automatic execution and sequencing of prelearned motor activity,[20] and more generally in the planning and modulating of ongoing behavior in the absence of external guidance.[21,22]

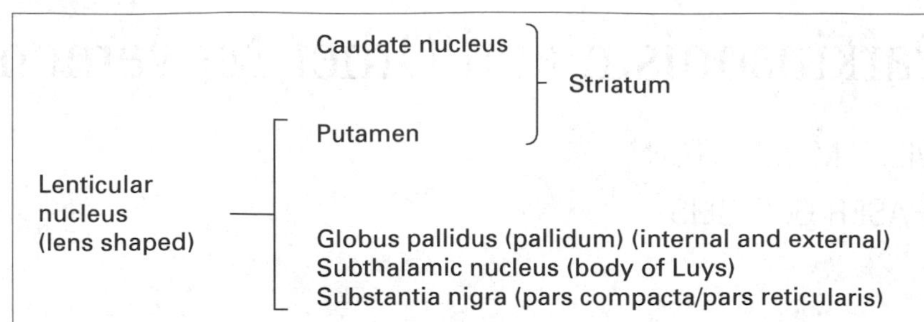

Figure 38-1 Schematic diagram of the basal ganglia.

Parkinsonism

Classification of Hypokinetic States

Parkinsonism is characterized by a variable combination of the clinical features of tremor, rigidity, bradykinesia, and impaired righting reflexes. There are many causes of this picture (Table 38-1), including the relatively rare akinetic-rigid syndromes, but the most common is idiopathic Parkinsonism (Parkinson's disease).[23–25]

Epidemiology

Parkinsonism is found worldwide in every country and in every ethnic group where studies have been conducted (Fig. 38-2). It principally affects old people and, although more insidious, ranks with stroke as a cause of severe disability.

The lack of uniform diagnostic criteria, the incomplete or imprecise ascertainment of cases, and reports based on atypical groups of patients have served to make the interpretation of data from studies difficult. Nonetheless, there have been well-conducted studies offering useful insights. Their value has been increased by recent worldwide[26] and European[27] reviews which have adjusted their data to a standard population to compensate for the differing age structures of communities at different points in time and in different parts of the world.

Table 38-1 Hypokinetic states

Parkinsonism
Primary
Idiopathic[a] (Parkinson's disease)
Secondary
Drug-induced[a]
Vascular[a]
Hydrocephalus
Tumor
Trauma
Postencephalitic
Associated with other neurological disorders
Alzheimer's disease[a]
Progressive supranuclear palsy[a]
Shy-Drager syndrome[a]
Olivopontocerebellar atrophy
Creutzfeld-Jakob disease
Parkinsonism-dementia (Guam)

[a] *These account for most cases of Parkinsonism.*[23–24]

From limited incidence data we can conclude that in different parts of the world from 2 to 24 new cases will appear each year for every 100,000 of the population.[26] The incidence is greatest in the eighth decade of life, and it is not clear whether the incidence of the disease is changing with time. More elderly people are now reported to have the disease, but this is probably because of a combination of demographic changes and greater interest in the health care of older people rather than because of any real change in the incidence of the disorder.

Prevalence studies indicate that the disease is at least as common in men as in women and may be more common in men. It mainly affects people over 50 years old, and a marked rise in prevalence with age is consistent throughout the world. Some studies suggest that the prevalence plateaus or falls above the eighth decade,[28] but others report a rising prevalence in the very old.[29,30] Poor case ascertainment and a tendency to dismiss clinical features of the disease as just "old age" may explain the apparent decline in some studies.

Over the next decade, in developed countries, if the shape of the age-specific prevalence graph is exponential, we can expect to see an increasing number of very old people with the disease since it is the over-eighty segment of the population that will increase most significantly. Such people tend to have many pathologies which, combined with disability from Parkinson's disease, have considerable implications for the provision of health and social support.

Recent reviews[26,27] have contributed to resolving the debate as to whether the prevalence of the disease truly varies in different parts of the world and in different ethnic groups (Fig. 38-2). Using age-standardized data from high-quality studies and stating confidence limits for age-adjusted prevalences, they agree that variations still remain but suggest that in Europe[27] and, indeed, worldwide,[26] much of the variation can be explained by differences in study methods and case ascertainment. Prevalences greater than 80 cases per 100,000 of the population have been reported in white, black American, Arab, and mixed racial communities but not in people of Asian descent. Significantly, low prevalence are consistently reported from Asian communities[31] and from the limited data available on black communities in Africa.[32] It remains unclear, however, whether the prevalence of the disease is low in these communities because of the action of protective factors, the absence of

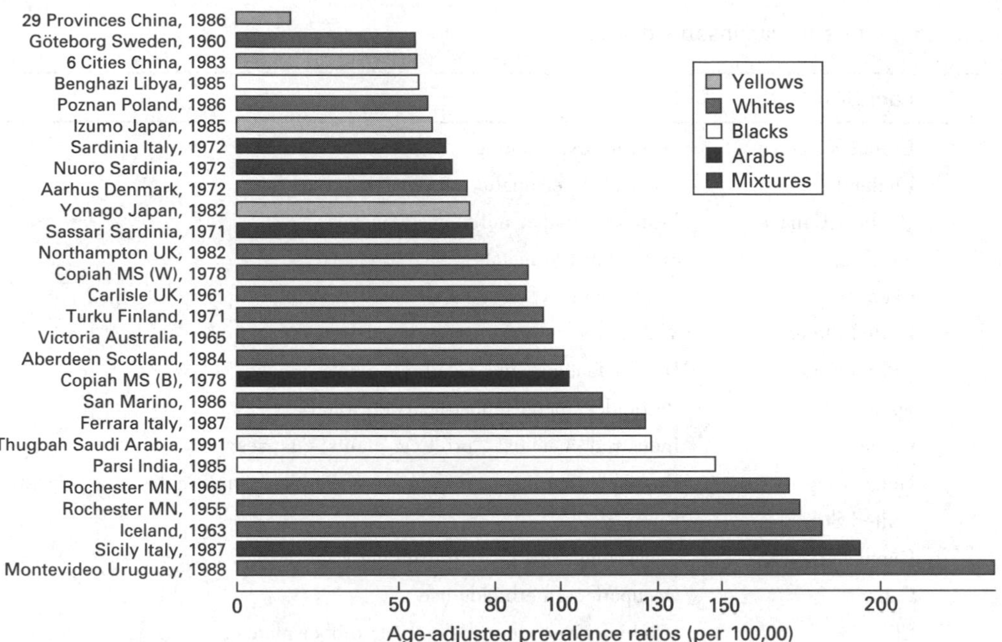

Figure 38-2 Worldwide comparisons of age-adjusted prevalence ratios, per 100,000, for Parkinson's disease by country for both sexes combined (adjusted to the 1970 U.S. population). (From Zhang and Roman,[26] with permission.)

environmental triggers for the disease, varying cultural or ethnic susceptibility, or even combinations of these factors. Research on migrant groups might help to clarify the contribution of ethnic factors to observed variations in the prevalence of the disease.

The reality of worldwide differences in the prevalence of the disorder and, by implication, susceptibility to it, is also an important public health issue, particularly for developing countries. It is they who will experience the most rapid growth (3 to 4 percent per year before 2020[33]) among individuals older than 65, the age group most associated with the disease.

Etiology

The cause of Parkinson's disease remains unknown.

Genetic

In 1949 Mjones[34] suggested that the disease was inherited as an autosomal dominant with incomplete penetrance, and indeed this belief has been supported by the findings of Golbe and colleagues[35] who have described a multiple case family with dopamine-responsive Parkinson's disease which they attribute to autosomal dominant inheritance with incomplete penetrance. There have been several family studies showing widely variable numbers of secondary cases in first-degree relatives,[36–41] however, these variable findings highlight methodologic differences among the studies. Family studies cannot readily control for the effect of common environmental exposure which can simulate inheritance. Studies on twins have been similarly compromised, although they offer a potentially powerful means of evaluating the contribution of genetic factors to disease.[42–45] Neuroimaging studies on twins using [^{18}F]dopa uptake have shown that preclinical disease is often present in the asymptomatic monozygotic twin of a discordant pair.[46] This might suggest that genes causing Parkinson's disease may be subject to variable penetrance and expressivity. Thus heritability may have been substantially underestimated in the past.

The development of idiopathic Parkinson's disease may be influenced by an inherited variation in the activity of the enzyme cytochrome P450IID6,[47,48] an xenobiotic metabolizing enzyme encoded by the gene CYP2D6. Poor metabolizer alleles of CYP2D6 are associated with a two- to threefold increase in the risk of developing the disorder. There is also evidence that poor metabolizers are more substantially over-represented in populations with early-onset Parkinson's disease compared to those with late-onset disease.[49] CYP2D6 is expressed in the substantia nigra, and its main function may be to protect the nigra by metabolizing potentially toxic chemicals. Other cytochrome enzymes may also have a role in protecting against the development of Parkinson's disease.

Environmental

In 1983 Langston[50] reported that an illicitly produced meperidine analog containing the substance l-methyl-4-phenyl-1,2,3,6-tetrahydropyridine (MPTP) produced apparently classic Parkinson's disease in young drug addicts. MPTP is, in fact, a protoxin which is converted to 1-methyl-4-phenylpyridine (MPP^+) by monoamine oxidase B (MAO-B). MPP^+ is highly toxic and is concentrated by the neuronal reuptake system in dopaminergic cells where it binds to neuromelamin. Neuromelamin is abundant in the substantia nigra,[51] has a high affinity for MPP^+, and is considered to enhance hydroxyl radical formation by reducing iron.[52] It has been shown that pigmented neurons are preferentially lost in patients with Parkinson's

Table 38-2 Possible environmental factors in Parkinson's disease

Study	Location	Factors
Godwin Austen et al. (1982)	United Kingdom	Head injury, smoking
Tedes CJ, Lees AJ (1985)	England	Premorbid personality
Barbeay A et al. (1986)	Quebec, Canada	Pesticides, paper mills, heavy metals
Aquilonius SM, Hartvig P (1986)	Sweden	Steel industry, metals
Rajput et al. (1986)	Canada	Rural living
Tanner CM et al. (1987)	United States	Well water
Golbe LI et al. (1988)	United States	Dietary factors, nuts, salad oil, plums protect
Jimenez-Jimenez FJ et al. (1988)	Spain	Pesticides, metal industries, well water
Tanner CM et al. (1989)	China	Industrial chemicals, printing, plants, quarries
Ho SC et al. (1989)	Hong Kong	Rural life, farming, previous use of herbicides/pesticides, raw vegetables
Koller W et al. (1990)	United States	Rural life
Duncan MW (1991)	Guam	Cycad flour, low Ca^{2+} in drinking water
Semchuck et al. (1992)	Canada	Occupational herbicide use
Wang Wen-Zhi et al. (1993)	China	Drinking river water, living near rubber plants
Hubble JP et al. (1993)	United States	Pesticides, family history of neurologic disease, depression

disease[53] and that the level of iron capable of generating free radicals is increased in postmortem studies of the disease.[54]

MPTP studies have generated a vast amount of information with wide-ranging implications. In particular, they stimulated a search for environmental factors that may cause Parkinson's disease, and in 1986 studies from Canada and Sweden suggested that Parkinson's sufferers were more commonly found in areas of high pesticide use, around paper mills,[55] and around metal industries.[56] Subsequent studies from many parts of the world have implicated many factors (Table 38-2), including the drinking of well water, diet, and the absence of protective factors (e.g., in the food chain) rather than an excess of toxins.

Reports of viral agents as a cause are inconsistent. However, the concept of intrauterine insult by influenza A, producing damage which subsequently presents as Parkinson's disease, has been both proposed and challenged.[57] More recent work has questioned the role of *Nocardia asteroides*[58] and pertussis.[59]

Smoking has previously been reported to have a negative association with Parkinson's disease, but a recent population-based study implies that the disorder simply reduces smoking, rather than smoking being protective.[62] In addition, people who smoke are more likely to die before Parkinson's disease becomes evident.

There have been remarkably few case-control studies, and frequently their data have been inconclusive or contradictory. Nonetheless, the idea that chemicals either in a rural or an urban setting may be involved in the etiology of the disease will not go away.[60,61] It is interesting to note, however, that in some case-control studies a family history of neurologic disease (e.g., tremor, Parkinson's disease, Alzheimer's disease) is also a significant, though weaker, risk factor.[61] It is possible that more than one environmental factor is involved. Studies with sufficient patient numbers possibly focusing on those with earlier-onset disease, whose memory of exposure to environmental factors is likely to be more intact, should yield useful results particularly if either multivariate analysis or multiple logistic regression techniques are used to assess the data. Finally, we should perhaps look more closely at dietary factors that might influence the development and/or progression of the disease.

Aging

The incidence of Parkinson's disease increases with age, and this has led to speculation that it occurs primarily as a component of normal aging or its exaggeration. Nigral dopaminergic cells,[63] levels of brain dopamine,[64] levels of tyrosine hydroxylase and dopa decarboxylase,[63] and measures of brain function such as reaction time[65] all decline with age but more markedly in Parkinson's sufferers when compared with age-matched controls. The significance of aging effects has been explored by Calne and Langston[66] who proposed that the disease results from a combination of environmental insult in early to middle adult life and later effects of aging. An alternative view that the aging brain is more susceptible to toxic effects has arisen from animal work using MPTP as a neuroprobe.[67] Age-related reasons include an increase in MAO activity, which may not heighten toxicity per se but rather may increase the catabolism of dopamine which, as a by product, generates destructive free radicals which can damage nigral tissue.[68]

On the basis of clinical and autopsy data comparing elderly age-matched postencephalitic cases and Parkinson's disease sufferers, Gibb and Lees[69] found evidence of active neuronal death in the Parkinson's disease sufferers but not in the postencephalitic patients, with the implication that the causative process was ongoing in elderly Parkinson's sufferers. This ongoing process was confirmed by Jenner's[70] group in London. To assess further the contribution of aging in the development of

Parkinson's disease, Fearnley and Lees[71] studied the microarchitecture of the substantia nigra in control patients of varying ages and patients with Parkinsonism. Control cases showed a linear fallout of pigmented neurons in the pars compacta with advancing age, but in Parkinson's disease patients of varying ages there was an exponential loss of pigmented neurons with a 45 percent loss in the first decade. Thus they concluded that age-related attrition of pigmented nigral cells is not an important factor in the pathogenesis of Parkinson's disease.

In addition, features of the disorder may also be influenced by other cerebral pathologies common in old age such as Alzheimer's disease and multiple infarcts, which, even if subclinical, may impair normal compensatory mechanisms that maintain dopaminergic functions. Such patients may therefore experience symptomatic disease at an earlier stage.[72]

Summary

Many investigators believe that environmental factors are an important causative or trigger factor for most people but that there must be an underlying susceptibility to these factors. While an age-related susceptibility seems less likely, it appears that genetic factors such as those described above may in fact play a role. Such genetic susceptibility may be inherited or result from mutations due to external or internally generated toxic effects.

It is possible that Parkinson's disease will be shown to be truly heterogeneous in terms of etiology. Factors might act individually or in combination to varying degrees in different people. Genetic and aging factors might also influence the progress of the disease despite its apparent self-sustaining nature.

Pathology

Parkinson's disease is characterized histologically by severe loss of neurons in the zona compacta of the substantia nigra, the locus coeruleus, the mesencephalic ventral tegmental area, the nucleus basalis of Meynert, and the dorsal nuclei of the vagus. Reports of cortical cell loss[73] are inconsistent.

Destruction of nigrostriatal neurons with the resulting decrease in striatal dopamine is the most distinctive biochemical feature of Parkinson's disease. It is not, however, pathognomonic.[13] Nigral projections to the striatum are topographically organized and result in the putamen showing the most marked depletion of dopamine. Clinical features appear when 80 percent of striatal dopamine has been lost.[74] Although loss of this substance is the characteristic biochemical abnormality of Parkinsonism, it is debatable whether it is the cause of the major motor symptoms. Jellinger[25] reports that rigidity and akinesia are correlated with progressive dysfunction of the nigrostriatal system, Jenner and Marsden[75] claim that striatal dopamine deficiency may contribute to tremor, and Ellenbroek et al.[76] believe that this deficiency does not contribute to rigidity.

Cell loss from the locus coeruleus leads to deficiency in the noradrenergic system, and loss from the nucleus basalis of Meynert to reduction of cholinergic input to the neocortex (frontal, temporal, occipital) and the amygdala and hippocampus of the limbic system.[77] The nucleus basalis is more severely involved in demented compared with nondemented Parkinson's sufferers,[13] but there is also evidence of subclinical involvement in the latter group.[78] Some cases show involvement of the Edinger-Westphal nucleus, which may explain some of the neuro-ophthalmic problems some Parkinson's sufferers experience.[79] Within the dopaminergic systems the degree of toxicity of the causative agent may determine the extent of involvement, with the nigrostriatal pathway involved first, followed by the mesocortical, the mesolimbic, and, less frequently, the hypothalamic dopaminergic system.[13] Peptide abnormalities have been reported,[15] but their significance is uncertain.[13] Thus a pattern is emerging of damage principally to the nigrostriatal dopaminergic system but also in varying degrees to other neurotransmitter systems with the possible exception of the dopaminergic innervation of the spinal cord. Other pathologies in the brain further alter the clinical picture and course of the disease.[80]

Although Lewy bodies[81] were first described in Parkinson's sufferers at the outbreak of World War I, only recently have they generated such intense interest. Essentially these bodies are eosinophilic intracytoplasmic inclusions with a darker central core and a paler halo. They indicate a cytoskeletal abnormality and are formed as cells degenerate and die. Their presence is characteristic but not pathognomonic of Parkinson's disease since Lewy bodies are found in cases attributable to other causes of Parkinsonism and in Alzheimer's disease. Also there are cases of Parkinson's disease without Lewy bodies.[82] Their distribution in Parkinson's disease is specific and includes the substantia nigra, locus coeruleus, nucleus basalis of Meynert, thalamus, and hypothalamus.[83] Nonetheless, it is the additional severe loss of pigmented nigral cells that distinguishes Parkinson's disease and correlates with the severity of the disorder. The prevalence of Lewy bodies increases with age in normal brains from 1.8 percent in the sixth decade to 18.2 percent in the ninth decade, and this increase is paralleled by the rise in age-specific prevalence of the disease.[84] Such people are regarded as being at risk of developing Parkinson's disease. Their state corresponds to a presymptomatic level of dopamine loss, and added insults, such as drugs,[85] could unmask the disease.

There has been a great debate about the relationship between Parkinson's disease and dementia. At autopsy 5 to 47 percent of Parkinson's patients show features of Alzheimer's disorder.[75] There is a six- to ninefold increase in Alzheimer's pathology in Parkinson's patients compared with controls of the same age.[86] Also, extrapyramidal signs[87] and Parkinsonian symptoms[88] are more common in Alzheimer's patients than in age-matched controls. Jellinger has reviewed the pathology of dementia in Parkinson's disease and concluded that mental impairment in this disorder cannot be related to pathology in a single neuronal or transmitter system. He supports the concept of three basic subtypes: (1) cortical dementia with neuronal and dendritic loss and Alzheimer's pathology in the neocortex, (2) limbic dementia with severe cell-specific Alzheimer's pathology leading to functional isolation of the hippocampus and amygdala, and (3) subcortical dementia due to dysfunction of the ascending cholinergic forebrain system (nucleus basalis of Meynert), the ascending noradrenergic system (locus coeruleus), the mesocorticolimbic system (ventral tegmental area), and the serotonergic and peptidergic system. Whether the latter two subtypes could produce a global impairment of intellect is debatable.[89,90] Nonetheless these subtypes may be found in various combinations with Parkinsonian pathology, thereby producing a wide range of clinical features and disease courses.

Agid et al.[13] and Jellinger[25] have extensively reviewed the biochemistry and pathology not only of Parkinson's disease but also of other causes of Parkinsonism, including a description of "senile Parkinsonism" which clinically shows Alzheimer's disease and Parkinson's disease signs but pathologically principally demonstrates Alzheimer's changes and minimal damage to pigmented brain stem nuclei.[91]

The cause of the selective neuronal loss in Parkinson's disease is unknown, but oxidative (free radical or redox) damage and mitochondrial dysfunctions are now considered important events.[92]

The brain is susceptible to oxidative damage because it has an enhanced requirement for oxygen, has a high iron content, and contains polyunsaturated fats as a major constituent.[93] A number of reports have now documented abnormalities in parameters of oxidative stress, implying increased free radical production in Parkinson's disease.[94,95] Some investigators believe that neuromelanin has a pivotal role. It may normally be cytoprotective in sequestering redox active metal ions but, under certain conditions related to increased iron levels, can have a cytotoxic role either by generating hydrogen peroxide or by releasing redox active metal ions if it loses its integrity. By overwhelming antioxidative defense mechanisms, the ensuing repeated oxidative stress could result in neuronal death.[96]

MPTP is thought to induce dopaminergic cell death through the inhibition of NADH COQ1 reductase (complex 1) by its metabolite MPP^+. Complex 1 is the proximal part of the mitochondrial transport chain, and its inhibition leads to a fall in adenosine triphosphate (ATP) production. Complex 1 deficiency has been identified in the substantia nigra of patients with Parkinson's disease and is thought to be specific to the disorder.[97] This deficiency, in combination with oxidative stress, could lead to a cycle of mitochondrial dysfunction and free radical production resulting in dopaminergic cell death. More recent work has reported loss of the α-ketoglutamate dehydrogenase complex (KGDHC) in the substantia nigra which, like complex 1 deficiency, could affect electron transport and ATP synthesis within mitochondria.[98] It is argued that the resulting respiratory failure increases free radical formation and consumes glutathione, which is an important antioxidant. The key point here is that the central defect is an energy crisis and that oxidative stress occurs secondary to this event.

Animal work has shown that L-dopa can cause a reversible 25 percent deficit of complex 1 activity. However, it appears that L-dopa does not cause complex 1 deficiency in Parkinson's disease striatum. It does not, however, preclude that it may enhance a pre-existing complex 1 deficit in the substantia nigra.[99] Glia may have a role in producing the mitochondrial and free radical changes in Parkinson's disease by releasing nitric oxide which is capable of inhibiting the mitochondrial respiratory chain.[100] The free radical hypothesis is, however, not universally accepted.[101]

The mechanism of neuronal death in Parkinson's disease is of interest. Apoptosis (programmed cell death) occurs in development, and in contrast to necrosis is an active process. There is in vitro and animal evidence that apoptosis can be induced by neurotoxins,[102] cycad ingestion,[103] and unopposed endogenous glutamate[104] (a transmitter found in the striatum). If apoptosis is involved in Parkinson's disease it would have significant implications for the development of new treatment strategies.

Diagnosis

The diagnosis of Parkinsonism is entirely clinical. It is therefore essential that clearly defined and agreed-on diagnostic criteria be used (Table 38-3). Data from the United Kingdom Parkinson's Disease Society Brain Bank, however, indi-

Table 38-3 Guideline diagnostic criteria for Parkinson's disease

A progressive usually nonfamilial disorder with bradykinesia (slowness of initiation of voluntary movement, progressive reduction in speed and amplitude of repetitive movement and difficulty switching smoothly from one motor program to the next) and at least one of the following:

Muscular rigidity,

Coarse 4 to 6-Hz resting tremor,

Impaired righting reflexes (not caused by primary visual, vestibular, cerebellar, or proprioceptive dysfunction)

Absolute exclusion criteria are the following:

Exposure to neuroleptic drugs within the year before the onset of symptoms, or to MPTP

Presence of cerebellar or corticospinal tract signs

Past history of encephalitis lethargica or viral encephalitis with oculogyric crises

Stepwise progression and/or a history of multiple strokes

Presence of communicating hydrocephalus or a supratentorial tumor

Presence of severe early autonomic failure

Supranuclear gaze palsy

Presence of severe early Alzheimer's type dementia

Negative response to large doses of L-dopa

(Modified from Lees and Gibb,[126] with permission.)

cate that even then 24 percent of cases diagnosed by committed neurologists and geriatricians do not have pathologic features of the disease at autopsy.[105] A negative response to L-dopa makes the diagnosis of Parkinson's disease suspect,[106] and some experts recommend a test dose of oral L-dopa or subcutaneous apomorphine.

Diagnosis can be a problem early in the disease. The disorder is insidious in onset and tends to fluctuate not only from day to day but also during the same day. Some patients present with subtle symptoms and signs; for example, rigidity may not be obvious on clinical examination until reinforcing maneuvers are used (synkinesis). About one-third of patients have a plethora of vague symptoms (fatigue, aches and pains, depression), some of which may even be sensory (paraesthesiae, numbness, burning sensations, and formication). They may be present for months or even years before the classic features appear.

Older patients also have more specific diagnostic difficulties. They may minimize their symptoms and say "It's just my age, doctor," and indeed the stooped posture, small, shuffling steps, and poor balance of the Parkinson's patient are regarded by many as natural concomitants of old age. The characteristic tremor may be minimal in the late-onset variant of the disease, and 15 percent of patients never have tremor.[107] Unilateral Parkinsonism with minimal tremor may be mistaken for a stroke; the immobility of demented or depressed patients may simulate bradykinesia; and rigidity with bradykinesia may simulate arthritis. The slowness and apathy of hypothyroidism may cause confusion. Despite these difficulties there are nonetheless regularly recurring complaints that should make one suspect Parkinson's disease. These include profound fatigue, a complaint of slowing down, unexplained falls, depression in the absence of a past history, painful frequent cramps, weakness or clumsiness with no stroke signs, and a decline in accustomed dexterity such as inability to manage small buttons, open jars, use a screwdriver, or crochet.

The role of positron emission tomography using [^{18}F]dopa as a tracer in the diagnosis of Parkinson's disease is being evaluated.[108] This investigative tool is limited in its availability at present but may prove of value in preclinical screening of individuals at risk of Parkinson's disease and for measuring disease progression.[109]

Clinical Features

Classic Parkinson's Disease

Tremor, rigidity, bradykinesia, and impaired righting reflexes are the principal features of the disease. The clinical features have been well described.[110,111] Of particular value is the recent description of the development of Parkinson's disease in a professional footballer.[112] I shall only add a few observations to emphasize certain points. All the features of Parkinson's disease can be made worse by anxiety, emotion, and intercurrent illness.

Tremor is essentially resting tremor but may carry over into action, leading to potential confusion with benign essential tremor. Instrumental analysis shows that it has a fundamental resting frequency of 4 to 5.3 Hz and a 6-Hz postural component.[113] Many patients report an inner tremulousness long before the sign appears clinically. Foot tremor may be missed unless the feet are examined hanging unsupported. While generally less disabling than bradykinesia, it is a major source of embarrassment to patients and leads to social isolation. Tremor may be due to an overactive long loop reflex pathway starting at the neuromuscular spindles and returning to muscles via the thalamus and motor cortex. This reflex may be triggered by a mechanism at the thalamic level which is itself influenced by peripheral afferents.[114]

Rigidity affects all muscles, but in the early stages is frequently best detected in the neck and proximal limb muscles.[115] Bradykinesia is the most disabling feature of Parkinson's disease and correlates well with loss of striatal dopamine.[116] It is a complex of various deficits which are outlined in Table 38-3. Rigidity may exacerbate the difficulties initiating movement and further reduce its speed and amplitude. Early signs are frequently seen in the face, with infrequent blinking and widening of the palpebral fissure. Spontaneous gestures are absent: patients lack body language. The voice is often hoarse and lacks resonance, and there is a loss of inflection or prosody.[117]

Many patients with Parkinson's disease experience significant pain, which is usually disease- or therapy-related and responds to manipulation of the therapy.[118]

Impairment of righting reflexes may lead to falls, particularly on getting up from a chair or bed and on turning. They are often present earlier in the disease course in older patients and are responsible for an increased risk of fracture, particularly of the proximal femur.[119] "Freezing" episodes are well recognized in Parkinson's suffers and may be independent of akinesia.[120]

Parkinson's patients may experience a range of visual problems, including blurring, due to impaired coordination of eye muscles, ocular lateropulsion (involuntary gaze drift), double vision, and impaired visual perception. They also experience more blepharitis and conjunctivitis because of reduced blinking.[111]

Autonomic symptoms such as impaired bladder function, constipation, and postural hypotension (usually due to treatment) are experienced and are particularly troublesome for old people.[121] Constipation may lead to impaction and frequent incontinence. Elderly women with Parkinson's may present as if they had features of prostatism. Swallowing problems are common at any stage of the disease, may be asymptomatic,[122] and have implications for nutrition, oral medication, and the risk of bronchopneumonia. Prominent autonomic symptoms at presentation should raise a suspicion of Shy-Drager syndrome.

Clinical Subgroups in Parkinson's Disease

Clinical experience suggests there are at least two subgroups of Parkinson's disease variously described as young versus old, classic versus late, benign versus malignant, and type I versus type II. All have in common a division according to age of onset somewhere within the seventh decade. There are differences in presentation, patients with younger-onset disease tending to present with tremor[123,124] that is more often asymmetric and severe than in older patients.[72] Bradykinesia may be a more common presentation in older individuals.[123] Gait disturbance affects more older-onset patients and appears earlier.[125,126] There is some debate about the progression of the disease, but most sources claim the younger-onset disease has a more benign[124,127] and less rapid course.[125,128] Dementia is thought to be more common in patients with older-onset disease,[125] even using DSM III criteria,[129] and they have more marked impairment of neuropsychologic function.[72,129] Some authors, however, find no difference in the prevalence of dementia, but that the onset is earlier in older-onset patients.[123] There is general agreement that dyskinesias, dystonia, and motor fluctuations are less common in older-onset patients.[130,131] The precise explanation for this is not clear but may be related to shorter disease duration and lower L-dopa doses. On pathologic examination, younger-onset patients have changes marked most in the substantia nigra and greater nigral cell loss, but those with older-onset disease have additional changes in the nucleus basalis of Meynert and the locus coeruleus.[125,126] This suggests that older-onset patients may have more widely distributed pathology. In addition, concurrent vascular or Alzheimer's pathologies may be present. This interplay of pathologies has already been referred to and may well explain some of the disparities observed. Caution is required, however, because most studies are based on relatively small numbers and are not community-based.

Table 38-4 Dependency (consistently requiring the help of at least one person) for various aspects of daily living

Dependent for	Parkinson's (n = 227) (%)	Controls (n = 227) (%)
Household tasks[a]		
Cleaning	54	44
Cooking meals	37	12
Laundry	55	34
Shopping	42	15
Control heat and light	13	5
Self-care		
Eating a meal	33	3
Drinking	5	<1
Toilet	17	5
Dressing	34	10
Bathing	57	24
Washing	18	3
Combing hair	10	3
Shaving	20[b]	2[b]
Bed		
Getting into	24	6
Getting out of	27	6
Turning in	29	7

[a] *These assessments were not applicable for many people who lived in institutions or were elderly men who never cooked, and so on. The percentages are therefore based on less than the 227 applicable elsewhere.*
[b] *These percentages are based on the 97 men in each sample.*

Burden of Disability

Five of the eight most common symptoms reported in studies from Aberdeen[132] and Tasmania[133] are related to mobility. Mobility is crucial to independence, and the loss of independence for Parkinson's sufferers compared with nonsufferers is seen over a wide range of day-to-day tasks (Table 38-4). For many activities the nature of the impairment is such that the disability cannot be adequately helped by material means. Patients need human help, and this has considerable implications both for caregivers and for the way we try to help sufferers achieve independence.[134]

Many patients are seen in clinics with lots of space and are assessed by methods such as timed walking. These procedures totally fail to come to terms with the reality of the elderly person at home. There much of their functioning depends on stop-start movements and there are short distances and a need for frequent changes in direction (e.g., in a modern small kitchen), all of which are difficult when bradykinesia and impaired righting reflexes are present.

Insomnia is more common in Parkinson's patients,[135] and it has been proposed that sleep abnormalities are related to a reduction in brain amine levels.[136] Sleep impairment may even be influenced by the severity of the disease[137] and is characterized by frequent waking and increased time awake. In addition, there are secondary reasons for disturbed sleep. Many patients must get up to go the toilet but find they cannot turn or get out of bed without help (Table 38-4). Many are in pain and, even when sleep comes, experience medication-induced vivid dreams and nightmares.[138] Sleep may have a beneficial effect on the next day's motor performance, but the universality of this sleep benefit has been challenged.[139] Nonetheless, insomnia and night-time discomfort and distress can hardly be a restful preparation for the next day or improve patients' morale.

Psychiatric Symptoms

Depression

The prevalence of the symptoms of depression in people with Parkinson's disease has been variously reported as 20 to 93 percent.[140–142] The clinical similarity of the features of depression and the bradyphrenia of Parkinson's disease makes the diagnosis of either difficult in the presence of the other.[143] The main symptoms encountered are pessimism, hopelessness, decreased motivation and drive, and increased concern with health,[144] but these are not specific to depression in Parkinson's disease.

Traditionally, depression is classified as reactive (e.g., to chronic disability) or endogenous. Not surprisingly, the nature of depression in Parkinson's disease has been debated, and Mindham et al.[145] and Taylor et al.[146] take the view that it is reactive. However, some studies report that the symptoms of depression are present prior to diagnosis,[147] and that there is an increased prevalence of depression in Parkinson's sufferers compared with other groups having a chronic disability, such as paraplegics and amputees.[148] Decreased activity of noradrenaline and serotonin have been implicated in depression, and levels of both these transmitters are reduced in Parkinson's disease.[149] Also the dexamethasone suppression test for depression, which when abnormal probably correlates with noradrenergic dysfunction,[150] was abnormal in Parkinson's patients.[151] The latter data are, however, somewhat tenuous. Common sense suggests that the depression has a reactive component, but the full extent of an endogenous component is not at present clear.

Anxiety

The problem of anxiety in Parkinson's disease is generally ignored, but talking to patients and their caregivers indicates that anxiety is increased in both.[152] Anxiety is significantly higher in Parkinson's sufferers compared with age- and sex-matched nonsufferers, and some have mixed anxiety and depression.[153] The diagnosis may be missed unless specifically sought and can have a significant effect on motivation and rehabilitation. As in the case of depression, there is no clear correlation with disease duration or severity; rather, specific happenings, for example, a decline in motor function, trigger both anxiety and depression. In general terms the cause of anxiety changes as the disease progresses, from fear of the unknown to concern about the loss of physical and financial independence. The judicious use of time to unburden, of therapists to provide practical help and advice, and of social assistance may be as effective as anxiolytics.

Toxic Confusional States and Hallucinations

All the drugs used in the management of Parkinson's disease can produce confusion and hallucinations. At greater risk are older patients, those with a past history of psychiatric disturbance, those with dementia, and those with drug-induced disease.[154] Tanner et al.[155] reviewed hallucinations and concluded they are not related to age or degree of disability but are associated with dementia. However, the presence of hallucinations does not imply a progressive dementing process.[156] Hallucinations are seen in 50 percent of patients after more than 2 years on L-dopa therapy,[157] are usually visual, recurrent, and nonthreatening, and generally occur at night. Insight is retained, and they are regarded as pseudohallucinations. Some individuals may progress to threatening hallucinations with a loss of insight, and such episodes may be associated with paranoia. Patients may also experience fixed paranoid delusions without other psychiatric features. L-Dopa confusion may be preceded for some time by sleep abnormalities, including vivid dreams, night terrors, and nightmares (which often have paranoid features).[154] It may be triggered by increased doses of L-dopa or the addition of a dopamine agonist or anticholinergic. In older people with concomitant brain pathology the threshold of confusion is lower, and multiple pathology, including chest, renal, cardiac, and infectious disease, may trigger confusion. It is therefore essential to diagnose and treat these other pathologies.

A high frequency of psychiatric toxicity is associated with the use of bromocriptine.[158] Confusion attributable to anticholinergics occurs at "therapeutic" doses in old people and in those with dementia. Anticholinergics are best avoided in older patients, and bromocriptine in older demented patients.

The significance of confusion in older people cannot be overestimated because of the high morbidity and the resultant high mortality. Despite being common, it is often poorly managed with an easy recourse to neuroleptics to control noisy or aggressive behavior in a busy hospital setting.

Cognitive Function

In a comprehensive review by Brown and Marsden[159] several difficulties have been highlighted. Treatment may affect cognitive function and its assessment. In addition, there is evidence that, just as with the physical problems of the disease, there is short-term improvement (more than 2 to 3 months) in cognition with L-dopa treatment, but this tails off with time (after 2 to 3 years) to pre-L-dopa levels of function.[160] Patients who have had stereotactic surgery develop a postoperative deficit which never fully recovers.[161]

Assessments may be influenced by factors related to disease and treatment. Most simply, Parkinson's is a disease of old age, and there is an age-related decline in performance on some neuropsychologic tests. Many such tests have a motor speed component which may be impaired in Parkinson's because of bradykinesia and fatigue due to the disease process. Dyskinesias that parasitize productive movement detract from performance, and all tests may be affected by depression, anxiety, and pain, all of which are common in Parkinson's sufferers. The predictive value of initial motor symptoms for subsequent cognitive decline remains controversial. Features associated with a higher risk of cognitive decline include bilateral presentation, a higher rate of decline in arm movement,[162] late-onset disease, a low percentage of improvement with L-dopa, and dystonic dyskinesias.[163]

The mean IQ of Parkinson's patients tends to be within the normal range, although the mean performance IQ, perhaps not surprisingly, is consistently lower than the verbal IQ.[159] Nonetheless, the consensus appears to be that, as a group, Parkinson's patients show evidence of impairment on a wide range of cognitive function tests.

Tests involving route finding, appreciation of body scheme, and judgments of visual and postural vertical have been used. Parkinson's disease is associated with marked deficits in both declarative (explicit) and procedural (implicit) memory.[164] There is thought to be impairment of the cortical-subcortical systems which may not necessarily be prefrontal or dopaminergic.[165]

Impairment of visuospatial functions has previously been reported.[166] More recent work, studying patients with Parkinson's disease at different stages, medicated and unmedicated, has shown deficits of spatial short-term and spatial working memory in more severely affected patients on medication. Patients in early stages of the illness and not on medication did not show impairment.[167] Interestingly, the putative role of dopamine in the retina and the suggestion of specific retinal dysfunction in Parkinson's disease have previously been examined.[168] Impairment of ideational fluency (ability to generate ideas) has also been reported.[169] Immediate and delayed free recall memory and frontal lobe functions such as behavior regulation (i.e., the planning and modulating of tasks based on internal cues) are impaired. The latter is of interest because it may depend on the complex cortex-caudate-pallidum/nigra-thalamus-frontal cortex loop.[170] This may explain the apathy and lack of drive in Parkinson's patients and their inability to respond to internal cues although they rapidly respond to external stimuli.

A topic of considerable interest has been whether cognitive deficits presage dementia. Hulley et al.[171] found no deterioration in cognitive function in a group of Parkinson's patients followed for 9 months, and other studies report a similar experience over 1 year[172] and up to 3 years of testing and more than 10 years after onset of the disease.[173] Porten and Rinne,[174] however, found a significant decline in the cognitive function of patients followed up for 8 or more years.

Dementia

There is a wide range in the reported prevalence of dementia in Parkinson's disease,[175,176] but a commonly quoted figure is one-third to one-half of patients. Some of the variation may be due to overinclusive criteria for the diagnosis of dementia; failure to discriminate confusion, depression, and simple forgetfulness; the inclusion of patients with Parkinsonism as opposed to Parkinson's disease; and selection bias in the sample studied.

Many of the reported prevalences are entirely based on MSQ scores with arbitrary cutoff points. When more appropriate criteria are introduced, incorporating the concept of social or occupational incompetence as in the DSM-III and DSM-IV criteria, the prevalence drops to 15 to 20 percent[175] compared with the range of rates (3 to 20 percent) reported in the general community for comparable age groups.[177] Thus it might appear that the risk has been overestimated, but when examined based on age at onset, increased risk certainly exists for older onset patients, while the state of younger patients is less clear (Table 38-5). A longitudinal study of the incidence of dementia in Parkinson's disease has shown a cumulative incidence of 19 percent over 54 months,[180] rising to 28 percent after 108 months.[181]

There is evidence that dementia and a generally poor prognosis in Parkinson's disease are associated with bradykinesia and gait disturbance[182,183] and that all are associated with a later onset of disease. In the Aberdeen study[184] age as well as age at onset was found to be a predictor of subsequent dementia, and given that Alzheimer's dementia is strongly associated with age, it may be that age at onset data are simply a corollary of age. If age is then controlled, the severity of features of Parkinsonian impairment—such as bradykinesia, rigidity, posture, arm swing, gait, and speech as measured by the Webster scale—also predict subsequent dementia, suggesting that in predictive terms the previously discussed conceptual division into only young and old onset is too simple. Those with more severe signs may have more severe pathology reflected by a greater spread outside the nigrostriatal system (e.g., to the mesocorticolimbic system or the cholinergic system), and this may independently increase their risk of dementia irrespective of age. Older people may be at greater risk of more widespread damage because of age-related changes in brain function or the effect of additional pathologies such as cerebral arteriosclerosis. A recent study has reported that significant predictors of dementia in Parkinson's disease are lack of education (less than a high school graduate), severity of motor deficit (UPDRS total motor score greater than 20), and onset of disease after 60 years of age. The predicted probability of dementia when all these variables were positive was 97.9 percent.[185]

Table 38-5 Dementia in Parkinson's disease (DSM III criteria)

Study	Earlier Onset (%)	Later Onset (%)
	<60	>60
Hictanen and Teravainen (n = 108)	2	25
Ebmeier et al[178a] (n = 106)	6	30
Reid[179] (n = 100)	8	39

There are many practical implications of dementia in Parkinson's disease. The psychiatric side effects of drugs become more prominent. Drug doses may have to be limited, resulting in a delicate balance between relieving motor symptoms and avoiding hallucinations or confusional states. Any intercurrent illness may upset this balance. Drug compliance may be more difficult, particularly if low, multiple doses are necessary. Rehabilitation becomes a greater challenge, and function declines more in demented compared with nondemented sufferers, even in those who are younger.[29] Of greater significance is the extra burden of care which can produce intolerable strain.

Mortality

Poor accuracy and the failure to take account of the secondary as well as the primary cause of death limit the value of data from death certificates when considering Parkinson's disease.

Cohort and case-control studies are available, but all data

suffer from the limitation that even neurologists who are experts in the field of movement disorders may make an incorrect diagnosis in 24 percent of cases.[105]

Nonetheless, the subject of mortality and Parkinson's disease has aroused considerable interest, not in the least because of the hope that the trebled mortality for Parkinson's sufferers in the pre-L-dopa[186] era might be improved by treatment.

With the introduction of L-dopa, mortality ratios of 0.95[187] to 2.59[188] have been reported in cohort studies, and ratios of 1.6[189] and 2.35[178] (95 percent confidence intervals 1.60 to 3.43) in the only case-control studies available. In a detailed analysis Clarke[190] concluded that overall mortality fell in the 1970s and rose in the 1980s as a result of the benefits of L-dopa in a cohort of frail elderly patients for whom death was delayed.

From the Aberdeen longitudinal study, which was conducted in the 1980s, it clearly emerged that the age of patients had a considerable influence on mortality since there was no statistical difference between patients and matched controls who were under 70 years of age, but a highly significant difference between those over 70 years of age.[178] Decreasing mortality in younger people with Parkinson's disease and increasing mortality in those over 75 years old have been reported in the United Kingdom,[191] Scandinavia,[192] and the United States[193] over the past two decades. This does not preclude a positive effect of L-dopa on the mortality of older patients with Parkinson's disease. It may be hidden by the impact of concomitant multiple pathology which is common in older people. L-Dopa probably improves the life expectancy in younger patients but may not for older patients, and additional carefully controlled studies are needed.

Other Causes of Parkinsonism

There are a number of conditions that may be mistaken for Parkinson's disease, and it is important to identify them since not only will management and prognosis be different, but L-dopa may be ineffective (Table 38-1).

Drug-induced Parkinsonism

Drugs are the most common cause of secondary Parkinsonism in older people.[194] The prevalence increases with age, and it may be higher in women. The condition is clinically indistinguishable from Parkinson's disease,[194,195] however, a helpful feature may be coexisting tardive dyskinesia.

The principal drugs responsible are the phenothiazines (particularly those with the greatest sedative properties) thioxanthenes, sulpiride, metoclopramide, and haloperidol. Rarely, methyldopa, calcium channel blockers, lithium, tetrabenazine, and tricyclic antidepressants also have been implicated.[196] In younger patients the evolution of the disease is dependent on the dosage and potency of the drug, but in older people it related to doses within the therapeutic range. The principal drugs act by blocking dopamine receptors; tetrabenazine depletes stores of dopamine.

In older people the most common causes are prochlorperazine and thioridazine prescribed for falls or vague postural instability, and restlessness and behavioral disturbances, respectively.[194] Interestingly, thioridazine is often regarded as a better choice of phenothiazine to avoid the problem. Many drugs are not mentioned during routine questioning, and it is therefore essential to remain vigilant to the possibility of drug-induced Parkinsonism. The use of drugs should be carefully monitored. Recovery usually occurs when the drug is discontinued, although it may take up to a year for this to happen.[197]

A proportion of patients with drug-induced Parkinsonism subsequently develop Parkinson's disease.[194] It is possible that in susceptible individuals these drugs may act as an environmental factor that unmasks the idiopathic disease. As observed by Rajput et al.[198] these patients may have Lewy bodies and simply be in a presymptomatic stage of the idiopathic disease. It has been reported that essential tremor is a predisposing factor for the development of cinnarazine-induced Parkinsonism.[199]

The first-line management is withdrawal of the drug or, if this is not possible, reduction of dosage. Anticholinergics are best avoided in older people, particularly if they are demented, and it is debatable whether L-dopa is useful.[195] Those patients who were helped by L-dopa may have had presymptomatic Parkinson's disease.

Vascular Parkinsonism

Arteriosclerosis was proposed as a cause of Parkinson's disease by Critchley[200] but subsequently rejected[201,202] as the concomitant occurrence of two common conditions in old age. Nonetheless, there is a well-recognized group of elderly patients who demonstrate features of Parkinsonism with long tract signs, upgoing plantars, and a broad-based military gait. They may also demonstrate pseudobulbar signs and emotional lability and have a history of hypertension, diabetes, and generalized vascular disease. The prevalence is about 6 percent of cases of Parkinsonism,[25] and the response to L-dopa is poor.

Multiple System Degenerations

Progressive supranuclear palsy[203] and Shy-Drager syndrome[204] are the principal degenerative conditions appearing in old age. Progressive supranuclear palsy accounts for nearly 6 percent of cases of Parkinsonism, as reported by Lees[205] in an extensive review. Features considered essential for the neuropathologic diagnosis are neurofibrillary degeneration of subcortical structures with involvement of the internal pallidum, the subthalamic nucleus, and the substantia nigra.[206] Disease onset occurs in middle and old age, and the characteristic supranuclear ophthalmoplegia affecting downgaze is the only diagnostic necessity. All other features are variable but include axial rigidity (leading to the head and neck being held in extension), bradykinesia, dystonia, pseudobulbar palsy, frontal lobe signs (often mistaken for dementia), and postural instability with a tendency to fall backward. Resting tremor may be present on occasion. Impaired mobility and falls are the usual mode of presentation, and psychiatric disturbance is common. Cognitive impairment and nonspecific affective and behavioral disturbances are commonly found, whereas frank psychosis and bipolar mood disorder are rare.[207] The variability of the features and the late appearance or, on occasion, complete absence of the classic eye signs can lead to major diagnostic problems.[205,208] Nonetheless Lees[205] has suggested that the following features are helpful in differentiating the condition from Parkinson's disease: symmetric onset, presentation with gait disturbance, rarity of resting tremor, presence of rigidity in extension, early behavioral symptoms, and lack of response to L-dopa. While most cases are sporadic, progressive supranuclear palsy occurring in three members of a family has been reported.[209] The disease is relentlessly progressive (mean survival 5 years, with no difference whether the patients is over 65 or under 65 years of age at presentation). There is no effective treatment, however, physiotherapists, occupational and speech therapists, and social workers can help to sustain the best possible quality of life.

In Shy-Drager syndrome features of Parkinsonism are associated with symptoms of autonomic failure such as postural hypotension and urinary frequency or retention. In addition, there may be a range of other findings such as iris atrophy, cerebellar ataxia, and corticospinal tract signs.[210] Hypotension and other signs may appear only in the later stages of the disease, but a marked antecollis may be a useful sign differentiating it from Parkinson's disease.[211] There is no consistent evidence of cognitive impairment, however, there are indications of a prominent frontal lobe-like component.[212] The pathologic changes are widespread, but cell loss in the intermediolateral column (which accounts for the autonomic features) is consistent. This syndrome is a rare condition but may be seen in the young elderly. L-Dopa may relieve the Parkinsonian signs but may worsen or cause postural hypotension. Treatment is therefore required. Elastic stockings, fludrocortisone, nonsteroidal anti-inflammatory drugs such as ibuprofen, and more recently the α-adrenergic agonist midodrine, are all useful in the management of postural hypotension.

Postencephalitic Parkinsonism

This condition was common in the earlier decades of this century following the ravages of the influenza A pandemics in the later part of the nineteenth century and the early years of the twentieth century. It is now very rare, although sporadic new cases do occur following viral infections. It is characterized by a history of an encephalitic illness and the development of oculogyric crises occasionally accompanied by marked autonomic disturbance.

Other Differential Diagnoses

Essential Tremor

Essential tremor is the most common movement disorder affecting older people. Its etiology and pathogenesis are not known, but attention has been focused on the role of the inferior olive and the olivocerebellorubral loop.[213] It is not a homogeneous disorder, which may explain why instrumental analysis reveals tremor frequencies in the range 6 to 12 Hz.[214] Findley[215] suggests division into two dominant groups, one between 7 and 11 Hz and another below 7 Hz. The former is regarded as enhanced physiologic tremor (classically 8 to 10 Hz); the other is of larger amplitude and distinct from physiologic tremor.

Prevalence figures vary enormously—from 0.5 to 5.6 percent of the general population.[216] A lack of common analytical methods and diagnostic criteria may account for differences in prevalence, but it is also possible that, just as in Parkinson's disease, prevalence varies in different parts of the world.[216] A recent study has found the age of onset to be bimodally distributed, with a median age of onset of approximately 15 years. The inheritance pattern is autosomal dominant with virtually full penetrance by the age of 65 years. Males and females were reported to be affected in equal proportions and with equal severity.[217] Previous reports have suggested that males are more commonly affected.[218]

The clinical features of essential tremor have been extensively reviewed.[219,220] It is essentially a distal, postural, and action tremor elicited by movements such as holding a cup or by maintaining the hands in an outstretched position. It is generally bilateral and assymetric in severity and disappears when the limb is completely relaxed. A marked titubant head tremor is common. It frequently affects the hands, leading to feeding and writing problems, and is therefore socially disabling. As such it is often far from benign. Hand tremor may be exaggerated when holding a finger in front of the nose, leading to confusion with intention (cerebellar or brain stem) tremor. Tremor of the legs, facial muscles, voice, tongue, and jaw may also coexist.[220] Trembling of the facial muscles may in itself have to be differentiated from geniospasm.[221]

Problems in differentiating essential tremor from Parkinson's disease may arise when stiffness due to concomitant arthritis is taken as rigidity or when patients are taking neuroleptics. A cogwheel phenomenon can be elicited with any tremor unless limbs are moved randomly through a range of movements. If the tremor amplitude is large, an apparent resting tremor may appear when the limb is lying in a supported position. The absence of features of bradykinesia is a helpful diagnostic point.

Parkinson's disease and essential tremor are not thought to be related,[222] however, a study has shown that the prevalence of Parkinson's disease in a group of patients with essential tremor was 24 times higher than expected.[223] More recent work suggests that susceptibility to cinnarizine-induced Parkinsonism is related to essential tremor and aging.[199]

There is no satisfactory treatment for essential tremor. It may be attenuated with alcohol, but this is not a practicable solution. Primidone is effective,[224] but side effects such as nausea, vomiting, and ataxia are particularly prevalent in older people. A slow increase from 62.5 mg daily to 250 mg twice a day may avoid this problem. Propranolol is also useful, with high-amplitude, low-frequency tremor being most responsive. Its use has been thoroughly reviewed by Findley.[215]

Other Conditions

Other conditions that may be confused with Parkinson's disease include normal pressure hydrocephalus which usually presents with the classic triad of apraxic gait, urinary incontinence, and dementia.[225,226] Confusion stems from the shared symptoms of difficulty in initiating movement and a wide-based shuffling gait. Indeed, some authorities believe the gait is due to a disorder of subcortical motor control rather than a classic gait apraxia, which is usually attributed to frontal cortical dysfunction.[227] On occasion, a history of head injury, previous meningitis, or subarachnoid hemorrhage is obtained. Shunting is the treatment of choice but often produces a poor result for elderly patients with concurrent cerebral atrophy or drowsiness.

Alzheimer's patients usually have a long history of dementia, toward the end of which mobility deteriorates and rigidity, accompanied by a stooping posture, appears. They are likely to have widespread primitive reflexes.

Senile Gait Disorder

The crucial issue in senile or essential gait disorder is whether one believes that abnormal neurologic signs in old age always indicate pathology or whether they can result from normal aging.[228] Sudarsky and Ronthal[229] identified elderly patients with short steps, a wide-based gait, and impaired righting reflexes. There was also minimal extrapyramidal rigidity, and only one member of the group was significantly demented. They appeared to represent a homogeneous group of unknown origin. Broe and Creasey[230] also described a senile gait disorder at the heart of which was a slowed, wide-based gait with short steps but no rigidity. Cognitive impairment was also noted. In addition, their patients more commonly had action tremor, impaired upward eye gaze, and absent ankle jerks. The core descriptions may be consistent with an element of an extrapyramidal disease process, but there was no pathologic confirmation and the condition was poorly responsive to L-dopa. Broe and Creasey postulated that the etiology was multifactorial—the result of a summation of subclinical pathologies.

Management of Parkinson's Disease

There is no cure for Parkinson's disease, but L-dopa can ameliorate its effects for a number of years. It is the single most effective treatment for improving function in young and old. Nonetheless, nondrug measures are also important and can add greatly to a patient's quality of life. This section will highlight rather than comprehensively review all management options.

Available Drugs

L-Dopa

We have a wealth of experience in the use of and the problems associated with L-dopa preparations,[231–234] and many papers focus on its use specifically in older people.[24,235–237] It is prescribed almost exclusively with a dopa decarboxylase inhibitor (benserazide/co-beneldopa or carbidopa/co-careldopa) to minimize peripheral side effects such as nausea and vomiting. The efficacy of these preparations is similar, and both are available in alternative formulations. Co-beneldopa comes in dispersible form, and co-careldopa tablets can be dissolved with a little effort. This can be useful for patients with swallowing problems and can help to reverse afternoon akinesia in some cases.[238] Controlled-release formulations were introduced to provide a more constant plasma level of L-dopa in the hope that this would minimize dyskinesias and predictable and nonpredictable (on/off) fluctuations in performance. Each dose produces a longer duration of action and hence fewer doses are required, but many patients prefer to take a standard preparation first thing in the morning because the time from taking a dose of controlled-release L-dopa to the onset of clinical benefit is longer. In general, to produce an adequate clinical response, the total dosage may need to be increased by about 15 to 35 percent compared with standard L-dopa preparations. This may not be necessary for older patients because of altered pharmacokinetic factors.[239]

Controlled-release preparations are useful when motor fluctuations such as "wearing-off" begin to appear, in relieving night-time akinesia and possibly in place of standard L-dopa, when new patients start therapy, to try and avoid later motor fluctuations and dyskinesias. L-Dopa helps 80 percent of patients and improves all features of the disease although occasionally tremor may be less responsive.[240] Since it is effective even with severe or long-standing disease, an absence of response, assuming compliance, should raise the question of other causes of Parkinsonism or an incorrect diagnosis.

The debate about early versus late use of L-dopa is sterile in regard to older people. When to start treatment is a matter to be discussed by patient and doctor, but it is likely to be when function is threatened. In older people this is often at presentation. L-Dopa should be commenced in low dosage and increased as required until function is restored. The dose should not be increased more often than every 5 to 7 days. The average maximum daily dose for elderly people is approximately 750 to 1000 mg.[241] Although, in general terms, a lower maintenance dose may be necessary in older patients, they are not a homogeneous group and may benefit from higher doses. The key is careful adjustment and regular review to avoid potentially harmful side effects.

Pharmacokinetics

Pharmacokinetic factors may be of particular relevance in old age. Geriatricians long ago reported that in older people a significant therapeutic effect could be achieved with doses of L-dopa markedly lower than those usually prescribed.[242] This may be because more of a dose of oral L-dopa is absorbed in older patients,[243] possibly as a result of an age-related reduction in gut decarboxylase and a consequent increase in proximal small bowel absorption.[244] This advantage should be lost with the addition of decarboxylase inhibitors, but with low-dose combinations their effect may be attenuated. Dopa decarboxylase is also active at the blood-brain barrier, but this observation appears to have no clinical relevance.

Older patients have delayed gastric emptying, which should reduce the rate of L-dopa absorption. However, in a small study on Parkinsonian patients without gastrointestinal pathology, gastric emptying was significantly reduced but drug absorption was only modestly slowed.[245] Antacids and achlorhydria enhance absorption, whereas meals retard it. Large neutral amino acids such as tryptophan, tyrosine, leucine, and methionine compete at the gut wall for the same transport system as L-dopa; thus low-protein meals can facilitate L-dopa absorption.[246] A similar effect can be achieved in older people by delayed gastric emptying acting to control the passage of protein. Competition also occurs at the blood-brain barrier but is not clinically significant. Patients should generally be advised to take their L-dopa prior to meals unless nausea is a prominent side effect.

Recently interest has focused on the metabolite 3-*O*-methyldopa, which is produced from l-dopa by the action of the enzyme catechol-*O*-methytransferase (COMT). This metabolic pathway is significant in the presence of decarboxylase inhibition. It is believed that the accumulation of this major metabolite reduces the bioavailability of L-dopa and dopamine in the brain and hence may contribute to later motor fluctuations. COMT inhibitors will soon be available for clinical use.[247,248]

Side Effects

The principal side effects of L-dopa are generally dose- and duration-related. They include dyskinesias, cardiovascular disturbance (e.g., postural hypotension), and gastrointestinal upsets, which may resolve in the first few weeks of treatment. Psychiatric manifestations occur in 20 to 38 percent of patients[237] and are more common when dementia coexists. Interestingly, the only reported prevalence of postural hypotension in elderly Parkinson's sufferers is 27 percent[237] and that in elderly nonsufferers is about 20 percent.[249] When L-dopa has to be discontinued, it is probably sensible to stop it slowly since there have been reports of a condition similar to the neuroleptic malignant syndrome when the drug is withdrawn abruptly.[250] This is particularly likely to happen in the later stages of the disease when end-of-dose phenomena are present and may be a risk during drug holidays. It is characterized by high fever, muscle stiffness, sweating, agitation, and confusion.

Other Drugs

Anticholinergics

Anticholinergics are often used in younger patients early in the disease before function is significantly impaired. They produce about a 25 percent improvement in all features of the disease. Unfortunately, in older people, in addition to the classic side effects of mydriasis, dry mouth, tachycardia, and increased tendency toward urinary retention and constipation, they tend to produce confusion and to potentiate dementia by their action on any cortical cholinergic deficit. Therefore, their routine use cannot be justified. There is no evidence that anticholinergics are better than L-dopa in the treatment of tremor. These drugs should not be discontinued suddenly, as this can precipitate a marked deterioration in the Parkinsonian state.

Amantadine

Pure serendipity led to the introduction of amantadine. A Parkinson's sufferer who developed influenza was treated with the antiviral agent and noted a marked improvement in Parkinsonian symptoms. It relieves all the major symptoms of the disease in almost 50 percent of patients, although it is not as effective as L-dopa and its benefits may be short-lived. The side effect profile is similar to that of anticholinergics with the addition of lower-limb edema and livedo reticularis.[251]

MAO-B inhibitors

Selegiline is a nonreversible selective MAO-B inhibitor. It is used in a dosage of 10 mg daily, either once a day or in divided dosage according to patient preference, and at that level has no "cheese effect" but has some alerting properties. It has no significant side effects per se, but its accepted role is to enhance the activity of dopamine by retarding its metabolism. L-Dopa side effects (in particular upper gastrointestinal bleeding in individuals with peptic disease, postural hypotension, and psychiatric symptoms) may therefore be experienced.[252] Selegiline can disturb sleep in some patients but improve it in others.

Given as monotherapy, the drug has only a mild anti-Parkinson's effect, but it may be sufficient to explain the observed L-dopa sparing effect.[253] Double-blind studies indicate it is beneficial in about 50 percent of patients on L-dopa who develop end-of-dose fluctuations.[254] Unfortunately the benefit often wanes over the first year of treatment. Recently there has been much speculation about a possible neuroprotective role for selegiline, which on balance has not been sustained (see below). Studies on humans are being conducted to assess the value of new potent, fully reversible, highly selective MAO-B inhibitors.[254]

Significant drug interactions have been reported with pethidine and fluoxetine.[255] With the former, delirium and marked muscle rigidity occurred.[256]

Dopamine agonists

Dopamine agonists are natural or synthetic compounds that directly activate dopamine receptors. Bromocriptine and lisuride act only on D_2 receptors, but pergolide and apomorphine act on D_2 and D_1 receptors, which should in theory increase their efficacy. Cabergoline is a potentially useful long-acting agonist which acts on both D_1 and D_2 receptor sites. The classic use of bromocriptine, lisuride, and pergolide is as oral adjuvant therapy to L-dopa in the later stages of the disease when motor fluctuations have become a problem or the effect of L-dopa as monotherapy is waning.[257] Although anecdotally some evidence is emerging that pergolide may be more helpful, direct comparisons do not indicate that one is superior to the other. Rather there are differences in individual patient responses. Switching from one agonist to another may therefore be useful.[258] They have been tried as de novo monotherapy for Parkinson's disease; unfortunately, while they are helpful for some patients, they are not as effective as L-dopa in improving function although they are less likely to be associated with later motor fluctuations and dyskinesias.[259] The side effects are similar those of L-dopa but may be more prominent.[258] In addition, they may occasionally cause pleural effusions and pulmonary fibrosis. Postural hypotention, hallucinations/agitation, and confusion are a problem with older patients, the latter especially so in those with coexisting dementia. These effects are dose-related and can be minimized by starting with a low dose (e.g., 1 mg bromocriptine or 50 μg pergolide at night) and increasing the dose slowly. Domperidone relieves the associated nausea. The maximum beneficial dose in older patients is about 15 mg daily for bromocriptine and 1.5 mg daily for pergolide.

In theory, the introduction of a dopamine agonist should allow a 20 to 40 percent reduction in the daily dose of L-dopa, but in practice, with older patients, if function is to be maintained, this may not always be possible.

Management Challenges

Fluctuations and Their Management

Unfortunately, after 5 to 6 years of L-dopa therapy, nearly two-thirds of patients who initially responded to the drug have returned to their pre-L-dopa level of function. In addition, they experience a wide range of motor problems including dyskinesias and predictable (end-of-dose failure) and nonpredictable (on-off) fluctuations in performance. These side effects are less common and generally less severe in older people. Nevertheless, dyskinesias have been found in to 3 to 26 percent of older patients and fluctuations in 3.3 to 10 percent,[237] and their management is just as problematic. Despite early debate it seems likely these effects are due to a combination of the shortening of therapeutic benefit after each dose, associated with a narrowing of the therapeutic window (i.e., the dose that gives benefit as opposed to causing dyskinesias[260]), the development of a critical threshold for turning patients on, the progressive loss of presynaptic dopamine storage capacity,[261] and changes in postsynaptic receptors.[261] As a result of these changes patients become extremely sensitive to plasma L-dopa levels which in turn can be affected by pharmacokinetic factors such as gut absorption. Early morning akinesia and wearing off—that is, the need for L-dopa before the next planned dose—herald the appearance of fluctuations. The standard response is to give smaller doses of L-dopa more often. Unfortunately, this may be impractical for older patients who are forgetful or demented. In addition, there is some evidence that lower doses under the circumstances of a critical threshold and a narrowed therapeutic window can lead to a failure to switch patients on or, at best, give a reduced duration of response. Fortunately this may be less of problem for older patients because they absorb more of a dose of L-dopa than younger patients. Nevertheless, it may explain why this maneuer produces only a short-lived benefit and emphasizes that there may be a need to maximize the absorption of L-dopa by giving it in liquid form, taking it before meals, or reducing associated dietary protein.[246] Intravenous infusions of L-dopa are effective but are not a feasible long-term strategy.

Other options that have been widely used include combining L-dopa with oral dopamine agonists,[257] which is most likely to help reduce dyskinesias, or with selegiline, the effects of which are seen within a few days.[254] More recently, controlled-release formulations of L-dopa have helped some patients,[262] but it may be necessary to continue with standard doses of L-dopa in the morning and afternoon to obtain the best benefit.[263] The most consistent benefit of these manipulations has been in patients with early fluctuations such as wearing off of the response to L-dopa. However no benefits, last, and it is unfortunate that dyskinesias, which are more common in older patients (up to 26 percent) are less likely to be improved.

Apomorphine

Patients with frequent and incapacitating "off periods" who have not responded to any of the regimes described above may benefit from apomorphine. Given as an intermittent subcutaneous injection using the Penject system or as a continuous subcutaneous infusion, it can consistently reverse off-period motor problems even after 5 years of continuous use.[264] It has no consistent effect on impaired speech or balance. Significant side effects include drowsiness which rapidly settles, local skin reactions which can be severe in patients using continuous infusions, increasingly severe on-period dyskinesias, and postural instability with falls.[264] Neuropsychiatric problems such as hallucinations and confusion can be troublesome. Rarely, an autoimmune hemolytic anemia occurs. Symptoms such as nausea and vomiting can be avoided by pretreatment with the peripheral dopamine antagonist domperidone, which can usually be withdrawn after several weeks although some patients require its long-term use. A limiting factor for the Penject system is the need for patients to anticipate off periods and to be able to inject themselves.

Published studies indicate that apomorphine has been used

long-term in patients up to 78 years of age. There is no suggestion that they were more liable to side effects or that their severity was greater in older patients. Elderly patients can be managed successfully when the circumstances are appropriate, but all should have specialist support and given the problems outlined above, it seems sensible to avoid its use in individuals with dementia, those with previous psychiatric problems (including those due to anti-Parkinsonian drugs), and those living alone who cannot manage the mechanics of the technique by themselves. The potential for rectal, sublingual, and intranasal routes of administration remains uncertain.

Are Fluctuations Avoidable?

Dopamine agonist monotherapy, early in the disease results in fewer dyskinesias and motor fluctuations later in the disease, but the functional benefit is significantly less than with L-dopa.[259] Function can be improved by increasing the dose of dopamine agonist, but most patients find the side effects intolerable.

Open studies have suggested that an early combination of tolerable doses of dopamine agonist with L-dopa not only maintains function but also results in fewer dyskinesias and fluctuations (especially of the end-of-dose variety) later in the disease than does L-dopa alone.[265] Critical reviews are less conclusive, however.[266,267] For older patients and even in low doses, the combination can lead to more side effects, particularly postural hypotension and mental changes. Also, given their much lower prevalence of motor fluctuations and the drawbacks of taking concomitant therapy for coexisting pathology, the risk may not be justified in the very old or in those with evidence of dementia or a significant psychiatric history.

Current treatment delivers the drug to target cells in the brain in pulses. Experimental work suggests that the physiologic mode of dopaminergic action is by sustained (tonic) release onto target cells.[268] This explains the observation that continuous intravenous or subcutaneous infusions can reduce established fluctuations.[269] It has been suggested that a similar tonic delivery of medication used from the start of treatment might reduce or even prevent fluctuations appearing later in the course of the disease. Continuous infusions are impractical at present, but longer-acting oral agents such as the dopamine agonist cabergoline or controlled-release L-dopa[270] might be useful. Long-term clinical trials using controlled-release L-dopa are under way. If successful, this seems to be a cleaner option for older patients.

Neuroprotection

In the past decade much of the interest in this issue has been centered on the use of selegiline (deprenyl) at the time of diagnosis of the disease.

In an open and retrospectively analyzed study Birkmeyer and colleagues[271] found a significant increase in the life expectancy of a group of patients treated with Madopar plus selegiline compared with that of a group treated only with Madopar.[271] Studies on the pathogenesis of the disease, in particular those on MPTP and mechanisms of free radical production (vide supra) suggested ways in which the drug might achieve such an effect.[272] Two randomized, prospective, double-blind trials involving patients with early Parkinson's disease were set up to determine whether selegiline could retard the progress of the disease.[273,274] Both reported favorable results, and the larger DATATOP study concluded that the onset of disability was delayed.[274] An intense debate followed as to whether the effects observed were due to symptomatic benefit or to a neuroprotective effect.

Subsequent reports from this group concluded there was evidence that selegiline delayed the need for L-dopa and had a symptomatic benefit on some features of the disease, but there was no conclusive evidence of a neuroprotective effect. They also found no beneficial effect from the free radical scavenger tocopherol.[275]

In addition, in an open prospective randomized trial in the United Kingdom, in which patients were allocated to Madopar alone or Madopar plus selegiline or bromocriptine alone, there was, over a 3-year period, "no evidence to support a differential rate of decline among the treatment groups.[276] More recently the same group has suggested that, contrary to Birkmeyer's experience, selegiline may even be harmful for some patients although the precise mechanism is not known.[253] This has not, however, been confirmed by other controlled studies around the world.

These results do not absolutely preclude a neuroprotective effect for selegiline. It may be a question of timing. Early in the symptomatic stage of the disease is late in the pathogenic process. It may be possible to produce only a marginal effect by this stage, but presymptomatic diagnosis could allow agents to be used earlier with possibly greater benefit. Such studies will require cheap, reliable, validated markers for both presymptomatic diagnosis and the progress of the disease.

Drug Holidays

Drug holidays have been the subject of much debate. Sweet et al.[277] first reported an enhanced response to L-dopa after a drug holiday,[277] and the mechanism was thought to be improved receptor function. Various reports appeared to confirm the benefit, but nonetheless it was recognized that there were significant risks of pneumonia, deep venous thrombosis, and severe psychological upset. More recent studies have concluded that the chances of lasting improvement do not merit the considerable discomfort, dangers, and cost of hospitalization.[278] They contend that the reduction of high doses to a more reasonable level is just as likely to produce an improvement as a full drug holiday, and this is certainly the experience of many geriatricians. Full assessment, review of all medications, and a reduction in L-dopa dosage are more appropriate for elderly patients.

Surgery

The role of neurotransplantation in Parkinson's disease has captured the imagination of both the media and the general public. The subject is complex and has been further complicated by the particular ethical issues relating to the use of human fetal nigral tissue. Recently, however, the 6-year-old ban on the use of fetal tissue in the United States was ended with the awarding of a grant specifically to support the implantation of fetal tissue in patients with Parkinson's disease.

Intrastriatal implants of embryonic ventral mesencephalic tissue, rich in dopamine neurons, reinervate the dopamine-denervated striatum of rodents and monkeys with experimental Parkinson's disease, form synaptic contacts with host striatal neurons, release dopamine, and improve motor and sensorimotor functions.[279,280]

In humans, adrenal autografts and human fetal mesencephalic tissue have been used as sources of dopamine. Adrenal grafts produce only modest symptomatic benefit, and survival of implants has been poor.[268,281] So far more than 150 patients have been grafted with human fetal tissue either unilaterally or, in a few cases, bilaterally in the caudate nucleus and/or putamen.[282] A general improvement in motor symptoms has been reported in almost all patients after transplantation,[283] but the mechanisms of improvement are unknown in most cases. Evidence of graft survival has been demonstrated,[284] perhaps most convincingly in the recent autopsy study reported by Kordower et al.[285]

Further avenues that may hold therapeutic promise include implantations into the stratum of cells genetically engineered to synthesize and release L-dopa.[286–288] Animal models also suggest that neurotrophic factors such as gangliosides (GUI) and brain-derived neurotrophic factor (BDNF) may in time also be useful.[289,290] With advances in stereotactic techniques neurosurgeons can lesion highly discrete areas of the brain. A lesion in the thalamic ventral intermediate nucleus (VIN), a technique used successfully in older people, relieves disabling tremor.[291] Lesions confined to the posteroventral pallidum can significantly relieve rigidity, bradykinesia, and tremor even when individuals have responded poorly to L-dopa.[292] Not all patients undergoing pallidotomy improve and, based on the current understanding of basal ganglia surgery, it does not produce all anticipated effects.[293] Rather than lesion the VIN of the thalamus, Benabid et al.[294] effectively relieved tremor by electrical stimulation.[294] None of these techniques is without potential significant morbidity.

Special Problems

Parkinsonism patients experience a wide range of problems, some of which are briefly reviewed in Table 38-6. The management of problems occurring at night is frequently overlooked and often unsatisfactory. Commonsense advice about the height of beds, the use of smooth, low-friction materials for bedding and nightclothes, and information on equipment such as rope ladders can all be useful. Techniques for getting into, turning in, and getting out of bed can be taught. Therapy encouraging truncal rotation can also be helpful. Symptomatic treatment, such as with hypnotics, sedatives, analgesics, and quinine tablets for cramp, are often prescribed and can be useful; however, in elderly people the side effects of the drugs may often detract from any significant benefit. Dopamine agonists and controlled-release L-dopa taken on retiring can help many patients, and some prefer to take a dose of standard L-dopa if they waken.

Table 38-6 Problems experienced by patients with Parkinson's disease

Problem	Management
Falls	Early: may respond to L-dopa; later: check postural hypotension, L-dopa; physiotherapist advice
Tremor	When resistant to L-dopa and disabling, anticholinergic or β-blocker
Painful dystonia	Baclofen, lithium, manipulated L-dopa
Myoclonus	Clonazepam
Postural hypotension	Review drug dose; support stockings; fludrocortisone (0.1–1 mg daily); nonsteroidal antiinflammatory drugs
Nocturnal cramps	Ensure anti-Parkinsonism treatment adequate; quinine sulfate
Dysphagia	Advice from speech therapist; ice, lemon to stimulate swallowing; if acute, IV anticholinergic
Drooling saliva	Anticholinergic unless contraindicated; DXT to salivary glands
Constipation	Ensure not hypothyroid; encourage regular exercise; ample fluids, fruit, bran; if necessary, laxatives
Nausea	Rule out other pathology; domperidone
Incontinence	Ensure no remediable cause (e.g., prolapse, constipation, prostatism, retention); consider associated brain failure; 2-hourly toileting; night-time bottles or commodes; consider oxybutynin; if not controllable, sheath urinals; if no alternative, urinary catheter
Depression	Tricyclic antidepressants (anticholinergic benefits) unless contraindicated; if nonresponsive, consider electroconvulsive therapy
Sleepiness	Reduce L-dopa; if altered sleep/wake cycle, stimulate by day and if necessary chlormethiazole at night
Drenching sweats	Rule out tuberculosis, bacterial endocarditis; β-blockers
Blepharitis	Saline eye wash
Loose dentures	Dentist
Freezing	Physiotherapy

Psychiatric Problems

Psychiatric manifestations occur in 20 to 38 percent of older patients[237] and are more common when dementia coexists. Sleep disturbance and hallucinations where insight is retained generally respond to adjustment of dopaminergic therapy. Persistent threatening hallucinations, paranoia, and drug-induced toxic confusional states can be extremely difficult to treat. Full assessment is essential to diagnose and treat any infective, metabolic, or other health problems that may exacerbate the situation, and admission to a hospital may be necessary. If anticholinergics or dopamine agonists are being used, they should be withdrawn gradually and avoided in the future. It may be necessary to reduce the dose of L-dopa, but this may threaten mobility and independence. A drug holiday, as an inpatient, over a period of 1 to 2 days appears to be beneficial and is indeed the only generally agreed-on indication for a drug holiday.[295] If symptoms persist or independence is threatened, it may be necessary to use a neuroleptic agent such as thioridazine in the lowest dose possible to manage psychotic symptoms. Some success has been reported using Risperidone to control hallucination,[296] and in some countries clozapine, a new benzobenzodiazepine derivative which is virtually free of extrapyramidal effects, is available.[297] The principal side effects of clozapine are sedation, drooling, postural hypotension, and, in 1 to 2 percent of cases, agranulocytosis.

Assessment

Successful management is only possible, however, with thorough and ongoing assessment of the patient's and caregivers' needs. Specialist assessment should include screening for dementia,[298] depression, and anxiety,[299] and the assessment of clinical features using the Hoehn and Yahr[186] and Webster scales.[300] Disability can be measured with the Northwestern University score.[301] Drug side effects should be screened for, and the need for treatment by therapists considered.

Nondrug Management

Hildick-Smith[302] and Andrews[303] have cogently reviewed the role of rehabilitation.[302,303] Physiotherapists, speech and occupational therapists, social workers, and nursing colleagues all have a role to play. At certain stages of the disease process their involvement can do more for the patient and their caregivers' quality of life than drugs per se. The need for[304] and value of intervention[305] by an occupational therapist has been demonstrated. Their role is by no means just to provide aids, important though that may be, but rather to assess fully the practical implications of situations and provide helpful and achievable solutions so that independence can be maintained.

Speech therapists can help by assessing swallowing as well as speech problems and give advice on communication difficulties. There is now considerable interest on the part of speech therapists in the problems of Parkinson's suffers,[306] and basic research has provided challenging modes of treatment[307] which can help over both the short and the long term.[305]

The role of physiotherapy has been questioned. In a controlled trial Gibberd et al.[308] concluded that physiotherapy in a day-hospital setting did not produce improvement in Parkinson's sufferers.[308] Steiner and Flewitt[309] and Franklyn and Stern,[310] however, found therapy to be beneficial. Banks and Caird[311] have demonstrated the benefits of physiotherapy in the patient's own home, and a randomized, single-blind, crossover study has shown that physiotherapy can help some patients but must be continued if benefit is to last.[312] Conductive education[313] and music therapy[314] have also been shown to be of benefit, the latter possibly because it increases sympathetic activity in the nervous system. Physiotherapists can advise on the suitability of mobility aids and teach the techniques of how to get up after a fall. Exercise in any reasonable form keeps the patient as fit and supple as possible; there is also the benefit of socialization within a group with stimulation and the maintenance of morale in patients who are often anxious, depressed, and isolated. Despite the benefits therapists can bring, patients often claim not to have seen them.[304,315]

Patients are likely to benefit most from care shared between a general practitioner and a specialist, with the latter based in a specific Parkinson's clinic. A specialist Parkinson's nurse may be useful.[316] Studies are needed to show that these changes in the way we care for patients can produce better outcomes and are cost-effective. The management of Parkinson's disease depends on a multidisciplinary approach, regular assessment, and a close integration of drug therapy with physical and social rehabilitation. Membership in the Parkinson's Disease Society is also helpful.

Other Movement Disorders

Hyperkinetic States

There are many hyperkinetic disorders of movement, some of which, until recently, have been diagnosed as psychiatric problems[317] Most occur principally in young people, but there are several that merit our attention.

Tardive Dyskinesia

This disorder is characterized by persistent, repetitive, choreiform movements affecting the lower orofacial muscles. Eye movements are less frequently involved. This is the most common presentation in older people and resembles lip smacking, chewing, and sucking. It may be accompanied by choreoathetoid movements of the limbs and truncal hyperkinesia (swaying, bending, twisting). Movements are abolished by sleep and made worse by anxiety and exercise. In severe forms respiration, speech, and swallowing may be impaired.

Neuroleptics (phenothiazines, butyrophenones) are the commonest cause, but metoclopramide,[318] particularly in doses above 30 mg daily, and L-dopa are also responsible. Rarely, antidepressants[319] and benzodiazepines[320] have been implicated. Twenty percent of patients taking a neuroleptic develop dyskinesia in the first year. Perversely, some patients experience dyskinesia only when the drug is stopped. Eight percent[321] to 13 percent[322] of cases occur spontaneously and may result from an age-related decline in D_2 receptors that alters the D_1/D_2 receptor ratio.[323]

Overall, the prevalence of dyskinesia rises with age to about 22 percent of those over 60 years of age taking neuroleptics.[321,322] It is more common in women over 70 years of age. Tardive dyskinesia is thought to be caused by a dopamine receptor blockade in the striatum, resulting in a compensatory receptor hypersensitivity. Management is particularly difficult since 50 percent of cases persist after the drug is discontinued; indeed, as already noted, the dyskinesia may be exacerbated for weeks afterward. Some may resolve after periods up to 5 years, and some never resolve, which is particularly sad since the drugs are often inappropriately prescribed. When the dyskinesia is socially or functionally disabling, tetrabenazine, which depletes striatal dopamine, has been used, but the side effects of Parkinsonism, sedation, depression, and postural hypotension limit its suitability for older people. A wide range of other treatments have been tried with little benefit.[324] Neuroleptics should be avoided where possible, but when they must be used, dose and duration should be kept to a minimum or a drug with less of an effect on D_2 receptors substituted. Clozapine, a new neuroleptic with fewer extrapyramidal side effects, may be indicated if ongoing neuroleptic treatment is required.[325] When all else has failed, increasing the dose of the offending drug may give temporary relief.

Akathisia or motor restlessness may occur in about 25 percent of patients with tardive dyskinesia. It is marked by a subjective feeling of restlessness, and objectively the patient may fidget, squirm, rub their limbs, pace, or even run around. Feelings of tension, irritability, and panic are expressed. It can be ameliorated by reducing the dose of neuroleptic. Diazepam or propranolol may also be helpful.

Choreoathetoid Movements

These movements occur in the elderly as a result of drug toxicity or degenerative or senile chorea, and very occasionally symptomatically, for example, due to polycythemia.[326] Choreiform movements are essentially jerky and nonrepetitive, whereas athetoid movements are slow, sinuous and repetitive with alternating flexion-extension at the wrists and other joints.

The drugs most frequently implicated are the neuroleptics and L-dopa. In addition, there are reports of dyskinesias due to tricyclic antidepressants, phenytoin, carbamazepine, and cimetidine.[324] Subclinical cerebral pathology may be present in some patients who develop dyskinesias.

Senile chorea is due to cell loss in the putamen and caudate. In some cases there is evidence of Alzheimer's pathology and/or multi-infarct vascular disease.[327] Senile chorea has previously been thought of as late-onset Huntington's disease with an undisclosed family history,[328] but it is now known that the molecular basis of Huntington's disease is CAG trinucleotide expansion and that this marker is highly sensitive and specific.[329] Not all cases of Huntington's disease, however, have CAG expansions.[330] In most cases people with 30 repeats are healthy, while those with 35 to 60 repeats follow the typical pattern of developing the disease in adulthood. Those with more than 60 repeats develop the disorder in childhood.[329] Worsening of the disease over successive generations (anticipatory) correlates with increasing expansion size.[331] A recent study of four patients with a clinical presentation of senile chorea found CAG repetition lengths to be normal, which supports the belief that senile chorea is a separate entity from late-onset Huntington's disease.[332]

Chorea is due to an excess of dopaminergic activity. When troublesome, treatment with tetrabenazine has been useful. Various other drugs, including clonazepam, valproate, and baclofen, have been tried but generally with little success.[333]

Ballismic movements are considered large-amplitude chorea. They occur sporadically in the elderly, usually as a result of a stroke affecting the contralateral subthalamic nucleus or multiple infarcts in the striatum. The prognosis for recovery over a period of months is generally good.

The "periodic movements of sleep" syndrome consists of brief myoclonic jerks during light sleep, "sleep starts," (i.e., large myoclonic jerks while falling asleep), and nocturnal myoclonus. Their prevalence increases with age to 29 percent of those over 50 years, and they may be associated with restless legs syndrome. Clonazepam or baclofen may be useful in treatment.[327]

Myoclonus is seen in the elderly following anoxia and in association with Alzheimer's disease, Jacob-Creutzfeld's disease, and progressive supranuclear palsy. It consists of sudden contractions of a muscle or group of muscles and may be treated with clonazepam or valproate.[334] Tics usually present in younger age groups but may be carried into old age. They may occur during treatment with L-dopa, neuroleptics, carbamazepine, and phenytoin, and also with stroke.[335] Clonazepam is useful when treatment is necessary.

Dystonia

Dystonia is defined as "a syndrome of sustained muscle contractions, frequently causing twisting and repetitive movements or abnormal postures."[336] Focal, segmental, and generalized dystonias are recognized, and they may have a familial basis.[337] Both focal and segmental dystonias may occur in old age. Examples of focal dystonias are blepharospasm, torticollis, and writer's cramp. The later the age of onset, the more likely is it that the severity will be less, the legs will not be involved, and the distribution of dystonia will be limited. Neuroleptics, anticonvulsants, metoclopramide, and L-dopa may produce dystonia in old people, as may stroke and Parkinson's disease.[338]

Sensory stimulation can lessen or eliminate dystonia, for example, touching periorbital skin in a blepharospasm. Treatment is otherwise unsatisfactory. High-dose anticholinergics have been used in young people, but this application is limited in the elderly because of confusion, hallucinations, and behavioral disturbances. Other useful therapies involve baclofen, benzodiazepines, and carbamazepine.[339] Focal dystonias such as blephorospasm and torticolis may be safely treated by local injections of botulinum toxin.[340] The toxin acts presynatptically at peripheral nerve terminals to prevent calcium-dependent release of acetylcholine.[341]

References

1. Pasik P, Pasik T, Di Figlia M: The internal organisation of the neostriatum in mammals. p. 5. In Divac I, Oberg REG (eds): The Neostriatum. Pergamon Press, Oxford, 1979
2. Graybiel AM, Ragsdale W: Biochemical anatomy of the striatum. p. 427. In Empson PC (ed): Chemical Neuroanatomy. Raven Press, New York, 1983
3. Alheid GF, Heimer L, Switzer III: Basal ganglia. p. 483. In Paxinos G (ed): The Human Nervous System. Academic Press, New York, 1990
4. Di Figlia M, Aronin N: Amino acid transmitters. p. 1115. Paxinos G (ed): The Human Nervous System. Academic Press, New York, 1990
5. Gerfen CR: The neostriatal mosaic: multiple levels of compartmental organisation in the basal ganglia. Ann Rev Neurosci 1992;15:285–320
6. Webster KE: The functional anatomy of the basal ganglia. p. 3. In Stern G (ed): Parkinson's Disease. Chapman and Hall Medical, London, 1990
7. Dray A: The striatum and substantia nigra; a commentary on their relationships. Neuroscience 1979;4:1407–1439
8. Graybiel AM: Neurochemically specified subsystems in the basal ganglia. p. 114. In Evered D, O'Connor M (eds): Functions of the basal ganglia. CIBA Foundation Symposium 107. Pitman, London, 1984
9. Hokfelt T, Martensson R, Bjorklund A: Distributional maps of tyrosine-hydroxylase-immunoreactive neurons in the rat brain. p. 277. In Bjorklund A, Hokfelt T (eds): Handbook of Chemical Neuroanatomy. Vol. 2. Elsevier, London, 1984
10. Bjorklund A, Lindvall O: Dopamine containing systems in the CNS. p. 55. In Bjorklund A and Hokfelt T (eds): Handbook of Chemical Neuroanatomy. Vol. 2, Elsevier, London, 1984
11. Tork I, Hornung JP: Raphe nuclei and the serotonergic system. p. 1001. In Paxinos G (ed): The Human Nervous System. Academic Press, San Diego, 1990
12. Pearson J, Halliday G, Sakamoto N, Michael JP: Catacholaminergic neurons. p. 1023. In Paxinos G (ed): The Human Nervous System. Academic Press, New York, 1990
13. Agid Y, Javoy-Agid F, Rubert M: Biochemistry of neurotransmitters in Parkinson's disease. p. 166. In Marsden CD, Fahn S (eds): Movement Disorders 2. Butterworths, London, 1987
14. McGeer EG, McGeer PL: Biochemical neuroanatomy of the basal ganglia. p. 113. In Calne DB (ed): Drugs for the treatment of Parkinson's Disease. Handbook of Experimental Pharmacology 88. Springer-Verlag, Berlin, 1989
15. Constantinidis J, Bouras C, Vallet PG: Neuropeptides in Alzheimer's and in Parkinson's disease. Mt Sinai J Med 1988; 55:102–115
16. Dahlstrom A, Fuxe K: Evidence for the existence of monoamine containing neurons in the central nervous system. Acta Physiol Scand 1964;232(suppl):1–55
17. Dahlstrom A, Fuxe K: Evidence for the existence of monoamine neurons in the central nervous system. II. experimentally induced changes in the intraneuronal amine levels of bulbospinal neuron systems. Acta Physiol Scand 1965; 247(suppl):1–36
18. Alexander GE, Delong MR: Parallel organisation of functionally segregated circuits linking basal ganglia and cortex. Ann Rev Neurosci 1986;9:357–381
19. Alexander GE, Crutcher MD, De Long MR: Basal ganglia-thalamocortical circuits: parallel substrates for motor, occulomotor, "prefrontal" and limbic functions. Prog Brain Res 1990;85:119–146
20. Marsden CD: The mysterious motor function of the basal ganglia: the Robert Wartenberg lecture. Neurology 1982;32: 514–539
21. Alexander GE, De Long MR: Microstimulation of the primate neostriatum. II. somatotopic organisation of striatal microexcitatory zones and their relationship to neuronal response properties. J Neurophysiol 1985;53:1417–1430
22. Stern Y, Mayeux R: Intellectual impairment in Parkinson's disease. p. 405. In Yahr MD, Bergmann KJ (eds): Advances in Neurology 45. Raven Press, New York, 1986
23. Rajput AH, Offord KP, Beard CM, Kurland LT: Epidemiology of Parkinsonism: incidence, classification and mortality. Ann Neurol 1984;16:278–282
24. Turnbull CJ, Aitken JA: Diagnosis and management of Parkinsonism in the elderly. Age Ageing 1983;12:309–316
25. Jellinger K: The pathology of Parkinsonism. p. 124. In Marsden CD, Fahn S (eds): Movement Disorders 2. Butterworths, London, 1987
26. Zhang Zhen-Xin, Roman GC: Worldwide occurrence of Parkinson's disease: an updated review. Neuroepidemiology 1993;12:195–208
27. de Petro Cuesta J: Parkinson's disease occurrence in Europe. Acta Neurol Scand 1991;84:357–365
28. D'Alessandro R, Gamberini G, Graniere F et al: Prevalence of Parkinson's disease in the Republic of San Marino. Neurology 1987;37:1679–1682
29. Mutch WJ, Dingwall-Fordyce I, Downie AW et al: Parkinson's disease in a Scottish city. Br Med J 1986;292:534–536
30. Hofman A, Ott A, de Rijk MC, Breteler MMB: Prevalence of Alzheimer's disease, vascular dementia, Parkinson's disease and epilepsy in a Dutch population study: the Rotterdam Study. Neuroepidemiology 1995;14:312
31. Li SC, Schoenberg BS, Wang CC: A prevalence survey of Parkinson's disease and other movement disorders in the People's Republic of China. Arch Neurol 1985;42:655–657
32. Schoenberg BS, Osuntokun BO, Adeuja AOG et al: Comparison of the prevalence of Parkinson's disease (PD) in black

populations in the rural U.S. and in rural Nigeria. Neurology 1987;37(suppl 1):120

33. Andrews GR: In Gerontology, Culture and Development. International Association of Gerontology Newsletter 1987;2:2–3
34. Mjones H: Paralysis agitans: a clinical and genetic study. Acta Psychiatr Neuro Scand 1949;25(suppl 54):1–195
35. Golbe LI, Do Iorio G, Bonavita V et al: Autosomal dominant Parkinson's disease. Ann Neurol 1990;27:276–282
36. Du voisin RC, Gearing F, Schweitzer M, Yahr MD: A family study of Parkinsonism. p. 492. In Barbeau A, Brunette JR (eds): Progress in Neurogenetics. Amsterdam, Excerpta Medica, 1969
37. Kondo K, Kurland LT, Schull WJ: Parkinson's disease, genetic analysis and evidence of a multifactorial aetiology. Mayo Clinic Proc 1973;48:465–475
38. Martilla RJ, Rinne UK: Arteriosclerosis, hereditary and some previous infections in the aetiology of Parkinson's disease. Clin Neurol Neurosurg 1976;79:46–56
39. Martin WE, Young WI, Anderson VE: Parkinson's disease: a genetic study. Brain 1976;96:495–506
40. Lang AE, Kierans C, Blair RDG: Family history of tremor in Parkinson's disease compared to controls and patients with idiopathic dystonia. Adv Neurol 1987;45:313–316
41. Marasganove DM, Harding AE, Marsden CD: A clinical and genetic study of Parkinson's disease. Mov Disor 1991;6: 205–211
42. Ward CD, Duvoisin RC, Ince SE et al: Parkinson's disease in 65 pairs of twins and in a set of quadruplets. Neurology 1983; 88:815–824
43. Marttila RJ, Kaprio J, Koskenvuo M, Rinne UK: Parkinson's disease in a nationwide twin cohort. Neurology 1988;38: 1217–1219
44. Marsden CD: Parkinson's disease in twins. J Neurol Neurosurg Psychiatry 1987;50:105–106
45. Vieregge P, Schiffte KA, Friedrich HJ et al: Parkinson's disease in twins. Neurology 1992;42:1453–1461
46. Burn DJ, Miles S, Sparr NK et al: Parkinson's disease in twin studies with ^{18}F-dopa and positron emission tomography. Neurology 1992;42:1894–1900
47. Armstrong M, Daly AK, Cholerton S et al: Instant debrisoquine hydroxylase genes in Parkinson's disease. Lancet 1992;339: 1017–1018
48. Smith CAD, Gough AC, Leigh PN et al: Debrisoquine hydroxylase polymorphism and susceptibility to Parkinson's disease. Lancet 1992;339:1375–1377
49. Gough AC, Mark MH, Playford ED et al: Identification of the primary gene defect of the cytochrome P450, CYP2D locus. Nature 1990;347:773
50. Langston JW: MPTP: the promise of a new neurotoxin. p. 73. In Marsden C D, Fahn S (eds): Movement Disorders 2. Butterworths, London, 1987
51. Graham DG: On the origin and significance of neuromelanin. Arch Pathol Lab Med 1979;103:359–362
52. Youdim MBH, Ben-Shachar D, Riederer P: Is Parkinson's disease a progressive siderosis of substantia nigra resulting from iron and melamin induced neurodegeneration? Acta Neurol Scand 1989;26:47–54
53. Hirsch E, Graybiel AM, Agid Y: Melanised dopaminergic neurones are differentially susceptible to degeneration in Parkinson's disease. Nature 1988;334:345–348
54. Dexter DT, Wells FR, Lees AJ et al: Increased nigral iron content and alterations in other metal ions occurring in brain in Parkinson's disease. J Neurochem 1989;52:1830–1836
55. Barbeu A, Roy M et al: Uneven prevalence of Parkinson's disease in the province of Quebec. Can J Neurol Sci 1985; 12:169–170
56. Aquilonius SM, Hartvig P: A Swedish county with unexpectedly high utilisation of anti-Parkinsonian drugs. Acta Neurol Scand 1986;74:379–382
57. Ebmeier KP, Mutch WJ, Calder SA et al: Does idiopathic Parkinsonism in Aberdeen follow intra-uterine influenza? J Neurol Neurosurg Psychiatry 1989;52:911–913
58. Kohbata S, Shimokawa K: Circulating antibody to *Nocardia* in the serum of patients with Parkinson's disease. Adv Neurol 1993;60:355–357
59. de Pedro Cuesta J, Petersen IJ, Stawiarz L et al: High levodopa use in periodically time-clustered, Icelandic birth cohorts: a vestige of Parkinsonian aetiology? Europarkinsonism Preparatory Activity Research Group. Acta Neurol Scand 1995;91: 79–88
60. Semchuk KM, Love EJ, Lee RG: Parkinson's disease and exposure to agricultural work and pesticide chemicals. Neurology 1992;42:1328–1335
61. Hubble JP, Cao BS, Hassanein RES et al: Risk factors for Parkinson's disease. Neurology 1993;43:1693–1697
62. Mayeux R, Tang MX, Mander K et al: Smoking and Parkinson's disease. Mov Disord 1994;9:207–212
63. McGeer PL, McGeer E, Suzuki JS et al: Aging and extrapyramidal function. Arch Neurol 1977;34:33–35
64. Carlsson A, Nyberg P, Winblad B: The influence of age and other factors on concentrations of monoamines in human brain. p. 53. In Nyberg P (ed): Brain Monoamines in Normal Ageing and Dementia. Umeo University, 1984
65. Euarts EV, Teravainen H, Calne DB et al: Reaction time in Parkinson's disease. Brain 1981;104:167–186
66. Calne DB, Langston JW: Aetiology of Parkinson's disease. Lancet 1983; ii:1457–1459
67. Ricaurte GA, Irwin I, Forno LS et al: Ageing and MPTP-induced degeneration of dopaminergic neurones in the substantia nigra. Brain Res 1987;403:43–51
68. Halliwell B: Oxidants and the central nervous system: some fundamental questions. Acta Neurol Scand 1989;80(suppl 126):23–33
69. Gibb WRG, Lees AJ: The progression of idiopathic Parkinson's disease is not explained by age related changes: clinical and pathological comparisons with post-encephalitic Parkinsonian syndrome. Acta Neuropathol 1987;73:195–201
70. Jenner P: Biochemistry of Parkinson's disease p. 10. In Chemistry or Surgery—Which Holds the Key? Parkinson's Disease Society, London, 1988
71. Fearnley JM, Lees AJ: Ageing and Parkinson's disease: substantia nigra regional selectivity. Brain 1991:114:2283–2301

72. Broe GA: Personal communication 1989

73. Alvord ED, Forno L, Kusske JA et al: The pathology of Parkinsonism: comparison of degeneration in cerebral cortex and brain stem. Adv Neurol 1974;5:175–193

74. Riederer P, Wuketich S: Time course of nigro-striatal degeneration in Parkinson's disease. J Neural Transm 1976;38: 227–301

75. Jenner P, Marsden CD: Neurochemical basis of parkinsonian tremor. p. 305. In Findley LJ, Capildeo R (eds): Movement disorders: tremor. Macmillan, London, 1984

76. Ellenbroek B, Schwarz M, Sontag KH et al: Muscular rigidity and delineation of a dopamine-specific neostriatal subregion: tonic EMG activity in rats. Brian Res 1985;345:132–140

77. Ezrin-Waters C, Resch L: The nucleus basalis of Meynert. Can J Neurol Sci 1986;13:8–14

78. Nakano I, Hirano A: Parkinson's disease: neuron loss in the nucelus basalis without concomitant Alzheimer's disease. Ann Neurol 1984;15:415–418

79. Guiloff RJ, George RJ, Marsden CD: Reversible supranuclear ophthalmoplegia associated with Parkinsonism. J Neurol Neurosurg Psychiatry 1980;43:352–354

80. Barbeau A: Parkinson's disease and etiopathology p. 87. In Vinken PJ, Bruyn GW, Klawans HL (eds): Handbook of Clinical Neurology. Elsevier, Amsterdam, 1986

81. Lewy FH: Zur pathologischen anatomie der paralysis agitans. Dtsch Z Nervheilk 1914;50:50–55

82. Forno LS: Pathology of Parkinson's disease. p. 25. In Marsden CD, Fahn S (eds): Movement Disorders. Butterworths, London, 1982

83. Bethlem J, den Hartogjager WA: The incidence and characteristics of Lewy bodies in idiopathic paralysis agitans (Parkinson's disease). J Neurol Neurosurg Psychiatry 1960;23: 74–80

84. Gibb WRG: The Lewy body and Parkinson's disease. p. 3. In Clifford Rose F (ed): Current Problems in Neurology 6. Parkinson's disease clinical and experimental advances. John Libbey, London, 1978

85. Rajput AH, Rozdilsky B, Hornykiewicz O et al: Reversible drug-induced Parkinsonism. Arch Neurol 1982;39:644–646

86. Boller F, Mizutani T, Roessmann U, Gambetti P: Parkinson's disease, dementia and Alzheimer's disease: clinicopathological correlations. Ann Neurol 1979;29:329–335

87. Morris JC, Drazner M, Fulling K, Berg L: Parkinsonism in senile dementia of the Alzheimer's type. p. 499. In Wurtman RJ, Corkin SJ, Growden JH (eds): Alzheimer's Disease: Advances in Basic Research and Therapies. Center for Brain Science and Metabolism Charitable Trust, Cambridge, 1987

88. Leverenz J, Sumi SM: Parkinson's disease in patients with Alzheimer's disease. Arch Neurol 1986;43:662–664

89. Lees AJ, Smith E: Cognitive deficits in the early stages of Parkinson's disease. Brain 1983;106:257–270

90. Snowden JS, Northen B, Neary D: The subcortical dementias. p. 157. In Griffith RA, McCarthy ST (eds): Degenerative neurological disease in the elderly. Wright, Bristol, 1987

91. Jellinger K, Riederer P: Dementia in Parkinson's disease and (pre) senile dementia of Alzheimer's type: morphological aspects and changes in the intracerebral MAO activity. Adv Neurol 1984;40:199–210

92. Shapira AH: Oxidative stress in Parkinson's disease. Neuropathol Appl Neurobiol 1995;21:3–9

93. Olanow CW: A radical hypothesis for neurodegeneration. Trends Neurosci 1993;16:439–444

94. Jenner P, Schapira AHV, Marsden CD: New insights into the cause of Parkinson's disease. Neurology 1992;42:2241–2250

95. Fahn S, Cohen G: The oxidant stress hypothesis in Parkinson's disease: evidence supporting it. Ann Neurol 1992;32: 804–812

96. Enochs WS, Sarna T, Zecca L et al: The roles of neuromelanin, binding of metal ions and oxidative cytotoxicity in the pathogenesis of Parkinson's disease: a hypothesis. J Neural Transm Basic Neurosci Neurol Sect Psychiatry Sect 1994; 7:83–100

97. Schapira AHV, Cooper JM, Dexter D et al: Mitochondrial complex I deficiency in Parkinson's disease. J Neurochem 1990; 54:823–827

98. Mizuno Y, Ikebe S, Hattori N et al: Role of mitochondria in the aetiology and pathogenesis of Parkinson's disease. Biochim Biophys Acta 1995;127:265–274

99. Cooper JM, Daniel SE, Marsden CD: L-Dihydroxyphenylalanine and complex I deficiency in Parkinson's disease brain. Mov Disord 1995;10:295–297

100. Cleeter MJW, Cooper JM, Darley-Usmar VM et al: Reversible inhibition of cytochrome C oxidase, the terminal enzyme of the mitochondrial respiratory chain, by nitric oxide: implications for neurodegenerative diseases. FEBS Lett 1994;345: 50–54

101. Calne DB: The free radical hypothesis in idiopathic Parkinsonism: evidence against it. Ann Neurol 1992;32:799–803

102. Walkinshaw G, Waters CM: Neurotoxin induced cell death in neuronal PC12 cells is mediated by induction of apoptosis. Neuroscience 1994;63:975–987

103. Gobe GC: Apoptosis in brain and gut tissue of mice fed a seed preparation of the cycad *Lepidozamia peroffskyana*. Biochem Biophys Res Commun 1994;205:327–333

104. Mitchell IJ, Lawson S, Moser B et al: Glutamate induced apoptosis results in a loss of striatal neurons in the Parkinsonian rat. Neuroscience 1994;63:1–5

105. Hughes AJ, Daniel SE, Kilford L, Lees AJ: Accuracy of clinical diagnosis of idiopathic Parkinson's disease: a clinico-pathological study of 100 cases. J Neurol Neurosurg Psychiatry 1992;55:181–184

106. D'Costa DF, Sheehan LJ, Phillips PA, Moore-Smith B: The levodopa test in Parkinson's disease. Age Ageing 1995;24: 210–212

107. Martin WE, Loewenson RB, Resch JA, Baker AB: Parkinson's disease: clinical analysis of 100 patients. Neurology 1973;23: 783–790

108. Eidelberg D: Positorn emission tomography in Parkinsonism. Neurol Clin 1992:10:421–433

109. Sawle GV: The detection of preclinical Parkinson's disease. Mov Disord 1993;8:271–277

110. Schwab RS, England AC: Parkinson's disease. J Chron Dis 1958;8:488–509

111. Duvoisin RC: Parkinson's disease: a guide for patient and family, 2nd Ed. Raven Press, New York, 1984

112. Lees AJ: Ray of Hope: The Ray Kennedy Story, Penguin, New York, 1994

113. Findley LJ, Gresty MA, Halmagyi GM: Tremor, the cogwheel phenomenon and clonus in Parkinson's disease. J Neurol Neurosurg Psychiatry 1981;44:534–536

114. Delwaide PJ, Gonce M: Pathophysiology of Parkinson's signs. p. 1. In: Jankovic J, Tolosa E (eds): Parkinson's disease and movement disorders. Urban and Schwarzenberg, Baltimore, 1988

115. Walshe FMR: A clinical analysis of the paralysis agitans syndrome. p. 245. In Critchley M (ed): James Parkinson, 1755–1824. Mcmillan, London, 1955

116. Bernheimer H, Birkmayer W, Hornykiewcz O et al: Brain dopamine and the syndromes of Parkinson and Huntington. J Neurol Sci 1973;20:415–455

117. Scott S, Caird FI: Speech therapy for Parkinson's disease. J Neurol Neurosurg Psychiatry 1983;46:140–144

118. Quinn NP, Lang AE, Koller WC, Marsden CD: Painful Parkinson's disease. Lancet 1986:i1366–1369

119. Johnell O, Melton III J, Atkinson EJ et al: Fracture risk in patients with Parkinsonism: a population based study in Olmsted County, Minnesota. Age Ageing 1992;21:32–38

120. Narabayashi H, Nakamura R: Clinical neurophysiology of freezing in Parkinsonism. p. 49. In Delwaide PJ, Agnoli A (eds): Clinical Neurophysiology in Parkinsonism 2. Elsevier, Amsterdam, 1985

121. Korczyn AD: Autonomic nervous system screening in patients with early parkinson's disease. p. 41. In Przuntek H, Riederer P (eds): Early Diagnosis and Preventive Therapy in Parkinson's Disease. Springer-Verlag, Vienna, 1989

122. Bird MR, Woodward MC, Gibson EM et al: Asymptomatic swallowing disorders in elderly patients with Parkinson's disease: a description of findings on clinical examination and videofluoroscopy in sixteen patients. Age Ageing 1994;23: 251–254

123. Tanner CM, Kinori I, Goetz CG et al: Clinical course in Parkinson's disease: relationship to age at onset. J Neurol 1985; 232(suppl):25

124. Goetz CG, Tanner CM, Stebbins GT, Buchman AS: Risk factors for progression in Parkinson's disease. Neurology 1988; 38:1841–1844

125. Godwin-Austen RB, Lowe J: The two types of Parkinson's disease. p. 79. In Clifford-Rose F (ed): Current Problems in Neurology: Parkinson's disease—Clinical and Experimental advances. John Libbey, London, 1987

126. Gibb WRG, Less AJ: A comparison of clinical and pathological features of young- and old-onset Parkinson's disease. Neurology 1988;38:1402–1406

127. Birkmayer W, Riederer P, Yondum JBA: Distinction between benign and malignant type of Parkinson's disease. Clin Neurol Neurosurg 1979;81:158–164

128. Diamond SG, Markham CH, Hoehn MM et al: Effect of age at onset on progression and mortality in Parkinson's disease. Neurology 1989;39:1187–1190

129. Hietanen M, Teravainen H: The effect of age of disease onset on neuropsychological performance in Parkinson's disease. J Neurol Neurosurg Psychiatry 1988;51:244–249

130. Pederzoli M, Girotti F, Scigliano G et al: L-Dopa long-term treatment in Parkinson's disease: age-related side effects. Neurology 1982;32:1518–1532

131. Hoehn MM: Parkinson's disease: progression and mortality. p. 457. In Yahr MD, Bergmann KT (eds): Advances in Neurology. Vol. 45. Raven Press, New York

132. Mutch WJ, Strudwick A, Roy SK, Downie AW: Parkinson's disease: disability review and therapy. Br Med J 1986;293: 675–677

133. Peterson GM, Nolan BW, Milligan KS: Survey of disability that is associated with Parkinson's disease. Med J Aust 1988; 149:66–70

134. Mutch WJ, Swallow MW, Baker M et al: A pilot survey of patient rated disability and the need for aids in Parkinson's disease. Clin Rehabil 1989;3:151–155

135. Kales A, Ansel RD, Markham CH et al:. Sleep in patients with Parkinson's disease and normal subjects prior to and following levodopa administration. Clin Pharmacol Ther 1971;12: 397–406

136. Jouvet M: Biogenic amines and the states of sleep. Science 1969;163:32–41

137. Friedman A: Sleep pattern in Parkinson's disease. Acta Med Pol 1980;21:193–199

138. Less AJ, Blackburn NA, Campbell VL: The night-time problems of Parkinson's disease. Clin Neuropharmacol 1988;11: 512–519

139. Sanchez-Ramos J, Factor SA, McAlarney T, Weiner WJ: The effect of sleep on motor symptomatology in Parkinson's disease. p. 70. Abstracts 9th International symposium on Parkinson's disease. World Federation of Neurology, Jerusalem, 1988

140. Mindham RHS: Psychiatric syndromes in Parkinsonism. J Neurol Neurosurg Psychiatry 1970;30:88–191

141. Patrick HT, Levy DM: Parkinson's disease: a clinical study of 146 cases. Arch Neurol 1922;7:711–720

142. Cummings JL: Depression in Parkinson's disease: a review. Am J Psychiatry 1992;149(4):443–454

143. Rogers D, Lees AJ, Smith E et al: Bradyphrenia in Parkinson's disease and psychomotor retardation in depressive illness. Brain 1987;110:761–776

144. Gotham AM, Brown RG, Marsden CD: Depression in Parkinson's disease: a quantitative and qualitative analysis. J Neurol Neurosurg Psychiatry 1986;49:381–389

145. Mindham RHS, Marsden CD, Parkes JD: Psychiatric symptoms during L-dopa therapy for Parkinson's disease and their relationship to physical disability. Psychol Med 1976;6: 23–33

146. Taylor AE, Saint-Cyr JA, Lang AE: Idiopathic Parkinson's disease: revised concepts of cognitive and affective status. Can J Neurol Sci 1988;15:106–113

147. Mayeaux R, Stern Y, Roson J, Leventhal J: Depression, intellectual impairment, and Parkinson's disease. Neurology 1981; 31:645–650
148. Robins AH: Depression in patients with Parkinsonism. Br J Psychiatry 1976;128:141–145
149. Mayeaux R, Stern Y, Sano M et al: The relationship of serotonin to depression in Parkinson's disease. Ann Neurol 1986;18: 149
150. Kawamura T, Kinoshita M, Iwasaki Y et al: Low-dose dexamethasone suppression test in Japanese patients with Parkinson's disease. J Neurol 1987;234:264–265
151. Kuhn W, Fuchs G, Laux G et al: Clinical and biochemical characteristics of early depression in Parkinson's disease. p. 49. In Przuntek H, Riederer P (eds): Early Diagnosis and Preventive Therapy in Parkinson's Disease. Vienna, Springer-Verlag, 1989
152. McMahon DG, Fletcher PJ: Psychiatric aspects of Parkinson's disease, letter. Br Med J 1989;299:388–389
153. Lindsay S, Mutch WJ: Depression and anxiety in fit old people and patients with Parkinson's disease and stroke disease. Personal communication, 1987
154. Klawans HL, Tanner CM. Management of psychiatric symptoms in Parkinson's disease. p. 957. In Calne DB (ed): Drugs for the treatment of Parkinson's disease. Handbook of Experiments Pharmacology 88. Springer-Verlag, Berlin, 1989
155. Tanner CM, Vogel C, Goetz CG, Klawans HL: Hallucinations in Parkinson's disease: a population study, abstracted. Ann Neurol 1983;14:136
156. Wilson RW, Tanner CM, Weingarten R, Goetz CG: Hallucinations in Parkinson's disease, abstracted. Neurology 1986; 36(suppl 1):216
157. Sweet RD, McDowell FH: Mental symptoms in Parkinson's disease during chronic treatment with levodopa. Neurology 1976;26:305–310
158. Parkes J, Debono A, Marsden CD: Bromocriptine in Parkinsonism: a long term treatment dose response and comparison with levodopa. J Neurol Neurosurg Psychiatry 1976;39: 1101–1107
159. Brown RG, Marsden CD: Neuropsychology and cognitive function in Parkinson's disease: an overview. p. 99. In Marsden C D, Fahn S (eds): Movement Disorders 2. Butterworths, London, 1987
160. Bowen FB, Burns MM, Yahr MD: Alterations in memory processes subsequent to short-and long-term treatment with L-dopa. p. 488. In Birkmayer W, Hornykiewicz O (eds): Advances in Parkinsonism. Roche, Basel, 1976
161. Christensen AL, Juul-Junsen P, Malmros R, Harmsen A: Psychological evaluation of intelligence and personality in Parkinsonism before and after stereotaxic surgery. Acta Neurol Scand 1970;46:527–537
162. Viitanen M, Mortimer JA, Webster DD: Association between presenting motor symptoms and the risk of cognitive impairment in Parkinson's disease. J Neurol Neurosurg Psychiatry 1994;57:1203–1207
163. Caparros-Lefebure D, Pecheux N, Petit V et al: Which factors predict cognitive decline in Parkinson's diseases. J Neurol Neurosurg Psychiatry 1995;58:51–55
164. Allain H, Lieury A, Quemener V et al: Procedural memory and Parkinson's disease. Dementia 1995;6:174–178
165. Allain H, Lieury A, Thomas V et al: Explicit and procedural memory in Parkinson's disease. Biomed Pharmacother 1995; 49(4):179–186
166. Boller F, Passafuime D, Keefe NC et al: Visuospatial impairment in Parkinson's disease. Arch Neurol 1984;41:485–490
167. Owen AM, James M, Leigh PN et al: Fronto-striatal cognitive deficits at different stages of Parkinson's disease. Brain 1992; 115:1727–1751
168. Bodis-Wollner, Onofrj N: The visual system in Parkinson's disease. p. 1. In Yahr M D, Bergmann K J (eds): Advances in Neurology. Vol 45. Raven Press, New York, 1986
169. Wilson RS, Gilley DW, Tanner CM, Goetz CG: Ideational fluency in Parkinson's disease. Brain Cogn 1992;20:236–244
170. Delong MR, Georgopoulos AP, Crutcher MD: Corticobasal ganglia relations and coding of motor performance. Exp Brain Res Suppl 1983;7:30–40
171. Hulley JL, Smith RJ, Cruickshank CA et al: A 9 month follow-up study of cognitive impairment in idiopathic Parkinson's disease. p. 297. In Crossman ARE, Sambrook MA (eds): Neural Mechanisms in Disorders of Movements. Current Problems in Neurology 9. John Libbey, London, 1989
172. Portin R, Rinne UK: Neuropsychological responses of Parkinsonian patients to long term levodopa therapy. p. 271. In Klinger M, Stamm G (eds): Parkinson's disease: Current Progress, Problems and Management. Elsevier, Amsterdam, 1980
173. Danielczyk W, Fischer P. Parkinson's disease, development of dementia in ageing. p. 9. In Przuntek H, Riederer P (eds): Early Diagnosis and preventive therapy in Parkinson's disease. Vienna, Springer-Verlag, 1989
174. Portin R, Rinne UK: Predictive factors for cognitive deterioration and dementia in Parkinson's disease. p. 413. In Yahr MD, Bergmann KL (eds): Parkinson's Disease. Raven Press, New York, 1986
175. Brown RG, Marsden CD: How common is dementia in Parkinson's disease? Lancet 1984;ii:1262–1265
176. Friedman A, Barcikowska M: Dementia in Parkinson's disease. Dementia 1994;5:12–16
177. Eastwood MR, Corbin SL: Epidemiology of mental disorders in old age. p. 17. In Arie T (ed): Recent Advances in Psychogeriatrics. Vol 1. Churchill Livingstone, Edinburgh, 1985
178. Ebmeier KP, Calder SA, Crawford JR et al: The prognosis of idiopathic Parkinson's disease: results from 3ϙfr1/2 years follow-up of a whole population sample. Acta Neurol Scand 1990;81:294–299

178a. Hietanen M, Teravainen H: The effect of age of disease onset on neuropsychological performance in Parkinson's disease. J Neurol Neurosurg Psychiatr 1988;51:244–249

179. Reid WGJ: The neuropsychology of de novo patients with idiopathic Parkinson's disease: the effect of age of onset. p. 9. Abstracts 9th International Symposium on Parkinson's disease. World Federation of Neurology, Jerusalem, 1988
180. Biggins CA, Boyd JL, Harrop FM et al: A controlled, longitudi-

nal study of dementia in Parkinson's disease. J Neurol Neurosurg Psychiatry 1992;55:566–571

181. Ross HF, Hughes TA, Biggins CA et al: A controlled, longitudinal study of dementia in Parkinson's disease: a continuation of the story. New Trends Clin Pharmacol 1994;8:252

182. Zetusky WJ, Jankovic J, Pirozzolo FJ: The heterogeneity of Parkinson's disease: clinical and prognostic implications. Neurology 1985;35:522–526

183. Huber SJ, Paulson GW, Shuttleworth EC: Relationship of motor symptoms, intellectual impairment, and depression in Parkinson's disease. J Neurol Neurosurg Psychiatry 1988;51: 855–858

184. Ebmeier KP, Calder SA, Crawford JR et al: Clinical features predicting dementia in idiopathic Parkinson's disease: a follow up study. Neurology 1990;40:1222–1224

185. Glatt SL, Hubble JP, Lyons K et al: Risk factors for dementia in Parkinson's disease: effect of education. Neuroepidemiology 1996;15:20–25

186. Hoehn MM, Yahr MD: Parkinsonism: onset, progression and mortality. Neurology 1967;17:427–442

187. Diamond SG, Markham CH: Long-term experience with L-dopa: efficacy, progression and mortality. p. 444. In Birkmeyer W, Hornykiewicz O (eds): Advances in Parkinsonism. Roche, Basel, 1976

188. Curtis L, Less AJ, Stern GM, Marmot MG: Effect of L-dopa on the course of Parkinson's disease. Lancet 1984;ii:211–212

189. Rajput AH, Offord KP, Beard CM, Kurland LT: Epidemiology of Parkinsonism: incidence, classification and mortality. Ann Neurol 1984;16:278–282

190. Clarke CE: Does Levodopa therapy delay death in Parkinson's disease? a review of the evidence. Mov Disord 1995;10: 250–256

191. Li TM, Swash M, Alberman E: Morbidity and mortality in motor neurone disease: comparison with multiple sclerosis and Parkinson's disease. J Neurol Neurosurg Psychiatry 1985;48: 320–327

192. Treves TA, de Petro Cuesta J: Parkinsonism mortality: time and space patterns. Acta Neurol Scand 1991;84:389–397

193. Lilienfeld DE, Chan A, Ehland J et al: Two decades of increasing mortality from Parkinson's disease among the U.S. elderly. Arch Neurol 1990;47:731–734

194. Stephen PJ, Williamson J: Drug-induced Parkinsonism in the elderly. Lancet 1984;ii:1082–1083

195. Hardie RJ, Lees AJ: Neuroleptic-induced Parkinson's syndrome: clinical features and results of treatment with levodopa. J Neurol Neurosurg Psychiatry 1988;51:850–854

196. Montastruc JL, Llau ME, Rascal O, Senard JM: Drug induced Parkinsonism: a review. Fundam Clin Pharmacol 1994;8: 293–306

197. Klawans HL, Bergen D, Bruyn GW: Prolonged drug-induced Parkinsonism. Confin Neurol 1973;35:368–377

198. Rajput AH, Rozdilsky B, Hornykiewicz O et al: Reversible drug-induced Parkinsonism. Arch Neurol 1982;39:644–646

199. Gimenez-Roldan S, Mateo D: Cinnarizine induced Parkinsonism; susceptibility related to ageing and essential tremor. Clin Neuropharmacol 1991;14:156–164

200. Critchley M. Arteriosclerotic Parkinsonism. Brain 1929;52: 23–83

201. Eadie MJ, Sutherland JM: Arteriosclerosis in Parkinsonism. J Neurol Neurosurg Psychiatry 1964;27:237–240

202. Martilla RJ, Rinne UK: Arteriosclerosis, heredity and some previous infections in the etiology of Parkinson's disease: a case control study. Clin Neurol Neurosurg 1976;79:46–56

203. Steel JC, Richardson JC, Olszewski J: Progressive supranuclear palsey: a heterogeneous degeneration involving the brain stem, basal ganglia and cerebellum with vertical gaze and pseudobulbar palsy, nuchal dystonia and dementia. Arch Neurol 1964;10:333–358

204. Shy GM, Drager GA: A neurological syndrome associated with orthostatic hypotension: a clinical-pathological study. Arch Neurol 1960;2:511–527

205. Lees AJ: The Steele-Richardson-Olszewski syndrome (progressive supranuclear palsy). p. 272. In Marsden CD, Fahn S (eds): Movement Disorders 2. Butterworths, London, 1987

206. De Bruin VM, Lees AJ: Subcortical neurofibrillary degeneration presenting as Steele-Richardson-Olszewski and other related syndromes: a review of 90 pathologically verified cases. Mov Disord 1994;9:381–389

207. Chiu HF: Psychiatric aspects of progressive supranuclear palsy. Gen Hosp Psychiatry 1995;17:135–143

208. Tolosa E, Valldeoriola F, Marti MJ: Clinical diagnosis and diagnostic criteria of progressive supranuclear palsy (Steele-Richardson-Olszewski syndrome). J Neurol Transm Suppl 1994;42:15–31

209. Brown J, Lantos P, Stratton M et al: Familial progressive supranuclear palsy. J Neurol Neurosurg Psychiatry 1993;56: 473–476

210. Jankovic J: Parkinsonian disorders. p. 1. In Appel S H (ed): Current Neurology. Vol 5. Wiley, New York, 1984

211. Quinn N: Disproportionate antecollis in multiple system atrophy. Br Med J 1989;1:844

212. Robbins TW, James M, Lange KW et al: Cognitive performance in multiple system atrophy. Brain 1992;115:271–291

213. Lee RG: The pathophysiology of essential tremor. p. 423. In Marsden CD, Fahn S (eds): Movement Disorders 2. Butterworths, London, 1987

214. Marshall J: Observations on essential tremor. J Neurol Neurosurg Psychiatry 1962;25:122–125

215. Findley LJ: The pharmacology of essential tremor. p. 438. In Marsden CD, Fahn S (eds): Movement Disorders 2. Butterworths, London, 1987

216. Schoenberg BS: Epidemiology of movement disorders p. 17. In Marsden CD, Fahn S (eds): Movement Disorders 2. Butterworths, London, 1987

217. Bain PG, Findlay LJ, Thompson PD et al: A study of hereditary essential tremor. Brain 1994;117:805–824

218. Dupont E: Parkinson's disease and essential tremor: differential diagnostic and epidemiological aspects. p. 165. In Rinne UK, Klingler M, Stamm G (eds): Parkinson's Disease: Current Progress, Problems and Management. Elsevier, Amsterdam, 1980

219. Critchley E: Clinical manifestations of essential tremor. J Neurol Neurosurg Psychiatry 1972;35:365–372
220. Larsen TA, Calne DB: Essential tremor. Clin Neuropharmacol 1983;6:185–206
221. Danek A: Geniospasm: hereditary chin trembling. Mov Disord 1993;8:335–338
222. Findley LJ, Cleeves L: The relation of essential tremor to Parkinson's disease. J Neurol Neurosurg Psychiatry 1985;48:192
223. Geraghty JJ, Jankovic J, Zetusky WJ: Association between essential tremor and Parkinson's disease. Ann Neurol 1985; 17:329–333
224. Findley LJ, Calzetti S, Cleeves L: Primidone in essential tremor of the hands and head: a double-blind controlled clinical study. J Neurol Neurosurg Psychiatry 1985;48:911–915
225. Adams RD, Fisher CM, Hakim S et al: Symptomatic occult hydrocephalus with "normal" cerebrospinal fluid pressure. N Engl J Med 1965;273:117–126
226. Sudarsky L, Sheldon S: Gait disorder in late-life hydrocephalus. Arch Neurol 1987;44:263–267
227. Curran T, Lange AE: Parkinsonian syndromes associated with hydrocephalus: case reports, a review of the literature and pathophysiological hypotheses. Mov Disord 1994;9:508–520
228. Paulson GW: Disorders of the central nervous system in the aged. Med Clin North Am 1983;67:345–359
229. Sudarsky L, Ronthal M: Gait disorder among elderly patients. Arch Neurol 1983;40:740–743
230. Broe GA, Creasey H: The neuroepidemiology of old age p. 51. In Tallis R (ed): Clinical Neurology of Old Age. John Wiley, London, 1989
231. McDowell FH, Cedarbaum JM: Natural history of dopa treated Parkinson's disease: 18 years follow-up. p. 119. In Clifford-Rose FS (ed): Parkinson's Disease: Clinical and Experimental Advances. Current Problems in Neurology. John Libbey, London, 1987
232. Le Witt PA: The pharmacology of levodopa in treatment of Parkinson's disease. p. 325. In Calne DB (ed): Drugs for the Treatment of Parkinson's Disease. Handbook of Experiment Pharmacology 88. Springer-Verlag, Berlin, 1989
233. Fahn S: Adverse effects of levodopa in Parkinson's disease. p. 385. In Calne D B (ed): Drugs for the treatment of Parkinson's Disease. Handbook of Experimental Pharmacology 88. Springer-Verlag, Berlin, 1989
234. Lees AJ: Levodopa substitution: the gold standard. Clin Neuropharmacol 1994;17(suppl 3):1–6
235. Sutcliffe RLG: L-Dopa therapy in elderly patients with Parkinsonism. Age Ageing 1973;2:34–38
236. White NJ, Barnes TRE: Senile Parkinsonism: a survey of current treatment. Age Ageing 1981;10:81–86
237. Wilson JA, Smith RG: The prevalence and aetiology of long-term L-dopa side effects in elderly Parkinsonian patients. Age Ageing 1989;18:11–16
238. Ziegler M, Ranoux D, Recondo J de: Clinical efficacy of a liquid formulation of levodopa (Madopar dispersible) in reversing afternoon "off" periods in Parkinson's disease. Clin Neuropharmacol 1994;17(suppl 3):21–25
239. Yeh KC, August TF, Bush DF et al: Pharmacokinetics and bioavailability of sinemet CR: a summary of human studies. Neurology 1989;39(suppl 2):20–24
240. Godwin Austen RB, Frears CC, Tomlinson EB, Kok HWL: Effects of L-dopa in Parkinson's disease. Lancet 1969;ii: 165–168
241. Anti-Parkinson drugs. p. 115. In Caird FI (ed): Drugs for the Elderly. WHO Regional Office for Europe, Copenhagen, 1985
242. Broe GA, Caird FI: Levodopa for Parkinsonism in elderly and demented patients. Med J Aust 1973;1:630–635
243. Evans MA, Triggs EJ, Broe GA, Saines N: Systemic availability of orally administered L-dopa in the elderly Parkinsonian patient. Eur J Clin Pharmacol 1980;17:215–221
244. Broe GA: Anti-Parkinsonian drugs. p. 473. In Swift CG (ed): Clinical Pharmacology in the Elderly. Marcel Dekker, New York, 1987
245. Evans MA, Broe GA, Triggs EJ et al: Gastric emptying rate and the systemic availability of levodopa in the elderly Parkinsonian patient. Neurology 1981;31:1288–1294
246. Pincus JH, Barry K: Protein redistribution diet restores motor function in patients with dopa-resistant "off" periods. Neurology 1987;38:481–483
247. Roberts JW, Cora-Locatelli G, Bravi D et al: Catechol-O-methyltransferase inhibitor tolcapone prolongs levodopa/carbidopa action in Parkinsonian patients. Neurology 1993;44: 2685–2688
248. Merello M, Lees AJ, Webster R et al: Effect of entacapone, a peripherally acting catechol-O-methyltransferase inhibitor, on the motor response to acute L-dopa administration in patients with Parkinson's disease. J Neurol Neurosurg Psychiatry 1994; 57:186–189
249. Exton-Smith AN: Disturbance of autonomic regulation. p. 85. In Isaccs B (ed): Recent Advances in Geriatric Medicine. Churchill Livingstone, Edinburgh, 1987
250. Gibb WRG, Griffith DNW: Levodopa withdrawal syndrome identical to neuroleptic malignant syndrome. Postgrad Med J 1986;62:59–60
251. Cederbaum JM: Clinical pharmacokinetics of anti-Parkinsonian drugs. Clin Pharmacokinet 1987;13:141–178
252. Lees AJ, Frankel J, Eatough V, Stern GM: New approaches in the use of selegiline for the treatment of Parkinson's disease. Acta Neurol Scand 1989;80:(suppl 126):139–145
253. Parkinson's Disease Research Group of the United Kingdom: Comparison of therapeutic effects and mortality data of levodopa and levodopa combined with selegiline in patients with early, mild Parkinson's disease. Br Med J 1995;311: 1602–1607
254. Tolosa E, Valldeoriola F: Mid-stage Parkinsonism with mild motor fluctuations. Clin Neuropharmacol 1994;17(suppl 2): 19–31
255. Suchowersky A, de Vries JD: Interaction of fluoxitene and selegiline. Can J Psychol 1990;35:571
256. Zornberg GL: Severe adverse interaction between pethidine and selegiline. Lancet 1991;337:246
257. Rabey JM: Late addition of dopamine agonists in Parkinson's disease. p. 283. In Rinne U K, Nagatsu T, Horowski R (eds): How to Proceed Today in Treatment. International Workshop

Berlin Parkinson's Disease. Medicom Europe BV: Bussum, 1991

258. Nutt JG, Hammerstad JP, Gancher ST: Therapy: Dopamine Agonists in Parkinson's Disease 100 Maxims. London, Edward Arnold, 1992

259. Rinne UK: Dopamine agonist in early Parkinson's disease. p. 343. In: Przuntek H, Riederer P (eds): Early Diagnosis and Preventive Therapy in Parkinson's Disease. Springer-Verlag, Vienna, 1989

260. Mouradian MM, Juncos JL, Fabbrini G et al: Motor fluctuations in Parkinson's disease: central pathophysiological mechanisms 11. Ann Neurol 1988;24:372–378

261. Sage JI, Mark MH: Basic mechanisms of motor fluctuations. Neurology 1994;44(suppl 6):10–14

262. Pahwa R, Busenbark RN, Huber SJ et al: Clinical experience with controlled-release carbidopa/levodopa in Parkinson's disease. Neurology 1993;43:677–681

263. Stocchi F, Patsalos PN, Berardelli A et al: Clinical implications of sustained dopaminergic stimulation. Clin Neuropharmacol 1994;17(suppl 2):7–13

264. Hughes AJ, Bishop S, Kleedorfer B et al: Subcutaneous apomorphine in Parkinson's disease: response to chronic administration for up to five years. Mov Disord 1993;8:165–170

265. Rinne UK: Strategies in the treatment of early Parkinson's disease. Acta Neurol Scand 1993;87(suppl 146):50–53

266. Weiner WJ, Factor SA, Sanchez-Ramos JR et al: Early combination (bromocriptine and levodopa) does not prevent motor fluctuations in Parkinson's disease. Neurology 1993;43:21–27

267. Goetz CG: Dopaminergic agonists in the treatment of Parkinson's disease. Neurology 1990;40(suppl 1):50–54

268. Sag JI, Mark MH: The rationale for continuous dopaminergic stimulation in patients with Parkinson's disease. Neurology 1992;42(suppl 1):23–28

269. Mouradian MM, Heuser IJE, Baronti F, Chase TN: Modifications of central dopaminergic mechanisms by continuous levodopa therapy for advanced Parkinson's disease. Ann Neurol 1990;27:18–23

270. Mouradian MM, Chase TN: Improved dopaminergic therapy of Parkinson's disease. p. 180. In Marsden CD, Fahn S (eds): Movement Disorders 3. Butterworth-Heinemann, Oxford, 1994

271. Birkmayer W, Knoll J, Riederer P et al: Increased life expectancy resulting from addition of L-deprenyl to Madopar treatment in Parkinson's disease: a long-term study. J Neural Transm 1985;64:113–127

272. Olanow CW: A scientific rationale for protective therapy in Parkinson's disease. J Neural Transm 1993;91:161–180

273. Tetrud JW, Langston WJ: The effect of deprenyl (selegiline) on the natural history of Parkinson's disease. Science 1989;245:519–522

274. The Parkinson Study Group: Effect of deprenyl on the progression of disability in early Parkinson's disease. N Engl J Med 1989;321:1364–1371

275. Parkinson Study Group: Effects of tocopherol and deprenyl on the progression of disability in early Parkinson's disease. N Engl J Med 1993;328:176–183

276. Parkinson's Disease Research Group of the United Kingdom: Comparisons of therapeutic effects of levodopa, levodopa and selegiline and bromocriptine in patients with early, mild Parkinson's disease: three year interim report. Br Med J 1993;307:469–472

277. Sweet RD, Lee JE, Spiegel HE, McDowell F: Enhanced response to low doses of levodopa after withdrawal from treatment. Neurology 1972;22:520–525

278. Mayeux R, Stern Y, Mulvey K, Cote L: Re-appraisal of temporary levodopa withdrawal ("drug holiday") in Parkinson's disease. N Engl J Med 1985;313:724–728

279. Dunnett SB: Transplantations of embryonic dopamine neurons: what we know from rats. J Neurol 1991;238:65–74

280. Dunnett SB, Annett LE: Nigral transplants in primate models of Parkinsonism. p. 27. In Lindvall O, Bjorklund A, Widner H (eds): Intracerebral Transplantation in Movement Disorders: Experimental Basis and Clinical Experiences. Amsterdam: Elsevier Science Publishers, Amsterdam, 1991

281. Lindvall O: Transplants in Parkinson's disease. Eur Neurol 1991;31(suppl 1):17–27

282. Lindvall O: Neural transplantation in Parkinson's disease. p. 103. In Dunnett SB, Bjorklund A (eds): Functional neural transplantation. Raven Press, New York, 1991

283. Lindvall O, Widner H, Rehncrona P et al: Transplantation of fetal dopaminergic neurons in Parkinson's disease: one year clinical and neuropsychological observations in two patients with putamenal implants. Ann Neurol 1992;31:155–165

284. Freed CR, Breeze RE, Rosenberg NL et al: Survival of implanted fetal dopamine cells and neurological improvement 12 to 46 months after transplantation for Parkinson's disease. N Engl J Med 1992;327:1549–1555

285. Kordower JH, Freeman TB, Snow BJ et al: Neuropathological evidence of graft survival and striatal reinervation after the transplantation of fetal mesencephalic tissue in a patient with Parkinson's disease. N Engl J Med 1995;332:1118–1124

286. Wolff JA, Fischer LJ, Xu L et al: Grarfting fibroblasts genetically modified to produce L-dopa in a rat model of Parkinson's disease. Proc Natl Acad Sci USA 1989;86:9011–9014

287. Horellou P, Brundin P, Kaben P et al: In vivo release of DOPA and dopamine from genetically engineered cells grafted to the rat striatum. Neuron 1990;5:393–402

288. Jiao S, Gurevich V, Wolff JA: Long-term correction of rat model of Parkinson's disease by gene therapy. Nature 1993;362:450–453

289. Schneider JS, Pope A, Simpson K et al: Recovery from experimental Parkinsonism in primates with GUI ganglioside treatment. Science 1992;256:843–846

290. Goetz CG, Delong MR, Penn RD, Bakay RAE: Neurosurgical lesions in Parkinson's disease. Neurology 1993;43:1–7

291. Shibazaki T, Hirai T, Hirato Y et al: Physiologically identified, selective ventrointermedius thalamotomy ameliorates, various kinds of tremor and other disorders of movement related to tremor. p. 393. In Crossman AR, Sambrook MA (eds): Neural Mechanisms in Disorders of Movement: Current Problems in Neurology 9. John Libbey, London, 1989

292. Laitinen LV, Bergenheimn AT, Hanz MI: Leskell's posteroventral pallidotomy in the treatment of Parkinson's disease. J Neurosurg 1992;76:53–61

293. Marsden CD, Obeso JA: The functions of the basal ganglia and the paradox of stereotactic surgery in Parkinson's disease. Brain 1994;117:877–897

294. Benabid AI, Pollak P, Gervason C et al: Long-term supression of tremor by chronic stimulation of the ventral intermediate thalamic nucleus. Lancet 1991;337:403–406

295. Marsden CD, Fahn S: Problems in Parkinson's disease and other akinetic-rigid syndromes. p. 65. In Marsden CD, Fahn S (eds): Movement Disorders 2. Butterworth, London, 1987

296. Meco G, Alessandri A, Bonifati V et al: Risperidone for hallucinations in levodopa treated Parkinson's disease patients. Lancet 1994;343:1370–1371

297. Greene P: Use of Clozapine in Parkinson's disease: focus Parkinson's Dis 1995;7:4–9

298. Folstein MF, Folstein SE, McHugh PR: Minimental state, a practical method for grading the cognitive state of patients for the clinician. J Psychiatr Res 1975;12:189–198

299. Snaith RP, Bridge GW, Hamilton M. The Leeds scales for the self-assessment of anxiety and depression. Br J Psychiatry 1976;128:156–165

300. Webster DD: Critical analysis of the disability in Parkinson's disease. Modern Treatment 1968;5:257–282

301. Canter C J, de la Torre R, Mier M: A method of evaluating disability in patients with Parkinson's disease. J Nerv Ment Dis 1961;133:143–147

302. Hildick-Smith M: Has rehabilitation a role in the treatment of Parkinson's disease. p. 105. In Clifford-Rose F (ed): Parkinson's Disease: Clinical and Experimental Advances. Current Problems in Neurology 6. John Libbey, London, 1987

303. Andrews K: Rehabilitation of the Older Adult. Edward Arnold, London, 1987

304. Mutch WJ, Strudwick A, Roy SK, Downie AW: Parkinson's disease: disability; review and therapy. Br Med J 1986;293: 675–677

305. Beattie A, Caird Fl: The occupational therapist and the patients with Parkinson's disease. Br Med J 1980;280: 1354–1355

306. Scott S, Caird FI, Williams BO: Communication in Parkinson's disease. Croom Helm, London, 1985

307. Scott S, Caird FI: The response of the apparent receptive speech disorder of Parkinson's disease to speech therapy. J Neurol Neurosurg Psychiatry 1984;47:302–304

308. Gibberd FB, Page NGR, Spencer KM et al: Controlled trial of physiotherapy and occupational therapy for Parkinson's disease. Br Med J 1981;282:1196

309. Steiner P, Flewitt B: Controlled trial of physiotherapy and occupational therapy for Parkinson's disease. Br Med J 1981; 282:1970

310. Franklyn S, Stern GM: Controlled trial of physiotherapy and occupational therapy for Parkinson's disease. Br Med J 1981; 282:1969–1970

311. Banks MA, Caird FI: Physiotherapy benefits patients with Parkinson's disease. Clin Rehabil 1989;3:11–16

312. Cornella CL, Stebbins GT, Brown-Toms N et al: Physical therapy and Parkinson's disease: a controlled clinical trial. Neurology 1994;44:376–378

313. Nanton V: Parkinson's disease. In Cottam P, Sutton A (eds): 1987 Conductive Education. Croom Helm, Kent, 1986

314. Swallow M: Can music help people with Parkinson's disease. In Clifford-Rose F (ed): Parkinson's Disease: Clinical and Experimental Advances. Current Problems in Neurology 6. John Libbey, London, 1987

315. Oxtoby M: Parkinson's disease patients and their social needs. London: Parkinson's Disease Society, London, 1981

316. Parkinson's Disease Society: Meeting a need? Parkinson's Disease Society, London, 1994

317. Lesser RP, Fahn S: Dystonia: A disorder often misdiagnosed as a conversion reaction. Am J Psychiatry 1978;153:349–352

318. L'e Orme M, Tallis RC: Metoclopramide and tardive dyskinesia in the elderly. Br Med J 1984;289:397–398

319. Fann WE, Sullivan JL, Richman BW: Dyskinesias associated with antidepressants. Br J Psychiatry 1976;128:490–493

320. Kaplan SR, Murkofsky C: Oral-buccal dyskinesia symptoms associated with low-dose benzodiazepine treatment. Am J Psychiatry 1978;135:1558–1559

321. Ramsay FM, Millard PH: Tardive dyskinesia in the elderly. Age Ageing 1986;15:145–150

322. Blowers AJ, Borison RJ: Dyskinesias in the geriatric population. Brain Res Bull 1986;11:175–178

323. Wolters EC, Calne DB: Current topics of interest in Parkinson's disease. p. 271. In Crossman AR, Sambrook MA (eds): Neural Mechanisms in Disorders of Movement. Current Problems in Neurology 9. John Libbey, London, 1989

324. Roos RAC, Buruma OJS: Drug-induced involuntary movements and tardive dyskinesia. p. 69. In Bruyn W, Roos RAC, Buruma OJS (eds): 1984 Actua Sandoz, Vol 7. Sandoz. Uden, 1989

325. Bennett JP, Landon ER, Dietrich S, Schuh LA: Suppression of dyskinesias in advanced Parkinson's disease: moderate daily clozapine doses provide long-term dyskinesia reduction. Mov Disord 1994;9:409–414

326. Padberg G: Symptomatic chorea. p. 61. In Bruyn W, Roos RAC, Buruma OJS (eds): Actua Sandoz. Vol 7. Sandoz, Uden, 1984

327. Marsden CD, Fahn S: Problems in the dyskinesias. p. 305. In Marsden CD, Fahn S (eds): Movement Disorders 2. Butterworths, London, 1987

328. Myers RH, Sax DS, Schoenfield M et al: Late onset of Huntington's disease. J Neurol Neurosurg Psychiatry 1985;48: 530–534

329. Kremer B, Goldberg P, Andrew SE et al: A worldwide study of Huntington's disease mutation: the sensitivity and specificity of measuring CAG repeats. N Engl J Med 1994;339: 1401–1406

330. Andrew SE, Goldberg YP, Kremer B et al: Huntington's disease without CAG expansion: phenocopies or errors in assignment? Am J Hum Genet 1994;54(5):852–863

331. La Spada AR, Paulson HL, Fischbeck KH: Trinucleotide

repeat expansion in neurological disease. Ann Neurol 1994; 36:814–822

332. Shimotoh H, Calne DB, Snow B et al: Normal CAG repeat length in the Huntington's disease gene in senile chorea. Neurology 1994;44:2183–2184
333. Fahn S: The medical treatment of movement disorders. p. 249. In Crossman AR, Sambrook MA (eds): Neural Mechanisms in Disorders of Movement. Current problems in Neurology 9. John Libbey, London, 1989
334. Playfer JR: Non-Parkinsonian movement disorders in the elderly. p. 50. In Grimley Evans J, Caird FI (eds): Advances Geriatric Medicine 7. Wright, London, 1988
335. Jankovic J: The neurology of TICS. p. 383. In Marsden CD, Fahn S (eds): Movement Disorders 2. Butterworths, London, 1987
336. Ad Hoc Committee Committee of the Dystonia Medical Research Foundation: Members Barbeau A, Calne DB, Fahn S, Marsden CD, Menkes J, Wooten GF, 1984
337. Gader T, Fahn S, Breakefield XO: The autosomal dominant dystonias. Brain Pathol 1992;2:297–308
338. Fahn S, Marsden CD, Calne DB: Classification and investigation of dystonia. p. 332. In Marsden CD, Fahn S (eds): Movement Disorders 2. Butterworths, London, 1987
339. Fahn S, Marsden CD: The treatment of dystonia. p. 359. In Marsden CD, Fahn S (eds): Movement Disorders 2. Butterworths, London, 1987
340. Fahn S, List T, Moskowitz C et al: Double-blind controlled study of botulinum toxin for blepharospasm. Neurology 1985; 35(suppl 1):271–272
341. Kao I, Drachman DB, Price DL: Botulinum toxin: mechanism of presynaptic blockage. Science 1976;193:1256–1258

CHAPTER 39

Disturbances of Gait, Balance, and the Vestibular System

REIN TIDEIKSAAR

Disturbances in gait and balance are prevalent in elderly people, especially as they advance in age. According to U.S. national survey statistics, although up to 85 percent of elderly, individuals aged 65 to 69 years report no difficulty in walking,[1,2] only about 66 percent of persons between 80 and 84 years old and 51 percent of persons over age 85 are capable of this level of ambulation.[1] Similarly, although approximately 13 percent of those aged 65 to 69 living in the community complain of balance problems or unsteadiness when walking or changing positions, about 46 percent of those 85 years old or older report such problems.[3,4] Gait and balance disturbances are associated with the risk of serious consequences. Beyond the loss of physical function and increased risk of falling, these kinds of disabilities may include psychosocial sequelae (e.g., loss of self-esteem and autonomy, depression, anxiety, fear of falling, and isolation).

Normal gait and balance involve sensory detection of body motions and execution of appropriate motor or musculoskeletal responses, a complex process. This chapter examines gait and balance from several perspectives: their function, age-related effects, common disease presentation, and clinical management.

Balance

The basic task of balance is to maintain the body's center of gravity (COG), located anterior to the second sacral vertebra, over its base of support (BOS) or limits of stability: the area surrounding or contained between the feet while standing [about 5 to 10 cm (1.95 to 3.9 in)] (Fig. 39.1). Balance or postural control is a complex process involving the coordinated efforts of afferent mechanisms or sensory systems (e.g., visual, vestibular, and proprioceptive) and efferent mechanisms or motor systems (e.g., upper- and lower-extremity muscle strength and joint flexibility). The afferent and efferent responses are organized through a variety of central mechanisms or central nervous system (CNS) functions which receive and organize sensory information and program appropriate motor system responses.

When the body's COG extends beyond its BOS, such as might occur when a person attempts to stand still on a moving bus, the limits of stability or postural control are exceeded and instability or loss of balance ensues. The resulting imbalance is detected by the sensory system—the visual, vestibular, and proprioceptive components—which sends signals to the motor system—consisting of stretch receptors located in the joints and muscles of the body—which in turn initiates a set of coordinated postural responses that act to reestablish stability or a realignment between the COG and BOS. Likewise, when an individual takes a step forward to walk or engages in other balance displacing activities (e.g., transferring, climbing steps or curbs, reaching, or stooping), the COG stretches beyond the BOS and the limits of stability and comparable postural control strategies are called into action to prevent loss of balance.

Afferent Mechanisms

The visual system provides information on the placement and distance of objects in the environment, the type of surface (stable versus unstable) on which movement will take place, and the position of body parts in relation to each other and to the environmental surroundings. Components of visual function deemed critical for balance include static and dynamic acuity, contrast sensitivity, depth perception, and peripheral vision. Proprioceptive input, emerging from muscle and tendon receptors, articular mechanoreceptors, and deep-pressure receptors in the plantar aspects of the feet also provide vital sensory data for postural control. Proprioceptors supply the body with information on the immediate environment, allowing it to orient itself as it stands and moves with respect to the support or ground surface and in relation to body segments (i.e., the head, trunk, and extremities).

The vestibular system works in conjunction with the visual and proprioceptive systems to achieve balance. It consists of three parts: a peripheral sensory component, a central processing component, and a motor control component. The sensory component, located in the inner ear, consists of semicircular canals and the otolith organs (utricle and saccule). It detects movement of the head (i.e., angular velocity and linear acceleration) and its orientation in space. This activity is triggered by specialized sensory (hair) cells located in the semicircular canals (cristae) and otolith (maculae) and supplied by branches of the eighth cranial nerve. The central processing component (pons and cerebellum) receives and integrates these signals and, after combining them with visual and propri-

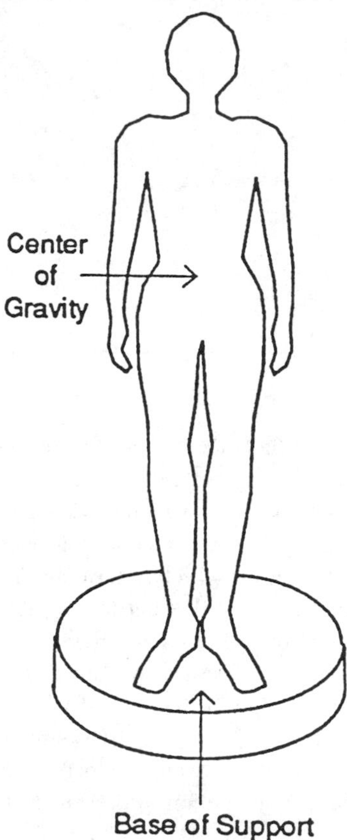

Figure 39-1 The center of gravity in relationship to the base of support when standing.

oceptive input, sends the information to the motor component (ocular muscles and spinal cord). In response, two important reflexes used by the body to regulate postural control are initiated: the vestibulo-ocular reflex (VOR) and the vestibulospinal reflex (VSR).

The VOR controls ocular stability (i.e., keeping the eyes fixed on the visual field) and orientation of the head as it moves about (i.e., knowledge of its position in space with respect to the direction of gravity and the surrounding environment). Without this reflex, visual images would change each time the head moved even slightly. Even performing an activity as simple as looking down, say, at a curb when walking, and up again, to visualize the walkway, might upset the control of balance (objects in the surrounding environment might appear to jiggle). The VSR influences skeletal muscles in the neck, trunk, and limbs and generates compensatory body movement which maintains head and postural control. This body orientating response, also referred to as the righting reflex, is exhibited when, following a loss of stability, an individual raises and stretches the arms away from the side of the body and into a forward outward position, a change of body posture employed to regain stability (i.e., realignment of the COG and BOS). The VOR and VSR are monitored by the central processing component and readjusted as needed.

Last, the vestibular system helps resolve conflicting sensory information when visual or proprioceptive inputs provide inaccurate feedback, as in the case of a moving visual field or a compliant ground surface. Under these circumstances, the vestibular system is quite adept in quickly rejecting the misleading information in order to preserve postural control.

Efferent Mechanisms

When a person's balance is disrupted, depending on the extent of displacement, one of three different postural control strategies is used to regain stability: an ankle strategy, a hip strategy, or a stepping or stumbling strategy. The ankle strategy is used in response to a slow, small disturbance of the BOS and is accomplished while maintaining the feet in place. This strategy is characterized by a continuous process of low-frequency anteroposterior (heel-to-toe) and lateral (side-to-side) motions or sway (rotating the body about the ankle joints with minimal activity of the hip and knee joints), movements designed to stretch or activate ankle muscles and realign the COG and BOS. The muscle sequence of activation occurs in distal-to-proximal order. During an unexpected displacement of the COG in the anterior direction (i.e., swaying or beginning to fall forward), the loss of stability triggers distal-to-proximal activation of the plantar flexor, knee flexor, gastrocnemius-hamstring, and trunk muscles. Conversely, during a displacement of the COG in the posterior direction (i.e., swaying or beginning to fall backward), the loss of stability activates the anterior muscles, including the dorsiflexors, knee extensors, quadriceps, and trunk flexors. These forward and backward muscles are activated rapidly about 100 milliseconds after a loss of stability—fast enough to prevent loss of balance.

The hip strategy repositions the COG by flexing or extending the hips. This technique is used for more forceful disturbances of the BOS and when the BOS is compliant or reduced, such as when a person attempts to stand on a foam-covered surface or a narrow beam or maintain balance with the feet placed in a tandem position. In this situation, the ankle strategy is inadequate, as the reduced size of the BOS limits the rotation that the ankle and foot can produce. In contrast to that for the ankle strategy, the order of muscle recruitment for the hip strategy is reversed: it is a proximal-to-distal sequence. During a forward displacement of balance, the trunk flexors and knee extensor muscles are activated first and proceed to trigger the ankle dorsiflexors. Last, the stepping strategy is used when the COG is displaced beyond the limits of the BOS. This strategy is required to regain equilibrium (i.e., realignment of the COG and BOS) when neither the ankle or hip strategy is sufficient, such as might be the case following an episode of tripping or being displaced backward. The stepping strategy is accomplished with a series of rapid steps, hops, or stumbles that establish the BOS under the COG.

Postural responses are either anticipatory adjustments preparatory to an imminent, predictable loss of balance (a feedforward activation) or compensatory reactions that restore equilibrium after an unexpected disturbance of balance (a feedback activation). The feedforward strategy is used in situations when a person expects a loss of stability, such as might occur while standing on a moving bus, walking on an ice-covered street, or reaching up (on tiptoes) to retrieve an object from a high shelf. In these instances the individual attempts to preserve balance by spacing the feet wider, a response that increases the BOS. Another example of this strategy is seen when an older person seeks additional support from a handrail or chair armrest (to increase their BOS) while climbing or descending a flight of stairs or rising from a chair, respectively. Often feedforward strategies reflect prior learning experiences involving situations that have led to instability. Conversely, feedback strategies are employed in situations in which the person unexpectently experiences a loss of stability, such as might occur after slipping on a wet floor or a sliding rug or after tripping on an uneven sidewalk or other ground elevation. In these circumstances balance is regained by taking a number of small steps in either the forward or the backward direction, a response that attempts to align the COG in relation to the BOS.

Central Mechanisms

The CNS plays an important role in the maintening balance. It assesses and integrates sensory information indicating instability provided by input from the visual, proprioceptive, and vestibular systems and, in response, selects the proper corrective postural strategy to be employed in situations of both unexpected and anticipatory loss of balance. Through the integration of motor and sensory commands, actual corrective responses that follow are formulated and initiated. If an individual is walking around in dim lighting, the CNS may rely less on information from visual input and more on information from other sensory components such as proprioceptive and vestibular input. Similarly, if an individual experiences an unexpected loss of balance (e.g., after slipping on a rug), the CNS triggers a set of corrective postural responses within a time interval shorter than that required for an anticipatory voluntary response such as reaching over to pick up a book.

Effects of Age on Balance

Numerous studies comparing healthy younger and older age groups have reported an age-related increase in unsteadiness or postural sway under both static conditions (i.e., standing still or a unilateral stance)[5–12] and dynamic circumstances (i.e., platform perturbations).[5,13,14] Some researchers have reported greater postural sway in women than in men, although others have not found that sway is affected by gender.[16–18] Wolfson et al.[19] found no gender differences in sway during quiet standing, although women tended to exhibit more sway and balance loss than men when deprived of visual and proprioceptive inputs. Other studies have shown that the direction of postural sway in older people is different from that of younger ones, with older individuals exhibiting greater posterior[20] and anteroposterior sway[7,21] than lateral sway.

The cause of age-related balance decline is related to a combination of decreased sensory input, slowing of motor responses, and musculoskeletal limitations. As evidenced by decreased cutaneous vibratory sensation and lower-extremity joint position sense, proprioceptive input has been shown to decline with increasing age.[11–24] Researchers have shown a relationship between decline in proprioceptive input and increased postural sway, although results vary widely. Brocklehurst et al.[11] found an inverse relationship between increased postural sway and impaired lower-extremity vibration sense in women 75 to 84 years old but not in women 65 to 74 years old or older than 85 years. MacLennan et al.[25] reported a significant association between vibration sense and postural sway in women 75 to 84 years old but no association in women aged 65 to 74 years or in men aged 65 to 84 years. Era and Heikkinen[6] found a positive association between sway and vibration sense in men 51 to 55 years old but not in men aged 71 to 75 years.

With respect to position sense, MacLennan et al.[25] measured proprioception in the toes but did not find an association with increased body sway. Duncan et al.[26] reported a strong relationship between impaired vibration sense and sway but not between passive joint movement and sway. Brocklehurst et al.[11] evaluated proprioception at the great toe and ankle and observed no significant correlation between joint position sense and sway. In contrast, Lord et al.[27] reported that poor joint position sense of the toes was strongly associated with increased body sway. Any lack of association between clinical findings of proprioceptive decline and postural sway may be due to imprecise testing methods (some clinical and laboratory measures of sway are better than others at revealing age-related differences in sway), or increased postural sway may have been caused by subtle declines in undetected visual and vestibular inputs which may have been falsely attributed to proprioceptive loss. Olney[22] suggested that despite the fact that vibration sense and proprioception are mediated via similar peripheral pathways, the neurons involved in vibration sense decline or degenerate independently of proprioceptive function and thus may not necessarily demonstrate age-related declines in a given individual.

Under conditions in which proprioceptive feedback is reduced or missing, visual input becomes more critical in maintaining balance.[9,28] Dornan et al.[29] compared a group of above-the-knee amputees (who had limited proprioception) with a nonamputee group and found that the amputee group had significant increases in sway. Woollacott and coworkers[30] observed that older persons were able to maintain balance when standing on a stable ground surface (i.e., receiving normal proprioceptive input), although when proprioceptive input was eliminated, they exhibited increased sway and about one-half experienced loss of balance once their eyes were closed. This response is demonstrated clinically when an older person with proprioceptive loss stands in place with their eyes closed or walks into a dimly lit room; in both cases, balance becomes unsteady. To compensate for poor balance, they rely on visual input to augment proprioceptive loss. Often individuals look down to view the correct placement of their feet when ambulating on ground and step surfaces.

When visual input is available, older people are generally

able to adapt to a loss of stability as well as younger individuals, however, this may not be the case when visual cues are absent. Studies have reported that age-related declines in visual acuity,[29,31] particularly near vision,[32] and decreased peripheral vision[33] are associated with increased postural sway. The effect of altered vision on postural control is most striking when proprioceptive input is decreased. Manchester et al.[34] observed that stability decreased significantly under conditions in which peripheral vision was occluded and ankle proprioception was limited. The effect of altered visual function, such as contrast sensitivity and visual acuity, and increased sway have been shown to be greater on compliant or absorptive support surfaces (when proprioceptive feedback is decreased).[35]

The vestibular system is subject to a number of age-related changes. Studies have demonstrated a 20 percent decline in hair cells in the otoliths and a 40 percent reduction of hair cells in the semicircular canals after the age of 70.[36,37] Reductions in vestibular function, as evidenced by VOR testing, have been observed by some investigators[38] but not by others.[39] Other important functions of visuo-ocular control, such as saccadic eye movements (i.e., small movements of both eyes simultaneously in changing the point of fixation on a visualized object), smooth pursuit, and optokinetic nystagmus, are affected as well. The latency of saccadic eye movements has been shown to increase with advancing age,[40,41] and smooth pursuit and optokinetic nystagmus both diminish with age, particularly at higher stimulus velocities.[42,43] Norre[44] showed that compensation was less effective for the VSR, as indexed by postural sway on posturography, than it was for the VOR, as measured by rotational tests.

Despite these changes, the effect of age-related vestibular decline on postural control is uncertain. Brocklehurst et al.,[11] employing a seat-tilting device, demonstrated that persons older than 85 years of age displayed impaired vestibular responses; however, no correlation with sway was found. They concluded that the tilt test used may have been affected by proprioception input from the buttock area and thus led to misleading information with respect to vestibular function. Lord et al.[27] failed to find an association between vestibular testing and body sway even though a large number of persons studied had evidence of vestibular impairment. Despite these findings, Woollacott et al.[45] reported that the inability of older people to stand while using primarily vestibular inputs (i.e., receiving decreased visual and proprioceptive feedback) may in part indicate impaired vestibular function. The lack of evidence on the association between vestibular dysfunction and postural control may be due to difficulty associated with experimental manipulation of the vestibular system, namely an inability to selectively stimulate the vestibular receptors.[46] Also, the role of the vestibular system in maintaining balance is difficult to define because this system provides only a portion of the inputs required.[47]

The coordination or initiation and execution of postural control strategies is affected by age as well. The initiation of postural muscular responses or latency (the speed of distal leg muscle activation) to balance displacements has been shown to be delayed (by about 20 to 30 milliseconds) in healthy older persons.[48,49] Also, in response to small balance disturbances, some individuals exhibited a reversal of the normal distal-to-proximal sequence of muscle activation: the proximal quadriceps muscles activated in advance of the distal tibialis anterior muscles. Further more, Manchester et al.[34] showed that older people used a hip strategy significantly more often than younger ones in reacting to small balance displacements, perhaps in response to decreased distal muscle strength or diminished proprioceptive inputs. Whereas younger persons take a single corrective step in reaction to sudden and significantly large displacements of balance (stepping strategies), older ones respond by talking multiple short steps.[50] This approach may represent a compensatory mechanism for maintaining balance, allowing them to correct early and faulty postural responses.

Similarly, voluntary postural responses to anticipatory balance disturbances decline with age. Mankovskii et al.[51] compared young and old age groups performing leg lifts by knee extension (at both slow and fast speeds) while standing. At slow speeds older individuals exhibited appropriate latency responses; however, when performing the task as quickly as possible, they showed a greater delay in muscle response latencies and increased instability in comparison to younger individuals. Ingin and Woollacott[52] reported that older persons, in comparison to younger ones, exhibited a significantly slower onset of postural muscle latencies when performing a reaction time task (e.g., pushing and pulling on a handle as quickly as possible when cued). In addition, a delay in the voluntary onset of postural muscle activity in response to anticipatory balance disturbances has been shown to be affected by decreased attention levels.[53,54]

Last, several age-related musculoskeletal changes can influence balance. Kyphosis (or stooping posture), due to either structural changes in the spine or to adaptive responses to instability (an approach aimed at maximizing balance by lowering COG in relation to BOS), can alter the body's balance threshold. The forward lean in posture shifts the COG forward past the BOS (the critical point of stability); as a result, maintaining standing balance becomes more difficult. Also, individuals with kyphotic posture may not be able to fully extend the muscles of the hips and knees when walking and to thrust the foot forward fast enough to preserve balance. Poor ankle muscle strength and loss of joint motion complicate the execution, making it difficult to adjust the COG in line with the BOS rapidly enough to prevent a fall.

With advanced age, the greatest decline in strength occurs in lower-extremity muscle groups.[55] Muscles most likely to show a decrease in strength are the active antigravity muscles such as the quadriceps, hip extensors, ankle dorsiflexors, and triceps. Also, there is an association between lower-extremity strength and balance. Older women with adequate hip abductor strength are more able to stand on one leg than those with less strength.[56] Any decline in muscle strength and joint flexibility of the lower extremities complicates the execution of postural strategies, making it more difficult to adjust the COG in line with the BOS.

In summary, despite any increase in postural sway occurring as a consequence of age, it appears that healthy older persons have enough sensory function reserve to maintain postural control. Normally, there is a great deal of redundancy in the sensory information necessary to maintain balance, and the failure of one source of input such as vision can be counteracted by feedback from an intact proprioceptive and vestibular system. However, deprivation in more than one system is likely to lower the balance threshold. Teasdale et al.[57] compared postural sway in a group of healthy older and younger persons and found that, with the exclusion or disruption of one sensory input (visual or proprioceptive feedback), body sway did not differ significantly in the young and the old. However, when both visual and proprioceptive input were eliminated, the older individuals exhibited substantially more sway than the younger ones. In addition, under conditions in which balance is maximally stressed, such as might occur when standing on one foot, climbing or descending steps or curbs, stepping onto a bus, and getting in and out of a bathtub (activities performed part of the time on one foot and with a reduced BOS), maintaining stability becomes more difficult, especially when any sufficient delay in a muscle sequence activating lower-extremity motor responses may lead to inappropriate postural responses and affect one's ability to maintain balance.

Gait

Gait, defined as manner or style of walking, is usually described in terms of the gait cycle, which consists of two phases: stance and swing (Fig. 39-2). The stance phase constitutes 60 percent of the gait cycle and occurs when one leg bears all the weight and in is contact with the ground. It permits the lower leg to support the weight of the body and allows advancement of the body over the supporting limb. The swing phase constitutes 40 percent of the gait cycle and occurs when the other non-weight-bearing leg is advanced forward to take the next step. Walking is accomplished by a series of reciprocal leg movements alternating between stance and swing: pushing off on the leg in the stance phase while at the same time swinging the other leg forward. As the lower extremities move alternately between stance and swing, the arms swing in a direction opposite that of the legs (i.e., the right arm swings forward with the forward swing of the left lower extremity while the left arm swings backward). This reciprocal movement of the upper extremities provides a counterbalancing action helping to maintain balance when walking.

During the stance phase, three major activities take place (Fig. 39-2). The initial contact (heel strike) represents the beginning of the gait cycle and stance phase, occurring imme-

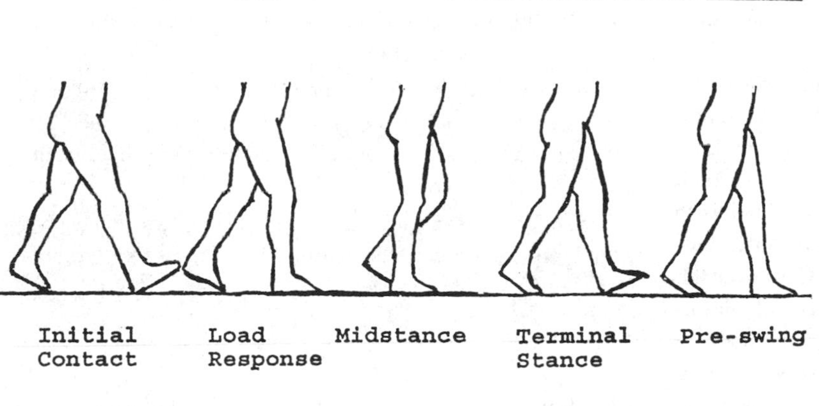

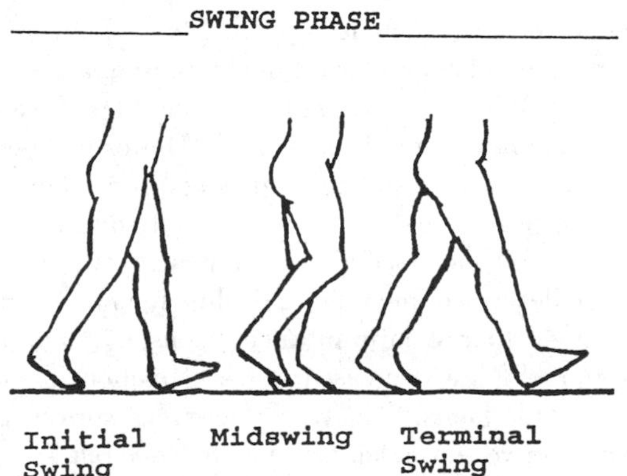

Figure 39-2 Phases of the gait cycle.

diately when the heel of the leading leg (in full extension) strikes the ground. The midstance (single-leg stance) occurs halfway through the stance phase and represents the point at which the body weight is directly over the supporting lower extremity. Last, the terminal stance (heel off), the final portion of the stance phase, represents the point at which the heel of the reference extremity leaves or pushes off the ground and advances the body forward.

The swing phase consists of three stages (Fig. 39-2). The initial swing (acceleration) occurs when the toe of the reference (ipsilateral) extremity leaves the ground and continues until the midswing or the point at which the swinging extremity is directly underneath the body. From this points, the accelerating stage, the leg then enters the midswing (swing-through). To allow for adequate ground clearance during the swing phase, the leg is flexed at the knee and dorsiflexed at the foot. The terminal swing (deceleration) occurs after the midswing when the leg prepares for initial contact with the ground or is in readiness for weight bearing (initial contact) as the stance phase begins again.

The stance and swing phases of gait are typically characterized by two basic variables, time and distance. Definitions of some of the basic variables are presented in the accompanying boxed list. Measurement of these variables provides a basic description of gait patterns.

When walking, the body moves forward in a smooth sinusodial curve. This is achieved through a series of pelvic movements (shift, tilt, and rotation) which to a large extent are responsible for controlling this motion. Pelvic shift effectively lengthens the lower extremity (the femur), thereby lengthening the stride and allowing the foot to make contact with the floor during heel strike, and at the same time minimizes the vertical displacement of the trunk. This maneuver allows the pelvis to shift toward the weight-bearing leg and helps to maintain balance by keeping the weight of the body and the COG over the stance leg. At the same time, the pelvis tilts vertically downward toward the weight-bearing leg and allows the body to keep the COG from moving up and down excessively during normal gait. Pelvic rotation lessens the angle between the femur and the ground, allowing a normal stride during ambulation. Together, pelvic movements help to minimize the up-and-down and side-to-side movements of the body that occur during walking and aid in maintaining balance.

Time and Distance Measurements of Gait

Time variables

- *Stance time*: amount of elapsed time that one foot spends in contact with the walking surface during one gait cycle
- *Swing time*: amount of elapsed time that one foot is not in contact with the walking surface during one gait cycle
- *Single-support time*: amount of time spent by one foot in the stance phase (i.e., in contact with the walking surface)
- *Double-support time*: amount of time spent with both feet on the walking surface during one gait cycle
- *Step time*: elapsed time spent on the walking surface by a single step
- *Cadence*: number or frequency of steps taken by an individual per unit of time (e.g., steps per second or minute)
- *Walking speed or velocity*: distance of forward motion of the body measured over time

Distance variables

- *Walking base width*: linear distance between two feet (the midpoint of the heel of one foot and the same point on the other foot)
- *Step length*: linear distance between the point of contact of one heel or toe with the walking surface and the point of contact of the contralateral heel or toe with the ground
- *Stride length*: linear distance between two successive events that are accomplished by the same leg during the gait cycle

Effects of Aging on Gait

There is considerable debate regarding the influence of age on gait, with some studies showing no difference.[58,59] However, when healthy older persons are compared with younger persons, certain gait characteristics become noticeable with increasing age. A slowing down or decline in average walking speed (5 to 15 percent) is the most common observation.[60,61] In a study of 289 men and 149 women from 19 to 102 years of age, Himann and colleagues[62] reported that between 19 and 62 years of age there was a 2.5 to 4.5 percent decline in normal speed of walking per decade for men and women, respectively. After the age of 62, however, subjects exhibited an accelerated decline in walking speed, a 16 percent and 12 percent decline for men and women, respectively. Decreases in walking speed are associated with a decline in step or stride length[63,64] and an increase in double-support time.[65] Both step and stride length and double-support time represent measures of gait velocity. Older women have been found to walk slower and take shorter steps than older men.[61,66] However, when gender differences in body weight and height are taken into account, gender differences in walking velocity disappear.[60]

Several factors that can influence walking velocity have been described, including a decline in lower-extremity muscle strength (particularly in knee extensors[67] and ankle plantar flexors),[68,69] a decreased range of motion in the hip, knee, and ankle joints,[70] the type of footwear worn by older persons (supportive shoes that facilitate balance but reduce ankle and foot movement),[71] and the nature of the walking surface (e.g., walking velocity is faster on carpeted than on vinyl surfaces).[72]

Some researchers have suggested that slower walking speeds are self-selected or else preferred by older persons.[31,73] During normal walking, the COG falls outside the boundaries of the BOS for 80 percent of the stride length,[74] which represents an unstable condition. As a result, many older people, especially those with a fear of falling, may walk more slowly to compensate for poor balance. Therefore, a decrease in stride length (taking shorter steps) might be a reasonable adaptation to unfavorable environmental surroundings. When asked to increase their walking speed, older persons are able to do so, but rather than increasing stride length as younger persons do to quicken their pace, they are more likely to respond by increasing the frequency of steps.[70]

Additional age-related gait changes include a loss of normal arm swing, reduced pelvic rotation, decreased hip and knee rotation, decreased cadence, increased stride width, and decreased steppage height or reduction in toe-floor clearance.[60,75,76] Also, decreased foot placement and clearance during stair descent in women[77] and difficulty negotiating ground surface obstacles, especially in persons with decreased step length,[78] have been described.

Whether gait changes are age-related or due to subtle pathology remains to be determined. In most gait studies limited information is available describing the criteria used to select subjects for observation. Thus, it is possible that samples included individuals with pathologic conditions. Several studies,[31,79] for example, have observed decreases in walking velocity, step length, and swing/stance ratio (increased double-support time) in older people but suggest that these gait changes were more strongly influenced by the onset of neuromuscular disease or use of multiple medications. Regardless, gait changes, especially a decline in walking velocity, are a marker of disability and dependency.[80,81] Also, investigators have shown that reductions in walking velocity are associated with difficulty in crossing street intersections before the light changes.[82,83]

Pathologic Disturbances

Diseases and their associated impairments play a more decisive role in gait and balance disturbances than age-related changes. However, in order to properly evaluate and treat older individuals, a clear understanding of the normal or usual age-related effects on gait and balance is critical. Unfamiliarity with this knowledge may have grave consequences. Age-related changes may be attributed to disease, leading to initiation of ineffective and possibly harmful treatments; or even worse, disease effects may erroneously be ascribed to normal aging changes and be neglected, allowing unrestrained progression of the disorder.

There are many causes of gait and balance disturbances in the elderly. Apart from dizziness and syncope due to acute or chronic cardiovascular abnormalities, most gait and balance disorders originate in the neuromuscular[84–86] and vestibular systems.[87,88] The following discussion considers some of the more characteristic gait and balance disturbances observed in the elderly and their associated diseases.

Senile Gait

Senile gait, also called essential or idiopathic gait, is characterized by a flexed posture and short, shuffling steps which are especially prominent when making turns, Typically, individuals move slowly and cautiously, uncertain of their step and foot placement. Patients often assume a widened stance (increased BOS) and are prone to retropulsion (toppling backward), particularly when turning. Women are especially predisposed to a narrow-based stance (decreased BOS), which increases their risk of loss of balance. Balance displacement may be elicited with a slight nudge on the sternum which results in posterior balance loss. While these changes in gait and balance are similar to those seen in a variety of disorders, such as normal pressure hydrocephalus (NPH) and Parkinson's disease, the cause of this gait disorder is uncertain. The condition is confirmed if the clinical and laboratory investigations are negative. It has been suggested that senile gait merely represents an exaggeration of age-related changes.[89]

Frontal Lobe Gait

Also referred to as frontal ataxia or apraxia, frontal lobe gait is characterized by a wide BOS, slightly flexed posture, and small, shuffling, hesitant steps. Gait initiation is often difficult. The feet appear to be stuck or glued to the floor, a condition referred to as magnetic gait. In an effort to lift the foot an individual may sway from side to side, although any excessive sway can easily produce loss of balance. Once they have begun walking, the person may suddenly come to a complete stop, be unable to move forward for several seconds, and then continue to walk. This is described as the "slipping clutch syndrome." Sometimes, after taking a few short steps, the gait inexplicably begins to improve. Similar problems can arise when the person attempts to change direction. One foot remains in place while the other initiates a series of small, uncertain steps during rotations. Turning around is accomplished in the same way, pivoting on both feet in a small circle. During this period the risk of balance loss is particularly great, as minor shifts-in BOS are difficult to correct.

In advanced forms of frontal lobe disorders, patients can develop truncal imbalance and as a result have great difficulty walking or standing without support. Some progress to the point of being unable to walk or take a step even with the assistance of others. Yet they are capable of initiating gait-related leg movements when they are lying in bed, which suggests the presence of gait apraxia.[90]

Patients with late stages of Alzheimer's disease, multiple cerebral infarcts, Binswanger's disease, and NPH typically demonstrate this type of gait disorder. In addition to gait disturbances, NPH is associated with mild forms of dementia and urinary incontinence, and these disorders are frequently the most prominent and earliest manifestation of NPH, sometimes preceding other features by as much as 3 to 4 years.[91] At times, the gait associated with NPH may be difficult to identify since it can take on many forms, including gait apraxia or a slow, shuffling gait similar to that of Parkinsonism. Clinical response to the removal of 40 to 50 mL of cerebrospinal fluid, manifested by an improvement in gait patterns, may be an acceptable screening test for NPH.[92]

Sensory Ataxic Gait

Sensory ataxic gait is characterized by a wide-based stance and a "foot stamping" walk. The legs are usually flung forward and outward in a high-stepping, stamping manner. The heel touches the ground first and a stamp of the foot may be heard. This gait pattern is a response to decreased lower-extremity proprioceptive input and the individual's not knowing where the feet are in relation to the ground or support surface. As a result, patients must constantly observe the position of their legs to ensure proper foot placement when walking, particularly on uneven surfaces. With good visual input, some individuals display a nearly normal gait, however, their gait becomes markedly worse when they walk under conditions of low illumination because of poor compensatory visual input. This is reflected by a positive Romberg's sign in which eye closure while standing in place elicits instability. Patients may manifest severe balance problems as well, such as reeling from side to side. Sensory ataxia is caused by disorders affecting the posterior column, peripheral nerve, or dorsal root of the spinal cord, such as thiamine deficiency, subacute combined degeneration (vitamin B_{12} deficiency), spinocerebellar degeneration, spinal cord compression, and diabetic neuropathy.

Cerebellar Ataxic Gait

A wide-based stance and small, irregular, unsteady steps characterize cerebellar ataxia gait. Sometimes this gait is accompanied by veering, staggering, and sudden lurching to either side, forward, or backward, giving the person the appearance of being drunk. In unilateral cerebellar disease, the patient may veer to ward one side only, typically to ward the side affected by the disease. In addition, control over trunk and leg movements is greatly impaired, which causes irregular steps and balance loss. Patients demonstrate truncal imbalance when walking and often lift their feet too high and place them down either too far apart or too close together. Typically, patients early on have difficulty walking on their heels and toes or in tandem gait (i.e., with a narrow BOS). Turning is accomplished en bloc and may give rise to loss of balance, particularly when the activity is performed too quickly. Ataxia is present whether the eyes are open or closed although in severe cases individuals are not able to remain standing even with their eyes open. The defect lies in the coordination of proprioceptive, labyrinthine, and visual information. This type of gait is associated with acute vestibular damage, stroke, chronic alcoholism, and degenerative conditions such as spinocerebellar atrophy and progressive supernuclear palsy. Modifiable causes of ataxia include thiamine and vitamin B_{12} deficiency, hypothyroidism, and hypnotic sedative toxicity.

Spastic Gait

Spastic gait is observed in patients with hemiplegia or hemiparesis, and paraparesis. In hemiplegia (or hemiparesis), the affected leg is stiff, slightly flexed at the hip, and extended at the knee, and the foot is plantar-flexed. The affected arm is maintained in a position of flexion at the elbow, stationed across the abdomen, and frequently supported by the good hand. When walking, arm swing on the affected side is impaired, and the toes of the involved leg scrape or drag across the floor, the result of decreased ankle dorsiflexion and reduced foot clearance. Examination of the patient's shoe usually shows excessive wear along the toe and outer side of the sole. To ensure proper ground clearance when walking, the patient must swing the affected leg slowly in an outward arc (circumduction) with each step. This is accomplished by a slight lateral flexion of the trunk toward the unaffected side, a posture that allows the affected leg to swing clear of the ground. At the same time, the hip on the affected side is hyperextended, elevating the plegic or paretic extremity and permitting foot-ground clearance. This maneuver is referred to as hip hiking.

Patients with hemiplegia or paresis frequently have poor balance. Leaning the trunk toward the unaffected side may lead to a narrow standing and walking BOS and increase the risk of balance loss. Most individuals, however, are able to maintain their balance by shifting the body weight (COG) to the intact or unaffected leg. Any loss of balance usually occurs toward the weaker side, the result of an inability to shift the COG sufficiently enough to counter instability. A loss of muscle strength and proprioceptive input in the affected leg has been shown to contribute to loss of balance.[93,94] Alterations in the sequence of postural muscle activation on the affected side have also been demonstrated to occur. During a displacement of balance, instead of the normal sequence of distal-to-proximal muscle activation occurring, the proximal muscles of the plegic or paretic extremity are activated first.[95] This can impair the ability to initiate quick postural responses and result in loss of balance. Poor postural control has also been attributed to vestibular dysfunction following stroke and affects both the VOR and VOS.[96] In addition, the presence of visual neglect (hemianopsia) and visuospatial impairment (hemi-inattention) following a stroke is quite common and can adversely influence gait and balance. Common causes of hemiplegic or paretic gait include contralateral cerebral infarction, mass lesions, and cerebral trauma.

In spastic paraparesis, each leg moves forward slowly in a stiff manner with short, labored steps and restricted movement at the hip and knee joints. In the course of walking, the legs rotate outward away from and then toward the trunk, tracing a semicircle (bilateral circumduction). Typically, ankle dorsiflexors are weak, causing the feet to scrape the ground. In severe cases of paraparesis, the legs are hyperextended and adducted close to the body (rubbing against each other), which results in a scissoring gait. This greatly compromises balance, as patients are forced to walk on a narrow base. Common causes include advanced cervical spondylitic myelopathy, pernicious anemia (vitamin B_{12} deficiency), chronic spinal cord compression, hyperthyroidism, and lacunar infarcts.

Steppage Gait

Steppage gait is characterized by lifting the feet high off the ground in order to keep the toes from scraping the floor. The toes strike the floor first and are followed by the heels, producing a slapping noise. This toe-to-heel slapping may be unilateral or bilateral. Steppage gait is caused by weakness or paralysis of the pretibial and peroneal muscles (foot drop) and decreased proprioceptive input. As a result, patients routinely need to observe the position of their legs in relation to the floor in order to determine proper foot placement. Frequently, these individuals complain of tripping over trivial objects such as cords or rug wrinkles, especially if they fail to lift their feet high enough to clear the ground surface. Common causes include peripheral neuropathies (e.g., resulting from diabetes mellitus, B_{12} deficiency, alcoholism).

Festinating Gait

Festinating gait involves a symmetric, rapid shuffling of the feet and is mostly associated with Parkinson's disease. When standing, the trunk of the patient is bent forward and the hips and knees are maintained in a position of flexion. As a result, the individual's COG is shifted forward, reaching the edge of their BOS. When walking, the patient's COG moves beyond the safe limits of their BOS, which leads to instability. Subsequently, the individual's steps become progressively quicker (festinating gait) in an attempt to regain postural control (i.e., alignment between the COG and BOS). In essence, the patient appears to be chasing and trying to overtake a displaced COG. Occasionally, they may have difficulty stopping and risk falling. Other causes of festinating gait include cerebral disease due to multiple small infarcts, dementia, and hydrocephalus.

Parkinson's disease is associated with several other gait and balance disturbances. Walking is frequently accomplished using a series of short, flat-footed shuffles, with the feet barely clearing the ground (marche a petits pas). Also, gait initiation may be delayed during the first few steps. As a result, the body sometimes moves forward before the feet start to move, placing individuals at a risk of losing their balance. At other times, the gait can "freeze"—halt immediately—particularly when the individual is approaching ground obstacles (e.g., curbs, steps, door thresholds). Sometimes a small lateral push allows patients to move their legs forward. In some cases, patients may display an inability to initiate or continue lateral shifts of the body when walking and instead rock the body from side to side, exhibiting excessive path deviation away from the normal smooth sinusoidal curve and lateropulsion (movement or instability toward one side). To preserve stability during walking and turning, patients typically assume a wide stance in order to increase the BOS. Turning is frequently accomplished using many small steps and a rigid trunk movement (en bloc turning). Additionally, late PD is associated with a loss of anticipatory and reactive postural control. If a small nudge is applied against the sternum, the patient may fall "in one piece" like a log (retropulsion). In addition, displacements in the anterior direction can lead to uncontrolled forward stability or propulsion.

Waddling Gait

Loss of strength involving the limb girdle muscles can lead to an unstable, waddling gait (a duck or a penguin's walk is an excellent example of this gait). Patients typically exhibit a characteristic lateral trunk movement away from the foot as it lifts, an exaggerated rotation of the pelvis, and a rolling of the hips with each step. These motions are the result of gluteal muscle weakness and an inability to stabilize the weight-bearing hip. In addition, patients commonly complain of difficulty climbing stairs and getting up from low-seated chairs or toilets because of proximal muscle weakness. Common conditions associated with this gait include hypo- and hyperthyroidism, polymyalgia rheumatica, polymyositis, osteomalacia, and proximal neuropathies.

Multisensory Deficit Gait

Abnormal gaits associated with multisensory deficits are ascribed to concurrent visual and proprioceptive impairment and vestibular dysfunction. Typically, patients complain of dizziness, unsteadiness, or lightheadedness experienced only when walking or turning around quickly. Individuals often use canes and walkers or touch walls and other furnishings while walking for both proprioceptive feedback and balance support. Diabetic patients are particularly prone to this gait because of visual and neuropathic complications.

Vestibular (Ataxic) Gait

Vestibular ataxia is characterized by a constant sensation of unsteadiness when walking. If the patient is stationary and standing still, typically there is no disequilibrium. The gait is broad-based, with frequent sidestepping. Patients display a drift toward the side of the vestibular impairment followed by a quick correction in the opposite direction. Unsteadiness is typically made worse by turning and progresses to staggering when the eyes are closed. Common conditions causing vestibular ataxia include labyrinthine disease, drug toxicity (e.g., from aminoglycosides), and cerebellopontile angle tumors.

Peripheral Vestibular Imbalance

Vestibular dysfunction is classified as either peripheral or central in origin. Peripheral disorders involve the end organs (semicircular canals, utricle, or saccule), the vestibular nerve, and vestibular nuclei, whereas central disorders mainly involve the brain stem and cerebellum. Peripheral vestibular disorders occur more commonly and are associated with more vertigo than central vestibular disorders, although acute vascular ischemia of the brain stem or cerebellum can cause acute, severe episodes of vertigo.

Benign paroxysmal positional vertigo (BPPV) is character-

Common Peripheral and Central Vestibular Disorders

Peripheral
- Benign paroxysmal positional vertigo (BPPV)
- Disequilibrium of aging
- Labyrinthitis (vestibular neuronitis)
- Ménière's disease
- Vestibulotoxic drugs
- Cervical vertigo
- Post-traumatic vertigo

Central
- Vertebrobasilar insufficiency
- Vestibular epilepsy
- Central brainstem/cerebellum lesions

ized by sudden, intense episodes of "spinning" lasting for 30 seconds or less and precipitated by a particular change in head position. These episodes often occur when the person is lying down, rolling over in bed, getting out of bed, bending over and straightening up, or extending the neck (as in looking up or reaching for an object from the top shelf of a kitchen cabinet). Complaints of nausea, usually mild, may accompany these activities. Symptoms are typically worse in the morning or earlier part of the day, and abrupt attacks sometimes cause the patient to fall to the ground. Posturographic measurements performed in patients with BPPV, in conjunction with their standing on a force platform and tilting their heads to elicit symptoms, demonstrate characteristic patterns of postural instability, most notably increased sway in the anterio posterior direction which becomes worse with the eyes closed.[97] Between episodes many patients become apprehensive, express a fear of recurrence, and exhibit mild disequilibrium. Hearing and neurologic examinations are normal, but a typical response to positional testing (rotatory nystagmus and symptoms of vertigo) provides objective evidence for the presence of this condition. BPPV can result from head injury (e.g., fracture of the temporal bone) and inner ear abnormalities or infections. In most patients, however, no underlying cause is found. It is felt that debris generated by degeneration of the utricle and semicircular canals becomes fixed to the cupula (located on the posterior aspect of the semicircular canal) and that moving the head from the erect position dislodges these deposits, thereby eliciting symptoms of BPPV or cupulolithiasis.[98]

This disorder is benign in that the patient improves with time. In many cases the symptoms of BPPV resolve either spontaneously or after a few days, particularly when the patient learns to recognize and avoid head movements that precipitate the episodes. Occasionally, however, symptoms may be intermittent, with exacerbations occurring over the course of several months to several years. When symptoms persist or recur, a program of habituation exercises (performing maneuvers that provoke symptoms) may be of benefit.[99] Vestibular depressants such as meclizine and diazepam are frequently prescribed for patients with BPPV, although there is no convincing evidence that these medications are of value. Furthermore, these drugs may cause undesirable side effects, preventing patients from exhibiting protective reflexes.

Age-related changes occurring in the vestibular portions of the inner ear may adversely affect balance, resulting in disequilibrium of aging. Degenerative changes occurring in the ampullary mechanism of the semicircular canal may cause episodes of vertigo associated with rotational head movements (ampullary disequilibrium). Patients typically experience symptoms of unsteadiness moments after rapidly turning their head to the right or left or while executing sudden neck flexion and extension activities. The sensation of unsteadiness may last for hours. Deterioration of the otolithic organs may lead to the onset of vertigo associated with changes in head position with respect to gravity (macular disequilibrium). This condition frequently occurs when patients stand up from bed and experience sensations of unsteadiness, and sitting on the side of the bed for a few minutes usually alleviates symptoms. Sometimes this type of clinical picture is confused with orthostatic hypotension although postural blood pressure measurements are normal. There is no specific treatment for disequilibrium of aging other than avoiding provoking activities.

Labyrinthitis or vestibular neuronitis may result in the sudden onset of vertigo, nausea, and vomiting and of episodes of unsteadiness. The vertigo usually lasts for a few days but may persist for several months in some elderly patients. Although the etiology is obscure, the condition usually occurs in epidemics (affecting several patients residing in close proximity), which suggests an infective cause which is most likely viral in origin. In many cases, a mild febrile illness or upper respiratory infection precedes the onset of vertigo. A few days after onset, without warning, the patient suddenly experiences severe disequilibrium and difficulty ambulating. Head movement exacerbates the vertigo, which often requires the individual to remain in bed for relief. For several weeks following onset, the patient may walk with exaggerated care and with eye movements replacing head movements so as to avoid provoking vertigo. At the height of the disorder spontaneous nystagmus may be noted, although if the condition is bilateral, nystagmus may be absent. There is no treatment for this disorder other than supporting the patient's mobility during the symptomatic and recovery phase.

Ménière's disease is a condition in which episodes of severe vertigo are accompanied and usually preceded by tinnitus and progressive low-frequency sensorineural hearing loss. Attacks of vertigo may last from 30 minutes to 12 hours, and each episode may be ushered in by an increase in tinnitus and hearing loss or a feeling of fullness in the ear. Spontaneous nystagmus may be present during the episode. The attacks subside when hearing loss is complete, although a mild ataxia may remain for a few days following an episode. The condition is associated with overdistension of the membranous endolymphatic system and degeneration of the cochlear cells. Ménière's disease is usually self-limiting, and treatment is directed toward providing symptomatic relief with vestibular suppressants. Occasionally, recurrent attacks of Ménière's disease may lead to chronic mild disequilibrium. A late feature of this disorder is Tumarkin's otolithic crisis,[100] which is characterized by drop attacks during which the patient feels pushed or driven to the ground. There is no loss of consciousness, and recovery is almost immediate. The condition is attributed to sudden abnormal stimulation of the otolith organ.

Most drugs that cause vertigo affect the labyrinthine and act peripherally. The main groups of drugs involved are aminoglycosides, which produce hair cell damage, and loop diuretics (e.g. ethacrynic acid and furosemide). Aminoglycosides damage the hair cells of the inner ear, and diuretics, in addition to producing hair cell injury, lead to an increase in sodium concentration in the inner ear. Other classes of medications commonly associated with drug-induced vertigo including anticonvulsants, benzodiazepines, and salicylates. Bilateral vestibular hypofunction, commonly caused by aminoglycoside ototoxicity, represents a manifestation of drug-induced vertigo. Patients may complain of spinning sensations but more frequently exhibit sudden unsteadiness of gait. Typically, balance is worse when walking in the dark or with the eyes closed. Sometimes patients complain of oscillopsia (i.e., objects in the visual field seeming to move back and forth) associated with head movements or walking. Diagnosis of bilateral vestibular hypofunction is confirmed with either caloric or rotational tests which reveal responses of below-normal intensity. Most instances of drug-induced vertigo are reversible, particularly if detected early enough before any permanent organ damage occurs.

Mild episodes of vertigo and unsteadiness may accompany head trauma (post-traumatic vertigo) such as might occur following a fall. Symptoms are present with or without evidence of temporal bone fracture and can occur days to weeks after the injury. Sometimes the disorder is accompanied by profound hearing loss. In most cases, the symptoms resolve after a few weeks, although in some patients BPPV may follow.

Last, cervical vertigo consists of brief attacks of disequilibrium induced by positional head and neck movements. Disorders of the cervical spine, such as cervical spondylosis and rheumatoid arthritis, interfere with somatosensory input from mechanoreceptors located in the spinal joints. The end result is difficulty with body balance and a tendency to stagger. A positive response to neck maneuvers may support the diagnosis, although it is important to exclude vertebrobasilar ischemia and carotid sinus hypersensitivity, both of which can cause symptoms of vertigo or lightheadedness. Treatment consists of teaching patients to avoid provoking positional movements. The use of a cervical collar to stabilize the neck is of little benefit in this condition.

Antalgic and Gonalgic Gait

Antalgic gait, which is caused by painful hip conditions, is characterized by a reluctance of the individual to place weight on the affected limb. The foot of the affected limb is placed flat on the ground, avoiding heel strike, in order to minimize jarring of impact. Similarly, push-off during the stance phase of the gait cycle is avoided to decrease transmission of ground forces to the involved hip. Attempts to keep weight off of the painful hip result in decreased stance and swing phases of gait and an overall decrease in walking velocity.

Osteoarthritic knee pain causing gonalgic gait can result in similar problems. Patients tend to walk with their knee and foot flexed in order to minimize the amount of time weight is placed on the affected leg. Individuals with osteoarthritis exhibit significantly less knee extension in the involved joint during gait,[101] which affects both heel strike and push-off. Patients with unilateral symptomatic osteoarthritis demonstrate decreased flexion and extension in the unaffected knee as well, although to a much lesser extent than in the symptomatic knee.[101] The reduced flexion and extension may represent either asymptomatic disease or a decrease in physical activity, leading to an altered range of motion.

Both antalgic and gonalgic gait may be viewed as being self-protective. Persons with irreversible disorders may benefit from the use of a cane on the uninvolved side, which reduces weight bearing on the painful hip or knee joint.

Leg length discrepancies caused by such problems as osteoarthritis of the hip and hip fracture repair can lead to gait and balance problems as well. As the foot prepares to make initial contact with the ground (heel strike), the pelvis on the side of the affected or shorter leg drops excessively in an attempt to extend the leg in order to reach the ground, causing the person to limp. To compensate, the joints of the unaffected leg typically exhibit exaggerated flexion in order to achieve swing-through, or else circumduction of the unaffected leg. Persons with leg length discrepancies following hip repair can usually be helped by supplying a heel lift for the affected leg.

Podalgic Gait

Foot disorders, including arthritic conditions, corns, calluses, thick, deformed toenails, hammertoes, bunions, and atrophy of plantar pads can lead to pain when walking and affect gait patterns.[102] Toe contact occurs for about three-quarters of the gait cycle,[103] thus any forefoot disorder may lead to mechanical problems and unsteady gait. Furthermore, foot disorders are associated with decreased proprioceptive input,[104] which contributes to gait and balance disturbances. Furthermore, loose- or tight-fitting footwear can lead to both foot disorders and gait disturbances.

Dementia-Related Gait

Dementia, especially the Alzheimer's type, is associated with disorders of gait and balance. Visser[105] showed that patients with moderately severe Alzheimer's disease had slower walking speeds, decreased step length, increased double-support time, increased step-to-step variability, and increased postural sway. Some patients with Alzheimer's disease display a marked flexion of posture and instability which appears insidiously and parallels the deteriorating course of the disease.[106] This change in posture may occur acutely as well. Rosenfeld et al.[107] described a series of five cases in which older patients with Alzheimer's disease who were admitted to a psychogeriatric ward experienced an acute onset of stooped posture. Previous to hospitalization all patients were able to walk in an erect manner. After the onset of stooping, however, they continued to walk but exhibited significant balance problems. The authors felt this acute change in posture was a reaction to fear because the patients had moved from small apartments to the wide, open space of the psychogeriatric ward.

Also, patients with moderate to severe degrees of Alzheimer's disease may exhibit apraxia, an inability to remember how to perform routine motor tasks, such as transferring and walking, in the absence of neuromuscular impairments. Patients with gait apraxia know they want to walk but are unable to ambulate correctly even though strength and sensation are intact. Sometimes patients with apraxia walk in place instead of moving ahead, or else they are unable to move their feet forward (as if the feet were glued to the floor). Typically, apraxia begins with clumsiness and eventually can progress to a profound lack of coordination in gait and balance. Other conditions associated with apraxia include frontal lobe lesions and NPH.

Cautious Gait

Patients with a fear of falling often display a cautious gait. Typically, posture is flexed forward, and ambulation is accomplished slowly (decreased stride length and walking speed) with the legs held in a slightly flexed position to maintain a low COG. This picture is very similar to that of someone attempting to walk on a sheet of ice. The gait is short-stepped with the feet held apart (slightly wide-based gait), a strategy used to maintain a greater BOS. Turning is accomplished en bloc, often with mild instability. Frequently, individuals hold onto walls and furnishings for balance support. This type of gait may be most dominant in persons with multiple falls, increased postfall lie times, and decreased sensory input. Most individuals are aware of impaired balance (even those with mild to moderate degrees of dementia) and express the need for caution. It is suggested that cautious gait represents a compensatory adaptation, "an appropriate response to real or perceived disequilibrium."[108] In some patients, gait may improve if they are allowed to walk while holding onto others or to a walker for support.

Management

For any older person with a gait and/or balance disturbance, an attempt should be made to determine the etiology of the problem and, when possible, treatment should be initiated. In particular, various medications such as benzodiazepines, tricyclic antidepressants, anticonvulsants, and hypnotic sedatives that affect stability should not be overlooked. Aside from the customary neuromuscular examination, a functional assessment of gait and balance may yield more useful clinical information.[109]

Components of Gait and Balance Assessment

Physical Examination

- *Mental status*: Dementia, depression, delirium
- *Blood pressure measurement*: Postural hypotension
- *Vision*: Visual fields, acuity, extraocular movements
- *Hearing*: Otoscopic and audiologic testing
- *Cardiac*: Arrhythmia, valvular disorders, bruits
- *Neurologic*: Position and vibration sense, DTRs, nystagmus, past pointing, finger-nose test, positional tests
- *Musculoskeletal*: Range of motion, strength

Diagnostic examination

- *Laboratory workup*: Serum chemistry profile, vitamin B_{12}, thyroid studies, drug levels
- *Radiologic*: Cervical spondylitic myelopathy, knee and hip osteoarthritis
- *Computed tomography/magnetic resonance imaging*: Infarction, hemorrhage, tumors, hydrocephalus, myelopathy
- *Electromyogram*: Peripheral neuropathy, neuromuscular disease

A simple mobility screen, such as the "get up and go" test,[110] can be used for this purpose. This test, performed in less than 2 minutes, examines the individual's ability to stand up from a chair, walk 10 feet, turn, walk back, and sit down again. Chair transfers (without the aid of armrests) are a reliable test of quadriceps and gluteal muscle strength and balance proficiency (i.e., ability to maintain one's COG over a shifting BOS). During the walking and turning maneuvers, the following should be observed: body posture, upper-extremity movements, gait initiation, step length and height, step continuity and symmetry, width of BOS, walking velocity, deviation of path, and degree of sway or unsteadiness. In addition, observing the patient walk in tandem, walking on the heels or toes, may reveal subtle deficits in gait.

Evaluation should also include observing the ability to maintain balance over dissimilar BOS: parallel, semitandem, tandem, and single-leg stance. These maneuvers progress from the least difficult (parallel stance) to the most challenging (single-leg stance) measure of balance. Additionally, a Romberg test (appraisal of sensory input) and a sternal nudge test (estimation of postural competence) should be given. A positive Romberg is indicative of altered proprioceptive and vestibular function; unsteadiness subsequent to nudging the sternum suggests Parkinson's disease, NPH, or cervical spondylosis. In cases in which a treatable disorder cannot be found, existing function should be supported. Targeted exercise regimens aimed at strengthening lower-extremity muscles, improving joint flexibility, and balance training designed to enhance sensory interaction can significantly improve gait and balance even in frail older persons.[111–113]

Regardless of the cause of gait and balance impairment, appropriate footwear (nonslip soles, minimal heel lift) should be encouraged. The use of canes, walkers, and assistive devices (e.g., bathroom grab bars and tub seats) to support gait and balance and the elimination of environmental hazards interfering with safe mobility should also be recommended. The importance of these strategies in the management of gait and balance disturbances can easily be underestimated. Although no direct evidence of their effectiveness exists, common sense dictates that they may of benefit and should be attempted.

References

1. Dawson D, Hendershot G, Fulton J: Aging in the eighties: functional limitations of individuals age 65 and over. Advance Data from Vital and Health Statistics. No. 113. Public Health Service, Hyattsville, MD, 1987
2. Cornoni-Huntley J, Brock DB, Ostfeld A et al: Established Populations for Epidemiologic Studies of Elderly: Resource Data Book. NIH 86–2443. National Institutes of Health, Bethesda, MD, 1986
3. Sixt E, Landahl S: Postural disturbances in a 75-year old population. I. prevalence and functional consequences. Age Ageing 1987;16:393–398
4. Gerson LW, Jarjoura D, McCord G: Risk of imbalance in elderly people with impaired hearing and vision. Age Ageing 1989;18:31–34
5. Baloh RW, Fife TD, Zwerling L et al: Comparison of static and dynamic posturography in young and older normal people. J Am Geriatr Soc 1994;42:405–412
6. Era P, Heikkinen E: Postural sway during standing and unexpected disturbance of balance in random samples of men of different ages. J Gerontol 1985;40:287–295
7. Lucy SD, Hayes KC: Postural sway profiles: normal subjects and subjects with cerebellar ataxia. Physiother Can 1985;37: 140–148
8. Jedrychowski W, Mroz E, Tobiasz-Adamczyk B, Jedrycnowksa I: Functional status of the lower extremities in elderly males: a community study. Arch Gerontol Geriatr 1990;10:117–122
9. Fernie GR, Holliday PJ: Postural sway in amputees and normal subjects. J Bone Joint Surg 1978;60:895–898
10. Bohannon RW, Larkin PA, Cook AC et al: Decrease in timed balance scores with aging. Phys Ther 1984;64:1067–1070
11. Brocklehurst JC, Robertson D, James-Groom P: Clinical correlates of sway in old age: sensory modalities. Age Ageing 1982; 11:1–10
12. Briggs RC, Gossman MR, Birch R et al: Balance performance among noninstitutionalized elderly women. Phys Ther 1989; 69:748–756
13. Holliday PJ, Fernie GR: Postural sway during low frequency floor oscillation in young and elderly subjects. pp. 66–69. In Igarashi M, Black FO (eds): Vestibular and Visual Control in Posture and Locomotor Equilibrium. Krager, Basel, 1985
14. Wolfson L, Whipple R, Derby CA et al: A dynamic posturography study of balance in healthy elderly. Neurology 1992;42: 2069–2075
15. Overstall PW, Exton-Smith AN, Imms FJ, Johnston AL: Falls in elderly related to postural imbalance. Br Med J 1977;1: 261–264
16. Fernie GR, Gryfe CI, Holliday PJ, Llewellyn A: The relationship of postural sway in standing to the incidence of falls in geriatric subjects. Age Ageing 1982;11:11–16
17. Maki BE, Holliday PJ, Fernie GR: Aging and postural control: a comparison of spontaneous and induced-sway balance tests. J Am Geriatr Soc 1989;38:1–9
18. Colledge NR, Cantley P, Peaston I et al: Ageing and balance: the measurement of spontaneous sway by posturography. Gerontology 1994;40:273–278
19. Wolfson L, Whipple R, Derby CA et al: Gender differences in the balance of healthy elderly as demonstrated by dynamic posturography. J Gerontol 1994;49:M160–M167
20. Lee WA, Deming LR: Age-related changes in the size of the effective support base during standing. Phys Ther 1988;68: 859
21. Ring C, Nayak USL, Isaacs B: The effect of visual deprivation and proprioceptive change on postural sway in healthy adults. J Am Geriatr Soc 1989;37:745–749
22. Olney RK: Age-related changes in peripheral nerve function. Geriatr Med Today 1985;4:76–86
23. Skinner HB, Barrack RL, Cook SD: Age-related decline in proprioception. Clin Orthop 1984;184:208–211
24. Kokmen E, Bossemeyer RW, Williams WT: Quantitative evaluation of joint motion sensation in an aging population. J Gerontol 1978;33:62–67
25. MacLennan WJ, Timothy JI, Hall MRP: Vibration sense, proprioception and ankle reflexes in old age. J Clin Exp Gerontol 1980;2:159–171
26. Duncan G, Wilson JA, MacLennan WJ, Lewis S: Clinical correlates of sway in elderly people living at home. Gerontology 1992;38:160–166
27. Lord SR, Clark RD, Webster IW: Postural stability and associated physiological factors in a population of aged persons. J Gerontol 1991;46:M69–M76
28. Paulus W, Straube A, Brandt TH: Visual postural performance after loss of somatosensory and vestibular function. J Neurol Neurosurg Psychiatry 1987;50:1542–1545
29. Dornan J, Fernie GR, Holliday PJ: Visual input: its importance in the control of postural sway. Arch Phys Med Rehabil 1978; 59:586–591
30. Woollacott MH, Shumway-Cook A, Nashner LM: Aging and postural control: changes in sensory organization and muscular coordination. Int J Aging Human Dev 1986;23:97–114
31. Imms FJ, Edholm OG: Studies of gait and mobility in the elderly. Age Ageing 1981;10:147–156
32. Lichtenstein MJ, Shields SL, Shiairi RG, Burger MC: Clinical determinants of biomechanics platform measures of balance in aged women. J Am Geriatr Soc 1988;36:996–1002
33. Paulus WM, Straube A, Brandt T: Visual stabilization of posture. Brain 1984;107:1143–1168
34. Manchester D, Woollacott M, Zederbauer-Hylton N, Marin O: Visual, vestibular and somatosensory contributions to balance control in the older adult. J Gerontol 1989;44:M118–M127
35. Lord SR, Clark RD, Webster IW: Visual acuity and contrast

sensitivity in relation to falls in an elderly population. Age Ageing 1991;20:175–181

36. Johnson LG, Hawkins JE: Sensory and neural degeneration with aging, as seen in microdissections of the inner ear. Ann Otol Rhinol Laryngol 1972;81:179–193
37. Rosenhall U, Rubin W: Degenerative changes in the human vestibular sensory epithelial. Acta Otolaryngol 1975;79: 67–81
38. DiZio P, Lackner JR: Age differences in oculomotor responses to step changes in body velocity and visual surround velocity. J Gerontol 1990;45:M89–M94
39. Peterka RJ, Black FO: Age-related changes in human posture control: motor coordination tests. J Vestib Res 1990;1:87–96
40. Carter JE, Obler L, Woodward S, Albert ML: The effect of increasing age on the latency for saccadic eye movements. J Gerontol 1983;38:310–320
41. Abel LA, Troost BT, Dell'Osso LF: The effects of age on normal saccadic characteristics and their variability. Vision Res 1983;23:33–37
42. Stefansson S, Imoto T: Age-related changes in optokinetic and rotational tests. Am J Otol 1986;7:193–196
43. Sharpe JA, Sylvester TO: Effect of aging on horizontal smooth pursuit. Invest Opthalmol Vis Sci 1978;17:465–468
44. Norre ME, Forrez G, Beckers A: Posturography measuring instability in vestibular dysfunction in the elderly. Age Ageing 1987;16:89–93
45. Woollacott M, Inglin B, Manchester D: Response preparation and posture control: neuromuscular changes in the older adult. Ann NY Acad Sci 1988;515:42–53
46. Stelmach GE, Worringham CJ: Sensorimotor deficits related to postural stability. Clin Geriatr Med 1985;1:679–694
47. Horak FB, Shupert CL, Mirka A: Components of postural dyscontrol in the elderly: a review. Neurobiol Aging 1989;10: 727–738
48. Stelmach GE, Teasdale N, DiFabio RP, Phillips J: Age-related decline in postural control mechanisms. Int J Aging Human Dev 1989;29:205–223
49. Woollacott MH: Changes in posture and voluntary control in the elderly: research findings and rehabilitation. Top Geriatr Rehabil 1990;5:1–11
50. Luchies CW, Alexander NB, Schultz AB, Aston-Miller J: Stepping responses of young and old adults to postural disturbances: kinematics. J Am Geriatr Soc 1994;42:506–512
51. Mankovskii NB, Mints AY, Lysenyuk VP: Regulation of the preparatory period for complex voluntary movement in old and extreme old age. Human Physiol 1980;6:46–50
52. Inglin B, Woollacott M: Age-related changes in anticipatory postural adjustments associated with arm movements. J Gerontol 1988;43:M105–M113
53. Zattara M, Bouisset S: Chronometric analysis of the posturokinetic programming of voluntary movement. J Motor Behav 1986;18:215–223
54. Woollacott MH, Manchester DL: Anticipatory postural adjustments in older adults: are changes in response characteristics due to changes in strategy? J Gerontol 1993;48:M64–M70
55. Grimby G, Saltin B: The ageing muscle. Clin Physiol 1983; 3:209–218
56. Probst C: The influence of hip abduction strength on postural sway in elderly females. Thesis, University of Pittsburgh, 1989
57. Teasdale N, Stelmach GE, Breunig A: Postural sway characteristics of the elderly under normal and altered visual and support surface conditions. J Gerontol 1991;46:B238–B244
58. Blanke DJ, Hageman PA: Comparison of gait of young men and elderly men. Phys Ther 1989;69:144–148
59. Gabell A, Nayak U: The effect of age on variability in gait. J Gerontol 1984;39:662–666
60. Elble RJ, Thomas SS, Higgins C, Colliver J: Stride-dependent changes in gait of older people. J Neurol 1991;238:1–5
61. Bendall MJ, Bassey EJ, Pearson MB: Factors affecting walking speed of elderly people. Age Ageing 1989;18:327–332
62. Hinmann JE, Cunningham DA, Rechnitzer PA, Paterson DH: Age-related changes in speed of walking. Med Sci Sports Exerc 1988;20:161–166
63. Hageman PA, Blanke DJ: Comparison of gait of young and elderly women. Phys Ther 1986;66:1382–1397
64. Ostrosky KM, VanSwearingen JM, Burdett RG, Gee Z: A comparison of gait characteristics in young and old subjects. Phys Ther 1994;74:637–646
65. Gillis B, Gilroy K, Lawley H et al: Slow walking speeds in healthy young and elderly females. Physiother Can 1986;38: 350–352
66. Chao EY, Laughman RK, Schneider E, Stauffer RN: Normative data of knee joint motion and ground reaction forces in adult level walking. J Biomech 1983;16:219–233
67. Aniansson A, Sperling L, Rundgren A, Lehnberg E: Muscle function in 75-year old men and women: a longitudinal study. Scand J Rehabil Med 1983d:92–102
68. Judge JO, Underwood M, Gennosa T: Exercise to improve gait velocity in older persons. Arch Phys Med Rehabil 1993;74: 400–406
69. Fiatarone MA, Marks EC, Ryan ND et al: High intensity strength training in nonagenarians. JAMA 1990;263: 3029–3034
70. Larish DD, Martin PE, Mungiole M: Characteristic patterns of gait in the healthy old. Ann NY Acad Sci 1988;515:18–32
71. Nigg BM, Skleryk BN: Gait characteristics of the elderly. Clin Biomech 1988;3:79–87
72. Willmott M: The effect of a vinyl floor surface and a carpeted floor surface upon walking in elderly hospital patients. Age Ageing 1986;15:119–120
73. Ferrandez AM, Pailhous J, Durup M: Slowness in elderly gait. Exp Aging Res 1990;16:79–89
74. Winter DA, Patla AE, Frank JS, Walt SE: Biomechanical walking pattern changes in the fit and healthy elderly. Phys Ther 1990;70:340–347
75. Wolfson L, Whipple R, Amerman P, Tobin JN: Gait assessment in the elderly: a gait abnormality rating scale and its relation to falls. J Gerontol 1990;45: M12–M19
76. Murray MP, Kory RC, Clarkson BH: Walking patterns in healthy old men. J Gerontol 1969;24:169–178
77. Simoneau GG, Cavanagh PR, Ulbrecht JS et al: The influence of visual factors on fall-related kinematic variables during stair descent by older women. J Gerontol 1991;46:M188–M195
78. Chen HC, Aston-Miller JA, Alexander NB, Schultz AB: Step-

ping over obstacles: gait patterns of healthy young and older adults. J Gerontol 1991;46:M196–M203

79. Finley FR, Cody KA, Finizie RV: Locomotion patterns in elderly women. Arch Phys Med Rehabil 1969;50:140–146

80. Friedman PJ, Richmond DE, Baskett JJ: A prospective trial of serial gait speed as a measure of rehabilitation in the elderly. Age Ageing 1988:17:227–235

81. Guralnik JM, Simonsick EM, Ferrucci L et al: A short physical performance battery assessing lower extremity function: association with self-reported disability and prediction of mortality and nursing home admission. J Gerontol 1994;49:M85–M94

82. Lundgren-Linquist B, Aniansson A, Rundgren A: Functional studies in 79-year-olds: walking performance and climbing capacity. Scand J Rehabil Med 1983;15:125–131

83. Hoxie RE, Rubenstein LZ, Hoeing H, Gallager BR: The older pedestrian. J Am Geriatr Soc 1994;42:444–450

84. Sudarsky L, Ronthal M: Gait disorders among elderly patients: a survey study of 50 patients. Arch Neurol 1983;40:740–743

85. Fuh JL, Lin KN, Wang SJ et al: Neurologic diseases presenting with gait impairment in the elderly. J Geriatr Psychiatry Neurol 1994;7:89–92

86. Hough JC, McHenry MP, Kammer LM: Gait disorders in the elderly. Am Fam Physician 1987;30:191–196

87. Weindruch R, Korper SP, Hadley E: The prevalence of dysequilibruim and related disorders in older people. Ear Nose Throat J 1989;68:925–929

88. McClure JA: Vertigo and imbalance in the elderly. J Otolaryngol 1986;15:248–252

89. Tinetti ME: Instability and falling in elderly patients. Semin Neurol 1989;9:39–45

90. Thompson PD, Marsden CD: Gait disorder of subcortical arteriosclerotic encephalopathy: Binswanger's disease. Mov Disord 1987;2:1–8

91. Cunha U: Differential diagnoses of gait disorders in the elderly. Geriatrics 1988;43:33–42

92. Sudarsky L: Geriatrics: gait disorders in the elderly. N Engl J Med 1990;322:1441–1446

93. Keenan MA, Perry J, Jordan C: Factors affecting balance and ambulation following stroke. Clin Orthop 1984;182:165–171

94. Dettman MA, Linder MT, Sepic SB: Relationship among walking performance, postural stability, and functional assessments of the hemiplegic patient. Am J Phys Med 1987;66:77–90

95. DiFabio RP, Badke MB, Duncan PW: Adapting human postural reflexes following localized cerebrovascular lesion: analysis of bilateral long latency responses. Brain Res 1986;363: 257-264

96. Catz A, Ron S, Solzi P, Korczyn AD: The vestibulo-ocular reflex and dysequilibrium after hemispheric stroke. Am J Phys Med Rehabil 1994;73:36–39

97. Brandt T, Dieterich M: Vestibular falls. J Vestib Res 1993; 3:3–14

98. Rees TS, Duckert LG: Auditory and vestibular dysfunction in aging. p. 443 In Hazzard WR, Andres R, Bierman EL, Blass JP (eds): Principles of Geriatric Medicine and Gerontology. 2nd Ed. McGraw-Hill, New York, 1990

99. Norre ME, Beckers A: Vestibular habituation training for positional vertigo in elderly patients. Arch Gerontol Geriatr 1989; 8:117–122

100. Black FO, Effron M, Burns DS: Diagnosis and management of drop attacks of vestibular origin: Tumarkin's otolithic crisis. J Otolaryngol Head Neck Surg 1982;90:256–262

101. Messier EL, Loeser RF, Hoover JL et al: Osteoarthritis of the knee: effect on gait, strength, and flexibility. Arch Phys Med Rehabil 1992;73:29–36

102. Albert SF, Jahnigen DW: Treating common foot disorders in older patients. Geriatrics 1983;38:42–55

103. Hughes J, Clark P, Klenerman L: The importance of the toe in walking. J Bone Joint Surg 1990;72B:245–251

104. Kosinski M, Ramcharitar S: In-office management of common geriatric foot problems. Geriatrics 1994;49:43–47

105. Visser H: Gait and balance in senile dementia of Alzheimer's type. Age Ageing 1983;12:296–301

106. Galasko D, Kwo-On-Yuen PF, Klauber R, Thal LJ: Neurological findings in Alzheimer's disease and normal aging. Arch Neurol 1990:47:625–627

107. Rosenfeld V, Lerman Y, Habot B: Acute stooped position in elderly with Alzheimer's disease. J Am Geriatr Soc 1993;41: 468

108. Nutt JG, Marsden CD, Thompson PD: Human walking and higher-level gait disorders, particularly in the elderly. Neurology 1993;43:268–279

109. Tinetti ME, Ginter SF: Identifying mobility dysfunctions in elderly patients. JAMA 1988;259:1190–1193

110. Mathias S, Nayak USL, Isaacs B: Balance in elderly patients: the "get-up and go" test. Arch Phys Med Rehabil 1986;67: 387–389

111. Fiatarone MA, O'Neill EF, Ryan ND et al: Exercise training and nutritional supplementation for physical frailty in very elderly people. N Engl J Med 1994;330:1769–1775

112. Hu MH, Woollacott MH: Multisensory training of standing balance in older adults. I. postural stability and one-leg stance balance. J Gerontol 1994;49:M52–M61

113. Lord SR, Lloyd DG, Nirui M et al: The effect of exercise on gait patterns in older women: a randomized controlled trial. J Gerontol 1996;51A:M64–M70

CHAPTER 40

Myasthenic Syndromes

WILLIAM J. K. CUMMING

Affecting all races, myasthenia gravis has a prevalence of 5 to 10 per 100,000.[1, 2] It presents most commonly with ocular signs, diplopia, and ptosis but any group of striated muscles may be affected as the disease becomes generalized. There is progressive weakness during sustained effort and nasal speech; difficulty in swallowing may occur. Electromyography (EMG) shows a reduction in the compound muscle action potential amplitude; a 10 percent decrement in compound muscle action potential amplitude at 3/s stimulation is diagnostic of myasthenia gravis. Single-fiber EMG is the most common electrophysiologic assessment for myasthenia gravis currently employed.[3–5]

Immunopathology

The immunopathology of myasthenia gravis is now almost fully understood.[6, 7] Antibodies, derived from the thymus, are directed to the acetylcholine receptor in the postsynaptic membrane. The interaction of these antibodies with the receptor leads to an increased degradation rate of the receptor (3 to 4 hours versus 72 to 96 hours in the normal), and, with time, the muscle cell is incapable of producing sufficient replacement receptor, leading to loss of total numbers and, hence, of functional capacity.

Major Types of Acquired Myasthenia Gravis

Early-onset myasthenia gravis, presenting under the age of 40 years with female predominance (4:1), accounts for 55 percent of cases.[2] These patients show the typical progression of involvement from eye muscles to oropharynx, to limb, to ventilatory muscles; they frequently have thymic hyperplasia. A strong association with HLA-B8 and a weaker association with DR3 has been detected. Histologically, the thymus contains lymphoid follicles with germinal centers that are not present in the normal thymus; follicles and T-cell areas invade the thymic medulla. Spontaneous antiacetylcholine-receptor antibodies are produced by thymic cell cultures in two-thirds of patients with T cells, and the myoid cells in the thymus are the target for the initial immune attack.[8, 9]

Myasthenia Gravis With Thymoma

In approximatly 10 percent of cases, a thymoma is associated with myasthenia gravis. The thymus has lymphoepithelial character and enrichment with acetylcholine-receptor-reactive T cells has been reported. Monoclonal antibodies against acetylcholine receptor proteins bind to acetylcholine-receptor-like determinants in thymomas.[10, 11] Antistriated muscle antibodies, including antititin antibodies, are present in 85 percent of thymoma patients.[12] Late-onset myasthenia gravis occurs more commonly in males than females and accounts for 20 percent of cases of the disease.[2] In these patients, the thymus is atrophic. They usually present with signs in the opposite order to early onset of myasthenia gravis, starting in the limbs. Initial presentation with ventilatory failure is not uncommon.

Investigation and Management

Detection of acetylcholine receptor antibodies greater than 0.5 nmol/L in the serum is specific for myasthenia gravis. In seronegative cases, the intravenous injection of edrophonium (Tensilon), leading to improvement of symptoms, may aid the diagnosis but this test is not specific. EMG, with a 10 percent decrement in compound muscle action potential amplitude at 3 s stimulation and single-fiber EMG, are of crucial importance in diagnosis.[5] In patients with thymoma, the tumor may be detected by computed tomography or magnetic resonance imaging and antistriated muscle antibodies are present in the serum in 85 percent of patients. Assay of anti-acetylcholine-receptor antibodies is by the use of isolated human acetylcholine receptors labeled with ^{125}I-bungarotoxin. Seronegativity in ocular disease probably reflects different epitopes on ocular muscles from limb muscles.

Muscle biopsy is rarely, if ever, used as a diagnostic test in myasthenia gravis, except to exclude other muscle disorders, particularly mitochondrial cytopathies. The changes in muscle in myasthenia gravis include the presence of small collections of lymphocytes, although this change is inconstant. The most common finding is atrophy of type 2 fibers but no definite signs of neurogenic atrophy are usually seen.

Treatment

Suppression of clinical symptomatology may be achieved with anticholinesterase agents such as pyridostigmine, but this does not address the underlying pathogenesis. Most patients eventually fail to distinguish between over and underdosage of anticholinergics, which may have fatal results. Thymectomy is now generally considered to be the treatment for the underlying condition.[13] Although there is some argument that this should be reserved for the younger age group of patients, clinical experience of the use of thymectomy in patients up to the age of 80 years has shown similar response rates as in younger patients. Certainly age per se does not seem to preclude effective surgery.

Plasma exchange is used to prepare the patient for thymectomy. It is preferable, in the elderly group of patients, to undertake this in intensive care units, where extensive monitoring is available. The aim of plasmapheresis is to improve the patient's functional status to Osserman grade 0 (asymptomatic) or 1 (eye symptoms only), and this usually requires 3 to 5 exchanges over a 1 to 2-week period. When thymectomy is undertaken within 24 hours of the last exchange, serious complications are rare and not life threatening. In the author's experience with more than 50 patients over the age of 60 years, no mortality has been experienced with this regimen. Steroids may be used to attain the same clinical situation. However, a proportion of patients will suffer significant deterioration in their clinical status within the first 14 days of treatment, and may require ventilation in addition to the usual complications of steroid therapy. Remission rates following thymectomy are high[14] and most patients become, at least, less dependent on anticholinsterase medication.

The treatment of subsequent relapse following thymectomy is commonly with either plasmapheresis or intravenous globulin,[15–17] although the possibility of a rise in serum viscosity associated with the latter therapy must be considered,[18] as this causes a risk of inducing thromboembolic events.

Lambert-Eaton Myasthenic Syndrome

The Lambert-Eaton myasthenic syndrome (LEMS) is characterized by difficulty in walking; autonomic symptoms such as dry mouth, constipation, and impotence[19, 20]; and, occasionally, respiratory failure.[21, 22] It is associated with small cell carcinoma of the lung in 40 to 50 percent of cases[20, 23] and the syndrome often presents before the tumor is obvious. Those cases that are not associated with cancer tend to occur in younger patients, but increasingly associations with other tumors and autoimmune disorders are being recognized.[24, 25]

On examination, there is mild bilateral ptosis and proximal limb weakness and, as a mark of distinction from myasthenia gravis, there is augmentation of muscle strength over the first few seconds of maximum effort. EMG was first used to distinguish this syndrome from myasthenia gravis[26, 27] and remains the principal investigation. Antibodies to the presynaptic calcium channels can be detected.[27–29]

Pathology

The primary defect is an antibody-mediated reduction in voltage-gated calcium channels at the motor nerve terminal.[24] Such channels are essential for the inflow of calcium into the nerve terminal, which induces the release of quanta of acetylcholine from the nerve terminal. The end-plate potential is reduced, but the quanta of acetylcholine released increase progressively during the first few impulses during muscle contraction. There is probably cross-linking of adjacent active-zone particles at the calcium channel by divalent antibody, leading to a reduction in density.

Voltage-gated calcium channels have been identified in small cell carcinomas of neuroectodermal origin in the lung. It thus appears that LEMS is an autoimmune response and removal of the tumor leads to improvement of symptomatology.[30] Most patients require therapy with 3, 4-diaminopyridine, which in modest doses leads to a significant clinical improvement.[31, 32]

References

1. Phillips LH: The epidemiology of myasthenia gravis. Neurol Clin N Am 1994;12:263–272
2. Newsom-Davies J: Myasthenia gravis and related syndromes. pp. 761–780. In Walton JN, Karpati G, Hilton-Jones D (eds): Disorders of Voluntary Muscle. Churchill Livingstone, Edinburgh, 1994
3. Wray D: Neuromuscular transmission. pp. 139–178. In Walton JN, Karpati G, Hilton-Jones D (eds): Disorders of Voluntary Muscle. Churchill Livingstone, Edinburgh, 1994
4. Magleby KL: Neuromuscular transmission. pp. 442–465. In Engel AG, Franzini-Armstrong C (eds): Myology. McGraw-Hill, New York, 1994
5. Kennett R, Fawcett PRW: Repetitive nerve stimulation of aconeus in the assessment of neuromuscular transmission disorders. Electroencephalogr Clin Neurophysiol Electromyogr Motor Control 1993;89:170–176
6. Lewis RA, Selwa JF, Lisak RP: Myasthenia gravis: immunological mechanisms and immunotherapy. Ann Neurol 1995;37: 51–62
7. Levinson AI, Wheatley LM: The thymus and the pathogenesis of myasthenia gravis. Clin Immunol Immunopathol 1996;78: 1–5
8. Willcox N: Myasthenia gravis. Curr Opin Immunol 1993;5: 910–917
9. Hohfield R, Wekerle H: The thymus in myasthenia gravis. Neurol Clin N Am 1994;12:331–342
10. Palmisani MT, Evoli A, Batocchi AP et al: Myasthenia gravis associated with thymoma: clinical characteristics and long-term outcome. Eur Neurol 1994;34:78–82
11. Tan PH, Sng ITY: Thymoma—a study of 60 cases in Singapore. Histopathology 1995;26:509–518

12. Gautel M, Takey A, Barlow AP et al: Titin antibodies in myasthenia gravis: identification of a major immunogenic region of titin. Neurology 1993;43:1581–1585
13. Blossom GB, Ernstoff RM, Howells GA et al: Thymectomy for myasthenia gravis. Arch Surg 1993;128:855–862
14. Olanow CW, Lane RJM, Roses AD: Thymectomy in late onset myasthenia gravis. Arch Neurol 1982;39:82–83
15. Genkins G, Sivak M, Tartter PI: Treatment strategies in myasthenia gravis. Ann NY Acad Sci 1993;681:603–608
16. Thornton CA, Griggs RC: Plasma exchange and intravenous immunoglobulin treatment of neuromuscular disease. Ann Neurol 1994;35:260–268
17. Gajdos P: Intravenous immune globulin in myasthenia gravis. Clin Exp Immunol 1994;97(suppl 1):49–51
18. Dalakas MC: High-dose intravenous immunoglobulin and serum viscosity: risk of precipitating thromboembolic events. Neurology 1994;44:223–226
19. Jablecki C: Lambert-Eaton myasthenic syndrome. Muscle Nerve 1983;7:250–257
20. O'Neill JH, Murray NMF, Newsom-Davies J: The Lambert-Eaton myasthenic syndrome: a review of 50 cases. Brain 1988; 111:577–596
21. Barr CW, Claussen G, Thomas D et al: Primary respiratory failure as the presenting symptom in Lambert-Eaton myasthenic syndrome. Muscle Nerve 1993;16:712–715
22. Beydoun SR: Delayed diagnosis of Lambert-Eaton myasthenic syndrome in a patient presenting with recurrent refractory respiratory failure. Muscle Nerve 1994;17:689–690
23. Anderson HJ, Churchill-Davidson HC, Richardson AT: Bronchial neoplasm with myasthenia. Lancet 1953;2:1291
24. Lang B, Newsom-Davis J: Immunopathology of the Lambert-Eaton myasthenic syndrome. Springer. Semin Immunopathol 1995;17:3–15
25. Maselli RA: Pathophysiology of myasthenia gravis and Lambert-Eaton syndrome. Neurol Clin N Am 1994;12:285–304
26. Howard JF, Sanders DB, Massey JM: The electrodiagnosis of myasthenia gravis and the Lambert-Eaton myasthenic syndrome. Neurol Clin N Am 1994;12:305–330
27. Rolfman CM et al: Reversal of chronic polymyositis following intravenous immune serum globulin therapy. JAMA 1987;258: 513–515
28. Lennon V, Lambert E: Autoantibodies bind solubilized calcium channel-w-conotoxin complexes from small-cell lung carcinoma: a diagnostic aid for Lambert-Eaton myasthenic syndrome. Mayo Clin Proc 1989;64:1498–1504
29. Lennon VA, Kriezer TJ, Griesmann GE et al: Calcium-channel antibodies in the Lambert-Eaton syndrome and other paraneoplastic syndromes. N Engl J Med 1995;332:1467–1474
30. Chalk CH, Murray NMF, Newson-Davies J et al: Response of the Lambert-Eaton myasthenic syndrome to treatment of associated small-cell lung carcinoma. Neurology 1990;40:1552–1556
31. McEvoy KM: Diagnosis and treatment of Lambert-Eaton myasthenic syndrome. Neurol Clin N Am 1994;12:387–400
32. Sanders DB, Howard JF Jr, Massey JM: 3,4-Diaminopyridine in Lambert-Eaton myasthenic syndrome and myasthenia gravis. Ann N Y Acad Sci 1993;681:588–590

CHAPTER 41

Peripheral Neuropathies in the Elderly

BRION D. REICHLER
DAVID M. SIMPSON

Peripheral neuropathy (PN) in the elderly presents a diagnostic challenge, as the peripheral nervous system (PNS) undergoes clinical and histologic changes with normal aging that are often similar to those seen with acquired pathology at all ages. The incidental discovery of absent ankle jerks or diminished vibration sensation in the toes, out of the proper clinical context, must be interpreted with caution. However, certain neuropathies occur more frequently in the older population, and others cause increased morbidity in the elderly because of lower "reserve" or complications in other organ systems. In general, the response to all varieties of nerve injury is impaired with age. Concomitant central nervous system (CNS) disease, which also is more common in the elderly, often complicates the diagnosis and obscures the extent of peripheral contribution to disability. This chapter summarizes the pathophysiologic and clinical changes in the PNS with aging, outlines a diagnostic approach to the patient with neuropathy, and provides an overview of neuropathies that occur with a higher incidence or are more significant in the geriatric population.

Normal Changes in Aging

The normal aging process involves alterations in clinical sensory, reflex, and motor function that resemble those seen in peripheral neuropathy. Possible causes of these changes include defects in neuronal transport mechanisms or protein synthesis, cumulative recurrent trauma, and endoneurial ischemia, as well as a purely biologic "axonopathy of aging."[1–3] Pathologic changes in the peripheral nerves that may be attributable to the aging process alone include neuronal loss, neuronal and Schwann cell pigment accumulation, demyelination-remyelination, and axon loss in both the peripheral nerves and the dorsal columns.[3,4] Nerve response to injury is limited in repertoire and becomes impaired with advancing age.[5–7]

Sensory System

Virtually all sensory modalities decline in acuity with age. Potvin et al.[8] reported a 97 percent decrease in quantitative vibratory sensation in the lower extremities of healthy patients between 20 and 80 years of age, but Verillo[9] found diminished sensation only at higher frequencies. Klawans et al.[10] reported that only 16 percent of poor urban outpatients older than 65 years had proprioceptive deficits, whereas 83 percent had impaired vibratory sensation. However, these data must be interpreted cautiously, because patients with diabetes mellitus (DM) and peripheral vascular disease (PVD) were not excluded.[10] Kokmen et al.[11] reported a slight, but statistically significant, increase in proprioceptive threshold (approximately 50 percent) at the toe in a "healthy" population older than age 60, as compared to younger subjects, but only at lower velocities of joint motion. Skinner et al.[12] demonstrated an age effect on joint position sense as far proximally as the knee. Age-related changes in temperature[13–15] and light touch sensation[15–18] have also been reported. There is a general consensus that threshold to deep pain sensation increases slightly with age, although this is confounded by the complex psychological component of pain perception.[1]

Deep tendon reflexes depend heavily on an intact sensory arc, involving muscle spindle fibers and large myelinated axons. Reflexes therefore become weaker with advancing age and are eventually lost, beginning at the ankles, and typically involving patellar reflexes last.[19] Klawans et al.[10] reported that ankle jerks were absent in 70 percent of their urban population over the age of 65. However, reflex loss in these patients correlated with the presence of DM and PVD, and was independent of age.

Lascelles and Thomas[20] described increased variability of internodal length in the sural nerve in patients over the age of 65. Asynchronous signal conduction due to the resulting temporal dispersion may explain the early and prominent deficits in reflexes and vibration sensation, which are the two modalities that depend most heavily on a coordinated impulse volley.[20] Other morphologic changes in the sensory system involve dorsal root ganglia, nerve, and dorsal columns (predominantly gracile tracts), and are reviewed elsewhere.[1,4,5]

Changes in somesthetic end-receptor organs probably contribute to perceptual decline with aging. Pacinian corpuscles, which subserve high-frequency vibratory sensation, undergo dropout and morphologic changes with age.[9,21] Meissner corpuscles, which mediate light touch and vibration at lower frequencies (less than 50 Hz), also degenerate with time.[22] Free nerve endings, which probably mediate temperature and pain sensation, begin to regress as early as the third decade.[1] Muscle spindles undergo capsular thickening, lamellar fibrosis, and a mild degree of intrafusal fiber loss.[23]

Motor System

Quantitatively evaluated muscle strength generally peaks in the third decade, with minimal decline until approximately age 50 and more rapid decline thereafter.[1,24] Muscles most likely to manifest weakness include foot dorsiflexors and intrinsic hand muscles. However, muscle endurance[25] remains relatively intact, possibly due to selective type II (fast-twitch) muscle fiber loss, with relative sparing of type I (slow-twitch) fibers.[25,26] This may lead to loss of power with rapid contraction,[26] although normal muscle shortening velocity is preserved.[1] Mild axial or limb rigidity and paratonia may occur with aging[24] and are presumably due to basal ganglia or "extrapyramidal" dysfunction. However, pyramidal signs, such as spastic hypertonia, hyperreflexia, and extensor plantar responses should always be regarded as pathologic,[24] as should asymmetry of motor findings. Mild atrophy, particularly in intrinsic hand, calf, and thigh muscles, is common even in the physically active elderly,[1,24] but asymmetry or the presence of marked fasciculations are pathologic.

Histologically, there is a modest degree of motor neuron loss with age, at the rate of about 200 cells per spinal segment per decade.[27] Similar findings occur in the aging mouse spinal cord.[1] This trend has been confirmed by electrophysiologic estimates of motor unit (MU) numbers, which suggest a greater than 50 percent decrease between ages 20 and 80 years, without loss of strength.[28–30] The absence of commensurate weakness is probably due to collateral reinnervation by surviving motor neurons. In support of this theory, Buchthal reported a twofold increase in mean MU duration between ages 3 and 75, reflecting an increase in remaining MU size.[31] However, there is no histologic evidence of increased axonal "terminal innervation ratio" with age, as would be predicted from this electrophysiologic observation.[32]

Fiber loss in the ventral root and motor nerve largely reflects loss of motor neurons, with a decrease of 350 fibers per decade in lumbar roots,[1] and a disproportionate decrease in the number of large-diameter myelinated motor axons with age.[33] Myelin changes due to aging include myelin bubbling, remyelination of axons, and onion bulb formation.[1] There is also a gradual decrease in mean internodal length.[33] Biopsy of striated muscle reveals evidence of mild denervation and type-2-specific myofiber loss,[25] with or without disuse atrophy.

Although not localized to the PNS, normal changes in extrapyramidal, cerebellar, and vestibular function may complicate and exacerbate deficits in peripheral motor function. The most conspicuous effect is on gait. These changes include decreased reaction time and balance, slowed rapid alternating movements, and mild dysmetria, and are discussed in separate chapters in this book.

Autonomic System

Manifestations of putative autonomic dysfunction with aging include postural hypotension, insufficiency of thermal regulation, decreased tearing and sluggish pupillary reaction.[34,35] These are similar to the autonomic symptoms that may occur with axonal, demyelinating, or pure autonomic neuropathies. However, not all of these age-related abnormalities are necessarily due to primary peripheral nerve dysfunction. The differential diagnosis of autonomic insufficiency includes medications, coincident non-neurologic illnesses, and other neurologic diseases such as Parkinson's disease and multiple system atrophy. Autonomic dysfunction is discussed at length elsewhere in this book.

Electrophysiology

A detailed discussion of electrodiagnostic principles is beyond the scope of this text. Briefly, the amplitude of the sensory or motor response correlates with the number and size of functioning axons. Conduction velocity (CV) reflects the fastest conducting nerve fibers, and can be diminished by either primary dysfunction of myelin or loss of the larger (faster conducting) axons. Late responses are antidromically stimulated potentials generating a reflex response at the spinal cord, and are therefore more sensitive to pathology along the entire length of the axon. There is a small and progressive decrease in sensory and motor amplitudes and CV from the third to the eighth decade,[36,37] with a fall in CV by about 0.15 m/s/y.[36] In contrast, central (dorsal column) CV declines only after age 60.[36]

Peripheral Neuropathy

Epidemiology

The paucity of published data on the overall incidence of PN in the elderly bespeaks the difficulty of clinically distinguishing normal from pathologic changes in this age group. Munoz et al.[38] estimated the prevalence of PN in a large French geriatric population to be about 1.6 percent. The most common causes of PN in the elderly include diabetes (17 to 27 percent) and neoplasia (12 to 13 percent), with alcoholism, medications, and idiopathic demyelination accounting for almost one-half of the remaining diagnosed cases.[39,40] The cause of PN could not be determined in approximately one-fourth of patients in these series.[39,40] However, Dyck et al.[41] reported that with intensive evaluation, 76 percent of such "undiagnosed" cases could be properly diagnosed, with the majority having either inherited or idiopathic inflammatory neuropathies.

Table 41-1 lists three different explanations for the higher prevalence of certain neuropathies in the elderly: (1) PN secondary to medical diseases that are more prevalent in the elderly, (2) PN attributable to progressive pathology or cumulative exposure/trauma, and (3) other neuropathies with a higher incidence in old age. Furthermore, subclinical neuropathy or neuropathy unrelated to age may have greater functional or neurophysiologic salience in the elderly because of (1) the additive effect of normal aging changes that resemble neuropathy, (2) decreased "reserve" of the elderly nervous system and impaired response to injury, (3) the presence of other causes of gait instability (e.g., extrapyramidal or vestibular disease), and (4) decreased sensory input (vision, hearing). Age may

Table 41-1 Mechanisms of increased incidence of neuropathy in the elderly

Neuropathies secondary to medical conditions more common in elderly
Diabetes, uremia, hypothyroidism
Malignancy
Dysproteinemia, paraproteinemia
Vasculitis, collagen vascular disease
Occlusive vascular disease, peripheral vascular disease
Neurotoxic medications
Cumulative effect of progressive disease or exposure over time
Progressive disease: inherited neuropathies
Progressive exposure: alcohol, industrial toxins
Progressive or repetitive trauma: entrapment neuropathies
Other neuropathies with higher incidence in elderly
Guillain-Barré syndrome, chronic inflammatory demyelinating polyneuropathy

also adversely affect prognosis in diseases such as the Guillain-Barré syndrome.[42] In general, Huang[40] did not find age to be an independent negative prognostic factor, but his conclusions were based on anecdotal data and a limited sample size.

Functional Implications of Neuropathy

One of the most important reasons to recognize and treat PN is the minimization of associated functional complications. Stride length and walking speed decrease modestly with age[43,44] and account for the majority of the changes in the syndrome often referred to as senile gait,[43,45] which is considered a "normal" aging phenomenon. Factors causing falls in the healthy elderly include decreased position sense, distal weakness, stooped posture, decreased postural reflexes or reaction time, and impaired balance. These may in part be due to changes in the visual and vestibular systems, basal ganglia, and cerebellum. The senile gait of PN is indistinguishable from that of other causes,[43] but PN is an independent risk factor for falls.[46] Other potential complications of PN include foot ulceration and fracture due to loss of pain sensation, deep vein thrombosis and contracture due to immobility from pain or weakness, and life-threatening respiratory compromise and cardiac arrhythmias. Autonomic dysfunction, such as incontinence, impotence, and orthostatic hypotension, poses a major risk to both lifestyle and health.

Classification of Neuropathies

Table 41-2 presents a schema for the classification of neuropathy based on pathologic mechanisms and electrophysiologic findings. Length-dependent, or "dying back," neuropathy first involves the distal part of the axon, usually on the basis of toxic, metabolic, or nutritional disorders, with subsequent myelin damage. Wallerian degeneration occurs with focal axonal disruption, leading to concurrent degeneration of the axon and myelin sheath distal to the lesion. Primary sensory neuron damage results in degeneration in both peripheral nerve and dorsal columns.[47] Table 41-3 outlines salient features of the major clinical subtypes. These patterns may exist in combination; for example, diabetes may be predominantly distal sensorimotor, with moderate small-fiber involvement, mild autonomic involvement, and superimposed focal entrapment.

Clinical Approach

A detailed history and physical examination are indispensable. The history should include inquiry into the use of alcohol and medication, travel and arthropod exposure, human immunodeficiency virus (HIV) risk factors, family history of progressive disability, and past vocational and athletic ability. Autonomic symptoms and neck or back pain should be noted. The examination should include inspection of the foot for high arches and palpation of nerves for hypertrophic enlargement

Table 41-2 Classification of neuropathies

Axonal
Distal symmetric ("dying back")
Diabetes
Uremia
Alcohol
Toxic/medication
Nutritional deficiency
Paraneoplastic
Paraproteinemic/dysproteinemic
CMT2
Sensory neuropathy
Paraneoplastic
Sjögren's syndrome
Cisplatin
Pyridoxine toxicity
Focal/multifocal (Wallerian degeneration)
Focal
Entrapment/compression (focal demyelination in early stage)
Ischemic: shunt, occlusive vascular disease, PVD
Diabetes
Herpes zoster
Multifocal (mononeuritis multiplex)
Vasculitic
Diabetes
Paraproteinemia
Infiltrative: leukemia, lymphoma
Infectious: Lyme, HIV
Demyelinating
Symmetric
GBS
CIDP
Paraproteinemic/dysproteinemic (also axonal)
CMT1
Multifocal
Multifocal motor neuropathy with conduction block
Hereditary liability to pressure palsies

Abbreviations: CMT, Charcot-Marie-Tooth; PVD, peripheral vascular disease; HIV, human immunodeficiency virus; GBS, Guillain-Barré syndrome; CIDP, chronic inflammatory demyelinating polyneuropathy.

Table 41-3 Clinical patterns of neuropathy

Distal sensorimotor (axonal)
Largest category
Symmetric distal sensory loss, usually large fiber first
Distal (ankle) reflex loss first
Weakness variable
Small-fiber sensory
Rarely exists by itself
Prominent pain: burning, dysesthetic
Autonomic dysfunction
Large-fiber sensory
Sensory "gangliononeuronopathies" (see Fig. 41-1)
Marked vibratory and proprioceptive loss
Proximal involvement
Sensory ataxia
Early reflex loss
Demyelinating
Acute, subacute, or chronic
May be distal symmetric, asymmetric, or proximal at onset
Motor signs often predominate (AIDP, CIDP, hereditary neuropathies)
Early reflex loss
Mononeuritis multiplex
Asymmetric, cranial, or peripheral nerve involvement (sensory and motor)
When confluent, may mimic distal polyneuropathy

Abbreviations: AIDP, acute inflammatory demyelinating polyneuropathy; CIDP, chronic inflammatory demyelinating polyneuropathy.

at the fibular head or ulnar groove. Vibratory sensation in the toes should be checked, and the pattern of muscle or sensory involvement should be evaluated for symmetry and for conformation to a pattern of multiple nerves or roots.

An algorithm for the diagnostic approach to peripheral neuropathy is presented in Figure 41-1. The first step is to determine that the problem is in the PNS. Features suggestive of CNS disease include an "upper motor neuron" pattern of weakness (extensor in arms, flexor in legs), normal or hyperactive tendon reflexes in weak muscles, and extensor plantar responses. Other causes of PNS disease (myopathy, neuromuscular junction disorders, and motor neuron disease) must be differentiated from PN. Features suggestive of these disorders include predominantly proximal weakness (including neck flexors), fatigable weakness on repetitive testing, prominent bulbar (cranial) symptoms, fasciculations, and brisk reflexes. It may be difficult to clinically distinguish confluent multifocal neuropathies from distal symmetric polyneuropathy, particularly with advanced disease, and certain disorders may present with either pattern.

After an initial clinical evaluation with attention to focality, time course, and sensory-motor predominance, electrodiagnostic testing provides valuable diagnostic information, especially in clinically difficult cases. The utility of electromyography and nerve conduction testing is several-fold: (1) to confirm neuropathy (versus myopathy, radiculopathy, motor neuron disease, etc.), (2) to distinguish axonal from demyelinating neuropathy and to subclassify demyelinating disease, (3) to distinguish symmetric polyneuropathy from mononeuritis multiplex, (4) to establish the approximate duration of nerve pathology, and (5) to grade severity, which is useful in monitoring progression of disease, gauging response to treatment, and determining prognosis.

Screening blood tests should be ordered even in the presence of a seemingly obvious etiology. For example, because diabetes is common in the elderly population, many cases of concomitant paraproteinemia, cancer, hypothyroidism, or hereditary neuropathy could be missed if not specifically searched for. A basic screening battery should include hemoglobin A1c, creatinine, thyroid function tests, erythrocyte sedimentation rate, antinuclear antibody, Venereal Disease Research Laboratory test, serum B_{12} and folate levels, serum and urine electropheresis, and Lyme and/or HIV titer if indicated. Further testing may include chest x-ray, cerebrospinal fluid (CSF) analysis, paraneoplastic autoantibodies, angiotensin converting enzyme level, cryoglobulins, heavy metal screen, antineutrophil cytoplasmic antibodies, antiganglioside or anti-myelin-associated glycoprotein antibodies, and anti-Ro and -La antibodies.

Specific Neuropathies by Etiology

Diabetes Mellitus

DM is the most common cause of peripheral nerve dysfunction in developed countries. Two-thirds of all diabetic patients have peripheral nerve dysfunction of some kind; more than 80 percent of these have evidence of sensorimotor polyneuropathy.[48] Patients with insulin-dependent and non-insulin dependent diabetes manifest no apparent difference in the incidence or spectrum of disease subtypes.[48,49] Approximately 70 percent of the diabetic population is over 55 years old, and age is an independent risk factor for the occurrence of peripheral neuropathy, as well as renal and retinal complications.[50]

Clinical syndromes

It is unclear whether the different forms of diabetic neuropathy represent discrete processes or a continuum,[51] and the tendency for syndromes to overlap renders this question even more difficult.[52] Distal symmetric sensory or sensorimotor polyneuropathy is the most common form of PN in DM, and occurs more frequently in the setting of poor glycemic control (see below). Because this neuropathy is length dependent, the distal lower extremities are involved first, followed by the proximal legs, distal arms, and eventually the trunk. The initial complaint is usually numbness or paresthesiae in the feet, which may be accompanied by a burning, stabbing, or dull pain at any point in its progression. There is usually prominent early involvement of large fibers, resulting in sensory ataxia and falling, which may be more prominent at night, when visual feedback is diminished. These features are all common to a

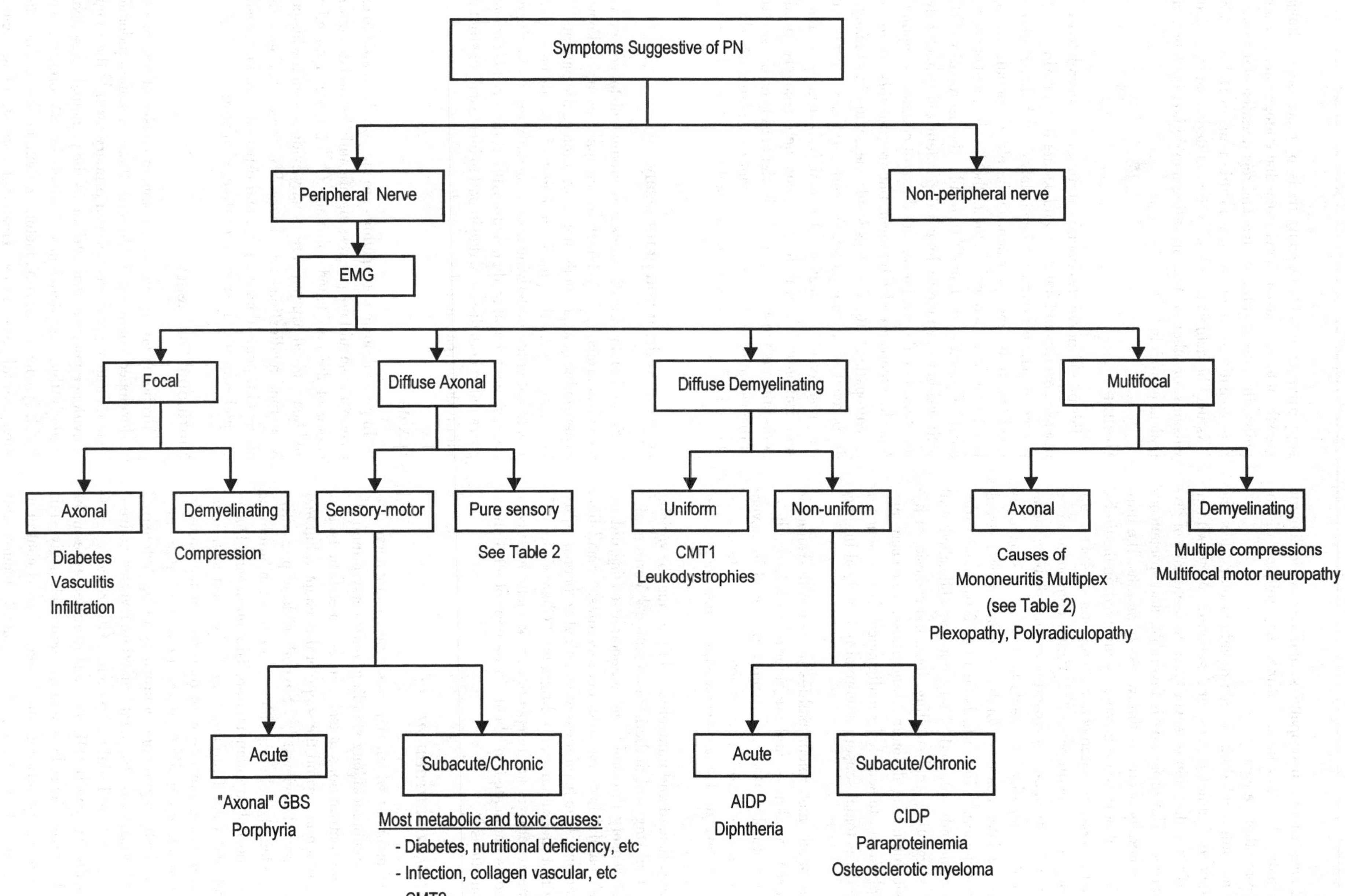

Figure 41-1 Algorithm for the clinical approach to the patient with peripheral neuropathy.

variety of sensorimotor neuropathies, and symmetric diabetic polyneuropathy does not have features that uniquely distinguish it from other causes.

Focal or multifocal diabetic neuropathies may affect the limbs, trunk, or cranial nerves, and generally occur without regard to disease duration or severity, or to the degree of glycemic control.[51] The prognosis is favorable, and spontaneous resolution generally occurs within weeks to months. The third and sixth cranial nerves are commonly involved. In the limbs, focal mononeuropathies often occur at common sites of entrapment or compression neuropathy.[51,53] Pain is common at onset.

Mononeuropathy of an intercostal nerve, or "diabetic thoracoabdominal neuropathy," presents as sudden or subacutely progressive unilateral pain and/or dysesthesia around the trunk or in the abdomen.[54] Individuals in their forties and fifties are most commonly affected. There may be abdominal wall weakness suggesting focal swelling, local hypesthesia, or hyperesthesia mimicking abdominal tenderness, which may mislead the physician to search for malignancy. The presence of a definite dermatomal sensory abnormality is helpful in diagnosis.

Predominantly motor neuropathies present with symmetric or asymmetric weakness, and are referred to historically as diabetic amyotrophy. Both are usually preceded by severe proximal leg or pelvic girdle pain, evolve over weeks to months, and typically have good spontaneous improvement or response to glycemic control.[51]

Small myelinated and unmyelinated fibers may be variably involved at all stages of diabetic neuropathy.[51] Veves et al.[55] found that sensory threshold and autonomic testing did not distinguish painful from painless neuropathies.[55] Small-fiber involvement may lead to painless mechanical or thermal injury, including foot ulceration and arthropathy ("Charcot's joint"). Clinical neuropathy is an independent risk factor for ulceration,[56] and is implicated in about 75 percent of all diabetic limb amputations.[57]

Pathogenesis and treatment

The mechanism by which DM causes peripheral nerve dysfunction is the subject of long-standing controversy, principally regarding the contributions of ischemic and metabolic factors. A full discussion is beyond the scope of this chapter, but may be found in recent reviews.[51,54] Several trials of preventive therapy have failed, including aldose reductase inhibition and dietary myo-inositol supplementation. The multicenter Diabetes Control and Complications Trial,[58] the most significant study to date on the prevention of diabetic complications by glycemic control, reported a 64 percent reduction in the incidence of clinically significant neuropathy using "intensive" (continuous infusion or frequent injections) versus conventional therapy in type I diabetic patients. Other trials suggest similar results for type II DM, the most prevalent type in the elderly.[59] However, the risks of insulin-induced hypoglycemia (seizures, coma) may outweigh the benefit of strict control in this population.[59] Focal neuropathies typically require only supportive treatment. Ongoing trials of recombinant human growth factor are based on evidence that endogenous neurotrophins affect the growth, survival and regeneration of neurons.[60] Symptomatic treatment of neuropathic pain in DM and other PNs may be achieved with tricyclic antidepressants, anticonvulsants, or other agents, including mexiletine, baclofen, and topical capsaicin.[51,61]

Uremia

Peripheral nerve dysfunction in uremia is correlated with disease severity and duration, and occurs in approximately 60 percent of patients requiring hemodialysis.[62] Although chronic renal failure is more prevalent in the elderly population, age is not an independent risk factor for the development of neuropathy.[63] Clinically, uremic PN resembles the neuropathy of DM, with insidious symmetric length-dependent sensorimotor dysfunction. Distal dysesthesias are the most common symptom.[64] Muscle cramps are also frequent, but are probably not related to neuropathy.[64] Restless legs syndrome occurs in as many as 40 percent of uremic patients[64] and correlates closely with the presence of neuropathy.[65] Hemodialysis usually results in stabilization of PN, with frequent complete recovery in mild cases, although response is variable, depending on the severity of disease at onset.[63] In contrast, renal transplantation almost always leads to significant or complete recovery of PN within a year.[66]

Hypothyroidism and Acromegaly

Several endocrine disorders may produce distal sensorimotor polyneuropathy.[67] Although the mechanisms are unknown, hypertrophic changes in the nerves of acromegalic patients[68,69] implicate in part the promitotic effect of growth hormone.[67] Treatment of the underlying disease usually results in clinical improvement. Focal median neuropathy at the wrist is far more prevalent in both diseases, due in part to increased constriction within the carpal tunnel.

Toxins

In general, toxic neuropathies are temporally related to exposure and should not progress significantly beyond discontinuation of the implicated substance.[70,71] Industrial chemical and heavy metal exposure are usually evident from the history. Numerous medications may cause PN, including isoniazid, phenytoin, penicillamine, gold, and especially antineoplastic chemotherapeutic agents (vincristine, cisplatin).

Nutritional Deficiency

Alcohol is one of the most common causes of neuropathy in developed countries.[49] Although there is some epidemiologic data to support alcohol as a primary toxin,[72] the weight of evidence points to malnutrition as the principal cause, particularly thiamine deficiency.[73] Alcoholic PN presents with distal, symmetric sensory, motor, and autonomic findings and often painful dysesthesia. Treatment consists of abstention from alcohol[74] and initiation of an adequate diet; thiamine supplementation alone is usually ineffective.[72,73] PN may also result from deficiencies of pyridoxine (B_6), cobalamin (B_{12}), niacin, folic acid, and vitamin E.[73] Generally, these result in a symmetric, predominantly sensory polyneuropathy, although B_{12} deficiency may present with subacute combined degeneration, involving corticospinal tracts,[75] and vitamin E deficiency often presents with associated spinocerebellar symptoms.[76] Pyridoxine deficiency is responsible for the neurotoxicity of isoniazid. Notably, excessive ingestion of pyridoxine can result in a "pure sensory" neuronopathy.[47] With the exception of alcoholism, malnutrition itself is an uncommon cause of polyneuropathy in the elderly.[2]

Ischemia and Vasculitis

Collagen vascular diseases may present either with symmetric sensorimotor neuropathy, which most likely results from cumulative ischemic lesions summated over the length of the nerve,[77] or more commonly, with mononeuritis multiplex. Vasculitic diseases include polyarteritis nodosa, rheumatoid arthritis, systemic lupus, and Wegener's granulomatosis. Vasculitic neuropathy may respond to corticosteroids with or without cyclophosphamide, although the prognosis is generally poor.[78] Sjögren's syndrome may present with a "pure sensory" ganglioneuronopathy.[47]

Large-vessel occlusion is an uncommon cause of PN because of the peripheral nerve's relative resistance to ischemic injury.[19] However, occlusion of the femoral or iliac artery for more than 5 hours may result in long-term dysesthesia and sensory loss in the foot.[19] Although chronic PVD is frequently associated with sensory abnormalities, the relationship between the two is uncertain.[19,49]

Cancer

Neoplasia is an important cause of neuropathy in the elderly, given the increased incidence of cancer with age. Paraneoplastic sensory neuronopathy features prominent proprioceptive loss and sensory ataxia, with minimal if any motor signs.[47] It may precede the diagnosis of cancer by a year or more[49,79] and usually does not respond to successful treatment of the primary tumor.[80] It is most commonly associated with primary malignancies of lung, breast, and gastrointestinal tract.[81] Distal sensorimotor neuropathy may rarely present later in the course of lung cancer.[49] Multiple mononeuropathy may result from leukemic or lymphomatous nerve infiltration, amyloid deposition in multiple myeloma, solid tumor compression of nerve or plexus, and possibly paraneoplastic vasculitis.[77]

Paraproteinemia

Neuropathies associated with monoclonal gammopathy most commonly occur in the older male population.[82] Associated diseases include multiple myeloma, osteosclerotic myeloma, cryoglobulinemia, Waldenström macroglobulinemia, and amyloidosis.[82] A monoclonal gammopathy of undetermined significance (MGUS) has no other disease association and accounts for the majority of cases of neuropathy presenting with a monoclonal protein.[82] A primary demyelinating neuropathy is typical of MGUS, although anti-myelin-associated glycoprotein antibodies may or may not be present.[83] There are reports of therapeutic benefit from plasmapheresis and chemotherapy.[82] Multiple myeloma rarely causes PN, and most such cases are attributable to amyloidosis.[82] Primary (AL) amyloidosis presents at a median age of 65[84] and may occur alone or in the setting of multiple myeloma. Typical neurologic presentations of amyloidosis include a small-fiber type neuropathy and carpal tunnel syndrome.[84]

Infection

Herpes zoster (HZV) infection occurs with greater frequency in elderly and immunocompromised populations.[85] Patients typically present with a painful dermatomal skin eruption associated with or preceded by pain and paresthesia. Dermatomal sensory loss may rarely be present even in the absence of rash. Postherpetic neuralgia and associated motor deficits are more common in the elderly.[85] With the exception of HZV, most infectious agents are not more prevalent in the elderly, but HIV, Lyme disease, and other entities should always be considered in the appropriate clinical setting.

Inflammatory Demyelination

Acute inflammatory demyelinating polyneuropathy

The incidence of acute inflammatory demyelinating polyneuropathy (AIDP), or Guillain-Barré syndrome (GBS), is bimodal, with the largest peak occurring between ages 40 and 80.[86] Antecedent conditions include upper respiratory (e.g., Epstein-Barr) or gastrointestinal (e.g., *C. jejuni*) infection, vaccination, and surgery.[86] There are numerous clinical variants of GBS[86] but the most common presentation is that of prominent weakness, usually in the distal lower extremities, which "ascends" to involve distal arms and proximal legs. Weakness may be asymmetric or even proximal at onset, and early involvement of facial muscles is common. Generalized vague pain in the limbs and trunk is common at onset, and sensory complaints, such as paresthesia, often outweigh objective findings. Sensory loss is usually distal, and reflexes are lost early. Autonomic instability, marked by cardiac arrhythmias and blood pressure lability, causes serious morbidity. Dysphagia occurs in as many as 40 percent of cases and may be a predictor of respiratory compromise requiring ventilatory support.[86] CSF analysis shows high protein with normal cell count, and electrodiagnostic testing suggests segmental demyelination. Older patients tend to have a significantly longer hospital stay[87] and worse prognosis for recovery[42] than younger patients.

Chronic inflammatory demyelinating polyneuropathy

The peak incidence of chronic inflammatory demyelinating polyneuropathy (CIDP) is in the fifth and sixth decades.[88] Weakness may develop over months or years, and follows a progressive or relapsing-remitting course, the former being more common in the elderly.[2] Clinical symptomatology and findings are similar to that of AIDP, although motor predominance may be less striking.[88]

Treatment

Plasmapheresis has therapeutic efficacy in the treatment of both AIDP[42,89] and CIDP.[90,91] The double-blind study of van Doorn et al.[92] showed improvement in CIDP patients with intravenous immunoglobulin (IVIg) therapy, as compared to placebo. The Dutch GBS Study Group[93] reported that IVIg treatment was at least as effective as plasmapheresis in the treatment of AIDP, but subsequent reports suggested an unacceptably high relapse rate.[94] Oral corticosteroid therapy is of no benefit over placebo in AIDP,[95,96] but has produced improvement in CIDP patients in a controlled trial.[97]

Hereditary Neuropathies

The two most common forms of hereditary motor and sensory neuropathy receive their current designation from the historic eponym Charcot-Marie-Tooth (CMT) disease. CMT1 is a usually dominantly inherited disorder that causes diffuse and uniform demyelination. Clinically, it is characterized by distal, symmetric, predominantly motor involvement, with marked wasting in muscles of the feet and calf ("inverted champagne bottle leg," pes cavus) and palpable nerve enlargement. There is early areflexia and stocking-glove sensory loss but usually absence of spontaneous sensory symptoms. Although disease onset is early in life, symptoms are often mild and slowly progressive, and most affected patients do not seek medical consultation.[98] CMT2 is similar to CMT1, but involves primary axon loss. CMT2 is characterized by relative sparing of hand muscles, a lesser degree of hyporeflexia, and later onset, as compared with CMT1. Due to the high incidence of undiagnosed cases of inherited neuropathy,[41] these entities should always be considered in the differential diagnosis of distal motor weakness in the elderly, and family members should be examined when possible.

A common diagnostic problem in the elderly is that of a chronic, slowly progressive, predominantly motor syndrome with distal muscle wasting and weakness. In addition to CMT2, CIDP, and multiple nerve entrapments, it is important to consider amyotrophic lateral sclerosis and cervical spondylosis, especially when upper motor neuron signs are present.

Conclusion

Current trends indicate a progressive increase in mean life span in developed countries, which will result in a higher incidence of neurologic disease, including peripheral neuropathy. Although PN is often overshadowed by concurrent systemic or CNS disease, it may be a major source of disability and discomfort. Appropriate diagnostic measures may establish the specific cause of PN, and may reveal unsuspected systemic disease. Symptomatic or specific therapies, including neurotrophic factors, may lead to substantial improvement in quality of life.

References

1. Schaumburg HH, Spencer PS, Ochoa J: The aging human peripheral nervous system. pp. 111–122. In Katzman R, Terry RD (eds): The Neurology of Aging. FA Davis, Philadelphia, 1983
2. Mitchell S: Aging in the peripheral nerves and peripheral neuropathy. pp. 433–439. In Brocklehurst JC, Tallis RC, Fillit HM (eds): Textbook of Geriatric Medicine and Gerontology. 4th Ed. Churchill Livingstone, Edinburgh, 1992
3. Thomas PK, Berthold C-H, Ochoa J: Microscopic anatomy of the peripheral nervous system. Nerve trunks and spinal roots. pp. 28–73, In Dyck PJ, Thomas PK, Griffin JW et al (eds): Peripheral Neuropathy. 3rd Ed. WB Saunders, Philadelphia, 1993
4. Thomas PK, Scaravilli F, Belai A: Pathologic alterations in cell bodies of peripheral neurons in neuropathy. pp. 476–513. In Dyck PJ, Thomas PK, Griffin JW et al (eds): Peripheral Neuropathy. 3rd Ed. WB Saunders, Philadelphia, 1993
5. Dyck PJ, Giannini C, Lais A: Pathologic alterations of nerves. pp. 514–595. In Dyck PJ, Thomas PK, Griffin JW et al (eds): Peripheral Neuropathy. 3rd Ed. WB Saunders, Philadelphia, 1993
6. Beal MF: Metabolic changes in aging peripheral nerve. pp. 135–140. In Thomas PK (ed): New Issues in Neurosciences. Vol. 1.
7. Spritz N, Singh H, Geyer B: Myelin from human peripheral nerves. Quantitative and qualitative studies in two age groups. J Clin Invest 1973;52:521–523
8. Potvin AR, Syndulko K, Tourtellotte WW et al: Human neurologic function and the aging process. J Am Geriatr Soc 1980; 28:1–9
9. Verillo RT: Age related changes in the sensitivity to vibration. J Gerontol 1980;35:185–193
10. Klawans HL, Tufo HM, Ostfeld AM et al: Neurologic examination in an elderly population. Dis Nerv Syst 1971;32:274–279
11. Kokmen E, Bossemeyer RW, Williams WJ: Quantitative evaluation of joint motion sensation in an aging population. J Gerontol 1978;1:62–67
12. Skinner HB, Barrack RL, Cook SD: Age-related decline in proprioception. Clin Orthop 1984;184:208–211
13. Dyck PJ, Curtis DJ, Bushek W, Offord K: Description of "Minnesota Thermal Disks" and normal values of cutaneous thermal discrimination in man. Neurology 1974;24:325–330
14. Jamal GA, Hansen S, Weir AI, Ballantyne JP: An improved automated method for the measurement of thermal threshold. I. Normal subjects. J Neurol Neurosurg Psychiatry 1985;48: 354–360
15. Kenshalo DR: Somesthetic sensitivity in young and elderly humans. J Gerontol 1986;41:732–742
16. Dyck PJ, Schultz PW, O'Brien PC: Quantitation of touch-pressure sensation. Arch Neurol 1972;26:465–473

17. Thornbury JM, Mistretta CM: Tactile sensitivity as a function of age. J Gerontol 1981;36:34–39

18. Dyck PJ, Karnes J, O'Brien PC, Zimmerman IR: Detection thresholds of cutaneous sensation in humans. pp. 706–728. In Dyck PJ, Thomas PK, Griffin JW et al (eds): Peripheral Neuropathy. 3rd Ed. WB Saunders, Philadelphia, 1993

19. Korthals JK: Neuropathies. pp. 283–293. In Barclay L (ed): Clinical Geriatric Neurology. Lea & Febiger, Philadelphia, 1993

20. Lascelles RG, Thomas PK: Changes due to age in internodal length in the sural nerve in man. J Neurol Neurosurg Psychiatry 1966;29:40–44

21. Cauna N, Mannan G: The structure of human digital Pacinian corpuscles (*corpuscula lamellosa*) and its functional significance. J Anat 1958;92:1–20

22. Bolton CF, Winkelmann RK, Dyck PJ: A quantitative study of Meissner's corpuscles in man. Neurology 1966;16:1–9

23. Swash M, Fox KP: The effect of age on human skeletal muscle: studies of the morphology and innervation of muscle spindles. J Neurol Sci 1972;16:417–432

24. Barclay L, Wolfson L: Normal aging: pathophysiologic and clinical changes. pp. 13–20. In Barclay L (ed): Clinical geriatric neurology. Lea & Febiger, Philadelphia, 1993

25. Larsson L: Morphological and functional characteristics of the ageing skeletal muscle in man. A cross-sectional study. Acta Physiol Scand Suppl 1978;457:1–36

26. Larsson L, Grimby G, Karlsson J: Muscle strength and speed of movement in relation to age and muscle morphology. J Appl Physiol 1979;46:451–456

27. Kawamura Y, O'Brien P, Okazaki H, Dyck PJ: Lumbar motoneurons of man II: the number and diameter distribution of large-and intermediate-diameter cytons in "motoneuron columns" of spinal cord of man. J Neuropathol Exp Neurol 1977; 36:861–870

28. Brown WF: A method for estimating the number of motor units in thenar muscles and the changes in motor unit count with ageing. J Neurol Neurosurg Psychiatry 1972;35:845–852

29. McComas AJ, Fawcett PRW, Campbell MJ, Sica REP: Electrophysiological estimation of the number of motor units within a human muscle. J Neurol Neurosurg Psychiatry 1971;34: 121–131

30. McComas AJ, Upton ARM, Sica REP: Motoneurone disease and ageing. Lancet 1973;2:1477–1480

31. Smith J: Clinical neurophysiology in the elderly. pp. 89–97. In Tallis R (ed): The Clinical Neurology of Old Age. John Wiley, Chichester, 1989

32. Coërs C, Telerman-Toppet N, Gerard JM: Terminal innervation ratio in neuromuscular disease. I. Methods and controls. Arch Neurol 1973;29:210–214

33. Stevens JC, Lofgren EP, Dyck PJ: Histometric evaluation of branches of peroneal nerve: technique for combined biopsy of muscle nerve and cutaneous nerve. Brain Res 1973; 52:37–59

34. Exton-Smith AN: Disorders of the autonomic nervous system. pp. 182–201. In Caird FI (ed): Neurological disorders in the elderly. Wright, Bristol, 1982

35. Lye M: Autonomic dysfunction and abnormal vascular reflexes. pp. 191–211. In Tallis R (ed): The Clinical Neurology of Old Age. John Wiley, Chichester, 1989

36. Dorfman LJ, Bosley TM: Age-related changes in peripheral and central nerve conduction in man. Neurology 1979;29:38–44

37. Bouche P, Cattelin F, Saint-Jean D: Clinical and electrophysiological study of the peripheral nervous system in the elderly. J Neurol 1993;240:263–268

38. Munoz M, Boutros-Toni F, Preux PM et al: Prevalence of neurological disorders in Haute-Vienne Department (Limousin Region—France). Neuroepidemiology 1995;14:193–198

39. George J, Twomey JA: Causes of polyneuropathy in the elderly. Age Ageing 1986;15:247–249

40. Huang CY: Peripheral neuropathy in the elderly: a clinical and electrophysiologic study. J Am Geriatr Soc 1981;29:49–54

41. Dyck PJ, Oviatt KF, Lambert EH: Intensive evaluation of referred unclassified neuropathies yields improved diagnosis. Ann Neurol 1981;10:222–226

42. McKhann GM, Griffin JW, Cornblath DR et al: Plasmapheresis and Guillain-Barré Syndrome: analysis of prognostic factors and the effect of plasmapheresis. Ann Neurol 1988;23:347–353

43. Elble RJ, Hughes L, Higins C: The syndrome of senile gait. J Neurol 1992;239:71–75

44. Wolfson L: Falls and gait. pp. 281–299. In R Katzman, JW Rowe (eds): Principles of Geriatric Neurology. FA Davis, Philadelphia, 1992

45. Koller WC, Glatt SL, Fox JH: Senile gait, a distinct neurologic entity. Clin Geriatr Med 1985;1:661–669

46. Richardson JK, Hurvitz EA: Peripheral neuropathy: a true risk factor for falls. J Gerontol 1995;50A:M211–M215

47. Smith BE: Inflammatory sensory polyganglionopathies. Neurol Clin 1992;10:735–759

48. Dyck PJ, Kratz KM, Karnes MS et al: The prevalence by staged severity of various types of diabetic neuropathy, retinopathy, and nephropathy in a population-based cohort: The Rochester Diabetic Neuropathy Study. Neurology 1993;43:817–824

49. Olney RK: Diseases of peripheral nerves. pp. 171–189. In Tallis R (ed): The clinical neurology of old age. John Wiley, Chichester, 1989

50. Naliboff BD, Rosenthal M: Effects of age on complications in adult onset diabetes. J Am Geriatr Soc 1989;37:838–842

51. Harati Y: Diabetes and the nervous system. Endocrinol Metab Clin North Am 1996;25:325–359

52. Harati Y: Diabetic peripheral neuropathies. Ann Intern Med 1987;107:546–559

53. Trautmann JC, Barnett CR: Diseases of the third, fourth, and sixth cranial nerves. pp. 785–800. In Dyck PJ, Thomas PK, Griffin JW, (eds): Peripheral Neuropathy. 3rd Ed. WB Saunders, Philadelphia, 1993

54. Thomas PK, Tomlinson DR: Diabetic and hypoglycemic neuropathy. pp. 1219–1250. In Dyck PJ, Thomas PK, Griffin JW et al (eds): Peripheral Neuropathy. 3rd Ed. WB Saunders, Philadelphia, 1993

55. Veves A, Young MJ, Manes C et al: Differences in peripheral and autonomic nerve function measurements in painful and

painless neuropathy: a clinical study. Diabetes Care 1994;17: 1200–1202

56. McNeely MJ, Boyko EJ, Ahroni JH et al: The independent contributions of diabetic neuropathy and vasculopathy in foot ulceration: how great are the risks? Diabetes Care 1995;18:216–219
57. Boulton AJ: End-stage complications of diabetic neuropathy: foot ulceration. Can J Neurol Sci 1994;21:S18–22
58. Diabetes Control and Complications Trial Research Group: The effect of intensive treatment of diabetes on the development and progression of long-term complications in insulin-dependent diabetes mellitus. N Engl J Med 1993;329:683–689
59. Skyler JS: Diabetic complications: the importance of glucose control. Endocrinol Metab Clin North Am 1996;25:243–254
60. Thomas PK: Growth factors and diabetic neuropathy. Diabet Med 1994;11:732–739
61. Max MB, Culnane M, Schafer SC et al: Amitriptyline relieves diabetic neuropathy pain in patients with normal or depressed mood. Neurology 1987;37:589–596
62. Bolton CF: Peripheral neuropathies associated with chronic renal failure. Can J Neurol Sci 1980;7:89–96
63. Asbury AK: Neuropathies with renal failure, hepatic disorders, chronic respiratory insufficiency, and critical illness. pp. 1251–1265. In Dyck PJ, Thomas PK, Griffin JW et al (eds): Peripheral Neuropathy. 3rd Ed. WB Saunders, Philadelphia, 1993
64. Nielsen VK: The peripheral nerve function in chronic renal failure. Acta Med Scand 1971;190:105–111
65. Thomas PK: Screening for peripheral neuropathy in patients treated by chronic hemodialysis. Muscle Nerve 1978;1: 396–399
66. Bolton CF, Baltzan MA, Baltzan RG: Effects of renal transplantation on uremic neuropathy. N Engl J Med 1971;284: 1170–1175
67. Pollard JD: Neuropathy in diseases of thyroid and pituitary glands. pp. 1266–1274. In Dyck PJ, Thomas PK, Griffin JW et al (eds): Peripheral Neuropathy. 3rd Ed. WB Saunders, Philadelphia, 1993
68. Stewart BM: The hypertrophic neuropathy of acromegaly: a rare neuropathy associated with acromegaly. Arch Neurol 1966;14: 107–110
69. Low PA, McLeod JG, Turtle JR et al: Peripheral neuropathy in acromegaly. Brain 1974;97:139–152
70. Fullerton PM: Toxic chemicals and peripheral neuropathy: clinical and epidemiological features. Proc R Soc Med 1969;62: 201–210
71. Schaumburg HH, Berger AR: Human toxic neuropathy due to industrial agents. pp. 1533–1548. In Dyck PJ, Thomas PK, Griffin JW et al (eds): Peripheral Neuropathy. 3rd Ed. WB Saunders, Philadelphia, 1993
72. Behse F, Buchthal F: Alcoholic neuropathy: clinical, electrophysiological, and biopsy findings. Ann Neurol 1977;2:95–110
73. Hillbom M, Wennberg A: Prognosis of alcoholic peripheral neuropathy. J Neurol Neurosurg Psychiatry 1984;47: 699–703
74. Windebank AJ: Polyneuropathy due to nutritional deficiency and alcoholism. pp. 1310–1321. In Dyck PJ, Thomas PK, Griffin JW et al (eds): Peripheral Neuropathy. 3rd Ed. WB Saunders, Philadelphia, 1993
75. Victor M, Lear AA: Subacute combined degeneration of the spinal cord. Current concepts of the disease process. Value of serum B_{12} determinations in clarifying some of the common clinical problems. Am J Med 1956;20:896–911
76. Harding AE, Muller DPR, Thomas PK, Willison HJ: Spinocerebellar degeneration secondary to chronic intestinal malabsorption: a vitamin E deficiency syndrome. Ann Neurol 1982;12: 419–424
77. Johnson PC, Rolak LA, Hamilton RH, Laguna JF: Paraneoplastic vasculitis of nerve: a remote effect of cancer. Ann Neurol 1979;5:437–444
78. Chalk CH, Dyck PJ, Conn DL: Vasculitic neuropathy. pp. 1424–1436. In Dyck PJ, Thomas PK, Griffin JW et al (eds): Peripheral Neuropathy. 3rd Ed. WB Saunders, Philadelphia, 1993
79. Horwich MS, Cho L, Porro RS, Posner JB: Subacute sensory neuropathy: a remote effect of carcinoma. Ann Neurol 1977;2: 7–19
80. Warenius HM: Paraneoplastic neurological syndromes. pp. 328–334. In Tallis R (ed): The clinical neurology of old age. John Wiley, Chichester, 1989
81. McLeod JG: Paraneoplastic neuropathies. pp. 1583–1590. In Dyck PJ, Thomas PK, Griffin JW et al (eds): Peripheral Neuropathy. 3rd Ed. WB Saunders, Philadelphia, 1993
82. Kyle RA, Dyck PJ: Neuropathy associated with the monoclonal gammopathies. pp. 1275–1287. In Dyck PJ, Thomas PK, Griffin JW et al (eds): Peripheral Neuropathy. 3rd Ed. WB Saunders, Philadelphia, 1993
83. Gosselin S, Kyle RA, Dyck PJ: Neuropathy associated with monoclonal gammopathies of undetermined significance. Ann Neurol 1991;30:54–61
84. Kyle RA, Dyck PJ: Amyloidosis and neuropathy. pp. 1294–1309. In Dyck PJ, Thomas PK, Griffin JW et al (eds): Peripheral Neuropathy. 3rd Ed. WB Saunders, Philadelphia, 1993
85. Baringer JR, Townsend JJ: Herpesvirus infection of the peripheral nervous system. pp. 1333–1342. In Dyck PJ, Thomas PK, Griffin JW et al (eds): Peripheral Neuropathy. 3rd Ed. WB Saunders, Philadelphia, 1993
86. Arnason BGW, Soliven B: Acute inflammatory demyelinating polyradiculopathy. pp. 1437–1497. In Dyck PJ, Thomas PK, Griffin JW et al (eds): Peripheral Neuropathy. 3rd Ed. WB Saunders, Philadelphia, 1993
87. Sridharan GV, Tallis RC, Gautam PC: Guillain-Barré Syndrome in the elderly. Gerontology 1993;39:170–175
88. McCombe PA, Pollard JD, McLeod JG: Chronic inflammatory demyelinating polyradiculoneuropathy. Brain 1987;110: 1617–1630
89. French Cooperative Group of Plasma Exchange in Guillain-Barré Syndrome: Efficiency of plasma exchange in Guillain-Barré syndrome: role of replacement fluids. Ann Neurol 1987; 22:753–761
90. Server AC, Lefkowith J, Braine H, McKhann GM: Treatment of chronic relapsing inflammatory polyradiculoneuropathy by plasma exchange. Ann Neurol 1979;6:258–261
91. Dyck PJ, Prineas J, Pollard J: Chronic inflammatory demyelinating polyradiculoneuropathy. pp. 1498–1517. In Dyck PJ, Thomas PK, Griffin JW et al (eds): Peripheral Neuropathy. 3rd Ed. WB Saunders, Philadelphia, 1993

92. van Doorn PA, Brand A, Strengers PFW et al: High-dose intravenous immunoglobulin treatment in chronic inflammatory demyelinating polyneuropathy: a double-blind, placebo-controlled, crossover study. Neurology 1990;40:209–212

93. van der Meché FGA, Schmitz PIM, Dutch Guillain-Barré Study Group: A randomized trial comparing intravenous immune globulin and plasma exchange in Guillain-Barré Syndrome. N Engl J Med 1992;326:1123–1129

94. Irani DN, Cornblath DR, Chaudhry V et al: Relapse in Guillain-Barré syndrome after treatment with human immune globulin. Neurology 1993;43:872–875

95. Hughes RAC, Newsom-Davis JM, Perkin GD, Pierce JM: Controlled trial of prednisone in acute polyneuropathy. Lancet 1978;2:750–753

96. Hughes RAC, Kadlubowski M, Hufschmidt A: Treatment of acute inflammatory polyneuropathy. Ann Neurol 1981;9(suppl): 125–133

97. Dyck PJ, O'Brien PC, Oviatt KF et al: Prednisone improves chronic inflammatory demyelinating polyradiculoneuropathy more than no treatment. Ann Neurol 1982;11:136–141

98. Dyck PJ, Chance P, Lebo R, Carney JA: Hereditary motor and sensory neuropathies. pp. 1094–1136. In Dyck PJ, Thomas PK, Griffin JW et al (eds): Peripheral Neuropathy. 3rd Ed. WB Saunders, Philadelphia, 1993

CHAPTER 42

Intracranial Tumors

DAVID H. ROSENBAUM

Intracranial tumor—"brain tumor"—is perhaps the diagnosis most feared by patients presenting for neurologic evaluation. Although neoplasms are less common than many of the other conditions that produce neurologic symptomatology, their importance in the elderly becomes proportionately greater because the incidence of brain tumor increases throughout adult life. Furthermore, the incidence and mortality of primary brain tumor have been increasing for the last 30 years, and this change also has been most evident in the elderly. Although the clinical presentation is often suggestive of the diagnosis, the manifestations of brain tumor are protean. The clinical picture may be even more obscure in the elderly. The introduction of noninvasive brain imaging modalities—computed tomography (CT) and magnetic resonance imaging (MRI)—in recent decades has greatly aided the diagnosis of tumors and intracranial disease in general. Although treatment options and prognosis are less favorable in the geriatric age group, recent advances in neurosurgery and radiation oncology have to some degree improved this outlook.

Classification and Epidemiology

Intracranial tumors are either primary or metastatic from systemic malignancies; although the incidence of the two is approximately equal in adults overall (8.2 to 8.3 per 100,00), metastatic lesions become more common in the elderly.[1] Of metastatic tumors, lung is the most frequent source (40 percent), whereas breast, melanoma, and miscellaneous (including gastrointestinal and renal) neoplasms each account for approximately 20 percent of the total.[2]

Primary tumors are either parenchymal, which are the majority in younger age groups but account for less than 50 percent in those over age 65,[1,2] or extra-axial. In adults, and particularly the elderly, parenchymal tumors are likely to be malignant, whereas extra-axial growths are nearly always benign. The relative incidence of the various tumor types varies widely from series to series, presumably depending on referral patterns. Tumors derived from glial cells account for approximately 90 percent of the primary parenchymal tumors; about 85 percent are astrocytomas and approximately one-half of these are classified as glioblastoma multiforme, the most malignant of brain tumors. Thirty percent are in the slightly less malignant category of anaplastic astrocytoma.[1–4] Glioblastoma and anaplastic astrocytoma together are classified as malignant gliomas. The most benign or "low-grade" tumors account for less than 10 to 15 percent of astrocytomas.[2] Oligodendrogliomas are also relatively benign and slow-growing glial tumors that have a tendency to calcify; they account for only 5 percent of adult parenchymal tumors and are rare in the geriatric population.[5] There is a decided shift in incidence toward the more malignant end of the spectrum with advancing age, and approximately 90 percent of gliomas in those over the age of 65 are glioblastomas.[6,7] Primary central nervous system (CNS) lymphoma (about 2 percent of parenchymal tumors) is quite uncommon in immunologically normal patients and occurs principally in the sixth and seventh decades.[8] Its incidence, however, is also increasing, not only in relation to acquired immunodeficiency syndrome and particularly in the elderly.[9]

Extra-axial tumors account for more than one-half of primary tumors in the older age group. About 80 percent are meningiomas, which become increasingly frequent with age and are as common as glioblastomas.[1,2] Approximately 10 percent are acoustic neuromas and 5 to 10 percent are pituitary adenomas.[1,2,4]

Epidemiologic studies indicate that brain tumors of all type are diagnosed with steadily increasing frequency throughout adult life up until the sixties, with a decline in incidence noted after the age of 75.[1,10] This apparent decrease may, however, be an artifact of relative diagnostic insensitivity or lack of diagnostic aggressiveness in the management of the elderly, because if asymptomatic tumors (discovered at autopsy) are included, the incidence continues to increase throughout life.[11] As noted above, the frequency with which certain tumor types are seen also increases with age: malignant lesions—metastatic tumors and malignant gliomas (especially glioblastoma multiforme)—become more common,[1] as do lymphomas[8] (although the latter remain uncommon). At the benign end of the spectrum, meningiomas (often discovered incidentally) show a striking increase in incidence.[1,11] Epidemiologic surveys have found a striking increase—between two- and eightfold—in deaths from brain malignancy over recent decades (1960s to 1980s), with the greatest increases in the oldest age groups (over 75 or 80 years).[12–14] Although some of the apparent increase is attributable to improved diagnosis consequent to availability of CT scanning beginning in the mid 1970s,[12] the trend was already established prior to this time. Changing attitudes toward medical care of the elderly may account for some portion of the change,[14] and environmental toxins or changes in global ecology may also be contributory.[13] A recent study has found that the increasing mortality rate from malignant primary brain tumor in the elderly is directly proportional to the increasing population size of this age group, and proposed a Darwinian differential survival mechanism operating in recent history—in this case, "survival of the less fit"—to account for the observation.[15]

Clinical Presentation

A brain tumor is a progressively expanding intracranial mass lesion, and its clinical hallmark is insidious progression of neurologic deficits. In up to 10 percent of cases, however, the onset may be abrupt, suggesting a stroke[16]; alternatively, stuttering or paroxysmal symptoms may appear during the course of the illness. These phenomena are occasionally related to intra- or peritumoral hemorrhage, secondary vascular compromise, or partial epileptic seizures, but often remain unexplained. On the other hand, fewer than 1 percent of those presenting with the clinical picture of stroke will be found to have a tumor.[17] Typically, brain tumors produce progressive dysfunction related to destruction or compression of eloquent areas of cortex and subcortical nuclei. With malignant tumors, symptoms develop over weeks to months, whereas meningiomas may present with insidious progression over months or years. Primary tumors, as a rule, involve the cerebral hemispheres in this age group[4] and manifestations may include changes in memory, mood, or personality with anterior frontal or temporal tumors; hemiparesis, hemisensory loss, and hemianopia with posterior frontal or parietal lesions; and aphasia with left-sided tumors in the region of the Sylvian fissure. Although primary tumors of the brain-stem and cerebellum are a rarity in the elderly, about 20 percent of metastatic tumors are located in the posterior fossa, more than three-fourths in the cerebellum.[18] They often present with ataxia or cranial nerve abnormalities. In addition to focal dysfunction, because the skull forms a rigid case and is further subdivided into fixed compartments (above and below the cerebellar tentorium that separates the cerebrum from the cerebellum and brain stem), an enlarging lesion may lead to increased intracranial pressure resulting in both diffuse and remote effects, and also creates the potential for herniation between compartments. Tumors within or adjacent to the cerebroventricular pathways often produce increased intracranial pressure early in their course by causing obstructive hydrocephalus. These effects include headache and mental changes, most importantly and ominously depressed level of consciousness, gait disturbance, etc.

Acoustic neuromas are very slow-growing Schwann cell tumors of the eighth nerve that produce unilateral hearing loss as the earliest symptom; the adjacent fifth and seventh cranial nerves may be subsequently involved. Only late in their course, with advancing size, do they produce the combination of brain stem and cerebellar signs implicit in their location at the cerebellopontine angle. Audiometric testing (including brain stem auditory potentials) reveals unilateral retrocochlear hearing loss and indicates the need for an imaging study, ideally MRI.[19] Pituitary adenomas may secrete adrenocorticotropic hormone, growth hormone, or prolactin, but are more commonly nonfunctioning and produce no symptoms.[20] With progressive enlargement, they may cause headache and can produce varying degrees of hypopituitarism. If the tumor grows into the suprasellar cistern, it may compress the optic chiasm and result in bitemporal hemianopia, an almost pathognomonic visual field defect.

Several factors modify the clinical picture of brain tumor in the elderly, tending to make the diagnosis less readily evident. The loss of brain parenchymal volume that occurs with age allows tumors to grow for a longer time and become larger without producing an increase in cerebrospinal fluid (CSF) pressure. Consequently morning headache, with projectile vomiting and papilledema, considered classic signs of brain tumor, are less likely to be prominent in the geriatric patient.[16] Furthermore, elderly individuals are prone to develop mental changes and delirium early in their course and these changes may be phenomenologically indistinguishable from similar states induced by toxic or metabolic disturbances. The clinical picture may at times be difficult to distinguish from degenerative dementia or even depression. Such changes in the absence of detectable motor or sensory abnormalities on examination are more likely to occur with tumors of the frontal lobes as well as with meningiomas, which because of their slow growth and extra-axial location allow neural structures to accommodate to their presence. Focal abnormalities on neurologic examination in a patient presenting with delirium should raise the suspicion of tumor, as should progression of a deficit that presents as a "stroke." The most frequent clinical manifestations of brain tumor in the elderly include motor signs in more than one-half, mental changes in one-third, and sensory changes, hemianopia, or speech abnormalities in one-fifth.[16] The incidence and prevalence of epilepsy and seizures (both partial and secondarily generalized) increase progressively with advancing age, and although vascular lesions account for more than one-half of the cases of epilepsy beginning after the age of 60, one-third are caused by brain tumors.[21]

It is conceptually useful to divide intracranial neoplasms into benign and malignant groups for purposes of prognosis and treatment, but it must be recognized that these terms have a different meaning than they do in general oncology, at least regarding the primary brain tumors. Malignancy in primary brain tumors is not defined by metastatic potential, which is virtually nil, or even by likely invasion of extraneural structures, but strictly by the ability of the tumor to invade normal neural structures and/or to be unresectable. In this scheme, meningiomas, pituitary adenomas, and acoustic neuromas are potentially benign and surgically curable. However, even these lesions, and meningiomas in particular, may not be surgically approachable because of their location in relation to vital structures (e.g., carotid artery). "Benign" tumors generally have indolent growth patterns, and even when they are not resectable, often allow for decades of good quality survival. Low-grade astrocytomas and oligodendrogliomas are *relatively* benign in this sense, though they are locally invasive, not surgically curable, and eventually, in most cases, result in the death of the patient.

Diagnosis

As is true in the field of neurology in general, a comprehensive history supplemented by a competent neurologic examination is likely to bring the clinician close to the correct diagnosis and to suggest the most efficient diagnostic plan. In the elderly, because of the complexities described above, it is essential that a high index of suspicion regarding the possibility of brain tumor be maintained, particularly because it is generally a treatable and often curable cause of disability.

Brain Imaging

Before CT scanning became widely available in the mid-1970s, a definitive evaluation to exclude or diagnose a brain tumor required hospitalization for invasive, uncomfortable, and risky procedures—specifically cerebral arteriography and/or pneumoencephalography. Clinicians were reluctant to submit patients, particularly the fragile elderly, to such risks in the absence of clear indications, and patients were often followed clinically without definitive testing as "brain tumor suspects." At the present time, most experienced neurologists would agree that an individual presenting with a new or progressive neurologic deficit or with dementia should, after appropriate clinical evaluation, undergo a definitive brain imaging study. Although CT scanning revolutionized the diagnostic evaluation of these patients, MRI has proven to be even more sensitive in the detection of focal brain lesions and is currently recognized as the optimal screening technique for the detection of most intracranial neoplasms, although it is not without its limitations.[19]

Specific details regarding the neuroimaging appearance of different types of tumors is beyond the scope of this chapter, and comprehensive reviews are readily available.[19] A few points are worth making here. By their nature as growing lesions, tumors generally exert mass effect and displace surrounding structures. They are also typically surrounded by a zone of edema, with characteristic appearance on CT and MRI, although in the case of gliomas, some of this zone also consists of "fingers" of tumor tissue.[22] Because the blood-brain barrier is defective in most tumors, contrast enhancement is an important diagnostic characteristic, although often lacking in the low-grade gliomas.[19] None of these features, of course, is pathognomonic, and each finding must be interpreted in its clinical context. Multiple lesions, often identified only with MRI, suggest metastatic disease, as does a cerebellar tumor, because primary cerebellar tumors are rare in the elderly. CNS lymphoma is often seen as a densely enhancing lesion in the deep periventricular white matter.[23] In patients with AIDS lymphomas are often small, multiple, and located in the basal ganglia, whereas in the non-AIDS (typically elderly) patient they tend to be solitary, greater than 2 cm, and located in the white matter of the parietal lobe.[24] Meningiomas are extra-axial in location, and usually have a broad base of attachment to the dura; they show extensive, uniform contrast enhancement.

Cerebrospinal Fluid Examination

Lumbar puncture is not usually indicated for the diagnosis of brain tumor. Although elevation of CSF protein is commonly seen, this is a nonspecific finding whose utility has been eclipsed by the advent of noninvasive imaging. Cytologic examination may reveal malignant cells and aid in pathologic diagnosis, particularly with primary lymphomas, leukemia, or metastases involving the meninges (meningeal lymphomatosis or carcinomatosis).[25] The usefulness of CSF tumor markers is also under investigation.[26] Rarely a glioma will present with a meningeal picture (meningeal gliomatosis) diagnosable by CSF cytology. Because there is a small but real risk that lumbar puncture will cause brain herniation, particularly in the presence of a large tumor and increased intracranial pressure, a CT or MRI should be performed first to rule out such a lesion.

Biopsy

The role of surgery and surgical tumor resection is discussed more fully in the section on treatment. As a rule, a definitive tissue diagnosis should be achieved when practically feasible. This is both because the particular treatment will depend on the tumor type and because not all space-occupying lesions seen on brain imaging prove to be neoplastic.[27,28] This statement must be conditioned, however, by the overall clinical context and the patient's medical and psychosocial status. A patient with known systemic malignancy and typical metastatic brain lesions does not usually require biopsy, nor does a frail patient with end-stage Alzheimer disease and a large, radiologically malignant lesion of the brain. In the patient with a single tumor or multiple brain lesions consistent with metastatic disease, workup to identify a primary source beyond complete physical examination (with testing for occult blood in stool) and CT scan of chest and abdomen is often unrevealing and probably not cost effective.[29] In this situation, biopsy (or resection, if appropriate—see below) would be the logical next step. When biopsy is indicated, the procedure of choice is a CT or MRI-guided needle biopsy, which has an overall morbidity of only 2 percent.[30]

Treatment

Surgery

The ideal treatment for brain tumor is total surgical resection resulting in cure. As indicated, this is generally possible only for the "benign" extra-axial lesions: meningioma, acoustic neuroma, and pituitary adenoma. Even here the anatomic location of the tumor or the general health of the patient may preclude aggressive surgery. Age itself is not a contraindication to neurosurgery and perioperative mortality and morbidity is not necessarily increased after the age of 65.[16] It has also been found, in another study, that patients over 65 years of age undergoing craniotomy for brain tumor, although sicker and having a higher rate of complications than those under 65, had similar outcomes, including quality-of-life scores.[31] However, because the elderly are more prone to suffer coexisting medical conditions that worsen their prognosis, the approach to treatment is usually balanced toward the less aggressive side, particularly in those who are frail. Because the natural history of "benign" tumors is often measured in decades, an incidentally discovered asymptomatic lesion may not require treatment, and partial removal of a tumor that cannot be completely resected may render the patient asymptomatic for the duration of the life span. Stereotactic radiosurgery for nonresectable tumors is proving to be an important option (see below). Pituitary adenomas can be treated with a high rate of success and low morbidity by transsphenoidal removal[32]; prolactin-secreting tumors are often effectively treated with bromocriptine;[33] tumors that are inoperable or incompletely removed should be treated with radiation. Radiation therapy may also useful in preventing recurrence of partially resected meningiomas or in treating recurrences.[34]

For malignant tumors and those that cannot be fully removed, and where the clinical situation does not contraindicate an aggressive approach (see discussion above in section on diagnostic biopsy), as much of the tumor as is readily accessible should be removed, with care taken not to disturb adjacent brain. Such "debulking" reduces mass effect, tends to decrease local and diffuse symptoms, often permits a reduction in steroid dose, and may allow the patient to better tolerate the edema that can accompany radiotherapy.[35] Postoperative morbidity is no greater in those undergoing large resections than in those having small resections or biopsies,[36] and large removals, in patients with malignant gliomas, have been shown to improve survival.[37–39] In patients with brain metastasis proven by MRI to be solitary and whose primary cancer is controlled, surgical removal followed by radiation has been shown to increase duration of life (40 versus 15 weeks) and to greatly prolong the period of functionally independent survival (38 versus 8 weeks) compared to only biopsy and radiation.[40] Unfortunately, the applicability of this study to geriatrics is unclear, because the median age of the patients was 60 years and none were over 74. As with gliomas, age is a negative prognostic factor for patients with brain metastases. Of note is that in this study of 54 patients with known systemic cancer and brain lesions diagnosed by CT or MRI as consistent with brain metastasis, 6 patients proved to have lesions that were *not* metastatic: two abscesses and one a nonspecific inflammatory reaction[40]—a cogent argument for tissue confirmation of diagnosis prior to radiation. Low-grade gliomas are uncommon in this population and require treatment only when they become symptomatic; this involves maximal feasible resection followed by local radiotherapy.

Adrenal Corticosteroids

Malignant glial tumors, metastatic tumors, and some meningiomas are surrounded by edema, which increases the mass effect, accentuates focal deficits and produces diffuse signs (headache, and mental and gait abnormalities). This "vasogenic" edema is caused by breakdown of blood-brain barrier secondary to abnormal fenestration of vascular endothelium in the tumor, allowing leakage of water and solutes into and around the tumor.[41] Glucocorticosteroids are effective at reversing this leakiness[42] and have been used as palliative and adjunctive therapy for more than 30 years. Significant symptomatic improvement occurs within 24 to 48 hours in the majority of patients and may be dramatic. Elderly patients respond as well as the young.[43] Primary CNS lymphoma often disappears when treated with steroids alone, but almost invariably recurs; best results are obtained with whole brain radiation,[8] perhaps with the addition of chemotherapy as well.[23] Dexamethasone is the standard preparation because of its potency, its relatively minimal mineralocorticoid effect, and because it may cause less psychiatric disturbance than other preparations. It has a prolonged biologic half-life that makes it suitable for twice a day dosing, and when given with meals, H2 blockers are needed only for patients with a history of peptic ulcer disease. The usual dose is 16 mg/d, with greater doses given if there is not a satisfactory response. A recent study, however, found that 4 mg/d was as effective as 16 (in patients without impending herniation), with significant reduction in toxicity.[44] The toxicity of glucocorticoids can be quite important, particularly when given for prolonged periods.[45] The most serious relate to immunosuppressive and antipyretic effects, which predispose to infection while masking some of its signs. Weight gain and the development of cushingoid habitus and facies adversely affect quality of life. Sleep disturbance and emotional lability may occur, the latter to the point of frank psychosis. Hyperglycemia, hypertension, increased gastric acid secretion, and osteoporosis can all lead to major complications. Steroid myopathy, manifesting with proximal muscle weakness, may be quite disabling.[46] The incidence of these toxicities increases with dose and duration of therapy, so that corticosteroids should be used at the lowest effective dose and tapered, if possible, once definitive therapy has been implemented.

Radiation Therapy

External beam radiotherapy is the most important modality in the treatment of malignant gliomas and metastatic disease; it more than doubles the median survival time in both conditions.[47,48] Unfortunately, radiation is toxic to normal brain, and there is evidence that the elderly may be more susceptible.[49] Higher doses are more effective, but also more toxic.[50] Particularly in the elderly, attempts should be made to restrict treatment to the "involved field" and to use the lowest effective dose. Primary CNS lymphoma is highly sensitive to radiation, and is generally treated, as noted earlier, with whole brain radiation,[8] often preceded by chemotherapy.[23] Low-grade gliomas are treated with localized radiation to the tumor bed following resection. Two relatively new techniques attempt to deliver very high radiation doses to a very localized field within a malignant tumor, often as an adjunct to lower dose external beam radiation. Interstitial or brachytherapy involves the placement (often stereotactically) of radioactive implants into the tumor. Although favorable results have been reported[51,52] the procedure remains experimental. Localized hyperthermia in combination with brachytherapy also shows some promise.[53] Stereotactic radiosurgery (by linear accelerator or gamma knife) is a widely available technique that also concentrates a high radiation dose into a restricted volume and is less invasive than brachytherapy. Once again, despite some promising preliminary results,[54] radiosurgery is still clearly an experimental treatment for malignant tumors. As mentioned above, it may be useful in the treatment of meningiomas and acoustic neuromas that cannot be completely removed by conventional surgery, although eventual recurrence is likely.[55]

Chemotherapy

The role of chemotherapy in the treatment of brain tumors, particularly in the geriatric population, is limited. It has no place in the therapy of benign extra-axial neoplasms or low-grade astrocytomas, nor have antineoplastic drugs proved to be of much use in the treatment of brain metastases. BCNU is the most widely used agent in the treatment of malignant gliomas, and a recent meta-analysis has shown it to have a definite but limited effect in prolonging life[56]; unfortunately even this modest benefit is much diminished in the elderly,[57,58] who also tend to tolerate antineoplastic drugs poorly. Overall, even with aggressive treatment (surgical excision, radiotherapy, and chemotherapy), median survival with glioblastoma is less than 1 year, and only slightly more than two with malignant astrocytoma. The outlook is even more dismal in the elderly.[59] On the other hand, chemotherapy does seem to prolong survival in CNS lymphoma,[60] although again the prognosis is significantly worse in the elderly.[61]

Experimental attempts to enhance the efficacy of chemotherapy have included intra-arterial administration (which, unfortunately, actually worsened survival in one large study)[62] and disruption of the blood-brain barrier.[63] Although some positive preliminary results have been reported, it does not seem that these approaches herald a major breakthrough. Even newer approaches include immunomodulation[64,65] and genetic manipulations.[66]

Conclusion

Although the manifestations of brain tumor in the elderly can be subtle and nonspecific, careful attention to the neurologic evaluation and appropriate use of brain imaging studies should minimize any delay in diagnosis. It is important to recognize that, ominous as the diagnosis may seem, the majority of primary brain tumors in this population are benign, eminently treatable, and usually curable. Even in the case of malignant tumors, advances in neurosurgical technique, radiation oncology, and chemotherapy have greatly improved the outlook for many elderly patients, in terms of both prolongation of life and enhanced quality of survival. Numerous experimental approaches are currently under investigation, and although a therapeutic breakthrough does not appear imminent, it is to be hoped that in the not-too-distant future more definitive treatments for malignant neoplasms of the brain will be found.

References

1. Walker AE, Robins M, Weinfeld FD: Epidemiology of brain tumors: the national survey of intracranial neoplasms. Neurology 1985;35:219–226
2. Jaeckle KA: Central nervous system tumors in the elderly. pp. 195–204. In Barclay L (ed): Clinical Geriatric Neurology, Lea & Febiger, Philadelphia, 1993
3. Walker MD: Malignant Brain Tumors. American Cancer Society, New York, 1975
4. Zulch KJ: Brain Tumors: Their Biology and Pathology. Springer-Verlag, New York, 1986
5. Salcman M: Brain tumors and the geriatric patient. J Am Geriatr Soc 1982;30:501–508
6. Werner MH, Schold CS: Primary intracranial neoplasms in the elderly. Clin Geriatr Med 1987;3:765–779
7. Trouillas P, Menaud G, De The G et al: Etude epidemiologique des tumeurs primitives de neuraxe dans la region Rhone-Alpes. Rev Neurol Paris 1975;131:691–708
8. Murray K, Kun L, Cox J: Primary malignant lymphomas of the central nervous system: results of treatment of 11 cases and review of the literature. J Neurosurg 1986;65:600–607
9. Eby NL, Grufferman S, Flannelly CM et al: Increasing incidence of primary brain lymphoma in the US. Cancer 1988;62: 2461–2465
10. Schoenberg BS, Christine BW, Whisnant JP: The descriptive epidemiology of primary intracranial neoplasms: the Connecticut experience. Am J Epidemiol 1976;104:499–510
11. Annegers JF, Schoenberg BS, Okazaki H, Kurland LT: Epidemiologic study of intracranial neoplasms. Arch Neurol 1981; 38:217–219
12. Greig NH, Ries LG, Rancik R, Rapoport SI: Increasing annual incidence of primary malignant brain tumors in the elderly. J Natl Cancer Inst 1990;82:1621–1624
13. Davis DL, Hoel D, Fox J, Lopez A: Epidemiology. International trends in cancer mortality in France, West Germany, Italy, Japan, England and Wales, and the USA. Lancet 1990;336: 474–481
14. Modan B, Wagener DK, Feldman JJ et al: Increased mortality from brain tumors: a combined outcome of diagnostic technology and change of attitude toward the elderly. Am J Epidemiol 1992; 135:1349–1357
15. Riggs JE: Rising primary malignant brain tumor mortality in the elderly: a manifestation of differential survival. Arch Neurol 1995;52:571–575
16. Tomita T, Raimondi AJ: Brain tumors in the elderly. JAMA 1981;246:53–55
17. Sandercock P, Molyneux A, Warlow C: Value of computed tomography in patients with stroke. BMJ 1985;290:193–197

18. Posner JB: Management of central nervous system metastases. Semin Oncol 1977;4:81–91
19. Manzione JV, Poe LB, Kieffer SA: Intracranial neoplasms. pp. 170–238. In Haaga JR, Lanzieri CF, Sartoris DJ, Zerhoumi EA (eds): Computed Tomography and Magnetic Resonance Imaging of the Whole Body. 3rd Ed. Mosby, St. Louis, 1994
20. Post KD, Jackson JMD, Reichlin S (eds): The Pituitary Adenoma. Plenum Medical Book, New York, 1980
21. Loiseau J, Loiseau P, Duche B et al: A survey of epileptic disorders in southwest France: seizures in elderly patients. Ann Neurol 1990;27:232–237
22. Halperin EC, Burger PC, Bullard DE: The fallacy of the localized supratentorial malignant glioma. Int J Radiat Oncol Biol Phys 1988;15:505–509
23. DeAngelis LM, Yahalom J, Heinemann MH et al: Primary CNS lymphoma: combined treatment with chemotherapy and radiotherapy. Neurology 1990;40:80–86
24. Schwaighofer BW, Hesselink JR, Press GA et al: Primary intracranial CNS lymphoma: MR manifestations. AJNR 1989;10:725–729
25. Posner JB, Chernik NL: Intracranial metastases from systemic cancer. pp. 579–592. In Schoenberg BS (ed): Neurological Epidemiology: Principles and Clinical Applications. Advances in Neurology. Vol. 19. Lippincott-Raven, Philadelphia, 1978
26. van Zanten AP, Twinjstra A, Ongerboer de Visser BW et al: Cerebrospinal fluid tumor markers in patients treated for meningeal malignancy. J Neurol Neurosurg Psychiatry 1991;54:119–123
27. Todd NV, McDonagh T, Miller JD: What follows diagnosis by computed tomography of solitary brain tumor? Audit of one year's experience in southeast Scotland. Lancet 1987;1:611–612
28. Patchell RA, Tibbs PA, Walsh JW et al: A randomized trial of surgery in the treatment of single metastasis to the brain. N Engl J Med 1990;322:494–500
29. Voorhies RM, Sundresan N, Thaler HT: The single supratentorial lesion: an evaluation of preoperative diagnostic tests. J Neurosurg 1980;53:364–368
30. Bullard DE: Role of streotaxic biopsy in the management of patients with intracranial lesions. Neurol Clin 1985;3:817–830
31. Layon JA, George BE, Hamby B, Gallagher TJ: Do elderly patients overutilize healthcare resources and benefit less from them than younger patients? A study of patients who underwent craniotomy for treatment of neoplasm. Crit Care Med 1995;23:829–834
32. Cohen LC, Bevan JS, Adams CBT: The presentation and management of pituitary tumors in the elderly. Age Ageing 1989;18:247–252
33. Besser GM: Medical management of prolactinomas. In Givens JR (ed): Hormone-Secreting Pituitary Tumors. Year Book Medical Publishers, Chicago, 1982
34. Wara WM, Sheline GE, Newman H et al: Radiation therapy of meningiomas. Am J Roentgenol Radium Ther Nucl Med 1975;123:453–458
35. Grossman SA, Zeltzman M: Practical considerations in the management of adults with malignant astrocytomas. Neurologist 1996;2:130–138
36. Fadul C, Wood J, Thaler H et al: Mortality and morbidity of craniotomy for excision of supratentorial gliomas. Neurology 1988;38:1374–1379
37. Ammirati M, Vick N, Liao YL et al: Effect of the extent of surgical resection on survival and quality of life in patients with supratentorial glioblastomas and anaplastic astrocytomas. Neurosurgery 1987;21:201–206
38. Devaux BC, O'Fallon JR, Kelly PJ: Resection, biopsy and survival in malignant glial neoplasms: a retrospective study of clinical parameters, therapy and outcome. J Neurosurg 1993;78:767–775
39. Simpson JR, Horton J, Scott C et al: Influence of location and extent of surgical resection on survival of patients with glioblastoma multiforme: results of three consecutive Radiation Therapy Oncology Group clinical trials. Int J Radiat Oncol Biol Phys 1993;26:239–244
40. Patchell RA, Tibbs PA, Walsh JW et al: A randomized trial of surgery in the treatment of single metastases to the brain. N Engl J Med 1990;322:494–500
41. Long DM: Capillary ultrastructure and the blood-brain barrier in human malignant tumors. J Neurosurg 1970;32:127–144
42. Delattre JY, Arbit E, Rosenblum MK et al: High dose versus low dose dexamethasone in experimental epidural spinal cord compression. Neurosurgery 1988;22:1005–1007
43. Graham K, Caird FI: High dose steroid therapy of intracranial tumor in the elderly. Age Ageing 1978;7:146–150
44. Vecht CJ, Hovestadt A, Verbiest HBC et al: Dose effect relationship of dexamethasone on Karnofsky performance in metastatic brain tumors: a randomized study of doses of 4, 8, and 16 mg per day. Neurology 1994;44:675–680
45. Weissman DE, Dufer D, Vogel V, Abeloff MD: Corticosteroid toxicity in neuro-oncology patients. J Neurooncol 1987;5:125–128
46. Dropcho EJ, Soong SJ: Steroid induced muscle weakness in patients with primary brain tumors. Neurology 1991;41:1235–1239
47. Borgelt B, Gelber R, Kramer S et al: The palliation of brain metastases: final results of the first two studies by the Radiation Therapy Oncology Group. Int J Radiat Oncol Biol Phys 1980;6:1–9
48. Walker MD, Green SB, Byar DP et al: Randomized comparisons of radiotherapy and nitrosoureas for the treatment of malignant glioma after surgery. N Engl J Med 1980;303:1323–1329
49. Stylopoulos LA, George AE, de Leon MJ et al: Longitudinal CT study of parenchymal brain changes in glioma survivors. Am J Neuroradiol 1988;9:517–522
50. Marks JE, Baglan RJ, Prassad SC, Blank WF: Cerebral radionecrosis: incidence and risk in relation to dose, time, fractionation and volume. Int J Radiat Oncol Biol Phys 1981;7:243–252
51. Gutin PH, Leibel SA, Wara WM et al: Recurrent malignant gliomas: survival following interstitial brachytherapy with high-activity iodine-125 sources. J Neurosurg 1987;67:864–873
52. Tian ZM, Liu ZH, Kang GQ et al: CT-guided stereotactic injection of radionuclide for treatment of brain tumors. Stereotact Funct Neurosurg 1992;59:169–173

53. Sneed PK, Stauffer PR, Gutin PH et al: Interstitial irradiation and hyperthermia for the treatment of recurrent malignant brain tumors. Neurosurgery 1991;28:206–215
54. Loeffler JS, Alexander E, Shea WM et al: Radiosurgery as part of the initial management of patients with malignant gliomas. J Clin Oncol 1992;10:1379–1385
55. Sawaya R: Neurosurgery issues in oncology. Curr Opin Oncol 1991;3:459–466
56. Fine HA, Dear KBG, Loeffler JS et al: Meta-analysis of radiation therapy with and without adjuvant chemotherapy for malignant gliomas in adults. Cancer 1993;71:2585–2597
57. Walker MD, Alexander E Jr, Hunt WE et al: Evaluation of BCNU and/or radiotherapy in the treatment of anaplastic gliomas: a cooperative clinical trial. J Neurosurg 1978;49:333–343
58. Green SB, Byar DP, Walker MD et al: Comparisons of carmustine, procarbazine and high dose methylprednisolone as additions to surgery and radiotherapy for the treatment of malignant glioma. Cancer Treat Rep 1983;67:121–132
59. Salcman M, Kaplan RS, Ducker TB et al: The effect of age and reoperation on survival in the combined modality treatment of malignant astrocytoma. Neurosurgery 1982;10:454–463
60. DeAngelis LM, Yahalom J, Thaler HT, Kher U: Combined modality therapy for primary CNS lymphoma. J Clin Oncol 1992; 10:635–643
61. Nelson DF, Martz KL, Bonner H et al: Non-Hodgkin's lymphoma of the brain: can high dose, large volume radiation therapy improve survival? Report on a prospective trial by the Radiation Tumor Oncology Group: RTOG 8315. Int J Radiat Oncol Biol Phys 1992;23:9–17
62. Shapiro WR, Green SB, Selker RG et al: A randomized comparison of intra-arterial versus intravenous BCNU, with or without intravenous 5-fluorouracil, for newly diagnosed patients with malignant glioma. J Neurosurg 1992;76:772–781
63. Gumerlock MK, Belshe BD, Madsden R, Watts C: Osmotic blood brain barrier disruption and chemotherapy in the treatment of high grade malignant glioma: patient series and literature review. J Neurooncol 1992;12:33–46
64. Jaeckle KA, Mittelman A, Hill FH: Phase II trial of *Serratia marescens* extract in recurrent malignant astrocytoma. J Clin Oncol 1990;8:1408–1418
65. Merchant RE, McVicar DW, Merchant LH, Young HF: Treatment of recurrent malignant glioma by repeated intracerebral injections of human recombinant interleukin-2 alone or in combination with systemic interferon-alpha: results of a phase I clinical trial. J Neurooncol 1992;12:75–83
66. Yung WK: New approaches in brain tumor therapy using gene transfer and antisense nucleotides. Curr Opin Oncol 1994;6: 235–239

CHAPTER 43

Disorders of the Spinal Cord and Nerve Roots

R. A. COWIE

The majority of the pathologic processes that affect the spinal cord in the elderly are related to degenerative diseases of the spinal column, or to insufficiency of the cord's blood supply. However, old age does not exclude many of the disorders that are more commonly seen in other age groups. In most patients, a definite clinical diagnosis can be reached by taking a thorough clinical history and performing a careful examination.

Neurologic assessment in the elderly is sometimes made difficult by failure to obtain a clear history, or by the presence of osteoarthritis of the limb joints and consecutive atrophy of the musculature, which masks weakness and reflex changes. Nonetheless, analysis of the way that a neurologic disorder develops and of the pattern of neurologic signs should provide a guide to the site of the lesion, both in the transverse plane and in the longitudinal segmental level. A lesion can usually be localized in the cervical, thoracic, lumbar, or sacral segments prior to specialized neuroradiologic investigations.

Cervical Radiculopathy and Myelopathy

The neuroradiologic sequelae of degenerative disease of the cervical spine were established in the 1950s.[1] The degenerative changes of cervical spondylosis begin with desiccation and fragmentation of the intervertebral discs. As the elasticity of the annulus is reduced, the disc height diminishes. Extremes of movement are less well tolerated, and the vertebral endplates are subjected to greater stress. Secondary osteophytic spurs develop circumferentially around the disc, projecting posteriorly into the spinal canal as bony ridges. Parallel degeneration of the hypophyseal joints combines with spurs from the vertebral bodies to reduce the size of the neural foraminae. In most patients there is progressive loss of movement between vertebrae, although in some cases excessive motion between vertebrae and a degree of subluxation may develop. Pathologic changes in the ligamentum flavum cause lack of elasticity and a tendency to buckle during extension. The compressive effects of the osteophytic spurs and buckled ligamentum flavum on the spinal cord are greatest when the neck is extended.

These changes bring about restriction of the natural motion of the spinal cord and nerve roots within the spinal canal. Repetitive compression and obstruction of the radicular arteries supplying the cord in the neural foraminae may further compromise cord function. This effect is aggravated if there is occlusive vascular disease of the proximal arteries in the neck. Occasionally, acute rupture of a cervical disc can follow sudden twisting or flexion/extension movements of the neck and cause cord or nerve root compression.[2]

The older the population the more these degenerative changes increase in severity and extent. It is clear from epidemiologic studies[3] that the prevalence of degenerative changes is increased when heavy laboring work has been undertaken.

Anatomic and radiologic studies have shown that the neurologic sequelae of cervical spondylosis are more prevalent when the natural size of the spinal canal and neural foraminae is restricted.[4] However, the presence of large osteophytic ridges and subluxation of the vertebrae aggravate the situation. The C5-C6 and C6-C7 levels are most commonly affected at the point of transition from a mobile spine to the fixed section in the upper part of thorax.[5]

Clinically, there is generally loss of lordosis so the head is held flexed and downward. However, if the natural kyphosis of the thoracic spine is exaggerated there may be a compensatory extension of the upper cervical spine to maintain forward gaze. Most patients complain of recurrent neck pain and stiffness, together with crepitus on movement. Pain radiates to the occiput, shoulders, and scapula regions.

Radiculopathy

Progressive narrowing of the neural foraminae results from osteophytic ridges alongside the intervertebral discs and hypertrophy of the facet joints, and causes compression and restriction of movement of the nerve root; pain radiates down the arm in the distribution of the nerve root(s) with a deep, boring quality, aggravated by activities such as lifting and reaching. The pain is generally accompanied by paresthesiae and some sensory loss in the affected dermatomes. In some patients sensory symptoms predominate. Muscular weakness is generally mild, but occasionally wasting can occur. The appropriate reflexes are lost.

Cervical Myelopathy

Cervical spondylosis is the most frequent cause of cord compression in the elderly. The clinical spectrum is wide, depending on many interrelating factors and the pathogenesis of cord damage. Compression leads to atrophy of the anterior horn cells, and the lateral and posterior funiculi of the cord.[6] Most commonly the onset of symptoms and signs is insidious, and a clinical history may extend for many months or years before help is sought. Most frequently there is a mixed picture of lower motor neurone features in the arms, together with long tract signs below.[7]

In the upper limbs, complaints of weakness, clumsiness, and loss of dexterity are common. Muscle wasting follows segmental anterior horn cell damage, affecting proximal muscles when compression is high in the neck, or the intrinsic muscles of the hand when compression is lower. The tendon reflexes reflect the segmental cord lesion and can either be lost or exaggerated. Inversion of the radial reflex occurs when the fifth cervical segment is affected.

In contrast, there is commonly a marked lower limb spasticity when the patient complains of a heavy, leaden weakness and a tendency to drag the limb. Some degree of ataxia may be present with reduction of vibration and joint position sense. Many patients complain of paresthesiae and intermittent numbness in the upper and lower limbs.

Occasionally, symptoms may rise abruptly due to trauma, or sudden extension of the neck; in this situation a central cord syndrome is common, with painless weakness of the upper limbs and spasticity in the legs. Rarely a Brown-Séquard syndrome can be identified. These neurologic disorders can be

Figure 43-1 Lateral cervical spine radiograph showing widespread spondylosis. Note the loss of disc height and large anterior osteophytes. This patient has a small spinal canal into which project osteophytes at the posterior margin of the C3-C4 of the 4-5 discs.

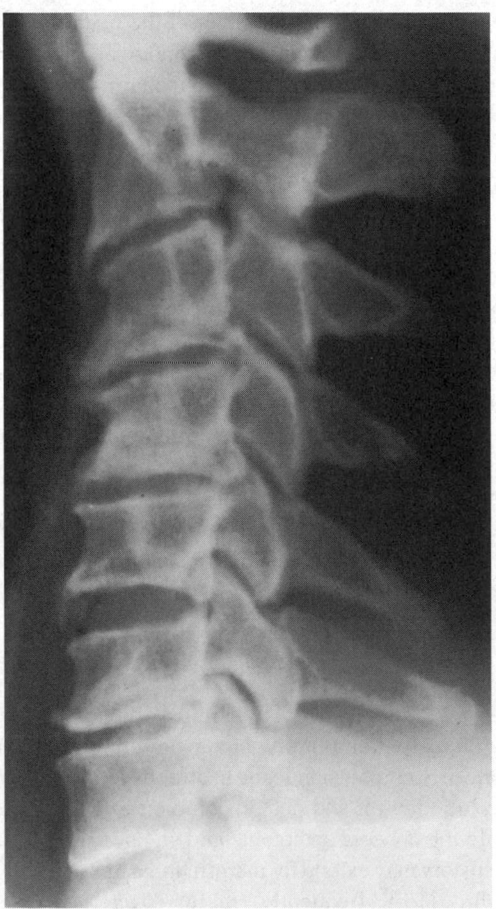

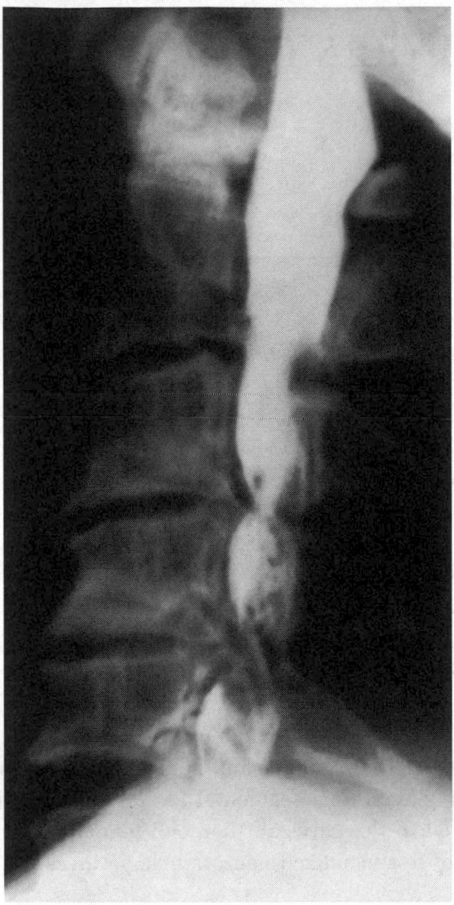

Figure 43-2 Cervical myelogram of the same patient as Figure 43-1. Note the indentations of the contrast column by the disc protrusions and osteophytes at C3-C4 and C4-C5. At C4-C5 the contrast fails to fill the subarachnoid space, indicating compression of the cord. The posterior indentation at C2-C3 is due to buckling of the ligamentum flavum.

associated with vertebrobasilar insufficiency, where symptoms are typically related to rotation and extension of the neck.

As the clinical presentation of spondylotic myelopathy varies it must be distinguished from other conditions with similar symptoms and signs including multiple sclerosis, cerebrovascular disease, cord tumor or syrinx, normal pressure hydrocephalus, amyotrophic lateral sclerosis, and peripheral neuropathies.

Investigation

Plain radiographs of the cervical spine reveal narrowing of the intervertebral disc space with sclerosis of adjacent cortical bone. Secondary anterior and posterior osteophytes are demonstrated in Figure 43-1, together with an indication of the size of the spinal canal. Oblique radiographs allow visualization of the neural foraminae. However, several authors 8 to 10 have shown that degenerative changes increase in frequency with age and that 70 to 90 percent of those over 65 years of age have radiologic abnormalities. There is poor correlation between symptomatic and asymptomatic groups and the structural changes revealed on plain radiographs.

When the clinical state suggests segmental cord or root compression and surgery is contemplated, then specialized neuroradiologic investigation is required. Figure 43-2 shows a myelogram using a water-soluble contrast medium, which reveals the degree of cord compression and nerve root pocket compression. This investigation can be supplemented by computerized tomography (CT) to clarify uncertain appearances. In addition, CT reveals the size and shape of the vertebral canals, but cannot given details of vertebral movements, disc protrusion, and corrugation of the bulging longitudinal ligament unless contrast medium has been injected. Magnetic resonance imaging (MRI), which has largely replaced myelography, reveals degeneration of intervertebral discs, the size of osteophytes, and the presence and degree of cord compression

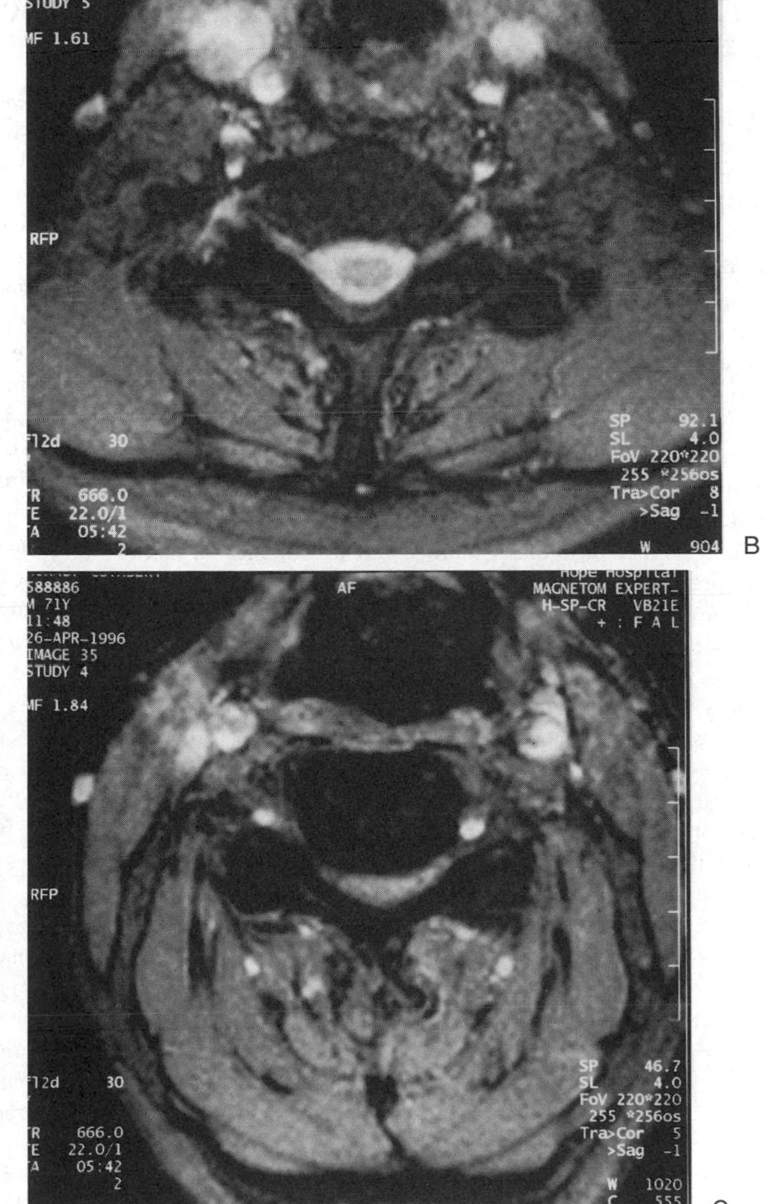

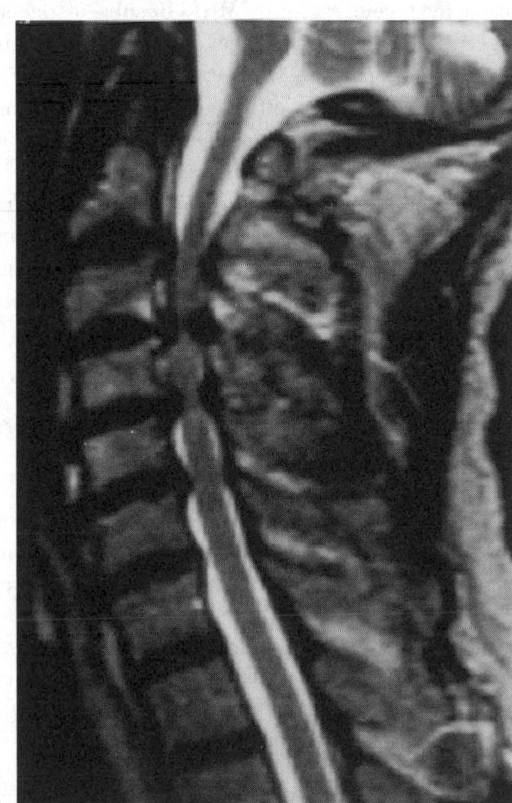

Figure 43-3 (**A**) Lateral magnetic resonance image of the cervical spine reveals compression of the spinal cord by posterior osteophyte and buckling of the ligamentum flavum. (**B**) Transverse image of normal cervical spine reveals spinal cord surrounded by cerebrospinal fluid. (**C**) Transverse image of patient seen in (**A**) shows severe narrowing of spinal canal and compression of the spinal cord.

(Fig. 43-3). It is the only method that allows visualization of intrinsic disorders of the spinal cord.

Management

Patients with neck pain and radiculopathy generally respond to a treatment regimen that includes a support collar, restriction of upper limb and shoulder movement, and nonsteroidal anti-inflammatory drugs, supplemented by other oral analgesics, if necessary. Physical methods of treatment and the application of local heat pads may be soothing. If the symptoms are severe, bed rest and cervical traction may relieve symptoms. Lees and Turner[12] showed that 22 of 51 patients were symptom-free within a few months and generally remained symptom-free during follow-up. These authors showed that patients with radiculopathy rarely progress to a myelopathic state.

Surgery is not generally required unless progressive motor and sensory deficits lead to loss of function of the upper limbs. Both anterior and posterior approaches can be used to decompress the nerve roots; each carries a good prognosis for neurologic recovery,[13–15] although recovery of muscle wasting is rarely satisfactory. The decision to operate is made after taking into account the severity of the disability, its effect on the patient's everyday life, and the patient's ability to withstand surgery.

The natural history of myelopathy complicating cervical spondylosis is variable and unpredictable; many patients run a chronic course characterized by episodes of deterioration separated by periods of stability.[7,12] The majority of elderly patients with cervical myelopathy will not need surgical intervention. Surgical treatment is indicated when the myelopathy interferes with daily activities, where there is a short progressive history, or when there is radiologic evidence of severe cord compression and/or instability. Anterior decompression of disc and osteophytic spurs is usually carried out when one or two intervertebral levels are affected, whereas laminectomy is indicated for more widespread stenosis and compression of the spinal cord. In general, the prime objective of surgery is to halt the decline in neurologic function before irreversible damage to the cord has occurred. There is poor correlation between the presenting severity, the duration of the symptoms, and the outcome.[4] Hukaka et al.[16] found that posterior decompression gave better results for more advanced myelopathy and that a short duration of symptoms was associated with better results, although these were not influenced by the age of the patient. Phillips[17] suggested that those patients with focal disease who underwent anterior surgery had a better outcome. However, some patients continued to deteriorate, in spite of adequate decompression, possibly because of vascular insufficiency.[7]

Spinal Cord Compression and Thoracic Disc Protrusion

The central protrusion of a thoracic intervertebral disc is an unusal cause of cord compression, but one that occurs in older age groups, as it is associated with degeneration of the disc annulus. Russell[18] noted that 67 percent occurred between the eighth and eleventh interspaces. The majority of patients present with a long history of gradually progressive myelopathy where sensory and motor symptoms are equally common. However, 49 percent of patients complained of radicular symptoms of pain and dysesthesiae. Sometimes the onset is more rapid, leading to a flaccid paraplegia.[19]

The presence of a thoracic disc protrusion is generally recognized when MRI is carried out to investigate the progressive neurologic deficit. Cord compression from this source carries a poor prognosis unless surgery is performed. The results of simple decompressive laminectomy are unsatisfactory and either costotransversectomy, transpedicular, or transthoracic approach is recommended.[18,20]

Cord Compression From Intradural Tumors

Intradural extramedullary tumors cause local compression of the spinal cord and nerve roots. Meningiomas represent approximately 25 percent of primary spinal cord tumors, and 80 percent of them occur in females. They are most commonly seen in the sixth decade, rather later than for neurofibromas; 80 percent occur in the thoracic spine. The majority of patients complain of local or radicular pain the significance of which often goes unrecognized for a long period until progressive spastic paraparesis, followed by sensory and bladder dysfunction, develops.[21]

Plain radiographs are rarely helpful, and the condition is only diagnosed by myelography or MRI. Results of decompressive surgery are generally good. Levy et al.[22] reported that one-third of paraplegic patients were able to walk after tumor excision. Neurofibromas are slightly more common than meningiomas, but because their peak incidence is in younger age groups, they are less frequently encountered in the elderly.[23] Radicular pain is more common, and enlargement of a neural foramen may be seen on plain radiographs if the tumor extends into the paravertebral tissues. Multiple tumors can be encountered in neurofibromatosis. As with meningiomas, surgical excision should be undertaken and carries a good prognosis for neurologic recovery.[24]

Metastatic Spinal Tumors

The most common extradural and spinal tumors to cause cord compression are those metastasizing from distant carcinomas or primary hematologic tumors. Spread may be hematogenous or via the vertebral venous plexus. Although myeloma and carcinomas of prostate and kidney seem to metastasize preferentially to the spine, in practice the most commonly encountered tumors are those that occur with the greatest frequency in the community. Therefore, primary lung, breast, kidney, and prostate tumors are seen, although in some patients the primary tumor cannot be identified. The thoracic section of the spine is most frequently involved, followed by the lumbosacral and cervical regions.

The majority of patients present with progressive walking difficulty, due to weakness and clumsiness, the significance of which may go unrecognized until the patient is no longer able to bear weight. Many patients have a history of preceding spinal pain, which should always lead to a suspicion of vertebral metastasis in a patient known to have malignant disease. The neurologic deficit may develop very rapidly, with collapse of the vertebra, or occlusion of the vascular supply to the cord. An analysis of the level of the sensory deficit helps in assessing the site of the spinal disease and planning the appropriate radiologic investigations. However, plain radiographs of all of the spine and chest should be carried out, and may reveal loss of outline of a pedicle, reduction in height of a vertebral body, or a soft tissue mass. MRI of the spine is the investigation of choice. However, CT may reveal evidence of bone destruction and allow percutaneous needle biopsy of the lesion.

There has been considerable debate about the value of decompressive surgery, as a laminectomy alone produces poor results.[25–27] If there has been collapse of the vertebral body, better results can be obtained by excision of the tumor, insertion of a bone graft, and stabilization of the spine.[28] Alternatively, radiotherapy under steroid cover can be carried out, particularly if the patient presents in the early stages of cord compression and cord compression is incomplete.[29] It has been shown that a long history is associated with a better prognosis after treatment, and that rapid loss of power is associated with a poor outcome.[30] Other features associated with a poor outcome are a paraplegia of greater than 24 hours' duration, collapse of the vertebral body, and metastasis from bronchogenic carcinomas. The prognosis is best in those whose neurologic function is preserved prior to surgery, or when there is compression of the cauda equina, rather than the spinal cord.[31]

Vascular Disorders of the Spinal Cord

The peculiar anatomic arrangement of the arterial blood supply of the spinal cord may protect it from the effects of occlusion of one feeding vessel. The anterior and posterior spinal arteries are fed by radicular arteries, which are branches of vessels arising from either the aorta or the subclavian arteries. There is generally a large feeding artery in the lower thoracic region, most commonly on the left at T10. A watershed lies at the second thoracic segment of the spinal cord, between areas supplied by thoracic vessels and those from the neck. Interruption of supply can occur in atheroma of the aorta,[32] in dissecting aneurysm,[33] or as a complication of aortic surgery.[34] The extent and severity of the spinal cord neurologic deficit varies considerably, probably depending on the anatomic variation of the spinal cord vessels in the individual patient.

The syndrome of the anterior spinal artery arises when this vessel is obstructed by thrombus. The posterior columns receiving a blood supply from the posterior spinal network are preserved, so that proprioception remains intact, whereas thermal and pain appreciation is impaired. In addition, a lower motor paralysis of the arms is associated with spastic paraparesis, or paraplegia. In some cases, the presence of cervical spondylosis and an osteophytic ridge has been implicated in local occlusion of the anterior spinal artery.[35]

Paget's Disease

Paget's disease is a generally progressive disorder of bone that causes neurologic sequelae of the brain, spinal cord, or peripheral nerves, depending on which bones are involved. It is important to recognize these complications, as many respond to treatment of the underlying disorder. In the spine, pagetic changes may affect one or several vertebrae. The disease is characterized by bony destruction followed by repair, which leads to flattening and expansion of the diameter of the vertebral bodies, and thickening of the pedicles and laminae. Bony projections in the vertebral canal cause spinal cord and nerve root compression. Neurologic symptoms may develop suddenly if collapse of a vertebral body occurs.

Spinal cord compression is most common in the thoracic region, and is generally slowly progressive, causing a spastic weakness of the lower limbs combined with sensory symptoms and signs. Pain may be due to local bony changes, malignant degeneration, or nerve root compression. In some patients progressive myelopathy occurs, yet myelography fails to reveal direct compression of the spinal cord. In these patients progressive ischemia may be the cause of neurologic deterioration.

When the disease affects the lumbar region, symptoms of single or multiple nerve root compression can develop, producing back pain and sciatica. When the spinal canal is constricted, neurogenic claudication may be the presenting symptom.

Surgical treatment is indicated only when medical treatment fails to control the progression of the neurologic sequelae of the condition. However, control of blood loss from the diseased bone during surgery can be very troublesome.[36,37]

Neurologic Complications of Degenerative Disease of the Lumbar Spine

Spondylosis of the lumbar spine increases in severity and extent with advancing age, often occurring simultaneously with disease in the cervical region.[3] Biochemical and pathologic changes are similar at both sites. Loss of disc height and the development of traction spurs and osteophytes are associated with sclerosis and enlargement of the vertebral bodies. Simultaneous changes in the facet joints occur, with destruction of articular cartilage, laxity of the joint capsule, and osteophytic enlargement of the joint surfaces.[38] This process may be asymmetric, so that rotational subluxation of one vertebra on the other can develop. The lowest intervertebral discs of the lumbar spine are most commonly affected at the point of transition from the mobile lumbar spine to the fixed sacrum.

A number of discrete neurologic conditions may complicate lumbar spondylosis, as follows.

Acute Nerve Root Entrapment

True herniation of an intervertebral disc can occur in the elderly and produce a pattern of symptoms and signs similar to that seen in younger patients.[39] However, the elderly have a higher incidence of motor deficit and are more likely to have a sequestrated disc nucleus compared with the average adult population.

Chronic Nerve Root Entrapment

Lumbar mono- and polyradiculopathy occur in the elderly, more commonly as a result of nerve root compression in the lateral recess of the spinal canal, and in the neural foramen, than from disc rupture. As degeneration of the intervertebral disc advances, there is loss of disc height and formation of osteophytes that bulge into the neural foramen; hypertrophy of the facet joint further compromises its capacity. At the same time, partial subluxation of the posterior joint with upward and forward movement of the superior articular surface narrows the lateral recess of the spinal canal.[40] At first extension and rotation of the spine aggravate the process, so that dynamic stenosis may produce intermittent compression and symptoms, although, as the condition advances, permanent compression occurs.

Typically, patients complain of pain and stiffness of the back, accompanied by the insidious onset of sciatic pain. These symptoms are generally aggravated by standing or walking and relieved by rest or lying, particularly when the spine is flexed. Patients complain of paresthesiae in the legs, which are also precipitated by the same types of activity. In chronic nerve root entrapment due to stenosis, coughing and straining aggravate the pain, and nerve root stretch tests are generally negative. Some patients show mild weakness of the legs, although objective sensory deficits are rare. The progression of symptoms and signs is generally much slower than for a herniated nucleus pulposus.[41–43]

Nerve root entrapment may complicate degenerative spondylolisthesis. This develops when degeneration of the facet joints and laxity of the disc annulus allow the upper vertebral body to slide forward on the lower. The L4-L5 intervertebral joint is most commonly affected, but other intervertebral levels can be involved[44] and produce sciatic pain and symptoms of nerve root compression.

Neurogenic Claudication

Narrowing of the central spinal canal can develop as a result of a combination of degenerative hypertrophy of the facet joints, hypertrophy and corrugation of the ligamentum flavum, and bulging of the disc and osteophytes. As the available space in the spinal canal narrows, there is compression of multiple nerve roots of the cauda equina and its circulation. The symptoms of claudication develop. Bilateral leg pain is precipitated by walking or standing and improved with rest, especially when the spine is flexed or when the patient sits or squats.[43]

Patients frequently develop a stooped posture. As the distance walked increases, a heavy leaden weakness builds up in intensity, accompanied by burning paresthesiae and a fear of the limb giving way.[45] Sometimes neurologic signs are present only after an exercise provocation test on a treadmill.

In the elderly the clinical picture is often confused with the effects of peripheral vascular disease. Sharr et al.[46] reported that urinary symptoms due to a neuropathic bladder often complicate central stenosis of the spinal canal.

Investigation

The extent and severity of degenerative changes of the discs and facet joints is revealed by plain radiographs. However, radiculography, using a water-soluble contrast agent, can be employed to confirm the presence of nerve root compression (Fig. 43-4). This investigation is indicated only when surgical treatment is planned, and has been superseded by CT and MRI, which reveal the cross-sectional anatomy of the spinal and neural canals, and can analyze the degree of degeneration

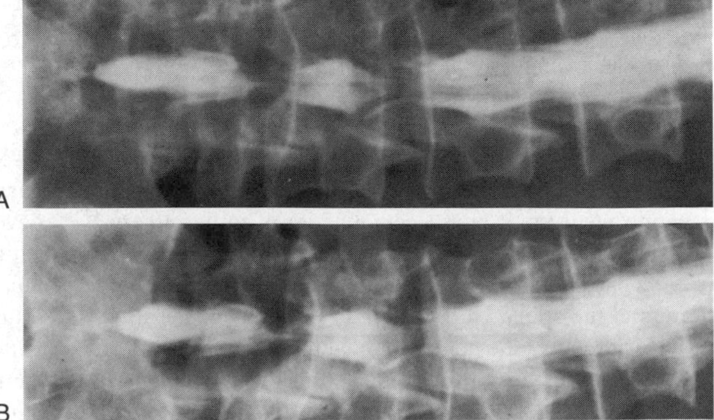

Figure 43-4 A lumbar radiculogram in an elderly patient with degenerative spondylosis and neurogenic claudication. The contrast column and root pockets fail to fill at the L3-L4 and L4-L5 levels.

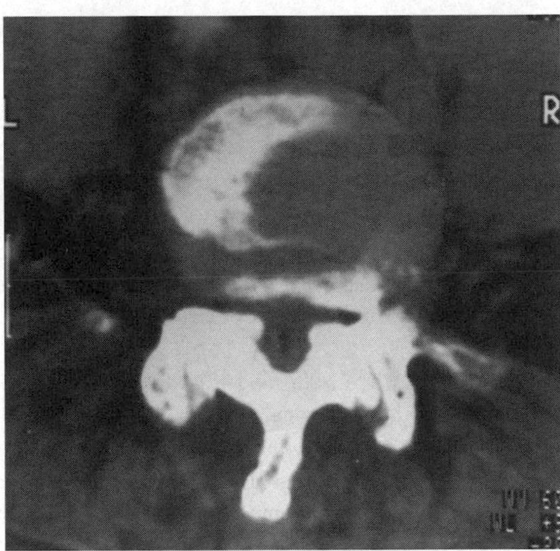

Figure 43-5 Computed tomography of the lumbar spine in a patient with advanced spondylosis and stenosis of the spinal canal. By a combination of disc bulging and hypertrophy of the hypophyseal joints, the spinal canal is reduced to a trefoil shape.

of the disc (Fig. 43-5). However, only MRI can adequately display detail of the neural structures.

Radionuclide scanning is generally not helpful, as increased uptake is common in areas of osteoarthritis, but can exclude spinal infection or neoplasm.

Management

The majority of elderly patients do not require surgical decompression, and their symptoms can be controlled by analgesic and anti-inflammatory medication and modification of their activities of daily living. Rest and physical treatment, combined with restriction of spinal movement, often produce satisfactory results. However, the elderly withstand surgery well, and age alone is rarely a contraindication to operation. Surgery is indicated when sciatic pain and other symptoms significantly reduce a patient's physical capacity, or cannot be controlled by medical treatment. Signs of severe nerve root compression, such as weakness or sensory loss, neurogenic claudication, and cauda equina compression are firm indications for surgical intervention. The aim of surgery is to decompress the spinal canal and neural foraminae, thus freeing the nerve roots. Getty et al.[47, 48] obtained satisfactory results in 85 percent of patients after a partial undercutting facetectomy. However, low backache persists after surgery in many patients, due to the background degenerative changes, and patients must be advised accordingly.[49, 50]

References

1. Brain WR, Northfield D, Wilkinson M: The neurological manifestations of cervical spondylosis. Brain 1952;75:187–225
2. Young S, O'Laoire S: Cervical disc prolapse in the elderly: an easily overlooked, reversible cause of spinal cord compression. Br J Neurosurg 1987;1:93–98
3. Lawrence JS: Disc degeneration. Its frequency and relationship to symptoms. Ann Rheum Dis 1969;28:121
4. Nurick G: The natural history and the results of surgical treatment of the spinal cord disorder associated with cervical spondylosis. Brain 1972;95:101–108
5. Henderson CM: Posterio-lateral foraminotomy as an exclusive operative technique for cervical radiculopathy: a review of 846 consecutively operated cases. Neurosurgery 1983;13:504–512
6. Ito T, Oyanagi K, Takahashi H, Takahashi ME: Cervical spondylotic myelopathy clinicopathologic study on the progression pattern and thin myelinated fibres of the lesions of seven patients examined during complete autopsy. Spine 1996;21: 827–833
7. Bernhardt M, Hynes RA, Blume HW, White AA: Current concepts review: cervical spondylotic myelopathy. J Bone Joint Surg 1993;75A:119–128
8. Pallis C, Jones AM, Spillaine JD: Cervical spondylosis: incidence and implications. Brain 1954;77:274–289
9. McRae DL: The significance of abnormalities of the cervical spine. AJR 1960;84:3–25
10. Gore DR, Sepic SB, Gardner GM: Roentgenographic findings of the cervical spine in asymptomatic people. Spine 1986;11: 521–524
11. Yu YL, du Boulay AH, Stevens JM, Kendall BE: Computed tomography in cervical spondylitic myelopathy and radiculopathy: visualisation of structures, myelographic comparison, cord measurements and clinical ability. Brain 1986;109:421–428
12. Lees F, Turner JW: Natural history and prognosis of cervical spondylosis. BMJ 1963;1:1607–1610
13. Dillin W, Booth R, Cuckler J et al: Cervical radiculopathy: a review. Spine 1985;11:998–991
14. Hunt WE: Cervical spondylosis: natural history and rare indications for surgical decompression. Clin Neurosurg 1980;27: 466–480
15. Lunsford DL, Bissonette DJ, Zorub PA, Zorub DS: Anterior surgery for cervical disease, part 2: treatment of cervical spondylotic myelopathy: 32 cases. J Neurosurg 1980;53:12–19
16. Hukaka S, Mochizuki T, Ogata M et al: Operations for cervical spondylotic myelopathy. J Bone Joint Surg 1985;67B:609–615
17. Phillips DG: Surgical treatment of myelopathy with cervical spondylosis. J Neurol Neurosurg Psychiatry 1973;36:879
18. Russell T: Thoracic intervertebral disc protrusion: experience of 67 cases and review of the literature. Br J Neurosurg 1989; 3:153–160
19. Perot PL: Thoracic disc disease. In Wilkins RH, Rengachary SS (eds): Neurosurgery. McGraw-Hill, New York, 1985
20. Young S, Karr G, O'Laoire S: Spinal cord compression due to thoracic disc herniation: results of microsurgical posterolateral costotransversectomy. Br J Neurosurg 1989;3:31–38
21. Zeidman SM, Ellenbogen RG, Ducker TB: Intradural tumours. Semin Spine Surg 1995;1:323–338
22. Levy WJ, Bay J, Dohn D: Spinal cord meningioma. J Neurosurg 1982;57:804–812
23. Gautier-Smith PC: Clinical aspects of spinal neurofibroma. Brain 1967;90:359–394

24. Nittner KM: pp. 177–322. In Vinker PJ, Bruyn GW eds: Handbook of Clinical Neurology. Vol. 20. North Holland, Amsterdam, 1976
25. Findlay GFG: Adverse effects of the management of malignant spinal cord compression. J Neurol Neurosurg Psychiatry 1984; 47:761–768
26. Findlay GFG: The role of vertebral body collapse in the management of malignant spinal cord compression. J Neurol Neurosurg Psychiatry 1987;50:151–154
27. Findlay GFG: Compressive and vascular disorders of the spinal cord. In Miller JD (ed): Northfield's Surgery of the Central Nervous System. 2nd Ed. Blackwell, Oxford, 1987
28. Black P: Spinal metastasis: current status and recommended guidelines for management. Neurosurgery 1979;5:726–746
29. Cobb CA, Leavens ME, Eckles N: Indications for non-operative treatment of spinal cord compression due to breast cancer. J Neurosurg 1977;47:653–658
30. Chade HO: pp. 415–434. In Vinken PJ, Bruyn GW (eds): Handbook of Clinical Neurology. Vol. 20. North Holland, Amsterdam, 1976
31. Seigal T, Seigal T: Neoplastic epidural spinal cord compression: pathophysiology and prognostic factors. Semin Spine Surg 7: 269–276
32. Kochar G, Kotler NN, Hartman J et al: Thrombosed aorta resulting in spinal cord ischaemia and paraplegia in ischaemia cardiomyopathy. Am Heart J 1987;113:1510–1513
33. Braunstein H: Pathogenesis of dissecting aneurysm. Circulation 1963;28:1071–1080
34. Hughes JT: Vascular disorders of the spinal cord. In Tolle JF (ed): Handbook of Clinical Neurology. Vol. 55. Vascular Diseases. Part III. Elsevier, Amsterdam, 1989
35. Hughes JT, Brownwell B: Cervical spondylosis complicated by anterior spinal artery thrombosis. Neurology 1964;14: 1073–1077
36. Douglas DL, Duckworth T, Kanis JA et al: Spinal cord dysfunction in Paget's disease of bone. J Bone Joint Surg 1981;63B: 495–503
37. Schmidek HH, Waters A: Neural dysfunction in Paget's disease of bone. In Wilkins RH, Rengachary SS (eds): Neurosurgery. McGraw-Hill, New York, 1985
38. Yong-Hing K, Kirlaldy-Willis WH: The pathophysiology of degenerative disease of the lumbar spine. Orthop Clin North Am 1983;14:491–504
39. Maistrelli GL, Vaughan PA, Evans DC, Barrington TW: Lumbar disc herniation in the elderly. Spine 1987;12:63–66
40. Reynolds AF, Weinstein PR, Wachter RD: Lumbar monoradiculopathy due to unilateral facet hypertrophy. Neurosurgery 1987;10:480–486
41. Ciric I, Mikhael MA, Tarkington JA, Vick NA: The lateral recess syndrome. A variant of spinal stenosis. J Neurosurg 1980;53: 433–443
42. Kirkaldy-Willis WH, Wedge JH, Yong-Hing K et al: Lumbar spinal nerve lateral entrapment. Clin Orthop 1992;169: 171–178
43. Dillin W, Watkins R: Natural history of lumbar spinal stenosis: clinical features. Semin Spine Surg 1994;6:84–89
44. Cauchoix J, Benoist M, Chassaing V: Degenerative spondylolisthesis. Clin Orthop 1976;115:122–129
45. Paine KWE: Clinical features of lumbar spinal stenosis. Clin Orthop 115:77–82
46. Sharr MM, Garfield JS, Jenkins JD: Lumbar spondylosis and neuropathic bladder: investigation of 73 patients with chronic urinary symptoms. BMJ 1976;1:695–697
47. Getty CJM, Johnson JR, Kirwan EOG, Sullivan MF: Partial undercutting facetectomy for bony entrapment of the lumbar nerve root. J Bone Joint Surg 1981;63B:330–335
48. Getty CJM: Lumbar spinal stenosis. The clinical spectrum and the results of operation. J Bone Joint Surg 1980;62B:481–485
49. Barr JS, Riseborough EJ: Treatment of low back and sciatic pain in patients over 60 years of age. Clin Orthop 1965;26: 12–18
50. Simon SD, Silver CM, Litchman HM: Lumbar disk surgery in the elderly (over the age of 60). Clin Orthop 1965;41:157–162

CHAPTER 44

Head Trauma in the Geriatric Patient

SHELDON JACOBSON

The problem of head injury in the geriatric patient looms as one of the key decision-making areas for the clinician. There is a significant potential for serious errors, and for this reason the clinician has to be ever vigilant for the patient with occult central nervous system (CNS) injury as well as the acutely injured and unstable patient. The incidence of head injuries for all ages is approximately 220/100,000 population/y.[1] The data on overall death rate is more difficult to find; however, brain injury is felt to be the major cause of death in 40 to 50 percent of all traumatic deaths. In 1990, there were approximately 150,000 traumatic deaths in the United States and thus about 60,000 brain injury deaths. The incidence of head injury peaks at ages 15 to 24 with incidences ranging from 250 to 400 cases per 100,000 per year and falls progressively until the late 60s to early 70s where there is a secondary but much lower peak incidence of approximately 250/100,000 population.[2] Whereas automobile accidents are the most frequent cause of head trauma in younger adults, the majority of head injuries in geriatric patients are due to falls.[3] Alcohol plays a major role in all types of accidents. In motor vehicle accidents, MacMillan[3] reports higher incidence in pedestrians (34 percent) compared to occupants of vehicles (29 percent).

Geriatric patients with head injuries enter the emergency or geriatric health care system in a number of characteristic ways: (1) acute presentation following a fall or other accident and/or after being assaulted; (2) subacute presentation in which the patient presents with headache, nausea, or vomiting, with or without a change in mental status several days following an injury;(3) patients presenting with a change in mental status who after workup are found to have a chronic subdural hematoma.

The evaluation of the geriatric patient with potentially significant head trauma is often difficult because of a pre-existing neurologic and cognitive impairment or there may be an acute change in mental status unrelated to the trauma. In the latter group, one would include delirium due to toxic and metabolic disturbances or cognitive deficits caused by a new cerebrovascular event. Obviously patients with delirium are more likely to sustain injury from falls and on more than one occasion patients will have both a delirium and evidence of a new intracranial injury. There is also epidemiologic evidence that previous head trauma is a risk factor for the development of Alzheimer's and Parkinson's diseases.[4–6]

A vexing and obfuscating problem is the relatively high incidence of small intracranial fluid collections in the elderly that are chronic and usually do not have any clinical significance. These include small subdural hematomas and subdural hygromas. Lesions should only be thought of as having pathophysiologic significance if the patient's presentation and the neurologic localization is consistent with the location of the lesion and the neuroimaging study shows localized brain swelling or evidence of mass effect.

The high incidence of underlying cardiopulmonary and neurologic diseases presents an added complexity in determining if the injury was sustained due to a "simple accident" or was caused by a preceding transient loss of consciousness. The patient's traumatic event was preceded by a syncopal episode, a transient cardiac rhythm disturbance, a seizure, or a hypoglycemic episode to name but a few common precipitating scenarios.

Classification of Head Trauma

Traditionally head trauma has been classified as open (compound) and closed depending on whether there has been a breach of the integrity of the cranial vault. Thus skull fractures associated with an overlying laceration are considered open injuries as are basilar skull fractures. In basilar skull fractures there is the potential for communication between the intracranial contents and a nasal sinus or the nasopharynx with the associated risk of infection. Skull fractures are also defined by whether they are simple (undisplaced) or whether they are depressed. Thus a patient with a closed head may have a compound depressed skull fracture or a linear undisplaced fracture. Another definition of head injury seeks to separate the wounding process into penetrating and nonpenetrating injuries (blunt head injury). Penetrating injuries are variants of open head injuries in which a wound has been created by a missile or sharp object that has violated both the cranium and the intracranial structures.

The patient with a skull fracture and/or a scalp laceration has to be considered with the context of the associated signs and symptoms as to whether there is an accompanying intracranial injury as well. In many patients, the scalp injury and the simple fracture merely indicate that the traumatic event caused tissue disruption in these structures but does not necessarily indicate underlying intracranial injury. Although these patients require careful investigation for a CNS injury, many do not have evidence of an associated intracranial injury as the energy delivered by the wounding mechanism of injury has been absorbed and dissipated by the scalp and the cranium, which have functioned, as designed, to protect the brain.

An exception to this is the situation that obtains with respect to depressed skull fractures. The energy associated with the mechanism of injury directed at the site(s) of injury is proportionately greater than that associated with undisplaced fracture and the likelihood of underlying brain injury is higher as is the incidence of post-traumatic epilepsy.

The classic categories of head injury include the following pathologic entities: concussion, brain contusion, laceration and hematoma, diffuse axonal injury, and epidural and subdural hematoma. In most patients, with the possible exceptions of the patient with a chronic subdural or epidural hematoma, a number of these pathologic entities are present simultaneously so that it would be unusual to see one of these significant conditions as an isolated entity.

Overview and Management of Important Pathologic and Pathophysiologic Entities

Scalp Laceration

The scalp consists of five tissue elements: skin, subcutaneous tissue, loose areolar layer, galea (the aponeurosis of the temporalis muscle), and the periosteum of the skull. It is involved in body temperature regulation and has a massive blood supply far in excess of the metabolic requirements of the local tissues and thus scalp lacerations are notorious for multiple simultaneous arterial bleeders with the potential of causing significant blood loss.

The bleeding can be controlled by direct pressure and then by infiltrating the wound edges with 1 or 2 percent lidocaine with epinephrine and everting the edges. Clamping and tying individual bleeders is futile. Ranney clips, which resemble plastic paper clips, can be applied to the wound edges. The wound is then irrigated until clear and digitally explored to palpate the underlying skull for depressed fracture and crepities and foreign bodies.

To facilitate closure of an uncomplicated scalp laceration, it is best to use longer stay sutures, #00 or #000, to coapt the edges to tamponade the bleeding, and then use fine suture material to close the wound edges. It is often necessary to clip hair away at the wound edges to facilitate placement of sutures. We prefer not to shave a large swatch of hair from about the laceration as this does not greatly help the closure and the impact to the patient of a large hairless defect adds to the psychic repercussions of the injury. If necessary, the hair can be parted and matted down with surgilube.

When closing a scalp laceration unassociated with an open or penetrating head injury, it is not necessary to close the galea as a separate layer using subcuticular sutures. If there is an open head injury, the laceration should not be sutured unless there is a delay in neurosurgical consultation. In all likelihood, when definitive neurosurgical care is completed the scalp will be closed in layers.

Concussion

Concussion is defined as a transient loss of consciousness following a direct blow to the head or following sudden deceleration or acceleration forces brought to bear on the head as the major mechanism of injury. These shearing forces may act to compress the reticular activating system directly or interfere with its blood supply. The period of unconsciousness is usually less than 5 minutes and is followed by gradual return to baseline functioning over the next hour or so. The patient will have retrograde amnesia for a period consisting of a few minutes to several hours preceding the accident. Prolonged unconsciousness or continued cognitive impairment should be considered to reflect possible structural brain injury until proven otherwise but is also compatible with a more protracted form of "simple concussion." Indeed it was formally believed that concussion syndrome was a functional entity unassociated with underlying injury. It is now known that the syndrome may be associated with permanent cognitive and functional impairments. This is an area of current controversy as the differentiation of premorbid deficits, litigation-related factors, and true trauma-related residual deficits is quite difficult to separate. It is probably fair to say that the greater the insult the greater will be the period of unconsciousness, and retrograde and anterograde amnesia. Following the acute concussion, most patients will have subacute to chronic sequelae consisting of persisting headaches, ataxia, vertigo, sleep abnormalities, and mild cognitive impairment. Finally there are clearly a number of patients with head injuries who have the acute syndrome and the late syndromes who were not unconscious during the period of injury.

Concussed patients who have had serious underlying pathology ruled out by computed tomography (CT) or magnetic resonance imaging (MRI) scans and who continue to have symptoms are a difficult group to manage. By and large they will also improve spontaneously over time but require support from their physicians, family, friends, and employers to tide them over very rough waters. A team approach to care of the patient is invaluable. The team should be managed by the patient's primary physician and include the neurologist, psychologist, neuropsychologist, and other rehabilitation professionals.

Diffuse Axonal Injury

Diffuse axonal injury is an entity that merges with and represents a progression from the milder injury of concussion. It too is felt to be caused by the angular or rotational acceleration or deceleration of the brain most often associated with automobile accidents. The neuronal elements of the white matter are stretched and/or torn. This injury is associated with a poor prognosis as it has a proclivity for evolving into a phase where vasogenic cerebral edema is the paramount issue. Patients with severe diffuse axonal injury are usually comatose or at least severely impaired following their injury and deteriorate progressively with the worsening cerebral edema. Management of these patients requires neurosurgical intensive care using intracranial pressure monitoring. Many of these patients will have other brain injuries requiring neurosurgical intervention such as acute subdural hematoma and large intracerebral hematomas, but the lesions of diffuse neural injury are managed nonsurgically.

Subdural Hematomas

Subdural hematomas[7] are classically divided into acute, subacute, and chronic categories. For the purposes of this discussion, acute and subacute subdural hematomas are considered together. These lesions result from angular or rotational effects where the shearing forces are vectored at the bridging arterioles and venules in the subdural space. The mechanism of injury for these lesions is similar to that of diffuse axonal injury and indeed they often coexist. Intracerebral hematomas and lacerations often have a polar location at the frontal, temporal, or occipital poles because they often are a part of a coup or contra coup lesion complex. These patients are usually very severely injured and will require neurosurgical intensive care and evacuation of the hematomas if they are thought to be a major cause of the patient's deterioration and they are felt to be salvagable.

Chronic subdural hematomas[8] are in a class by themselves because they are in adults almost uniquely a disease of the geriatric patient. The initial traumatic event is usually trivial or completely unnoticed by the patient and his or her family. Predisposing factors include brain atrophy, atheroscleroses, seizure disorders, and primary or iatrogenic coagulopathy. The initial subdural hemorrhage is usually a small collection located over the hemispheres and goes unnoticed perhaps because brain atrophy provides some initial space for hematoma expansion without significantly affecting the underlying brain. A capsule forms about the hematoma and the hematoma becomes chronic and breaks down to "motor oil" consistency. At this point the hematoma may resolve spontaneously or continue to grow in volume. The capsule that forms about the hematoma becomes vascularized. Expansion of the fluid collection when it occurs is either due to microhemorrhages from the fragile capsular vessels, osmotic shifts of fluid into the hematoma, or both mechanisms. As the hematoma progressively enlarges, it eventually reaches a critical size where the intracranial pressure becomes elevated and results in brain compression and shift and neurologic dysfunction becomes overt.

The most common presentation of this group of patients is with progressive dementia usually unassociated with other focal neurologic signs. Less common presentations include generalized seizures and isolated focal neurologic deficits. Late in the course the patient can develop a herniation syndrome, either uncal or central syndromes or both. These patients become lethargic, somnolent, and develop acute focal neural deficits, usually a homolateral dilated and fixed pupil and a contralateral hemiparesis. At this point, the process is life threatening and immediate evacuation of the hematoma is mandatory.

Epidural Hematomas

Epidural hematomas are thought to be caused by direct contact with the scalp of the wounding object resulting in skull fractures or shearing stress to the meningeal vessels that run in concavities of the inner table of the skull. The injury results in arterial bleeding into the epidural space. About 70 percent of epidural hematomas occur in the temporal area from injury to the middle meningeal artery or vein. Interestingly, epidural hematomas are less frequent in the geriatric population either due to a different mechanism of injury or to the more adherent attachment of the dura to the calvarium in the elderly. Because of the rapid ingress of blood into the epidural space, this process is fast moving following the initial injury and in the concussive period the patient is lucid and deteriorates rapidly. However, some patients with epidural hematomas never have a noticeable lucid interval, enter the hospital in coma, and continue to decline inexorably without evacuation of the hematoma.

Missile Injuries

The material in this chapter deals with the closed head injured patient because the survival of all patients who sustain gunshot wounds to the head is quite poor. Kaufman et al.[9] reported that 60 percent of cranial gunshot victims died in the field and only 38 percent of those hospitalized eventually were discharged from the hospital. The mortality rates for hospitalized patients in other studies ranges between 50 and 60 percent. The mortality of geriatric patients with these injuries is substantially higher. The management of these patients requires neurosurgical and intensive care resources, discussions of which are beyond the scope of this chapter.

Associated Spinal Injuries

A patient with an acute significant head injury has to be considered to have an associated spinal injury until proven otherwise.[10] The exact incidence varies with the series; however, an incidence of about 6 percent is usually given. The vast majority of these are cervical spine injuries. In a series of patients arriving in the emergency department with predominant spinal injuries, 24 percent had associated head injuries. Some of the spinal injuries are potentially unstable but have not as yet affected the spinal cord. Thus the potentially at-risk spinal cord must be protected by full spinal immobilization until the spine has been cleared by physical examination as well as appropriate imaging studies. High-dose methylprednisolone has been found to have a modest effect in lowering the ultimate deficit in spinal-cord-injured patients when administered within 8 hours of injury. This is yet another, albeit less compelling, reason for early detection of associated spinal injuries.

Initial Evaluation and Management

The material in this section is in two subsections because of the markedly different presentation management options and differential diagnoses of acute and subacute head trauma versus chronic subdural hematomas.

Acute and Subacute Head Trauma

Patients with acute and subacute head trauma will present to the physician with a history of a recent injury or be brought to an emergency department by ambulance following the injury. For all but the most trivial injuries, the patient should receive stereotypic and algorithmic initial trauma management until the resultant CNS injury can be identified and stabilized. Thus the patient should be immobilized to a long board and fitted with an extrication type cervical collar (e.g., Philadelphia collar). A clear airway may be established and stabilized and the vital signs monitored and supported. The respiratory rate depth rhythm and pattern of breathing are evaluated next as key elements of the neurologic evaluation. Cardiac and rhythm vital sign and pulse oximetry is monitored continuously. An initial cardiopulmonary examination looking for aspiration, pneumothorax, congestive heart failure, or rhythm disturbance is the next priority. If the blood pressure is low suspect an acute myocardial infarction, occult blood loss, usually within the abdomen, or an associated high spinal cord injury and begin infusing electrolyte solution and if necessary blood rapidly until the pressure is stabilized.

The trauma examination seeks to establish the patient's level of orientation and response to stimulation using the standard Glasgow Coma Scale (GCS)[12–14] (Table 44-1) as well as noting the patient's level of neurologic functioning and whether there are focal deficits or a sensory or motor level is present. For example, the patient may be said to be in light coma that is, grimaces when a noxious stimulus is applied to the head and to the extremities and has semipurposeful movement with the right hand and decorticates with the left arm and legs (i.e., extends the leg and inverts foot, flexes elbow with hand all on the left side). This patient has a GCS of 8. This is calculated as follows: eye opening—none, score = 1; best verbal response—uncomprehensible sounds, score = 2; and best motor response—localizes painful stimulus, score = 5. Recording pupillary size and reaction is also critical. A basilar fracture should be sought by examining the eyes for a periorbital ecchymosis, the area behind the ear for a hematoma (Battle sign), spinal fluid and otorrhea and hemotypanum, and the nose for spinal fluid rhinorrhea. Spinal fluid contains glucose whereas nasal secretions do not, thus a dipstick or glucose stick test is very useful in differentiating these fluids. The back of the head and the entire spine should be palpated for swelling, crepitus, and discongruities (stepoffs). A rapid examination of the cranial nerves and the muscle tone of all four extremities is then carried out. Motor strength and reflexes are recorded as is rectal tone. Spinal cord injury is suspected when there is loss of rectal tone, loss of reflexes, hypotension, or priapism.

Table 44-1 Glasgow coma scale

Eye opening	
Spontaneously	4
To verbal command	3
To pain	2
Never	1
Best verbal response	
Oriented and converses	5
Disoriented and converses	4
Inappropriate words	3
Incomprehensible sounds	2
None	1
Best motor response	
Obeys verbal command	6
Localizes painful stimulus	5
Flexion withdrawal	4
Abnormal flexion (decorticate rigidity)	3
Extension (decerebrate rigidity)	2
No response	1

The key signs (e.g., pupillary size and reaction, patient's mental state and response to stimulation, as well as the formal Glasgow Coma Scale) are repeated every 15 minutes for the first few hours and then every hour as the patient's condition becomes known in order to follow the patient's stability and to identify early deterioration.

The patient's oxygenation is key to limiting neuronal loss and must be carefully monitored. Patients with coma or severe agitation following a head injury will usually require endotracheal intubation to maintain the airway, prevent aspiration, permit imaging studies under sedation, and allow hyperventilation when necessary. Intubation is carried out with the head immobilized and using an organized, rapid sequence protocol[15] to minimize aspiration and elevation of intracranial pressure.

During the initial evaluation, the head and trunk should be elevated at about 30° if possible to decrease intracranial pressure. The patient's fluid status should be purposefully kept on the side of slight dehydration (free water, i.e., dextrose in water should be minimized as well). A Foley catheter should be inserted into the bladder to monitor output and a gastric tube should be placed after endotracheal intubation to decompress the stomach. In patients with penetrating or open head injuries, a short course of broad-spectrum antibiotics is indicated as is tetanus prophylaxis. Patients with severe injuries will usually receive phenytoin for seizure prophylaxis.

Laboratory and Imaging Studies

In patients with moderate head injury, a baseline complete blood count, SMA7, coagulation profile, and toxicologic screen are usually obtained.

To rule out suicidal intent and drug toxicities, toxocologic screening is indicated for drugs of abuse and for specific intoxicants if known. Clues to suicidal behavior include a single-vehicle accident during good weather and lack of skid marks on the road, indicating that the patient did not apply the brakes. The same clues can also be seen in patients whose accident is caused by loss of consciousness, as in hypoglycemia, epilepsy, or cardiac rhythm disturbances. The cardiopulmonary evaluation includes an electrocardiogram and subsequent electrophysiologic studies where indications are that the injury may have been precipitated by a cardiac rhythm disturbance.

Imaging studies[16,17] for these patients are carried out once they are initially stabilized and for most patients include a complete cervical spine series: anteroposterior (AP) lateral, and odontoid (or open mouth) views; if these are normal and there is no evidence of a spinal cord injury the patients can be demobilized. An initial lateral film of the cervical spine is taken at the bedside and if all seven cervical vertebrae are seen and appear normal, the AP and open mouth views are obtained. Often the plain films of the neck are inadequate or show varying degrees of pre-existing subluxation and degenerative changes, abnormalities that will require CT in order to clear the spine. Almost all geriatric patients that have been concussed and patients with moderate or more severe head injuries should have an unenhanced head CT. Plain skull films are useful if a penetrating or depressed skull fracture is suspected, but an unenhanced CT of the head will still be required to evaluate the underlying brain and the skull films are redundant at that point.

Classification of Head Injury

A minor head injury is defined as a patient with a GCS of 15 who is alert and back to his or her baseline, but who may have some residual mild cognitive impairment (e.g. retrograde amnesia). A patient with a moderate head injury has a GCS of 9 to 13, loss of consciousness for more than 5 minutes, and may have a focal neurologic deficit. A severe head injured patient has a GCS of 8 or less and will usually be stuporous or comatose.

Disposition

Head injured patients seen in the emergency department who have a mild head injury and a negative CT are back to baseline and can be sent home if there is a very stable and supportive home situation. More often it is our preference to admit these patients for 24 to 48 hours for monitoring neurologic checks and a thorough medical evaluation.

Patients with moderate head trauma are confused or sleepy and are admitted even with a normal head CT. If the CT is abnormal, neurosurgical consultation and observation in a neurologic neurosurgical intensive care unit is mandatory is most cases. Patients with severe head injury will require neurosurgical intensive care. Most of these will be intubated and require a neurosurgical procedure within the first 48 hours. The issue of survivability of the patient with a severe head injury raises the ethical issues of resource utilization and medical futility. These issues are discussed elsewhere in this text as well as in the section on prognosis at the end of this chapter.

Critical Care Issues on the Management of the Head Injured Patient

Early in their stay in the hospital, the patient's nutritional status and fluid and electrolyte balance have to be considered.[11] Although we wish to decrease brain swelling by keeping those patients slightly dehydrated, we are also concerned about the rapid loss of nitrogen that occurs due to protein breakdown secondary to the stress of trauma and immobilization. To minimize negative nitrogen balance, 10,500 J/d (2,500 calories/d) of carbohydrate and a source of nitrogen are required. Basic fluid replacement consists of about 2,500 cc of fluid per day to cover urine output and insensible losses. Maintenance electrolyte requirements are at least 40 mEq of potassium, 50 to 100 mEq of sodium per day. Skin care, bowel and bladder function, as well as thrombophlebitis prophylaxis are even more important in these patients than in other types of acute bedbound patients because of their immobility.

In the emergency management of patients with actual or incipient herniation, medical reduction of intracranial pressure consists of hyperventilation to a PCO_2 of 25 to 30 mm, mannitol 0.5 to 1 g/kg via rapid infusion, and furosemide 1 mg/kg as temporizing measures while hematoma evacuation via burr hole or craniotomy or removal of ventricular cerebrospinal fluid can be carried out.

Patients with head trauma may develop transient or permanent diabetes insipidus manifested by polyuria and severe hypernatremia and prerenal azotemia. This is treated by administering vasopressin (desmopressin) and replacing free water. Other patients will develop the syndrome of dilutional hyponatremia due to the syndrome of inappropriate secretion of antidiuretic hormone. This is managed by restricting fluids and infusing furosemide. Adjunctive treatments with demeclocycline, phenytoin, and lithium may be helpful to supplement water restriction.

Prognosis

Aside from the severity of injury, age constitutes perhaps the single most important variable influencing outcome.[1,18–21] Patients over age 65 have nearly twice the mortality of younger patients with similar injury levels[2] The issues relating to this worsened prognoses in the elderly is also seen in all categories of major trauma involving other organ systems. In a recent series of geriatric head injured patients,[22] 40 percent of patients with a GCS of 9 or less on admission had a mortality of 85 percent.

Age does not appear to be a factor in the severity of injury, thus for each level of injury the mortality, morbidity, and failure to return to baseline function are significantly increased in the geriatric population. In the study of Vollmer et al.[23] of all patients who had a period of coma following head injury in the 25 to 35 age group, approximately 30 percent of patients died within 6 months. This mortality rose to 80 percent in patients over age 55.

In patients 55 years of age or older sustaining acute head injury complicated by a large extracerebral collection (greater than 15 ml), 89 percent resulted in death or a vegetative state compared to 50 percent in the 16 to 25 age group.[4] In patients over age 60 with moderate head injury defined as an initial GCS of 9 to 13, 24 percent made a good recovery, 10 percent has residual moderate disability, 10 percent severe disability, and 55 percent dead or in a vegetative state.

Some of the premorbid factors in the geriatric patients thought to adversely affect outcome are underlying medical diseases that predispose to pulmonary infection, skin breakdown, and thrombophlebitis. The aging process itself is associated with a reduced rate of wound healing, slower recovery from injury, and chronic and acute deconditioning and greater requirement for intensive rehabilitation.

Other studies[24] suggest that the release of neuroexcitatory transmitters, glutamate and aspartate, may play a role given the diminished neuronal pool and altered receptor availability and sensitivity. Another group of investigators[25] have published a series of experiments on the propensity of the aging brain to respond to direct injury with more gliosis and fibrosis than immature brains. Vascular factors that are thought to be important in prejudicing outcome in the elderly include amyloidangiopathy, atherosclerosis, and fibrosis of vessels, causing them to be less tolerant to shearing forces. Cerebral atrophy, while surrounding the brain with more cerebrospinal fluid, does not adequately protect the brain from the shearing forces if sustained from abrupt accelerating and decelerating forces.

Diagnosis of brain death in head injured patient–standard criteria[20,27]

Clinical criteria for cerebral unresponsiveness:

- Patient unresponsive to deep pain
- Patient apneic (There must be a formal test for apnea by preoxygenating the patient and withdrawing the patient from a ventilator for approximately 12 minutes or until the $PaCo_2$ is greater than 60 mm.)
- Brain stem reflexes are absent
- Hypothermia and exogenous substances, (e.g., alcohol and barbiturates) are absent
- The mechanism and result of the head injury have been documented and are unsurvivable

Confirmatory tests of brain death

Used to shorten period of observation or to help define the patient's status when other factors are involved.

- Four vessel angiography: no cerebral blood flow
- Electroencephalogram: electrocerebral silence
- Cerebral radionuclide angiogram: no isotope in cerebral arteries

Summary

The challenge of rapidly and accurately diagnosing head injured geriatric patients is based on creating a rapid medical database that includes early detection of intracranial hematomas and intracranial hypertension and leads to prompt medical and neurosurgical management. It also requires us to quickly evaluate the patient for underlying and predisposing medical, psychiatric, toxicologic, and neurologic conditions that may have been the initiating factors in causing the injury. This type of comprehensive assessment and rapid management can improve what is currently a rather poor prognosis for the geriatric patient with a serious head injury. The team approach to the problem should maximize the potential for limiting mortality and lowering the morbidity for these vulnerable patients.

For patients with serious or critical head injury who do not rapidly improve with intensive management over the first few days, there is a dismal prognosis. This situation is no different from other terminal care situations faced by primary physicians every day and for which there are accepted approaches to limiting futile care. In the head injured patient, brain death criteria[26,27] (see Boxes) are obviously key elements in helping the family and friends in coming to grips with the loss of their loved one. Patients who are successfully resuscitated from the acute insult to the CNS will require intensive physical and emotional rehabilitation, with a slow response toward baseline the optimum result that can be expected.

References

1. Krauss JF, McArthur DL, Silverman TA: Epidemiology of brain injury. p. 14. In Nayoyou (ed): Neurotrauma. McGraw-Hill, New York, 1996
2. Krauss JF: Epidemiology of head trauma. In Cooper PR (ed): Head Injury, 3rd Ed. Williams & Wilkins, Baltimore, 1993
3. Strong L, Moe Millen R, Jennet B: Head injuries in accident and emergency departments in Scotland. Injury 1978;10:154–159
4. Gravis AB, White E, Kopssell TD: The association between head trauma and Alzheimer's disease. Am J Epidemiol 1990; 131:491–501
5. Chaudra V, Kokman E, Schoenberg BS: Head trauma with loss of consciousness as a risk factor for Alzheimer's disease. Neurology 1989;39:1576–1578
6. Rassmussen DX, Brandt J, Martin DB: Head injury as a risk factor in Alzheimer's disease. Brain Inj 1995;9:213–219

7. Fell DA, Fitzgerald S, Maid RH: Acute subdural hematomas, review of 144. J Neurosurg 1973;42:37–42
8. Cameron M: Subacute and chronic subdural hematoma. J Neurol Neurosurg Psychiatry 1978;41:834–839
9. Kaufman HH, Layola WP, Makela ME: Civilian gun shot Wounds—The Limits of salvagability. Acta Neurochir 1983; 67:115–125
10. O'Malley KF, Ross SF: The incidence of injury to the cervical spine in patients with craniocerebral injury. J Trauma 1988; 28:1476–1478
11. White R, Likovec M: The diagnosis and initial management of head injury. N Engl J Med 1992;327:1507–1511
12. Teasdale G, Jennett B: Assessment of coma and impaired consciousness: a Practical scale. Lancet 1974;2:81–84
13. Oppenheim JS: Predicting outcome in brain-injured patients using the Glasgow Coma Scale in primary care. Postgrad Med, 1992;91:261
14. Jennett B, Teasdale G: Aspects of coma after severe head injury. Lancet 1977;23:878–881
15. Tabicci RC, Shaikh KA, Schnab CW: Rapid sequence induction with oral endotracheal intubation in the multiply injured patient. Ann Surg 1988;54:185–187
16. Stern SC, Ross SE: The value of computed tomographic scans in patients with low risk head injuries. Neurosurgery 1990;26: 638–640
17. Yealy DM, Hagan DE: Imaging after head trauma: who needs what? Emerg Med Clin North Am 1991;9:707–717
18. Conroy C, Kraus JF: Survival after brain injury: cause of death, length of survival and prognostic variables in a cohort of brain injured people. Neuroepidemiology 1988;7:13–22
19. Becker DP, Miller JD, Ward JD: The outcome from severe head injury with early diagnosis and intensive management. J Neurosurg 1977;47:491–502
20. Penthand B, Jones PA, Ray CW: Head injury in the elderly. Age Aging 1986;15:193–202
21. Luerssen TG, Klauber MR, Marshall LF: Outcome from head injury related to patient's age—a longitudinal prospective study of adult and pediatric head injury
22. Kotwica Z, Jakubowski JK: Acute head injuries in the elderly: an analysis of 136 consecutive patients. Sita Neurochiv Wien 1992;118:98–102
23. Vollmer DJ, Torner JC, Jane JA: Age and outcome following traumatic coma: why do older patients fare worse? J Neurosurg 1991;75:537–549
24. Olneg JW: Excitotoxin medical. Neuronal death in youth and old age. Prog Brain Res 1990;86:37–51
25. Rudge JS, Smith GM, Silver J: An in-vitro model of wound healing in the CNS: analysis of cell reaction and interaction of different ages. J Exp Neurol 1989;103:1–16
26. Guidelines for the Determination of Death. Report of the Medical Consultants on the Diagnosis of Death to the President's Commission for the Study of Ethical Problems in Medicine and Biomedical and Behavioral Research. JAMA 1981;246: 2184–2186
27. Bleak PM: Conception and practical issues in the declaration of death by brain criteria. Neurosurg Clin Nh Am 1991;2: 490–501

CHAPTER 45

Infections of the Central Nervous System

STEVEN L. BERK
JAMES W. MYERS

Bacterial meningitis is a disease that presents particular challenges in the elderly patient. The mortality rate from bacterial meningitis is higher in the elderly than in younger adults. Bacterial meningitis has become a more common problem in elderly patients over the past two decades. In 1973, Fraser et al.[1] reported that the mean age of death from meningitis in Olmstead County, Minnesota, had gone from 11.5 years in the period 1935 to 1946 to 64 years during the period of 1959 to 1970. In the later period more than one-half of all deaths from meningitis occurred in those over 60 years of age. The incidence of bacterial meningitis rose from 5 cases per 100,000 to 15 cases per 100,000.[1] A Centers for Disease Control survey performed between 1978 and 1981 showed an increasing incidence of meningitis in older patients[2] as did a survey on the incidence of meningitis conducted in Rhode Island.[3] In a recent review of 445 adults treated for bacterial meningitis at the Massachusetts General Hospital, 56 percent of community-acquired meningitis occurred in patients over 50 years of age.[4] In this recent study as well as all previous studies the mortality rate was much higher in older patients. The mortality rate in the Massachusetts General Hospital study was 37 in those over 60 years of age compared to 17 in younger adults. In the Rhode Island study, 55 percent of elderly patients died compared with an overall mortality rate of 10.[3]

The increased incidence of meningitis in this age group probably is explained, in part, by the more aggressive care given to elderly patients including more rigorous evaluation of fever, change in mental status, and coma. Nosocomial meningitis particularly related to neurosurgical procedures is also a cause of the increasing incidence of meningitis in this age group. Durand et al.[4] have shown that nosocomial meningitis has increased from 28 percent of all meningitides between 1962 and 1970 to 45 percent of all cases of meningitis from 1980 to 1988. Many of these cases occur in the chronically ill, frequently hospitalized elderly.

Bacteria may reach the subarachnoid space of the elderly patient by several different mechanisms.[5] Elderly patients with focal infections may develop bacteremia and seed the meninges. This occurs, for example, in the elderly patient with pneumococcal pneumonia, or less frequently in the patient with pyelonephritis and gram-negative meningitis. Meningitis develops by way of direct inoculation of bacteria into the meninges such as occurs in head trauma or after a neurosurgical procedure. Elderly patients are prone to frequent falls and head injuries. *Staphylococcus aureus*, coagulase-negative staphylococci, and gram-negative bacilli are responsible for most cases of meningitis secondary to head trauma or neurosurgery. Meningitis may occur from contagious spread of infection to the meninges as in patients with otitis media, sinusitis, or mastoiditis. This mechanism of infection is probably somewhat less common in the elderly as compared with younger adults.

In the bacteremic, elderly patient, symptoms of fever, chills, and rigors will usually be present but afebrile bacteremia in the elderly is well described. Patients with contiguous spread of infection usually complain of localized findings such as ear or facial pain. Bacteria in the subarachnoid space will cause an inflammatory reaction in the pia and arachnoid matter that will manifest itself as neck pain and stiffness with protective reflexes that cause the Kernig and Brudzinski signs. Structures that lie within the subarachnoid space are involved in the inflammatory reaction. Pial arteries and veins may become inflamed and cranial nerve roots damaged.

A diffuse encephalopathy may occur. Abnormal mental status results from cerebral ischemia, edema, or toxic encephalopathy. Confusion, headache, or lethargy is a manifestation of this diffuse, inflammatory process. Papilledema, hydrocephalus, and other focal findings may occur as a result of pus occluding the foramina of Luschka and Magendie resulting in increased intracranial pressure.

The clinical features of meningitis in elderly patients are more subtle than in younger adults. This is a recurring theme in almost all studies that involve older patients with meningitis.[6,7] Most, but not all, studies have found that elderly patients with bacterial meningitis are less likely to have neck stiffness and meningeal signs. At the same time, older patients often have cervical spine disease and poor neck mobility, making interpretation of clinical signs more difficult. Berman et al.[8] found meningismus present in only 58 percent of elderly patients with meningitis. Gorse et al.[9] compared signs and symptoms of patients with meningitis above 50 years of age to those in patients below 50. Older patients had more mental status abnormalities and were more likely to have seizures, neurologic deficits, and hydrocephalus. Berk,[6] Roos,[10] Massanari[11] and others have noted that a delay in diagnosis is frequently associated with meningitis in the elderly and this delay may explain the high mortality rate noted in this group of patients.

Elderly patients with bacterial meningitis may not have as pronounced fever or may at times be afebrile. The change in mental status that occurs in the elderly may be attributed to senility, delirium, psychosis, transient ischemia, or stroke. In the elderly patient who has undergone neurosurgery, postoperative lethargy may be mistakenly attributed to an expected postoperative course. A stiff neck in an elderly patient may not arouse the same concern that it would in a young adult.

Physical examination is a critical part of the evaluation of an elderly patient with suspected meningitis. Nuchal rigidity is reported in between 56 and 92 percent of elderly patients depending on the series.[7] When neck stiffness is the result of meningeal irritation, the neck will resist flexion but can be rotated from side to side. A funduscopic and cranial nerve examination are mandatory to alert the clinician to associated increased intracranial pressure or brain abscess. Mental status should be carefully described and followed. Lethargy and coma are poor prognostic signs. Examination of the head should include a search for skull fracture, avulsion, or hematoma. Careful otoscopic examination is also a necessity as otitis media may be missed in the elderly patient, particularly when mental status is abnormal and a history cannot be obtained. The elderly patient may present with pneumonia and concomitant meningitis. Gorse et al.[9] found pneumonia to be much more common in older adults with meningitis. The elderly patient may not complain of respiratory symptoms so examination of the lung may be the first clue to pneumonia. Examination of the heart is necessary to detect underlying valvular heart disease that might predispose the elderly patient to endocarditis with seeding of the meninges. Examination for costovertebral tenderness, decubitus ulcers, and petechial lesions will also provide important information in determining the source and etiologic agent in meningitis.

Performance of a lumbar puncture without delay is the critical element in the diagnosis of bacterial meningitis in both young and old. About 35 percent of elderly patients with meningitis present with focal neurologic findings.[9] Because lumbar puncture is contraindicated in patients with brain abscess, computed tomography (CT) or magnetic resonance imaging (MRI) will be necessary in some older patients. However, the high mortality rate from meningitis in the elderly makes time of the essence in the diagnosis and treatment of meningitis in this group. Many infectious disease experts now support the strategy of beginning empirical antibiotic therapy, pending lumbar puncture, particularly when a delay of hours is anticipated due to an imaging study. (The combination of ampicillin and a third-generation cephalosporin has been recommended to cover all pathogens likely to occur in the elderly.)

There is very little in the literature to suggest that the cerebrospinal fluid (CSF) findings in elderly patients with meningitis differ from young adults with meningitis. Lumbar puncture will show purulent fluid with white blood cell counts between about 500 and 10,000 cu/mm. Polymorphonuclear leukocytes predominate usually making up more than 90 percent of total cell count. Meningitis caused by *Listeria monocytogenes* sometimes has a mononuclear cell predominance. At least one study has shown that elderly patients with meningitis are more likely to have a lack of cellular response in CSF than younger adults.[12] Those elderly patients with meningitis who have few cells in CSF but many bacteria have a poor prognosis.[13] CSF glucose levels are usually low in bacterial meningitis. CSF to serum glucose ratios are usually less than 50 percent. Seventy percent of patients with meningitis will have a ratio less than 31 percent.[14] Spinal fluid protein is elevated above 50 mg/dl. Very high protein levels are associated with poor prognosis. Gram stain of CSF will be positive in 60 to 90 percent of all patients with meningitis.[14] In the study by Berman et al.[8] only 50 percent of elderly patients with meningitis had a positive Gram stain. The Gram stain is most likely to be negative in patients who have received prior antibiotic therapy. In those patients whose Gram stain is negative, a variety of methods to detect bacterial antigen are now in common use. These include latex fixation, coagglutination, and counterimmunoelectrophoresis. The limulus lysate assay has been used to detect gram-negative meningitis, an important cause of meningitis in the elderly. Other tests such as lactic acid levels and measurement of C-reactive protein have been recommended to help distinguish bacterial from viral meningitis but clinical decisions are rarely based on them.

Blood cultures are recommended in all patients in whom bacterial meningitis is suspected. In the study by Berman et al.[8] almost one-half of all elderly patients with meningitis had concomitant bacteremia. In addition, other cultures such as sputum, urine, and wound may be extremely helpful in determining etiologic agent and source of infection.

Streptococcus pneumoniae is the most common organism to cause meningitis in elderly patients.[5] *S. pneumoniae* was responsible for more than one-half of all cases of meningitis in the elderly in several studies.[15–17] The organism caused 43 percent of all cases in the study of Berman et al.[8] and 24 percent of cases in the study of Gorse et al.[9] Gram-negative bacilli cause meningitis in elderly patients both by bacteremic spread of infection such as in urinary tract infection or pneumonia, and as a nosocomial infection after neurosurgery.[18,19] *Escherichia coli* is the most common organism to cause meningitis secondary to bacteremic spread. *E. coli* and *Klebsiella* pneumonia are the more common gram-negative bacilli to cause meningitis after neurosurgery but more unusual organisms, particularly *Acinetobacter*[20–22] have been more commonly reported. In a review of 581 cases of bacterial meningitis in elderly patients between 1967 and 1980, about 8 percent of cases were caused by gram-negative bacilli[6] (Fig. 45-1). However, more recent studies have shown gram-negative bacilli to be responsible for 20 to 25 percent of cases.[8,9] This increase is not unexpected in light of the reported increase in nosocomial meningitis in all age groups. Gram-negative meningitis occurs at the extremes of life, in the neonate and the debilitated elderly. In a study of 158 patients with gram-negative meningitis in New York City over one-half of the patients were over 60 years of age. Almost all of these elderly patients died.[23] However, third-generation cephalosporins have replaced chloramphenicol for treatment of gram-negative meningitis with improvement in overall survival.

L. monocytogenes is also an organism more likely to cause meningitis in the elderly than the younger adult. Because this infection is T-cell-mediated, it is possible that immunologic

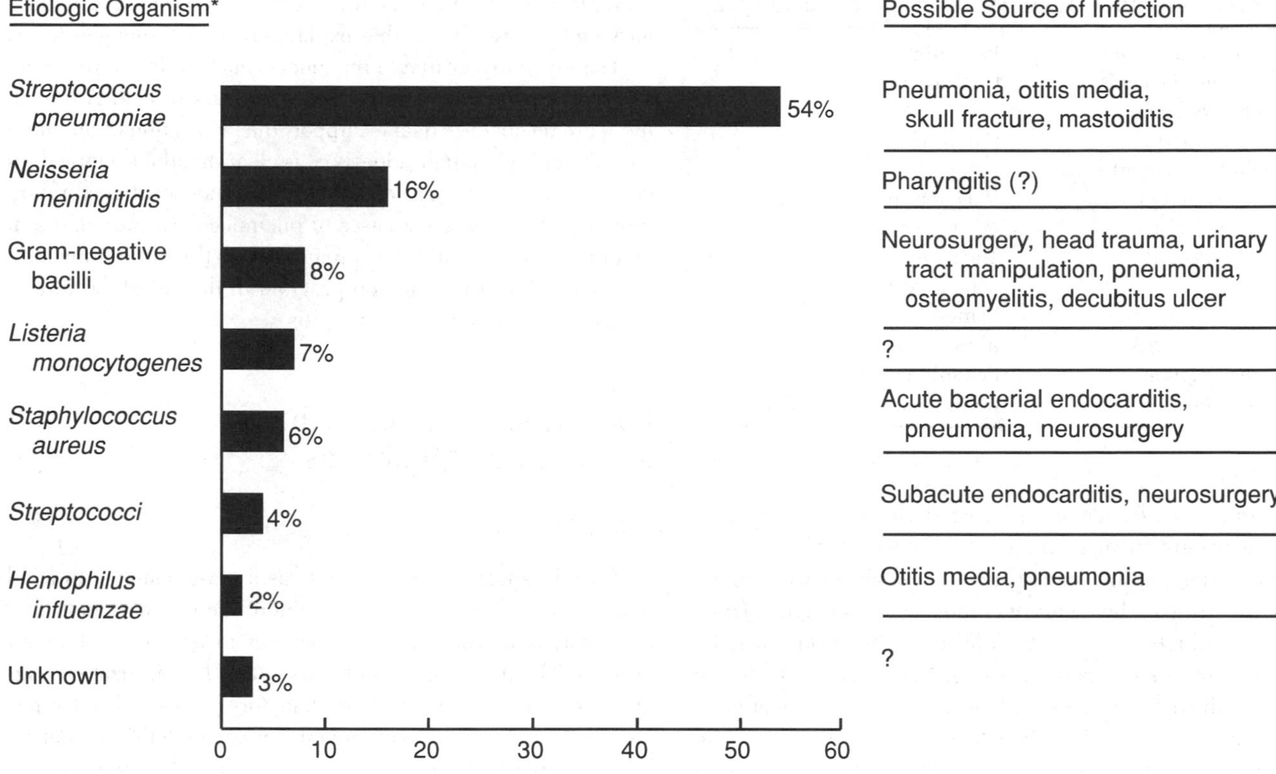

Figure 45-1 Bacterial meningitis in elderly patients. (Modified from Berk and Smith,[5] with permission.)

senescence of this system may explain the predisposition of the elderly to this infection. Although *Listeria* accounts for 4 to 8 percent of all cases of meningitis in the elderly, it is an extremely rare cause of meningitis in young healthy adults. Of 53 cases of *L. monocytogenes* meningitis in New York City, 77 percent of patients were older than 50 and 87 percent of these elderly patients died.[23]

Meningococcal meningitis is the most common cause of meningitis in young adults, but a less common cause of meningitis in the elderly. The incidence of meningococcal meningitis in the elderly patient population varies from one study to another, reflecting the epidemic nature of the disease. Outbreaks have occurred in nursing homes and institutional settings.[24] The infection should be considered in elderly patients who present with meningeal signs and have a petechial or macular rash. No focus of infection will be noted.

S. aureus was the most common cause of meningitis in the elderly in a Mayo Clinic study between the years 1948 and 1958.[25] All cases were secondary to neurosurgery. Overall the organism is probably responsible for about 10 percent of cases of meningitis in older patients, either as a neurosurgical infection or part of a complicated staphylococcal sepsis secondary to pneumonia or endocarditis. Coagulase-negative staphylococci have become a more common cause of meningitis in the elderly, being associated with CSF shunts and other neurosurgical procedures.

β-Hemolytic streptococci are a relatively rare cause of meningitis in the elderly. However, this appears to be another organism that causes life-threatening infection and meningitis at the extremes of life.[26] *Hemophilus influenzae*, the most common cause of meningitis in children, is unusual in adults and the elderly. When *H. influenzae* does occur in older patients, it is usually a nonencapsulated organism.[27] This is in contrast to children, where the type B encapsulated organism is most likely to cause infection.

The treatment of bacterial meningitis requires prompt initiation of antibiotic therapy. The antibiotic chosen must have excellent activity against the etiologic agent. Information from the history and physical examination in combination with a careful review of the CSF Gram stain will be the foundation on which the etiologic agent will be determined and the optimal antibiotic chosen. An infectious disease specialist, when possible, should be involved in the case as the mortality rate from the disease is high and the margin of error is small. The antibiotic chosen should be bactericidal for the etiologic agent and must diffuse across the blood-brain barrier. Table 45-1 lists the etiologic agent and the antibiotic generally recommended. However, the particular epidemiology of the hospital or community of the patient will take on increasing importance in determining antibiotic of choice. The rapid emergence of penicillin-resistant pneumococci in the United States has created some uncertainty in regard to the initial treatment of pneumo-

Table 45-1 Antibiotic of choice for bacterial meningitis

Organism	Antibiotic
Streptococcus pneumoniae	Penicillin
Streptococcus pneumoniae (penicillin-resistant)	Ceftriaxone (see text)
Staphylococcus aureus (methicillin-sensitive)	Nafcillin
Staphylococcus aureus (methicillin-resistant)	Vancomycin
Gram-negative bacilli	Third-generation cephalosporin (see text)
β-Hemolytic streptococci	Penicillin
Listeria monocytogenes	Ampicillin
Neisseria meningitides	Penicillin
Hemophilus influenzae	Ceftriaxone or cefotaxime

coccal meningitis. In communities where high-level penicillin resistance occurs in more than 1 to 2 percent of isolates, a third-generation cephalosporin such as ceftriaxone will likely become the drug of choice for pneumococcal meningitis. However, the antibiotic sensitivity profile to the isolate will be very important as some penicillin-resistant strains will also be resistant to third-generation cephalosporins. A combination of vancomycin and rifampin might then be considered. In the treatment of gram-negative meningitis, the antibiotic sensitivity pattern of gram-negative bacilli at a particular hospital is also critically important. If the infection has occurred after a neurosurgical procedure, the organisms responsible for prior neurosurgical infections should be noted. If *Pseudomonas aeruginosa* is suspected as the etiologic agent, ceftazidime is the antibiotic of choice. Cefotaxime or ceftriaxone are generally used for other gram-negative bacilli including *H. influenzae*. Ampicillin is the drug of choice for *L. monocytogenes*. Oxacillin or nafcillin are drugs of choice for methicillin-sensitive staphylococci; vancomycin is the antibiotic of choice for methicillin-resistant staphylococci and most coagulase-negative staphylococci. As previously noted, ampicillin plus a third-generation cephalosporin is recommended for treatment of meningitis in the elderly when the etiologic agent is unknown. Although corticosteroids are now recommended in the treatment of acute bacterial meningitis in children, there is no evidence at present to establish their use in the adult or elderly patient. Elderly patients with meningitis are generally admitted to an intensive care unit, where vital signs and neurologic status can be carefully monitored. Some patients will be severely dehydrated or volume depleted, and others will be in septic shock. Colloid or crystalloid may be necessary to improve blood pressure and urine output. Inappropriate antidiuretic hormone secretion may accompany central nervous system (CNS) infections but should be self-limited if hypotonic solutions are avoided.

The comatose, elderly patient requires specialized care. The patient may need frequent suctioning, particularly if pneumonia is present. The patient should be turned frequently to avoid decubiti. A condom catheter is preferable to a Foley, unless urinary retention develops. In patients who develop relapsing or prolonged fever, a repeat lumbar puncture is necessary. Drug fever, phlebitis, urinary tract infection, and pulmonary emboli are all possible explanations for prolonged fever.

The currently available pneumococcal vaccine is routinely recommended in all patients over 65 years of age. Although there are no specific data to support the prevention of pneumococcal meningitis in the elderly, it is clear that the vaccine does decrease the incidence of serious pneumococcal respiratory infection. Because most cases of pneumococcal meningitis in older patients are caused by pneumonia as the initial infection, it is likely that a vaccination program in the elderly would be of benefit in preventing meningitis.

Focal Lesions, Encephalitis, and Chronic Meningitis

Brain Abscess

A brain abscess often presents as a mass lesion with focal neurologic deficits. Since the advent of the CT scan, mortality has decreased from 30 to 50 percent to as low as 4 to 20 percent. The duration of symptoms before hospitalization usually has a mean of 15 days.[28] Risk factors for adverse outcomes include a severe change of mental status on admission, neurologic abnormalities on admission, and a short duration between the first symptoms and presentation suggesting a rapid progression. Fever may be absent in 40 to 50 percent of patients; common symptoms such as headache, change of mental status, and focal neurologic deficits may be misdiagnosed as cerebral tumors or cerebral vascular accidents, which are very common in the elderly.

The white blood cell count is ordinarily normal to slightly elevated. A lumbar puncture, which may be dangerous particularly in patients with focal neurologic signs, reveals nonspecific findings. Seventeen percent of patients may have a white count greater than 500, suggesting a bacterial meningitis. Cultures of the spinal fluid, however, are usually negative.[28] Because 15 to 40 percent of patients with brain abscesses may die within 24 to 48 hours of a diagnostic lumbar puncture, this should be avoided in most cases.

The radiologic appearance of a "doughnut ring" lesion may be detectable in the majority of patients with brain abscesses. However, ring-enhanced lesions can also be seen with necrotic tumors and cerebral infarction. Surrounding edema may also be seen on CT scan and might be an indication for corticosteroids.[29,30] In cases of a single abscess, the most common location is generally that of the frontal lobe or parietal lobe rather than the occipital or temporal. Sites of brain abscesses are often independent from presumed origin of infection except for the possibility of ear and sinus infections more often leading to abscesses within the frontal brain.

Generalized seizures can prompt hospitalization of many patients including the elderly. Often 50 percent of patients with a brain abscess may have a focal neurologic sign such as a hemiparesis or focal seizure. Patients may also present with a diffuse neurologic dysfunction such as a coma, generalized seizure, or neuropsychiatric manifestations. Funduscopic examination may also reveal papilledema. In Seydoux and Francioli's study[28] of 39 cases of brain abscesses, predisposing factors were not equally distributed in the different age groups in contrast to previous studies. They were more common in patients less than 50 years of age. Direct spread from a sinus or otologic focus appears to be more common with brain abscesses in younger adults, and was infrequently noted in patients older than 60 years of age. A short duration of symptoms before hospitalization also characterized patients between 20 and 60 years of age and was often associated with a poor outcome. The microbiology of brain abscesses does not appear to be significantly different between younger and older patients. Often viridans streptococcus and *Streptococcus milleri* are the most frequently isolated aerobes. *Fusobacterium* and other anaerobes were also common isolates.

Surgery is the only procedure that allows optimal microbiologic documentation. Several authors recommend medical therapy, particularly in cases in which abscess is less than 2 cm in diameter and when the lesion is of high density, suggesting a cerebritis.[31,32]

A combination of a β-lactam agent with chloramphenicol or metronidazole generally has been recommended as standard therapy for brain abscesses. Microbiologic data obtained from a stereotaxic biopsy will be a further guide to therapy. The optimal duration of brain abscesses has been variable.[33] Usually most authors recommend approximately 4 to 6 weeks of antibiotics including the combination of parenteral and oral agents. Neurologic sequela can be quite high occurring in as much as 46 percent of cases.[28]

Subdural Empyema

Subdural empyema may arise as a complication of a sinusitis or otitis media. Presenting symptoms can often mimic a brain abscess. A contrasted study of the CNS is indicated and neurologic drainage is mandatory. Antibiotic therapy is targeted at many of the same organisms that cause brain abscess. Length of therapy is generally several weeks with intravenous antibiotics.

Chronic Meningitis

Tuberculosis of the elderly is a serious disorder. Previously this was thought to be a diagnosis of the pediatric age group but recent reports indicate a rising incidence in the elderly.[35] Tuberculosis meningitis is often an insidious disease and may be especially difficult to diagnosis in the elderly. Nonspecific symptoms of fatigue, anorexia, nausea, and an altered mental status may suggest dementia in an elderly patient. A miliary picture on chest x-ray may be the only feature that is useful to distinguish tuberculosis meningitis from cryptococcal meningitis. Duration of symptoms may range from 2 days to 6 months. Hospitalization is often precipitated by change in mental status, headache, or fever. Meningeal signs are present in less than one half of the cases. Ocular palsies, particularly due to involvement of nerve VI, are found in 30 to 70 percent of cases.

CSF findings often reveal a protein level above 50 and a low glucose below 40. Acid-fast positivity varies among the studies but can range anywhere from 10 to 80 percent depending on how many spinal taps were performed. A chest x-ray and purified protein derivative should be routinely obtained. Several attempts have been made to develop a rapid, common, and specific method for diagnosing tuberculous meningitis. Adenosine deaminase activity has been detected in the spinal fluid. At levels greater than 9 units/L, the test was found to be sensitive and specific. Levels can also be increased in patients with sarcoid or lymphoma. Levels appear to perhaps correlate with disease activity. Radioimmunoassay has been used for detecting a *Mycobacterium tuberculosis* antigen. The assay becomes negative after therapy.

Tuberculostearic acid, a structural component of *M. tuberculosis*, can be identified by gas-liquid chromatography and may also be useful to diagnosis tuberculosis.[36] Recent methodologies such as polymerase chain reaction (PCR) testing and immunomagnetic enrichment may also prove to be useful for cases of tuberculosis including tuberculosis meningitis.[37,38]

Prognosis is influenced by age, duration of symptoms, and neurologic deficits. Mortality is greatest in patients younger than age 5 and older than 50 (60 percent). Clinical staging is often based on neurologic status: stage I—rational, no focal neurologic signs or hydrocephalus; stage II—confusion, depression, or focal neurologic deficits; stage III—stuporous or dense paraplegia or hemiplegia. Isoniozid (INH), pyrazinamide (PZA), and rifampin penetrate the blood-brain barrier to achieve adequate CSF concentrations. Multidrug-resistant tuberculosis may require several drugs.[39] Many authorities recommend the adjunctive use of corticosteroids for stage II and III patients, beginning with the dose of prednisone at 80 mg/d, which may be gradually tapered over 4 to 6 weeks as guided by the patient's symptoms. If hydrocephalus is present, ventricular shunting procedures may be beneficial.

Cryptococcal Meningitis

Cryptococcal meningitis may present in a manner very similar to tuberculosis. Between 20 and 50 percent of patients with *Cryptococcus* may have no underlying disease such as human immunodeficiency virus (HIV). Spinal fluid findings are very similar to tuberculosis in that there is a lymphocyte predominance. The India ink may be positive in 50 percent or more of cases. A cryptococcal antigen is often positive in 90 percent of cases by rapid simple latex fixation test. A CT scan may be helpful to rule out hydrocephalus, which is not uncommon in cryptococcal meningitis.

Poor prognostic signs for cryptococcal meningitis may be related to a high CSF opening pressure, low CSF glucose, fewer than 20 white blood cells in the CSF, and high titers of cryptococcal antigen in a positive India ink and the presence of HIV disease.

Amphotericin B is the traditional drug of choice for cryptococcal meningitis.[40] Flucytosine can serve as a useful adjunct, particularly when trying to lower the dose of amphotericin B to prevent renal insufficiency. However, flucytosine has bone marrow suppressive toxicities. Fluconazole is particularly useful for maintenance therapy but may also be useful as an acute therapy for patients with cryptococcal meningitis as well, particularly for those patients with less poor prognostic parameters.[41] Liposomal amphotericin B is also a new modality that may prove to be useful for treatment for cryptococcal meningitis. Combination therapy with fluconazole and flucytosine has also been investigated in patients with acquired immunodeficiency syndrome.

Coccidiomycosis is another common cause of chronic meningitis syndrome and a careful travel history may be an important clue to disease. Residents of the southwestern United States and Mexico appear to be at increased risk for this disease. Two-thirds of the patients, however, may have no risk factors. Blacks, Filipinos, pregnant women, and patients with HIV disease appear more likely to disseminate. CSF parameters are very similar to cryptococcal and tuberculosis meningitis. Detection of complement fixation antibody in the CSF is specific and sensitive for the diagnosis. Amphotericin B has been the traditional drug of choice. Many experts often recommend the use of an Ommaya reservoir for intraventricular therapy. Newer data suggest that fluconazole may be helpful as an alternative to amphotericin B for long-term treatment of *Coccidioides* meningitis.[42]

Herpes Simplex Encephalitis

Herpes simplex encephalitis is a serious infection of the CNS most commonly caused by herpes simplex virus type I. Mortality of untreated biopsy proven cases is 60 to 80 percent, with fewer than 10 percent of the patients being left without any neurologic sequelae. This illness occurs in all age groups with an equal number of cases between the sexes. It has no seasonal association. Mortality may be higher in patients over 50 years of age.[43]

Patients may present with an abrupt onset of personality change, altered mental status, fever, and headache. Localizing signs such as speech deficits, olfactory hallucinations, temporal lobe seizures, hemiparesis, and nasal field defects are common and may suggest the diagnosis. The spinal fluid findings are nonspecific with an elevated number of lymphocytes. An elevated number of polymorphonuclear leukocytes may be found early in the disease process. This will later change to a mononuclear site cell predominance as the disease progresses. An elevated red blood cell count can be suggestive of the diagnosis but is not required. The electroencephalogram pattern may consist of slow wave complexes at regular to 2- to 3-second intervals, usually localized to the temporal lobe. CT scanning eventually becomes positive in more than 70 percent of the patients but MRI is more sensitive and results are abnormal earlier in the course of the disease.

The virus cannot usually be isolated from the spinal fluid but newer PCR-based methodology may be helpful in making the diagnosis.[44] The definitive diagnosis of herpes simplex encephalitis can be made by brain biopsy and appropriate culture and histology. Effective therapy usually consists of acyclovir at a dose of 10 mg/k every 8 hours for 10 days, which must be adjusted for renal function in the elderly patients as acyclovir can cause nephrotoxicity, particularly in patients that are dehydrated. Survivals correlate with the patient's level of consciousness at the initiation of treatment. Neurologic sequelae is higher if treatment is delayed or the patient is comatose. A high index of suspicion is often required to make the diagnosis and to begin effective therapy for herpes simplex encephalitis.

Spirochetal Infections

Neurosyphilis

Several studies have suggested that neurosyphilis remains an important and frequently encountered entity. An estimated two symptomatic cases of neurosyphilis occur per 100,000 patients yearly. Syphilis is often the cause of reversible dementia in an elderly patient. Although neurosyphilis is often felt to be a late manifestation of syphilis, spirochetes invade the nervous system throughout the entire course of syphilis. Syphilitic meningitis may occur at the same time as the rash of the secondary syphilis. Most patients with cerebrovascular syphilis have had a duration of approximately 5 to 10 years. This can manifest as a stroke in a young person. Elderly patients typically have a presentation of paretic neurosyphilis or tabes dorsalis. The interval between infection and symptoms often ranges from 20 to 30 years for these syndromes. Both races appear easily susceptible. Men, however, have an increased risk as compared to women. The neurologic examination may be entirely normal with neurosyphilis, and the diagnosis may only be made by an abnormal CSF examination. As the disease progresses, intellectual function can decline and psychotic changes can occur. Symptoms include irritability, fatigability, personality changes, impaired judgment, depression, confusion, and delusions. Patients may have coarse, movement-induced facial, lingular, and labial tremors. Patients also may have difficulty with distorted handwriting and abnormal reflexes and focal findings may also occur.[45] Untreated, the disorder is fatal within a few months to 3 or 4 years. Penicillin treatment can effectively reverse the CSF abnormalities and arrest the disease, but the neurologic outcome depends on the degree of structural CNS damage that had occurred at the time of therapy.[46] CSF findings in general paresis include an opening pressure between 50 and 300. The cell count is usually less than 100 in 90 percent of the cases. The glucose may be normal or moderately reduced. The protein is greater than 100 in 25 percent of cases. CSF and blood serology are generally positive in greater than 95 percent of cases.[45]

Tabes dorsalis continues to be a common form of CNS syphilis, although the percentage seems to be decreasing. This disease, again, is much more common in men than in women. It has the longest incubation period, being as high as 50 years in some patients. A triad of symptoms including lightning pains, dysuria, and ataxia may be seen in patients. A triad of signs including Argyll Robertson pupils, areflexia, and a loss of proprioception are characteristic of this disorder. Lightning pains last for a few seconds to minutes at a time and usually occur in the lower extremities. These can be separated by interval-free periods of a few months. Pain sensation is often strikingly impaired compared to that of hot and cold sensation.[46] Reduction or loss of ankle or knee jerks can occur in approximately 80 to 90 percent of patients. Pupillary abnormalities are noted in 79 percent of patients and consist of pupils that accommodate but do not react. In the elderly patient, diabetes can mimic tabes. Other rare causes mimicking tabes include Wernicke's encephalopathy and Charcot-Marie-Tooth disease. As the disease progresses, sensory ataxia becomes a problem. Many patients may have a positive Romberg sign. Less common abnormalities include syphilitic optic atrophy and gastric crises. Characteristic CSF findings of tabes usually include a normal opening pressure in 90 percent of the patients. Only 9 to 10 percent of patients have a cell count greater than 160. The protein is usually normal to moderately elevated. The majority of patients have an abnormal serum and CSF Verereal Disease Research Laboratory test. In the series by Merritt[45] completely normal findings including an unreactive CSF and blood serology occurred in 2 of the 100 cases reported. In "burned-out" tabes, the fluid may be entirely normal. Penicillin treatment should clear the CSF and arrest progression of the disease; however, findings such as urinary incontinence, lighting pains, and gastric crises may not completely respond to penicillin therapy.

An unreactive peripheral blood FTA-ABS usually excludes the diagnosis of neurosyphilis, and in most cases a CSF examination would not be warranted. Any patient with a positive blood serology for syphilis and neurologic symptoms would warrant a lumbar puncture. An abnormal CSF VDRL test would constitute proof of neurosyphilis. Patients with only an abnormal protein or cell count might also be strongly considered for penicillin therapy. In patients with signs of neurosyphilis but with an unreactive CSF (normal cells and protein), such as in "burned out" neurosyphilis, the neurologic deficit is probably due to fixed structural damage and will probably not respond to additional penicillin.[46] A treponemicidal level has been assumed to be 0.3 IU/ml. Comparisons of serum and CSF penicillin levels after benzathine penicillin suggest that benzathine penicillin may not reach adequate treponemicidal levels in the CSF. Adequate levels are achieved by adequate intravenous penicillin doses given for neurosyphilis. This author generally tends to treat patients with neurosyphilis with 18 to 24 million units per day for approximately 10 to 14 days. Adequate therapy is suggested by a normal spinal fluid cell count and a falling protein count at 6 months following treatment. Repeat CSF examination should be performed every 6 months for the next 2 years during which time the protein count should fall and the cell count should remain normal. The VDRL will probably also disappear during this time period or reach a low-level "serofast" state. Any increase in the cell count or major deviation from this response would require retreatment with high-dose penicillin. Neurosyphilis is often an indication to consider desensitization if the patient has a penicillin allergy. Ceftriaxone may be a reasonable alternative in some patients. Penicillin allergy would be an indication for infectious diseases and allergy consultation. Many patients who have a positive serum test and no symptoms could potentially be treated with three injections of benzathine penicillin over a 3-week period. However, this would only be warranted if the physician is sure there is no symptoms of neurosyphilis. A negative CSF would be reassuring to the patient and physician before embarking on this treatment course. Hypothyroidism, cryptococcal and tuberculous meningitis, or other causes of reversible dementia need to be considered in the differential diagnosis of neurosyphilis.

Lyme Disease

The CNS effects of Lyme disease are receiving increasing attention in the literature. Lyme disease can cause a meningitis in the second stage weeks to months after the tick exposure. Bell's palsy and peripheral neuropathy syndromes are quite common. A CSF pleocytosis is often found with an elevated protein and a normal to low CSF sugar. Local CSF antibody production occurs. A positive enzyme-linked immunosorbent assay test for Lyme disease is usually recommended to be followed by a Western blot test. Ceftriaxone is generally considered the treatment of choice for the CNS manifestations of syphilis.[47] An exception might possibly be the use of doxycycline for facial nerve palsy.

References

1. Fraser DW, Henke CE, Feldman RA: Changing patterns of bacterial meningitis in Olmstead County, Minnesota, 1935–1970. J Infect Dis 1973;128:300–307
2. Schlech WF III, Ward JI, Band JD: Bacterial meningitis in the United States, 1978 through 1981: The National Bacterial Meningitis Surveillance study. JAMA 1985;253:1749
3. Aronson SM, DeBuono BA, Buechner JS: Acute bacterial meningitis in Rhode Island: a survey of the years 1976 to 1985. Rhode Island Med J 1991;74:33
4. Durand ML, Calderwood SB, Weber DJ: Acute bacterial meningitis in adults. A review of 493 episodes. N Engl J Med 1993; 328:21–28
5. Berk SL, Smith JK: Infectious diseases in the elderly. Med Clin North Am 1983;67:273–293
6. Berk SL: Bacterial meningitis. pp. 235–253. In Gleckman RA, Gantz NM (eds): Infections in the Elderly. Little Brown, Boston, 1989
7. Choi C: Bacterial meningitis. Clin Geriatric Med 1992;8: 889–902
8. Berman RE, Meyers BR, Mendelson MH: Central nervous system infections in the elderly. Arch Intern Med 1989;149: 1596–1599
9. Gorse GO, Trupp LD, Needlewoman KL: Bacterial meningitis in the elderly. Arch Intern Med 1984;144:1603–1607

10. Roos KL: Meningitis as it presents in the elderly: diagnosis and care. Geriatrics 1990;45:63–75
11. Massanari RM: Purulent meningitis in the elderly. Geriatrics 1977;32:55–59
12. Jonson M, Alvin A: A 12 year review of acute bacterial meningitis in Stockholm. Scand J Infect Dis 1971;3:141–150
13. Quaade F: Meningitis in the aged. Geriatrics 1963;18:860–864
14. Marton KI, Gean AD: The spinal tap: a new look at an old test. Ann Intern Med 1986;104:840–848
15. Newton JE, Wilczynski PJG: Meningitis in the elderly. Lancet 1979;1:157–158
16. Swartz MN, Dodge PR: Bacterial meningitis—a review of selected aspects. N Engl J Med 1965;272:725–731
17. Quaade F, Kristensen KP: Purulent meningitis. A review of 658 cases. Acta Med Scand 1962;171:543–550
18. Berk SL, McCabe WR: Meningitis caused by gram-negative bacilli. Ann Intern Med 1980;93:253–260
19. Mangi RJ, Quintiliani R, Andriole VT: Gram-negative bacillary meningitis. Am J Med 1975;59:829–836
20. Berk SL, McCabe WR: Meningitis caused by *Acinetobacter Calcoaceticus var. Antitratus*. A specific hazard in neurosurgical patients. Arch Neurol 1981;38:95–98
21. Nguyen MH, Harris SP, Muder RR, Pasculle AW: Antibiotic-resistant *Acinetobacter* meningitis in neurosurgical patients. Department of Medicine and Pathology, University of Pittsburgh School of Medicine, Pennsylvania. Neurosurgery 1994;35:851–855
22. Siegman IY, Bar-Yosef S, Gorea A, Avram J: Nosocomial *Acinetobacter* meningitis secondary to invasive procedures: report of 25 cases and review. Department of Neurosurgery, Tel Aviv Sourasky Medical Center and Sackler Faculty of Medicine, Tel Aviv University, Israel. Clin Infect Dis 1993;17:843–849
23. Cherubin CE, Marr JS, Sierra MD, Becker S: *Listeria* and gram-negative bacillary meningitis in New York City 1972–1979. Am J Med 1981;71:199–209
24. Young LS, LaForce FM, Head JJ: A simultaneous outbreak of meningococcal and influenza infections. N Engl J Med 1972;287:5–9
25. Eigler JO, Wellman WE, Rooke ED: Bacterial meningitis—a general review. Proc Mayo Clin 1961;26:357–365
26. Dunne DW, Quagliarello V: Group B streptococcal meningitis in adults. Medicine 1993;72:1–10
27. Van Dijk K, Burger A: *Hemophilus influenzae* meningitis in the elderly. J Am Geriatr Soc 1986;34:530–532
28. Seydoux CH, Francioli P: Bacterial brain abscesses: factors influencing mortality and sequelae. Clin Infect Dis 1992;15:394–401
29. Scheld WM, Brodeur JP: Effect of methylprednisolone on entry of ampicillin and gentamicin into the cerebrospinal fluid in experimental pneumococcal and E. coli meningitis. Antimicrob Agents Chemother 1983;23:108–112
30. Kourtopoulous H, Holm SE, Norrby SR: The influence of steroids on the penetration of antibiotics into brain tissue and brain abscess. An experimental study in rats. J Antimicrob Chemother 1983;11:245–249
31. Rosenblum ML, Hoff JT, Norman D et al: Nonoperative treatment of brain abscesses in selected high-risk patients. J Neurosurg 1980;52:217–225
32. Garvey G: Current concepts of bacterial infections of the central nervous system. J Neurosurg 1983;59:735–744
33. Sjölin J, Lilja A, Eriksson N et al: Treatment of brain abscess with cefotaxime and metronidazole: prospective study of 15 consecutive cases. Clin Infect Dis 1993;17:857–863
34. Warner JF, Perkins RL, Cordero L: Metronidazole therapy of anaerobic bacteremia, meningitis and brain abscess. Arch Intern Med 1979;139:167–169
35. Weir MR, Thornton GF: Extrapulmonary tuberculosis: experience of a community hospital and review of the literature. Am J Med 1985;79:467–478
36. French GL, Teoh R, Chan CY et al: Diagnosis of tuberculosis meningitis by detection of tuberculostearic acid in cerebral spinal fluid. Lancet 1987;2:117–119
37. Shankar P, Manjunath N, Mohan K et al: Rapid diagnosis of tuberculosis meningitis by polymerase chain reaction. Lancet 1991;337:5–7
38. Mazurek GH, Reddy V, Murphy D, Ansari T: Detection of mycobacterium tuberculosis in cerebrospinal fluid following immunomagnetic enrichment. J Clin Microbiol 1996;34:450–453
39. Centers for Disease Control and Prevention: Initial therapy for tuberculosis in the era of multidrug resistance: recommendations of the Advisory Council for the elimination of tuberculosis. JAMA 1993;270:694–698
40. Bennett JE, Dismukes WE, Duma RT et al: A comparison of amphotericin B alone and combined with flucytosine in the treatment of cryptococcal meningitis. N Engl J Med 1979;301:126–131
41. Larsen RA, Leal MAE, Chan LS: Fluconazole compared with amphotericin B plus flucytosine for cryptococcal meningitis in AIDS: a randomized trial. Ann Intern Med 1990;113:183–187
42. Dewsnup DH, Galgiani JN, Graybill JR et al: Is it ever safe to stop azole therapy for *Coccidioides immitis* meningitis? Ann Intern Med 1996;124:305–310
43. Whitley RJ, Soong SJ, Linneman C Jr et al: Herpes simplex encephalitis: clinical assessment. JAMA 1982;247:317–320
44. Aurelius E, Johansson B, Skoldenberg B et al: Rapid diagnosis of herpes simplex encephalitis by nested polymerase chain reaction of cerebrospinal fluid. Lancet 1991;337:189
45. Merritt HH: A Textbook of Neurology. 2nd Ed. pp. 129–153. Lea & Febiger, Phildelphia, 1950
46. Simon RP: Neurosyphilis. Arch Neurol 1985;42:606–613
47. Dattwyler RJ, Halperin JJ, Volkmann DJ, Luft BJ: Treatment of late Lyme borreliosis—randomized comparison of ceftriaxone and penicillin. Lancet 1988;1:1191

C H A P T E R 46

Aging and Disorders of the Eye

SCOTT E. BRODIE

Loss of vision, one of the most feared forms of medical disability, falls disproportionately on the elderly. Unfortunately, the damage to the delicate tissues of the eye from the various metabolic insults that may occur throughout life is generally cumulative. Consequently, most forms of ocular pathology occur ever more frequently, and in more debilitating forms, with increasing age.

Estimates of the prevalence of blindness from all causes vary by perhaps a factor of 13 between industrialized and Third World societies.[1] Nevertheless, regardless of the degree of economic development, the prevalence rate for blindness in any society is typically 100-fold greater among individuals over 65 years of age than among children in the same society.[2] In developed countries, the major causes of blindness are primarily cataract, glaucoma, and retinal disease (mostly macular degeneration and diabetic retinopathy), all of which are strongly related to advancing age. In the Third World, the major causes of blindness are cataract, corneal scarring, glaucoma, and retinal disease.[2]

Delivery of adequate eye care to elderly individuals remains an unsolved problem, even in wealthy countries. Recent surveys in the United States have identified significant rates of untreated eye disease among the elderly. The nursing home population appears to be notably underserved.[3,4]

Discussion of age-related ocular problems is conveniently organized by considering the visual apparatus in anatomic order from anterior to posterior.

Eyelids

The eyelids are vital for the proper circulation of tears and maintenance of the smooth ocular surface necessary for clear image formation by the eye. With increasing age, the skin of the eyelids, as elsewhere, loses elasticity, and the lids become more loosely apposed to the globe. Atrophy of the fascial planes within the eyelids may lead to herniation of the orbital fat into the lid tissue, producing the "bags under the eyes" frequently seen in the elderly. Atrophy or disinsertion of the aponeurosis of the levator palpebrae muscle, which ordinarily supports the upper eyelid, may cause the opened lid to fail to uncover the pupil, as seen in senile ptosis, despite normal levator muscle function (Fig. 46-1; see also Plate 46-1). Senile ptosis must be differentiated from ptosis due to mechanical and neuromuscular causes, such as oculomotor nerve palsies and myasthenia gravis.[5]

Laxity of the lower lid may allow the free lid margin to rotate away from the eyeball, a condition known as ectropion. If severe, the lacrimal punctum may fail to make contact with the pool of tears adjacent to the lower lid. This prevents the normal conduction of tears into the lacrimal sac, which may result in persistent tearing (epiphora) even in the absence of lacrimal duct obstruction. More dangerous is entropion, in which a loosening of the adhesions between tissue planes in the lid allows the muscle tone of the orbicularis oculi to rotate the lid margin inward.[6] Frequently, the lashes come to rub directly against the cornea or conjunctiva, producing irritation or scarring.

The treatment of eyelid malpositions is generally surgical. For senile ptosis, resection of the levator aponeurosis is generally performed.[7] Ectropion and entropion are generally treated by resection of redundant lid tissue.[8]

Of the tumors of the eyelid skin, basal cell carcinomas are the most common. These tumors are frequently a consequence of lifetime exposure to sunlight. If the lesions are detected early, a curative local resection is often possible. In advanced cases, the tumor may cause massive destruction of facial structures by local extension. Metastases are very rare.[9]

Lacrimal Apparatus

The lacrimal apparatus consists of the lacrimal glands, which secrete the tears, and the lacrimal ducts, which convey the tears into the nasal cavity. Secretory function of the lacrimal glands declines with age, and many elderly individuals develop "dry eye" syndrome. (This nonspecific reduction in tear production is much more common than the full-fledged Sjögren syndrome, which is an autoimmune disease process affecting both salivary and lacrimal secretion.[10]) Paradoxically, many tear-deficient patients complain of excess tearing, because the chronically irritated eyes may stimulate reflex tear production. Dry eyes are treated with artificial tear eyedrops, as often as needed. In patients whose eyes dry out overnight, lubricant ointment at bedtime may be helpful. In severe cases, surgical occlusion of the lacrimal puncta may conserve the available tears.

Obstruction of the lacrimal ducts also leads to epiphora. Uncomplicated mechanical stenosis may occasionally be relieved with simple probing, but severe cases (often following bacterial infection of the lacrimal sac) are treated surgically: a dacryocystorhinostomy is performed to anastamose the mu-

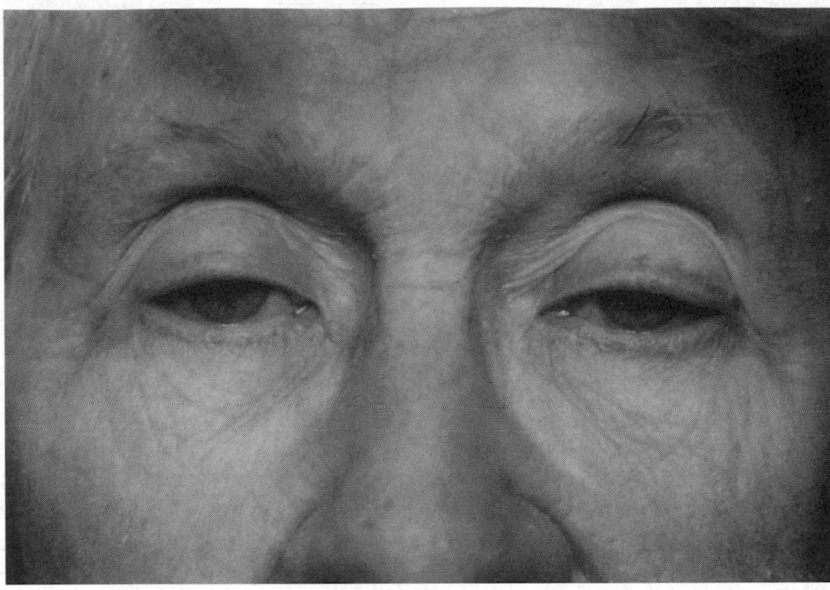

Figure 46-1 Senile ptosis. Note the low lid level and the loss of the normal lid folds. (Courtesy of Murray Meltzer, MD.)

cosa of the nasal cavity to the lacrimal sac through an osteotomy made in the lacrimal bone.[11]

Conjunctiva

Subconjunctival hemorrhage, a localized accumulation of blood seen between the conjunctiva and the globe, is frequently seen in the elderly, either following minor trauma, or occurring spontaneously (Fig. 46-2; see also Plate 46-2). Such hemorrhages are rarely of any consequence, but are often alarming in appearance. They resolve spontaneously without treatment over a period of several days. Occasionally, recurrent hemorrhages may suggest an underlying disease such as hypertension or a coagulation disorder.

Chronic exposure to sunlight, particularly at tropical latitudes, may cause a degeneration of the connective tissue in the exposed sector of the conjunctiva between the eyelids, leading to thickening of the conjunctiva (pingueculum), which may grow over the cornea from the periphery toward the pupil (pterygium). If the growth threatens to cover the visual axis, surgical excision may be indicated. Recurrence after surgery is, unfortunately, not uncommon.[12]

Tumors such as squamous cell carcinoma and melanoma may arise from the conjunctiva. Local excision and cryoablation may be adequate in early cases, but advanced cases may require orbital exenteration.[13]

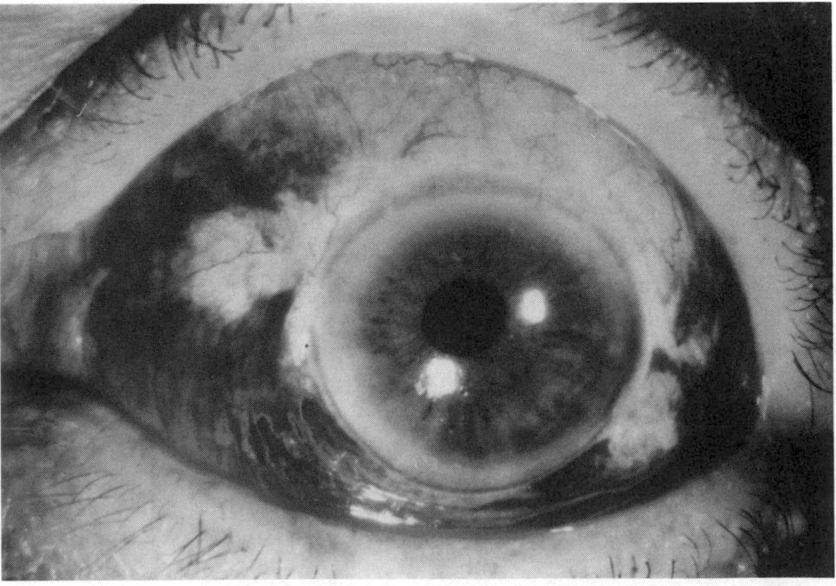

Figure 46-2 Subconjunctival hemorrhage. This small hematoma, seen through the transparent conjunctiva, is benign, unless recurrent.

Cornea

The eye is unique in its requirement for transparent tissues: the cornea and crystalline lens. The need for transparency places many constraints on the architecture and metabolism of these ocular structures. In particular, the eye must nourish these tissues with a cell-free fluid, as red blood cells preclude transparency. Similarly, the transparent tissues must rely primarily on anaerobic glycolytic metabolism, as the enzyme systems required for oxidative phosphorylation (aptly named cytochromes) strongly absorb visible light. Even in the absence of these absorbent components, the tissues must be constructed in a highly compact and regular manner, so that light scattering from tissue organelles does not cause a white, opaque appearance. This requirement is met in the case of the cornea by an active metabolic pump in the corneal endothelial cell layer, which acts to dehydrate the corneal stroma. (Absence of this dehydration mechanism is the main reason that the sclera, which is otherwise histologically very similar to the cornea, is opaque.)[14]

The corneal endothelial cells, on which the dehydration critical for corneal transparency depends, do not divide during adulthood. Indeed, the endothelial cell density declines slowly with age.[15] If the number of endothelial cells falls below a critical level, the cornea imbibes fluid, swells, and becomes cloudy (Fig. 46-3; see also Plate 46-3). Edema fluid percolates to the epithelial surface, and may coalesce into subepithelial bullae. Mild cases may be managed with the use of hypertonic saline eyedrops and ointment to withdraw fluid from the cornea osmotically. If these measures fail, a full-thickness corneal graft, which replaces the deficient endothelium, is necessary to restore vision.[16]

Bacterial ulcers of the cornea (Fig. 46-4; see also Plate 46-4). are particularly common in the elderly, perhaps reflecting impairments of tear secretion, epithelial integrity, and cellular and humoral immunity. Intensive antibiotic therapy is generally required.[17]

The ring-shaped deposition of lipid in the far periphery of the cornea, referred to as *arcus senilis*, is completely benign.

Uveal Tract

The uveal tract ("uvea") comprises the iris, ciliary body, and chorioid, which form a continuous, highly vascular layer inside the sclera. Inflammation of the uvea occurs frequently, as a primary disease process, or in response to infections, in many patients with collagen-vascular disease, and as a sequela to accidental or surgical trauma. Clinically, inflammatory cells are seen in the aqueous or vitreous humor. These inflammatory reactions can cause ocular injury by many mechanisms. They may occlude the trabecular meshwork, causing glaucoma. They may accumulate on the inner surface of the cornea as keratic precipitates, where they may injure or destroy the corneal endothelial cells and cause corneal edema. Inflamed tissues often develop pathologic adhesions, which may derange normal ocular function. Adhesions between the anterior surface of the peripheral iris and the anterior chamber angle (peripheral anterior synechiae) may occlude the trabecular meshwork, leading to chronic angle-closure glaucoma. Adhesions between the posterior surface of the iris and the anterior surface of the crystalline lens can seal off access of the aqueous humor to the anterior chamber (pupillary block), forcing the iris to bow forward (iris bombé). In cases where the peripheral iris becomes apposed to the trabecular meshwork, the egress of aqueous humor from the eye is blocked, resulting in angle-closure glaucoma. In the posterior segment, inflammatory cells in the vitreous humor may obscure vision, and may lead to fibrovascular proliferation that may distort the retina, or even cause a retinal detachment.

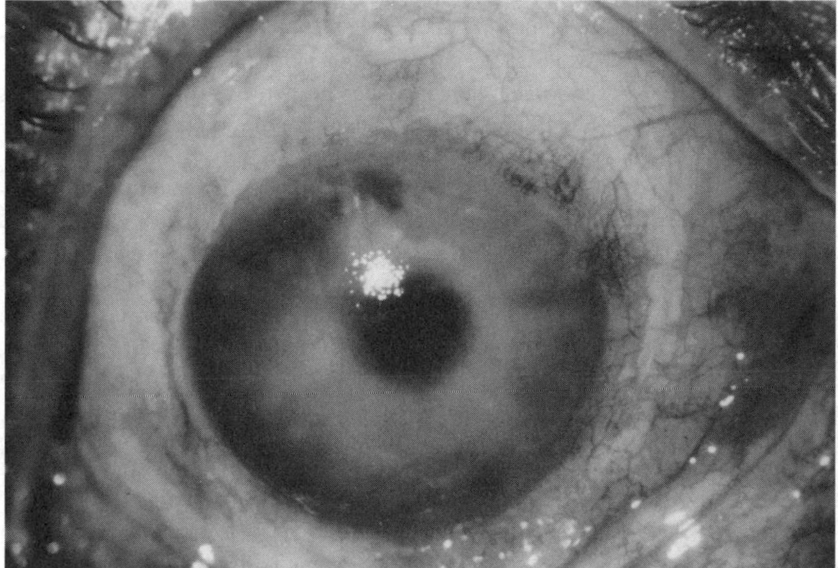

Figure 46-3 Corneal edema. The cornea is thickened and cloudy due to failure of the corneal endothelium to adequately dehydrate the tissue. (Courtesy of Calvin Roberts, MD.)

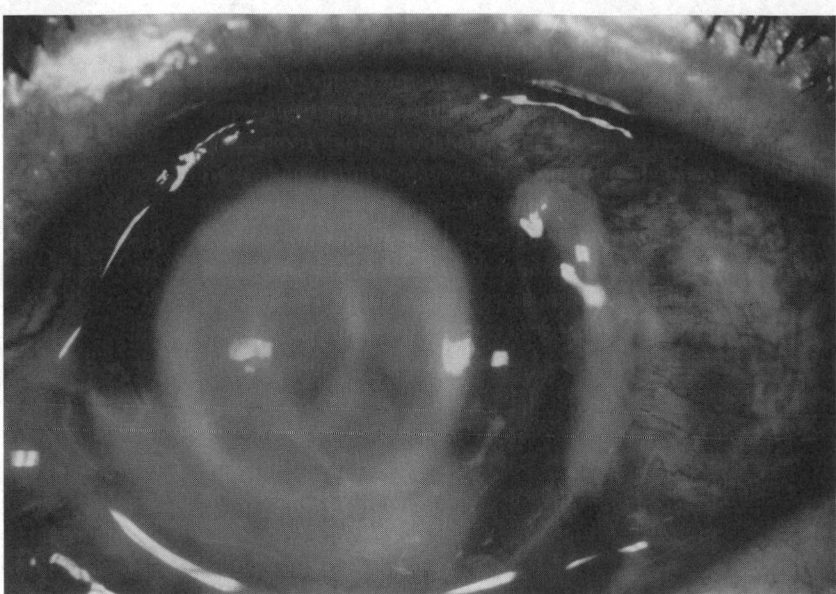

Figure 46-4 Corneal ulcer. A localized infection causes an epithelial defect, and attracts an infiltrate of white blood cells. (Courtesy of Michael Newton, MD.)

Treatment in most cases of uveitis is generally empirical. Dilation of the pupil with cycloplegic eyedrops is generally advisable to prevent posterior synechiae and pupillary block, and to relieve the discomfort (photophobia) caused by light-induced miosis of the inflamed iris. If the inflammation is confined to the anterior segment, topical steroid eyedrops are usually sufficient. In cases involving the posterior segment, retrobulbar steroid injections or systemic administration of steroids are frequently required. In recalcitrant or recurrent cases, a workup for underlying systemic disease is appropriate. If a treatable systemic condition is discovered, such as syphilis or tuberculosis, specific treatment for the underlying condition may simultaneously cure the uveitis. In refractory cases, some success has been achieved with systemic administration of cytotoxic medications and cyclosporine A.[18]

Intraocular tumors in the elderly occur most frequently within the uveal tract. Melanomas are the most common primary tumor. Treatment is controversial; although prompt enucleation (surgical removal of the eyeball) has been the traditional management, retrospective studies have suggested that there is an excess mortality which appears to be associated with the enucleation procedure itself, perhaps due to manipulation of the globe during surgery.[19] Many authorities now recommend that, because they have only a very low propensity for metastasis, small uveal melanomas be followed closely, rather than enucleated. (Enucleation is still recommended in cases where tumor enlargement is observed.)[20] Larger tumors have been successfully treated in many cases with irradiation, either by temporary implantation of a radioactive plaque applied to the overlying sclera,[21] or administered by external beam. Primary enucleation is recommended for large tumors. Metastatic melanoma is usually detected initially in the liver. Regular physical examinations and monitoring of hepatic enzyme activity in the serum are advisable for patients at risk.

Tumors metastatic to the choroid are not uncommon. Lung primaries predominate in men, breast primaries in women.[22] As the eye is seldom the sole site of metastasis, these patients generally require systemic chemotherapy directed at the primary cancer.

Glaucoma

Glaucoma is a form of progressive atrophy of the optic nerve, frequently associated with increased intraocular pressure (Figs. 46-5 and 46-6; see also Plates 46-5 and 46-6).

Open-Angle Glaucoma

In many cases, the primary pathology is presumed to lie in the trabecular meshwork, the ring of porous tissue located in the anterior chamber angle through which aqueous humor drains from the eye. Impaired facility of aqueous outflow through the trabecular meshwork is generally idiopathic (so-called primary open-angle glaucoma). This condition is generally reported to increase in prevalence with increasing age, at least in most Western populations.[23] Loss of outflow facility may also arise from various insults to the trabecular meshwork, including trauma, uveitis, hemorrhage, and dispersion of intraocular pigment.

Visual impairment from open-angle glaucoma is generally insidious and chronic, with visual field damage occurring initially in the far periphery, where it is rarely noticeable except by formal testing. Our ability to diagnose this condition in its early stages is quite imperfect. The actual risk of visual field loss in untreated individuals with modestly elevated intraocular pressure is only 1 to 2 percent per year[24]; conversely, histologic studies have shown that as many as 40 percent of the optic nerve fibers must be destroyed before any abnormality of the visual field is detectable by standard techniques.[25]

Initial treatment is usually medical. The goal of therapy is to lower the intraocular pressure with topical or systemic medications, to a level that is tolerated by the optic nerve, as

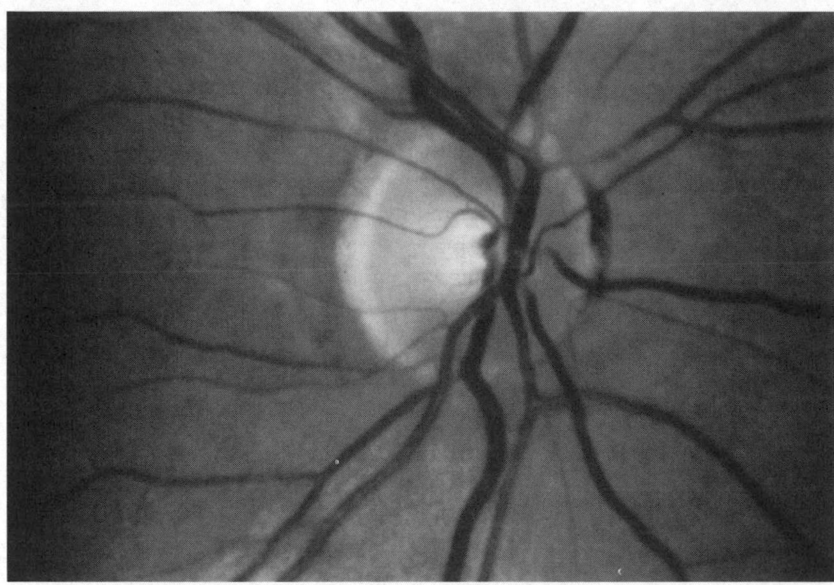

Figure 46-5 Normal optic nerve head. Cup to disc ratio is about 0.3.

demonstrated by the cessation of progressive visual field loss. Available medications include parasympathomimetic miotics, anticholinesterase miotics, sympathomimetics, β-adrenergic blockers, carbonic anhydrase inhibitors, and prostaglandin analogs. The potential side effects of the various topical and systemic pressure-lowering drugs are occasionally serious, particularly in elderly patients (see Systemic Complications of Ophthalmic Medications, below). If medical treatment is unsuccessful, or poorly tolerated, intraocular pressure may be further lowered by laser treatments to the trabecular meshwork, or by "filtering surgery," which creates a fistula between the anterior chamber and the subconjunctival space, allowing easier egress of aqueous humor. Complications of filtering surgery are not infrequent, including hypotony, choroidal effusion, and cataract. Supplementary medical treatment after filtering surgery is often also required. The optimal stage in the disease process for surgical intervention is unclear. Some authors have reported better long-term visual results with earlier surgery.[26]

A recent study has suggested that laser treatment to the trabecular meshwork may also be suitable as initial therapy.[27]

Angle-Closure Glaucoma

Occasionally, alterations in intraocular anatomy may predispose the iris to cover the trabecular meshwork, suddenly preventing aqueous outflow, and causing an acute elevation of the intraocular pressure. Frequent scenarios include adhesions between iris and lens (pupillary block), which may cause the iris to bow forward so as to occlude the trabecular meshwork, and dilation of the pupil, such as may occur spontaneously in the dark, or following pharmacologic mydriasis. Gradual enlargement of the lens with increasing age or cataract forma-

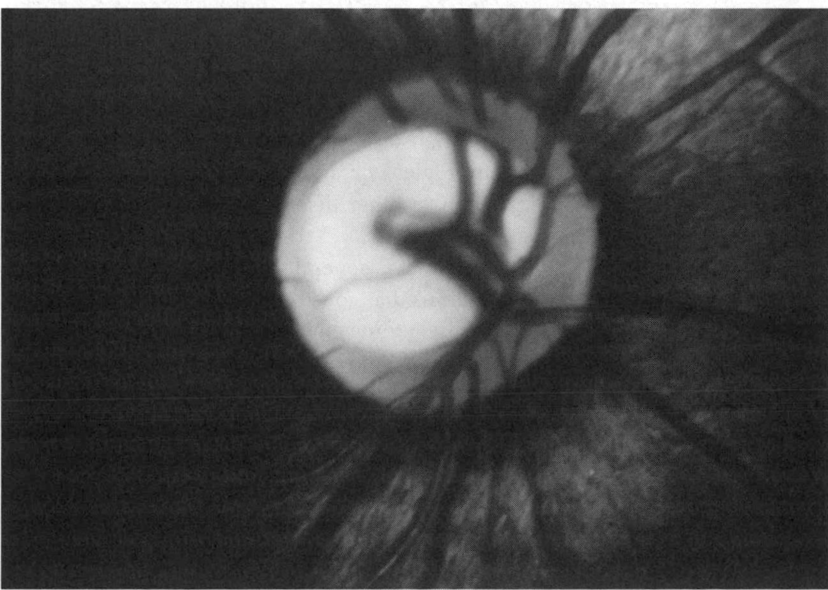

Figure 46-6 Glaucomatous optic nerve head cupping. Loss of neural tissue is seen as narrowing of the neural rim of the optic disc, and enlargement of the central cup. (Compare with Fig. 46-5.)

tion is an important factor that predisposes the eye to this process in the elderly. Acute angle-closure glaucoma is generally a dramatic event, with symptoms including severe pain, blurring of vision, perception of colored haloes around lights, nausea, and vomiting. Diagnosis of acute angle closure is easy once attention is directed to the eye, but may be missed if attention is diverted to the gastrointestinal symptoms. Cases have been reported from the emergency departments of general hospitals where concentration on the nausea and vomiting of a patient with acute angle closure has led to exploratory laparotomy!

The massive elevation of intraocular pressure following acute angle closure (often to triple the normal upper limit of 21 mmHg) may cause permanent optic nerve damage within a matter of weeks. Acute angle closure is generally treated by lowering the intraocular pressure with systemic and topical medications, including miotic eyedrops and systemic osmotic agents. In cases of pupillary block, a small hole (peripheral iridectomy) is made in the iris by laser or invasive surgery to bypass the pupillary block and allow passage of aqueous humor from the posterior segment into the anterior chamber. This prevents subsequent angle-closure attacks. Because the anatomic factors that predispose an eye to acute angle closure are generally found bilaterally, it is usually considered prudent to perform a peripheral iridectomy prophylactically in the fellow eye after an attack of angle closure.

Prolonged episodes of angle closure may result in permanent damage to the trabecular meshwork, or even adhesions between the iris and sectors of the trabecular meshwork, leading to chronic angle-closure glaucoma. If the angle is sufficiently compromised, filtering surgery may be necessary.

Although elevated intraocular pressure has historically been the hallmark of the diagnosis of glaucoma, it has become clear in recent decades that many patients with otherwise typical glaucomatous optic atrophy and visual field loss seldom if ever are found to have elevated intraocular pressure. Identification and treatment of this so-called low-tension glaucoma (or perhaps more accurately normal-tension glaucoma) remains problematic, although even in this cohort, reduction of intraocular pressure is thought to convey some benefit. This entity is probably more common than previously thought, as population-based surveys have demonstrated a substantial incidence of otherwise typical glaucomatous field loss in patients with normal intraocular pressures.[28]

Crystalline Lens

The crystalline lens of the eye is a unique ectodermal structure that develops entirely within the primordial lens vesicle. Only the cells on the extreme periphery of the lens divide, adding cells to the outer surface of the growing lens. Thus the center of the adult lens represents the earliest tissue laid down during embryonic development. There is no mechanism by which these cells can turn over, unlike the situation in typical ectodermal structures, such as the skin. The metabolism of the lens is largely confined to anaerobic glycolysis, as neither hemoglobin-mediated oxygen transport nor cytochrome-mediated oxidative phosphorylation is available owing to the need for transparency. The lens is at a further metabolic disadvantage due to the need to maintain a state of great disequilibrium with its surroundings, as the lens must maintain the highest protein concentration, and one of the lowest water concentrations, of any tissue in the body. Thus, relatively modest metabolic insults or osmotic stresses may overwhelm the lens metabolism, resulting in protein denaturation and cataract formation.[29]

The lens of the eye continues to grow and mature throughout life. As the lens ages, it becomes more rigid, and responds less effectively to changes in ciliary muscle tone, decreasing the effectiveness of accommodation, the eye's mechanism for focusing from distant to near objects. This loss of accommodation (presbyopia) is managed with reading glasses or bifocals, or other refractive strategies.

The lens responds to virtually any mechanical or metabolic insult by loss of optical clarity, resulting in the formation of a cataract (Fig. 46-7; see also Plate 46-7). Several patterns of opacities are recognized.

Oxidation ("browning reactions") of lens proteins, particularly in the older, central portions of the lens, is referred to as *nuclear sclerosis*, which may result in alterations in the refractive index of the lens as well as frank opacity. The most common refractive change is in the direction of an increase in myopia or decrease in hyperopia. In some instances, this refractive shift will allow the patient to read without reading glasses (so-called second sight). This improvement in visual performance is usually only temporary, and often heralds the development of a more debilitating lens opacity. Refractive changes in the lens need not be uniform. Patients will occasionally report monocular diplopia due to inhomogeneous refraction by distinct portions of the lens resulting in two distinct images being formed on the retina. (The notion that monocular diplopia is generally indicative of hysteria is incorrect.)

Denaturation of lens proteins in a sector of adjacent cortical lens fibers results in a wedge-shaped cuneiform or cortical opacity. These are often found in the far periphery of the lens, but frequently spare the optical zone near the center.

Aberrant proliferation of lens fibers on the posterior lens capsule produces a posterior subcapsular cataract. These are often induced by topical or systemic steroid treatment, and are frequently seen in other disease states, such as retinitis pigmentosa.

Treatment of cataract is generally surgical. With rare exceptions, the lens proteins that constitute the opacity are irreversibly denatured, precluding medical treatment.[30] Surgical strategies for removal of the lens material have evolved greatly over recent years. In all cases, an incision must be made in the eyeball—a cataract cannot be removed solely "with a laser." The simplest operation is to remove the entire lens intact within its lens capsule, a so-called intracapsular procedure. At present, the extracapsular procedure, in which the opaque lens tissue is carefully aspirated from within the lens capsule, has returned to favor, as retention of the capsule to

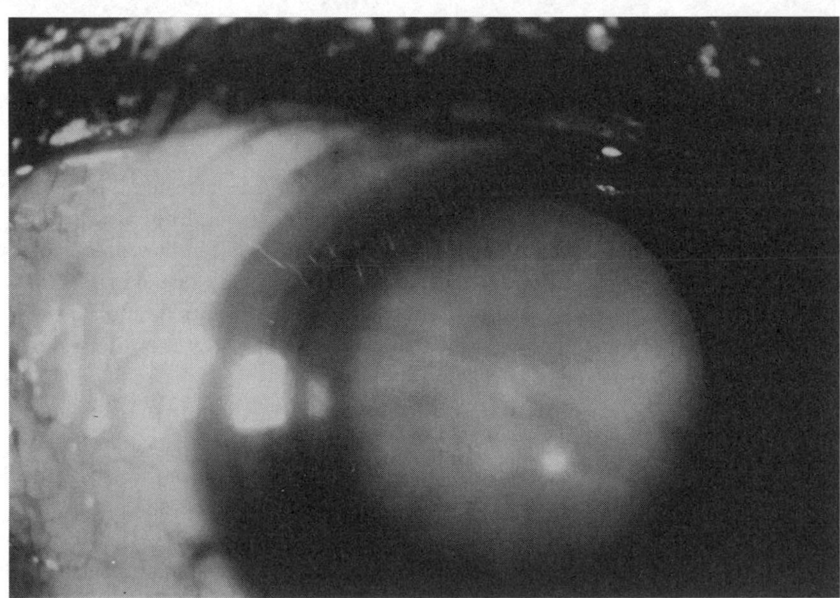

Figure 46-7 Cataract. Loss of transparency of the crystalline lens impairs visual acuity. (Courtesy of Calvin Roberts, MD.)

serve as a barrier between the anterior and posterior segments of the eye appears to reduce the rate of complications. Recently, greater emphasis has been placed on the development of minimally invasive surgical methods for cataract extraction. Often, the cataract can be liquefied by the mechanical action of a rapidly vibrating needle (phacoemulsification), and aspirated from the eye through an incision only 3 to 4 mm in length.[31] In favorable cases, such wounds can be constructed to be self-sealing, eliminating the need for sutures.[32]

Indications for cataract surgery should be determined in relation to the visual needs of each individual patient. Occasionally, cataract extraction is recommended for technical reasons, such as those rare cases when the lens is itself causing injury to the eye (as in phacolytic glaucoma, when lens proteins leak from a cataractous lens and occlude the trabecular meshwork), or when a cataractous lens prevents adequate visualization or treatment of disease of the posterior segment of the eye, such as diabetic retinopathy. Otherwise, cataract surgery is appropriate whenever the anticipated improvement in visual function would be of benefit to the patient. In general, a visual result of 6/12 (20/40) or better may be anticipated in 90 to 95 percent of cases without other known concurrent ocular disease; thus, surgery is generally recommended only when the acuity has fallen to the level of 6/15 (20/50) or worse. In some patients, difficulties with glare, contrast sensitivity, diplopia, or occupational demands may justify cataract extraction regardless of the visual acuity.

Optical rehabilitation of the aphakic eye requires replacement of the focusing power of the cataractous lens that was removed. Where economic conditions permit, this is usually provided by means of a plastic intraocular lens prosthesis, which is generally implanted at the time of the primary cataract operation. Alternatives include contact lenses (often worn on an extended-wear basis) and thick "aphakic" spectacles, which subject the patient to substantial optical distortions, and (if the aphakia is unilateral) may cause substantial difficulties due to unequal perceived image size in the two eyes. (Indeed, the difficulties with spectacle correction of unilateral aphakes are sufficiently severe that, if spectacle correction is the only modality of optical rehabilitation available, most surgeons recommend deferral of surgery until visual acuity in the *better* eye falls to 6/18 [20/60] or worse.) In some Third World countries, local custom may discourage the use of spectacles after cataract surgery. In these situations, the attitudes of the patient must be taken into account in the decision as to whether or not to perform a cataract extraction.

Some yellowing of the lens proteins is nearly universal with aging. Sufficient opacity to impair visual acuity results in over 1 million cataract extractions each year in the United States, the vast majority in individuals over 65 years of age. In developing countries, the rate of cataract formation appears to be even higher, so that untreated cataract typically forms the largest single cause of acquired blindness. In India, for example, even at the present rate of millions of cataract procedures each year, present surgical efforts continue to fall behind the rate of new cataract formation in the general population.

Cataract formation may occasionally reflect an underlying metabolic abnormality, such as galactosemia or renal failure. Cataract formation is accelerated in diabetic patients, and may be triggered by various drugs (particularly topical or systemic steroids). In addition to these specific associations, several studies have shown a nonspecific excess mortality among cataract patients, compared with age-matched control patients undergoing other elective surgical procedures.[33] These studies suggest that development of cataracts may reflect a generalized reduction in metabolic competence in these elderly individuals.

Retina and Vitreous

Diseases of the retina, particularly diabetic retinopathy and so-called age-related macular degeneration (formerly referred to as "senile macular degeneration") constitute the most frequent cause of acquired blindness, at least in developed countries.

Diabetic retinopathy shows a steady increase in incidence and severity with increasing duration of diabetes mellitus, with significant visual complications rarely occurring before 10 to 15 years after the onset of the disease.[34] Thus, while juvenile-onset (type I) patients may develop severe retinopathy as early as the third decade, the retinal burden of adult-onset (type II) patients is borne largely by the elderly. The disease seems to attack primarily the retinal capillary circulation. Initially, small, innocuous microaneurysms are noted ophthalmoscopically. With time, the retinal capillaries begin to leak fluid into the surrounding tissue, causing retinal edema and precipitation of exudates into the retinal tissue, with a concomitant reduction in visual acuity (Fig. 46-8; see also Plate 46-8) At this stage of the disease, loss of visual acuity may be reduced through the use of laser treatments, directed at leaking microaneurysms or, if the leakage is diffuse, placed in a grid pattern over the leaky segments of the retinal capillary bed.[35]

In later stages, perfusion of small sectors of the retinal capillary bed fails (capillary dropout), leading to localized retinal infarctions, which may be seen ophthalmoscopically as cotton-wool spots. The remaining capillaries are often seen to become dilated, irregular, and leaky. Ultimately, in many patients, the ischemic retina develops a neovascular proliferative response, sprouting new blood vessels that may grow along the retinal surface or along the posterior surface of the vitreous body. These aberrant blood vessels are prone to leaking and hemorrhages. Vision may also be lost through traction exerted on the retina by fibroblastic membranes that accompany the neovascular proliferation (Fig. 46-9; see also Plate 46-9). In severe cases, the neovascular response may extend to the anterior segment, producing neovascularization on the surface of the iris (rubeosis iridis). If the fibrovascular membrane extends over the anterior chamber angle, it obstructs filtration of aqueous humor through the trabecular meshwork, producing a refractory neovascular glaucoma.

Proliferative retinopathy may often be arrested through the ablation of a large fraction of the peripheral retina with laser photocoagulation.[36] In severe cases, blood in the vitreous cavity and fibrovascular membranes may be removed surgically, typically by introducing mechanized suction-cutter instruments through small scleral incisions over the ciliary body (pars plana vitrectomy).

The benefit of tight control of blood glucose in the management of diabetic retinopathy depends on the stage of the disease. Many attempts to retard the progression of established retinopathy by improving the degree of glucose control have been disappointing.[37] Indeed, in some studies, tight control has been associated with a worsening of retinopathy. Similarly, in one study, successful pancreatic transplantation, with near-perfect normalization of blood glucose levels, failed to improve diabetic retinopathy, compared to the retinal disease in fellow pancreatic transplant patients whose allografts failed, requiring resumption of daily insulin injections, with the usual deficiencies in control of blood glucose.[38] However, it has recently been demonstrated (albeit in a study enrolling only type I diabetic patients) that better glucose control in recent-onset diabetic patients may retard the onset of diabetic retinal disease.[39]

Age-related macular degeneration is a common cause of impaired vision, although rarely total blindness, in the elderly population. In the "atrophic" form, the retinal pigment epithelium and choriocapillaris underlying the macula appear to degenerate, resulting in dysfunction of the overlying photorecep-

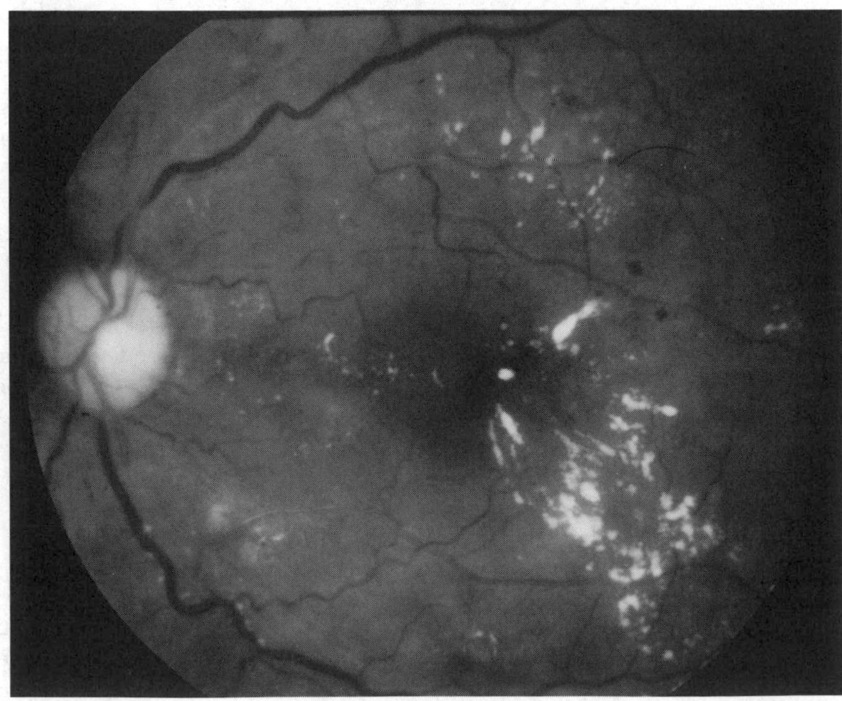

Figure 46-8 Background diabetic retinopathy. Microaneurysms ("dot hemorrhages"), intraretinal hemorrhages ("blot hemorrhages"), and "hard" exudates indicate deterioration of the retinal microcirculation.

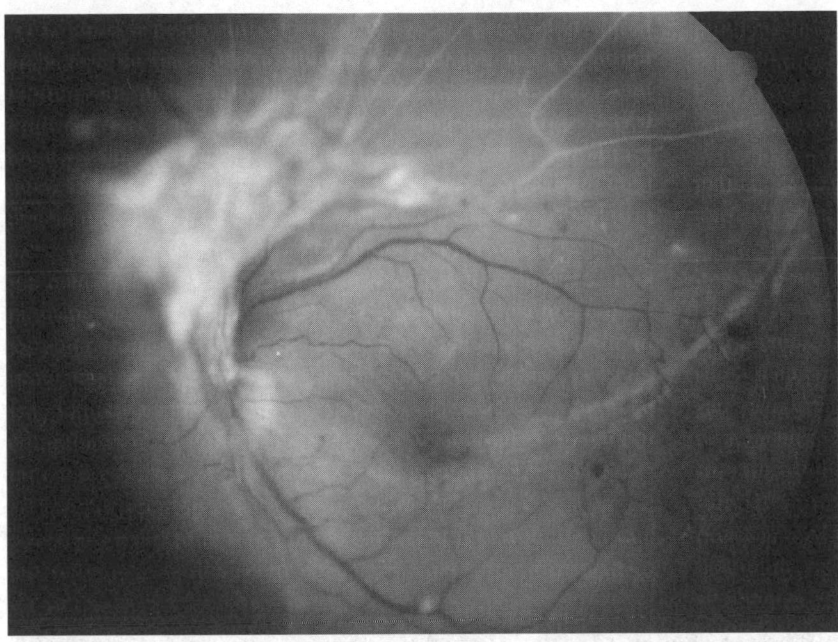

Figure 46-9 Proliferative diabetic retinopathy. A membrane of fibrovascular tissue has sprouted from the optic disc in response to prolonged retinal ischemia.

tors (Fig. 46-10; see also Plate 46-10). There is no known treatment. In the "exudative" form, a neovascular net emanates under the macular region of the central retina from the choroidal circulation, proliferating between the retina and the underlying retinal pigment epithelium.[40] Leakage of plasma components and frank subretinal hemorrhage cause loss of vision (Fig. 46-11; see also Plate 46-11). In a small portion of cases, laser treatment of neovascular membranes outside of the foveal region may arrest the growth of these membranes before they undermine the central macula, thus helping to preserve central vision.[41]

Some authors have even recommended laser treatment of subfoveal membranes, on the theory that it may be possible to thus limit the size and severity of the central scotoma (blind spot) that ultimately results from leakage and scarring. This treatment has gained only limited acceptance, as the immediate effects of the laser treatment frequently include acute loss of central vision, and a net benefit is not apparent until about 2 years after laser treatment.[42]

In both atrophic and exudative types of macular degeneration, the pathologic process appears to be confined to the posterior pole. These diseases thus spare the peripheral retina in nearly all cases, so that most affected patients indefinitely retain sufficient vision for independent ambulation, and may

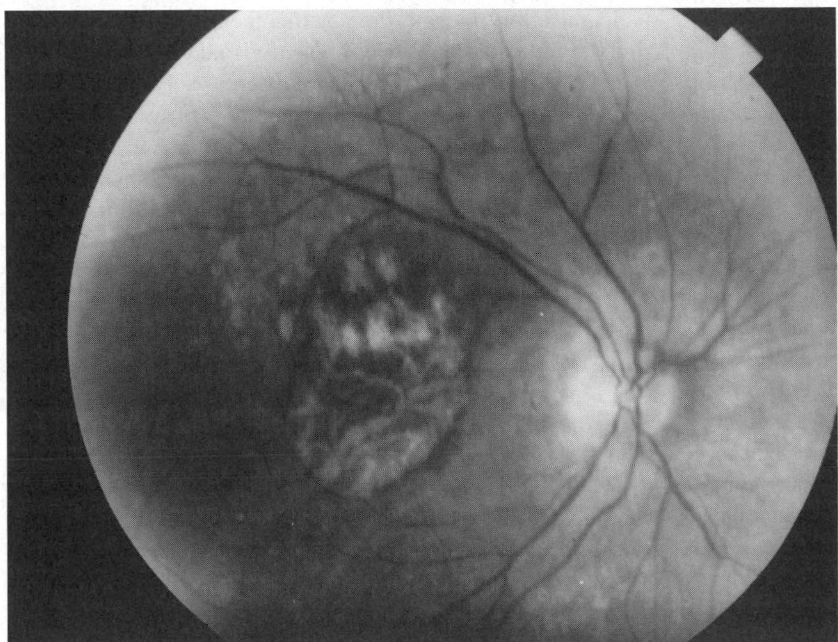

Figure 46-10 Atrophic ("dry") age-related macular degeneration. Geographic atrophy of the retinal pigment epithelium causes loss of central vision.

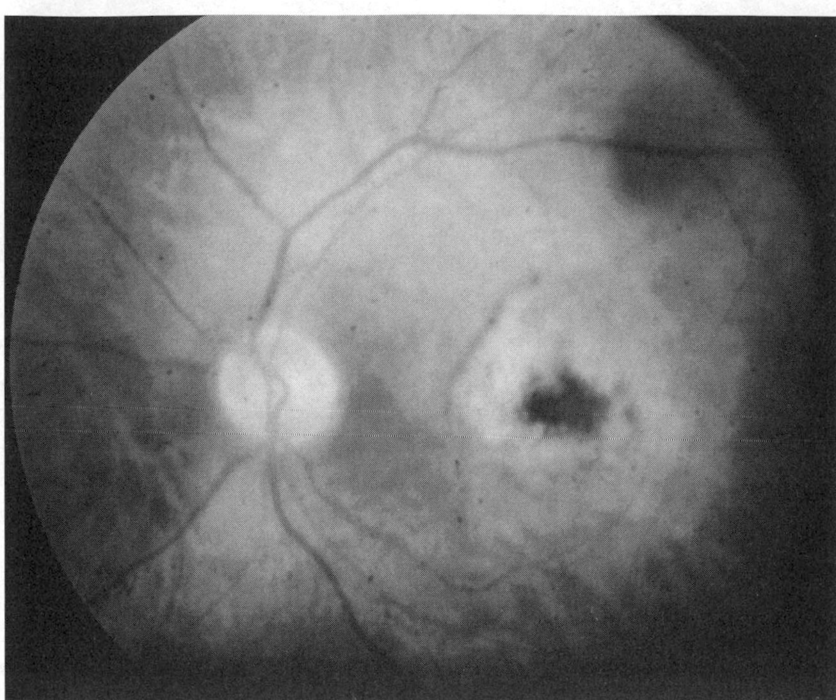

Figure 46-11 Exudative ("wet") age-related macular degeneration. Leakage and scarring from a subretinal neovascular membrane destroys central retinal function.

be reassured that they are not going to go completely blind.

The pale white dots known as *drusen*, frequently seen in the retinas of older patients, are usually quite benign. They correspond to small deposits of amorphous hyaline material seen histologically between Bruch's membrane and the retinal pigment epithelium. However, these lesions appear to serve as a predisposing factor in the evolution of exudative macular degeneration.[43] Elderly patients with drusen, or who have lost vision in one eye to age-related macular degeneration, may be advised to check their vision every day by examination of an Amsler grid, a 10-cm square of ruled graph paper. Any abnormality or distortion of the central vision should prompt an immediate examination of the retina. This will maximize the chance that a subretinal neovascular net will be discovered before it undermines the fovea, when laser treatment is most effective.

Retinovascular Occlusive Disease

Both retinal arteries and retinal veins are subject to sudden occlusive events, particularly in the elderly. Retinal artery occlusions are usually either embolic or arteritic in nature. Embolic occlusions are due to the occlusion of a retinal artery by a small particle derived from the more proximal circulation, most commonly a cholesterol fragment from an ulcerated atherosclerotic plaque. A small refractile cholesterol crystal may often be visualized within a retinal artery (Hollenhorst plaque). The affected sector of the retina appears pale. Various measures to encourage migration of the occlusive plaque toward the retinal periphery have been recommended, including lowering of intraocular pressure by medical means or by withdrawal of a small amount of fluid from the anterior chamber with a fine needle, and dilation of the retinal arterial tree by breathing an elevated concentration of carbon dioxide. No convincing benefit of these maneuvers has been demonstrated.[44]

Transient obscurations of vision, typically lasting less than 10 minutes (amaurosis fugax) are generally believed to represent embolic arterial occlusions that are quickly dislodged into the far retinal periphery.[45] These attacks indicate an elevated risk of occlusive stroke.[46]

Arteritic disease (e.g., temporal arteritis) may also cause occlusion of the arteries of the retina or optic nerve head. An elevated erythrocyte sedimentation rate is commonly, but not invariably, observed. The diagnosis is usually confirmed by temporal artery biopsy. Prompt treatment with systemic steroids is indicated, and may prevent visual loss in the fellow eye.[47] If the diagnosis of temporal arteritis is suspected, most authorities recommend immediate initiation of systemic steroid treatment; it is unwise to wait until the erythrocyte sedimentation rate and the results of a temporal artery biopsy can be obtained, as the fellow eye may lose vision in the interim. If the tests are negative, the steroid treatment can usually be stopped promptly without a period of tapering doses.

Retinal vein occlusions result in a pattern of vascular tortuosity and intraretinal hemorrhage in the affected sector of the retina. Most retinal vein occlusions seem to be due to compression of a retinal vein by an adjacent retinal artery, frequently exacerbated by hypertension, arteriosclerosis, or glaucoma. Although there is no treatment for the occlusion itself, retinal vein occlusion carries a significant risk of subsequent neovascular complications, particularly glaucoma. In cases where retinal ischemia can be demonstrated (typically by fluorescein angiography or electroretinography), retinal ablation by laser photocoagulation can substantially reduce the risk of subsequent neovascularization.[48]

Optic Nerve

The elderly are particularly susceptible to ischemic injury to the optic nerve. Infarctions of the entire optic nerve head cause sudden obscuration of vision in one eye, and present ophthalmoscopically with optic nerve head swelling and hemorrhages. Many patients present with infarction of only a portion of the optic nerve head, resulting in sudden onset of an altitudinal visual field defect. As with retinal artery occlusions, it is important to distinguish between arteritic and nonarteritic occlusions,[49] as only the former respond well to systemic steroids.

Ischemic optic neuropathy is also occasionally seen in the period following otherwise uncomplicated cataract extraction. Visual recovery is rare, and the benefit of steroids in this setting is unproved.[50]

The term *papilledema* is reserved in ophthalmic usage for optic disc swelling due to increased intracranial pressure. In these patients, visual acuity is rarely impaired (at least initially); the only visual field abnormality is typically an enlarged blind spot. In chronic papilledema, optic atrophy may ensue, with progressive visual impairment. Treatment is directed at the underlying intracranial cause of the increased pressure. In occasional cases of idiopathic intracranial pressure, elevations (pseudotumor cerebri), medical treatment with carbonic anhydrase inhibitors, or surgical decompression of the central nervous system via a shunt or fenestration of the optic nerve sheath, may be of value.[51] Other causes of optic disc swelling that must be distinguished from papilledema include ischemic optic neuropathy, malignant hypertension, and severe uveitis.

Neuro-Ophthalmology

The oculomotor nerves and the posterior visual pathways are frequently targets in the elderly for ischemic injury and for compressive injuries due to intracranial mass lesions (typically tumors or aneurysms) and shifts of the intracranial contents. Sudden loss of function of a *single*, isolated cranial nerve is quite common. An isolated trochlear or abducens nerve palsy in a patient otherwise susceptible to atherosclerotic disease is usually a benign event, and spontaneous recovery is frequently seen.[52] Ischemic insults to the oculomotor nerve typically spare the pupillary fibers.[53] Patients with *multiple* cranial nerve deficits, or in whom pupillary dilation has occurred, require a thorough neurologic evaluation, preferably including computed tomography or magnetic resonance imaging, if available.

Abnormalities of the visual field should be thoroughly investigated. Scotomas that affect only one eye, or that respect the horizontal meridian, are generally due to injury to the retina, optic disc, optic nerve, or, of course, to glaucoma. Injuries at or posterior to the level of the optic chiasm will impair vision in both eyes. Of particular importance are bitemporal hemianopsias, which suggest compression of the optic chiasm, typically by a pituitary tumor, and highly congruous homonymous field defects, which suggest an injury of the occipital cerebral cortex.

Orbit

Tumors of the orbit generally present with horizontal, vertical, or anterior displacement of the globe (proptosis). In the elderly, the most frequently diagnosed entities include orbital pseudotumor (idiopathic inflammation of one or more orbital tissues, typically the extraocular muscles, lacrimal gland, or infiltration of the orbital fat), hemangiomas and lymphangiomas, lymphomas, and primary tumors of the lacrimal gland. Management frequently requires orbital exploration for anatomic correction, as well as histopathologic diagnosis.[54]

Thyroid ophthalmopathy (Graves' disease) is a well-known orbital problem. The impairment of ocular motility, lid retraction, and exophthalmos are largely due to the infiltration of the extraocular muscles. The orbital fat is rarely, if ever, involved.[55] Progression of the orbital disease is poorly correlated with the actual thyroid hormone levels, and restoration of the euthyroid state, although desirable for many reasons, is not particularly effective as a tool in the management of the ocular complications. Early cases respond well to systemic steroids. In long-standing cases, patients should be monitored closely for signs of optic nerve compression, and should be promptly offered surgical decompression (generally achieved by fracturing the orbital bones to provide greater room for the swollen orbital contents) if the optic nerve is at risk.[56]

Ophthalmic Complications of Systemic Diseases

The vision of elderly patients is at risk, not only from primary ocular diseases, but from the effects of systemic diseases as well. In addition to the effects of diabetes mellitus and thyroid disease mentioned above, a few of the more prominent disease entities with serious ophthalmic sequelae include hematologic disorders (such as leukemia and polycythemia), collagen-vascular diseases (including rheumatoid arthritis, ankylosing spondylitis, and systemic lupus erythematosus), Marfan syndrome, and renal failure. Treatment is usually directed at the primary disease process, but topical or systemic steroids may be needed to control ocular inflammation.

In addition to the local, mechanical effects of metastasis to the eye or orbit, systemic malignancy may also exert a remote deleterious effect on retinal function, greatly impairing vision.[57] Chemotherapy directed at the primary malignancy has occasionally led to visual improvement.

Ophthalmic Complications of Systemic Medications

Many elderly patients receive several concurrent medications, some of which may frequently cause ocular symptoms. A few of the more common problems are described below.[58]

Tricyclic antidepressants have a mild parasympatholytic action, which may cause mydriasis and paralysis of accommodation. Major tranquilizers, such as chlorpromazine, may also cause mydriasis and interfere with accommodation, and may cause a pigmentary retinopathy. Significant visual impairment has generally been reported only with protracted, chronic use. Chloroquine may also cause a "bull's-eye" maculopathy with impairment of central vision, particularly after prolonged use with a total dosage exceeding 100 g of the chloroquine base. Hydroxychloroquine appears to be substantially less retinotoxic than chloroquine.

Systemic steroids may precipitate an open-angle glaucoma (which frequently does not abate until several weeks after cessation of the drug), as well as accelerate the formation of cataracts. Digitalis derivatives may produce various visual disturbances, in addition to the classic "yellow vision" (xanthopsia). Ethambutol is also reported to produce dyschromatopsia, as well as optic atrophy and visual field defects.

Precipitation of an acute angle-closure attack by the mydriatic action of systemic medications is extremely rare.

Systemic Complications of Ophthalmic Medications

Because the dosages of topical eye medications are generally much smaller than the dosages used in systemic treatment, systemic complications from these applications are very rare. However, these drugs are rapidly absorbed across the conjunctiva and nasal mucous membranes, and occasionally cause systemic complications. Of course, it is also sometimes necessary to treat localized eye disease with systemic medications, which may cause further systemic problems.[58]

The topical anticholinergics used as mydriatic/cycloplegics may occasionally cause the full spectrum of systemic atropinic complications. Of the drugs in common use, cyclopentolate appears to cause these problems most frequently. Conversely, the parasympathomimetics, such as pilocarpine, carbachol, and the anticholinesterases, such as echothiophate, may cause such side effects such as abdominal cramps, diarrhea, and nausea.

Topical adrenergic agents, such as neosynephrine, may cause tachycardia, hypertension, and even frank arrhythmias. Conversely, topical β-blockers, such as timolol maleate, may cause the full spectrum of side effects of β-blockade, including bradycardia, asthma, and hypotension. The use of "cardioselective" β-blockers, such as betaxolol, has not completely eliminated these problems.

Topical use of chloramphenicol has resulted in a few reported cases of aplastic anemia, generally after prolonged treatment. There have also been rare reports of Stevens-Johnson syndrome following topical administration of sulfa antibiotics. Otherwise, there are very few reports of serious systemic toxicity from topical antibiotics, other than hypersensitivity reactions.

Mannitol and glycerine are frequently administered as osmotic agents to lower intraocular pressure in acute glaucoma. The fluid shifts that result may also cause congestive heart failure, renal shutdown, and altered mentation. Patients undergoing repeated treatments should be closely monitored for electrolyte imbalances and signs of renal decompensation.

Systemic carbonic anhydrase inhibitors, such as acetazolamide and methazolamide, are frequently used to treat glaucoma. These are difficult drugs for many patients, frequently causing anorexia, depression, impotence, and paresthesias, in addition to such rare complications as bone marrow depression, gout, and acidosis. Recently, carbonic anhydrase inhibitors have become available in topical formulations, which may reduce or eliminate many of these complications. Patients whose quality of life is intolerable on these medications should be offered medical or surgical alternatives.

Low-Vision Rehabilitation

The rehabilitation of individuals who have sustained an irremediable loss of vision is an important component of effective medical care, particularly among the elderly. In the United States, over two-thirds of individuals with acuity less than 6/18 are over 65 years of age. Conversely, of individuals over 65 years of age, 7.8 percent are reported to have acuity worse than 6/18, a fraction that increases to 25 percent among individuals over 85 years old. Loss of vision has been ranked as the third most common chronic condition (after arthritis and heart disease) for which individuals over the age of 70 require assistance with the activities of daily living.[59]

Low-vision rehabilitation attempts to allow vision-impaired individuals to make the most effective use of whatever vision they retain, so as to facilitate activities of daily living, prolong independence, and enhance self-confidence. Successful rehabilitation frequently requires the coordinated efforts of a team of care providers, including the ophthalmologist, optometrist, and occupational therapist, as well as the assistance and understanding of the patient's family and friends, or caretakers. Rehabilitation is generally most successful if it is begun as soon as permanent visual disability has been diagnosed. Critical to the functional outcome is the acceptance by the patient of the need to adopt compensatory visual strategies to cope with the loss of vision, rather than to continue vain attempts to reverse the visual loss.

Rehabilitation programs should center on the needs of the patient. A thorough functional history should be obtained. Emphasis should include the patient's perceptions of the impact of the visual disability on accustomed activities, and on goals for the future. Every attempt should be made to identify specific tasks that the patient's visual limitations have curtailed, and whose recovery would be particularly valued. Typical problems include inability to read, mend, or pay bills; loss of independent mobility, and difficulty with distance vision, such as watching television or reading signs.

The severity of the visual deficit should be determined, including measurements of visual acuity, visual fields, and contrast sensitivity. It is often helpful to be more specific in identifying the level of visual acuity that is typical in general ophthalmic practice. Placement of eye charts as close as 1 m may be used to expand the range of acuity testing. It is frequently essential to allow a substantially greater amount of time than usual for visual assessment in low-vision patients, especially the elderly.

Rehabilitation may then proceed.[60] A comprehensive program frequently entails the dispensing and instruction in the use of optical aids (such as spectacles, telescopes, and magnifiers) and nonoptical aids (such as improved lighting, large-print reading materials, high-contrast guides for reading and writing, and closed-circuit television magnifiers). Training in the use of residual vision, such as eccentric viewing for individuals who have lost central macular function, may be attempted, but may require many hours of practice over many months in order to obtain optimal performance. Training in adaptations for activities of daily living, and the introduction of suitable equipment, such as needle threaders or large-print playing cards, can help recapture self-confidence and facilitate independence. Professional counseling, often in a group setting, can play an important role in helping patients deal with the emotional impact of visual disabilities.

It is important that the patient adopt reasonable goals for low-vision rehabilitation. In nearly every case, it is impossible to recover the efficiency enjoyed prior to the loss of visual function. Each patient must individually decide whether the results achieved are worth the extra effort that will remain necessary to perform most visual tasks. The best results are achieved when specific tasks, of great value to the patient and the patient's independence, are targeted.

References

1. World Health Organization: Methods of Assessment of Avoidable Blindness. Geneva, WHO Offset Pub. No. 54, 1980
2. Foster A: Patterns of Blindness. Ch. 53. In Tasman W Jaeger EA (Eds): Duane's Clinical Ophthalmology Vol. 5. Lippincott-Raven, Philadelphia, 1984
3. Klein R, Klein BEK, Linton KLP et al: The Beaver Dam Eye Study: visual acuity. Ophthalmology 1991;98:1310
4. Tielsch JM, Javitt JC, Coleman A et al: The prevalence of blindness and visual impairment among nursing home residents in Baltimore. N Engl J Med 1995;332:1205–1209
5. Frueh BR: The mechanistic classification of ptosis. Ophthalmology 1980;87:1019–1021
6. Dryden RM, Leibsohn J, Wobig J: Senile entropion: pathogenesis and treatment. Arch Ophthalmol 1978;96:1883–1885
7. Berlin AJ, Vestal KP: Levator aponeurosis surgery. A retrospective review. Ophthalmology 1989;96:1033–1036
8. Smith B: The "lazy-T" correction of ectropion of the lower punctum. Arch Ophthalmol 1976;94:1149–1150
9. Mohs FE: Micrographic surgery for the microscopically controlled excision of eyelid cancers. Arch Ophthalmol 1986;104: 901–909
10. van Bijsterveld OP, Mackor AJ: Sjogren's syndrome and tear function parameters. Clin Exp Rheumatol 1989;7:151–154
11. Rosen N, Sharir M, Moverman DC, Rosner M: Dacryocystorhinostomy with silicone tubes: evaluation of 253 cases. Ophthalmic Surg 1989;20:115–119
12. Vorkas AP: Pterygium. Choice of operation. Trans Ophthal Soc UK 1981;101:192–194
13. Fraunfelder FT, Wingfield D: Management of intraepithelial conjunctival tumors and squamous cell carcinomas. Am J Ophthalmol 1983;95:359–363
14. Edelhauser HF, Van Horn DL, Records RE: Cornea and sclera. Ch. 1. In Tasman W, Jaeger EA (eds): Duane's Clinical Ophthalmology Vol. 2. Lippincott-Raven, Philadelphia, 1989
15. Carlson KH, Bourne WM, McLaren JW, Brubaker RF: Variations in human corneal endothelial cell morphology and permeability to fluorescein with age. Exp Eye Res 1988;47:27–41
16. Olson RJ, Waltman SR, Mattingly TP, Kaufman HE: Visual results after penetrating keratoplasty for aphakic bullous keratoplasty and Fuchs' dystrophy. Am J Ophthalmol 1979;88: 1000–1004
17. Baum J, Barza M: Topical vs. subconjunctival treatment of bacterial corneal ulcers. Ophthalmology 1983;90:162–168
18. Nussenblatt RB, Palestine AG, Chan C-C: Cyclosporine A treatment of intraocular inflammatory disease resistant to systemic corticosteroids and cytotoxic agents. Am J Ophthalmol 1983; 96:275–282
19. McLean IW, Foster WD, Zimmerman LE: Uveal melanoma: location, size, cell type, and enucleation as risk factors in metastasis. Hum Pathol 1982;13:123–132
20. Gass JD: Observation of suspected choroidal and ciliary body melanomas for evidence of growth prior to enucleation. Ophthalmology 1980;87:523–528
21. Shields JA, Augsburger JJ, Brady LW, Day JL: Cobalt plaque therapy of posterior uveal melanomas. Ophthalmology 1982;89: 1201–1207
22. Stephens RF, Shields JA: Diagnosis and management of cancer metastatic to the uvea: a study of 70 cases. Ophthalmology 1979;86:1336–1349
23. Shiose Y: Intraocular pressure: new perspectives. Surv Ophthalmol 1990;34:413–435
24. Yablonski ME, Zimmerman TJ, Kass MA, Becker B: Prognostic significance of optic disk cupping in ocular hypertensive patients. Am J Ophthalmol 1980;89:585–592
25. Quigley HA, Addicks EM, Green R: Optic nerve damage in human glaucoma III. Quantitative correlation of nerve fiber loss and visual field defect in glaucoma, ischemic neuropathy, papilledema, and toxic neuropathy. Arch Ophthalmol 1982;100: 135–146
26. Jay JL, Murray SB: Early trabeculectomy versus conventional management in primary open angle glaucoma. Br J Ophthalmol 1988;72:881–889
27. The Glaucoma Laser Trial (GLT) and Glaucoma Laser Trial Follow-up Study: 7. Results. Glaucoma Laser Trial Research Group. Am J Ophthalmol 1995;120:718–731
28. Katz J, Tielsch JM, Quigley HA et al: Automated suprathreshold screening for glaucoma: the Baltimore Eye Survey. Invest Ophthalmol Vis Sci 1993;34:3271–3277
29. Olson L: Anatomy and embryology of the lens. Ch. 71. In Tasman W, Jaeger EA, (eds): Duane's Clinical Ophthalmology. Vol. 1. Lippincott-Raven, Philadelphia, 1978.

30. Cotlier E, Fagadau W, Cicchetti DV: Methods for evaluation of medical therapy of senile and diabetic cataracts. Trans Ophthalmol Soc UK 1982;102,3:416–422

31 Kelman CD: Phaco-emulsification and aspiration of senile cataracts: A comparative study with intra-capsular extraction. Can J Ophthalmol 1973;8:24–32

32. Spaeth GL: No-stitch surgery: good, bad, or both? editorial. Ophthalmic Surg 1991;22:630–631

33. Benson WH, Farber ME, Caplan RJ: Increased mortality rates after cataract surgery. A statistical analysis. Ophthalmology 1988;95:1288–1292

34. Frank RN, Hoffman WH, Podgor MJ et al: Retinopathy in juvenile-onset diabetes of short duration. Ophthalmology 1980;87: 1–9

35. Early Treatment Diabetic Retinopathy Study Research Group: Treatment techniques and clinical guidelines for photocoagulation of diabetic macular edema. ETDRS Report No. 2. Ophthalmology 1987;94:761–774

36. Diabetic Retinopahy Study Research Group: Indications for photocoagulation treatment of diabetic retinopathy: DRS report No. 14. Int Ophthalmol Clin 1987;27:239–253

37. Kroc Collaborative Study Group: Blood glucose control and the evolution of diabetic retinopathy and albuminuria. N Engl J Med 1984;311:365–372

38. Ramsey RC, Goetz FC, Sutherland DE et al: Progression of diabetic retinopathy after pancreas transplantation for insulin-dependent diabetes mellitus. N Engl J Med 1988;318:208–214

39. The Diabetes Control and Complications Trial Research Group: The effect of intensive treatment of diabetes on the development and progression of long-term complications in insulin-dependent diabetes mellitus. N Engl J Med 1993;329:977–986

40. Gass JDM: Pathogenesis of disciform detachment of the neuroepithelium, III. Senile disciform macular degeneration. Am J Ophthalmol 1967;63:617–644

41. Macular Photocoagulation Study Group: Argon laser photocoagulation for neovascular maculopathy. Three-year results from randomized clinical trials. Arch Ophthalmol 1986;104: 694–701

42. Macular Photocoagulation Study Group: Laser photocoagulation of subfoveal neovascular lesions in age-related macular degeneration. Results of randomized clinical trial. Arch Ophthalmol 1991;109:1220–1231

43. Gass JDM: Drusen and disciform macular detachment. Trans Am Ophthalmol Soc 1972;70:409–436

44. Augsburger JJ, Magargal LE: Visual prognosis following treatment of acute central retinal artery obstruction. Br J Ophthalmol 1980;64:913–917

45. Bernstein EF (ed): Amaurosis Fugax. Springer-Verlag, New York, 1988

46. Poole CJM, Ross Russel RW: Mortality and stroke after amaurosis fugax. J Neurol Neurosurg Psychiatry 1985;48:902–905

47. Keltner JL: Giant-cell arteritis. Signs and symptoms. Ophthalmology 1982;89:1101–1110

48. Magargal LE, Brown GC, Augsburger JJ, Donoso LA: Efficacy of pan-retinal photocoagulation in preventing neovascular glaucoma following ischemic central retinal vein occlusion. Ophthalmology 1982;89:780–784

49. Glaser JS: Topical diagnosis: pre-chiasmal visual pathways. Ch 5. In Tasman W, Jaeger EA (eds): Duane's Clinical Ophthalmology Vol. 2. Lippincott-Raven, Philadelphia, 1989

50. Hayreh SS: Anterior ischemic optic neuropathy, IV. Occurrence after cataract extraction. Arch Ophthalmol 1980;98: 1410–1416

51. Sergott RC, Savino PJ, Bosley TM: Modified optic nerve sheath decompression provides long-term visual improvement for pseudotumor cerebri. Arch Ophthalmol 1988;106:1384–1390

52. Rush JA, Younge BR: Paralysis of cranial nerves III, IV, and VI. Cause and prognosis in 1000 cases. Arch Ophthalmol 1981; 99:76–79

53. Glaser JS: Infranuclear disorders of eye movement. Ch. 12. In Tasman W, Jaeger EA (eds): Duane's Clinical Ophthalmology. Vol. 2. Lippincott-Raven, Philadelphia, 1988

54. Jones IS, Jakobiec FA, Nolan BT: Patient examination and introduction to orbital disease. Ch. 21. In Tasman W, Jaeger EA (eds): Duane's Clinical Ophthalmology. Vol. 2. Lippincott-Raven, Philadelphia, 1976

55. Trokel SL, Jakobiec FA: Correlation of CT scanning and pathologic features of ophthalmic Graves' disease. Ophthalmology 1981;88:553–564

56. Schorr N, Seiff SR: The four stages of surgical rehabilitation of the patient with dysthyroid ophthalmopathy. Ophthalmology 1986;93:476–483

57. Thirkill CE, Roth AM, Keltner JL: Cancer-associated retinopathy. Arch Ophthalmol 1987;105:372–375

58. Fraunfelder FT: Drug-Induced Ocular Side Effects and Drug Interactions. 3rd Ed. Lea & Febiger, Philadelphia, 1989

59. Eaglestein A, Rapaport S: Prediction of low vision aid usage. J Vis Impair Blindness 1991;85:31–33

60. Rehabilitation: The Management of Adult Patients with Low Vision. American Academy of Ophthalmology, Preferred Practice Pattern, 1995

CHAPTER 47

Disorders of Hearing

BARBARA E. WEINSTEIN

Epidemiology of Hearing Loss

As people age the likelihood of experiencing one or more chronic condition increases. Overall, it is estimated that 80 percent of persons 65 years of age and older experience at least one chronic condition. The high prevalence of chronic conditions and the increased prevalence of chronic disease with age lead to comorbidity of chronic disease in large numbers of older adults. Specifically, 49 percent of persons 60 years of age and older have two or more chronic conditions, 23 percent have three or more, and 8 percent have four or more. The three most prevalent chronic conditions include arthritis, hypertension, and hearing impairment. These conditions have remained the most prevalent for several years.

The 10 most prevalent chronic conditions among persons 65 years of age and older in the United States are displayed in Table 47-1. It is evident that according to the 1991 survey, the prevalence of hearing impairment, 295.2 of 1,000 persons, was demonstrably higher than the prevalence of visual impairment, 79.2 of 1,000 persons. It is noteworthy that tinnitus was the ninth most prevalent chronic condition among respondents 65 years of age and older in the 1991 survey. Note in Table 47-1 that this hierarchy of chronic conditions is similar, albeit not identical, for persons 75 years of age and older, and that the prevalence of each condition increases dramatically with age. For example, the prevalence of hearing impairment among persons 75 years of age and older of rises to 354.3 of 1,000 whereas the prevalence of visual impairment rises to 113.3 of 1,000 persons. According to results of the 1989 survey conducted by the National Center for Health Statistics, the prevalence of chronic conditions tends to vary somewhat with race.[1] As is evident from Table 47-2, hearing loss is more prevalent among whites than blacks whereas hypertension is more prevalent among blacks than whites. Finally, with the rapid growth in the population over 75 years, it is estimated that there will be approximately 11 million elderly people with hearing loss in the United States by the year 2000.

As the prevalence of hearing loss is nearly 40 percent among persons aged 65 years and older, it is no surprise that the majority of persons purchasing hearing instruments are in this age bracket. In fact, 65 percent of hearing instrument consumers are 65 years of age or older whereas only 6 percent are under 18 years of age.[2] Despite the fact that the vast majority of hearing aid users are over 65 years of age, the majority of older adults with handicapping hearing impairment do not use hearing aids. Given the significant communicative and psychosocial effects of hearing loss, and the efficacy of hearing aids in reducing the latter consequences of hearing impairment, audiologists are working hard to promote hearing aid use early before hearing loss becomes an intolerable burden and less responsive to intervention.

Age-Related Anatomic and Physiologic Changes

The inner ear is composed of several functional components that are vulnerable to the effects of aging. These components comprise the sensory, neural, vascular, supporting, synaptic, and/or mechanical structures within the peripheral and/or central auditory systems.[3] The organ of Corti, which extends spirally from the basal convolution to the cupula or apex of the cochlea, houses the sense organ of hearing. It is the structure most susceptible to age-related histopathologic changes. The cochlea rests atop the basilar membrane and is composed of sensory cells (outer and inner hair cells along with their stereocilia), supporting cells, the Reisner's membrane, the tectorial membrane, and stria vascularis, among other structures. The fact that various frequencies are registered in different parts of the cochlea is the basis for the tonotopic organization of the auditory system. The organ of Corti is the site of transduction of mechanical to neural energy, and age-related atrophy interferes with the transduction process integral to the reception of sound.[3]

The most critical risk factor for the auditory sense organ is age.[4] The changes the aging ear undergoes have been studied most extensively by Schuknecht.[5–8] In general, hair cell loss is the rule rather than the exception in older adults. Loss of both types of hair cells is most severe in the basal region of the cochlea, with apical and midcochlear involvement of the outer hair cells, as well. Although both outer and inner hair cells tend to degenerate with age, the outer hair cells are more vulnerable than inner hair cells and their degeneration accounts in large part for the "normal" decline in hearing with age.[3]

Recent research[9] clearly demonstrates a relation between age and loss of ganglions cells. As would be expected, neural histopathologic studies suggest that age-related loss in ganglions cells is greatest near the base of the cochlea. Similarly,

Table 47-1 Prevalence of selected chronic conditions per 1,000 persons over 65 years of age (1991)

Condition	65 Years and Older	65–74 Years	75 Years and Older
Arthritis	484.8	425.6	575.2
Hypertension	372.2	376.6	365.5
Hearing impairment	295.2	256.4	354.3
Heart disease	320.5	266.2	403.6
Deformity or orthopaedic impairment	177.5	167.1	193.3
Cataracts	173.0	127.6	242.3
Sinusitis	139.5	156.4	113.7
Diabetes	99.3	103.8	92.6
Tinnitus	82.4	95.3	62.6
Visual impairment	79.2	56.8	113.3

(From Adams and Benson,[43] with permission.)

age is associated with a decrease in the average number of fibers in the cochlear nerve with nerve fiber loss greatest within the basal 10 mm of the cochlea.[10] A number of histopathologic studies have revealed that neural degeneration can occur before and/or independently of sensory cell loss. That is, loss of nerve fibers in one turn of the cochlea or in all turns has been noted without severe hair cell loss.[3] Stated differently, loss of inner or outer hair cells is not a condition for age-related pathology of ganglion cells.[3] In conclusion, two major age-related structural changes have been observed histologically in the inner ear and auditory nerve. These include extensive atrophy and degeneration of the hair cells, numerous supporting cells, and of the stria vascular, as well as a reduction in the number of functional spiral ganglia and nerve fibers that comprise the auditory portion of the eighth nerve.

Table 47-2 Ten most prevalent chronic conditions by race: 1989 (number per 1,000 persons)

Condition	White	Black
Arthritis	483.2	522.6
Hypertension	367.4	517.7
Hearing impairment	297.4	174.5
Heart disease	286.5	220.5
Cataracts	160.7	139.8
Deformity or orthopaedic impairment	156.2	150.8
Chronic sinusitis	157.1	125.2
Diabetes	80.2	165.9
Visual impairment	81.1	77.0
Varicose veins	80.3	64.0

(From National Center for Health Statistics,[1] with permission.)

Histologic studies of the central auditory nervous system suggest that portions undergo age-related changes as well.[11] These apparent changes, which predominate in the auditory brain stem pathways and the auditory cortex, are not universal across individuals, nor are they universal across the nuclei or tracts within the auditory brain stem. These changes within the central auditory nervous system have profound implications for speech understanding in less than optimal listening conditions and interfere with hearing aid benefit.

In addition to age-related degeneration, a number of other factors can lead to hearing loss in older adults. These include excessive exposure to occupational or recreational noise; genetic factors; acoustic neuroma; trauma; metabolic disease such as kidney problems; vascular disease; infections; and ingestion of ototoxic agents most notably aminoglycosides, ethacrynic acid, and salicylates. Impacted cerumen, otitis media, glossopharyngeal tumors, or otosclerosis are not uncommon. These diseases that are associated with conductive hearing loss can occur in the presence of cochlear involvement. Finally, affective disorders such as depression and cognitive disorders such as senile dementia of the Alzheimer's type are associated with hearing loss. In fact, the prevalence of hearing loss is higher among persons with dementia than among those without it. In addition, inattention or confusion related to depression or dementia may give the impression of significant hearing loss and should be considered in a systematic geriatric assessment. Complete audiometric studies can help identify the etiology of hearing loss in older adults.

Behavioral Implications of Anatomic and Physiologic Changes

The aforementioned age-related changes are associated with decrements in hearing for pure-tone and speech stimuli. In fact, it appears that age and frequency effects emerge in most cross-sectional and longitudinal studies of hearing loss, such that air conduction thresholds became poorer as age or frequency increase.[4,12,13] The majority of recent studies on hearing loss characterizing noninstitutionalized older adults confirm that age-related hearing loss commonly referred to as "presbycusis" has several distinct features. First, pure-tone hearing sensitivity tends to decline with increasing age and the hearing loss tends to be greatest in the frequencies above 1,000 Hz. Further, the hearing loss tends to be bilateral, symmetric, and sensorineural in origin, associated with damage to the sensory structures within the cochlea. The decline in high-frequency sensitivity appears to be greatest in males whereas the decline in low-frequency thresholds tends to be greatest in females of comparable age.[4] The average hearing loss in males can be described as mild to moderately severe, bilateral, and sensorineural with a sharply sloping configuration, whereas women tend to present with a mild to moderate gradually sloping bilaterally symmetric sensorineural hearing loss. Among residents of nursing facilities, the sensorineural hearing loss tends to be more significant, moderately severe sloping to severe, and more prevalent, affecting approximately 70 to 80 percent of residents. The fact that nursing home residents are older accounts for the high prevalence of more severe hearing loss among residents.

The pure-tone hearing loss and site of involvement within the cochlea, eighth nerve, auditory brain stem pathways, and auditory cortex determine in large part the nature of the speech understanding problems experienced by older adults. The classic complaint of older adults with presbycusis, namely "I can hear people talking but cannot understand what they are saying especially in noisy situation," very aptly describes the problems that derive from the reduction in transmission, reception, and perception of the speech signal attributable to sensorineural hearing loss. In fact, these difficulties can easily be predicted from the speech bananna and audiograms depicted in Figure 47-1. The speech bananna shown in the left panel displays the frequency and intensity levels of typical sounds necessary for speech understanding. Ordinary conversation or the normal speech spectrum is carried out within the range of frequencies from 250 to 6,000 Hz and within the range of decibels from 20 to 60 dBHL. Consonant sounds and diphthongs such as "s," "sh," "th," "k," "t," "p," and "g" are relatively high in frequency or pitch and low in intensity or loudness. Conversely, vowel sounds such as "a," "i," "o," and "u" are concentrated in the lower frequencies and are somewhat higher in intensity.[14] Environmental noise is high in intensity and low in frequency as well. Audibility of the consonant sounds is critical to the understanding of speech. The middle panel depicts a typical hearing loss characterizing older adults suffering from presbycusis.[14]

Those sounds falling below threshold symbolized by the connected circles are audible (e.g., m, n, e, r, p) whereas those falling above are inaudible (s, t, th). For most older adults with age-related hearing loss, consonants with energy in the high frequencies are frequently inaudible, rendering speech understanding difficult. This difficulty comprehending ordinary conversation is exacerbated in a noisy room, as background noise tends to be audible given good low-frequency hearing, yet consonant sounds important to understanding are inaudible. Further, older adults with good low-frequency hearing can perceive vowels well, even though they may have difficulty with consonant sounds.[14] As a result, older adults claim that they can hear people talking (vowels audible) but they cannot make out the words (consonants inaudible). The goal of hearing aids is to bring consonants into the audible range without amplifying the already audible noise and vowel sounds. This is shown in the right-hand panel in Figure 47-1. Note that the circles in the frequencies above 1,000 Hz, which represent aided air conduction thresholds, are now better than (above) the speech sounds depicted in the bananna. The hearing aid has rendered the high-frequency sounds audible.

Psychosocial Consequences of Decrements in Pure-Tone Sensitivity and Speech Understanding

The behavioral implications of the speech understanding difficulties characterizing older adults are numerous for the individual, family members, the functioning of nursing facilities, and potentially for society at large. In general, hearing loss in older adults restricts one or more dimensions of quality of life including physical functional status, and cognitive, emotional, and social function.[15–18] Specifically, hearing impairment has been shown to:

- Negatively impact on communicative behavior
- Alter psychosocial behavior
- Strain family relations
- Limit the enjoyment of daily activities
- Jeopardize physical well-being

Figure 47-1 Air conduction thresholds of typical presbycusic hearing loss shown relative to typical speech sounds. Also shown are aided air conduction thresholds. (From Bess and Humes[14] with permission.)

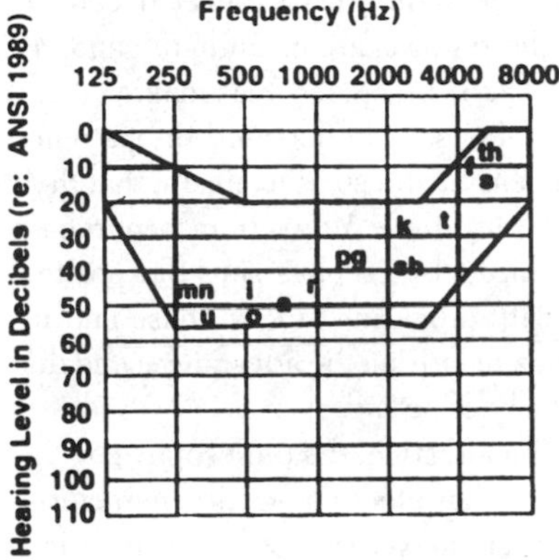

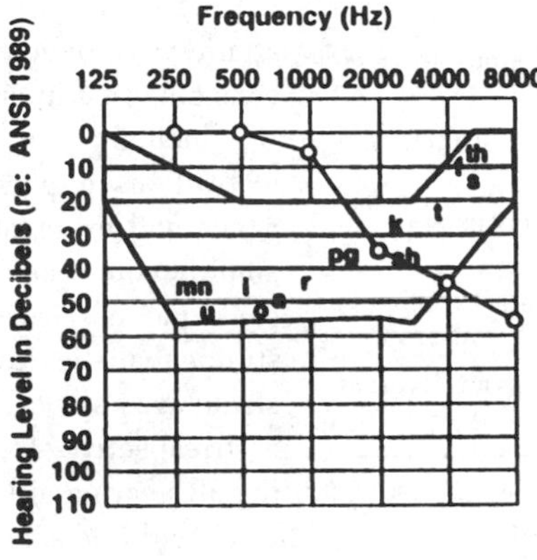

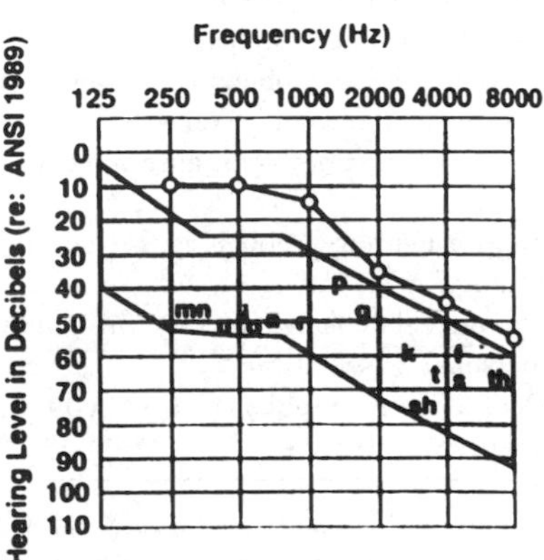

- Interfere with the ability to live independently and safely
- Interfere with long distance contacts on the telephone, potentially jeopardizing safety and security
- Interfere with medical diagnosis, treatment, and management
- Interfere with compliance with pharmacologic regimens, and
- Interfere with therapeutic interventions across all disciplines including social work, speech-language therapy, and physical or occupational therapy

An interesting aspect of the hearing impairment that afflicts older adults is the large variability in response to a given hearing loss. Two individuals with the same level of hearing loss (e.g., mild) will react very differently and will experience different behavioral consequences. Accordingly it is imperative that included in the complete hearing assessment is quantification of the perceived handicapping effects of a given hearing loss on communication and social and emotional function. Items comprising the long or shortened versions of the Hearing Handicap Inventory for the Elderly (HHIE) are ideal for assessing the perceived handicapping effects of hearing loss. Table 47-3 contains the items comprising the 10-item screening version (HHIE-S).[19] The HHIE/HHIE-S have high test-retest reliability, excellent internal consistency reliability and adequate content, construct, and predictive validity.[19,20] Scores on the questionnaire are highly predictive of hearing aid use such that individuals obtaining a score of 18 or greater on the HHIE-S are considered hearing aid candidates who are likely to purchase and benefit from hearing aid use, irrespective of hearing loss severity.

Table 47-3 Screening version of the hearing handicap inventory for the elderly (HHIE-S)

Instructions: Answer Yes (4 points), Sometimes (2 points), or No (0 points) for each question. If you are a hearing aid user answer questions according to how you hear with the hearing aid. If the question does not apply merely enter no as your response.

E-1. Does a hearing problem cause you to feel embarrassed when meeting new people?

E-2. Does a hearing problem cause you to feel frustrated when talking to members of your family?

S-1. Do you have difficulty hearing when someone speaks in a whisper?

E-3. Do you feel handicapped by a hearing problem?

S-2. Does a hearing problem cause you difficulty when visiting friends, relatives, or neighbors?

S-3. Does a hearing problem cause you to attend religious services less often than you would like?

E-4. Does a hearing problem cause you to have arguments with family members?

S-4. Does a hearing problem cause you difficulty when listening to TV or radio?

E-5. Do you feel that any difficulty with your hearing limits or hampers your personal or social life?

S-5. Does a hearing problem cause you difficulty when in a restaurant with relatives or friends?

Abbreviations: S, items probe social/situational consequences of hearing loss; E, items probe emotional consequences of hearing loss.

Audiologic Rehabilitation

Once hearing loss is documented, the etiology determined, and the handicap quantified, an older adult should undergo some form of rehabilitation, assuming medical treatment has been ruled out. Audiologic rehabilitation consists of several components: (1) provision of a custom hearing aid and/or assistive listening devices to make sounds audible, comfortable, tolerable, and comprehensible; (2) orientation to the use and maintenance of the hearing aids; and (3) patient and family counseling/education to promote adjustment to hearing loss and the use of hearing aids. The greatest barrier to audiologic rehabilitation is lack of awareness or acceptance of hearing loss combined with societal ageism about the necessity to hear well as we age. Of the components of audiologic rehabilitation, the provision of a hearing aid in the context of a brief counseling session is the most beneficial, improving hearing-related quality of life.[21]

Hearing Technologies

Hearing Aids

A host of audiologic and nonaudiologic variables interact to determine hearing aid candidacy, hearing aid satisfaction, and hearing aid benefit. These include but are not limited to the following: auditory, physical, sociological, psychological, cognitive, and environmental factors. With regard to auditory variables, sensorineural hearing loss of nearly any degree can be remediated via a hearing aid assuming the client is interested in pursuing amplification. Clinical experience suggests that motivation is one of the most important, yet least well understood, psychological factors that affects rehabilitation potential in general and hearing aid candidacy.[22] It explains why behavior is initiated, why it persists, and why it is attenuated. Motivation to pursue intervention is optimal when an individual (1) knows what he or she wants; (2) expects it can be attained; (3) believes that the rewards are meaningful; and (4) considers that intervention takes place at a reasonable cost.[22] It is incumbent on the audiologist to understand the patient's motivations for pursuing a hearing aid so as to ensure that their needs and expectations are fulfilled. Motivation to purchase amplification can be optimized by emphasizing the positive consequences associated with a hearing aid purchase and instilling realistic expectations regarding the advantages and disadvantages associated with hearing aid use.

Irrespective of the hearing aid style, the philosophy governing all hearing aid fittings is that electroacoustic characteristics should be selected that (1) maximize speech recognition,

Table 47-4 Hearing aid components

Components	Function
Microphone	Converts incoming acoustic signals to electrical signals
Amplifier	Amplifies and selectively processes the microphone output signals
Receiver	Converts the amplified and processed electrical signal back to an acoustic signal
Battery	Provides power as needed for all the above components
Earmold/tubing	Delivers the acoustic signal to the hearing aid user's ear(s)

(From Preves,[44] with permission.)

(2) provide good sound quality, and (3) provide for amplification that is comfortable and compensates for the loss of loudness resulting from the impaired hearing.[23] Simply put, an optimal hearing aid fitting is one that makes speech audible without exceeding the listener's loudness discomfort level and restores the normal loudness relations for speech and other environmental sounds.[24] Prior to selecting the electroacoustic characteristics, hearing aid style and arrangement must be mutually agreed upon.

All hearing aids, irrespective of their style, include the components listed in Table 47-4. The amplifier, along with the microphone, receiver, and battery, make up the central core. In large part, the quality of the signal processing accomplished by the amplifier determines how well a person with handicapping hearing impairment will function with a hearing instrument. An important function of the amplifier, in combination with the receiver and earmold/molded piece, which deliver sound to the ear, is to limit the maximum amount of amplification the user receives. This function is critical as it will minimize the possibility of hearing aid rejection because sound is uncomfortably loud. The size, style, and amplifier type determine which battery powers the hearing aid. All hearing aids take 1.4 V batteries and at the time the hearing aid is dispensed, the audiologist will advise consumers on the correct battery type for particular unit. The American Association of Retired Persons is one of the least expensive sources of batteries.

A variety of hearing aid styles is available to the hearing-impaired older adult once it is mutually decided that hearing aids are the appropriate intervention. The variety of styles available to the consumer is listed in Table 47-5. As would be expected from the description accompanying the hearing aid style, body aids and eyeglass hearing aids are the least popular units dispensed whereas custom in-the-ear (ITE) hearing aids represent the largest market share. According to a recent survey of hearing instrument dispensers, 84 percent of all hearing aids sold in 1995 were ITE units.[2] Specifically, 15 percent were behind the ear, 41 percent were custom (ITE), 29 percent were in-the-canal (ITC), and 15 percent were completely in-the-canal (CIC) units. Approximately, 5 to 10 percent of all hearing aids sold in 1995 were programmable. Programmable hearing aids have greater flexibility and range over all of the traditional frequencies and intensities typically amplified.[25] In general, programmable instruments employ different circuit options to achieve a variety of sound qualities and performance characteristics. With programmable instruments, hearing aid users have the ability to custom tailor the hearing instrument to their lifestyle, enabling them to benefit from amplification in situations in which previously a hearing aid may have been unusable.[25] Similarly, the dispenser can adjust

Table 47-5 Hearing aid styles

Style	Description
Behind-the-ear	Crescent-shaped device that hooks over the ear. A small tube connects the hearing aid to a custom earmold. Microphone, amplifier and receiver are housed within plastic crescent-shaped case that rests behind the ear. Sound is conveyed to the ear via a coupling system that includes tubing and the custom earmold.
In-the-ear	One-piece custom-fitted to the contour of the ear. Components are built into the shell of a custom ear mold from an impression of the hearing impaired user's ear(s).
In-the-canal	All components are housed within a plastic shell that occupies the outer one-third or cartilaginous part of the external auditory canal.
Completely in-the-canal	All components housed within a plastic shell molded to fit deep within the ear canal extending into the bony portion. Deep insertion of the ear tip into the bony portion of the ear canal allows for higher real ear gain relative to the actual gain of the amplifier. Allows for comfortable listening at low volume control settings with less chance of feedback.
Body hearing aids	A large plastic case worn on the body houses the microphone, amplifier, and battery, which is connected via a cord to a circular plastic external receiver that is connected to an earmold.
Eyeglass hearing aids	The microphone, amplifier, and receiver are contained within the temple portion of the eyeglass. A piece of tubing connects the temple piece to the earmold, which delivers the sound to the user's ears.

Each of the above styles is available as a programmable unit from selected manufacturers and some digital hearing aids are available in most of these styles.

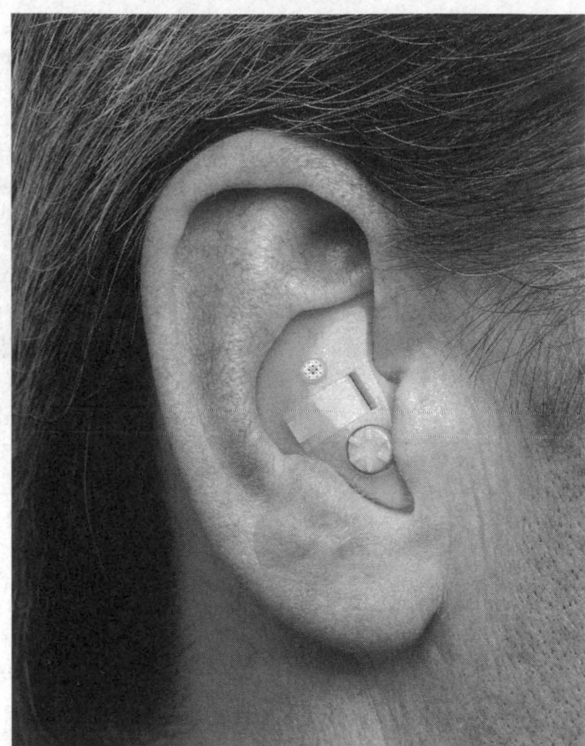

Figure 47-2 In-the-ear hearing aid shown in a user's ear. (Courtesy of Rexton, Inc.)

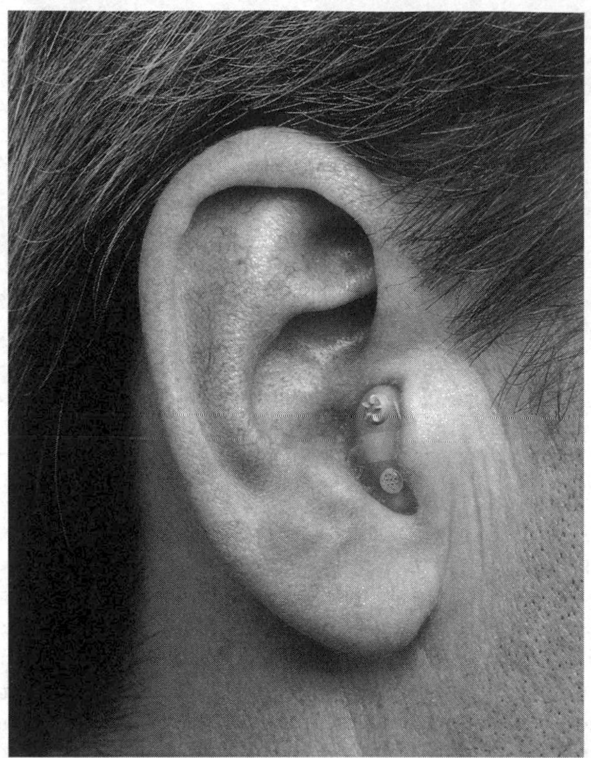

Figure 47-3 Canal hearing aid shown in a user's ear. (Courtesy of Rexton, Inc.)

the low frequencies independent of the high frequencies depending on the hearing configuration and the nature of the input sound, providing for improved speech understanding in favorable and unfavorable listening environments.[25]

Custom ITE hearing aids range in size and are identified according to their physical location and their dimensions within the concha of the outer ear or pinna. For example, a full concha ITE hearing aid, shown in Figure 47-2, completely occupies the external portion of the pinna known as the concha. In contrast, a low-profile unit provides for less protrusion from the concha and a half concha only fills a portion of the concha, namely the concha cavum and the ear canal. Half conchas are smaller and less flexible in that they contain less complicated circuitry and take a smaller size battery (e.g., 312 batteries). Full conchas, on the other hand, are larger, allow for more complex circuit designs, and take a larger battery cell (e.g., #13). ITC hearing aids are smaller than ITE units, having most of their components within the cartilaginous portion of the ear canal. Figure 47-3 shows a canal hearing aid in the user's ear. For the most part ITCs use small 312 batteries or even smaller size cells (i.e., #10). CIC hearing aids have all of their electronic components deep within the external auditory canal terminating close to the tympanic membrane. Figure 47-4 displays a CIC hearing aid with its tiny components relative to a dime and Figure 47-5 shows a CIC in the user's ear. The only piece visible is the thin piece of plastic extending outward from the faceplate of the hearing aid, which is used to remove the unit. The microphone of CIC hearing aids is located deep in the ear canal providing for a natural high frequency boost, less wind noise, and theoretically better speech understanding because of the acoustic advantage provided by the outer ear.

Until very recently behind-the-ear (BTE) hearing instruments were the hearing aid of choice for hearing impaired consumers. Presently they tend to be reserved for persons with severe to profound hearing impairment or persons with milder loss and manual dexterity problems. BTEs are ideal for hearing-impaired persons who require high gain (50 to 70 dBSPL), a strong telecoil for telephone use, and or larger controls for independent manipulation. Two additional advantages include

Figure 47-4 Completely in-the-canal hearing aid. (Courtesy of Rexton, Inc.)

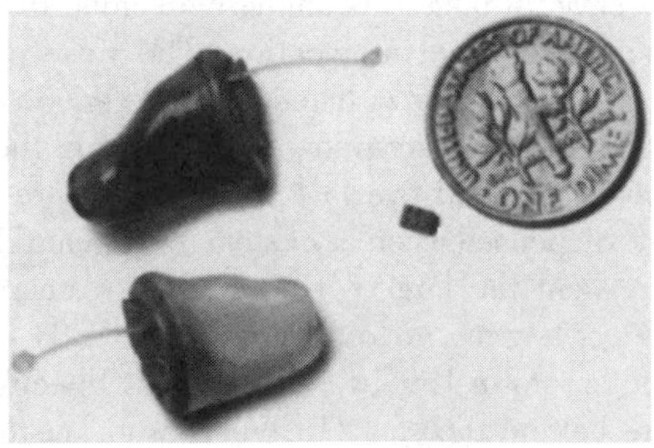

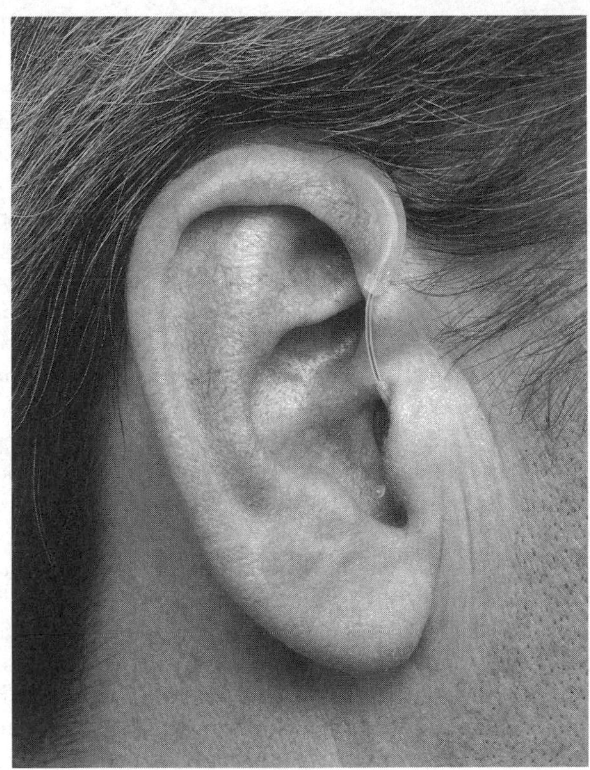

Figure 47-5 Completely in-the-canal hearing aid shown in a user's ear. (Courtesy of Rexton, Inc.)

their flexibility and compatibility with direct audio input microphones. Often, residents of nursing facilities use BTE hearing instruments because of a long history of hearing aid use and because some individuals consider them easier to manipulate and insert comfortably in the ear. It is important to ensure that the earmold is comfortable and rests securely in the ear. New earmolds should be made by the audiologist when the mold routinely becomes unseated or when acoustic feedback is consistently audible. The earmold and hearing aid arrangement should be checked annually to make sure that the hearing-impaired individual is still using the hearing aid and that it is still operating according to manufacturer specifications. Ideally, the check should be scheduled after 11 months of hearing aid use, as this is within the 1-year warranty period and the consumer is entitled to a free hearing aid overhaul. The latter applies to all hearing aid styles and users.

Overall, the average price for a monaural hearing aid was $794 in 1995.[26] It is noteworthy that the cost of hearing aids differs dramatically by dispenser, clinical setting, and style of hearing aid. The average price of a hearing aid purchased from a hearing instrument specialist is $826 versus $783 when purchased from an audiologist. In part, hearing aids are more costly from hearing instrument specialists because dispensing audiologists (42 percent) tend to charge a separate dispensing fee (approximately $133 per patient fitted in 1995).[26] Table 47-6 summarizes the price

Table 47-6 Price of hearing instruments by style and dispenser

Hearing Aid Style	Dispensing Audiologist	Hearing Instrument Specialist	Average
Behind-the-ear	$747	$756	$751
In-the-ear	805	721	763
In-the-canal	964	930	947
Completely in-the-canal	1,466	1,557	1,512
Programmable	1,639	1,845	1,742

(From Skafte,[27] with permission.)

of hearing instruments by style according to the 1996 Hearing Review Survey.[27] It is evident that overall, programmable hearing instruments are the most and conventional BTE instruments the least expensive. High-end programmable hearing instruments range from $1,619 for a BTE unit to $1,906 for a CIC hearing aid. It is worthwhile noting that persons who obtain two hearing aids, one for each ear, function much better in terms of speech understanding, but the cost of the hearing aids is nearly double the aforementioned prices. Thus, the price for CIC hearing aids may reach $3,500 to $4,000. The considerable financial investment associated with the purchase of hearing aids underlines the importance of referring the consumer to a qualified professional who spends time dispensing the product and orienting the individual and family members to the hearing aid in an effort to optimize the fit. Finally, with the exception of cochlear implant surgery for severely and profoundly impaired individuals, support for hearing care is modest or unavailable in most health plans. However, recently selected managed care plans have introduced some, albeit minimal, coverage (e.g., $500) toward the purchase of a hearing instrument.

Despite some limitations in their ability to separate out speech from noise, hearing aids have been shown to provide short- and long-term quality-of-life improvements. Hearing aids reduce the social, emotional, and communication dysfunction perceived by older adults with mild to moderately severe sensorineural hearing loss after 6 weeks of hearing aid use and these benefits are sustained after 1 year of use.[15] Compared with the waiting list group, those older adults who received hearing aids demonstrated an 85 percent improvement in social and emotional function, a 68 percent improvement in communication function, and a 26 percent improvement in depressive symptoms as assessed by the Geriatric Depression Scale.[15] Another group of investigators has demonstrated that hearing aids, in conjunction with audiologic rehabilitation, effectively improve psychosocial well-being of persons with handicapping hearing loss.[28] Finally, it has recently been demonstrated that improvements in psychosocial well-being and communication function associated with short-term hearing aid use are comparable for older and younger adults.[29] This finding is an important step toward dispelling the myth that older adults cannot derive significant benefits from hearing aids.

Counseling/Hearing Aid Orientation

When people first put hearing aids in the ear, their own voice and that of others sound very strange.[30] Their own voices tend to have a hollow booming quality as if talking from the bottom of a barrel. The audiologist can make the necessary adjustments to eliminate this sensation. To ensure maximal benefit from hearing aids, older adults must have realistic expectations and patience. Of utmost importance, the new hearing aid user must understand that hearing aids "are not very smart," that they do not always do a good job of discriminating between desirable sounds persons want to hear (i.e., speech) and those undesirable sounds they want to ignore (i.e., background noise).[30] However, this situation is slowly changing with the advent of digital hearing aids and the development of more sophisticated electronics. New hearing aid users should not expect to suddenly hear normally. They should, however, expect to have a reduction in the degree of difficulty they have been having, depending on the acoustics of the listening situation.

Hearing aid users must understand that it takes time to realize the potential benefit from hearing aids, and thus should not become discouraged early. Their ears and their brains must become "re-educated" to hearing selected patterns of sounds that have been made louder by the hearing aid.[30] In a sense new hearing aid users are suddenly being exposed to or "bombarded with" a world of sounds they have forgotten existed, such as the blare of street noises in the city, and must become reoriented to or acquain-ed with the location and source of these "new" sounds. To facilitate adaptation to the hearing aid, new hearing users should wear the hearing aids for as many hours during the day that they feel comfortable with the units in their ears. It is advisable that new hearing aid users wear their hearing aids in restricted situations at first, such as while at home with family members, while watching the television, or while eating dinner. Once the individual feels comfortable with amplified sound at home, he or she should venture into new hearing situations, at all times experimenting with the volume control to maintain speech input at a comfortable level and noise at a minimum. Although full-time use should be the goal, there are some exceptions. Persons with mild hearing loss may find their hearing aids useful in business meetings, but may find them burdensome in noisy situations such as restaurants or parties. If patients complain that some intense sounds produce an uncomfortably loud hearing sensation, they should alert the dispensing audiologist at the follow-up visit as a simple adjustment can usually be made to the hearing aid. Many hearing aid users report that although at first they prefer "natural sounding" louder sounds as their ears and mind adjust, they tend to prefer a boost in the high-frequency response of the hearing aid that makes the consonants of speech crisper and easier to understand.[30] It is of utmost importance that new hearing aid users schedule and keep all follow-up appointments (a minimum of 2 to 4 weeks following receipt of the hearing aid) so that the audiologist can make the necessary adjustments to ensure that sounds are comfortable, audible, tolerable, and understandable. At these visits, the audiologist and new hearing aid user work together to modify the response of the hearing aid for optimal speech understanding. Finally, new hearing aid users should accept their hearing loss and not continue to consider it a disgrace or a stigma. They should not cover their hearing aids as a way of hiding the hearing loss, as hearing aids serve as a signal to others that a hearing loss exists and that they should speak clearly to facilitate speech understanding. According to Ross,[30] an experienced and successful hearing aid user and audiologist, the hearing impaired should not worry about people seeing their hearing aids. If the hearing aid users accept their hearing loss and hearing aids, so will persons to whom they are speaking. In short, acceptance of hearing loss, and motivation to overcome its consequences, are conditions for hearing aid satisfaction and success.

The points mentioned above are typically discussed at the individual hearing aid follow-up appointment but are also emphasized in a group hearing aid orientation program made available to consumers upon the purchase of hearing instruments. Although not all professionals provide orientation programs, the consumer organization Self Help For Hard of Hearing People, Inc. (SHHH) recently recommended that all hearing aid dispensers make available and encourage participation in group programs. Group orientation programs should be short term, 3 to 6 weeks, and should provide sufficient time for an instructional component and for the emergence of group exchanges.[31] The instructional component should include (1) discussions about hearing loss and the audiogram; (2) instructions in troubleshooting with hearing aids; (3) discussions about the availability of assistive listening devices to supplement hearing aids; (4) an introduction to speech reading/auditory training; and (5) an overview of coping and conversational repair strategies to facilitate communication. Recently, a few investigators have demonstrated that short-term group programs do in fact promote hearing aid benefit among new hearing aid users above that achieved with just one orientation session.

Assistive Listening Devices

Very often hearing aids do not provide for the easy clear listening one desires in all communication environments. The major reason for the lack of a clear acoustic signal in selected situations is that the speech signal (S) is much louder than the background noise (N) yielding an unfavorable S/N ratio.[32] People with normal hearing require the signal to be twice as intense as background noise for speech to be intelligible, whereas people with hearing loss require the primary signal to be 10 times more intense than background sounds to enable them to detect word/sound distinctions, etc. Well-fit hearing aids can provide a favorable S/N ratio if the environment is free of distractions and if the speaker is close to the person with hearing impairment. For the most part, however, the hearing aid microphone at the listener's ear is typically some distance from the sound source, making speech difficult to understand. In essence, the further away from the sound source one is, the softer the sound pressure and the less clear the speech signal.[32] For the most part the listening environments we live in are demanding, and hearing aids alone are insufficient to access auditory events that are not close to the person who is hearing impaired. The use of alternative hearing technologies, known as assistive listening devices, has proven invaluable in overcoming some of the environmental barriers to successful communication. Four categories of devices are available including (1) sound enhancement technology, (2) television enhancement technology, (3) telecommunications technology, and (4) signal alerting technology.[32]

Sound enhancement technologies enable a person with hearing impairment to understand speech clearly when the speaker is at a considerable distance from the listener. This is accomplished by transmitting the signal directly to the ear of the listener, thereby overcoming the barriers posed by distance and environmental noise. Sound enhancement technologies include a remote microphone, placed close to the sound source (within 6 inches), which picks up the signal via one of several modes of transmission, sends the signal to the listener's ear(s). Signals can be transmitted to the listener via a hard-wired connection between the microphone/amplifier/receiver and the headphones, via wireless radio transmission of signals (i.e., FM unit), via an induction loop system, or via infrared light.

Hard-wired systems that are commercially available and relatively inexpensive (under $50) are ideal in one to one situations as in a physician's office, or when being interviewed by a nurse or social worker.[18] Personal FM systems that must be fit by an audiologist are more costly (i.e., greater than $500) yet can facilitate large and small group communication as well as classroom listening. FM systems can be used outdoors and when the speaker and listener are in different rooms. BTE/FM hearing aids have recently been introduced and represent a cosmetically appealing way to enhance speech understanding in a noisy backgound using an ear level array (otherwise FM systems require a body-worn receiver that connects in one of several ways to a personal hearing aid). In this arrangement the FM receiver and a conventional hearing aid are both incorporated in a BTE case such that the BTE/FM system can be used as a regular hearing aid, as an FM receiver, or as both together.[33] Older hearing-impaired adults with severe sensorineural hearing loss and/or auditory processing problems should inquire about the availability of BTE/FM systems. They have proven beneficial in restaurants, at lectures, in cars, and at noisy receptions. With this arrangement the FM microphone transmitter is worn close to the source of speech (speaker), and the signal is delivered via FM signals to the listener's ears free of environmental noise. Finally, infrared systems use invisible light, the wavelength of which is outside the range of human visibility, to transmit signals indoors in a single room from the speaker to the listener.[18]

The sound enhancement technology described above can be used with different forms of media including television, stereo systems, and video cassette recorders. Infrared systems provide the best quality sound for radio and television, and are widely used in theaters and concert and lecture halls. Essentially the remote microphone of the system is placed within 6 inches of the media speaker to provide a favorable S/N ratio. Telecaptioning or dialogue in the form of captions that run across the bottom of the television screen can also assist in television enjoyment for persons with severe to profound hearing loss. All new televisions manufactured today include telecaptioning capabilities.

Telecommunication technology facilitates communication over the telephone. Options include portable or built-in amplifiers, speakerphones, FAX machines, and telecommunication systems for the deaf (TDD). TDDs are invaluable to persons with severe to profound hearing loss for whom it is impossible to discriminate speech over the telephone. TDDs are approximately the size of a typewriter. Individuals communicating over the telephone merely type in their message, or use a relay operator who types in a message, and it is displayed across the listener's TDD. The telephone company provides relay service free of charge for persons wishing to speak with a TDD user. E-mail is also an excellent form of telecommunication technology for persons with hearing impairment unable to communicate comfortably over the telephone. Finally, signal-alerting technology includes any system that warns, signals, or alerts a person with a hearing loss. They use loud sounds, visual signals, or tactile signals to alert the hearing impaired to sounds in the environment. For example, a vibrator placed under the pillow can awaken the person with hearing loss in the morning, or a strobe light attached to a smoke alarm can alert the hearing impaired person to a fire.[32] Signal-alerting devices are commercially available and are invaluable for hearing impaired persons who are homebound, for persons with cognitive impairments, and for residents of nursing facilities who cannot hear external events due to hearing loss. Audiologists are well equipped to guide persons and institutions about the system(s) that will best meet their needs and to arrange for the purchase of the necessary assistive listening devices.

Screening Protocols

In light of the psychosocial consequences of acquired hearing loss, and the variety of technologies available to overcome communication difficulties, a variety of major authorities have recently advocated routine screening for hearing impairment among older adults. The American Academy of Family Physicians and U.S. Preventive Services Task Force recommend that persons over 65 years of age undergo periodic hearing evaluations and counseling regarding the availability of hearing aids.[34,35] The Canadian Task Force on the Periodic Health Examination suggests that a hearing screen be considered part of the periodic health examination.[36] Finally, the U.S. Public Health Service recommends that older adults should be questioned about signs of hearing loss.[37] They suggest that a screening questionnaire may be used to screen for communication problems, and social and emotional handicaps stemming from hearing loss. Questionnaires have the advantage of identifying patients who perceive hearing loss to be a problem and who therefore may be particularly motivated to use a hearing aid. They strongly recommend that persons found to have evidence of hearing loss by screening be considered for referral to a specialist, not a hearing aid dealer, for comprehensive audiologic evaluation especially if they feel handicapped by the hearing loss. Because the point of entry into the hearing health care system usually involves the primary care physician, he or she has a critical role to play in identifying older persons with handicapping hearing impairments.

A simple, reliable, and valid screening program has been advocated by a number of investigators.[19,38,39] The procedure entails a pure-tone screen and administration of the 10-item screening version of the Hearing Handicap Inventory for the Elderly (HHIE-S). The purpose of the screen should be to identify older persons with handicapping hearing impairment who require audiologic testing and intervention.[40] The pure-tone screen involves use of the Audioscope, a hand-held otoscope combined with a screening audiometer that delivers pure tones at 40 dBHL at four frequencies: 500, 1,000, 2,000, and 4,000 Hz. The current cost of the Audioscope is within the range of $500 to $600. A patient fails the screen if he or she does not hear the tones at 1,000 or 2,000 Hz in one or both ears. The patient is instructed to raise his or her finger or hand when the tone is heard. The patient's response should be time-locked to the presentation of the stimulus signaled by a red indicator light on the Audioscope. If otoscopic examination indicates the presence of cerumen impaction, this necessitates a failure and a referral.

Prior to or following the pure-tone screen, the patient should complete the HHIE-S using a face to face, paper and pencil or computer-assisted presentation. A score of 10 or greater signifies the necessity of a referral. More specifically, scores of 0 to 8 signify no handicap, scores of 10 to 22 signify a mild to moderate handicap, and scores of 24 to 40 suggest significant self-perceived handicap. Scores on the HHIE-S are directly correlated to hearing aid uptake and have been shown to improve after the initiation of hearing aid use.[15] Primary care physicians with first-hand experience with this screening protocol consider it to be simple, cost-effective, quick, and easy to administer.[39]

Fino et al.[41] were among the first investigators to demonstrate that hearing aid candidacy is directly linked to the prefitting score on the HHIE-S.[41] Specifically, they found that the extent of self- perceived hearing handicap on the 10-item (HHIE-S) is predictive of hearing aid candidacy, in that it reliably distinguishes between hearing aid users and nonusers. Irrespective of hearing level (e.g., mild or moderate sensorineural hearing loss), persons who obtained hearing aids were more handicapped as evidenced by higher scores on the HHIE-S, than those who did not. Similarly, on the average scores on the HHIE-S for new hearing aid users were approximately 18, irrespective of mean hearing level and mean word recognition ability.[42] Persons with mild and moderately severe hearing levels presented with comparable scores on the HHIE-S (i.e., 18). Similarly, persons with excellent and those with poor scores on a test of word recognition emerged with mean prefitting HHIE-S scores ranging from 16 to 18. Following 3 weeks of hearing aid use all subjects experienced a dramatic improvement in scores on the HHIE-S such that average postfitting scores were approximately 3.[42] The latter studies demonstrate that self-perceived handicap, identified using a simple and easy screening tool, is linked to hearing aid use and is dramatically reduced following intervention.

When and to Whom to Refer

Audiologists and otolaryngologists are hearing health care specialists who provide assistance to persons with hearing problems. The otolaryngologist is a medical doctor whose goal is to identify and treat medical diseases of the ear that may be causing a hearing problem. If medical treatment in the form of antibiotic therapy or surgery is not indicated, the person with hearing loss should be seen by an audiologist.[40] The audiologist has a master's or doctoral degree and is trained to evaluate hearing sensitivity/auditory function and to provide services that will improve the ability to communicate. They administer pure-tone tests of middle and inner ear function and measures of speech understanding that help uncover peripheral or central auditory processing problems. Audiologists fit hearing aids in an attempt to help the hearing impaired overcome some of their speech understanding difficulties. Audiologists work in private practice, hospitals, clinics, or rehabilitation centers. Although audiologists can represent the point of entry into the hearing health care system, older adults referred to the audiologist by their physician are most likely to purchase audiologic services in the form of hearing tests and hearing aids. The latter underlines the role of the physician in assisting older adults in overcoming the effects of hearing loss.

Concluding Remarks

Approximately 30 to 50 percent of older adults suffer from handicapping hearing impairment that can interfere with the quality of their lives. The advent of technologically sophisticated hearing aids that are more effective than ever before in separating out the speech from noise are a boon to older adults who are living longer and retiring early yet continue to be confronted by difficulty understanding the speech of others, especially in noise. Further, the availability of assistive listening devices that compensate for the shortcomings remaining with hearing aids is another avenue for persons with hearing impairment to pursue. The physician has a responsibility and tools in the form of a hand-held Audioscope or reliable and valid questionnaires to identify persons with hearing problems who require and can benefit from the expertise of audiologists. Physicians and audiologists are encouraged to work together to promote the quality of life of the increasing population of older adults suffering from handicapping hearing impairment.

References

1. National Center for Health Statistics: Current Estimates from the National Health Interview Survey, 1989. Vital and Health Statistics Series, 10, No. 176 (October, 1990)
2. Strom K: An analysis of 1995 hearing instrument sales. Hearing Rev 1996;3:8–36
3. Willott J: Aging and the Auditory System. Singular Publishing, San Diego, 1991
4. Moscicki E, Elkins E, Baum H, McNamara P: Hearing loss in the elderly: an epidemiologic study of the Framingham Heart Study Cohort. Ear Hearing 1985;6:184–190
5. Schuknecht H: Presbycusis. Laryngoscope 1955;65:402–419
6. Schuknecht H: Further observations on the pathology of presbycusis. Arch Otolaryngol 1964;80:369–382
7. Schuknecht H: Pathology of presbycusis. In Goldstein J, Kashima H, Koopman C (eds): Geriatric Otorhinolaryngology. B C Decker, Toronto, 1989
8. Schuknecht H: Pathology of the Ear, 2nd Ed. Lea & Febiger, Philadelphia, 1993
9. Otte J, Schuknecht H, Kerr A: Ganglion cell populations in normal and pathological human cochleae. Implications for cochlear implantation. Laryngoscope, 1978;88:1231–1246
10. Crowe S, Guild S, Polvogt L: Observations on the pathology of high-tone deafness. Johns Hopkins Hosp Bull 1934;54: 315–380
11. Hansen C, Reske-Nielsen E: Pathological studies in presbycusis. Arch Otolaryngol 1965;82:115–132
12. Cooper J: Health and Nutrition Examination Survey of 1971–75: Part I. Ear and race effects in hearing. J Am Acad Audiol 1994;5:30–36
13. Gates G, Cooper J, Kannel W, Miller N: Hearing in the elderly: the Framingham Cohort, 1983–1985. Part 1. Basic audiometric test results. Ear Hearing 1991;4:247–256
14. Bess F, Humes L: Audiology, the Fundamentals. 2nd Ed. Williams & Wilkins, Baltimore, 1995
15. Mulrow C, Aguilar C, Endicott J et al: Quality of life changes and hearing impairment: results of a randomized trial. Ann Intern Med 1990;113:188–194
16. Bess F, Lichtenstein M, Logan S: Hearing impairment as a determinant of function in the elderly. J Am Geriatr Soc 1989; 37:123–128
17. Uhlmann R, Larson E, Koepsell T: Hearing impairment and cognitive decline in senile dementia of the Alzheimer's type. J Am Geriatr Soc 1986;34:207–210
18. Weinstein B: Auditory testing and rehabilitation of the hearing impaired. In Lubinski R (ed): Dementia and Communication. Singular Publishing San Diego, 1995
19. Ventry I, Weinstein B: Identification of elderly individuals with hearing problems. ASHA 1983;25:37–42
20. Ventry I, Weinstein B: The hearing handicap inventory for the elderly: a new tool. Ear Hearing 1982;3:128–134
21. Lavizzo-Mourey R, Siegler F: Hearing impairment in the elderly. J Gen Intern Med 1992;7:191–198
22. Kemp B: The psychosocial context of geriatric rehabilitation. In Kemp K, Brummel-Smith K, Ramsdell J (eds): Geriatric Rehabilitation, Little Brown, Boston, 1990
23. McCandless G: Overview and rationale of threshold based hearing aid selection procedures. In Valente M (ed): Strategies for Selecting and Verifying Hearing Aid Fittings. Thieme-Medical Publishers, New York, 1996
24. Cox R, Alexander G: The abbreviated profile of hearing aid benefit. Ear Hearing 1995;16:176–186
25. Radcliffe D: Programmable hearing aids: digital control comes to analog amplification. Hearing J 1991;44:9–12
26. Kirkwood D: Dispensers report expanding practices, predict additional growth in 1996. Hearing J 1996;49:13–23
27. Skafte M: The 1995 hearing instrument market—the dispenser's perspective. Hearing Rev 1996;3:16–34
28. Abrams H, Chisolm T, Guerreiro S, Ritterman S: The effects of intervention strategy on self perception of hearing handicap. Ear Hearing 1992;13:371–377
29. Primeau R: Hearing aid benefit in adults and older adults. In Weinstein B (ed): Seminars in Hearing. Thieme, NY, 1997
30. Ross M: You've done something about it! Helpful hints to the new hearing aid user. SHHH J 1996;17:7–11
31. Self Help for Hard of Hearing People, Inc: Position statement on group hearing aid orientation programs. SHHH J 1996;17: 29
32. Flexer C: Access to communication environments through assistive listening devices. Hearsay 1991;6:9–14
33. Ross M: Developments in research and technology. SHHH J 1995;16:32–34
34. American Academy of Family Physicians, Commission on Public Health and Scientific Affairs: Age Charts for Periodic Health Examination. American Academy of Family Physicians, Kansas City, MO, 1993
35. U.S. Preventive Services Task Force: Screening for hearing impairment. Ch. 33. In Guide to Clinical Preventive Services. Williams & Wilkins, Baltimore, 1989
36. Canadian Task Force on the Periodic Health Examination: The periodic health examination monograph. Quebec: Ministry: 2. 1984 update. Can Med Assoc J 1984;130:1278–1285
37. U.S. Public Health Service: The Clinician's Handbook of Preventive Services. International Medical Publishing, Virginia, 1994
38. Weinstein B: Validity of a screening protocol for identifying elderly people with hearing problems. ASHA 1986;28: 41–45

39. Lichtenstein M, Bess F, Logan S: Validation of screening tools for identifying hearing-impaired elderly in primary care. JAMA 1988;259:2875–2878
40. Jerger J, Chmiel R, Wilson, Luchi R: Hearing impairment in older adults: new concepts. J Am Geriatr Soc 1995;43:928–935
41. Fino M, Bess F, Lichtenstein M, Logan S: Factors differentiating elderly hearing aid wearers and non-wearers. Hearing Instrum 1991;43:6–10
42. Newman C, Jacobson G, Hug G et al: Practical method for quantifying hearing aid benefit in older adults. J Am Acad Audiol 1991;2:70–75
43. Adams P, Benson V: Current Estimates from the National Health Interview Survey. 1991; National Center for Health Statistics. Vital Health Statistics, 10 (1984)
44. Preves D: The role of the hearing instrument amplifier. Hearing Rev 1996;3:34–3

CHAPTER 48

Delirium

A. J. D. MACDONALD

The Importance of Delirium

Delirium is a frequent (Table 48-1), frightening, dangerous, and costly[1] condition that is often missed in the elderly medical patient[2], yet often has a remediable cause and is amenable to simple care and treatment. It sits in the hinterland between medicine and psychiatry, less neglected now largely thanks to Lipowski[3], whose masterly account published in 1990 has no equal. It is important as a "window" onto the mind/brain problem as well as a practical, albeit complex everyday problem for physicians. This chapter is therefore divided into two sections, describing theoretical and practical matters.

Theoretical Issues in Delirium

Definitions

The "semantic muddle"[3] of delirium is gradually clearing as ICD-10[4] takes hold, but many other terms still pepper the literature and clinical talk. The most common *apparent* synonyms are "acute confusional state," and "acute brain syndrome"; apparent, because some still distinguish these and other terms from delirium. The most frequently used standardized criteria for delirium fall into two groups: those created by committee (American Psychiatric Association,[5] World Health Organization[4]) and those emanating from researchers. The former are subject to compromise and political pressure. The latter are mostly derived from the former, particularly, *Diagnostric and statistical Manual of Mental Disorders*, 3rd edition, revised (DSM-IIIR) criteria.[5] Whatever their source, all current criteria have intrinsic problems. The most basic of these is that although they correlate well with traditional clinical concepts of delirium, they are poorly validated against independent criteria—only mortality has been systematically used in a few studies.[6] Mortality is a distant surrogate for delirium, the main confounder being comorbid, mortal conditions. Criteria based on DSM-IIIR also suffer from the stipulation of an "organic" etiologic factor; this has no place in the delineation of a syndrome at all[7], let alone one that is known to be multifactorial.

Delirium and dementia

A further problem is the relationship of delirium to dementia syndromes. It is a frequent observation that delirium arises during dementia and thereafter may disappear altogether, leaving patients exactly as they were before, worse, or not leave the patient at all. Criteria that demand resolution exclude these states. Furthermore, Lewy Body dementia has characteristics that are very similar to delirium—particularly abrupt changes, fluctuation, and visual hallucinations.[8] The concept of "sundowning" (agitation in demented patients at dusk)[9], has taken root in the literature but its status is uncertain. It seems likely that this represents a combination of day-night reversal of dementia and delirium, but it is described too loosely to allow critical evaluation.

Standardized Measures

Two tasks face standardized assessments in delirium: ascertainment of the presence of the syndrome, and, for outcome purposes, ascertainment of its severity. A further measurement task for research is that of the severity of underlying physical illness.

Ascertaining the presence of delirium

The short measures of cognitive assessment used until recently for delirium research, such as the Mini-Mental State Examination MMSE, the Mental Status Questionnaire, and the Short Portable Mental Status Questionnaire, are not specific enough for the syndrome[10] as they cannot distinguish it from dementia. Specific measures such as the Delirium Rating Scale[11], the Confusion Assessment Method[12], the Clinical Assessment of Confusion[13], the Delirium Symptom Interview[14], and the Confusion Rating Scale and NEECHAM Confusion Scale[15] have been developed, validated against DSM-IIIR criteria or independent psychiatric interview. This is somewhat circular, in that DSM-IIIR criteria and prevalent concepts of delirium are similar, although ICD-10 seems to identify a different, smaller set of delirious subjects.[16] The author and a colleague have recently argued that the best independent validating criterion is outcome[6], and this seems feasible using repeated tests of cognitive function, because fatigue and practice effects do not seem to be significant.[17]

Subtle cognitive changes may require more sensitive tests such as the High Sensitivity Cognitive Screen.[18] Direct application of DSM-IIIR criteria may be useful in prospective studies; studies involving retrospective (chart) review diagnosis of delirium have been shown to be biased by inaccurate recording.[19] Other approaches deserve consideration in delirium research. The IQCODE is a standardized cognitive history, taken

Table 48-1 Prevalence of delirium in elderly populations

Population	Age (y)	Assessment	N	Prevalence (%)	Year of Publication	Study Reference
Hospitalized	70+	DSM-IIIR	229	22	1990	25
Community residents	55+	DSM-IIIR	810	1.1 (85+ : 13.6)	1991	26
Acute medical patients	72–99	DSM-IIIR	106	23	1991	27
Acute geriatric patients	60–97	DSM-IIIR	184	22	1992	28
General medical emergencies	70+	DSM-IIIR	331	14	1993	29
Geriatric patients	65+	Symptom Rating Scale	168	18	1993	30
Medical or surgical inpatients	65+	DSM-IIIR	432	15	1994	31
Elective orthopaedic patients	60+	Confusion Assessment Method	80	17.5	1995	32
Emergency room patients	70+	Confusion Assessment Method	188	39.9	1995	33

Abbreviation: DSM-IIIR, Diagnostic and Statistical Manual of Mental Disorders, *3rd edition, revised.*

from a relative or caregiver.[20] Writing impairment may be very specific for delirium. Slow eye movements have been reported as showing good correlation with the electroencephalogram EEG changes of drowsiness.[21] The hand-held tachistoscope has been disappointing, because many elderly delirious subjects cannot see it at all.

Measuring the severity of delirium

The Delirium Assessment Scale has been suggested as useful for assessing severity as opposed to presence of the syndrome, although, as yet, this has not been so validated.[22] The MMSE does not appear suitable for the assessment of mild cognitive impairment or change.[23] As yet, the measurement of change in delirium has not been specifically studied. This is not surprising, because change is a characteristic of the syndrome itself (see below).

Measuring the severity of any underlying illness

The confounding effect of underlying physical illness on outcome demands a separate assessment of its severity. Commonly used dependency (activities of daily living [ADL]) measures are a distant proxy for this. The Cumulative illness Rating Scale[24] may offer the prospect of such assessment.

Prevalence and Incidence

Table 48-1 shows more recent estimates of prevalence in various populations of older people. A high rate was found in the accident and emergency study, whereas the lowest rate was in the community. It seems reasonable to suggest that between 1 in 6 and 1 in 4 of older (in patients) on medical and surgical wards are delirious at any one time. Incidence studies are rare. Ninety-one (31 percent) of 291 nondelirious elderly patents admitted for acute medical conditions developed delirium during their stay[34] and more patients had symptoms of delirium falling short of DSM-IIIR criteria.[35] Of 107 medical patients, neither demented nor delirious initially, who were assessed daily, 27 percent developed delirium.[36] A recent structured review of postoperative delirium in all ages estimated the incidence at 36.8 percent (range, 0 to 73.5 percent).[37] In a more recent study of older surgical patients 15 percent developed delirium on their third postoperative day.[38]

We can conclude that delirium is a common problem in medical settings. Whether its frequency in other settings is sufficient to warrant attention remains to be seen; it does look as if it is relatively infrequently found in community subjects. However, the DSM-IIIR criterion of "organicity" is very difficult to meet in these subjects.

Risk Factors

Studies of risk factors for delirium are important in increasing our understanding of it, and may lead to strategies that may reduce its impact. Several risk factors have emerged for delirium in medical settings as well as for perioperative delirium.

General risk factors

In 325 elderly medical patients admitted to a teaching hospital, advanced age was a risk factor in community residents but not in those admitted from institutions.[35] In 323 elderly medical and surgical patients, pre-existing cognitive impairment, comorbid conditions, depression, and alcoholism were associated with the development of delirium.[31] Urinary tract infection, low serum albumin, and high white blood cell count or proteinuria were associated with chart diagnosis of delirium in 471 of 1,285 patients discharged from a teaching hospital over 2 years, and these factors predicted delirium in subsequent discharges.[39] However, the inaccuracy of the chart diagnosis of delirium is likely to have caused bias in these correlations. Delirium was a common presenting symptom in 50 consecutive cases of bacteremia in a geriatric unit, with 24 percent from a urinary tract source.[40] Of the 91 previously nondelirious elderly patients admitted for acute medical care who developed the syndrome more were cognitively impaired, aged more than 80, had a fracture, had a symptomatic infection, were of male sex, or were taking a neuroleptic or narcotic drug than those who did not. Taking anticholinergic drugs did not appear to be a risk factor.[34] When 107 medical patients, who were neither demented nor delirious initially, were assessed daily, 27 percent developed delirium. Risk factors were vision impairment, severity of medical illness, cognitive impairment, and high urea/nitrogen ratio. These factors predicted delirium in subsequent patients.[36] In a psychiatric sample of 70 patients with delirium, 81 percent had structural brain disease.[41] Surprisingly, visual impairment does not seem to have been systematically assessed as a risk factor for delirium in the elderly.

Risk factors for perioperative delirium in the elderly

In 1,341 patients over 50 years of age admitted for elective surgery, being over 70 years old; alcohol abuse; preoperative cognitive impairment; abnormal sodium, potassium, or glucose; and type of surgery was associated with delirium, and these risk factors predicted delirium in subsequent cases.[42] Surgery in patients with Parkinson's disease appears to carry an increased risk of postoperative delirium; there was a relative risk of 2.8 to 8.1 in one study.[43] Previous suggestions that preoperative anxiety might predict delirium were not confirmed in a study of 45 elderly patients undergoing elective hip replacement[44], and anticholinergic drugs were not associated with delirium in 91 elderly patients undergoing elective orthopaedic surgery[32], although benzodiazepines were. However, a structured review of postoperative delirium in patients of all ages found that age, preoperative cognitive impairment, and the use of anticholinergic drugs were significantly associated with postoperative delirium, whereas gender, type and route of anesthesia, and sleep deprivation were not.[37] An earlier, structured review of this problem specifically in elderly patients found only age and female gender as risk factors, but bemoaned the lack of standardization and the failure of studies to meet elementary methodologic criteria.[45] Mention must be made of "black patch disease"—delirium after cataract surgery. This appears to be a very rare event, both considering the literature and in routine practice. The author participated in a trial of local versus general anesthetic in relation to delirium after cataract surgery in the elderly that was abandoned due to the absence of postoperative delirium in elderly patients in a tertiary ophthalmologic center.

Conclusions: risk factors for delirium

A simple model of risk for delirium in the elderly can be constructed that would crudely fit the research findings, incorporating degree of structural brain disorder and severity of the physical illness or insult. The question of whether aging is inevitably linked to structural brain disorder remains unclear; if it is not, then it would also need to be incorporated as an independent factor. Figure 48-1 demonstrates how brain disorder and physical insult severity seem to be related to risk of developing delirium. Of course, it does not explain the whole picture—for example, the mildly cognitively impaired patient who has a fulminating delirium with a urinary tract infection and acute urinary retention, and then, within a few weeks, experiences a septicemia from an infected injury without any clouding of consciousness or cognitive decrement at all.

Etiology

No one understands how apparently trivial physical illnesses or minor toxins can provoke relatively sudden global impairment of cognitive, perceptual, affective, and psychomotor functioning, nor why this impairment fluctuates, nor why

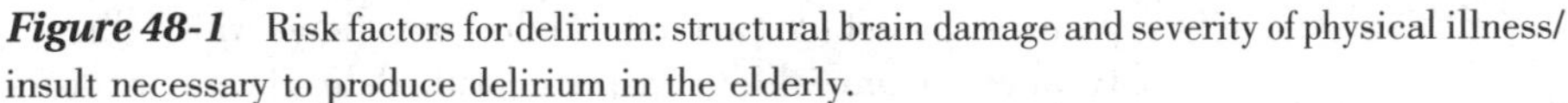

Figure 48-1 Risk factors for delirium: structural brain damage and severity of physical illness/ insult necessary to produce delirium in the elderly.

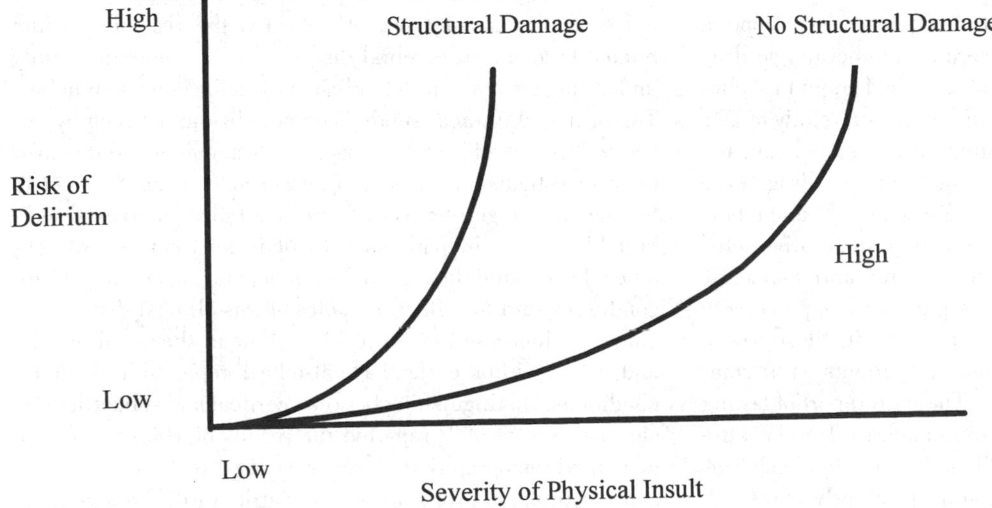

the syndrome often lasts longer than the stimulus that provoked it. Present attention to the problem is focused on three main areas: that occasioned by the EEG changes that have long been known to accompany delirium, the evidence that there is disturbance of the hypothalamic-pituitary-adrenal axis in delirium, and the evidence that anticholinergic drugs impair cognitive functioning. There are a number of other, less studied, avenues of research as well.

Electroencephalogram and ictal concepts of delirium

The original findings by Engel and Romano[46] of characteristic EEG changes in delirium have been extended by the use of modern electrical mapping techniques. Two-channel EEGs may eventually be performed at the bedside as part of the assessment of psychiatric disturbance in medical wards.[47] Nonconvulsive status epilepticus is a rare cause of delirium itself.[48] Epilepsy may present with delirium in old age, and interictal delirium is a recognized feature of epilepsy in older people. The action of intravenous (IV) benzodiazepines in certain kinds of withdrawal delirium may also be connected with their anticonvulsant properties.[49] Somatosensory evoked potential studies suggest a significant subcortical, as well as cortical, origin of the disturbances in hepatic delirium.

Hypothalamic-pituitary-adrenal axis malfunction in delirium

The dexamethasone suppression test has been used to show abnormalities in delirious patients with lower respiratory tract infections, and it may predict delirium risk during illness.[50] Dexamethasone itself reduces mortality in younger delirious patients with typhoid,[51] although this benefit is not necessarily produced by direct action on the mechanisms of delirium itself. It is known that in delirium associated with stroke there is massive adrenocorticotropic hormone (ACTH) release[52] and also, perhaps, hypercortisolism.

Cholinergic disruption and delirium

There is some evidence of a relationship between postoperative delirium in the elderly and serum anticholinergic drug levels,[53] although doubts have been expressed about the "cholinergic score" used in this work. In a follow-up study of 291 nondelirious elderly patients admitted for acute medical care, in which 91 developed delirium, anticholinergic drugs were not found to affect risk of delirium significantly,[34] and others have also failed to find an association with postoperative delirium.[54] However, in another study total serum anticholinergic activity was elevated in 11 delirious patients compared with 11 controls 60 years of age and older, and in those whose delirium persisted compared with that in patients with "complete resolution" of the syndrome.[55] The case report of lasting visual hallucinations in clear consciousness after IV atropine,[56] and the influence of small doses of scopolamine as premedication on cognitive functioning in elderly subjects[57] is also suggestive of a possible relationship. Ten of the 25 medications most commonly prescribed in elderly people had significant anticholinergic levels judged by radioceptor assay.[58]

A rat model of delirium has been proposed, based on EEG responses of animals to atropine, as opposed to saline. The syndrome produced is described as "lack of focused direction, irritability, fluctuating levels of activity, and excessive random sniffing."[59]

Other possible physical etiologic mechanisms

Koponen and colleagues have reported, over 4 years, changes in cerebrospinal fluid β-endorphin-like immunoreactivity, somatostatin, acetylcholinesterase, and 5HIAA associated with delirium. In general surgery patients, mean arterial oxygen saturation one night prior to post-thoracotomy delirium was lower than in controls.[60] However, the cholinergic physostigmine apparently increases cerebral blood flow and oxygenation in rats[61]; postulated anticholinergic and low oxygenation mechanisms may therefore be linked. Neuroanatomic theories of delirium are few. One, based on delirium in a patient with right middle cerebral artery infarction, proposed that delirium was due to lesions in convergence areas for the association areas in the cortex.[62]

Psychological theories

Psychological theories are sparse and difficult to sustain. Delirium has been described as a semivoluntary "denial of reality," and one author has suggested a voluntary component to delirium in terminal cancer.[63]

Imaging Studies

There is little published work in the area of imaging studies. The necessity for stillness in most neuroimaging techniques is, perhaps, thought to preclude studies of patients with delirium. However, many elderly patients with delirium are hypoactive.[64] Research has been conducted on the imaging characteristics of clinical subtypes of delirium, the risk of delirium related to localized cerebral disease, and attempts to identify underlying mechanisms of delirium using imaging techniques. The principal clinical subdivision of delirium between hyperactive ("activated") and hypoactive ("somnolent") states has been investigated by Hemmingsen et al.[65] using Xenon-133 inhalation tomography. They found generalized increased cerebral blood flow in patients with delirium tremens, whereas others have found decreased flow in hepatic encephalopathies, conditions said to reflect the poles of this clinical distinction. However, increased cerebral blood flow in the basal ganglia and right occipital cortex have also been reported in the latter conditions. Distinguishing between cortical and subcortical lesions, Brown et al.[66] reported the results of 100 consecutive computed tomography (CT) requests of patients referred with acute neurologic problems on a geriatric ward. Twenty-one of these patients had "acute confusional states." Of these 21, 7 had major cerebral pathology (4 subdural hematomas, 1 midline oligodendroglioma, 1 cerebellar hemorrhage, 1 no result given) and 4 had other pathology that would not have changed management. Most subdural hematomas were in the group with "acute confusional states." However, small numbers and other methodologic problems limit what can be ascertained from this work. Subcortical (particularly thalamic) infarcts have largely been reported as single cases. Magnetic resonance imaging (MRI) evidence of subcortical disease appears, however, to be consistently associated with an increased risk of electroconvulsive therapy (ECT) and antidepressant-induced delirium in the depressed elderly. Trzepacz[67] has reviewed position emission tomography (PET) and single photon emission computed tomography (SPECT) studies of delirium in younger patients with hepatic encephalopathy, delirium tremens, and traumatic brain injury. The results are inconclusive, and sample sizes are small. Brain electrical activity maps (BEAM) offer a means of visualizing cortical EEG activity.[68] However, they allow only crude localization. Jacobson et al.[69] reported BEAM results on a sample of 15 delirious, 10 demented, and 8 control subjects examined by repeated MMSE results, and reported a high correlation between initial scores and ratings of increased relative and absolute slow-wave power maps, the latter also being associated with change in scores over time. This seems a promising line of enquiry, as examination times are mercifully short. However, at present, there appear to be no grounds for using imaging techniques clinically as part of the investigation of possible underlying causes, given the discomfort caused to the patient by many of these procedures.

Causes of Delirium

Medication

A serious difficulty confronts anyone reviewing the medication causing delirium. There are hundreds of reports in the literature of delirium associated with medications, singly or in combination, but evaluation of their impact is almost always impossible. First, there is the problem of the illness for which the medication is given. For instance, intrathecal amphotericin B was associated with delirium.[70] The patient had coccidioidal meningitis, a condition that seems highly likely to have its own association with delirium. Second, delirium, by definition, fluctuates and may abate abruptly; such changes can easily be attributed to the removal of a medication when the relationship is, in fact, one of chance. "N of 1" trials are very difficult to carry out in this condition. Third, publication bias operates to heighten the profile of certain medications that are unexpectedly related to delirium, hiding those that are frequent, expected accompaniments and thus suspected with more reason. For example, the infrequency of reports of delirium associated with L-DOPA or β-blockers in the elderly bears little relation to its frequency in clinical practice. Fourth, medication is frequently quoted as the most "important" or "common" cause of delirium in the elderly, but controlled studies of risk factors (see above) do not all confirm this; medication appears low in the risk tables, if it is found to be a factor at all. Finally, some medications attract a deliriogenic reputation because of their effect in overdose, whereas they may be blameless in therapeutic doses. A list of medications that have been associated with delirium in the elderly is almost coterminous with pharmacopeia. Such a list is not useful. While we await definitive studies of relative risk, it is preferable to concentrate on those medications that may be associated with delirium in a surprising way, and those that are often used in elderly patients.

Topical preparations The clinician must be aware that topical medications are absorbed in sufficient concentrations to have systemic effects. Ophthalmic homatropine eyedrops have long been associated with delirium,[71] and transdermal analgesic medication has also been implicated,[72] as has topical scopolamine[73] and topical podophyllin.[74]

Psychotropic medication Psychotropic medications are frequently implicated in delirium in the elderly, particularly tricyclic antidepressants at high and low[75] plasma levels. However, there was a low prevalence of delirium in 43 geriatric patients on tricyclics over 18 months.[76] Benzodiazepine withdrawal seems a well-established factor in delirium in the elderly, and it may be unresponsive to diazepam[77]; it is possibly mediated by sudden γ-aminobutyric acid reduction.[78] Interestingly, IV benzodiazepines may themselves provoke delirium.[79] A structured review of the relationship of triazolam to delirium suggested that it was no stronger than for any other benzodiazepine.[80] A high serum lithium level in the elderly is often reported as causing delirium, but the latter is also reported (as are other signs of toxicity) at therapeutic levels.[81] Delirium with lithium may be mediated by hypothyroidism, and there are reports of delirium when combined with thioridazine. Thioridazine is a potent anticholinergic, but does not appear to be widely reported as a sole cause of delirium in the elderly, despite being, as discussed below, widely used in the management of mild delirium and agitation in dementia in the United Kingdom. Neuroleptic-induced delirium is rarely reported, but neuroleptic malignant syndrome, sometimes difficult to distinguish from delirium, is discussed below. Despite widespread suspicion of the adverse effects of anticholinergic medication on cognitive function in the elderly, reports of delirium caused by anticholinergics given for parkinsonian side effects of major tranquilizers are uncommon.

Digoxin Digoxin was frequently mentioned as deliriogenic in reports until the late 1980s.[82] Since then, presumably because it is widely recognized as a problem, reports appear to have ceased, although there has been a recent report of delirium with therapeutic serum concentrations when the drug is combined with quinidine.[83]

Other medications It is reported that antibiotics cause delirium, but assessment of this risk is problematic because the infections they are treating may be an equally important cause. Ciprofloxacin, tobramycin, and ofloxacin have specifically been implicated recently. A report of delirium caused by influenza vaccine[84] is epidemiologically highly likely to be a chance finding, given its widespread use. Histamine-2 receptor blockers may cause delirium, usually within 2 weeks of starting, and resolving within 3 days of cessation.[85] There is one report of physostigine reversing cimetidine delirium.[86] For several years there have been reports of delirium caused by chronic salicylate poisoning.[87] Finally, nonsteroidal anti-inflammatory drugs such as tiaprofenic acid[88] have been implicated in the genesis of delirium.

Other substances This section would not be complete without mention of more esoteric causes of delirium, such as paint fumes[89], typewriter correction fluid[90] (now obsolete), deadly nightshade berries,[91] thallium,[92] nasal decongestants,[93] and over-the-counter sleep remedies.[94]

Procedures

Electroconvulsive therapy ECT in Parkinson's disease[95] is suggested as particularly likely to provoke delirium, as it may do in patients with any structural brain changes other than stroke.[96] ECT after stroke appears not to carry any special risk of delirium, except, it has been suggested, if damage involves the caudate nucleus.[97] Post-ECT delirium does not appear to be related to electrode placement, although the relationship between cognitive impairment and ECT is confounded by many other factors such as age, anesthetic, oxygenation, and other concurrent morbid conditions.

Other procedures Arteriography contrast agents have been reported as provoking delirium, although, as before, the condition under investigation may well have contributed significantly. Contrast agents used in myelography may also be deliriogenic, although their use has declined significantly with the advent of better alternative imaging techniques.

Physical disorders

Just as the list of medications apparently implicated in delirium encompasses the pharmacopeia, so a list of physical diseases and disorders that may cause delirium resembles the index to this textbook. How can they be ordered in terms of importance? Clearly, to gain some appreciation of their relative importance, the frequency of their occurrence must be multiplied by the frequency with which they cause delirium. Unfortunately, the former rate differs according to the population under consideration; sampling from family practice patients medical outpatients, patients at a day hospital, acute medical in patients, surgical patients, those referred to a psychiatric or neurologic consultation service, or those attended by, or admitted by, psychiatrists will all produce different rates of the physical conditions described below. It is also quite possible that, whatever its prevalence in the particular sample, the same physical condition will be associated with different risks of delirium in different circumstances (e.g., in response to isolation). In matched patients with less than 60 percent burns, 40 percent of those isolated for laminar air-flow treatment developed delirium, compared with 7 percent of the nonisolated patients.[98] It follows that, in the absence of estimates of frequency using standardized criteria in well-defined populations, any classification of the medical causes of delirium in the elderly is likely to be shaped by the particular experience of the author. Consequently, the reader should bear in mind that the author is a psychiatrist working in a community-based service.

Infections In community-based psychogeriatric practice, urinary tract infections UTIs probably cause more delirium than any other single disorder (or medication), and studies in psychiatric inpatients reflect this.[99] Only a minority of such patients with UTI volunteer urinary symptoms, so diagnosis is made difficult without a high degree of suspicion. Urinary retention causing delirium, the so-called cystocerebral syndrome,[100] is also important, although the two are often linked. Lower respiratory tract infections are perhaps the next most frequent cause. Delirium appears to occur without frank septicemia, or even systemic signs of infection, in the majority of cases. The mechanism is unknown. At the other end of the spectrum of infective causes lie malaria, brucellosis, and psittacosis.

Metabolic Electrolyte disturbance,[101] uremia,[102] and dehydration[103] are all important factors in delirium in the elderly. Correction of these is an important prerequisite to recovery, whatever other factor may be at play. Magnesium deficiency in inflammatory bowel disease[104] and other disorders is a rare cause.

Cerebrovascular disorder Cerebrovascular accidents were infrequently found to cause delirium in a series of patients referred to a neurologic consultation service for sudden mental changes,[105] but a study of 661 stroke patients indicates that 3 percent presented with delirium,[106] and at least 9 percent had delirium in a smaller study.[107] Delirium appears to be less common after anterior cerebral artery infarction,[108] but more common with posterior cerebral infarctions[109] and almost universal with rostral basilar artery syndrome.[110] In a study of 79 patients with subdural hematoma 58 percent had mental changes, particularly delirium,[111] and this may be the presenting feature.[112] Multiple cerebral infarcts may cause delirium[113]; indeed, delirium is not infrequent in vascular dementia.

Other cerebral disorders Head injury[114] and normal pressure hydrocephalus[115] may present with delirium in the elderly.

Endocrine disorders Hypoglycemia as part of the presentation of maturity onset diabetes, or as part of unstable established diabetes is not an infrequent cause. Other endocrine disorders such as thyrotoxicosis, and hyperparathyroidism may also present with delirium.[116] A rare syndrome of hypocorticalism with low ACTH has been described, presenting with delirium in an elderly man.[117]

Cardiopulmonary Congestive cardiac failure and chronic obstructive airways disease are potent causes of delirium in older patients. In a study of 777 patients aged 65 to

100 years with myocardial infarct, a tendency for patients over the age of 85 years to present with delirium rather than chest pain has been reported.[118] Heart block in the elderly may also present in this way,[119] and although pacing may lead to clinical recovery, psychological testing of cognitive function may show lasting deficits.[120] Pulmonary embolism may present as delirium in the elderly.

Nutritional Thiamine deficiency was found to be associated with delirium in patients admitted to a geriatric unit,[121] and hypoalbuminemia was the most common laboratory abnormality in 100 patients with delirium referred to a psychiatric consultation service.[122] Hector and Burton[123] have reviewed the relationship between vitamin B_{12} deficiency and various psychiatric conditions, including delirium.

Epilepsy Godfrey et al.[124] found that 11 of 81 elderly patients with epilepsy had ictal and interictal delirium lasting up to 8 days. Epilepsy may present in this way in the elderly,[125] and Primavera and colleagues[126] report five elderly patients presenting with delirium whose EEGs showed non-convulsive status.

Cancer Cancer is associated with delirium principally at two stages: in the terminal phase, when other factors such as powerful narcotics may be playing a part, and in the paraneoplastic encephalopathies. Newman and colleagues[127] have reported a 76-year-old man with recurrent delirium whose underlying malignancy was not found in life. Hyponatremia caused by inappropriate antidiuretic-hormone-secreting tumors can also present with delirium in the elderly, as may cerebral metastases or, very rarely, primary cerebral tumors.

Other physical causes of delirium Systemic lupus erythematosus, polycythemia rubra vera, and giant cell arteritis can all present with delirium in the elderly, as can acute intermittent porphyria.

Psychosocial causes of delirium

Psychiatric disorders, in the absence of any underlying structural brain disease or medical illness, are probably unusual causes of delirium syndromes in the elderly. Occasional cases of acute psychiatric disorder presenting in clouded states are reported,[128] but problems in diagnosis only really arise when early dementia is present as well as psychiatric disorder. However, testing of orientation, memory, and consciousness in acute "functional" disorder is often cursory, and anecdotal evidence suggests that clouded states are more common than suspected. It must be kept in mind that water intoxication[129] caused by psychiatric disorder may lead to life-threatening hyponatremia and delirium. Again, psychosocial factors such as bereavement and relocation as sole causes of delirium are rare.[130] "Intensive care delirium"[131] is very difficult to assess because of the absence of controls and the serious illnesses concerned. An unusual case of delirium in an 88-year-old research subject apparently provoked by a battery of psychological tests prior to a drug trial ("the endless inquiry," as she later called it) has been reported.[132]

The Outcome of Delirium

Transient delirious episodes

Brief delirious episodes may herald the onset of frank dementia. Baker and colleagues[133] found that 25 percent of 122 patients with clinically diagnosed Alzheimer's disease had had a delirious episode within the 2 years prior to its presumed onset.

Full delirium

Lipowski[3] suggested in 1990 that although patients with delirium do not always recover, full recovery is the most common outcome. However, there is growing evidence that full and permanent recovery from delirium may not occur with the great frequency that we have previously supposed. In a study of 168 geriatric patients with delirium followed for 12 months, only 52 percent had made a complete recovery.[30] In a meta-analysis of outcome of delirium in elderly patients, it was estimated that 55 percent improved within a month; however, at 6 months 43 percent were in institutions. However, methodologic problems in all the studies were considerable; no study met all inclusion criteria.[134] Those elderly patients with delirium during admission for hip fractures remained significantly more disabled at 6 months than those without.[135] Follow-up, over 4 years, of 70 delirious elderly psychiatric patients revealed declining cognition and ADL functioning.[136] Francis and Kapoor[137] found that only 11 of 50 delirious elderly patients were at home after 2 years, and many of them were cognitively impaired. Levkoff et al.[35] concluded from their follow-up of 91 elderly patients with delirium at 6 months, when only 18 percent had resolution of all new symptoms, that "delirium may be substantially less transient than currently believed." One explanation for the difference in prognosis between these more recent studies and those reported before 1990 is changing demography; severe delirium can be caused by trivial illness in the demented, of whom there are ever-increasing numbers. These cases may be increasingly outnumbering cases of severe delirium, with arguably a better long-term prognosis, caused by critical illness in cognitively intact elderly patients. The latter may not carry with them the cognitive prognosis of an underlying dementing illness. In those patients in whom improvement does occur, it frequently lags behind resolution of the underlying physical condition—for example, in recovery from lithium toxicity.[138]

Death remains, however, a relatively frequent outcome of delirium in the elderly. Rabins and Folstein's[139] important study of mortality at 1 year of demented and delirious patients confirms the excess risk for the latter, and validated the distinction; this is the only study yet published to validate the syndrome against an independent criterion. Two studies have linked the excess mortality of delirium in the elderly to the severity of the underlying physical illness rather than the delirium itself,[25,140] which may weaken this method of validation. Self-harm and even suicide during hyperactive delirium is a possibility that must be considered and guarded against.[141]

There are occasional reports of "chronic" delirium, for example after stroke,[142] but it now seems likely that these would be better regarded as examples of Lewy body dementia.

Practical Aspects of Delirium in the Elderly

Phenomenology

Cardinal features of most common presentations

Cognitive decrement from the pre-existing level always occurs. There is decrement also in conscious level ("clouding", drowsiness, sleep/wake cycle disturbance), and in attention and concentration, (which is often confined to the immediate space around the patient and/or cannot be controlled by the patient). Decrement also occurs in orientation in time and place, and in short- and long-term memory. Clarity of thought is often impaired, with loosening of associations; delusions (fixed abnormal beliefs) are usually transient, often taking the form of being an impotent witness to unspeakable or terrifying events. Perceptual changes occur, particularly in the visual or tactile rather than other sense modalities. Illusions and hallucinations, particularly of small creeping things, shimmering water, or fluids, are common; or example, a patient may spend all night standing on a chair in the kitchen thinking that it is flooded. Visual hallucinations and illusions are most prominent in those with poor eyesight, and, together with tactile hallucinations, may lead to secondary delusions of infestation.[143] Mood changes may be the most prominent feature, with anxiety (even terror), perplexity, anger, or outrage. Depressed mood and tearfulness may alert physicians to the delirium. Movement is usually retarded (late) and slow; overactivity and agitation are slightly less common than hypoactivity,[144] but may lead to accusations by staff of "aggression," and being "uncooperative," especially where there is shouting, removal of drips, etc. Plucking at clothes, bedclothes, at the floor (perhaps in response to illusions), and at the air (in response to hallucinations) has been observed from ancient times. "Occupational delirium" may occur, with inappropriate motor acts related to habitual activity. Incontinence may occur de novo,[145] or worsen if the patient was already demented.

The central features of delirium are relatively abrupt onset of decrement (over days or hours see below), fluctuation of any or all abnormalities from minute to minute or hour to hour (usually worse in the evening or night), altered thinking, and altered consciousness.

Other less common features of delirium

Sleepwalking, movement disorder,[146] autoscopy (seeing a replica of oneself, "Doppelganger") and Lilliputian hallucinations have been reported. Delirium may be a factor in crescendo pain in cancer.[147]

Mode of onset

Delirium may present initially with brief episodes of nocturnal anxiety, disorientation, or visual phenomena that wax and wane for several nights, with normality during the day, before the full-blown picture emerges. For a few days before the onset of delirium, patients have reported a prodromos, with restlessness, difficulty thinking clearly, sensory hypersensitivity, insomnia, daytime somnolence, and vivid dreams.[148] Usually, however, the mode of onset is abrupt, over 24 hours.

Duration and course

Classically, the syndrome abates within a few days of onset, but, as discussed above, there is a lag between recovery from the underlying illness and recovery from the delirium. Chronic, subacute delirious states occur, which may take weeks to resolve.

Immediate sequelae of delirium

Patients may have a retrograde amnesia for the delirious episode, but it may occasionally leave persistent delusions.[149] Delirium may be regarded in the same way as incidents of awareness during anesthesia: post-traumatic stress disorder or depression may succeed it, despite amnesia, after recovery. Mackenzie and Popkin[150] suggest that careful follow-up explanation may be beneficial.

Recognition and Screening: How to Miss Delirium

The following steps will guarantee that the delirium syndrome is missed in an elderly patient. First, keep any talk with patients to a minimum, and especially do not assess cognitive function. If they are crying, start an antidepressant, or if they are noisy or disturbed a benzodiazepine. Second, do not take a history of cognitive or ADL decline from a relative or other informant: assume that any problems are long-standing. Third, do not take a medication or alcohol[151] history. Fourth, ensure that medical and nursing staff do not talk to each other. Doctors and nurses together have shown reasonable accuracy in recognizing the syndrome, but not separately.[152] Finally, ensure that no nurse is ever on duty in the same ward long enough to note the fluctuation in the patient, and that handover arrangements are sufficiently casual for this not to happen.

Differential Diagnosis of the Syndrome

Dementia

Delirium can occur without pre-existing dementia, in which case it may resolve completely or progress to dementia, or, in geriatric and psychogeriatric practice, delirium often may occur in established dementia. These relationships produce difficulties for the usual textbook tables distinguishing the two states. For instance, vascular dementias may have an abrupt onset with the first stroke, and may also be associated with perceptual abnormalities. Lewy Body dementia fluctuates and visual hallucinations are common. Sleep/wake cycle disturbance occurs in advanced dementia. Nevertheless, the distinction is critical, because the search for a remediable cause for delirium is much more likely to be successful than for dementia.[153] The cardinal features of fluctuation and altered consciousness should always lead to the working hypothesis of delirium.

Depressive illness

As discussed above, a purely "functional" psychiatric disorder such as depression is a rare cause of a full delirium syndrome. It appears that because clinicians expect delirious older patients to demonstrate all the features of the classic "typhoid state" seen in younger patients,[154] the hypoactive patient with mood disturbance is likely to be regarded as depressed. Depressive disorder may be accompanied by subtle cognitive changes, but the severe problems shown in delirium are highly unusual. Visual phenomena are very rare in depression, as is thought disorder, clouding of consciousness, and incontinence.[155] A cognitive assessment, a brief history from an informant, and nursing observations are all that are usually required to distinguish the two.

Delusional disorders and acute schizophrenia

In these conditions the delusions are fixed, and hallucinations rarely visual. In young, very acute schizophrenic patients clouding of consciousness may occur, but this is very rare in old age. There may, however, be cultural differences in this relationship with age, and, as discussed above, failure to discover attentional deficits and impairment of consciousness in the older paranoid patient may well be due to failure to seek them out with any great enthusiasm.

Charles Bonnet syndrome

Charles Bonnet syndrome is characterized by the presence of complex, repetitive, visual hallucinations without cognitive impairment, delusional elaboration, or hallucinations in other modalities.[156] The mood may be one of exasperation, but patients with this syndrome may tolerate the experiences (e.g., a full circus in the living room) with extraordinary sangfroid. Its origin and prognosis is unclear. A cognitive state examination should clarify the diagnosis.

Peduncular hallucinosis

Complex visual hallucinations also occur in lesions of the cerebral peduncles and midbrain.[157] However, they appear to occur in clear consciousness, and almost all have localizing neurologic signs.

Neuroleptic malignant syndrome

Neuroleptic malignant syndrome has many features of a delirium in the elderly, and, combined with the pyrexia, seems highly likely to provoke investigation for infection.[158] A careful drug history will be helpful, although the syndrome can develop after long exposure. A high creatinine phosphokinase (CPK) level is strongly suggestive of this syndrome. The use of antipsychotics to manage a delirium-like state caused by this condition may prove fatal.

Differential Diagnosis of the Causes of Delirium

The search for a physical illness or toxic drug causing delirium in the elderly can be as cursory or extensive as for any other condition. Certain practical steps, however, should be considered mandatory.

Taking the history

A history should be attempted from the patient, and **always** from an informant. The former may need to be taken in short bursts. The latter may reveal pre-existing, established cognitive impairment, the course of the present decrement, its fluctuation, and the temporal relationship between the development of the delirium and any symptoms of causative physical illness or exposure to medications or injury. Central to the questioning is the assessment of change. A medication history, including over-the-counter and herbal remedies, is best gathered in conjunction with the primary care physician, preferably with the actual medication bottles in hand. Alcohol consumption should be firmly but tactfully established. A history of relevant life events such as foreign travel, moving house, bereavement, or changes in family relationships may help in the differential diagnosis.

Examination

A physical examination, which in the agitated patient may have to be done piecemeal, should include, if possible, a rectal examination because there is anecdotal evidence of an association of constipation with delirium in dementia. A simple assessment of cognitive functioning such as the abbreviated mental test score[159] or the MMSE[160] will identify any cognitive impairment and will serve as a baseline for future reference. Consciousness can be assessed by a test of attention and concentration, in reverse order of ease, asking the patient to recount the months of the year backward or the days of the week backward. Even patients with well-established dementia, without delirium, can do these tasks.

Investigations

Basic protocol A basic protocol should include a full blood count, electrolytes, random blood sugar, and urine microbiology. If this is not possible (e.g., in the patient's home), a reagent strip for urinalysis may show phosphate levels that predict infection.[161] A chest x-ray, erythrocyte sedimentation rate, thyroid function tests, and an electroencephalogram should be carried out routinely. Drug levels should be carried out if the patient is on digoxin, anticonvulsants, lithium, or certain tricyclic antidepressants.

Extended protocol An extended protocol might include vitamin B_{12}, folate, magnesium, calcium, and, if the patient has been exposed to neuroleptics, CPK estimation. Blood culture may be necessary. A dexamethasone suppression test should be considered. An EEG may help confirm the delirium,[162] and, rarely, suggest a cause. CT scan may reveal stroke, cortical atrophy, or normal pressure hydrocephalus. Rarely, MRI may be needed to clarify CT abnormalities. Lumbar puncture without specific indication is not recommended in delirium.[163] A physostigmine test may be helpful if an anticholinergic cause is suspected.[164]

Management of the Delirious Patient

Management consists of managing the underlying physical illness, once found, and managing the distressing mental state, and its consequences.

General management

There is now evidence that long advocated general measures have a beneficial effect on delirium.[165] These include maintaining adequate food and fluid intake, maintaining a balance between over- and understimulation, minimizing the unfamiliarity of the environment, particularly staff, minimizing iatrogenic complications, and minimizing disorientation. To this should be added careful support and guidance for the patient's family. Because many of these general factors are easiest to sustain at home, domiciliary management is preferred if adequate support can be arranged, and the underlying physical illness can be both diagnosed and treated without recourse to hospital facilities.

Pharmacologic management

Not all patients with delirium require pharmacologic treatment, but it is likely that their levels of distress are likely to be high even when hypoactive,[166] and the distress that the agitated delirious patient can cause their visitors, other patients, and staff needs to be taken into account. In the United Kingdom, a traditional approach has been to use thioridazine (10 to 200 mg daily in divided doses) in mild delirium in the elderly, although, as discussed above, this is theoretically questionable as it is the most anticholinergic of all the major tranquilizers. Haloperidol is one of the least anticholinergic, and is usually thus recommended (2 to 30 mg daily in divided doses), although it may be fatal in neuroleptic malignant syndrome, and produces extrapyramidal effects in a high proportion of patients. Both these medications may cause cardiac arrhythmia. Benzodiazepines are usually avoided in the management of delirium in the elderly, because withdrawal states are often associated with the syndrome. However, younger patients with severe delirium requiring IV psychotropics apparently have fewer extrapyramidal side effects from a combination of butyrophenone and benzodiazepine than butyrophenone alone.[167] Other approaches mentioned in the literature, often in connection with younger patients, are a combination of carbamazepine and buspirone[168] continuous IV butyrophenone infusion[169] and continuous subcutaneous midazolam.[170] There is a suggestion that IV or slow-release physostigmine may be useful in benzodiazepine withdrawal delirium,[171] but toxicity may restrict its use in the elderly. Finally, psychostimulants have been suggested for hypoactive delirium.[172]

Electroconvulsive therapy

ECT is used occasionally in severe delirium; its use in Nordic countries has not declined over the years.[173] The use of ECT in dementia is a controversial issue; as delirium may often occur in the setting of structural brain disease, it seems that ECT should be reserved for extreme cases of delirium with no underlying dementia or central nervous system disorder.

Ethical and Legal Aspects of Delirium

The ethical and legal aspects of delirium are occasionally problematic. In the United Kingdom, the duty of care under common law obliges action in serious emergency, and delirium is usually managed, in the face of the incompetence of the patient, within this rubric.[174] Nursing and medical staff may need support in carrying out treatment procedures without the explicit consent of the patient, and the involvement of relatives is crucial in this. Occasionally, disturbed behavior is of a nature or degree that requires formal psychiatric inpatient treatment. A delirium is a mental disorder within the meaning of the Mental Health Act 1993, so that admissions can be formally arranged against the patient's apparent wishes. The benefits of this must be balanced against the disadvantages of stigmatization, and the problem of managing essentially medical illnesses in a psychiatric setting. It is technically possible in the United Kingdom to detain patients under the Mental Health Act in general medical wards; again, the advantages of this unusual step must be balanced against the administrative chaos produced by lack of familiarity with formal, legalistic procedures by often very busy medical and nursing staff. If admitting the delirious elderly patient from home in the United Kingdom difficult, an older piece of legislation is sometimes used: Section 47 of the National Assistance Act. However, it does not permit treatment, and has few legal safeguards, is cumbersome to arrange, and should not be used. Increasingly, advanced directives are being prepared by older people who may develop delirium at some stage in the future. Medical and nursing staff may find themselves in difficulty if it can be shown that they ignored such directives, although their legal status is, as yet, unclear in the United Kingdom.

Delirium in Depression

Interestingly, there have been reports that tricyclic- and anticholinergic-induced delirious states may, upon clearing, leave the depressive syndrome markedly improved, and the author has seen this at least once.[175]

Delirium Tremens in the Elderly

Delirium following alcohol withdrawal should always be suspected in cases developing a few days after admission. There is a dearth of reports in the literature on this problem in the elderly, and management is the same as for younger patient with alcohol dependence.

Conclusions

Major challenges are to be faced in relation to both the theoretical and practical aspects of delirium. The syndrome's characteristics need validating against criteria other than convention, especially in discriminating the disorder from dementia.[6] The validated syndrome's relationship to putative causes on the one hand, and underlying mechanisms on the other needs elucidation, using standardized assessments. Protocols for routine investigation need to be established on sound epidemiologic and cost-benefit principles. There need to be more treatment trials in the elderly. In the meantime, recognition and management of delirium in older patients needs attention; there is evidence that recognition of delirium can be improved by a simple training program for medical and nursing staff.[176] In the United Kingdom perhaps, the poor knowledge of psychiatric conditions among medical staff[177] will improve, especially now that the General Medical Council has changed the emphasis of undergraduate medical education toward development of the skills, knowledge, and attitudes necessary for trainees to function as house physicians.

References

1. Saravay SM, Lavin M: Psychiatric comorbidity and length of stay in the general hospital. A critical review of outcome studies. Psychosomatics 1994;35:233–252
2. McCartney JR, Palmateer LM: Assessment of cognitive deficit in geriatric patients. A study of physician behavior. J Am Geriatr Soc 1985;33:467–471
3. Lipowski Z: Delirium: Acute Confusional States. Oxford University Press, New York, 1990
4. World Health Organization: The ICD-10 Classification of Mental and Behavioural Disorders. World Health Organization, Geneva, 1992
5. American Psychiatric Association: Diagnostic and Statistical Manual of Mental Disorders. 3rd Ed., revised. American Psychiatric Association, Washington, DC 1987
6. Macdonald AJD, Treloar A: Delirium and dementia: are they distinct? J Am Geriatr Soc 1997;44:1001–1002
7. Spitzer RL, First MB, Williams JB et al: Now is the time to retire the term "organic mental disorders." Am J Psychiatry 1992;149:240–244
8. Perry RH, Irving D, Blessed G et al: Senile dementia of Lewy body type. A clinically and neuropathologically distinct form of Lewy body dementia in the elderly. J Neurol Sci 1990;95: 119–139
9. Bliwise DL, Carroll JS, Lee KA et al: Sleep and "sundowning" in nursing home patients with dementia. Psychiatry Res 1993; 48:277–292
10. Nelson A, Fogel BS, Faust D: Bedside cognitive screening instruments. A critical assessment. J Nervous Mental Dis 1986;174:73–83
11. Trzepacz PT, Dew MA: Further analyses of the Delirium Rating Scale. Gen Hosp Psychiatry 1995;17:75–79
12. Inouye SK, van Dyck CH, Alessi CA et al: Clarifying confusion: the confusion assessment method. A new method for detection of delirium. Ann Intern Med 1990;113:941–948
13. Pompei P, Foreman M, Cassel CK et al: Detecting delirium among hospitalized older patients. Arch Intern Med 1995;155: 301–307
14. Albert MS, Levkoff SE, Reilly C et al: The delirium symptom interview: an interview for the detection of delirium symptoms in hospitalized patients. J Geriatr Psychiatry Neurol 1992;5: 14–21
15. Williams MA: Delirium/acute confusional states: evaluation devices in nursing. Int Psychogeriatr 1991;3:301–308
16. Liptzin B, Levkoff SE, Cleary PD et al: An empirical study of diagnostic criteria for delirium. Am J Psychiatry 1991;148: 454–457
17. Sands LP, Katz IR, Doyle S: Detecting subclinical change in cognitive functioning in older adults: II. Initial validation of the method. Am J Geriatr Psychiatry 1993;1:275–287
18. Fogel BS: The high sensitivity cognitive screen. Special Issue: Delirium advances in research and clinical practice. Int Psychogeriatr 1991;3:273–288
19. Johnson JC, Kersc NM, Gottlieb G et al: Prospective versus retrospective methods of identifying patients with delirium. J Am Geriatr Soc 1992;40:316–339
20. Jorm AF: A short form of the Informant Questionnaire on Cognitive Decline in the Elderly (IQCODE): development and cross-validation. Psychol Med 1994;24:145–153
21. Kojima T, Shimazono Y, Ichise K et al: Eye movement as an indicator of brain function. Folia Psychiatrica Neurol Jap 1981;35:425–435
22. O'Keeffe, ST: Rating the severity of delirium: The Delirium Assessment Scale. Int J Geriatr Psychiatry 1994;9:551–556
23. Wettstein RM: The mini-mental state in mild cognitive dysfunction. Am J Psychiatry 1986;143:128
24. Parmelee PA, Thuras PD, Katz IR, Lawton MP: Validation Of the Cumulative Illness Rating Scale in a geriatric residential population. J Am Geriatr Soc 1995;43:130–137
25. Francis J, Martin D, Kapoor WN: A prospective study of delirium in hospitalized elderly. JAMA 1990;263:1097–1101
26. Folstein MF, Bassett SS, Romanoski AJ, Nestadt G: The epidemiology of delirium in the community: the Eastern Baltimore Mental Health Survey. Int Psychogeriatr 1991;3:169–176
27. Ramsay R, Wright P, Katz A et al: The detection of psychiatric morbidity and its effects on outcome in acute elderly medical admissions. Int J Geriatr Psychiatry 1991;6:861–866
28. Jitapunkul S, Pillay I, Ebrahim S: Delirium in newly admitted elderly patients: a prospective study. Q J Med 1992;83: 307–314

29. Kolbeinsson H, Jonsson A: Delirium and dementia in acute medical admissions of elderly patients in Iceland. Acta Psychiatr Scand 1993;87:123–127

30. Rockwood K: The occurrence and duration of symptoms in elderly patients with delirium. J Gerontol 1993;48: M162–M166

31. Pompei P, Foreman M, Rudberg MA et al: Delirium in hospitalized older persons: outcomes and predictors. J Am Geriatr Soc 1994;42:809–815

32. Fisher BW, Flowerdew G: A simple model for predicting postoperative delirium in older patients undergoing elective orthopedic surgery. J Am Geriatr Soc 1995;43:175–178

33. Naughton BJ, Moran MB, Kadah II et al: Delirium and other cognitive impairment in older adults in an emergency department. Ann Emerg Med 1995;25:751–755

34. Schor JD, Levkoff SE, Lipsitz LA et al: Risk factors for delirium in hospitalized elderly. JAMA 1992;267:827–831

35. Levokoff SE, Evans DA, Liptzin B et al: Delirium. The occurrence and persistence of symptoms among elderly hospitalized patients. Arch Intern Med 1992;152:334–340

36. Inouye SK, Viscoli CM, Horwitz RI et al: A predictive model for delirium in hospitalized elderly medical patients based on admission characteristics. Ann Intern Med 1993;119: 474–481

37. Dyer CB, Ashton CM, Teasdale TA: Postoperative delirium. A review of 80 primary data-collection studies. Arch Intern Med 1995;155:461–465

38. Ni Chonchubhair A, Valacio R, Kelly J, O'Keefe S: Use of the abbreviated mental test to detect postoperative delirium in elderly people. Br J Anaesth 1995;75:481–482

39. Levkoff SE, Safran C, Clearly PD et al: Identification of factors associated with the diagnosis of delirium in elderly hospitalized patients. J Am Geriatr Soc 1988;36:1099–1104

40. Windsor AC: Bacteraemia in a geriatric unit. Gerontology 1983;29:125–130

41. Koponen H, Stenback U, Mattila E et al: Delirium among elderly persons admitted to a psychiatric hospital: clinical course during the acute stage and one-year follow-up. Acta Psychiatr Scand 1989;79:579–585

42. Marcantonio ER, Goldman L, Mangione CM et al: A clinical prediction rule for delirium after elective noncardiac surgery. JAMA 1994;271:134–139

43. Golden WE, Lavender RC, Metzer WS: Acute postoperative confusion and hallucinations in Parkinson disease. Ann Intern Med 1989;111:218–222

44. Simpson CJ, Kellett JM: The relationship between pre-operative anxiety and post-operative delirium. J Psychosom Res 1987;31:491–497

45. Cryns AG, Gorey KM, Goldstein MZ: Effects of surgery on the mental status of older persons. A meta-analytic review. J Geriatr Psychiatry Neurol 1990;3:184–191

46. Engel GL, Romano J: Delirium: a syndrome of cerebral insufficiency. J Chronic Dis 1959;9:260–277

47. Katz IR, Mossey J, Sussman N et al: Bedside clinical and electrophysiological assessment: assessment of change in vulnerable patients. Int Psychogeriatr 1991;3:289–300

48. Wells CE: Transient ictal psychosis. Arch Gen Psychiatry 1975;32:1201–1203

49. van Sweden B, Mellerio F: Toxic ictal delirium. Biol Psychiatry 1989;25:449–458

50. O'Keeffe ST, Devlin JG: Delirium and the dexamethasone suppression test in the elderly. Neuropsychobiology 1994;30: 153–156

51. Hoffman SL, Punjabi NH, Kumala S et al: Reduction of mortality in chloramphenicol-treated severe typhoid fever by high-dose dexamethasone. N Engl J Med 1984;310:82–88

52. Fassbender K, Schmidt R, Mossner R et al: Pattern of activation of the hypothalamic-pituitary-adrenal axis in acute stroke. Relation to acute confusional state, extent of brain damage, and clinical outcome. Stroke 1994;25:1105–1108

53. Tune L, Carr S, Cooper T et al: Association of anticholinergic activity of prescribed medications with postoperative delirium. J Neuropsychiatry Clin Neurosci 1993;5:208–210

54. Marcantonio E, Juarez G, Goldman L et al: The relationship of postoperative delirium with psychoactive medications. JAMA 1994;272:1518–1522

55. Mach JR Jr, Dysken MW, Kuskowski M et al: Serum anticholinergic activity in hospitalized older person with delirium: a preliminary study. J Am Geriatr Soc 1995;43:491–495

56. Fisher CM: Visual hallucinations on eye closure associated with atropine toxicity. A neurological analysis and comparison with other visual hallucinations. Can J Neurol Sci 1991;18: 18–27

57. Miller PS, Richardson JS, Jyu CA et al: Association of low serum anticholinergic levels and cognitive impairment in elderly presurgical patients. Am J Psychiatry 1988;145: 342–345

58. Tune L, Carr S, Hoag E, Cooper T: Anticholinergic effects of drugs commonly prescribed for the elderly: potential means for assessing risk of delirium. Am J Psychiatry 1992;149: 1393–1394

59. Trzepacz PT, Leavitt M, Ciongoli K: An animal model for delirium. Psychosomatics 1992;33:404–415

60. Aakerlund LP, Rosenberg J: Postoperative delirium: treatment with supplementary oxygen. Br J Anaesth 1994;72:286–290

61. Hoffman WE, Albrecht RF, Miletich DJ et al: Cerebrovascular and cerebral metabolic effects of physostigmine, midazolam, and a benzodiazepine antagonist. Anesth Analg 1986;65: 639–644

62. Mesulam MM, Waxman SG, Geschwind N, Sabin TD: Acute confusional states with right middle cerebral artery infarctions. J Neurol Neurosurg Psychiatry 1976;39:84–89

63. Sirois F: Psychosis as a mode of exitus in a cancer patient. J Palliat Care 1993;9:16–18

64. Ross CA, Peyser CE, Shapiro I, Folstein MF: Delirium: phenomenologic and etiologic subtypes. Int Psychogeriatr 1991;3: 135–147

65. Hemmingsen R, Vorstrup S, Clemmesen L et al: Cerebral blood flow during delirium tremens and related clinical states studied with Xenon-133 inhalation tomography. Am J Psychiatry 1988;145:1384–1390

66. Brown G, Warren M, Williams JE et al: Cranial computed

tomography of elderly patients: an evaluation of its use in acute neurological presentations. Age Ageing 1993;22:240–243

67. Trzepacz PT: The neuropathogenesis of delirium. A need to focus our research. Psychosomatics 1994;35:374–391
68. Leuchter AF, Jacobson SA: Quantitative measurement of brain electrical activity in delirium. Int Psychogeriatr 1991;3: 231–247
69. Jacobson SA, Leuchter AF, Walter DO: Conventional and quantitative EEG in the diagnosis of delirium among the elderly. J Neurol Neurosurg Psychiatry 1993;56:153–158
70. Winn RE, Bower JH, Richards JF: Acute toxic delirium. Neurotoxicity of intrathecal administration of amphotericin B. Arch Intern Med 1979;139:706–707
71. Tune LE, Bylsma FW, Hilt DC: Anticholinergic delirium caused by topical homatropine ophthalmologic solution: confirmation by anticholinergic radioreceptor assay in two cases. J Neuropsychiatry Clin Neurosci 1992;4:195–197
72. Steinberg RB, Gilman DE, Johnson F III: Acute toxic delirium in a patient using transdermal fentanyl. Anesth Analg 1992; 75:1014–1016
73. Rozzini R, Inzoli M, Trabucchi M: Delirium from transdermal scopolamine in an elderly woman. JAMA 1988;260:478
74. Stoudemire A, Baker N, Thompson TL II: Delirium induced by topical application of podophyllin: a case report. Am J Psychiatry 1981;138:1505–1506
75. Kutcher SP, Shulman KI: Desipramine-induced delirium at "subtherapeutic" concentrations: a case report. Can J Psychiatry 1985;30:368–369
76. Meyers BS, Mei-Tal V: Psychiatric reactions during tricyclic treatment of the elderly reconsidered. J Clin Psychopharmacol 1983;3:2–6
77. Zipursky RB, Baker RW, Zimmer B: Alprazolam withdrawal delirium unresponsive to diazepam: case report. J Clin Psychiatry 1985;46:344–345
78. Cowen PJ, Nutt DJ: Abstinence symptoms after withdrawal of tranquillising drugs: is there a common neurochemical mechanism?. Lancet 1982;2:360–362
79. Minichetti J, Milles M: Hallucination and delirium reaction to intravenous diazepam administration: case report. Anesth Prog 1982;29:144–146
80. Rothschild AJ: Disinhibition, amnestic reactions, and other adverse reactions secondary to triazolam: a review of the literature. J Clin Psychiatry 1992;53(suppl):69–79
81. Brown AS, Rosen J: Lithium-induced delirium with therapeutic serum lithium levels: a case report. J Geriatr Psychiatry Neurol 1992;5:53–55
82. Grubb BP: Digitalis delirium in an elderly woman. Postgrad Med 1987;81:329–330
83. Eisenman DP, McKegney FP: Delirium at therapeutic serum concentrations of digoxin and quinidine. Psychosomatics 1994;35:91–93
84. Boutros N, Keck BP: Delirium following influenza vaccination. Am J Psychiatry 1993;150:1899
85. Cantu TG, Korek JS: Central nervous system reactions to histamine-2 receptor blockers. Ann Intern Med 1991;114: 1027–1034
86. Jenike MA, Levy JC: Physostigmine reversal of cimetidine-induced delirium and agitation. J Clin Psychopharmacol 1983; 3:43–44
87. Steele TE, Morton was Jr: Salicylate-induced delirium. Psychosomatics 1986;27:455–456
88. Allison N, Shantz I: Delirium related to tiaprofenic acid. Can Med Assoc J 1987;137:1022–1023
89. Atkinson L, Ince P, Smith NM, Taylor R: Toxic reaction to inhaled paint fumes. Postgrad Med J 1989;65:559–561
90. Levy AB: Delirium induced by inhalation of typewriter correction fluid. Psychosomatics 1986;27:665–666
91. Trabattoni G, Visintini D, Terzano GM, Lechi A: Accidental poisoning with deadly nightshade berries: a case report. Hum Toxicol 1984;3:513–516
92. Saddique A, Peterson CD: Thallium poisoning: a review. Vet Hum Toxicol 1983;25:16–22
93. Blackwood GW: Severe psychological disturbance resulting from abuse of nasal decongestants. Scott Med J 1982;27: 175–176
94. Allen MD, Greenblatt DJ, Noel BJ: Self-poisoning with over-the-counter hypnotics. Clin Toxicol 1979;15:151–158
95. Figiel GS, Hassen MA, Zorumski C et al: ECT-induced delirium in depressed patients with Parkinson's disease. J Neuropsychiatry Clin Neurosci 1991;3:405–411
96. Figiel GS, Botteron K, Zorumski CF et al: The treatment of late age onset psychoses with electroconvulsive therapy. Int J Geriatr Psychiatry 1992;7:183–189
97. Martin M, Figiel G, Mattingly G et al: ECT-induced interictal delirium in patients with a history of a CVA. J Geriatr Psychiatry Neurol 1992;5:149–155
98. May SR, Ehleben CM, DeClement FA: Delirium in burn patients isolated in a plenum laminar air flow ventilation unit. Burns 1984;10:331–338
99. Manepalli J, Grossberg GT, Mueller C: Prevalence of delirium and urinary tract infection in a psychogeriatric unit. J Geriatr Psychiatry Neurol 1990;3:198–202
100. Blackburn T, Dunn M: Cystocerebral syndrome. Acute urinary retention presenting as confusion in elderly patients. Arch Intern Med 1990;150:2577–2578
101. Koizumi J, Shiraishi H, Ofuku K, Suzuki T: Duration of delirium shortened by the correction of electrolyte imbalance. Jp J Psychiatry Neurol 1988;42:81–88
102. Fraser CL, Arieff AI: Nervous system complications in uremia. Ann Intern Med 1988;109:143–153
103. Seymour DG, Henschke PJ, Cape RD, Campbell AJ: Acute confusional states and dementia in the elderly: the role of dehydration/volume depletion, physical illness and age. Age Ageing 1980;9:137–146
104. Galland L: Magnesium and inflammatory bowel disease. Magnesium 1988;7:78–83
105. Benbadis SR, Sila CA, Cristea RL: Mental status changes and stroke. J Gen Intern Med 1994;9:485–487
106. Dunne JW, Leedman PJ, Edis RH: Inobvious stroke: a cause of delirium and dementia. Aust N Z J Med 1986;16:771–778

107. Reding MJ, Gardner C, Hainline B, Devinsky O: Neuropsychiatric problems interfering with inpatient stroke rehabilitation. J Neurol Rehabil 1993;7:1–7

108. Bogousslavsky J, Regli F: Anterior cerebral artery territory infarction in the Lausanne Stroke Registry. Clinical and etiologic patterns. Arch Neurol 1990;47:144–150

109. Devinsky O, Bear D, Volpe BT: Confusional states following posterior cerebral artery infarction. Arch Neurol 1988;45: 160–163

110. Mehler MF: The rostral basilar artery syndrome: diagnosis, etiology, prognosis. Neurology 1989;39:9–16

111. Black DW: Mental changes resulting from subdural haematoma. Br J Psychiatry 1984;145:200–203

112. Velasco J, Head M, Farlin E, Lippmann S: Unsuspected subdural hematoma as a differential diagnosis in elderly patients. South Med J 1995;88:977–979

113. Balter RA, Fricchione G, Sterman AB: Clinical presentation of multi-infarct delirium. Psychosomatics 1986;27:461–462

114. Galbraith S: Head injuries in the elderly. BMJ 1987;6568: 325

116. Gambert SR, Escher JE: Atypical presentation of endocrine disorders in the elderly. Geriatrics 1988;43:69–71, 76–78

117. Fang VS, Jaspan JB: Delirium and neuromuscular symptoms in an elderly man with isolated corticotroph-deficiency syndrome completely reversed with glucocorticoid replacement. J Clin Endocrinol Metab 1989;69:1073–1077

118. Bayer AJ, Chadha JS, Farag RR, Pathy MS: Changing presentation of myocardial infarction with increasing old age. J Am Geriatr Soc 1986;34:263–266

119. Fearon MP, LaPalio L: Complete heart block presenting as intermittent delirium: case report and review of the literature on cardiac disease in the elderly. J Am Geriatr Soc 1992;40: 507–509

120. Rockwood K, Dobbs AR, Rule BG et al: The impact of pacemaker implantation on cognitive functioning in elderly patients. J Am Geriatr Soc 1992;40:142–146

121. O'Keeffe ST, Tormey WP, Glasgow R, Lavan JN: Thiamine deficiency in hospitalized elderly patients. Gerontology 1994; 40:18–24

122. Dickson LR: Hypoalbuminemia in delirium. Psychosomatics 1991;32:317–323

123. Hector M, Burton JR: What are the psychiatric manifestations of vitamin B12 deficiency? J Am Geriatr Soc 1988;36: 1105–1112

124. Godfrey JW, Roberts MA, Caird FI: Epileptic seizures in the elderly: II. Diagnostic problems. Age Ageing 1982;11:29–34

125. Laudadio S, Crisci M, de Carolis P et al: Acute psychosis and epileptic seizures as the presenting symptom of late-onset epilepsy. Acta Neurol Scand 1994;89:77–79

126. Primavera A, Giberti L, Scotto P, Cocito L: Nonconvulsive status epilepticus as a cause of confusion in later life: a report of 5 cases. Neuropsychobiology 1994;30:148–152

127. Newman NJ, Bell IR, McKee AC: Paraneoplastic limbic encephalitis: neuropsychiatric presentation. Biol Psychiatry 1990;27:529–542

128. Swartz MS, Henschen GM, Cavenar JO Jr, Hammett EB: A case of intermittent delirious mania. Am J Psychiatry 1982; 139:1357–1358

129. Cosgray RE, Hanna V, Davidhizar RE, Smith J: The water-intoxicated patient. Arch Psychiatr Nurs 1990;4:308–312

130. Rabins PV: Psychosocial and management aspects of delirium. Int Psychogeriatr 1991;3:319–324

131. Wilson LM: Intensive care delirium. The effect of outside deprivation in a windowless unit. Arch Intern Med 1972;130: 225–226

132. Rozzini R, Zanetti O, Trabucchi M: Delirium induced by neuropsychological tests. J Am Geriatr Soc 1989;37:666

133. Baker FM, Kokmen E, Chandra V, Schoenberg BS: Psychiatric symptoms in cases of clinically diagnosed Alzheimer's disease. J Geriatr Psychiatry Neurol 1991;4:71–78

134. Cole MG, Primeau FJ: Prognosis of delirium in elderly hospital patients. Can Med Assoc J 1993;149:41–46

135. Brannstrom B, Gustafson Y, Norberg JA, Winblad B: ADL performance and dependency on nursing care in patients with hip fractures and acute confusion in a task allocation care system. Scand J Caring Sci 1991;5:3–11

136. Koponen HJ, Riekkinen PJ: A prospective study of delirium in elderly patients admitted to a psychiatric hospital. Psychol Med 1993;23:103–109

137. Francis J, Kapoor WN: Prognosis after hospital discharge of older medical patients with delirium. J Am Geriatr Soc 1992; 40:601–606

138. DePaulo JR Jr, Folstein MF, Correa EI: The course of delirium due to lithium intoxication. J Clin Psychiatry 1982;43: 447–449

139. Rabins PV, Folstein MF: Delirium and dementia: diagnostic criteria and fatality rates. Br J Psychiatry 1982;140:149–153

140. van Hemert AM, van der Mast RC, Hengeveld MW, Vorstenbosch M: Excess mortality in general hospital patients with delirium: a 5-year follow-up of 519 patients seen in psychiatric consultation. J Psychosom Res 1994;38:339–346

141. Younger SC, Clark DC, Oehmig-Lindroth R, Stein RJ: Availability of knowledgeable informants for a psychological autopsy study of suicides committed by elderly people. J Am Geriatr Soc 1990;38:1169–1175

142. Mullally WJ, Ronthal M, Huff K, Geschwind N: Chronic confusional state. N J Med 1989;86:541–544

143. O'Keeffe ST: Delusions of infestation during delirium in a patient with restless legs syndrome. J Geriatr Psychiatry Neurol 1995;8:120–122

144. Liptzin B, Levkoff SE: An empirical study of delirium subtypes. Br J Psychiatry 1992;161:843–845

145. Rousseau P, Fuentevilla-Clifton A: Urinary incontinence in the aged, Part 1: patient evaluation. Geriatrics 1992;47: 22–26, 33–34

146. Reed SM, Wise MG, Timmerman I: Choreoathetosis: a sign of lithium toxicity. J Neuropsychiatry Clin Neurosci 1989;1: 57–60

147. Coyle N, Breitbart W, Weaver S, Portenoy R: Delirium as a contributing factor to "crescendo" pain: three case reports. J Pain Symptom Manage 1994;9:44–47

148. Levkoff SE, Liptzin B, Evans DA et al: Progression and resolution of delirium in elderly patients hospitalized for acute care. Gerontological Society of America Meetings (1991, San Francisco, California). Am J Geriatr Psychiatry 1994;2:230–238

149. Edmands MS: "Murder:" she said: a case of iatrogenic delirium. Issues Mental Health Nurs 1995;16:109–116

150. Mackenzie TB, Popkin MK: Stress response syndrome occurring after delirium. Am J Psychiatry 1980;137:1433–1435

151. Naik PC, Jones RG: Alcohol histories taken from elderly people on admission. BMJ 1994;308:248

152. Bowler C, Boyle A, Branford M et al: Detection of psychiatric disorders in elderly medical inpatients. Age Ageing 1994;23: 307–311

153. Draper B: Potentially reversible dementia: a review. Aust N Z J Psychiatry 1991;25:506–518

154. Verghese A: The "typhoid state" revisited. Am J Med 1985; 79:370–372

155. Berrios GE: Temporary urinary incontinence in the acute psychiatric patient without delirium or dementia. Br J Psychiatry 1986;149:224–227

156. Ball CJ: The vascular origins of the Charles Bonnet syndrome: four cases and a review of the pathogenic mechanisms. Int J Geriatr Psychiatry 1991;6:673–679

157. Serra Catafau J, Rubio F, Peres Serra J: Peduncular hallucinosis associated with posterior thalamic infarction. J Neurol 1992;239:89–90

158. Nicklason FN, Finucane PM, Pathy MJ, Sutton DA: Neuroleptic malignant syndrome: an unrecognized problem in elderly patients with psychiatric illness? Int J Geriatr Psychiatry 1991;6:171–175

159. Hodkinson HM: Evaluation of a mental test score for assessment of mental impairment in the elderly. Age Ageing 1972; 1:233–238

160. Folstein MF, Folstein SE, McHugh PR: Mini-mental state—a practical method for grading the cognitive state of patients for the clinician. J Psychiatric Res 1975;12:189–198

161. Evans PJ, Leaker BR, McNabb WR, Lewis RR: Accuracy of reagent strip testing for urinary tract infection in the elderly. J R Soc Med 1991;84:598–599

162. Zisook S, Braff DL: Delirium: recognition and management in the older patient. Geriatrics 1986;41:67–70

163. Warshaw G, Tanzer F: The effectiveness of lumbar puncture in the evaluation of delirium and fever in the hospitalized elderly. Arch Fam Med 1993;2:293–297

164. Brizer DA, Manning DW: Delirium induced by poisoning with anticholinergic agents. Am J Psychiatry 1982;139:1343–1344

165. Cole MG, Primeau FJ, Bailey RF et al: Systematic intervention for elderly inpatients with delirium: a randomized trial. Can Med Assoc J 1994;151:965–970

166. Platt MM, Breitbart W, Smith M et al: Efficacy of neuroleptics for hypoactive delirium. J Neuropsychiatry Clin Neurosci 1994;6:66–67

167. Menza MA, Murray GB, Holmes VF, Rafuls WA: Controlled study of extrapyramidal reactions in the management of delirious, medically ill patients: intravenous haloperidol versus intravenous haloperidol plus benzodiazepines. Heart Lung 1988; 17:238–241

168. Pourcher E, Filteau MJ, Bouchard RH, Baruch P: Efficacy of the combination of buspirone and carbamazepine in early posttraumatic delirium. Am J Psychiatry 1994;151:150–151

169. Frye MA, Coudreaut MF, Hakeman SM, Shah BG et al: Continuous droperidol infusion for management of agitated delirium in an intensive care unit. Psychosomatics 1995;36:301–305

170. Stiefel F, Fainsinger R, Bruera E: Acute confusional states in patients with advanced cancer. J Pain Symptom Manage 1992; 7:94–98

171. Blitt CD, Petty WC: Reversal of lorazepam delirium by physostigmine. Anesth Analg 1975;54:607–608

172. Stiefel F, Bruera E: Psychostimulants for hypoactive-hypoalert delirium? J Palliat Care 1991;7:25–26

173. Stromgren LS: Electroconvulsive therapy in the Nordic countries, 1977–1987. Acta Psychiatr Scand 1991;84:428–434

174. Fogel BS, Mills MJ, Landen JE: Legal aspects of the treatment of delirium. Hosp Commun Psychiatry 1986;37:154–158

175. Borchardt CM, Popkin MK: Delirium and the resolution of depression. J Clin Psychiatry 1987;48:373–375

176. Perez EL, Silverman M: Delirium: the often overlooked diagnosis. Int J Psychiatry Med 1984;14:181–189

177. Cohen-Cole SA, Bird J, Freeman A et al: An oral examination of the psychiatric knowledge of medical housestaff: assessment of needs and evaluation baseline. Gen Hosp Psychiatry 1982; 4:103–111

CHAPTER 49

Dementia: Basic Neurosciences

JANET E. CARTER
DECLAN M. McLOUGHLIN

The advent of DNA technology and its ready availability and applicability has revolutionized our ability to investigate the basic molecular biology of the nervous system and to unravel the DNA-encoded genetic information stored within the cell's nucleus in the form of genes. It is now possible experimentally to manipulate individual proteins and their DNA and, by applying these techniques, study a protein's structure, interactions, and function from the cellular to the animal model level. The explosion in molecular neuroscience in the final decades of the 20th century bears witness to the power of these new research tools and nowhere has this been more evident than in the study of neurodegeneration. This chapter focuses on the recent advances made in our understanding of the molecular pathology and genetics of the common primary neurodegenerative diseases that cause dementia and how these advances may lead to the development of rational therapies for these devastating disorders.

Alzheimer's Disease

β-Amyloid Peptide, Amyloid Formation, and Neuritic Plaques

Alzheimer's disease (AD) is characterized neuropathologically by widespread extracellular amyloid deposition, intraneuronal neurofibrillary tangle (NFT) formation, reactive gliosis, astrocytosis, neuronal cell death, and synaptic loss (Fig. 49-1A; see also PLATE 49-1). It is important always to bear in mind that these abnormalities represent the end stages of pathologic processes that have for years, if not decades, been underpinning the neurodegeneration seen in AD. When sufficient neuronal damage accrues, nerve cell dysfunction and neurotransmitter deficits ensue (for review, see Ref. 1), giving rise to the clinical features of dementia that worsen as the neurodegenerative mechanisms relentlessly progress.

Amyloid deposition is one of the first abnormalities to be observed in the brains of individuals developing AD.[2] Amyloid is an abnormal accumulation of protein fibrils that, due to its secondary structure, when stained with Congo red, displays green-red birefringence under polarized light. The extracellular "mature" neuritic plaque (NP) is one of the hallmark lesions in AD and comprises a relatively insoluble dense core of 8 to 10-nm β-pleated amyloid fibrils surrounded by dystrophic neurites, reactive astrocytes, and activated microglia (Fig. 49-1B). These amyloid fibrils are also deposited within the walls of cerebral blood vessels creating a coexisting amyloid angiopathy (Fig. 49-1C). Biochemical analyses of these amyloid deposits led to the identification of its major constituent, a 4-kd 39–43 amino acid peptide known as the β-amyloid peptide (Aβ).[3,4] Antibodies raised to Aβ revealed that Aβ was actually more widely deposited in AD brains than previously considered but in diffuse amorphous deposits without the associated cytopathology that surrounds NPs[5] (Fig. 49-1C). In fact, these amorphous entities are the first type of Aβ deposits to be seen in early AD brains, initially occurring in the basal regions of the isocortex,[2] and are considered to be preamyloid "immature" plaques. This possibility is supported by the finding of diffuse plaques in the brains of young persons with Down syndrome (trisomy 21), in whom AD neuropathology almost invariably occurs, before the advent of NP and NFT formation.[6]

Structure and Function of the Amyloid Precursor Protein

Soon after it was identified Aβ was discovered to be a proteolytic breakdown product of a much larger membrane-spanning protein, the amyloid precursor protein (APP),[7,8] which itself is a member of a highly conserved protein family including amyloid precursor-like proteins 1 and 2.[9] Alternative splicing of mRNA for APP, the gene for which resides on chromosome 21, results in the production of a set of at least 10 different APPs ranging in size from 365 to 770 amino acids, APP_{695} and APP_{770} being the predominant isoforms in, respectively, human brain and non-neuronal tissues.[10] Ubiquitously expressed and highly evolutionarily conserved, APP is an integral glycosylated protein comprising a large extracellular amino (N)-terminal domain wherein resides most of the variation between the different isoforms of APP, a single membrane-spanning domain and a short 47 amino acid intracellular carboxyl (C)-terminal domain (Fig. 49-2). The Aβ sequence starts 28 amino acid residues external to the membrane and extends for the first 11 to 15 residues into the transmembranous domain.

The biologic function of APP remains relatively unclear. Several putative functions for secreted forms of APP have been identified but it is difficult to implicate definitively any of these in the etiology of AD.[11] Secreted APPs encoding a 56 amino acid sequence near the N-terminus for a Kunitz protease inhibitor domain have been identified as a fibroblast-derived growth factor and serine protease inhibitor, protease nexin II, and as inhibitors of coagulation factor XIa. Secreted forms

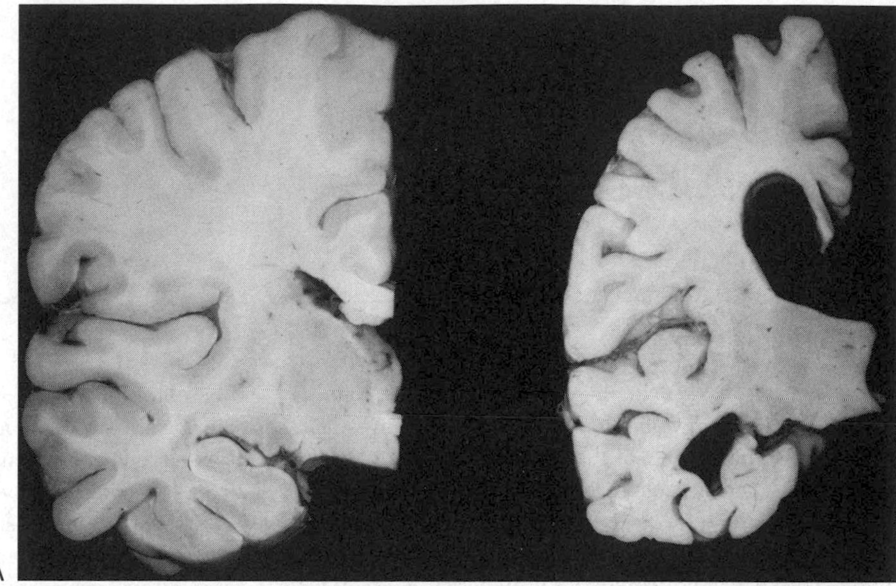

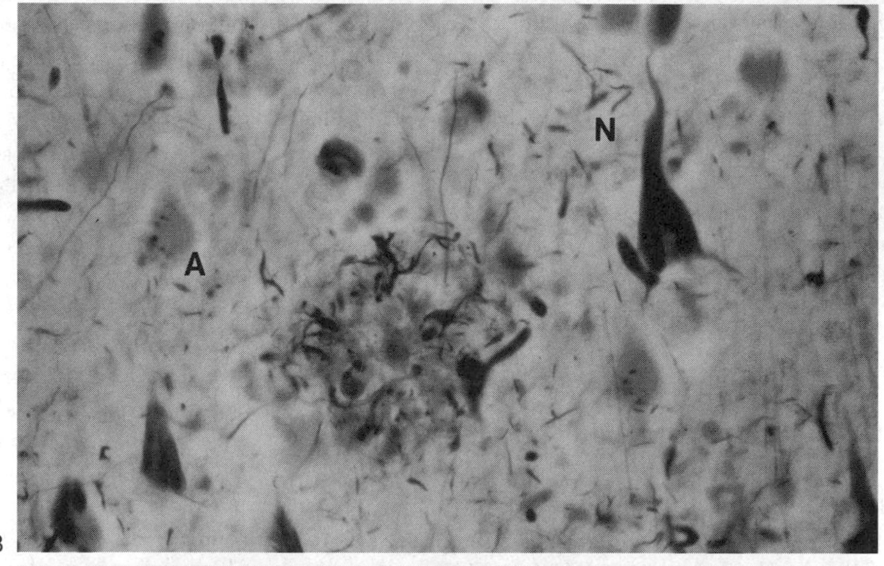

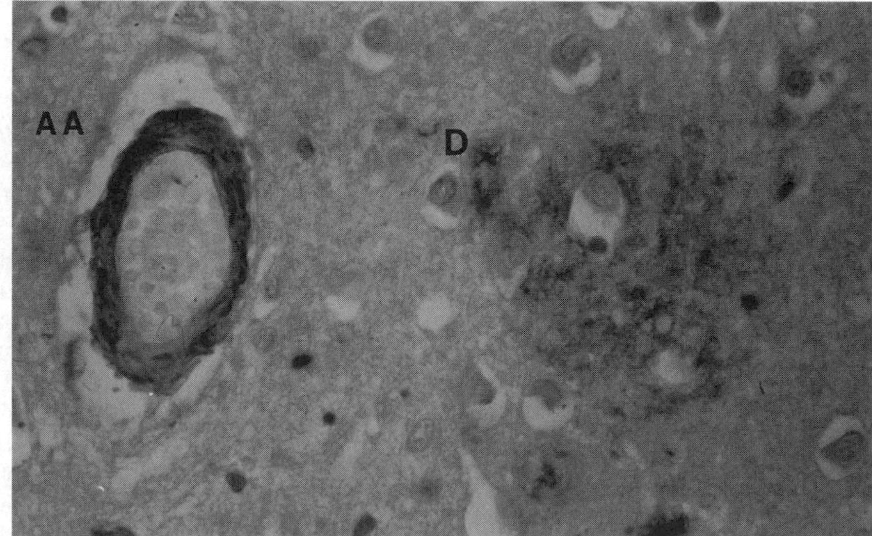

Figure 49-1 Characteristic features in Alzheimer's disease (AD) brain. (**A**) Cerebral atrophy due to AD in a 78-year-old female, featuring narrowed gyri, widened sulci, and dilated ventricles. The normal hemisphere on the left, from a nondemented 77-year-old female, is for comparison. (**B**) An extracellular neuritic plaque with a dense amyloid core (A) and a typical flame-shaped pyramidal cell occupied by darkly stained NFTs (N), demonstrated by a Glees and Marsland stain (magnification ×400). (**C**) Amyloid angiopathy (AA) and a diffuse amyloid plaque (D), stained with an antibody to ApoE (magnification ×400).

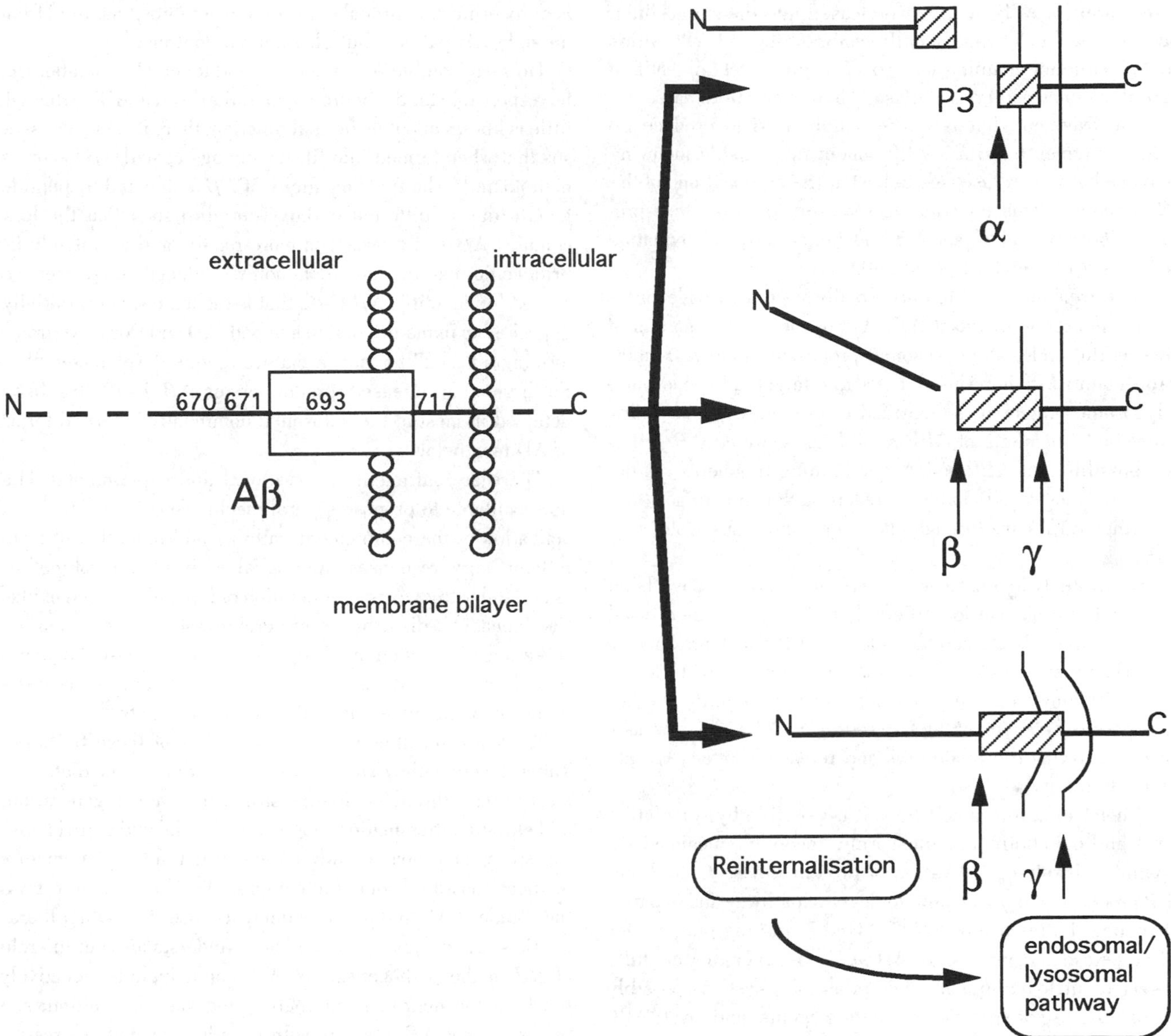

Figure 49-2 Schematic diagram indicating the sites of mutations in APP (APP 770 isoform), flanking and within Aβ, and the pathways for APP metabolism. Only the lower two pathways are capable of generating intact Aβ. α, β, and γ denote the cleavage sites for the respective secretases.

of APP have also been demonstrated to regulate cell growth, mediate neurite outgrowth, promote cell-cell and cell-matrix adhesion, and lower intraneuronal Ca^{2+} levels and maintain synaptic integrity and plasticity. These partial functions support the notion of a cellular "housekeeping" function for APP in facilitating neuronal and other cell-type growth and survival. It could be that somehow loss of the normal functions of APP contributes to AD pathology.

APP's structure and location are suggestive of it being a cell surface receptor.[7] A 20 amino acid sequence in the intracytoplasmic domain of APP has been demonstrated to couple with the GTP-binding protein G_o[12] endorsing a role for APP in signal transduction. Further study of the role of APP in intracytoplasmic signaling may provide the much sought after link between APP and NFT pathology, particularly as the latter is dependent on kinase and protease activities governed by various intracytoplasmic signaling cascades and pathways.

Processing and Trafficking of Amyloid Precursor Protein and the Generation of Aβ

The proteolytic processing and intracellular trafficking of APP is complex (Fig. 49-2). Aberrant processing of APP causing either increased production of Aβ, decreased removal of Aβ, or the production of abnormally amyloidogenic Aβ isoforms is possibly the primary pathogenic event in AD.[11] Secreted forms of APP (APP_s) are released into the extracellular space following cleavage of cell membrane-bound APP within the Aβ sequence at amino acid 16/17 by the as yet unidentified proteolytic enzyme(s) α-secretase,[13] leaving a 10-kd carboxyl-terminal fragment that is further catabolized to produce P3 (a 3-kd fragment) and a 7-kd fragment presumably following cleavage by γ-secretase (see below) at the carboxyl end of the Aβ sequence. This constitutive secretory pathway thus precludes formation of intact Aβ and hence amyloid formation (i.e., it is a nonamyloidogenic pathway).

There are, however, alternative pathways that provide routes for the generation of intact Aβ. One of the most important of these is the endosomal/lysosomal processing pathway: membrane-bound APP is re-internalized and targeted in endosomes to lysosomes where it is degraded to produce Aβ-containing C-terminal fragments of APP as well as secreted Aβ.[11] It is also possible that APP and Aβ-containing fragments are degraded in lysosomes before ever reaching the cell surface (i.e., following trafficking through the Golgi and trans Golgi network).

Two proteolytic enzymes, or enzyme systems, have been described, but not yet identified, that allow Aβ to be excised from within APP. β-Secretase cleaves APP just proximal to the Aβ sequence, releasing a truncated form of APP_s and a potentially amyloidogenic Aβ-containing fragment.[14] The latter is possibly cleaved at the C-terminus of Aβ by γ-secretase, thereby allowing the production and release of intact Aβ into the medium.[10]

Of note, in cultured cell lines it is possible by stimulation of m1 and m3 cholinergic muscarinic receptors, mediated via a pathway involving activation of protein kinase C, to direct APP processing to the nonamyloidogenic pathway and in parallel reduce the release of Aβ.[15,16] One intriguing prospect for a therapeutic intervention for AD would be, once they are fully dissected out, to manipulate these processing systems, possibly through the use of specific cholinergic agents, and divert APP metabolism away from the amyloidogenic pathways and thereby reduce production and secretion of Aβ.

The Role of Aβ in Neurodegeneration and the Implications for Rational Therapies

Although Aβ deposition and amyloid formation are indisputably key features of AD, it remains uncertain how these events might lead to neuronal dysfunction and cell death. Furthermore, it has been thought for some time that Aβ deposition in the brain does not correlate with dementia severity as closely as the presence of dystrophic neurites and NFTs. This view, however, may be changing as more recent computerized image analysis studies of the entorhinal cortex, measuring total area occupied by β-amyloid immunopositive deposits rather than plaque numbers, are indicating a closer relationship between the clinical features of AD and plaque pathology.[17] Initially considered to be pathologic in origin, Aβ is now known to be a normal metabolic product of APP that can be detected in healthy primary neuronal cultures and cerebrospinal fluid from not only AD patients but also normal controls.[18]

How can soluble Aβ, a normal product of APP metabolism, be responsible for the neurodegeneration seen in AD? Although little is known about its normal function, there is now a consensus that when formed into fibrils and aggregated Aβ becomes neurotoxic.[19] The fibrillogenicity of Aβ is dictated by peptide length (due to different carboxyl-termini) such that the less common Aβ 1–42 variant is more readily and completely fibrillogenic than the more commonly produced but shorter Aβ 1–40.[20] In fact, it is Aβ 1–42 that is the main species initially deposited in immature plaques in both AD and Down syndrome forming a "seed" for future mature plaque development.[21,22] Furthermore, increased production of Aβ 1–42 has been detected in most of the autosomal dominantly inherited forms of AD (see below).

There are sufficient observational and experimental data now available to propose several mechanisms for Aβ toxicity: activation of the complement pathway and induction of local inflammatory responses, microglial activation, cytokine release, and astrocytosis[23]; generation of free radicals and oxidative damage[24]; disturbance of cerebrovascular regulation via Aβ-induced production of superoxide ions in vascular endothelial cells[25]; and disruption of local calcium homeostasis rendering cells more vulnerable to excitotoxicity.[26]

What are the therapeutic implications of these findings? Taken together they suggest that Aβ-toxicity is mediated, at least in part, through oxidative stress, free radical generation, and chronic inflammation. Some clinical trial and co-twin control study data have already indicated that anti-inflammatory medications afford some protection in that they can slow down the course of AD and possibly delay its onset.[27,28] Other therapeutic strategies, based on a clearer understanding of the role of Aβ in the pathogenesis of AD, could include selectively blocking the neuronal, microglial, and vascular cell-surface receptors that Aβ interacts with to induce oxidative stress[29]; antioxidants and free radical scavenging agents; selective neuronal agents to modify calcium channel activity and maintain calcium homeostasis; and the development of drugs that in the first instance could decrease production of the longer Aβ 1–42 isoform, reduce its fibrillogenicity, and enhance the degradation of Aβ and its clearance.

Neurofibrillary Tangles

The neurofibrillary lesions of AD include NFTs, neuritic plaques, and dystrophic neurites (Fig. 49-1B; see also Plate 49-1). The burden of such neurofibrillary lesions is closely correlated to the degree of clinical dementia whereas similar correlations traditionally have not been observed between total amyloid deposits and AD.[30,31] This may no longer be the case.[17] The structural building blocks of the neurofibrillary lesions are paired helical filaments (PHF) of which the protein tau is the major integral constituent,[32] so called PHF-tau.

Paired Helical Filaments and Normal Tau Protein

In the adult human brain, tau protein exists in six isoforms generated from a single gene on chromosome 17 by alternative splicing.[33,34] Tau expression is developmentally regulated with all six isoforms being found in the adult brain but only the smallest isoform in fetal brain. All six tau isoforms are phosphorylated but PHF-tau of AD brains was originally reported to be abnormally phosphorylated or "hyperphosphorylated" at sites not found in normal adult human tau isolated from postmortem brain samples.[35,36] This hyperphosphorylated form renders tau protein relatively insoluble and of apparently larger molecular weight on electrophoretic gels.[37,38] This finding generated the hypothesis that excessive or abnormal phosphorylation of tau is a key event in the transformation of normal tau into PHF-tau. Enormous energy has thus been directed at identifying significant phosphorylation sites and the responsible phosphorylating kinases (for review see Ref. 39).

Tau is a microtubule-associated protein that is involved in the stabilization and assembly of axonal microtubules, the integrity of which is required for axonal transport of material between the cell body and axonal synapses. Studies have demonstrated that reversible phosphorylation/dephosphorylation of tau regulates its binding to microtubules, and that in the hyperphosphorylated state tau's capacity to bind to microtubules is reduced. Significantly, in terms of the disease process the possible result of this may be impaired microtubule assembly.[40,41] Identification of significant phosphorylation sites that may be involved in regulation of tau binding to microtubules has been greatly aided by the development of recombinant wild-type and mutant tau proteins for use in vitro.[41]

However, new evidence has now emerged that adult tau isolated from rapidly processed human biopsy brain samples or rat brain is, in fact, phosphorylated at the same sites as fetal tau and almost all the same sites as PHF-tau. This finding, therefore, suggests that many of the so-called abnormal phosphorylation sites previously identified in PHF-tau are actually normal sites of tau phosphorylation. Rapid dephosphorylation of adult tau in brain tissue samples, during brief postsurgical or postmortem delays in isolating tau, is the most plausible explanation for the previous discrepancy.[42] However, quantitative immunochemical analysis does confirm that none of these sites in normal adult human tau is phosphorylated to the same extent as in PHF-tau. Thus it is the extent of tau phosphorylation rather than the abnormal phosphorylation of disease-specific sites that is distinctive in AD. These observations have led to a reassessment of current hypotheses about the pathogenesis of neurofibrillary lesions in AD brain, switching the emphasis from aberrant phosphorylation to defective dephosphorylation cascades. They imply that activities of specific phosphatases may be downregulated or defective in neurones in the AD brain that accumulate PHF-tau.

Candidate Kinases and Phosphatases for Tau Phosphorylation

To date many protein kinases, including glycogen synthase kinase 3α and 3β, protein kinase A, p110^{mark}, and both Ca and calmodulin-dependent kinase II, have been implicated as candidate kinases that phosphorylate tau in vitro. Likewise many protein phosphatases (PPs) including PP2A, PP2B have been implicated as candidate phosphatases in dephosphorylation. The research emphasis ultimately lies, however, in identifying the enzymes that phosphorylate/dephosphorylate tau within neurones in vivo.

Mechanisms of Neurofibrillary Tangle Formation

New information concerning the possible mechanism of NFT formation in the disease process derives from in vitro studies. Hyperphosphorylated tau from the AD brain is shown to disassemble microtubules and act as a nucleation center to assemble normal tau into filaments.[43] In addition to hyperphosphorylation, tau protein is abnormally glycosylated in AD, a modification that may stabilize PHF.[44] It has been postulated that hyperphosphorylation and glycosylation act in tandem, with the former disrupting microtubules and causing the initial polymerization of tau into straight filaments, which are then cross-linked by glycosylation into PHF. Despite this experimental evidence the primary cause of the post-translational modifications of tau that lead to NFT formation remains unresolved.

Linking the Two Major Pathologies of Alzheimer's Disease

The precise role of tau in the disease mechanism requires clarification and any theoretical framework for AD must naturally explain the link between the two cardinal pathologic features of the disease (Fig. 49-3). As yet, this remains to be elucidated but some insights concerning direct links come from in vitro studies that suggest that Aβ fibril formation, known to confer neurotoxicity, can induce tau hyperphosphorylation and consequently cytoskeletal disruption (see above).[45] Further, oxidative stress, a mechanism by which Aβ may generate toxicity, may act in a contributory manner because it also induces formation of PHF.[46] Finally, a common rather than direct link may be provided by the susceptibility gene for ApoE4 (see below). ApoE3 binding to tau protein protects tau from becoming hyperphosphorylated in vitro, whereas ApoE4 does not afford this protection.[47] Subsequent aggregation of hyperphosphorylated tau to form PHF, perhaps providing a nucleation center into which normal tau is sequestered, would lead to microtubule disassembly, loss of integrity of the neuronal cytoskeleton, and ultimately lead to neuronal death.

The Amyloid Precursor Protein Gene and Alzheimer's Disease

Although the final common pathways leading to the characteristic neuropathologic features are similar in most cases, AD is a heterogeneous condition with a multifactorial etiology in-

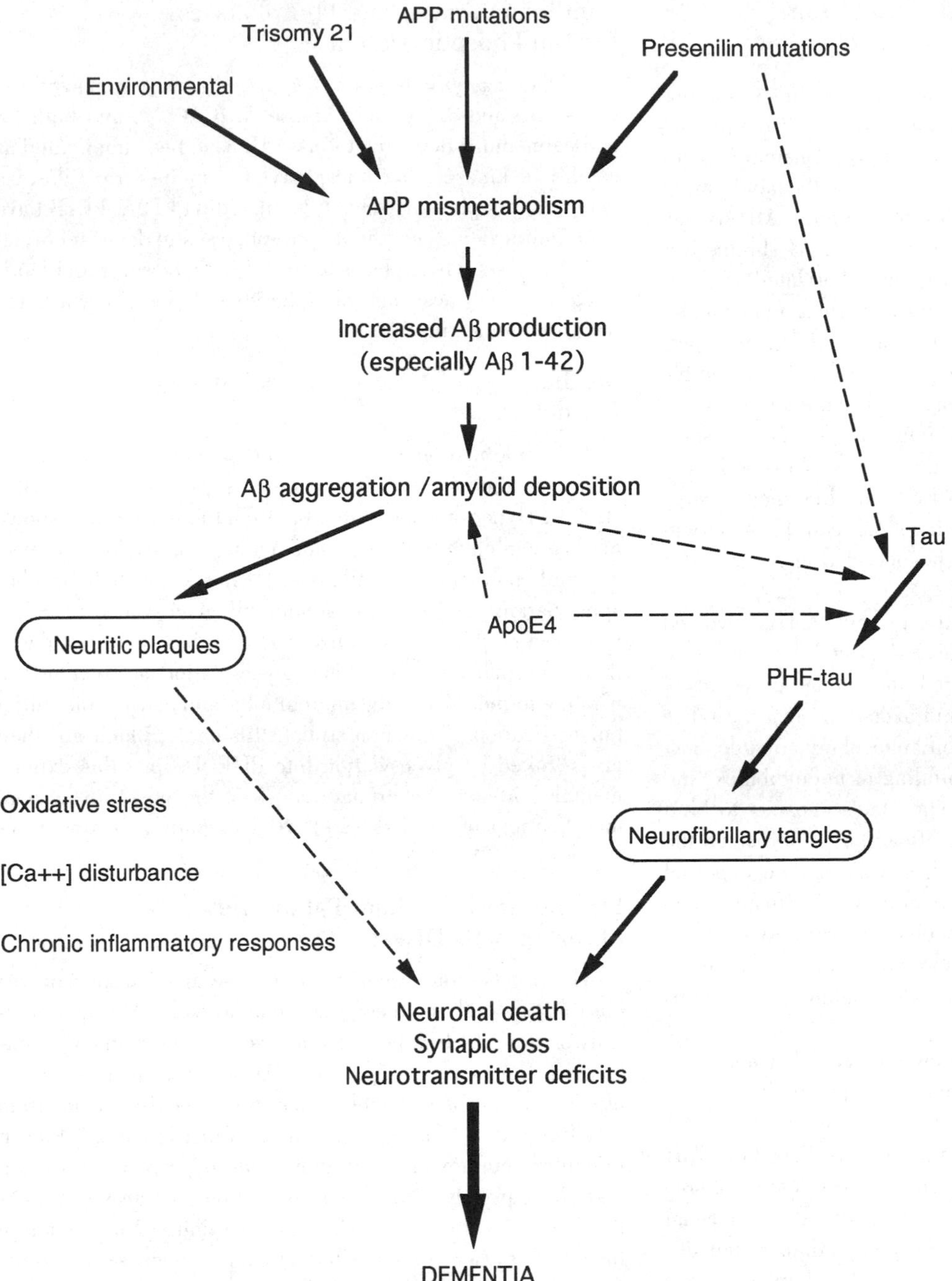

Figure 49-3 Pathogenic mechanisms in Alzheimer's disease. The broken lines indicate possible, but not definitively proven, pathways. PHF, paired helical filament; ApoE, apolipoprotein E.

fluenced by both genetic and environmental factors. To date the major risk factors identified for AD include old age, head injury, and perhaps most important family history.

Soon after $A\beta$ was found to be derived from APP the gene for APP was localized to chromosome 21.[8] It was already well recognized that AD neuropathology occurred almost invariably in adults with Down syndrome (trisomy 21) and that dementia supervened in the majority surviving into their fifties.[6] This has been attributed to a gene dosage effect resulting in excess $A\beta$ production, the consequence of having an extra chromosome 21 and hence an extra APP gene and a surfeit of APP.

Studying large single pedigrees with autosomal dominant early-onset (50 to 60 years) familial AD (EOFAD) eventually led to the discovery of missense point mutations (single nucleotide base changes that alter the DNA code for a particular amino acid) in the APP gene. These mutations cosegregate with the disease and are considered to be causative in these rare instances, only 20 families worldwide having so far been identified. The first defect to be reported was a single nucleotide change of cytosine to a thymine causing a substitution of isoleucine for valine in the APP molecule at amino acid 717 (numbering is for the APP 770 isoform).[48] This position is just two amino acids after the carboxyl-terminus of the Aβ sequence. Two other similar mutations at APP 717 were subsequently reported resulting in valine being substituted by phenylalanine[49] and by glycine.[50]

A double mutation occurs in the APP gene in a Swedish family affecting the two amino acids (APP670 and 671) immediately preceding the amino-terminus of Aβ so that lysine is substituted by asparagine and methionine by leucine.[51] A point mutation has also been found within the middle of the Aβ sequence causing a glutamine for glutamic acid substitution in APP 693.[52] Individuals with this mutation develop hereditary cerebral hemorrhage with amyloidosis, Dutch type (HCHWA-D) in which recurrent cerebral hemorrhages occur due to Aβ deposition weakening cerebral and meningeal blood vessel walls. A similar point mutation resulting in substitution of alanine into glycine at codon 692 has been reported in a Flemish family with presenile dementia and cerebral hemorrhage due to cerebral amyloid angiopathy.[53]

Given the location of these mutations, either flanking or within Aβ, it is not surprising to learn that they appear to exert their pathogenic effects by their influence on processing of APP. Cultured cells that express the valine to isoleucine APP717 mutant produce an increased amount of the highly amyloidogenic Aβ 1-42 isoform.[54] The Swedish double mutations cause an up to eight-fold increase in Aβ production in transfected cells,[55,56] a finding that was confirmed in studies of primary skin fibroblasts from patients with these mutations.[57] In vitro aggregation studies have shown that the mutation within Aβ responsible for HCHWA-D enhances the fibrillogenicity of Aβ.[58] The neuropathologic findings in a patient with the APP717 valine to isoleucine mutation are essentially the same as that seen in common sporadic late-onset AD, suggesting that the APP mutation is somehow responsible for not only the attendant increased production of Aβ and amyloid deposition but also for the cytoskeletal changes.[59]

The Presenilins and Alzheimer's Disease

Genetic linkage to chromosome 14 was established in the early 1990s for the majority (60 to 80 percent) of autosomal dominant inherited cases of EOFAD,[60,61] a particularly aggressive form of AD with an age of onset ranging from 30 to 60. The responsible gene, Presenilin-1 (*PS-1*), was cloned in 1995.[62,63] At roughly the same time that this remarkable finding was being made a locus for EOFAD in the rare Volga German kindred (Germans who emigrated in the mid-18th century to the district around the Volga river in Russia and whose descendants then emigrated in the late 19th century to the United States) was found on chromosome 1[64] and the gene, Presenilin-2 (*PS-2*), was subsequently cloned and its product found to be highly homologous to PS-1 (63 percent overall; 95 percent in some of the transmembrane regions)[65,66] and to have a similar predicted protein structure. More than 30 missense mutations and one in frame splice-site mutation, causing an exonic deletion, have been reported in *PS-1* that cosegregate with EOFAD and are considered to be causative, whereas only 2 missense mutations have so far been identified in *PS-2*.[67] In addition, an intronic polymorphism (a normal sequence variant) in the *PS-1* gene has been reported to be associated with increased risk for late-onset AD.[68] This potentially important finding, relating to the group most commonly affected by AD, remains to be confirmed and elaborated on in larger studies.

The PS-1 and PS-2 proteins have, respectively, 467 and 448 amino acids each and their predicted structure is a 7 (possibly 9) transmembrane domain protein, a serpentine structure that is often found in receptor proteins. Many of the reported mutations in *PS-1* cluster around the predicted second transmembrane region and a large extracellular hydrophilic loop domain between transmembrane domains 6 and 7.

The normal functions of the PS proteins are currently unknown. Potential functions, based on their common structure and the established functions of other proteins to which the PS proteins bear some degree of homology, include roles in intracellular protein trafficking, inhibiting apoptosis, acting as a calcium channel and signaling from the cell surface to the nucleus.[67] The latter function is of interest in that it may provide a link between the presenilins and cytoskeletal pathology in that some of these intracellular signaling pathways are thought to be involved in the aberrant phosphorylation of tau protein ultimately causing NFT formation.

The pathogenic functions of the PS proteins in AD remain to be fully elucidated. However, an indirect link to APP has already been discovered. Elevated levels of Aβ 1–42 can be detected in both plasma samples and cultured fibroblast cells obtained from carriers of the presenilin mutations.[69] Therefore, the mechanism common to all genetic causes of AD so far identified is increased production of Aβ, particularly the longer fibrillogenic Aβ 1–42 isoform.

Apolipoprotein E and Susceptibility Genes for Alzheimer's Disease

The vast majority of cases of AD are of late onset (i.e., over 65 years), and many, perhaps up to 50 percent, have a family history for dementia indicating that late-onset AD (LOAD) is not as "sporadic" as commonly believed. The genetic contribution to LOAD is complex and is probably influenced by several genes and modified by environmental factors yet to be established.

The first susceptibility gene to be identified was the $\epsilon 4$ allele of the gene for apolipoprotein E (ApoE) located on chromosome 19, to which linkage had previously been detected in familial LOAD.[70–72] ApoE is a polymorphic protein with three common isoforms E2, E3, and E4 encoded by the $\epsilon 2$, $\epsilon 3$, and $\epsilon 4$ alleles whose frequencies in the general population are 7, 78, and 15 percent, respectively. This situation is dramatically different in LOAD, in which up to 60 percent of patients have at least one $\epsilon 4$ allele.

A gene dosage effect is apparent in both familial and sporadic LOAD. It has been demonstrated in numerous clinical case series and family studies, and confirmed in autopsy-proven and population studies (although with some differences reported in various ethnic groups, notably African-Americans) that the presence of the $\epsilon 4$ allele is associated with an increased risk for AD, an earlier age of onset, and a greater accumulation of neuritic plaques.[73] In broad terms the possession of one $\epsilon 4$ allele elevates the risk for AD by lowering the age of onset by 5 years and for two $\epsilon 4$ alleles by 10 years. Interestingly, it appears that the $\epsilon 2$ allele confers some protection against AD in Caucasian populations by delaying the age of onset.[74] It has been demonstrated that $\epsilon 4$ predicts a negative response to the cholinomimetic agent tacrine,[75] an intriguing preliminary finding that paves the way for pharmacogenetic studies and that could have major clinical implications for tailoring drug treatments not only to patients' phenotypes but also their genotypes.

There are many people homozygous for $\epsilon 4$ who do not develop AD, plus many people with AD do not have any $\epsilon 4$ alleles. Therefore, possession of the $\epsilon 4$ allele is neither necessary nor sufficient to develop AD. Although possession of $\epsilon 4$ modifies the age of onset of AD in APP mutation families and also in Down syndrome, this effect is not apparent in families with presenilin mutations.[76]

The normal function of ApoE is to mediate phospholipid and cholesterol mobilization and distribution, and the E4 isoform has long been recognized as a major risk factor for hypercholesterolemia and atherosclerosis. ApoE is the major type of apolipoprotein in the human brain where it is produced by astrocytes in response to neuronal injury and is active in membrane remodeling and maintenance of synaptic plasticity. It could be that ApoE4 performs these reparative functions less effectively than the E3 or E2 isoforms, thereby bringing forward the onset of dementia in persons developing AD.[77] Other possible ApoE4-related pathogenic mechanisms could be due to isoform-specific activity. For example, ApoE4 has been shown in vitro to have a greater avidity for binding Aβ compared to the other isoforms[72,78] and a lower efficacy for interacting with tau and protecting it from hyperphosphorylation and NFT formation.[47,79] It is of interest that in addition to other elements, ApoE is found within NPs and is also internalized by neurones containing NFTs. However, whether it is subsequently able to gain access to intracytoplasmic tau protein remains unknown.

Apolipoprotein E and Predictive Testing for Alzheimer's Disease

Functional neuroimaging studies using positron emission tomography to study regional cerebral glucose metabolism in normal middle-aged subjects homozygous for the $\epsilon 4$ allele have indicated that it is possible to detect patterns of abnormal metabolism similar to that seen in persons with AD.[80] Such preclinical findings could be used to identify individuals at greatest risk for developing AD and initiating neuroprotective treatments, if and when available, prior to the onset of dementia. However, caution is required as predictive testing using *APOE* is complex and not to be undertaken lightly. At the moment there is a consensus that *APOE* genotyping is not indicated for predictive testing but that it may be of use as an adjunct to other diagnostic tests.[81] Individuals from families with autosomal dominant AD are in a different situation as identification of a mutation will provide, in most instances, a definitive prediction. The discovery and confirmation of further susceptibility genes for AD and improved neuroimaging techniques to detect preclinical cerebral changes will yield further insights into its etiology and probably allow the development of improved algorithms to more precisely assess individual risk. Such discoveries will clearly have enormous medical, legal, and ethical implications and will necessitate establishing suitable genetic counseling services.[82]

Transgenic Animal Models of Alzheimer's Disease

In order to study in vivo the molecular and cellular processes underlying neurodegeneration in AD and test novel therapies, much effort has been expended on identifying animal models of AD. The best strategy for this is to construct manipulable transgenic animal models in which it is possible to replicate the same pathologic features of AD that occur in humans.[83] Transgenic animals, usually mice, are created by stably transferring new or altered genes into the germ line of the mouse and breeding the mouse to produce lines of transgenic offspring carrying a new genetic identity. Such an approach allows selective disruption of specific molecular and cellular systems, shedding light on the function of the altered gene and its product.

The most promising transgenic mouse model developed so far expresses full-length human complementary DNA with the APP717 Val→Phe mutation but at levels 10 times that of endogenous mouse APP.[84] By the age of 6 to 9 months these mice display progressive neuropathology very similar in character and distribution to that seen in AD: Aβ deposits, neuritic plaques, synaptic loss, microgliosis, and astrocytosis. To some extent this mouse model can be considered to provide further evidence for the central role of APP and amyloid formation in AD. However there is as yet no evidence of any NFT formation suggesting that either NFTs are not crucial to the evolution of AD or, more likely, that this transgenic mouse is an incomplete model of AD. Attempts to produce transgenic animal models of PHF have demonstrated that mice overexpressing the largest tau isoform do not have NFTs.[85] Similarly, knockout mice, where expression of the gene of interest is prevented, lacking tau protein, demonstrate no obvious phenotype.[86] APP and ApoE "knockout" mice have been developed and are under investigation. The construction of presenilin transgenic mice is already under way.

Lewy Body Disease

Lewy bodies are associated with a spectrum of disease varying from those presenting with motor Parkinson's disease to those presenting with dementia. As with AD the pathologic

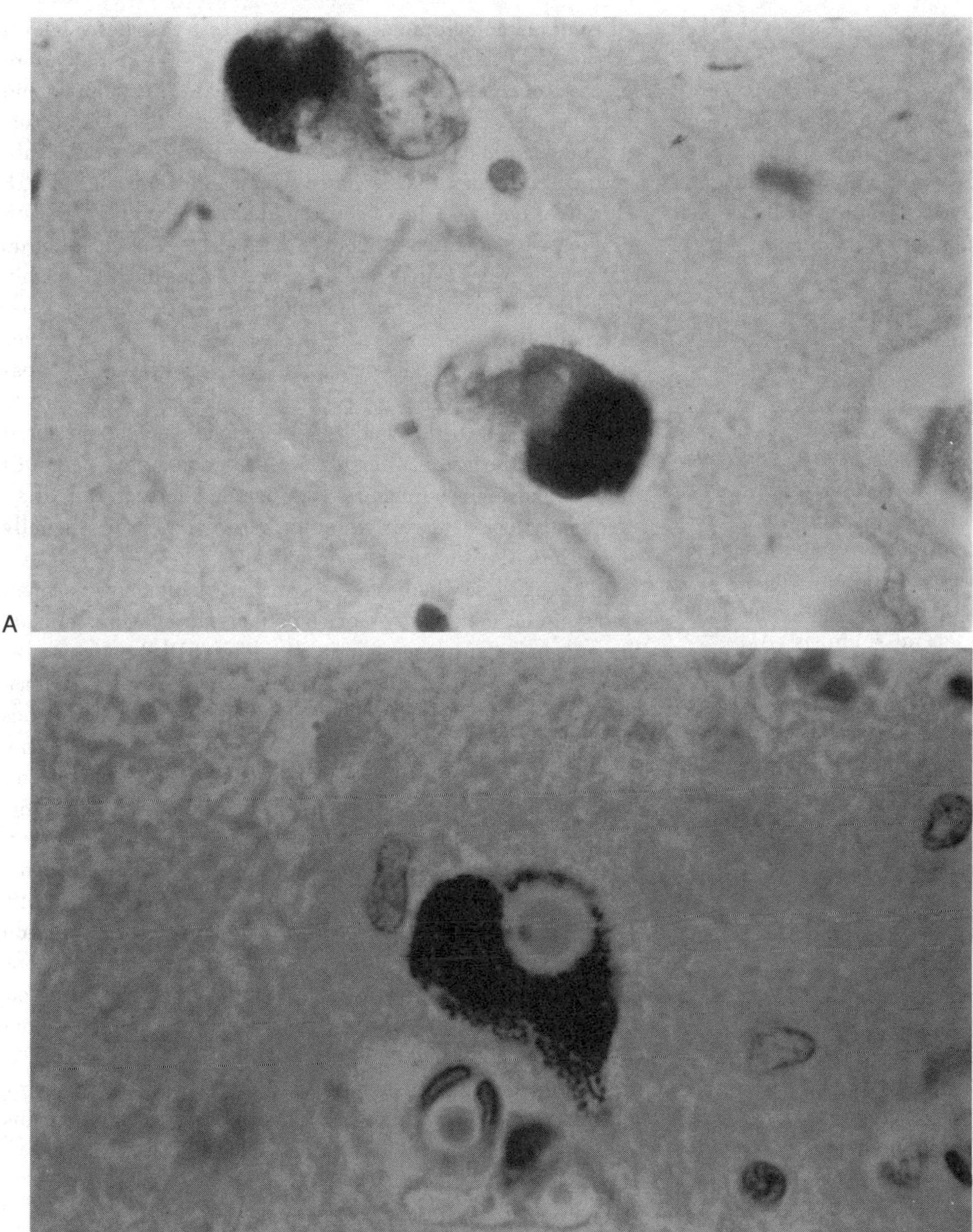

Figure 49-4 High-power photomicrograph demonstrating (**A**) ubiquitin staining of cortical Lewy bodies; (**B**) Hematoxylin and eosin staining of substantia nigra Lewy bodies.

hallmark of these diseases is an inclusion body derived from a component of the neuronal cytoskeleton.

Structure and Cell Biology of Lewy Bodies

Lewy bodies are intracytoplasmic eosinophilic inclusion bodies consisting of two morphologic types (for review see Ref. 87). The term brain stem or *classical* Lewy body refers to inclusions with a hyaline core and pale halo typically seen in the substantia nigra and locus ceruleus. The term *cortical* Lewy body refers to less well-defined inclusions, lacking a peripheral halo seen in the cortex (Fig. 49-4; see also Plate 49-2). Bulk isolation and characterization of Lewy bodies has proved difficult because of their relatively small numbers. Understanding of their biology has, therefore, come almost exclusively from immunohistochemical analyses using well-characterized antibodies.[88–91] These confirm that the most abundant LB components are neurofilaments but a variety of other cytoskeletal elements including B-crystallin, ubiquitin, and enzymes associated with ubiquitin-mediated proteolysis are also present.

Neurofilaments are neurone-specific cytoskeletal elements measuring 10 to 12 nm in diameter that together with microtubules and actin filaments form the neuronal cytoskeleton. Neurofilaments are composed of three distinct polypeptide subunits differing in molecular weight and designated NF-L (light), NF-M (medium), and NF-H (heavy).[92] All three subunits are present in both cortical and brain stem Lewy bodies.[93] In particular, antibodies to phosphorylated neurofilaments immunostain Lewy bodies directly and this has been taken to indicate that phosphorylation of neurofilaments is important in the formation of Lewy bodies.[94] Convincing evidence that the microtubule-associated protein tau is associated with Lewy bodies is lacking.[90,94]

Neurofilament Pathology in Neurodegenerative Disease

Neurofilaments are synthesized in the neuronal cell body and assembly occurs at the time of entry into the axon. Disruption of neurofilament organization such that neurofilaments misaccumulate in proximal axons and neuronal cell bodies to form an intraneuronal inclusion is a characteristic pathologic hallmark of a variety of neurodegenerative conditions including dementia with Lewy bodies (DLB),[90,95,96] Parkinson's disease (PD),[88,89] and amyotrophic lateral sclerosis (ALS).[97,98] The mechanism underlying neurofilament accumulation remains unknown although cell culture, chemical, and transgenic animal models of neurofilament accumulation have advanced understanding of this phenomenon.[99–102]

Transgenic Animal Models of Neurofilament Accumulation

Evidence from transgenic animal models of ALS has confirmed that neurofilament accumulations per se are a key intermediary in the pathogenic process leading to neuronal dysfunction and death in these diseases. For example, manipulating expression of human NF-H and mouse NF-L in a transgenic mouse to produce neurofilament accumulation in motor neurones results in both the clinical and pathologic phenotype of human ALS (for review see Refs. 100 and 101). Similarly, expression of mutant NF-H[103] results directly in neurofilament accumulation in cell bodies with subsequent loss of axons in ventral roots suggesting slow degeneration of the motor neurones. Although the initiating mechanism that produces neurofilament accumulation in human neurodegenerative disease is unlikely to be overexpression of neurofilament subunits[104] and remains unknown, the likely consequence of such accumulation is understood. In transgenic animals overexpressing the human NF-H gene, defects in axonal transport of newly synthesized proteins are detectable, indicating that accumulations of neurofilaments cause axonal degeneration by impeding the transport of components required for axonal maintenance.[105]

Dementia with Lewy Bodies and Parkinson's Disease

The finding that the majority of patients with PD have cortical Lewy bodies in addition to subcortical pathology[106] and the recognition of their association with a form of dementia, DLB, has led to increased interest in the Lewy body.

Neuropathologic autopsy series suggest that Lewy bodies are found in the brain stem and cortex of 15 to 25 percent of all cases of elderly demented patients, making them the second most common neurodegenerative pathology.[107,108] The majority of dementia cases with cortical Lewy bodies also have subcortical pathology that is indistinguishable from that of PD. However, one case has been reported of an individual with progressive dementia, numerous cortical Lewy bodies, but no PD pathology, so-called cerebral type.[109] Thus the relationship between PD and dementia is complicated. It is suggested that a quantitative difference in the number of cortical Lewy bodies may differentiate nondemented patients with PD and DLB patients because there is a direct correlation between the density of cortical Lewy bodies and the severity of dementia measured late in the disease. Cortical Lewy body containing neurones in DLB have been identified as pyramidal cells and these frequently coexist with ubiquitin-positive neurites usually found in CA2–3 of the hippocampus.[91]

Although Lewy bodies may be the only pathology in a small subgroup of, generally younger, patients, nosologic confusion has arisen because the majority of (elderly) DLB patients also have coexisting AD pathology at postmortem. Quantitative assessment of this AD pathology confirms that it distinguishes patients from age-related controls.[110] Typically, this AD-type pathology consists of diffuse, rather than neuritic plaques and furthermore NFTs are rarely observed. This has attracted differing interpretations from various authors including the suggestion that DLB is a variant of AD. Current terminology favors the use of the generic term *dementia with Lewy bodies* with three pathologic subtypes according to the relative distribution of LB in the brain stem, limbic, and neocortical regions. Consensus criteria (report of the CLBD Workshop)[111] are based on the supposition that DLB exists as a disorder with discernible pathologic and clinical boundaries. However, exact clarification of the position with respect to other conditions causing dementia, especially to AD, is necessary and this aim remains a focus for current research (for review see Ref. 111).

Susceptibility Genes and Dementia With Lewy Bodies

As yet no familial cases of DLB have been found and no specific genetic markers exist. However, the frequency of the desbrisoquine hydroxylase CYP2D6B allele, a known risk factor for PD is also raised in DLB and the apolipoprotein $\epsilon 4$ allele frequency is raised in cases of DLB and AD but not in PD or "pure Lewy body disease."[112,113] One explanation for the loss of this latter association is that the ApoE risk factor is mediated through tau phosphorylation and in the absence of NFT and tau pathology, this association disappears.[114]

Therapeutic Implications

Many DLB patients are clinically misdiagnosed; the search for diagnostic markers must therefore continue. The cortical Lewy body remains the most important pathologic marker for diagnosis. Understanding the mechanism underlying Lewy body pathogenesis provides a major focus of current research and may ultimately lead to new therapeutic approaches targeted to limit neuronal loss in these diseases.

Asymmetric Cortical Degeneration Syndromes

Recognition of the increasing clinical and genetic heterogeneity of the neurodegenerative diseases has resulted in renewed focus on the relationship between topography of the disease and clinical phenotype. Thus the term *asymmetric cortical degeneration* has been coined to provide a clinically based classification system that encompasses the majority of atypical cortical dementia patterns.

Frontotemporal Dementia

Non-Alzheimer frontotemporal lobar atrophy probably accounts for 20 percent of cases of primary cerebral atrophy and clinically presents most commonly with the syndrome of frontotemporal dementia (FTD). The nosologic status of FTD currently remains uncertain in relationship to other frontal syndromes such as progressive aphasia (PA), semantic dementia (SD), "Pick's disease," and frontotemporal dementia–motor neuron disease (FTD-MND) and refinement of this issue may come from molecular genetics.

Genetic Markers and Heterogeneity in Frontotemporal Dementia

Fifty percent of patients presenting with FTD have a first degree relative with the disorder and an autosomal mode of inheritance has been suggested in some families. A recent study mapped the linkage to chromosome 3.[115] Genetic heterogeneity is demonstrated by linkage to markers on chromosome 17 in other families with the disinhibition-dementia-Parkinsonism-amyotrophy complex,[116] a familial neurodengenerative overlap syndrome including frontal lobe dementia, Parkinsonism, and ALS.

Inclusion Bodies and Frontal Lobe Syndromes

The histologic changes of frontal lobe degeneration (i.e., neuronal loss, spongiform change, and astrocytic gliosis), which are common to the syndromes of progressive aphasia, semantic dementia, and FTD serve to distinguish them from the histologic changes characterized as Pick's type. Here, intense astrocytic gliosis with or without ubiquitinated and tau-positive inclusions (Pick bodies) and swollen neurons (Pick cells) are present. These findings have lent support to the concept that FTD, PA, and SD represent distinct clinical manifestations of a common disease process with the topographic distribution dictating the clinical syndrome: bilateral symmetric temporal pathology in FTD, left-sided frontotemporal pathology in PA, and bilateral temporal lobe pathology in SD.

In recent years an association between FTD and MND has been recognized with reports of frontal lobe dysfunction in MND patients. However, the presence of ubiquitinated inclusions in the frontal cortical neurons in FTD-MND sets this disorder apart not only from the frontal lobe degeneration of FTD, PA, and SD, but also from Pick-type pathology. It remains to be clarified as to whether FTD-MND represents a separate disease entity or represents an interface between FTD and "classic" (nondementing) motor neuron disease.

Huntington's Disease and Trinucleotide Repeat Disorders

Huntington's disease (HD) is a neurodegenerative autosomal dominant condition characterized by progressive chorea, dementia, and psychiatric disorders. Although the mean age of onset is 35 to 40 years it can present in later life. The gene for HD is on the short arm of chromosome 4. The responsible abnormality is an unstable and expanded cytosine-adenine-guanosine (CAG) trinucleotide repeat sequence in the upstream noncoding region of the gene that codes for an unknown protein named "huntingtin."[117] Individuals having less than 35 CAG repeats do not develop HD whereas those with more than 35 copies do.

In general, the greater the number of repeats the earlier is the age of onset and the more severe the disorder.[118] Several trinucleotide triplet repeat disorders have now been identified and they are all neurologic/psychiatric conditions: spinal and bulbar muscular atrophy (Kennedy's disease), fragile X syndrome, myotonic dystrophy, spinocerebellar ataxia type 1, dentatorubral-pallidoluysian atrophy, Machado-Joseph disease, and Friedreich's ataxia. Several of these conditions, including HD, demonstrate "anticipation" (ie, the disease becomes more severe with an earlier age of onset in successive generations within a family). This is due to the inherent instability of abnormally expanded trinucleotide repeat sequences that further expand in miosis during gamete production. For HD this miotic instability is more prominent in sperm than in ova and hence the risk of inheriting an even further expanded repeat sequence is greater with paternal transmission.

Genetic Counseling

As a result of these remarkable advances a relatively straightforward molecular diagnostic/predictive test is now available that is much more reliable than the previously used linkage analysis studies, which required the cooperation of a large number of family members. Guidelines for predictive testing and the need for specialized counseling have been agreed upon[119] and provide a helpful model of genetic counseling for those seeking either predictive or risk assessment genetic testing for AD.

Following an initial assessment appointment, the counseling sessions usually take place over a period of several months, providing the testees with a "cooling off" period in which they can reconsider the choices available to them. The aim of counseling is to enable the testee to make an informed decision about having the test done, to explore the reasons and the need to have the test done at this particular time, to prepare the testee for the result, and to anticipate any adverse consequences.

Prion Disorders

The prion disorders are transmissible diseases of the central nervous system (CNS) that affect both animals and humans. Clinically they are characterized by a long incubation period followed by a rapidly progressive dementia leading to death within several months to a few years. Histopathology of the CNS usually reveals extensive neuronal vacuolation, giving a "sponge-like" appearance to the brain (hence the term *spongiform encephalopathy*), neuronal loss, gliosis, and the deposition of a modified partially protease-resistant form of a normal cellular protein, known as the prion protein (PrP^c).[120]

Four relatively rare prion disorders have been described in humans: Creutzfeldt-Jakob disease (CJD; the most common with an incidence of only 0.5 to 1 case per million population per annum and average age of onset 63 years), Gerstmann-Straussler-Scheinker disease, fatal familial insomnia, and kuru. The latter was caused by ingestion of infected CNS tissues by the Fore people of Papua New Guinea during ritual cannibalism, a practice abandoned only in the late 1950s.

The exact mechanism of infection for these transmissible disorders is controversial. Despite initial skepticism the most widely accepted hypothesis is that it is a modified form of the prion protein, PrP^{sc} (named after scrapie, the naturally occurring prion disease in sheep), that, alone and in the absence of any nucleic acid, is the responsible infectious agent—the "*pro*teinaceous *in*fectious particle," hence the term *prion*.[121] Intriguingly, both PrP^c and PrP^{sc} have identical amino acid sequences. The pathologic properties of PrP^{sc} have been attributed to conformational changes in the protein following post-translational modification. These changes render the protein resistant to degradation, which eventually leads to PrP^{sc} accumulation within the brain. The conversion of PrP^c to the protease-resistant PrP^{sc} isoform is brought about either by direct exposure of PrP^c with exogenous infectious PrP^{sc} or by genetic mutations.

About 5 to 10 percent of cases of CJD are familial with an autosomal dominant inheritance and are associated with mutations in the gene coding for PrP, located on chromosome 20. Iatrogenic transmission of CJD has occurred following corneal transplantation, neurosurgery, and therapeutic use of hormones derived from human pituitary. Otherwise, the majority of cases appear to be sporadic. Both sporadic and iatrogenic CJD occur predominantly in genetically susceptible persons homozygous for a common methionine-valine polymorphism at codon 129 of PrP.[122,123]

Recently a new variant of CJD has been detected in more than 10 cases in the United Kingdom.[124] These cases have an earlier age of onset (mean of 24 years) but slower progression, prominent psychiatric symptoms as early clinical features, absence of the characteristic electroencephalogram pattern of CJD, plus extensive PrP plaque formation and a pattern of PrP deposition more similar to that seen in kuru. The route of transmission in these new cases has not been definitively ascertained but is thought to be due to a new strain of infectious PrP^{sc} possibly linked to the United Kingdom epidemic of bovine spongiform encephalopathy (BSE) and the entrance of contaminated meat products into the human food chain. The development of BSE in the mid-1980s is thought to be due to the introduction of infectious scrapie-contaminated material into cattle feed following changes in the rendering procedures for these materials in the early 1980s.[125] The question of how BSE might cross the species barrier from cattle to humans remains to be answered.

Conclusion

The progress of neuroscience in the last decade toward unraveling the molecular mechanisms that underlie the major dementing illnesses brings closer a future in which therapeutic approaches will ultimately target the disease process itself rather than act simply to alleviate disease symptoms. In combination with advances in the early detection and diagnosis of neurodegenerative conditions, the new millenium heralds the prospect of an age in which individuals at risk can be identified and preventative strategies implemented. The realization of such a future for dementia patients and their caregivers presents a major challenge for molecular medicine now and into the 21st century.

Acknowledgments

JEC is supported by the Wellcome Trust and DMM by the Alzheimer's Disease Society. We are indebted to Dr. Nigel Cairns of the MRC Brain Bank at the Institute of Psychiatry, London, for histopathologic slides.

References

1. Francis PT, Pangalos MN, Bowen DM: Animal and drug modelling for Alzheimer synaptic pathology. Prog Neurobiol 1992; 39:517–545
2. Braak H, Braak E: Neuropathological staging of Alzheimer-related changes. Acta Neuropathol 1991;82:306–315
3. Glenner GG, Wong CW: Alzheimer's disease: initial report of the purification and characterization of a novel cerebrovascular amyloid protein. Biochem Biophys Res Commun 1984; 120:885–890
4. Masters CL, Simms G, Weinman NA et al: Amyloid core plaque protein in Alzheimer's disease and Down Syndrome. Proc Natl Acad Sci USA 1985;82:4245–4249
5. Yamaguchi H, Hirai S, Morimatsu M et al: Diffuse type of

senile plaques in the brains of Alzheimer-type dementia. Acta Neuropathol 1988;77:113–119

6. Mann DMA, Royston MC, Ravindra CR: Some morphometric observations on the brains of patients with Down's syndrome: their relationship to age and dementia. J Neurol Sci 1990;99: 153–164
7. Kang J, Lemaire H-G, Unterbeck A et al: The precursor of Alzheimer's disease amyloid A4 protein resembles a cell-surface receptor. Nature 1987;325:733–736
8. Goldgaber D, Lerman MI, McBride OW et al: Characterization and chromosomal localization of a cDNA encoding brain amyloid of Alzheimer's disease. Science 1987;235:877–880
9. Wasco W, Gurubhagavatula S, Paradis MD et al: Isolation and characterization of *APLP2* encoding a homologue of the Alzheimer's associated amyloid β protein precursor. Nature Genet 1993;5:95–100
10. Octave J-N: The amyloid peptide and its precursor in Alzheimer's disease. Rev Neurosci 1995;6:287–316
11. Selkoe DJ: Cell biology of the amyloid β-protein precursor and the mechanism of Alzheimer's disease. Annu Rev Cell Biol 1994;10:373–403
12. Nishimoto I, Okamoto T, Matsuura Y et al: Alzheimer amyloid protein precursor complexes with brain GTP-binding protein G_o. Nature 1993;362:75–79
13. Esch FS, Keim PS, Beattie EC et al: Cleavage of amyloid beta peptide during constitutive processing of its precursor. Science 1990;248:1122–1124
14. Seubert P, Oltersdorf T, Lee MG et al: Secretion of ß-amyloid precursor protein cleaved at the amino terminus of the ß-amyloid peptide. Nature 1993;361:260–263
15. Nitsch RM, Slack BE, Wurtman RJ, Growdon JH: Release of Alzheimer amyloid precursor derivatives stimulate by activation of muscarinic acetylcholine receptors. Science 1992;258: 304–307
16. Slack BE, Breu J, Petryniak MA et al: Tyrosine phosphorylation-dependent stimulation of amyloid precursor protein secretion by the m3 muscarinic acetylcholine receptor. J Biol Chem 1995;270:8337–8344
17. Cummings BJ, Cotman CW: Image analysis of β-amyloid load in Alzheimer's disease and relation to dementia severity. Lancet 1996;346:1524–1528
18. Haass C, Schlossmacher MG, Hung AY et al: Amyloid ß-peptide is produced by cultured cells during normal metabolism. Nature 1992;359:322–325
19. Pike CJ, Burdick D, Walencewicz AJ et al: Neurodegeneration induced by β-amyloid peptides in vitro: the role of peptide assembly state. J Neurosci 1993;13:1676–1687
20. Jarrett JT, Berger EP, Lansbury PT Jr: The carboxy terminus of the β amyloid protein is critical for the seeding of amyloid formation: implications for the pathogenesis of Alzheimer's disease. Biochemistry 1993;32:4693–4697
21. Iwatsubo T, Odaka A, Suzuki N et al: Visualization of Aβ42(43) in senile plaques with end-specific Aβ monoclonals: evidence that an initially deposited species is Aβ42(43). Neuron 1994;13:45–53
22. Teller JK, Russo C, DeBusk LM et al: Presence of soluble amyloid β-peptide precedes amyloid plaque formation in Down's syndrome. Nature Med 1996;2:93–95
23. Aisen PS, Davis KL: Inflammatory mechanisms in Alzheimer's disease: implications for therapy. Am J Psychiatry 1994;151: 1105–1113
24. Hensley K, Butterfield DA, Hall N et al: Reactive oxygen species as causal agents in the neurotoxicity of the Alzheimer's disease-associated amyloid beta peptide. Ann NY Acad Sci 1996;786:120–134
25. Thomas T, Thomas G, McLendon C et al: β-amyloid-mediated vasoactivity and vascular endothelial damage. Nature 1996; 380:168–171
26. Mattson MP, Barger SW, Cheng B et al: ß-Amyloid precursor protein metabolites and loss of neuronal Ca^{2+} homeostasis in Alzheimer's disease. Trends Neurosci 1993;16:409–414
27. Rogers J, Kirby LC, Hempelman SR et al: Clinical trial of indomethacin in Alzheimer's disease. Neurology 1993;43: 1609–1611
28. Breitner JCS, Gau BA, Welsh KA et al: Inverse association of anti-inflammatory treatments and Alzheimer's disease: initial results of a co-twin study. Neurology 1994;44:227–232
29. Yan DS, Chen X, Fu J et al: RAGE and amyloid-β peptide neurotoxicity in Alzheimer's disease. Nature 1996;382: 685–691
30. Arriagada PA, Growdon JH, Hedley-White ET, Hyman BT: Neurofibrillary tangles but not senile plaques parallel duration and severity of Alzheimer's disease. Neurology 1992;42: 631–639
31. Dickson DW, Crystal HA, Mattiace LA et al: Identification of normal and pathological ageing in prospectively studied nondemented elderly humans. Neurobiol Ageing 1991;13: 179–189
32. Lee VM-Y, Balin BJ, Otvos L, Trojanowski JQ: A68: a major subunit of paired helical filaments and derivatised forms of normal tau. Science 1991;252:675–678
33. Goedert M, Spillantini MG, Potier MC et al: Cloning and sequencing of the cDNA encoding an isoform of microtubule-associated protein tau containing four tandem repeats: differential expression of tau protein mRNA's in human brain. EMBO J 1989;8:393–399
34. Lee G, Nerve RL, Kosik KS: The microtubule binding domain of tau protein. Neuron 1989;2:1615–1624
35. Goedert M, Jakes R, Crowther RA et al: The abnormal phosphorylation of tau protein at serine^{202} in Alzheimer's disease recapitulates phosphorylation during development. Proc Natl Acad Sci 1993;90:5066–5070
36. Goedert M, Spillantini MG, Cairns NJ, Crowther RA: Tau proteins of Alzheimer paired helical filaments: abnormal phosphorylation of all six isoforms. Neuron 1992;8:159–168
37. Brion JP, Hanger DP, Couck AM, Anderton BH: A69 proteins in Alzheimer's disease are composed of several tau isoforms in a phosphorylated state which affects their electrophoretic mobilities. Biochem J 1991;279:831–836
38. Hanger DP, Brion JP, Gallo JM et al: Tau in Alzheimer's disease and Down's syndrome is insoluble and abnormally phosphorylated. Biochem J 1991;275:99–104

39. Trojanowski JQ, Lee VM-Y: Phosphorylation of neuronal cytoskeletal proteins in Alzheimer's disease and Lewy body dementia. Ann NY Acad Sci 1994;747:92–109
40. Bramblett GT, Goedert M, Jakes R et al: Abnormal tau phosphorylation at ser[396] in Alzheimer's disease recapitulates development and contributes to microtubule binding. Neuron 1993;10:1089–1099
41. Biernat J, Gutstke N, Drewes G et al: Phosphorylation of ser 262 strongly reduces binding of tau to microtubules: distinction from PHF-like immunoreactivity and microtubule binding. Neuron 1993;11:153–163
42. Matsuo ES, Shin R-W, Bilingsley ML et al: Biopsy-derived adult human brain tau is phosphorylated at many of the same sites as Alzheimer' disease paired helical filaments. Neuron 1994;13:989–1002
43. Alonso A, Grundke-Iqbal I, Iqbal K: Alzheimer's disease hyperphosphorylated tau sequesters normal tau into tangles of filaments and disassembles microtubules. Nature Med 1996; 2:783–787
44. Wang J-Z, Grundke-Iqbal I, Iqbal K: Glycosylation of microtubule-associated protein tau: An abnormal post-translational modification in Alzheimer's disease. Nature Med 1996;2: 871–875
45. Busciglio J, Lorenzo A, Yeh J, Yankner BA: Beta-amyloid fibrils induce tau phosphorylation and loss of microtubule binding. Neuron 1995;14:879–888
46. Schweers O, Mandelkow E-M, Biernat J, Mandelkow E: Oxidation of cysteine-322 in the repeat domain of microtubule-associated protein tau controls the in vitro assembly of paired helical filaments. Proc Natl Acad Sci USA 1995;92: 8463–8467
47. Strittmatter WJ, Weisbgraber KH, Goedert M et al: Microtubule instability and paired helical filament formation in the Alzheimer disease brain are related to apolipoprotein E genotype. Exp Neurol 1994;125:163–171
48. Goate A, Chartier-Harlin M-C, Mullan M et al: Segregation of a missense mutation in the amyloid precursor protein gene with familial Alzheimer's disease. Nature 1991;349: 704–706
49. Murrell J, Farlow M, Ghetti B, Benson MD: A mutation in the amyloid precursor protein associated with hereditary Alzheimer's disease. Science 1991;254:97–99
50. Chartier-Harlin M-C, Crawford F, Houlden H et al: Early onset Alzheimer's disease caused by mutations at codon 717 of the ß-amyloid precursor gene. Nature 1991;353:844–846
51. Mullan M, Crawford F, Axelman K et al: A pathogenic mutation for probable Alzheimer's disease in the APP gene at the N-terminus of ß-amyloid. Nature Genet 1992a;1:345–347
52. Levy E, Carman MD, Fernandez-Madrid IJ et al: Mutations of the Alzheimer's disease amyloid gene in hereditary cerebral hemorrhage, Dutch-type. Science 1990;248:1124–1126
53. Hendriks L, van Duijn CM, Cras P et al: Presenile dementia and cerebral haemorrhages linked to a mutation at codon 692 of the β-amyloid precursor protein gene. Nature Genet 1992; 1:218–221
54. Suzuki N, Cheung TT, Cai X-D et al: An increased percentage of long amyloid β protein secreted by familial amyloid β protein precursor (βAPP717) mutants. Science 1994;264: 1336–1340
55. Citron M, Vigo-Pelfrey C, Teplow DB et al: Excessive production of amyloid ß-protein by peripheral cells of symptomatic and presymptomatic patients carrying the Swedish familial Alzheimer's disease mutation. Proc Natl Acad Sci USA 1994; 91:1993–11997
56. Cai X-D, Golde TE, Younkin SG: Release of excess amyloid ß protein from a mutant amyloid ß protein precursor. Science 1993;259:514–516
57. Citron M, Oltersdorf T, Haass C et al: Mutation of the ß-amyloid precursor protein in familial Alzheimer's disease increases ß-protein production. Nature 1992;360:672–674
58. Wisniewski T, Ghiso J, Frangione B: Peptides homologous to the amyloid protein of Alzheimer's disease containing a glutamine for glutamic acid substitution have accelerated amyloid fibril formation. Biochem Biophys Res Commun 1991; 179:1247–1254
59. Lantos PL, Luthert PJ, Hanger D et al: Familial Alzheimer's disease with the amyloid precursor protein position 717 mutation and sporadic Alzheimer's disease have the same cytoskeletal pathology. Neurosci Lett 1992;137:221–224
60. Schellenberg GD, Bird TD, Wijsman E et al: Genetic linkage evidence for a familial Alzheimer's disease locus on chromosome 14. Science 1992;258:668–671
61. Mullan M, Houlden H, Windelspecht M et al: A locus for familial early onset Alzheimer's disease on the long arm of chromosome 14 proximal to the alpha 1-antichymotrypsin gene. Nature Genet 1992b;2:340–342
62. Sherrington R, Rogaev EI, Liang Y et al: Cloning of a gene bearing missense mutations in early-onset familial Alzheimer's disease. Nature 1995;375:754–760
63. Alzheimer's Disease Collaborative Group: The structure of the presenilin 1 (S182) gene and the identification of six novel mutations in early onset AD families. Nature Genet 1995;11: 219–222
64. Levy-Lahad E, Wijsman EM, Nemens E et al: A familial Alzheimer's disease locus on chromosome 1. Science 1995a;269: 970–973
65. Levy-Lahad E, Wasco W, Poorkaj P et al: Candidate gene for the chromosome 1 familial Alzheimer's disease locus. Science 1995b;269:973–977
66. Rogaev EI, Sherrington R, Rogaeva EA et al: Familial Alzheimer's disease in kindreds with missense mutations in a gene on chromosome 1 related to the Alzheimer's disease type 3 gene. Nature 1995;376:775–778
67. Cruts M, Hendricks L, Van Broeckhoven C: The presenilin genes: a new gene family involved in Alzheimer disease pathology. Hum Mol Genet 1996;5:1449–1455
68. Wragg M, Hutton M, Talbot C, and the Alzheimer's Dice Collaborative Group: Genetic association between intronic polymorphism in presenilin-1 gene and late-onset Alzheimer's disease. Lancet 1996;347:509–512
69. Scheuner D, Eckman C, Jensen M et al: Secreted amyloid β-protein similar to that in the senile plaques of Alzheimer's disease is increased *in vivo* by the presenilin 1 and 2 and APP mutations linked to familial Alzheimer's disease. Nature Med 1996;2:864–870

70. Pericak-Vance MA, Bebout JL, Gaskell PC et al: Linkage studies in familial Alzheimer's disease: evidence for chromosome 19 linkage. Am J Hum Genet 1991;48:1034–1050

71. Saunders AM, Strittmatter WJ, Schmechel D et al: Association of apolipoprotein E allele ϵ4 with late-onset familial and sporadic Alzheimer's disease. Neurology 1993;43:1467–1472

72. Strittmatter WJ, Saunders AM, Schmechel D et al: Apolipoprotein E: high-avidity binding to ß-amyloid and increased frequency of type 4 allele in late-onset familial Alzheimer disease. Proc Natl Acad Sci USA 1993a;90:1977–1981

73. Strittmatter WJ, Roses AD: Apolipoprotein E and Alzheimer's disease. Annu Rev Neurosci 1996;19:53–77

74. Corder EH, Saunders AM, Risch NJ et al: Protective effect of apolipoprotein E type 2 allele for late-onset Alzheimer disease. Nature Genet 1994;7:180–184

75. Poirier J, Delisle M-C, Quirion R et al: Apolipoprotein E4 allele as a predictor of cholinergic deficits and treatment outcome in Alzheimer's disease. Proc Natl Acad Sci 1995;92: 12260–12264

76. Van Broeckhoven C, Backhovens H, Cruts M et al: ApoE genotype does not modulate age of onset in families with chromosome 14 encoded Alzheimer's disease. Neurosci Lett 1994; 169:179–180

77. Poirier J: Apolipoprotein E in the brain and its role in Alzheimer's disease. J Psychiatry Neurosci 1996;21:128–134

78. Strittmatter WJ, Weisgraber KH, Huang DY et al: Binding of human apolipoprotein E to synthetic amyloid ß peptide: isoform-specific effects and implications for late-onset Alzheimer disease. Proc Natl Acad Sci USA 1993b;90:8098–8102

79. Strittmatter WJ, Saunders AM, Goedert M et al: Isoform-specific interactions of apoliprotein E with microtubule-associated protein tau: implications for Alzheimer disease. Proc Natl Acad Sci USA 1994;91:1183–11186

80. Reiman EM, Caselli RJ, Lang SY et al: Preclinical evidence of Alzheimer's disease in persons homozygous for the ϵ4 allele for apolipoprotein E. N Engl J Med 1996;334:752–758

81. National Institute of Aging/Alzheimer's Association Working Group: Apolipoprotein E genotyping in Alzheimer's disease. Lancet 1996;347:1091–1095

82. Post SG: Genetics, ethics, and Alzheimer disease. J Am Geriatr Soc 1994;42:782–786

83. Higgins LS, Cordell B: Transgenic mice and modelling in Alzheimer's disease. Rev Neurosci 1995;6:87–96

84. Games D, Adams D, Alessandrini R et al: Alzheimer-type neuropathology in transgenic mice overexpressing V717F β-amyloid precursor protein. Nature 1995;373:523–527

85. Goetz J, Probst A, Spillantini MG et al: Somatodendritic localisation and hyperphosphorylation of tau protein in transgenic mice expressing the longest human tau isoform. EMBO J 1995; 14:1304–1313

86. Harada A, Oguchi K, Okabe S et al: Altered microtubule organisation in small-caliber axons of mice lacking tau protein. Nature 1994;369:488–491

87. Lowe J: Lewy bodies. pp. 51–69. In: Neurodegenerative Diseases. WB Saunders, Philadelphia, 1994

88. Goldman J, Yen S-H, Chiu F, Peress N: Lewy bodies of Parkinson's disease contain neurofilament antigens. Science 1983; 221:1082–1084

89. Forno LS: The Lewy body in Parkinson's disease. pp. 35–43. In Yahr NM, Bergmann KJ (eds): Parkinson's Disease, Advances in Neurology. Lippincott-Raven, Philadelphia, 1986

90. Schmidt ML, Murray J, Lee VM-Y et al: Epitope map of neurofilament protein domains in cortical and peripheral nervous system Lewy bodies. Am J Pathol 1991;139:53–65

91. Dickson DW, Ruan D, Crystal H et al: Hippocampal degeneration differentiates diffuse Lewy body disease (DLBD) from Alzheimer's disease: light and electron microscopic immunocytochemistry of CA2-3 neurites specific to DLBD. Neurology 1991;41:1402–1409

92. Julien JP, Grosveld F: Structure and expression of neurofilament genes. pp. 215–231. In Burgoyne R (ed): The Neuronal Cytoskeleton. Wiley-Liss, New York, 1991

93. Hill WD, Lee VM-Y, Hurtig HI et al: Epitopes located in spatially separate domains of each neurofilament subunit are present in Parkinson's disease. J Comp Neurol 1991;309: 150–160

94. Bancher C, Lassmann H, Budka H et al: An antigenic profile of Lewy bodies: immunocytochemistry indication for protein phosphorylation and ubiquitination. J Neuropathol Exp Neurol 1989;48:81–93

95. Sima A, Clarke A, Sternberger N, Sternberger L: Lewy body dementia without Alzheimer changes. Can J Neurol 1986;13: 490–493

96. Pollanen MS, Bergeron C, Weyer L: Detergent-insoluble cortical Lewy body fibrils share epitopes with neurofilaments and tau. J Neurochem 1992;58:1953–1956

97. Manetto V, Sterberger NH, Perry G et al: Phosphorylation of neurofilaments is altered in amyotrophic lateral sclerosis. J Neuropathol Exp Neurol 1988;47:642–653

98. Munoz DG, Greene C, Perl DP, Selkoe DJ: Accumulation of phosphorylated neurofilaments in anterior horn motor neurones of amyotrophic lateral sclerosis patients. J Neuropathol Exp Neurol 1988;47:9–18

99. Carter J, Gallo JM, Anderson VE et al: Aggregation of neurofilaments in NF-L transfected neuronal cells: regeneration of a filamentous network by a protein kinase C inhibitor. J Neurochem 1997;67:1997–2004

100. Cote F, Collard JF, Julien JP: Progressive neuronopathy in transgenic mice expressing the human neurofilament heavy gene: a mouse model of amyotrophic lateral sclerosis. Cell 1993;73:35–46

101. Xu Z, Cork LC, Griffin JW, Cleveland DW: Increased expression of neurofilament subunit NF-L produces morphological alterations that resemble the pathology of human motor neuron disease. Cell 1993;73:23–33

102. Griffin JW, Hoffman PN, Clark A et al: Slow axonal transport of neurofilament proteins: impairment by β, β' iminodipropionitrile. Science 1978;202:633–635

103. Eyer J, Peterson A: Neurofilament-deficient axons and perikaryal aggregates in viable transgenic mice expressing a neurofilament β-galactosidase fusion protein. Neuron 1994;12: 389–405

104. Muma NA, Cork LC: Alterations in neurofilament mRNA in hereditary canine spinal muscular atrophy. Lab Invest 1993; 69:436–442

105. Collard JF, Cote F, Julien JP: Defective axonal transport in a transgenic mouse model of amyotrophic lateral sclerosis. Nature 1995;375:61–64

106. Hughes AJ, Daniel SE, Kilford L, Lees AJ: Accuracy of clinical diagnosis of idiopathic Parkinson's disease. J Neurol Neurosurg Psychiatry 1992;55:181–184

107. Kosaka K, Yoshimura M, Ikeda K et al: Diffuse type of Lewy body disease: progressive dementia with abundant cortical and senile changes of varying degree—a new disease. Clin Neuropathol 1984;185:185–192

108. Perry RH, Irving D, Blessed G et al: Senile dementia of the Lewy body type. A clinically and neuropathologically distinct type of Lewy body dementia in the elderly. J Neurol Sci 1990; 95:119–139

109. Kosaka K, Iseki E, Odawara T, Yamamoto T: Cerebral type of Lewy body disease—a case report. Neuropathology 1996; 16:72–75

110. Ince PG, Irving D, McArthur F et al: Quantitative neuropathological study of Alzheimer-type pathology in the hippocampus: comparison of senile dementia of Alzheimer type, senile dementia of Lewy body type, Parkinson's disease and nondemented controls. J Neurol Sci 1991;106:142–152

111. McKeith I, Galasko D, Kosaka K et al: Clinical and pathological diagnosis of dementia with Lewy bodies (DLB): report of the CDLB international workshop. Neurology 1996;47: 1113–1124

112. Benjamin R, Leake A, Edwardson JA et al: Apolipoprotein genes in Lewy body and Parkinson's disease. Lancet 1994; 343:1565

113. Galasko D, Saitoh T, Xia T et al: The apolipoprotein E allele $\epsilon 4$ is over-represented in the Lewy body variant of Alzheimer's disease. Neurology 1995;44:1950–1951

114. Strong C, Anderton BH, Perry RH et al: Abnormally phosphorylated tau protein in senile dementia of the Lewy body type: evidence that the disorders are distinct. Alzheimer Dis Assoc Disord 1995;9:218–222

115. Brown J, Ashworth A, Gysdesen L et al: Familial non-specific dementia maps to chromosome 3. Hum Mol Genet 1995;9: 1625–1628

116. Wilhelmsen KC, Lynch T, Nygaard TG: Localisation of disinhibition-dementia-parkinsonism-amyotrophy complex to 17q21-22. Am J Hum Genet 1994;55:1159–1165

117. The Huntington's Disease Collaborative Research Group: A novel gene containing a trinucleotide repeat that is expanded and unstable on Huntington's disease chromosomes. Cell 1993;72:971–983

118. Paulson HL, Fischbeck KH: Trinucleotide repeats in neurogenetic disorders. Annu Rev Neurosci 1996;19:79–107

119. Simpson SA, Harding AE: Predictive testing for Huntington's disease: after the gene. J Med Genet 1993;30:1036–1038

120. Prusiner SB, DeArmand SJ: Prion diseases and neurodegeneration. Ann Rev Neurosci 1994;17:311–339

121. Prusiner SB: Novel proteinaceous particles cause scrapie. Science 1982;216:136–144

122. Palmer MS, Dryden AJ, Hughes JT, Collinge J: Homozygous prion protein genotype predisposes to sporadic Creutzfeldt-Jakob disease. Nature 1991;352:340–342

123. Collinge J, Palmer MS, Dryden AJ: Genetic predisposition to iatrogenic Creutzfeldt-Jakob disease. Lancet 1991;337: 1441–1442

124. Will RG, Ironside JW, Zeidler M et al: A new variant of Creutzfeldt-Jakob disease in the UK. Lancet 1996;347:921–925

125. Anderson RM, Donnelly CA, Ferguson NM et al: Transmission dynamics and epidemiology of BSE in British cattle. Nature 1996;382:779–788

C H A P T E R 5 0

Classification of the Dementias

DAVID NEARY

JULIE S. SNOWDEN

Dementia is not the name of a disease. It is a generic term that refers to the cognitive and behavioral disorder resulting from chronic brain disease or encephalopathy. Chronic encephalopathies may be nonprogressive, occurring, for example, as a consequence of brain trauma or cerebral hypoxia; or progressive, arising as a result of intrinsic, extrinsic, or metabolic cerebral disorder. The major focus of this chapter are the dementia syndromes that result from progressive intrinsic degenerative and vascular disease. However, extrinsic and metabolic causes of chronic encephalopathy are also considered, because they are important for differential diagnosis.

Dementia Syndromes

Traditionally, dementia has been construed as a global deterioration of intellectual function, yet there are good grounds for assuming such a definition to be erroneous. Cerebral diseases do not affect the brain uniformly, but preferentially affect certain brain regions and spare others. Moreover, psychological processes themselves are regionally organized and depend on the functioning of specific brain regions. It follows that different cerebral diseases should be associated with distinctive characteristic neuropsychological syndromes, whose identification can lead to a high degree of accuracy in clinical diagnosis. A useful empirical classification of progressive encephalopathies leading to dementia can be made on the basis of the major distribution of pathology within the brain. This classification is as follows: Cortical, Subcortical, Cortico Subcortical, Multifocal. Some disorders chiefly affect the cerebral cortex whereas others predominantly affect subcortical structures. Others affect both cortex and subcortex together. Only a minority have a multifocal distribution, having no respect for functional anatomic systems. These anatomic distinctions are reflected in highly distinct patterns of cognitive and behavioral change, and neurologic symptoms and signs. Within the classificatory framework, prototypical syndromes are described in terms of neurologic findings, the precise nature of the psychological breakdown, the distribution of cerebral pathology as demonstrated by functional single-photon emission computed tomographic (SPECT) imaging and the results of the associated electroencephalographic (EEG) recordings. This process of syndrome analysis permits a differential diagnosis of the different forms of dementia.

Cortical Encephalopathies

Functional Topography of the Cortex

Psychological functions are regionally organized in the cerebral cortex (Fig. 50-1). The posterior hemispheres are critical for perceptual and spatial functions, that is, appreciation of the identity of visual percepts (e.g., objects in the environment) and of their spatial relationship with respect to each other and to the individual. Breakdown in visual perception leads to a failure to recognize objects (agnosia) and faces (prosopagnosia), whereas spatial impairment leads to inability to navigate external surroundings (spatial disorientation). Language is dependent on the areas around the sylvian fissure, extending from the frontal into the parietal and temporal lobes in the left hemisphere. Breakdown of language leads to an inability to express and comprehend spoken and written language (aphasia) and to communicate by gesture (gestural apraxia). Parietal lesions of the left hemisphere may be associated with an inability to calculate (acalculia). The superior parietal areas are important for the organization of skilled movements. Failure of executive motor functions leads to difficulties in the purposeful use of the limbs, face, and mouth (apraxia). The medial portion of both hemispheres, designated the limbic system, which includes the hippocampus and amygdala, is essential for the acquisition and retention of information. Damage to limbic structures leads to a failure to learn new information and to recall past experience (amnesia). The anterior, or prefrontal, cortex is essential for the regulation of mental life, including strategic planning and monitoring and evaluation of actions taking place over time. Breakdown in regulatory processes leads to aberrant personal and social behavior, change in personality, and an inability to conceive of and successfully achieve behavioral goals.

Cortical encephalopathies give rise to distinct dementia syndromes, reflecting the topographic distribution of pathologic change within anterior, medial, and posterior cortices (Fig. 50-2).

Alzheimer's Disease

Alzheimer's disease is a cortical dementia,[1] in which the earliest symptom is commonly memory failure, reflecting medial temporal pathology. Patients have difficulty learning new information and are forgetful of day-to-day events. As the disease progresses past memories are also affected, although in-

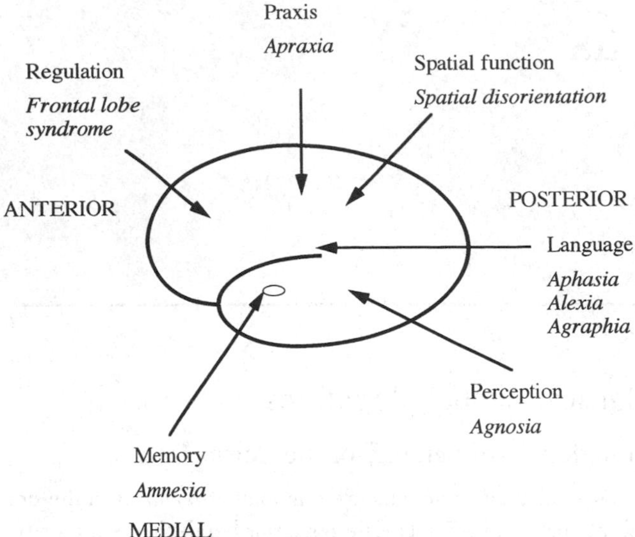

Figure 50-1 Functional topography of the cerebral cortex and the various psychological syndromes arising from breakdown of function of particular cortical areas.

formation from the distant as opposed to the recent past may appear to be relatively well preserved. Amnesia may, in a minority of patients, be the exclusive psychological symptom for many years, reflecting a relatively circumscribed distribution of pathologic change within medial temporal lobe structures. Additional cognitive deficits in such patients may emerge only at the late stages.

Visuospatial impairment is a characteristic feature of Alzheimer's disease, reflecting pathologic involvement of posterior cerebral hemispheres. Patients have difficulty aligning cutlery when laying a table, folding clothes, and orienting clothing when dressing, because of failure to appreciate spatial relationships. They become lost in their surroundings, and eventually spatially disoriented even within their own home. Spatial difficulties may dominate the clinical presentation and in some patients precede symptoms of memory breakdown. Failure of patients to recognize faces, including their own face in the mirror, and misidentification of objects often occurs late in the disease secondary to visuoperceptual disorder. Spatial problems, however, usually outweigh perceptual problems in the early and middle phase: patients have difficulty locating objects in the environment, which once located are recognized accurately.

Figure 50-2 Topographic distribution of impaired function in cortical encephalopathies.

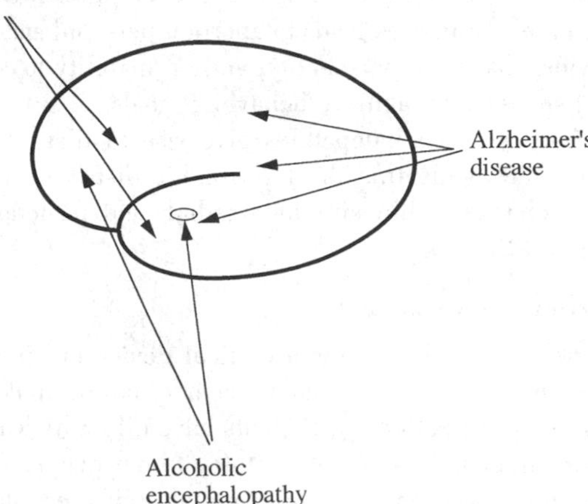

When language areas around the perisylvian fissure are involved, language skills are affected. Utterances are halting, reflecting difficulty in finding words and failure to maintain a line of thought. Repetition and comprehension, reading, and writing and calculation are impaired. Alexia, agraphia, and acalculia are compounded by spatial difficulties, because the written word and numerals are poorly organized in space. Breakdown of skilled movements of the arms and legs may be secondary to spatial disorientation, which results in difficulty with copying drawings and designs (constructional apraxia) and with dressing (dressing apraxia). Sometimes there may be severe motor executive difficulties, disproportionate to perceptuospatial impairment, that are sufficient to prevent the manual use of objects and the adoption of postures and appropriate movements on attempted walking.

In contrast to the severe cognitive deficits social graces are well preserved into the advanced stages of the disease. Indeed, the magnitude of the cognitive disorder is often masked by the patient's normal social facade. Patients rarely complain of symptoms spontaneously, although they may be aware of difficulties when confronted by test failures, and show signs of agitation and distress. The extent of insight is variable and seems to be inversely related to the severity of the patient's amnesia.

Neurologic signs in Alzheimer's disease consist of akinesia, rigidity, and myoclonus, which emerge with the gradual involvement of subcortical structures. Physical problems, however, are dwarfed by the momentous psychological disturbance and may be totally absent until the relatively late stages of disease.

The EEG exhibits progressive slowing of wave forms. Computed tomography (CT) reveals nonspecific cerebral atrophy but functional imaging techniques, such as positron emission tomography (PET) and SPECT, reveal characteristic abnormalities of the parietal regions. Abnormalities may be present in the anterior regions, but typically these emerge relatively late in the disease and invariably in the context of posterior hemisphere deficits. Demographic features, the nature and distribution of pathologic change, and genetic characteristics are summarized in Table 50-1.

Frontotemporal Lobar Degeneration

Frontotemporal lobar degeneration refers to a cortical degeneration pathologically distinct from Alzheimer's disease associated with circumscribed atrophy of the frontal and temporal lobes.[2] It encompasses distinct subsyndromes determined by

Table 50-1 Alzheimer's disease: demographic features, pathology, and genetics

Age of onset	
	Any age from 30 years onward. Most common after 65 years of age
Sex incidence	
	Affects females more than males
Duration	
	Variable, mean 7 years, range 2–12 years
Gross pathological features	
	Generalized cortical atrophy with temporal lobe preference
	Ventricular dilatation
Histopathology	
	Numerous deposits of amyloid β/A4 protein in the cerebral cortex, many with dystrophic neurites (neuritic plaques)
	Amyloid β/A4 protein deposits in cerebellar cortex and basal ganglia
	Numerous neurofibrillary tangles in cerebral cortex and hippocampus containing tau and ubiquitin
	Amyloid angiography; β/A4 protein in vessel walls
	Hirano bodies and granulovacuolar degeneration in hippocampus
Genetics	
	Point mutations in codons 670/671 and codon 717 of gene for amyloid precursor protein, located on the long arm of chromosome 21
	Other genetic loci on chromosome 14, 19 (apolipoprotein E), and 22 segregate with the disease
	Autosomal dominant inheritance

the distribution of pathology within the anterior hemispheres (Fig. 50-3). Bilateral frontal and anterior temporal lobe involvement is characterized by a prominent behavioral disorder (frontotemporal dementia). Asymmetric involvement predominantly of the left dominant anterior hemisphere leads to the syndrome of progressive nonfluent aphasia. Predominant involvement of both temporal lobes leads to a syndrome of fluent aphasia with associative visual agnosia (semantic dementia). These syndromes may be complicated by the development of the amyotrophic form of motor neuron disease. Demographic, pathologic, and genetic features are summarized in Table 50-2.

Figure 50-3 The clinical syndromes of lobar atrophy.

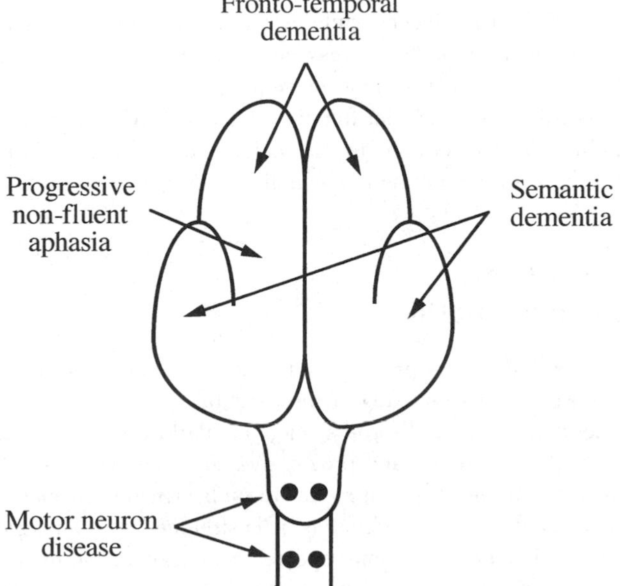

Frontotemporal Dementia

Frontotemporal dementia,[3,4] although less common than Alzheimer's disease, accounts for approximately 20 percent of cases of primary cerebral atrophy occurring in the presenium. The striking characteristic is of change in personality and social and personal behavior. Patients rapidly become incapable of managing their own affairs and lose their jobs through irresponsibility and impaired judgment. They may appear apathetic and lacking in motivation, or overactive and disinhibited. Insight is lost and, in contrast to those with Alzheimer's disease, patients show no distress or concern when confronted with task failures. Stereotyped and perseverative behaviors may occur, ranging from simple repetitive actions such as hand rubbing to complex rituals surrounding activities of daily living. Gluttony, food fads, and a preference for sweet foods are common. Speech is economic and concrete, and verbatim copying of what is said by others (echolalia) and repetition of their own responses (perseveration) occur particularly in more apathetic patients. Patients eventually become mute. Severe difficulties in abstraction, mental set shifting, organizational, and strategic skills are elicited on psychological tests sensitive to frontal lobe dysfunction. Despite the severity of their behavioral disorder, patients remain oriented in their environment and show no spatial abnormalities into the terminal stages of the disorder. Neurologic signs are minimal and consist of primitive reflexes in the early stages. Akinesia and rigidity occur very late in the disease. The EEG is normal. CT confirms cerebral atrophy, which may be more evident in frontal regions. Preferential involvement of frontal and anterior temporal lobes is typically demonstrable on magnetic resonance imaging (MRI). SPECT confirms selective abnormalities in the frontal and temporal lobes.

Progressive Nonfluent Aphasia

In this form of lobar degeneration a progressive decline in language occurs in the relative absence of other psychological deficits.[5] Speech is nonfluent, effortful, and lacking in prosody, with resemblance to a Broca-type aphasia. Repetition, series speech, and reading aloud are also impaired, with effortful production and phonemic (literal) paraphasic errors (e.g., "tig" for "big"). Word finding difficulties are prominent. Writing and oral spelling are impaired. However, auditory and reading comprehension are relatively preserved. Structural brain imaging using CT and MRI reveals atrophy of the left cerebral hemisphere. Asymmetric left hemisphere abnormalities are also apparent on SPECT imaging. The EEG may be normal or show asymmetric slow waves over the dominant cerebral hemispheres. Behavioral change akin to that of frontotemporal

Table 50-2 Frontotemporal lobar degeneration: demographic features, pathology, and genetics

Age of onset
Usually 45–65 years, range 21–75
Sex incidence
Equal sex incidence
Duration
Variable. Median duration 8 years, range 2–20
Gross features
Atrophy particularly affecting the frontal and/or temporal lobes
Bilateral frontal lobe and anterior temporal atrophy (frontotemporal dementia)
Asymmetric atrophy of left hemisphere, particularly involving frontal and temporal regions (progressive nonfluent aphasia)
Bilateral atrophy of temporal lobes (semantic dementia)
Histopathology
Affected areas of cortex show loss of pyramidal cells, microvacuolation of outer cortical laminae, and mild astrocytosis. No inclusion bodies or swollen neurons
or
Affected cortex shows severe loss of pyramidal cells and severe astrocytosis, sometimes with inclusion (Pick) bodies and swollen (Pick) neurons
Genetics
Up to 50% of patients have a positive family history of dementia; with linkage to chromosome 3 or 17. Autosomal dominant inheritance is demonstrable in some families

dementia may develop late in the disease, reflecting a spread of pathology to both frontotemporal lobes.

Semantic Dementia

Patients with semantic dementia exhibit a multimodal loss of meaning, affecting understanding of words, and face and object identity.[2] Spontaneous speech is fluent, effortless, and grammatically correct, but empty of content and there are semantic (verbal) paraphasias (e.g., "dog" for "pig"), but no sound-based errors. There is a profound anomia and lack of comprehension for spoken and written words. Repetition, reading aloud, and writing to dictation of regularly spelled words are essentially intact, reflecting preservation of phonologic and articulatory skills. The pattern of language disturbances closely resembles the transcortical sensory aphasia of focal lesions. Failure to recognize the significance of objects and the identity of faces occurs despite a preserved ability to copy accurately and match objects and faces (associative agnosia). The relative prominence of the semantic disorder for verbal and visual material reflects the relative involvement of left and right temporal lobes.

In contrast to patients with Alzheimer's disease visuospatial skills are invariably normal. Moreover, day-to-day memorizing is well preserved, contrasting with the striking loss of "semantic" knowledge. Behavioral alterations are common, although they are typically less prominent and socially disruptive than those seen in frontotemporal dementia, and have a more compulsive quality. CT reveals either nonspecific cerebral atrophy or more selective widening of the interhemispheric and sylvian fissures suggesting frontotemporal atrophy, especially involving the temporal lobes. Prominent temporal lobe atrophy is invariably detected by MRI. SPECT shows reduced uptake of tracer in anterior regions. The EEG is normal.

Lobar Atrophy and Motor Neuron Disease

Frontotemporal lobar degeneration, in particular the syndrome of frontotemporal dementia, can be complicated by the development of motor neuron disease.[6] This is of the amyotrophic form with bulbar palsy, weakness, wasting, and fasciculations of the limbs, in the absence of significant spasticity of the muscles. Typically the neurologic symptoms and signs commence after the development of the dementia and lead to death within 3 years from respiratory complications. In longer-surviving patients, the extrapyramidal signs seen in the late stages of frontotemporal dementia can make an appearance. Electrophysiologic studies demonstrate widespread denervation of muscles.

Alcoholic Encephalopathy

Both the frontal lobes and limbic system suffer damage from alcohol abuse and therefore alcoholics may exhibit a medial or anterior cortical syndrome, or both. The medial cortical or amnesic syndrome usually arises as the aftermath of an acute neurologic crisis (Wernicke's encephalopathy).[7] The patient sinks into stupor or coma, develops ocular palsies, irregular pupils, and ataxia. A proportion of individuals who survive are left with profound amnesia in the absence of the posterior cortical symptoms of aphasia, spatial disorientation, or apraxia (Korsakoff's amnesia or Wernicke-Korsakoff syndrome). They may perform normally on tests sensitive to frontal lobe dysfunction. A proportion of chronic alcohol abusers who neglect their diet present with a progressive dementing syndrome in which there are features both of frontal lobe disturbance and amnesia. The Korsakoff's amnesic syndrome is associated with gradual improvement although this may not be complete in all cases, whereas the more insidious presentation is associated with chronic decline in mental function. CT and MRI evidence of cerebral atrophy is seen in the majority of individuals with both the acute and chronic alcoholic syndromes.

Subcortical Encephalopathies

Several diseases predominantly affect subcortical structures with relative sparing of the cerebral cortex.[1] These include degenerative disorders such as Parkinson's disease, Huntington's disease, and progressive supranuclear palsy. A similar syndrome also occurs when the subcortical white matter is destroyed by multiple infarcts or is stretched and damaged as a consequence of chronic repeated head trauma and hydrocephalus. Subcortical structures and their projections to the cerebral cortex exert a quantitative and regulatory effect on the pace and organization of psychological functions. Patients with subcortical disorders exhibit slowness and rigidity of thinking (bradyphrenia) with inflexibility and difficulty in switching responses (perseveration). Although forgetful they do not exhibit a severe amnesia. They have difficulties in planning and sequencing mental events and may fail on tests sensitive to frontal lobe dysfunction, thus showing similarities to patients with anterior cortical disease. They do not, however, show the specific abnormalities of language, visual perception, and spatial functioning seen in cortical disorders. Nor do they typically show the gross behavioral disorder of frontal cortical disease. The exception to this is Huntington's disease, in which personality change and bizarre behavior are not uncommon. Progressive supranuclear palsy represents the prototypical subcortical dementia.[8]

In subcortical disorders the neuropsychological deficits are overshadowed by profound and characteristic neurologic symptoms and signs: akinesia, rigidity, and tremor in Parkinson's disease; involuntary and purposeless jerking movements in Huntington's disease, and paralysis of eye movements in progressive supranuclear palsy. The EEG may be normal or show slight slowing of wave forms but is of no diagnostic significance. CT and MRI may be normal or show nonspecific cerebral atrophy. In progressive supranuclear palsy, PET and SPECT reveal abnormalities in frontal cortex similar to those of frontotemporal dementia.

Corticosubcortical Encephalopathy

Two disorders show features of both cortical and subcortical syndromes determined by the spread of pathology to both structures. In Lewy body disease the distribution of pathology is symmetric whereas in corticobasal degeneration it is highly asymmetric.

Cortical Lewy Body Disease

Lewy body disease[9] is a disorder of the elderly without reported familial incidence. Mental changes develop before or after parkinsonian symptoms and signs of akinesia, rigidity, and tremor, which are responsive to the administration of L-dopa. Changes in the cerebral cortex may give rise to cortical symptoms of aphasia, agnosia, and apraxia but the dominant feature of the illness is a fluctuating mental state with visual illusions and hallucinations leading to secondary delusions. Such fluctuations, which are presumably due to simultaneous disorder of cortex and subcortex, are highly diagnostic, because they are not characteristic of the cortical or subcortical encephalopathies. When "confusion" does occur in these latter disorders it usually relates to systemic complications, drug toxicity, anesthesia, or the relative sensory deprivation of nighttime or unfamiliar surroundings. The EEG in Lewy body disease characteristically reveals severe slowing of wave forms and sometimes periodic wave complexes. CT reveals cerebral atrophy. SPECT reveals reductions of uptake in the cerebral cortex especially in the posterior hemispheres. Demographic features, the nature and distribution of pathologic change, and genetic characteristics are summarized in Table 50-3.

Table 50-3 Lewy body disease: demographic features, pathology, and genetics

Age of onset
Any age after 40 years
Most common after 75 years
Sex incidence
Affects males and females equally
Duration
Variable, usually a few years
Gross features
Mild generalized cortical atrophy
Depigmentation of substantia nigra
Histopathology
Lewy inclusion bodies in cerebral cortical neurons, usually layers V and VI mostly in cingulate and entorhinal cortex
Ubiquitin protein
Lewy bodies in substantia nigra
Numerous cortical deposits of amyloid β/A4 protein in 40% of patients
A few tangles present, more in the hippocampus and entorhinal cortex, and such patients have an amyloid angiopathy
Genetics
Appears to be spontaneous; no confirmed familial cases yet reported

Corticobasal Degeneration

Corticobasal degeneration[10] is a rare condition in which a cortical neuropsychological syndrome (apraxia) is superimposed on a subcortical dementia and neurologic signs of basal ganglia disorder. There is significant left-right asymmetry with respect to the severity of neurologic signs and extent of apraxia, reflecting an asymmetric distribution of pathology within cortical and subcortical sites.

Asymmetric akinesia and rigidity affect predominantly the upper limbs, which are also the site of tremor, dystonic movements, and myoclonus. Psychologically there is slowing, inflexibility, and preservation concordant with a subcortical syndrome. The cortical syndrome is characterized by a profound, asymmetric apraxia, typically most marked in the upper limbs, but gradually involving buccofacial, lower limb, and whole body movements. The limbs progressively lose all executive functions and may develop autonomous movements (alien limb). Additional features of parietal lobe disease, namely visuospatial deficits, may also emerge. CT reveals cerebral atrophy. Functional imaging (PET and SPECT) reveals asymmetric abnormalities of the basal ganglia and associated frontoparietal cortex. EEG changes are of nonspecific asymmetric slow waves.

Vascular Encephalopathy

Recurrent completed strokes lead to an accumulated neurologic and psychological deficit. The ictal nature of the evolution of the disorder, together with evidence of multiple infarctions or hemorrhages on brain imaging, is not likely to lead to diagnostic confusion.

When vascular lesions predominantly affect the subcortical white matter,[1] a characteristic subcortical syndrome (subcortical arteriosclerotic dementia) emerges that is often progressive and lacking ictal events. This syndrome requires differentiation from subcortical neurodegenerative diseases and from communicating hydrocephalus.

In a proportion of patients vascular events occur both in the cortex and the subcortex, but again without evident historic stroke-like events. The clinical picture of multiple (cortical and subcortical) infarct dementia may superficially resemble Alzheimer's disease. CT, MRI, and functional brain imaging reveals asymmetrically distributed focal lesions in the cerebral hemispheres. Demographic features, the nature and distribution of pathologic change, and genetic characteristics are summarized in Table 50-4.

Multifocal Encephalopathy

Subacute spongiform encephalopathies (prion disease), such as Creutzfeldt-Jakob disease,[11] are rapidly progressive disorders, with low familial incidence, which are often terminal

Table 50-4 Vascular dementia: demographics, pathology, and genetics

Age of onset
Any age after 40 years
More common over 70 years of age
Sex incidence
Males affected more often than females
Duration
Variable, up to 12 years
Gross features
Multiple completed infarcts in cerebral cortical and subcortical grey matter and internal capsule
or
White matter demyelination, often with lacunae, usually in frontal and temporal cortex. Incomplete infarction
Histopathology
Completed infarcts, many cases with histopathology of Alzheimer's disease
or
Fibrous and hyaline degeneration of arteries. Stenosis of lumen. Microcystic degeneration around blood vessels sometimes confluent leading to incomplete infarction of white matter. Reactive astrocytosis
Genetics
Spontaneous (associated with atherosclerosis of extracerebral arteries or hypertension and cigarette smoking)

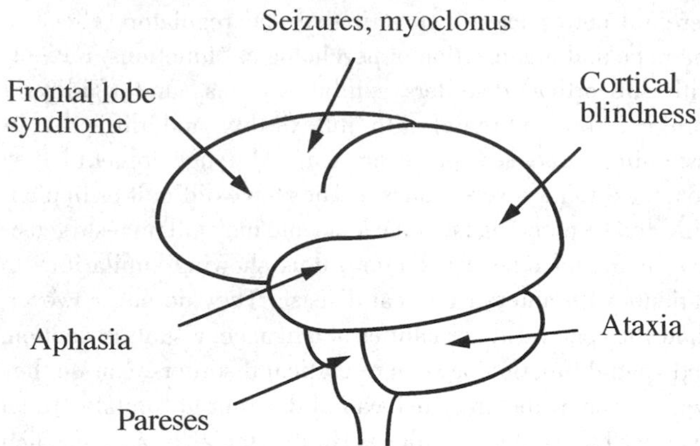

Figure 50-4 Neurologic and cognitive disorders associated with multifocal encephalopathy. The figure illustrates the potential widespread cerebral involvement, including cerebellum and brain stem as well as cortical and subcortical areas, resulting in ataxia (unsteadiness) and paresis (paralysis).

within approximately 6 months. Longer survival may occur in familial disease forms such as Gerstmann-Straussler-Scheinker syndrome.

The aggressive disease process seems not to respect anatomic boundaries or functional systems so that a wide variety of psychological and neurologic deficits rapidly emerge (Fig. 50-4). Some patients present with neurologic symptoms such as a cerebellar syndrome, cortical blindness, sensory motor deficits, myoclonus, and epileptic seizures. Focal psychological syndromes such as aphasia and ataxia may herald the onset of the disease. When thalamic structures are preferentially involved the predominant picture may be one of progressive somnolence. Despite the apparent heterogeneity of symptoms, in the early stages of the disease there is a characteristic disorder rarely seen in other encephalopathies. Dramatic fluctuations are seen in the patient's responsiveness. For long periods there may be immobility with open staring eyes and catatonic posturing of the limbs. Following these periods of unresponsiveness patients begin to move and speak, cease posturing, and are able to comment on events occurring during their nonresponsive states, indicating that they are conscious. With progression of the disease these islands of responsiveness become progressively attenuated until akinetic mutism supervenes.

The severe neurologic and psychological disorder is reflected in the grossly disturbed EEG in which there is profound slowing of wave forms and characteristic periodic triphasic wave complexes emerge. CT is either normal or reveals nonspecific cerebral atrophy. SPECT imaging reveals a patchy reduction of uptake of tracer in the cerebral cortex.

Diagnostic Considerations

Cortical, subcortical, corticosubcortical, and multifocal encephalopathies differ with respect to the relative prominence of associated mental and physical changes in the evolution of

Table 50-5 Nature and relative severity of psychological, neurologic, and electroencephalographic (EEG) disorders associated with forms of encephalopathy

Encephalopathy	Cognitive Disorder	Neurologic Disorder	EEG
Cortical	Severe, specific	Mild, specific	Slow (AD); normal (FTLD)
Subcortical	Mild, specific	Severe, specific	Nonspecific
Corticosubcortical	Severe, specific	Severe, specific	Periodic complexes (CLBD)
Multifocal	Severe, nonspecific	Severe, nonspecific	Periodic complexes (CJD)

Abbreviations: AD, Alzheimer's disease; FTLD, frontotemporal lobar degeneration; CLBD, cortical Lewy body disease; CJD, Creutzfeldt-Jakob disease.

disease (Table 50-5), providing a further basis for differential diagnosis of these disorders. Cortical encephalopathies are characterized by profound mental changes in the relative absence of early neurologic signs, whereas subcortical encephalopathies are associated with striking physical signs while mental changes may be of relatively lesser significance and tend to emerge later in the disease. In corticosubcortical and multifocal encephalopathies physical symptoms and signs emerge along with the psychological disturbance.

The EEG is also of diagnostic significance. In Alzheimer's disease the standard EEG often shows mild slowing of wave forms in the moderately advanced stages of the disease. Frontotemporal dementia is unique in that a normal record is preserved until the latest stages of the disease. Gross slowing of wave forms and periodic complexes are characteristic of the subacute spongiform encephalopathies and also of cortical Lewy body disease. Whereas CT is useful in delineating structural changes such as the presence of vascular disease or hydrocephalus, it is less useful in differential diagnosis in neurodegenerative disorders because scans may be normal or reveal nonspecific cerebral atrophy. However, high-resolution MRI may be useful in highlighting prominent areas of atrophy, complementing the clinical and SPECT findings. SPECT imaging demonstrates functional change in the brain which is of high diagnostic value in the neurodegenerative disorders, because the abnormalities on imaging closely reflect the topographic distribution of pathology within the cerebrum (Table 50-6).

Table 50-6 SPECT abnormalities in dementia

Syndrome	Disease	Abnormality
Anterior cortical	Frontotemporal dementia	Anterior deficit
Posterior cortical	Alzheimer's disease	Posterior deficit
Subcortical	Progressive supranuclear palsy	Anterior subcortical deficits
Corticosubcortical	Corticobasal degeneration	Asymmetric frontoparietal deficits
Multifocal	Subacute spongiform encephalopathy	Diffuse and focal deficits

The radioactive tracer crosses the blood-brain barrier and is taken up by cerebral tissue reflecting the cerebral blood flow and perfusion, and hence regional metabolic function. In frontotemporal dementia the characteristic abnormality in the frontotemporal lobes contrasts strikingly with the bilateral parietal defects seen in Alzheimer's disease (see Plate 50-1). An asymmetric dominant hemispheric defect characterizes progressive nonfluent aphasia, whereas predominantly bitemporal defects underlie the "semantic" dementia of fluent aphasia and associative agnosia. Subcortical disorders such as progressive supranuclear palsy display an anterior cerebral defect that is less severe than in lobar atrophy. An asymmetric frontoparietal defect is seen in corticobasal degeneration, whereas multifocal lesions are demonstrated in subacute spongiform encephalopathy.

Extrinsic Encephalopathy

Extrinsic brain disorders describe the neurosurgical conditions that lead to mechanical compression of the brain and increased space occupation within the cranium, requiring surgical decompressive relief. Two major clinical syndromes are associated with extrinsic compressive disease. The most common results from a space-occupying and expanding lesion within or on the surface of the brain such as a neoplasm, abscess, or hematoma. Here a focal and unilateral neuropsychological syndrome (e.g., aphasia and right hemiparesis) related to the specific site of the lesion in the cerebral cortex or subcortex is compounded by the symptoms and signs of raised intracranial pressure, namely headache and papilledema and progressive confusion and obtundation leading to coma and eventually death due to brain stem failure.

The second extrinsic cortical syndrome is that of hydrocephalus[1] in which, due to obstruction of the flow and absorption of cerebrospinal fluid (CSF), the cerebral ventricles expand under the increased pressure of the CSF. A characteristic syndrome emerges in which bilateral neurologic signs reflect the progressive change to the subcortical white matter and nuclei, especially those immediately adjacent to the ventricles. The gait is characteristically slow, shuffling, and wide-based with the feet seemingly rooted to the ground. There is corticospinal (pyramidal) weakness and spasticity of the lower limbs often with akinesia and rigidity. The upper limbs are less affected, although clumsy and incoordinate, and speech is slow, slurred, and indistinct. Mental function is slowed and inefficient, with response perseverations. Concentration and memory become progressively impaired but "cortical functions" are unaffected, so that aphasia, agnosia, apraxia, and spatial disorientation are absent. This syndrome shares commonalities with the "subcortical dementia" described above. However, in the case of obstructive hydrocephalus usually due to a tumor, progress is rapid and confusion, obtundation, and coma occur early. In the case of "communicating" hydrocephalus due to impaired CSF absorption the cause is more chronic, consciousness is disrupted later, and therefore the differential diagnosis from neurodegenerative and vascular forms of dementia can be more difficult and requires both structural and functional imaging and physiologic studies of the CSF pathways.

Metabolic Encephalopathy

Another important group of disorders of general medical significance that must be distinguished from progressive dementia syndromes are those arising when systemic disorders attack a potentially intact nervous system.[12] Cerebral impairment fluctuates in degree as a function of the severity of the general medical disorder, and constitutes a distinct clinical syndrome, referred to as a *confusional state*, intermediate between full arousal and unresponsive coma. The reduced level of arousal leads secondarily to reduced cognitive efficiency. Mental and physical tasks are carried out more slowly, and the ability to sustain attention and attend selectively in the face of distraction are severely compromised. Drowsiness and sleepiness may be evident. Rapid fluctuations of alertness occur. Before coma supervenes behavior may be overactive and purposeless (delirium). Language is not frankly dysphasic insofar as grammatical and phonemic paraphasic errors are absent, but patients are unable to maintain a coherent train of thought so that content of speech is irrelevant and often incomprehensible. Written expressions are typically even more incoherent than spoken utterances, and may contain perseverations of words and individual pencil strokes. Naming errors occur, with verbal substitutions and perseverations, although these are inconsistent over repeated trials.

Misperception leads to illusions and hallucinations, often of a fearful aspect. Patients have difficulty carrying out all tasks requiring organizational skills. Constructional tasks such as copying drawings and spatial tasks such as maze-trailing are failed. There is disorientation particularly for time, but often also for place, but never for personal identity. The purposeful regulation of behavior becomes impossible leading to erratic responses and motiveless wandering. Neurologic signs frequently accompanying metabolic encephalopathy are postural tremor, asterixis, and myoclonus. The EEG typically reveals diffuse slow wave large-amplitude wave forms. Metabolic encephalopathy may be produced by a variety of systemic diseases (Table 50-7). In addition to the characteristic neuropsychological syndrome there is evidence of systemic disease on clinical examination and hematologic, biochemical, and endocrine investigation.

Table 50-7 Causes of metabolic encephalopathy

Toxic state
Systemic infection
Alcohol, drug overdose
Deficiency state
Vitamin B_{12} deficiency
Hepatic encephalopathy
Renal encephalopathy
Cardiorespiratory encephalopathy
Endocrine disorder
Diabetic ketoacidosis
Hypoglycemia
Hypothyroidism
Electrolyte imbalance
Hyper- and hyponatremia
Hyper- and hypocalcemia

Metabolic encephalopathy is likely to account only for a small proportion of the chronic encephalopathies typically encountered by specialists working with the elderly. Nevertheless, recognition of its features is essential so that it can be accurately distinguished from dementia due to progressive intrinsic brain disease. The clinical differentiation is of high therapeutic import because the metabolic encephalopathies are essentially treatable. Diagnosis and treatment of systemic disease, especially in the early stages, can lead to a complete resolution of the metabolic encephalopathy. Moreover, patients with dementia due to intrinsic brain disease, in whom an inexorable decline is inevitable, are themselves not immune, but indeed are more susceptible, to the development of metabolic encephalopathy because they have less cerebral reserve and are more likely to be old and frail. The development of fluctuations in arousal and especially nocturnal confusion in patients with dementia should instigate a search for systemic complications such as drug intoxication and infection.

Conclusion

Dementia is a generic term embracing a number of neuropsychological syndromes characteristic of different brain diseases. Dementia is not a nonspecific end-stage intellectual failure, nor is it a synonym for brain disease. Hierarchical descriptions at the levels of neurologic and psychological behavior taken together with the results of brain imaging and electrophysiology permit a rational classification of disorders leading to forms of dementia.

References

1. Cummings JL, Benson DF: Dementia. A Clinical Approach. Butterworth-Heinemann, Boston, 1992

2. Snowden JS, Neary D, Mann DMA: Fronto-Temporal Lobar Degeneration: Fronto-Temporal Dementia, Progressive Aphasia, Semantic Dementia. Churchill Livingstone, New York, 1996

3. Gustafson L: Frontal lobe degeneration of non-Alzheimer type. II. Clinical picture and differential diagnosis. Arch Gerontol Geriatr 1987;6:209–223

4. Neary D, Snowden JS, Northen B, Goulding PJ: Dementia of frontal lobe type. J Neurol Neurosurg Psychiatry 1988;51: 353–361

5. Mesulam M-M: Slowly progressive aphasia without generalized dementia. Ann Neurol 1982;11:592–598

6. Neary D, Snowden JS, Mann DMA, Northern B: Frontal lobe dementia and motor neurone disease. J Neurol Neurosurg Psychiatry 1990;53:23–32

7. Victor M, Adams RD, Collins GH: The Wernicke-Korsakoff Syndrome. Blackwell, Oxford, 1971

8. Albert ML, Feldman RG, Willis AL: The subcortical dementia of progressive supranuclear palsy. J Neurol Neurosurg Psychiatry 1974;37:121–130

9. Lennox G, Lowe EJ, Landon M: Diffuse Lewy body disease: clinical features in 15 cases. J Neurol Neurosurg Psychiatry 1989;52:709–717

10. Gibb WRG, Luthert PT, Marsden CD: Corticobasal degeneration. Brain 1989;112:1171–1192

11. Matthews WB: Creutzfeldt-Jakob disease. pp. 289–299. In Frederiks JAM (ed): Handbook of Clinical Neurology. Elsevier, Amsterdam, 1985

12. Albert MS, Moss MB: Acute confusional states. pp. 100–114. In Geriatric Neuropsychology. Guilford Press, New York, 1988

CHAPTER 51

Presentation and Clinical Management of Dementia

EVELYN M. RUSSELL
ALISTAIR BURNS

The purpose of this chapter is to provide an overview of the presentation and clinical management of dementia. The clinical manifestations of dementia can be described in three categories: (1) *neuropsychological*: memory loss (amnesia) is universal and often associated with aphasia, apraxia, and agnosia; (2) *neuropsychiatric*: psychiatric symptoms and behavioral disturbances have become increasingly recognized as important expressions of the syndrome, are distressing to caregivers, and often determine the need for institutionalization; (3) *activities of daily living*: loss of abilities to care for oneself can lead to practical difficulties in management of patients and loss of independence is probably what people fear most.

Discussions of the management of dementia usually revolve around drugs to ameliorate the progression of cognitive impairment. Although there are agents that have a positive impact on memory loss, there is no curative treatment. This inevitably encourages a pervasive attitude of therapeutic nihilism. However, there is much that can be done for patients and their families in terms of diagnosis, education, alleviation of excesses of behavior and distressing symptoms, advice, and practical help. These are of enormous help and are greatly appreciated.

Diagnosis

Dementia is defined[1] as "an acquired global impairment of intellect, memory and personality, but without impairment of consciousness." It is almost always of long duration, usually progressive, and often irreversible, but these latter features, according to Lishman,[1] are not generally included as part of the definition. Some classification systems such as the International Classification of Diseases, 10th Edition (ICD-10) state that the impairment must be of at least 6 months duration.

A diagnosis of dementia does not carry any etiologic implication. Dementia defines a clinical syndrome affecting brain function in a similar way that jaundice defines a clinical syndrome affecting the liver. As with jaundice, dementia has a number of causes both intra- and extracranial (cf. intrahepatic and extrahepatic). The list of causes is long and includes infection (e.g., Creutzfeld-Jakob disease), metabolic (e.g., thyroid disease), nutritional (e.g., B_{12} deficiency), vascular (e.g., multi-infarct dementia), inflammatory (e.g., systemic lupus erythematosus), malignancy (e.g., meningioma), obstructive (e.g., normal pressure hydrocephalus), and degenerative (e.g., Alzheimer's disease and Lewy body dementia).

Differential Diagnosis

The most important differential diagnoses of dementia in older people are delirium and depression. The situation is complicated by the fact that patients may have one or even both of these conditions superimposed on a dementia. Delirium can be recognized by the presence of marked fluctuations in the clinical picture of the patient (a change over a day may encourage relatives and even staff to suppose a degree of control is being exercised by the patient) and characteristically is associated with impaired concentration, poor attention, overarousal and changes in behavior, fearful affect, and perceptual abnormalities such as visual hallucinations. Clouding of consciousness was previously the hallmark by which delirium was diagnosed but it is a difficult sign to detect and disorders of attention and concentration tend to be used as proxy measures. It can be difficult to differentiate between delirium and a dementia characterized by fluctuating cognitive performance such as vascular dementia or Lewy body dementia (see Corey Bloom[2] for review).

Depression can mimic dementia and the term *pseudodementia* was coined to describe patients who presented with cognitive impairment in the context of depressive symptoms. Recent studies using computed tomography (CT) scans have shown that such patients often have evidence of brain atrophy intermediate between normal age-matched controls and patients with dementia. Patients with depression and no associated brain abnormalities may also present with self-neglect and loss of interest and may perform poorly on formal testing of cognitive function, often giving depressive "don't know" answers to questions rather than providing an incorrect answer. The diagnosis of depression can be reached if patients are questioned about their mood, associated neurovegetative symptoms (e.g., diurnal mood variation, poor appetite, early morning wakening), poor concentration, anergia, and negative thoughts about the future and their own self-worth. Older people may not present with feelings of low mood but will admit to experiencing a loss of pleasure (anhedonia) and to giving up their interests over and above what might be normally expected for an older person. Such changes may be explained away by the patient as a natural reaction to growing old or to limitations imposed by physical disability. An informed account of the situation from a relative or caregiver may be invaluable in teasing apart the history.

Clinical Presentation of Dementia

Initial presentation

Patients with dementia tend to present to specialist services only when their symptoms are moderately severe and have started to impair daily functioning. By that stage the patient will be usually unable to give an accurate history, and indeed may deny any difficulties. A collateral history should be obtained from anyone available, preferably a family member. Although dementia may appear to have had a sudden onset, perhaps coinciding with the death of a spouse or a move from a familiar neighborhood, such an impression may have merely brought the condition to the notice of others. Support of the patient by a spouse or other caregiver can minimize problems that become evident to others only after a bereavement. A good history from a son or daughter usually describes the true nature of the sequence of events. Failing cognitive function can be minimized by adherence to rigid routines that are disrupted when the patient moves away from familiar surroundings.

Symptoms of Alzheimer's disease

Common early symptoms of Alzheimer's disease are memory impairment and disorientation in time and place. Oppenheim[3] found that in one-third of patients a psychiatric problem was the presenting complaint. Memory impairment particularly affects short-term memory, and the significance of such a change is sometimes not fully appreciated by families and others (including professionals), being dismissed as a "normal" age-related change. Changes in personality may, retrospectively, be regarded as one of the earliest signs of dementia and are well documented in the later stages. Blessed et al.[4] described 11 types of personality change that are seen, including increased rigidity, increased egocentricity, impairment of regard for the feelings of others, coarsening of affect, impairment of emotional control, hilarity in inappropriate situations, diminished emotional responsiveness, sexual misdemeanor, hobbies relinquished, diminished initiative or growing apathy, and purposeless hyperactivity.

Impairment of judgment is an important symptom that may put the patient at risk and cause concern to families.

In addition to the changes in personality and judgment the symptoms of Alzheimer's disease can be summarized[5] as the "five A's": amnesia (memory loss), aphasia (language disturbance), apraxia (inability to perform motor actions), agnosia (failure to recognize persons and objects), and associated symptoms. The associated symptoms are collectively described as the noncognitive (neuropsychiatric) features to distinguish them from the cognitive features (the first four of the A's). Neuropsychiatric features include psychiatric symptoms and behavioral disturbances. Examples of the former include disorders of mood (depression and elation), disorders of thought content (delusions and paranoid ideas), and disorders of perception (hallucinations, misidentification). Behavioral disturbances include aggression, wandering, hoarding, sexual disinhibition, and eating disturbances. It is often the appearance of the noncognitive features of the dementia that caregivers find so difficult to cope with and that results in referral to specialist services.

The overall course of Alzheimer's disease is usually steadily and smoothly progressive with death following usually within 5 to 7 years when the onset is in later life.[6]

Symptoms of vascular dementia

Differentiation between Alzheimer's disease and vascular dementia can be difficult during life in elderly people and an accurate diagnosis often depends on a reliable informant supplying a collateral history. Classically the onset of a vascular dementia is sudden and follows a clearly definable cerebrovascular accident. The course is usually described as a stepwise progression with episodes of clouding of consciousness and subsequently a fluctuating level of cognitive impairment. Apoplectiform features punctuate the progress of the disorder and are due to episodes of infarction. Commonly they consist of abrupt episodes of hemiparesis, sensory change, dysphasia, or visual disturbances. At first they can be transient and followed by gradual restitution of function but later permanent neurologic deficits appear. When the onset is more gradual, noncognitive changes are said to predate the impairments of memory and intellect. There is greater mood lability and a greater tendency toward depression and anxiety than is commonly seen in Alzheimer's disease. Very occasionally lacunar infarcts can be associated with gradual mental deterioration without focal signs. Other early features include somatic symptoms such as headache, dizziness, tinnitus, and syncope, which may be the main complaints for some time prior to diagnosis. The patchy nature of the psychological deficits in contrast to the global impairment of Alzheimer's disease is said to distinguish between the two types of dementia with relative preservation of personality and insight in the vascular dementias.

The key features that distinguish between Alzheimer's disease and vascular dementia were described by Hachinski et al.[7] and made into a checklist from which a score (the Hachinski score) is derived. The original score was based on features of vascular dementia in a textbook of psychiatry and studies of the cerebral blood flow in patients with dementia. The initial study group were relatively young and more mildly affected by their illness than are patients seen in most old age psychiatry services. A bimodal distribution of scores was found and suggested that patients with a score below 4 had a dementia of the Alzheimer's type and those having a score of 7 or above

Table 51-1 The Hachinski Score

	Points
Abrupt onset	2
Stepwise deterioration	1
Fluctuating course	2
Nocturnal confusion	1
Preserved personality	1
Depression	1
Somatic complaints	1
Emotional incontinence	1
Hypertension	1
History of strokes	2
Associated atherosclerosis	1
Focal neurologic signs	2
Focal neurologic symptoms	2

a vascular dementia. Patients scoring between 4 and 7 were thought to have a mixed picture. These key features are shown in Table 51-1. More recently the validity of using the Hachinski score to differentiate between vascular dementias and other types of dementias has been questioned. The Hachinski score has been criticized as not being sufficiently sensitive. Moreover, higher scores on the Hachinski do not mean that a diagnosis of vascular dementia is more likely and the checklist does not take into account results from neuroradiologic examinations. Infarctions are common in older people, including those with Alzheimer's disease, and thus a mixed picture is common.

The features that have been found to be most accurate in differentiating vascular and Alzheimer-type dementia include neurologic signs and symptoms, history of strokes, hypertension, and abrupt onset.[5]

Symptoms of Lewy body dementia

Lewy body dementia is characterized by a fluctuating course with distressing psychotic symptoms and marked behavioral disturbance interspersed with periods of lucidity where the degree of cognitive impairment seems relatively minor in relation to the severity of the behavioral disturbance. There are two sets of diagnostic criteria currently published: those from the Newcastle group and those from the Nottingham group.[8,9] In summary, the Newcastle criteria[8] require the presence of a fluctuating cognitive state, affecting both memory and other higher cortical functions, and at least one of the following: (1) visual/auditory hallucinations, (2) extrapyramidal signs (primary or secondary to neuroleptics), or (3) falls. Fluctuation tends to persist over weeks or months (unlike delirium) and there is no evidence of physical illness detectable to account for the disorder, specifically vascular disease.

The Nottingham criteria[9] describe the presence of Lewy body dementia as indicated by the gradual onset of dementia, the presence of Parkinsonian features, or both. Stroke, focal neurologic signs, and other causes of dementia must be absent and three or more of the following features must be present: tremor, rigidity, postural change, bradykinesia, or gait abnormality.

The psychiatric symptoms may be the presenting feature or may appear in the context of long-standing Parkinson's disease. Sleep disturbance, autonomic lability, and marked sensitivity to neuroleptic drugs are also characteristic of the illness. At times it can be difficult to differentiate between a vascular dementia and a Lewy body dementia and as with Alzheimer's disease and vascular dementias a mixed picture is not uncommon.

Investigation

The aim of the medical investigation is to establish a diagnosis and to determine the presence of coexisting disorders. An accurate diagnosis allows informed discussion of further management and prognosis with the patient and the family. For example, a diagnosis of dementia in a family member may arouse anxieties about the genetic implications and it may be that informed reassurance or referral for genetic counseling is needed and this depends on the diagnosis. Differentiating between Alzheimer's disease and vascular dementia allows the clinician to give the family information about the course of the illness.

History

The most important investigation is obtaining a full history from the patient together with further information from suitable informants. These will include members of the patient's family and close friends and other professionals involved with the patient. The family doctor will be a valuable source of information about the patient's family history, past medical and personal history, premorbid personality, social circumstances, and dynamics of family relationships.

Discussion with an informant will usually establish the onset and duration of the presenting problem. Difficulties with memory and changes in personality are usual. Problems encountered with hobbies such as following a complicated knitting pattern or playing bridge may be the first change noted. Difficulties may have become apparent after a change in social or personal circumstances when support was removed. The course of the illness is also of importance in distinguishing between vascular dementia and Alzheimer's disease. A detailed account of the difficulties that patients experience in their activities of daily living is important with due attention paid to preserved abilities.

Evidence of memory impairment can be obtained from the patient telling the same story or asking the same questions during the interview as well as from specific questions about whether the patient forgets, unless reminded, family anniversaries or important appointments. Reports of episodes where patients become lost are also important. Language difficulties may be apparent during the interview but are often elicited only on direct questioning. Evidence of dyspraxia can be obtained by judging the patient's ability to use a knife and fork and to dress. Changes in personal habits or interactions with family or friends may indicate a change in personality. Evidence of hallucinations or delusions can also be obtained from family members who may describe the situation when the patient appears to talk to someone when there is no one there, to see things when no one else can, or to have odd ideas, for example, accusing others of stealing from him or her or of not being who they claim.

Other details from the history can be of importance in establishing factors that may be of etiologic importance, such as a family history of dementia or vascular risk factors such as hypertension, diabetes, ischemic heart disease, or cerebrovascular disease.

Examination of Mental State

Appearance and behavior

Evidence of self-neglect is relevant as is the presence of disinhibited or otherwise inappropriate behavior. Guarded or hostile behavior may indicate paranoid ideas or personality change. Clouding of consciousness is an important clinical sign in differentiating between a delirium and a dementia. It can be difficult to detect and usually a deficit in attention span is taken as indicating clouded consciousness. The patient may look physically ill. Signs that may indicate depression, such as agitation or retardation, may be apparent at interview.

Speech

The patient's speech may reveal evidence of aphasia or dysarthria. Abnormalities of speech such as perseveration (when the patient continues to give the answer to the previous question in response to new questions), palilalia (when the last word of a question is repeated with increasing frequency), logoclonia (when the last syllable is repeated), or logorrhea (a meaningless outpouring of words) should be noted. The patient may echo the examiner's speech (echolalia) or actions (echopraxia). Often in dementia, speech may be fluent but somewhat banal, giving the impression of lack of content.

Thought content

The content of thought is often impoverished in dementia but careful questioning may reveal the presence of delusions or depressive ideas and the patient may elaborate on psychotic experiences.

Mood

Mood disturbances are often found in association with dementia and can be the presenting feature. Objective evidence of agitation, anxiety, irritability, or low mood should be noted. Subjective symptoms of depression are less likely to be forthcoming but should be sought.

Perceptions

Some patients may be hallucinating at interview but as psychotic symptoms are common in dementia they should be inquired about in all patients by a nondirective question such as "Does your imagination play tricks on you?"

Assessment of cognitive state

Much of the assessment of cognitive function is carried out before formal testing but a quantitative assessment is also important. Two of the most commonly used measures are the Mini-Mental State Examination (MMSE)[10] and the Abbreviated Mental Test Score (AMTS).[11] An amalgam of the two tests is shown in Table 51-2. The AMTS is used widely by geriatricians and the longer MMSE is commonly used by geriatric psychiatrists. The MMSE is scored out of 30 points of which 10 are given for orientation in time and place and the remainder for tests of attention, registration, recall, language, manipulating information, and praxis. It has been suggested that a cutoff of 23 or 24 on the MMSE is a satisfactory discriminator between cognitive dysfunction and normality. The MMSE is a useful screening instrument in clinical assessment but is not a substitute for a full history and mental state examination. Normal scores on the MMSE can be found in patients with quite marked frontal lobe abnormalities as the screen does not include tests of frontal lobe dysfunction. If the history includes symptoms such as loss of interest, poor motivation, or personality change without evidence of a mood disorder then it is worthwhile adding some tests of frontal lobe function. Such tests include asking patients to name four-legged animals or words beginning with F (where 12 or more words in a minute would be considered normal) and asking them to copy sequences of simple hand actions (when patients with frontal lobe problems often have difficulties changing set from one sequence to another).

The MMSE is a useful screen in patients referred with a possible dementia. It is quick and easy to complete and sensitive to changes over time with an expected decline of approximately 3 points each year in a patient with Alzheimer's disease.

Physical examination

Physical examination include a search for the signs of conditions known to cause dementia. Assessment of vision and hearing is important, not necessarily as causal factors in cognitive impairment but as exacerbating factors. A neurologic examination will detect focal neurologic signs that are more commonly found in vascular dementias and will detect the presence of primitive reflexes that are found in dementia.

There is some controversy as to the extent to which patients with dementia should be investigated. The argument against so doing is the assumed relatively low prevalence of treatable dementias compared to the cost of the investigations. The prevalence of different forms of dementia remains unknown and data from different studies vary greatly because of the way in which cases are selected.[12] Investigations that are most useful

Table 51-2 Cognitive function

NAME .... DATE .... NO: ....

	MMSE	AMTS
1. What time is it? (To nearest hour)		____
2. Day of the week	____	
3. Date (Correct day of the month +/− one)	____	
4. Month	____	
5. Season	____	
6. Year	____	____
"I would like you to remember this name and address: John Brown, 42 Church Street, Bedford"		
7. Name of place/hospital	____	____
8. Name of two nearby streets	____	
9. Name of town	____	
10. Name of district/county	____	
11. Floor of building	____	
12. How old are you? (exact year)		____
13. What is your date of birth?		____
14. In what year did the First World War begin?		____
15. Who is on the throne at the moment?		____
16. Can you count backwards from 20 to 1?		____
17. Spell WORLD backwards (or serial 7's × 5) (Max = 5)	____	
What is this:		
18. Pencil	____	
19. Watch	____	
20. Repeat "No ifs ands or buts"	____	
21. Three stage command: "I am going to give you a piece of paper. When I do, take it in your *right* hand, fold it in half and put in on your lap" (Max = 3)	____	
22. Can you tell me the name and address I asked you to remember a few minutes ago? John Brown, 42 Church Street, Bedford		____
23. Read the sentence "Close your eyes"	____	
24. Write any complete sentence	____	
25. Copy the drawing	____	
26. Repeat the following words: apple penny table (Repeat up to five times) (Max = 3)	____	
27. Recognition of two persons (e.g. neighbors, relatives, name photographs in room)		____
28. Can you remember the words I just said? (Max = 3)	____	
TOTAL: MMSE		30
AMTS		10

Abbreviations: MMSE, Mini-Mental State Examination; AMTS, Abbreviated Mental Test Score.

are minimally invasive and relatively inexpensive. A standard screen would include full blood count, erythrocyte sedimentation rate, serum B_{12} and folate, urea and electrolytes, liver function tests, thyroid function tests, and serologic tests for syphilis. More detailed investigation by a physician may be indicated in patients with cerebrovascular disease in order to try to prevent further strokes.

Memory clinics

The establishment of memory clinics is likely to be useful in encouraging early referral of patients with cognitive impairment. A survey of memory clinics carried out in 1993[13] showed that 20 clinics were active in the United Kingdom. Many were established in teaching hospitals in which there was an interest in testing treatments for dementia and therefore also served to provide patients with the opportunity to participate in drug trials. However, most clinics regularly referred patients on to district health and social services and 60 percent said that they themselves initiated and monitored nonresearch treatments. Published descriptions show the clinics to be broadly similar in that they are hospital-based, multidisciplinary services that provide a detailed first assessment for a small number of patients. Advocates of memory clinics argue that they will play an increasingly important role both in the assessment of patients with possible dementia referred from primary care and in the treatment of dementia.

Neuroimaging

For reviews of the role of neuroimaging in dementia, the reader is referred to Burns and Pearlson,[14] Burns,[15] and Forstl and Hentschl.[16] There are two main types of brain imaging:

structural imaging, which reflects the anatomy of the brain, and functional imaging, which assesses cerebral function in relative or absolute terms. This division is useful in attempting to understand the two types of brain imaging, but increasingly there is an integration of the two methods (e.g., by functional magnetic resonance imaging [MRI]). Structural imaging includes CT and MRI, whereas the two examples of functional imaging are single photon emission computed tomography (SPECT) and positron emission tomography (PET).

Computed Tomography

The main use of CT is to exclude intracranial lesions such as tumors (primary or secondary), cerebral infarctions, subdural or extradural hematomata, cerebral abscess, and normal pressure hydrocephalus. Two other features of the CT scan are of particular interest: cerebral atrophy and ventricular enlargement, both as a result of brain shrinkage. Cerebral atrophy (also referred to as sulcal, surface, or cortical atrophy) represents a diminution of the cortex whereas ventricular enlargement (subcortical or central atrophy) indicates swelling of the ventricular system. The CT scan in dementia can provide useful information on the following: (1) the distribution of cerebral atrophy (frontal atrophy may suggest frontotemporal dementia); (2) the size of the caudate nuclei (gross shrinkage would support a clinical diagnosis of Huntington's disease); and (3) white matter changes (indicative of small vessel vascular disease).

Guidelines for performing CT scans have been discussed by Bradshaw et al.[17] and Larson et al.[18] Alexander et al.[19] performed a study of patients over the age of 65 who had been referred for CT brain scans, reporting the presence of subdural hematoma, hydrocephalus, and intracranial tumor (which was not obviously metastatic). They found that these potentially treatable lesions were rare (145 in 137,100 person years at risk) and most presented in a way that was clearly distinguishable from typical Alzheimer's disease. Of 59 patients who presented with cognitive impairment, the following clinical features determined the likelihood of finding a lesion with over 90 percent sensitivity: cognitive impairment for 1 month or less, head trauma in the week before mental state change, rapid onset of change over 48 hours, history of cerebrovascular accident, seizures or incontinence, focal neurologic signs, papilledema, visual field defects, gait abnormalities, postural instability, or headaches.

Many people mistakenly regard the failure to find a treatable structural lesion as indicating that the scan is superfluous. However, it is important to exclude small vascular lesions such as lacunar infarctions. It is also important to evaluate the distribution of cerebral atrophy and observe the presence of leukoariaosis, which may indicate small vessel disease.

Structural brain imaging reveals the extent of cerebral atrophy. There is considerable overlap between Alzheimer's disease and normal aging. The precision with which brain scans can differentiate, in groups, between normal aging and Alzheimer's disease varies with the method of interpretation. Visual ratings have relatively low discriminatory power whereas more sophisticated, computer-assisted assessments are superior.[20] Specific analyses of certain cerebral regions have been undertaken in an attempt to improve this discriminatory power (e.g., measurements of the temporal lobe region may be particularly accurate in discriminating patients from normal controls).[21] Volumetric CT scans measurements of lateral ventricular and sylvian fissure size achieve satisfactory sensitivity and specificity distinctions between normal aging and mild Alzheimer's disease.[22,23] The entorhinal cortex is known to be affected early in Alzheimer's disease[24] and several studies have concentrated on this area as a site where differences can be found. Jobst et al.[25] found that in 44 patients with Alzheimer's disease, the minimum width of the medial temporal lobe was approximately half that of normal controls.

Magnetic Resonance Imaging

MRI scanning has several advantages: no radiation is involved, resolution is superior to CT, and there is no bone artifact. There is prolongation of the T1 relaxation in patients with Alzheimer's disease and multi-infarct dementia compared with nondemented age-matched controls.[26] However, the ability of this technique to differentiate Alzheimer's disease from multi-infarct dementia is poor and it is possible that prolongation times represent small infarcts or white matter changes that can occur in both disorders. O'Brien et al.[27] examined MRI scans in 43 patients with Alzheimer's disease and compared them with scans of 32 subjects with major depression. Atrophy ratings (on a four-point scale) were made of temporal lobe structures—hippocampus, amygdala, entorhinal cortex, parahippocampal gyrus, and cerebral cortex—and correct allocation of patients to their respective diagnostic groups was achieved in nearly 90 percent of cases. Within the dementia group, entorhinal cortex atrophy was significantly correlated with length of history.

White matter changes have been investigated extensively in Alzheimer's disease and normal aging. The exact nature of white matter changes or leukoaraiosis is still uncertain. Subcortical white matter lesions appear to be age related whereas periventricular lesions are more associated with cognitive decline and are found in Alzheimer's disease.[28,29] The prevalence of leukoaraiosis varies from 20 percent to over 60 percent and specific relationships have been found between the severity of the white matter change and the degree of cognitive impairment, particularly deficits of attention and comprehension.[30]

Single Photon Emission Computed Tomography

SPECT involves the administration (usually intravenously) of single photon emitting element (e.g., Technetium-99, Xenon-133, iodoamphetamine-123) attached to compounds (e.g., hexamethylpropyleneamineoxime) that are distributed in the brain according to cerebral blood flow. The compound crosses the blood-brain barrier and is trapped within functioning brain cells. The amount of radioactivity present can be measured by a rotating gamma camera (which can be used for any nuclear medicine examination) or by multiple scintillation counters in a machine dedicated to brain imaging. Image reconstruction allows sagittal, coronal, and transverse planes to be viewed, enabling localization of radionucleotide distribution to be made.

The pattern of distribution of tracer in Alzheimer's disease is temporoparietal hypoperfusion and comparative measures of temporoparietal blood flow (often presented as a ratio compared to the cerebellum, traditionally regarded as being unaffected in dementia) have been used to differentiate dementia from normal aging.[31,32]

Patchy distribution of tracing can often demonstrate marked abnormalities in blood flow that may not be apparent on a CT or even MRI scan. Normal pressure hydrocephalus demonstrates a pattern of blood flow reflecting the underlying structural changes (i.e., a thin area of preservation of blood flow in the cortical rim). Correlations have been found between areas of regional hypoperfusion and cognitive impairment.[33]

Specific relationships have been evaluated and associations have been found between amnesia and temporal hypoperfusion, between apraxia and decreased posterior parietal hypoperfusion, and between aphasia and hypoperfusion throughout the left hemisphere.[33] Other associations have included level of previous education, occupation,[34] and delusions and hallucinations.[35] The technique has also been used to define dementia of the frontal lobe type[36] when anterior deficits in blood flow are prominent, quite different from the posterior hypoperfusion seen in Alzheimer's disease. Diminished uptake in the caudate nuclei has been shown in Huntington's disease. Although SPECT methodology has been used for some time to image the brain and the development of new compounds and imaging systems has greatly advanced the technique, SPECT still remains to be established as a widely used and applicable neuroimaging modality in the diagnosis of dementia. It can be used to assess the response to drug treatment.[37,38] The combination of functional and structural imaging can increase diagnostic power in relation to the early assessment of Alzheimer's disease.[25]

Positron Emission Tomography

PET can be used to measure regional cerebral metabolism (as opposed to purely blood flow) in vivo. However, the practicalities of performing a PET scan have thus far precluded use in clinical diagnosis in psychiatry and the value is still primarily as a research tool.[33] The two most common positron emission compounds are ^{15}O and ^{18}F-deoxyglucose.

Frackowiak et al.[39] were the first to use ^{15}O in the investigation of dementia and showed that in Alzheimer's disease there was diminished oxygen consumption in the frontotemporal and parietal lobes with prominent frontal lobe diminution in severe dementia. Parietal lobe deficits characterized vascular dementia (possibly because of the greater frequency of infarcts in the middle cerebral artery territory). A close link between cerebral blood flow and cerebral oxygen consumption was demonstrated, suggesting that there was no chronic ischemia (which would have led to increased oxygen consumption relative to blood flow) in either vascular or degenerative dementia. Generally, the findings of PET scan studies in dementia have shown the following: there is a decrease in metabolism with increasing age; temporoparietal deficits have been found in Alzheimer's disease; less commonly frontal lobe defects occur in Alzheimer's disease; focal deficits have been described in vascular disease; specific associations have been demonstrated between clinical features and regional blood flow metabolism (e.g., between apraxia and right-sided hypometabolism, between aphasia and lower left frontotemporal metabolism, and between personality changes and decreased metabolism in frontal regions).

Asymmetric temporoparietal hypometabolism may indicate the development of cognitive impairment in previously nondemented patients but there is no real evidence that the metabolic changes occur in the absence of detectable cognitive deficits. The two tend to run in parallel, thus reducing the additional value of PET scanning in early diagnosis in Alzheimer's disease.

Electroencephalography

Electroencephalography (EEG) has been used to differentiate dementia from normal aging and more recently quantified EEG studies have been reported. In normal aging the EEG tracing is symmetric and four characteristic wave forms have been described: delta (less than 4 Hz), theta (4 to 7 Hz), alpha (8 to 13 Hz), and beta (14 to 30 Hz). Delta waves predominate in the newborn, theta waves are apparent until age 18 years, and both disappear with increasing age although some delta activity may occur in the normal adult especially during sleep. Thus, the faster rhythms (predominantly alpha and beta activity) predominate in the young adult. After the age of 60 years the EEG changes. There is slowing of the alpha rhythm from a mean rate of 10 Hz to a rate of about 9 Hz at age 80 years. Theta and delta activity increase after age 75 (theta activity is mostly focal on the left temporal region and delta activity occurs bilaterally in the anterior regions). Beta activity tends to increase throughout adult life until about age 60 and does not diminish significantly until age 80. There is evidence that increased slow activity may be associated with a number of nonspecific symptoms in the elderly, such as dizziness and headache.

In dementia, the earliest studies of the EEG showed gross abnormalities with a regular slow wave activity. However, many of these patients had advanced disease. When studies of less advanced cases were reported, the abnormalities seen were inconsistent and poorly correlated with the degree of dementia. The EEG then largely fell into disrepute as a diagnostic instrument for dementia. Cummings and Benson[40] describe the situation where a normal EEG in the presence of severe dementia was likely to be indicative of Alzheimer's disease whereas an abnormal tracing in mild impairment was associated with delirium. The EEG is usually normal in very early stages of Alzheimer's disease but diffuse slowing of the tracing can occur thereafter. As the disease progresses there is progressive slowing of the tracing with alpha and beta activity decreasing symmetrically and delta and theta waves increasing. Soininen et al.[41] found that EEG abnormalities were present in 52 percent of 62 patients with Alzheimer's disease but only 1 of 90 in age-matched controls. The average dominant frequency was 7 Hz in the patient group and 9 Hz in the control group. Another important feature in dementia is the presence of paroxysmal bifrontal delta waves, which are more common in dementia than normal aging. It has been shown in Alzheimer's disease that there was a decrease in the mean frequency of dominant occipital activity[42] of the alpha-theta ratio and an increase of the relative or absolute theta power whereas delta power increases in the later stages of the illness.[43,44]

Treatments in Dementia

Treatments can be divided into pharmacologic therapies for the cognitive and noncognitive features of dementia and nonpharmacologic interventions.

Pharmacologic Treatments

Treatment of cognitive deficits in Alzheimer's disease

Modification of cholinergic systems Among the neurotransmitter abnormalities found in Alzheimer's disease, deficits in the acetylcholine system have been the most consistently found.[45] The synthesis and degradation of acetylcholine is shown in Figure 51-1.

There are three ways in which the concentration of acetylcholine can be increased as indicated above: (1) loading the substrate, (2) actions on the receptors for acetylcholine, and (3) inhibiting the enzyme responsible for the breakdown of acetylcholine.

SUBSTRATE LOADING Attempts to replace acetylcholine by loading with one of the precursors of acetylcholine, choline, produced disappointing results.[46] Increasing the level of the other precursor, Acetyl CoA, has been more successful and a small double-blind study of L-acetylcarnitine versus placebo in patients with Alzheimer's disease has shown some benefit in slowing the progression of the disease.[47] L-Acetylcarnitine, in addition to its effects on acetyl-coenzyme A, also affects the enzyme that catalyzes the formation of acetylcholine and affects the uptake of choline and the release of acetylcholine.

ACETYLCHOLINE RECEPTOR AGONISTS There are two main types of receptors in the cholinergic system: muscarinic receptors such as those found at the neuromuscular junction and nicotinic receptors including those found at synapses within ganglia. In the brain, the system seems even more complicated with at least five different subgroups of muscarinic receptors having been identified. Early animal studies using direct agonists appeared promising when used in animals but did not produce the expected improvements in cognitive function in humans. Moreover, the need to administer some of these drugs parenterally made them unsuitable for clinical use. Overall, studies with muscarinic agonists have produced disappointing results.[48] There is some suggestion that agonists of nicotinic receptors may have some benefit. Individuals who smoke have a reduced risk of developing Alzheimer's disease.[49] Studies have used only small samples of patients and have not shown consistent changes although subcutaneous nicotine may have some effect on cognitive function.

ACETYLCHOLINESTERASE INHIBITORS More success has been obtained with acetylcholinesterase inhibitors. Physostigmine appears reliably to improve memory in some patients[50] but the short half-life, narrow therapeutic index, and poor oral absorption of the compound make it unsuitable for clinical use.

Tetrahydroaminoacridine (THA, tacrine or Cognex) has been the most extensively studied of the anticholinesterases and is presently the only drug available for treatment of cognitive features in Alzheimer's disease although it is not licensed in the United Kingdom at the time of writing. Initial doubts about the clinical efficacy of tacrine resulted from methodologic problems. The initial study by Summers and colleagues[51] in 1986 was hailed, in the journal in which it was published—the *New England Journal of Medicine*—as "a triumph for scientific method." The effects of THA in 17 patients with moderate to severe Alzheimer's disease were reported. The trial was in three phases: a nonblind assessment, a double-blind placebo-controlled crossover study, and an assessment of the long-term effects of the drug over a period of 1 year. Dramatic improvements were reported during the third phase of the trial in the absence of serious side effects. A number of questions about the methodology of the trial were raised in subsequent correspondence in the journal, and the American Food and Drug Administration was prompted to investigate the matter when an application to license the drug was submitted. This investigation uncovered methodologic flaws in the design

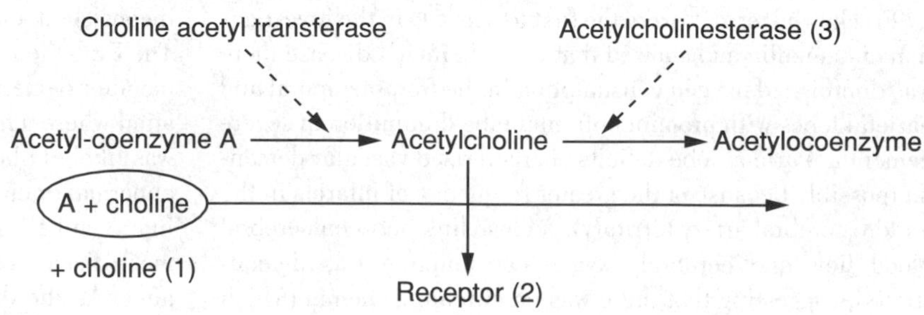

Figure 51-1 Synthesis and degradation of acetylcholine.

of the study and the assignment of patients to drug and placebo groups. The accompanying publicity prompted the research community into designing more methodologically sound trials. These have consistently shown a significant advantage for tacrine over placebo on both cognitive tests and on observations made by clinicians and caregivers.[52–55] However, the response to tacrine is variable and only 20 to 30 percent of patients show a significant response with up to one-half of patients withdrawing from trials due to adverse events, including gastrointestinal effects (e.g., nausea, vomiting, diarrhea, loss of appetite), aggression and irritability, skin rashes, and headaches. The major problem found with the drug was elevation of liver transaminases, indicating some liver damage[56] and this occurred in 40 percent of individuals. In about one-quarter of patients who have taken the drug the level was raised to three times normal. The effect was dose related and reversed after withdrawal of the drug. Tacrine without a doubt offers significant benefits to a subgroup of Alzheimer's disease patients; however, it is not possible to predict who will respond positively to THA and how long the effect will last.

Modification of other neurotransmitter systems Although most early research concentrated on developing drugs that modify transmission in the cholinergic pathways in the brain, there is evidence that all the main neurotransmitters are reduced with increasing age and in patients with Alzheimer's disease.[57] However, neither treatment with noradrenergic receptor agonists[58] nor with serotonin reuptake inhibitors (SRI) has been successful in altering cognitive function. It has been suggested[59] that Citalopram, one of the newer selective serotonin reuptake inhibitors (SSRIs) may be of some benefit in Alzheimer's disease but the evidence suggests that it is helpful in relieving symptoms of irritability, anxiety, and restlessness rather than having any significant effect on cognitive function per se.

Drugs acting on the dopamine system have also been investigated and of these selegiline has shown the most promise with both cognitive and noncognitive effects.[60,61]

Cerebroactive compounds Other cerebroactive compounds can be divided into the cerebral vasodilators and the nootropics. There is no evidence from double-blind placebo trials of any benefit on cognitive function from cerebral vasodilators. Schneider and Olin[62] reviewed the efficacy of Hydergine and found the drug to be more effective than placebo but to have a very modest benefit.

The nootropics are a chemically heterogeneous group of compounds that are thought to directly activate higher integrative brain mechanisms with the results that there is enhanced cortical vigilance and restoration of deficient higher nervous activity. The "original" nootropic is the compound Piracetam, which is a cyclic derivative of GABA and is thought to work by converting adenosine diphosphate to adenosine triphosphate, thus increasing the intracellular energy levels. Double-blind placebo studies, although failing to show any improvement, did demonstrate a reduction in the rate of progression of the dementia in the active drug group.[63] Results from other compounds remain inconclusive and overall the role of nootropics in the management of dementia is unproven.

Other mechanisms Research on animal models has yielded important information about the role of neurotrophic factors in regulating cholinergic neurons and of the mechanisms involved in the deposition of amyloid protein in degenerative disorders, but to date these findings have not led to the development of strategies for treatment of Alzheimer's disease. For a review of biologic nonpharmacologic treatments, the reader is referred to Wilcock and Dawbarn.[64]

In summary, the only pharmacologic agent available (in some countries) for treatment of the cognitive impairment occurring in Alzheimer's disease is tetrahydroaminoacridine (trade name, Cognex) but other classes of compounds are being evaluated and other compounds are awaiting approval by the regulatory authorities. Treatments to slow down the progress of the disease by blocking the formation of amyloid or tau phosphorylation are not currently available but offer the hope of prevention.

Management of noncognitive symptoms of dementia

Mood disorders Depressive symptoms in a patient with dementia should be treated vigorously. Such symptoms include low mood, anhedonia, pessimism about the future, irritability, sleep disturbance, diurnal variation in mood or behavior, weight loss, and appetite changes. Treatments include tricyclic antidepressants (e.g., amitriptyline, lofepramine, trazodone); SSRIs (e.g., fluoxetine, sertraline, citalopram, paroxetine, fluvoxamine), and monoamine oxidase inhibitors (e.g., Phenalzine). About 60 to 70 percent of depressed patients derive benefit from treatment regardless of the choice of drug. The side effect profile and individual preference of the clinician normally govern the choice of drug. The anticholinergic effects of the tricyclics are said to further impair cognitive function but this is rarely a problem in practice. Toxic confusional states can be a result of treatment with tricyclics (as with many drugs in patients with dementia); therefore, starting doses need to be much lower than in younger adults and the patients need careful monitoring for adverse side effects. Clinical experience shows that a good response to the drug is often found with doses of tricyclics (e.g., amitriptyline 10 mg three times a day), which would be considered well below the therapeutic dose in younger adults. SSRIs seem to be well tolerated in older people and are preferable in patients with cardiac problems or where the anticholinergic effects make tricyclics inadvisable. Some clinicians would choose an SSRI as their first choice of antidepressant and some a tricyclic regardless of the patient's age. The atypical antidepressants such as trazodone, the newer selective reversible monoamine oxidase inhibitors such as moclobemide, and drugs acting on both noradrenergic and serotonin receptors such as venlafaxine, also all have a role in the treatment of depression in patients with dementia. Restlessness and an inner feeling of being driven can also be helped by small doses of a sedating tricyclic antidepressant such as amitriptyline.

In patients with vascular dementia emotional lability can be a problem both for patients and their families and there is some suggestion that SSRIs may be helpful in dealing with this symptom.

Behavioral disturbances Drugs are commonly prescribed for agitation in dementia.[65] Neuroleptics are widely used for agitation and aggression regardless of the cause of the symptom.[66] These drugs are very useful but do not replace the need for appropriate investigation and treatment of patients and attention to physical factors such as constipation or a urinary tract infection that may produce a deterioration in behavior. Most studies have shown neuroleptics to be better than placebo in the treatment of symptoms of agitation, overactivity, and restlessness. A meta-analysis of the literature suggests that about 18 percent of agitated patients benefit from treatment with neuroleptics.[66] Thioridazine and haloperidol have been shown to be equally efficacious.[67] However, both drugs have significant side effects and the lowest effective dose should always be used. Side effects include extrapyramidal symptoms of stiffness, tremor and gait disturbance that mimic the symptoms of Parkinson's disease, tardive dyskinesia, postural hypotension, agranulocytosis, liver and cardiac toxicity, sedation, and anticholinergic side effects. Some side effects such as the postural hypotension and the anticholinergic effects can be a problem clinically whereas others such as sedation can be beneficial in some patients.

Anticholinergic drugs such as procyclidine that are used in younger patients to counteract the extrapyramidal side effects of neuroleptic drugs are best avoided in elderly people with dementia as they can significantly impair cognitive function. Instead the drug dosage should be reduced or the drug stopped completely if side effects are bothersome.

Newer neuroleptics such as risperidone are also useful in the treatment of patients with agitation or other behavioral disturbances, particularly in patients who have had marked side effects when treated with conventional neuroleptics.[68]

Aggression and irritability can also be helped in some patients by SSRIs or trazodone.[69] These effects on aggression and irritability are often seen much earlier than would be expected from an antidepressant effect and it is likely that antidepressant drugs have specific effects in addition to their antidepressant actions. Trazodone also seems to be of benefit in a minority of patients in stopping apparently purposeless shouting.

Psychotic symptoms Psychotic symptoms are common in dementia and if they are distressing or result in disturbances of behavior it is appropriate to treat them. Paranoid ideas are common, often relate to members of the family or other caregivers, and respond well to neuroleptics. Low doses of trifluoperazine are often helpful in this situation as the side effects are relatively mild; haloperidol is also useful. The treatment of the psychotic symptoms and disturbed behavior in patients with Lewy body dementia needs to be considered carefully in view of the increased mortality resulting from neuroleptic treatment.[70] Recommendations from the Committee for Safety of Medicines[71] have emphasized the need for caution. Chlormethiazole can be useful either alone or in conjunction with lorazepam, which is an effective anxiolytic and sedative.

In some patients with a less marked sensitivity to neuroleptics, a very cautious introduction of an atypical neuroleptic such as risperidone may be worthwhile.

Nonpharmacologic Treatments

Specific treatments for some of the symptoms of dementia have been developed and both patients and their families benefit. To maximize the benefit, these treatments should be administered with empathy and understanding of the patient's predicament and a recognition of their past experiences. Patients, even those with quite severe dementias, should be encouraged to participate as fully as they are able with the activities of daily living, to make choices, to engage in activities, and to interact socially. Providing such an environment of care requires considerable time and expertise and has financial implications.

Memory training

At present, most patients with dementia are referred to specialist services when their illness is too severe for any benefit to be gained from memory training. However, for people with mild memory impairment the maxim "use it or lose it" is relevant. Techniques to aid memory, for example, by making visual associations, together with the use of prompts have been shown to be helpful. Often, over the early stages of the development of the memory impairment, patients and their families have put such ideas into practice but there are some patients who can benefit from the formal teaching of such techniques either individually or in groups.[72,73]

Behavior modification

The basis of the technique is often described as the ABC of behavior where A is the antecedent, B the behavior itself, and C the consequences of the behavior. Behavior modification can be useful with a range of undesirable behaviors such as aggression, wandering, screaming, incontinence, lack of cooperation when personal care is being provided, repetitive or stereotyped behavior, and some types of incontinence.

Caregivers are first asked to give a detailed description of the type and circumstances of the undesired behavior. From that information, it is usually possible to establish a treatable cause such as constipation. A valuable part of the therapy is the hope that it offers caregivers that something can be done to improve the lives of both the patient and the caregivers.

Reality orientation

Disorientation to time and place is an early symptom of dementia and there are two forms of reality orientation, an informal or a 24-hour reorientation when all opportunities are taken to orient the patient to time and place.[74] Orientation boards common in most institutions are examples. A more formal structured reality orientation session consists of a small number of patients undergoing a program of discussion exploring topics of interest. Exponents of formal reality orientation emphasize that these sessions are intended as a supplement to, as opposed to an alternative for, 24-hour reality orientation. It is fundamental in both types of reality orientation that staff or caregivers do not collude with patients in situations where the patient is clearly mistaken.

Although the relationship between patient and therapist is fundamental to all psychotherapeutic interventions including behavioral therapy and reality orientation, such techniques in practice may not encompass important features such as empathy, support, and nonjudgmental listening. Reality orientation may degenerate to sharply worded information about today's date with a lack of sensitivity to the patient's feelings and cognitive impairment. It has been criticized as a "dehumanizing" behavior modification technique solely preoccupied with targeting symptom management. However, evaluations of reality orientation have clearly demonstrated improvements in verbal orientation and have a positive effect on staff and caregivers.[74]

Validation therapy

Validation therapy is a more patient-centered therapy that was designed to validate the patient's past and present experiences and feelings. It was designed for use in elderly patients with dementia and emphasizes the need to interact in "whatever reality they are in, in order to ease distress and restore self-worth."[75] Thus, for example, if a patient became anxious about the need to collect her children from school, the therapist would start by sharing the anxiety associated with these thoughts and then gradually move the patient through that phase of their life to the present day. The precise date is of less importance in this therapy than the patient's stage in the life cycle and a sharing of their past experiences. As with reality orientation these techniques can be used formally in groups or can be incorporated into round-the-clock care for the patient. Although widely used in institutions, especially in the United States, the evidence that they are useful is solely anecdotal.

Reminiscence therapy

A range of other techniques have been used with patients with dementia with the aim of increasing their quality of life. Reminiscence therapy is widely used. It has its roots in psychodynamic theory and ideas about the process of life review in later life where past experiences are reviewed and past conflicts can be looked at again and re-integrated. Most often the technique is applied as a group therapy. Groups of patients normally meet with a therapist and various techniques are used to help patients recall parts of their personal memory. Photographs of past times, music, or other sensory experiences such as smells are used as triggers to memory and then the therapist aims to facilitate discussion. Specifically designed packages of audiovisual material have been produced for use in reminiscence therapy. According to King[76] meeting in groups allows opportunity for socialization and social re-integration, resolution of old conflicts through life review, identification of current concerns and struggles, recognition of self as a survivor, and appreciation of one's own achievements and those of others.

Much of the published work on reminiscence therapy is anecdotal and many of the studies have not included a control group. Reminiscence therapy groups are reported as often being enjoyed by both staff and patients and are important in giving both groups a sense of mastery. The groups are also said to increase staff knowledge of their patients and to increase the quality of interactions between patients and staff. It is not clear to what extent these positive benefits are nonspecific or related to the reminiscence therapy. No lasting effects on memory have been reported in controlled trials.

Expressive therapies

Other techniques are used with patients with dementia, not only to provide interest and occupation, but also to reduce anxiety and aid self-expression, often through nonverbal routes. Art and music are used as are techniques involving physical contact. Hand massage and aromatherapy using specific oils are increasingly used and are likely to have at least some nonspecific benefit. The Snoezelen technique, used for people with mental handicap,[77] has also been used in severely demented patients with the aim of providing input through a range of senses.

Longer term management of patients with dementia

Dementia affects not only the patient but predominantly the patient's family. Many spouses caring for patients with dementia are elderly and frail themselves and many are reluctant to accept help until a crisis point is reached and they can no longer cope. An emergency or unplanned admission to institutional care then becomes the only solution. Nonmedical professionals, including community psychiatric nurses, occupational therapists, physiotherapists, psychologists, speech therapists, and social workers all have important roles in the management of dementia. It is important that one professional takes over the role of key worker and is responsible for maintaining good communication between members of the team so that a package of care is delivered.

The initial assessment of patients will include their physical, psychological, and social environment. Care will be required for their self-care, shopping, and food preparation. Activity will often be needed and this may be provided within the circle of family and friends; within the wider community, for example, by church or voluntary groups; at a social services day center, or at a day hospital. If the patient is being cared for at home the needs of the family must be considered and it may be important to provide some day care and/or respite care to allow the caregiver to have a break and to encourage the

Table 51-3 Services available

Primary care team
General practitioner
District nurse
Health visitor
Practice nurse
Counseling/psychology
Social services
Domiciliary care (elderly care team)
Social work assessment
Home help
Meals on wheels
Sitting services
Continence service
Chiropody
Laundry service
Other
Day centers
Residential care
Respite care
Housing
Hospital services
Geriatric psychiatrist
Geriatrician
Psychologist
Domiciliary assessment
Hospital admission
Long-term/respite care
Community psychiatric nurses
Day hospitals
Multidisciplinary team assessment
Physiotherapy
Occupational therapy
Speech therapy
Voluntary agencies
Alzheimer's Disease Society
Age Concern
Housing associations
Others
Private nursing/residential homes
DSS—attendance allowance

caregiver to join a support group, such as one run by the Alzheimer's Disease Society. Table 51-3 outlines the services that are potentially available to an individual with dementia. The provision of such a package of care requires time and effort to understand the needs of both the patient and his or her family and to tailor the care to those needs. The needs of patients and their caregivers will change over time and the provision of care should be flexible to cope with these changes. New symptoms or behaviors may develop in the course of the illness and these need to be dealt with using the treatments already discussed. Although many patients wish to stay at home and care should be provided for them, institutional care can be beneficial for other patients and should not always be seen as the last resort. Removing the daily burden of care from a relative may enhance the relationship between patient and family and allow both to enjoy the patient's last years or months of life.

Conclusions

The management of dementia is complex, including many techniques ranging from highly technologic neuroimaging to hand massage. The first stage in the management is to obtain a definitive diagnosis. Where a treatable etiology is identified this should be treated. For the majority of patients with a progressive and untreatable dementia a long-term management plan needs to be drawn up that employs general therapeutic principles supplemented by specific pharmacologic, psychological, and social interventions as necessary to meet the needs of the individual patient and the family. Teamwork is essential for the delivery of such a service. Due recognition must be given to the skills and knowledge both of the various professionals in the team and also of others such as members of the family, friends, community members, caregivers such as home helpers, and voluntary workers, all of whom have important contributions to make to the care of the patient.

References

1. Lishman WA: Organic Psychiatry: The Psychological Consequences of Cerebral Disorder. 2nd Ed. Blackwell Scientific Publications, Oxford, 1987
2. Corey Bloom J, Thal L, Galasko D et al: Diagnosis and evaluation of dementia. Neurology 1995;45:211–218
3. Oppenheim G: The earliest signs of Alzheimer's disease. J Geriatr Psychiatry Neurol 1994;7:118–122
4. Blessed G, Tomlinson B, Roth M: The association between quantitative measures of dementing and senile change in cerebral grey matter of elderly subjects. Br J Psychiatry 1968;114: 797–811
5. Burns A, Howard R, Pettit W: Alzheimer's disease: A Medical Companion. Blackwell Scientific Publications, Oxford, 1995
6. Burns A, Lewis G: Survival in Dementia. pp. 125–143. In Burns A (ed): Ageing and Dementia: A Methodological Approach. Edward Arnold, London, 1993
7. Hachinksi V, Iliff L, Zilkha E et al: Cerebral blood flow in dementia. Arch Neurol 1975;32:632–637
8. McKeith I, Perry R, Fairbairn A et al: Operational criteria for senile dementia of the Lewy body type. Psych Med 1992;22: 911–922
9. Byrne EJ, Lennox GG, Goodwin-Austen RB et al: Dementia associated with cortical Lewy bodies: proposed diagnostic criteria. Dementia 1991;2:283–284
10. Folstein MF, Folstein SE, McHugh PR: Mini-Mental State Examination—a practical method for grading the cognitive state of patients for the clinician. J Psychiatr Res 1975;12:189–198
11. Hodkinson M: Mental impairment in the elderly. J R Coll Phys 1973;7:305–317
12. Philpot M, Burns A: Reversible dementias. In Katona C (ed): Dementia Disorders: Advances and Prospects. Chapman & Hall, London, 1989

13. Wright N, Lindesay J: A survey of memory clinics in the British Isles. Int J Geriatr Psychiatry 1995;10:379–385
14. Burns A, Pearlson G: Computed tomography. In Burns A, Levy R (eds): Dementia. Chapman & Hall, London, 1994
15. Burns A: Cranial computed tomography in dementia of the Alzheimer type. Br J Psychiatry 1990;157(suppl 9):10–15
16. Forstl H, Hentschl F: Contributions to the differential diagnosis of dementia 2: neuroimaging. Rev Clin Gerontol 1994;4: 317–341
17. Bradshaw J, Thomas J, Campbell M: Computed tomography in the investigation of dementia. BMJ 1983;286:277–280
18. Larson E, Reifler B, Featherstone J, English D: Dementia in elderly outpatients: A prospective study. Ann Intern Med 1984; 100:417–423
19. Alexander E, Wagner E, Buchner D et al: Do surgical brain lesions present as isolated dementia? A population based study. J Am Geriatr Soc 1995;43:138–143
20. De Carli C, Kaye J, Horowitz B, Rapoport S: Critical analysis of the use of CT to study human brain in ageing and dementia of the Alzheimer type. Neurology 1990;40:872–873
21. Jobst K, Smith A, Szatmari M et al: Detection in life of confirmed Alzheimer's disease using a simple measurement of medial temporal lobe atrophy by computed tomography. Lancet 1992;340: 1179–1183
22. Burns A, Jacoby R, Philpot M, Levy R: CT in Alzheimer's disease—methods of scan analysis comparison with normal controls and clinico-radiological correlations. Br J Psychiatry 1991;159:609–614
23. Forstl H, Zerfass R, Geiger-Kabisch C et al: Brain atrophy in normal ageing and Alzheimer's disease. Br J Psychiatry 1995
24. Braak H, Braak E: Neuropathological staging of Alzheimer-related changes. Acta Neuropathol 1991;82:239–259
25. Jobst K, Smith A, Barker C et al: Association of atrophy of the medio-temporal lobe with reduced blood flow in the posterior parieto-temporal cortex in patients with a clinical and pathological diagnosis of Alzheimer's disease. JNNP 1992;55:190–194
26. Besson J, Corrigan F, Foreman E et al: NMR imaging in dementia. Br J Psychiatry 1985;146:31–36
27. O'Brien J, Desmond P, Ames D et al: The differentiation of depression from dementia by temporal lobe magnetic resonance imaging. Psych Med 1994;24:633–640
28. McDonald W, Krishnan K, Doraiswamy P et al: Magnetic resonance findings in patients with early onset Alzheimer's disease. Biol Psychiatry 1991;29:799–810
29. Matsubayashi K, Shimada K, Kawamoto A, Ozawa T: Incidental brain lesions on magnetic resonance imaging and neurobehavioural functions in the apparently healthy elderly. Stroke 1992; 23:175–180
30. Kertesz JP, Nalciolglu O, Cotman CW: Cognition and white matter changes on magnetic resonance imaging in dementia. Arch Neurol 1990;47:387–391
31. Burns A, Tune L, Steele C, Folstein M: Positron emission tomography in dementia—a clinical review. Int J Geriatr Psychiatry 1989;4:67–72
32. Gemmil H, Sharpe P, Smith F et al: Cerebral blood flow measured by SPET as a diagnostic tool in the sudy of dementia. Psychiatry Res 1989;27:327–329
33. Burns A, Philpot MP, Costa DC et al: The investigation of Alzheimer's disease with single photon emission tomography. J Neurol Neurosurg Psychiatry 1989;52:248–253
34. Stern Y, Alexander G, Prohovnik I et al: Relationship between lifetime occupation and parietal flow. Neurology 1995;45: 55–60
35. Starkstein et al. 1991
36. Neary D, Snowden J, Northen B, Goulding P: Dementia of frontal lobe type. J Neurol Neurosurg Psychiatry 51:353–361
37. Geaney D, Soper N, Shepstone B, Cowan P: Effect of central cholinergic stimulation on regional cerebral blood flow in Alzheimer's disease. Lancet 1990;335:1484–1487
38. Hunter R, McLuskie R, Wyper D et al: The pattern of function related regional cerebral blood flow investigated by SPET with 99 mTc HMPAO in patients with presenile Alzheimer's disease and Korsakoff's psychosis. Psych Med 1989;19:847–855
39. Frackowiak R, Pozzilli C, Legg N et al: Regional cerebral oxygen supply and utilisation in dementia. Brain 1981;104: 753–758
40. Cummings J, Benson DF: Laboratory aids in the diagnosis of dementia. pp. 285–308. In Cummings JL, Benson DF (eds): Dementia—A Clinical Approach. Butterworths, Boston, 1983
41. Soininen H, Partinen VJ, Helkala EL, Riekkinen PJ: EEG findings in senile dementia and normal ageing. Acta Neurol Scand 1982;65:59–70
42. Prinz PN, Vitello MV: Dominant occipital (alpha) rhythm frequency in early stage Alzheimer's disease and depression. EEG Clin Neurophysiol 1989;73:427–432
43. Prichep LS, John ER, Ferris SH et al: Quantitative EEG correlates of cognitive deterioration in the elderly. Neurobiol Aging 1994;15:85–90
44. Coben LA, Danziger WL, Berg L: Frequency analysis of the resting awake EEG in mild senile dementia of Alzheimer type. EEG Clin Neurophysiol 1983;55:372–380
45. Bowen D, Smith C, White P, Davidson A: Neurotransmitter transmitted enzymes as indices of hypoxia in senile dementia and other abiotrophies. Brain 1976;459–496
46. Little A, Levy R, Kidd P et al: A double-blind placebo controlled trial on high dose lecithin in Alzheimer's disease. JNNP 1985; 48:736–742
47. Livingstone G, Sax K, McClenahan Z et al: Acetyl L carnitine in dementia. Int J Geriatr Psychiatry 1991;6:853–860
48. Spiegel R, Azcona A, Wettstein A: First results with RS86, an orally active muscarinic agonist in healthy subjects and in patients with dementia. pp. 391–405. In Wurtman S, Corkin S, Growdon J (eds): Alzheimer's disease: Advances in Basic Research and Therapy. Center of Basic Sciences and Metabolism Charitable Trust, Cambridge, MA, 1987
49. van Duijn CM, Hofman A: Relation between nicotine intake and Alzheimer's disease. BMJ 1991;302:1491–1494
50. Thal et al. 1983
51. Summers W, Haovskil M, Marsh G: Oral THA in the long term treatment of senile dementia of the Alzheimer type. N Engl J Med 1986;315:1241–1245
52. Eagger S, Levy R, Sahakian B: Tacrine in Alzheimer's disease. Lancet 1991;337:989–992
53. Farlow M, Gracon S, Hershey L et al: A controlled trial of tacrine in Alzheimer's disease. JAMA 1992;268:2523–2529

54. Davies K, Thal L, Gamzu E et al: A double-blind placebo controlled multicentre study of tacrine for Alzheimer's disease. N Engl J Med 1992;327:1253–1259
55. Wilcock G, Surmon D, Scott M et al: An evaluation of the efficacy and safety of THA without lecithin in the treatment of Alzheimer's disease. Age Ageing 1993;22:316–324
56. Watkins P, Zimmerman H, Knapp N et al: Hepatotoxic effects of tacrine administration in patients with Alzhemier's disease. JAMA 1994;271:992–998
57. de Deyn PP, Verslegers W, Saerens J et al: Treatment strategies in Alzheimer's disease. pp. 177–194. In Gottfries CG, Levy R, Clincke G, Tritsmans L (eds): Diagnostic and Therapeutic Assessments in Alzheimer's Disease. Wrightson Biomedical Publishing, Petersfield, England, 1994
58. Knezevic S, Bogdanovic N, Spilich G, Chundy D: Pharmacological treatment of Alzheimer's dementia: a review. pp. 384–394. In Kostovic I, Knezevic S, Wisniewski HM, Spilich GJ (eds): Neurodevelopment, Ageing and Cognition. Birkhauser, Boston, 1992
59. Gottfries CG: Use of Citalopram in syndromes related to 5-HT disturbance. Rev Contemp Pharmacother 1995;6:307–313
60. Tariot P, Cohen R, Sunderland T et al: L deprenyl in Alzheimer's disease. Arch Gen Psychiatry 1987;44:427–433
61. Schneider L, Olin J, Pawluczyk S: A double blind cross over pilot study of selegiline combined with cholinesterase inhibitor in Alzheimer's disease. Am J Psychiatry 1993;150:321–323
62. Schneider L, Olin J: Overview of clinical trials of hydergine in dementia. Arch Neurol 1994;51:787–798
63. Croisile B, Trillet M, Fondarai J et al: Long-term and high-dose piracetam treatment of Alzheimer's disease. Neurology 1993; 43:301–305
64. Wilcock G, Dawburn D: Nerve growth factor and other biological treatments: an overview. pp. 477–492. In Burns A, Levy R (eds): Dementia. Chapman & Hall, London, 1994
65. Cohen-Mansfield J: Agitation in the elderly. Adv Psychosom Med 1989;19:101–113
66. Schneider LS, Sobin P: Treatments for psychiatric symptoms and behavioral disturbances in dementia. In Burns A, Levy R (eds): Dementia. Chapman & Hall, London, 1994
67. Steele C, Lucas M, Tune L: Haloperidol -v- thioridazine in the treatment of behavioural symptoms in senile dementia of the Alzheimer's type. J Clin Psychiatry 1986;47:310–312
68. Oberholzer A, Hendriksen C, Monsch A et al: Safety and effectiveness of low dose clozapine in psychogeriatric patients. Int Psychogeriatr 1992;4:187–195
69. Wilcock G, Stevens J, Perkins A: Trazodone/tryptophan for aggressive behaviour. Lancet 1987;1:929–930
70. McKeith I, Fairburn A, Perry R et al: Neuroleptic sensitivity in patients with senile dementia of Lewy body type. BMJ 1992; 305:673–678
71. Committee on Safety of Medicine: Neuroleptic sensitivity in patients with dementia. Curr Prob Pharmacovigilance 1994; 20(6)
72. Twining C: Can we train the brain. pp. 139–150. In Levy R, Howard R, Burns A (eds): Treatment and Care in Old Age Psychiatry. Wrightson Biomedical Publishers, Petersfield, England 1993
73. West R: Compensatory stategies for age associated memory impairment. In Baddely A, Wilson B, Watts F (eds): Handbook of Memory Disorders. John Wiley & Sons, Chichester, 1995
74. Bleathman C, Morton I: Psychological treatments. In Burns A, Levy R (eds): Dementia. Chapman & Hall, London, 1994
75. Morton I, Bleathman C: The effectiveness of validation therapy in dementia—a pilot study. Int J Geriatr Psychiatry 1991;6: 327–330
76. King K: Reminiscing psychotherapy with ageing people. J Psychosoc Nurs Ment Health Serv 1982;20:21–25
77. Haggar L, Hutchinson R: Snoezelen: an approach to the leisure resource for people with profound mental handicap. Ment Handicap 1991;19:51–55

C H A P T E R 5 2

Functional Psychiatric Illness in Old Age

VIVIENNE WATKIN
CORNELIUS KATONA

Older people may suffer a wide range of psychiatric difficulties in late life; those with concurrent physical illness are particularly vulnerable. Although these conditions tend to be underdetected and undertreated, their outcome with appropriate management is often excellent. In this chapter the clinical presentation, epidemiology, management, and outcome of depression, the schizophrenia-like psychoses and delusional disorders, mania, the anxiety disorders, alcohol-related problems, and disorders of personality in old age are discussed in some detail, with briefer discussion also of obsessive-compulsive disorder, somatoform disorders, post-traumatic stress disorder, and bereavement.

Depression

Depression is common and disabling in old age. It is often missed, ignored, or not managed adequately. This is in part a consequence of widely held "agist" misconceptions that depression is intrinsic to the aging process, and that treatment is inappropriate, excessively risky, or unlikely to be effective.

Epidemiology

The prevalence of depression in older people varies widely depending on sample selection, instruments used, and "caseness" criteria. The clinical features of depressive disorder may be complicated by its less than obvious presentation as well as by coexisting medical problems and/or cognitive impairment. It is possible that elderly individuals with clinically significant depression may not be identified as suffering from major depression defined by standard diagnostic criteria. Elderly subjects in the community appear to have a lower prevalence of major depression than their younger counterparts.[1] In an early United Kingdom community study, a 10 percent prevalence for depression in community residents was found, but only 1.3 percent met criteria for what would correspond to major depression.[2] In a recent Australian study,[3] which included individuals living in both community and institutional settings, the rate for depressive episodes as defined by Draft ICD-10 criteria[4] was 3.3 percent. The rate found using DSMI-IIR criteria[5] was somewhat higher at 11 percent. Within DSM criteria, rates for dysthymia (chronic mild depression) are far from consistent; whereas in the Epidemiologic Catchment Area Study of United States communities, the prevalence for dysthymia was only 1 to 1.5 percent in those aged over 65,[6] a Finnish study[7] reported a rate for dysthymia as high as 23 percent.

More consistent results have been achieved using semi-structured interviews and diagnostic algorithms designed to detect depression in the elderly. The most extensively validated of these is the Geriatric Mental State (GMS) interview and associated AGECAT computerized diagnostic system.[8] An alternative instrument, the SHORT-CARE,[9] is also specifically designed for the elderly and is an extensively validated diagnostic interview. It generates very similar findings. The GMS has been used in Hobart, Tasmania, with a reported prevalence of 14.2 percent for moderate to severe depression,[10] as well as in Liverpool,[11] where the prevalence was 11.3 percent, and in a two-center transatlantic study that found rates of 16.2 percent in New York City and 19.5 percent in London.[12] In these studies, the overall depression prevalence rates for women were about 50 percent greater than for men. The rates for severe depression were, however, similar in male and female subjects. An inner London community-based study using the SHORT-CARE[13] reported a prevalence of pervasive depression of 15.9 percent; this study also involved a follow-up that revealed an annual new incidence rate of 3.8 percent.

The prevalence of depressive illness appears higher among those elderly people who attend their general practitioner (GP). Rates as high as 31 and 34 percent have been reported.[14,15] There is an established inter-relationship between depression, physical disability, and contact with services.[16] Livingston et al.[13] noted a statistically significant association in community subjects between depression and frequency of GP attendance, suggesting that frequent attendance may be a "marker" of increased likelihood of depression. Not all studies, however, report higher prevalence of depression in primary care attenders.[17]

In the hospitalized elderly, the prevalence of depression rises further, with a reported range between 12 and 45 percent.[18] Similarly, the prevalence of depressive disorders among elderly people in long-term institutional care is in excess of 20 percent.[19]

Depression in old age may be complicated by underlying cerebral pathologies. The range of reported depression in people with Alzheimer's disease varies between 19 and 87 percent.[20] Studies that screen out individuals with cognitive impairment may miss clinically significant depression, although such depressive symptoms may be relatively likely to remit spontaneously.[21]

Etiology

The relationship between depression and age itself within the elderly population is not clear-cut; some studies find depression to be more common in the very old,[10] whereas others find the reverse to be true.[22] Demographic, social, and biological factors have all been implicated in the etiology of depression in old age.

Genetic susceptibility

Genetic factors are generally reported to be less important in elderly patients with depression than in their younger counterparts.[23] However, some studies have found a positive family history for depression in about one-third of patients whose depression had its first onset after the age of 60 years.[24]

Neurobiologic risk factors

Brain electrical activity has shown some discriminatory power in elderly patients with depression. A study using sleep electroencephalogram recordings found depression in older subjects to be associated with reduced rapid eye movement (REM) latency and increased proportion of REM sleep.[25] A study of auditory evoked potentials[26] demonstrated increased P300 variability in older subjects with depression.

Neuroendocrine responses, such as the dexamethasone suppression test (DST), are more likely to be abnormal in older than in younger patients with depression.[27] The DST is, however, unhelpful in distinguishing depression from dementia because it may be abnormal in both conditions.[28]

In both depression and aging, there may be decreased nonadrenergic responsiveness with compensatory increases in postsynaptic receptor number. A positive correlation has been noted between age and platelet α-2 adrenergic binding capacity in controls but not in subjects with depression.[29] Aging may enhance depression-associated changes in serotonergic responsiveness as evidenced by reduced platelet ^{3}H-imipramine binding[30] and blunted prolactin responses to the 5HT precursor L-tryptophan.[31] It has been hypothesized that cholesterol might be an important factor in the relationship between serotonergic dysfunction and depression, through alterations in synaptosomal membrane properties. However, a recent meta-analysis of the outcome of elderly patients participating in clinical trials of cholesterol-lowering agents revealed no significant associations between low cholesterol concentration and severity of depressive symptoms.[32]

Imaging techniques have been widely used in the study of depression in old age. A recent review of structural imaging studies in depression in old age concluded that ventricular enlargement, and arteriosclerotic and ischemic changes are more frequently found in patients whose first onset of depression was after age 60.[33] An important study using single-photon emission computed tomography (SPECT) demonstrated that at rest elderly patients with depression had lower regional cerebral blood flow (rCBF) than controls, particularly in the left hemisphere.[34] However, rCBF failed to correlate with severity of depressed mood but there was a positive correlation between rCBF and severity of psychotic symptoms and negative correlations with somatic symptoms and anxiety. Reduced anterior frontal and temporal blood flow but an increase in occipital flow have also been shown in elderly depressed patients.[35] Studies using positron emission tomography (PET) reveal that depression in the elderly is associated with a reduction in whole brain glucose metabolic rate.[36]

Physical health

Depression is more common in physically ill than in healthy older people. The prevalence range varies from 6 to 25 percent when diagnostic interviews validated among elderly people are used.[37] The main predictors of depression appear to be the severity of physical illness and a positive past psychiatric history. Physical disability seems to be particularly strongly associated with depression in institutional settings.[19] Depression in elderly medical patients frequently becomes chronic, and in turn appears to have an adverse effect on the physical prognosis, especially in terms of likelihood of successful rehabilitation.[38] In addition, older medical patients with depression consume more health care resources, have longer admissions, a higher mortality, and are more likely to be transferred to residential care.[39] However, depression in elderly medical patients is frequently overlooked by medical staff, despite high rates of depressive symptomatology.[40] Its detection may be facilitated by simple screening tests such as the Geriatric Depression Scale.[41] The management of depression in physically ill elderly patients is difficult but there is some clinical trial evidence to suggest that newer antidepressants may be of value.[42] Patients with depression should be discouraged from making decisions about life-sustaining therapy until after their depression is treated.[43]

Personality

Those individuals with late-onset depressive illness have more robust personalities than those with recurrent depression arising earlier.[44] Dependent, anxious, and avoidant personality traits have, however, been reported to be associated with late life depression.[45]

Life events

Life events often precipitate depression in old age.[46] Several community studies have emphasized the importance of the concept of loss in understanding the depressions of old age. Illness, chronic disability, social isolation, bereavement, and poverty are correlates of depressive symptoms.[47] The importance of physical illness has already been discussed. Those individuals who are separated, divorced, or widowed exhibit more depressive illness than single or married subjects.[48]

Depression is associated with recent deaths and accidents in near relatives.[49]

Social supports and intimacy

Social losses have been implicated in the etiology of depressive illness; a confidant may act as a buffer against such loss-related depression, particularly in women.[46] This research area is particularly problematic because of the lack of cause/effect clarity: Does poor support render persons liable to depression, or does depression lead to the loss of supports? Personality variables are likely to be important mediators.

Clinical Features

Depression often presents in a less typical fashion in old age. This clearly has implications for the under- or misdiagnosis of depression in the elderly. Older patients tend to have an increase in somatic complaints, sleep disturbance (initial insomnia), and agitation.[50] Depressive symptomatology is often found in older subjects without frank depressive illness; the psychological symptoms frequently elicited include dysphoria, sleep disturbance, thoughts of death, anergy, impaired concentration, agitation, and retardation.[51]

Symptom patterns have been found to differ by gender. Depressed mood, guilt, anxiety, and diurnal mood variation were found to be more common in women with depression than in men with depression.[52] Age-related differences in symptom patterns have been reported within the elderly. Items relating to low self-esteem showed an inverse relationship with age, whereas the presence of hypochondriasis was positively correlated with age.[53] Subjects whose first episode of depression occurred in late life are less likely to display psychotic features, and are also more likely to display cognitive impairment.[54] However, the latter finding may be a reflection of the greater age of the late first-onset group.

Cognitive impairment is frequently found in association with depression in older subjects. Its presence may be important not only in terms of hindering diagnosis, but more positively, as an etiologic and prognostic pointer and an element in a possible specific approach to the subtyping of depression in old age. Prominent cognitive dysfunction that initially reverses with successful antidepressant treatment is the essential clinical feature in the minority of elderly depressed patients with "depressive pseudodementia."[55] Subtle cognitive impairment may, however, be present in a broad spectrum of the elderly depressed and may in any case not be as consistently reversible as had been thought.[56] Conventional teaching suggests that "don't know" responses are helpful in distinguishing such depressive pseudodementia from true dementia but a recent study suggests that this may not be so.[57]

The evolution of cognitive and depressive symptoms in subjects in whom these coexist is not always straightforward. In a study of people aged over 75 years with declining cognitive function, mood disturbance first increased, then decreased.[58] Lack of motivation increased sharply with decreasing cognitive function, and increasing disability was associated with deterioration in both mood and motivation symptoms. Cognitive impairment in elderly inpatients with depression tended to be associated with late-onset depression. This suggests that subjects with the combination of cognitive impairment and late first onset of depression may represent a distinct subgroup whose depression reflects neurodegenerative change. This is further supported by the finding that subjects becoming depressed for the first time in late life have a distinct pattern of symptoms and are less likely to have first-degree relatives with depression.[50] In addition, late first-onset depression has been reported to be associated with more frequent cognitive impairment, suboptimal treatment response, and a higher rate of brain imaging abnormalities.[36]

Depression may also be an important cause of disability in people with primary dementia. It frequently presents as part of the prodrome of Alzheimer's disease as well as complicating both early and late stages of dementia.[20] Depression within dementia appears to be clinically relevant and amenable to treatment.[59] The detection of depression in subjects with dementia is difficult. The subject finds it difficult as dementia progresses to articulate emotional distress. There are, however, rating scales specifically designed to detect depression in subjects with dementia; the best of these is probably the Cornell Scale.[60]

In view of the differences in symptom pattern found in older people with depression compared with their younger counterparts, screening instruments specific for depression in the elderly may be useful even in the absence of cognitive impairment. The Geriatric Depression Scale[43] is sensitive and specific in both the hospital[42] and primary care[61] settings, is quick to administer and highly acceptable to patients,[61] and has been extensively validated.[62]

The Management of Depression in Old Age

Community and primary care studies suggest that only a small minority of older patients with depression receive treatment. A community study found that only 13 percent of subjects with depression were being treated with antidepressants; at follow-up the figure remained virtually the same at 14 percent.[13] Similarly, only 10 percent of patients with depression identified from consecutive primary care attenders were receiving treatment for depression.[14] However, their general practitioners were aware of depression in 95 percent of cases. This suggests that GPs may conceptualize depression in old age as a legitimate and unavoidable consequence of aging and associated adversity, which is recognizable but not seen as treatable.

This failure to treat depression in old age is unfortunate because treatment is clearly efficacious. Reviews of the many controlled trials of tricyclic and newer antidepressants against each other and against placebo[63] have consistently demonstrated superior efficacy for active drug (response rate about 50 percent) over placebo (about 25 percent). No particular drug has emerged as being more effective than any other. Cardiotoxicity was minimum at therapeutic doses. Further trials[64] have been carried out with the newer antidepressants such as the serotonin specific reuptake inhibitors (SSRIs). They have no advantage over tricyclics in terms of efficacy, but have a better side effect and safety profile that may be more relevant in "real life" patients than in the "super-fit, super-depressed" subjects eligible for clinical trials. There is some evidence that antidepressants may take as long as 10 to 12 weeks to show clinical improvement in older subjects.[65]

The safety profile of electroconvulsive therapy (ECT) in older patients with depression is very good.[66] A wide spectrum of clinical response, including anxiety symptoms, have been demonstrated. A meta-analysis of published studies revealed a 62 percent recovery and 21 percent substantial improvement.[67] Unilateral electrode placement appears as effective as bilateral in older patients, but there is clearer evidence that unilateral electrode placement is associated with fewer memory-related side effects in this age group.[68]

Psychological treatments are also underused in old age. This is partly because their availability is often limited. There is also a misconception that older people lack the psychological flexibility to benefit from psychotherapeutic interventions.[69] Elderly people appear to respond particularly well to cognitive therapy for depression; this is effective both in an individual setting and (more economically) in groups. The focus is often on real or threatened losses (bereavement, physical health, financial security) and on fears of impending death.

Depression in old age frequently fails to respond to initial treatment. Pharmacologic strategies for treatment-resistant depression may be useful despite the toxicity risk. Lithium augmentation in particular is often associated with a favorable outcome despite the increased risk of neurotoxicity in old age.[70]

Suicide and Depression in Old Age

Suicide in old age is far from rare. Suicide rates in most countries are highest in the elderly.[71] In the United Kingdom the rate in those over 65 years is approximately three times that in the 15 to 24 year age group, and in men, continues to rise into the ninth decade. In the United Kingdom suicide attempts in old age are usually by overdose. Violent means (hanging, firearms, etc.) are more frequently used by men to commit suicide.[72] Suicide is much more closely associated with depression in older than in younger subjects. Other factors associated with suicide in old age include bereavement, increasing social isolation, deteriorating physical health, and pain.

Attempted suicide closely resembles completed suicide in the elderly.[73,74] Psychiatric illness is prominent in most cases. The predominant psychiatric diagnosis is depression. Comorbid diagnoses include delirium and mild dementia. Minor depression and personality dysfunction are associated with suicide attempts of relatively low intent and higher levels of psychosocial stresses. There is an interaction with physical illness, psychosocial stress, age, and gender. Hopelessness persisting after remission of other depressive symptoms is associated with suicide attempts and completed suicide.[75]

Suicide in old age is often associated with undetected or untreated depression and is thus potentially preventable. The close association between depression and deliberate self-harm in old age carries a clear message that all such behavior in older patients should be taken seriously with particular attention to the exclusion or treatment of underlying depressive illness.

The Prognosis of Depression in Old Age

It has been suggested as a rule of thumb that one-third of patients get better, one-third stay the same, and one-third get worse.[76] However, there is considerable dispute about outcome. Some studies have reported relatively favorable outcomes with up to 60 percent of patients either remaining well or having relapses that are successfully treated.[77] The mortality rate is considerably higher in elderly patients with depression than in age- and sex-matched controls,[78] although this in large part reflects pre-existing health problems that are significantly more common in these patients whose depression has a poor outcome.

The prognostic significance of cognitive impairment within elderly depressed patients remains unclear. Depression does not appear to be associated with increased incidence of dementia in elderly subjects whose depression is not complicated by cognitive impairment at the start.[79] However, in patients presenting with "pseudodementia," not only do computed tomography (CT) scan abnormalities seem to be significantly more common, but this subgroup of patients has a poorer prognosis.[80]

In older people with depression, physical illness, cognitive impairment, and severe depressive symptoms rather than social factors seem more robustly related to poor prognosis.[81] There is conflicting evidence regarding the role of age of onset, advanced age, and duration of illness in terms of prognosis. Family problems including psychiatric symptoms in the spouse or adult child and poor physical health adversely influence prognosis.[82] Chronic health problems and acute new physical illness predict poor outcome, with the combination of depressive symptoms and physical disability together initiating a spiraling decline in physical and psychological health.

Although depression in old age does not necessarily have a worse prognosis than earlier in life, there is considerable room for improvement. This improvement could result from optimizing treatment. Continuing treatment appears to have a protective effect against relapse. This has been shown most clearly for maintenance antidepressant drugs[83] but the efficacy of supportive group psychotherapy has also been shown.[84]

Late Life Psychosis

The onset of schizophrenia-like psychotic illness later in life not due to an organic or affective disorder has been referred to as *paraphrenia*, *late paraphrenia*, and *late-onset schizophre-*

nia. The term *paraphrenia* is used to describe these conditions within this chapter. More circumscribed delusional disorders also occur in late life; these are referred to below as *late life delusional disorders*. In addition, the challenges posed by patients with long-standing psychotic illness (usually schizophrenia) who "graduate" to old age are also considered within this section.

Paraphrenia

The original concept of paraphrenia referred to the first onset of persecutory delusions and associated hallucinations after the age of 60 years in the absence of an affective or organic psychosis.[85] It may thus be viewed as schizophrenia or a schizophrenia-like illness in old age.

Epidemiology

In an early (1961) study, paraphrenia was estimated to account for 10 percent of psychogeriatric admissions[85]; this is probably an overestimate. Data from admissions to psychiatric units reveal an age-related increase in first admission rates for schizophrenia and paranoid states from 8.7 per 100,000 in subjects aged 65 to 74 years to 14.5 per 100,000 in the 75-plus age group.[86] Community studies, however, usually find either no cases at all or prevalence rates of less than 2 percent.[87] There is clearly a problem with epidemiologic survey data because patients with paraphrenia will, by the very nature of the condition, be far less likely than the rest of the population to cooperate with survey investigators. This probably results in gross underestimation of the true community prevalence. Hospital admission data also probably underestimate prevalence because patients with paraphrenia tend only to be admitted compulsorily and in the context of particularly severe behavioral disturbance. There is relatively good consensus that late-onset schizophrenia is more common in women than in men.[86]

Etiology

About 10 percent of the relatives of patients developing schizophrenia in middle age also have the disease; this is similar to the proportion for patients with early-onset schizophrenia.[88] In family studies of paraphrenia, however, the rate of schizophrenia in first-degree relatives is much lower, generally less than 5 percent.[89] Standardized instruments were not used in the paraphrenia studies, however, so the data are not directly comparable to those from fully operationalized family studies of younger subjects.

The influence of personality, social, and environmental factors, in association with genetic predisposition is clearly complex.[90] Patients with paraphrenia are often socially isolated and live alone.[91] They are more likely to have paranoid and/or schizoid premorbid personalities that are characterized by suspicion, sensitivity to setback and disappointment, and preoccupation with what others may think about them. Their isolation is often chronic and may well be secondary to personality traits. They are predominantly unmarried women without close family or personal attachments. Those who do marry often end up divorced or separated. Fertility seems markedly reduced. This social isolation creates an environment allowing the individual to become preoccupied in her own world.

The social isolation can be further accentuated by sensory impairment. There is a confirmed association between deafness and late paraphrenia in particular. Many paraphrenics suffer conductive hearing loss contracted in early life to such a degree as to impair social interaction resulting in "social deafness."[92] Visual impairment may be present but is probably no more common than in normal elderly people.[85,89] Patients with paraphrenia have been found to come from the lower social classes and/or socioeconomic groups[91]; this may result from social deterioration secondary to the disease, as also occurs in younger people with schizophrenia.

Presentation and clinical features

Patients often come to the attention of services because they complain to the police and neighbors with bizarre accusations over a period of time or because of neighborly concern triggered by extreme self-neglect. On mental state assessment there are no qualitative differences between the symptoms of early-onset schizophrenia and of paraphrenia. The clinical presentation of paraphrenia is quite varied. Patients are in clear consciousness. Usually their affective state is normal although occasionally a secondary depressive mood is found. The history may be difficult to elicit from patients with paraphrenia who tend to be distrustful and hostile.

Delusions are central. Persecutory delusions are particularly common. Sexual themes are common in women. The patient usually accuses a man or men of entering her bed at night and molesting her sexually. Delusions of influence and passivity phenomena are frequently reported.[93] Patients may describe their bodies as being controlled, or complain that some power affects them and they are made to do things against their will. Thought insertion, withdrawal, and broadcasting are, however, fairly rare, and formal thought disorder is almost nonexistent.

Hallucinations are frequently experienced.[91] Paraphrenics experience a great number of different types of hallucinations. Auditory hallucinations are the most common and usually have an accusatory and/or insulting content. The voices speak in the second or the third person with "running commentary" occasionally encountered. Hallucinations of bodily sensation are also found. Patients complain of being vibrated, raped, or forced to have sexual intercourse. Olfactory hallucinations often relating to poisonous gas are encountered. Visual hallucinations are rare in paraphrenia and if present should raise the strong suspicion of an underlying organic state.

At the time of initial presentation, the cognitive function of patients with paraphrenia is often mildly impaired on formal testing. Although such impairment is to a much lesser degree than found in dementia, it is nevertheless significantly greater than in psychiatrically healthy age-matched controls.[92] Decline is usually very slowly progressive, with only a small group of patients entering the dementia range at 3-year follow-up.

Brain imaging studies

A representative CT study has reported increased mean ventricle to brain ratio with cortical sulcal appearances remaining within normal limits.[92] Magnetic resonance imaging (MRI) has demonstrated an excess of deep white matter changes,[94] although these findings have failed to be consistently replicated[95] and may have reflected the over-representation of individuals with cerebrovascular disease risk factors. SPECT studies have found significant abnormalities in rCBF in late-onset psychotic patients compared to controls.[96]

A number of studies using PET have shown increased basal ganglia dopamine D2 receptors in late-onset schizophrenia.[87] However, these findings have not been consistently replicated, particularly in drug-naive subjects, suggesting that some of the differences initially reported may have reflected treatment, rather than disease-induced receptor alteration.

Neuropsychological testing

Patients with paraphrenia have been shown to perform less well on the Mental Test Score and Digit Copying Test than age-matched controls. Deficiencies have also been shown on full-scale IQ tests, tests of frontal lobe function, and verbal memory tasks.[92] The presence of brain abnormalities was not associated with particularly low neuropsychological test scores.

Assessment, treatment, and course

The initial management of late paraphrenia involves evaluation and engagement.[91] Patients should be assessed at home (rather than in a clinic) both because they are unlikely to comply with outpatient appointments and because their psychopathology may be strongly triggered by cues within their normal environment and less obvious away from it. It is also not surprising on this basis that hospital admission commonly results in an apparent complete remission followed by relapse on return home. Health workers may initially find it difficult to gain access to the home of a patient with paraphrenia. Once initial access is gained, patients are often glad to gain a new audience for the expression of their delusional beliefs.

Paraphrenia tends to run a chronic course.[97] Attempts at treatment should begin in the community wherever possible, with hospital admission reserved for patients with particularly severe or dangerous behavioral disturbance or poor self-care. Medication, psychosocial intervention, and ECT have all been reported to produce temporary remission. Adequate neuroleptic treatment produces improvement in psychotic symptoms but not much improvement to the patient's pretreatment level of social functioning. Dosages of neuroleptics are much lower than those used in younger patients with schizophrenia; people with paraphrenia are often very sensitive to extrapyramidal side effects.[98] Compliance is a major problem in these patients who usually live alone and do not have any insight into treatment necessity. Even when compliance is assured, many patients with paraphrenia remain psychotic, although they may be less distressed by their symptoms and less disturbed in their behavior.[87] Community psychiatric nurses administering depot preparations are most likely to ensure a favorable response.

An attempt should be made to correct remediable physical or environmental contributory factors, particularly through alleviating sensory and/or social isolation. A flexible approach is required, and patients' characteristic insistence on remaining isolated (as they have often been for much of their lives) must be respected. Patients' importuning requests for rehousing should, if secondary to delusional beliefs, be resisted; although symptoms improve or even abate in a new home setting this is usually a temporary respite. Old "tormentors" re-emerge and new ones may be acquired. Antipsychotic medication is a vital component of the total therapeutic package but is far from the whole answer; improvisation and ingenuity in engaging these patients and then retaining them in long-term follow-up is crucial to maintain both compliance and an optimal level of social functioning and to reduce risk of symptomatic relapse. The benefits of long-term neuroleptics in reducing relapse rate must be weighed against the increased risk of tardive dyskinesia in old age.

Late Life Delusional (Paranoid) Disorder

Persecutory ideas are common in older people. It has been estimated that 4 percent of a community-living elderly population experience some persecutory beliefs of delusional intensity.[99] Such beliefs are commonly associated with a neuropsychiatric disorder. A primary delusional disorder is present when there is evidence of persistent, nonbizarre delusions that are not attributable to another psychiatric disorder or any organic cause.[100] Delusional disorder refers to persistent delusions without evidence of schizophrenia, schizophreniform, or mood disorders. Hallucinations are not prominent. There is no evidence of organic dysfunction. The distinction between such disorders and paraphrenia reflects the relative absence of schizophrenia-like features other than delusions in the late life delusional group. Delusional disorder occurs in middle as well as late life. Men tend to be affected earlier than women (40 to 49 years versus 60 to 69 years).

Pathogenesis and etiology

An increased evidence of schizophrenia has been observed in families of patients with late life delusional disorder.[101] Individuals with avoidant, paranoid, or schizoid personality disorders may be more susceptible to developing a delusional disorder. There is an association between hearing loss and delusional disorder in the elderly.[102] Immigration or low socioeconomic status may also predispose individuals to delusional disorder.[103] There is an increased frequency of women, immigrants, or children of immigrants with somatic delusions diagnosed as part of a delusional disorder. There may be a possible association of early life trauma and the failure to reproduce progeny with the development of delusions in later life.[104]

Management and outcome

The optimal approach encompasses drug treatment, psychotherapy, and environmental change.[105] Neuroleptics may be effective in decreasing the intensity of the delusions, but (as in paraphrenia) noncompliance is a common problem. Intramuscular depot neuroleptics may be preferable. Antidepressant drugs and ECT have been used with variable success in delusional patients, particularly those with coexistent depressive symptoms. The provision of alternative explanations for patients' delusional beliefs may be a useful psychotherapeutic approach. There are few outcome data available, but the overall outcome is often poor.[100]

Graduates

The term *graduates* is used to refer to patients with longstanding mental illness who have "graduated" to elderly status.[106] Many graduates entered a mental hospital when relatively young and remained in institutional care. Many such patients are now returning to the community as the large psychiatric hospitals close. There is no separate term for people with psychiatric illness enduring from adulthood into old age who have received or will receive care in the community. Although the latter group is likely to be less institutionalized, there is likely to be considerable overlap in terms of both current clinical presentation and care needs, and these people may also usefully be considered as graduates.

The largest subgroup of graduates have schizophrenia. Most of the remainder have primary diagnoses of affective psychoses, learning disability, or personality disorder. Disability in the graduate population is varied. Some patients may require total nursing care whereas others remain physically fit and relatively competent in daily living skills. Many have some degree of cognitive impairment. There are associations between negative symptoms (social withdrawal, slowness, underactivity, poverty of speech, lack of interest, and poor self-care), cognitive deficit, and structural brain abnormality. This highlights the issue of the long-term cognitive effects of schizophrenic illness. Some of the deficits of chronic schizophrenia are probably integral to the illness process and may manifest at a relatively early stage in the evolution of the illness over time. It must also be borne in mind that increasing social disability may be due not only to the effects of the illness itself but secondary to the deleterious effects of institutional care on the capacity to return to independent living. It has been suggested that in some patients a phenomenon of "burn-out" in schizophrenia (an amelioration of positive symptoms after the age of 55) may occur, but this is still disputed.[107] The lowered prevalence of positive symptoms in this group may be due to reduced exposure to the stresses and strains of everyday life rather than either the effects of medication or the natural history of schizophrenia.

There is a high prevalence of physical disability and handicap among long-stay patients. This increases with age but is not confined to elderly patients or those with the longest duration of stay. The presence of neurologic abnormalities referred to as "soft" neurologic signs, including disorders of posture and tone, motor performance, inappropriate activity, abnormal movements, automatic movements, and speech production, seem to be intrinsic to the schizophrenic process and cannot be attributed to hospitalization, physical treatment, or undiagnosed neurologic illness.[108] Incontinence of urine and less often of feces is a problem in long-stay patients. Likely contributory factors include physical disability, inefficient bladder emptying, and colonic fecal stasis.[109] These problems, particularly constipation, are difficult to manage and require individual assessment and particularly tailored programs. Graduates may also suffer from the range of physical problems to which their age range is vulnerable. Cardiovascular and respiratory disease is found relatively frequently reflecting the heavy smoking in this patient group. The mortality of long-stay patients is disputed. Patients with schizophrenia are considered either to have a life expectancy similar to the general population or a higher mortality attributable to the suicide rates or to the effects of rapid and inadequately planned transfers from their familiar hospital surrounding into the community.[110]

The care of graduate patients encompasses elements of good practice within old age psychiatry, psychiatric rehabilitation, and medicine of the elderly.[106] It is vital for the multidisciplinary teams caring for such patients in the hospital setting, and now, increasingly, in the community, to overcome the negative attitudes traditionally held about elderly long-stay patients. The needs of graduates are very different from those of patients with severe dementia and they should not be cared for in the same settings. Patients' skills should be identified and cultivated as part of a rehabilitative process, in the context of working toward an improved quality of life by improving the physical and social environment. Residential options in the community are varied and should be determined by the individual's present and likely future physical and mental health needs. Medication regimens often need review, and many patients benefit from cautious reduction or withdrawal of antipsychotic drugs that have often been prescribed in substantial amounts over the years.

Mania

Epidemiology

The reported prevalence and new incidence of mania in old age varies widely; studies to date are reviewed by Shulman.[111] Several studies have suggested that mania only rarely occurs de novo in old age, with approximately 90 percent of patients with a manic episode in old age having been identified as bipolar by 50 years of age. National statistics from the United States for first admission to psychiatric hospitals, however, suggest that the number of first admissions with mania does not reduce with age but rather increases in older men. The initial Epidemiologic Catchment Area (ECA) data revealed no manic cases in the community[112] and a more recent ECA study reported a prevalence of only 0.1 percent compared with 1.4 percent in young adults.[113] This does not reflect clinical experience, however, because manic and hypomanic illnesses are quite commonly encountered on psychogeriatric units, representing 12 percent of all admissions with affective disorders.[111] The discrepancies between these results may reflect that mania in old age has different clinical features than those found in younger people; this is reviewed below.

Older patients with mania typically had their first manic episode in their mid- to late fifties.[114] People with mania of earlier onset are under-represented in these hospitalized samples; possible explanations for this include effective treatment with lithium, "burn-out" after many years, and higher mortality rates among younger patients with bipolar disorder. In about one-half of elderly patients with mania, the first episode of mental illness is depression,[115] with many years latency before mania becomes manifest.

Clinical Features

Many of the clinical features of mania are similar to those found in younger patients but dramatic physical overactivity, violence, criminal behavior, infectious euphoria, and grandiosity are less common.[116] Clinical experience suggests that mixed mood states are more commonly found in older subjects, but this has not been substantiated in a controlled study.[117] Adverse life events, particularly episodes of illness, more commonly appeared to precipitate mania in older subjects. Subjective confusion or perplexity is relatively prominent in the elderly. First episode mania in very late life with no previous psychiatric history was frequently associated with comorbid neurologic disorder.

Secondary Mania

This concept refers to an episode of mania causally associated with medical illness, exogenous substances, and organic cerebral dysfunction.[116] First-onset mania in old age should be considered to have an underlying organic cause until proven otherwise. The frequent presence of some degree of nonprogressive cognitive impairment in secondary mania reflects its heterogeneous etiology. Even if no acute cause is discovered there is still a greater prevalence of coexisting neurologic illness. Stroke is the most characteristic precipitant of secondary mania, and long-standing cerebrovascular disease is also overrepresented, with white matter hyperintensities often found on MRI scanning. Family history and prior psychiatric disturbance are uncommon in secondary mania.

The Treatment of Mania in Old Age

The drug treatment of elderly people with mania is similar to that in younger patients.[111] However, drug doses will generally be smaller. Neuroleptics are the mainstay of acute treatment. In secondary mania treatment is also directed at the underlying medical cause. Prophylactic treatment is with lithium although the risks of neurotoxicity are higher, even at relatively low serum lithium levels.[70] The acute antimanic effect may also be useful in older people. The anticonvulsants carbamazepine and sodium valproate are increasingly widely used for their mood stabilizing effects, but few data have been reported in older people with mania. The long-term use of neuroleptics should be avoided due to the increased risks of tardive dyskinesia with increasing age. Family involvement is important in ongoing management. The risk of marital and family breakup is high. The range of skills available within a multidisciplinary team are often needed to deal with the complexities of managing bipolar disorder in old age.

Outcome

The acute and long-term outcome is similar to that in younger patients. Mania with first onset in old age may, however, have a poorer prognosis than mania recurring in old age. This may be due to the greater likelihood of comorbid physical disease and/or cognitive impairment.[116]

Anxiety Disorders

Epidemiology

Several studies have examined the prevalence of anxiety disorders in community-based populations.[118–120] The prevalence rates for phobias range between less than 1 and 11.7 percent; for generalized anxiety the range is between 1.4 and 7.1 percent. The variability in these findings probably reflects the use in some of specific case-finding instruments designed for elderly subjects. There is good consensus that panic disorder is extremely rare in old age.

Phobic Disorders

Phobic disorders consist of persistent or recurrent irrational fear of an object, activity or situation that results in the compelling desire to avoid the phobic stimulus.[121] In old age they are associated with higher rates of medical and of other psychiatric morbidity, but are frequently found in the absence of other psychiatric disorder.[118] Agoraphobia is often triggered by the traumatic experience of acute physical ill-health.[121]

The longitudinal course of phobic disorders in old age is unclear. Individuals with one phobia may develop another. Fear of crime is particularly common in old age, leading to fear of going out and to night-time fearfulness. Social phobias in old age have usually developed earlier in life and persisted; they tend to be chronic and unremitting.[122] Comorbidity with agoraphobia, specific phobia, depression, and alcohol abuse is common.[123] The elderly rarely seek treatment. Cognitive-behavioral treatment is favored over pharmacologic interventions, although antidepressants may be useful. Anxiolytics provide only symptomatic relief and are best avoided because of their dependency potential.[121]

Generalized Anxiety Disorder

Generalized anxiety disorder consists of generalized, persistent anxiety, with motor tension, autonomic symptoms, apprehensiveness and hypervigilance.[124] It usually runs a chronic course.[123] It is hard to diagnose in the elderly because of its high degree of comorbidity with depression. Coexistent medical conditions can complicate the situation. Benzodiazepines have been the mainstay of treatment, but dependence and adverse effects should limit their use to very short-term management only. Antidepressants may be useful, and cognitive-behavioral strategies may be effective.

Panic Disorder

Panic disorder is characterized by recurrent attacks of panic, with intense fear accompanied by severe somatic anxiety symptoms, and usually runs a chronic course[125] but may remit spontaneously or become less disabling secondary to reduced rates of social interaction in old age. It may, albeit rarely, occur de novo in older people.[126] Panic disorder with onset earlier in life is associated with depression,[127] alcohol abuse,[128] increased suicide risk,[129] and higher cardiovascular morbidity.[130] Part of the explanation for the low prevalence in the elderly may be that sufferers may not survive into old age. Antidepressants are the pharmacologic antipanic agents of choice with SSRIs increasingly used in preference to tricyclics.[123] Benzodiazepines are efficacious for symptom control, but can only be used very short term because of undesirable side effects and dependence. Cognitive-behavioral therapy can be effective. Long-term outcome is improved by combination drug and cognitive-behavioral approach.

Post-Traumatic Stress Disorder and Bereavement

Post-traumatic stress disorder (PTSD) occurring earlier in life can be associated with disabilities persisting into old age; traumatic events in old age can trigger similar PTSD reactions to those occurring in younger victims.[123] The intensity of the physiologic response to the original trauma may be the most significant predictor of a poor outcome. Further stressful life events can slow recovery, which may also be hindered by drug and alcohol abuse, which may themselves be triggered by PTSD.[131] PTSD probably responds best to a combination of supportive therapeutic relationship, antidepressants, and cognitive-behavioral therapy.

Bereavement is, sadly, an all-too-common experience for older people. Although depressive symptomatology is very common in the weeks immediately after bereavement, most subjects experience a gradual diminution of these symptoms without developing a full-blown depressive illness. Persistent, severe depression following bereavement is most strongly associated with a past history of depression. Surprisingly, only weak statistical associations are found with quality of the relationship with the lost partner or with level of postbereavement social support.[132]

Obsessive-Compulsive Disorder

Obsessive-compulsive disorder (OCD) has a prevalence rate of 1.5 percent in older people.[119] The onset is usually earlier in life, with persistence into old age.[123] OCD is often resistant to treatment, but the use of clomipramine, SSRIs, and cognitive-behavioral techniques has improved the outlook.[133] In the elderly, it is important to bear in mind that obsessive-compulsive phenomena frequently occur within a primary depressive illness, and the development of obsessional orderliness may indicate the onset of dementia.[134]

Somatoform Disorders

Older people often develop exaggerated bodily complaints in the context of real physical illness. Physically ill patients may also present with generalized anxiety or panic symptoms. The common medical disorders producing anxiety symptoms are endocrine, cardiovascular, pulmonary, and neurologic conditions. A thorough history must be taken in an attempt to establish the temporal relationship of psychiatric symptomatology and the onset of medical illness.

Somatoform disorders are those in which physical symptoms occur in the absence of any or sufficient organic pathology to account for them. Psychological contributory factors can usually be identified. Although the onset of somatoform disorder is usually in early life and runs a chronic course, somatizing patients avoid psychiatrists in youth and adulthood and so not uncommonly present for the first time in old age.[134] Such patients usually have clear symptoms of depression and/or anxiety; their bodily complaints tend to be restricted to one or two body organs or systems. They are preoccupied with the possibility of serious physical illness. They demand investigation rather than treatment. In contrast, hypochondriacal preoccupation presenting for the first time in old age is likely to be secondary to anxiety and depression. Elderly patients only rarely present with hysterical amnesia or conversion reactions in response to stressful experience.

Alcoholism

The average alcohol intake of older people is less than that of younger adults. Fewer drink regularly[135] and abstinence is more common.[136] Social and psychological factors may contribute to a decrease in alcohol intake with age, including reduced social opportunities and financial constraints. Older people are, however, more vulnerable to the effects of alcohol because of physiologic changes and the increased presence of pathologic processes. Despite the general downward trend, drinking is an important contributor to mental and physical ill health in some old people.[137]

Epidemiology and Etiology

American studies suggest that the prevalence of abusive or dependent drinking is about 5 percent in the population aged 65 years and over, with a male preponderance of about 4: 1.[138] A recent British community study reported a 1 percent prevalence of problem drinking.[139] In the hospital setting, elderly patients who abuse alcohol are concentrated in general medical settings; one study[140] identified 14 percent of elderly emergency admissions as having current alcohol abuse. Cultural, ethnic, and socioeconomic factors; differences between countries; and regional variation may influence drinking behavior and related problems resulting in variable prevalence.

The rates of alcohol abuse in the elderly are related to the levels of consumption by the community as a whole.[141] Psychiatric disorder and personality attributes predispose to alcohol abuse. In particular, those older people with a late onset of alcohol abuse tend to have a past history of harmless drinking patterns, with consumption increased in the context of depression, bereavement, lack of social support, and/or deteriorating physical health.[137,142] Elderly people with insomnia and/or chronic pain, those previously dependent on alcohol, and those with current depression or dementia seem particularly vulnerable to develop alcohol-related problems in old age.[143] Persisting social problems perpetuate the cycle of loneliness and further drinking.[141]

Clinical Features

The diagnosis of alcohol abuse may be difficult because the presentation may be masked, unsuspected, or atypical.[144] In a general medical setting the prevalence is higher and the index of suspicion should be raised.[145] In particular, alcohol abuse must be suspected in the assessment of otherwise unexplained falls. Alcohol abuse may present with a wide range of neuropsychiatric complications.[135] Patients can present with cognitive impairment, problems due to mixed intoxication with drugs, or unrecognized withdrawal states. Alcohol abuse is also associated with functional psychiatric disorder.[146] Up to one-third of elderly persons who break the law abuse alcohol or are dependent on it.[147] They are often under the influence of alcohol when the crime is committed.

There is little information regarding the clinical course and prognosis. Light to moderate use of alcohol is associated with a decreased mortality in the elderly. The benign course of "normal" drinking seems very different, however, from that of the problem drinkers in old age, who often present when brain damage or social breakdown supervenes. A past history of alcohol-related problems is associated with both depression and dementia in later life. Depression and anxiety are major comorbid diagnoses.

Management

Alcohol abuse in older people is probably often undetected,[148] particularly in patients presenting with medical conditions. Screening at-risk groups[143] may identify individuals at risk of alcohol abuse. Screening instruments used for younger people are probably limited in their value in the elderly; a recent review by Beresford[138] presents one such screening test designed for older people, the Michigan Alcoholism Screening Test—Geriatric Version, although this has yet to be extensively validated.

When an individual is recognized as having an alcohol-related problem, several services may need to be involved. Home visits are often invaluable in the initial assessment.[149] Hospital admission may be needed to break the drinking routine, reduce risks associated with acute alcohol withdrawal,[150] and allow for full physical and psychiatric assessment. Alcohol withdrawal symptoms become more severe with age, and detoxification is more likely to be complicated by intercurrent illness. Withdrawal seizures occur within 24 hours if at all. Tremor, tachycardia, hypertension, anxiety, nausea, and insomnia are prominent features of the alcohol withdrawal syndrome in old age. The patient should be nursed in a calm, well-lit environment. Shorter acting benzodiazepines and chlormethiazole are preferred for sedation. The dosage for older patients undergoing detoxification should begin at about one-third of that used for a fit younger person and should then be titrated against the clinical response.

A long-term management plan needs to be formulated with either abstinence or controlled drinking as a goal. The elderly respond better to social intervention than intensive confrontation. Amelioration of social stresses, group socialization, family work, medical treatment, and management of depression are all part of the approach needed. Disulfiram is not recommended in older people because of increasing medical risks involved with ingesting alcohol while taking the drug.[151]

Personality Disorders in Old Age

Personality disorders are generally recognizable by adolescence or earlier and continue throughout most of adult life, although they become less obvious in middle or old age.[152] Some patients with life-long subclinical personality traits may present clinically in old age as a result of experiencing increasing stress and adversity. Global well-being, life satisfaction, and capacity to cope with illness and loss in old age are also critically influenced by personality and its adaption to old age.[153] Personality traits may be critical in adapting to the adverse life events all too often encountered by older people.

Epidemiology

An individual's personality is essentially stable over time.[154] Introversion has, however, been shown to increase with age,[155] whereas extraversion, neuroticism, and openness to experience decrease.[156] Older people tend to have higher scores on scales for orderliness, social conformity, and emotional stability and lower scores for activity and energy.[157] A decline in sociopathy and criminality has been documented.[158]

Few large-scale studies of personality disorder in old age have been performed. An early epidemiologic survey[2] reported a prevalence of 3.6 to 10.6 percent for personality disorders in subjects aged 65 years and over. More recent surveys of older community-living individuals using standardized diagnostic schedules have found lifetime prevalence rates for personality disorder ranging between 2.1 and 18 percent.[159]

Senile Self-Neglect (Diogenes Syndrome)

Patients with senile self-neglect often present to units for medicine of the elderly. The syndrome can best be understood as an expression of abnormal personality traits, in reaction to stress and loneliness or as the end stage of long-standing reclusiveness.[160] The clinical picture is of very gross self-neglect unaccompanied by any psychiatric or physical disorder sufficient to account for the squalor in which the individual lives. Some early organic cerebral impairment or mild depressive symptoms may be present. The prognosis of such cases is not good. Compulsory hospitalization is difficult to accomplish and mortality is high; apparently successful rehabilitation is usually followed by relapse.[161] Day care might maintain an individual but some form of institutional care usually becomes necessary.

Outcome of Personality Disorder in Old Age

Clinical experience suggests that patients with personality disorders do not cause as much trouble for themselves, their families, and health care professionals by the time they reach old age.[152] Formal long-term follow-up studies are, however, sparse. Immature personality disorders including antisocial, impulsive, histrionic, dependent, and narcissistic improve with time. Mature personality disorders, including anancastic, paranoid, schizoid, and schizotypal, tend to persist into later life. Deterioration may become evident in the obsessive-compulsive patient as increased rigidity, in the paranoid patient as more suspicious and isolated and, in the schizotypal/schizoid patient as more withdrawn and anxious. This view, however, has not been adequately substantiated by follow-up studies.

The high suicide rate of patients with borderline personality precludes their frequent graduation to the care of geriatric psychiatrists. In those who do survive into old age, the criteria for borderline personality disorder are still rare because self-mutilation is so uncommon. Good global outcome in such patients is associated with high intelligence, attractiveness, artistic talent, and coexisting obsessive-compulsive traits.[162] The highly subjective "likeability" seems also to confer good prognosis. Poor outcome is associated with a history of parental brutality, impulsivity, poor premorbid functioning, and coexistent schizotypal/antisocial personality disorder.[163]

In patients with antisocial personality disorder, there is a tendency toward spontaneous remission so that these individuals are rarely encountered over the age of 60.[152] Patients with schizotypal and schizoid personality disorder rarely seek treatment, so little is reported on their long-term outcome but the outlook is probably poor.[164] There is also little information on the outcome of histrionic, narcissistic, obsessive-compulsive, and depressive personality disorders.[152]

Management of Personality Disorder in Old Age

There has been little formal study of treatment approaches to personality disorders in old age.[152] The psychotherapeutic treatment of elderly patients is unpromising for individuals with long-standing personality disorders who realistically cannot be expected to resolve a lifetime of failed relationships and missed opportunities. However, the general principles of psychiatric treatment of older people apply to patients with primary personality psychopathology. Concurrent disorders should be optimally treated with medication or other means. The use of medication per se in geriatric personality disorders has not been formally studied.

References

1. Myers JK, Weissman MM, Tischler GL et al: Six-month prevalence of psychiatric disorders in three communities. Arch Gen Psychiatry 1984;41:959–967
2. Kay DWK, Beamish P, Roth M: Old age mental disorders in Newcastle upon Tyne. Part I: a study of prevalence. Br J Psychiatry 1964;110:146–158
3. Henderson AS, Jorm AF, Mackinnon A et al: The prevalence of depressive disorders and the distribution of depressive symptoms in later life: a survey using draft ICD-10 and DSM-III R. Psychol Med 1993;23:719–729
4. World Health Organization: International Classification of Mental Disorders. 10th Ed. World Health Organization, Geneva, 1992
5. American Psychiatric Association: Diagnostic and Statistical Manual of Mental Disorders. 3rd Ed. revised. American Psychiatric Association, Washington DC, 1987
6. Weissman MM, Leaf PJ, Bruce ML, Florio L: The epidemiology of dysthymia in five communities—rates, risks, co-morbidity and treatment. Am J Psychiatry 1988;145:815–819
7. Kivela S-L, Pahkala K, Laippala P: Prevalence of depression in an elderly population in Finland. Acta Psychiatr Scand 1988;78:401–413
8. Copeland JRM, Dewey ME, Griffiths-Jones HM: A computerized psychiatric diagnostic system and case nomenclature for elderly subjects: GMS and AGECAT. Psychol Med 1986;16: 89–99
9. Gurland BJ, Golden RR, Teresi JA, Challop J: The SHORT-CARE: an efficient instrument for the assessment of depression, dementia and disability. J Gerontol 1984;39:166–169
10. Kay DWK, Henderson AS, Scott R et al: Dementia and depression among the elderly living in the Hobart community: the effect of a diagnostic criteria on the prevalence rates. Psychol Med 1985;15:771–778
11. Copeland JRM, Dewey ME, Wood N et al: Range of mental illness among the elderly in the community: prevalence in

Liverpool using the GMS-AGECAT package. Br J Psychiatry 1987;150:815–823

12. Copeland JRM, Gurland BJ, Dewey ME et al: Is there more dementia, depression and neurosis in New York? A comparative community study of the elderly in New York and London using the community diagnosis AGECAT. Br J Psychiatry 1987b;151:466–473

13. Livingston G, Hawkins A, Graham N et al: The Gospel Oak Study: prevalence rates of dementia, depression and activity limitation among elderly residents in inner London. Psychol Med 1990;20:137–146

14. Macdonald AJD: Do general practitioners "miss" depression in elderly patients? BMJ 1986;292:1365–1367

15. Evans S, Katona CLE: The epidemiology of depressive symptoms in elderly primary care attenders. Dementia 1993;4: 327–333

16. Iliffe S, Tai SS, Haines A et al: Assessment of elderly people in general practice. 4. Depression, functional ability and contact with services. Br J Gen Pract 1993;431:371–374

17. Callahan MC, Hui SL, Niebauer NA et al: Longitudinal study of depression and health service use among elderly primary care patients. J Am Geriatr Soc 1994;42:833–838

18. Koenig HG, Meador KG, Cohen HJ, Blazer D: Depression in elderly hospitalised patients with medical illness. Arch Intern Med 1988;148:1929–1936

19. Ames D: Depression among elderly residents of local-authority residents homes: its nature and the efficacy of intervention. Br J Psychiatry 1990;156:667–676

20. Wragg RE, Jeste DV: Overview of depression and psychosis in Alzheimer's disease. Am J Psychiatry 1989;146:577–586

21. Ballard CG, Patel A, Solis M et al: A one-year follow-up study of depression in dementia sufferers. Br J Psychiatry 1996; 168:287–291

22. Heeren TJ, van Hemert AM, Lagaay AM, Rooymans HGM: The general population prevalence of non-organic psychiatric disorders in subjects aged 85 years and over. Psychol Med 1992;22:733–738

23. Mendlewicz J: The age factor in depressive illness: some genetic considerations. J Gerontol 1976;31:300–303

24. Baldwin R: Age of onset of depression in the elderly. Br J Psychiatry 1990;156:445–446

25. Reynolds CF, Kupfer DJ, Houck PR et al: Reliable discrimination of elderly depressed and demented patients by electroencephalographic sleep data. Arch Gen Psychiatry 1988;45: 258–264

26. Patterson JV, Michalewski HJ, Storr A: Latency variability of the components of auditory event-related potentials to infrequent stimuli in aging, Alzheimer-type dementia and depression. Electroencephalogr Clin Neurophysiol 1988;71: 450–460

27. Schneider LS: Biologic features of geriatric affective disorder. Clin Geriatr Med 1992;8:253–265

28. Katona CLE, Aldridge CR: The dexamethasone suppression test and depressive signs in dementia. J Affect Disord 1985; 8:83–89

29. Stahl SM, Lemoine PM, Ciaranello RD, Berger PA: Platelet adrenergic receptor sensitivity in major depressive disorders. Psychiatry Res 1983;10:157–164

30. Mellerup ET, Plenge P: Imipramine binding in depression and psychiatric conditions. Acta Psychiatr Scand 1988;78(suppl 345):61–68

31. Heninger GR, Charney DS, Sternberg GE: Serotonergic function in depression: prolactin response to intravenous tryptophan in depressed patients and healthy subjects. Arch Gen Psychiatry 1984;41:398–402

32. Guraluik JM, Kohout FJ: Low cholesterol concentrations and severe depressive symptoms in elderly people. BMJ 1994;308: 1328–1332

33. Philpot MP, Banerjee S, Needham-Bennett H et al: tc-HMPAO single photon emission tomography in late-life-depression: a pilot study of regional cerebral blood flow at rest and during a verbal fluency task. J Affect Disord 1993;28:233–240

34. Beats B, Levy R: Imaging and affective disorder in the elderly. Clin Geriatr Med 1992;8:267–274

35. Kumar A: Functional brain imaging in late-life depression. J Clin Psychiatry 1993;54(suppl):21–25

36. Baldwin RC: Late life depression and structural brain changes: a review of recent magnetic resonance imaging research. Int J Geriatr Psychiatry 1993;8:115–123

37. Kok RM, Heeren TJ, Hooijer C et al: The prevalence of depression in elderly medical inpatients. J Affect Disord 1995;33: 77–82

38. Koenig HG, Shelp F, Goli V et al: Survival and health care utilization in elderly medical inpatients with major depression. J Am Geriatr Soc 1989;37:599–606

39. Cooper B: Psychiatric disorders among elderly patients admitted to hospital medical wards. J R Soc Med 1987;80:13–16

40. Koeing HG, Meador KG, Cohen HJ et al: Self-rated depression scales and screening for major depression in the older hospitalized patient with medical illness. J Am Geriatr Soc 1988;36: 699–706

41. Yesavage JA, Brink TL, Rose TL, Lum O: Development and validation of a geriatric depression screening scale: a preliminary report. J Psychiatric Res 1983;17:37–49

42. Tan RSH, Barlow RJ, Abel C et al: The effect of low dose lofepramine in depressed elderly patients in general medical wards. Br J Clin Pharmacol 1994;37:321–324

43. Ganzini L, Lee MA, Heintz RT et al: The effect of depression treatment on elderly patients' preferences for life-sustaining medical therapy. Am J Psychiatry 1994;151:1631–1636

44. Roth M: The natural history of mental disorder in old age. J Ment Sci 1955;101:281–301

45. Abrams RC, Alexopoulos GS, Young RC: Geriatric depression and DSMIII R personality disorder criteria. J Am Geriatr Soc 1987;35:383–386

46. Murphy E: Social origins of depression in old age. Br J Psychiatry 1982;141:135–142

47. Kennedy GJ, Kelman HR, Thomas C et al: Hierarchy of characteristics associated with depressive symptoms in an urban elderly sample. Am J Psychiatry 1989;146:220–227

48. Murrell SA, Himmelfarb SA, Wright K: Prevalence of depression and its correlates in older adults. Am J Epidemiology 1983;117:173–185

49. Linn MW, Hunter K, Harris R: Symptoms of depression and recent life events in the community elderly. J Clin Psychology 1980;36:675–682

50. Brown RP, Sweeney J, Loutsch E et al: Involutional melancholia revisited. Am J Psychiatry 1984;137:439–444

51. Fredman L, Schoenbach VJ, Kaplan BH et al: The association between depressive symptoms and mortality among older participants in the Epidemiologic Catchment area—Piedmont Health Survey. J Gerontol 1989;44:S149–S156

52. Kivela SL, Pahkala K: Symptoms of depression in old people in Finland. Z Gerontol 1988;21:257–263

53. Wallace J, Pfohl B: Age-related differences in the symptomatic expression of major depression. J Nerv Ment Dis 1995;183: 99–102

54. Burvill PW, Hall WD, Stampfer HG, Emmerson JP: A comparison of early-onset and late-onset depressive illness in the community. Br J Psychiatry 1989;155:673–679

55. Alexopoulos GS: Late-life depression and neurological brain disease. Int J Geriatr Psychiatry 1989;4:187–190

56. Abas MA, Sahakian BJ, Levy R: Neuropsychological deficits and CT scan changes in elderly depressives. Psychol Med 1990;20:507–520

57. O'Boyle M, Amadeo M: "Don't know" responses in elderly demented and depressed patients. J Geriatr Psychiatr Neurol 1989;2:83–86

58. Forsell Y, Jorm AF, Winblad B: Association of age, sex, cognitive dysfunction and disability with major depressive symptoms in an elderly sample. Am J Psychiatry 1994;151: 1600–1604

59. Allen NHP, Burns A: The non-cognitive features of dementia. Rev Clin Gerontol 1995;5:57–75

60. Alexopoulos GS, Abrams RC, Young RC, Shamoian CA: Cornell Scale for Depression in Dementia. Biol Psychiatry 1988; 23:271–284

61. D'Ath P, Mullan M, Katona P et al: Screening, detection and management of depression in elderly primary care attenders. 1: the acceptability and performance of the 15 item Geriatric Depression Scale (GDS15) and the development of short versions. Fam Pract 1994;11: 260–266

62. Katona CLE: Screening for depression: the Geriatric Depression Scale. In Philp I (ed): Assessing Elderly Patients. Farrand Press, London, 1994

63. Rockwell E, Lam RW, Zisook S: Antidepressant drug studies in the elderly. Psychiatr Clin N Am 1988;11:215–233

64. Anstey K, Brodaty H: Antidepressants and the elderly: double-blind trials 1987–1992. Int J Geriatr Psychiatry 1995;10: 265–279

65. Georgotas A, McCue RE, Cooper TB et al: Factors affecting the delay of anti-depressant effect in responders to nortriptyline and phenelzine. Psychiatr Res 1989;28:1–9

66. Benbow SM: The role of electroconvulsive therapy in the treatment of depressive illness in old age. Br J Psychiatry 1989; 155:147–152

67. Mulsant BH, Rosen J, Thornton JE, Zubenko GS: A prospective naturalistic study of electroconvulsive therapy in late-life depression. J Geriatr Psychiatry Neurol 1991;4:3–13

68. Fraser RM, Glass IB: Unilateral and bilateral ECT in elderly patients: a comparative study. Acta Psychiatr Scand 1980;62: 13–31

69. Morris RG, Morris LW: Cognitive and behavioural approaches with the depressed elderly. Int J Geriatr Psychiatr 1991;6: 407–413

70. Finch EJL, Katona CLE: Lithium augmentation of refractory depression in old age. Int J Geriatr Psychiatry 1989;4:41–46

71. Lindesay J: Suicide in the elderly. Int J Geriatr Psychiatry 1991;6:355–361

72. Pierce D: Deliberate self-harm in the elderly. Int J Geriatr Psychiatry 1987;2:105–110

73. Barraclough BM, Bunch J, Nelson B et al: One hundred cases of suicide—clinical aspects. Br J Psychiatry 1974;125: 355–373

74. Draper B: Suicidal behaviour in the elderly. Int J Geriatr Psychiatry 1994;9:655–661

75. Rifai AH, George CJ, Stack JA et al: Hopelessness in suicide attempters after acute treatment of major depression in late life. Am J Psychiatry 1994;151:1687–1690

76. Millard P: Depression in old age. BMJ 1983;267:375–376

77. Baldwin RC, Jolley DJ: The prognosis of depression in old age. Br J Psychiatry 1986;149:574–583

78. Murphy E, Smith R, Lindesay J, Slattery J: Increased mortality rates in late-life depression. Br J Psychiatry 1988;152: 347–353

79. Murphy E: The prognosis of depression in old age. Br J Psychiatry 1983;142:111–119

80. Alexopoulos GS, Meyers BS, Young RC et al: The course of geriatric depression with "reversible dementia": a controlled study. Am J Psychiatry 1993;150:1693–1699

81. Cole MG: The prognosis of depression in the elderly. Can Med Assoc J 1990;142:633–639

82. Hinrichsen GA, Hernandez NA: Factors associated with recovery from and relapse into major depressive disorders in the elderly. Am J Psychiatry 1993;150:1820–1825

83. Old Age Depression Interest Group: How long should the elderly take antidepressants? A double-blind placebo-controlled study of continuation/prophylaxis therapy with dothiepin. Br J Psychiatry 1993;162:175–182

84. Ong YK, Martineau F, Lloyd C, Robbins I: A support group for the depressed elderly. Int J Geriatr Psychiatry 1987;2: 119–123

85. Kay DWK, Roth M: Environmental and hereditary factors in the schizophrenias of old age ("late paraphrenia") and their bearing on the general problems of causation in schizophrenia. J Ment Sci 1961;107:649–686

86. DHSS (Department of Health and Social Security): Mental Health Statistics. HMSO, London, 1985

87. Howard R: Late paraphrenia. Int Rev Psychiatry 1993;5: 455–460

88. Castle D, Howard R: What do we know about the aetiology of late-onset schizophrenia? Eur Psychiatry 1992;7:99–108
89. Herbert ME, Jacobson S: Late paraphrenia. Br J Psychiatry 1967;113:461–469
90. Howard R, Levy R: Personality structure in the paranoid psychoses of later life. Eur Psychiatry 1993;8:59–66
91. Naguib M, Levy R: Paranoid states in the elderly and late paraphrenia. pp. 758–778. In Jacoby R, Oppenheimer C (eds): Psychiatry in the Elderly. Oxford University Press, Oxford, 1991
92. Naguib M, Levy R: Late paraphrenia—neuropsychological impairment and structural brain abnormalities on computed tomography. Int J Geriatr Psychiatry 1987;2:83–90
93. Levy R, Naguib M: Late paraphrenia. Br J Psychiatry 1985; 146:451
94. Miller BL, Lesser IM, Boone K et al: Brain white matter lesions and psychosis. Br J Psychiatry 1991;158:76–82
95. Krull AJ, Press G, Dupont R et al: Brain imaging in late onset schizophrenia and related psychoses. Int J Geriatr Psychiatry 1991;6:651–658
96. Lesser IM, Miller BL, Schwartz TR et al: Brain imaging in late-life schizophrenia and related psychoses. Schizophr Bull 1993;19:773–782
97. Post F: Persistent Persecutory States of the Elderly. Pergamon Press, Oxford, 1966
98. Jeste DV, Harris MJ, Pearlson GD et al: Late onset schizophrenia. Studying clinical validity. Psychiatr Clin N Am 1988;11: 1–13
99. Christenson R, Blazer D: Epidemiology of persecutory ideation in an elderly population in the community. Am J Psychiatry 1984;141:1088–1091
100. Lacro JP, Harris MJ, Jeste DV: Late-life psychosis. pp. 231–244. In Murphy E, England, Alexopoulou G (eds): Geriatric Psychiatry. Vol. 18. John Wiley, Chichester, England, 1995
101. Kendler S, David KL: The genetics and biochemistry of paranoid schizophrenia and other paranoid psychoses. Schizophr Bull 1981;7:689–709
102. Cooper AF, Curry AR: The pathology of deafness in the paranoid and affective psychoses of later life. J Psychosom Res 1976;20:97–105
103. Rockwell E, Krull AJ, Dimsdale J, Jeste DV: Late-onset psychosis with somatic delusions. Psychosomatics 1992;35: 66–72
104. Gurian BS, Wexler D, Baker EH: Late-life paranoia: possible association with early trauma and infertility. Int J Geriatr Psychiatry 1992;7:277–284
105. Greene JA, Taylor SE: Paranoid states in the elderly. Clin Rep Aging 1989;3:8–11
106. Campbell P: Graduates. pp. 779–818. In Jacoby R, Oppenheimer C (eds): Psychiatry in the Elderly. Oxford University Press, Oxford, 1991
107. Bridge TP, Cannon HE, Wyatt RJ: Burned-out schizophrenia: evidence for age effects on schizophrenia symptomatology. J Gerontol 1978;33:835–839
108. Rogers D: The motor disorders of severe psychiatric illness: a conflict of paradigms. Br J Psychiatry 1985;147:221–232
109. Carrick J, Ramchurn L, Malone-Lee D: Urinary incontinence in a large psychiatric hospital. Health Trends 1988;20: 118–119
110. Ciompi L: Aging and schizophrenic psychosis. Acta Psychiatri Scand 1985;136:413–420
111. Shulman KI: Mania in the elderly. Int Rev Psychiatry 1993; 5:445–453
112. Kramer M, German PS, Anthony JC et al: Patterns of mental disorders among the elderly residents of Eastern Baltimore. J Am Geriatr Soc 1985;33:236–245
113. Weissman MM, Leaf PJ, Tichler GL et al: Affective disorders in five United States communities. Psychol Med 1988;18: 141–153
114. Winokur G: The lowa 500: heterogeneity and course in manic depressive illness (bipolar) Compr Psychiatry 1975;16: 125–131
115. Shulman K, Tohen M, Satlin A et al: Mania compared to unipolar depression in old age. Am J Psychiatry 1992;149:341–345
116. Collins CC: Affective disorders in old age. pp. 257–280. In Joyce PR, Romans SE, Ellis PM, Silverstone TS (eds): Affective Disorders. University of Otago, Christchurch, New Zealand, 1995
117. Young RC, Kleinman GL: Mania in late life: focus on age at onset. Psychiatry 1992;149:867–876
118. Manela M, Katona C, Livingston G: How common are the anxiety disorders in old age? Int J Geriatr Psychiatry 1996; 11:65–70
119. Myers JK, Weissman M, Tischler GL: Six month prevalence of psychiatric disorders in three communities—1980–1982. Arch Gen Psychiatry 1984;959–967
120. Lindesay J, Briggs C, Murphy E: The Guy's/Age Concern Survey. Prevalence rates of cognitive impairment, depression and anxiety in an urban elderly community. Br J Psychiatry 1989; 155:317–329
121. Lindesay J: Phobic disorders in the elderly. Br J Psychiatry 1991;159:531–541
122. Blazer D, George LK, Hughes D: The epidemiology of anxiety disorders: an age comparison. pp. 17–30. In Salzman C, Lebavitz BD (eds): Anxiety in the Elderly. Springer, New York, 1991
123. Sheikh JI, Salzman C: Anxiety in the elderly. Psychiatr Clin N Am 1995;18:871–883
124. Lindesay J: Anxiety disorders in the elderly. pp. 735–757. In Jacoby R, Oppenheimer C (eds): Psychiatry in the Elderly. Vol. 22. Oxford University Press, Oxford, 1991
125. Sheikh JI, King RJ, Taylor CB: Comparative phenomenology of early-onset versus late-onset panic attacks: a pilot survey. Am J Psychiatry 1991;148:1231–1233
126. Sheikh JI, Taylor CB, King RJ et al: Panic attacks and avoidance behaviour in the elderly. In Proceedings of the 141st Annual Scientific Meeting of the American Psychiatric Association, Montreal, 1988
127. Katon W, Vitiliane P, Anderson et al: Panic disorder: residual symptoms after the acute attacks abate. Compr Psychiatry 1987;28:151–158

128. Kushner MG, Sher KJ, Beitman BD: The relation between alcohol problems and the anxiety disorders. Am J Psychiatry 1990;147:685–695

129. Weissman MM, Kleinman GL, Markovitz JS et al: Suicidal ideation and suicide attempts in panic disorder and attacks. N Engl J Med 1989;321:1209–1214

130. Coryell W: Mortality of anxiety disorders. pp. 311–320. In Noyes R Jr, Roth M, Burrows GP (eds): Handbook of Anxiety. Vol. 2. Classification, Etiological Factors and Associated Disturbances. Elsevier Science, Amsterdam, 1988

131. Van der Kolk B: Psychopharmacological issues in post-traumatic stress disorder. Hosp Commun Psychiatry 1983;34: 683–691

132. Katona CLE: The aetiology of depression in old age. pp. 43–62. In Katona CLE (ed): Depression in Old Age. John Wiley, Chichester, England, 1994

133. Rasmussen SA, Eisen JL, Pato MT: Current issues in the pharmacological management of obsessive compulsive disorder. J Clin Psychiatry 1993;54(suppl 6):4–9

134. Lindesay J: Neurotic disorders in the elderly. Int Rev Psychiatry 1993;5:461–467

135. Wattis JP: Alcohol and old people. Br J Psychiatry 1983;143: 306–307

136. Busby WJ, Campbell AJ, Borrie MJ, Spears GFS: Alcohol use in a community-based sample of subjects aged 70 years and older. J Am Geriatr Soc 1988;36:301–305

137. Brody JA: Aging and alcohol abuse. J Am Geriatr Soc 1982; 30:123–126

138. Beresford TP: Alcoholism in the elderly. Int Rev Psychiatry 1993;5:477–483

139. Saunders PA, Copeland JRM, Dewey ME et al: Alcohol use and abuse in the elderly: findings from the Liverpool Longitudinal Study of continuing health in the community. Int J Geriatr Psychiatry 1989;4:103–108

140. Adams WL, Magruder-Habib K, Trued S, Broome HL: Alcohol abuse in elderly emergency department patients. J Am Geriatr Soc 1992;40:1236–1240

141. Ticehurst S: Alcohol and drug abuse. pp. 172–192. In Lindesay J (ed): Neurotic Disorders in the Elderly. Vol. 10. Oxford University Press, Oxford, 1995

142. Rosin AJ, Glass MM: Alcohol excess in the elderly. Q J Studies Alcohol 1971;32:53–55

143. King MB: Alcohol abuse and dementia. Int J Geriatr Psychiatry 1983;1:31–36

144. Zimburg S: Diagnosis and management of the elderly alcoholic. pp. 23. In Atkinson RM (ed): Alcohol and Drug Abuse in Old Age. American Psychiatric Press, Washington, DC, 1984

145. Wattis JP: Alcohol problems in the elderly. J Am Geriatr Soc 1981;24:131–134

146. Schuckit MA, Pastor PA: The elderly as a unique population: alcoholism. Alcoholism Clin Exp Res 1978;2:31–38

147. Taylor J, Parrott JM: Elderly offenders. Br J Psychiatry 1988; 152:340–346

148. Zimberg S: Diagnosis and treatment of the elderly alcoholic. Alcoholism Clin Exp Res 1978;2:27–29

149. Jolley D, Hodgson S: Alcoholism in the elderly: a tale of women and our times. pp. 3–12. In Isaacs B (ed): Recent Advances in Geriatric Medicine. 3rd Ed. Churchill Livingstone, Edinburgh

150. Liskow BI, Rinck C, Campbell J, De Souza C: Alcohol withdrawal in the elderly. J Studies Alcohol 1989;50:414–421

151. Dunne FJ, Schipperheijn JAM: Alcohol and the elderly. BMJ 1989;298:1660–1661

152. Howard R, Bergmann K: Personality disorders in old age. Int Rev Psychiatry 1993;5:469–475

153. Abrams RC: Personality disorders. pp. 154–171. In Lindesay J (ed): Neurotic Disorders in the Elderly. Vol. 9. Oxford University Press, Oxford, 1995

154. Costa PT, McCrae RR: Still able after all these years: personality as a key to some issues in adulthood and old age. In Baltes PB, Brinn OG (eds): Lifespan Development and Behavior. Academic Press, New York, 1980

155. Gutman GM: A note on the MMPI: age and sex differences in extroversion and neuroticisms in a Canadian sample. Br J Social Clin Psychol 1996;5:128–129

156. Costa PT, McCrae RR, Zonderman AB et al: Cross-sectional studies of personality in a national sample: 2. Stability in neuroticism, extroversion and openness. Psychol Aging 1986; 1:149

157. Stoner SB, Panek PE: Age and sex differences with the Courey Personality Scales. J Psychol 1985;119:137–142

158. Vaillant GE, Vaillant CO: Natural history of male psychosocial health XII. A 45 year study of predictors of successful aging at age 65. Am J Psychiatry 1990;147:31–37

159. Casey P: The epidemiology of personality disorder. In P Tyrer (ed): Personality Disorders: Diagnosis, Management and Care. Wright, London, 1988

160. Post F: Functional disorders. Description, incidence and recognition. In Levy R, Post F (eds): The Psychiatry of Later Life. Blackwell, Oxford, 1982

161. Bergmann K: Psychiatric aspects of personality in older patients. pp. 852–871. In Jacoby R, Oppenheimer C (eds): Psychiatry in the Elderly. Vol. 24. Oxford University Press, Oxford, 1991

162. Woolcott P: Prognostic indicators in the psycho-therapy of borderline patients. Am J Psychother 1985;39:17–29

163. Links P, Mittan JE, Steiner M: Predicting outcome for borderline personality disorder. Compr Psychiatry 1990;31:490–498

164. Stone MH: Long-term outcome in personality disorders. Br J Psychiatry 1993;162:299–313

CHAPTER 53

Characterization and Management of Behavioral Disturbances in the Elderly

GEORGE FULOP

New approaches to managing agitated and disturbing behaviors in the elderly have evolved over the past decade. Increased emphasis is now placed on strategies targeting environmental factors or caregiver and family members' reactions to disturbed behaviors. In contrast, earlier management interventions focused on identifying distressing patient behaviors, diagnosing the underlying pathophysiologic disease processes, treating with psychotropic medication, and using environmental limitations such as institutionalization and physical restraints. This chapter goes beyond the traditional focus on disease and pharmacotherapy by highlighting creative behavioral and social/environmental manipulations that augment the therapeutic armamentarium.

The process of evaluating and managing the typical problem affects, behaviors, and cognitions that present as behavioral disturbances in the elderly (with a special emphasis on the geriatric medical patient) will be outlined including (1) identification and characterization of the nature and intensity of disturbed behaviors; (2) diagnosis of commonly associated conditions—the "5D's" (Delirium, Dementia, Depression, Drugs of abuse/interactions/adverse effects, and DSM-IV[1] Psychiatric Disorders); (3) implementation of appropriate behavioral and environmental interventions; (4) judicious utilization of pharmacotherapy, physical restraints, and restrictive settings; and (5) referral of caregivers to support groups and respite. The impact of problem behaviors on general medical resource use, and interventions to ameliorate disturbed behaviors while reducing medical expenditures, are also described.

Categories of Disturbing Behaviors: Identification and Characterization of the Nature and Intensity of Disturbed Behaviors

Like beauty, disturbed behaviors are in the eye of the beholder. Perceptions vary by observer. Ratings by physicians may differ markedly from those of patients, family members, and caregivers. Health care providers should exercise caution against minimizing the caregiver's assessments and complaints of disturbing behavior on the one hand, and overemphasizing the caregiver's needs at the expense of the elder with the "disturbed behavior" on the other hand. Balancing competing needs and interests—patients versus caregivers—requires ongoing compromise, creativity, and fairness to satisfy all involved parties. The health care provider's primary responsibility, however, remains to advocate the best quality of life for the elder in the least restrictive environment.

A wide range of behavioral disturbances require medical attention and vary by setting. In medical settings, the three most common reasons for a behavioral consultation worldwide were threats of suicide, homicide, and disturbing behaviors.[2] A psychiatric screening evaluation of all 140 admissions to a Geriatric Medicine Evaluation and Treatment Unit at The Mount Sinai Hospital in 1 year found that among 28 possible disturbed behaviors requiring geriatric psychiatric involvement, depression (36 percent), noncompliance (23 percent), coping with chronic illness (15 percent), unclear medical or psychiatric diagnosis (14 percent), behavior management (9 percent), and test refusal (4 percent) were the important behavioral problems that affected the delivery of medical care.[3] In a nursing home, Rovner et al.[4,5] identified the most common behavioral disturbances of dementia as agitation/combativeness, insomnia, irritability, over-reaction to minor annoyances or changes in environment, restlessness, wandering, inappropriate sexual behavior, and misidentification syndrome. On a geropsychiatry unit, Greenwald et al.[6] noted the importance of treating disruptive vocalizations (screaming) and banging. In long-term care settings, psychiatric consultation is most frequently requested for pacing, wandering, verbal abusiveness, disruptive shouting, physical aggression and resistance to necessary care.[7] At home, family members are most distressed by patients who wander, present with insomnia, psychomotor agitation, irritability, incontinence, disinhibition (inappropriate or lewd comments or sexual behaviors) or physical threats. Disturbed behaviors combined with inability to perform basic activities of daily living were the most common reasons for admission to nursing homes among demented elderly.[8]

Conceptually, Kolanowski[9] identified five meaningful clusters of disturbing behaviors in demented elders: (1) aggressive psychomotor behavior; (2) nonaggressive psychomotor behavior; (3) verbally aggressive behavior; (4) passive behavior; and

(5) functionally impaired behavior. Cohen-Mansfield et al.[10] similarly characterized agitation in nursing home elderly as (1) verbally agitated behaviors—constant requests for attention, negativism, repetitious sentences and questions, screaming, and complaining; (2) physically nonaggressive behaviors—pacing, inappropriate dress, movement, handling objects, restlessness, and mannerisms; and (3) aggressive behavior—hitting, kicking, and pushing.

Whereas much has been written regarding behavioral disturbances in dementia and in nursing homes,[4,5] there is a need to expand the conceptualization of behavioral disturbances beyond the demented and elderly in nursing homes in order to remain relevant to other geriatric populations. For example, the author proposes expansion of the above categories of disturbances to the elderly medically ill, as problem affects, behaviors, and cognitions.

Disturbed Behaviors in the Medically Ill—"Problem Affects, Behaviors and Cognitions"

In order to intervene effectively, there is a need to identify categories of disturbed behaviors that may be independent of psychiatric disorders. Target problem behaviors may be defined using criteria employed by cognitive/behavioral scientists as (1) internal mental processes (dysphoric affects [e.g., anxiety, depression]); (2) motor behaviors (e.g., agitation); and (3) cognitions (e.g., thoughts or beliefs about illness or treatment necessity).[11] Problem behaviors may impede required medical diagnostic and therapeutic treatment plans, and interfere with the efficient delivery of medical services. "Effective care should result when medical practice (problem recognition, appropriate diagnostic and therapeutic maneuver, and reassessments) and patient behaviors (utilization, acceptance, understanding and compliance) converge appropriately for episodes of acute need. . . . In large part, medical practice affects outcome through its influence on the behavior of patients."[12]

Behavioral disturbances and psychiatric disorders coexisting with medical disorders in geriatric medical patients are associated with increased medical resource use and prolonged medical hospital length of stays (1.3 to 2 times the stay of inpatients without psychiatric comorbidity).[13,14] This prolongation in stay is associated with numerous medical and psychiatric diagnostic categories.[15] Medical inpatients *with* a psychiatric disorder (e.g., a cooperative demented patient), *may not* exhibit problem behaviors, whereas medical inpatients *without* a psychiatric disorder (e.g., depressed mood and diminished compliance) *may* manifest problem behaviors that interrupt medical care delivery.

Patient behaviors contribute to a wide range of delays in hospital care delivery such as refusal of diagnostic tests (defined as a problem when not reflecting sound judgment or personal preference), food, medication and rehabilitation.[16,17] Noncompliant behaviors of patients impede effective and efficient medical care and contribute to increased health care costs.[18] Behavioral withdrawal or immobility leads to diminished functional status and even secondary complications such as emboli, malnutrition, and immune compromise.[17,19,20] Daily nursing care is disrupted by patients pulling out intravenous lines or resisting toileting, washing, or feeding. Disposition plans are delayed as patients fail to learn self-care routines (e.g., insulin self-administration), unrealistically assess their independence; or deny their need for supportive care or nursing home placement. Although several researchers have examined patient attitudes/motivation, coping, and staff–patient conflicts, only limited systematic evaluation and direct observation of problem behaviors in the medically ill have been undertaken.[20,21]

Instruments to Assess Behavioral Disturbances in Nondemented Elderly Medically Ill

Disease-specific behavior disturbance inventories (e.g., Dementia Behavior Disturbance Scale[22]) and agitation inventories in nursing home populations (e.g., Cohen-Mansfield Agitation Inventory[10]) are available. Most notably, Cohen-Mansfield et al.[10] developed a 29-item agitation inventory for demented and nondemented nursing home elderly that the caregiver rates on a seven-point scale, from 1 (never) to 7 (a few times an hour), as the highest frequency of occurrence. The term *agitation* rather than disturbed behavior was chosen because the former was more commonly used in long-term care settings. Agitation was defined as inappropriate verbal, vocal, or motor activity that is not explained by confusion or needs.[23] Although relevant to up to one-half of the geriatric medically ill, these instruments do not adequately emphasize nondemented or less severely demented elderly problem behaviors.

Given the need for an interviewer-rated, objective inventory of elderly medical inpatient behaviors, a consensus panel (geriatricians, geriatric psychiatrists, health economist, psychologists, and social worker) reviewed items from well-tested instruments (e.g., Alzheimer Disease Assessment Scale [ADAS],[24] Brief Psychiatric Rating Scale [BPRS][25,26]) and suggested inclusion of the following behaviors (source of operationalization of term, and/or item number on original questionnaire) for each problem behavior category: (1) problem affects for example, depressed affect (DSM-IV),[1] appears sad (ADAS), somatic concern (BPRS 1), anxiety (BPRS 2), emotional withdrawal (BPRS 3) hostility (BPRS 10), suspiciousness (BPRS 11), and morale[27]; (2) problem behaviors, for example, motor retardation (BPRS 13), excitement (BPRS 17), tension (BPRS 5), and uncooperative to treatment; and (3) problem cognition/capacity, for example, concentration/distractibility (ADAS 14), attitude (uncooperativity to testing/staff [ADAS 15], uncooperativeness [BPRS 14]), assessment of insight (CERAD C3),[28] comprehension of spoken language (ADAS 2), delayed word recall, and self-efficacy.[29]

In a feasibility study among 30 geriatric medical inpatients,[29] these categories combined with the Sandoz Clinical Assessment-Geriatrics (SCAG)[30]—a measure extensively used in geriatric clinical trials—showed promise in capturing a wide range of problem behaviors on medical wards, and an association (Pearson's $r = 0.3, P < .05$) with increased medical resource use. Using the Microcomputer Clinical Research Administrative and Educational System (MICRO-CARES),[31] a software program for consultation/liaison psychiatry database management at the interface of psychiatry and medicine, a retrospective review of 450 elderly medical/surgical referrals to psychiatry revealed that the available problem affect, behavior, and cognition items and psychiatric conditions among reasons for psychiatric referral included depression (35 percent), organic mental disorder (30 percent), behavior management (23 percent), suicide risk (15 percent), coping (15 percent), judgment (15 percent), refusing test (9 percent), and anxiety/fear (11 percent).[32] Compared to the 12.9 (days) average length of stay of 30,095 elderly inpatients admitted during 2 years to The Mount Sinai Hospital in New York City, the average length of stay (days) for elderly inpatients referred to psychiatry for the following, problems were depression (26), organic mental disorder (27), by diagnosis, behavior management (23), suicide risk (20), judgment/informed consent (25), anxiety/fear (30), and alcohol (31).[32] Disturbed behaviors and psychiatric disorders are associated with increased medical resource use, but the utility of the problem behavior instrument in the elderly medically ill requires further development.

Diagnosis of Conditions Commonly Associated With Behavioral Disturbances in the Elderly Medically Ill—The "5 D's"

Because diagnosis drives management, it is critical to search for the etiology of disturbed behaviors (Table 53-1). In an inpatient geriatric evaluation and treatment unit, 47 percent of admissions had two "D's", Delirium and Dementia, during the hospital stay.[33] Both delirium and dementia are characterized by global cognitive impairment, but are differentiated by the presence or absence of impaired level of consciousness/attention, respectively. Delirium represents the single most important consideration because the behavioral symptoms mask an underlying medical emergency. Delay in recognition and treatment of the medical/surgical etiology of the neuropsychiatric manifestations may in part explain the increased risk of death associated with delirium.[34] Useful mnemonics of the important conditions that may result in death or severe disability if not detected early are WHHHHIMP (Wernicke's disease, Hypertensive encephalopathy, Hypoglycemia, Hypoperfusion, Hypoxia, Intracerebral hemorrhage, Meningitis-encephalitis, and Poisoning/medications) and I WATCH DEATH (infectious, withdrawal, acute metabolic, Trauma, CNS pathology, Hypoxia, Deficiencies [vitamins], Endocrinopathies, Acute vascular, Toxins/Drugs, and Heavy Metals).[35] By 4 weeks, most deliria should have resolved, increasing the likelihood that the continued presence of cognitive impairment represents a pre-existing comorbid dementia, or the transformation of an acute insult into a permanent deficit.

Table 53-1 The 5 "D's" of behavioral disturbances in the geriatric patient

Disorder/ Category	Description/ Distinguishing Feature
1. *D*elirium	Global cognitive impairment *with* altered level of consciousness/attention
2. *D*ementia	Global cognitive impairment *without* altered level of consciousness/attention
3. *D*epression	Depressed mood or diminished interest, with up to 15% of elderly denying mood symptoms but complaining only of somatic distress or irritability
4. *D*rugs	Prescription and nonprescription pharmaceuticals—adverse effects, interactions, and withdrawal; and substances of abuse (primarily alcohol in men, and benzodiazepines in women)
5. *D*SM-IV	All other diagnostic categories in the Diagnostic and Statistical Manual of Mental Disorders, Fourth Edition (DSM-IV), especially anxiety and psychosis.

Depression was the third, and Drugs the fourth most common "D" among the geriatric medical inpatients. The diagnosis of depression is helped by applying another useful mnemonic SIG: E CAPS (impairments in Sleep, Interest, Guilt [and hopelessness, helplessness, worthlessness],":" ["colon" represents somatizations common in the elderly such as preoccupation with constipation, and gastrointestinal disturbances], Energy, Concentration, Psychomotor Agitation/Retardation, and Suicidal Ideation.[36] Drugs comprise iatrogenic (prescription), over-the-counter, and substances of abuse (e.g. alcohol and benzodiazepines) that contribute to neuropsychiatric adverse effects, drug-drug interactions, intoxication, and withdrawal. The fifth "D" is the remainder of the psychiatric conditions included in the Diagnostic and Statistical Manual of Mental Disorders (DSM-IV)[1] and range from anxiety and psychotic disorders, to personality disorders.

The prevalence of the "5 D's" varies by setting. In an outpatient medical setting, anxiety (panic, generalized anxiety, and phobic disorders) and depression (major depression, dysthymia) predominate. In an inpatient psychiatric unit, depression and dementia or psychosis may be most prevalent depending on referral patterns and unit specialization. In a nursing home, dementia predominates. Whatever the setting, careful consideration of the "5 D's" generally leads to the correct diagnosis underlying behavioral disturbances.

Management of Disturbed Behaviors—Behavioral and Environmental/Social Manipulations in General Medical, Long-Term Care, and Home Settings

The implementation of appropriate behavioral and environmental interventions follows the careful characterization and search for an underlying diagnosis of behavioral disturbances and precedes judicious utilization of pharmacotherapy, physical restraints, and restrictive settings. Numerous reports focus on management of disturbed behavior in demented elderly and nursing home populations, with few data on geriatric medical inpatient behavior management.

Psychiatric Management Strategies in the Elderly Medically Ill—Staff Factors in the Geriatric Medical Inpatient Setting

Psychiatric management strategies for the hospitalized elderly medically ill with behavioral disturbances should address, at a minimum, the following staff or provider related factors associated with delays that prolong patient suffering and increase medical stays: (1) delay in recognition of behavioral or psychological symptoms; (2) misidentification of a mental disorder as a physical disorder; (3) undertreatment or mistreatment of behavioral disturbances; (4) delay in requesting a mental health consultation; and (5) failure to implement psychiatric recommendations (Table 53-2). Timely identification and initiation of a treatment plan are associated with improved patient well-being and reduced costs, and assume increased importance in the current cost containment environment.[37] Examples of the type and frequency of management recommendations made by a psychiatrist on a geriatric medicine unit are described in (Table 53-3).[3]

Behavioral Management Strategies—Nursing Home Setting

The Omnibus Budget Reconciliation Act of 1987 OBRA-87 reacted to the problem of the extensive and excessive reliance on antipsychotics by requiring dose reviews, gradual reductions, drug holidays, and behavioral interventions. Physical restraints are used in 25 to 85 percent of nursing homes, and chemical restraints in 11 to 58 percent of institutionalized patients.[38] Similarly, 35 percent of residents in board and care facilities received psychotropics, with 30 percent receiving two to four different agents.[39] Burgio and Bourgeois[40] note that OBRA-87 was a catalyst for the initiation of nonpsychotropic behavioral management strategies of disruptive behavior in the nursing home.[40]

Several creative behavior management strategies have been reported in nursing home settings, including the "AGE" dementia care program (Activities, Guidelines for psychotropic medication, Educational rounds).[5] In a randomized clinical trial with 6-month follow-up of 81 residents in a nursing home with dementia and behavior disorders, the efficacy of the "AGE" program versus standard nursing home care was described: (1) at 6 months 29 percent of 42 intervention patients exhibited behavior disorders compared to 50 percent of 39 controls; (2) intervention patients were much more likely to

Table 53-2 Staff or provider factors associated with unnecessary delay in addressing behavioral disturbances in the elderly and with excess medical resource use

1. *Delay in recognizing behavioral and psychological symptoms* results in a disruption in the medical diagnosis and treatment plan. Lyons et al.[37] observed that increased lagtime (days from admission to recognition of need to address behavioral problems) was associated with longer hospital stays and a delay in instituting treatment plan for the behavioral disturbance.
2. *Misidentification of signs and symptoms of a mental disorder as a medical disorder* (e.g., depression misdiagnosed as hypothyroidism) results in reduced diagnostic certainty and therapeutic delay. Further delays are caused by pursuing futile diagnostic tests that forestall therapeutic actions that would address the underlying psychiatric disturbance.[71]
3. *Undertreatment or mistreatment of behavior disturbance* by primary care physicians is common.[72,73] General physicians tend to prescribe anxiolytics rather than antidepressants for depression, or ineffective, nontherapeutic dosages of antidepressants.[74] The accurate identification and labeling of problem behaviors would result in a more timely psychiatric/behavioral evaluation and initiation of effective treatment.
4. *Delays in calling for mental health consultation* or addressing behavioral problems, even if the primary physician appropriately recognizes the importance of behavior problems, commonly occur. As mentioned above, psychiatric consultations tend to be called in the later half or even last day of a hospital stay, severely limiting the potential impact of psychiatric treatment of the behavior problem.[37] These delays may reflect the following: (1) therapeutic nihilism (no effective psychiatric treatments for behavioral problems in elderly); (2) ageism; (3) a physician's wish to care for the disturbance without a psychiatrist; (4) accession to a patient's wish not to be evaluated by a psychiatrist due to stigma; or (5) resistance to psychiatric care.[75] Presenting the behavioral evaluation and treatment as part of the medical workup on the medical unit may result in diminished stigma and increased compliance, especially in the elderly.
5. *Failure to implement psychiatric recommendations* is a problem even if a psychiatrist is consulted, because there is a lack of concordance with the consulting psychiatrist's recommendation for diagnostic assessments, treatment plan, and medication management.[76] There may even be a concern that treatment of depression would prolong the patient's stay on the medical unit, although transfer to a psychiatric unit may be indicated and would result in a second, diagnosis-related-group exempt hospitalization. Similar to the General Health Questionnaire in the outpatient setting, behavioral inventories may provide feedback of psychiatric data to the primary care physician and may facilitate increased physician compliance in treating problem behaviors.[77]

participate in activities; and (3) controls were more than twice as likely to receive antipsychotics, and to be restrained during activity times and on nursing units.[5] Management strategies are suggested by Malone et al.'s[41] observation that 94 reports of aggressive behavior among 350 residents in a 1-year period were related to patients with cognitive impairment, decreased activities of daily living, poor or infrequent social interactions, poor communication between patient and staff, and new staff or inadequate staffing ratios, and that six patients accounted for 44 percent of the aggressive behaviors.

Jarrett et al.[42] suggested combining pharmacotherapy and alternative behavioral treatments such as (1) environmental changes—calming background music, soothing color scheme, and plants—to form a tranquil milieu to reduce stimuli; (2) restraints and/or behavior modification; (3) regular exercise programs; (4) bright-light treatment; and (5) music and/or pet therapy. A simple, yet effective strategy to reduce wandering was to use masking tape as a visual grating pattern that demented patients will not cross.[43] Severe behavioral disturbances may respond to antecedent and consequent interventions and environmental redesign.[40]

Winograd and Jarvik[44] present the "Seven I's" as a framework for the care of the institutionalized demented patient by the practicing physician (Intellectual impairment, Insomnia/Wandering/Agitation, Immobility, Instability, Incontinence, Iatrogenic conditions, and Involvement of families), and offer helpful environmental manipulations. These interventions in the institutionalized elderly represent a clear move from dependence on pharmacologic and physical restraints, to behavioral, environmental, and social strategies that emphasize increased patient socialization, stimulation, interaction, and activity.

Psychiatric Management Strategies—Home Management of the Behaviorally Disturbed Elderly

Two examples of recently reported strategies to facilitate the care of the community-dwelling elderly are highlighted. A geriatric community mental health outreach program observed that cognitive impairment, behavioral disturbances, physical/medical problems, and depression were the most common reasons for referral.[45] Stolee et al.[45] intervened with a program that included a multidisciplinary consultation team, specialized information/resource service, educational efforts, and a coordinating role in the health care system. Most of the referred patients did not require management at higher levels of care. Development of caregiver and other local resources, as well as program activities such as focused educational initiatives in the community and institutions, were initiated.

Especially after a hospital stay, Grieco[46] recommends a "perihospital" home care "review of systems" that includes examining the adequacy of the home environment, the patient's capability, and the family's ability and accuracy of medication management. The physician should support the home caregiver's central tasks: providing emotional support and physical assistance to the patient; making observations and calling for help; rendering housekeeping/household chores; and, participating in the treatment regimen.[46] Physicians need to evaluate how the family members react to home care responsibility and to determine if they can handle the burden. If not, physicians may need to refer them to self-help groups or appropriate home health aide services. In order to facilitate return to home after hospitalization, the primary home caregiver of the patient should be involved in treatment in order to readily assimilate their future roles. Grieco[46] concludes that coordination of care among the patient, family, hospital staff, home care agency, and the physician is important to ensure that the patient maintains maximum functional ability at home.

Table 53-3 Psychiatric treatment and management recommendations made by a geriatric psychiatrist screening 140 consecutive geriatric medicine inpatients in a university hospital in a 1-year period

Treatment Recommendation	Number (%)
To be completed by unit staff	
Constant nursing observation	5 (4%)
Diagnostic tests	71 (51%)
Other consultation required	48 (34%)
To be completed by consulting psychiatrist	
Psychotherapy	30 (21%)
Transfer to psychiatry	10 (7%)
Outpatient treatment	30 (21%)
Impaired judgment	23 (16%)

Pharmacologic Management of Disturbed Behavior

There is increased recognition of the limited to moderate efficacy of psychotropics in reducing behavioral disturbances, with few randomized, placebo-controlled studies, or specification of which behaviors respond best to different categories of drugs.[47–49] In general, the efficacy of neuroleptics, and to a lesser degree, short half-life benzodiazepines, have demonstrated benefit, but often only for a minority of patients and with adverse side effects that even contribute to worsening of the behavioral disturbance.[50] For example, a meta-analysis revealed that neuroleptics benefited only 18 of 100 demented patients.[47] In fact, withdrawal from neuroleptics was paradoxically associated with improved behavior.[51] Novel antipsychotics, such as risperidone, may offer hope for improved efficacy. Anticonvulsants, β-adrenergic antagonists, buspirone, estrogen, lithium, and trazodone may also play a role in managing disturbed behaviors.[52]

Maletta[53] described behaviors responsive to psychotropics as anxiety, psychosis (delusions and hallucinations), physical or verbal assault, and regression. Behaviors usually not amenable to medication include wandering, hoarding, stealing, difficult personalities, repetitive/annoying activities and hypersexuality, and inappropriate voiding.[53] Billig and colleagues[54] conducted a medical chart survey of the use of psychotropics by 408 nursing home residents in the previous week and found that antipsychotics (major tranquilizers, e.g., haloperidol and thioridazine) were more commonly utilized in agitated demented elderly (21 percent), and benzodiazepines (minor tranquilizers, e.g., alprazolam) were used in agitated nondemented elderly (14 percent), whereas fewer antidepressants (e.g., doxepin, trazodone) were used in agitated versus nonagitated residents (12 percent). A particular strength of this report is the association of the psychotropic prescribed with the type of agitation. Neuroleptics were used approximately twice as often as benzodiazepines, and four times as often as sedative/hypnotics and antidepressants in aggressive, physically nonaggressive, and verbal agitation subtypes.[54] Much of pharmacotherapeutic treatment employed to date remains empirical.

Pharmacologic management has often been the initial step in the medical caregiver's attempt to relieve a patient's distress. An extensive literature exists on the selection, dose, and titration of psychopharmacotherapeutics.[23,55–57] Rovner[5] describes the role of psychotropics in the initial treatment of behavioral disturbances when the patient is extremely agitated or if the agitation prevents medical evaluation. The next steps are (1) the need to complete medical and psychiatric evaluations to determine differential diagnoses; and (2) identify and treat underlying physical symptoms.[5] Rovner[5] also recommends consideration of antidepressants with few anticholinergic side effects, antipsychotics, and education for the family and caregiver.

Caregiver Burden

An important trend is the growing emphasis on the needs of family caregivers in support of their care of behaviorally disturbed elders. Increased rates of depression, insomnia, headaches, and irritability are commonly noted among caregivers. The characteristics of caregivers who institutionalize family members include the need for increased social support before, and stress-reducing medications after institutionalization.[58] "The 36-hour Day" provides welcome attention to the caregiver's burden, and at times respite from the daily workload.[59] Rabins[60] also highlights the strategies and benefits of family-directed therapy to reduce the burden of caregivers. In addition to lower caregiver distress,[61] Brodaty et al.[62,63] reported a dramatic difference in survival at home (53 versus 13 percent) and fewer deaths (20 versus 41 percent) among patients whose caregivers had an intensive 10-day residential training program for dementia caregivers. Outpatient geriatric assessment compared to usual medical care also resulted in less caregiver stress at 1 year in a randomized multisite trial.[64] In general, educational support group interventions predominate, followed by problem-solving approaches, therapeutic skill training, and psychotherapy.[65]

Larson et al.[66] offer practical suggestions for health care professionals to aid caregivers and patients: (1) anticipate future problems; (2) determine the patient's wishes;(3) discuss emotional reactions;(4) pay attention to communications with patients and families; and (5) attend to practical details of care. By extrapolation, nursing home staff and home aides also may benefit from similar strategies and support offered to family caregivers.

Psychiatric/Behavioral Interventions Reduce Medical Resource Use in the Elderly Medically Ill

Psychiatric interventions in the medically ill are associated with reduced cost of medical care. Mumford et al.[67] noted a 2-day reduction in hospital stay, especially evident among elderly women, in their meta-analysis of psychosocial interventions in the medically ill. Smith and colleagues[68] described a 50 percent reduction in medical services use following a psychiatric evaluation for somatization disorder. Strain et al.[69] reported a 2-day reduction in hospital stay following a screening psychiatric intervention among elderly hip fracture patients. The shorter stays were not followed by increased outpatient medical resource use, and in fact, total episode of care (inpatient and outpatient) costs were 9 percent less for those receiving psychiatric intervention. The mechanisms for reducing stays included (1) prescribing only short-acting hypnotic medication to avoid daytime sedation and facilitate fuller participation in physical rehabilitation; (2) teaching families, nursing homes, and other caretakers how to manage behavioral disturbances in the medically ill elderly; and (3) initiating treatment of mental disorders early in the hospital course. Strain and Huyse[20,21] also helped operationalize problem-focused psychiatric interventions in the medically ill. These studies found a high concordance (staff's implementation of the consulting psychiatrist's recommendations) with medication administration, but lower concordance for diagnostic testing.

Angell[70] noted that rationing of health care resources may not be necessary if inefficient modes of medical care delivery can be identified. A careful inventory of problem affects, behaviors, and cognitions and patient–staff interactions is an important step in dissecting the major behavioral factors associated with patient distress and inefficient health services delivery. Targeted behavioral interventions then can be identified and implemented to reduce both disturbed and disturbing behaviors, as well as medical resource use, and improve the quality of life for the elderly.

References

1. Diagnostic and Statistical Manual of Mental Disorders. American Psychiatric Association, Washington, DC, 1994
2. Krakowski AJ: Consultation psychiatry, present global status. Psychother Psychosom 1974;23:78–86
3. Fulop G, Strain JJ, Bronheim H: Psychiatric consultation versus

screening on a geriatric medicine unit abstracted. Psychosom Med 1989;51:261–262

4. Rovner BW, Steele CD, Shmuely Y et al: A randomized trial of dementia care in nursing homes. J Am Geriatr Soc 1996;44: 7–13
5. Rovner BW: Behavioral disturbances of dementia: overview of disorders and treatments. Curr Approaches Dementia 1995;1: 1–6
6. Greenwald BS, Marin DB, Silverman SM: Serotonergic treatment of screaming and banging in dementia. Lancet 1985;20: 1464–1465
7. Streim JE, Katz IR: Clinical psychiatry in the nursing home. pp. 413–432. In Busse EW, Blazer DG (eds): Textbook of Geriatric Psychiatry. American Psychiatric Press, Washington DC, 1996
8. Steele C, Rovner BW, Chase GA et al: Psychiatric symptoms and nursing home placement in Alzheimer's Disease. Am J Psychiatry 1990;147:1049–1051
9. Kolanowski AM: Disturbing behaviors in demented elders: a concept synthesis. Arch Psychiatr Nurs 1995;9:188–194
10. Cohen-Mansfield J, Marx MS, Rosenthal AS: A description of agitation in a nursing home. J Gerontol 1989;44:M77–M84
11. Lazarus AA, Fay A: Behavior therapy. pp. 483–538. In Karasu TB (ed): The Psychiatric Therapies Part II. The Psychosocial Therapies. American Psychiatric Association, Washington, DC, 1984
12. Starfield B: Health services research: a working model. N Engl J Med 1973;289:132–136
13. Fulop G, Strain JJ, Vita J et al: Impact of psychiatric comorbidity on length of hospital stay of medical/surgical inpatients: a preliminary report. Am J Psychiatry 1987;144:878–882
14. Fulop G, Strain JJ, Fahs MC et al: A prospective study of the impact of psychiatric comorbidity on length of hospital stays of elderly medical/surgical inpatients. Psychosomatics (in press).
15. Fulop G, Strain JJ, Hammer JS et al: DRGs, psychiatric comorbidity, and prolonged hospital stay. Hosp Commun Psychiatry 1989;40:80–82
16. Fillit H: The Geriatric Evaluation and Treatment Unit: A model for the development of excellent care for the hospitalized frail elderly. Report to the Mount Sinai Auxiliary Board, 1987
17. Fillit H, Miller M: The geriatric evaluation and treatment unit: a model site for acute geriatric care, education and research. Mount Sinai J Med 1993;60:6:475–481
18. Lipowski ZJ: Review of consultation psychiatry and psychosomatic medicine: II. Clinical aspects. Psychosom Med 1967;29: 201–224
19. Saravay SM, Lavin M: Psychiatric comorbidity and length of stay in the general hospital: a critical review of outcome studies. Psychosomatics 1994;35:233–252
20. Huyse FJ: Systematic Interventions in Consultation/Liaison Psychiatry. Free University Press, Amsterdam, 1989
21. Huyse FJ, Strain JJ, Hengeveld MW et al: Interventions in consultation-liaison psychiatry: the development of a schema and a checklist for operationalized interventions. Gen Hosp Psychiatry 1988;10:88–101
22. Baumgarten M, Becker R, Gathier S: Validity and reliability of the Dementia Behavior Disturbance Scale. J Am Geriatr Soc 1990;38:221–226
23. Cohen-Mansfield J, Billig N: Agitated behaviors in the elderly: I. A conceptual review. J Am Geriatr Soc 1986;34:10:711–721
24. Rosen WG, Mohs RC, Davis KL: A new rating scale for Alzheimer's disease. Am J Psychiatry 1984;141:1356–1364
25. Overall JE, Gorham DE: The Brief Psychiatric Rating Scale. Psychol Rep 1962;10:799–812
26. Gottlieb GL, Gur RE, Gur RC: Reliability of psychiatric scales in dementia of the Alzheimer's type. Am J Psychiatry 1988; 145:7:857–860
27. Lawton MP: The Philadelphia Geriatric Center Morale Scale: a Revision. J Gerontol 1975;30:85–89
28. Tariot PN, Mack JL, Patterson MB et al: The Behavior Rating Scale for Dementia of the Consortium to Establish a Registry for Alzheimer's Disease. Am J Psychiatry 1995;152:1349–1357
29. Fulop G, Strain JJ, Mohs RC et al: The Mount Sinai Hospital Consensus Panel and Feasibility Trial of a Problem Affect, Behavior, Cognition (PABC) Inventory in the Elderly Medically Ill. Mt. Sinai Hospital, New York, 1995
30. Venn RD: The Sandoz Clinical Assessment-Geriatric (SCAG) Scale. A general-purpose psychogeriatric rating scale. Gerontology 1983;29:185–198
31. Hammer JS, Hammond D, Strain JJ et al: Microcomputers and consultation psychiatry in the general hospital. Gen Hosp Psychiatry 1985;7:119–124
32. Fulop G, Strain JJ, Blank E: Phases of late life development and referral to psychiatry, abstracted. J Am Geriatr Soc 1987; 5:35
33. Fulop G, Strain JJ, Bronheim H: Psychiatric consultation versus screening modalities on a geriatric medicine unit abstracted. Psychosom Med 1989;51:261–262
34. Rabins PV, Folstein MF: Delirium and dementia: diagnostic criteria and fatality rates. Br J Psychiatry 1982;140:149–153
35. Wise MG: Delirium. pp. 89–106. In Hales RE, Yudofsky SC (eds): The American Psychiatric Press Textbook of Neuropsychiatry. American Psychiatric Press, Washington DC, 1987
36. Jenike MA: Geriatric Psychiatry and Psychopharmacology. Year Book Medical Publishers, New York, 1990
37. Lyons JS, Hammer JS, Strain JJ, Fulop G: The timing of psychiatric consultation and the length of hospital stay. Gen Hosp Psychiatry 1986;8:159–162
38. Sloane PD, Mathew LJ, Scarborough M et al: Physical and pharmacologic restraint of nursing home patients with dementia. Impact of specialized units. JAMA 1991;265:1278–1282
39. Spore D, Mor V, Hiris J et al: Psychotropic use among older residents of board and care facilities. J Am Geriatr Soc 1995; 43:1403–1409
40. Burgio LD, Bourgeois M: Treating severe behavioral disorders in geriatric residential settings. Behav Resident Treatment 1996;7:145–168
41. Malone ML, Thompson L, Goodwin JS: Aggressive behaviors among the institutionalized elderly. J Am Geriatr Soc 1993;41: 853–856
42. Jarrett PG, Rockwood K, Mallery L: Behavioral problems in nursing home residents. Safe ways to manage dementia. Postgrad Med 1995;97:189–196
43. Hussian RA, Brown DC: Use of two-dimensional grid patterns to limit hazardous ambulation in demented patients. J Gerontol 1987;42:558–560

44. Winograd CH, Jarvik LF: Physician management of the demented patient. J Am Geriatr Soc 1986;34:295–308
45. Stolee P, Kessler L, Le Clair JK: A community development and outreach program in geriatric mental health: four years' experience. J Am Geriatr Soc 1996;44:314–320
46. Grieco AJ: Physician's guide to managing home care of older patients. Geriatrics 1991;46:49–60
47. Schneider L, Pollock VE, Lyness SA: A metaanalysis of controlled trials of neuroleptic treatment in dementia. J Am Geriatr Soc 1990;38:553–563
48. Barnes R, Veith R, Okimoto J et al: Efficacy of antipsychotic medications in behaviorally disturbed dementia patients. Am J Psychiatry 1982;139:1170–1174
49. Coccaro EF, Kramer E, Zemishlany Z et al: Pharmacologic treatment of noncognitive behavioral disturbances in elderly demented patients. Am J Psychiatry 1990;147:1640–1645
50. Risse SC, Barnes R: Pharmacologic treatment of agitation associated with dementia. J Am Geriatr Soc 1986;34:368–376
51. Raskind MA, Risse SC, Lampe TH: Dementia and antipsychotic drugs. J Clin Psychiatry 1987;48:16–18
52. Lake JT, Grossberg GT: Management of Psychosis, Agitation, and Other Behavioral Problems in Alzheimer's Disease. Psychiatr Ann 1996;26:274–279
53. Maletta GJ: Pharmacologic treatment and management of the aggressive demented patient. Psychiatr Ann 1990;20:446–455
54. Billig N, Cohen-Mansfield J, Lipson S: Pharmacological treatment of agitation in a nursing home. J Am Geriatr Soc 1991; 39:1002–1005
55. Cassem NH: Massachusetts General Hospital Handbook of General Hospital Psychiatry. Third Ed. Mosby-Year Book, St. Louis, 1991
56. Busse EW, Blazer DG: Textbook of Geriatric Psychiatry. American Psychiatric Press, Washington DC, 1996
57. Salzman C: Anxiety in the Elderly: Treatment & Research. Springer, New York, 1991
58. Colerick EJ, George LK: Predictors of institutionalization among caregivers of patients with Alzheimer's disease. J Am Geriatr Soc 1986;34:493–498
59. Mace NL, Rabins PV: The 36 Hour Day: A Family Guide to Caring for Persons with Alzheimer's Disese, Related Dementing Illnesses, and Memory Loss in Later Life, Revised Edition. Johns Hopkins University Press, Baltimore, 1991
60. Rabins PV: Family-Directed Therapy. pp. 225–233. In Cummings JL, Miller BL (eds): Alzheimer's Disease Treatment and Long-Term Management. Marcel Dekker, New York, 1990
61. Brodaty H, Gresham M: Effect of a training programme to reduce stress in carers of patients with dementia. Br Med J 1989;299: 1375–1379
62. Brodaty H, Petere KE: Cost effectiveness of a training program for dementia carers. Int Psychogeriatr 1991;3:11–22
63. Brodaty H, McGilchrist C, Harris L et al: Time until institutionalization and death in patients with dementia. Arch Neurol 1993;50:643–650
64. Silverman M, Musa D, Martin DC et al: Evaluation of outpatient geriatric assessment: a randomized multi-site trial. J Am Geriatr Soc 1995;43:733–740
65. Toseland RW, Rossiter CM: Group interventions to support family caregivers: a review and analysis. Gerontologist 1989;29: 438–448
66. Larson EB, Lo B, Williams ME: Evaluation and care of elderly patients with dementia. J Gen Int Med 1986;1:116–125
67. Mumford E, Schlesinger HS, Glass GV et al: A new look at evidence about reduced cost of medical utilization following mental health treatment. Am J Psychiatry 1984;141: 1145–1158
68. Smith GR, Monson RA, Ray BS: Psychiatric consultation in somatization disorder: a randomized controlled study. N Engl J Med 1986;22:1407–1413
69. Strain JJ, Lyons JS, Hammer JS et al: Cost offset from a psychiatric consultation-liaison intervention with elderly hip fracture patients. Am J Psychiatry 1991;148:1044–1049
70. Angell M: Cost containment and the physician. JAMA 1985; 254:1203–1207
71. Fulop G, Strain JJ: Psychiatric emergencies in the general hospital. Gen Hosp Psychiatry 1986;8:425–431
72. Strain JJ: Dilemmas of the psychiatrist in the medical setting—generalist or specialist. In The Medical Patient. Psychiatr Clin N Am 1981;4:2:199–201
73. Strain JJ: Diagnostic considerations in the medical setting. Psychiatr Clin N Am 1981;4:2:287–300
74. Fulop G, Reinhardt J, Strain JJ et al: Identification of alcoholism and depression in a geriatric medicine outpatient clinic. J Am Geriatr Soc 1993;41:737–741
75. Pasnau RO: Consultation-liaison psychiatry: progress, problems, and prospects. Psychosomatics 1988;29:1:4–15
76. Popkin MK, Mackenzie TB, Callies AL: Consultees' concordance with consultants' recommendations for diagnostic action. J Nerv Ment Dis 1980;168:9–12
77. Shapiro S, German PS, Skinner EA et al: An experiment to change detection and management of mental morbidity in primary care. Med Care 1987;25:327–339

CHAPTER 54

Psychology in the Diagnosis and Treatment of the Dementias

RAJENDRA JUTAGIR

The primary role of the psychologist working with older patients is evaluation and treatment of cognitive and emotional disorders. The prevalence of dementia in the community increases with age. One estimate was 3 percent for ages 65 to 74 years and as high as 47 percent beyond age 85.[1] Apart from dementia there may be cognitive impairment that is not pervasive or does not include memory loss. For example, in vascular disease there is a continuum of cognitive impairment, which may range from subtle, subclinical cognitive loss, up to and including dementia.[2] If one includes more subtle deficits, the rate of cognitive impairment would be very high in older people. Thus the psychologist working with a geriatric population must be knowledgeable about cognitive disorders. This requires a background in neuropsychology, beyond expertise in working with emotional disorders. The first part of this chapter focuses on neuropsychological evaluation of the dementias in geriatric patients. The second part addresses psychological treatment of dementing individuals and their families.

Cognitive Impairment

Memory loss is one of the most common reasons for referral of geriatric patients for neuropsychological testing, and often leads to a diagnosis of dementia. Dementia is defined as global intellectual impairment, operationalized as memory loss and impairment in at least one other domain of higher cortical functioning (aphasia, apraxia, agnosia, executive functioning), decline in social or occupational functioning, with exclusion of delirium and possible nonorganic causes of cognitive loss.[3] These criteria rely heavily on evaluation of intellectual deficits, which are best documented by neuropsychological testing. The nature and degree of cognitive impairment is uncovered by a test battery that should minimally evaluate the following domains: attention and orientation, learning and memory, language, motor, visuospatial, and executive functions.[4] Additional tests, such as calculations, are helpful in evaluating older people. The neuropsychological profile, consisting of intact and impaired cognitive domains, is used to arrive at a diagnosis. For example, if it shows circumscribed impairment one might suspect a focal event. More widespread deficits in intellectual functioning would suggest a dementia.

The first task in developing the profile is to differentiate impairment from normal aging. Both cross-sectional and longitudinal studies indicate that many cognitive abilities, including memory, undergo normative decline with age.[5–8] Therefore care must be taken to avoid overdiagnosing impairment in older people by attributing normative change to disease, especially in memory disorders where positive findings can be distressing to both patient and family. To avoid this problem, a patient's performance on neuropsychological tasks is compared with normative data derived from others in the same age group. This allows the clinician to judge the likelihood that the patient belongs to a "normal" or "impaired" population. The use of normative data by itself is not always sufficient to make this discrimination. Early in a dementing process, for example, individuals may function below their usual capacity even though they still fall within normal limits for their age group. This is especially likely to occur in individuals of high intellectual capacity.[9] When this occurs, premorbid capacity is estimated from the patient's level of educational or occupational achievement. Premorbid functioning can also be inferred from standardized reading tests or tests of crystallized intelligence such as vocabulary or general information. Even though these show early and progressive decline in dementia,[10–12] they are thought to be less affected by organic deterioration than other tests. Discrepancies between premorbid and current capacity can suggest whether decline has occurred.

Once the neuropsychological profile of intact and impaired cognitive domains is established, it is used to identify the disease process that gave rise to it. There are compelling reasons to differentiate among the dementias. As treatments proliferate, improved diagnosis will ensure appropriate treatment. Iatrogenic illness may be avoided, as in the case of neuroleptic treatment in Lewy body disease.[13] The correct prognosis is valuable in patient management, and improves counseling for families. Finally, accurate diagnosis enhances research, which holds the promise of further improvement in diagnosis and treatment.

Differential diagnosis of the dementias is complicated by the overlap of deficits in different syndromes, which compromises the specificity of the diagnosis. Cortical disorders may have some subcortical involvement, posterior disorders may have some anterior involvement, and different disorders that involve the same regions of the brain (especially degenerative disorders that spread progressively) can show convergence of symptoms. Furthermore, a patient may present with more than one disorder, as in the case of mixed vascular and Alzheimer's dementia,[14] mixed Alzheimer's and Lewy body dementia,[15,16] or mixed Alzheimer's and Parkinson's disease.[17] In addition to clinical ambiguity, there are deficiencies in research efforts to differentiate the dementias. Many studies have failed to control for the severity of dementia, making it unclear whether the findings represent true differences between disorders, or are merely due to the stage of the disorder. Furthermore, absence of neuropathologic confirmation in many studies makes it uncertain whether cases were correctly classified.

The complexity of dementing disorders is matched by the complexity of memory itself. Different theoretical memory systems have been proposed, and attempts made to relate these to underlying brain structures and processes. Memory is broadly divided into primary (short-term) and secondary (long-term) memory. The former refers to temporary storage of material in memory for periods of up to about 30 seconds, whereas secondary memory refers to storage for longer periods. Primary memory has been extensively investigated in the context of "working memory," which is described as a central executive system that integrates and coordinates slave subsystems, two of which are the articulatory loop system and the visuospatial scratch pad.[18]

Secondary memory has been divided into explicit (or declarative) memory, and implicit[19] (or nondeclarative) memory, based on whether stored information is available to conscious awareness or not. Implicit memory consists of unconscious processing, such as occurs in conditioning, priming, or using information (which may be motoric, perceptual, or cognitive) that enables performance in the world. Explicit memory has been further subdivided into episodic and semantic memory. Tulving[20] proposed that memory consists of three systems that are monohierarchically arranged. Procedural memory is necessary for adaptation to the environment, and stands at the bottom of the hierarchy. Semantic memory has the additional capability of internally representing knowledge of words, concepts, and facts of the world, and constructing mental models. On top of that, episodic memory has the additional capacity of storing autobiographical experiences with specific reference to the time when they occurred. Each system requires the system below it. The distinction between episodic and semantic memory has been criticized, but is regarded as heuristically productive.[21] Secondary memory has also been subdivided into recent and remote memory, the latter referring to the more distant past. These theoretical subdivisions of memory are not universally agreed upon. They have been reviewed elsewhere.[22–24]

The complexity of the brain, its functions, and diseases make the neuropsychological profile a valuable tool in specifying and quantifying the patterns of deficits seen in brain disorders, especially when combined with information derived from detailed inquiry into the nature, onset, duration, and course of symptoms. For this reason it is often included in research diagnostic criteria for the dementias.[14,25–27] Neuropsychological evaluation is perhaps the most sensitive instrument for the detection of early or mild dementia, when deficits are not grossly apparent, and are too subtle for detection by screening tests. It may also be of value in identifying progressive dementia in the preclinical stage.[28] An interdisciplinary approach to differential diagnosis has also become increasingly necessary, combining neuropsychological testing with medical and neurological evaluation, and neuroradiologic procedures.

Dementias have been grouped according to cortical and subcortical symptoms,[29,30] although there is not universal agreement about this distinction. Alzheimer's disease and the focal lobar atrophies[31] would be considered cortical, whereas Parkinson's disease, progressive supranuclear palsy, and Huntington's disease would be considered subcortical. However, some disorders such as Lewy body disease and vascular dementia may span these categories, producing lesions in both cortical and subcortical areas. Cortical dementias have been grouped along a topographic axis from anterior to posterior regions of the cortex according to presumed location of lesions.[32] Frontotemporal dementias and Pick's disease would be considered anterior, whereas Alzheimer's disease would be posterior. Neuropsychological profiles of the most common dementias found in the elderly are described below. Studies were selected for review with a bias toward the early detection of dementia.

Alzheimer's Disease

Alzheimer's disease (AD) is the most common dementia in the elderly.[33] In AD there is progressive degeneration of cortical tissue in the temporal and parietal lobes, and damage to the hippocampus is considered responsible for memory deficits. For clinical diagnosis, the Diagnostic and Statistical Manual of the American Psychiatric Association (DSM-IV) requires, beyond documentation of a dementia, that there be insidious onset and gradual progression of symptoms.[3] Research criteria for *probable* AD established by the National Institute of Neurologic and Communicative Disorders (NINCDS) and the Alzheimer's and Related Disorders Association (ADRDA) are dementia established by clinical examination, documented by a screening test for dementia and confirmed by neuropsychological testing; deficits in two or more areas of cognition; progression of memory and other cognitive deficits; no disturbance of consciousness; onset between ages 40 and 90 years; and exclusion of systemic disorders or other brain diseases that could account for progressive cognitive deficits. A diagnosis of *possible* AD is made if there is a concurrent systemic or brain disorder that could produce dementia, or if only one progressive cognitive deficit can be identified.[25] Using these criteria, clinical classification of AD, which included neuropsychological evaluation, was found to be 80 to 90 percent accurate when compared with the results of postmortem neuropathologic testing.[34] As AD remains a diagnosis of exclusion, the requirement that other brain disorders be excluded takes on increased significance with the documentation of "new" dementias such as frontal lobe dementia and diffuse Lewy body disease.

Memory

Episodic memory

By definition, episodic memory is impaired in AD. There is abundant documentation of impairment on a wide variety of episodic memory tasks in AD relative to normal elderly subjects (NE). Numerous studies have shown impairment in immediate and/or delayed recall of word lists.[28,35–45] Using a grocery list that may have better ecological validity, similar deficits were found.[46] Patients with mild AD retain the capacity to learn new information, although not to the same degree as NE; their learning curve declines as the severity of dementia increases.[47–49] Recognition testing for word list items is also impaired in AD.[28,35,36,50] Overall, word lists that evaluate episodic memory appear to be particularly sensitive in identifying AD.

Impaired performance has also been documented in episodic memory when memoranda consist of stories.[44, 51–56] Although patients with mild AD are able to learn to associate pairs of words, performance is deficient relative to NE.[51] This ability is sensitive to severity of dementia, as patients with moderate dementia do not show a learning curve. Only NE and a group of patients who had very mild cognitive deficits showed a learning curve for difficult associates.[57]

Serial-position effects in recall of word lists is different in AD than in NE. In normal recall, more words are retrieved from the beginning (primacy) and end (recency) than from the middle of a word list. In AD, a smaller number of items are recalled from the beginning of lists, indicating that the primacy effect is weaker in AD than in NE.[35,36,42,48] Closer inspection reveals that in AD there is a primacy effect on shorter lists, which is lost as the list gets longer.[58] This may represent an extension of the finding of impaired immediate recall in AD, because a list that is longer than seven words would exceed the capacity of working memory, necessitating transfer to secondary memory.[59] The weakening of the primacy effect is related to the severity of dementia.[49,60] Not everyone has found an attenuated primacy effect in AD relative to NE.[61]

Numerous studies of patients with AD have shown a liberal response bias, and retrieval errors on learned word lists such that they allow intrusion of items that are not on the list. Patients with AD made more intrusions on cued recall than NE, and this effect was also statistically significant in a small subsample of preclinical AD cases.[28] The same effect was found for immediate and delayed free recall in AD.[35,36] Intrusion errors are also more frequent in visual reproduction tasks in patients with AD.[62]

There is disagreement about the mechanism that results in poorer performance in patients with AD on tests of episodic memory. Some investigators believe that there is a more rapid rate of forgetting in AD. Studies that purport to demonstrate this have used a "savings score," which represents the percent of learned material recalled or recognized after delay. This is problematic; even if both groups forget the same number of items, it would appear that patients with AD forget a higher proportion, because they initially learn fewer items (i.e., the denominator is smaller). A number of studies that have attempted to equate the amount of learning in AD and NE failed to find evidence of an increased rate of forgetting in learned material, and lend support to the hypothesis that encoding rather than storage is impaired in AD.[41,63–65] Nonetheless "savings scores" may have clinical value as an index of the amount of material learned and forgotten. Empirically, they have demonstrated efficacy in discriminating patients with AD from NE subjects.[53,54]

Episodic memory for visual stimuli is also impaired in AD. Deficient reproduction of geometric shapes has been noted in very mild AD, becoming worse with severity of dementia.[66] Patients with mild but not moderate AD showed a learning curve for visual stimuli.[49] Delayed recall of visual material is worse in patients with AD than in NE,[41,52,56,63–65, 67] regardless of severity of dementia.[45] Recognition memory for faces is impaired in AD,[50] as is learning to associate names with faces.[46]

Semantic memory and semantic knowledge

There is widespread impairment of semantic memory in AD. Store of general information is impaired,[44] as is vocabulary[37,68] Word finding (confrontation naming) deficits have consistently been found in AD[37,43,55,68,69] and increase with severity of dementia.[44] Word finding difficulty occurs even in mild AD.[70]

In category fluency tests of semantic memory, subjects are required to name as many exemplars within a given category (animals, fruits, vegetables) as they can within a fixed period of time, usually 1 minute. Performance on this task is quite impaired in AD[43,68,71–74] and has discriminated between mild AD and NE with 100 percent sensitivity and 92.5 percent specificity.[75] It has even successfully differentiated NE from patients with mild and preclinical AD[28,45] and people at risk for developing dementia.[69] One prospective study, although limited by a small sample size, found that generating words to category cue was impaired more than 2 years prior to diagnosis of AD.[76] A recent study showed that patients with mild AD generated not only fewer words, but fewer clusters (subcategories) within the category tested. This was interpreted as evidence that semantic knowledge is lost as opposed to difficulty accessing an intact store of semantic information.[77] Patients with AD are also impaired in making associations to words.[78]

Additional findings suggest impairment in semantic memory in AD. Patients with mild AD are impaired in reading low-frequency words with irregular spelling-to-sound correspondence (e.g., ache), and degree of impairment increases with severity of dementia. Patients with AD are also impaired on nonword reading.[11] Impairment in reading skill has been found in the earliest stage of clinically detectable AD.[12] Performance on a picture vocabulary test was impaired in mild and moderate

AD.[79] Picture matching was reported to be impaired in minimal AD.[45]

In an extensive review of semantic memory in AD, Nebes[80] concluded that word finding and certain aspects of concept formation are deficient in patients with AD and that they benefit less than NE from the effect of semantic context when contextual cues are subtle. Patients with AD may be able to use semantic information to facilitate episodic memory, but perform less well on tests of general world knowledge than do normal individuals.

Remote and autobiographical memory

Patients with AD recalled fewer important life events than normal subjects, but they showed the same distribution of recalled events throughout the life span.[81] With increasing severity of dementia not only were memories lost, but also memories that were elicited contained fewer details.[82] Patients with mild AD were better at locating places on a map of the area where they were raised than using a map of the area where they resided, suggesting temporally graded retrograde amnesia.[83]

Working memory

Deficits due to AD in the components of working memory have been reviewed. The articulatory loop system is essentially intact in AD, and it remains unclear whether the visuospatial scratchpad is impaired. However, there is considerable evidence of dysfunction of the central executive system, which may account for the observed decrement in memory span and vulnerability to distraction in AD.[84] A neural network basis for this dysfunction has been proposed, namely the disruption of fibers that connect the anterior and posterior regions of the brain.[85]

Visuospatial Functions and Calculations

Copying of a clock and geometric figures was found to be impaired relative to NE.[69] Visuoconstructional skills are correlated with severity of impairment in other cognitive domains, and with overall severity of dementia.[86] Visuospatial performance is worse in patients with AD who are disoriented or wander.[87,88] Arithmetic calculations are also impaired in early to moderate AD.[51] In one sample of mildly demented patients with AD (mean MMS = 22), the majority fell below the cutoff for normal performance in calculations. Scores did not correlate with episodic memory score for verbal material, which may indicate that working memory is more important than episodic memory in this skill.[89]

Executive Functions

Some executive functions begin to decline early in the disease. Letter fluency, measured by the number of words generated for a given letter in a limited period of time, is impaired in AD.[69,74,75,90] It is impaired very early in the disease process, as even preclinical cases do less well than NE.[28,69] One study found that letter fluency was not worse in mild AD; however, all but two patients performed below the mean for NE.[73] Measures of attention such as digit span are also impaired in mild AD.[28,69] Studies that have not found reduced spans tend to use small samples,[51,91] suggesting that the effect size in early dementia is small. Verbal and visual continuous performance tests are deficient in AD.[43] Divided attention is impaired in AD.[84] Ability to shift mental set is impaired in mild AD, both on a trailmaking task, and on a card sorting test.[28,69] Abstraction is impaired on a similarities task that requires grouping of stimuli according to abstract criteria, even in preclinical cases.[28,51] Performances on a delayed alternation task and a subject-ordered pointing task were also impaired in mild AD.[90] Planning and anticipation are impaired in AD, as measured by performance on a maze task.[43]

Cognitive Markers of Alzheimer's Disease

Many neuropsychological tests show differences between AD and NE, but of significance is whether they can differentiate between *mild* AD and NE, with adequate sensitivity *and specificity*. A few studies have addressed this issue, using discriminant function analysis to identify which combination of neuropsychological tests would optimally differentiate AD from NE. They have done so with sensitivity ranging from 82 to 98 percent, and specificity ranging from 92 to 100 percent. Two recently published investigations that prospectively followed healthy elderly subjects arrived at similar conclusions about tests that are good cognitive markers of AD. Principal components extracted from indices derived from a verbal learning test were able to accurately classify 94 percent of AD and NE subjects. Of particular interest were the NE subjects misclassified as having AD. They went on to develop AD at a subsequent evaluation. In addition, subjects who had a first-degree relative with progressive dementia performed statistically worse on almost all indices than those whose family history was negative.[28] A second study found that four tests selected by a statistical procedure from among a battery of tests were good predictors of healthy elderly persons who would develop dementia over a 4-year period (positive predictive value was 68 percent), and a very good predictor of those who would not (negative predictive value of 88 percent). They were delayed recall from yet another verbal learning test, immediate recall from an object memory test, a category fluency test, and the digit symbol subtest of the Wechsler Adult Intelligence Scale.[92] Category fluency and digit symbol tests were also found to differentiate statistically between NE and preclinical cases in the first study, although they were not used in the discriminant function analysis.

Additional studies using discriminant function analysis are somewhat difficult to compare as the rationale for inclusion of variables is not always clear, and the battery of neuropsychological tests used at different sites varied. Nonetheless, consistent findings have emerged. Delayed word list recall again appears as a sensitive discriminator in mild AD[39,40,69,70] and beyond this delayed visual recall added to discrimination.[69] One study found that a measure of forgetting was the best discriminator between AD and NE; it is likely that this capitalized on impairment in delayed recall.[36] Immediate verbal[10,93] and visual[94] recall were good discriminators in earlier studies, but later studies appear to show that delayed recall is a better measure. Other tests that have shown some discriminative power are trailmaking,[69,93] naming,[10,69] and word fluency.[93,94]

In summary, features in the neuropsychological profile that are the most useful in making an early diagnosis of AD are impaired episodic memory in both verbal and visual modalities, in particular poor delayed recall; attenuated primacy effect, such that more words are recalled from the end of a long word list or set of memoranda than from the beginning; a liberal response bias and a high rate of intrusions; and poor performance on category fluency tasks, indicating impairment in semantic memory. Given the relentless progression of AD, all neuropsychological skills are devastated by the later stages of the disorder, and the neuropsychological profile may become similar to that of other degenerative diseases. Therefore specificity is enhanced when the diagnosis is made early in the course of the disease.

Vascular Dementia

A variety of cerebrovascular diseases can cause ischemic damage to the brain. The neuropsychological presentation depends on the extent and region of the brain that is affected. Strokes can produce focal deficits, and an accumulation of small strokes can lead to dementia. Lesions may be cortical and/or subcortical.[95] Large vessel disease is caused by occlusion of the major cerebral arteries, resulting in cortical impairment. Small vessel disease (Binswanger's, lacunar state, thalamic dementia) damages subcortical tissue.[96] These conditions are all classified as vascular dementia (VaD), which has come to replace the term "multi-infarct dementia."

DSM-IV clinical criteria for VaD are memory loss and impairment in at least one other domain of higher cortical functioning (aphasia, apraxia, agnosia, executive functioning), decline in social or occupational functioning, focal neurologic signs and symptoms or laboratory evidence of cerebrovascular disease, and exclusion of delirium.[3] Research criteria for VaD (from the National Institutes for Neurological Disorders and Stroke and the Association Internationale pour la Recherche et l'Enseignement en Neurosciences) require a decline in memory and intellectual abilities that is associated with impaired functioning in daily living; the existence of cerebrovascular disease as shown by focal signs consistent with stroke, a temporal relationship with symptom onset, and neuropsychological documentation of cognitive decline demonstrated by loss of memory and deficits in at least two other cognitive domains; brain imaging that shows nontrivial infarcts or extensive and diffuse white matter changes, and that correlates with clinical evidence; and supportive clinical features such as abrupt decline within 3 months of a stroke, gait disorder or falls, psychiatric changes, urinary infrequency or incontinence, or other neurologic signs and symptoms.[26]

Unfortunately these criteria do not differentiate among types of VaD, which complicates efforts to delineate a neuropsychological profile.[2] The continuum of impairment in cerebrovascular disease[2,96,97] is a further complication, as the profile may vary depending on the severity of impairment. As AD is the most common dementia in the elderly, many investigations of VaD have compared its profile to that of AD. Only those that matched patient groups for severity of dementia are included here.

Memory

Episodic, semantic, and remote memory

Studies that equated severity of dementia (usually by matching on a screening test for dementia) have found that episodic memory is less impaired in VaD than in AD. On each of three different word lists and an object memory task, performance was worse on immediate recall in patients with AD.[98–101] It was also worse on delayed recall.[98–100] Using stories, patients with Binswanger's disease were found to have better recall than patients with AD,[102] as did patients with VaD more broadly defined.[43,101] One study found that the primacy effect in word list recall was intact in VaD but diminished in AD, whereas the recency effect was spared in both groups.[24] These findings need to be replicated. Patients with VaD have fewer intrusions than patients with AD.[103] Visual reproduction fails to differentiate VaD from AD.[43,99,100,104] One study found that recognition of novel faces did not differ between VaD and AD.[105]

The findings with regard to semantic memory are less clear-cut. Some studies report that naming is better in VaD[43,103] and Binswanger's disease,[106] whereas others have found no statistical difference.[98,101,104] Category fluency is consistently found to be no different in VaD and AD.[43,101–103]

NE performed better on a remote memory recognition test of faces of famous people. Patients with VaD did better than patients with AD, but this finding needs replication as AD patients were also slightly more demented.[105] Store of general information did not differ between these two patient groups.[104]

Working memory

Relative to NE, spans were found to be the same,[99] or lower[107] in VaD. Backward span was better in NE in one study.[43] Patients with VaD do not differ from patients with AD on verbal and spatial memory spans forward and backward.[43,99,104,107] Auditory and visual continuous performance tasks were found to be worse in VaD than in AD.[43] Overall, the findings indicate no difference between VaD and AD except for vigilance tasks, where patients with VaD were more impaired. This pattern may be due to an executive function deficit.

Visuospatial Functions

Mild to moderately demented patients with VaD have been reported to be impaired on tests of visual organization, analysis, and synthesis relative to NE. They do not differ from patients with AD on block design,[104] copying,[43,99,103] or visual organization.[43] However, they were found to be worse on timed subtests of the Wechsler Adult Intelligence Scale-Revised (WAIS-R) that require copying symbols and putting together puzzle-like pieces.[104]

Speech and Language

There are mixed findings with regard to language functions in VaD. One study failed to find any differences between patients with dementia and NE on a lengthy aphasia battery, nor could patients with VaD be discriminated from those with AD.[108] On the other hand, mechanical problems of speech have been reported to be worse in VaD, whereas linguistic changes were more marked in AD.[109] Dysarthria was more common in a sample of patients with subcortical lacunae than in NE.[97] More recently, in patients with VaD with subcortical lesions only, severity of white matter ischemia was highly correlated with verbal output disturbance consisting of expressive and articulatory deficits.[110]

Executive Functions

Frontal subcortical structures are preferentially affected in VaD,[111] with concomitant decrement in executive functions that is well documented. Using a pair of unstructured tasks designed to elicit spontaneity and initiative, patients with VaD performed poorly relative to both AD and NE.[98] Ability to shift mental set is impaired in VaD,[97,98] but no difference has been found relative to AD.[101,103] Perseveration, difficulty inhibiting responses, and semantic clustering were worse in VaD than in NE.[97] Patients with VaD have also been shown to be impaired on mazes, pattern completion and auditory and visual continuous performance tests, and they are also worse than patients with AD on these tasks. Orientation to time and place was impaired in VaD, but better than in AD.[43] Letter fluency is impaired in VaD relative to NE,[97] but does not differ from AD.[98,99,103] Closing-in responses on copying tasks, and global or odd responses to a visual conceptualization task were found to be more frequent in AD than in VaD.[99] Tasks that tap motor or cognitive speed are more impaired in VaD than AD, suggesting subcortical involvement.[104] A motor performance index that tapped executive functions, writing, and arrangement of cartoon pictures into stories was found to be more impaired in VaD than AD.[112]

Behavioral Disorder

Apathy was observed more frequently in a well-defined sample of patients with subcortical lacunae than in NE.[97] Patients with Binswanger's disease also showed more apathy than severity-matched patients with AD.[113] More symptoms of depression are also reported in VaD.[114] A sample of patients with pure subcortical VaD was rated with the Neurobehavioral Rating Scale, a test designed to assess behavioral change following head injury.[115] The severity of white matter lesions was correlated with overall score, and also with anxiety/depression.[110] In a separate study using the same scale, patients with VaD were reported to show more motor retardation, and more anxiety and depression than patients with AD who were matched for severity of dementia. Patients with VaD also had more subjectively experienced symptoms of depression and anxiety, and more neurovegetative signs, as measured by the Hamilton Depression Scale. They were more impaired on a motor inventory that tapped speech, psychomotor speed, posture, gait, and movement.[116] On a personality inventory that was also initially developed for use in head injury, spouses of patients with VaD reported more change in personality traits than did spouses of NE before and after their retirement.[117]

In summary, immediate recall is impaired in mild VaD, but not as much as in early AD. The same is true of delayed recall. This pattern of memory deficit may reflect relative sparing of the hippocampus, as VaD lesions tends to occur anteriorly. The primacy effect may be intact in VaD, but attenuated in AD. Some executive functions are more impaired in VaD than in early AD, such as vigilance, orientation to time and place, ability to manage in unstructured situations, and motor or cognitive speed. There may be more problems with mechanics of speech in VaD, whereas in mild AD language impairment is likely to be at a deeper, linguistic level. There are also more behavioral symptoms, such as depression. Overall, impairment in VaD reflects frontal-subcortical lesions, whereas deficits in early AD reflect temporal and parietal lobe lesions.

Spectrum of Lewy Body Disease

In the last decade the presence of Lewy bodies in both brain stem and neocortex has been increasingly identified as a source of dementia. Until recently, VaD was thought to be the second most common type of dementia, but recent studies indicate that senile dementia Lewy body type (SDLT) may be more common.[118] An early review of published cases found that dementia, psychosis, and Parkinsonism were frequently reported.[119] Attempts at disease classification tend to conceptualize this as a spectrum of disorders ranging from preclinical states with mild subcortical Lewy body disease, through Parkinson's disease (PD), up to SDLT, which has cortical involvement.[16,120]

Parkinson's Disease

Cognitive decline in PD has been cited as an example of subcortical dementia, as it is associated with Lewy bodies in the locus ceruleus and substantia nigra. There may be distinct subgroups of PD, with and without dementia. The neuropsychological features of PD have been studied extensively, and the following is drawn from comprehensive reviews of the profile of patients with PD.[121,122]

Episodic memory, semantic memory, and semantic knowledge

Learning and immediate recall of words is impaired in PD. Delayed recall may also be impaired, but recognition memory is generally preserved. The findings are mixed with respect to delayed recognition. Recall of stories is impaired in PD, as is paired associate learning. Recall of visual material is impaired. Vocabulary is preserved in PD, but not store of information. Category fluency has generally been found to be impaired.

Visuospatial functions

Visuospatial functioning is impaired in PD, even on tasks that do not require a motor response. Visual analysis and synthesis is impaired on matching and embedded figures tasks. Personal orientation is impaired, such as changing direction to follow a map. Facial recognition is compromised as is constructional praxis. Mental rotation is preserved, except in patients with unilateral left-sided symptoms.

Executive functions

Patients with PD have difficulty with delayed response tasks. Their ability to shift mental set is impaired, so that it takes longer for them to complete a trailmaking task, and they acquire fewer categories on card sorting tasks. They have a central deficit in motor planning. This is shown on neuropsychological tests of initiating and sequencing finger movements, making bimanual motor movements, and difficulty with ideomotor apraxia. Finger tapping speed is often compromised. Motor difficulties interfere with many tests that require motor responses, such as writing and drawing. Qualitative signs of motor impairment in PD on neuropsychological tests include slowness, tremor, and micrographia. Memory span for digits shows mixed results in PD. Abstract reasoning is generally intact, as is letter fluency. It has been suggested that poor executive functions in PD are due to disrupted connections between the basal ganglia and frontal lobes.

Language

Speech is dysarthric. The rate of speech output is reduced, and there are deficits in prosody and a loss of voice amplitude. However, patients with PD are intact on linguistic tasks requiring processing and comprehension.

Behavioral disorder

The rate of depression is high in PD, estimated at 46 percent. This may be related to a decrease of serotonin in patients with PD.

Several investigations have contrasted neuropsychological profiles in AD and PD. Patients with AD performed better than patients with PD matched for severity of dementia on letter fluency and visual conceptualization tasks. They did worse than the PD group on digit span, remote memory, confrontation naming, and block design. Patients with PD were significantly more depressed.[123] When matched for severity of memory loss, there was poorer visual reproduction, letter and category fluency, and drawing in PD, but patients with AD showed more loss of learned verbal material after a delay.[124] Immediate and delayed recall of a word list did not differentiate patients with AD from a group with PD matched for severity of dementia, nor did amount of learning over five trials. Patients with AD showed characteristic attenuation of the primacy effect, whereas patients with PD did not. False-positive responses on delayed recognition testing did not distinguish between the patient groups.[35] Discriminant function analysis based on characteristics of a verbal learning task showed that patients with PD could be discriminated from patients with AD and Huntington's disease. AD had more intrusions than any other patient group, and more perseverations than the PD group.[125]

Senile Dementia of Lewy Body Type

Significant proportions of patients with SDLT may be misclassified as having VaD or AD.[118] Retrospective analysis of medical records of 21 cases of SDLT with neuropathologic confirmation showed patients with SDLT to be more demented at presentation than patients with AD and equivalent on tests of temporal and parietal lobe function.[13] The authors proposed clinical criteria for diagnosis. These include fluctuating cognitive impairment affecting both memory and other higher cortical functions, as documented by performance on tests of cognition or activities of daily living; at least one of the following: hallucinations, mild extrapyramidal symptoms, or exaggerated adverse response to neuroleptic medication; clinical features that fluctuate over a long period, unlike delirium; exclusion of physical illness that could account for cognitive changes, and exclusion of cerebrovascular disease by history or structural brain imaging. A later study of 20 neuropathologically confirmed cases showed that when these clinical criteria were applied retrospectively to patients' medical records, trained raters could classify cases with 73 percent sensitivity and 95 percent specificity.[126] One investigation, however, did not find support for these clinical criteria.[127]

One of the first studies with good neuropsychological data found a significant subgroup of patients who met clinical and neuropathologic criteria for AD also had Lewy body disease (36 percent). Episodic and semantic memory tasks were similar to matched patients with AD, but Lewy body patients showed poorer attention span, letter fluency, visuospatial processing, and conceptualization, suggestive of a more frontal-subcortical profile. Writing from dictation was also impaired. Masked facies, bradykinesia, and essential tremor were more common. These cases were seen as a Lewy body variant of AD, rather than as combined AD and PD.[128]

Neuropsychological testing of 15 patients with SDLT who were later identified on neuropathologic grounds showed dysphasia, dyscalculia, and visuospatial, constructional, and ideomotor dyspraxia.[129] However, there was no comparison group, and it is unclear whether cognitive status was assessed at different stages of severity of the disorder. The primary symptom at presentation was about equally divided between Parkinsonism and dementia, but eventually all cases progressed to dementia.

A series of investigations of spatial working memory was conducted using seven patients with SDLT who were identified by the proposed clinical criteria for SDLT.[126] Their performance was compared to patients with AD matched for severity of dementia, and NE. Patients with SDLT were more impaired than patients with AD on a task that required them to associate patterns with specific locations,[130] and on a visual delayed matching-to-sample task.[131] On a task of self-ordered pointing that required subjects to find hidden tokens, patients with SDLT made more errors and were slower than patients with AD.[132] On all tasks SDLT did worse than NE.

Behavioral disorder

Depression and hallucinations are reported early in the disease, but behavioral changes have not yet been formally studied relative to other dementias.

SDLT may be differentiated from other dementias by its fluctuating course, early Parkinsonism or poor response to neuroleptic medication, and possible early psychotic features. Relative to AD, one might expect subcortical features such as slowed processing speed. There is also evidence that working memory is worse than in AD. Further characterization relative to other dementias is not attempted, as SDLT has not yet been adequately investigated from a neuropsychological standpoint.

Frontal Lobe (Frontotemporal) Dementias

Several degenerative cortical diseases preferentially afflict the anterior regions of the brain, leading to a dementia syndrome. Recently, attention has focused on one of these that is variably called frontal lobe degeneration of non-Alzheimer type,[133] dementia lacking distinctive histology,[134] frontotemporal dementia,[27] or dementia of the frontal type.[31] This disorder is neuropathologically distinct from AD, Pick's disease, and dementia with motor neuron disease.[133,135] Functional neuroimaging has demonstrated a reduction in cerebral metabolism in the frontal and anterior temporal lobes,[136] although some cortical tissue in posterior temporal and parietal regions may be simultaneously hypoperfused.[137] Clinical symptoms reflect the topographic distribution of cortical lesions, which may be be unilateral on either side, or bilateral. Onset is between age 40 and 70.[32,137,138] The widely used designation of *frontal lobe dementia* (FLD) is adopted here.

Proposed diagnostic criteria for FLD have emphasized progressive behavioral and affective symptoms preceding or exceeding cognitive impairment, memory deficit less prominent than personality change, possible language impairment, and preservation of visuospatial and other posterior functions. Frontally mediated executive functions should be shown by neuropsychological tests to be impaired. Structural or functional neuroimaging should show abnormalities of frontal or anterior temporal regions.[14,27,31] Diagnosis is best made early in the disorder, when the relative salience of anterior and posterior deficits can be more clearly observed. Eventually most domains of cognitive functioning become severely impaired,[139] as in AD.

The following profile is generated from six studies that reported details of neuropsychological testing in patients in whom FLD was confirmed by measurement of cerebral metabolism. They represent a total of 61 patients. Unfortunately, only two studies compared FLD statistically to NE,[140,141] and only one study made a comparison to AD.[141] Nonetheless, combined with information from brain imaging procedures, behavioral symptoms, and the course of the disease, the findings may advance the cause of differential diagnosis.

Executive Functions

Investigations that reported impaired executive functions in FLD are shown in the accompanying box. The most frequently cited deficits are in sorting and shifting mental set, word generation to letter and category cue, divided attention, and anticipation and planning. Studies that used similar test batteries tended to agree with regard to the skills that were impaired. Deficient executive functions are necessary for a diagnosis of FLD, but not sufficient, because positive findings with executive tests are not specific to FLD.[142,143]

Memory

Memory is thought to be only mildly or moderately impaired in early FLD, because the hippocampal area is not the focus of disease. Two studies that evaluated episodic memory supported this.[139,140] In one study poor performance on memory tests was exaggerated by qualitative factors such as poor use of strategies, reflecting executive deficits rather than inability to acquire and retain new information.[138] Patients with right frontotemporal hypoperfusion showed mild to moderate impairment of immediate story recall, and a severe deficit in delayed recall.[137] Semantic memory was found to be intact early on, but later in the course of the disease became severely impaired.[139] In another group of mildly demented patients (MMS scores ranged from 21 to 30) tested with a similar task (confrontation naming), semantic memory was impaired.[137] Interestingly, there was temporal lobe hypoperfusion in each patient in the latter series.

Memory in FLD is thought to be less severely impaired than

Reports of executive dysfunction in frontal lobe dementia

- Sorting and shifting set[134,137,139,140,144]
- Letter fluency[134,137,139,140]
- Category fluency[137,140]
- Divided attention[137,140]
- Anticipation and planning[134,139]
- Disinhibition[137]
- Interpretation of proverbs[139]
- Arranging pictures in a meaningful sequence[139]

in AD. One study that made this comparison, controlling for severity of dementia, showed relative sparing of episodic nonverbal memory. An episodic verbal memory task did not differentiate the groups, which was interpreted as an artifact of language impairment in patients with FLD.[144]

Language

There is general agreement that language functions are impaired in FLD, manifested by deficits in expressive rather than receptive ability.[32,138] Stereotypy and impoverishment of speech, progressing to mutism, are commonly reported.[32] Paradoxically, some patients may exhibit verbal aspontaneity, and others logorrhea. One study found comprehension to be intact in early FLD.[139] In another study of patients with right frontal hypometabolism only, language functions were preserved, reflecting damage to the nondominant hemisphere.[137] Left frontal hypometabolism with severe progressive language deterioration has been observed. This is reviewed below under the rubric of primary progressive aphasia.

Visuospatial Functions

Drawings and block designs are generally intact or only mildly deficient,[137–140] which reflects minimal parietal or occipital involvement. However, these become severely impaired later in the disease.[139]

Behavioral Disorder

There is significant behavioral impairment in FLD, and it is often the first symptom observed. The proportion of patients showing behavioral disturbance and functional level inconsistent with level of memory loss was found to be higher in FLD than in AD; on the other hand, a statistically higher proportion of patients with AD had memory disturbance at onset of decline, functional impairment consistent with level of memory loss, and spatial disorientation. Observation of qualitative differences show speech and social graces preserved in AD, whereas impulsive, unempathic, or inappropriate behavior was found in FLD.[144] The box lists behavioral disturbances that have been noted. Apathy, bizarre or psychotic behavior early in the course of the disease, disinhibition, agitation, and hyperorality are commonly reported. The wide range of observed behaviors, which may sometimes seem mutually exclusive, is likely due to the heterogeneity of the disease. Onset of behavioral change is insidious, and there is progressive deterioration of the personality.

Differential diagnosis of FLD and AD would focus on the relative neuropsychological deficits that are known to correlate with the distribution of cortical lesions in these disorders. In FLD, where deterioration is frontal and anterior temporal, alteration in behavior is marked early in the course of the disease, and is out of proportion to the amount of memory loss. Mechanics of language may be impaired. In AD, which is due to temporal and parietal lobe degeneration, there is instead profound episodic and semantic memory loss early in the course of the disease, with preserved behavior. Whereas the primacy effect is impaired in AD, one might speculate that it would be preserved in FLD, because the hippocampus is relatively spared. Visuospatial impairment would suggest AD, as would deficits in deeper aspects of language.

Thus far FLD has not been formally compared to VaD. Differential diagnosis may be difficult because both disorders can share frontal features with impairment in executive functions, impairment in mechanics of speech/language, and memory loss milder than in AD. Marked behavioral disturbance early in the disease would be a strong indicator of FLD, as would functional impairment out of proportion to memory loss. Features that would incline toward a diagnosis of VaD include impairment in visuospatial function, a "patchy" distribution of cortical deficits, abrupt onset, focal neurologic signs soon after onset, a subcortical picture with slowed processing speed, gait disorder and incontinence, and structural imaging with infarcts.

Reports of behavioral disturbance in frontal lobe dementia

- Apathy, social withdrawal[32,138,140]
- Early presentation of psychosis or bizarre behavior[32,137,140]
- Disinhibition, disruption of social conduct[32,137,140,144]
- Lack of insight or empathy for others[32]
- Poor planning and judgment[140]
- Remoteness, blunted affect[137]
- Irritability, aggression, restlessness, agitation[32,138,144]
- Depression[32,140]
- Kluver-Bucy syndrome or hyperorality (e.g., hypersexuality, changes in oral or dietary behavior)[32,138,144]
- Obsessive-compulsive behavior[32,137]
- Wandering[140]

Pick's Disease

Like FLD, Pick's disease results in progressive cortical degeneration of anterior regions. Therefore it produces similar deficits, even though it is neuropathologically distinct. At present it is unknown whether its neuropsychological profile is distinguishable from FLD. Future investigation should use sensitive neuropsychometric tests longitudinally, determine group membership postmortem, then compare test profiles. Given the relatively low incidence of both of these diseases, it may be some time before this question can be answered. In the meantime, it is assumed that some patients with Pick's disease are included in samples of FLD.

Primary Progressive Aphasia

Primary progressive aphasia (PPA) was initially described as slowly progressing anomic aphasia.[145] Since then numerous additional cases have been reported, and two patterns have been distinguished, a fluent and a nonfluent syndrome.[31] Longitudinal testing revealed that naming, word fluency, and repetition of words and sentences declined over 3 to 5 years, whereas episodic memory, visuospatial skills, and conceptualization remained intact.[146] It has been suggested that this is a left-sided FLD, as brain imaging implicates the left perisylvan area. A study of eight cases showed that naming declined more precipitously over serial test administrations whereas memory and other cognitive functions declined more slowly. However, after 5 years, most of these cases met criteria for a mild dementia.[147] A recent study that compared patients with PPA, AD, and aphasia using an aphasia test battery found that spontaneous speech and object naming were worst in PPA. Aphasia deepened over time, and eight patients later developed global dementia. Postmortem examination of two cases found evidence of Pick's disease and AD, leading to the conclusion that there may be heterogeneous underlying disease processes, but a specific lesion site.[148] Reviews of many of these cases also found that cognitive impairment eventually becomes global, and that symptoms are caused by a variety of diseases, including Pick's disease, AD, Creutzfeldt-Jakob disease, and focal spongiform degeneration.[149,150] This raises doubt that PPA is a distinct clinical entity.

Depression

Depression is known to produce cognitive changes that can be confused with mild dementia. Because depression is treatable, it is important that it be differentiated from dementia. The term "pseudodementia" has been used to describe this condition, but has come under increasing criticism, in part because it implies that the cognitive loss seen in depression is not real.[151–153] Recent thinking and research challenge the implied distinction between functional and organic disease.

Numerous studies have shown that depressed patients have deficits in episodic memory. Immediate recall of word lists by severely depressed patients is impaired relative to NE,[42,154,155] but is consistently better than in patients with dementia.[42,156,157] Delayed recall also falls between NE and AD patients.[42] On recognition testing, patients with dementia have more intrusions and random errors than patients with depression.[156–158] Similar patterns have been found for visual stimuli.[159,160] Immediate recall of stories is also worse in dementia than in depression.[67,155,156]

The major neuropsychological findings in depression have been reviewed.[152] Rate of forgetting, which has been shown to be very rapid in AD, is no different in patients with depression relative to NE subjects.[42,161] This suggests that impairment in depression is not due to difficulty with retention, but rather appears to be related to response style and motivational state. Patients with depression make conservative responses that result in more false negatives than patients with AD, who have a liberal response bias that produces more false positives.[42,156,159,162] This difference is best elicited by delayed recognition tasks which allow observation of response style while minimizing effort. Responses of patients with AD also favor items at the end of a word list over items at the beginning of the list, whereas patients with depression are more like normal subjects in showing both primacy and recency effects,[42] the implication being that secondary memory is basically intact in depression. Semantic memory as measured by confrontation naming was found to be better in patients with depression than in AD, but no different from NE,[163] and better in depressed patients with cognitive loss relative to dementia patients with depression.[164] Category fluency is impaired in depression relative to NE,[67] but not as deficient as in AD.[155] Recall of events from autobiographical memory showed the same distribution in patients with depression as in AD and NE, but the group with depression recalled more negative memories in recent years.[81]

On an aphasia battery, language functions were invariably better in NE and patients with depression than in AD patients, whereas patients with depression showed worse performance than NE on word fluency, reading comprehension, and on a test of syntactic complexity.[163] Difficulty with letter fluency in patients with depression is a consistent finding,[67,155] and may be due to deficient psychomotor speed.

Performance is sometimes worse on tasks that require effort, leading to the conclusion that patients with depression are less motivated than NE.[165] They may do better when challenged, giving rise to the clinical observation that they are sometimes inconsistent, performing better on difficult items than on easy ones.

There is a growing body of evidence suggesting that a frontal-subcortical substrate mediates the cognitive changes observed in depression.[166] Support for this theory comes from various sources. Patients with depression were successfully classified into two subgroups, one that performed similarly to NE on a verbal learning task, and another that was similar to patients with a subcortical dementia (Huntington's disease).[154] Depression is common in other dementias with known subcortical lesions, such as vascular dementia and Parkinson's disease.[96,121,122] Finally, recent investigations using functional brain imaging show a decrease in cerebral metabolism in anterior paralimbic and prefrontal cortex in primary depression.[167] These converging lines of evidence suggest that depression of different etiologies may reflect the same neuroanatomic substrate. However, there is some disagreement.[168]

In summary, patients with depression have mild cognitive deficits, but their performance on a variety of cognitive tasks is more like that of healthy subjects than patients with mild dementia. Thus the rate of forgetting learned material is similar to that of NE in being less rapid than in patients with AD, and the primacy effect is also preserved, unlike in AD. Patients with depression are more likely to show a conservative response bias on delayed recognition testing, with more false negatives, but fewer false positives than patients with AD. Their language functions are also superior to patients with AD, and confrontation naming may be slightly worse in early AD than in depression. Additional data that facilitate the differential diagnosis of depression and mild AD come from the patient's history. Sometimes it can be determined that onset of memory loss preceded symptoms of depression. Often true symptoms of depression can be distinguished from apathy or withdrawal secondary to cognitive decline, which are often interpreted by family members as depression.

Age-Associated Memory Impairment

Benign senescent forgetfulness,[169] and more recently, the concept of age-associated memory impairment (AAMI) are attempts to describe older people with memory loss due to non-disease-related cognitive decline relative to the person's level of functioning at an earlier age. Proposed criteria for AAMI include subjective complaints of memory loss in everyday living, memory test performance at least one standard deviation below the mean established for young adults, adequate intellectual function (verbal IQ estimated to be above the 37th percentile), with exclusion of dementia and psychiatric or other disorders that might impair cognition.[170]

These criteria have psychometric deficiencies, and remain controversial.[171,172] They are heir to some of the problems associated with diagnosing dementia. Very early dementia is difficult to differentiate from normative change with aging, as memory loss may be below the threshold that would enable sensitive detection. Using the above criteria, these cases would be falsely identified as having AAMI. Classification could be improved by the use of tests and indices that have demonstrated some promise in detection of preclinical or very early AD. These include delayed recall or savings scores,[28,54] category fluency,[76] and reading lists of low-frequency words with irregular spelling-to-sound correspondence.[11] Word lists should be used because semantic clustering, recognition, and serial position effects (blunted primacy effect or elevated percent recall from recency) have shown good discrimination of very early AD.[28] Use of delayed word list recall, visual memory, digit symbol, and verbal fluency are suggested by data from follow-up studies in which subjects thought to be cognitively intact or to have AAMI went on to develop dementia.[28,173,174]

Additional false-positive errors would occur by inclusion of dementing people of high premorbid intellectual capacity who, despite decline, still function within normal limits. Older people of average intellectual capacity whose memory is unchanged might also be falsely identified as having AAMI by the existing criteria because their performance falls one standard deviation below the average for young adults, which would approximate the 80th percentile for the person's own age group. The second problem could be avoided by the use of appropriate age-referenced norms,[175] and both problems could be addressed by incorporation of educational or occupational achievement as indices of premorbid functioning.[176] Finally, requirement of a subjective complaint of memory loss is likely to include people whose symptoms are due to masked depression or anxiety.[177]

Concerns about diagnostic specificity are borne out by the finding that up to 41 percent of cases identified by these criteria were no longer classified as AAMI after an average of 3.6 years of follow-up; 9 percent developed dementia, and another 7 percent showed mild decline but had not yet progressed to dementia.[174] A follow-up study of patients complaining of memory loss who were initially thought to have benign senescent forgetfulness also found that about 9 percent were demented 3 years later.[178] Clearly better psychometric criteria are needed to improve the classification of AAMI.

Interventions

A critical moment in the care of the elderly patient with dementia occurs immediately following evaluation, when the provider and patient meet to review the findings. This contact is important because it lays the groundwork that determines the success of later interventions. There is some debate about the wisdom of telling the patient her diagnosis when she has an irreversible dementia, AD in particular. In favor of disclosure are the patient's right to self-determination and the need for her full participation in formulating advance directives, financial planning, and other personal affairs while she is still competent to express her wishes. A recent questionnaire study of older people living in a retirement community supported this point of view. It found that 79 percent of respondents would want to know if they had AD, and 65 percent would want their spouse to be told if the spouse had the disease.[179] Having the opportunity to do advance and financial planning, to settle family matters, and to get a second opinion were the major reasons cited for wanting to know the diagnosis. Because the subjects were not patients undergoing evaluation for AD, it remains unknown whether they would respond similarly if actually faced with this situation.

Arguing against disclosure has been the uncertainty of the diagnosis, the perceived paucity of therapeutic options, and the fear that the stress of the diagnosis may exacerbate the patient's symptoms. The uncertainty of the diagnosis no longer appears tenable, because antemortem diagnosis of dementia has become increasingly sophisticated. Clinical classification of AD may be 80 to 90 percent accurate when compared to neuropathologic evidence,[34] and there is a growing literature on differential diagnosis of the dementias.[13,26,32] Regarding therapeutic options, treatment is available in the form of psychological and psychosocial interventions, which provide significant reduction of excess disability and enhance the quality of life for both patient and family. In addition, pharmacologic agents such as tacrine and hydrochloride donepezil, although not curative, may be of help to some patients. Unless the diagnosis is discussed, it is difficult to utilize these interventions to maximum effect. The fear that stress caused by knowing the diagnosis may be damaging to the patient deserves consideration. Although the majority of respondents to a survey indicated that they would want to know if they had AD, about 11 percent said they would not want to know, and 2.5 percent would want to know if they had AD so they could consider suicide.[179]

These are complex issues in need of future study. Should not wanting to know the diagnosis be accepted at face value, or treated as denial? What is the rate of suicide upon receiving a poor medical prognosis? Currently many patients are aware of the public debate about assisted suicide, and may reasonably wonder whether this is an alternative they should consider.

This author takes the position that the benefits of frankness in disclosing the diagnosis outweigh the disadvantages. It is generally in the patient's best interest, facilitating adaptation to disability while promoting both self-determination and confidence in the health care provider. The diagnosis is best presented by a professional who has established a relationship with the patient, and to whom the patient can turn for follow-up care. Family members should be present for support. If a patient indicates that she does not want to know the diagnosis, the reasons should be discussed, with exploration of both pros and cons. In the end her wishes should be respected. Often the patient will allow family involvement, so that interventions to guarantee the patient's health and safety can be implemented anyway.

Clinical judgment regarding the patient's mental status should determine how the diagnosis is presented. If the patient is suicidal or otherwise acutely emotionally disturbed, it would be preferable to withhold the findings until she has been stabilized. If the patient is likely to have a less extreme but nonetheless adverse reaction to disclosure, caution should be used. For example, with a few very anxious or depressed patients it may be better to describe a degenerative disorder by using words such as "cognitive impairment," "memory disorder," or even "dementia," which are less alarming than "Alzheimer's disease." If the patient asks if she has AD, she can be told that her symptoms have to be followed in subsequent months to document whether they progress. This allows work to proceed to address the patient's deficits. At a later date, when the patient has become accustomed to the idea of having a disability, a treatment alliance has been formed, and social supports are in place, the exact diagnosis can be presented. This strategy should be used sparingly, and deception should be avoided. In all cases the provider should be sensitive to the patient's anxiety about the information she is going to receive, and attentive to her response.

Psychotherapy

Psychotherapy can help the dementing patient with the immediate tasks of adjusting to the diagnosis, and becoming engaged in planning for the future. Treatment necessarily includes a psychoeducational component. Thus the professional provides information about the diagnosis and the disease, and makes recommendations, while simultaneously responding to the patient's emotional reactions and mobilization of defenses. When the diagnosis is made early in the dementing process, long-term psychotherapy is also feasible for some patients. Deeper psychodynamic exploration of the personality structure and defenses can help the patient come to terms with unresolved life conflicts. There is a complex interaction between internalized psychic structure and brain deterioration. For example, a chronic weak sense of self could explain some AD patients' inability to accept the loss of capacity, because it would be too severe a narcissistic injury to tolerate. It could also account for the agitation seen in some as they lose the capacity to hold themselves together.

Psychotherapy must be adapted to the stage of the disease.[180] With progression there is increased emphasis on loss of function. Having someone to discuss this with is reassuring to the patient and can lead to better coping with deficits. The psychologist may have to be empathic in verbalizing the patient's feelings as self-expression diminishes. Still later, reality testing may become compromised, with evidence of delusions or hallucinations. Knowing that certain experiences are merely the product of her difficulty interpreting reality can reduce a patient's anxiety. For example, one patient stated that he knew that the bomb next to his bed was probably not real; instead of becoming agitated and trying to flee the bedroom, he turned over and went back to sleep. Psychopharmacologic intervention becomes increasingly helpful in this stage of the disorder, although drug holidays are necessary to identify when medication can be discontinued.

Some aspects of family psychoeducational treatment developed for mental illness[181] can be adapted for use with the families of patients with dementia. Examining how family members react to the patient's symptoms can help to manage stresses of caregiving and minimize family burden. The professional also serves an important educational function. What is dementia? What tests were done and what did they show? What are the implications for the future? Will the patient have to go to a nursing home? Will the disease be inherited by family members? These questions are commonly raised by families and can be addressed in this context. Structured recommendations regarding future planning and use of respite or home aides can also be made and clarified. Providing continuity of care is critical so that the family feels supported and knows where to turn for help. Given the multiple needs of the patient with dementia, the establishment of a treatment team is helpful in ensuring that the patient receives comprehensive care. Even when professionals are in private practice, they can establish relationships with health care providers in other disciplines who, through consultations and referrals, serve as a team. Connecting family members with a support network (e.g., psychotherapy groups, social agencies) helps to reduce isolation and the sense they often have of enduring difficult times alone.[182]

Dementia bears some similarity to chronic mental illness, and some of the concepts developed in the latter may put the disorder into perspective for the health care provider. In one view,[183] families must adapt to chronic mental illness in three primary areas: interpersonal, instrumental, and life course. Interpersonally, many feelings are aroused in family members toward the patient. They may express anger at her because of her behavior, thinking that she could perform normally if she tried harder. Their anger may be exacerbated by feeling frustrated and let down by the health care system that often fails to diagnose dementia adequately, or to provide adequate support. The psychologist can address family anger by clarifying that the patient is functioning as best she can, which may require providing concrete evidence of organic dysfunction in the form of test results. Another emotional strain commonly encountered in families when the disease progresses is mourning the loss of the person they knew. Because the patient often remains physically healthy while her personality disintegrates under the onslaught of the disease process, families may not readily become aware of their sense of loss and the emotions that accompany it. The psychologist can bring this feeling into awareness and help the family deal with their grief.

Instrumentally, the family must adapt to behavioral problems. A major source of burden to dementia caregivers is the patient's daily difficulty in functioning (e.g., losing things, inability to get dressed), and problem behaviors (e.g., wandering, combativeness). The psychologist can make practical suggestions about how to deal with these, while at the same time exploring aspects of the caregiver's circumstances or personality that make certain behaviors particularly difficult to cope with. Finally, life course issues are raised because patients can live for many years with a dementia. A common pattern is for a close family member to become completely consumed by the caregiving task. With support and planning the disease process can become better integrated into family life so that it does not demand the end of a normal existence for this person. Family treatment can explore family resources, build a sense of perspective with regard to the disease, and engender optimism in family members who may have felt that they were unable to continue.

References

1. Evans DA, Fukenstein HH, Albert MS et al: Prevalence of Alzheimer's disease in a community population of older persons. JAMA 1989;262:2551–2592
2. Hachinski V: Vascular dementia: a radical redefinition. Dementia 1994;5:130–132
3. American Psychiatric Association: Diagnostic and Statistical Manual of Mental Disorders. 4th Ed. American Psychiatric Association, Washington, DC, 1994
4. White RF: Clinical Syndromes in Adult Neuropsychology: The Practitioner's Handbook. Elsevier Science, New York, 1992
5. Schaie KW: Intellectual development in adulthood. pp. 266–286. In Birren JE, Schaie KW (eds): Handbook of the Psychology of Aging. Academic Press, San Diego, 1996
6. Shock NW, Greulich RC, Costa PT: Normal human aging: the Baltimore Longitudinal Study of Aging. Department of Health and Human Services, Rockville, MD 1984
7. Salthouse T: Age-related changes in basic cognitive processes. pp. 5–40. In Storandt M, VandenBos G (eds): The Adult Years: Continuity and Change. American Psychological Association, Washington, DC, 1989
8. Schaie KW: The optimization of cognitive functioning in old age: predictions based on cohort-sequential and longitudinal data. pp. 94–117. In Baltes PB (ed): Successful Aging. Cambridge University Press, Cambridge, 1990
9. Naugle R, Cullum CM, Bigler ED: Evaluation of intellectual and memory function among dementia patients who were intellectually superior. Clin Neuropsychol 1990;4:355–374
10. Storandt M, Hill RD: Very mild senile dementia of the Alzheimer type: II. Psychometric test performance. Arch Neurol 1989;46:383–386
11. Patterson KE, Graham N, Hodges JR: Reading in dementia of the Alzheimer type: a preserved ability? Neuropsychology 1994;8:395–407
12. Storandt M, Stone K, LaBarge E: Deficits in reading performance in very mild dementia of the Alzheimer type. Neuropsychology 1995;9:174–176
13. McKeith IG, Perry RH, Fairbairn AF et al: Operational criteria for senile dementia of Lewy body type (SDLT). Psychol Med 1992;22:911–922
14. Brun A, Englund B, Gustafson L et al: Clinical and neuropathological criteria for frontotemporal dementia. J Neurol Neurosurg Psychiatry 1994;57:416–418
15. Kosaka K, Yoshimura M, Ikeda K, Budka H: Diffuse type of Lewy body disease: progressive dementia with abundant cortical Lewy bodies and senile changes of varying degree—a new disease? Clin Neuropathol 1984;3:185–192
16. Olichney JM, Galasko D, Corey-Bloom J, Thal LJ: The spectrum of diseases with diffuse Lewy bodies. Adv Neurol 1995; 65:159–170
17. Leverenz J, Sumi S: Parkinson's disease in patients with Alzheimer's disease. Arch Neurol 1986;43:662–664
18. Baddeley A: The concept of working memory: a view of its current state and probable future development. Cognition 1981;10:17–23
19. Schacter DL: Implicit memory: history and current status. J Exp Psychol Learn Mem Cogn 1987;13:501–518
20. Tulving E: How many memory systems are there? Am Psychol 1985;40:385–398
21. Tulving E: Precis of elements of episodic memory. Behav Brain Sci 1984;7:223–268
22. Butters N, Delis DC, Lucas JA: Clinical assessment of memory disorders in amnesia and dementia. Annu Rev Psychol 1995; 46:493–523
23. Morris RG, Kopelman MD: The memory deficits in Alzheimer-type dementia: a review. Special Issue: Human memory. Q J Exp Psychol 1986;38A:575–602
24. Gainotti G, Marra C: Progress and controversies in neuropsychology of memory. Second Congress of the Pan European Society of Neurology (1991 Vienna, Austria). Acta Neurol 1992;14:561–577
25. McKhann G, Drachman D, Folstein M et al: Clinical diagnosis of Alzheimer's disease: report of the NINCDS-ADRDA Work Group under the auspices of Department of Health and Human Services Task Force on Alzheimer's disease. Neurology 1984; 34:939–944
26. Roman GC, Tatemichi TK, Erkinjuntti T et al: Vascular dementia: diagnostic criteria for research studies: report of the NINDS-AIREN International Workshop. Neurology 1993;43: 250–260
27. Kumar A, Gottlieb G: Frontotemporal dementias. A new clinical syndrome? Am J Geriatr Psychiatry 1993;1:95–107

28. Bondi MW, Monsch AU, Galasko D et al: Preclinical cognitive markers of dementia of the Alzheimer type. Neuropsychology 1994;8:374–384
29. Albert ML: The "subcortical dementia" of progressive supranuclear palsy. J Neurol Neurosurg Psychiatry 1974;37: 121–130
30. Cummings JL: Vascular subcortical dementias: clinical aspects. Special issue: vascular dementia: etiological, pathogenetic, clinical and treatment aspects. Dementia 1994;5: 177–180
31. Gregory CA, Hodges JR: Dementia of frontal type and the focal lobar atrophies. Int Rev Psychiatry 1993;5:397–406
32. Gustafson L: Frontal lobe degeneration of non-Alzheimer type: II. Clinical picture and differential diagnosis. Eric K. Fernstrom Foundation Symposium: frontal lobe degeneration of non-Alzheimer type (1986, Lund, Sweden). Arch Gerontol Geriatr 1987;6:209–223.
33. Larson EB, Reifler BV, Sumi SM et al: Diagnostic tests in the evaluation of dementia. A prospective study of 200 elderly outpatients. Arch Intern Med 1986;146:1917–1922
34. Tierney MC, Fisher RH, Lewis AJ et al: The NINCDS:ADRDA Work Group criteria for the clinical diagnosis of probable Alzheimer's disease: a clinicopathologic study of 57 cases. Neurology 1988;38:359–364
35. Tierney MC, Nores A, Snow WG et al: Use of the Rey Auditory Verbal Learning Test in differentiating normal aging from Alzheimer's and Parkinson's dementia. Psychol Assess 1994;6: 129–134
36. Incalzi RA, Capparella O, Gemma A et al: Effects of aging and of Alzheimer's disease on verbal memory. J Clin Exp Neuropsychol 1995;17:580–589
37. Pillon B, Deweer B, Agid Y, Dubois B: Explicit memory in Alzheimer's, Huntington's, and Parkinson's diseases. Arch Neurol 1993;50:374–379
38. Moss MB, Albert MS, Butters N, Payne M: Differential patterns of memory loss among patients with Alzheimer's disease, Huntington's disease, and alcoholic Korsakoff's syndrome. Arch Neurol 1986;43:239–246
39. Welsh K, Butters N, Hughes J et al: Detection of abnormal memory decline in mild cases of Alzheimer's disease using CERAD neuropsychological measures. Arch Neurol 1991;48: 278–281
40. Knopman DS, Ryberg S: A verbal memory test with high predictive accuracy for dementia of the Alzheimer type. Arch Neurol 1989;46:141–145
41. Carlesimo GA, Sabbadini M, Fadda L, Caltagirone C: Forgetting from long-term memory in dementia and pure amnesia: role of task, delay of assessment and aetiology of cerebral damage. Cortex 1995;31:285–300
42. Gainotti G, Marra C: Some aspects of memory disorders clearly distinguish dementia of the Alzheimer's type from depressive pseudo-dementia. J Clin Exp Neuropsychol 1994;16:65–78
43. Villardita C: Alzheimer's disease compared with cerebrovascular dementia. Neuropsychological similarities and differences. Acta Neurol Scand 1993;87:299–308
44. Mitrushina M, Drebing C, Uchiyama C et al: The pattern of deficit in different memory components in normal aging and dementia of Alzheimer's type. J Clin Psychol 1994;50: 591–596
45. Hodges JR, Patterson K: Is semantic memory consistently impaired early in the course of Alzheimer's disease? Neuroanatomical and diagnostic implications. Neuropsychologia 1995; 33:441–459
46. Larrabee GJ, Youngjohn JR, Sudilovsky A, Crook TH: Accelerated forgetting in Alzheimer-type dementia. J Clin Exp Neuropsychol 1993;15:701–712
47. Mitrushina M, Satz P, Drebing CE et al: The differential pattern of memory deficit in normal aging and dementias of different etiology. J Clin Psychol 1994;50:246–252
48. Simon E, Leach L, Winocur G, Moscovitch M: Intact primary memory in mild to moderate Alzheimer disease: indices from the California Verbal Learning Test. J Clin Exp Neuropsychol 1994;16:414–422
49. Pollmann S, Haupt M, Romero B, Kurz A: Is impaired recall in dementia of the Alzheimer type a consequence of a contextual retrieval deficit? 36th Annual Meeting of the German Society of Neuropathology and Neuroanatomy (1991 Dusseldorf, Germany). Dementia 1993;4:102–108
50. Diesfeldt HF: Recognition memory for words and faces in primary degenerative dementia of the Alzheimer type and normal old age. J Clin Exp Neuropsychol 1990;12:931–945
51. Pillon B, Dubois B, Lhermitte F, Agid Y: Heterogeneity of cognitive impairment in progressive supranuclear palsy, Parkinson's disease, and Alzheimer's disease. Neurology 1986; 36:1179–1185
52. Cullum CM, Butters N, Troster AI, Salmon DP: Normal aging and forgetting rates on the Wechsler Memory Scale—Revised. Arch Clin Neuropsychol 1990;5:23–30
53. Butters N, Salmon DP, Cullum CM et al: Differentiation of amnesic and demented patients with the Wechsler Memory Scale—Revised. Special issue: initial validity studies of the new Wechsler Memory Scale—Revised. Clin Neuropsychol 1988;2:133–148
54. Troster A, Butters N, Salmon DP et al: The diagnostic utility of savings scores: differentiating Alzheimer's and Huntington's diseases with logical memory and visual reproduction tests. J Clin Exp Neuropsychol 1993;15:773–788
55. van der Hurk PR, Hodges JR: Episodic and semantic memory in Alzheimer's disease and progressive supranuclear palsy: a comparative study. J Clin Exp Neuropsychol 1995;17: 459–471
56. Becker JT, Boller F, Saxton J et al: Normal rates of forgetting of verbal and non-verbal material in Alzheimer's disease. Cortex 1987;23:59–72
57. Duchek JM, Cheney M, Ferraro FR, Storandt M: Paired associate learning in senile dementia of the Alzheimer type. Arch Neurol 1991;48:1038–1040
58. Bemelmans KJ, Goekoop JG: The contribution of list length to the absence of the primacy effect in word recall in dementia of the Alzheimer type. Psychol Med 1991;21:1047–1050
59. Morris RG, Baddeley AD: Primary and working memory functioning in Alzheimer-type dementia. J Clin Exp Neuropsychol 1988;10:279–296

60. Pepin EP, Eslinger PJ: Verbal memory decline in Alzheimer's disease: a multiple-processes deficit. Neurology 1989;39: 1477–1482
61. Martin A, Browers P, Cox C, Fedio P: On the nature of the verbal memory deficit in Alzheimer's disease. Brain Lang 1985;25:323–341
62. Jacobs D, Salmon DP, Troster AI, Butters N: Intrusion errors in the figural memory of patients with Alzheimer's and Huntington's disease. Arch Clin Neuropsychol 1990;5:49–57
63. Huppert FA, Kopleman MD: Rates of forgetting in normal ageing: a comparison with dementia. Neuropsychologia 1989; 27:849–860
64. Kopelman MD: Multiple memory deficits in Alzheimer-type dementia: implications for pharmacotherapy. Psychol Med 1985;15:527–541
65. Freed DM, Corkin S, Growdon JH, Nissen MJ: Selective attention in Alzheimer's disease: characterizing cognitive subgroups of patients. Neuropsychologia 1989;27:325–339
66. Robinson-Whelen S: Benton Visual Retention Test performance among normal and demented older adults. Neuropsychology 1992;6:261–269
67. Hart RP, Kwentus JA, Taylor JR, Harkins SW: Rate of forgetting in dementia and depression. J Consult Clin Psychol 1987; 55:101–105
68. Martin A, Fedio P: Word production and comprehension in Alzheimer's disease: the breakdown of semantic knowledge. Brain Lang 1983;19:124–141
69. Cahn DA, Salmon DP, Butters N et al: Detection of dementia of the Alzheimer type in a population-based sample: neuropsychological test performance. J Int Neuropsychol Soc 1995; 1:252–260
70. Welsh K, Butters N, Hughes JP et al: Detection and staging of dementia in Alzheimer's disease: use of the neuropsychological measures developed for the Consortium to Establish a Registry for Alzheimer's disease. Arch Neurol 1992;49: 448–452
71. Bayles KA, Trosset MW, Tomoeda CK et al: Generative naming in Parkinson disease patients. J Clin Exp Neuropsychol 1993;15:547–562
72. Randolph C, Braun AR, Goldberg TE, Chase TN: Semantic fluency in Alzheimer's, Parkinson's, and Huntington's disease: dissociation of storage and retrieval failures. Neuropsychology 1993;7:82–88
73. Mickanin J, Grossman M, Onishi K et al: Verbal and nonverbal fluency in patients with probable Alzheimer's disease. Neuropsychology 1994;8:385–394
74. Monsch AU, Bondi MW, Butters N et al: A comparison of category and letter fluency in Alzheimer's disease and Huntington's disease. Neuropsychology 1994;8:25–30
75. Monsch AU, Bondi MW, Butters N et al: Comparisons of verbal fluency tasks in the detection of dementia of the Alzheimer type. Neurology 1992;49:1253–1258
76. Weingartner HJ, Kawas C, Rawlings R, Shapiro M: Changes in semantic memory in early stage Alzheimer's disease patients. Gerontologist 1993;33:637–643
77. Binetti G, Magni E, Cappa S et al: Semantic memory in Alzheimer's disease: an analysis of category fluency. Neuropsychology 1995;17:82–89
78. Abeysinghe SC, Bayles KA, Trosset MW: Semantic memory deterioration in Alzheimer's subjects: evidence from word association, definition, and associate ranking tasks. J Speech Hear Res 1990;33:574–582
79. Knotek PC, Bayles KA, Kaszniak AW: Response consistency on a semantic memory task in persons with dementia of the Alzheimer type. Brain Lang 1990;38:465–475
80. Nebes RD: Semantic memory in Alzheimer's disease. Psychol Bull 1989;106:377–394
81. Fromholt P, Larsen P, Larsen SF: Effects of late-onset depression and recovery on autobiographical memory. J Gerontol 1995;50B:P74–P81
82. Fromholt P, Larsen SF: Autobiographical memory in normal aging and primary degenerative dementia (dementia of Alzheimer type). J Gerontol 1991;46:P85–P91
83. Beatty WW, Salmon DP: Remote memory for visuospatial information in patients with Alzheimer's disease. J Geriatr Psychiatr Neurol 1991;4:14–17
84. Baddeley A, Logie R, Bressi S et al: Dementia and working memory. Special issue: human memory. Q J Exp Psychol 1986; 38A:603–618
85. Morris RG: Working memory in Alzheimer-type dementia. Special section: working memory. Neuropsychology 1994;8: 544–554
86. Reichman WE, Cummings JL, McDaniel KD et al: Visuoconstructional impairment in dementia syndromes. Behav Neurol 1991;4:153–162
87. Henderson VC, Mack W, Williams BW: Spatial disorientation in Alzheimer's disease. Arch Neurol 1989;46:391–394
88. de Leon MJ, Potegal M, Gurland B: Wandering and parietal signs in senile dementia of Alzheimer's type. Neuropsychobiology 1984;11:155–157
89. Deloche G, Hannequin D, Carlomagno S et al: Calculation and number processing in mild Alzheimer's disease. J Clin Exp Neuropsychol 1995;17:634–639
90. Bhutani GE, Montaldi D, Brooks DN, McCulloch J: A neuropsychological investigation into frontal lobe involvement in dementia of the Alzheimer type. Neuropsychology 1992;6: 211–224
91. Lines CR, Dawson C, Preston GC et al: Memory and attention in patients with senile dementia of the Alzheimer type and in normal elderly subjects. J Clin Exp Neuropsychol 1991;13: 691–702
92. Masur DM, Sliwinski M, Lipton RB et al: Neuropsychological prediction of dementia and the absence of dementia in healthy elderly persons. Neurology 1994;44:1427–1432
93. Storandt M, Botwinick J, Danzinger WL et al: Psychometric differentiation of mild senile dementia of the Alzheimer type. Arch Neurol 1984;41:497–499
94. Eslinger PJ, Damasio AR, Benton AL, Van Allen M: Neuropsychologic detection of abnormal mental decline in older persons. JAMA 1985;253:670–674
95. Erkinjuntti T: Types of multi-infarct dementia. Acta Neurol Scand 1987;75:391–399

96. Mahler ME, Cummings JL: Behavioral neurology of multi-infarct dementia. Special issue: dementia. Alzheimer Dis Assoc Disord 1991;5:122–130

97. Wolfe N, Linn R, Babikian VL et al: Frontal systems impairment following multiple lacunar infarcts. Arch Neurol 1990; 47:129–132

98. Mendez MF, Ashla Mendez M: Differences between multi-infarct dementia and Alzheimer's disease on unstructured neuropsychological tasks. J Clin Exp Neuropsychol 1991;13: 923–932

99. Gainotti G, Parlato V, Monteleone D, Carlomagno S: Neuropsychological markers of dementia on visual-spatial tasks: a comparison between Alzheimer's type and vascular forms of dementia. J Clin Exp Neuropsychol 1992;14:239–252

100. Zimmer NA, Hayden S, Deidan C, Lowenstein DA: Comparative performance of mildly impaired patients with Alzheimer's disease and multiple cerebral infarctions on tests of memory and functional capacity. Int Psychogeriatr 1994;6:143–154

101. Libon DJ, Swenson RA, Malamut BL et al: Periventricular white matter alterations, dementia, and Bingswanger's disease. Dev Neuropsychol 1993;9:87–102

102. Bennett DA, Gilley DW, Lee S, Cochran EJ: White matter changes: neurobehavioral manifestations of Binswanger's disease and clinical correlates in Alzheimer's disease. Dementia 1994;5:148–152

103. Barr A, Benedict R, Tune L, Brandt J: Neuropsychological differentiation of Alzheimer's disease from vascular dementia. Int J Geriatr Psychiatry 1992;7:621–627

104. Almkvist O, Backman L, Basun H, Wahlund LO: Patterns of neuropsychological performance in Alzheimer's disease and vascular dementia. Cortex 1993;29:661–673

105. Ricker JH, Keenan PA, Jacobson MW: Visuoperceptual-spatial ability and visual memory in vascular dementia and dementia of the Alzheimer type. Neuropsychologia 1994;32: 1287–1296

106. Grosse DA, Gilley DW, Bernard BA et al: Semantic and episodic memory in Binswanger's versus Alzheimer's disease. J Clin Exp Neuropsychol 1991;13:70

107. Carlesimo GA, Fadda L, Lorusso S, Caltagirone C: Verbal and spatial memory spans in Alzheimer's and multi-infarct dementia. Acta Neurol Scand 1994;89:132–138

108. Erkinjuntti T, Laaksonen R, Sulkava R et al: Neuropsychological differentiation between normal aging, Alzheimer's disease and vascular dementia. Acta Neurol Scand 1986;74:393–403

109. Powell AL, Cummings JL, Hill MA, Benson DF: Speech and language alterations in multi-infarct dementia. Neurology 1988;38:717–719

110. Sultzer DL, Mahler ME, Cummings JL et al: Cortical abnormalities associated with subcortical lesions in vascular dementia. Arch Neurol 1995;52:773–780

111. Ishii N, Nishihara Y, Imamura T: Why do frontal lobe symptoms predominate in vascular dementia with lacunes? Neurology 1986;36:340–345

112. Kertesz A, Clydesdale S: Neuropsychological deficits in vascular dementia vs Alzheimer's disease: frontal lobe deficits prominent in vascular dementia. Arch Neurol 1994;51:1226–1231

113. Bernard BA, Wilson RS, Gilley DW et al: The dementia of Binswanger's disease and Alzheimer's disease. Neuropsychiatry Neuropsychol Behav Neurol 1994;7:30–35

114. Fischer P, Simanyi M, Danielczyk W: Depression in dementia of the Alzheimer type and in multi-infarct dementia. Am J Psychiatry 1990;147:1484–1487

115. Levin HS, High WM, Goethe KE et al: The neurobehavioural rating scale: assessment of the behavioural sequelae of head injury by the clinician. J Neurol Neurosurg Psychiatry 1987; 50:183–193

116. Sultzer DL, Levin HS, Mahler ME et al: A comparison of psychiatric symptoms in vascular dementia and Alzheimer's disease. Am J Psychiatry 1993;150:1806–1812

117. Dian L, Cummings JL, Petry S, Hill MA: Personality alterations in multi-infarct dementia. Psychosomatics 1990;31: 415–419

118. McKeith IG, Fairbairn AF, Perry RH, Thompson P: The clinical diagnosis and misdiagnosis of senile dementia of Lewy body type (SDLT). Br J Psychiatry 1994;165:324–332

119. Burkhardt CR, Filley CM, Kleinschmidt-DeMasters BK et al: Diffuse Lewy body disease and progressive dementia. Neurology 1988;38:1520–1528

120. Filley CM: Neuropsychiatric features of Lewy body disease. Special issue: neuropsychological issues in Lewy body disease and related disorders. Brain Cogn 1995;28:229–239

121. Raskin SA, Borod JC, Tweedy J: Neuropsychological aspects of Parkinson's disease. Neuropsychol Rev 1990;1:185–221

122. Levin BE, Tomer R, Rey GJ: Cognitive impairments in Parkinson's disease. Neurologic Clinics 1992;10:471–485

123. Huber SJ, Shuttleworth EC, Friedenberg DL: Neuropsychological differences between the dementias of Alzheimer's and Parkinson's disease. Arch Neurol 1989;46:1287–1291

124. Stern Y, Richards M, Sano M, Mayeux R: Comparison of cognitive changes in patients with Alzheimer's and Parkinson's disease. Arch Neurol 1993;50:1040–1045

125. Kramer JH, Levin BE, Brandt J, Delis DC: Differentiation of Alzheimer's, Huntington's and Parkinson's disease patients on the basis of verbal learning characteristics. Neuropsychology 1989;3:111–120

126. McKeith IG, Fairbairn AF, Bothwell RA, Moore PB et al: An evaluation of the predictive validity and inter-rater reliability of clinical diagnostic criteria for senile dementia of Lewy body type. Neurology 1994;44:872–877

127. Forstl H, Burns A, Luthert P et al: The Lewy-body variant of Alzheimer's disease: clinical and pathological findings. Br J Psychiatry 1993;162:385–392

128. Hansen L, Salmon D, Galasko D et al: The Lewy body variant of Alzheimer's disease: a clinical and pathologic entity. Neurology 1990;40:1–8

129. Byrne EJ, Lennox G, Lowe J et al: Diffuse Lewy body disease: clinical features in 15 cases. J Neurol Neurosurg Psychiatry 1989;52:709–717

130. Galloway PH, Sahgal A, McKeith IG et al: Visual pattern recognition memory and learning deficits in senile dementias of Alzheimer and Lewy body types. Dementia 1992;3:101–107

131. Sahgal A, Galloway PH, McKeith IG et al: Matching-to-sample deficits in patients with senile dementias of the Alzheimer and Lewy body types. Arch Neurol 1992;49:1043–1046

132. Sahgal A, McKeith IG, Galloway PH et al: Do differences in visuospatial ability between senile dementias of the Alzheimer and Lewy body types reflect differences solely in mnemonic function? J Clin Exp Neuropsychol 1995;17:35–43

133. Brun A: Frontal lobe degeneration of non-Alzheimer type revisited. 2nd International Conference: frontal lobe degeneration of non-Alzheimer type (1992, Lund, Sweden). Dementia 1993;4:126–131

134. Knopman DS, Mastri AR, Frey WH et al: Dementia lacking distinctive histologic features: a common non-Alzheimer degenerative dementia. Neurology 1990;40:251–256

135. Mitsuyama Y: Presenile dementia with motor neuron disease. Dementia 1993;4:137–142

136. Risberg J, Passant U, Warkentin S, Gustafson L: Regional cerebral blood flow in frontal lobe dementia of non-Alzheimer type. 2nd International Conference: frontal lobe degeneration of non-Alzheimer type (1992, Lund, Sweden). Dementia 1993; 4:186–187

137. Miller BL, Chang L, Mena I et al: Progressive right frontotemporal degeneration: clinical, neuropsychological and SPECT characteristics. Dementia 1993;4:204–213

138. Neary D, Snowden JS, Northen B, Goulding P: Dementia of frontal lobe type. J Neurol Neurosurg Psychiatry 1988;51: 353–361

139. Elfgren C, Passant U, Risberg J: Neuropsychological findings in frontal lobe dementia. 2nd International Conference: frontal lobe degeneration of non-Alzheimer type (1992, Lund, Sweden). Dementia 1993;4:214–219

140. Miller BL, Cummings JL, Villanueva-Meyer J et al: Frontal lobe degeneration: clinical, neuropsychological, and SPECT characteristics. Neurology 1991;41:1374–1382

141. Frisoni GB, Trabucchi M, Pizzolato G: Frontal lobe dementia. Int J Geriatri Psychiatry 1993;8:357

142. Stuss D: Assessment of neuropsychological dysfunction in frontal lobe degeneration. Dementia 1993;4:220–225

143. Benson DF: Progressive frontal dysfunction. Dementia 1993; 4:149–153

144. Frisoni GB, Pizzolato G, Geroldi C et al: Dementia of the frontal type: neuropsychological and [^{99}Tc]-HM-PAO SPET features. J Geriatr Psychiatry Neurol 1995;8:42–48

145. Mesulam MM: Slowly progressive aphasia without generalized dementia. Ann Neurol 1982;11:592–598

146. Weintraub S, Rubin NP, Mesulam MM: Primary progressive aphasia: longitudinal course, neuropsychological profile, and language features. Arch Neurol 1990;47:1329–1335

147. Green J, Morris JC, Sandson J et al: Progressive aphasia: a precursor of global dementia? Neurology 1990;40:423–429

148. Karbe H, Kertesz A, Polk M: Profiles of language impairment in primary progressive aphasia. Arch Neurol 1993;50: 193–201

149. Duffy JR, Petersen RC: Primary progressive aphasia. Aphasiology 1992;6:1–15

150. Kirshner HS: Progressive aphasia and other focal presentations of Alzheimer disease, Pick disease, and other degenerative disorders. pp. 108–122. In Emery VO, Oxman TE (eds): Dementia Presentations, Differential Diagnosis, and Nosology The Johns Hopkins University Press, Baltimore 1994

151. Poon LW: Toward an understanding of cognitive functioning in geriatric depression. Special issue: 1991 IPA Research Awards in Psychogeriatrics: winning papers and selected outstanding submissions. Int Psychogeriatr 1992;4(suppl 2): 241–266

152. Lamberty GJ, Bieliauskas LA: Distinguishing between depression and dementia in the elderly: a review of neuropsychological findings. Arch Clin Neuropsychol 1993;8:149–170

153. Folstein MF, Rabins PV: Replacing pseudodementia. Neuropsychiatry Neuropsychol Behav Neurol 1991;4:36–40

154. Massman PJ, Delis DC, Butters N et al: The subcortical dysfunction hypothesis of memory deficits in depression: neuropsychological validation in a subgroup of patients. J Clin Exp Neuropsychol 1992;14:687–706

155. Hart RP, Kwentus JA, Taylor JR, Hamer RM: Productive naming and memory in depressed and Alzheimer's type dementia. Arch Clin Neuropsychol 1988;3:313–322

156. Whitehead A: Verbal learning and memory in elderly depressives. Br J Psychiatry 1973;123:203–208

157. Taylor R, Gilleard CJ: Encoding preferences in memory in dementia. Br J Clin Psychol 1990;29:243–244

158. LaRue A, D'Elia LF, Clark EO et al: Clinical tests of memory in dementia, depression, and healthy aging. J Psychol Aging 1986;1:69–77

159. Miller E, Lewis P: Recognition memory in elderly patients with depression and dementia: a signal detection analysis. J Abnorm Psychol 1977;86:84–86

160. Abas MA, Sahakian BJ, Levy R: Neuropsychological deficits and CT scan changes in elderly depressives. Psychol Med 1990;20:507–520

161. Hart RP, Kwentus JA, Harkins SW, Taylor JR: Rate of forgetting in mild Alzheimer's-type dementia. Brain Cogn 1988;7: 31–38

162. Niederehe G, Camp CJ: Signal detection analysis of recognition memory in depressed elderly. Exp Aging Res 1985;11: 207–213

163. Emery OB, Breslau LD: Language deficits in depression: comparisons with SDAT and normal aging. J Gerontol Med Sci 1989;44:M85–92

164. Hill CD, Stoudemire A, Morris R et al: Dysnomia in the differential diagnosis of major depression, depression-related cognitive dysfunction, and dementia. J Neuropsychiatry Clin Neurosci 1992;4:64–69

165. Weingartner H: Automatic and effort-demanding cognitive processes in depression. pp. 218–225. In Poon L (ed) Handbook for Clinical Memory Assessment of Older Adults. American Psychological Association, Washington, DC 1986

166. Nussbaum PD: Pseudodementia: a slow death. Neuropsychol Rev 1994;4:71–90

167. Ketter TA, George MS, Kimbrell TA et al: Functional brain imaging, limbic function, and affective disorders. Neuroscientist 1996;2:55–65

168. Sahakian BJ: Depressive pseudodementia in the elderly. Special issue: affective disorders in old age. Int J Geriatr Psychiatry 1991;6:453–458
169. Kral VA: Senescent forgetfulness: benign and malignant. Can Med Assoc J 1962;86:257–260
170. Crook T, Bartus RT, Ferris SH et al: Age-associated memory impairment: proposed diagnostic criteria and measures of clinical change: report of a National Institute of Mental Health work group. Dev Neuropsychol 1986;2:261–276
171. O'Brien JT, Levy R: Age-associated memory impairment. Int J Geriatr Psychiatry 1993;8:779–780
172. Coria F: Clinical and molecular aspects of age-associated memory impairment. Ann Med 1994;26:85–88
173. Masur EM, Sliwinski M, Lipton RB et al: Neuropsychological prediction of dementia and the absence of dementia in healthy elderly persons. Neurology 1994;44:1427–1432
174. Hanninen T, Hallikainen M, Koivisto K et al: A follow-up study of age-associated memory impairment: neuropsychological predictors of dementia. J Am Geriatr Soc 1995;43: 1007–1015
175. Smith G, Ivnik RJ, Petersen RC et al: Age-associated memory impairment diagnoses: problems of reliability and concerns for terminology. Psychol Aging 1991;6:551–558
176. Larrabee GJ, McEntee W: Age-associated memory impairment: sorting out the controversies. Neurology 1995;45: 611–614
177. Bolla KI, Lindgren KN, Bonaccorsy C, Bleecker ML: Memory complaints in older adults. Fact or fiction? Arch Neurol 1991; 48:61–64
178. O'Brien JT, Beats B, Hill K et al: Do subjective memory complaints precede dementia? A three-year follow-up of patients with supposed 'benign senescent forgetfulness". Int J Geriatr Psychiatry 1992;7:481–486
179. Holroyd S, Snustad D, Chalifoux Z: Attitudes of older adults on being told the diagnosis of Alzheimer's disease. J Am Geriatr Soc 1996;44:400–403
180. Solomon K, Szwabo P: Psychotherapy for patients with dementia. pp.295–319. In Morely J, Coe R, Strong R, Grossberg G (eds): Memory Function and Aging-Related Disorders. Springer, New York 1992
181. McFarlane WR: Family psychoeducational treatment. pp.363–395. In Gurman AS, Kniskern DP (eds): Handbook of Family Therapy. Vol. 2. Brunner/Mazel, New York 1991
182. Zarit SH, Zarit JM: Families under stress: interventions for caregivers of senile dementia patients. Psychother Theory Res Prac 1982;19:461–471
183. Smyer MA, Birkel RC: Research focused on intervention with families of the chronically mentally ill elderly. pp.111–130. In Light E, Lebowitz B (eds): The Elderly With Chronic Mental Illness. Springer, New York 1991

C H A P T E R 5 5

Overview: Geriatric Gastroenterology

ROBERT E. TEPPER
SEYMOUR KATZ

Since more than 20 percent of our population is expected to exceed 65 years of age by 2030,[1] the practicing gastroenterologist in the twenty-first century will be increasingly confronted with digestive diseases in elderly patients. Gastrointestinal disease is the second most common indication for hospital admission of elderly patients,[2] who account for four times as many hospitalizations as do younger patients.[1] In the outpatient setting, patients 75 and older visit internists six times more frequently than do younger adults.[2]

Normal Physiology of Aging

With few notable exceptions, the digestive system maintains normal functioning in the elderly. In order to distinguish between the expected age-related alterations of the gut and symptoms referable to pathologic conditions, the clinician must have an understanding of the normal physiology of aging. With this knowledge, it will become apparent that most new gastrointestinal complaints in otherwise healthy older people are due to disease rather than to aging alone and therefore merit appropriate investigation and treatment.

Up to 40 percent of healthy elderly people subjectively complain of a dry mouth. Although baseline salivary flow probably decreases with aging, stimulated salivation is unchanged in both healthy and edentulous geriatric patients.[3–6] Gustatory and olfactory sensations, however, do tend to decrease with aging.[7–8] Chewing power is diminished, probably because of decreased bulk of the muscles of mastication,[9–10] though perhaps attributable in part to preclinical manifestations of neurologic disease rather than to the normal aging process.[6]

Despite early data to the contrary, the physiologic function of the esophagus in otherwise healthy individuals is well-preserved with increasing age, with the exception of very old patients.[11–12] Studies from the early 1960s introduced the concept of the "presbyesophagus" based on cineradiographic and manometric data,[13–14] but a subsequent study that excluded patients with diabetes or neuropathy found no increase in dysmotility in elderly men.[15] More recently, investigators have found that minor alterations may occur in some octogenarians, including decreased pressure and delayed relaxation of the upper esophageal sphincter and reduction in the amplitude of esophageal contractions.[16–17]

Most studies on gastric histology have found evidence of an increased prevalence of atrophic gastritis in people over 60.[18] Consequently, it has been suggested that aging results in an overall decline in gastric acid output.[11,19–20] However, more recent data have demonstrated that gastric atrophy and hypochlorhydria are not normal processes of aging. Rather, *Helicobacter pylori* infestation, which is common in the elderly, not advancing age itself, appears to be the more likely cause of these histologic and acid secretory changes.[21–24] The literature remains in conflict over the issue of whether aging alone, rather than factors such as increased *H. pylori* infestation and decreased smoking, leads to altered pepsin secretion.[23,25] Intrinsic factor secretion is usually maintained into advanced age and is retained longer in the setting of gastric atrophy than is acid or pepsin secretion.[26] Finally, gastric emptying of solids remains intact in the elderly, although liquid emptying is prolonged.[27–29]

Small bowel histology[30–31] and transit time[32–34] do not appear to change with age in humans, although increased epithelial proliferation in response to cellular injury has been found in a rodent model.[35] Small bowel absorptive capacity for most nutrients remains intact, but there are some exceptions. No change with aging was found in duodenal brush border membrane enzyme activity of glucose transport.[36] D-Xylose absorption testing remains normal after correction for renal impairment, except perhaps in octogenarians.[37–38] Jejunal lactase activity decreases with age, while that of other disaccharidases remains relatively stable, declining only during the seventh decade.[39] Protein digestion and assimilation[11] and fat absorption remain normal with aging, although the latter has a more limited adaptive reserve capacity.[40–43] Absorption of the fat-soluble vitamin A is increased in the elderly,[44] while vitamin D absorption may be impaired.[45–46] Absorption of the water-soluble vitamins B_1 (thiamine),[47] B_{12} (cyanocobalamin),[40,42,48] and C (ascorbic acid)[49] remains normal, while conflicting data exist on folate absorption with aging.[50–51] Iron absorption is maintained in the healthy elderly who are not hypochlorhydric,[52] but absorption of zinc[53] and calcium[54–56] declines with age.

Several histologic changes have been demonstrated in the colon, including atrophy of the muscularis propria with an increase in the amount of fibrosis and elastin,[11,57] and an increase in proliferating cells especially at the superficial portions of the crypts.[35,58] Some studies have found that colonic transit time decreases with aging to varying degrees,[59] while others have not shown any decline.[60–61]

Anorectal physiologic changes have been well-documented in the elderly. Aging is associated with decreased resting anal sphincter pressure in both sexes and decreased maximal sphincter pressure in women.[62] This may be due in part to age-related changes in muscle mass and contractility and in part to pudendal nerve damage associated with perineal descent in elderly women.[63] The closing pressure, that is, the difference between the maximum resting anal pressure and the rectal pressure, also falls in elderly women.[64] Maximum squeeze pressure declines with age, particularly in postmenopausal women,[3] as does rectal wall elasticity.[65] An age-dependent increase in rectal pressure threshold producing an initial sensation of rectal filling has also been demonstrated.[66] Histologic[67] and endosonographic[68] studies on anorectal structure have revealed that the internal anal sphincter develops fibrofatty degeneration and increased thickness, respectively, with aging.

The pancreas undergoes minor histologic changes with aging.[11] There also appears to be a steady increase in the caliber of the main pancreatic duct, with other branches showing areas of focal dilatation or stenosis without any apparent disease.[69] Aging reduces exocrine pancreatic flow rate and secretion of bicarbonate and enzymes, and the rate falls significantly with repeated stimulation.[3,70]

Anatomic studies on the liver reveal an age-related decrease in weight, both absolute and relative to body weight, as well as in the number and size of hepatocytes.[71–72] Lipofuscin accumulation, bile duct proliferation, fibrosis, and nonspecific reactive hepatitis are histologic changes more common in the elderly.[72] The major functional changes in older patients are reduction in hepatic blood flow, altered clearance of certain drugs, and delayed hepatic regeneration after injury.[73] The altered drug clearance is due to age-related reductions in phase I reactions (e.g., oxidation, hydrolysis, reduction), first-pass hepatic metabolism, and serum albumin binding capacity. Phase II reactions (e.g., glucuronidation, sulfation), however, remain unaffected by aging.[71–74]

While an early cholecystographic study found that gallbladder emptying remained stable with increasing age,[75] more recent data showed that gallbladder contraction may be less responsive to cholecystokinin in the elderly.[76] Increases in the proportions of the phospholipid and cholesterol components of bile raise the lithogenicity index,[77–78] leading to increased occurrence of gallstones in the aged.[11]

Altered Manifestations of Adult Gastrointestinal Disease

While there are certain disorders that occur almost exclusively in the elderly, the majority of diseases afflicting older people are those that affect younger adults as well. However, these illnesses may have atypical features which must be recognized by clinicians and represent a formidable challenge. In a study of elderly people with an "acute abdomen," the initial diagnostic impression was incorrect in up to two-thirds of patients.[79]

Acute abdominal pain appears to mute with age.[26] Theories explaining this phenomenon include increased endogenous opiate secretion, a decline in nerve conduction, and mental depression.[80] Pain localization is often atypical in elderly patients. For example, in a study on acute appendicitis, 21 percent of patients over 60 years of age presented with atypical pain distribution, while this occurred in only 3 percent of patients under 50 years of age.[81] The causes of acute abdominal pain differ as well. A multicenter review found that 25 percent of emergency patients over the age of 70 had cancer as the etiology of pain, whereas patients below age 50 had malignancy as the explanation in less than 1 percent of cases.[82]

Acute appendicitis may have few overt abdominal signs[81,83] and may therefore progress more frequently to gangrene and perforation.[84] Other intra-abdominal inflammatory conditions, such as diverticulitis, may have rather nonspecific symptoms including anorexia, altered mental status, low-grade fever or absence of fever, relatively little tenderness, and late-stage complications, for example, hepatic abscess. Even perforation of a viscus may lack the typical dramatic manifestations.[80,85] Possible explanations for the paucity of tenderness in some cases include altered sensory perception, use of psychotropic drugs, and absence of chemical peritonitis if the patient is hypochlorhydric.[26]

Gastroesophageal reflux disease (GERD) has a higher prevalence rate and a greater number of associated complications in the elderly.[12] Severe esophagitis is much more common in patients beyond the age of 65 than in young people. The magnitude of the symptoms does not correlate well with the severity of mucosal disease, and so very severe esophagitis may be associated with a relative paucity of symptoms. Therefore, manifestations of GERD are more likely to be late-stage complications such as bleeding from hemorrhagic esophagitis, dysphagia from a peptic stricture, or adenocarcinoma in the setting of Barrett's esophagus. GERD-induced chest pain may mimic, or occur concomitantly with, cardiac disease. Thus, reflux must be excluded in any elderly patient with all but very typical angina.[12] Finally, aspiration from occult GERD should be considered in elderly patients with recurrent pneumonia or exacerbations of underlying chronic obstructive pulmonary disease.[12]

Gastroduodenal ulcer disease has a severalfold greater incidence, hospitalization rate, and mortality in the elderly,[86–87] with 85 to 90 percent of ulcer-related mortality in the United States occurring in patients over 65.[88] This is due to an increase in injurious agents (e.g., *H. pylori*, nonsteroidal anti-inflammatory drugs [NSAIDs]) and to impaired defense mechanisms (e.g., lower levels of mucosal prostaglandins[89]). There may be a paucity or distortion of classic burning epigastric pain, temporal features related to food intake, and typical patterns of radiation.[26] Pain was absent in one-third of elderly hospitalized patients with peptic ulcer disease.[90] As a result, elderly patients more frequently develop complications like bleeding or perforation. Giant benign ulcers of the elderly can mimic malignancy by presenting with weight loss, anorexia, hypoalbuminemia, and anemia.

The manifestations of celiac sprue differ considerably in the elderly since features are generally more subtle than in young patients.[26] Only one-fourth of newly diagnosed elderly patients with celiac disease present primarily with diarrhea and weight loss.[91] Vague symptoms including dyspepsia or an isolated folate or iron deficiency may be the patient's sole manifestation. Severe osteopenia and osteomalacia and a bleeding diathesis due to hypoprothrombinemia are more common in the elderly than in the young.[26] Small bowel lymphoma may be particularly common when celiac disease occurs in the elderly.[92]

Constipation may be manifested in unusual ways in the elderly. When it leads to excessive defecatory straining in patients with underlying cerebrovascular disease or impaired baroreceptor reflexes, it can appear to be syncope or a transient ischemic attack. When unrelieved constipation progresses to fecal impaction, an overflow "paradoxical" diarrhea may occur, even in patients with relatively normal anal sphincter pressures. If the clinician does not recognize this and prescribes standard antidiarrheal therapy, the underlying impaction will only worsen and potentially lead to other serious complications, for example, stercoral ulcers and bleeding.

Crohn's disease of new onset in the elderly is more commonly limited to the colon than it is in young patients.[93] The colitis is more often left-sided in the elderly, whereas proximal colonic involvement is more common in the young.[94] Elderly patients with Crohn's disease may suffer fewer relapses,[26] and their postoperative recurrence rate is lower than, or equal to, that of young people.[93] Whereas those few young Crohn's disease patients who die do so of their disease, death in older patients tends to have unrelated causes.[93]

The manifestations of ulcerative colitis are generally the same in the young and the old. In the elderly, proctosigmoiditis is more common, while pancolitis and the need for surgery are less common.

The most common manifestations of gallstone disease in the elderly are acute cholecystitis and cholangitis.[26] Cholecystitis in the elderly may have nonspecific symptoms including vague mental and physical disability.[95–96] Pain may be muted or absent even in the presence of gallbladder empyema, leading to a delay in hospitalization.[97] Typical features of cholangitis may be absent. Therefore, blood cultures are critical to exclude bacteremia as the sole evidence of an infected biliary tract which can result in greater mortality in the elderly.[98–99]

The clinical course of liver disease in the elderly is usually similar to that in the young, though complications are tolerated less well.[26,100] Viral hepatitis more commonly has a more prolonged and cholestatic picture in the elderly, although data are equivocal on whether older people are more or less likely to suffer severe or fulminant hepatitis.[72] Certain liver diseases are often initially seen in more advanced stages in older patients. These include alcoholic liver disease, hemochromatosis, primary biliary cirrhosis, and hepatocellular carcinoma.[72]

Gastrointestinal Problems Unique to the Elderly

Certain gastrointestinal symptoms and diseases occur primarily, or even exclusively, in the elderly.

In the esophagus, a posterior hypopharyngeal (Zenker's) diverticulum may form because of incomplete upper esophageal sphincter opening due to reduced muscle compliance.[101] Neurologic disorders, particularly cerebrovascular accidents and Parkinson's disease, account for 80 percent of cases of oropharyngeal dysphagia in the elderly.[102] Dysphagia aortica is a syndrome in which symptoms are caused by extrinsic compression of the esophagus by a large thoracic aneurysm or a rigid atherosclerotic aorta.[17] While cervical osteophytes are common in the elderly, they are thought to be a very rare cause of dysphagia.[17]

Stomach disorders generally confined to the elderly include atrophic gastritis, with or without pernicious anemia. As mentioned previously, prolonged *H. pylori* infection rather than aging alone may be responsible for this condition. A Dieulafoy's lesion, resulting from a nontapering ectatic submucosal artery, may be an obscure etiology of upper gastrointestinal bleeding in patients of all ages but is particularly frequent in the elderly.[103]

The prevalence of small bowel diverticulosis increases greatly in older people. The condition may be limited to a single large duodenal diverticulum or may be characterized by numerous diverticula throughout the jejunum. While most cases are completely asymptomatic, some lead to perforation, hemorrhage, or bacterial overgrowth-induced malabsorption.[26] Chronic mesenteric ischemia, manifested by intestinal angina, is a very rare form of mesenteric vascular disease seen in elderly patients with atherosclerosis. Aortoenteric fistula, an uncommon cause of life-threatening gastrointestinal hemorrhage, occurs in elderly patients with prior graft placement for an abdominal aortic aneurysm (AAA) or, rarely, with an untreated AAA.

Several colonic disorders are seen far more commonly in old patients than in young patients. These include colonic diverticulosis, a condition found on postmortem examination in more than half of people over the age of 70[104]; sigmoid volvulus; vascular ectasia of the cecum[105]; stercoral ulcer in the setting of fecal impaction; and fecal incontinence, a common reason for institutionalization among the elderly.[63]

The majority of elderly patients with jaundice have biliary tract obstruction as the cause, rather than hepatocellular disease. Malignancy is more common than choledocholithiasis as the etiology of the obstruction. When hepatitis occurs, it is more commonly drug-induced and not viral as in young people.[72]

General Principles

Clinicians should consider the following principles when evaluating and treating gastrointestinal symptoms and diseases in the elderly.

- Normal physiologic changes in the aged gastrointestinal tract are few. Therefore, one must seek out and actively treat gastrointestinal disorders of the elderly (e.g., oropharyngeal dysphagia, malabsorption, abnormal liver enzymes) and not ascribe disease symptoms to the aging process.[3,106]
- Elderly patients have diminished reserve capacity to accommodate illness and should be thoughtfully evaluated and treated early in the course of the disease to prevent irreversible deterioration.[107]
- Goals of treatment must be realistic and individualized, with an emphasis on returning the patient to a functional pre-existing lifestyle.
- Comorbid conditions and concomitant medications have a dramatic effect on the presentation and prognosis of gastrointestinal disease in the elderly.
- In order to improve medicinal compliance, one must avoid prescribing medications that are expensive and/or are taken frequently throughout the day if alternatives are available since elderly patients may be on a fixed income, subject to "polypharmacy," and have memory impairment.
- One should avoid prescribing drugs more likely to cause adverse effects in the elderly (e.g., isoniazid, corticosteroids, opiates, mineral oil, NSAIDs, anticholinergics) if reasonable alternatives are available and avoid *over*prescribing drugs (e.g., tranquilizers, antidepressants) for symptoms thought to be due to somatization.
- While irritable bowel syndrome of new onset may occur in the elderly, 90 percent of cases first appear before the age of 50.[108] Therefore, the diagnosis should be rendered only after thorough evaluation to exclude other diseases including malignancy and ischemia.
- Endoscopy and abdominal surgery can be performed safely in the elderly; morbidity and mortality are related to the degree of concomitant disease and the emergent or elective nature of the procedure. An unnecessary delay in surgery is often lethal.
- Chronologic age need not be an absolute contraindication to aggressive therapeutic measures (e.g., chemotherapy, organ transplantation), as the tolerance of these interventions correlates more with the overall physiologic condition.

References

1. Katz S: Gastrointestinal diseases of the elderly: introduction to the series. Practical Gastroenterol 1993;17:9
2. Almy TP: The gastroenterologist and the graying of America. Am J Gastroenterol 1989;84:464–468
3. Lovat LB: Age related changes in gut physiology and nutritional status. Gut 1996;38:306–309
4. Shern RJ, Fox PC, Li SH: Influence of age on the secretory rates of the human minor salivary glands and whole saliva. Arch Oral Biol 1993;38:755–761
5. Gilbert GH, Heft MW, Duncan RP: Mouth dryness as reported by older Floridians. Community Dent Oral Epidemiol 1993; 21:390–397
6. Baum BJ, Bodner L: Aging and oral motor function: evidence for altered performance among older persons. J Dent Res 1983; 62:2–6
7. Doty RL, Shaman P, Applebaum SL et al: Smell identification ability: changes with age. Science 1984;226:1441–1443
8. Weiffenbach JM, Baum BJ, Burghauser R: Taste thresholds: quality-specific variation with human aging. J Gerontol 1982; 37:372–377
9. Karlsson S, Persson M, Carlsson GE: Mandibular movement and velocity in relation to state of dentition and age. J Oral Rehabil 1991;18:1–8
10. Newton JP, Yemm R, Abel RW et al: Changes in human jaw muscles with age and dental state. Gerodontology 1993;10: 16–22
11. Baime MJ, Nelson JB, Castell DO: Aging of the gastrointestinal system. pp. 665–681. In Hazzard WR, Bierman EL, Blass JP et al (eds): Principles of Geriatric Medicine and Gerontology. 3rd Ed. McGraw-Hill, New York, 1994
12. Brandt LJ: In Capell MS: Upper gastrointestinal diseases and the elderly: an interview. Intern Med World Rep 1995;10 (suppl):1–2.
13. Soergel KH, Zboralske FF, Amberg JR: Presbyesophagus: esophageal motility in nonagenarians. J Clin Invest 1964;43: 1972–1979
14. Zboralske FF, Amberg JR, Soergel KH: Presbyesophagus: cineradiographic manifestations. Radiology 1964;82: 463–464
15. Hollis JB, Castell DO: Esophageal function in elderly men: a new look at "presbyesophagus." Ann Intern Med 1974;80: 371–374
16. Fulp SR, Dalton CB, Castell JA et al: Aging related alterations in human upper esophageal sphincter functions. Am J Gastroenterol 1990;85:1569–1572
17. Schroeder PL, Richter JE: Swallowing disorders in the elderly. Practical Gastroenterol 1994;18:19–41
18. Bird T, Hall MR, Schade RO: Gastric histology and its relation to anaemia in the elderly. Gerontology 1977;23:309–321
19. Baron JH: Studies of basal and peak acid output with an augmented histamine meal. Gut 1963;4:136–144
20. Grossman MI, Kirsner JB, Gillespie IE et al: Basal and histolog-stimulated gastric secretion in control subjects and in patients with peptic ulcer or gastric ulcer. Gastroenterology 1963;45:14–26
21. Dooley CP, Cohen H, Fitzgibbons PL et al: Prevalence of *Helicobacter pylori* infection and histologic gastritis in asymptomatic persons. N Eng J Med 1989;321:1562–1566
22. Goldschmiedt M, Barnett CC, Schwarz BE et al: Effect of age on gastric acid secretion and serum gastrin concentrations in healthy men and women. Gastroenterology 1991;101: 977–990
23. Feldman M, Cryer B, McArthur KE et al: Effects of aging and gastritis on gastric acid and pepsin secretion in humans: a prospective study. Gastroenterology 1996;110:1043–1052
24. Kawaguchi H, Haruma K, Komoto K et al: *Helicobacter pylori*

infection is the major risk factor for atrophic gastritis. Am J Gastroenterol 1996;91:959–962

25. McCloy RF, Arnold R, Bardhan KD et al: Pathophysiological effects of long-term acid suppression in man. Dig Dis Sci 1995; 40(suppl):96S–120S
26. Holt P: Approach to gastrointestinal problems in the elderly. pp.882–899. In Yamada T (ed): Textbook of Gastroenterology. Lippincott-Raven, Philadelphia, 1991
27. Moore JG, Tweedy C, Christian PE et al: Effect of age on gastric emptying of liquid-solid meals in man. Dig Dis Sci 1983;28:340–344
28. Riezzo G, Pezzolla F, Giorgio I: Effects of age and obesity on fasting gastric electrical activity in man: a cutaneous electrogastrographic study. Digestion 1991;50:176–181
29. Kao CH, Lai TL, Wang SJ et al: Influence of age on gastric emptying in healthy Chinese. Clin Nucl Med 1994;19: 401–404
30. Warren PM, Pepperman MA, Montgomery RD: Age changes in small-intestinal mucosa. Lancet 1978;ii:849–850
31. Corazza GR, Frazzoni M, Gatto MR et al: Ageing and small-bowel mucosa: a morphometric study. Gerontology 1986;32: 60–65
32. Kim SK: Small intestine transit time in the normal small bowel study. Am J Roentgenol 1968;104:522–524
33. Kupfer RM, Heppell M, Haggith JW et al: Gastric emptying and small bowel transit rate in the elderly. J Am Geriatr Soc 1985;33:340–343
34. Nobles LB, Marcuard SP, Farrior ES et al: No effect of fiber and age on oral cecum transit time of liquid formula diets in women. J Am Diet Assoc 1991;91:600–602
35. Atillasoy E, Holt P: Gastrointestinal proliferation and aging. J Gerontol 1993;48:B43–B49
36. Wallis JL, Lipski PS, Mathers JC et al: Duodenal brush-border mucosal glucose transport and enzyme activities in aging man and effect of bacterial contamination of the small intestine. Dig Dis Sci 1993;38:403–409
37. Kendall MJ: The influence of age on the xylose absorption test. Gut 1970;11:498–501
38. Montgomery RD, Haeney MR, Ross IN et al: The ageing gut: a study of intestinal absorption in relation to nutrition in the elderly. Q J Med 1978;47:197–224
39. Welsh JD, Poley JR, Bhatia M et al: Intestinal disaccharidase activities in relation to age, race, and mucosal damage. Gastroenterology 1978;75:847–855
40. Webster SG, Wilkinson EM, Gowland E: A comparison of fat absorption in young and old subjects. Age Ageing 1977;6: 113–117
41. McEvoy A: p. 100. In Evans JG, Laird FI (eds): Advanced Geriatric Medicine. Pitman, London, 1982
42. Arora S, Kassarjian Z, Krasinski SD et al: Effect of age on tests of intestinal and hepatic function in healthy humans. Gastroenterology 1989;96:1560–1565
43. Holt PR, Balint JA: Effects of aging on intestinal lipid absorption. Am J Physiol 1993;264:G1–G6
44. Krazinski SD, Russell RM, Dallal GE et al: Aging changes vitamin A absorption characteristics, abstracted. Gastroenterology 1985;88:1715
45. Barragry JM, France MW, Corless D et al: Intestinal cholecalciferol absorption in the elderly and in younger adults. Clin Sci Mol Med 1978;55:213–220
46. Gallagher JC, Riggs BL, Eisman J et al: Intestinal calcium absorption and serum vitamin D metabolites in normal subjects and osteoporotic patients: effect of age and dietary calcium. J Clin Invest 1979;64:729–736
47. Thomson AD: Thiamine absorption in old age. Gerontol Clin 1966;8:354
48. McEvoy AW, Fenwick JD, Boddy K et al: Vitamin B_{12} absorption from the gut does not decline with age in normal elderly humans. Age Ageing 1982;11:180–183
49. Booth JB, Todd GB: Subclinical scurvy—hypovitaminosis C. Geriatrics 1972;27:130
50. Elsborg L: Reversible malabsorption of folic acid in the elderly with nutritional folate deficiency. Acta Haematol 1976;55: 140–147
51. Baker H, Jaslow SP, Frank O: Severe impairment of dietary folate utilization in the elderly. J Am Geriatr Soc 1978;26: 218–221
52. Marx JJ: Normal iron absorption and decreased red cell uptake in the aged. Blood 1979;53:204–211
53. Turnlund JR, Durkin N, Costa F et al: Stable isotope studies of zinc absorption and retention in young and elderly men. J Nutr 1986;116:1239–1247
54. Bullamore JR, Wilkinson R, Gallagher JC et al: Effect of age on calcium absorption. Lancet 1970;ii:535–537
55. Ireland P, Fordtran JS: Effect of dietary calcium and age on jejunal calcium absorption in humans studied by intestinal perfusion. J Clin Invest 1973;52:2672–2681
56. Ambrecht HJ, Zenser TV, Bruns ME, et al: Effect of age on intestinal calcium absorption and adaption to dietary calcium. Am J Physiol 1979;236:E769
57. Yamajata A: Histopathological studies of the colon due to age. Jpn J Gastroenterol 1965;62:224
58. Roncucci L, Ponz de Leon M, Scalmati A et al: The influence of age on colonic epithelial cell proliferation. Cancer 1988; 62:2373–2377
59. Madsen JL: Effects of gender, age, and body mass index on gastrointestinal transit times. Dig Dis Sci 1992;37:1548–1553
60. Melkerssen M, Andersson H, Bosaeus I et al: Intestinal transit time in constipated geriatric patients. Scand J Gastroenterol 1983;18:593–597
61. Merkel IS, Locher J, Burgio K et al: Physiologic and psychologic characteristics of an elderly population with chronic constipation. Am J Gastroenterol 1993;88:1854–1859
62. McHugh SM, Diamant NE: Effect of age, gender, and parity on anal canal pressures. Dig Dis Sci 1987;32:726–736
63. Wald A: Managing constipation and fecal incontinence in the elderly. Practical Gastroenterol 1994;18:28H–37H
64. Haadem K, Dahlstrom JA, Ling L: Anal sphincter competence in healthy women: clinical implications of age and other factors. Obstet Gynecol 1991;78:823–827
65. Ihre T: Studies on anal function in continent and incontinent patients. Scand J Gastroenterol 1974;25:1–64

66. Akervall S, Nordgren S, Fasth S et al: The effects of age, gender, and parity on rectoanal functions in adults. Scand J Gastroenterol 1990;25:1247–1256
67. Klosterhalfen B, Offner F, Torf N: Sclerosis of the internal anal sphincter—a process of ageing. Dis Colon Rectum 1990; 33:606–609
68. Papachrysostomou M, Pye SD, Wild SR et al: Significance of the thickness of the anal sphincters with age and its relevance in faecal incontinence. Scand J Gastroenterol 1994;29: 710–714
69. Sahel J, Cros RC, Lombard C et al: Morphometrique de la pancreatographie endoscopique normal du sujet age. Gastroenterol Hepatol 1979;15:574–577
70. Gullo L, Ventrucci M, Naldoni P et al: Aging and exocrine pancreatic function. J Am Geriatr Soc 1986;34:790–792
71. Mooney H, Roberts R, Cooksley WG et al: Alterations in the liver with aging. Clin Gastroenterol 1985;14:757–771
72. Keefe EB: Abnormal liver tests and liver disease in the elderly. Practical Gastroenterol 1993;17:16A–17A
73. Popper H: Aging and the liver. pp. 659–683. In Popper H, Schaffner F (eds): Progress in Liver Disease. Vol. VIII. Grune and Stratton, Orlando, FL, 1986
74. Kenichi K: Aging and the liver. pp. 603–623. In Popper H, Schaffner F (eds): Progress in Liver Diseases. Vol. IX. WB Saunders, Philadelphia, 1990
75. Boyden EA, Grantham SA Jr: Evacuation of the gallbladder in old age. Surg Gynecol Obstet 1936;62:34
76. Khalil T, Walder JP, Wiener I et al: Effect of aging on gallbladder contraction and release of cholecystokinin-33 in humans. Surgery 1985;98:423–429
77. Trash DB, Ross PE, Murison J et al: Proceedings: the influence of age on cholesterol saturation of bile. Gut 1976;17:394
78. Valdivieso V, Palma R, Wunkhaus R et al: Effect of aging on biliary lipid composition and bile acid metabolism in normal Chilean women. Gastroenterology 1978;74:871–874
79. Oliver N: Abdominal pain in the elderly. Aust Fam Physician 1984;13:402–404
80. Phillips SL, Burns GP: Acute abdominal disease in the aged. Med Clin North Am 1988;72:1213–1224
81. Arnbjornsson E: Recognizing appendicitis in the elderly. Geriatr Med Today 1984;3:72
82. Telfer S, Fenyo G, Holt PR et al: Acute abdominal pain in patients over 50 years of age. Scand J Gastroenterol 1988;23: 47–50
83. Hangos G, Thurzo R: Appendicitis in the aged. Gerontol Clin 1961;3:55–67
84. Arnbjornsson E, Adren-Sandberg A, Bengmark S: Appendicectomy in the elderly: incidence and operative findings. Ann Chir Gynaecol 1983;72:223–228
85. Narayanan M, Steinheber FU: The changing face of peptic ulcer in the elderly. Med Clin North Am 1976;60:1159–1172
86. Schoon IM, Mellstrom D, Oden A et al: Incidence of peptic ulcer disease in Gothenburg, 1985. BMJ 1989;299: 1131–1134
87. Holt PR: Are gastrointestinal disorders in the elderly important? J Clin Gastroenterol 1993;16:186–188
88. Holt PR: Perspectives on upper gastrointestinal disease in the elderly: symposium on perspectives on upper GI diseases in the elderly—Strategies for treatment. Practical Gastroenterol 1988;12:5–12
89. Cryer B, Redfren JS, Goldschmiedt M et al: Effect of aging on gastric and duodenal mucosal prostaglandin concentrations in humans. Gastroenterology 1992;102:1118–1123
90. Clinch D, Banerjee AK, Ostick G: Absence of abdominal pain in elderly patients with peptic ulcer. Age Ageing 1984;13: 120–123
91. Swinson CM, Levi AJ: Is coeliac disease underdiagnosed? BMJ 1980;281:1258–1260
92. Swinson CM, Clavin G, Coles EC et al: Coeliac disease and malignancy. Lancet 1983;i:111–115
93. Kadish SL, Reinus J: Inflammatory bowel disease in the elderly. Practical Gastroenterol 1994;18:23–30
94. Carr N, Schofield PF: Inflammatory bowel disease in the older patient. Br J Surg 1982;69:223–225
95. Croker JR: Biliary tract disease in the elderly. Clin Gastroenterol 1985;14:773–809
96. Cobden I, Lendrum R, Venables CW et al: Gallstones presenting as mental and physical disability in the elderly. Lancet 1984;i:1062–1064
97. Thornton JR, Heaton KW, Espiner HJ et al: Empyema of the gallbladder—reappraisal of a neglected disease. Gut 1983; 24:1183–1185
98. Madden JW, Croker JR, Beynon GP: Septicaemia in the elderly. Postgrad Med J 1981;57:502–506
99. Esposito AL, Gleckman RA, Cram S et al: Community acquired bacteremia in the elderly: analysis of 100 consecutive episodes. J Am Geriatr Soc 1980;28:315–319
100. Gibinski K, Fojit E, Suchan S: Hepatitis in the aged. Digestion 1973;8:254–260
101. Cook IJ, Gabb M, Penagopoulos V et al: Pharyngeal (Zenker's) diverticulum is a disorder of upper esophageal sphincter opening. Gastroenterology 1992;103:1229–1235
102. Pulliam JT, Richter JE: Dysphagia and esophageal obstruction. pp. 428–436. In Renkel RE (ed): Conn's Current Therapy. WB Saunders, Philadelphia, 1990
103. Wootton FT, Johnson DA: Gastrointestinal bleeding in the elderly. Practical Gastroenterol 1994;18:11–19
104. Almy TP, Howell D: Diverticular disease of the colon. N Engl J Med 1980;302:324–331
105. Boley SJ, DiBiase A, Brandt LJ et al: Lower intestinal bleeding in the elderly. Am J Surg 1979;137:57–64
106. Holt PR: Introduction: gastrointestinal and liver disease in the elderly. Semin Gastrointest Dis 1994;5:151–153
107. Snape WJ Jr: Gastrointestinal disorders in the elderly. II. bowel dysfunction in the elderly: a growing problem. Intern Med World Rep 1995;10(13):14–24
108. Schuster MM: Irritable bowel syndrome. pp. 1402–1418. In Sleisinger MH, Fordtran JS (eds): Gastrointestinal Disease. WB Saunders Philadelphia, 1989

CHAPTER 56

Aging and the Orofacial Tissues

HUGH DEVLIN
MARK W. J. FERGUSON

Some of the world's greatest artists have depicted the face of old age. Leonardo Da Vinci's sketchbooks and Rembrandt's self-portraits over a lifetime illustrate the gnarled features, the wrinkles, the compressed lips, the sunken, jaws and prominent chin the changes in pigmentation, and the moles that mark the aging face. Indeed, it would be surprising if the tissues in and around the mouth did not suffer the abuses of wear and tear. A lifetime of eating and drinking, of talking and breathing, of smiling and frowning, and of exposure to heat, cold, wind, and rain—as well as a lifetime's vigilance in warding off threats to the body at its main portal of entry—is bound to leave a mark, even on tissues that are uniquely equipped for self-preservation and defense of the body. Oral tissues have high rates of turnover and repair, rich sensory and motor networks for testing the environment and reacting appropriately, and elaborate general and specific immune defenses, while the teeth themselves contain highly specialized and unique tissues such as enamel, dentine, pulp, cementum, and the periodontal ligament, all of which have their own specific diseases and aging changes. Moreover, the oral cavity can serve as a window to the rest of the body. Many age changes and disorders that occur elsewhere in the body affect the oral tissues, often first, making them useful diagnostic indicators. The accessibility and variety of the oral tissues makes them useful model systems for investigating a number of issues related to aging from the clinical to the molecular and from the physiologic to the pathologic.

Despite a rapidly emerging body of literature, the ease of examination of the oral cavity, and recent significant improvements in dental health, even in the elderly, there remain large reservoirs of ignorance and neglect of the oral tissues among both the public and health care providers. Many believe that tooth loss in old age, either through caries or periodontal diseases, is inevitable. Many believe that alterations of tooth color, dry mouth, burning sensations, and changes in oral function such as speech, mastication, and swallowing are inevitable consequences of aging. Nothing could be further from the truth. All too often, elderly patients with head or neck cancer undergo life-saving chemotherapy or radiation only to suffer unnecessary pain, rampant tooth decay, and gum infection that lead to the loss of all their teeth. Serious tooth and gum disorders also plague individuals who may otherwise lead full, active lives but whose daily medication to control blood pressure, heart problems, depression, or other systemic conditions has adverse oral effects. The side-effects of dry mouth (xerostomia) associated with approximately 500 over-the-counter and prescription drugs may go completely unmentioned by the patient or be dismissed by the examining physician, an oversight that indicates how little is appreciated about the role of saliva in protecting, preserving, and lubricating the oral tissues. Most people recognize the beneficial effects of fluoride treatment—in the water supply, by self-medication (e.g., mouthwashes, toothpaste, tablets), or by professional administration—in controlling and preventing dental diseases in children. What is not generally appreciated is that these beneficial effects extend into old age and that similar preventative programs are required to care for the aging dentition in elderly patients who have lost some of their natural defenses. The diet of many elderly people is often soft, mushy, and carbohydrate-rich, which renders their teeth more susceptible to periodontal disease and caries—often of a unique kind (e.g., root caries) not seen commonly in younger patients.

Therefore, this chapter summarizes the effects of normal aging on the principal cells and tissues of the oral cavity and suggests how the effect of these changes on the functional capacity of the tissues can be minimized. It also summarizes epidemiologic data outlining the extent of oral problems in the elderly, concentrating on American data, which are the most up to date and comprehensive in the world. Common conditions affecting the oral cavity in the elderly, including those induced iatrogenically, are described, as are the oral effects of systemic aging. Whenever possible, recent developments and future changes in the clinical management of dentistry for the elderly are mentioned: geriatric dentistry is a rapidly emerging speciality as evidenced by the recent establishment of university chairs, consultancies, and departments of gerodontology, and the publication of journals and textbooks (e.g., Drummond, Newton and Yemm Colour Atlas and Text of Dental Care of the Elderly.[1])

Tissues of the Oral Cavity

The mucous membrane (epithelium and underlying connective tissue) of the gingivae covers the roots of the teeth and their surrounding alveolar bone. The outside of the crown of each tooth is covered by hard, dense, white enamel (the most highly mineralized tissue—97 percent—in the body). The cells that form the enamel are present on its outermost surface before eruption but are lost on eruption; consequently, once erupted in the oral cavity, enamel contains no living cells. The inorganic enamel matrix does, however, participate in mineral exchange with the saliva and oral contents and is capable of limited chemical repair (remineralization) after acid attack (e.g., in dental caries). This property is the biologic basis for topical fluoride therapy and the evolution of caries-minimizing dietary regimes.

Beneath the enamel lies the yellow dentine. It contains no cell inclusions (only nerve fibers and odontoblast processes) but is resilient in nature and forms the basic shape outline of the crown and root. Dentine is permeated by millions (30,000/ mm^2) of tiny tubules which contain the cytoplasmic processes of the cells that form the dentine (odontoblasts, whose cell bodies lie in the pulp) together with tissue fluid and nerves. Movement of fluid within the dentinal tubule stimulates the nerve endings, which accounts for dentine's extreme sensitivity (to hot, cold, osmotic, or pressure stimuli) which is usually perceived as pain. As dentine contains the living cellular processes of the odontoblasts, it undergoes a number of age changes and reparative responses to injury. Covering the external surface of the dentine on the root lies a thin layer of cementum which resembles bone in composition. The collagen fibers of the periodontal ligament attach the tooth to the bone inserted into the cementum on one side and to bone on the other side. Cementum contains living cells and is continually deposited throughout life. The periodontal ligament consists mostly of collagen fibers, blood vessels, nerves, and lymphatics. Most of the collagen fibers run obliquely from the bone toward the apex of the root of the tooth. The periodontal ligament is thin (0.2 mm) and has the highest rate of collagen turnover anywhere in the body. It also contains numerous proprioceptive nerve endings essential for precise regulation of oral function in eating, speaking, swallowing, and so on. At the apex of the root of the tooth, vessels and nerves pass into the central pulp via the apical foramen. The pulp of the tooth contains a rich supply of blood vessels, sensory nerves, lymphatics, fibroblasts, undifferentiated mesenchyme cells, extracellular matrix, and cell bodies of the odontoblasts adjacent to the dentine.

The alveolar bone completely surrounds the roots of the teeth and is contiguous with the underlying basal bone of the mandible. Alveolar bone develops from part of the embryonic dental follicle and is critically dependent on the presence of teeth for its persistence in the adult—when teeth are extracted the alveolar bone disappears.

The soft tissues of the gum and the hard tooth tissues meet at the gingival margin. This junction is highly specialized and critical for maintenance of the dentition. Close apposition of the gum to the tooth depends on many factors but chiefly on an intact network of supporting collagen fibers from the tooth root and bone to the overlying gingival cuff. The epithelium adjacent to the tooth is highly specialized and very permeable—numerous immunoglobulins and leukocytes pass out in the continual flow of gingival (crevicular) fluid from the gum margin. This junction between living, rapid-turnover gingiva and dead, highly mineralized enamel must be tight at the micrometer level to prevent ingress of microorganisms or food debris.

Elsewhere the tissues of the oral cavity are covered by mucous membrane, the structure of which varies according to the region of the oral cavity. The epithelium covering the hard palate is nonpermeable, keratinized, stratified squamous with a thick lamina propria densely bound down to the alveolar bone, whereas that lining the floor of the mouth (beneath the tongue) is thin, permeable, and nonkeratinized, with a loose elastic submucosa. These marked regional variations in oral epithelial differentiation are regulated by the underlying fibroblasts and stroma via epithelial mesenchymal interactions.

Injury to the oral mucosa usually results in a regenerative scar-free mode of wound healing typical of the embryo.[2] There is usually little inflammation, and healing occurs rapidly. Fibroblasts from the papillary region of the gingiva resemble embryonic mesenchymal cells[3] in the way they migrate into the three-dimensional matrices of collagen gels and produce migration stimulating factor (MSF). This protein has sequence homology with the gelatin-binding domain of fibronectin.[4] MSF-producing fibroblasts in the gingival papillae may contribute to the advantageous healing pattern in the mouth. Healthy adult skin fibroblasts and larger fibroblasts from the deeper, reticular region of the gingiva do not exhibit a fetal-like migratory phenotype or produce MSF. The matrix of the gingival papillary layer also differs from that of the reticular layer in having a greater predominance of collagen type III fibers (which are also more abundant in fetal than in adult skin).

Saliva is secreted from the parotid, submandibular, and sublingual salivary glands and from a multitude of minor salivary glands in the cheeks and palate. It is a complex secretion with the unique feature that 70 percent of the secreted protein comprises salivary-specific, proline-rich proteins.[5] Saliva is rich in mucin; lubricating proteins; immunoglobulins; blood group antigens; antibacterial, antifungal, and antiviral agents (e.g., lactoferrin, lysozyme, histatins); amylase enzymes; and proteins which protect against dietary factors (e.g., tannins,[6] epidermal growth factor, and nerve growth factor). Of special importance are remineralization proteins which allow calcium and phosphate salts to exist in a supersaturated solution, thereby preventing teeth from dissolving in saliva by the law of mass action. Saliva has a neutral or alkaline pH, with buffers to neutralize proton production by cariogenic bacteria, and is an aqueous solvent of appropriate viscosity for such functions as dissolving tastants, hydrating the oral mucosa, and contributing to food bolus formation.

Age Changes in the Oro-facial Tissues

Teeth

Many of the changes encountered in teeth are not due to age changes alone but are the result of incremental effects of wear, habit, and disease (Fig. 56-1). The most conspicuous

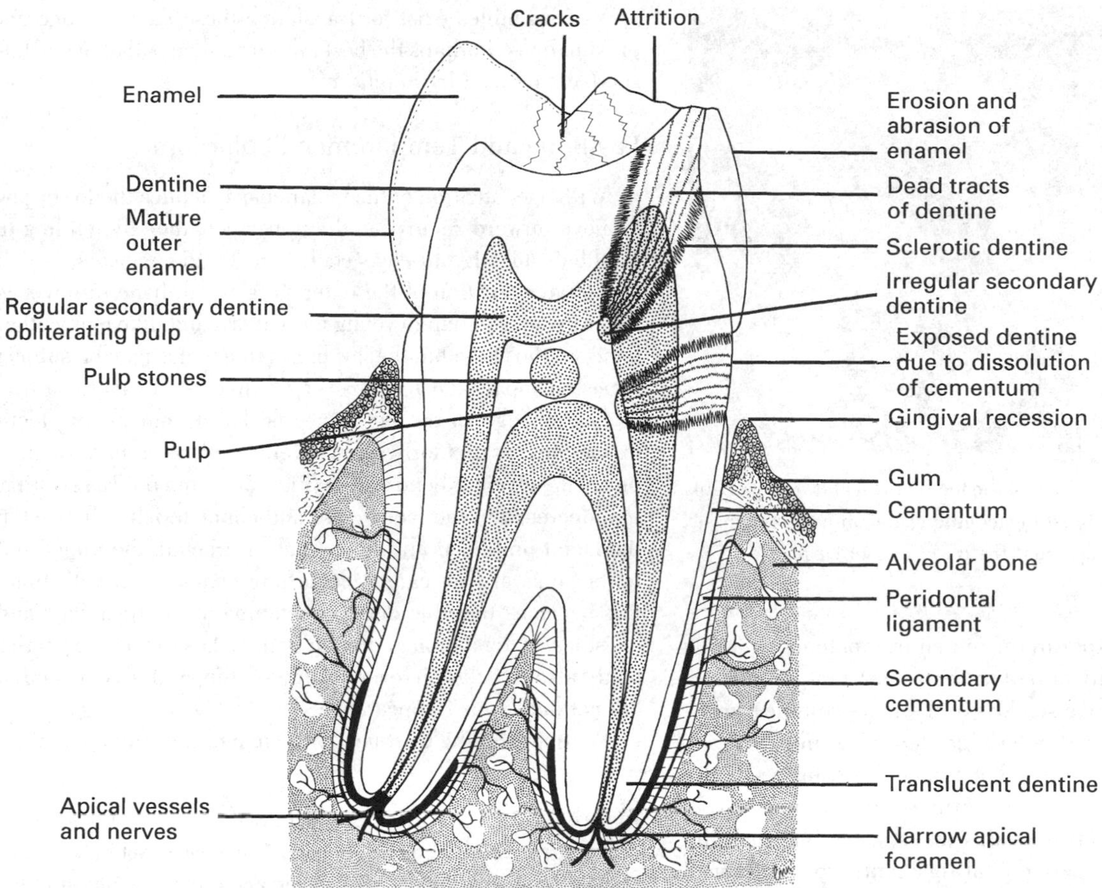

Figure 56-1 Age changes in teeth and surrounding bone and gums. (Adapted from Ferguson,[14] with permission.)

feature is loss of tooth substance due to wear. Tooth surface wear is extremely variable and is related to diet, occlusion, habits, occupation, and the composition of the enamel itself. Occlusal wear may be due to attrition (tooth-tooth contact), abrasion (tooth-food contact or contact with other exogenous particles, e.g., abrasive toothpaste) or erosion (acid). Occlusal attrition gradually increases the occlusal areas of the teeth that are in direct contact; it is claimed that this relates to more efficient food processing in older dentition. The length of the tooth is maintained by deposition of cementum, which is thickest on the apical surface of the root. The thickness of apical cementum on single rooted teeth is approximately tripled between 10 and 70 years.[7] Attrition also occurs at contact points between teeth because of their movement during mastication. Interproximal attrition may result in the loss of as much as 1 cm from the overall arch circumference by the age of 40, the teeth maintaining their contacts through mesial drift. Abrasion of the buccal and lingual surfaces of the enamel tends to thin the enamel, allowing the underlying yellowish dentine to show through (Fig. 56-2). This, together with extrinsic staining of the enamel means that teeth tend to darken with age.

Loss of tooth substance by erosion is caused by acids in the diet or in medicines, or as a result of regurgitation. Regurgitation erosion may occur in older patients as a result of esophageal reflux or hiatus hernia. Hydrochloric acid replacement therapy, vitamin C, aspirin, or pure fruit juices used habitually can all cause tooth erosion.

Vertical hairline cracks running from the occlusal surface of the enamel are prevalent in older teeth. These are probably the result of age changes in the dentine which result in it becoming less aqueous, shrinking, and also becoming less resilient, consequently becoming unsupportive of the overlying enamel. Importantly, the fluoride content of surface enamel increases with age.[8] This has important implications for resistance to dental caries and for restorative dental procedures.

Two age changes take place in dentine: continued growth, called regular secondary dentine formation, which progressively reduces the volume of the pulp chamber, and gradual obliteration of the dentinal tubules by deposition of intratubular dentine (called dentine sclerosis).[7] What remains of the diminishing dental pulp tends to become less cellular, more fibrous, less vascular, and less innervated with increasing age.[9,10] Dystrophic calcification, often in the form of pulp stones, frequently occurs in the pulps of older teeth. Collectively, these changes result in the teeth being less sensitive (elderly patients may require no anesthesia for restorative dental procedures) and more brittle with increasing age.[9]

With increasing age, the gingival margin tends to migrate

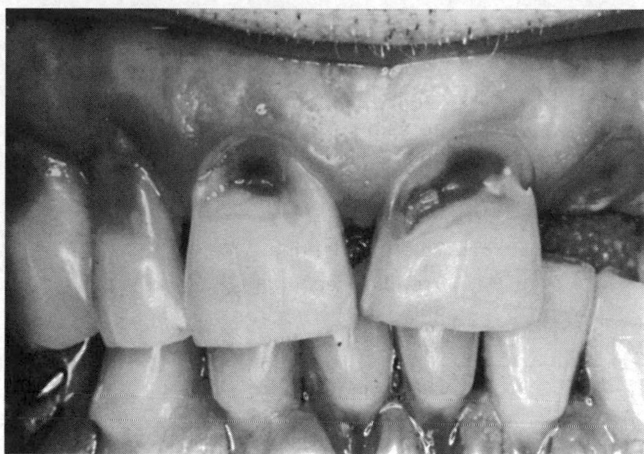

Figure 56-2 Severe abrasion of the tooth crown and root, probably caused by incorrect tooth brushing technique and abrasive toothpaste. The dark stained areas represent the onset of root caries.

apically, leading to exposure of the entire anatomic crown of the tooth and eventually of part of the cementum-covered root (Fig. 56-2). This often causes loss of the more soluble cementum and exposure of the underlying dentine which, if rapid, results in marked sensitivity to hot and cold substances. It also results in a dental disease—root caries—almost unique to old people (Fig. 56-2). Severson et al.[11] investigated histologically the age changes in 80 periodontal ligaments from 24 human cadavers aged 20 to 90 years and found that the older specimens had a decreased fiber and fibroblast content and an increase in the size of interstitial compartments but no change in collagen orientation. Diffuse calcification is also frequent.[12] The rate of collagen synthesis decreases, and the collagen fibers become thicker and more stable, exhibiting increased insolubility, thermal stability, and mechanical strength.[12,13] Investigations of changes in the width of the periodontal ligament with age yield equivocal data,[12] probably because of differences in the functional loading of the teeth studied.

Teeth are exceptionally useful in determining the age of mutilated or otherwise unrecognizable bodies and also in archaeologic studies. Up to the age of 20, the developing and erupting teeth provide a useful estimate of an individual's age.[14] Beyond that age or when only individual teeth are available, an estimate can be made by considering a number of parameters from longitudinal ground sections of the teeth, particularly the following.

1. Degree of attrition
2. Degree of secondary dentine formation
3. Presence or absence of translucent dentine and its extent
4. Position of the epithelial attachment
5. Thickness of cementum on the root of the tooth
6. Condition of the apical foramen
7. Size and shape of the pulp cavity

Various tables exist for translating these data into age approximations. Perhaps the best known method is that of Gustafsen (summarized by Ferguson[14]).

Jaw Bone and Temporomandibular Joint

With age, attrition of the molar cusps enables the lower jaw to move forward relative to the upper jaw, thereby tending to establish an edge-to-edge occlusion for the incisors, which accelerates attrition of the latter. In general, bone turnover is lower in old age than in young individuals and, like many other bones in the skeleton, the jaw bones in females may be subject to postmenopausal osteoporosis.[15,16] However, by far the greatest age change in the jaw bones is that accompanying tooth extractions, particularly when several teeth are removed: atrophy of the alveolar bone occurs (Figs. 56-3 and 56-4), resulting in a decrease in the face height and characteristic changes in the facial profile. If all the teeth are extracted, the upper and lower gums at first cannot come into contact but, with time, this becomes possible due to stretching of the ligaments and capsules of temporomandibular joints. Loss of the posterior teeth also results in overclosure of the oral cavity and a "Punch-and-Judy" appearance.

Patients seeking treatment of symptoms attributable to their

Figure 56-3 Comparison between dried mandibles from elderly dentate (top) and edentulous (bottom) individuals. Note the loss of alveolar bone with the mental foramen approaching the crest of the jaw bone in the edentulous specimen, the thinning of the coronoid process, the narrowing of the ramus of the mandible, and the characteristic notching at the inferior border of the edentulous mandible.

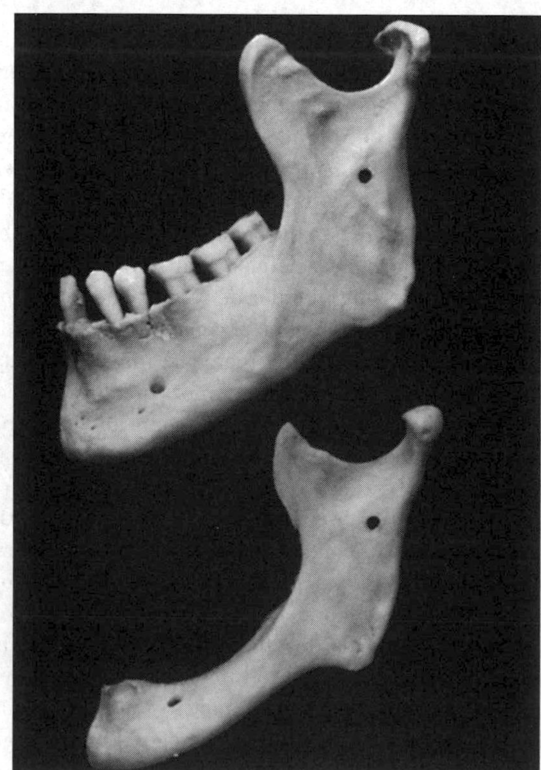

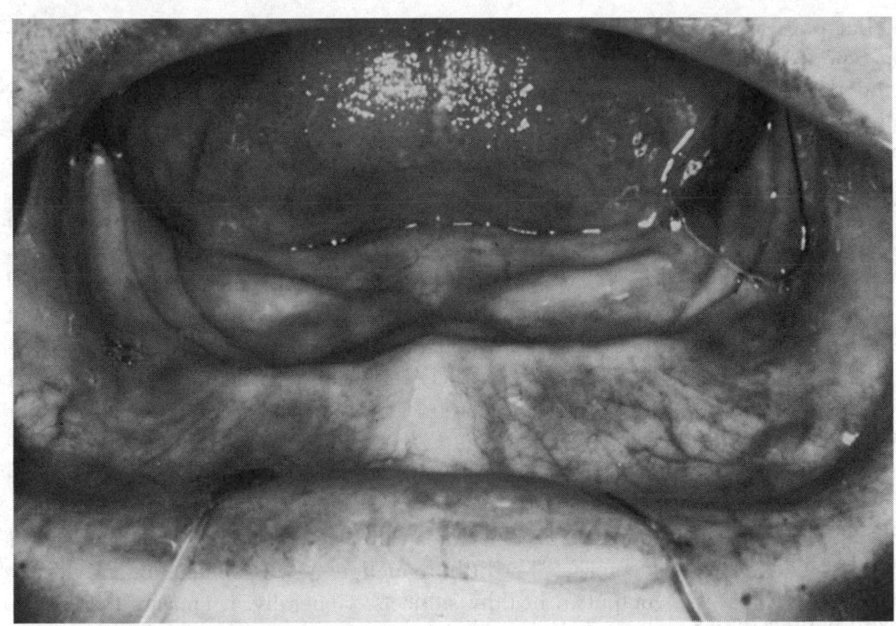

Figure 56-4 Intraoral view of the edentulous lower jaw of an elderly patient. Note that there is almost no dental ridge on which to construct a denture. This massive loss of alveolar bone contributes to the difficulties of denture wearing and can be further compounded by tranquilizers and other drugs that reduce the amount of lubricating saliva.

temporomandibular joint are normally young. The prevalence of disk displacement and osteoarthritis of this joint increases with age but is not usually accompanied by an increase in patient symptoms.[17] However, some surveys of selected elderly populations have found a high prevalence of joint symptoms.[18] Perhaps the elderly assume that painful temporomandibular joints, deviation of the jaw to one side on opening, or joint noises are all part of growing old and therefore do not seek treatment.[19] Osteoarthritis of the temporomandibular joint is characterized by erosion and flattening of the condylar surface and is a common finding in radiographic surveys of elderly cadaver specimens.[20]

Continued resorption of the jaw bones following tooth extraction is especially severe in the mandible, often resulting in a pencil-thin mandible. Loss of mandibular teeth usually results in atrophy of the muscles of mastication and the muscular processes of the bones concerned; for example, the coronoid process becomes narrow and pointed and the mandibular angle widens (Fig. 56-3). There is a measurable reduction in masseter and medial pterygoid muscle bulk with age.[21] Old people are also less precise in their contraction of masticatory muscles,[22] suggesting that, overall, masticatory muscles become less efficient with age.

These changes in bone and muscle, together with associated age changes in the dermis and epidermis, give rise to the typical appearance of the drooping, aged face and lips: numerous plastic surgical procedures have been devised to "lift" the appearance of the aging face to resemble that of its young predecessor.[23,24]

The Soft Tissues

Clinically, the oral mucosa and skin differ between young and old subjects. With age, the oral mucosa becomes increasing thin, smooth, and dry,[25] has a satinlike, edematous appearance with loss of elasticity and stippling,[26] and is more susceptible to injury.[27] Often, the tongue appears smooth, with the loss of filiform papillae, apparent disturbance of taste, and occurrence of occasional burning sensations. Perceived alterations in taste may relate not only to structural changes and atrophy in the taste buds but also to alterations in diet and masticatory efficiency. Sodium chloride detection levels increase with age,[28] but early reports exaggerated the loss of salt taste acuity. The elderly rarely complain that they are unable to detect tastes (probably because of the small changes in perceived threshold) but report alterations in the intensity of the stimulation. Perceived taste intensity rises more steeply with stimulus concentration in young adults than in the elderly.[29] Age reduces the perceived intensity of taste sensations, but the changes are small. Age-related changes in taste perception are not uniform for all taste qualities, for all taste performances, or for all populations of elderly individuals.[30] Apparently, the mechanisms underlying the four basic taste qualities age independently, but deficits reflect age-related sensory loss.[30] Further, aging alters not only chemosensory sensitivity but also chemosensory preference,[31] which may be significant in the context of nutrition of the elderly. Dietary deficiencies, for example, lack of iron or B vitamins can also lead to atrophic changes of the oral mucosa. In postmenopausal women, mucosal atrophy and the associated clinical symptoms, (e.g., a burning mouth) may be reversed by estrogen therapy,[32] suggesting systemic influences rather than intrinsic age changes. Changes in the blood vessels with age, particularly the development of varicosities in the cheeks, lips, and especially sublingually are part of the normal aging process and are not associated with cardiovascular disease.[33]

Elderly patients often complain of a burning sensation in the tongue, palate, and denture bearing area, but the tissues appear normal. This condition is termed burning mouth syndrome (BMS). In one form of this condition, the patient is rarely wakened by pain during the night, but pain severity increases during the day (type 1 BMS). In type 2 BMS, the burning sensation is present on waking and throughout the day. Patients with type 3 BMS have symptom-free periods.[34]

Allergy to food preservatives or flavoring agents, as well as emotional instability, are important in the etiology of type 3 BMS. The symptoms can also be caused by local denture trauma, nutritional inadequacies, diabetes, or anemia. The patient may consult their medical practitioner suspecting that they have oral cancer. It is important that the medical practitioner liaise with dental colleagues to investigate and treat BMS.

Structural changes in human oral epithelia with aging include thinning of the epithelial cell layers (e.g., thinning of the lingual epithelial,[35]) diminished keratinization, and simplification of epithelial structure.[36] In addition there are alterations in the morphology of the connective tissue-epithelial interface, with a more papillary (rather than ridge) architecture[37] of shortened rete pegs.[13] Age changes in the rate of cell renewal in human oral epithelia are controversial, with both increases and decreases reported.[12] The age of the patient per se does not affect the results of surgical periodontal therapy,[38] suggesting that the healing capacity of healthy oral mucosa is not functionally impaired with increasing age (as reviewed elsewhere[39]).

Many clinically apparent changes in the oral mucosa with age are probably the result of changes in the dermis rather than the epithelia, particularly as the connective tissue lamina propria is considered responsible for signaling and maintaining the regional specific epithelial differentiation patterns of the oral mucosa.[35,40] A thickening of the collagen and elastin fibers[41] probably reduces flexibility and resilience with age, while changes in staining characteristics suggest alterations in the proteoglycan composition.[12] The fibroblasts appear reduced in size, and the matrix collagen denser and more heavily cross-linked. Gingival fibroblasts derived from donors of different ages show a decrease in proliferative activity, proteoglycan synthesis,[42] and protein and collagen synthesis.[43] The concept of heterogeneity in a population of fibroblasts is now receiving much attention, with the description of differentiation of human skin fibroblasts along a seven-stage lineage, each with distinctive phenotypes.[44] Fibroblast populations aged in vitro or obtained from old donors have higher proportions of stage 7 large, epithelioid-like cells. Such changes in fibroblast heterogeneity with aging are particularly relevant to the oral mucosa which already shows marked differences in fibroblast morphology, growth requirements, metabolism of steroid hormones, and biosynthetic activity according to site of origin in the oral cavity.[45,46] Alterations in fibroblast clonal heterogeneity are probably important in the development, aging, and pathogenesis of various diseases.[47] Much more is known about age changes in the skin than in the oral mucosa.[12]

Saliva

The stereotype that growing old is associated with decreased salivary flow, dry mouth, and its associated pathologies has its basis in several clinical studies conducted 30 to 40 years ago. These investigations did not distinguish among healthy, diseased, or drug-consuming individuals and had numerous methodologic and analytical errors.[48] The decreased salivary gland function reported in nearly all studies before 1980 probably reflects pathologic or pharmacologic-induced gland dysfunction and not normal aging.[48]

Histologic studies of aging salivary glands show a gradual loss of acinar elements, a relative increase in the proportion of ductal elements, an increase in inflammatory infiltrates, and an increase in fibrofatty tissue.[49–51] These changes are present not only in the submandibular gland (where up to half of the acini may be lost between youth and old age), the sublingual gland, and the parotid gland but also in the numerous minor salivary glands.[52–55] Despite these structural changes, the effects of aging on salivary flow rate are still controversial. Since 1981, several reports[48,53] have indicated no reduction in parotid salivary flow rates with age; others have reported marked decreases[56] or little reduction[57,58] in submandibular salivary output in healthy subjects. Generally, it appears that in the major salivary glands, extensive secretory tissue is lost with age but without significant decreases in salivary flow, presumably because of the large secretory reserve in the major glands. However, the function of the numerous minor salivary glands is reduced[52,57] which may be of considerable functional significance in view of their unique biochemical constituents.[56] Studies on the composition of either major or minor gland saliva with aging are scanty[58–62] but indicate a diminution in sodium concentration and no alteration in potassium concentration, total protein concentration, or anionic proline-rich protein content. The perception of xerostomia probably results from reduced minor gland function, nutritional disturbances, side effects of medication, or oral or systemic diseases.[63] For patients with real xerostomia induced by any of these factors, commercially available artificial saliva may be useful.

Systemic Disorders and the Oral Cavity

Many systemic diseases have oral manifestations which often appear before the full-blown systemic condition; as such the oral cavity provides a unique diagnostic window. Jones and Mason[64] provide an excellent analysis of the oral manifestations of systemic diseases; what follows is a brief summary of the more important age-related diseases and disorders.

Osteoporosis

The mandible is largely composed of thick cortical plates and a thin sandwich of trabecular bone. Age-related bone loss in both the edentulous mandible[65] and long bones[66] consists of a thinning of the cortex rather than an increase in cortical porosity.

Generalized skeletal osteoporosis results in an increased incidence of hip, vertebral, and wrist fractures as the study population ages. Age-related loss of bone is a normal feature of advancing years, but this atrophy does not affect the skeleton uniformly at all sites.

Several groups of clinical investigators have suggested a relationship between severe mandibular atrophy of edentulous subjects and metabolic bone disease.[67,68] Cadaver studies have demonstrated relationships between the specific gravity of femoral bone and edentulous alveolar bone[69] and between the specific gravity of slices of edentulous mandible and the radius.[15] Clinical studies have used quantitative computed tomography and have shown significant relationships between the bone mineral density of the buccal (outer) mandibular cortex and that of the femur and lumbar spine.

Many radiographs are taken by dentists investigating patients' complaints unrelated to osteoporosis. It would be beneficial if radiographic investigations undertaken by a dental surgeon could provide a useful screening function, allowing referral of those suspected of osteoporosis to specialist centers for definitive investigation. Measurement of bone loss from the jaws is handicapped by the methodologic problems of obtaining accurate reproducible data. Routine radiographic diagnosis of bone loss is too insensitive since a reduction of less then 20 percent of bone calcium cannot be detected radiographically. The condition of the cortical part of the mandible is more predictive of the general bone status than that of the trabecular portion,[70] but measurement of mandibular cortical width has low sensitivity and specificity and cannot accurately predict osteoporosis risk.[71]

Diabetes Mellitus

In cross-sectional randomized surveys, the proportion of diabetics in the population increases with age. Surprisingly high numbers of patients with symptoms of altered taste, burning, dryness, or gingival tenderness have glucose intolerance. Unfortunately, the correlation of blood glucose levels with those of glucose in the saliva is poor. Some diabetics with xerostomia may have a measurable reduction in salivary flow, and others have no change in salivary flow rate. Despite one-third of patients, in one study, complaining of a dry mouth, none had alterations in salivary flow rate.[12] Changes in salivary flow rate may be due to increased urination, dehydration, or atherosclerosis of the salivary blood vessels; enlargement of the parotid gland (sialosis) is sometimes present. Diabetics have an increased incidence and severity of periodontal diseases, possibly because of gingival microangiopathy, altered polymorphonuclear leukocyte function, or an increased rate of collagen breakdown.

Iron Deficiency Anemia

Hypochromic anemia is a significant problem in elderly people. The oral mucosa has a yellowish pallor and may be associated with atrophy and aphthous ulceration, angular cheilitis, dysphagia, or candidiasis. In the tongue, atrophy of the filiform papillae occurs, followed by atrophy of the fungiform papillae. This produces the characteristic raw, red, painful tongue.

If the patient has an unsatisfactory dentition or dentures, they may choose easily masticated, poorly nutritious food, which can only exacerbate anemia (see later).

Benign Mucous Membrane Pemphigoid

Benign mucous membrane pemphigoid is a disease that principally affects those over 40 years of age. Subepidermal vesiculobullous blisters may appear on the oral cavity, conjunctiva, or skin and on the mucous membranes of the vagina, penis, anus, or pharynx. The oral blisters eventually rupture, leaving a raw, ulcerated surface.

Lichen Planus

Lichen planus has both oral and skin manifestations, with most patients in the 30 to 60-year age group. About three-quarters of patients with oral lichen planus are over the age of 50 years. Many different types of lesions have been described, but the most common (the reticular type) is characterized by a white lacework pattern on the buccal mucosa (Fig. 56-5).

Other variations in presentation are seen with the predominance of either papular, plaque, atrophic, or ulcerative lesions. The painful erosions of lichen planus are treated by local steroid application.

Drug-Induced Problems

The tongue undergoes changes in color or texture in a number of age-related disorders and also as a result of pharmacologic therapy, for example, antibiotic administration may result in elongation of the filiform papillae which become darkly stained, the so-called black hairy tongue.

A number of drugs (e.g., salicylates, corticosteroids, pancreatic enzymes, emepromium, tetracycline, clindamycin) can cause ulcerations of the oral mucosa, particularly if they are not swallowed immediately.[73] Oral herpes often occurs during immunosuppressive treatment; similarly, oral candidal infections during therapy with corticosteroids and antibiotics, as well as in a variety of compromising systemic conditions.

The dental complications of drug-induced decreased salivary secretion and consequent dry mouth include rampant dental caries (Fig. 56-6), loss of fillings, poorly fitting dentures,[74] oral ulcers, glossitis, stomatitis, acute parotitis, candida, and other mucosal infections. Dry mouth occurs during therapy with drugs with an anticholinergic effect, for example antihistamines, cyclic antidepressants (particularly amitriptyline, imipramine, and doxepin), high doses of neuroleptics, some opiates, and disopyramide.[75] Lithium also induces dry mouth and thirst, owing to its diuretic effect. Management of tricyclic-induced dry mouth may include dose reduction or substitution of a nonanticholinergic drug, for example, fluoxetine, as well as artificial salivary substitutes.[76]

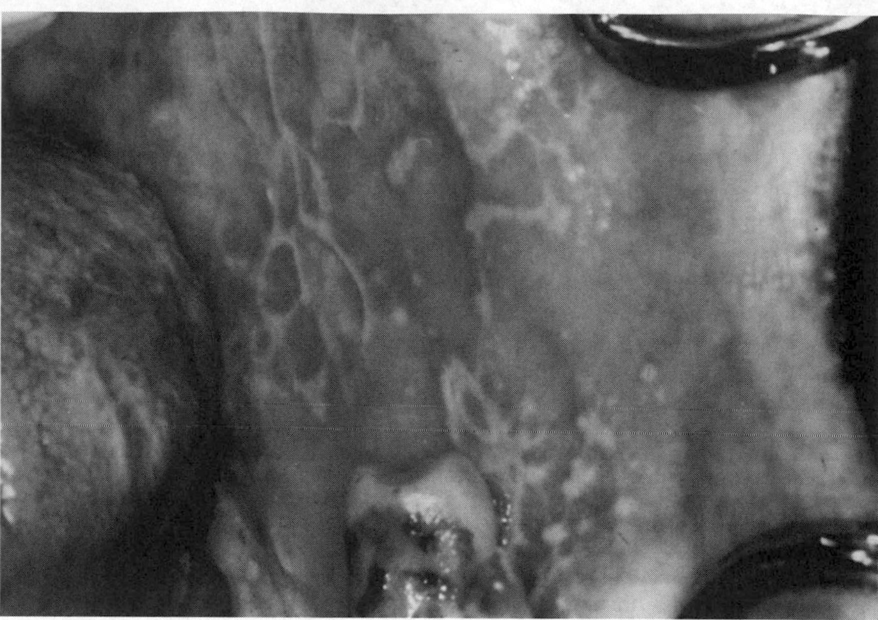

Figure 56-5 Typical reticulated pattern of nonerosive lichen planus on the inside of the cheek of an elderly patient.

Systemic diseases and therapies in the elderly may markedly affect the nature and type of dental treatment.[73–78]

Age-Related Diseases of the Oral Cavity

Surveys of elderly people have shown that a large percentage have some pathologic lesion present in their mouth, ranging in severity from localized inflammation, ulceration, and leukoplakia to carcinoma. Hoad-Reddick[79] examined 233 elderly subjects living in Cheshire, England, and found 41 percent of the sample had an oral pathologic lesion. The highest incidence of oral pathology was present in those living in the community with no assistance (over 60 percent). Medical practitioners and all those caring for the elderly must therefore be aware of the oral problems of older people and educate them to the value of regular oral examination.

Oral Cancer

The oral cavity is easily examined, and oral cancer can therefore be diagnosed early (Fig. 56-7). The prognosis for patients with oral cancer improves dramatically when the lesion is small and there is an absence of metastases to the lymph nodes in the neck. Unfortunately though, about half of patients with oral cancer will die from it. Oral cancer is often painless, has a variable clinical appearance, and can mimic

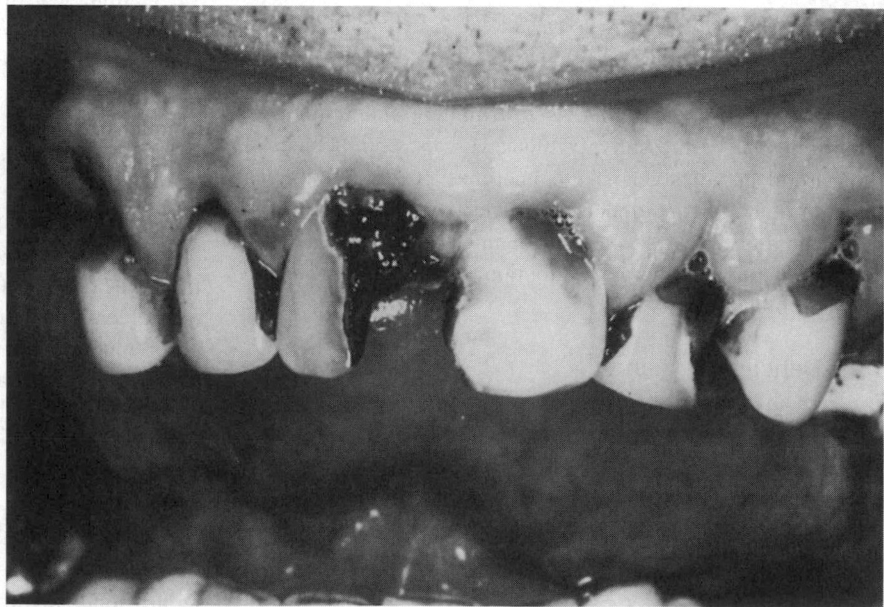

Figure 56-6 Advanced, rapidly destructive dental caries in an elderly person. This caries was almost certainly induced by the damaging effects of reduced salivary gland secretion as a result of oral tranquilizer use.

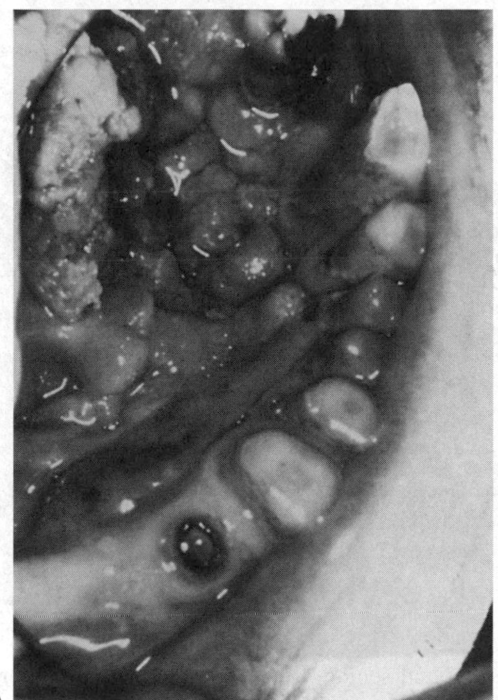

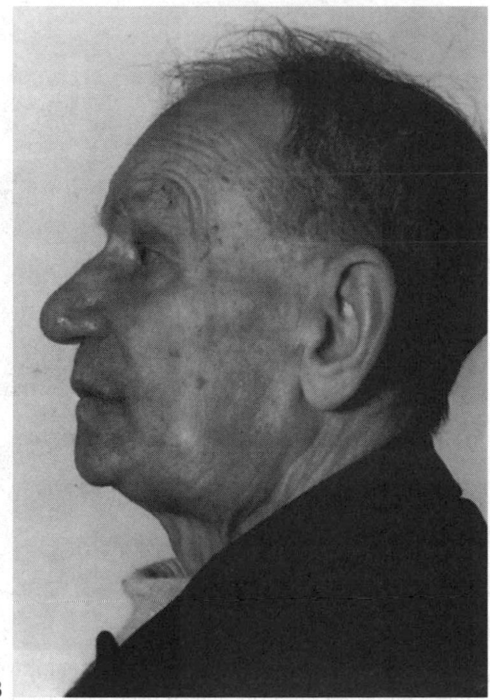

Figure 56-7 (A) Intraoral and (B) extraoral views of an advanced squamous cell carcinoma of the anterior floor of the mouth. Note the fungating appearance of the carcinoma in the intraoral view and the hard, fixed lump on the lower border of the mandible, visible in the external view.

denture trauma. Chronic lesions with associated induration or fixation to underlying tissue should be investigated urgently.

Squamous cell carcinoma is the most common oral malignant tumor; its incidence increases sharply with age, most cases occurring in the 60+ age group.[80] The lower lip is the most commonly affected site, the tumor manifesting in a variety of ways—large exophytic growth, deep ulcer, swelling of the vermilion border, crusty inconspicuous lesion.[80] An important feature of oral mucosal cancers is the induration palpable at the periphery of the tumor. After the lip, the tongue is the next most common site of cancer, with a variety of clinical manifestations: leukoplakia, exophytic growth, ulcer, asymptomatic; 75 percent arise on the lateral borders and inferior surface of the anterior two-thirds of the tongue; the highest incidence is in the sixth to eighth decades. Cancer of the buccal mucosa and floor of the mouth is common in the seventh decade, usually as an ulcerated lesion with raised and indurated margins near the frenum. All oral cancers are more frequent in men than in women, but the pattern is changing: in Manchester, United Kingdom, the male/female ratio decreased from 13:1 in 1932 to 1939 to 4:1 in 1960 to 1969, probably because of an increased consumption of cigarettes and alcohol by women.[81] Both smoking and alcohol consumption (and sunlight for lip cancer) are important risk factors, with a synergistic effect occurring between the two. Regular oral examination, every year or two, provides an efficient screening service for intraoral lesions and vastly improves the patient's prognosis. Both the incidence and mortality from oral cancer vary widely: for example, the 1985 male mortality per 100,000 population for oral cancer was 19.6 in France and 3.0 in the Netherlands.[82] Importantly, white (leukoplakia) or red (erythroplakia) patches in the mouth are important early signs and must be regarded as premalignant lesions until proven otherwise.

Treatment of oral cancer usually involves either surgery and/or radiotherapy. Surgical reconstruction techniques have been revolutionized by the use of titanium implants, which have done much to minimize aesthetic and functional defects.

Denture-associated Pathology

Denture stomatitis are inflammatory lesions of varying severity beneath upper dentures and may occur in up to 60 percent of elderly denture-wearing patients.[80] Causes include ill-fitting, dirty dentures, often with superimposed yeast, especially candida, infection. Treatment involves adjustment or replacement of the denture, instructing the patient to remove the denture at night and clean it, and, occasionally, fungistatic ointment applied to the denture.

Elderly denture wearers often develop painful lateral lip fissures (prevalence about 16 percent), which are frequently infected by *Candida albicans* and *Staphylococcus aureus* (Fig. 56-8). Predisposing factors include flaccid, sagging cheeks, deepened labial angles constantly moistened by saliva, and a decreased vertical dimension of occlusion.

Denture irritation hyperplasia manifests itself as folds and excesses of oral mucosa at the periphery of the dentures, which have usually been ill-fitting over a long period of time. Its incidence varies from 3 to 26 percent.[80,82]

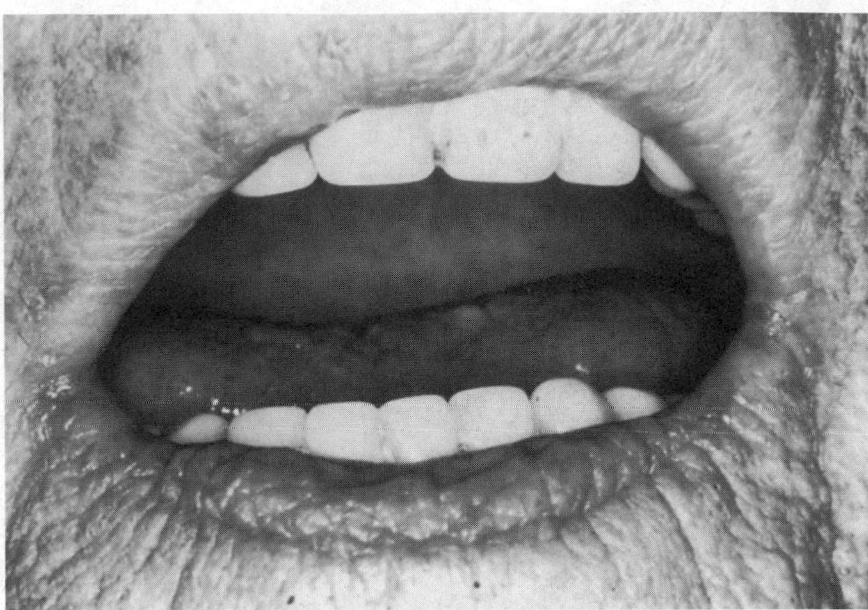

Figure 56-8 Angular cheilitis in an elderly patient. This condition is often associated with denture stomatitis, candida infection, and poorly fitting dentures.

In extensive surveys of the elderly, generally less than one-third of dentures examined have been considered acceptable by the examining clinicians.[72,83] Most have been worn for a considerable time without replacement—60 percent were at least 10 years old and a further 30 percent in excess of 20 years old.[84,85] It is generally accepted among dentists that dentures need regular checking and replacement every 5 to 10 years. Health professionals must communicate this message more clearly to patients.

Dental Health in the Elderly

Practical Oral Health Care

Numerous surveys have demonstrated that the main problems associated with aging are loss of teeth, periodontal disease, oral mucosal lesions,[86] and root surface caries.[87,88] Professionals from all branches of medicine, politicians, and the elderly people themselves all have a role to play in dental health promotion. Good oral hygiene, avoidance of a confectionary or a starchy diet, and regular visits to the dentist will improve dental health. Chlorhexidine rinses are recommended for confused and physically handicapped elderly people.[89] Rinsing with fluoride solutions may encourage remineralization of early carious lesions.[90] Fluoridation of the public water supply is inexpensive, does not require active cooperation from those who benefit, and at optimal levels has no harmful effects. Deaths from oral cancer could be reduced with regular oral examination of elderly people because diagnosis could be made while the lesions are small.

Epidemiology and Demography

The comparison of data and trends is often marred by numerous methodologic problems, but the best recent data set is from an extensive national survey of the oral health of U.S. employed adults and seniors from 1985 to 1986, which provides estimates of the prevalence of oral disease for approximately 150 million Americans.[91] These data show that in the employed population between 18 and 64 years of age, 37 percent had all their teeth, 49 percent had at most one tooth missing, and 4 percent were edentulous. By contrast, in the senior population (65 to 80+ years), 41 percent were edentulous and only 2 percent had all their teeth. However, the prevalence of edentulism at every age interval had dropped significantly from the previous survey 25 years ago (Fig. 56-9). This trend can be predicted to accelerate as the older (55+) cohort diminishes and younger ones fill their places—the "new elderly" (Fig. 57-9). The prevalence of coronal caries has dropped, but the number of root surface caries has increased. The percentage of persons with at least one carious or filled root

Figure 56-9 Percentage of edentulous individuals among the population of adult U.S. citizens. Two study periods are indicated: 1960 to 1962 (dotted line) and 1985 (solid line). Note the general improvement in edentulousness in this 23-year period. (From Oral Health of U.S. Adults.[91])

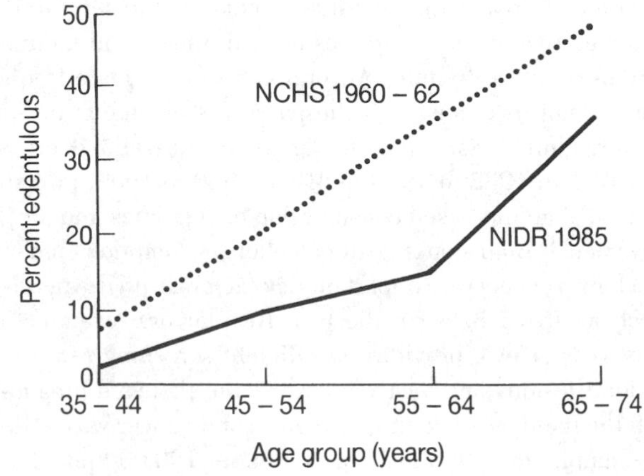

surface ranged from 7 percent in 20-year-olds to 67 percent of males and 61 percent of females in the senior population. Interestingly, 66 percent of these root lesions were unrestored in males but only 38 percent in females, who clearly had received more dental care. The incidence of root caries is decreased by using a fluoride-containing (1,100 ppm fluoride) toothpaste.[92]

Periodontal diseases were much more prevalent in the senior population, with about twice the prevalence of calculus (62 percent), gingival bleeding (53 percent), loss of gingival attachment (98 percent), deep pockets (22 percent), and gingival recession (88 percent). Similar high prevalences of periodontal diseases in the elderly British have also been reported.[83,85]

Regional variations are present, as in the United Kingdom where the percentage of elderly people with no natural teeth varies from 57 percent in the north of England to 33 percent in the south.[93] The presence of 20 or 21 teeth has been used as an oral health goal by the World Health Organization.[94] Even within a particular region, variations in the level of dental health correlate with income, social class, pattern of visits to the dentist, and degree of social independence of the elderly group.[95] Several subgroups (e.g., the mentally ill or extremely elderly) may have a yet higher dental treatment need.

Care of natural dentition is generally poor, with 98 percent of elderly dentate patients requiring some form of restorative treatment, 50 percent of elderly patients wearing their prostheses at night, and a gradual deterioration of oral hygiene with age. Moreover, when the last remaining tooth is lost, the proportion of the elderly who do not wear, or even possess, a denture may reach 25 percent.[86]

Elderly people have an increased incidence of illness but consult their medical practitioners less than might be expected.[96] Similarly, less than 20 percent of the elderly visit the dentist regularly, and over 30 percent have not visited a dentist for more than 20 years.[86] Moreover, although some surveys indicate a huge need for dental treatment in the elderly, other surveys recording self-assessment reveal a markedly low level of demand for dental care (e.g., 60 to 90 percent were satisfied with dentures that clinically were ranked unacceptable). One conclusion could be that old people accept the degeneration of oral tissues as part of the normal aging process and do not seek dental treatment, perhaps because of apathy or financial and logistical considerations and because dental treatment is perceived as irrelevant by a person of limited life expectancy. Denture usage decreases as patients' dependence on others increases, with those living at home leading more active lives and caring more about their appearance and eating ability than those in institutions.

The large differences between dentist-assessed and patient-perceived needs for dental care are of the utmost importance in planning geriatric dental health education and preventative or curative procedures.

The medical practitioner should be aware that dentures require regular assessment of their function and appearance. They should be inspected by a dental surgeon at least every 2 years. Successive surveys have shown that chronic trauma and poor denture hygiene account for an astonishing amount of oral pathology in the elderly. Nursing staff and dental hygienists can be invaluable in instructing and assisting with oral hygiene. For example, surprisingly few elderly patients realize that dentures should be removed, cleaned, and left in water overnight. In nursing homes, elderly patients' dentures can be mislaid or jumbled with others. Proprietary denture-marking kits are available to mark the patient's name on their surface. Other easy temporary methods are available for marking dentures for identification where no proprietary kit is available. For example, the patient's name can be written on the roughened denture surface in pencil and protected with clear nail varnish.

Barriers to Care: The Low Demand for Dental Services

Radical new approaches to the organization and delivery of dental care to elderly people (both in the community and in institutions) are being pioneered worldwide.[97] The implementation of such schemes is being expedited by financial and demographic changes, including a reduction in the birthrate and marked improvements in the dental health of children (thereby allowing diversion of labor and resources from children to old people), the increasing number of old people, and the emergence of the new elderly—better educated, healthier, and more demanding of dental services. These individuals will reach old age with more teeth at risk of dental decay, further straining government-funded dental services. From this emerging group of old people, large increases in demand for an increasingly wide range of complex dental restorative treatments (e.g., implants for tooth replacement, aesthetic procedures) are predicted.

Oral Disease and the Quality of Life

The aim of dental care is a healthy, functional dentition providing good aesthetics and speech. The established approach has been to restore as many teeth as possible and provide dentures routinely where extractions have been necessary. However, this treatment approach for elderly people has undergone re-examination recently because of the costs involved to patients and to the health care systems.[98] Anterior and premolar teeth are essential for speech and good aesthetics,[99] and restorative care should be concentrated on preserving these strategic parts of the dentition.[100] Elderly people can function satisfactorily with a reduced dentition consisting of 10 or fewer occluding teeth.[101]

There are important correlations between oral health and the psychological and social functioning of an elderly individual. Smith and Sheiham[102] reported that 40 percent of elderly individuals with inadequate dentition claimed that the length of time they took to eat a meal was a source of embarrassment to them, 32 percent reported oral discomfort, and 30 percent had difficulty chewing. In many cases, individuals were so concerned about their dental state that they avoided eating in company, which in turn led to social isolation and depression. These difficulties often cause dentally handicapped patients to avoid particular foods, many of which contain high levels of protein and vitamins.[103] Recent studies[103,104] indicate that, following dental treatment, 75 percent of elderly patients felt that they had benefited, with greatest improvements in self-image and social interaction. Recent surveys of the new elderly indicate a change of attitude, with a high percentage perceiving the loss of teeth and the provision of dentures as requiring high levels of psychosocial readjustment.[105] Unfortunatley, though, it is not always possible to restore the dentition to satisfactory levels of function. For example, gross bone resorption of the jaws, poor neuromuscular control, and a lack of displaceable tissue can limit an individual's ability to wear dentures.

Finally, when planning geriatric health care programs, the quality of life of elderly people could be improved with more attention to the present high levels of oral disease in this group.[106] Patients with oral disease may have signs indicating an underlying systemic disease. A team approach involving dental and medical specialists will therefore provide the best outcome for patients.

References

1. Drummond J, Newton J, Yemm R: Colour Atlas and text of Dental Care of the Elderly. Mosby-Wolfe, London, 1995
2. Longaker MT, Whitby DJ, Ferguson MW et al: Adult skin wounds in the fetal environment heal with scar formation. Ann Surg 1994;219:65–72
3. Irwin CR, Picardo M, Ellis I et al: Inter- and intra-site heterogeneity in the expression of fetal-like phenotypic characteristics by gingival fibroblasts: potential significance for wound healing. J Cell Sci 1994;107:1333–1346
4. Schor SL, Grey AM, Ellis I et al: Migration stimulating factor: its structural homology to the gelatin-binding domain of fibronectin, mode of action and possible function in health and disease. Symp Soc Exp Biol 1993;47:235–251
5. Bennick A: Structural and genetic aspects of proline rich proteins. J Dent Res 1987;66:457–461
6. Mehansho H, Butler LG, Carlsson DM: Dietary tannins and salivary proline-rich proteins: interaction, induction and defence mechanisms. Ann Rev Nutr 1987;7:423–440
7. Mjor IA: Age changes in the teeth. pp. 94–101. In Holm-Pedersen P, Loe H (eds): Geriatric Dentistry. Munksgaard, Copenhagen, 1986
8. Arends J: Enamel. pp. 47–62. In Reaction Patterns in Human Teeth. CRC Press, Boca Raton, FL, 1983
9. Fried K: Changes in innervation of dentine and pulp with age. pp. 63–84. In Ferguson DB (ed): The Aging Mouth. Karger, Basel, 1987
10. Nielsen CJ: Collagen changes in dental pulp. pp. 111–125. In Ferguson DB (ed): The Aging Mouth. Karger, Basel, 1987
11. Seversen JA, Moffett BC, Kokich V et al: A histological study of age changes in the adult human periodontal joint (ligament). J Periodontol 1987;49:189–200
12. MacKenzie IC, Holm Pedersen P. Karring T: Age changes in the oral mucous membranes and periodontium. pp. 102–113. In Holm-Pedersen P, Loe H (eds): Geriatric Dentistry. Munksgaard, Copenhagen, 1986
13. Shklar G: The effects of ageing upon oral mucosa. J Invest Dermatol 1986;47:115–120
14. Ferguson MWJ: The dentition through life. pp. 1–48. In Elderton RJ (ed): The Dentition and Dental Care. Heinneman, Oxford, 1990
15. Henrikson PA, Wallenius K: The mandible and osteoporosis. J Oral Rehabil 1974;1:67–74
16. Wowern NV, Stoltze J: Pattern of age-related bone loss in mandible. Scand J Dent Res 1978;88:134–146
17. Ow RKK, Loh T, Neo J, Khoo J: Symptoms of craniomandibular disorder among elderly people. J Oral Rehabil 1995;22: 413–419
18. Galan D, Odlum O, Grymoupre R, Brecx M: Medical and dental status of a culture in transition, the case of the Inuit elderly of Canada. Gerodontology 1993;10:44–50
19. Penreira FJ Jr, Lundh H, Westesson PL: Morphologic changes in the temporomandibular joint in different age groups: an autopsy investigation. Oral Surg, Oral Med, Oral Pathol 1994; 78:279–287
20. Ebner KA, Otis LL, Zakhary R, Danforth RA: Axial temporomandibular joint morphology: a correlative study of radiographic and gross anatomic findings. Oral Surg, Oral Med, Oral Pathol 1990;69:247–252
21. Newton JP, Abel KW, Robertson EM et al: Changes in human masseter and medial pterygoid muscle with age: a study using computed tomography. Gerodontics 1987;3:151–154
22. Yemm R, Newton JP, Lewis GR: Age changes in human muscle performance. pp. 17–25. In Lisney SJW, Matthews B (eds): Current Topics in Oral Biology. University of Bristol Press, Bristol, 1985
23. Fanous N: Ageing lips: aesthetic analysis and correction. Facial Plast Surg 1987;4:179–183
24. Gonzalez-Ulloa M: The Ageing Face. Williams & Wilkins, Baltimore, MD, 1987
25. Kydd WL, Daly CH: The biological and mechanical effects of stress on oral mucosa. J Prosthet Dent 1982;47:317–329
26. Pickett HG, Appleby RG, Osborn MO: Changes in denture supported tissues associated with ageing. J Prosthet Dent 1972;27:35–42
27. Corbet EF, Holmgren CJ, Phillipsen HP: Oral mucosal lesions in 65–74 year old Hong Kong Chinese. Community Dent Oral Epidemiol 1994;22:392–395
28. Grzegorczyk PB, Jones SW, Mistretta CM: Age related differences in salt taste acuity. J Gerontol 1979;34:834–840
29. Bartoshuk LM, Rifkin B, Marks LE et al: Taste and ageing. J Gerontol 1986;41:51–57
30. Weiffenbach JM: Taste perception mechanisms. pp. 151–167. In Ferguson DB (ed): The Ageing Mouth. Karger, Basel, 1987

31. Murphy C: Ageing and chemosensory perception. pp. 135–150. In Ferguson DB (ed): The Ageing Mouth. Karger, Basel, 1987

32. Belding JH, Tate WH: Evaluation of epithelial maturity in hormonally related stomatitis. J Oral Med 1978;33:17–19

33. Ettinger RL, Manderson RD: A clinical study of sublingual varices. Oral Surg 1974;40:540–545

34. Lamey PJ, Lewis MAO: Oral medicine in practice: burning mouth syndrome. Br Dent J 1989;167:197–200

35. MacKenzie IC: Epithelial connective tissue relationships and development and maintenance of structure. pp. 119–139. In Meyer J, Squier CA, Gerson SJ (eds): The Structure and Function of the Oral Mucosa. Pergamon Press, New York, 1984

36. Scott J, Valentine JA, Hill CA et al: A quantitative analysis of the effect of age and sex on human lingual epithelium. J Biol Bucal 1983;11:303–315

37. Loe H, Karring T: The three dimensional morphology of the epithelium-connective tissue interface of the gingiva as related to age and sex. Scand J Dent Res 1971;79:315–326

38. Lindhe J, Socransky S, Nyman S et al: Effect of age on healing following periodontal therapy. J Clin Periodontol 1985;12: 774–787

39. Ashcroft GS, Horan MA, Ferguson MW: The effects of ageing on cutaneous wound healing in mammals. J Anat 1995;187: 1–26

40. Mackenzie IC, Binnie WH: Recent advances in oral mucosal research. J Oral Pathol 1983;12:389–416

41. Rossa B: Quantitative changes in the elastic fibres of the human oral mucosa of the hard palate and cheek of various ages. Zahn Mund Kieferhalbid 1984;72:217–222

42. Bartold PM, Boyd RR, Page RC: Proteoglycans synthesized by gingival fibroblasts derived from human donors of different ages. J Cell Physiol 1986;126:37–46

43. Johnson BD, Page RC, Narayanen AS et al: Effects of donor age on protein and collagen synthesis in vitro by human diploid fibroblasts. Lab Invest 1986;55:490–496

44. Bayreuther K, Roredmann HP, Hommel R et al: Human skin fibroblasts in vitro differentiate along a terminal cell lineage. Proc Natl Acad Sci USA 1988;85:5112–5116

45. Otsuka K, Pitarn S, Overall CM et al: Biochemical comparison of fibroblast populations from different periodontal tissues: characterisation of matrix protein and collagenolytic enzyme synthesis. Biochem Cell Biol 1988;66:167–176

46. Somerman MJ, Archer SY, Imm GR et al: A comparative study of human periodontal ligament cells and gingival fibroblasts in vitro. J Dent Res 1988;67:66–70

47. Schor SL, Schor AM: Clonal heterogeneity in fibroblast phenotype: Implications for the control of epithelial-mesenchymal interactions. Bioassays 1988;7:200–204

48. Baum BJ: Saliva secretion and composition. pp. 126–134. In Ferguson DB (ed): The Ageing Mouth. Karger, Basel, 1987

49. Scott J: Structure and function in ageing human salivary glands. Gerodontology 1986;5:149–158

50. Scott J: Structural age changes in salivary glands. pp. 40–62. In Ferguson DB (ed): The Ageing Mouth. Karger, Basel, 1987

51. Drummond JR: Morphological changes in human salivary glands. pp. 31–39. In Ferguson DB (ed): The Ageing Mouth. Karger, Basel, 1987

52. Drummond JR, Chisholm DM: A qualitative and quantitative study of ageing human labial salivary glands. Arch Oral Biol 1984;29:151–155

53. Baum BJ: Salivary gland function during ageing. J Am Geriatr Soc 1989;37:453–458

54. Pederson W, Izutsu K, Schubert M: Age dependent decreases in human submandibular gland flow rates as measured under resting and post stimulation conditions. J Dent Res 1985;64: 822–825

55. Tylenda CA, Ship JA, Baum BJ: Evaluation of submandibular flow rate in different age groups. J Dent Res 1988;67: 1225–1228

56. Slomiany BL, Zolebska E, Murty VLN et al: Lipid composition of human labial salivary gland secretions. Arch Oral Biol 1981; 28:711–714

57. Gandara BK, Izutsu KT, Truelore EL et al: Age related salivary flow rate changes in controls and patients with oral lichen planus. J Dent Res 1985;64:1149–1151

58. Baum BJ, Kousrelari EE, Oppenheim FG: Exocrine protein secretion from human parotid glands during ageing; stable release of the acidic proline rich proteins. J Gerontol 1982; 37:392–395

59. Dagogo JS: Epidermal growth factor EGF in human saliva: effect of age, sex, race, pregnancy and sialogogue. Scand J Gastroenterol Suppl 1986;124:47–54

60. Fox PC, Heft MW, Herrerd M et al: Secretion of antimicrobial proteins from the parotid glands of different aged healthy persons. J Gerontol 1987;42:466–469

61. Kim SX: Protein synthesis in salivary glands as related to ageing. pp. 90–110. In Ferguson DB (ed): The Ageing Mouth. Karger, Basel, 1987

62. Smith DJ, Taubman MA, Ebersile JL: Ontogeny and senescence of salivary immunity. J Dent Res 1987;66:451–456

63. Wavazesh M: Xerostomia in the aged. Dent Clin North Am 1989;33:75–80

64. Jones JH, Mason DK: Oral manifestations of systemic disease. 2nd Ed. Bailliere Tindall, London, 1990.

65. Bras J, van Ooij CP, Abraham-Inpijn L et al: Radiographic interpretation of the mandibular angular cortex: a diagnostic tool in metabolic bone loss. I. normal state and postmenopausal osteoporosis. Oral Surg Oral Med Oral Pathol 1982;53: 541–545

66. Thompson DD: Age changes in bone mineralization, cortical thickness, and Haversian canal area. Calcif Tissue Int 1980; 31:5–11

67. Bays RA, Weinstein RS: Systemic bone disease in patients with mandibular atrophy. J Oral Surg 1982;40:270–272

68. Bras J, Ooij CPV, Duns JV et al: Mandibular atrophy and metabolic bone disease: a radiographic analysis of 126 edentulous patients. Int J Oral Surg 1983;12:309–313

69. Dyer MRY, Ball J: Alveolar crest recession in the edentulous. Br Dent J 1980;149:290–292

70. Klemetti E, Kolomakov S, Heiskanen P et al: Panoramic man-

dibular index and bone mineral densities in postmenopausal women. Oral Surg Oral Med Oral Pathol 1993;75:774–779

71. Klemetti E, Kolmakov S, Kroger H: Pantomography in assessment of the osteoporosis risk group. Scand J Dent Res 1994; 102:68–72
72. Stuck AE, Chappuis C, Flury H et al: Dental treatment needs in an elderly population referred to a geriatric hospital in Switzerland. Community Dent Oral Epidemiol 1989;17: 267–272
73. Molhulm-Hansem P, Kampmann D: Pharmacology and ageing pp. 195–204. In Holm-Pedersen P, Loe H (eds): Geriatric Dentistry. Munksgaard, Copenhagen, 1986
74. Kreher JM, Graser GN, Handelman SL: The relationship of drug use to denture function and saliva flow rate in a geriatric population. J Prosthet Dent 1987;57:631–638
75. Baker KA, Ettinger RL: Intra-oral effects of drugs in elderly persons. Gerodontics 1985;1:111–116
76. Borson S, Finkel SI: Essentials of geropsychiatry for the dental profession. pp. 205–217. In Holm-Pedersen P, Loe H (eds): Geriatric Dentistry. Munksgaard, Copenhagen, 1986
77. Irvine PW: Diseases in the elderly with implications for oral stratum and dental therapy. pp. 179–186. In Holm-Pedersen P, Loe H (eds): Geriatric Dentistry. Munksgaard, Copenhagen, 1986
78. Gottfries CG: Psychiatric disorders in old age. pp. 187–194. In Holm-Pedersen P, Loe H (eds) Geriatric dentistry. Munksgaard, Copenhagen, 1986
79. Hoad-Reddick GA: Oral pathology and prostheses—are they related? Investigation in an elderly population. J Oral Rehabil 1989;16:75–87
80. Pindborg JJ: Pathology and treatment of diseases in oral mucous membranes and salivary glands. pp. 290–306. In Holm-Pedersen P, Loe H (eds): Geriatric Dentistry. Munksgsaard, Copenhagen, 1986
81. Easson EC, Palmer MK: Prognostic factors in oral cancer. Clin Oncol 1976;2:191–202
82. Hamilton FA, Sarl DW, Grant AA et al: Dental care for elderly people by general dental practitioners. Br Dent J 1990;168: 108–112
83. Wilson GN, Salway DJ, McLaughlin EA: The dental needs and demands of an elderly population living in care in South Cumbria. Community Dent Health 1987;4:395–405
84. Farmer PE, Drummond JR, Yemm R: Dental state, dental needs and demands of an elderly population of residential homes in Tayside: a pilot study. J Dent Res 1986;65: 1151–1156
85. Hoad-Reddick GA, Grant AA, Griffiths C: Knowledge of dental service provided: investigations in an elderly population. Community Dent Oral Epidemiol 1987;15:137–140
86. Kandelman D, Bordear JM, Simard P et al: Dental needs of the elderly a comparison between some European and North American surveys. Community Dental Health 1986;3:19–39
87. Banting DW: Epidemiology of root caries. Gerodontology 1986;5:5–11
88. Wallace MC, Retief DH, Bradley EL: Prevalence of root caries in a population of older adults. Gerodontics 1988;4:84–89
89. de Baat C, Kalk W, Schuil GR: The effectiveness of oral hygiene for elderly people—a review. Gerodontology 1993;10: 109–113
90. Youngs G: Risk factors for and the prevention of root caries in older adults. Spec Care Dentist 1994;14:68–70
91. Oral Health of U.S. Adults: National Findings 1987. US Department of Health and Human Services, National Institutes of Health. NIH Publication 87–2868. U.S. Government Printing Office, Washington DC, 1987
92. Jensen ME, Kohout F: The effect of a fluoridated dentifrice on root and coronal caries in an older population. J Am Dent Assoc 1988;117:829–832
93. Steele JG, Walls AWG, Ayatollahi SMT, Murray JJ: Major clinical findings from a dental survey of elderly people in three different English communities. Br Dent J 1996;180:17–23
94. WHO: A Review of Current Recommendations for the Organisation and Administration of Community Oral Health Services in Northern and Western Europe. World Health Organization, Copenhagen, 1982
95. Hoad-Reddick GA, Grant AA, Griffiths C: Knowledge of dental service provided: investigations in an elderly population. Community Dent Oral Epidemiol 1987;15:137–140
96. Cartwright A, Smith C: In Conclusion. Elderly People, Their Medicines, and Their Doctors. Routledge, London, 1988 p. 140.
97. Holm-Pedersen P, Loe H (eds): Geriatric Dentistry. Munksgaard, Copenhagen, 1986
98. Kayser AF, Meeuwissen R, Meeuwissen JH: An occlusal concept for dentate geriatric patients. Community Dent Oral Epidemiol 1990;18:319
99. Kayser AF: The shortened dental arch: a therapeutic concept in reduced dentitions and certain high-risk groups. Int J Perio Rest Dent 1989;9:427–438
100. Kayser AF, Witter DJ: Oral functional needs and its consequences for dentulous older people. Community Dent Health 1985;2:285–291
101. Kayser AF: How much reduction of the dental arch is functionally acceptable for the ageing patient? Int Dent J 1990;40: 183–188
102. Smith JM, Sheiham A: How dental conditions handicap the elderly. Community Dent Oral Epidemiol 1979;7:305–310
103. Ettinger RL: Oral disease and its effect on the quality of life. Gerodontics 1987;3:103–106
104. Friske J, Gillier S, Watson RM: The benefit of dental care to an elderly population assessed using a sociodental measure of oral handicap. Br Dent J 1990;168:153–156
105. Bergendal B: The relative importance of tooth loss and denture wearing in Swedish adults. Community Dent Health 1989;6: 103–111
106. Beck JD, Hunt RJ: Oral Health status in the United States: problems of special patients. J Dent Educ 1985;49:407–426

CHAPTER 57

The Upper Gastrointestinal Tract

JOHN F. REINUS
LAWRENCE J. BRANDT

Symptoms of gastrointestinal disorders are frequently mentioned by older Americans during visits to the doctor, and the digestive diseases producing these symptoms are among the most common hospital discharge diagnoses for elderly patients in the United States.[1,2] As the elderly population expands and the demand by older individuals for medical care grows, it becomes increasingly important for physicians to be acquainted with the manifestation of diseases of the upper gastrointestinal tract in members of this age group.

The Oral Cavity

The most proximal of the digestive organs traditionally is considered to be the esophagus; patients with complaints thought to originate within the oral cavity or pharynx are referred to a dentist or a specialist in disorders of the ear, nose, and throat. The oral cavity, however, is examined easily by the general practitioner and may reveal the cause of unexplained or apparently unrelated abnormalities; thus evaluation of the upper gastrointestinal tract should begin with the mouth.

The Mouth and Nutrition

Changes in the oral cavity occasionally limit the ability of the elderly to eat and enjoy a normal diet. Problems with eating sometimes are severe enough to cause malnutrition and prompt a search for a wasting illness.[3,4]

A variety of abnormalities of oral structure and function may contribute to malnutrition. The muscles of mastication may become impaired during aging as the result of a decrease in (lean) body mass.[5] Eating occasionally becomes difficult because of tooth loss due to periodontal disease, poor dentition, or loosening of dentures caused by resorption of mandibular bone.[6]

A reduction in food intake by elderly individuals is sometimes related to a change in taste perception. The number of taste buds decreases after age 45, resulting in a decrease in taste sensation, especially the ability to appreciate salty and sweet foods.[7–10] Diminished perception of sour and bitter tastes is associated with palatal defects and typically occurs in patients who wear dentures. Taste sensation may also be altered directly by medications or indirectly affected by a drug's unpleasant flavor. Agents associated with abnormal taste perception (dysgeusia) include tricyclic antidepressants, sulfasalazine, clofibrate, L-dopa, gold salts, lithium, and metronidazole. Medications with anticholinergic properties interfere with taste by reducing salivary gland secretions and producing xerostomia. Age alone, however, is not associated with a reduction in stimulated saliva flow in nonmedicated subjects.[11]

While abnormal perception may lead to deficient nutrition, some primary nutritional disorders may be responsible for dysgeusia and glossitis. For example, vitamin B_{12} and niacin deficiency are associated with a "bald" or magenta-colored tongue, respectively. Taste sensation and eating habits also are disturbed by processes that interfere with the sense of smell.

Vascular Lesions

Diminutive vascular lesions of the upper gastrointestinal tract are poorly understood and rarely reported. The nomenclature for these lesions is confusing, and the terms *arteriovenous malformation, vascular ectasia, angiodysplasia*, and *telangiectasia* are usually used interchangeably with little regard as to their true meanings.

The lips are a frequent site of senescent vascular lesions resembling those of hereditary hemorrhagic telangiectasia (Osler-Weber-Rendu disease), and involvement often includes the upper gastrointestinal tract. In addition to this form of small vascular abnormality, patients often have sublingual varices, or "caviar lesions" (Fig. 57-1). The walls of these dilated vessels are thick, but the endothelial lining is hypoplastic.[12] In males, sublingual varices may be associated with the occurrence of capillary phlebectasias, or Fordyce lesions, of the scrotal skin (Fig. 57-2).

Because vascular abnormalities are often responsible for cryptogenic gastrointestinal bleeding, their presence in the mouth should suggest that similar lesions elsewhere in the gastrointestinal tract may be responsible for blood loss in such cases.[13] Not every individual, however, with bleeding vascular lesions of the gastrointestinal tract has involvement of oral structures, and the presence of oral lesions does not preclude existence of an unrelated distal bleeding lesion.

The Oral Mucosa

A number of abnormalities of the oral mucosa are encountered in elderly patients. These changes may be the result of medical therapy, signify the presence of a systemic disease, or represent premalignant changes.

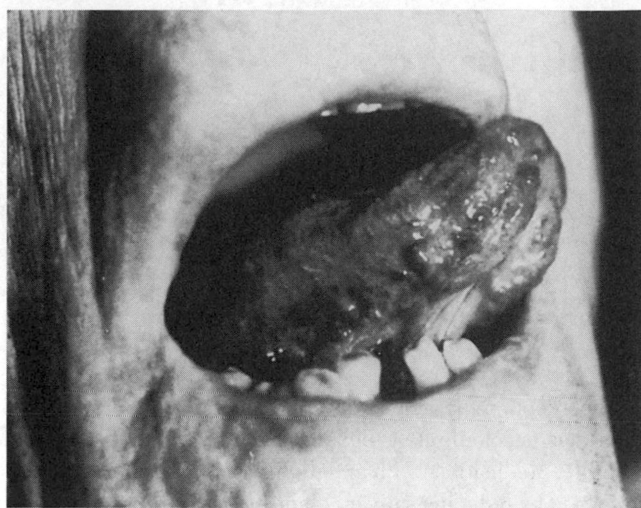

Figure 57-1 Caviar lesion (sublingual varices) in a patient with occult upper gastrointestinal bleeding. (From Brandt,[154] with permission.)

Candidiasis

Candidiasis is usually caused by the fungus *Candida albicans*. This organism is part of the normal gastrointestinal flora, and its presence is not sufficient by itself to produce disease. Mucosal candidiasis occurs only after a change in other constituents of the normal flora or in the presence of an immunologic abnormality. In elderly patients, the widespread use of antibiotics and immunosuppressive chemotherapy for malignancies is most often responsible for the development of mucosal candidiasis.

The typical oral lesions of candidiasis are soft, white plaques which resemble cottage cheese. Characteristically, these plaques can be peeled from the mucosa, leaving the underlying surface raw and bleeding. This observation is important because most other white, plaquelike lesions, for example, leukoplakia, cannot be stripped off of the mucosa.

A diagnosis of candidiasis is made by smearing scrapings of the lesion on a glass slide, macerating them with 20 percent potassium hydroxide, and examining this preparation under a microscope for the presence of typical hyphae. A definitive diagnosis can be made by culture on selected media.

Therapy usually consists of re-establishing the normal microbiologic flora by discontinuing antibiotics. In the immunocompromised host and the individual with significant morbidity, topical therapy with nystatin suspensions or troches is usually successful, although treatment with absorbable oral agents may be required. Antifungal agents may be supplemented by the use of topical anesthetics to provide symptomatic relief (see below).

Stomatitis

Cancer patients treated with radiation or chemotherapy frequently develop painful inflammation and erosions of the oropharyngeal mucosa. Stomatitis complicating cancer therapy is the direct consequence of drug and radiation toxicity to susceptible, rapidly dividing cell populations of the upper gastrointestinal tract and the indirect consequence of neutropenia, which impairs regeneration of injured tissues. Radiation to the head and neck also causes xerostomia secondary to fibrosis of the salivary glands. An absence of lubrication by saliva further aggravates mucosal damage, and a lack of salivary IgA permits overgrowth of bacteria and fungi. Oral lesions may become infected, contributing to persistent injury, discomfort, and poor nutrition and posing a risk of more widespread infection in immunocompromised individuals.

The initial therapy for stomatitis is promotion of good oral hygiene. Brushing and flossing are contraindicated in neutro-

Figure 57-2 Phlebectasias in the scrotum of the same patient as in Figure 57-1. (From Brandt,[154] with permission.)

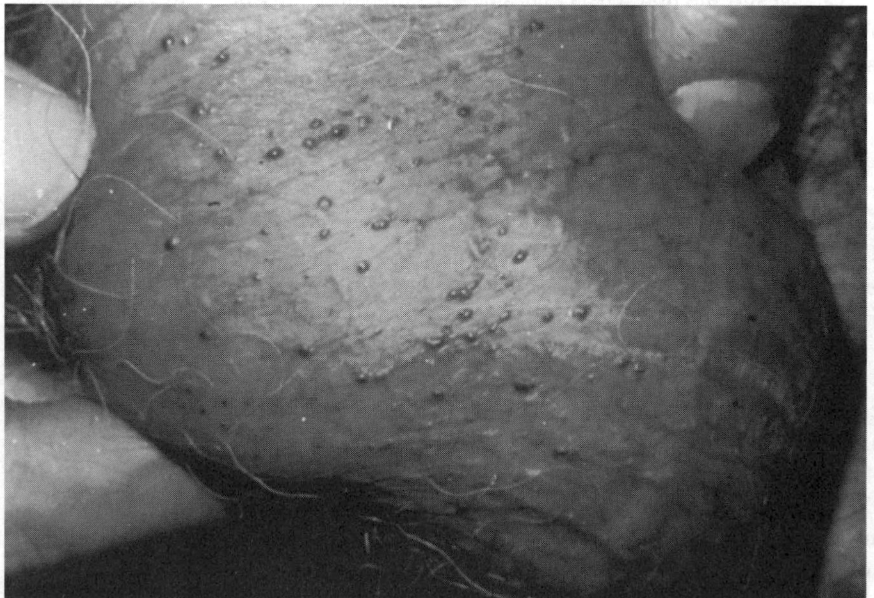

penic patients because of the risk of disseminated infection. Instead, mouthwashes containing dilute hydrogen peroxide or a salt and soda solution are used to reduce mucosal bacterial and fungal colonization.

A number of therapeutic mouthwash "cocktails" have been recommended to relieve symptoms, promote healing, and treat superficial mucosal infection in patients with stomatitis.[14,15] Some of these cocktails have been tested in controlled trials, but the use of most is empirical, based on the known analgesic, antibiotic, and protective effects of widely available liquid medicines. Viscous lidocaine (2 percent) is frequently used as a topical anesthetic, as is diphenhydramine, which is often mixed with Maalox, Mylanta, or kaolin-pectin. Many recipes include sucralfate suspension because it coats damaged epithelium and promotes the production of mucus and protective prostaglandins.[15] Antibiotics used alone or in combination in mouthwash cocktails to treat superficial infection include chlorhexidine gluconate, nystatin, tetracycline, neomycin, vancomycin, and clindamycin. Hydrocortisone and other glucocorticoids also have been added to reduce inflammation, but rapid absorption across the denuded oral mucosa into the systemic circulation may compromise the patient's immune defenses. Artificial saliva replacements (Salivart, Moi-Stir, Xero-Lube) are also available for patients with xerostomia.

"Hairy tongue"

"Hairy tongue" is characterized by hypertrophy of the filiform papillae of the tongue and a lack of normal desquamation. In this condition, the color of the tongue varies from yellow to brown or black, depending on staining by exogenous substances such as tobacco or food and on the presence of various chromogenic microorganisms. Hairy tongue is frequently seen in patients who have had extensive radiotherapy to the head and neck. While these individuals are usually asymptomatic, some complain of nausea, dysgeusia, and halitosis. On occasion, the lingual papillae reach such considerable length that they brush against the soft palate, gagging the patient.

Many organisms have been cultured from papillary scrapings from this entity; there is, however, no proof of a cause-and-effect relationship with any microorganism, and invasion of the lingual epithelium has not been demonstrated. Species of microorganisms that have been isolated are, in all probability, simply colonizing an already abnormal, excessively papillated tongue.

Therapy for this disorder consists of vigorous brushing of the tongue to promote desquamation and to remove accumulated debris. In extreme cases, topical treatment with podophyllin, an alcoholic extract of the mayapple, may result in a dramatic response.

Leukoplakia

The term *leukoplakia* was introduced by Schwimmer in 1877 to describe any white plaque. Today, some authors use this term to refer to histologic zones of hyperkeratosis, acanthosis, and chronic inflammation, while others reserve it to describe malignant dyskeratosis and epithelial atypia. Although leukoplakia is considered by many clinicians to be a premalignant condition, its natural history is uncertain because of a lack of uniform definition in case selection. The term should be abandoned because of its lack of specificity. Any persistent white lesion of the oral mucosa should be biopsied in an attempt to make a specific histologic diagnosis.

Leukoplakia is more common in men than in women, and most often occurs during the sixth and seventh decades.[16] It can be found anywhere in the oral cavity, although it is most common on the buccal mucosa, tongue, and floor of the mouth. Leukoplakia varies in appearance, partly depending on the age of the lesion. Some investigators consider verrucous patches to be of higher malignant potential than smooth plaques, whereas others believe that granular pinkish-gray to red islands, also called erythroplakia, are most likely to be associated with carcinoma in situ or even invasive malignancy. Such controversy stresses the importance of biopsy in the management of all such lesions. Approximately 10 percent of patients with leukoplakia have or will develop invasive carcinoma in the lesion.[16–18]

Once the diagnosis of leukoplakia has been substantiated by microscopic examination of a biopsy specimen, therapy is initiated. When dysplasia is present, or when the lesion fails to resolve after a source of physicochemical trauma has been eliminated, treatment consists of ablation.

Epidermoid Carcinoma

Approximately 5 percent of human cancers arise in the mouth; 95 percent of oral malignancies are epidermoid carcinomas.[19] The lower lip is the most common site of malignancy in the area of the oral cavity. Epidermoid carcinoma of the lip occurs almost exclusively in elderly men; etiologic factors include actinic radiation, syphilis, and tobacco use, especially pipe smoking.

Carcinoma of the lip varies in clinical appearance and may be bulky or ulcerated. It metastasizes slowly, usually to the ipsilateral submental or submaxillary lymph nodes. Surgical resection or radiation therapy produces equally good results, with cures in approximately 80 percent of affected individuals. Successful treatment depends on the duration of symptoms, size of lesion, and presence of metastases.

Within the oral cavity, one-half of epidermoid carcinomas originate in the tongue, and the rest arise with equal frequency in the palate, buccal mucosa, floor of the mouth, and gingiva. The disease is seen mainly in older individuals and occurs most often in males. Factors suspected of contributing to the development of oral cancer include tobacco, alcohol, nutritional deficiencies, syphilis, and miscellaneous forms of physicochemical trauma, such as irritation from pipe stems and dentures.[20] Almost 90 percent of patients have a combination of predisposing factors.

Intraoral epidermoid carcinomas display a considerable amount of histologic variation, although lesions tend to be moderately well differentiated. Early carcinomas arising in the tongue typically are painless, even though they may ulcerate.

Pain develops later, as the lesions grow, especially if they become secondarily infected. Tumors are usually located on the lateral or ventral surface of the tongue. The site of the primary lesion is of prognostic importance because cancers of the posterior aspect of the tongue tend to be more malignant. Nodal metastases are located on either or both sides of the neck. Tumors also spread by direct invasion. Early detection is mandatory if patients are to survive more than a year after diagnosis.

Keratoacanthoma is a spontaneously resolving benign lesion often mistaken for epidermoid carcinoma. It occurs most frequently in adults 50 to 70 years of age, involves the upper and lower lips equally, and usually presents as a painful umbilicated lesion seldom more than 1 to 1.5 cm in diameter. It initially appears as a small nodule which reaches full size within 4 to 8 weeks. It persists as a static lesion for another 4 to 8 weeks, after which the keratin core is expelled and the mass resorbed over a period of 6 to 8 weeks. Recurrence is rare.

The Oropharynx

The oropharyngeal phase of swallowing is exceedingly complex, requiring the participation of multiple distinct structures in the mouth, pharynx, and esophagus coordinated by six cranial nerves and orchestrated by the swallowing center of the central nervous system. After food has been masticated and moistened with saliva, the tongue initiates swallowing by thrusting the food bolus into the oropharynx. The soft palate prepares for the arrival of the bolus by elevating, so that material from the mouth cannot enter the nasal passages. The glottis also shuts, and the epiglottis tilts downward to prevent the bolus from entering the trachea. Relaxation of the upper esophageal sphincter in association with contraction of the pharyngeal muscles allows propulsion of food into the esophagus.[21]

Striated muscle involved in the oropharyngeal phase of swallowing, like the muscles of mastication, may be impaired during aging by a decrease in lean body mass. A radiographic study of 100 individuals beyond the age of 65 suggested that 22 had pharyngeal muscle weakness as well as abnormal cricopharyngeal relaxation with pooling of barium in the valleculae and pyriform sinuses.[22] Several individuals also were noted to have tracheal aspiration of barium. All the subjects, however, were asymptomatic. Thus, although functional changes in the oropharyngeal phase of swallowing may occur with aging, these changes have not been identified as a cause of morbidity in the elderly.

Oropharyngeal Dysphagia

Patients with oropharyngeal (cervical or "transfer") dysphagia complain of difficulty shifting food from the front of the mouth into the back of the throat, or of trouble initiating a swallow once the food bolus has been positioned in the oropharynx. Symptoms may be most severe when the patient attempts to swallow liquids. Signs of transfer dysphagia include nasal regurgitation or aspiration of oral contents during swallowing as a result of a failure to seal the nasopharynx or the trachea by appropriate muscle contraction. Inasmuch as oropharyngeal dysphagia may be due to a neuromuscular disorder, the patient may display other signs of neuromuscular dysfunction including dysarthria, nasal speech, cranial nerve dysfunction, weakness, or sensory abnormalities.[23]

> ***Causes of oropharyngeal dysphagia in the elderly***
>
> Malignancy—pharyngeal carcinoma
> Central nervous system disease—tumor, Parkinson's disease, stroke
> Peripheral nervous system disease—diabetes mellitus
> Muscle disease—hypothyroidism
> Mechanical—strictures, osteophytes, thyromegaly
> Postoperative—laryngectomy
> Medication
> Motility disorders of the upper esophageal sphincter

A variety of conditions interfere with the transfer of food from the mouth to the esophagus.[24] Mechanical lesions, including tumors, abscesses, and strictures, may block passage of the food bolus or disrupt structures that directly mediate the oropharyngeal phase of swallowing. A neoplasm, infection, or cerebrovascular accident may damage the central nervous system, producing brain stem or pseudobulbar palsy and associated transfer dysphagia. The initiation of swallowing also may be impaired by degenerative diseases of the central or peripheral nervous system, the motor end plate, or the muscle itself. Finally, oropharyngeal dysphagia is often caused by a failure of upper esophageal sphincter function. Many of these problems are encountered in older individuals.

Cricopharyngeal achalasia

The term *cricopharyngeal achalasia*, partly derived from the Greek word meaning "absence of slackening," is a misnomer, as the cricopharyngeus muscle of patients with this disorder is capable of relaxing. The problem in circopharyngeal achalasia is failure of the muscle to function in synchrony with other elements of the swallowing mechanism. As a result, the pharyngeal muscles propel all or part of the food bolus against a closed sphincter, producing symptoms of cervical dysphagia.

Cricopharyngeal achalasia is usually encountered in elderly individuals. Many disorders may cause this problem, but central nervous system diseases predominate. The clinical features are those of oropharyngeal dysphagia in general. Depending on the cause, the onset of symptoms may be sudden, as with a cerebrovascular accident, or intermittent, as with more insidious disorders such as diabetic neuropathy. The natural history of cricopharyngeal achalasia is also variable, again probably reflecting its many causes: dysphagia may diminish, remain unremitting, or follow a relapsing, remitting course. Most individuals with this disorder have more difficulty swallowing liquids than solids. Many patients have a pulmonary presentation with laryngitis, bronchitis, recurrent pneumonia, bronchiectosis, and pulmonary abscesses as the sequelae of otherwise quiet cricopharyngeal dysfunction.[23] In some patients, symptoms result in such a fear of eating that weight loss, malnutrition, and psychological problems overshadow the motility disorder.

Postintubation dysphagia

Special mention must be made of cervical dysphagia occurring as a sequela of endotracheal intubation. Unilateral vocal cord weakness is a common complication of endotracheal intubation and, because the vocal cords are important to the formation of a tight laryngeal seal during the oropharyngeal phase of glutition, patients with vocal cord weakness may experience coughing and aspiration with swallowing. Individuals who have undergone a tracheostomy also may develop symptoms of oropharyngeal dysphagia. Scar formation from a tracheostomy occasionally prevents normal elevation and anterior rotation of the larynx, causing decreased pharyngeal contraction and incomplete upper esophageal sphincter relaxation during swallowing.

Management of oropharyngeal dysphagia depends only in part on its etiology. Any underlying disorder, such as Parkinsonism, should be treated. If dysphagia persists despite such therapy, or if significant complications result from impairment of the swallowing mechanism, treatment can be directed at the esophagus itself.

Bougienage of the upper esophageal sphincter with mercury-weighted rubber dilators is beneficial to some patients but often gives only temporary relief. This technique is contraindicated by the presence of a pharyngoesophageal diverticulum because of the high risk of perforation (see below).

Many individuals with cricopharyngeal achalasia benefit from surgical interruption of the upper esophageal sphincter.[26] Failure to respond is observed most often in patients with central nervous system disease or peripheral neuropathy, although even these individuals are occasionally relieved of symptoms by this procedure. Serious complications following cervical myotomy are rare. Gastroesophageal reflux or severe distal esophagitis indicating reflux is an absolute contraindication to cricopharyngeal myotomy unless the lower esophageal defect is corrected first.

Pharyngeal Diverticula

Zenker's diverticulum

Zenker's diverticulum (Fig. 57-3) is a posterior herniation of the hypopharynx through the triangular area just above the upper esophageal sphincter where the oblique and transverse fibers of the cricopharyngius muscle join. It is seen once in every 1,000 routine upper gastrointestinal series and is more frequent in males. Approximately 85 percent of cases occur in individuals over the age of 50.[27]

Symptoms of Zenker's diverticulum usually develop insidiously. An annoying irritation in the back of the throat is an early complaint which may be followed later by the more classic symptoms of oropharyngeal dysphagia. Occasionally, an affected individual complains of a noise like the "roar of the ocean" or a "washing machine" during swallowing. Postcibal and nocturnal regurgitation of undigested food are common complaints. Obstructive symptoms may be caused by associated cricopharyngeal achalasia or, rarely, by compression of the esophagus by a large diverticulum.

Incoordination and incomplete relaxation of the upper

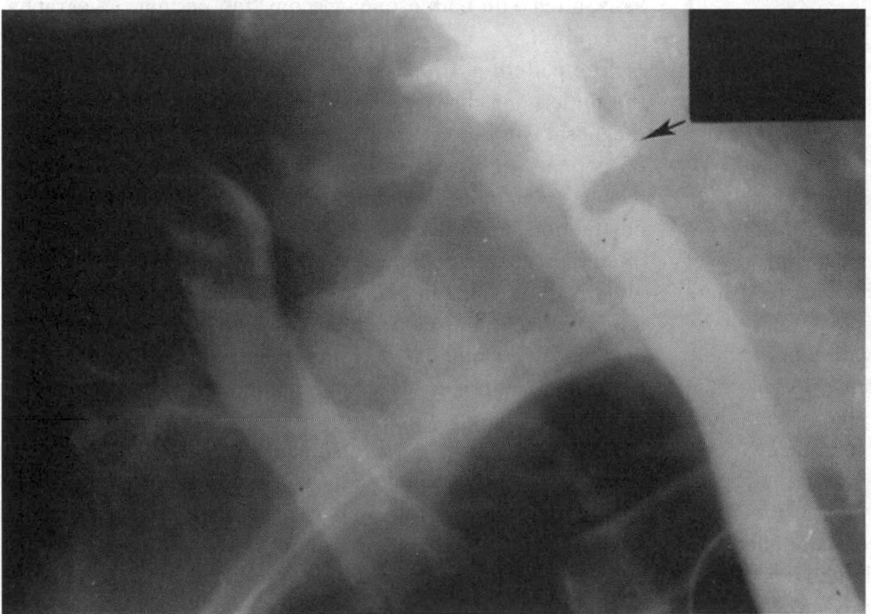

Figure 57-3 Oblique view of a barium-filled esophagus showing a small Zenker's diverticulum (arrow) proximal to a hypertrophied cricopharyngeus. (From Brandt,[154] with permission.)

esophageal sphincter during swallowing have been described in association with Zenker's diverticulum, lending support to the theory that circopharyngeal dysfunction leads to high pharyngeal pressures which result in the formation of hypopharyngeal diverticula. Many patients with a Zenker's diverticulum, however, have normal function of the upper esophageal sphincter or even reduced upper esophageal sphincter pressure, suggesting that high pharyngeal pressures may be due to stiffening of the pharyngeal muscles with loss of compliance.[28]

Zenker's diverticula most often are seen during x-ray examination but when small may be missed in the posteroanterior view because of superimposition over the main column of barium in the esophagus; this problem can be avoided by rotating the patient during the study (Fig. 57-3). Endoscopic examination of the upper gastrointestinal tract in the presence of a hypopharyngeal diverticulum may be associated with an increased risk of perforation; however, this danger is minimized by passage of the instrument under direct vision.

Complications include compression and obstruction of the distal esophagus by a large diverticulum, respiratory difficulties caused by aspiration of diverticular contents, and diverticulitis with perforation. Rarely, carcinoma may develop in a Zenker's diverticulum.[29] Worsening of dysphagia, weight loss, and the appearance of blood in regurgitated material suggest the development of a malignant neoplasm.

The therapy for a symptomatic Zenker's diverticulum includes surgical excision alone or cricopharyngeal myotomy with or without removal of the diverticulum.[30,31]

Lateral pharyngeal diverticula

Lateral pharyngeal diverticula, or pharyngoceles, occur with increased frequency in the elderly and are especially common in men.[32] They develop in the gap between the superior and middle pharyngeal constrictors. Symptoms are the same as those of a Zenker's diverticulum. In addition, patients may complain of a neck mass that enlarges with a Valsalva maneuver. Increased intrapharyngeal pressure may be an important etiologic factor, as exemplified by the frequency of this entity in muezzins and wind instrument players. Surgical repair is safe and effective.

The Esophagus

The muscularis propria of the esophagus is composed of striated muscle fibers proximally and smooth muscle fibers distally. The central nervous system governs the activity of the striated muscle by means of sequential activation of extrinsic nerves. In humans, the dominant mechanism for control of the smooth muscle of the esophagus is unknown; both central and intramural neural pathways have been demonstrated. Orderly peristaltic contractions of esophageal muscle are necessary for normal esophageal function.

Although no information is available about the effects of aging on the regulation of esophageal muscle activity, alterations in esophageal muscle function have been identified manometrically in elderly individuals. These changes were described first in 1964 by Soergel and colleagues,[33] who referred to motility disturbances in the elderly as "presbyesophagus." Soergel and his coworkers studied 15 subjects beyond the age of 90 and found a variety of abnormalities; 13 of their patients, however, had diseases known to affect esophageal motility. Subsequent studies have confirmed that, in the absence of other disorders, esophageal motility may be abnormal in elderly individuals, but the only manometric change identified in all the published work is a reduction in the amplitude of muscle contraction after a swallow.[34–36]

The elderly also may be noted to have disordered motility, or "tertiary contractions," during a barium esophagram, but this finding is rarely associated with symptoms.[37] Because motility changes that develop with aging do not appear to have clinical importance, the diagnosis of presbyesophagus should be abandoned. Elderly patients with dysphagia should be evaluated for the presence of disease processes involving the esophagus, and complaints should not be ascribed to motility changes occurring as a result of age alone.

Dysphagia and Heartburn

Dysphagia and heartburn (pyrosis) are the principal symptoms of esophageal diseases; patients with esophageal disorders, especially the elderly, also may complain of respiratory difficulties, painful swallowing (odynophagia), chest pain resembling the pain of myocardial ischemia, regurgitation, and vomiting.[38–40]

Dysphagia is caused by impaired passage of food through the esophagus and is experienced immediately after the act of deglutition. Patients often complain that food "sticks on the way down." Since sensation in the esophagus is referred proximally, lesions at the gastroesophageal junction often appear as symptoms experienced at the level of the sternal notch. When a patient has symptoms apparently originating in the area of the proximal esophagus, evaluation of the entire esophagus, often with both esophagoscopy and barium radiography, is required.

The pattern of dysphagia frequently suggests the nature of the underlying disease.[41] Schatzki[42] observed that a correct diagnosis can be made after taking a careful history in up to 85 percent of patients with this complaint. Thus, intermittent dysphagia connotes a motility disorder or a pliant mechanical obstruction such as an esophageal web. Progressive dysphagia often represents a neoplasm. Individuals who experience difficulty in swallowing liquids as well as solid foods usually have a primary neuromuscular abnormality and disordered esophageal motility, while dysphagia produced only by solid foods is associated with mechanical obstruction of the esophagus.

Heartburn is a manifestation of the reflux of gastric contents into the esophagus and, as its name suggests, is described as being a hot sensation behind the sternum or in the left parasternal area. Pyrosis is relieved by antacids and intensified by bending at the waist or lying supine, especially when the stomach is full. Pyrosis also may be aggravated by some medications, smoking, and ingestion of alcohol, fruit juices, caffeine, chocolate, or peppermint. Discomfort is often accompanied by regurgitation of gastric contents, belching, vomiting, or secretion of saliva (water brash). The nature or extent of esophageal abnormalities associated with gastroesophageal reflux and heartburn cannot be predicted on the basis of the intensity of symptoms, especially in the elderly; severe reflux disease as evidenced by esophageal ulcers may be present in the absence of substantial symptoms.[43]

Esophageal Motility Disorders

After individuals with structural lesions have been excluded, over 50 percent of adults of all ages with a complaint of dysphagia are found to have esophageal motility disorders.[44,45] These abnormalities may be primary or secondary and are classified according to their manometric signatures. Most often, adults with dysphagia have disordered motility with nonspecific and inconsistent manometric features.

Nonspecific secondary motility disorders

In the elderly, nonspecific disorders of esophageal motility frequently are secondary to a systemic disease. Examples of generalized disorders sometimes responsible for esophageal dysmotility are myxedema, amyloidosis, connective tissue diseases, and diabetes mellitus.

Approximately 50 percent of patients with diabetic neuropathy have abnormal esophageal motility. Findings in these individuals include a decrease in the amplitude of muscle contraction, delayed esophageal emptying, esophageal dilation, and reduced lower esophageal emptying sphincter pressure. In patients with diabetes, the severity of motility changes correlates with the severity of other neuropathic complications; however, affected individuals usually do not have significant dysphagia. For this reason, esophageal symptoms in a diabetic must be fully evaluated and not simply attributed to diabetes.

Primary and secondary achalasia

Primary achalasia is the second most common motility disorder diagnosed in patients with nonstructural dysphagia, but it is rare in the elderly.[46] In persons beyond the age of 50, achalasia is most often secondary to gastric adenocarcinoma (Fig. 57-4); pancreatic adenocarcinoma, oat cell carcinoma, reticulum cell sarcoma, and anaplastic lymphoma are responsible for isolated cases.[47,48] Manometric findings in secondary achalasia are identical to those in the primary disorder: absence of esophageal peristalsis, usually in association with elevation of resting lower esophageal sphincter pressure and failure of the lower esophageal sphincter to relax following an appropriate stimulus. The elevation of resting lower esophageal sphincter pressure typical of achalasia is less pronounced in the elderly, who also experience less chest pain in association with this disorder than do younger patients.[49]

Patients with both primary and secondary achalasia may experience progressive difficulty in swallowing.[50] Food collects in the esophagus, which may become distended and tortuous even when the patient has an underlying carcinoma. In the absence of proximal dilation of the esophagus, a diagnosis of malignancy is favored. When the patient reclines, pooled food flows out of the esophagus back into the pharynx, resulting in coughing and aspiration. Affected individuals, therefore, may present with aspiration pneumonia. In addition to an infiltrate, a chest x-ray may reveal an air-fluid level in the esophagus and absence of the gastric air bubble. Because the presentations of primary and secondary achalasia may be identical, malignancy must be excluded in an elderly patient with this syndrome. Computed tomographic x-rays of the chest and upper abdomen, as well as endoscopy with biopsy of the distal esophagus, are recommended. Endoscopic ultrasound may be helpful in differentiating primary from secondary achalasia.

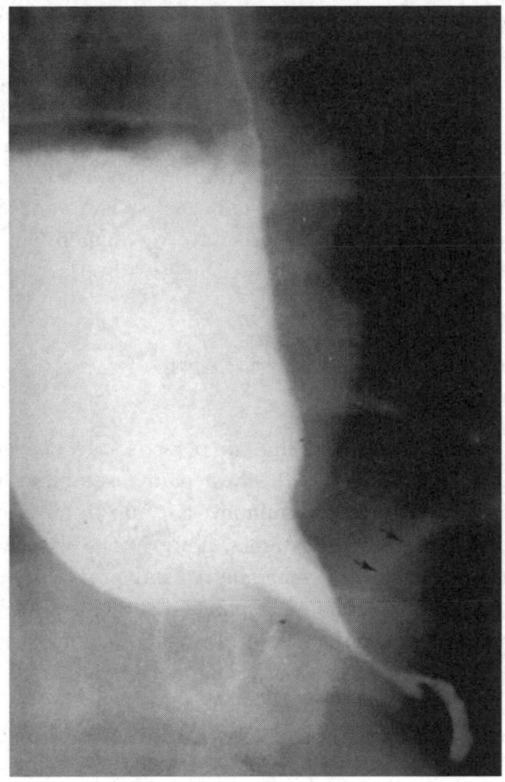

Figure 57-4 Barium esophagram showing tapering of the distal esophagus simulating achalasia. The subtle presence of a mass in the gastric fundus (arrows) suggested a diagnosis of carcinoma. (From Brandt,[154] with permission.)

The pathogenesis of secondary achalasia is unknown. Submucosal infiltration of the distal esophagus by tumor has been noted in some cases and normal histology in others.[51] It is possible that, in the absence of tumor infiltration, the motility disorder reflects a paraneoplastic neuropathy; manometric and roentgenographic abnormalities may disappear after resection of a gastric carcinoma or therapy for a lymphoma.[52,53]

Diffuse esophageal spasm

Although primary esophageal motility disorders usually occur in middle-aged individuals, manometric recordings in elderly persons with intermittent dysphagia occasionally display the pattern of diffuse esophageal spasm.[38] In this motility disturbance, the patient has simultaneous, repetitive muscle contractions of prolonged duration occurring spontaneously or after a swallow. Normal peristalsis is present most of the time, explaining the intermittent nature of symptoms, which may be triggered by hot or cold foods, pills, or carbonated beverages. The pathogenesis of diffuse esophageal spasm is obscure; on the basis of case reports, experts have speculated that in some cases this disorder represents a stage in the development of achalasia.

"Nutcracker" esophagus and noncardiac chest pain

It is usually assumed that in persons free of significant coronary artery disease with chest pain resembling the pain of myocardial ischemia, symptoms are due to an esophageal motility disorder. Such patients, however, rarely have chest pain during esophageal manometry, and provocative testing may be used to precipitate symptoms. Provocative testing with intravenous edrophonium chloride and infusion of acid into the esophagus causes chest pain in about 30 percent of subjects with a history of noncardiac chest pain.[54] A similar number of patients with noncardiac chest pain have been found to have an esophageal motility disorder, but only 25 percent of these individuals have symptoms during provocative testing.[44] It is often difficult, therefore, to prove that the esophagus is the source of the patient's complaints.

The most common motility disorder found in patients with noncardiac chest pain is "nutcracker" esophagus.[44] This abnormality is characterized by peristaltic muscle contractions of extremely high amplitude and long duration in the distal portion of the esophagus. A defect in esophageal transit can be demonstrated in many affected patients using a radionuclide marker. In one large series of individuals with noncardiac chest pain, 50 percent of patients with a motility disorder had nutcracker esophagus; other symptomatic individuals were found to have diffuse esophageal spasm.[44] A causal role for these motility defects in the production of chest pain has not been proved. In recent studies, many patients with noncardiac chest pain were found to have musculoskeletal disorders.

A number of medicines have been used to treat primary esophageal motility disorders, especially diffuse esophageal spasm and nutcracker esophagus. Nitrates, anticholinergics, calcium channel blockers, or sedatives are occasionally effective in relieving symptoms of dysphagia and chest pain; their benefit in this setting, however, has never been evaluated in an appropriately designed trial. Some patients also obtain relief from dysphagia after bougienage. Forceful dilation is the treatment of choice for primary achalasia.

Hiatus Hernia

The incidence of hiatus hernia (Fig. 57-5) increases with each decade of life from less than 10 percent of those under age 40 to approximately 40 percent in the sixth and seventh decades and 70 percent in patients beyond the age of 70.

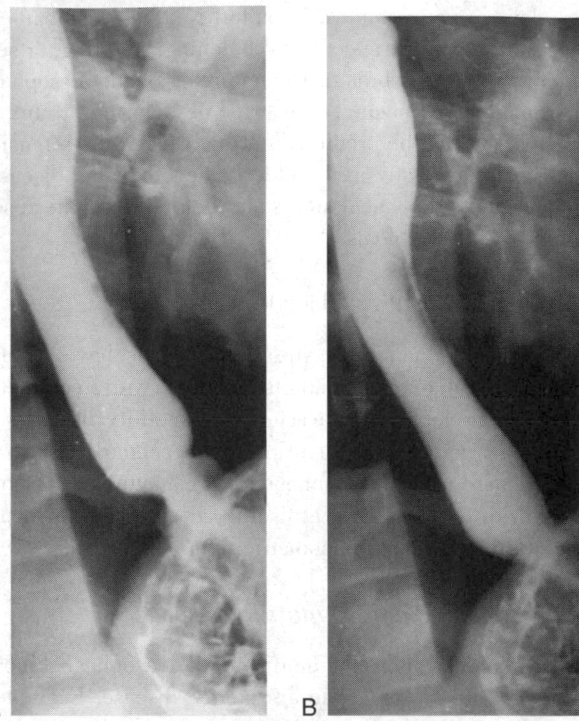

Figure 57-5 A small hiatus hernia **(A)** sliding in and **(B)** out of the thorax. The esophagogastric junction is seen above the diaphragm. (From Brandt,[154] with permission.)

Symptoms such as pyrosis and regurgitation formerly attributed to the hernia are now known to be due to lower esophageal sphincter dysfunction. Sphincter dysfunction and gastrointestinal reflux are independent of the presence of a hiatus hernia, and the common "sliding" hiatus hernia is not considered by itself to be pathogenic.

One type of hiatus hernia that deserves special mention is the paraesophageal hernia (Fig. 57-6), an uncommon hernia that occurs most often in persons between the ages of 60 and 70. Paraesophageal hernias often result in significant complications and therefore are of major importance. These hernias are frequently asymptomatic or cause only nagging discomfort until mechanical entrapment occurs. Such a catastrophe is associated with progressive distension of the incarcerated segment, vascular embarrassment, hemorrhage, gangrene, and perforation. In the absence of contraindications, a paraesophageal hernia demands surgical repair.

Reflux Esophagitis

The only notable change in the lower esophageal sphincter seen with aging is a reduction in the amplitude of postdeglutative contraction or relaxation. Nevertheless, because the secretion of gastrin, which potentiates contraction of the lower esophageal sphincter, increases with age, and because gastric acid secretion declines with age in many individuals, it is unusual for reflux esophagitis to appear for the first time in the elderly. The nature or extent of esophageal injury associated with gastroesophageal reflux cannot be predicted on the basis of the intensity of symptoms in older patients.[43] Complications of chronic, asymptomatic reflux such as stricture formation may be the initial clinical presentation of esophagitis in about 20 percent of affected elderly patients. When an aged individual complains of the recent onset of pyrosis, other causes of esophageal symptoms, such as candidiasis, must be considered. The therapy of reflux in the elderly is the same as in younger patients, however, attention must be paid to the potential development of adverse effects of medications (see below).[55]

Barrett's Metaplasia

In patients with Barrett's metaplasia, the lower esophagus is lined for a variable distance by columnar, rather than the usual stratified squamous, epithelium.[56,57] The metaplastic columnar epithelium may be continuous with the columnar epithelium of the stomach and extend in tongues into the distal esophagus, or it may be present in islands surrounded by normal sequamous epithelium. The importance of Barrett's metaplasia lies in its association with reflux esophagitis, (deep) esophageal ulcers, (high) esophageal strictures (Fig. 57-7), and adenocarcinoma. The metaplastic columnar lining is believed to develop as a consequence of gastroesophageal reflux.

Figure 57-6 Barium esophagram demonstrating a paraesophageal hernia with the gastric fundus above the diaphragm. The esophagogastric junction is at the level of the diaphragm. (From Brandt,[154] with permission.)

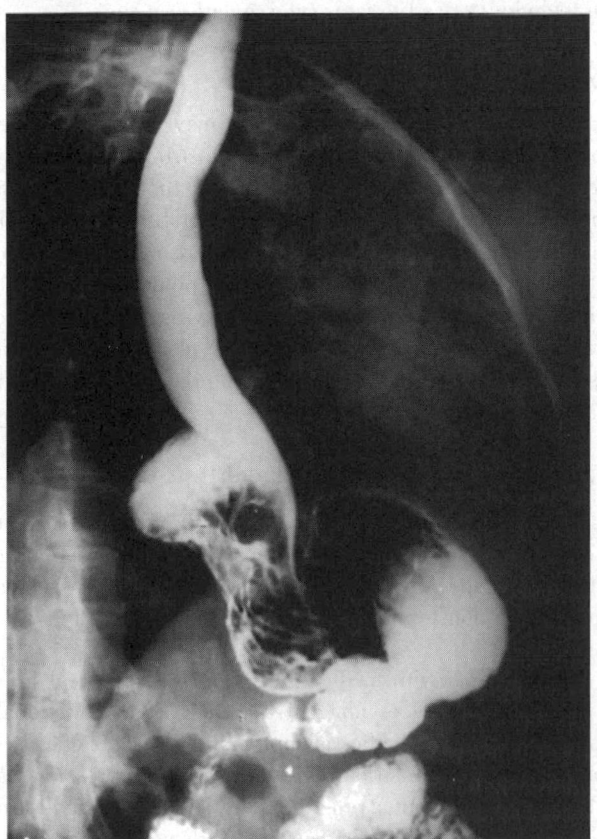

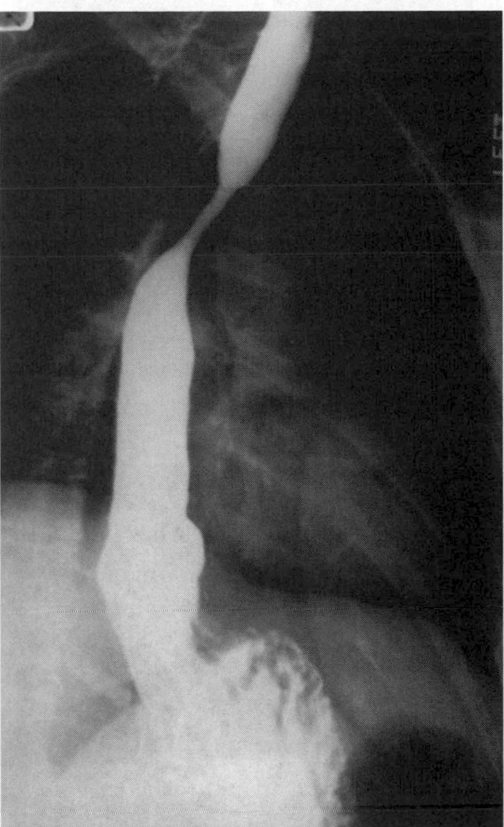

Figure 57-7 Barium esophagram revealing a stricture of the esophagus at the level of the aortic arch in a patient with Barrett's esophagus. A hiatus hernia is also present. (From Brandt,[154] with permission.)

Esophageal squamous epithelium damaged by exposure to gastric contents is replaced by a specialized columnar epithelium (intestinal metaplasia), a junctional-type epithelium, or a gastric fundic-type epithelium. Each of these three cell types may be seen alone or in combination with the others.

Most cases of Barrett's esophagus probably occur between the ages of 50 and 70; the exact incidence is unknown. The most common symptoms are those related to the reflux of stomach contents, and the entity is diagnosed best by esophagoscopy with multiple biopsies. The presence of specialized columnar epithelium establishes the diagnosis of Barrett's esophagus.[57] If the columnar epithelium in the biopsy specimen is one of the other two types, the biopsy must have been made at least 3 cm above the gastroesophageal junction to make the diagnosis. Intestinal metaplasia can be recognized in situ by staining with Alcian blue.

Stricture and neoplasia are long-term complications of Barrett's esophagus. There is increasing evidence that cancer arises only in specialized columnar epithelium. By careful screening using esophagoscopy with directed biopsy and cytology every 1 to 2 years, premalignant dysplastic changes can usually be detected.[58,59] The development of severe dysplasia or carcinoma in situ requires resection of the involved esophagus. Therapy of reflux usually results in symptomatic improvement, but regression of the columnar epithelium does not occur without surgery.

Lower Esophageal Ring

A lower esophageal or Schatzki ring (Fig. 57-8) is a thin, annular ridge of mucosa projecting perpendicularly into the esophageal lumen at or near the squamocolumnar junction.[60–62] A Schatzki ring may be asymptomatic, found incidentally during evaluation of the upper gastrointestinal tract for unrelated reasons, or it may cause intermittent episodes of dysphagia and an uncomfortable sticking or pressing sensation due to food lodging above the ring. Episodes commonly occur during hurried meals, meals requiring a great deal of mastication, or meals consumed with alcohol, hence the appellation "steakhouse syndrome." As the lumen of the ring diminishes to less than 12 mm (0.047 in.) in diameter, attacks become more frequent. Attacks usually last several minutes or more until the patient regurgitates the food bolus or flushes it into the stomach with a beverage.

Figure 57-8 A Schatzki ring prevents passage of a barium pill in a patient with intermittent dysphagia. (From Brandt,[154] with permission.)

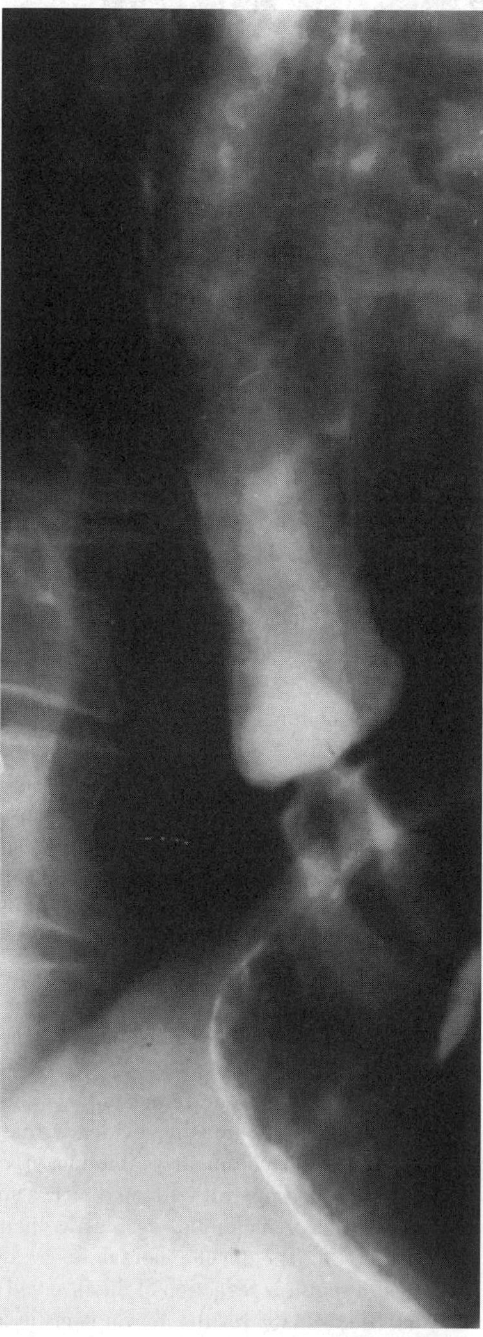

Total obstruction of the esophagus secondary to food impaction frequently brings patients to the emergency department. Papain solution (meat tenderizer) may be administered to digest enough of the impacted bolus to allow it to pass. The solution can be made by adding a tablespoon of crude papain powder to 25 mL of warm water; 1 ounce is administered every 30 minutes. Anaphylaxis to papain has been described, and digestion with papain should be attempted only within a few hours of the onset of the attack. Many experts do not recommend papain because its use has been associated with esophageal perforation in cases where severe esophagitis is present. Relaxation of the esophagus by administration of a small dose of intravenous benzodiazepine or 1 mg of glucagon also is occasionally effective in relieving the impaction. If the impacted bolus does not pass, it must be removed by esophagoscopy. Alternatively, it may be gently nudged into the stomach if a patent lumen can be seen distally, the esophageal mucosa is intact, and there is no bone or other sharp object present. Multiple biopsies to disrupt the ring or dilation with bougies are techniques used to treat symptomatic rings.

Dysphagia Aortica

Degenerative changes in the aorta may produce compression of the esophagus and dysphagia. Obstruction of the upper esophagus is occasionally caused by a thoracic aneurysm, while the distal esophagus may be squeezed between an atherosclerotic aorta posteriorly and the heart or esophageal hiatus anteriorly. Most patients are women beyond the age of 70.[63–65] Symptoms are usually prevented by having the patient thoroughly masticate solid foods, but occasionally the obstruction is severe enough to warrant surgical mobilization of the esophagus at the hiatus.[66]

Medication-Induced Esophageal Injury

Esophageal injury can occur as a result of the local caustic effects of medications.[67,68] The most frequent offenders are antibiotics, especially tetracyclines, potassium chloride, ferrous sulfate, nonsteroidal anti-inflammatory drugs, and quinidine.

Most patients with medication-induced esophageal injury have no underlying esophageal disorder. Some individuals, however, have nonspecific, asymptomatic disorders of esophageal motility, peptic strictures, esophageal compression from left atrial enlargement, a prominent aortic knob, or mediastinal adhesions following thoracic surgery. Pills commonly lodge in the esophagus at the level of the aortic knob or the lower esophageal sphincter without the patient's knowledge. Many cases of pill-induced esophageal injury probably remain unrecognized with full recovery. The most frequent symptoms of medication-induced esophageal injury are odynophagia and retrosternal pain. Symptoms usually resolve within 6 weeks of stopping the medication or changing it to a liquid formulation; damage, however, may result in esophageal stricture formation or, occasionally, hemorrhage or perforation. Pills should always be taken with a generous amount of water, and elderly patients should not take pills immediately before bedtime, as a decrease in salivation and esophageal motor activity accompanies sleeping.[69]

Esophageal Diverticula

Diverticula of the esophagus are much less common than diverticula of other parts of the gastrointestinal tract. In a review of 20,000 barium studies on the upper gastrointestinal tract, Wheeler[70] noted only six midesophageal (traction-type) and three epiphrenic (pulsion-type) diverticula, as compared with 1,020 duodenal diverticula. The terms *traction* and *pulsion* refer to commonly accepted theories regarding the pathogenesis of esophageal diverticula. Traction diverticula are thought to be caused by the effects of fibrotic disease in structures contiguous with the esophagus, while pulsion diverticula are hypothesized to result from increased intraluminal pressure. Pseudodiverticulosis of the esophagus also has been described.

Midesophageal diverticula (traction diverticula)

Traction diverticula occur most commonly in the middle third of the esophagus, where a large group of lymph nodes lies in direct contact with the esophageal wall. Nodal inflammation of this area may lead to periesophagitis, fixation of the esophagus to the lymph nodes, and distortion of the esophageal wall. In the past, tuberculosis was the most common etiology for this process; any infection with lymph node involvement, however, may lead to the formation of a traction diverticulum.

Traction diverticula usually occur in patients of middle age or older and are slightly more common in men. They rarely cause symptoms, perhaps because they are small, have a broad neck, and can contract and empty because they contain all the layers of the esophageal wall including muscle.

Epiphrenic diverticula (pulsion diverticula)

Pulsion diverticula are found in the lower 10 cm of the esophagus, usually on the right wall. Like traction diverticula, they contain all the layers of the esophageal wall; the muscular layer, however, may be quite attenuated.

Epiphrenic diverticula usually develop in males during middle age. Patients may complain of dysphagia or chest pain, but symptoms are probably due to an associated esophageal motor abnormality such as achalasia or diffuse esophageal spasm.[71] The occurrence of an epiphrenic diverticulum without an underlying motility disorder or a hiatus hernia appears to be rare.

Many epiphrenic diverticula are asymptomatic, and in these instances no therapy is required.[72] Treatment of esophageal reflux or an underlying motility disorder may afford the patient symptomatic relief.[73,74] In cases of larger diverticula, surgical resection may be necessary.[75]

Intramural pseudodiverticulosis

In esophageal pseudodiverticulosis, dilation of the excretory ducts of submucosal glands causes multiple small (1 to 3 mm) invaginations of the esophageal wall.[76] These defects involve all, or segments of, the esophagus in a circumferential fashion. Pseudodiverticula are best detected by barium contrast studies; their roentigenographic appearance is quite characteristic (Fig. 57-9). Pseudodiverticulosis is usually diagnosed during the seventh decade of life in patients with dysphagia. In at least 20 percent of cases, gastroesophageal reflux, a motility disorder, or a malignancy is found, and in approximately one-half of patients, smears or cultures of the esophageal mucosa reveal *Candida albicans*. Stenoses, or areas of reduced distensibility, are found in up to 90 percent of cases of pseudodiverticulosis and preferentially seem to involve the upper esophagus. Surprisingly, there is no fixed relationship between the narrowed area and the segment involved with pseudodiverticula.

The etiology of pseudodiverticulosis is unknown. The term *adenosis* has been used to refer to this entity because the number of deep esophageal mucous glands is markedly increased.[77] Therapy consists of treatment of associated abnormalities. Coexisting strictures should be evaluated to ensure that they are benign.

Esophageal Candidiasis

Infection of the esophagus is rare in patients without acquired immunodeficiency syndrome, with the exception of infection with *C. albicans*. *Candida albicans* is a normal inhabitant of the alimentary tract; the yeast form is found in almost 50 percent of oral washings and 80 percent of stool samples.[78] The population of *C. albicans* is suppressed in healthy adults by other intestinal flora. Comparison of fecal specimens from subjects aged 70 to 100 with those of individuals aged 20 to 69 have revealed fungi to be more common in the elderly group. This finding may be explained by a diminution in esophageal peristalsis, a reduction in gastric acid secretion, and age-related alterations in cellular and humoral immunity.

In the absence of antibiotic therapy or an underlying immune disorder, esophageal candidiasis is a disease of the elderly. Most cases in this age group, however, occur in association with predisposing conditions, including malignancy, therapy with immunosuppresive or cytotoxic drugs, diabetes mellitus, malnutrition, and treatment with broad-spectrum antibiotics.[79,80]

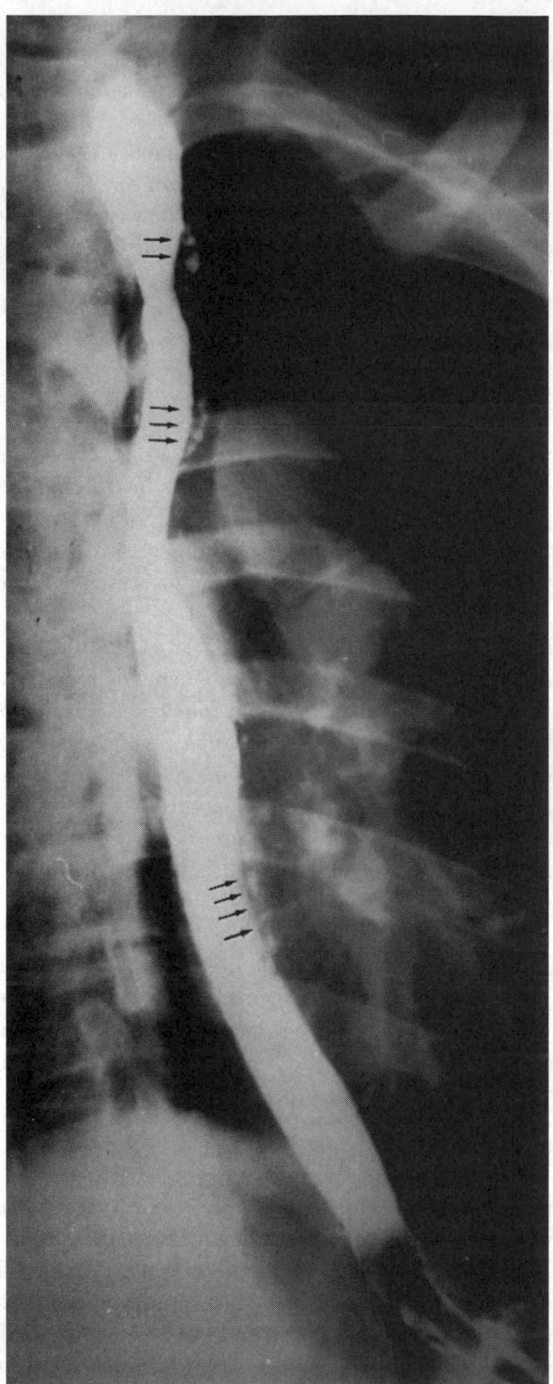

Figure 57-9 Intramural pseudodiverticulosis with multiple outpouchings (arrows) on a barium esophagram. (From Brandt,[154] with permission.)

In the proper clinical setting, dysphagia, odynophagia, substernal burning, or an awareness of food passing down the esophagus should suggest the possibility of candida infection, although even in the presence of infection with *C. albicans*, up to one-half of patients may be asymptomatic. Esophageal candidiasis often results from the extension of oral lesions, and a careful examination of the oral cavity is important in any debilitated patient complaining of esophageal symptoms.

A diagnosis of candida esophagitis may be suggested by an abnormal barium esophagram, although a normal study does not exclude the presence of this organism. Esophagoscopy is the best method for detecting candida infection; raised white plaques, hyperemia, ulceration, and friability are characteristic. The gross appearance of candida esophagitis may be confused with that of exudative esophagitis, and therefore the diagnosis must be confirmed by brushings and biopsies. Typical hyphae are revealed under the microscope in scrapings placed on a glass slide and macerated with 20 percent potassium hydroxide.

In the appropriate setting, a trial of therapy may be initiated without attempting an invasive diagnosis. As in oral and vaginal candidiasis, therapy usually consists of promoting the reestablishment of normal microbiologic flora by discontinuing antibiotics. In an immunocompromised host or in an individual with significant morbidity, topical therapy with a suspension of nystatin or the use of nystatin troches is usually successful. Odynophagia can be treated with viscous lidocaine or with a "swish-and-swallow" preparation of the type used to treat stomatitis (see above). Failure to respond to simple treatment necessitates endoscopic confirmation of the diagnosis and, often, systemic therapy with antifungal agents.

Esophageal Neoplasms

Esophageal cancer (Fig. 57-10) occurs most frequently after age 55 and is three times more common in males than in females in the United States, and two times more common in males than in females in the United Kingdom.[1] In the United States, it accounts for approximately 2 percent of all reported cancers. Factors associated with the development of esophageal cancer include alcohol and tobacco use, thermal irritation, poor oral hygiene, and esophageal stasis.[1,81,82] Furthermore, an association has been noted with certain esophageal diseases, notably achalasia, Barrett's esophagus, lye stricture, and Plummer-Vinson syndrome, and also with previous gastric surgery.[83–85]

Surveillance, epidemiology, and end results (SEER) data show an increase in adenocarcinoma from 8 to 18 percent of all esophageal cancers during the years 1973 to 1984.[86] Esophageal adenocarcinoma is either cancer of the gastric fundus or a malignancy that has developed in a segment of Barrett's esophagus. Squamous cell carcinoma most commonly involves the middle third of the esophagus. Local spread occurs early, and, because the esophagus dilates so readily, dysphagia, the most common complaint at the time of diagnosis, is a late symptom.

In the elderly an important manifestation of esophageal cancer is an achalasia-like syndrome. Primary achalasia is uncommon in patients beyond the age of 50. Elderly individuals who present with symptoms of achalasia of less than 1 year's duration associated with marked weight loss should be suspected of having a malignancy, most often gastric adenocarcinoma. The pathogenesis of secondary achalasia is unknown; in some

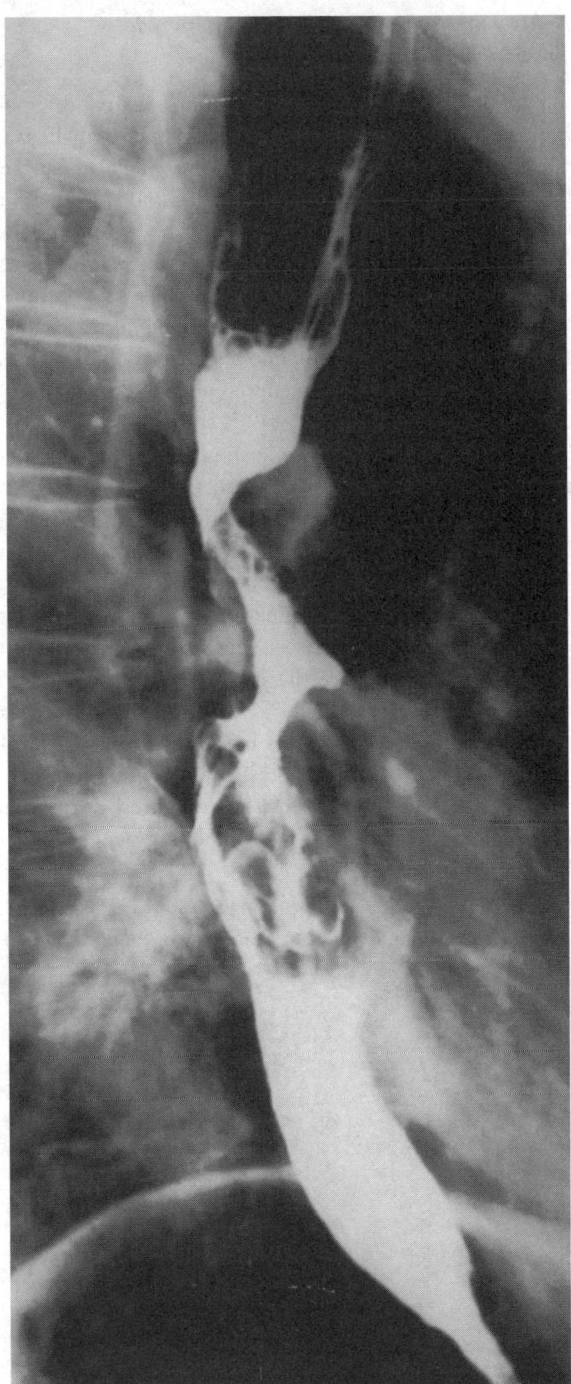

Figure 57-10 Barium esophagram demonstrating an ulcerating esophageal carcinoma. (From Brandt,[154] with permission.)

cases the lower esophagus is infiltrated with tumor cells, but in other cases achalasia may reflect a paraneoplastic process.

The prognosis for esophageal cancer is dismal. Management is directed at relieving progressive obstruction.[87–89] Surgical resection and radiation are the accepted modes of treatment. Surgical resection offers the only chance for long-term survival, but fewer than half of all patients presenting with esophageal cancer have a respectable lesion. If there is evidence of nodal or distant metastases, a thoracotomy should be avoided. Thoracic radiation, while useful, may be followed by the development of esophagitis, usually within 3 weeks of initiating therapy and continuing for several weeks after its completion. Chemotherapy may result in symptomatic improvement but does not substantially prolong survival. New chemotherapeutic agents should be administered under an investigational protocol. Palliative therapy with endoscopically placed stents or with a laser to burn away obstructing tumor is often very useful and has improved the quality of life for many patients, albeit without prolonging survival.

The Stomach

Aging is associated with alterations in both the motor and secretory functions of the stomach but, as in other parts of the gastrointestinal tract, changes in gastric physiology attributable to age alone rarely are responsible for symptoms.

The motor activity of the stomach allows it to behave as two individual, albeit coordinated, organs: one that processes liquids and another that processes solids. The fundus and proximal body of the stomach serve as a reservoir for liquids. In contrast, the distal gastric body and the antrum grind solids into small particles and pump them into the duodenum. The activities of both the proximal and distal stomach are controlled by complex neural and hormonal mechanisms. Studies employing food labeled with radioactive isotopes suggest that gastric emptying of liquids is prolonged in elderly persons, while emptying of solids is unaffected by age.[90,91]

Changes in gastric secretion also occur in individuals as they grow older. In the past, almost every study on gastric acid production showed a decline in basal and stimulated acid output with advancing age.[92] Work by Goldschmiedt and colleagues,[93] however, suggests that, in the absence of *Helicobacter pylori* infection, aging is actually associated with an increase in gastric acid secretion. Previous confusion about the effect of aging on gastric acid secretion is probably related to the high incidence of *H. pylori* infection and chronic atrophic gastritis with secondary achlorhydria in older individuals (see below).[94]

Gastric and Duodenal Mucosal Injury

Advances in our understanding of the pathobiology of gastric and duodenal mucosal injury, and improvements in our ability to examine the upper gastrointestinal tract and detect diseases responsible for mucosal injury, make it important for physicians to use descriptive and diagnostic terminology carefully in clinical practice.[95,96] Unless diagnostic findings are reported with a precision that accurately reflects current understanding of mucosal injury, the benefits of medical advances made during the past two decades may be lost to patients.

In usual cases of gastric or duodenal mucosal injury, endoscopic inspection often reveals the presence of gross epithelial defects. Small epithelial defects, or erosions, do not penetrate the muscularis mucosae. Ulcers are defined as being larger than 3 mm in diameter and extend a variable distance through the muscularis mucosae, in some instances freely perforating into the peritoneal cavity or penetrating into an adjacent organ. A typical ulcer is composed of four layers or zones: a superficial layer of fibrinopurulent debris overlying a zone of inflammation, a layer of granulation tissue, and, at its base, a collagenous scar. Both erosions and ulcers may be sources of bleeding.

Diffuse mucosal erythema, a common finding at endoscopy, in most instances represents microvascular congestion and, although it is interpreted by many endoscopists as indicating the presence of "gastritis," this conclusion is unjustified. Mucosal erythema due to microvascular congestion is caused by a variety of factors and is without any specific etiologic significance or clinical association.[96] Conversely, patients often have histologic gastritis without the presence of mucosal erythema.

The term *gastritis* implies the presence of inflammation and should not be used unless examination of a biopsy specimen has revealed typical mucosal inflammatory changes, including infiltration of the lamina propria with polymorphonuclear leukocytes and mononuclear cells. Neutrophils are seen early in the course of inflammation (acute gastritis). With the passage of time mononuclear cells, mainly plasma cells, and eosinophils appear in increasing numbers (chronic gastritis). Most patients with gastritis have a predominance of mononuclear cells in the lamina propria with a lesser number of neutrophils (chronic active gastritis).[97] The inflammatory changes of gastritis are accompanied by signs of cell injury and regeneration. Cell damage and death cause submucosal hemorrhage and edema and lead to development of epithelial defects. Hemorrhage and edema may be grossly visible at endoscopy as well as evident on microscopic examination of biopsy specimens, as are erosions and ulcers. In response to injury, the epithelium regenerates by proliferation and differentiation of mucous neck cells, a process that leads to elongation and tortuosity of the gastric pits (foveolar hyperplasia). The vast majority of cases of gastritis are caused by infection with *H. pylori* (type B gastritis). Gastritis also may be due to other less common bacterial infections, granulomatous disease, autoimmune disease (type A gastritis), and hypersensitivity reactions.

Other agents of gastric injury damage the mucosa without exciting an inflammatory response. This gastropathy is sometimes referred to as type C gastritis, an unfortunate misnomer given the noninflammatory nature of the process.[98] Microscopic examination of biopsy specimens from patients with gastropathy typically reveals vascular congestion and edema of the lamina propria, hypertrophy of the muscularis mucosae, and mucosal regenerative changes with foveolar hyperplasia.[99] As in gastritis, cell damage and death are accompanied by submucosal hemorrhage and edema and lead to the development of epithelial defects. The latter changes are all often grossly visible on endoscopy. The most common causes of gastropathy are ingestion of nonsteroidal anti-inflammatory drugs (NSAIDs) and ethanol.

Helicobacter pylori, gastritis, and peptic ulcer disease

Infection with *H. pylori*, a spiral gram-negative microaerophilic rod, is the most common chronic bacterial disease in humans. This organism attaches to receptors on the surface of gastric mucous neck cells and is also found on metaplastic gastric epithelium in the duodenum but not on the duodenal mucosa itself or on metaplastic duodenal mucosa in the stomach (Fig. 57-11).[100] *Helicobacter pylori* causes alterations in cell structure and function, inflammation, metaplasia, and cell death.[101] A number of virulence factors, including urease, make it possible for the organism to colonize the stomach and produce disease.[102]

Helicobacter pylori infection is the most common cause of chronic gastritis (type B antral gastritis) and is one of the two principal causes of peptic ulcer disease, the other being ingestion of NSAIDs. More than 90 percent of patients with duodenal ulcer and more than 75 percent of patients with gastric ulcer also have *H. pylori* infection and chronic active gastritis.[1] The relationship between ulcer disease and gastritis was recognized long before the etiologic role of *H. pylori* in the pathogenesis of peptic ulcer disease was understood. *Helicobacter pylori* infection also has been linked to the development of gastric cancer, another gastritis-associated disease.[103]

Infection with *H. pylori* is usually acquired during childhood and occurs most often in persons living under conditions

Figure 57-11 Gastric biopsy showing *H. pylori* in the surface mucous layer (Giemsa stain, 1000×). (Courtesy of Sumi Mitsudo.)

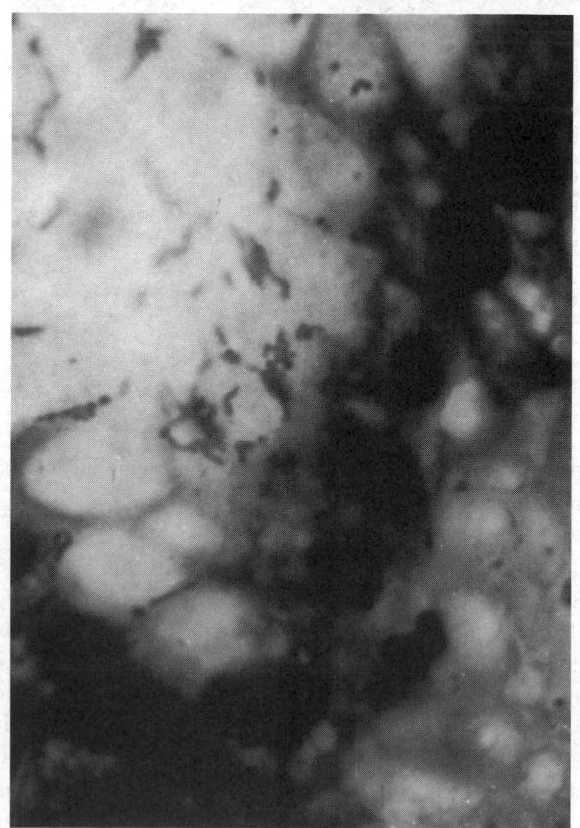

of poverty, crowding, and inadequate sanitation.[104] The prevalence of *H. pylori* infection in the United States and in the nations of western Europe increases with advancing age, a result of the poorer living conditions in these countries during the early years of the twentieth century.[105] Thus, regardless of present socioeconomic status, infection is most prevalent in older individuals. The incidence of peptic ulcer disease also increases progressively with advancing age, reflecting the age-related increase in *H. pylori* infection.

Under experimental conditions, acute infection with *H. pylori* causes transient dyspeptic symptoms accompanied by the development of active antral gastritis.[106] Mucosal inflammation apparently may resolve spontaneously in the minority of patients or become chronic, gradually spreading proximally into the body and fundus of the stomach. As the disease progresses, inflammation extends into the deeper, glandular part of the epithelium containing the gastric secretory cells; these include parietal cells which make hydrochloric acid and intrinsic factor, chief cells which make pepsin, pylorocardiac gland cells which make mucus, and endocrine G cells which make gastrin. Normal glands are gradually destroyed and replaced by metaplastic glands (intestinal metaplasia) or by atrophic gastric mucosa (atrophic gastritis), a process that takes many years. Atrophic gastritis often is associated with low serum gastrin levels and antibodies to gastrin-secreting cells. Patients with chronic active gastritis frequently also have submucosal hemorrhage, edema, epithelial erosions (erosive gastritis), and peptic ulcers.

Individuals with active gastritis and gastric mucosal atrophy are usually asymptomatic but may complain of intermittent dyspepsia, abdominal pain, distension, nausea and vomiting (nonulcer dyspepsia). The relationship, if any, between symptoms of nonulcer dyspepsia and gastritis is unclear (see below); many persons with dyspepsia do not have gastritis, and many persons with gastritis do not have dyspepsia.[107] Dyspeptic symptoms may be due to the development of a gastric or duodenal ulcer, although, at least 50 percent of patients with acute ulcers are asymptomatic.

Helicobacter pylori infection may be diagnosed by a transendoscopic pinch biopsy of the stomach. Microscopic examination of biopsy specimens from infected individuals reveals chronic active gastritis and typical spiral gram-negative rods in the mucus coating the surface epithelium (Fig. 57-11). The absence of gastritis strongly argues against *H. pylori* infection, while its presence suggests that a failure to identify *H. pylori* is due to sampling error. Tissue also may be implanted in commercially available agar plates containing urea and a pH indicator. If *H. pylori* is present in the tissue specimen, bacterial urease will split the urea into bicarbonate and ammonia, raising the pH and producing a color change. Because infection may be patchy, testing several specimens obtained from different parts of the stomach improves the sensitivity of the assay.

Noninvasive diagnosis of *H. pylori* infection can be made by detecting serum antibody to bacterial antigens. This method of diagnosis is satisfactory—presuming there is no indication for endoscopy—if the patient has not previously been treated with antibiotics to which *H. pylori* is sensitive. Antibody titers decrease gradually after eradication of infection, but qualitative serology remains positive for a number of years, leaving what has been referred to as an "immunologic scar." The presence of an immunologic scar makes it impossible to use antibody testing to assess the effectiveness of therapy or the occurrence of reinfection. This problem is avoided by using the urea breath test, which is positive only in a setting of active infection. In the urea breath test, the patient is given an oral dose of urea labeled with either a stable (^{13}C) or unstable (^{14}C) isotope of carbon. If the patient is infected with *H. pylori*, the urea will be metabolized by bacterial urease to ammonia and bicarbonate, and bicarbonate containing the isotopic tracer will be converted to CO_2 and expired. The presence of labeled CO_2 in samples of expired gas indicates active *H. pylori* infection.

Simultaneous treatment with three antibiotics is the most consistently effective means of curing *H. pylori* infection.[108] *Helicobacter pylori* is sensitive to a variety of antimicrobial agents, including metronidazole, tetracyclines, macrolides, some quinolones, β-lactams, and bismuth preparations, as well as to proton pump inhibitors. The most commonly used regimen is a combination of a bismuth preparation, metronidazole, and either tetracycline or amoxicillin; therapy with tetracycline achieves a significantly higher cure rate (90.3 percent) than treatment with amoxicillin (69.9 percent). These regimens have the advantage of low cost but are limited by the frequent occurrence of bacterial resistance to metronidazole. The use of a proton pump inhibitor has the triple benefit of promoting ulcer healing and palliating symptoms of active ulcer disease at the same time that it treats *H. pylori* infection, but regimens including proton pump inhibitors are very expensive. Because of the morbidity caused by *H. pylori* infection, the National Institutes of Health Consensus Development Panel has published guidelines mandating treatment of all *H. pylori*-infected ulcer patients, including those currently without an active ulcer crater or dyspeptic symptoms.[109] The significant treatment failure rate makes it desirable to document cure by conducting a urea breath test 4 weeks after the completion of therapy. In addition to antibiotic therapy for *H. pylori* infection, patients with acute ulcers should be treated with an antisecretory agent to promote ulcer healing.

Nonsteroidal anti-inflammatory drugs, gastropathy, and peptic ulcer disease

Nonsteroidal anti-inflammatory drugs (NSAIDs) are among the most frequently prescribed medicines in the world. Approximately 3 million people in the United States, or 1.2 percent of the population, take at least one NSAID daily. Uncounted others regularly use over-the-counter NSAID preparations, including aspirin. As a result, NSAID-related morbidity is exceedingly common; each year 2 to 4 percent of chronic NSAID users have a serious drug-induced complication involving the gastrointestinal tract.[110] The use of NSAIDs and complications of NSAID use are most prevalent in the elderly.[111–113] In the United Kingdom, NSAID prescription rates for the entire population increased steadily from 1967 to 1985 and did so in direct proportion to the age of the recipient, with progressively more prescriptions being written for progressively older patients.[114] Thus, in 1985, an astonishing 1,400 NSAID prescriptions were written for every 1,000 women in the United Kingdom aged 65 years or older. These chronic NSAID users are estimated to have a two-to threefold greater mortality than nonusers because of drug-related gastrointestinal complications.[111]

Each and every NSAID is capable of injuring the gastrointestinal mucosa and does so in a dose-dependent fashion roughly proportional to its anti-inflammatory effect. Virtually 100 percent of patients who take a NSAID preparation, including aspirin, develop acute gastropathy during the first 1 to 2 weeks of therapy.[115] This gastropathy has the typical histologic features described above and characteristically is associated with submucosal hemorrhage and some degree of edema both of which are often grossly visible at endoscopy. Many NSAIDs, like aspirin, are weak acids which remain nonionized as the tablets break up and are dispersed in low-pH gastric secretions. Because they are nonionized, NSAIDs move easily across the membranes of epithelial cells and then ionize at the neutral pH of the cytoplasm. In the ionic form, they interact with cell constituents and cause cell damage and death.[116] Dead epithelial cells leave shallow mucosal defects (erosions) which may bleed. Patients often have dyspeptic symptoms during this acute phase of injury.

In a significant minority of chronic NSAID users, mucosal defects enlarge and form true ulcers; approximately 12 to 30 percent of patients develop a gastric ulcer, and 2 to 19 percent of patients develop a duodenal ulcer.[117] The elderly seem to be particularly vulnerable to the harmful effects of NSAIDs. In a study of peptic ulcer disease in persons aged 65 and older, Griffin and colleagues[118] found that almost 30 percent of ulcers diagnosed in these individuals may have been caused by NSAIDs. The principal mechanism by which NSAID use leads to the development of peptic ulcers is dose-dependent systemic inhibition of prostaglandin synthesis.[119] Prostaglandins protect the upper gastrointestinal mucosa by stimulating the secretion of bicarbonate and mucus, increasing mucosal blood flow, and promoting a number of cellular processes crucial to mucosal defense and repair. A decrease in prostaglandin synthesis tips the balance between defensive and aggressive factors in the upper gastrointestinal tract in favor of those that injure the mucosa, leading to the formation of ulcers and the possible development of complications including hemorrhage, obstruction, perforation, and penetration into an adjacent organ.

A variety of treatment strategies for preventing the development of gastric and duodenal ulcers in patients on chronic NSAID therapy have been tested.[120] Many commonly used medicines are without any demonstrable prophylactic benefit in this setting. Ranitidine and omeprazole have been shown to prevent duodenal but not gastric ulcers in arthritis patients taking NSAIDs.[120–122] Similar results were obtained by Taha and coworkers[123] in arthritis patients treated with prophylactic famotidine, however, in the same study high-dose famotidine reduced the incidence of both duodenal and gastric ulcers.[123] An alternative approach to ulcer prevention in patients who require chronic NSAID therapy is prostaglandin replacement with an oral synthetic prostaglandin E analog. The prostaglandin E_1 analog, misoprostol, like famotidine, has been shown to prevent development of both duodenal and gastric ulcers.[124] This agent also reduces the incidence of bleeding, perforation, and gastric outlet obstruction in patients on chronic NSAID therapy.[112] The use of misoprostol has been limited by its tendency to cause loose stools, abdominal cramps, and flatulence in a significant minority of individuals during initiation of treatment.

The large number of eligible patients makes it impossible to prescribe prophylactic famotidine or misoprostol for every NSAID user. Instead, an effort should be made to identify and treat those who both require chronic NSAID therapy and are at greatest risk for developing a significant NSAID-related complication. Included in this high-risk group are the elderly, as well as persons with a history of peptic ulcer disease or previous upper gastrointestinal bleeding, individuals also taking steroids, and patients with cardiovascular disease.[112,113] Once an ulcer develops, a serious complication is often the first sign of its presence in as much as approximately 50 percent of persons with ulcers have no dyspeptic symptoms. Patients taking NSAIDs who have dyspeptic symptoms require evaluation for ulcer disease as well as possible *H. pylori* infection, and those with ulcers should be treated with an antisecretory agent and also antibiotics, if indicated.

Peptic ulcer disease in the elderly

Ulcer disease, whether due to *H. pylori* infection, NSAID use, or some other less common cause, frequently exhibits a virulent course in the elderly with more complications and mortality than in the young.[125–127] Duodenal ulcer occurs two to three times more frequently than gastric ulcer, but the latter is responsible for two of every three deaths from peptic ulcer disease in older individuals, and the death rate increases with advancing age.

The presentation of ulcer disease in the elderly tends to be acute, often with bleeding or perforation, but symptoms may be subtle; this is particularly true of gastric ulcers. Gastric ulcers produce chronic blood loss more commonly than duodenal ulcers, and resultant anemia may lead to cardiac or neurologic symptoms. Weight loss and fatigue suggesting malignancy may be the only complaints, a presentation characteristic of giant ulcers. So-called geriatric ulcers (Fig. 57-12) high in the cardia may cause misleading symptoms such as dysphagia mimicking esophageal neoplasm or chest pain suggesting angina. A history of NSAID use is commonly obtained from elderly patients with peptic ulcer disease.

The complication rate of peptic ulcer disease rises progressively from 31 percent in patients 60 to 64 years of age to 76 percent in those 75 to 79 years of age. Surgery should not be withheld or delayed solely because of advanced age because it is often life-saving in older patients. Bleeding, the most

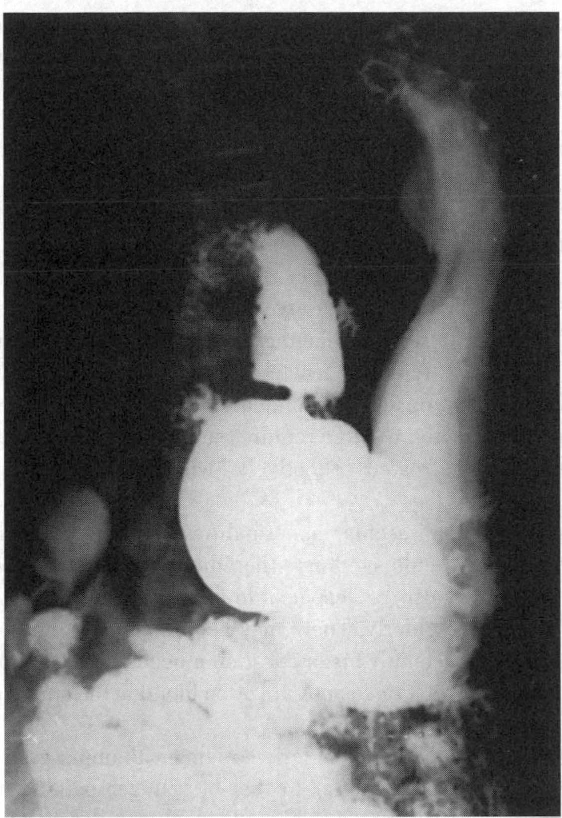

Figure 57-12 Upper gastrointestinal series revealing a large benign "geriatric ulcer" high on the lesser curvature. (From Brandt,[154] with permission.)

common complication, accounts for one-half to two-thirds of all fatalities (see below). Perforation is the second most common complication of peptic ulcers in the elderly. The presentation of a perforated ulcer is subtle in this age group, delaying the correct diagnosis and contributing to the high mortality. Gastric outlet obstruction complicates ulcer disease in 10 to 15 percent of patients beyond 60 years of age, generally occurring in those with a long history of disease; an obstructing malignant lesion must be excluded in such patients.

Duodenal ulcers greater than 2 cm in diameter were once considered a distinct entity because of their poor prognosis, but it is probable that most of these "giant" duodenal ulcers are caused by either *H. pylori* infection or NSAID use, just like smaller lesions. Giant duodenal ulcers occur most often in men over 70 years of age who have no prior history of peptic ulcer disease. The most frequent complaint is of abdominal pain radiating to the back or right upper quadrant, suggesting pancreatic or biliary disease. Pain may be relieved by antacids, but aggravated by eating, and is often accompanied by significant weight loss. The ulcer crater is so large that it sometimes is mistaken for the duodenal bulb on an upper gastrointestinal series (Fig. 57-13). While giant duodenal ulcers were often fatal 30 years ago, today they usually respond to therapy with histamine antagonists or proton pump inhibitors and with antibiotics when indicated by the presence of *H. pylori* infection.

Giant gastric ulcers have a diameter of over 3 cm.[128,129] They also are most likely caused by either *H. pylori* infection or NSAID use. Giant gastric ulcers are slightly more common in males and are usually seen in patients over 65 years of age. Pain is not a prominent complaint, but only about 10 percent of patients are completely free of pain. Pain may radiate to the chest, periumbilical region, or lower abdomen. Morbidity and mortality rates are high, with hemorrhage being the most common complication. These ulcers are usually benign and can be treated with histamine antagonists or proton pump inhibitors as well as with antibiotics when there is documented *H. pylori* infection. Patients should be followed carefully with endoscopy to demonstrate healing. Candidiasis of the ulcer crater may delay healing and requires adjunctive antifungal therapy.

The etiology of nonulcer dyspepsia is unknown; numerous explanations have been proposed for this syndrome, including psychosocial factors, altered sensation, abnormal gastrointestinal motility and compliance, and *H. pylori* infection. Gas washout studies show that individuals with nonulcer dyspepsia do not have increased gas in their digestive tracts, and therefore complaints of bloating are probably explained by sensitivity to normal volumes of gas; in some, the transit of infused gas is abnormal, suggesting a motility disorder. Gastric antral hypomotility and impaired gastric emptying of solids have been observed in 40 to 50 percent of patients with nonulcer dyspepsia, and treatment with drugs that affect upper gastrointestinal motility relieves symptoms in many patients.[132–134] Thirty to 50 percent of patients with symptoms of nonulcer dyspepsia have chronic active gastritis, even when the gastric mucosa appears grossly normal at endoscopy.[107] It has been suggested that nonulcer dyspepsia is part of the spectrum of disease caused by *H. pylori*, which includes chronic active gastritis, duodenitis, and peptic ulcer disease. The successive develop-

Figure 57-13 Upper gastrointestinal series demonstrates a giant duodenal ulcer resembling the duodenal bulb (arrows). (From Brandt,[154] with permission.)

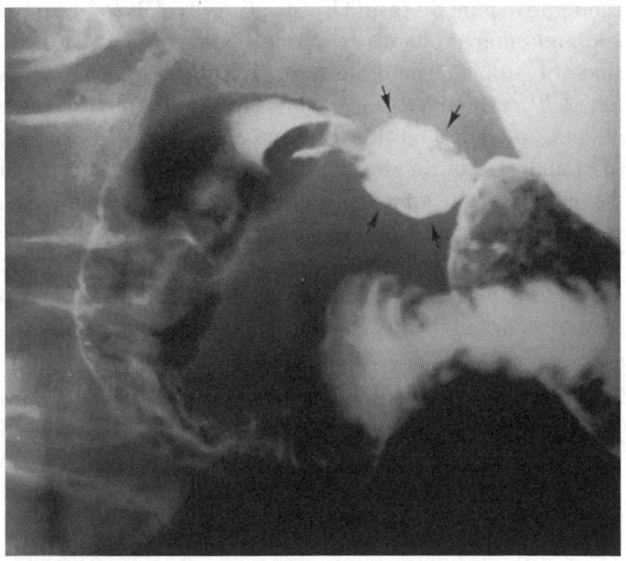

ment of nonulcer dyspepsia, duodenitis, and duodenal ulcer disease has been termed Moynihan's disease.[135] *Helicobacter pylori* infection, however, has not been shown to be the etiology of nonulcer dyspepsia, nor has a definite relationship between nonulcer dyspepsia and peptic ulcer disease been proved.[136]

In practice, therapy for nonulcer dyspepsia is the same as for peptic ulcer disease, despite the fact that in double-blind, placebo-controlled trials, histamine antagonists are only a little better than a placebo in treating this disorder, and the role of gastric acid hypersecretion in nonulcer dyspepsia is unproved by formal measurements of basal and peak acid outputs.[137,138] Peptic ulcer disease, NSAID use, *H. pylori* infection, and gastric cancer must be excluded in elderly patients who present with dyspeptic complaints.

Upper Gastrointestinal Bleeding in the Elderly

Thirty-five to 45 percent of all cases of acute upper gastrointestinal hemorrhage occur in patients beyond age 60, and of these, half are caused by peptic ulcer disease.[139–141] Other important causes of gross upper gastrointestinal bleeding in the elderly are gastric erosions and esophagitis; these two entities in combination with peptic ulcer disease account for 70 to 80 percent of hospital admissions for upper gastrointestinal bleeding in older patients.

It is unclear whether elderly patients with upper gastrointestinal hemorrhage frequently have a long history of underlying acid-peptic disease, for example, chronic peptic ulcer disease, or whether they usually bleed from newly developed lesions. In one series, 36 percent of older individuals admitted to the hospital with acute upper gastrointestinal bleeding gave no history of preceding symptoms.[140] Alternatively, some patients complain of prior epigastric pain, pain in other parts of the abdomen, anorexia, dyspepsia, pyrosis or, simply, weight loss. Elderly patients with acute upper gastrointestinal bleeding usually present with hematemesis, although 30 percent of patients have only melena.[140] Hemorrhage is often seen in persons with chronic medical illnesses, the most common being degenerative joint disease. Therapy with NSAIDs for rheumatologic and other problems has been found to be an important cause of upper gastrointestinal bleeding in elderly patients.[141,142] Other causes include disease found in younger patients, as well as entities seen almost exclusively in older individuals. Geriatric ulcers and giant duodenal ulcers are not associated with an unusually high incidence of hemorrhage, while giant gastric ulcers frequently do bleed.[129]

Aortoenteric fistula is an uncommon cause of gastrointestinal hemorrhage seen most often in men during the seventh and eighth decades of life. The most common etiology is rupture of an arteriosclerotic abdominal aortic aneurysm. Other causes of aortoenteric fistulas include graft-enteric fistula, aortitis, mycotic aneurysm, carcinoma, trauma, foreign body, and peptic ulceration.[143–145] The overwhelming majority of fistulas between the aorta and the alimentary tract occur in the duodenum and, as a result, usually produce upper gastrointestinal bleeding. Other reported sites of communication include the esophagus, stomach, distal small bowel, and colon. Most patients experience an initial self-limited or "sentinel" bleed, followed hours to days later by massive hemorrhage. Mortality is very high but may be reduced by early endoscopic detection of the fistula during investigation of the cause of bleeding. An elderly patient with an aortic graft who has upper gastrointestinal bleeding, no matter how trivial, must undergo immediate endoscopy because of the possible presence of a graft-enteric fistula.

Another rare cause of massive upper gastrointestinal hemorrhage in the elderly is a dilated gastric artery with an overlying mucosal defect, typically located within 2 cm of the cardioesophageal junction. This lesion, called exulceratio simplex, or the ulcer of Dieulafoy, often requires surgical therapy, although it has been treated effectively with electrocautery or laser.[146,147]

Occasionally, vascular abnormalities of the type found in Osler-Weber-Rendu syndrome (hereditary hemorrhagic telangiectasia) may also be responsible for upper gastrointestinal bleeding in the elderly. There may be no history of childhood epistaxis and no family history of similar occurrences, although typical telangiectactic lesions are often found in the oral cavity, lips, nailbeds, and skin.

The hospital course of elderly patients with upper gastrointestinal bleeding is similar to that of younger patients with respect to duration, amount of blood transfused, and frequency of surgery.[140,148] Older patients, however, suffer significantly more morbidity than do younger patients; complications include cardiac, neurologic, and renal disease, sepsis, and reactions to medications and transfusions. Elderly patients are more likely than young patients to die during a hospital admission for gastrointestinal bleeding, especially if peptic ulcer is the cause.

The evaluation and treatment of upper gastrointestinal bleeding in the elderly is the same as in younger individuals. Age per se is not a contraindication for surgery; the decision to operate on an individual patient must be made in the context of the clinical setting. Early surgery should be contemplated for elderly patients who have bled from ulcers, who have signs of major hemorrhage (e.g., hypotension), and when endoscopic findings imply a significant risk of recurrent bleeding.

Volvulus of the Stomach

Volvulus of the stomach is a relatively rare condition occurring most often after age 50 and requires relaxation of the gastric ligaments for its development.[149,150] Gastric volvulus may be responsible for chronic abdominal symptoms or may be manifested acutely with strangulation and gangrene.

Gastric volvulus is classified according to the axis around which the stomach rotates: torsion about a longitudinal axis formed by a line connecting the cardia and pylorus is known as organoaxial volvulus; rotation about a vertical axis passing through the middle of the lesser and greater curvatures is referred to as mesenteroaxial volvulus. Approximately 60 percent of affected patients have the organoaxial type, 30 percent have

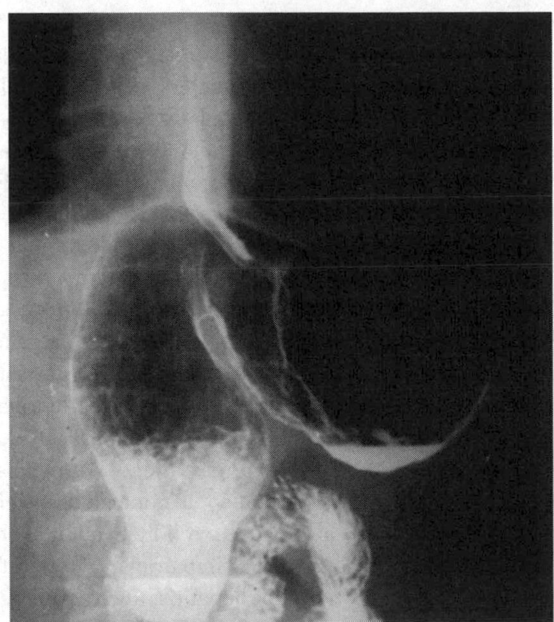

Figure 57-14 An organoaxial volvulus of the stomach identified on upper gastrointestinal series. (From Brandt,[154] with permission.)

the mesenteroaxial type, and 10 percent have a combination form. Rotation may be partial or complete; complete twists often severely impair gastric blood flow and may cause gangrene, while partial twists may be asymptomatic or responsible for chronic symptoms.

Organoaxial volvulus usually has an acute presentation and often is associated with the presence of a large paraesophageal hiatus hernia or eventration of the diaphragm. Patients complain of the abrupt onset of upper abdominal or lower thoracic pain. Vomiting gives way to retching, and it is difficult to pass a nasogastric tube beyond the gastroesophageal junction. This group of symptoms and signs has been referred to as Borchardt's triad. Roentgenograms may reveal a gas-filled viscus in the chest or an "upside-down stomach" in the upper abdomen (Fig. 57-14). Gangrene ensues in approximately 5 percent of cases, mostly in individuals with a traumatic diaphragmatic hernia. Organoaxial volvulus usually requires surgical correction.

Mesenteroaxial volvulus is often intermittent and incomplete. Affected persons complain of chronic postprandial pain, belching, bloating, vomiting, and early satiety; strangulation is rare. Diagnosis is made by barium roentgenogram. Decompression with a nasogastric tube may return the stomach to its normal position. Surgery is indicated for persistent symptoms. Some patients have been successfully treated by fixation of the stomach with two percutaneous endoscopic gastrostomy tubes; these are removed after adhesions fix the stomach to the anterior abdominal wall.

Benign Gastric Tumors

The incidence of benign gastric tumors increases with age. A hyperplastic polyp accounts for 75 to 90 percent of such growths and typically is a small, solitary lesion at the junction of the gastric body and antrum.[151] Hyperplastic polyps are not considered true neoplasms and are not premalignant. They rarely produce symptoms and thus are found incidentally in an evaluation of the upper gastrointestinal tract. In contrast, adenomatous polyps are true neoplasms and account for 10 to 25 percent of gastric polyps. The mean incidence of malignant change in gastric adenomas is reported to be anywhere from 6 to 75 percent, probably reflecting their heterogeneity in size, age, and histology (tubular, villous, or mixed).

Gastric polyps may occur in some gastrointestinal polyposis syndromes, but the only one appearing in older individuals is the Cronkhite-Canada syndrome. This disorder is acquired, not inherited, and is characterized by diffuse gastrointestinal polyposis, protein-losing enteropathy, and ectodermal abnormalities, including hyperpigmentation, alopecia, and dystrophic nail changes. Polyps in this syndrome are hamartomas composed of tubules and mucus-filled cysts.

Mesenchymal tumors, including leiomyomas, fibromas, and tumors of neural origin, account for a significant percentage of benign gastric tumors. Symptoms of these tumors are usually related to their size and not their type. Pain and bleeding are the most common manifestations.

Malignant Gastric Tumors

Gastric adenocarcinoma

Inexplicably, the incidence of gastric cancer is decreasing in the elderly, while relatively more cases are being diagnosed in younger patients.[152,153] Nevertheless, the vast majority of gastric cancers occur in patients beyond 60 years of age.[1] Carcinoma of the stomach is usually incurable by the time symptoms appear because symptoms often do not develop until the tumor is large. Initial symptoms are often mild and nonspecific. The tendency to treat dyspepsia in older patients without a diagnostic evaluation prompted Sir Heneage Ogilvie to say in the early 1900s, "in carcinoma of the stomach, alkalis are the undertaker's best friend."

Vague epigastric discomfort, anorexia, early satiety, and weight loss are the most frequent symptoms of gastric cancer. Physical examination may reveal enlarged left axillary and supraclavicular lymph nodes, an umbilical nodule, or a hard palpable left hepatic lobe. Rarely, the patient develops acanthosis nigricans, dermatomyositis, or an explosive outbreak of skin tags or keratotic lesions (sign of Leser-Trélat), raising the suspicion of a visceral neoplasm. Laboratory abnormalities are nonspecific.

Surgical excision is the only potentially curative treatment. Seventy to 90 percent of patients with gastric cancer are considered suitable for laparotomy, but only half are found to be eligible for potentially curative resections and death occurs in most of these individuals within 1 year. Five-year survival rates are 5 to 15 percent. Combined chemotherapy and irradiation may be of some benefit, but irradiation alone is ineffective except for palliation of bone pain from metastases.

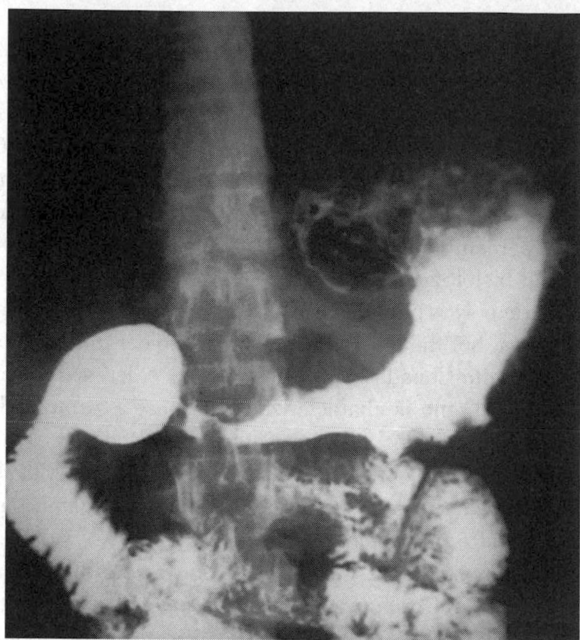

Figure 57-15 Upper gastrointestinal series showing a gastric lymphoma with antral narrowing mimicking an adenocarcinoma. (From Brandt,[154] with permission.)

Gastric lymphoma

The stomach is the most frequent site of primary, extranodal lymphoma and accounts for one-half to three-fourths of patients with lymphoma of the gastrointestinal tract. Gastric lymphoma produces nonspecific symptoms, but epigastric pain with weight loss and a palpable mass in a patient who is otherwise well is typical. Radiographically, lymphoma resembles carcinoma in up to two-thirds of cases (Fig. 57-15). Large, ulcerated masses, hyperrugosity, polypoid lesions, or antral narrowing suggests lymphoma. A definitive diagnosis cannot be made from gastroscopic brush cytology and biopsy, and laparotomy may be necessary. Therapy is wide excision followed by radiation and leads to a 5-year survival of about 40 to 50 percent.

Systemic Diseases

Diabetes mellitus

Patients with long-standing diabetes mellitus often have profound abnormalities of gastrointestinal motility, including delayed gastric emptying of solids. Such abnormalities are frequently without clinical manifestations, although difficulty controlling plasma glucose, due to an inconstant and unpredictable rate of gastric emptying, may be a subtle indication of gastroparesis. Gastric atony may be manifested by a gradual onset of upper abdominal fullness, satiety, and vomiting. Gastroparesis and accompanying hypochlorhydria probably underlie the development of gastric bezoars and bacterial and fungal overgrowth in this population.

A number of potential problems must be considered in prescribing acid-suppressive therapy for elderly patients with peptic ulcer disease. Many antacid preparations contain large amounts of mineral salts which may produce undesirable effects, such as fluid retention, diarrhea, or constipation. Aluminum hydroxide forms insoluble chelates with a number of drugs, including digoxin, quinidine, and tetracycline, interfering with their absorption. Histamine antagonists variably inhibit the oxidative metabolism of many drugs, prolonging their duration of action. Cimetidine impairs the elimination of lidocaine, nifedipine, phenytoin, propranolol, quinidine, theophylline, and warfarin, to mention a few. Ranitidine is a less potent inhibitor of mixed-function oxidases than cimetidine, and alterations in drug metabolism caused by ranitidine are usually not associated with pharmacologic effects. Famotidine has no effect on the oxidative metabolism of drugs. Intravenous administration of cimetidine in elderly patients with impaired renal function may produce mental confusion in a dose-related fashion. Cimetidine may also cause a mild elevation of serum creatinine levels unassociated with impairment of renal function. Ranitidine is a rare cause of hepatitis, and ranitidine and famotidine may cause headache. Sucralfate frequently causes constipation in elderly individuals. The National Institutes of Health Consensus Development Panel has published guidelines mandating antibiotic treatment of all ulcer patients infected with *H. pylori*, including those without an active ulcer crater or dyspeptic symptoms.[109]

Nonulcer Dyspepsia

Patients with nonulcer dyspepsia suffer from chronic, recurrent upper abdominal pain and nausea which may or may not be related to meals and which occurs in the absence of an ulcer crater.[130] Nonulcer dyspepsia is at least twice as common as true peptic ulcer disease. Most patients with this problem have no recognizable pathologic abnormality, although many have histologic gastritis.[107] Nonulcer dyspepsia is further defined by the absence of reflux esophagitis, disease of the biliary tract or pancreas, or most symptoms of irritable bowel syndrome. The criteria used to select patients for inclusion in clinical studies of nonulcer dyspepsia are very inconsistent, perpetuating confusion about this diagnosis among physicians and patients.[131]

Diabetic gastroparesis is caused by an abnormality of the autonomic nervous system almost always associated with peripheral or autonomic neuropathy. Metoclopramide has been used to improve gastric motility and relieve symptoms but causes intolerable central nervous system effects in many patients. Cisapride, a prokinetic agent that acts mainly by facilitating acetylcholine release, is better tolerated but may cause cramping and diarrhea.

Amyloidosis

The gastrointestinal tract is involved in 50 to 75 percent of patients with amyloidosis, and in approximately one-half of these cases the stomach is affected. It is unusual for signs and symptoms of gastrointestinal involvement to be directly attributable to the amyloidosis per se. Outlet obstruction may be caused by an obstructing mass of amyloid in the distal stomach. Amyloid may also diffusely infiltrate the gastric wall, making surgery difficult, and may be associated with giant gastric ulcers resistant to medical therapy. Prognosis is related to that of the primary disease.

References

1. Everhart JE (ed): Digestive Diseases in the United States: Epidemiology and Impact. US Department of Health and Human Services, Public Health Service, National Institutes of Health, National Institute of Diabetes and Digestive and Kidney Diseases. NIH Publication 94–1447. U.S. Government Printing Office, Washington, DC, 1994
2. Cohen RA, Van Nostrand JF: Trends in the Health of Older Americans: United States, 1994. National Center for Health Statistics. 1995; Vital Health Stat 3(30)
3. Shafar J: Dysgeusia in the elderly. Lancet 1965;i:83–84
4. Henkin RI, Schiechter PJ, Hoye R et al: Idiopathic hypogeusia with dysgeusia, hyposmia and dysosmia. JAMA 1971;217: 434–440
5. Finch CE, Hayflick L: Muscle. p. 709. Handbook of the Biology of Aging. Van Nostrand Reinhold, New York, 1977
6. Nordin B: Clinical significance and pathogenesis of osteoporosis. BMJ 1971;1:571
7. Busse EW: How mind, body and environment influence nutrition in the elderly. Postgrad Med 1978;63:118
8. Henkin RI, Graziadei PPG, Bradley DF: The molecular basis of taste and its disorders. Ann Intern Med 1969;71:791–821
9. Griffith IP: Abnormalities of smell and taste. Practitioner 1976;217:907–913
10. Guerrier Y, Uziel A: Clinical aspects of taste disorders. Acta Otolaryngol (Stock) 1979;87:232–235
11. Baum BJ: Evaluation of stimulated partoid saliva flow rate in different age groups. J Dent Res 1950;29:686
12. Bean WB: The changing incidence of certain vascular lesions of the skin with aging. Geriatrics 1956;11:97–102
13. Shiffman MA, Rappaport I: Multiple phlebectasia. Arch Surg 1967;94:771–775
14. Carnel SB, Blakeslee DB, Oswald SG et al: Treatment of radiation- and chemotherapy-induced stomatitis. Otolaryngol Head Neck Surg 1990;102:326–330
15. Barker G, Loftus L, Cuddy P, Barker B: The effects of sucralfate suspension and diphenhydramine syrup plus kaolin-pectin on radiotherapy-induced mucositis. Oral Surg Oral Med Oral Pathol 1991;71:288–293
16. Shafer WG, Waldron CA: A clinical and histopathologic study of oral leukoplakia. Surg Gynecol Obstet 1961;112:411–420
17. Pindborg JJ, Jolst O, Renstrup G et al: Studies in oral leukoplakia based on a follow-up study of 248 patients. J Am Dent Assoc 1968;76:767–771
18. Shafer WG et al: A Textbook of Oral Pathology. 4th Ed. WB Saunders, Philadelphia, 1984
19. Shklar G: Oral Cancer: The Diagnosis, Therapy, Management, and Rehabilitation of the Oral Cancer Patient. WB Saunders, Philadelphia, 1983
20. Wynder EL, Bross IJ, Feldman RM: A study of the etiological factors in cancer in the mouth. Cancer 1957;10:1300–1323
21. Buchholz DW, Boxma JF, Donner MW: Adaptation, compensation, and decompensation of the pharyngeal swallow. Gastrointest Radiol 1985;10:235–239
22. Piaget F, Fouillet J: Le pharynx et l'oseuphage séniles: stude clinique radiogique et radiocinematographique. J Med Lyon 1959;40:951
23. Cattau EL, Castell DO: Symptoms of esophageal dysfunction. Adv Intern Med 1982;27:151–181
24. Hurwitz AL, Newlson JA, Haddad JK: Oropharyngeal dysphagia. Am J Dig Dis 1975;20:313–324
25. Belsey R: Pulmonary complaints of esophageal diseases. Br J Dis Chest 1960;54:342–348
26. Hurwitz AL, Duranceau A: Upper esophageal sphincter dysfunction: pathogenesis and treatment. Am J Dig Dis 1978;23: 275–281
27. Holinger PH, Schild JA: The Zenker's (hypopharyngeal) diverticulum. Ann Otol 1969;78:679–688
28. Knuff TE, Benjamin SB, Castell DO: Pharyngoesophageal (Zenker's) diverticulum: a reappraisal. Gastroenterology 1982;82:734–736
29. Huang B, Unni KK, Payne WS: Long-term survival following diverticulectomy for cancer in pharyngoesophageal (Zenker's) diverticulum. Ann Thorac Surg 1984;38:207
30. Huang B, Payne WS, Cameron SJ: Surgical management for recurrent pharyngoesophageal (Zenker's) diverticulum. Ann Thorac Surg 1984;37:189
31. Einarsson S, Hallen O: On the treatment of esophageal diverticula. Acta Otol Laryngol 1967;64:30
32. Norris CW: Pharyngoceles of the esophagus. Laryngoscope 1979;89:1788–1807
33. Soergel KH, Zboralske FF, Amberg JR: Presbyesophagus: esophageal motility in nonagenarians. J Clin Invest 1964;43: 1472
34. Hollis JB, Castell DO: Esophageal function in elderly men: a new look at "presbyesophagus." Ann Intern Med 1974;80: 371
35. Khan TA, Shragge BW, Crispin JS, Lind JF: Esophageal motility in the elderly. Am J Dig Dis 1977;22:1049–1054
36. Richter JE, Wu WC, Johns DN et al: Esophageal manometry in 95 healthy adult volunteers: variability of pressures with age and frequency of "abnormal" contraction. Dig Dis Sci 1987;32:583–592
37. Castell DO: The aging esophagus, letter. Dig Dis 1978;23: 667
38. Castell DO: Dysphagia. Gastroenterology 1979;76: 1015–1024
39. Richter JE: Heartburn, dysphagia, odynophagia, and other esophageal symptoms. p. 331. In Sleisenger MH, Fordtran JS (eds): Gastrointestinal Disease: Pathophysiology, Diagnosis and Management. 5th Ed. WB Saunders, Philadelphia, 1993
40. Raiha I, Hietanen E, Sourander L: Symptoms of gastro-oesophageal reflux disease in elderly people. Age Ageing 1991;20: 365–370

41. Edwards DAW: Discriminative information in the diagnosis of dysphagia. J R Coll Physicians Lond 1975;9:257
42. Schatzki R: Panel discussion on diseases of the esophagus. Am J Gastroenterol 1959;31:117–119
43. Collen MJ, Abdulian JD, Chen YK: Gastroesophageal reflux disease in the elderly: more severe disease that requires aggressive therapy. Am J Gastroenterol 1995;90:1053–1057
44. Katz PO, Dalton CB, Richter JE et al: Esophageal testing of patients with noncardiac chest pain or dysphagia: results of three year's experience with 1161 patients. Ann Intern Med 1987;106:593–597
45. Russell COH, Hill LD, Holmes ER III et al: Radionuclide transit: a sensitive screening test for esophageal dysfunction. Gastroenterology 1981;80:887–892
46. Mayberry JF, Atkinson M: Studies on the incidence and prevalence of achalasia in the Nottingham area. Q J Med 1985;56: 451–456
47. Kahrilas PJ, Kishik SM, Helm JF et al: Comparison of pseudoachalasia and achalasia. Am J Med 1987;82:439
48. Sandler RS, Bozymsky EM, Orlando RC: Failure of clinical criteria to distinguish between primary achalasia and achalasia secondary to tumor. Dig Dis Sci 1982;27:209–213
49. Clouse RE, Abramson BK, Todorczuk JR: Achalasia in the elderly: effects of aging on clinical presentation and outcome. Dig Dis Sci 1991;36:225–228
50. Goulbourne IA, Walbaum PR: Long-term results of Heller operation for achalasia. J R Coll Surg Edin 1985;30:101–103
51. Kolodny M, Schrader ZR, Rubin W: Esophageal achalasia probably due to gastric carcinoma. Ann Intern Med 1968;69: 569–572
52. Menin R, Fisher RS: Return of esophageal peristalsis in achalasia secondary to gastric cancer. Dig Dis Sci 1981;26: 1038–1044
53. Davis JA, Kantrowitz PA, Chandler HL et al: Reversible achalasia due to reticulum cell sarcoma. New Engl J Med 1975; 293:130–132
54. Richter JE, Hackshaw BT, Wu WC et al: Edrophonium: a useful provocative test for esophageal chest pain. Ann Intern Med 1985;103:14–21
55. Wesdorp ICF: Treatment of reflux esophagitis. Scand J Gastroenterol 1982;79:106–119
56. Spechler SJ, Goyal RK: Barrett's esophagus. New Engl J Med 1986;315:362–371
57. Spechler SJ, Goyal RK: The columnar-lined esophagus, intestinal metaplasia, and Norman Barrett. Gastroenterology 1996; 110:614–621
58. Spechler SJ: Endoscopic surveillance for patients with Barrett esophagus: does the cancer risk justify the practice? Ann Intern Med 1987;106:902–904
59. Achkar E, Carey W: The cost of surveillance for adenocarcinoma complicating Barrett's esophagus. Am J Gastroenterol 1988;83:291
60. Schatzki R, Gary JE: Dysphagia due to a diaphragm-like localized narrowing in the lower esophagus ("lower esophageal ring"). Am J Radiol 1953;70:911
61. Goyal RK, Bauer JL, Spiro HM: The nature and location of lower esophageal ring. New Engl J Med 1971;284:1775
62. Hendrix TR: Schatzki ring, epithelial junction, and hiatal hernia—an unresolved controversy. Gastroenterology 1980;79: 584
63. Birnholz JC, Ferrucci TT Jr, Wyman SM: Roentgen features of dysphagia aortica. Radiology 1974;111:93–96
64. Mucklow EH, Smith OE: Dysphagia and unusual radiographic appearances associated with the variable relationships of the aorta and lower oesophagus. J Fac Radiol 1954;6:88–95
65. Pearson RH, Bessell EM, Bowely NB: Compression of oesophagus by toruous dilated aorta. BMJ 1981;282:1032–1033
66. McMillin IKR, Hyde I: Compression of the oesophagus by the aorta. Thorax 1969;24:32–38
67. Kikendall JW, Friedman AC, Oyewole M et al: Pill-induced esophageal injury: case reports and review of the medical literature. Dig Dis Sci 1983;28:174–182
68. Bott S, Prakash C, McCallum RW: Medication-induced esophageal injury: survey of the literature. Am J Gastroenterol 1987; 82:758
69. Channer KS, Virjee JP: The effect of size and shape of tablets on their esophageal transit. J Clin Pharmacol 1986;26:141
70. Wheeler D: Diverticula of foregut. Radiology 1947;49: 476–481
71. Debas HT, Payne WS, Cameron AJ et al: Physiopathology of lower esophageal diverticulum and its implications for treatment. Surg Gynecol Obstet 1980;151:593–600
72. Habein H, Moersch H, Kirklin J: Diverticula of the lower part of the esophagus. Arch Intern Med 1956;97:768–777
73. Bender MK, Haddad JK: Disappearance of multiple esophageal diverticula following treatment of esophagitis. Gastrointest Endosc 1973;20:19–22
74. Hurwitz AL, Way LW, Haddad JK: Epiphrenic diverticulum in association with an unusual motility disturbance: report of surgical correction. Gastroenterology 1975;68:795–798
75. Payne WS, Clagett OT: Pharyngeal and esophageal diverticula. pp. 25–26. In Current Problems in Surgery. Year Book Medical Publishers, Chicago, 1965
76. Cho SR, Sanders MM, Turner MA et al: Esophageal intramural pseudodiverticulosis. Gastrointest Radiol 1981;6:9–16
77. Lupovitch A, Tippins R: Esophageal intramural pseudodiverticulosis: a disease of adnexal glands. Radiology 1974;113: 271–272
78. Gorback SL, Nahas L, Lerner PI et al: Studies of intestinal microflora. I. Effects of diet, age and periodic sampling on numbers of fecal microorganisms in man. Gastroenterology 1967;53:845–855
79. Kodsi BE, Wickremesinghe PC, Kozinn PJ et al: Candida esophagitis: a prospective study of 27 cases. Gastroenterology 1976;71:715–719
80. Scott BB, Jenkins D: Gastro-oesophageal candidiasis. Gut 1982;23:137–139
81. Wienbeck M, Berges W: Oesophageal lesions in the alcoholic. Clin Gastroenterol 1981;10:375

82. La Vecchia CL, Liati P, Decarli A et al: Tar yields of cagarettes and the risk of oesophageal cancer. Int J Cancer 1986;38:381

83. Carter R, Brewer LA: Achalasia and esophageal carcinoma: studies in early diagnosis for improved surgical management. Am J Surg 1975;130:114

84. Appelqvist P, Salmo M: Lye corrosin carcinoma of the esophagus. Cancer 1980;45:2655

85. Hameeteman W, Tytgat GN, Houthoff HJ et al: Barrett's esophagus: development of dysplasia and adenocarcinoma. Gastroenterology 1989;96:1249–1256

86. Sondik EJ, Dessler LG, Ries LA: Cancer Statistics Review 1973–1986, Including a Report on the Status of Cancer Control. National Cancer Institute, Division of Cancer Prevention and Control, Surveillance Program. NIH Publication. 89–2789. U.S. Government Printing Office, Washington DC, 1989

87. Lawrence WL Jr: Surgical management of gastrointestinal cancer. Clin Gastroenterol 1976;5:703

88. Cooper JD, Jamieson WRE, Blair N et al: The palliative value of surgical resection for carcinoma of the esopahgus. Can J Surg 1981;24:145

89. Payne WS: Palliation of esophageal carcinoma. Ann Thorac Surg 1979;28:208

90. Evans MA et al: Gastric emptying rate in the elderly: implications for drug therapy. J Am Geriatr Soc 1981;29:201

91. Moore JG et al: Effect of age on gastric emptying of liquid-solid meals in man. Dig Dis Sci 1983;28:340

92. Blackman AH, Lambert DL, Thayer WR et al: Computed normal values for peak acid output based on age, sex and body weight. Am J Dig Dis 1970;15:783–789

93. Goldschmiedt M, Barnett CC, Schwarz BE et al: Effect of age on gastric acid secretion and serum gastrin concentrations in healthy men and women. Gastroenterology 1991;101: 977–990

94. Kekki M, Samloff IM, Ihamaki T et al: Age- and sex-related behavior of gastric acid secretion at the population level. Scand J Gastroenterol 1982;17:737–743

95. Misiewixz JJ, Price AB, Tytgat GNJ: Working party report to the World Congresses of Gastroenterology, Sydney, 1990. J Gastroenterol Hepatol 1991;6:207–234

96. Carpenter HA, Talley NJ: Gastroscopy is incomplete without biopsy: clinical relevance of distinguishing gastropathy from gastritis. 1995;108:917–924

97. Yoshida N, Granger DN, Evans DJ Jr et al: Mechanisms involved in *Helicobacter pylori*-induced inflammation. Gastroenterology 1993;105:1431–1440

98. Hawkey CJ, Hudson N: Mucosal injury caused by drugs, chemicals, and stress. pp. 656–699. In Haubrich WS, Schaffner F (eds): Bockus, Gastroenterology. 5th Ed. WB Saunders, Philadelphia, 1995

99. Wyatt JL, Dixon MF: Chronic gastritis—a pathogenetic approach. J Pathol 1988;154:113–124

100. Boren T, Falk P, Roth KA et al: Attachment of *Helicobacter pylori* to human gastric epithelium mediated by blood group antigens. Science 1993;262:1892–1895

101. Blaser MJ: *Helicobacter pylori* and the pathogenesis of gastroduodenal inflammation. J Infect Dis 1990;161:626–633

102. Rathbone BJ, Heatley RV: Possible pathogenic mechanisms in *Helicobacter pylori* infection. p. 217. In Rathbone BJ, Heatley RV (eds): *Helicobacter pylori* and Gastroduodenal Disease. Blackwell Scientific Publications, Oxford, 1992

103. Parsonnet J, Freiedman GD, Vandersteen DP et al: *Helicobacter pylori* infection and the risk of gastric carcinoma. N Engl J Med 1991;325:1170–1171

104. Dooley CP, Cohen H, Fitzgibbons PL et al: Prevalence of *Helicobacter pylori* infection and histologic gastritis in asymptomatic persons. N Engl J Med 1989;321:1562–1566

105. Banatvala N, Mayo K, Megraud F et al: The cohort effect and *Helicobacter pylori*. J Infect Dis 1993;168:219–221

106. Morris A, Nicholson G: *Helicobacter pylori*: human ingestion studies. p. 209. In Rathbone BJ, Heatley RV (eds): *Helicobacter pylori* and Gastroduodenal Disease. Blackwell Scientific Publications, Oxford, 1992

107. Shallcross TM, Rathbone BJ, Heatley RV: *Helicobacter pylori* and non-ulcer dyspepsia. p. 165. In Rathbone BJ, Heatley RV (eds): *Helicobacter pylori* and Gastroduodenal Disease. Blackwell Scientific Publications, Oxford, 1992

108. Chiba N, Rao BV, Rademaker JW et al: Meta-analysis of the efficacy of the antibiotic therapy in eradicating *Helicobacter pylori*. Am J Gastroenterol 1992;87:1716–1726

109. NIH Consensus Development Panel on *Helicobacter pylori* in Peptic Ulcer Disease: *Helicobacter pylori* in peptic ulcer disease. JAMA 1994;272:66–69

110. FDC Reports. November 29, 1987:8

111. Armstrong CP, Blower AL: Nonsteroidal anti-inflammatory drugs and life threatening complications of peptic ulceration. Gut 1987;28:527–532

112. Silverstein FE, Graham DY, Senior JR et al: Misoprostol reduces serious gastrointestinal complications in patients with rheumatoid arthritis receiving nonsteroidal anti-inflammatory drugs. Ann Intern Med 1995;123:241–249

113. Gabriel SE, Jaakkimainen L, Bombardier C: Risk for serious gastrointestinal complications related to use of nonsteroidal anti-inflammatory drugs. Ann Intern Med 1991;115: 787–796

114. Walt R, Katschinski B, Logan R et al: Rising frequency of ulcer perforation in elderly people in United Kingdom. Lancet 1986;2:489–492

115. Graham DY, Smith JL, Spjut HJ, Torres E: Gastric adaptation: studies in humans during continuous aspirin administration. Gastroenterology 1988;95:327–333

116. Graham DY, Smith JL: Aspirin and the stomach. Ann Intern Med 1986;104:390–398

117. Fries JF, Miller SR, Spitz PW et al: Toward an epidemiology of gastropathy associated with nonsteroidal anti-inflammatory drug use. Gastroenterology 1989;96:647–655

118. Griffin MR, Piper JM, Daughterty JR et al: Nonsteroidal anti-inflammatory drug use and increased risk for peptic ulcer disease in elderly persons. Ann Intern Med 1991;114: 257–263

119. Soll AH, Kurata J, McGuigan JE: Ulcers, nonsteroidal anti-

inflammatory drugs, and related matters. Gastroenterology 1989;96:561–568

120. Dajani EZ, Agrawal NM: Prevention and treatment of ulcers induced by nonsteroidal anti-inflammatory drugs: an update. J Physiol Pharmacol 1995;46:3–16

121. Ehsanullah RSB, Page MC, Tildesley G, Wood JR: Prevention of gastroduodenal damage induced by non-steroidal anti-inflammatory drugs: controlled trial of ranitidine. BMJ 1988; 297:1017–1021

122. Robinson MG, Griffin JW Bowers J et al: Effect of rnaitidine gastroduodenal (sic) mucosal damage induced by nonsteroidal antiinflammatory drugs. Dig Dis Sci 1989;34:424–428

123. Taha AS, Hudson N, Hawkey CJ et al: Famotidine for the prevention of gastric and duodenal ulcers caused by nonsteroidal anti-inflammatory drugs. N Engl J Med 1996;334: 1435–1439

124. Graham DY, White RH, Moreland LW et al: Duodenal and gastric ulcer prevention with misoprostol in arthritis patients taking NSAIDs. Ann Intern Med 1993;119:257–262

125. Permutt RP, Cello JP: Duodenal ulcer disease in the hospitalized elderly patient. Dig Dis Sci 1982;27:1

126. Levrat M, Pasquier J, Lambert R et al: Pepteic ulcer in patients over 60: experience in 287 cases. Am J Dig Dis 1966;11: 279–285

127. Elashoff JD, Grossman MI: Trends in hospital admissions and death rates for peptic ulcer in the United States from 1970 to 1978. Gastroenterology 1980;78:280–285

128. Barragry TP, Blatchford JW III, Allen MO: Giant gastric ulcers: a review of 49 cases. Ann Surg 1986;203:255–299

129. Strange SL: Giant innocent gastric ulcer in the elderly. Geront Clin 1963;5:171–189

130. Talley NJ, Phillips SF: Non-ulcer dyspepsia: potential causes and pathophysiology. Ann Intern Med 1988;108:865–879

131. Barbara L, Camilleri M, Corinaldesi R et al: Definition and investigation of dyspepsia—consensus of an international *ad hoc* working party. Dig Dis Sci 1989;34:1272–1276

132. Camilleri M, Malagelada JR, Kao PC, Zinsmeister AR: Gastric and autonomic responses to stress in functional dyspepsia. Dig Dis Sci 1986;31:1169–1177

133. Greydanus MP, Vassallo M, Camilleri M et al: Neurohormonal factors in functional dyspepsia: insights on pathophysiological mechanisms. Gastroenterology 1991;100:1311–1318

134. Halter F, Miazza B, Brignoli R: Cisapride or cimetidine in the treatment of functional dyspepsia. Scand J Gastroenterol 1994; 29:618–623

135. Spiro HM: Moynihan's disease? the diagnosis of duodenal ulcer. N Engl J Med 1974;291:567–569

136. Talley NJ: A critique of therapeutic trials in *Helicobacter pylori*-positive functional dyspepsia. Gastroenterol 1994;106: 1174–1183

137. Dobrilla G, Comberlato M, Steele A, Vallaperta P: Drug treatment of functional dyspepsia: a meta-analysis of randomized controlled clinical trials. J Clin Gastroenterol 1989;11: 169–177

138. Collen MJ, Loebenberg MJ: Basal gastric acid secretion in nonulcer dyspepsia with or without duodentitis. Dig Dis Sci 1989;34:246–250

139. Antler AS, Pitchumoni CS, Thomas E et al: Gastrointestinal bleeding in the elderly: morbidity, mortality and cause. Am Surg 1981;142:271

140. Cooper BT, Weston CFM, Neuman CS: Acute upper gastrointestinal haemorrhage in patients aged 80 years or more. Q J Med 1988;258:765

141. Beard K, Walker AM, Perera DR et al: Nonsteroidal antiinflammatory drug use and hospitalization for gastroesophageal bleeding in the elderly. Arch Intern Med 1987;147:1621

142. Griffin MR, Ray WA, Schaffner W: Nonsteroidal antiinflammatory drug use and death from peptic ulcer in elderly persons. Ann Intern Med 1988;109:359

143. Champion MC, Sullivan SN, Coles JC et al: Aortenteric fistula: incidence, presentation, recognition, and management. Ann Surg 1982;195:314

144. Connolly JE, Kwaan JHM, McArt PM et al: Aortoenteric fistula. Ann Surg 1981;194:402

145. Schramek A, Weisz GM, Erlik D: Gastrointestinal bleeding due to arterio-enteric fistula. Digestion 1971;4:103

146. Pointer R, Schwab G, Konigsrainer A et al: Endoscopic treatment of Dieulafoy's disease. Gastroenterology 1988;94:563

147. Veldhuyzen van Zanten SJO, Bartelsman JFWM, Schipper MEI et al: Recurrent massive haematemesis from Dieulafoy vascular malformations—a review of 101 cases. Gut 1986; 27:213

148. Silverstein FE, Gilbert DA, Tedesco FJ et al: The National ASGE Survey on Gastrointestinal Bleeding. II. clinical prognostic factors. Gastrointest Endosc 1981;27:80

149. Carter R, Brewer LA III, Hinshaw DB: Acute gastric volvulus: a study of 25 cases. Am J Surg 1980;140:99–106

150. Patel NM: Chronic gastric volvulus: report of a case and review of literature. Am J Gastroenterol 1985;80:170

151. Ming SC, Goldman H: Gastric polyps: a histogenetic classification and its relation to carcinoma. Cancer 1965;18:721–726

152. Cancer statistics: Cancer J Clin 1981;31:13

153. Keppen M: Upper gastrointestinal malignancies in the elderly. Clin Geriatr Med 1987;3:637

154. Brandt LJ: Gastrointestinal Disorders of the Elderly. 1st Ed. Lippincott-Raven, New York

CHAPTER 58

The Pancreas

JOAN M. BRAGANZA
N. M. SHARER

Consult the current[1] or previous[2] pancreatic bible, examine the proceedings of symposia,[3–6] or read influential reviews[7–13] and it will become apparent that diseases of the exocrine pancreas have defied two centuries of therapeutic endeavor. An attack of pancreatitis causes up to 20 percent of patients to die of multiorgan dysfunction syndrome (MODS); resective pancreatic surgery is the palliative answer when the pain from chronic pancreatitis becomes unbearable; most patients with pancreatic cancer die within 6 months of the first symptom; the risk of this dreaded tumor is amplified by pre-existing chronic pancreatitis[14] and seemingly also by its surest antecedent illness, cystic fibrosis,[15] or even an isolated attack of pancreatitis.[16]

Clinicians and experimentalists have been reluctant to face up to the prospect that the bleak outlook for patients with pancreatitis might indicate shaky pathogenetic premises.[17] These tenets and the current consensus on management are discussed in the first section of this chapter. Thereafter we will focus on a "radical" approach that has already fulfilled its therapeutic potential in patients with chronic pancreatitis, is poised to offer first-line treatment for acute pancreatitis and holds out opportunities for prophylaxis. The new concept may be especially germane to the idiosyncrasies of pancreatic disease in the elderly.[18–29]

Acute Pancreatitis

Definition and Natural History

The phrase *acute pancreatitis* describes sudden inflammation of the pancreas. The histologic spectrum is wide, ranging from interstitial pancreatitis, with pancreatic edema, inflammatory cells and foci of interstitial and/or pancreatic fat necrosis, to necrotizing pancreatitis, when portions of the gland become devitalized and may be overrun with hemorrhages.[30] These features have for a long time been taken to represent autodigestion due to premature activation of trypsinogen; formerly an intraductal location of this problem was favored, from contact with enterokinase in refluxed duodenal juice or abnormal bile; more recently an intra-acinar location has been proposed, via excessive contact between the zymogen and the lysosomal enzyme cathepsin B.[1]

Pancreatitis is rapidly self-limiting in most cases, but approximately 40 percent of patients develop local or systemic complications and up to half of them die. The main local complications are infected necrosis, with bacterial or fungal invasion of devitalized tissue; pseudocyst, a sterile collection of pancreatic juice localized in the lesser sac or within the gland substance and indicating disruption of a pancreatic duct or ductule; infected pseudocyst; and pancreatic abscess, a bacterially infected collection of purulent fluid bounded by adjacent organs.[31] In about 10 percent of patients, death from MODS, usually including adult respiratory distress syndrome (ARDS), occurs so rapidly that pancreatitis may only be recognized as the cause at autopsy; a further 10 percent succumb 3 to 4 weeks later when colonic bacteria have translocated to the pancreas.[32] These risks are revisited if the etiological agent is not eliminated.

The terms *acute pancreatitis* and *chronic pancreatitis* are histologic definitions.[1,2,6,30] The former describes a gland that was previously normal and will return to normal when (and if) it recovers from the active lesions of edema and/or hemorrhage and/or necrosis. The latter indicates that the attack or recurrence occurred against a background of smoldering destruction, such that the stigmata of patchy acinar loss and replacement fibrosis remain as indelible evidence after the lesions of active damage have healed. However, in clinical jargon *pancreatitis* describes any painful attack of active pancreatic damage and should be—but in practice seldom is—further qualified on the basis of morphologic and functional tests done 6 weeks after full recovery. If both aspects are within normal limits a retrospective diagnosis of acute pancreatitis is retained; if one or other modality is unequivocally abnormal a diagnosis of chronic pancreatitis is revealed.[1,2,6,17] It has been regarded as axiomatic that acute pancreatitis, even if it recurs, does not progress to chronic pancreatitis except when the main pancreatic duct is severed during a virulent attack; in this rare event the lesions of chronic pancreatitis develop upstream. Implicit in this concept is that the two diseases are fundamentally different etiologically and pathogenetically. Furthermore, clinicians have been exhorted to exclude from any discussion on pancreatitis the lesions associated with cystic fibrosis, kwashiorkor, and metal storage diseases.[1,2,6]

Demography and Etiological Factors

Figures cited for the incidence of acute pancreatitis range between 0.01 and 0.5 percent. This variability reflects differences in the source of information, whether extrapolated from hospital admissions or unselected autopsies, dissimilar end points for diagnosis, and esoteric factors such as geography, culture, ethnicity, and even season of data collection.[2,18,33]

The risk factors[1,2] are conveniently grouped as follows: (1) conditions that impede pancreatic drainage (e.g., migrating gallstone, periampullary tumor), (2) conditions that compromise the pancreatic microcirculation (e.g., hypertriglyceridemia, oligemic shock), and (3) conditions that interfere with acinar cell metabolism (e.g., prescribed drugs, industrial toxins, infective agents).[34,35] More than one ignition route may be involved in certain circumstances. Thus, an alcoholic debauch causes spasm of the sphincter of Oddi and has multifarious effects on the metabolism of the acinar cell[1,35]; the high frequency of acute pancreatitis after coronary artery bypass grafting (CABG) has been ascribed to pancreatic ischemia and also to perturbation of calcium homeostasis[36]; and the inevitability of acinar cell dysfunction after pancreatic transplantation, progressing to frank pancreatitis in a third of cases, could reflect the previous two factors and also the use of immunosuppressive drugs.[37] No etiological factor is identified in up to 50 percent of cases, but it has been argued that microlithiasis may be responsible for a substantial number, in that endoscopic sphincterotomy and/or the use of ursodeoxycholic acid may prevent relapses.[38]

In the older age group, gallstones are the overriding risk factor and are present in more than 75 percent of patients over the age of 80 years.[19] Pancreatic ischemia is another important consideration, from atherosclerosis or arteritis,[18] aortic or renal grafting, or CABG. Operative trauma has been implicated in about 12 percent of cases.[19] Prescribed drugs (e.g., diuretics, steroids, tetracycline), unusual infections (e.g., aspergillosis, tuberculosis, candidiasis),[28] and invasive tests such as endoscopic retrograde cholangiopancreatography (ERCP) account for a few cases. Hypothermia and smoke inhalation[39] should not be forgotten since these are hazards to which the elderly are particularly susceptible. Alcoholism, blunt trauma to the abdomen, viral infection, and metabolic disturbances are under-represented among the elderly. The disease is idiopathic in at least 30 percent of cases.

Clinical Features

Clinical features depend on the time that has elapsed and on disease severity. The classic manifestation is as an attack of excruciating upper abdominal pain accompanied by an abrupt rise in blood levels of amylase, lipase, and all the other normal secretory constituents of the gland. The pain may pass through to the back or radiate into the lower chest on the left side and sometimes into the left shoulder or right hypochondrium. Nausea and vomiting occur in many cases. In elderly patients the following peculiarities should be borne in mind: the pain may be predominantly in the lower abdomen; an acute confusional state or even coma may be the presenting feature; the condition may be "silent," especially after major surgery when analgesics are given; infarction or major organ failure may result.[20,24]

There may be little to find on abdominal examination if the patient reports soon after the onset of pain. Tenderness and guarding with reduced bowel sounds accompany an established attack. Pyrexia and/or icterus suggest a stone in the common bile duct with cholangitis. In a very severe attack the patient is quickly propelled into a state of shock. Subcutaneous fat necrosis is an extremely rare feature. So too is bluish discoloration of the periumbilical region or flanks (Cullen's sign or Grey Turner's sign, respectively), indicating hemorrhagic necrosis. The clinician must be vigilant for signs of alimentary (intestinal obstruction, hemorrhage, perforation), hepatobiliary (obstructive or hepatocellular jaundice), metabolic (hyperglycemia, hypocalcemia, hypoalbuminemia), hematologic (coagulation disorders), renal (prerenal failure, tubular necrosis), neurologic (confused state, coma), cardiovascular (electrocardiogram [ECG] changes suggesting infarction, circulatory failure), and pulmonary complications (hypoxemia, shock lung). By the end of the second week an epigastric mass may be discernible, representing a pancreatic pseudocyst or abscess.

Diagnosis

The clinical value of any test depends on its sensitivity (positivity in disease), specificity (negativity in the absence of disease), and laboratory performance. However useful these characteristics may be, the predictive value of a positive result (the chance that an abnormal result truly indicates the disease) is governed by the local prevalence of the disease, remaining low when the disease is rare. By contrast, prevalence has little impact on the predictive value of a negative result (the chance that a normal result reliably excludes the disease).[40] Application of these Bayesian principles shows that the simple blood amylase test is far from ideal[2,41] for several reasons: (1) Serum amylase represents the sum of pancreatic and salivary isoenzymes, and their proportion differs among ethnic groups.[17] (2) Even if the level of pancreatic isoenzyme is measured, its increment depends on the time that has elapsed and the amount of viable pancreatic tissue. (3) Hyperlipidemic serum contains an inhibitor that should be diluted out to avoid a spuriously low amylase measurement.[1,2] (4) Conditions that mimic acute pancreatitis (e.g., perforated peptic ulcer, mesenteric infarction) may be accompanied by high blood levels of pancreatic enzymes, representing their absorption across devitalized gut. (5) Unsuspected chronic renal failure is another potential explanation, but nothing is gained by analyzing the urinary amylase/creatinine clearance ratio.[41] (6) In patients with intracranial bleeding, a substantial increase in blood levels of amylase and lipase appears to represent altered central control of pancreatic enzyme discharge, not pancreatitis.[42] (7) Salivary hyperamylasemia occurs in numerous conditions including chronic abdominal pain syndrome.[1]

The bottom line is that there is no hard and fast threshold of blood amylase level for diagnosing pancreatitis and no advantage in measuring another pancreatic secretory component. A previous history of pancreatitis is suggestive, as is the presence of an air-filled loop of upper intestine ("sentinel" loop) but without air under the diaphragm on a plain x-ray of the abdomen; diffuse enlargement of the gland on an ultrasound scan or a computed tomography (CT) scan offers strong diagnostic support. However, the absence of these signs does not exclude pancreatitis, and laparotomy should not be delayed when there is serious suspicion of a surgically correctable cause of an "acute abdomen."

Prognostic Aids

The goal is to identify at the time of admission the subset of patients whose disease is likely to pursue a downward spiral toward death from MODS (Table 58-1). There are two assumptions here: first, severity is proportional to the degree of pancreatic necrosis; second, necrotizing pancreatitis is synonymous with extensive autodigestion. These tenets are denied by the evidence. Thus, a review of autopsy series showed only interstitial pancreatitis in a quarter of cases.[2,23] The primacy of autodigestion is questioned by the interval of about 48 hours before any active trypsinogen was detected in patients who died.[43]

The high frequency of pre-existing disease in the elderly, and hence the ease with which they are tipped into MODS, explains the very high mortality in this age group.[21,24,44] It also devalues clinical instinct and objective measures of disease severity (Table 58-1). Numerical data can be manipulated in order to exclude patients who are unlikely to do badly (high predictive value of negatives) but not in identifying those at risk (low predictive value of positives). The APACHE II system has the advantage that the prognostic information is available at admission (Table 58-1).

Among global measures of the inflammatory response, the blood white cell count is not discriminatory at any stage of the illness, and the C-reactive protein concentration is only helpful after 48 hours when a value greater than 150 mg/dl portends a severe outcome. Recent European studies emphasize the prognostic value of neutrophil elastase-α_1-protease inhibitor complexes in admission plasma samples obtained as early as 2 hours after the first symptom: the levels were substantially higher in every patient whose disease pursued a severe course.[45] Several studies have shown that α_2-macroglobulin is grossly depleted by the fifth day in patients with severe disease despite high levels of α_1-protease inhibitor[3,41,45]; this discrepancy is explained by the ability of the former antiprotease, but not the latter, to bind cytokines. Unfortunately, measurement of cytokines[46] and antiproteases is beyond the resources of most hospitals.

It has been recommended that any suspicion of severe disease (Table 58-1) should serve as the cue for contrast enhanced CT of the pancreas (Fig. 58-1): nonenhancement of 50 percent or more of the gland indicates extensive necrosis.[47] This recommendation has been questioned recently following experimental evidence that intravenous contrast may actually increase tissue damage.[48] The finding of blood-stained aspirate on diagnostic peritoneal lavage is a clear pointer to severe disease, but the technique is invasive. A brilliant innovation for detecting the presence of a substantial amount of trypsin in the circulation at about 48 hours, by measuring the amount of trypsinogen activation peptide (TAP) in urine, looks promising[49] and is undergoing exhaustive investigation in animal studies.

Table 58-1 Adverse prognostic factors in acute pancreatitis

At admission		
Clinical	Advanced age and/or obesity and/or abdominal ecchymoses	
	Systolic BP <90 mm Hg and/or respiratory strain and/or urine volume <50 ml/h	
	APACHE II score ≥8	
	Bloody peritoneal lavage	
Biochemical	Blood urea >7.4 mmol/L and/or glucose >11 mmol/L	
	Huge increase in plasma PMN elastase-α_1PI complexes	
	Huge increase in plasma IL-6, IL-8	
Radiologic	≥50% nonperfusion in contrast-enhanced CT	
Within 48 hours		
Biochemical package	Blood urea >16 mmol/L (45 mg/dl urea N)	Modified Glasgow package (≥3)
	Blood glucose >10 mmol/L (180 mg/dl)	
	Arterial pO_2 <8.0 kPa (60 mmHg)	
	Serum albumin <32 g/L	
	Serum calcium <2.0 mmol/L (8.0 mg/dl)	
	White cell count >15 × 10^9/L	
	AST >200 U/L	
	LDH >600 U/L	
Urinalysis	Substantial amount of TAP	

Abbreviations: BP, blood pressure; IL, interleukin; CT, computed tomography, AST, aspartate transaminase; LDH, lactate dehydrogenase; PMN, polymorphonuclear leucocytes; α_1PI, alpha-1 proteinase inhibitor; TAP, trypsinogen activation peptide

Management

The objectives are the same in any age group: to control pain; to replace protein, fluid, and electrolytes lost into the pancreatic bed; to maintain the pancreatic microcirculation; to be vigilant for the earliest signs of ARDS and infection. Pre-existing medical conditions leave elderly patients vulnerable to the hemodynamic, respiratory, and septic complications of acute pancreatitis.

Blood samples are taken at admission (Table 58-1) to check the hematocrit, white cell count, liver function profile and levels of urea and electrolytes, blood gases, amylase, and glucose. These measurements should be repeated 12 hours later and then daily until the patient is asymptomatic, with regular checks on serum calcium after the first 24 hours by which time any fall due to hypoalbuminemia should have been rectified. The blood clotting and platelet count determinations should be repeatedly monitored. An admission chest x-ray and ECG are mandatory in older patients.

The control of pain requires injections of strong analgesics.

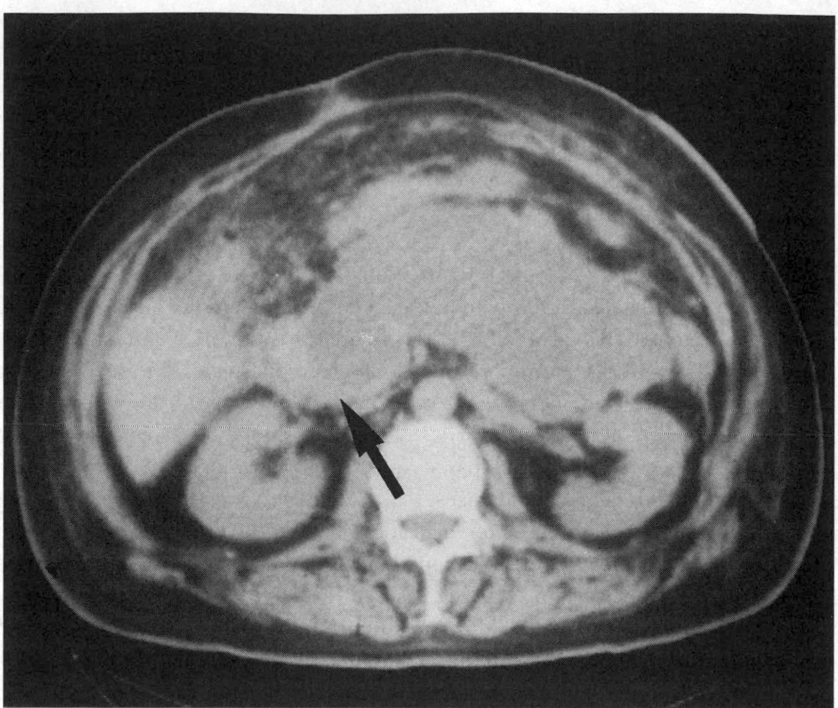

Figure 58-1 Contrast-enhanced CT scan in a patient with acute necrotizing pancreatitis. Note the nonperfusion of all but a rim of the swollen pancreas.

Morphine is best avoided because it contracts the sphincter of Oddi; pentazocine is a better choice, but some elderly patients react unfavorably. There is no evidence that continuous nasogastric suction accelerates recovery, and the oft-repeated recommendation to "rest the pancreas" is unfounded; however, patients often prefer to remain without food or drink.

The aggressive but safe replacement of fluid and electrolytes in older patients necessitates the use of a central venous pressure gauge and urinary catheter. Colloid is required in the form of plasma, purified protein derivative, albumin, or blood. Recent evidence that the microcirculation quickly becomes disorganized, not just in the pancreas but also in the liver, lung, and kidney,[3] supports the recommendation that dextran or mannitol be given routinely.[50] The need for potassium, insulin, and oxygen will be evident from blood measurements. A Swann-Ganz catheter should be inserted to monitor pulmonary arterial pressure in patients with cardiopulmonary disease or marked fluid shifts. Antacids have been recommended to prevent gastrointestinal hemorrhage from acute ulceration. A recent study suggests that a second-generation cephalosporin should be used routinely to prevent pancreatic infection.[32]

An abdominal ultrasound scan should be performed as soon as possible to look for gallstones, especially in icteric or pyrexic patients and when blood levels of liver enzymes are elevated. In these circumstances blood cultures are needed. ERCP with sphincterotomy under appropriate antibiotic cover (e.g., imipenem, piperacillin, or ciprofloxacin with gentamicin) should not be delayed if there is any suspicion of gallstones. Not only is it remarkably well tolerated, but it accelerates recovery and reduces the threat of biliary sepsis.[51,52]; subsequent cholecystectomy is considered unnecessary in this age group. We do not subscribe to the view that sphincterotomy should be performed in patients with idiopathic disease on the assumption that occult microlithiasis is responsible. However, we perform ERCP, after full clinical recovery, to look for small neoplasms that are readily missed on ultrasound and CT.

A self-limiting course of pancreatitis is heralded by an exponential fall in the serum amylase level such that by 72 hours it is within the reference range and the patient is pain-free. The decline in amylase level may be delayed if there has been a substantial "acute fluid collection" in the peripancreatic area or pleural space. This is merely part of the inflammatory response and should not be confused with a pseudocyst. If there is no sign that the blood amylase level is falling by the end of the first week, the following possibilities should be considered: overzealous use of analgesics that contract the sphincter of Oddi, pre-existing or impending renal failure, an evolving pancreatic pseudocyst or abscess. An impacted gallstone or periampullary tumor may cause the same phenomenon but will be excluded by ERCP. A pseudocyst is easily located and aspirated under ultrasound guidance but tends to recur. If the patient is asymptomatic, then a "wait and see" approach is justified irrespective of the size of the pseudocyst. Such patients can safely be discharged provided they are able to tolerate food, and they should be reviewed about 6 weeks later in the light of further assessment by ultrasound. If a sizable pseudocyst is still present and is symptomatic, CT will facilitate internal drainage. If the percutaneous or endoscopic route is successful, the need for surgery is obviated.

Fever, leukocytosis, and high plasma levels of C-reactive protein are expected in patients with extensive pancreatic necrosis in the absence of infection (Fig. 58-1). Formerly, an aggressive surgical approach was advocated to lay open the pancreatic bed and attach an abdominal wall zipper to allow repeated irrigation and repacking of the bed under general anesthesia, but nowadays intensive medical treatment is favored.[50] However, if fever and leukocytosis persist into the second week, infected pancreatic necrosis or pancreatic abscess should be suspected. The CT scan should be repeated and may show the characteristic gas-filled pockets of an abscess. This abscess, and the pancreatic bed also, should be aspirated percutaneously under ultrasound or CT guidance. Microbiology findings consistent with either diagnosis indicate the need for immediate open drainage under appropriate antibiotic cover to include antifungal agents.

The substantial mortality from acute pancreatitis, despite the best efforts of pancreatobiliary and intensive care teams, underlines the absence of specific medical treatment. Controlled clinical trials have not shown any benefit from glucagon, high or low molecular weight antiproteases, or fresh frozen plasma. A recent meta-analysis suggests a therapeutic advantage from treatment with somatostatin, apparently reflecting its immunomodulatory properties rather than an inhibitory effect on pancreatic protein synthesis.[53] Exchange transfusion, hemofiltration, or plasmapharesis has been used anecdotally to treat hypertriglyceridemia or to remove the burden of toxins. The current fashion is to employ anticytokine treatment. A few years ago the focus was on antitumor necrosis factor and now it is on antiplatelet activating factor,[54] but so far claims of improvement in outcome are unconvincing.

Chronic Pancreatitis

Definition and Natural History

This chronic inflammatory process is peculiar in that it has lithogenic potential. Indeed, it is this potential that governs the "ductal obstruction" theory of pathogenesis. The proposal is that intraductal deposits of protein steadily become impregnated with calcium carbonate so that calculi eventually develop. These ulcerate adjacent epithelium, leading to periductal strictures and ductal hypertension triggering attack after attack of pancreatitis. It has further been argued that reduced secretion by pancreatic acinar cells of lithostatin, a calcium-solubilizing protein formerly called pancreatic stone protein, lies at the heart of the problem. There is no evidence supporting this orthodox hypothesis. Indeed, it is illogical in that patchy loss of secretory parenchyma and irregular fibrosis are the prerequisites for diagnosis but ductal involvement is not.[34] Each inflammatory wave is followed by destruction of a further population of acinar cells. While foci of fat necrosis seem to determine the location and intensity of the fibrotic reaction,[55] perineural clusters of inflammatory cells and nesidioblastosis are other features of the established disease. Complete effacement of acinar tissue and intense fibrosis draws to a close the natural history of chronic pancreatitis, but pancreatic cancer may have developed well before then.[14]

Demography and Etiologic Factors

It is impossible to be precise about the incidence or prevalence of chronic pancreatitis because tests that distinguish acute from chronic pancreatitis are seldom applied after an attack[33] and because patients with chronic pain are often misdiagnosed as having peptic ulcer disease or spastic colon syndrome. Despite these difficulties, there is no doubt that disease frequency is much lower in developed countries (maximum prevalence 0.025 percent in Scandinavia[56]) than in countries of the Third World where it may be as high as 0.5 percent.[34] These statistics exclude cystic fibrosis, in which chronic pancreatitis-like lesions develop in utero.[34] Excluding this subgroup, the mean age at presentation is about 35 years in developed countries. However, in the Far East the disease starts in childhood and runs an aggressive course to pancreatic calculi, glandular effacement, and diabetes mellitus.[34]

Alcoholism is documented in about 50 percent of cases as a whole, but it is a weak factor in that the first symptom is generally preceded by an average of 12 to 15 years of drinking more than 150 g alcohol daily. An excess of dietary protein, an excess or deficiency of dietary fat, and exposure to cigarette smoke are confounding influences. In perhaps 10 percent of patients the disease occurs against a background of hyperparathyroidism, longstanding diabetes, inflammatory bowel disease, or drug therapy (azathioprine, sodium valproate, estrogens).[56] The condition is idiopathic in at least 30 percent of patients overall. Our large case-controlled investigation pinpointed close exposure to volatile hydrocarbons in the occupational environment as an independent risk factor in a substantial number of patients;[33] an earlier study had disclosed a similar relationship among ex-alcoholics who continued to experience painful attacks.[57] Males outnumber females when alcoholism is the dominant etiological factor, but gender distribution is equal otherwise.

The aging process itself seems to be a risk factor for chronic pancreatitis in developed countries.[58,59] A Japanese study of routine autopsies showed that the frequency of pancreatic calculi increased from 0 percent under 69 years to 4.2 percent, 7.7 percent, and 16.7 percent in the next three decades.[59] The rarer condition of primary inflammatory pancreatitis is different, affecting elderly women and being characterized by hypergammaglobulanemia with mononuclear cell infiltration of the gland.[2] Recent reports show that milder variants of cystic fibrosis may appear for the first time in elderly patients.[60]

The endemicity of calcific chronic pancreatitis in the Far East is not due to alcoholism. It has been proposed that the pancreas is slowly poisoned by hydrogen cyanide because the dietary supply of inorganic sulfate is insufficient to detoxify the load of cyanogenetic glycosides from dietary staples.[1,2,34] The endemicity of the disease among blacks of southern Africa has traditionally been equated with alcoholism.[6] However, recent studies showed that in southern India and southern Africa, as in the United Kingdom,[33,57] patients were closely exposed to volatile chemicals in their occupational and/or domestic environment.[61,62]

Clinical Features

Most patients present with an attack of pancreatitis, and further attacks follow with increasing frequency. Occasionally the pattern mimics that of peptic ulcers or gallstones. Sooner or later background pain sets in, and its intensity increases relentlessly until all exocrine secretory parenchyma is effaced. Only then does steatorrhea occur, together with weight loss, because the gland has a huge secretory reserve. Painless disease characterized by steatorrhea and/or diabetes is recorded in 10 percent of cases overall but in a much higher proportion of elderly patients and in those in tropical zones. The development of diabetes is influenced by genetic factors. Complications of the disease include obstruction of the gastric outlet, duodenum, or bile duct; true pancreatic cysts and pseudocysts; portal hypertension from local venous thromboses; hemorrhage from an inflammatory arterial aneurysm, and problems due to diabetes. Psychological disturbances eventually occur as a result of regular use of narcotic analgesics, alcoholism, job loss, and disrupted family life,[40] so that there is a real risk of suicide. Chronic pancreatitis increases the risk of pancreatic cancer.[14]

Diagnosis

Diagnosis of chronic pancreatitis is easily made if pancreatic calculi are found on the first plain x-ray of the abdomen or CT scan, as is the case in about 30 percent of patients in developed countries but in a much higher proportion of patients in the Third World. Otherwise a pancreatic function test as well as ERCP is needed to detect acinar loss or ductal distortion, respectively, because these changes do not go hand in hand.[17] In patients under the age of 60 years, ERCP findings of a moderately dilated main duct or small cystlike endings of second-order ducts support the diagnosis. However, since these are normal findings in elderly people, an ERCP diagnosis requires evidence of a clear stricture with upstream dilatation, complete ductal obstruction, large cysts, or a "chain-of-lakes" transformation of the main duct.[63] In about 15 percent of patients the diagnosis is missed at the first assessment because the early lesions are patchy.[17]

In elderly patients with painless steatorrhea the functional aspect is particularly relevant. Duodenal intubation tests, involving analysis of aspirates after stimulation with hormones or a Lundh test meal, are over-rated and uncomfortable.[64] Fortunately, they are unnecessary now that a tubeless test has been validated. This is based on the hydrolysis by pancreatic chymotrypsin of a synthetic peptide, *N*-benzoyl-l-tyrosyl *p*-aminobenzoic acid (BT-PABA). In the Manchester version the fasted patient is given 500 mL of a flavored drink containing 0.5 g BT-PABA, an internal marker to correct for problems of intermediate metabolism, and 25 g casein as a competitive substrate for chymotrypsin. Formerly, ^{14}C-PABA was used as the internal marker, but *p*-aminosalicylic acid (PAS) is currently employed. The outputs of PABA and the internal marker are measured in urine collected for 6 hours while the patient continues to fast. The PABA/^{14}C excretion index, or PABA/PAS index, is compared with the reference range.[65] The fluorescein dilaurate test is based on similar principles but is less specific.[17] Serum isoamylase analysis helps to identify patients with exocrine pancreatic failure (low pancreatic isoenzyme levels) and those with salivary hyperamylasemia-chronic pain syndrome.[17]

Management

The control of pancreatic pain is the main objective in management. Its cause is multifactorial: an increase in interstitial fluid pressure irrespective of ductal anatomy; irritation of nociceptive nerve endings; an inflammatory mass, as tends to occur in the head of the gland in about 30 percent of patients; creeping periductal fibrosis leading to ductal hypertension. Nonsteroidal anti-inflammatory drugs (NSAIDS) soon become ineffective, necessitating the use of potent but addictive narcotic analgesics. Regular counseling is an important part of overall management. For a long time pancreatoduodenectomy has been the standard treatment for a mass lesion in the head of the gland. For diffuse disease without main duct dilatation, near-total pancreatectomy is the only answer, but at the expense of gross maldigestion and brittle diabetes. Many patients with large duct disease also require this procedure when previous duct drainage operations fail to control pain.[13]

In older patients the control of steatorrhea and malnutrition is especially important. Microencapsulated preparations of pancreatic extracts have simplified management. The newer high-potency preparations have been banned for use in patients with cystic fibrosis because they result in colonic strictures, but there is no reason to question their use in other settings of chronic pancreatitis. If steatorrhea remains troublesome, a gastric acid inhibitor should be tried.[1] If this does not resolve the problem, the intake of long-chain fat should be reduced to about 30 g, avoiding fat deficiency by using a supplement of medium-chain triglycerides. Injections of fat-soluble vitamins should be given at appropriate intervals. The absorption of vitamin B_{12} requires the presence of pancreatic proteases in the intestinal lumen, and so patients with exocrine pancreatic failure may need a periodic injection of vitamin B_{12}. Diabetes may initially respond to dietary manipulation and oral hypoglycemic drugs but eventually most patients require insulin.

Cancer of the Pancreas

Origin

There is a school of thought claiming that all pancreatic tumors originate in centroacinar cells and then either acquire a ductal phenotype via dedifferentiation or retain an acinar phenotype.[1] In human beings a ductal phenotype is the rule, and the bulk of tumors are in the head of the pancreas. They are generally adenocarcinomas with varying degree of differentiation and mucinous or cystic change. Experimental cancer in hamsters follows this pattern, but acinar characteristics predominate in rats.[1]

Demography and Etiologic Factors

The incidence of pancreatic cancer approximates its prevalence, currently 0.1 percent, because patients usually die within 6 months of the first symptom. There is a clear correlation with age: approximately 80 percent of cases occur between the age of 60 and 80 years. Other risk factors include cigarette smoking and high fat intake. Heavy coffee consumption has probably been exonerated, but alcoholism, exposure to volatile hydrocarbons, and long-standing diabetes remain under suspicion.[1] There is undeniable evidence that chronic pancreatitis increases cancer risk[14] and some evidence, too, that an isolated episode of acute pancreatitis or cystic fibrosis does the same.[15,16] Of relevance in the elderly age group, patients with Alzheimer's disease appear to run an increased risk of pancreatic cancer.[66]

Clinical Features

The classic features of a periampullary tumor are painless jaundice with steatorrhea (silver stools) and a palpable gallbladder (Courvoisier's sign), but it may declare itself as an attack of pancreatitis. A tumor in the head of the gland may also manifest itself in this way, but ever-increasing pain is characteristic. Tumors in the body or tail of the pancreas tend to be associated with pain passing through to the back, a change in bowel habits, and diabetes: on examination there may be a palpable mass with a bruit due to compression of the splenic artery. Liver enlargement is common and does not necessarily imply metastases. Migrating thrombophlebitis (Trousseau's sign) is a rare mode of presentation. Dyspepsia and neuropsychiatric syndromes are cited as other common but nonspecific features. Elderly patients may present with symptoms from metastases rather than from the primary tumor.[67] The onset of diabetes in an elderly patient, or instability when diabetes was previously well controlled, should raise suspicion of cancer.[68]

Diagnosis

In patients with jaundice, ultrasound scanning should be the first test, followed by endoscopic or percutaneous cholangiography if there is evidence of bile duct obstruction. If the scan shows a pancreatic mass, fine-needle aspiration provides material for cytology. Because of sampling problems, however, the absence of malignant cells does not exclude the diagnosis. A deliberate search should be made for an ampullary cancer, an intraductal mucin-hypersecreting tumor[69] (Fig. 58-2), or a cystadenocarcinoma, using a combination of ERCP and CT, because these lesions are amenable to curative resection. When steatorrhea is the presenting feature, a pancreatic function test is the logical first choice, followed, if it is abnormal, by ERCP. Every effort should be made to confirm the diagnosis by histology or cytology. Preliminary reports suggest that the difficult distinction from chronic pancreatitis may be facilitated by the finding in pancreatic juice or pancreatic tissue of Kirsten (K)-*ras* mutations, using appropriate gene amplification techniques.[70] Another recent study suggests that the combination of ultrasonography findings and high blood levels of a mucin-based tumor marker, CAM 17.1, may be especially useful.[71] In elderly patients with atypical clinical features the diagnosis may be made only at autopsy.

Management

The cardinal problem in pancreatic cancer is the long presymptomatic period of tumor growth. Laparoscopy, angiography, and CT scanning are useful in assessing whether a tumor that looks small on ultrasound scanning is truly resectable. Even when the chances look good, surgery is poorly tolerated in frail elderly patients and those with pre-existing medical problems. Jaundice is easily palliated by cutting through an ampullary lesion during the course of ERCP or by inserting an endoscopic stent to bridge a low bile duct stricture (Fig. 58-2). If stenting fails, the percutaneous transhepatic route is still available, as is a combined percutaneous-endoscopic approach, before resorting to surgery. A gastric bypass operation will be needed if the tumor obstructs the pylorus. The combination of an NSAID with sublingual buprenorphine helps to relieve pain in the early stages. Chemical destruction of nerve fibers offers further help in the short term, but narcotic analgesics are eventually needed. Chemotherapy is probably contraindicated in elderly patients. Considering that the 5-year survival rate of less than 5 percent is largely due to the late presentation of the tumor, efforts have been made to find a screening test for pancreatic cancer. Unfortunately, none is sufficiently reliable to justify population studies.

A "Radical" Approach to Pancreatic Disease

Dilemmas

Orthodox theories regarding the pathogenesis of acute and chronic pancreatitis leave many fundamental questions unanswered. (1) Why is an attack of pancreatitis so stereotyped despite the etiologic diversity and differences in the underlying disease process? (2) Why does an increase in the blood level of pancreatic enzymes, including zymogens, precede an attack? (3) Why do some people recover spontaneously but others die from MODS? (4) What is the stimulus to inflammation in pancreatitis when the inciting agent is neither infective nor traumatic in most cases? (5) Why is the exocrine pancreas the primary target in cystic fibrosis with lesions that are indistinguishable from those of chronic pancreatitis and lead to neonatal hypertrypsinogenemia as a diagnostic clue? (6) Why do chronic pancreatitis, acute pancreatitis, and cystic fibrosis increase the risk of pancreatic cancer? (7) Why is the aging process associated with calcific chronic pancreatitis and pancreatic cancer?

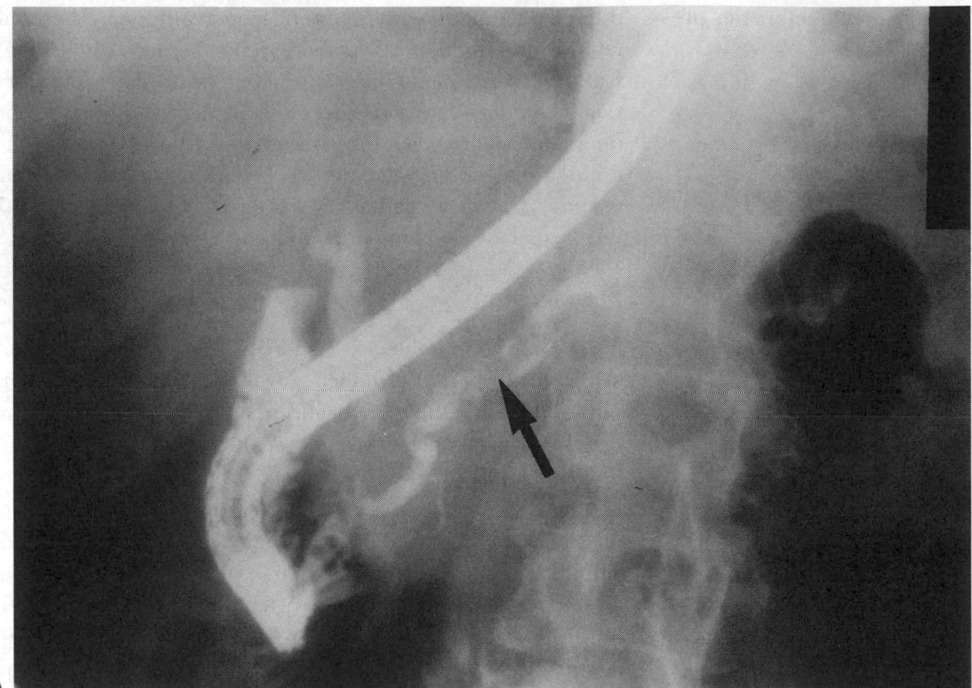

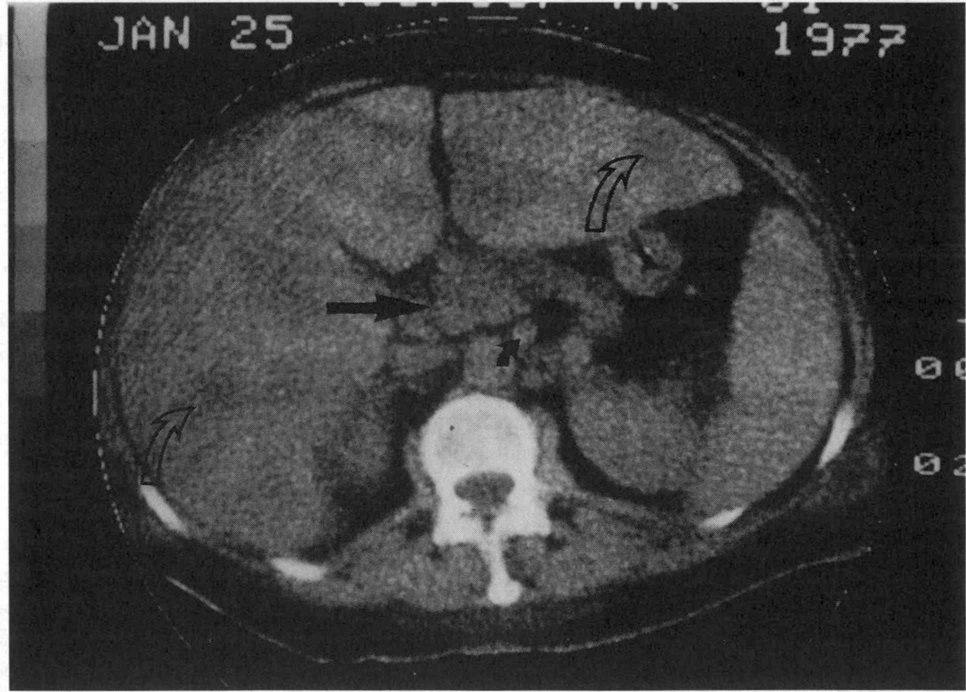

Figure 58-2 (**A**) ERCP showing serpiginous filling defects in the pancreatic duct of a 53-year-old woman with relapsing pancreatitis. These appearances are now known to be typical of mucin-secreting tumors. She died with metastases 12 months later. (**B**) CT scan of a 72-year-old woman with a 3-month history of increasing epigastric pain and weight loss. Note the irregular expansion of the pancreatic head, lateral displacement of the superior mesenteric artery, and metastatic deposits in the liver. *(Figure continues.)*

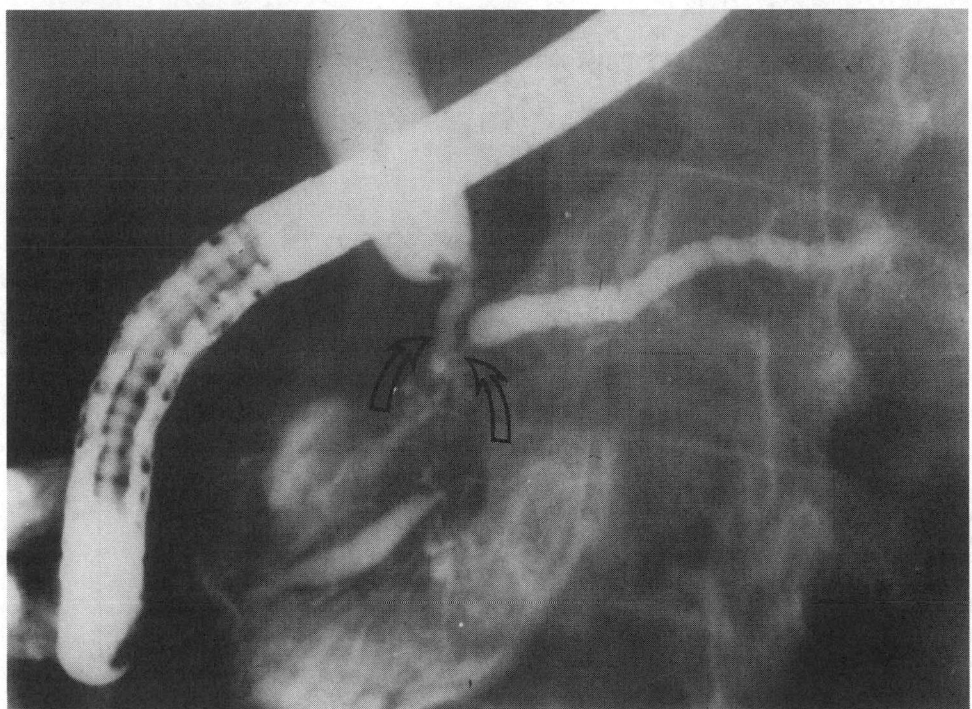

Figure 58-2 *(Continued)* (**C**) ERCP images of a 74-year-old man with a 4-month history of steatorrhea and weight loss; the BT-PABA/[^{14}C] PABA excretion index was only 0.14 (normal > 0.75). Note the double duct sign, contiguous strictures in bile and pancreatic ducts due to the tumor in the neck of the gland. When the patient became jaundiced, a palliative bile duct stent was inserted endoscopically.

Oxidative Stress: The Common Denominator

The phrase *oxidative stress* describes the potential for tissue injury when free radical load exceeds antioxidant availability.[72] The problem may arise from an absolute increase in free radical production, depletion of antioxidant stores, or an imbalance in favor of radicals although their production rates and antioxidant supply remain within the broad limits of normal.[73] Electron spin resonance and chemiluminescence studies can pinpoint a free radical burst and characterize the species involved, but these methods are inapplicable, by and large, in human disease. Instead, the presence of oxidative stress is inferred from increases in the concentrations of free radical oxidation products (FROPs) in biologic materials, prevention of acute disease by pretreatment with an inhibitor of the suspected free radical source and/or free radical scavengers, or amelioration of chronic disease with concomitant reduction in levels of FROPs by long-term treatment with micronutrient antioxidants. These micronutrients constitute the third line of antioxidant defense in tissues. Primary protection is afforded by proteins that sequester transition metals or hold them in the oxidized state, thus limiting the production of reactive oxygen species. Antioxidant enzymes, including superoxide dismutase, catalase, and glutathione (GSH) peroxidase, provide secondary protection.[72–74] Micronutrient antioxidants may function in the aqueous phase (e.g., sulfur amino acids and their metabolic end products including GSH)[34,35] or in the lipid phase (e.g., vitamin E and β-carotene) or may contribute to protection in both media (e.g., ascorbate, the bioactive form of vitamin C).

Every organelle in every cell type seems to have the potential to generate reactive oxygen species because these species subserve vital functions such as signal transduction,[75] cellular respiration, biotransformation of endogenous and exogenous lipophilic substrates (xenobiotics),[34,35,72] scavenging by lysosomes, phagocytosis,[72] and membrane turnover by controlled lipid peroxidation.[76]

A range of experimental and clinical observations in the 1980s suggested that oxidative stress may be the common pathogenetic denominator in exocrine pancreatic disease.[17] Over the next decade, this unorthodox concept received steady support.[17,55,77] The weight of evidence suggests that a burst of oxygen radical activity[34] underlies acute pancreatitis, while nonbiologic species produced during the metabolism of xenobiotics are relevant in chronic pancreatitis and pancreatic cancer.[33,35,78]

An attack of pancreatitis (Fig. 58-3) appears to be precipitated when oxidative stress compromises exocytosis by interfering with the methionine transulfuration pathway.[34,35,77] This route provides cells with critical methyl groups and GSH, and it conserves stores of high-energy phosphate and adenosine. Choline, vitamin B_{12}, folate, and ascorbate interact closely at various stages in the pathway. Acinar cells respond in two ways: pent-up granules are resorbed by crinophagic processes

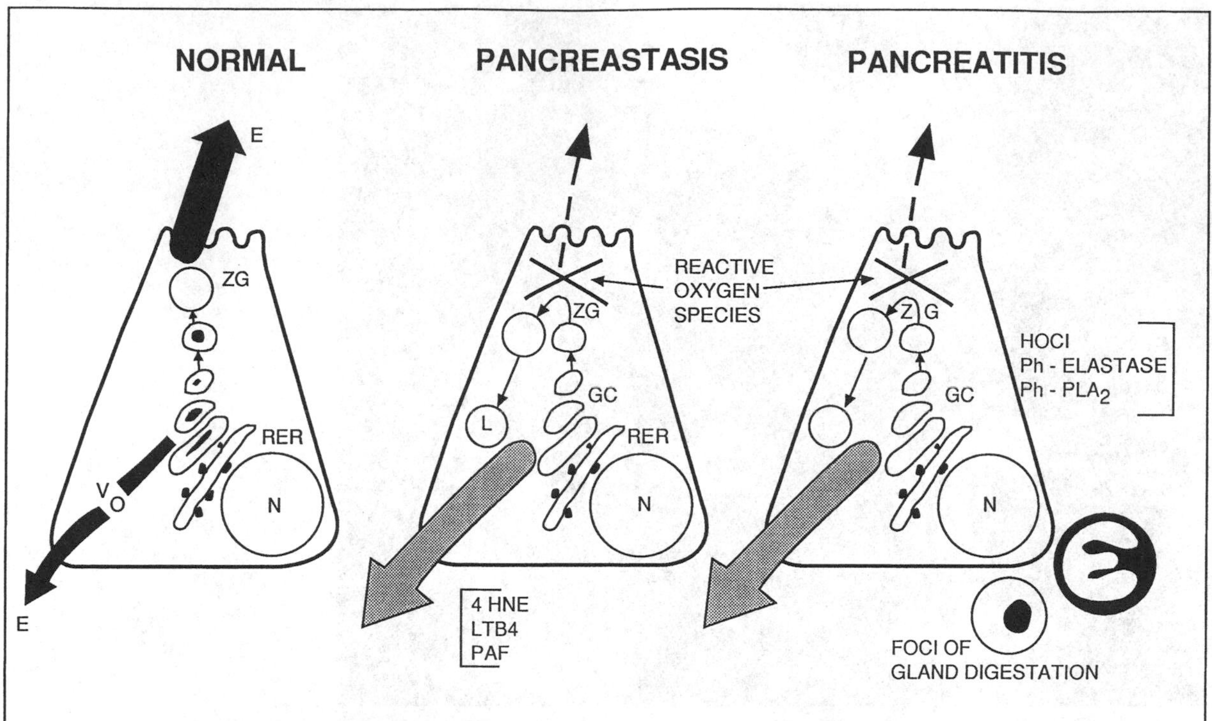

Figure 58-3 Schematic representation of the evolution of an attack of pancreatitis. The arrows indicate the direction of pancreatic enzyme secretion in the normal acinar cells and in pancreatitis. The cross indicates impedence to exocytosis. N, Nucleus; RER, rough endoplasmic reticulum; GC, Golgi complex; ZG, zymogen granules; L, lysosomes; 4-HNE, 4-hydroxynonenal; LTB-4, leucotriene B-4; PAF, platelet activating factor; HOCl, hypochlorous acid produced via activated leucocytes; Ph-PAL$_2$, phagocyte-derived phospholipase A$_2$. (Modified from Braganza et al.,[94] with permission.)

involving lysosomes, and less mature products are discharged via the basolateral membrane into the bloodstream and lymphatics (Fig. 58-3). The critical point is that relatively long-lived FROPs, codiverted into the interstitium as part of the reversal in secretory polarity, provoke the intense inflammatory response. The response is inherently disregulated, veering toward MODS with its component causes of frustrated phagocytosis and premature immunosuppression, because radicals have assumed the role of conductor in the inflammatory orchestra when they were intended to be just one class of players.[77] There is increasing evidence that the wholesale extracellular discharge of elastase and phospholipase A$_2$ from activated neutrophils initiates necrotizing pancreatitis and, furthermore, that the secondary but rapid activation of trypsinogen and pancreatic phospholipase A$_2$ may be brought about by plasmin and thrombin, respectively.[34]

Thus, the real conundrum is why any patient with acute pancreatitis can recover spontaneously. The evidence suggests that prior antioxidant status is an important factor; if this is poor, the stage is set for a severe outcome, and whether or not this happens depends on the speed with which the exocytosis blockade is lifted. The burst of free radical activity that imposes the blockade may arise from from a variety of causes, for example, transient obstruction to drainage of pancreatic secretions by a migrating gallstone, ischemia-reperfusion injury during CABG or pancreas transplantation, or hyperstimulation of the gland after a prolonged fast.[34] It has been proposed[78a] that another critical factor in determining outcome is the genetic influence on production of cytokines, in that an innate anti-inflammatory cytokine profile may set the stage for MODS pancreatitis and other fulminant inflammatory states.

In relation to chronic pancreatitis, there is now unequivocal evidence incriminating pancreatic drug metabolizing enzymes, the so-called cytochromes P450. These enzymes are induced by chronic exposure to alcohol, constituents of cigarette smoke, and dietary unsaturated fatty acids. Xenobiotics are generally detoxified when metabolized by cytochromes P450, but sometimes highly reactive metabolites are produced and their yield is higher if the relevant cytochrome P450 isoenzymes were induced to start with. In these circumstances, oxidative stress increases with time, so that recurrent attacks of pancreatitis are only to be expected. Likewise, the steady increase in collagen deposition and irritation of nociceptive nerve endings can also be expected, as wave upon wave of FROPs enters the interstitium (Fig. 58-3).[55] The inhalation route of xenobiotic exposure ensures a direct strike at the pancreas, whereas ingested substances are channeled to the liver which is best equipped to deal with them. Should the products of xenobiotic metabolism be mutagenic, the seeds for cancer would be sown, explaining the increased risk in patients with chronic pancreatitis.[78]

Recent studies also help to explain why cystic fibrosis invariably leads to chronic pancreatitis.[34] The abnormal genotype results in forms of the cystic fibrosis transmembrane regulator protein (CFTR) that cannot function as a cyclic adenosine monophosphate (cAMP)-driven chloride channel in membranes or cannot find their way to the appropriate membrane domains. Not only is it now recognized that the wild-type protein is involved in macromolecule trafficking[79,80] but also that there is evidence that CFTR malfunction may be conducive to oxidative stress.[81] The corollary that possession of a mutant CFTR allele renders people vulnerable to chronic pancreatitis, and hence pancreatic cancer, is borne out by recent work.[82,83]

The new disease template accommodates the regularity of exocrine pancreatic damage in kwashiorkor and metal storage diseases. The first link is rationalized on the basis of profound antioxidant deficiencies, and the second by the free radical-promoting effects of transition metals.[34]

Relevance to Pancreatic Disease in the Elderly

These arguments resonate with the free radical theory of aging.[74,75] Poor antioxidant intake in the face of normal drug metabolizing capability seems to be the basic problem. Thus, it has been recognized for some time that many elderly people have subclinical deficiencies of macronutrients[84] and vitamin C.[85] Furthermore, a recent study of elderly people showed that although serum concentrations of folate, vitamin B_{12}, and vitamin B_6 were within normal limits, supplements of these vitamins improved the levels of methionine metabolites.[86] A deficiency of choline jeopardizes methionine metabolism; hence it is interesting that choline deficiency has been implicated in Alzheimer's disease and that both experimental pancreatitis and pancreatic cancer can be produced by denial of choline along with methionine.[35] Considering all this evidence, it is perhaps not surprising that experimental deprivation of different antioxidants results in pancreatic changes that show histologic similarities to the pancreatopathy of aging.[35]

The Therapeutic Corollary

Treatment with oral antioxidants, including average daily doses of 0.54 g vitamin C with 2 g methionine and 600 μg organic selenium, controls background pain in chronic pancreatitis and prevents further attacks of acute or acute-on-chronic pancreatitis.[87–90] Indeed, pancreatic surgery for pain is now virtually obsolete at our institution. Restoration of GSH sufficiency is the best explanation for the success of treatment insofar as normalization of plasma GSH levels reflects adequate concentrations of the antioxidant in organs of active GSH synthesis and turnover.[35] The pancreas seems to be extremely active in these respects,[91] such that rapid depletion of pancreatic GSH can of itself cause experimental pancreatitis.[92] The failure of GSH precursor therapy to alter the outcome of acute pancreatitis in a controlled clinical trial[93] could in retrospect be rationalized by the very low concentrations of ascorbate and also selenium in the baseline blood samples.[94] We and other investigators are now considering a trial of an antioxidant combination but, because of the time lag of about 15 hours before treatment can begin in developed countries, it would be best if it could be initiated by the primary care physician in a manner analogous to, but much safer than, the use of streptokinase in myocardial infarction. It seems to us that hemofiltration or plasma exchange may be the best way to debulk injurious cytokines and enzymes from activated phagocytes if deterioration toward MODS is not aborted within 12 hours of treatment.

The Prophylactic Corollary

Collaborative studies suggest that chronic pancreatitis, and hence pancreatic cancer, may be avoidable in underprivileged populations of the Third World by fortifying dietary staples with the deficient antioxidants or by providing these supplements in the form of a daily tablet beginning in childhood.[61,62] Should the oxidative stress philosophy for the pathogenesis of gallstones be substantiated,[95] communities with a high prevalence of gallstones, and hence acute pancreatitis, could benefit in the same way. Meanwhile, the finding of pre-existent oxidative stress in patients awaiting CABG[96] suggests that supplements of oral antioxidants in the months leading up to the operation may protect against postoperative pancreatitis. Considering the association of aging with atherosclerosis, gallstones, and severe pancreatitis, there may be a case for supplying a compound antioxidant tablet to all elderly individuals on a daily basis. In these cost-conscious days the dividends, quite apart from humane considerations, should far outweigh the cost.

Acknowledgments

We thank Rosie Shearburn for superb secretarial assistance and Sandra Roe for preparing Figure 58-3.

References

1. Go VLW, DiMagno EP, Gardner JD et al (eds): The Pancreas: Biology, Pathobiology and Disease. 2nd Ed. Lippincott-Raven, New York, 1993
2. Howat HT, Sarles H (eds): The Exocrine Pancreas. WB Saunders, London, 1979
3. Johnson CD, Imrie CW (eds): Pancreatic Disease: Progress and Prospects. Springer-Verlag, London, 1993
4. Beger HG, Büchler M, Ditschuneit H, Malfertheiner P (eds): Chronic Pancreatitis. Springer-Verlag, Berlin, 1990
5. Hollander LF (ed): Controversies in Acute Pancreatitis. Springer-Verlag, Berlin, 1982
6. Gyr KE, Singer MV, Sarles H (eds): Pancreatitis: Concepts and Classification. Excerpta Medica, Amsterdam, 1984
7. Weatherall DJ, Ledingham JGG, Warrell DA (eds): New Oxford Textbook of Medicine. 3rd Ed. pp. 2027–2045. Oxford University Press, Oxford, 1996
8. Slesinger M, Fordtran J (eds): Gastroinstestinal Disease. 5th Ed. pp. 1573–1721. WB Saunders, Philadelphia, 1993
9. Calleja GA, Barkin JS: Acute pancreatitis. Med Clin North Am 1993;77:1037–1056

10. Thompson DG, Hawkey C (eds): Gastroenterology Medicine International 1994;287–296
11. Steinberg W, Tenner S: Acute pancreatitis. N Engl J Med 1994; 330:1198–1210
12. Steer ML, Waxman I, Friedman S: Chronic pancreatitis. N Engl J Med 1995;332:1482–1490
13. Frey CS: Current management of chronic pancreatitis. Adv Surg 1995;28:337–370
14. Lowenfels AB, Maisonneuve P, Cavallini G et al: Pancreatitis and the risk of pancreatic cancer. N Engl J Med 1993;328: 1433–1437
15. Neglia JP, Fitzsimmons SC, Maisonneuve P et al: The risk of cancer among patients with cystic fibrosis. N Engl J Med 1995; 332:494–499
16. Bansal P, Sonnenberg A: Pancreatitis is a risk factor for pancreatic cancer. Gastroenterology 1995;109:247–251
17. Braganza JM: The pancreas. pp. 251–280. In Pounder R (ed): Recent Advances in Gastroenterology. Vol. 6. Churchill Livingstone, London, 1988
18. Rittenbury M: Pancreatitis in the elderly patient. Am Surg 1961; 27:475–494
19. Park J, Fromkes J, Cooperman M: Acute pancreatitis in elderly patients. Am J Surg 1986;152:638–642
20. Fan ST, Choi TK, Lai CS, Wong J: Influence of age on the mortality from acute pancreatitis. Br J Surg 1988;75:463–466
21. Gross JS, Neufeld RR, Libow LS et al: Autopsy study of the elderly institutionalised patient: review of 234 autopsies. Arch Intern Med 1988;148:173–176
22. Wilson C, Imrie CW, Carter DC: Fatal acute pancreatitis. Gut 1988;29:782–788
23. Kimura W, Ohtsubo K: Clinical and pathological features of acute interstitial pancreatitis in the aged. Int J Pancreatol 1989; 5:1–10
24. Fan ST: Causes and prognosis of acute pancreatitis in the geriatric patient. Geriatr Med Today 1988;8:46–55
25. Ingbar S, Jacobson IM: Biliary and pancreatic disease in the elderly. Gastroenterol Clin North Am 1990;19:433–457
26. Browder W, Patterson MD, Thompson JL, Walters DN: Acute pancreatitis of unknown aetiology in the elderly. Ann Surg 1993; 5:469–475
27. Gullo L, Sipalvi HM, Pezzilli R: Pancreatitis in the elderly. J Clin Gastroenterol 1994;19:64–68
28. Banks PA: Pancreatic disease in the elderly. Semin Gastrointest Dis 1994;5:189–196
29. Lillemore KD: Pancreatic disease in the elderly patient. Surg Clin North Am 1994;74:317–344
30. Kloppel G, Heitz PU (eds): Pancreatic Pathology. Churchill Livingstone, London, 1984
31. Frey CF, Bradley EL, Beger HG: Progress in acute pancreatitis. Surg Gynecol Obstet 1988;167:282–286
32. Sainio V, Kemppainen E, Puolakkainen P et al: Early antibiotic treatment in acute necrotising pancreatitis. Lancet 1995;ii: 663–667
33. McNamee R, Braganza JM, Hogg J et al: Occupational exposure to hydrocarbons and chronic pancreatitis: a case-referent study. Occup Environ Med 1994;41:631–637
34. Braganza JM (ed): The Pathogenesis of Pancreatitis. Manchester University Press, Manchester, 1991
35. Braganza JM: Toxicology of the pancreas. pp. 663–714. In Ballantyne B, Turner P, Marrs TC (eds): Textbook of General and Applied Toxicology. Macmillan, New York, 1993
36. Fernandez del Castillo C, Harringer W, Warshaw AL et al: Risk factors for pancreatic cellular injury after cardiopulmonary bypass. N Engl J Med 1991;325:382–387
37. Büsing M, Hopt UT, Quacken M et al: Morphological studies of graft pancreatitis following pancreas transplantation. Br J Surg 1993;8:1170–1173
38. Ros E, Navarro S, Bur C et al: Occult microlithiasis in "idiopathic" acute pancreatitis: prevention of relapses by cholecystectomy or ursodeoxycholic acid therapy. Gastroenterology 1991;101:1701–1709
39. Ryan CM, Sheridan RL, Shoenfeld DA et al: Postburn pancreatitis. Ann Surg 1995;222:163–170
40. Galen RS, Gambino SR: Beyond normality. John Wiley, New York, 1975
41. Malfertheiner P, Ditschuneit H (eds): Diagnostic Procedures in Pancreatic Disease. Springer-Verlag, Berlin, 1986
42. Justice AD, DiBenedetto RJ, Stanford E: Significance of elevated pancreatic enzymes in intracranial bleeding. South Med J 1994;87:889–893
43. Durie PR, Gaskin KJ, Ogilvie JE et al: Serial alterations in the forms of immunoreactive pancreatic cationic trypsin in plasma from patients with acute pancreatitis. J Pediatr Gastroenterol Nutr 1985;4:199–207
44. Corfield AP, Cooper MJ, Williamson RCN: Acute pancreatitis: a lethal disease of increasing incidence. Gut 1985;26:724–729
45. Viedma JA, Perez Mateo M, Agullo J et al: Inflammatory response in the early prediction of severity in human acute pancreatitis. Gut 1994;35:822–827
46. Gross V, Andreesen R, Leser HC et al: Interleukin-8 and neutrophil activation in acute pancreatitis. Eur J Clin Invest 1992; 22:200–203
47. Bradley EL: A clinically based classification system for acute pancreatitis. Arch Surg 1993;128:586–590
48. Foitzik J, Bassi DG, Fernandez del Castillo C et al: Intravenous contrast medium impairs oxygenation of the pancreas in acute necrotising pancreatitis in the rat. Arch Surg 1994;129: 706–711
49. Gudgeon AM, Heath DI, Hurley P et al: Trypsinogen activation peptides assay in the early prediction of severity of acute pancreatitis. Lancet 1990;i:4–8
50. Bradley EL, Allen K: A prospective longitudinal study of observation versus surgical intervention in the management of necrotising pancreatitis. Am J Surg 1991;161:19–25
51. Neoptolemos JP, Carr-Locke DL, London NJ et al: Controlled trial of urgent endoscopic retrograde cholangio-pancreatography and endoscopic sphincterotomy versus conservative treatment for acute pancreatitis due to gallstones. Lancet 1988;ii: 979–982

52. Shemesh E, Czerniak A, Schenabaum S, Nass S: Early endoscopic sphincterotomy in the management of acute gallstone pancreatitis in elderly patients. J Am Geriatr Soc 1990;38: 893–896

53. Jenkins SA, Berein A: The relative effectiveness of somatostatin and octreotide therapy in pancreatic disease. Aliment Pharmacol Ther 1995;9:349–361

54. Kingsnorth AN, Galloway SN, Formela LJ: Randomised double blind phase II trial of Lexipafant, a platelet-activating factor antagonist in human acute pancreatitis. Br J Surg 1995;82: 1414–1420

55. Braganza JM: The pathogenesis of chronic pancreatitis. Q J Med 1996;89:243–250

56. Worning H: Chronic pancreatitis. Clin Gastroenterol 1984;13: 871–894

57. Braganza JM, Jolley JE, Lee WR: Occupational volatile chemicals and pancreatitis: a link? Int J Pancreatol 1986;1:9–19

58. Ammann RW, Sulser H: Die "senile" chronische pankreatitis—cine neue nosologische einheit? Schweiz Med Wochenschr 1976;106:429–437

59. Nagai H, Ohtsubo K: Pancreatic lithiasis in the aged: its clinicopathology and pathogenesis. Gastroenterology 1984;86: 331–338

60. Su CT, Beanblossom B: "Typical" cystic fibrosis in an elderly woman. Am J Med 1989;86:701–703

61. Braganza JM, John S, Padmalayam I et al: Xenobiotics and tropical chronic pancreatitis. Int J Pancreatol 1990;6:231–245

62. Segal I, Braganza JM, Gut A et al: Alcohol, nutritional factors and occupational xenobiotics in chronic calcific pancreatitis: a case control study. S Afr Med J 1993;83:A780

63. Jones SN, McNeil NI, Lees WR: The interpretation of retrograde pancreatography in the elderly. Clin Radiol 1984;40:393–396

64. Hunt LP, Braganza JM: On optimising the yield from secretin pancreozymin tests. Clin Chim Acta 1990;186:91–108

65. Braganza JM, Kay GH, Tetlow VA, Herman KJ: Observations on the BT-PABA/^{14}C-PABA tubeless test of pancreatic function. Clin Chim Acta 1983;130:339–347

66. Burke WJ, McLaughlin JR, Chung HD et al: Occurrence of cancer in Alzheimer and elderly controlled patients: an epidemiologic necropsy study. Alzheimer Dis Assoc Disord 1994;8: 22–28

67. Hartviet F, Maartman-Moe H: Pancreatic cancer—a hidden disease in the elderly? Clin Oncol 1982;8:223–229

68. Girelli CM, Reguzzoni G, Limido E et al: Pancreatic carcinoma: differences between patients with or without diabetes mellitus. Recenti Prog Med 1995;86:143–146

69. Lichtenstein DR, Carr-Locke DL: Mucin secreting tumours of the pancreas. Gastrointest Clin North Am 1995;5:237–258

70. Van Lathem JL, Vertongen P, Deviere J et al: Detection of c-Ki-ras gene codon 12 mutations from pancreatic duct brushings in the diagnosis of pancreatic tumours. Gut 1995;36:781–787

71. Yiannakou JY, Newland P, Calder F et al: Prospective study of CAM 17.1 mucin assay for serological diagnosis of pancreatic cancer. Lancet 1997;349:389–392

72. Sies H (ed): Oxidative Stress. Academic Press, London, 1985

73. Braganza JM: Towards antioxidant therapy for gastrointestinal disease. Curr Med Lit Gastroenterol 1989;8:99–106

74. Gutteridge JM: Ageing and free radicals. Med Lab Sci 1992; 49:313–318

75. Joseph JA, Cutler RC: The role of oxidative stress in signal transduction changes and cell loss in senescence. Ann N Y Acad Sci 1994;738:37–43

76. Dormandy TL: In praise of peroxidation. Lancet 1988:ii: 1126–1128

77. Braganza JM, Chaloner C: Acute pancreatitis. Curr Opin Anaesthesiol 1995;8:126–131

78. Foster JR, Idle JR, Hardwick JP et al: Induction of drug metabolising enzymes in human pancreatic cancer and chronic pancreatitis. J Pathol 1993;169:457–463

78a. Rinderknecht H: Genetic determinants of mortality in acute necrotising pancreatitis. Int J Pancreatol 1994;16:11–15

79. Jaran AS, Braganza JM, Quesnel LB: Abnormal antibiotic accumulation by cystic fibrosis cells. Med Sci Res 1993;21: 733–737

80. Morris AP, Frizzell RA: Vesicle targetting and ion secretion in epithelial cells: implications for cystic fibrosis. Ann Rev Physiol 1994;56:371–397

81. Jones M, Shiel N, Summan M et al: Application of breath pentane analysis to monitor age-related change in free radical activity. Biochem Soc Trans 1993;21:485S

82. Sharer NM, Schwarz MJ, Maloney GM et al: CFTR gene mutations in chronic pancreatitis. Gut 1996;39:A42

83. Aygalenq AU, Eugene P, Fingerhut A: Pancréatite chronique non alcholique: la mutation delta E508 du gène CFTR pourrait-elle être considèrée un factor de risque? Gastroenterol Clin Biol 1994;18:907–908

84. Paxton-Smith AN: Nutritional status: diagnosis and prevention of malnutrition. pp.66–76. In Smith AN, Carid F (eds): Metabolic and nutritional disorders in the elderly. Wright, Bristol, 1993

85. Burr ML, Hurley RJ, Sweetnam PM: Vitamin C supplementation of old people with low blood levels. Gerontol Clin 1975;17: 236–243

86. Naurath HJ, Joosten E, Riesler R et al: Effects of vitamin B_{12}, folate and vitamin B_6 supplements in elderly people with normal serum vitamin concentrations. Lancet 1995;ii:85–89

87. Uden S, Bilton D, Nathan L et al: Antioxidant therapy for recurrent pancreatitis: placebo-controlled trial. Aliment Pharmacol Ther 1990;4:357–371

88. Bilton D, Schofield D, Mei G et al: Placebo-controlled trials of antioxidant therapy including *S*-adenosylmethionine in patients with recurrent non-gallstone pancreatitis. Drug Invest 1994;8: 10–20

89. Whiteley GSW, Kienle APB, Lee S et al: Micronutrient antioxidant therapy in the non-surgical management of painful chronic pancreatitis: long-term observations. Pancreas 1994;9:A807

90. Whiteley GSW, Kienle APB, Lee SH et al: Recurrent pancreatitis in children and adolescents. Gut 1995;37:A38

91. Githens S. Glutathione metabolism in the pancreas compared with that in the liver, kidney and small intestine. Int J Pancreatol 1991;8:97–109
92. Lüthen R, Grendell JH, Haüssinger D, Niederau C: Susceptibility of the exocrine pancreas to GSH oxidation in vivo. Digestion 1995;56:A302
93. Sharer NM, Scott PD, Dearden DJ et al: Clinical trial of 24 hours' treatment with glutathione precursors in acute pancreatitis. Clin Drug Invest 1995;10:147–157
94. Braganza JM, Scott P, Bilton D et al: Evidence for early oxidative stress in acute pancreatitis: clues for correction. Int J Pancreat 1995;17:69–81
95. Braganza JM, Worthington H: A radical view of gallstone etiogenesis. Med Hypoth 1995;45:510–516
96. Gu M, Schofield D, Sharer NM et al: Coronary artery bypass grafting (CABG) as a risk factor for acute pancreatitis: shared predisposition to oxidative stress. Pancreas 1994;9: A789

CHAPTER 59

The Liver

OLIVER F. W. JAMES

Structure And Age

The liver reaches maximum size in early adult life, and thereafter there is a decrease in liver volume, both in absolute terms and in relation to body weight, which is more marked from about the age of 60 onward. This reduction has been recently estimated to be about 37 percent between ages 24 and 90.[1] The number and conformation of the hepatic lobes and other aspects of gross hepatic architecture remain unaltered throughout life. Liver blood flow also declines by about 35 percent from early adult life to the age of 90.[2] Furthermore, liver perfusion (liver blood flow per unit volume liver) also falls over this age range by about 10 percent. The liver becomes a darker brown color with advanced age as a result of the accumulation of fluorescent brown pigmented lipofuscin granules in lysosomes within hepatocytes. The deposition of this protein is due to decreased intracellular proteolysis with age. Lipofuscin is also deposited elsewhere in advanced age—notably in the brain.[3,4]

Although liver size declines with age, human hepatocytes increase in size, unlike the situation in liver atrophy accompanying starvation. Liver cell nuclei show polyploidy and increased nuclear size; as in other organelles, mitochondria are also enlarged.[5-7] It is unclear whether the increased intracellular protein is functionally active or whether it represents the accumulation of "junk" within liver cells. In the absence of disease, hepatocytes divide only two or three times during the human life span. The space of Disse between liver cells is enlarged in aging, and there is a corresponding increase in the amount of collagen. However, the nature of the collagen appears unaltered.[8]

Liver Function

As with the morphologic changes described above, it is useless to extrapolate alterations in hepatic function found in aging from experimental animals to humans. Conventional liver blood tests do not change with age. There has been little examination of the changes in hepatic synthetic function with age, but there is a significant negative correlation between peak urea synthesis and age[9]; and hepatic conversion of α-aminonitrogen to urea nitrogen—functional hepatic nitrogen clearance—declines by about 50 percent in advanced age. This appears to be greater than the concomitant decline in liver volume.[10] Hepatic synthesis of cholesterol is reduced in old age, and there is a reduction in total bile acid pool and possibly synthesis of bile acid from cholesterol.[11] With normal aging, galactose elimination, a cytosolic function, is reduced at the same rate as liver size.[2]

It is conceivable that the capacity of the liver for regeneration is impaired in advanced age, and this may reduce its ability to "repair" itself. It has recently been shown that there is an age-related decline in mitogen-activated protein kinase activity in rat hepatocytes stimulated by epidermal growth factor, which provides a possible explanation, at least in part, for the decline in liver regeneration and repair.[12] Furthermore, an age-associated twofold increase in DNA bases damaged by oxidative modification has recently been observed in the rat liver, which was similar to modification induced by carcinogens and seen in experimental hepatocellular cancers. Thus, hepatic synthetic function, regenerative capacity, and susceptibility to external insults such as potential carcinogens may all be impaired in normal advanced age.[13]

Drug Metabolism

This is the most widely studied aspect of aging and the human liver. The clearance of drugs whose metabolism is dependent on the cytochrome P450 group of liver enzymes declines variably anywhere between 0 and 50 percent according to age.[14] Furthermore, there is a widely described increase in the variance of drug clearance with advancing age. It seems probable that when such lifetime environmental variables as diet, smoking, and nutrition are taken into account, there is a broad decline in hepatic drug metabolism of between 5 and 30 percent from adulthood to old age.[15,16] It is probable that the decline in metabolism of such model drugs as antipyrene, aminopyrene, and caffeine can be largely accounted for by the decline in liver blood flow already mentioned.[17]

Investigations of Hepatobiliary Disease

A good history, including a history of medications, and a clinical examination are of paramount importance in the diagnosis of possible liver disease in the elderly. While there are no major differences in this respect between old and young patients, selection of appropriate investigations, particularly those that are invasive, may differ according to age. Specific points relating to history and examination will arise in relation to the diseases discussed below. It is the purpose of this section to propose a rational system for the investigation of elderly patients with possible hepatobiliary disease. For further more detailed accounts of individual modes of investigation, readers are referred to major texts on liver disease.[18–20]

Laboratory Investigations

Serum biochemistry

Routine serum biochemical tests—liver function tests (LFTs)—include determinations of serum bilirubin, serum alkaline phosphatase (ALP), and serum aspartate aminotransferase (AST) or alanine aminotransferase (ALT). In general, elevated ALP indicates cholestasis, whereas elevated transaminase indicates liver cell damage. In addition, serum γ-glutamyl transpeptidase (γ-GT) can be used to evaluate cholestasis. Since ALP originates not only in the biliary tree but also in bone and intestine—relevant sources in some elderly patients—measurement of γ-GT may confirm or refute suspected cholestasis in a patient with isolated elevated ALP. γ-GT activity may be increased by a wide range of enzyme inducers, hence care must be taken in interpreting elevated γ-GT. Since alcohol is itself a hepatic enzyme inducer, elevated γ-GT has been used as a possible marker for alcoholism. Unfortunately this test has limited specificity and sensitivity.

Serum transaminases are elevated in most liver diseases. The highest occur with severe liver cell necrosis—whether toxin-induced by, for example, paracetamol (acetaminophen) overdose, in acute viral hepatitis, or as a result of ischemic damage to the liver. Elevation of serum bilirubin leads to the most obvious sign of clinical liver disease—jaundice. This condition is normally clinically detectable when serum bilirubin is elevated above about 50 mmol/L or 3 mg percent (three times the normal range). Bilirubin may be elevated in cholestatic or hepatocellular disease; unfortunately, as with other biochemical LFTs, its degree of elevation does not correspond closely with the severity of liver disease. Furthermore, hemolysis—leading to increased red cell breakdown and formation of bilirubin—which may accompany some liver diseases, may also contribute to elevation of serum bilirubin.

Blood tests for suspected liver disease (the liver screen)

Blood count and film
LFTs (alkaline phosphatase, transaminase, bilirubin)
Proteins (albumin, total globulin)
HBsAg, anti-HBc
Anti-HCV
Autoimmune profile (AMA, SMA, ANA)
Ferritin
Random blood ethanol
Urea, creatinine, electrolytes

Serum albumin is often reduced in chronic liver disease. Although albumin is synthesized by the liver, serum albumin level reflects not only synthesis but also dietary protein intake and absorption. Nonetheless, since serum albumin reflects hepatic synthetic function, it should be regarded as one of the most important LFTs.

Serum globulin levels do not reflect liver function. Persistent elevation of total globulin and particularly γ-globulin is associated with autoimmune liver disease, elevated IgA with alcoholic liver disease (ALD), and elevated IgM with primary biliary cirrhosis (PBC). None of these is more than indicative.

Probably the best routine test of hepatic synthetic function is prothrombin time (or ratio), since the liver synthesizes clotting factors I (fibrinogen), II (prothrombin), V, VII, IX and X. Because these factors are normally present in excess in human serum, impairment of coagulation dependent on one or more of them may indicate quite profound liver cell dysfunction. In cholestasis or in circumstances in which steatorrhea occurs, coagulation may be deficient not because of impairment of the clotting factors themselves but because of lack of procoagulant function. In these circumstances parenteral vitamin K (usually one or two 10-mg injections) should restore normal clotting function. Indeed in patients with moderate impairment of prothrombin time correction by parenteral K is itself highly suggestive of a cholestatic, usually obstructive, cause of the liver disease under investigation.[21]

Hepatic Metabolic Capacity

A variety of metabolic tests dependent on model substrates have been used to assess more accurately the true function of the liver. None need be used in routine clinical practice, indeed none have been widely adopted for this purpose. Advances in other investigational modalities, particularly in imaging, have rendered such metabolic tests redundant except in a research context.

How to Use LFTs in the Elderly

All elderly patients with suspected liver disease should have routine LFTs and serum proteins examined. In any individual with significant liver disease prothrombin time (or ratio) should be added to this first-line list. In the presence of elevated serum ALP, γ-GT is probably more reliable than ALP electrophoresis in confirming cholestasis (i.e., intra- or extrahepatic obstruction). It should be emphasized that these tests are not an end in themselves but part of a group of investigations that should be routinely used in suspected hepatobiliary disorders. Faced with apparently isolated abnormalities of one or more LFTs but with no clinical indication of significant liver disease, careful exclusion of heart failure and occult infection should be made. The other blood tests considered part of the "liver screen" in the preceding box should be carried out. It is important to remember that mild abnormalities in one or more of these enzymes are present in diabetes, in a variety of generalized inflammatory disorders (e.g., rheumatoid arthritis, polymyalgia rheumatica), in a variety of malignancies not directly affecting the liver, and in obesity. Faced with an apparently isolated LFT abnormality and in the absence of any other positive information from the liver screen, the clinician may well decide to reassure their elderly patient after a period of time, particularly if ultrasound examination of the hepatobiliary system shows no abnormality. It is poor practice, however, merely to ignore abnormal LFTs in an elderly patient who is otherwise well and not consider further investigation or follow-up.

Hematology

Blood count and blood film are mandatory in the investigation of suspected liver disease. In chronic liver disease with hypersplenism associated with portal hypertension, there is depressed erythropoesis and shortened red cell life. Splenic enlargement may lead to reduced platelet levels and in severe instances to reduced white blood cell count and anemia. The toxic effects of ALD result from a combination of the direct effect of alcohol on the bone marrow, the liver disease and portal hypertension, and the frequent concomitant undernutrition. Macrocytosis, frequently with normal serum folate and red blood cell folate, is seen in all forms of chronic liver disease, not just in patients with ALD. Blood loss from esophageal varices or portal gastropathy can occur in all forms of chronic liver disease, while bleeding from esophagitis, gastritis, and duodenitis occurs particularly in ALD or in severe acute or chronic liver damage associated with impaired clotting. The hematology of liver disease is complex, and readers are referred to an excellent monograph by Berk.[21]

Hepatobiliary Radiology and Scanning

Ultrasound

In patients with signs, symptoms, or LFTs suggesting biliary obstruction, ultrasound examination should be the first imaging procedure employed. It is fast, safe, and noninvasive. Ultrasound in experienced hands is reliable in detecting extrahepatic obstruction, usually giving a good indication of the site of such obstruction.[22] Nonetheless, normal-sized intrahepatic or extrahepatic bile ducts do not necessarily exclude bile duct obstruction. Furthermore, while ultrasound is excellent in detecting gallstones within the gallbladder, it appears to be relatively insensitive in detecting gallstones in the common hepatic and bile ducts. Ultrasound can also be used to detect tumors of the gallbladder and within the biliary tree (cholangiocarcinomas). If despite negative ultrasound findings there is reasonable clinical suspicion of extrahepatic biliary disease, then further radiology with either endoscopic retrograde cholangiopancreatography (ERCP) or CT scanning, or if available, MR cholangiography should be carried out. Routine oral cholecystography has no real place in modern imaging, however, plain upper abdominal radiographs are still of great value in detecting hepatic or biliary tree calcification—usually indicating gallstones. The appearance of air in the biliary tree in a patient who has not had previous endoscopic sphincterotomy is highly suggestive of biliary sepsis.

Modern color ultrasound with Doppler and (increasingly) other modalities such as three-dimensional imaging and vascular enhancements will increasingly enable more sophisticated noninvasive evaluation of the liver and its circulation.[23,24] At present ultrasound may be carried out for three reasons: (1) to detect space occupying lesions within the liver, (2) to assess the texture, size, and shape of the liver, (3) to assess the patency of the hepatic vascular tree. Ultrasound is able to detect liver masses as small as 1 to 2 cm in diameter, and expert hands over 95 percent of such lesions can be visualized. Nonetheless, it is best to be cautious about overconfident interpretation of the appearances of lesions within the liver.[25] For example, the distinction between a small tumor and a regeneration nodule in a patient with cirrhosis may be extremely difficult.

While claims have been made that ultrasound examination can reliably distinguish between cirrhosis and, for example, fatty liver or acute hepatitis, these claims are usually made in reference to selected patients at extremely specialized centers using the most sophisticated equipment. In routine clinical practice ultrasound is still seldom helpful in making an histologic diagnosis beyond reporting the existence of a shrunken irregular liver highly suggestive of cirrhosis, particularly in conjunction with an enlarged spleen, distended portal vessels, or ascites. As indicated, ultrasound examination of the abdomen may also detect other helpful diagnostic features apart from the appearance of the liver and biliary tree; thus enlarged abdominal lymph nodes or pancreatic abnormalities, as well as enlarged or abnormal intra-abdominal vessels, can readily be detected.[24]

Radionucleide scanning

This form of scanning has largely been replaced by other imaging techniques, but it is still useful in the evaluation of liver disease.[26] In particular, since the radiolabeled colloid used in scanning is taken up by the reticuloendothelial system, radionucleide scanning acts as a test of function of the Kupffer cells within the liver. In severe cirrhosis, particularly in severe alcoholic cirrhosis with alcoholic hepatitis, uptake of the colloid is very poor indeed, which may lead to a so-called white-out appearance—essentially nonvisualization of the liver. This result may, however, also lead to some false positive and false negative reports of space occupying lesions within the liver.

Computed tomography

Computed tomography (CT) is currently the best noninvasive imaging technique for the liver. CT with vascular enhancement is particularly useful in detecting tumors within the liver or in the biliary tree. In the evaluation of primary hepatocellular cancer (HCC) CT is carried out 1 to 2 weeks following lipiodol angiography (see below).[27]

CT should be regarded as a complementary investigation to ultrasound. Neither is entirely reliable in detecting small stones within the common duct, however, CT is particularly useful in revealing small ampullary tumors.

Magnetic resonance imaging

Until recently magnetic resonance imaging (MRI) had no major advantage over CT scanning since the process was slower, leading to more movement artifact in the images.[28] Newer, faster MRI scanners can now produce images similar in definition to the best CT scans. Furthermore, gadolinium enhancement provides information about direction of vascular flow more reliably than all but the very best Doppler ultrasound and is a great deal less operator-dependent.[29,30] Soon MR cholangiography may reduce the need for ERCP. MRI also provides information about the texture of the liver, especially in the detection of hemochromatosis in which excessive iron deposition is particularly easily observed.[31]

Guided liver biopsy

Liver biopsy is now very frequently carried out under the guidance of one of the above imaging techniques, usually ultrasound. With the advent of portable ultrasound machines, it is now perceived as good practice for most liver biopsies, not just those carried out to detect specific focal lesions within the liver, to be carried out under ultrasound guidance. It should, however, be stated that to optimize the benefit of ultrasound guided biopsy the procedure (ultrasound and biopsy) must be carried out by an experienced operator.

Angiography

In clinical practice in older patients, angiography involving the liver has two purposes—diagnostic and therapeutic. Therapeutic angiography will be considered below with respect to clinical indications. Angiography is an invasive and uncomfortable procedure which carries morbidity and (extraordinarily rarely) mortality risks. It should not, therefore, be undertaken except after the use of other imaging techniques or in circumstances where specific information available only from angiography is required.[32] It is particularly useful in the assessment of patients who may have liver tumors. Most tumors, whether benign or malignant, primary or secondary, exhibit an abnormal vascular pattern within the liver. The diagnostic value of hepatic angiography has been enormously enhanced by the use of intrahepatic injection of the radiodense contrast medium Lipiodol. Lipiodol is selectively retained in or around tumor tissue in the liver and can best be detected 1 to 2 weeks after angiography by obtaining a subsequent CT scan.[32] The Lipiodol is retained only in relation to tumor tissue within the liver, hence can be visualized on a CT scan. This technique is sensitive and specific and is particularly important where resection of small primary liver cancers is being considered. Angiography may also be used to assess the portal venous system of the liver, which becomes visible on later films following mesenteric angiography. The direction of blood flow within the portal system can be examined in this way. Increasingly, however, Doppler ultrasound is being used for this purpose. Angiography is mandatory before major hepatic surgery.

Venography of the vessels associated with the liver is now less commonly used. Occasionally, in the assessment of suspected hepatic vein occlusion (Budd Chiari syndrome), inferior venacavography or hepatic venography is used, although color Doppler is now superseding its use.[33] Hepatic venous catheterization is also used to assess free and wedged hepatic vein pressures, which are of considerable interest in patients with portal hypertension, but the technique is of little diagnostic or therapeutic value in older patients except in relation to transjugular intrahepatic portal systemic shunt (TIPSS) (see below).

Transjugular intrahepatic portal systemic shunt

This new radiologic technique, in which a stent is placed angiographically between a major branch of the portal vein and the hepatic vein within the liver, thus creating the equivalent of a surgical portosystemic shunt, has received a great deal of attention and evaluation in the past few years. This treatment should be carried out only at highly experienced centers. The place of TIPSS in the treatment of bleeding varices is still controversial.[34,35] It is currently recommended for treatment of intractable repeated bleeding from esophageal varices where injection and/or banding has been unsuccessful or of repeated bleeding from portal gastropathy where these techniques are inapplicable. In patients with resistant ascites this procedure may also represent an alternative to repeated abdominal paracentesis. In both instances advanced age is an independent risk factor for mortality. In patients with Child's grade C status, mortality following TIPSS is in excess of 70 percent at 6 months. The place of TIPSS in the management of elderly patients with complications of portal hypertension is thus unproven. Nonetheless, in patients with a previous good quality of life who develop intractable bleeding from portal hypertension, this treatment may be highly effective.

ERCP

This technique is not only the best method for visualizing the biliary tree but also offers an opportunity for immediate therapeutic intervention (see below).[36] ERCP allows inspection of the duodenum and ampulla together with outlining of the pancreatic duct system, thus providing information concerning the possible cause of obstruction of the biliary system at its lower end. Injection of contrast, opacifying the biliary tree, reveals the anatomy of the common bile duct, common hepatic duct, and intrahepatic biliary tree together with the cystic duct and gallbladder. It is the gold standard in diagnosis of stones in the biliary tree (apart from the gallbladder itself), as well as in the diagnosis of sclerosing cholangitis. In patients who have not had previous gastric surgery, particularly polyagastrectomy, the common bile duct can be outlined satisfactor-

Color Plates

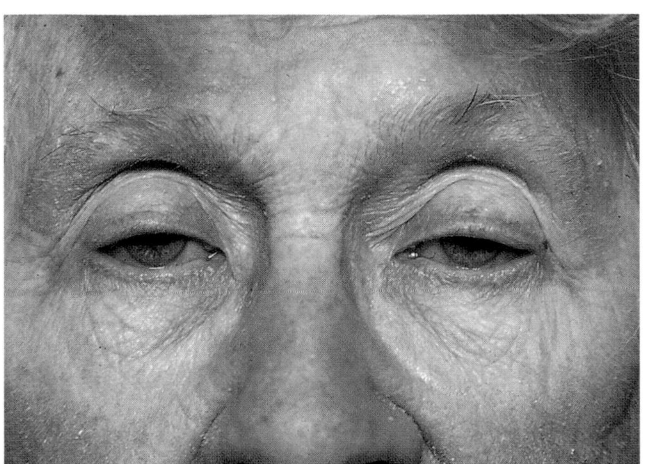

Plate 46-1

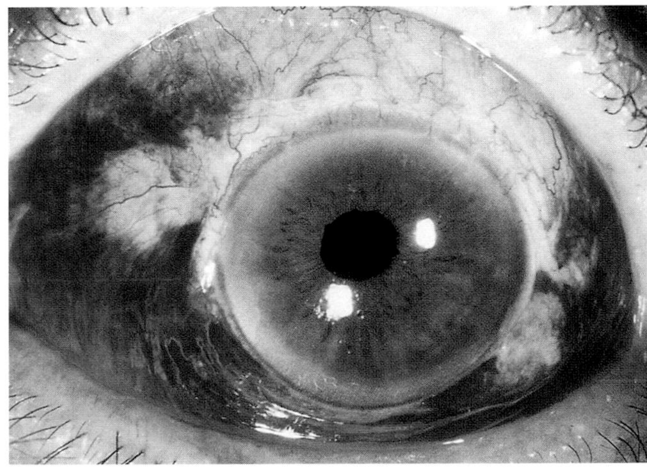

Plate 46-2

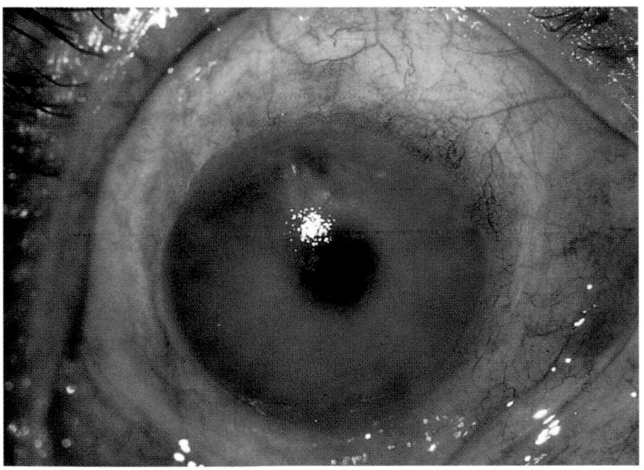

Plate 46-3

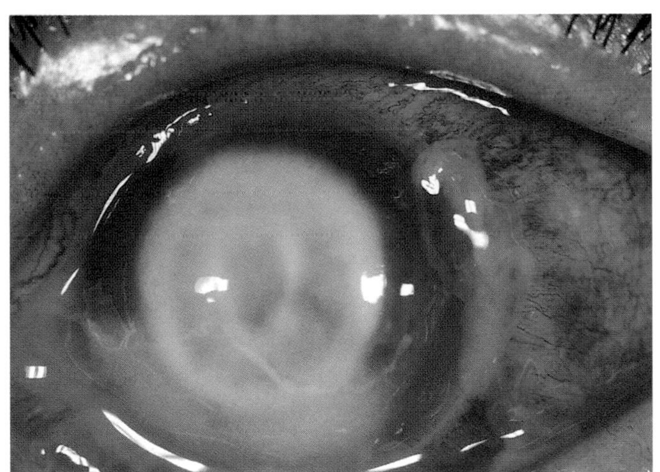

Plate 46-4

Plate 46-1 Senile ptosis. Note the low lid level and the loss of the normal lid folds. (Courtesy of Murray Meltzer, MD.)

Plate 46-2 Subconjunctival hemorrhage. This small hematoma, seen through the transparent conjunctiva, is benign unless recurrent.

Plate 46-3 Corneal edema. The cornea is thickened and cloudy due to failure of the corneal endothelium to adequately dehydrate the tissue. (Courtesy of Calvin Roberts, MD.)

Plate 46-4 Corneal ulcer. A localized infection causes an epithelial defect and attracts an infiltrate of white blood cells. (Courtesy of Michael Newton, MD.)

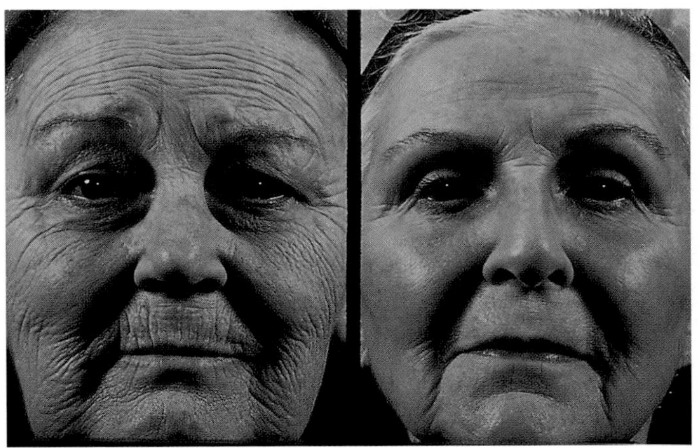

Plate 90-1

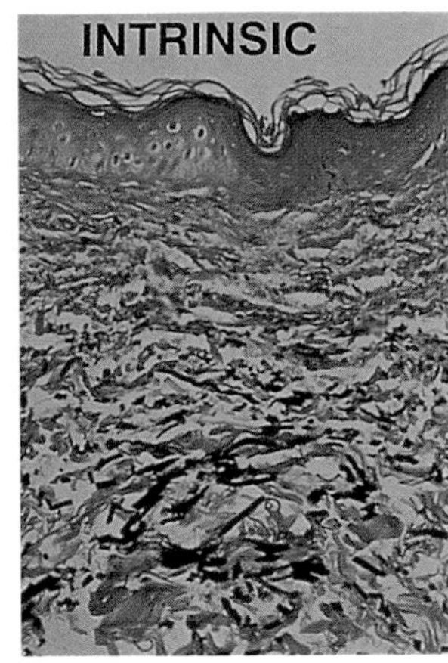

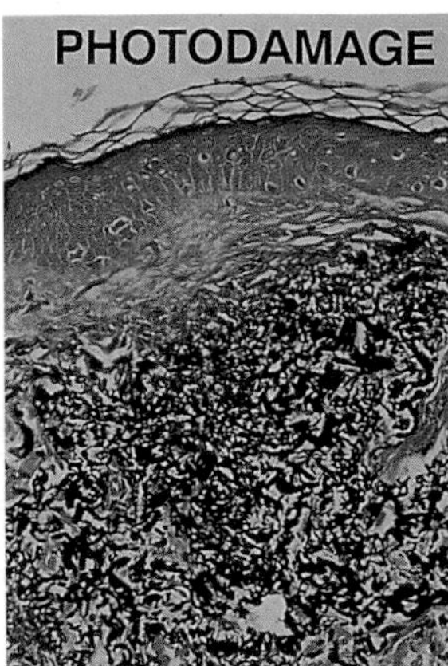

Plate 90-2

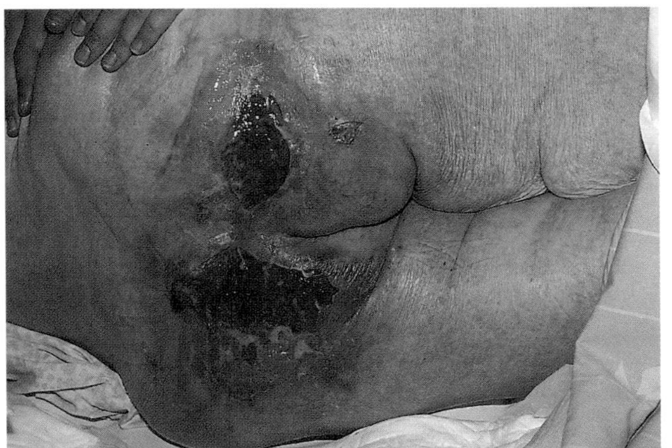

Plate 97-1

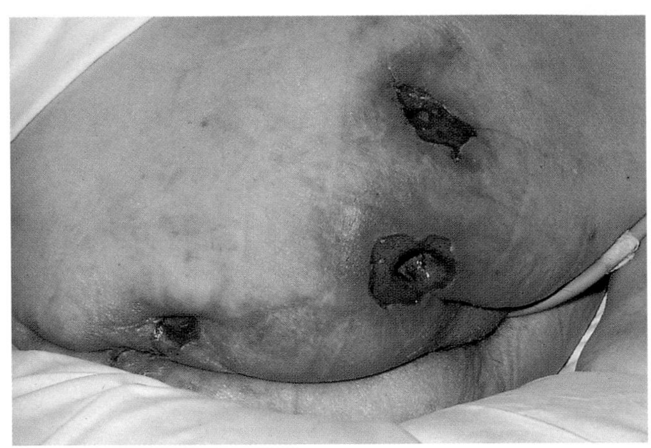

Plate 97-2

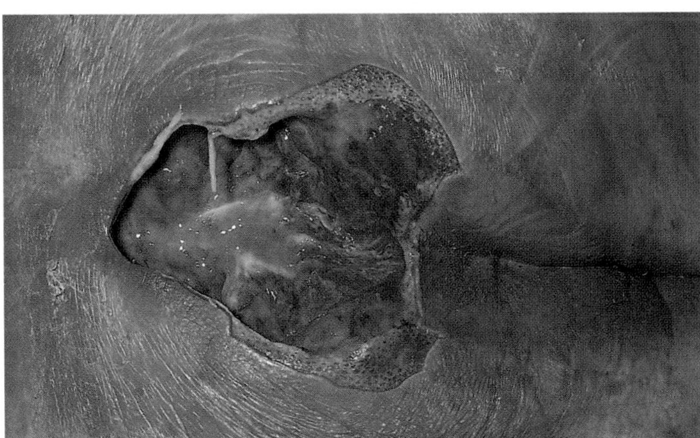

Plate 97-3

Plate 90-1 Faces of two 71-year-old women. The woman on the right has avoided sun exposure for most of her life and the changes are mostly those of intrinsic, chronologic aging. The woman on the left has suffered a great deal of sun exposure and the wrinkles and thickened skin are evidence of photoaging. To the untrained observer the woman on the left appears older than her stated age.

Plate 90-2 Photomicrographs of histologic sections of intrinsic and extrinsically aged skin stained with Verhoeff van Giesen stain for elastin. The salient difference is the gross increase in black-staining, elastotic material in the reticular dermis of extrinsic, photoaged skin (× 40).

Plate 97-1 Superficial sore.

Plate 97-2 Deep sore.

Plate 97-3 Full-thickness sacral sore.

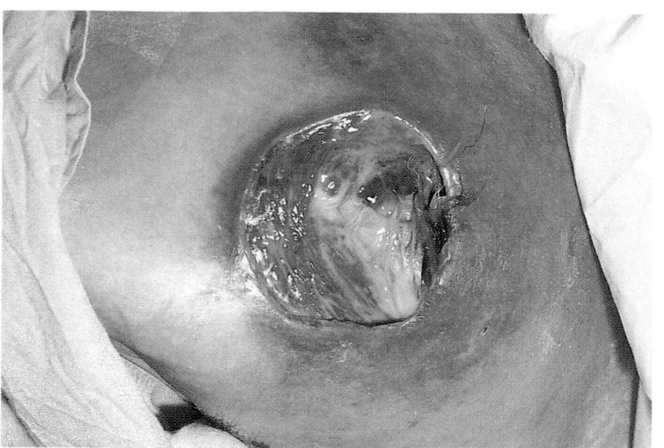

Plate 97-4

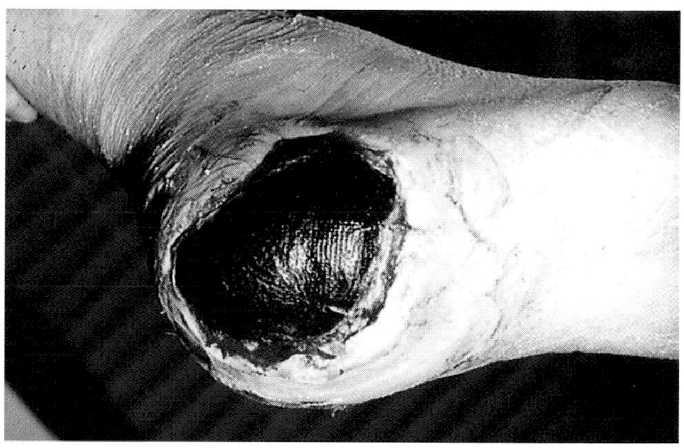

Plate 97-5

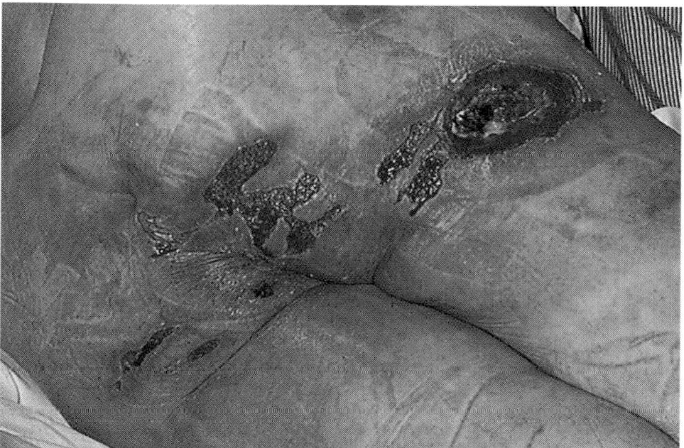

Plate 97-6

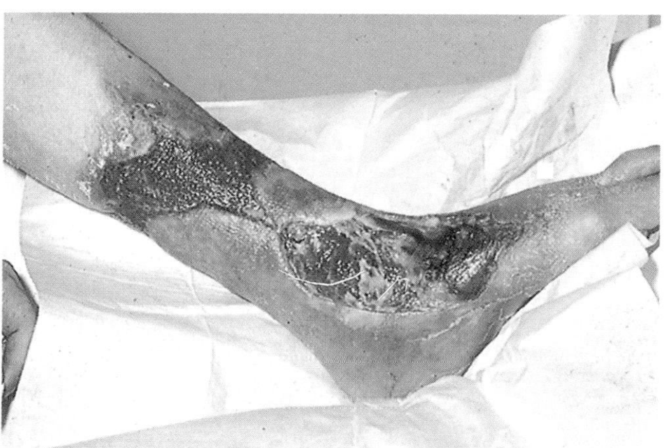

Plate 97-7

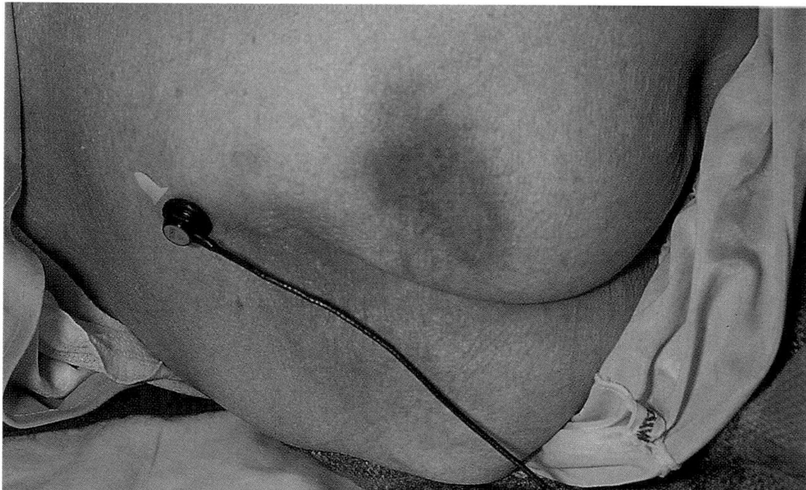

Plate 97-8

Plate 97-4 Deep sore over the greater trochanter.

Plate 97-5 Heel sore.

Plate 97-6 Chair sores.

Plate 97-7 Pressure sore caused by a bandage. Note characteristic deep necrosis over the instep.

Plate 97-8 Measurement of transcutaneous gas tension.

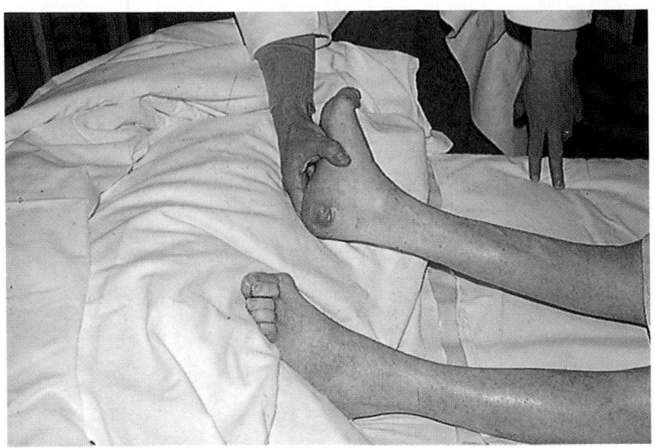

Plate 98-1

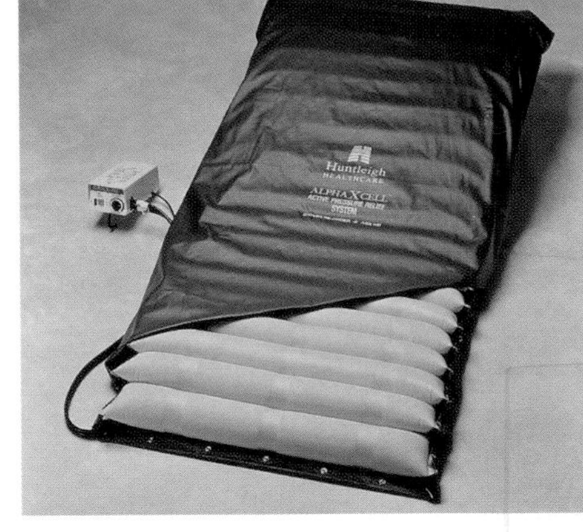

Plate 98-2

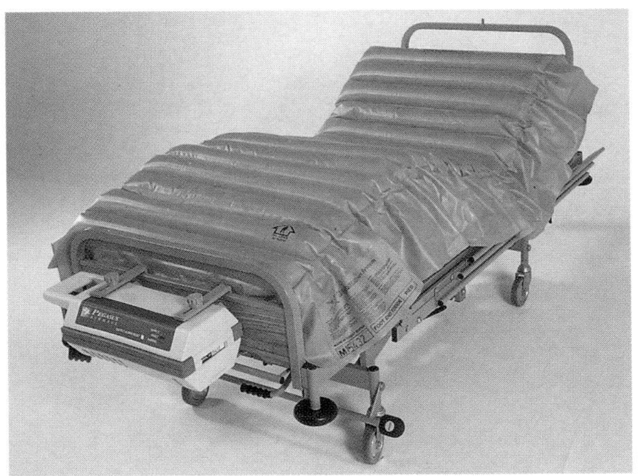

Plate 98-3

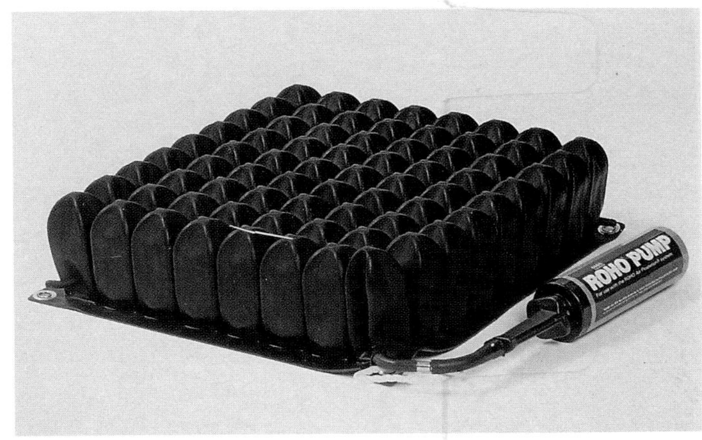

Plate 98-4

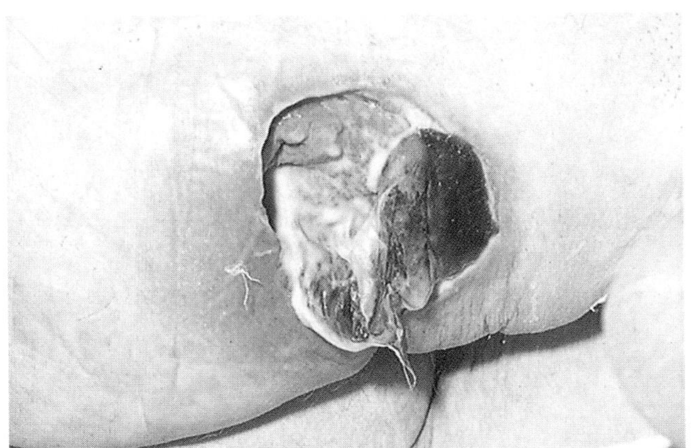

Plate 98-5

Plate 98-1 Persistent erythema—grade 1 pressure sore.

Plate 98-2 Large-cell alternating-pressure overlay.

Plate 98-3 Deep alternating-pressure mattress replacement.

Plate 98-4 Roho cushion.

Plate 98-5 Natural debridement of a necrotic slough.

ily in 90+ percent of examinations by a good investigator.[37] In patients with biliary obstruction and jaundice, care should be taken concerning hydration, and it is recommended that all elderly patients undergoing ERCP have an intravenous crystalloid infusion started before the procedure. In cases where biliary obstruction is suspected, a single shot of broad-spectrum antibiotic (gentamycin or cephalosporin) should be given just prior to the procedure.

Percutaneous transhepatic cholangiography

In circumstances in which the anatomy of the upper gastrointestinal tract makes successful ERCP unlikely, or where ERCP has already been attempted and has failed, percutaneous transhepatic cholangiography (PTC) is the investigation of choice in examination of the biliary tree, particularly if there is ultrasound evidence of an obstructed and dilated biliary tree. Complications including septicemia, biliary leak, and intraperitoneal hemorrhage are not uncommon and, as in the case of ERCP, it is recommended that prophylactic intravenous antibiotics be given.[38]

Clinicians investigating the possibility of biliary obstruction or intrahepatic lesions in the elderly must steer a course between investigative and therapeutic nihilism on the one hand—which may merely be an excuse for ignorance of the range of diagnostic and therapeutic techniques now available—and the overuse of invasive investigative techniques in extremely elderly individuals on the other. Therapeutic uses of the above imaging procedures will be discussed in the clinical section below.

Laparoscopy

Laparoscopy, like other invasive investigational techniques already described, is increasingly being used in elderly patients because it offers opportunities for immediate therapeutic intervention where appropriate.[39] It should be carried out only at a center where the technique is in routine use. Its particular virtues are in (1) direct visualization of lesions within or adjacent to the liver, (2) enhancing or speeding up diagnosis of some disseminated intra-abdominal condition (e.g., metastases or infections), and (3) undertaking biopsies with direct vision.

Liver Biopsy

The histologic assessment of liver disease is fundamental to understanding its pathogenesis and thus its treatment. Physicians caring for elderly patients with liver disease must not hesitate to carry out needle biopsies of the liver. With appropriate safeguards concerning clotting and, where appropriate, under ultrasound-guided control, the procedure is extremely safe. Complications include hemorrhage, perforation of the gallbladder with biliary peritonitis, pneumothorax, and septicemia.[40,41]

In a recent survey of 1,500 liver biopsies from district hospitals throughout England and Wales, the median age for biopsy was 60 to 69 years, 6 percent of the patients were over the age of 80, and mortality was 0.13 percent. Accurate pathologic assessment of liver histology is critical in the following circumstances.[42]

1. *Documentation of neoplastic disease*: This is critical both in confirming the nature of a disease and in planning treatment. In the recent England and Wales study 50 percent of liver biopsies in persons over 65 years old were carried out because of suspected malignant disease.[42] Tissue diagnosis of tumor within the liver is often justifiable and necessary, however, there are two important exceptions to this rule. First, if surgical excision of a focal lesion within the liver is contemplated, then biopsy, with its risk of tumor spread, is best avoided. Characterization of the lesion should be carried out with the scanning and angiographic procedures described above. Serum α-fetoprotein is elevated in 70+ percent of primary HCCs and can be regarded as diagnostic in a patient with a focal intrahepatic lesion at a level of above 500 IU/L. Exceptionally, in patients over the age of 65 liver transplantation for primary hepatic malignancies is again being carried out after exhaustive exclusion of extrahepatic spread. Again, preoperative biopsy is contraindicated. Second, biopsy of intrahepatic neoplastic disease should be avoided in cases in which widespread disseminated malignancy is already established or where the likely nature of the hepatic lesion is already known because of previous histologic diagnosis of a distant primary neoplasm.
2. *Classification of chronic liver disease*: In chronic viral or autoimmune liver disease, while serologic markers are extremely important, the gold standard is liver histology. It is particularly in the area of classifying liver disease and staging progressive liver diseases that sampling errors may occur. Current treatment strategies (with interferon) for hepatitis C are based on histologic assessment of both inflammatory activity and degree of fibrosis.
3. *Staging liver disease*: It is often invaluable in estimating prognosis and formulating strategy to know the histologic stage of a specific progressive liver disease—ALD and PBC are cases in point.
4. *Evaluation of treatment programs*: Again the gold standard for evaluation of the success of treatment is a baseline biopsy (for the reasons stated above) with a follow-up biopsy or biopsies after a defined period of treatment. Even in relatively elderly patients this practice may be desirable and justifiable, particularly in evaluating new therapies or in monitoring possible drug hepatotoxicity.
5. *Evaluation of abnormal LFTs*: In patients with consistently abnormal LFTs or in whom there is diagnostic doubt concerning the nature of their liver disease, liver biopsy is clearly vital.

Table 59-1 Second-line tests for suspected liver disease

In hepatitis	HAV IgM; plus if HBsAg positive, then e antigen or e antibody; anti-HCV
In hyperbilirubinemia	Conjugated vs unconjugated
To confirm cholestasis	γ-Glutamyl transpeptidase
For HCC	α-Fetoprotein
For immune disease	Immunoglobulins; anti-M_2AMA, LKM, ANA, SMA
α_1-Antitrypsin deficiency	α_1-Antitrypsin phenotype

Other Serologic Tests (Table 59-1)

Viral Markers

Hepatitis A

HAV IgM is a reliable marker for recent or current infection with hepatitis A virus (HAV).[43]

Hepatitis B

HBsAg indicates the presence of the surface protein of hepatitis B virus (HBV) in the serum. In patients with acute type B hepatitis this protein is often associated with the presence of the whole virus in the blood and thus infectivity. In patients with chronic liver disease, after incorporation of the viral genome into hepatic nuclear material, production of the HBsAg protein and its presence in the serum give no indication of infectivity or of stage of illness. Anti-HBs is usually present in low titer following initial infection with HBV. It may or may not persist for months or years following an initial infection. Anti-HBc—an antibody to the core of the virus—is the most reliable indicator of past infection. It gives no indication of current infectivity or of when initial infection took place. HBeAg, the e antigen, is distinct from HBsAg and anti-HBc but is closely associated with the virion core. Presence of the e antigen in the serum is indicative of the presence of whole virus and thus of infectivity. Anti-HBe usually indicates disappearance of whole HBV and thus loss of infectivity. Until recently it was thought that absence of e antigen in the serum indicated a low risk of infectivity, but new strains of HBV not expressing e antigen but which are nonetheless infective have now been described, particularly in Mediterranean countries; thus the mere absence of HBeAg does not necessary indicate a lack of infectivity. Levels of HBV DNA can now be measured in the serum, and this is the most direct method of estimating infectivity and presence of the whole virus. The test is available only at a very limited number of centers and at present is probably unnecessary except in the context of transplantation.

Hepatitis C

Anti-HCV merely indicates past or present infection with the hepatitis C virus (HCV), giving no indication of either prognosis or infectivity.[44] Anti-HCV does not become detectable in the serum for up to 6 months after initial exposure. Anti-HCV RIBA is a more recently developed second-generation test that uses multiple immunodominant regions of structural and nonstructural HCV to provide confirmatory tests for the "screening" anti-HCV enzyme-linked immunoabsorbent assay (ELISA). The HCV RNA test, which allows viral RNA to be detected and quantified by a polymerase chain reaction (PCR), is still a nonroutine test.[45]

Hepatitis D (delta virus)

Anti-HDAg IgM and IgG responses are used to investigate hepatitis D virus (HDV), and tests are available from central laboratories. HDV requires HBV for replication and thus is found only in patients with simultaneous acute or chronic HBV infection.

Hepatitis E and hepatitis G

No routine serologic testing is yet available for these newly described viruses.

Autoimmune Markers

Autoimmune markers are summarized in Table 59-1.

Antimitochondrial antibody

Antimitochondrial antibody (AMA) is non-tissue and non-species-specific but is highly disease-specific for PBC. The group of antigens against which AMAs are directed have recently been isolated, and the current indirect immunofluorescent test is being replaced by more specific radioimmunoassay or ELISA tests at some centers.[46]

Smooth muscle antibody and liver kidney microsomal antibody

Smooth muscle antibody (SMA) and liver kidney microsomal antibody (LKM) are usually indicators of autoimmune chronic hepatitis, particularly in titers greater than 1 in 40.

Antinuclear antibody

Antinuclear antibodies (ANAs) are a group of antibodies detected by various indirect immunofluorescent techniques. They are seen in the full spectrum of autoimmune liver diseases, particularly in so-called autoimmune cholangiopathy (AMA-negative PBC), in autoimmune chronic hepatitis, and in up to half of patients with sclerosing cholangitis.

Serum α-fetoprotein

This marker is elevated in about 70 percent of patients with primary HCC. Normally values are less than 10 mmol/L in adults; in patients with chronic liver disease and cirrhosis this level may rise to 50 mmol/L. Values above 500 mmol/L in the context of an elderly patient with chronic liver disease or a possible liver tumor are virtually diagnostic of primary liver cancer. A rising value above about 50 mmol/L over a period of months in a patient with cirrhosis is highly suggestive of the development of primary HCC. Unfortunately, about one-third of primary hepatic tumors do not synthesize this fetal protein, and a normal serum value by no means excludes such a tumor.

α_1-Antitrypsin

This acute phase α_1-globulin is a normal protease inhibitor. It is present in the serum in several phenotypes. The measurement of total serum α_1-antitrypsin is an unreliable method for indentifying patients with abnormal phenotypes who may have associated liver disease since its level rises as part of the normal acute phase protein response in, for example, infections. Thus, in patients in whom α_1-antitrypsin deficiency is a suspected cause of liver disease, serum phenotyping must be undertaken in a specialized laboratory. Usually this takes place after the detection of periodic acid-Schiff (PAS)-positive diastase resistance granules in periportal hepatocytes found on liver biopsy in patients with hitherto cryptogenic chronic liver disease.

Serum ferritin and iron binding capacity

Serum ferritin is markedly elevated in patients with hemochromatosis; the normal value for men and postmenopausal women is up to 300 ng/mL. Hemochromatosis should be considered in elderly patients with chronic liver disease whose level is above about 800 ng/mL.[47] Unfortunately this increased level reflects only an increase in total body iron. Furthermore, liver damage itself can cause a nonspecific rise in serum ferritin, and thus patients with secondary hemochromatosis or hemosiderosis (e.g., after many blood transfusions) or patients with severe (particularly alcoholic) active liver disease may show very elevated serum ferritin levels. If hemochromatosis is suspected, then serum iron, total iron binding capacity (TIBC), or transferrin and ferritin concentrations should be determined. Transferrin saturation of over 70 percent is suggestive of hemochromatosis. Until recently a certain diagnosis of hemochromatosis depended on liver biopsy with measurement of liver iron concentration and histologic assessment of iron overload. Recently, the gene for hemochromatosis has been detected on chromosome 6. This discovery will form the basis of a reliable diagnostic test for homozygous hemochromatosis and for the presence of the heterozygous state, at least in individuals of Celtic origin (HLA-H).

Specific Diseases of the Liver in the Elderly

Toxic Damage: ALD in the Elderly

Although ALD is perceived as being uncommon in older people, a British series showed that 28 percent of patients with this disease presented for the first time over the age of 60 and 7 percent over the age of 70.[48] In France a large retrospective study found that 20 percent of patients were over the age of 70.[49] In the United States one study among white males showed that the peak decade for presentation with cirrhosis was the seventh.[50] In our own series, older patients presented with a higher proportion of signs and symptoms suggestive of the complications of severe liver disease—jaundice, hypoproteinemia, ascites, or bleeding from esophagogastric varices. Almost all patients over the age of 70 who are referred to hospitals for the first time have cirrhosis, against a proportion of less than 50 percent among under 50 year olds. Prognosis is related to age. Mortality among those under 60 years old at presentation was 5 percent at 1 year and 24 percent at 3 years, whereas of those presenting at over 70 years of age, 75 percent were dead at 1 year and 90 percent at 3 years. It is generally true that age-specific mortality from cirrhosis, whatever the cause, rises strikingly with age. It is unclear why older patients present with more severe clinical features and have a worse prognosis. It may be that family doctors are more reluctant to refer elderly individuals with minor signs or symptoms of possible ALD to hospitals; this may be understandable—even correct—in the social context in which patients find themselves. Older patients presumably present further down the clinical path than younger ones; for one reason or another they have not received medical attention until the disease has become decompensated.

It has also been suggested that with advanced age there is increased susceptibility of the liver to the toxic effects of alcohol. Recent careful pharmacokinetic studies have shown that blood ethanol area under curve (AUC) in both men and women is significantly greater in older subjects following ingestion of ethanol in the fasting state but, interestingly, not when ethanol is given following a meal.[51] This observation may imply a decline in one or more mechanisms responsible for rapid ethanol metabolism within the first hour after ingestion, but the reason for this is unclear, particularly as there are no age-related changes in the specific activity of total hepatic alcohol dehydrogenase.

Investigation

Elderly patients with ALD usually have deranged LFTs, but there is no characteristic diagnostic pattern. As with other parenchymal liver diseases, the LFTs may be rather more cholestatic than in younger individuals. Routine investigation of an old person with suspected ALD should also include serum albumin, blood film (note raised mean corpuscular volume [MCV]), and clotting screen. Random blood or urine ethanol estimation is also useful, as is γ-GT. Liver biopsy provides useful diagnostic and prognostic information and should be carried out except where there is marked ascites or where clotting is impaired or platelets markedly reduced (prothrombin time prolonged by 4 seconds or more, platelet count below 60,000). In the presence of ascites a diagnostic tap should be carried out since spontaneous bacterial peritonitis (SBP) is a common complication of advanced cirrhosis in these patients and carries a high mortality. A polymorphonuclear white cell count of more than 250/cm^3 ascitic fluid is considered diagnostic of SBP. Fluid should also be submitted for aerobic and anaerobic culture. Liver imaging with ultrasound or CT is particularly important in elderly patients with suspected alcoholic cirrhosis since a high proportion may have complicating HCC. Liver pathology can be regarded in terms of three stages, but two or all three may coexist.

1. *Fatty liver*: Some patients merely show fatty change alone; this is usually reversible, but where significant fibrosis or alcoholic hepatitis coexists, the prognosis is worse. In the few individuals who, despite drinking to great excess for many years, have only mildly abnormal LFTs with liver histology showing only fatty change, the prognosis is relatively good, and for an old person advice concerning future alcohol consumption need not be too prescriptive.
2. *Alcoholic hepatitis*: This condition may have a mild to an extremely aggressive histologic appearance and concomitantly may occur in individuals who have few clinical symptoms or signs as well as those with deep jaundice who are very seriously ill. In general, alcoholic hepatitis usually accompanies cirrhosis in elderly patients. The histologic appearance is of a polymorph infiltrate of the liver parenchyma, often with fibrosis. Continuing ethanol consumption, particularly in women, leads to a poor prognosis. Although alcohol hepatitis alone is potentially reversible, the vast majority of patients progress to cirrhosis.
3. *Alcoholic cirrhosis*: This is an irreversible condition. Recent population surveys have suggested that even among the elderly up to 40 percent of individuals with alcoholic cirrhosis may have few signs or symptoms. Once decompensation occurs, however, the prognosis is poor.[52]

Clinical findings

The clinical findings in elderly patients with ALD are shown in Table 59-2. They are the same as for other patients with chronic liver disease.

Table 59-2 Clinical findings in alcoholic liver disease

Compensated	Decompensated
Telangiectasia	Encephalopathy
Parotid enlargement	Alcohol withdrawal symptoms
Spider naevi	Jaundice
Loss of body hair	Fetor hepaticus
Gynecomastia	Ascites
Hepatomegaly ±	Dilated abdominal veins
Splenomegaly ±	Asterixis
Vertebral (plus rib) fractures	Peripheral edema
Liver palms	
Clubbing plus leuconychia	
Muscle wasting	
Testicular atrophy	

Treatment

By far the most important treatment for ALD is abstinence or, in the case of mild disease, a return to sensible drinking levels. By far the single most important prognostic factor in ALD is drinking behavior.

Acute alcohol withdrawal should be treated with chlordiazepoxide, up to 20 mg QDS, although elderly patients may need less. The β-blocker atenolol is beneficial in preventing peripheral manifestations of alcohol withdrawal—tremor and hypertension in particular—and 50 mg daily is the recommended dose for the first week in the hospital. Benzodiazepines should be withdrawn before or shortly after hospital discharge.[53] The only study that examined alcohol withdrawal specifically in elderly subjects suggested that it was more severe and that higher doses of chlordiazepoxide were required to control symptoms. The reason for this increased severity is not clear.

If liver disease is assessed to be very severe on clinical and biochemical grounds, particularly if bilirubin is markedly elevated and there is significant impairment of clotting, consideration should be given to treatment with corticosteroids—40 mg prednisolone daily for 4 weeks. This is based on several studies showing benefit in survival for up to 1 year in patients with severe alcoholic hepatitis defined by a discriminant function of less than 32 (a formula based on elevation of bilirubin and prolongation of clotting). Intercurrent infection or coincident variceal bleeding are absolute contraindications to initiation of steroid treatment.[54] No other treatment has currently been shown to be of proven benefit in acute alcoholic hepatitis. Nutritional support, initially with intravenous vitamins (particularly thiamine), together with maintenance of blood glucose is vital. Longer-term restoration of normal nutrition with a high-protein diet containing sufficient calories is also important.

No studies on long-term treatment of ALD, specifically in elderly patients, have been conducted. It is recommended that elderly patients with established ALD receive frequent follow-up for the following reasons: (1) to encourage abstinence, (2) to check on therapy for complications (diuretics, lactulose, and so on), (3) to maintain biochemical and nutritional supervision, and (4) to monitor for possible development of HCC in cirrhotic patients. This is particularly important since a very high proportion of patients with alcoholic cirrhosis presenting at or surviving past the age of 65 ultimately develop HCC.[48]

Drug-induced Liver Disease

Hepatic drug reactions are common in the elderly and may be responsible for up to 40 percent of cases involving elderly patients with acute hepatitic LFTs.[55] Although adverse drug reactions (ADRs) are said to be commoner in the elderly, it is possible that much of this impression is created by increased prescribing for elderly individuals and the increased number of drugs they receive.[56] Furthermore, older patients have more intercurrent illness with impaired cardiac or renal function which may directly or indirectly potentiate the adverse effects of some drugs on the liver. In a major Swedish study on hepatic ADRs, which examined the effects of age and corrected for

Drugs used in the elderly that have well-recognized hepatic adverse side effects

Analgesics and NSAIDs
- Paracetamol (acetaminophen)
- Salicylates (at consistent high levels)
- Several NSAIDs
- Dextropropoxyphene (Propoxythene)

Antibiotics
- Ampicillin plus clavulinic acid (Augmentin)
- Flucloxacillin
- Rifampicin
- Tetracyclines
- Isoniazid

Cardiovascular
- Amiodarone (Cordarone)
- Captopril
- Methyldopa
- Nifedipine
- Perhexiline
- Quinidine

Psychiatric
- Most phenothiazines
- Most monoamine oxidase inhibitors
- Most tricyclics

Other
- Anabolic and other steroids
- Antineoplastic drugs
- Halothane and other halogenated anesthetics
- Several anticoagulants

age-related prescribing variables, no increased frequency of reactions to a variety of medications was observed, although a variety of frequently used medications for which ADRs are recognized were not included in the study.

While it is not appropriate to review the whole range of potential hepatic ADRs here, it is likely that mild dose-related abnormalities of LFTs are more frequent than is recognized, particularly in patients with intercurrent illnesses. Because most severe hepatic ADRs are idiosyncratic, however, age-related decline in drug clearance is probably irrelevant. The accompanying boxed list contains a number of drugs used particularly in elderly patients in whom hepatic ADRs have been well described.

Viral Hepatitis

Hepatitis A

Probably because of a cohort effect due to improved sanitation, the proportion of the older adult population in western countries who have not acquired immunity to hepatitis A is rising. With increased world travel to areas of high endemicity of the disease, screening of elderly travelers for hepatitis A IgG antibodies and vaccination of those who are negative is strongly indicated, although the effectiveness of the vaccine has not been specifically tested in the elderly.[57] Mortality from HAV is age-related. In Britain, while the number of deaths compared to the number of reported cases was about 7 per 10,000 in patients aged 15 to 24, it was over 400 per 10,000 in those over the age of 65.[58] In all forms of viral hepatitis, if fulminant hepatic failure develops, increased age is an adverse prognostic factor.

Hepatitis B

Routine testing for HBsAg in donor blood and blood products for over 20 years, together with the fact that the major risk groups for acute hepatitis B in Europe and the United States (homosexuals, intravenous drug abusers) are not highly represented in the elderly population, means that acute hepatitis B among the elderly has become much less common. When it occurs, the disease is more cholestatic, and one report of an outbreak in an nursing home for the elderly reported a resultant carrier rate of 59 percent.[59]

HBV vaccination is progressively less satisfactory with advancing age, producing a lower antibody response. This does not appear to be due to failure of nonresponders to recognize HBsAg but rather to a lack of antibody-producing B cells, presumably a facet of failure of the immune response in old age.[60] Again, elderly travelers to the Far East, Africa, and other areas of high endemicity of hepatitis B should be vaccinated despite lack of evidence as to the efficacy of the vaccine.[61]

Hepatitis D (delta virus) is able to replicate only in the presence of HBV and can thus be termed a satellite virus. It is common in southern Europe and the Middle East, and infection may occur simultaneously with hepatitis B infection (coinfection) or, more commonly, it may infect a patient with chronic HBV liver disease (superinfection). HDV is responsible for increased severity of acute hepatitis or for unexpected "hepatitic" deterioration of patients with known chronic liver disease. It is extraordinarily rare except in areas of the Mediteranean basin.

Chronic hepatitis B Older patients may present with signs and symptoms of chronic liver disease in which chronic HBV infection is the underlying factor. Such patients are usually HBsAg-positive, e antigen-negative, and often e antibody-positive, thus indicating lack of great infectivity.[62]

In considering treatment of elderly patients with chronic HBV infection, the objectives and the nature of the treatment, as well as its likelihood of success, should be borne in mind. In precirrhotic patients in general the two goals of the treatment are to prevent progression to cirrhosis and to reduce or abolish infectivity. In precirrhotic chronic HBV infection, interferon (usually given subcutaneously three times weekly for 6 months) is the standard treatment and can be accompanied by malaise, weight loss, transient flulike symptoms, and occasionally depression. It produces a good clinical and immunologic effect in 30 to 40 percent of patients, however, no specific studies on elderly patient groups have been reported.[63] Patients with relatively recently acquired HBV infection, but with evidence of chronicity, who are e antigen-positive and have high transaminase levels, have the best likelihood of successful treatment. Once cirrhosis has supervened or there is serologic evidence of HBV incorporation into the liver cell genome, interferon treatment is of no value in elderly patients. It is my opinion that elderly patients fulfilling the criteria for suitability for interferon treatment are rare. It is emphasized that steroid treatment at an acute phase of the illness is strongly contraindicated since it may lead to persistence of HBV infection and deterioration in clinical status. It should also be noted that age is an independent adverse prognostic variable in the natural history of chronic HBV infection.[64] Possibly the major complication of chronic HBV infection with cirrhosis in the elderly is the development of HCC. This outcome is particularly common in men (see section on HCC below).

Hepatitis C The natural history of hepatitis C in older people is at present controversial. One study on community-acquired hepatitis C in the United States suggested that at least a proportion of mainly elderly patients have a rather benign course.[65] In contrast, in a hospital-based study on hepatitis C in Britain, of 25 patients presenting over the age of 65, 18 of the 20 patients who had a liver biopsy showed cirrhosis (12 patients) or cirrhosis with HCC (6 patients) and 4 further patients developed HCC.[66] These differences are probably related to the fact that the American study was a wide, community-based survey while the British study examined a highly selected group of elderly patients presenting to hospitals. Nonetheless, hepatitis C with alcoholic cirrhosis and PBC, is now the commonest cause of chronic liver disease in elderly people in western countries. An Italian study has suggested that the prevalence of HCV infection in a residential community for the elderly was greater than that in the younger population in the same region.[67] Since HCV is a parenteral virus—often acquired following blood transfusion until introduction of the anti-HCV antibody test in the early 1990s, or associated with the communal use of poorly sterilized needles in small communities in earlier times—cohort effects for prevalence of HCV in several communities cannot be excluded.

Following acute acquisition of HCV the long-term prognosis for the disease is still controversial. It seems likely that over a 20-year period following infection, cirrhosis ultimately develops in more than a third of individuals. It is for this reason that we can expect hepatitis C-associated cirrhosis to increase as a problem in our elderly population in the next decade before beginning to decline following the routine use of anti-HCV screening of blood donors in the early 1990s.

Because of the cholestatic presentation and the relative rarity of acute viral hepatitis (whether A, B, or C) in older age, delay in diagnosis or misdiagnosis as possible extrahepatic obstruction occurs too frequently. The availability of reliable serologic tests for all three viruses now means that all older patients with jaundice or abnormal LFTs should be screened for acute or chronic infection at the time of first presentation. In the case of hepatitis C the clinical course is often indolent and asymptomatic for many years with fluctuations of LFTs—sometimes normal and sometimes with raised transaminase. Diagnosis is based on liver biopsy as well as serology.

As in the case of HBV chronic liver disease, the current treatment for chronic HCV infection is with interferon. Again, controlled trials suggest that about 30 percent of patients may benefit from interferon treatment in terms of prevention of progression to cirrhosis and/or elimination of the HCV itself.[68] Again, no specific studies have been carried out on older individuals, and again, there is a price to be paid for 6 months' interferon treatment—the side effects of the drug and the cost to the community. It is emphasized that there is little point in offering interferon treatment to elderly patients who have already developed cirrhosis. Soon Lamivudine and other antiviral agents will be added to interferon to provide a treatment "cocktail."[69]

Other viral liver disease Recently another enteral hepatitis virus—hepatitis E—has been described which is responsible for epidemics of enterally transmitted viral hepatitis, particularly on the Indian and South American subcontinents. Still more recently another hepatotrophic virus—hepatitis G—has been described, but at this stage it is not clear whether it is pathogenic. In my opinion, neither of these viruses will frequently trouble physicians attending elderly patients.

Pyogenic Liver Abscess

Almost 50 percent of European and North American patients presenting with pyogenic liver abscess are aged 70 or older.[70–72] Such patients frequently have very nonspecific symptoms—epigastric pain, weight loss, shortness of breath, and rigors—although the last mentioned symptoms have been reported as being less common in the very elderly. General malaise, nausea and vomiting, diarrhea, and pleuritic pain may also be encountered in an elderly patient with pyogenic liver abscess. The conditions most commonly associated with liver abscess are now biliary tract obstruction and cholangitis, but distant abdominal sepsis—often associated with paracolic abscess—is still seen in many elderly patients with "cryptogenic" liver abscess. There appears to be an increased incidence in individuals with diabetes mellitus and metastasic cancer.

Diagnosis

The diagnosis of pyogenic liver abscess is often delayed or missed. Many patients have anemia, and over 75 percent have an elevated leukocyte count. Serum ALP is elevated in almost all patients, but other LFTs are more inconsistent; serum albumin is often low and globulin elevated. On examination the liver or lower ribs over the liver are often tender. Diagnosis should be made by high-quality ultrasound, often followed by CT scanning. The abscess is often loculated or multiple and ill-formed. Sometimes debris is shown in the middle of the abscess, and these features can make distinction from multicentric tumor more difficult. In most series of elderly patients *Escherischia coli* is the organism most commonly isolated.

Treatment

Several recent series have shown that, excluding individuals with associated malignancy and those in whom the abscess was found only at postmortem, prognosis for older patients is no different from that for younger ones. The strong consensus of many series describing the management of liver abscess is that percutaneous needle aspiration, usually (in patients with well-delineated abscess) with subsequent continuous catheter drainage is now the treatment of choice rather than open surgical drainage.[73] Antibiotic treatment, which should initially be intravenous, may be carried out with, for example, third-generation cephalosporin or ciprofloxacin and metronidazole. This treatment should be continued intravenously for about 2 weeks and then followed by 2 to 3 months of oral treatment. The catheter should be removed when drainage becomes negligible, usually after a few days, and the treatment progress monitored with repeated ultrasound examinations. Subsequent investigation, first of the hepatobiliary tree and then (if indicated) of the colon, should be carried out to detect the source of primary infection. Rapid treatment of pyogenic liver abscess by drainage and antibiotics is vital since in untreated cases mortality is extremely high. It is emphasized that in sick elderly patients with nonspecific symptoms, such as those referred to above, and with abnormal LFTs (particularly serum ALP) together with a raised white cell count, the index of suspicion should be high and early ultrasound of the liver is mandatory.

Liver Abnormalities in Systemic Infections

Abnormal LFTs may be associated with systemic infections of almost all types. In addition, distant localized infections in which there is no overt evidence of bacteremia may be associated with hepatic abnormalities. Sites of infection include appendicitis, diverticulitis, renal disease, endocarditis, or soft tissue abscesses.[74,75] In lobar pneumonia, raised serum ALP and sometimes jaundice (particularly with pneumococcal infection) are extremely frequent, however, the reasons for this are quite unclear. In gram-negative bacterial infection endotoxinemia may be contributory.

In an elderly person with a known infection (e.g., pneumonia), nonspecific abnormalities of LFTs need not be investigated unless they persist following the treatment and resolution of the infective illness. In one unselected series of mainly elderly general hospital patients with abnormal LFTs, the abnormality was ascribed to nonhepatic bacterial infection in almost 15 percent.[76]

Autoimmune Liver Disease

Primary Biliary Cirrhosis

PBC must now be recognized as an important disease in middle-aged and elderly women. The mean age of presentation was 55 to 60 years in various large series. Increasing age has been shown to be an independent prognostic indicator for PBC even when deaths from liver disease alone are considered.[77] In a major epidemiologic study in the United Kingdom involving 111 new incident cases of PBC diagnosed in a specific population over the age of 65 with a mean follow-up of 5 years, 26 percent of patients died of liver-related causes. In northern England the point prevalence of PBC in women over 65 years old was about 1 in 1,000 in 1994.[78]

Asymptomatic disease

Physicians now make a diagnosis of PBC in asymptomatic patients either based on the finding a positive AMA on an autoimmune profile for some other suspected disease—usually because of joint pains or suspected thyroid disease—or based on the unexpected finding of persistently elevated serum ALP on biochemical screening. Occasionally a diagnosis is based on the clinical finding of liver enlargement on a routine abdominal examination. In women over the age of 50 with positive AMA and persistently elevated serum ALP, the diagnosis of asymptomatic PBC is highly likely but, assuming no major contraindication, this should be confirmed by liver biopsy. Recently it has been shown that strongly positive AMA alone, even in the absence of raised serum ALP or signs or symptoms of liver disease, is a strong indication that an individual will ultimately develop biochemically and clinically apparent PBC.[79] At present it appears that the prognosis for patients with asymptomatic PBC is close to that for normal individuals matched for age and gender. However, from the moment of development of symptoms suggestive of liver disease, the prognosis for that individual becomes the same as that for other symptomatic patients.[80] With no firmly established treatment for presymptomatic patients with PBC available and with the usually excellent prognosis, no treatment beyond occasional review is presently indicated for those over 65 year old in whom asymptomatic PBC is detected by chance.

Symptomatic disease

Most patients present with symptoms of malaise, lethargy, upper abdominal pain, or, more specifically, pruritus or jaundice. Again, in an individual, particularly a woman, over the age of 50 with one or more of these symptoms and a positive AMA with deranged LFTs, a diagnosis of PBC is very likely indeed. This should be confirmed by liver biopsy after any conceivable extrahepatic biliary obstruction has been excluded by ultrasound examination.[81]

In addition to age, other factors with prognostic importance in symptomatic patients are serum bilirubin, presence or absence of cirrhosis on liver biopsy, presence or absence of complications of portal hypertension, and serum albumin. About 50 percent of PBC patients presenting with or developing symptoms of liver disease will die within 5 years without therapeutic intervention. Death usually arises from complications of portal hypertension or sepsis; very rarely primary HCC supervenes.[81]

Complications

Apart from the complications of portal hypertension (bleeding varices and ascites) and of hepatocellular failure (encephalopathy, undernutrition, and susceptibility to infections), the prolonged cholestasis of PBC and possibly additional malabsorption due to associated pancreatic hyposecretion lead to weight loss and increased likelihood of osteoporosis.[81] Gallstones are also more common in PBC patients. A wide variety of autoimmune diseases have been associated with PBC, the most important of which are Sjögren's syndrome, rheumatoid arthritis, thyroid disease (hypo or hyper), mixed connective tissue disease or scleroderma, and fibrosing alveolitis.[81]

Treatment

The treatment for late-stage PBC in cirrhotic patients with complications is liver transplantation. Indeed, PBC is one of the major indications for transplantation in a person over the age of 60. Several studies have now shown that in very carefully selected patients over the age of 60 overall 1-year graft and patient survival rate equal those achieved in younger patients.[82] Only a few patients over the age of 70 with PBC have now received successful transplants. Such patients must undergo an exhaustive assessment to ensure that they have no other medical contraindications to very major surgery.[83] As technology and technique advance, debate as to the ethical and economic consequences of more widespread availability of liver transplantation for patients over 70 years old must take place.

Analysis of several major published trials involving ursodeoxycholic acid (Urso) treatment (12 to 15 mg/kg body weight) has suggested improved survival in patients receiving this treatment.[84] There appears to be little long-term beneficial effects on symptoms and, paradoxically, no slowing of histologic progression of the disease with Urso treatment has yet been shown. Nonetheless, since this treatment appears almost free of adverse affects, beyond dose-related looseness of bowels, it should be considered in patients with symptomatic disease or possibly in those with "active" LFTs and biopsies. Other treatments under current evaluation include prednisolone and methotrexate. Pruritus is usually effectively treated with cholestyramine, 4-12gm daily. Symptoms of malabsorption with weight loss and diarrhea may be helped by a low-fat diet with supplements of fat-soluble vitamins. Prophylaxis against the development of accelerated osteoporosis should be considered using bisphosphonates. Recently hormone replacement treatment has also been introduced with no cholestatic adverse effect but, thus far, no proof of benefit in PBC patients.

Autoimmune Hepatitis

Chronic autoimmune hepatitis (AIH) is defined as chronic inflammation of the liver with an inflammatory infiltrate, mainly of lymphocytes and plasma cells, expanding outward from the portal tracts into the liver lobules with accompanying piecemeal necrosis of liver cells. In severe disease fibrotic scarring and fibrotic bridging between portal tracts and central veins are seen—the precursors of cirrhosis. In addition to these histologic features chronic AIH is accompanied by the presence of one or more autoantibodies in the serum (usually AMA and/or ANA).

AIH has been thought to be uncommon in the elderly, but recently a group of patients over the age of 65 presenting with this disease have been described.[85] While this group had a more severe initial histologic grade, their overall prognosis was no different from that for patients presenting at a younger age. Interestingly, the diagnostic score (based on very strict internationally agreed-on criteria for diagnosis) was lower in the older patients. Presenting symptoms are usually insidious, arising over a few weeks or months. Fatigue, fluid retention, and jaundice are usually prominent. Biochemical test results are variable, but serum transaminase values are usually twice normal values. Immunoglobulins are usually markedly elevated, and serum albumin decreased. The disease may be associated with arthralgia or hemolytic anemia. A very careful drug history must be taken to exclude a drug-related cause for this chronic liver disease. Recently, for example, AIH has been described as being triggered by the antibiotic minocycline.[86] In this instance withdrawal of the medication was enough to reverse the disease.

In all cases of chronic hepatitis the full diagnostic blood test screen (Table 59-1) should be carried out. The diagnosis of AIH is thus one of inclusion (compatible histologic and immunologic pictures) and exclusion (absence of markers for hepatitis C, for example). Physical signs of AIH are similar to those for other chronic liver diseases.

Prognosis and treatment

In a recently published series prognosis for older AIH patients was similar to that for younger ones.[85] Interestingly, in clinically mild cases prednisolone treatment was not given, and this did not appear to adversely effect prognosis. In the absence of "evidence" it is recommended that in patients with clinically, histologically, and/or biochemically severe disease, standard treatment with prednisolone plus azathioprine should be given, and maintenance treatment should be continued to maintain LFTs near normal. In patients with an histologic picture of AIH but with no confirmatory autoimmune markers, a trial of steroid treatment (20 mg daily, falling to 10 mg daily) is worthwhile for 1 to 2 months. If there is no response, treatment can be discontinued.

It is increasingly clear that there is an overlap among the autoimmune liver diseases, particularly PBC and AIH. The next few years will see the dissection of a number of different causes giving rise to this spectrum of diseases.

Primary Sclerosing Cholangitis

Primary sclerosing cholangitis (PSC) is rare in individuals over the age of 65, the mean age of onset being about 40 years. PSC is often associated with ulcerative colitis and may be an indolent disease. Thus, occasionally an elderly patient, usually a man, presents with persistent LFT abnormalities—usually cholestatic—together with symptoms and signs of chronic liver disease and usually ulcerative colitis. The diagnosis rests on (1) diagnostic appearance of the biliary tree on ERCP, (2) compatible liver histology, (3) persistent LFT abnormalities, usually cholestatic, with exclusion of other possible causes of liver disease. Patients entering old age with indolent PSC appear to have a good prognosis. At present, despite numerous clinical trials no treatment has been shown to be of definite benefit. If a "critical stricture" of the extrahepatic biliary tree is demonstrated, it can be stented. Recurrent attacks of cholangitis should be energetically treated with antibiotics.

Inherited Diseases of the Liver

There are only two inherited diseases of the liver that are of importance in the elderly: hemochromatosis and α_1 antitypsin deficiency. Wilson's disease is unknown to occur in individuals over the age of 50, and other important inborn errors of metabolism causing liver injury usually lead to death well before the age of 60.

Hemochromatosis

Genetic hemochromatosis[47] results from increased inappropriate absorption of iron with increased hepatic uptake of iron from transferin. The hemochromatosis gene, recently described, is located on the short arm of chromosome 6. Abnormalities in this single gene appear to be responsible for most cases of genetic hemochromatosis, at least in populations of Celtic origin. It is the most common autosomal recessive gene of importance.[87]

The mean age of presentation with first symptoms attributable to hemochromatosis is probably just over 50 years, but in individuals with no previously known family history detection may be made up to 75 years. Similarly, screening of families in which newly detected cases have been observed can reveal asymptomatic subjects over the age of 65 or 70.

Typically, symptoms are weakness, abdominal pain, and lethargy. Arthralgia, loss of libido or impotence, cardiac failure, and symptoms of diabetes represent nonhepatic manifestations of the illness. Clinical diabetes is present in over 50 percent of older patients. Occasionally, older patients present for the first time with the complications of portal hypertension or liver failure superimposed on evidence of cirrhosis, often associated with the development of HCC. In general, elderly patients presenting with cirrhosis rapidly develop severe complications of portal hypertension and liver cell failure. Suspicion should be extremely high that these individuals already have or will shortly develop HCC.[47] For this reason family screening, even for elderly family members, is mandatory after detection of an individual with hemochromatosis and may be carried out simply by measurement of serum ferritin. Routine genotyping will shortly be available.[87]

Treatment is with venesection. About 500 mL of blood should be removed at 2-week intervals until serum ferritin levels fall into the normal range. Despite this frequent venesection anemia very seldom occurs. Once serum ferritin has been returned to normal, follow-up may be two or three times a year with repeat venesection if serum ferritin rises again significantly. Venesection prevents progression to cirrhosis in precirrhotic patients. In cirrhotic patients it reduces the likelihood of hepatocellular failure, but unfortunately it does not prevent subsequent development of HCC. Up to 30 percent of patients with hemochromatosis die of HCC. Venesection prevents the onset of nonhepatic complications of hemocromatosis if they have not already occurred.

α_1-Antitrypsin Deficiency

α_1-Antitrypsin, synthesized in the liver, is the serum α_1-globulin whose function is to inhibit proteases. It is genetically controlled by a single autosomal dominant gene situated on the long arm of chromosome 14. Although there are many phenotypic alleles, the normal protease inhibitory protein PiM is associated with normal serum levels. Very low serum levels, even in response to circumstances in which an acute phase protein would be expected, are associated with the homozygous form of the abnormal protein PiZZ. Either severe emphysema or development of cirrhosis, frequently in childhood, is associated with this phenotype. Most commonly in elderly individuals α_1-antitrypsin deficiency is suspected only following liver biopsy when periportal hepatocytes are seen to contain granules of PAS-positive, diastase-resistant material. These granules are probably composed of abnormal α_1-antitrypsin protein whose transport out of the cell is impaired.[88] It is still unclear whether the presence of moderate quantities of these granules and heterozygosity for one of the abnormal α_1-antitrypsin phenotypes is associated with increased risk of development of chronic liver disease (e.g., increased susceptibility to cirrhosis in alcoholics or a worse prognosis in hepatitis C). It has been suggested that among elderly individuals with cirrhosis α_1-antitrypsin deficiency, usually among Z heterozygotes, might in some way be the cause of cryptogenic cirrhosis of an indolent nature.[89,90] In view of the frequency of the heterozygous state in the general population and the lack of a definite mechanism whereby mere accumulation of this effete protein within liver cells could cause occult liver damage, it appears unlikely that this is in fact a cause of "senile" cirrhosis. This is in marked distinction to the situation for ZZ homozygotes, most of whom die of emphysema or liver disease, often with HCC, before the age of 50.

Liver Cysts

It is unclear whether many cysts within the liver are congenital or arise during life. It is convenient to consider them under this section on inherited disorders. Liver cysts are defined for this purpose as a liver enclosed space or spaces that may contain air, liquid, or a small amount of solid.[91]

Solitary cysts

These cysts are now being detected much more frequently because of increased use of ultrasound. They are almost always under low pressure, seldom grow with any speed, and are only rarely associated with symptoms. Occasionally an elderly patient with abdominal pain of unknown origin may be shown to have a solitary liver cyst, or two or three such cysts. It may be worth aspirating such a cyst by percutaneous needle aspiration, under local anesthetic, on one occasion. If the treatment produces relief of symptoms, consideration can be given to marsupialization since, following aspiration, cysts almost always reform. Unfortunately the connection between right-sided upper abdominal pain and liver cysts, even of moderate size, is still quite unclear.

Adult fibropolycystic disease

Multiple cysts, from three or four up to several hundred, within the liver are frequently associated with polycystic kidneys. There is an overlap among the conditions of congenital hepatic fibrosis, intrahepatic biliary cystic disease (Caroli's disease), and simple polycystic disease. Occasionally, such cystic diseases of the liver appear in elderly adults, and there may be a question of distinguishing between such cysts and malignant lesions. Polycystic disease of the liver is compatible with long life, and no specific treatment is indicated. These cysts are usually filled with clear fluid, and aspiration confirms the innocent nature of the lesions. In extraordinarily rare circumstances there may be malignant transformation of such cysts.

Cryptogenic Chronic Liver Disease

While perhaps 20 percent of elderly patients with chronic liver disease have no identified cause at present, it seems likely that the discovery of new autoantigens and the emergence of understanding as to which environmental factors, usually infections or foreign compounds (xenobiotics), can initiate chronic liver disease, together with the continuing detection of markers for further hepatotrophic viruses, will further reduce the proportion of liver disease currently labeled "cryptogenic." Nonetheless, the importance of this group was emphasized by a study of factors influencing survival in patients with cirrhosis. It showed that the most important independent adverse factor was increased age and that death was due largely to hepatic causes not merely to nonhepatic age-related diseases. The group with the worst prognosis was that with cryptogenic cirrhosis.[92]

The Liver in Systemic Conditions

It has already been mentioned that in conditions such as severe cardiac failure and severe systemic (essentially nonhepatic) bacterial infections the liver may become involved, showing abnormal blood tests, impaired function, and abnormal histology. In addition, there are several systemic diseases in which, while the liver is not the origin of the illness nor indeed the prime target organ, clinically important or vital hepatic abnormalities may occur, occasionally being life-threatening in their own right. These conditions will be briefly reviewed specifically in relation to liver disease of old age.

Liver in Heart Failure

Hepatomegaly is present in over 90 percent of patients with chronic right heart failure, and since splenomegaly, peripheral edema, pleural effusions, and ascites may also be present in chronic right heart failure, as well as in cirrhosis, there are occasionally difficulties in making a differential diagnosis in an elderly patient with these signs. With improved treatments for severe heart failure now available, the development of fibrosis (so-called nutmeg liver) and ultimately cirrhosis now very rarely occurs.[83] In patients with acute left heart failure accompanied by hypotension, hepatic hypoperfusion may occur, giving rise to a sudden, very sharp elevation in liver enzymes, particularly transaminases. So-called ischemic hepatitis is said to be most frequent in elderly patients—particularly in the setting of acute myocardial infarction or following major abdominal surgery. A proportion of patients with ischemic hepatitis have transient hyperglycemia, usually lasting up to 2 weeks and occasionally requiring insulin therapy. Treatment should be directed at the underlying cause of hypotension or hypoperfusion.[83,93]

Connective Tissue Diseases

While certain specific liver diseases (like PBC) are found in association with a variety of connective tissue disease (e.g., rheumatoid arthritis and primary Sjögren's syndrome), in many instances more nonspecific abnormalities in LFTs and histology are noted. In particular, elevations of serum ALP may be observed in up to 50 percent of patients with rheumatoid arthritis. In some of these individuals the ALP may be of bony origin, in some it may be related to medications, and in some it may be attributable to asymptomatic PBC. Nonetheless, variable elevation of serum ALP over time is seen in elderly patients with rheumatoid arthritis for whom none of the above explanations are applicable.[94] Liver histology in such patients shows mild nonspecific (and largely nonprogressive) changes. Similar abnormalities in LFTs and liver histology are frequently found in elderly patients with polymyalgia rheumatica. Unless an additional separate liver disease is suspected, therefore, it is unnecessary to investigate mild abnormalities of LFTs in other patients with collagen vascular disorders.

Hodgkin's Lymphoma and Non-Hodgkin's Lymphomas

The liver is significantly involved in perhaps 5 percent of patients with Hodgkin's lymphoma and in a higher proportion (about 25 percent) with non-Hodgkin's lymphomas. Such liver involvement can vary from mild abnormalities in serum ALP (seen in up to 40 percent of Hodgkin's disease patients), but with no clinical significance, to gross hepatic enlargement due to massive infiltration of the liver or obstructive jaundice due to hilar lymph node enlargement.[95] Occasionally in the investigation of pyrexia of unknown origin, liver biopsy reveals the presence of the Reed-Sternberg cells of Hodgkin's disease or the highly abnormal lymphocytes of non-Hodgkin's lymphoma. The treatment of such patients is the same as for other elderly patients with lymphoma (see Ch. 89).

Complications of Cirrhosis

Portal Hypertension

The pathogenesis and anatomy of portal hypertension are well described in standard major texts on liver disease. This section will deal with acute and longer-term management of the two major complications of portal hypertension—bleeding varices and ascites. Portal hypertension may result from cirrhosis of any cause and may also occur following occlusion of the hepatic vein (Budd-Chiari syndrome) or occlusion of the portal vein (portal vein thrombosis). Budd-Chiari syndrome is extremely rare in elderly patients but may occasionally occur in association with a hypercoagulable state associated with a myeloproliferative disorder. Far more common is the development of portal hypertension in an elderly patient as a result of portal vein thrombosis. This may occur following abdominal sepsis (e.g., a diverticular abscess) or abdominal surgery with associated hypotension. Portal vein thrombosis is manifested by ascites, LFTs that are often normal or near normal, and liver biopsy revealing no serious hepatic abnormality. Diagnosis can now be made by Doppler ultrasound and confirmed by MRI.

Bleeding Esophageal and Gastric Varices

The definitive cause of bleeding in a patient who may have had esophageal varices for several years is still unclear. What can be said is that large varices are more likely to bleed than smaller ones, as are varices in patients with more severe liver disease (as reflected by Child's classification). Finally, the appearance of red wale markings on the varices suggests increased likelihood of hemorrhage. Varices may also form in the stomach, often after endoscopic obliteration of esophageal varices. Effectively, these varices merge into so-called portal hypertensive gastropathy in which there is increased gastric mucosal blood flow associated with increased portal pressure, often following obliteration of other varices. In its severe form cherry-red spots and a granular mucosa are seen. In severe gastropathy chronic blood loss may occur, as well as the sudden blood loss associated with true varices.[96]

Patients bleeding from varices may present with sudden hematemasis or melaena, and occasionally only with the signs and symptoms of severe anemia. Probably about 5 percent of first-time upper gastrointestinal bleeders admitted to general hospitals are bleeding from varices. If it is assumed that on admission to the hospital bleeding has been recent and overt, the twin tracks of diagnosis and treatment run side by side. Acute treatment of bleeding from varices is as for other upper gastrointestinal hemorrhage, with emergency resuscitation initially with plasma expander until blood has been cross-matched and is available. In severe circumstances this may need to be via a central venous line which, in patients with chronic liver disease and potential clotting abnormalities, should be placed by a highly experienced person. Once blood pressure has been restored in a patient with suspected varices still actively bleeding, upper gastrointestinal endoscopy should take place. If bleeding is confirmed, start intravenous infusion of either the somatostatin analog octreotide (50 mg/hr for up to 48 hours intravenously) or, if it is not available, vasopressin (0.4 unit/min).[97] If bleeding does not stop with the above treatment, balloon tamponade with a Sengstaken-Blakemore triple lumen tube should be used. There is a high rate of complications with the use of this or a similar device (the Minnesota tube), and placement should preferably take place at an experienced center following at least partial control of bleeding with octreotide infusion. If possible at the time of first endoscopy, direct injection of the varices should be made with sclerosant (see below for details).[98]

Longer-term treatment

Following initial control and preliminary treatment of bleeding varices in an elderly patient, the question arises as to what further treatment is necessary, if any. Each of four main treatment options have their advocates, and it is probable that there is little difference among them provided each is carried out properly at an experienced center. Briefly, treatment options are as follows.

1. *Pharmacologic*: If patients have no contraindications to the use of β-blockers, propranalol may be given prophylactically in a sufficient dose to lower the resting pulse rate by 20 percent. This has been shown in meta-analysis of control trials to reduce the risk of recurrent bleeding and death from bleeding by about 40 percent.[99] In patients with known varices that have never bled, prophylactic use of propranolol has been shown to substantially reduce risk of bleeding, and its use should, therefore, be considered unless contraindications exist.[100]
2. *Sclerotherapy*: A course of injection sclerotherapy into the varices at roughly weekly intervals until the veins are eradicated has, until relatively recently, been the most popular treatment. The problems with sclerotherapy are more frequent hospital inpatient stays and the development of portal gastropathy. Its effectiveness in preventing rebleeding and in improving mortality at least 1 year following an initial bleed is probably very similar to that of propranalol.[101] A combination of sclerotherapy and β-blockers may give marginally better results in regard to rebleeding and mortality than either treatment alone.[102]

3. *Banding*: In the past few years ligation of varices using an endoscopic ligation apparatus has been suggested to further reduce rebleeding rates, as well as the number of complications, compared with sclerotherapy.[103]
4. *TIPSS*: This procedure has been largely dealt with earlier in the chapter. Complications include long-term stenosis of the shunt (which should be reviewed using high-quality Doppler ultrasound or hepatic venography at 6-month intervals) and the development of hepatic encephalopathy. This technique is highly effective in reducing rebleeding from varices if wedged hepatic pressure is maintained below 12 mmHg.[104]

Although the prognosis for upper gastrointestinal bleeding is generally worse in the elderly, at centers with experience in treating this condition, immediate mortality and the proportion of elderly patients leaving the hospital following admission with bleeding esophageal varices are little different than for younger ones. In one recent study overall admission fatality for patients over 65 years old with varices was 26 percent, compared with 19 percent for those under 65 years old. It is therefore emphasized that older patients benefit from the same intensive specialist management of portal hypertension as younger ones even if the longer-term outlook appears worse.[105,106]

Cirrhotic Ascites

Ascites may be classified conveniently in terms of its causation as transudate or exudate. Transudative causes include severe right-sided heart failure, tricuspid incompetence and constrictive pericarditis, uncomplicated cirrhosis, and portal venous obstruction. Ascites is clearly a transudate if ascitic fluid protein is less than about 15 g/L. Exudative causes include intraperitoneal carcinomatosis, intraperitoneal infectious chylous ascites, and pancreatic ascites; these are unequivocal above about 25 g/L. Unfortunately there is considerable overlap among many of the above conditions, but the distinction is still of value.

Investigation

Investigation of liver ascites starts with a diagnostic tap which can be carried out with a small (venipuncture-type) needle. Fluid should be submitted for protein content, microscopy, cytology, and culture. In the investigation of ascites of unknown origin, the overwhelming majority of cases are caused by (1) cirrhosis, (2) right-sided heart failure, (3) hepatic venous or portal venous obstruction, and (4) disseminated intra-abdominal carcinomatosis.

Bacterial infection of ascitic fluid without an overt primary source of infection—SBP—is a common complication in patients with cirrhosis and carries a serious prognostic implication. All patients admitted to a hospital with ascites should have a diagnostic tap to exclude SBP on admission. Up to 20 percent of patients admitted to a hospital with alcoholic cirrhosis and ascites may have occult SBP, is now thought to be due to translocation of bacteria from the gut lumen. Specific signs and symptoms of infection are rather lacking, although fever, abdominal pain, and tenderness in a patient with ascites are highly suggestive. The diagnosis is made by examination of ascitic fluid. If it contains more than 250 polymorph cells per cubic millimeter, the diagnosis is highly likely.[107] Fever and peripheral leukocytosis may be seen in most patients, sometimes with positive blood cultures. Culture of ascitic fluid is not always reliable, and the need for urgent antibiotic treatment is so great that if a raised polymorph count is found in the fluid, treatment should be started immediately. Treatment with a third-generation cephalosporin (e.g., cephotaxime) or with ciprofloxacin has been shown to be highly effective and should be continued for 7 days.[108] If SBP has occurred in an individual on more than one occasion, long-term prophylactic treatment with low-dose cephalosporin or a nonabsorbable antibiotic should be considered. Over 75 percent of patients developing SBP die within 1 year of its first occurrence.

Ascites treatment

Ascites treatment should not necessarily be aimed at completely abolishing all ascitic fluid. Such an objective often leads to overtreatment, with consequent risk of electrolyte imbalance and renal impairment. This is particularly true in older patients. Cirrhotic ascites is often accompanied by sodium retention, hence the first step in its treatment is moderate restriction of sodium intake. In ill elderly patients with cirrhosis, malnutrition and ascites often go hand in hand, and a high-protein intake is desirable. Hence, a balancing act must be carried out between providing enough salt to make protein palatable and not giving an excess, thus worsening a tendency toward ascites. Since impaired water excretion frequently accompanies cirrhotic ascites, paradoxical hyponatremia may also develop—particularly in patients treated with diuretics. Patients in whom serum sodium falls below 125 mmol (125 mEq/L) should have water intake restricted to 1 L/d. Intravascular volume can be replaced in these patients with modest infusions of salt-poor albumin (2 units every 2 days until serum sodium rises and water restriction can be lifted).

The two mainstays of therapy for ascites are diuretic treatment and abdominal paracentesis. Because hyperaldosteronism is a concomitant of cirrhotic ascites, the use of spironolactone, which opposes the action of aldosterone and blocks tubular reabsorption of sodium, is the recommended first-line treatment in ascites. Dosage should be cautiously increased from 50 mg/d up to a maximum of 600 mg/d (normally 200 to 400 mg/d is sufficient). In patients with peripheral edema as well as ascites, a loop diuretic such as frusemide might be added. Thiazide diuretics, which cause natriuresis as well as excretion of potassium and metabolic alkalosis, are not recommended for cirrhotic patients. The progress of diuretic therapy must be monitored by daily weighing. A patient with abdominal ascites and without peripheral edema should not lose more than about 1/2 kg/d, or the risk of renal impairment or development of encephalopathy will be greatly increased. Bed rest adds to the likely efficacy of this treatment.

Large-volume abdominal paracentesis with simultaneous intravenous infusion of albumin is now the most commonly used treatment for severe ascites. This procedure has been shown to be followed by no greater incidence of side effects than conventional diuretic treatment.[109] Its advantage is that it relieves the patient of discomfort more quickly and may shorten their hospital stay. In elderly patients with end-stage liver disease, repeated 24-hour hospital stays with abdominal paracentesis followed by moderate diuretic treatment at home seem sensible and pragmatic. In the abdominal paracentesis technique 4 to 6 L of fluid are removed over 1 to 2 hours and replaced with an infusion of 40 g albumin intravenously. This procedure can be repeated on two or three occasions to remove all readily accessible ascites. Strict aseptic technique is, of course, vital. A peritoneal dialysis catheter is used but must be removed immediately following the paracentesis since leaving it in place greatly increases the risk of subsequent infection.[110]

Two further treatments are now available for treatment of intractable ascites. The first—TIPSS—has already been mentioned in connection with treatment of bleeding varices. This procedure is also highly effective in treatment of ascites, although a small residual volume of ascitic fluid usually remains after stabilization. Again, in patients with very severe liver disease as reflected by Child's grade C status, complications of infection, encephalopathy, other manifestations of hepatocellular failure, or renal failure frequently supervene in the months following the TIPSS procedure. The advantage of this treatment is that, if successful, it is a "one off." Following TIPSS, patients should receive prophylactic lactulose (10 to 30 ml/d) to reduce the likelihood of overt encephalopathy. Modest diuretic treatment is often required, and 6-month checks of TIPSS patency are also advised. If ascites reaccumulates, it is likely that the TIPSS has become occluded. This can frequently be redilated. It is stressed that this procedure is extremely technically demanding and should be carried out only at an experienced center.[111]

In elderly patients for whom there is no question of transplantation, some form of peritoneovenous shunt can be used, essentially as a palliative procedure, in intractable ascites.[112] It has been my experience that a saphenoperitoneal shunt is effective and has less complications than the more commonly used shunts between the peritoneal cavity and the superior vena cava (of the Le Veen type). When successful, these shunts also need follow-up treatment with moderate doses of diuretics. Complications include diffuse intravascular coagulation, central venous thrombosis, peritonitis, and vascular hemorrhage. Previous SBP or bilirubin more than 50 mmol/L (3 m/100 ml), is a strong contraindication to shunt placement.

Hepatic Encephalopathy

Hepatic encephalopathy is the reversible decrease in consciousness seen in patients with severe liver disease; at the worse end of the spectrum it results in coma. Encephalopathy may be acute, chronic, or episodic. In patients with cirrhosis it is usually precepitated by an adverse event—infection, gastrointestinal bleeding, constipation, electrolyte disturbance, or incorrect medication. In hepatic encephalopathy lethargy, confusion, and stupor are characteristic. At an early stage the characteristic asterixis (flapping tremor) may be seen, although it is not specific to hepatic encephalopathy—occasionally being seen in other metabolic encephalopathies. It is sometimes important to distinguish encephalopathy from the confusion of alcohol withdrawal. In the latter, agitation and anxiety with sweating, tachycardia, hypertension, and tremulousness are important features. The clinical course of hepatic encephalopathy depends on the rapidity with which steps are taken to reverse it, the nature of the precipitating cause, and the severity of the underlying liver disease. The greater the depression of concious level, the greater the corresponding risks.The pathogenesis of hepatic encephalopathy is still controversial, but although increased levels of such toxins as ammonia and mercaptans may well be contributory or sensitizing factors, it is becoming clear that the major mechanism involved in induction of encephalopathy concerns the inhibitory neurotransmitter γ-aminobutyric acid (GABA) and its receptor.[113] The GABA receptor, whose molecular structure has recently been described, also appears to be the receptor for benzodiazepines and benzodiazapine-like substances.[114] It is conceivable that there is an increased number or sensitivity of GABA-benzodiazepine receptors in the brain of individuals developing encephalopathy. It has even been suggested that in hepatic encephalopathy there is a circulating benzodiazepine-like substance which may be largely responsible for the onset of coma.[115] The site of production of this putative coma-causing substance is speculative.

Hepatocellular Cancer

It is becoming increasingly clear that primary HCC is largely a disease of aging in western countries. It is usually associated with cirrhosis, regardless of the underlying cause, and it is probable that the length of time for which an individual has had cirrhosis is an important determining factor. In Britain about half of HCC patients with cirrhosis present over the age of 65. Although the vast majority of these individuals do have cirrhosis, a recent U.K. study found that in only a quarter of those over 65 years old was the underlying cirrhosis known prior to presentation with HCC. The main underlying causes of cirrhosis among elderly HCC patients varies from country to country. In the United Kingdom, an area with low prevalence of HBV infection, 34 percent of younger HCC patients showed HBV markers against only 23 percent of those over 65 years old.[116] Conversely, up to 40 percent of elderly cirrhotic patients with HCC in the United Kingdom have evidence of previous presumed HCV infection. In a Korean study on HCC this same change in the ratio of HBV to HCV among patients with HCC has also been shown, the ratio being 29:7 in patients under the age of 60 and 0.9 in those over the age of 60. Thus, in this Far Eastern population the age of acquisition of HVB (usually infancy) is contrasted with the presumed acquisition of HCV later in life, as in European populations.[117] In European populations the combination of alcohol consumption with markers for previous HBV or HCV infection appears to be particularly potent in leading to the development of HCC in elderly cirrhotics. In addition, European war veterans with exposure to service in the Far East or Africa are presenting in late life with HCC. While some of these patients have a life history and histology suggesting that alcohol is now at least a contributory factor to their cirrhosis, early exposure during military service to HBV, HCV, or the known hepatic carcinogen aflatoxin seems very possible.[116]

Presentation and management

Elderly patients with HCC frequently present with the complications of cirrhosis —bleeding varices, ascites, and encephalopathy—and it is only during subsequent investigation of the underlying cause of their liver disease and the reason for its sudden decompensation that HCC becomes apparent. Thus, in patients with previously unknown hemochromatosis, stable compensated alcoholic cirrhosis, or cirrhosis associated with hepatitis C, once the cause of the underlying cirrhosis has been recognized a complicating HCC can frequently be found. There should be high suspicion of underlying HCC in all individuals over 70 year old presenting for the first time with complications of what is clearly cirrhosis. Patients with known cirrhosis, particularly men, should now be followed to try to detect the development of very early HCC. Routine screening with serum α-fetoprotein at 6-month intervals is a minimal requirement. If possible, this should be accompanied by annual liver ultrasound screening.[118] Otherwise patients may present with weight loss, abdominal pain, and symptoms of hepatic enlargement—often dyspnea—or even because they have noted an abdominal mass. Ascites is a frequent complication of HCC and is more difficult to treat since the portal vein is often obstructed. The prognosis for HCC in elderly patients is dreadful.[119] In the recent U.K. review mean survival following diagnosis was 10.5 weeks in patients over 65 years old versus 18.5 weeks in younger patients.[110] Perhaps not surprisingly, older patients presented with worse prognostic features (raised bilirubin, ascites, extrahepatic spread, multiple and larger tumors). Investigation of HCC has been described earlier. As implied by the very poor survival figures, treatment is still very unsatisfactory. In patients with small (less than 5 cm) lesions percutaneous injection with ethanol can occasionally be extremely effective and should be carried out on several occasions to obliterate the tumor or tumors. Very rarely, in extremely fit elderly patients, surgical excision may be considered, in which case prior biopsy should not be carried out for reasons described above.[120] In larger, often multiple, tumors consideration should be given to infusion into the hepatic artery branches of chemotherapy—Adriamycin or cisplatin, using Lipiodol as a vehicle to deliver the chemotherapy to the lesion. Except in patients with Child's grade A status, almost no improvement in survival has been shown with this treatment in this desperately ill group of patients.[119] It is my view that unless treatment is demanded, no chemotherapy should be given to HCC patients with poor prognostic features. (Even intrahepatic therapy can lead to profound malaise and the complications of infection, bleeding, and encephalopathy, requiring a prolonged hospital stay).

Metastatic Cancer

Hepatic metastases from distant primary sources, often in the gut, are far more common in elderly individuals than primary tumors. Such metastases are usually detected in one of three ways: (1) as part of routine screening following detection of a primary tumor elsewhere—before colonic surgery for carcinoma of the colon; (2) in the investigation of an ill elderly patient with abnormal LFTs, and (3) in the investigation of a patient presenting with an abdominal mass revealed to be an enlarged liver. In any event histologic confirmation of a lesion detected by one imaging technique or another must be obtained unless the source of a presumed distant primary tumor is already established or unless surgical resection of the hepatic lesion is contemplated. The reason for biopsy is that, whereas multiple metastases from pancreatic or gastric primary adenocarcinomas carry an extremely poor prognosis, this is not the case for some ovarian tumors, carcinoid tumors, or lymphoma. The management of these conditions is considered elsewhere in this book.

References

1. Wynne HA, Cope E, Mutch E et al: The effect of age upon liver volume and apparent liver blood flow in healthy man. Hepatology 1989;9:297–301
2. Marchesini G, Bua V, Brunori A et al: Galactose elimination capacity and liver volume in aging man. Hepatology 1988;8: 1079–1083
3. Kitani K: Aging and the liver. pp. 603–623. In Popper H, Schaffner F (eds): Progress in Liver Diseases. Vol. 9. WB Saunders, Philadelphia, 1990
4. Ivy GO, Schottler F, Baudrey M et al: Inhibition of lysosomal enzymes: accumulation of lipofuscin-like dense bodies in the brain. Science 1984;226:85–987
5. David H, Reinke P: Liver morphology with aging. pp. 143–159. In Bianchi L, Holt P, James OFW, Butler RN (eds): Aging in Liver and Gastro-intestinal tract. MTP, Lancaster, UK, 1988
6. Watanabe T, Tanaka Y: Age-related alterations in the size of human hepatocytes: study of mononuclear and binuclear cells. Virchows Archiv 1982;39:9–20
7. Sato T, Tauchi H: The formation of enlarged and giant mitochondria in the aging process of human hepatic cells. Acta Pathol Jpn 1975;25:403–412
8. Popper H:1986. Aging and the liver. pp. 659–683. In Popper H, Schaffner F (eds): Progress in Liver Diseases Vol. VIII. Grune & Stratton, New York, 1986
9. Marchesini G, Bianchi GP, Fabbri A et al: Synthesis of urea after a protein rich meal in normal man in relation to ageing. Age Ageing 1990;19:4–10

10. Fabbri A, Marechesini A, Bianchi G et al: Liver 1994;14:288
11. Einarsson K, Nilsell K, Leijd B, Angelin B: Influence of age on secretion of cholesterol and synthesis of bile acids by the liver. N Engl J Med 1985;313:277–282
12. Liu Y, Guyton KZ, Gorospe M et al: Age-related decline in mitogen activated protein kinase activity in epidermal growth factor-stimulated rat hepatocytes. J Biochem 1996;271: 3604–3607
13. Wang E: Senescent human fibroblasts resist programmed cell death and failure to suppress bc 12 is involved. Cancer Res 1995;55:2284–2292
14. Greenblatt DJ, Sellers EM, Shader RI: Drug disposition in old age. N Engl J Med 1982;306:1081–1088
15. Woodhouse KW, James OFW: Hepatic drug metabolism and ageing. Br Med Bull 1990;46:22–35
16. Vestal RE: Aging and determinants of hepatic drug clearance. Hepatology 1989;9:331–334
17. Schnegg MI, Lauterberg BH: Quantitative liver function in the liver assessed by galactose elimination capacity, aminopyrine demethylation and caffeine clearance. J Hepatol 1986;3: 164–171
18. Zakim D, Boyer TD (eds): Hepatology: A Textbook of Liver Disease. 3rd Ed. WB Saunders, Philadelphia, 1996
19. Sherlock S, Dooley JS: Diseases of the Liver and Biliary System. 10th Ed. Blackwell, Oxford, 1997
20. McIntyre N, Benhamou JP, Bircher J et al: Oxford Textbook of Clinical Hepatology. 2nd Ed. Oxford Medical Publications, Oxford, 1997
21. Berk PD: Hematologic issues in contemporary hepatology. Semin Liver Dis 1987;7:169–277
22. Friedman LS, Martin P, Munoz SJ: Liver function tests and objective evaluation of the patient with liver disease. pp. 791–832. In Zakim D, Boyer TD (eds): Hepatology: A Textbook of Liver Disease. 3rd Ed. WB Saunders, Philadelphia, 1996
23. Taylor KJW, Holland S: Doppler ultrasound 1. basic principles, instrumentation and pitfalls. Radiology 1990;174: 297–308
24. Scoutt IM: Doppler ultrasound. 2. clinical applications. Radiology 1990;174:309–330
25. Sheu JC, Sung JL, Chen DS et al: Ultrasonography of small hepatic tumours using high resolution linear array real-time instruments. Radiology 1984;150: 797–801
26. Rosenthal S: Are hepatic scans overused? Am J Dig Dis 1976; 21:659–666
27. Bernardino ME, Erwin BC, Steinberg HV et al: Delayed hepatic CT scanning: increased confidence and improved detection of hepatic metastases. Radiology 1986;159:71–76
28. Heiken JP, Lee JKT, Glazer HS et al: Hepatic metastases studied by MR and CT. Radiology 1985;156:153–158
29. Edelman RR, Warach S: Magnetic resonance imaging. N Engl J Med 1993;328: 785–792
30. Bernardino ME, Young SW, Kee JKT et al: Hepatic MR imaging: safety, image quality and sensitivity. Radiology 1992;183: 53–60
31. Stark DD, Moseley M, Bacon BR et al: Magnetic resonance imaging and spectroscopy of hepatic iron overload. Radiology 1984;154:137–140
32. Raby N, Karani R, Mitchell M et al: Lipiodol enhanced CT scanning in assessment of hepatocellular carcinoma. Clin Radiol 1989;40:480–485
33. Ralls PW, Johnson MB, Radins DR et al: Budd-Chiari syndrome: detection with color Doppler sonography. Am J Radiol 1992;159:112–117
34. Roessle M, Haag K, Ochs A et al: The transjugular intrahepatic portosystemic stent-shunt procedure for variceal bleeding. N Engl J Med 1994;330:165–171
35. Simpson KJ, Chalmers N, Redhead DN et al: Transjugular intrahepatic portasystemic shunting for control of acute and recurrent upper gastrointestinal hemorrhage related to portal hypertension. Gut 1993;34:968–973
36. Kasmin FE, Siegel JH: Biliary disease in the elderly. pp. 185–212. In Gelb AM (ed): Clinical Gastroenterology in the Elderly. Dekker, New York, 1996
37. Leung JWC: Endoscopic management of gallstone disease. pp. 87–100. In Cotton PB, Tytgat GNJ, Williams CB (eds): Annual of Gastrointestinal Endoscopy. Current Science, London, 1989
38. Harbin WP, Mueller PR, Ferrucci JT: Transhepatic cholangiography: complications and use patterns of the fine-needle technique. Radiology 1980;135:15–20
39. Lightdale CJ: Laporoscopy. pp. 833–844. In Zakim D, Boyer TD (eds): Hepatology: A Textbook of Liver Disease. WB Saunders, Philadelphia, 1996
40. Popper H: General pathology of the liver: light microscopic aspects serving diagnosis and interpretation. Semin Liver Dis 1986;6:175–205
41. MacSween RNM, Anthony PP, Scheuer PJ: Pathology of the Liver. 2nd Ed. Churchill Livingstone, Edinburgh, 1987
42. Gilmore IT, Burroughs A, Murray-Lyon IM et al: Indications, methods and outcomes of percutaneous liver biopsy in England and Wales. Gut 1995;30:437–441
43. Robinson WS: Biology of human hepatitis viruses in hepatology. pp. 1146–1205. In Zakim D, Boyer TD (eds): Hepatology: A Textbook of Liver Disease. 3rd Ed. WB Saunders, Philadelphia, 1996
44. Bradley DW: Virology, molecular biology and serology of hepatitis C virus. Transfus Med Rev 1992;VI:93–125
45. Zaaijer HL, Cuypers HTM, Reesink HW et al: Reliability of polymerase chain reaction for detection of hepatitis C virus. Lancet 1993;341:722–724
46. Leung PSC, Coppel RL, Ansari A et al: Serology of PBC in PBC. In Gershwin ME (ed): Semin Liver Dis 1997;17:61–70
47. Bacon BR, Tavill AS: Haemochromatosis. pp. 1439–1472. In Zakim D, Boyer TD (eds): Hepatology—A Textbook of Liver Disease. 3rd Ed. WB Saunders, Philadelphia, 1996
48. Potter JR, James OFW: Clinical features and prognosis of alcoholic liver disease in respect of advancing age. Gerontology 1987;33:380–387
49. Aron E, Dupin M, Jobard P: Les cirrhoses du troisieme age. Ann Gastroenterol Hepatol 1979;15:558–563
50. Garagliano CF, Lilienfeld AM, Mendelhof AI: Incidence rates of liver cirrhosis and related diseases in Baltimore and

selected areas of the United States. J Chron Dis 1979;32: 543–554

51. Beresford TP, Lucey MR: Ethanol metabolism and intoxication in the elderly. pp. 117–127. In Beresford TP and Gomberg E (eds): Alcohol and Ageing. Oxford University Press, New York, 1995
52. James OFW, Bridgewater R, Gilder F et al: Alcoholism, alcoholic liver disease and its mortality among the elderly in England. pp. 359–370. In Kitani K (ed): Liver and Aging, Elsevier, Amsterdam, 1986
53. Kraus ML, Gottlieb LD, Horwitz RI et al: Randomised clinical trial of atenolol in patients with alcohol withdrawal. N Engl J Med 1985;313:905–909
54. Ramond MJ, Poynard T, Rueff B et al: A randomised trial of prednisolone in patients with severe alcoholic hepatitis. N Engl J Med 1992;326:507–510
55. Benhamous JP: Drug induced hepatitis: clinical aspects. pp. 23–30. In Fillastre JP (ed): Hepatotoxicity of Drugs. University of Rouen, Rouen, France, 1986
56. Woodhouse KW, Mortimer O, Wiholm BE: Hepatic adverse drug reactions—the effect of age. pp. 75–80. In Kitani K (ed): Liver and Aging. Elsevier, Amsterdam, 1986
57. Parry JV, Farrington CP, Perry KR et al: Rational programme for screening travellers for antibodies to hepatitis A virus. Lancet 1988;i:1447
58. Forbes A, Williams R: Increasing age—an important adverse prognostic factor in hepatitis A virus infection. J R Coll Physicians Lond 1988;22:237–239
59. Kondo Y, Tsukada K, Takeuchi I et al: Higher carrier rate after hepatitis B infection in the elderly. Hepatology 1993;18: 768–774
60. Cook JM, Gualde M, Hessel L et al: Alterations in the human immune response to the hepatitis B vaccine among the elderly. Cell Immunol 1987;109:89–96
61. Vandervelde EM, Millard JM, Parry JV et al: Time for action on hepatitis B immunisation. BMJ 1987;294:1031–1033
62. Chiaramonte M, Floreani A, Naccarato R: Hepatitis B infection in homes for the aged. J Med Virol 1982;9:247–255
63. Hoofnagle JH: Therapy of acute and chronic viral hepatitis. Adv Intern Med 1994;39:241–250
64. Weisberg JI, Andres LL, Smith CI et al: Survival in chronic hepatitis B: an analysis of 379 patients. Ann Intern Med 1984; 101:613–619
65. Alter MJ, Margolis HS, Krawczynski K et al: The natural history of community-acquired hepatitis C in the United States. N Engl J Med 1992;327:1899–1905
66. Brind AM, Watson JP, James OFW, Bassendine MF: Hepatitis C infection in the elderly. Q J Med 1996;89:291–296
67. Floreani A, Berlin T, Soffiati G et al: Anti-hepatitis C virus in the elderly: a sero-epidemiological study in a home for the aged. Gerontology 1992;38:214–216
68. Pagliano L, Craxi A, Cammaa C et al: Interferon-alpha for chronic hepatitis: a analysis of pretreatment clinical predictors of response. Hepatology 1994;19:820–825
69. Di Bisceglie AM, Hoofnagle JH: Chronic viral hepatitis. pp. 1299–1329. In Zakin D, Boyer TD (eds): Hepatology: A Textbook of Liver Disease. 3rd Ed. WB Saunders, Philadelphia, 1996
70. Sridharan GV, Wilkinson SP, Primrose WR: Pyogenic liver abscess in the elderly. Age Ageing 1990;19:199–203
71. Smoger et al: Liver abscess in the elderly. Age and Ageing 1997;26 (in press)
72. Greenstein AJ, Lowenthal D, Hammer GS et al: Continuing changing patterns of disease in pyogenic liver abscess: a study in 38 patients. Am J Gastroenterol 1984;79:217–222
73. Bertel CR, Van Heerden JA, Sheedy PF: Treatment of pyogenic hepatic abscess: surgical vs. percutaneous drainage. Arch Surg 1986;121:554–562
74. Zimmerman HJ, Fang M, Utili R et al: Jaundice due to bacterial infection. Gastroenterology 1979;77:362–369
75. Miller DJ, Keeton GR, Webber GL et al: Jaundice in severe bacterial infection. Gastroenterology 1976;71:94–98
76. Parker SG, James OFW, Young ET: Causes of raised serum alkaline phosphatase in elderly patients. Mod Trends Aging Res 1986;147:153–157
77. Grambsch PM, Dickson ER, Kaplan MM et al: Extramural cross-validation of the Mayo PBC model. Hepatology 1989; 10:846–850
78. Metcalfe JV, Bhopal RS, Gray J et al: The incidence and prevalence of PBC in the city of Newcastle upon Tyne. Int J Epidemiol 1997 (in press)
79. Metcalfe JV, Mitchison HC, Palmer JM et al: Natural history of early primary biliary cirrhosis. Lancet 1997;348:1399–1402
80. Mitchison HC, Lucey MR, Kelley PJ et al: Symptom development and prognosis in primary biliary cirrhosis. Gastroenterology 1990;99:778–784
81. O'Donahue J, Williams R: Primary biliary cirrhosis. Q J Med 1996;89:5–14
82. Emry S, Mor E, Schwartz ME et al: Liver transplantation in patients beyond 60. Tranplant Proc 1993;25:1075–1076
83. Clain DJ: Liver disease in the elderly. pp. 167–183. In Gelb AM (ed): Clinical Gastroenterology in the Elderly. Dekker, New York, 1996
84. Heathcote EJ, Cauch-Dubek K, Walker V et al: The Canadian multi-center double-blind randomized controlled trial of ursodeoxycholic acid in PBC. Hepatology 1994;19:1149–1158
85. Newton JL, Burt AD, Park JB et al: Autoimmune hepatitis in the elderly. Age and Ageing 1997;26 (in press)
86. Malcolm A: Minocycline induced liver injury. Am J Gastroenterol 1996;91:1641–1643
87. Feder JN, Gnirke A, Thomas W et al: A novel MHC class I like gene is mutated in patients with hereditary hemochromatosis. Nature Genet 1996;13:399–408
88. Brind AM, Bassendine MF, Bennett MK, James OFW: Are alpha-1-antitrypsin granules in the liver always important. Q J Med 1990;76:699–710
89. Roggli VL, Hausner RJ, Askew JB: Alpha-1-antitrypsin globules in hepatocytes of elderly persons with liver disease. Am J Clin Pathol 1981;75:538–542
90. Battle WM, Matarazzo A, Selhat GF et al: Alpha-1-antitrypsin deficiency—a cause of cryptogenic liver disease in the elderly. J Clin Gastroenterol 1982;4:269–273
91. Summerfield JA, Nagafuchi Y, Sherlock S et al: Hepatobiliary fibropolycystic disease: a clinical and histological review of 51 patients. J Hepatol 1986;2:141–149

92. Johnson P, Hayllar K, Metivier E et al: Survival in cirrhosis: importance of age as an indicator of disease duration, abstracted. J Hepatol 1989;9:546

93. Gitlin N, Serio KM: Ischaemic hepatitis: widening horizons. Am J Gastroenterol 1992;87:831–834

94. Thompson PW, Houghton BJ, Clifford C et al: The source and significance of raised serum enzymes in rheumatoid arthritis. Q J Med 28:869–881

95. Jaffe ES: Malignant lymphomas: pathology of hepatic involvement. Semin Liver Dis 1987;7:257–270

96. Rector WG, Reynolds TB: Risk factors for haemorrhage from esophageal varices and acute gastric erosions. Clin Gastroenterol 1985;14:139–144

97. Sung JJ, Chung SC, Lai W et al: Octreotile infusion or emergency sterotherapy for variceal haemorrhage. Lancet 1993; 342:637–639

98. Paquet KJ, Feussner H: Endoscopic sclerosis and balloon tamponade in acute hemorrhage from esophagogastric varices: a prospective controlled randomised trial. Hepatology 1985;5: 580–584

99. Poynard T, Cales P, Pasta L et al: Beta-adrenergic antagonist drugs in the prevention of gastrointestinal bleeding in patients with cirrhosis and oesophageal varices. N Engl J Med 1991; 324:1532–1535

100. Pagliano L, D'Amea G, Sorensen T et al: Prevention of first bleeding in cirrhosis: a meta analysis of randomized trials of non-surgical treatment. Ann Intern Med 1992;117:59–66

101. Westaby D, MacDougall BRD, Williams R: Improved survival following sclerotherapy for esophageal varices: final analysis of a controlled trial. Hepatology 1985;5:827–832

102. Vinel JP, Lamouiliatte H, Cales P: Propandol reduces the rebleeding rate during endoscopic sclerotherapy before variceal obliteration. Gastroenterology 1992;102:1764–1766

103. Gimson AES, Ramage JK, Paros ML et al: Randomised trial of variceal banding ligation versus injection sclerotherapy for bleeding oesophageal varices. Lancet 1993;342:391–395

104. Roessle M, Haag K, Ochs A et al: The transjugular intrahepatic portosystemic shunt procedure for variceal bleeding. N Engl J Med 1994;330:165–171

105. Bullimore DW, Miloszewski KJA, Losowsky MS: The prognosis of elderly subjects with oesophageal varices. Age Ageing 1989;18:35–38

106. Roberts CM, Carey H, Faizallah R et al: Injection sclerotherapy for oesophageal varices in the elderly. Age Ageing 1983; 12:139–143

107. Reynolds TB: Rapid presumptive diagnosis of spontaneous bacterial peritonitis. Gastroenterology 1986;90:1294–1295

108. Felisart J, Rimola A, Arroyo V et al: Cefotaxime is more effective than is ampicillin-tobramycin in cirrhotics with severe infections. Hepatology 1985;5:457–461

109. Gines P, Arroyo V, Quintero E et al: Comparison of paracentesis and diuretics in the treatment of cirrhotics with tense ascites. Gastroenterology 1987;93:234–240

110. Tito LI, Gines P, Arroyo V et al: Total paracentesis associated with intravenous albumin in the management of patients with cirrhosis and ascites. Gastroenterology 1990;98:146–154

111. Somberg K, Lake JR, Tomlanovitch et al: Transjugular intrahepatic portosystemic shunts for refractory ascites. Hepatology 1995;21:709–716

112. Gines P, Arroyo V, Vargas V et al: Paracentesis with intravenous infusion of albumin as compared with pentoneovenous shunting in cirrhosis with refractory ascites. N Engl J Med 1991;325:829–835

113. Schofield PR, Darlison MG, Fujita N et al: Sequence and functional expression of the GABA receptor shows a ligand gated receptor super family. Nature 1987;328:221–222

114. Schaffer D: Hepatic coma: studies on the target organ, editorial. Gastroenterology 1987;93:1131–1133

115. Basile AE, Gemmal SH, Mullen KD et al: Hepatic encephalopathy: evidence for the involvement of an endogenous benzodiazepine receptor ligand. Hepatology 1987;7:1103–1110

116. Collier JD, Curless R, Bassendine MF, James OFW: Clinical features and prognosis of hepatocellular carcinoma in Britian in relation to age. Age Ageing 1994;23:22–28

117. Lee HS, Hans CJ, Kim CV: Predominant etiologic association of hepatitis C virus with hepatocellular carcinoma compared with hepatitis B virus in elderly patients. Cancer 1993;72: 2564–2567

118. Liaw YF, Tai DI, Chu CM et al: Early detection of hepatocellular carcinoma in patients with chronic type B hepatitis. Gastroenterology 1986;90:263–270

119. Kew MC: Tumours of the liver. pp. 1513–1548. In Zakim D, Boyer TD (eds): Hepatology: A Textbook of Liver Disease. 3rd Ed. WB Saunders, Philadelphia 1996

120. Fortner JG, Lincer RM: Hepatic resection in the elderly. Ann Surg 1990;211:141–145

CHAPTER 60

Biliary Tract Disease

JOHN CROKER

Gallstones and malignancy are the two most common disease processes affecting the biliary tree in elderly patients.

Gallstones

Gallstones are more common in women than in men, being present in 30 percent of elderly women.[1] Seventy to 90 percent of gallstones obtained at cholecystectomy from patients in a western society are cholesterol stones consisting of more than 50 percent cholesterol.[2] Cholesterol gallstones are thought to arise because of a triple hepatobiliary defect[3,4]: (1) Cholesterol-supersaturated gallbladder bile, (2) increased rate of cholesterol crystal nucleation, and (3) reduced gallbladder contractility. Diet, rapid weight loss, major surgery, cirrhosis, inflammatory bowel disease, and abnormalities in intestinal transit have all been implicated. Pigment stones result from the supersaturation of bile with calcium bilirubinate, typically in hemolytic states. The increased prevalence of gallstones in the elderly seems most likely to reflect the probability of lithogenic bile producing stones with increasing age. Most common bile duct stones migrate from the gallbladder, and these types of stones are present in approximately 12 percent of patients with gallbladder stones at the time of cholecystectomy.[5] Both surgical and endoscopic studies have shown that most common bile duct calculi are brown pigment stones (less than 50 percent cholesterol). Stasis and infection both contribute to stone type. Pigment stones are more common in the presence of juxtapapillary diverticula.[6] The same authors have shown that duodenal diverticula are found with growth of β-glucuronidase-producing bacteria and subsequent deconjugation of bilirubinate glucuronides, which lead to pigment precipitation and stone formation. Both juxtapapillary diverticula and bacterial overgrowth are more common in elderly patients. It is quite likely that a cholesterol stone migrating from the gallbladder acts as a nucleus for the precipitation of pigment. In patients with recurrent gallstones after cholestectomy, bile infection in the presence of stasis can certainly give rise to primary choledochal stones.[7]

Presentation

Most gallbladder stones are asymptomatic and remain undiagnosed until necropsy. However, the increasing use of ultrasound imaging in the investigation of abdominal symptoms has led to an increased finding of asymptomatic gallstones. Most stones that are asymptomatic remain so, and most people with gallstones usually die of unrelated causes.[8] Ten percent of patients with asymptomatic stones develop symptoms within 5 years of diagnosis, and 20 percent by 20 years.[9,10] The difficulty with these studies is the evaluation of symptoms due to gallstones. Although biliary colic, acute cholecystitis, jaundice, and pancreatitis are readily accepted as symptoms of stones, upper abdominal pain not clearly due to another cause is often ascribed to gallstones when these stones are present. Such symptomatic patients may not be helped by cholecystectomy.[11] Indeed, patients who know they have gallstones tend to be more symptomatic than those who are happily ignorant. Of those patients with symptomatic gallstones, 25 percent go on to develop complications within 10 to 20 years. Symptom progression is greatest in the early years after diagnosis. Acute cholecystitis caused by cystic duct obstruction leads to hospital admission and can cause abscess formation, perforation, or mucocele. The presentation of patients with empyema of the gallbladder may be insidious and diagnosis difficult.[12] Occult gallstone disease may simply lead to nonspecific physical and mental disability,[13] and such deterioration may be marked by an abnormality in liver function. In 100 consecutive patients with symptomatic choledocholithiasis pain was present in 75 percent of cases, and Charcot's triad was present in only 40 percent of cases. Jaundice was found in 70 percent of cases, but abnormality of liver function was almost universal, with elevation of serum alkaline phosphatase level being the most common finding.[14] In a series of patients with choledochal stones referred for endoscopic sphincterotomy, 10 percent presented with isolated elevation of alkaline phosphatase level.[15] Acute pancreatitis is an uncommon condition in the elderly and should always prompt a search for gallstones. Stones and cancer together account for between one-half and three-quarters of cases of jaundice in the elderly.[16] Jaundice is first misdiagnosed as cancer in about 20 percent of cases. Gallstone disease is uncommon in patients with serum bilirubin levels above 200 μmol/L (11.7 mg/dl) whereas malignant disease is less likely with sepsis or a fluctuating clinical picture. A palpable gallbladder should be specifically investigated.

Diagnosis

Imaging is required initially to distinguish medical from surgical jaundice and can be done by ultrasound scanning in 96 percent of cases in experienced hands. The sensitivity and specificity of ultrasonography in the detection of gallbladder

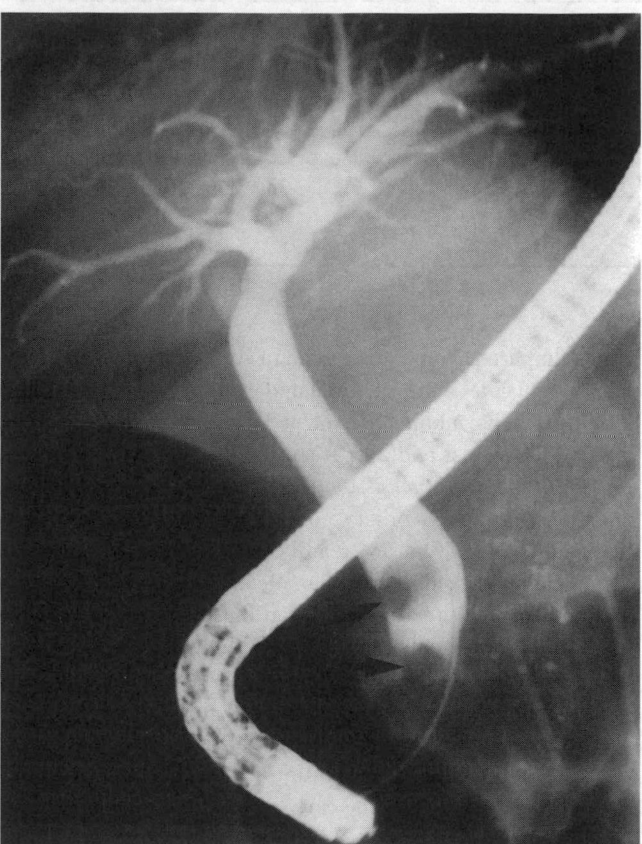

Figure 60-1 Cholangiogram showing two stones in dilated common bile duct (arrow). Note pancreatic calcification.

stones exceeds 90 percent. Stones in the common bile duct are more difficult to detect. False negatives are usually caused by gallstones that produce intermittent obstruction by a ball valve effect. One-third of patients with choledocholithiasis have ducts of normal size, and imaging must therefore be considered in the clinical context. Endoscopic retrograde cholangiopancreatography (ERCP) supplements ultrasound and facilitates therapy. Acute cholecystitis is diagnosed on clinical grounds and supported by ultrasound findings of gallbladder stones together with abnormality of the gallbladder wall. Radionuclide biliary scanning is a sensitive technique which can be used to diagnose acute cystic duct obstruction and therefore acute cholecystitis.

Treatment of Common Bile Duct Stones

Endoscopic sphincterotomy (ES) was developed over 20 years ago by Classen and Demling.[17] ES and gallstone retrieval with a basket or balloon is the treatment of choice for removing stones from the bile duct in elderly patients. In this population of individuals with diminished physiologic reserve, the mortality for common bile duct exploration may reach 9 percent, particularly when sepsis and jaundice are present.[18] Comparison of surgical data with those from ES is difficult because of selection criteria.[19] The endoscopic approach is usually completed within 30 to 45 minutes, and most patients can be discharged from the hospital within 2 to 6 days. Gallstone clearance is achieved in more than 80 to 85 percent of patients, although many require more than one procedure.[20] Complications such as pancreatitis, cholangitis, perforation, and bleeding occur in about 7 percent of patients. Mortality is about 1 percent although some series do not distinguish procedural rates from those at 30 days. Large gallstones greater than 15 mm in diameter can be more difficult to remove. Anatomic problems (periampullary diverticulum, polya gastrectomy, stone above a stricture) limit success. When unable to extract stones, most endoscopists insert temporary biliary stents to ensure adequate drainage.[21,22] Retained common bile duct stones may be further treated by surgery or by lithotripsy employing extracorporeal shock wave, pulsed laser, and electrohydraulic approaches. Bile duct irrigation with solvents (monooctanoin or methyl-*tert*-butyl ether [MTBE]) has been disappointing. It is our policy to attempt mechanical lithotripsy in fitter patients and to resort to long-term biliary stenting where this fails or when patients are very frail. Long-term follow-up of these patients is not easy to obtain. Up to 20 percent of them may experience further biliary problems, but nonbiliary morbidity and mortality are high, emphasizing the extreme frailty of such subjects.[21–23] ES is increasingly being performed on elderly patients with gallbladders still present. The role of elective cholecystectomy after ES is debated. It seems that only between 10 and 15 percent of patients require cholecystectomy during a 5-year follow-up.[24,25] Generally, then, an expectant policy is to be recommended in an elderly population. Unfortunately it does not seem possible at present to identify those factors that predict a requirement for later surgery. Identifying such patients would allow a more accurate evaluation of the risk and role of surgery and indeed of nonsurgical alternatives to cholecystectomy.

Cholecystectomy

Cholecystectomy carries a higher mortality rate in elderly patients compared to younger patients, particularly when performed as an emergency procedure.[26] Open cholecystectomy has been superseded by laparoscopic cholecystectomy as the standard treatment for gallstones in developed countries. It will be interesting to see whether laparoscopic cholecystectomy is any safer for elderly patients when compared with open surgery. To date no figures have been published. Laparoscopic cholecystectomy is less painful and facilitates a shorter hospital stay than formal surgery. The risk of bile duct injury is higher, however[27,28] In elderly and unfit patients with acute cholecystitis, a laparoscopic or open approach may be dangerous. In these situations the gallbladder can be drained under local anesthesia by inserting a drain under ultrasound control.[29] After an acute gallbladder has been drained there is usually an immediate resolution of symptoms. It is then possible to proceed to laparoscopic cholecystectomy, or, if the patient is very unfit, to percutaneous cholecystolithotomy under local anesthesia.[30] Other treatment options for gallbladder

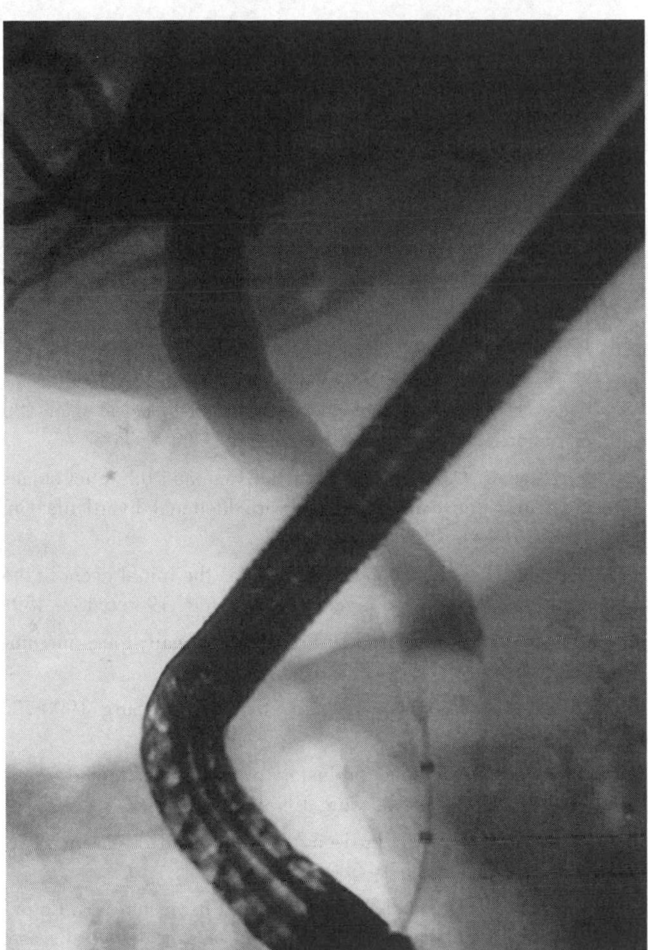

Figure 60-2 Balloon cholangiogram in same patient as in Figure 60-1 after endoscopic sphincterotomy confirming stone clearance.

stones include solvent dissolution therapy, endoscopic basket removal, and extracorporeal shock wave lithotripsy.

Silent Gallstones

Elective cholecystectomy for asymptomatic gallstones has not been cost-effective and is rarely indicated, particularly for elderly subjects.[31] Although laparoscopic cholecystectomy may be safer than open cholecystectomy, the total number of deaths following cholecystectomy may not be reduced because of the increased number of operations being performed. Thus the health care impact of laparoscopic cholecystectomy is unclear.[32] Until more data are available there appears to be no justification in operating electively on silent gallstones in an elderly population. A further argument advanced for prophylactic cholecystectomy is that it may prevent gallbladder cancer. However, for patients with asymptomatic stones, the risk of developing carcinoma of the gallbladder is less than the mortality of surgery, with the exception of the rare porcelain or calcified gallbladder. A link between previous cholecystectomy and colonic carcinoma remains unconfirmed.[33] In frail and elderly subjects the message is clear: leave the silent gallbladder alone.

Malignant Jaundice

Over 50 percent of elderly patients presenting with obstructive jaundice have malignant disease. The most common lesions causing jaundice are carcinomas of the head of the pancreas, followed by tumors of the gallbladder, the bile duct itself, and the papilla of Vater. Other gastrointestinal cancers may produce jaundice by nodal compression of the biliary system. The outlook for such patients is appalling whatever their age; for patients with pancreatic cancer, the average length of survival from the time of diagnosis is about 6 months, and overall 5-year survival is less than 1 percent. Survival after resection for carcinoma in the head of the pancreas has historically been dismal, with reported 5-year survival rates of about 5 percent.[34] A similar outcome is found in patients with gallbladder cancer.[35] Aggressive surgery for cholangiocarcinoma can yield better results at specialized centers, although resectability rates are low and there is considerable morbidity and mortality.[36] Carcinoma of the papilla carries a better prognosis, and younger patients should always be considered for resection. However, surgical resection is almost never an option

Figure 60-3 Cholangiocarcinoma (arrow).

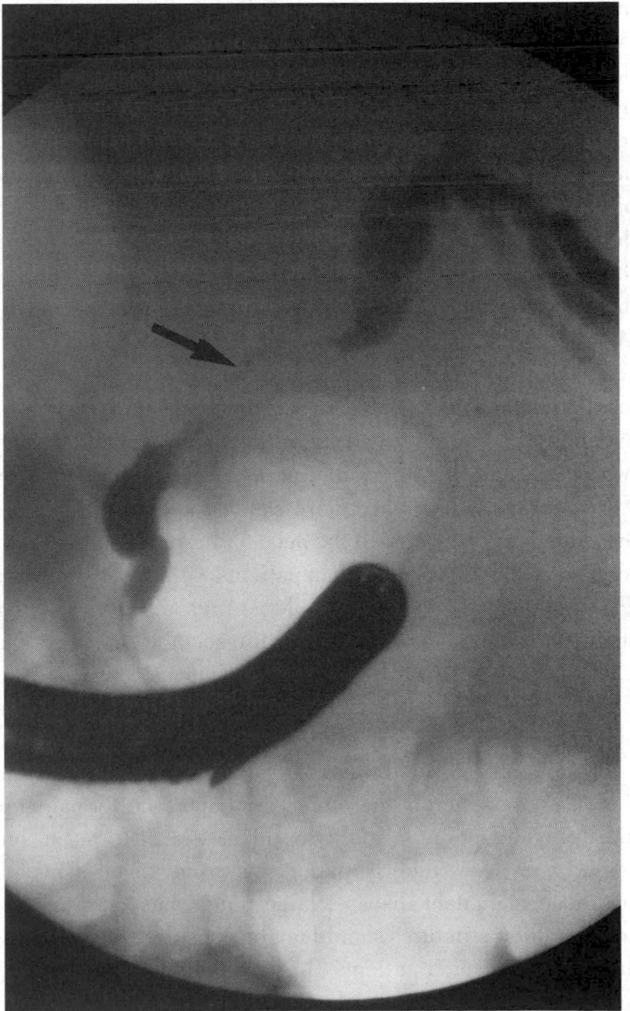

in elderly patients with malignant jaundice. Patients can be palliated by bypass surgery, although again this approach is not usually relevant for a geriatric population. Endoscopic stenting by placing plastic tubes across strictures can provide useful palliation. Following retrograde cholangiography and sphincterotomy, a guide wire enclosed in a radio-opaque polyethylene catheter is passed via the endoscope and through the biliary stricture. The stricture is dilated using endoscopic visual and radiologic control by passing another tube over the catheter and guide wire. This large polyethylene tube is then used to push the endoprosthesis, which is the same diameter, over the guide wire and through the now dilated stricture. Once a satisfactory position is obtained, the guide wire, catheter, and pushing tube are removed through the endoscope, leaving the prosthesis in situ. In a randomized study at Middlesex Hospital comparing surgical bypass to endoscopic stenting in 200 patients deemed fit for surgery, the early morbidity and 30-day mortality rates were much lower for endoscopy. The long-term outlook was of course not affected.[37] Endoscopic relief of jaundice is seen in over 85 percent of patients, and similar results can be achieved outside specialized centers.[38] Endoscopic biliary stenting is safer than the percutaneous route,[39] although this approach can be very useful in the treatment of difficult hilar strictures and when endoscopic access is impossible. The major problem with plastic stents is that they become blocked with sludge and bacteria, and impregnating them with antibiotics has not improved their patency. The internal diameter of a stent has been shown to be the critical factor in the development of stent occlusion. The maximum possible diameter of the prosthesis is of course determined by the diameter of the endoscope instrumentation channel. Two-thirds of patients die with their first stent in place, but one-third need a stent change within an average time of 4.5 months. Metal self-expanding stents can now be inserted either endoscopically or percutaneously and, when released, expand to a maximum diameter of 1 cm. In a recent open study metal self-expanding stents performed superiorly to plastic ones. Twenty-two of 28 patients were still free of jaundice at 14 months. Although metal stents are more expensive than plastic ones, they can be cost-effective if the need for hospital readmission is reduced.[40] The trick is to select patients with a good prognosis, although this can be very difficult. At present the use of metal stents is restricted to patients with unresectable ampullary malignancy and those with cholangiocarcinomas.

Most elderly patients with malignant jaundice are unsuitable for any kind of surgery. Endoscopic stenting can be helpful, but results vary considerably with the site and cause of obstruction. Case selection is therefore very important, for palliation must provide improved quality of life as well as technical success. In my view elderly patients with advanced dementia, advanced malignant disease, large tumor masses, ascites, or complex hilar strictures should not be considered for palliative therapy. In selected patients effective palliation and early return to the community can be achieved.

References

1. Bates T, Harrison M, Lowe D et al: Longitudinal study of gall stone prevalence at necropsy. Gut 1992;33:103–107
2. Vitetta L, Sali A, Chou ST et al: Gall stones at autopsy and cholecystectomy: a comparative study. Aust N Z J Surg 1988; 58:561–168
3. Hatsushika S, Tazuma S, Kajiyama G: Nucleation time and fatty acid composition of lecithin in human gall bladder bile. Scand J Gastroenterol 1993;28:131–136
4. Paumgartner G, Sauerbruch T: Gall stones: pathogenesis. Lancet 1991;338:1117–1121
5. Glenn F, Beil AR: Choledocholithiasis demonstrated at 586 operations. Surg Gynecol Obstet 1964;118:499–506
6. Sandstad O, Osnes T, Skar V et al: Common bile duct stones are mainly brown and associated with duodenal diverticula. Gut 1994;35:1464–1467
7. Cetta FM: Bile infection documented as the initial event in the pathogenesis of brown pigment. Hepatology 1986;6:482–489
8. Bateson MC, Bouchier IAD: Prevalence of gall stones in Dundee: a necropsy study. BMJ 1975;IV:437–430
9. Gibney EJ: Asymptomatic gall stones. Br J Surg 1990;77: 368–372
10. Friedman GD: The natural history of asymptomatic and symptomatic gall stones. A J Surg 1993;165:399–404
11. Bates T, Mercer JC, Harrison M: Symptomatic gall stone disease. Gut 1984;25:579–580
12. Thornton JR, Heaton KW, Espiner HJ, Eltringham WK: Empyema of the gall bladder—reappraisal of a neglected disease. Gut 1983;24:1183–1185
13. Cobden I, Lendrum R, Venables CW, James OFW: Gall stones presenting as mental and physical debility in the elderly. Lancet 1984;ii:1062–1064
14. Anciaux ML, Pelletier G, Attali P et al: Prospective study of clinical and biochemical features of symptomatic choledocholithiasis. Dig Dis Sci 1986;31:449–453
15. Mee AS, Vallon AG, Croker JR, Cotton PB: Nonoperative removal of bile duct stones by duodenoscopic sphincterotomy in the elderly. BMJ 1981;283:521–523
16. Croker JR: Biliary tract disease in the elderly. Clin Gastroenterol 1985;14:773–809
17. Classen M, Demling L: Endoskopiche sphinkerotomie der papilla vateri und steinextraction aus dem ductus choledochus. Dtsch Med Wochenschr 1974;99:496–497
18. Roukem JA, Carol FJ, Lieu F, Jakimowicz JJ: A retrospective study of surgical common bile duct exploration: ten years experience. Neth J Surg 1986;38:11–14
19. Cotton PB: Endoscopic management of bile duct stones (apples and oranges). Gut 1984;25:587–597
20. Vaira D, D'Anna L, Ainley C et al: Endoscopic sphincterotomy in 1000 consecutive patients. Lancet 1989;ii:431–433
21. Cairns SR, Dias L, Salmon PR, Russell RCG: Additional endoscopic procedures instead of urgent surgery for retained common bile duct stones. Gut 1989;30:535–540
22. Maxton DG, Tweedle DEF, Martin DF: Retained common bile

duct stones after endoscopic sphinterotomy: temporary and long term treatment with biliary stenting. Gut 1995;36:446–449

23. Croker JR, Williams SG, Charlton M et al: Endoscopic therapy for bile duct stones in a geriatric population. Postgrad Med J 1992;68:457–460
24. Ingoldby CJH, El-Saadi J, Hall RI, Denyer ME: Late results of endoscopic sphincterotomy for bile duct stones in elderly patients with gall bladders in situ. Gut 1989;30:1129–1131
25. Hansell DT, Millar MA, Murray WR et al: Endoscopic sphincterotomy for bile duct stones in patients with intact gall bladders. Br J Surg 1989;76:856–858
26. McSherry CK, Glenn F: The incidence and causes of death following surgery for non malignant biliary tract disease. Ann Surg 1980;191:271–275
27. McMahon AJ, Fullarton G, Baxter JN, O'Dwyer PJ: Bile duct injury and bile leakage in laparoscopic cholecystectomy. Br J Surg 1995;82:307–313
28. Hobbs KEF: Laparoscopic cholecystectomy. Gut 1995;36: 161–164
29. Melin MM, Sarr MG, Bender CE, Van Heerden JA: Percutaneous cholycystostomy: a valuable technique in high risk patients with presumed cholecystitis. Br J Surg 1995;82:1274–1277
30. Cheslyn-Curtis S, Gillams ARG, Russell RCG et al: Selection, management and early outcome of 113 patients with symptomatic gall stones treated by percutaneous cholecystolithotomy. Gut 1992;33:1253–1259
31. Ranshoff DF, Gracie WA: Treatment of gall stones. Ann Intern Med 1993;119:606–619
32. Lam CM, Murray FE, Cuschieri A: Increased cholecystectomy rate after the introduction of laparoscopic cholecystectomy in Scotland. Gut 1996;38:282–284
33. Turunen MJ, Kivilaakso EO: Increased risk of colorectal cancer after cholecystectomy. Ann Surg 1981;194:639–641
34. Warren KW, Christophi C, Armendariz R: Current trends in the diagnosis and treatment of carcinoma of the pancreas. A J Surg 1983;145:813–818
35. Cubertafond P, Gainant A, Cucchiaro G: Surgical treatment of 724 carcinomas of the gall bladder: results of the French Surgical Association Survey. Ann Surg 1994;219:275–280
36. Blumgart LH, Hadjus NS, Benjamin IS, Beazley R: Surgical approaches to cholangiocarcinoma at confluence of hepatic ducts. Lancet 1984;i:66–70
37. Hatfield ARW: Palliation of malignant obstructive jaundice—surgery or stent. Gut 1990;31:1339–1340
38. Rao KJM, Varghese NM, Blake H, Theodossi A: Endoscopic biliary stenting in a district general hospital. Gut 1995;37: 270–283
39. Speer AG, Cotton PB, Russell RCG et al: Randomized trial of endoscopic versus percutaneous stent insertion in malignant obstructive jaundice. Lancet 1987;ii:57–62
40. O'Brien S, Hatfield ARW, Craig PI, Williams SP: A three year follow up of self expanding metal stents in the endoscopic palliation of long term survivors with malignant biliary obstruction. Gut 1995;36:618–621

C H A P T E R 6 1

The Small Bowel

CHRISTOPHER RODRIGUES

Diseases of the small bowel can be divided into two categories for clinical purposes. Diffuse processes such as celiac disease interfere with nutrient absorption and result in the malabsorption syndrome, whereas discrete diseases like small bowel tumors produce focal manifestations. Some diseases like Crohn's disease and radiation enteritis can result in a combination of malabsorption and focal features. The true prevalence of malabsorption in elderly people is not known, but it occurred in 7 percent of elderly residents of a home[1] and in 30 percent of elderly patients in a hospital series.[2] A department of geriatric medicine with a special interest in malnutrition found that 55 of their 490 elderly inpatients were undernourished, 24 of whom (5 percent) had malabsorption.[3] Three conditions account for the majority of cases of malabsorption in the elderly: bacterial overgrowth syndrome, chronic pancreatitis, and celiac disease. The causes of malabsorption in three series are shown in Table 61-1.

Steatorrhea, the typical symptom of fat malabsorption, is much less likely to occur in elderly patients[6] who may even be constipated despite an increased stool volume. This is probably due to low dietary fat intake and slower transit of intestinal contents. Steatorrhea is more common in pancreatic insufficiency than in small bowel disease. Carbohydrate malabsorption causes watery diarrhea, abdominal distention, borborygmi and flatulence. These symptoms are due to the action of bacteria on carbohydrate residues in the colon. Lactose intolerance can occur with many diffuse small bowel diseases and should be suspected when such symptoms occur after the ingestion of milk or milk products.

The classic malabsorption syndrome of steatorrhea, weight loss, anemia, osteomalacia and other mineral, vitamin, and trace element deficiencies is rare in elderly people. The typical symptoms of malabsorption in this age group are much more likely to be general ill health, poor mobility, anorexia, weight loss, and mental symptoms such as depression and confusion.[1,3] This insidious picture is due to the gradual development of protein-calorie malnutrition frequently accompanied by nutritional anemia due to malabsorption of folate, vitamin B_{12}, or iron. Vague generalized body ache and muscle weakness may be early symptoms of osteomalacia. Though abdominal discomfort and distention are common symptoms in patients with malabsorption, abdominal pain is relatively rare. Recurrent abdominal pain can be due to chronic pancreatitis, inflammation as in Crohn's disease, or subacute obstruction due to strictures.

The diagnosis of malabsorption should therefore be considered in elderly patients with clinical and anthropometric evidence of undernutrition even in the absence of gastrointestinal symptoms. A dietary assessment is important in determining whether the malnutrition can reasonably be attributed to inadequate nutrient intake. The details of previous surgical procedures should be ascertained as far as possible: gastric surgery or intestinal bypass procedures can result in the bacterial overgrowth syndrome, and extensive small bowel resection can cause malabsorption because of critical reduction in the mucosal absorptive surface area.

Investigation of Small Bowel Disorders

Screening Tests

Routine blood tests are often helpful in the diagnosis of small bowel disease. The full blood count and blood film may show anemia with macrocytosis, an iron deficient picture, or a dimorphic film. Leukopenia and thrombocytopenia with macrocytosis suggest a diagnosis of megaloblastic anemia. Iron studies and measurement of vitamin B_{12} and red cell folate levels should be done in patients with suspected malabsorption even with a normal blood film, as typical changes may not be present in early deficiency. A low vitamin B_{12} level and a normal or increased red cell folate level raise the possibility of small bowel bacterial overgrowth. The blood film may also show evidence of splenic atrophy which occurs in celiac disease, with target cells, Howell-Jolley bodies, and thrombocytosis. Osteomalacia results in a raised alkaline phosphatase level with low calcium and phosphate levels. Vitamin K malabsorption may have bleeding manifestations associated with a prolonged international normalized ratio (INR). A low serum albumin level is not helpful in diagnosis, as it also occurs with dietary undernutrition, injury, sepsis, and malignancy. Malabsorption is unlikely if these screening tests are completely normal.

Tests of Absorption

Fat absorption

Detection of excess fecal fat in stool samples by Sudan staining is simple and inexpensive but is reliable only in patients with moderate or severe steatorrhea. The steatocrit is the relative quantity of fat in a stool sample expressed as a percentage of total stool solids. It has been validated in adults

Table 61-1 Causes of malabsorption in three series of patients more than 65 years old[a]

Cause	Montgomery[4] (1986)	McEvoy[3] (1983)	Price[5] (1977)
Pancreatic insufficiency	14 (20%)	2 (8%)	7 (44%)
Celiac disease	8 (11%)	2 (8%)	4 (25%)
Bacterial overgrowth	48 (69%)	17 (71%)	3 (19%)
Small bowel diverticula	12	9	1
Postgastric surgery	11	4	2
Normal small bowel	15	4	
Crohn's disease	3		
Scleroderma	2		
Miscellaneous	5		
Short bowel syndrome		1 (4%)	
Tropical sprue			2 (13%)
Unknown (refused further investigation)		2 (8%)	
Total	70	24	16

[a] *Percentages do not add up to 100 because of rounding.*

as a test of malabsorption—when fat excretion exceeds 10 g/day[7]—and may therefore be a useful screening test in elderly patients.

Measurement of fecal fat over a 72-hour period with the patient taking a 100-g fat diet is the standard method of quantifying fat malabsorption. Values of less than 7 g (20 mmol) of stool fat per day are normal. The test is unpopular with patients and staff, and older patients are often unable to tolerate a high-fat diet. The [^{14}C]triolein breath test is more appropriate for frail elderly patients, as it does not involve either a special diet or stool collection.[8] This radiolabeled triglyceride releases $^{14}CO_2$ after undergoing digestion, absorption, and metabolism. After an overnight fast, 5 μCi of [^{14}C]triolein are administered with a test meal, and $^{14}CO_2$ is measured in breath samples collected hourly for 6 to 8 hours. The test cannot be used where there are coexistent disorders, such as diabetes mellitus, that alter the conversion of fatty acids to CO_2 and in chronic lung diseases which lower breath CO_2 excretion. The results are affected by age, probably because of delayed rather than decreased absorption with aging; however, normal reference ranges have been defined for the elderly.[9] Fecal fat estimation and the triolein breath test do not distinguish between fat malabsorption due to small bowel disease and maldigestion resulting from pancreatic insufficiency.

Carbohydrate absorption

Xylose is a pentose sugar absorbed unchanged in the proximal jejunum. The amount absorbed is proportional to the area of normal mucosa. After an overnight fast 25 g of d-xylose is administered orally, urine is collected for 5 hours, and a 1-hour venous blood sample taken. Abnormal function is indicated by a 5-hour urinary excretion of less than 4 g or a serum level of less than 25 mg/dl.[10] Urinary xylose excretion declines with age because of declining renal function.[11–13] This can be corrected for by performing oral and intravenous xylose tolerance tests on separate days since renal function affects both tests to the same degree,[11–13] however, this is impractical for clinical use. The alternative is to use the 1-hour serum level, either after 25 g of xylose[10] or after a 5-g dose with a correction for body surface area.[14] Earlier studies found decreased xylose absorption in hospital inpatients beyond 70 years of age even after correcting for altered renal function,[13,15] but more recent work in healthy elderly people showed no change in absorption up to the ninth decade.[16,17] The xylose breath hydrogen test is another method of measuring xylose absorption and is independent of renal function.[18] After an oral dose of 25 g, end-expiratory breath samples are collected every 30 minutes for 5 hours. Malabsorption of xylose results in fermentation of the sugar by colonic flora, producing a rise in breath hydrogen at about 3 hours. A rise in breath hydrogen also occurs in patients with small bowel bacterial overgrowth, though usually much earlier than in patients with jejunal mucosal disease. Three to 25 percent of individuals are not colonized by hydrogen-producing colonic flora and hence have a false negative test.

Lactose intolerance can be confirmed by a wide variety of tests.[19] In the lactose tolerance test, blood glucose levels are measured at half-hourly intervals for 2 hours after the ingestion of 50 g of lactose. A rise of less than 1.1 mmol/L indicates lactose intolerance. Lactose absorption can also be assessed using the breath test described above for xylose, after the ingestion of 15 to 25 g lactose.

Vitamin B_{12} absorption

The Schilling test distinguishes vitamin B_{12} malabsorption due to terminal ileal disease from that due to lack of intrinsic factor. A modification of the procedure requires only a single 24-hour urine collection, as two separate radioisotopes of cobalt are used—one to label vitamin B_{12} and the other to label the vitamin B_{12}-intrinsic factor complex.[20]

Tests for Bacterial Overgrowth

The gold standard for the diagnosis of small bowel bacterial overgrowth is quantitative aerobic and anaerobic culture of fasting small bowel fluid: normal jejunal bacterial counts are less than 10^5/mL, and ileal counts less than 10^8/mL.[21,22] Collection of jejunal fluid can be carried out either by intubation under radiologic control[23] or, more convieniently, during upper gastrointestinal endoscopy.[3,24,25] The invasive procedure and cumbersome culture techniques involved have led to the development of noninvasive tests. In the [^{14}C]glycocholate breath test[26,27] 5 to 10 μCi of glycocholic acid, a conjugated bile acid, radiolabeled with ^{14}C is administered with a test meal. Bacterial deconjugation results in separation of [^{14}C]glycine from cholic acid, and $^{14}CO_2$ produced from the former is measured in breath samples collected over the next 4 to 8 hours. Terminal ileal disease or resection also results in a positive test since the bile acid is not reabsorbed and is then metabolized by colonic flora. The two conditions can be distinguished by measuring fecal ^{14}C radioactivity,[26] but this complicates an otherwise simple, convenient test. The alternative is to use the ^{75}Se-homotaurocholate (SeHCAT) test, an isotopic method for diagnosing bile acid malabsorption.[28] False negative results with the glycocholate breath test have been reported in as many as 30 to 40 percent of patients with culture-proven overgrowth.

Breath hydrogen measurement after ingestion of 50 to 80 g of glucose or 10 to 12 g of lactulose can also be used in the diagnosis of small bowel bacterial overgrowth.[21,29] The timing of the hydrogen rise is crucial for the lactulose test since this sugar is not absorbed in the small bowel and produces a second "colonic" hydrogen peak. Breath hydrogen tests have relatively low sensitivity and specificity rates,[21,23] and false negative results occur in individuals not colonized by hydrogen-producing flora. The [^{14}C]xylose breath test[30] was developed to avoid these problems and is more accurate than the hydrogen breath test.[31] Xylose is a better substrate than glycocholic acid or lactulose since it is absorbed in the jejunum with no risk of false positive results due to the action of colonic flora. Elevated CO_2 levels appear in breath samples within 60 minutes of taking 10 μCi of [^{14}C]xylose with 1 g of unlabeled xylose by mouth. However, studies in patients with bacterial overgrowth have produced conflicting results,[28,31,32] and in more recent work in patients with "simple colonization"[33,34] and motility disorders[35,36] the test failed to detect overgrowth reliably. Thus the search for the ideal breath test continues.

Radiology and Endoscopy

Double-contrast barium follow-through examination and enteroclysis (small bowel enema) are the two radiologic contrast techniques used to investigate the small bowel. Enteroclysis is probably more accurate but is more invasive. The role of abdominal computed tomography (CT) scanning and mesenteric angiography is described in the relevant sections. Upper gastrointestinal endoscopy is the usual method for collecting fluid for culture and for obtaining biopsies from the distal duodenum. Small bowel enteroscopy is beginning to be used more widely, and two methods are available. The push enteroscope can visualize most of the jejunum and can be used to take biopsies and perform polypectomy. The Sonde enteroscope can be intubated up to the distal ileum but has no biopsy channel and involves a much longer procedure.

Small Bowel Diseases

In this section, the five common clinical conditions affecting elderly patients will be discussed.

Celiac Disease

In celiac disease, sensitivity to dietary gluten in cereals like wheat, barley, and rye leads to a characteristic small bowel mucosal lesion, hyperplastic villous atrophy. The disease affects the proximal small bowel, decreases in severity distally, and may spare the distal jejunum and ileum. This variation in extent of affected bowel results in a wide clinical spectrum ranging from asymptomatic individuals to patients with full-blown malabsorption. Celiac disease is being increasingly recognized in older people. A bimodal age distribution has been described, with an earlier peak in women in the fourth decade and a later peak in men in the sixth and seventh decades.[37] The proportion of people with celiac disease who are elderly has increased from 2 to 7 percent in series reported about 30 years ago[38] to 19 to 27 percent more recently.[39,37] Celiac disease is present in 8 to 25 percent of patients over the age of 65 years who have malabsorption (Table 61-1).[3–5]

Many elderly patients with celiac disease are either asymptomatic or have trivial or nonspecific symptoms. In a recent series, only 45 percent of patients had diarrhea, the rest presenting with abdominal distension and flatulence, fatigue, anemia, or dermatitis hepetiformis.[39] The diagnosis should be considered in patients with unexplained anemia, macrocytosis, or evidence of splenic atrophy on the blood film.[38] Folate deficiency is the most common cause of anemia, but celiac disease can result in malabsorption of iron alone or of vitamin B_{12} when the terminal ileum is involved. Osteoporosis and osteomalacia are common, the former occurring in about 50 percent of patients with untreated celiac disease.

The diagnosis is confirmed by proximal small bowel biopsy. The mucosal surface is flattened as a result of subtotal or total villous atrophy, with stunting of or an absence of the brush border and hyperplastic crypts. The intraepithelial lymphocyte count is increased, and the lamina propria is infiltrated mainly with plasma cells and lymphocytes. These changes, accompanied by a clinical response to a gluten-free diet, are adequate to establish the diagnosis. A repeat biopsy to confirm histologic remission is now not considered necessary, and rarely changes management of the disease. Tests of nutrient absorption are unhelpful, but serologic markers are useful for screening patients for biopsy. Currently, antiendomysial antibody is the best test[40] and is probably as reliable in the elderly.[41] Antibody titers decrease or disappear with treatment, thus adding support to the diagnosis as well as being useful in monitoring dietary compliance.

Most elderly patients respond to a well-balanced gluten-free diet and cope well with the change in life-long eating habits.[39] Lactose intolerance can cause apparently resistant disease in some patients. However, milk and milk products are an important source of calcium and should be restricted only if they exacerbate symptoms, ideally after confirming the diagnosis with an objective test. Patients should receive supplements to correct nutrient deficiencies, as complete recovery of mucosal function can take months. All elderly patients with celiac disease should be given multivitamins and a calcium supplement for the first few months, and those with osteomalacia need vitamin D as well.[42] A few individuals with refractory disease fail to respond to gluten withdrawal or relapse after an initial remission. Some of these patients improve on corticosteroids or immunosuppressives but most have a poor prognosis and develop progressive malabsorption.

Malignancy occurs more frequently in patients with celiac disease. T-cell lymphoma of the small intestine is the commonest tumor, but there is an increased risk of developing squamous cell carcinomas of the esophagus, mouth, and pharynx and adenocarcinoma of the small bowel.[43,44] The incidence of lymphoma rises with age, and patients in their sixth, seventh, and eighth decades have a 1 in 10 chance of developing the tumor.[45] Lymphoma may be the first manifestation of celiac disease, but the diagnosis should also be considered in patients known to have celiac disease whose condition is either resistant to, or relapses on, a strict gluten-free diet. Weight loss is the commonest symptom, and patients also experience profound lethargy and muscle weakness, abdominal pain, and diarrhea. A gluten-free diet, adhered to for at least 5 years, has a protective effect against the development of malignancy in celiac disease.[43,46] Small intestinal ulceration and stricture formation occur in a small proportion of patients.[47,48] A few respond to steroids, but most patients need a laparotomy with resection of the involved segment.

Bacterial Overgrowth Syndrome

Bacterial counts in the gastrointestinal tract increase aborally (as one moves away from the mouth): the jejunum is normally colonized by gram-positive aerobes and facultative anaerobes, ileal flora contain some strict anaerobes as well, and the colon is heavily populated by predominantly anaerobic bacteria.[21,22] Malabsorption can occur when these populations increase, partly because of bacterial injury to the intestinal mucosa but also because of uptake or binding of major nutrients and vitamin B_{12} by bacteria. Fat absorption is also affected by an increase in anaerobic bacteria which deconjugate bile salts, resulting in impaired micelle formation. Folic acid and vitamin K are synthesized by bacteria, and folate levels are often normal or raised when bacterial overgrowth is present. Two factors are largely responsible for regulating bacterial proliferation: gastric acid and intestinal motility.[21,22,49] Gastric acid secretion destroys microorganisms ingested with food and saliva. The interdigestive migrating motor complex, a cyclic motility pattern, regularly propels luminal contents toward the colon, thus preventing stagnation and bacterial overgrowth.[50] Gut immune defenses[49] and interactions between microbial populations[22] also play a part in limiting bacterial growth.

Overgrowth of bacteria in the small bowel occurs under conditions that impair gastric acid secretion—such as atrophic gastritis, treatment with acid-reducing drugs, or after surgery for peptic ulcer disease. The prevalence of atrophic gastritis rises with age, largely as a result of *Helicobacter pylori* infection,[51] and probably affects 20 to 30 percent of otherwise healthy elderly people.[52,53] Nutrient malabsorption occurs only in a minority,[33,34] probably in those with an additional risk factor that results in the proliferation of anaerobic or gram-negative flora. Simple colonization[52] without malabsorption is common in elderly people, occurring in 16 to 56 percent of healthy individuals[17,54,55] and in 17 to 50 percent of hospital patients.[54,55] Simple colonization was present in 53 percent and 17 percent of patients receiving omeprazole and cimetidine, respectively.[56] Since 1977, bacterial overgrowth and malabsorption have been reported in small numbers of elderly patients with an anatomically normal small bowel (Table 61-1).[3,4,57] These individuals have normal gastric acid secretion and a prolonged mouth-to-cecum transit time.[24] Asymptomatic small bowel stasis is common in healthy elderly people[58] and appears to be more important than atrophic gastritis in the pathogenesis of this unique syndrome, though the two conditions must coexist in some cases.

Grossly disordered intestinal motility in conditions such as diabetic autonomic neuropathy, late radiation enteropathy, collagen diseases such as scleroderma, and the numerous causes of chronic intestinal pseudo-obstruction also results in the proliferation of bacteria. Partial small bowel obstruction due to strictures, radiation damage, or adhesions has a similar effect. Bacterial overgrowth occurs in abnormal reservoirs that permit stagnation of luminal contents, for example, small bowel diverticula and the afferent limb of a Billroth II gastrectomy. Abnormal communications between the proximal and distal intestine result in contamination of the former by denser, more anaerobic bacterial populations. Examples of this group include gastrocolic and jejunocolic fistulas, resection of the ileocecal valve, and surgical bypass of obstructed or diseased intestinal segments.

As already noted, bacterial overgrowth is the commonest cause of malabsorption in elderly patients (Table 61-1)[3,4] Apart from overgrowth associated with a normal small bowel, some of the predisposing conditions, such as small bowel diverticula, become more common with increasing age. Most patients who have undergone surgical procedures for peptic ulcer disease are now elderly.[59] Hence, a surgical history is particularly important, and all patients with suspected overgrowth should have a small bowel x-ray series to look for abnormal communications or reservoirs. The next steps are to confirm the presence of increased bacterial proliferation and to exclude simple colonization, preferably by assessing both carbohydrate and fat absorption. The nonspecific manifestations and the presence of malnutrition may otherwise lead to an erroneous diagnosis of overgrowth with malabsorption and to unnecessary and possibly harmful treatment with antibiotics.

The conditions underlying bacterial overgrowth are rarely amenable to surgical correction, and the mainstay of treatment is antibiotics. Tetracycline was traditionally used to reduce bacterial flora, but about two-thirds of patients do not benefit from this drug. Chloromycetin and clindamycin are rarely used now because of their toxicity. Co-amoxyclav in doses containing 250 to 500 mg of amoxycillin three times a day for a week is probably the drug of choice, with metronidazole and one of the cephalosporins as alternatives. Oral penicillin, ampicillin, and aminoglycosides are not effective. In some patients, a single course produces a satisfactory response lasting for months, but many patients need cyclic courses given at monthly intervals for 4 to 6 months.[24] Prokinetic agents may play a role in the management of bacterial overgrowth, particularly in elderly patients with prolonged small bowel transit.[49]

Crohn's Disease

Crohn's disease is characterized by chronic transmural inflammation and ulceration occurring in a segmental distribution. Intestinal ulceration ranges from superficial aphthoid ulcers to deep fissures, and the disease is often complicated by the formation of strictures, abscesses, and fistulas. This disease predominantly affects young adults, but there is a second smaller peak in the seventh and eighth decades.[60,61] The proportion of patients with Crohn's disease aged 60 years or more at the time of diagnosis ranges from 7 to 26 percent,[62] and these figures are likely to increase. Small bowel involvement is less common in this age group, occurring in 40 to 67 percent of elderly patients with Crohn's disease[63–66] compared to the overall frequency of 75 to 80 percent.

The clinical features of Crohn's disease,[64–66] including the extraintestinal manifestations,[65] are no different in elderly patients. Extensive small bowel disease is rare,[63] but the terminal ileum is affected in most individuals. Right iliac fossa pain, diarrhea, weight loss, fever, and an abdominal mass are typical features. Stricture formation can lead to subacute or acute obstruction, and fistulas to a wide variety of manifestations. In some series[63,65,66] elderly patients have presented more frequently with acute complications, such as obstruction and perforation, needing early or emergency surgery. This may be due to delays in diagnosis,[66,67] which is made only when a stricture, severe inflammation, or perforation results in acute illness. Terminal ileal Crohn's disease mimics acute appendicitis or an appendiceal abscess. The differential diagnosis in older patients should also include cecal diverticulitis, colonic carcinoma, and small bowel ischemia.

The radiologic features of Crohn's disease in the elderly do not differ from those in younger patients.[64] The distribution, extent, and severity of disease are usually well visualized on a double-contrast barium follow-through or enteroclysis. Abdominal CT scanning demonstrates bowel wall thickening, delineates fistulas not picked up by barium studies, and accurately outlines abscess cavities. Ultrasound is also used to detect inflammatory masses and abscesses. Labeled leukocyte scanning is a noninvasive method of assessing the extent and severity of disease and complements other imaging techniques in the detection of intra-abdominal abscesses.

Elderly patients with small bowel disease respond as well to medical treatment as younger patients.[64,65] Aminosalicylates are used in mild or moderate disease, but sulfasalazine is not effective in small bowel Crohn's disease without colonic involvement. This is probably because the active component, mesalazine or 5-aminosalicylate, is released from its "carrier" sulfapyridine by the action of colonic bacteria. Asacol, Claversal, and Pentasa consist of mesalazine alone in formulations that start to release the drug in the small bowel. They are effective both in achieving and in maintaining remission in patients with small bowel disease.[68] Corticosteroids are the most effective drugs for acute disease but do not maintain remission and cause many side effects. Newer topically active steroids such as budesonide have a better side effect profile[69] and could therefore be important in elderly patients. Immunosuppressive agents such as azathioprine and 6-mercatopurine are used as steroid sparing agents when it proves difficult or impossible to decrease the steroid dose. They should be used cautiously in the elderly given their potential for serious toxicity. Metronidazole is not effective in Crohn's disease limited to the small bowel, but other antibiotics such as ciprofloxacin may have a role in ileitis.[68]

Malnutrition is common in small bowel Crohn's disease and is due to a combination of reduced nutrient intake, intestinal failure, and increased energy requirements resulting from inflammation, sepsis, or surgery. In most patients nutrient intake can be increased by using small, frequent, low-fiber meals and supplementary polymeric sip feeds. Some patients benefit from tube feeding, and a few need parenteral nutrition. Parenteral and enteral nutrition are also effective in inducing remission in active disease.

Elderly patients usually tolerate surgery well,[63,64,70] except those presenting more acutely with severe disease, among whom postoperative mortality is high.[66] Thus early surgery, usually a limited right hemicolectomy and terminal ileal resection, is advisable in elderly patients not responding to medical treatment. Postoperative recurrence rates are lower than those in younger patients.[63,64,70] Adenocarcinoma of the small bowel can complicate small bowel Crohn's disease and is more likely to arise in the distal ileum.[71–73] Mortality rates in elderly people with Crohn's disease are similar to those in age-matched controls.[73]

Small Bowel Ischemia

Small bowel ischemia is predominantly a disease of the elderly. The superior mesenteric artery supplies the entire small bowel and the right half of the colon, and hence irreversible occlusion of this vessel has catastrophic effects. Patients who survive frequently require long-term nutritional support and may need parenteral nutrition depending on the length of residual jejunum.

Acute mesenteric ischemia

Acute arterial mesenteric ischemia is due to embolism, thrombus formation, or nonocclusive ischemia of the superior mesenteric artery or its territory. Embolism accounts for 40 to 50 percent of cases and usually occurs in elderly people with predisposing causes such as atrial fibrillation, left-sided cardiac chamber enlargement, or myocardial infarction. Nonocclusive mesenteric ischemia occurs in 20 to 30 percent of cases and is due to intense vasoconstriction of the mesenteric circulation following a low-output state or circulatory collapse, for example, severe congestive cardiac failure (CCF), hypotension, cardiac arrhythmias, following major surgery or cardiac arrest. Thrombosis (20 to 30 percent) occurs in the setting of widespread vascular disease, and 20 to 50 percent of patients have a history of abdominal angina in the proceeding weeks to months.

The mortality rate of about 70 to 80 percent has changed very little in the last 40 years and is even higher in the elderly.[74] Patients present with colicky central or upper abdominal pain, diarrhea, vomiting, and sweating. Elderly patients may have none of these features, and about a third may present with an acute confusional state.[75] Abdominal examination is initially either normal or reveals only tenderness. Distention develops later on, and definite signs of localized or generalized peritonitis and hypotension occur only with irreversible infarction. Patients usually have a marked leukocytosis and metabolic acidosis, and up to one-half have a raised level of serum amylase. Elevation in serum phosphate level[76] has not yet been confirmed as a reliable early marker of mesenteric infarction. Fluid levels and dilated loops of bowel on plain abdominal films occur in up to a third of patients, but more specific radiologic features such as gas in the intestinal wall or portal vessels are very rare. Mesenteric angiography should ideally be performed before signs of infarction appear. It can, however, be difficult to differentiate between acute and long-standing vascular changes on an angiogram. Abdominal CT scanning is being increasingly used in suspected mesenteric infarction.

Management warrants aggressive measures in the appropriate patients, and initial resuscitation includes monitoring of central pressures, correction of hypovolemia, and inotropic support if needed. Broad-spectrum antibiotics are given to treat the septicemia resulting from passage of intestinal flora across infarcted bowel. Patients with established signs of infarction need emergency surgery with resection of infarcted bowel and embolectomy, thrombectomy, or arterial reconstruction. A second-look operation is often indicated 12 to 24 hours later to differentiate between viable and nonviable intestine. When the diagnosis is suspected before clinical signs of infarction have developed, emergency angiography should be performed first. Intra-arterial infusions of the vasodilator papaverine relieve the associated mesenteric arterial spasm and improve perfusion perioperatively. One group has achieved a reduction in mortality to less than 50 percent using early angiography and vasodilator infusion as part of an intensive treatment plan.[74] Full anticoagulation with heparin is usually started 48 hours after surgery. There are a few anecdotal accounts of successful intra-arterial thrombolysis.

Focal segmental ischemia causes localized infarction, often at multiple sites, and can be due to vasculitis, cholesterol, or atheromatous emboli and various nonvascular diseases. In 5 to 10 percent of patients acute mesenteric infarction is due to mesenteric vein thrombosis.[77]

Chronic mesenteric ischemia

The syndrome of "abdominal angina," pain of ischemic origin precipitated by meals, has been assumed to have the same basis as other ischemic processes such as angina pectoris and intermittent claudication. However, individuals with advanced atherosclerotic disease can have severe stenosis or occlusion of two or even all three main mesenteric arterial trunks and remain asymptomatic.[78] The pain of chronic mesenteric ischemia begins within 30 minutes of a meal, lasts for up to 3 hours, and is gnawing or cramping in character. In some individuals it is relieved by lying prone or by squatting. Patients may miss or restrict meals in order to avoid pain and hence lose weight. Diagnosis therefore depends on history as well as angiographic findings of proximal stenosis in at least two of the main mesenteric trunks with a collateral circulation indicating chronic ischemia. It is important to exclude atypical angina pectoris and other causes of recurrent abdominal pain such as gallstone colic, and peptic ulcer disease. Doppler duplex scanning is an accurate, noninvasive screening test for imaging celiac and superior mesenteric artery stenosis and may help select patients for angiography.[79] Surgical arterial reconstruction relieves symptoms in most patients who fulfill the above criteria and prevents acute thrombotic occlusion.[80] Angioplasty may play a role in management by clarifying the indications for surgery. Chronic mesenteric ischemia remains a rare cause of abdominal pain, even in elderly patients.

Small Bowel Tumors

Small bowel tumors are relatively rare, accounting for only 2 to 3 percent of all gastrointestinal neoplasms. Adenomas, leiomyomas, and lipomas are the most common benign tumors. Adenomas usually arise in the duodenum and proximal jejunum, whereas leiomyomas and lipomas are more frequent in the ileum. These tumors can either be asymptomatic or can cause obstructive symptoms, intussuception, or occult bleeding. Adenomas situated within reach of an endoscope should be snared and removed, as lesions larger than 1 cm (0.39 in) in diameter have malignant potential. The treatment of distal adenomas and leiomyomas is surgical resection, but asymptomatic lipomas discovered incidentally can be left in situ.

Malignant small bowel tumors increase in frequency with age, with a peak incidence in the sixth and seventh decades.[81,82] Four histologic types account for most malignancies: carcinoid tumors (27 to 41 percent of tumors), adenocarcinomas (24 to 42 percent), lymphomas (20–22 percent), and leiomyosarcomas (11 percent). The overall 5-year survival in a population-based study of 328 tumors over a 25-year period was 54 percent,[81] which is much better than the figure of about 20 percent in most hospital-based reports.

Abdominal pain, bleeding, and intestinal obstruction are the main manifestations with weight loss and a palpable abdominal mass being less frequent.[83,84] With small bowel carcinoids, the carcinoid syndrome comprising flushing, diarrhea, and less commonly right heart failure, occurs only when hepatic metastases are present.[85] Diagnosis is often delayed because of the nonspecific history and an absence of clinical signs.[84,86] Barium studies to visualize the small bowel are usually performed when investigation of the upper and lower gastrointestinal tracts is negative. Abdominal CT scanning is also accurate in visualizing larger tumors. Small bowel enteroscopy should be reserved for patients whose lesions remain undetectable. Mesenteric angiography, used in the workup of patients with obscure gastrointestinal bleeding, detects some small bowel tumors that present in this way.

Carcinoid tumors, lymphomas, and sarcomas are distal tumors occurring more frequently in the ileum, whereas adenocarcinomas usually arise in the duodenum and proximal jejunum and decrease in frequency aborally. Carcinoid tumors grow slowly and are compatible with prolonged survival even with incurable disease. The 5-year survival rate after surgical resection is 80 percent, and even patients with hepatic metastases have a median survival of 3 years with 30 percent alive at 5 years.[85] Octreotide, a long-acting analog of somatostatin, is an effective, albeit temporary, palliative treatment for the carcinoid syndrome. Cyproheptadine, an antihistamine with antiserotonergic activity, is useful for relieving diarrhea, as are the standard antidiarrheal agents, codeine, and loperamide. The place of chemotherapy and hepatic artery embolization in treating metastases has not yet been established, but combinations of these therapies are being developed for patients with disseminated disease.

Most primary small bowel lymphomas[87] are of the B-cell type, T-cell lymphomas usually being associated with enteropathy, mainly celiac disease. About 20 percent of B-cell lymphomas are low-grade tumors of mucosa-associated lymphoid tissue (MALT lymphomas). Weight loss and a palpable abdominal mass are more common as presenting features of small bowel lymphomas compared with other tumors. Treatment is primarily by surgical resection which is possible in up to 80 percent of cases. T-cell tumors have a worse prognosis, with 5-year survival rates of 25 percent compared to 75 percent for low-grade B-cell lymphomas.

Adenocarcinomas and leiomyosarcomas are both treated by surgical resection in the appropriate patients without disseminated disease. The prognosis is poor for these tumors compared with that for small bowel carcinoids. Five-year survival rates are only 24 to 34 percent for adenocarcinoma and 20 to 45 percent for sarcomas.[81,83]

References

1. Pelz KS, Gottfried SP, Soos E: Intestinal absorption studies in the aged. Geriatrics 1968;23:149–153
2. Montgomery RD, Haeney MR, Ross IN et al: The ageing gut: a study of intestinal absorption in relation to nutrition in the elderly. Q J Med 1978;47:197–211
3. McEvoy A, Dutton J, James OFW: Bacterial contamination of the small intestine is an important cause of malabsorption in the elderly. BMJ 1983;287:789–793
4. Montgomery RD, Haboubi NY, Mike NH et al: Causes of malabsorption in the elderly. Age Ageing 1986;15:235–240
5. Price HL, Gazzard BG, Dawson AM: Steatorrhoea in the elderly. BMJ 1977;1:1582–1584
6. Ryder JB: Steatorrhoea in the elderly. Gerontol Clin 1963;5:30–37
7. Sugai E, Srur G, Vazquez H et al: Steatocrit: a reliable semiquantitative method for the detection of steatorrhoea. J Clin Gastroenterol 1994;19:206–209
8. Newcomer AD, Hofmann AF, DiMagno EP et al: L-Triolein breath test: a sensitive and specific test for fat malabsorption. Gastroenterology 1979;76:6–13
9. Mylvaganam K, Hudson PR, Herring A, Williams CP: ^{14}C triolein breath test: an assessment in the elderly. Gut 1989;30:1082–1086
10. Craig RM, Atkinson AJ Jr: D-Xylose testing: a review. Gastroenterology 1988;95:223–231
11. Kendall MJ: The influence of age on the xylose absorption test. Gut 1970;11:498–501
12. Kendall MJ, Nutter S: The influence of sex, body weight, and renal function on the xylose test. Gut 1970;11:1020–1023
13. Webster SGP, Leeming JT: Assessment of small bowel function in the elderly using a modified xylose tolerance test. Gut 1975;16:109–113
14. Haeney MR, Culank LS, Montgomery RD, Sammons HG. Evaluation of xylose absorption as measured in blood and urine: a one-hour blood xylose screening test in malabsorption. Gastroenterology 1978;75:393–400
15. Mayersohn M: The "xylose test" to assess gastrointestinal absorption in the elderly: a pharmacokinetic evaluation of the literature. J Gerontol 1982;37:300–305
16. Johnson SL, Mayersohn M, Conrad K: Gastrointestinal absorption as a function of age: xylose absorption in healthy adults. Clin Pharmacol Ther 1985;38:331–335
17. Arora S, Kassarjian Z, Krasinski SD et al: Effect of age on tests of intestinal and hepatic function in healthy humans. Gastroenterology 1989;96:1560–1565
18. Casellas F, Chicharro L, Malagelada JR: Potential usefulness of hydrogen breath test with D-xylose in clinical management of intestinal malabsorption. Dig Dis Sci 1993;38:321–327
19. Arola H: Diagnosis of hypolactasia and lactose malabsorption. Scand J Gastroenterol Suppl 1994;29:26–35
20. Bell TK, Bridges JM, Nelson MG: Simultaneous free and bound radioactive vitamin B_{12} urinary excretion test. J Clin Pathol 1965;18:611–613
21. King CE, Toskes PP: Small intestine bacterial overgrowth. Gastroenterology 1979;76:1035–1055
22. Simon GL, Gorbach SL: Intestinal flora in health and disease. Gastroenterology 1984;86:174–193
23. Corazza GR, Menozzi MG, Strocchi L et al: The diagnosis of small bowel bacterial overgrowth. Gastroenterology 1990;98:302–309
24. Haboubi NY, Montgomery RD: Small-bowel bacterial overgrowth in elderly people: clinical significance and response to treatment. Age Ageing 1992;21:13–19
25. Bardhan PK, Gyr K, Beglinger C et al: Diagnosis of bacterial overgrowth after culturing proximal small-bowel aspirate obtained during routine upper gastrointestinal endoscopy. Scand J Gastroenterol 1992;27:253–256
26. Fromm H, Hofmann AF: Breath test for altered bile-acid metabolism. Lancet 1971;ii:621–625
27. James OFW, Agnew JE, Bouchier IAD: Assessment of the ^{14}C-glycocholic acid breath test. BMJ 1973;3:191–195
28. Suhr O, Danielsson A, Horstedt P, Stenling R: Bacterial contamination of the small bowel evaluated by breath tests, ^{75}Se-labelled homocholic-tauro acid, and scanning electron microscopy. Scand J Gastroenterol 1990;25:841–852

29. Rhodes JM, Middleton P, Jewell DP: The lactulose hydrogen breath test as a diagnostic test for small-bowel bacterial overgrowth. Scand J Gastroenterol 1979;14:333–336
30. King CE, Toskes PP, Spivey JC et al: Detection of small intestinal bacterial overgrowth by means of a ^{14}C-D-xylose breath test. Gastroenterology 1979;77:75–82
31. King CE, Toskes PP: Comparison of the 1-gram [^{14}C]xylose, 10-gram lactulose-H_2, and 80-gram glucose-H_2 breath tests in patients with small intestine bacterial overgrowth. Gastroenterology 1986;91:1447–1451
32. Rumessen JJ, Gudmand-Hoyer E, Bachmann E, Justesen T: Diagnosis of bacterial overgrowth of the small intestine. Scand J Gastroenterol 1985;20:1267–1275
33. Husebye E, Skar V, Hoverstad T, Melby K: Fasting hypochlorhydria with Gram positive organisms is highly prevalent in healthy old people. Gut 1992;33:1331–1337
34. Saltzman JR, Kowdley KV, Pedrosa MC et al: Bacterial overgrowth without clinical malabsorption in elderly hypochlorhydric subjects. Gastroenterology 1994;106:615–623
35. Husebye E, Skar V, Hoverstad T et al: Abnormal intestinal motor patterns explain enteric colonization with Gram-negative bacilli in late radiation enteropathy. Gastroenterology 1995; 109:1078–1089
36. Valdovinos MA, Camilleri M, Thomforde GM, Frie C: Reduced accuracy of ^{14}C-D-xylose breath test for detection of bacterial overgrowth in gastrointestinal motility disorders. Scand J Gastroenterol 1993;28:963–968
37. Swinson CM, Levi AJ: Is coeliac disease underdiagnosed? BMJ 1980;281:1258–1260
38. Anonymous: Coeliac disease in the elderly. Lancet 1984;i: 775–776
39. Hankey GL, Holmes GKT: Coeliac disease in the elderly. Gut 1994;35:65–67
40. Ferreira M, Lloyd Davies S, Butler M et al: Endomysial antibody: is it the best screening test for coeliac disease? Gut 1992; 33:1633–1637
41. Attia L, Holt PR: Serological testing for celiac disease in the elderly. Gastroenterology 1995;109:2053
42. Walters JRF: Bone mineral density in coeliac disease. Gut 1994;35:150–151
43. Holmes GKT, Prior P, Lane MR et al: Malignancy in coeliac disease—effect of a gluten free diet. Gut 1989;30:333–338
44. Swinson CM, Slavin G, Coles EC, Booth CC: Coeliac disease and malignancy. Lancet 1983;i:111–115
45. Cooper BT, Holmes GKT, Cooke WT: Lymphoma risk in coeliac disease of later life. Digestion 1982;23:89–92
46. Collin P, Reunala T, Pukkala E et al: Coeliac disease—associated disorders and survival. Gut 1994;35:1215–1218
47. Baer AN, Bayless TM, Yardley JH: Intestinal ulceration and malabsorption syndromes. Gastroenterology 1980;79:754–765
48. Robertson DAF, Dixon MF, Scott BB et al: Small intestinal ulceration: diagnostic difficulties in relation to coeliac disease. Gut 1983;24:565–574
49. Holt PR: Clinical significance of bacterial overgrowth in elderly people. Age Ageing 1992;21:1–4
50. Vantrappen G, Janssens J, Hellemans J, Ghoos Y: The interdigestive motor complex of normal subjects and patients with bacterial overgrowth of the small intestine. J Clin Invest 1977; 59:1158–1166
51. Lovat LB: Age related changes in gut physiology and nutritional status. Gut 1996;38:306–309
52. Holt PR, Rosenberg IH, Russell RM: Causes and consequences of hypochlorhydria in the elderly. Dig Dis Sci 1989;34: 933–937
53. Saltzman J: Epidemiology and natural history of atrophic gastritis. pp. 31–47. In Holt PR, Russell R (eds): Chronic Gastritis and Hypochlorhydria in the Elderly. CRC, Boca Raton, 1993
54. Lipski PS, Kelly PJ, James OFW: Bacterial contamination of the small bowel in elderly people: is it necessarily pathological? Age Ageing 1992;21:5–12
55. Hellemans J, Joosten E, Ghoos Y et al: Positive $^{14}CO_2$ bile acid breath test in elderly people. Age Ageing 1984;13:138–143
56. Thorens J, Froehlich F, Schwizer W et al: Bacterial overgrowth during treatment with omeprazole compared with cimetidine: a prospective randomised double blind study. Gut 1996;39: 54–59
57. Roberts SH, James O, Jarvis EH: Bacterial overgrowth syndrome without "blind loop": a cause for malnutrition in the elderly. Lancet 1977;ii:1193–1195
58. Haboubi NY, Hudson P, Rahman Q et al: Small-intestine transit time in the elderly. Lancet 1988;i:933
59. Mellstrom D, Rundgren A: Long-term effects after partial gastrectomy in elderly men. Scand J Gastroenterol 1982;17: 433–439
60. Rose JDR, Roberts GM, Williams G et al: Cardiff Crohn's disease jubilee: the incidence over 50 years. Gut 1988;29: 346–351
61. Stowe SP, Redmond SR, Stormont JM et al: An epidemiologic study of inflammatory bowel disease in Rochester, New York. Gastroenterology 1990;98:104–110
62. Grimm IS, Friedman LS: Inflammatory bowel disease in the elderly. Gastroenterol Clin North Am 1990;19:361–389
63. Fabricius PJ, Gyde SN, Shouler P et al: Crohn's disease in the elderly. Gut 1985;26:461–465
64. Shapiro PA, Peppercorn MA, Antonioli DA, et al: Crohn's disease in the elderly. Am J Gastroenterol 1981;76:132–137
65. Softley A, Myren J, Clamp SE et al: Inflammatory bowel disease in the elderly patient. Scand J Gastroenterol Suppl 1988;23: 27–30
66. Lee FI, Giaffer M: Crohn's disease of late onset in Blackpool. Postgrad Med J 1987;63:471–473
67. Foxworthy DM, Wilson JAP: Crohn's disease in the elderly: prolonged delay in diagnosis. J Am Geriatr Soc 1985;33: 492–495
68. Elton E, Hanauer SB: Review article: the medical management of Crohn's disease. Aliment Pharmacol Ther 1996;10:1–22
69. Sachar DB: Budesonide for inflammatory bowel disease—is it a magic bullet? N Engl J Med 1994;331:873–874
70. Tchirkow G, Lavery IC, Fazio VW: Crohn's disease in the elderly. Dis Colon Rectum 1983;26:177–181

71. Ribeiro MB, Greenstein AJ, Heimann TM, et al: Adenocarcinoma of the small intestine in Crohn's disease. Surg Gynecol Obstet 1991;173:343–349

72. Hawker PC, Gyde SN, Thompson H, Allan RN: Adenocarcinoma of the small intestine complicating Crohn's disease. Gut 1982;23:188–193

73. Munkholm P, Langholz E, Davidsen M, Binder V: Intestinal cancer risk and mortality in patients with Crohn's disease. Gastroenterology 1993;105:1716–1723

74. Reinus JF, Brandt LJ, Boley SJ: Ischaemic diseases of the bowel. Gastroenterol Clin North Am 1990;19:319–343

75. Finucaine PM, Arunachalam T, O'Dowd J, Pathy MSJ: Acute mesenteric infarction in elderly patients. J Am Geriatr Soc 1989;37:355–358

76. Jamieson W, Marchuk S, Rowsom J, Durand D: The early diagnosis of massive acute mesenteric ischaemia. Br J Surg 1982; 69:S52–S53

77. Grendell JH, Ockner RK: Mesenteric venous thrombosis. Gastroenterology 1982;82:358–372

78. Croft RJ, Menon GP, Marston A: Does "intestinal angina" exist? A critical study of obstructed visceral arteries. Br J Surg 1981; 68:316–318

79. Moneta GL, Lee RW, Yeager RA et al: Mesenteric duplex scanning: a blinded prospective study. J Vasc Surg 1993;17:79–86

80. Marston A, Clarke JMF, Garcia Garcia J, Miller AL: Intestinal function and intestinal blood supply: a 20 year surgical study. Gut 1985;26:656–666

81. DiSario JA, Burt RW, Vargas H, McWhorter WP: Small bowel cancer: epidemiological and clinical characteristics from a population-based registry. Am J Gastroenterol 1994;89:699–701

82. Gabos S, Berkel J, Robson D, Whittaker H: Small bowel cancer in western Canada. Int J Epidemiol 1993;22:198–206

83. Frost DB, Mercado PD, Tyrrell JS: Small bowel cancer: a 30-year review. Ann Surg Oncol 1994;1:290–295

84. Maglinte DDT, Chernish SM, Bessette J et al: Factors in the diagnostic delays of small bowel malignancy. Indiana Med 1991;84:392–396

85. Moertel CG: An odyssey in the land of small bowel tumours. J Clin Oncol 1987;5:1503–1522

86. Ciresi DL, Scholten DJ: The continuing clinical dilemma of primary tumours of the small intestine. Am Surg 1995;61: 698–703

87. Domizio P, Owen RA, Shepherd NA, et al: Primary lymphoma of the small intestine: a clinicopathological study of 119 cases. Am J Surg Pathol 1993;17:429–442

C H A P T E R 62

The Large Bowel

ARNOLD WALD

Anatomy

The colon is a large, hollow organ that is derived embryologically from the primitive mid- and hindguts.[1] The appendix and transverse and sigmoid colons have mesenteries, whereas the ascending and descending colons do not. Like the stomach and small intestine, the colon has both circular and longitudinal smooth muscle layers, but uniquely, the longitudinal muscle of the colon is separated into three bundles known as taenia. The configuration of the taenia causes the colon to be divided into haustral folds which presumably help to slow the passage of fecal material and thus facilitate absorption.

The superior mesenteric artery supplies the right colon to the midtransverse colon, whereas the inferior mesenteric artery supplies the left colon.[2] The anorectum derives its blood supply from branches of the internal iliac arteries.[3] In the distal transverse to middescending colon, the superior and inferior mesenteric arteries are linked by a series of anastomoses known as the marginal artery of Drummond. This anatomic arrangement increases the vulnerability of this area to ischemic damage.

Innervation of the colon is via the autonomic nervous system and the enteric neurons.[4] Parasympathetic innervation is by the vagus nerve in the right colon and by sacral parasympathetics from the second, third, and fourth sacral nerves. Sympathetic innervation is derived from the lowest cervical to the third lumbar nerves via the splanchnic nerves. However, colon function may persist even after vagal or splanchnic interruption because of the presence of a well-developed enteric nervous system which can function in the absence of extrinsic innervation.

Functions and Symptoms

The principal functions of the colon and rectum are to store fecal wastes for prolonged periods of time and to expel them in a socially appropriate manner. Storage is facilitated by adaptive compliance of the bowel and by muscular contractions of colonic smooth muscle, which retard the forward movement of stool, thereby promoting electrolyte and water absorption and reducing stool volume. Forward movement occurs principally by relatively infrequent peristaltic contractions which move intraluminal contents over long distances. Continence is maintained by recognition of rectal filling and coordinated function of the anal sphincters and pelvic floor muscles to defer defecation until socially appropriate. Colonic motility and transit in healthy elderly are similar to that in younger individuals,[5] whereas aging is associated with diminished anal sphincter tone and strength as well as a less compliant rectum.[6,7] The latter changes may lead to greater susceptibility to fecal incontinence in the elderly (see Ch. 93).

The major symptoms of colonic and rectal disorders are constipation, diarrhea, pain, and rectal bleeding. The conditions that produce these symptoms are not unique to the elderly population; those occurring with increased frequency in the elderly include diverticulosis, neoplasms, ischemic colitis, vascular ectasias, fecal incontinence, constipation, and antibiotic-associated diarrhea and colitis. Inflammatory bowel diseases occur in all age groups, but onset of these diseases is less likely in the elderly population.

Diagnostic Testing

Radiology

Contrast studies

Contrast examination of the large intestine is done by using barium sulfate in either a single- or a double-contrast technique in which a thickened barium suspension is used to coat the mucosa followed by insufflation to expand the viscus. Alternatively, water-soluble contrast agents can be used if perforation is suspected.

The single-contrast technique is preferred when studying patients with suspected obstruction, diverticulitis, or fistula, whereas the double-contrast technique is preferred for demonstrating fine mucosal lesions and neoplasms. There continues to be controversy concerning the choice of barium contrast or colonoscopy when investigating colonic diseases, although most clinicians favor colonoscopy for its greater sensitivity and opportunity for biopsy and therapy. Contrast studies may be indicated in cases where severe stricturing disease or adhesions make colonoscopy hazardous, where conditions such as diverticulitis are suspected, if the location and nature of a colonic obstruction requires assessment, and if functional as well as structural information is required. A barium enema should not be attempted when increases in colon pressure may worsen the patient's condition, for example, in patients with suspected toxic megacolon or those with peritoneal signs that suggest ischemic colitis.

When patients complain of constipation or a recent change

in bowel habit, barium radiographs complement sigmoidoscopy in detecting organic causes and are also useful in diagnosing functional megacolon and megarectum. Complete filling of the colon with barium is neither necessary nor desirable in patients with megacolon. However, conventional barium studies provide limited information about colonic motor function in most patients with chronic constipation.[8] Moreover, they are frequently inadequate in frail or hospitalized elderly patients.[9,10]

Imaging techniques

Abdominal computed tomography This procedure allows visualization of the thickness of the bowel wall, the solid viscera within the abdomen, the mesenteries, and soft tissues adjacent to the bowel. It offers a modest advance in the diagnosis of diverticulitis by demonstrating inflammation of pericolic fat, abscesses that may contain collections of fluid and gas, and intramural sinus tracts. Fistulas to other organs can be identified when gas is found within the bladder or vagina. It also can identify extension of disease at a distance from the colon, including unsuspected intra-abdominal abscesses.

Computed tomography is also valuable when evaluating and managing complications of Crohn's disease, including abscesses, fistulas, and involvement of psoas muscles and ureters, and occasionally for percutaneous drainage of collections. Other complications, including sacral osteomyelitis, cholelithiasis, nephrolithiasis, and vascular necrosis of the femoral head associated with corticosteroid therapy, can also be diagnosed.

In appendicitis (and cecal diverticulitis, which is usually misdiagnosed as appendicitis), computed tomography may augment the clinical diagnosis by showing the periappendicular inflammatory process and differentiating phlegmon from abscess.[11] Occasionally, appendicoliths are identified, which are considered pathognomonic of appendicitis when associated with periappendicular inflammatory signs.

Anal and rectal endosonography This new technique accurately delineates the layers of the rectal wall, the internal and external anal sphincters, and the levator muscles.[12] Several studies suggest that endosonography is potentially useful in evaluating pelvic floor structures in many patients with fecal incontinence to detect occult sphincter injuries arising from childbirth or other conditions associated with potential injury to continence mechanisms.[13,14]

Endoscopic ultrasonography has been used to image rectal polyps, focal malignancy within polyps, tumor masses penetrating into the bowel wall, and extramural lesions such as prostatic tumors and ovarian lesions. Perirectal fistuals and abscesses can also be evaluated (including determining whether there is destruction of pelvic muscles).

Colonoscopy and Flexible Sigmoidoscopy

These procedures are usually performed in the prepared colon except when evaluating diarrheal illnesses. Colonoscopic examinations provide unparalleled evaluation of the mucosal surfaces and opportunities for biopsy and therapy. These include diagnosis and determining extent of inflammatory bowel disease, evaluation of patients with overt or occult gastrointestinal bleeding, evaluation of chronic watery diarrhea, endoscopic sampling and removal of polyps, decompression of sigmoid volvulus or functional megacolon, and ablation of vascular lesions. Colonoscopy is generally done under conscious sedation, whereas flexible sigmoidoscopy usually is not.[15] In many elderly patients, the physician must be aware of their increased sensitivity to sedatives and analgesic medications. As the elderly are susceptible to hypotension and respiratory depression, careful monitoring of the patient during the procedure is especially important. Even in elderly patients, such procedures are generally safe in experienced hands and when done in units that monitor blood gases and cardiorespiratory functions. Major complications include bleeding and perforation, which should not occur more than 2 or 3 times in 1,000 routine procedures.

Histopathology

Mucosal biopsies are often indicated when evaluating undiagnosed diarrhea, in long-standing ulcerative colitis during surveillance for precancerous dysplasia, in obtaining tissue for viral culture, and in evaluating polypoid or ulcerated lesions. In inflammatory disorders of the colon and rectum, biopsies serve to establish the presence, extent, and distribution of colitis and to differentiate ulcerative from Crohn's colitis and these disorders from other inflammatory conditions such as infectious colitis. Biopsies should be obtained from endoscopically normal as well as abnormal areas, as characteristic changes may be patchy and therefore missed if too few biopsies are obtained. This is especially true in pseudomembranous, collagenous, and lymphocytic colitis in which the distal colon may be spared. As hypertonic phosphate enemas and purgative laxatives may induce mucosal changes that can be mistaken for mild colitis, they should be avoided when evaluating suspected inflammation of the colon.

Fecal Occult Blood Testing

Fecal occult blood tests (FOBTs) identify hemoglobin or altered hemoglobin compounds in the stool. Foods containing peroxidases, such as melon and uncooked broccoli, horseradish, cauliflower, and turnips, may produce false positive results, whereas reducing agents such as ascorbic acid may decrease sensitivity.[16] Tests that extract the protoporphyrin from hemoglobin, such as Hemo Quant, are more specific and are quantitative but are also more time-consuming and expensive. Rehydration of Hemoccult slides increases sensitivity but decreases specificity and is not recommended. A weakly positive slide may become negative after 2 to 4 days of storage. Oral iron supplements do not interfere with any of these tests.

Colonic Diverticulosis

Colonic diverticula are herniations of colonic mucosa through the smooth muscle layers. Diverticula occur in areas of anatomic weakness of the circular smooth muscle created by penetration of blood vessels to the submucosa. They are most commonly found in the sigmoid and descending colons and rarely, if ever, in the rectum.[17]

This disorder has been recognized with increasing frequency in modern western countries.[18] Dietary fiber insufficiency and the increased longevity of modern western populations have been hypothesized to explain the increased prevalence of diverticulosis. Dietary factors may promote increased colonic motor activity and intraluminal pressures, whereas aging may lead to structural weakness of the colonic muscle.[17] As diverticula are asymptomatic in most individuals, caution must be taken before attributing nonspecific gastrointestinal symptoms to them.[19]

Painful Diverticular Disease

Painful diverticular disease is characterized by crampy discomfort in the left lower abdomen. Symptoms are often associated with constipation or diarrhea as well as with tenderness over the affected areas. These symptoms are similar to those of irritable bowel syndrome as well as partial bowel obstruction due to tumors or ischemia. In contrast to diverticulitis, there is no fever, leukocytosis, or rebound tenderness.

Diverticulitis

Diverticulitis develops in approximately 10 to 25 percent of individuals with diverticulosis who are followed for 10 years or more; however, less than 20 percent of these patients require hospitalization. Inflammation begins at the apex of the diverticulum when the opening of a diverticulum becomes obstructed (e.g., with stool), leading to micro- or macroperforation of a diverticulum.[20] The presence of a palpable mass, fever, leukocytosis, and/or rebound tenderness indicates an inflammatory process which often remains localized in the adjacent pericolic tissues but may progress to a peridiverticular abscess.[21] Other complications include fibrosis and bowel obstruction, fistula formation to the bladder, vagina, or adjacent small intestine, and free perforation with peritonitis. The frequency of complications rises to about 60 percent with recurrent attacks of diverticulitis.

Making a clinical distinction between painful diverticular disease and diverticulitis carries a sizable rate of error.[20] In an elderly or debilitated patient, the absence of fever, leukocytosis or rebound tenderness does not exclude diverticulitis.[21]

Bleeding

Bleeding associated with diverticula is typically brisk and painless and usually arises in the right colon. Bleeding is thought to occur when a fecalith erodes into a vessel in the neck of the diverticulum or there is rupture of the penetrating arteriole in its course around the diverticular sac.[17]

Other disorders such as carcinoma, inflammatory bowel disease, and ischemia may mimic symptomatic diverticular disease. Diagnostic studies include barium enema, computerized tomography, ultrasonography, and colonoscopy. In most cases of suspected diverticulitis, barium enema should be delayed for about a week to allow some resolution of the inflammatory process. A single-contrast study should be performed cautiously to minimize the risk of perforation. Radiographic findings suggesting diverticulitis include longitudinal fistulas connecting diverticula over segments of colon, fistula into adjacent organs, a fixed eccentric defect in the colon wall, contrast outside the lumen of the colon or diverticulum, and intraluminal defects representing abscesses.[17] Computed tomography and ultrasonic imaging of the abdomen provide superior definition of colonic wall thickness and extraluminal structures and are preferred at the time of initial evaluation. Colonoscopy is a less attractive option during an acute episode and is best employed to exclude tumors or other conditions if other diagnostic tests are inconclusive.

An important indication for emergent colonoscopy is to identify the source of bleeding in patients with diverticula, as other lesions not seen by contrast studies may be the actual source.[22] If bleeding is brisk, a bleeding scan or selective mesenteric angiography can locate the site of bleeding, and the latter can be used to infuse vasoactive substances to control bleeding (see Lower Gastrointestinal Bleeding).

The treatment of painful diverticular disease is designed to reduce symptoms based on smooth muscle spasm, in contrast to the treatment of diverticulitis which is designed to treat bacterial infection (Table 62-1).

Surgery is recommended for patients with diverticulitis who fail to respond to medical therapy within 72 hours, often for those who have had two or more attacks of diverticulitis, and for immunocompromised patients.[23] A one-stage operation, in which the diseased segment of bowel is resected and continuity restored by a primary anastomosis, is preferred.[24] In cases of generalized peritonitis or emergent surgery for perforation with abscess or high-grade obstruction, a two-stage procedure requiring a diverting colostomy should be used.[25] Large abscesses can often be drained percutaneously by an interventional radiologist using computerized tomography or ultrasonography as a guide.[26,27] Elective surgery can then be performed after 2 to 3 weeks of antibiotic therapy.

Emergent surgery is required for generalized peritonitis or persistent high-grade bowel obstruction. Most patients with complicated diverticular disease require surgery, even if clinical recovery occurs, since there is a high risk of recurrent attacks.

Appendicitis

Elderly patients with appendicitis are at increased risk (about 60 percent) for perforation. They have a higher mortality and often do not exhibit a fever or elevated white blood cell count.[28]

The onset of abdominal pain is abrupt, begins in the midabdomen, relocates to the right lower quadrant, and is often associated with nausea, vomiting, and fever. Physical examination characteristically reveals signs of local peritonitis in the right

Table 62-1 Medical treatment of diverticular disease

Measure	Painful Diverticulosis	Diverticulitis
Diet	Increase fiber	Reduce fiber (or NPO)
Bulk laxatives	Sometimes effective	Not indicated
Analgesics	Avoid narcotics	Avoid morphine; meperidine is best
Antispasmodics	Propantheline bromide (15 mg tid); dicyclomine hydrochloride (20 mg tid); hyoscyamine sulfate (0.125–0.250 mg q4h)	Not indicated
Antibiotics	Not indicated	Oral: amoxicillin/clavulanate K^+ (750 mg tid) Parenteral: (1) gentamycin or tobramycin (5 mg/kg/d) plus clindamycin (1.2–2.4 g/d) or (2) cefoxitin (4–6 g/d) or (3) ampicillin/sulbactam sodium (6–12 g/d)

(Modified from Wald,[17] with permission.)

lower quadrant, and the white blood cell count is frequently elevated. The differential diagnosis includes pyelonephritis, Crohn's disease, gastroenteritis, pelvic inflammatory disease, ovarian cyst, and cecal diverticulitis. In the elderly, appendicitis may occur in association with colon cancer in which low-grade obstruction results in distention of the appendix and mimics true appendicitis.

If the diagnosis is uncertain, ultrasonography has been shown to have positive and negative predictive values of about 90 percent for appendicitis and is also useful in identifying another cause of symptoms in patients with right lower quadrant pain.[29] One sonographic criterion for acute appendicitis is visualization of a noncompressible appendix with a diameter of greater than 6 mm.

Infectious Diseases

Clostridium difficile

The vast majority of cases are associated with two protein exotoxins (A and B) produced by *Clostridium difficile*. Toxin A is an enterotoxin which triggers diarrhea, epithelial necrosis, and a characteristic inflammatory process in animals, whereas toxin B is a cytoxin in tissue culture but does not by itself cause toxicity in animals.[30] The disease spectrum ranges from mild diarrhea, with little or no inflammation, to severe colitis, often associated with pseudomembranes which are adherent to necrotic colonic epithelium. Acquisition of *C. difficile* occurs most frequently in elderly persons in hospitals or nursing homes, potentially because of environmental contamination with *C. difficile* and spores carried on the hands of hospital or institutional personnel.[31] Acquisition is often asymptomatic but may have clinical consequences if elderly patients receive certain antibiotics or chemotherapeutic agents. Other possible risk factors include surgery, intensive care, nasogastric intubation, and length of hospital stay. A smaller number of patients have antibiotic-associated diarrhea but no evidence of *C. difficle* infection.

Although virtually all antibiotics have been implicated, the most common are cephalosporins, ampicillin or amoxicillin, and clindamycin.[32] Less commonly mentioned antibiotics include other penicillins, erythromycin, and trimethoprim sulfamethoxazole.

The typical clinical picture of *C. difficile*-associated colitis includes nonbloody diarrhea, lower abdominal cramps, fever, and leukocytosis. Fever is usually low grade although, on occasion, it can be quite high. In severe cases, dehydration, hypotension, hypoproteinemia, toxic megacolon, or even colonic perforation may occur.

In severely ill patients, the diagnostic test of choice is flexible sigmoidoscopy or colonoscopy. As the distal colon is involved in the majority of cases, flexible sigmoidoscopy is usually satisfactory; however, changes may be confined to the right colon in up to one-third of cases, making colonoscopy necessary if less extensive procedures do not confirm a suspected diagnosis. The yellowish-gray pseudomembranes are densely adherent to the underlying colonic mucosa, interspersed with mucosa that appears normal. Mucosal biopsies may exhibit characteristic findings of epitheilial necrosis and micropseudomembranes ("volcano lesions") even when pseudomembranes are not grossly visible. Endoscopy should be performed in severely ill patients who present atypically and therefore require a rapid diagnosis.[33]

Several tests identify *C. difficile* or its toxin. The enzyme immunoassay is the preferred test to detect toxin, whereas stool cultures for *C. difficile* require selective growth media and an experienced laboratory. Moreover, it is difficult to implicate *C. difficile* as the cause of antibiotic-associated diarrhea in the absence of an identifiable cytotoxin.

The offending drug should be discontinued if possible. If symptoms persist or are severe, patients should receive oral metronidazole 250 mg qid for 7 to 14 days or oral vancomycin 125 mg PO qid for 7 to 14 days. If oral intake is not possible, metronidazole 500 mg IV q6h is given until oral administration can be accomplished. Metronidazole and vancomycin appear to be therapeutically comparable, but metronidazole costs less.[34] In general, fever resolves within 24 hours and diarrhea decreases within 4 to 5 days.

Relapses average about 20 to 25 percent following successful treatment with either agent,[35] often involving sporulation which leads to relapse within 4 weeks after completion of successful treatment. These episodes invariably respond to another course of antibiotic therapy. About 5 to 10 percent of patients have multiple relapses. In such individuals metronidazole or vancomycin in conventional doses should be followed by a 3-week course of cholestyramine 4 g tid and/or Lactinex 500 mg PO qid, or vancomycin 125 mg PO every other day. Others advocate a 6-week schedule consisting of a 2-week course of vancomycin or metronidazole given daily in the standard dose, a 2-week course in the same dose given every other day, followed by a 2-week course at the same dose given every third day. Currently, trials are being conducted to explore the efficacy of a nonpathogenic yeast, *Saccharomyces boulardii*, and preliminary results appear to be promising.[36] It has been show that this yeast inhibits the binding of toxin A to rat ileum, with consequent prevention of enterotoxicity.

Shigella

These organisms consist of four groups: A (*Shigella dysenteriae*), B (*S. flexneri*), C (*S. boydii*), and D (*S. sonnei*), the last of which accounts for most clinical infections in western countries. In contrast to other enteric pathogens, very few organisms are needed to produce infection, which is spread by fecal-oral transmission between humans and which continues to occur despite high standards of water purification and sewage disposal. The precise virulence factor(s) of this organism is (are) unknown. Disease is caused by invasion of colonic epithelial cells, perhaps in part mediated by cytotoxins produced by *S. dysenteriae* and *S. flexneri*, but enterotoxins may also contribute to early symptoms of nondysenteric diarrhea. Enterotoxins have also been hypothesized to mediate the hemolytic-uremic syndrome associated with severe colitis caused by *S. dysenteriae* type I.

Symptoms

Colitis is heralded by the passage of bloody mucoid stools associated with urgency, tenesmus, abdominal cramping, fever, and malaise. The frequency of stools is highest during the first 24 hours of illness and gradually diminishes thereafter.

Diagnosis

Stool examination reveals numerous polymorphonuclear cells, and leukocytosis is common. Stool culture grown on selective media is the definitive diagnostic study. Sigmoidoscopy is usually not necessary, but if done, will demonstrate a friable hyperemic mucosa. Barium contrast studies are not indicated.

Treatment

If the illness is mild and self-limited, antibiotics can be withheld. As resistance to sulfonamides, ampicillin, and tetracycline is now common, treatment with trimethoprim-sulfamethoxazole or a fluoroquinolone (e.g., ciprofloxacin 500 mg twice daily for 5 days) is indicated in elderly or debilitated patients with acute disease to shorten the illness and the period of fecal excretion of the organism.[38] Antidiarrheal agents prolong the clinical illness and carrying of the organism and should not be administered.[39] The development of a chronic carrier state is rare and difficult to treat.

Toxigenic *Escherichia coli*

This organism commonly causes disease in developed countries and is a major cause of diarrhea in tourists visiting underdeveloped countries. As older individuals increasingly engage in overseas travel, this organism can be come a major impediment to a successful trip.

Low-grade fever, anorexia, and watery diarrhea are characteristic and are caused by plasmid-controlled enterotoxins which are both heat-stable and heat-labile. Strictly speaking, this organism does not affect the colon directly. The presence of dysentery or other manifestations of colitis should suggest another cause of diarrhea. Preventive measures include eating cooked food only while it is still hot and avoiding local water, including fruits and vegetables washed with local water. In elderly tourists, the disease can be shortened by prompt use of trimethoprim-sulfamethoxazole or a fluoroquinolone.[40]

Escherichia coli 0157:H7

This organism has been identified as a major pathogen in the United States and Canada.[41] Epidemics have been traced to consumption of undercooked and raw ground beef, and infections have also been associated with exposure to patients with bloody diarrhea, contaminated water supplies, and nonpreserved apple cider. Clinical manifestations include nonbloody diarrhea, hemorrhagic colitis, and hemolytic-uremic syndrome (HUS).[42] Unlike most bacterial enteric diseases, *E. coli* 0157:H7 is often characterized by low-grade fever or the absence of a fever.[43] The pathogenesis of colitis has been linked to Shiga-like toxins (verocytotoxins 1 and 2) which bind to a glycolipid on the surface of colonocytes, but adherence factors may also play a role. Older age is both a risk factor for this infection and increases the risk of HUS and death. It is generally believed that antibiotics are not indicated for active infections.[42]

Campylobacter Species

Campylobacter jejuni and *C. coli* are among the most common bacterial causes of diarrhea and can be manifested by gastroenteritis, pseudoappendicitis, or colitis. These organisms are usually transmitted from animals to humans through contaminated food and water and sometimes by direct contact with pets. Constitutional symptoms usually precede diarrhea and abdominal cramps by up to 24 hours, and colitis may be characterized by fever and dysentery lasting for a week or more. Convalescent carriage up to a mean of 5 weeks is common after the onset of illness and is significantly reduced by antimicrobial treatment.

Although the infection is usually self-limited, antibiotics may be given if the illness is severe or in patients who are immunosuppressed.[44] Treatment consists of erythromycin or fluoroquinolones; newer macrolides such as azithromycin and clarithromycin show excellent in vitro activity. Resistance to fluoroquinolones has been reported in Europe.

Entamoeba histolyticia

This organism remains a primary cause of dysentery which may be complicated by fulminant colitis, toxic megacolon, bleeding, stricture, and perforation. Severe disease is more common in the elderly and in patients who are immunosuppressed or debilitated.[45] The disease is typically acquired by ingesting cysts from contaminated water or fresh vegetables but can also be transmitted venereally through sexual practices that promote fecal-oral transmission. Studies on germ-free animals suggest that intestinal disease does not develop unless bacteria are present. This may partly account for the effectiveness of metronidazole, which is also active against anaerobic bacteria.

Three separate stool specimens should be examined if the diagnosis is suspected. A wet preparation should be performed within 30 minutes of passage to look for motile trophozoites which may contain ingested red blood cells. A Formalin-ethyl acetate concentration preparation should be examined for cysts. Barium, bismuth, kaolin compounds, magnesium hydroxide, castor oil, and hypertonic enemas all interfere with the ability to detect the parasite in stools.[45]

Colonoscopy may reveal erythema, edema, friability of the mucosa, and scattered ulcers 5 to 15 mm in diameter, covered with a yellow exudate. These ulcers may occur anywhere in the colon but are most common in the cecum and ascending colon. Biopsies from the edge of these ulcers may reveal typical "hour-glass" ulcers containing trophozoites. Cathartics and enemas should not be used because they interfere with identification of the parasite.

As these techniques may miss identifying the parasite, serologic tests for antiamebic antibody should also be obtained in suspected cases. The indirect hemagglutination assay (IHA) is positive in almost 90 percent of patients with amebic dysentery and in virtually all patients with amebic liver abscesses. The IHA remains positive for years after treatment of invasive amebiasis.[46]

Treatment of acute amebic dysentery consists of metronidazole 750 mg three times daily for 10 days or, if not tolerated orally, by the intravenous route. This should be followed by luminal acting oral drugs such as paromomysin 500 mg three times daily for 7 days or iodoquinol 650 mg three times daily for 20 days to eliminate all cysts and prevent possible relapse.[47]

Cytomegalovirus

Cytomegalovirus (CMV) is a member of the herpes virus family which enters a lifelong latent phase after primary infection in immunocompetent persons. In patients who are immunocompromised with diminished T-cell function, reactivation may occur and may become persistent, with reappearance of IgM anti-CMV antibodies in the serum. Among the gastrointestinal syndromes associated with CMV are focal and diffuse colitis.

CMV colitis is associated with severe small-volume diarrhea, abdominal pain, and fever. Colonoscopy may reveal variable degrees of focal erythema, petechial hemorrhage, erosions, and in advanced cases, scattered ulcers. Mucosal biopsy may reveal characteristic intranuclear inclusions ("owl-eye" lesions) or cytoplasmic inclusions in vascular endothelial cells. In cases in which biopsy is not diagnostic, immunohistologic or in situ hybridization techniques may be helpful, together with serum IgM anti-CMV antibodies.

The treatment of choice is ganciclovir (5 mg/kg IV q12h for 21 days) to achieve remission.[48] For patients who relapse after discontinuation of the drug, chronic maintenance therapy (6 mg/kg five times per week) may be instituted. As the drug has hematologic side effects such as neutropenia, regular blood counts should be obtained. Human immunodeficiency virus (HIV)-infected patients with CMV colitis should be placed on maintenance therapy indefinitely. Foscarnet is used in patients who do not respond to ganciclovir or who cannot tolerate its toxicity.

Inflammatory Bowel Disease

Both ulcerative colitis and Crohn's disease are more common in early adulthood but are found with increased frequency in the elderly population. In part, this is because increasing numbers of patients with inflammatory bowel disease (IBD) now live into old age. In addition, both ulcerative colitis and Crohn's disease exhibit a bimodal age of onset,[49,50] the peak incidence occurring in the third decade and the second between the ages of 50 and 80 years; over 10 percent of cases have their onset after the age of 60. This pattern persists even when other diseases that mimic inflammatory bowel disease, such as ischemic colitis and infectious causes, have been excluded. The reasons for this bimodal pattern are unknown.

Ulcerative Colitis

Ulcerative colitis is a chronic inflammatory process of unknown etiology which affects the mucosa and submucosa of the colon in a continuous distribution.

Histopathology

Histologically, there are diffuse ulcerations and epithelial necrosis, depletion of mucin from goblet cells, and a polymorphonuclear and lymphocytic infiltration involving the superficial layers of the colon to the muscularis mucosa.[51] The finding of crypt microabscesses is characteristic but not pathognomonic. The inflammatory process invariably involves the rec-

Table 62-2 Proposed criteria for assessment of disease activity in ulcerative colitis

Factor	Severe[a]	Mild
Bowel frequency	≥6 daily	≤4 daily
Blood in stool	+ +	±
Temperature	>37.5°C on 2 of 4 days	Normal
Pulse rate (beats/min)	>90	Normal
Hemoglobin (allow for transfusion)	≤75%	Normal or near normal
Erythrocyte sedimentation rate (mm in 1 h)	>30	≤30

[a] *Moderate disease is intermediate between severe and mild classifications.*
(Data from Truelove and Witts.[119]*)*

tum and extends proximally for variable distances but does not involve the gastrointestinal tract proximal to the colon.

Symptoms and Signs

Symptoms in the elderly are similar to those seen in younger persons.[52] The severity of ulcerative colitis may be classified as mild, moderate, and severe and is generally proportional to the extent of colonic inflammation (Table 62-2). Most patients exhibit diarrhea, with or without blood in the stools, although older patients with proctitis only occasionally present with constipation or hematochezia. Systemic manifestations occur during more severe attacks and carry a poorer prognosis. Indeed, despite the occurrence of less extensive disease in older patients, elderly persons more often present with a severe initial attack and have higher mortality and morbidity than do younger patients.[53]

Toxic megacolon is a feared complication of ulcerative colitis which occurs more frequently in elderly patients. Abdominal radiographs show colonic dilatation, often to impressive proportions, and patients may exhibit mental confusion, high fever, abdominal distension, and overall deterioration.[54]

Extraintestinal manifestations may occur in ulcerative colitis, including arthralgias, erythema nodosum, pyoderma gangrenosum, uveitis, and migratory polyarthritis. These disorders occur less frequently than in Crohn's disease and are generally associated with increased disease activity.

Diagnosis

The diagnosis is made by sigmoidoscopy and rectal mucosal biopsies since the disorder invariably involves the rectum. The extent of the disease is determined by colonoscopy or barium radiography, both of which should be avoided in patients who are severely ill because of the danger of inducing perforation or toxic megacolon. The characteristic findings are diffuse erythema, granularity, and friability of the mucosa without intervening areas of normal mucosa. Inflammatory pseudopolyps indicate more severe erosion of the mucosa and must be distinguished from true polyps.

Particularly in the elderly, it is important to exclude other diseases that may mimic ulcerative colitis, including Crohn's colitis (see below), ischemic colitis, radiation proctocolitis, and diverticulitis. In acute presentations, infectious agents should be excluded with appropriate stool cultures, including *Salmonella*, *Campylobacter*, *Shigella*, amebiasis, *Yersinia*, and *E. coli* 0157:H7. Finally, *C. difficile*-associated diarrhea and pseudomembranous colitis should be considered in elderly persons, particularly those who have recently been treated with antibiotics, reside in institutions, or have recently been hospitalized.

Treatment

The treatment of ulcerative colitis is based on the extent and the severity of the disease (Table 62-3). Medical therapy consists of a number of effective drugs which are administered intravenously, orally, or rectally. The major classes of drugs are corticosteroids, 5-aminosalicylate (5-ASA) products, and immunosuppressive agents.[55] In the elderly, some drugs must be used more carefully than in younger patients. For example, corticosteroids have a higher risk of complications, whereas sulfasalazine, 5-ASA products, and immunosuppressive agents are generally tolerated well.[53]

Severe Disease

Patients with severe or fulminant disease, including toxic megacolon, should be hospitalized for intravenous therapy. This treatment consists of hydrocortisone or adrenocortico-

Table 62-3 Medical treatment of ulcerative colitis

Indication	Drug	Dosage
Active distal disease	Hydrocortisone enemas	hs
	5-ASA (mesalamine) enemas	hs
	Sulfasalazine	2–4 g/d PO
Mild to moderate disease (proximal to sigmoid)	Sulfasalazine	2–4 g/d PO
	Mesalamine[a]	2.4–4.8 g/d PO
	Prednisone	40–60 mg/d PO
Severe disease (recently receiving steroids)	Prednisolone	60–80 mg/d IV
	Hydrocortisone	300 mg/d IV
Severe disease (not recently receiving steroids)	Corticotropin (ACTH)	120 units/d IV
Maintenance of remission		
Distal disease	5-ASA (mesalamine) enemas	o.n. or q 3rd night
Pancolonic		
	Sulfasalazine	2 g/d PO
	Olsalazine[a]	1 g/d PO

Abbreviations: ASA, aminosalicylate; ACTH, adrenocorticotrophic hormone.
[a] *If patient is intolerant of sulfasalazine.*

trophic hormone (ACTH) infused in fluids containing sufficient amounts of potassium to avoid hypokalemia. One study suggests that ACTH is superior for treating patients who have not previously received corticosteroids, whereas hydrocortisone tends to be more effective in those who have.[56] If ACTH or hydrocortisone does not produce significant improvement within 2 to 3 days, IV cyclosporin may be attempted with close monitoring of renal function, an especially important consideration in an elderly patient. Once improvement is noted, the patient should be converted to oral therapy (see below). However, in most cases, surgery should be preferred unless the patient is an extremely poor operative risk.

Moderately severe disease

Oral corticosteroids are used to achieve remission or to sustain remission after intravenous therapy. Initial therapy should be 40 to 60 mg/d in divided doses, followed by conversion to a single morning dose. Corticosteroids should be viewed as acute phase drugs and should not be used as long-term maintenance therapy because of significant side effects related to both the dose and duration of therapy. Diabetes, congestive heart failure, osteoporosis, and hypertension are common in the elderly and may be exacerbated by corticosteroids.[53] Corticosteroid reduction should be accomplished in stepwise fashion while monitoring clinical activity and appropriate laboratory studies.

5-ASAs should be started together with oral corticosteroids. Sulfasalazine is quite effective and inexpensive but is somewhat limited by side effects which are often dose-dependent and occur in as many as 30 percent of patients. Side effects include nausea, anorexia, headache and, less commonly, a generalized rash; in most cases, these conditions are due to the inactive sulfapyridine carrier rather than the 5-ASA moiety. If side effects occur, patients should be switched to the more expensive 5-ASA products such as olsalazine or mesalamine. Diarrhea is a potential side effect of all 5-ASA drugs.

If patients fail to respond to 5-ASA drugs and cannot be weaned from oral corticosteroids, a trial of azathioprine or 6-mercaptopurine should be considered an alternative to surgery.[57] These drugs act slowly and have a response time ranging from 2 to 6 months. Complete blood counts should be monitored frequently when these agents are used.

Mild disease

Patients with mild disease can be treated effectively with 5-ASA drugs which can be administered orally, by enema in cases of left-sided disease, or by suppositories in patients with proctitis. Corticosteroid enemas are also effective in left-sided disease but in general are not more effective than 5-ASA products. As up to 60 percent of the rectal corticosteroid may be absorbed, they also are less suitable for maintenance therapy. Several poorly absorbed steroid enemas or steroids that do not affect the adrenal-pituitary-hypothalamic axis are currently under investigation.[55]

Maintenance therapy

For patients in remission, long-term maintenance with a 5-ASA product reduces the frequency of relapses.[58] The usual maintenance dose of sulfasalazine is 1 g bid with little or no long-term adverse effects. For patients who are intolerant to sulfasalazine, olsalazine 500 mg bid with meals is also effective. For those with ulcerative proctitis or left-sided colitis, 5-ASA suppositories and enemas are very effective when given every night to every third night. Nonsteroidal anti-inflammatory drugs have been reported to activate quiescent inflammatory bowel disease and should be avoided if possible.[59]

Surgery

Indications for surgery include failure of medical therapy for acute fulminant disease, inability to wean patients from long-term corticosteroid therapy, development of precancerous colonic lesions identified during surveillance studies, and suboptimal response to medical therapy in chronic ulcerative colitis.

The surgical procedure most commonly performed for acute fulminant colitis in all age groups is subtotal colectomy and ileostomy. In the elderly patient, proctocolectomy and ileostomy also remains the most popular choice for chronic failure of medical treatment or because of the development of premalignant changes. Although procedures that avoid ileostomy, such as the ileoanal reservoir, are a viable choice for many younger patients, the increased morbidity of the treatment minimizes its use in the elderly who also are at greater risk for fecal incontinence because of age-associated changes in anal sphincter function.

Risk of colon cancer

The risk of developing colorectal cancer in elderly patients with ulcerative colitis is approximately nine times that of the general population of that age group.[60] The risk in all age groups increases substantially about 8 years after the onset of the disease and is greatest in those with universal colitis. Carcinoma almost always develops many years after quiescent disease has been present and occurs at an earlier age than in the general population. For this reason, yearly colonoscopy has been recommended to detect severe mucosal dysplasia, which is considered a premalignant lesion in ulcerative colitis. Biopsies are obtained randomly throughout the colon and in areas that appear suspicious. Despite some shortcomings in the interpretation of biopsies and in the outcome of surveillance programs, all patients with long-standing ulcerative colitis should receive periodic colonoscopy and biopsy to look for evidence of mucosal dysplasia. The presence of high-grade dysplasia is an indication for proctocolectomy.[59]

Crohn's Disease

Crohn's disease is a chronic inflammatory process of unknown etiology which most often affects the terminal ileum and/or colon and is characterized by transmural inflammation of the bowel wall, often with linear ulcerations and granulomas.

Histopathology

Histologically there is transmural inflammation affecting all layers of the bowel and often associated with submucosal fibrosis. Other features that serve to distinguish this disease from ulcerative colitis are linear ulcerations, fissures, fistulas, discrete mucosal ulcers, granulomas, skip areas, and frequent rectal sparing.[51] The disease can involve all areas of the gastrointestinal tract, from the mouth to the anus, but most frequently involves the ileum and colon. According to most published series, Crohn's disease confined to the colon (Crohn's colitis) occurs more frequently in the elderly than in younger persons, and left-sided colitis appears to be prevalent in elderly women.[53]

Symptoms and signs

As with ulcerative colitis, the clinical picture in the elderly is similar to that in younger individuals and includes rectal bleeding, diarrhea, fever, abdominal pain, and weight loss. In patients with colorectal involvement, perianal disease, including fistulas, may be an early manifestation. The prevalence of extraintestinal manifestations such as migratory arthritis, pyoderma gangrenosum, iritis, and erythema nodosum is similar to that in younger patients. Common laboratory abnormalities such as anemia, leukocytosis, hypoalbuminemia, and elevated sedimentation rate vary with the severity of the illness. Rarely, the disease may be manifested by peritonitis duc to bowel perforation, but this occurs more commonly with ileal disease. In the elderly, peritonitis may occur atypically with mild abdominal pain, often minimal abdominal findings, and mental confusion. Uncommonly, Crohn's colitis is characterized by massive lower gastrointestinal bleeding or bowel obstruction.

Diagnosis

Prolonged delays in diagnosis probably occur more frequently in the elderly. It has been speculated that there is a tendency for Crohn's colitis to appear in a more indolent fashion than does ileal or ileocolonic involvement.[53]

As the disease may often not involve the rectum and the distribution in the colon is often not confluent, colonoscopy and barium radiography are the diagnostic tests of choice. Both procedures can identify the characteristic ulcerations, skip lesions, and areas of colonic narrowing. Barium studies are superior for identifying fistulas from the intestine to adjacent visceral organs, whereas colonoscopy provides superior examination of the mucosa and allows mucosal biopsies to be obtained. Biopsies should also be obtained from grossly normal appearing mucosa to help distinguish Crohn's colitis from other diseases that may mimic it. This is particularly important because of the increased frequency with which diverticula occur in the elderly and because of the tendency for ischemic colitis to occur in a discontinuous distribution.

Computed tomography provides superior definition of the wall of the colon and can identify extraintestinal abdominal pathology, such as abscesses in patients with fever or palpable masses. Computed tomography and ultrasonography can also identify renal lithiasis or ureteral obstruction, which often occur silently.

Perianal involvement is a well-recognized manifestation of Crohn's disease and may be characterized by rectal or anal strictures, fissures, fistulas, abscesses, prominent skin tags, and ulcers. Venereal disease (uncommon in the elderly) and carcinoma should be excluded, particularly as the latter may complicate long-standing Crohn's proctitis. Infectious agents should be excluded by appropriate studies.

Treatment

As with ulcerative colitis, treatment of Crohn's disease is based on its extent and severity as well as its distribution. Medical therapy encompasses all the drugs used in treating ulcerative colitis[55]; in addition, selected antibiotics are helpful in some patients (Table 62-4).

Ileocolitis and colitis

Patients with mild to moderate disease often respond to sulfasalazine, or if they are intolerant to the drug, to one of the newer 5-ASA products in doses similar to those used for ulcerative colitis. If the disease remains mild or only moderate in severity but responds inadequately to 5-ASA drugs, metroni-

Table 62-4 Medical treatment of Crohn's colitis

Indications	Drug	Dosage
Ileocolitis or colitis	Sulfasalazine	2–4 g/d PO
	Mesalamine[a]	2.4–4.8 g/d PO
	Metronidazole	10–20 mg/kg/d PO
	Prednisone	40–60 mg/d PO
Perineal disease	Metronidazole	1–2 g/d PO
	6-Mercaptopurine or	50 mg/d up to 1.5 mg/kg/d
	Azathioprine or	50 mg/d up to 2 mg/kg/d PO
	Ciprofloxacin	500 mg bid PO
Refractory disease	6-Mercaptopurine or	50 mg/d to 2 mg/kg/d PO
	Azathioprine	50 mg/d up to 2 mg/kg/d PO
Maintenance of remission	Sulfasalazine or	2 g/d PO
	Mesalamine[a]	500 mg/d PO
	6-Mercaptopurine or azathioprine	50 mg/d up to 2 mg/kg/d
	Olsalazine[a]	500 mg bid PO

[a] *If patient is intolerant of sulfasalazine.*

dazole 125 to 250 mg three times daily or ciprofloxacin 500 mg once or twice daily can be tried before using immunosuppressive agents.[61]

If the disease worsens despite conservative therapy or if the patient has moderate to severe symptoms, corticosteroids are begun in doses similar to those used in ulcerative colitis. After remission is induced, prednisone is tapered at rate of 5 to 10 mg/wk until a dose of 20 mg/d is achieved. Subsequently, prednisone should be reduced by 5 mg/d every 3 weeks while monitoring clinical activity and laboratory studies.

Approximately 60 percent of patients who cannot be weaned from oral corticosteroids respond to azathroprine (up to 2 mg/kg/d) or 6-mercaptopurine (up to 1.5 mg/kg/d). Responses may not occur for 6 to 9 months.[62] These drugs can be continued indefinitely, but at least one attempt should be made to discontinue them after 1 year of therapy to see if quiescence can be maintained.

Perianal disease

Perianal fistulas and abscesses can be terribly debilitating and frustrating to treat. Although perianal disease often improves with standard therapy for bowel inflammation and control of diarrhea, some patients continue to have persistent symptoms. Short-term success has been reported with metronidazole in doses of 1.5 to 2 g/d, but side effects at these doses are not uncommon and relapses occur when the drug is discontinued or tapered.[63] Ciprofloxacin 500 mg twice daily is a more expensive alternative, albeit one with fewer side effects, but again there is a high relapse rate when the drug is discontinued. If an abscess develops, incision and drainage should be performed.

If perianal disease remains unresponsive to therapy, surgical diversion of the colon may be performed in an attempt to allow healing, but this too may be unsuccessful. Azathroprine or 6-mercaptopurine may be helpful in some patients with refractory disease.[64]

Surgery

Unlike ulcerative colitis, Crohn's disease cannot be cured by surgery. Therefore, surgical procedures should be reserved for patients who do not respond to medical therapy.[65]

Protocolectomy with ileostomy is the best surgical option for patients with extensive Crohn's colitis. In elderly patients who are debilitated or malnourished, an initial subtotal colectomy with ileostomy is less debilitating and permits weight gain and improved physical well-being. If proctectomy is subsequently required, it can be done with a low complication rate but may not be necessary if rectal disease is mild or absent. More limited colonic resections may be appropriate if severe disease is localized or obstructive symptoms are caused by relatively circumscribed bowel involvement.

Colonic Ischemia

The blood supply to the colon is derived mainly from branches of the superior and inferior mesenteric arteries and is characterized by a rich collateral circulation, except for the potentially susceptible marginal artery of Drummond and the arc of Riolan located at the peripheral junction of the two mesenteric arteries.[66] Occlusion of a major artery results in immediate opening of collateral vessels to maintain an adequate blood supply to the bowel. Intestinal ischemia may occur as a result of generalized reduction of blood flow (nonocclusive ischemia), redistribution of blood flow (e.g., vessel obstruction with poor collateral circulation), or a combination of the two. Colonic ischemia is the most common vascular disorder of the intestines in the elderly population and one that is often misdiagnosed unless there is a high index of suspicion and an aggressive diagnostic approach is used in patients suspected of having this disorder.[67]

The clinical spectrum of colonic ischemia includes a vast array of presentations and may be associated with a number of potentiating factors. Ischemia may be classified as reversible and irreversible; the former may present with submucosal or intramural hemorrhage or transient ischemic colitis which completely resolves within weeks to months, depending on the severity of the process. Irreversible ischemia may be characterized by chronic ulcerations, strictures of varying lengths, colonic gangrene, or fulminant transmural colitis.[68]

In most cases, the etiology of colonic ischemia cannot be established with certainty and no vascular occlusions can be identified. A significant minority of patients are found to have a potentially obstructing process in the colon such as a benign stricture, diverticulitis, or carcinoma. Other contributing factors include hypotension, dehydration, congestive heart failure, use of digitalis, polycythemia, volvulus, and cardiac arrhythmias.

Symptoms and signs

The most common manifestation is the sudden onset of mild to moderately severe left lower abdominal cramping pain; this is often accompanied by bloody diarrhea or hematochezia which may not appear until 24 hours later. Frank hemorrhage is not characteristic of ischemia. Physical examination reveals tenderness at the site of the involved bowel; these sites encompass the distal transverse, splenic flexure, and/or descending colons in about two-thirds of patients. Peritoneal signs may last for several hours, but persistence beyond that time suggests a transmural process. Fever, leukocytosis, absence of bowel sounds, and abdominal distension also suggest the possibility of bowel infarction.

Diagnosis

If the diagnosis is suspected on clinical grounds, a gentle barium enema or colonoscopy with minimal insufflation with air should be performed within 48 hours. Barium studies may reveal "thumbprinting" in the affected areas of the colon, which represents submucosal or mucosal hemorrhages and edema during the early phase of the process. This corresponds to the purplish blebs noted on colonoscopic examination of the bowel. Later radiographic findings include segmental ischemia which may or may not return to normal within weeks or months;

such findings correspond to segmental necrosis, inflammation, ulcerations, or mucosal sloughing on endoscopic studies. There is no meaningful role for mesenteric angiography in patients with colon ischemia, in contrast to those with suspected mesenteric ischemia of the small intestine.

Treatment

Patients should be managed with bowel rest, intravenous fluids, or plasma expanders, and in severe cases, systemic antibiotics such as gentamycin and clindamycin.[69,70] Corticosteroids are of no benefit and should not be administered. In mild disease, symptoms resolve within several days, and radiologic healing occurs within several weeks, although some patients may not heal for up to 6 months.

If the patient continues to have diarrhea, bleeding, or significant obstructive symptoms for more than several weeks, surgical resection is usually indicated. If colonic infarction is suspected, emergency laparotomy with resection of nonviable bowel is needed.[69]

Prognosis

Recurrent episodes of colonic ischemia occur in less than 10 percent of patients. Attempts should be made to correct or remove underlying conditions that predispose to this disorder.

Colonic Pseudo-obstruction

Acute colonic pseudo-obstruction, sometimes termed Ogilvie's syndrome, is characterized by nonobstructive, nontoxic dilatation of the colon.[71] This condition may develop after surgical procedures, especially orthopedic ones, and also occurs in a setting of serious coexisting illness, including sepsis, pneumonia, acute pancreatitis, spinal cord injury, or administration of anticholinergic, narcotic, or psychotropic drugs. This disorder can compromise respiratory status and cause cecal perforation. The risk of cecal perforation is said to rise when the diameter of the cecum increases beyond 10 cm. A variant of this disorder is "megasigmoid syndrome," often described in psychotic patients[72] but not exclusively seen within this group.

After obstruction has been excluded, treatment includes correction of electrolyte imbalances, discontinuation of offending drugs, treatment of underlying infection or inflammation, nasogastric suction, a rectal or colonic decompression tube with positioning of the patient on the right and left sides at intervals of several hours, or decompression with colonoscopy if there is severe dilatation.[73] Surgical decompression under local anesthesia using a stab-wound cecostomy can be performed if other measures fail. Postdecompression x-ray films should be obtained for several days to document continued resolution.

Chronic colonic pseudo-obstruction, with or without colonic dilatation (megacolon), may be associated with amyloidosis, muscular dystrophy, myxedema, dementia, multiple sclerosis, Parkinson's disease, quadriplegia, and schizophrenia, as well as idiopathic visceral neuropathy and myopathy. There may be esophageal, gastric, small intestinal, and genitourinary dysfunction. Although most patients have constipation, diarrhea occurs if there is small bowel bacterial overgrowth or overflow around a fecal impaction.

Subtotal colectomy may be necessary in some patients with refractory symptoms and if anorectal function is normal. If anorectal dysfunction is present, proctocolectomy with ileostomy is indicated. Sigmoid resection may be all that is necessary in patients with megasigmoid syndrome. Most patients can be treated conservatively.

Volvulus

Factors thought to contribute to colonic volvulus include increasing age, chronic constipation, fecal retention, poor peritoneal fixation during embryologic rotation of the hindgut, and, in some areas of the world, diets very high in fiber.[1] The clinical setting typical of a sigmoid volvulus is an elderly institutionalized individual with a history of chronic constipation or laxative abuse.[74]

The sigmoid colon, with its copious mesentery, is most commonly involved, but cecal volvulus can occur when fixation to the posterior parietal wall is incomplete. Volvulus of the transverse colon is by far the least common. Patients have a sudden onset of severe abdominal pain, followed by rapid and marked abdominal distension. Compromise of blood flow occurs as a result of twisting of the mesentery and marked distension of the loop.

Abdominal x-rays reveal massive distention of a single loop of bowel; the obstructed loop frequently is shaped like a coffee bean, with the concavity marking the point of torsion. The concavity points to the left lower quadrant in patients with sigmoid volvulus, and to the right lower quadrant when cecal volvulus is present. Administering contrast through the rectum confirms the diagnosis by the appearance of the pointed twist of the contrast column.

Closely related to a cecal volvulus is a cecal bascule in which malfixation allows the cecum to fold anteriorly and in a cephalad direction, which can result in a flap-valve obstruction with cecal distension. Abdominal x-rays reveal distension of the cecum, but no "bird beak" is seen on a barium enema, as in volvulus. However, treatment is identical to that for conventional cecal volvulus.

Attempts to untwist a sigmoid volvulus may be made by gently inserting an endoscope as far as the twisted segment.[75] Successful detorsion must be followed by careful observation should the bowel continue to be ischemic. Nonoperative decompression is more successful with a sigmoid than with a cecal volvulus; indeed, attempts to treat a cecal volvulus by nonoperative means can be dangerous. Opinion is divided as to whether the first episode of sigmoid volvulus should be treated with resection. Fixation without resection is not considered a useful option. Certainly, patients with more than one episode of sigmoid volvulus should have resection.

In patients with cecal volvulus, early surgical intervention to untwist the volvulus followed by cecal fixation (cecopexy) is frequently all that is necessary unless bowel necrosis is present. If the latter is present, resection with ileostomy is indicated.

Neoplastic Lesions

Colonic polyps may be classified into (1) neoplastic polyps which include adenomatous polyps and carcinomas; (2) non-neoplastic polyps which include hyperplastic, inflammatory, and hamartomatous types; and (3) submucosal tumors such as lipomas, leiomyomas, hemangiomas, fibromas, lymphoid polyps, and carcinoids.[76]

Most (80 to 90 percent) colonic polyps are either adenomatous or hyperplastic, and of these about 75 percent are adenomas. However, when only polyps less than 5 mm are considered, half are hyperplastic and most are found in the rectosigmoid colon. Current evidence suggests that hyperplastic polyps are not of clinical importance.[77] In contrast, it is widely accepted that most carcinomas arise from adenomas.

Adenomatous Polyps

These polyps arise from mucosal glandular epithelium and can be described based on the following characteristics.

1. *Size*: Approximately 25 percent of adenomas are larger than 1 cm, and over 80 percent of large adenomas occur in the left colon and rectum.
2. *Architecture*: Over 80 percent of adenomas are tubular, 3 to 6 percent are villous, and the rest are tubulovillous. Those with a higher proportion of villous elements tend to be larger and carry a higher risk of malignant transformation.
3. *Dysplasia*: All adenomas are dysplastic, but high-grade dysplasia is strongly associated with malignancy.

In the United States, prevalence rates in men and women are similar. Except in familial syndromes, colonic adenomas are rare before the age of 40, increase steadily, and reach a peak after the age of 60. Population studies suggest that the environment strongly contributes to adenoma prevalence and probably to the frequency of colon cancer as well.[78]

It is logical to identify and remove all benign adenomas at an early stage to prevent progression to carcinoma. In one study, screening and polyp removal by rigid sigmoidoscopy during the previous 10 years resulted in a 70 percent reduction in the risk of fatal cancer of the rectum and distal colon compared to the outcome in nonscreened subjects.[79] In the National Polyp Study, colonoscopic polypectomy reduced the incidence of colorectal cancer by 76 to 90 percent during a follow-up of almost 6 years.[80] These findings form the basis for current screening recommendations.

There is epidemiologic evidence that aspirin and other, nonsteroidal anti-inflammatory drugs (NSAIDs) may reduce the risk of colorectal cancer.[81] Several large studies, although not all, have found a significant reduction in death rates from colon cancer among both men and women who use NSAIDs on a regular basis. Such observations are supported by laboratory studies demonstrating that aspirin and other cycloxygenase inhibitors demonstrate chemopreventive effects in animal models of colon carcinogenesis. There currently are insufficient data supporting the use of NSAIDs as colorectal cancer chemopreventive agents outside appropriately designed trials.

Management of Polyps

Criteria for the adequacy of colonoscopic polypectomy are well established for pedunculated malignant polyps.[82,83] In patients having favorable criteria, the risk of residual tumor is 0.3 percent for pedunculated lesions and 1.5 percent for sessile lesions, whereas the risk is 8.5 percent for those having unfavorable criteria. Surgery is therefore strongly considered in the latter situation, although recommendations should be individualized based on patient age and comorbid conditions.

The following recommendations for treatment after polypectomy are based on recent information.[84]

1. Patients should undergo complete colonoscopy at the time of polypectomy and removal of all synchronous polyps.
2. In 3 years the first follow-up colonoscopy should be performed to check for missed synchronous and or metachronous adenomas. It has been suggested that if the results are negative, subsequent surveillance intervals may be increased to 5 years.
3. Selected patients with multiple adenomas or those with suboptimal initial clearing examinations may require colonoscopy at 1 year or sooner and then again 3 years later if the colon is clear.

Screening Strategies

A clear consensus does not exist concerning recommendations for screening of asymptomatic subjects at *average risk* for colorectal cancer. Although a yearly FOBT for all patients 50 years and older has been suggested, controversy exists regarding the cost and benefits of such a policy. The sensitivity of Hemoccult II tests for detecting asymptomatic colorectal cancer ranges from 45 to 80 percent in mass-screened populations and is less than 25 percent for detecting polyps 1 cm or larger in diameter.[85,86] Thus, a FOBT is a relatively effective way to screen for asymptomatic cancers but is ineffective in detecting even sizable premalignant polyps.[87] Moreover, at least 50 percent of screened individuals over the age of 40 are false positive or have an upper gastrointestinal source of bleeding. However, the specificity of an unrehydrated FOBT is about 98 to 99 percent.

More recent data suggest that an annual FOBT with rehydration and colonoscopy in patients who screen positive for FOBT has a 90 percent sensitivity in detecting colorectal cancer and is associated with a decrease of 33 percent in 13 years' cumulative mortality from colorectal cancer.[88] This benefit was largely lost by increasing the screening interval to 2 years. However, rehydration resulted in a decrease of specificity to 90 percent with a positive predictive value (true positive/true positive plus false positive) of only 2.2 percent. As almost 10 percent of the screened population had a positive FOBT when rehydrated, cost-effectiveness was significantly and adversely affected.

Existing recommendations apply to screening asymptomatic subjects in the context of an individual doctor-patient relationship rather than to entire populations as part of a public health policy. The American Cancer Society currently recommends an annual FOBT and flexible sigmoidoscopy every 3 to 5 years. Some studies suggest that colonoscopy should be performed only when flexible sigmoidoscopy detects high-risk adenomas, tentatively defined as adenomas larger than 1 cm and all tubulovillous or villous adenomas, as well as subjects with multiple adenomas.

Colorectal Cancer

Colorectal cancer is the second most common cause of cancer death in the United States (138,000 new cases and 55,000 deaths annually). Epidemiologic evidence strongly suggests that colon cancer is an acquired genetic disease produced by chronic exposure to environmental carcinogens. Thus, deaths from colon cancer increase slowly by middle age and rise steeply thereafter. Moreover, immigrants from areas of low incidence acquire, within a single generation, the increased risks of the indigenous population in areas of higher incidence.[89] Except for the increased risk for colorectal cancer among individuals with ulcerative colitis and those with a family history of colorectal cancer, no high-risk exposures have consistently been identified in the United States. However, epidemiologic evidence implicates both decreased dietary fiber and increased consumption of animal protein and fat. That colorectal cancer is caused by cumulative alterations in the cellular genome, and not by a single genetic alteration, may explain the long latency period between initial exposure to carcinogen(s) and the appearance of cancer.[90]

Somatic mutations in the APC gene on chromosome 5 are the earliest recognized genetic alterations in sporadic colonic carcinogenesis and are found in the smallest adenomas. These mutations permit unregulated proliferation at the base of the colonic crypt. A multistep genetic model for sporadic colorectal tumorigenesis involves sequential mutations in cellular oncogenes (e.g., the *ras* gene) and tumor suppressor genes.[90,91] Two cellular proteins associated with the APC gene have recently been identified and appear to be involved in cell adhesion, which may provide an important clue to the mechanism of tumor initiation.

Recently, a colon cancer "susceptibility gene" on the short arm of chromosome 2 has been identified in patients with families with hereditary nonpolyposis colon cancer (HNPCC) and in sporadic colon cancers as well. Widespread mutations in short, repeated DNA sequences due to defective or mutant DNA mismatch repair enzymes have been identified on chromosome 2p. At least four such repair genes have now been identified in the pathogenesis of colon cancer.[92] These tumors appear to have a genetic pathogenesis different from that of the hereditary polyposis syndromes that probably result in different clinical features and less aggressive behavior.

Colonic cancers can be classified by gross appearance, histology (well to poorly differentiated, mucinous, signet-ring type) or by DNA content.[89] In general, poorly differentiated carcinomas have a somewhat worse prognosis than well-differentiated tumors. More helpful is staging, for example, by the modified Dukes (Dukes-Turnbull) classifications: A, tumor extends no further than muscularis mucosa; B1, tumor penetrates muscularis propria or, B2, extends through serosa into pericolic fat; C1, four or fewer regional lymph node metastases or, C2, greater than four nodes involved; and D, distant metastases. Actuarial 5-year survival rates diminish from 99 percent for Dukes A lesions to less than 20 percent for Dukes D lesions. As expected, prognosis is much poorer when there is vascular or neural invasion.

The primary treatment for colorectal cancer is surgical resection. Preoperative studies include a complete evaluation of the colon, preferably by colonoscopy, chest x-ray, and measurement of carcinoembryonic antigen (CEA). The CEA is not useful as a primary screening test, but serial measurements have been advocated to detect early recurrences after surgery. However, in a recent study, cancer cures attributable to CEA monitoring were infrequent.[93] The investigators questioned whether such a practice was justified in view of the substantial cost or the emotional stress that CEA testing may cause patients. Abdominal imaging studies are most useful for detecting advanced disease (i.e., hepatic metastases) but are less useful in finding localized extracolonic spread. However, such information can be obtained directly at the time of surgery, and the presence of metastases does not influence the need for surgery or the type of surgery that is performed. In contrast, rectal endosonography appears to be superior to computed tomography and magnetic resonance imaging in staging rectal cancers.[94]

There is no benefit from adjunctive radiation therapy for colon cancer outside the rectum. However, adjuvant chemotherapy with fluorouracil and levamisole[95] or fluorouracil and leucovorin has been associated with a significant reduction in tumor recurrence and enhanced survival in patients with Dukes C colon cancer.[96] A more recent study suggests that the postoperative adjuvant therapeutic combination of fluorouracil and leucovorin also enhances disease-free survival and overall survival in Dukes B colon cancer. These data support the use of postoperative adjuvant chemotherapy in both Dukes B and C colon cancers. In contrast, adjuvant combined radiotherapy and chemotherapy improve postsurgical survival in patients with rectal carcinoma, albeit with increased and often severe toxicity.[97] Some patients with unresectable rectal cancer may become surgical candidates following radiation therapy.

Table 62-5 Clinical presentation of common causes of lower gastrointestinal bleeding

Symptom	Young Adult	Middle Age	Elderly
Abdominal pain	IBD	IBD	Ischemia, IBD
Painless	Meckel's diverticula, polyp	Diverticulosis, polyp, cancer	Angiodysplasia, diverticulosis, polyp, cancer
Diarrhea	IBD, infection	IBD, infection	Ischemia, infection, IBD
Constipation	Hemorrhoids, fissure, rectal ulcer	Hemorrhoids, fissure	Cancer, hemorrhoids, fissure

Abbreviation: IBD, inflammatory bowel disease.

Lower Gastrointestinal Bleeding

The two most frequent causes of acute lower gastrointestinal bleeding in the elderly, defined as originating below the ligament of Trietz, are diverticulosis and vascular ectasias (angiodysplasia).[98] These two entities account for two-thirds of hemodynamically significant lower gastrointestinal bleeding (Table 62-5). The most common causes of chronic lower gastrointestinal bleeding are hemorrhoids, angiodysplasia, and colonic neoplasms. Known causes of acute lower gastrointestinal bleeding other than angiodysplasia and diverticulosis make up perhaps 25 percent of all bleeding episodes. These include neoplasm; radiation enterocolitis; ischemic, ulcerative, and Crohn's colitis; solitary rectal ulcer syndrome; and internal hemorrhoids. Less frequently reported causes of bleeding include small intestinal and Meckel's diverticula, vasculitis, and Dieulafoy lesions of the small intestine and colon.

Angiodysplasia

Angiodyplasia are small clusters of dilated and tortuous veins which appear in the mucosa of the colon as well as in the small intestine.[99] They are thought to result from age-associated degeneration of colonic submucosal veins, are often multiple, and are an important cause of lower gastrointestinal bleeding in the elderly population; two-thirds of patients with angiodysplasia are over 70 years of age. The principal theory concerning their development is that repeated episodes of low-grade partial obstruction of submucosal veins occur during muscular contraction or from increased intraluminal pressure, resulting in dilatation and tortuosity of the vein.[100] This process may extend to the mucosal veins which are drained by the submucosal vein. Finally, the precapillary sphincter becomes incompetent, and a small arteriovenous communication with an ectatic tuft of vessels develops. The tendency of vascular ectasias to occur in the right colon is best explained by the greater tension on the bowel wall, as expressed by Laplace's law relating tension to the diameter of the bowel lumen. A recent review of the literature casts doubt on a causal association between vascular ectasias and aortic stenosis.[101] Nevertheless, it has been reported that recurrent bleeding from these lesions decreases after replacement of a stenotic aortic valve.[102]

Vascular ectasias remain asymptomatic in most individuals. The usual manifestation is that of painless subacute or recurrent bleeding which stops spontaneously in most cases. Bleeding may consist of bright red blood, maroon stools or (rarely) melena, or may be occult.[98] About 10 to 15 percent of patients have episodes of brisk blood loss, and up to half exhibit iron deficiency anemia.

Diagnosis may be made by colonoscopy or angiography; of the two, colonoscopy is preferred since it can exclude other causes of bleeding and can be used for therapeutic interventions.[103,104] As lesions are small, often multiple, and difficult to see, thorough cleansing of the colon is necessary to provide adequate visualization of the mucosa. Colonoscopy is usually performed after bleeding has stopped and within 48 hours to permit identification of other bleeding sources.

Mesenteric angiography is the diagnostic procedure of choice when acute bleeding is brisk. The finding of tortuous, densely opacified clusters of small veins that empty slowly represents the advanced ectatic process. Early filling of the vein, indicative of the presence of an arteriovenous communication, is found in most patients who are studied for bleeding. Extravasation of contrast into the bowel lumen is seen when there is active bleeding at a rate of at least 0.5 ml/min; as bleeding is often intermittent, a bleeding site is identified by angiography in only a minority of patients.

Bleeding can be controlled acutely by intra-arterial administration of vasopressin in doses ranging from 0.2 to 0.6 units/min. This often permits stabilization of the patient and appears to be more effective when bleeding is from the right colon. When bleeding cannot be controlled, surgery is required. Colonoscopic therapeutic modalities generally involve thermal ablation techniques, but rebleeding remains a significant problem.[105] A right hemicolectomy is performed if bleeding from the right colon has been identified by angiography or colonoscopy and if other sources of bleeding have not been identified. The extent of resection should not be influenced by the presence of left colonic diverticulosis. Recurrent bleeding, probably due to undetected ectasias, occurs in up to 20 percent of patients who may require either more extensive colonic resection or exploratory laparotomy.

Treatment should be conservative whenever possible and consists of blood or iron replacement as appropriate. For recurrent bleeding, transcolonoscopic electrocoagulation or laser coagulation may be attempted; difficulties include identifying the ectatic lesion(s) and excluding other causes of blood loss if bleeding has stopped. Perforation of the right colon with coagulation therapy is a hazard.[106]

The development of small bowel enteroscopy may eventually reduce the need for diagnostic laparotomy in patients with recurrent bleeding from obscure sites.

Vasculitis

Inflammation and necrosis of blood vessels may lead to ischemia and ulceration, resulting in pain and/or bleeding. Polyarteritis nodosa, Churg-Strauss syndrome, Henoch-Schonlein purpura, systemic lupus erythematosus, rheumatoid vasculitis, Behcet's disease, and essential mixed cryoglobulinemia have all been reported to produce gastrointestinal bleeding and are best diagnosed with endoscopic procedures in the appropriate clinical setting.

Dieulafoy Lesions

Recently, these lesions have been reported to cause bleeding, in several cases massive, in the small intestine and colon.[107] They are characterized by a small mucosal defect with minimal inflammation and a congenitally large, tortuous, thick-walled arteriole at the base which ruptures into the bowel lumen. The histology of these vessels is normal, and their abnormality is their size relative to their superficial location. Bleeding can be localized with angiography, although occasionally colonoscopy can identify the lesion if bleeding has stopped and the colon is well prepared. Surgical resection or embolization therapy is the treatment of choice.

Evaluation and Management of Lower Gastrointestinal Bleeding

The first goal of management is to rapidly assess the severity of bleeding and cardiovascular status of the patient and to resuscitate those with major blood loss (Fig. 62-1). Vital signs reflecting orthostatic changes and other signs of hypovolemia should be checked immediately and at frequent intervals thereafter. If signs of shock or hypovolemia are present, one or two large-bore intravenous catheters should be placed to facilitate fluid resuscitation. Initial blood work, including hemogram, platelet count, coagulation profiles, routine blood chemistries, and type and cross-match should be obtained immediately. Only after these critical tasks are completed should a more detailed history and physical examination be performed to help determine the site of bleeding and potential etiologies. Another important step is to distinguish acute bleeding from active bleeding superimposed on chronic blood loss—this is best done with the hematocrit and mean corpuscular volume; if the latter is low, chronic bleeding should be suspected.

The third step is to consider the location of the gastrointestinal bleed based on characteristics of the bleeding and a BUN/creatinine ratio.[108] Although hematochezia, defined as the passage of red blood through the rectum, suggests a lower gastrointestinal source, up to 20 percent of patients with upper gastrointestinal bleeding may present with hematochezia because of the rapid passage of large amounts of blood through the small and large intestines.[109] Such patients always show evidence of severe hemodynamic compromise, and most have a BUN/creatinine ratio greater than 25 on initial evaluation.[108] On the other hand, melena is often characteristic of upper gastrointestinal bleeding but can also be seen in patients with bleeding from the small intestine or right colon when colonic transit is slow. Fresh unclotted blood dripping into the toilet after defecation suggests a very distal anorectal source, whereas blood streaking the stool suggests origin in the left colon.

Exclusion of an upper gastrointestinal site begins with passage of a nasogastric tube and examination of gastric contents for red blood, coffee ground material, and bile. The presence of bile and an absence of blood or coffee ground materials significantly diminishes but does not exclude bleeding proximal to the duodenojejunal junction; thus, an upper endoscopy should be performed in a setting compatible with an upper gastrointestinal source. There is no role for occult blood testing of a nasogastric aspirate in the absence of coffee grounds or bloody material. Finally, hemorrhoidal and low rectal bleeding should be excluded by sigmoidoscopy in patients thought to have lower gastrointestinal hemorrhage.

When evaluating stable patients with acute lower gastrointestinal hemorrhage, colonoscopy preceded by oral bowel preparation is preferred in identifying and potentially treating a colonic bleeding source.[22] If an emergency colonoscopy is to be considered, the nasogastric tube should be left in place to permit rapid administration of a polyethylene glycol electrolyte solution to cleanse the colon.

If bleeding is active and bowel preparation cannot be done, scintigraphy with ^{99m}Tc-labeled red blood cells can be used to locate a bleeding site. This technique detects active bleeding at rates of 0.05 to 0.1 mL/min, and the patient can be serially scanned for up to 36 hours if bleeding is intermittent. Site localization may be impaired if delayed films are taken too infrequently and, of course, the patient must be actively bleeding at the time of the study. Although there were initial enthusiastic reports of an approximately 90 percent rate of detection of active bleeding, subsequent studies have yielded conflicting results.[110,111] These latter reports have raised serious concerns regarding a rigid policy of routinely performing nuclear scintigraphy prior to mesenteric angiography, particularly in high-risk patients for whom rapid diagnosis is preferred. It may be more accurate if upper gastrointestinal bleeding has been excluded.[111] If bleeding is active and severe and/or scintigraphy is not diagnostic, selective mesenteric angiography can be used to detect extravasated contrast into the bowel when bleeding rates are 0.5 to 1.0 mL/min, or to demonstrate vascular lesions, neovascularity, or tumors in the absence of extravasation.[112] Sensitivity declines when bleeding is recurrent or chronic. Attempts have been made to increase diagnostic sensitivity and accuracy by using systemic heparinization, intra-arterial vasodilators, or thrombolytic agents during angiography if the initial study is negative.[113] More extensive experi-

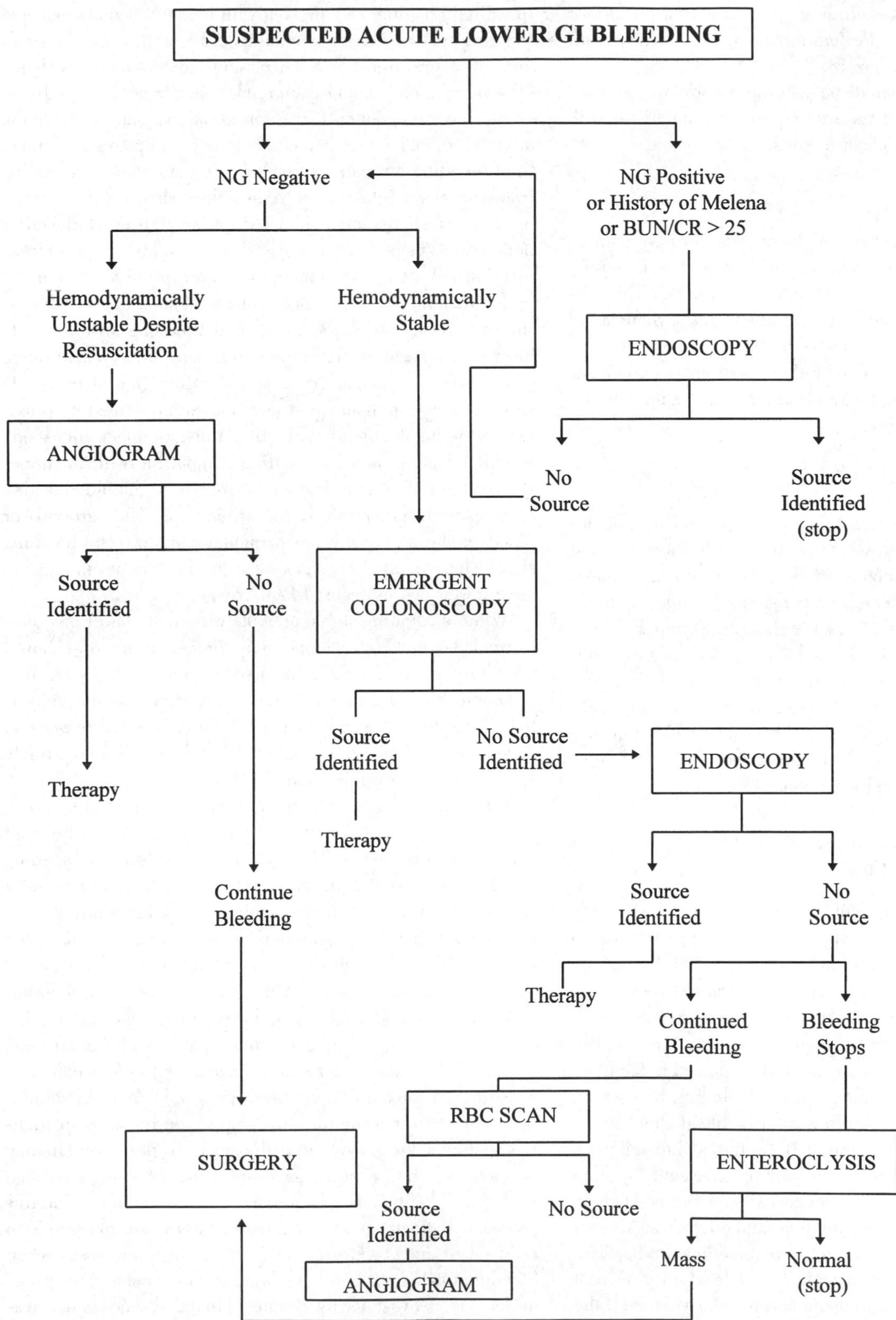

Figure 62-1 Suspected acute lower gastrointestinal bleeding.

ence is needed to determine whether the increased yield justifies the increased risk of bleeding complications.

Angiography also offers the potential for local therapy, provided selective catheterization can be achieved. These modalities include infusion of vasopressin to control acute arterial bleeding in colonic diverticular disease or angiodysplasia,[114] as well as selective embolization of an identified bleeding site with a gelatin sponge, vascular coils, or polyvinyl alcohol particles.[115] Complications include electrolyte disturbances, cardiovascular complications, and bowel ischemia with vasopressin infusion and bowel infarction following embolization. The latter should be attempted only at centers that have the expertise to perform superselective catheterization. Some investigators report that urgent colonoscopy is superior to selective mesenteric angiography in identifying the source of severe lower gastrointestinal bleeding. If bleeding is massive, emergent surgery with or without intraoperative endoscopy may be the best option. There is little or no place in modern surgical practice for blind colonic resection.

If no source of bleeding is detected by colonoscopy and no further bleeding occurs, a small bowel enteroscopy and/or enteroclysis should be performed. Enteroscopes can often be passed to 60 to 100 cm past the ligament of Treitz if the procedure is done by experienced personnel.[116] The diagnostic yield has varied from 30 to 60 percent, with arteriovascular malformations accounting for most of the causes of bleeding.

Barium enema has no role in the evaluation of patients with acute lower gastrointestinal bleeding. It is unable to demonstrate active bleeding and interferes with attempts to perform colonoscopy or mesenteric angiography. Even if a lesion is detected, there is no proof that it is the source of the acute bleed.

References

1. Cohn SM, Birnbaum EH: Colon: Anatomy and structural anomalies. pp. 1735–1747. In Yamada T (ed). Textbook of Gastroenterology. 2nd Ed. JB Lippincott, Philadelphia, 1995
2. Sonneland J, Anson B, Beaton L: Surgical anatomy of the arterial supply to the colon from the superior mesenteric artery based upon a study of 600 specimens. Surg Gynecol Obstet 1958;106:385
3. Boxall TA, Smart P, Griffiths JD: The blood supply of the distal segment of the rectum in anterior resection. Br J Surg 1963;50:399
4. Smith TK, Sanders KM: Motility of the large intestine. pp. 234–261. In Yamada, T (ed): Textbook of Gastroenterology. 2nd Ed. JB Lippincott, Philadelphia, 1995
5. Merkel IS, Locher J, Burgio K et al: Physiologic and psychologic characteristics of an elderly population with chronic constipation. Am J Gastroenterol 1993;88:1854–1859
6. McHugh SM, Diamant NE: Effect of age, gender and parity on anal canal pressure: contribution of impaired anal sphincter function to fecal incontinence. Dig Dis Sci 1987;32: 726–736
7. Bannister JJ, Abouzekry I, Read NW: Effect of aging on anorectal function. Gut 1987;28:353–357
8. Patriquin H, Martelli H, Devroede G: Barium enema in chronic constipation: is it meaningful? Gastroenterology 1978;75: 619–622
9. Tinetti ME, Stone L, Cooney L, Kapp MC: Inadequate barium enemas in hospitalized elderly patients. Arch Intern Med 1989;149:2014–2016
10. Gurwitz JH, Noonan JP, Sanchez M, Prather W: Barium enemas in the frail elderly. Am J Med 1992;92:41–44
11. Mulholland MW: Approach to the patient with acute abdomen. pp. 783–796. In Yamada T (ed): Textbook of Gastroenterology. 2nd Ed. JB Lippincott, Philadelphia, 1995
12. Law PL, Bartram CI: Anal endosonography: technique and normal anatomy. Gastrointest Radiol 1989;14:349–353
13. Cuesta MA, Meijer S, Derksen EJ et al: Anal sphincter imaging in fecal incontinence using endosonography. Dis Colon Rectum 1992;35:59–63
14. Sultan AH, Kamm MA, Hudson CN et al: Anal sphincter disruption during vaginal delivery. N Engl J Med 1993;329: 1905–1911.
15. Foutch PG: Flexible fiberoptic sigmoidoscopy. Pract Gastroenterol 1988;12:25–31
16. Ransohoff DF, Lang CA: Improving the fecal occult-blood test. N Engl J Med 1996;334:189–190
17. Wald A: Colonic diverticulosis. pp. 34.1–34.18. In Winawer SJ (ed): Management of Gastrointestinal Diseases. Gower Medical Publishing, New York, 1992
18. Painter NS, Burkitt DP: Diverticular disease of the colon: a 20th-century problem. Clin Gastroenterol 1975;4:3–25
19. Thompson WG: Do colonic diverticula cause symptoms? Am J Gastroenterol 1986;81:613–614
20. Morson BC: Pathology of diverticular disease. Clin Gastroenterol 1974;4:37–52
21. Wahlby L, Knutsen OH: Leukocyte counts, ESR and fever in the diagnosis of diverticulitis. Acta Chir Scand 1982;148: 623–624
22. Jensen DM, Machicado GA: Diagnosis and treatment of severe hematochezia: the role of urgent colonoscopy after purge. Gastroenterology 1988;95:1569–1574
23. Perkins JD, Shield CF, Chang FC, Farha GJ: Acute diverticulitis: comparison of treatment in immunocompromised and nonimmunocompromised patients. Am J Surg 1984;745–748
24. Rodkey GV, Welch CE: Changing patterns in the surgical treatment of diverticular disease. Ann Surg 1984;200: 466–478
25. Veidenheimer MC: Surgical management of diverticulitis and its complications. pp. 117–130. In Kodner IJ, Fry RD, Roe JP (eds): Colon, Rectal and Anal Surgery. CV Mosby, St. Louis, 1985
26. vanSonnenberg E, Mueller PR, Ferrucci JT Jr: Percutaneous drainage of 250 abdominal abscesses and fluid collections. I. results, failures and complications. Radiology 1984;151: 337–341
27. Saini S, Mueller PR, Wittenberg J: Percutaneous drainage of diverticular abscess. Arch Surg 1986;121:474–478

28. Lewis FR, Holcroft JW, Boey J, Dunphy JE: Appendicitis: a critical review of diagnosis and treatment in 1000 cases. Arch Surg 1975;110:677
29. Puylaert JBCM, Rutgers PH, Lalisang RI et al: A prospective study of ultrasonography in the diagnosis of appendicitis. N Engl J Med 1987;317:666–669
30. Kelly CP, Pothoulakis C, LaMont JT: *Clostridium difficile* colitis. N Engl J Med 1994;330:257–262
31. McFarland LV, Mulligan ME, Kwok RYY, Stamm WE: Nosocomial acquisition of *Clostridium* infection. N Engl J Med 1989;320:204–210
32. Miller PD, LaMont JT: Antibiotic-induced diarrhea: the role of *C. difficile*. Pract Gastroenterol 1989;13:45–51
33. Fekety R, Shah AB: Diagnosis and treatment of *Clostridium difficile* colitis. JAMA 1993;269:71–75
34. Teasley DG, Gerding DN, Olson MM et al: Prospective randomized trial of metronidazole versus vancomycin for *Clostridium difficile*-associated diarrhea and colitis. Lancet 1983;2: 1043–1046
35. Walters BAJ, Roberts R, Stafford R, Seneviratne E: Recurrence of antibiotic associated colitis: endogenous persistence of *C. difficile* during vancomycin therapy. Gut 1983;24: 206–212
36. McFarland LV, Surawicz CM, Greenberg RN et al: A randomized placebo-controlled trial of *Saccharomyces boulardii* in combination with standard antibiotics for *Clostridium difficile* disease. JAMA 1994;271:1913–1918
37. LaMont JT: Bacterial infections of the colon. pp. 1891–1911. In Yamada T (ed): Textbook of Gastroenterology. 2nd Ed. JB Lippincott, Philadelphia 1995
38. Bennish ML, Salam MA, Khan AM: Treatment of shigellosis. III. comparison of one- or two-dose ciprofloxacin with standard 5-day therapy: a randomized blinded trial. Ann Intern Med 1992;117:727
39. DuPont HL, Hornick RB: Adverse effect of Lomotil therapy in shigellosis. JAMA 1973;226:1525
40. Ericsson CD, Johnson PC, DuPont HL et al: Ciprofloxacin or trimethoprim-sulfamethoxazole as initial therapy for traveler's diarrhea. Ann Intern Med 1987;106:216
41. MacDonald KL, O'Leary MJ, Cohen ML et al: *Escherichia coli* 0157:H7, an emerging gastrointestinal pathogen: results of a one year, prospective, population based study. JAMA 1988; 259:3567–3570
42. Boyce, TG, Swerdlow DL, Griffin PM: *Escherichia coli* 0157: H7 and the hemolytic-uremic syndrome. N Engl J Med 1995; 333:364–368
43. Griffin PM, Ostroff SM, Tauxe RV et al: Illnesses associated with *Escherichia coli* 0157:H7 infections: a broad clinical spectrum. Ann Intern Med 1988;109:705–712
44. Cornick NA, Gorbach SL: *Campylobacter*. Infect Dis Clin North Am 1988;2:643
45. Hill DR, Petri WA, Guerrant RL: Parasitic diseases: protozoa. pp. 2343–2348. In Yamada T (ed): Textbook of Gastroenterology. 2nd Ed. JB Lippincott, Philadelphia, 1995
46. Kagan IG. Serologic diagnosis of parasitic diseases. N Engl J Med 1970;282:685–686
47. Kozarsky PE, Jernigan JA: Amebiasis. pp. 66–69. In RE Rakel (ed): Conn's Current Therapy. WB Saunders, Philadelphia, 1996
48. Meyers JD: Prevention and treatment of cytomegalovirus infections. Ann Rev Med 1991;42:179
49. Garland CF, Lilienfeld AM, Mendeloff AM et al: Incidence of rates of ulcerative colitis and Crohn's disease in fifteen areas of the United States. Gastroenterology 1981;81:1115
50. Kyle, J: An epidemiological study of Crohn's disease in Northeast Scotland. Gastroenterology 1971;61:826
51. Kirsner JB, Shorter RG: Inflammatory Bowel Disease. 3rd Ed. Lea and Fibiger, Philadelphia, 1988
52. Softley A, Myren J, Clamp SE et al: Inflammatory bowel disease in the elderly patient. Scand J Gastroenterol 1988; 23(suppl 144):27
53. Holt PR: Approach to gastrointestinal problems in the elderly. pp. 968–988. In Yamada T (ed): Textbook of Gastroenterology. 2nd Ed. JB Lippincott, Philadelphia, 1995
54. Danovitch SH: Fulminant colitis and toxic megacolon. Gastroenterol Clin of North Am 1989;18:73
55. Peppercorn MA: Advances in drug therapy for inflammatory bowel disease. Ann Intern Med 1990;112:50–60
56. Meyers S, Sachar DB, Goldberg JD, Janowitz HD: Corticotropin versus hydrocortisone in the intravenous treatment of ulcerative colitis. Gastroenterology 1983;85:351–357
57. Adler DJ, Korelitz BI: The therapeutic efficacy of 6-mercaptopurine in refractory ulcerative colitis. Am J Gastroenterol 1990;85:717–722
58. Azad Khan AK, Howes DT, Piris J, Truelove SC: Optimum dose of sulphasalazine for maintenance treatment in ulcerative colitis. Gut 1980;21:232–240
59. Kaufman HJ, Taubin HL: Nonsteroidal anti-inflammatory drugs activate quiescent inflammatory bowel disease. Ann Intern Med 1987;107:513–516
60. Korelitz BI: Considerations of surveillance, dysplasia and carcinoma of the colon in the management of ulcerative colitis and Crohn's disease. Med Clin North Am 1990;74: 189–199
61. Sutherland L, Singleton J, Sessions J et al: Double-blind placebo controlled trial of metronidazole in Crohn's disease. Gut 1991;32:107–105
62. Present DH, Korelitz BI, Wisch N et al: Treatment of Crohn's disease with 6-mercaptopurine. N Engl J Med 1980;302: 981–987
63. Brandt LJ, Bernstein LH, Boley SJ, Frank MS: Metronidazole therapy for perineal Crohn's disease: a follow-up study. Gastroenterology 1982;83:383–387
64. Korelitz BI, Present DH: Favorable effect of 6-mercaptopurine on fistulae of Crohn's disease. Dig Dis Sci 1985;30:58–64
65. Block GE: Surgical management of Crohn's colitis. 1980;302: 1068–1070
66. Binns JC, Isaacson P: Age related changes in the colonic blood supply: their relevance to ischemic colitis. Gut 1978;19: 384–390

67. Robert JH, Mentha G, Rohner A: Ischemic colitis: two distinct patterns of severity. Gut 1993;34:4–6

68. Marston A: Ischemia. Clin Gastroenterol 1985;14:847–862

69. Kaleva RN, Boley SJ: Colonic ischemia. pp. 324–329. In Fazio VW (ed): Current Therapy in Colon and Rectal Surgery. BC Decker, Toronto, 1990

70. Bower TC: Ischemic colitis. Surg Clin North Am 1993;73: 1037–1053

71. Rex DK: Acute colonic pseudo-obstruction (Ogilvie's syndrome). Gastroenterologist 1994;2:233–238

72. Ehrentheil OF, Wells EP: Megacolon in psychotic patients. Gastroenterology 1955;29:285–294

73. Nano D, Prindiville T, Pauly M et al: Colonoscopy therapy of acute pseudoobstruction of the colon. Am J Gastroenterol 1987;82:145–148

74. Ballantyne GH, Brandner MD, Beart RW et al: Volvulus of the colon: incidence and mortality. Ann Surg 1985;202:83–92

75. Morrissey KP: Sigmoid volvulus: is it a difficult twist to manage. pp. 543–550. In Barkin JS, Rogers A (ed): Difficult Decisions in Digestive Diseases. Yearbook Medical Publishers, Chicago, 1989

76. O'Brien M, Winawer SJ, Waye JD: Colorectal polyps. pp. 26.1–26.45. In Winawer, SJ (ed): Management of Gastrointestinal Diseases. Gower Medical Publishing, New York, 1992

77. Provenzale D, Garrett JW, Condon SE, Sandler RS: Risk for colon adenomas in patients with rectosigmoid hyperplastic polyps. Ann Intern Med 1990;113:760–763

78. Correa P: Epidemiology of polyps and cancer. pp. 126–152. In Morson BC (ed): The Pathogenesis of Colorectal Cancer. WB Saunders, Philadelphia, 1978

79. Selby JV, Friedman GD, Quesenberry CP, Weiss NS: A case-control study of screening sigmoidoscopy and mortality from colorectal cancer. N Engl J Med 1992;326:653–657

80. Winawer SJ, Zauber AG, Ho MN et al: Prevention of colorectal cancer by colonoscopic polypectomy. N Engl J Med 1993;329: 1977–1981

81. Thun MJ, Namboodiri MM, Heath CW: Aspirin use and reduced risk of fatal colon cancer. N Engl J Med 1991;325: 1593–1596

82. Cranley JP, Petras RE, Carey WD et al: When is endoscopic polypectomy adequate therapy for colonic polyps containing invasive carcinoma? Gastroenterology 1986;91:419–427

83. Cooper HS, Deppish LM, Gourley WK et al: Endoscopically removed malignant colorectal polyps: clinicopathologic correlations. Gastroenterology 1995;108:1657–1665

84. Winawer SJ, Zauber AG, O'Brien MJ et al: Randomized comparison of surveillance intervals after colonoscopic removal of newly diagnosed adenomatous polyps. N Engl J Med 1993; 328:901–906

85. Allison JE, Tekawa IS, Ransom LJ, Adrain AL: A comparison of fecal occult-blood tests for colorectal cancer screening. N Engl J Med 1996;334:155–159

86. St John DJB, Young GP, Alexeyeff MA et al: Evaluation of new occult blood tests for detecting colorectal neoplasia. Gastroenterology 1993;104:1661–1668

87. Selby JV, Friedman GD, Quesenberry CP, Weiss NS: Effect of fecal occult blood testing on mortality from colorectal cancer. Ann Intern Med 1993;118:1–6

88. Mandel JS, Bond JH, Church TR et al: Reducing mortality from colorectal cancer by screening for fecal occult blood. N Engl J Med. 1993;328:1365–1371

89. Winawer SJ, Enker WE, Levin B. Colorectal cancer. pp. 27.1–27.40. In Winawer SJ (ed): Management of Gastrointestinal Diseases. Gower Medical Publishing, New York, 1992

90. Vogelstein B, Fearson ER, Hamilton SR et al: Genetic alterations during colorectal tumor development. N Engl J Med 1988;319:525–532

91. Scott N, Quirke P: Molecular biology of colorectal neoplasia. Gut 1995;34:289–292

92. Rustgi AK: Hereditary gastrointestinal polyposis and nonpolyposis syndromes. N Engl J Med 1994;331:1694–1702

93. Moertel CG, Fleming TR, Macdonald JS et al: An evaluation of the carcinoembryonic antigen (CEA) test for monitoring patients with resected colon cancer. JAMA 1993;270:943–947

94. Milsom JW, Graffner H: Intrarectal ultrasonography in rectal cancer staging and in the evaluation of pelvic disease: clinical uses of rectal ultrasound. Ann Surg 1990;212:602–606

95. Moertel CG, Fleming TR, Macdonald JS et al: Levamisole and fluorouracil for adjuvant therapy of resected colon carcinoma. N Engl J Med 1990;322:352–358

96. Moertel CG: Chemotherapy for colorectal cancer. N Engl J Med 1994;330:1136–1142

97. O'Connell MJ, Martenson JA, Wieand HS et al: Improving adjuvant therapy for rectal cancer by combining protracted-infusion fluorouracil with radiation therapy after curative surgery. N Engl J Med 1994;331:502–507

98. Sharma R, Gorbien MJ: Angiodysplasia and lower gastrointestinal bleeding in elderly patients. Arch Intern Med 1995;155: 807–812

99. Duray PH, Marcel JM Jr, Livolsi VA et al: Small intestinal angiodysplasia in the elderly. J Clin Gastroenterol 1984;6: 311–319

100. Boley SJ, Brandt LJ, Frank MS: Severe lower intestinal bleeding: diagnosis and treatment. Clin Gastroenterol 1981;10: 65–91

101. Imperiale TF, Ransohoff DF: Aortic stenosis, idiopathic gastrointestinal bleeding and angiodysplasia: is there an association? Gastroenterology 1988;95:1670–1676

102. Cappell MS, Lebwohl O: Cessation of recurrent bleeding from gastrointestinal angiodysplasias after aortic valve replacement. Ann Intern Med 1986;105:54–57

103. Richter JM, Hedbert SE, Athanasoulis CA et al: Angiodysplasia: clinical presentation and colonoscopic diagnosis. Dig Dis Sci 1984;29:481–485

104. Trudel JL, Fazio VW, Sivak MV: Colonoscopic diagnosis and treatment of arteriovenous malformations in chronic lower gastrointestinal bleeding: clinical accuracy and efficacy. Dis Colon Rectum 1988;31:107–110

105. Richter JM, Christensen MR, Colditz GA, Nishioka NS: Angio-

dysplasia: natural history and efficacy of therapeutic interventions. Dig Dis Sci 1989;34:1542–1546

106. Foutch PG: Angiodysplasia of the gastrointestinal tract. Am J Gastroenterol 1993;80:807–808
107. Abdulian JD, Santor MJ, Chen YK et al: Dieulafoy-like lesions of the rectum presenting with exsanguinating hemorrhage: successful endoscopic sclerotherapy. Am J Gastroenterol 1993; 88:1939–1941
108. Snook JA, Holdstock GE, Bamforta J: Value of a simple biochemical ratio in distinguishing upper and lower sites of gastrointestinal hemorrhage. Lancet 1986;1:1064
109. Wara P, Stodkilde H: Bleeding pattern before admission as a guideline for emergency endoscopy. Scand J Gastroenterol 1985;20:72–78
110. Hunter JM, Pezim ME: Limited value of technetium^{99m} labelled red cell scintigraphy in localization of lower gastrointestinal bleeding. Am J Surg 1990;159:504–506
111. Dusold R, Burke K, Carpentier W, Dyck WP: The accuracy of technetium^{99m} labeled red cell scintigraphy in localizing gastrointestinal bleeding. Am J Gastroenterol 1994;89: 345–348
112. Schapiro MJ: The role of the radiologist in the management of gastrointestinal bleeding. Gastroenterol Clin North Am 1994;23:123–181
113. Risch J, Keller FS, Wawrukiewicz AS et al: Pharmacoangiography in the diagnosis of recurrent massive lower gastrointestinal bleeding. Radiology 1982;145:615–619
114. Gomes AS, Lois JF, McCoy RD: Angiographic treatment of gastrointestinal hemorrhage: comparison of vasopressin infusion and embolization. Am J Gastroenterol 1986;146: 1031–1037
115. Lawler G, Bircher M, Spencer J et al: Embolization in colonic bleeding. Br J Radiol 1985;58:83–84
116. Waye JD: Endoscopy of the small bowel: push, Sonde and intraoperative. Endoscopy 1994;26:60–63
117. Truelove SC, Witts LJ: Cortisone in ulcerative colitis: final report on a therapeutic trial. BMJ 1955;2:1041–1048

CHAPTER 63

Nutrition

ANITA J. THOMAS

The diagnosis and treatment of malnutrition in adult medicine is inadequately taught[1,2] and practiced.[3] Institutional malnutrition is a particular concern.[4] Older people are more at risk because, with advancing age, reduction in food intake may be accompanied by disadvantageous changes in gut function, inefficient metabolism, failing homeostasis, and defective nutrient utilization. The coincidence of acute or chronic illness, trauma, hypercatabolic states, infection, and drug therapy changes nutrient requirements and may cause a critical deterioration in nutritional status which impairs tissue repair and immune function and from which recovery is difficult if not impossible.

The U.K. Department of Health and Social Services multicenter study on nutrition and health in old age[5] cited a 7 percent incidence of malnutrition diagnosed on clinical and biochemical grounds in well subjects living in their own homes. The incidence doubled in those aged 80 years and over. Homebound individuals are particularly vulnerable,[6,7] and incidence and prevalence in ill older people can be expected to be much higher. A recent survey of elderly people living in private households revealed that over half reported a longstanding illness or disability, 1 in 5 reporting difficulty seeing even with glasses, 1 in 10 was unable to walk down the road or manage stairs, 1 in 6 was unable to manage household shopping, 1 in 10 had been visited by their doctor at home in the preceding 3 months, and 1 in 5 had seen a hospital doctor. Approximately 50 percent of women and 25 percent of men aged 85 years and over were unable to cook a main meal without help, yet only 10 percent received Meals on Wheels.[8] Malnutrition in hospitals is well documented, and nutritional support has improved the clinical outcome in older patients, for example, with a fractured femur.[9] The true extent of malnutrition in the institutionalized elderly population is little researched yet is fundamental to clinical management, rehabilitation, and recovery.

Nutritional influences in fetal and infant life have been linked to some of the major diseases of middle and late life. In the United Kingdom, Barker and colleagues have provided evidence suggesting that heart disease, stroke, diabetes, hypertension, and obstructive pulmonary disease may be determined by programming in early life. The death rate from ischemic heart disease in men from one area of the United Kingdom whose body weight at 1 year of age was 18 lb or less was three times that of men from the same area who attained 27 lb or more.[10,11] Swedish work supports the association of impaired fetal growth with adult hypertension, particularly in those who become obese, and it is suggested that this may be mediated by metabolic disturbances such as insulin resistance.[12]

Assessment of Nutritional Status

A simplified hypothetical model of a nutrient deficiency suggests an evolution from predisposition through subclinical deficiency to clinical disease. An early stage may be dietary inadequacy revealed by dietary assessment, which may then be followed by a decrease in tissue reserves, body fluids, or nutrient-dependent enzymes or function revealed by biochemical or anthropometric methods. Clinical symptoms and signs are the last manifestation of nutrient deficiency.

In clinical practice, deficiencies of more than one nutrient often coexist, sometimes at different stages of evolution. For individual nutrients some methods of detection are better researched than others, and in some instances biochemical tests are a research tool not routinely available. Gibson[13] provides an authoritative account of nutritional assessment, but a basic summary is provided below to allow interpretation of the often sparse information available for the senior age group.

Estimates of nutrient requirements and thus guidelines for adequate intake are derived from various sources including metabolic balance studies, prevention or cure of deficiency states, and biochemical or enzymatic indexes of adequacy.[14]

The nutritional status of individuals and of populations therefore can be assessed by the following.

- Dietary assessment
- Laboratory tests of biochemical status or of function
- Measurements of body size and composition (including anthropometry)
- Clinical assessment

Dietary Assessment

Food consumption can be assessed at the national, group, or individual level. Information is collected on the food available per capita nationally and at the household level as in the U.K. National Food Survey. Food consumption of individuals can be measured over a defined time period either qualitatively (a dietary history or food frequency questionnaire) or quantitatively (recall, written or weighed record). Such methods require

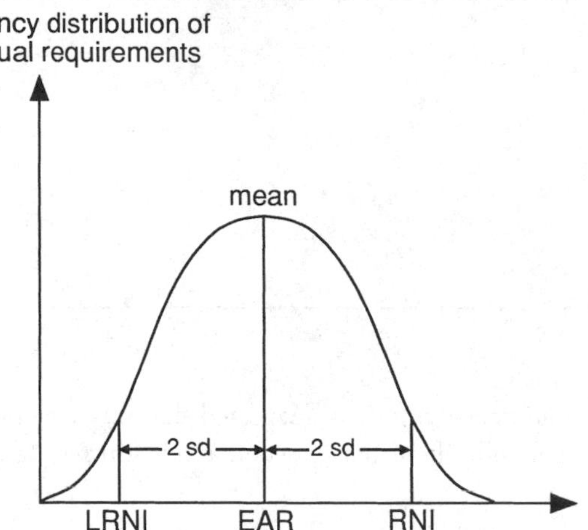

Figure 63-1 Dietery reference values. SD, standard deviation; EAR, estimated average requirement; LRNI, lower reference nutrient intake; RNI, reference nutrient intake.

the subject to have a good memory, to be numerate and literate, and to have a stable diet during the study period. Interpretation necessitates reference to food tables[15] that have been compiled over many years with changing methods of food preparation, preservation, and analysis and which are probably reliable for macronutrients though not accurate for some micronutrients. Chemical analysis of duplicate meals is the most accurate method of assessing actual intake of nutrients and forms part of the metabolic balance study in which all output is also chemically analyzed (including urine, feces and sometimes sweat, menstrual loss, and semen). Such information has been used to estimate human requirements for individual nutrients, for example, nitrogen, iron, and calcium.

In 1970 the Committee on Medical Aspects of Food (COMA) panel on nutrition of the elderly drew attention to the fall in dietary intake with age and the links between poor socioeconomic status, disease, and overt malnutrition in hospitals.[5] The multicenter survey in England and Scotland in 1967/8 using dietary recall and diaries provided data on 764 people over 65 years old. In 1972–1973 the 365 traceable survivors from the 1967–1968 study were re-examined. These studies, which excluded people in institutional care, showed that well older people in general ate a diet that was similar to that of younger people and identified several risk factors for the development of malnutrition. The Dietary and Nutritional Survey of British Adults[16] studied people aged 16 to 64 years and is about to publish a similar survey of the older population reporting weighed dietary intakes, and anthropometric data. A European community project called Survey in Europe on Nutrition in the Elderly—A Concerted Action (SENECA) has collected anthropometric, laboratory, dietary, health, and lifestyle data on almost 2,000 subjects longitudinally.[17]

COMA has a new set of guidelines for dietary intake of food energy and nutrients for all ages with a comprehensive literature review[14] in which dietary reference values (DRVs) replace the earlier recommended dietary allowances (RDAs). Figure 63-1 shows the derivation of DRVs: assuming a normal distribution, the notional mean requirement is designated the estimated average requirement (EAR). The mean plus two standard deviations is the reference nutrient intake (RNI), and intakes above this amount "will almost certainly be adequate." The lower reference nutrient intake (LRNI) represents intakes that are at or below the mean minus two standard deviations and that are "almost certainly inadequate for most individuals." The data available for formulating these recommendations vary in amount and quality and are sparse for the older population. Historically many recommendations depended on extrapolation from data for younger age groups. Table 63-1 summarizes the dietary recommendations for energy, protein, and most minerals, and DRVs for older people for vitamins can be found in Table 6-3. In 1992 COMA published a more specialized and detailed review entitled, "The Nutrition of Elderly People," which endorsed the DRVs for the population aged 50+ years and made specific recommendations.[18]

Laboratory Tests of Biochemical Status or of Physiological Function

Static biochemical tests measure the concentration of a nutrient in biologic tissue or fluid, the most common being blood or a blood component (such as plasma, erythrocytes, or leukocytes). Plasma and serum levels tend to reflect acute changes in nutritional status and are affected by many factors as varied as recent dietary intake, diurnal variation, concomitant medication, infection, inflammation, and stress. Erythrocyte nutrient levels are difficult to analyze and seldom useful. Leukocyte levels may be helpful, but laboratory analysis is time-consuming and requires relatively large blood samples. Biopsy of tissue storage sites such as bone for calcium, adipose tissue for vitamin E or liver, and bone marrow for iron is useful in some clinical settings but is invasive.

Trace element analysis is particularly challenging, and the use of hair or nails is not generally acceptable. Urinary excretion of the nutrient or a metabolite may reflect acute nutritional status and can be useful for vitamin C and water-soluble B vitamins as well as for some minerals and nitrogen.

Functional tests vary from in vivo responses (such as dark adaptation for vitamin A), in vitro and in vivo induced responses, and loading tests to the more familiar measurements of change in enzymatic activity or of a blood component concentration dependent on the nutrient (such as hemoglobin concentration for iron or erythrocyte transketolase activity for thiamin).

Measurements of Body Size and Composition

Body weight is one of the simplest and most neglected clinical parameters. Baseline measurements and a regular check can identify significant weight loss or gain at an early stage. Dependence on late and subjective visible identification of significant weight loss is unscientific and clinically unsound.

The translation of body weight into a useful measure of body fatness, which takes account of height and body shape, has produced a series of anthropometric indexes, the first of which

Table 63-1 UK dietary reference values[14]

Nutrient	Gender and Age Group (yr)	Lower Reference Nutrient Intake, LRNI	Estimated Average Requirement, EAR	Reference Nutrient Intake, RNI
Energy, MJ/d (kcal/d)	M 65–74		9.71 (2,330)	
	75+		8.77 (2,100)	
	F 65–74		7.96 (1,900)	
	75+		7.61 (1,810)	
Protein, g/d	M 50+			53.3
	F 50+			46.5
Calcium, mmol/d	M 50+, F 50+	10	13.1	17.5
Phosphorus, mmol/d	M 50+, F 50+			17.5
Magnesium, mmol/d	M 50+	7.8	10.3	12.3
	F 50+	6.2	8.2	10.9
Sodium, mmol/d	M 50+, F 50+	25		70
Potassium, mmol/d	M 50+, F 50+	50		90
Chloride, mmol/d	M 50+, F 50+			70
Iron, μmol/d	M 50+, F 50+	80	120	160
Zinc, μmol/d	M 50+	85	110	145
	F 50+	60	85	110

Abbreviations: M, male; F, female.

was the indice ponderale (weight^{-3}/height) derived from physical scaling principles (as the size of a spherical body increases, the weight varies according to the cube of the diameter).[19] Hydrodensitometry (underwater weighing) allowed calculation of body fat content. Assuming a lean body mass (LBM) with a constant density of 1.10, weighing individuals in air and then under water with a correction for residual lung volume allows body volume and percentage of body fat to be calculated.[20] It is not surprising to find that few older people were included in these studies.

Skinfold thickness measurements from different sites (triceps, biceps, subscapular, suprailiac) were first used as an estimate of subcutaneous fat by Jelliffe[21] in the Third World and have shown a close correlation with hydrodensitometric measurements in youth and middle life. Mean arm muscle circumference (MAMC) with triceps skinfold thickness (TSF) allows calculation of muscle area (assuming the arm to be circular in cross section) and thence a derivation of fat-free mass (FFM). Corrections for "bone-free" FFM and for gender are available.[22,23] Comparisons of body mass indexes (BMIs) are valid within groups of the same gender and ethnic origin, though there may be inter-regional differences.[24]

Population studies on adults in the western world provide reference data; for example, the Dietary and Nutritional Survey of British Adults in the United Kingdom (age range 16 to 64 years),[16] the U.S. National Health and Nutrition Examination Surveys (age range 25 to 74 years), and the Nutrition Canada National Survey (age range 20 to 69 years).[13]

The use of anthropometry in ill older people has presented some problems,[25] though some information is available for TSF and conventional BMI values.[26] Low BMIs in older people have been associated with an increased mortality risk in general[27–29] and specifically after fracture of the femur.[9,30]

Modifications of anthropometric indexes for use in an older population may improve interpretation. Height may be difficult to measure or unreliable because of kyphosis, vertebral collapse, or unsteadiness. Demispan shows a close correlation with height and is measured from the finger web to the sternal notch with the arm outstretched.[31] Indexes have been developed for use in older men and women using demispan as a measure of stature in the United Kingdom[32] and Canada.[33] Demiquet (weight[kg]/demispan^2) is used for men and Mindex (weight[kg]/demispan) for women. The Nottingham Ageing and Activity Survey[32] provides information on a randomly selected sample of 890 free-living people aged 65 to 74 years and 75 to 94 years and is summarized in Table 63-2.

Age-related changes in body composition, with a fall in FFM[34,35] and a relative increase in deposition of internal rather than subcutaneous fat,[36] taken with the relative paucity of hydrodensitometric reference values and methodologic problems with skinfold calipers prompt caution in interpretating anthropometric variables such as TSF and MAMC in older populations. However, it is suggested that the interindividual differences observed in a comparison of various methods of measuring body composition in a group of 60 individuals predominantly under 75 years of age may not be of practical significance.[37]

Body composition has been measured in the laboratory. Direct chemical analysis of cadavers earlier this century provided some information, though most subjects had had a

Table 63-2 Weight, demispan, and derived ratios in elderly people: Nottingham Activity and Ageing Survey

Age Range (yr)	Number	Weight (kg)[a]	Demispan (cm)[a]	Demiquet (kg/m^2)[a]	Mindex (kg/m)[a]
Men					
65–74	205	72.5 ± 12.6	81.6 ± 4.05	108.8 ± 17.2	
75–91		(39–114)	(71.5–92.7)	(68.6–162.6)	
	153	68.6 ± 11.4	80.4 ± 4.1	106.0 ± 15.1	
		(43–94)	(71.5–91.3)	(72.0–153.6)	
Women					
65–74	257	64.5 ± 13.3	73.8 ± 3.6		87.3 ± 17.4
75–94		(35–124)	(63.3–84.0)		(49.9–168)
	275	59.7 ± 11.6	72.7 ± 3.5		82.1 ± 15.2
		(35–102)	(64.2–84.8)		(49.3–86.8)

[a] *Mean values ±1 standard deviation is shown in parentheses.*
(Data from Department of Health[18] *and Lehmann et al.*[32]*)*

chronic illness and more recent work has shown that fat-free tissue contained approximately 72 percent water, 20 percent protein, and 69 mmol/kg potassium with a variable amount of fat.[38]

Other methods measuring specific components of body composition depend on either a two-compartment model (body fat and FFM) or a four-compartment model (water, protein, minerals, and fat). Estimation of total body potassium measures the γ-radiation emitted by naturally occurring ^{40}K as a measure of FFM. One study has used multi-isotope dilution and elimination kinetics in older people.[39] Total body water can be measured with a stable isotope dilution technique using ^{18}O, ^{3}H, and ^{2}H, and since all body water comprises approximately 73.2 percent FFM, both FFM and body fat can be estimated. Total body nitrogen measured by neutron activation analysis estimates total body protein because there is a fixed relationship between the mass of protein and that of nitrogen (1 g N to 6.25 g protein). Plethysmography estimates body volume without underwater weighing, the disadvantages of which were mentioned above. Differences in the electric conductivity of fat and FFM allow the development of total body electric conductivity and bioelectric impedance as measures. Imaging techniques such as ultrasound, computed tomography (CT) and magnetic resonance imaging (MRI) are currently under review.[40–42] These more recently developed methods are still research tools and have not yet been validated in clinical practice.

Little information from older subjects is available, and many of the inherent assumptions regarding the use of anthropometry in older people have been challenged. The development of simple, noninvasive methods for measuring body composition in this age group would be an important advance.[37,43]

Clinical Assessment

Clinically evident malnutrition represents the culmination of months or years of nutrient deficiency. Multiple pathology and nonspecific presentation of disease complicate the diagnosis of specific nutrient deficiencies which rarely exhibit pathognomonic features even in a younger population. A proper clinical (including social) history and examination also reveals the presence of risk factors for malnutrition.[5] Factors influencing nutritional status in older people are summarized as follows.

- *Acquisition of food:* poverty, immobility, social isolation, and choice may be limited by dietary traditions, by impaired appetite, taste, smell, vision, and hearing, and by inadequate cooking facilities.
- *Ingestion of food:* affected by dentition and oral health[44] as well as conditions such as dysphagia.
- *Digestion and absorption:* influenced by previous surgery (e.g., partial gastrectomy and malabsorption syndromes).
- *Utilization of nutrients and tissue requirements:* may vary with age, physical activity, drugs and disease.

Physical examination should therefore note conditions that may affect individual ability to acquire, ingest, digest, absorb, and efficiently utilize nutrients, as well as physical signs arising as a consequence of poor nutrition. The factors predisposing to malnutrition and some clinical cosequences are represented in Figure 63-2. Single indexes used in nutritional assessment, such as serum transferrin or delayed cutaneous hypersensitivity, have low sensitivity, specificity, and predictive value. Indexes based on a composite of several parameters such as prognostic nutritional index (PNI) and hospital prognostic index (HPI) have been used in some clinical settings. Subjective global assessment based on history and physical examination may be as effective.[13]

Specific Nutrients

Energy

Energy requirements, and thus the dietary intake needed to meet them, are determined by the level of energy expenditure. Total energy expenditure (TEE) is determined by basal

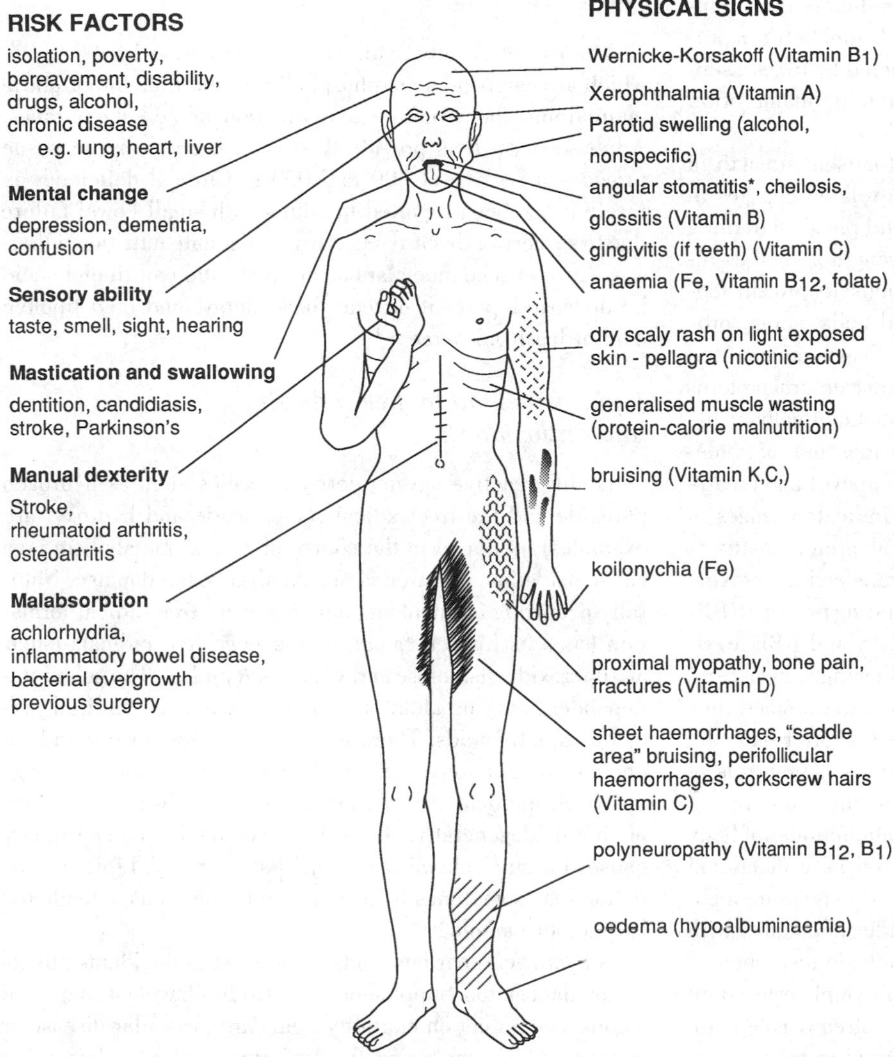

Figure 63-2 Clinical assessment of nutritional status. Parentheses indicate associated nutrient deficiency. *Angular stomatis refers to ill-fitting dentures are the most common cause of angular stomatitis.

metabolic rate (BMR) and physical activity (with a small contribution from thermogenesis). A decrease in the mass of metabolically active tissue and a reduction in physical activity result in a fall in TEE with increasing age.[45] Energy requirements may decrease by about a third between the ages of 30 and 80 years, mainly because of reduced physical activity, the moderate decline in BMR being a consequence of a decrease in total FFM.[46] There is no fall in BMR per kilogram FFM, and the interindividual variation in energy intake and expenditure seen earlier in life persists into old age.[47,48] Neuromuscular inefficiency with age[49] or disability[50] may increase the energy cost of apparently light physical activity though adaptation may occur.[51] Declining energy expenditure may compromise adequate intake of nutrients, and maintaining an active lifestyle has other potential benefits for older individuals.[52]

Malnutrition and a negative energy balance are common in hospitalized older people[53–55] in comparison to healthy older people.[7] The coexistence of low intake and increased BMR, such as may occur with surgery, acute infection, and disability producing mechanical inefficiency in activities of daily living, contribute to the vulnerability of the hospital patient. Nutritional supplementation can improve immune function[56] and recovery from chest infection[57] and reduce mortality in both general[58] and specific conditions, such as fracture of the neck of the femur, even after 6 months of follow-up.[30] Weight loss in psychogeriatric patients may be due to an intermittently negative energy balance, perhaps during sepsis.[59] Energy expenditure may be increased in chronic obstructive pulmonary disease,[60] and there may be a negative energy balance in patients with Parkinson's disease who lose weight despite increased energy intake.[61]

Protein

Total body protein in LBM declines with age, and the rates of protein synthesis, turnover, and degradation decrease.[62–64] Utilization of protein and homeostatic mechanisms such as increased albumin synthesis with adequate dietary protein intake may also be inefficient.[65,66] The equilibrium between protein synthesis and degradation may be affected by illness, sepsis, trauma, and immobility.[64,67,68] Protein malnutrition impairs cellular and humoral immunity.[69]

The decline in functional capacity and muscle strength in old age may be largely attributable to age-related changes in body composition but is not irreversible, and physical training may produce profound improvement in strength as well as increased protein requirement.[70] Skeletal muscle protein (somatic protein) and visceral protein (blood cells, serum proteins, and solid organs such as heart and liver) comprise the metabolically available protein. Noncellular structural proteins (e.g., cartilage) in skeletal tissue are not metabolically available. Total body nitrogen and potassium are measures of whole-body protein; anthropometric indexes (see above) and creatinine and 3-methylhistidine excretion can indicate changes in somatic (skeletal muscle) protein. Visceral protein status is estimated from serum levels of albumin, transferrin, thyroxine binding prealbumin (TBPA), and retinol binding protein (RBP) which are all of hepatic origin. Serum TBPA and RBP levels are most reliable for monitoring short-term changes in visceral protein status during recovery from acute illness since they have a relatively smaller body pool, have a shorter half-life, and are less confounded by the often coexistent problems of sepsis, stress, and dehydration than albumin and transferrin.[13] Nitrogen balance is an example of one metabolic index of body protein, and muscle strength has been used as a functional measure though handgrip dynamometry used to measure muscle strength has obvious problems in an older population with a high prevalence of joint disease. Immunologic tests such as delayed cutaneous hypersensitivity and T-lymphocyte count are affected by protein malnutrition but, as already noted, are of low sensitivity and specificity as functional indexes.

Nitrogen balance studies have been the traditional method of estimating protein requirements, and metabolic equilibrium for protein in elderly people has been observed with daily intakes of between 0.59 and 0.80 g/kg body weight[71,72] though 0.80 g/d was found inadequate by others.[66] Healthy older people living at home and eating a self-selected diet in the United Kingdom were in equilibrium with daily intakes equivalent to 0.97 g/kg body weight.[7] Hospitalized elderly patients studied by the same methods had inadequate energy and protein intakes.[53] Current DRVs are shown in Table 63-1 and agree with the WHO/FAO/UNU recommendation of not less than 0.75 g good-quality protein per kilogram body weight per day. However, these recommendations have been challenged with more recent work suggesting that a safe protein intake for older people is 1.0 to 1.25 g/kg body weight/d.[73,74] In recent years the model for protein metabolism has undergone a conceptual re-evaluation, and it is proposed that dietary amino acids not only function as a substrate for protein synthesis but also have a regulatory role, exerting an anabolic drive.[75] Isotopic studies on amino acid oxidation are prompting reassessment of current recommendations for protein adequacy as well as enabling organ-specific measures of protein turnover.[76,77]

Fats

The essential fatty acids are linoleic and α-linoleic acid, which are components of phospholipids and thus important in maintaining the structure and function of cell membranes. Adult western diets provide 8 to 15 g/d, and adipose tissue provides a reserve of 500 to 1,000 g. Clinical deficiency is rare but has been reported in adults with small bowel failure due to surgery or disease receiving inadequate nutritional therapy. Current recommendations are that intake of linoleic acid be at least 1 percent of total food energy, and of α-linoleic acid at least 0.2 percent.[14]

Lipid peroxidation, free radicals, and antioxidants

Highly reactive oxygen-derived species such as hydrogen peroxide and the free radicals (superoxide and hydroxyl are examples) produced in the course of normal metabolism may cause oxidation, and iron is one catalyst of the damage. Naturally occurring antioxidants either prevent free radical formation (such as iron chelators) or scavenge free radicals (such as superoxide dismutase and vitamins A and C.) The selenium-dependent enzyme glutathione peroxidase converts lipid peroxides to fatty acids. There is a balance between free radical and antioxidant activity in healthy tissue. Free radical damage has been implicated in normal aging[78] and in the pathology of chronic degenerative disease and is thought to be a primary cause of tissue ischemia or reoxygenation injury. Lipid peroxidation may sometimes be a sequel to tissue damage mediated by another pathology.[79]

It is not yet clear how dietary intake of antioxidants affects antioxidant status. Supplementation studies have not suggested a consistent effect on mortality from cardiovascular disease or cancer and re-emphasize the importance of complementing observational and epidemiologic studies with clinical trials and empirical research.[80]

Insofar as dietary fat is considered, COMA recommend that saturated fat provide an average of 10 percent of the population's total dietary intake. Despite recent concerns, there is no clear evidence that a higher intake of polyunsaturated fatty acid (PUFA) contributes to human disease, but the current COMA recommendation is that PUFA constitute not more than 10 percent total food intake.[14] The biologic effects of isomeric fatty acids are unclear, and the current recommendation is that daily intake not exceed 5 g or 2 percent of dietary energy.[14]

The major environmental risk factors for coronary heart disease (CHD) are smoking, hypertension, and serum cholesterol. International differences in mortality from CHD relate to dietary fat intake and correlate most strongly with saturated fat intake which in turn correlates with serum cholesterol. Contrary to earlier beliefs, serum cholesterol level remains predictive of mortality from CHD in older people, justifying the recommendation that "older people adopt a diet that moderates their serum cholesterol."[18] Since long-chain fatty acids may reduce thrombogenicity and there are some clinical and epidemiologic data suggesting a possible cardioprotective effect of a higher intake of $n-3$ fatty acid, it has also been suggested that older people eat more oily fish.[18]

Carbohydrates (Sugars and Complex Carbohydrates)

Sugars

Glucose, fructose, and galactose (monosaccharides) and sucrose, lactose, and maltose (disaccharides) are soluble carbohydrates (sugars) and a valuable source of energy. Classified according to their metabolic availability, intrinsic sugars are those naturally integrated into the cellular structure of food, and extrinsic sugars are those that are free in food or added to it. Extrinsic sugars comprise milk sugars found in milk and milk products (e.g., lactose) and nonmilk sugars (e.g., honey, fruit juices, added sugar). The COMA panel on dietary sugars[81] recommended a reduction in the intake of nonmilk extrinsic sugars, noting the association with dental caries and (at intakes above 30 percent of total food energy) adverse metabolic responses. The most recent figures from the 1972–1973 survey of older people in the United Kingdom indicated that 12 percent of dietary energy intake came from added sugars.[5] Older people probably consume more nonmilk extrinsic sugar than younger ones, and though edentulousness increases with age, remaining teeth are important and abnormal metabolic responses to a sucrose load more common.[18] As the quantity of food eaten falls with age, the quality is all the more important, and consumption of large amounts of sugar may threaten the adequacy of the diet overall. Nutrient density expresses the nutrient content of food as a ratio of the energy content and is a helpful index of dietary quality.

Complex carbohydrates

Dietary polysaccharides comprise starches (long-chain or branched α-glucan polysaccharides) and nonstarch polysaccharides (nondigestible and nonabsorbable plant cell wall carbohydrates). The latter represent the majority of what was previously described as "dietary fiber," a term now considered obsolete because of imprecision in definition and analysis.[14]

Starches Information regarding the intake of starches will soon be available from the British National Diet and Nutrition Survey of older people, but the 1972–1973 survey indicated that bread accounted for 24 percent of food energy and potatoes for 8 percent, with an extra amount from cakes and biscuits. Current recommendations for adults, which are probably equally beneficial for older individuals, suggest that starches and intrinsic and milk sugars contribute 37 percent of the total dietary energy for the population.[81]

Nonstarch polysaccharides Increasing daily dietary intake of nonstarch polysaccharides from 12 g to 18 g benefits older people in the prevention of constipation, diverticular disease, and colonic cancer though other potential benefits are not yet proven.[18] The consumption of large amounts of raw bran can reduce bioavailability of essential minerals such as iron, calcium, zinc, and copper because phytate binds to divalent mineral cations.

Vitamins

Table 63-3 summarizes the metabolic role, features of clinical deficiency states, and reference nutrient intakes for vitamins A, B_1 (thiamin), B_2 (riboflavin), niacin, B_6 (pyridoxine), B_{12}, folic acid, C (ascorbic acid), D, and E. Detailed discussions of measures of status,[13] deficiency states,[82] and illustrations of clinical signs[83] can be found in other texts. Clinical deficiencies of vitamins D and C, folic acid, and vitamins B_{12} and B_1 are seen in older people, particularly in institutions,[84] but are rare or undefined for the other vitamins. Metabolic evidence of vitamin deficiencies may be seen with normal serum levels.[85] Comparison of the U.K. and U.S. literature should be made with the knowledge that the use of vitamin supplements is more common in the United States. The 1979 study on nutrition and health in old age did not estimate vitamin A or E status, but low intakes were rare. Statutory fortification of yellow fats other than butter is endorsed since it provides an additional source of intake from a group of foods favoured by older people.[18] Since deficiencies of vitamins A and E are rare in the western world and there is no substantial literature relating to older people, no further discussion is presented here except to note that, with increasing interest in the antioxidant role of these two vitamins, it is noteworthy that toxicity may occur at doses 10 times the recommended intake for vitamin A.

Vitamin B_1 (thiamin) The mean thiamin intake for elderly men and women in the 1972–1973 study was half that for an adult population aged 16 to 64 years.[5,16] Fortified cereals are an important source.[86] Thiamin intake is closely related to dietary energy intake, and assessment of biochemical adequacy is limited. Thiamin intake may become inadequate if energy intake falls in ill institutionalized older people,[87–89] and it was suggested that confusional states in older orthopedic patients might be partly attributable to poor thiamin status.[90] Thiamin deficiency does not appear common in elderly patients with cardiac failure.[91] Interactions occur between thiamin and other B vitamins, as well as with drugs. Alcohol abuse is associated with thiamin deficiency and the clinical syndromes of Korsakoff's psychosis (short-term memory loss, confabulation) and Wernicke's encephalopathy (acute confusion, opthalmoplegia, and ataxia).

Vitamin B_2 (riboflavin) Dietary intake levels of riboflavin in the 1972–1973 study.[5] were in keeping with current recommendations,[14] and though some indication of biochemical insufficiency was found in this[5] and other[87] studies, the relationship between vitamin intake and biochemical status is complex,[92] with other information suggesting that inadequate riboflavin status is a not a common problem for older subjects.[93]

Niacin Pellagra is the clinical syndrome of niacin deficiency and is rare in the western world. Adequate protein in-

Table 63-3 Vitamins

Vitamin	Reference Nutrient Intake[a]	Metabolic Role	Laboratory Test	Clinical Features of Deficiency
A: retinol	M, 700 μg/d; F, 600 μg/d	Formation of rhodopsin	Dark adaptation, colorimetric or fluorimetric assay, serum retinol	Night blindness, follicular hyperkeratosis, xeropthalmia
B: thiamin	M, 0.9 mg/d; F, 0.8 mg/d	Thiamin pyrophosphate (TPP) is coenzyme for oxidative decarboxylation of pyruric acid	Erythrocyte transketolase activity before/after TPP	Polyneuropathy (dry beri beri), cardiomyopathy (wet beri beri), encephalopathy (Wernicke-Korsakoff syndrome)
Niacin: nicotinic acid equivalent	M, 16 mg/d; F, 12 mg/d	Component of respiratory enzymes (NAD, NADP)	HPLC urinary excretion of *N*-methylnicotinamide	Pellagra—symmetric, pruritic erythema on light-exposed skin, chronic dry scaly dermatitis, delirium, dementia, neuropathy
B_2: riboflavin	M, 1.3 mg/d; F, 1.1 mg/d	Component of flavin adenine dinucleotide (FAD), oxidation reduction reactions	Erythrocyte glutathione reductase activity before/after FAD	Angular stomatitis, glossitis, cheilosis, nasolabial seborrhea
B_6: pyridoxine	M, 1.4 mg/d; F 1.2 mg/d	Coenzyme for amino acid decarboxylation and transamination reactions	Plasma pyridoxal 5-phosphate	Peripheral neuropathy (e.g., isoniazid)
B_{12}: cyanocobalamin	M, 1.5 μg/d; F, 1.5 μg/d	Synthesis of thymine (DNA base) from deoxyuridine, proprionate metabolism	Serum vitamin B_{12} (radioassay)	Macrocytic anemia, subacute combined degeneration of cord
Folate	M, 200 μg/d; F, 200 μg/d	Thymine synthesis	Serum, erythrocyte folate (microbiologic or radioassay)	Macrocytic anemia
C: ascorbic acid	M, 40 mg/d; F, 40 mg/d	Antioxidant	Colorimetric or fluorimetric assay, plasma or (better) leukocyte ascorbic acid	Scurvy—gingvitis (if not edentulous), perifollicular petechiae, corkscrew hairs, bruises, sheet hemorrhages in skin, ocular hemorrhage, femoral neuropathy, sudden death
D: cholecalciferol	M and F 65+ years, 10 μg/d	Promotes calcium and phosphate absorption, calcium release from bone (PTH-dependent)	Competitive binding assay of 25-OHD	Bone tenderness, spontaneous fractures, proximal myopathy

Abbreviations: M, male; F, female; HPLC, high-pressure liquid chromatography; PTH, parathormone.
[a] *Aged 50+ years unless otherwise stated. RNI assumes protein = 14.7% EAR for energy.*

take usually ensures adequate niacin intake, and flour is fortified with niacin. Intakes appeared adequate in the 1972–1973 study.[5] No functional measure of niacin status exists.

Vitamin B_6 Plasma levels of pyridoxal phosphate (PLP) fall with age, but the activity of erythrocyte aspartate aminotransferase (for which PLP is a coenzyme) does not. While there may be a higher absolute requirement in elderly subjects[94] COMA found that there was no evidence supporting a higher recommended intake.[14]

Vitamin B_{12} Dietary inadequacy is relatively rare, and deficiency is more commonly caused by absorption dysfunction, whether due to pernicious anemia and absence of the specific binding protein gastric intrinsic factor or to small intestinal malabsorption secondary to disease, surgery, or bacterial overgrowth. Vitamin B_{12} absorption does not decline with age,[95] and healthy older populations in general do not seem to have lower serum vitamin B_{12} levels than younger groups[96] though almost a fifth of the U.K. 1972–1973 study had serum vitamin B_{12} levels between 100 and 200 pg/mL and 2.5 percent had levels below 100 pg/mL.[5] Vitamin B_{12} deficiency may appear as macrocytic anemia or subacute combined degeneration of the cord, but current diagnostic methods are insensitive indexes of status and atypical presentation in older people may lead to important delays in diagnosis and treatment.[97] Microbiologic methods and radioassay are the most commonly used techniques.

Folic acid Folic acid is destroyed by prolonged cooking, and the dietary lifestyle of some disabled or ill older people may not allow a sufficient intake of folate-rich foods. Malabsorption can occur, as in the case of vitamin B_{12}. Serum folate levels reflect recent dietary intake, and erythrocyte levels reflect tissue status. Metabolism of vitamin B_{12} and of folate are interrelated,[98] and since vitamin B_{12} deficiency can result in low erythrocyte folate levels, it is important to measure both serum and erythrocyte folate levels. Metabolic consequences of folate deficiency in advance of macrocytic anemia are indicated by abnormal deoxyuridine suppression tests on bone marrow and peripheral blood lymphocytes.[13] Borderline erythrocyte folate levels were seen in a fifth of the healthy older people studied in the 1972–1973 study, and 1 in 20 had subnormal levels. Dietary folate deficiency is not considered a major factor in anemia in healthy elderly people but may be important in patients who abuse alcohol, in the prescription of certain drugs (e.g., phenytoin), or in hospitalization.[99]

Vitamin C Vitamin C is a water-soluble antioxidant which is rapidly oxidized with prolonged heating. Over 20 years ago it was reported that food provided by Meals on Wheels lost over 90 percent of its vitamin C content before delivery,[100] and foods high in vitamin C content often require preparation and chewing, thus making them relatively less accessible for some older people. In the 1972–1973 U.K. study mean daily intake of vitamin C was at the level of the RNI with 2 percent of men and 6 percent of women eating less than the LRNI of 10 mg[5] and three cases of frank scurvy in a community-based study. In the United States intakes were higher, reflecting the more widespread use of supplements.[101] Patients in continuing-care settings are vulnerable.[102] Chronic marginal vitamin C status may have quite different pathophysiologic effects on acute severe deficiency.[103] Vitamin C intake has been related to cognitive impairment, atherogenesis,[104] and death from stroke,[105] and serum ascorbate levels have been shown to have a strong inverse correlation with plasma fibrinogen and factor VIIC, providing a possible mechanism for the suggestion that a high intake of vitamin C may be cardioprotective.[106]

Vitamin D Vitamin D_3 (cholecalciferol) is synthesized in the skin by the action of sunlight (ultraviolet radiation of wavelength 290 to 310 nm) on 7-dehydrocholesterol and converted in the liver to 25-hydroxyvitamin D (25-OHD). This compound is then further hydroxylated in the kidney to 1,25-dihydroxyvitamin D (1,25[OH]$_2$D), the active form of the vitamin which promotes intestinal calcium and phosphate absorption and ensures adequate bone mineralization via its effects on bone resorption and renal reabsorption of calcium and phosphate. Dietary sources of vitamin D include eggs and margarine (which is statutorily fortified with vitamins A and D) and oily fish. Vitamin D_3 from the skin is the major source of the vitamin in U.K. adults, with diet contributing an approximate average of 3 μg/d (DRV). Solar radiation varies with season, latitude, and time of day. Limited skin exposure makes dietary contribution relatively more important, and older people, particularly those who are institutionalized and housebound, are vulnerable to subclinical and clinical vitamin D deficiency. Malabsorption, gastric surgery, anticonvulsant therapy, and hepatic disease can compromise vitamin D status. Levels of 25-OHD$_3$ reflect vitamin D status[13] and decline with age,[107] probably reflecting less exposure to the sun. Levels of 25-OHD below 10 nmol/L (4.1 ng/ml) (with an associated rise in parathormone levels) are seen in osteomalacia. Plasma 25-OHD levels are maintained above the level associated with osteomalacia when daily dietary intake is 5 to 10 μg in the absence of skin synthesis of the vitamin.[108] Seasonal postmenopausal bone loss can be favorably influenced by vitamin D supplementation.[109] The COMA recommendation that elderly people seek some exposure to sunlight from May to September is complemented by advice to provide supplements ensuring a total daily intake of 10 μg vitamin D for homebound or institutionalized individuals.[14,18] Recent European work supports this concept and considers older people to be at substantial risk of vitamin D deficiency.[110]

Minerals

Calcium

Ninety-nine percent of body calcium is found as a vital structural component of bone, and the remaining 1 percent is found in tissues and serum involved with enzyme activity, blood clotting, and the expression of hormonal effects via cyclic adenosine monophosphate. Milk is an important source of dietary calcium, particularly in older people, and the recognition that milk consumption in this age group is falling has led to the recommendation that doorstep deliveries of milk continue.[18] Intestinal absorption of calcium declines with age,[111,112] probably partly as a consequence of vitamin D status[113–115] since this is the major factor controlling calcium absorption. Phytate, oxalates, and fiber also reduce calcium absorption, and bioavailability must be taken into account when assessing adequacy of calcium in the diet. Aging is accompanied by reduced ability to adapt to low calcium intake.[116]

The current RNI for daily calcium intake is 17.5 mmol (700 mg) for all adults over 50 years of age, assuming a mean intestinal absorption of 30 percent, but it is recognized that the data on which this recommendation is based are particularly sparse for people over 60 years of age.[14,117] Elderly subjects in the community were found to be in metabolic equilibrium with an intake of 25 mmol (1,000 mg) daily,[7] and calcium requirements determined by metabolic balance may rise to as much as 37 mmol (1,480 mg) daily perimenopausally.[118] There is no convenient biochemical test for estimating calcium status; serum calcium concentrations are homeostatically tightly controlled, and serum ionized calcium levels are not widely available. Measurement of bone mineral mass by absorptiometry or imaging techniques indicates body calcium stores.

Hypocalcemia may result in cardiac arrhythmias and neuromuscular dysfunction. Adequate dietary calcium intake is important in the achievement of peak adult bone mass,[119] but the relevance of calcium in the diet to the development of osteoporosis in later life and the place of dietary calcium supplements in the management of osteoporosis remain unclear.[120–124]

Magnesium

Mean national daily intake of 10 mmol magnesium accords with the level at which balance was seen in a healthy elderly group.[125,7] Dietary magnesium deficiency is rare, and malabsorption due to surgery or gut dysfunction or increased losses, such as occur with diuretic therapy,[126,127] are a more common cause of a clinical deficiency. Magnesium deficiency may occur in alcoholism and congestive cardiac failure, and physical signs of deficiency include muscle weakness, cardiac arrhythmias, and neurologic signs such as muscle fasiculation, spasm, and fits. Serum magnesium levels are of low specificity and sensitivity but may be a guide to magnesium status in clinical practice though leukocyte and muscle magnesium levels are probably a better reflection of total body status.[13] Older people may be vulnerable to deficiencies because of the coincidence of poor diet, disease, and drug treatment.

Sodium

The U.K. RNI for sodium is 70 mmol (4 g), and average daily intakes for adults in the United Kingdom are 9 g, well above current WHO guidelines for population intakes. Hypertension is related to dietary salt intake,[128] and convenience foods have a high salt content. It is recommended that older people follow the same guidelines as other adults in reducing their level of salt consumption.[18]

Iron

Heme iron in the diet is better absorbed than nonheme iron, and vitamin C enhances absorption. Cereals and meat are important dietary sources in the United Kingdom. Achlorhydria and previous gastric surgery may reduce dietary iron absorption, and bioavailability may be lower with diets containing complex carbohydrates, phytate, or even tannins in tea.[14] Gut mucosal absorption of iron is responsive to body iron status, and different mechanisms may operate in the iron-sufficient and iron-deficient states.[129,130] Advancing age is associated with reduced iron absorption[131] and inefficient tissue utilization of iron perhaps as a result of ineffective erythropoiesis or increased hepatic retention of iron.[132] The DRV for iron for men and women over 50 years of age (daily EAR and RNI = 120 μmol and 160 μmol) is the same as for younger men, though older women may have depleted iron stores from their premenopausal years. Hospitalized and homebound older people, particularly women, may have low intakes compared to free-living healthy subjects even with comparable dietary iron densities.[133]

The hypochromic microcytic anemia of iron deficiency is the best recognized of any micronutrient deficiency, but iron deficiency can result in other less well-defined effects such as muscle dysfunction, tiredness, impaired cellular immunity, and abnormalities in catecholamine metabolism.[134] Progressive changes in the indexes of iron status in the development of deficiency begin with depletion of storage iron manifested by low serum ferritin levels but normal hemoglobin and transport iron levels indicated by normal transferrin saturation. Later, iron-deficient erythropoeisis is seen, accompanied by a decrease in transferrin saturation. Last, frank iron deficiency anemia occurs.[135] Serum ferritin is the most sensitive index of early iron deficiency but may be raised in chronic inflammation. Simultaneous measurement of iron binding capacity reveals a low level of transferrin saturation, and thus it may be important in some circumstances to use two or more indexes of iron status. Iron deficiency without anemia may be a common but unrecognized problem in homebound older women and hospitalized older people.[133] Gastrointestinal blood loss is a major cause of iron deficiency in hospitalized elderly people[136] and is often due to a remediable pathology,[137] justifying a careful evaluation before attributing anemia to dietary deficiency.

Zinc

Zinc is essential for the function of major metabolic pathways because it is involved in many enzymatic reactions, in maintaining the integrity of biomembranes, and in DNA and RNA synthesis. Zinc deficiency in the adult can cause hypoguesia (reduced or abnormal taste), neuropsychiatric symptoms, dermatitis, and impaired cellular immunity. Deficiency may be seen in clinical practice as a complication of other conditions such as alcoholic liver disease and inflammatory bowel disease. The daily RNI for zinc (145 μmol for men and 110 μmol for women aged 50+ years) is of a order of magnitude similar to that of iron (160 μmol) but clinical deficiency is rarely recognized, perhaps partly because of difficulties with biochemical assessment (serum levels are of low specificity and sensitivity) and poorly defined symptoms and signs.[13] Institutionalized older people are at risk of zinc deficiency.[52,138] Supplementation in a proven state of zinc deficiency improves wound healing, but indiscriminate use of zinc supplements may produce adverse effects such as gastritis.[18]

References

1. Department of Health: The Health of the Nation. Nutrition: Core Curriculum for Nutrition in the Education of Health Professionals. HMSO, London 1994
2. Garrow J: Starvation in hospital. BMJ 1994;308:934
3. McWhirter JP, Pennington CR: Incidence and recognition of malnutrition in hospital. BMJ 1994;308:945–948
4. Bender AE: Institutional malnutrition. BMJ 1984;288:92–93
5. Department of Health and Social Services: Nutrition and Health in Old Age. Report on Health and Social Subjects. 16. HMSO, London, 1979

6. Exton-Smith AN, Stanton BK, Windsor ACM: Nutrition of Housebound Old People. King Edward's Hospital Fund, London, 1972
7. Bunker VW, Clayton BE: Research review: studies in the nutrition of elderly people with particular relevance to essential trace elements. Age Ageing 1989;18:422–429
8. Office of Population Census and Surveys: Living in Britain. Results from the 1994 General Household Survey. OPCS Social Survey Division. HMSO, London, 1996
9. Bastow MD, Rawlings J, Allison SP: Benefits of supplementary tube feeding after fractured neck of femur: a randomised controlled trial. BMJ 1983;287:1589–1592
10. Barker DJP: Fetal origins of coronary heart disease. BMJ 1995; 312:171–174
11. Barker DPJ, Osmond C, Winter PD et al: Weight in infancy and death from ischaemic heart disease. Lancet 1989;ii: 577–580
12. Leon DA, Koupilova I, Lithell HO et al: Failure to realise growth potential in utero and adult obesity in relation to blood pressure in 50 yr old Swedish men. BMJ 1996;312:401–410
13. Gibson RS: Principles of Nutritional Assessment Oxford University Press, New York, 1990
14. DH: Dietary Reference Values for Food Energy and Nutrients for the United Kingdom. Report on Health and Social Subjects 41. HMSO, London, 1991
15. Paul NA, Southgate DAT: McCance and Widdowson's The Composition of Foods. 4 Ed. HMSO, London, 1985
16. Office of Population Census and Surveys: The Dietary and Nutritional Survey of British Adults. OPCS Social Survey Division. HMSO, London, 1990
17. SENECA: Nutrition and the elderly in Europe. Eur J Clin Nutr 1991;45(suppl 3):1–196
18. Department of Health: The Nutrition of Elderly People: Report on Health and Social Subjects. 43. HMSO, London, 1992
19. Micozzi MS, Albanes D, Jones Y, Chumlea WC: Correlations of body mass indices with weight, stature, and body composition in men and women in NHANES I and II. Am J Clin Nutr 1986;44:725–731
20. Durnin JVGA, Rahaman MM: The assessment of the amount of fat in the human body from measurements of skinfold thickness. Br J Nutr 1967;21:681–689
21. Jelliffe DB: The assessment of the nutritional status of the community. WHO Monograph. 53. World Health Organization, Geneva, 1966
22. Frisancho AR: Triceps skinfold and upper arm muscle size norms for assessment of nutritional status. Am J Clin Nutr 1974;27:1052–1058
23. Heymsfield SB, McManus C, Smith J et al: Anthropometric measurement of muscle mass: revised equations for calculating bone free arm muscle area. Am J Clin Nutr 1982;36:680–690
24. Delarue J, Constans T, Malvy D et al: Anthropometric values in an elderly French population. Br J Nutr 1994;71:295–302
25. Kemm JR, Allcock J: The distribution of supposed indicators of nutritional status in elderly patients. Age Ageing 1984;13: 21–28
26. Burr ML, Phillips KM: Anthropometric norms in the elderly. Br J Nutr 1984;51:165–169
27. Freidman PJ, Campbell AJ, Caradoc-Davies TH: Prospective trial of a new diagnostic criterion for severe wasting malnutrition in the elderly. Age Ageing 1985;14:149–154
28. Mattila K, Haavisto M, Rajala S: Body mass index and mortality in the elderly. BMJ 1986;292:867–868
29. Campbell AJ, Spears GFS, Brown JS et al: Anthropometric measurements as predictors of mortality in a community population aged 70 years and over. Age Ageing 1990;19:131–135
30. Delmi M, Rapin CH, Bengoa JM et al: Dietary supplementation in elderly patients with fractured neck of the femur. Lancet 1990;335:1013–1016
31. Bassey EJ: Demispan as a measure of skeletal size. Ann Hum Biol 1986;13:499–502
32. Lehmann AB, Bassey EJ, Morgan K, Dalluso HM: Normal values for weight, skeletal size and body mass indices in 890 men and women aged over 65 years. Clin Nutr 1991; 10:18–22
33. Smith WDF, Cunningham DA, Paterson DH, Koral JJ: Body mass indices and skeletal size in 394 Canadians aged 55–86 years. Ann Hum Biol 1995;22:305–314
34. Snead DB, Birge ST, Kohrt WM: Age related differences in body composition by hydrodensitometry and dual x-ray absorptiometry. J Appl Physiol 1993;74:770–775
35. Paolisso G, Gambardella A, Balbi V et al: Body composition, body fat distribution and resting metabolic rate in healthy centenarians. Am J Clin Nutr 1995;62:746–750
36. Durnin JVGA, Womersley J: Body fat assessment from total body density and its estimation from skinfold thickness measurement in 481 men and women aged 16–72 years. Br J Nutr 1974;32:77–92
37. Reilly JJ, Murray LA, Wilson J, Durnin JVGA: Measuring the body composition of elderly subjects. Br J Nutr 1994;72: 33–44
38. Garrow JS: Indices of adiposity. Nutr Abstr Rev 1983;53: 697–708
39. Fulop T, Worum I, Csongor J et al: Body composition in elderly people. Gerontology 1985;31:6–14
40. Lukaski HC: Methods for the assessment of human body composition: traditional and new. Am J Clin Nutr 1987;46: 537–556
41. Fuller MF, Fowler PA, McNeill G, Foster MA: Body composition: the precision and accuracy of new methods and their suitability for longitudinal studies. Proc Nutr Soc 1990;49: 423–436
42. Campbell IT, Watt T, Withers D et al: Muscle thickness, measured with ultrasound may be an indicator of lean tissue wasting in multiple organ failure in the presence of oedema. Am J Clin Nutr 1995;62:533–539
43. Bergsma-Kadijk JA, Baumeister B, Deurenberg P: Measurement of body fat in young and elderly women: comparison between a four compartment model and widely used reference methods. Br J Nutr 1996;75:649–657
44. Moynihan PJ: The relationship between diet, nutrition and dental health: an overview and update for the 90's. Nutr Res Rev 1995;8:193–224
45. Shock NW: Energy metabolism, caloric intake and physical

activity in the aging. pp. 12–23. Symposia of the Swedish Nutrition Foundation. X. Nutrition in Old Age Swedish Nutrition Foundation. Upsala, Sweden, 1972

46. McGandy KB, Barrows CH Jr, Spanias A et al: Nutrient intake and energy expenditure in men of different ages. J Gerontol 1966;22:581–587
47. Durnin JVGA: Body composition and energy expenditure in elderly people. Bibl Nutr Dieta 1983;33:16–30
48. Prentice AM: Energy expenditure in the elderly. Eur J Clin Nutr 1992;46(suppl 3):521–528
49. Bassey EJ, Terry AM: The oxygen cost of walking in the elderly. J Physiol 1986;373:42P
50. Isakor E, Suzak Z, Becker E: Energy expenditure and cardiac responses in above knee amputees while using prostheses with open and locked knee mechanisms. Scand J Rehabil Med Suppl 1985;12:108–111
51. Didier JP, Mourey F, Brondel L et al: The energetic cost of some daily activities: a comparison in a young and old population. Age Ageing 1993;22:90–96
52. Fiatarone MA, O'Niell EF, Ryan ND et al: Exercise training and nutritional supplementation for physical frailty in very elderly people. N Engl J Med 1994;330:1769–1775
53. Thomas AJ, Bunker VW, Hinks LJ et al: Energy, protein, zinc and copper status of twenty-one elderly inpatients: analysed dietary intake and biochemical indices. Br J Nutr 1988;59: 181–191
54. Roberts M, Reilly JJ, Klipstein K, Potter J: The nutritional status and clinical course of acute admissions to a geriatric unit. Age Ageing 1995;24:131–136
55. Klipstein-Grobusch, Reilly JJ, Potter J, Edwards CA, Roberts MA: Energy intake and expenditure in elderly patients admitted to hospital with acute illness. Br J Nutr 1995;73:323–334
56. Roebothan BV, Chandra RK: Relationships between nutritional status and immune function of elderly people. Age Ageing 1994;23:49–53
57. Woo J, Ho SC, Mak YT et al: Nutritional status of elderly patients during recovery from chest infection and the role of nutritional supplementation assessed by a prospective randomised single-blind trial. Age Ageing 1994;23:40–48
58. Larsson J, Unosson M, Ek AC et al: Effect of dietary supplement on nutritional status and clinical outcomes in 501 geriatric patients—a randomised study. Clin Nutr 1990;9:179–184
59. Prentice AM, Leavesley K, Murgatroyd PR et al: Is severe wasting in elderly mental patients caused by an excessive energy requirement? Age Ageing 1989;18:158–167
60. Wilson DO, Rogers RM, Hoffmann RM: Nutrition and chronic lung disease. Am Rev Resp Dis 1985;132:1347–1365
61. Davies KN, King D, Davies H: A study of the nutritional status of elderly patients with Parkinson's disease. Age Ageing 1994; 23:142–145
62. Uauy R, Winterer JC, Bilmazes C et al: The changing pattern of whole body protein metabolism in aging humans. J Gerontol 1978;33:663–671
63. Golden MHN, Waterlow JC: Total protein synthesis in elderly people: a comparison of results with ^{15}N glycine and ^{14}C leucine. Clin Sci Mol Med 1977;53:277–288
64. Lehmann AB, NM Johnston C, James OFW: The effects of old age and immobility on protein turnover in human subjects with some observations on the possible role of hormones. Age Ageing 1989;18:148–157
65. World Health Organisation: Energy and Protein Requirements: Report of a Joint FAO/WHO/UNU Expert Consultation. WHO Technical Reports Series 724. World Health Organisation, Geneva, 1985
66. Gersovitz M, Motil K, Munro HN et al: Human protein requirements: assessment of the adequacy of the current recommended allowance for dietary protein in elderly men and women. Am J Clin Nutr 1982;35:6–14
67. Reeds PJ, James WPT: Protein turnover. Lancet 1983;i: 571–574
68. Rennie M, Harrison R: Effect of injury, disease and malnutrition on protein metabolism in man: unanswered questions. Lancet 1984;i:323–325
69. Chandra RK: The relation between immunology, nutrition and disease in elderly people. Age Ageing 1990;19:S25–S31
70. Fielding RA: Effects of exercise training in the elderly: impact of progressive—resistance training on skeletal muscle and whole-body protein metabolism. Proc Nutr Soc 1995;54: 665–675
71. Uauy R, Scrimshaw NS, Young VR: Human protein requirements: nitrogen balance response to graded levels of egg protein in elderly men and women. Am J Clin Nutr 1978;31: 779–785
72. Zanni E, Calloway DH, Zezulka AY: Protein requirements of elderly men. J Nutr 1979;109:513–524
73. Young VR: Amino acids and proteins in relation to the nutrition of elderly people. Age Ageing 1990;19:S10–S24
74. Campbell WW, Crim MC, Dallal GE et al: Increased protein requirement in elderly people: new data and retrospective reassessments. Am J Clin Nutr 1994;60:501–509
75. Millward DJ, Price GM, Pacy PJH, Halliday D: Maintenance protein requirement: the need for conceptual re-evaluation. Proc Nutr Soc 1990;49:473–487
76. Millward DJ, Price GM, Pacy PJH, Halliday D: Whole body protein and amino acid turnover in man: what can we measure with confidence? Proc Nutr Soc 1991;50:197–216
77. Garlick PJ, Wernerman J, McNurlan MA, Heys SD: Organ specific measurements of protein turnover in man. Proc Nutr Soc 1991;50:217–225
78. Meydani SN, Wu D, Santos MS, Heyck MG: Antioxidants and immune response in aged persons, an overview of present evidence. Am J Clin Nutr 1995;62:1462S–1476S
79. Halliwell B, Gutteridge JMC: Free Radicals in Biology and Medicine. 2nd Ed. Clarendon Press, Oxford, 1989
80. Greenberg ER, Sporn MB: Antioxidant vitamins, cancer and cardiovascular disease. N Engl J Med 1996;334:1189–1190
81. Department of Health: Dietary Sugars and Human Disease. Report on Health and Social Subjects 37. HMSO, London, 1989
82. Thurnham DI: The interpretation of biochemical measurements of vitamin status in the elderly. pp. 46–67. In Kemm J, Ancill R (eds): Vitamin Deficiency in the Elderly. Blackwell, London, 1985

83. McLaren DS: A Colour Atlas of Nutritional Disorders. Wolfe Medical Publications, London, 1981
84. Baker H, Frank O, Thind IS et al: Vitamin profiles in elderly persons living at home or in nursing homes versus profile in healthy young subjects. J Am Geriatr Soc 1979;XXVII: 444–449
85. Naurath HJ, Joosten E, Reizler R et al: Effects of vitamin B_{12}, folate and vitamin B_6 supplements in elderly people with normal serum vitamin concentrations. Lancet 1995;346: 85–89
86. Anderson SH, Vickery CA, Nicol AD: Adult thiamine requirements and the continuing need to fortify processed cereals. Lancet 1986;ii:85–89
87. Vir SC, Love AHG: Nutritional status of institutionalised aged in Belfast, Northern Ireland. Am J Clin Nutr 1979;32: 1934–1947
88. Thomas AJ, Finglas P, Bunker VW: The B vitamin content of hospital meals and potential low intake by elderly inpatients. J Hum Nutr Diet 1988;1:309–320
89. O'Rourke NP, Bunker VW, Thomas AJ et al: Thiamine status of healthy and institutionalised elderly subjects: analysis of dietary intake and biochemical indices. Age Ageing 1990;19: 325–329
90. Older MJW, Dickerson JWT: Thiamine and the elderly orthopaedic patient. Age Ageing 1982;11:101–197
91. Kwok T, Falconer Smith JF et al: Thiamine status of elderly patients with cardiac failure. Age Ageing 1992;21:67–71
92. Rutishauser IHE, Bates CJ, Paul AA et al: Longterm vitamin status and dietary intake of healthy elderly subjects. Br J Nutr 1979;42:33–42
93. Garry PJ, Goodwin JS, Hunt WC: Nutritional status in a healthy elderly population: riboflavin. Am J Clin Nutr 1982; 36:902–909
94. Vir SC, Love AHG: Vitamin B_6 status of hospitalised aged. Am J Clin Nutr 1978;31:1383–1391
95. McEvoy AW, Fenwick JD, Boddy K, James OFW: Vitamin B_{12} absorption from the gut does not decline with age in normal elderly humans. Age Ageing 1982;11:180–183
96. Garry PJ, Goodwin JS, Hunt WC: Folate and B_{12} status in a healthy elderly population. J Am Geriatr Soc 1984;32: 719–726
97. van Goor LP, Woiski MD, Lagaay AM et al: Review: cobalamin deficiency and mental impairment in elderly people. Age Ageing 1995;24:S36–S42
98. Shane B, Stokstad ELR: Vitamin B_{12} folate interrelationships. Ann Rev Nutr 1985;5:115–141
99. Rosenberg IH, Bowman BB, Cooper BA et al: Folate nutrition in the elderly. Am J Clin Nutr 1982;36:1060–1066
100. Stanton BR: Meals for the Elderly. King Edward's Hospital Fund for London, London, 1971
101. Garry PJ, Goodwin JS, Hunt WC, Gilbert BA: Nutritional status in a healthy elderly population. Am J Clin Nutr 1982;36: 332–339
102. Andrews J: Vitamin C status of elderly long stay hospital patients. Gerontol Clin 1973;15:221–226
103. Ginter E: Chronic marginal vitamin C deficiency: biochemistry and pathophysiology. World Rev Nutr Diet 1979;33:104–141
104. Gale CR, Martyn CN, Cooper C: Cognitive impairment and mortality in a cohort of elderly people. BMJ 1996;312: 608–611
105. Gale CR, Martyn CN, Winter PD, Cooper C: Vitamin C and risk of death from stroke and coronary heart disease in a cohort of elderly people. BMJ 1995;310:1563–1565
106. Khaw KT, Woodhouse P: Interrelation of vitamin C, infection, haemostatic factors and cardiovascular disease. BMJ 1995; 310:1559–1563
107. Dattani JT, Exton Smith AN, Stephen JM: Vitamin D status of the elderly in relation to age and exposure to sunlight. Hum Nutr Clin Nutr 1984;38C:131–137
108. Krall EA, Sahyoun N, Tannenbaum S et al: Effect of vitamin D intake on seasonal variations in parathyroid hormone secretion in post-menopausal women. N Engl J Med 1989;321: 1777–1783
109. Dawson-Hughes B, Dallas GE, Krall EA et al: Effect of vitamin D supplementation in winter-time and overall bone loss in healthy post-menopausal women. Ann Intern Med 1991;115: 505–512
110. van der Wielen RPJ, Lowik MRH, Van der Berg H et al: Serum vitamin D concentrations among healthy elderly people in Europe. Lancet 1995;346:207–210
111. Avioli LV, McDonald JE, Lee SW: The influence of age on the intestinal absorption of ^{47}Ca in women and its relation to ^{47}Ca absorption in postmenopausal osteoporosis. J Clin Invest 1965;44:1960–1967
112. Bullamore JR, Wilkinson R, Gallagher JC et al: Effect of age on calcium absorption. Lancet 1970;ii:535–537
113. Francis RM, Peacock M, Storer JH et al: Calcium malabsorption in the elderly: the effect of treatment with oral 25 hydroxyitamin D. Eur J Clin Invest 1983;13:391–396
114. Francis RM, Peacock M, Barkworth SA: Renal impairment and its effects on calcium metabolism in elderly women. Age Ageing 1984;13:14–20
115. Nordin BEC, Baker MR, Horsman A, Peacock M: A prospective trial of the effect of vitamin D supplementation on metacarpal bone loss in elderly women. Am J Clin Nutr 1985;42: 470–474
116. Ireland P, Fortran JS: Effect of dietary calcium and age on jejunal calcium absorption in humans studied by intestinal perfusion. J Clin Invest 1973;52:2672–2682
117. Wood RJ, Suter PM, Russell RM: Mineral requirements of elderly people. Am J Clin Nutr 1995;62:493–505
118. Heaney RP, Recker RR, Saville PD: Menopausal changes in calcium balance. J Lab Clin Med 1978;92:953–963
119. Matkovic V, Kostial K, Simonovic I et al: Bone status and fracture rates in two regions of Yugoslavia. Am J Clin Nutr 1979;32:540–549
120. Hegsted DM: Calcium and osteoporosis. J Nutr 1986;116: 2316–2319
121. Stevenson JC, Whitehead MI, Padwick M et al: Dietary intake of calcium and postmenopausal bone loss. BMJ 1988;297: 15–17
122. Kanis JA, Passmore R: Calcium supplementation of the diet I. BMJ 1989;298:137–140

123. Kanis JA, Passmore R: Calcium supplementation of the diet II. BMJ 1989;298:205–208
124. Nordin BEC, Heaney RP: Calcium supplementation of the diet: justified by present evidence. BMJ 1990;300: 1056–1060
125. Lewis J, Buss DH: Trace nutrients. 5. minerals and vitamins in the British household food supply. Br J Nutr 1988;60: 413–424
126. Lim P, Jacob E: Magnesium deficiency in patients on longterm diuretic therapy for heart failure. BMJ 1972;3:620–622
127. Dykner T, Wester PO: The relation between intra and extracellular electrolytes in patients with hypokalaemia and/or diuretic treatment. Acta Med Scand 1978;204:269–282
128. Elliott P, Stamler J, Nichols R et al: Intersalt revisited: further analysis of 24 hour sodium excretion and blood pressure within and across populations. BMJ 1996;312:1249–1253
129. Bjorn Rasmussen E: Iron absorption: present knowledge and controversies. Lancet 1983;i:914–916
130. Valberg LS, Flanagan PR: Intestinal absorption of iron and related metals. pp. 41–66. In Sarkar B (ed): Biological Aspects of Metals and Metal-Related Diseases. Raven Press, New York, 1983
131. Jacobs AM, Owen GM: The effect of age on iron absorption. J Gerontol 1969;24:95–96
132. Marx JJM, Dinant HJ: Ferrokinetics and red cell iron uptake in old age: evidence for increased liver iron retention. Haematologica 1982;67:161–168
133. Thomas AJ, Bunker VW, Stansfied MF et al: Iron status of hospitalised and housebound elderly people: dietary intake, metabolic balance, haematological and biochemical indices. Q J Med 1989;262:175–184
134. Dallman PR: Manifestation of iron deficiency. Semin Hematol 1982;19:19–29
135. Cook JD, Finch CA: Assessing iron status of a population. Am J Clin Nutr 1979;32:2115–2119
136. Croker JR, Beynon G: Gastrointestional bleeding—a major cause of iron deficiency in the elderly. Age Ageing 1981;10: 40–43
137. Calvey HD, Castleden CM: Gastrointestinal investigations for anaemia in the elderly: a prospective study. Age Ageing 1987; 16:399–404
138. Senapati A, Jenner G, Thompson RPH: Zinc in the elderly. Q J Med 1989;70:81–87

CHAPTER 64

Obesity

CYRIL WEINKOVE

The effects and causes of obesity in elderly people are little different from those in younger adults, and the subject has been well reviewed[1] in other texts. This chapter should be read in conjunction with Ch. 63, nutrition, which defines the body compartments, the nutritional requirements of elderly people, and methods of measuring body adiposity.

In this chapter I will stress the clinical importance of obesity in elderly people, describe the difficulties in helping patients lose weight, correct some of the obesity mythology, and explain the pivotal role of the medical profession in the management of overweight and obese elderly patients.

Definition

By convention, the weights of males and females of different heights as shown by the 1983 Metropolitan Life Insurance Company tables have been accepted as normal. These tables, however, offer no correction for the age of the subjects.

In the United Kingdom people weighing in excess of 110 percent of the accepted normal weight for their height are referred to as overweight, those weighing in excess of 120 percent of the accepted normal weight are referred to as obese, and those weighing more than 130 percent of the accepted limit are described as suffering from morbid obesity.

It is now generally agreed that it is not only the degree of obesity that determines the pathologic outcome but also the distribution of the excess fat (see later). Central obesity with fat concentrated around the abdominal viscera (an "apple shape") is accepted as being more hazardous than excess fat concentrated around the buttocks, hips, and thighs (a "pear shape").

Measurement

Instead of referring to standard tables of heights and weights, most clinicians quote a patient's body mass index (BMI) or Quetelet's index. This figure is calculated by dividing the patient's weight in kilograms by the square of their height in meters (kg/m^2). In Europe patients with a BMI between 25 and 30 kg/m^2 are considered overweight. In this text, as in many publications, the BMI units (kg/m^2) will be omitted. Individuals with a BMI greater than 30 are obese, and those with a BMI greater than 40 are regarded as suffering from morbid obesity. In the United States the cutoff point for overweight is 27.8 in men and 27.3 for women, with severe overweight occurring in men with a BMI greater than 31.1 and in women with a BMI greater than 32.3. In the United States morbid obesity has been defined as a BMI of 39 or greater.[2] In this text I will use the European cutoff points of 25 and 30 to separate the overweight from the obese.

Body Fat Distribution

Both obesity and central body fat distribution are related to multiple adverse changes in cardiovascular risk factors. By dividing the waist circumference, at the level of the umbilicus, by the hip circumference at the level of the iliac crest, the waist/hip ratio[3] (WHR) can be calculated. This ratio correlates positively with the amount of visceral fat mass, which has metabolic characteristics that are unique in comparison with other adipose tissues.[4]

Visceral adipose tissue is associated with hyperinsulinism, insulin resistance, and high, amounts of free fatty acids.[5] This leads to an impairment of glucose tolerance,[6] high total triglyceride and low high-density lipoprotein (HDL) cholesterol concentrations[7] and hypertension.[8]

Thus central body fat distribution is associated with an increased risk for non-insulin-dependent diabetes mellitus (NIDDM) in middle-aged subjects even after accounting for overall obesity.[9,10] In the same population central body fat distribution has been consistently shown to be associated with an increased risk of coronary heart disease, again independently of obesity.[11,12]

Although the effect of obesity and fat distribution on glucose tolerance and cardiovascular risk factor levels has been thoroughly investigated in middle-aged subjects, little is known about this effect in the elderly.

Mykkänen and coworkers[13] have re-examined the relationship between obesity and waist/hip ratio in elderly people. They concluded that obesity per se rather than its distribution was a more significant determinant of glucose and insulin as well as total triglyceride and HDL cholesterol levels in elderly subjects. This observation could be explained by the fact that, with advancing age, fat tends to be distributed around the abdomen in both males and females.

Prevalence of Obesity

One of the Health of the Nation policy targets is "to reduce the percentages of men and women aged 16–64 who are obese by at least 25% for men and at least 33% for women by 2005 (from 8% for men and 12% for women in 1986/87 to no more than 6% and 8% respectively)."[14] It is interesting to note that elderly people are excluded from these goals.

Obesity is more prevalent among the "young old" (65 to 75 years), with the National Centre for Health Statistics (1987) finding just over 10 percent to be severely overweight[19] and 25 percent of men and 35 percent of women overweight.

The prevalence of obesity is rising in developed and developing countries, and this trend is affecting the older population as well. Two cross-sectional surveys,[15] involving residents aged 50 or more in a Jerusalem neighborhood showed a higher mean BMI and an increased prevalence of obesity in 1986 compared with 1970. It is interesting to note that the prevalence of obesity peaked in the 55 to 64-year-old group and fell progressively to the lowest level in the 75 to 84-year-old group. This trend was observed in both 1970 and 1986 and was reflected in both men and women, although the prevalence of obesity was higher in women.

Causes of Obesity

Overweight and obesity arise when the total energy intake exceeds the energy output. There is *no* other cause. Many patients attending obesity clinics feel that they are unique in that they eat little and yet continue to gain weight, ascribing this abnormality to an abnormally low metabolic rate. In a comprehensive summary of the causes of and associations with obesity, Kopelman[16] points out that less than 10 percent of patients have a primary endocrine condition or a secondary endocrine disorder associated with obesity.

In general only two endocrine causes of obesity need be considered: hypothyroidism and Cushing's syndrome. The latter should be clinically apparent from the history and physical signs. Weight gain after steroid treatment is more common. Hypothyroidism is also more common than Cushing's syndrome but impossible to exclude on clinical grounds. Thyroid function tests should be done on *all* overweight individuals prior to medical treatment. We have identified two new covert hypothyroid patients attending our weight management clinic. Like other known obese hypothyroid patients, they require a restricted caloric intake as well as thyroxine, to help them lose weight.

To understand the mechanism of excessive weight gain one must review the two components of the metabolic equation, energy expenditure and energy intake.

Energy Expenditure

Three components of energy expenditure can be easily identified by measuring the metabolic rate under varying conditions.

Resting metabolic rate

The lowest or the basal metabolic rate (BMR)[17] occurs transiently during the early morning hours of deep sleep. In clinical practice this transient basal rate has little influence on total energy requirements and is often impractical to measure. Another state of metabolism is the resting metabolic rate (RMR) which occurs while a person is resting and fasting. The RMR is the best predictor of the person's overall requirements and usually approximates 65 to 70 percent of the daily energy requirements of most ambulatory humans; it also reflects almost all the energy requirements of bedridden hospitalized patients.[18] In healthy elderly people body weight alone predicted RMR when compared with other indexes of body composition. The influence of age on RMR was trivial, and regional distribution of fat had no influence. There were wide 95 percent confidence limits of RMR in both lean and obese subjects. Thus metabolic efficiency was not necessarily or exclusively related to obesity.

Dietary-induced thermogenesis

Dietary-induced thermogenesis (DIT) is the increase in energy associated with eating and digesting a meal and accounts for 10 percent of total daily energy expenditure.

Thermic effect of physical activity

The thermic effect of physical activity is the most variable component of daily energy expenditure and includes less conscious muscular activity, such as shivering and fidgeting, as well as purposeful exercise.

Poehlman[19] has shown that all these components of daily expenditure decline with age. Energy intake also declines with age, but intake and expenditure do not decline proportionally, leading to an energy imbalance characterized by obesity or leanness. This is at variance with the findings of Owen[18] mentioned above.

Energy Intake

Until recently it has been impossible to obtain a true measure of a patient's dietary intake. In the past we were dependent on the patient providing an accurate dietary history or else observing the individual under unnatural conditions, such as in a metabolic unit. Now, using a doubly labeled water ($^2H_2{}^{18}O$) technique, it is possible to measure total daily energy expenditure in free-living subjects. Prentice[20] and others using this method have convincingly demonstrated that, despite claims to the contrary, the obese grossly misreport their caloric intake. Dietary histories can no longer be accepted as accurate since the obese underestimate their dietary intake by as much as 40 percent.[21]

Consequences of Obesity

Obesity causes, or is associated with, many complications (Table 64-1), all generally recognized to increase mortality and morbidity. In the absence of complicating factors the clinician has to decide whether treating obesity is warranted, particularly in light of some evidence that longevity is increased

Table 64-1 Risks associated with obesity

Disorders Directly Caused by Obesity	Disorders Aggravated by Obesity
Diabetes mellitus (NIDDM)[39]	All cardiorespiratory disorders
Hypertension	Esophagitis
Ischemic heart disease	Anesthetic risks
Hernias and uterine prolapse	Postoperative complications
Sleep apnoea (Pickwickian syndrome)	Arthritis
Malignant disease	Hyperlipidemia

Abbreviation: NIDDM, non-insulin-dependent diabetes mellitus.

in the overweight. For example a 5-year longitudinal study performed by Matilla et al.[22] (1986) in 526 people over the age of 85 showed that the overweight elderly (BMI greater than 30, 53 percent mortality) survived longer than those with the lowest weight (BMI less than 20, 87 percent mortality).

Similarly, in another study on the hypertensive elderly, total mortality and cardiovascular and noncardiovascular terminating events were highest in patients in the leanest BMI quintile. Thus these workers report that the association between BMI and cardiovascular end points was U-shaped.[23]

Kinney and Caldwell[24] have pointed out that not all mortality studies on elderly people have controlled for cigarette smoking, hypertension, glucose intolerance, or subclinical disease. When early deaths were excluded (presumably due to subclinical disease) in subjects over 75 years old, the only variable significantly related to survival was age. Interestingly they concluded that there was no ideal weight per se for aged men. The lowest BMI was associated with decreased survival, but none of the aged men had a BMI greater than 36.5. They suggest that men with a high BMI might die before reaching 75 years of age.

Most clinicians agree that obesity in diabetic and hypertensive patients requires treatment, but they may hesitate before treating the "healthy" obese. Hubert[25] has reviewed publications concerned with the relationship between obesity and cardiovascular disease. It is well established that obesity is associated with elevated blood pressure and high levels of blood lipids, lipoproteins, and blood glucose and that changes in body weight are accompanied by changes in these risk factors for cardiovascular disease. Both clinical and epidemiologic evidence suggests that even mild obesity may "lie at the beginning of the chain of events leading to disease causation" and that preventive strategies that include weight control need to be encouraged.

Some studies suggest that the increased risk observed in heavier individuals is due primarily to the influence of the associated risk factors and not to the degree of obesity per se. This has been interpreted as suggesting that obesity is benign when it exists without other major risk factors for disease.

The Framingham Study[26] and other long-term prospective studies[27,28] concerned with the independent role of obesity in cardiovascular risk challenge this notion. Some may argue that the physician treating the elderly patient is not primarily concerned with disease prevention and that managing obesity is the work of others.

The Value of Treating Obesity in Elderly Patients

Clinicians and patients demand evidence of the benefits of medical intervention. However, it is impossible to conduct "placebo-controlled" double-blind trials demonstrating the long-term benefits of weight loss, and whether the healthy obese should be treated is an unresolved issue.

According to Garrow,[29] "obesity is associated with serious morbidity and mortality, and the more overweight and the younger the patient the more severe the health implications. Since many of the diseases related to obesity are crippling rather than killing diseases, so the mortality figures tend to underestimate the importance of obesity as a public health problem."

My experience running an obesity clinic for 9 years leads me to believe that healthy obese patients are the exception rather than the rule. Obesity, like hypothyroidism, has a gradual onset, and most obese patients remain unaware of their increasing incapacity. Even in the absence of overt cardiovascular or respiratory disease, these patients all comment on improved breathing, exercise tolerance, and well-being following a small (5 percent) reduction in weight (unpublished data).

Results in elderly patients are no different from those in younger patients. We found that elderly patients responded just as well as younger patients to a very low-calorie treatment regimen (Table 64-2) provided they gained some clinical advantage to offset the inconvenience of weekly visits to the clinic. The prospect of hip or knee replacement is a strong motivating factor. In our experience minimal weight loss leads to an improvement in patients' breathing, angina, diabetes, and hypertension, with a corresponding reduction in drug dosage. Olefsky and coworkers[30] found a 33 percent decrease in insulin resistance and a 40 percent decrease in very low-density triglyceride production in obese subjects after weight reduc-

Table 64-2 The effect of age on the response to a very low-calorie diet[a]

Age	Total No.	Percentage Weight Loss			
		<0	0–10%	10–20%	>20%
<65 years	559	33 (6%)	280 (50%)	152 (27%)	94 (17%)
>65 years	47	1 (2%)	23 (49%)	17 (36%)	6 (13%)

[a] *The number (and percentage) of obese patients, below and above the age of 65, losing varying percentages of their initial body weight. All subjects were managed on a very low calorie diet (Lipotrim, Howard Research Foundation, Cambridge, UK) at the Hope Hospital Weight Management Clinic.*

tion.[30] They observed no difference in this objective biochemical response between the five most and the five least obese men in their experimental group after an average weight loss of 11 kg. They concluded that modest decreases in weight can initiate profound metabolic changes. Thus patients do not have to achieve their ideal body weight to benefit clinically and biochemically from weight loss.

Practical Management of the Obese Elderly

In getting patients to lose weight, one must examine both parts of the energy equation, energy intake and energy output.

Increasing energy output appears to be a reasonable way to get elderly people to lose weight. However, to dissipate 420 kJ (100 kcal) the patient would have to walk or run 1 mile, which is not an easy option in a less mobile elderly patient.

A study by Reed et al.[31] measured physical exercise by questionnaire, body adiposity by anthropometry and bioelectric impedance, and muscle strength using a hand-held dynamometer in 213 healthy ambulatory patients over the age of 60 (mean age 70). Muscle strength increased with the increase in physical exercise. However, the level of reported physical exercise over the range of 0 to 6,418 kJ/d [0 to 1,520 Kcal/d] did not predict body adiposity in the healthy elderly population. Those exercising were probably eating more, and the authors conclude that "to decrease body fat without modifying caloric consumption in elderly individuals would require a more intensive exercise regimen."

Decreasing energy intake is not an easy option. In 1958 Stunkard[32] summarized the results of the previous 30 years of experience of treating obesity as follows: "Most obese persons will not stay in treatment for obesity. Of those who stay in treatment, most will not lose weight, and of those who do lose weight, most will regain it."

This depressing finding continues to be the experience of clinicians referring their obese patients to dietitians for treatment on conventional diets. It is not surprising that few doctors are interested in directly managing their obese patients despite the fact that, as with other lifestyle changes (e.g., smoking cessation and blood pressure control), even minimal physician involvement may enhance outcome.[33]

However, there is some good news. Reviewing the results of clinical research trials, Wadden[34] revealed that patients treated in randomized trials using a conventional 5,040-kJ/d (1,200-kcal/d) reducing diet, combined with behavior modification, lost approximately 8.5 kg in 20 weeks, maintaining approximately two-thirds of this weight loss 1 year later. Patients treated under medical supervision using a very low-calorie diet (1,680 to 3,360 kJ/d [400 to 800 kcal/d]) lost approximately 20 kg in 12 to 16 weeks and maintained one-half to two-thirds of this loss in the following year. These results are certainly better than the earlier experience of Stunkard.

Two other issues need to be addressed: why patients fail to lose weight and whether repeated dieting can lead to weight gain by decreasing the lean body mass (LBM), thereby reducing the patient's caloric requirement.

Why Patients Fail to Lose Weight

Most doctors do not understand why many of their obese patients fail to lose weight on conventional low-calorie diets. They and their patients are too ready to accept the idea that the obese suffer from some abnormality in metabolic rate. This problem has been thoroughly dealt with by Kreitzman,[35] who makes the following points.

- The rapid initial weight loss on any reduced-calorie diet consists predominantly of water, with every pound of glycogen (7,560 kJ [1,800 kcal]) catabolized releasing 4 lb of water. To lose an equivalent weight (5 lb) of fat would require a 73,500-kJ (17,500-kcal [5 × 3,500]) deficit.
- Any restriction of caloric intake is countered by up to a 15 percent reduction in RMR.
- The RMR is linearly related to the patient's weight. Hence with increasing weight loss the RMR decreases, and even further reductions in caloric intake are necessary to maintain weight loss.
- Dietitians, let alone patients, cannot accurately calculate the caloric content of a conventional food diet. In one study[36] 4,200-kJ (1,000-kcal) diet sheets prepared by hospital dietitians were found, after careful examination by nutrition experts, to provide 4,305 to 6,917 kJ (1,025 to 1,647 kcal).

It is easy to see why many dieting patients lose heart rather than weight. The initial encouraging weight loss (predominantly fluid) is followed by a much slower weight loss which diminishes even further with time. Excessive fluid loss in the early phases of dieting may lead to a diminished circulating blood volume and a fall in blood pressure. The patient may feel "faint" and "weak," erroneously attributing this to a need for food rather than a requirement for fluid. It is therefore important that the dieting patient understand the pathophysiology of weight loss and that fluid intake be carefully monitored, especially if very low-calorie diets are used.

The calorie content of a "natural" diet varies enormously with the type of food eaten. Any unintentional miscalculation of dietary caloric content may cause patients to gain weight, which makes them depressed and unhappy. They begin to overeat in earnest and then blame dieting for damaging their metabolic rate permanently and being the *cause* of their obesity. It is for this reason that I favor the use of commercially prepared, prepackaged, very low-calorie diets in elderly patients who fail to lose weight on normal diets. No calculation of calories is required, the macro- and micronutrient content of the diet is known, and portions do not have to be carefully weighed. Thus the dieting process is considerably simplified.

Effects of Weight Cycling on Body Composition

Many patients seeking help for weight loss give a history of weight regain being substantially greater after periods of successful weight loss. It has been argued that it is the repeated cycles of weight loss and regain that make people fat,[37] the mechanism allegedly being an inappropriate and irreversible loss of LBM. Prentice and colleagues[38] present good animal and human, clinical and experimental evidence against this commonly accepted myth. They have shown that natural weight cycling in a rural Gambian population does not lead to a more rapid age-related loss of lean mass than occurs in better nourished, noncycling populations. Furthermore, the substantial published animal studies, which they review, are remarkable in agreeing that body composition is unaffected by weight cycling. Their own study of experimental yo-yo dieting in humans revealed no evidence of excessive lean tissue loss and in fact provided some indication of the reverse.

Why then do patients tend to regain more weight after bouts of restricted intake? The majority of overweight people look forward to returning to their "normal" diet once they have lost weight. They fail to appreciate that having lost weight they can never go back to their previous eating habits. Doctors and dietitians do not stress the simple physiologic fact that lighter people need fewer calories to maintain their weight than do heavier subjects. The previously obese patient who returns to their normal eating habits rapidly regains weight, becomes depressed, eats even more and, as already noted, attributes their failure to loss of LBM and a damaged metabolism.

Summary

Obesity is not as common in elderly people as in younger adults, perhaps because obesity is associated with a higher mortality in the young. Excessive weight is more incapacitating in elderly people than in the young because of the general decrease in muscle mass and the additional pathology associated with aging. Clinicians are less willing to subject elderly patients to rigorous dietary regimens because they feel that the risks outweigh the advantages and because most overweight patients (regardless of age) do badly on diets. The negative attitude of the physician (and dietitian) is readily apparent to the patient, and failure is guaranteed.

Elderly obese patients should see some clinical advantage in weight loss. They must appreciate that dietary restriction is the only really effective way to lose a significant amount of weight. Commercial prepackaged vitamin- and mineral-supplemented meal replacements are the only way to ensure that elderly patients receive adequate replacement of micronutrients. The author has successfully used very low-calorie diets (less than 3,360 kJ/d [800 kcal/d]) in such patients. It is important to maintain careful medical monitoring at weekly intervals of the patients' weight, blood pressure, fluid intake, and drug therapy, which will need alteration with weight loss. These diets may or may not be supplemented by small (prepackaged) standard meals of known macronutrient content.

There is no need to aim for a BMI of 25 kg/m^2 since the lower the final weight, the more difficulty the patient will have maintaining this weight. Caloric intake can be increased once the patient feels better and the desired effect on blood pressure, angina, or breathing has been obtained. The patient will then need to be re-educated regarding their eating habits and seen regularly at a weight maintenance clinic. Increased exercise can help to maintain the weight loss.

If physicians took a more active, positive role in the management of obesity in elderly patients, patients' hospital stays and medication could be reduced and the quality of their life improved. Those caring for elderly people must accept that obesity is a chronic recurrent problem requiring lifelong management and that even minimal but sustained weight loss has clinical benefits, fully justifying their efforts.

References

1. Morley JE, Glick Z: Obesity. pp. 245–255. In Morley JE, Glick Z, Rubinstein LZ (eds): Geriatric Nutrition. Raven Press, New York, 1995
2. Kuczmarski RJ: Prevalence of overweight and weight gain in the United States. Am J Clin Nutr 1992;55:495S–502S
3. Kalkoff RK, Hartz AH, Rupley D et al: Relationship of body fat distribution to blood pressure, carbohydrate tolerance and plasma lipids in healthy obese women. J Lab Clin Med 1983; 102:621–627
4. Seidell JC, Björntorp P, Sjöström L et al: Regional distribution of muscle and fat mass in men—new insight into the risk of abdominal obesity using computed tomography. Int J Obes 1989;13:289–303
5. Reaven GM: Role of insulin resistance in human disease. Diabetes 1988;37:1595–1607
6. Fujioka S, Matsuzawa Y, Tokunaga K, Tarui S: Contribution of intra-abdominal fat accumulation to the impairment of glucose and lipid metabolism in human obesity. Metabolism 1987;36: 54–59
7. Despres JP, Moorjani S, Lupien PJ et al: Regional distribution of body fat, plasma lipoproteins and cardiovascular disease. Arteriosclerosis 1990;10:497–511
8. Peiris AN, Sothmann MS, Hoffmann RG et al: Adiposity, fat distribution, and cardiovascular risk. Ann Intern Med 1989; 110:867–872
9. Ohlson LO, Larsson B, Svärdsudd K et al: The influence of body fat distribution on the incidence of diabetes mellitus: 13.5 years of follow-up of participants in the study of men born in 1913. Diabetes 1985;34:1055–1058
10. Lundgren H, Bengtsson C, Blohme G et al: Adiposity and adipose tissue distribution in relation to incidence of diabetes in women: results from a prospective population study in Gothenburg, Sweden. Int J Obes 1989;13:413–423
11. Larsson B, Svärdsudd K, Welin L et al: Abdominal adipose tissue distribution, obesity and risk of cardiovascular disease and death: 13 year follow-up of participants in the study of men born in 1913. BMJ 1984;288:1401–1404
12. Lapidus L, Bengtsson C, Larsson B et al: Distribution of adipose tissue and risk of cardiovascular disease and death: a 12 year follow-up of participants in the population study of women in Gothenburg, Sweden. BMJ 1984;289:1257–1261
13. Mykkänen L, Laakso M, Pyörälä K: Association of obesity and distribution of obesity with glucose tolerance and cardiovascular risk factors in the elderly. Int J Obes 1992;16:695–704

14. The Health of the Nation: A Strategy for Health in England. HMSO, London, 1992
15. Gofin J, Abramson JH, Kark JD, Epstein L: The prevalence of obesity and its changes over time in middle-aged and elderly men and women in Jerusalem. Int J Obes 1996;20:260–266
16. Kopelman PG: Investigation of obesity. J Clin Endocrinol 1994; 41:703–708
17. Ravussin E, Burnand B, Schutz Y, Jequier E: Twenty-four-hour energy expenditure and resting metabolic rate in obese, moderately obese and control subjects. Am J Clin Nutr 1982; 35:566–573
18. Owen OE: Resting metabolic requirement of men and women. Mayo Clin Proc 1988;53:503–510
19. Poehlman ET: Energy expenditure and requirements in aging humans. J Nutr 1992;122:2057–2065
20. Prentice AM: Assessing food intake in obese people. Micrographia 1994;16:29–32
21. Bandini LG, Schoeller DA, Cyr HN, Dietz WH: Validity of reported energy intake in obese and non-obese adolescents. Am J Clin Nutr 1990;52:421–425
22. Matilla K, Haavisto M, Rajala S: Body mass index and mortality in the elderly. BMJ 1986;292:867–868
23. Tuomilehto J: Body mass index and prognosis in elderly hypertensive patients: a report from the European Working Party on High Blood Pressure in the Elderly. Am J Med 1991;90(suppl 3A):34S–41S
24. Kinney EL, Caldwell JW: Relationship between body weight and mortality in men aged 75 years and older. Southern Med J 1990;83:1256–1258
25. Hubert HB: The nature of the relationship between obesity and cardiovascular disease. Int J Cardiol 1984;6:268–274
26. Hubert HB, Feinleib M, McNamara PM et al: Obesity as an independent risk factor for cardiovascular diseases: a 26 year followup of participants in the Framingham Heart Study. Circulation 183;67:968–977
27. Manson JE, Colditz GA, Stampfer MJ: A prospective study of obesity and risk of coronary heart disease in women. N Engl J Med 190;332:882–889
28. Rabkin SW, Mathewson FAL, Hsu PH: Relation of body weight to development of ischaemic heart disease in a cohort of young North American men after a 26 year observation period: the Manitoba Study. Am J Cardiol 1977;39:452–458
29. Garrow JS: Obesity and Related Diseases. Churchill Livingstone, Edinburgh, 1988
30. Olefsky J, Reaven GM, Farquhar JW: Effects of weight reduction on obesity: studies of lipid and carbohydrate metabolism in normal and hyperlipoproteinaemic subjects. J Clin Invest 1974;53:64–76
31. Reed RL, Yochum K, Pearlmutter L et al: The interrelationship between physical exercise, muscle strength and body adiposity in a healthy elderly population. J Am Geriatr Soc 1991;39: 1189–1193
32. Stunkard AJ: The management of obesity. N Y State J Med 1958;58:79–87
33. Blackburn GL: Comparison of medically supervised and unsupervised approaches to weight loss and control. Ann Intern Med 1993;119:714–718
34. Wadden TA: Treatment of obesity by moderate and severe caloric restriction: results of clinical research trials. Ann Intern Med 1993;119:688–693
35. Kreitzman SN: Why patients fail to lose weight. pp. 430–433. In Brown JS, Gray DJP, Horne RA, McBride M (eds): The Royal College of General Practitioners Members' Reference Book 1993. Sabrecrown Publishing, London, 1993
36. Stordy BJ: Data presented at Physician Conference on Obesity Management. Swiss Cottage, London, 1991
37. Cannon G, Einzig H: Dieting makes you fat. Century Publishing, London, 1983
38. Prentice AM, Jebb SA, Goldberg GR et al: Effects of weight cycling on body composition. Am J Clin Nutr 1992;56: 209S–216S
39. West KM: Epidemiology of diabetes and its vascular complications. Elsevier, New York, 1978

CHAPTER 65

Aging of the Urinary Tract

VANITA JASSAL
HOWARD FILLIT
DIMITRIOS G. OREOPOULOS

The study of the aging process in the kidney is beset by difficulties. One major problem, as in all gerontologic research, is to distinguish between changes influenced by "normal" aging, and those influenced by disease. With the possible exception of the lung, the changes in kidney function with normal aging are the most dramatic of any human organ or organ system. In a normal young adult, renal capacity far exceeds the ordinary demands for solute and water conservation and excretion. In old age, renal function, while substantially diminished, still provides, under ordinary circumstances, for adequate regulation of the volume and composition of extracellular fluid. However, the reduced function of the kidney has important clinical implications for diagnosis and treatment of many disorders and clearly reduces the individual's capacity to respond to a variety of physiologic and pathologic stresses.

Epidemiology and symptomatology of renal disease in the elderly, diagnostic difficulties, and response to treatment are problems about which there is still a lack of basic information. In general, renal disease in the aged is often caused by several concomitant pathoanatomic changes. Atherosclerosis, infection, and age-induced changes might occur simultaneously. The diagnostic entities are not so clear cut as in younger individuals.

Anatomic Changes

Changes in the Nephron

Age-induced renal changes are manifested macroscopically by a reduction in weight of the kidney and a loss of parenchymal mass. According to Oliver,[1] the average combined weight of the kidneys in different age groups is as follows: 60 years, 250 g; 70 years, 230 g; 80 years, 190 g. The decrease in weight of the kidneys corresponds to a general decrease in the size and weight of all organs.[2] Microscopically, the most impressive changes are reductions in the number and size of nephrons. Loss of parenchymal mass leads to a widening of the interstitial spaces between the tubules. There is also an increase in the interstitial connective tissue with age.

The total number of identifiable glomeruli falls with age, roughly in accord with the changes in renal weight.[3] The number of sclerotic glomeruli identified on light microscopy increases from 1 to 2 percent during the third to fifth decades, to 12 after age 70.[4,5]

Aging is associated with a loss of lobulation of the glomerular tuft, thus decreasing effective filtering surface. Although the total number of nuclei per glomerulus is unchanged with age, the filtering surface is diminished by a progressive increase in the number of mesangial cells after age 40, and a reciprocal decrease in the number of epithelial cells. The mesangium, which accounts for roughly 8 percent of total glomerular volume at age 45, increases to nearly 12 percent by age 70.[6] Glomerular basement membrane thickening may occur during aging.[7] Biochemical changes of significance also occur, such as changes in the degree of sulfation of basement membrane glycosaminoglycans.[8] However, despite these changes, studies of glomerular filtration characteristics show no differences in permeability with aging.[9]

Darmady et al.[7] have shown an interesting change in the distal convoluted tubule. They observed that the number of diverticula in the distal convoluted tubules increased with age. They reasoned that these diverticula might play a part in the production of pyelonephritis, through harboring organisms and causing and maintaining recurrence of renal infection in the aged. It has been suggested that these diverticula represent the origin of the simple retention cysts commonly seen in the elderly.[3]

Vascular Changes

Changes in the intrarenal vasculature with age, independent of hypertension or other renal diseases, are probably responsible for most clinically relevant changes in renal function with age. Normal aging is associated with variable sclerotic changes in the walls of the larger renal vessels. These sclerotic changes do not encroach on the lumen, and are augmented in the presence of hypertension.[4] Smaller vessels appear to be spared, with fewer than 20 percent of senescent kidneys from nonhypertensive individuals displaying arteriolar changes.[10]

Combined microangiographic and histologic studies have identified very distinctive patterns of change in arteriolar-glomerular units with senescence.[11,12] In the cortex, hyalinization and collapse of the glomerular tuft is associated with obliteration of the lumen of the preglomerular arteriole and a resultant loss in blood flow. Changes in the juxtamedullary area are

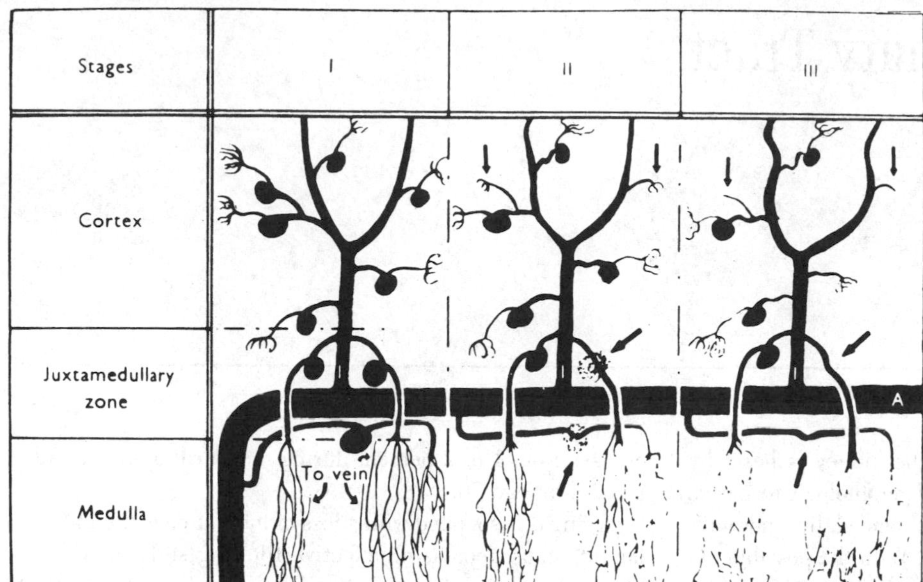

Figure 65-1 Changes in the intrarenal arterial pattern with age. (A, arcuate artery. 1, interlobular artery.) Stage I—basic adult pattern showing glomerular arterioles; stage II—partial degeneration of some glomeruli. Two cortical afferent arterioles ramify into remnants of glomerular tufts (small arrows). Two juxtamedullary arterioles pass through partially degenerated glomeruli (large arrows). There is slight spiraling of interlobular arteries and afferent arterioles. Stage III—two cortical afferent arterioles now end blindly (small arrows), and two juxtamedullary arterioles are agromerular (large arrows). The corresponding glomerular tufts have degenerated completely. The spiraling of interlobular arteries and afferent arterioles is now more pronounced. (From Ljungqvist and Lagergren,[12] with permission.)

characterized by the development of anatomic continuity between the afferent and efferent arterioles during glomerular sclerosis. The end point is thus loss of the glomerulus and shunting of blood flow from afferent to efferent arterioles. Blood flow is maintained to the arteriolar rectae verae, the primary vascular supply of the medulla, which are not decreased in number with age (Fig. 65-1).

In humans, it is difficult to differentiate between age-induced changes and changes caused by past renal disease. Changes due to arteriosclerosis in connection with hypertension, diabetes, and pyelonephritis are very common. The histologic appearance of kidney structure in the elderly without any evidence of pathology is rare. According to Brocklehurst,[13] an analysis of 100 consecutive autopsies on geriatric patients at Farnborough Hospital, England, showed normal histology in only 3 percent of the cases.

Functional Changes

Renal Blood Flow

A progressive reduction in renal plasma flow of approximately 10 percent per decade from 600 mL/min. in young adulthood to 300 mL/min by 80 years of age is well-established.[15,16] Detailed studies indicate selective loss of cortical vasculature with preservation of medullary flow. These cortical vascular changes likely account for the patchy cortical defects commonly seen on renal scans in healthy older adults. This histologic and functional demonstration of selective decrease in cortical flow may explain the observation that filtration fraction (the fraction of renal plasma flow that is filtered at the glomerulus) actually increases with advancing age, since outer cortical nephrons have a lower filtration fraction than juxtamedullary nephrons.

As local changes in the vascular tone of both afferent and efferent renal arterioles control renal blood flow and glomerular filtration rate (GFR), any alteration in renal vascular reactivity to circulating and local mediators, including endothelin, endothelin-derived relaxing factor (EDRF), and the renin angiotensin system, would cause the hemodynamic alterations seen in aged kidneys. Renal responsiveness to vasoconstrictor stimuli including angiotensin II, endothelin, and EDRF-blockers (for example L-NAME and L-NMME) cause exaggerated responses in aging rat kidneys.[17–19] In contrast, responses to vasodilators, including angiotensinogen-converting enzyme (ACE) inhibitors and losartan (an angiotensin-II blocker), are normal. A relative increase in endogenous EDRF activity preserves the renal blood flow and GFR, but reduces the vasodilatory reserve and adaptation to superimposed hemodynamic insults. Although the literature is incomplete, and in some cases contradictory, an overall picture of increased vasoconstriction and decreased vasodilator reserve of the renal vascular bed is seen with age.

Glomerular Filtration Rate

The major clinically relevant renal function defect arising from these histologic and physiologic changes is a progressive decline after maturity in the GFR whether estimated by the clearance of inulin or creatinine. Age-adjusted normative standards for creatinine clearance have been established.[20] Creatinine clearance is stable until the middle of the fourth decade when a linear decrease of about 8.0 mL/min per 1.73 m^2/decade begins (Fig. 65.2).

The decrease in GFR with age is not matched by an elevation in serum creatinine.[20] Because muscle mass, from which creatinine is derived, falls with age at roughly the same rate as GFR, the rather drastic age-related loss of renal function is not reflected in an elevation of serum creatinine. Thus, serum creatinine often overestimates GFR in the elderly.

Although methods for estimating creatinine clearance based on normative data employing various formulae have been developed,[21,22] the reliability of these formulae has recently been questioned.[23,24] Up to one-third of elderly patients may have no decline in glomerular filtration rate with aging, and some individuals actually demonstrate an increase in glomerular filtration rate with aging.[25] As the individual rate of decline cannot be predicted, creatinine clearance should not be estimated using only the serum creatinine. Even the most commonly used formula, published by Cockcroft and Gault,[21] leads to a mean underestimation of measured creatinine clearance of 12.1 mL/min in a healthy group of patients.[24] In a comparison of 15 equations used to estimate creatinine clearance in healthy elderly patients, none correlated closely to measured clearance. The average bias ranged from −33.1 mL/min to + 19.6 mL/min. Equations were variable in their erroneous placement of individuals into renal function categories.[24] Elderly patients with apparently normal serum creatinine and blood urea nitrogen levels may have clearances of 60 mL/min or less, even in the ambulatory and healthy elderly. Individual variation may be very high. In severely ill elderly patients on medications, the reliability of such estimations may be low, and because the frail elderly are the most susceptible to the dangers of overestimation of creatinine clearance when prescribing medications, the formulae should be used with caution. Timed urine collections, of short duration, for creatinine clearance are therefore recommended.[24,26] Depressions of GFR, so severe as to result in elevation of serum creatinine above 132 mmol/L (1.5 mg/dL), are rarely due solely to normal aging, and generally indicate the presence of an additional disease state.

Renal reserve function, a measure of the ability of the kidney to increase GFR in response to an increased protein or amino acid load, appears to be well preserved in the elderly.[27,28]

Tubular Function

Both excretory and reabsorptive capacities of the renal tubules decrease as age increases.[29–31] The decrease in tubular secretion of diodrast and para-amino-hippuric acid in the aged

Figure 65-2 Cross-sectional differences in standard creatinine clearance with age. The number of subjects in each age group is indicated above the abscissa. Values plotted indicate mean − SEM. The data represent creatinine clearance determinations based on measure of true creatinine. Creatinine autoanalyzer determinations in common clinical use will yield creatinine clearance values approximately 20 to 25 percent lower than results shown here. Values in women are approximately 20 percent lower than men. (From Rowe et al,[20] with permission.)

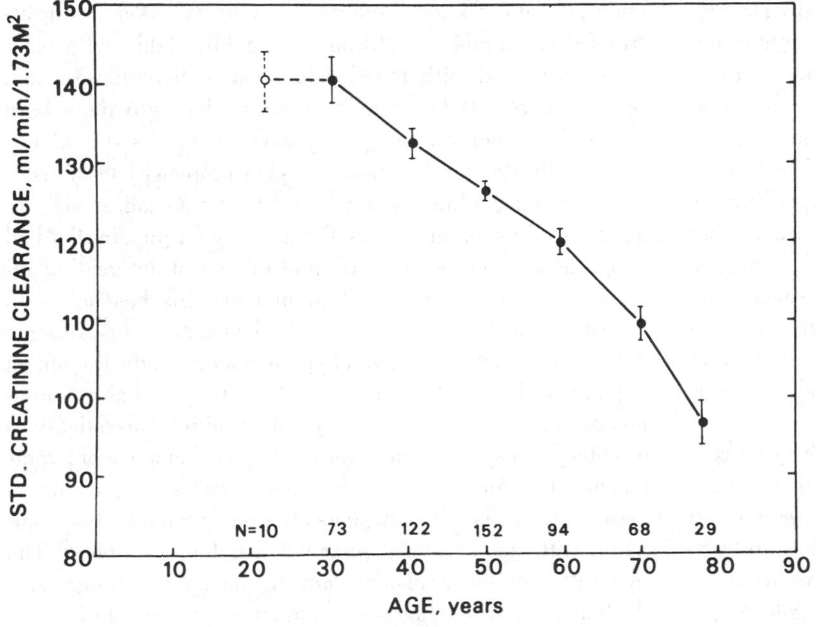

reveals a decrease in tubular function. The kidney of an old individual is, however, generally capable of maintaining a normal electrolyte and acid-base balance unless stressed.

Salt and water handling is impaired in stress states in the elderly individual. The ability to both conserve and excrete sodium is impaired. Animal and human studies show abnormal resorption of salt in the ascending loop of Henle,[32] reduced serum aldosterone secretion[33,34] and a relative resistance to both aldosterone and angiotensin-II.[35] Animal studies suggest a reduced renal Na-K-ATPase activity,[36] although this is not confirmed in human studies. The resultant effect is that older persons can maintain sodium balance in steady state but, when under stress, for example salt depletion or dehydration, they are unable to defend their intravascular and intracellular volume and osmolality. Antidiuretic hormone levels tend to be higher with increasing age, yet the maximal osmolality of urine falls by 5 percent every 10 years. The diluting capacity is decreased, but the overall free water clearance remains proportional to the GFR.

As with sodium balance, the elderly individual has difficulty maintaining potassium balance in stress states. An overall reduction in total body potassium by around 20 percent[37] presdiposes the individual to hypokalemia when given diuretics.

An acid load in the elderly patient causes a prolonged decrease in the pH and pCO^2 compared to younger individuals. Basal ammonium excretion appears unchanged, although a slower adaptive response is seen.[38–40]

Mechanisms of Age-Related Reductions in Renal Function

The precise causes of age-related changes in the kidney have not been fully elucidated. The proposed theories include the hyperfiltration theory,[41–43] based on the presence of a reduced nephron mass,[44] and progressive glomerulosclerosis.

Within the glomerulus, capillary blood flow rate and intracapillary hydraulic pressure are finely regulated by changes in vascular tone, to maintain a stable filtration pressure gradient. The term "single-nephron glomerular filtration rate" (SNGFR) has been coined to describe the filtration rate across the basement membrane of each individual nephron. A reduction in nephron number causes increased blood flow to each nephron and, therefore, increased SNGFR. The hyperfiltration hypothesis[42] proposes that, in a kidney with a reduced number of glomeruli, there is increased capillary blood flow through each glomerular capillary bed and, thus, a correspondingly high intracapillary pressure. This high pressure (often referred to as shear stress) results in local endothelial cell damage and resultant glomerular injury. Contrary to initial reports there is no alteration in systemic hemodynamics.[43]

As small increases in blood flow seen with increased SNGFR lead to disproportionate increases in pressure, endothelial cell damage occurs, causing platelet aggregation and thrombin production. Activation of platelets leads to release of growth factors including platelet-derived growth factor (PDGF), epidermal growth factor (EGF), fibroblast growth factor (FGF) and tumor necrosis factor-β (TNF-β), which are associated with increased fibroblast collagen production and mesangial cell sclerosis.[45–47] At the same time, shear stresses cause a disruption in the ion exchange, changes in cell membrane voltage, and altered protein transcription within the endothelial cells.[48] Alterations in the endothelin-derived relaxing factor (EDRF)/endothelin axis upset vascular hemodynamics and increase angiotensin II secretion. As glomeruli become sclerosed, the amount of blood flow directed to each of the remaining nephrons increases, further potentiating the damage.

In support of this theory, a reduction in glomerular capillary pressure associated with restricted protein intake decreases glomerular injury and can prolong the time to doubling of serum creatinine in patients with impaired creatinine clearances.[49,50] Similarly, antihypertensives, which reduce single-nephron GFR (e.g. ACE inhibitors and angiotensin-II blockers) reduce glomerular injury more than antihypertensives that solely control systemic blood pressure at comparable levels.[50] Experimentally, both reduced protein intake and ACE inhibitors cause local hemodynamic changes and decrease angiotensin-II. As angiotensin-II is a known growth factor causing increased mesangial hypercellularity and sclerosis, there is unresolved debate about whether the reduced glomerular injury is because of reduced local endothelial wall stress or because of reduced mitogenic stimulation.

Other factors, including sodium restriction, hyperglycemia, female gender, castration, adrenalectomy, and hypophysectomy have also been demonstrated to ameliorate age-related glomerular sclerosis in aging animals.

A reduced nephron mass at the time of birth is believed to contribute to the natural progression of renal disease. In animal models, renal ablation, resulting in a reduction in the number of functioning nephron units, causes single nephron hyperfiltration, progressive systemic hypertension, proteinuria, and renal failure associated with glomerular sclerosis.[41,49] Patients with congenital unilateral renal agenesis invariably show focal and segmental glomerulosclerosis on biopsy,[51–55] a finding attributed to chronic hyperfiltration from birth (although not always associated with the development of hypertension and renal impairment). One may hypothesize that individuals born with reduced nephron mass may have an increased tendency to hyperfiltrate and thus have a higher propensity for a faster rate of renal decline as illustrated by Lindeman et al.[25] In animal studies, pregnant rats fed a restricted protein diet had offspring with fewer glomeruli and tubular structures but increased connective tissue.[56] In humans this has not been shown, although epidemiologic data demonstrate a correlation between low-birth weight and hypertension.[57] In the transplant population, low nephron mass has been proposed as a nonimmunogenic cause of chronic transplant failure. Investigations of kidney transplant donors show a higher incidence of hypertension and proteinuria, and in some cases biopsy-proven glomerular sclerosis, 10 to 30 years after nephrectomy when compared with age- and sex-matched matched controls.[58] The hyperfiltration theory also explains the nonspecific progressive decline of renal function seen in many chronic renal diseases.

In patients with chronic poststreptococcal glomerulonephritis,[59] vesicoureteric reflux,[60] and diabetes mellitus,[61] once renal failure has reached a threshold level (estimated at a glomerular filtration rate of 30 mL/min or less), progression of renal failure may occur despite control of the underlying disease.

Some have questioned whether the hyperfiltration hypothesis truly accounts for glomerular sclerosis in aging humans.[31] Studies in animals suggest that neuroendocrine or immune mechanisms may play more important role in glomerular sclerosis than hyperfiltration.[62,63] Finally, the role of processes associated with normal aging, such as age-related changes in the vasculature, blood pressure, and serum glucose, and age-related diseases and syndromes, including atherosclerosis, hypertension, diabetes, and polypharmacy, on the progressive glomerular sclerosis seen in humans remains unclear.

References

1. Oliver J: Urinary system. In Cowdry EV (ed): Problems of Aging. Williams & Wilkins, Baltimore, 1952
2. Roessle R, Roulet F: Mass und Zahl in der Pathologie. Springer, Berlin, 1932
3. McLachlan MSF: The ageing kidney. Lancet 1978;ii:143–143
4. McLachlan MSF, Guthric JC, Anderson CK: Vascular and glomerular changes in the aging kidney. J Pathol 1977;121:65–65
5. Kaplan C, Pasternack B, Shah B: Age-related incidence of sclerotic glomeruli in human kidneys. Am J Pathol 1975;80:227
6. Sorenson F: Quantative studies of the renal corpuscles. Acta Med Scand 1977;85:356
7. Darmady EM, Offer J, Woodhouse MA: The parameters of the aging kidney. J Pathol 1973;195–209
8. Cohen MR, Kin L: Age-related changes in sulfation of basement membrane glycosaminoglycans. Exp Gerontol 1983;18: 461–469
9. Artursen G, Groth T, Grotte G: Human glomerular membrane porosity and filtration pressure: dextran clearance data analyzed by theoretical models. Clin Sci 1971;10:137
10. Mortiz AR, Oldt MR: Arteriolar sclerosis in hypertensive and non-hypertensive individuals. Am J Pathol 1973;13:679
11. Takazakura E, Sawabu N, Handa A et al: Intrarenal vascular changes with age and disease. Kid Int 1972;2:224
12. Ljungqvist A, Lagerggen C: Normal intrarenal arterial pattern in adult and aging human kidney. J Anat (London) 1962;96: 285
13. Brocklehurst JC: Clinical geriatrics. p. 227. In Rossman 1 (ed): Lippincott-Raven, Philadelphia, 1971
14. Wesson LG: Physiology of the Human Kidney. Grune & Stratton. New York, 1969
15. Holtenberg NK, Adams DF, Solomon HS, et al: Senescence and the renal vasculature in normal man. Circ Res 1974;34: 309–316
16. Hollenberg NK, Moore TJ: Age and the renal blood supply: renal vascular responses to angiotensin converting enzyme inhibition in healthy humans. J Am Geriatr Soc 1994;42:805–808
17. Sharma K, Ziyadeh FN: The emerging role of transforming growth factor-β in kidney diseases. Am J Physiol 1994;266: F829–F842
18. Mulkerrin EC, Brain A, Hampton D et al: Reduced renal haemodynamic response to atrial natriuretic peptide in elderly volunteers. Am J Kidney Dis 1993;22:538–544
19. Reckelhoff JF, Manning RD: Role of endothelium-derived nitric oxide in control of renal microvasculature in aging male rats. Am J Physiol 1993; 265:R1126–R1131
20. Rowe JW, Andres R, Tobin JD et al: The effect of age on creatinine clearance in man: a cross-sectional and longitudinal study. J Gerontol 1976;31:155–163
21. Cockcroft DW, Gault MH: Prediction of creatinine clearance from serum creatinine. Nephron 1976;16:31–41
22. Lott RD, Hayton WL: Estimation of creatinine clearance from serum creatinine concentration: a review. Drug Intell Clin Pharm 1978;12:140
23. Friedman JR, Norman DC, Yoshikawa TT: Correlation of estimated renal function parameters versus 24 hour creatinine clearance in ambulatory elderly. J Am Geriatr Soc 1989;37: 145–149
24. Malmrose LC, Gray SL, Pieper CF et al: Measured versus estimated creatinine clearance in a high-functioning elderly sample: MacArthur Foundation study of successful ageing. JAGS 1993;41:715–721
25. Lindeman RD, Tobin JD, Shock NW: Longitudinal studies on the rate of decline in renal function with age. J Am Geriatr Soc 1985;33:278–285
26. Goldberg TH, Finkelstein MS: Difficulties in estimating glomerular filtration rate in the elderly. Arch Intern Med 1987;147: 1430
27. DeSanto NG, Anastasio P, Coppola S et al: Age related changes in renal reserve and tubular changes in healthy humans. Child Nephrol Urol 1991;11:33–40
28. Bohler J, Gloer D, Reetze-Bonorden P, Keller E, Schollmeyer: Renal functional reserve in elderly patients. Clin Nephrol 1993; 39:145–150
29. Shock NW, Powers JH: The physiology of aging. WB Saunders, London, 1968
30. Frocht A, Fillit H: Renal disease in the geriatric patient. J Am Geriatr Soc 1984;32:28–43
31. Meyer BR: Renal function in aging. J Am Geriatr Soc 1989; 37:791–800
32. Macias Nunez JF, Garcia lglesias C, Bondia Roman A et al: Renal handling of sodium in old people: a functional study. Age Ageing 1978;7:178–181
33. Sambhi MP, Crane MG, Genest J: Essential hypertension: new concepts about mechanisms. Ann Int Med 1973;79:411–424
34. Tsunoda K, Abe K, Goto T et al: Effect of age on the renin-angiotensin-aldosterone system in normal subjects: simultaneous measurement of active and inactive renin, renin substrate, and aldosterone in plasma. J Clin Endocrinil Metabol 1986;62: 384–389
35. Duggan J, Nussberger J, Kilfeather S, O'Malley K: Aging and human hormonal and pressor responsiveness to angiotensin II infusion with similtaneous measurement of exogenous and endogenous angiotensin II. Am J Hypertens 1993;6:641–647
36. Benegle HH, Mathias R, Perkins JH et al: Impaired renal and

extrarenal potassium adaptation in old rats. Kidney Int 1983; 23:684–690

37. Cox JR, Shalaby WA: Potassium changes with age. Gerontology 1981;27:340–344
38. Adler S, Lindeman RD, Yiengst MJ et al: Effects of acute acid loading on urinary acid excretion by the aging kidney. J Lab Clin Med 1968;72:278–289
39. Agarwal BN, Cabebe FG: Renal acidification in elderly subjects. Nephron 1980;26:291–295
40. Shuck O, Nadvornikova H: Short acidification test and its interpretation with respect to age. Nephron 1987;46:215–216
41. Hostetter TH, Olson JL, Renneke HG et al: Hyperfiltration in remnant nephrons: a potentially adverse response to renal ablation. Am J Physiol 1981;241:F85–F93
42. Brenner BM: Nephron adaptation to renal injury or ablation. Am J Physiol 1985;249:F324–F337
43. Neuringer JR, Brenner BM: Haemodynamic theory of progressive renal disease: a 10 year update in brief review. Am J Kid Dis 1993;22:98–104
44. Brenner BM, Chertow GM: Congenital oligonephropathy and the etiology of adult hypertension and progressive renal injury. Am J Kid Dis 1994;23:171–175
45. Klahr S: Chronic renal failure management. Lancet 1991;338: 423–427
46. Wardle EN: Cytokine growth factors and glomerulonephritis. Nephron 1991;57:257–261
47. Wardle EN: Cellular biology of glomerulosclerosis. Nephron 1992;61:125–128
48. LaBarbera M: How fluid dynamics channel natural selection. Sci NY Acad Sci 1991;31:30–37
49. Brenner BM, Meyer TW, Hostetter TH: Dietary protein intake and the progressive nature of kidney disease: the role of haemodynamically mediated glomerular injury in the pathogenesis of progressive glomerular sclerosis in aging, renal ablation and intrinsic renal disease. N Engl J Med 1982;307:652–659
50. Zucchelli P, Zuccala A, Borghi M et al: Long-term comparison between captopril and nifedipine in the progression of renal insufficiency. Kid Int 1992;42:452–458
51. Thorner PS, Arbus GS, Celermajer DS, Baumal R: Focal segmental glomerulosclerosis and progressive renal failure associated with a unilateral kidney. Pediatrics 1984;73:806–810
52. Bhathena DB, Julian BA, McMorrow RG, Baehler RW: Focal sclerosis of hypertrophied glomeruli in solitary functioning kidneys of humans. Am J Kid Dis 1985;5:226–232
53. Weinstein T, Zevin D, Gafter U et al: Proteinuria and chronic renal failure associated with unilateral renal agenesis. Isr J Med Sci 1985;21:919–921
54. Rugiu C, Oldrizzi L, Lupo A et al: Clinical features of patients with solitary kidneys. Nephron 1986;43:10–15
55. Gutierrez-Millet V, Nieto J, Praga M et al: Focal glomerulosclerosis and proteinuria in patients with solitary kidneys. Arch Int Med 1986;146:705–709
56. Zeman FJ: Effects of maternal protein restriction on the kidney of the newborn young of rats. J Nutr 1968;94:111–116
57. Simpson A, Mortimer JG, Silva PA et al: Correlates of blood pressure in a cohort of Dunedin seven-year old children. pp. 191–205. In Onesti G, Kim KE (eds): Hypertension in the Young and Old. Grune & Startton, New York 1981
58. McKay DB, Milford EL, Sayegh MH: Clinical aspects of renal transplantation. pp. 2602–2632. In Brenner BM (ed): The Kidney. WB Saunders, 1996
59. Baldwin DS: Chronic glomerulonephritis: nonimmunologic mechanisms of progressive glomerular damage. Kid Int 1982; 21:109–120
60. Cotran RS: Glomerulosclerosis in reflux nephropathy. Kid Int 1982;21:258–627
61. Morgensen CE, Christensen CK: Predicting diabetic nephropathy in insulin-dependent patients. N Engl J Med 1984;311: 89–93
62. Wyndham JR, Everitt AV, Eyland A, Major J: Inhibitory effect of hypophysectomy and food restriction on glomerular basement membrane thickening, proteinuria and renal enlargement in aging male Wistar rats. Arch Gerontol Geriatr 1987;6:323–337
63. Yared A, Miyazawa H, Puckerson ML et al: Effect of diet, age and sex on the renal response to immune injury in the rat. Kid Int 1988;33:561–570

CHAPTER 66

Disturbances of Homeostasis

MICHAEL LYE

The milieu interieur of Claude Bernard is more a hypothetical concept than a palpable entity.[1] Knowledge and understanding of its composition and function have been constantly refined and elaborated on since the mid-17th century, as newer investigative tools and more experiments have led to a better understanding of what Bernard later called "integrated physiology".[2] Cells require a precisely determined microenvironment—the milieu interieur—to operate optimally. The milieu interieur envelopes, supports, and protects cells both from each other and from a potentially harmful milieu exterieur. Maintenance of such an environment requires integrated function by all the body systems,[3] including the so-called higher order behavioral systems.[4] Consideration of this vast area of normal and pathologic homeostasis requires discussion of virtually the whole of human physiology and medicine. In the context of aging, many of these topics are dealt with throughout this book under the various systematic chapter headings. In this section the milieu interieur and homeostasis will be discussed only in the context of whole body or intersystem regulation and will thus span that area of integrative physiology lying across and between classic body systems. It is often difficult to isolate aging changes in clinical physiology from the impact of age-related diseases. The two areas are inter-related, and to some extent are interdependent upon each other.

Since the time of Bernard, a vast literature covering the interieur milieu and homeostasis has evolved. Most of the research reported in this area has been derived from studies of young adults, often for the sole reason that young subjects are readily available in research environments. Many research reports which include "old" or "elderly" in their titles limit their studies to individuals below the sixth decade. Recently, however, there has been a heartening increase in studies of old age as witnessed by the number of specialist journals devoted to aging in both man and other species. Much of gerontologic research is still at the stage of descriptive study. Thus, in an aging study the average value or normal range of some variable is compared in young and old healthy individuals. While age differences in such descriptive studies may be important, how the young and old respond if the variable is perturbed is much more important especially for the clinical practitioner.[5]

Degradation or instability of homeostatic control mechanisms underlie many of the observed age differences (Fig. 66-1). Thus, observation of how quickly and in what manner an old person's system responds to perturbation may answer many questions and pose others, leading to greater understanding of "specific age lesions". The acquisition of more quantifiable data from experiments as opposed to observation would allow much better formulation and testing of hypotheses. Indeed, the elaboration of mathematical models (Fig. 66-1) of complicated aging homeostatic mechanisms would advance clinical medicine and biology.[6] The most frequent stress for the elderly human is produced by disease. It should be remembered that in elderly people psychological and social trauma may disturb homeostasis as much as pathology. Degradation of homeostatic mechanisms will have important secondary effects on the pharmacokinetics and pharmacodynamics of drugs in old age.

Body Composition

From the moment of conception to extreme old age the human body undergoes a considerable change in shape, size, and composition.[7] The most dramatic changes take place during the first fraction of life, in utero, but change (maturation, development, senescence) is a continuous process and changes occurring in the latter half of the life span may have considerable impact on the physiology, pathology, and pharmacology of the older individual.[8]

Body Weight

There are many reports of cross-sectional studies of the effects of aging on body weight in humans. Many of these reports reach variable or even conflicting conclusions. This is probably due to differences in culture or genetic makeup of populations studied. Overall, however, beyond middle age changes in body weight well into old age are not gross.

In healthy individuals, body weight generally reaches a plateau in middle life and is maintained to approximately the sixth decade, to be followed by a progressive decrease.[9–12] Over the whole adult life span the average changes in body weight are slight. Thus, because of the more rapid loss of weight in old age, 30- and 80-year old men will show similar body weights, the elderly having shed their "middle-aged spread" over the 5 decades. Women, on the other hand, are not so efficient and over the same age range old women may seem to have gained weight. However, on average they were still heavier in their middle age. In old age the body weights of men and women are similar (Fig. 66-2). In general, men achieve a

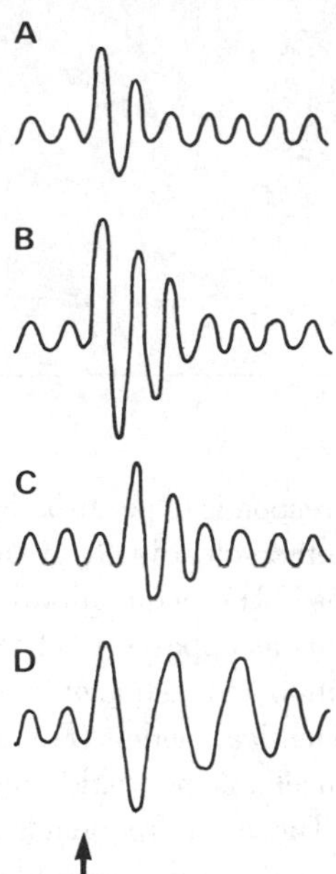

Figure 66-1 Response to perturbation of a hypothetical system under feedback control. (**A**) Young individual; (**B–D**) effects of aging; (**B**) amplitude exaggerated; (**C**) initiation of response delayed; (**D**) phase of response delayed. The simplified function is of the form $f(x) = A + A_o \sin(\omega + \pi) + A_1 e^{-6+} \sin(\omega_2 t + \pi_2)$. Examination of age-changes in the parameters of such a function may provide insight as to where the "age lesion" acts.

higher peak weight than women and tend to start to lose weight earlier, but at approximately the same rate as women. This rate is around 0.45 kg/year (1 lb/year) beyond the age of 45 to 50 years. Caution, however, needs to be applied to these cross-sectional studies because of secular changes and selective survivorship.[13]

Fat and Fat-Free Mass

Within the somewhat minor age changes that are occurring in body weight, major redistributions of tissue proportions are taking place (Fig. 66-2). The weight of the body can be considered to be composed of only two simple components—fat and the rest—fat-free mass. Lean body mass is that component of the fat-free mass less the weight of bone and nonadipose fat.[14] While precise definitions of lean body mass vary slightly depending on measurement methods, for the purposes of this review of whole body composition the fat-free and lean body mass will be treated as equivalent. Age changes in lean body mass and bones are essentially parallel so that no significant systematic errors will be introduced.[15] Fat is a relatively inert consumer of body energetics, while the fat-free mass is a measure of active organ and especially muscle mass.[16] Thus, several studies of elderly subjects have shown that fat-free mass is a better predictor of physical fitness and muscle strength than body weight.[17] Similarly, lean body mass is closely related to the metabolic rate because muscle is the major consumer of oxygen.[18,19] This applies even into extreme old age. It is suggested that the lean body mass or fat-free mass should be

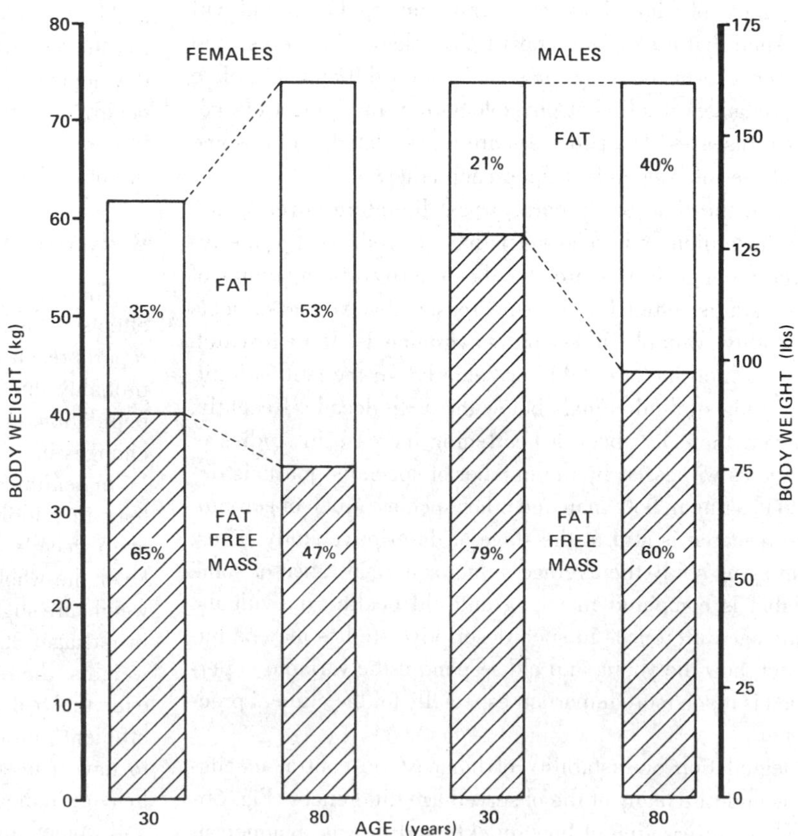

Figure 66-2 Effects of age on body composition in healthy adults.

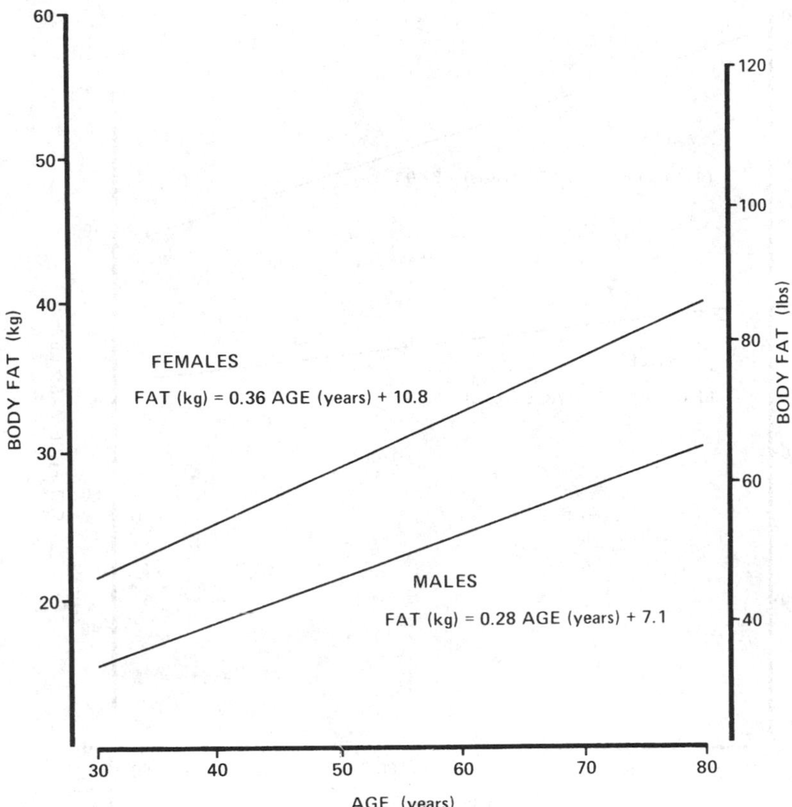

Figure 66-3 Linear increase in body fat of males and females with increasing age.

used as a normalizing factor for many physiologic variables such as cardiac output,[20] body potassium,[21] and physical fitness.[22-25] Lean body mass can also be used as a predictor of the daily requirement for thyroid hormone replacement in the elderly.[26]

Aging Fat and Fat-Free Mass

Body fat

Cross-sectional studies in small mammals have given rise to conflicting reports of the effect of aging on body fat stores. In the Osborne-Mendel rat, perirenal adipose tissue increases by hypertrophy throughout the lifespan,[27] whereas in the Fischer 344 rat the increase in perirenal fat is due to hyperplasia of adipocytes and not hypertrophy.[28] In the same rat, however, epididymal fat increases by hyperplasia, but the increase plateaus after midlife.[29] In the C57B mouse epididymal fat increases into midlife by hypertrophy and not hyperplasia.[30] Total fat mass in the Fischer 344 rat strain increases for the first two-thirds of the life span, then decreases significantly.[31] Thus, fat changes with age in small mammals vary considerably both between species, between strains and between different anatomical sites.

Numerous cross-sectional studies using different techniques have consistently demonstrated significant increase in the body fat of humans with increasing age.[32-36] These results have been confirmed in a small number of longitudinal studies, though the rates of increase of body fat are somewhat less than in longitudinal studies, indicating a secular trend in body fat change.[37-39]

In spite of differences in technique and subject selection, the increase in body fat that occurs in Caucasians is remarkably similar in the different studies. Thus, using the data in the studies quoted above, weighted regression coefficients can be calculated to show that, on average, healthy males and females accumulate body fat at the approximate rate of 2.8 and 3.6 kg/decade (6.2 and 8.0 lb/decade), respectively (Fig. 66-3). These results, however, cannot be applied to non-Caucasians. In studies of primitive populations no increase in body fat with age has been observed.[40,41]

Fat-free mass

Few studies of the effects of aging on lean body or fat-free mass have been reported for small mammals. Lesser, Deutsch, and Markofsky[42] report that longitudinal studies in the rat show no change in lean body mass and this was the conclusion also of Yu and Masoro.[31] However, inspection of the latter's data does suggest quite a marked decrease in lean body mass of their very old rats, though this may have been a preterminal event. It is well-recognized that small mammals kept in animal houses invariably show a sudden decline in body weight preterminally.[43] In this case, it would indeed be surprising if such mammals did not show some loss of lean body mass.

In the human, the situation is more clear. The majority of studies (for references see above) show a consistent decline in lean body or fat-free mass with increasing age (Fig. 66-4). Even in primitive populations that demonstrate no increase in

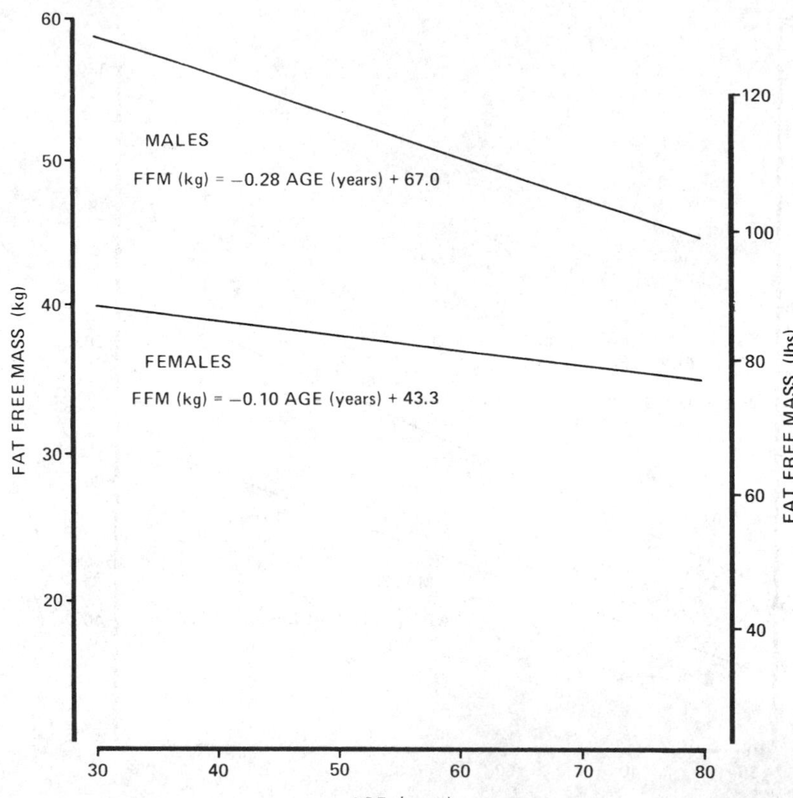

Figure 66-4 Linear decrease in fat-free mass of males and females with increasing age.

body fat because body weight tends to fall, especially in extreme old age, fat-free mass must decrease, *pari passu*.[40] Moore[16] has summed up the phenomenon pithily, "The engine shrinks within the chassis". From the literature the rate of decline in fat-free mass can be calculated approximately as 2.8 kg/decade (6.2 lb/decade) in males and 1.0 kg/decade (2.2 lb/decade) in females (Fig. 66-4). Clearly, men lose lean body mass at twice the rate of women. Therefore, sex differences in fat-free mass become much less in old age because middle-aged men start from a higher peak fat-free mass than women.

Significance of Fat and Fat-Free Mass Changes

The basal metabolic rate of man declines with increasing age.[44,45] However, if the basal metabolic rate is related to fat-free mass, the age effect is almost removed.[46] Similarly, it has been shown in cross-sectional[47] and longitudinal studies[48,49] that maximal oxygen consumption during exercise decreases as a function of increasing age. Miller and Blyth[50] showed that most of this decrease in metabolic rate could be accounted for by the aging decrease in fat-free mass. Later, Tzankoff and Norris[51] demonstrated that the decrease in metabolic rate could be more closely related to the decrease in muscle mass as determined from 24 hour creatinine excretion. These authors also showed that the proportion of oxygen consumption derived from nonmuscle tissues (heart, liver, kidneys, brain, etc.) did not change with increasing age.

Thus, because the "engine" of the body is shrinking, it is no surprise that physical fitness and working capacity also decline.[48,52,53] The decline in physical fitness with age is less in physically active individuals[54–56] and can be halted or even reversed in some part at least by physical training.[48,57] Regular physical exercise preserves the engine (fat-free mass) and slows fat accumulation.[19] This important recent study confirms again the benefits of physical exercise even in the "old old."

Cardiac output decreases with increasing age, both at rest[58] and during exercise.[59,60] If, however, the cardiac output is related to fat-free mass, then the output is appropriate to the mass. This is because body fat that is increasing with age requires very little of the cardiac output for metabolism. The age-related accumulation of body fat has significant effects on halothane pharmacokinetics. Saraiva et al.[61] demonstrated that individuals with higher body fat stores, measured from skinfold thicknesses, had an increased uptake of halothane and prolonged recovery times following anesthesia. Similar observations have now been reported for a more modern anesthetic, thiopental.[62] If body weight is used as a predictor of thyroid replacement requirements and no correction is made for the increased proportion of fat accumulated by an elderly patient, overdosage is likely.[26] Similarly, estimates of body fat: fat-free mass ratio, are better measures than body weight of nutritional status[63,64] and indeed of subsequent dependency[65] and mortality in the elderly.[63,66,67]

Etiology of Changes

The reason for the decrease in fat-free mass and corresponding accumulation of body fat with increasing age is not obvious. Research in this area is hampered by the lack of any suitable animal model in which hypotheses can be tested. The situation is further confounded by the problem of determining which is cause and which is effect.

Inactivity in whatever form leads to disuse atrophy,[68] and this is likely to affect muscle bulk, the main component of fat-free mass. Is inactivity a consequence of increasing age? Certainly, with increasing age there is a decrease in physical activity in both mammals and healthy humans.[69,70] Even in individuals continuing physical training into extreme old age, there is an inevitable reduction in physical fitness and fat-free mass with increasing age.[19,52] Alternatively, does the loss of lean body mass cause the decrease in physical fitness?[60] Does the decrease in cardiac output lead to muscle anoxia, and hence, reduction in fat-free mass or is the decrease in cardiac output secondary to the reduced demands of a fat-free mass? What are the roles of subnutrition or pathologic processes?[71–73] Before answers to these questions can be formulated, more longitudinal studies of body composition need to be carried out. With the advent of nontoxic, noninvasive methods for measuring body composition such studies should be pursued in the near future.

Body Compartments

Classic teaching divides the body fluid (total body water, TBW) into two primary compartments, extracellular fluid (ECF) and intracellular fluid (ICF), neatly separated by a cell wall. This somewhat simplistic division was modified by Robinson and McCance,[74] who suggested that the two fluid compartments are, in physiochemical terms, similar to two phases of an emulsion, where ECF represents the continuous phase and ICF the disperse phase, thus emphasising that ECF is a transport medium serving the metabolic needs of the ICF. The ECF can be subdivided further into intravascular and extravascular components, though apart from slight protein differences the two are identical in composition.

In Figure 66-5 the classic cation/anion balance between ECF (plasma) and ICF is depicted. There are differences between the chemical composition of ECF and ICF, but also some similarities. The main cation in the ECF is sodium whereas in the ICF it is mainly potassium plus magnesium. It was suggested by MacCallum[75] that this ionic difference was related to the fact that mammals had evolved from a "primeval soup", though this simple evolutionary idea has been questioned by Conway.[76]

Total Body Water

In view of the age changes in fat and fat-free mass proportions discussed above it would be surprising if TBW did not fall with increasing age. However, studies have reported variable results. Edelman et al.[77] and Shock and colleagues[46] using antipyrine to measure TBW, report significant age decrements. Similarly, Olbrich and Woodford-Williams[78] reported a decrease in TBW, but this was quite small. Young and colleagues[79] reported an overall average decrease with increasing age, but there was considerable intersubject variation. Steele and colleagues[80] found no significant decrease. Two studies from Scandinavia are pertinent. In a longitudinal study, Steen, Isaksson, and Svanborg[81] found that 70-year old healthy, elderly subjects showed a decrease in TBW measured with tritiated water over 5-year intervals. Thus, males and females decrease by 3.0 and 2.0 L, respectively, while body weight decreased by 2.9 and 1.7 kg (6.4 and 3.7 lb), respectively over the same period. In a larger cross-sectional study of healthy elderly subjects (N = 134 males and 342 females), the same group reported that TBW decreased, but in relation to body weight changed little.[82] These studies and others,[45,83] suggest that TBW does decrease significantly with increasing age, but this is in keeping with loss of body tissue (in particular, fat-free mass) and does not represent a form of aging "dehydration".[84,85] Albala and colleagues[84] derived prediction equations for TBW based entirely on anthropometric measurements that did not require age as a predictor variable.

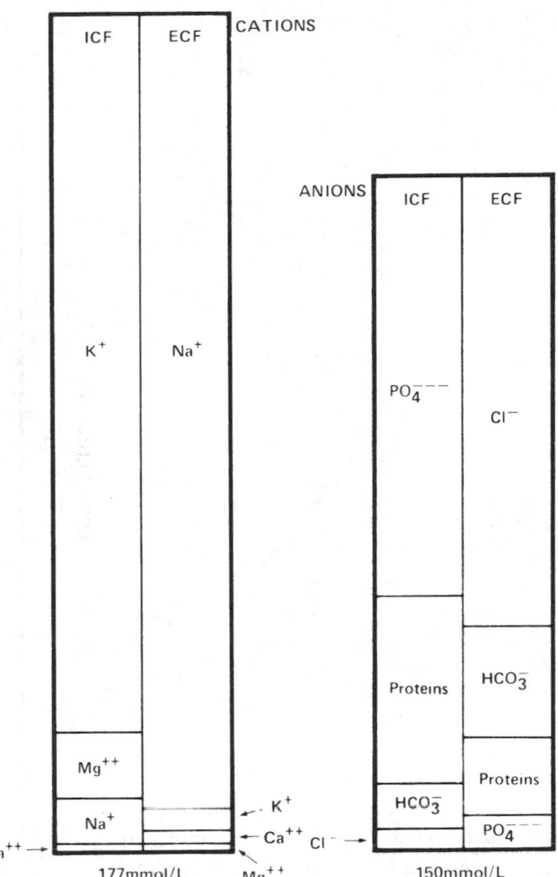

Figure 66-5 The ionic composition of intracellular and extracellular fluids.

Intra-and extracellular fluids

In the early days of body composition study it was thought that ECF increased with age[86] until Shock and colleagues[46] suggested from their own and other workers' data that there

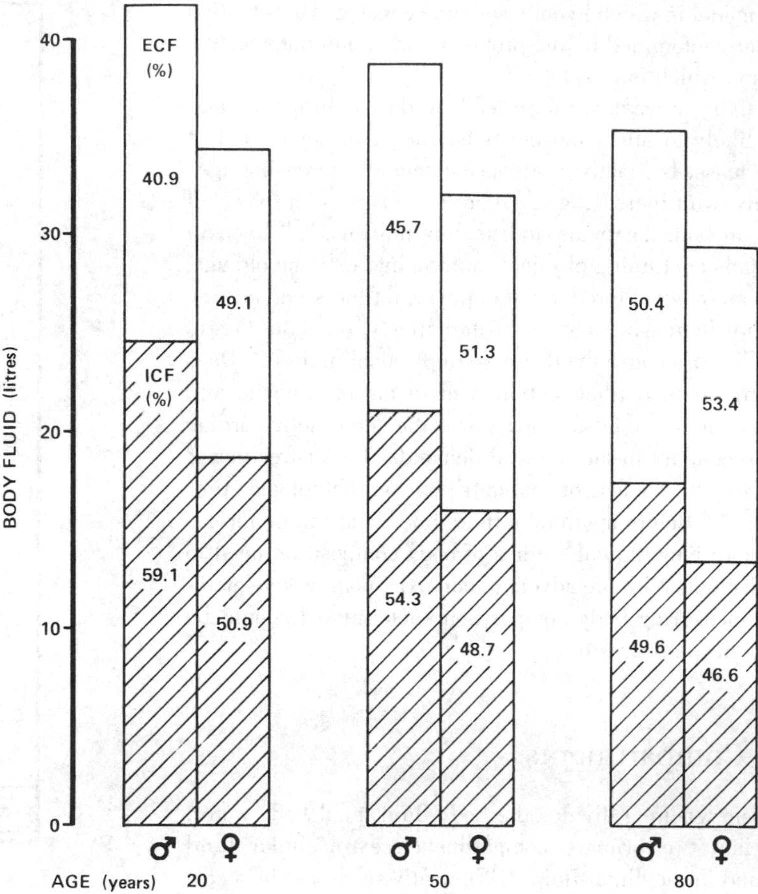

Figure 66-6 Effects of age on absolute and relative proportions of intra- and extracellular fluid volumes in men and women.

was no significant change in ECF after the age of 40 years though TBW continued to decrease (Fig. 66-6). Inspection of Table 66-1 reveals that the decrease in TBW does occur over the whole adult age range, but is much steeper before the fifth decade than after due to a marked reduction in rate of loss of ECF after this age. Shock and colleagues suggested that after the fifth decade no further change occurs in ECF so that the decrease in TBW is accounted for by loss of ICF only.

Table 66-1 Total body water, extracellular fluid, and intracellular fluid by age group

Age (years)	TBW (liters)	ECF (liters)	ICF (liters)	ECF/ICF
20–29	39.8	16.0	23.8	0.67
30–39	38.3	13.9	24.4	0.57
40–49	34.7	12.0	22.7	0.53
50–59	35.0	12.4	22.6	0.55
60–69	32.9	11.4	21.5	0.53
70–79	31.6	11.8	19.8	0.60
80–89	30.8	11.8	19.0	0.62
90–99	30.1	11.4	18.7	0.61

Abbreviations: TBW, total body water; ECF, extracellular fluid; ICF, intracellular fluid.
(Data from Shock et al.[46])

Bruce and colleagues[82] used tritiated water to measure TBW and derived ICF from whole body or exchangeable potassium measurements. They confirmed the trends in ECF and ICF found in the earlier nonisotopic studies. Their results differ in absolute values from the earlier reports, probably because the earlier thiocynate method of measuring ECF tends to overestimate the true value. Thus, the ratio ECF:ICF is higher in the Scandinavian studies[81,82] and the fall in ECF more marked. Steen[87] has commented on the fall in TBW occurring especially in subjects in their eighth decade. The recent wider availability of bioelectrical impedance providing accurate, noninvasive measurement of ECF in populations of healthy individuals has confirmed the relative stability of ECF in old age.[88,89]

Blood and plasma volume

Both the total blood and plasma volumes in healthy man are remarkably constant in spite of varying salt intake and cardiovascular activity.[90] Classic studies failed to show any systematic change in blood volume with increasing age.[91,92] Chien and colleagues[39] confirmed these earlier cross-sectional studies in a 16 to 17 year longitudinal follow-up study. A very recent study[93] using invasive measures in surgical, but otherwise healthy individuals, demonstrated decreases in blood volume with increasing age, but attributed the changes to decreasing body weight. It also confirmed large deviations between observed and predicted blood volumes in this population. A constant blood volume gives stability and is particularly important for optimum performance of the circulatory system so lack of major and/or systematic change with age is reassuring.

Regulation of body fluids

There are a number of mechanovolume (pressoreceptors and volume) receptors located throughout the vascular tree. The main receptors are located within the thorax,[94–96] arterial tree (baroreceptors),[97] and in the kidneys.[98] Any decrease in volume sensed by these receptors is followed by a prompt increase in renal reabsorption of sodium. Similarly, an increase in blood volume causes sodium excretion. The renal response is brought about by changes in glomerular filtration rate,[99] aldosterone, and angiotensin.[100,101] Changes in volume or pressure also control the secretion of renin and arginine vasopressin (AVP), the latter is also under the control of plasma osmolality, see below. For an excellent discussion of body fluid homeostasis, the reader is referred to the review by Skorecki and Brenner.[102] Human antidiuretic hormone (AVP) plays a crucial role in regulating water balance in mammals, including man.[103] Basal levels of AVP are not altered by increasing age.[104,105] The stimulus to secretion of AVP may be either osmotic or volume-mediated.[106,107] The effects of aging on the AVP response to osmotic stress (dehydration or ethanol infusion) is *enhanced* by increasing age.[104,108,109] Alternatively, some workers have found the AVP response to volume change is *attenuated* by increasing age,[110] while others have reported the opposite.[111] The renal response to AVP is impaired even in healthy elderly subjects.[112–114]

The situation in the human is further complicated by age-related changes in higher cortical and/or neurohormonal responses to the sensation of thirst. It has been known for a long time that endogenous levels of angiotensin II, increased by volume depletion (or indeed by hypotension), determine the "drinking response", that is, thirst.[115] Studies have shown that plasma angiotensin II levels on average fall moderately with increasing age in man.[116,117] Similarly, healthy elderly subjects are less responsive in exogenous angiotensin II.[118] It would not be surprising, therefore, to find the sensation of thirst decreased with age. A number of studies, particularly from one group of workers, has indeed demonstrated that the elderly appreciate the sensation of thirst less, or respond to experimentally induced thirst, less than young subjects.[119–123]

There is one recent contradictory report based on carefully screened healthy subjects suggesting no change with age in thirst.[109] Previously, these workers had reported impaired thirst reflexes in elderly patients.[124–126] For the clinician the lesson is clear—whatever the aging effects on thirst in healthy individuals, elderly patients do not respond to thirst and are at risk of dehydration.

The control of water balance involves interaction between several neurohumoral mechanisms.[102] Changes in cardiovascular and renal function are also important. The finding that apparently healthy elderly subjects living in the community are chronically hyperosmolar cannot be explained solely by age changes in AVP control.[127] Latent or undiscovered pathology may be a factor.[124,128] It is likely that minor degrees of cardiovascular dysfunction, so common in old age, elicit changes in neurohumoral parameters affecting fluid balance.[129,130] For example, atrial natriuretic peptide (ANP) is intimately involved in fluid and electrolyte balance.[131] This hormone, like AVP, shows systematic increase in mean basal levels with increasing age[132] and additionally seems to lose diurnal variation.[133] The hormone is increased in patients with cardiac failure.[134] It is further increased in elderly patients with chronic cardiac failure.[135] The effects of increasing age on homeostatic mechanisms controlling fluid and electrolyte status need to be further explored. It is essential however, to disentangle the effects of age-related disease(s) (subclinical or overt) from "normal aging". This requires prolonged follow-up of subjects to exclude unsuspected pathology that may only present at a later date.

Blood Constituents

The ionic composition of the ICF and ECF differ considerably (Fig. 66-5), but in clinical practice the composition of the ECF is assumed to be in equilibrium with the intravascular compartment and this is used in the assessment of overall electrolyte homeostasis, both in health and disease. The ionic differences between the ECF and ICF are maintained by energy-dependent processes operating in the cell wall. The integrity of the cell wall is not impaired by aging unaccompanied by disease. Any difference found in old people in the ionic concentrations of ICF and ECF are likely to be due to latent or overt pathologic processes[136] or secondary to the action of drugs.[137]

Electrolytes

Sodium

The normal range of serum sodium does not change with increasing age in healthy individuals.[111,138,139] There is, however, a small but significant increase in serum sodium around the time of the menopause.[140] Values in elderly hospitalized patients tend to be lower than age-matched healthy controls, though a few patients may exhibit hypernatremia.[136]

Potassium

A number of cross-sectional reports have stated that the mean value of serum or plasma potassium in healthy adults does not change with increasing age.[136,138,141] However, Wilding, Rollason, and Robinson[140] in their survey of 4,800 healthy individuals did demonstrate a systematic trend with age (Figs. 66-7 and 66-8). Their figures are in very good agreement with the results published by Leask, Andrews, and Caird,[138] who

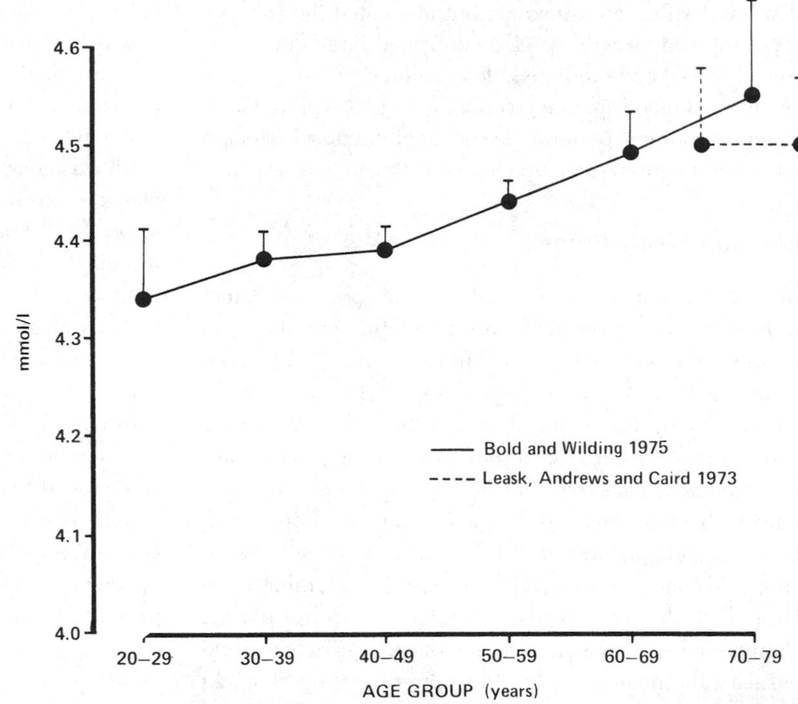

Figure 66-7 Age changes in serum potassium of healthy males.

confined their measurements to healthy individuals over the age 65 living in the community. Similarly, in a longitudinal study, Haavisto and colleagues[142] showed an increase, though not statistically significant, in serum potassium over 5 years in old people. Support for the idea that the serum potassium, especially in men, tends to rise with increasing age is provided by Hodkinson.[136] He showed that serum potassium levels are lower in ill old people compared with healthy age-matched controls. Thus, if unrecognized disease in the healthy populations studied was operating then the age trend would be toward a decrease and not, as observed, an increase in serum potassium. The acute rise and fall in serum potassium around the

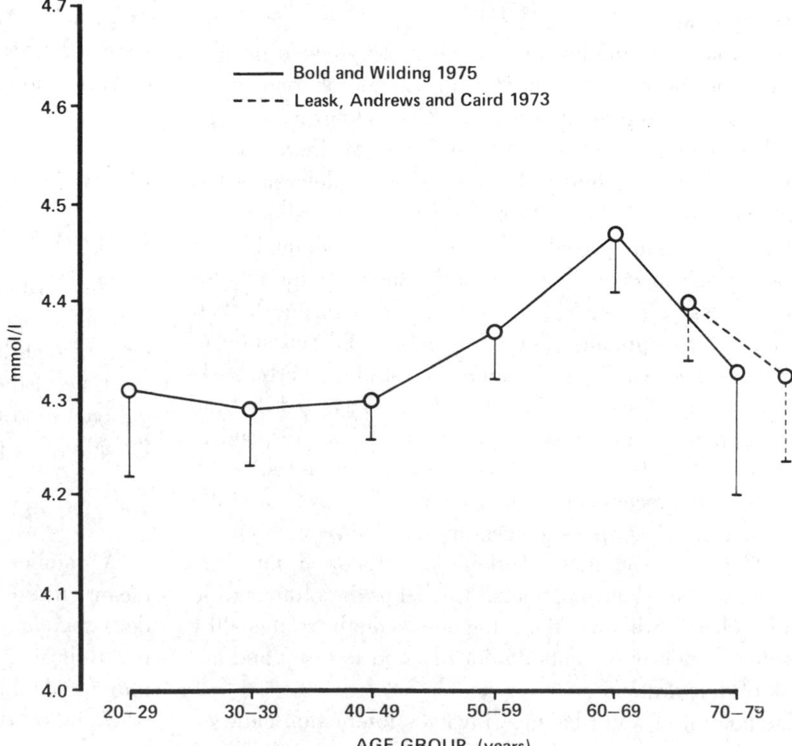

Figure 66-8 Age changes in serum potassium of healthy females.

menopause is unexplained, though may be related to the simultaneous increase in blood urea and creatinine occurring at the same time.

Chloride and bicarbonate

Measurements of the serum chloride and bicarbonate levels have shown no consistent trends with increasing age in healthy populations.[136,138,141] Thus, the normal ranges applicable to young adults (98 to 108 and 22 to 26 mmol (mEq)/L, respectively) should be used for assessment of elderly subjects and patients. Hale and colleagues[137] confirmed these normal ranges in the healthy elderly, but also showed that both ranges were significantly altered if subjects were taking drugs.

Urea and creatinine

In general, the blood urea is reported consistently to increase with increasing age in both sexes, though average values in women are lower than in men.[138,140,143,144] There is an accelerated increase in blood urea of women around the menopause, but in contradistinction to potassium it does not decline thereafter.[140,145] Thus, the sex difference is less in the elderly but is still significant.[137] The approximate upper level for blood urea in elderly individuals (greater than 65 years of age) in both sexes is 10.0 mmol/L (60 mg/100 mL). It is necessary to realize that blood urea is log normally distributed and mean values and normal ranges have been determined on the transformed values. This is particularly relevant in the consideration of ranges for hospital patients.[138,146]

The serum creatinine follows the same pattern as urea with age. However, the sex difference is greater and the rise with age much less than that occurring with the blood urea.[138,142,145,147] The upper limits for serum creatinine are given in Table 66-2. While blood urea and serum creatinine are both related to renal function and, in particular, the glomerular filtration rate, the relationship in *healthy individuals* is not very precise. Thus, urea, and particularly creatinine, measurements are influenced by the dietary intake of protein, the size of the muscle mass, the general state of catabolism, and prior level of exercise. The attenuated increase in creatinine with age compared with that of urea can be attributed to these factors and especially the reduction in lean body mass discussed previously.[145,148,149] The net result of these changes invalidates the use of serum creatinine as a measure of renal function in old people.[150,151] Similarly, it has been shown to be a poor predictor of dehydration in ill old people.[152] In such patients the impact of pathology, especially affecting the cardiovascular and renal systems, and drugs cause difficulties in interpreting plasma creatinine levels.[147]

Table 66-2 Normal ranges for serum creatinine

	Age (years)	
	65–74	75+
mmol/L		
Males	0.06–0.14	0.06–0.15
Females	0.04–0.12	0.04–0.14
mg/100 mL		
Males	0.65–1.60	0.70–1.70
Females	0.50–1.40	0.50–1.60

Acid-Base Balance

In health, the hydrogen ion content of the arterial blood, usually measured as pH, is kept constant in spite of changes in acid load produced by many metabolic processes and exercise—the normal range being between 36 and 43 mmol/L (pH 3.45 to 3.35).[141] This resting basal level is the same in healthy elderly individuals as in youth.[153] Acid-base balance is regulated by rapidly acting changes in respiration and longer term adjustment is by renal excretory mechanisms.[154] Disturbances in acid-base balance may be produced by primary changes in respiration, that is, increased ventilation leading to respiratory acidosis and vice versa, producing respiratory acidosis. Acid loads from excess catabolism or exercise cause primary metabolic acidosis whereas loss of acid, often in the elderly via gastrointestinal fluid, leads to primary metabolic alkalosis. In the clinical situation, however, it is unusual to have a single primary disturbance of acid-base balance because the response of the body to a primary disturbance is toward compensation by the unaffected system. Thus, a primary metabolic acidosis due to renal failure is in part compensated by a secondary respiratory alkalosis brought about by increased ventilation in response to the lowered pH. Thus, the interpretation of changes in acid-base balance and pH require a consideration of the clinical circumstances—reliance upon laboratory results in isolation is fraught with danger.

Moderate exercise imposes an acid load on the body from working muscles, which, if exercise becomes severe enough may be supplemented by a lactic acid load due to utilization of the pyruvate/lactate anaerobic shunt.[155] There is some evidence that the healthy elderly take longer to clear this metabolic load after exercise than young individuals.[156,157] Whether the elderly produce more acid for the same exercise stress is not known. The decrease in cardiac output and blood distribution to muscle, brought about by aging, leads to anoxia at an earlier stage during exercise and thus more lactic acid will be generated. Unfortunately, it is difficult to control for the effects of training and physical fitness when comparing age effects on aerobic or anaerobic metabolism. It is likely that both respiratory and metabolic compensatory responses following changes in acid-base status are impaired with increasing age. Thus, the response to inhaled CO_2 is attenuated in the elderly,[158] probably due to mechanical changes within the lung rather than changes in sensitivity of chemodetectors or to the output of "respiratory centers".[159] Similarly, the ability of the aged kidney to respond to acid/alkali loads and to drugs is impaired.[151] In the clinical sphere it is important that acid-base function be closely monitored in the sick elderly because general principles and clinical experience suggest that the elderly tolerate such disturbances less than younger patients. It is also important not to be too enthusiastic in correcting pH disturbances, especially metabolic acidosis, by the injudicious use of fluids. Correction of the underlying cause of the disturbance usually resolves the problem. Only with life-threatening acidosis is direct correction with bicarbonate warranted. The formula proposed by Hazard and Griffin[160] (0.5 $PCO_2 - HCO_3^-$) × 0.5 body weight) is a good guide to replacement requirements in geriatric practice.[161] Dichloroacetate may be safer in elderly patients with impaired cardiac function where the danger of precipitating heart failure with sodium bicarbonate infusion is very real.[162]

Major Electrolyte Problems in the Elderly

The maintenance, particularly under stress, of a constant milieu interieur is vital to the survival of all mammals, including man. Evolutionary processes have ensured that successful species are those who have developed effective and efficient homeostatic mechanisms to counter pathologic and environmental insults. Evolutionary pressure exerts less force on postfertile humans so the elderly have less compensatory mechanisms to cope with insults. The substance of this volume deals with these aspects in a systematic or organ-specific fashion. The precise regulation of salt, water, and potassium involve integrated responses by the cardiovascular, renal, and neuroendocrine systems and thus represent inter- or multisystem disorders of homeostasis. They present a paradigm of "age changes" for the clinical doctor looking after elderly patients.

Salt and Water Homeostasis

Disturbances of plasma sodium concentration are common in elderly patients and are associated with an increased mortality.[163, 164] Alterations of ECF volume are compensated by changes in sodium excretion with water usually acting as a passive agent, only moving to maintain a constant plasma sodium or plasma osmolality. Age effects on the mechanisms regulating salt and water balance have been quite well studied in the recent past and have provided explanations as to why hypo- and hypernatremia are so common in elderly patients, and further point the way to the rational management of these serious disturbances.

Total body water decreases with age so the loss or gain of 1 L of water represents proportionately a much larger change in older subjects compared with young subjects. Alteration of the thirst threshold with increasing age has been discussed earlier (see above). In addition, elderly patients usually suffer from multiple pathology so they may be unable to communicate their need for water or because of immobility, unable to obtain access.[165, 166]

Alterations in renal function with increasing age affect salt and water balance.[167] The aged kidney is less able to excrete a water load[111,168] and alternatively, less able to retain water when depleted.[169] As discussed previously, even though the release of AVP is enhanced by increasing age,[108] because of an age-related attenuation of renal tubular responsiveness to the hormone,[170,171] the elderly patient is less able to retain water especially in the presence of dehydration. The contribution of altered activity of the sympathetic nervous system[172,173] and the renin-angiotensin-aldosterone axis[172,174] to altered water homeostasis in healthy elderly people is not as yet clear.

Hyponatremia

There is no single syndrome of hyponatremia, rather the plasma-sodium concentration is a measure of the ratio of sodium:body water.[175,176] Detailed biochemical investigation of the elderly patient with hyponatremia is not indicated.[177] Meddlesome investigation and treatment is not necessary and may even be dangerous.[178] In most cases the condition is self-limiting especially if the degree of hyponatremia is moderate, that is, plasma-sodium concentration more than 125 mmol (mEq)/L.[178] Some healthy ambulatory elderly people may exhibit chronic mild hyponatremia for no other reason than being old and additionally show no detrimental effects.[179] A detailed history of the circumstances leading up to the condition, the underlying pathology, and the time course of events will indicate appropriate etiology and management.[161] Morbidity and mortality are related to underlying pathology rather than the degree of hyponatremia, per se.[180]

Dilutional Hyponatremia

In this situation there is excess body water with a normal body sodium. The condition may occur rapidly or over a period of time. The most common cause in the elderly patient is due to the administration of hypotonic fluids in the postoperative period[181,182] when the stress of operation has lead to an increased secretion of AVP. Thus, postoperative hyponatremia in elderly patients is invariably iatrogenic and can be prevented by the administration of isotonic fluid[183] or restricting hypotonic fluid to 1 L or less per day.[184] Rightly, junior hospital doctors are aware of the dangers of precipitating cardiac failure in elderly postoperative patients by administering saline fluids, but the pendulum has swung too far in the direction of caution favoring hyponatremia.[161]

Chronic water excess with normal body sodium is common in the elderly. This condition was called "the syndrome of inappropriate antidiuretic hormone secretion (SIADH)" by Bartter and Schwartz.[185] A number of conditions cause an elevation of AVP in the absence of gross salt and water depletion. Acute respiratory infection in the elderly patient is the most common cause.[186,187] In most cases the hyponatremia does not require direct treatment; even in the symptomatic patient with a plasma sodium less than 125 mmol (mEq)/L fluid restriction is unnecessary as treatment of the pulmonary infection will rapidly resolve the hyponatremia.[187]

Malignant tumors, particularly bronchial, in the elderly may cause persistent symptomatic hyponatremia.[188,189] The secre-

Etiology of hyponatremia in the elderly with excess AVP without gross disturbance of body fluids

- Respiratory infections
- Malignant tumors
  - Bronchial
  - Pancreatic
  - Prostatic
  - Duodenal
- Neurologic
  - Stroke
  - Tumor
  - Meningitis
  - Encephalitis
  - Guillain-Barré
- Acute stress
  - Accidental
  - Surgical
  - Psychological
- Drugs

tion of AVP is usually uncontrolled though occasionally there may be some feedback.[190] Treatment by water restriction is not well tolerated by the elderly and demeclocycline 600 to 1,200 mg/day is to be preferred.[189] Demeclocycline produces a form of nephrogenic diabetes insipidus and may worsen renal function especially in the presence of liver dysfunction.[191] Occasionally, a chronic mildly hyponatremic patient may precipitate severe hyponatremia by consuming excess hypotonic fluid, especially beer.[192] In this emergency situation, hypertonic saline intravenously is required. In an elderly patient, frusemide should be administered concurrently to increase free water clearance and prevent cardiac failure.[166,193] Hypertonic saline does not correct chronic hyponatremia due to SIADH because the extra sodium is rapidly excreted in the urine.

Acute stress following neurologic trauma or surgery[184,194] is a common cause of hyponatremia. In elderly patients the addition of coma[195] or intermittent positive pressure ventilation[196] further depresses the plasma sodium. A common cause of usually transient hyponatremia in elderly patients is an acute cerebrovascular accident.[197] It has long been recognized that emotional stress may precipitate hyponatremia without gross disturbance of body fluid or body salt.[198] Pain, not always severe,[199] or psychosis[200] are often particular factors. Clinch[201] described prolonged hyponatremia in a 86-year-old female following bereavement, which reappeared following a minor fall and hospital admission. Hypothyroidism may present in the elderly as hyponatremia.[189,202]

Water Excess with Lesser Salt Excess

It may seem to be paradoxical that hyponatremia may exist in the presence of increased total body sodium, but where AVP is increased by a nonosmotic stimulus, the condition is not uncommon. The most frequent nonosmotic stimulus to AVP seen in the elderly is effective intravascular volume depletion due to chronic cardiac failure. Less common causes of a reduction in effective blood volume in the elderly include nephrotic syndrome and hepatic cirrhosis.[203,204] Pregnancy in the elderly as a cause of hyponatremia has not been reported, as yet.

Hyponatremia in elderly patients with chronic cardiac failure has been attributed to diuretic usage. With the possible exception of the so-called potassium-sparing agents,[205,206] diuretics are not usually the cause of a low-plasma sodium.[207] Indeed, hyponatremia is common in patients with chronic cardiac failure who are not receiving diuretics.[208–210] The mechanisms involved in the pathogenesis of hyponatremic cardiac failure include enhanced sympathetic tone, reduced renal blood flow and glomerular filtration, augmented thirst secondary to angiotensin secretion, nonosmotic stimulation of AVP, and enhanced reabsorption by proximal tubules.[211–213] The effects of "normal aging" and of cardiac failure combine to increase the likelihood of hyponatremia in elderly patients.

Treatment in the main should be aimed at increasing renal blood flow and function by treating the failure and improving cardiac function. Changing from a thiazide to a loop diuretic and stopping potassium-sparing agents is worthwhile.[214–216] An angiotensin-converting enzyme inhibitor (ACEI) is often very effective in reducing the high angiotensin levels and increasing renal blood flow[217,218] leading to resolution of the hyponatremia.[219] This approach should be limited to mild degrees of hyponatremia. Hypotension, which may be profound, after the first dose of ACEI in an elderly hyponatremic patient requires that this treatment should only be started in hospital.[220]

Salt Depletion with Normal Water

Loss of sodium leads to contraction of the ECF and intravascular volumes, thus providing a powerful nonosmotic stimulus to AVP. If water alone is replaced and not supplemented with salt, hyponatremia will occur. In elderly patients, vomiting and diarrhea are common causes.[221,222] The hyponatremia may be aggravated by the use of diuretics. A few elderly individuals, usually frail and female, given diuretics for chronic cardiac failure may develop rapid hyponatremia and hypokalemia.[223] The mechanism is not understood, though it has been suggested that sodium moves into cells to replace lost potassium.[224,225]

Diuretics, particularly thiazide agents, may lead to hyponatremia with or without hypokalemia.[223,225,226] Invariably, however, there are other contributing factors, such as high water intake, restricted sodium diet, or loss of sodium in vomit or diarrhea.[224,227] Hyponatremia is a particular problem with amiloride[205,228] though is also seen with other potassium-sparing agents such as triamterene[229] and spironolactone.[230] These agents should not be used in the elderly.[206,216] Another drug that should not be used in the elderly, chlorpropamide, acts synergistically with diuretics to produce hyponatremia.[231] Elderly patients with CNS diseases are particularly at risk of developing significant hyponatremia,[197,232] so it is no surprise that "psychoactive" drugs often precipitate hyponatremia.[233] Particular concern relates to antidepressants, including imipramine[234] and the newer, and otherwise safer, 5-HT reuptake inhibitors.[235] The antiepileptic, carbamazapine, often also used for trigeminal neuralgia and sometimes used for diabetic neuropathy in older patients, is commonly implicated.[236] The nonsteroidal anti-inflamatory drugs (NSAIDs), often overprescribed to elderly people, have been noted to cause serious hyponatremia through their prostaglandin-synthetase inhibitory activity.[225,237]

Redistribution Hyponatremia

Excess of large molecules in the plasma may lead to hyponatremia though the "activity" of the sodium ions is normal.[238] In the elderly the most common cause of what may be termed pseudohyponatremia is excess of paraproteins in multiple myeloma.[239] Occasionally, hyperlipidemia in diabetics or alcoholics can produce pseudohyponatremia.[240,241] Measurement of sodium using an ion-selective electrode gives a true result.[242,243] In hyperglycemia the apparent hyponatremia is related to the blood sugar level and can be corrected by a simple formula.[244]

Hyponatremia is common in severely sick elderly patients and may be in part a manifestation of the so-called "sick cell syndrome".[245] According to this hypothesis, cellular membrane permeability is increased due to metabolic failure leading to a loss of intracellular solute. In order to maintain osmolality, water accompanies the solute and "hyponatremia" ensues.[246] Experimental data are not available to allow interventions to be recommended. Treatment of the underlying pathology usually restores normal metabolic function.

Hypernatremia

Hypernatremia, usually defined as a serum sodium concentration of more than 145 mmol (mEq/L) or a serum osmolality greater than 290 mOsm/kg, may be due to an increased body sodium or an absolute or relative decrease in body water.[175] Hypernatremia occurs in between 0.3[247] and 3.3[248,249] of all hospital admissions aged over 65 years and is associated with a mortality of nearly 50 percent.[247,250,251] The high mortality of hypernatremia in the elderly is undoubtedly a reflection of the underlying pathology. Clinically, the most common cause of hypernatremia is absolute water lack associated with an acute febrile illness.[252,253] Paradoxically, chest infections, which often produce hyponatremia, are also the most common cause of hypernatremia in elderly patients. Where both hyponatremia and hypernatremia coexist, the patient would undoubtedly be normonatremic, but probably moribund. Pre-existing use of diuretic agents (all types) is common[247] and chronic cognitive impairment an additional risk factor.[254,255] Other causes of hypernatremia follow obvious excessive fluid loss. Thus, fluids lost from the gastrointestinal tract, and acute or chronic diarrhea, may be insufficiently replaced. A high solute load on the kidney as produced by uncontrolled diabetes mellitus and glycosuria soon leads to dehydration and hypernatremia. Nonketotic hyperosmolar hypernatremia is a medical emergency.[256] Other causes of dehydration may be more subtle. Thus, the increased ventilation produced by nonfebrile mild respiratory infections in the elderly leads to excess fluid loss from the lungs.[252] Similarly, steroid therapy by increasing protein catabolism leads to increased urea production which provides another high renal solute load.

As detailed above, the elderly are particularly at risk of becoming dehydrated and not replacing fluid loss because of age-related diminution in the thirst threshold[120,257] combined with renal insensitivity to endogenous AVP.[112–114] Equally, the kidney's ability to conserve water also becomes impaired with age. The elderly are also more likely than the young to develop nephrogenic diabetes insipidus because of the age-related change in kidney function.[175] In the elderly, diabetes insipidus is usually nephrogenic in origin though partial pituitary diabetes insipidus is also seen.[113] The differentiation of the causes of hypernatremia in an elderly patient is usually quite straightforward. Measurements of urinary osmolality or specific gravity and volume are all that are usually required. Sometimes an elderly dehydrated patient may show little or no increase in urine osmolality because of inability to concentrate the urine. However, the urine output will always be low. Pituitary and nephrogenic diabetes insipidus can be separated by the response to exogenous AVP. Thus, the patient with pituitary diabetes insipidus will show a response by increasing urine osmolality and decreasing urine volume. Those with the nephrogenic type will show no such change. If plasma AVP levels can be measured, then low or absent levels would suggest a pituitary origin whereas in the nephrogenic form AVP levels tend to be high. In the elderly the fluid deprivation test[258] or saline load[259] are too dangerous to be recommended for diagnostic purposes.

The symptoms of hypernatremia with or without ECF volume depletion are often nonspecific in the early stages and are mimicked by many conditions prevalent in the elderly. Thus, the two prime symptoms, weakness and lethargy, are so common in geriatric practice as not to alert one to the presence of hypernatremia. Severe (more than 155 mmol/L) hypernatremia may cause drowsiness leading to coma, muscular rigidity, and fits. If the hypernatremia is due to dehydration, then symptoms may be ascribed to the disease causing the dehydration. This is particularly likely to occur in elderly patients with respiratory infections. Depression of conscious level or fits demands that treatment be instituted promptly. Treatment of dehydration hypernatremia is relatively straightforward—give water either orally or, if this is not feasible, by the intravenous route using 5 percent dextrose. In the confused or agitated patient, subcutaneous fluids can provided up to 2 L daily and are tolerated better than intravenous methods.[260] Careful monitoring of serum electrolytes, especially sodium and potassium, urine flow, and central venous pressure should be carried out at frequent intervals. Prophylaxis requires the prescription of

Table 66-3 Etiology of diabetes insipidus in the elderly

Pituitary	Nephrogenic
Idiopathic	Obstructive uropathy
Tumor	Myeloma
Metastases	Amyloidosis
Primary	Potassium deficiency
Vascular accident	Hypercalcemia
Trauma	Renal failure
Surgical	Hyperthyroidism
Fracture	Drugs
Aneurysm	Lithium
Encephalitis	Demeclocycline
Meningitis	Amphotericin
Tuberculosis	Vinblastine
Sarcoidosis	Colchicine
Guillain-Barré syndrome	

fluids as elderly patients will not respond to simple provision and encouragement.[257] As with any other drug, the nurse must ensure compliance. It is a personal view that where an elderly patient is at risk of developing dehydration hypernatremia due to an inadequate fluid intake they should be admitted to hospital where it can be administered and monitored regularly.[261]

Patients with diabetes insipidus require detailed investigation, bearing in mind the potential etiologies outlined in Table 66-3. The treatment of diabetes insipidus is of the underlying cause wherever possible.

Unfortunately, in geriatric practice this may sometimes be difficult. Pituitary diabetes insipidus responds to AVP administered parenterally or by nasal insufflation. The analog 1-desaminodearginine vasopressin is less sensitizing and is now the drug of choice.[262] If hypersensitivity does develop, chlorpropamide and carbamazapine can be tried. Nephrogenic diabetes insipidus can best be treated by reducing the ECF with salt restriction or thiazide diuretic. Contraction of the ECF enhances proximal absorption of sodium, thus reducing urinary flow and relieving to a greater or lesser extent the symptoms of polyuria. Indomethacin, which acts directly on the distal tubule, tends to cause excessive fluid retention and precipitate cardiac failure in the elderly.

Potassium Homeostasis

Potassium plays a key role in many metabolic and enzymatic processes, especially those involved in neuroexcitatory mechanisms and energy—dependent cell membrane functions. The cation is uniquely placed within cells to perform these roles with very little potassium being extracellular. Overall body content of potassium decreases with increasing age, though much of this loss can be accounted for by loss of potassium containing cell mass (see above) The relationship between intra- and extracellular content is not fixed, though it is controlled.[263,264] Because 98 percent of body potassium is intracellular, and most metabolic functions of potassium depend upon the ratio between intra- and extracellular content, knowledge of body content is not as important as was once thought. Thus, in clinical practice knowledge of the concentration in the ECF, which is the same as the plasma, is sufficient for most purposes. In very general terms, a repeated plasma level of 3.0 mmol (mEq)/L in the absence of acid-base disturbance represent approximately 100 to 200 mmol (mEq) body loss.[265] Potassium homeostatic mechanisms operate to maintain a constant ECF concentration of potassium using the intracellular mass as a reserve or buffer.

The control of potassium homeostasis involves a number of systems that regulate distribution between extra- and intracellular compartments and modulate urinary and fecal excretion of potassium. Thus, a rise in ECF or plasma potassium increases potassium secretion by the colon.[266] With a decrease in pH (acidosis), potassium migrates out of cells raising the plasma concentration and vice versa with an increase in pH.[267] The control parameter for this mechanism is probably not hydrogen-ion concentration itself, but the plasma bicarbonate level.[268] Insulin and noradrenaline both favor the transfer of potassium from the extracellular compartment into cells and insulin has been used therapeutically for many years to lower elevated plasma potassium.[269,270] Approximately 90 percent of potassium filtered by the glomerulus is passively reabsorbed by the proximal tubule and loop of Henle. In the distal nephron, potassium is actively absorbed or secreted by an energy-dependent mechanism that acts as a fine regulator of plasma potassium.[271,272] In potassium depletion there remains an obligatory potassium excretion of 5 to 10 mmol (mEq)/day that cannot be reduced[265] There is no evidence that this level changes with age. The final mechanism by which the body can regulate potassium is via the colon, the mucosa of which acts very much like the distal renal tubule actively varying potassium secretion.[273]

Hyperkalemia

The upper limit for the plasma potassium is set at 5.5 mmol (mEq)/L. Levels above this value result in abnormalities of the cardiovascular, neuromuscular, and gastrointestinal systems.[265] Marked hyperkalemia (more than 8.0 mmol (mEq)/L) produces severe neuromuscular and cardiac dysfunction. Initially, these include generalized and nonspecific weakness and later, ascending paralysis. Flaccid quardriplegia has been reported with severe hyperkalemia.[274] In the elderly, cardiac conduction defects are the most feared and every elderly patient with hyperkalemia requires continuous ECG monitoring.[275] The elderly patient with less severe hyperkalemia may present with nonspecific acute or acute on chronic confusion.[276]

Hyperkalemia may be caused by a shift of potassium from the intracellular to the extracellular compartment or alternatively due to overall body retention of the cation. In practice, redistribution of potassium is the most common cause of hyperkalemia as no case of excess body potassium has ever been recorded.[277] This may, however, be due to difficulty in defining the "normal" body content of an individual.[278] Occasionally, factitious hyperkalemia may be due to in vitro hemolysis following prolonged storage of blood or increased red cell fragility. Blood specimens are sometimes taken downstream of intravenous infusions containing potassium. Hyperkalemia occurs in nearly 2 percent of elderly people admitted to the hospital.[248] In the elderly the most common cause of hyperkalemia is related to the use of potassium-sparing diuretics or spironolactone.[216] Not uncommonly, patients may continue to take potassium supplements when their diuretic is changed to a potassium-sparing one. It is estimated that 12 percent of patients taking a triamterene/hydrochlorothiazide diuretic will develop hyperkalemia.[279] A similar proportion become hyperkalemic with spironolactone even without the addition of potassium supplements.[280] Because of the dangers of hyperkalemia coupled with the observation that potassium-sparing agents lower glomerular filtration rate,[277,281] these agents should not be used if the creatinine clearance rate is less than 30 mL/min.[282] Many elderly patients have creatinine clearances of this order and a superadded infection perhaps with dehydration (see above) causes further deterioration leading to rapid, and possibly fatal, hyperkalemia.[283–286] The widespread use of potassium-sparing diuretics cannot therefore be recommended in the elderly.[206,216] ACEI may rarely by themselves induce hyperkalemia,[287,288] but if prescribed with potassium-sparing diuretics or potassium supplements the risk becomes considerable.[289,290] Indeed, such combinations may prove fatal.[291] Occasionally, severe and sudden hyperkalemia may be an idiosyncratic reaction.[292]

The plasma potassium rises with both respiratory and metabolic acidosis due to a shift of the cation from the intracellular compartment.[293] Tissue necrosis may release a large quantity of potassium, which may not be eliminated fast enough if renal function is reduced by age or disease. In the elderly this may be seen following arterial surgery and restoration of blood flow to near-necrotic limbs. The hyperkalemia is partly caused by potassium release from severely damaged cells, but the accompanying acid load also contributes to potassium shift. Many forms of renal failure lead to hyperkalemia, especially if there is oliguria. In milder forms of renal failure, excretion of potassium by the gut can often compensate.[294] Less common causes of hyperkalemia in elderly patients include Addison's disease,[295] ileal conduit diversion,[296] and multiple myeloma.[297] As always, iatrogenic drug causes should be considered. Not only potassium-sparing diuretics or potassium supplements but also ACEI (see above) NSAIDs,[298] and trimethoprim-sulphamethoxazole combinations.[234,299] In some cases the hyperkalemia may only be apparent during or immediately after exercise.[287,300] Paradoxically, this is more likely to occur in those regularly physically active rather than the sedentary—so-called master athletes are particularly at risk because of age-related impairment of β-2-adrenoceptors.[301] Other causes of hyperkalemia in the elderly such as intravascular hemolysis, hyperkalemic periodic paralysis, and hypoaldosteronism are rare.

Hypokalaemia

A plasma potassium of less than 3.0 mmol (mEq)/L is usually considered to be abnormal.[265] Hypokalemia, however, is not synonymous with body potassium depletion though the likelihood of depletion being present rises if several consecutive plasma values are low.[263,264] A shift of potassium from the ECF into cells is probably the most common cause of hypokalemia in all age groups. The lower body potassium of the elderly female compared with elderly males probably explains their higher frequency of hypokalemia.[302] In the elderly of both sexes, persistent minor hypokalemia may present with apathy, nonspecific weakness, or confusion.[303] At values less than 2.5 mmol (mEq)/L more widespread and severe manifestations are apparent with paresis and ileus or constipation leading to fecal impaction.[304,305] Cardiac conduction defects, especially in the presence of digoxin or acute myocardial infarction; may be prominent and require urgent treatment.[306–308] Mild to moderate hypokalemia, especially if nonacute, is not associated with increases in cardiac arrhythmias[309,310] though some authors may disagree.[311] Chronic hypokalemia can lead to significant impairment of renal tubular function, which is initially reversible, but if prolonged may become permanent.[312,313]

Hypokalemia may be a prominent feature of conditions giving rise to extensive fluid loss from the gastrointestinal tract. Such conditions in the elderly include vomiting, diarrhea from any cause, gastric aspiration, and laxative abuse.[314–317] Villous adenomas of the colon or rectum often present with profuse diarrhea and hypokalemia.[318] It has been assumed that the hypokalemia that develops in these conditions is secondary to the loss of the cation along with the gastrointestinal fluid. However, other factors are important. Thus, loss of gastric fluid causes metabolic alkalosis, which in turn causes increased uptake of ECF potassium by cells.[267] Equally, fluid loss leads to volume depletion which stimulates AVP and aldosterone secretion (see above). Argine vasopressin, by favoring water retention, is likely to produce a dilutional component to hypokalemia and increased aldosterone secretion produces increased urinary potassium excretion. These hormonal factors may be more important than the direct loss of electrolyte from the gut.[319,320] The kaliuretic action of thiazide and loop diuretics may lead to potassium depletion and hypokalemia, particularly in elderly individuals with chronic cardiac failure.[321,322] Early studies demonstrated that the total exchangeable potassium of patients with cardiac failure was between 13 and 37 percent below the normal range.[263,323–327] Others who measured body potassium directly by whole body counting showed a much smaller decrease of around 5 to 10 percent.[328–331] The difference between the studies can be accounted for by the observation that exchangeable measurements of body potassium underestimate the body content in patients with a history of fluid retention,[332,333] including elderly patients with edema-free cardiac failure.[334] Most of the remaining "depletion" of body potassium in both young and old patients can be explained by loss of potassium-rich body tissue.[331,335] Thus, there is little evidence of significant loss of body potassium due to cardiac failure or its treatment in old people and attention should be focused on plasma measurements. Estimates of the prevalence of hypokalemia with thiazide diuretics average around 20 percent.[336,337] The prevalence with loop diuretics is lower because of the smaller kaliuretic action of these drugs.[338] There is evidence that the elderly are less likely to develop hypokalemia with diuretic therapy than the young.[339,340] This is perhaps not surprising in view of the fact that plasma potassium tends to rise with increasing age (Figs. 66-7 and 66-8). In elderly patients taking diuretics who develop hypokalemia other causes for the low potassium should be sought. In particular, minor degrees of diarrhea should be considered. In the minority of patients with diuretic-induced hypokalemia in whom no other cause for potassium wasting can be found, potassium supplements should be prescribed. The dose required should be titrated against the response as often large doses of potassium are needed.[341] Occasionally, diuretic—induced hypomagnesemia may produce refractory hypokalemia, which only responds to magnesium supplements.[342]

Hypokalemia may be associated with low thyrothopin levels as well as overt thyrotoxicosis.[343] Tumors of nonendocrine organs may produce ectopic ACTH and present with severe hypokalemic alkalosis.[344] In the elderly the most common tumor is an oat cell carcinoma of the bronchus, which may be small and difficult to detect.[345] Locally administered acetozolamide used in the management of chronic glaucoma may produce persistent hypokalemia in elderly patients.[346] Other causes of hypokalemia, such as primary hyperaldosteronism, Cushing's disease, Bartter's syndrome, and renal tubular acidosis, are thought to be uncommon in the elderly. Multiple pathology is common in old people and more than one cause of hypokalemia is often found with detailed assessment and investigation. Thus, hypokalemia in a patient taking diuretics may be exacerbated by latent purgative abuse. Volume depletion of the ECF by excess diuretic dosage may lie behind hypokalemia rather than simple potassium wasting. Hypokalemia is not a diagnosis by itself. Efficient management requires full assessment and alleviation of underlying and contributory mechanisms. In this respect, the elderly are the same as the young—there is no evidence that elderly patients have deficient potassium homeostatic control systems by virtue of age alone. Any higher prevalence of hypokalemia is secondary to the higher disease load borne by the elderly.

References

1. Bernard C: Introduction à l'Étude de la Medicine Experimentale. Ballìere, Paris, 1865
2. Bernard C: Léçons sur les Phenomenes de la Vie. Cours de Physiologie Generale de Musée d'Histoire Naturelle, Paris, 1878
3. Adolph EF: Origins of Physiological Regulations. Academic Press, New York; 1968
4. Pavlov IP: Conditional Reflexes. Oxford University Press, London, 1927
5. Lye M, Vargas E, Faragher EB et al: Haemodynamic and neurohumoral responses in elderly patients with postural hypotension. Eur J Clin Invest 1990;20:90–96
6. Donbal S: Theory of reliability, biological systems and aging. Mech Ageing Dev 1982;18:339–353
7. Canon WB: The Wisdom of the Body. Norton, New York, 1932
8. Finch CE: Enzyme activities, gene function and aging in mammals. Exp Gerontol 1972;7:53–75
9. Damon A, Seltzer CC, Stoudt HW, Bell B: Age and physique in healthy white veterans at Boston. J Gerontol 1972;27: 202–208
10. Frisancho AR: New standards of weight and body composition by frame size and height for assessment of nutritional status of adults and the elderly. Am J Clin Nutr 1984;40: 808–819
11. Prothro JW, Rosenbloom CA: Body measurements of black-and-white elderly persons with emphasis on body-composition. Gerontology 1995;41:22–38
12. Lehmann AB, Bassey EJ, Morgan K, Dallosso HM: Normal values for weight. Clin Nutr 1991;10:18–22
13. Borkan GA, Hults DE, Glynn RJ: Role of longitudinal change and secular trend in age differences in male body dimensions. Hum Biol 1983;55:629–641
14. Bevier WC, Wiswell RA, Pyka G: Relationship of body composition, muscle strength, and aerobic capacity to bone mineral density in older mem and women. J Bone Min Res 1989;4: 421–432
15. Munro HN: Nutrition and ageing. Br Med Bull 1981;37:83–88
16. Moore FD, Olsen KH, MacMurrey JD et al: The Body Cell Mass and its Supporting Environment. WB Saunders, London, 1963
17. Boddy K, Hume R, King PC et al: Total body, plasma and erythrocyte potassium and leucocyte ascorbic acid in "ultra-fit" subjects. Clin Sci Mol Med 1974;46:449–456
18. Owen OE: Resting metabolic requirements of men and women. Mayo Clin Proc 1988;53:503–510
19. Horber FF, Kohler SA, Lippuner K, Jaeger P: Effect of regular physical-training on age-associated alteration of body composition in men. Eur J Clin Invest 1996;26:279–285
20. Adams GM, DeVries HA: Physiological effects of an exercise training regimen upon women aged 52 to 79. J Gerontol 1973; 28:50–55
21. Lye M: Body potassium content and capacity of elderly individuals with and without cardiac failure. Cardiovasc Res 1982; 16:22–25
22. Pearson MB, Bassey EJ, Bendall MJ: Muscle strength and anthropometric indices in elderly men and women. Age Ageing 1985;14:49–54
23. Meyers DA, Goldberg AP, Bleecker ML et al: Relationship of obesity and physical fitness to cardiopulmonary and metabolic function in healthy older men. J Gerontol 1991;46: M57–65
24. Marti B, Howald H: Long-term effects of physical training on aerobic capacity: controlled study of former elite athletes. J Appl Physiol 1990;69:1451–1459

25. Danneskiold-Samsoe B, Kofod V, Munter J et al: Muscle strength and functional-capacity in 78-81-year-old men and women. Eur J Appl Physiol 1984;52:310–314
26. Cunningham JJ, Barzel US: Lean body mass is a predictor of the daily requirement for thyroid hormone in older men and women. J Am Geriatr Soc 1984;32:204–207
27. Schemmel R, Mickelsen O, Mostosky U: Influence of body weight, age, diet and sex on fat depots in rats. Anat Rec 1970; 166:437–445
28. Bertrand HA, Masoro EJ, Yu BP: Increasing adipocyte number as the basis for perirenal depot growth in adult rats. Science 1978;201:1234–1235
29. Stiles JW, Francendese AA, Masoro EJ: Influence of age on size and number of fat cells in the epididymal depot. Am J Physiol 1975;229:1561–1568
30. Greenwood MRC, Johnson PR, Hirsch J: Relationship of age and cellularity to metabolic activity in C57B mice. Proc Soc Exp Biol Med 1970;133:944–947
31. Yu BP, Masoro EJ: Age-related changes in the total body mass, lean body mass and adipose tissue mass. Gerontologist 1978; 18:140
32. Novak LP: Aging, total body potassium, fat free mass and cell mass in males and females between ages 18 and 85 years. J Gerontol 1972;27:438–443
33. Durnin JVGA, Womersley J: Body fat assessed from total body density and its estimation from skinfold thickness: measurements on 481 men and women aged from 16 to 72 years. Br J Nutr 1974;32:77–79
34. Lye M: Distribution of body potassium in healthy elderly subjects. Gerontology 1981;27:286–292
35. Shimokata H, Tobin JD, Muller DC: Studies in the distribution of body fat. I. Effects of age, sex and obesity. J Gerontol 1989; 44:M66–73
36. Silver AJ, Guillen CP, Kahl MJ, Morley JE: Effect of aging on body-fat. J Am Geriatr Soc 1993;41:211–213
37. Forbes GB, Reina JC: Adult lean body mass declines with age: some longitudinal observations. Metabolism 1970;19: 653–663
38. Parizkova J, Eiselt E: A further study on changes in somatic characteristics and body composition of old men followed longitudinally for 8-10 years. Hum Biol 1971;43:318–326
39. Chien S, Peng MT, Chen KP et al: Longitudinal measurements of blood volume and essential body mass in human subjects. J Appl Physiol 1975;39:818–824
40. Bourliere F, Parot S: Le vieillissement de deux populations blanches vivant dans des conditions ecologiques tres differentes, etude comparative. RF Etud Clin Biol 1962;7:629–635
41. Glanville EV, Geerdink RA: Skinfold thickness, body measurements and age changes in Trio and Wajana Indians of Surinam. Am J Phys Anthropol 1970;32:455–461
42. Lesser GT, Deutsch S, Markofsky J: Aging in the rat: longitudinal and cross-sectional studies of body composition. Am J Physiol 1973;225:1472–1478
43. Rowlatt C, Chesterman FC, Sheriff MU: Lifespan age changes and tumour incidence in an aging C57BL mouse. Lab Anim 1976;10:419–442
44. Boothby WM, Berkson J, Dunn HL: Studies of the energy metabolism of normal individuals: a standard for basal metabolism with a nomogram for chemical application. Am J Physiol 1936;116:468–484
45. Fukagawa NK, Bandini LG, Dietz WH, Young JB: Effect of age on body water and resting metabolic rate. J Gerontol Ser A 1996;51A:M71–73
46. Shock NW, Watkin DM, Yiengst MJ et al: Age differences in the water content of the body as related to basal oxygen consumption in males. J Gerontol 1963;18:1–8
47. Poehlman ET, Melby CL, Badylak SF: Relation of age and physical exercise status on metabolic rate in young and older healthy men. J Gerontol 1991;46:B54–58
48. Robinson S, Dill DB, Tzankoff SP et al: Longitudinal studies of aging in 37 men. J Appl Physiol 1975;38:263–267
49. Holden S-H, MacRae HSH, Dennis SC et al: Effects of training on lactate production and removal during progressive exercise in humans. J Appl Physiol 1992;72:1649–1656
50. Miller AT, Blyth CS: Estimation of lean body mass and body fat from basal oxygen consumption and creatinine excretion. J Appl Physiol 1952;5:73–78
51. Tzankoff SP, Norris AH: Effect of muscle mass decrease on age-related BMR changes. J Appl Physiol 1977;43: 1001–1006
52. Grimby G, Saltin B: Physiological analysis of physically well-trained middle aged and old athletes. Acta Med Scand 1966; 179:513–526
53. Drinkwater BL, Horvath SM, Wells CL: Aerobic power of females ages 10 to 68. J Gerontol 1975;30:385–394
54. Wilmore JH, Miller HL, Pollock ML: Body composition and physiological characteristics of active endurance athletes in their eighth decade of life. Med Sci Sports Exer 1974;6:44–48
55. Robinson S, Dill DB, Robinson RD et al: Physiological aging of champion runners. J Appl Physiol 1976;41:46–51
56. Spirduso WW, Clifford P: Replication of age and physical activity effects on reaction and movement time. J Gerontol 1978;33:26–30
57. Dill DB, Yousef MK, Vitez TS et al: Metabolic observations on Caucasian men and women aged 17 to 88 years. J Gerontol 1982;37:565–571
58. Brandfonbrenner M, Landowne M, Shock NW: Changes in cardiac output with ageing. Circulation 1955;12:557–566
59. Granath A, Jonsson B, Strandell T: Circulation in healthy old men studied by right heart catheterisation at rest and during exercise in supine and sitting position. Acta Med Scand 1964; 176:425–446
60. Hossack KF, Bruce RA: Maximal cardiac function in sedentary normal men and women: comparison of age-related changes. J Appl Physiol 1982;53:799–804
61. Saraiva RA, Lunn JN, Mapleson WW et al: Adiposity and the pharmacokinetics of halothane. Anaesthesia 1977;32: 240–246
62. Avram MJ, Sanghvi R, Henthorn TK et al: Determinants of thiopental induction dose requirements. Anesth Analg 1993; 76:10–17

63. Constans T, Bacq Y, Brechot JF et al: Protein energy malnutrition in elderly medical patients. J Am Geriatr Soc 1992;40: 263–268

64. Morgan DB, Newton HMV, Schorah CJ et al: Abnormal indices of nutrition in the elderly: a study of different clinical groups. Age Ageing 1986;15:65–76

65. Galanos AN, Pieper CF, Cornoni-Huntley JC: Nutrition and function: is there a relationship between body mass index and the functional capabilities of community dwelling elderly. J Am Geriatr Soc 1994;42:368–373

66. Mattila K, Haavisto M, Rajala S: Body mass index and mortality in the elderly. Br Med J 1986;292:868

67. Muhlethaler R, Stuck AE, Minder CE, Frey BM: The prognostic-significance of protein-energy malnutrition in geriatric-patients. Age Ageing 1995;24:193–197

68. Lehmann AB: Nutrition in old age: an update and questions for future research: Part 2. Rev Clin Gerontol 1991;1:231–240

69. Jones DC, Kimeldorf DJ, Rubadeau DO, Castanera TJ: Relationship between volitional activity and age in the male rat. Am J Physiol 1953;172:109–114

70. Sidney KH, Shephard RJ: Activity patterns of elderly men and women. J Gerontol 1977;32:25–32

71. Friedman PJ, Campbell AJ, Caradoc-Davies TH: Hypoalbuminaemia in the elderly is due to disease not malnutrition. J Clin Exp Gerontol 1985;7:191–205

72. Durrieu G, Llau M-E, Rascol O et al: Parkinson's disease and weight loss: a study with antrhopomctric and nturitional assessment. Clin Auton Res 1992;2:153–157

73. Elmstahl E, Petersson M, Lilja B et al: Body composition in patients with Alzheimer's disease and healthy controls. J Clin Exp Gerontol 1992;14:17–31

74. Robinson JR, McCance RA: Water metabolism. Annu Rev Physiol 1952;14:115–122

75. MacCallum AB: The paleochemistry of the body fluids and tissues. Physiol Rev 1926;6:316–357

76. Conway EJ: The chemical evolution of the ocean. Proc Irish Med Acad 1943;8:161–212

77. Edelman IS, Haley HB, Schloerb PR et al: Further observations on total body water. I. Normal values throughout life span. Surg Gynecol Obstet 1952;95:1–12

78. Olbrich O, Woodford-Williams E: Water distribution in the aged in correlation to cardiac and renal function. pp. 236–245. In: Experimentelle Alternsforschung. Birkhauser Verlag, Basel, 1956

79. Young CM, Blondin J, Tensuan R, Fryer JH: Body composition studies of "older" women thirty to seventy years of age. Ann NY Acad Sci 1963;110:589–607

80. Steele JM, Berger EY, Dunning MF, Brodie BB: Total body water in man. Am J Physiol 1950;162:313–317

81. Steen B, Isaksson B, Svanborg A: Body composition at 70 and 75 years of age: a longitudinal population study. J Clin Exp Gerontol 1979;1:185–200

82. Bruce A, Andersson M, Arvidsson B, Isaksson B: Body composition. Prediction of normal body potassium, body water and body fat in adults on the basis of body height, body weight and age. Scand J Clin Lab Invest 1980;40:461–473

83. Cleland JGF, Dargie HJ, Robertson I et al: Total body electrolyte composition in patients with heart failure: a comparison with normal subjects and patients with untreated hypertension. Br Heart J 1987;58:230–238

84. Albala C, Yanez M, Salazar G, Vio F: Body composition in the elderly: total body water and anthropometry. Nutr Res 1994;14:1797–1809

85. Mazariegos M, Wang ZM, Gallagher D et al: Differences between young and old females in the 5 levels of body composition and their relevance to the two-compartment chemical model. J Gerontol Ser A 1994;49:M201–208

86. Lowry OH, Hastings AB: Quantitative histochemical changes in aging. pp. 105–138. In Lansing AI (ed) Cowdry's Problems of Aging. 3rd Ed. Williams & Wilkins, Baltimore, 1952

87. Steen B: Body water in the elderly. Lancet 1985;1:101

88. Sergi G, Bussolotto M, Perini P et al: Accuracy of bioelectrical impedance analysis in estimation of extracellular space in healthy subjects and in fluid retention states. Ann Nutr Metab 1994;38:158–165

89. Tagliabue A, Cena H, Deurenberg P: Comparative study of the relationship between multifrequency impedance and body water compartments in 2 European populations. Br J Nutr 1996;75:11–19

90. Strauss MB, Lamdin E, Smith WP, Bleifer DJ: Surfeit and deficit of sodium: a kinetic concept of sodium excretion. Arch Intern Med 1958;102:527

91. Gibson JG, Evans WAJ: Clinical studies of the blood volume. II. The relation of plasma and total blood volume to venous pressure, blood velocity, physical measurements, age and sex in 90 normal humans. J Clin Invest 1937;16:317–318

92. Cohn JE, Shock NW: Blood volume studies in middle-aged and elderly males. Am J Med Sci 1949;217:388–391

93. Gunnarsson L, Tokics L, Brismar B, Hedenstierna G: Influence of age on circulation and arterial blood gases in man. Acta Anaesthesiol Scand 1996;40:237–243

94. Epstein M, Duncan DC, Fishman LM: Characterization of the natriuresis caused in normal man by immersion in water. Clin Sci 1972;43:275–287

95. Paintal AS: Vagal sensory receptors and their reflex effects. Physiol Rev 1973;53:159–227

96. Epstein M: Cardiovascular and renal effects of head-out water immersion in man: application of the model in the assessment of volume homeostasis. Circ Res 1976;39:619–628

97. Keeler R: Natriuresis after unilateral stimulation of carotid receptors in unanaesthetised rats. Am J Physiol 1974;226: 507–511

98. Burnett JCJ, Knox FG: Renal interstitial pressure and sodium excretion during renal vein constriction. Am J Physiol 1980; 238:F279–282

99. DeWardner HE, Mills IH, Clapham WF, Hayter CJ: Studies on the efferent mechanism of the sodium diuresis which follows the administration of intravenous saline in the dog. Clin Sci 1961;21:249–258

100. Johnson MD, Malvin RL: Stimulation of renal sodium reabsorption by angiotensin II. Am J Physiol 1977;232:F298–306

101. Young DB, Guyton AC: Steady state aldosterone dose-response relationships. Circ Res 1977;40:138–142

102. Skorecki KL, Brenner BM: Body fluid homeostasis in man: a contemporary overview. Am J Med 1981;70:77–88

103. Bie P: Osmoreceptors, vasopressin, and control of renal water excretion. Physiol Rev 1980;60:961–1048

104. Helderman JH, Vestal RE, Rowe JW et al: The response of arginine vasopressin to intravenous ethanol and hypertonic saline in man: the impact of aging. J Gerontol 1978;33: 39–47

105. Duggan J, Kilfeather S, Lightman SL, O'Malley K: The association of age with plasma arginine vasopressin and plasma osmolality. Age Ageing 1993;22:332–336

106. Robertson GL, Athar S: The interaction of blood osmolality and blood volume in regulating plasma arginine vasopressin in man. J Clin Endocrinol Metab 1976;42:613–620

107. Hammer M, Ladefogerd J, Olgoord K: Relationship between plasma osmolarity and plasma vasopressin in human subjects. Am J Physiol 1980;238:E313–317

108. Kirkland JL, Lye M, Goddard C et al: Plasma arginine vasopressin in dehydrated elderly patients. Clin Endocrinol 1984; 20:451–456

109. Davies I, O'Neill PA, McLean KA et al: Age-associated alterations in thirst and arginine vasopressin in response to a water or sodium load. Age Ageing 1995;24:151–159

110. Rowe JR, Minaker KL, Sparrow D, Robertson GL: Age-related failure of volume-pressure medited vasopressin release. J Clin Endocrinol Metab 1982;54:661–664

111. Ishikawa S, Fujita N, Fujisawa G et al: Involvement of arginine-vasopressin and renal sodium handling in pathogenesis of hyponatremia in elderly patients. Endocrinol J 1996;43: 101–108

112. Wilson PD, Dillingham MA: Age-associated decrease in vasopressin-induced renal water transport: a role for adenylate cyclase and G protein malfunction. Gerontology 1992;38: 315–321

113. Faull CM, Holmes C, Baylis PH: Water balance in elderly people—is there a deficiency of vasopressin? Age Ageing 1993;22:114–120

114. Sonnenblick M, Algur N: Hypernatremia in the acutely ill elderly patients: role of impaired arginine-vasopressin secretion. Min Electrol Metab 1993;19:32–35

115. Johnson AK, Mann JFE, Rascher W et al: Plasma angiotensin II concentrations and experimentally induced thirst. Am J Physiol 1981;240:R229–234

116. Skott P, Ingerslev J, Damkjaer Nielsen M, Giese J: The renin-angiotensin-aldosterone system in normal 85 year old people. Scand J Clin Lab Invest 1987;47:69–74

117. Duggan J, Kilfeather S, O'Brien E: Effects of aging and hypertension on plasma angiotensin II and platelet angiotensin II receptor desnity. Am J Hypertens 1992;5:687–693

118. Duggan J, Nussberger J, Kilfeather S, O'Malley K: Aging and human hormonal and pressor responsiveness to angiotensin II infusion with simultaneous measurement of exogenous and endogenous angiotensin II. Am J Hypertens 1993;6: 641–647

119. Phillips PA, Rolls BJ, Ledingham JGG et al: Reduced thirst in the elderly after 24-hour water deprivation. Clin Sci 1983; 64:61P–62P

120. Phillips PA, Rolls BJ, Ledingham JGG et al: Reduced thirst after water deprivation in healthy elderly men. N Engl J Med 1984;311:753–759

121. Rolls BJ, Phillips PA, Phil D: Aging and disturbances of thirst and fluid balance. Nutr Rev 1990;48:137–144

122. Phillips PA, Bretherton M, Johnston CI, Gray L: Reduced osmotic thirst in healthy elderly men. Am J Physiol 1991;261: R166–171

123. Mack GW, Weseman CA, Langhans GW et al: Body-fluid balance in dehydrated healthy older men: thirst and renal osmoregulation. J Appl Physiol 1994;76:1615–1623

124. O'Neill PA, Davies I, Wears R, Barrett JA: Elderly female patients in continuing care: why are they hyperosmolar? Gerontology 1989;35:205–209

125. Duggan J, Catania J, O'Neill P, Davies I: Response to dehydration in long term care elderly patients. Clin Sci 1991;81:27

126. O'Neill PA, Davies I, Fullerton KJ, Bennett D: Fluid balance in elderly patients following acute stroke. Age Ageing 1992; 21:280–285

127. McLean KA, O'Neill PA, Davies I: Are the elderly dehydrated? A study to determine plasma osmolality in a community population. Clin Sci 1989;77:7

128. Davies I: A physiological approach to ageing. p. 84–104. In: Horan MA, Brouwer A (eds): Gerontology—Approaches to Biomedical and Clinical Research. Edward Arnold, London, 1990

129. Lye M: Electrolyte disorders in the elderly. Clin Endocrinol Metab 1984;13:377–398

130. Phillips PA, Hodsman GP, Johnston CI: Neuroendocrine mechanisms and cardiovascular homeostasis in the elderly. Cardiovasc Drugs Ther 1991;4(suppl 6):1209–1213

131. Needleman P, Greenwald JE: Atriopeptide: a cardiac hormone intimately involved in fluid, electrolyte, and blood-pressure homeostasis. N Engl J Med 1986;314:828–834

132. O'Hashi M, Fujio N, Nawata H et al: High plasma concentration of human atrial natriuretic polypeptide in aged men. J Clin Endocrinol Metab 1987;64:81–85

133. Cugini P, Lucia P, Dipalma L et al: Effect of aging on circadian rhythm of atrial natriuretic peptide, plasma renin activity, and plasma aldosterone. J Gerontol Ser A 1992;47:B214–219

134. Richards AM: Human plasma atrial natriuretic peptide concentrations in health and disease. Curr Opin Cardiol 1987;2: 660–670

135. Ezaki H, Matsushita S, Shiraki M: Clinical evaluation of the plasma levels of immunoreactive atrial natriuretic peptide in elderly patients with heart diseases. J Am Geriatr Soc 1988; 36:537–541

136. Hodkinson HM: Biochemical Diagnosis of the Elderly. Chapman and Hall, London, 1977

137. Hale WE, Stewart RB, Marks RG: Haematological and

biochemical laboratory values in an ambulatory elderly population: an analysis of the effects of age, sex and drugs. Age Ageing 1983;12:275–284

138. Leask RGS, Andrews GR, Caird FI: Normal values for sixteen blood constituents in the elderly. Age Ageing 1973;2: 14–23

139. Osterlind PO, Alafuzoff I, Lofgren A-C et al: Blood components in an elderly population. Gerontology 1984;30:247–252

140. Wilding P, Rollason JG, Robinson D: Patterns of change for various biochemical constituents detected in well population screening. Clin Chim Acta 1972;41:375–387

141. Bold AM, Wilding P: Clinical Chemistry. Blackwell Scientific Publications, Oxford, 1975

142. Haavisto MV, Heikinheimo RJ, Mattila KJ, Rajala SA: Living conditions and health of a population aged 85 years or over: a five-year follow-up study. Age Ageing 1985;14:202–208

143. Roberts LB: The normal ranges, with statistical analysis for seventeen blood constitutents. Clin Chim Acta 1967;16: 69–78

144. Keating FR, Jones JD, Elveback LR, Randall RV: The relation of age and sex to distribution of values in healthy adults of serum calcium, inorganic phosphorus, magnesium, alkaline phosphatase, total proteins, albumin and blood urea. J Lab Clin Med 1969;73:825–834

145. Bowker LK, Briggs RSJ, Gallagher PJ, Robertson DRC: Raised blood urea in the elderly: a clinical and pathological study. Postgrad Med J 1992;68:174–179

146. Denham MJ, Hodkinson HM, Fisher M: Glomerular filtration rate in sick elderly inpatients. Age Ageing 1975;4:32–36

147. Salive ME, Jones CA, Guralnik JM et al: Serum creatinine levels in older adults: relationship with health-status and medications. Age Ageing 1995;24:142–150

148. Rowe JW, Andres R, Tobin JD et al: The effect of age on creatinine clearance in men: a cross-sectional and longitudinal study. J Gerontol 1976;31:155–163

149. Rowe JW, Andres R, Tobin JD et al: Age-adjusted standards for creatinine clearance. Ann Intern Med 1976;84:567–569

150. Sica DA: Renal disease, electrolyte abnormalities, and acid-base imbalance in the elderly. Clin Geriatr Med 1994;10: 197–211

151. Lubran MM: Renal function in the elderly. Ann Clin Lab Sci 1995;25:122–133

152. Bahemuka M, Hodkinson HM, Denham MJ, Padmore GRA: Serum creatinine in a geriatric inpatient population. Age Ageing 1974;3:43–48

153. Shock NW, Yiengst M: Age changes in the acid-base equilibrium of the blood of males. J Gerontol 1950;5:1–4

154. Guyton AC: Parathyroid hormone, calcitonin, calcium and phosphate metabolism, vitamin D, bone and teeth. pp. 1052–10 In Guyton AC (ed) Textbook of Medical Physiology. 5th Ed. WB Saunders, London, 1976

155. Langfort J, Pilis W, Zarzeczny R et al: Effect of low-carbohydrate-ketogenic diet on metabolic and hormonal responses to graded-exercise in men. J Physiol Pharmacol 1996;47: 361–371

156. Dill DB, Phillips EE, MacGregor D: Training: youth and age. Ann NY Acad Sci 1966;134:760–775

157. Bouhuys A, Pool J, Binkhorst RA, van Leeuwen P: Metabolic acidosis of exercise in healthy males. J Appl Physiol 1966; 21:1040–1046

158. Altose MD, McCauley WC, Kelsen SG, Cherniack NS: Effects of hypercapnia and inspiratory flow resistive loading onrespiratory activity in chronic airways obstruction. J Clin Invest 1977;59:500–507

159. Rubin S, Tack M, Cherniack NS: Effect of aging on respiratory responses to CO_2 and inspiratory resistive loads. J Gerontol 1982;37:306–312

160. Hazard PB, Griffin JP: Calculation of sodium bicarbonate requirement in metabolic acidosis. Am J Med Sci 1982;283: 18–22

161. Solomon LR, Sangster G, Lye M: Hyponatraemia in the elderly patient. Geriatr Nephrol Urol 1992;2:63–74

162. Stacpoole PW, Wright E, Baumgartner TG et al: A controlled clinical trial of dichloroacetate for treatment of lactic acidosis in adults. N Engl J Med 1992;327:1564–1569

163. Anderson RJ: Hospital-associated hyponatraemia. Kidney Int 1986;29:1237–1247

164. Parameshwar J, Sparrow J, Sutton G, Poole-Wilson PA: Prediction of outcome in severe chronic heart failure. Br Heart J 1991;66:58

165. Himmelstein DU, Jones AA, Woolhandler S: Hypernatremic dehydration in nursing home patients: an indicator of neglect. J Am Geriatr Soc 1983;31:466–471

166. Solomon LR, Lye M: Hypernatraemia in the elderly patient. Gerontology 1990;36:171–179

167. Mimran A, Ribstein J, Jover B: Aging and sodium homeostasis. Kidney Int 1992;37:S107–113

168. Crowe MJ, Forsling ML, Rolls BJ et al: Altered water excretion in healthy elderly men. Age Ageing 1987;16:285–293

169. Rowe JW, Shock NW, DeFronzo RA: The influence of age on the renal response to water deprivation in man. Nephron 1976; 17:270–278

170. Anonymous: Thirst and osmoregulation in the elderly. Lancet 1984;1:1017–1018

171. Davies AB, Williams I, John R et al: Diagnostic value of thyrotrophin releasing hormone tests in elderly patients with atrial fibrillation. Br Med J 1985;291:773–776

172. Vargas E, Lye M, Faragher EB et al: Cardiovascular haemodynamics and the response of vasopressin, aldosterone, plasma renin activity and plasma catecholamines to head-up tilt in young and old healthy subjects. Age Ageing 1986; 15:17–28

173. Fukagawa NK, Bandini LG, Lee MA, Young JB: Effect of age on dopaminergic responses to protein feeding. Physiol-Renal Fluid Electrol Physiol 1995;37:F613–625

174. Hayduk K, Krause DK, Kaufman W: Age dependent changes of plasma renin concentrations in humans. Clin Sci 1975;45: 273S–278S

175. Bay WH, Ferris TF: Hypernatraemia and hyponatraemia: disorders of tonicity. Geriatrics 1976;31:53–64

176. Berl T, Anderson RJ, McDonald KM, Schrier RW: Clinical disorders of water metabolism. Kidney Int 1976;10:117–132

177. Kennedy PGE, Mitchell DM, Hoffbrand BI: Severe hyponatraemia in hospital inpatients. Br Med J 1978;2:1251–1253

178. Morgan DB, Thomas TH: Water balance and hyponatraemia. Clin Sci 1979;56:517–522

179. Miller M, Hecker MS, Friedlander DA, Carter JM: Apparent idiopathic hyponatremia in an ambulatory geriatric population. J Am Geriatr Soc 1996;44:404–408

180. Tanneau RS, Bourbigot B, Richard P et al: Prognosis and neurologic outcome of severe hyponatremia in elderly patients. Eur J Intern Med 1993;4:311–318

181. Chung HM, Kluge R, Schrier RW, Anderson RJ: Post-operative hyponatremia. Arch Intern Med 1986;146:333–336

182. Everitt NJ: Severe hyponatremia in elderly patients: cause for concern. Ann R Coll Surg Engl 1996;78:73

183. Burrows FA, Shautack JG, Crone RK: Inappropriate secretion of antidiuretic hormone in a postsurgical pediatric population. Crit Care Med 1983;11:527–531

184. Bouzarth WF, Shenkin HA: Is "cerebral hyponatraemia" iatrogenic? Lancet 1982;1:1061–1062

185. Bartter FC, Schwartz WB: The syndrome of inappropriate secretion of antidiuretic hormone. Am J Med 1967;42:790–806

186. Charles R, Rees JR: Inappropriate secretion of antidiuretic hormone in pneumonia. Postgrad Med J 1975;51:663–664

187. Thomas TH, Morgan DB, Swaminathan R et al: Severe hyponatraemia. A study of 17 patients. Lancet 1978;1:621–624

188. Verbalis JG: Tumoral hyponatremia. Arch Intern Med 1986; 146:1686–1687

189. Arieff AI: Fortnightly review: management of hyponatraemia. Br Med J 1993;307:305–308

190. Padfield PL, Morton JJ, Brown J et al: Plasma arginine vasopressin in the syndrome of antidiuretic hormone excess associated with bronchogenic carcinoma. Am J Med 1976;61: 825–831

191. Carrilho F, Bosch J, Arroyo V et al: Renal failure associated with demeclocycline in cirrhosis. Ann Intern Med 1977;85: 336–337

192. Daggett P: Endocrine emergencies. Br J Hosp Med 1979;21: 38–44

193. Hartman D, Rossier B, Zohlman R: Rapid correction of hyponatraemia in the syndrome of inappropriate secretion of antidiuretic hormone. Ann Intern Med 1973;78:870–875

194. Mather HM, Ang V, Jenkins JS: Vasopressin in plasma and CSF of patients with subarachnoid haemorrhage. J Neurol Neurosurg Psych 1981;44:216–219

195. Auger RG, Zehr JE, Siekert RG, Segar WE: Position effect on antidiuretic hormone. Arch Neurol 1970;23:513–517

196. Hemmer M, Viquerat CE, Suter PM, Vallotton MB: Urinary antidiuretic hormone excretion during mechanical ventilation and weaning in man. Anesthesiology 1980;52:395–400

197. Joynt RJ, Feibel JH, Sladek CM: Antidiuretic hormone levels in stroke patients. Ann Neurol 1981;9:182–184

198. Rydin H, Vernay EB: The inhibition of water diuresis by emotional stress and muscular exercise. J Exp Physiol 1938;27: 343–374

199. Moran WH, Miltenberger FW, Shuayb WA, Zimmerman B: The relationship of antidiuretic hormone secretion to surgical stress. Surgery 1964;56:99–108

200. Dubovsky SL, Groban S, Berl T, Schrier RW: Syndrome of inappropriate secretion of antidiuretic hormone with exacerbated psychosis. Ann Intern Med 1973;79:551–554

201. Clinch D: Syndrome of inappropriate antidiuretic hormone secretion associated with stress. Lancet 1982;1:1131–1132

202. Skowsky WR, Kikuchi TA: The role of vasopressin in the impaired water excetion of myxedema. Am J Med 1978;64: 613–621

203. White AG, Rubin G, Leiter L: Studies in edema. IV. Water retention and the antidiuretic hormone in hepatic and cardiac disease. J Clin Invest 1953;32:931–939

204. Stein M, Schwartz R, Mersky IA: The antidiuretic activity of plasma of patients with hepatic cirrhosis, congestive heart failure, hypertension and other clinical disorders. J Clin Invest 1954;33:77–81

205. Sunderam SG, Mankikar GD: Hyponatraemia in the elderly. Age Ageing 1983;12:77–80

206. Fidler HM, Goldman J, Bielawska CA et al: A study of plasma sodium-levels in elderly people taking amiloride or triamterene in combination with hydrochlorothiazide. Postgrad Med J 1993;69:797–799

207. Dzau VJ, Hollenberg NK: Renal response to captopril in severe heart failure: role of furosemide in natriuresis and reversal of hyponatremia. Ann Intern Med 1984;100:777–782

208. Weston RE, Grossman J, Borun ER, Hanenson IB: The pathogenesis and treatment of hyponatremia in congestive heart failure. Am J Med 1958;25:558–572

209. Takasu T, Lasker N, Shalhoub RJ: Mechanisms of hyponatremia in chronic congestive heart failure. Ann Intern Med 1961;55:368–383

210. Lembo NJ, Dell'Italia LJ, Crawford MH, O'Rourke RA: Bedside diagnosis of systolic murmurs. N Engl J Med 1988;318: 1572–1578

211. Hamilton RW, Buckalew VM: Sodium, water and congestive heart failure. Ann Intern Med 1984;100:902–904

212. Dzau VJ: Renal and circulatory mechanisms in congestive heart failure. Kidney Int 1987;31:1402–1415

213. Schrier RW: Pathogenesis of sodium and water retention in high-output and low-output cardiac failure, nephrotic syndrome, cirrhosis, and pregnancy. N Engl J Med 1988;319: 1127–1134

214. Decaux G, Waterlot Y, Genette F et al: Inappropriate secretion of antidiuretic hormone treated with frusemide. Br Med J 1982; 285:89–90

215. Szatalowicz VL, Miller PD, Lacher JW et al: Comparative effective of diuretics on renal water excretion in hyponatraemic oedematous disorders. Clin Sci 1982;62:235–238

216. Levy DW, Lye M: Diuretics and potassium in the elderly. J R Coll Phys London 1987;21:148–152

217. Montgomery AJ, Shepherd AN, Emslie-Smith D: Severe hyponatraemia and cardiac failure successfully treated with captopril. Br Med J 1982;284:1085–1086

218. Packer M, Medina N, Yushak M: Correction of dilutional hyponatremia in severe chronic heart failure by converting- enzyme inhibition. Ann Intern Med 1984;100:782–789

219. Elisaf M, Theodorou J, Pappas C, Siamopoulos K: Successful treatment of hyponatremia with angiotensin-converting enzyme-inhibitors in patients with congestive heart failure. Cardiology (Basel) 1995;86:477–480

220. Yodfat Y, Yodfat O: First-dose response and long-term effect of the ACE-inhibitor spirapril in hypertensive patients formerly treated with a diuretic. J Drug Develop Clin Pract 1995;7: 91–95

221. Baran D, Hutchinson TA: The outcome of hyponatraemia in a general hospital poulation. Clin Nephrol 1984;22:72–76

222. Anderson RJ, Chung HM, Kluge R, Schrier RW: Hyponatremia: a prospective analysis of its epidemiology and the pathogenetic role of vasopressin. Ann Intern Med 1985;102: 164–168

223. Ashraf N, Locksley R, Arieff AI: Thiazide-induced hyponatremia associated with death or neurologic damage in outpatients. Am J Med 1981;70:1163–1168

224. Fichman MP, Vorherr H, Kleeman CR, Telfer N: Diuretic-induced hyponatraemia. Ann Intern Med 1971;75:853–863

225. Clark BA, Shannon RP, Rosa RM, Epstein FH: Increased susceptibility to thiazide-induced hyponatremia in the elderly. J Am Soc Nephrol 1994;5:1106–1111

226. Chan TYK: Indapamide-induced severe hyponatremia and hypokalemia. Ann Pharmacother 1995;29:1124–1128

227. Solomon LR, Atherton JC, Bobinski H, Green R: Effect of dietary sodium chloride and posture on plasma immunoreactive atrial natriuretic peptide concentrations in man. Clin Sci 1987;72:201–208

228. Tarssanen L, Huikko M, Rossi M: Amiloride induced hyponatraemia. Acta Med Scand 1980;208:492–494

229. Roberts CJC, Channer KS, Bungay D: Hyponatremia induced by a combination of hydrochlorothiazide and triamterene. Br Med J 1984;288:1962

230. Walters EG, Barnes IC, Price SA, Ali Akbar F: Hyponatraemia associated with diuretics. Br J Clin Pract 1987;41:841–844

231. Zalin AM, Hutchinson CE, Jong M, Matthews K: Hyponatraemia during treatment with chlorpropamide and Moduretic. Br Med J 1984;289:659

232. Miller M, Morley JE, Rubenstein LZ: Hyponatremia in a nursing-home population. J Am Geriatr Soc 1995;43:1410–1413

233. Sharma H, Pompei P: Antidepressant-induced hyponatremia in the aged: avoidance and management strategies. Drugs Aging 1996;8:430–435

234. Colgate R: Hyponatremia and inappropriate secretion of antidiuretic-hormone associated with the use of imipramine. Br J Psych 1993;163:819–822

235. Tenholt WL, Vaniperen CE, Schrijver G, Bartelink AKM: Severe hyponatremia during therapy with fluoxetine. Arch Intern Med 1996;156:681–682

236. Kamiyama T, Iseki K, Kawazoe N et al: Carbamazepine-induced hyponatremia in a patient with partial central diabetes-insipidus. Nephron 1993;64:142–145

237. Rault RM: Hyponatremia associated with nonsteroidal antiinflammatory drugs. Am J Med Sci 1993;305:318–320

238. Waugh WH: Utility of expressing serum sodium per unit of water in assessing hyponatraemia. Metabolism 1969;18: 706–712

239. Frick PG, Schmid JR, Kestler JH, Hitzig WM: Hyponatraemia associated with hyperproteinaemia in multiple myeloma. Helv Med Acta 1966;33:317–329

240. Frier BM, Steer CR, Baird JD, Bloomfield S: Misleading plasma electrolyte in diabetic children with severe hyperlipidaemia. Arch Dis Child 1980;55:771–775

241. Elisaf M, Merkouropoulos M, Tsianos EV, Siamopoulos KC: Acid-base and electrolyte abnormalities in alcoholic patients. Min Electrol Metab 1994;20:274–281

242. Swaminathan R, Morgan DB: Pseudohyponatraemia. Lancet 1985;1:96

243. Worth HGJ: A comparison of the measurement of sodium and potassium by flame photometry and ion-selective electrode. Ann Clin Biochem 1985;22:343–350

244. Katz MA: Hyperglycemia-induced hyponatremia: calculation of expected serum sodium depression. N Engl J Med 1973; 289:843–844

245. Flear CTG, Singh CM: Hyponatraemia and sick cells. Br J Anaesthesiol 1973;45:976–994

246. Inaba H, Hirasawa H, Mizuguchi T: Serum osmolality gap in postoperative patients in intensive care. Lancet 1987;1: 1331–1335

247. Long CA, Marin P, Bayer AJ et al: Hypernatremia in an adult inpatient population. Postgrad Med J 1991;67:643–645

248. Molaschi M, Macchione C, Bertagna B et al: Fluid and electrolyte disorders in the elderly: a statistical and clinical study. Arch Gerontol Geriatr 1991;(S2):583–587

249. Borra SI, Beredo R, Kleinfeld M: Hypernatremia in the aging: causes, manifestations and outcome. J Nat Med Assoc 1995; 87:220–224

250. Arieff AI, Guisado R: Effects on the central nervous system of hypernatraemic and hyponatraemic states. Kidney Int 1976; 10:104–116

251. Visser L, Devuyst O: Physiopathology of hypernatremia following relief of urinary-tract obstruction. Acta Clin Belgica 1994; 49:290–295

252. Mahowald JM, Himmelstein DU: Hypernatremia in the elderly: relation to infection and mortality. J Am Geriatr Soc 1981;29:177–180

253. Weinberg AD, Pals JK, Levesque PG et al: Dehydration and death during febrile episodes in the nursing-home. J Am Geriatr Soc 1994;42:968–971

254. Macdonald NJ, McConnell KN, Stephen MR, Dunnigan MG: Hypernatraemic dehydration in patients in a large hospital for the mentally handicapped. Br Med J 1989;299:1426–1429

255. O'Neill PA, Davies I: Hypernatraemic dehydration in patients in a large hospital for the mentally handicapped. Br Med J 1990;300:396–397

256. Lorber D: Nonketotic hypertonicity in diabetes mellitus. Med Clin North Am 1995;79:39–52

257. Miller PD, Krebs RA, Neal BJ, McIntyre DO: Hypodipsia in geriatric patients. Am J Med 1982;73:354–356

258. Dashe AM, Cramm RE, Crist CA et al: A water deprivation test for the differential diagnosis of polyuria. J Am Med Assoc 1963;185:699–703

259. Jadresic A, Maira J: A simple test for the diagnosis of diabetes insipidus. Lancet 1962;1:402–403

260. O'Keeffe ST, Lavan JN: Subcutaneous fluids in elderly hospital patients with cognitive impairment. Gerontology 1996;42: 36–39

261. Bang A: Towards better oral rehydration. Lancet 1993;342: 755–765

262. Schrier RW, Leaf A: Effect of hormones on water, sodium chloride and potassium metabolism. pp. 1032–1046. In Williams RH (ed): Textbook of Endocrinology. 6th Ed. WB Saunders, Philadelphia, 1981

263. Moore FD, Edelman IS, Olney JM et al: Body sodium and potassium III. Inter-related trends in alimentary, renal and cardiovascular disease; lack of correlation between body stores and plasma concentration. Metabolism 1954;3:334–350

264. Flear CTG, Cooke WT, Quinton A: Serum potassium levels as an index of body content. Lancet 1957;1:458–459

265. Kliger AS, Hayslett J: Disorders of potassium balance. pp. 168–204. In Brenner BM, Stein JH (eds): Acid-Base and Potassium Homeostasis. Churchill Livingstone, London, 1978

266. Schon DA, Silva P, Hayslett JP: Mechanism of potassium excretion in renal insufficiency. Am J Physiol 1974;227: 1323–1330

267. Mudge GH, Vislocky K: Electrolyte changes in human striated muscle in acidosis and alkalosis. J Clin Invest 1949;28: 482–486

268. Fraley DS, Adler S: Isohydric regulation of the plasma potassium by bicarbonate in the rat. Kidney Int 1976;9:333–343

269. Andres R, Baltzan MA, Cader G, Zierler KL: Effect of insulin on carbohydrate metabolism and on potassium in the forearm of man. J Clin Invest 1962;41:108–115

270. Todd EP, Vick RL: Kalemotropic effect of epinephrine: analysis with adrenergic agonists and antagonists. Am J Physiol 1971;220:1964–1969

271. Davidson DJ, Levinsky NG, Berliner RW: Maintainence of potassium excretion despite reduction of glomerular filtration during sodium diuresis. J Clin Pathol 1958;37:548

272. Malnic G, Klose RM, Giebisch G: Micropuncture study of distal tubular potassium and sodium transport in rat nephron. Am J Physiol 1966;211:529–559

273. Berger EY: Intestinal absorption and excretion. p.249–286. In Comar CL, Bronner F (eds): Mineral Metabolism—An Advanced Treatise. Academic Press, New York, 1960

274. Bull AM, Carter AB, Lowe KG: Hyperpotassaemic paralysis. Lancet 1953;2:60–63

275. Ettinger PO, Regan TJ, Oldewurtel HA: Hyperkalaemia, cardiac conduction and the EKG: a review. Am Heart J 1974; 88:360–371

276. Adams KRH, Vargas E, Lye M: Electrolyte abnormalities and diuretics in the elderly. J Clin Exp Gerontol 1988;10:171–180

277. Wan HH, Lye M: Moduretic induced metabolic acidosis and hyperkalaemia. Postgrad Med J 1980;56:348–350

278. Lye M, Faragher EB: Can body potassium of old people be predicted from anthropometric data? Clin Physiol 1982;2: 345–350

279. Bender AD, Carter CL, Hansen KB: Use of a diuretic combination of triamterene and hydrochlorothiazide in elderly patients. J Am Geriatr Soc 1967;15:166–173

280. Greenblatt DJ, Koch-Weser J: Adverse reactions to spironolactone. A report from the Boston Collaborative Drug Surveillance Program. J Am Med Assoc 1973;225:40–43

281. Bailey RR: Adverse renal reactions to non-steroidal anti-inflammatory drugs and potassium-sparing diuretics. Adver Drug React Bull 1988;131:492–495

282. Bennett WM, Muther RS, Parker RA et al: Drug therapy in renal failure: dosing guidelines for adults. Part II. Ann Intern Med 1980;93:286–325

283. Herman E, Rado J: Total hyperkalaemic paralysis associated with spironolactone. Observation on a patient with severe renal disease and refractory oedema. Arch Neurol 1966;15: 74–77

284. Knight AH, Parkinson T: Diuretic induced hypokalaemia. Lancet 1967;1:446–447

285. Jaffey L, Martin A: Malignant hyperkalaemia after amiloride/ hydrochlorothiazide treatment. Lancet 1981;1:1271

286. Zimran A, Kramer M, Plaskin M, Hershko C: Incidence of hyperkalaemia induced by indomethacin in a hospital population. Br Med J 1985;291:107–108

287. Frost L, Bottcher M, Botker HE: Enalapril and exercise-induced hyperkalemia. A study of patients randomized to double-blind treatment with enalapril or placebo after acute myocardial infarction. Int J Cardiol 1992;37:401–405

288. Barnes JN, Drew PJT, Furniss SS et al: Effect of angiotensin converting-enzyme inhibition on potassium-mediated aldosterone secretion in essential hypertension. Clin Sci 1985;68: 625–630

289. Shionoiri H: Pharmacokinetic drug interactions with ACE inhibitors. Clin Pharmacokinet 1993;25:20–58

290. Borra S, Shaker R, Kleinfeld M: Hyperkalemia in an adult hospitalized population. Mt Sinai J Med (NY) 1988;55: 226–229

291. Johnston RT, De Bono DP, Nyman CR: Preventable sudden death in patients receiving angiotensin converting enzyme inhibitors and loop/potassium sparing diuretic combinations. Int J Cardiol 1992;34:213–215

292. Barnes JN, Davies ES, Gent CB: Rash, eosinophilia, and hyperkalaemia associated with enalapril. Lancet 1983;2:41–42

293. Scribner BH, Fremont-Smith K, Burnell JM: The effect of acute respiratory acidosis on the internal equilibrium of potassium. J Clin Invest 1955;34:1276–1285

294. Hayes CPJ, McLeod ME, Robinson RR: An extrarenal mechanism for the maintenancebof potassium balance in severe chronic renal failure. Trans Assoc Am Phys 1967;80: 207–216

295. Pollen RH, Williams RH: Hyperkalaemic neuromyopathy in Addison's disease. N Engl J Med 1960;263:273–276

296. Tak PP, Diamant Z: Hyponatremia, hyperkalemia and hypercalcemia after ileal conduit diversion. Scand J Urol Nephrol 1993;27:271–274

297. Shaked Y, Blau A, Shpilberg O, Samra Y: Hyporeninemic hypoaldosteronism associated with multiple-myeloma: 11 years of follow-up. Clin Nephrol 1993;40:79–82

298. DeJong PE: Incidence of hyperkalaemia induced by indomethacin. Br Med J 1985;291:1047

299. Perlmutter EP, Sweeney D, Herskovits G, Kleiner M: Case-report: severe hyperkalemia in a geriatric-patient receiving standard doses of trimethoprim-sulfamethoxazole. Am J Med Sci 1996;311:84–85

300. Crake T, Poole-Wilson PA: Effect of bicycle exercise on plasma potassium in man. Clin Sci 1988;74:9P

301. Ford GA, Blaschke TF, Wiswell R, Hoffman BB: Effect of aging on changes in plasma potassium during exercise. J Gerontol Ser A 1993;48:M140–145

302. Kleinfeld M, Borra S, Gavani S, Corcoran A: Hypokalemia: are elderly females more vulnerable? J Nat Med Assoc 1993; 85:861–864

303. Judge TG: Hypokalaemia in the elderly. Gerontol Clin 1968; 10:102–107

304. Welt LG, Hollander WJ, Blythe WB: The consequences of potassium depletion. J Chron Dis 1960;11:213–254

305. Pick A: Arrhythmias and potassium in man. Am Heart J 1966; 72:295–306

306. Allison SP, Morley CJ, Burns-Cox CJ: Insulin, glucose, and potassium in the treatment of congestive heart failure. Br Med J 1972;3:675–678

307. Steiness E, Olsen KH: Cardiac arrhythmias induced by hypokalaemia and potassium loss during maintenance digoxin therapy. Br Heart J 1976;38:167–172

308. McCarthy ST, Vandenburg MJ, McCarthy G et al: Potassium and cardiac arrhythmias in elderly patients treated with diuretics. Clin Sci 1983;65:47P

309. Saggarmalik AK, Cappuccio FP: Potassium supplements and potassium-sparing diuretics: a review and guide to appropriate use. Drugs 1993;46:986–1008

310. Papademetriou V: Effect of diuretics on cardiac arrhythmias and left ventricular hypertrophy in hypertension. Cardiol (Basel) 1994;84:43–47

311. Hoes AW, Grobbee DE, Peet TM, Lubsen J: Do non-potassium sparing diuretics increase the risk of sudden cardiac death in hypertensive patients. Recent evidence. Drugs 1994;47: 711–733

312. Relman AS, Schwartz WB: The nephrology of potassium depletion: a clinical and pathophysiological entity. N Engl J Med 1956;255:195–203

313. Schwartz WB, Relman AS: Effects of electrolyte disorders on renal structure and function. N Engl J Med 1967;276: 383–389

314. Schwartz WB, Relman AS: Metabolite and renal studies in chronic potassium depletion resulting from over use of laxatives. J Clin Invest 1953;32:258–271

315. Crane CW: Observations on the sodium and potassium content of mucus from the large intestine. Gut 1965;6:439–443

316. Fleischer N, Brown H, Graham DY, Delenna S: Chronic laxative-induced hyperaldosteronism and hypokalaemia simulating Bartter's syndrome. Ann Intern Med 1969;70: 791–798

317. Copeland PM: Renal-failure associated with laxative abuse. Psychother Psychosomat 1994;62:200–220

318. Shields R: Absorption and secretion of electrolytes and water by the human colon with particular reference to benign adenoma and papilloma. Br J Surg 1966;53:893–897

319. Shields R, Miles JB: Absorption and secretion in the large intestine. Postgrad Med J 1965;41:435–439

320. Paraskevaidis IA, Kremastinos DT, Kassimatis AS et al: Increased response of diastolic blood pressure to exercise in patients with coronary artery disease: an index of latent ventricular dysfunction. Br Heart J 1993;69:507–511

321. Anonymous: Diuretics in the elderly. Lancet 1978;1: 1092–1093

322. Ibrahim IK, Ritch AES, MacLennan WJ, May T: Are potassium supplements for the elderly necessary? Age Ageing 1978;7: 165–170

323. Aikawa JK, Fitz RA: Exchangeable potassium content of the body in congestive failure. Circulation 1956;34:1093–1098

324. Flear CTG, Quinton A, Carpenter JG et al: Exchangeable body potassium and sodium in patients in congestive heart failure. Clin Chim Acta 1966;13:1–12

325. White RJ, Chamberlain DA, Hamer J et al: Potassium depletion in severe heart disease. Br Med J 1969;2:606–610

326. Cox JR, Horrocks P, Speight CJ et al: Potassium and sodium distribution in cardiac failure. Clin Sci 1971;41:55–61

327. Olsen KH, Valentin N: Total exchangeable potassium sodium and chloride in patients with severe valvular heart disease during preparation for cardiac surgery. Scand J Thorac Cardiovasc Surg 1973;7:37–44

328. Delwaide PA, Rorive GL: Interet de la determination du potassium total en cardiologie. Acta Cardiol (Brux) 1973 (suppl 17):282–290

329. Davidson C, Burkinshaw L, McLachlan MSF, Morgan DB: Effect of long-term diuretic treatment on body-potassium in heart-disease. Lancet 1976;2:1044–1047

330. Lawson DH, Boddy K, Gray JMB et al: Potassium supplements in patients receiving long-term diuretics for oedema. Q J Med 1976;45:469–478

331. Thomas RD, Silverton NP, Burkinshaw L, Morgan DB: Potassium depletion and tissue loss in chronic heart failure. Lancet 1979;2:9–11

332. Boddy K, King PC, Lindsay RM et al: Exchangeable and total body potassium in patients with chronic renal failure. Br Med J 1972;1:140–142

333. Boddy K, Davies DL, Howie AD et al: Total body and

exchangeable potassium in chronic airways obstruction: a controversial area? Thorax 1978;33:62–66

334. Lye M, Winston B: Whole body potassium and total exchangeable potassium in elderly patients with cardiac failure. Br Heart J 1979;42:568–572

335. Lye M: The prediction of body potassium in the elderly. Age Ageing 1982;11:108–112

336. Manner RJ, Brechbill DO, DeWitt K: Prevalence of hypokalaemia in diuretic therapy. Clin Med 1972;79:15–18

337. Leemhuis MP, Struyvenburg A: Significance of hypokalaemia due to diuretics. Neth J Med 1973;16:18–28

338. Morgan DB, Davidson C: Hypokalaemia and diuretics: an analysis of publications. Br Med J 1980;1:905–908

339. Skovbo P, Bjerregaard P, Hvidt R: Diuretika og hypokaliaemi. Ugeskr Laeger 1972;134:1043–1047

340. Krakauer R, Lauritzen M: Diuretic therapy and hypokalaemia in geriatric outpatients. Dan Med Bull 1978;25:126–129

341. Schwartz AB, Swartz CD: Dosage of potassium chloride elixir to correct thiazide-induced hypokalaemia. J Am Med Assoc 1974;230:702–704

342. Sheehan J, White A: Diuretic associated hypomagnesaemia. Br Med J 1982;285:1157–1159

343. Hickey PM, Harp JB: Hypokalemia is associated with low thyrotropin levels in the elderly. J Invest Med 1996;44:A5

344. Rees LH: The biosynthesis of hormones by non-endocrine tumours: a review. J Endocrinol 1975;67:143–175

345. Azzopardi JG, Williams ED: Pathology of non-endocrine tumours associated with Cushing's syndrome. Cancer 1968;22: 274–286

346. Davis AR, Diggory P, Seward HC: Prevalence of chronic hypokalemia amongst elderly patients using acetozolamide and diuretics. Eye 1995;9:381–382

CHAPTER 67

Diseases of the Aging Kidney

VANITA JASSAL
HOWARD FILLIT
DIMITRIOS G. OREOPOULOS

Diagnostic Problems of Renal Disease in the Aged

The diagnosis of renal disease in the elderly poses a unique challenge to the clinician and indeed calls for sensitivity and attention to detail. Some of the difficulties in diagnosis are

1. The unspecifiable nature of symptoms and often even the complete absence of the classic symptoms found in younger patients
2. The concomitant occurrence of diseases other than renal—diabetes, cardiac failure, arteriosclerotic vascular disease—confuse both the clinical picture and the symptomatology, and as a result the clinical diagnosis often overlooks renal disease
3. The interpretation of clinical findings, urinary findings and clearance estimations, is often difficult without special knowledge of alterations induced by the aging process.

These diagnostic difficulties indicate the need for a high index of suspicion for renal disease in the elderly. A high prevalence of renal disease has been well-documented in this age group.[1,2] The basic examinations that must be performed as a matter of routine on all patients are as follows: hemoglobin (or hematocrit), blood urea nitrogen and/or serum creatinine, urinalysis for albumin, sugar, pH, microscopic examination of the urinary sediment, and screening for bacteria.

Collection of Urine Samples

Obtaining a clean urine sample for examination is of special importance because, in elderly women, there is frequent contamination of the sample. The bedridden female patient of advanced age is the most difficult subject, and therefore the nursing staff needs special training in collecting urine samples. According to Roberts and colleagues,[3] the best method is to clean the periurethral area with water without adding any disinfecting agent. The specimen is best obtained in the morning when the urine has been in the bladder for some time. A large diuresis might reduce the concentration of bacteria, and therefore impede interpretation of the bacteria count. It is of the utmost importance that the laboratory data be obtained under controlled conditions.

The incontinent elderly patient can, with careful nursing care, sometimes provide a clean catch specimen of urine.[4,5] However, occasionally single or intermittent catheterization is necessary. The use of a sterile technique provides no superior benefit over the standard clean method of catheterization.[6] Catheterization must only be performed if necessary as it can itself infect the urinary tract in up to 5.6 percent of cases.[7] As a last resort, bladder puncture and suprapubic aspiration may be used. Suprapubic aspiration is both safe and accurate, but it is technically difficult in the elderly and has a consistent success rate of only 65 percent, making it impractical as a routine procedure.[8] According to these investigators, the mid stream urine (MSU) has an incidence of doubtful results between 17.5 percent and 28 percent, while frankly contaminated results may be as high as 31 percent.

Interpretation of Urinary Sediment

As with younger patients, the interpretation of urinary sediment helps identify glomerular disease and vasculitis. Casts, dysmorphic red cells, and high levels of proteinuria and hematuria all call for further investigation by a nephrologist. The addition of salicylic acid to urine causes precipitation of protein, not normally identified with albumin dipsticks, if light-chain protein excretion in myeloma is significant. In the elderly, however, most commonly, microscopic examination of sediment reveals an increased number of leukocytes, and epithelial cells. If the bacteriologic findings reveal a mixed infection, then contamination must be suspected, although mixed infection may occur especially in patients with indwelling catheters. In these cases, the urinary tests should be repeated. An increase in the number of leukocytes—more than 10/ml—is regarded as pathologic in younger patients, but is not always a sign of an infection of the urinary tract in the elderly. Conversely, the occurrence of a normal number of leukocytes does not exclude the possibility of infection. It should be recognized that there are several sources of error in the examination of the urinary sediment.[9] These include the volume of urine being sampled; the presence of bacteria in the urinary sediment, with a negative culture, suggesting the presence of lactobacilli and corynebacteria; variations in the number of white blood cells seen under the microscope, which depends upon (1) how the specimen was obtained (i.e., the degree of vaginal or urethral contamination); (2) the urine flow rate at the time of collection; (3) the intensity of the tissue reaction of the uroepithelial surfaces to the disease process; (4) the volume, time, and speed of centrifugation; and (5) the volume in which the observer suspends the sediment. According to Stamey,[9] "... the number of WBC present in the spun sediment can vary so markedly as to be meaningless." Thus, the presence or absence of pyuria in the urinary sediment cannot be used alone as a criterion for infection. However, in an investigational study in whom these variables were presumably well-controlled,[10] a random sample of 405 elderly inhabitants were examined for significant bacteriuria and the correlation between significant bacteriuria and increased number of leukocytes in the high-power field of urinary sediment was found to be significant.

Screening for Bacteria

Screening for bacteria in the urine is traditionally done using the colony count method described by Kass and colleagues.[11] In this series of young healthy women a bacterial count of more than 10^5 organisms/mL was associated with a 80 percent probability of representing true bacteriuria rather than contamination. Strictly speaking, the definition applies only to *Escherichia coli* and *Proteus* spp., which do not grow in clumps or chains. However, the definition has traditionally become synonymous with the presence of a urinary tract infection. As urine samples are more difficult to obtain in elderly persons, a high false-positive rate is seen when this definition is used[12] and the use of urine culture as a screening test for urinary tract infection has been brought into question.[13] Lower counts of bacteriuria may also be significant and bacterial invasion of the bladder wall has been recorded with fewer than 10^5 colonies of bacteria/mL.[14]

A number of chemical and microscopic methods for rapid screening of urine for infection are in use. These include dipstick testing for urinary nitrites, leukocyte esterase, and ward-based urine microscopy for urinary leukocytes. No one screening test has adequate sensitivity and specificity, however, the use of two or more tests together increase the sensitivity to over 90 percent when one or more tests is positive and over 95 percent specificity when all are negative.[5] These tests should not be used after urinary catheterization or any urological procedure as they have unacceptably low sensitivity and specificity rates.[15]

Diseases of the Kidney in the Aged

The elderly are prone to the same diseases of the kidney as younger patients. The difference lies in the presentation, which may be less overt or confounded by the presence of multisystem disease. As with all renal pathology, the main problems will be divided into those affecting the interstitium and tubules, those affecting the glomeruli, and disorders of the vasculature.

Diseases of the Interstitium

Urinary Tract Infections and Pyelonephritis

The significance of Bacteriuria in the Elderly

Significant bacteriuria occurs very often in the aged. Four categories describing the relationship between bacteriuria and urinary tract infection include symptomatic infection, asymptomatic infection (asymptomatic bacteriuria), relapsing or persisting infection, and reinfection.[16] The relationship between bacteriuria, lower urinary tract infection, and upper urinary tract infection (or pyelonephritis) in these categories of patients is not clear, and methods for making the distinction between upper and lower urinary tract infection are not completely reliable.

In an epidemiologic study in Finland, Sourander[10] showed that significant bacteriuria occurred in 20 percent of the population aged 65 and over. Similar findings were observed by Brocklehurst.[17] In an examination 5 years later Sourander et al.[18] found that the infection continued in 35 percent of the patients—in 14 percent of men and 41 percent of women. New infection had developed in 7 percent of the men and in 13 percent of the women. Again a similar prevalence of urinary tract infection of 16.5 percent (24 percent of women and 8 percent of men) was found. The infected cases had not increased in number, though over the 5-year period some of the previously noninfected patients had become infected.

In the institutionalized patients the incidence of bacteriuria has been shown to increase to 43 percent in noncatheterized patients[19] and 50.6 percent in patients intermittently catheterized.[20] The risk of bacteriuria increases with age, non-self-catheterization (in males) and infrequently practiced catheterization routines.[20] Although the presence of immobility, urinary, and fecal incontinence is associated with a high rate of bacteriuria, treatment of the bacteriuria does not appear to improve the functional status.[17,21]

The relationship between bacteriuria and hypertension in the aged also remains an unresolved issue. In younger age groups the occurrence of hypertension in connection with chronic pyelonephritis is well-established.[22] Marketos[23] studied the relationship between bacteriuria and hypertension in the elderly. Although he reports a higher incidence of both bacteriuria and hypertension in elderly institutionalized patients when compared with ambulant residents (the average occurrence of bacteriuria in the first-mentioned groups was 18.7 percent and in the second group 57.9 percent and of hypertension, respectively, 25.6 and 48.7 percent) this association is now believed to be more coincidental than causative, reflecting a more ill, bedridden population at higher risk of urinary infections.

No long-term sequelae of bacteriuria are seen in the elderly.[13,21,24–26] The older, sicker and less mobile patients are more prone to urinary infections leading to an initial impression of a causal relationship between increased mortality and bacteriuria.[27] This has since been disproven and the occurrence of bacteriuria is known to reflect how sick an individual is. Antimicrobial therapy does not improve mortality and neither screening for, nor treatment of, asymptomatic urinary tract infections is warranted in elderly patients. The exception to this rule is the presence of asymptomatic bacteriuria at the time of removal of a urinary catheter, or prior to urologic and gynecologic instrumentation. Bacteriuria, in this case, is strongly associated with a high incidence of subsequent infection and a single dose of antimicrobial therapy (for example, 320 to 1,600 mg of trimethoprim/sulphamethoxazole) is recommended.[28] Treatment of chronic bacteriuria may be of value in selected male patients with predisposing identifiable conditions, such as nephrolithiasis, pyelonephritic scarring, and enterococal infections in whom long-term therapy may delay recurrence of bacteriuria and reduce morbidity.[29]

The most common organisms seen on urine culture in uncomplicated urinary tract infections are *E. coli*, *Klebsiella* spp., *Staphylococcal saphrophyticus*, *Enterococcus* spp., and *Proteus* spp. Catheter-associated infections with *Pseudomonas* and *Candida* species are not uncommon.

Prevalence of pyelonephritis

The prevalence of pyelonephritis in the aged has been extensively studied in autopsy series. Raaschou[30] studied an autopsy series of 3,107 patients aged 10 years and over. He reported pyelonephritis in 28 percent of the patients. Kimmelstiel[31] studied the result of 3,393 autopsies and detected chronic pyelonephritis in 2.8 percent of patients. Baumanis and Russell,[32] who studied a series of 900 autopsies obtained from a hospital for chronic disease, reported chronic pyelonephritis in 185 instances, or 20 percent of the patients. Ascending infection is most common, with only 12 percent being acquired by hematogenous spread. The ages of the subjects varied from 50 to 101 years. Bruckel and Wincker[33] reported that pyelonephritis occurred in 28 percent of an autopsy series obtained from a hospital for chronic diseases. Numerous other authors reported a prevalence of acute and chronic pyelonephritis varying between these percentages.[34–39] Discrepancies in the reports are due to the different populations studied and the various interpretations placed on the findings. It has now been proven without doubt, that women with urinary symptoms may have low, but significant, bacterial counts in bladder urine and that organisms other than those traditionally accepted as aerobic pathogens can cause urinary symptoms.[40] Low bacterial counts may result from early urinary infection with progression or subsequent infection over a period of a few days,[41–43] because of infection with fastidious organisms or because of invasion and inflammation of the bladder wall when shedding of bacterial material into the urine is minimal. The concept of fastidious bacteria has been studied by Maskell and colleagues.[44] In a cohort of 51 women with a history of recurrent urinary symptoms and negative culture, he showed an increased presence of fastidious organisms, principally lactobacilli, associated with symptoms. Infection with these organisms persisted for some time after symptoms disappeared suggesting a slower return to normal commensal flora than with the more common aerobic organisms. Other fastidious organisms seen include *Ureaplasma urealyticum*,[45] *Gardnerella vaginalis*,[46,47] *Staphylococcus saphrophyticus*,[48] *Corynebacteria* spp.,[49,50] and certain strains of *Streptococcus* spp.[51,52]

An important feature of chronic pyelonephritis in the old is the asymptomatic course of the disease. Kass[53] claimed that pyelonephritis is clinically diagnosed in one-fifth of those patients detected at autopsy. Many cases of chronic pyelonephritis in the aged are detected when the patients have been admitted into hospital for other reasons and the disease has often attained an advanced level with uremia. In a few cases viruses may have caused the infections, although such cases presumably are rare. Endotoxins and immunologic mechanisms, producing free-oxygen radical species, cytokines, and other mediators of inflammation such as leucotrienes, thromboxanes, prostacyclins, and prostaglandins can induce prolonged damage in the renal interstitium after the disappearance of detectable bacteria in the tissue.[54]

Predisposing factors causing urinary tract infections

Escherichia coli causing urinary tract infection mostly originate in the intestine. Because of special affinity for the urogenital mucosa or abundance in the stool flora,[55–57] bacteria proceed to colonize the outer genital[58] and periurethral areas[59] and ascend the urinary tract. Bacteria ascend and remain in the urinary tract despite the urine flow. Predisposing factors include structural and functional abnormalities, invasive manipulation of the urinary tract, underlying disease causing relative immunosuppression, and bacterial virulence. Postmenopausal changes in women with estrogen deficiency are probably important in decreasing the mucosal resistance to infection in elderly women. A relationship has been shown between ability to attach to human uroepithelial cells in vitro and severity of infection produced in vivo.[60] Capacity to attach to the epithelium is a virulence factor for *E. coli* causing urinary tract infection. This attachment is specific for the epithelium of the urogenital tract. *Proteus mirabilis* strains show an adhesion pattern different from *E. coli*. They attach only to squamous and not to transitional epithelial cells. Recent studies indicate that genetically determined uroepithelial receptors for uropathogenic organisms may play an important role in recurrent urinary tract infections in women.[61] Other markers that appear to correlate with bacterial virulence include the presence of *P. fimbriae*, *S. fimbriae*, hemolysin, aerobactin, and urease.[62]

Another important predisposing factor causing urinary tract infection and pyelonephritis in the aged is urinary obstruction. In men prostatic hypertrophy and carcinoma of the prostate account for the vast majority of infections.[10] Digital examination of the prostate is not satisfactory—even an apparently normal finding does not exclude enlargement of the prostate and bladder neck obstruction. Obstruction can also be promoted by changes in the bladder neck, malformations, nephro- and ureterolithiasis, and neoplasms. In women, prolapse conditions and even slight descensus of the vagina increase the possibility of urinary tract infection.[63] In both sexes neurologic disorders and diabetes are important factors in the development of urinary tract infection, because an atonic bladder is at risk of infection. This is of particular importance in patients with stroke, Parkinson's disease, motor neuron disease, and spinal injury.

In women, however, the vast majority of infected patients show no evidence of obstruction. Some of these patients have coexistent prolapse conditions.[63] The occurrence of recurrent and therapy-resistant infections correlate with the presence of laxity of the vaginal wall and definite vaginal or uterine prolapse. Cases established as having recurrent urinary tract infection are, apparently, influenced by anatomic changes of the bladder, and frequently have a cystocele caused by vaginal descensus of uterine prolapse. Bladder capacity is often decreased in such patients, as is shown by cystometry. Patients established as therapy-resistant are less influenced by these changes and are represented in equal proportions in all groups. The similarity in the amount of residual urine both in correlation to gynecologic findings and to infection suggest the minor significance of this factor in promoting urinary tract infection in elderly females. The authors believed that anatomical prolapse conditions were important in promoting urinary tract infection in female hospital patients of advanced years, but not significant in patients with a continuous therapy-resistant infection—these apparently having a true pyelonephritis. The patients considered to have pyelonephritis formed one-third of the total of all patients with urinary tract infection.

An important factor promoting urinary tract infection is the use of indwelling catheters in the aged.[64] In a prospective series of patients in a nursing home, urinary catheterization was significantly associated with urinary tract infection.[65] The duration of catheterization was associated with increasing prevalence of bacteriuria, polymicrobial bacteriuria, chronic pyelonephritis, and chronic renal inflammation. The prevalence of chronic pyelonephritis at death was 10 percent for patients catheterized more than 90 days during their last year of life and 0 percent when catheterized less than or equal to 90 days. Chronic pyelonephritis was significantly associated with renal stones and hydronephrosis. The prevalence of chronic renal inflammation without chronic pyelonephritis was greater than that of chronic pyelonephritis (43 percent when catheterized more than 90 days and 18 percent when less than or equal to 90 days). More recent studies have confirmed the relationship between indwelling catheters and pyelonephritis,[66] suggesting that one mechanism by which catheters cause pyelonephritis is through the selection of specific pathogenic bacteria (*Providencia stuartii*) that are capable of adhering to the catheter.[67]

Reflux may play a role in the pathogenesis of pyelonephritis. Parvinen and colleagues[68] studied the correlation between radiographic findings at micturition cystography and evidence of urinary infection in a group of elderly, hospitalized women. A unilateral, ureteral reflux was observed in 3 patients out of 37 with urinary tract infection. Among the 22 patients without urinary tract infection no cases of reflux were found. Diverticula, trabeculation, and deformation were present in both groups, and normal cystographic findings were not significantly more frequent in the group without infection. These findings support the opinion that vesicoureteral reflux and urinary tract infection are concomitant features in a small number of elderly women.

The increased incidence and severity of urinary tract infections in geriatric patients may be related to an impaired immune response in the elderly.[69] Mucosal immunity may be altered in old age.[70] Sepsis from gram-negative pathogens is a grave disorder that must be considered possible in all aged patients with unexplained fever. Seneca and Grant[71] have claimed that older patients are more susceptible to the consequences of instrumentation and surgical operations involving the genitourinary tract. An early diagnosis and vigorous treatment decreases the mortality dramatically. Repeated urine and blood cultures from samples drawn during the rise of fever are essential in establishing the diagnosis and allowing appropriate antibiotic therapy.

Treatment of urinary tract infections

In both complicated and uncomplicated urinary tract infections the main therapeutic objectives should be to eradicate microorganisms invading the renal parenchyma and blood and to prevent chronic infection and scarring. In uncomplicated infections cotrimoxazole or amoxycillin are recommended.[72] Catheter-associated infections require both penicillin and aminoglycoside therapy, or treatment with a quinolone, because of the increased chance of *Pseudomonas* infection. Acute pyelonephritis is traditionally treated with intravenous antibiotics given for a 2-week period. Recently, patients without sepsis have been successfully treated with oral therapy only.[73] Antibiotic therapy with ampicillin and an aminoglycoside, a third generation cephalosporin or a quinolone is recommended. As in younger patients, an evaluation for reversible causes of urinary tract infection and pyelonephritis should be sought, including obstruction, nephrolithiasis, cysts, and neoplasms.

The treatment of patients with asymptomatic bacteriuria has been criticized by Petersdorf and colleagues[74] according to whom elderly patients with asymptomatic bacteriuria should not be treated. Petersdorf claims that these patients have relatively normal renal function, have few acute flare-ups, and are unlikely to have shortened life spans as a result of urinary infection. Furthermore, Petersdorf points to the fact that the toxic side effects of drugs, the risk of superinfection, and the expense involved, in addition to the high failure rate of therapy, all argue against therapy of asymptomatic urinary infections in this group.

Brocklehurst et al.[12,75] have studied the problem of treating urinary tract infections in the elderly and are of the opinion that patients without subjective complaints of urinary infections should not be treated, though patients who have various distressing symptoms should, as is the case with younger age groups, be given adequate therapy with antimicrobial drugs. These opinions are in accord with the present interpretation of the relationship between significant bacteriuria and renal involvement in the aged. Therapy for significant bacteriuria is unnecessary in protecting against renal damage, but is helpful in mitigating distressing symptoms. There are, however, some patients with significant bacteriuria and nonspecific symptoms, like fatigue, dizziness, and cognitive deterioration, who perhaps can benefit from treatment of the urinary infection. A short-term course of antibiotic therapy for elderly patients manifesting significant bacteriuria for the first time seems indicated regardless of the symptoms. Foul smell and social handicap can be important problems for the aged, and successful treatment of urinary tract infection is of great importance for these patients.

An important question is the indication for long-term treatment of urinary tract infections in the aged. This applies only to a relatively small group of patients—those with distressing symptoms and a high recurrence rate. The benefits are, of course, quite limited. The urine remains sterile a little longer than it would without treatment. With a long-acting sulfonamide, Sourander and Kasaren[76] found that 65 percent of patients were free of bacteriuria after a 6-month course of treatment. In a corresponding group of patients without treatment, 35 percent were free of bacteriuria. The bacterial strain that caused the reinfection was in all cases a strain that was resistant to the drug used in long-term treatment. The benefit derived from long-term treatment with a combination of sulfamethoxazole and trimethoprim was investigated by Sourander and colleagues.[77] In two similar groups of geriatric hospital patients with significant bacteriuria, one received short-term sulfamethoxazole-trimethoprim treatment and the other short-term treatment with ampicillin. After sterilizing the patients' urine, they administered to the first group long-term treatment with sulfamethoxazole-trimethoprim (sulfamethoxazole 800 mg and trimethoprim 160 mg daily, divided into two doses), while the second group received long-term treatment with a placebo. The urine of the patients in the first group was sterile for an average of 195 days, and in the placebo-treatment group for an average of 113 days. Of course, the development of superimposed infection and drug reactions during antibiotic treatment is quite frequently seen in geriatric practice.

Urinary bacteria commonly originate in the intestinal flora.[55,78] Lincoln and colleagues[79] have claimed that treatment with sulfonamides may cause a change in the resistance pattern of the intestinal flora which then plays a part in subsequent urinary infection. In their series of children the resistance patterns of urinary bacteria in recurrent infections closely reflected preceding changes in the intestinal flora. The authors point out that the use of potent new antibiotics also causes profound changes in the intestinal flora. The discrepancy between urinary and fecal flora is explained according to Lincoln et al. by serial cultures from feces and urethra which showed how an acquired, resistant strain disappeared from the feces but persisted in the urethra. This is in keeping with the isolation of fastidious bacteria in the urine from patients with "culture negative" urethritis.

There is obviously a great need for a critical attitude and a restrictive treatment policy for the use of antibiotics in hospitals. Gruenberg and Bendall[57] reported a hospital outbreak of plasmid-borne trimethoprim resistance in pathogenic coliform bacteria, which was associated with heavy use of cotrimoxazole, sulfonamides, and ampicillin, but was controlled by isolation of the patients and restriction of antibiotic use. These observations have not been confirmed in old age, but it seems highly probable that the frequent occurrence of multiply-resistant *E. coli* strains causing urinary tract infections and pyelonephritis in the aged is not simply a result of treatment of urinary infections with antibiotics and chemotherapeutic agents, but is also related to the treatment of other infections, with a change in the fecal bacterial resistance-pattern and subsequent reinfection of the urinary tract. This might explain the high degree of recurrent urinary tract infection with multiply-resistant bacterial strains in geriatric hospitals, and also explain the failure of the long-term administration of sulfonamides to prevent reinfection.

Failure of therapy is mostly because of reinfection with a new pathogen, bacterial resistance, or the use of appropriate antibiotics for a insufficient period of time. Reinfection with a new pathogen can be responsible for up to 20 percent of the failures observed.[54] Resistance, identified after culture of the organism, should prompt the clinician to change to a more suitable antibiotic. The organisms more often associated with resistance are *Pseudomonas*, *Enterobacter*, *Citrobacter*, *Serratia*, *Proteus*, and *Klebsiella* spp. Treatment with aminoglycosides, the newer third generation cephalosporins, carbapenems (including imipenem), quinolones, and monobactams has reduced this problem significantly.[80] Tissue penetration of the various antibiotics used in the management of pyelonephritis cannot be predicted from blood or urine samples.[54,81] Intracellular concentrations should be above the minimum inhibitory concentrations for effective therapy. Bergeron and Marois[82] have shown that the accumulation of tissue aminoglycoside or quinolone concentration is increased during pyelonephritis or endotoxemia. In contrast, betalactams have lower tissue levels and high tubular secretion. Pharmacologic synergism may have an important role in the therapy of pyelonephritis. When ampicillin was administered after a short course of intravenous aminoglycoside therapy, in a randomized controlled study, the results were equivalent to those seen with intravenous and oral quinolones suggesting synergism. Over 80 percent of patients had clinical and bacteriologic cure with both regimes. The ideal duration of therapy is not well-determined, but most reports suggest a course of treatment lasting between 5 and 14 days.[83–85]

Other Interstitial Nephropathies

Allergic interstitial nephropathy

Medication use is a common and important cause of renal disease in the elderly, particularly frail elderly patients who are subject to polypharmacy. A wide variety of medications may cause interstitial nephropathies, in addition to various forms of glomerular disease. Presenting features include renal impairment, often with urinary white blood cells in the absence of infection. Classically, patients also show features of allergy-eosinophilia, rash, and pruritus, temporally associated with the introduction of a new drug. The most common medications causing interstitial nephropathy are antibiotics, particularly the penicillin and sulfonamide derivatives, analgesics, and anti-inflammatory medications[86,87] although other offending agents include anticoagulants, diuretics, anticonvulsants, allopurinol, various metals (particularly lithium), and azathioprine and other immunosuppressives.[88] Nonsteroidal anti-inflammatory drugs (NSAIDs) have been demonstrated to induce renal dysfunction via several mechanisms, including interference with renal prostaglandin release, particularly in patients with underlying renal impairment. In addition, NSAIDs may cause an acute or chronic allergic interstitial reaction often without the classic features of allergy or eosinophilia. Intersititial nephritis should be considered as a differential diagnosis in patients with heavy proteinuria and taking anti-inflammatory medication on a regular basis. Withdrawal of the offending drug is usually sufficient, though a trial of steroid therapy may be warranted in some situations.

Radiocontrast nephrotoxicity

Radiocontrast materials cause vacuolization of the cells in the proximal tubule and hence, interstitial disease, possibly by inducing intense local vasoconstriction. The healthy kidney does not appear to be at risk of damage. However, as age increases the incidence of subclinical renal disease, a higher incidence of radiocontrast nephrotoxicity is seen in the older patient. Age itself is not a risk factor for the nephrotoxic effects of radiocontrast materials.[89] Predisposing factors include diabetes,[90–92] particularly if associated with reduced renal function,[93,94] severe congestive cardiac failure[95] dehydration, the volume of contrast used[91,96] (higher volumes causing increased risk), and the use of high osmolality nonionic contrast media.[97,98] The literature describing an increased risk of contrast mediated nephrotoxicity with the administration of contrast media to patients with multiple myeloma is weak. Often the renal impairment can be attributed to the myeloma or the complications of the disease and its treatment.[99] The overall incidence of contrast-associated nephropathy varies according to the population studied and the definition used, but most data report 1 to 7 percent incidence of radiocontrast-mediated nephrotoxicity.[100] Nephrotoxicity can be prevented with prior hydration with saline or hypotonic saline for a minimum of 12 hours.[101–104] The use of agents to increase intratubular urine flow rates, for example mannitol or frusemide, or the use of renal vasodilatory agents, including theophylline or calcium-channel blockers, does not improve outcome and in some studies is associated with a poorer prognosis.[101] Interstitial nephritis can also be caused by multiple myeloma, with light-chain nephropathy and uric acid nephropathy.

Renal papillary necrosis

Renal papillary necrosis is not an uncommon complication of urinary infection in the aged. The disease can be defined as a severe form of chronic pyelonephritis with ischemic necrosis of the papillae and the medullary pyramid. Necrotic papillae migrate through the urinary passages and are often detected microscopically in the urine. The patients suffer from hematuria, urinary colic, and very often from fever, which may be high. The disease often has a quite rapid course resulting in uremia and death. Diabetes and vascular diseases, including unilateral renal artery stenosis, are of importance as etiological factors.[105] Consumption of analgesics—especially phenacetin—may play an important role. Clinical experience favors the opinion that continuous prolonged use of analgesics is connected with the development of papillary necrosis in the aged. In the majority of cases, relief of the obstruction caused by the necrotic papilla leads to improved renal function. On rare occasions, patients present with end stage renal disease and may require renal replacement therapy.

Glomerular Diseases

Although glomerular disease was previously believed to be rare in older patients, this may have reflected a lack of routine urine testing and a reluctance to refer older individuals to a nephrologist. More recent data indicate a similar or slightly higher incidence of primary glomerular disease in elderly people (8.5 patients per 10^5 population per year in the over 75-year-old compared with 8.4 per 10^5 population per year in younger adults).[106] The disease spectrum seen in the older individual is as diverse as in the younger population. As in the younger population, the main presenting features of glomerular disease are proteinuria and hematuria with or without hypertension and renal dysfunction. The clinical syndromes often used to describe the common patterns include the terms nephritic, nephrotic, and secondary diseases. These, though useful in some settings, often do not correlate with etiology or histologic features, resulting in complex classifications. To simplify the schema we use the following terminology—nephrotic syndrome (describing a predominantly proteinuric presentation), proliferative syndromes including cresentic nephritis (which describe a clinical picture of hematuria and proteinuria, often with cellular casts), and systemic disorders causing glomerular disease.

Diagnosis is often based on the clinical features of disease and serology, however the "gold standard" for diagnosis is renal biopsy. Renal biopsy is safe in the over 60-year-old. Most attempts at biopsy are successful and reported complication rates vary from 2.2 to 9.8 percent.[107,108] Interpretation of the tissue is more difficult, as arteriolar sclerosis and global sclerosis associated with chronic ischemia and aging may be difficult to differentiate from previously healed proliferative glomerulonephritis (GN) or focal sclerosing GN. The largest biopsy series published is from the Medical Research Council

(UK) database.[109] Data were collected over a 13-year period. From a database of 7,086 cases, 825 biopsies were from patients aged over 65 years old. One striking finding was that a renal biopsy was 3.5 times less likely to be done in older patients in the earlier years than in more recent years. In general, the older patients were less likely to have asymptomatic urinary abnormalities, and correspondingly more likely to have impaired renal function and heavier proteinuria at the time of biopsy. At all ages idiopathic GN was the most common underlying diagnosis, secondary GN, and unclassified being the next most common diagnoses seen in the older cohort. Few elderly patients were biopsied to help establish a diagnosis of diabetic nephropathy. Of the patients diagnosed as having histologic features suggestive of idiopathic GN, membranous nephropathy was the most common, with focal segmental GN and minimal change GN coming a close second. Disorders associated with a proliferative picture on histology, including cresentic GN, were rarer. IgA was reported much less frequently in the older patients than in a corresponding younger group in this series.

Nephrotic Syndrome

Nephrotic syndrome is one of the most common reasons given for performing a renal biopsy in the over 75-year-old.[110] The most common cause of nephrotic syndrome is membranous nephropathy. Minimal change disease (MCD) and nephrotic syndrome secondary to amyloidosis and myeloma are the next most common diagnoses. Based on data from a 15-year prospective study[111] in patients aged 60 years or more, the annual incidence of membranous nephropathy was 2.5 patients per 10^5 population per year, a figure almost three times as high as the overall incidence of membranous nephropathy. Bias, arising from a reluctance to biopsy older patients, may have been present, but this would tend to skew the data toward an even higher incidence in elderly patients. Focal segmental glomerulosclerosis and IgA nephropathy are less common than in younger patients.

Membranous nephropathy

Seventy-five to 80 percent of cases of membranous nephropathy are idiopathic, with the remaining 20 to 25 percent being secondary to solid organ tumors and drugs. The clinical presentation is fairly typical with proteinuria, often greater than 3 g/24 hours. In contrast to younger patients, 40 percent of older patients have associated hypertension, 30 to 90 percent hematuria, and 15 percent renal impairment at the time they are first seen. A mortality rate of 34 percent has been derived from the available data, although because of varied follow-up periods, the validity of this value may be questioned.[111] As the absolute numbers of patients are low, and the reported studies small, it is difficult to ascertain if age affects the overall prognosis. In a small retrospective study, older patients with membranous nephropathy responded favorably to treatment with prednisone and chlorambucil.[112] The time to remission was often longer, and the incidence and severity of side effects higher than in younger patients. In contrast, remission rates were lower. Response rates for patients treated conservatively or with corticosteroids alone were poor. On this basis, the recommended treatment for the older patient is corticosteroid therapy and low-dose chlorambucil (0.1 mg/kg/day) for a 3 to 6 month period.

Minimal change nephropathy

Minimal change nephropathy, as with younger patients, typically presents with the features of the nephrotic syndrome. The incidence of microscopic hematuria, hypertension, and renal impairment at the time of presentation is much higher than in younger patients. Oliguria usually heralds a poor prognosis with progression to death or renal replacement therapy. Further complications, resulting from hypoalbuminemia, hyperlipidemia, and hypercoagulability include thrombotic events, infection, and progressive cardiovascular disease. As with membranous nephropathy, standard therapeutic regimes can be used. Treatment with oral corticosteroid therapy frequently needs to be prolonged for up to 16 weeks. Corticosteroid-resistant cases may benefit from the introduction to chlorambucil, cyclophosphamide, or cyclosporine A, although the risk of bone marrow depression is high.

A history of nonsteroidal usage should be actively sought as minimal change nephropathy secondary to drugs may partially remit without aggressive immunosuppressive therapy.

Focal and segmental glomerulosclerosis

Focal and segmental glomerulosclerosis is much less commonly seen in the elderly. It can be difficult to distinguish from ischemic changes without electron microscopy. Patients present with heavy proteinuria and often have some degree of renal insufficiency. A trial of corticosteroids or immunosuppressive medication may be offered on the basis of the results of a small study of focal segmental glomerulosclerosis (FSGS) in the older patient.[113] Therapy should be gradually withdrawn after a 3-month trial period unless partial remission has occurred. Angiotensin-converting enzyme (ACE) inhibitors and nonsteroidal inflammatory agents are both effective antiproteinuric drugs, but can lead to significant elevations in serum creatinine and must be used with caution.

Proliferative Syndromes

Proliferative GN includes glomerular diseases caused by immune complex deposition, the antineutrophil cytoplasmic antibody (ANCA) associated syndromes, and also antiglomerular basement membrane (anti-GBM) antibody-mediated disease. The clinical characteristics and rate of deterioration are similar to those seen in younger patients, though the diagnosis is best confirmed with renal biopsy. The older patient tends to present with much higher serum creatinine levels and at a later stage of the disease. Immunosuppression is not well studied in this population and no randomized controlled studies of therapy in the over 65-year-old exist. Most therapeutic studies are small, but appear to show a good short-term prognosis with standard regimes of therapy. Observational data suggest that older patients are at higher risk of septic and gastrointestinal complications with immunosuppression.[114] Some also report a higher incidence of refractory renal impairment and hypertension compared to younger patients.

Cresentic GN is a pathologic lesion that occurs in a range of renal and systemic disorders. In some series it is more common in older individuals than the younger patient.[108,114–115] The clinical presentation is variable with nonspecific complaints of nausea, anorexia, malaise, edema, arthalgia, and myalgia. Symptoms of pyrexia, rash, and hemoptysis are more typical of systemic vasculitis. The renal manifestations include microscopic (and macroscopic) hematuria, hypertension, and oliguria. The majority of patients present with significant renal failure and become dialysis-dependent in the early course of their disease. The differential diagnoses should include idiopathic cresentic GN, Wegener's granulomatosis, anti-GBM disease, systemic lupus erythematosus, polyarteritis nodosa, and mesangiocapillary GN. Henoch-Schönlein disease and IgA nephropathy, though recognized in older patients, are less commonly seen. Cryoglobulinemia should always be suspected in patients presenting with a palpable purpuric rash. Serum ANCA levels, anti-GBM levels, antinuclear factor, complement, immunoglobulin levels, and renal biopsy help distinguish the different syndromes.

Systemic Disorders Causing Glomerular Disease

Many systemic diseases can be associated with glomerular disease, in particular diabetes, myeloma, and systemic lupus erythematosus. The presentation and course of these diseases are similar in both old and young patients.

Although the classic description of temporal arteritis does not include renal disease, glomerular involvement has been described in the literature from as early as 1958.[116–118] Azotemia in giant cell arteritis is recognized, although renal disease may also be secondary to involvement of the aorta, with dissection of the renal artery or renal artery thrombosis. Azotemia and renal involvement in giant cell arteritis is responsive to immunosuppressive therapy.

Chronic or acute systemic bacterial infection may cause immune complex formation and thus, active glomerular proliferative disease. Acute poststreptococcal glomerulonephritis (APSGN) has also been reported in the elderly.[119–122] However, APSGN in the elderly tends to originate more often from pyodermal streptococcal infections rather than streptococcal throat infections. Since the antistreptolysin O titer may fail to rise after a pyodermal infection, anti-deoxyribonuclease B titers may be of more value in assessing precedent streptococcal infections in elderly patients with APSGN. In addition, oliguria may be more common in elderly patients with APSGN, perhaps because of underlying age-related changes. However, the outcome of APSGN in the elderly is similar to younger age groups, with most patients recovering renal function. Thus, dialysis is generally of value, when required, in elderly patients with APSGN and acute renal failure.

Renovascular Disease

Nephrosclerosis

Hypertension, diabetes, and atherosclerosis are common in the elderly, and their long-term effects on the renal vasculature result in characteristic pathologic changes termed *nephrosclerosis*. Together with end-stage renal disease (ESRD) of unknown etiology, nephrosclerosis remains the most common cause of ESRD in the elderly.[123,124] The clinical diagnosis is often overlooked because of the scarce urinary findings. Isothenuria and a usually slight proteinuria, granular casts, and hyaline cylinders in the high-power field of the urinary sediment, are typical laboratory findings. Progression of the disease is often slow, and once renal disease is established, its progression can be further slowed with strict blood pressure control. It remains unclear if antihypertensive therapy prevents the development of nephrosclerosis, but regardless, treatment of hypertension is imperative. The ideal treatment regime remains unclear although the first line therapy still recommended by most bodies remains diuretic therapy. Progression of renal disease, once established, is retarded by ACE inhibitors. Studies using improved morbidity as an end point, have only been done using diuretic and β-blocker therapy.

Renal Arterial Emboli, Stenosis, and Thrombosis

Atheroembolism is an important cause of both acute and chronic renal failure in the elderly.[126] Renal arterial emboli occur in any setting associated with peripheral embolization, such as acute myocardial infarction, chronic atrial fibrillation, subacute bacterial endocarditis, and aortic surgery or aortography. Renal embolization in the elderly varies from a clinically silent event to a full-blown syndrome of severe flank pain and tenderness, hematuria, hypertension, spiking fevers, marked reduction in renal function, and elevations of serum lactate dehydrogenase. Small emboli are very difficult to detect since renal scans may show focal perfusion defects in many apparently normal elderly patients. Major emboli are suggested by findings of differential contrast excretion on pyelography and confirmed by renal scanning and aortography. Thrombolytic therapy, given intra-arterially, is now the treatment of choice and few cases warrant surgical intervention.[127] The degree and duration of occlusion does not affect outcome and the final level of renal function often correlates with the degree of collateral renal blood flow.[127] In patients where renal function is discernibly impaired, improvement may occur over several days to weeks. When atheroembolism causes acute renal failure, dialysis can maintain the patient through the critical period of recovery.

Renal dysfunction secondary to cholesterol embolism is seen in older individuals with diffuse atheromatous disease. The classic presentation is with a sudden increase in serum creatinine, typically after arterial catheterization or systemic heparinization. As urine microscopy is often bland, and clinical examination unremarkable, the diagnosis can be easily overlooked. On occasion, an active urinary sediment, signs of peripheral embolism in the limbs, fluctuating confusional state, gut ischemia, and peripheral eosinophilia can be seen. The diagnosis is confirmed if intravascular cholesterol crystals are seen on renal biopsy, skin biopsy, or muscle biopsy.

Thrombotic renal arterial disease or renal artery stenosis frequently complicate severe aortic and renal arterial atherosclerosis, especially in the setting of decreased renal blood flow caused by congestive heart failure or volume depletion. Renal artery stenosis is an increasingly important cause of renal impairment in the elderly patient. It should be suspected in patients with widespread atheromatous disease, severe hypertension, or with renal impairment worsening with ACE inhibitor therapy. As fibromuscular hyperplasia is almost unheard of in this age group, there is no preponderance of the female sex. True prevalence data is not available, and the reported incidence varies from 4 percent in a general hypertensive population to 37 percent in patients referred to a tertiary center for management of severe hypertension. Screening for unilateral renal artery stenosis is recommended when the clinical risk is high.[128] Although numerous methods of investigation are available (Table 67-1), the currently recommended screening test is captopril renal scintigraphy.[128,129] The introduction of magnetic resonance arteriography may herald a noninvasive but highly sensitive diagnostic test without the attendant risk from intravenous contrast or irradiation.[130–132]

Surgical or endovascular revascularization is advised as renal impairment continues to progress to ESRD in a higher percentage of patients managed with medical therapy, regardless of blood pressure control. Progression of the stenotic lesion is seen in up to 30 to 40 percent of cases over a 4-year period with corresponding decreases in renal size if the lesion is left untreated. Numerous interventional techniques are available, among them percutaneous transluminal renal angioplasty (PTRA) and stenting. Older patients with diffuse atheromatous disease present a particularly challenging problem. In the majority of these patients the stenotic lesion is close to or at the ostium of the renal artery precluding PTRA. The recent introduction of metallic stents has allowed these lesions to be treated without surgery, however the technique is still in the early stages and not always widely available. Surgical methods traditionally used included aortorenal bypass surgery and transaortic renal endarterectomy. However, newer methods include hepatorenal or gastroduodenal renal bypass for right sided stenoses, splenorenal bypasses for left-sided lesions, extra-anatomic revascularisation or exvivo reconstruction, and autotransplantation.[133]

Other Renal Disease in the Aged

Diabetic Nephropathy

Nephropathy is a common complication of diabetes at all ages. In the elderly, non-insulin dependent diabetes mellitus (NIDDM) is more commonly seen, and the incidence of nephropathy at the time of diagnosis is high. It is usual for the nephropathy to present with microalbuminuria or, more commonly, proteinuria. Although the cost-benefit ratio of screening for microalbuminuria in patients with non-insulin-dependent diabetes is not established, the National Kidney Foundation recommend that all individuals, aged 70 years or less with NIDDM have their urine tested for microalbuminuria at yearly

Table 67-1 Screening and diagnostic tests for renal artery stenosis

	Sensitivity (%)	**Specificity (%)**	**Comments**
Rapid sequence intravenous pyelogram	74.5	86.2	
Nuclear imaging with or without captopril	83 75	93 85	Improved sensitivity and specificity with captopril challenge
Renal artery duplex scanning	89.5	90.7	Low detection of accessory renal artery if present Requires technical expertise
Selective renal vein renin sampling	77–80	62–75	Not useful for bilateral disease but may help predict hypertensive response to revascularization
Peripheral plasma renin sampling with or without captopril	52–100 44–62	85–95 17–93	High false negative and false positive results, but good for detection of bilateral disease, esp. in transplant renal artery stenosis
Split renal function tests	—	—	Rarely performed, variable results, very invasive
Angiography			
Standard angiography	Gold standard		
Carbon dioxide angiography	—	—	
Magnetic resonance angiography	83–100	91–97	
Spiral computed angiography	82	86	

intervals.[134] Albuminuria, predicting the onset of diabetic nephropathy, is present if at least two urine samples, evaluated within a 6 to 12-week period, show an albumin excretion of 30 mg or more over a 24-hour period. Strict glycemic control, the introduction of ACE-inhibitor therapy and reduction of blood pressure to less than 130/85 mmHg are advised if microalbuminuria or proteinuria is present. Diabetic dyslipidemia has been proposed as a further independent risk factor in the progression of renal disease, however, a reduced rate of disease progression has not been demonstrated with the introduction of lipid lowering agents. Although the disease course can be modified by the early introduction of ACE inhibitors[135] the elderly diabetic patient is at a high risk of subclinical renal artery stenosis and close monitoring of serum creatinine and serum potassium levels is mandatory.

Multiple Myeloma

Multiple myeloma is seen predominantly in the older population and is the primary renal disease in 1 percent of patients on chronic renal replacement therapy.[124] Renal failure is estimated to occur in 20 to 60 percent of patients with myeloma[136–138] and can be caused by myeloma glomerulopathy, tubular toxic effects of light chains, light-chain cast formation with intratubular obstruction (myeloma kidney), hypercalcemia, hyperuricemia, cryoglobulinemia, and the additive effect of dehyration and nephrotoxic drugs. In a large proportion of patients the renal failure is reversible and careful attention should be paid to the prevention of further renal insult. Hyperuricemia secondary to chemotherapy, hypercalcemia, and radiocontrast nephrotoxicity should be avoided by adequate hydration and the use of allopurinol if needed. Although successful case reports of both hemodialysis and peritoneal dialysis (PD) are published, some authors recommend PD as the treatment of choice.[139] Peritoneal dialysis has the advantage of clearing a small fraction of the immunoglobulin load, particularly if rapid exchanges are used. This may confer a theoretical benefit with a reduction in tubular toxic effect of the light chains, the incidence of hyperviscosity syndrome and amyloidosis.[140,141] The long-term survival of patients with myeloma commenced onto renal replacement therapy has improved as a result of better chemotherapeutic regimes. Recent studies have shown that the presence and degree of azotemia does not correlate with outcome and that the survival of patients with myeloma on chronic dialysis is good.[142–146] On this basis, patients with multiple myeloma should be offered renal replacement therapy, if needed, at least for a trial period.

Obstructive Nephropathy

The most common cause of urinary obstruction in old age is prostatic hypertrophy.[126,147] Olbrich et al.[148] reported a 30 to 50 percent decrease of glomerular filtration rate and renal plasma flow in aged males with prostatic hypertrophy. After prostatectomy, renal plasma flow increased slightly, but glomerular filtration rate did not change.

The increased intrapelvic pressure caused by urinary obstruction has been considered to be transmitted back through the tubular lumina and induce pressure atrophy of the renal parenchyma. Renal failure caused by obstruction is, however, restored after removal of obstruction if the renal trauma is not irreversible.

Age does not have a major effect on the likelihood or clinical presentation of nephrolithiasis, renal tumors, or renal tuberculosis. Renal disease occasionally presents in old age with hematuria, recurrent urinary infections, or azotemia. The progress is usually slow. Treatment of urinary tract infection and hypertension is indicated in patients with this disorder.[149]

Renal Failure in the Elderly

Acute Renal Failure

Acute renal failure (ARF) is seen more frequently in older patients probably because of common inciting events. These include hypotension associated with marked volume depletion, major surgery, sepsis, major angiographic procedures, and the injudicious use of antibiotics often in multiply-impaired patients with pre-existing moderate renal insufficiency. The disease is often due to multifactorial causes. In addition, age-related changes in renal function, including changes in tubular function such as alterations in water and electrolyte balance, predispose the elderly to acute renal failure.

The incidence of acute renal insufficiency is estimated to be around 6 to 10 percent of all elderly admissions to an acute medical service. In a prospective study, of patients over 65 years of age, 6.8 percent of all hospital admissions had a serum urea equal to or greater than 17 mmol/L (48 mg/dl urea N) and/or creatinine equal to or greater than 160 μmol/L at presentation.[150] Fifty-five percent of patients had a prerenal etiology and had an excellent rate of renal recovery. The majority of patients had mild renal impairment with only 24 percent of patients presenting with serum urea equal to or greater than 31 mmol/L and/or creatinine equal to or greater than 400 μmol/L. Patients with intrinsic renal failure had a higher mortality rate (48 percent) than expected, possibly because of a delay in recognition of the disease. In contrast to other studies, however, a higher mortality was seen in patients with obstructive renal disease. This appears to be because of a disproportionately high number of patients with pelvic neoplasia and may reflect some sampling bias.

The causes of ARF seen in patients admitted to an intensive care unit include cardiogenic or septic shock in 17 percent of cases, postsurgical causes in 13 percent, and ischemia and hypovolemic shock in 22 percent.[151] Other causes included primary renal disease, contrast and nephrotoxin-induced ARF, postrenal causes, and hepatic failure. Overall, mortality rates correlate with the severity of the clinical disease state and range between 40 and 60 percent. The highest mortality is seen with hepatic failure, shock, renal parenchymal, and renovascular disease. The prognosis for patients with ARF resulting from aortic aneurysm repair is poor, with a 100 percent mortality in some series.[152] Good recovery is expected when ARF is caused by hypercalcemia or medication. Mortality appears to correlate closely to the serum creatinine and urea levels. Where dialysis is started, the prescription should be tailored to ensure serum blood urea nitrogen (BUN) levels are maintained lower than 15 mmol/L.[153,154] Age itself does not have a significant impact on the prognosis of the patient with ARF.[151,154–159] Hypophosphatemia and hypokalemia are associated with an unexpectedly high death rate and it remains unclear if this reflects the severity of the underlying disease or malnutrition. Of those patients who survive to discharge, 58 percent have complete recovery of renal function and 39 percent have some degree of renal impairment but do not require dialysis.[151]

The management of ARF in the elderly is complex and demanding. The aged kidney retains the capacity to recover from acute ischemic or toxic insults over the course of several weeks. Additional insult during recovery from acute tubular necrosis (ATN), for example, with further administration of nephrotoxins (including aminoglycoside antibiotics) or radiocontrast agents can prolong recovery. Renal function, as reflected in serum BUN and creatinine levels, is impaired for several days after a brief hypotensive episode associated with surgery, sepsis, overmedication, or volume depletion, or after the administration of nephrotoxic radiographic contrast agents. After a brief period of azotemia, renal function gradually returns to its previous level. Despite this transient and reversible loss of renal function, oliguria is not a prominent component of the clinical picture, although if present is associated with a poorer outcome. Because the clinical hallmark of renal failure is generally thought to be a dramatic reduction in urine output, cases of nonoliguric ARF may go unrecognized. This may result in the inadvertent overdose of patients during the period of impaired renal function with medications excreted predominately via renal mechanisms, including digitalis preparations and aminoglycoside antibiotics such as gentamicin.

Aside from the initiation of dialysis, careful attention to the balance of several factors is necessary. Water and salt balance must be monitored carefully. Due to catabolism, the usual patient with ARF will lose about 0.5 kg of body mass per day. Attempts to keep body weight constant will result in the gradual expansion of the extracellular fluid, and consequently cause increase in blood pressure and risk of precipitation of cardiac failure. Similarly, overzealous fluid restriction will impair the patients' general condition and CNS function and may delay the recovery of renal function. Nutritional support should be implemented at an early stage.

Standard intermittent hemodialysis, peritoneal dialysis, or slow continuous methods of hemodialysis are all reported to be successful in older patients, however no data exist as to the most preferable method.

Chronic Renal Failure and End-Stage Renal Disease

The most common primary diagnoses in newly treated elderly ESRD patients are nephrosclerosis, diabetes, and renal disease of unknown etiology. The incidence of tubulointerstitial disease, glomerulonephritis, and polycystic kidney disease is lower in the over 65-year-old patient group than in the age group 15 to 65 years.[124,160,161,162]

Predialysis management

As the number of older patients with advanced renal failure increases, the importance of continued follow-up at a predialysis clinic grows. Early referral to a nephrologist is recognized to improve long-term survival,[163,164] and family physicians and general internists are encouraged to refer all patients, regardless of age, for specialist follow-up at an early stage. Although the literature suggests an age-related bias still persists in referral patterns, the tendency to deny older patients specialist access is less with increasing awareness of the benefits of dialysis in the elderly. In the ideal situation patients are reviewed in predialysis clinics where the four main aims are

- To optimize the rate of renal deterioration
- To control predialysis uremic complications including hyperkalemia, fluid balance, anemia, and renal osteodystrophy early in the disease course
- To educate and prepare both the patient and family for dialysis
- To identify a suitable time to start dialysis and prevent an acute event precipating dialysis

The rate of deterioration of renal function is stable with time. Shorter kidney survival is seen in patients with glomerulonephritis, diabetes mellitus, and nephrosclerosis, while those with tubulointerstitial disease have a slower renal decline. Like their younger counterparts, strict control of blood pressure, prevention of hyperglycemia and moderate protein restriction in the elderly is essential in the preservation of residual renal reserve. Recent studies addressing the question of protein restriction have only been able to demonstrate a small benefit from moderate protein restriction in patients with mildly impaired renal function (defined as a GFR of 25 to 55 ml/min).[164,165] Blood pressure control is of greater benefit than dietary restriction especially when ACE inhibitors are used. As the older patient is more prone to malnutrition, dietary restriction to less than 1 g/kg body weight is not recommended.

The assessment and control of symptoms in the older patient with advanced renal disease is confounded by the poor correlation between serum creatinine and glomerular filtration rate. More frequent monitoring of creatinine clearance is necessary, therefore clinicians are advised to place increased emphasis on symptom control. Furthermore, as the elderly are increasingly prone to minor changes in sodium and fluid balance precipating either dehydration or symptoms of pulmonary edema, close attention to fluid balance is required. Regular weight records are an easy and quick guide to the state of hydration, particularly in the inpatient setting. Fluid overload can usually be controlled by the use of high-dose loop diuretics (e.g., 80 to

120 mg frusemide) although in some patients addition of metolazone is necessary to augment the diuretic effect of either frusemide or ethacrynic acid.

Severe, and often refractory, constipation can exacerbate the hyperkalemia of chronic renal failure as a larger percentage of potassium is lost via the gastrointestinal system. In such situations, simple therapies directed toward correction of the constipation are often sufficient. If ion-exchange resins are required they must be given with sufficient doses of sorbitol (for example a dose of 30 ml of 70 percent sorbitol with each 15 g of calcium resonium).

With the introduction of human recombinant erythropoeitin (rh-Epo), anemia is less frequently encountered in the dialysis patient. Few studies have been directed specifically at the over 65-year-old population, nevertheless, the older patient appears to have similar dose responses to those seen in younger patients. The use of rh-Epo in predialysis patients is well-established in practice, although there are valid concerns regarding the theoretical deleterious effect of rh-Epo on blood pressure and renal function.[166] Data from a number of studies show an improvement in left ventricular mass and quality of life with rh-Epo. Current National Kidney Foundation recommendations[166] suggest commencing rh-Epo in predialysis patients, if symptoms attributable to anemia (fatigue, decreased exercise tolerance, angina, congestive heart failure, diminished work performance, and symptomatic peripheral vascular disease) are present in patients with a GFR greater than 15 mL/min. Anemia associated with chronic renal failure often requires more aggressive management in elderly patients because of coexisting cardiac disease. Red cell indices are not a reliable estimate of iron deficiency in uremia. Iron deficiency should be excluded by evaluation of serum iron and ferritin and oral or parenteral iron supplements administered if indicated. Uremic patients, especially the aged, should be very cautiously treated with blood transfusions to avoid the development of acute pulmonary edema. Packed red cells are better tolerated than whole blood. Ideally, hemoglobin should be maintained around 10.5 g/dl to achieve the optimal cost-benefit ratio.[166]

The predialysis patient remains at risk of renal osteodystrophy and malnutrition. As serum phosphate rises, phosphate-binding antacids (e.g., calcium carbonate) should be given, with meals, in order to suppress hyperphosphatemia, hypocalcemia, and the resultant adverse effects on bone. As serum phosphate falls in response to treatment, serum calcium will generally rise toward the normal range. If hypocalcemia persists after normalization of phosphate, this should be treated with preparations of vitamin D or its active metabolites. As aluminium toxicity is well-recognized, aluminium hydroxide should no longer be used as a phosphate binder.

Dietary management of elderly people with chronic renal failure is often overdone, compounding the nutritional impact of the disease. Protein and salt restriction is often needed in young individuals to suppress the volume expansion and BUN elevations. Many elderly patients ingest only 60 to 70 g of protein daily and 4 to 5 g of salt under normal conditions, and strict limitation of these dietary constituents is often unnecessary. Similarly, hyperkalemia should be avoided and dietary potassium controlled, but the reductions required in the elderly are often moderate. Acidosis should be controlled with the addition of oral sodium bicarbonate tablets with the aim to keep serum bicarbonate levels near normal. The best approach to these modifications is careful alteration of the diet to the proven needs of the individual patient.

Pruritus is a major problem in elderly uremic patients, especially in the presence of coexisting xerosis. In addition to skin moisteners, ultraviolet light treatments have been found effective and safe. Administration of so-called "antipruritic" agents such as antihistamines is rarely helpful, because they act primarily by causing sedation and may have adverse nervous system effects in the elderly.

Chronic Dialysis Therapy

As renal replacement therapy becomes increasingly common in the elderly there is a growing awareness that this population poses a unique set of problems. Many types of dialysis are available—in center hemodialysis (IHD), home hemodialysis, continuous ambulatory peritoneal dialysis (CAPD), intermittent peritoneal dialysis (IPD), and nocturnal peritoneal dialysis (NIPD). All forms of PD and home hemodialysis are grossly underused in this age group, especially within the US.[167–169] The provision of transplantation as a means of treatment for the elderly patient with ESRD remains limited, despite its demonstrated success.

The acceptance criteria used for older patients worldwide have been liberalized over the years. This is reflected by an increased number of older patients accepted onto renal replacement therapy programs. The percentage of patients who start dialysis therapy when aged 65 years or more ranges from 32 percent in the UK to 46 percent in Italy, with a mean worldwide acceptance rate of 34 patients aged over 65 years per million population per year.[168] In fact, the 65- to 74-year-old age group show the fastest rate of growth of all age groups, and by the year 2000 it is projected that over 60 percent of all ESRD patients will be over the age of 65 years.[167,170] Acceptance rates across the world differ for many reasons. Some differences result from resource restrictions (for example in the UK where dialysis is funded by the government), but some differences are due to selection bias (for example Japan and New Zealand where there is a high overall acceptance rate but a relatively lower population of aged dialysis patients). There is a growing concern that without adequate provision of specialized services targeted at the elderly a medical and ethical crisis is imminent.[169,171]

One year survival rates vary from 65 to 95 percent in maintenance hemodialysis patients aged 65 years or more.[172–184] Patients on peritoneal dialysis have an average survival rate of 41 and 22 percent at 3 and 5 years, respectively.[181–183,185–190] As most national databases define chronic dialysis patients as patients who are dialysis-dependent for "more than 90 days," early deaths are not accounted for. Hence, the true mortality rate in older patients is much higher than reported. Eleven percent of patients aged 65 to 69 years die within the first 90 days of treatment.[191] As expected, the early mortality rate increases linearly with age (14, 18, 19, and 26 percent for age groups 70 to 74, 75 to 79, 80 to 84, and 85 or more years, respectively).[169] In the US, a 40 percent higher mortality risk is seen in older patients compared with Japanese patients of equal age. A similar, but less marked, survival advantage is seen in European patients even after adjustment for age and diabetes. The reason for this survival advantage is not known.

The choice of dialysis modality (usually IHD versus CAPD) is based on the clinical history, functional capabilities, and the social circumstances. Most studies show similar survival in both hemodialysis and PD patients, despite differences in comorbidity, however, recent data have led to some doubt about the effectiveness of CAPD in the long term. The CANUSA study[192] showed a marginal survival advantage in elderly patients managed on hemodialysis. In contrast, however, a 0.76 risk advantage (confidence interval 0.69 to 0.83) was seen in Canadian patients aged 65 or more on PD, even after correction for age and the number of comorbid illnesses.[124] Diabetic patients appear to have better outcome if treated with hemodialysis.[124,193] Unlike younger patients, technique failure is no higher with PD.[124,185] Peritoneal dialysis is ideal for patients with good family support, where a family member is prepared to assist with dialysis exchanges. The introduction of NIPD, where a preprogrammed machine performs the exchanges during the night, provides more flexibility for family members who may work during the day. Peritoneal dialysis has been performed successfully in the nursing home.[194]

Medical advantages of PD include better cardiovascular stability, reduced dialysis-induced arrhythmias, easier control of hypertension, and preservation of residual renal function. The physician may favor PD if vascular access difficulties arise repeatedly. In contrast, the increased intra-abdominal pressures associated with CAPD reduce diaphragmatic movements and may compromise respiratory function. Other disadvantages of PD in the elderly include poor tissue turgor and wound healing, which cause abdominal wall herniae and catheter leaks. Protein losses in dialysate exacerbate malnutrition and may increase abnormal bone mineralization and reduce immune function.

Hospitalization rates are higher in the elderly dialysis patient. The median number of days spent in hospital for the 65 years or older dialysis patient was 15 days per year compared with 9.75 days for younger patients. The frequency of hospitalization was also higher (1.89 and 1.43 admissions per year for 65 year or older patients and 45 to 64-year-old patients, respectively).[173,175,195–197] Most admissions are precipitated by fluid overload or access-related problems, although cardiac disease accounts for over 25 percent of admissions.[161] In PD, the rate of peritonitis is similar to that of the center where the patient is based,[198–200] however, patients over 80 years of age tend to have a prolonged hospital stay with peritonitis.[201] There is no difference in admission rates between HD and PD patients.

Comorbidity increases with increasing age.[124,125] This does not appear to impact on the initial choice of dialysis modality among elderly patients, but does influence the long-term outcome of the individual, regardless of age. Mortality increases with increasing comorbid conditions. The strongest predictors of survival are high predialysis functional state, good nutritional status, and low comorbidity[125]. Diabetes, cardiac disease, and underdialysis are predictors of poor outcome.

The experience with vascular access creation in the older patient is variable and may reflect partly the skill and enthusiasm of the surgeon and the patient selection criteria. There is conflicting data about the success rate for AV fistulae creation, with over 80 percent of patients having a functional access creation in some series[202,203] and 25 to 30 percent in others.[161,196,203] Fistula survival rates are poor, with a less than 10 percent success rate at 1 year.[202,203] In contrast, prosthetic graft survival averages around 60 to 80 percent at 1 year, and 50 to 70 percent at 2 years.[202–206] One problem, more common in the elderly, is poor wound healing after fistula or graft creation.[205] Elective vascular access surgery should be considered as early as possible in the elderly patient to allow adequate healing and maturation of the fistula or graft. Although the guidelines suggest access creation when the creatinine clearance reaches 10 to 12 mL/min, in patients with cardiac disease or diabetes access creation should be planned when creatinine clearance reaches close to 15 mL/min.[169] Despite the apparently poor patency rate of fistulae, in the elderly patient, some suggest an initial attempt at access creation should be with a native vessel fistula rather than prosthetic graft. As with younger dialysis patients, temporary hemodialysis access can be gained using double-lumen catheters placed in the internal jugular vein, femoral vein, or (less commonly) subclavian vein.

Specific problems resulting from the vascular access are rare, but include high-output cardiac failure and steal syndrome. The incidence of high-output cardiac failure as a result of fistula or graft creation is low. Temporary occlusion of the fistula leading to a reduction in heart rate or increase in ejection fraction, as measured by two-dimensional echocardiogram, may help to identify those few patients who would benefit from banding or ligation of the fistula. Steal syndrome is seen in patients with severe peripheral vascular disease where small arterial vessels have compromised perfusion. In these cases, the creation of a fistula or graft further exacerbates the problem by diverting blood away from the extremity. This may result in gangrenous changes which, often only partially, respond to ligation of the access.

Intradialytic problems are similar in the elderly to those seen in younger patients. However, two complications (hypotension and hypoxemia) occurring during hemodialysis and one (protein loss) during PD merit mention here. Both hypotension and hypoxemia, though temporary, may reduce functional independence in an older compromised patient and may affect the rate of rehabilitation. Hypotension may be reduced or minimized by frequent assessment of dry weight, maintaining hemoglobin greater than or equal to 100 g/L (or hematocrit greater than 30 percent), and the avoidance of rapid ultrafiltration and of antihypertensive medications prior to dialysis. The consumption of food during and immediately before dialysis may exacerbate hypotension. Dialysis prescriptions with sequential ultrafiltration and sodium ramping may be used. In addition, both hyperparathyroidism and uremia can cause a functional cardiomyopathy and, consequently, hypotension. Hypoxemia can be prevented by the use of biocompatible membranes and bicarbonate-buffered dialysate and is less frequently seen nowadays. Hemodialysis-related arrhythmias are more common in the older patient.[207]

High protein loss in PD is recognized, and may contribute to hypoalbuminemia, malnutrition, and hyperlipidemia of renal failure. Malnutrition has been reported in up to 20 percent of older hemodialysis patients[208] and 30 to 35 percent of PD patients.[209,210] Predisposing factors include low income, social isolation, ill-fitting dentures, depression, uremic anorexia and impaired taste acuity, constipation, frequent and prolonged hospitalization, and underdialysis. It may remain unrecognized for some time and be very profound at the time of diagnosis. Consequently active assessments should be performed at 6-month intervals. The recommended nutritional intake is more than 35 Kcal/kg/day for energy expenditure and 1.0 to 1.2 g/kg/day protein. Fluid restriction, traditionally, is imposed to prevent more than 5 percent interdialytic weight gain. This is being brought into question as current data show improved nutritional indices in patients with higher intradialytic weight gain.[211] Vitamin supplementation should be introduced early, as dialysis causes a loss of water soluble vitamins. Weight loss remains the simplest and most accurate indicator of malnutrition, although measurement scales, for example, the subjective global assessment scale, are highly recommended as formal measures of nutritional status. Other indices include body weight less than 80 percent of ideal body weight, serum albumin less than 35 g/L, serum cholesterol concentration less than 2.6 mmol/L, and a low serum creatinine or serum urea in patients without residual renal function. Low predialysis serum potassium, phosphorus, and a protein catabolic rate less than 0.8g/kg/day are also useful nonspecific biochemical markers of malnutrition. Recent studies reveal an early alteration in growth hormone and insulin-like growth factor-1 (IGF-1) function,[212] with clinical evidence of growth hormone resistance despite normal or increased serum levels. Newer techniques to improve nutrition include amino acid-based peritoneal dialysate,[213,214] parenteral nutrition (containing amino acid, lipid, and dextrose solutions) given during hemodialysis,[215] the use of anabolic steroids,[216] and subcutaneous injection of human-recombinant growth hormone or recombinant human IGF-1.[212] Some of these methods are in clinical use and seem promising, although further randomized controlled studies are needed to establish an improvement in long-term outcome.

Other complications in dialysis patients include gastric bleeding, hyperparathyroidism, malnutrition, rapidly progressive cardiac disease, left ventricular hypertrophy, and falls. Falls, particularly those occurring postdialysis, may cause subdural bleeding because of the heparin used during hemodialysis. Accelerated athlerosclerosis is seen in all patients with advanced renal disease, and recent research data implicate advanced glycosylation end-products (AGE) in the pathogenesis of the rapidly progressive disease course.[217] These glycosylation products nonenzymatically bind to amine groups and can increase oxidative damage, cause cellular growth and matrix formation via cytokine activation, or cause protein crosslinks and increased connective tissue rigidity.[218–221] In animal studies, the administration of AGE-peptides cause increased vascular permeability and impaired vasodilatation responses. Normally AGEs are detected and cleared by scavenger cells including endothelial cells, macrophages, monocytes, T cells, and renal mesangial cells among others. However, in diabetes, the hyperglycemic milieu allows an increased generation of AGEs, while in renal failure the clearance of the AGEs is impaired.[222,223] Advanced age is associated with increased levels of AGE. Although promising, further research into AGEs and aminoguanide (which inhibits the final stages of the glycosolation pathway) is required before its role in advanced athlerosclerosis can be fully understood.[224,225]

Functional independence is one of the strongest predictors of outcome in the elderly patient starting renal replacement therapy.[125] It can be measured using the Karnofsky scale, which records physical capacity and can identify whether one can perform routine living chores with or without assistance. In a randomly selected population of hemodialysis patients, with a mean age of 56 years (range 21 to 92 years), 36 percent were unable to perform routine living chores without assistance.[226] Diabetic patients were more likely to have decreased functional independence regardless of age. In the elderly this figure rises to 68 percent.[227] The majority of older patients feel so weak that they become housebound, leaving the house only to report for dialysis. Despite improved dialysis techniques and increased survival, renal replacement therapy does not appear to restore patients to their premorbid level of functioning.[227]

Most elderly ESRD patients can be managed in the home setting, although over 25 percent require a home attendant.[227] Other studies report even higher levels of social assistance.[228] Although dialysis does not restore the patients to their previous level of independence, further decline is not seen after dialysis treatment is started.[228] An estimated 0.4 to 0.6 percent of dialysis patients are residents of a nursing home at any one time. Anderson and colleagues[229] have shown that elderly dialysis patients are less likely to be in institutional care than nondialysis patients matched for age. Social workers surveyed in this study report transportation difficulties to and from dialysis, financial difficulties, and a reluctance of the nursing homes to take dialysis patients due to the main difficulties encountered. Rehabilitation and chronic care facilities specifically for dialysis patients are currently under evaluation and preliminary data suggest a 40 percent successful discharge rate. Cost-benefit analyses show an average saving of $76 US per person per day with specialized chronic care and rehabilitation facilities for dialysis patients.[230]

The quality of life of elderly patients on dialysis depends on the comparison group used. When compared with younger dialysis patients, older patients have more disability but show a more positive psychological outlook and higher satisfaction with life.[231–235] Westlie et al.[174] report that 40 percent of respondents felt they were in better health than other 70-year-old people. In contrast, in studies using objective measures of quality of life in an age-matched control population, older dialysis patients had significantly lower life satisfaction[236] and it is now recognized that age is one of the main determinants of quality of life.[237]

Transplantation

Transplantation is becoming an increasingly favored option for renal replacement therapy in the younger age group. The ethical dilemma revolving around the paucity of cadaver kidneys continues and some nephrologists still advocate the restriction of transplantation to younger individuals. The recent literature, however, is in favor of the use of cadaver kidneys harvested from older donors as well as transplantation as a therapy for ESRD in elderly patients.

The use of kidneys from older donors for cadaveric transplantation is well established.[238–248] Although the best results are seen with donor kidneys from patients aged 16 to 45 years of age, the outcome from kidneys from donors over the age of 55 years is good. As the incidence of concomitant disease is higher with increasing age, the number of patients aged over 60 years at the time of death who are suitable for organ donation is lower than in a comparable, but younger population. Nevertheless, the criteria used for acceptance of a kidney is the same as that applied to younger donors. In particular, there should be no past history of renal disease, normal serum creatinine, and an inactive urinary sediment. In cases of doubt, a renal biopsy, done at the time of harvesting, is helpful. Kidneys with less than 20 percent glomerulosclerosis are acceptable.[247] Biopsies showing more than 20 percent sclerosis are predictive of an increased incidence of delayed graft function, a lower baseline renal function, and need for early transplant nephrectomy. Graft survival ranges from 62 to 94 percent at 1 year[248–261] and patient survival 80 to 91 percent at 1 year.[248,256,260] Variations reflect the different age groups studied and the differing criteria for patient acceptance. No difference is seen in graft survival or function when the outcome of transplantation with kidneys from donors aged 55 to 64 compared with donors aged 65 years or more.[244]

The use of older kidneys is associated with a similar incidence of primary nonfunction, delayed graft function, acute rejection, and ATN to that seen in kidneys from younger donors.[238–242,244,248] The baseline serum creatinine tends to be higher in patients receiving older cadaveric transplant kidneys, suggesting reduced functional renal reserve.[250] If transplanted into highly sensitized patients, older kidneys appear to have a higher risk of rejection and their sensitivity to prolonged ischemia is greater.[246] As older individuals are less immunologically efficient, they tend to have a lower incidence of high sensitization and some authors advocate the use of older kidneys for older patients.[246] The reverse philosophy has also been proposed—the avoidance of older, higher risk, kidneys in older (also higher risk) patients. Neither practice has been validated and the restriction of certain kidneys to particular age groups of donors is not recommended. Age matching of the donor kidney to within 5 years of the age of the recipient does not change outcome.[252] Results from living related donors aged 65 years or more are similar to those from younger living related donors.

Kidney transplantation is increasingly offered to elderly patients.[248,255] In the pre-cyclosporin era, the patient and graft outcomes were significantly poorer than those of younger patients[259] and transplantation was not recommended in those over 55 years of age.

More recent data show comparable censored graft survival rates (calculated as graft loss not including loss due to patient death with a functioning graft) in both the under 65-year-old and over 65-year-old populations.[248,256,262] In comparison, patient survival is lower in older patients. Both transplant recipients aged 40 to 55 and those aged 55 years or more have a higher risk of death compared with patients aged 18 to 40 years (relative risk of death of 1.94 and 4.86, respectively).[256] The incidence of acute rejection is lower, possibly because of compromised immunocompetence with increasing age.[263,264] Live donor transplants still have the best outcome, though as with cadaveric donors, the baseline serum creatinine is higher in older recipients.[243,245]

The increased rate of patient death is mostly attributable to higher rates of infection and cardiac disease. Additionally, older patients treated for acute rejection have almost twice the mortality rate of those without rejection.[256] Sepsis is not only more common, but also associated with increased mortality. Altered immune function results in increased sensitivity to immunosuppressive therapy with age and centers with higher reported patient survival often use lower doses of immunotherapy.[265] The most appropriate regime for immunosuppression has not been studied, but the general opinion is that older patients should be treated with lower doses of immunosuppression, particularly low-dose steroids.[266] Cyclosporin A has been recommended and is shown to reduce the number of episodes of acute rejection. Patient survival rates with cyclosporin A are not reported.[251]

The acceptance criteria for transplantation in the over 65-year-old remain poorly defined and although the frequency of transplantation in the elderly is increasing, services remain restricted. The published literature illustrates a definite sociodemographic selection bias with fewer diabetic patients, fewer over 70-year-old patients, and fewer patients with one or more concomitant illnesses being transplanted. Increased comorbidity alone does not account for the reduced numbers of elderly patients reaching transplantation.[266–268] Most reports compare the survival rates of older patients with younger patients and are therefore of limited use in the clinical setting. In contrast, Schaubel et al.[255] compared the survival of older patients treated with transplantation with similarly aged patients remaining on dialysis. The study shows a lower mortality rate in transplanted patients, although the comparison groups (dialysis and transplant patients) were dissimilar. Subgroup analysis, of a better matched group of patients without comorbid illness, showed the survival advantage was still present. No information regarding psychosocial data or dialysis adequacy was included and a selection bias cannot be excluded.

Physical fitness and strength does not appear to improve with transplantation possibly because of corticosteroid-related myopathy.[269] Increased quality of life,[263] and freedom for the patient is, however, well-recognized and transplantation should be a considered option in the older dialysis patient.

Ethical Issues Associated with the Provision of Renal Replacement Therapy in Elderly Patients

The ethical issues surrounding the question of renal replacement therapy in the elderly are complex and are influenced by society as well as by personal experiences. No answers exist and, to date, no guidelines outlining the most suitable patients for either dialysis or transplantation have been published.

Political arguments revolve around limited health care resources and increasing costs, with the elderly often being the first group to be considered expendable. Recent surveys show that financial limitations have a powerful impact on patient selection for dialysis: for example, in a survey of dialysis directors, 10 percent would reject patients on the basis of age alone, while 85 percent indicated that they would do so under significant scarcity.[270,271] Is this a valid argument? Should we, as physicians, be involved in the allocation of finances as well as having primary responsibility for the care of the individual?

The elderly are a heterogeneous group of individuals in whom chronologic age does not match physiologic age. No two patients are alike and each should be assessed individually. Few would argue that renal replacement therapy has little role in a patient in whom treatment is futile or where the quality of life is felt, by the patient, to be unacceptable. The problem lies in identifying these patients. There are no criteria for futility, and the assessment of quality of life is so individualized that we, as health care workers, are unable to accurately assess life satisfaction on behalf of our patients. It is interesting to note that in one ethicist's eyes, dialysis in the elderly was, "at the price of a doubtful or poor quality of life."[272] This assumption is false, and in fact, most elderly dialysis patients see their lives as better than, or at least as good as, those not on dialysis.[170,233–235]

So what is the best management of the elderly patient with ESRD? Should we offer dialysis or transplantation to our older patients? One dogma is that, "individualism should give way to a community-based and affirmed notion of the value of the aged in the society. . . ."[272] Is our role to serve society or is our responsibility to the patient? This question remains unanswered. Our recommendation is that a treatment trial should be offered to all patients, and that appropriate outcome objectives be established from the outset.[273] If, after such a trial, treatment is not beneficial, the physician can discontinue dialysis and direct their energy to reducing uremic symptoms and easing the patient to a more dignified end. Careful attention to symptom relief, psychological support of the patient, and support for the patient's family and the nursing staff is essential.

The question of stopping therapy also arises in those patients well-established on chronic dialysis. Respect for the patient's autonomy dictates that dialysis be withdrawn at his or her own request. Indeed, dialysis withdrawal is becoming one of the leading causes of death in the ESRD patient.[274] However, the case is less clear when the patient suffers some catastrophic medical event (e.g., a severe disabling stroke) and has not previously expressed their wishes. The discussion and introduction of an "advance directive" or "living will" at an early stage of treatment helps, both the physician and the patient, plan therapy in such an event. Strict guidelines in the preparation and execution and frequent review of the directive can prevent abuse by either the physician or the family.

Physicians, as their patients advocates, have an obligation to advocate for the needs of their elderly patients and each must strive to avoid discrimination or "ageism."

References

1. Sourander L, Kasanen A, Pasternack A, Kaarsalo E: Uraemia in the aged in south-western Finland. A longitudinal study. pp. 540–546. In Orimo H, Shimada K, Iriki M, Maeda D (eds): Recent Advances in Gerontology. International Congress Series 469. Excerpta Medica, Amsterdam, 1979
2. Guillen Llera F, Gil Gregorio P: Incidence of renal diseases in a geriatric unit. pp. 208–236. In Macias Nunez JF, Cameron JS (eds): Renal Function and Disease in the Elderly. Butterworths, London, 1987
3. Roberts AP, Robinson RE, Beard RW: Some factors affecting bacterial colony counts in urinary tract infection. Br Med J 1967;1:400–403
4. Ouslander JG, Schapira M, Fingold S, Schnelle J: Accuracy of rapid urine screening tests among incontinent nursing home residents with asymptomatic bacteriuria. J Am Geriatr Soc 1995;43:772–775
5. Ouslander JG, Schapira M, Schnelle JF et al: Does eradicating bacteriuria affect the severity of chronic urinary incontrinence in nursing home residents? Ann Intern Med 1995;122: 749–754
6. Duffy LM, Cleary J, Ahern S et al: Clean intermittent catheterisation: safe, cost-effective bladder management for male residents of VA nursing homes. J Am Geriatr Soc 1995;43: 865–870
7. Bakke A, Vollset SE, Hoistaeter PA, Irgens LM: Physical complications in patients treated with clean intermittent catheterisation. Scand J Urol Nephrol 1993;27:55–61
8. Moore-Smith B: The treatment of urinary tract infections in elderly women. Mod Geriatr 1974;4:408–414
9. Stamey TA: Diagnosis, localization and classification of urinary infections. pp. 1–51. In Stamey TA (ed): Pathogenesis and Treatment of Urinary Tract Infections. Williams & Wilkins, Baltimore, 1980
10. Sourander LB. Urinary tract infection in the aged. An epidemiological study. Ann Med Intern Fenn 1966;55(suppl 45): 1–55

11. MacDonald RA, Levitin H, Mallory GK, Kass EH: Relation between pyelonephritis and bacterial counts in the urine: an autopsy study. N Engl J Med 1957;256:915–922

12. Brocklehurst JC, Bee P, Jones D, Palmer M: Bacteriuria in geriatric hospital patients: its correlates and management. Age Ageing 1977;6:240–245

13. Clague JE, Horan MA: Urine culture in the elderly: scientifically doubtful and practically useless? Lancet 1994;344: 1035–1036

14. Dontas AS, Parasaki I, Petrikkos G, Giamarellou H: Diuresis bacteriuria in physically dependent women. Age Ageing 1977; 6:240–245

15. Mills SJ, Ford M, Gould FK, Burton S, Neal DE: Screening for bacteriuria in urological patients using reagent strips. Br J Urol 1992;70:314–317

16. Choudhury SL, Brocklehurst JC: Urinary tract infection in old age. pp. 254–281. In Macias-Nunez JF, Cameron JS (eds): Renal Function and Disease in the Elderly. Butterworths, London, 1987

17. Brocklehurst JC, Dillane JB, Griffiths L, Fry J: The prevalence and symptomatology of urinary infection in an aged population. Gerontol Clin 1968;10:242–253

18. Ruikka I, Sourancer LB: Phenacetin consumption, occurrence of urinary tract infection and renal function in a series of aged hospital patients. Gerontol Clin 1967;9:99–102

19. Eberlye CM, Winsemius SE: Risk factors and consequences of bacteriuria in non-catheterized nursing home residents. J Gerontol 1993;48:M266–M271

20. Bakke A, Vollset SE: Risk factors for bacteriuria and clinical urinary tract infection in patients treated with intermittent catheterisation. J Urol 1993;149:527–531

21. Nicolle LE, Mayhew WJ, Bryan L: Prospective randomized comparison of therapy and no therapy for asymptomatic bacteriuria in institutionalized elderly women. Am J Med 1987;83: 27–33

22. Kass EH, Miall WE, Stuart KL: Relationship of bacteriuria to hypertension; an epidemiological study. J Clin Invest 1961; 40:1053

23. Marketos SG, Dontas AS, Papanayiotou P, Economous P: Bacteriuria and arterial hypertension in old age. Geriatrics 1970; 25:136–146

24. Kirkland JL, Robinson JM: Bacteriuria and survival in old age. N Eng J Med 1981;305:586–587

25. Nordenstam GR, Ake Brandenberg O, Oden AS et al: Bacteriuria and mortality in an elderly population. N Eng J Med 1986; 314:1152–1156

26. Abrutyn E, Mossey J, Berlin JA et al: Does asymptomatic bacteriuria predict mortality and does antimicrobial treatment reduce mortality in elderly ambulent women? Ann Intern Med 1994;120:827–833

27. Dontas AS, Kasavaki-Charvati P, Papanayiotou PC, Marketos SG: Bacteruria and survival in old age. N Eng J Med 1981; 304:939–943

28. Harding GK, Nicolle LE, Ronald AR et al: How long should catheter-acquired urinary tract infection in women be treated? A randomized controlled study. Ann Intern Med 1991;114: 713–719

29. Freeman RB, Smith WM, Richardson JA et al: Long-term therapy for chronic bacteriuria in men. Ann Intern Med 1975;83: 133–147

30. Raaschou F: Studies of chronic pyelonephritis with special reference to kidney function. Munksgaard, Copenhagen, 1948

31. Kimmelstiel P: The nature of chronic pyelonephritis. Geriatrics 1964;19:145–157

32. Baumanis J, Russell HK: Pyelonephritis in a chronic disease hospital. Geriatrics 1959;14:25–37

33. Bruckel RW, Wincker HJ: Clinical aspects of urinary tract infections in Geriatrics. 6th International Congress of Gerontology (Excerpta Medica Congress Series 57), Copenhagen 1963

34. Lieberthal F: Pyelonephritic contracture of the kidney. Surg Gynecol Obstet 1939;69:159–171

35. Bell ET: Exudative interstitial nephritis (pyelonephritis). Surgery 1942;II:261–280

36. Prewitt G: Pyelonephritis. West J Surg 1943;51:393–393

37. Jackson GG, Dallenbach FD, Kipnis GP: Symposium on clinical advances in medicine; pyelonephritis; correlation of clinical and pathologic observations in antibiotic era. Med Clin North Am 1955;39:297

38. Sanjurjo LA: The problem of chronic pyelonephritis. Med Clin North Am 1959;43:1601–1610

39. Kleeman SE, Freedman LR: The finding of chronic pyelonephritis in males and females at autopsy. N Eng J Med 1960; 263:988–992

40. Maskell R: Broadening the concept of urinary tract infection. Br J Urol 1995;76:2–8

41. Fihn SD, Johnson C, Stamm WE: *Escherichia coli* urethritis in women with symptoms of acute urinary infection. J Infect Dis 1988;157:196–199

42. Kunin CM, White Lvm Tong HH: A reassessment of the importance of "low-count" bacteruria in young women with acute urinary symptoms. Ann Intern Med 1993;119:454–460

43. Arav-Boger R, Leibovici L, Danon YL: Urinary tract infections with low and high colony counts in young women. Arch Intern Med 1994;154:300–304

44. Maskell R, Pead L, Sanderson RA: Fastidious bacteria and the urethral syndrome: a 2-year clinical and bacteriological study of 51 women. Lancet 1983;2:1277–1280

45. Fairley KF, Birch DF: Detection of bladder bacteriuria in patients with acute urinary symptoms. J Infect Dis 1989;159: 226–131

46. Savige JA, Birch DF, Fairley KF: Comparison of mid catheter collection and suprapubic aspiration of urine for diagnosing bacteriuria due to fastidious micro-organisms. J Urol 1983; 129:62–63

47. Wilkins EGL, Payne SR, Pead PJ et al: Interstitial cystitis and urethral syndrome: a possible answer. Br J Urol 1989; 64:39–44

48. Pead L, Maskell R, Morris J: *Staphyloccus saphrophyticus* as a urinary pathogen: a six year prospective survey. BMJ 1985; 291:1157–1159

49. Maskell R, Pead L: Corynebacteria as urinary pathogens. J Infect Dis 1990;162:782–783

50. Soriano F, Fernandez-Roblas R: Infections caused by antibiotic-resistant *Corynebacterium* Group D2. Eur J Clin Microbiol Infect Dis 1988;7:337–341

51. Brumfitt W, Gargan RA, Hamilton-Miller JMT: Diagnosis and cure of recurrent urinary infection with microaerophilic and anaerobic bacteria. Br Med J 1980;281:909–910

52. Collins LE, Clarke RW, Maskell R: Streptocci as urinary pathogens. Lancet 1986;2:479–481

53. Kass EH: Chemotherapeutic and antibiotic drugs in management of infection of urinary tract. Am J Med 1955;18:764–781

54. Bergeron MG: Treatment of pyelonephritis in adults. Med Clin North Am 1995;79:619–649

55. Turck M, Petersdorf RG, Fournier MR: The epidemiology of non-enteric *Escherichia coli* infections: prevalence of serological groups. J Clin Invest 1962;41:1760–1765

56. Lidin Janson G, Hanson LA, Kaijser B: Comparison of *Escherichia coli* from bacteriuric patients with those from faeces of healthy school children. J Infect Dis 1977;136:346–353

57. Gruneberg RN, Bendall MJ: Hospital outbreak of trimethoprim resistance in pathologenic coliform bacteria. BMJ 1979;2:7–9

58. Stamey TA, Timothy M, Miller M, Mihara G: Recurrent urinary infections in adult women. The role of introital enterobacteria. California Med 1971;115:1–19

59. Bollgren I, Winberg J: The periurethral aerobic flora in girls highly susceptible to urinary infection. Acta Paediatr Scand 1976;65:81–87

60. Svanborg EC: Attachment of *Escherichia coli* to human uroepithelial cells. An in vitro test system applied in the study of urinary tract infection. Scand J Infect Dis 1978;15(suppl): 1–74

61. Sheinfeld J, Schaeffer AJ, Cordon-Cardo C et al: Association of the Lewis blood-group phenotype with recurrent urinary tract infections in women. N Eng J Med 1989;320: 773–777

62. Mobley HL, Island MD, Massad G: Virulence determinants of uropathogenic *Escherichia coli* and *Proteus mirabilis*. Kidney Int Suppl 1994;47:S129–136

63. Sourander LB, Ruikka I, Gronroos M: Correlation between urinary tract infection, prolapse conditions and function of the bladder in the aged female hospital patient. Gerontol Clin 1965;7:179–184

64. Carty M, Brocklehurst JC, Carty J: Bacteriuria and its correlates in old age. Gerontology 1981;27:72–75

65. Warren JW, Muncie HL, Jr, Hebel JR, Hall-Craggs M: Long-term urethral catheterization increases risk of chronic pyelonephritis and renal inflammation. J Am Geriatr Soc 1994;42: 1286–1290

66. Warren JW, Muncie HL, Jr, Hall-Craggs M: Acute pyelonephritis associated with bacteriuria during long-term catheterization: a prospective clinicopathological study. J Infect Dis 1988;158:1341–1346

67. Mobley HLT, Chippendale GR, Tenney JH et al: MR/K hemagglutination of *Providencia stuartii* correlates with adherence to catheters and with persistence in catheter-associated bacteriuria. J Infect Dis 1988;157:264–271

68. Parvinen M, Sourander LB, Vuorinen P: Cystographic studies of old women. Gerontol Clin 1965;7:343–347

69. Saltzman RL, Peterson PK: Immunodeficiency of the elderly. Rev Infect Dis 1987;9:1127–1139

70. Wade AW, Szewczuk MR: Changes in the mucosal-associated B cell response with age. pp. 95–127. In Goidl EA (ed): Aging and the Immune Response. Marcel Dekker, New York, 1987

71. Seneca H, Grant JP, Jr: Urologic sepsis/shock. J Am Geriatr Soc 1976;24:292–300

72. Isada CM, Kasten BL, Goldman MP et al: Infectious Diseases Handbook, LexiComp Inc, Hudson, Cleveland, 1995–1996

73. Pinson AG, Philbrick JT, Lindbeck GH, Schorling JB: Oral antibiotic therapy for acute pyelonephritis: a methodologic review of the literature. J Gen Int Med 1992;7:544–553

74. Petersdorf RG, Ingelfinger FJ, Relman AS, Findland M: Controversy in Internal Medicine. WB Saunders, Philadelphia, 1966

75. Brocklehurst JC, Dillane JB, Griffiths L, Fry J: A therapeutic trial in urinary infection of old age. Gerontol Clin 1968;10: 345–347

76. Sourander LB, Kasanen A: En dos langtids' sulfonamid i veckan (4-sulfanilamido-5-6-dimetoxypyrimidin) vid behandling av urinvagsinfektioner hos aldringar. Nord Med 1965; 74:1229–1230

77. Sourander LB, Saarimaa H, Arvilommi H: Treatment of sulfonamide-resistant urinary tract infections with a combination of sulfonamide and trimethoprim. Acta Med Scand 1972;191: 1–3

78. Vahlne G: Serological typing of the colon bacteria. Acta Pathol Microbiol Scand 1945;62(suppl)

79. Lincoln K, Lidin-Janson G, Winberg J: Resistant urinary infections resulting from changes in resistance pattern of faecal flora induced by sulphonamide and hospital environment. BMJ 1970;3:305–309

80. Chamberland S, L'Ecuyer J, Lessard C et al: Antibiotic susceptibility profiles of 941 gram negative bacteria isolated from septicaemic patients throughout Canada. Clin Infect Dis 1992; 15:615–628

81. Bergeron MG. Therapeutic potential of high renal levels of aminoglycosides in pyelonephritis. J Antimicrob Chemother 1985;15:4–8

82. Bergeron MG, Marois Y: Benefit form high levels of gentamycin in the treatment of *E. coli* pyleonephritis. Kidney Int 1986;30:481–487

83. Mouton Y, Ajana F, Chidiac C et al: A multicenter study of lomefloxacin and trimethoprim/sulfamethoxazole in the treatment of uncomplicated acute pyelonephritis. Am J Med 1992; 92:87S–90S

84. Cox CE, Gentry LO, Rodriguez-Gomez G: Multicenter open-label study of parenteral ofloxacin in treatment of pyelonephritis in adults. Urology 1992;39:453–456

85. Bailey RR, Lynn KL, Robson RA et al: Comparison of ciprofloxacin with netilmicin for the treatment of acute pyelonephritis. N Z Med J 1992;105:102–103

86. Cove-Smith JR, Knapp MS: Analgesic nephropathy: an impor-

tant cause of chronic renal failure in the elderly. Q J Med 1978;47:49–69

87. Clive DM, Stoff JS: Renal syndromes asociated with nonsteroidal anti-inflammatory drugs. N Engl J Med 1984;310: 563–572
88. Heptinsall RH: Interstitial nephritis: a review. Am J Pathol 1976;83:214–236
89. Moore RD, Steinberg EP, Powe NR et al: Frequency and determinants of adverse reactions induced by high-osmolality contrast media. Radiology 1989;170:727–732
90. Weisberg LS, Kurnik PB, Kurnik BR: Risk of radiocontrast nephropathy in patients with and without diabetes mellitus. Kidney Int 1994;45:259–265
91. Manske CI, Sprafka JM, Strong JT, Wang Y: Contrast nephropathy in diabetic patients undergoing coronary angiography. Am J Med 1990;89:615–620
92. Weinrauch LA, Healy RW, Leland OS et al: Coronary angiography and acute renal failure in diabetic azotemic nephropathy. Arch Int Med 1977;86:56
93. Berkseth RO, Kjellstrand CM: Radiolic contrast-induced nephropathy. Med Clin North Am 1984;68:351–370
94. Cochran ST, Wong WS, Roe DJ: Predicting angiographic-induced acute renal impairment: clinical risk model. Am J Radiol 1983;141:1027–1033
95. Taliercio CP, Vlietstra R, Fisher LD, Burnett JC: Risks of renal dysfunction with cardiac angiography. Ann Intern Med 1986;104:501–504
96. Porter GA: Contrast associated nephropathy. Am J Cardiol 1989;64:22E–26E
97. Barrett BJ, Carlisle E: A meta-analysis of the relative nephrotoxicity of high and low-osmolality contrast media. J Am Soc Nephrol 1992;3:719
98. Moore RD, Steinberg EP, Powe NR et al: Nephrotoxicity of high-osmolality versus low-osmolality contrast media: randomised clinical trial. Radiology 1992;182:649–655
99. McCarthy CS, Becker JA: Multiple myeloma and contrast media. Radiology 1992;183:519–521
100. Porter GA: Contrast-associated nephropathy: presentation, pathophysiology and management. Min Electrolyte Metab 1994;20:232–243
101. Solomon R, Werner C, Mann D et al: Effects of saline, mannitol, and furosemide to prevent acute decreases in renal function induced by radiocontrast agents. N Eng J Med 1994;331: 1416–1420
102. Weinstein JM, Heyman S, Brezis M: Potential deleterious effect of furosemide in radiocontrast nephropathy. Nephron 1992;62:413–415
103. Weisberg LS, Kurnik PB, Kurnik BR: Dopamine and renal blood flow in radiocontrast-induced nephropathy in humans. Ren Fail 1993;15:61–68
104. Erley CM, Duda SH, Schlepckow S et al: Adenosine antagonist theophylline prevents the reduction of glomerular filtration rate after contrast media application. Kidney Int 1994;45: 1425–1431
105. Eknoyan G: Renal papillary necrosis. pp. 1910–1916. In: Massry SG, Glassock RJ (eds): Textbook of Nephrology. Wilkins & Wilkins, Baltimore, 1989
106. Simon P, Charasse C, Autuly V et al: Epidemiology of primary glomerular disease in the elderly: a prospective study during a 15 year period. pp. 161–166. In Sessa A, Meroni M, Battini G (eds): Glomerulonephritis in the Elderly. Contributions in Nephrology. S. Karger, Basel 1993
107. Diaz-Buxo JA, Donadio JV, Jr: Complications of percutaneous renal biopsy: an analysis of 1000 consecutive biopsies. Clin Nephrol 1975;4:223–227
108. Levison SP. Renal disease in the elderly: the role of the renal biopsy. Am J Kidney Dis 1990;16:300–306
109. Johnston PA, Coulshed SJ, Davison AM: Renal biopsy findings in patients older than 65 years of age presenting with the nephrotic syndrome. A report from the MRC Glomerulonephritis Registry. pp. 127–132. In Sessa A, Meroni M, Battini G (eds) Glomerulonephritis in the Elderly. Contributions in Nephrology. S. Karger Basel, 1993
110. Labeeuw M, Caillette A, Colon S et al: Renal biopsy in elderly adults over 75 years of age. Geriatr Nephrol Urol 1995;4: 177–181
111. Bolton KW: Nephrotic syndrome in the aged. pp. 523–554. In Cameron JS, Glassock RJ (eds): The Nephrotic Syndrome. Marcel Dekker, New York, 1988
112. Passerini P, Como G, Vigano E: Idiopathic membranous nephropathy in the elderly. Nephrol Dial Trans 1993;8: 1324–1325
113. Nagai R, Cattran DC, Pei Y: Steriod therapy and prognosis of focal segmental glomerulosclerosis. Clin Nephrol 1994;42: 18–21
114. Jeffrey RF, Gardiner DS, More IA et al: Cresentic glomerulonephritis: experience of a single unit over a five year period. Scott Med J 1992;37:175–178
115. Donadio JV: Treatment of glomerulonephritis in the elderly. Am J Kidney Dis 1990;16:307–311
116. Wagener HP, Hollenhorst RW: The ocular lesions of temporal arteritis. Am J Opthalmol 1958;45:617–630
117. Truong L, Kopelman RG, Williams GS, Pirani CL: Temporal arteritis and renal disease. Case report and review of the literature. Am J Med 1985;78:171–175
118. Pascual J, Quereda C, Liano F et al: End-stage renal disease after necrotising glomerulonephritis in an elderly patient with temporal arteritis. Nephron 1994;66:236–237
119. Samily AG, Field RA, Merrill JP: Acute glomerulonephritis in elderly patients: report of seven cases over sixty years of age. Ann Intern Med 1961;54:603–609
120. Moorthy AV, Zimmerman SW: Renal disease in the elderly: clinicopathologic analysis of renal diseases in 115 elderly patients. Clin Nephrol 1980;14:223–229
121. Montoliu J, Darnell A, Torras A, Revert L: Primary acute glomerular disorders in the elderly. Arch Intern Med 1980;140: 755–756
122. Melby PC, Musick WD, Luger AM, Khanna R: Poststreptococcal glomerulonephritis in the elderly; report of a case and review of the literature. Am J Nephrol 1987;7:235–240
123. Roy AT, Johnson LE, Lee DBN et al: Renal failure in older people. J Am Geriatr Soc 1990;38:239–253
124. Canadian Organ Replacement Register 1993 Annual Report,

Canadian Institute for Health Information, Don Mills, Ontario, 1995

125. Jassal SV, Douglas JF, Stout RW: Prognostic markers for one year survival in elderly dialysis patients. Nephrol Dial Trans 1996 Nephrol Dial Transplant 1996;11:1052–1057
126. Frocht A, Fillit H: Renal disease in the geriatric patient. J Am Geriatr Soc 1984;32:28–43
127. Gasparini M, Hofman R, Stoller M: Renal artery embolism: clinical features and therapeutic options. J Urol 1992;147: 567–572
128. Mann SJ, Pickering TG: Detection of renovascular hypertension. State of the Art 1992. Ann Intern Med 1992;117: 845–853
129. Canzanello VJ, Textor SC: Noninvasive diagnosis of renovascular disease. Mayo Clin Proc 1994;69:1172–1181
130. Grist T: Magnetic resonance angiography of the aorta and renal arteries. MRI Clin North 1993;1:253–269
131. Grist T, Kennel T, Sproat I, McDermott JC et al: Prospective evaluation of renal angiography: Comparison with conventional angiography in 35 patients. Radiology 1993;189:190
132. Grist TM: Magnetic resonance angiography of renal artery stenosis. Am J Kidney Dis 1994;24:700–712
133. Sicard GA, Reilly JM, Picus DD, Allen BT: Alternatives in renal vascularisation. Curr Probl Surg 1995;32:571–652
134. Bennet PH, Haffner S, Kasiske BL et al: Screening and management of microalbuminuria in patients with diabetes mellitus: Recommendations to the scientific advisory board of the National Kidney Foundation from an ad hoc committee of the council on diabetes mellitus of the National Kidney Foundation. Am J Kidney Dis 1995;25:107–112
135. Lewis EJ, Hunsicker LG, Bain RP, Rohde RD: The effect of angiotensin converting enzyme inhibition on diabetic nephropathy. N Eng J Med 1993;329:1456–1462
136. Kyle RA: Multiple myeloma: review of 869 cases. Mayo Clin Proc 1975;59:29–40
137. Ganeval D, Cathomen M, Noel LH, Grunfeld JP: Kidney involvement in multiple myeloma and related disorders Contrib Nephrol 1982;33:210–222
138. Fang LST: Light chain nephropathy. Kid Int 1985;27: 582–592
139. Shetty A, Oreopoulos DG: CAPD in the treatment of end stage renal disease in myeloma patients. Geriatr Nephrol Urol 1995; 5:3–8
140. Rosansky SJ, Richards FW: Use of peritoneal dialysis in the treatment of patients with renal failure and paraproteinemia. Am J Nephrol 1985;5:361–365
141. Solling K, Solling J: Clearances of Bence Jones proteins during dialysis or plasmapheresis in myelomatosis associated with renal failure. Contrib Nephrol 1988;68:259–262
142. Misiani R, Tiraboschi G, Mingardi G, Mecca G: Management of myeloma kidney: an anti-light chain approach Am J Kidney Dis 1987;10:28–33
143. Nissenson AR, Port FK: Outcome of ESRD in patients with rare causes of renal failure. I. Inherited and metabolic disorders. Q J Med 1989;73:1055–1061
144. Port FK, Nissenson AR: Outcome of ESRD in patients with rare causes of renal failure. II. Renal systemic neoplasms. Q J Med 1989;73:1162–1166
145. Alexanian R, Baslogie B, Dixon D: Renal failure in multiple myeloma. Arch Intern Med 1990;150:1693–1695
146. Iggo N, Parsons V: Renal disease in multiple myeloma: Current perspectives. Nephron 1990;56:229–233
147. Mukamel E, Nissenkorn I, Boner G: Occult progressive renal damage in the elderly male due to benign prostatic hypertrophy. J Am Geriatr Soc 1979;27:403–406
148. Olbrich O, Woodford-Williams E, Irvine RE, Webster D: Renal function in prostatism. Lancet 1957;i:1322
149. Ralston AJ: Renal disease. Mod Geriatr 1975;5:10–14
150. Mclnnes EG, Levy DW, Chaudhuri MD, Bhan GL: Renal failure in the elderly. Q J Med 1987;64:583–588
151. Druml W, Lax F, Grimm G et al: Acute renal failure in the elderly 1975–1990. Clin Nephrol 1994;41:342–349
152. Gornick CC, Kjellstrand CM: Acute renal failure complicating aortic aneurysm surgery. Nephron 1983;35:145–157
153. Hakim RW, Lazarus JM: Haemodialysis in acute renal failure. pp. 767–807. In Brenner BM, Lazarus JM (eds): Acute Renal Failure. Churchill Livingstone, New York, 1988
154. Bellomo R, Farmer M, Boyce N: The outcome of critically ill elderly patients with severe renal failure treated by continuous hemodiafiltration. Int J Artif Org 1994;17:466–472
155. Lamiere H, Dekeyterk N, Pauwels W: Acute renal failure in the elderly. pp. 461–484. In Oreopoulos DG (ed): Geriatric Nephrology. Dordrecht Martinus Nijhof, 1987
156. Lamiere N, Matthys E, Vanholder R et al: Causes and prognosis of acute renal failure in elderly patients. Nephrol Dial Trans 1987;2:316–322
157. Rosenfeld JB, Shobat J, Grosskopf I, Borner G: Acute renal failure: a disease of the elderly. Adv Nephrol 1987;16: 159–168
158. Pascual J, Orofino L, Liano F: Incidence and prognosis of acute renal failure in older patients. J Am Geriatr Soc 1990; 38:25–30
159. Gentric A, Cledes J: Immediate and long term prognosis in acute renal failure in the elderly. Nephrol Dial Trans 1991; 6:86–90
160. Blagg CR: Chronic renal failure in the elderly. pp. 117–126. In Oreopoulos DG (ed) Geriatric Nephrology. Martinus Nijhoff, Boston, 1986
161. Challah S, Wing AJ, Bauer R et al: Negative selection of patients for dialysis and transplantation in the United Kingdom. Br Med J 1984;288:1119–1122
162. Porush JG, Faubert PF: Chronic renal failure in the elderly. pp. 285–313. In Porush JG, Faubert PF (eds): Renal disease in the Aged. Little Brown, Boston, 1991
163. Dalzeil M, Garrett C: Intraregional variation in treatment of end stage renal failure. Br Med J 1987;294:1382–1383
164. Klahr S, Levey AS, Beck GJ et al: The effects of dietary protein restriction and blood pressure control on the progression of chronic renal disease. N Eng J Med 1994;330:877–884

165. Peterson JC, Adler S, Burkart JM et al: Blood pressure control, proteinuria and the progression of renal disease. The modification of diet in renal disease study. Ann Intern Med 1995;123: 754–762

166. Muirhead N, Cattran DC, Zaltzman J et al: Safety and efficacy of recombinant human erythropoietin in correcting the anaemia of patients with chronic renal allograft dysfunction. J Am Soc Nephrol 1994;5:1216–1222

167. Nissenson AR: Chronic peritoneal dialysis in the elderly. Geriatr Nephrol Urol 1991;1:3–12

168. D'Amico G, Striker GE: Proceedings from the symposium on renal replacement therapy throughout the world: the registries. Comparibility of the different registries on renal replacement therapy. Am J Kidney Dis 1995;25:113–118

169. Ismail N, Hakim R, Oreopoulos DG, Patrikarea A: Renal replacement therapies in the elderly. Part 1. Hemodialysis and chronic peritoneal dialysis. Am J Kidney Dis 1993;22: 759–782

170. US Renal Data System: USRDS 1989 Annual Report. Bethesda, Maryland, The National Institutes of Health, National Institute of Diabetes and Digestive and Kidney Diseases. August, 1989, pp. 17–20

171. Agodoa LY, Eggers PW: Renal replacement therapy in the United States: data from the United States Renal Data System. Am J Kidney Dis 1995;25:119–133

172. Chester AC, Rakowski TA, Argy WP, Jr et al: Hemodialysis in the eighth and ninth decades of life. Arch Intern Med 1979; 139:1001–1005

173. Mion C, Oules R, Canaud B et al: Maintenance dialysis in the elderly: a review of 15 years' experience in Languedoc-Roussilon. Proc Eur Dial Trans Assoc 1984;21:490–509

174. Westlie L, Umen A, Nestrud S, Kjellstrand CM: Mortality, morbidity and life satisfaction in the very old dialysis patient. ASAIO J 1984;30:21–30

175. Schaefer K, Asmus G, Quellhorst E et al: Optimum dialysis treatment for patients over 60 years with primary renal disease. Survival data and clinical results from 242 patients treated by either hemodialysis or hemofiltration. Proc Eur Dial Trans Assoc 1985;21:510–523

176. Rotellar E, Lubelza RA, Rotellar C et al: Must patients over 65 be dialyzed. Nephron 1985;41:152–156

177. Port FK, Novello AC, Wolfe RA: Outcome of treatment modalities for geriatric end-stage renal disease. pp. 199–152. In Micheles MF, Davis BB, Preuss HG (eds): Geriatric Nephrology. Field Rich and Associates, New York, 1986

178. Tapson JS, Rodger RSC, Mansy H et al: Renal replacement therapy in patients aged over 60 years. Postgrad Med J 1987; 63:1071–1077

179. Loew H: Long term dialysis treatment in advanced age. J Gerontol 1987;20:52–55

180. Husebye DG, Kjellstrand CM: Old patients and uraemia. Rates of acceptance to and withdrawal from dialysis. Int J Artif Org 1987;10:166–172

181. Panarello G, DeBaz H, Cecchin E, Tesis F: Dialysis for the elderly: survival and risk factors. Adv Perit Dial 1985;5: 49–51

182. Benevent D, Benzakour M, Peyronnet P et al: Comparison of continuous ambulatory peritoneal dialysis and haemodialysis in the elderly. Adv Perit Dial 1990;6(suppl):68–71

183. Walls J: Dialysis in the elderly. Some UK experience. Adv Perit Dial 1990;6(suppl):82–85

184. Park MS, Lee HB: Outcome of dialysis in the elderly. Geriatr Nephrol Urol 1992;1:173–179

185. Picolli G, Quarello F, Salomone M et al: Dialysis in the elderly: comparison of different dialytic modalities. Adv Perit Dial 1990;6(suppl):72–81

186. Nissenson AR, Gentile DE, Soderblom R: CAPD in the elderly. Southern California/Southern Nevada experience. Adv Perit Dial 1990;6(suppl):51–55

187. Gokal R: CAPD in the elderly. European and UK experience. Adv Perit Dial 1990;6(suppl):38–40

188. Williams AJ, Nicholl JF, El-Nahas Am et al: Continuous ambulatory peritneal dialysis and haemodialysis in the elderly. Q J Med 1990;274:215–223

189. Segoloni GP, Salamone M, Piccoli GB: CAPD in the elderly. Italian multicenter study experience. Adv Perit Dial 1990; 6(suppl):41–46

190. Nebeel M, Finke K: CAPD in patients over 60 years of age. Adv Perit Dial 1990;6(suppl):56–60

191. Khan IH, Catto GR, Edward N, MacLeod AM: Death during the first 90 days of dialysis: a case control study. Am J Kidney Dis 1995;25:276–280

192. Churchill DN, Thorpe KE, Vonesh EF, Keshaviah PR: Patient survival on CAPD: comparison between Canada and the United States (USA). CANUSA Peritoneal Dialysis Study Group. J Am Soc Nephrol 1995;6:507

193. Lunde NM, Port FK, Wolfe RA, Guire KE: Comparison of mortality risk by choice of CAPD versus hemodialysis among elderly patients. Adv Perit Dial 1991;5:68–72

194. Michel C, Bindi P, Viron B: CAPD with private home nurses: an alternative treatment for elderly and disabled patients. Adv Perit Dial 1990;6(suppl):92–94

195. Carlson DM, Duncan DA, Naessens JM, Johnson WJ: Hospitalisation in dialysis patients. Mayo Clin Proc 1984;59: 769–775

196. Gokal R, Jakubowski C, King J et al: Outcome in patients on chronic ambulatory peritoneal dialysis and hemodialysis: 4 year analysis of a prospective multicenter study. Lancet 1987; 2:1105–1109

197. US Renal Data System: 1991 Annual Data Report. Bethesda, Maryland, The National Institutes of Diabetes and Digestive and Kidney Diseases, 1991. Excerpts in Am J Kidney Dis 1991;18(suppl 2):38–48

198. Gokal R: CAPD in the elderly. European and UK experience. Adv Perit Dial 1990;6(suppl):38–40

199. Nissenson AR, Gentile DE, Soderblom R: CAPD in the elderly: Southern California/South Nevada experience. Adv Perit Dial 1990;6(suppl):51–55

200. Nolph KD, Lindblad AS, Noval JW, Steinberg SM: Experiences with the elderly in the national CAPD registry. Adv Perit Dial 1990;6(suppl):33–37

201. Jagose JT, Afthentopoulos IE, Shetty A, Oreopoulos DG: Successful use of CAPD in octogenarians. Adv Perit Dial 1996; 12:126–131

202. Wing AJ, Brunner FP, Brynger H: Combined report on regular dialysis and transplantation in Europe, IX 1978. Proc Eur Dial Trans Assoc 1979;13:2–52

203. Hinsdale JG, Lipcouritz GS, Hoover EL: Vascular access in the elderly: Results and perspectives in a geriatric population. Dial Trans 1985;14:560–562

204. Pourchez T, Moriniere P, St Priest A: Outcome of vascular access for haemodialysis in the elderly (<75 years). Proc Eur Dial Trans Assoc 1990;27:160

205. Palder SB, Kirkman RL, Whittemore AD, et al: Vascular access for hemodialysis: patency rates and results of revision. Ann Surg 1985;202:235–239

206. Munda R, First MR, Alexander JW et al: Polytetrafluoro-ethylene graft survival in hemodialysis. JAMA 1983;249:219–222

207. Gruppo Emodialisi e Pathologie Cardiovascolari: Multicentre cross-sectional study of ventricular arrhythmias in chronically haemodialysed patients. Lancet 1988;6:305–308

208. Marckmann P: Nutritional staus and mortality of patients on regular dialysis therapy. J Intern Med 1989;226:429–432

209. Fenton SSA, Johnston N, Delmore T et al: Nutritional assessments of CAPD patients. ASAIO Trans 1987;33:650–653

210. Young GA, Kopple JD, Lindholm B et al: Nutritional assessment of chronic ambulatory peritoneal dialysis: an international study. Am J Kidney Dis 1991;17:462–471

211. Sherman RA, Cody RP, Rogers ME, Solanchick JC: Interdialytic weight gain and nutritional parameters in chronic haemodialysis patients. Am J Kidney Dis 1995;25:579–583

212. Blake PG: Growth hormone and malnutrition in dialysis patients. Perit Dial Int 1995;15:210–216

213. Jones MR, Martis L, Algrim CE et al: Amino acid solutions for CAPD: rationale and clinical experience. Min Electrolyte Metab 1992;18:309–315

214. Kopple JD, Bernard D, Messana J et al: Amino acid solutions for CAPD patients with an amino acid based dialysate. Kidney Int 1995;47:1148–1157

215. Chertow GM, Ling J, Lew NL et al: The association of intradialytic parenteral nutrition administration with survival in haemodialysis patients. Am J Kidney Dis 1994;24:912–920

216. Dombros NV, digenis GE, Soliman G, Oreopoulos DG: Anabolic steroids in the treatment of malnourished patients: a retrospective study. Perit Dial Int 1994;14:344–347

217. Bucala R, Vlassara H: Advanced glycosylation end products in diabetic renal and vascular disease. Am J Kidney Dis 1995; 26:875–888

218. Schnider SI, Kohn RR, Cerami A: Effects of age and diabetes mellitus on the solubility of collagen from human skin, tracheal cartilage and dura mater. Exp Gerontol 1982;17:185–194

219. Monnier VM, Vishwantath V, Frank KE et al: Relation between complications of type I diabetes mellitus and collagen-linked fluorescence. N Eng J Med 1986;314:403–408

220. Skolnik EY, Yang Z, Makita Z et al: Human and rat mesangial cell receptors for glucose-modified proteins: potential role in kidney tissue remodelling and diabetic nephropathy. J Exp Med 1991;174:931–938

221. Doi T, Vlassara H, Kirstein M et al: Receptor-specific increase in extracellular matrix production in mouse mesangial cells by advanced glycosylation end products is mediated via platelet-derived growth factor. Proc Natl Acad Sci USA 1992;89: 2873–2877

222. Sell DR, Monnier VM: End stage renal disease and diabetes catalyse the formation of a pentose-derived crosslink from aging human collagen. J Clin Invest 1990;685:380–384

223. Makita Z, Radoff S, Rafield EJ et al: Advanced glycosylation endproducts in patients with diabetic nephropathy. N Eng J Med 1991;325:836–842

224. Vlassara H, Fuh H, Makita Z et al: Endogenous advanced glycosylation end products induce complex vascular dysfunction in normal animals; a model for diabetic and aging complications. Proc Natl Acad Sci USA 1992;89:12043–12047

225. Fuh H, Yang D, Striker G, Vlassara H: In vivo AGE-peptide injection induces kidney enlargement and glomerular hypertrophy in rabbits; prevention by aminoguanidine. Diabetes 1992;41(abstract):9A

226. Ifudu O, Paul H, Mayers JD, et al: Pervasive failed rehabilitation in center-based maintenance haemodialysis patients. Am J Kidney Dis 1994;23:394–400

227. Ifudu O, Mayers J, Matthew J et al: Dismal rehabilitation in geriatric inner-city haemodialysis patients. JAMA 1994;271: 29–33

228. Jassal SV, Douglas JF, Stout RW: Increasing dependency on dialysis: an age old problem. Fourth International Conference in Geriatric Nephrology and Urology, Abstract 7, 1996

229. Anderson JE, Kraus J, Sturgeon D: Incidence, prevalence and outcomes of end stage renal disease patients placed in nursing homes. Am J Kid Dis 1993;6:619–627

230. Roscoe JM: Haemodialysis in the nursing home. Presented at the 4th International Conference on Geriatric Nephrology, Toronto, April 19–2 1996

231. Evans RW, Manninen DL, Garrison LP et al: The quality of life of patients with end stage renal disease. N Eng J Med 1985;312:553–559

232. United States Congress Office of Technology Assessment: Life sustaining technologies and the elderly: Excerpts of Congressional OTA study. Nephrol News Issues 1989;35:31–34

233. Stout JP, Gokal R, Hillier VF et al: Quality of life of high risk and elderly dialysis patients in the UK. Dial Trans 1987;16: 674–677

234. Moody H, Moody C, Szabo E et al: Are old dialysis patients happy and can they fend for themselves or not? XII Int Congr Nephrol (abs) Jerusalem 1993

235. Horina JH, Holzer H, Reisinger EC et al: Elderly patients and chronic haemodialysis. Lancet 1992;339:183

236. Kutner NG, Brogan DJ: Assisted survival, aging and rehabilitation needs: comparison of older dialysis patients and age-matched peers. Arch Phys Med Rehab 1992;73:309–315

237. Neves PL: Chronic haemodialysis in elderly patients. Nephrol Dial Trans 1995;10(suppl):69–71

238. Wyner LM, McElroy JB, Hodge EE et al: Use of kidneys from older cadaver donors for renal transplantation. Urology 1993; 41:107–110

239. Kumar MS, Stephan R, Chui J et al: Donor age and graft outcome in cadaver renal transplantation. Trans Proc 1993; 25:3097–3098
240. Cacciarelli TV, Sumrani N, Scriven R et al: Influence of donor and recipient age on renal allograft survival time. Trans Proc 1993;25:3140–3142
241. Lloveras J, Arais M, Puig JM et al: Long-term follow-up of recipients of cadaver kidney allografts from elderly donors. Transp Proc 1993;25:3175–3176
242. Phillips AO, Bewick M, Snowdon SA et al: The influence of recipient and donor age on the outcome of renal transplantation. Clin Nephrol 1993;40:352–354
243. Shmueli D, Nakache R, Lustig S et al: Renal transplant from live donors over 65 years old. Trans Proc 1994;26:2139–2140
244. Alexander JW, Bennett LE, Breen TJ: Effect of donor age on outcome of kidney transplantation. A two-year analysis of transplants reported to the United Network for Organ Sharing Registry. Transplantation 1994;57:871–876
245. Hayashi T, Koga S, Higashi Y, et al: Living related renal transplantation from elderly donors (older than 66 years of age). Trans Proc 1995;27:984–985
246. Cecka JM, Terasaki PI: Optimal use for older donor kidneys: older recipients. Trans Proc 1995;27:801–802
247. Gaber LW, Moore LW, Alloway RR et al: Glomerulosclerosis as a determinant of posttransplant function of older donor renal allografts. Transplantation 1995;60:334–339
248. Albrechtsen D, Leivestad T, Sodal G et al: Kidney transplantation in patients older than 70 years of age. Trans Proc 1995; 27:986–988
249. Cofan F, Oppenheimer F, Campistol JM et al: Advanced age donors in the evolution of renal transplantation. Trans Proc 1995;27:2248–2249
250. Andreu J, de laTorre M, Oppenheimer F et al: Renal transplantation in elderly recipients. Trans Proc 1992;24:120–121
251. Ismail N, Hakim RM, Helderman JH: Renal replacement therapies in the elderly. Part II. Renal transplantation. Am J Kidney Dis 1994;23:1–5
252. Cardella CJ, Harding ME, de Veber GA: A controlled trial comparing sequential anti-lymphocyte serum and cyclosporine therapy in renal transplant patients. Trans Proc 1987;19: 1996–1998
253. Newstead CG, Dyer PA: The influence of increased age and age matching on graft survival after first cadaveric renal transplantation. Transplantation 1992;54:441–443
254. Cardella CJ, Oreopoulos DG, Uldall R et al: Renal transplantation in patients 60 years of age or older. Trans Proc 1986;18: 151–152
255. Schaubel D, Desmeules M, Mao Y et al: Survival experience among elderly end stage renal disease patients. Transplantation 1995;60:1389–1394
256. Cole EH, Farewell VT, Aprile M et al: Renal transplantation in older patients: the University of Toronto experience. Geriatr Nephrol Urol 1995;5:85–92
257. Evans DB: Renal transplantation in patients over the age of 55 years. pp. 295–300. In Touraine JL, Traeger J, Betuel H et al. (eds): Transplantation and Clinical Immunology XVIII. Risk factors in Organ Transplantation. Excerpta Medica, Amsterdam, 1986
258. Jordan ML, Novick AC, Steinmuller D et al: Renal transplantation in the older recipient. J Urol 1985;134:243–246
259. Ost L, Groth CG, Lindholm B et al: Cadaveric renal transplantation in patients of 60 years and above. Transplantation 1980; 30:339–340
260. Pirsch JD, Stratto RJ, Armburst MJ et al: Cadaveric renal transplantation with cyclosporin in patients more than 60 years of age. Transplantation 1989;47:259–261
261. Schulak JA, Mayes JT, Johnson KH, Hrieik DE: Kidney transplantation in patients aged sixty years and older. Surgery 1990; 108:726–733
262. Tesi RJ, Elkhammas EA, Davies EA et al: Renal transplantation in older people. Lancet 1994;343:461–464
263. Benedetti E, Matas AJ, Hakim N et al: Renal transplantation for patients 60 years or older. A single-institution experience. Ann Surg 1994;220:445–460
264. Hestin D, Frimat L, Hubert J et al: Renal transplantation in patients over sixty years of age. Clin Nephrol 1994;42: 232–236
265. Vivas CA, Hickey DP, Jordan ML et al: Renal transplantation in patients 65 years old or older. J Urol 1992;147:990–993
266. Briggs JD. Should older patients receive renal transplants? Nephrol Dial Trans 1995;10:18–20
267. Gaylin DS, Held PJ, Port FK et al: The impact of comorbid and sociodemographic factors on access to renal transplantation. JAMA 1993;269:603–608
268. McMillan MA, Briggs JD: Survey of patient selection for cadaveric renal transplantation in the United Kingdom. Nephrol Dial Trans 1995;10:855–858
269. Nyberg G, Hallste G, Norden G et al: Physical performance does not improve in elderly patients following successful kidney transplantation. Nephrol Dial Trans 1995;10:18–20
270. McKenzie JM: Decisions for dialysis: survey of Canadian directors. Canadian Society of Nephrology, Vancouver, September 1–12, 1993
271. Kilner JF: Selecting patients when resources are limited: a study of US medical directors of kidney dialysis and transplantation facilities. Am J Pub Health 1988;78:144–147
272. Callaghan D: Setting Limits: Medical Goals in an Aging Society. Simon and Schuster, New York, 1987
273. Oreopoulos DG: Should the elderly be denied dialysis? Ger Nephrol Urol 1994;4:67–70
274. Churchill DN, Taylor DW, Cook RJ et al: Canadian haemodialysis morbidity study. Am J Kidney Dis 1992;19:214–234

C H A P T E R 6 8

The Prostate

N. J. R. GEORGE

The prostate gland lies between the bladder base and pelvic floor and is intimately associated with each structure. Secretions of the seminal vesicle and vas deferens are conducted through its substance to the ejaculatory duct, which terminates in the urethra at the verumontanum. Exocrine secretion products, largely under androgenic control, are discharged into prostatic acini and include zinc, citric acid, and numerous enzymes—acid phosphatase, coagulases, fibrinolysins, and proteolytic enzymes—that form a significant part of the seminal plasma acting to support the physiologic changes required for transport of spermatozoa.

Development

The embryonic prostate differentiates in response to androgen secretion by the fetal testis commencing about the eighth week of intrauterine life.[1] Adrogenic activity at the time of puberty results in rapid growth to a weight of approximately 20 g by the age of 20 years. Thereafter, weight remains reasonably constant until 40 to 50 years of age when growth of benign adenomatus (prostatic) hyperplasia (BPH) becomes increasingly common with advancing years. Autopsy studies reveal BPH in more than 40 percent of men in their 50s and almost 90 percent of men in their 80s;[2] figures are confirmed by community-based studies involving transrectal ultrasound estimation of prostatic volume.[3]

Castration prior to puberty prevents prostatic development as well as the later emergence of both BPH and prostate cancer. Removal of testes in the adult leads to involution of the gland,[4] but replacement reactivates growth though only to and not beyond the normal adult size.

The action of androgen on the prostate cell is highly complex and only partially understood. Within the prostate testosterone is converted to its active metabolite, 5α-dihydrotestosterone (DHT) by the 5α-reductase enzyme located on the nuclear membrane. Most evidence suggests that prostatic epithelial cells per se are unresponsive to DHT, which acts via signaling between stromal and epithelial components of the tissue; epidermal growth factor (Fig. 68-1) and transforming growth factor-α (TGFα) providing the most potent mitogenic stimulus.[5] The importance of DHT to prostatic growth has been illustrated by the studies of Imperato-McGinley and colleagues[6] into males from the Dominican Republic with an autosomal recessive form of male pseudohermaphroditism caused by deficiency of the 5α-reductase enzyme. These children develop phenotypically into men at puberty with normal serum testosterone, but with prostates that remain impalpable.[6] These observations form the basis of the development of the 5α-reductase inhibitors presently widely prescribed for men with early symptomatic BPH.

Morphology

Early work by Lowsley[7] concerning the anatomy of the prostate has been superseded in recent years by the extensive studies of McNeal and associates.[8] They described peripheral and central zones of the gland (Fig. 68-2) as distinct from earlier lobe terminology; the central zone, approximately one-third of the gland mass, completely surrounds the ejaculatory ducts while the peripheral zone extends to the apex and wraps around the central zone like an egg cup. The benign prostatic hypertrophy mass arises from the periurethral zone (within the transitional zone) and this extends from the bladder neck to the region of the veromontanum, but never caudal to that structure. By contrast, prostate cancer usually arises from the peripheral zone, explaining the difficulties in identifying early disease endoscopically via the urethra (see below).

Much confusion has been created by this conflicting prostatic terminology over the years. Surgeons refer to "lateral" and "middle" lobes at operation, but clearly these are all contained within the periuretheral transitional zones. The true exocrine prostate is not removed in operations for BPH, although patients frequently assume—not unnaturally—that "prostatectomy" means removal of the entire gland. The operation of radical prostatectomy for cancer does, however, involve extirpation of all prostatic tissue—each zone and contained BPH tissue en bloc.

The substance of the prostate consists of glandular tissue, stroma, and smooth muscle. The preprostatic sphincter lies at the bladder neck (Fig. 68-2) and is responsible for preventing retrograde ejaculation during intercourse. This α-adrenergic muscle is inevitably damaged during the operation of transurethral resection (TUR) for BPH, but lack of leakage following the procedure shows, however, that this sphincter is not normally responsible for urinary continence. α-Adrenergic fibers are present throughout the gland and may be implicated in the etiology of chronic inflammatory conditions of the gland (see below); pharmacologic manipulation by α-adrenergic blocking agents provides a useful therapeutic approach to patients with mild prostatic obstruction.

The continence mechanism lies intimately related to the

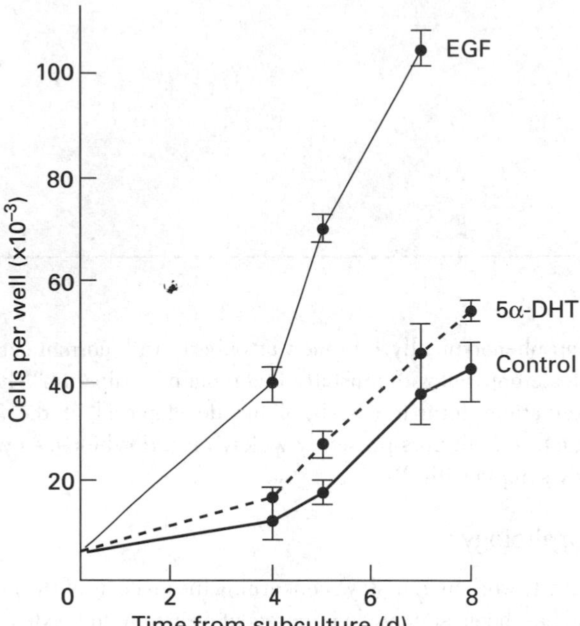

Figure 68-1 Prostate epithelial cells (CAPE-1) in culture. 5-α-DHT stimulation is no greater than control while EGF stimulation leads to significantly enhanced stimulation.

apex of the prostate at the level of the pelvic floor. Studies by Gosling[10] and coworkers clearly show that the true external urethral sphincter lies within a sleeve of connective tissue, which separates it from the periurethral striated (levator ani) pelvic floor muscle. This latter muscle is innervated via the pudendal nerve and is responsible for emergency continence requiring extra voluntary effort such as occurs during laughing, coughing, or sneezing. The nerve supply to the (slow twitch) specialized external urethral sphincter remains debatable; horseradish peroxidase techniques have suggested it travels via the pelvic nerve to terminate in the ventral horn of S2-S3 on Onuf's Nucleus X.[11] Damage to this sphincter, which by anatomical definition must be distal the veromontanum, during TUR by inexperienced surgeons will inevitably lead to postoperative genuine stress incontinence.

Assessment of the Prostate

The prostate is relatively accessible to a number of techniques that may confirm normal or abnormal morphologic features. In a broader sense, prostatic investigations may also encompass assessment of vesicourethral dysfunction, the gland being intimately involved in the storage and voiding disorders of the lower urinary tract.

Rectal Examination

Digital rectal examination can by definition only assess the posterior aspect of the peripheral zone of the prostate. The periphery of the gland and the midline sulcus, as well as the texture of the gland may be recorded, but inevitably the experience of the examiner is crucial for accuracy of diagnosis. Rectal examination gives a poor indication of prostatic size; glands may protrude variably into the rectal lumen and other factors, such as a full bladder in acute or chronic retention of urine, may displace the bladder base and prostate downward leading to an erroneous assessment of volume. Additionally, prostatic

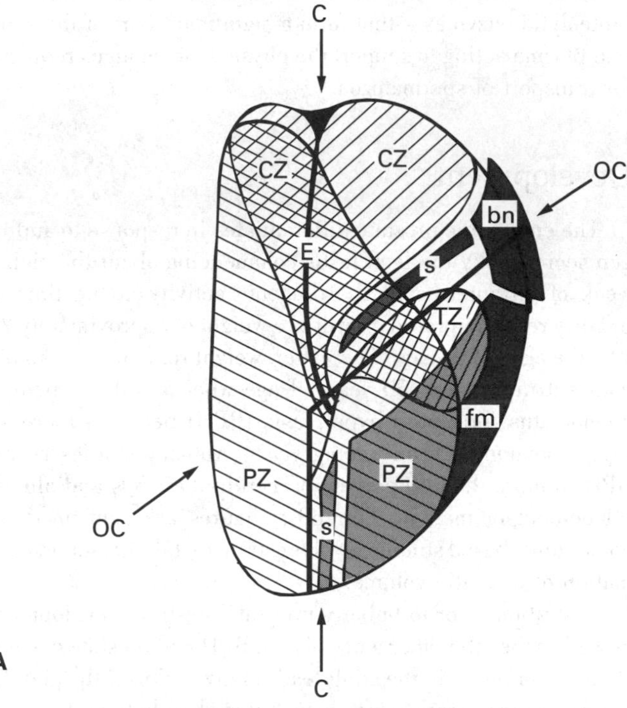

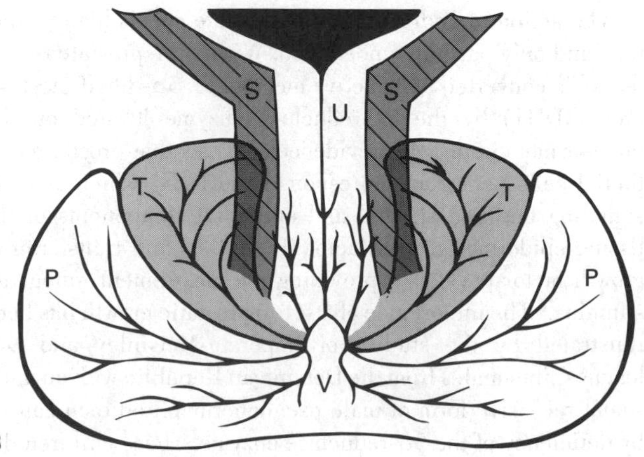

Figure 68-2 (**A**) Sagittal section through prostate showing zonal architecture relative to urethra. PZ, peripheral zone; CZ, central zone; TZ, transitional zone; bn, bladder neck; fm, fibromuscular stroma; s, pre-prostatic, and distal striated sphincter; E, ejaculatory ducts; C, true coronal plane; OC, oblique coronal plane (**B**) Section through oblique coronal plane as shown in Fig. A showing site of origin of BPH tissue surrounding proximal urethra—the periuretheral zone. U, urethra; S, preprostatic sphincter; T, transitional zone; P, peripheral zone; V, verimontanum; (Data from McNeal.[9])

size is not related to the presence or absence of outflow tract obstruction,[12] but nevertheless the examination remains an essential technique of assessment, particularly with regard to the detection of neoplastic change.

Plain X-Ray of Abdomen

A single film showing kidneys, ureter, and bladder (KUB) may frequently be performed prior to prostatic surgery, chiefly to exclude bladder stone. Although the size of the gland cannot be assessed on these films, abnormalities such as calcification may be seen within the gland substance, perhaps indicating past inflammatory disease within the prostatic ducts.

Intravenous Urogram

For many years urography was routinely performed prior to prostatectomy,[13] and although it is now accepted that this is unnecessary in the majority of cases,[14] radiologists continue to report on the size of the prostate as judged by shadows on bladder films (Fig. 68-3). Clinical experience suggests that such assessment can be very misleading, not only because of other causes of intravesical impressions (i.e., bladder tumor), but because of technical factors such as the variable angle of incidence of the X-rays through the pelvis.

Transrectal Ultrasound

Transrectal ultrasound (TRUS) imaging of a prostate is now accepted as the principal methodology by which accurate anatomic detail of the gland may be obtained. Modern machines linked to sophisticated software packages may give high resolution in both multiple transverse and sagittal planes. Additionally, computer-assisted guided needle biopsies may retrieve tissue from exactly specified areas of the gland to distinguish between benign and malignant disease.

In practice, TRUS technology is rarely applied unless it is necessary to exclude or confirm the presence of carcinoma. Patients with straightforward symptom complexes thought on the basis of tests including prostate-specific antigen (PSA) to be due to BPH are likely to be offered therapy without the need further to image the gland and its appendices.

By contrast, TRUS is an essential preoperative investigation in patients with suspicious prostate on rectal examination and in those—often younger—patients in whom PSA tests indicate the possibility of cancer. Most cancers are seen as hypoechoic lesions although approximately one-fourth may be isoechoic. Additionally, the images may identify capsular bulge (Fig. 68-4) or extension indicating tumorous spread that will restrict treatment options.[15,16] Spread of cancer to the seminal vesicles can also be imaged with relative ease. TRUS-guided biopsies have been shown to be more accurate than digitally guided biopsies for both palpable and impalpable tumors.

Computed Tomography

Computed tomography (CT) scanning is not commonly employed in the diagnosis of prostatic disorders. Although relatively good resolution may be obtained with modern machines, the technique does not offer major advantages over other radio-

Figure 68-3 Bladder film from intravenous urogram series. Shadows at base of bladder (arrows) are a poor indicator of prostatic size and may represent bladder tumor or other intravesical pathology.

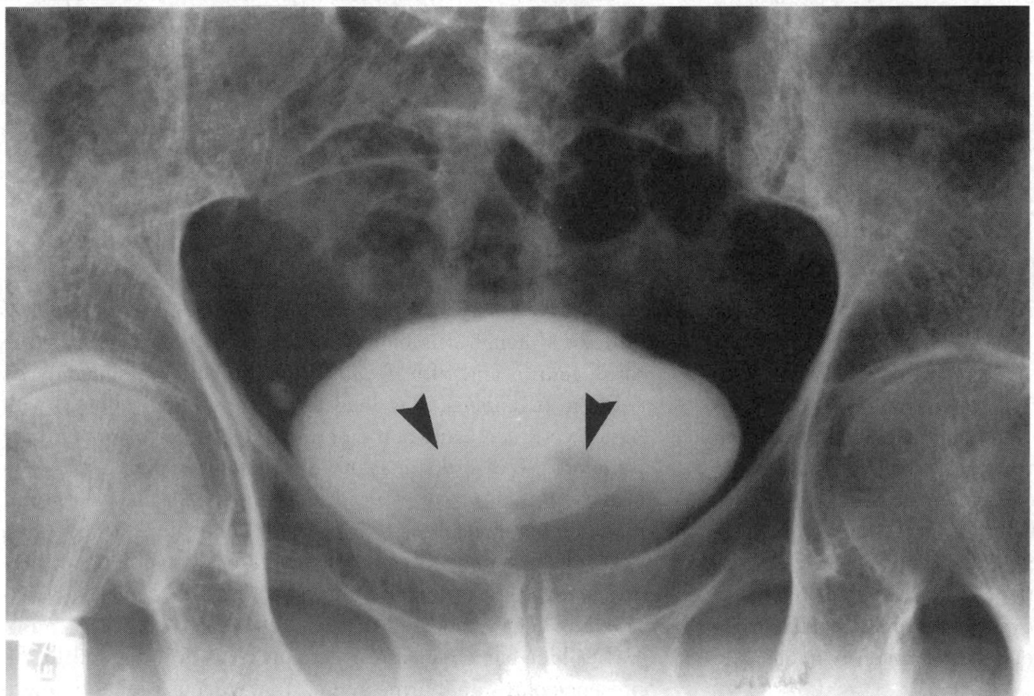

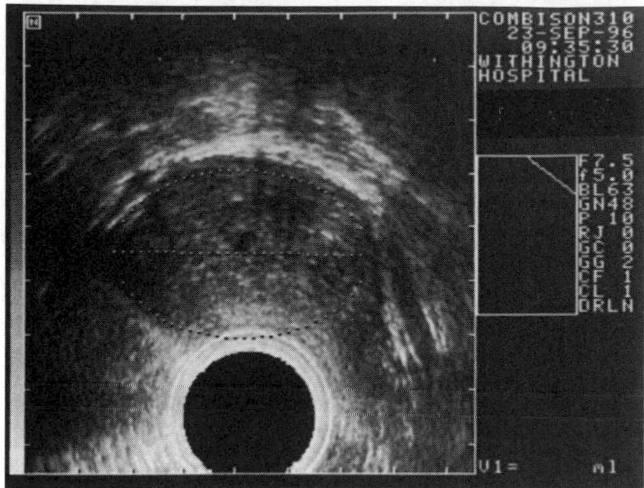

Figure 68-4 Transrectal ultrasound scan of prostate showing relatively homogeneous pattern within, but with loss of capsular definition on the left. Biopsy from this area showed well-differentiated prostatic cancer.

logical investigations and precise interpretation of capsular spread and seminal vesicle invasion has been difficult.[17]

Magnetic Resonance Imaging

In recent years developing magnetic resonance imaging (MRI) technology has been used extensively in an attempt to make an early and reliable diagnosis of prostate cancer. Magnetic resonance images give a reasonably clear capsular outline (Fig. 68-5), although the accuracy of local staging is presently no better than TRUS.[18] T2-weighted images show internal architecture of the gland, but disappointingly it has not proved possible with accuracy to distinguish carcinoma from other disorders such as inflammatory foci of prostatitis. Nevertheless, within the UK, MRI is commonly used as part of the objective database assembled for patients undergoing therapeutic trials in early prostate cancer.

Serum Markers of Prostatic Disease

Acid Phosphatase

Since the report of Gutman and Gutman[19] noting high acid phosphatase levels in men with metastatic prostate disease, acid phosphatase estimations have been widely used in the staging of prostate cancer. Unfortunately, lack of sensitivity with regard to localized disease precluded its use for cancer detection and the test has now effectively been replaced by PSA, although it is still employed by some authorities to monitor results of therapy in patients with proven bony metastatic disease.

Prostate-Specific Antigen

This serum protease was isolated from prostatic tissue in 1979 by Wang and associates[20] and has rapidly emerged as the most important marker of prostatic epithelial activity. Contrary to widespread public opinion, this marker is not cancer-specific (Fig. 68-6), but may be elevated in other pathologies such as inflammation or benign hyperplasia. Prostate-specific antigen varies with the proportion of ductal epithelial cells, so it is not surprising that higher values are found in patients with larger glands and that age-adjusted ranges have been proposed.[21] Damage to epithelial cells either by inflammation or other means such as elective prostate biopsy may elevate levels markedly, often for some weeks, making interpretation difficult in an already cancer-anxious patient.

Other problems surround the rapidly expanding PSA biotechnology industry. In 1996 in Europe alone there were more than 40 firms manufacturing PSA assay kits, each with different standards and reference ranges. Although attempts are being made to establish quality control systems, it is incumbent upon each physician to establish the normal values and ranges of the PSA kit being used in the local laboratory.

Free and bound prostate-specific antigen

Recent studies have extended the utility of PSA by showing that it may exist in the serum in two modes—free and bound or complexed forms.[22] Determination of these fractions has added new impetus to the search for a test that can distinguish between BPH and cancer; tumor cells may stimulate production of α-chymotrypsin (ACT) with which binding may occur, leading to higher levels of complexed PSA-ACT than is detected in patients with simple BPH.[23] Once again, however, the new assays may need to be interpreted with caution due to different sensitivities relating to the free and complexed forms and further work is required to clarify the clinical relevance of these important observations.

Clinical Aspects of Prostatic Disease

Prostatitis

Inflammation of the prostatic ducts and acini may occur at any age although it is more common in its typical form in the third, fourth, and fifth decades. The infection, commonly by coliform organisms, may lead to severe systemic illness with high fever, rigors, and acute perineal discomfort. More chronic forms of the disorder may be difficult to eradicate and it is suggested that spasm of α-adrenergic smooth muscle as well as general pelvic floor tension may contribute to poor duct drainage, and hence, persisting symptoms. Combination therapy using both antibiotics and smooth/striated muscle relaxants has been advocated in such cases.[24]

In older men, prostatic infection is usually related to the presence of residual urine and outflow tract obstruction. Infec-

A

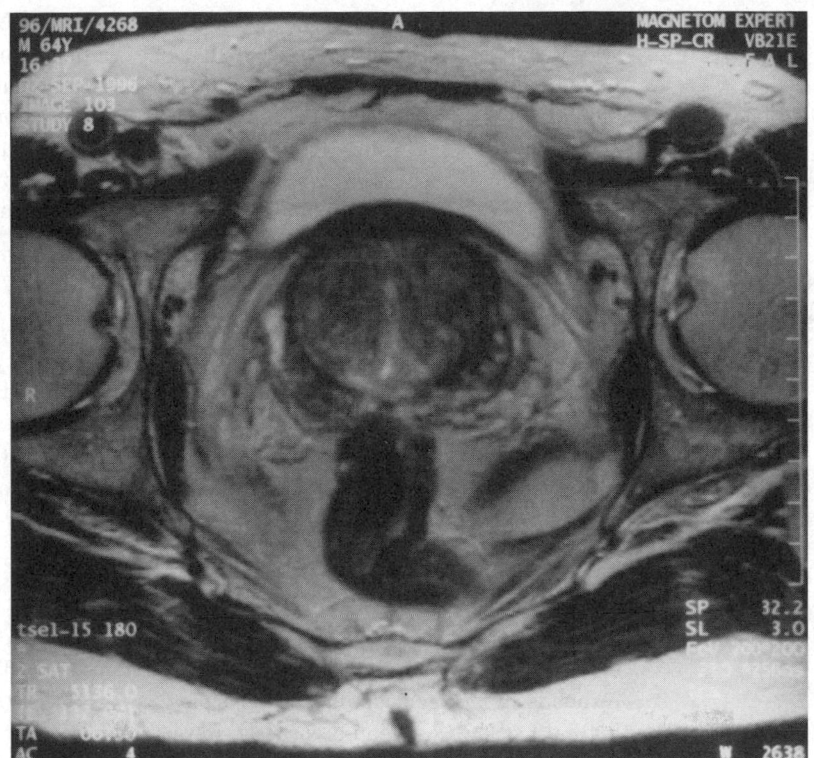

B

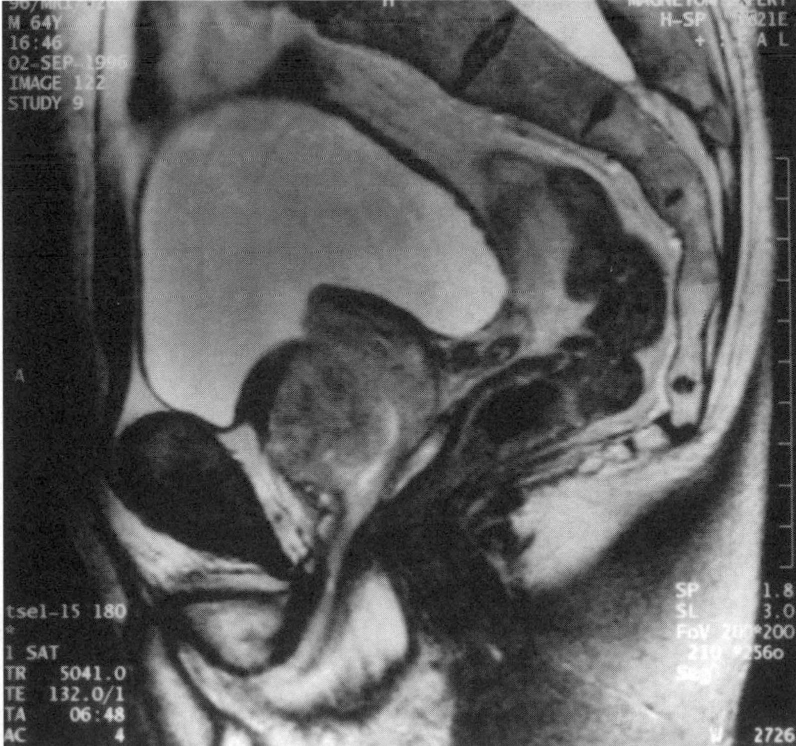

Figure 68-5 MRI scans. (**A**) Transverse (axial) section through prostate. In the peripheral zone on the left a 1.5-cm lesion is identified adjacent to, but probably not penetrating, the capsule. (**B**) Sagittal section through same case as in Fig. A. The architecture and relations of bladder, prostate, and urethra are clearly shown.

tion commonly spreads distally down the vas deferens leading to epididymo-orchitis; in earlier times bilateral vasectomy was commonly performed at the time of (open) prostatic surgery to prevent this almost inevitable consequence of the infected residual. In general, the presence of lower urinary tract infection associated with poor bladder emptying will demand surgical intervention after a period of suitable antibiotic treatment so as to reduce the residual volume. In some cases in whom surgery is inappropriate or contraindicated, direct instalation of antibiotics into the bladder by a self-catheterization has been described[25] and tried in the elderly with some success.

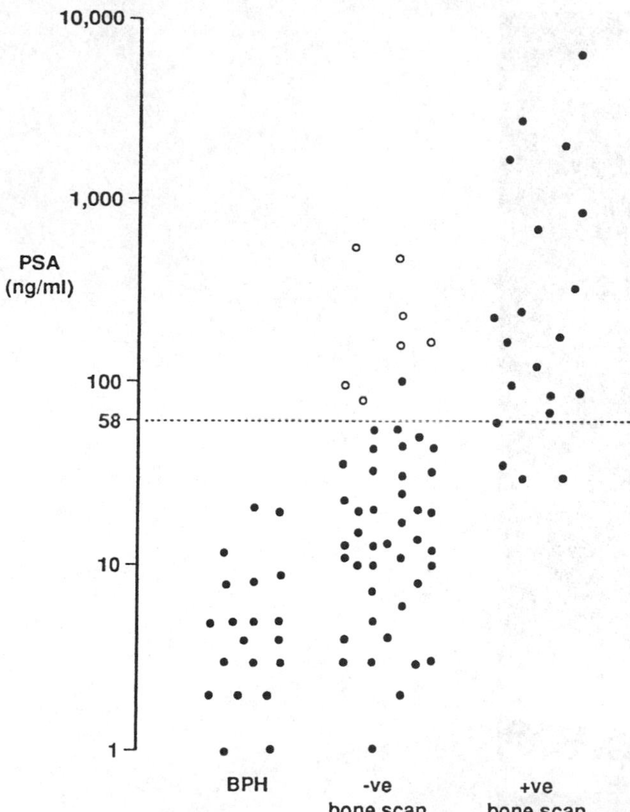

Figure 68-6 Prostate-specific antigen levels in patients with benign prostatic hyperplasia, localized prostate cancer (bone scan negative), and metastatic prostate cancer. Open circles: seven patients with raised acid phosphatase suggesting metastatic disease despite apparently negative scans. The degree of overlap between the values can be clearly seen, illustrating that PSA is a marker of prostate epithelium and not a specific indicator of prostate cancer. Dotted line: discriminant analysis identifies 58 ng/ml as optimum cut off distinguishing between skeletal and nonskeletal disease. See text for details. (Data from Pantilides et al.[54])

Benign Prostatic Hyperplasia

Symptom complexes and terminology

It has already been noted that BPH arises chiefly in the periurethral zone and affects a high proportion of men as part of the aging process. It is essential to appreciate, however, that the presence of hyperplasia per se does not imply either significant obstruction to the lower urinary tract or association with particular clinical symptom complexes that may be related to vesicourethral dysfunction rather than the enlarged prostate gland.

These three components—hyperplasia, symptoms, and obstruction—have been brought together in a classic diagram by Hald[26] (Fig. 68-7) demonstrating that while all three may be found in a minority of cases, each may exist alone or with one other in a random association.

Urologists have argued for many years against the usage of the common phrase "prostatism" employed to describe a wide range of symptoms relating to the male lower urinary tract. Not only does this imply, often wrongly, that the symptoms may be due to the hyperplasia, but it also suggests that therapeutic attention to the gland will cure the patient. "Obstruction" should be reserved for those patients proven to be obstructed by urodynamic tests—lower urinary tract symptoms (LUTS) more exactly describe the symptom complex that may or may not be associated with the gland.[27]

Detrusor Dysfunction Associated with Benign Prostatic Hyperplasia

The reaction of the bladder to the presence of emergent BPH is responsible for the symptom complexes which are associated with the condition. These changes are best understood if the filling and voiding segments of the micturition cycle are considered independently.

Filling phase

The bladder, receiving urine at 1 mL/min from the kidneys under normal circumstances in temperate climates, normally responds by accommodating the physiological volume (400/500 mL) at low (less than 5 cm H_2O) intrinsic detrusor pressure. This normal reaction to filling may be observed even in the presence of significant outflow obstruction.

More commonly, however, the growth of the emerging gland may give rise to *bladder instability*—abnormal intrinsic detrusor pressure waves during filling that lead the patient to experience frequency, nocturia, urgency, and possibly urge incontinence. Unfortunately, not all bladder instability is related to prostatic obstruction, there being a significant association with old age and neurologic disorder (when instability is correctly called detrusor hyper-reflexia). Careful studies have shown that approximately two-thirds of older men being investigated for "prostatic" symptoms have bladder instability and of these only two-thirds will lose their instability following prostatectomy.[28] Unfortunately, there is no test at present that can detect preoperatively which patients will not lose their bladder instability postoperatively. Persistence of the disorder following surgery leaves a very unhappy patient with significantly worse urge symptoms that may take many months to settle.

Voiding phase

As with the filling phase, significant prostatic hyperplasia may not necessarily affect vesicourethral function. This observation presumably explains in part the large number of elderly men who have apparently enlarged glands on rectal examination, but who deny any impairment to micturition performance. More typically, however, two types of bladder dysfunction are found in association with BPH—typical *high pressure* obstructed voiding or relatively *low pressure* underactive detrusor function.

High pressure/low flow voiding is the classic reaction to mechanical blockage of the urethra by BPH leading to typical symptoms of hesitancy, poor stream, and gradually increasing

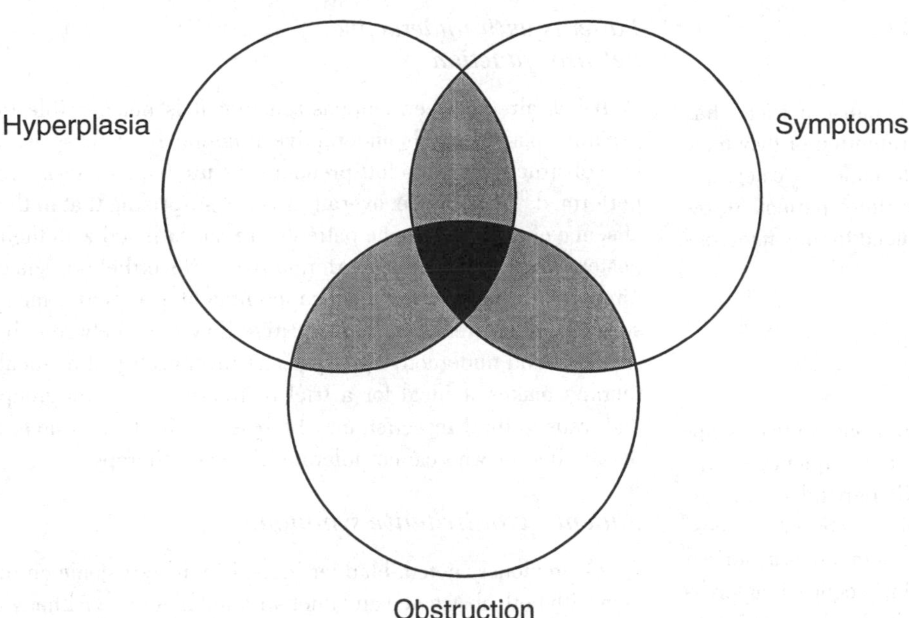

Figure 68-7 Interlocking diagram demonstrating the interdependence of lower urinary tract symptoms, outflow tract obstruction, and hyperplastic tissue when considering symptoms of patients with "prostatism." Significant volumes of hyperplasia may not necessarily be associated either with obstruction or symptoms, while all three may be present in some cases. (Adapted from Hald,[26] with permission.)

frequency by day and night. Additionally (see above) symptoms of bladder instability may superimpose problems related to urgency and urge incontinence.

Low pressure/low flow underactive bladders have been recognized only relatively recently, but may account for 20 to 25 percent of patients with outflow tract symptomatology. The reason for the abnormal detrusor function remains unknown, although the condition has been likened to a nonobstructive myopathy.[29] Men with low flow voiding also complain of frequency and poor stream (often prolonged and interrupted), which is impossible to separate from high pressure/low flow voiding except by invasive urodynamic tests. It has been recognized increasingly that inclusion of such low pressure/low flow patients in prostatectomy series leads to poor outcomes from the procedure.[30,31]

Retention and Bladder Dysfunction

Sudden increase in prostate size, such as may occur during hemorrhage or infarction, may cause acute (painful) retention of urine, but these conditions are unusual. It is a common observation that patients on urological waiting lists for outflow tract obstruction rarely present in acute retention; by contrast men admitted with this condition have usually not seen their general practitioner previously and the precipitating factor seems often to relate to acute fluid loading and subsequent overstretching of the unrelieved bladder—as happens for example during a long coach trip.

Chronic (painless) retention of urine is broadly divided into two forms: the low pressure "floppy" bladder, which may become complicated by infection, but which has normal upper tracts; and the high-pressure "tense" bladder, which frequently is seen in patients with few if any lower tract symptoms, but which usually is associated with bilateral upper tract dilatation and obstructive uropathy.[32]

Investigation of the Patient with Benign Prostatic Hyperplasia

In recent years, audit studies have lead to rationalization of investigations required to assess the patient with BPH. Frequency/volume charts filled in by the patient at home are helpful in revealing nonprostatic causes of urinary tract disorders such as fluid excretion patterns related to cardiovascular disease or excessive tea drinking. Following urine microscopy and culture, rectal examination, and palpation of the abdomen for chronic retention of urine, plain X-ray of the abdomen (KUB) will detect potential operative problems such as bladder calculus. An independent flow rate test, correctly performed (greater than 150 mL voided, no valsalva pushes permitted) is mandatory. Intravenous urography is no longer advised unless the patient complains of, or is found on urine testing to suffer from, significant hematuria. Five percent of patients with high-pressure obstruction develop upper tract dilatation and may be uremic[32,33]; for this reason if a residual urine of greater than 300 mL is detected abdominally, upper tract ultrasound is advised to assess renal anatomy. In summary, audit studies suggest that patients without blood in their urine or significant residual urine do not require any form of upper tract studies prior to consideration for surgery.

Management of Patients with Benign Prostatic Hyperplasia

Many patients come to their doctor because a friend has recently been admitted in acute painful retention or they have seen a television program about prostate cancer. A negative workup followed by reassurance permits these patients to return to their normal lifestyle without the need for any intervention.

Patients with high pressure/low flow voiding

Advice for patients with uncomplicated obstructive symptoms—hesitancy, poor stream, and moderate frequency/nocturia (no urge or urge incontinence)—will depend to a large extent on the patient's own circumstances and preferences. Frequency may not trouble a retired man as much as a clerical officer at his desk. Reassurance, particularly concerning prostate cancer, may be all that is required and it is tempting to propose that the reduction in α-adrenegic periprostatic tone might be responsible for the noted improvement.

More usually, however, active intervention will be required, and typically the choice will be between medical therapy and operation-transurethral resection of the prostate. Two forms of medical therapy are presently in common use, but both suffer from a relatively slow onset of action with resultant modest increment in urine flow rate. Nevertheless, for patients with smaller prostates who have equivocal symptoms or for those who wish to avoid the risks of operation, these drugs can be effective. A number of α-blockers are available with varying degrees (see list below) of uroselectivity.[34] Most of the α-blockers exert their full effect within 1 month whereas the α-reductase inhibitors[35] may take up to 3 months for clinical effect to be noticeable. Recently, a controversial report has considered α-blockade to be significantly superior to α-reductase inhibition, which was equal in efficacy only to placebo.[36]

For patients with severe "simple" obstruction, TUR offers the unquestioned "gold standard" in terms of measured outcomes. Despite the significant comorbidity of the elderly treatment population, a rapid resolution of symptoms ensures that the great majority are delighted with the results of treatment.

- Non-selective α-blockers
  - Phenoxybenzamine
- Selective α-blockers
  - Prazosin
  - Alfusozin
  - Indoramin
- Selective long-acting α-blockers
  - Terazosin
  - Doxazosin
  - Tamsulosin

Patients with underactive detrusor function

It has already been emphasized that it is not possible to separate patients with underactive function from those with true obstruction unless full preoperative urodynamic tests are performed,[30] and hence, overall, it is not surprising that in the absence of such tests some patients are not satisfied with their postoperative micturition performance.[31] Nevertheless, some improvement is seen and the disappointment is a relative measure of the difference in postoperative flow rates between obstructive and underactive groups. The reversibility of medical therapy makes it ideal for a trial of treatment in this group and transurethral resection may be reserved for those who are dissatisfied or who cannot tolerate blockade therapy.

Patients with irritative symptoms

As previously noted, bladder instability is very common in men with both obstructed and unobstructed bladders. Although a complete diagnostic picture may be obtained by urodynamic tests on each patient, few units can afford the academic luxury of this purist approach and hence, trials of therapy are commonly practiced in elderly patients with the frequency urge syndrome.

Physiologic bladder contraction is mediated by stimulation of postganglionic parasympathetic cholinergic receptors on detrusor smooth muscle. Hence, atropine and atropine-like agents will induce a lessening of the contraction wave with corresponding decrease in detected urgency by the patient. Trials of such agents[37] or musculotropic relaxation agents such as oxybutynin chloride[38] show reasonable efficacy, although many will be familiar with the statement about any treatment for instability: "one is always surprised when it works."

New Modalities for Treatment of Benign Prostatic Hyperplasia

While it is accepted that transurethral resection remains the gold standard for treatment of patients with obstructive BPH,[39] a number of new modalities have been introduced, including prostate incision, laser therapy, stent therapy, and varieties of thermotherapy. All these techniques have their vociferous supporters, but all agree that for the patient with a significant volume of hyperplastic tissue obstructing the bladder outlet, endoscopic transurethral resection remains the treatment of choice. The need for critical evaluation of the new technology in terms of outcome measures continues to be debated in urologic circles.

Prostatic Surgery in the Elderly

Recent advances in anesthetic techniques have allowed a complete reappraisal of treatment options in the elderly and it is now rare for a patient to be refused prostatectomy on anesthetic grounds alone. While many patients over a 100 years of age have been treated satisfactorily—an unnecessary urethral catheter is undesirable at any age—the chief contraindication to operation is presently the inability of the patient mentally to appreciate what is being offered to alleviate his symptoms. Hence, apart from a very few seriously compromised patients, modern anesthesia permits straightforward decisions to be made about the elderly patient and "lesser" operative techniques such as urethral stent insertion[40] hold little advantage over simple transurethral resection.

Incontinence

Stress incontinence is very rare in neurologically normal males and when observed is usually the result of prostatic surgery where the sphincter mechanism has been damaged during the procedure. By contrast, urge incontinence is common, particularly in the older age group and is chiefly related, in the presence of sterile urine, to bladder instability. The therapeutic approach to instability has been mentioned above and is discussed more fully in Chapter 94.

Prostate Cancer

Introduction

In recent years, prostate cancer has developed into a significant and increasing health problem.[41,42] Presently second only to lung cancer as a cause of cancer mortality, greater public awareness and the development of cancer detection programs utilizing PSA have ensured that the problem will not diminish in the foreseeable future.

However, the increasing age of the population and the very slow growth of some tumors means that, unlike many other neoplasms, not every cancer is a life-threatening event for the patient. Many older men die *with* rather than *of* their prostate cancer, but the prediction as to whether the disease as identified in any one individual patient carries a good prognosis remains extremely difficult. This problem is not helped by the very wide difference between the *incidence* and *mortality* of the disease in many western countries. In the US in 1995 the incidence/mortality ratio was 1:7.8, and in Holland, 1:2.1 (Holtgrewe, Schröder, personal communication, 1996), demonstrating that the diagnostic tests were detecting many more cancers than were later dying of the disease. The essential question relates to whether or not all detected cancers are capable of progressing and leading eventually to the death of the patient.

Site of disease

Anatomically, most cancers (70 to 75 percent) are found in the peripheral zone of the gland (Fig. 68-2). Approximately 20 percent of lesions are thought to originate in the transitional zone while the remainder are located in the central zone. As such, most nodules or palpable lesions should be detected by the educated finger on rectal examination, while in a minority the transurethral resection of the transitional zone (i.e., for an obstructive lesion thought to be "BPH") may occasionally eradicate unsuspected tumor in that area.

Epidemiologic studies

Prostatic disease is rare in the Far East, Japan, and China. Migratory studies have clearly shown, however, that the incidence of the disease increases as males move to a more western lifestyle. Significant racial differences also exist; within the San Francisco Bay area Japanese Americans are eight times less likely to suffer from the disease than African Americans.[43]

Prostate cancer and the elderly

It has already been mentioned that the disease is presently being diagnosed at an earlier stage in younger men. At the present time, the question of whether to screen for prostate cancer and which treatment to offer for the cases so detected remains at the forefront of medical debate. Views are strongly expressed because a tumor discovered at age 53, however indolent its growth pattern, is likely to lead to death within the patient's natural life span. For the older person, however, the decision criteria are different and it is in this context that the following variants of disease presentation are discussed.

Localized Prostate Cancer

Localized prostate cancer may be detected incidentally or it may be discovered as part of the investigation of a man with developing lower urinary tract symptoms. Prostate-specific antigen led ultrasound biopsy may reveal carcinoma (stage T^1C, Table 68-1) in a patient who merely presented with anxiety, no symptoms, and a normal rectal examination (i.e., BPH in texture). However, in the elderly, lower urinary tract symptoms—irritation or obstruction—are more often the reason for a first visit to his primary physician. At this time, digital rectal examination may or may not reveal obvious neoplastic change and it is likely that histologic confirmation will need to await specialist referral and subsequent TRUS biopsy or transurethral resection. The absence of bony metastatic disease may be confirmed by isotope bone scan, but it has been recently suggested that PSA is a superior predictor of a negative scan if levels are less than 20 ng (Hybritech assay) and thus, the time-consuming and expensive scan may be avoided.[44]

Treatment of local disease

Three options are available for a treatment of older men with apparently localized disease—watchful waiting, radical radiotherapy, or radical prostatectomy. The therapeutic choice will depend on the histologic grade of the tumor, the PSA level at diagnosis, and the biological age of the patient.

Watchful waiting

Studies from Scandinavia[45] and England[46] have shown that long symptom-free intervals may be obtained by observation policies if histologic grade is favorable. Originally, the concept of "latent" cancer was introduced for cancers that apparently failed to progress, but the observational studies have clearly demonstrated that local advance, albeit slow, does occur in

Table 68-1 TNM Classification (1992 revision) compared to Whitmore-Jewett system

TNM 1992		Whitmore-Jewett
Incidental finding; no tumor palpable		
T1a	Tumor <5% of excised tissue	A1
T1b	Tumor >5% of excised tissue	A2
T1c	Tumor found on needle biopsy (raised PSA)	
Tx	Local tumor cannot be evaluated	
To	No local tumor detectable	
Intracapsular palpable tumor		
T2a	Tumor limited to half of one lobe or less	B1
T2b	Tumor spread to half of one lobe, but not to both	B2
T2c	Tumor spread into both lobes	B3
Extracapsular tumor		
T3a	Unilateral extracapsular spread	C1
T3b	Bilateral extracapsular spread	C2
T3c	Tumor spread to one or both seminal vesicles	
T4	Tumor is attached or has invaded adjacent structures other than the seminal vesicles	
Disseminated tumor		
N0	No lymph node involvement	
N1	Lymph nodes <2 cm in diameter	
N2	One node only >2 cm or <5 cm; multiple <5 cm	
Nx	Lymph nodes cannot be evaluated	D1
M0	No distant metastases	
M1	Distant metastases present	
Mx	Distant metastases cannot be evaluated	D2
		D3 resistant to hormonal therapy

nearly all prostate cancers.[46] These findings have been confirmed in the last 8 years by PSA data that are requested at 6-month intervals during routine follow-up. Histologic grade is acknowledged as the most important prognostic indicator for progression; Figure 68-8 shows survival and time to metastasis data for patients from Northwest England on a watchful waiting protocol. In this series[46] the mean age at presentation was 74.5 years and it can be seen that patients with well-differentiated tumors have not yet reached the median point at 10 years. The survival data also emphazise that many moderate and all high-grade tumors are not suited to a watch and wait policy.

Radiotherapy

In the UK radiotherapy has traditionally been the mode of treatment for those patients with localized disease in whom markers, grade or stage (as judged by rectal examination), pointed to the need for local primary control. Recently, the efficacy of this treatment modality has been questioned, particularly in the context of younger patients. Additionally, results of comparative trials with surgery have not been favorable, but it is generally agreed that patients entered to the radiotherapy arm of such trials are poorly staged when compared to those submitted to radical surgery. Nevertheless, for the older man in whom watchful waiting or radical surgery is contraindicted, radiotherapy remains a reasonable method of treatment without serious short- or long-term complications.

Radical surgery

Radical prostatectomy has always been the first choice in the US for the treatment of localized prostate cancer. Recently, however, enthusiasm has been taken to extremes with a rapid increase in the numbers of procedures performed even in men over 75 years old.[47] Most would regard this as overtreatment as the complications of surgery—incontinence and impotence—are not insignificant in the elderly, particularly when the procedure is performed by an inexperienced surgeon.

In summary, the observational studies incorporating histologic grade have shown that the biological age of the patient is the most important factor in making a decision between the three treatment options. Whereas there is little doubt that the man of 55 years of age should be offered surgery on the basis of the 10 to 15 year predicted survival data, for the same reason this is the incorrect choice for most men over 70 years. A few fit men 70 to 75 years of age with long life expectancy might just be included in the operative group, but the remainder are better served by a more conservative balanced approach.

Extensive Local Disease

Occasionally, patients are discovered who have quite large ($T3^+$) local tumors, but an apparently normal bone scan. Prostate-specific antigen data may show these lesions to be slow-growing, but it is most likely that treatment should be offered—usually in addition to transurethral resection to cure outflow tract symptoms. Hormone manipulation by medical (LHRH) or surgical (bilateral subcapsular orchidectomy) means is usually found to be very satisfactory in these cases. Resection or estrogen therapy (i.e., IV Honvan) may be required occasionally when local tumor advance leads to blockage of the lower ends of the ureters with resultant abnormalities of renal function.

Metastatic Disease

It is an unfortunate fact that until very recently the majority of patients with prostate cancer presented with bone metastases, and thus, treatment could be regarded only as palliative rather than curative. Worldwide it is accepted that even with immediate treatment the survival for such patients is approximately 50 percent at 2 years and 10 to 14 percent at 5 years.[46,48]

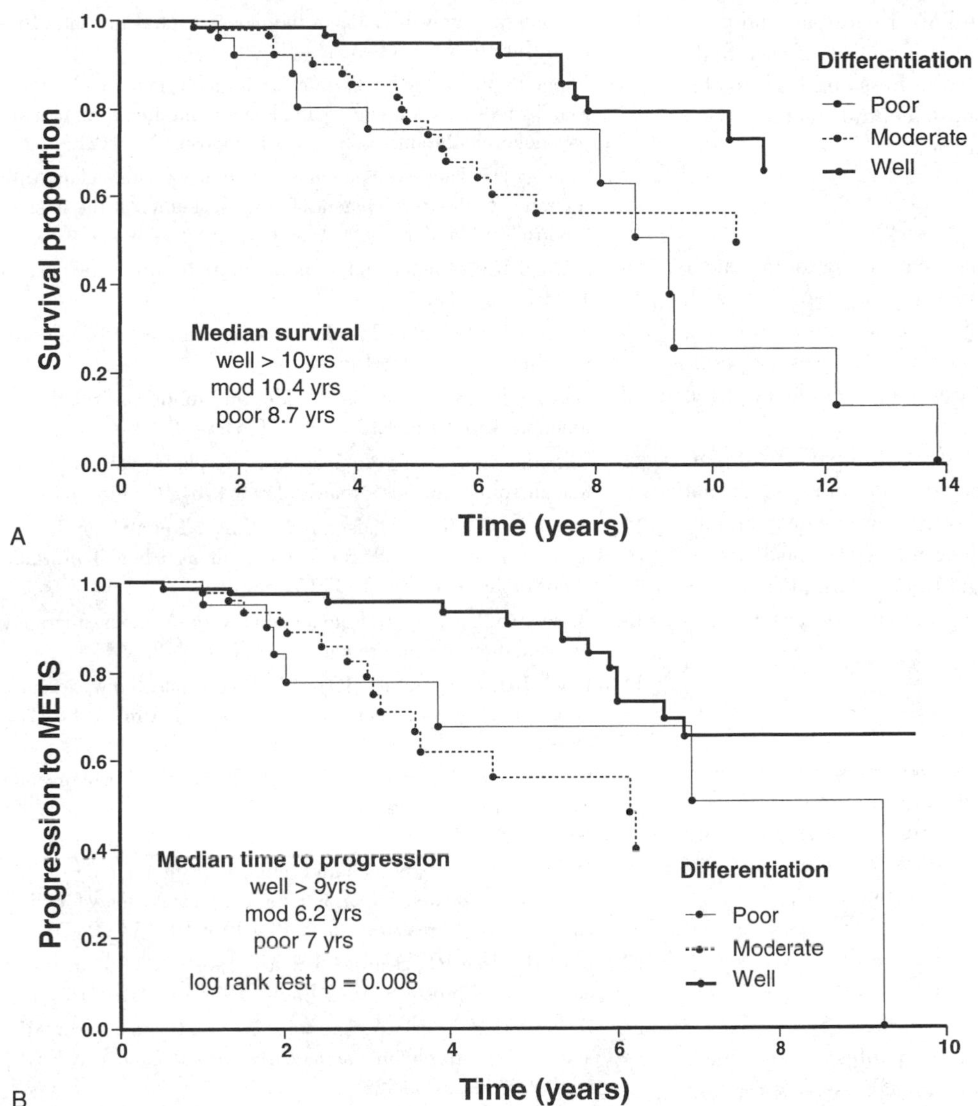

Figure 68-8 Disease-specific Kaplan-Maier analysis of localized prostate cancer in the Manchester series. (1980–1995). The importance of histologic grade can be seen, as (**A**) the median times to survival and (**B**) progression to bony metastases (the most significant cause of morbidity, Figure 8B) has not yet been reached for patients with well-diferentiated tumors.

Treatment by hormonal manipulation

Androgen deprivation has, since 1940 when Huggins discovered the hormone-dependent nature of the tumor, been the mainstay of treatment for metastatic prostate cancer. Remission occurs for a variable period—usually 9 to 12 months—before prostate markers, which usually fall following treatment, start to rise again. Approximately 10 to 15 percent of patients fail to respond significantly to the hormonal manipulation, which may be achieved by either medical or surgical means. Bilateral subcapusular orchidectomy has been the traditional approach to androgen deprivation and the serum testosterone rapidly falls into the "castrate" range. Medical therapy by LHRH analog[49] has, however, become widely established,[50] although the injections are expensive and the serum testosterone does not fall for 8 to 10 days, which may be of clinical importance. It has to be emphasized to the patients that the side effect profile of these two treatments—impotence and hot flushes—is identical, a point not always well made by the manufacturers. Diethylstilboestriol (DES) 5 mg was for many years used to achieve the required hormonal manipulation. Well-publicized cardiac toxicity, however, has led many to avoid this medication even at the lower 1 mg dose, although some continue to advocate the approach in combination with daily aspirin.

Nonsteroidal antiandrogens

Nonsteroidal antiandrogens have the attraction of blocking the action of testosterone peripherally without the major side effect problems associated with traditional hormonal manipulations. Each compound, however, has particular drawbacks.

Flutamide leads to significant gastrointestinal upset and diarrhea while nilutamide, which has the attraction of once daily dosage,[51] also causes some breast tenderness and leads to elevation of serum testosterone due to a central agonist action effecting a rise in luteinizing hormone.

Timing of treatment

Some debate has surrounded the ideal timing for treatment of metastatic prostate cancer. Surprisingly, some patients with positive bone scans remain entirely asymptomatic, and it was argued that, as the patients were feeling well, it was not possible to improve their situation and treatment should await the onset of symptoms.

The Medical Research Council Early/Delayed Treatment Trial has addressed this issue. Although a formal report has not yet been published, early indications are that, while treatment delay does not affect survival it does affect the incidence of morbidity (i.e., bone pain, pathologic fracture) and it has been suggested for this reason that therapy should be commenced at the time of diagnosis.

Bone pain

Bone pain remains the most troublesome aspect of the disease for the patient and it is often difficult to manage. Radiotherapy remains the basis of local control, although promising results[52] have been noted with strontium[89] and disphosphonate (antiosteoclast) infusions[53] among other approaches.

Conclusion

In the elderly, prostate cancer may manifest as an almost benign slow-growing local tumor or as an aggressive spreading disease that almost invariably leads to a painful and distressing death. Surgical relief of obstruction plays a major part in each of these variants, but for the latter group an approach involving hospital specialists, the palliative care team, and the general practitioner is most likely to result in meaningful support for both the patient and his family.

References

1. Cunha GR, Donjacour AA, Cooke PS et al; The endocrinology and developmental biology of the prostate. Endocr Rev 1987; 8:338–362
2. Berry SJ, Coffey DS, Walsh PC et al; The development of human benign prostatic hypertrophy with age. J Urol 1984;132: 474–477
3. Garraway WM, Collins GN, Lee RJ: High prevelance of benign prostatic hypertrophy in the community. Lancet 1991;338: 469–471
4. Lee C: Physiology of contraction induced regression in rat prostate. pp. 145–159. In Murphy GP, Sandberg AA, Carr JP (eds): Prostate Cell: Structure and Function. Alan R Liss, New York
5. Hiramatsu M, Kashimata M, Minami N: Androgenic regulation of epidermal growth factor in the mouse ventral prostate. Biochem Int 1988;17:311–314
6. Imperato-McGinley J, Guerrero L, Gautier T, Peterson RE: Steroid 5α reductase deficiency in men: an inherited form of male psuedohermaphroditism. Science 1974;186:1213–1215
7. Lowsley OS: The development of the human prostate gland with reference to the development of other structures at the neck of the urinary bladder. Am J Anat 1912;13:299–304
8. McNeal JE: Normal histology of the prostate. Am J Surg Pathol 1988;12:619–626
9. McNeal JE: Origin and evolution of benign prostatic hypertrophy. Invest Urol 1978;15:340
10. Gosling J: Structure of the bladder and urethra in relation to function. Urol Clin North Am 1979;6:31–38
11. Schroder HD: Onuf's Nucleus X: a morphological study of a human spinal nucleus. Anat Embryol 1981;162:443–453
12. Simonsen O, Moller-Madsen B, Dorflinger T et al: Significance of age on symptoms and urodynamic findings in bengin prostatic hypertrophy. Urol Res 1987;15:355–361
13. Butler MR, Donnelly B, Komaranchat A: Intravenous urography in evaluation of acute retention. Urology 1978;12:464
14. Pinck BD, Corrigan MJ, Jasper P: Preprostatectomy excretary urography: does it merit the expense? J Urol 1980;123: 390–394
15. Scardino PT, Shinohara K, Wheeler TM et al: Staging of prostate cancer: value of ultrasonography. Urol Clin North Am 1989; 16:713–734
16. Ohori M, Egawa S, Shinohara K et al: Detection of microscopic extra capsulor extension prior to radical prostatectomy for clinically localised prostate cancer. Br J Urol 1994;74:72–79
17. Platt IF, Bree RL, Schwab RE: Accuracy of CT in staging of carcinoma of prostate. Am J Radiol 1987;149:315–318
18. Rifkin MD, Zerlouri EA, Gatsonis CA et al: Comparison of MRI and ultrasonography in staging early prostate cancer. N Engl J Med 1990;323:611–625
19. Gutman AB, Gutman EB: An "acid" phosphatase occuring in the serum of patients with metastatic carcinoma of the prostate gland. J Clin Invest 1938;17:473–477
20. Wang MC, Valenzuela LA, Murphy GP et al: Purification of a human prostate specific antigen. Invest Urol 1979;17:159
21. Oesterling JE, Jacobsen SJ, Chute CG et al: Serum prostate specific antigen in a community based population of healthy men: establishment of age specific reference ranges. JAMA 1993;270:840–864
22. Lilja H, Christensson A, Dahlen U et al: Prostate specific antigen in serum occurs predominantly in complex with an alpha 1 chymotrypsin. Clin Chem 1991;37:9–14
23. Christensson A, Bjork T, Nilsson O et al: Serum PSA complexed to alpha 1 chymotrypsin as an indicator of prostatic cancer. J Urol 1993;150:100–105
24. George NJR, Reading C: Sympathetic nervous system and dysfunction of the lower urinary tract. Clin Sci 1986;70:69–76
25. McGuire EJ, Savastano JA: Treatment of intractable bacterial cystitis with intermittent catherterization and antimicrobial installation. J Urol 1987;137:495–496
26. Hald T: Urodynamics in benign prostatic hypertrophy. A survery. The Prostate 1989;suppl 2:69–77

27. Abrams PH: New words for old: lower urinary tract symptoms for "prostatism". Br Med J 1994;308:929
28. Abrams PH, Farrar DJ, Turner-Warwick RT et al: The results of prostatectomy: A symptomatic and urodynamic analysis of 152 patients. J Urol 1979;121:640–642
29. Holm-Bentzen M, Larsen S, Hainan B, Howells T: Non obstructive detrusor myopathy. Scand J Urol Nephrol 1985;19:21–26
30. Jensen K-ME, Jorgensen JP, Mogensen P: Urodynamics in prostatism II: prognostic value of pressure flow study. Scand J Urol Nephrol 1988;114:72–77
31. Neal DE, Ramsden PD, Sharples L: Outcome of elective prostatectomy. Br Med J 1989;299:762–767
32. George NJR, O'Reilly PH, Barnard RJ, Blacklock NJ: High pressure chronic retention. Br Med J 1983;286:1780–1783
33. Abrams PH, Roylance J, Fenerley RCL: Exceretion urography in the investigation of "prostatism". Br J Urol 1976;48: 681–684
34. Kirby RS, Coppinger SWC, Corcoran MO et al: Prazosin in the treatment of prostatic obstruction. Br J Urol 1987;60:136–142
35. Stoner E, Finasteride Study Group: Three year safety and efficacy data on the use of finasteride in the treatment of BPH. Urology 1994;43:284–292
36. Lepor H, Willford W, Barry MJ et al: Efficacy of terazosin, finasteride or both in BPH. N Engl Med J 1996;335:533–539
37. Benson GS, Sarshik SA, Baezer DM: Comparison of the effects and mechanisms of action of atropine, propantheline, flavoxate and imipramine. Urology 1977;9:31–37
38. Moisey C, Stephenson TR, Brendler C: The urodynamic and subjective result of treatment of detrusor instability with oxybutimin chloride. Br J Urol 1980;52:472–475
39. Holtgrewe HL: Transurethral prostatectomy. Urol Clin N Am 1995;22:357–368
40. Milroy E, Chapel CR: The UroLume stent in the managment of BPH. J Urol 1993;150:1630–1635
41. Carter HB, Coffey DS: The prostate: an increasing medical problem. The Prostate 1990;16:39–48
42. CRC Fact Sheet No. 20. London, 1994
43. Waterhouse JA, Murir CS, Shanmugaratuam K et al: IARC Scientific Publication No. 15. Lyon, 1982
44. Chybowski FM, Larson-Keller JJ, Bergstrath EJ et al: Predicting bone scan findings in patients with newly diagnosed untreated prostate cancer: PSA is superior to all other parameters. J Urol 1991;145:313–318
45. Johansson J, Adami H, Andersson S et al: High ten year survival rate in patients with early untreated prostate cancer. JAMA 1992;267:2191–2196
46. George NJR: Natural history of localised prostate cancer treated by conservative therapy alone. Lancet 1988;1:494–497
47. Lu-Yao GL, McClerran D, Wasson J et al: An assessment of radical prostatectomy. JAMA 1993;269:2633–2636
48. Sandhu DPS, Mayor PE, Sambrook P, George NJR: Increased survival of patients with massive lymphadenopathy and prostate cancer: evidence of heterogenous tumorur behaviour. Br J Urol 1990;66:415–419
49. Peeling WB: Phase III Studies to compare Goserelin (Zoladex) with orchidectomy and DES in the treatment of prostatic carcinoma. Urology 1989;33:45–52
50. Cassileth BR: Patients choice of treatment in Stage D prostatic cancer. Urology 1989;33:57–59
51. Furr BA, Valcaccia B, Curry B: ICI 176334: a novel non-steroidal peripherally selective anti-androgen. J Endocrinol 1987; 113:R7–R9
52. Crawford ED, Balmar C, Kozlowski JM et al: Strontium^{89} for palliation of pain for bone metatases associated with hormone refractory prostate cancer. Urology 1994;44:481–485
53. Clarke NW, Halbrook J, McClure J et al: Effects of osteoclast inhibition by pamidronate in metastatic bone disease from prostate cancer. Br J Cancer 1991;63:420–423
54. Pantilides ML, Bowman SP, George NJR: Levels of PSA that predicts skeletal spread in prostate cancer. Br J Urol 1992;17: 299–303

CHAPTER 69

Gynecologic Disorders in the Elderly—Sexuality and Aging

ALAN D. G. BROWN
TARA K. COOPER

Age Changes in the Genital Tract

The female physiologic aging process accelerates after menopause, particularly in the genital tract.

Hormone Changes

In the reproductive years the ovary has three compartments for steroid biosynthesis the maturing follicle, functioning corpus luteum, and stroma. After menopause the remaining follicles fail to respond to greatly increased pituitary stimulation so that the stroma is the only source of estrogen.

Estrone is the major postmenopausal estrogen and it is derived from the conversion of androgens, mainly androstenedione, produced by the ovaries and adrenal glands. The efficiency of this process increases with age and estrone levels rise to four times that found in young women (45 pmol/L to 180 pmol/L). This conversion correlates with body weight as fat has the ability to aromatize androstenedione to estrone.[1] Ovarian androgen output increases postmenopausally[2] while its adrenal production remains the same.

Ovarian estradiol secretion is minimal postmenopausally[3] with blood levels being reduced by about 90 percent. However, as estrone has one-tenth the biological activity of estradiol it is likely that the latter is more important in maintaining hormone-dependent tissues,[4] particularly as body weight does not correlate with vaginal estrogenization. Estriol is a weak estrogen that does not seem to have a significant role; progesterone is derived mainly from the adrenal glands and levels fall steadily.

In perimenopausal women the ovary becomes increasingly resistant to follicular stimulating hormone (FSH) and secretes less estrogen, which reduces the negative feedback to the pituitary gland. FSH begins to rise and may reach postmenopausal levels (greater than 15 IU/L), but there are marked daily variations and therefore serum FSH is a poor diagnostic test. Luteinizing hormone (LH) concentrations can remain normal until menopause but eventually there are 10 to 20 and threefold increases in FSH and LH, respectively, reaching peaks 3 to 5 years after menopause; thereafter there is a gradual, slight decline to premenopausal values 20 years later.[5]

Anatomic Changes

The major change is atrophy, which results in smaller and smoother structures, flattened epithelial surfaces, and fibrous stroma with much reduced vascularization and fat content.

Ovary

The postmenopausal ovary is small and sclerotic; atretic follicles disappear, the cortex involutes, and germinal inclusion cysts are found. Lipid droplets may be seen in the stroma as evidence of continuing steroidogenesis.

Uterus

There is a marked reduction in size of the uterus so that the uterine body to cervix ratio reverts from 4:1 in reproductive life to the 2:1 of childhood. In the myometrium there is interstitial fibrosis and thickened blood vessels due to obliterative, subintimal sclerosis. The endometrium is a single layer of fat or cuboidal cells with a few inactive glands that are often dilated due to blocked ducts.

Cervix and vagina

The cervix becomes flush with the vaginal vault as the fornices disappear and the squamocolumnar junction recedes into the endocervical canal, which sometimes causes stenosis of the external os. Vaginal atrophy results in a pale foreshortened, and narrow structure and the external urethral meatus retracts along the anterior wall. Reduced estrogen produces a thinner squamous epithelium and less intracellular glycogen to interact with lactobacilli; thus lactic acid production diminishes, which causes reduced vaginal secretion, an alkaline pH, and the loss of a potent defense mechanism.

Vulva

Postemenopausal changes are characterized by skin shrinkage, loss of prominent landmarks, and sparse, graying hair. The epidermis is thinner although there is increased keratinization. These changes may coincide with a vulval epithelial disorder (see below).

Pelvic floor

Aging produces pelvic floor weakness. Damage to the nerve supply starts with partition[6] and further progressive enervation is found with prolapse.[7] An important element of pelvic floor support is collagen, which also diminishes after the climacteric.

Menopause

The cessation of ovarian function at menopause has many short- and long-term consequences. Early menopausal symptoms (e.g., mood swings, hot flushes, and night sweats) affect most women to varying degrees and those who have problems are treated effectively by hormone replacement therapy (HRT).

More relevant here is the prolonged effect of estrogen deficiency postmenopausally. The average age of menopause has remained around 51 years for centuries. With female life expectancy now reaching over 80 years there has been a massive increase in postmenopausal women, and the morbidity/mortality resulting from ovarian failure becomes increasingly important. At present there is poor correlation between early symptoms and late consequences; therefore it is not possible to select women for prophylactic HRT on the basis of the most beneficial outcome. Widespread hormonal use has been advocated to improve quality of life and slow down the female aging process,[8] but it is not accepted universally. The protective influence of HRT against deranged connective tissue in bones and skin as well as cardiovascular disease is well documented.

Osteoporosis

In postmenopausal women there is accelerated bone loss so that by 70 years 50 percent of bone mass is lost, whereas men lose 25 percent by 80 years.[9] This is due to increased bone absorption by osteoclasts by a mechanism that is uncertain. Altered calcium metabolism may be a factor, but the primary defect is generalized connective tissue loss with reduced bone mineral content following breakdown of the organic collagen matrix.[10] The resultant osteoporosis increases dramatically the postmenopausal fracture rate compared with men. The most common sites are wrists, vertebral bodies, and neck of femur, and in women aged 75 years 50 percent will have sustained one or more of these. Fractured neck of femur is the most significant consequence of osteoporosis because of its high morbidity and mortality; there is a 20 percent death rate within the first year and 50 percent of patients fail to gain their independence.[11]

Two years of hormone treatment results in a 66 percent reduction in hip fracture in the subsequent 2 years,[12] and HRT for 10 years results in a 60 percent reduction in the estimated mortality rate associated with osteoporotic hip fractures.[13]

Cardiovascular disease

Heart disease is five times more common in men than in premenopausal women but by 70 years there is no sex difference. In younger women the cardioprotective effect of estrogen is mediated through lipoprotein metabolism. Ovarian failure causes increased levels of cholesterol, triglyceride, and low-density lipoprotein (LDL) and a reduction in high-density lipoprotein (HDL). These changes result in an increased predisposition to ischemic heart disease.[14] Estrogen therapy increases HDL, lowers LDL,[15] and may have a vasodilatory effect through the release of peptides in blood vessels. HRT produces a 30 to 50 percent reduction in mortality from ischemic heart disease and stroke.[13]

Skin

Skin changes have been attributed to the aging process but estrogen deficiency and light exposure are the main cause. Skin thickness declines postmenopausally by 30 percent in the first 10 years, which is comparable to bone loss over the same time.[16] When HRT is started early there is no decline in skin collagen or thickness.

Postmenopausal Bleeding

Postmenopausal bleeding (PMB) is defined as bleeding from the genital tract after 1 year's amenorrhea. Frequently the cause is not determined but it should be considered to be due to malignancy until proved otherwise. One and 10 percent of isolated and recurrent episodes, respectively, have a malignant etiology, predominantly endometrial carcinoma.[17] Benign causes include atrophic vaginitis (greater than 40 percent), endometrial and cervical polyps, decubital ulceration secondary to prolapse, and vaginal infection. Rarer problems are vulval or vaginal carcinoma and hormone-secreting ovarian tumors that produce endometrial hyperplasia and hence bleeding.

The medical history should include details of recent drug treatment because exogenous estrogen may cause breakthrough bleeding; examination is sometimes difficult in an elderly and often obese patient. Investigation consists of a cervical smear if appropriate and outpatient aspiration (e.g., Pipelle de Cornie DM) or curettage under general anesthesia. Hysteroscopy (where an endoscope is passed into the uterine cavity distended with an aqueous solution or carbon dioxide) is becoming standard practice, especially with recurrent bleeding; it may be carried out in the clinic but usually under anesthesia in the elderly.

Vaginal ultrasound measurement of endometrial thickness may be helpful in patients unsuitable for the above techniques, for example the very elderly, unfit patient or those with a stenosed cervix. Thickness of less than 5 mm is reassuring.[17] Cystoscopy and sigmoidoscopy are necessary when appropriate or if there is doubt about the bleeding source.

Treatment depends on the cause and is outlined in the appropriate section. Recurrent bleeding requires detailed reassessment including hysteroscopy, laparoscopy, or hysterectomy, which may be the only way to exclude a small ovarian tumor. Bleeding after hysterectomy is usually due to vaginal vault granulation tissue or atrophic vaginitis.

Hormone Replacement Therapy

Estrogen therapy is the appropriate treatment for ovarian failure and it may be given orally or parenterally (i.e., transvaginally, transdermally, or subcutaneously). Also there is the need for progesterone in women with a uterus because prolonged, unopposed estrogen causes endometrial hyperplasia, which may lead to adenocarcinoma. Oral progestogen for 12 to 14 days each month abolishes these risks[18] and it is required whichever technique is used for long-term estrogen replacement. Progestogens are less important in hysterectomized women because their protective role against breast cancer is in doubt[19] and there is concern that they may attenuate the cardiovascular benefits of HRT.[20] This issue remains unresolved but it is unlikely to be a problem in that only 30 percent of estrogen benefits are mediated through lipid effects.

When progesterone is given sequentially a withdrawal bleed occurs at the end of each course; newer regimens incorporate a continuous, low-dose progestogen that prevents endometrial proliferation, so there is no bleeding.

Oral Estrogen

Oral estrogen is the most widely used route and many combinations of estrogen and progesterone are available commercially (e.g., Prempak-C, Nuvelle, and Trisequens). Continuous combined preparations include Premique and Kliofem. The disadvantage of the oral method is that estrogen passes directly to the liver, where it is inactivated and partially metabolized to the less effective estrone; this is called the "first-pass" effect.

These preparations, therefore, are given in higher doses than parenteral therapy; this may result in altered hepatic metabolism with changes in clotting factors and increased renin substrate that predisposes to hypertension. However, oral preparations increase cardioprotective HDL and are useful for women with abnormal lipid profiles; they are also convenient to use and generally well tolerated.

Topical Estrogen

Vaginal estrogen creams and pessaries, such as Ortho-Gynest, are used primarily for treating atrophic vaginitis. Absorption is rapid and if the hormone is continued for more than 2 months cyclical progesterone should be given. In general a short course is adequate: the maximum response occurs after 2 weeks and there is a carry-over effect of 2 weeks following therapy. An initial 14-day course should be followed by two nights' application each week thereafter. A problem with this regimen in the elderly is reduced acceptability and the fact that manual dexterity is required for self-administration. The district nurse may therefore be required to insert or teach the use of cream or pessary with the vaginal applicator. Alternatives include vaginal tablets (Vagifem), which has a finer applicator, or a slow-release vaginal ring (Estring), which provides 3 months' therapy.

Transdermal Patches

Transdermal patches may be reservoir or matrix in type (Estraderm, Evorel) and deliver estradiol at controlled rates depending on the surface area used. The first-pass effect is avoided and appropriate estradiol plasma levels are obtained without affecting hepatic metabolism, thus avoiding the risk of hypertension or thrombosis. Patches are changed once or twice weekly and cause transient skin redness in up to 30 percent of patients, but the matrix type causes less irritation. Estrogen may also be given transdermally as a gel using a metered dose applicator and this is rapidly absorbed.

Subcutaneous Implants

Estradiol implants are inserted using local anesthesia. Gonadotrophin levels fall within 2 weeks and estradiol rises to a peak at 2 to 3 months and is sustained for several months depending on the dose. There is increased bone mass in these women compared with oral therapy,[21] due to the higher estradiol level from the implant.

Contraindications to Hormone Replacement Therapy

There are few contraindications to HRT, which provides estrogen replacement at below the normal premenopausal plasma concentrations and high-dose synthetic estradiols used in the oral contraceptive pill. Women with such hormone-dependent tumors as breast or endometrial cancer should not be treated unless symptoms are debilitating and there is specialist supervision. Controlled hypertensive patients are eligible and the progesterone may lower the blood pressure.[22] Moreover, natural estrogen causes less disturbance to fibrinolytic and coagulation mechanisms and is suitable for patients at risk of thromboembolism. HRT may be given where there are preexisting problems (e.g., fibroids) which may fail to shrink, thus causing heavy withdrawal bleeds.

Duration of Treatment

There is no limit to the duration of HRT as it is given to women in their seventies and eighties for the first time if they have significant osteoporosis. The benefits are well proven so the question is no longer whether HRT should be given but when it should be stopped. Long-term therapy requires regular screening of blood pressure and breast screening using mammography.

The chief concern with HRT is that studies have shown a modest increase in breast cancer risk related to prolonged use (i.e., greater than 10 years).[23] Although this is not conclusive and the cardioprotective benefits and reduction in mortality from osteoporosis outweigh the cancer problem, it is reasonable to advocate HRT for 5 to 10 years and only continue thereafter in patients willing to accept the risk.

Compliance with HRT is poor, in that 40 percent of patients at risk of osteoporosis do not take it 8 months after starting treatment.[24] The main reasons for stopping are the persistence of withdrawal bleeds and breast malignancy fears. Compliance should improve with the wider variety of HRT available, including the newer "no bleed" continuous combined therapies, and improved data analysis concerning breast cancer risk.

Vulval Disorders

The vulva is affected by many conditions particular to the area or as part of a general problem, for example, psoriasis. Vulval skin is more sensitive than other epithelium, because it is subjected to increased heat, friction, and occlusion.[25] Aging is also a factor and some chronic vulval disorders represent an advanced stage of atrophic change.

It is necessary to diagnose accurately vulval pathology, in particular malignancy and infection because, even in the elderly, genital warts, herpes, and chlamydia may be detected. Therefore, local/general examination and investigation of urine, vaginal discharge, and biopsies of abnormal areas may be required. Vulval epithelial disorders are important because of the severity and chronicity of symptoms (the most common is pruritus) and the association with carcinoma. For years there have been conflicting views concerning pathogenesis, diagnosis, and terminology but a classification (see accompanying box) has been agreed on by the two International Societies for the Study of Vulvar Disease and of Gynaecological Pathologist[25] for non-neoplastic epithelial disorders of vulval skin and mucosa.

Lichen Sclerosis

Lichen sclerosis (LS) is a common problem affecting the aging vulva. The etiology is uncertain but there is an association with genetic and hormonal factors, and autoimmune disease.[26] In a study of 350 women with LS these authors found that lesions were noted at the vulva and elsewhere (97.5 percent), vulva and perianal skin only (44 percent), and vulva alone (38 percent). The vulva appearance varies but the characteristic lesions are a figure of eight configuration around the vulval appearance of white plaques of keratin with purple areas where it is much reduced; the condition does not extend into the vagina. Fusion of tissue occurs: for example the prepuce to the clitoris, and the labia minora which may lead to introital stenosis. The picture is complicated by chronic scratching, so the skin may become thickened (i.e., lichenified). Although the clinical appearance varies there are characteristic histologic features, including an atrophic epidermis with hyalinization and areas of thickening (hyperkeratosis), and inflammation.

The histologic pattern varies throughout the vulva. Biopsies of any suspicious areas are therefore necessary to exclude atypicality; these may be obtained under local anesthesia in the outpatient clinic. The most effective treatment is anti-inflammatory topical steroids, for example betamethasone valerate 0.1 percent or, if necessary, clobetasol propionate 0.05 percent, which arrest epithelial reaction. Although the condition is associated with atrophy, topical estrogen is ineffective and should be considered only for vaginal use. Simple vulvectomy has been used for intractable problems but it is contraindicated because the epithelial changes and symptoms invariably recur.

The risk of LS undergoing malignant change to squamous cell carcinoma is 5 to 10 percent[26]; these patients therefore should report any symptom changes and be seen regularly to detect alterations requiring biopsy.

Non-neoplastic epithelial disorders of vulval skin and mucosa

1. Lichen sclerosis
2. Squamous cell hyperplasia (Squamous cell hyperplasia is used for those instances in which hyperplasia is not attributable to another cause.)
3. Other dermatoses (Dermatosis describes a noninfective, non-neoplastic skin condition that is recognized as a dermatologic entity.)

Vulval Discomfort (Vulvodynia)

Chronic pain or burning in the vulva, vagina, and perineum is a well-recognized problem in elderly women. The discomfort is often exacerbated by sitting and relieved by standing or lying down. Etiology is largely unknown but subclinical infection and a neurologic cause should be excluded. Depression is a possible factor as these patients often live alone. Assessment includes neurologic and local examinations with urethral, vaginal, and endocervical swabs to exclude infections. Pathology is rarely found.

Treatment consists of local applications used empirically but under strict control and in the short term, such as estrogen topical steroid and anesthetic cream. The use of pelvic floor exercises to improve muscle tone and blood supply is helpful, as is sitting on a rubber ring to relieve pressure. Antidepressants should be considered and in intractable cases referral to a psychiatrist or a pain clinic may be necessary.[27] Surgery is rarely, if ever, indicated as it is likely to aggravate the situation.

Uterovaginal Prolapse

Prolapse of the anterior and posterior vaginal walls occurs independently or together, resulting in any combination of urethrocele, cystocele, rectocele, and enterocele, which are displacements of the underlying urethra, bladder, rectum, and pouch of Douglas (and any contents), respectively. Uterine descent may predominate but usually this is associated with some degree of vaginal laxity. Prolapse is most commonly associated with childbirth and postmenopausal hormone deficiency when lack of estrogen causes collagen loss and ligament atrophy.[28] Congenital weakness of sustaining structures and the natural aging process are other factors.

Supports of the Genital Organs

The main supports of the uterus and upper vagina are the transverse cervical, or cardinal, ligaments, which arise from the supravaginal cervix and upper vagina and are inserted into the pelvic side walls. These ligaments extend anteriorly to form the pubocervical fascia, which supports the bladder base, urethra, and anterior vaginal wall as it travels to insertion in the symphysis pubis; their posterior extensions—the uterosacral ligaments—contribute minimally to uterine support. The lower vagina is buttressed by fibers of the levator ani muscles that are inserted into its side walls, the urogenital diaphragm, and perineal muscles. In the erect posture the anterior vagina rests on the posterior wall, which is strengthened by the rectovaginal fascia and perineal body.

Major degrees of prolapse are less common now because of lower parity and improved obstetric management. The patient presents with a dragging, or bearing down, sensation of gradual onset that is worse with activity and settles with rest, and a lump may be seen or felt. Urinary symptoms such as frequency, urgency, incontinence, and incomplete/slow emptying result from distortion of the prolapsed bladder and urethra but they may also be due to atrophy, infection, or detrusor instability. Digital replacement of the anterior or posterior vaginal wall is sometimes necessary before micturition or defecation, respectively, may proceed.

With prolonged uterine descent edema occurs due to interference with venous and lymphatic drainage, leading to epithelial hyperkeratinization and decubital ulceration; bleeding may result but carcinoma rarely develops.

The management of prolapse depends on severity of symptoms, degree of incapacity, and the patient's operative fitness. Surgery is most effective and includes, as appropriate, anterior colporrhaphy, amputation of the elongated cervix or vaginal hysterectomy, and posterior colpoperineorrhaphy. It is now standard practice to give subcutaneous heparin pre- and postoperatively to reduce venous thromboembolism risk. Most patients tolerate surgery well because of improved anesthetics and minimal postoperative morbidity, and the procedures lead to improved mobility and return to an independent life.

When surgery is contraindicated or declined conservative measures may be used. A polyvinyl ring pessary is inserted and inspection and cleaning/renewing every 4 to 6 months are necessary because mucosal ulceration occurs; in this event the ring should be removed for a few weeks and estrogen cream or pessaries used daily to allow epithelial healing. Vaginal douching is no longer used.

Urinary Incontinence

Urinary incontinence is particularly disabling and distressing in the elderly, but with modern investigation and treatment symptoms may be alleviated if not cured (see also Ch. 94). Uninhibited detrusor muscle contraction (detrusor instability) is usually the cause in geriatric patients, due to age-related changes in the central nervous system. Brading and Turner[29] have recently shed light on this troublesome condition. Leakage may be due also to weakness or dysfunction of the urethral closure mechanism (i.e., genuine stress incontinence, which is a common cause in reproductive and early postmenopausal years). Assessment has reached a high degree of sophistication; for example, combined video cystourethrography with pressure and flow studies to diagnose detrusor instability with/without outlet obstruction.[30] However, static cystometry is known to have poor sensitivity and specificity compared with ambulatory monitoring[31] but the significance of the increased incidence of unstable contractions detected with this new technique is unclear. In the elderly, however, such simple and noninvasive tests as daily urination and incontinence chart[32] are particularly important, because the patient or attendants can provide accurate and objective information about bladder habit and function (Table 69-1).

The treatment of genuine stress incontinence should be nonoperative initially and the best results for mild/moderate leakage are with pelvic floor exercises.[33] The urethra has two striated muscles within and immediately adjacent to it, so regular, active contraction has been shown to improve leakage and reduce frequent urination. The use of estrogen therapy for leakage is of limited value.[34]

Gynecologic Cancer in the Elderly

Female genital cancer affects four main sites: the vulva, vagina, uterus, and ovary.

Vulva

Vulval carcinoma is seen most frequently in the 60 to 70 year age group and accounts for about 5 percent of genital neoplasia. Elderly patients often ignore or conceal this problem

Table 69-1 24-Hour frequency/volume chart[a]

	Time	Volume (ml)
	01.00	300
	06.00	275
	08.20	175
	09.30	100
	12.40	200
	13.20	300
	15.25	150
	20.40	300
	22.35	200
	23.55	150
Totals	10	2150

[a] *Data from a 61-year-old woman who had typical detrusor instability symptoms. The chart shows frequency, nocturia, consistently reduced bladder capacities, and excessive output with no history of infections. There was marked symptom improvement with a tailored dose of oxybutynin (2.5 mg bid) and reasonable fluid restriction (mean output of 1,300 ml/24 h).*

because of embarrassment, so they may present with advanced disease that causes bleeding and/or a foul-smelling discharge. Early symptoms are pruritus and the discovery of a lump. Usually the lesion arises on the labium majus and spreads by direct infiltration to the regional lymph glands—the superficial inguinal and prefemoral nodes. Tumors in the outer vulva spread to the ipsilateral nodes whereas more central growths may involve the contralateral groin.

Radical vulvectomy with bilateral groin node dissections is performed. This extensive surgery is generally well tolerated, as there are few postoperative complications and it is curative in 80 to 90 percent of patients because most present with early stage disease. The large butterfly incision, incorporating the tumor and groin nodes, has been abandoned because of infection and wound healing problems.

Wide excision of advanced or recurrent lesions may be used as palliation in patients unfit for radical surgery. When there is a large defect nurse management is difficult, so with appropriate help a myocutaneous flap, using rectus abdominus or gracilis muscle, may be used. Pelvic radiotherapy is needed when there is extensive nodal involvement but dosage determination is difficult because of the anatomy. Chemotherapy is not commonly used in this condition but recently regimens have been developed following successful experience in treating anal carcinomas.

Vagina

Primary vaginal squamous cancer is rare but tends to occur in the elderly. Vaginal malignancy is usually metastatic adenocarcinoma with blood or lymphatic spread from uterus and, rarely, kidney, breast, or colon. Direct invasion occurs from bladder, cervical, or vulval lesions. Presenting symptoms are postmenopausal bleeding, offensive discharge, and, eventually, fistula formation. Diagnosis is by biopsy and the treatment is radiotherapy. Endometrial metastases respond to progesterone, but urinary diversion may be required if there is a fistula. Occasionally palliative colpocleisis is performed.

Uterus

The management of gynecologic cancer patients is becoming centralized in units staffed by experienced gynecologic oncologists where the care and outcome is improved. Cervical and corpus cancer prognosis is encouraging due to early diagnosis and accurate treatment selection.[35]

Cervix

Worldwide, cervical carcinoma is the most common gynecologic malignancy. In developed countries it ranks the sixth most frequent female cancer, well behind breast and lung tumors. In young women there is an increasing incidence and in the elderly who may never have been screened it often presents as an advanced lesion. Squamous cell cancer accounts for more than 80 percent of cases. Etiologic factors are early age of coitus, many sexual partners, and a history of sexually transmitted disease. The human papilloma virus (HPV) types 16 and 18 have been incriminated in the pathogenesis of invasive squamous carcinoma and are detectable in over 90 percent of cases. Comprehensive cytologic screening programs are in place in most developed countries and these are achieving reductions in death rates from this disease.[37]

Elderly patients presenting with advanced disease have such symptoms as offensive vaginal discharge, and postmenopausal or postcoital bleeding. Pain is experienced late and is related usually to diffuse pelvic infiltration or bony metastases; the first sign of cervical cancer may be obstructive renal failure resulting from hydronephrosis due to advanced disease.

Diagnosis is by biopsy of suspicious areas at colposcopy or, preferably, under general anesthesia that permits precise clinical staging and evaluation of tumor grade from the histology, Lymphatic metastases occur quickly so that up to 30 percent of early lesions have pelvic node spread at presentation. Tumors confined to the cervix may be treated by radical hysterectomy and pelvic node dissection or radiotherapy. At the same stage both treatments carry similar 5-year survival rates but, in the elderly, radiotherapy is preferred because of the radical surgery complications. In advanced disease the tumor may infiltrate the vagina, parametrium, and finally bladder and/or rectum, which results in a fistula. As in other squamous carcinomas the success of chemotherapy is limited.

Corpus uteri

Endometrial adenocarcinoma is the most common gynecologic malignancy in the elderly with a mean age at presentation of 62 years.[38] Postmenopausal bleeding is the most frequent symptom and occurs early, so prognosis is good. There are significant associations with celibacy, nulliparity, late menopause, and also with obesity, hypertension, and diabetes mellitus (Saint's Triad). The etiologic role of estrogen is established, for example, with polycystic ovary syndrome, hormone-producing ovarian tumors, and unopposed exogenous estrogen endometrial proliferation occurs that may result in carcinoma.[39] This process is opposed by adding cyclical progesterone.[18] In contrast to simple (benign) endometrial hyperplasia, atypical endometrial change predisposes to cancer, more rarely, sarcomatous and mixed mesodermal tumors occur. The latter have a bad prognosis.

Clinical staging and diagnosis are achieved using examination under anesthesia with or without hysteroscopy, and fractional curettage identifies cervical involvement; histologic tumor grading helps to determine treatment and prognosis. Early cancers require total hysterectomy and bilateral salpingo-oophorectomy and postoperative vaginal radiotherapy may be given as vault recurrence occurs in up to 12 percent.[35] External radiotherapy is used when the myometrium is deeply invaded or there is poor differentiation, and tumors extending to the cervix require irradiation pre- and postoperatively. Wertheim hysterectomy may be used but there is significant morbidity, for example, pulmonary embolus or urinary fistula, with no improvement in results.

Advanced cancers are treated with radiotherapy and then surgery if the response is good. Progestational agents cause regression of endometrial hyperplasia and carcinoma in situ and are used as adjunctive therapy; they may control vaginal bleeding associated with advanced disease and reduce pain due to bony metastases.

Ovary

Ovarian cancer remains the most common fatal gynecologic malignancy. The incidence in the Western world is about 12 per 100,000 women and although 25 percent of gynecologic cancers are of ovarian origin they account for over 50 percent of deaths. The onset and progress of these tumors is often insidious so that 70 percent of patients present with late stage disease. The peak age incidence is in the fifth and sixth decades so this cancer is seen frequently in the elderly population. Despite the use of chemotherapy, prognosis is poor. A high index of suspicion is therefore necessary in postmenopausal women who develop ovarian enlargement. Ninety percent of ovarian malignancies in older women are epithelial adenocarcinomas but the other ovarian components may become malignant and give rise to such histologic types as sex cord and germ cell tumors, and metastases may be seen from elsewhere.

Granulosa cell tumor is the most common sex cord malignancy and up to 60 percent occur after menopause. It arises from adult medullary cells and hormone production may result in vaginal bleeding due to endometrial hyperplasia. Generally they are malignant and clinical presentation is similar to other ovarian neoplasms. A thecoma is more characteristic of the aging female and arises from cortical stroma. Often it is benign and estrogen is produced so that endometrial adenocarcinoma may result.

The cryptic development of many ovarian malignancies results in patients presenting to nongynecologic specialties. The principal symptoms are nonspecific such as abdominal discomfort/distension, malaise, and weight loss, although ascites may lead to weight gain. The tumor may cause pain from torsion or hemorrhage and symptoms related to compression of vital structures by the enlarging mass. In a postmenopausal woman with ascites ovarian cancer should be high on the list of differential diagnoses.

Investigation includes hematologic and biochemical profiles, chest x-ray, intravenous urogram, and ultrasound screening, which is often diagnostic as ascites and solid areas suggest malignancy. The tumor marker CA12541 is a sensitive and specific indicator of ovarian malignancy and is elevated in about 90 percent of carcinomas. Ultrasound and marker studies have been incorporated into screening programes particularly in young women with a high family incidence of breast and ovarian cancer.

Laparotomy establishes the diagnosis and examination of abdominal contents provides accurate staging, this will influence treatment and prognosis. Total hysterectomy, bilateral salpingo-oophorectomy, and omentectomy are required; complete tumor removal may be difficult but the greater the reduction of tumor bulk the more effective is adjuvant therapy and ascites better controlled. Invariably, postoperative chemotherapy is required because of this cancer's propensity for disseminating widely. Further, most patients have residual disease after surgery. Cis-platinum and carboplatin are used but they are toxic and have unpleasant side effects in that they cause myelosuppression and nephro- and neurotoxicity, and are severely emetogenic. They are given by intermittent intravenous therapy with sufficient antiemetics and intravenous fluids to minimize problems. Forty to 50 percent of patients with extensive disease will have complete remission with platinum but the majority relapse within 2 years.[41]

A less aggressive option is the oral alkalating agent, chlorambucil, which is used frequently in the elderly. Failure of first-line treatment is ominous as recurrent disease is often resistant to further therapy. Newer agents, for example Taxanes, offer hope in all groups of patients. Recurrent ascites is a major problem and repeated hospital admissions and paracenteses are required; diuretics (e.g., spironolactone) may reduce the fluid and limit recurrence. Occasionally a peritoneal venous shunt is inserted but often it becomes blocked or infected and requires removal. Radiotherapy is limited to the unresectable, symptomatic recurrence and is used only for palliation.

Sexuality and Aging

There is a view that sexuality in the elderly is irrelevant and unnecessary. The facts are, however, that sexual drive is not exhausted with aging, and as life expectancy increases it is necessary to recognize that continued sexual activity is an important requirement of old age to promote satisfactory relationships, personal well-being, and quality of life. Also from this age group there will be an increasing demand for advice and expert help on sexual matters.[42] Many older people have problems because they grew up in sexually restricted times so that ignorance is widespread.[43] Society has an obsession with youth and its sexuality while largely stereotyping the elderly and ignoring their difficulties in this area. In addition, as is generally the case with disabled people, the organization of institutions for the elderly does not recognize their sexuality, so their needs, for example opportunities for privacy, are ignored.[45] Many factors contribute to changing sexuality with age, and the evidence is reviewed below.

Sexual Behavior and Age

In the male

A steady reduction in male sexual activity from early and middle years has been observed.[45] Brecher (see Ref. 57) noted that 75 percent of 70-year-old men continued to have some sexual activity. Figure 69-1 shows that in Danish men aged 51 to 95 years the related phenomena of sexual interest and morning erections diminished similarly with age[46]; coital activity declined dramatically whereas masturbation did to a lesser extent, indicating that the latter is the most common outlet in the very old.

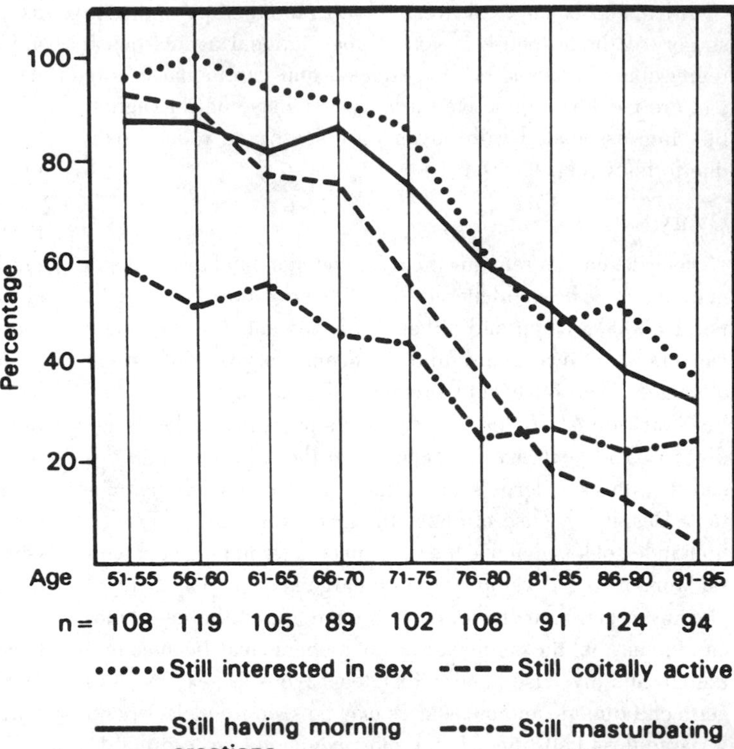

Figure 69-1 Sexuality and aging in 936 Danish men aged 51 to 96 years. (Data from Hegelar and Mortensen.)[46]

Waning sexuality with age is also a function of previous activity.[47] High levels of interest in early life produced lesser changes with age, compared with young men having low activity, which was associated with increased problems later. Continued male activity is also said to be associated with a feeling of well-being, good health, and a nondogmatic personality.[48]

In the female

An early study observed little change in women's capacity until later life.[49] However, questionnaires[50,51] from both sexes between ages 45 and 71 were analyzed. A greater reduction was noted in sexual interest and activity in women; the most significant effect was between 50 and 60 years. At 66 to 71 years 50 and 10 percent of women and men, respectively, had no sexual interest. Persson[52] noted that only 16 percent of 70-year-old women were having intercourse compared with 46 percent of men at the same age. A similar relationship was found in women as in men concerning the decrease in sexuality with age, which appeared to depend on the level of activity in early life.[53]

Interest also relates to the availability of a partner; women, having tended to marry older men who die before them, are often left alone and may experience difficulty finding a new partner.[43] Thus masturbation may become a more regular activity. It has been found that female sexual activity was highest in those currently married and progressively fell away in the divorced, widowed, and never married.[54] Resumption of interest a year after widowhood is more likely when death was expected, there had been extramarital experience, and in younger women; activity diminished when the marriage had been sexually satisfying and there was still a strong attachment to the lost partner.[55]

The role of menopause has been studied[56] in 800 Swedish women aged 38 to 54 years. With advancing age there was reduced sexual interest, orgasmic capacity, and coital frequency. It was shown that decline in interest was the cause rather than the result of infrequent coitus, and diminished activity was due significantly to menopause and not aging.

A common problem following postmenopausal lack of estrogen is vaginal atrophy and dryness causing dyspareunia[57] which leads to loss of interest and activity. It has been observed[58] that the more sexually active women (with coitus and masturbation) have less vaginal atrophy, suggesting that activity protects the vagina by stretching and possibly stimulating hormone production. The use of HRT has been studied.[59] Estrogen, androgen, a combination of both, and placebo were compared in oophorectomized women. The results indicated a beneficial effect of androgen alone or with estrogen on sexual motivation and coital frequency. Thus the evidence suggests that female sexuality is affected by aging but initially less so than by menopause, and the hormones involved are estrogen and androgen. Although testosterone implants have been recommended for some postmenopausal women[60] it is unlikely that they have much place in elderly women because of their limited success and the risk of masculinizing effects.

Sexual Response and Aging

It has been noted[60] that with age vasocongestive changes following sexual stimulation develop more slowly in both sexes; these alterations are gradual, so that the couple adjusts to activity that is less intense but may be as enjoyable. In older men morning erections are less frequent, they develop slowly, and psychic stimulation is less effective, so direct tactile stimulation is often required although sensitivity to touch is reduced.[43] Maintenance of the erection is not as good and if lost it is more difficult to regain. Also ejaculation is less forceable with a small volume and fewer contractions; scrotal and testicular changes are reduced, the postorgasmic resolution phase is rapid, and the refractory period prolonged.

In women vaginal lubrication diminishes and takes longer, there is less vaginal elasticity so that there is shrinkage in the absence of coitus. There are changes elsewhere, for example, nipple erection and breast engorgement is less marked, and orgasm is associated with fewer contractions but orgasmic capacity may not be reduced.[57]

Management of Sexual Problems

The management of these disorders involves the same principles whatever the age and condition, but the emphasis may vary. Both partners must take part in therapy because although one usually presents a problem the other invariably contributes to it, and treatment is facilitated by their cooperation. After an initial discussion the couple should be seen separately so that a confidential interview is obtained including information not to be disclosed to the partner, for example concerning extramarital affairs. A preliminary medical and social history may suggest contributory factor(s) and helps rapport to be established before turning to more sensitive questions.

The sexual history concerns the couple's problems, their duration, and current activity; their past life together is relevant, particularly the emotional relationship, which has a profound effect on sexual function. Information is required about adolescent experience and thereafter regarding masturbation, other activity, difficulties with previous partners, and incidence of sexual assault which is most important. Also negative parental and religious sexual attitudes have a profound effect on development and are often major factors causing future disorder. Examination and investigation will depend on whether a physical basis is suggested, particularly in men where sexuality is more commonly affected by such problems. For example, in a study[61] where 262 patients with erectile dysfunction were investigated, 52 percent had organic disease, the most common being arterial and urologic disorders.

The principles of management include stressing the couple's mutual responsibility for shared problem, and changing negative attitudes resulting from parental or religious influences or past experiences. Ignorance about sexuality is common, so there is a need for basic education and permission to experiment, for example, with different methods of stimulation and coital positions. Couples, particularly older ones, frequently have difficulty talking to each other about sexual anxieties or needs, and discussion with the therapist increases their mutual understanding and ability to communicate.

A series of touching exercises called "sensate focus"[43,60] have been devised to improve lovemaking and analyze the couple's emotional response. An initial ban on intercourse and fondling the breasts and genitals is enforced to reduce performance anxiety because many problems relate to difficulties with erection, intercourse, and orgasm. The initial exercises, therefore, are not goaloriented, and they allow each partner to experiment with touching the other in a pleasurable and nondemanding way and to communicate through touch. The sensations and any problems encountered are discussed together and later with the therapist, and when difficulties are overcome progress is allowed slowly with genital contact and then coitus. Thus sensate focus is a gradual relearning of sexual or courting behavior, which initially involves touching and kissing, leading to intercourse. It forms the basis for treatment of most disorders and the results are generally good.[61]

Acknowledgments

We wish to acknowledge the help of Dr. G. J. Beattie for his advice with the gynecologic cancer section, and Pamela Stirling for her secretarial skills and unfailing patience.

References

1. Upton GV: The menopause; physiologic correlates and clinical management. J Reprod Med 1982;27:1–27
2. Greenblatt Colle ML, Mahesh VB: Ovarian and adrenal steroid production in postmenopausal women. Obstet Gynaecol 1976; 47:383
3. Judd HL, Lucas WE, Yen SSC: Serum 17-estradiol and estrone levels in postmenopausal women with and without endometrial cancer. J Clin Endocrinol 1976;43:272–278
4. Morse AR, Hutton JD, Jacob HS et al: Relation between karyopyknotic index and plasma oestrogen concentrations after the menopause. Br J Obstet Gynaecol 1979;86:981–983
5. Speroff L, Glass RH, Kase NG: Clinical Gynaecology Endocrinology, and Infertility. 5th Ed. pp. 108–111. Williams and Wilkins, Baltimore, 1994
6. Smith ARB, Hosker GL, Warrell DW: Partial denervation of the pelvic floor in the aetiology of genital tract prolapse. J Obstet Gynaecol 1989;96:25–29
7. Allan RE, Hosker GL, Smith ARB, Warrell DW: The role of pregnancy and childbirth and partial denervation of the pelvic floor. Neurol Urodyn 1988;7:237–239
8. Whitehead MI, Studd JWW: Selection of patients for treatment. Which therapy and for how long? Menopause 1988;10:116–129
9. Grimley Evans J: The significance of osteoporosis. pp. 1–8. In Smith R (ed): Osteoporosis. Royal College of Physicians, London, 1990
10. Savvas M, Brincat M, Studd JWW: Postmenopausal osteoporosis. Br J Hosp Med 1987;38:16–18, 22, 24
11. Cummings SR, Kelsey JL, Nevitt MC, O'Dowd KJ: Epidemiology of osteoporosis and osteoporotic fractures. Epidemiol Rev 1985;7:178–208
12. Kiel DP, Felson DP, Anderson JJ et al: Hip fracture and the use of estrogens in postmenopausal women. The Framingham Study. N Engl J Med 1987;317:1169–1174
13. Ross RK, Pike PC, Henderson BE et al: Stroke prevention and oestrogen replacement therapy. Lancet 1989;1:505

14. Whitehead MI: The climacteric. pp. 338–339. In Studd JWW (ed): Progress in Obstetrics and Gynaecology. Vol. 3. Churchill, London, 1985
15. Crook D, Godsland IF, Wynn V: Ovarian hormones and plasma lipoproteins. Menopause 1988;15:168–180
16. Brincat M, Moniz CJ, Studd JWW et al: Long term effects of the menopause and sex hormones on skin thickness. Br J Obstet Gynaecol 1985;92:256–259
17. McKay Hart D: Postmenopausal bleeding. In Medical Dialogue No. 362, 1992
18. Studd JWW, Magos A: Ostrogen therapy and endometrial pathology. Menopause 1988;18:197–212
19. Miller WR, Anderson TJ: Oestrogens, progestogens and the breast. Menopause 1988;21:234–246
20. Studd JWW: Complications of HRT and postmenopausal women. J R Soc Med 1992;85:376–378
21. Savvas M, Studd JWW, Fogelman I et al: Skeletal effects of oral oestrogen compared with subcutaneous oestrogen and testosterone in postmenopausal women. BMJ 1988;297:331–333
22. Rylance PB, Brincat M, Lafferty K et al: Natural progesterone and antihypertensive action. BMJ 1985;290:13–14
23. Sillero-Arenas M, Delgado-Rodriguez M, Rodigues-Conteras R et al: Menopausal hormone replacement therapy and breast cancer: a meta-analysis. Obstet Gynecol 1992;79:286–294
24. Ryan et al: Br J Obstet Gynaecol 1992;99:325
25. Ridley CM: Dermatological conditions of the vulva. pp. 317–339. In Stanton SL (ed): Clinical Obstetrics and Gynaecology. Bailliere Tindall, London, 1988
26. Meyrick Thomas RH, Ridley CM, McGibbon DH, Black MM: Lichen sclerosis et atrophicus and autoimmunity—a study of 350 women. Br J Dermatol 1988;118:41–46
27. Bradley JJ, Ridley CM: Historical and psychological considerations: subjective and traumatic conditions of the vulva. In Ridley CM (ed): The Vulva. Churchill Livingstone, London, 1988
28. Brincat M, Moniz CF, Studd JWW et al: Sex hormones and skin collagen content in postmenopausal women. BMJ 1983;287: 1337–1338
29. Brading AF, Turner WH: The unstable bladder: towards a common mechanism. Brit J Urol 1994;73:3–8
30. Bates CP, Whiteside CG, Turner-Warwick RT: Synchronous cine-pressure flow cystourethrography with special reference to stress and urge incontinence. Br J Urol 1970;42:714–723
31. Bristow SE, Neal DE: Ambulatory urodynamics. Br J Urol 1996; 77:333–338
32. Brown ADG: The GP's role in the management of female urinary incontinence. Practitioner 1988;232:768–769
33. Wilson PD, Al Samarrai T, Deakin M et al: An objective assessment of physiotherapy for female genuine stress incontinence. Br J Obstet Gynaecol 1987;94:575–582
34. Wilson PD, Faragher B, Butler B et al: Treatment with oral piperazine oestrone sulphate for genuine stress incontinence in postmenopausal woman. Br J Obstet Gynaecol 1987;94: 568–574
35. Kilstad P: Advances in the treatment of carcinoma of the cervix and corpus uteri. pp. 325–340 In Bonnar J (ed): Recent Advances in Obstetrics and Gynaecology. Vol. 14. Churchill Livingstone, Edinburgh, 1982
36. Royal College of Obstetricians and Gynaecologists: In Whitfield CR (ed): Report of Working Party on Further Specialisation within Obstetrics and Gynaecology, p. 65,1982
37. Hakama M: Trends in the incidence of cervical cancer in the Nordic countries. pp. 279–292. In Magnus K (ed): Trends in Cancer Incidence. Hemisphere Publishing, Washington DC, 1982
38. Studd JWW, Thom M: Oestrogens and endometrial cancer. pp. 182–188. In Studd JWW (ed): Progress in Obstetrics and Gynaecology. Churchill Livingstone, London, 1981
39. Whitehead MI, Lane G, Dyer G et al: Estradiol: the predominent intranuclear estrogen in the endometrium of estrogen-treated postmenopausal women. Br J Obstet Gynaecol 1981;88: 914–918
40. Oram DH, Bridges JE, Jacobs IJ: Disorder of the ovaries. pp. 220–221. In Grudzinskas JG, Beedham T (eds): Obstetrics and Gynaecology, Treatment and Prognosis. Heinemann Professional Publishing, 1988
41. Wiltshaw E, Kroner T: Phase II study of cis-diaminodichoroplatinum (III) 9NSC 119875) in advanced adenocarcinoma of the ovary. Cancer Treat Rep 60:55–60
42. Webster L: Sex and ageing. Br J Sex Med 1992;19:124–126
43. Bancroft J: Human Sexuality and Its Problems. 2nd Ed. Churchill Livingstone, Edinburgh, 1989
44. White CB: Sexual interest, attitudes, knowledge and sexual history in relation to sexual behaviour in the institutionalised aged. Arch Sexual Behav 1982;11:11–22
45. Kinsey AC, Pomoroy WB, Martin CE: Sexual Behaviour in the Human Male. WB Saunders, Philadelphia, 1948
46. Hegelar S, Mortensen M: Sexuality and ageing. Br J Sexual Med 1978;5:16–19
47. Martin CE: Factors affecting sexual functioning in 60–79 year old married males. Arch Sexual Behav 1981;10:399–420
48. Vallery Masson J, Valleron AJ, Poitrenaud J: Factors related to sexual intercourse frequency in a group of French pre-retirement managers. Age Ageing 1981;10:53–59
49. Kinsey AC, Pomoroy WB, Martin CE, Gebhard PH: Sexual Behaviour in the Human female. WB Saunders, Philadelphia, 1953
50. Pfeiffer E, Davis GC: Determinants of sexual behaviour in middle and old age. J Am Geriatr Soc 1972;20:151–158
51. Pfeiffer E, Verwoerdt A, Davis GC: Sexual behaviour in middle life. Am J Psychiatry 1972;128:1262–1267
52. Persson G: Sexuality in a 70-year-old urban population. J Psychosom Res 1990:24:335–342
53. Christenson CV, Gagnon JH: Sexual behaviour in a group of older women. J Gerontol 1965;20:351–356
54. Corby N, Solnick RL: Psychosocial and physiological influences on sexuality in the older adult. In Birren JE, Sloane RE (eds): Handbook of Mental Health and Ageing. Prentice-Hall, Englewood Cliffs, NJ, 1980
55. Kansky J: Sexuality of widows: a study of sexual practices of widows during the first fourteen months of bereavement. J Sex Marital Ther 1986;12:307–321
56. Halstrom T: Mental Disorders and Sexuality in the Climacteric. Scandinavian University Books, Goteborg, 1973
57. Brecher EM: Love, Sex and Aging: A Consumer's Union Report. Little Brown, Boston, 1984
58. Leiblum S, Bachman G, Kemmann E et al: Vaginal atrophy in the postmenopausal woman. The importance of sexual activity and hormones. JAMA 1983;249:2195–2198

59. Sherwin BB, Gelfand MM: The role of androgen in the maintenance of sexual functioning in oophorectomised women. Psychosomat Med 1987;49:397–409

60. Griffin M: The sexual health of women after the menopause. Sex Marital Ther 1995;10:277–291

61. Masters WH, Johnson VE: Human Sexual Response. Churchill Livingstone, London, 1966

62. Warner P, Bancroft J, and members of Edinburgh Human Sexuality Group: A regional clinical service for sexual problems: a three-year survey. 1987;2:115–126

CHAPTER 70

Carcinoma of the Breast

R. E. MANSEL
R. N. L. HARLAND

Management of elderly patients with cancer of the breast is often directed toward preservation of quality of life, with less emphasis on "cure" than is usual with younger patients. Achieving a balance between minimizing intervention, which may reduce quality of life temporarily, and securing lasting relief from local and systemic effects of the cancer can present the clinician with several difficulties.

Presentation, Diagnosis, and Staging

Carcinoma of the breast can present in various ways, as follows.

Painless Lump

Any discrete mass within the breast of a patient over 65 years old is likely to be malignant whether it displays overt signs of malignancy or not. Cysts are uncommon as the normal age range for these is 35 to 60 years. A "cyst" in a patient over the age of 65 is more likely to be a cancer with a necrotic center. Ancient fibroadenomas may present as the surrounding breast tissue undergoes involution but these are normally heavily calcified and easily visible on mammography. The incidence of inflammatory masses related to duct ectasia decreases from the seventh decade onward.[1] Fat necrosis can simulate a malignant mass, but is usually preceded by a history of trauma and extensive bruising.

Discharge From the Nipple

A persistent serous or blood-stained discharge from a single duct is usually associated with a benign ductal papilloma, but the proportion of patients with such a discharge who have a carcinoma rises to about 30 percent in the seventh decade.[2]

Persistent Localized Pain

Five to 15 percent of carcinomas present with pain or tenderness.[1,3] Most will also have a palpable mass.

Paget's Disease

Any eczema-like eruption on the nipple should be viewed with suspicion. Although there may be no palpable mass, all cases are associated with ductal carcinomas. If neglected the rash spreads outward onto the skin of the breast.

Fungation

A majority of patients presenting with neglected, locally advanced tumors are elderly. The appearance may vary from a shrunken ulcerated plaque (automastectomy) to a cavitating mass with bleeding, purulent exudate, slough, and offensive odor.

Effects of Metastasis

Rarely patients may present with symptoms due to metastases (e.g., bone pain or shortness of breath).

Diagnosis

With fine-needle aspiration cytology, needle biopsy, and mammography it is usually possible to confirm malignancy without the need for open biopsy. Modern triple assessment using ultrasound imaging has increased the accuracy of preoperative diagnosis. The stage of the tumor can be assessed clinically (Table 70-1) and is a guide to the prognosis (Fig. 70-1).

Screening by Mammography

The initial design of the National Health Screening Programme imposed an upper limit of 64 years on women invited for screening and there have been recent calls for extension of the program to older women. Women who reach 64 years while in the program can elect to continue to be screened. Recent studies indicate that older women do respond to screening invitations as readily as younger women. Extending screening to older women has major financial implications in view of the growing proportion of elderly women in the population. The detection rate for elderly women is higher than that for women under 65 years (13.1 cancers per 1,000 mammograms versus 5.9; NHS Screening Programme Review, 1996).

Treatment

Early (Stage I and II) Cancer

The standard surgical treatment in the past for "early" cancer of the breast was some form of mastectomy. More recently there has been a trend for reducing the extent of surgery be-

Table 70-1 Clinical staging of cancer of the breast

Stage I: Only breast parenchymal tissue is involved	Palpable tumour in breast, not involving skin or fixed to deep structures; no palpable nodes
Stage II: Breast parenchymal + ipsilateral axillary node involvement	Primary tumour as stage I, with palpable, mobile, discrete, ipsilateral axillary nodes[a]
Stage III: Local extension beyond breast or axillary nodes	Deep fixation or involvement of skin of breast (infiltration, ulceration, oedema, or satellite nodules) and/or axillary nodes fixed to chest wall or to skin of axilla or matted to each other
Stage IV: Distant spread	Any more distant disease

[a] *Histologic confirmation of nodal involvement gives better prognostic discrimination*

cause studies have shown that wide excision of the cancer with postoperative radiotherapy gives similar results in terms of local recurrence and mortality as does mastectomy.[4] This approach is also relevant in the older woman provided that she is fit for a general anesthetic.

Simple (total) mastectomy

Simple mastectomy comprises removal of all breast tissue without dissection of axillary nodes. It is unsuitable as sole treatment for patients with suspiciously enlarged axillary nodes. With retention of axillary nodes, locoregional recurrence occurs in 30 to 40 percent of patients within 10 years of primary treatment.[5] For patients aged 80 years or over this is less than the risk of death in the same period,[6,7] and so the balance of probability is that simple mastectomy would be the only treatment needed. For younger patients this balance of risk is reversed. Simple mastectomy carries no significant morbidity or mortality in patients who are otherwise fit for surgery.

Modified radical (Patey) mastectomy

In this operation axillary nodes are cleared in continuity with a total mastectomy but without the extensive removal of skin and muscle of the classic Halsted radical mastectomy. This results in a low incidence of local recurrence, which is usually confined to the skin flaps. The disadvantage is related to the extensive axillary dissection that results in longer admissions than simpler procedures, and a risk of reduced mobility at the shoulder joint. With attention to postoperative exercises the risk of long-term disability is low. Although published evidence suggests that elderly patients tolerate extensive surgery well, radical surgery is used selectively in patients over 75 years of age.

Local excision

Although local excision alone is superficially attractive as a treatment for operable cancer in elderly patients, experience has shown that local relapse occurs in 29 to 40 percent of patients within 5 years of presentation.[8–11] For this reason local excision is usually offered in combination with either radiotherapy or endocrine treatment to enhance control. Rare exceptions include localized in situ carcinoma, and small tubular pattern lesions, which have an excellent prognosis.

Local excision and radiotherapy

The high local recurrence rate after excision alone can be reduced by postoperative radiotherapy, providing adequate surgical clearance has been obtained and the disease is not

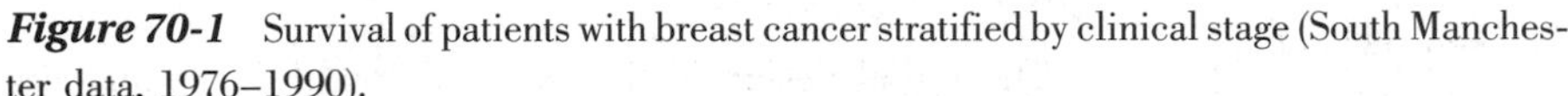

Figure 70-1 Survival of patients with breast cancer stratified by clinical stage (South Manchester data, 1976–1990).

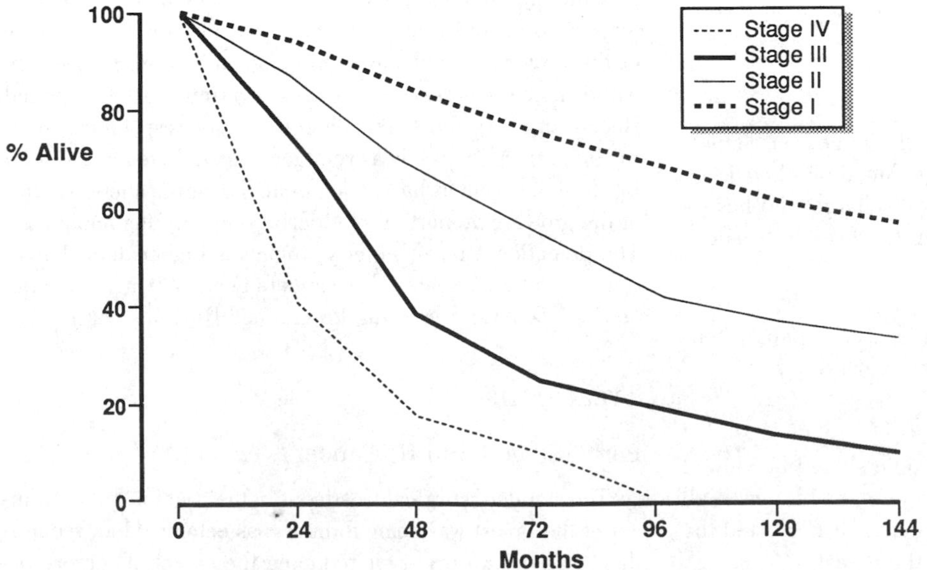

multifocal.[12] When surgical clearance of axillary nodes is carried out, radiotherapy can be confined to the residual ipsilateral breast. Axillary node clearance virtually abolishes the risk of uncontrolled axillary recurrence seen from time to time with other treatments but carries the same problems of rehabilitation discussed earlier. This program of therapy may need to be abandoned in favor of mastectomy when the histologic margins are positive after local excision. In addition, some radiotherapists enforce an upper age limit for treatment because radiotherapy is not tolerated well by the elderly.

Local excision and tamoxifen

Tamoxifen is effective as a treatment for advanced disease, and as an adjuvant agent.[13,14] There are few data on the value of tamoxifen after local excision but it is reasonable to assume that patients with endocrine-responsive tumors will benefit.

Tamoxifen as sole agent in operable breast cancer

The efficacy of tamoxifen in advanced disease has led to its use as sole agent initially in patients unfit for surgery and lately in fit elderly patients. Early studies have reported regression rates of 61 to 81 percent in this context,[15–18] while surgical salvage remains possible for patients who show no sign of response within 3 to 6 months. Formal trials comparing tamoxifen alone with surgery have produced differing conclusions. In one study there was no difference in rates of local relapse although surgical management was inadequate relying on local excision alone.[19] In another, subtotal "anterior" mastectomy was superior to tamoxifen although the ultimate prevalence of relapse was higher than would be expected after total mastectomy.[9]

With median durations of response of 18 to 25 months,[15,17] even responders are likely to suffer further progression of disease and present for surgery eventually. A recent randomized trial comparing surgery against primary tamoxifen showed higher rates of local failure in the tamoxifen-treated arm although there was no demonstrable effect on survival.[21] This suggests that tamoxifen alone is appropriate only in patients with a very limited expectation of life for other reasons.

Adjuvant treatment

Adjuvant treatment is given after potentially curative treatment to reduce the rate of relapse. Cytotoxic treatment is tolerated poorly and offers little benefit over hormone therapy in postmenopausal patients.[14,20] Recent updating of the overview of breast cancer treatments confirms the benefit of tamoxifen in mortality at 10 years.

Locally Advanced (Stage III) Disease

There are two aims of treatment of patients with locally advanced disease: control of primary disease and systemic control.

Surgical clearance may be possible when the disease is not fixed firmly onto the chest wall or involving skin widely. Radiotherapy is also valuable, particularly for localized unresectable tumors. Irrespective of primary treatment, dissemination and local relapse occur frequently. Endocrine therapy reduces the rate both of relapse and mortality. In hormone-sensitive tumors tamoxifen may produce a dramatic response in advanced tumors.

Metastatic (Stage IV) Cancer

Palliation is the principal aim. The best management should be decided by consultation between surgeon, oncologist, and primary care palliation team. There are three treatment modalities that can be used, as follows.

Radiotherapy

Radiotherapy is particularly useful for painful bone deposits. A single treatment to a painful area usually relieves pain within 10 to 14 days. Spinal deposits that threaten paraparesis can also be treated, although preliminary decompression is necessary when symptoms are severe or progress rapidly. Bony disease is improved by bisphosphonates, which are also the agents of choice in hypercalcemia secondary to bony metastases.

Endocrine therapy

About half of patients who have endocrine therapy will benefit. Tamoxifen is the first choice. Megestrol acetate (160 mg od) is a useful alternative but causes fluid retention. Second-line endocrine therapy is achieved by suppression of peripheral synthesis of estrogens by aromatases. Aminoglutethamide was the first-line aromatase inhibitor but side effects including adrenocortical suppression were common. Newer agents such as formestane 250 mg by injection every 2 weeks or anastrozole 1 mg daily given orally are highly effective suppressants of aromatase but without the side effects of adrenal suppression. These second-line agents can produce useful complete responses especially where there was a previous documented first-line response to tamoxifen or another hormonal agent. About one-half of patients who have responded once (regression or stability) respond again.

Cytotoxic chemotherapy

Cytotoxic chemotherapy is tolerated poorly by elderly patients. Although recent developments of less morbid forms of treatment, for example, oral combination of cyclophosphamide, methotrexate, and fluorouracil, are tolerated better than intravenous therapy,[21] such treatment is generally reserved for younger patients with visceral metastases, and for symptomatic patients who fail to respond to endocrine therapy.

References

1. Haagensen CD: Disease of the Breast. 3rd Ed p.357. WB Saunders, Philadelphia 1986
2. Seltzer MH, Perloff LJ, Kelly RI et al: The significance of age

in patients with nipple discharge. Surg Gynecol Obstet 1970; 131:519–522

3. Yorkshire Breast Cancer Group: Symptoms and signs of operable breast cancer 1976–1981. Br J Surg 1983;70:350–351
4. Fisher B, Redmond C, Poisson R et al: Eight year results of a randomised clinical trial comparing total mastectomy and lumpectomy with or without radiation in the treatment of breast cancer. N Engl J Med 1989;320:822–828
5. Murray JG, Mitchell JR, Gresham GA: Management of early cancer of the breast: report on an international multicentre trial supported by the Cancer Research Campaign. BMJ 1976;1: 1035–1037
6. Office of Population Census and Surveys (OPCS): Mortality Statistics for 1985. HMSO, London
7. Herbsman H, Feldman J, Seldera J et al: Survival following breast cancer in the elderly. Cancer 1981;47:2358–2363
8. Reed MWB, Morrison JM: Wide local excision as the sole primary treatment in elderly patients with carcinoma of the breast. Br J Surg 1989;76:898–900
9. Robertson JFR, Todd JH, Ellis IO et al: Comparison of mastectomy with tamoxifen for treating elderly patients with operable breast cancer. BMJ 1988;297:511–514
10. Fisher B, Bauer M, Margolese R et al: Five year results of a randomised clinical trial comparing total mastectomy and segmental mastectomy with or without radiation in the treatment of breast cancer. New Engl J Med 1985;312:665–673
11. Tagart R, Bratherton D, Hartley L, Sikora K: Partial mastectomy alone in early breast cancer. BMJ 1985;290:434
12. Schnitt SG, Connolly JL, Harries JR et al: Pathological predictors of early local recurrence in stage I and stage II breast cancer treated by primary radiation therapy. Cancer 1984;53: 1049–1057
13. Nolvadex Adjuvant Trial Office (NATO): Controlled trial of tamoxifen as single adjuvant agent in the management of early breast cancer. Lancet 1985;1:836–839
14. Early Breast Cancer Trialists Group: Systemic treatment of early breast cancer by hormonal, cytotoxic or immune therapy. Lancet 1992;339:1–15,71–85
15. Bradbeer JW, Kyngdon J: Primary treatment of breast cancer in elderly women with tamoxifen. Clin Oncol 1983;9:31–34
16. Preece PE, Wood RAB, Mackie CR, Cuschieri A: Tamoxifen as initial sole treatment of localised breast cancer in elderly women: a pilot study. BMJ 1982;284:869–870
17. Allan SG, Rodger A, Smyth JF et al: Tamoxifen as primary treatment of breast cancer in elderly or frail patients: a practical management. BMJ 1985;290:358
18. Helleberg A, Lundren B, Norin T, Sanders S: Treatment of early localised breast cancer in elderly patients by tamoxifen. Br J Radiol 1982;55:511–515
19. Gazet J-C, Markopoulos C, Ford HT et al: Prospective randomised trial of tamoxifen versus surgery in elderly patients with breast cancer. Lancet 1988;1:679–681
20. Howell A, Bush H, George WD et al: Controlled trial of adjuvant chemotherapy with cyclophosphamide, methotrexate and fluorouracil for breast cancer. Lancet 1984;2:307–311
21. Bates T, Riley D, Houghton J et al: Breast cancer in elderly women; a Cancer Research Campaign trial comparing treatment with tamoxifen and optimal surgery with tamoxifen alone. Br J Surg 1991;78:591–594

CHAPTER 71

Aging and the Endocrine System

IOAN DAVIES

The endocrine system detects and integrates humoral and sensory information to regulate physiologic function—the process of homeostasis. Age-associated declines in physiologic performance are well-documented and it is accepted that the basis of this decline is a *failure of homeostasis*. The conventional view is that "normal" aging changes predispose to age-related disease, and contribute to the poor recovery of elderly patients after intercurrent illness, or severe stresses such as surgery. The results of early studies of age-changes in endocrine function were frequently contradictory because investigators often failed to take sufficient account of other interfering factors (see box). This subject has been dealt with at length elsewhere.[1,2] Researchers using human subjects are employing increasingly more sophisticated selection procedures, particularly when attempting to define normative measures,[3] and subject selection and screening is rightly becoming a high priority for quality research.

The endocrine system may be involved in the progressive decline in function after sexual maturity, but whether it is the cause of these changes is not easy to determine. However, what currently are considered to be age-changes in the endocrine system can lead to pathologies that are very important; for example, modifications in mineral, glucose, water, and electrolyte metabolism are common in the elderly. Perhaps surprisingly, the equilibrium concentrations of the principal hormones are not necessarily altered with age,[4] but what may differ as we get older is the way we achieve equilibrium hormone levels, which implies changes in regulatory control. Thus, with advancing age, significant alterations in hormone production, metabolism, and action are found. The scale of the age-related changes is highly variable and sex-dependent. Whereas only subtle changes occur in pituitary dynamics, adrenal gland physiology, and thyroid function, the changes in glucose homeostasis, reproductive function, and calcium metabolism are more apparent.[4]

This chapter is about changes in the way that certain components of the endocrine system are regulated in old age, and how this may affect other functions in the body. It focuses on the hypothalamus and pituitary, or the neuroendocrine system, and examines the regulation of growth hormone secretion and the thyroid gland.

The Hypothalamus and Pituitary

Measurement of Function

The hypothalamus has a central homeodynamic role, although direct examination of its function in the living human subject, is difficult. Advances in molecular biologic techniques have given us better probes than ever before for the measurement of hypothalamic hormones. Measuring hypothalamic or pituitary function by assessing suppression, or stimulation, of secretion is a matter of routine. However, the importance of the confounding effect of serious illness must be appreciated.[5] Many changes in the pituitary gland are related to illness and laboratory reference ranges for pituitary function obtained from young ambulatory subjects are not appropriate for hospital in patients over the age of 75 years.[6] More sophisticated testing of pituitary function has involved repeated administration of releasing hormones in healthy young and elderly men.[7] Combined testing of the pituitary gland by administration of growth hormone-releasing hormone (GHRH), corticotropin-releasing hormone (CRH), gonadotropin-releasing hormone (GnRH), and thyrotropin-releasing hormone (TRH) has been proposed for clinical studies.[7] In one study elderly men had lower testosterone, free tri-iodothyronine (FT_3), and somatomedin-C levels than young men, while 17β-estradiol and inhibin were not significantly different, with all values being within normal laboratory limits. However, after challenge with a cocktail of intravenous GHRH, CRH, GnRH, and TRH, the elderly men differed from young men only for growth hormone (GH) and prolactin release at one time point.[7]

Some components of the neuroendocrine system increase in performance with age. The clearest example, in my view, is the increased sensitivity of the release of the antidiuretic hormone, arginine vasopressin (AVP) from the posterior pituitary, under osmotic challenge.[8,9] The secretion of AVP is significantly increased in health status defined old people, suggesting that their reduced water conservation is due to defects in the kidney.[9] Changes in the thirst response are controversial. Some investigators find a decline in thirst[10] and others no change.[9]

Hypothalamic Morphology

Most of the principal neuroendocrine nuclei in the hypothalamus are structurally intact in old age, although there is some loss of morphologic integrity of the suprachiasmatic nucleus (SCN) (see below).[11] Morphometric variables associated with increased cellular functional activity have been measured in several hypothalamic nuclei—supraoptic (SON), lateral tuberal (LTN), and lateral mammillary (LMN) nuclei—and some age-related declines were observed in all investigated structures, most obviously in the LTN. However, the size of neuron cell bodies and the number of neurons did not change signifi-

The aging endocrine system–potential interfering factors:

- Subject age—what age is old?
- Health status
- Method used to stimulate the endocrine axis under study
- The choice of stimulating ligand (i.e., is recombinant human material more effective than factors extracted from other species?)

cantly with age in any of these nuclei.[12] Earlier studies in laboratory rodents and humans of the numbers of neurons in the hypothalamus have found no consistent, age-related loss of cells in this region of the brain.

Certain neurons in the human paraventricular nucleus (PVN) seem activated.[13] The neurons that produce AVP increase in size, and the number of neurons that express both AVP and CRH, increase with age.[13] These data have important implications for vasopressinergic innervation of the brain, the modulation of neuronal function in the CNS, and possibly the endocrine control of water metabolism. Neuronal hypertrophy in a subpopulation of neurons in the infundibular nucleus also correlates with changes in the sex hormone secretion of postmenopausal women.[14] Studies in rodents have shown a reduced sensitivity of the hypothalamic–pituitary system to ovarian sex steroid feedback with increasing age and recent research suggests that in postmenopausal women a similar process is taking place.[15,16] It has been argued that the hypothalamus of postmenopausal women shows impaired negative feedback sensitivity to ovarian sex steroids, which interferes with the central neurotransmitter activity governing GnRH secretion.[16] However, despite the development of intrinsic age-related defects, at all levels of the hypothalamic-pituitary-testicular axis reproductive capacity is maintained in most healthy, elderly men,[17] but the frequency of sexual activity declines dramatically with age.

The Regulation of Circadian Rhythms

Morphologic alterations in the hypothalamus suggest disruption of hypothalamic nuclei that control circadian rhythms. One autopsy study showed alterations in the diurnal oscillations of AVP immunoreactive neurons in the SCN of old people.[11] Others have investigated the circadian rhythms of plasma melatonin, ACTH, cortisol, and oral temperature in healthy young and old women.[18] Elderly subjects exhibited a reduction of the mean level, and of the amplitude of the circadian rhythm of oral temperature. The mean level of ACTH and cortisol rhythms increased, and nocturnal melatonin secretion was selectively impaired in old women. Elderly subjects also showed a reduced sensitivity to the dexamethasone suppression test. These changes could depend either on CNS modification, or on alterations of the hormonal metabolic clearance.[18]

Many studies of the anterior pituitary show unchanged output of stimulating hormones, although the peripheral levels of target hormones have decreased (see below). The evidence suggests those age-changes in hormone levels are not simply related to concentrations of hormones in the hypothalamus, anterior pituitary, or peripheral circulation, but also with rhythms in their secretion. Twenty-four-hour profiles of cortisol, thyroid-stimulating hormone (TSH), melatonin, prolactin, and GH levels were compared in healthy young and old men.[19] Mean cortisol levels in the older men were normal, but the amplitude of the circadian rhythm was reduced. Circulating levels of day- and nighttime levels of both TSH and GH were greatly diminished in old age. In contrast, prolactin and melatonin concentrations were decreased during the night only. The circadian rises of cortisol, TSH, and melatonin occurred 1 to 1.5 hours earlier in elderly subjects, and the distribution of rapid eye movement (REM) stages during sleep was similarly advanced, suggesting that circadian timekeeping is modified during normal senescence. Despite perturbations of sleep, sleep-related release of GH and prolactin occurred in all elderly men. Age-related decreases in hormonal levels were associated with a decrease in the amplitude, but not the frequency, of secretory pulses. These findings suggest that aging influences those central mechanisms controlling the timing of hormone release.[19]

Hypothalamic Regulation—Receptors and Neurotransmitters

As well as morphologic robustness, there is some degree of receptor stability in the hypothalamus. For example, the distribution and properties of $\alpha 2$-adrenoreceptors in many regions of the brain, including the hypothalamus, are not affected by age.[20] However, there are many gaps in our knowledge regarding age changes in neurotransmitter function. Most of the data have been derived from the study of laboratory rodents, but uncertainties far outnumber demonstrated causative relationships between changes in neurotransmitter release and age-associated changes in hormone secretion. A decline in function of the tuberoinfundibular dopamine system is responsible, in part, for the age-related elevation in prolactin secretion, and may be involved in the decline in luteinizing hormone (LH) secretion. An age-associated reduction in hypothalamic noradrenaline turnover plays a role in the reduced LH and GH secretion, and may be involved in altered TSH secretion with age. A postulated decline in the circadian activity of SCN serotoninergic neurons may account for the age-associated blunting of circadian rhythms of several anterior pituitary hormones.[21] Other areas of hypothalamic regulation are becoming more accessible to study with the arrival of new molecular probes.

Clearly, a qualitative preservation of hypothalamic and pituitary secretion has emerged from these investigations, but the critical aspect of hypothalamopituitary regulation is the timing and size of the secretory bursts. The temporal organization of the secretory patterns of this axis is usually critical and this is what may be affected in both rodents and humans. The female reproductive cycle depends on carefully timed surges of hormone secretion, as does growth in the early stages of development. Is it this aspect of endocrine regulation that is most affected with age? The remainder of this chapter is a discussion of two hormone systems that are crucial in the early stages of development for the correct growth of bodily components. The importance of these hormone systems later in the life span has been revealed through conventional treatment of old people with hormone supplements.

Growth Hormone and Aging

The somatotrophic effects of GH are mediated through the actions of either circulating insulin-like peptides and/or, local insulin-like peptides (by autocrine or paracrine effects). Most, if not all, of the circulating somatomedin activity in humans can be accounted for by insulin-like growth factors I and II (IGF-I, IGF-II). Levels of circulating IGF-I and IGF-II are affected by GH, but the former is more sensitive. Levels of circulating IGF-I in humans are low at birth, rise progressively during childhood, and peak during mid-adolescence. The normal increase in stature during adolescence, is probably the result of the increase in circulating IGF-I. Following adolescence levels of circulating IGF-I fall progressively with age, and is associated with a decreased secretion of GH. Changes in IGF-II are small as a function of increasing age.[22] Low levels of GH are also a feature of old age in other primates,[23] and rats, although the decrease is seen at an earlier age in females.[24,25]

Circulating GH concentrations in man fluctuate widely due to pulsatile GH secretion by the pituitary. Time series analysis of plasma GH levels show dynamic fluctuations of more than three orders of magnitude.[26] GH pulses occur with an average frequency of about 13 per day in both sexes, with a dominant, but not strictly periodic, 2-hour rhythm. Thus, the pulsatile secretion of GH in man is oscillatory rather than episodic.[26] Somatomedin levels decrease substantially with age in healthy men, which may be partially responsible for the age-associated catabolic effects on muscle and bone.[27,28] It has been proposed that the declining activity of the GH-IGF-I axis with advancing age may contribute to the age-associated decrease in lean body mass, and the increase in adipose tissue mass.[27]

Replacement Therapy with Growth Hormone

The reduction in muscle mass with age can be increased by treatment with GH.[29] Treatment of men, with GH levels below 350 U/L, by subcutaneous injections of biosynthetic human GH for 6 months, led to significant increases in plasma IGF-I, lean body mass, and lumbar vertebral bone density, and a decrease in adipose tissue mass. Skin thickness tended to increase. However, no significant change in bone density of the radius or proximal femur was detected. In controls, lean body mass, the mass of adipose tissue, skin thickness, and bone density during treatment remained unchanged.[29] Malnourished elderly people (weight 20 percent below average body weight, and serum albumin less than 3.8 g/dl) benefitted from daily intramuscular injections of recombinant human GH for 21 days.[30] During this period mid-arm muscle circumference increased an average of 0.6 cm in the treated group, compared with a fall in saline injected controls. Weight increased by an average of 2.2 kg in the group treated with GH, but decreased by an average of 2.2 kg in the controls. Urinary nitrogen retention occurred only in the GH-treated subjects. IGF-I rose significantly in those treated with GH, but was unchanged in the controls. Furthermore, there was a significant association between weight change and IGF-I concentration. Neither clinical edema nor hyperglycemia was noted. These findings suggest GH may be an effective way of maintaining and enhancing weight in malnourished older people.[30] Furthermore, aged muscle tissue can respond to GH stimulation by increasing in mass, although to my knowledge, strength has not been assessed.

Growth Hormone Regulation

The mean basal plasma GH level is similar in healthy young and old men. However, the total GH peak area, and the amplitude of the peaks, is significantly lower in old men, although the frequency of secretory pulses is unchanged. This suggests that a threshold level of GH is not being reached in older people. Plasma somatomedin-C levels are significantly lower in old men.[19,31] However, despite sleep perturbations the sleep-related release of GH occurred in all elderly men. These, and other data related to age-associated diurnal variations in neuroendocrine control, suggest that circadian timekeeping is modified with age.[19] Similarly, aged nonhuman primates (rhesus monkeys) experience a reduction in plasma GH and fewer nocturnal GH pulses.[32]

The effect of age on GH secretory responses to indirect,[33–36] and direct stimulation by GHRH-mediated GH secretion in healthy older men, is controversial. Serum levels of somatomedin-C were significantly lower in older men both before, and 24 hours after, a single intravenous injection of GHRH.[37] However, others claim that GHRH-induced increases of GH are unchanged. Priming GH-secretion with a β-blocker (propranalol) caused a significant rise in both basal and peak GHRH-stimulated increases in GH despite age.[38] This treatment is likely to affect the basal GH secretory tone and not GHRH-stimulated GH-secretion. A priming dose of human pituitary GHRH (hpGHRH) also increased the GH response to GHRH. This suggests an age-associated decline in the sensitivity of somatotrophs to GHRH stimulation, and that repetitive administration of GHRH could restore the attenuated response.[39] Oral administration of GHRP-6 in normal elderly subjects over 4 days shows a trend toward an increase in IGF-I levels after treatment.[40] Furthermore, low doses of either intravenous or oral arginine can enhance the GH response to GHRH in elderly subjects.[41] The response is dose-dependent and the authors argue that combined administration of GHRH and arginine may be a useful approach to restore the impaired function of the GH-IGF axis in aging. A subsequent study suggested that a dosing regime involving intravenous injection of arginine combined with GHRH maintained a high GH response up to 15 days later.[42]

The age-associated decrease in GH may be due to either increased hypothalamic somatostatin release, or to decreased secretion of GHRH. Somatostatin secretion is inhibited by the cholinergic system, and several investigators have tried to manipulate "central cholinergic tone".[43,44] GH secretion, after treatment with physostigmine, a cholinergic agonist, is increased with age.[45] α-Glyceryl-phosphorylcholine (a putative acetylcholine precursor) has a potentiating effect on GH secretion that is more pronounced in elderly people.[46] Others have examined the effect of intravenous injection of GHRH, either alone, or in combination with pyridostigmine (a cholinesterase inhibitor), or arginine, on GH release.[47] Serum IGF-I levels were significantly lower in the old subjects, and the GHRH-induced GH increase was lower in elderly people.[47] Pyridostigmine significantly increased the GH response to GHRH in both groups, but the response was lower in the old subjects. Simultaneous administration of arginine potentiated the GHRH-induced release of GH, in both young and old groups. The increase was greater than that found after pyridostigmine and GHRH in the elderly, but not in young subjects. Of the elderly subjects 61.3 percent had a GH peak below the limit observed for normal young adults after combined pyridostigmine and GHRH administration, while arginine with GHRH elicited a normal GH peak in all but one old person. Finally, it has been shown that pyridostigmine treatment followed by an intravenous injection of TRH can stimulate the release of GH in euthyroid, old subjects.[48] In healthy elderly men (65 to 88 years), the GH response to G-DAMME (a guanyl derivative of the opioid analog D-ala2,MePhe4-Met-enkephalin-(o)-ol) was reduced or absent, while prompt GH release was found in all young men.[49]

In rodents, the marked decline in pituitary response to GHRH contributes to the decline in amplitude of GH pulses with age.[50] At the receptor-signal transduction level in the anterior pituitary, a diminished cAMP response to GHRH has been recorded[51], and GHRH-stimulated adenylate cyclase activity is reduced by 50 percent in senescent rats.[52] The data suggest an age-associated, selective loss of functional GHRH receptors, but much of the postreceptor signal transduction mechanism was intact.[52] The GH response to an intravenous bolus of GHRH, morphine, and clonidine is dramatically reduced, or absent in old male and female rats.[25] Age-associated changes in GHRH-binding sites may precede, or even initiate the GH impairment.[53]

In aged rats, major alterations in brain neurotransmitters and neuropeptides are present in hypothalamic and extrahypothalamic structures, especially in catecholaminergic and acetylcholinergic neurons.[54] These alterations are probably due to defects in neurosecretory GHRH and somatostatin neurons. Although the expression of somatostatin seems to decrease with age in the rat hypothalamus, secretion and activity of this hormone is increased, resulting in an altered relationship between GHRH and somatostatin gene expression and secretion. Age-associated variations in the mRNAs of GH and somatostatin have been measured in rats of both sexes by quantitative in situ hybridization with cDNA probes.[55,56] Because a gradual decline in somatostatin mRNA was observed in middle-aged and aging rats of both sexes, it has been suggested that middle age and aging are probably not a consequence of an increase of somatostatin activity.[56] Furthermore, the GHRH-induced GH secretion is differentially affected by the inhibiting action of somatostatin, suggesting a loss of pituitary sensitivity to somatostatin in the presence of a high concentration of GHRH. Old rats stimulated with both GHRH and a synthetic GHRH-6, show a robust and immediate GH secretion when compared with animals challenged only with GHRH. These data suggest that the cellular processes involved in GH secretion are intact in old rats, and that age-related decrements in GH secretion may result from inadequate stimulation, rather than defective GH release.[57]

Somatotrophic effects are mediated through binding proteins. Although the number and size of serum IGF-binding proteins (IGF-BPs) do not change with age, the IGF-BP binding ratios for certain of the binding proteins were lower in older subjects. In contrast, the 34K IGF-BP binding ratio was significantly greater in the elderly than in the young and correlated closely with advancing age. In vitro several IGF-BPs are known to modulate the mitogenic activity of IGF-I; the age-associated changes in serum IGF-BP may be an important factor in the regulation of connective tissue, muscle, and bone with age.[58] However, the role of GH in regulating GH-binding protein (GHBP) and GH-receptor concentration in humans is not clear.[59]

Thyroid Function and Aging

Changes in Thyroid Hormones

Thyroid disease in the elderly is common, but often has an insidious onset with symptoms that mimic those of normal aging.[60] Because of this similarity in symptoms, the significance of thyroid function tests takes on new importance, and their interpretation requires a recognition of the so-called "normal" physiologic variations of aging and the complicating effects of diseases and medications. Screening for thyroid disease in the elderly has been advocated by some reviewers.[61]

A series of longitudinal studies from Sweden established the pattern of thyroid hormone changes in old people, at least for this Scandinavian population. The results suggested that while valuable information can be obtained by screening, the clinical signs and symptoms of thyroid disease in the elderly may be too subtle for diagnosis.[62] Two other surveys of thyroid function in subjects with a greater range ages were also conducted. In one large study of 81-year-olds it was shown that of 144 men only 2 had markedly abnormal values of serum

TSH and serum-free thyroxine (FT_4). In these two cases L-thyroxine treatment had been prescribed for both, one because of primary hypothyroidism (concentrations at screening were high for TSH and low for FT_4) and one because of panhypopituitarism (low FT_4 at screening). Among 250 women, 10 had TSH concentrations greater than 10 m U/L; L-thyroxine therapy had been prescribed for 3 of them. Only one woman, who had not been treated with L-thyroxine, had a high FT_4 concentration, and she had few clinical signs and symptoms of hyperthyroidism (mainly weight loss), and multinodular goiter. However, her records showed that "T_4-toxicosis" had been present for at least 11 years without evidence of progression of her hyperthyroidism.[63] The data led to the conclusion that most elderly individuals with low-serum TSH concentrations are not hyperthyroid, and that abnormal thyroxine-binding globulin (with drug treatment or nonthyroidal illness), is not a common cause of low thyrotropin concentration.[64]

T_3 and T_4 have been implicated in age-related changes for many years. The success of treatment for hypothyroidism (myxoedema) using synthetic thyroid hormones generated considerable interest in the possible role of thyroid deficiency with increasing age. The thyroid gland undergoes a progressive decrease in size with aging, although enlargement due to the presence of nodules is not uncommon. These nodules consist of sites of focal tissue proliferation with overlapping areas of cell involution. The prevalence of multinodular goiter may be as high as 70 percent in women more than 60 years of age. Evaluation of these nodules shows that although they are more frequent they are likely to be benign, but thyroid cancer has been reported in about 5 percent of patients with nodular goiter, regardless of age.[65]

The concentration of thyroid hormones found in the blood of old human subjects is still a matter of some debate.[66] It has been suggested that aging changes are due to the variability of responses to various stimuli, and the confounding influence of disease (see box). T_4 is the hormone most in doubt. Total and FT_4, levels may be unchanged, decreased, or increased depending on age, sex, and health status.[67] However, many studies of T_4 concentrations show no change with age though thyroid secretion may have decreased by upward of 50 percent.[68] On the other hand, it is generally accepted that plasma T_3 decreases with age,[66,69] although it is also argued that this decline is only found in old people with disease or a poor diet.[66,70]

Factors influencing age-associated changes in thyroid hormone concentrations

- A simultaneous decreased T3 secretion from the thyroid gland and increased degradation, metabolism, and excretion of the hormone
- Reduced T4 to T3 conversion in peripheral tissues
- A simultaneous reduction in secretion and metabolic clearance of T4 which results in essentially normal plasma levels of this hormone

Aging Changes

Despite the relative normality of the pituitary-thyroid axis in normal subjects under experimental conditions, there is a wealth of evidence arguing for an altered thyroid state in old people. One common feature of many studies of the endocrine system is aged-associated alterations in the responsiveness of target tissues. Several investigations have focused on the target cell signaling responses to endocrine stimulation. In the case of the thyroid, the receptors for T_3 are in the nucleus, mitochondria, plasma membrane, and cytosol. Studies of age-associated changes in receptor number have suggested no decrease with age, although in the light of declining levels of T_3 in the plasma, an increase in receptor number would have been anticipated. Timiras[66] argues that an age-related reduction in the ability of aged tissues to increase receptor numbers in response to a reduction in hormone levels suggests a fundamental alteration in cellular responsiveness with age. This is a field that requires much more research.

The reduction in thyroid hormone levels with increasing age is correlated with many physiologic and pathologic sequelae. The major actions of thyroid hormones are in directing growth and development, although these functions cease upon maturity. This seems an unlikely scenario, and clearly, the removal of thyroid hormones has important effects on physiologic function. Although there is a decline in basal metabolic rate with age, the role of thyroid hormones are not fully understood. The thyroid is heavily implicated in the age-associated impairment in thermoregulation. The reduced cellular demand reflected in a loss of lean body mass has been debated for many years, but there is uncertainty about whether the changes observed are due to reduced hormonal secretion or reduced cellular demand. Changes in cholesterol metabolism accompany hypothyroidism, and the implications for the cardiovascular system is obvious. However, the effect of reduced thyroid hormone output extends beyond cholesterol metabolism. Thyroid hormones interact with catecholamines to affect cardiac output by influencing heart rate and the strength of contraction. Finally, the frequency of antithyroid antibodies that are directed against the TSH receptors on thyroid cells is increased with age, particularly in women more than 70-years-old. The incidence of Grave's and Hashimoto's diseases, putative autoimmune diseases of the thyroid, increases with age. The cause of these diseases is unknown but the immune system is strongly implicated.[66,71]

Thyroid Function Tests

The secretion of TSH by the anterior pituitary is modulated by TRH and the plasma concentrations of T_3 and T_4. Administration of exogenous TRH to subjects increases the concentrations of circulating TSH and the thyroid hormones. This test shows that TSH responses are maintained into old age in women,[72,73] although this is not necessarily the case for men.[66,73] One study reported decreased basal and stimulated TSH secretion in healthy elderly men without thyroid antibodies.[74] In these subjects the total 24-hour secretion of TSH was reduced, and the pituitary was less responsive to stimulation by TRH. However, the chronobiologic modulation was preserved. These alterations could reflect an adaptive mechanism to the reduced need for thyroid hormones in old age, but that the thyroid maintains a capacity to respond to acute increases in TSH concentration.[74] Others suggest a role for dopaminergic regulation in the pulsatile secretion of TSH.[75] The baseline thyroid function tests include serum T_3, T_3 resin uptake, TSH, and the response of TSH to TRH, and were all within normal limits in both the young and old subjects. Antimicrosomal and antithyroglobulin antibodies were absent in all participants.[75] Pulsatile TSH secretion was identified in all subjects, and as a group there were significant increases in nocturnal peak height, amplitude, and mean TSH. However, the night time amplitude of the TSH pulse did not increase significantly in old subjects. After the administration of metoclopramide there was a significant increase in peak height, amplitude, and mean TSH, but the effect of metoclopramide was different in young and old subjects. In the young subjects, daytime administration of metoclopramide increased both TSH pulse height and the mean TSH, but the pulse parameters remained unchanged at night. In the old subjects after metoclopramide, pulse parameters were unchanged during the day, but pulse amplitude increased significantly at night.[75] It has also been shown that glucocorticoids have an inhibitory role on the thyrotropic axis and that normal elderly men are hyporesponsive to this suppressant effect of corticosteroids.[76]

Clearly, the issues surrounding aging and thyroid function have extensive implications for the clinician. However, the fundamental question for aging relates to whether the thyroid undergoes a decline in function, or whether it is responding to altered cell and tissue requirements in target organs. Sadly, there is not any progress regarding this question. Much of the research centers on the clinical component of the thyroid in aged people, and this is clearly related to several different factors, of which age is a component.

However, one study is of interest in this regard.[77] This investigation examined the influence of age and endurance training on metabolic rate and hormones in healthy men. The associations among ages, maximal aerobic capacity (VO_{2max}), and body composition with resting metabolic rate (RMR), and fasting plasma hormones were examined in endurance-trained, and untrained younger and older men. A significantly higher RMR, normalized per kilogram of fat-free weight (FFW), was found in endurance-trained younger and older men compared with untrained men. VO_{2max}, independent of FFW, accounted for a significant portion of the variation in RMR. Fasting insulin and the fasting insulin-to-glucose ratios were higher in older men compared with younger men. This difference was diminished when differences in percent body fat were taken into account. Plasma thyroid hormones and glucagon were not associated with age, VO_{2max}, or percent body fat and the investigators concluded that endurance-trained and older men have a higher RMR than untrained younger and older men independent of differences in FFW.[77] I have not found any follow-up to this study, but it highlights the potential beneficial effect of exercise and careful diet in the maintenance of good physiologic function and suggests strongly that plasma levels of thyroid hormones are not influenced by age, VO_{2max}, or adiposity in healthy nonobese men.

Conclusion

The evidence discussed above gives support to the idea that manipulation of the endocrine milieu can influence some aspects of age-associated change. It is also evident, at least circumstantially, that neurotransmitters and neuroendocrine factors regulating hypothalamic function, and thus, anterior pituitary hormone secretion, must be intimately involved in aging. The age-related decrease in turnover of hypothalamic noradrenaline is involved in the decline of LH and GH secretion. The age-associated decline in circadian activity of 5-HT neurons in the SCN may account for altered circadian rhythms in the secretions of several anterior pituitary hormones with age. Administration of drugs that increase hypothalamic noradrenaline and dopamine activity can delay, or reverse, these events.[21] The hyposomatotropism of aging has been linked to a progressive defect in hypothalamic neurons producing GHRH, although alterations of somatostatin-producing neurons have also been implicated.[78,79]

Some aspects of the age-associated changes in body composition can be reversed by GH therapy. However, even though the benefits of treating adults with GH deficiency are well recognized, the criteria for deciding on which patients to treat are not clear,[80] and the standard insulin stress test (IST) is unpleasant and potentially dangerous. Furthermore, careful long-term clinical trials are necessary with development of specific targeting criteria before conclusions regarding efficacy and benefits can be decided.[81] In addition, it is still not clear what role the thyroid gland has in the metabolism of the healthy old person. In health there does not seem to be a major defect, but in ill health the matter is very different.

The neuroendocrine system seems to be a major factor in the age-associated failure in homeostasis. The maintenance of life relies on correct gene expression, and in order to function appropriately the organism also has to integrate gene expression in a large number of systems simultaneously. Although neuroendocrine and endocrine effects may not be the primary cause of the age-associated decline in function, they are capable of modifying certain of the associated phenomena, and can restore certain functions. The introduction of therapeutic measures designed to re-establish homeostatic control may ameliorate the rate of deterioration in older organisms leading to modification of the effects of advancing age and improving the quality of life of the elderly. However, if the current ideas about the cellular and molecular mechanisms of aging are correct, then the effects of these manipulations can only be temporary.

References

1. Rowe JW: Clinical research on aging: strategies and directions. N Engl J Med 1977;297:1332–1336
2. Minaker KL, Meneilly GS, Rowe JW: Endocrine systems. pp. 433–456. In Finch CE, Schneider EL (eds): Handbook of the Biology of Aging. Van Nostrand Reinhold, New York, 1985
3. Lighthart GJ, Corberand JX, Fournier C et al: Admission criteria for immunogerontological studies in man: the Senieur protocol. Mech Ageing Dev 1984;28:47–55
4. Mooradian AD, Morley JE, Korenman SG: Endocrinology in aging. Dis Mon 1988;34:393–461
5. Van den Berghe G, de Zegher F, Lauwers P, Veldhuis JD: Luteinizing hormone secretion and hypoandrogenaemia in critically ill men: effect of dopamine. Clin Endocrinol 1994;41: 563–569
6. Impallomeni M, Yeo T, Rudd A et al: Investigation of anterior pituitary function in elderly in-patients over the age of 75. J Med 1987;63:505–515
7. Pontiroli AE, Ruga S, Maffi P et al: Pituitary reserve after repeated administration of releasing hormones in young and in elderly men: reproducibility on different days. J Endocrinol Invest 1992;15:559–566
8. Davies I, O'Neill PA: Aging in the hypothalamo-neurohypophysial-renal system. Geriatr Nephrol Urol 1993;3:93–106
9. Davies I, O'Neill PA, McLean KA et al: Age-associated alterations in thirst and arginine vasopressin in response to a water or sodium load. Age Ageing 1995;24:151–159
10. Phillips PA, Johnston CI, Gray L: Disturbed fluid and electrolyte homoeostasis following dehydration in elderly people. Age Ageing 1993;22:S26–S33
11. Hofman MA, Swaab DF: Alterations in circadian rhythmicity of the vasopressin-producing neurons of the human suprachiasmatic nucleus (SCN) with aging. Brain Res 1994;651:134–142
12. Morys J, Dziewiatkowski J, Switka A et al: Morphometric parameters of some hypothalamic nuclei: age-related changes. Folia Morphol (Warszaw) 1994;53:221–229
13. Raadsheer FC, Hoogendijk WJ, Stam FC et al: Increased numbers of corticotropin-releasing hormone expressing neurons in the hypothalamic paraventricular nucleus of depressed patients. Neuroendocrinology 1994;60:436–444
14. Rance NE: Hormonal influences on morphology and neuropeptide gene expression in the infundibular nucleus of postmenopausal women. Prog Brain Res 1992;93:221–235
15. Rossmanith WG, Reichelt C, Scherbaum WA: Neuroendocrinology of aging in humans: attenuated sensitivity to sex steroid feedback in elderly postmenopausal women. Neuroendocrinology 1994;59:355–362
16. Rossmanith WG: Gonadotropin secretion during aging in women: review article. Exp Gerontol 1995;30:369–381
17. Tsitouras PD, Bulat T: The aging male reproductive system. Endocr Metab Clin North Am 1995;24:297–315
18. Ferrari E, Magri F, Dori D et al: Neuroendocrine correlates of the aging brain in humans. Neuroendocrinology 1995;61: 464–470
19. van Coevorden A, Mockel J, Laurent E et al: Neuroendocrine rhythms and sleep in aging men. Am J Physiol 1991;260: E651–661
20. Meana JJ, Barturen F, Garcia-Sevilla JA: Characterization and regional distribution of alpha 2-adrenoceptors in postmortem human brain using the full agonist [3H]UK 14304. J Neurochem 1989;52:1210–1217
21. Meites J: Neuroendocrine biomarkers of aging the rat. Exp Gerontol 1988;23:349–358
22. Hammerman MR: Insulin-like growth factors and aging. Endocrinol Metab Clin North Am 1987;16:995–1011
23. Wheeler MD, Schutzengel RE, Barry S, Styne DM: Changes in basal and stimulated growth hormone secretion in the aging rhesus monkey: a comparison of chair restraint and tether and vest sampling. J Clin Endocrinol Metab 1990;71:1501–1507
24. Takahashi S, Gottschall PE, Quigley KL et al: Growth hormone secretory patterns in young, middle-aged and old female rats. Neuroendocrinology 1987;46:137–142
25. Millard WJ, Romano TM, Simpkins JW: Growth hormone and thyrotropin secretory profiles and provocative testing in aged rats. Neurobiol Aging 1990;11:229–235
26. Winer LM, Shaw MA, Baumann G: Basal plasma growth hormone levels in man: new evidence for rhythmicity of growth hormone secretion. J Clin Endocrinol Metab 1990;70: 1678–1686
27. Rudman D: Growth hormone, body composition and aging. J Am Geriatr Soc 1985;33:800–807
28. Florini JR, Prinz PN, Vitiello MV, Hintz RL: Somatomedin-C levels in healthy young and old men: relationship to peak and 24-hour integrated levels of growth hormone. J Gerontol 1987; 40:2–7
29. Rudman D, Feller AG, Nagraj HS et al: Effects of human growth hormone in men over 60 years old. N Engl J Med 1990;323: 1–6
30. Kaiser FE, Silver AJ, Morley JE: The effect of recombinant human growth hormone on malnourished older individuals. J Am Geriatr Soc 1991;39:235–240
31. Vermeulen A: Nyctohemeral growth hormone profiles in young and aged men: correlation with somatomedin-C levels. J Clin Endocrinol Metab 1987;64:884–888
32. Kaler LW, Gliessman P, Craven J et al: Loss of enhanced nocturnal growth hormone secretion in aging rhesus males. Endocrinology 1986;119:1281–1284
33. Zadik Z, Chalew SA, McCarter RJ Jr et al: The influence of age on the 24-hour integrated concentration of growth hormone in normal individuals. J Clin Endocrinol Metab 1985;60: 513–516
34. Muggeo M, Moghetti P, Querena M et al: Effect of aging on growth hormone, ACTH and cortisol response to insulin-induced hypoglycemia in type I diabetes. Acta Diabet Lat 1985; 22:159–168
35. Giusti M, Lomeo A, Marini G et al: Role of aging on growth hormone and prolactin release after growth hormone-releasing hormone and domperidone in man. Horm Res 1987;27: 134–140
36. Monteleone P, Iovino M, Orio F, Steardo L: Impaired growth

hormone response to sodium valproate in normal aging. Psychopharmacology (Berlin) 1987;91:10–13

37. Pavlov EP, Harman SM, Merriam GR et al: Responses of growth hormone (GH) and somatomedin-C to GH-releasing hormone in healthy aging men. J Clin Endocrinol Metab 1986;62:595–600

38. Lang I, Kurz R, Geyr G, Tragl KH: The influence of age on human pancreatic growth hormone releasing hormone stimulated growth hormone secretion. Horm Metab Res 1988;20:574–578

39. Iovino M, Monteleone P, Steardo L: Repetitive growth hormone-releasing hormone administration restores the attenuated growth hormone (GH) response to GH-releasing hormone testing in normal aging. J Clin Endocrinol Metab 1989;69:910–913

40. Ghigo E, Arvat E, Rizzi G et al: Growth hormone-releasing activity of growth hormone-releasing peptide-6 is maintained after short-term oral pretreatment with the hexapeptide in normal aging. Eur J Endocrinol 1994;131:499–503

41. Ghigo E, Ceda GP, Valcavi R et al: Low doses of either intravenously or orally administered arginine are able to enhance growth hormone response to growth hormone releasing hormone in elderly subjects. J Endocrinol Invest 1994;17:113–117

42. Ghigo E, Ceda GP, Valcavi R et al: Effect of 15-day treatment with growth-hormone-releasing hormone alone or combined with different doses of arginine on the reduced somatotrope responsiveness to the neurohormone in normal aging. Eur J Endocrinol 1995;132:32–36

43. Giusti M, Marini G, Sessarego P et al: Growth hormone secretion in aging. Effect of pyridostigmine on growth hormone responsiveness to growth hormone-releasing hormone. Rec Prog Med 1991;82:665–668

44. Giusti M, Marini G, Sessarego P et al: Effect of cholinergic tone on growth hormone-releasing hormone-induced secretion of growth hormone in normal aging. Aging (Milano) 1992;4:231–237

45. Raskind MA, Peskind ER, Veith RC et al: Differential effects of aging on neuroendocrine responses to physostigmine in normal men. J Clin Endocrinol Metab 1990;70:1420–1425

46. Ceda GP, Ceresini G, Denti L et al: Alpha-glycerylphosphorylcholine administration increases the GH responses to GHRH of young and elderly subjects. Horm Metab Res 1992;24:119–121

47. Ghigo E, Goffi S, Arvat E et al: A neuroendocrinological approach to evidence an impairment of central cholinergic function in aging. J Endocrinol Invest 1992;15:665–670

48. Giusti M, Giovale M, Sessarego P et al: Cholinergic modulation of growth hormone, prolactin and thyroid stimulating hormone responses to thyrotropin-releasing hormone in normal aging. Rec Prog Med 1995;86:341–344

49. Giusti M, Delitala G, Marini G et al: The effect of a met-enkephalin analogue on growth hormone, prolactin, gonadotropins, cortisol and thyroid stimulating hormone in healthy elderly men. Acta Endocrinol (Copenhagen) 1992;127:205–209

50. Sonntag WE, Gough MA: Growth hormone releasing hormone induced release of growth hormone in aging male rats: dependence on pharmacological manipulation and endogenous somatostatin release. Neuroendocrinology 1988;47:482–488

51. Ceda GP, Valenti G, Butturini U, Hoffman AF: Diminished pituitary responsiveness to growth hormone-releasing factor in aging male rats. Endocrinology 1986;118:2109–2114

52. Robberecht P, Gillard M, Waelbroeck M et al: Decreased stimulation of adenylate cyclase by growth hormone-releasing factor in the anterior pituitary of old rats. Neuroendocrinology 1986;44:429–432

53. Abribat T, Deslauriers N, Brazeau P, Gaudreau P: Alterations of pituitary growth hormone-releasing factor binding sites in aging rats. Endocrinology 1991;128:633–635

54. Müller EE, Cella SG, De Gennaro Colonna V et al: Aspects of the neuroendocrine control of growth hormone secretion in ageing mammals. J Reprod Fertil 1993;46:99–114

55. Crew MD, Spindler SR, Walford RL, Koizumi A: Age-related decrease of growth hormone and prolactin gene expression in the mouse pituitary. Endocrinology 1987;121:1251–1255

56. Martinoli MG, Ouellet J, Rheaume E, Pelletier G: Growth hormone and somatostatin gene expression in adult and aging rats as measured by quantitative in situ hybridization. Neuroendocrinology 1991;54:607–615

57. Walker RF, Yang SW, Bercu BB: Robust growth hormone (GH) secretion in aged female rats co-administered GH-releasing hexapeptide (GHRP-6) and GH-releasing hormone (GHRH). Life Sci 1991;49:1499–1504

58. Donahue LR, Hunte SJ, Sherblom AP, Rosen C: Age-related changes in serum insulin-like growth factor-binding proteins in women. J Clin Endocrinol Metab 1990;71:575–579

59. Davila N, Alcaniz J, Salto L et al: Serum growth hormone-binding protein is unchanged in adult panhypopituitarism. J Clin Endocrinol Metab 1994;79:1347–1350

60. Francis T, Wartofsky L: Common thyroid disorders in the elderly. Postgrad Med J 1992;92:225–230

61. Martinez-Weber C, Wallack PF, Lefkowitz P, Davies TF: Prevalence of thyroid autoantibodies in ambulatory elderly women. Mt Sinai J Med 1993;60:156–160

62. Sundbeck G, Lundberg PA, Lindstedt G et al: Screening for thyroid disease in the elderly. Serum free thyroxine and thyrotropin concentrations in a representative population of 81-year-old women and men. Aging (Milano) 1991;3:31–37

63. Sundbeck G, Lundberg PA, Lindstedt G et al: Incidence and prevalence of thyroid disease in elderly women: results from the longitudinal population study of elderly people in Gothenburg, Sweden. Age Ageing 1991;20:291–298

64. Sundbeck G, Jagenburg R, Johansson PM et al: Clinical significance of low serum thyrotropin concentration by chemiluminometric assay in 85-year-old women and men. Arch Intern Med 1991;151:549–556

65. Sampson RJ, Woolner LB, Bahn RC, Kurland LT: Occult thyroid carcinoma in Olmsted County, Minnesota: prevalence at autopsy compared with that in Hiroshima and Nagasaki, Japan. Cancer 1974;34:2072

66. Timiras PS: Hormones of the thyroid and parathyroid glands. pp. 85–106. In Timiras PS, Quay WD, Vernadakis A (eds): Hormones and Aging. CRC Press, Boca Raton, 1995

67. Cavalieri TA, Chopra A, Bryman PN: When outside the norm is normal: interpreting lab data in the aged. Geriatrics 1992;47:66

68. Gregerman RI, Solomon N: Acceleration of thyroxine and triiodothyronine turnover during bacterial pulmonary infections and fever: implications for the functional state of the thyroid during stress and in senescence. J Clin Endocrinol Metab 1967;27:93

69. Mobbs CV: Neuroendocrinology of aging. pp.234–282. In Schneider EL, Rowe JW (eds): Handbook of the Biology of Aging. Academic Press, San Diego, 1995

70. Goichot B, Schlienger JL, Grunenberger F et al: Thyroid hormone status and nutrient intake in the free-living elderly. Interest of reverse triiodothyronine assessment. Eur J Endocrinol 1994;130:244–252

71. Levy EG: Thyroid disease in the elderly. Med Clin North Am 1991;75:151–167

72. Jaques C, Schlienger JL, Kissel C et al: TRH-induced TSH and prolactin responses in the elderly. Age Ageing 1987;16:181

73. Targum SD, Marshall LE, Magac-Harris K, Martin D: TRH tests in a healthy elderly population. Demonstration of gender differences. J Am Geriatr Soc 1989;37:533–536

74. van Coevorden A, Laurent E, Decoster C et al: Decreased basal and stimulated thyrotropin secretion in healthy elderly men. J Clin Endocrinol Metab 1989;69:177–185

75. Greenspan SL, Klibanski A, Rowe JW, Elahi D: Age-related alterations in pulsatile secretion of TSH: role of dopaminergic regulation. Am J Physiol 1991;260:E486–E491

76. Iovino M, Steardo L, Monteleone P: Impaired sensitivity of the hypothalamo-pituitary-thyroid axis to the suppressant effect of dexamethasone in elderly subjects. Psychopharmacology (Berlin) 1991;105:481–484

77. Poehlman ET, McAuliffe TL, Van Houten DR, Danforth E Jr: Influence of age and endurance training on metabolic rate and hormones in healthy men. Am J Physiol 1990;259:E66–E72

78. Simpkins JW, Millard WJ: Influence of age on neurotransmitter function. Endocrinol Metab Clin North Am 1987;16:893–917

79. Cocchi D: Age-related alterations in gonadotropin, adrenocorticotropin and growth hormone secretion. Aging Clin Exp Res 1992;4:103–113

80. Bates AS, Evans AJ, Jones P, Clayton RN: Assessment of GH status in adults with GH deficiency using serum growth hormone, serum insulin-like growth factor-I and urinary growth hormone excretion. Clin Endocrinol 1995;42:425–430

81. Shetty KR, Duthie EH Jr: Anterior pituitary function and growth hormone use in the elderly. Endocrinol Metab Clin North Am 1995;24:213–231

CHAPTER 72

Pituitary and Adrenal Disorders in Old Age

PAUL E. BELCHETZ

PETER HAMMOND

Adrenal Cortical Disorders

The need for normal adrenal function continues into old age. After decades of speculation, there is now firm evidence that the patterns of basal and stimulated levels of cortisol secretion are substantially unchanged in the healthy aging population compared with younger people. Subtle age-related changes have been described regarding the metabolism of adrenal hormones and morphologic features such as nodules appear quite commonly in the aging adrenal glands. Their importance arises from much readier and often serendipitous recognition as advanced imaging techniques are more widely used. It is, therefore, relevant to open this chapter with a resumé of the physiologic and biochemic actions of adrenal steroids, mechanisms controlling their secretion, and techniques available for assessing the function and anatomy of the adrenal glands.

Physiological Responses to Adrenocortical Steroids

Of the multitude of steroids found in the adrenal cortex, only the secretion of cortisol and aldosterone have undisputed and vital endocrine roles. The distinction between glucocorticoid and mineralocorticoid hormone actions is based on physiologic observations, backed by differential effects on critical enzyme systems in target tissues.

Glucocorticoids

Cortisol (hydrocortisone) is the natural glucocorticoid of man and most other mammals (but not the rat, which is unable to synthesize cortisol and uses corticosterone instead). It has been long recognized that cortisol, especially in high doses, has mineralocorticoid properties and this has led to the widespread use of dexamethasone, a synthetic glucocorticoid, effectively without mineralocorticoid properties as the "benchmark" glucocorticoid.[1]

This practice has passed from laboratory experiments to clinical investigation as will be discussed below. There are growing reasons to question the validity of such assumptions although the pragmatic clinical tests have proven value. There has previously been a tendency to subdivide the actions of glucocorticoids into those seen at low doses and termed physiologic, and those seen with high doses, classically causing cushingoid side effects, as pharmacologic. There is no sound scientific basis for this differentiation as new effects are not seen with high doses, although the clinical sequelae are, of course, striking.

The term *glucocorticoid* derives from the effects on carbohydrate metabolism: antagonism of insulin action, promotion of hepatic glycogen synthesis, and participation in the defenses against hypoglycemia. It may affect resource utilization by virtue of tissue differences in response of the key glycolytic enzyme, phosphoenol pyruvate carboxykinase.[2] Glucocorticoids have many other actions, often permissive in nature. These include vascular and renal responses affecting control of blood pressure and extracellular water content. Other critical roles include actions on protein and lipid synthesis and complex interactions with the immune system. In addition there is the well-recognized but poorly characterized function that enhanced glucocorticoid secretion plays in combating stress. The stimuli recognized as stressful and capable of evincing enhanced cortisol secretion are numerous, including: fever, trauma, hemorrhage, and plasma-volume depletion, hypoglycemia, and even psychological disturbance. A unifying hypothesis is thus hard to achieve, but with regard to inflammatory processes, it is now widely believed that the role of glucocorticoids is to curtail the effects of the rapidly responding cytokine and acute phase protein production, which if protracted could be potentially damaging.[3]

Mineralocorticoids

The action of aldosterone is ostensibly simpler, operating primarily via renal mechanisms to control extracellular sodium and potassium levels with secondary consequences on fluid balance and blood pressure. The effects of mineralocorticoids on other tissues such as the colon, brain, and pituitary are documented, but their significance is much less certain. The secretion of aldosterone and its circadian rhythm are maintained in the elderly despite a decrease in tonic levels of renin, its principal regulator.[4]

Adrenal androgens

The adrenal cortex also synthesizes androgens. These include androstenedione and dehydroepiandrosterone; much of the latter is conjugated and secreted as the sulfate. The function of adrenal androgens remains obscure, although much has been made of the phenomenon in childhood of the so-called adrenarche, when enhanced amounts are made from about the age of 7 years. By contrast with cortisol production, there is a well-documented fall in adrenal androgen production in old age, to as little as 5 percent of young adult levels, with decreased ACTH responsiveness, which has been termed the adrenopause.[5]

Apart from effects on body hair, it is not at all clear what function the secretion of adrenal androgens serves in normal adults. It has been postulated that the decline in dehydroepiandrosterone levels is, in part, responsible for the increased atherogenesis and, hence, cardiovascular disease in old age, but recent evidence does not support this hypothesis.[6] It appears more likely that dehydroepiandrosterone has an immunomodulatory, and possibly antioncogenic, action. Dehydroepiandrosterone replacement in the elderly increases natural killer (NK) cell cytotoxicity and is claimed to dramatically improve the sense of physical and psychological well being.[7]

Biochemical Actions of Steroid Hormones

The effects of hormones on tissues depend on the distribution of specific receptors. Recent advances in knowledge have simultaneously clarified aspects of steroid hormone action and raised paradoxes that await definitive resolution. Steroids are lipophilic and readily enter cells: steroid receptors are intracellular. The classic model of steroid action is that steroid hormones bind to cytoplasmic receptors, forming activated complexes that are translocated to the nucleus where specific genes are activated, leading eventually to protein products as the end point of hormone influence.[8] A similar pattern was proposed for the structurally dissimilar thyroid hormones. Molecular cloning techniques have not only revealed that all steroid hormone receptors show strong homologies to each other and the proto-oncogene *c*-erb A, but that the latter actually appears to be a thyroid-hormone receptor. All these receptors share homologies, both in the hormone and the DNA-binding domains, and can be regarded as constituting a superfamily of genes, whose products are transcriptional regulatory proteins evolved from a common ancestor gene.[9] The steroid-hormone receptor is bound to a protein complex containing the heat shock proteins hsp 90, hsp 70, and hsp 65. Exposure to steroid hormone leads to dissociation of the receptor from the complex so that the receptor is able to bind the hormone.[10]

The new complex of hormone plus receptor adopts a different molecular conformation, exposing the DNA-binding domain of the receptor. Thus far, the generalized scheme for steroid hormones applies to glucocorticoids. When it comes to identifying the molecular basis for mineralocorticoid and glucocorticoid actions, difficulties arise. The type-1 receptor —originally considered to bind mineralocorticoids with higher affinity than glucocorticoids—show no such distinction with more modern techniques. Indeed, there is a marked kinship shown at the molecular level as well.[11,12] A possible explanation for the failure of the great molar excess of cortisol to swamp the type-1 receptor with regard to aldosterone binding has been suggested for tissues such as kidney, gut, and salivary glands. These tissues posses a potent 11-hydroxysteroid dehydrogenase enzyme system, which rapidly converts cortisol to cortisone, and cortisone does not bind measurably to the receptor.[13]

Acting through the genome, glucocorticoids enhance several key metabolic enzymes such as hepatic tyrosine aminotransferase[14] and tryptophan oxygenase.[15] In addition to this classic mode of action, it has also been suggested that many of the actions of glucocorticoids on the immune system are mediated by a specific protein product termed lipocortin, which acts as a second messenger.[16] The major site of action of lipocortin is thought to be on phospholipase A_2 and blocking the arachidonic acid pathways to prostaglandins and other inflammatory mediators.

Regulation of Adrenal Function

Regulation of glucocorticoid production

Cortisol secretion is under the immediate control of pituitary ACTH secretion acting to promote the conversion of cholesterol to pregnenolone by the removal of the six-carbon fragment from the cholesterol side-chain. These steps occur within the mitochondrion. A complex cascade of cytochrome-P450 variants has been implicated as steroidogenesis proceeds, shuttling from mitochondrion to endoplasmic reticulum and back. The chronic effects of ACTH affect many more steps in steroidogenesis than just cholesterol side-chain cleavage.[17]

Physiologic control of ACTH secretion involves three major areas: circadian rhythms, stress, and negative feedback inhibition by cortisol. ACTH is synthesized as part of a large 31-kDA precursor polypeptide pro-opiomelanocortin.[18] This is cleaved and the major fragments, including ACTH and β-endorphin, are usually cosecreted in equimolar proportions. The stimulus to ACTH release is from the hypothalamus by way of the hypothalamopituitary portal vessels conveying corticotrophin-releasing factors.[19]

These are a complex of polypeptides, the major constituent of which is a 41-residue moiety, corticotrophin-releasing hormone (CRH). However, this alone has less potent ACTH-releasing properties than crude hypothalamic extracts. It has been shown that vasopressin (AVP) and probably other, as yet unidentified, compounds act synergistically with CRH.[20] The secretion of these corticotrophin-releasing factors appears to be pulsatile-driving pulses —driving pulses of ACTH and cortisol in turn. The circadian rhythm is composed of pulses of varying amplitudes and frequency, with a nadir reached at midnight, but the onset of activity at about 03.00 to 04.00 hours reaching a peak at 08.00 to 09.00 hours. The pulses of ACTH and cortisol decline in size and frequency thereafter, although there is often a secondary rise at about lunchtime which seems to be related to food ingestion.[21]

As mentioned earlier, there is a formidable array of apparently unrelated stressors that can stimulate the release of ACTH and cortisol. There is preliminary evidence that the relative importance of CRH, AVP, and oxytocin varies according to the stimulus.[22] Where inflammation is involved, there is growing evidence for interleukin-1, interleukin-6, and tumor necrosis factor (TNF) having the capacity to stimulate the hypothalamo-pituitary-adrenal axis, thus providing a loop to suppress their own production.[23]

Reports suggesting extrahypothalamic production of ACTH secretagogues lack confirmation of authenticity or physiologic significance.

Negative feedback of cortisol on ACTH production constitutes a sensitive homeostatic regulatory mechanism. The sites of negative feedback include not only the ACTH-producing cells of the anterior pituitary itself, but also higher centers including the hypothalamus and CA3 field of the hippocampus.[24]

Regulation of aldosterone production

Aldosterone is produced by the distinct outer part of the adrenal cortex, the zona glomerulosa. In man this is found in cell clusters rather than in a distinct zone. The main regulation of aldosterone is by the renin-angiotensin system. The stimuli to renin release from the juxtaglomerular cells of the kidney are low-renal perfusion pressure, sodium depletion, and hypokalemia, although hyperkalemia acting directly on the zona glomerulosa is a more potent stimulus to aldosterone release than hypokalemia. Renin acts on renin substrate or angiotensinogen, released into the circulation from the liver, to form angiotensin-I. This decapeptide is converted to the octapeptide angiotensin-II by angiotensin-converting enzyme (ACE), which is of widespread distribution, but most importantly found in the pulmonary bed.[25]

Angiotensin-II, apart from being a powerful arteriolar vasoconstrictor, stimulates aldosterone secretion from the adrenal cortex. Aldosterone, as mentioned earlier, acts powerfully to retain salt (and obligatorily water), but promotes kalliuresis, hence closing the homeostatic feedback loop. There are other minor influences recognized as acting on aldosterone secretion, including ACTH, dopamine, and serotonin.

Adrenocortical Function in Normal Aging

Numerous studies indicate that basal, circadian, and stimulated cortisol secretion remains intact well into old age.[26–32] This is particularly important with regard to the ability to withstand stress and the cortisol response to exogenous ACTH has been shown to be normal in elderly patients following myocardial infarction.[33] There are well-documented changes in the metabolism of corticosteroids with age-related decrease in the catabolism of cortisol.[34,35] Because of the intact negative feedback mechanisms there is a commensurate reduction in cortisol production rate. Aldosterone secretion is also normally well-preserved in the healthy geriatric population.[36] The recognized decline in adrenal androgen production[29,37–40] has been referred to earlier.

Tests of Adrenal Function

Tests of adrenal function in the elderly are for the foregoing reasons largely those established for the younger adult population. The diminishing reliance on urinary collections is beneficial for practical reasons, and also means that some of the physiologically irrelevant changes alluded to earlier will not prove distracting. The key to successful and safe investigation is careful selection.

Adrenal insufficiency

To investigate possible adrenal insufficiency, the basal measurement of greatest value is the plasma cortisol, measured at the circadian peak of 08.00 to 09.00 hours. Measurement of midnight cortisol is uninformative. If the 09.00 cortisol is less than 150 nmol/L, the diagnosis of adrenal insufficiency is made, and if greater than 450 nmol/L the patient is normal. For values inbetween, adrenal reserve should be assessed by measuring plasma cortisol before the intramuscular administration of 250 mcg tetracosactrin (synthetic $ACTH_{1-24}$) and then 30 minutes after. If secondary adrenal insufficiency is suspected, central mechanisms need assessing. While the insulin-induced hypoglycemia test is still the "gold standard" for younger patients, and indeed, has been used successfully in the elderly,[41] there are serious hazards attending its use. If the 09.00-hour plasma cortisol is not greater than 180 nmol/L, if there is a history of epilepsy, or if there is a significant risk of ischemic heart disease (surely present in all elderly patients), the test is contraindicated.

Alternative test have been suggested, including several varieties of the metyrapone (metopirone) test. This drug blocks the 11-hydroxylase enzyme, which is a crucial step in cortisol biosynthesis. If negative feedback mechanisms are intact, metyrapone provokes enhanced ACTH secretion, which drives adrenal synthesis of 11-desoxycortisol. In the classic version, the adrenal response is measured by urinary 17-oxogenic steroid excretion,[42,43] but altered production of urinary metabolites in old age plus the nonstandardized assays used for the measurements diminish the value of this approach. Other investigators have proposed measurement of the plasma 11-desoxycortisol response, but this, too, has not been fully validated, especially in the elderly.[44–46] Finally, it has been proposed that the ACTH level should be directly monitored, and this has been evaluated in a geriatric population.[47] The difficulties of ACTH measurements are many, standardization nonexistent, and the assay is costly and not widely available; thus, as a practical test this version does not bear further consideration. Most importantly, it does not assess what one needs to know: the capacity to secrete cortisol adequately in the face of stress. It is popular in North America, but for reasons of tradition rather than sound science.

A test by which contrast has much to recommend is the glucagon stimulation test. In the most widely used version, 1 mg glucagon is injected subcutaneously and blood samples then taken basally at 90 minutes and thereafter at 30-minute intervals up to 240 minutes. As with the insulin test, the patient fasts overnight. There is no correlation between the cortisol response (or growth hormone response, because it is a reliable test of reserve of this hormone) and blood glucose changes. The diagnostic power of the test closely approaches the insulin stress test.[48] Glucagon is, however, safe to use even in the presence of heart disease and in epilepsy. The length of sampling period is dictated by the variable time taken to reach peak cortisol secretion—this adds inconvenience and expense. The use of intramuscular glucagon has been a simpler, more reliable version requiring samples only at 0, 150, and 180 minutes.[49] It is a more reliable test than the short Synacthen test when compared to the insulin tolerance test as the reference.[50] As with the insulin tolerance test, a peak plasma cortisol of 550 nmol/L or higher is regarded as a satisfactory response to glucagon.

Another useful aid in distinguishing primary and secondary hypoadrenalism is the long ACTH-stimulation test using depot tetracosactrin 1 mg intramuscularly and sampling at 0, 30, and 60 minutes as with the short test, but taking further samples at 4, 8, 16, and 24 hours.[51] The atrophied adrenals following ACTH deficiency can usually be stimulated, albeit subnormally, over this time span in contrast to the flat response in Addison's disease.

Glucocorticoid excess

Adrenal hyperfunction usually means cortisol excess or Cushing's syndrome. Conventional methods of investigation are employed first to establish the presence of the syndrome. The 24-hour urine-free cortisol is a simple and reliable test.[52,53] Its value derives from the fact that at normal levels of plasma cortisol is much bound to a high-affinity cortisol-binding globulin (CBG). The free cortisol level (though thought to be the biologically active fraction) is generally small, and is readily excreted in the urine. Because the capacity of CBG is limited, and saturated with even minor degrees of cortisol hypersecretion, there tends to be a nonlinear and marked rise in urinary-free cortisol. The overnight dexamethasone suppression test is much used, but also much criticized for unacceptable error rates.[54] If a patient is genuinely thought to have Cushing's syndrome, inpatient investigation is usually required. The low-dose dexamethasone test (0.5 mg orally taken strictly every 6 hours for 48 hours) and high-dose dexamethasone test (2 mg every 6 hours for 48 hours) were originally described in terms of suppression of urinary cortisol metabolites and proved useful in the differential diagnosis of pituitary-dependent Cushing's syndrome from other causes of the syndrome, namely adrenal tumors (benign and carcinoma) and ectopic ACTH secretion from a wide variety of neoplasms.[55] More commonly, the plasma cortisol response is relied upon these days.[56] The basis of this test is that in Cushing's syndrome the pituitary lesion, most commonly a microadenoma only a few millimeters in diameter, is not truly autonomous, but shows blunted suppression of ACTH secretion, especially with high-dose dexamethasone. The plasma cortisol is an accurate index of ACTH secretion because its measurement is not affected by the concomitant presence of dexamethasone. (This useful property of dexamethasone can be used to assess adrenal reserve in seriously ill patients with suspected Addison's disease in whom glucocorticoid therapy may need to be given empirically, and the cortisol response to tetracosactrin assessed at the same time to establish diagnosis.) There is increasing use of synthetic CRH, either of ovine or human composition.[57,58] Though many investigators find this a helpful and safe test, as with all tests used in Cushing's syndrome it is not infallible.[59] Nevertheless, it is useful to know that there is a preservation of response in the healthy elderly population.[32]

In cases of adrenal carcinoma it is not unusual to have mixed patterns of steroid excess. Virilization in women is not uncommon, and plasma testosterone is raised. A striking rise in dehydroepiandrosterone sulfate is characteristic of adrenal carcinoma[60] and this large production of a weak androgen may greatly raise the urinary 17-oxosteroid excretion.[61]

Mineralocorticoids

The mineralocorticoid status can be monitored by measurement of plasma aldosterone and also plasma renin activity both lying and standing (if clinically possible). The latter measurement of renin requires prior consultation with the laboratory so that rapid handling can be arranged to prevent artefactual results. Primary hyperaldosteronism is very uncommon in the elderly and is diagnosed by raised aldosterone and suppressed plasma renin activity in hypertensive patients who usually exhibit hypokalemic alkalosis. The much more frequent occurrence of secondary hyperaldosteronism is indicative of disease outside the adrenals, such as renal artery stenosis, cardiac failure, or hepatic cirrhosis leading to raised renin, driving the normal zona glomerulosa to secrete high levels of aldosterone.

Hyporeninemic hypoaldosteronism occurs predominantly in the elderly and is characterized by hyperkalemia, a hyperchloremic metabolic acidosis and moderate hyponatremia. It is more common in men, and is often associated with diabetes mellitus, particularly in the presence of autonomic failure or renal impairment. It is aggravated by potassium-sparing diuretics, β-blockers and nonsteroidal anti-inflammatory drugs.[62]

Imaging techniques in adrenal disease

The adrenal glands are readily visualized using CT scanning, especially if the patient is at all obese. Ultrasound can be useful, but is much less valuable than CT.[63] There is growing experience with magnetic resonance imaging (MRI), which may provide an indication of the likely functional status of any lesion. However, potential pitfalls arise with the exquisite sensitivity, but nonspecificity of this and advanced CT scanning techniques.[64]

There remains a small role for isotopic scintigraphy in the diagnosis of adrenal hyperfunction, perhaps more for extra-adrenal or bilateral pheochromocytomas using metaiodobenzylguanidine than the use of selenocholesterol or its variants in Cushing's and Conn's syndromes.[64] Angiography is invasive, but much less so with the advent of digital venous imaging (DVI), which can be useful in adrenal disease. The pituitary may require imaging in Cushing's disease—often the tiny size of the tumor defies even the latest generation CT scanners,[66] but it does seem that MRI with Gadolinium enhancement offers a slight edge.[67] In cases of hypopituitarism, CT scanning may be valuable.

As a final resort, venous sampling under radiographic control may be useful in the diagnosis of adrenal, pituitary, or ectopic sites of hormone production.[68] This approach in the elderly patient should be undertaken only if, after the most careful consideration, a balance of cost-benefit factors point inescapably in this direction. In practice this will rarely be the case.

Clinical Patterns

The patterns of adrenal disease are not greatly different in the elderly than in younger adults. Because these are well-described in standard textbooks of clinical medicine and endocrinology, full descriptions will not be given in all cases. Instead, emphasis will be placed on points particularly relevant to the elderly.

Adrenal insufficiency

Primary adrenal failure, Addison's disease, characteristically begins insidiously with nonspecific symptoms, although gastrointestinal features, including weight loss, are often prominent and in the elderly functional status may be diminished.[69] Though the characteristic ACTH-mediated pigmentation is a useful feature if present, it is occasionally absent.[70] A large survey suggested that in elderly patients Addison's disease was not only more likely to be tuberculous than in younger patients, but likely to prove fatal and the diagnosis be made postmortem.[71] Other rarer causes of adrenal failure, such as hemorrhage and amyloid, should be borne in mind.[72]

Though metastases are commonly found in the adrenal glands, they only exceptionally compromise cortisol secretion.[73] The therapeutic dividend from diagnosing Addison's disease is so great that the cortisol response to tetracosactrin should be assessed at the slightest suspicion. It is emphatically not necessary for the electrolytes to be disturbed or random cortisol to be "subnormal" for the significant adrenal insufficiency to be present. Secondary adrenal insufficiency is considered later.

Cushing syndrome and adrenal carcinomas

Cushing syndrome is rare in the elderly. It is most frequently due to ectopic ACTH production, usually by small cell carcinoma of the lung, but these patients typically present with cachexia and profound hypokalemia, rather than the characteristic cushingoid appearance. If due to pituitary-dependent disease, transsphenoidal surgery may be considered because it causes little constitutional disturbance. Nevertheless, in mild cases medical treatment with metyrapone alone may suffice and be more appropriate. This mode of treatment is certainly appropriate with other forms of Cushing syndrome, e.g., ectopic ACTH secretion. The mixed picture of Cushing syndrome and virilization in adrenal carcinoma may be difficult to recognize: the hirsuties and thinning of capital hair may be much more prominent than the features of cortisol excess (Fig. 72-1). Indeed, the main features of Cushing's syndrome may be skin atrophy and fragility with spontaneous bruising. Obesity and plethora may be conspicuously absent. In the elderly certain features are more marked, particularly impaired cognitive function, myopathy, osteoporosis, and diabetes. Hypokalemia is common in all forms of Cushing's syndrome other than pituitary-dependent, although a patient with the nodular hyperplasia variety of Cushing's disease was diagnosed following an

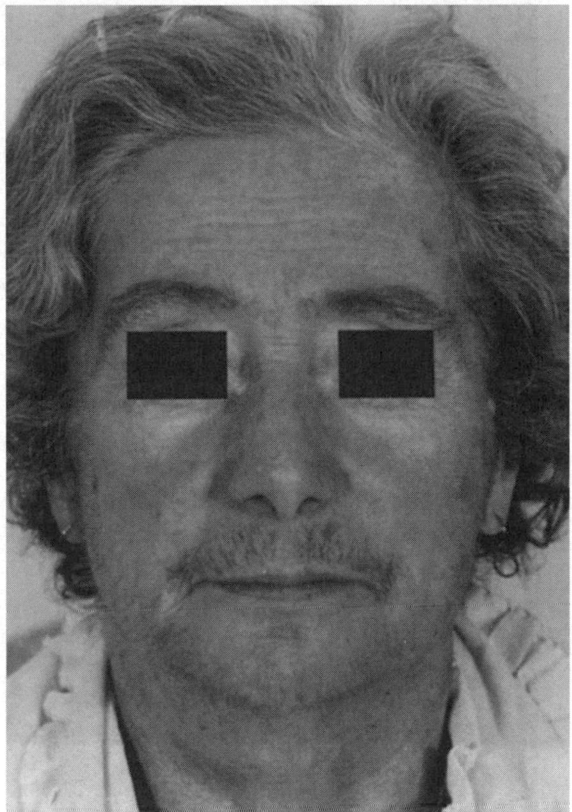

Figure 72-1 Patient with a metastasizing adrenal carcinoma causing virilization and Cushing syndrome. Note hirsuties, slight scalp recession, but absence of cushingoid facies.

admission precipitated by an acute diarrheal illness in which the plasma potassium fell to 1.2 mmol/L.

Adrenal carcinomas may occasionally secrete estrogen. This was retrospectively recognized in a youthful looking elderly woman with Cushing syndrome (Fig. 72-2) following removal of her large adrenal tumor (Fig. 72-3) when she had a brisk vaginal blood loss. Rescue of preoperative urine specimens revealed high estrogen levels. Treatment is primarily surgical unless there are widespread metastases. The use of opDDD is probably helpful, but may be associated with severe side effects in which case it should not be persevered with.[74]

Iatrogenic glucocorticoid excess

The most common cause of Cushing syndrome in the elderly is the exogenous administration of steroids for a variety of medical disorders. The side effects of steroid therapy, often aggravating pre-existing problems, are usually more marked in the elderly. Particular problems include decreased cognitive function, emotional lability, and dysphoria; osteoporotic fractures; myopathy and muscle wasting with limitation of mobility; skin fragility; and impaired glucose tolerance. Furthermore, patients on maintenance steroids ($>$ 10 mg prednisolone daily or equivalent for more than 2 weeks) are at risk of adrenal insufficiency in the event of intercurrent illness, and the daily

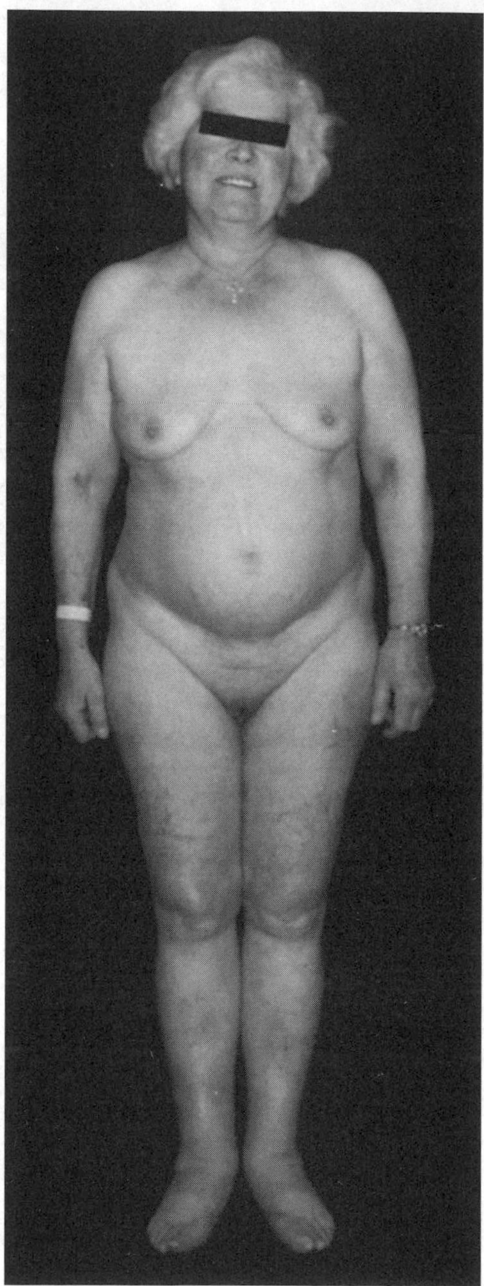

Figure 72-2 Patient with adrenal carcinoma causing Cushing syndrome and feminization.

steroid dose should be doubled for at least 3 days in these circumstances.

Incidentalomas

Last, but very far from least, is the vexed problem of what to do with a patient who for usually quite unrelated reasons has an abdominal ultrasound or CT scan that reveals an unsuspected adrenal mass.[75,76] Because about 20 percent of adrenocortical carcinomas are nonfunctioning in the absence of any clinical endocrine syndrome, it is probably prudent to repeat the scans at intervals, particularly for lesions greater than 3 cm in diameter, since lesions progressing to greater than 6 cm in diameter are almost always malignant. However, the problem must be kept in proportion. Adrenal cancer is rare, with an annual incidence approximately two per million.[77] Autopsy studies show benign nodules are extremely common, especially with advancing age, and particularly in hypertensives.[78] Most are microscopic, but lesions of greater than 1 cm are found in approximately 1 percent of patients undergoing abdominal CT.[64] Clearly, there is a need for biochemical screening to exclude pheochromocytoma, Conn, and also Cushing syndrome. Hypertension and hypokalemia are particularly good indicators of functioning lesions. It has been estimated that the frequency of these conditions in 100,000 patients with an adrenal incidentaloma would be 6,500 pheochromocytomas, 7,000 Conn syndrome, and only 35 Cushing syndrome. However, subclinical cortisol hypersecretion has been reported in up to 25 percent of patients with adrenal tumors incidentally discovered on CT in a number of studies.[79,80]

Pituitary Disorders

Pituitary Tumors

Pituitary tumors are increasingly uncommon in the elderly, with the exception of nonfunctioning (null-cell) adenomas, which increase in incidence over the age of 50. These tumors present with local complications—usually due to compression

Figure 72-3 Intravenous pyelogram showing large right-sided adrenal mass depressing the right kidney.

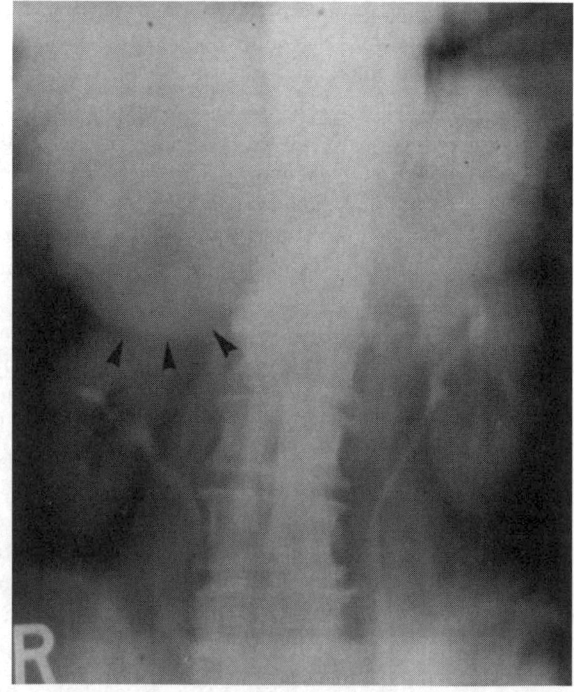

of the optic chiasm causing bitemporal hemianopia, or more rarely due to invasion into surrounding structures, such as the cavernous sinus—or with features of hypopituitarism (see below). Functioning pituitary tumors are associated with the characteristic syndromes of hormone excess, notably, acromegaly and Cushing's disease, and behave in a similar fashion to tumors in younger patients, although it has been suggested that the somatotroph adenomas causing acromegaly are more benign in the elderly, and thus medical therapy could be considered as a first-line option.[81] However, advances in neurosurgical techniques mean that almost all tumors can be at least debulked by the transphenoidal approach, and the relative simplicity, and low morbidity and mortality of this procedure make it the treatment of choice for even the very elderly.

Other sellar lesions are very rare, although two occur more commonly in the elderly: pituitary metastases may present like nonfunctioning tumors; pituitary incidentalomas—adenomas, usually less than 1 cm in diameter, without clinical sequelae—may be identified on CT or MRI scan performed for other indications, in the same way as adrenal incidentalomas, and have a prevalence of up to 10 percent in the over-80 age group, but intervention is not required in such cases.

Hypopituitarism

Hypopituitarism may be caused by pituitary adenoma as in younger age groups. A valuable clue in postmenopausal women is finding inappropriately low gonadotrophin levels, although it has been reported that these can be depressed in nonspecific illness in the extremely elderly.[47] More important, because subtler and more difficult to diagnose, is idiopathic hypopituitarism, in which the pituitary fossa is normal in size. Key features may be orthostatic hypotension, hyponatremia (reflecting adrenal and thyroid insufficiency causing water overload, possibly from inappropriate ADH secretion), or hypothyroidism with inappropriately low TSH.[82] Computed tomograph scanning may indicate a number of abnormalities ranging from a thickened pituitary stalk to empty sella.[83] Replacement therapy with hydrocortisone and thyroxine is gratifyingly effective. As with patients on steroid therapy, those patients needing replacement hydrocortisone should be advised to double the dose of hydrocortisone for 3 days with intercurrent illnesses, and need parenteral steroids if they cannot tolerate oral medication while unwell.

Growth hormone deficiency

Growth hormone secretion declines by about 15 percent per decade from a peak at about 30 years of age,[84] and stimulated growth hormone secretion, both using pharmacologic agents and physiologic stimuli, such as exercise, is diminished in the elderly. This fall in growth hormone secretion is due to a decline in the frequency[84] and amplitude[85] of growth hormone pulses, probably the result of an increase in somatostatinergic tone. Furthermore, there is a decrease in circulating levels of insulin-like growth factor-I (IGF-I), the peripheral mediator of the somatic effects of growth hormone, although, in contrast to young adults, the IGF-I levels do not show as strong a correlation with 24-hour growth hormone secretion.[86]

Some of the features of aging are similar to the characteristics of adult growth hormone deficiency, such as the decrease in lean body mass and bone mineral density, the increase in fat mass,[87] and possibly, neuropsychological sequelae and increased cardiovascular mortality.[88] The availability of recombinant growth hormone has made the treatment of adult growth hormone deficiency possible, and recently there has been interest in its effects on the healthy elderly. In individuals with low IGF-I levels, administration of growth hormone increases lean body mass, skin thickness, lumbar spine bone density, and nitrogen retention, and decreases adipose tissue. No effect was seen on bone density at other sites or on serum cholesterol, and nonsignificant increases in blood pressure and fasting glucose have been reported. Side effects of fluid retention, in some cases causing bloating or carpal tunnel syndrome, arthralgia, headaches, lethargy, and gynecomastia may occur.[87,89]

At present, the only group for whom growth hormone therapy can be recommended are those with pituitary disease, requiring at least one form of pituitary hormone replacement therapy, in whom growth hormone deficiency has been demonstrated using a pharmacologic stimulation test and who have symptoms of growth hormone deficiency.

Isolated ACTH deficiency

Less frequent is the development of isolated ACTH deficiency. This has been seen in an octogenarian who developed frequent hypoglycemic comas associated with raised insulin levels. The clue that this was not due to an insulinoma came from the equimolar secretion of insulin and C-peptide. Replacement therapy with hydrocortisone completely abolished the hypoglycemic episodes.

References

1. Funder JW: On mineralocorticoid and glucocorticoid receptors. pp. 86–95. In Anderson DC, Winter JSD (eds): Adrenal Cortex. Butterworth, London, 1985
2. Feldman D, Funder JW, Loose D: Is the glucocorticoid receptor identical in various target organs? J Steroid Biochem 1978;9: 141–145
3. Munck A, Guyre, Holbrook NJ: Physiological functions of glucocorticoids in stress and their relation to pharmacological actions. Endocrinol Rev 1984;5:25–44
4. Cugini P, Lucia P, Di Palma L et al: Effect of aging on circadian rhythm of atrial natriuretic peptide, plasma renin activity, and plasma aldosterone. J Gerontol 1992;47:214–219
5. Dewis P, Anderson DC: The adrenarche and adrenal hirsutism. pp. 96–119. In Anderson DC, Winter JSD (eds): Adrenal Cortex. Butterworth, London, 1985
6. Casson PR, Andersen RN, Herrod HG et al: Oral dehydroepiandrosterone in physiologic doses modulates immune function in postmenopausal women. Am J Obstet Gynecol 1993;169: 1536–1539

7. Morales AJ, Nolan JJ, Nelson JC, Yen SS: Effects of replacement dose of dehydroepiandrosterone in men and women of advancing age. J Clin Endocrinol Metab 1994;78:1360–1367
8. Gorski J, Gannon F: Current models of steroid hormone action: a critical review. Ann Rev Physiol 1976;38:425–450
9. Green S, Chambon P: A superfamily of potentially oncogenic hormone receptors. Nature 1986;324:615–617
10. Joab I, Radanyi C, Renoir M et al: Common non-hormone binding component in non-transfonned chick oviduct receptors of four steroid hormones. Nature 1984;308:850–853
11. Gustafsson J-A, Carlstedt-Duke J, Poellinger L et al: Biochemistry, molecular biology, and physiology of the glucocorticoid receptor. Endocrinol Rev 1987;8:185–234
12. Arriza JL, Weinberger C, Cerelli G et al: Cloning of human mineralocorticoid receptor complementary DNA: structural and functional kinship with the glucocorticoid receptor. Science 1987;237:268–275
13. Edwards CRW, Burt D, Stewart PM: The specificity of the human mineralocorticoid receptor: clinical clues to a biological conundrum. J Steroid Biochem 1989;32:213–216
14. Ernest MJ, Feigelson P: Multihormonal control of tyrosine transferase in isolated liver cells. pp. 219–241. In Baxter JD, Rousseau GG (eds): Glucocorticoid Hormone Action. Springer-Verlag, Heidelberg, 1979
15. Schultz G, Beato M, Feigelson P: Messenger RNA for hepatic tryptophan oxygenase: its partial purification, its translation in a heterologous cell-free system, and its control by glucocorticoid hormones. Proc Natl Acad Sci USA 1973;70:1218–1221
16. Flower RJ: Background and discovery of lipocortins. Agents Actions 1986;17:255–262
17. Waterman MR, Simpson ER: Cellular mechanisms involved in the acute and chronic actions of ACTH. pp. 57–85. In Anderson DC, Wmter JSD (eds): Adrenal Cortex. Butterworth, London, 1985
18. Eipper BA, Mains RE: Structure and biosynthesis of proadrenocorticotropin/endorphin and related peptides. Endocrinol Rev 1980;1:1–27
19. Harris GW: Neural control of the pituitary gland. Physiol Rev 1948;28:139–173
20. Gillies GE, Linton EA, Lowry PJ: Corticotropin releasing activity of the new CRF is potentiated several times by vasopressin. Nature 1982;299:355–357
21. Weitzman ED, Fukushima D, Nogeire C et al: Twenty-four hour pattern of the episodic secretion of cortisol in normal subjects. J Clin Endocrinol Metab 1971;33:14–22
22. Antoni FA: Hypothalamic control of adrenocorticotropin secretion: advances since the discovery of 41-residue corticotropin-releasing factor. Endocrinol Rev 1986;7:351–378
23. Tsagarikis S, Gillies G, Rees LH et al: Interleukin-1 directly stimulates the release of corticotropin-releasing factor from rat hypothalamus. Neuroendocrinology 1989;49:98–101
24. Sopolsky RM, Krey IC, McEwen BS: The neuroendocrinology of stress and aging: the glucocorticoid cascade hypothesis. Endocrinol Rev 1986;7:284–301
25. James VHT: Adrenal cortex physiology. pp. 6.2–6.10. In Besser GM, Cudworth AG (eds): Clinical Endocrinology: An Illustrated text. Gower, London, 1987
26. West C, Brown H, Simons E et al: Adrenocortical function and cortisol metabolism in old age. J Clin Endocrinol Metab 1961;21:1197–1207
27. Touitou YK, Sulon J, Bogdan A et al: The adrenocortical hormones, aging and mental condition: seasonal and circadian rhythm of plasma 18-OH-11-DOC total and free cortisol and urinary corticosteroids. J Endocrinol 1983;96:53–64
28. Grad B, Rosenberg G, Liberman H et al: Diurnal variation of serum cortisol level of geriatric subjects. J Gerontol 1971;26:351–357
29. Serio M, Piolanti P, Cappelli G et al: The miscible pool and turnover rate of cortisol with aging and variations in relation to time of day. Exp Gerontol 1969;4:95–101
30. Tourigny-Rivard M, Raskind M, Rivard D: The dexamethasone suppression test in an elderly population. Biol Psych 1981;16:1173
31. Ohashi M, Kato K, Nawata H, Ibayashi H: Adrenocortical responsiveness to graded ACTH infusions in normal young and elderly human subjects. Gerontology 1986;32:43–51
32. Ohashi M, Fujio N, Kato K et al: Aging is without effect on the pituitary adrenal axis in men. Gerontology 1986;32:335–339
33. Jensen BA, Sanders S, Frlund B, Hjortrup A: Adrenocortical function in old age as reflected by plasma cortisol and ACTH test during the course of acute myocardial infarction. Arch Gerontol Geriatr 1988;7:289–296
34. Romanoff LP, Morris CW, Welch P et al: The metabolism of cortisol-4-14C in young and elderly men. I: Secretion rate of cortisol and daily excretion of tetrahydrocortisol, allotetrahydrocortisol, tetrahydrocortisone and cortolone (20α and 20β). J Clin Endocrinol Metab 1961;21:1413–1425
35. Abbo FE: The 17-ketosteroid/17-hydroxycorticosteroid ratio as a useful measure of the physiological age of the human adrenal cortex. J Gerontol 1966;21:112–114
36. Lebel M, Grose JH: angiotensin II effect on plasma steroids in selective hypoaldosteronism. Horm Metab Res 1982;14:432–436
37. Hamburger C: Normal urinary excretion of neutral 17-ketosteroids with special reference to age and sex variations. Acta Endocrinol (Copenhagen) 1948;1:19–37
38. Migeon C, Keller A, Lawrence B, Shepard T: DHA and androsterone levels in human plasma. Effect of age and sex: day-to-day and diumal variations. J Clin Endocrinol Metab 1957;17:1051–1061
39. Parker LN, Odell WD: Decline of adrenal androgen production as measured by radioimmunoassay of urinary unconjugated dehydroepiandrosterone. J Clin Endocrinol Metab 1978;47:600–602
40. Vermeulen A, Deslypere JP, Schelflhout W et al: Adrenocortical function in old age: response to acute adrenocorticotropin stimulation. J Clin Endocrinol Metab 1982;54:187–191
41. Muggeo M, Fedele D, Tiengo A et al: Human growth hormone and cortisol response to insulin stimulation in aging. J Gerontol 1975;30:546–551
42. Liddle GW, Estep HL, Kendall JW Jr et al: Clinical application of a new test of pituitary reserve. J Clin Endocrinol Metab 1959;19:875–894
43. Gold EM, DeRaimondo VC, Forsham PH: Quantitation of pitui-

tary corticotropin reserve in man by use of adrenocortical 11 β-hydroxylase inhibitor (SU-4885). Metabolism 1960;9:3–20

44. Jubiz W, Matsukara S, Meikle AW: Plasma metyrapone, adrenocorticotropic hormone, cortisol, and deoxycortisol levels. Sequential changes during oral and intravenous metyrapone administration. Arch Int Med 1970;125:468–471
45. Nattrass M, Smith J, Wood PJ, Marks V: Plasma corticosteroid determinations for assessment of pituitary response to metyrapone. Lancet 1972;ii:903–904
46. Blicher-Toft M, Hummer L: Serum immunoreactive corticotropin and response to metyrapone in old age in man. Gerontology 1977;23:236–243
47. Impallomeni M, Yeo T, Rudd A et al: Investigation of anterior pituitary function in elderly in-patients over the age of 75. Q J Med 1987;63:493–503
48. Spathis GS, Bloom SR, Jeffcoate WJ et al: Subcutaneous glucagon as a test of the ability of the pituitary to secrete GH and ACTH. Clin Endocrinol 1974;3:175–186
49. Rao RH, Spathis GS: Intramuscular glucagon as a provocative stimulus for the assessment of pituitary function: growth hormone and cortisol responses. Metabolism 1987;36:658–663
50. Orme SM, Peacey SR, Barth JH, Belchetz PE: Comparison of tests of stressreleased cortisol secretion in pituitary disease. Clin Endocrinol 1996;45:135–140
51. Galvao-Teles A, Burke CW, Fraser RT: Adrenal function tested with tetracosactrin depot. Lancet 1971;i:557–560
52. Burke CW, Beardwell CG: Cushing's syndrome: an evaluation of the clinical usefulness of urinary free cortisol and other urinary steroid measurements in diagnosis. Q J Med 1973;42: 175–204
53. Crapo L: Cushing's syndrome: a review of diagnostic tests. Metabolism 1979;28:955–977
54. Cronin C, Igoe D, Duffy MJ et al: The overnight dexamethasone test is a worthwhile screening procedure. Clin Endocrinol 1990; 33:27–33
55. Liddle GW: Tests of pituitary-adrenal suppressibility in the diagnosis of Cushing's syndrome. J Clin Endocrinol Metab 1960;20:1539–1560
56. Ashcraft MW, van Herle AJ, Vener SL, Geffner DL: Serum cortisol levels in Cushing's syndrome after low and high-dose dexamethasone suppression. Ann Int Med 1982;96:21–26
57. Chrousos GP, Schulte HM, Oldfield EH et al: The corticotropin releasing factor stimulation test. An aid in the evaluation of patients with Cushing's syndrome. N Engl J Med 1984;310: 622–626
58. Hermus AR, Picters GF, Pesman GJ et al: The corticotropin-releasing hormone test versus the high-dose dexamethasone test in the differential diagnosis of Cushing's syndrome. Lancet 1986;ii:540–544
59. Orth DN: The old and the new in Cushing's syndrome. N Engl J Med 1984;310:649–651
60. Freeman DA: Steroid hormone-producing tumors in man. Endocr Rev 1986;7:204–220
61. Hutter AM Jr, Kayhoe DL: Adrenal cortical carcinoma. Clinical features of 138 patients. Am J Med 1966;41:572–580
62. Holland OB: Hypoaldosteronism: disease or normal response? N Engl J Med 1991;324:488
63. Abrams HL, Siegelman SS, Adams DF et al: Computed tomography versus ultrasound of the adrenal: a prospective study. Radiology 143:121–128
64. Glazer GM, Francis IR, Quint LE: Imaging of the adrenal glands. Invest Radiol 1989;23:3–11
65. Hawkins LA, Britton KE, Shapiro B: Selenium 75 selenomethyl cholesterol: a new agent for quantitative functional scintigraphy of the adrenals: physical aspects. Br J Radiol 1980;53:883–889
66. Semple CG, Thomson JA, Teasdale GM: Transsphenoidal microsurgery for Cushing's disease. Clin Endocrinol 1984;21: 621–629
67. Kulkarni MV, Lee KF, McArdle CB et al: 1.5-T MR imaging of pituitary microadenomas: technical considerations and CT correlation. AJNR 1988;9:5–11
68. Findling JW, Aron DC, Tyrrell JB et al: Selective venous sampling for ACTH in Cushing's syndrome. Differentiation between Cushing's disease and the ectopic ACTH syndrome. Ann Intern Med 1981;94:647–652
69. Tobin MV, Aldridge SA, Morris AI et al: Gastrointestinal manifestations of Addison's disease. Am J Gastroenterol 1989;84: 1302–1305
70. Nerup J: Addison's disease: clinical studies. A report of 108 cases. Acta Endocrinol (Copenhagen) 1974;76:127–141
71. Mason AS, Meade TW, Lee JAH, Morris JN: Epidemiological and clinical picture of Addison's disease. Lancet 1968;ii: 744–747
72. Edwards OM: Adrenal apoplexy: the silent killer. JR Soc Med 1993;86:1–2
73. Cedermark BJ, Sjoberg HE: The clinical significance of metastases to the adrenal glands. Surg Gynaecol Obstet 1981;152: 607–610
74. Luton J-P, Cerdas S, Billaud L et al: Clinical features of adrenocortical carcinoma, prognostic factors, and the effects of mitotane therapy. N Engl J Med 1990;322:1195–1201
75. Geellhoed GW, Druy EM: Management of the adrenal 'incidentaloma'. Surgery 1982;92:866–874
76. Prinz RA, Brookes MH, Churchill R et al: Incidental asymptomatic adrenal masses detected by computed tomographic scanning: is operation required? JAMA 1982;248:701–704
77. Dobbie JW: Adrenocortical nodular hyperplasia: the aging adrenal. J Pathol 1969;99:1–18
78. Virkkala A, Valimaki M, Pelkonen R et al: Endocrine abnormalities in patients with adrenal tumours incidentally discovered on computed tomography. Acta Endocrinol (Copenhagen) 1989; 121:67–72
79. Osella G, Terzolo M, Borretta G et al: Endocrine evaluation of incidentally disovered adrenal masses (incidentalomas). J Clin Endocrinol Metab 1994;79:1532–1539
80. Reincke M, Nieke J, Krestin GP et al: Preclinical Cushing's syndrome in adrenal "incidentalomas": comparison with adrenal Cushing's syndrome. J Clin Endocrinol Metab 1992;75: 826 832
81. Lamberts SWJ: Medical treatment of acromegaly. In Wass JA (ed): Treating Acromegaly. Society for Endocrinology, Bristol, 1992
82. Belchetz PE: Idiopathic hypopituitarism in the elderly. Br Med J 1985;291:247–248

83. Belchetz PE: Clinical recognition of idiopathic hypopituitarism in the geriatric patient. Geriatr Med Today 1987;6:27–42

84. Iranmanesh A, Lizarraide G, Veldhuis JD: Age and relative adiposity are specific negative determinants of the frequency and amplitude of growth hormone (GH) secretory bursts and the half-life of endogenous GH in healthy men. J Clin Endocrinol Metab 1991;73:1081–1088

85. van Coevorden A, Mookel J, Laurent E et al: Neuroendocrine rhythms and sleep in aging men. Am J Physiol 1991;260: E651–E656

86. Rudman D, Vintner MH, Rogers CM et al: Impaired growth hormone secretion in the adult population. Relation to age and adiposity. J Clin Invest 1981;67:1361–1369

87. Rudman D, Feller AG, Nagray HS et al: Effects of human growth hormone in men over 60 years old. N Engl J Med 1990;323: 1–6

88. Rosen T, Bengtsson B-A: Premature mortality due to cardiovascular disease in hypopituitarism. Lancet 1990;336:285–288

89. Thompson JL, Butterfield GE, Marcus R et al: The effects of recombinant human insulin-like growth factor-1 and growth hormone on body composition in elderly women. J Clin Endocrinol Metab 1995;80:1845–1852

C H A P T E R 7 3

Disorders of the Thyroid

MYRON MILLER

Although thyroid disorders occur over the entire age range, many appear to be increasingly common with advancing age. It is important to recognize that the clinical features of thyroid disease may be significantly altered in the aged individual so that symptoms and physical findings typical in young persons may be modified, different, or absent in the elderly.

The diagnosis of thyroid disorders may be further influenced by the age of the patient as a consequence of normal aging-associated changes in thyroid physiology. Of even greater importance is the impact of nonthyroidal illnesses that frequently occur in the elderly on many of the tests used to assess thyroid function.[1]

Normal Aging

Morphology

The normal aging process is accompanied by changes in the gross and microscopic appearance of the thyroid gland. It has been stated that overall mass begins to decline from the normal range of 15 to 25 g so that with increasing age a progressively larger proportion of individuals will have glands weighing less than 20 g.[2] More recent data obtained by ultrasound in healthy subjects indicate that aging results in little change in size of the thyroid.[3]

With advancing age, there is progressive fibrosis, the appearance of lymphocytes, a decrease in follicle size, and a reduction in the amount of colloid.[4] Although these changes are common in the elderly, they are by no means characteristic of all aged persons. More importantly, there does not appear to be a decline in thyroid function concomitant to the morphologic changes and neither weight nor histologic appearance correlate with common measures of thyroid function.[5]

Hypothalamic-Pituitary-Thyroid Regulation

The production of thyroid hormones is regulated by the hypothalamic-pituitary-thyroid axis. Thyrotropin-releasing hormone (TRH) is synthesized in the hypothalamus and functions to stimulate release of thyroid-stimulating hormone (TSH) from the anterior pituitary by binding to receptors on the cell membrane of TSH-producing thyrotropes. Thyroid-stimulating hormone is regulated by the negative feedback of the thyroid hormones thyroxine (T4) and triiodothyronine (T3) acting on the pituitary gland.

The neuroendocrine mechanisms controlling TSH release may be altered during the normal aging process. Thus, serum TSH concentration, which undergoes circadian variation, exhibits smaller fluctuations in elderly than in young men.[6] The ability of TRH to stimulate TSH release may be affected by both the age and gender of the individual. Several studies have documented that elderly men have an impaired TSH response to TRH stimulation with peak serum TSH values in men over the age of 60 showing approximately a 40 percent reduction compared with young men.[7–12] In women, however, there does not appear to be an effect of age on TSH responsiveness.[13]

The ability of the pituitary gland to synthesize TSH does not appear to be diminished by the aging process as reflected by observation that pituitary TSH content undergoes no significant change over the life span.[14] The 24-hour TSH secretion has been reported to be decreased in healthy elderly men,[10] but the secretion rate of TSH has also been reported to be higher in elderly subjects than in young individuals.[15] However, circulating levels of TSH remain constant with advancing age and the elevations that are commonly seen in elderly persons must be considered as evidence for failing thyroid function.[16]

Thyroid-stimulating hormone exerts its effects by binding to the membrane of thyroid follicular cells. The response of these cells to TSH stimulation is not impaired by aging as reflected by T4 and T3 release into the circulation following either TRH or TSH administration.[17]

Within the thyroid gland, T4 and T3 synthesis results from the trapping of iodide by follicular cells, subsequent oxidation of iodide leading to iodination of tyrosine and coupling of two iodinated tyrosines. In the normal adult, approximately 80 μg of T4 and 30 μg of T3 are produced daily.[18] In elderly individuals, T4 and T3 production decline to approximately 60 and 20 μg per day, respectively. These changes may be related to the decrease in thyroidal iodide accumulation, which has been observed with aging.[19]

Thyroid Hormone Secretion and Metabolism

In response to TSH stimulation, T4 and T3 stored in thyroid follicles are hydrolyzed from thyroglobulin and released into the circulation where they are bound to albumin, thyroid-binding prealbumin (TBPA), and thyroid-binding globulin (TBG) with less than 0.1 percent of the hormones circulating in the free form. Thyroid-binding globulin is the primary thyroid hormone transport protein, carrying about 70 percent of bound hormone, and its levels do not appear to differ between healthy young and old individuals.[9] A greater T4-binding capacity of TBG has been observed in the elderly.[20,21]

The small proportion of T4 and T3 in the free state (FT4 and FT3) are the biologically active forms of the hormones and are responsible for peripheral thyroid hormone action and metabolism. Circulating levels of both FT4 and FT3 remain constant over the age span and a decrease in concentration, especially FT3, should be considered a consequence of illness rather than due to normal aging.[9,16,17,20,22] Approximately 20 to 30 percent of circulating T3 is directly secreted by the thyroid gland with the remaining 70 to 80 percent resulting from 5′-monodeiodination of the outer ring of T4 in peripheral tissues.[18] T4-degradation is decreased with advancing age so that by age 90, the degradation rate is approximately 50 percent that of young subjects.[17,23,24] This change appears to be due to an age-related reduction in the activity of monodeiodinase enzymes in peripheral tissue.[25] T3 degradation is less affected by aging.[17,25] A consequence of these changes is a decline in T4 metabolic clearance rate and an increase in half-life of circulating T4 from approximately 6 days in young persons to over 9 days in individuals who have reached their ninth decade.[23,24,26]

Part of T4 degradation involves 5-monodeiodination of the inner ring of the molecule and results in the generation of the biologically inactive reverse T3 (rT3).[18,27] The outer ring 5′-monodeiodinase is sensitive to a variety of influences including starvation, febrile illness, elevation of glucocorticoid concentration, and drugs such as propranolol, amiodarone, and iodinated contrast materials.[18,28] As a result of inhibition of the enzyme activity, there is impaired T4 conversion to T3, with a decline in serum T3 concentration and a parallel rise in rT3 concentration. Serum rT3 is not affected by normal aging, and an increase must be considered to be a consequence of illness or drug-induced alteration in T4 degradation.[22,25] Figure 73-1 shows the structures of T4, T3, and rT3.

Thyroid Hormone Action

The primary thyroid hormone acting on peripheral tissue and responsible for the broad range of thyroid actions is FT3. FT3, and to a lesser amount FT4, act on peripheral tissue cells by binding to specific nuclear receptors and subsequently affect DNA transcription, RNA formation, and new protein synthesis.[29,30] There are two T3 receptor genes, located on chromosomes 17 and 3, whose products are a group of T3 receptors.[31] Protein products coded for by the c-*erb*-A gene family, the cellular counterpart of the viral oncogene v-*erb*-A, have been demonstrated to be nuclear receptors for thyroid hormone.[32,33] At the level of the pituitary, thyroid hormone action results in inhibition of synthesis and release of TSH.[34,35]

Figure 73-1 Structures of thyroxine (T4), triiodothyronine (T3), and reverse triiodothyronine (rT3).

Thyroxine, T4

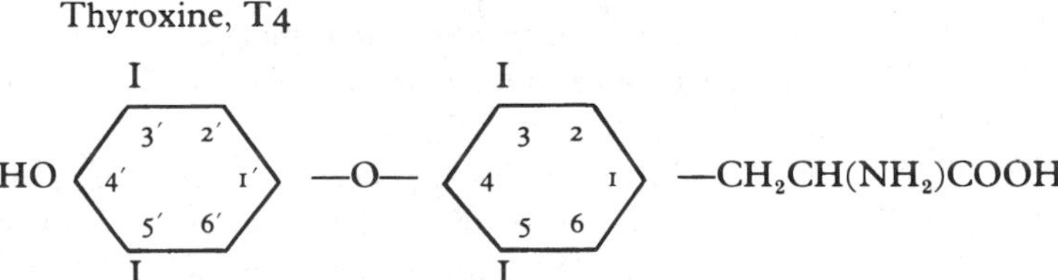

T4 is 3 : 5 : 3′ : 5′-tetra-iodothyronine

Tri-iodothyronine, T3

HO —O— —$CH_2CH(HN_2)COOH$

T3 is 3 : 5 : 3′-tri-iodothyronine

Reverse Tri-iodothyronine, rT3

HO —O— —$CH_2CH(NH_2)COOH$

rT3 is 3 : 3′ : 5′-tri-iodothyronine

Thyroid hormone action appears to be diminished as part of the aging process, as reflected by diminished oxygen expenditure[36] and decreased ability to stimulate hepatic enzyme synthesis following exposure to thyroid hormone.[37] Clinical support for diminished thyroid hormone action is provided by the observation that typical features of hyperthyroidism are often absent in the elderly.

Thyroid Function in Advanced Aging

Recent studies in healthy centenarians ranging in age from 100 to 110 years provide further information regarding the extent to which aging alone contributes to change in measures of thyroid function. There was no difference in serum FT4 of the centenarians as compared to both healthy elderly (age 65 to 80 years) and healthy younger adults (age 20 to 64 years), but serum FT3 was reduced in the centenarians. Serum TSH was also lower in the centenarians, and for the older groups as a whole there was an inverse relationship between serum TSH and age. Serum rT3 was increased in the centenarians, suggesting that there was reduced outer-ring deiodination of T4. Thus, in healthy aging persons, thyroid function was preserved into the eighth decade, while advanced old age was associated with reduced thyroid activity likely due to a decrease in TSH secretion and impairment of peripheral 5′-deiodination.[1,38]

Assessment of Thyroid Function

Circulating Thyroid Hormones

Screening of the secretory status of the thyroid gland can be accomplished by measurement in the blood of TSH, total circulating T4 and T3 concentrations, and FT4 and FT3 concentrations through use of radioimmunoassay or immunometric assays.[12] The development of "super sensitive" immunoassays for TSH have allowed differentiation of normal from suppressed levels of the hormone so that this single measurement can provide evidence supporting a diagnosis of primary hypothyroidism, secondary hypothyroidism, and hyperthyroidism.[39–41] It now appears that this assay may be the best initial test of thyroid function in evaluating patients for suspected under- or overactivity of the thyroid gland.[39] There is some suggestion that the generally accepted value of 5 mIU/L as the upper limit of normal for the adult population may actually be as high as 10 mIU/L in individuals who have reached their eighth decade.[41]

Total and free concentrations of T4 and T3 are commonly used to document the status of thyroid secretory activity. It appears to be well supported that the normal range for these hormones is unaffected by aging and that deviations from normal must be considered as evidence for thyroid disease or for other illness or states that may affect hormone measurement.[16,17,20,22,25,42]

Serum-free T4 is best measured by equilibrium dialysis.[43,44] Less reliable estimates of FT4 concentration can be obtained from the FT4 index, which involves measurement of both total T4 and a measure of thyroid hormone-binding protein capacity such as the T3 resin uptake. Because the free thyroxine index is derived from two separate tests, it is subject to significant technical error. It also loses reliability in clinical states associated with marked alteration of thyroid hormone-binding proteins.[12] Methods have been developed for direct measurement of FT4 using T4-specific antibodies immobilized on solid surfaces such as test tubes or microbeads. Results obtained by these procedures appear to correlate well with FT4 measured by equilibrium dialysis.[45,46]

Low T4 States

In addition to the expected reduction in total T4 seen in primary or secondary hypothyroidism, total T4 may be low due to a variety of other causes. Levels of TBPA may be acutely lowered in the presence of infectious disease, protein wasting states, surgery, and malnutrition with accompanying decline in total T4. More importantly, TBG levels can be depressed as a result of X-linked congenital deficiency, severe catabolic illness, chronic hepatic disease, glucocorticoids, and androgen administration.[47] Binding of T4 to TBG can be inhibited by drugs such as phenytoin and high-dose salicylates.[48] In from 20 to 74 percent of patients with nonthyroidal illness, an inhibitor of T4 binding to TBG has been detected, which may contribute to the measurement of a low T4 in these patients.[47,49]

The finding of a low T4 concentration in the presence of nonthyroidal illness has been termed the euthyroid sick syndrome.[50] In mild to moderate forms, measurement of FT4 will be normal even though total T4 concentration is reduced.[44,47] However, severe illness can result in marked reduction of both total and free T4 concentrations. When this circumstance occurs, the prognosis of the patient is poor with a mortality rate of approximately 80 percent having been reported.[51] The ability to differentiate these patients from those with hypothyroidism can be difficult.[52] Although serum TSH is usually in the normal range, occasionally mild to moderately elevated concentrations are found. This is especially true in the recovery phase of the illness when values can rise to as high as 20 mIU/L. Within 4 to 20 weeks after clinical recovery, all measures of thyroid function usually will have returned to normal.[53]

Low T3 States

The serum concentration of total T3 is easily affected by many nonthyroidal illnesses and low values are often seen in elderly ill patients, giving rise to the "low T3 syndrome." This consequence of systemic illness is the earliest and most common of the alterations in thyroid hormone levels.[16,17,28,42,47,52,54,55] In response to many acute illnesses, there is decreased peripheral 5′-monodeiodination of T4 to T3 with consequent reduction in serum T3 concentration and increase in serum rT3. Lowering of TBPA and TBG in the presence of acute and chronic illness further contributes to the marked fall in serum T3 characteristic of the sick elderly.

Often, the possibility of a diagnosis of hypothyroidism is raised and can usually be excluded by the absence of an increase in TSH and by the demonstration of normal or increased serum levels of rT3.

Cytokines such as interleukin-1, interleukin-6, and tumor necrosis factor (TNF) could be involved as intermediaries in the development of low T4 and T3 states. Many patients with nonthyroidal illnesses and low T4 and/or T3 also have elevated serum concentrations of cytokines.[56,57] Experimental increase of TNF-α has been observed to induce low serum concentrations of T4, T3, and TSH.[58]

High T4 States

Although less common than low thyroid hormone states, nonthyroidal factors can result in elevation of serum T4 concentration.[52,59] A euthyroid increase in total T4 can occur as a result of overproduction of TBG, a disorder that may be familial.[60] More commonly, TBG is increased due to exposure to estrogen or as a transient phase during acute hepatocellular injury. In these circumstances, serum-free T4 will be normal. Frequently, with mild to moderate levels of illness, an increase in FT4 is found in the patient with euthyroid sick syndrome as a result of impaired T4 monodeiodination by peripheral tissues.[47,50]

Thyrotropin-Releasing Hormone Test

The response of serum TSH to exogenously administered TRH is a useful method of assessing the dynamics of the pituitary-thyroid axis. In the normal individual, the bolus intravenous administration of 500 μg TRH results in a prompt rise in serum TSH, with peak values achieved in 30 minutes.[7,8] The minimal normal response should be an increase of greater than 2 mIU/L over the basal value, with many normal subjects reaching peak concentrations up to 30 mIU/L.[12] As previously stated, many elderly males respond less well to TRH stimulation than younger subjects or women at all ages.[7–13] Failure to respond to TRH is supportive of a diagnosis of hyperthyroidism, while a normal response will exclude the diagnosis. Subnormal responses may be seen in patients with severe illness, depression, or hypercortisolism as well as in euthyroid patients with thyroid adenomas or multinodular goiter. An exaggerated response of serum TSH is characteristic of primary hypothyroidism.[41]

Measures of Iodine Uptake

The ability of the thyroid gland to trap iodide and other ions such as technetium (Tc), has been the basis for assessment of both thyroid gland function and morphology. The oral administration of ^{131}I to normal individuals results in accumulation of 5 to 25 percent of the dose in the gland by 24 hours.[61,62] Because of considerable overlap between normal and hypothyroid subjects, low values for 24-hour ^{131}I uptake are of lesser diagnostic usefulness in establishing a diagnosis of hypothyroidism. Further, exposure to increased amounts of iodide in the diet or to iodine-containing drugs or radiographic contrast media will result in marked reduction of ^{131}I uptake. Elevated values are useful in supporting a diagnosis of hyperthyroidism, although some patients with toxic nodules may have 24-hour ^{131}I uptake values within the normal range. The 24-hour ^{131}I uptake is usually obtained in a patient with an established diagnosis of hyperthyroidism in order to calculate the dose of ^{131}I to be given for ablation therapy.

Thyroid scanning with ^{99m}Tc is useful in the evaluation of the patient with a palpable single thyroid nodule where demonstration of activity within the nodule markedly reduces the likelihood of the nodule representing an area of malignancy. In the elderly patient, scanning can be used to differentiate a diffusely overactive thyroid from the gland with single or multiple toxic nodules as the basis for hyperthyroidism.[63]

Other Thyroid Imaging Procedures

High-quality anatomic detailing of thyroid structure can be achieved by currently available imaging techniques, including realtime ultrasonography, CT, and MRI. These procedures can be useful in evaluating patients with single and multiple nodules by identifying cysts, areas of hemorrhage, and tissue calcification. Ultrasonography may be of value in determining which regions of the thyroid are most appropriate for fine-needle aspiration. Both CT and MRI are expensive and have few clinical indications at present, but may be of occasional value in assessing extent of tracheal compression by a thyroid mass and in determining extent of local invasion by thyroid cancers.[64]

Antithyroid Antibodies

Many thyroid disorders including hyperthyroidism of the Graves' disease type[65] and hypothyroidism of the Hashimoto type are believed to be the result of autoimmune disease.[12,66] As a consequence, high levels of serum antibodies to both thyroglobin and to microsomes are commonly found in patients with thyroid disease. Low levels of antithyroglobulin antibody (titer less than 1:100) may be present in patients without clinical sign of thyroid disorder. Moderate to high titers (1:1600 to 1:25600) can be found in patients with nonthyroid autoimmune disorders.[12]

Thyroid antibodies in the serum increase in incidence progressively with increasing age, reaching a peak incidence of 20 to 25 percent in women above the age of 50 years and 5 to 10 percent in similarly aged men.[67,68] However, in a highly selected population of healthy elderly ranging from 65 to 110 years, the prevalence of antithyroid antibodies was low and did not differ from the prevalence in healthy young persons.[1] This finding suggests that the high incidence of antithyroid antibodies in aging populations is a reflection of disease, and is not a consequence of normal aging. In many patients, the findings of high-serum antithyroglobulin and/or antimicrosomal antibody titers is accompanied by elevation of basal serum TSH concentration and reduced levels of serum T4, suggesting the presence of an autoimmune thyroiditis and a failing thyroid gland.[69]

From a diagnostic standpoint, high titers of antithyroid antibodies are commonly found in patients with documented hypothyroidism and suggest a diagnosis of chronic lymphocytic or Hashimoto's thyroiditis. In patients with hyperthyroidism, elevated antithyroglobulin and antimicrosomal antibody titers are more characteristic of patients with Graves' disease than of those with toxic nodules.

Thyroid-Stimulating Hormone Receptor Antibodies

Thyroid-stimulating activity similar to that of TSH can be found in the IgG portion of serum obtained from many patients with hyperthyroidism due to Graves' disease. These immunoglobulins have been demonstrated to be antibodies directed against the TSH receptor.[65] Thyroid-stimulating hormone-receptor antibodies can be detected by both radioreceptor assays utilizing radiolabeled TSH and by bioassay based on stimulation of cyclic AMP release from isolated thyroid cell cultures.[70–73] Both methods reveal positive tests for TSH receptor antibodies in over 85 percent of patients with untreated Graves' disease and in essentially 100 percent of patients with severe Graves' ophthalmopathy. Positive tests are infrequent in Hashimoto's disease and rare in nodular thyroid disease, including toxic nodular goiter. Monitoring of antibody levels may be useful in predicting likelihood of sustained remission in patients with Graves' disease who are treated with antithyroid drugs.[74]

Serum Thyroglobulin

Thyroglobulin involved in intrathyroidal synthesis of T4 and T3 can gain entry to the circulation where it can be detected in normal individuals at low levels by means of immunometric assays.[75] Normal individuals have been found to have serum concentrations of thyroglobulin of less than 5 μg/L. Concentrations can be increased in patients with hyperthyroidism, benign nodules, and inflammatory disorders, such as subacute thyroiditis. High levels are found in the majority of patients with thyroid cancer.

In patients with thyroid cancer previously treated by surgical or radioiodine ablation, measurement of serum thyroglobulin appears to be a sensitive indicator of tumor recurrence, either locally or by metastases. However, caution must be observed in interpreting blood levels because elevations above normal can be found in patients whose ablation has not been complete and have been left with small remnants of nonmalignant thyroid tissue.[75]

Hyperthyroidism

Overproduction of thyroid hormone leads to the clinical condition of hyperthyroidism. This disorder, also referred to as thyrotoxicosis, is accompanied by a broad array of symptoms and signs that can differ markedly between young and old patients.

Demography

In the past, hyperthyroidism has been regarded as a disorder with preferential expression in young to middle-aged individuals, especially women. It is now clear that this disorder is also common in the elderly population. The proportion of patients with hyperthyroidism who are over 60 years of age is estimated to be 15 to 20 percent.[76,77] Several studies of prevalence indicate the presence of hyperthyroidism in 1 to 2 percent of community-residing individuals. In a study of the population of Whickham, England, hyperthyroidism was identified in 19 per 1000 women, a prevalence rate 10 times greater than in men. The mean age at diagnosis was 48 years and the estimate of new cases was 2 to 3 per 1,000 women per year.[78] A survey of 968 ambulatory home-residing individuals over the age of 55 years in an urban, midwestern US community identified suppressed serum TSH levels in 2.5 percent with a prevalence of 2.7 percent in women compared to 1.8 percent in men. Based on suppressed serum TSH and unresponsiveness to TRH stimulation, the calculated prevalence of hyperthyroidism in this population over the age of 55 was 2.0 percent.[79] Many studies confirm that hyperthyroidism is far more common in women than men, with estimates of female preponderance ranging from 4:1 to as high as 10:1.[76,78,80]

Etiology

In young persons, Graves' disease remains the most common cause of hyperthyroidism and is the consequence of thyroid receptor antibodies, which have stimulatory effects on the thyroid gland.[65,71,73] With increasing age, there is a change in etiology so that more cases are due to multinodular toxic goiter and fewer to Graves' disease.[76] It is estimated that more than 50 percent of hyperthyroid patients over the age of 60 years have thyroxicosis due to multinodular toxic goiters. Multinodular goiters are common in the elderly and may not be clinically apparent.[5] Many clinical observations support the concept that long-standing multinodular goiters after many years of documented euthyroid activity may undergo change to become overproductive of thyroid hormones.[76]

Another less common cause of hyperthyroidism in the elderly is toxic adenoma (Plummer's disease), usually identifiable on thyroid scanning by the demonstration of a solitary hyperfunctioning nodule with suppression of activity in the remainder of the thyroid gland.[81,82] Hyperthyroidism can occur in a previously euthyroid person following ingestion of iodide or iodine-containing substances (Jod Basedow phenomenon). This is usually a self-limiting disorder lasting several weeks to several months.[83]

The possibility of hyperthyroidism must always be considered in the elderly person who is receiving thyroid hormone, especially if the dose is greater than 0.15 mg of L-thyroxine daily. Patients who have received such doses for many years without evidence for hyperthyroidism may insidiously develop features of hyperthyroidism as they age past 60 years due to age-associated slowing in thyroid hormone metabolism.[84]

Rare causes of hyperthyroidism in the elderly include TSH-producing pituitary tumors[85,86] and ectopic TSH production by nonpituitary tumors. These can be recognized by the finding of non-suppressed levels of serum TSH in the presence of increased amounts of circulating thyroid hormone. An additional uncommon cause of hyperthyroidism is overproduction of thyroid hormone by metastatic follicular carcinoma.

Occasionally, transient hyperthyroidism may occur in patients with subacute thyroiditis as a result of increased discharge of thyroid hormone into the circulation during the inflammatory phase of the illness.[87] In a similar fashion, radiation injury to the thyroid can be accompanied by transient increase in circulating thyroid hormone levels with associated symptoms.

T3 Toxicosis

In a small proportion of cases of hyperthyroidism, measurement of serum thyroid hormone concentrations will result in the expected increase in serum T3, but with the finding that serum T4 is within the normal range, although often at the upper end. This circumstance has been designated as T3 toxicosis and can occur with any type of hyperthyroidism, but most commonly in patients with solitary toxic adenoma.[82] The diagnosis will not be missed if T3 is measured in patients with clinically suspected hyperthyroidism who do not demonstrate elevated levels of serum T4.

Subclinical Hyperthyroidism

The finding of suppressed or absent serum TSH along with serum T4 and/or T3 in the upper end of the normal range has led to the recognition of subclinical hyperthyroidism. Individuals with these thyroid function values generally do not have clinical features suggestive of hyperthyroidism. However, these persons are at increased risk of developing atrial fibrillation as reflected by a cumulative incidence of 28 percent over a 10-year period in individuals over the age of 60 years, representing a threefold increase in risk.[88] The finding of subnormal TSH concentrations in the elderly is not infrequent. In a study of 1,210 persons in England, low TSH was found in 6.3 percent of women and 5.5 percent of men.[89] However, repeat measurements of serum TSH 1 year later showed a return of TSH to the normal range in the majority of cases. Similarly, in a US population of 2,575 persons over the age of 60 years, 101 were found to have low TSH and, of these, 30 had no history of past or present thyroid disease. Over a 4-year follow-up period, most had normal TSH on subsequent testing, but two became overtly hyperthyroid with an increase in serum T4 to above normal values.[90] Thus, the natural history of subclinical hyperthyroidism is variable, usually diappearing over time but becoming clinically manifest as atrial fibrillation or overt hyperthyroidism in a small munber of elderly individuals. Therefore, the finding of suppressed TSH and normal T4 in an asymptomatic elderly person calls for periodic retesting of thyroid function, including measurement of FT4. Subsequent development of atrial fibrillation or increased thyroid hormone production should then be treated by appropriate measures.

Table 73-1 Frequency of symptoms and signs of hyperthyroidism

	Kawabe et al.[91] (%)		Davis and Davis[76] (%)
Symptom/Sign	**Young (n = 48)**	**Elderly (n = 45)**	**Elderly (n = 85)**
Palpitation	100	60	63
Goiter	98	58	64
Tremor	96	71	55
Excessive perspiration	92	66	38
Weight loss	73	85	69
Eye signs	71	28	57
Arrhythmias (atrial fibrillation and VPC)	4.6	16.4	62

(From Griffin and Solomon,[92] with permission.)

Clinical Presentation

As with other disorders occurring in the elderly person, the clinical presentation of hyperthyroidism often differs from the classic description of the disease in younger individuals[76,77,91–93] (Table 73-1). Presenting features may be progressive functional decline, including weakness, fatigue, changes in mental status, loss of appetite, weight loss, cardiac arrhythmia, and congestive heart failure. A symptom complex peculiar to the geriatric hyperthyroid patient is "apathetic hyperthyroidism," in which the patient lacks the hyperactivity, irritability, and restlessness common to the young patient with thyrotoxicosis and presents instead with weakness, lethargy, listlessness, depression, and the appearance of a chronic, wasting illness. Often, the initial impression in such patients is that of depression, malignancy, or cardiovascular disease.[94,95]

The elderly patient with Graves' disease often differs from younger patients in nature and severity of expected classic symptoms and in physical findings. Clinically detectable thyroid enlargement, present in almost all younger patients, is absent in as many as 37 percent of elderly patients. Infiltrative ophthalmopathy with severe proptosis and exophthalmos occur infrequently in the elderly. Thus, none of the elements of the classic triad of Graves' disease (clinical hyperthyroidism, diffuse goiter, and infiltrative ophthalmopathy) may be recognizable in the elderly patient in whom the diagnosis may be suspected only on the basis of laboratory studies.[76,91,92]

Several reports have attempted to compare symptoms and objective physical findings in young and elderly patients with hyperthyroidism. Symptoms less commonly present in the elderly include nervousness, increased sweating, tremor, increased appetite, and increased frequency of bowel movements. Symptoms more common in the elderly include marked weight loss, present in over 80 percent of patients, poor appetite, worsening angina, edema, agitation, and confusion. Similarly, physical findings differ in elderly patients. In addition to absence of palpable goiter and eye signs of exophthalmos, pulse rate is slower, and reflexes are often not hyper-reflexic. Cardiac arrhythmias, especially atrial fibrillation and ventricular premature beats, are more common. Lid lag and lid retraction are frequently seen.[76,91–95]

The spectrum of symptoms and findings due to thyroid hormone excess is broad and can involve almost all body systems. Thyroid hormones act on the myocardium to sensitize the heart to β-adrenergic stimulation with resultant increase in heart rate, stroke volume, cardiac output, and shortened left ventricular ejection time.[96,97] These changes underlie the clinical consequences of increased risk of atrial fibrillation, often with a slow ventricular response, exacerbation of angina in patients with pre-existing coronary artery disease, and precipitation of congestive heart failure, which responds less readily to digoxin treatment due to increased renal clearance of the drug.

Gastrointestinal consequences of hyperthyroidism in the elderly include weight loss, poor appetite, and occasionally abdominal pain, nausea, and vomiting.[76,77] Diarrhea and increased frequency of bowel movements resulting from thyroid hormone action on intestinal motility can occur, but are often absent in the elderly in whom constipation is likely to be present. Hepatic actions of thyroid hormone can lead to alterations in liver enzymes, including elevation of alkaline phosphatase and γ-glutamyl transpeptidase levels, which return to normal following restoration of thyroid function to normal.

Weakness, especially of the proximal muscles, is a major feature of hyperthyroidism in the elderly and is often accompanied by muscle wasting.[76,95] As a consequence, disorders of gait, postural instability, and falls can be significant symptoms. Tremor occurs in over 70 percent of elderly thyrotoxic patients, but this sign must be distinguished from other causes of tremor common in the elderly.[91,92] A rapid relaxation phase of the deep tendon reflexes is common in young patients, but is often difficult to assess in the older patient. Central nervous system manifestations may be a prominent component of the symptom complex of the elderly patient and include confusion, depression, forgetfulness, irritability, and a shortened concentration span.[98] These cognitive impairments may point to a diagnosis of dementia and failure to consider the presence of hyperthyroidism.

Other clinical manifestations of hyperthyroidism in the elderly may include glucose intolerance and, ocassionally, the unmasking of latent diabetes mellitus. Mild elevations of serum calcium can occur along with development of osteoporosis.

Diagnosis

Because of the altered clinical presentation of hyperthyroidism in the elderly, suspicion must always be high and the laboratory should used in any patient with possible symptoms. It is not uneconomical to employ screening tests for thyroid status in all geriatric patients undergoing initial clinical evaluation.[99,100]

Serum T4 and measurement of serum TSH by modern ultrasensitive methods are the preferable screening procedures for thyroid dysfunction.[41,101] The findings of a normal serum T4 with suppressed serum TSH raises the possibility of T3 toxicosis and calls for measurement of serum T3. Determination of FT4 concentration by one of the direct measurement techniques may be useful when there is reason to suspect an alteration in thyroid-binding proteins.[43,46] Demonstration of anti-TSH receptor antibodies can be helpful in making a diagnosis of Graves' disease.[65,71]

The TRH stimulation test can be useful in evaluating the patient with borderline laboratory tests.[8,12] A significant rise in serum TSH will exclude the likelihood of hyperthyroidism, but an inadequate rise of TSH can only be considered as supportive of the diagnosis.

Thyroid scanning with ^{99m}Tc and measurement of ^{131}I uptake can be useful in establishing the presence of hyperfunctioning thyroid nodules.[61–63] Scanning may demonstrate the presence of a small diffusely active goiter that could not be detected on physical examination. Very low ^{131}I uptake in a patient with elevated circulating thyroid hormone levels suggests exogenous thyroid hormone ingestion (factitious hyperthyroidism), the hyperthyroid phase of subacute thyroiditis or iodine-induced hyperthyroidism.

Management

The first step in management of the patient with hyperthyroidism is determination of the underlying etiology to exclude the possibility of one of the transient forms that may require supportive therapy directed toward the primary process (hormone ingestion, iodine exposure, subacute thyroiditis). The vast majority of patients, with Graves' disease or multinodular toxic goiter, can be treated using antithyroid drugs, radioactive iodine, or surgery.[102,103]

In the patient with suspected hyperthyroidism who is still undergoing investigation, a useful initial step in treatment is the administration of β-adrenergic blocking agents such as propranolol or atenolol. These agents are especially indicated in patients who have palpitations, tachycardia, angina, or agitation as symptoms. These features of thyrotoxicosis can be quickly controlled with use of the β-blockers. These drugs act by interfering with some peripheral actions of thyroid hormone, but do not correct the hypermetabolic state. The drugs, however, do not interfere with laboratory assessment of thyroid function and can allow control of symptoms until definitive treatment can be undertaken.

Once a diagnosis of Graves' disease or a toxic nodular state is established, treatment should be started with one of the antithyroid drugs, propylthiouracil or methimazole.[104] These agents impair biosynthesis of thyroid hormone and will lead to depletion of intrathyroidal hormone stores and consequently to decreased hormone secretion. A decline in serum-T4 concentration can be seen by 2 weeks after initiation of antithyroid drug therapy, and the dose can be tapered once thyroid hormone levels reach the normal range in order to avoid development of hypothyroidism. In 1 to 5 percent of patients, the antithyroid drugs may cause fever, rash, and arthralgia. More serious is drug-induced agranulocytosis, which is most likely to occur within the first 2 months of treatment. Periodic monitoring of the white blood cell count should be done and the drugs discontinued if there is evidence of a fall. Although long-term antithyroid drug administration can be used as a primary therapy in young patients in an attempt to induce a long-lasting remission of Graves' disease, this approach is rarely successful in the elderly, and especially in patients with a nodular etiology.

The desired definitive treatment in the elderly is ablation of thyroid tissue through use of ^{131}I therapy.[103] Once the patient has been rendered euthyroid by antithyroid drugs, these agents can be stopped for 3 to 5 days, following which ^{131}I is given orally. Therapy with β-blockers can be maintained and antithyroid agents can be restarted 5 days after radiotherapy and continued for 3 to 4 weeks until the effect of radioiodine is achieved. Many therapists will attempt to calculate a dose that will render the patient euthyroid without subsequent development of hypothyroidism. These calculations are based on clinical estimate of thyroid gland size, 24-hour ^{131}I uptake, and whether the gland is diffusely overactive or contains toxic nodules. In spite of this approach, many patients will still develop permanent hypothyroidism following ^{131}I therapy.[105] It is not unreasonable to treat all elderly patients with a large dose of ^{131}I to assure ablation of thyroid tissue and avoid the possibility of recurrance of hyperthyroidism. Using this approach, patients are monitored following treatment until their serum thyroid hormone levels reach the hypothyroid range and are then put on permanent replacement therapy with exogenous thyroid hormone. Hypothyroidism may be evident as early as 4 weeks after treatment and can occur at any time after treatment. With all dosing regimens, by 12 months post-therapy 40 to 50 percent of patients are hypothyroid and hypothyroidism continues to occur thereafter at the rate of 2 to 3 percent per year.[106] Periodic monitoring of thyroid status is a necessity for any patient treated with ^{131}I who has not yet become hypothyroid.

Surgery is not recommended as a primary choice for treatment of hyperthyroidism in the elderly. The accompaniment of hyperthyroidism by many other disorders, including cardiac, pulmonary, and CNS disease, puts the patient at increased operative risk. In addition, postoperative complications of hypoparathyroidism and recurrent laryngeal nerve damage represent significant problems, especially when surgery is performed by surgeons not highly experienced in thyroidectomy.[107] Surgery may be of value for the rare patient with tracheal compression secondary to a large goiter.

Thyroid Storm

Acute hyperthyroidism or "thyroid storm" can occur in the patient with either known or undiagnosed hyperthyroidism who is subjected to acute stress such as an operative procedure, trauma, or infection. It can also occur in the elderly patient treated with ^{131}I who did not receive adequate antithyroid medication prior to therapy.[108] In these patients, features of severe hyperthyroidism may develop over several hours and include fever, tachycardia, vomiting, diarrhea, dehydration, severe restlessness, and disorientation. Acute heart failure can be precipitated. Thyroid storm is a life-threatening condition and must be treated vigorously and promptly.[109,110] Immediate treatment involves administration of iodide and antithyroid drugs to interfere with thyroid hormone synthesis, β-blockers and high-dose corticosteroids to blunt peripheral action of thyroid hormones, and supportive measures including sedation, fluids, antipyretics, and antibiotics if infection is present.

Hypothyroidism

Hypothyroidism is the clinical state that results from inadequate peripheral tissue response to thyroid hormone action. Most commonly, this occurs as a consequence of decreased thyroid hormone production from the thyroid gland,[111,112] but in rare instances can result from tissue unresponsiveness to the presence of adequate amounts of thyroid hormone in the circulation.[113,114] Deficient thyroid hormone release most commonly is the result of disease or dysfunction of the thyroid gland itself and is referred to as primary hypothyroidism. In some patients, pituitary TSH release is inadequate, leading to failure of the thyroid gland and secondary hypothyroidism. Rare cases of tertiary hypothyroidism have been identified in which the underlying mechanism is failure of synthesis or release of hypothalamic TRH.

Demography

Hypothyroidism is relatively common in the general population and shows a clear sex and age relationship. The Whickham, England study identified hypothyroidism, based on measurement of serum TSH, in 19 per 1,000 women with a mean age at diagnosis of 57 years and a prevalence tenfold more common in women than in men. The incidence rate of elevated serum TSH showed a direct relationship to age in women, increasing from 4.0 to 5.7 percent of women under age 45 to 17.4 percent of women over the age of 75 years. In men, elevated serum TSH was present in 1.6 to 3.5 percent of those under age 65 and increased to 3.5 to 6.9 percent in persons over the age of 65 years.[78] Similarly, study of the Framingham population in the US revealed clear elevation of serum TSH in 5.9 percent of women between the ages of 60 and 89 years and borderline elevation in an additional 7.7 percent. Men of the same age had elevated serum TSH in 2.4 percent of subjects, with another 3.3 percent showing borderline levels.[115]

In a US study of urban, community-dwelling individuals over the age of 55 years, elevated serum TSH levels were found in 8.5 percent of women and 4.4 percent of men, with a higher prevalence in whites (8.8 percent) than in blacks (4.4 percent). Abnormal values increased with age, rising from 5.3 percent of the 55 to 64 year group to 9.8 percent in those over 75 years.[79]

Many other population studies carried out in Great Britain, Sweden, Switzerland, West Germany, Japan, and in the US confirm the high frequency of hypothyroidism in the population, its predominance in women, and its progressive increase with advancing age.[100,116–121] Hypothyroidism may be especially common in elderly patients who seek geriatric evaluation. Among patients admitted to geriatric hospital units in the UK, 2.3 to 3.8 percent were found to have biochemical evidence for hypothyroidism, usually not suspected on clinical grounds. Similar results have been found in surveys of patient populations in the US and New Zealand.[99,122] Based on the clear influence of age on the risk of development of hypothyroidism, it is reasonable to screen all elderly individuals for the possible presence of the disorder through measurement of serum TSH.[100]

Etiology

Hypothyroidism can arise as a consequence of inborn or acquired disorders/diseases of the thyroid gland, from exposure to agents affecting thyroid-hormone synthesis and from disease or disturbance of hypothalamic-pituitary production of TRH and TSH. In the elderly population, the most common cause of thyroid failure is Hashimoto's disease.[112] This autoimmune disorder is characterized histologically by continuous replacement of normal thyroid tissue with lymphocytic and fibrous tissue, ultimately leading to a reduced mass of functional thyroid elements and decline in hormone production.[4] Many patients can be identified by demonstrating the presence of antithyroglobulin and antimicrosmal antibodies in their serum.[66,67,70] Much evidence has accumulated for the presence of another family of immunoglobulins that are capable of blocking the action of TSH on thyroid cells either by interfering with TSH binding to its receptor or by blocking both pre- and postreceptor processes.[66,123]

There is question whether or not the presence of antithyroid antibodies in the serum can predict the subsequent development of hypothyroidism.[124] In a study of subjects with demonstrated thyroid antibodies, hypothyroidism developed at a rate of 5 percent per year. Other reports do not support the predictive value of antithyroid antibodies, although they document the strong association of the antibodies with the presence of increased serum TSH and clinical hypothyroidism.[125]

Some patients with previously diagnosed Graves' disease may go on to develop an autoimmune hypothyroidism.[126] This consequence may be related to the presence of TSH-blocking antibodies. Other forms of thyroiditis, such as subacute and silent thyroiditis, may progress from a transient hyperthyroid state to euthyroidism, and finally, to permanent hypothyroidism.

A major cause of hypothyroidism is the prior treatment of hyperthyroidism, especially Graves' disease, by either radioiodine[105,106] or subtotal thyroidectomy.[127] Both treatments have been demonstrated to be followed by a continuous, life-long risk of development of hypothyroidism, with a rate 1 year after initial treatment of 20 to 40 percent and an annual incidence of 2 to 4 percent each year thereafter. Any patient with a prior history of surgical or radioiodine treatment of hyperthyroidism should have yearly monitoring of thyroid status with serum TSH and/or T4.

Iodide and iodine-containing drugs can result in inhibition of thyroid-hormone synthesis (Wolff-Chaikoff effect) with ensuing hypothyroidism, which is usually reversible when the source of exogenous iodine or iodide is removed.[128] Common sources of iodine ingestion are expectorants (potassium iodide), topical antifungal or antiseptic agents (betadine), iodine-containing radiographic contrast agents, and the antiarrhythmic agent, amiodarone.[129]

Impairment of production or release of TSH from the anterior pituitary or of TRH from the hypothalamus leads to secondary and tertiary hypothyroidism, respectively. These alterations can be the consequence of pituitary or hypothalamic tumors, surgical or traumatic injury, radiotherapy, or infiltrative diseases such as histiocytosis, sarcoidosis, tuberculosis, or amyloidosis. These patients may have isolated abnormalities of the TRH-TSH-thyroid axis or, more commonly, other associated disorders of hypothalamic, anterior, and posterior pituitary function.

Iodine deficiency in the past accounted for many cases of hypothyroidism, usually with an accompanying goiter. With the routine use of iodized salt and common exposure to many iodinecontaining agents in the diet, this is now a rare cause of hypothyroidism in the US. However, in many underdeveloped parts of the world, iodine deficiency remains as a common cause of failure of thyroid hormone production.

Clinical Presentation

Hypothyroidism, particularly in the elderly, is a disorder with insidious onset characterized by the emergence of symptoms and signs over many years, so that neither the patient nor close associates may be aware of the process.[130,131] Consequently, the manifestations of hypothyroidism are often attributed to "old age" or to other disorders common in the elderly person. Depending on recognition of the "classic" clinical features of hypothyroidism will invariably result in failure to make the diagnosis in many symptomatic patients. In one study, only 10 percent of patients with a laboratory-confirmed diagnosis were recognized as being hypothyroid on clinical examination.[132] Similar results have been found in other investigations.[115,116,118]

Central nervous system manifestations are a significant consequence of hypothyroidism in the elderly. Mental slowing is common along with complaints of fatigue and excessive sleepiness. The possibility of psychiatric disorder is raised by patients who present with depression, delerium, or paranoid ideation.[116,133,134] So-called "myxedema madness" with psychotic behavior is infrequent. Alterations in level of consciousness can occur with confusion and coma. An acute decline in mental status may be precipitated by the stress of infection or trauma, exposure to the cold, or to drugs such as sedatives and narcotics.[135] Seizures can occasionally be due to severe hypothyroidism. The possibility that hypothyroidism may be a cause of reversible dementia has led to much study of patients undergoing dementia evaluation. Most reports confirm that while hypothyroidism is common in patients with dementia, only rarely is the dementia truly reversible with thyroid hormone therapy, although there may be overall improvement in the patients' functional state.[116]

Classic cold intolerance and diminished sweating are often present in the elderly hypothyroid patient, but these symptoms are also common in euthyroid elderly. Hypothermia may be found. Dry skin, puffiness of the face, periorbital edema, coarsened and thinned hair, thinning of the outer parts of the eyebrows, brittle nails, and yellowing of the skin are common features of the patient, but also occur with great frequency in patients of advanced age whose thyroid function appears normal.

Coarsening of the voice with slow and sometimes slurred speech should increase the awareness of possible hypothyroidism. Hearing impairment may be due to thyroid insufficiency or, more commonly, hypothyroidism may aggravate a hearing disorder of other cause.

An important feature of thyroid deficiency in the elderly is physical slowing with accompanying symptoms of fatigue, weakness, and occasionally muscle stiffness. Arthralgia can also lead to physical slowing. Entrapment neuropathy with paresthesias can occur, especially involving the carpal tunnel.[136] Other aspects of neurologic involvement in hypothyroidism include impairment of reflex function leading to the classic delayed or "hung-up" relaxation phase of the reflex. Not infrequently, there may be hyporeflexia or complete loss of reflexes, especially of the achilles tendon.

In the elderly patient, assessment of changes in weight may give little insight into a possible diagnosis of hypothyroidism. Weight gain may occur, but decrease in appetite may be sufficient to result in weight loss. Bowel motility may be slowed with resultant constipation but, here again, this is a common complaint of the nonhypothyroid elderly.

The myocardium is affected by thyroid-hormone deficiency, so that slowing of the heart rate can occur along with stroke volume decrease, leading to reduced cardiac output.[137] The myocardium may undergo myxedematous infiltration with resultant cardiac enlargement, symptoms of ischemic heart disease, and development of pericardial effusion.[138] Electrocardiographic abnormalities may be seen including slow heart rate, low voltage of the QRS complex, and flattening or inversion of T waves. Alterations in peripheral vascular resistance can lead to hypertension. Reduced cardic output results in decrease of glomerular filtration rate, and consequent renal retention of sodium and water, so that peripheral edema may develop even in the absence of overt congestive heart failure.

Hematologic, metabolic, and other systemic impacts of hypothyroidism are more likely to be detected by laboratory evaluation than by clinical examination.[139] Anemia of the normocytic or macrocytic type can be found in about one-third of patients,[116] appears to be mediated by insufficient production of erythropoietin and is directly attributable to the lack of thyroid hormone. Serum iron may be low in some patients, but serum levels of folic acid and B12 are usually normal. Pernicious anemia occurs frequently in association with autoimmune forms of hypothyroidism and should be looked for in hypothyroid patients with persistent anemia after hormonal treatment or in patients with macrocytosis and low serum B12.

Hyponatremia occurs frequently in elderly individuals and may be found in patients with hypothyroidism. The clinical picture is that of the syndrome of inappropriate antidiuretic-hormone secretion, that is, dilutional hyponatremia, concentrated urine, normal or expanded intravascular volume, and sodium excretion in the urine. The mechanism appears to be due to increased release of antidiuretic hormone as well as to altered renal blood flow with increased tubular reabsorption of sodium and water.

Evidence suggestive of myopathy is provided by elevated levels of serum-creatine phosphokinase (CPK), which may be striking high. The increased levels are largely contributed to by decreased renal clearance of the enzyme.

Subclinical Hypothyroidism

As a result of a number of large laboratory survey studies, a significant population of individuals has been identified who have serum levels of TSH above the accepted upper limits of normal, but in whom serum concentrations of T4 and T3 are normal, and symptoms of hypothyroidism are usually lacking. This syndrome has been termed *subclinical hypothyroidism* and is most commonly found in women above the age of 60 years.[140–142] It is thought that the failing thyroid gland responds with an increase in TSH secretion which, in turn, is capable of further driving the thyroid to maintain normal levels of T4 and T3 until true thyroid failure ensues. In the Framingham study, 61 percent of subjects over the age of 60 years with clearly elevated serum-TSH concentrations (>10 mIU/L) had normal serum T4 levels and of those with slightly elevated serum TSH (5 to 10 mIU/L), 87 percent had normal serum T4.[115] Other studies have established a prevalence rate of between 25 and 104 per 1,000 persons with the highest rate occuring in women over age 55 years. The incidence in women between 40 and 60 years of age may be as high as 10 percent.[100]

Data from the Whickham study indicate that 60 percent of subjects with serum TSH values greater than 6 mIU/L and 80 percent of those with TSH values greater than 10 mIU/L had demonstrable antithyroid antibodies in their serum. Of the entire population of women, 5 percent had both elevated TSH levels and antithyroid antibodies.[78]

Of primary clinical importance is the question of what is the likelihood that the person with laboratory criteria for subclinical hypothyroidism will go on to develop clinical hypothyroidism. In a long-term follow-up study, women who initially had antithyroglobulin and antimicrosomal antibodies along with a serum TSH of greater than 6 mIU/L developed overt hypothyroidism at the rate of 5 percent per year. No cases developed in women with borderline elevation of TSH only (6 to 10 mIU/L) and only 1 case developed in the 67 women who had antithyroid antibodies with normal TSH levels.[141] Other studies support progression to overt hypothyroidism at the rate of 7 percent per year in women with elevated serum TSH and high titers of antithyroid antibodies with ranges from 1 percent to 20 percent per year.[100,143,144] It is clear that the presence of antithyroid antibodies constitutes a significant risk factor for the development of clinically apparent hypothyroidism in women who are found to have isolated elevated values of serum TSH.

Patients with subclinical hypothyroidism have been noted to have a relative increase in low-density lipoprotein and decrease in high-density lipoprotein with a higher prevalence of ischemic heart disease.[145] Thus, attention must be given to the question of whether or not the detection of subclinical hypothroidism warrants treatment. Several studies have reported that treatment with L-thyroxine results in improvement in left-ventricular ejection fraction with exercise, increase in serum high-density lipoproteins and decrease in low-density lipoproteins and apolipoprotein B, and some sense of improved well-being and performance on psychometric testing.[146–150] At present, a conservative approach dictates that patients identified with the syndrome should be monitored with serum TSH and T4 at 6 to 12 month intervals. Replacement therapy with thyroxine should be given to those patients with serum TSH greater than 10 mIU/L and to those in whom serum T4 has fallen below normal limits.

Myxedema Coma

Myxedema coma is an extreme, life-threatening form of hypothyroidism that occurs almost exclusively in the elderly. Presentation is that of an elderly person with rapid development of stupor, seizures, or coma, often in association with infection, stress, exposure to the cold, or following administration of sedatives, tranquilizers, or narcotics.[135] History or symptoms of hypothyroidism may have been present for a long time period. Hypothermia of profound degree is often present along with more common signs of hypothyroidism. Respiratory depression with hypoxia and carbon dioxide retention is commonly present and may necessitate intubation and ventilatory assistance. Blood pressure may be low, along with bradycardia and features of shock. Laboratory data will reveal, in addition to marked hypothyroxinemia, hyponatremia, hypoglycemia, elevation of serum CPK, and evidence of respiratory acidosis with increase in pCO_2. Recognition of the syndrome and prompt initiation of therapy is essential to avoid a mortality rate which may be in excess of 50 percent. If the diagnosis is suspected, therapy must be started at once, even though laboratory confirmation has not yet been obtained.[110,151]

Laboratory Diagnosis of Hypothyroidism

The findings of low-serum T4 concentration along with elevation of serum TSH clearly establish a diagnosis of primary hypothyroidism and these two findings require no further investigation.[41] Measurement of serum T3 in the elderly is of little diagnostic value because many disorders or drugs common in this age group lead to reduced concentrations of T3.[28] Conversely, in some patients with hypothyroidism, serum T3 levels may remain in the normal range.

The failure to find elevation of serum TSH in a patient with reduced serum T4 and/or T3 concentrations and clinical features suspicious for hypothyroidism requires that more extensive laboratory evaluation be carried out. The differentiation between secondary or tertiary hypothyroidism and the various "sick euthyroid" syndromes may be difficult. Normal values of FT4 point against hypothyroidism, but low FT4 may be seen in both conditions. Measurement of rT3 may be useful because its concentration will be low in true hypothyroidism and is generally normal or increased in nonthyroidal illness.[28]

The TRH test may be of value because patients with secondary hypothyroidism will show blunted or absent rise in TSH, while the sick euthyroid individual usually will respond to TRH with a rise. The measurement of antithyroid antibodies may provide indirect support for a diagnosis of hypothyroidism if the titers are high, but the levels themselves cannot indicate the functional state of the thyroid gland.

Therapy

The establishment of a diagnosis of hypothyroidism generally calls for initiation of thyroid hormone replacement. In the vast majority of patients, the preferred form of treatment is with synthetic L-thyroxine. There is little role for treatment with T3 because peripheral conversion of T4 to T3 is capable of providing adequate amounts of T3.

It is now well-established that the usual replacement dose of T4 is lower in the elderly than in the young patient, largely as a result of age-related reduction in rate of T4 clearance.[152–156] The mean daily dose of T4 for patients over the age of 65 years has been estimated to be 0.110 mg (1.6 μg/kg), but varies in individual patients from 0.05 to 0.2 mg. Determination of optimum T4 dose is based on monitoring of serum TSH and is defined as the dose of T4 that will reduce serum TSH into the normal range.[157] There is suggestion that the magnitude of initial serum TSH elevation correlates with the final T4 replacement dose.[156]

Excessive thyroid hormone replacement should be avoided. Elderly patients treated with L-thyroxine in standard doses and with serum T4 in the normal range have often been found to have suppressed serum TSH. Even though clinically evident features of hyperthyroidism are not detectable, metabolic effects of increased thyroid hormone can occur, and include increased nocturnal heart rate, shortened systolic time interval, increased urinary sodium excretion, and increased hepatic and muscle enzyme activity.[158,159] Of even greater consequence is the observation that patients on thyroid hormone replacement who have suppressed serum TSH also have evidence for increased bone resorption with consequent risk of accelerated rate of osteoporosis and, possibly, increased risk of fracture.[159–161]

In the elderly patient, initiation of hormone replacement should be with small doses, which are then slowly increased until full replacement has been achieved.[152,153] For most older patients, a dose of 0.025 mg daily of L-thyroxine is an appropriate starting amount. Subsequent increases can be in increments of 0.025 mg daily at 4 to 8 week intervals until normalization of serum TSH has been accomplished. It is not usual for the decline in TSH to lag behind the attainment of normal values for serum T4. This approach to treatment will minimize the risk of possible adverse effects of thyroid therapy, which include provocation of anginal pain, myocardial infarction, congestive heart failure, and arrhythmias.

Special attention must be given to the patient who, in addition to hypothyroidism, has an established diagnosis of ischemic heart disease. In this circumstance, it may be different to achieve full hormone replacement without provoking cardic symptoms. Attempt should be made to maximize the antianginal regimen, including administration of β-blockers, vasodilator agents, and calcium-channel blockers.[162,163] Should this approach fail, the patient should undergo evaluation for the possibility of angioplasty or coronary artery bypass surgery.[164]

In the patient who is thought to have secondary or tertiary hypothyroidism, consideration must be given to the possibility that there may be coexistent ACTH deficiency with resultant hypoadrenalism. Because the increased metabolic state resulting from thyroid replacement can precipitate the clinical picture of adrenal insufficiency, glucocorticoid replacement should be started concomitantly with thyroid hormone if there is any likelihood that ACTH deficiency is present. Some patients with long-standing, severe primary hypothyroidism may also develop signs of adrenal insufficiency following initiation of thyroid hormone due to metabolic impairment of adrenal hormone production from the hypothyroidism itself. Should any features of hypoadrenalism be suspected, prompt treatment with physiologic doses of glucocorticoids should be started. After a euthyroid state has been acheived, the steroid dose may be tapered and discontinued. In some patients, it may be prudent to start treatment with both thyroid and glucocortocoid hormones and discontinue the later as the patient approaches euthyroidism.

The treatment of myxedema coma warrants special consideration. In this life-threatening condition, treatment must be started promptly whenever the diagnosis is suspected, even before laboratory confirmation. The patient should be cared for in an intensive-care unit setting. Thyroid hormone must be given immediately by the intravenous route because both intestinal and intramuscular absorption are likely to be unreliable.[110,151] Although the type and amount of thyroid hormone has been the subject of some controversy, current recommendations are for intravenous L-thyroxine in an initial dose of 0.3 to 0.5 mg to replace the depleted total body thyroid hormone pool. Once evidence of clinical response has taken place, the daily dose should be reduced to 0.05 to 0.1 mg with subsequent dosage adjustments made in the conventional manner. Pharmacologic doses of glucocorticoids should also be given intravenously until evidence of clinical improvement and stabilization has occured. Supportive measures include slow, passive external rewarming if severe hypothermia is present, treatment of infection or other underlying illness, vasopressors for hypotension, and avoidance of CNS active drugs. Intubation with respiratory assistance may be necessary for management of hypoxia, acidosis, and bicarbonate retention.

Nodular Thyroid Disease and Neoplasia

The development of thyroid nodules clearly is an age-related process that occurs more commonly in women than in men. Autopsy studies have demonstrated that thyroid nodules are frequently found in the elderly, even when clinical examination of the neck has failed to reveal abnormality.[165] Autopsy data reveal that an increase in frequency of nodules is evident in women and men over age 30 with a rapid increase to a frequency of 90 percent in women and 50 percent in men over age 70 years. In the Whickham study, clinically detectable nodules were found in 0.8 percent of males, without a relationship to age. In women, however, 5.3 percent had nodules and the frequency increased from about 4 percent in those under age 50 years to 9.1 percent in those aged 75 years or more.[78] The Framingham study disclosed a 4.2 percent overall incidence of thyroid nodules with 6.4 percent in women and 1.5 percent in men.[166] New nodules become clinically recognizable at the rate of 0.1 percent per year. By means of ultrasonographic study, thyroid nodules have been found in approximately 50 percent of individuals beyond the age of 50 years.[167]

Clinical Presentations

Thyroid nodules most commonly are asymptomatic and may be discovered accidently by the patient or are found by the physician during the course of a physical examination. Of greatest concern is the finding of a single palpable nodule, which raises the possibility of thyroid malignancy. In many such patients, further evaluation will reveal the presence of multiple nodules. Although a single nodule is more likely to harbor a malignancy than a multinodular thyroid, only approximately 10 percent of clinical single nodules will, in fact, be malignant.

It is essential that the patient be questioned for the history of external radiation exposure of the head, neck, and upper thorax. It is well-established that radiation of the thyroid results in a marked increase in risk of developing thyroid malignancy. In the US, it was common practice for many years up to the 1950s to treat facial acne, tonsillar enlargement, cervical adenitis, and thymic enlargement with external radiation. It is estimated that several million people were irradiated, many of whom are entering or are now in the over-60 year age group. Although a history of irradiation in a patient with nodular thyroid increases the likelihood of malignancy, it is important to note that irradiation also increases the development of benign nodules. Of individuals who as children received low-dose head and neck irradiation, from 16 to 29 percent will develop palpable thyroid nodules and, of these, approximately one-third will be malignant. Nodules are apparent after a latency of 10 to 20 years and the incidence of malignant nodules reaches a peak 20 to 30 years after exposure.[168]

Ocassionally, a thyroid nodule will be associated with acute onset of neck pain and tenderness. This circumstance may be the result of acute or subacute thyroiditis or hemorrhage into a pre-existing nodule.

The finding of multinodular thyroid is increased in areas of iodine deficiency. Often there is a history of goiter dating back to childhood or young adult years. Very large multinodular goiter, particularly those with a sizeable substernal component, may compress the trachea and lead to complaints of dyspnea. Disturbances of swallowing may also occur. This presentation is most common in older women. A large substernal goiter sometimes is first recognized when the patient has had a chest radiogram and is noted to have compression or deviation of the trachea or a superior mediastinal mass.[169]

Differential Diagnosis

The entities that present as thyroid nodules are many. The vast majority are the result of benign thyroid lesions and include follicular and colloid adenomas, acute and subacute thyroiditis, Hashimoto's thyroiditis, and thyroid cysts. Malignant thyroid neoplasms include papillary, follicular, medullary, and anaplastic carcinomas as well as sarcoma and lymphoma of the thyroid. Nonthyroid lesions may also present as apparent thyroid nodules and include lymph nodes, aneurysms, parathyroid adenomas and cysts, and thyroglossal duct cysts.[170]

The likelihood that a single nodule is malignant is increased if there is a history of radiation exposure, if it occurs in a man, has been observed to undergo increase in size, is accompanied by hoarseness of the voice suggestive of impingement on the recurrant laryngeal nerve, and is stony hard on palpation. Age is a factor in predicting histologic type of malignancy.[171] More than 60 percent of thyroid malignancies are papillary carcinomas and these tend to occur in individuals under the age of 40 years. In patients over the age of 64 years, papillary carcinoma accounts for approximately 35 percent of thyroid cancers. Follicular carcinoma, the next most common histologic type, occurs with equal frequency in young and older persons and makes up approximately 20 percent of the thyroid malignancies in the over-64 year population. Medullary carcinoma accounts for 5 percent of thyroid cancers and is more commonly found in older than young persons, making up about 15 percent of thyroid cancers in the elderly.

Anaplastic carcinoma of the thyroid is almost exclusively a disease of older persons and accounts for approximately 20 percent of thyroid cancers in this age group. It is invariably fatal in a short period of time from its first diagnosis. Clinically, it often arises in an area of previous thyroid disease and is recognized by its rapid growth, rock-like consistency, and local invasiveness with recurrent laryngeal nerve involvement and tracheal compression.

Lymphoma, sarcoma, and metastatic cancers make up the remaining thyroid maligancies of the older person. Both lymphoma and sarcoma are characterized by a rapidly enlarging neck mass and initially may be difficult to differentiate from anaplastic carcinoma on clinical appearance alone. A history of Hashimato's thyroiditis is commonly present in patients with lymphoma.[172]

The rapid onset of a painful, tender thyroid mass with accompanying fever and leukocytosis is highly suggestive of acute suppurative thyroiditis. Similarly, the development of a painful, tender, firm thyroid mass without fever and leukocytosis points toward a diagnosis of subacute or granulomatous thyroiditis. History of an antecedent upper-respiratory tract infection with sore throat is further supportive of the diagnosis. This disorder may be accompanied in its acute phase by transient hyperthyroidism as a result of leakage of thyroid hormones from damaged follicular cells. Another consideration in the patient with acute onset of a painful, tender neck mass is hemorrhage into a previously asymptomatic thyroid cyst or adenoma.

Evaluation

A major consideration in the patient who is found to have a thyroid nodule, especially an apparently single nodule, is that of malignancy. A number of diagnostic modalities are available.

Blood tests of thyroid function will usually give normal results with the exception of the patient with a hyperfunctioning adenoma or toxic multinodular goiter. In some patients with nodular disease secondly to Hashimato's thyroiditis, serum TSH may be increased. Measurement of serum thyroglobulin is often elevated in patients with thyroid cancer, but cannot reliably differentiate malignancy from benign adenoma or thyroiditis.[75] Its major usefulness is in the early recognition of recurrance or metastasis in patients with papillary or follicular carcinoma who had previously undergone total thyroidectomy. Elevation of serum calcitonin concentration is highly supportive of a diagnosis of medullary carcinoma.[173]

Determination of functional status of a nodule by isotope imagining is useful. Malignant tissue rarely is able to take up iodine so that identification of a nodule as "warm" or "hot" by ^{123}I or technetium scanning makes the likelihood of malignancy in the nodule remote. In addition, scanning may reveal that an apparent single nodule is, in fact, part of a multinodular thyroid, again decreasing the risk of malignancy. The finding of a nonfunctioning or "cold" nodule does not establish a diagnosis of malignancy because the majority of thyroid nodules are cold and, of these, the incidence of malignancy is 10 to 15 percent.[174] For this reason, isotopic scanning is no longer considered as an initial diagnostic test.

High-resolution ultrasonography can detect lesions as small as 2 mm and can permit classification of a nodule as solid, cystic, or mixed solid-cystic.[175] The technique will often demonstrate multinodularity in a gland with a single palpable nodule. The value of ultrasongraphy in establishing a diagnosis of malignancy is limited because there is considerable overlap in the ultrasound characteristics of benign and malignant nodules. The procedure may be useful in detecting recurrent or residual thyroid cancer and in screening individuals who have had a history of irradiation exposure.

Computed tomograph and MRI can provide detailed information on thyroid anatomy. These procedures are expensive and appear to add little to clinical assessment for malignancy.[64]

In the past, thyroid hormone has been used to suppress TSH on the assumption that benign lesions were more likely to be TSH-dependent and, therefore, likely to decrease in size. The procedure involves giving L-thyroxine in a dose sufficient to suppress serum TSH and monitoring of size of the thyroid nodule for a period of 3 to 6 months. Because of the subjective nature of assessment of thyroid nodular size and the recent demonstration that suppressive therapy had no significant effect on nodule size during a 6-month, well-controlled, double-blind trial of L-thyroxine, there does not appear to be justification for future use of this procedure.[176] In addition, the administration of suppressive doses of L-thyroxine to elderly patients carries substantial risk for precipitation or aggrevation of ischemic heart disease and for acceleration of bone loss.

At the present time, fine needle aspiration (FNA) of the thyroid to obtain tissue for cytologic or histologic examination appears to be the most reliable and accurate method of separating benign from malignant disease.[177–179] In skilled hands, the procedure is safe, inexpensive, and capable of determing presence or absence of malignancy with 95 percent accuracy. The reliability of FNA can be further increased if done in conjunction with real-time sonographic guidance. The cytopathologic findings from FNA are assigned to four categories: positive for malignancy, suspicious for malignancy, negative for malignancy, and nondiagnostic. Surgery is recommended for all patients with a malignant cytologic diagnosis. For patients with a suspicious interpretation of the FNA, thyroid scanning is recommended with surgical excision to follow if the lesion is hypofunctioning. In the case of a nondiagnostic aspirate, a repeat FNA is recommended.

Management

The management of thyroid nodules is largely dependent on the results of the diagnostic evaluation, especially the determination as to whether or not the nodule has a high risk of being malignant.[179] Nodules identified as being "warm" and with associated normal thyroid hormone production and no compressive symptoms warrant only observation with examination at intervals of 6 to 12 months. "Hot" nodules are managed similarly as long as thyroid function is normal. If evidence for hyperthyroidism is found, then appropriate treatment for this condition should be initiated.

Large compressive goiters respond to ablation doses of ^{131}I with significant shrinkage of the thyroid and accompanying relief of compressive symptoms such as stridor, dyspnea, and dysphagia.[169] In these patients, replacement doses of L-thyroxine should be given following radioiodine treatment to maintain suppression of thyroid tissue and to avoid the late development of hypothyroidism.

If acute, suppurative thyroiditis is suspected, treatment with antibiotics is called for. The microorganisms most commonly responsible are *Staphyloccus aureus*, *Streptococus hemolyticus*, *Escherichia coli*, *Pneumococcus*, and *Salmonella*. Rarely, surgical drainage of a fluctuant mass will be necessary. Nodules found in association with subacute thyroiditis require no special care and may diminish in size as the disease resolves.

Management of the "cold" nodule is more complex. When possible, FNA biopsy should be performed.[177–179] Demonstration of benign cytology in either a solid or cystic nodule indicates that the patient can be managed subsequently by observation. The combination of suspicious cytology by FNA and cold appearance on scanning should lead to recommendation of surgical excision. If FNA reveals malignant cells, operation is recommended with little need for further study.

Surgery for thyroid carcinoma should be performed only by a surgeon experienced in the procedure. If a diagnosis of malignancy has not been firmly established preoperatively, the nodule should be removed with a wide margin of uninvolved tissue and examined by frozen section. If a diagnosis of papillary or follicular carcinoma is confirmed or has been made prior to surgery, near total thyroidectomy should be carried out because of the high frequency of multicentricity of malignancy and the need to remove functional thyroid tissue in order to monitor the patient with isotope scanning in the future.[180–182] Regional lymph nodes should be explored and removed if there is evidence of metastatic involvement. Postoperatively, attention must be paid to the possible complications of recurrent largngeal nerve injury and hypoparathyroidism, which may be transient or permanent. Almost certainly, patients will become hypothyroid following surgery and will require hormone replacement, which should be in a dose sufficient to suppress serum TSH to levels below normal, if clinically tolerated.

Postoperatively, and at 6 to 12 month intervals thereafter, it will be necessary to discontinue thyroid replacement for a period of up to 6 weeks to allow endogenous serum TSH levels to rise sufficiently high to promote tissue uptake of ^{131}I. At that time, blood is obtained for measurement of thyroglobulin and then large scanning doses of ^{131}I are administered and neck and total body scans are performed at 24, 48, and 72 hours. If serum thyroglobulin is elevated, or if areas of uptake are found, large ablative doses of ^{131}I are then administered and replacement therapy reinstituted 48 hours later. This approach reduces the recurrence rate of both papillary and follicular carcinoma and prolongs survival.[181–183] The 10-year survival for patients over the age of 40 years with papillary carcinoma is estimated to be 90 percent, while 10-year survival falls to 84 percent in patients with follicular carcinoma and 75 percent for medullary carcinoma.[171] In patients with follicular carcinoma, increased size (greater than 3 cm) was associated with increased recurrence and distant metastases at time of diagnosis predicted high-risk of subsequent death. Age at time of diagnosis was not an adverse risk factor for death.[184]

If thyroid malignancy has been determined to be due to medullary carcinoma, the operative procedure of choice is total thyroidectomy because the disease is often multicentric. Routine dissection of the lymph modes is also recommended. The majority of medullary carcinomas do not respond to ^{131}I therapy so that patients with inoperable residual or recurrent disease are treated palliatively with external irradiation. The sur-

Table 73-2 Occurence and survivorship of thyroid malignancy in the older patient

Cancer Type	% of Patients with Type >Age 40	% of Patients with Type >Age 64	10-Year Survival (%)
Papillary/mixed	58	35	90
Follicular	26	20	84
Medullary	3	15	75
Anaplastic	10	20	0
Other (lymphoma, metastatic sarcoma)	3	10	0

vival declines with increase in age at time of initial diagnosis, being substantially lower in patients over age 50 years. In patients in their seventh decade, approximately two-thirds will have persistent disease after surgery.[185] The efficacy of surgery can be monitored postoperatively by measurement of blood calcitonin concentration, both in the basal state and after stimulation.[173] Occurrence and survival rates for thyroid malignancy are given in Table 73-2.

The management of anaplastic carcinoma of the thyroid remains unsatisfactory.[183] Relief of symptoms of compression can sometimes be achieved by surgery followed by high-dose (45–60Gy) external irradiation.[186] Chemotherapy with doxorubicin may be beneficial in combination with surgery and external irradiation.[187]

References

1. Mariotti S, Franceschi C, Cossarizza A, Pinchera A: The aging thyroid. Endocrinol Rev 1995;16:686–715
2. Mochizuki Y, Mowafy R, Pasternak B: Weights of human thyroids in New York City. Health Phys 1963;9:1299–1301
3. Hegedus L, Perrild H, Poulsen LR et al: The determination of thyroid volume by ultrasound and its relationship to body weight, age and sex in normal subjects. J Clin Endocrinol Metab 1983;56:260–263
4. Blumenthal HT, Perlstein IB: The aging thyroid. I. A description of lesions and an analysis of their age and sex distribution. J Am Geriatr Soc 1987;35:843–854
5. Denham MJ, Wills EJ: A clinco-pathological survey of thyroid glands in old age. Gerontology 1980;26:160–166
6. Barreca T, Franceschini R, Messina U et al: 24-hour thyroid-stimulating hormone secretory pattern in elderly men. Gerontology 1985;31:119–123
7. Snyder PJ, Utiger RD: Response to thyrotropin releasing hormone (TRH) in normal man. J Clin Endocrinol Metab 1972; 34:380–385
8. Utiger RD: Thyrotropin-releasing hormone and thyrotropin secretion. J Lab Clin Med 1987;109:327–335
9. Harman SM, Whemann RE, Blackman MR: Pituitary-thyroid hormone economy in healthy aging men: basal indices of thyroid function and thyrotropin responses to constant infusion of thyrotropin releasing hormone. J Clin Endocrinol Metab 1984;58:320–326
10. Van Coevorden A, Laurent E, Decoster C et al: Decreased basal and stimulated thyrotropin secretion in healthy elderly men. J Clin Endocrinol Metab 1989;69:177–185
11. Targum SD, Marshall LE, Magac-Harris K, Martin D: TRH tests in a healthy elderly population. Demonstration of gender differences. J Am Geriatr Soc 1989;37:533–536
12. Hay ID, Klee GG: Thyroid dysfunction. Endocrinol Metab Clin North Am 1988;17:473–509
13. Snyder PJ, Utiger RD: Thyrotropin response to thyrotropin releasing hormone in normal females over forty. J Clin Endocrinol Metab 1972;34:1096–1098
14. Ryan M, Kovaks K, Ezrin C: Thyrotrophs in old age: an immunologic study of human pituitary glands. Endokrinologie 1979; 73:191–198
15. Cuttelod S, Lemarchand-Beraud T, Magnenat P et al: Effect of age and role of kidneys and liver on thyrotropin turnover in man. Metabolism 1974;23:101–113
16. Olsen T, Laurberg P, Weeke J: Low serum triiodothyronine and high serum reverse triiodothyronine in old age: An effect of disease not age. J Clin Endocrinol Metab 1978;47:1111–1115
17. Hermann J, Heinen E, Kroll HJ et al: Thyroid function and thyroid hormone metabolism in elderly people. Low T3-syndrome in old age? Klin Wochenschr 1981;59:315–323
18. Chopra IJ, Solomon DH, Chopra U et al: Pathways of metabolism of thyroid hormones. Rec Prog Horm Res 1978;34: 521–567
19. Hansen JM, Skovsted L, Siersboek-Nielsen K: Age dependent changes in iodine metabolism and thyroid function. Acta Endocrinol (Copenhagen) 1975;79:60–65
20. Braverman LE, Dawber NA, Ingbar SH: Observations concerning the binding of thyroid hormones in serum of normal subjects of varying age. J Clin Invest 1966;45:1273–1279
21. Hesch RD, Gatz J, Juppner H, Stubbe P: TBG dependency of age-related variations of thyroxine and triiodothyronine. Horm Metab Res 1977;9:141–146
22. Kabadi UM, Rosman PM: Thyroid hormone indices in adult healthy subjects: no influence of aging. J Am Geriatr Soc 1988; 36:312–316
23. Gregerman RI, Gaffney GW, Shock NW: Thyroxine turnover in euthyroid man with special reference to changes with age. J Clin Invest 1962;41:2065–2074
24. Ingbar SH: Effect of aging on thyroid economy in man. J Am Geriatr Soc 1976;24:49–53
25. Nishikawa M, Inada M, Naito K et al: Age-related changes of serum 3, 3′-diiodothyronine, 3′–5′-diiodothyronine, and 3,5-diiodothyronine concentrations in man. J Clin Endocrinol Metab 1981;52:517–552
26. Gambert SR, Tsitouras PD: Effect of age on thyroid hormone physiology and function. J Am Geriatr Soc 1985;33:360–365
27. Engler D, Burger AG: The deiodination of the iodothyronines and of their derivatives in man. Endocrinol Rev 1984;5: 151–184
28. Chopra IJ, Hershman JM, Pardridge MD et al: Thyroid function in nonthyroidal illnesses. Ann Intern Med 1983;98:946–957
29. Dillman WH: Mechanism of action of thyroid hormones. Med Clin North Am 1985;69:849–861

30. Oppenheimer JH: Thyroid hormone action at the nuclear level. Ann Intern Med 1985;102:374–384
31. Brent GA: The molecular basis of thyroid hormone action. N Engl J Med 1994;331:847–853
32. Kohrle J, Hesch RD, Leonard JL: Intracellular pathways of iodothyronine metabolism. pp. 144–189. In Braverman LE, Utiger RD (eds): The Thyroid. 6th Ed. Lippencott-Raven, Philadelphia, 1991
33. Larsen PR, Silva JE, Kaplan MM: Relationships between circulating and intracellular thyroid hormone: physiological and clinical implications. Endocrinol Rev 1981;2:87–102
34. Sap J, Munoz A, Damm K et al: The *c-erb*-A protein is a high affinity receptor for thyroid hormone. Nature 1986;324: 635–640
35. Weinberger C, Thompson CC, Ong ES et al: The *c-erb*-A gene encodes a thyroid hormone receptor. Nature 1986;324: 641–646
36. Denckla WD: Role of the pituitary and thyroid glands on the decline of minimal oxygen consumption with age. J Clin Invest 1974;53:572–581
37. Gambert SR, Ingbar SH, Hagen TC: Interaction of age and thyroid hormone status on Na^+-K^+ ATPase in rat renal cortex and liver. Endocrinology 1980;108:27–30
38. Mariotti S, Barbesino G, Caturegli P et al: Complex alteration of thyroid function in healthy centenarians. J Clin Endocrinol Metab 1993;77:1130–1134
39. Spencer CA: Clinical utility and cost effectiveness of sensitive thyrotropin assay in ambulatory and hospitalized patients. Mayo Clin Proc 1988;63:1214–1222
40. Franklyn JA, Black EG, Betteridge J, Sheppard MC: Comparison of second and third generation methods for measurement of serum thyrotropin in patients with overt hyperthyroidism, patients receiving thyroxine therapy, and those with nonthyroidal illness. J Clin Endocrinol Metab 1994;78:1368–1371
41. Klee GG, Hay ID: Assessment of sensitive thyrotropin assays for an expanded role in thyroid function testing: proposed criteria for analytic performance and clinical utility. J Clin Endocrinol Metab 1987;64:461–471
42. Burrow AW, Shakespear RA, Hesch RD et al: Thyroid hormones in the elderly sick: "T4 euthyroidism". Br Med J 1975; 4:437–439
43. Kaptein EM, MacIntyre SS, Weiner JM et al: Free thyroxine estimates in nonthyroidal illness: comparison of eight methods. J Clin Endocrinol Metab 1981;52:1073–1077
44. Surks MI, Hupart KH, Pan C, Shapiro LE: Normal Free thyroxine in critical nonthyroidal illnesses measured by ultrafiltration of undiluted serum and equilibrium dialysis. J Clin Endocrinol Metab 1988;67:1031–1039
45. Csako G, Zweig MH, Benson C, Ruddel M: On the albumin dependence of measurements of free thyroxine. I. Technical performance of seven methods. Clin Chem 1986;32:108–115
46. Spencer CA: Clinical evaluation of free T4 techniques. J Endocrinol Invest 1986;9(suppl 4):57–66
47. Kaptein EM: Thyroid hormone metabolism in illness. pp. 297–333. In Hennemann G (ed): Thyroid Hormone Metabolism. Marcel Dekker, New York, 1986
48. Wenzel KW: Pharmacological interference with in vitro tests of thyroid function. Metabolism 1981;30:717–732
49. Chopra IJ, Huang T-S, Beredo A et al: Serum thyroid hormone binding inhibitor in nonthyroidal illnesses. Metabolism 1986; 35:152–159
50. Wartofsky L, Burman KD: Alterations in thyroid function in patients with systemic illnesses: the "euthyroid sick syndrome". Endocrinol Rev 1982;3:164–217
51. Slag MF, Morley JE, Elson MK et al: Hypothyroxinemia in critically ill patients as a predictor of high mortality. JAMA 1981;245:43–45
52. Gavin LA: The diagnostic dilemmas of hyperthyroxinemia and hypothyroxinemia. Adv Int Med 1988;33:185–203
53. Hamblin PS, Dyer SA, Mohr VS et al: Relationship between thyrotropin and thyroxine changes during recovery from severe hypothyroxinemia of critical illness. J Clin Endocrinol Metab 1986;62:717–722
54. Tibaldi JM, Surks MI: Effects of nonthyroidal illness on thyroid function. Med Clin North Am 1985;69:899–911
55. Simmons RJ, Simon JM, Demers LM, Santen RJ: Thyroid dysfunction in elderly hospitalized patients. Effect of age and severity of illness. Arch Intern Med 1990;150:1249–1253
56. Bartalena L, Brogioni S, Grasso L et al: Relationship of the increased serum interleukin-6 concentration to changes of thyroid function in nonthyroidal illness. J Endocrinol Invest 1994; 17:269–274
57. Rogy MA, Coyle SM, Oldenburg HSA et al: Persistently elevated soluble tumor necrosis factor receptor and interleukin-1 receptor antagonist levels in critically ill patients. J Am Coll Surg 1994;178:132–138
58. Pang XP, Hershman JH, Mirell CJ, Pekary AE: Impairment of hypothalamic-pituitary-thyroid function in rats treated with human recombinant tumor necrosis factor-α (cachectin). Endocrinology 1989;125:76–84
59. Borst CG, Eil C, Burman KD: Euthyroid hyperthyroxinemia. Ann Intern Med 1983;98:366–378
60. Ruiz M, Rejatanavin R, Young RA et al: Familial dysalbuminemic hyperthyroxinemia: a syndrome that can be confused with thyrotoxicosis. N Engl J Med 1982;306:635–639
61. Khafagi FA, MacFarlane DJ, Shapiro B, Gross MD: Nuclear medicine. pp. 451–492. In Moore WT, Eastman RC (eds): Diagnostic Endocrinology. 2nd Ed. Mosby-Year Book, St. Louis, 1996
62. Robertson JS, Nolan NG, Wahner HW, McConahey WM: Thyroid radioiodine uptakes and scan in euthyroid patients. Mayo Clinic Proc 1975;50:79–84
63. Sarkar SD, Becker DV: Thyroid uptake and imaging. pp. 284–289. In Becker KL (ed): Principles and Practice of Endocrinology and Metabolism. Lippincott-Raven, Philadelphia, 1990
64. Blum M: Thyroid sonography, computed tomography, and magnetic resonance imaging. pp. 289–293. In Becker KL (ed): Principles and Practice of Endocrinology and Metabolism. Lippincott-Raven, Philadelphia, 1990
65. Zakarija M, McKenzie JM: The spectrum and significance of autoantibodies reacting with the thyrotropin receptor. Endocrinol Metab Clin North Am 1987;16:343–363
66. Dussault JH, Rousseau F: Immunologically mediated hypothyroidism. Endocrinol Metab Clin North Am 1987;16:417–429

67. Robuschi G, Safran M, Braverman LE et al: Hypothyroidism in the elderly. Endocrinol Rev 1987;8:142–153
68. Blumenthal HT, Perlstein IB: The aging thyroid. II. An immunocytochemical analysis of the age-associated lesions. J Am Geriatr Soc 1987;35:855–863
69. Spaulding SW: Age and the thyroid. Endocrinol Metab Clin North Am 1987;16:1013–1025
70. Delespesse G, Hubert C, Gausset P, Govaerts A: Radioimmunassay for human antithyroglobulin antibodies of different immunoglobulin classes. Horm Metab Res 1976;8:50–54
71. Massart C, Hody B, Mouchel L et al: Assay for thyrotropin-receptor binding and thyroid-stimulating antibodies in sera from patients with Graves' disease. Clin Chem 1986;32: 1332–1335
72. Kasagi K, Konishi J, Iida Y et al: A sensitive and practical assay for thyroid-stimulating antibodies using FRTL-5 thyroid cells. Acta Endocrinol (Copenhagen) 1987;115:30–36
73. Rees Smith B, McLachlan SM, Furmaniak J: Autoantibodies to the thyrotropin receptor. Endocrinol Rev 1988;9:106–121
74. Wilson R, McKillop JH, Henderson N et al: The ability of the serum thyrotropin receptor antibody (TRAB) index and HLA status to predict long term remission of thyrotoxicosis following medical therapy for Graves' disease. Clin Endocrinol (Oxford) 1986;25:151–156
75. Spencer CA, Wang C-C: Thyroglobulin measurement: techniques, clinical benefits, and pitfalls. Endocrinol Metab Clin North Am 1995;24:841–863
76. Davis PJ, Davis FB: Hyperthyroidism in patients over the age of 60 years: clinical features in 85 patients. Medicine 1974; 53:161–182
77. Ronnov-Jessen V, Kirkegaard C: Hyperthyroidism: a disease of old age? Br Med J 1973;1:41–43
78. Tunbridge WMG, Evered DC, Hall R et al: The spectrum of thyroid disease in a community: the Whickham survey. Clin Endocrinol (Oxford) 1977;7:481–493
79. Bagchi N, Brown TR, Parish JD: Thyroid dysfunction in adults over age 55 years. A study in an urban US community. Arch Intern Med 1990;150:785–787
80. Furszyfer J, Kurland LT, McConahey WM et al: Epidemiologic aspects of Hashimoto's thyroiditis and Graves' disease in Rochester, Minnesota (1935–1967), with special reference to temporal trends. Metabolism 1972;21:197–204
81. Ferriman D, Hennebry TM, Tassopoulos CN: True thyroid adenoma. Q J Med 1972;41:127–139
82. Marsden P, Facer P, Acosta M, McKerron CG: Serum triiodothyronine in solitary autonomous nodules of the thyroid. Clin Endocrinol (Oxford) 1975;4:327–330
83. Fradkin JE, Wolff J: Iodine induced thyrotoxicosis. Medicine 1983;62:1–20
84. Banovac K, Papic M, Bilsker MS et al: Evidence of hyperthyroidism in apparently euthyroid patients treated with levothyroxine. Arch Intern Med 1989;149:809–812
85. Smallridge RC: Thyrotropin-secreting pituitary tumors. Endocrinol Metab Clin North Am 1987;16:765–792
86. Beck-Peccoz P, Mariotti S, Guillausseau PJ et al: Treatment of hyperthyroidism due to inappropriate secretion of thyrotropin with the somatostatin analog SMS 201–995. J Clin Endocrinol Metab 1989;68:208–214
87. Hay ID: Thyroiditis: a clinical update. Mayo Clin Proc 1985; 60:836–843
88. Sawin CT, Geller A, Wolf PA et al: Low serum thyrotropin concentrations as a risk factor for atrial fibrillation in older persons. N Engl J Med 1994;331:1249–1252
89. Parle JV, Franklyn JA, Cross KW et al: Prevalence and follow-up of abnormal thyrotropin (TSH) concentrations in the elderly in the United Kingdom. Clin Endocrinol (Oxford) 1991;34: 77–83
90. Sawin CT, Geller A, Kaplan MM et al: Low serum thyrotropin (thyroid-stimulating hormone) in older persons without hyperthyroidism. Arch Intern Med 1991;151:165–168
91. Kawabe T, Komiya I, Endo T et al: Hyperthyroidism in the elderly. J Am Geriatr Soc 1979;27:152–155
92. Griffin MA, Solomon DH: Hyperthyroidism in the elderly. J Am Geriatr Soc 1986;34:887–892
93. Trivalle C, Doucet J, Chasogne P et al: Differences in the signs and symptoms of hyperthyroidism in older and younger patients. J Am Geriatr Soc 1996;44:50–53
94. Thomas FB, Mazzaferri EL, Skillman TG: Apathetic thyrotoxicosis: a distinctive clinical and laboratory entity. Ann Intern Med 1970;72:679–685
95. Tibaldi JM, Barzel US, Alben J et al: Thyrotoxicosis in the very old. Am J Med 1986;81:619–622
96. DeGroot LJ: Thyroid and the heart. Mayo Clin Proc 1972;47: 864–871
97. Forfar JC, Muir AL, Sawers SA, Toft AD: Abnormal left ventricular function in hyperthyroidism: evidence for a possible reversible cardiomyopathy. N Engl J Med 1982; 307: 1165–1170
98. Salzman C, Shader RI: Depression in the elderly. I. Relationship between depression, psychologic defense mechanisms and physical illness. J Am Geriatr Soc 1978;26:253–260
99. Livingston EH, Hershman JM, Sawin CT, Yoshikawa TT: Prevalence of thyroid disease and abnormal thyroid tests in older hospitalized and ambulatory persons. J Am Geriatr Soc 1987; 35:109–114
100. Helfand M, Crapo LM: Screening for thyroid disease. Ann Intern Med 1990;112:840–849
101. Bayer MF, Macoviak JA, McDougall IR: Diagnostic performance of sensitive measurements of serum thyrotropin during severe nonthyroidal illness: their role in the diagnosis of hyperthyroidism. Clin Chem 1987;33:2178–2184
102. Solomon B, Glinoer D, Lagasse R, Wartofsky L: Current trends in the management of Graves' disease. J Clin Endocrinol Metab 1990;70:1518–1524
103. Orgiazzi J: Management of Graves' hyperthyroidism. Endocrinol Metab Clin North Am 1987;16:365–389
104. Cooper DS: Antithyroid drugs. N Engl J Med 1984;311: 1353–1362
105. Sridama V, McCormick M, Kaplan EL et al: Long-term follow-up study of compensated low-dose ^{131}I therapy for Graves' disease. N Engl J Med 1984;311:426–432
106. Holm LE: Changing annual incidence of hypothyrodism after iodine-131 therapy for hyperthyroidism, 1951–1975. J Nucl Med 1982;23:108–112
107. Palestini N, Valori MR, Carlin R et al: Mortality, morbidity and long-term results in surgically treated hyperthyroid patients. Review of 597 cases. Acta Chir Scand 1985;151:509–513

108. McDermott MT, Kidd GS, Dodson LE et al: Radio-iodine induced thyroid storm. Am J Med 1983;75:353–359
109. Hoffenberg R: Thyroid emergencies. Endocrinol Metab Clin North Am 1980;9:503–513
110. Nicoloff JT: Thyroid storm and myxedema coma. Med Clin North Am 1985;69:1005–1017
111. Havard CWH: The thyroid and aging. Endocrinol Metab Clin North Am 1981;10:163–178
112. Hurley JR: Thyroid disease in the elderly. Med Clin North Am 1983;67:497–516
113. Refetoff S, DeGroot LJ, Barsano CP: Defective thyroid hormone feedback regulation in the syndrome of peripheral resistance to thyroid hormone. J Clin Endocrinol Metab 1980;51: 41–45
114. Cooper DS, Ladenson PW, Nisula BC et al: Familial thyroid hormone resistance. Metabolism 1982;31:504–509
115. Sawin CT, Castelli WP, Hershman JM et al: The aging thyroid. Thyroid deficiency in the Framingham study. Arch Intern Med 1985;145:1386–1388
116. Bahemuka M, Hodkinson HM: Screening for hypothyroidism in elderly impatients. Br Med J 1975;1:601–603
117. Falkenberg M, Kogedal B, Norr A: Screening of an elderly female population for hypo and hyperthyroidism by use of a thyroid hormone panel. Acta Med Scand 1983;214:361–365
118. Riniker M, Tiechl M, Lupi GA et al: Prevalence of various degrees of hypothyroidism among patients of a general medical department. Clin Endocrinol (Oxford) 1981;14:69–74
119. Herrmann J: Prevalence of hypothroidism in the elderly in Germany. A pilot study. J Endocrinol Invest 1981;4:327–330
120. Inada M, Nisikawa M, Kawai I: Hypothyroidism associated with positive results of the perchlorate discharge test in elderly patients. Am J Med 1983;74:1010–1015
121. Okamura K, Ueda K, Sone H et al: A sensitive thyroid stimulating hormone assay for screening of thyroid functional disorder in elderly Japanese. J Am Geriatr Soc 1989;37:317–322
122. Campbell AJ, Reinken J, Allan BC: Thyroid disease in the elderly in the community. Age Ageing 1981;10:47–52
123. Konishi J, Iida Y, Kasagi K et al: Primary myxedema with thyrotrophin-binding inhibitor immunoglobulins: Clinical and laboratory findings in 15 patients. Ann Intern Med 1985;103: 26–31
124. Tunbridge WMG, Brewis M, French J: Natural history of autoimmune thyroiditis. Br Med J 1981;282:258–262
125. Sawin CT, Bigos ST, Land S, Bacharach P: The aging thyroid. Relationship between elevated serum thyrotropin level and thyroid antibodies in elderly patients. Am J Med 1985;79: 591–595
126. Hirota Y, Tamai H, Hayashi Y et al: Thyroid function and history in forty-five patients with hyperthyroid Graves' disease in clinical remission more than 10 years after thionamide drug treatment. J Clin Endocrinol Metab 1986;62:165–169
127. Max MH, Scherm M, Bland KI: Early and late complication after thyroid operations. South Med J 1983;76:977–980
128. Roti E, Vagenakis AG: Effect of excess iodide: clinical aspects. pp. 390–402. In Braverman LE, Utiger RD (eds): The Thyroid. 6th Ed. Lippincott-Raven, Philadelphia, 1991
129. Martino E, Safran M, Aghini-Lombardi F et al: Environmental iodine intake and thyroid dysfunction during chronic amiodarone therapy. Ann Intern Med 1984;101:28–34
130. Tachman ML, Guthrie GP: Hypothyroidism: diversity of presentation. Endocrinol Rev 1984;5:456–465
131. Bastenie PA, Bonnyns M, Vanhaelst L: Natural history of primary myxedema. Am J Med 1985;79:91–100
132. Lloyd WA, Goldberg IJL: Incidence of hypothyroidism in the elderly. Br Med J 1961;2:1256–1259
133. Hall RCW: Psychiatric effects of thyroid hormone disturbance. Psychosomatics 1983;24:7–18
134. Logotheis J: Psychiatric behavior as the initial indicator of adult myxedema. J Nerv Ment Dis 1963;136:561–568
135. Zellman HE: Unusual aspects of myxoedema. Geriatrics 1968; 23:140–148
136. Rao SN, Katiyar BC, Nair KRP, Misra S: Neuromuscular status in hypothyroidism. Acta Neurol Scand 1980;61:167–177
137. Buccino RA, Spann JF, Pool PE et al: Influence of the thyroid state on the intrinsic contractile properties and the energy stores of the myocardium. J Clin Invest 1967;46:1669–1682
138. Vanhaelst L, Neve P, Chailly P, Bastenie P: Coronary artery disease in hypothyroidism. Lancet 1967;2:800–802
139. Horton L, Coburn RJ, England JM, Himsworth RL: The haematology of hypothyroidism. QJ Med 1976;45:101–124
140. Evered DC, Ormston BJ, Smith PA et al: Grades of hypothyroidism. Br Med J 1973;1:657–662
141. Tunbridge WMG, Brewis M, French J et al: Natural history of autoimmune thyroiditis. Br Med J 1981;282:258–262
142. Jayme JJ, Ladenson PW: Subclinical thyroid dysfunction in the elderly. Trends Endocrinol Metab 1994;5:79–86
143. Lazarus JH, Burr ML, McGregor AM et al: The prevalence and progression of autoimmune thyroid disease in the elderly. Acta Endocrinol 1984;106:199–202
144. Rosenthal MJ, Hunt WC, Garry PJ, Goodwin JS: Thyroid failure in the elderly. Microsomal antibodies as discriminant for therapy. JAMA 1987;258:209–213
145. Althous BU, Staub JJ, Ryff-de-Leche A et al: LDL/HDL changes in subclinical hypothyroidism: possible risk factors for coronary heart disease. Clin Endocrinol (Oxford) 1988;28: 157–163
146. Bell GM, Todd WTA, Forfar JC et al: End-organ responses to thyroxine therapy in subclinical hypthyroidism. Clin Endocrinol (Oxford) 1985;22:83–89
147. Cooper DS, Halpern R, Wood LC et al: L-Thyroxine therapy in subclinical hypothyroidism. A double blind placebo-controlled trial. Ann Intern Med 1984;101:18–24
148. Nystrom E, Caldahl K, Fager G, et al: A double-blind crossover 12 month study of l-thyroxine treatment of women with "subclinical" hypothyroidism. Clin Endocrinol (Oxford) 1988; 29:63–75
149. Arem R, Patsch W: Lipoprotein and apolipoprotein levels in subclinical hypothyroidism. Effect of levothyroxine therapy. Arch Intern Med 1990;150:2097–2100
150. Caron P, Calazel C, Parra HJ et al: Decreased HDL cholesterol in subclinical hypothyroidism: the effect of L-thyroxine therapy. Clin Endocrinol (Oxford) 1990;33:519–523
151. Ridgway EC, McCammon JA, Benotti J, Maloof F: Acute meta-

bolic responses in myxedema to large doses of intravenous L-thyroxine. Ann Intern Med 1972;77:549–555

152. Rosenbaum RL, Barzel US: Levothyroxine replacement dose for primary hypothyroidism decreases with age. Ann Intern Med 1982;96:53–55

153. Sawin CT, Herman T, Molitch ME et al: Aging and the thyroid. Decreased requirement for thyroid hormone in older hypothyroid patients. Am J Med 1983;75:206–209

154. Davis FB, LaMantia RS, Spaulding SW et al: Estimation of a physiologic replacement dose of levothyroxine in elderly patients with hypothyroidism. Arch Intern Med 1984;144: 1752–1754

155. Cunningham JJ, Barzel US: Lean body mass is a predictor of the daily requirement for thyroid hormone in older men and women. J Am Geriatr Soc 1984;32:204–207

156. Kabadi UM: Optimal daily levothyroxine dose in primary hypothyroidism. Its relation to pretreatment thyroid hormone indexes. Arch Intern Med 1989;149:2209–2212

157. Mandel S, Brent GA, Larsen PR: Levothyroxine therapy in patients with thyroid disease. Ann Intern Med 1993;119: 492–502

158. Toft AD: Thyroxine therapy. N Engl J Med 1994;331:174–180

159. Oppenheimer JH, Braverman LE, Toft A, et al: Thyroid hormone treatment: when and what? J Clin Endocrinol Metab 1995;80:2873–2883

160. Stall GM, Harris S, Sokoll LJ, Dawson-Hughes B: Accelerated bone loss in hypothyroid patients overtreated with L-thyroxine. Ann Intern Med 1990;113:265–269

161. Solomon BL, Wartofsky L, Burman KD: Prevalence of fractures in postmenopausal women with thyroid disease. Thyroid 1993; 3:17–23

162. Steinberg AD, Schrader ZR: Myxoedema with angina pectoris treated with propranolol and triiodothyronine. Lancet 1971;2: 213

163. Levine HD: Compromise therapy in the patient with angina pectoris and hypothyroidism. Am J Med 1980;69:411–418

164. Becker C: Hypothyroid and atherosclerotic heart disease: pathogenesis, medical management and the role of coronary artery bypass surgery. Endocrinol Rev 1985;6:432–440

165. Mortensen JD, Woolner LB, Bennett WA: Gross and microscopic findings in clinically normal thyroid glands. J Clin Endocrinol Metab 1955;15:1270–1280

166. Vander JB, Gaston EA, Dawber TR: The significance of nontoxic thyroid nodules. Final report of a 15-year study of the incidence of thyroid malignancy. Ann Intern Med 1968;69: 537–540

167. Horlocker TT, Hay JE, James EM et al: Prevalence of incidental nodular thyroid disease detected during high-resolution parathyroid ultrasonography. pp. 1309–1312. In Medeiros-Neto G, Gaitan E (eds): Frontiers in Thyroidology. Vol 2. Plenum, New York, 1986

168. DeGroot LJ: Clinical review II. diagnostic approach and management of patients exposed to irradiation to the thyroid. J Clin Endocrinol Metab 1989;69:925–928

169. Huysmans DAKC, Hermus ARMM, Corstens FHM et al: Large, compressive goiters treated with radioiodine. Ann Intern Med 1994;121:757–762

170. Mazzaferri EL: Management of a solitary thyroid nodule. N Engl J Med 328;1993:553–559

171. Molitch ME, Beck JR, Dreisman M et al: The cold thyroid nodule: an analysis of diagnostic and therapeutic options. Endocrinol Rev 1984;5:185–199

172. Holm L-E, Blomgren H, Lowhagen T: Cancer risks in patients with chronic lymphocytic thyroiditis. N Engl J Med 1985;312: 601–604

173. Rude RK, Singer R: Comparison of serum calcitonin levels after a 1-minute calcium injection and after pentogastrin injection in the diagnosis of medullary thyroid carcinoma. J Clin Endocrinol Metab 1977;44:980–985

174. Burch HB: Evaluation and management of the solid thyroid nodule. Endocrinol Metab Clin North Am 1995;24:663–710

175. James EM, Charboneau JW: High frequency (10 MHz) thyroid ultrasonography. Sem Ultrasound CT MR 1985;6:294–309

176. Gharib H, James EM, Charboneau JW et al: Suppressive therapy with levothyroxine for solitary thyroid nodules: a double-blind controlled clinical study. N Engl J Med 1987;317:70–75

177. Gharib H, Goellner JR: Evaluation of nodular thyroid disease. Endocrinol Metab Clin North Am 1988;17:511–526

178. Gharib H, Goellner JR: Fine-needle aspiration biopsy of the thyroid: an appraisal. Ann Intern Med 1993;118:282–289

179. Ashcraft NW, Van Herle AJ: Management of thyroid nodules. I: History and physical examination, blood tests, X-ray tests, and ultrasonography. II: Scanning techniques, thyroid suppressive therapy, and fine needle aspiration. Head Neck Surg 1981;3:297–322

180. Hay ID, Grant CS, Taylor WF, McConahcy WM: Ipsilateral lobectomy versus bilateral lobar resection in papillary thyroid carcinoma: a retrospective analysis of surgical outcome using a novel prognostic scoring system. Surgery 1987;102: 1088–1095

181. Beierwaltes WH: The treatment of thyroid carcinoma with radioactive iodine. Sem Nucl Med 1978;8:79–94

182. Robbins J, Merino MJ, Boice JD Jr et al: Thyroid cancer: a lethal endocrine neoplasm. Ann Intern Med 1991;115: 133–147

183. Thoresen SO, Akslen LA, Glattre E et al: Survival and prognostic factors in differentiated thyroid carcinoma: a multivariate analysis of 1055 cases. Br J Cancer 1989;59:231–240

184. DeGroot LJ, Kaplan EL, Shukla MS et al: Morbidity and mortality in follicular thyroid cancer. J Clin Endocrinol Metab 1995;80:2846–2953

185. De Bustros AC, Baylin SB: Medullary carcinoma of the thyroid. pp. 1166–1183. In: Braverman LE, Utiger RD (eds): The Thyroid. 6th Ed. Lippincott-Raven, Philadelphia, 1991

186. Simpson WJ: Anaplastic thyroid carcinoma: a new approach. Can J Surg 1980;23:25–27

187. Kim JH, Leeper RD: Treatment of locally advanced thyroid carcinoma with combination doxorubicin and radiation therapy. Cancer 1987;60:2372–2375

CHAPTER 74

Disorders of the Parathyroids

PAUL E. BELCHETZ
PETER HAMMOND

There are usually four parathyroid glands, but a larger number may sometimes be found, which poses potential problems for the surgeon. The usual positions are behind the upper and lower poles of the thyroid in each side of the neck, but they may be enwrapped by thyroid tissue. The normal parathyroid gland weighs about 35 mg, and thus, may be quite inconspicuous. In embryonic life the glands originate from the third and fourth branchial pouches, but the initial upper glands migrate to a final lower position, and indeed, may be taken into the mediastinum with the associated descent of the thymus.

Regulation of Parathyroid Hormone Synthesis and Secretion

The normal parathyroid is largely regulated by the circulating level of ionized calcium acting directly on the parathyroid tissue. Advances in molecular biology have led to a deeper understanding of normal functioning parathyroid tissue and pathophysiology of adenomas. It is now known in some detail that the parathyroid hormone gene consists of three exons and these transcribe to form a large messenger RNA species with a polyadenylate tail. Following a series of specific splicings, this is translated outside the nucleus on ribosomes to form the large precursor pre-proPTH. This undergoes a series of cleavages before and after reaching the Golgi apparatus where the 84-residue parathyroid hormone (PTH) is packaged into granules for storage prior to secretion.[1]

Raised levels of ionized calcium suppress the messenger RNA for PTH in normal bovine parathyroid glands and adenomatous tissue, but PTH secretion is unsuppressed from adenomas in vitro.[2] It has recently been demonstrated that calcium ions act to suppress PTH synthesis and secretion via specific cell membrane G-protein coupled receptors. Inactivating mutations of this receptor elevate the set point for PTH secretion, causing familial hypocalciuric hypercalcemia, a benign condition associated with mild hypercalcemia.[3]

The normal parathyroid mRNA production is also regulated by 1,25 dihydroxy-vitamin D levels, but adenomatous cell also fail to give this response.[4] It is possible that at normal levels of ionized calcium the rate of gene transcription is maximal, and thus, the response to hypocalcemia may be regulated by liberating a normally inaccessible pool of mRNA bound to riboprotein, hence increasing the rate of translation without changes in steady-state levels in mRNA.

Parathyroid Hormone Secretion in the Elderly and Age-Related Bone Loss

Serum PTH concentrations increase in the elderly by about 30 percent. This increase correlates with a decline in vitamin D levels and treatment with 1,25 dihydroxy-vitamin D results in a decrease in circulating PTH levels.[5] The age-related increase in PTH levels is thought to account for age-related bone loss, and this is supported by the observation that the hypoparathyroid state protects against such loss.[6] This provides the rationale for using vitamin D, with or without calcium supplements, in elderly people with osteoporosis (type-II osteoporosis). This treatment has proved effective in reducing the risk of hip fractures in elderly populations.[7]

Actions of Parathyroid Hormone

Parathyroid hormone raises the ionized calcium levels in the blood through actions on the kidney, gut, and bones. The major renal action is to increase tubular reabsorption of calcium via activation of adenylate-cyclase mechanisms.[8] This mediation can be uniquely observed because of the liberation of cyclic AMP into the tubular luminal fluid, allowing its ready measurement in the excreted urine. Parathyroid hormone also exerts a phosphaturic effect enhancing tubular secretion of phosphate. Parathyroid hormone has a complex action on bone, which is partly dose-dependent. High levels are catabolic with increased bone resorption, but lower levels may exert an overall anabolic effect. This is discussed in greater detail below.

The gastrointestinal absorption of calcium is enhanced by PTH. Some of these effects are mediated by the promotion of 25-hydroxy-vitamin D 1-hydroxylation to form the active metabolite 1:25 dihydroxy-vitamin D,[9] which has actions on gut absorption, bone, and indeed on many tissues. Parathyroid hormone has complex relationships with magnesium, and it enhances magnesium absorption. Hypomagnesemia can significantly suppress PTH secretion, however.[10] Low magnesium levels can also inhibit renal production of 1:25 dihydroxyvitamin D, blocking this important action of PTH.[11] Finally, it appears that PTH may have independent and important effects on vascular tone.

Hyperparathyroidism

It is commonly believed that hyperparathyroidism is rare and that the nature of the disease is changing. The disease which Fuller Albright described over half a century ago was a fulminating disorder with devastating effects on bone, which led to its ready recognition. This form of the disease is indeed exceedingly rare today—as it almost certainly was when the early cases were being collected. With time came diagnostic refinement and the recognition of the frequent causative role of hyperparathyroidism in renal calculus formation associated with hypercalciuria. The most dramatic change came with the wide, and almost indiscriminate availability of accurate plasma calcium measurements.[12]

Currently, the great majority of cases of hyperparathyroidism are detected by accident or screening. This trend may be reversed if economic pressures restrict chemical tests performed to the few specifically requested by the clinician. The definitive audit has yet to be performed as to whether this would matter. It is indisputable that most of these cases have only modest degrees of hypercalcemia, especially in the elderly female population where the incidence of hyperparathyroidism soars to about 2 per 1,000.[13]

Etiology

Hyperparathyroidism is most commonly caused by a single benign adenoma. Involvement of two glands is not uncommon, and when it occurs the histologic appearance in the two glands may be strikingly different. There is some dispute whether involvement of more than one gland in fact represents parathyroid hyperplasia—histologic distinction of adenoma from hyperplasia based on the presence of a rim of normal, if sometimes compressed gland, is not totally reliable.[14] True hyperplasia is an important diagnosis because surgery must be radical if early relapse is to be avoided. The presence of hyperplasia is a pointer to possible multiple endocrine neoplasia type-1 (MEN-1), which is inherited as an autosomal dominant trait with high penetrance.[15] In this syndrome, hyperparathyroidism is very much the rule affecting 97 to 100 percent of subjects at risk in affected families.[16]

The other associated lesions are gastroenteropancreatic tumors, with insulinoma and gastrinoma the most frequently occurring types, and adenomas of the anterior pituitary gland where functionless tumors and prolactinomas occur most often, but acromegaly is not rare.[17] As might be anticipated, there is evidence for a circulating factor leading to parathyroid gland hyperplasia, which has been partially characterized.[18]

Molecular biology is proving informative in both the sporadic adenomatous and hyperplastic forms of hyperparathyroidism. In the case of tumors appearing in the context of MEN-1, it is proposed that the MEN-1 gene, found on the long arm of chromosome 11 in the region q 11.13, acts as a tumor suppressor and loss of one allele from the germ-line leads to hyperplasia.[19,20] A further somatic loss of the corresponding allele from the second chromosome 11 may occur later, and is associated with larger, clonal tumor development. In the case of the more common sporadic parathyroid adenomas there appear to be somatic mutations involving both chromosomes 11. The gene for parathyroid hormone itself is localized to the short arm of chromosomes 11, and in at least some cases of sporadic parathyroid adenoma, there is a rearrangement of genetic material on chromosome 11 between regions containing the MEN-1 gene and the locus for the parathyroid hormone.[21] In other cases of sporadic hyperparathyroidism, no obvious changes in chromosome 11 have been observed.

Clinical Features

Symptoms attributable to hyperparathyroidism range widely and nonspecifically. Overall, 50 percent of patients have minimal or no symptoms, although elderly patients more often have neuropsychiatric or neuromuscular symptoms or suffer osteoporotic fractures. Common features caused by the ensuing hypercalcemia include polyuria and the consequent polydipsia. The increased urine volume partly results from the overall increased urinary calcium excretion exerting an osmotic diuresis—hypersecretion of PTH increases tubular reabsorption, but this does not compensate for the greatly raised glomerular filtration of calcium caused by the hypercalcemia. Hypercalcemia also can induce varying degrees of tubular resistance to vasopressin, leading to nephrogenic diabetes insipidus. Sustained hypercalcemia may lead to nephrocalcinosis with impaired renal function, or promote the formation of renal calculi. Calculi may be passed or impact, for example at the vesicoureteric junction, causing pain and hematuria. Stones may be associated with pyelonephritis, which is difficult to eradicate, especially if stag horn calculi form and may require removal surgically or by lithotripsy.

Symptoms of fatigue, lethargy, loss of vitality, and varying degrees of mental impairment are also common in hyperparathyroidism. These symptoms are nonspecific and common in the aging community in general, and it is often hard to predict in which cases surgical cure of the hyperparathyroidism will improve such problems. This is a vexed question as a causal relationship has been claimed even in cases with biochemically mild disease, yet it is clearly true that resection of a parathyroid adenoma with restoration of normocalcemia is not invariably successful. This problem is further discussed below. Rare patients show a marked and reversible neuromuscular syndrome, characterized histologically by type-II muscle fiber atrophy.[22]

More florid manifestations of hyperparathyroidism are less common, including gastrointestinal features of anorexia and nausea. This rarely can proceed to vomiting with a danger of a hypercalcemic crisis when loss of extracellular fluid exacerbates the hypercalcemia and vomiting, causing a vicious spiral that can prove fatal. Hypercalcemia, per se, may increase gastrin secretion and gastric acid production with dyspepsia and peptic ulceration. This occurs separately from the independent association with gastrinomas (Zollinger-Ellison syndrome). There is a well-recorded, but fortunately rare, association with acute pancreatitis.

Hyperparathyroidism is also associated with cardiovascular disease, especially hypertension. It is far from certain what the nature of this link is, and whether the cure of the hyperparathyroidism has any beneficial effect on the blood pressure control.[23] It has been suggested that there are delayed benefits on mortality from cardiovascular disease following surgery for hyperparathyroidism.[24]

Hyperinsulinism reflecting insulin resistance is being increasingly recognized as a cardiovascular risk factor, and this has been linked with hyperparathyroidism.[25] It is not certain whether this is a function of hypercalcemia, or may be an independent effect of hypophosphatemia, whether or not it is part of primary hyperparathyroidism.[26]

Occasionally, hyperparathyroidism may be masked by a coexistent hypocalcemic disorder, usually involving vitamin D-deficiency, such as coeliac disease. Such problems are more likely to occur in the elderly. These patients usually present with bone pain and marked elevation of alkaline phosphatase due to a combination of osteomalacia and parathyroid bone disease.

Asymptomatic Disease

The management of asymptomatic disease, diagnosed following request for a biochemical profile, continues to cause heated, if not always illuminated, discussion. The frequently cited need for controlled prospective randomized trials combined with quite varied criteria for determining a conservative approach versus surgery are the main reasons for this continuing uncertainty.[27] At one extreme lie the advocates for surgery in virtually all cases of hyperparathyroidism, who invoke prevention or arrest of bone disease among their arguments.[28] This is highly dubious as discussed below. Several reviews conclude that mild disease is stable and does not lead to progressive renal failure or bone disease.[29,30] Judging mild hyperparathyroidism truly asymptomatic may be difficult as the features may be slight and nonspecific even in severe cases, and those labeled asymptomatic may feel better following parathyroidectomy.

Case report

A 70-year-old woman developed profuse diarrhea for a week while away from home on holiday. She had a long history of angina and having an attack, collapsed following use of her nitrolingual spray. On admission to hospital she was dehydrated and found to be in hyperosmolar nonketotic precoma with blood glucose 33 mmol/L. Subsequent routine biochemical screen revealed plasma calcium 4.32 mmol/L, which only fell to 3.73 mmol/L after vigorous rehydration, but intravenous pamidronate lowered the level to 2.5 mmol/L. She then developed a massive anterior myocardial infarction and pump failure, dying despite prompt thrombolysis and resuscitative measures. Prior to this, systematic enquiry did not reveal any specific features of hypercalcemia. Autopsy revealed a not unexpected severe triple coronary artery disease. It also disclosed a massive parathyroid adenoma weighing 52 g in the right side of her neck (Fig. 74-1). Her bones showed osteitis fibrosa (Fig. 74-2) and there was widespread nephrocalcinosis (Fig. 74-3).

Comment This patient had severe hyperparathyroidism, which would certainly have been treated surgically had she survived. There was, nevertheless, a striking lack of symptoms that could be directly attributed to her hyperparathyroidism. It is noteworthy that her hypercalcemia responded rapidly to the bisphosphonate pamidronate.

The consensus opinion is that in elderly patients with asymptomatic hyperparathyroidism, serum calcium less than 3 mmol/L, normal renal function, no stones, and no obvious bone disease, then a conservative approach has much to commend it with serum calcium and renal function being monitored at 6-month intervals.

Bone Disease

As mentioned above, the possibility of developing bony complications has been cited as a reason for ready surgical intervention. It is generally believed that hyperparathyroidism particularly affects the cortical bone of the appendicular skeleton. There have been studies indicating a lack of continued accelerated bone loss in hyperparathyroidism or excess of vertebral fractures,[31] and indeed there may be preservation of cancellous bone structure,[32] consonant with the demonstration of increased bone mass in osteoporotic patients actually treated with PTH.[33] However, although this appears true for the majority, certain individuals unpredictably lose bone at a much faster rate,[34] and in individuals with low-bone mineral density, parathyroidectomy restores bone mass at a variety of skeletal sites,[35] so that continued monitoring of bone mineral density is necessary. The apparent diminishing frequency of severe bone complications such as giant cell or brown tumors is incompletely explained, but has been linked with improving nutrition leading in particular, to less concomitant vitamin D-deficiency.

Mental Symptoms

The spectrum of mental symptoms that has been attributed to hypercalcemia is wide and includes fatigability, failing memory, poor concentration, sleep disturbance, aggression, and depression. It is generally agreed that elderly patients are especially susceptible to such changes even with modest degrees of hyperparathyroidism. This may be particularly true when there is multiple pathology.

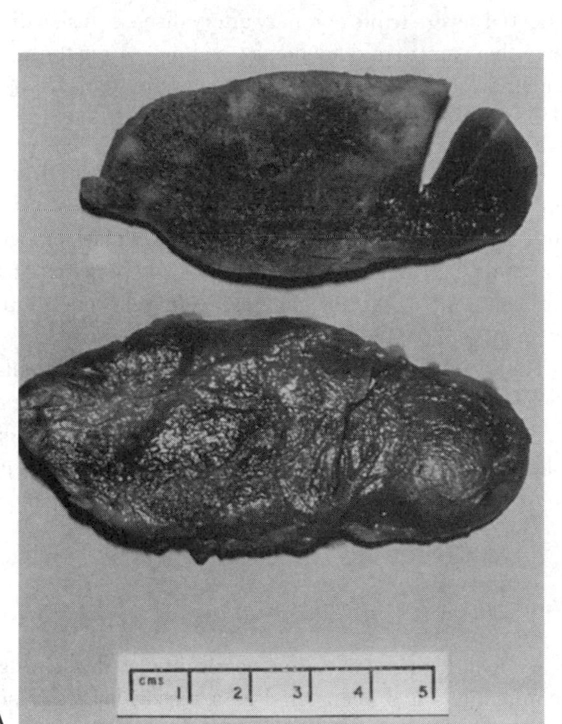

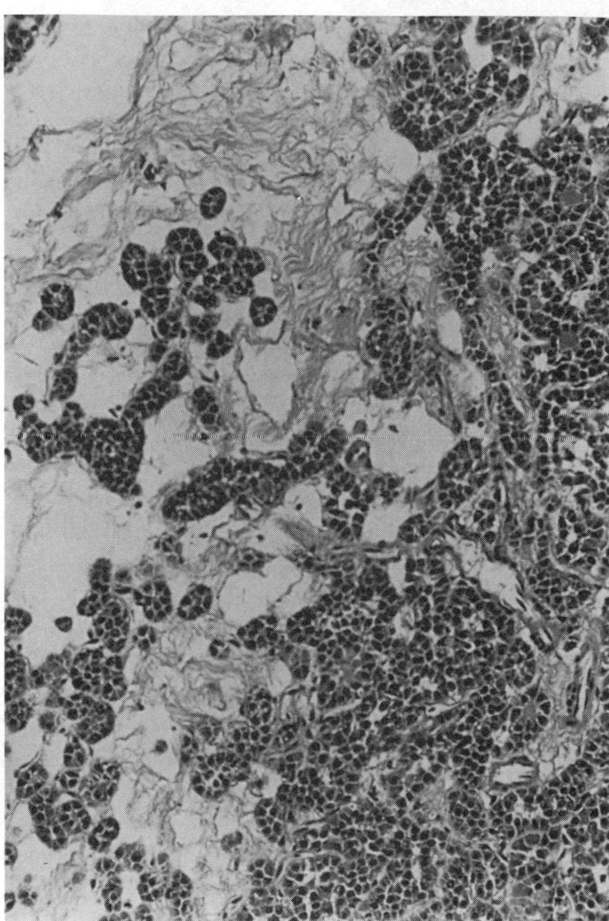

Figure 74-1 (**A**) Macroscopic view of massive parathyroid adenoma—cut surface (top) uncut surface (bottom). (**B**) Parathyroid (H&E, × 78)—loose trabeculae of oxyphilic "chief cells" extend into an edematous matrix.

Case reports

A 70-year-old man developed acute confusion. Hydrocephalus was diagnosed, and a ventriculoperitoneal shunt relieved symptoms. Mild hyperparathyroidism was detected during follow-up. He then suddenly became euphoric and disorientated in time and space. Neurosurgical causes were excluded. Surgical correction of his hypercalcemia normalized his mental state. Formal psychometric assessment reported, "Intellectually he is functioning within the high average range of intelligence. Compared to his pre-operative state, the mild confusion, poor remote memory, slight disorientation and confabulation have all improved. In addition there is now no evidence of the short-term memory impairment previously reported."

A 46-year-old woman developed noncirrhotic portal hypertension and underwent portacaval anastomosis. Thirteen years later she developed confusion, anemia, and mild hyperparathyroidism was also diagnosed, but a conservative approach was adopted. After 5 years, serum calcium rose to 2.94 mmol/L. She was widowed, living alone and had frequent falls. She was encephalopathic with hyperammonemia. A year later she fractured her left humerus. After a further 2 months, right-upper parathyroid adenomectomy rendered her normocalcemic and greatly improved her mental state.

Diagnosis

Hyperparathyroidism is now a relatively straightforward diagnosis to make with the advent of sensitive immunoradiometric assays for PTH.[36] These have largely overcome the problems posed by circulating PTH fragments without biological activity, but which were sometimes read in the older radioimmunoassays. A normal PTH level is inappropriate in the face of hypercalcemia and confirms hyperparathyroidism, although using intact PTH assays, serum PTH levels are usually unequivocally raised as parathyroid adenoma cells secrete a higher proportion of intact molecule than normal cells. The latter secrete more PTH fragments. The combination of inappropriately elevated PTH measurements using these techniques in the presence of bona fide hypercalemia is highly reliable evidence. It may be prudent to check urinary calcium excretion to exclude hypocalciuric hypercalcemia.[37,38] The other major cause of hypercalcemia is malignancy—with or without bony metastases. The clinical diagnosis is usually not difficult and common causes include carcinomas of the lung (usually squamous), and breast and kidney hematological malignancies, including multiple myeloma. It must be remembered that malignancy and hyperparathyroidism may occasionally coincide.[39]

Treatment

It is often helpful to localize the parathyroid tumor preoperatively. Favored methods include CT scanning, ultrasound, and isotopic scanning. None is universally accurate, but the last means is probably the most specific. Thallium-technetium subtraction scanning is commonly used; it may possibly be improved by three-dimensional emission tomography.[40] However, recent evidence indicates that scanning with ^{99m}Tc-Sestamibi is superior, with high sensitivity and specificity.[41] Selective venous sampling for high PTH levels is now usually restricted to cases where the first neck exploration has failed to identify the tumor. The normal parathyroid gland can usually be identi-

Figure 74-2 (**A**) Lumbar vertebrae (H&E, × 78)—there is a prominent bony resorption with osteitis fibrosa. (**B**) Lumbar vertebrae (H&E, × 250)—there is a lacunar reabsorption of the bony trabeculum with small osteoclasts.

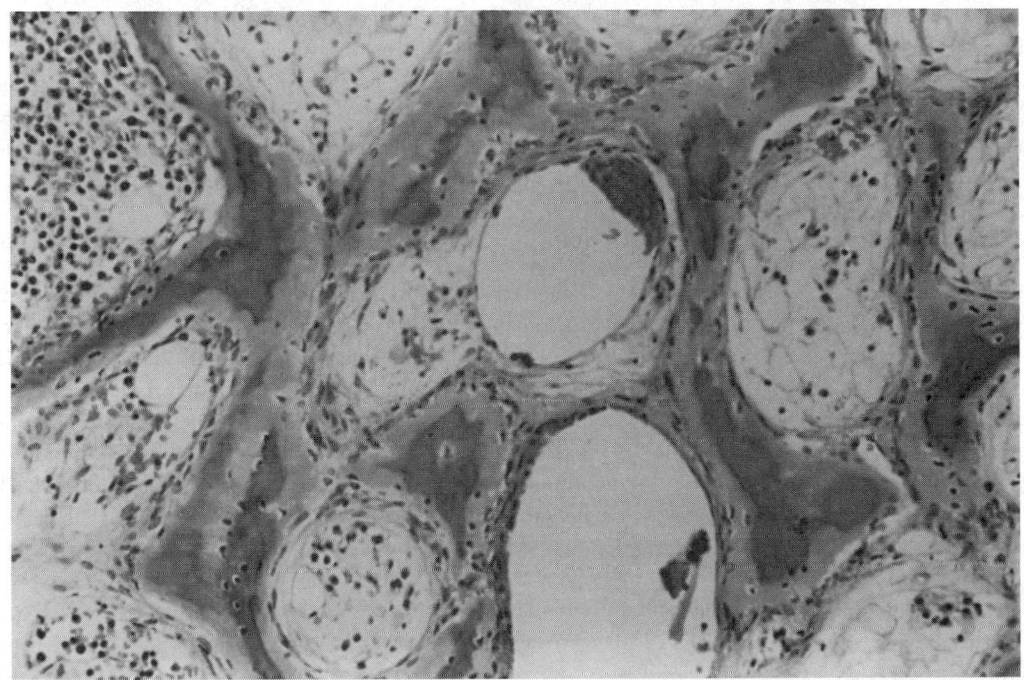

A

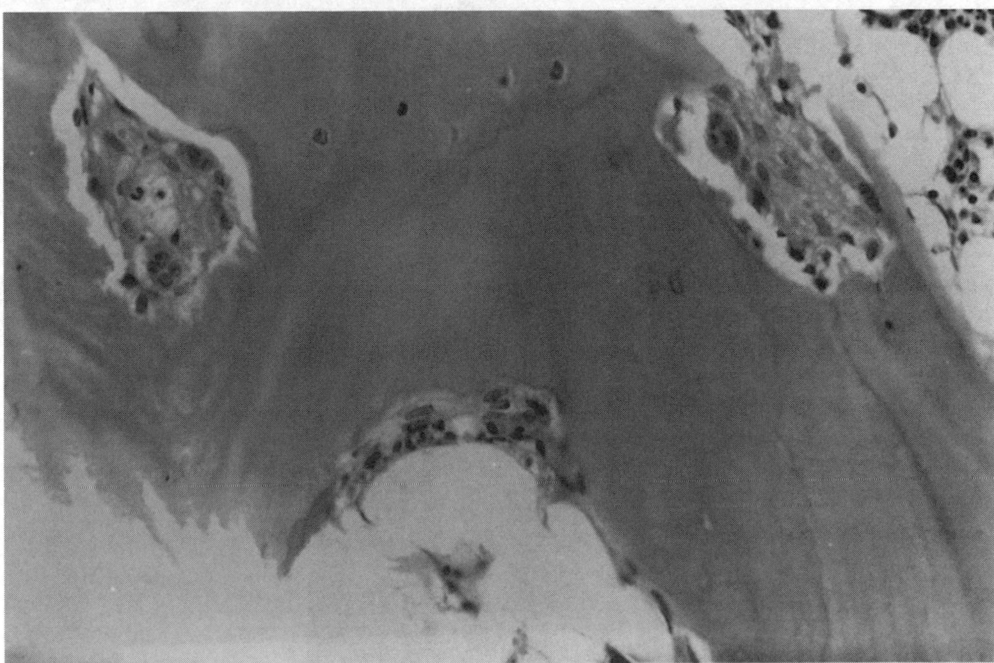

B

fied by the experienced surgeon. Scanning techniques are often unhelpful, with the smaller tumors weighing less than 400 mg, which is just when their assistance is most needed. The surgery for a single adenoma is straightforward. In hyperplasia, the intraoperative frozen section reports may not always easily provide conclusive information. It is common practice to remove 3.5 out of 4 identified glands.

Medical treatment is increasingly sought in cases of relatively mild hyperparathyroidism in the elderly, and estrogen has been used in women in the past. Bisphosphonates, such as pamidronate or clodronate, can control hypercalcemia acutely, but a rebound increase in PTH secretion occurs, so repeated doses are necessary.[42] Calcium receptor agonists have been developed, which suppress PTH secretion from normal parathyroid cells. Preliminary studies suggest that they may be valuable in treating mild hyperparathyroidism.[43] Interventional radiology, with ultrasound-guided ethanol injection of parathyroid adenomas, also has its advocates.

Hypoparathyroidism

Hypoparathyroidism leads to hypocalcemia and hyperphosphatemia. The clinical hallmark of low-ionized calcium is tetany. This neuromuscular hyperexcitability can cause carpopedal spasm and rarely, but dangerously, laryngeal spasm causing stridor and even respiratory arrest. Mild forms present with paresthesiae, which are characteristically perioral. Latent tetany may be elicited by Trousseau's sign: inflating a sphygmomanometer cuff above systolic pressure for up to 3 minutes. Discomfort is to be expected, but the involuntary flexion of the fingers and thumb or "main d'accoucheur," which constitutes a positive response (Fig. 74-4) is intensely painful and the cuff must be immediately deflated when this sign is elicited. Chvostek's sign is elicited by tapping the facial nerve just as it emerges into the cheek in front of the parotid gland. The positive response of ipsilateral twitching of the corner of the mouth is too commonly seen in normal people for this sign to have much value. It must be recalled that tetany may also result from hypomagnesemia, hypokalemia, and hyperventilation. Hypocalcemia may cause central problems with mental depression, fits,[44] and even reversible Chronic cognitive impairment in elderly people[45] The most common cause of hypoparathyroidism is iatrogenic following neck surgery. An idiopathic variety is increasingly recognized in the elderly. Two forms of pseudohypoparathyroidism exist where there is end-organ resistance to the action of PTH. In the first, the generation of cyclic AMP is impaired and in the second, this is normal and the defect lies distal to this within the target cells.

Treatment of Hypoparathyroidism

When hypoparathyroidism occurs after neck surgery, it is often transient and the postoperative administration of short-term calcium supplementation may be all that is needed. If it persists, then vitamin D administration is required. This is commonly given as one of the 1-α-hydroxylated preparations, which act rapidly and directly. There is no justification for the continued use of pharmacologic doses of cholecalciferol. This is because the ever-present danger in vitamin D therapy is

Figure 74-3 Kidney (H&E, × 160)—there is advanced interstitial fibrosis and ischemic contracture of the glomerular tuft with periglomerular fibrosis. A dilated tubule contains a granular deposit of calcium phosphate (arrow).

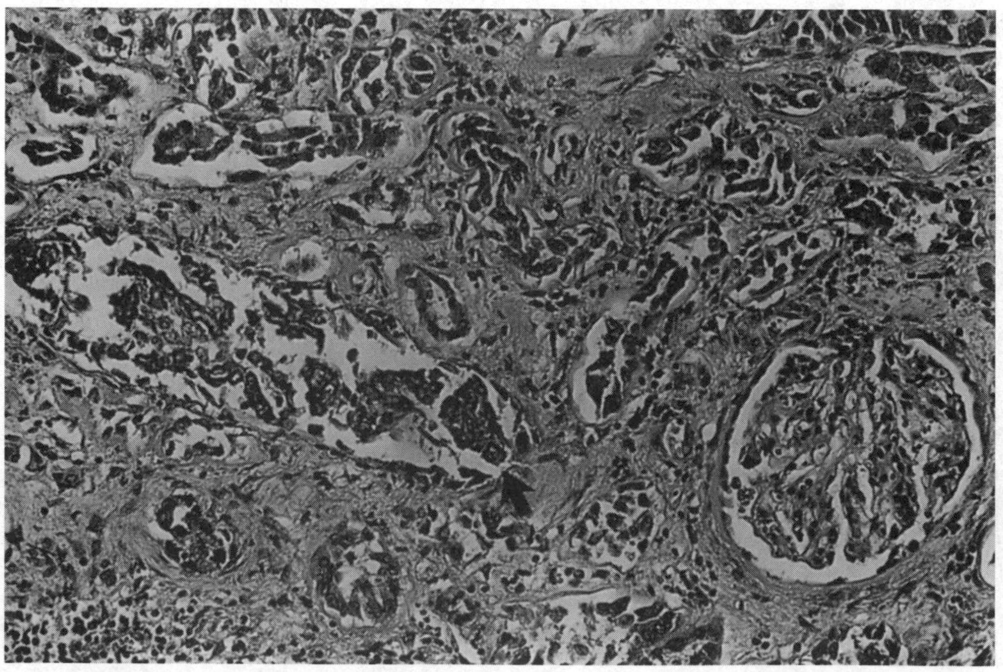

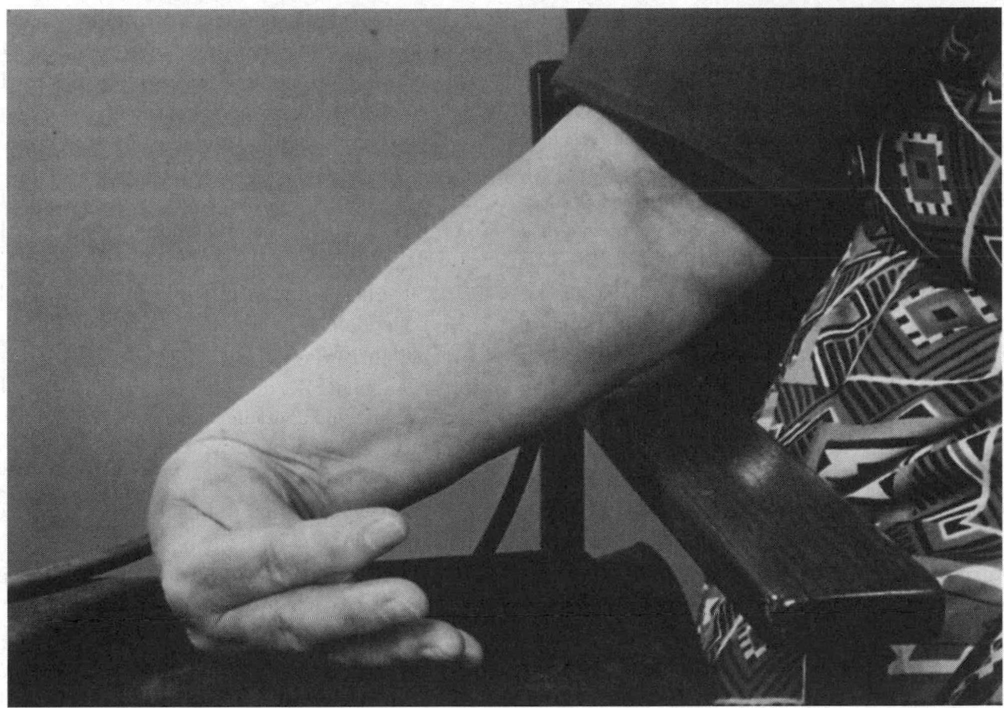

Figure 74-4 Hand held in position "main d'accocheur"—positive Trouseau's sign.

unpredictable hypercalcemia. Cholecalciferol is a fat soluble prohormone and it is difficult to remove from stores if calcium levels rise excessively.[46] Reversibility is normal, easy, and quick withdrawal of the more polar 1-hydroxylated compounds. It must be emphasized that dangerous hypercalcemia can develop quite asymptomatically with potentially disastrous effects on renal function. It is, therefore, mandatory to measure serum calcium levels regularly— approximately every 2 months is a reasonable routine interval—lifelong for patients treated in this way for hypoparathyroidism.

References

1. Farrow SM, O'Riordan JLH: Regulation of parathyroid hormone gene expression. Bone (Clin Biochem News Rev) 1990;7:51–53
2. Farrow SM, Karmali R, Gleed JH et al: Regulation of preproparathyroid hormone messenger RNA and hormone synthesis in human parathyroid adenomata. J Endocrinol 1988;117: 133–138
3. Brown EM, Pollak M, Seidman CE et al: Calcium-ion-sensing cell-surface receptors. N Engl J Med 1995;333:234–239
4. Karmali R, Farrow S, Hewison M et al: Effects of 1,25-dihydroxyvitamin D, and cortisol on bovine and human parathyroid cells. J Endocrinol 1989;123:137–142
5. Quesada JM, Coopmans W, Ruiz B et al: Influence of vitamin D on parathyroid function in the elderly. J Clin Endocrinol Metab 1992;75:494–501
6. Fujiyama K, Kiriyama T, Ito M et al: Attenuation of postmenopausal high bone loss in patients with hypoparathyroidism. J Clin Endocrinol Metab 1995;80:2135–2138
7. Chapuy MC, Arlot ME, Duboeuf F et al: Vitamin D_3 and calcium to prevent hip fractures in elderly women. N Engl J Med 1992; 333:1437–1443
8. Agus ZS, Wasserstein A, Goldfarb S: PTH, calcitonin, cyclic nucleotides, and the kidney. Ann Rev Physiol 1981;41: 583–595
9. Garabedian M, Holick MF, De Luca HF, Boyle IT: Control of 25-hydroxycholecalciferol metabolism by the parathyroid glands. Proc Natl Acad Sci USA 1972;69:1673–1676
10. Anast CS, Mohs JM, Kaplan SL, Burns PW: Evidence for parathyroid failure in magnesium deficiency. Science 1972;177: 606–608
11. Fraser DR, Kodicek E: Unique biosynthesis by kidney of a biologically active vitamin D metabolite. Nature 1979;228: 764–766
12. Mundy GR, Cove DH, Fisken RA: Primary hyperparathyroidism: changes in the pattern of clinical presentation. Lancet 1980;i:1317–1320
13. Heath H, Hodgson SF, Kennedy MA: Primary hyperparathyroidism. Incidence, morbidity and potential economic input in a community. N Engl J Med 1980;302:189–193
14. Black WC III, Utley JR: The differential diagnosis of parathyroid adenoma and chief cell hyperplasia. Am J Clin Pathol 1968; 49:761–775
15. Trump D, Farren B, Wooding C et al: Clinical studies of multiple endocrine neoplasia type 1 (MEN 1). Q J Med 1996;89: 653–669
16. Jung RT, Grant AM, Davie M et al: Multiple endocrine adenomatosis (type I) and familial hyperparathyroidism. Postgrad Med J 1978;54:92–94
17. Leshin M: Multiple endocrine neoplasia. pp. 1274–1289. In Wilson JD, Foster DW (eds): Williams Textbook of Endocrinology. 7th Ed. WB Saunders, Philadelphia, 1985

18. Brandi ML, Aurbach GD, Fitzpatrick LA et al: Parathyroid mitogenic activity in plasma from patients with familial multiple endocrine neoplasia type I. N Engl J Med 1986;314:1287–1293
19. Friedman E, Sakaguchi K, Bale AE et al: Clonality of parathyroid tumors in familial multiple endocrine neoplasia type I. N Engl J Med 1989;321:213–218
20. Thakker RV, Bouloux P, Wooding C et al: Association of parathyroid tumors in multiple endocrine neoplasia type I with loss of alleles on chromosome 11. N Engl J Med 1989;321:218–224
21. Arnold A, Staunton CE, Kim HG: Monoclonality and abnormal parathyroid hormone genes in parathyroid adenomas. N Engl J Med 1988;318:658–662
22. Patten BM, Bilezikian JP, Mallette LE et al: The neuromuscular disease of hyperparathyroidism. Ann Intern Med 1974;80: 182–194
23. Posen S, Clifton Bligh P, Reeve T et al: Is parathyroidectomy of benefit in primary hyperparathyroidism? Q J Med 1985;54: 241–251
24. Palmer M, Adami H-O, Bergstrom R et al: Mortality after surgery for primary hyperparathyroidism: a follow-up of 441 patients operated on from 1956 to 1979. Surgery 1987;102:1–7
25. Kim H, Kalkhoff RK, Costrini NV et al: Plasma insulin disturbances in primary hyperparathyroidism. J Clin Invest 1971;50: 2596–2605
26. DeFronzo RA, Lang R: Hypophosphatemia and glucose intolerance: evidence for tissue insensitivity to insulin. N Engl J Med 1980;303:1259–1263
27. Potts JR Jr: Management of asymptomatic hyperparathyroidism. J Clin Endocrinol Metab 1990;70:1489–1493
28. Stevenson JC, Lynn JA: Time to end a conservative treatment for mild hyperparathyroidism. Br Med J 1988;296:1016–1017
29. Paterson CR, Burns J, Mowat E: Long term follow-up of untreated primary hyperparathyroidism. Br Med J 1984;289: 1261–1263
30. Sampson MJ, van't Hoff W, Bicknell EJ: The conservative management of primary hyperparathyroidism. Q J Med 1987;65: 1009–1014
31. Rao DS, Wilson RJ, Kleerekoper M, Parfitt AM: Lack of biochemical progression or continuation of accelerated bone loss in mild asymptomatic primary hyperparathyroidism: evidence for biphasic disease course. J Clin Endocrinol Metab 1988;67: 1294–1298
32. Parisien M, Silverberg SJ, Shane E et al: The histomorphometry of bone in primary hyperparathyroidism: preservation of cancellous bone structure. J Clin Endocrinol Metab 1990;70:930–938
33. Reeve J, Meunier PJ, Parsons JA et al: Anabolic effect of human parathyroid hormone fragment on trabecular bone in involutional osteoporosis: a multicentre trial. Br Med J 1980;280: 1340–1344
34. Silverberg SJ, Gartenberg F, Jacobs TP et al: Longitudinal bone density measurements in untreated primary hyperparathyroidism. J Clin Endocrinol Metab 1995;80:723–728
35. Silverberg SJ, Gartenberg F, Jacobs TP et al: Increased bone mineral density following parathyroidectomy in primary hyperparathyroidism. J Clin Endocrinol Metab 1995;80:729–734
36. Nussbaum SR, Zahradnik RJ, Lavigne JR et al: Highly sensitive two-site immunoradiometric assay of parathyrin, and its clinical utility in evaluating patients with hypercalcemia. Clin Chem 1987;8:1364–1367
37. Paterson CR, Gunn A: Familial benign hypercalcaemia. Lancet 1981;ii:61–63
38. Marx SJ, Spiegel AM, Levine MA et al: Familial hypocalciuric hypercalcemia: the relation to primary parathyroid hyperplasia. N Engl J Med 1982;307:416–426
39. Drezner MK, Lebovitz HE: Primary hyperparathyroidism in paraneoplastic hypercalcaemia. Lancet 1978;i:1004–1006
40. Jenkins BJ, Newell MS, Goode AW et al: Impact of conventional and three-dimensional thallium-technetium scans on surgery for primary hyperparathyroidism. J Roy Coll Phys 1990;83: 427–429
41. Heath DA: Localization of parathyroid tumours. Clin Endocrinol 1995;43:523–524
42. Hamdy NAT, Gray RES, McCloskey E et al: Clodronate in the medical management of hyperparathyroidism. Bone 1987; 8(suppl 1):569–577
43. Silverberg SJ, Thys-Jacobs S, Locker FG et al: The effect of the calcimimetic drug NPS R-568 on parathyroid hormone secretion in primary hyperparathyroidism. J Bone Min Res 1996; 11(suppl 1):87
44. Graham K, Williams BO, Rowe MJ: Idiopathic hypoparathyroidism: a cause of fits in the elderly. Br Med J 1979;i: 1460–1461
45. Eraut D: Idiopathic hypoparathyroidism presenting as dementia. Br Med J 1974;i:429–430
46. Hossain M: Vitamin-D intoxication during treatment of hypoparathyroidism. Lancet 1970;i:1149–1151

CHAPTER 75

Diabetes Mellitus in the Older Adult

ALAN J. SINCLAIR
SIMON C. M. CROXSON

There is ample proof of the economic, social, and health burden of diabetes in the elderly.[1–4] Despite this recognition, there has been relative neglect in the medical literature, with few detailed studies of older diabetic patients being published.[1,5] For example, published articles dealing with diabetes research involving specific studies in older patients accounted for less than 5 percent of those published between 1978 and 1988.[5] Partly as a consequence of this scientific neglect and an emphasis on insulin-dependent diabetes in younger patients by specialists in diabetic care, the present state of diabetic care for older adults is essentially unstructured, poorly coordinated, often inappropriate, and therefore in great need of reorganization.[6]

Recent initiatives, however, justify optimism that care is improving.[7] In particular, there is more recognition that older patients with diabetes may be different than younger counterparts[8]; for example, they have a high degree of comorbidity, an age-related impairment of functional ability, and an increased vulnerability to hypoglycemia and its consequences. They may also require a different approach to management, which involves spouses and other carers to a greater extent.[9] Along with these developments has come an appreciation of new aims of care for the older patient[6], which are far more comprehensive than previous aims that focused only on avoiding hypoglycemia and keeping the patient symptom-free! This chapter will provide an account of the scientific and clinical basis of managing older people with diabetes and enable the reader to implement practical steps to improve care.

Impairment of Glucose Tolerance With Aging

The prevalence of diabetes mellitus is known to increase with advancing age and is predominantly of the noninsulin-dependent type. As early as 1921, Spence[10] reported observations relating to an impairment of glucose tolerance (IGT) in subjects aged 60 years and over. This age-related impairment has been confirmed by more recent studies that indicate that glucose intolerance begins in the third decade and continues throughout adulthood.[11–13] The magnitude of the rise has been estimated to be 0.33 to 0.72 mmol/L (5.9 to 13.0 mg/dl) per decade in 1- and 2-hour postglucose ingestion samples. The rise is more pronounced in women (about 0.55 mmol/L [9.9 mg/dl] higher than in men).[14] The National Health and Nutrition Examination Survey (NHANES II) of over 15,000 subjects from a stratified sample of households throughout the US found a rise in prevalence of IGT of 2.1 percent in those aged 20 to 44 years to 9.2 percent in those aged 65 to 74 years[15]; this survey also demonstrated increasing prevalence rates of diabetes with age (Table 75-1).

In the Bedford study,[16] varying diagnostic criteria were used to define the percentage of adults with abnormal glucose tolerance following a 50-g oral glucose tolerance test (OGTT). In the group classed as "borderline" diabetics, whose 2-hour capillary glucose ranged from 6.7 to below 11.1 mmol/L (120 to below 200 mg/dl), there was an age-related increase in the percentage of individuals for each criterion of glucose measured; for example, at the lowest criterion used (6.7 mmol/L [120 mg/dl]) the percentage rose from 7.3 percent at ages 20 to 29 years to 40.2 percent at 70 years and above. Using the 75-g OGTT (which is the currently accepted version to diagnose diabetes mellitus), the Islington diabetes survey,[17] which was a general practice survey of more than 1,000 adults aged 40 years and over, identified 43 subjects with IGT (4.1 percent) of which 63 percent were aged 60 years and over. Of 27 subjects with IGT who were retested (mean follow-up of 8.5 months), 9 subjects had reverted to normal glucose tolerance, 3 subjects were classified as diabetic, and 4 subjects could not be easily classified. In the Melton Mowbray diabetes screening survey[18] of 583 subjects aged 65 to 85 years, 44 subjects were identified as having IGT (7.6 percent) with predominantly more cases of IGT seen in the age range 65 to 75 years compared with 80- to 85-year-olds. This may have underestimated the true prevalence of IGT in the very old subjects because of a high refusal rate amongst this group for the OGTT.

Mechanisms of Age-Related Glucose Intolerance

There are several possible mechanisms that may contribute to glucose intolerance during aging and these are listed below. A detailed description of each mechanism is outside the scope of this chapter. The impairment is clearly multifactorial, being characterized by delays in glucose-mediated insulin secretion, insulin-induced suppression of hepatic glucose output, and a rise in insulin-mediated glucose uptake. From the results of glucose clamp techniques,[19–20] the major disturbance appears

Aims in managing diabetes in the elderly

1. To promote freedom from symptoms of hyperglycemia
2. To assess the impact of coexisting disease, for example, ischemic heart disease
3. To prevent undesirable weight loss
4. Avoidance of hypoglycemia and other adverse drug reactions
5. To screen for and prevent complications
6. To recognize disability and limit handicap
7. To maintain patient well-being and quality of life

Mechanisms of decreased glucose tolerance in old age

- Delayed/decreased glucose-induced insulin secretion
- Impaired insulin-mediated glucose uptake in skeletal muscle and in adipose tissue
  - Reduction in number of insulin receptors (±)
  - Post-receptor defect
- Influence of other factors
  - Increased body fat
  - Physical inactivity
  - Reduced dietary carbohydrate
  - Impaired renal function
  - Hypokalemia
  - Increased sympathetic nervous system activity
  - Diabetogenic drugs, for example, thiazides

to be impaired insulin-mediated glucose uptake, with skeletal muscle being the principal site of this defect.[14] Because insulin receptor number or binding are not generally affected by age, the impairment is due primarily to a postreceptor defect. Of the factors indicated in the accompanying list that may modify muscle uptake of glucose, none appears to exert a major influence. The postreceptor defect may comprise abnormalities of glucose transport within the cell, or defective insulin internalization and intracellular metabolism. Age-associated glucose intolerance has been considered to be specific for the aging process and distinct from those defects that are seen in obesity and noninsulin-dependent diabetes mellitus, but others disagree.[21] A detailed description of the mechanisms mentioned above is available.[22]

Epidemiology of Diabetes Mellitus in the Elderly

It is difficult to review the epidemiology of diabetes in the elderly because approximately 50 percent of the elderly diabetic subjects are undiagnosed.[15] However, even studies of subjects with previously diagnosed diabetes can provide useful information; for instance the surveys of Poole, Oxford, and Southall of caucasian subjects with diagnosed diabetes[23] reveals that 60 percent of known diabetic subjects are aged 60 years or more. However, when considering the overall prevalence of diabetes, one should include only studies using adequate survey methods, and these must include ascertainment of cases using the glucose tolerance test. Different investigators have studied different age groups. Some have not analyzed the result by the different ethnic groups in their sample and presentation of results is quite variable. In the past, studies used different diagnostic criteria,[24,25] and some studies prescreened with a simple test, for example, urinalysis, to select subjects for further study.

Table 75-1 Changing prevalence of diabetes with age from NHANES 2 screening survey

	Prevalence of Diabetes (%)	
Age Group (years)	**White**	**Nonwhite**
20–44	1.7	3.2
45–54	8.2	12.9
55–64	12.5	22.5
65–74	17.9	26.4

(Data from Harris et al.[15])

The prevalence of diabetes rises from youth to old age (see Table 75-1). However, the Melton screening survey,[18] East & West Finland screening survey,[26] and a survey of Pima Indians[27] found static prevalences from age 65 to 85, suggesting that the age-related increase in diabetes prevalence levels off after age 65. The prevalence of diabetes in different elderly populations is given in Table 75-2, from which we can see that most most developed countries have a prevalence of approximately 17 percent in their elderly white population and around 25 percent in nonwhite populations. The prevalence in white British elderly is only around 9 percent, although the prevalence in nonwhite British elderly is still approximately 25 percent.

The prevalence of previously diagnosed diabetes in the UK elderly has increased over the last few decades being approximately 3 percent recently,[23] although it was only 1.9 percent in Edinburgh in 1968.[31] On reinterpreting the Ibstock survey of 1958[32] and Birmingham screening surveys of the early 1960s[33,34] to allow for the effect of prescreening by urinalysis, and the effect of the change in diagnostic criteria, it is likely that the previous overall rate of diabetes in the British elderly was around 10 percent. Thus, the increase in prevalence of diagnosed diabetes in the UK is almost certainly due to increased rate of diagnosis rather than a true increase in prevalence.

The risk of developing NIDDM is increased by parental history,[15,39] obesity,[15,37,39] hypertension,[37] and lack of exercise.[37] In subjects with these risk factors, exercise seems to

Table 75-2 Prevalence of diabetes in different screened elderly populations

Study	Year	Ref.	Age	Sex	Ethnic Origin	Diabetes Rate (%)	IGT Rate (%)
Melton, UK	1991	18	65–85	M+F	White	9.1	7.1
Coventry, UK	1988	28	60–79	M+F	White	7.0	—
Coventry, UK	1988	28	60–79	M+F	South Asian	27.8	—
NHANES II US	1976–1980	15	65–74	M+F	White	17.9	23.0
NHANES II US	1976–1980	15	65–74	M+F	Nonwhite	26.4	14.5
California US	1972–1974	29	60–89	M+F	White	16.1	—
Tampere, Finland *(F)*	1977	30	85+	M+F	White	17.0	—
Fredericia, Denmark *(F)*	1981–1982	31	60–74	M+F	White	7.2	—
Glostrup, Denmark *(U)*	1967	32	70	M+F	White	10.0	25
Glostrup, Denmark *(U)*	1977	32	80	M+F	White	12.0	36
East/West Finland *(pm gtts)*	1984	26	65–84	M	White	29.8	31.8
Gothenburg, Sweden	1980	33	67	M	White	10.8	14.2
Amsterdam, Holland *(D)*	1985	34	65+	M+F	White	23.6	—
Kuopio, Finland	1986–1988	35	65–74	M+F	White	17.8	20.8

Abbreviations: F, FBG based survey; *D*, recruitment details scanty; *pm gtts*, testing performed in afternoon, which may increase diabetes prevalence; *U*, previously undiagnosed diabetic subjects only recorded.

protect against the development of diabetes to a certain extent. This is important when advising the offspring of patients severely affected by specific and nonspecific complications; they are told to stay slim, avoid refined carbohydrates, to exercise more (climb 15 flights stairs per day), and to be aware of their risk of diabetes and hypertension.[40]

Thus, many subjects with known diabetes are elderly, and many elderly people are diabetic. An increased prevalence of diabetes in the elderly is associated with nonwhite race, family history of diabetes, obesity, hypertension, and lack of exercise.

Diabetes Definition, Classification, and Diagnosis

The majority of elderly diabetic people will have noninsulin-dependent diabetes mellitus (NIDDM); this is defined by hyperglycemia and the tendency to develop specific complications. Thus, a venous plasma glucose level equal to or exceeding 11.1 mmol/L (200 mg/dl)[24,41] predicts those subjects who have a dramatically increased chance of retinopathy.[16,42–44] This cut-off value is derived from Whitehall civil servants,[44] residents of Bedford,[16] and Pima Indians of all ages.[42,43] If one examines populations with a very high incidence of NIDDM, such as the Pima Indians or Nauru Islanders, who have not previously been diagnosed as diabetic, then the results of mass glucose tolerance testing reveal a bimodal distribution of 2 h-glucose values at all ages including the elderly, which is not seen in other populations due to their small numbers of undiagnosed diabetic subjects.[45,46] The cut-off value of 11.1 mmol/L (200 mg/dl) does actually separate normoglycaemic and diabetic populations (each with a Gaussian distribution of 2 hour values) in different age groups, suggesting that the WHO criteria apply in the elderly as well as the young. However, the 11.1 mmol/L (200 mg/dl) cut-off has never been subjected to long-term follow-up in the elderly to confirm the tendency to specific complications.

Not all diabetes in the elderly is noninsulin-dependent; insulin-dependent diabetes mellitus (IDDM) does occur and diabetes may be secondary to or exacerbated by other conditions such as pancreatic disease, endocrine disease such as Cushing syndrome, acromegaly, or thyrotoxicosis, and most commonly, drug therapy such as high-dose thiazide diuretics, oral glucocorticosteroids, and oral β-blockers; a comprehensive list of diabetogenic drugs is given in the NDDG criteria.[24] A simple classification is given in the list describing classes of diabetes mellitus in the elderly.

Impaired glucose tolerance is a state between normal and diabetic glucose tolerance; in itself it does not lead to diabetic-specific complications, but is a significant risk factor for large vessel disease and over 10 years, 10 percent will progress to diabetes in British residents,[47] but far more will progress in populations with a high prevalence of diabetes, such as the Pima Indians[48] in whom 6 percent convert per year. Although the cut-off between diabetic and nondiabetic glucose tolerance is based on the risk of specific complications, the cut-off between IGT and normal glucose tolerance is more arbitrary and was reached by consensus of experts.[25] One should note that diabetic complications are divided into specific complications, for example, retinopathy, which are related to degree and duration of hyperglycemia, and nonspecific complications, such as large vessel disease, which occur in normal glucose tolerant subjects, but are more common with any degree of abnormal

Classification of diabetes mellitus in the elderly

Primary
- Insulin-dependent
- Non-insulin-dependent
  - Non-obese
  - Obese
- Insulin-treated, noninsulin-dependent

Secondary
- Drugs (glucocorticosteroids, thiazide diuretics, oral β-blockers, oral β-agonists)
- Pancreatic disease
- Endocrine disease (Cushing's syndrome, acromegaly, thyrotoxicosis, phechromocytoma).

glucose tolerance, including IGT.[47,49] The WHO criteria for diabetes and IGT are given in Table 75-3.

Impact of Diabetes Mellitus in the Elderly

Older patients with diabetes appear to burden the hospital care system 2 to 3 times more than the general population[50] and use primary care services 2 to 3 times more than non-diabetic controls.[51] Damsgaard's primary care study from Denmark[51] indicated that insulin-treated patients accounted for more than half of the service provision, mainly due to chronic vascular disease with a correspondingly high number of hospital clinic visits. The average number of bed-days occupied per person per year was 6.8 for males and 8.2 for females, whereas the figures for insulin-treated NIDDM patients was 23.9, which was considerably higher than for insulin-treated patients with IDDM (15.2).[50] Similar bed-occupancy rates for patients with known diabetes have been reported by others.[52]

Several studies have focused on defining the prevalence of elderly patients in hospital diabetic populations.[2,53] In a study from Edinburgh Royal Infirmary, elderly patients with diabetes aged 65 years and over accounted for 60 percent of the bed-occupancy due to diabetes giving a mean hospital prevalence of 4.6 percent.[2] A Cardiff-based study of three district general hospitals found a hospital prevalence (pooled data) of 8.4 percent with a mean age of 65 years.[53]

Table 75-3 Diagnostic values for 2-hour post-75-g glucose load blood sample (mmol/L)

	Plasma		Whole Blood	
	Venous	Capillary	Venous	Capillary
Diabetes	11.1+	12.2+	10.0+	11.1+
IGT	7.8–11.0	8.9–12.1	6.7–9.9	7.8–11.0

Diabetes in older subjects is associated with considerable morbidity mainly due to the long-term complications.[54–57] A population-based study from Oxford[54] measured the incidence of complications over a median period of 6 years in 188 patients aged 60 years and over by using a structured questionnaire and clinical examination. Incidence rates of ischemic heart disease, stroke, and peripheral vascular disease (PVD) were 56, 22, and 146 per 1,000-person-years, which are comparable to rates found in the Framingham study,[58] but slightly higher since the Oxford study involved an older age group. Retinopathy occurred at a rate of 60 and cataract at 29 per 1,000-person-years, while proteinuria (albumin concentration greater than 300 mg/L) was 19 per 1,000-person-years. Incidence rates appeared to be unrelated to sex or duration of diabetes, but stroke and PVD rose significantly with age.

In Poole, a coastal town in Southern England, the prevalence of diabetic neuropathy, an important cause of foot ulceration and amputation, was determined in 1,077 diabetic subjects,[55] which comprised 94 percent of the known diabetic population. Neuropathy was diagnosed, using a single-observer approach, by the presence of neuropathic symptoms plus one or more physical findings such as loss of light touch or impairment of pain sensation. The overall prevalence of neuropathy was 16.3 percent (compared with 2.9 percent in non-diabetic controls) with similar values in both IDDM and NIDDM patients, with three-quarters of patients reporting symptoms. In this study, duration of diabetes and metabolic control were significant predictors of neuropathy. The prevalence of neuropathy increased with age in all groups with one in four NIDDM patients aged 80 years and over being affected.

A community survey from Nottingham, England,[56] of 98 elderly diabetic patients (mean age 73 years) registered with two inner-city general practices, studied the impact of diabetes in terms of complications and frequency of hospital and general practice contacts. Figure 75-1 shows that diabetic subjects had significantly higher prevalences of stroke, cognitive impairment, diminished leg pulses, visual impairment, and absent vibration senses (perceptive threshold greater than 50 V at one or more sites, as a marker of neuropathy) compared with nondiabetic controls. Disability was present in four out of five patients. Cataract was the most common cause of disability associated with visual impairment.

The prevalence of some diabetic complications have been reported to increase with advancing age.[42,59–61] In a cross-sectional study of NIDDM patients aged 53 to 80 years,[61] the prevalence of retinopathy, peripheral neuropathy, and hypertension were evaluated at different ages. Logistic regression demonstrated a significant increase in the prevalence of retinopathy with aging, independent of the effects of metabolic control, duration of disease, and other risk variables. Age was also related to the prevalence of peripheral neuropathy, hypertension, and impotence. The independent contribution of age, per se, to retinopathy was not seen in a study by Ballard et al.[60] in 1988 in Minnesota, who found a positive relationship

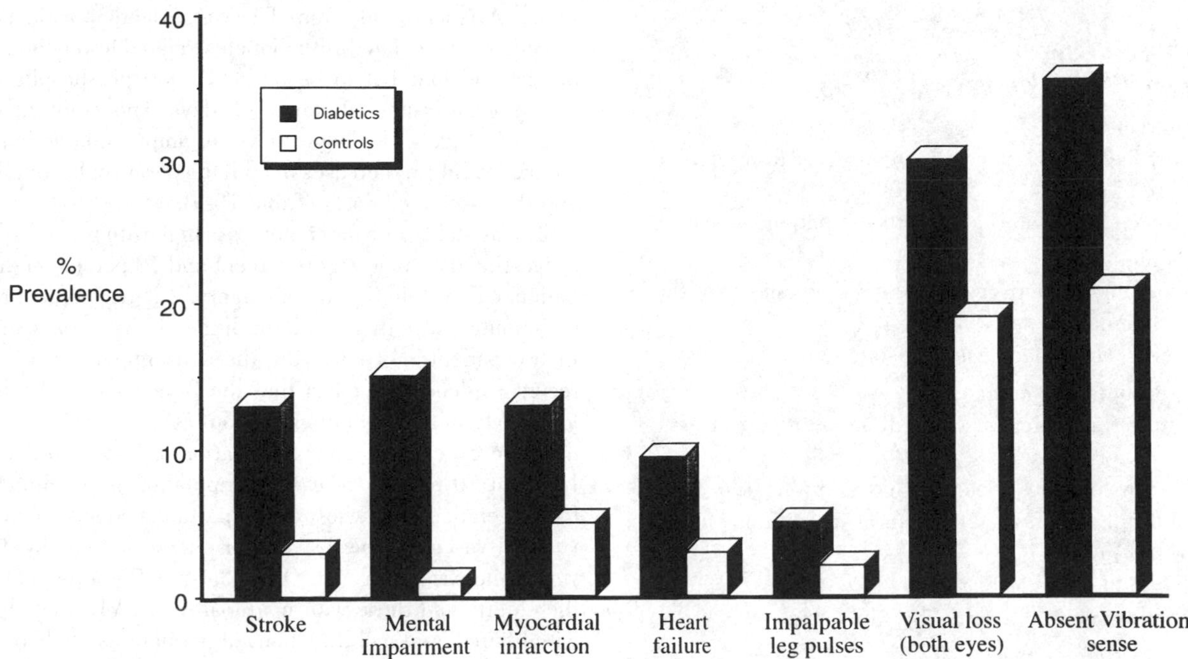

Figure 75-1 Comparison of morbidity between patients with diabetes and nondiabetic controls (see Dornan et al.[56]).

with persistent proteinuria only, or in a study in 1986 by Knuiman et al.[59] who studied both IDDM and NIDDM patients and found independent associations of age with renal impairment, macrovascular complications, and sensory neuropathy only.

Visual Loss Due to Diabetic Eye Disease

Diabetic retinopathy was the third main cause of blindness and partial sight registration in one epidemiologic study in Avon, UK;[62] however, the diabetic person also has a greater risk of cataract, glaucoma, retinal artery thrombosis, and retinal vein thrombosis. Thus, it is no surprise that blind registrations for diabetic subjects in Nottingham are eight times higher than the subjects not known to have diabetes,[56] with 16 percent of elderly diabetic subjects having blind or partial sight registrations. The diabetic blind registration is predominately due to maculopathy, which is treatable, unlike age-related macular degeneration, the main cause of blind registration in the elderly.

The underlying problem in diabetic retinopathy is capillary occlusion[63]; this may cause a hypoxic area of retina with new vessel formation. However, other capillaries become dilated; this causes microaneurysms if focal, or leakage from the capillaries if generalized. It is this capillary leakage that causes exudative and edematous maculopathies that are the main forms of sight-threatening retinopathy in the older subject with NIDDM.

Many cross-sectional studies show that good glycemic control is associated with less chance of developing retinopathy.[64,65] Unfortunately, association does not mean causation and there are no intervention studies in elderly NIDDM subjects to determine whether good control itself prevents retinopathy from developing. Duration of disease is also associated with increased risk of retinopathy. Because the elderly diabetic subject has often had NIDDM for some 5 to 7 years before diagnosis,[66] it is not surprising that diabetic retinopathy is already present at diagnosis in 10.5 percent of elderly subjects in whom only one pupil was dilated[67]; 23.8 percent of subjects of all ages in the United Kingdom Prospective Diabetes Study (UKPDS) had retinopathy at presentation.[68]

Laser photocoagulation can preserve vision in edematous and exudative maculopathies if visual acuity is 6/9 or better,[69,70] and it has been calculated that screening and treating diabetic retinopathy would precent 56 percent of blind registrations due to diabetic retinopathy.[70] Cataract has been shown to be more common in diabetic subjects[72,73] even at the time of diagnosis,[74] and its presence predicts increased mortality.[75]

Although some studies show an association of diabetes with open angle glaucoma,[76] many other studies refute this.[77–79] There is some evidence that glaucoma is associated with worse retinopathy,[80] and neovascularization is associated with glaucoma.[81] It is well accepted that retinal venous thrombosis is a complication of diabetes,[82] and there is some evidence that retinal artery thrombosis is associated with diabetes.[74,83]

Age-related macular degeneration (ARMD) seems very common in our diabetic patients in clinical practice; theoretical reasons why ARMD should be associated with diabetes are discussed in the paper by Klein et al.[84] However, most studies show no such association,[85–87] and only one study has shown such an association in men aged 75 or more.[84]

Reasons to refer to an ophthalmologist

1. Cataract
   Any cataract preventing the observer from viewing the fundus
   Any cataract interfering with the patient's vision
2. Maculopathy
   Exudates around or within 1 disc diameter of the macula
   Unexplained decrease in visual acuity
3. Preproliferative change
   Intraretinal microvascular abnormalities (flat new vessels)
   Venous changes (beading, loops, duplication)
   Multiple cotton wool spots (6 or more in one quadrant)
   Large blot hemorrhages
   Replacement of arteries by white line
4. Proliferative changes
   Visible new vessels
   Vitreous hemorrhage
5. Blind registration

The gold standard ophthalmologic assessment is slit lamp examination by an experienced user;[88] however, this is often not practicable. Mydriatic retinal photography has a sensitivity of detection of eye disease of 89 percent which is significantly better than the sensitivity of direct ophthalmoscopy of 65 percent.[88] If photography is not available, subjects need measurements of visual acuity and dilated fundoscopy by experienced observers each year; this is probably worth doing anyway opportunistically because even photography misses 11 percent of retinopathy. Although exudative maculopathy is easy to spot in the dilated eye (exudates around or within one disc's diameter of the macula), macular edema is practically impossible to distinguish from a normal eye by ophthalmoscopy; hence, the importance of measuring the corrected visual acuity. The reasons for referral to an ophthalmologist are set out in the accompanying box.

Diabetic Foot Disease

Limb amputation remains an important health problem in the diabetic population with the rate of lower limb amputation being 15 times higher than for nondiabetic patients.[89] It is three times higher in diabetic men than in women.[90] The elderly are particularly affected.[91] Management of diabetic limb disease is expensive. Even 10 years ago, the total annual cost of major leg amputations in diabetic patients in the UK was estimated to be in excess of £13.0 million,[92] while in the US, the direct medical care costs for all amputations in the diabetic populations, not including rehabilitation, exceeded $500 million.[93] A recent study from The Netherlands[94] estimated the direct costs associated with diabetes-related lower-limb amputations and found it to be over £10,000 per hospitalization with a mean in-patient stay of 42 days. This study identified increasing age and a higher level of amputation as important factors leading to increases in both the period of hospitalization and the associated costs (Table 75-4).

The mortality rate for amputees is high with previous studies suggesting that between 40 percent and 70 percent of diabetic patients die within 5 years of surgery.[95] Thirty percent require an amputation of the remaining limb within 3 years with one in two patients not surviving the subsequent 5 years. More recent evidence indicates that the 3-year survival following lower extremity amputation is about 50 percent,[96] with a median life expectancy after amputation of less than 2 years.[90] In about 70 percent of cases, amputation is precipitated by foot ulceration,[97,98] whose principal antecedents include peripheral vascular disease and peripheral neuropathy, both of which increase with age. Other "at-risk" groups apart from the elderly and those with neuropathy or PVD, include those with limited joint mobility, bony abnormalities, diabetic nephropathy, excess alcohol intake, visual impairment, and patients living alone.[91]

Various risk factors have been identified that increase the likelihood of foot ulceration (see list below). Peripheral sensorimotor neuropathy is the primary cause or contributory factor in 90 percent of cases.[99,100] Both small (often unmyelinated) and large (usually myelinated) nerve fibers are affected, which leads to the common symptoms of numbness, lancinating, and burning pain, "pins and needles", and hyperesthesia, which is typically worse at night.[91] Physical examination reveals a glove and stocking loss of pain, fine touch and thermal sensation (small fibers), with coexisting vibration and proprioceptive loss (large fibers). Small muscle atrophy in the foot can also occur due to motor fibers loss, which can cause flexor/extensor muscle inbalance resulting in clawed toes, prominent metatarsal heads, and forward displacement of the metatarsal foot pads.[101] This can lead to abnormally high foot pressures developing, which can increase the risk of foot ulceration and lead to gait disturbances. In elderly patients with peripheral neurop-

Table 75-4 Duration of hospitalization for lower extremity amputations and mean costs of hospitalization (including hospital stay and surgery) by age group in the diabetic population

Age Group	Duration of Hospitalization[a]	Mean Costs of Hospitalization (£-sterling)	Number of Cases
<45	25.5 ± 20.5	6,516	53
45–64	38.7 ± 36.0	9,734	346
65–74	43.5 ± 37.2	10,996	521
75+	43.3 ± 42.9	10,928	655
Total	41.8 ± 39.1	10,531	1,575

[a] *Results expressed as mean ± SD in days.*

Risk factors for foot ulceration in the elderly

- Peripheral sensorimotor neuropathy
- Automatic neuropathy
- Peripheral vascular disease
- Limited joint mobility
- Foot pressure abnormalities
- Other risk factors
  - History of previous foot problems
  - Reduced resistance to infections
  - Smoking and alcohol

athy, this may give rise to further foot injuries and falls. The presence of visual loss may exacerbate the situation.[102] A trivial foot injury in a patient with severe neuropathy can eventually lead to the development of a Charcot joint, which is a chronic neuroarthropathy whose prevalence varies from as low as 0.15 to 7 percent depending on the study populations.[91] The majority of cases have had diabetes for at least 10 years and most are elderly.

Peripheral blood flow in patients with diabetes is disturbed, with loss of blood flow autoregulation, increased arteriovenous shunting, and changes in capillary blood flow. Some of these abnormalities may be reversible or ameliorated by improved glycemic control.[103] Chronic change in peripheral blood vessels is usually manifested by atherosclerosis with the pattern of PVD tending to involve vessels below the knee more often in diabetic than in nondiabetic individuals.[104] Risk factors for PVD include smoking, hypertension, and hypercholesterolemia, with prevalence increasing with both advancing age and duration of diabetes. Symptoms include intermittent claudication and/or rest pain with lower limb ulceration or gangrene being important clinical outcomes. Radiologic investigation may show medial arterial calcification, which has been reported to be associated with both diabetic peripheral somatosensory and autonomic neuropathy.[105] Objective assessment of limb blood flow by Doppler ultrasound can be affected by extensive medial calcification, giving rise to a misleadingly high ankle-pressure index.[106]

A schematic diagram of the interplay of factors leading to foot ulceration is shown in Figure 75-2. It seems logical that interventions designed to prevent diabetic foot disease and amputations in patients with diabetes should be directed to the prevention of peripheral neuropathy and PVD and the prevention, early detection, and treatment of foot lesions. Several studies using staff and patient education and a multidisciplinary approach to foot care have demonstrated a reduction in diabetes-related amputations.[107–109] By incorporating an intensive multidisciplinary approach in a diabetes foot clinic,[107] a London-based study demonstrated a 44 percent decline in amputation rate after 2 years. By use of suitable-fitting shoes, the recurrence rate of foot ulcers was reduced from 83 to 26 percent. At the University Hospital of Geneva, an 85 percent reduction in the rate of below-knee amputations was seen over a 4-year observation period by a combination of education and training in foot care in patients with diabetes.[108] A 12-year retrospective study from Sweden[98] evaluated the changes in diabetes-related lower extremity amputations following the introduction of a multidisciplinary program for preventing and treating diabetic foot ulcers. The number of major amputations decreased by 75 percent, the number of minor amputations rose from 28 to 53 percent, and the reamputation rate de-

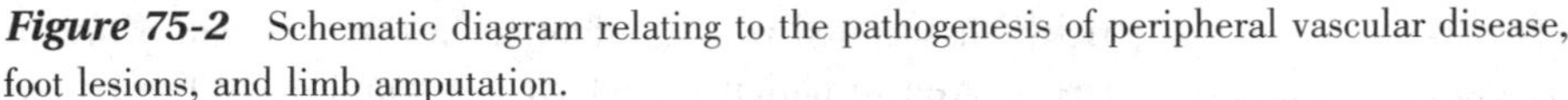
Figure 75-2 Schematic diagram relating to the pathogenesis of peripheral vascular disease, foot lesions, and limb amputation.

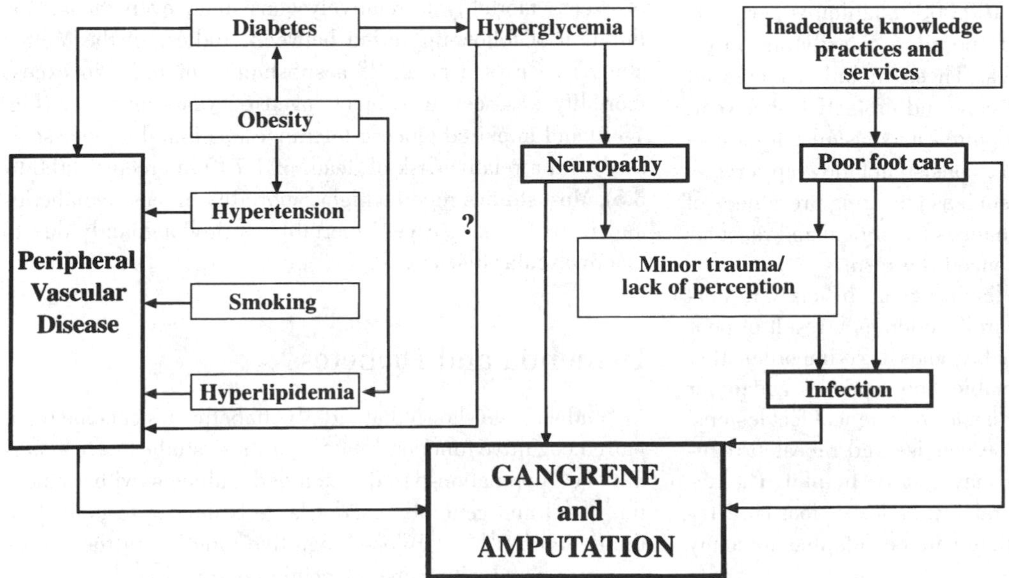

General principles of foot care education

1. Target the level of information to the needs of the patient. Those not at risk may require only general advice about foot hygiene and shoes.
2. Assess the ability of the patient to understand and perform the necessary components of foot care. If this is limited, then the spouse or carer should be involved at the beginning of the process.
3. Suggest a positive approach to foot care with "do's" rather than "don'ts" as the principle of active rather than passive foot care is more likely to be successful and acceptable to the patient.
   - Inspect the feet daily.
   - Report any problems immediately.
   - Have your feet measured every time new shoes are bought.
   - Buy shoes with a square toe box and laces.
   - Inspect the inside of shoes for foreign objects every day before putting them on.
   - Attend a fully trained chiropodist regularly.
   - Cut your nails straight across and not rounded.
   - Keep your feet away from heat (fires, radiators, and hot water bottles) and check the bath water before stepping into it.
   - Always wear something on your feet to protect them and never walk barefoot.
4. Repeat the advice at regular intervals and check that it is being followed.
5. Disseminate advice to other family members and other health care professionals involved in the care of a patient.

creased from 36 to 22 percent. The incidence of major amputations fell from 16.1 to 3.6 per 100,000 inhabitants per year. Many factors were identified as possible contributing influences on the observed changes. These included increased availability of preventative foot care and protective shoewear, new healing strategies, use of noninvasive vascular tests, use of strict amputation criteria, and a consistent follow-up service. Along with these, other factors such as changing prevalence of diabetes, smoking habits, and changes in surgical and vascular techniques will also have influenced the results.

With many elderly patients having great difficulty in performing the most routine foot care[109] often as a result of poor vision and reduced mobility, it becomes very important that strategies are designed that enable both spouses and other carers to have a role in prevention and treatment of foot lesions. Educational material needs to be concise and repeated regularly[91] and video presentations may also be helpful. The accompanying box provides general principles of foot care reflecting a positive approach that can be adapted to many patients in clinical settings.

Mortality in Elderly Diabetic Patients

It is a widely held belief that diabetes mellitus confers little or no excess mortality risk in older patients, with life expectancy being similar after age 70 to 75 years.[110–112] This was explained by a shorter life in elderly subjects with other competing causes of death minimizing the effect of diabetes. In line with this, most early reports indicated that the ratio of death rates in diabetics to rates in the general population falls progressively with age especially in those aged 65 years and over, though it remains above unity up to the age 80 years.[113] More recently, one study actually found a significantly lower mortality in patients aged 75 (mortality ratio 0.88) years and over compared with the general population[114] and these contradictory findings have created uncertainty about the true impact of this metabolic disorder on the older diabetic population.

Few of the studies that have looked at diabetic mortality in the population employed universal screening using an oral glucose tolerance test (or other methods of confirming the presence of diabetes). It is possible that actual mortality in any given population may be underestimated because many patients will be undiagnosed. Other methodologic variations have prevented consistent comparisons being made across different diabetic populations. It is important to determine whether premature death due to diabetes is observable in elderly patients because this evidence would provide guidance to those responsible for providing health services on how best to focus their resources. An unequivocal finding of increased mortality would argue for a more sustained commitment to diabetic health care provision and research. Alternatively, the absence of excess mortality could redirect care strategies toward reducing morbidity and disability only.

A recent literature review by the present authors has confirmed that diabetes in later life imposes an excess mortality risk[115] associated with a reduction in life expectancy in both sexes, even in patients aged 75 years and over. The pattern of excess mortality is relatively consistent, even though the duration of follow-up varied between studies. In the Melton study by Croxson et al.,[116] a substantial increase in excess mortality was seen in subjects aged 65 years and over (Fig. 75-3) and impaired glucose tolerance was found to be associated with a relative risk of death of 1.7 (95 percent CI:0.8 to 3.5). Most studies report a higher mortality in female diabetics and in both sexes, excess mortality is predominantly due to macrovascular disease.

Dementia and Diabetes

Studies have shown that elderly diabetic subjects have impaired cognitive function,[117–121] but these studies were generally not population-based, excluded subjects with dementia,[118–121] and generally used a large battery of tests to show the deficit.[117,119–121] Worse cognitive function in these tests was associated with worse glycemic control.[117–121]

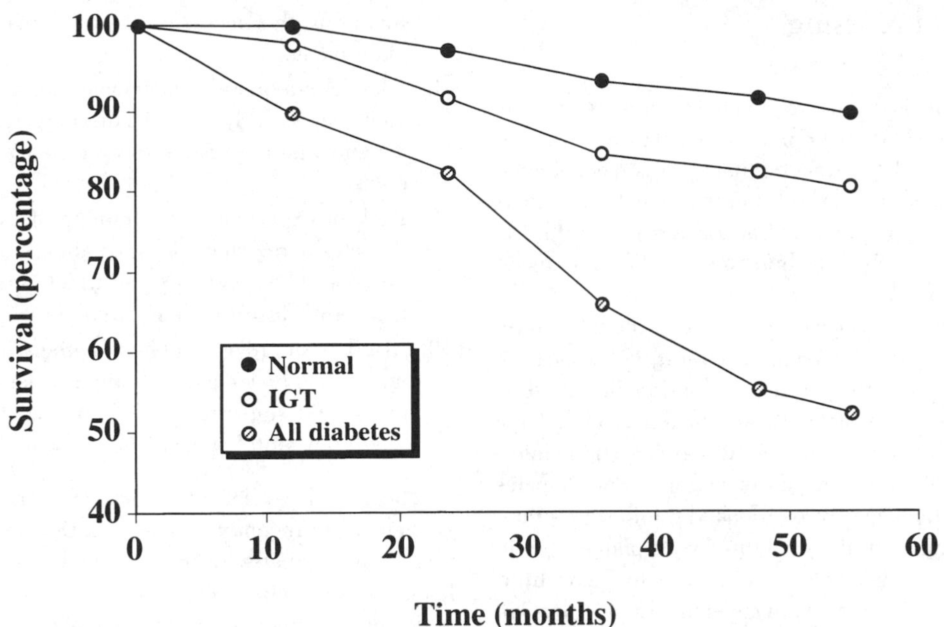

Figure 75-3 Survival curves for subjects in the Melton study showing increased mortality in patients with diabetes. (Data from Croxson et al.[116])

Community-based studies in both Melton Mowbray[122] and Nottingham[56] have shown worse cognitive function in elderly diabetic subjects using simple tests such as the Folstein MMSE and Hodkinson AMT. Data from the Melton surveys[122] suggest that in comparison with subjects with normal glucose tolerance, subjects with known diabetes are more likely to have a low Folstein MMSE score (odds ratio 3.3, 95 percent CI 1.29 to 8.48), and subjects with newly diagnosed diabetes are less likely to have a low MMSE (upper 95 percent CI of odds ratio 0.003) compared with normal glucose tolerance subjects. However, other workers have either found no decreased cognitive function in elderly diabetic subjects,[123–124] or that the decreased cognitive function in diabetic subjects is partly explained by depression in the diabetic subjects.[125]

There are several possible explanations for the lower cognitive function in the known diabetic subjects, apart from abnormal plasma glucose levels. First, depression, a cause of cognitive impairment, has been found to be associated with known diabetes.[125–126] Second, hypertension is associated with diabetes and insulin resistance,[127] and is itself associated with decreased cognitive function[128]; there is even evidence to suggest that among hypertensive subjects, hyperinsulinemia is associated with worse cognitive function.[129] Third, cerebrovascular disease is 2 to 3 times more common in people with known diabetes,[56,130] which again might be associated with cognitive impairment. Fourth, there is evidence that cortical atrophy is associated with diabetes. A small population-based study found temporal atrophy to be more marked in diabetic subjects, which was most marked for drug-treated rather than diet-treated diabetic subjects[131]; a second study of routine CT scans of hospital patients found that diffuse cerebral and cortical atrophy was associated with diabetes allowing for the effect of age, hypertension, and cerebrovascular disease.[132]

From a management point of view, does hyperglycemia contribute to cognitive impairment? Two studies have shown that tightening control in poorly controlled subjects does improve cognitive function, but the degree of hyperglycemia was quite high. Many studies show an association between cognitive function, and indices of long-term glycemic control. Some studies have shown that cognitive impairment is increased by increasing duration of diabetes, and cognitive impairment may be associated with peripheral neuropathy, which is a specific complication associated with duration of disease and glycemic control[118,133–134]; thus, cognition may be impaired as a diabetic-specific complication. Although cognitive impairment in younger subjects with insulin-dependent diabetes is associated with hypoglycemia,[133–134] the high levels of glycemia found in community studies of the elderly diabetic person[56] suggest that this is not a major contributory factor in the elderly, but there is little research on this area.

Whatever the reason, known diabetic subjects appear to have poorer cognitive function than subjects not known to have diabetes. It is interesting to note the two studies that suggest that improving glycemic control improves cognitive function.[135–136] Impaired cognitive function should be borne in mind when treating elderly diabetic subjects because it has implications for their safe treatment; this may cause difficulty with glycemic control due to erratic taking of diet and medication, and may present with hypoglycemia where patients forget that they have medication and repeat the dose. One should enlist the help of family and services to optimize glycemic control to see if this makes any difference, and then accept that one has to change goals from good control to less strict, but safer control.[137] It is, however, important to consider to screen for other treatable causes of cognitive impairment.

Residential and Nursing Home Care

Little information is available about the quality of care, treatment, and nature of diabetic patients living within institutions. A study from the US estimated that 14.5 percent of nursing home residents had diabetes,[138] but this may be an underestimate. A screening program in Canada led to one-third of residents in an old people's home being reclassified as diabetic over a 3-year period.[139]

In the UK and other European countries[140] there has been a rapid expansion in residential and nursing home care for elderly people with a corresponding reduction in long-term hospital care. Many of the residents are disabled, and a large percentage are likely to have diabetes, although accurate information is not available. The needs of patients with diabetes living within institutions may be overlooked if follow-up strategies have been terminated, if a structured care plan is absent, if no "nominated" carer is available, or if care staff have little knowledge of basic diabetes management. In addition, in smaller institutions, the number of residents with diabetes may be relatively small and care staff accordingly have little opportunity for gaining experience in diabetes care.

Management Problems

Various common problems make diabetes management more complex in these patients[141] and include:

1. Irregular oral intake due to: (a) confusion and/or a poor appetite due to concurrent illness; (b) dysphagia due to stroke or other neurologic or gastroenterologic disorders. Lack of regular calorific intake can be particularly troublesome for insulin-treated patients.
2. Recurrent urine, chest, and other infections rendering the diabetic person liable to hyperglycemia, and possibly ketosis with poor metabolic control.
3. Leg ulcers and pressure sores that may rapidly deteriorate in diabetic patients.
4. Dysphasia, dysarthria, or deafness and blindness, which may make it difficult to communicate—needs are thus unrecognized and unmet.
5. Increased vulnerability to hypoglycemia (especially those taking sulfonylureas or insulin) due to poor appetite and difficulties in ensuring sufficient and regular calorific intake (as in 1), lack of glucose monitoring (urine or blood), lack of knowledge of symptoms and signs of hypoglycemia that may be attenuated in older people with diabetes, polypharmacy (multiple drug therapy), and recurrent acute illness.
6. Concurrent pathology in any resident (especially cardiac and renal failure) increasing the likelihood of adverse drug reactions to prescribed medications. This may be exacerbated by infrequent review of existing medications.
7. Inadequate facilities within institutions to cater for the dietary needs of residents with diabetes including inadequate knowledge of catering staff on what and how to provide appropriate and varied food for diabetic residents including the necessity of provisions of snacks outside main meals.
8. Lack of adequate arrangements for regular diabetes review, particularly for those discharged from hospital clinics and who are unable to visit their primary care physician.
9. Lack of experience and training of institutional staff in diabetes care, which does not allow glucose monitoring to be undertaken correctly and which prevents useful assistance with insulin administration.
10. Insufficient provision of health professional input, particularly specialist nurses, dietitians, dental surgeons, opticians, and state-registered chiropodists and doctors, including hospital specialists.

The British Geriatrics Society (Special Interest Group in Diabetes) has recently published a Document of Care for patients with diabetes residing in both residential or nursing homes,[142] which lists several strategies to improve overall diabetic care for this vulnerable group of people (see accompanying box).

Management of Diabetes Mellitus in the Older Adult

Despite the advent of modern dietary therapy and pharmacologic approaches, it remains common clinical experience that the majority of diabetic subjects exhibit poor glycemic control and the incidence of microangiopathic complications such as nephropathy, retinopathy, and neuropathy is unacceptably high. The Diabetes Control and Complications Trial (DCCT) has confirmed that longer-term "tight" glycemic control leads to a delay in the onset of microangiopathy and a fall in the rate of progression of established complications in IDDM,[143] and it is hoped that this benefit will also be seen

Improving care within residential and nursing home settings

1. Each resident should have an individual diabetes care plan agreed between patient (or relative), doctor (who is responsible for diabetic care), and home care staff.
2. There should be increased community support from experienced health professionals such as diabetes specialist nurses and dieticians.
3. Diabetic patients living in residential and nursing homes should have ready access to other specialist health professionals.
4. Each resident with diabetes should be reviewed by either the family doctor or a hospital consultant physician/geriatrician at least once a year.
5. Patients in residential and nursing homes should be included in any local audit of diabetic care.

in patients with NIDDM where large-vessel (macroangiopathy) complications are predominantly the major cause of mortality. The efficacy of available treatments for NIDDM in terms of metabolic control and complications incidence may be answered in 1998 when the UK Prospective Diabetes Study[144] reports the long-term outcome in more than 5,000 patients.

Several surveys have identified that more than half of patients with NIDDM are treated by diet and oral agents, with treatment by diet alone or by insulin accounting for about one in five in each case[55–56]: older patients tend to have insulin less often than younger patients with NIDDM. Details of a comprehensive strategy for the care of older patients with diabetes have recently been published,[145] and only specific comments relating to nonpharmacologic and pharmacologic therapeutic approaches will be discussed in this section.

Pathologic Basis for the Treatment of NIDDM

Noninsulin-dependent diabetes mellitus accounts for more than 90 percent of cases of diabetes in old age[146] with the remainder being IDDM.[147] NIDDM has been characterized by a combination of insulin resistance (at both hepatic and peripheral tissue levels) due to a potentially decreased number of insulin receptors and a postreceptor defect, and β-cell dysfunction characterized by defective insulin secretion.[148] In association with hyperglycemia, other disturbances often occur and include hypertension and dyslipidaemia. In addition, patients may be obese and have evidence of coronary heart disease, a combination which has sometimes been referred to as Syndrome X.[149] In these circumstances, the main objectives of treatment would include reducing hyperglycemia, as well as treatment of these other metabolic defects, those are, the use of antihypertensive treatment and lipid-lowering agents (where appropriate), and weight reduction.

Specific treatments must, therefore, aim to reverse or ameliorate these metabolic defects by one or more of the following ways: Improve β-cell dysfunction—this may be achieved by:

1. Stimulating pancreatic β-cells to secrete more insulin, for example, by use of sulfonylureas.
2. Lowering circulating levels of glucose, by, for example, dietary modification.

Decrease insulin resistance by enhancing the biological response of insulinsensitive tissues to circulating insulin—this may be accomplished by:

1. Direct actions of certain oral antihyperglycaemic drugs, such as sulfonylureas or metformin.
2. The use of insulin sensitizers which are being evaluated.
3. Directly reducing hyperglycemia, by, for example, dietary modification.

Limit the dietary intake of monosaccharides, which:

1. Prevents rapid peaks in blood glucose levels after meals (postprandial hyperglycemia).
2. Lessens β-cell secretory dysfunction and enhances insulin sensitivity of target tissues. This may be achieved by taking smaller meals more frequently and reducing the content of certain foodstuffs rich in monosaccharides as part of a recommended dietary program. This is more effective if foods are selected that have slower rates of absorption (poly- and oligosaccharides). Alternatively, drugs that delay the intestinal absorption of monosaccharides would also be of potential value, for example, α-glucosidase inhibitors.

Initial Treatment

An 8- to 12-week course of dietary instruction by a trained dietitian is suggested in patients whose random glucose values are less than 20 mmol/L (360 mg/dl) and who are not troubled significantly by symptoms. For patients with significant symptoms of diabetes or initial random glucose of greater than 20 mmol/L (360 mg/dl), or who fail to respond to diet alone, oral agents should be used. The goals are adapted for each individual patient and agreed with them and/or their carer (see list of care plan steps). Patients and carers should be educated about the indications for referral to hospital as an outpatient and when admission is likely to be required.

Oral Antidiabetic Therapy

Oral agents are required when dietary therapy alone is no longer sufficient to control symptoms of hyperglycemia, or random blood glucose levels are greater than 20 mmol/L (360 mg/dl), or control is unacceptable as estimated by long-term measures of diabetic control, for example glycosylated hemoglobin. In general, the lowest effective dose of an oral agent should be used. Treatment options can be related to the following categories of patients.

Normal weight patients (BMI >20 kg/m^2 and <26 kg/m^2)

Therapy is usually started with a sulfhonylurea agent, such as tolbutamide or gliclazide. Tolbutamide is least potent and has the least risk of causing hypoglycemia. It can be started

Initial care plan for the older adult with diabetes

- Set realistic glycemic goals.
- Agree upon the frequency of diabetic follow-up by primary or secondary healthcare.
- Organize monitoring of glycemic control by the patient and/or carer, for example, by home urine or blood glucose monitoring or, if the patient cannot manage this, by regular review.
- Refer to social or community services as appropriate.
- Advise on stopping smoking, on exercise (ideally a minimum of three weekly brisk walks of 30 to 45 min duration) and on alcohol intake.

at 500 mg bid prior to the main meals. Gliclazide or glipizide can be used if tighter control is required and are started at 40 to 80 mg (gliclazide) or 2.5 to 5.0 mg (glipizide) daily before breakfast. The recently introduced α-glucosidase inhibitor, acarbose, may also be used. To lessen gastrointestinal side effects, the starting dose should be 50 mg per day for 1 week with the first mouthful of the main meal, slowly increasing the dose over the next 2 to 3 weeks to a dose of 50 mg tid. Further increases in the dose to a maximum of 100 mg tid may be considered according to the patient's tolerance and the therapeutic benefit obtained. Metformin can be used alone or if necessary in addition to a sulfonylurea if glucose levels remain unacceptably high, noting the cautions mentioned in the next section.

Overweight patients (BMI>26 kg/m²)

In the absence of cardiac, renal, or hepatic failure and alcohol abuse, critical limb ischemia or acute illness, metformin may be given as monotherapy starting at a dose of 500 mg with the main meals and gradually increasing to a maximum of 850 mg bid with meals depending on the diabetic control (see accompanying box). When metformin is ineffective in producing adequate control, a sulfonylurea preparation can be added. Although metformin does not generally cause hypoglycemia at therapeutic doses, it may be associated with lactic acidosis if the above conditions are present. It is recommended that all patients receiving metformin are monitored closely with tests of renal and hepatic function. Sulfonylureas can be used in overweight patients following the instructions above in combination with metformin or alone. An increase in body weight often results when sulpfonylureas are used alone.

Hypoglycemia in the Older Patient

A recent study showed that up to one in five patients with NIDDM treated with sulfhonylureas experienced a symptomatic episode of hypoglycemia in the previous 6 months.[150] In older patients, susceptibility to hypoglycemia is pronounced,[151–152] and this is exacerbated by some people having little knowledge of the symptoms and signs of hypoglycaemia.[153] Patients with cognitive impairment and those with loss of the warning symptoms of hypoglycemia (e.g., those with autonomic dysfunction) are vulnerable because they may not recognize impending hypoglycemia and/or fail to communicate their feelings to their carers. They are often incapable of treating hypoglycemia themselves.[145] The educational program should include advice and information relating to the detection and treatment of hypoglycemia, including the criteria for admission in cases of unresponsive hypoglycemia.

Suggested oral agents for older adults with diabetes

- Tolbutamide 500 mg od to 1 g bid
- Gliclazide 40 mg od to 160 mg bid
- Glipizide 2.5 to 5.0 mg od to 40 mg daily
- Acarbose 50 mg od to 100 mg tid
- Metformin 500 mg od to 850 mg bid

Hypoglycemia with sulfonylureas

Sulfonylureas are metabolized in the liver to metabolites with minimal hypoglycemic activity, which are cleared via urinary excretion. For this reason, sulfonylureas are contraindicated in hepatic and renal disease, both of which increase the risk of hypoglycemia. Sulfonylurea-induced hypoglycemia (SIH) is much less common than insulin-induced hypoglycemia. The incidence of severe SIH with coma has been estimated at 0.19 to 0.25 per 1,000 patient years[154,155] in contrast with insulin-induced hypoglycemia coma with an incidence of 100 per 1,000 patient years.[156] The incidence of less severe symptoms is considerably higher with as many as one in five subjects experiencing hypoglycemia regularly.[150]

Prolonged hypoglycemia with glibenclamide (glyburide) and chlorpropamide is a worrying clinical problem and these drugs should be avoided in elderly diabetic patients. Glibenclamide-induced hypoglycemia may be more pronounced because the drug accumulates within β-cells and its metabolites retain some hypoglycemic activity. Due to the long elimination half-life (35 hours) of chlorpropamide, continued dosing results in drug accumulation (steady state being achieved by 7 to 10 days). In the presence of impaired renal function, further prolongation of hypoglycemia occurs. In the elderly, hypoglycemia is often mistaken for transient neurologic or cardiac events, and appears to have a worse prognosis: 10 percent of those admitted to hospital die and 3 percent have permanent neurologic damage,[157] presumably because, in some cases, cerebral function is already compromised.

Most sulfonylureas have caused fatal hypoglycemia, although this is often associated with chlorpropamide or glibenclamide.[158] Other factors apart from old age, that predispose to fatal hypoglycemia, are alcohol consumption, poor food intake, renal impairment, potentation of hypoglycemia by other drugs and prescription of sulfonylureas with prolonged actions in patients with only marginal elevations of blood glucose levels.[159] Many, if not all, these factors are directly relevant in the elderly patient with NIDDM.

Treatment of sulfonylurea-induced hypoglycemia

Sulfonylurea-induced hypoglycemia (blood glucose level less than 3.0 mmol/L) may be prolonged (up to a week) and requires hospital admission. A bolus intravenous injection of 20 to 50 mL of 50 percent dextrose should be given immediately, followed by an intravenous infusion of 10 or 20 percent dextrose to maintain the plasma glucose level between 6 to 12 mmol/L until residual hypoglycemic effects of the drug are minimal. Diazoxide, which has a direct inhibitory effect on insulin secretion, may be used as an adjunct to treatment. In the unconscious patient, diazoxide can be given as a slow intravenous infusion of 300 mg over 30 minutes, and can be repeated every 4 hours if necessary.

Glucagon is widely used to reverse hypoglycemia in insulin-induced hypoglycemic coma in patients with NIDDM. Because glucagon may stimulate insulin secretion, it is usually contraindicated in patients with NIDDM who may have a residual β-cell function.

Insulin therapy

Insulin is required for:

- Patients with IDDM.
- Noninsulin-dependent patients with poor control in spite of oral agents used at maximum tolerated dose. For these patients insulin is used on a trial basis for 6 to 12 weeks, observing the effect on diabetic control, how the patient and carer cope with insulin, and noting the frequency of hypoglycemia. If the patient does not wish to continue insulin at the end of the trial, then oral agents can be resumed.
- Acute conditions such as severe illness, hyperosmolar states, surgery, diabetic amyotrophy, or peripheral neuropathy.
- The development of a ketosis-prone state.

The decision to use insulin depends on the following:

- The ability of the patient and carer to recognize and manage hypoglycemia.
- The availability of community support to educate patient and carer on use of insulin.
- Cognitive impairment of the patient and/or carer or other disability affecting the administration of insulin.

Practical Aspects of Insulin Administration

Starting insulin

Insulin is best started at home for those with poor control using the experience of the diabetes specialist nurse and the support of a community dietitian and involving if necessary, the district (community) nurse. The general practitioner should always be involved.

Type and frequency of insulin

The insulin regimen with a lower risk of hypoglycemia for noninsulin-dependent diabetes is twice daily isophane insulin, although many patients use a mixture of short and intermediate acting insulins, for example, Mixtard or the Humulin M range of insulins. Some patients, however, may have reasonable control, with infrequent hypoglycemia, using once daily animal isophane insulin or human or animal insulin zinc suspension (e.g., Humulin Zn, Human Ultratard, or beef lente insulin). A once-a-day regimen is particularly appropriate where tight control is not needed, for example, in patients who have a terminal illness or dementia.

Insulin-related equipment

Insulin pens or prefilled syringes stored in the refrigerator and glucometers with a memory, a large figure display, or which speak out results are particularly helpful for disabled patients who are blind or have hand problems. Training in the use of such equipment is given by the diabetes-trained nurse.

Home Monitoring of Diabetic Control

Patients using insulin

Blood glucose monitoring is recommended for patients with insulin-dependent diabetes and for those with noninsulin-dependent diabetes being treated with insulin, though at present there is no definite evidence that this improves control or reduces complications. This should be performed by the patient or principal carer.

Patients on diet therapy and/or oral agents

For patients with noninsulin-dependent diabetes who are taking diet therapy and/or oral agents, home blood glucose monitoring should be offered, although it is not essential. Blood glucose monitoring is important for those patients who have poor metabolic control or who are at risk of hypoglycemia, for example, those taking sulfonylurea drugs or insulin. Urine monitoring in the fasting state and preprandially once per week is adequate for some patients so long as the renal threshold is normal. Monitoring is of more value when a patient or carer is able to interpret and react to the results.

Timing of glucose monitoring

Blood glucose monitoring should be carried out on at least two occasions per day for those patients who are in poor metabolic control, but for stable patients a four-point profile once per week is adequate. The timing of blood glucose estimations is before meals and at bedtime.

Targets for blood glucose

Targets for metabolic control will depend on the circumstances of the patient. In general, a fasting glucose level of 7 to 9 mmol/L, and a random level of 8 to 11 mmol/L will be sufficient to avoid the symptoms of hyperglycemia and to avoid the risk of hypoglycemia. In some situations, for example, those aged less than 70 years and mentally and physically fit, much tighter metabolic control can be achieved and, in fact, may be warranted to prevent the onset and progression of chronic complications of diabetes. Glucometers are helpful for those using blood glucose monitoring who have adequate visual acuity and dexterity. For those patients who are blind, a large figure meter or a glucometer that speaks and/or has a memory is valuable.

Hyperglycemic Comas

Diabetic ketoacidosis (DKA) may occur at any age, while hyperglycemic hyperosmolar nonketotic (HONK) comas occur predominantly in subjects aged over 50 years old.[160] Although DKA is not considered to be a disease of elderly people, 203 out of 929 admissions (22 percent) with DKA in Birmingham were aged 60 years or more[161]; DKA may occur in subjects with NIDDM if severely ill,[160] but has occasionally occurred in subjects with NIDDM who later return to oral agents and have no apparent precipitant for their DKA.[162]

It appears that in hyperglycemic comas most subjects with NIDDM have just enough residual insulin secretion to suppress lipolysis and ketogenesis, thus avoiding DKA, and develop a HONK coma instead. The tendency to hyperosmolarity in HONK comas may worsen in elderly people who may not appreciate thirst well, may have difficulty drinking enough to compensate for their osmotic diuresis,[160,163] and may also be on diuretics.[164] It also appears that hyperosmolarity not only worsens insulin resistance, but may also inhibit lipolysis.[163]

Diabetic ketoacidosis may be defined as hyperglycemia occurring in conjunction with ketoacidosis as evidenced by significant ketosis (3+ Ketostix in urine or plasma) and significant acidosis (venous plasma bicarbonate less than 15 mmol/L or arterial pH below 7.2). HONK comas may be defined as hyperglycemia occurring in conjunction with raised plasma osmolarity (greater than 350 mosm/L) with no evidence of ketoacidosis. The osmolarity may be measured directly in the laboratory using a freezing point depression technique, or can be estimated approximately by calculating the sum of $2 \times (Na^+ + K^+) +$ urea + glucose concentrations in mmol/L.

All studies of hyperglycemic comas show a progressive increase in mortality with age.[161,165,166] In Birmingham, the mortality due to DKA rose from 5 percent at age 60 to 69 to 100 percent at age 90,[161] although the number of 90-year-old subjects was small. Most studies suggest that death is primarily due to acute illnesses such as pneumonia and myocardial infarction.[161,165–166] There has been no apparent decrease in mortality over the past 15 to 21 years.[161,165]

The cause of the hyperglycemia may be infection, myocardial infarction, inadequate hypoglycemic treatment or inappropriate drug treatment. Often, a particular cause cannot be identified;[161,165] for instance there was no apparent cause in 354 out of 929 admissions with DKA in Birmingham.[161] Thiazide diuretics and steroids are known to increase blood glucose levels and may precipitate DKA; thiazide diuretics and frusemide may be particularly likely to precipitate HONK coma.[164]

Immediate management of hyperglycemic comas

1. Be aware of hyperglycemic coma as a possibility.
2. Test for hyperglycemia, ketosis, and acidosis.
3. Screen for any precipitating illness (for example, infection, cerebral or myocardial infarction, inadequate treatment).
4. A slow insulin infusion guided by frequent bedside blood glucose monitoring to halve glucose level over 4 hours.
5. Prompt, adequate fluid replacement with 0.9 percent saline (if Na^+ less than 155 mmol/L) or 0.45 percent saline (if Na^+ greater than 155 mmol/L) at 500 mL/h over first 4 hours.

Management of Hyperglycemic Comas

The history and examination should pay special attention to previous diabetic symptoms and treatment, any precipitating infection, infarction or medication, evidence of heart failure and the degree of dehydration (see accompanying box). Blood should be taken for glucose, urea and electrolytes, creatinine, cardiac enzymes, and cultures. Urine and sputum should also be cultured and an electrocardiogram and chest X-ray obtained.

Arterial blood gas samples are should be taken to measure pH. Urine (or plasma from blood in a lithium heparin tube left to stand) should be tested for ketone bodies with any proprietary testing stick, for example, Ketostix. A blood sample to measure the arterial or venous bicarbonate level should be taken, depending on local practice. Intravenous (IV) fluid replacement should be at a rate of 500 mL/h over the initial 4 hours, reducing to 250 mL/h. The patient needs more rapid infusion where there is shock due to hypovolemia, and here a central line is invaluable to monitor aggressive infusions, particularly in the presence of cardiac failure or recent myocardial infarction. There is a wide choice of IV fluid depending on the condition of the patient. In DKA or a HONK coma with a plasma sodium level less than 155 mmol/L, use 0.9 percent saline. If the plasma sodium level rises above 155 mmol/L, then use 0.45 percent saline,[160,163] although if the plasma glucose level is less than 15 mmol/L, five percent dextrose could be used. If the patient is shocked due to hypovolemia, then a plasma volume expander such as Haemacel may be needed.

An insulin pump (50 units human soluble insulin in 50 mL 0.9 percent saline) is undoubtedly the easiest way to deliver the required insulin, and syringe pumps are now very reliable. The dose of insulin infused is varied according to the result of blood glucose testing, which is initially performed hourly, and then less frequently as the readings stabilize.

Subjects with a HONK coma may need very small doses of insulin to reduce plasma glucose levels; however, if the patient is in hypercatabolic state or has marked insulin resistance, as in obesity or some subjects with NIDDM, larger doses of insulin may be required. The plasma glucose should halve over 4 hours; if it does not, check that the insulin is actually being given, and increase the insulin infusion rate as necessary, For example, initially by 25 percent, aiming to reduce the plasma glucose level by 5 to 10 mmol/L per hour.

The potassium level needs to be checked 2 hours after starting treatment, and then 4 hourly until stable; if the level is 4.0 to 5.0 mmol/L add 20 mmol/L of KC1 to each liter of IV fluid, and add 40 mmol/L if the potassium level is below 4.0 mmol/L.

Thrombotic complications may occur, or may well have occurred before hospitalization in subjects with a HONK coma. Most authors recommend prophylaxis against deep venous thrombosis with heparin 5,000 units t.d.s. subcutaneously.[160,163] If there is decreased conscious level, one must pay particular attention to pressure areas and use pressure relieving mattresses and bootees because heels in particular are very prone to ulceration. Unconscious diabetic subjects with hyperglycemia should have a nasogastric tube passed. As the subject improves and the plasma glucose falls below 15 mmol/L, one can either change to 5 percent dextrose, or feed the patient, to further reduce ketone bodies in DKA. The immediate management of these comas is summarized in the accompanying box.

Hypoglycemic Comas

Hypoglycemic episodes should be suspected in any subject taking insulin or sulfonylurea therapy who has a "funny turn" or "dizzy do", any episode of confusion, fitting or neurologic deficit or a low glycosylated hemoglobin. Hypos present classically as episodes of sweating, pallor, hunger, tremor, and anxiety. The relationship between symptoms and low blood glucose level is not strong, with biochemical hypoglycemia present in 29 percent of symptomatic episodes, and symptomatic hypoglycemia present in 16 percent of biochemical episodes in younger Danes with IDDM.[167] Silent nocturnal hypoglycemia should also be considered in any subject taking more than 1 unit insulin per kilogram body weight.[168] Elderly people may not recognize hypoglycemia as well as the young do[169] so hypoglycemic treatment must only be used in this age group following failure of dietary control, and must be used cautiously and carefully.

After the patient has recovered from am hypoglycemic episode, the cause needs to be ascertained. A missed meal, unusual exercise, excess or inappropriate hypoglycemic medication or displacement of sulfonylurea from plasma protein binding due to other drugs are the likely causes.[170] In their study of subjects with NIDDM taking oral agents, Jennings and colleagues[150] found that 24 percent of patients with hypoglycemic episodes were taking other agents that would potentiate sulfonylureas. The cause may not, however, be identified; in one study 37 percent of hypoglycemic episodes in subjects with IDDM had no obvious cause.[171] The patient's cognitive function should be assessed after recovery, since chronic confusion may lead to repetition of doses of hypoglycemic medication or missing meals.

Lactic Acidosis

This is an uncommon complication of metformin therapy and is a disease of elderly people with the modal age of victims being 65 to 70 years.[172] It is largely preventable by observing the contraindications (see list on contraindications to metformin).[173–174]

Contraindications to metformin

1. Renal impairment
2. Cardiac failure, even if treated
3. Severe peripheral vascular disease
4. Hepatic impairment
5. Alcohol abuse
6. Severe infections or trauma

Diagnosis is based on demonstrating acidosis (arterial pH less than 7.2), and a raised lactate level (either plasma lactate greater than 5 mmol/L or anion gap greater than 18 mmol/L). The anion gap ($Na^+ + K^+$) − ($CL^- - HCO_3$) may also be raised by ketones, salicylates, urea, methanol, and ethylene glycol.

The standard treatment is to infuse 1.4 percent sodium bicarbonate until the pH reaches 7.2[174–175]; however, the evidence that this improves mortality (60 to 70 percent unless shocked, when mortality approaches 100 percent) is lacking.[176] Survival correlates more with plasma lactate levels than with the degree of acidosis.[176]

Care Issues and Future Initiatives

Diabetes mellitus in old age is increasingly recognized to be a specialist area and demands skills and committment often not available to hard-pressed physicians attempting to cope with the dramatic increase in scientific knowledge and the invariable escalation of clinical involvement required by most employers whether in hospital or primary care settings. In this final section we explore several topical themes within the discipline of "geriatric diabetology."[177]

Models of Care

Four models of care are usually defined in relation to managing older adults with diabetes.[178] In the first, there is effectively a breakdown in patient and doctor education and communication and the patient is essentially self-caring. In one survey, about 7 percent of elderly patients were managed in this way.[3] This model should be avoided. A primary care-only approach is a common and often an acceptable model as long as there is an enthusiastic committment to diabetes care. It has several advantages including increased convenience for both patients and relatives, familiarity with practice staff, and continuity of care. Disadvantages such as lack of on-site specialist input and unstructured follow-up practices may lead to suboptimal care. In one group of patients discharged to primary care,[179] 14 percent were not followed-up at all and 20 percent apparently thought they were cured! In another study of patients similarly discharged,[180] only 5 percent achieved acceptable glycemic control and mortality was three times higher than those followed up in a hospital specialist clinic.

Hospital service only is a third model and has the advantage of regular specialist input, but has two main disadvantages. These are the lack of clinic time to deal with the vast numbers of patients needed to be seen and the fact that junior medical staff are often expected to provide this "expert" opinion. The extra inconvenience for patient travelling large distances and the excessive waiting times discourage many patients from being involved in this practice. In our view, primary care physicians should always be involved.

The fourth model is our favored one and consists of a "shared care" approach between the hospital (diabetologist or geriatrician) and primary care. Joint management policies are essential for this to be a worthwhile partnership with an emphasis on early referral to secondary care when problems develop. Good communication is important and a common diabetes record card is mandatory. Clear boundaries of responsibility need to be established and educational strategies should form the basis of a common approach to management.

Diabetes Specialist Nurses for the Elderly

Diabetes specialist nurses are an invaluable addition to a diabetes service and can form an integral link between primary and secondary care sectors.[145] They have many other roles (see accompanying box) and we feel strongly that these specialist nurses should be appointed specifically to manage older patients with diabetes. In conjunction with the primary care physician, community dietician, social worker, chiropodist, geriatric liaison sister and geriatrician (or diabetologist), they should constitute a "Community Diabetes Team" that will provide multiprofessional diabetes healthcare.

The role of the diabetic specialist nurse for the elderly

1. To teach, advise, and counsel patients and carers both in the clinic and in the patient's home
2. Where possible, to educate patients to achieve self-care
3. To teach self-monitoring of blood glucose (or urinalysis, if appropriate) and instruct in the use of special monitoring techniques for patients with physical problems, partial-sightedness or blindness.
4. Teaching and advising on insulin administration
5. To liaise with and refer to other health professionals, chiropodists, community nurses, general practitioners, etc.
6. To commence insulin treatment in the patient's home
7. To advise and guide residential and nursing home staff to manage patients with diabetes
8. To provide continuing support and advice to patients and health care providers when specific problems relating to diabetes arise

Role of geriatricians in elderly diabetic care

- To assess coexisting disease that impacts on diabetes management
- To manage increasing dependency and disability
- To recognize and manage cognitive impairment
- To assess and treat urinary incontinence
- To liaise between hospital and community support services
- To provide respite programs for spouses and carers
- To be a member of hospital diabetic clinic team

Role of Geriatricians in Elderly Diabetic Care

The specialist geriatric service can also provide important care provision for elderly diabetic patients.[141] Geriatricians with experience in diabetic care can contribute in a number of ways (see list on role of geriatricians) and often are in an ideal position to liaise with specialist nurses to coordinate the care a patient receives both inside and outside of the hospital. Both authors participate in older adult diabetic clinics that see patients on the basis of need and dependency levels rather than age alone. In these clinics, functional status is measured as routinely as a blood glucose level and only senior doctors attend.

Diabetes mellitus remains an exciting challenge for all health professionals involved in clinical geriatrics and progress is being made in improving all aspects of the care of this common and serious condition.

References

1. Tattersall RB: Diabetes in the elderly: a neglected area? Diabetologia 1984;27:167–73
2. Harrower ADB: Prevalence of elderly patients in a hospital diabetic population. Br J Clin Pract 1980;34:131–133
3. Neil HAW, Thompson AV, Thorogood M et al: Diabetes in the elderly: the Oxford community diabetes study. Diab Med 1989;6:608–613
4. Damsgaard EMS: Known diabetes and fasting hyperglycaemia in the elderly. Prevalence and economic impact upon health services. Dan Med Bull 1990;37:530–546
5. Sinclair AJ: Initial management of non-insulin-dependent diabetes mellitus in the elderly. In Finucane P, Sinclair AJ (eds): Diabetes in Old Age. John Wiley & Sons, Chichester, 1995
6. Sinclair AJ, Barnett AH: Special needs of elderly diabetic patients. BMJ 1993;306: 1142–1143

7. Sinclair AJ: Diabetes care in the aged: time for reappraisal. Pract Diab 1994;11:60–63

8. Hendra TJ, Sinclair AJ: Improving the care of the elderly diabetic patients: the final report of the St. Vincent Joint Task Force for Diabetes. Age Ageing 1996 (in press)

9. Sinclair AJ, Woodhouse KW: Meeting the challenge of diabetes in the aged. (Editorial: Diabetes in the aged.) J R Soc Med 1994;87:607–608

10. Spence JW: Some observations on sugar tolerance with special reference to variations found at different ages. Q J Med 1921; 14:314–326

11. Davidson MB: The effect of ageing on carbohydrate metabolism: a review of the English literature and a practical approach to the diagnosis of diabetes mellitus in the elderly. Metabolism 1979;28:688–705

12. Andres R: Aging and diabetes. Med Clin N Am 1971;55: 835–845

13. Jackson RA, Blix PM, Matthews JA et al: Influence of ageing on glucose homeostasis. J Clin Endocrinol Metab 1982;55: 840–848

14. Jackson RA: Mechanisms of age-related glucose intolerance. Diabetes Care 1990;13(suppl 2):9–19

15. Harris MI, Hadden WC, Knowler WC, Bennett PH: Prevalence of diabetes and impaired glucose tolerance and plasma glucose levels in U.S. population aged 20–74 years. Diabetes 1987; 36:523–534

16. Jarrett RJ, Keen H: Hyperglycaemia and diabetes mellitus. Lancet 1976;1009–1012

17. Forrest RD, Jackson CA, Yudkin JS: Glucose intolerance and hypertension in North London: the Islington Diabetes Study. Diab Med 1986;338–342

18. Croxson SCM, Burden AC, Bodlington M, Botha JL: The prevalence of diabetes in elderly people. Diab Med 1991;8:28–31

19. De Fronzo RA: Glucose intolerance and aging. Evidence for tissue insensitivity to insulin. Diabetes 1979;28:1095–1101

20. Fink RI, Kolterman OG, Griffin J, Olefsky JM: Mechanisms of insulin resistance in aging. J Clin Invest 1983;71:1523–1535

21. Villareal DT, Morley JE: Prevention of diabetes in elderly people. pp. 45–67. In Finucane P, Sinclair AJ (eds): Diabetes in Old Age. John Wiley & Sons, Chichester, 1995

22. Stout RW: Ageing and glucose tolerance. pp. 21–44. In Finucane P, Sinclair AJ (eds): Diabetes in Old Age. John Wiley & Sons, Chichester, 1995

23. Neil HAW, Gatling W, Mather HM et al: The Oxford Community Diabetes Study: evidence for an increase in the prevalence of known diabetes in Great Britain. Diab Med 1987;4: 539–543

24. National Diabetes Data Group: Classification and diagnosis of diabetes mellitus and other categories of glucose intolerance. Diabetes 1979;28:1039–1057

25. WHO Study Group: Diabetes Mellitus. Technical Report Series 646. WHO, Geneva, 1980

26. Tuomilehto J, Nissinen A, Kiveiä S-L et al: Prevalence of diabetes mellitus in elderly men aged 65 to 84 years in eastern and western Finland. Diabetologia 1986;29:611–615

27. Knowler WC, Bennett PH, Hamman RF, Miller M: Diabetes incidence and prevalence in Pima Indians: a 19-fold greater incidence than in Rochester, Minnesota. Am J Epidemiol 1978;108:497–505

28. Simmons D, Williams DRR, Powell MJ: Prevalence of diabetes in a predominantly Asian community: preliminary findings of the Coventry diabetes study. BMJ 1989;298:18–21

29. Wingard DL, Sinsheimer P, Barrett-Connor EL, McPhillips JB: Community based study of prevalence of NIDDM in older adults. Diab Care 1990;13(suppl 2):3–8

30. Haavisto MV, Mattila KJ, Rajala SA: Blood glucose and diabetes mellitus in subjects aged 85 years or more. Acta Med Scand 1983;214:239–244

31. Falconer DC, Duncan LJP, Smith C: A statistical and genetical study of diabetes: 1. Prevalence and mortality. Ann Hum Genet 1971;34:347–369

32. Walker JB, Kerridge D: Diabetes in an English Community. Leicester University Press, Leicester, 1961

33. College of General Practitioners: A diabetes survey. Br Med J 1962;1:1497–1503

34. College of General Practitioners: Glucose tolerance and glycosuria in the general population. BMJ 1963;2:655–659

35. Damsgaard EM, Faber OK, Frøland A et al: Prevalence of fasting hyperglycaemia and known non-insulin-dependent diabetes mellitus classified by plasma C-peptide. Diab Care 1987;10:26–32

36. Agner E, Thorsteinsson B, Eriksen M: Impaired glucose tolerance and diabetes mellitus in elderly subjects. Diab Care 1982;5:600–605

37. Ohlson LO, Larsson B, Eriksson H et al: Diabetes mellitus in Swedish middle aged men. Diabetologia 1987;30:386–393

38. Cromme PVM, van der Veen EA, Bezemer PD, Kuik DJ: Serum fructosamine assessment as a screening test for diabetes mellitus. Neth J Med 1987;30:202–203

39. Mykkänen L, Laakso M, Uusitua M, Pyörälä K: Prevalence of diabetes and impaired glucose tolerance in elderly subjects and their association with obesity and family history of diabetes. Diab Care 1990;13:1099–1105

40. Helmrich SP, Ragland DR, Leung RW, Paffenbarger RS Jr: Physical activity and reduced occurrence of non-insulin-dependent diabetes mellitus. N Engl J Med 1991;325:147–152

41. WHO Study Group: Diabetes Mellitus. Technical Report Series 727. WHO, Geneva, 1985

42. Dorf A, Ballintine EJ, Bennett PH, Miller M: Retinopathy in Pima Indians: relationships to glucose level, duration of diabetes, age at diagnosis of diabetes, and age at examination in a population with a high prevalence of diabetes mellitus. Diabetes 1976;25:554–560

43. Pettitt DJ, Knowler WC, Lisse JR, Bennett PH: Development of retinopathy and proteinuria in relation to plasma glucose concentrations in Pima Indians. Lancet 1980;2:1050–1052

44. Sayegh HA, Jarrett RJ: Oral glucose-tolerance tests and the diagnosis of diabetes. Lancet 1979;2:431–433

45. Zimmet P, Whitehouse S: The effect of age on glucose tolerance: studies in a Micronesian population with a high prevalence of diabetes. Diabetes 1979;28:617–623

46. Rushforth NB, Bennett P, Steinberg A et al: Diabetes in the Pima Indians. Diabetes 1971;20:756–765

47. Jarrett RJ, Keen H, McCartney P: The Whitehall study: ten

year follow-up report on men with impaired glucose tolerance with reference to worsening to diabetes and predictors of death. Diab Med 1984;1:279–283

48. Saad MF, Knowler WC, Pettitt DJ et al: The natural history of diabetes mellitus in the Pima Indians. N Engl J Med 1988; 319:1500–1506
49. Jarrett RJ, McCartney P, Keen H: The Bedford Survey: ten year mortality rates in newly diagnosed diabetics, borderline diabetics and normoglycaemic controls and risk indices for coronary heart disease in borderline diabetics. Diabetologia 1982;22:79–84
50. Damsgaard EM, Froland A, Green A: Use of hospital services by elderly diabetics and fasting hyperglycaemic patients aged 60–74 years. Diab Med 1987;4:317–322
51. Damsgaard EM, Froland A, Holm A: Ambulatory medical care for elderly diabetics: the Fredericia survey of diabetic and fasting hyperglycaemic subjects aged 60–74 years. Diab Med 1987;4:534–538
52. Williams DRR: Hospital admissions of diabetic patients: information from hospital activity analysis. Diab Med 1985;2: 27–32
53. Hudson CN, Lazarus J, Peters J et al: An audit of diabetes care in three district general hospitals in Cardiff. Pract Diab Intern 1996;13:29–32
54. Cohen DL, Neil HAW, Thorogood M, Mann JL: A population based study of the incidence of complications associated with Type 2 diabetes in the elderly. Diab Med 1991;8:928–933
55. Walters DP, Gatling W, Mullee MA, Hill RD: The prevalence of diabetic distal sensory neuropathy in an English Community. Diab Med 1992;9:349–353
56. Dornan TL, Peck GM, Dow JDC, Tattersall RB: A community survey of diabetes in the elderly. Diab Med 1992;9:860–865
57. Watkins PJ: Chronic complications of diabetes. pp. 119–127. In Finucance P, Sinclair AJ (eds): Diabetes in Old Age. John Wiley & Sons, Chichester, 1995
58. Kannel WB, McGee DL: Diabetes and cardiovascular disease: the Framingham Study. JAMA 1979;241:2035–2038
59. Knuiman MW, Welborn TA, McCann VJ et al: Prevalence of diabetic complications in relation to risk factors. Diabetes 1986;35:1332
60. Ballard DJ, Humphrey LL, Melton LJ et al: Epidemiology of persistent proteinuria in type II diabetes mellitus: population based study in Rochester, Minnesota. Diabetes 1988;37: 405–412
61. Naliboff BD, Rosenthal M: Effects of age on complications in adult onset diabetes. JAGS 1989;37:838–842
62. Grey RHB, Burns-Cox CJ, Hughes A: Blind and partial sight registration in Avon. Br J Ophthalmol 1989;73:88–94
63. Kohner EM: Diabetic retinopathy. Br Med J 1993;307: 1195–1199
64. Howard-Williams J, Hillson RM, Bron A et al: Retinopathy is associated with higher glycaemia in maturity onset type diabetes. Diabetologia 1984;27:198–202
65. Nathan DM, Singer DE, Godine JE et al: Retinopathy in older type 2 diabetics. Diabetes 1986;35:797–801
66. Harris MI, Klein R, Welborn TA, Knuiman MW: Onset of NIDDM occurs at least 4–7 yr before clinical diagnosis. Diab Care 1992;15:815–821
67. Soler NG, Fitzgerald MG, Malins JM, Summers ROC: Retinopathy at diagnosis of diabetes with special reference to patients under 40 years of age. BMJ 1969;3:567–569
68. Aldington SJ, Kohner EM, Nugent Z: Retinopathy at entry in the United Kingdom Prospective Diabetes Study (UKPDS) of maturity onset diabetes. Diab Med 1987;4 (abstr A41):355
69. British Multicentre Study Group: Photocoagulation for diabetic maculopathy. Diabetes 1983;32:1010–1016
70. Kohner EM, Barry PJ: Prevention of blindness in diabetic retinopathy. Diabetologia 1984;26:173–179
71. Rohan TE, Frost CD, Wald NJ: Prevention of blindness by screening for diabetic retinopathy: a quantitative assessment. BMJ 1989;299:1198–1201
72. Hiller R, Sperduto RD, Ederer F: Epidemiologic associations with cataract in the 1971–1972 National Health and Nutrition Survey. Am J Epidemiol 1983;118:239–249
73. Caird FI, Hutchinson M, Pirie A: Cataract and diabetes. BMJ 1964;2:665–668
74. Croxson SCM: Complications in screened diabetic subjects. BGS Autumn meeting 1994. Age Ageing 1995;24(suppl 1) (abstr 2):30
75. Cohen DL, Neil HAW, Sparrow J et al: Lens opacity and mortality in diabetes. Diab Med 1990;7:615–617
76. Klein BE, Klein R, Jensen SC: Open-angle glaucoma and older-onset diabetes. The Beaver Dam Eye Study. Ophthalmology 1994;101:1173–1177
77. Wormald RP, Basauri E, Wright LA, Evans JR: The African Caribbean Eye Survey: risk factors for glaucoma in a sample of African Caribbean people living in London. Eye 1994;8: 315–320
78. Leske MC, Connell AM, Wu SY et al: Risk factors for open-angle glaucoma. The Barbados Eye Study. Arch Ophthalmol 1995;113:918–924
79. Tielsch JM, Katz J, Quigley HA, Javitt JC, Sommer A: Diabetes, intraocular pressure, and primary open-angle glaucoma in the Baltimore Eye Survey. Ophthalmology 1995;102:48–53
80. Schranz AG, Zarabinska L: Retinopathy in Maltese type 2 diabetic patients. Diab Med 1995;12:441–444
81. Sanders RJ, Wilson MR: Diabetes-related eye disorders [Review]. J Nat Med Assoc 1993;85:104–108
82. Newell FW: Ophthalmology: Principles and Concepts. CV Mosby, St Louis, 1986
83. Duker JS, Sivalingam A, Brown GC, Reber R: A prospective study of acute central retinal artery obstruction. Arch Ophthalmol 1991;109:339–342
84. Klein R, Klein BE, Moss SE: Diabetes, hyperglycemia, and age-related maculopathy. The Beaver Dam Eye Study. Ophthalmology 1992;99:1527–1534
85. Gibson JM, Shaw DE, Rosenthal AR: Senile cataract and senile macular degeneration: an investigation into possible risk factors. Trans Ophthalmol Soc UK 1986;105:463–468
86. Hyman LG, Lilienfeld AM, Ferris FL, Fine SL: Senile macular degeneration: a case control study. Am J Epidemiol 1983;118: 213–227
87. Ferris FL: Senile macular degeneration: review of epidemiologic features. Am J Epidemiol 1983;118:132–151
88. Harding SP, Broadbent DM, Neoh C et al: Sensitivity and

specificity of photography and direct ophthalmoscopy in screening for sight threatening eye disease: the Liverpool Diabetic Eye Study. BMJ 1995:311:1131–1135
89. Most RS, Sinnock P: The epidemiology of lower extremity amputations in diabetic individuals. Diab Care 1983;6:87–91
90. Deerochanawong C. Home PD, Alberti KGMM: A survey of lower limb amputation in diabetic patients. Diab Med 138–179. 1992;9:942–946
91. Young MJ, Boulton AJM: The diabetic foot. pp. 139–179. In Finucane P, Sinclair AJ (eds): Diabetes in Old Age. John Wiley & Sons, Chichester, 1995
92. Connor H: The economic impact of diabetic foot disease. pp. 150–159. In Connor H, Boulton AJM, Ward JD (eds): The Foot in Diabetes. John Wiley & Sons, Chichester, 1986
93. Bild DE, Selby JV, Sinnock P et al: Lower-extremity amputation in people with diabetes. Epidemiology and prevention. Diab Care 1989;12:24–31
94. Van Houtum WH, Lavery LA, Harkless LB: The costs of diabetes-related lower extremity amputations in the Netherlands. Diab Med 1995;777–781
95. Silbert S: Amputation of the lower extremity in diabetes mellitus. Diabetes 1952;1:297–299
96. Palumbo PJ, Melton LJ: Peripheral vascular disease and diabetes. pp. 1–21. In Diabetes in America; Diabetes Data. Compiled 1984. U.S. Government Printing Office, Washington DC, (NIH publ. no. 85–1468) 1985
97. Pecoraro RE, Reiber GE, Burgess EM: Pathways to diabetic limb amputation. Basis for prevention. Diab Care 1990;13: 513–521
98. Larsson J, Apelqvist J, Agardh DD, Stenstrom A: Decreasing incidence of major amputation in diabetic patients: a consequence of a multidisciplinary footcare team approach? Diab Med 1995;12:770–776
99. Assal JP, Gfeller R, Ekoe JM: Patient education in diabetes. pp. 276–289. In Recent Trends in Diabetic Research. Almquist and Wiksell, Stockholm, 1982
100. Thomson FJ, Veves A, Ashe H et al: A team approach to diabetic foot care: the Manchester experience. Foot 1991;1: 75–82
101. Cavanagh PR, Young MJ, Adams JE et al: Correlates of structure and function in the diabetic foot. Diabetologia 1991; 34(suppl 2):A39
102. Cavanagh PR, Simoneau GG, Ulbrecht JS: Ulceration, unsteadiness and uncertainty: the biomechanical consequences of diabetes mellitus. J Biomech 1993;26(suppl 1):23–40
103. Flynn MD, Boolell M, Tooke J, Watkins PJ: The effect of insulin infusion on capillary blood flow in the diabetic neuropathic foot. Diab Med 1992:9:630–634
104. Logerfo FW, Coffman JD: Vascular and microvascular disease of the foot in diabetes: implications for foot care. N Eng J Med 1984;25:1615–1961
105. Euerhart JE, Pettitt DJ, Knowler WC et al: Medial arterial calcification and its association with mortality and complications of diabetes. Diabetologia 1988;31:16–23
106. Dormandy J (ed): European Consensus Document on Critical Limb Ischaemia. Springer-Verlag, Berlin, 1989
107. Edmonds ME, Blundell MP, Morris HE et al: The diabetic foot: impact of a foot clinic. Q J Med 1986;232:763–771
108. Assal JP, Muhlhauser I, Pernet A et al: Patient education as a basis for diabetes care in clinical practice. Diabetologia 1985;28:602–613
109. Thomson FJ, Masson EA: Can elderly diabetic patients cooperate with routine foot care? Age Ageing 1992;21:333–337
110. Panzram G: Mortality and survival in type 2 (non-insulin-dependent) diabetes mellitus. Diabetologia 1987;30:123–131
111. Fitzgerald MG, Kilvert A: Diabetes mellitus. pp. 715–730. In Brocklehurst JC (ed): Textbook of Geriatric Medicine and Gerontology. 3rd Ed. Churchill Livingstone, Edinburgh, 1985
112. Krolewski AS, Warram JH, Christlieb AR: Onset, course, complications, and prognosis of diabetes mellitus. pp. 251–277. In Marble A, Krall LP, Bradley RF et al (eds): Joslin's Diabetes Mellitus. 12th Ed. Lea & Febiger, Philadelphia, 1985
113. Keen H, Fuller JH: The epidemiology of diabetes. pp. 146–160. In: Exton-Smith AN, Caird FI (eds): Metabolic and Nutritional Disorders in the Elderly. John Wright and Sons, Bristol, 1980
114. Wong JSK, Pearson DWM, Murchison LE et al: Mortality in diabetes mellitus: experience of a geographically defined population. Diab Med 1991;8:135–139
115. Sinclair AJ, Robert IE, Croxson SCM: Mortality in older people with diabetes mellitus. (in press 1996)
116. Croxson SCM, Price D, Burden M et al: Mortality of elderly people with diabetes. Diab Med 1994;11:250–252
117. Reaven GM, Thompson LW, Nahum D, Haskins E: Relationship between hyperglycaemia and cognitive function in older NIDDM patients. Diab Care 1990;13:16–21
118. Perlmuter LC, Hakami MK, Hodgson-Harrington C et al: Decreased cognitive function in aging non-insulin-dependent diabetic patients. Am J Med 1984;77:1043–1048
119. U'Ren RC, Riddle MC, Lezak MD, Bennington-Davis M: The mental efficiency of the elderly person with type 2 diabetes mellitus. J Am Geriatr Soc 1990;38:505–510
120. Mooradian AD, Perryman K, Fitten J et al: Cortical function in elderly non-insulin dependent diabetic patients: behavioural and electrophysiological studies. Arch Intern Med 1988; 148:2369–2372
121. Jagust W, Cramon DY, Renner R, Hepp KD: Cognitive function and metabolic state in elderly diabetic patients. Diab Nutr Metab 1992;5:265–274
122. Croxson S, Jagger C: Diabetes and cognitive impairment: a community based study of elderly subjects. Age Ageing 1995; 24:421–424
123. Richardson-Tchabo EA: A longitudinal study of cognitive performance in non-insulin dependent (type 2) diabetic men. Exp Gerontol 1986;21:459–467
124. Atiea JA, Moses JL, Sinclair AJ: Neuropsychological function in older subjects with non-insulin-dependent diabetes mellitus. Diab Med 1995;12:679–685
125. Tun PA, Perlmuter LC, Russo P, Nathan DM: Memory self-assessment and performance in aged diabetics and non-diabetics. Exp Aging Res 1987;13:151–157
126. Palinkas LA, Barrett-Connor E, Wingard DL: Type 2 diabetes and depresive symptoms in older adults: a population based study. Diab Med 1991;8:532–539
127. Reaven GM: Role of insulin resistance in human disease. Diabetes 1988;37:1595–1607

128. Kalra L, Jackson SHD, Swift CG: Review: neuropsychological test performance as an indicator of silent cerebrovascular disease in elderly hypertensives. Age Ageing 1994;23:517–523
129. Kuusisto J, Koivisto K, Mykkanen L et al: Essential hypertension and cognitive function: the role of hyperinsulinemia. Hypertension 1993;22:771–779
130. Palumbo PJ, Elveback LR, Whisnant JP: Neurologic complications of diabetes mellitus: transient ischemic attack, stroke and peripheral neuropathy. Adv Neurol 1978;19:593–601
131. Soininen H, Puranen M, Helkala E-L et al: Diabetes mellitus and brain atrophy: a computed tomography study in an elderly population. Neurobiol Ageing 1992;13:717–721
132. Pirtilla T, Jarvenpaa R, Laippala P, Frey H: Brain atrophy on computerized axial tomography scans: interactions of age, diabetes and general morbidity. Gerontology 1992;38: 285–291
133. Amiel S: Diabetes and dementia: a causal association? Diab Med 1994;11:430–431
134. Ryan CM, Williams TM, Finegold DN, Orchard TJ: Cognitive dysfunction in adults with type 1 (insulin dependent) diabetes mellitus of long duration: effects of recurrent hypoglycaemia and other chronic complications Diabetologia 1993;36: 329–334
135. Jagust W, Cramon DY, Renner R, Hepp KD: Tight metabolic control improves cerebral function in older type 2 diabetic patients. Diabetologia 1987;30(abstract 245):535A
136. Gradman TJ, Laws A, Thompson LW, Reaven GM: Verbal learning and/or memory improves with glycaemic control in older subjects with non-insulin dependent diabetes mellitus. JAGS 1993;41:1305–1312
137. Bayer AJ, Johnston J, Sinclair AJ: Impact of dementia on diabetic care in the aged. J Roy Soc Med 1994;87:619–621
138. National Center for Health Statistics: The National Nursing Home survey, 1977. Summary for the United States (DHEWH publication no. PHS-79–1794) (Vital and Health Statistics, Ser. 3, No. 143). U.S. Government, Hyattsville, Maryland 1979
139. Gobin W: Diabetes in the aged: under-diagnosis and overtreatment. Can Med Assoc J 1970;103:915–923
140. Laing W: Living environments for the elderly. 3: The mixed economy in longterm care. pp. 235–248. In Wells, Freer C (eds): The Ageing Population: Burden or Challenge? Macmillan Press, Basingstoke, 1988
141. Turnbull CJ, Sinclair AJ: Modern perspectives and recent advances. In Finucane P, Sinclair AJ (eds): Diabetes in Old Age. John Wiley & Sons, London, 1995
142. Sinclair AJ, Croxson SCM, Turnbull CJ: Document of diabetes care for residents in residential and nursing homes. 1997 Postgrad Med J (in press)
143. The Diabetes Control and Complications Trial Research Group: The effect of intensive treatment of diabetes on the development and progression of long-term complications in insulin-dependent diabetes mellitus. N Eng J Med 1993;329: 977–986
144. UK Prospective Diabetes Study Group: UK Prospective Diabetes Study 16. Overview of 6 years' therapy of Type II Diabetes: a progressive disease. Diabetes 1995;44:1249–1258
145. Sinclair AJ, Turnbull CJ, Croxson SCM: Document of care for older people with diabetes. Postgrad Med J 1996;72:334–338
146. Laakso M, Pyorala K: Age of onset and type of diabetes. Diab Care 1985;8:114–117
147. Kilvert A, Fitzgerald MG, Wright AD, Natrass M: Clinical characteristics and aetiological classification of insulin-dependent diabetes in the elderly. Q J Med 1986;60:865–872
148. De Fronzo RA: Pathogenesis of Type 2 (non-insulin-dependent) diabetes mellitus: a balanced overview. Diabetologia 1992;35:389–397
149. Reaven GM: Resistance to insulin-stimulated glucose uptake and hyperinsulinanaemia. Role of non-insulin-dependent diabetes, high blood pressure, dyslipidaemia and coronary heart disease. Diab Metab 1991;17:78–86
150. Jennings AM, Wilson RM, Ward JD: Symptomatic hypoglycaemia in NIDDM patients with oral hypoglycaemic agents. Diab Care 1989;12:203–208
151. Asplund K, Wilholm BE, Lithner F: Glibenclamide-associated hypoglycaemia: a report of 57 cases. Diabetologia 1983;24: 412–417
152. Campbell IW: Sulphonylureas and metformin: efficacy and inadequacy. pp. 33–51. In Bailey CJ, Flatt PR (eds): New Antidiabetic Drugs. Smith-Gordon, London, 1990
153. Thomson FJ, Masson EA, Leeming JT, Boulton AJM: Lack of knowledge of symptoms of hypoglycaemia by elderly diabetic patients. Age Ageing 1991;20:404–406
154. Berger W: Incidence of severe side-effects during therapy with sulphonylureas and biguanides. Horm Metab Res 1985;15: 111–115
155. Campbell IW: Metformin and the sulphonylureas: the comparative risk. Horm Metab Res 1985;15:105–111
156. Gerich J: Oral hypoglycaemic agents. N Eng J Med 1989;34: 1231–1245
157. Williams G: Management of non-insulin-dependent diabetes mellitus. Br Med J 1994;343:95–100
158. Ferner RE, Neil HAW: Sulphonylureas and hypoglycaemia. Br Med J 1988;296:949–950
159. Seltzer HS: Drug-induced hypoglycaemia: a review of 1418 cases. Endocrinol Metab Clin North Am 1989;18:163–183
160. Alberti KGGM: Diabetic emergencies. Br Med Bull 1989;45: 242–263
161. Basu A, Close CF, Jenkins D et al: Persisting mortality in diabetic ketoacidosis. Diab Med 1993;10:282–284
162. Leutscher PDC, Svendsen KN: Svaer ketoacidose hos en ikke-insulinkraevende diabetes mellitus patient. Ugeskr Laeger 1991;253:2634–2635
163. Berger W, Keller U: Treatment of diabetic ketoacidosis and non-ketotic hyperosmolar diabetic coma. Bailliere's Clin Endocrinol Metab 1992;6:1–22
164. Fonseca V, Phaer DN: Hypersomolar non-ketotic diabetic syndrome precipitated by treatment with diuretics. BMJ 1982; 284:36–37
165. Hamblin PS, Topliss DJ, Chosich N et al: Deaths associated with diabetic ketoacidosis and hyperosmolar coma. Med J Aust 1989;151:439–444
166. Barnett DM, Wilcox DS, Marble A: Diabetic coma in persons over 60. Geriatrics 1962;17:327–336
167. Pramming S, Thorsteinsson B, Bendtson I, Binder C: The relationship between symptomatic and biochemical hypoglycae-

mia in insulin dependent diabetic patients. J Intern Med 1990; 228:641–646

168. Gill CV, Alberti KGGM: Diabetic hypoglycaemia. Pract Diab 1985;2:5–10
169. Brierley FJ, Broughton DL, James OFW, Alberti KGGM: Awareness of hypoglycaemia in the elderly. Age Ageing 1993; 22(suppl 3):9–10
170. Gale E: Causes of hypoglycaemia. Br J Hosp Med 1985;33: 159–162
171. Potter J, Clarke P, Gale EAM et al: Insulin-induced hypoglycaemia in an accident and emergency department: the tip of an iceberg? BMJ 1982;1180–1182
172. Luft D, Schmulling RM, Eggstein M: Lactic acidosis in biguanide-treated patients. Diabetologia 1978;14:75–87
173. Joint Formulary Committee: British National Formulary, No. 26, British Medical Association and Royal Pharmaceutical Society of Great Britain, London, 1993;249–284
174. Monson JP: Selected side-effects: 11. Metformin and lactic acidosis. Prescribers J 1993;33:170–173
175. Robinson R, Stott R: Medical Emergencies: Diagnosis and Management. 5th Ed. Heinnemann Medical Books, London, 1987
176. Stacpoole PW: Lactic acidosis: the case against bicarbonate therapy. Ann Intern Med 1986;105:276–279
177. Sinclair AJ: Geriatric Diabetes: Concerns and Celebrations. State of the Art Lecture, Autumn Meeting, Medical and Scientific Section, British Diabetic Association. October 5, 1995, Harrogate, England
178. Hill RD: Models of care for the elderly diabetic. J Roy Soc Med 1994;87:617–619
179. Wilkes E, Laughton EE: The diabetic, the hospital and primary care. J Roy Coll Gen Pract 1980;30:199–206
180. Hayes T, Harries J: Randomised control trial of routine hospital clinic care versus routine general practice care for type 2 diabetics. BMJ 1984;289:728–730

C H A P T E R 7 6

Age-Related Changes in the Respiratory System

MARTIN J. CONNOLLY

In common with all organ and control systems there are both structural and functional changes in the respiratory system associated with the aging process. An understanding of such changes is essential to the understanding of respiratory pathology. However, before such changes can themselves be understood it is necessary to have a grasp of normal respiratory function in younger adults.

Respiratory Function Tests

This section provides a brief introduction to the most commonly used nonradiologic investigations in respiratory disease together with the typical patterns seen in different classes of respiratory pathology in younger adults.

The most commonly used "breathing tests" are as follows:

FEV_1—the forced expiratory volume in 1 second (liters). The volume of air expired during the first second of a forced expiratory maneuver from vital capacity.

FVC—forced vital capacity (liters). The total volume of air expired during forced expiration from vital capacity. This is usually identical to slow vital capacity (SVC) (i.e. that expired during a nonforced maneuver). However, in severe emphysema with loss of elastic support FVC may fall disproportionately more than SVC.

PEFR (or PEF)—peak expiratory flow rate (L/min). A simple measure of maximal expiratory flow rate.

TL_{co}—transfer factor (mmol/min). A measure of the ability of the lung to oxygenate hemoglobin. It usually measured as a single breath technique using carbon monoxide.

K_{co}—transfer coefficient (mmol/min/k/Pa/L_{STPS}). Essentially TL_{co} corrected for lung volume.

In addition to the above, blood gas measurements are frequently performed in the investigation of patients with respiratory problems. Their purpose is to assess acid-base balance and oxygenation. The most important measures are therefore partial pressure of oxygen (PO_2), partial pressure of carbon dioxide (PCO_2), and pH.

Acutely rising PCO_2 (type 2 respiratory failure) will result in a fall in pH. This is most commonly seen in chronic obstructive pulmonary disease COPD. A chronically high PCO_2 (also common in COPD) will be compensated for by renally mediated mechanisms and will thus be associated with a normal or near normal pH. Hyperventilation (e.g., panic attacks, pulmonary embolism, Cheyne-Stokes respiration) will sometimes produce a high pH (alkalosis) due to "blowing off" of CO_2.

There are essentially two characteristic "patterns" of abnormal respiratory function:

Obstructive pattern. This is most commonly found in asthma and COPD and is characterized by the following:

1. Reduced FEV_1 and PEF.
2. Reduced FVC although proportionately less so than FEV_1.
3. Reduced FEV_1/FVC ratio (normal approximately 70 percent).
4. PO_2 usually normal in asthma (apart from severe exacerbation) but may be low in moderate to severe COPD (either chronically or more commonly during acute exacerbations).
5. PCO_2 may be raised in chronic severe COPD or in acute exacerbations of COPD.
6. pH may be low during acute exacerbations of COPD (respiratory acidosis).

PCO_2 is usually normal in asthma although it may *fall* in acute episodes. A rising PCO_2 (due to patient exhaustion) in acute asthma (or a falling pH) is an adverse prognostic sign suggesting the need for assisted ventilation.

Restrictive pattern (e.g. interstitial fibrotic lung disease):

1. Reduced FVC.
2. Similarly reduced FEV_1.
3. Normal or sometimes high FEV_1/FVC ratio.
4. Reduced TL_{co} and K_{co}.
5. Reduced PO_2.
6. Normal or low PCO_2 (secondary to hyperventilation).
7. Normal or high pH.

Age-Related Changes in the Respiratory System

Having established normal patterns and the most common abnormalities seen in young adults, this section provides a summary of the relatively sparse data available on age-related changes in the respiratory system. It is theoretically important to distinguish between changes *due to* aging itself and those merely *associated with* old age. In other words, it is necessary to distinguish between "aging" changes and "age-related" changes.

Age-related changes in structure and in function (excluding those in respiratory control and monitoring) may have an enormous number of potential causes. In Western populations the effects of disease far outweigh any effects due to aging itself. In particular the effects of smoking (probably including passive smoking[1]) are of most importance. Much interest is currently focused on reactive oxidants in the lung both in terms of smoking-related pathology and aging changes. Reactive oxidants reduce the capacity of amino acid proteinase inhibitor (A-1-proteinase inhibitor) to prevent elastase damaging collagen elastin fibers. Smoking is thought to increase levels of reactive oxidants in the lung.[2] A variety of inconclusive studies have suggested a relationship between antioxidant status and preservation of respiratory function with aging. However high antioxidant levels or a high antioxidant diet may be merely an epiphenomenon (possibly a socially related marker).

Other theories of decline of respiratory function with age include previous respiratory infection (particularly in childhood), nutritional status, environmental pollution, and increased bronchial responsiveness to irritants. It is difficult to distinguish here between "disease effects" and aging effects and such mechanisms are discussed in more detail in Chapter 77.

There is, similarly, debate about the possibility that asthma in particular is an age-related disease. Age-related abnormalities in β_2-adrenoceptor status are recognized in a variety of bodily systems including the lung and are similar to those seen in young patients with asthma. This is also discussed in more detail in the following chapter as is the possibility that atopic status may have implications for respiratory function even in the absence of clinically apparent atopic disease in the elderly.

There is an absence of longitudinal studies (following subjects into old age) in this area. Our information on the differences in the respiratory system of elderly and young people comes therefore from cross-sectional studies (comparing a group of young people to a group of elderly people). Because no other internal organ is so intimately exposed to external environmental influences as the lung, it is difficult even in the absence of disease, to differentiate clearly between physical and physiologic changes of aging itself and those brought about by a lifetime sum of diverse inspired "environmental" insults. These changes comprise physical (structural) changes and physiologic (functional) changes, in the lung, in ventilatory control, and in oxygen exchange and uptake.

Age-Related Structural Changes

The most important age-related change in the large airways is a reduction in the number of glandular epithelial cells. This results in reduced production of protective mucus and thus impaired defense against respiratory infection. There are few changes in the bronchi but the area of the alveoli falls and the alveoli and alveoli ducts enlarge. Function residual capacity, residual volume, and compliance increase. There is deposition of amyloid in lung vasculature and alveolar septa although the significance of this, if any, is unclear.

Small airways suffer qualitative and quantitative changes in the supportive elastin and collagen with coiling and rupture of fibers and consequent dilatation of alveolar ducts and air spaces (so-called senile emphysema),[3] and an increased tendency for small airways to collapse during expiration (see below). These changes may be exacerbated by reduced mobility (often consequent upon acute illness) with reduction in deep breaths, hypoventilation of dependent zones, failure to clear dependent sputum, and thus further risk of lower respiratory infection. There is up to a 20 percent reduction in alveolar surface area with consequent reduction in respiratory reserve, although this is of little or no significance in healthy elderly individuals.

The respiratory muscles comprise the diaphragm (responsible for perhaps 85 percent of respiratory muscle activity), the intercostals, the anterior abdominal muscles, and the accessory muscles of the neck, back, and upper chest. The accessory muscles can be brought into action only by splinting of the arms (trapezius is an exception to this). In normal breathing, expansion of the chest (inspiration) is brought about by the action of these muscles whereas expiration is a passive phenomenon. Under increased demands the accessory muscles are brought into play for inspiration and expiration becomes at least partially active. All respiratory muscles are made up of type I (slow), type IIA (fast-fatigue resistant), and type IIB (fast-fatiguable) fibers. This differentiation is based on adenosine triphosphate activity in the myofibrils, and confers differing physiologic properties.

The major age-related change in the respiratory muscles is a reduction in the proportion of type IIA fibers with consequent impairment of strength and (more importantly) endurance.[4]

In addition to age-related changes in muscle strength and endurance the situation is complicated by changes brought about by systemic and respiratory pathologies common in the elderly. Overall "lack of fitness" (deconditioning) will exacerbate age-related changes detailed above. Clearly musculoskeletal disorders can affect all striated muscles but other common although less immediately obvious pathologies (e.g., osteomalacia) may also cause significant impairment of strength and endurance. Medications (particularly corticosteroids) may also cause problems particularly in respiratory muscle strength. Acute infection including, but not exclusively respiratory infection is often associated with muscle weakness due to toxemia.

Ossification of costal cartilages,[5] loss of vertebral disc space, increased anteroposterior diameter, and calcification of rib articulatory surfaces combine with muscle changes to produce impaired mobility of the thoracic cage. These "normal" changes may be compounded by osteoporotic vertebral collapse (leading to kyphosis) and/or rib or even sternal fracture. Atraumatic sternal fracture is indeed a recognized cause of "atypical" chest pain in the frail elderly.

Age-Related Functional Changes

Lung volumes (both static lung volumes and expiratory volumes) fall gradually with age. Until recent years there have been no large studies of elderly patients in this regard and apparent falls in FEV_1 and FVC have been extrapolated from younger patients. However, it is clear that this has produced an underestimate in rate of decline in these indices with age as hard data are now available for elderly populations.[6] Earlier studies by Milne[7] and Milne and Williamson[8] had also suggested this and in addition had produced longitudinal rather than cross-sectional data in support of the above. The FEV_1/FVC ratio falls by approximately 0.2 percent per year from 70 percent at the age of 40 to 45 years.[9]

There are sex differences in these age-related functional changes. The FEV_1/FVC ratio declines less rapidly in older men than in older women.[10] Maximal expiratory flow and maximum voluntary ventilation decline less rapidly in women.[10]

Flow in the small airways also declines with age.[11] However, the most clinically important functional changes in the aging respiratory system are (1) the increased tendency for small airways to collapse sooner (at higher lung volumes) during expiration (increased "closing volume"); (2) reduction in respiratory muscle strength and endurance; and (3) changes in the monitoring and control of breathing.

Increased closing volume results from degeneration of the collagen and elastin support structure of small airways. In the normal elderly person airway closure in the dependent zones takes place during tidal breathing,[12] with consequent impaired ventilation of the dependent areas, ventilation-perfusion mismatch, and reduced resting arterial oxygen tension.[13] Conversely, because of the sigmoid shape of the oxygen dissociation curve, percentage oxygen saturation is not significantly affected by normal aging, at least until oxygen tension falls below 8 kPa (60 mmHg). Although small airway closure and ventilation mismatch is the *main* reason for the fall in oxygen tension, minor structural alveolar changes also contribute to impaired gas transfer.

At least partially because of the rise in pulmonary artery pressure, blood flow in the healthy elderly lung is increased toward the apices.[14] This further enhances the tendency to mismatch in that ventilation follows the pattern seen in young adults (i.e., greater ventilation at the bases than the apices).

Respiratory muscle strength and endurance fall, in major part as a consequence of type IIA fiber atrophy. Such changes may again be of little or no functional significance in the healthy elderly person but lead to impaired reserve to combat respiratory challenges consequent upon acute respiratory disease. Although there is a wide range of normal, maximal inspiratory mouth pressures (an indirect measure of inspiratory muscle strength) fall by up to 35 percent in men from 20 to 75 years.[15]

Functional changes

A variety of age-related changes produce relative inefficiency in control and monitoring and of ventilation. The much quoted study of Kronenberg and Drage[16] suggested impaired ventilatory responses to both hypoxia and hypercapnia at rest in old age. More recent Anglo-Canadian work[17,18] has challenged some of these data by showing a normal response to resting eucapnic hypoxia, but an impaired response to hypoxia during sustained hypercapnia. The elderly show *increased* ventilatory response to exercise-induced carbon dioxide production.[19] Conversely episodes of sleep apnea are more common in the healthy elderly population.[20] The significance of this latter observation is unclear. Other nonrespiratory diseases (e.g., stroke) may further interfere with respiratory control, producing, for example, posture-dependent hypoxia.[21]

Elderly people are less able to perceive acute bronchoconstriction.[22] This may in part be due to the altered sensitivity of chemoreceptors to hypoxia as discussed above. Other possible mechanisms include the reduced ability to perceive elastic or resistive loads on inspiration or expiration,[23,24] impaired perception of tactile sensation and joint movement,[25–27] or age-associated abnormalities in central processing.[28–30] Such impaired perception of bronchoconstriction, whatever its cause, may have important clinical implications in terms of the awareness of respiratory symptoms, self-referral and access to medical care, and mortality from acute respiratory problems.[22]

Mucociliary clearance is reduced in old age.[31] However, recent limited evidence suggests that the cough reflex is unaffected by the aging process.[32]

Maximal oxygen uptake declines with age (with a consequent decline in "reserve" and in exercise capacity). Although this is partly the result of cardiovascular changes (fall in maximum heart rate and cardiac output[13]), a fall in diffusing capacity[13] and alveolar capillary volume together with ventilation-perfusion mismatch (see above) are also implicated. The decline in maximal oxygen uptake with age can be attenuated but not abolished by regular aerobic exercise.[33]

In addition to "aging" changes specific to the respiratory system there are significant changes in host defense that predispose elderly patients to more frequent and severe bacterial, viral, and fungal infection. Many of these changes (especially local changes) are not specific to aging but occur in consequence of the pathologies seen more commonly in older subjects.

Colonization of the upper respiratory tract (pharynx) by potential pathogens is not uncommon in the elderly, particularly those in institutions.[34,35] In particular, colonization may occur with gram-negative enterobacteria. Colonization of the stomach may in fact precede airway colonization. Stomach colonization is facilitated by achlorhydria, which is itself more common in old age and may be further precipitated by antacids or H_2-blockers.[36–38] Swallowing disorders especially in association with stroke and other neurologic diseases together with tracheal intubation or the presence of nasogastric tubes may facilitate aspiration. The mucous layer itself may be altered by smoking or chronic lung disease and the respiratory epithelium breached by the effects of chronic lung disease.[39]

Aging is characterized by increasing immune deficiency. The degree of change in immune function varies dramatically between individuals and a large part of so-called aging changes may be the results of chronic disease, poor nutrition, and a variety of other factors not specific to aging itself. Defects occur in both cell-mediated immunity and humoral immunity, the latter probably secondary to T-cell dysfunction. Defects in humoral immunity predispose to bacterial infections and may partly explain the increased frequency of pneumonias, particularly pneumococcal pneumonia in the elderly. Humoral changes include both a reduction in the peak antibody response to immunization and a reduction in the duration of antibody response following immunization. These defects may in part explain why beneficial effects of pneumococcal and influenza immunization have been more difficult to prove in elderly populations.

Cell-mediated changes include reduction in a number of active peripheral T cells with a corresponding increase in the proportion of circulating immature T cells, a reduced thymic mass; a reduced T-cell response to interleukins; a reduced T-cell response to mitogens; and a reduction in the generation of cytotoxic T cells.[40]

Summary

Data on aging or age-related changes in respiratory structure and function are surprisingly limited. The most clinically important changes so far recognized are functional rather than structural changes, the majority of the latter serving only to reduce the vast reserve capacity present in the young mature respiratory system. Further research should therefore probably concentrate on functional changes, changes in control and monitoring of respiratory function, and on the effects of depression of immune response (both local and systemic) on the predisposition to respiratory infection and neoplasia.

References

1. Kauffman F, Tessier JF, Oriol P: Passive smoking: a risk factor for chronic airflow limitation. Am J Epidemiol 1983;117: 269–280
2. Richards GA, Theron AJ, Van der Merwe CA, et al: Spirometric abnormalities in young smokers correlate with increased chemiluminescence responses of activated blood phagocytes. Am Rev Respir Dis 1989;139:181–187
3. Verbeken EK, Cauberghs M, Mertens I et al: The senile lung. Comparison with normal and emphysematous lungs. 1. Structural aspects. Chest 1992;101:793–799
4. Brook MH, Kaiser KK: Muscle fiber-types: how many and what kind. Arch Neurol 1970;23:369–379
5. Teale C, Romaniuk C, Mulley G: Calcification on chest radiographs: the association with age. Age Ageing 1989;18:333–336
6. Enright PL, Kraonma RA, Higgins M et al: Spirometry reference values for men and women aged 65 to 85 years of age. Cardiovascular health study. Am Rev Respir Dis 1993;147:125–133
7. Milne JS: Longitudinal respiratory studies in older people. Thorax 1978;33:547–554
8. Milne JS, Williamson J: Respiratory function tests in older people. Clin Sci 1972;42:371–381
9. Tager IB, Segal MR, Speizer FE, Weiss ST: The natural history of forced expiratory volumes. Effect of cigarette smoking and respiratory symptoms. Am Rev Respir Dis 1988;138:837–849
10. Young RC, Borden DL, Rachel RE: Aging of the lung: pulmonary disease in the elderly. Age 1987;10:138–145
11. Knudson RJ, Slatin RC, Leibowitz MD, Burrows B: The maximal expiratory flow-volume curve, normal standards, variability and effects of age. Am Rev Respir Dis 1976;113:587–560
12. Anthoniesen NR, Danson J, Roberton PC et al: Airway closure as a function of age. Respir Physiol 1970;8:58–65
13. Young RC, Borden DL, Rachel RE: Aging of the lung: pulmonary disease in the elderly. Age 1987;10:138–145
14. Kronenberg RS, L'Heureux P, Ponto RA et al: The affect of ageing on lung perfusion. Ann Intern Med 1972;76:413–421
15. Dow L, Carroll M: The ageing lung: structural and functional aspects. pp. 2–17. In Connolly MJ (ed): Respiratory Disease in the Elderly Patient. Chapman & Hall, London, 1996
16. Kronenberg RS, Drage CW: Attenuation of the ventilatory and heart responses to hypoxia and hypercapnia with ageing in normal men. J Clin Invest 1973;52:1812–1819
17. Smith WDF, Cunningham DA, Paterson DH, Poulin MJ: Ventilatory responses to sustained isocapnic hypoxia in the eighth decade. Age Ageing 1995;24 (suppl 2):P12
18. Poulin MJ, Cunningham DA, Paterson DH et al: Ventilatory sensitivity to CO_2 in hyperoxia and hypoxia in older aged humans. J Appl Physiol 1993;75:2209–2216
19. Brischetto MJ, Millman RP, Peterson DD et al: Effect of ageing on ventilatory response to exercise and CO_2. J Appl Physiol 1984;56:1143–1150
20. Hayward L, Mant A, Eyland A et al: Sleep disordered breathing and cognitive function in a retirement village population. Age Ageing 1992;21:121–128
21. Elizabeth J, Singarayar EJ, Bearer D, Lye M: Arterial oxygen saturation and posture in acute stroke. Age Ageing 1993;22: 269–272
22. Connolly MJ, Crowley JJ, Charan NB et al: Reduced subjective awareness of bronchoconstriction provoked by methacholine in elderly asthmatic and normal subjects as measured on a simple awareness scale. Thorax 1992;47:410–413
23. Tack M, Altose MD, Cherniack NS: Effects of ageing on respiratory sensations produced by elastic loads. J Appl Physiol 1981; 50:844–850
24. Tack M, Altose MD, Cherniack NS: Effects of aging on the perception of resistive ventilatory loads. Am Rev Respir Dis 1982;126:463–467
25. Dyck PJ, Schultz PW, O'Brien PC: Quantitation of touch pressure sensation. Arch Neurol Chicago 1972;26:465–473
26. Kormen E, Bossemeyer RW, Williams WJ: Quantitative evaluation of joint motion in an aging population. J Gerontol 1978; 33:62–67
27. Levin HS, Benton AL: Age effects in proprioceptive feedback performance. Gerontol Clin 1973;15:161–169

28. Walsh DA: Age differences in central perceptual processing: a dichoptic backward masking investigation. J Gerontol 1976;31: 178–185
29. Walsh DA, Williams MV, Hertzog CK: Age-related differences in two stages of central perceptual processes; the effects of short duration targets and criterion differences. J Gerontol 1979;34: 234–241
30. Till RE, Franklin LD: On the locus of age differences in visual information processing. J Gerontol 1981;36:200–210
31. Goodman RM, Yergin BM, Landa JF et al: Relationship of smoking history and pulmonary function tests to tracheal mucous velocity in non-smokers, young smokers, ex-smokers and patients with chronic bronchitis. Am Rev Respir Dis 1978;117: 205–214
32. Katsumata U, Tagasugi R, Kotaku K et al: Cough reflex does not decline with age. Am Rev Respir Dis 1991;143:A535
33. Bortz WM: Disuse and aging. JAMA 1982;248:1203–1208
34. Valenti WM, Trudell RG, Bentley DW: Factors predisposing to oropharyngeal colonisation with gram-negative bacilli in the aged. N Engl J Med 1978;298:1108–1111
35. Crossley KB, Thurn JR: Nursing home-acquired pneumonia. Semin Respir Infect 1989;4:64–72
36. Du Moulin GC, Paterson DG, Hedley-Whyte J, Lisbon A: Aspiration of gastric bacteria in antacid-treated patients: a frequent cause of post-operative colonisation of the airway. Lancet 1982; 1:242–245
37. Heyland D, Mandell LA: Gastric colonisation by gram-negative bacilli and nosocomial pneumonia in the intensive care unit patient. Chest 1992;101:187–193
38. Inglis TJJ, Sherratt MJ, Sproat LJ et al: Gastroduodenal dysfunction and bacterial colonisation of the ventilated lung. Lancet 1993;341:911–913
39. Goodman RM, Yergin BM, Landa JF: Relationship of smoking history and pulmonary function tests to tracheal mucus velocity in non-smokers, young smokers, ex-smokers and patients with chronic bronchitis. Am Rev Respir Dis 1978;117: 205–214
40. Schwalo R, Walters CA, Weksler ME: Host defense mechanisms and ageing. Semin Oncol 1989;16:20–27

CHAPTER 77

Respiratory Diseases

MARTIN J. CONNOLLY

Respiratory diseases result in great morbidity and potentially avoidable mortality in elderly people. The burden of many respiratory diseases (asthma, chronic obstructive pulmonary disease [COPD], pulmonary tuberculosis) is increasing in this age group. The elderly themselves regard respiratory conditions as second only to musculoskeletal disorders as a cause of severe disability, general practitioners can expect 700 respiratory consultations per year from every 1,000 elderly patients on their list, and at least 8 percent of all hospital admissions among the elderly in England are attributable to respiratory conditions.[1–3]

In addition to the burden of respiratory problems in this age group the likelihood of atypical and nonspecific presentation of respiratory problems is becoming increasingly recognized. The sensitivity and specificity of physical signs may be diminished. There is an age-related reduction in the cardiovascular response to hypoxia together with an age-related impairment of the subjective appreciation of bronchoconstriction and probably breathlessness in general. There are age-related differences in the presentation and progression of fibrotic lung diseases, tuberculosis, pneumonias, asthma, and bronchogenic carcinomas.

The recognition of such differences has been relatively recent and has both occurred because of and in turn stimulated interest and research into the specific respiratory problems of elderly patients. Within the confines of the present chapter a comprehensive review is impossible, and reference is made to both original research and recent more extensive reviews.

Patterns of Physical Signs

Despite the fact that respiratory diseases in the elderly may present nonspecifically in terms of both symptoms and physical signs, there remain classic features of the history and more particularly of examination that can be grouped into "patterns" suggestive of specific diagnoses or of more general diagnostic areas.

Airway Obstruction

The following signs refer to chronic obstruction, although many will also apply to acute obstruction (acute asthma or acute exacerbation of smoking-related airways obstruction).

1. Audible wheeze
2. Use of accessory muscles (often with arms fixed on the hips, chair, or bed)
3. High shoulders
4. Increased anteroposterior (AP) diameter of chest
5. Prolonged expiration time
6. Inward movement of the costal margin
7. Absent (or downwardly displaced) liver dullness
8. Rhonchi and impaired air entry (in severe obstruction air entry may be so poor that rhonchi are absent)

Collapse

The following are signs of collapse:

1. Reduced movement of the affected side, tracheal deviation to the affected side, and displacement of the apex toward the collapse
2. Diminished breath sounds

Consolidation

Consolidation can be recognized by the following signs:

1. Dullness to percussion
2. Reduced vocal fremitus
3. Increased vocal resonance (aegophony)
4. Bronchial breathing
5. Signs of collapse often coexist
6. Crepitations

Pneumothorax

Pneumothorax (air in the pleural space) displays the following signs:

1. Reduced or absent breath sounds
2. Pleural click (left-sided pneumothoraces only)

When a pneumothorax occurs with tension, other signs may occur in addition. "Tension" indicates increasing accumulation of air in the pleural space with each inspiration, due to a "flap" of pleura producing a one-way valve effect. Other signs include the following:

3. Displacement of the apex and trachea *away* from the affected side
4. Hyper-resonance to percussion
5. Absent breath sounds
6. Tachycardia
7. Hypotension
8. Respiratory distress
9. Cyanosis
10. Sweating
11. Raised jugular venous pressure (JVP)

Pleural Effusion

Signs of pleural effusion include the following:

1. Reduced chest movement over the effusion
2. Profound dullness to percussion ("stony dullness")
3. Reduced breath sounds
4. Reduced vocal fremitus and vocal resonance
5. Displacement of apex and trachea *away from* the effusion (if large)

Diffuse Lung Fibrosis

Diffuse lung fibrosis (e.g., fibrosing alveolitis) can be recognized by the following signs:

1. Fine, late inspiratory or pan-inspiratory crepitations (velcro-creps)
2. Clubbing (often)
3. Cyanosis

Asthma

Epidemiology

The true prevalence of asthma in elderly people is complicated by problems with diagnostic labeling. Epidemiologic studies suggest a prevalence of between 6.5 and 17 percent, with one recent preliminary report suggesting a prevalence of 25 percent.[4–8] Despite the fact that most subjects revealed in these studies to have asthma are symptomatic, the prevalence rate of *diagnosed* asthma in clinical practice falls after the age of 65 years, suggesting underdiagnosis and undertreatment.[4,9] This probably relates to a combination of reduced mobility (less exertion-related dyspnea), reduced expectation on the part of patient and physician, impaired subjective awareness of acute bronchoconstriction,[10] and the poor predictive value of "typical," respiratory symptoms in old age.[112] Whether screening tests in primary care (possibly as part of the "over-75 check" in the United Kingdom) or elsewhere is justified has not been studied.

Pathogenesis

Most elderly patients with asthma have developed the disease as adults, not in childhood[5,13] (i.e., have late-onset asthma), and in contrast to those with juvenile-onset asthma, are rarely atopic. The pathogenesis of such "intrinsic" disease is hotly debated. Absence of clinical atopy does not imply absence of the airway inflammation that is pathognomonic of asthma at all ages. The pathology underlying asthma in elderly patients has been little studied, but intrinsic asthma in younger patients displays similar patterns of cellular immune response and eosinophil activation to those in atopic asthma.[14,15]

The search for the trigger for inflammation has produced several theories of pathogenesis that are not necessarily mutually exclusive. There is debate in the medical[16,17] and lay press about the relevance of atmospheric pollution in asthma *pathogenesis* (as opposed to exacerbating asthma in those with the condition). This debate is no less relevant to the elderly especially in view of their greater lifelong exposure to a greater variety of potentially atmospheric pollutants. Agents hypothesized in this regard include smoke particulates (indoors from heating systems and outdoors from diesel engines), oxides of sulfur, nitrogen, and low-level ozone, and even "new" crops such as oil-seed rape and soya-bean. Most publicity has centered on outdoor pollution, with emphasis on the internal combustion engine; however recent evidence suggests that nitrogen dioxide (from gas cookers) may reach significant levels indoors.[18] A recent preliminary report has indicated that women (not men) who use a gas stove or have an open gas fire have significant impairment of lung function compared with women who do not.[19] Elderly people have, by virtue of relative poverty, tended to live in well-ventilated (drafty) homes. The otherwise laudable trends to home insulation and draft exclusion may have unwittingly increased indoor pollution levels, and the persistent relative poverty of elderly people may mean they are likely to use older, less well-maintained cooking and heating appliances that might exacerbate these effects.

Second, despite lack of obvious clinical atopic disease (including atopic-related exacerbations and elevated serum IgE levels) an atopic etiology cannot be entirely dismissed. IgE levels are recognized to fall with age,[20] but remain a predictor of lung function in elderly populations independent of the presence or absence of asthma.[21] Although the possibility of a relationship between IgE levels and bronchial responsiveness (airway irritability, high levels of which characterize asthma) is not as clear, in studies of older subjects as it is in the young, such a relationship may indeed exist.[20,22]

Possible imbalances between β-adrenergic, cholinergic, and α-adrenergic receptor pathways have also been suggested as possible causes. Most work in this area has concentrated on β-adrenergic receptors with evidence of exaggeration of the "normal" age-related changes in β-adrenoceptor activity being seen in elderly late-onset patients with asthma,[23,24] and being directly associated not only with imbalance in autonomic regulation of airway smooth muscle[24] but also with the increased leukocyte activation necessary for airway inflammation.[25] Down-regulation of glucocorticoid receptors in the elderly[26] may also be implicated as the β-adrenoceptor adenylyl cyclase pathway is modulated by corticosteroid activity.[27–30]

Presentation

The classic presenting symptoms of asthma seen in young patients (intermittent cough, breathlessness, wheezing, tight chestedness, often in association with viral infection and nonspecific respirable irritants, exercise and emotion) are also seen in elderly patients with asthma.[31–35] However, as well as the problems of diagnostic confusion (specificity) with other conditions common in this age group (e.g., COPD, cardiac failure, angina) and some rare ones (e.g., myasthenia gravis[36]) the sensitivity of symptoms is reduced in the elderly. Acute bronchoconstriction is poorly perceived by elderly people whether asthmatic or not.[10] The same is true of other symptoms characteristic of asthma[34] and in particular the predictive value of the so-called bronchial irritability syndrome (wheeze, cough, and chest tightness on exposure to respirable irritants such as cold air and traffic fumes) is much less in the elderly than in the young.[11] Furthermore the intrinsic nature of asthma in older people together with a reduced tendency to diurnal variation, "reversed" seasonal variation (elderly asthma patients tend to be worse in the winter), and the chronic nature of the condition (i.e., even with maximal treatment bronchoconstriction is rarely completely reversible), may result in considerable diagnostic confusion with smoking-related COPD. Even the presence of right-sided cardiac failure (cor pulmonale), usually taken as evidence of COPD rather than asthma, does not exclude a diagnosis of the latter.[37]

As both COPD and asthma are common they are not mutually exclusive,[35] but misdiagnosis and bias because of differences in age, sex, and social class is well recognized. Elderly men[38] and those of lower social class[39] seem more likely to receive a diagnosis of emphysema or COPD than one of asthma irrespective of clinical features. This probably adversely influences treatment in that patients in general practice with a label of asthma are much more likely to receive inhaled bronchodilators than those with a label of COPD.[40] A survey in Northern Ireland recently revealed that over one-quarter of all deaths in the 56 to 75 year age group registered as being due to COPD were in fact probably the result of asthma.[41] The same survey confirmed frequent misdiagnosis of sudden death from asthma being recorded as myocardial infarction or cardiac failure.

However, in contrast to a strong relationship between general practice (GP) prescribing and hospital admission in young adults with asthma there is some evidence that lack of appropriate GP prescribing in elderly patients with asthma does not increase the risk of hospital admission, although this in itself may reflect lack of diagnostic accuracy in the elderly.[42]

Management

In light of the above, the first step is clearly accurate diagnosis and assessment of severity. Spirometry with reversibility assessment to inhaled or nebulized bronchodilators is essential. Although the reversibility detected may be less than in the young it is usually in excess of 20 percent. For those without significant immediate reversibility a course of inhaled or oral corticosteroid (for 6 weeks or 2 weeks, respectively) followed by repeat reversibility assessment may be helpful. It is possible that diurnal peak flow monitoring with reversibility assessment (at least four times daily[43]) may be useful but as well as potential problems of unsupervised inhaler technique the meters may prove difficult to read for elderly people with poor vision. Even if the figures on the meters themselves are readable those on the peak flow graphs usually supplied with mini-peak flow meters can be very difficult even for younger people to read and understand. It is a recommendation of this author that low reading peak flow meters (peak flow ranging between 30 and 350 L/min) should be used because the scale is both appropriate and easier for elderly people to read. Patients should not be expected to chart a graph but should merely be asked to record their peak flow in simple tabular form.

A diurnal variability in peak flow of 15 percent or more suggests asthma, but (particularly in old age) lack of such variability does not exclude it. Measurement of peak flow less than four times daily significantly reduces the likelihood of detecting variability.[43]

Assessment of bronchial responsiveness to methacholine may be helpful in a few cases (especially those in whom pulmonary function is normal or equivocal) but in addition to the lack of an accepted normal range of responsiveness in the elderly the test is not generally available and will probably remain chiefly a research tool. Chest radiography and electrocardiography should be performed to exclude pulmonary edema and help exclude ischemic heart disease. Allergy testing is usually not helpful and rarely necessary.

Management of the chronic condition

Guidelines[44] on asthma management have been published by the British Thoracic Society (BTS) and are widely accepted in the United Kingdom. They suggest stepwise increments in treatment depending on severity of the condition as judged chiefly (although not exclusively) by patient-reported symptoms. The principles of these guidelines are just as applicable to elderly patients with asthma but there are arguable differences in application. The first step in the BTS guidelines is "on demand" use of regular bronchodilators. This is probably inappropriate for elderly patients who are less able to appreciate acute bronchoconstriction,[10] and the prophylactic use of regular low-dose inhaled corticosteroids should be considered as a first step. Whether one should also give *prescribed* (as opposed to "on demand") regular inhaled bronchodilators is unclear (i.e., there is no available research to guide the decision). The possibility and likely clinical significance of down-regulation (tachyphylaxis) of airway β-adrenoceptors due to regular use of inhaled β-agonists is discussed below under COPD. The subsequent incremental steps (higher dose inhaled steroids, followed by additional regular β-agonists, followed finally by oral corticosteroids) are appropriate. Emphasis should be placed on *objective* outcome measures (e.g., home peak flow measures) over subjective complaints (or more likely lack of these) in order to guide transitions between steps in management. Only a very small minority of elderly patients with asthma should require regular oral corticosteroid therapy for adequate control. It is likely that the expected revision of the BTS guidelines (1997) will address age-related differences in management.

Patients with asthma with psychotic illness have greater risk of asthma death.[45] This presumably relates to poor personal control of the condition among patients with psychiatric problems. It is likely that similar difficulties in control will be found in chronically confused patients or those acutely confused for reasons other than their asthma. In addition there is evidence that the demented may *perceive* bronchoconstriction less well.[46] These factors may go part of the way to explaining the increased differential mortality from asthma in elderly people. Particular care must be taken over the chronic management of the condition in elderly psychotic or chronically confused patients.

Inhaler management must be simplified as much as possible. This involves not just choosing the correct inhaler device for optimum technique (see below) but simplifying the inhaler *regimen*. Longer acting inhaled β-agonists (salmeterol and eformoterol) may be administered twice instead of four times daily. They have been shown to be effective and safe in elderly patients.[47,48] Although twice the dose of inhaled steroid given once daily may not provide as tight control as the normal dose administered on a twice daily basis, it can provide reasonable control in more stable patients,[49] and may on occasion make home management with once daily family support more feasible for the mildly demented elderly patient with asthma.

There has been enormous amount of debate regarding inhaler technique in elderly people. The standard metered-dose inhaler (MDI) is probably obsolete when used in isolation for elderly patients. Patients with reduced hand-grip strength find difficulty coordinating inhalation and triggering of the device and even mildly confused elderly patients find MDI technique difficult to learn and retain.[50] The addition of a large volume spacer device (Volumatic, Allen and Hanbury's Ltd. or Nebuhaler, Astra Pharmaceuticals Ltd.) involves a technique that removes the problem of coordination, is easier for patients to learn and retain, and is preferred by elderly patients.[51] In addition, such devices ameliorate the problem of systemic absorption of significant quantities of inhaled corticosteroid when using high doses of such drugs.[52] Furthermore, large volume spacers can be triggered by caregivers or relatives if the patients themselves find them difficult to use. Any consequent delay between triggering and inhalation in such circumstances is unlikely to have a major effect on deposition of the drug in the airways.[53]

A large number of breath-actuated devices are available. There is limited literature on inhaler technique with these devices; however, the Turbohaler and the Autohaler seem relatively successful in the elderly whereas the Rotahaler and the Diskhaler seem more difficult for the elderly to use.[54,55]

Whichever inhaler is employed it is important that where possible different drugs are given through the same type of device and that the patient has frequent demonstration and reinstruction on techniques. More tuition and reinstruction together with *inpatient* first prescription of inhalers and consequent opportunity for nurse-led reinforcement both improve inhaler technique in elderly people.[50,56]

Assessment and management of the acute condition

Mortality rates for asthma are much higher in old age.[57] Most asthma mortality occurs during acute exacerbations and is frequently due to potentially avoidable factors.[58] Elderly patients with asthma underestimate the severity of acute bronchoconstriction[10] and take on average three times as long to get to the hospital as their young counterparts during exacerbations.[59] The elderly also develop less tachycardia and pulsus paradoxus than the young with the same degree of bronchoconstriction,[59] and are thus more likely to be perceived by their medical attendants as having less severe exacerbations.

The BTS guidelines for the management of acute asthma[44] are generally applicable to the elderly patient with asthma. However, in light of the above, even more emphasis must be given to *objective* assessment rather than reliance on misleadingly "minor" symptoms and the "reassuring" absence of worrying physical signs. All patients should have peak flow estimated and compared to their predicted level or previous known best.[60] Patients at the hospital should also have arterial blood gas estimations (preferably when breathing room air). Chest radiography should look for evidence of pneumothorax, pulmonary edema, and infections. Unsuspected abnormalities (often of immediate clinical significance) occur on the majority of chest X-rays in elderly patients with acute asthma.[61]

Immediate treatment should include high-flow oxygen and nebulized β-agonists and ipratropium. Ipratropium should not be given in conjunction with β-agonists in patients with diagnosed or suspected glaucoma. High doses of systemic corticosteroids (initially intravenously) are needed. A dose of 200 mg of hydrocortisone should be given followed by 30 to 40 mg of prednisolone daily.

Objective measurement of response should comprise regular peak flow monitoring (including response to nebulizers) and if this is not clearly improving, repeat blood gas measurements. Blood gases should in any case be repeated at least once or if there is *any* suspicion of a clinical deterioration.

For patients who do not respond to the above treatment intravenous salbutamol and/or aminophylline should be considered. A rising PCO_2 (or even a normal PCO_2) may be an indication of impending patient exhaustion. Mechanical ventilation may be more often considered for the elderly patient with asthma than for one with end-stage COPD. Advanced age is not a barrier to intensive care entry or to mechanical ventilation. The decision whether to ventilate an elderly patient is usually a difficult one and needs to be made in conjunction with the patient (if possible), relatives, the full multidisciplinary team, and the patient's own general practitioner if available. An enlightened discussion of this area is given in a review by Nielson.[62]

Other treatment

Respiratory infection may or may not be present in patients with severe asthma. If there is objective evidence of infection (raised white blood cell count, pyrexia, infiltration on the chest x-ray) then antibiotics should be chosen as discussed for COPD. Many will need judicious intravenous rehydration and maintenance.

Chronic Obstructive Pulmonary Disease

Epidemiology

The British Thoracic Society Guidelines on COPD[63] define the condition as "a chronic slowly progressive disorder characterised by airways obstruction . . . which does not change markedly over several months." COPD is almost always the result of cigarette smoking, and a smoking history of less than 10 pack years (1 pack year = 20 cigarettes per day for 1 year) strongly suggests the possibility of an alternative diagnosis (e.g., chronic asthma, bysinnosis). Following a long asymptomatic phase of decline in respiratory function, initial presentation of COPD usually occurs between the ages of 50 and 60 years. Epidemiologic surveys reveal a high prevalence of COPD in the elderly, much of which is undetected clinically (probably for reasons similar to those discussed above for asthma) and thus untreated. Our own recent studies suggest that nearly 30 percent of Caucasian inner-city community dwellers over the age of 65 years have airways obstruction (COPD plus asthma), and that nearly two-thirds of these receive no treatment.[4] Other British, European, and United States epidemiologic studies from less industrialized areas with lower rates of cigarette smoking report COPD prevalence of between 7 and 16 percent,[1,64,65] although a British survey of the more dependent elderly reported a prevalence (COPD plus asthma) of over 40 percent.[31] Smoking rates appear to be falling, or at least leveling off, in men in Western nations but are still increasing in women.[66] The fall in smoking prevalence has been smaller in the less well educated, in ethnic minorities, and in those from poorer socioeconomic groups.[67] The cohort of people making up today's elderly have had the highest uptake of cigarette smoking[68] and thus should be expected to have a higher prevalence of COPD than younger cohorts.[4] Indeed it is likely that the health care burden caused by COPD (particularly in women) in the Western world will continue to rise in absolute terms paralleling the rise in the elderly population.[69] There is some evidence that this latter is in fact the case, and certainly COPD is no less common in the elderly than in the middle-aged,[4] and although it is less frequently diagnosed and treated,[4,9] COPD produces major morbidity and impairment of quality of life in old age.[70]

Presentation

COPD is characterized by a variable phase (usually several years) of minimal symptoms (perhaps except "smokers cough") or physical signs before the onset of wheeze and/or breathlessness. Most patients who subsequently develop COPD will qualify for the label of chronic bronchitis (the production of sputum each day for at least 3 months on 2 consecutive years), but often do not regard sputum production as abnormal. The essential abnormality of lung function in COPD is obstructive (a reduced forced expiratory volume in 1 second [FEV_1] and FEV_1/forced vital capacity [FVC] ratio), and it is only when FEV_1 falls below 60 percent of predicted (or even lower in the elderly) that breathlessness and wheeze on exertion become troublesome. Other presenting symptoms include general malaise, fatigue (often neglected), cough and sputum production (as for chronic bronchitis), and possibly sleep disturbance. As the condition progresses (FEV_1 below 40 percent predicted) breathlessness and wheeze worsen and hyperinflation of the chest, cyanosis, and signs of right heart strain appear (due to pulmonary vasoconstriction from chronic hypoxia): right ventricular heave, raised JVP, and peripheral edema. Secondary polycythemia affects some sufferers. Sleep disturbance and daytime somnolence become more common. Nocturnal hyperventilation and hypoxia may interfere with sleep pattern.[71–74] It is usually only in this latter phase (FEV_1 below 40 percent predicted) that patients become known to the hospital, generally because of emergency admission with intermittent exacerbations (see below). Gradual weight loss is common secondary to a combination of increased energy demands of breathing and in the latter stages reduced intake because of breathlessness on eating.[75] Prognosis is inversely related to age and to lung function (particularly to postbronchodilator lung function.[76]

Management of the Chronic Condition

Smoking cessation is the corner stone of management at all levels of severity. The argument that this is not possible in elderly patients is specious. Cessation is as successful in the motivated elderly[77] and possibly even more so,[78] with 1 year quit rates of 10 to 15 percent. However, research studies looking at quit rates by necessity have examined a subgroup of elderly patients (the motivated) that may not be representative of elderly smokers in general and there is strong anecdotal evidence that elderly smokers overall are less motivated to join smoking cessation groups. This phenomenon needs further study. Nicotine replacement for the highly motivated including the elderly[78,79] may improve 1 year quit rates to about 20 percent. Sudden cessation is more effective than gradual reduction.[80] The benefits of smoking cessation upon rate of loss in lung function decline with age but probably remain valuable up to the age of 80 years (particularly in women).[81]

Lung function testing (FEV_1 and FVC) is essential for diagnosis. Peak expiratory flow rate (PEFR) measurement can be misleadingly high in COPD.[63] Bronchodilator reversibility testing should be carried out in all patients (FEV_1 before and 30 minutes after 2.5 to 5 mg nebulized salbutamol and 0.5 mg nebulized ipratropium). Classically a 15 percent improvement in FEV_1 was until recently considered significant; however, this can be misleading when baseline FEV_1 is very low, and current recommendations are that a significant improvement in FEV_1 comprises a 15 percent increase *and* an absolute improvement of 200 ml.[63] Response to oral steroids (30 mg of prednisolone daily for 2 weeks) or inhaled steroids (for 6 weeks) should be examined by repeating reversibility testing at the end of the steroid course. Objective response indicates the need for regular inhaled steroid prescription.

Drug treatment

The use of on demand β-agonist treatment is not appropriate for the elderly in whom reduced appreciation of bronchoconstriction may impair demand.[10] Such impaired demand with consequent failure to respond to worsening bronchoconstriction is recognized as contributary to increased mortality from asthma.[82] Some authorities argue that regular β-agonists are associated with an increased risk of mortality or near death episodes from acute asthma. The mechanism for this is believed to be tachyphylaxis (down regulation) of lung β-receptors. The majority of the evidence for this comes from studies of fenoterol, a relatively nonselective (compared to salbutamol and terbutaline) β-agonist.[83–85] However, most of the excess mortality in these studies was in younger patients and the Committee of Safety of Medicines and the Royal Society of Medicine both recently concluded that the evidence against β-agonists is limited and not sufficient to recommend changes in their use.[86,87]

Inhaled medication usage (both technique and dosage compliance) is variable and probably worse in the elderly. It is improved by regular follow-up visits and by the provision of feedback about inhaler use and technique.[88] In patients with compliance problems a safe and effective (although expensive) alternative may be the long-acting inhaled β-agonists salmeterol and eformoterol,[47,48] although there is an increasing suggestion that such long-acting β-agonists may produce a small loss of bronchodilator effect with prolonged use together with a more rapid and significant decline in *bronchoprotective* effect that is not prevented by concurrent use of inhaled corticosteroids.[89] Inhaled corticosteroids should be given only to those with a documented steroid response (i.e., objective improvement in lung function). Large-scale trials are awaited concerning the possible benefits of inhaled steroids on COPD progression, but at present there is no evidence to support their use in those patients without documented objective response. Similarly an apparent response to steroids during an acute exacerbation does not necessarily imply response between exacerbations. There is little or no place for oral corticosteroids in the chronic management of COPD. β-Blockers should be avoided because they may exacerbate bronchoconstriction. Even β-blocker eye drops used for the treatment of glaucoma are recognized to produce bronchoconstriction, which is reversible on stopping treatment. Where β-blocker eye drops are essential a "cardioselective" medication such as betaxolol should be used in preference to timolol (Timoptol) or carteolol.[90,91]

The optimal dose of inhaled anticholinergic agent for the stable patient is surprisingly not yet established with certainty. There is recent evidence, from a small study including patients up to the age of 76 years, that a dose of ipratropium of at least 160 μg (four times the standard dose) is necessary for maximal bronchodilation and that such doses are needed before any improvement in exercise tolerance is seen.[92] This work needs confirmation in larger numbers of older subjects.

Inhaler technique is discussed above. Although nebulizers do have a place for inhaled drug administration in COPD they have too frequently been prescribed without objective evidence of benefit, and even more frequently are employed in an unsupervised fashion.[93] Elderly patients in particular may find nebulizers difficult to manage, and often need the help of a caregivers for effective use.[94] This, among other things, implies that nebulizers should not be seen as the simple alternative to inhalers in the patient with inadequate inhaler technique. Hospital-based assessment of benefit from nebulizers is probably inadequate and domiciliary assessment may be preferable.[95,96] Nebulizers need regular servicing and replacement of filters, and patients or caregivers should be aware of who to contact about this. There is evidence from a recent preliminary report that compliance with nebulized therapy is surprisingly low (of the order of 50 percent) despite the fact that good compliance was associated in the same study with better quality of life.[97]

Theophyllines are beneficial both as bronchodilators and in improving respiratory muscle strength. Unfortunately their side effects are often prohibitive in elderly patients, particularly as clinically significant benefit is only obtained when plasma concentrations are at the upper end of the therapeutic range.[98] Sustained-release preparations reduce the incidence of side effects. Both theophyllines and oral β-agonist preparations may be useful in the small number of patients (often the demented) who are unable to use any form of inhaled bronchodilator.

Long-term oxygen therapy

Long-term oxygen therapy (LTOT) is proven to prolong survival in COPD. The only other measure for which this claim can be made is smoking cessation. LTOT implies the delivery of oxygen (usually by oxygen concentrator) for at least 15 hours per day in order to alleviate or prevent right ventricular failure (cor pulmonale), which results from pulmonary hypertension precipitated by chronic hypoxia. It must be distinguished from giving intermittent oxygen for palliation of symptoms. The two studies that indicated a reduction in mortality on LTOT did not include large numbers of the elderly, and one, the MRC LTOT Trial, *excluded* patients over 70 years of age.[99,100] Nonetheless, if assessment follows established criteria (as an inpatient at least overnight) there is no reason to suppose that the elderly are less likely to benefit. In brief, criteria for selection for LTOT are:

- Persistent irreversible airflow obstruction
- Nonsmoker
- No hypercapnia
- PO_2 less than 55 mmHg (7.3 kPa) on two sequential estimations at least 1 month apart, and not during an acute exacerbation
- LTOT leads to increased PO_2 without dangerous fall in pH or rise in PCO_2

Noninvasive nasal positive pressure ventilation

Noninvasive nasal positive pressure ventilation (NIPPV) has recently been shown in studies including a few patients over the age of 70 years,[772] to be of benefit, as an adjunct to LTOT, in selected patients with COPD. In addition to patient compliance, motivation, and good cognitive function, criteria for possible benefit from NIPPV comprise documented nocturnal hypoventilation (hypoxia), reversible with NIPPV, together with daytime hypercapnia. Considerable improvement in quality of life in terms of reduced sleep disturbance, activity, and psychosocial factors may be possible.[71,72] Patients should have stable disease, and NIPPV should not be seen as a last resort in rapidly deteriorating end-stage disease.[73] This area has recently been the subject of an excellent review,[74] and may provide further hope for elderly patients in the future. However, studies to date are small scale, and further work needs to be done in larger numbers of elderly patients before the technique can be widely recommended in this age group.

Short-burst oxygen therapy may be symptomatically beneficial for relief of breathlessness. Opiates (including nebulized morphine) and diazepam are not of proven value in the alleviation of breathlessness.

Depression is extremely common in moderate or severe COPD, particularly in the elderly.[101,102] Treatment of depression may produce significant improvement in quality of life.[101]

Pulmonary rehabilitation

Pulmonary rehabilitation is the subject of an enormous amount of recent and current research, although with a few exceptions elderly patients have not been included in such studies.[103] Pulmonary rehabilitation programs are a multidisciplinary effort comprising education, optimization of medical therapy, nutritional assessment and modification, psychological evaluation and support, relaxation techniques, smoking cessation support, and (essentially) exercise training and reconditioning.

Although exercise reconditioning comprising aerobic training (both of arms and legs) and expiratory and inspiratory resistive training (respiratory muscle training) is recognized to improve exercise tolerance in the short term, there are questions that need unequivocal answers in this area. Most frail elderly COPD patients *seem* able to perform the relatively intensive protocols needed to obtain improved exercise tolerance.[104,105] These data need confirmation. There is debate, however, even in younger patients, about the duration of benefit with some studies claiming that improvement in exercise tolerance persists for up to 1 year in the absence of maintenance therapy, but others contradicting this.[106,107] Arguably of most importance is the question of whether improvement in exercise tolerance translates to improvement in quality of life. The data on this area in the elderly are scanty.[108] There is currently no evidence that respiratory rehabilitation reduces mortality or frequency of hospital admission in elderly patients, although there are some older data suggesting the latter in younger patients.[108] Our own recent data in the elderly (unpublished) also suggest that elderly patients who have completed a pulmonary rehabilitation program are less likely to be admitted to the hospital in the subsequent 12 months, and that most of the improvement in exercise tolerance gained during the program is maintained at 12 months irrespective of whether the patient performs maintenance exercises.

Greater evaluation of respiratory rehabilitation is, however, needed in elderly patients, and depending on the results it may become an expanding area of rehabilitation in geriatric medicine. Certainly, elderly patients with irreversible COPD and chronic asthma (provided they are able to exercise to a sufficient intensity to produce an aerobic training effect) should be considered for referral to existing respiratory rehabilitation programs. Home-based pulmonary rehabilitation programs may prove especially suitable for elderly subject.[108,109]

All patients should be advised to remain as physically active as possible and the obese given advice on weight reduction (which will reduce oxygen requirements of exercise). Conversely, malnutrition is common and correlates with mortality, but beneficial effects of nutritional supplements are unproven. Wheeled walking frames may improve exercise tolerance in the severely disabled.[110] In a recent study the use of wheeled frames did not improve distance walked but was associated with a major and significant reduction in breathlessness in patients (including the elderly) with severe COPD.[111]

Influenza vaccination is recommended for all patients with COPD, not just the elderly,[112] and reduces mortality by over two-thirds.[113,114] However, the rate of uptake of influenza vaccination in those in whom it is indicated is only around 50 percent,[115–117] with failure to offer the vaccine and refusal of the offer being almost equally common.[117] The value of polyvalent pneumococcal vaccine is not absolutely proven although early studies in elderly patients are encouraging with 45 to 80 percent protection over 3 years.[118] Its indications are similar to those for influenza vaccine.

Quality of life

In the context of what is an incurable disease, where the management aim should arguably shift toward enhancing quality of life, it is perhaps surprising that there remains considerable debate about the factors most affecting quality of life in patients with COPD.[119–126] Most authors have concluded that the patient's emotional reactions to his or her condition is a significant if not the most important quality of life determinant, and that perhaps surprisingly absolute level of respiratory function (spirometry) is of limited help in assessment. Whether age and socioeconomic status are independent variables continues to tax the minds of investigators. Our own preliminary data lead us to conclude that as well as optimum medical management, therapy should be directed at helping patients come to terms with their illness and develop coping strategies for everyday use. Much more research is needed here.

Management of the Acute Exacerbation

Although most exacerbations are managed effectively in the community it is during an acute exacerbation of COPD (AECOPD) that the patient is most likely to present to the hospital. The peak age for hospital admissions for AECOPD is approximately 70 years.[127] Many, but not all, are the result of bacterial infections, acute infective bronchitis, and pneumonia which will be considered separately. Other causes include viral infection, pulmonary edema, peripheral edema, or pulmonary embolus. Symptoms may include fever, increased sputum volume and/or purulence, increased breathlessness and wheeze, fluid retention, confusion, and somnolence. The BTS Guidelines[63] list the criteria for determining which AECOPD patients need hospital admission. These criteria include severe breathlessness; poor or deteriorating general condition; cyanosis; increasing peripheral edema; confusion or impaired consciousness; inability to cope at home; and patients already receiving LTOT. Further indications for admission are pulmonary infiltration on the chest x-ray, arterial pH less than 7.35, arterial pO_2 on air less than 7 kPa, or infiltration present on chest x-ray. Immediate hospital investigation should include chest x-ray and blood gas estimation (preferably when breathing room air).

The cause of death in AECOPD is usually hypoxia and the aim is thus to achieve adequate oxygenation (PO_2 of 6.6 kPa) greater without a rise in PCO_2 or worsening acidosis. Oxygen delivery by nasal cannula is not controlled (i.e., percentage of inspired oxygen is not predictable) and thus Venturi masks should be used if at all possible. When the patient cannot tolerate a Venturi mask (not uncommon in the elderly) and nasal cannulae are employed, blood gas monitoring needs to be more frequently performed, and should be done within 30 minutes of commencement of supplemented oxygen. When delivery by a Venturi mask is possible a 28 percent mask should be used initially and blood gases rechecked within 1 hour, adjusting the inspired oxygen delivery (different Venturi mask) as indicated by the results. Blood gases should be repeated if there is any change in conscious level or other clinical deterioration.

Not all patients with AECOPD require antibiotic treatment, but antibiotics are indicated if two or more of the following are present: increased sputum volume, increased sputum purulence, or increased breathlessness. For the majority of infective episodes that develop in the community amoxycillin, tetracycline, or co-amoyclav will be appropriate choices.[63] Episodes beginning in the hospital may need different antibiotics depending on local sensitivities, and the choice(s) should cover gram-negative bacilli (e.g., co-amoyclav, cefuroxime). Unfortunately such broad-spectrum antibiotics are prone to produce the potentially serious complication of pseudomembranous colitis in the elderly. Any diarrhea in such circumstances, particularly if accompanied by abdominal pain and bloating, should be taken very seriously, samples sent for culture including that of *Clostridium difficile* (and toxin estimation), and treatment with oral metronidazole and/or vancomycin commenced upon local microbiological advice.

Bronchodilators should be given by nebulizer (driven by compressed air not by oxygen) every 4 hours, beginning at 6 to 7 AM and including overnight if the patient is awake. Salbutamol 2.5 to 5 mg and ipratropium 0.5 mg are usually given together, but the latter should be omitted in patients with glaucoma because of the risk of an anticholinergic-precipitated acute episode.

For patients with severe bronchoconstriction who fail to respond to nebulized treatment, intravenous aminophylline (0.5 mg/kg/h) may be valuable although research is contradictory and has mainly been performed in acute asthma rather than in AECOPD.[128–132] Intravenous aminophylline should be avoided in a patient already receiving methylxanthine therapy unless serum theophylline levels are available. Intravenous or subcutaneous β-agonists may be an alternative in the patient with severe bronchoconstriction when nebulized drugs may penetrate poorly. Clinical experience suggests their usefulness but controlled trials in the elderly are lacking.

It is common practice to administer systemic corticosteroids to patients with AECOPD. However, their value in this condition is unclear.[63] The BTS guidelines suggest the administration of a 1- to 2-week course if the patient has been previously shown to respond to steroids, is on maintenance steroid therapy, is presenting for the first time with AECOPD, or fails to respond to high-dose bronchodilators. It is important to recognize that steroid response in the acute episode does not necessarily justify maintenance inhaled steroid therapy.

In patients with severe respiratory acidosis (arterial pH less than 7.25) intravenous doxapram may be useful. Close supervision with regular blood gas estimation is needed and doxapram is contraindicated in the presence of coexisting ischemic heart disease (an all too common association).

If intermittent positive pressure ventilation (IPPV) is available, it is valuable for some patients with respiratory acidosis. Old age is not a contraindication but the acutely confused patient responds less well.[133,134] Mechanical ventilation is similarly not precluded by age alone but is beyond the scope of this chapter. It has been reviewed recently elsewhere.[135]

Objective assessment of the severity of airways obstruction in AECOPD (by means of regular blood gas and peak flow estimation) is essential in all age groups but most particularly in the elderly. The absence of pulsus paradoxus and of tachycardia are common in severe airways obstruction in the elderly and are not reassuring.[59] Similarly the assertion by patients themselves that their dyspnea is not particularly troublesome or is improving may be unreliable, as the elderly patient may have impaired perception of bronchoconstriction.[63]

Nebulized treatment should be changed to inhalers (unless the patient uses a home nebulizer) at least 2 days before discharge to allow time for monitoring of inhaler technique and exclusion of deterioration on dosage reduction. Inhaler technique should be demonstrated, checked repeatedly, and documented as adequate prior to discharge.

Nonmycobacterial Respiratory Infection

Epidemiology and Pathogenesis

Respiratory infection is probably more common in older people. Certainly *death* from respiratory infection is more common in the elderly. However, epidemiologic studies are patchy and many specifically exclude elderly people. The best estimate is that the death rate from respiratory infection for the age group over 65 years approaches 500 per 10,000 people per year. This figure is 50 times higher than that in young adults.[136]

Factors that increase the risk of respiratory infection in old age have been detailed in an earlier chapter. Briefly these comprise a depressed immune response, increased closing volume, an increased prevalence of chronic lung disease (in turn producing impairment of the mucociliary escalator, impaired respiratory muscle strength and endurance, breaches of the respiratory epithelium, and alteration in the mucous layer), institutionalization leading to greater proximity to other potentially infected individuals, and colonization of the upper respiratory tract by potential pathogens (gram-negative enterobacteria are particularly likely in some circumstances).[137] In addition other medical conditions common in elderly people also predispose to increased infection (stroke and other neurologic conditions increasing the risk of aspiration, achlorhydria, and impaired nutritional status further depressing immunity).

Influenza

Influenza is not more common in the elderly. However its complication rate, morbidity, and mortality are much greater. Hospitalization as a result of influenza is up to 20 times more common in old people and even more so than those with other chronic illness.[138,139] Approximately one-quarter of elderly patients suffer complications from influenza.[140] Acute infective bronchitis is up to 20 times more common after influenza in elderly people and pneumonia nearly 10 times more common.[141] The well-recognized complication of staphylococcal pneumonia following influenza in fact only accounts for about one-quarter of postinfluenza pneumonias even during epidemic periods and the most common bacterial pathogen following influenza is *Streptococcus pneumoniae*.[142] Pneumonia directly due to the influenza virus rather than bacterial superinfection is a not uncommon complication.

Influenza epidemics are associated with the peak of death from pneumonia and acute bronchitis in elderly people. However, there is also a large increase in deaths from cerebrovascular and cardiovascular disease that are precipitated by the influenza infection.[143]

Influenza vaccination is recommended in the United Kingdom for residents of nursing or residential homes as well as those with diabetes, chronic renal failure, or chronic respiratory conditions.[112,144] The vaccine is modified each year to cover serotypic changes. In Canada, the United States, and the majority of European countries government recommendations are that influenza vaccination should be given to all elderly persons irrespective of their state of health.[145–147]

The main benefit of vaccination is in reducing the incidence of hospitalization (and other complications) and mortality. It is estimated that mortality is reduced at least 60 percent.[139,148] Unfortunately on the relatively tight criteria in the United Kingdom a large proportion of the elderly population of the Western world would be suitable for vaccination. Currently only a small minority receive it.[149] A variety of factors are recognized to influence uptake of influenza vaccination. These include the presence and absence of recognized risk factors,[116,150] the perception of side effects[117] versus the perceived threats of developing influenza and its complications,[151] income, marital status, and racial origin.[115,152]

The only effective antiviral drugs for influenza are the adamantane group (e.g. amantadine). This is effective only against influenza A, and reduces the illness severity in almost all those to whom it is given. However it rapidly leads to the production of drug-resistant strains. It might be useful to limit the spread of influenza during outbreaks in nursing or residential homes or even in hospital rehabilitation wards where the residents or patients have not previously been vaccinated.

Pneumonia

Pneumonia is much more common in the elderly than younger adults. European studies suggest an incidence approaching 20 cases per 1,000 population per year in the 70 to 79 age group compared with one or two per 1,000 in young adults.[153,154] The vast majority (over 90 percent) of deaths from pneumonia in developed countries occur in the elderly. National figures in the United Kingdom suggest pneumonia is a primary cause in over 5 percent of deaths in the over 65 age group.[155]

In Britain *Haemophilus influenzae* and *Pneumococcus* are the most common causes of community-acquired pneumonia in the elderly.[156,157] "Atypical" pneumonias in the elderly seem rare in the United Kingdom[157] although less so in the United States. The exception to this is that mycoplasma infection is common in the United Kingdom during epidemics that tend to occur approximately every 4 years and peak between January and March.[156] Gram-negative enterobacteria are thought to be uncommon as a cause of community-acquired pneumonia in Britain.

The elderly, particularly those who are cognitively impaired,[158] are more likely to present with atypical (nonrespiratory) symptoms. The most common of these is confusion (up to 70 percent of cases versus 30 percent of young adults[156,157,159,160]). Indeed confusion is so common as a nonspecific presenting feature that a chest x-ray will reveal the diagnosis in nearly one-quarter of cases of elderly patients presenting with acute confusion and no physical signs.[161] A tachypnea (greater than 24/min) is a very early although equally nonspecific feature of pneumonia in the elderly.[162] Signs of cardiac failure are present in nearly one-quarter of patients.[163] Pleuritic chest pain and rigors are very uncommon[164] but although oral or axillary temperature may not be raised, core temperature is almost always elevated in the first 24 hours after hospital admission,[160] (i.e., the suggestion that elderly people do not develop a pyrexia is erroneous). Although most elderly patients with pneumonia will have localizing crackles on chest auscultation, the presence of isolated (especially bilateral) pulmonary basal crackles is a nonspecific finding in the ill elderly.[165] Similarly dehydration, although much more common in older people than in younger people with pneumonia, may be difficult to detect clinically. Our own studies have shown that the presence of axillary sweating is highly suggestive that the patient is not dehydrated although its absence is not as helpful.[166]

Investigations and Management

Investigations of pneumonia in the hospital are not unique to the elderly and comprise urgent urea and electrolyte estimation, full blood count, chest x-ray, blood gas estimation, and (if possible) peak flow estimation. Measurement of erythrocyte sedimentation rate or C-reactive protein may give further evidence of infection in uncertain cases. However, this apparently simple scenario frequently does not apply in old age where the investigations may be aimed at detecting the cause of an acute confusional state, and will initially therefore include more wide-ranging tests.

Blood cultures should also be taken before institution of antibiotic therapy. However, antibiotic therapy should not be delayed by waiting for a sputum sample, because in the early stages less than one-half of patients are able to produce sputum. Microbiologic identification is even more difficult in the elderly.[163,167,168] Indeed attempts to establish bacterial etiology of pneumonia fail in over 60 percent of cases without apparently affecting prognosis in the majority. Gram staining is almost as valuable as culture of sputum[169] but not available in all centers. Blood cultures should always be taken and should be positive in almost one-third of patients with pneumococcal pneumonia.[156,157] Where bacteriologic diagnosis is deemed essential, counter current-immune-electrophoresis of sputum or urine is sensitive in the detection of pneumococcal capsular antigen.[156,157] However, it may give false-positive results in patients with chronic lung disease who are often colonized with pneumococcus.

General supportive measures include careful intravenous rehydration (necessary in the majority of patients) and oxygen treatment (often high-flow oxygen) as indicated by blood gases. Even if the patient is not initially dehydrated intravenous fluids are often necessary to maintain hydration in a patient with reduced intake (secondary to anorexia and possibly confusion) and increased needs due to pyrexia and tachypnea.

Bacterial etiology and antibiotic treatment

Pneumococcus is the most common cause of community-acquired pneumonia in people, causing 30 to 60 percent of cases.[157,170] It is less well recognized that viral pneumonia is the second most common cause (most particularly influenza viruses); the third is *Haemophilus influenzae*. The incidence of *Legionella pneumonia* in the elderly is low, with less than 100 cases per year in England and Wales.[171] Similarly mycoplasma pneumonia in the absence of an epidemic is extremely rare in the elderly.[172] In contrast staphylococcal pneumonia, although not common, affects the elderly as well as the young, most particularly following influenza.[173] Chlamydia infection is not uncommon with about 15 percent of all cases of psittacosis occurring in elderly people.[174]

Gram-negative enterobacteria are the most commonly identified cause of nosocomial pneumonia accounting for over one-half of cases.[175] This probably relates to prior usage of antibiotics both in the individual patient and in the hospital. The relevance of gram-negative enterobacteria in community-acquired pneumonia is uncertain. There is some suspicion that it may be more common in patients admitted from nursing homes, particularly if antibiotics have been recently given to that patient, but evidence for this is limited.[167] Staphylococcal infection is the second most common cause of nosocomial pneumonia in Britain and there is now increased appreciation of the relevance of aspiration pneumonia, particularly in the elderly with neurologic impairment. Although patients most commonly aspirate mouth and oropharyngeal commensal bacteria (including anaerobes), gram-negative enterobacteria may also be important, particularly in patients who have been in the hospital for a few days, because oropharyngeal colonization with gram-negatives is common following hospitalization of elderly patients.

Overall nosocomial pneumonia is second only to urinary tract infection as a cause of hospital-acquired infection. Crude incidence rates are between 1.5 and 8 percent in the acute sector and about 8 percent in long-term care[165,176] although there is a dearth of studies in this area. Pre-existing chest disease and recent antibiotics *do not* appear to increase the overall risk of nosocomial pneumonia.[176] Caution in diagnosis is needed here as a recent preliminary report has suggested that in about one-third of cases urinary tract infection may be misdiagnosed as respiratory infection,[177] with implications on choice and duration of antibiotic therapy.

Initial antibiotic therapy for pneumonia in the elderly differs greatly between community-acquired pneumonia and nosocomial pneumonia. For relatively mild community-acquired infection, ampicillin, amoxycillin, or erythromycin are the drugs of first choice. The dose of erythromycin will need to be reduced in patients with renal impairment. For the more severely ill patient with community-acquired pneumonia a second- or third-generation cephalosporin (e.g., cefuroxime) plus erythromycin is the best first-line combination. For nosocomial pneumonia a quinolone (e.g., ciprofloxacin) *plus* an aminoglycoside *or* a second- or third-generation cephalosporin *plus* an aminoglycoside should be employed. For patients with suspected aspiration, ampicillin or amoxycillin plus metronidazole is the usually accepted treatment. However some authorities now recommend cefuroxime plus metronidazole in order to reliably "cover" gram-negative aspirates. Ciprofloxacin should never be used alone in the primary treatment of pneumonia as it does not reliably kill pneumococcus.

Modification of antibiotic treatment may prove necessary once the results of sputum or blood culture are available.

Mortality from pneumonia in the elderly is high. Most studies suggest mortality rates of 15 to 35 percent or even higher in the most frail elderly.[157,163,168,170,178] As well as death directly related to pneumonia some patients (probably a minority) die of complications such as stroke and pulmonary embolus. Factors predicting death include tachypnea, dehydration, and hypotension.[179] Patients may spend prolonged periods in hospital and take many months to resume full activity.[157] The resolution of radiologic abnormalities may be extremely slow with nearly one-third remaining abnormal 3 months after admission.[156] Thus a "slowly resolving" persistingly abnormal chest x-ray should not necessarily prompt further investigation in the medium term, especially invasive investigation, unless there are accompanying persisting clinical features, or worsening radiology (particularly progressive collapse).

Bronchiectasis and Infection

The true prevalence of bronchiectasis in the elderly is unknown but overall in the population it is a relatively rare condition affecting 1 to 2 per 1,000 population. For most patients the condition is merely a nuisance or a social embarrassment. However, a minority (particularly those colonized by *Pseudomonas aeruginosa*) will have rapidly progressive disease with repeated severe exacerbations.

The definition of bronchiectasis is pathologic with dilated bronchi and bronchioles and ciliary absence or dysfunction. Its causes are varied and include congenital causes (e.g., Kartagener syndrome: bronchiectasis in association with dextrocardia), cystic fibrosis (patients under 40 years); postinfective (following bronchial obstruction, following tuberculosis or whooping cough); obstructive (e.g., foreign body, carcinoma); and rarely in association with pulmonary eosinophilia and aspergillus infection.

Pathology comprises replacement of the bronchial wall with squamous epithelium often with ulceration. There is usually destruction of the bronchial walls and cartilage with significant infiltration of the lumen with inflammatory cells particularly neutrophils. There is hypertrophy of the bronchial arterial tree.

Typical clinical features are cough and the production of large amounts of purulent sputum (often deeply green). Hemoptysis is common (usually only streaks or small amounts but occasionally severe). Halitosis may produce profound social embarrassment in a minority. There is often associated airways obstruction and severe bronchiectasis may produce a restrictive ventilatory deficit. In such cases the patient will complain of dyspnea and/or wheeze. Clubbing is common and there are usually coarse or midcharacter crepitations chronically present in the affected region(s). For any patient with more than mild disease early stages of infection may be difficult to identify as they only involve a slight qualitative or quantitative change in the production of already purulent sputum, perhaps with recurrence of exacerbation of hemoptysis.

The interpretation of microbiological results is made difficult for several reasons. Most patients are chronically colonized by a variety of organisms (most commonly *Haemophilus influenzae*[180]). Second, different areas of the abnormal bronchial tree may harbor different bacterial pathogens making sputum sampling somewhat patchy and possibly unrepresentative. Third, some patients with bronchiectasis harbor forms of *Haemophilus* difficult to identify on sputum culture because of absence of a cell wall.[181] Preventative therapy essentially comprises regular postural drainage. Supportive treatment for established exacerbation is similar to that discussed above for pneumonia with the addition of increased postural drainage (possibly using oxygen via nasal cannula because postural changes may produce hypoxia). Even in the absence of *Pseudomonas* infection there is need for broad-spectrum antibiotics with β-lactamase activity. Supranormal doses may be needed to achieve sputum penetration with some evidence of increased efficacy and longer exacerbation-free interval.[182,183]

Patients who have infective relapses frequently may respond to nebulized antibiotics as prophylaxis.[183] Recurrent infection with *Pseudomonas aeruginosa* is particularly problematic. Oral ciprofloxacin is a first-line treatment but in most cases the organism develops early resistance to this agent.

Mycobacterial Infections

The prevalence of tuberculosis is once again increasing in the Western world with a disproportionate rise in prevalence in elderly people.[184–187] This may partly be due to increasing urban deprivation, which also disproportionately affects the elderly,[188] and to relative ease of transmission in nursing and residential homes.[189] Whatever the reason for the increase, tuberculosis is more common in the elderly with notification rates approximately five times those in young adults, in the 65 to 75 year age range (approximately 20 per 10,000 population), and up to 12 times those in young adults in the over 75 age range (approximately 60 per 10,000).[186,187]

Presentation

Most cases of tuberculosis in the elderly represent reactivation of previous (often unrecognized) disease. This may be precipitated by the depressed immunocompetence of normal aging, malnutrition (often in association with alcohol excess), human immunodeficiency virus (HIV) infection, diabetes mellitus, corticosteroid therapy, gastrectomy,[190] and even cigarette smoking.[191]

Presenting features of tuberculosis in old age are similar to those in younger patients and include weight loss, cough, hemoptysis, pyrexia, and night sweats. However, in addition the elderly are more likely to have hypoalbuminemia, abnormal liver function tests, hypokalemia, and hyponatremia.[192] Miliary tuberculosis seems more common in the elderly, this presentation occurring in up to 1 in 20 cases.[185] Presentation in such cases may be atypical and subacute.

Renal and genitourinary tuberculosis is less common in older people[185] but when present is often asymptomatic. Bony and joint tuberculosis affects approximately 5 percent of elderly patients with the disease.[185] It most commonly involves the spine often with paravertebral infection.[193]

A failure to diagnose the condition during life in the elderly is evidenced by an up to 20-fold disparity (versus the young) in the number of cases diagnosed at postmortem.[185,194] Although this may in part reflect a reluctance on the part of elderly procedures such as bone marrow aspiration and bronchoscopy, it also suggests a low index of suspicion among physicians.

The radiologic features of tuberculosis in the elderly are similar to those in younger patients but with a greater prevalence of mid- and lower zone shadowing.[185,195] The most common radiologic appearance is that of old healed disease with a peripheral calcified primary complex and calcified hilar nodes together with upper zone patchy calcification and possibly pleural thickening ("capping"). Cavitation is present in 20 to 30 percent and pleural effusions in approximately 15 percent.[185,195] In such cases it may be difficult to differentiate tuberculosis from primary lung malignancy especially in apical disease. The computed tomography (CT) scan may be of use here when more invasive tests are thought inappropriate. A normal chest x-ray almost excludes tuberculosis with a very rare exception of endobronchial postprimary disease.[196]

Besides radiography other useful screening investigations include C-reactive protein or ESR estimation and tuberculin skin test, although the latter must be interpreted with caution in elderly patients with possible postprimary disease. Biochemical abnormalities (as discussed above) are common as is a normochromic normocytic anemia and mildly raised peripheral white blood cell count.

A grade 3 or 4 positive Heaf skin test (a ring of six confluent papules filled-in in the center with induration with or without ulceration) or a greater than 10-mm reaction on Mantoux skin testing is diagnostic of present *or past* tuberculous infection. Thus the emergence or "conversion" from skin test negativity to skin test positivity suggests active disease. However, repeated skin testing is known to produce a "booster" effect. This phenomena occurs in those individuals who have suffered previous (often asymptomatic) infection but whose skin test reactivity has fallen over many years and is subsequently stimulated once again by skin testing so that a first test is negative but a second or subsequent test may be positive.[197] More commonly a tuberculin skin test may be falsely negative in association with other infections (bacterial or viral), corticosteroids, sarcoidosis, lymphoma, malnutrition, or even massive overwhelming tuberculous infection.

Isolation of *Mycobacterium tuberculosis* is the only absolute confirmation of active infection. The organism is isolated from approximately two-thirds of elderly patients treated for active disease, a slightly lower percentage than that in younger patients.[185] Smear positivity (identification of the organism by simple Ziehl-Neelsen or Kinyoun staining of sputum) in an untreated patient is very highly suggestive of infectivity. More commonly, sputum culture in a Lowenstein-Jensen medium is necessary and may require up to 8 weeks. Common practice is to send at least three good sputum samples for microscopy and culture before any antituberculous therapy is given. This is important not only for confirmation of diagnosis but also to establish antimicrobial sensitivities. Where sputum production is difficult this may be aided by physiotherapy and inhalation of ultrasonically nebulized saline. Bronchoscopy and washings of radiologically affected areas may occasionally be required as may aspiration of pleural fluid together with pleural biopsy. When renal or genitourinary infection is suspected then three samples of early morning urine should be sent for microscopy and culture. Bone marrow aspiration, liver biopsy, synovial aspiration, or lymph node biopsy may be helpful in disseminated disease.

Treatment

The British Thoracic Society has published recommendations on the treatment of tuberculosis.[198] For those patients with pulmonary disease 6 months of treatment with rifampicin and isoniazid together with pyrazinamide and ethambutol for the first 2 months is advised. This is generally applicable to the elderly with a possible omission of ethambutol because of the increased risk of eye toxicity in old age. The same drugs may be appropriate to nonpulmonary disease although the duration of chemotherapy may need to be longer. Combined preparations are recognized to improve medication compliance, which may be particularly problematic in the elderly.

Other agents may be helpful or even essential in a small minority of cases depending on sensitivity results. These may include thiacetazone, para-aminosalicylic acid, capreomycin, kanomycin, cycloserine, prothionamide, and viomycin. Streptomycin is occasionally used but may produce vestibular damage and for this reason is usually avoided in the elderly.

Liver function tests should be checked before commencement of therapy. However, a transient hepatic enzyme rise is common and does not indicate the need for modification of treatment unless hepatitis or jaundice occur. If ethambutol is used visual acuity should be checked by an ophthalmologist before and during treatment. Isoniazid-related peripheral neuropathy is preventable by pyridoxine 10 mg daily. Treatment side effects seem to be more common in old people.[185,199] Overall almost 1 in 5 elderly people will experience treatment side effects.

Patients with a positive smear should be isolated from other hospitalized patients until they have received adequate chemotherapy for at least 2 weeks. Local infection control policy should be adhered to.

The treatment of tuberculosis is not complete without contact tracing, which is performed by public health departments. Tuberculosis is a notifiable condition. Prophylaxis is usually given to children who have not been previously immunized, have been in contact with a proven case of active disease, and have a positive skin test. It may seem logical that the same criteria should apply to elderly patients especially those in nursing homes.[200]

Atypical mycobacterial infection is relatively rare in Britain. There is no direct evidence that it is more common in older people although some atypical mycobacteria seem to be more likely to cause infection in patients with pre-existing respiratory conditions that may be more common in the elderly.[201] Clinical features of mycobacterial infection are similar to those of true tuberculosis although upper lobe and pleural involvement appears more common.[202] Culture of nontuberculous mycobacteria may take longer than that of *Mycobacterium tuberculosis* and sensitivity patterns are often unusual. Treatment guidelines have been published by the American Thoracic Society.[202]

Lung Cancer and Other Thoracic Neoplasms

Aging is a major and independent risk factor for the development of malignant disease. Both lung cancer and pleural mesothelioma are most common in older people. However, partly because of a nihilistic attitude toward diagnosis and treatment the management of thoracic neoplasms in the elderly has not advanced at the same rate as that of the same conditions in younger patients.

Bronchogenic Carcinoma

Lung cancer mortality is highest in the aged. In elderly men mortality has, in common with that in younger men, fallen slightly in the last decade although it continues to rise in women over the age of 60.[203] Almost 95 percent of lung cancer is caused by cigarette smoking with the highest rates not surprisingly occurring in those with the highest uptake of smoking habit (men born between 1910 and 1920).[68] Asbestos exposure is a contributory factor in a minority of cases and is multiplicative to the risk caused by cigarette smoking.[204]

Presentation

Presenting symptoms of lung cancer in the elderly do not differ from those in younger patients (chest pain, cough, hemoptysis, breathlessness, weight loss, etc.). However, elderly patients tend to present with more advanced disease.[205] In contrast with many other respiratory and nonrespiratory conditions in elderly people, nonspecific presentation is unusual unless patients present with infective complications. On the other hand the existence of multiple pathology in many elderly patients means that lung cancer may be discovered as a consequential finding during investigation of other conditions.

Cytologic confirmation of cancer type may be invaluable in management (see below). The first step is cytologic examination of expectorated sputum. Success, however, is critically dependent on not only the patient's ability to expectorate but also upon the skill and experience of the cytologist. The use of nebulized saline may aid sputum expectoration. Cytologic examination of fine-needle aspirates under CT scan control may also be helpful. Flexible bronchoscopy is well tolerated and safe even in very old patients.[206] The advantages of accurate histologic diagnosis are discussed below but in at least one series 60 percent of bronchoscopies resulted in the exclusion of a tumor and diagnosis of insignificant or curable pathology (e.g., tuberculosis) instead.[206]

Apart from histologic diagnosis the other indication for bronchoscopy may be for tumor staging (e.g., carinal widening suggesting mediastinal lymph node involvement). CT scanning of the thorax may be invaluable in this process.

There is considerable evidence that elderly patients are less likely to be referred for bronchoscopy with current rates of histologic confirmation (40 to 60 percent) falling well below those in younger patients (more than 80 percent).[207] It may be, however, that some of this discrepancy is not inappropriate as relatively fit elderly patients with possible lung cancer as a single pathology are more likely (appropriately) to be referred to respiratory physicians or even thoracic surgeons, whereas those with multiple pathology who are perhaps less fit for investigation or treatment are more likely (appropriately) to be referred to geriatricians.

Non-Small Cell Lung Cancer

Squamous cell carcinoma is the most common form of lung cancer in old age accounting for 45 to 70 percent of cases.[206] Other non-small cell types (adenocarcinoma, bronchoalveolar carcinoma, and large cell carcinoma) together account for 20 to 25 percent of cases.

As surgical resection is at present the only chance of cure for non-small cell lung cancer, staging is vital in assessment. Full details of staging criteria are beyond the scope of this chapter.[208] However, the single most important factor in staging is mediastinal lymph node involvement. Mediastinal lymph node size can be accurately assessed by CT scanning and/or bronchoscopy, although enlarged mediastinal nodes should if possible be biopsied if there is no other evidence that the tumor is inoperable because lymphadenopathy does not always indicate metastatic spread.

Distant (extrathoracic) spread is in theory a contraindication to surgical intervention. However, there is no evidence that ultrasonic or invasive search for distant metastases is valuable unless physical examination or simple biochemical or hematologic testing suggests their presence.

Staging by uncomfortable and/or invasive methods is difficult to justify if the patient is unfit for surgical intervention. Age alone, however, is not a contraindication to surgery. The presence of comorbid multiple pathology should be assessed in the same way as in younger patients. Particular attention must be given to respiratory function and in borderline cases lung isotope scanning may help determine whether the patient has sufficient respiratory reserve to undergo pneumonectomy (is the involved lung contributing a significant proportion of the patient's vital capacity or FEV_1?). In most centers elderly patients are much less likely to undergo pneumonectomy or indeed any form of surgical intervention. However, studies from several centers have indicated 5-year survival rates of between 35 and 50 percent, little different than those in younger patients.[209–211] A recent report has also shown that solitary brain metastasis in non-small cell lung cancer may be successfully treated with surgical intervention with prolonged (years) survival.[212] Although all the patients in this study were under 65 years of age it provides some evidence that single brain metastasis should not be generally regarded as uniformly fatal and should stimulate further research in this area in older patients.

A recent meta-analysis of chemotherapy for non-small cell carcinoma has concluded that there is no benefit in terms of long-term survival and any small benefit to be gained in short-term (6 months) survival is probably more than outweighed by high levels of toxicity. Almost all the studies in this analysis included cisplatin in their treatment regimens. This drug is highly nephrotoxic (potentially more so in the elderly with pre-existing renal impairment). There is currently no justification for advocating the use of chemotherapy in non-small cell carcinoma in elderly patients.[213]

Radiotherapy for non-small cell lung cancer is similarly controversial. There is limited evidence that radical radiotherapy may be particularly suitable for the 70- to 80-year-old age group;[214] however the data are very limited. Radiotherapy is most commonly used for symptom palliation both of local disease (especially the treatment of hemoptysis)[215] and metastatic spread (particularly bony pain). There is now good evidence that the use of only two fractions of radiotherapy 1 week apart is equally effective in symptom palliation as multiple fractions spread over a longer period.[216] This is a particularly important finding in terms of improving quality of life of patients by reducing hospitalization time or trips to outpatient radiotherapy departments.

Small Cell Lung Cancer

Small cell lung cancer accounts for about one-quarter of all lung cancers in the elderly. The over 70 age group comprises about 20 percent of all small cell lung cancer patients.[217] Small cell lung cancer has very different growth patterns and clinical characteristics than non-small cell lung cancer. It is a rapidly growing tumor and is almost always metastasized by the time of diagnosis; thus surgery has little or no place in its management. Conversely it is highly sensitive to therapeutic agents but responders have a very high relapse rate. Combination chemotherapy has improved median survival but produces long-term survival in only a minority of patients. Extending the duration of chemotherapy or using "maintenance chemotherapy" in cyclical form has produced little significant advance.

The use of multiagent "high-intensity" chemotherapy is generally advocated in younger patients. However, such regimens have high levels of toxicity in the elderly without significant extra survival benefit and single-agent "low-intensity" regimens using etoposide or other podophylotoxins produce similar survival rates with less toxicity. Untreated small cell lung cancer has a median survival of approximately 3 months. Patients with limited disease (no spread outside one hemithorax) treated with podophylotoxins have median survival of approximately 12 months whereas for those with extensive disease median survival is approximately 9 months.[218–220] Furthermore etoposide is administered orally reducing the need for hospitalization or frequent outpatient attendance.

Pleural Mesothelioma

Pleural mesothelioma is caused by air-borne respirable asbestos (particularly blue asbestos) dust usually over a period of years. In the United Kingdom it primarily occurs in response to occupational exposure (shipyard workers, plumbers, gas fitters and central heating engineers, electricians, builders, demolition workers, asbestos factory workers). However, it is most common in the elderly, particularly the 65- to 74-year-old age group,[221] as clinical manifestations occur only after a latent period of between 20 and 40 years.

Presentation

Mesothelioma most commonly presents with breathlessness due to pleural effusion or with chest wall pain. Pleural aspiration and conventional pleural biopsy only yield positive results in approximately 50 percent of patients.[222] Thoracoscopy with direct visualization of the pleura and hence the tumor (well tolerated in the elderly) almost always provides diagnostic material on biopsy.[223]

Mesothelioma is uniformly fatal but more rapidly so in the elderly in whom median survival is less than 12 months.[224] Mesothelioma is uniformly insensitive to chemotherapy or radiotherapy and only very rarely resectable (pleurectomy). Treatment is almost always palliative. Mesothelioma is a compensatable condition even without definite histologic confirmation. However, such confirmation may aid claims through the courts, which usually result in much higher levels of settlement. Local trade union representatives can offer advice and support in the pursuit of legal claims.

Other Lung Tumors

Lymphomas

Although lymphomas are rarely confined to the thorax, mediastinal involvement and parenchymal infiltration are not uncommon. There has been a rise in incidence of lymphoma since the 1960s. The incidence of non-Hodgkins lymphoma increases directly with age with about one-third of patients being over the age of 70 years. Conversely Hodgkins disease has a bimodal incidence with peaks at about 30 and 65 years.[225] Increasing age adversely affects survival.[226,227]

There have recently been promising advances in the development of intensive therapy regimens specific to the elderly with Hodgkin's disease.[228] Elderly patients seem less able to tolerate standard regimens.[229]

Non-Hodgkin's lymphoma can be divided into three subgroups in terms of prognosis. High-grade disease responds well to multiagent chemotherapy in younger patients but the elderly treated with similar combinations suffer unacceptable levels of toxicity. Recently regimens including podophyllotoxins have been developed for the elderly and seem to produce useful response with minimal toxicity.[230] The use of α-interferon may improve survival but further studies in the elderly are necessary.

Carcinoid tumors

About 20 percent of all cases of carcinoid tumors occur in the elderly. However they are rare, accounting for less than 1 percent of all thoracic tumors. Age adversely affects prognosis in most studies.[231] Resection or laser ablation is the treatment of choice with the latter being particularly suitable for elderly patients especially those with multiple other pathologies.[232] Occasionally carcinoid tumors may metastasize. In such cases there is no effective treatment.

Squamous papillomas

Squamous papillomas are relatively rare tumors usually occurring in smokers. They may be solitary or multiple and vary in histology from completely noninvasive to invasive and metastatic carcinoma. Endoscopic removal is the treatment of choice.

Other thoracic tumors

These comprise hamartomas and other benign lung tumors, mediastinal tumors (mainly teratomas and neurogenic tumors), salivary gland tumors, and thymomas. All are rare in the elderly and are not discussed further.

Palliative Therapy and Quality of Life in Lung Neoplasms in the Elderly

It is logical to assume that response to chemotherapy or radiotherapy (as assessed, for example, by radiologic tumor shrinkage) will be associated with improved quality of life and levels of activity. However, this has not been carefully assessed in the elderly. The performance scores used to measure activity and quality of life in cancer are usually not appropriate for elderly patients, and there is a need for appropriate methods of measurement.

The palliative use of radiotherapy for treatment of bony pain and hemoptysis has already been discussed. Laser photocoagulation[233] or cryotherapy[234] of large endobronchial tumors may improve stridor and breathlessness. Insertion of endobronchial stents can dramatically improve breathlessness in patients with large airway obstruction, and can now be accomplished during bronchoscopy without the need for general anesthetic.[235] A recent preliminary report has shown that cryotherapy not only improves breathlessness but also produces a significant improvement in quality of life, fatigue, physical activity, and depression.[236]

The judicious use of nonsteroidal anti-inflammatory agents may improve bone pain. There is a wealth of literature on pain control in cancer that is beyond the scope of this chapter; however, it is a disturbing fact that approximately one-third of cancer patients still suffer pain and/or other distressing physical symptoms (e.g., nausea) in the latter stages of their illness. Referral to pain control teams, palliative care teams, and inpatient or outpatient hospice care should always be considered. Macmillan nurses play an invaluable role both in physical palliation and emotional support in the United Kingdom.

As in many aspects of care of elderly patients the physician often needs to communicate not only with the patients themselves but also with relatives. The request that the doctor does "not tell the patient the bad news" is frequently heard from caring relatives. Such a request must always be taken seriously as the relatives will usually have deep insights into the emotional needs and capabilities of the patient. However, it is vital to remember that the primary relationship is between physician and patient and if the physician is perceived by the patient to be withholding information this will seriously damage the doctor/patient relationship and erode trust. A general policy of open access to (without insistence upon) information from doctor to patient should operate regardless of the patient's age.

Pulmonary Embolic Disease

Pulmonary embolic disease is common in the elderly particularly the ill elderly. It is estimated that over one-half of subjects with pulmonary embolism are over the age of 65.[237] Age-associated risk factors include immobility, hemiplegia, cancer, surgery, and hip fracture. Clinical features of pulmonary embolism in elderly patients differ little from those in the young.[238] These are usually acute and comprise breathlessness, severe central constricting chest pain (in large hemodynamically compromising emboli), pleuritic chest pain (in more peripheral emboli), and hemoptysis. Occasionally symptoms may be chronic or subacute due to multiple emboli and comprise gradual onset of breathlessness and right-sided cardiac failure. Only about one-fifth of patients present atypically (usually with radiologic abnormalities, most commonly linear atelectasis). Patients with very large emboli will present with chest pain, breathlessness, and severe hypotension often with right ventricular heave and signs of right-sided cardiac strain.

Physical signs as well as those of right-sided strain include tachypnea, cyanosis, tachycardia, localized crepitations, pleural rub, and (particularly in a patient with pre-existing asthma or COPD) wheeze.

Unfortunately diagnosis based on clinical features or on investigations short of pulmonary angiography is inaccurate with high false-positive and false-negative rates.[237,239] Diagnosis may be particularly difficult in patients (often the elderly) with previous respiratory disease. The accuracy of the ventilation-perfusion (V/Q) scan may be particularly compromised by this. Simple screening tests may do little other than enhance clinical suspicion. Electrocardiograms will show right-sided strain in a minority of cases. Abnormalities include right bundle branch block, P "pulmonale", S wave in lead 1 and Q wave and T wave inversion in lead 3 (S_1 Q_3 T_3). Pulmonary embolism may also precipitate atrial fibrillation. Blood gas estimation frequently reveals hypoxia in association with hypocapnia. These findings are not specific. The chest x-ray may be normal (thus helping to exclude other pathologies) or occasionally may show effusions, basal atelectasis, or wedge-shaped areas of hypoperfusion.

An entirely normal V/Q scan essentially excludes pulmonary embolism. The presence of multiple perfusion defects with normal ventilation (a mismatched scan) is highly suggestive of pulmonary embolic disease. However, matched ventilation perfusion defect(s) will occur if the scan has been delayed for 24 hours or more. Such a scan may be classified as having a low or intermediate probability for pulmonary embolism but up to one-third of patients with scans so classified will have pulmonary embolism.[237]

Arguably the absolute diagnosis of pulmonary embolism is less critical in the presence of a proven diagnosis of deep venous thrombosis (DVT). Ultrasound and impedance plethysmography is the investigation of choice for potential DVT. It is as accurate as venography without the complications.[238]

However, the only absolutely definite diagnostic investigation for pulmonary embolism is pulmonary angiography. This may be difficult or impossible in ill, frail elderly patients and is not without risk although the limited evidence available suggests that the risks are no higher in elderly patients.[238,240]

Treatment

Immediate supportive therapy comprises supplemental oxygen (usually high inspired percentage as dictated by blood gas measurement) and analgesia in patients with pleuritic chest pain. Anticoagulation, initially with intravenous or subcutaneous heparin, should aim to keep the activated partial thromboplastin time at about twice the control value. Following 5 to 7 days of heparinization, maintenance therapy should be with oral anticoagulation, usually warfarin, aiming for an international normalized ratio of between 2 and 3. Recent evidence suggests that the classic duration of anticoagulation is excessive and that for pulmonary emboli 3 months anticoagulation is adequate, 1 month being adequate for DVT.[241]

Anticoagulation will need frequent hematologic monitoring. Patients should receive written and verbal information regarding side effects and what to do should these arise as well as information on drug interactions and which drugs to avoid. Access to outpatient warfarin clinics may prove difficult for elderly patients and domiciliary phlebotomy may need to be provided in some cases.

A small proportion of patients who suffer recurrent pulmonary emboli despite anticoagulation may benefit from the insertion of a filter device into the inferior vena cava. These can now be inserted by a minimally invasive percutaneous procedure.

For patients with catastrophic acute pulmonary emboli associated with circulatory collapse the prognosis is dire with a mortality rate of over 80 percent.[241] Thrombolysis may be beneficial and the minority of patients may be appropriate for surgical pulmonary embolectomy. This latter can be performed as an open procedure or by percutaneous suction catheterization. It is clear that many frail elderly patients may not be suitable for such aggressive invasive measures. This is probably particularly true of those with medical conditions that put them at the highest risk of pulmonary embolic disease (stroke, cancers, the frail elderly female patient with fractured neck of femur).

Fibrotic (Interstitial) Lung Diseases

Fibrotic (interstitial) lung diseases comprise a wide variety of pathologies and etiologies and are generally taken not to include carcinomas, lymphomas, other neoplasms, and infection.

Epidemiology

Many fibrotic interstitial lung diseases have a higher prevalence in elderly people. These include the more common conditions of fibrosing alveolitis in association with connective tissue disorders, cryptogenic fibrosing alveolitis, and the pneumoconioses associated with industrial dust exposures. Some of the rarer conditions are also more common in the elderly. These include Wegener's granulomatosis, amyloidosis, and cryptogenic organizing pneumonia. Conversely sarcoidosis is extremely rare as a primary presentation in elderly people and chronic eosinophilic pneumonia less common than in younger adults.

The mortality rate from all causes of pulmonary fibrosis is

increasing in both men and women.[242] Peak of death from all fibrotic causes (both absolute numbers of deaths and percentage of deaths per head of age [stratified population]) occurs in the 75- to 84-year-old age group.[242]

Investigations

Fibrotic interstitial lung diseases classically produce a restrictive ventilatory defect on spirometry (relatively preserved forced expiratory flow with a reduced forced vital capacity and thus a normal or raised FEV_1/FVC ratio). Wegener's granulomatosis, however, usually produces an obstructive pattern (low FEV_1/FVC ratio). Total lung capacity is reduced as is the transfer factor (TL_{co}). The transfer coefficient (K_{co}), which is essentially the transfer factor corrected for lung volumes, is generally affected later than the TL_{co}. Blood gas analysis commonly reveals hypoxia often with hypocapnia (the latter secondary to hyperventilation).

Chest X-ray may be normal in early disease, and even in some more advanced cases.[243] More commonly characteristic parenchymal shadowing in the form of reticular, nodular, reticulonodular, linear, or ground-glass appearances may be present. The distribution of such shadowing may be a clue to diagnosis. For example a "reversed bat's wing" appearance (i.e., peripheral shadowing) is commonly seen in chronic pulmonary eosinophilia and cryptogenic organizing pneumonia. The presence of nonparenchymal abnormalities on chest x-ray (e.g., eggshell calcification of hilar lymph nodes in silicosis or pleural involvement in association with asbestosis) may be helpful. However, diagnosis based on the type of distribution of shadowing on chest x-rays is possible in less than 20 percent of cases.[244]

Conversely CT or high-resolution CT scanning has a high diagnostic accuracy.[244–246] Classification of CT scan abnormalities is based both on the site of the abnormality and its nature. Abnormalities may be classified as occurring in three separate sites or compartments: the peripheral compartment (the pleura and interlobular sector); the middle compartment (most of the central areas of the lung); and the axial compartment (immediately surrounding the mediastinum and extending along the lymphatics, and vascular and bronchial structures). A variety of characteristic abnormalities is seen including a ground-glass appearance suggesting very active disease, a nodular appearance often associated with sarcoidosis and pneumoconiosis, and a cystic appearance of end-stage alveolitis.

CT patterns may be so helpful (both in diagnosis and estimation of disease activity and progression[246]) as sometimes to render other investigations (e.g., lung biopsy) redundant. Occasionally bronchoalveolar lavage may be indicated for differential diagnosis and characteristic patterns of cellular abnormality have been described in different conditions.[247] However, bronchoalveolar lavage remains more commonly a research tool.

Lung biopsy may be by means of transbronchial technique, a percutaneous drill technique, or an open technique. Any of these procedures involves morbidity and a small risk of mortality (see below) and thus should not be undertaken lightly. Even if the patient is fit for biopsy it is probably unnecessary in those with stable or mild disease or those with a typical presentation. When biopsy *is* necessary, transbronchial lung biopsy is less invasive and can be performed in patients who would be unfit for open biopsy. Multiple transbronchial biopsies are usually taken with a high diagnostic rate[248] especially in a disease with a characteristic histologic pattern. Mortality rate of transbronchial biopsy in one very large series was only 0.2 percent, the most common complications (overall rate less than 10 percent) being pneumothorax and bleeding.[249]

Percutaneous drill biopsy has been little studied and is not commonly used. This may reflect its slightly higher complication rate and lower diagnostic yield when compared with transbronchial biopsy.

Open lung biopsy is a surgical procedure, requiring a general anesthetic. It is most commonly employed when transbronchial biopsy has failed to achieve a diagnosis, and as well as producing a large enough material for increased diagnostic yield the larger sample is usually able to produce a good estimate of disease activity. The mortality rate, however, is 1 to 2 percent. Other complications include infection and persistent pneumothorax in approximately one in six patients.[250,251]

Specific Conditions

Pneumoconioses

Pneumoconiosis results from an abnormal lung parenchymal reaction to respirable *inorganic* dusts usually in an occupational context. The most common dusts involved are coal (producing coal workers pneumoconiosis), silica (producing silicosis), and asbestos (producing asbestosis).

Coal workers pneumoconiosis is the result of fibrosis in alveoli and interlobular sector with compensatory dilatation of other alveoli leading to centrilobular emphysema. This may progress (even after cessation of occupational exposure) to the insidious complicated pneumoconiosis or progressive massive fibrosis (PMF). PMF mainly affects the upper lobes, which contain large fibrotic masses several centimeters across often with necrotic centers. PMF is associated with the increased likelihood of autoimmune antibodies such an antinuclear antibody and rheumatoid factor.[252] Occasionally, in patients with rheumatoid arthritis, Caplan's syndrome may result. This takes the form of flitting radiologic lesions in the lung that occasionally necrose or calcify. These may be associated with pleural effusion.

An obstructive ventilatory picture is common in patients with simple pneumoconiosis especially where there is associated central alveolar emphysema. PMF produces both restrictive and obstructive defects, the restrictive defects in part being the result of reduced lung volume. Progression to cor pulmonale and respiratory failure is not uncommon.

Symptoms usually comprise those of chronic bronchitis together with the production of coal-stained black sputum (melanoptysis). Patients often erroneously feel that they have coughed up blood, although true hemoptysis is indeed common in PMF. Patients are not clubbed. Complicated pneumoconiosis is a compensatable industrial disease. There is no specific treatment other than supportive therapy and treatment of any reversibility of airways obstruction.

Silicosis

High occupational risk occurs in quarrying, sand blasting, mining (copper, tin, gold) boiler workers, and some forms of brick manufacture.

Acute silicosis may occur after intense brief exposure to silica dust, and this is rare in old age. It is associated with extreme dyspnea and a chest x-ray appearance similar to that of pulmonary edema. It may be fatal within weeks or months. More commonly, chronic silicosis has similar pathologic features to coal workers pneumoconiosis with fibrosis of lymphatics, blood vessels, and bronchi and some degree of secondary emphysema. Active chronic silicosis predisposes to pulmonary tuberculosis.

There are usually mixed obstructive and restrictive ventilatory defects, hypoxia, and cor pulmonale in the later stages. Radiologic abnormalities usually comprise miliary or nodular lesions throughout all the lung fields especially in the middle and upper zones. In addition there may be larger, sometimes cavitated, shadowing. "Eggshell" calcification of the hilar lymph nodes is pathognomonic.

Symptoms are gradually progressive over several years. They are similar to those of chronic bronchitis and chronic obstructive pulmonary disease together with occasional hemoptysis, cachexia, and weight loss. In such circumstances tuberculosis needs to be actively excluded.

Treatment is once again supportive and the disease is notifiable and compensatable.

Asbestosis

Asbestosis is a fibrotic condition of the lungs due to usually prolonged occupational exposure to asbestos dust. Occupations at greatest risk comprise shipyard workers, asbestos factory workers, plumbers and gas fitters, insulation workers, rail workers, electricians, demolition workers, and builders. Asbestosis must be distinguished from asbestos-related pleural thickening and calcification, mesothelioma, and bronchogenic carcinoma—all of which can also be precipitated by asbestos exposure. Fibrosis originates in the alveoli and bronchioles. It is most marked in the lung bases but may spread to involve the whole of the lungs. Progressive massive fibrosis is not a common feature.

A recent survey has shown that there may be a nihilistic attitude to the development of fibrotic interstitial lung disease in those previously exposed to asbestos, with approximately 5 percent of such individuals in fact having another treatable interstitial lung disease.[253]

In common with mesothelioma and bronchial carcinoma, the latent period after exposure before the development of asbestosis may be in excess of 20 years and it is not unusual for symptoms to appear for the first time in the elderly. Smokers with asbestosis should be counseled strongly about smoking cessation because smoking and asbestosis have a synergistic effect on the development of bronchial carcinoma.

The major ventilatory defect is restrictive with reduced transfer factor and reduced total lung compliance. Radiologic appearance include fine mottling and patchy streaky fibrosis often with associated pleural lesions (a diagnostic clue), most commonly on the diaphragm (coin lesions).

Symptoms initially comprise breathlessness on exertion and later cough, weight loss, and fatigue. Patients are usually clubbed with fine bilateral basal crepitations. Treatment is oncc again supportive. Asbestosis is a notifiable and compensatable disease.

Extrinsic allergic alveolitis

Extrinsic allergic alveolitis is essentially a type III immunologic reaction to organic dusts at the alveolus level. It follows chronic repeated exposure and is associated with the formation of systemic precipating antibodies (precipitins). An acute form (type I reaction) can occur more rarely, with shivers, acute dyspnea, and cough. Budgerigar-Fancier's lung is probably the most common form.[254] There is some suggestion that the keeping of budgerigars as pets is more common in the elderly but that, independent of this, age is an important prognostic indicator.[255] Other extrinsic alveolitides include farmer's lung (secondary to molds in damp straw and hay), ventilation pneumonitis (due to thermophylic actinomycetes in air conditioning systems), and mushroom workers lung (from mushroom spores). Symptoms comprise breathlessness on exertion progressing to breathlessness at rest with production of sputum. Clubbing is uncommon but when present may be associated with a poorer prognosis.[256] Weight loss (often marked) is not unusual.

A diffuse ground-glass or micronodular pattern is the most common radiologic abnormality and etiologic diagnosis is by identification of the appropriate serum precipitins. Treatment comprises removal of or from the offending antigen. This may prove difficult in a patient who is particularly attached to his or her pets. Furthermore it is recognized that in some affected patients the disease is not progressive despite continued exposure to the offending antigen whereas in others removal of the antigen does not prevent progression.[257] Some patients may require corticosteroid or immunosuppressive therapy as discussed below for cryptogenic fibrosing alveolitis.

Cryptogenic fibrosing alveolitis

Cryptogenic fibrosing alveolitis is the most common interstitial lung disease in the elderly. Estimates of the peak age at presentation have increased recently to a mean of about 60 years.[258] There may be a slight male excess in prevalence.[259] Overall the estimated prevalence is about 5 cases per 100,000 population. There is a rare familial form of the disease but otherwise its etiology is unknown. Histologic appearances are many and varied. The two ends of the spectrum of histology are a fibrotic pattern in which the alveoli are replaced by collagen and there is very little active inflammation and a cellular pattern with infiltration of lymphocytes, neutrophils, and eosinophils into the interstitium with the alveolar spaces containing larger numbers of macrophages. It is possible but not certain that the cellular form *progresses* to the fibrotic form. However, the cellular appearance is certainly associated with an increased chance of steroid responsiveness and with a better prognosis.[259,260]

Typical presentation is with breathlessness on exertion progressing to breathlessness at rest. There is some suspicion that elderly patients present later than younger patients possibly because of reduced appreciation of breathlessness.[10] Many patients complain of a productive cough and the volume of sputum produced relates negatively to prognosis.[261] Minor hemoptysis is fairly common. Patients will have fine crepitations ("velcro" crepitations) at the bases possibly extending to mid and even upper zones. The majority are clubbed and hypertrophic pulmonary osteoarthropathy is described. In most patients the disease progresses slowly and insidiously with an untreated 50 percent mortality at about 5 years.[258] In the rarer, although classically described Hamman-Rich syndrome progression is more rapid (over 6 months or so to death if untreated). In such cases there may be pyrexia, cough, and purulent sputum.

There is a strong association with progression to bronchial carcinoma. Advanced age seems to be associated with a poorer prognosis and with a recently recognized rise in overall mortality from the condition.[262]

Chest x-rays vary from normal to ground-glass appearance or miliary mottling. Abnormalities may be diffuse but are most common in the lower zones.

In addition to supportive treatment, as for the pneumoconioses specific treatment regimens are advocated for the cryptogenic fibrosing alveolitis. There is, however, limited consensus on when to start treatment even in younger patients, although in practice the decision is often based on evidence of progressive disease. A relatively old survey suggested that elderly patients tend to receive less corticosteroid therapy than the young.[263] The response rate to high-dose corticosteroid therapy is up to 30 percent overall but possibly less in the elderly. The addition of azathioprine to high-dose corticosteroid therapy increases the response rate to perhaps as much as 50 percent but there seems to be little benefit in using immunosuppressive therapy in a steroid-sparing role.[264,265] The standard dose of prednisolone in high-dose regimens is up to 100 mg daily for up to 6 to 8 weeks reducing by approximately 20 mg/day, per month to a maintenance dose of 10 mg/day. Any response is usually seen within 3 months.

Fibrosing alveolitis in association with autoimmune disorders

Autoimmune disorders, particularly rheumatoid arthritis but also Sjögrens syndrome, systemic sclerosis and celiac disease can lead to fibrotic lung disease in up to 5 percent of cases. Occasionally respiratory problems precede other manifestations of the disease. The association with rheumatoid arthritis and fibrotic lung disease seems stronger for elderly rheumatoid patients and the condition is more common in men (2:1 M:F ratio). Pathology and clinical features are very similar to those of cryptogenic fibrosing alveolitis although pleural changes are more common on chest x-rays. Treatment regimens and response rates are very similar, although there is less evidence for the value of cyclophosphamide and azathioprine.

Wegener's granulomatosis

Wegener's granulomatosis is a relatively rare condition that is more common in the elderly with a peak age of onset at about 55 years. It is a granulomatous and vasculitic condition principally affecting the lung, upper respiratory tract, and kidneys. Patients present with upper and lower respiratory symptoms including breathlessness, pleuritic chest pain, cough, hemoptysis, epistaxis, sinusitis, rhinitis, and otitis. However, upper respiratory problems are less common in the elderly and renal involvement at this initial diagnosis is more common in this age group.[266] Central nervous system involvement (vasculitis usually presenting with acute confusion or fits) is relatively common in old age.[266] The prevalence of infective complications is not more common in the elderly although mortality from infection is significantly more common in this age group.[266]

Diagnosis is usually by biopsy of the upper and lower respiratory tract or kidneys.[267–269] Circulating antineutrophyl cytoplasmic antibodies are usually positive in the majority of patients including the elderly.[266]

Usual treatment regimens comprise cyclophosphamide and high-dose steroids with initially up to a 90 percent response rate at about 6 to 12 months. However, relapse rates are high (up to 50 percent).[270] There is no evidence that elderly patients with Wegener's granulomatosis show a less aggressive form of the disease and intensive chemotherapy is usually indicated. Although infection is the cause of mortality in a large proportion of elderly patients, this does not seem to correlate with immune suppression due to chemotherapy.[266,271] Indeed there is no evidence that the elderly are more likely to suffer complications of treatment for this condition.

Drug-induced interstitial lung disease

Despite an overall incidence of adverse drug reactions of 10 to 25 percent in elderly people[272] there is little evidence that the elderly are more prone to adverse drug reactions producing inflammatory lung disease.[273,274] However, such iatrogenic disease is more common in the elderly probably by virtue of their increased exposure to multiple drugs. Perhaps the most commonly prescribed are carbamazepine, phenytoin, nitrofurantoin, and amiodarone. Others comprise the cytotoxic agents methotrexate, bleomycin, and busulfan together with gold salts, penicillamine, and sulfasalazine. Treatment comprises withdrawal of the offending drug with occasionally recourse to specific anti-inflammatory therapies.

Cryptogenic organizing pneumonia

Cryptogenic organizing pneumonia is a rare condition but is again slightly more common in the elderly with a peak age of onset of 50 to 60 years. It is characterized by the appearance of buds of connective tissue in the alveoli and small bronchioles. Presenting features comprise breathlessness on exertion and cough and in the majority of patients pyrexias, weight loss, and general malaise. Clubbing is unusual. Radiologic appearances are usually patchy and peripheral. Its importance lies in its rapid (sometimes within days) and frequent (60 percent or more) response to high-dose corticosteroid therapy. Over one-half of the responders will relapse on discontinuing corticosteroids.

Chronic eosinophilic pneumonia

Once again, chronic eosinophilic pneumonia is a rare disease and probably even rarer in the elderly. Most patients have an atopic history.

Sarcoid lung disease

Over the whole population sarcoidosis is the most common idiopathic interstitial lung disease. However, the appearance of sarcoidosis for the first time in an elderly patient is extremely unusual. There is limited evidence that when this does occur the prognosis is slightly worse.

Summary

The diagnosis and investigation of fibrotic interstitial lung disease is relatively complex and specialized. Furthermore even the less rare of these conditions are by no means common. For both of these reasons elderly patients with suspected interstitial lung disease who do not respond to the withdrawal of potential iatrogenic agents (e.g., drugs, budgies) should be referred to a specialist respiratory physician for assessment, diagnosis, and management.

References

1. Lung and Asthma Information Agency: The burden of respiratory disease. Factsheet 95/3, London, 1995
2. Department of Clinical Epidemiology, National Heart and Lung Institute: Respiratory disease in England and Wales. Thorax 1988;43:949–954
3. Hunt A: The elderly at home. A study of people aged sixty-five and over living in the community in England in 1976. HMSO, 1976
4. Renwick DS, Connolly MJ: Prevalence and treatment of chronic airflow obstruction in adults over the age of 45. Thorax 1996;51:164–168
5. Burr ML, Charles TJ, Roy K, Seaton A: Asthma in the elderly: an epidemiological survey. BMJ 1979;1:1041–1044
6. Dodge RR, Burrows B: The prevalence and incidence of asthma and asthma-like symptoms in a general population sample. Am Rev Respir Dis 1980;122:567–575
7. Braman SS, Kaemmerlen JT, Davis SM: Asthma in the elderly. A comparison between patients with recently acquired and long-standing disease. Am Rev Respir Dis 1991;143:336–340
8. Parameswaran K, Bansal SK, Chadda D et al: Asthma in the elderly—underdiagnosed and undertreated? Thorax 1995; 50(suppl 2):A58
9. Roberts SJ, Bateman DN: Which patients are prescribed inhaled anti-asthma drugs? Thorax 1994;49:1090–1095
10. Connolly MJ, Crowley JJ, Charan NB et al: Reduced subjective awareness of bronchoconstriction provoked by methacholine in elderly asthmatic and normal subjects as measured on a simple awareness scale. Thorax 1992;47:410–413
11. Dow L, Coggon D, Holgate ST: Respiratory symptoms as predictors of airways lability in an elderly population. Respir Med 1992;86:27–32
12. Renwick DS, Connolly MJ: Do symptoms predict chronic airflow obstruction and bronchial hyperresponsiveness in older adults? abstracted. Age Ageing 1996;25(suppl 1):8
13. Rackemann FM: Studies in asthma 1. A clinical survey of 1074 patients with asthma followed for two years. J Lab Clin Med 1927;12:1185–1197
14. Walker C, Bode E, Boer L et al: Allergic and nonallergic asthmatics have distinct patterns of T-cell activation and cytokine production in peripheral blood and bronchoalveolar lavage. Am Rev Respir Dis 1992;146:109–115
15. Bentley AM, Menz G, Storz CHR et al: Identification of T lymphocytes, macrophages and activated eosinophils in the bronchial mucosa in intrinsic asthma. Am Rev Respir Dis 1992;146:500–506
16. Environmental and Occupational Health Assembly of the American Thoracic Society: State of the art. Health effects of outdoor air pollution. Am J Respir Crit Care Med 1996;153: 3–50
17. Tattersfield AE: Altounyan Address. Air pollution: brown skies research. Thorax 1996;51:13–22
18. Coggon D: Air pollution in homes, editorial. BMJ 1996;312: 1316
19. Jarvis D, Burney P, Chinn S et al: The association of respiratory symptoms and lung function with the use of domestic gas appliances. Thorax 1990;50(suppl 2):A34
20. Barbee RA, Halon M, Kaltenborn W et al: A longitudinal study of serum IgE in a community cohort: correlations with age, sex, smoking, and atopic status. J Allergy Clin Immunol 1987; 79:919–927
21. Dow L, Coggon D, Campbell MJ et al: The interaction between immunoglobulin E and smoking in airflow obstruction in the elderly. Am Rev Respir Dis 1992;146:402–407
22. Burrows B, Martinez FD, Halonen M et al: Association of asthma with serum IgE levels and skin-test reactivity to allergens. N Engl J Med 1989;320:271–277
23. Connolly MJ, Crowley JJ, Nielson CP et al: Peripheral mononuclear leucocyte beta adrenoceptors and non-specific bronchial

responsiveness to methacholine in young and elderly normal subjects and asthmatic patients. Thorax 1994;49:29–32

24. Connolly MJ, Crowley JJ, Charan NB et al: Impaired bronchodilator response to albuterol in healthy elderly men and women. Chest 1995;108:401–406
25. Nielson CP, Crowley JJ, Vestal RE, Connolly MJ: Impaired beta-adrenoceptor function, increased leucocyte respiratory burst and bronchial hyperresponsiveness. J Allergy Clin Immunol 1992;90:825–832
26. Chang W, Roth G: In vitro biosynthesis of adipocyte proteins having the characteristics of glucocorticoid receptors. Biochim Biophys Acta 1980;632:58–72
27. Besse JC, Bass AD: Pretentiation by hydrocortisone of responses to catecholamines in vascular smooth muscle. J Pharmacol Exp Ther 1966;154:224–238
28. Scarpace PJ, Abrass IB: Desensitization of adenylate cyclase and the downregulation of beta adrenergic receptors after in vivo administration of beta agonist. J Pharmacol Exp Ther 1982;223:327–331
29. Hui KK, Conolly MB, Tashkin DP: Reversal of the human lymphocyte beta-adrenoceptor desensitisation by glucocorticoids. Clin Pharmacol Ther 1982;32:566–571
30. Rimo G, Hanski E, Braun S, Levitski A: Mode of coupling between hormone receptors and adenylate cyclase elucidated by modulation of membrane fluidity. Nature 1978;276: 394–396
31. Banergee DK, Lee GS, Malik SK, Daly S: Underdiagnosis of asthma in the elderly. Br J Dis Chest 1987;81:23–29
32. Lee HY, Stretton TB: Asthma in the elderly. BMJ 1972;4: 93–95
33. Allen SC: Missed asthma: a study of 13 old people. Br J Clin Pract 1988;42:158–160
34. Bailey WC, Richards JM Jr, Brooks CM et al: Features of asthma in older adults. J Asthma 1992;29:21–28
35. Burrows B, Barbee RA, Cline MG et al: Characteristics of asthma among elderly adults in a sample of the general population. Chest 1991;100:935–942
36. Putman MT, Wise RA: Myasthenia gravis and upper airway obstruction. Chest 1996;109:400–404
37. Corris PA, Gibson GJ: Asthma presenting as cor pulmonale. BMJ 1984;288:389–390
38. Dodge R, Cline MG, Burrows B: Comparisons of asthma, emphysema and chronic bronchitis diagnoses in a general population sample. Am Rev Respir Dis 1986;133:981–986
39. Littlejohns P, Ebrahim S, Anderson R: Prevalence and diagnosis of chronic respiratory symptoms in adults. BMJ 1989;298: 1556–1560
40. Littlejohns P, Ebrahim S, Anderson R: Treatment of adult asthma: is the diagnosis relevant? Thorax 1989;44:797–802
41. Smyth ET, Wright SC, Evans AE et al: Death from airways obstruction: accuracy of certification in Northern Ireland. Thorax 1996;51:293–297
42. Griffiths C, Naish J, Sturdy P, Pereira F: Prescribing in hospital admissions for asthma in East London. BMJ 1996;312: 481–482
43. Gannon PFG, Newton DT, Pantin CFA, Burge PS: Effect of the number of peak expiratory flow readings a day on diurnal variation. Thorax 1992;48:845
44. British Thoracic Society and others: Guidelines on the management of asthma. Thorax 1993;48(suppl):S1–S24
45. Joseph KS, Blaisl Ernst P, Suissa S: Increased morbidity and mortality related to asthma among asthmatic patients who use major tranquillisers. BMJ 1996;312:79–82
46. Connolly MJ, Jarvis EH, Hendrick DJ: Late-onset asthma in a demented elderly patient; the value of methacholine challenge in diagnosis. J Geriatr Soc 1990;38:539–541
47. Starke ID, Luce P: The efficacy and safety of inhaled salmeterol 50μg in older patients with reversible airflow obstruction. Age Ageing 1995;25:67–71
48. Cazola M, Matera MG, Santagelo G et al: Salmeterol and formoterol in partially reversible severe chronic obstructive pulmonary disease: a dose-response study. Respir Med 1995;89: 357–362
49. Weiner P, Weiner M, Azgad Y: Long term clinical comparison of single versus twice daily administration of inhaled budesonide in moderate asthma. Thorax 1995;50:1270–1273
50. Allen SC, Prior A: What determines whether an elderly patient can use a metered-dose inhaler correctly? Br J Dis Chest 1986; 80:45–49
51. Connolly MJ: Large volume spacer devices and inhaler technique in elderly patients. Age Ageing 1995;24:190–192
52. Selroos O, Halme M: Effect of a Volumatic spacer and mouth rinsing on systemic absorption of inhaled corticosteroids from a metered-dose inhaler and dry powder inhaler. Thorax 1991; 46:891–894
53. Newman SP, Woodman G, Moren F, Clarke SW: Bronchodilator therapy with nebuhaler; how important is the delay between firing the dose and inhaling. Br J Dis Chest 1988;82:262–267
54. Diggory P, Bailey R, Vallon A: Effectiveness of inhaled bronchodilator delivery systems for elderly patients. Age Ageing 1991;20:379–382
55. Harvey J, Williams JG: Randomised cross-over comparison of five inhaler systems for bronchodilator therapy. Br J Clin Pract 1992;46:249–251
56. Armitage JM, Williams SJ: Inhaler technique in the elderly. Age Ageing 1988;17:275–278
57. Lung and Asthma Information Agency: Trends in asthma mortality in the elderly. Factsheet 92/1, London, 1992
58. Model D: Preventable factors and death certification in death due to asthma. Respir Med 1995;21–25
59. Petheram IS, Jones DA, Collins JV: Assessment and management of acute asthma in the elderly: a comparison with young asthmatics. Postgrad Med J 1982;58:149–151
60. Cook NR, Evans DA, Scherr PA et al: Peak expiratory flow rate and 5-year mortality in an elderly population. Am J Epidemiol 1991;133:785–794
61. Connolly MJ, Renwick DS, Gibson HN, Taylor PM: Admission chest radiograph (CXR) in elderly patients admitted to hospital with acute severe asthma. Age Ageing 1995;24(suppl 2):p13
62. Nielson C: Critical care. pp. 209–230. In Connolly MJ (ed): Respiratory Disease in the Elderly Patient. Chapman & Hall, London, 1996

63. British Thoracic Society et al. Guidelines for the Management of Chronic Obstructive Pulmonary Disease. Thorax 1997 (in press).
64. Horsley JR, Sterling IJ, Waters WE, Howell JB: Respiratory symptoms among elderly people in the New Forest area as assessed by postal questionnaire. Age Ageing 1991;20: 325–331
65. Isoaho R, Puolijoki H, Huhti E et al: Prevalence of chronic obstructive pulmonary disease in elderly Finns. Respir Med 1994;88:571–580
66. Lung and Asthma Information Agency: Trends in lung cancer and smoking. Factsheet 93/1, 1993
67. Davis RM, Novotny TE: The epidemiology of cigarette smoking and its impact on chronic obstructive pulmonary disease. Am Rev Respir Dis 1989;140:S82–84
68. Lee PN, Fry JS, Forey BA: Trends in lung cancer, chronic obstructive lung disease, and emphysema death rates for England and Wales 1941–85 and their relation to trends in cigarette smoking. Thorax 1990;45:657–665
69. Feinleib M, Rosenberg HM, Collins JG et al: Trends in COPD morbidity and mortality in the United States. Am Rev Respir Dis 1989;140:9–18S
70. Renwick DS, Connolly MJ: Quality of life in older adults: the impact of obstructive airways disease. Thorax 1996;25(suppl 1):P8
71. Elliot MW, Simonds AK, Carroll MP et al: Domicilliary nocturnal nasal positive pressure ventilation in hypercapnic respiratory failure due to chronic obstructive lung disease. Thorax 1992;47:342–348
72. Mecham Jones DJ, Paul EA, Jones PW, Wedzicha JA: Nasal pressure support ventilation plus oxygen compared to oxygen therapy alone in hypercapnic COPD. Am J Respir Crit Care Med 1995;152:538–544
73. Mecham Jones DJ, Wedzicha JA: Non-invasive positive pressure ventilation in advanced progressive chronic respiratory failure due to COPD. Am Rev Respir Dis 1993;147:A322
74. Wedzicha JA, Meecham Jones DJ: Domicilliary ventilation in advanced chronic obstructive pulmonary disease: where are we? editorial. Thorax 1996;51:455–457
75. Schols AMWJ, Soeters PB, Mostert R et al: Energy balance in chronic obstructive pulmonary disease. Am Rev Respir Dis 1991;143:1248–1252
76. The Intermittent Positive Pressure Breathing Trial Group: Intermittent positive pressure therapy of chronic obstructive pulmonary disease. Ann Intern Med 1983;99:612–620
77. Vetter NJ, Ford D: Smoking prevention among people aged 60 and over: a randomized controlled trial. Age Ageing 1990; 19:164–168
78. Campbell IA, Prescott RJ, Tjeder-Burton SM: Transdermal nicotine plus support in patients attending hospital with smoking-related diseases: a placebo-controlled study. Respir Med 1996;90:47–51
79. Russel MAH, Stapleton JA, Feyerbend C et al: Targeting heavy smokers in general practice: randomised controlled trial of transdermal nicotine patches. BMJ 1993;306:1308–1312
80. Flaxman J: Quitting smoking now or later: gradual, abrupt, immediate and delayed quitting. Behav Ther 1978;9:260–270
81. Burchfiel CM, Marcus EB, Curb D et al. Effects of smoking and smoking cessation on longitudinal decline in pulmonary function. Am J Respir Crit Care Med 1995;151:1778–1785
82. Stableforth DE: Asthma mortality and physician competence. J Allergy Clin Immunol 1987;80:463–466
83. Crane J, Pearce N, Flatt N et al: Prescribed Fenoterol and death from asthma in New Zealand, 1981–83: case-control study. Lancet 1989;1:917–922
84. Grainger J, Woodman K, Pearce N et al: Prescribed Fenoterol and death from asthma in New Zealand, 1981–7: further case control study. Thorax 1991;46:105–111
85. Sears MR, Taylor DR, Print CG et al: Regular inhaled beta-agonist treatment in bronchial asthma. Lancet 1990;336: 1391–1396
86. Kuitert LM: Beta-agonists in asthma — state of the art: report on a Royal Society of Medicine seminar. Thorax 1992;47: 568–569
87. Committee on Safety of Medicines: Report of the Beta-agonist Working Party. Medicines Control Agency, London, 1992
88. Simmons MS, Nides MA, Rand CS et al: Trends in compliance with bronchodilator use between follow-up visits in a clinical trial. Chest 1996;109:963–968
89. Sears MR: Long-acting beta-agonists, tachyphylaxis and corticosteroids, editorial. Chest 1996;109:862–864
90. Diggory P, Cassels-Brown A, Vail A et al: Avoiding unsuspected respiratory side-effects of topical timolol with cardioselective or sympathomimetic agents. Lancet 1995;345: 1604–1606
91. Diggory P, Franks WA: Glaucoma therapy may take your breath away. Age Ageing 1997;26:63–67
92. Ikeda A, Nishimura K, Koama H et al: Dose response study of ipratropium bromide aerosol on maximum exercise performance in stable patients with chronic obstructive pulmonary disease. Thorax 1996;51:48–53
93. Anon: The nebuliser epidemic. Lancet 1984;2:789–790
94. Teale C, Jones A, Patterson CJ et al: Community survey of home nebulizer technique by elderly people. Age Ageing 1995; 24:276–277
95. O'Driscoll BR, Kay EA, Taylor RJ, Bernstein A: Home nebulisers: can optimal therapy be predicted by laboratory studies? Respir Med 1990;84:471–477
96. Teale C, Morrison JFJ, Jones PC, Muers MF: Reversibility tests in chronic obstructive airways disease: their predictive value with reference to benefit from domiciliary nebuliser therapy. Respir Med 1991;85:281–284
97. Bosley CM, Corden ZM, Cochrane GM: Home nebulized therapy for patients with chronic obstructive airways disease (COAD): patient adherence to nebulized treatment and its relation to quality of life. Thorax 1995;50(suppl 2):A29
98. McKay SE, Howie C, Thomson AH et al: Value of theophylline treatment in patients handicapped by chronic obstructive lung disease. Thorax 1993;48:227–232
99. Nocturnal Oxygen Therapy Trial Group: Continuous or nocturnal oxygen therapy in hypoxic chronic obstructive lung disease. Ann Intern Med 1980;93:391–398

100. Report of the Medical Research Council Oxygen Working Party: Long-term domiciliary oxygen therapy in chronic hypoxic cor pulmonale complicating chronic bronchitis and emphysema. Lancet 1981;1:681–685

101. Light RW, Merrill EJ, Despars JA et al: Prevalence of depression and anxiety in patients with COPD: relationship to functional capacity. Chest 1985;87:35–38

102. Yohannes AM, Roomi J, Connolly MJ: Depression in elderly outpatients (OPs) with disabling chronic airways disease. Thorax 1995;50(suppl 2):A55

103. Chauhan AJ, Leahy BC: Pulmonary rehabilitation in the elderly patient. pp. 261–295. In Connolly MJ (ed): Respiratory Disease in the Elderly Patient. Chapman & Hall, London, 1996

104. Roomi J, Johnson MM, Waters K et al: Respiratory rehabilitation, exercise capacity and quality of life in chronic airways disease in old age. Age Ageing 1996;25:2–16

105. Roomi J, Yohannes A, Connolly MJ: Respiratory rehabilitation improves exercise capacity in elderly patients with chronic airflow limitation. Thorax 1995;50(suppl 2):A56

106. Swerts PM, Kretzers LM, Terpstra-Windevan E et al: Exercise reconditioning in the rehabilitation of patients with chronic obstructive pulmonary disease: a short and long-term analysis. Arch Phys Med Rehab 1990;71:570–573

107. Vale F, Reardon JZ, Zuwallack RL: The long-term benefits of out-patient pulmonary rehabilitation on exercise endurance and quality of life. Chest 1993;103:42–45

108. Ries AL: Position paper of the American Association of Cardiovascular and Pulmonary Rehabilitation. Scientific basis of pulmonary rehabilitation. J Cardiopulmon Rehab 1990;10: 418–441

109. Wijkstra PJ, van der Mark TW, Kraan J et al: Long-term effects of home rehabilitation on physical performance in chronic obstructive pulmonary disease. Am J Respir Crit Care Med 1996; 153:1234–1241

110. Grant BJB, Capel H: Walking aid for pulmonary emphysema. Lancet 1972;2:1125–1127

111. Dalton G, Ashley J, Rudkin ST, White RJ: The effect of walking aids on walking distance, breathlessness and oxygenation with patients with severe chronic obstructive pulmonary disease (COPD). Thorax 1995;50(suppl 2):A57

112. Department of Health: Immunisation against infectious disease. HMSO, London, 1992

113. Howells CHL, Vesselinova-Jenkins CK, Evans AD, James J: Influenza vaccination and mortality from bronchopneumonia in the elderly. Lancet 1985;1:381–383

114. Gross PA, Quinnan GV, Rodstein M et al. Association of influenza immunisation with reduction in mortality in an elderly population. A prospective study. Arc Intern Med 1988;148: 562–565

115. van der Wulp CG, Perenboom RJM, Davidse W: Ontwikkelingen in de griepvaccinatie in Nederland. Maandbericht Gezondheid (CBS) 1995;2:4–9

116. Nicholson KG: Immunization against influenza among people aged over 65 living at home in Leicestershire during winter 1991–2. BMJ 1993;306:974–976

117. Frank JW, Henderson M, McMurray L: Influenza vaccination in the elderly: 1. Determinance of acceptance. Can Med Assoc J 1995;132:371–375

118. Shapiro ED, Berg AT, Austrian R et al: Protective efficacy of polyvalent pneumococcal polysaccharide vaccine. N Engl J Med 1991;325:1453–1456

119. Dudley DL, Glasser EM, Jorgenson Logan DL: Psychosocial and psychological concomitants to rehabilitation in COPD. Part 1. Psychosocial considerations. Chest 1980;77: 413–420

120. Dudley DL: Coping with chronic obstructive pulmonary disease: therapeutic options. Geriatrics 1981;36:69–74

121. Cockcroft AE: Randomised controlled trial of rehabilitation in chronic respiratory disability. Thorax 1981;36:200–203

122. McSweeney AJ, Grant I, Heaton RK et al: Life quality of patients with chronic obstructive pulmonary disease. Arch Intern Med 1982;142:473–478

123. Prigatano GP, Wright EC, Levin D: Quality of life and its predictors in patients with mild hypoxemia and chronic obstructive pulmonary disease. Arch Intern Med 1984;144: 1613–1619

124. Williams SJ: Chronic respiratory illness and disability: a critical review of the psychosocial literature. Soc Sci Med 1989; 28:791–803

125. Cutris JR, Deyo RA, Hudson LD: Health-related quality of life among patients with chronic obstructive pulmonary disease. Thorax 1994;49:162–170

126. Okubadejo AA, Jones PW, Wedzicha JA: Quality of life in patients with chronic obstructive pulmonary disease and severe hypoxaemia. Thorax 1996;5144–5147

127. Vilkman S, Keistinen T, Tuuponen T, Kivela SL: Age distribution of patients treated in hospital for chronic obstructive pulmonary disease. Age Ageing 1996;25:109–112

128. Seigel D, Sheppard D, Gelb A, Weinberg PE: Aminophylline increases the toxicity but not the efficacy of an inhaled beta-adrenergic agonist in the treatment of acute exacerbations of asthma. Am Rev Respir Dis 1985;132:283–286

129. Self TH, Abou-Shala N, Burns R et al: Inhaler albuterol and oral prednisone in hospitalised adult asthmatics. Does aminophylline add any benefit? Chest 1990;98:1317–1321

130. Wrenn K, Slovis CM, Murphy F, Greenberg RS: Aminophylline therapy for acute bronchospastic disease in the emergency room. Ann Intern Med 1991;115:241–247

131. Murphy DC, McDermott MJ, Rydman RJ et al: Ainophylline in the treatment of acute asthma when β_2-adrenergics and steroids are provided. Arch Intern Med 1993;153: 1784–1788

132. Huang D, O'Brian RG, Harman E et al: Does aminophylline benefit adults admitted to hospital for an acute exacerbation of asthma? Ann Intern Med 1993;119:1155–1160

133. Bott J, Carroll MP, Conway J et al: Randomised controlled trial of nasal ventilation in acute ventilatory failure due to chronic obstructive airways disease. Lancet 1993;341: 1555–1567

134. Brochard C, Mancebo J, Wysocki M et al: Non invasive ventila-

tion for acute exacerbations of chronic obstructive pulmonary disease. N Engl J Med 1995;338:817–822

135. Nielson C: Critical care. pp. 209–230. In Connolly MJ (ed): Respiratory Disease in the Elderly Patient. Chapman & Hall, London, 1996

136. Cockburn WC: The importance of infections of the respiratory tract. J Infect 1979;1(suppl 2):3–8

137. Valenti WM, Trudell RG, Bentley DW: Factors predisposing to oropharyngeal colonisation with gram-negative bacilli in the aged. N Engl J Med 1978;298:1108–1111

138. Barker WH, Mullooly JP: Influenza vaccination of elderly persons. Reduction in pneumonia and influenza hospitalisations and deaths. J Am Med Soc 1980;244:2547–2549

139. Glezen WP, Decca MD, Joseph SW, Mercready RG: Acute respiratory disease associated with influenza epidemics in Houston 1981–83. J Infect Dis 1987;155:1119–1126

140. Nicholson KG, Baker DJ, Farquhar A et al: Acute upper respiratory tract virol illness and influenza immunisation in homes for the elderly. Epidemiol Infect 1990;105:609–618

141. Connolly AM, Salmon RL, Lervy V, Williams DH: What are the complications of influenza and can they be prevented? Experience from the 1989 epidemic of H3N2 Influenza A in general practice. BMJ 1993;306:1452–1454

142. Schwarzmann SW, Adler JL, Sullivan RJ, Marine WM: Bacterial influenza during the Hong Kong influenza epidemic 1968–69. Arch Intern Med 1971;127:1037–1041

143. Curwan M, Dunnell K, Ashley J: Hidden influenza deaths. BMJ 1990;300:896

144. Guideline on the Control of Infection in Residential and Nursing Homes: Public Health Medicine Environmental Group Department of Health, Wetherby, 1996

145. National Advisory Committee on Immunization (NACI): Statement on influenza vaccination for the 1991–1992 season. Can Dis Weekly Rep 1991;17–24:121–126

146. Centers for Disease Control and Prevention and Controls of Influenza: Recommendations of the immunization practices advisory committee (ACIP). MMWR 1992;40:1–17

147. Nicholson KG, Snacken R, Palache AM: Influenza immunization policies in Europe and the United States. Vaccine 1995; 4:365–369

148. Howells CHL, Vesselinova-Jenkins CK, Evans AD, James J: Influenza vaccination and mortality from broncho-pneumonia in the elderly. Lancet 1985;1:381–383

149. Nicholson KG, Wiselka MG, May A: Influenza vaccination of the elderly: perceptions and policies of General Practitioners and outcome of the 1985–86 Immunisation Programme in Trent, UK. Vaccine 1985;5:302–306

150. Gillick MR, Ditzion B: Influenza vaccination. Are we doing better than we think? Arch Intern Med 1991;151:1742–1744

151. Carter WB, Beach LR, Inui TS et al: Developing and testing a decision model for predicting influenza vaccination compliance. Health Serv Res 1986;20:897–932

152. Pearson DC, Thompson RS: Evaluation of group health cooperative of Puget Sound's senior influenza immunization program. Public Health Rep 1994;109:571–578

153. Ortquist A, Sterner G, Nilsson JA: Severe community-acquired pneumonia: factors influencing need of intensive care treatment and prognosis. Scand J Infect Dis 1985;17:377–386

154. Woodhead MA: Studies on pneumonia in the community and in hospital in Nottingham. DM Thesis. University of Nottingham, 1988

155. Office of Population Censuses and Surveys: Mortality Statistics HMSO, London, 1990

156. The British Thoracic Society and the Public Health Laboratory Service: Community-acquired pneumonia in adults in British hospitals in 1982–1983: a survey of aetiology, mortality, prognostic factors and outcome. Q J Med 1987;239:195–230

157. Venkatesan P, Gladman J, MacFarlane JT et al: A hospital study of community acquired pneumonia in the elderly. Thorax 1990;45:254–258

158. Harper C, Newton P: Clinical aspects of pneumonia in the elderly veteran. J Am Geriatr Soc 1989;37:867–872

159. Starczewski AR, Allen SC, Vargas E, Lye M: Clinical prognostic indices of fatality in elderly patients admitted to hospital with acute pneumonia. Age Ageing 1988;17:181–186

160. Esposito AL: Community-acquired bacteremic pneumococcal pneumonia. Effect of age on manifestations and outcome. Arch Intern Med 1984;144:945–948

161. Puxty JAH, Andrews K: The role of chest radiography in the evaluation of "Geriatric Giants." Age Ageing 1986;15: 174–176

162. McFadden JP, Price RC, Eastwood HD, Briggs RS: Raised respiratory rate in elderly patients: a valuable physical sign. BMJ 1982;284:626–627

163. Marrie TJ, Durant H, Yates L: Community-acquired pneumonia requiring hospitalization: 6-year prospective study. Rev Infect Dis 1989;11:586–599

164. La Croix AZ, Lipson S, Miles TP, White L: Prospective study of pneumonia hospitalizations and mortality of U.S. older people: the role of chronic conditions, health behaviors and nutritional status. Public Health Rep 1989;104:350–360

165. Connolly MJ, Crowley JJ, Vestal RE: Clinical significance of crepitations in elderly patients following acute hospital admission: a prospective survey. Age Ageing 1992;21:43–48

166. Eaton D, Bannister P, Mulley GP, Connolly MJ: Axillary sweating in clinical assessment of dehydration in ill elderly patients. BMJ 1994;308:1271

167. Garb JL, Brown RB, Garb JR, Tuthill RW: Differences in etiology of pneumonias in nursing homes and community patients. JAMA 1978;240:2169–2172

168. Marrie TJ, Haldane EV, Faulkner RS et al: Community-acquired pneumonia requiring hospitalization: is it different in the elderly? J Am Geriatr Soc 1985;33:671–679

169. Levy M, Dromer F, Brion N et al: Community-acquired pneumonia. Importance of initial noninvasive bacteriologic and radiographic investigations. Chest 1988;92:42–48

170. Ausina V, Coll P, Sambeat M et al: Prospective study on the aetiology of community-acquired pneumonia in children and adults in Spain. Eur J Clin Microbiol Infect Dis 1988;7: 343–347

171. Report from the PHLS Communicable Disease Surveillance Centre. BMJ 1988;296:778–779

172. Noah ND: *Mycoplasma pneumoniae* infection in the United Kingdom—1967–73. BMJ 1974;1:554–556

173. Kaye MG, Fox MJ, Bartlett JG et al: The clinical spectrum of *Staphylococcus aureus* pulmonary infection. Chest 1990;97: 788–792

174. Yung AP, Grayson ML: Psittacosis—review of 135 cases. Med J Aust 1988;148:228–233

175. Horan TC, White JW, Jarvis WR et al: Nosocomial infection surveillance 1984. MMWR 1986;34:17ss–29ss

176. Harkness GA, Bentley DW, Roghmann KJ: Risk factors for nosocomial pneumonia in the elderly. Am J Med 1990;89: 457–463

177. Barkham TMS, Martin FC: The respiratory presentation of urinary tract infection in older patients. Age Ageing 1995; 24(suppl 2):P18–19

178. Ebright JR, Rytel MW: Bacterial pneumonia in the elderly. J Am Geriatr Soc 1980;18:220–223

179. British Thoracic Society: Community-acquired pneumonia in adults in British hospitals in 1982–1983; a survey of aetiology, mortality, prognostic factors and outcome. Q J Med 1987;62: 195–220

180. Roberts DE, Cole PJ: Use of selective media in bacteriological investigation of patients with chronic suppurative lung infection. Lancet 1980;1:796

181. Roberts D, Higgs E, Rutman A, Cole PJ: Isolation of spheroplastic forms of *Haemophilus influenza* from sputum in conventionally treated chronic bronchial sepsis using selective medium supplanted with N-acetyl-D-glucosamine: possible reservoir for re-emergence of infection. BMJ 1984;289:1409

182. Cole PJ, Roberts DE: High dose antibiotic is logical, effective and economical in treatment of severe bronchial sepsis. Lancet 1983;1:248

183. Hill SL, Morrison HM, Burnett D, Stockley RA: Short term response of patients with bronchiectasis to treatment with amoxycillin given in standard or high doses orally or by inhalation. Thorax 1986;41:559–565

184. Powell KE, Farer LS: The rising age of the tuberculosis patient. J Infect Dis 1980;142:946–948

185. Teale C, Goldman JM, Pearson SB: The association of age with the presentation and outcome of tuberculosis—a 5 year survey. Age Ageing 1993;22:289–293

186. Duffield JS, Adams WH, Anderson M, Leitch AG: Increasing incidence of tuberculosis in the young and the elderly in Scotland. Thorax 1996;51:140–142

187. Leitch AG, Iubilar M, Kurnow J et al: Scottish national survey of tuberculosis notifications 1993 with special reference to the prevalence of HIV seropositivity. Thorax 1996;51:78–81

188. Kearney HT, Wanklyn PD, Goldman JM et al: Urban deprivation and tuberculosis in the elderly. Respir Med 1994;88: 703–704

189. Morris CDW, Nell H: Epidemic of pulmonary tuberculosis in geriatric homes. S Afr Med J 1988;74:117–120

190. Snider DE: Tuberculosis after gastrectomy. Chest 1985;87: 414–415

191. Dull R, Peto R: Mortality in relation to smoking: 20 years observations on male British doctors. BMJ 1976;2:215–225

192. Morris CDW, Bird AR, Nell H: Haematological and biochemical changes in severe pulmonary tuberculosis. Q J Med 1989; 73:1151–1159

193. Gorse GJ, Pais PJ, Kusske JA et al: Tubercular spondylitis: a report of six cases and review of the literature. Medicine 1983;62:1788–1784

194. Counsell S, Tan JS, Dittus RS: Unsuspected pulmonary tuberculosis in a community teaching hospital. Arch Intern Med 1989;149:1274–1278

195. Morris CDW, Nell H: Epidemic pulmonary tuberculosis in geriatric homes. S Afr Med J 1988;74:117–125

196. Ip MSM, Yo SY, Lam WK, Mok CK: Endo-bronchotuberculosis revisited. Chest 1986;89:727–729

197. Snider DE: The tuberculin skin test. Am Rev Respir Dis 1982; 125:108–114

198. Joint Tuberculosis Committee of the British Thoracic Society: Chemotherapy and the management of tuberculosis in the United Kingdom: recommendations of the Joint Tuberculosis Committee of the British Thoracic Society. Thorax 1990;45: 403–408

199. The British Thoracic Society Research Committee and the Medical Research Council: Cardio-thoracic Epidemiology Research Group. The management of pulmonary tuberculosis in adults notified in England and Wales in 1988. Respir Med 1991;85:319–324

200. Yoshikawa TT: Tuberculosis in aging adults. J Am Geriatr Soc 1992;40:178–187

201. Connolly MJ, Magee JG, Hendrick DJ: *Mycobacterium malmoense* in the North-East of England. Tubercle 1985;66: 211–217

202. American Thoracic Society: Diagnosis and treatment of disease caused by non tuberculous mycobacteria. Am Rev Respir Dis 1990;142:940–953

203. Lung and Asthma Information Agency: Trends in lung cancer and smoking. Factsheet 1993.1, London, 1993

204. Muscat JE, Wynder EL: Cigarette smoking, asbestos exposure and malignant mesothelioma. Cancer Res 1991;51: 2263–2267

205. O'Rourke MA, Feussner JR, Feigle P, Laslo J: Age trends in lung cancer: stage at diagnosis. JAMA 1987;258:921–926

206. Knox AJ, Mascie-Taylor H, Page RL: Fibreoptic bronchoscopy in the elderly: 4 years' experience. Br J Dis Chest 1978;82: 290–293

207. Joslin C, Rider L: Cancer in Yorkshire: 1. Lung Cancer. Cancer Registry Special Report Series, Leeds Graphic Press Limited, Leeds, England, 1993

208. Mountain CF: A new international staging system for lung cancer. Chest 1983;89(suppl):225–233

209. Sherman S, Guido CE: The feasibility of thoracotomy for lung cancer in the elderly. JAMA 1982;258:927–930

210. Shirakusa T, Tsutsui M, Iriki N et al: Results of resection for bronchogenic carcinoma in patients over the age of 80. Thorax 1989;44:189–191

211. Mâné JM, Estapé J, Sánchez-Lloret J et al: Age and clinical characteristics of 1433 patients with lung cancer. Age Ageing 1994;23:28–31

212. Shahidi H, Kvale PA: Long-term survival following surgical treatment of solitary brain metastasis in non-small cell lung cancer. Chest 1996;109:2.71–76

213. Soquet PJ, Chauvin F, Boissel JP et al: Poly-chemotherapy in advanced non small cell lung cancer: a meta-analysis. Lancet 1993;342:19–21

214. Coy P, Kennelly GM: The role of curative radiotherapy in the treatment of lung cancer. Cancer 1980;45:698–702

215. Patterson CJ, Hocking M, Bond M, Teale C: Evaluation of radiotherapy for non-small cell bronchial carcinoma in the elderly. Thorax 1995;50(suppl 2):A26

216. Blehan NM, Girling DJ, Fayers PM et al: Inoperable non-small cell lung cancer (NSCLC): a medical research Council (MRC) randomised trial of palliative radiotherapy with two fractions or ten fractions. Cancer 1991;68:265–270

217. Smit EF, Carney DN, Harford P et al: A phase II study of oral etoposide in elderly patients with small cell lung cancer. Thorax 1989;44:631–633

218. Allan SG, Gregor A, Cornbleet ME, Leonard RCF: Phase II trial of Vindesine and VP16:213 in the palliation of poor-prognosis patients and elderly patients with small cell lung cancer. Cancer Chemother Pharmacol 1984;13:106–108

219. Carney DN, Grogan L, Smit EF et al: Single-agent oral etoposide for elderly small cell lung cancer patients. Semin Oncol 1990;17(suppl 2):49–53

220. Tummarallo D, Isidori P, Pasini G et al: Tenoposide as single agent drug therapy for elderly patients affected by small cell lung cancer. Eur J Cancer 1992;28a:1081–1084

221. Lung and Asthma Information Agency: Pleural mesothelioma. Fact sheet 92/3. Department of Public Health Sciences, St George's Hospital Medical School, London, 1992

222. Boutin C, Rey F: Thoracoscopy in pleural malignant mesothelioma. A prospective study of 188 consecutive patients. Part 1: diagnosis. Cancer 1993;72:389–393

223. Boutin C, Rey F, Viallat JR et al: Thoracoscopy in pleural malignant mesothelioma: a prospective study of 188 consecutive patients. Part 2: prognosis and staging. Cancer 1993;92: 394–404

224. De Pangher Manzini V, Brollo A, Franchesi S et al: Prognostic factors of malignant mesothelioma of the pleura. Cancer 1993; 72:410–417

225. Cartwright RA, McKinney PA, Barnes M: Epidemiology of the lymphomas in the United Kingdom: recent developments. Baillieres Clin Haematol 1987;1:59–76

226. Guinee VF, Giacco GG, Durand M et al: The prognosis of Hodgkins disease in older adults. J Clin Oncol 1991;9: 947–953

227. Vose JM, Armitage JO, Weisenburger D et al: The importance of age in survival of patients treated with chemotherapy for aggressive non-Hodgkins lymphoma. J Clin Oncol 1988;6: 1838–1844

228. Levis A: Recent advances in the therapy of Hodgkin's disease in elderly patients. Haematol Oncol 1993;11(suppl):78–84

229. Erdkamp FL, Breed WP, Bosch LJ et al: Hodgkin's disease in the elderly. Cancer 1992;70:830–840

230. Tiralli U, Zagonel V, Errante D et al: A prospective study of a new combination therapy regimen in patients older than 70 years with unfavourable non-Hodgkin's lymphoma. J Clin Oncol 1992;10:228–232

231. Greenberg RS, Baumgarten DA, Clark WS et al: Prognostic factors for gastro-intestinal and bronchopulmonary carcinoid tumours. Cancer 1987;60:2476–2483

232. Diaz-Jimenez JP, Canela-Cardona M, Maestro-Alcader J: Nd: YAG laser photoresection of low-grade malignant tumours of the tracheobronchial tree. Chest 1990;97:920–922

233. Dumon JF, Reboud E, Garbc L ct al: Treatment of tracheobronchial lesions by laser photoresection. Chest 1982;81:278–284

234. Maiwand MO: Cryotherapy for advanced carcinoma of the trachea and bronchi. BMJ 1986;293:181–182

235. Wilson GE, Walsha MJ, Hind CRK: Treatment of large airways obstruction in lung cancer using expandable metal stents inserted under direct vision via the fibreoptic bronchoscope. Thorax 1996;51:248–252

236. Maiwant MO, Tai YP, Straughan S: Survival and quality of life following cryotherapy for carcinoma of the bronchus. Thorax 1995;50(suppl 2):A26

237. PIOPED Investigators: Value of the ventilation/perfusion scan in acute pulmonary embolism. Results of the prospective investigation of pulmonary embolism diagnosis (PIOPED). JAMA 1990;263:2753–2759

238. Stein PD, Facc AG, Saltzmann HA, Terrin ML: Diagnosis of acute pulmonary embolism in the elderly. J Am Cardiol Clin 1991;18:145–147

239. Dalen JE: Clinical diagnosis of acute pulmonary embolism. When should a V/Q scan be ordered?, editorial. Chest 1991; 100:1185–1186

240. Raskob GE, Hull RD: Diagnosis and management of pulmonary embolism. Q J Med 1990;76:787–789

241. Research Committee for the British Thoracic Society: Optimum duration of anticoagulation for deep vein thrombosis and pulmonary embolism. Lancet 1992;340:873–876

242. Mannino DM, Etzel RA, Parrish RG: Pulmonary fibrosis deaths in the United States, 1979–1991. An analysis of multiple-cause mortality data. Am J Respir Crit Care Med 1996; 153:1548–1552

243. Epler GR, McLoud TC, Gaensler AE et al: Normal chest roentgenograms in chronic infiltrative lung disease. N Engl J Med 1978;298:934–939

244. Mathiesom JR, Mayo JR, Staples CA, Muller ML: Chronic diffuse infiltrative lung disease: comparison of diagnostic accuracy of CT and chest radiography. Radiology 1989;181: 111–116

245. Padley SP, Adler B, Hansell DM et al: High-resolution computerised tomography of drug-induced lung disease. Clin Radiol 1992;46:232–236

246. Muller NL, Miller RR: Computed tomography of chronic diffuse infiltrative lung disease. Am Rev Respir Dis 1990;142: 1206–1215

247. Booth HL, Walters EH: Interstitial lung disease in the elderly patient. pp. 171–207. In Connolly MJ (ed): Respiratory Disease in the Elderly Patient. Chapman & Hall, London, 1996

248. Poe RH, Israel RH, Utell MJ, Hall WJ: Probability of positive transbroncheal lung biopsy result in sarcoidosis. Arch Intern Med 1979;139:761–763

249. Herf SM, Suratt PM: Complications of transbroncheal lung biopsies. Chest 1978;73:759–760

250. Warner DO, Warner MA, Divertie MB: Open lung biopsy in patients with diffuse pulmonary infiltrates and acute respiratory failure. Am Rev Respir Dis 1988;137:90–94

251. Venn GE, Kay PH, Midwood CJ, Goldstraw P: Open lung biopsy in patients with diffuse pulmonary shadowing. Thorax 1985;40:931–935

252. Soutar CA, Turner-Warwick M, Parkes WR: Circulating antinuclear antibody and rheumatoid factor in coal pneumoconiosis. BMJ 1974;3:145

253. Gaensler EA, Jedelinic PJ, Churg A: Idiopathic pulmonary fibrosis in asbestos-exposed workers. Am Rev Respir Dis 1991;144:689–696

254. Hendrick DJ, Faux JA, Marshall R: Budgerigar-Fancier's lung: the commonest variety of allergic alveolitis in Britain. BMJ 1978;2:81–84

255. Allen DH, Williams GV, Woolcock AJ: Bird breeders hypersensitivity pneumonitis: progress studies and lung function after cessation of exposure to the provoking antigen. Am Rev Respir Dis 1976;114:555–566

256. Sansores R, Sales J, Chapela R: Clubbing in hypersensitivity pneumonitis. Arch Intern Med 1990;150:184–151

257. Kokkarinen JL, Tukiainen HO, Terho EO: Effective corticosteroid treatment and the recovery of pulmonary function in farmer's lung. Am Rev Respir Dis 1992;145:3–5

258. Crystal RG, Bitterman PB, Rennard SI et al: Interstitial lung disease of unknown cause. Disorders characterised by chronic inflammation of the lower respiratory tract. N Engl J Med 1984; 310:154–166

259. Wright PH, Heard BE, Steel SJ, Turner-Warwick M: Cryptogenic fibrosing alveolitis: assessment by graded trephine lung biopsy: histology compared with clinical radiographic and physical features. Br J Dis Chest 1981;75:61–70

260. Stack BHR, Choo-Kang YFJ, Heard BE: The prognosis of cryptogenic fibrosing alveolitis. Thorax 1972;27:535–542

261. Hiwitari N, Shimura F, Sasaki T et al: Prognosis of idiopathic pulmonary fibrosis in patients with mucus hypersecretion. Am Rev Respir Dis 1991;143–145

262. Johnson I, Britton J, Kinnear W, Logan R: Rising mortality from cryptogenic fibrosing alveolitis. BMJ 1990;301: 1017–1021

263. Turner-Warwick M, Burrows B, Johnson A: Cryptogenic fibrosing alveolitis: response to corticosteroid treatment and its effect on survival. Thorax 1980;35:593–599

264. Johnson MA, Kwan S, Snell NJC et al: Randomized control trial comparing prednisolone alone with cyclophosphamide and low dose prednisolone in combination in cryptogenic fibrosing alveolitis. Thorax 1989;44:280–288

265. Ragu G, Depaso WJ, Cain K et al: Azathioprine combined with prednisolone in the treatment of idiopathic pulmonary fibrosis: a prospective double-blind randomized placebo-controlled clinical trial. Am Rev Respir Dis 1991;144:219–226

266. Krafcik SS, Cobin RB, Lynch JP, Sitrin RG: Wegener's granulomatosis in the elderly. Chest 1996;109:430–437

267. Devaney KO, Travis WD, Hoffman GS et al: Interpretation of head and neck biopsies in Wegener's granulomatosis. Am J Surg Pathol 1990;14:555–564

268. Travis WD, Hoffman GS, Leavitt RY et al: Surgical pathology of the lung in Wegener's granulomatosis. Am J Surg Pathol 1991;15:315–333

269. Andrassy K, Erb A, Koderisch J et al: Wegener's granulomatosis with renal involvement: patient survival and correlations between initial renal function, renal histology, therapy and renal outcome. Clin Nephrol 1991;35:139–147

270. Fauci AS, Haynes BF, Katz P, Wolff SM: Wegener's granulomatosis: prospective clinical and therapeutic experience with 85 patients for 21 years. Ann Intern Med 1983;98:76–85

271. Bradley JD, Brandt KD, Katz BP: Infectious complications of cyclophosphamide for vasculitis. Arthritis Rheum 1989;32: 415–453

272. Seidl LG, Thornton GF, Smith JW, Cluff LE: Studies on the epidemiology of adverse drug reactions. III. Reactions in patients on a general medical service. Bull. Johns Hopkins Hosp 1966;119:299–315

273. Hurwitz N: Predisposing factors in adverse reactions to drugs. BMJ 1969;1:536–539

274. Levy M, Kewitz H, Altwein W et al: Hospital admissions due to adverse drug reactions: a comparative study from Jerusalem and Berlin. Eur J Clin Pharmacol 1980;17:25–31

CHAPTER 78

Muscle Strength

STUART BRUCE

Like wrinkled skin and white hair, loss of muscle strength is part of the stereotyped image of old age. And beneath the wrinkles of the caricature, shriveled muscles testify to the accompanying wasting, raising questions as to its cause and whether the remaining muscle is as strong, proportionately, as it was in youth or is further weakened by age. If the weakness is greater than we would expect for the degree of wasting, what might be the causes of the additional weakness? What does a knowledge of possible causes tell us about approaches to prevention or reversal of the changes?

"Strength" has no precise physiologic definition, although it is often used synonymously with "force." The maximum force that a muscle can produce may be measured under isometric conditions, when the muscle's length is constant, or during dynamic contractions, when the muscle is shortening (concentric) or stretching (eccentric). These laboratory conditions have functional counterparts: the maintenance of posture depends largely on isometric contractions; climbing stairs involves shortening contractions whereas descending necessitates muscle lengthening.

Methodologic Considerations

The maximal force produced by a muscle should be proportional to its cross-sectional area (CSA) taken at right angles to the individual fibers. Thus to compare the force produced between individuals of different sizes we need to measure their muscle CSAs and relate force to CSA. Measuring CSA is particularly important in aging studies because both muscle size and force are known to be changing. Because interpreting anatomic CSA measurements is not straightforward, some authors have related muscle force measurements to estimates of overall muscle bulk. However this is unsatisfactory because bulk and force measurements are not likely to be directly proportional and because different muscles may waste to different extents.

Speed of contraction and the product of the velocity of shortening and force (muscle power) are both important in activities such as climbing stairs and getting up from a low seat. Muscle power, unlike force, should be proportional to overall muscle bulk, at least of those muscles involved in the movement observed, but these parameters do not seem to have been compared in any study of aging.

Methods for measuring muscle force in the clinical setting have been established since the 1950s.[1,2] These vary from simple devices measuring hand grip, to motorized dynamometers that may be used to measure isometric or dynamic contractions, for example of quadriceps. Maximal grip strength is a popular measurement because it is a simple technique that is easy to explain to subjects. However, the movement is a complex mixture of isometric and dynamic contractions of forearm and hand muscles and although it is possible to get repeatable measurements in an individual it is impossible to normalize the measurements between individuals because there is no reliable method of measuring the CSAs of the muscles involved. Even if there were such a method it would still be difficult to assess the relative contributions of the hand and forearm muscles used and thus how their properties might change with aging.

Another method of assessing strength that is difficult to interpret is maximum weight-lifting for one repetition (1-RM), which has been used in some American studies. Weight-lifting requires the complex coordinated action of muscles, other than the group being studied, to stabilize the body. There is a large central learning component to this.[3] In one study 1-RM overestimated changes in strength of knee extensors and flexors by up to 10 times compared with isokinetic testing in the same subjects; although repeatable measurements were obtained using both methods there was no correlation between them.[4] Weight-lifting is one situation where "strength" is decidedly not synonymous with "force."

The Extent of the Weakness

Figure 78-1 shows age-related changes in grip strength in men taken from four cross-sectional studies published over the past 150 years.[5–8] Despite the caveats above, grip is the most extensively reported measurement in both cross-sectional and longitudinal studies. Overall declines from youth are consistently between 30 and 40 percent. However, in the more recent studies, maximum strength is attained earlier and preserved longer into middle age, suggesting that environmental or behavioral factors can modify the underlying trend.

Similar declines are seen in other muscle groups and in both sexes. Figure 78-2 shows an example redrawn from a recent study of quadriceps;[9] isometric and concentric contractions show declines of 26 to 37 percent, with those in women starting earlier than in men. However, there is no significant change in eccentric strength in either sex. Similar age-related changes in the force-velocity relationship (relative sparing of

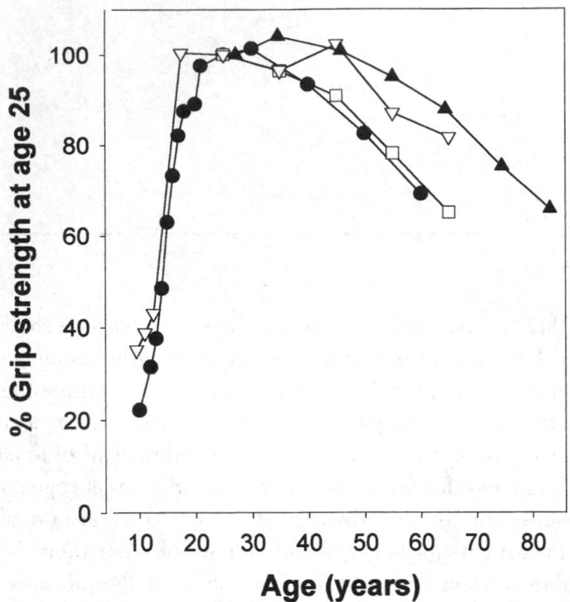

Figure 78-1 Age-related changes in male grip strength in studies from the early nineteenth century to the present day. (Data from Quetelet,[5] [•], Ufland[6] [□], Shephard[7] [∇], and Kallman et al.[8] [▲].)

Figure 78-2 Age-related changes in maximal isometric and dynamic contractions of quadriceps in women (open symbols and solid lines) and men (black symbols and dotted lines). ○,●: isometric; ∇, ▼: concentric; □, ■: eccentric. (Data from Hortobágyi et al.[9])

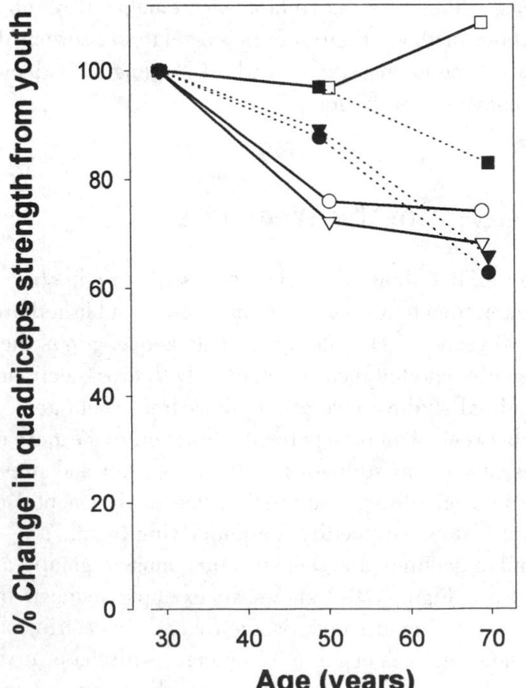

eccentric strength by aging) are seen in abductor pollicis and in mouse muscle.[10]

The examples given so far have been from cross-sectional studies and, unless otherwise stated, this is true for the remainder of this chapter. Comparisons between cross-sectional and longitudinal measurements of strength have been surprisingly inconsistent. In one large study of grip strength in subjects aged over 65 years, the cross-sectional decline over 4 years (2 percent per year) underestimated the longitudinal decline in men (3 percent per year) and even more so in women (5 percent).[11] However in the Baltimore study, where longitudinal and cross-sectional measurements of grip in men are compared in decades from the third to the eighth, cross-sectional declines were consistently steeper.[8] Two longitudinal studies of quadriceps also give disparate results.[12,13]

Muscle Mass, Reserve Capacity, and Thresholds

Estimates of total muscle mass from measurements of total body potassium,[14] body density,[15] and creatinine excretion shown in Figure 78-3 demonstrate that a large part of the decline in muscle force after middle age can be accounted for by loss of muscle mass. The greater apparent decline seen in the older subjects in the Baltimore creatinine excretion data[16] (Fig. 78-3A) may be partly explained by the youngest and oldest groups having relatively few subjects and consequently large standard errors.

Figure 78-3B also shows that, from adolescence, muscle mass is lower in females than males.[14,15] The functional reserve is thus likely to be lower in women than in men. For example, tasks such as rising unaided from the toilet may require maximal quadriceps contractions for women in their eighties,[3] their quadriceps strength being approximately 50 percent that of men. Such observations have been generalized into the concept of "thresholds" below which any further decline renders everyday activities impossible.[3] A period of illness and recumbency may be sufficient to cross the threshold to dependence.

Is the Weakness All Due to Wasting?

Figure 78-4 shows declines in maximum voluntary isometric force (MVF) and in CSA from studies of a variety of muscles in women[17–21] (Fig. 78-4A) and men[18,20–23] (Fig. 78-4B). In all except one influential study of quadriceps in women by Young's group[17] where no age-related differences between the declines in MVF and in CSA were found, the declines in MVF are greater than can be accounted for by the respective declines in CSA. There is also greater variation in the CSA measurements between studies, particularly in women. Although wasting may affect some muscles more than others there is also variation between investigators even for the same muscle group, pointing to error in the CSA measurements. This makes

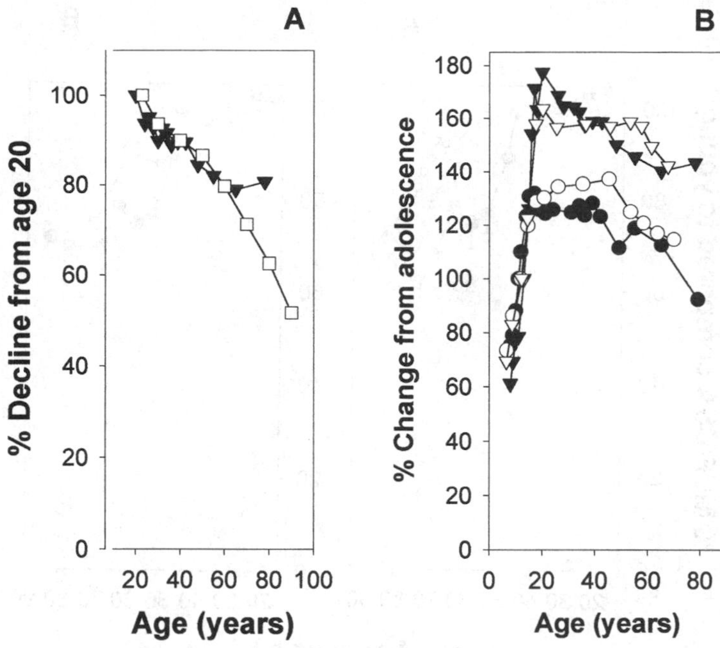

Figure 78-3 Age-related changes in estimates of total muscle bulk. (**A**) Declines in total muscle bulk from age 20 years in men. (Data from studies of total body potassium[14] [▼], and creatinine excretion[16] [□]. (**B**) Age-related changes in total muscle bulk from adolescence in males (inverted triangles) and females (circles). Data from studies of total body potassium[14] (black symbols) and body density[15] (white symbols).

the interpretation of regression analyses of force against CSA difficult because of the assumption in the analysis that all the error is in the force measurements. It is better to assume that MVF is proportional to CSA and compare the means of the ratio MVF/CSA for the individual subjects, knowing that this is an approximation because of the errors in both force and CSA measurements. The time course of the decline in this ratio has been studied in abductor pollicies (AP) in both sexes[24] (Fig. 78-5A) and in quadriceps in women[19] (Fig. 78-5B). In women there are significant declines in MVF/CSA around the time of the menopause in both quadriceps and AP. In AP this is strikingly different from men, in whom the decline starts later and is more gradual. By the eighth decade the decline in MVF/CSA in both studies is of the order of 25 percent and about one-half the overall declines in strength of these muscles are accounted for by decline in force/CSA.

Fiber Numbers, Fiber Types, and Motor Units

Muscles are composed of fibers with differing biochemical and mechanical properties. In mammalian muscle the main subdivision is into type I (slow) and type II (fast). Aging results in loss of type I and type II fibers from upper and lower limb muscles[25] and in the loss of motor units.[26] Figure 78-6 shows

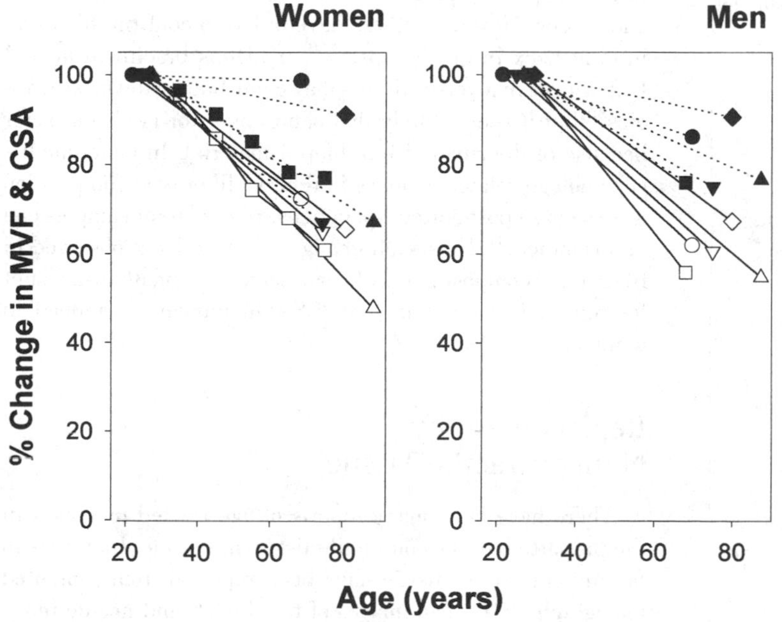

Figure 78-4 Age-related declines in MVF (open symbols) and CSA (black symbols) in women and men. CSA was measured by ultrasound: ▽, ▼ (quadriceps: female,[17] male[22]); △, ▲ (triceps surae[18]); by CT scanning: □, ■ (quadriceps: female,[19], male[23]); and by anthropometry: ○, ● (triceps surae[20]); ◇, ◆ (adductor pollicis[21]).

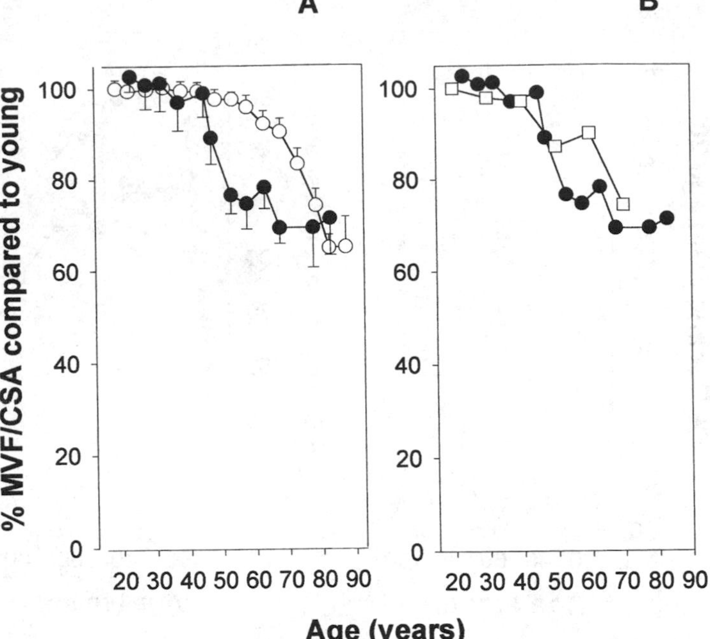

Figure 78-5 Age-related declines in MVF/CSA. (**A**) Adductor pollicis in women (●) and men (○). (Data from Phillips et al.[24]) (**B**) Adductor pollicis (●) and quadriceps (□) in women. (Data from Phillips et al.[24] and Rutherford et al.,[19] respectively.)

that in soleus the decline in motor units estimated electrophysiologically[18] is comparable with the numbers in histologic sections of S1/2 spinal cord segments.[26] In quadriceps the decline in muscle fiber numbers[27] is greater than the decline in L3/4 motor units.[26] This may again be due to some muscles being affected to a greater extent than others but there may also be other factors that result in the loss of muscle fibers (e.g., decline in the local production of growth factors).

Figure 78-6 Age-related declines in motor units and fiber numbers. Motor units in postmortem spinal cord sections[26] (○: L3/4 segments; △: S1/2 segments); ▲: motor unit numbers in soleus muscle (supplied by S1/2 roots) estimated by incremental stimulation[18]; ●: muscle fiber numbers in postmortem cross-sections of vastus lateralis[27] (supplied by L3/4 roots).

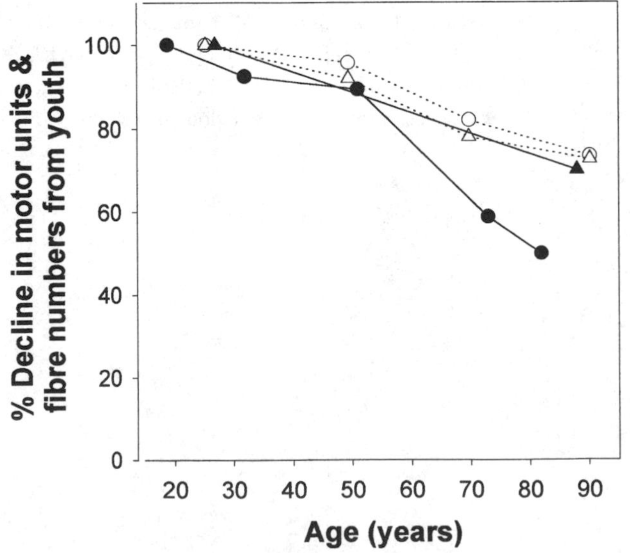

Wasting may also be due to the remaining fibers getting smaller. That fiber atrophy also occurs is demonstrated by a significant decline in alkali soluble protein per unit DNA content of muscle.[28] This atrophy appears to affect type II fibers but not type I.[27,29,30] Since type II fibers are recruited during more strenuous contractions this might relate to decline in activity. Type II fibers have been reported to produce greater force/CSA than type I although uncertainties remain about the size of this difference.[31] A decline in the proportion or size of type II fibers with age might therefore account for decline in force/CSA as well as for some of the decline in muscle bulk. In addition to decline in type II fiber area, studies by Larsson[29] also found a progressive decrease in the proportion of type II fibers in quadriceps biopsies of men between their twenties and sixties. However, others have failed to confirm this trend in either sex in quadriceps,[23,30] or biceps brachii in men.[23] Differences in levels of fitness may contribute to the discrepancies[30] but it seems likely that sampling error is also a factor because of the small size of biopsy material. In male quadriceps no age-related changes in relative fiber type composition were seen in postmortem specimens, where larger samples can be examined.[27] Thus such changes as have been observed in fiber type composition with age seem too small to account for reported changes in force/CSA in humans or indeed in animals.[31]

Replacement by Noncontractile Tissue

There have been many reports of age-related increases in the proportion of noncontractile tissue in muscle. Increases in fat and connective tissue have been reported from computed tomography (CT) scan images of the thigh[32] and needle biop-

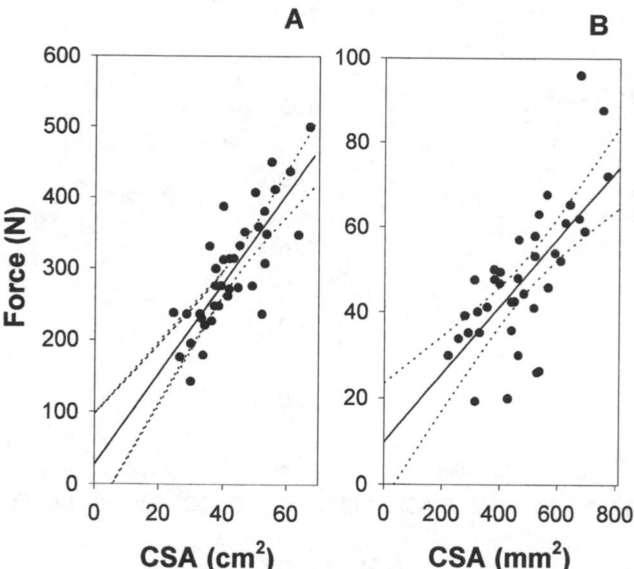

Figure 78-7 Relationship between MVF and CSA in elderly male and female subjects. (**A**) Quadriceps (ages 70 to 81 years). (Data from Young et al.[17,22], (**B**) Adductor pollicis (ages 74 to 90 years). Regression lines and 99 percent confidence intervals are shown. (Data from Phillips et al.[21])

sies of quadriceps,[28] although a surface nuclear magnetic resonance (NMR) study of flexor digitorum superficialis found no increases in fat content in older men or women.[33] Where there is a good correlation between force and CSA measurements, as in elderly subjects from the studies of quadriceps[17,22] and AP[21] shown in Figure 78-7, the absence of significant positive intercepts on the x-axis, when force is plotted against CSA, argues against the presence of noncontractile tissue significantly affecting force/CSA measurements in humans. The magnitude of the reported changes in noncontractile tissue is also unlikely to account for observed declines in force/CSA in animals.[34]

Failure of Activation

A simple explanation for the decline in force/CSA would be that older people are unable to activate their muscles completely due to loss of motivation or to reflex inhibition, secondary to arthropathy, which may result in muscle weakness even in the absence of pain.[35] Obviously in individual circumstances these factors may be important. However, studies using supramaximal tetanic stimulation in triceps surae,[20] and the technique of superimposing stimulated twitches during voluntary contractions[1] in calf muscles,[18] quadriceps,[19] and AP,[21] suggest that failure of voluntary activation is not a general cause of reduced force/CSA with age.

Metabolic Changes

The most everyday example of decline in force/CSA is muscle fatigue. In fatigue this is at least partly due to buildup of metabolites, especially inorganic phosphate (P_i). The decline in force/CSA in fatigued animal muscle is absent in eccentric contractions.[36] Because we have seen (Fig. 78-2) that force produced by eccentric contractions is also unaffected by age, it is attractive to postulate that metabolic changes might contribute to the age-related decline in isometric force/CSA. Mitochondrial respiration rates[37] and muscle carnitine,[38] an essential cofactor for the transport of long-chain fatty acids into mitochondria, have been shown to decline with age. However, NMR studies in humans[33] and mice[39] found no age-related changes in P_i or in pH, another known metabolic influence on force/CSA.

Disuse and Training

It is obvious that the majority of us become less active as we get older. Disuse leads to muscle wasting, and detraining to decline in force/CSA.[40] Isometric force of triceps surae has been found to be significantly correlated with walking speed (i.e., with an objective measure of activity)[41]; it is especially attractive to postulate that detraining might be a major cause of the weakness of aging because of the potential for prevention. However, if it were as simple as this, the trend in Figure 78-1 would be reversed; that is, the weakness would be observed to start at an earlier age in more recent studies, because most of us are becoming more sedentary than our forebears. Observations on aging runners and swimmers show that these activities do not protect against loss of strength or decline in type II fiber area, although strength training maintained into old age apparently does so.[23] As well as force, leg extensor power has been shown to correlate with functional variables in elderly men and women[42] but also to decline faster in men than women despite elderly men remaining more active.[43] Thus neither muscle force nor power in older subjects is consistently related to activity.

Studies testing whether training can reverse age-related changes rather than prevent them have been particularly beset by methodologic inadequacies. However, a carefully conducted controlled study of women over the age of 75 years has recently reported a 27 percent increase in isometric quadriceps strength after 12 weeks of strength training.[44] The hypothesis tested in this study was that function would improve purely by increasing strength and the training regimen thus avoided functional tasks. Unfortunately tests of functional ability showed little change, but in another study in which elderly subjects were given specific task-oriented training for 8 weeks, functional improvements were more impressive, although the gains in muscle force were not as great.[45] This suggests that in order to improve function, central motor programming may be at least as important as increasing strength. However, there was another difference between these two studies in that the subjects in the second study were more frail. It may be easier to show functional improvements with strength training where the degree of initial disability is greater; another controlled study demonstrated functional improvements, after 10 weeks of resistance training, in very frail nursing home patients, al-

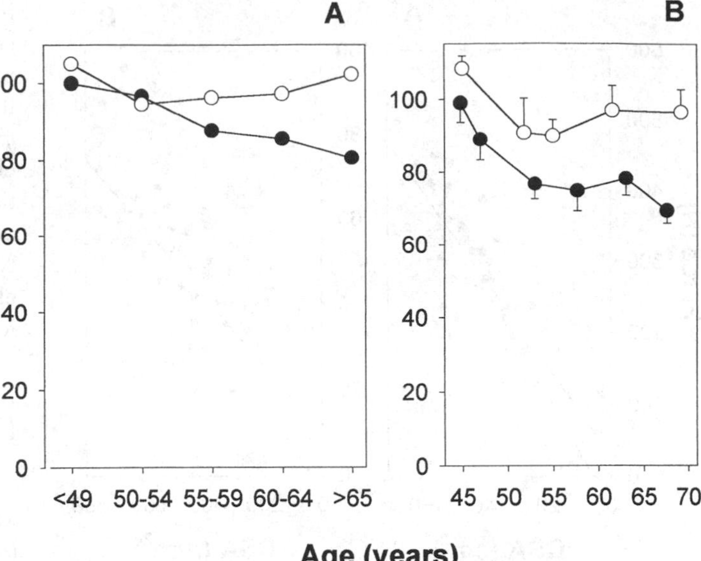

Figure 78-8 Percent change in strength compared with young nonusers of hormone replacement therapy. Women users are represented by open symbols; nonusers, by black symbols. (**A**) Grip strength. (Data from Cauley et al.[52]) (**B**) Adductor pollicis. (Data from Phillips et al.[24])

though the relationship between these and the reported changes in strength is tenuous because 1-RM was used as the strength measurement.[46]

Hormones

Hormones may influence muscle force by increasing the number of cross-bridges (anabolic action), influencing the amount of force the cross-bridges exert when they are attached (inotropic action) and by influencing the rates of force development or relaxation (chronotropic action).[10] Growth hormone (GH); insulin-like growth factor-1, and male sex hormones have well-known actions on muscle and are also known to decline with age. Actions of female sex hormones on muscle force have recently been postulated.[10,47]

GH administered to GH-deficient young adults results in increases in quadriceps size and strength[48] followed by declines on discontinuation of therapy.[49] These changes are in proportion (i.e., no change in MVF/CSA). In the elderly, although increases in muscle size have been reported,[50] so far no group has been able to demonstrate increases in strength.

In a small study of testosterone replacement in hypogonadal elderly men, grip strength increased approximately 10 percent after 3 months.[51] In women hormone replacement therapy (HRT) is, of course, much better established. HRT has been shown to protect against the age-associated decline in grip strength.[52] (Fig. 78-8A) and in MVF/CSA in AP[24] (Fig. 78-8B). In the study of grip strength estrogen dose was positively associated with strength but the number of subjects over 65 years of age was very small; in a large follow-up study of women over 65 years of age the protective effect seemed to be lost.[53]

Summary

Muscle strength declines with age due to a number of factors whose respective contributions probably differ from one individual to another and from one muscle to another. Irreversible loss of motor units and muscle fibers accounts for about one-half of this decline. Strength and power have been related to functional variables[41,42] and old muscle is undoubtedly trainable resulting in both increases in strength[4,43] and in fiber hypertrophy.[4] It is therefore attractive to think that activity maintained into old age would prevent the decline in muscle function. The paradox is that so far only strength training, hardly a universal indulgence nor likely to become so, has been shown to prevent decline in strength and fiber atrophy.[23]

Hormone treatment may have a role but conclusive benefits of GH replacement remain tantalizingly elusive and, despite the apparent benefits,[24,52] many questions remain about sex hormone replacement therapy with regard to muscle function: as to how long the protective effects persist, whether sex hormone related changes are reversible, whether the benefits shown in strength translate into function, whether the effects shown in the hand are present in other muscles, and the extent to which men as well as women might benefit.

References

1. Merton PA: Voluntary strength and fatigue. J Physiol 1954;123:553–564
2. Edwards RHT, Young A, Hosking GP, Jones DA: Human skeletal muscle function: description of tests and normal values. Clin Sci Mol Med 1977;52:283–290
3. Young A: Strength and power. pp. 599–600. In Evans JG, Williams FT (eds): Oxford Textbook of Geriatric Medicine. Oxford University Press, Oxford, 1992
4. Frontera WR, Meredith CN, O'Reilly KP et al: Strength conditioning in older men: skeletal muscle hypertrophy and improved function. J Appl Physiol 1988;64:1038–1044
5. Quetelet A: A Treatise on Man and the Development of His Faculties. p. 69. Chambers, Edinburgh, 1842
6. Ufland JM: Einfluss des Lebensalters, Geschlechts, der Konstitution und des Berufs auf die Kraft verschiedener Muskelgruppen. Arbeitsphysiologie 1933;6:653–663

7. Shephard RJ: Endurance Fitness. pp. 107–108. University of Toronto Press, Toronto, 1969
8. Kallman DA, Plato CC, Tobin JD: The role of muscle loss in the age-related decline of grip strength: cross-sectional and longitudinal perspectives. J Gerontol Med Sci 1990;45:M82–88
9. Hortobágyi T, Zheng D, Weider M et al: The influence of aging on muscle strength and muscle fiber characteristics with special reference to eccentric strength. J Gerontol Biol Sci 1995;50: B399–B406
10. Phillips SK, Rutherford OM, Birch K et al: Hormonal influences on muscle force: evidence for an inotropic effect of oestrogen. Sports, Exercise Injury 1995;1:58–63
11. Bassey EJ, Harries UJ: Normal values for handgrip strength in 920 men and women over 65 years, and longitudinal changes over 4 years in 620 survivors. Clin Sci 1993;84:331–337
12. Aniansson A, Hedberg M, Henning G-B, Grimby G: Muscle morphology, enzymatic activity and muscle strength in elderly men: a follow-up study. Muscle Nerve 1986;9:585–591
13. Greig CA, Botella J, Young A: The quadriceps strength of healthy elderly people remeasured after eight years. Muscle Nerve 1993; 16:6–10
14. Allen TH, Andersen EC, Langham WH: Total body potassium and gross body composition in relation to age. J Gerontol 1960; 15:348–357
15. Barlett HL, Puhl SM, Hodgson JL, Buskirk ER: Fat-free mass in relation to stature: ratios of fat-free mass to height in children, adults, and elderly subjects. Am J Clin Nutr 1991;53:1112–1116
16. Tzankoff SP, Norris AH: Effect of muscle mass decrease on age-related BMR changes. J Appl Physiol 1977;43:1001–1006
17. Young A, Stokes M, Crowe M: Size and strength of the quadriceps muscles of old and young women. Eur J Clin Invest 1984;14: 282–287
18. Vandervoort AA, McComas AJ: Contractile changes in opposing muscles of the human ankle joint with aging. J Appl Physiol 1986;61:361–367
19. Rutherford OM, Jones DA: The relationship of muscle and bone loss and activity levels with age in women. Age Ageing 1992; 21:286–293
20. Davies CTM, Thomas DO, White MJ: Mechanical properties of young and elderly human muscle. Acta Med Scand 1986;suppl 711:219–226
21. Phillips SK, Bruce SA, Newton D, Woledge RC: The weakness of old age is not due to failure of muscle activation. J Gerontol Med Sci 1992;47:M45–M49
22. Young A, Stokes M, Crowe M: The size and strength of the quadriceps muscles of old and young men. Clin Physiol 1985;5: 145–154
23. Klitgaard H, Mantoni M, Schiaffino S et al: Function, morphology and protein expression of ageing skeletal muscle: a cross-sectional study of elderly men with different training backgrounds. Acta Physiol Scand 1990;140:41–54
24. Phillips SK, Rook KM, Siddle NC et al: Muscle weakness in women occurs at an earlier age than in men, but strength is preserved by hormone replacement therapy. Clin Sci 1993;84: 95–98
25. Jennekens FGI, Tomlinson BE, Walton JN: Histochemical aspects of five limb muscles in old age: an autopsy study. J Neurol Sci 1971;14:259–276
26. Tomlinson BE, Irving D: The numbers of limb motor neurons in the human lumbosacral cord throughout life. J Neurol Sci 1977; 34:213–219
27. Lexell J, Taylor CC, Sjöström M: What is the cause of ageing atrophy? Total number, size and proportion of different fibre types studied in whole vastus lateralis muscle from 15- to 83-year-old men. J Neurol Sci 1988;84:275–294
28. Forsberg AM, Nilsson E, Werneman J et al: Muscle composition in relation to age and sex. Clin Sci 1991;81:249–256
29. Larsson L: Morphological and functional characteristics of the ageing skeletal muscle in man. A cross-sectional study. Acta Physiol Scand 1978;suppl 457:1–36
30. Grimby G, Aniansson A, Zetterberg C, Saltin B: Is there a change in relative muscle fibre composition with age? Clin Physiol 1984; 4:189–194
31. Larsson L, Ansved T: Effects of ageing on the motor unit. Prog Neurobiol 1995;45:397–458
32. Overend TJ, Cunningham DA, Paterson DH, Lefcoe MS: Thigh composition in young and elderly men determined by computed tomography. Clin Physiol 1992;12:629–640
33. Taylor DJ, Crowe M, Bore PJ et al: Examination of the energetics of aging skeletal muscle using nuclear magnetic resonance. Gerontology 1984;30:2–7
34. Faulkner JA, Brooks SV, Zerba E: Skeletal muscle weakness and fatigue in old age: underlying mechanisms. p. 153. In Cristofalo VJ (ed): Annual Review of Gerontology and Geriatrics. Vol. 10. Springer, New York, 1991
35. Stokes M, Young A: The contribution of reflex inhibition to arthrogenous muscle weakness. Clin Sci 1984;67:7–14
36. Flitney FW, Jones DA: The effects of stretch on force production in fresh and fatigued skeletal muscle, abstracted. J Muscle Res Cell Motil 1990;11:75–76
37. Trounce I, Byrne E, Marzuki S: Decline in skeletal muscle mitochondrial respiratory chain function: possible factor in ageing. Lancet 1989;1:637–639
38. Costell M, O'Connor JE, Grisolia S: Age-dependent decrease in carnitine content in muscle of mice and humans. Biochem Biophys Res Commun 1989;161:1135–1143
39. Phillips SK, Wiseman RW, Woledge RC, Kushmerick MJ: Neither changes in phosphorus metabolite levels nor myosin isoforms can explain the weakness in aged mouse muscle. J Physiol 1993; 463:157–167
40. Narici MV, Roi GS, Landoni L et al: Changes in force, cross-sectional area and neural activation during strength training and detraining of the human quadriceps. Eur J Appl Physiol 1989; 59:310–319
41. Bassey EJ, Bendall MJ, Pearson M: Muscle strength in the triceps surae and objectively measured customary walking activity in men and women over 65 years of age. Clin Sci 1988;74:85–89
42. Bassey EJ, Fiatrone MA, O'Neill EF et al: Leg extensor power and functional performance in very old men and women. Clin Sci 1992;82:321–327
43. Skelton DA, Greig CA, Davies JM, Young A: Strength, power and related functional ability of healthy people aged 65–89 years. Age Ageing 1994;23:371–377
44. Skelton DA, Young A, Greig CA, Malbut KE: Effects of resistance training on strength, power, and selected functional abilities of

women aged 75 and older. J Am Geriatr Soc 1995;43:1081–1087

45. Skelton DA, McLaughlin AW: Training functional ability in old age. Physiotherapy 1996;82:159–166
46. Fiatrone MA, O'Neill EF, Ryan ND et al: Exercise training and nutritional supplementation for physical frailty in very elderly people. N Engl J Med 1994;330:1769–1775
47. Sarwar R, Beltran Niclos B, Rutherford OM: Changes in muscle strength, relaxation rate and fatiguability during the human menstrual cycle. J Physiol 1995;493:267–272
48. Cuneo RC, Salomon F, Wiles CM et al: Growth hormone treatment in growth hormone-deficient adults. I. Effects on muscle mass and strength. J Appl Physiol 1991;70:688–694
49. Rutherford OM, Jones DA, Round JM et al: Changes in skeletal muscle and body composition after discontinuation of growth hormone treatment in growth hormone deficient young adults. Clin Endocrinol 1991;34:469–475
50. Rudman D, Feller AG, Hoskote SN et al: Effects of human growth hormone in men over 60 years old. New Engl J Med 1990;323:1–6
51. Morley JE, Perry HM III, Kaiser FE et al: Effects of testosterone replacement therapy in old hypogonadal males: a preliminary study. J Am Geriatr Soc 1993;41:149–152
52. Cauley JA, Petrini AM, LaPorte RE et al: The decline of grip strength in the menopause: relationship to physical activity, estrogen use and anthropometric factors. J Chronic Dis 1987;40:115–120
53. Seeley DG, Cauley JA, Grady D et al: Is postmenopausal estrogen therapy associated with neuromuscular function or falling in elderly women? Arch Intern Med 1995;155:293–299

CHAPTER 79

Aging and Neuromuscular Disease

WILLIAM J. K. CUMMING

Age Changes

Skeletal muscle fibers are the "end organ" of the anterior horn cell. A single motor neuron, associated with the many muscle fibers it innervates, is known as the motor unit. This motor unit is not static throughout life, and changes occur as a consequence of disease or aging. Muscle fibers are subdivided into two main groups: type I or "slow-twitch" fibers and type II or "fast-twitch" fibers. The proportions of each fiber type differ according to the specialization of the individual muscle. Fast and slow muscle fibers have different patterns of energy metabolism. Fast fibers either rely on glycolysis alone (type IIB) or in combination with oxidative pathways (type IIA), whereas slow fibers rely on oxidative pathways only.[1,2] These different metabolic properties can be used to distinguish the fiber types by histochemical techniques and form the basis for the histochemical analysis of muscle biopsies.

Motor neurons also show diversity of form and function, large motor neurons innervating large motor units and, conversely, small motor neurons innervating small motor units.[1,2] The muscle fiber differentiation into fast and slow also depends on the parent neuron, which is either fast or slow.

In muscle the most common changes seen with advancing age, in the absence of any signs of associated disease, are those of muscle atrophy both in terms of overall muscle bulk and of the size of individual fibers.[3,14] These changes are to some extent dependent on the fallout of anterior horn cells that occurs with age, but this does not completely explain the process of aging atrophy. In detailed studies it has been shown that the progressive reduction that occurs in muscle volume with aging can be detected from age 25 years and that up to 10 percent of muscle volume is lost by age 50 years. Thereafter the rate of muscle volume atrophy increases, so that by 80 years almost half the muscle has wasted.[15] These changes are not usually accompanied by any change in functional ability or major loss of strength.[16,17]

Both reduction in fiber number and fiber size are implicated in the loss of muscle volume. Type II fibers seem particularly vulnerable to atrophy; however this is a nonspecific reaction, similar type II atrophy being seen in association with disease states.[18] It seems probable, but as yet unproven, that the loss of anterior horn cells leads to denervation of muscle fibers in that motor unit.[19,20] Initially, reinnervation from surrounding normal terminal axons is possible; however, this process diminishes with time so that the fibers are permanently denervated. This loss of functioning motor units can be shown electrophysiologically.[21]

There are now several studies that show that mitochondrial abnormalities occur in skeletal muscle fibers in both the aged rat and human.[22–28] These abnormalities are of a respiratory chain type and are mostly associated with mitochondrial DNA deletions. Abnormalities of the mitochondrial genome, for example deletion at site[4374], which normally leads to the development of the MELAS syndrome (multiple stroke-like episodes with a mitochondrial myopathy), can be shown to be present as a normal finding in aged muscle.[29] Up to 50 percent of the muscle fibers of the elderly population have been shown to contain abnormalities of mitochondrial DNA. However, these abnormalities in the mitochondrial genome are not regularly associated with major evidence of mitochondrial dysfunction as judged by histochemical stains for mitochondrial function or by studies of mitochondrial respiratory chain function.[23,30]

In the mitochondrial myopathies, where clear ultrastructural change within the mitochondria is seen, it has been suggested that the abnormal mitochondria in some way contributes to the muscle weakness that the patient experiences. The same is also true in myotonic dystrophy, where there is an increasing amount of abnormal mitochondrial DNA with advancing muscle weakness. However, in myotonic dystrophy, the gene abnormality is in the nuclear genome[31,32] and the findings of mutant mitochondrial DNA in limb muscle remain to be explained.

Although there is persuasive evidence to suggest that increased abnormalities of peroxidation can lead to increasingly damaged mitochondrial DNA,[33] this may well occur in the anterior horn cell and could be a contributing factor to anterior horn cell loss in association with aging.[34] However, it is more difficult to understand the mechanism whereby increased mitochondrial genomic deletions in muscle fibers would lead to abnormalities within the muscle fiber in terms of its loss of size and volume and consequent loss of strength. The exact relationship, therefore, between mitochondrial DNA deletions and skeletal muscle of aging remains to be elucidated.

It would appear therefore that at the present time the most prominent mechanism in the loss of muscle fiber bulk with age relates to anterior horn cell changes leading to denervation with ineffective reinnervation within the muscle.

The constant remodeling at the microscopic level of the

limb muscles, which is the inevitable consequence of the above process, implies that any changes that are said to occur in a muscle as a consequence of disease must be set in the context of what is normal for that muscle.[35] Such studies are infrequent, particularly with respect to the elderly, and should be the focus of further research.

Clinical Aspects of Neuromuscular Disease

The major manifestations of neuromuscular disease are, at all ages, muscle weakness and, to a lesser extent, pain and stiffness. The clinical symptomatology of the cardinal features varies according to age. Thus minor symptoms will prompt consultation in the young athlete and the development of proximal weakness will soon prompt consultation in the young fit adult; however, older patients will generally tolerate moderate symptoms given that their expectations for mobility and stamina are reduced. Because of this, neuromuscular disease in the elderly may well be advanced before they seek medical advice. Once neuromuscular disease is suspected, the same principles apply to the delineation of the disorder and its investigation, irrespective of the age group of the patient involved. Only the emphasis differs with age, inherited disorders being of greater significance in younger patients and neuromuscular disorders associated with metabolic disease, malignancy, and drugs being of more significance in elderly patients.

Investigative Approach to the Patient With Neuromuscular Disease

It is often difficult to determine the duration of weakness in an individual, not only because of the patient's expectations, but also because the rate of progression of the majority of neuromuscular diseases is slow. Increasing weakness may be present for months and it is only the loss of the ability to perform some well-established task that brings the severity of the weakness to the patient's attention. In general, proximal weakness will be tolerated longer than distal weakness. Proximal lower limb weakness, as manifested by difficulty in rising from a low chair and difficulty climbing stairs, may be tolerated as "normal" whereas symptoms of distal lower limb weakness, for example catching the foot on stairs or experiencing difficulty in depressing the pedals while driving, are more quickly recognized as abnormal. Similarly in the upper limbs, symptoms suggestive of proximal weakness such as reaching up to a shelf or combing hair are tolerated whereas difficulty in turning a key or opening a bottle, suggestive of distal weakness, will often prompt the patient to seek medical advice. The presence of pain or stiffness in addition to weakness may initially be attributed to arthritis and it is only the failure of standard remedies to relieve the pain that will force the patient to seek advice. In many cases it will be the family who will initiate the referral on the basis that their relative is "slowing up." Although this is a highly nonspecific complaint, the presence or absence of neuromuscular disease can be determined on the basis of history, examination, and simple investigations.

History

The most common presenting symptoms of muscle disease are weakness and pain, but the patient may require a lot of help in describing the history correctly, and the full history will sometimes be obtained only after several consultations with the patient and interviews with relatives.[36–38]

Although slowness in walking and increasing falls can be due to primary neuromuscular disease this is relatively uncommon, and the more common disorders of gait must be excluded before considering the neuromuscular system as at fault.[39]

Many of the neuromuscular diseases are inherited, and it is important therefore to inquire specifically about other family members. The remarkable explosion of knowledge in the field of molecular biology has led to the recognition of disease states that in the past defied diagnosis. This underscores the need to examine first-degree relatives in a family suspected of having inherited neuromuscular disorder. The history may not suggest that the elderly relative is affected, whereas this can be confirmed by examination.

The identification of the gene locus for spinal muscular atrophy[40] will widen the scope of this anterior horn cell disease. Although most common in children and young adults, late adult and elderly onset of disease have been described.[41] In families it will become increasingly important that the grandparents are screened for evidence of muscle weakness and minor evidence of the disease on muscle biopsy. This is exemplified by the finding of a family with an Xp21 (Duchenne and Becker muscular dystrophy) deletional myopathy where the grandfather showed only minor weakness even though he had the same deletion as his son and grandson who were more severely affected.[42–44]

Myotonic dystrophy, because of its marked variability in expression, and the presence of anticipation, may present in older patients with minor manifestations only (e.g., cataracts), compared with major symptoms in siblings.[45] The gene defect, which is an expansion of the trinucleotide repeat,[46] is unstable and tends to be magnified from generation to generation particularly via the female line, leading to anticipation[47] (i.e., the development of the disease earlier in siblings).

Weakness is commonly found in the proximal upper and lower limbs in disease of the muscle fibers per se (myopathic weakness) and also in many of the inherited spinal muscular atrophies (neurogenic weakness). Distal weakness is seen mainly in myotonic dystrophy and to a lesser extent in myopathic and neurogenic disease. Weakness of the cervical muscles will often lead to a complaint of the head falling forward, and some patients will report the necessity of using the hand to support the head.

Muscle pain is a relatively nonspecific feature seen in the majority of patients with progressive muscular disease. It is often poorly described and in many patients is related to exercise. As a presenting feature it is commonly seen only in inflammatory myopathy of acute or subacute onset, in polymyalgia rheumatica, and in "metabolic myopathies." In myasthenia gravis, power is reported as being normal at rest with weakness developing with exercise (which in the elderly often means toward the end of the day), the clear association with exercise being more commonly encountered in younger patients. The classic presentation of myasthenia gravis (with initial involvement of the eyes, then the oropharynx, then the limbs, and then ventilation) is not often seen in the group of patients with late onset (55 to 75 years). In this group limb weakness is usually the presenting feature, then spreading to the oropharynx and less commonly to the eyes. Ventilatory failure can occur at any stage of this progression and is not uncommonly the mode of presentation in the elderly. This presentation of myasthenia gravis in the elderly is difficult to distinguish from Lambert-Eaton myasthenic syndrome (LEMS), which has the same mode of onset at all ages (i.e., legs to oropharynx) and in which a history of improving strength with exercise is rarely encountered in the elderly.

Myotonia (delayed relaxation) is an uncommon complaint in the older patient. When present it usually signifies myotonic dystrophy or, more commonly, drug-induced disease. Fasciculation (involuntary contraction of individual motor units) is seen in patients with motor neuron disease/amyotrophic lateral sclerosis (MND/ALS) and rarely in the other late-onset denervating conditions of anterior horn cell origin.

Examination

The aim of examination of the neuromuscular system is to determine the distribution of muscle weakness and to assess its degree.[48] It has become apparent over the past decade that the terms limb girdle dystrophy (LG) and facioscapulohumeral dystrophy (FSH) do not adequately describe the patient's disease. They are only descriptive terms that convey the pattern of weakness in an individual and do not in any sense describe the underlying pathology.[18,49] It is now recognized that many different muscle diseases will produce weakness in a limb girdle or facioscapulohumeral distribution and therefore LG and FSH should be referred to as "syndromes," which more fully describes their varied etiology. In a patient with LG syndrome, the muscles involved are those of the proximal upper and lower limb girdles with preservation of strength in the distal muscles of arms and legs. In FSH the involved muscles are those of the obicularis oculi and oris and the proximal muscles of the upper limbs. With progression of the underlying disorder lower limb muscles will become involved. LG and FSH syndromes account for the majority of patients with neuromuscular disease. Two other patterns may be encountered, scapuloperoneal (SP) and distal. In SP, weakness is seen in the proximal upper limb muscles and the distal lower limb muscles.

SP disease is associated with a virtually normal life span, but the majority of patients develop cardiac conduction defects requiring the insertion of a pacemaker. The elderly patient who presents in heart block should be examined carefully to exclude the presence of an underlying SP disorder. Distal weakness, with involvement of the forearm and hand muscles in the upper limb and the anterior and posterior tibial compartment in the lower limb, is seen in some forms of spinal muscular atrophy and in myotonic dystrophy.

Having established the pattern of weakness, the symmetry of involvement is often a guide to the underlying etiology. In myopathic diseases (those involving the muscle fiber per se) symmetry is seen between right and left. In addition, around a joint, all of the muscles will be involved to about the same degree. In neurogenic diseases (in which the abnormality lies in the anterior horn cell or in the peripheral nerve) asymmetry and unequal involvement around a joint are seen. For example, in polymyositis the right and left deltoid, supra and infraspinatus, pectorals, and biceps may all be around MRC grade 4 strength, whereas in MND/ALS the right deltoid may be normal and the left MRC grade 3 with a normal supraspinatus, but weak infraspinatus on the left.

With the exception of MND/ALS, tone and reflexes in muscle diseases are either normal or, as in the majority of diseases, reduced. A careful search should be made for fasciculations in all patients with muscle disease. Although they will be seen most frequently in MND/ALS, they are a feature of any denervating neuromuscular disease. Difficulty is often encountered in observing fasciculations in the tongue. This is best seen with the tongue lying at rest in the floor of the mouth. Apparent fasciculation may be seen in the normal individual when the assessment is made with the tongue in any other position.

Investigations

Although it is possible on the basis of history and examination to make an accurate diagnosis in the majority of cases of neuromuscular disease, confirmation of that diagnosis requires the application of electrophysiologic, pathologic, and biochemical techniques.[18] In most cases this involves (1) estimation of the serum enzymes, (2) electromyography (EMG) and nerve conduction studies, and (3) muscle biopsy.

Although in previous years, various enzymes including serum glutamic oxaloacetic transamianse and aldolase were used as markers for muscle cell damage, it has become generally recognized that estimation of serum creatine kinase (CK) is the most sensitive index of muscle necrosis. This applies not only to primary muscle necrosis, as in polymyositis, but also to secondary myopathic change in long-standing denervation. CK consists of three separate isoenzymes: MM derived from skeletal muscle, MB derived largely from cardiac muscle, and BB derived mainly from brain. In normal serum the major isoenzyme is MM with about 6 percent MB. The proportion of the latter rises after acute myocardial injury. Alterations in serum CK are discussed in the appropriate sections.

Electrophysiology

A detailed description of electrophysiologic techniques in the diagnosis of neuromuscular disease is outside the scope of this chapter but will be found in appropriate textbooks.[50–52]

The most common method of electrophysiologic sampling of muscle is with concentric needle electromyography (CNEMG), which produces characteristic patterns that can be used to distinguish neurogenic and myopathic disorders.

Lower motor neuron lesions, due to damage to anterior horn cells or peripheral nerves, produce positive sharp wave and fibrillation potentials. A motor unit consists of those muscle fibers supplied by a single neuron; following the loss of motor neuron units, surviving units show abnormally high firing rates. Quantification of motor unit potential by Turns analysis and measurement of amplitude shows a reduction of the Turns/amplitude ratio in denervation. If an axon degenerates, neighboring intact axons may sprout to innervate the denervated muscle fibers. With such collateral innervation of denervated fibers, the number of muscle fibers per motor unit increases and "giant" motor units are detected by electrophysiology.

Primary myopathies are characterized by high-frequency discharges and by positive sharp waves and fibrillations. With the developments of so-called secondary myopathic changes in neurogenic muscle disease, CNEMG may be unable to resolve the question of whether the disease is primarily neurogenic with secondary myopathic changes, or primarily myopathic.

Single-fiber EMG (SFEMG) is of particular value in assessing end-plate disorders and is increasingly used to determine the nature of myopathic disorders.

Nerve conduction studies, in which the conduction velocity of peripheral nerves is measured, are used to detect primary pathology in peripheral nerves. Thus, very significant slowing of nerve conduction velocities suggests demyelination, whereas a reduction in amplitude and moderate slowing of conduction velocity is indicative of axonal degeneration.

Despite advances in biochemistry and neurophysiology, the final diagnosis in patients with muscle disease can be made only on muscle biopsy. The development of the technique of needle muscle biopsy,[53] which can be performed as an outpatient, has led to a greater understanding of the changes that occur with time in any given disease because sequential biopsies on the same patient are now available. Of even greater significance has been the application of histochemical techniques to fresh frozen muscle. This permits the differentiation of muscle fiber types (see above) and can be used to study the distribution of cellular enzymes and metabolic reserves.

Routine histologic stains can also be used with fresh frozen material and therefore the information obtained from paraffin-embedded muscle is not lost but rather is supplemented by the addition of histochemistry. The problems involved in both the processing and interpretation of muscle biopsies makes the technique unsuitable for routine laboratories and it is important therefore that muscle samples are sent to special neuromuscular laboratories or to experienced pathology centers.[18] Further descriptions of the pathologic changes seen on biopsy are given with the descriptions of the individual diseases. Developments in the field of radiology are beginning to have an impact on neuromuscular investigation. These relate to scanning of muscle (computed tomography [CT], magnetic resonance imaging [MRI]).[54,55] CT/MRI scan of the muscle can be used to assess the loss of muscle bulk and also the distribution of muscle involvement. This is important in obtaining a muscle biopsy where CT/MRI guided biopsies have a much greater yield of diagnostic information than those carried out "blind."[56]

Neuromuscular Diseases in the Elderly

This chapter is concerned only with those diseases that are common in the older age groups of patients. A description of the nosology of muscle diseases is therefore not appropriate because detailed recent reviews are available.[18,57,58] The majority of patients with inherited neuromuscular disease will have been identified at a younger age and details of these diseases will be found in standard textbooks.

Inflammatory Myopathy

The inflammatory myopathies can be broadly subdivided into those in which an infective agent can be demonstrated (bacterial, viral, and parasitic) and those in which an autoimmune basis is presumed (idiopathic). Although the first group is the most common worldwide, in Western societies idiopathic inflammatory myopathy is the most common variety and accounts for the greatest proportion of "acquired" primary myopathies.

The idiopathic group comprises polymyositis (PM), dermatomyositis (DM), PM-DM in association with connective tissue disorders, PM-DM in association with malignancy, and inclusion body myositis (IBM). There has been considerable debate as to the correct classification of this group. However, given that the response to therapy is similar in both PM and DM it seems advisable to adhere to the classification into group 1 "pure" PM-DM, group 2 PM-DM in association with other autoimmune diseases, and group 3 PM-DM associated with malignancy.[60–63]

Polymyositis-dermatomyositis complex

PM-DM has been considered to belong to the group of autoimmune disorders, mainly because of its association with other conditions, for example systemic lupus erythematosus. In addition, mononuclear cells are frequently seen in muscle biopsy. It is rare, however, to find circulating antibodies and evidence is increasing that cell-mediated immunity is the main basis of pathogenesis.

Clinical features PM-DM can occur at any age but there appear to be peaks in both childhood and late middle age. The overall incidence is 4 to 5 per million population[60,61,63] and women are more frequently affected than men. Initial presenting symptoms are weakness, skin rash, and joint or muscle pain. Progression is usually over weeks to months rather than years and on rare occasions hyperacute presentation with subcutaneous edema, intense muscle pain, and myoglobinuria may be seen.[64]

Weakness occurs during the course of the disease in every case. The pattern is usually that of limb girdle syndrome with symmetric proximal upper and lower limb girdle weakness. Wasting is seen in about 50 percent of cases. Involvement of distal muscles, in addition to proximal, is seen in about 30 percent and pharyngeal involvement leading to dysphagia and dysphonia in about 50 percent.[60,61,63,64] Weakness of respiratory muscles is rare. Rare presentations include predominantly distal weakness,[65] FSH weakness,[66] and localized nodular myositis.[67–71] In this variant, painful nodules recur in various muscles prior to the onset of proximal myopathy. When these occur in the gastrocnemius-soleus group they can be misdiagnosed as deep venous thrombosis.

The rash of DM occurs in about one-third of cases (range 15 to 40 percent). Typically it involves the face in a butterfly distribution and may spread to periorbital areas. In the arms and legs, the extensor surfaces are more commonly involved, dusky red patches being found over the elbows, knuckles, and to a lesser extent the knees and medial malleoli. Grottron's papules and periungal telangiectasis are uncommon skin manifestations.

Evidence of joint involvement is seen in 25 percent of patients with PM-DM. In some patients with long-standing rheumatoid arthritis, proximal myopathy with evidence of muscle necrosis on biopsy may develop as a late complication. It is probable that in general, dysphagia, Raynaud's phenomenon, and articular symptoms are more common in PM-DM associated with systemic collagen-vascular disease.[72] Involvement of other organ systems is rare in PM-DM. Cardiac involvement with heart block has been described,[73,74] as has parenchymal lung involvement with fibrosing alveolitis.[64,75]

PM-DM and malignancy The reported incidence of malignancy in PM-DM varies from 5 to 35 percent of all cases.[76,77] This disparity is not unexpected because many case reports are anecdotal rather than prospective and/or retrospective studies, the criteria for the diagnosis of PM-DM have differed between reports, and muscle biopsy has not been employed to confirm the presence of necrosis. In one series[78] the incidence of malignancy was 7.7 percent, the majority of patients having DM. The series of Bohan et al.[79] showed an incidence of 19 percent in male and 18 percent in female patients over the age of 50 years. In this group of patients PM was seen as frequently as DM. In most cases associated with malignancy, the onset of symptoms of the malignancy coincides with symptoms of PM-DM. Barnes[80] has, however, reported that myopathy can precede malignancy by months or years. The most common sites of malignancy in women are breast, ovary, uterus, and colon and, in men, lung, prostate, and colon.[80,81] The response of PM-DM to treatment in these cases associated with malignancy has been reported as similar to uncomplicated PM-DM and as being dependent on the malignancy. It would appear that clarification of this issue depends on prospective series that adopt the same criteria for diagnosis.

Investigation The investigations are those of any myopathy (i.e., serum enzymes, EMG, and muscle biopsy). In the majority of patients, serum CK will be elevated often into the range 1,000 to 2,000 IU/L and sometimes higher. There has been considerable interest in the possibility of using serum myoglobin as a marker of disease state (see below); however, this has not proved to be as useful in practice as was first thought.

The EMG shows a triad of features in classic PM-DM[50] with spontaneous activity and fibrillation, positive potentials, and increased insertional activity; small amplitude, short-duration polyphasic potentials on volitional activity, and "pseudomyotonic" discharges provoked by mechanical stimulation.

Muscle biopsy shows characteristic changes of PM/DM in about 70 percent of cases.[48] The diagnostic yield of biopsy can be greatly enhanced by the use of CT/MRI-guided biopsies.[56]

There is increasing evidence that pathologically the diseases vary in their etiology. In PM there is predominantly scattered involvement of necrosis whereas in DM necrosis is classically perifascicular in distribution. It has been suggested that these divergent appearances on muscle biopsy are of importance in etiology.[61,82] This remains a major point of discussion in the field of myology, but as indicated previously, treatment regimens as yet have not changed on the basis of the pathologic appearances and for practical purposes treatment should be considered as being the same in both PM and DM.

Treatment The treatment of PM-DM in the majority of cases is oral steroid (e.g., prednisone) in high dose and for an adequate period. The usual initial dose levels are 1 to 2 mg per kg body weight daily. These levels must be maintained until there is clear clinical evidence of improvement, when a change to alternate-day therapy is indicated.[60,61,83]

It is important that clinical criteria of improvement rather than CK levels are used because, although initial CK levels are significantly related to the degree of muscle necrosis, this is not the case when treatment has been started.[84] Serial testing of muscle strength has been shown to parallel metabolic function studies of muscle breakdown and repair and is therefore a simple but reliable indicator of disease activity. It has been demonstrated that steroids produce a nonspecific fall in the serum CK and therefore reliance cannot be attached to this investigation. In most patients, the steroid dose can be tapered to maintenance levels of 10 to 15 mg within 9 to 12 months of commencing therapy and treatment at that level may be required for several years. During the course of treatment, diminution in muscle strength may indicate recrudescence of myositis or the development of a steroid myopathy. It is important to distinguish these two possibilities on repeat muscle biopsy because late secondary steroid myopathy appears to be a major contributor to the poor prognosis recorded in some series of PM-DM. Recently, there has been increasing interest in the use of azathioprine in the treatment of PM-DM. In doses of 1 to 2 mg/kg there is evidence of improved functional ability over a period of 3 years, and in addition there is a considerable steroid-sparing effect.[83]

It is apparent that using such doses of steroids carries with it in any patient the risk of steroid-induced side effects and this risk may well increase in the elderly population. It is to be expected, therefore, that the patient will develop gastrointestinal symptomatology and therefore will require gastric protection with an H_2 antagonist. Changes in the serum glucose level will occur and will require therapy in its own right as will changes in serum potassium.

With the use of azathioprine, careful hematologic monitoring is required and, on occasion, bone marrow studies are required if there is evidence of excessive marrow suppression. However, in clinical practice the number of patients who must discontinue immunosuppressant therapy is very low.

There have been advocates for the use of methotrexate, cyclophosphamide, and cyclosporin A as adjuvant chemotherapy, but these carry a higher rate of side effects and have not been shown to be superior to azathioprine.

In general, patients with PM/DM respond relatively well to therapy and in the author's personal experience, excluding those cases associated with malignancy (see below), only 20 percent of patients are, at the end of an appropriate course of therapy (3 to 5 years), left with handicap, although they may require continuing clinical support. There remain, however, patients whose disease is refractory to therapy and in that group use of intravenous high-dose steroids (methylprednisolone), intravenous globulin therapy, thymectomy, total body radiation, and total nodal radiation have all been employed.[48,83] Patients requiring such therapy should be referred to specialist centers who have experience in dealing with refractory myositis.

A small group of patients develop a hyperacute form of either PM or DM. Their symptoms develop over a period of 48 to 72 hours, are usually associated with marked subcutaneous edema and marked muscle pain, and there may be evidence of widespread myocarditis. In some patients associated thyroid disorders have been seen and occasionally patients have been described with associated myasthenic component.[85] The majority of these patients have underlying malignancy and therapy is rarely if ever successful.

In all patients with PM/DM the initial response to therapy is by far the most important prognostic indicator and patients who "relapse" are much more difficult to treat on a second occasion.

It is this group of patients who commonly require the alternative therapies described above. This underlines the importance of determining appropriate therapy on the first occasion and pursuing this even in the face of apparent adverse events.

Prognosis In uncomplicated PM-DM the prognosis has been improved by the use of steroids (with or without azathioprine), particularly in those patients in whom treatment was initiated early in the course of the disease. Bohan et al.[79] found a mortality rate of 14 percent overall, the poorest response being found in those patients with malignancy and in the older age groups.

In general terms, apart from acute PM/DM, mortality is confined to those patients with underlying neoplasia or is determined by the underlying autoimmune disorder if that is present. In the idiopathic form of the disease the major risk is that of cardiac disease, which may develop up to 5 years after the completion of treatment.

The majority of patients (more than 75 percent) will achieve normal walking or will require only a cane for support. There remain a small group of patients in whom a significant disability persists despite therapy and it is in that group that further investigation should be undertaken to ensure that the diagnosis is not that of inclusion body myositis[83] (see below).

Inclusion body myositis

IBM has been increasingly recognized as a cause of slowly progressive myopathy, particularly in males over the age of 60 years.[86–90] It differs from PM-DM complex in that myalgia and dysphagia are uncommon and there is usually significant distal weakness that may at times predominate. The course of the disease is slow (up to 6 years) and there is no association with malignancy. A familial form of the disorder has been described.[91,92] Pathologically the features are those of a necrobiotic myopathy with, in addition, the presence of "rimmed" vacuoles.

The vacuoles are classically subsarcolemmal, but may be associated with the nucleus. They contain a proteinaceous material that shows positive staining for amyloid and ubiquitin.[93,94] Many patients are erroneously diagnosed as having PM-DM complex, particularly because the vacuoles are often few and widely scattered in the biopsy material. However, failure to respond to steroid and/or immunosuppressive therapy should alert the attending physician to the possibility of IBM. It may be that a second, third, or occasionally fourth biopsy is required to confirm the presence of IBM.

Strict criteria encompassing clinical and pathologic features have been described.[95] Various therapies have been tried including steroids and steroids plus immunosuppression,[96,97] neither of which has produced any sustained improvement in the underlying condition; however, most of these reports have been anecdotal. There are single case reports and a single study that indicate that, potentially, intravenous globulin therapy may be of benefit.[98–100]

Neuromuscular Diseases in Malignancy

In the aging population the frequency of carcinoma increases and therefore the incidence of neuromuscular disorders associated with malignancy also increases. The incidence of these disorders is 5 percent in unselected patients with cancer. Three major groups of these disorders have been defined: (1) polymyopathy, (2) disorders of neuromuscular transmission (LEMS), and (3) PM-DM complex.

The subdivisions into LEMS and PM-DM complex are discussed in Chapter 102 and above, and will not be further considered in this section.

Polymyopathy has traditionally been subdivided into cachectic myopathy and proximal myopathy. In cachectic myopathy the clinical features are loss of subcutaneous fat with greater than 10 percent loss of body weight, and muscles being diffusely wasted, the wasting involving proximal and distal muscles equally. Despite the degree of wasting, muscle strength is well maintained until the final stages of the disease when weakness becomes profound.

In proximal myopathy (previously termed carcinomatous neuromyopathy), weakness in the proximal and axial muscles is found, initially with little evidence of wasting. The weakness may precede the symptoms of carcinoma by months or years. The common tumor sites are lung, breast, and gastrointestinal tract. In a prospective study of neuromuscular symptoms associated with carcinoma of the lung, the pathologic features of both conditions were those of selective type II fiber atrophy that was of greater severity than could have been accounted for by age, and it was impossible to distinguish the clinical subdivisions on the basis of the histopathology.[101] Similarly, pathologic evidence of necrobiosis, with or without associated clinical feature of the PM-DM complex, were seen in both subdivisions of clinical presentation. These results suggest that the remote effects of the tumor on the motor unit cannot be assessed by clinical evidence alone.[102]

Polymyalgia rheumatica

Polymyalgia rheumatica (PMR) may be mistaken for PM-DM complex because the painful restriction of movement, which characterizes the disorder, may be incorrectly attributed to muscle weakness. PMR is one of the group of arteritides and rarely presents under the age of 50 years. The average age of onset is 65 years. The clinical features are those of painful stiffness predominantly affecting the proximal limb girdle musculature (often with the upper limbs more affected than the lower) and the axial musculature.[103,104] The clinical presentation is over weeks to months and the pain is usually increased by movement.[105] Stiffness is conversely increased by rest, often making it difficult for the patient to turn over in bed or to get out of the bed in the morning. Apparent muscle weakness is most commonly due to pain, because formal myometer testing shows no evidence of overt weakness. Some 10 percent of patients may present with focal, unilateral symptomatology in either the upper or lower limb. About 25 percent of patients have coincident symptoms of temporal arteritis[106] (see Ch. 45) and the majority of patients have constitutional symptoms of general malaise, low-grade fever, and mild anemia. The characteristic finding is that of an elevated erythrocyte sedimentation rate (ESR) with often marked elevation to values in excess of 60 mm in the first hour. The serum CK, EMG studies, and muscle biopsy are all normal. The response of patients to steroid therapy is almost diagnostic in that, even with modest amounts of prednisolone (10 to 20 mg), there is usually resolution of symptoms within the first 24 to 48 hours of therapy.[107] Low-dose therapy may not, however, prevent serious complications due to associated temporal arteritic (e.g., blindness) and this complication has been reported in up to 42 percent of patients. In the absence of symptoms suggestive of cranial arteritis, in order to reduce the risk of steroid complications, it is suggested that low-dose steroids (10 to 15 mg/day) should be employed. If the ESR fails to fall within the first 2 weeks, or if the patient has symptoms suggestive of cranial arteritis, the doses of 40 to 60 mg/day should be employed, in both cases reducing the dose gradually as the ESR and clinical symptoms improve. Alternate day therapy is rarely helpful, and the majority of patients require therapy for up to 3 years.

Drug-Induced Myopathy

Clinically significant drug-induced myopathy is uncommon. However, this is thought to reflect the substantial functional reserve of muscle rather than a low incidence of drug-induced muscle damage. It is clear that the muscle cell may become affected at different subcellular sites, depending on the class of drug involved; however, such specificity is not seen in the resulting clinical syndromes. These can be subdivided into focal myopathy; acute and subacute painful myopathy; rhabdomyolysis; chronic, painless proximal myopathy; and myotonia.[108–112]

Focal myopathy

Focal myopathy is a consequence of the intramuscular injection of many types of drugs, including benzodiazepines, opiates, phenothiazines, and antibiotics. Chronic focal injections may lead to fibrosis in the underlying muscle, but this is usually only a problem with opiates. The nature of the drug vehicle appears to be important in determining the extent of associated muscle damage, oil-based vehicles being less toxic than aqueous.[113,114] The possibility that a rise in CK, as part of the evaluation of patients with chest pain, could be influenced by intramuscular injection has been investigated. The problem only seems to occur in a very small number of patients and is not of practical significance. However, following the trauma of concentric needle EMG, the CK may be significantly elevated for up to 72 hours.

Acute and subacute painful myopathy

Acute and subacute painful myopathy may be due to the direct toxic effect of the drug or may be a consequence of the drug's inducing hypokalemia or an inflammatory response in the muscle.

The clinical syndrome is that of a rapidly progressive proximal limb girdle myopathy with muscle pain and tenderness. The serum CK is elevated, often to considerable degree, the EMG is myopathic, and the muscle biopsy shows necrosis. Such reactions may be seen with alcohol and opiates, epsilon-aminocaproic acid, clofibrate, and emetine. A less severe syndrome of vague weakness with myalgia and fatiguability is seen with β-blocking drugs. The statin drugs, used in the treatment of elevated cholesterol, may produce myalgia, with a rise in CK, and can go on to produce a profound necrotizing myopathy.[111,112]

Acute, profound hypokalemia (with serum K^+ levels of 1 to 2 mmol) leads to a painful myopathy that may be severe. Pathologic evidence of necrobiosis is prominent. The majority of cases have been described following treatment with diuretics and ingestion of large amounts of licorice.

Drug-induced myositis, which clinically and pathologically resembles the PM-DM complex, is seen with drugs that have a demonstrable effect on the immune system. The most common causative drug in this regard is D-penicillamine,[109,115] although the drug more commonly causes myasthenia gravis as its principal side effect[116] (see Ch. 102). The other common drug in this situation is procaineamide.[111]

The increasing use of high-dose intravenous steroids has led to the recognition of a profound, acute myopathy, associated with massive rise in CK and gross necrobiosis, in the muscle biopsy.[112,117] A similar situation has been described in association with neuromuscular blocking drugs, both on their own[118] and in association with modest doses of steroid, both oral and parenertal.[119] In these situations a policy of supportive therapy is required until the drug effects have remitted, which may be a considerable time, measured in weeks.

Chronic, painless proximal myopathy

Chronic, painless proximal myopathy is the most common form of drug-induced disease. It is often missed both by patients and their attending physicians. Clinically the syndrome is that of a slowly progressive, proximal painless myopathy (with a curious tendency to affect the lower limb girdle before the upper limb girdle), usually of mild degree, which is not associated with elevation of serum CK. The muscle biopsy shows only a type II fiber atrophy.[111] The degree of atrophy may be difficult to distinguish from that attributable to age.

The most common drugs that produce this syndrome are steroids, alcohol, chronic hypokalemia usually due to diuretics, β-blockers, chloroquine, perhexilene maleate, and amiodarone. The mechanism of steroid-induced weakness is unknown. The syndrome is most commonly seen with long-term therapy and with relatively high levels of drug dosage (30 to 60 mg/day), although this association is not proven.

Myotonia

Myotonia is rarely of clinical significance and is due to drugs that have an effect on the muscle membrane (e.g., chloroquine, clofibrate, and propranolol).[109,110] The importance of these drugs is that they can unmask clinically significant myotonia in genetically susceptible individuals (e.g., those with myotonic dystrophy).

Metabolic Myopathies

Muscle not only provides power for movement, it is the largest protein store and hence plays an important role in gluconeogenesis. The relationship between the force-generating and metabolic functions of muscle is of importance in the genesis of muscle disorders associated with endocrine abnormalities.[120–123] The majority of the syndromes associated with abnormalities of the intermediary metabolism of muscle, particularly those associated with defects in glycogen metabolism, will have been determined in childhood, and presentation in later life would be exceptional. However, some of the disorders of mitochondrial and hence lipid metabolism are seen in the more elderly population, and it is probable that the incidence of these disorders is greatly underestimated if reliance is placed solely on clinical findings.

Endocrine myopathies

Endocrine myopathies are seen predominantly in patients with under- or overactivity of the adrenal or thyroid glands, and in disturbances of Ca^{++} metabolism. In adrenal overactivity (Cushing's disease) the myopathy is exactly that of iatrogenic steroid myopathy. In adrenal insufficiency (Addison's disease) there is generalized muscle weakness often associated with muscle pain and cramp. Serum CK, EMG, and muscle biopsy are all normal.[122,123]

In thyroid overactivity, due either to natural or iatrogenic excess of thyroxine, muscle weakness, which is usually generalized, occurs in up to 60 percent of patients. This is often associated with complaints of fatigue and fasciculations. The latter may be of sufficient frequency that the history of weakness with fasciculations suggests a diagnosis of MND. Muscle investigation with serum CK, EMG, and muscle biopsy is unhelpful because there are no diagnostic features of the condition.[123,124]

In hypothyroidism muscle manifestations may predominate in the clinical picture and may also predate the development of overt biochemical abnormalities. Whereas muscle weakness is the main feature of hyperthyroid myopathy, muscle pain and stiffness, associated with frequent painful cramps (Hoffman's syndrome), is the most common presentation, although a proximal limb girdle myopathy with wasting is also seen.[122,125] The rise in serum CK may be massive, and its fall may be used as a guide to replacement therapy. Muscle biopsy shows glycogen accumulation at the periphery of the muscle fiber. The exact relationship between the muscle biopsy and clinical features remains unexplained.

Disorders of calcium metabolism In these disorders, muscle symptoms of fatigue, cramp, and proximal weakness are frequently encountered. There are, however, no typical changes in serum CK, EMG, or muscle biopsy.[126] The nonspecificity of the changes in the majority of endocrine myopathies is underlined by the above descriptions. It is important, therefore, that the relatively simple biochemical tests that confirm or exclude the appropriate condition are undertaken in all patients presenting with muscle pain, cramp, and/or weakness.

Disorders of mitochondrial function These have, for the most part, been considered as being diseases of childhood and early adult life. However, as muscle biopsy has become more common in the evaluation of patients in the older age group, so the recognized incidence of these disorders is increasing.

The first descriptions of lipid myopathy (where, probably due to a defect in the mitochondrion, the carrier protein for lipid in the muscle cytosol, carnitine, is deficient) were in patients considered to have PM-DM complex.[127] Given that carnitine deficiency may be helped by the provision of carnitine supplementation, to the point where the patients may regain independent function, the importance of muscle biopsy in the workup of all patients with muscle weakness is underlined.

The most common form of "pure" mitochondrial disorder in the elderly is chronic progressive external ophthalmoplegia (CPEO). Because of the familial nature of the mitochondrial disorders and the variability of clinical expression, there will frequently be the need to investigate all members of the family where mitochondrial abnormalities are suspected.[128] In addition to CPEO, proximal, painless myopathy may also be found to be on the basis of mitochondrial dysfunction. In the majority of cases there is elevation of the resting serum lactate and this estimation should be added to the "routine" evaluation of elderly patients with myopathy.

Amyotrophic Lateral Sclerosis Motor Neuron Disease

Motor neuron disease (MND, generally known as amyotrophic lateral sclerosis [ALS] in the United States) is a relentlessly progressive disease of the nervous system in which motor neurons die over a relatively short period. Patients become progressively paralyzed and death occurs usually as a consequence of respiratory failure. MND/ALS has an incidence of 1 to 3 per 100,000 and a prevalence of 4 to 6 per 100,000.[129,130] Familial MND/ALS accounts for 10 percent of cases and one-fifth of these (2 percent of all cases) have an SOD1 gene mutation.[131] Clinically, MND/ALS is the most common presenting form of the disease, characterized by progressive weakness and wasting of limb musculature that most frequently starts in the legs and less frequently in the arms. It is usually asymmetric at the onset and if one leg is involved first, then the contralateral leg is the next area to become involved. Fasciculations are widespread and patients frequently complain of excessive cramps. Deep tendon reflexes are exaggerated and at some stage of the disease, the plantar responses will be extensor. There is steady progression of the weakness in all limbs and eventually the bulbar musculature becomes involved. The mean age of onset is 52.6 years,[132] 50 percent of patients die within 3 years of onset and 90 percent within 5 years.[129]

There are several varieties of presentation of MND/ALS. Progressive muscular atrophy (PMA) was first described by Aran in 1850 as "atrophie musculaire progressive" (cited in Ref. 132, and presents with atrophy of skeletal muscles involving the upper limbs initially (40 percent of cases), and then progressing to the lower limbs. In the "bulbar" form the presentation is with difficulty in swallowing and with indistinct speech. In the majority of these cases, the progression will be to MND/ALS within 1 to 2 years; however, there are occasional patients whose disease remains confined to the bulbar musculature for 5 to 10 years before becoming generalized. Primary lateral sclerosis is by far the least common presentation, and because of the difficulty in differentiating cord signs from muscular involvement, it may take many years before the diagnosis is secure.

In general terms, irrespective of clinical presentation, the vast majority of patients with MND/ALS will follow a final common pathway, with more widespread neuromuscular involvement and progression, with time, to the common presenting form of MND/ALS.[133] To date no form of therapy has been shown to have a convincing effect on the progression of the disease. Although there may appear to be "step-downs" in the patient's ability, this is usually due to the loss of a particular muscle group (e.g., quadriceps), which, by loss of knee bracing properties, appears to lead to a rapid loss of muscle function. However, sequential studies of loss of muscle functional ability have shown a linear progression in the majority of patients.[134,135]

Treatment is therefore supportive.[136,137] Baclofen is of benefit in the early stages of the disease to reduce muscle spasm and hence cramp. However, with progression of the underlying disorder, eventually baclofen becomes counterproductive, leading to hypotonia. The use of percutaneous gastrotomy prevents the patients from dying from inanition,[138,139] and should be initiated at the time of first presentation of swallowing difficulty, to prevent secondary parenchymal lung disease from aspiration. Respiratory support, either with central positive airways pressure or ventilation, remains a controversial issue.[140–143]

The future prospect of gene therapy[144,145] remains speculative at present. Drug therapy with thyrotropin-releasing hormone, administered either per orum or intrathecally, has not been shown to be of long-term benefit.[146–149] Attempts to relieve fatigue with 3,4-diaminopyridine have been variable.[150,151] The possibility that riluzole may be helpful in slowing the progression of the disease, in other than patients with progressive bulbar palsy, awaits further evaluation.[152,153]

Previously, therapeutic trials in MND/ALS were beset with methodologic problems. Guidelines for the future conduct of drug trials should overcome such problems.[154–156] Criteria for the diagnosis of the disorder have been established and validated.[157] Treatment with intravenous globulin[158] and immunosuppression by total lymphoid irradiation[159] have been unsuccessful.

A small proportion of patients with otherwise typical MND/ALS will be found to be suffering from multifocal conduction block, or to be associated with elevated levels of anti-GM1 antibodies, and/or elevated levels of immunoglobulins into the paraproteinemic range.[160] It is potentially worth considering immunosuppressive therapy in such patients, provided therapy is not prolonged beyond the point of obvious clinical deterioration.[161,162] Drug therapy will undoubtedly play a part in the treatment of MND/ALS in the future, particularly the use of ciliary neurotrophic factor,[163,164] but at present a degree of skepticism regarding claims for given drug remains appropriate.

A small proportion of patients will exhibit evidence of dementia, of frontal lobe type.[165–169]

Investigation

It is of crucial importance that the diagnosis of MND/ALS is based on appropriate investigation to confirm the diagnosis positively and to exclude potential mimics,[170,171] given the prognosis for the disorder. Electrophysiology is valuable in identifying MND as a neurogenic muscle disorder from the presence of spontaneous fibrillations and fasciculations, together with enlarged polyphasic motor units.[172] Serum CK levels may be moderately increased in 40 percent of patients,[48] other investigations have largely failed to show consistent diagnostic data.

With such a devastating prognosis as MND/ALS, muscle biopsy should be performed to confirm the neurogenic nature of the muscle wasting and to exclude other disorders, particularly late-onset glycogenoses. This is particularly important in the early stages of the disease when the clinical signs may be less certain. Muscle biopsies in this disease are characterized by neurogenic changes, with atrophy of both type I and type II fibers forming groups of angulated fibers. If the major damage is to the upper motor neuron tracts, then type II fiber atrophy only may be seen. Hypertrophic fibers are common in the early stages of MND/ALS and especially type II fiber hypertrophy. Most of the groups of atrophic fibers are small and in 25 percent of cases fiber type grouping is seen, indicating reinnervation. Degeneration and sprouting of nerve fibers is also observed in muscle biopsies. In a survey of 745 muscle biopsies from patients with typical MND/ALS denervation was absent in 2.2 percent, mild in 28.1 percent, moderate in 42.8 percent, and severe in 26.9 percent. Reinnervation was observed in 54.3 percent and inflammation in 9 percent.[129] In some 25 percent of cases, degenerating or regenerating muscle fibers may be present but there is usually little fibrosis; such changes may cause confusion with myopathy. There is no correlation between the severity of denervation and the clinical progression of the disease.[173]

Etiology of motor neuron disease

The last decade has seen considerable advances in the understanding of the pathogenesis of MND/ALS. Excitotoxicity is the best defined parameter in the pathogenesis of MND/ALS; glutamate metabolism is altered but it is not known whether this is an essential factor in the pathogenesis or part of the progression of the disease. It is postulated that chronically elevated levels of glutamate may overstimulate glutamate postsynaptic receptors and induce activation of calcium-dependent enzymes, protein degradation, and neuronal death.[174,175] An imbalance between functional sodium and potassium channels has been proposed,[176] and a possible disorder in the neuronal glutamate transporter gene has also been investigated.[177] Autoimmune factors may also play a role in the pathogenesis of MND/ALS.[178] In some 10 percent of patients, there may be monoclonal paraproteinemia, antibodies to GM1, multifocal motor neuropathy with conduction block, and lymphoproliferative disease.[179]

Familial motor neuron disease

In some 10 percent of patients with MND, the disorder is familial with an autosomal dominant pattern of inheritance.[132] The responsible gene maps to chromosome 21[131] and missense mutations in the copper/zinc superoxide dismutase 1 (SOD1) gene have been identified.[180,181] This is a gene of approximately 15 kd comprising 5 exons.[181] Although it was proposed that superoxide injures cells, studies of transgenic mice with SOD1 mutations suggest that other factors in addition to superoxide toxicity may be involved.[182] Some cases of familial MND have a juvenile onset and the disease may be prolonged.

References

1. Slater CR, Harris JB: The anatomy and physiology of the motor unit. pp. 3–32. In Walton JN, Karpati G, Hilton-Jones D (eds): Disorders of Voluntary Muscle. Churchill Livingstone, Edinburgh, 1994
2. Burke RE: Physiology of motor units. pp. 464–484. In Engel AG, Franzini-Armstrong C (eds): Myology. McGraw-Hill, New York, 1994
3. Grimby G, Danneskiold-Samse B, Hvid K, Saltin B: Morphology and enzyme capacity in arm and leg muscles in 78–81 year old men and women. Acta Physiol Scand 1982;115:125–134
4. Munsat TL: Aging of the neuromuscular system. pp. 404–424. In Albert ML (ed): Clinical Neurology of Aging. Oxford University Press, New York, 1984
5. Jennekens FGI: Disuse, cachexia and aging. pp. 763–767. In Mastaglia FL, Walton JN (eds): Skeletal Muscle Pathology. Churchill Livingstone, Edinburgh, 1992
6. Lexell J, Downham DY: The occurrence of fibre-type grouping in healthy human muscle: a quantitative study of cross-sections of whole vastus lateralis from men between 15 and 83 years. Acta Neuropathol (Berl) 1991;81:377–381
7. Lexell J, Downham D: What is the effect of ageing on type 2 muscle fibres? J Neurol Sci 1992;107:250–251
8. Lexell J, Downham D, Sjöström M: Distribution of different fibre types in human skeletal muscles: fibre type arrangements in m. vastus lateralis from three groups of healthy men between 15 and 83 years. J Neurol Sci 1986;72:211–222
9. Lexell J, Henriksson-Larsen K, Sjöström M: Distribution of different fibre types in human skeletal muscle: 2. A study of cross sections of whole m. vastus lateralis. Acta Physiol Scand 1983;117:115–122
10. Lexell J, Henriksson-Larsen K, Winblad B, Sjöström M: Distribution of different fibre types in human skeletal muscles: effects of aging studied in whole muscle cross section. Muscle Nerve 1983;6:588–595
11. Lexell J, Henriksson-Larsen K, Winblad B, Sjöström M: Distribution of different fiber types in human skeletal muscles: effects of aging studied in whole muscle cross sections. Muscle Nerve 1983;6:588–595
12. Lexell J, Sjoestroem M, Nordlund A-S, Taylor CC: Growth and

development of human muscle: a quantitative morphological study of whole vastus lateralis from childhood to adult age. Muscle Nerve 1992;15:404–409

13. Lexell J, Taylor CC: Variability in muscle fibre areas in whole human quadriceps muscle: effects of increasing age. J Anat 1991;174:239–249
14. Cumming WJK: Ageing in muscle. In Burns A (ed): Ageing. Cambridge University Press, Cambridge, 1996
15. Lexell J, Taylor CC, Sjostrom M: What is the cause of ageing atrophy? Total number, size and proportion of different fiber types studied in whole vastus lateralis muscle from 15-to-83-year-old men. J Neurol Sci 1988;84:275–294
16. Vandervoort AA, Hayes KC, Belanger AY: Strength and endurance of skeletal muscle in the elderly. Physiother Canada 1986;38:167–173
17. Young A, Stokes M, Crowe M: The size and strength of the quadriceps muscles of old and young men. Clin Physiol 1985; 5:145–154
18. Cumming WJK, Fulthorpe J, Hudgson P, Mahon M: Colour Atlas of Muscle Pathology. Mosby Year Book, London, 1994
19. Tomlinson BE, Irving D: The number of limb motor neurones in the human lumbosacral cord throughout life. J Neurol Sci 1977;34:213–219
20. Hashizume K, Kanda K: Neuronal dropout is greater in hindlimb motor nuclei than in forelimb motor nuclei in aged rats. Neurosci Lett 1990;113:267–269
21. Campbell MJ, McComas AJ, Petito F: Physiological changes in ageing muscles. J Neurol Neurosurg Psychiatry 1973;36: 174–182
22. Schonk D, Van DP, Riegmann P et al: Assignment of seven genes to distinct intervals on the midportion of human chromosome 19q surrounding the myotonic dystrophy gene region. Cytogenet Cell Genet 1990;54:15–19
23. Cooper JM, Mann VM, Schapira AHV: Analyses of mitochondrial respiratory chain function and mitochondrial DNA deletion in human skeletal muscle: effect of ageing. J Neurol Sci 1992;113:91–98
24. Katayama M, Tanaka M, Yamamoto H et al: Deleted mitochondrial DNA in the skeletal muscle of aged individuals. Biochem Int 1991;25:47–56
25. Mueller-Hoecker J: Cytochrome c oxidase deficient fibres in the limb muscle and diaphragm of man without muscular disease: an age-related alteration. J Neurol Sci 1990;100:14–21
26. Mueller-Hoecker J, Seibel P, Schneiderbanger K, Kadenbach B: Different in situ hybridization patterns of mitochondrial DNA in cytochrome c oxidase-deficient extraocular muscle fibres in the elderly. Virch Arch A Pathol Anat Histopathol 1993;422:7–15
27. Miquel J: An integrated theory of aging as the result of mitochondrial-DNA mutation in differentiated cells. Arch Gerontol Geriatr 1991;12:99–117
28. Edstroem L, Larsson H, Larsson L: Neurogenic effects on the palatopharyngeal muscle in patients with obstructive sleep apnoea: a muscle biopsy study. J Neurol Neurosurg Psychiatry 1992;55:916–920
29. Zhang C, Baumer A, Maxwell RJ et al: Multiple mitochondrial DNA deletions in an elderly human individual. FEBS Lett 1992;297:34–38
30. Byrne E, Dennett X: Respiratory chain failure in adult muscle fibres: relationship with ageing and possible implications for the neuronal pool. Mutat Res DNA Aging Genet Instability Aging 1992;275:125–131
31. Sahashi K, Tanaka M, Tashiro M et al: Increased mitochondrial DNA deletions in the skeletal muscle of myotonic dystrophy. Gerontology 1992;38:18–29
32. Ptacek LJ, Johnson KJ, Griggs RC: Mechanisms of disease: genetics and physiology of the myotonic muscle disorders. N Engl J Med 1993;328:482–489
33. Hruszkewycz AM: Lipid peroxidation and mtDNA degeneration. A hypothesis. Mutat Res DNAging Genet Instability Aging 1992;275:243–248
34. Wallace DC: Mitochondrial genetics: a paradigm for aging and degenerative diseases. Science 1992;256:628–632
35. Froes MMQ, Kristmundsdottir F, Mahon M, Cumming WJK: Muscle morphometry in motor neuron disease. Neuropathol Appl Neurobiol 1987;13:405–419
36. Lane RJM, Fuller GN: Clinical presentation. pp. 1–17. In Lane RJN (ed): Handbook of muscle disease. Marcel Decker, New York, 1996
37. Gardner-Medwin D: Neuromuscular disorders in infancy and childhood. pp. 781–835. In Walton JN, Karpati G, Hilton-Jones D (eds): Disorders of Voluntary Muscle. Churchill Livingstone, Edinburgh, 1994
38. Gomez MR: The clinical examination. pp. 746–765. In Engel AG, Franzini-Armstrong C (eds): Myology. McGraw-Hill, New York, 1994
39. Lacomis D, Chad DA, Smith TW: Myopathy in the elderly: evaluation of the histopathologic spectrum and the accuracy of clinical diagnosis. Neurology 1993;43:825–828
40. Thomas NH, Doboweitz V: Spinal muscular atrophies pp. 28–44. In Williams AC (ed): Motor Neurone Disease. Chapman & Hall Medical, London, 1994
41. Rietschel M, Rudnik-Schoeneborn S, Zerres K: Clinical variability of autosomal dominant spinal muscular atrophy. J Neurol Sci 1992;107:65–73
42. Nicholson LVB, Johnson MA, Bushby KMD et al: Integrated study of 100 patients with Xp21 linked muscular dystrophy using clinical, genetic, immunochemical, and histopathological data. Part 1. Trends across the clinical groups. J Med Genet 1993;30:728–736
43. Nicholson LVB, Johnson MA, Bushby KMD et al: Integrated study of 100 patients with Xp21 linked muscular dystrophy using clinical, genetic, immunochemical, and histopathological data. Part 2. Correlations within individual patients. J Med Genet 1993;30:737–744
44. Nicholson LVB, Johnson MA, Bushby KMD, et al: Integrated study of 100 patients with Xp21 linked muscular dystrophy using clinical, genetic, immunochemical, and histopathological data. Part 3. Differential diagnosis and prognosis. J Med Genet 1993;30:745–751
45. Harper PS: The myotonic disorders. pp. 595–618. In Walton JN, Karpati G, Hilton-Jones D (eds): Disorders of Voluntary Muscle. Churchill Livingstone, Edinburgh, 1994
46. Pizzuti A, Friedman DL, Caskey CT: The myotonic dystrophy gene. Arch Neurol 1993;50:1173–1179

47. Teisberg P: The genetic background of anticipation. J R Soc Med 1995;88:185–187
48. Weller RO, Cumming WJK, Mahon M: Neuromuscular disease. In Grahan D (ed): Greenfield's Neuropathology. Churchill Livingstone, Edinburgh
49. Gardner-Medwin D, Walton JN: The muscular dystrophies. pp. 543–594. In Walton JN, Karpati G, Hilton-Jones D (eds): Disorders of Voluntary Muscle. Churchill Livingstone, Edinburgh, 1994
50. Fawcett PRW, Barwick DD: The clinical physiology of neuromuscular disease pp. 1033–1104. In Walton JN, Karpati G, Hilton-Jones D (eds): Disorders of Voluntary Muscle. Churchill Livingstone, Edinburgh, 1994
51. Kennett RP: Electromyography. pp. 41–52. In Lane RJN (ed): Handbook of Muscle Disease. Marcel Decker, New York, 1996
52. Daube JR: Electrodiagnosis of muscle disorders. pp. 764–794. In Engel AG, Franzini-Armstrong C (eds): Myology. McGraw-Hill, New York, 1994
53. Edwards RHT, Jackson MJ, Helliwell TR: Muscle biopsy techniques. pp. 53–59. In Lane RJN (ed): Handbook of Muscle Disease. Marcel Decker, New York, 1996
54. de Visser M, Reimers CD: Muscle Imaging. pp. 795–806. In Engel AG, Franzini-Armstrong C (eds): Myology. McGraw-Hill, New York, 1994
55. Walton JN, Karpati G, Hilton-Jones D (eds): Disorders of Voluntary Muscle. Churchill Livingstone, Edinburgh, 1994
56. Schweitzer ME, Fort J: Cost effectiveness of MR imaging in evaluating polymyositis. Am J Roentgenol 1995;165: 1469–1471
57. Walton JN, Rowland LP: Clinical examination, differential diagnosis and classification. pp. 499–542. In Walton JN, Karpati G, Hilton-Jones D (eds): Disorders of Voluntary Muscle. Churchill Livingstone, Edinburgh, 1994
58. Vinken PJ, Bruyn GW, Klawans HL et al (eds): Myopathies. Elsevier, Amsterdam, 1992
59. Engel AG, Franzine-Armstrong C (eds): Myology. McGraw Hill, New York, 1994
60. Lane RJM, Hudgson P: Idiopathic inflammatory myopathies. pp. 539–574. In Lane RJN (ed): Handbook of Muscle Disease. Marcel Decker, New York, 1996
61. Engel AG, Hohlfeld R, Banker BQ: Inflammatory myopathies. pp. 1335–1383. In Engel AG, Franzini-Armstrong C (eds): Myology. McGraw Hill, New York, 1994
62. Dalakas MC (ed): Polymyositis and Dermatomyositis. Butterworths, Boston, 1988
63. Byrne E, Dennett X: Idiopathic inflammatory myopathies: clinical aspects. pp. 499–526. In Mastaglia FL (ed): Baillière's Clinical Neurology. Baillière Tindall, London, 1993
64. Dalakas MC: Inflammatory myopathies. pp. 369–390. In Vinken PJ, Bruyn GW, Klawans HL (eds): Handbook of Clinical Neurology. Elsevier, Amsterdam, 1992
65. Hollinrake K: Polymyositis presenting as distal muscle weakness. J Neurol Sci 1969;8:479–484
66. Bates D, Stevens JC, Hudgson P: "Polymyositis" with involvement of the facial and distal musculature. One form of the facioscapulohumeral syndrome. J Neurol Sci 1973;19: 105–108
67. Cumming WJK, Weiser R, Teoh R et al: Localised nodular myositis: a clinical and pathological variant of polymyositis. Q J Med 1977;46:531–546
68. Isaacson G, Chan KH, Heffner RR: Focal myositis: a new cause for the pediatric neck mass. Arch Otolaryngol Head Neck Surg 1991;117:103–105
69. Flaisler F, Blin D, Asencio G et al: Focal myositis: a localized form of polymyositis? J Rheumatol 1993;20:1414–1416
70. Toti P, Catella AM, Benvenuti A: Focal myositis—a pseudotumoral lesion. Histopathology 1994;24:171–173
71. Caldwell CJ, Swash M, Van der WJD, Geddes JF: Focal myositis: a clinicopathological study. Neuromuscul Disord 1995;5: 317–322
72. Mastaglia FL, Walton JN: Inflammatory myopathies. pp. 453–492. In Mastaglia FL, Lord Walton of Detchant (eds): Skeletal Muscle Pathology. Churchill Livingstone, Edinburgh, 1992
73. Henderson A, Cumming WJK, Williams DO, Hudgson P: Cardiac complications of polymyositis. J Neurol Sci 1981;47: 425–428
74. Lie JT: Cardiac manifestations in polymyositis/dermatomyositis: how to get to the heart of the matter. J Rheumatol 1995; 22:809–810
75. Bamanikar S, Mathew M: Focal myositis of the tongue—a pseudotumoral lesion. Histopathology 1995;26:291–292
76. Callen JP: The relationship of dermatomyositis/polymyositis to malignancy. J Rheumatol 1991;18:1645–1646
77. Callan JP: Myositis and malignancy. pp. 117–130. In Ansell BM (ed): Inflammatory Disorders of Muscle. WB Saunders, London, 1984
78. Hudgson P, Walton JN: Polymyositis and other inflammatory myopathies. pp. 51–93. In Vinken PJ, Bruyn GW (eds): Handbook of Clinical Neurology. North-Holland, Amsterdam, 1979
79. Bohan A, Peter JB, Bowman RL, Pearson CM: A computer-assisted analysis of 153 patients with polymyositis and dermatomyositis. Medicine (Baltimore) 1977;56:255–286
80. Barnes BE: Dermatomyositis and malignancy: a review of the literature. Ann Intern Med 1976;84:68–76
81. Sigurgeirsson B, Lindeloef B, Edhag O, Allander E: Risk of cancer in patients with dermatomyositis or polymyositis—a population-based study. N Engl J Med 1992;326:363–367
82. Karpati G, Currie GS: The inflammatory myopathies. pp. 619–646. In Walton JN, Karpati G, Hilton-Jones D (eds): Disorders of Voluntary Muscle. Churchill Livingstone, Edinburgh, 1994
83. Cumming WJK: Steroids in polymyositis. pp. 247–257. In Capildeo R (ed): Steroids in Diseases of the Central Nervous System. Wiley, London, 1989
84. Bunch TW, Worthington JW, Combs JJ et al: Azathioprine with prednisone for polymyositis. A controlled clinical trial. 1980;92:365–369
85. Venables GS, Bates D, Cartlidge NEF, Hudgson P: Acute polymyositis with subcutaneous oedema. J Neurol Sci 1982;55: 161–164
86. Rose M, Lane RJM: Inclusion body myositis and other rimmed vacuolar myopathies. pp. 575–590. In Lane RJN (ed): Handbook of Muscle Disease. Marcel Decker, New York, 1996

87. Schlesinger I, Soffer D, Lossos A et al: Inclusion body myositis: atypical clinical presentations. Eur Neurol 1996;36:89–93
88. Garlepp MJ, Mastaglia FL: Inclusion body myositis. J Neurol Neurosurg Psychiatry 1996;60:251–255
89. Mikol J, Engel AG: Inclusion body myositis. pp. 1384–1398. In Engel AG, Franzini-Armstrong C (eds): Myology. McGraw Hill, New York, 1994
90. Chou SM: Inclusion body myositis. pp. 557–577. In Mastaglia FL (ed): Baillière's Clinical Neurology. Baillière Tindall, London, 1993
91. Neufeld MY, Sadeh M, Assa B et al: Phenotypic heterogeneity in familial inclusion body myopathy. Muscle Nerve 1995;18: 546–548
92. Mitrani-Rosenbaum S, Argov Z, Blumfeld A et al: Hereditary inclusion body myopathy maps to chromosome 9p1-q1. Hum Mol Gene 1996;5:159–163
93. Askanas V, Alvarez RB, Engel WK: Beta-amyloid precursor epitopes in muscle fibers of inclusion body myositis. Ann Neurolo 1993;34:551–560
94. Albrecht S, Bilbao JM: Ubiquitin expression in inclusion body myositis: an immunohistochemical study. Arch Pathol Lab Med 1993;117:789–793
95. Griggs RC, Askanas V, DiMauro S et al: Inclusion body myositis and myopathies. Ann Neurol 1995;38:705–713
96. Barohn RJ, Amato AA, Sahenk Z et al: Inclusion body myositis: explanation for poor response to immunosuppressive therapy. Neurology 1995;45:1302–1304
97. Leff RL, Miller FW, Hicks J et al: The treatment of inclusion body myositis: a retrospective review and a randomized, prospective trial of immunosuppressive therapy. Medicine (Baltimore) 1993;72:225–235
98. Soueidan SA, Dalakas MC: Treatment of inclusion-body myositis with high-dose intravenous immunoglobulin. Neurology 1993;43:876–879
99. Amato AA, Barohn RJ, Jackson CE et al: Inclusion body myositis: treatment with intravenous immunoglobulin. Neurology 1994;44:1516–1518
100. Salvarani C, Boiardi L, Maldini MC et al: High dose immunoglobulin therapy in a case of inclusion body myositis: clinical and immunologic aspects. J Rheumatol 1993;20:1455–1456
101. Gomm S, Thatcher N, Barber P, Cumming W: A clinicopathological study of the paraneoplastic neuromuscular syndromes associated with lung cancer. Q J Med 1990;75:577–595
102. Gomm SA, Thatcher N, Barber PV, Cumming WJK: A clinicopathological study of the paraneoplastic neuromuscular syndromes associated with lung cancer. Q J Med 1990;75: 577–595
103. Cohen M, Ginsberg W: Polymyalgia rheumatica. Rheum Dis Clin North Am 1990;16:325–339
104. Pountain G, Hazleman B: ABC of rheumatology: polymyalgia rheumatica and giant cell arteritis. BMJ 1995;310:1057–1059
105. Orrell RW: Polymyalgia rheumatica. pp. 595–598. In Lane RJN (ed): Handbook of Muscle Disease. Marcel Decker, New York, 1996
106. Turnbull J: Temporal arteritis and polymyalgia rheumatica: nosographic and nosologic considerations. Neurology 1996; 46:901–906
107. Di MO, Imbimbo B, Mazzantini M et al: Deflazacort versus methylprednisolone in polymyalgia rheumatica: clinical equivalence and relative antiinflammatory potency of different treatment regimens. J Rheumatol 1995;22:1492–1498
108. Kakulas BA, Mastaglia FL: Drug-induced, toxic and nutritional myopathies. pp. 511–540. In Mastaglia FL, Lord Walton of Detchant (eds): Skeletal Muscle Pathology. Churchill Livingstone, Edinburgh, 1992
109. Mastaglia FL: Toxic myopathies. pp. 595–622. In Vinken PJ, Bruyn GW, Klawans HL, (eds): Handbook of Clinical Neurology. Elsevier, Amsterdam, 1992
110. Argov Z, Mastaglia FL: Drug-induced neuromuscular disorders in man. pp. 989–1029. In Walton JN, Karpati G, Hilton-Jones D (eds): Disorders of Voluntary Muscle. Churchill Livingstone, Edinburgh, 1994
111. Lane RJM: Toxic and drug-induced myopathies. pp. 379–390. In Lane RJN (ed): Handbook of Muscle Disease. Marcel Decker, New York, 1996
112. Jain KK: Drug-induced myopathies. pp. 245–264. In Jain KK (ed): Drug-induced Neurological Disorders. Hogrefe & Huber Publishers, Seattle, 1996
113. Wagner JM, Cohen S: Fibrous myopathy from butorphanol injections. J Rheumatol 1991;18:1934–1935
114. Louis ED, Bodner RA, Challenor YB, Brust JCM: Focal myopathy induced by chronic intramuscular heroin injection. Muscle Nerve 1994;17:550–552
115. Aydintug AO, Cervera R, D'Cruz D et al: Polymyositis complicating D-penicillamine treatment. Postgrad Med J 1991;67: 1018–1020
116. Bever CT Jr, Asofsky R: Augmented lgG anti-acetylcholine receptor response following chronic penicillamine administration. Neuroimmunol 1991;35:131–137
117. Hirano M, Ott BR, Raps EC et al: Acute quadriplegic myopathy: a complication of treatment with steroids, nondepolarizing blocking agents, or both. Neurology 1992;42:2082–2087
118. Gooch JL: AAEM case report #29: prolonged paralysis after neuromuscular blockade. Muscle Nerve 1995;18:937–942
119. Barohn RJ, Jackson CE, Rogers SJ et al: Prolonged paralysis due to nondepolarizing neuromuscular blocking agents and corticosteroids. Muscle Nerve 1994;17:647–654
120. Hudgson P, Kendall-Taylor P: Endocrine myopathies. pp. 493–510. In Mastaglia FL, Lord Walton of Detchant (eds): Skeletal Muscle Pathology. Churchill Livingstone, Edinburgh, 1992
121. Kissel JT, Mendell JR: The endocrine myopathies. pp. 527–551. In Vinken PJ, Bruyn GW, Klawans HL (eds): Handbook of Clinical Neurology. Elsevier, Amsterdam, 1992
122. Moxley RT: Metabolic and endocine myopathies. pp. 647–716. In Walton JN, Karpati G, Hilton-Jones D (eds): Disorders of Voluntary Muscle. Churchill Livingstone, Edinburgh, 1994
123. Kaminski HF, Ruff RL: Endocrine myopathies. pp. 1726–1753. In Engel AG, Franzini- Armstrong C (eds): Myology. McGraw Hill, New York, 1994
124. Ramsey ID: Muscle dysfunction in hyperthyroidism. Lancet 1966;2:931
125. Lochmueller H, Reimers CD, Fischer P et al: Exercise-induced myalgia in hypothyroidism. Clin Invest 1993;71: 999–1001

126. Yamaguchi H, Okamoto K, Shooji M et al: Muscle histology of hypocalcaemic myopathy in hypoparathyroidism. J Neurol Neurosurg Psychiatry 1987;50:8177

127. Bindoff LA, Jackson S, Turnbull DM: Mitochondrial and lipid storage disorders of muscle. pp. 717–738. In Walton JN, Karpati G, Hilton-Jones D (eds): Disorders of Voluntary Muscle. Churchill Livingstone, Edinburgh, 1994

128. Pavlakis SG, Rowland LP, DeVivo DC et al: Mitochondrial myopathies and encephalomyopathies. pp. 95–133. In Plum F (ed): Advances in Contemporary Neurology. FA Davies, Philadelphia, 1988

129. Haverkamp LJ, Appel V, Appel SH: Natural history of amyotrophgic lateral sclerosis in a database population. Validation of a scoring system and a model for survival prediction. Brain 1995;118:707–719

130. Brooks BJ: Clinical epidemiology of amyotrophic lateral sclerosis. pp. 399–420. In Riggs JE (ed): Neurologic Clinics. WB Saunders, Philadelphia, 1996

131. Siddique T: Molecular genetics of familial amyotrophic lateral sclerosis. Adv Neurol 1991;56:227–231

132. Campbell MJ, Munsat TL: Motor neurone diseases. pp. 879–919. In Walton JN, Karpati G, Hilton-Jones D (eds): Disorders of Voluntary Muscle. Churchill Livingstone, Edinburgh, 1994

133. Tandan R: Clinical features and differential diagnosis of classical motor neurone disease. pp. 3–27. In Williams AC (eds): Motor Neurone Disease. Chapman & Hall Medical, London, 1994

134. Guiloff RJ, Goonetilleke A: Natural history of amyotrophic lateral sclerosis—observations with the Charing Cross Amyotrophic Lateral Sclerosis Rating Scales. Adv Neurol 1995;68: 185–198

135. Munsat TL, Hollander D, Andres P, Finison L: Clinical trials in ALS: measurement and natural history. Adv Neurol 1991; 56:515–519

136. Heafield T, Powell A: Early management. pp. 193–202. In Williams AC (ed): Motor Neurone Disease. Chapman & Hall Medical, London, 1994

137. Howard RS, Wiles CM, Loh L: Respiratory complications and their management in motor neuron disease. Brain 1989;112: 1155–1170

138. Hull MA, Rawlings J, Murray FE et al: Audit of outcome of long-term enteral nutrition by percutaneous endoscopic gastrostomy. Lancet 1993;341:869–872

139. Rawlings JK, Allison SP: Nutritional support. pp. 265–280. In Williams AC (ed): Motor Neurone Disease. Chapman & Hall Medical, London, 1994

140. Hayashi H, Kato S: Total manifestations of amyotrophic lateral sclerosis (ALS) in the totally locked-in state. J Neurol Sci 1989;93:19–35

141. Hayashi H, Kato S, Kawada A: Amyotrophic lateral sclerosis patients living beyond respiratory failure. J Neurol Sci 1991; 105:73–78

142. Moss AH, Casey P, Stocking CB et al: Home ventilation for amyotrophic lateral sclerosis patients: outcomes, costs, and patient, family, and physician attitudes. Neurology 1993;43: 438–443

143. Shneerson JM: Motor neurone disease—some hope at last for respiratory complications. BMJ 1996;313:244–245

144. Aebischer P, Kato AC: Treatment of amyotrophic lateral sclerosis using a gene therapy approach. Eur Neurol 1995;35: 65–68

145. Finiels F, Ribotta MG, Barkats M et al: Specific and efficient gene transfer strategy offers new potentialities for the treatment of motor neurone diseases. Neuroreport 1995;6:2473–2478

146. Brooke MH: A summary of the current position of TRH in ALS therapy. Ann N Y Acad Sci 1989;553:431–461

147. Brooks BR, Lewis D, Rawling J et al: The natural history of amyotrophic lateral sclerosis. pp. 131–169. In Williams AC (ed): Motor Neurone Disease. Chapman & Hall Medical, London, 1994

148. Goonetilleke A, Guiloff RJ: Continuous response variable trial design in motor neuron disease: long term treatment with a TRH analogue (RX77368). J Neurol Neurosurg Psychiatry 1995;58:201–208

149. Munsat TL, Taft J, Jackson IMD et al: Intrathecal thyrotropin-releasing hormone does not alter the progressive course of ALS: experience with an intrathecal drug delivery system. Neurology 1992;42:1049–1053

150. Aisen ML, Sevilla D, Gibson G et al: 3,4-diaminopyridine as a treatment for amyotrophic lateral sclerosis. J Neurol Sci 1995;129:21–24

151. Aisen ML, Sevilla D, Edelstein L, Blass J: A double-blind placebo-controlled study of 3,4-diaminopyridine in amytrophic lateral sclerosis patients on a rehabilitation unit. J Neurol Sci 1996;138:93–96

152. Couratier P, Sindou P, Esclaire F et al: Neuroprotective effects of riluzole in ALS CSF toxicity. Neuroreport 1994;5: 1012–1014

153. Rowland LP: Riluzole for the treatment of amyotrophic lateral sclerosis—too soon to tell? N Engl J Med 1994;330:636–637

154. Azulay JP: The design of clinical trials in amyotrophic lateral sclerosis. Adv Neurol 1995;68:225–227

155. Bossuyt PMM, Louwerse ES, Weverling GJ, De JJMBV: Baseline assessments in amyotrophic lateral sclerosis trials. J Neurol Sci 1995;129(suppl):28

156. Munsat TL: Airlie House Guidelines—therapeutic trials in amyotrophic lateral sclerosis. J Neurol Sci 1995;129(suppl): 1–10

157. Chaudhuri KR, Crump S, AI-Sarraj S et al: The validation of EI Escorial criteria for the diagnosis of amyotrophic lateral sclerosis: a clinicopathological study. J Neurol Sci 1995; 129(suppl):11–12

158. Dalakas MC, Stein DP, Otero C et al: Effect of high-dose intravenous immunoglobulin on amyotrophic lateral sclerosis and multifocal motor neuropathy. Arch Neurol 1994;51: 861–864

159. Drachman DB, Chaudhry V, Cornblath D et al: Trial of immunosuppression in amyotrophic lateral sclerosis using total lymphoid irradiation. Ann Neurol 1994;35:142–150

160. Boucraut J: Amyotrophic lateral sclerosis with paraproteins and autoantibodies—a discussion. Adv Neurol 1995;68: 107–111

161. Feldman EL, Bromberg MB, Albers JW, Pestronk A: Immuno-

supressive treatment in multifocal motor neuropathy. Ann Neurol 1991;30:397–401

162. Lacomblez L, Bensimon G, Leigh PN et al: Dose-ranging study of riluzole in amyotrophic lateral sclerosis. Lancet 1996;347: 1425–1431

163. Miller RG, Petajan JH, Bryan WW et al: A placebo-controlled trial of recombinant human ciliary neurotrophic (rhCNTF) factor in amyotrophic lateral sclerosis. Ann Neurol 1996;39: 256–260

164. Festoff BW: Amyotrophic lateral sclerosis—current and future treatment strategies. Drugs 1996;51:28–44

165. Caselli RJ, Windebank AJ, Petersen RC et al: Rapidly progressive aphasic dementia and motor neuron disease. Ann Neurol 1993;33:200–207

166. Deymeer F, Smith TW, DeGirolami U, Drachman DA: Thalamic dementia and motor neuron disease. Neurology 1989;38: 58–61

167. Gallassi R, Montagna P, Morreale A et al: Neuropsychological electroencephalogram and brain computed tomography findings in motor neuron disease. Eur Neurol 1989;29:115–120

168. Kato S, Hayashi H, Yagishita A: Involvement of the frontotemporal lobe and limbic system in amyotrophic lateral sclerosis: as assessed by serial computed tomography and magnetic resonance imaging. J Neurol Sci 1993;116:52–58

169. Kiernan JA, Hudson AJ: Frontal lobe atrophy in motor neuron diseases. Brain 1994;117:747–757

170. Belsh JM, Schiffman PL: Misdiagnosis in patients with amyotrophic lateral sclerosis. Arch Intern Med 1990;150: 2301–2305

171. Chancellor AM: Diagnosing motor neurone disease—its many mimics and grave prognosis make confident diagnosis essential. BMJ 1996;312:650–651

172. Bradley W: Recent views on amyotrophic lateral sclerosis with emphasis on electrophysiological studies. Muscle Nerve 1987; 10:490–502

173. Froes MMQ, Kristmundsdottir F, Mahon M, Cumming WJK: Motor neurone disease and evaluation of muscle pathology. Neuropathol Appli Neurobiol 1987;13:405–419

174. Rothstein JD: Excitotoxic mechanisms in the pathogenesis of amyotrophic lateral sclerosis. pp. 7–20. In Serratrice GT, Munsat TL (eds): Pathogenesis and Therapy of Amyotrophic Lateral Sclerosis. Lippincott-Raven, Philadelphia, 1995

175. Kato AC: Excitotoxic mechanisms in the pathogenesis of amyotrophic lateral sclerosis: a discussion. pp. 21–27. In Serratrice GT, Munsat TL (eds): Pathogenesis and therapy of amyotrophic lateral sclerosis. Lippincott-Raven, Philadelphia, 1995

176. Bostock H, Sharief MK, Reid G, Murray NMF: Axonal ion channel dysfunction in amyotrophic lateral sclerosis. Brain 1995;118:217–225

177. Meyer T, Lenk U, Küther G et al: Studies of the coding region of the neuronal glutamate transporter gene in amyotrophic lateral sclerosis. Ann Neurol 1995;37:817–819

178. Appell SH, Smith RG, Alexianu MF et al: Autoimmunity as an etiological factor in sporadic amyotrophic lateral sclerosis. pp. 47–57. In Serratrice GT, Munsat TL (eds): Pathogenesis and therapy of amyotrophic lateral sclerosis. Lippincott-Raven, Philadelphia, 1995

179. Rowland LP: Amyotrophic lateral sclerosis with paraproteins and autoantibodies. pp. 93–105. In Serratrice GT, Munsat TL (eds): Pathogenesis and therapy of amyotrophic lateral sclerosis: Lippincott-Raven, Philadelphia, 1995

180. Deng H-X, Hentati A, Tainer JA et al: Amyotrophic lateral sclerosis and structural defects in Cu, Zn superoxide dismutase. Science 1993;261:1047–1051

181. Rosen DR, Siddique T, Patterson D et al: Mutations in Cu/Zn superoxide dismutase gene are associated with familial amyotrophic lateral sclerosis. Nature 1993;362:59–62

182. Borchelt DR, Lee ML, Slunt HH et al: Superoxide dismutase 1 with mutations linked to familial amyotrophic lateral sclerosis possess significant activity. Proc Natl Acad Sci USA 1994; 91:8292–8296

CHAPTER 80

Bone and Joint Aging

PAUL DIEPPE
JONATHAN TOBIAS

The musculoskeletal system serves three primary functions: (1) it enables an efficient means of limb movement; (2) it acts as an endoskeleton thereby providing overall mechanical support and the protection of soft tissues; and (3) it serves as a reservoir of mineral for calcium homeostasis. In the elderly, the first two of these functions frequently become compromised, as illustrated by the fact that musculoskeletal problems are the major cause of pain and physical disability in people over the age of 65 years,[1] and by observations that fracture incidence rises steeply with age (Fig. 80-1).

Several factors contribute to the age-related decline in musculoskeletal function, including the following (see also the accompanying box):

- Aging effects on components of the musculoskeletal system (i.e., articular cartilage, the skeleton, and soft tissues). These effects are responsible for the increasing incidence of osteoporosis and osteoarthritis with age, for the reduced range of joint movement, and for the stiffness and difficulty in initiating movement that occurs in the elderly.
- The age-related rise in the prevalence of common musculoskeletal disorders that begin in young adulthood or in middle age, and cause increasing pain and disability without shortening life span.
- The high incidence of certain musculoskeletal disorders in the elderly, such as polymyalgia rheumatica and Paget's disease of bone.

A number of interrelated hypotheses have been advanced to explain the high prevalence of bone, muscle, and joint problems in older humans[2–5]

- The long life span of humans results in increasing accumulation of mechanical damage to the musculoskeletal system in older people.
- There is a lack of genetic investment in the repair of age-related tissue damage that develops in the postreproductive phase of life.
- The musculoskeletal system in humans has not adapted fully to the upright posture and prehensile grip because of lack of evolutionary pressure to do so, with the result that many of our bones and joints are inappropriately shaped and "underdesigned" to be able to cope with the stresses applied.
- By virtue of their sedentary lifestyle, modern humans tend to be exposed to less mechanical stress than their ancestors. Because musculoskeletal strength is governed by the mechanical inputs to which that individual is exposed, this may result in modern humans having a weaker musculoskeletal system, which is not well adapted for episodes of sudden major stress.

Several different mechanisms are apparently involved in musculoskeletal tissue aging,[6] including:

- Reduced synthetic capacity of differentiated cells such as osteoblasts and chondrocytes, with a consequent loss of ability to maintain matrix integrity.
- A decline in the mesenchymal stem cell populations.
- Post-translational modification of structural proteins such as collagen.
- The accumulation of degraded molecules, such as proteoglycan fragments, in musculoskeletal tissue matrices.
- Decreased circulating and local levels of trophic hormones, growth factors, and cytokines, such as insulin-like growth factor-1 (IGF-1), involved in maintaining tissue integrity.
- A decreased capacity for wound healing and tissue repair, which may be the result of some or all of the mechanisms described above.

The major tissues that have received the most attention, and which are pivotal to the integrity of the system, are articular cartilage, the skeleton, and soft tissues. Age-related changes in these structures are now described in more detail.

Aging and Articular Cartilage

The structure of a mammalian synovial joint is summarized in Figure 80-2. Much of its function owes itself to the properties of articular cartilage, which cushions the subchondral bone and provides a low friction surface necessary for free movement. Articular cartilage contains very few cells, is aneural

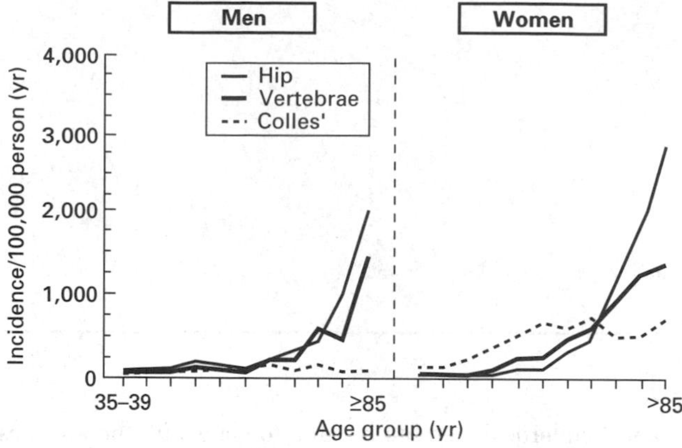

Figure 80-1 Age-specific incidence rates for hip, vertebral, and distal forearm fracture (Colles') fracture in Rochester, Minnesota, men and women. (From Cooper and Melton,[18] with permission.)

and avascular, and yet its integrity is maintained throughout a lifetime of biomechanical stress. With increasing age the cartilage surface often starts to break down, leading to osteoarthritis (OA). This is associated with changes in other tissues of the joint (Fig. 80-3). Whether the latter directly cause OA, are a necessary predisposition to OA, or are unrelated to the disorder remains controversial, but current opinion favors some relationship between the two processes.

With age articular cartilage thins and changes color from a glistening white to a dull yellow. In addition, the mechanical features of the tissue change. There is a decrease in tensile

Some of the factors contributing to the high prevalence of musculoskeletal problems in the elderly

Aging effects on components of the musculoskeletal system, leading to osteoarthritis and osteoporosis
- The skeleton
- Articular cartilage
- Soft tissues (i.e., muscle, ligaments, tendons, joint capsule)
- Neurologic function (e.g., joint proprioception)

Common disorders with peak incidence in younger adults, but which cause increasing pain and disability with age, without shortening life span
- Rheumatoid arthritis
- Seronegative spondarthritides
- Musculoskeletal trauma

Other disorders of the musculoskeletal system with a high incidence in the elderly
- Paget's disease of bone
- Crystal-related arthropathies
- Polymyalgia rheumatica

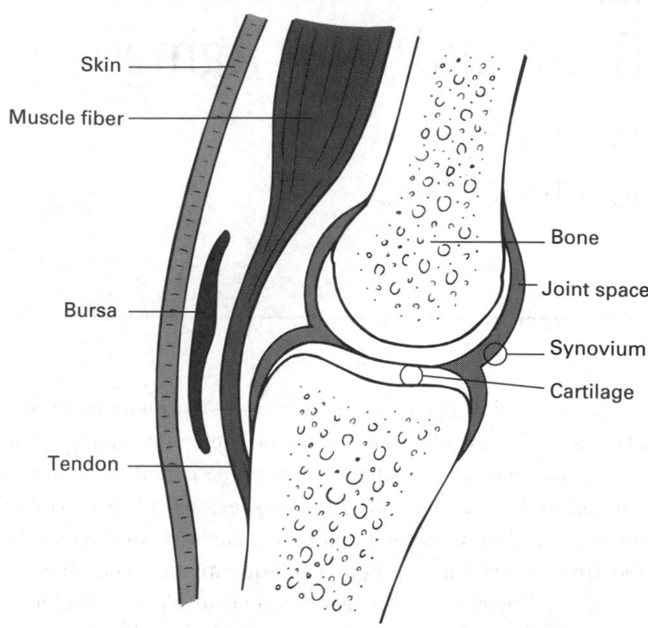

Figure 80-2 The synovial joint. The histologic appearances of the main tissues are highlighted. (Courtesy of Drs. J. H. Klippel and P. A. Dreppe.)

stiffness, fatigue resistance, and strength, but no significant change in the compressive properties. These changes are partly caused by the decrease in water content that accompanies aging.

The morphology and function of the cells (chondrocyte) and nature of the two main matrix components, aggrecan and type II collagen, also change with age. The density of cells in the tissue changes little, but their morphology alters with an increase in intracytoplasmic filaments, and they change their secretion of matrix components, producing more variable proteoglycans. Aging is also associated with alterations in the response of the chondrocytes to anabolic and catabolic stimuli such as the cytokine interleukin-1.

The main proteoglycan—aggrecan—binds with hyaluronan to form massive, hydrophilic aggregates that expand the collagen framework of the tissue, to provide it with its compressive and tensile strength. With age there is reduced proteoglycan aggregation and smaller proteoglycans are synthesized with an increase in keratin sulfate and reduced chondroitin sulfate content. The collagen also changes, with some increase in fiber diameter, as well as an increase in cross-linking. Less is known about the age-related changes in minor components of the cartilage, such as small molecular weight proteoglycans and noncollagenous proteins.

Aging and the Skeleton

Structural Changes

Weight-bearing bones consist of an outer shell of cortical bone, an arrangement that is designed for maximum strength. In addition, certain sites, such as vertebrae and metaphyses,

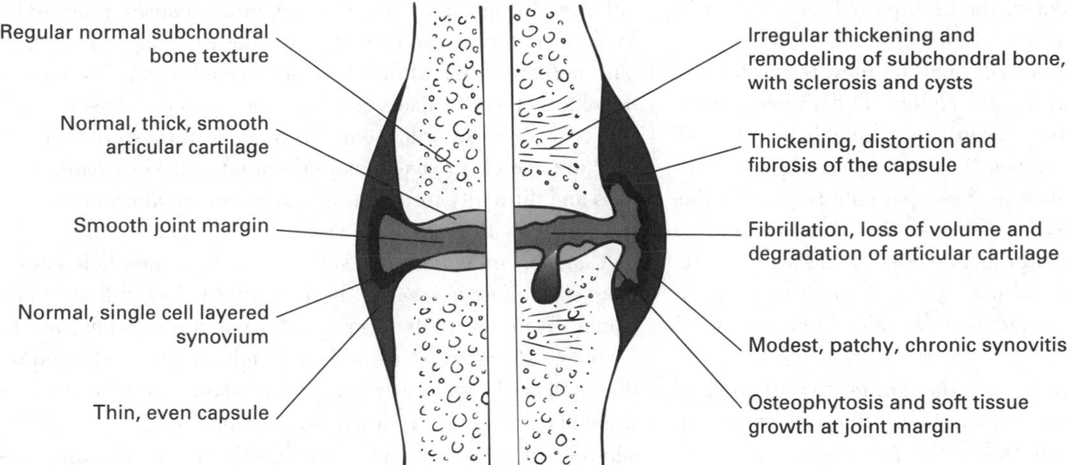

Figure 80-3 Normal versus osteoarthritic synovial joint. (Courtesy of Drs. J. H. Klippel and P. A. Dreppe.)

contain an inner meshwork of trabecular bone to act as an internal scaffold. Microscopically, the skeleton is made up of interconnecting fibrils of type I collagen, which provide tensile strength. Hydroxyapatite crystals, which are made up of calcium and phosphate, are desposited in holes within the collagen fibrils, giving bone its rigidity.

Once middle age is reached, the total amount of calcium in the skeleton (i.e., bone mass) starts to decline with age, a process that is accelerated during the first 5 years following the menopause in women.[7] This is associated with changes in skeletal structure, resulting in it becoming weaker and more prone to sustaining fractures. For example, the bony cortex becomes thinner due to expansion of the inner medullary cavity, the trabecular network disintegrates, and there is an accumulation of microfractures.[8]

Pathophysiology

Adult bone continuously undergoes self-renewal. This process, which is known as bone remodeling, occurs at discrete sites throughout the skeleton called bone remodeling units. Bone remodeling involves the coordinated activity of those cells responsible for bone formation and resorption (i.e., osteoblasts and osteoclasts, respectively) (Fig. 80-4). Bone loss in the elderly is largely a result of excess osteoclast activity,[9] which causes both an expansion in the total number of remodeling sites and an increase in the amount of bone resorbed per individual site.

The rise in osteoclast activity in older women partly reflects the decline in ovarian hormone production following the menopause, because estrogens exert an important restraining influence on bone resorption,[10] an effect that is largely thought to reflect an inhibitory action of estrogen on osteoclast recruitment.[11] Androgens are thought to exert a similar protective effect on the skeleton to estrogen,[12] deficiency of which is also common in the elderly. However, that estrogen deficiency is universal in women following the menopause presumably ex-

Figure 80-4 The bone remodeling sequence. This commences with osteoclastic bone resorption, following which a cement line is laid down (reversal phase). Osteoblasts then fill up the resorption cavity with osteoid, which subsequently mineralizes, the bone surface finally being covered by lining cells and a thin layer of osteoid.

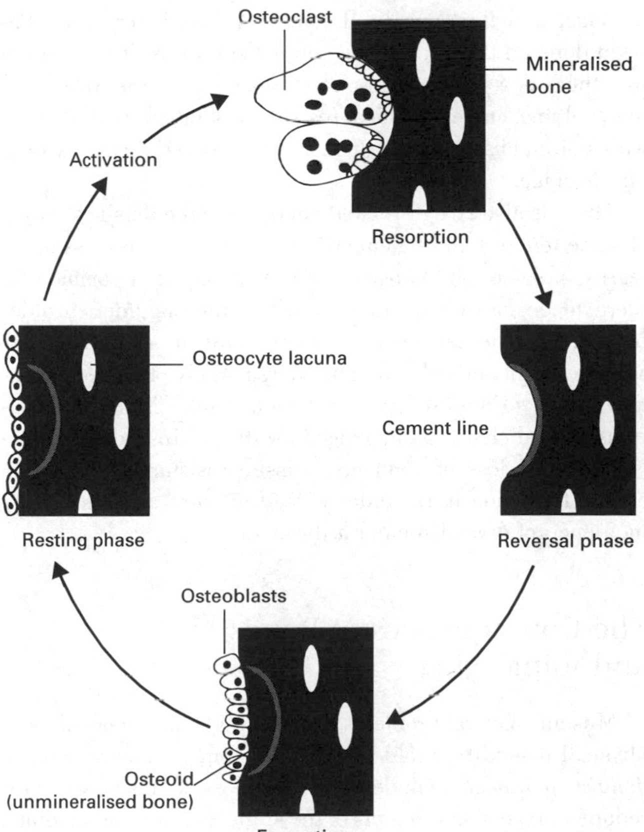

plains the fact that, in women, the lifetime risk of fractures is approximately three times that of men.[13]

In addition, osteoclast activity may be elevated in the elderly as a consequence of dietary vitamin D deficiency combined with reduced sunlight exposure, which leads to mild secondary hyperparathyroidism.[14] Despite subclinical evidence of osteomalacia, many of these patients present in the same way as osteoporosis, for example, with fractures of the femoral neck. Other metabolic bone diseases associated with osteoclast stimulation may also be present, such as primary hyperparathyroidism, the incidence of which increases with advancing age.

Bone loss in the elderly is also thought to involve an age-related decline in the recruitment and synthetic capacity of osteoblasts. This may partly reflect the reduction in physical activity associated with aging, thereby reducing the quality and quantity of mechanical inputs into the skeleton that are important in maintaining osteoblast activity. Additionally, age-related changes in the production of sex steroids, and in the bioavailability of other important regulatory factors such as IGF-1, have been suggested to contribute to impaired osteoblast function in the elderly.[15,16]

Aging and Soft Tissues

Back and neck pain and stiffness are common complaints in the elderly, as are periarticular problems. These might be due to age-related changes in intervertebral discs, ligaments, tendons, and the capsule of joints. Although less work has been done on the effect of age on these tissues, it is apparent that there is a gradual age-related decrease in the water content, volume, and mechanical resistance of intervertebral discs, with similar changes in the matrix to those described for articular cartilage.

There is also an age-related decrease in the tensile strength of some tendons and ligament-bone complexes and loss of integrity of some joint capsules. For example, it is common for there to be loss of the rotator cuff of the shoulder in older people, with the development of communications between the shoulder joint and subachromial bursa. Many of these changes may relate to alterations in collagen synthesis and to post-translational changes in collagens with age. In addition, there is a gradual loss of connective tissue resistance to calcium crystal formation in the elderly, leading to an increase in the incidence of crystal-related arthropathies.

The Consequences of Bone and Joint Aging

Musculoskeletal problems cause a huge burden of pain and physical disability in older people. The most important *functional impairments* include the marked loss of muscle strength, reduced range of movements of the spine and peripheral joints, and loss of joint proprioception contributing to problems of balance. In addition, spinal osteoporosis causes progressive kyphotic deformity and height loss. The key *symptoms* include pain and stiffness. Although pain thresholds may increase in the elderly there is also a very high prevalence of musculoskeletal pain. For example, some 25 percent of those individuals over the age of 55 years complain of current knee pain. Stiffness and difficulty in initiating movement are almost universal in those over the age of 70 years.

Changes in the bone and soft tissues make the whole system more *susceptible to trauma*. Periarticular pain syndromes and spinal disorders related to minor trauma are common, but by far the most important result is the high incidence of fractures (Fig. 80-1). These partly reflect the age-related increase in skeletal fragility that characterizes osteoporosis, and partly the age-related increase in falls, which is thought to be multifactorial (see Ch. 86).

The extent of the *disability and handicap* related to musculoskeletal changes in the elderly is well described in community surveys. Problems with reaching and with locomotion are particularly frequent, the latter contributing extensively to the isolation of older people. In addition, it is well recognized that in the elderly who sustain a hip fracture the majority fail to regain their previous level of functioning, and there is also an appreciable excess mortality.[17]

References

1. Martin J, White A: The prevalence of disability among adults. OPCS survey of disability in Great Britain, Report 1. HMSO, London, 1988
2. Hutton CW: Generalised osteoarthritis: an evolutionary problem? Lancet 1987;1:1463–1465
3. Lim KKT, Rogers J, Shepstone L, Dieppe PA: The evolutionary origins of osteoarthritis: a comparative skeletal study of hand disease in two primates. J Rheumatol 1995;22:2132–2134
4. Dieppe PA: Therapeutic targets in osteoarthritis. J Rheumatol 1995;22(suppl 43):136–139
5. Alexander C: Relationship between the utilisation profile of individual joints and their susceptibility to primary osteoarthritis. Skeletal Radiol 1989;18:199–205
6. Buckwalter JA, Woo S L-Y, Goldberg VM et al: Soft tissue aging and musculoskeletal function. J Bone Jt Surg 1993;75A: 1533–1548
7. Pouilles JM, Tremollieres F, Ribot C: Effect of menopause on femoral and vertebral bone loss. J Bone Miner Res 10: 1531–1536
8. Todd RC, Freeman MAR, Price CJ: Isolated trabecular fatigue fractures in the femoral neck. J Bone Jt Surg 1972;54B:723–728
9. Garnero P, Sornay-Rendu E, Chapuy MC, Delmas PD: Increased bone turnover in late postmenopausal women is a major determinant of osteoporosis. J Bone Miner Res 1996;11:337–349
10. Stepan JJ, Presl J, Broulik P, Pacovsky V: Serum ostecalcin levels and bone alkaline phosphatase isoenzyme after oophorectomy and primary hyperparathyroidism. J Clin Endocrinol Metab 1987;64:1079–1084
11. Jilka RL, Hangoc G, Girasole G et al: Increased osteoclast development after oestrogen loss: mediation by interleukin-6. Science 1992;257:88–91

12. Bellido T, Jilka RL, Boyce BF et al: Regulation of osteoclastogenesis and bone mass by androgens, JCI 1995;95:2886–2895
13. Melton LJ, Chrischilles EA, Cooper C et al: How many women have osteoporosis? J Bone Miner Res 1992;7:1005–1010
14. Chapuy MC, Arlot ME, Duboeuf F et al: Vitamin D3 and calcium to prevent hip fractures in elderly women. N Engl J Med 1992; 327:1637–1642
15. Chow J, Tobias JH, Colston KW, Chambers TJ: Estrogen maintains bone volume in rats not only by suppression of bone resorption but also by stimulation of bone formation. JCI 1992;89: 74–78
16. Rosen C, Donahue LR, Hunter S et al: The 24/25-k-Da serum insulin-like growth factor-binding protein is increased in elderly women with hip and spine fractures. JCEM 1992;74:24–27
17. Keene GS, Parker MJ, Pryor GA: Mortality and morbidity after hip fractures. BMJ 1993;307:1248–1250
18. Cooper C, Melton LJ: III. Epidemiology of osteoporosis. Trends Endocrinol Metab 1992;3:224–229

CHAPTER 81

Metabolic Bone Disease

R. M. FRANCIS

Although the popular image of the skeleton is of an inert structure supporting the rest of the body, bone is a dynamic tissue that undergoes constant remodeling throughout life. This remodeling is necessary to allow the skeleton to increase in size during growth, respond to the physical stresses placed on it, and repair structural damage due to structural fatigue or fracture. In addition to its mechanical properties, bone also plays an important role in calcium homeostasis, acting as a mineral reservoir that can be drawn upon to maintain normocalcemia. The skeleton comprises two types of bone: cortical or compact, and trabecular or cancellous bone. The respective proportion of cortical and trabecular bone varies with the anatomic site, although overall the skeleton is composed of 80 percent cortical and 20 percent trabecular bone. Cortical bone is predominantly found in the shafts of the long bones, whereas trabecular bone is mainly located in the vertebrae, pelvis, and the ends of long bones, where it forms a lattice-like structure within bone. Trabecular bone has a larger surface area, undergoes greater remodeling, and is therefore more responsive to changes in mineral metabolism than cortical bone.

The three major cell types involved in bone remodeling are osteoclasts, osteoblasts, and osteocytes. Osteoclasts are multinucleate cells derived from macrophage-monocyte precursors that resorb bone, releasing mineral and removing degraded organic material. Osteoblasts are derived from fibroblast precursors and synthesize bone matrix or osteoid, which is subsequently mineralized around foci of crystal formation known as matrix vesicles. The matrix vesicles are extruded from osteoblasts by exocytosis and contain promoters of crystal formation such as alkaline phosphatase and pyrophosphatase. Osteocytes are mature osteoblasts that become trapped within calcified bone. These are interconnected by long dendritic processes, possibly providing a communication network to transmit information about mechanical forces and direct bone resorption and formation.

Bone remodeling is initiated by a period of bone resorption lasting about 2 weeks, when osteoclasts erode an area of bone. Osteoblasts are then attracted to the resorption cavity, where over the subsequent 3 months new bone matrix is deposited and mineralized. The processes of bone resorption and bone formation are usually closely coupled, probably through local humoral factors, although bone formation exceeds resorption during skeletal growth and resorption outstrips bone formation after involutional bone loss starts. Bone remodeling may be influenced by mechanical forces applied to the skeleton, by local humoral factors, and by circulating hormones such as estrogen, testosterone, calcitonin, parathyroid hormone (PTH), and 1,25-dihydroxyvitamin D ($1,25(OH)_2D$).

Bone mass changes throughout life in three major phases: growth, consolidation, and involution.[1,2] Up to 90 percent of the ultimate bone mass is deposited during skeletal growth, which lasts until the closure of the epiphyses. There is then a phase of skeletal consolidation lasting for up to 15 years, when bone mass increases further until the peak bone mass is achieved in the mid-thirties. Involutional bone loss then starts between the ages of 35 and 40 in both sexes, but in women there is an acceleration of bone loss in the decade after the menopause. Overall, women lose 35 to 50 percent of trabecular and 25 to 30 percent of cortical bone mass with advancing age, whereas men lose 15 to 45 percent of trabecular and 5 to 15 percent of cortical bone.[1,2]

Osteoporosis

Osteoporosis is characterized by a reduction in the amount of bone in the skeleton, associated with skeletal fragility and an increased risk of fracture after minimal trauma. The three major osteoporotic fractures are those of the forearm, vertebral body, and femoral neck, although fractures of the humerus, tibia, pelvis, and ribs are also common in osteoporosis.[3] There is a strong inverse relationship between bone mass and fracture risk, with a two- to threefold increase in fracture incidence for each standard deviation reduction in bone density.[4,5]

Prior to the development of techniques that accurately measure bone density, osteoporosis was usually detected only after a fracture had occurred. The term *osteoporosis* was therefore reserved for the fracture syndrome resulting from reduced bone density. With the advent of bone densitometry and the therapeutic possibility of preventing bone loss, the term osteoporosis is now increasingly used to describe reduced bone density before fractures have occurred. The World Health Organization (WHO) has quantitatively defined osteoporosis as a bone density 2.5 standard deviation units or more below the mean value for young adults, whereas the term severe or established osteoporosis indicates that there has also been one or more fragility fractures.[6]

Prevalence of Osteoporosis

Using the WHO definition, the prevalence of osteoporosis in the hip increases in white women in the United States from 8 percent in the seventh decade to 47.5 percent in the ninth decade, whereas the prevalence of osteoporosis in the forearm, spine, or hip rises from 21.6 to 70 percent.[6] An alternative approach is to determine the prevalence of osteoporotic fractures. It has been estimated that the lifetime risk of fracture for a 50-year-old white woman in the United States is 16.0 percent for the forearm, 15.6 percent for the vertebra, and 17.5 percent for the proximal femur, whereas the corresponding figures for a 50-year-old man are 2.5, 5.0, and 6.0 percent.[7] The cumulative prevalence of these fractures in women and men is shown in Figure 81-1.

Pathogenesis of Osteoporosis

Bone mass at any age and therefore the risks of fracture is determined by the peak bone mass, the age at which bone loss starts, and the rate at which it progresses.[1,2] An individual with a high peak bone mass who starts to lose bone late in life and loses it slowly is unlikely to sustain osteoporotic fractures, whereas someone with a suboptimal peak bone mass who starts to lose bone earlier in life or loses bone rapidly is more likely to develop osteoporosis and its attendant fractures.

Peak bone mass

Genetic factors account for as much as 80 percent of the variance in peak bone mass.[8] Negroid populations have a higher bone mass than Caucasians or Asians, and men have bigger, denser skeletons than women.[9,10] There is also greater concordance of bone mass between monozygotic than dizygotic twins, and the daughters of osteoporotic women have a lower than expected bone density.[11,12] Recent work suggests that polymorphism of the vitamin D receptor gene may have an important effect on bone density in women.[13] Other potential determinants of peak bone mass include exercise, diet, smoking, alcohol consumption, and hormonal factors. Bone mass is greater in young adults who exercise regularly than in more sedentary individuals, emphasizing the importance of mechanical factors in the determination of bone mass.[14] Several studies suggest that a high dietary calcium intake during skeletal growth and consolidation may also be beneficial to the skeleton.[15–17] The combination of regular exercise and high dietary calcium intake may act together to produce an optimal peak bone mass.[15] In contrast, smoking and alcohol consumption during adolescence and early adult life may have an adverse effect on peak bone mass.[18] Endocrine factors also affect peak bone mass, as early menarche, pregnancy, and the use of the oral contraceptive pill are associated with higher bone mass.[19]

Involutional bone loss

Bone loss starts between the ages of 35 and 40 years in both sexes, possibly related to impaired new bone formation, due to declining osteoblast function. The onset of bone loss is likely to be genetically predetermined, and the subsequent rate of bone loss may also be influenced by genetic factors, as there is a greater concordance of bone loss, $1,25(OH)_2D$, PTH, calcium absorption, and biochemical markers of bone remodeling in monozygotic than dizygotic twins.[20,21] Bone loss increases at the menopause, due to the marked reduction in the circulating concentrations of estradiol and progesterone. Other causes of age-related bone loss include low body weight, smoking, excess alcohol consumption, physical inactivity, nutritional factors, and declining calcium absorption.[22,23]

Body weight is another important determinant of bone mass, because bone loss is more rapid in postmenopausal women with low body weight and osteoporotic subjects with femoral or vertebral fractures are lighter than expected.[24,25] The protective effects of high body weight on bone mass may be due to the mechanical effects of body weight on bone formation or to increased conversion of adrenal androgens to estrone in fat.

Smoking may increase bone loss by reducing the age at menopause by several years, decreasing plasma estrogen levels by increasing their metabolism, and possibly depressing osteoblast function.[26–28] The deleterious effect of smoking on the skeleton may also be due in part to the association with low body weight. Although alcoholism is a recognized cause of osteoporosis,[29] the result of modest alcohol consumption is unclear, as different studies show adverse and beneficial effects on bone density.[18,30]

The decline in physical activity with advancing age is also likely to cause further bone loss. Physical activity is important to the skeleton because the associated weight-bearing and muscular activity stimulates bone formation and increases bone mass, whereas immobilization leads to rapid bone loss.[31,32] The importance of physical activity is underlined by several case control studies, which show that patients with femoral fracture are habitually less physically active than control subjects.[33–35]

The role of dietary calcium intake in the pathogenesis of bone loss remains controversial. Although there is a relationship between dietary calcium in adolescence and bone mass,[15,16] other studies show no correlation between calcium intake and bone density or bone loss in postmenopausal women.[36,37] Other nutrients that have been suggested as potential determinants of the rate of bone loss include fluoride, protein, and sodium, although their importance is still uncertain.[38]

There is a reduction in circulating 25 hydroxyvitamin D (25OHD) and $1,25(OH)_2D$ concentrations with advancing age, due to decreased cutaneous production and impaired metabolism of vitamin D.[39,40] This is likely to contribute to the observed decline in calcium absorption and increase in circulating PTH with age.[41,42] If there is no compensatory increase in dietary calcium intake or reduction in urinary calcium, then the decline in calcium absorption might be expected to cause bone loss. There is a weak relationship between serum 25OHD and bone density in middle-aged women, with an inverse correlation between bone density and serum PTH, suggesting that vitamin D status may influence bone loss.[43] Vitamin D supplementation reduces bone loss during the winter months in postmenopausal women, suggesting that relative vitamin D deficiency and secondary hyperparathyroidism may contribute to bone loss.[44]

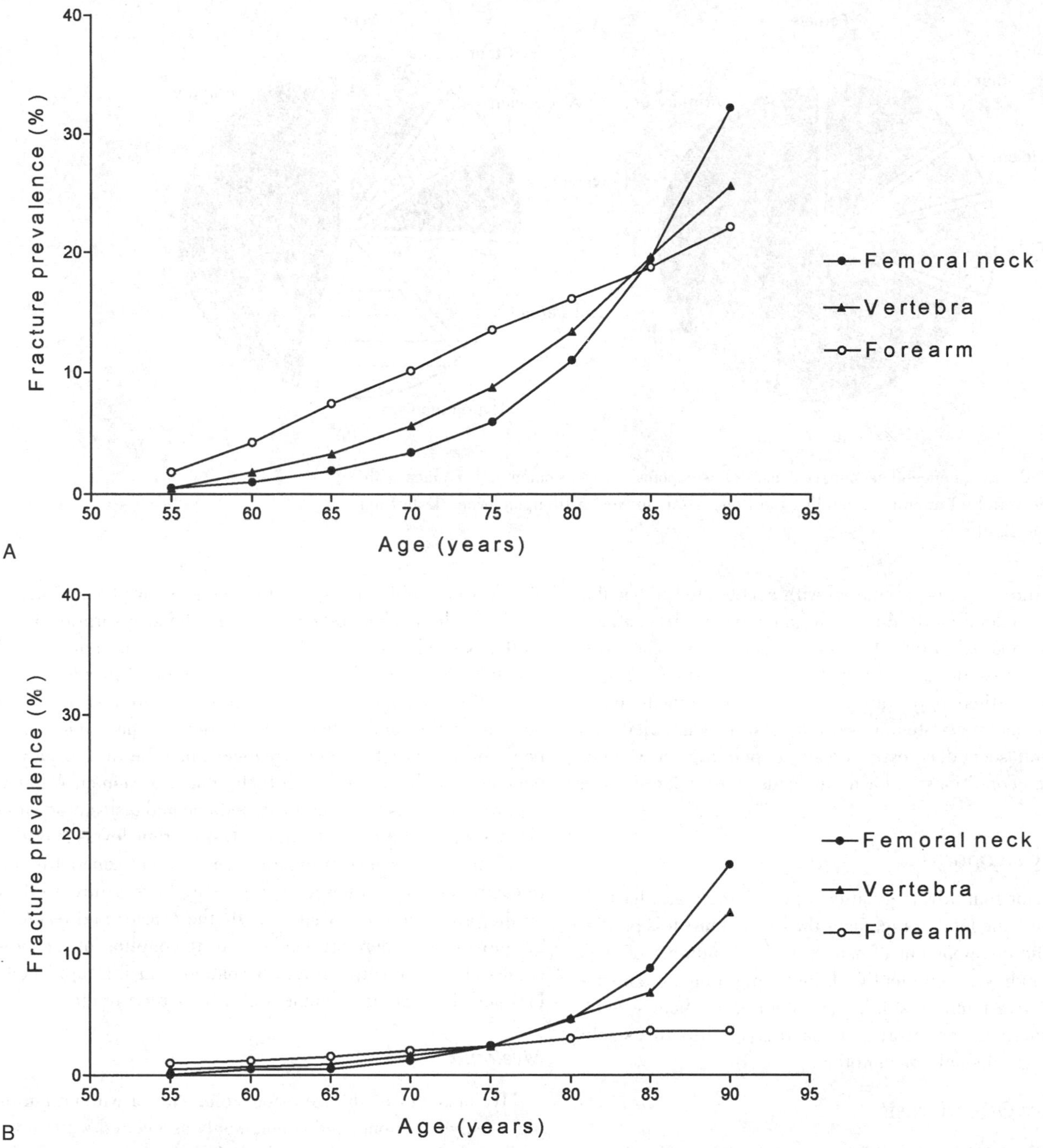

Figure 81-1 Cumulative prevalence of osteoporotic fractures with age in (**A**) women and (**B**) men. Prevalence calculated by F. H. Anderson and R. M. Francis from the incidence data of Melton.[7]

Secondary causes of osteoporosis

In addition to the factors influencing the attainment of peak bone mass and subsequent involutional bone loss, there are a number of conditions that may accelerate the development of osteoporosis. Secondary causes of osteoporosis may be found in up to 35 percent of women and 55 percent of men with symptomatic vertebral crush fractures.[45,46] (Fig. 81-2). The most frequently encountered are steroid therapy, myeloma, skeletal metastases, gastric surgery, anticonvulsant therapy, thyrotoxicosis, male hypogonadism, and immobilization.[45,46]

Classification of Osteoporosis

Riggs[1,47] has postulated that there are two distinct osteoporotic syndromes: type I or postmenopausal osteoporosis and type II or senile osteoporosis. Type I osteoporosis presents between the ages of 51 and 75 years with forearm and vertebral

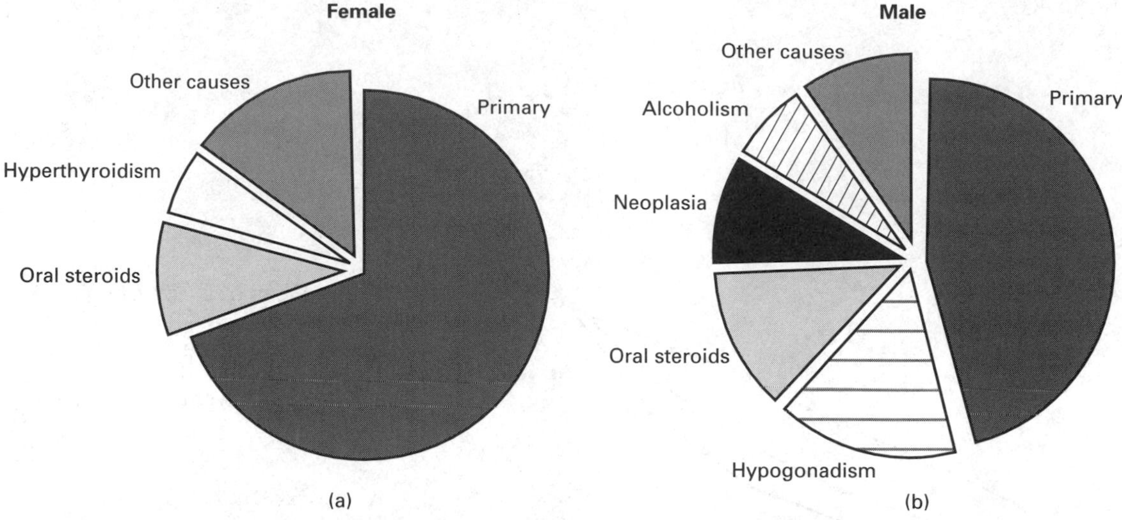

Figure 81-2 Prevalence of secondary causes of osteoporosis in (**A**) women and (**B**) men with symptomatic vertebral fractures attending the Bone Clinic in Newcastle upon Tyne. (Data from Caplan[45] and Baillie.[46])

crush fractures, and is associated with accelerated trabecular bone loss predominantly due to the menopause. In contrast, type II osteoporosis presents over the age of 70 years with femoral fractures and wedging of the vertebrae, and is characterized by cortical and trabecular bone loss due to other age-related factors. Osteoporosis may also be classified into primary and secondary osteoporosis, depending on whether underlying conditions known to cause osteoporosis are present.[2]

Primary Osteoporosis

Any factor that adversely affects peak bone mass, hastens the onset of bone loss, or increases the rate of bone loss predisposes to the development of osteoporosis. A number of such risks factors have been identified, including premature menopause, positive family history, short stature, low body weight, low calcium intake or absorption, inactivity, nulliparity, smoking, and high alcohol consumption.[1,2]

Secondary Osteoporosis

As mentioned earlier, a number of conditions may accelerate the development of osteoporosis. The most common causes of secondary osteoporosis are steroid therapy, myeloma, skeletal metastases, gastric surgery, anticonvulsant therapy, thyrotoxicosis, male hypogonadism, and immobilization[45,46] (Fig. 81-2).

Steroid therapy

Steroid therapy is the most common cause of secondary osteoporosis, occurring in 10 to 20 percent of patients with crush fractures.[45,46] Steroids decrease calcium absorption by a direct effect on the bowel mucosa, thereby increasing circulating PTH and $1{,}25(OH)_2D$, both of which are potential bone resorbing agents.[48] They also suppress the adrenal production of androgens, which consequently leads to low plasma estrone levels.[48] These changes may increase bone resorption indirectly, but cell culture techniques suggest that steroids may also have a direct effect on bone resorption.[49] In addition to their effects on bone resorption, steroids may also suppress bone formation and collagen production.[48] The reduction in bone formation with steroid treatment may be due in part to decreased androgen levels in both men and women. Adrenal suppression leads to low androstenedione and testosterone levels in women, whereas reduction in testosterone levels may also occur in men, because of impaired secretion of gonadotrophin releasing hormone. Steroid therapy may have a direct effect on the production of sex steroids by the ovaries and testes.[50] Steroid therapy therefore leads to an uncoupling of the processes of bone resorption and formation, causing rapid bone loss and the early development of osteoporotic fractures.

Myeloma

Myeloma causes diffuse osteopenia, with or without multiple osteolytic lesions, and is commonly associated with vertebral crush fractures and pathologic fractures elsewhere.[2] The myeloma cells stimulate bone resorption by secreting an osteoclast-activating factor. It is probably worthwhile performing serum and urine immunoelectrophoresis in all osteoporotic patients even in the absence of anemia, raised erythrocyte sedimentation rate (ESR), hypercalcemia, or radiologic evidence of osteolytic lesions. Establishing the diagnosis of myeloma is important, as treatment with melphalan and steroids may improve the prognosis, particularly when given early in the course of the disease. Radiotherapy may also be helpful in patients with localized bone pain. Recent evidence suggests that bisphosphonates such as clodronate and pamidronate may be useful in the management of bone disease in patients with myeloma.[51]

Skeletal metastases

Tumors commonly metastasize to bone, and the most frequent sites of skeletal metastases are the spine, femur, pelvis, ribs, sternum, and humerus.[52] Skeletal metastases may have either an osteolytic or osteoblastic appearance, with carcinomas of the lung, thyroid, kidney, and large bowel producing osteolytic metastases, whereas carcinoma of the prostate, carcinoid tumors, and Hodgkin's lymphoma are associated with osteoblastic deposits in bone.[52] Skeletal metastases from carcinoma of the breast may be either osteolytic or osteoblastic. Bone destruction associated with metastases may be due to the resorption of bone by tumor cells or to stimulation of osteoclasts by local humoral factors released by the metastatic cells.[2] The possibility of skeletal metastases should be considered in all osteoporotic patients with severe bone pain, other clinical features of malignancy, anemia, raised ESR, persistently elevated plasma alkaline phosphatase, or hypercalcemia. X-rays may show osteolytic or osteoblastic lesions, and isotope bone scan may reveal multiple areas of increased isotope uptake. The histologic examination of bone that appears radiologically abnormal may also be useful in the diagnosis of skeletal metastases on occasions.

Gastric surgery

Gastrectomy is a well-established cause of osteomalacia, but gastric surgery may also be a risk factor for the development of osteoporosis.[2] A number of pathogenic mechanisms may lead to bone loss after gastric surgery, including decreased absorption of vitamin D, reduced food intake, and malabsorption of calcium due to marginal vitamin D deficiency, the absence of gastric acid, and intestinal hurry.[2]

Anticonvulsant therapy

Although the association between anticonvulsant medication and osteomalacia is widely accepted, the relationship between anticonvulsant therapy and osteoporosis is less clear. Vertebral crush fractures are not uncommon in epileptic patients receiving anticonvulsant drugs, but this may be related to trauma during convulsions rather than to underlying osteoporosis. Nevertheless, bone mass in patients receiving anticonvulsants is 20 to 30 percent lower than expected, suggesting that it is a genuine risk factor for the development of osteoporosis.[53]

Anticonvulsant drugs decrease calcium absorption by a direct effect on the bowel mucosa and by lowering plasma 25OHD. The reduction in plasma 25OHD is probably due to stimulation of hepatic microsomal metabolism of vitamin D, leading to the formation of polar biologically inactive metabolites.[2] Anticonvulsant treatment during bone growth and consolidation may also reduce peak bone mass, thereby predisposing to osteoporotic fractures early in adult life.[54]

Thyrotoxicosis

Hyperthyroidism is a well-established cause of osteoporosis, although the diagnosis may not always be apparent in elderly osteoporotic patients, because the other clinical features of thyrotoxicosis may be absent.[2] Thyrotoxicosis stimulates both bone formation and resorption, although resorption exceeds formation such that bone is lost from the skeleton.[55] Increased bone resorption in thyrotoxicosis suppresses PTH production, leading to low plasma $1,25(OH)_2D$ and malabsorption of calcium, all of which are reversed when the patient is rendered euthyroid by treatment.[2] Treatment may also increase bone formation further, and the parallel increase in bone formation and plasma $1,25(OH)_2D$ suggests that the initial disparity between bone formation and resorption may be due to low plasma $1,25(OH)_2D$ levels.[2] The apparent uncoupling of bone formation and resorption during treatment of thyrotoxicosis may persist for up to a year, and might be expected to increase bone mass and at least in part reverse the osteoporotic process.

Male hypogonadism

Hypogonadism is a common cause of osteoporosis in men, occurring in up to 20 percent of men with vertebral crush fractures and 50 percent of elderly men with femoral neck fractures.[23] The pathogenesis of bone loss in hypogonadal men remains uncertain, although histologic studies show evidence of increased resorption and decreased bone formation, which has been attributed to androgen or estrogen deficiency, low plasma $1,25(OH)_2D$ concentrations, malabsorption of calcium, or reduced calcitonin levels.[23] The diagnosis of hypogonadism may not always be readily apparent in men with osteoporosis, particularly in elderly patients when the condition may have developed insidiously; routine measurement of serum testosterone and gonadotrophins may therefore be worthwhile. Treatment with androgens decreases bone resorption and stimulates bone formation, and may therefore increase bone mass.[23]

Immobilization

Immobilization leads to rapid bone loss of about 1 percent per week, which then stabilizes after about 6 months when a new steady state is reached.[31,32,56] Bone loss in immobilization is due to a stimulation of bone resorption and a decrease in bone formation,[56] and the more rapid loss in weight-bearing bones suggests that bone loss is due to mechanical factors rather than changes in circulating PTH, $1,25(OH)_2D$, thyroxine, or cortisol.[57] Where practicable, remobilization should be encouraged, as this appears to increase trabecular bone mass by 0.25 percent per week and may partially replace the lost bone.[32]

Clinical Features of Osteoporosis

Osteoporosis is generally considered to be asymptomatic until fractures occur. Fractures of the forearm and femur are usually easy to diagnose, but vertebral crush fractures are more difficult to detect clinically. Only 30 percent of patients come to medical attention after a vertebral fracture[58] and there are many other causes of acute back pain. Classically, however, a crush fracture is associated with an acute episode of back pain lasting for 6 to 8 weeks before settling to a more chronic backache. The pain may radiate anteriorly but rarely radiates to the hips or legs. Osteoporotic subjects may also be aware of loss of height of several inches and notice the development of a kyphosis. Physical signs include a kyphosis, local tenderness over the spine, and horizontal skin creases and abdominal protrusion due to the loss of trunk height.

Investigation of Osteoporosis

As mentioned above, patients with osteoporosis present with fractures or their sequelae. In patients with forearm or femoral fractures, radiography is performed to confirm that a fracture has occurred and to determine its position prior to subsequent fixation. As vertebral crush fractures are more difficult to diagnose, spine x-rays should be considered in patients with acute back pain, loss of height, or kyphosis, to look for evidence of vertebral deformation (Fig. 81-3), degenerative arthritis, or other pathology. Such x-rays may also show lytic or sclerotic lesions that suggest the possibility of neoplastic disease. Although spine x-rays are useful in the diagnosis of vertebral fracture, they are unreliable in the assessment of bone density.[59]

Whereas alkaline phosphatase may rise transiently after a fracture, other investigations are generally normal in primary osteoporosis, although they may indicate the presence of a secondary cause of osteoporosis. As secondary osteoporosis is common in individuals with vertebral crush fractures,[45,46] and specific treatment of the underlying condition may prevent or reduce further bone loss in many cases, it is worthwhile performing full blood count, ESR, plasma biochemical profile, thyroid function tests, and serum and urine electrophoresis in all such patients, together with serum testosterone and gonadotrophins in males.[45,46] Anemia, raised ESR, persistent elevation of alkaline phosphatase, or hypercalcemia suggests the possibility of myeloma or skeletal metastases and requires further investigation, including isotope bone scan and bone marrow examination. Thyroid function tests, serum testosterone, and gonadotrophins may also reveal unsuspected thyrotoxicosis and hypogonadism, respectively. Serum and urine immunoelectrophoresis should probably be performed in all patients with vertebral crush fractures, as the condition may be present even in the absence of other abnormal laboratory findings.[45,46]

Prevention of Osteoporosis

Ideally the prevention of osteoporosis should include the promotion of an optimal peak bone mass, the delay of the onset of bone loss, and the retardation of the subsequent rate of bone loss.

Increasing peak bone mass

Although the extent to which the attainment of peak mass can be modified is uncertain, it seems prudent to encourage children and young adults to eat a balanced diet rich in calcium

Figure 81-3 (**A**) X-ray of the thoracic spine of a woman with osteoporosis, showing vertebral deformation. (**B**) X-ray of the lumbar spine of a woman with osteoporosis, showing biconcavity and vertebral deformation.

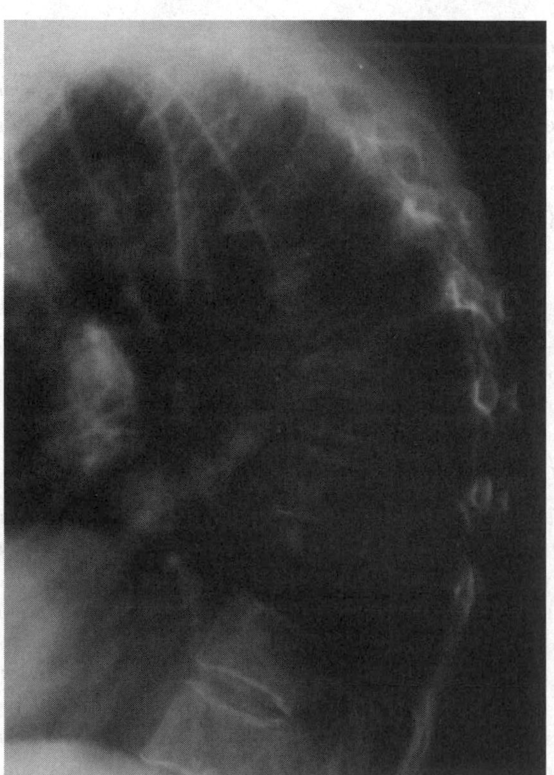

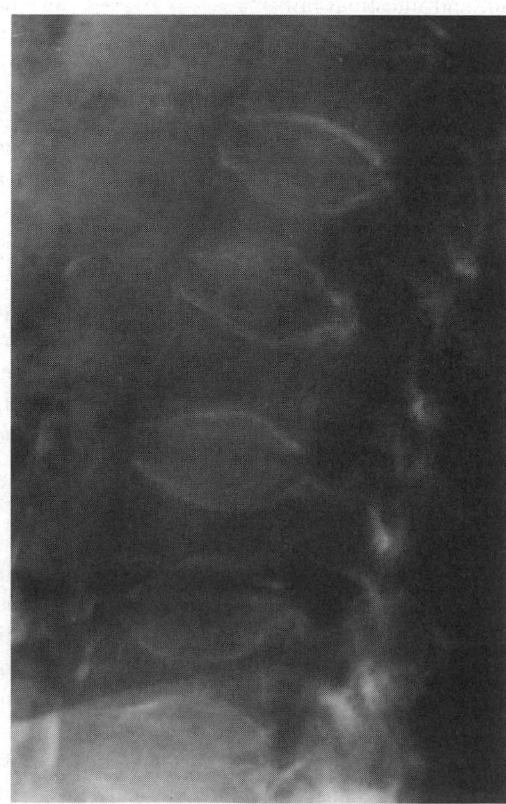

and to avoid excessive dieting, because of the association between low body weight and osteoporosis.[60] Regular exercise should be encouraged, although females should avoid exercising to the point where they become amenorrheic, as this has a deleterious effect on bone mass.[61] Secondary amenorrhea due to other causes is common in young women, and should be investigated and treated as rapidly as possible, because of the adverse effects of the associated estrogen deficiency on bone mass.[62]

Delaying the onset of bone loss—hormone replacement therapy

The most effective way of delaying the onset of bone loss is by the use of hormone replacement therapy (HRT) at the time of the menopause. HRT prevents bone loss and may increase bone density in the hip and spine by up to 3 percent in normal postmenopausal women.[63–65] If given for 5 to 10 years at the time of the menopause, HRT significantly decreases the risk of osteoporotic fractures by up to 50 percent.[63,64] Bone loss recommences after HRT is discontinued, so that the benefits of previous treatment may diminish with advancing age. A recent study shows that women over the age of 75 years who have previously taken HRT for at least 7 years have only 3.2 percent higher bone density than those who have never taken such treatment.[66]

In addition to the benefits on the skeleton, HRT controls menopausal symptoms such as hot flushes, nocturnal sweats, vaginal dryness, and dyspareunia. It also improves the lipid profile and reduces the risk of cardiovascular disease.[67] There are a number of potential complications of HRT. Early studies showed that unopposed estrogen treatment increased the risk of endometrial hyperplasia and carcinoma, but the addition of a cyclical progestogen for 12 days each cycle appears to abolish this increased risk.[68,69] Although the role of estrogen treatment in the pathogenesis of carcinoma of the breast remains controversial, it seems that there may be some increased risk of breast carcinoma after prolonged estrogen treatment, which is not reduced by concomitant progestogen therapy.[70] Nevertheless, if the increased risk of breast cancer is weighed against the benefits of estrogen treatment on the skeleton and cardiovascular and cerebrovascular disease, the balance favors HRT.[71] Other side effects of HRT include nausea, fluid retention, breast tenderness, and headaches. The regular vaginal bleeding experienced by many women receiving an estrogen and cyclical progestogen preparation may also be inconvenient and poorly tolerated, particularly in older individuals.[72,73] The advent of continuous combined estrogen/progestogen preparations may improve the situation, as it offers a woman the benefits of HRT without the need for a regular monthly bleed. Furthermore, such treatment appears to have a significantly greater effect on spine bone density than a conventional estrogen and cyclical progestogen preparation, presumably because of the independent action of continuous progestogen on bone.[74]

Reduction of bone loss

Although prolonged HRT prevents bone loss and reduces the subsequent risk of fracture, treatment is less well tolerated with advancing age, and is rarely continued for more than 10 to 15 years.[72] Is there anything that can be done to reduce the subsequent rate of bone loss? Metabolic balance studies show an apparent increase in the dietary requirement for calcium at the menopause from 1,000 to 1,500 mg/day,[75] but there is little relationship between dietary calcium intake and bone loss at this time,[36,37] suggesting that increasing dietary calcium is unlikely to produce a major effect on the rate of bone loss. Nevertheless, the reduction in calcium absorption later in life may increase the dietary calcium requirements further,[41] so it seems wise to advise postmenopausal women to take a diet rich in calcium. Stopping smoking and reducing alcohol consumption might also be expected to reduce bone loss, although there is no definite evidence to confirm this. In view of the benefits of weight-bearing and exercise on bone, and the deleterious effects of immobilization on the skeleton, regular exercise and physical activity should be encouraged throughout life.[31,32] As the decline in calcium absorption is in part due to decreased plasma 25OHD concentrations, efforts should be made to ensure that elderly people are vitamin D replete by encouraging adequate sunlight exposure and considering vitamin D supplementation in housebound or institutionalized individuals.

Screening for Osteoporosis

There is considerable interest in the early detection of asymptomatic osteoporosis, as effective treatments are now available to prevent further bone loss. Although accurate measurements of lumbar spine and femoral bone density can be made using dual energy x-ray absorptiometry, population-based bone density screening cannot be advocated for the prevention of osteoporotic fractures. Nevertheless, bone density measurements may be useful in the management of individuals at particularly high risk of osteoporosis, because of factors such as early menopause, prolonged oral steroid therapy, or family history of the condition. Bone densitometry may also be helpful in patients with history of peripheral fractures after minimal trauma or those with apparent reduced bone density on x-ray.

An alternative approach is to identify individuals who are losing bone rapidly, using biochemical tests. Christiansen et al.[24] have described the use of a combination of serum alkaline phosphatase, fasting urine hydroxyproline/creatinine and calcium/creatinine, and body weight to classify individuals into fast bone losers, slow bone losers, and an intermediate group. Newer biochemical markers may improve patient classification, but it is likely that these techniques will be used as an adjunct to bone densitometry, rather than replace it.

Treatment of Established Osteoporosis

Treatments for osteoporosis may be classified into antiresorptive agents, such as estrogens, progestogens, calcium supplements, calcitonin, and bisphosphonates, which prevent or reduce further bone loss, and anabolic agents such as sodium fluoride and anabolic steroids, which appear to increase bone mass.[73] As antiresorptive agents lead to a transient uncoupling of bone resorption and formation, there may be a small increase in bone mass before a new equilibrium is reached.[73] Although anabolic agents may increase bone mass, they do not necessarily improve bone strength, particularly when the trabecular architecture has been disrupted by the osteoporotic process.

Estrogen

In addition to increasing bone mass in normal postmenopausal women, HRT has also been shown to increase spine bone density by 5 percent in postmenopausal women with established osteoporosis.[76,77] One of these studies also showed a 60 percent reduction in the number of further vertebral fractures.[77] HRT is the treatment of choice in the younger woman with osteoporosis, because of its beneficial effect on climacteric symptoms and on the risk of ischemic heart disease. Estrogen treatment appears to be less well tolerated with advancing age, because of an increased incidence of side effects and the inconvenience of withdrawal bleeds if the uterus is still present.[72]

Other hormones

Norethisterone and tibolone appear to prevent bone loss as effectively as estrogens, without the need for regular vaginal bleeding.[78,79] Nevertheless, these agents are not licensed for the prevention and treatment of osteoporosis and there is no information on their effect on fracture incidence. Their use cannot therefore be advocated at present.

Although tamoxifen is used in the management of breast cancer because of its action as an estrogen antagonist, it acts as an estrogen agonist on the skeleton and cardiovascular system, reducing bone loss and decreasing the risk of ischemic heart disease.[80] Other estrogen analogs such as raloxifene are under investigation in the management of osteoporosis.

Bisphosphonates

Biphosphonates are powerful antiresorptive agents, which although poorly absorbed by mouth, localize preferentially in bone. They bind to hydroxyapatite crystals and reduce osteoclast recruitment and function. As bisphosphonates persist in the skeleton for many months, their duration of action is prolonged beyond the period of administration.[81] Intermittent cyclical etidronate therapy and continuous alendronate treatment both increase spine bone density in women with osteoporosis by 5 to 8 percent over 3 years, and this is associated with a reduction in the incidence of further vertebral fractures of about 60 percent.[82–85] Alendronate appears to have a more rapid effect on femoral neck bone density, increasing this by 5.9 percent in 3 years, compared with 1.4 percent with cyclical etidronate.[84,85] Nevertheless, there is no definite evidence that any bisphosphonate treatment will decrease the risk of femoral neck fractures.

Bisphosphonates are particularly useful in older women with osteoporosis who are unwilling or unable to take HRT. Intermittent cyclical etidronate therapy is particularly indicated in the management of women with spinal osteoporosis and vertebral fractures, whereas alendronate may be more appropriate where there is a marked reduction in bone density at other sites. Other bisphosphonates are being evaluated at present, including clodronate, pamidronate, tiludronate and risedronate.[81]

Calcitonin

Calcitonin is a peptide hormone secreted by the C cells of the parathyroid glands, although its precise role in human physiology is unclear. Nevertheless, calcitonin is a potent antiresorptive agent, having a rapid but short-lived effect on osteoclast function. A dose response study of intranasal calcitonin in the treatment of women with reduced forearm bone density showed increases in spine bone density of 1 to 3 percent over 2 years, associated with a 64 percent reduction in the number of vertebral fractures.[86] Another study in postmenopausal women with vertebral crush fractures showed that cyclical intramuscular calcitonin and calcium supplements decreased the incidence of vertebral fractures by 60 percent over 2 years, compared with an increase in 35 percent in a group receiving calcium alone.[87] Calcitonin is expensive and associated with side effects such as flushing, nausea, vomiting, diarrhea, dizziness, and headache. These side effects may be less with the intranasal route of administration, although this is not currently available in the United Kingdom.

Calcium supplements

Although calcium supplements were previously used alone in the treatment of osteoporosis, this is probably no longer appropriate as a number of more effective treatments are now available. Calcium supplements decrease bone loss, but not to the same extent as other antiresorptive agents.[88,89] There is no convincing evidence that calcium supplements alone decrease the risk of vertebral or hip fractures.

Vitamin D

With advancing age there is a reduction in cutaneous production and subsequent metabolism of vitamin D. This leads to a decrease in calcium absorption and PTH-mediated bone resorption. A French study in nursing homes and apartment blocks for the elderly showed that 800 IU of vitamin D_3 and 1.2 g of elemental calcium daily reduces the risk of hip fracture by 43 percent.[90] It is unclear if the benefits of treatment seen in this study were due to vitamin D, calcium, or the combination of both, but a Finnish study showed that an annual injection of 150,000 to 300,000 IU vitamin D decreases the risk of long bone fractures in elderly people.[91] Nevertheless, there is no evidence that vitamin D and calcium supplementation decreases spine bone loss or the incidence of vertebral fractures. Vitamin D supplementation is therefore most appropriate in frail and housebound elderly people, who are at high risk of vitamin D deficiency and hip fractures.

Vitamin D metabolites

Patients with established osteoporosis have lower calcium absorption than age-matched control subjects, which may be due to reduced serum $1{,}25(OH)_2D$ concentrations or to relative resistance to the action of vitamin D metabolites on the bowel.[92] Malabsorption of calcium in osteoporosis can be overcome by pharmacologic doses of parent vitamin D or by low doses of the vitamin D metabolites, calcitriol and alfacalcidol. Studies of the effect of treatment with vitamin D metabolites on bone loss and fractures in established osteoporosis have produced conflicting results.[92] A recent study comparing calcitriol with calcium supplementation has shown a significantly lower vertebral fracture incidence with calcitriol, although this was due to an increase in fracture rate with calcium rather than a reduction with calcitriol.[93] Treatment with the vitamin D metabolites is associated with an increased risk of hypercalcemia, but this did not appear to be a major problem in this study.[93]

Fluoride

Initial studies showed that sodium fluoride increased spine bone density by up to 35 percent over 4 years in women with vertebral osteoporosis, although this appeared to be at the expense of cortical bone loss.[94,95] There was no reduction in vertebral fracture incidence, whereas the number of nonvertebral fractures increased with fluoride.[94,95] These studies also showed that sodium fluoride is potentially toxic, causing nausea, vomiting, indigestion, and lower extremity bone pain.[94,95] A more recent study using lower dose, slow-release sodium fluoride shows smaller increases in spine and hip bone density, without adverse effects on forearm bone mass.[94,95] This study also showed a significant reduction in vertebral fracture incidence, without the side effect profile described with the higher dose treatment. Nevertheless, the therapeutic window for fluoride appears narrow and this agent cannot yet be advocated for the management of osteoporosis.

Anabolic steroids

Anabolic steroids such as stanozolol and nandrolone increase bone mass in osteoporosis by 5 to 10 percent.[97,98] This has previously been attributed to increased bone formation, but may be due to decreased bone resorption. Anabolic steroids may be associated with androgenic side effects and fluid retention, whereas prolonged administration may lead to abnormal liver function tests and even hepatocellular tumors. Their use in the management of osteoporosis cannot be advocated, particularly as there is no evidence of a reduction in fracture incidence.

Osteomalacia

Osteomalacia is a generalized bone disorder characterized by an impairment of mineralization leading to accumulation of unmineralized matrix or osteoid in the skeleton.[99,100] There are a number of causes of osteomalacia but the majority of cases are due to vitamin D deficiency, abnormal vitamin D metabolism, or hypophosphatemia (Table 81-1).

Table 81-1 Classification of the major causes of osteomalacia

Deficiency	Cause	Clinical Form
Vitamin D	↓ Sunlight exposure ↓ Dietary vitamin D Malabsorption	Housebound elderly Asian immigrants Small bowel disease
25OHD	Abnormal vitamin D metabolism	Anticonvulsants Liver disease
$1{,}25(OH)_2D$	↓ 1α-hydroxylase activity	Renal failure
Phosphate	↓ Tubular reabsorption	Familial Tumoral Sporadic
	Phosphate depletion	Use of phosphate binders

Adequate amounts of calcium and phosphate are essential for mineralization of osteoid to proceed normally, and although vitamin D is important in the homeostasis of calcium and phosphate, the precise role of the vitamin D metabolites in mineralization remains uncertain. The major source of vitamin D is from cutaneous production, following the exposure of the precursor 7-dehydrocholesterol to ultraviolet irradiation.[101–103] The diet provides much smaller amounts of vitamin D, but this becomes essential when cutaneous production is limited.[102,103] Vitamin D itself has little biological activity, and is metabolized in the liver to 25OHD, the major circulating form of vitamin D. This undergoes further hydroxylation in the kidneys to form $1{,}25(OH)_2D$, the hormonally active metabolite of vitamin D, which regulates calcium absorption from the bowel, influences bone remodeling, and affects muscle function.[101,104,105]

Vitamin D deficiency osteomalacia predominantly occurs because of reduced cutaneous production of vitamin D due to lack of exposure to sunlight or increased skin pigmentation. It is therefore particularly seen in the housebound elderly or Asian immigrants, particularly when the dietary intake of vitamin D is poor.[99,100] Vitamin D deficiency osteomalacia is also seen with malabsorption or after gastric surgery, and is related to reduced sunlight exposure, decreased absorption of vitamin D, and malabsorption of calcium or phosphate.[99,100] Anticonvulsant therapy and hepatic disease are also associated with low plasma 25OHD levels and the development of vitamin D deficiency osteomalacia.[99,100]

Anticonvulsants induce liver enzymes that metabolize vitamin D to biologically inactive polar metabolites, whereas liver disease may be associated with impaired 25 hydroxylation of vitamin D.[2] In addition, patients with epilepsy or liver disease may be less exposed to sunlight and therefore have reduced cutaneous production of vitamin D.

Renal impairment leads to the development of osteomalacia

because of reduced production of $1,25(OH)_2D$; malabsorption of calcium, and low plasma calcium, although plasma 25OHD concentration may also be low because of reduced sunlight exposure. Hypophosphatemic osteomalacia may result from decreased renal tubular reabsorption of phosphate as in familial, tumor-associated, and sporadic cases, or from phosphate depletion associated with the use of phosphate binders.[99,100]

Osteomalacia in the Elderly

Vitamin D deficiency is the most common cause of osteomalacia in the elderly. Renal failure is a smaller but significant cause in this age group. There is a reduction in plasma 25OHD with advancing age,[39] which is mainly due to reduced sunlight exposure, although decreased capacity for cutaneous production, low dietary intake, poor absorption, and impaired hepatic hydroxylation of vitamin D may also contribute to this.[102,103,106,107] Plasma 25OHD concentrations are lower in individuals living in residential care than in people living in the community, and lowest in residents of long-term geriatric wards.[108,109] The reduction in renal function with age is associated with decreased plasma $1,25(OH)_2D$ concentrations, which may contribute to the development of osteomalacia in the elderly.[110]

Osteomalacia is essentially a histologic diagnosis, so there is little information on its overall prevalence in the elderly. Nevertheless, as mentioned above, low 25OHD concentrations are common in the elderly, particularly in subjects who are housebound or institutionalized. As about 10 percent of the elderly are housebound, a significant proportion of the elderly are at risk of developing osteomalacia because of absent cutaneous production of vitamin D, and several investigators have shown that osteomalacia occurs in about 4 percent of elderly people admitted to the hospital.[111,112] A histologic study from Leeds suggested that up to 40 percent of patients with femoral fracture have evidence of osteomalacia, although the criteria used for this diagnosis were either excess osteoid or decreased calcification fronts.[113] Using the stricter diagnostic criteria of the combination of increased osteoid and decreased calcification fronts, the prevalence of osteomalacia in this group was nearer 20 percent.[113]

Clinical Features of Osteomalacia

The presentation of osteomalacia may be variable, and the diagnosis may be easily missed in the early stages of the disease, because of the vague nature of the symptoms. The patient may complain of aches and pains, aggravated by muscular contraction, but tending to persist after rest. Although there is a propensity for fracture in osteomalacia, the soft elastic bone also deforms easily, leading to kyphosis, scoliosis, and deformity of the rib cage, pelvis, and long bones. The patient may also develop a proximal myopathy, causing a waddling gait and difficulties rising from a chair or climbing stairs. Occasionally, the hypocalcemia associated with osteomalacia leads to latent tetany, with paresthesiae of the hands and around the mouth, cramps, a main d'accoucheur appearance of the hands, and positive Chvostek and Trousseau signs.

Radiology in Osteomalacia

The classic radiologic appearances of osteomalacia are relatively rare and may not be found in the early stages of the disease. Osteomalacic bone is softer than normal and so becomes easily deformed. The intervertebral discs balloon out and deform the adjacent vertebrae to give them a uniformly biconcave cod-fish appearance. Similar deformity may occur in osteoporosis, but the biconcavity is more regular in osteomalacia than with osteoporosis, where the extent of vertebral deformity is variable. There may be radiologic evidence of deformity of the rib cage, pelvis, and long bones (Figs. 81-4 and 81-5). A characteristic finding in osteomalacia is the Looser's zone or pseudofracture, which consist of a large area of osteoid. These appear as bands of decalcification surrounded by more dense bone, which occur perpendicular to the bone surface, often where nutrient arteries enter bone (Fig. 81-6). Looser's zones are seen particularly in the proximal femur, humeral neck, pubic rami, ribs, metatarsals, and the outer border of the scapula. There may also be radiologic evidence of secondary hyperparathyroidism, with subperiosteal erosions in the metacarpals or phalanges.

Biochemical Findings in Osteomalacia

The biochemical findings in the major types of osteomalacia are shown in Table 81-2. In vitamin D deficiency osteomalacia the plasma calcium tends to be low, because of reduced calcium absorption due to low plasma 25OHD and $1,25(OH)_2D$ concentrations. The hypocalcemia leads to secondary hyperparathyroidism, which in turn stimulates the renal tubular re-

Figure 81-4 Chest x-ray of a woman with osteomalacia, showing deformity of rib cage due to bone softening.

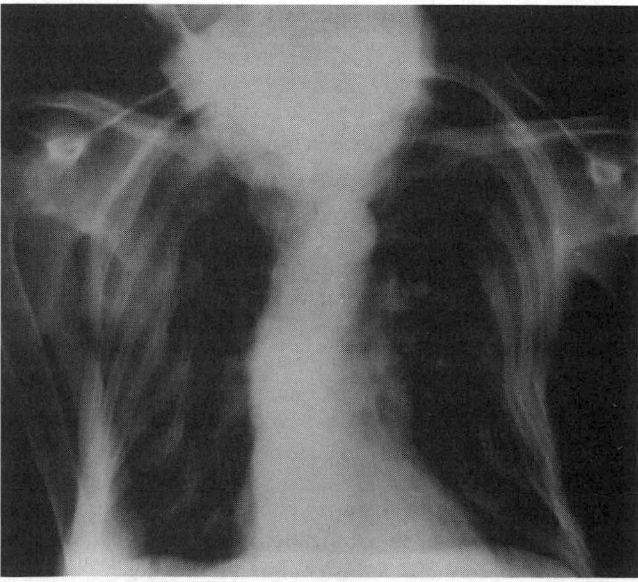

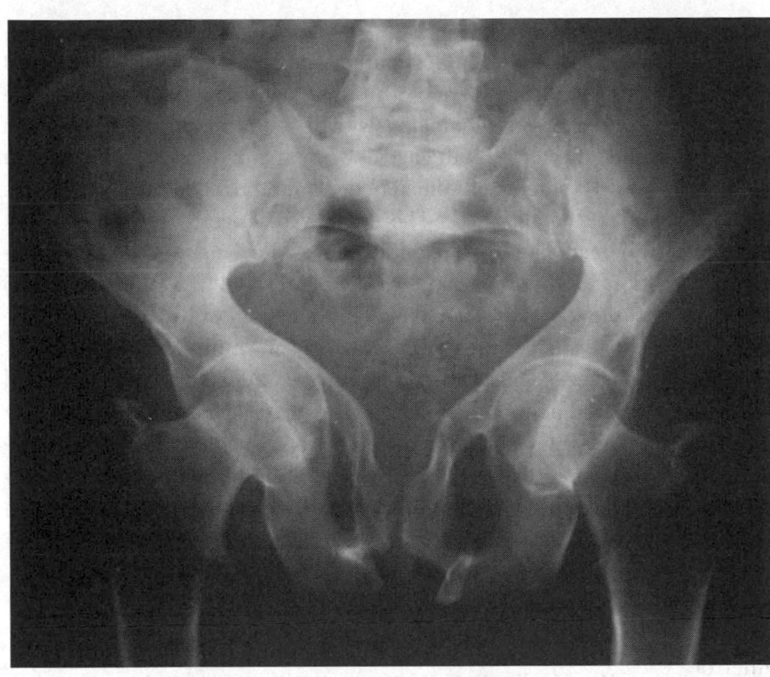

Figure 81-5 X-ray of the pelvis of a woman with osteomalacia, showing deformity of the pelvic bones due to bone softening.

absorption of calcium and reduces tubular reabsorption of phosphate. Plasma phosphate is therefore often low in osteomalacia because of reduced absorption from the bowel and decreased renal tubular reabsorption. The secondary hyperparathyroidism also increases bone remodeling, which is reflected in elevation of the plasma alkaline phosphatase and urine hydroxyproline excretion. Not all patients with vitamin D deficiency osteomalacia will have hypocalcemia, hypophosphatemia, and raised alkaline phosphatase, and these abnormalities may occur individually in the elderly with intercurrent illness, so they lack specificity in the diagnosis of osteomalacia in the elderly.[114]

Figure 81-6 X-ray of the pelvis of a woman with osteomalacia, showing Looser's zones in the public rami.

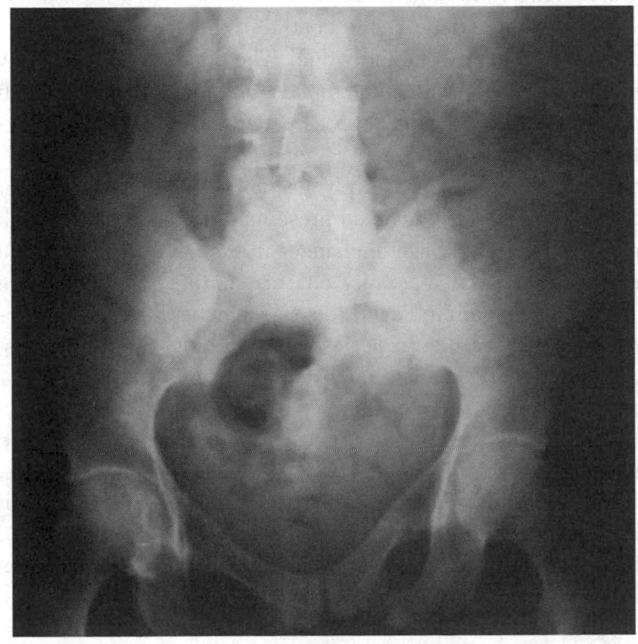

In osteomalacia associated with renal failure, hypocalcemia is seen in the majority of cases, although the plasma phosphate is normal or high because of reduced urinary excretion of phosphate. The plasma $1{,}25(OH)_2D$ is low because of impaired production by the kidneys, although the plasma 25OHD may also be reduced because of inadequate exposure to sunlight. Plasma alkaline phosphatase is raised in the vast majority of cases and serum PTH is invariably elevated.

In hypophosphatemic osteomalacia the major biochemical abnormality is a low plasma phosphate, although this may vary in severity. A few cases may also show hypocalcemia, low plasma $1{,}25(OH)_2D$, and elevation of serum PTH (Table 81-2).

Table 81-2 Biochemical abnormalities in major types of osteomalacia

	Vitamin D Deficiency (%)	Renal Failure (%)	Hypo-phosphatemic (%)
Hypocalcemia	59	63	9
Hypophosphatemia	68	0	73
↑ Alkaline phosphatase	88	88	27
↓ 25OHD	80	58	0
↓ $1{,}25(OH)_2D$	75	81	36
↑ PTH	90	100	11

(Data from Peacock.[99])

Diagnosis of Osteomalacia in the Elderly

The only definite way of diagnosing osteomalacia is by histologic examination of undecalcified bone and demonstrating excess osteoid and reduced calcification fronts or mineralization rate. Histologic confirmation of the diagnosis is required only in the minority of cases, however. In patients with a typical history of bone pain and muscle weakness, with radiologic evidence of Looser's zones or typical biochemical changes, there is little indication for bone biopsy. When the diagnosis is less clear-cut, measurement of plasma 25OHD and serum PTH may be useful, as the combination of low plasma 25OHD and elevated PTH is a strong indicator of the presence of osteomalacia.[99] An alternative approach is to use a therapeutic trial of vitamin D in subjects likely to have osteomalacia, and to monitor any subsequent clinical and biochemical improvement.

Treatment of Osteomalacia

In cases of vitamin D deficiency osteomalacia, the condition will heal with ultraviolet irradiation or vitamin D treatment. Treatment with vitamin D is more practical and can either be given orally in a regular daily dose of 25 μg (1,000 units) or as a single intramuscular injection of 7.5 mg (300,000 units) vitamin D, which should be repeated every 6 to 12 months to prevent recurrence. In patients with osteomalacia associated with malabsorption, the metabolites of vitamin D should be given, in a dose of 1 to 4 μg daily of either alfacalcidol or calcitriol. Calcium supplements containing 1 g elemental calcium may also be required, along with magnesium supplements if hypomagnesemia is present. If malabsorption is due to bacterial overgrowth, pancreatic insufficiency, or celiac disease, appropriate treatment of the underlying disorder with antibiotic therapy, pancreatic enzyme supplements, or gluten-free diet should be instituted. In patients with osteomalacia and renal impairment, either alfacalcidol or calcitriol should be used in a dose of 1 μg daily.

Treatment of osteomalacia leads to a resolution of the proximal myopathy and any symptoms of hypocalcemia within a few weeks, although the bone pain may take longer to improve. The biochemical abnormalities also persist for up to 6 months after treatment is started, and the bone remains histologically and structurally abnormal during this time. Care should therefore be taken to avoid falls during rehabilitation, as these may easily lead to fractures of the abnormal bone. The plasma calcium and phosphate returns to normal within a few weeks, whereas the plasma alkaline phosphatase rises further on treatment and may take many months to return to normal.[99] Serum PTH also remains elevated for up to 6 months. Ultimately, radiologic abnormalities such as Looser's zones and changes of secondary hyperparathyroidism will resolve on treatment, although deformity will persist despite the remodeling of bone.

Paget's Disease

Paget's disease of bone (osteitis deformans) is a common but poorly understood condition that causes significant morbidity in elderly patients.[115] Studies of its prevalence are limited by the fact that many cases are asymptomatic, but radiographic surveys in hospital patients over age 55 years suggest an overall prevalence of up to 4 percent in England and the United States, compared with less than 0.1 percent in Asia and Africa.[116] By the age of 85 years, up to 20 percent of men and 10 percent of women in the United Kingdom have evidence of the condition.[117] The etiology of Paget's disease remains unclear. There is a significant genetic component to the condition, as there is some evidence of HLA linkage and about 25 percent of patients have a family history of the condition. The clustering of cases of Paget's disease within families includes spouses, so may reflect not only genetic factors but also shared environment. It has been suggested that Paget's disease may result from a slow virus infection, which either causes the disease or triggers it in a susceptible individual.[118,119] Inclusion bodies resembling paramyxoviruses have been seen in affected osteoclasts, but their role in the pathogenesis of Paget's disease remains uncertain.[117,119]

Pathophysiology of Paget's Disease

Paget's disease is characterized by increased bone resorption mediated by enlarged, hyperactive osteoclasts.[120] This leads secondarily to increased osteoblastic activity and new bone formation. The rapid bone turnover leads to the deposition of woven bone, which is structurally weak, more vascular, and prone to fracture.

Clinical Features of Paget's Disease

Paget's disease may present at any age over 30 years, but is most often diagnosed in the sixth decade of life. The condition is more common in men than women. The majority of people with radiologic evidence of Paget's disease are asymptomatic and do not come to medical attention. The condition is therefore often an incidental finding in patients having radiographs for an unrelated reason.

It is characteristic of the condition that only a few bones are affected in any one individual. The bones most commonly involved are the skull, spine, pelvis, and long bones, although the distribution of the disease is usually asymmetric. The extent of skeletal involvement is generally constant, with previously unaffected bones rarely becoming involved long after diagnosis. The most common presentation is with pain, which may be due to the Pagetic changes in the bone itself or to the effects of skeletal deformity on surrounding structures. The cause of bone pain in Paget's disease may be difficult to determine. It may be due to periosteal stretching, microfractures, or to direct nerve stimulation by substances released by osteoclasts during bone resorption.

Paget's disease may also cause skeletal deformity, as the affected bones thicken, enlarge, and become more elastic. Classically, this causes frontal bossing of the skull, bowing of the long bones and deformity of the pelvis (protrusio acetabuli). Pagetic bone is more likely to fracture and fissure fractures may also occur on the outer aspect of bowed long bones.

Thickening of the skull may cause compression of the cranial nerves, particularly the auditory nerves, resulting in deafness. Other cranial nerves are only rarely involved in Paget's disease. The increased vascularity of Pagetic bone may also result in neurologic deficit because of a "vascular steal" syndrome. Softening of the base of the skull may rarely lead to basilar invagination, causing brain stem compression. Vertebral involvement may result in crush fractures or more rarely spinal cord compression.

A major management problem is the development of secondary degenerative arthritis in joints adjacent to involved bone. This is frequently more disabling than the Paget's disease itself, and will not respond to treatment of the underlying bone disease. Other complications of Paget's disease include high output cardiac failure, due to the increased vascularity of the affected bone, which although often described is rarely seen. Sarcomatous change also occurs only rarely, but has a poor prognosis.[121]

Diagnosis and Investigation of Paget's Disease

The diagnosis of Paget's disease is reached through a combination of clinical assessment and selected investigations. Although the history rarely leads directly to a diagnosis of Paget's disease, it is very important to seek clues to other conditions that may coexist with or masquerade as it. Examination may reveal skeletal deformity, especially of the skull or long bones, which may feel warm to the touch. There may also be signs of associated degenerative arthritis. A full neurologic assessment is advisable in symptomatic patients, although abnormalities other than deafness are not often found.

The diagnosis of Paget's disease is usually confirmed radiologically. X-rays may show an increase in size of affected bones, alteration of bone texture with areas of sclerosis and lucency, skeletal deformity, and evidence of degenerative arthritis in adjacent joints. The radiologic appearances are often said to be pathognomonic, but skeletal metastases from occult carcinoma of the prostate or breast should be considered in the differential diagnosis. Prostate-specific antigen should therefore be measured in all men with probable Paget's disease. Rarely, bone biopsy may be required if the diagnosis remains uncertain.

The extent of the bone disease can be assessed by isotope bone scan, although x-rays of areas with increased uptake may be advisable, if there is any doubt about the diagnosis. Serum alkaline phosphatase and fasting urine hydroxyproline are often markedly raised in Paget's disease, reflecting increased osteoblast and osteoclast activity, respectively, so may be used to assess the activity of the condition and its response to treatment.

Treatment of Paget's Disease

Treatment of Paget's disease is directed at suppressing the overactivity of osteoclasts, thereby decreasing bone turnover. Although calcitonin has been used for several decades in the management of Paget's disease, bisphosphonates have now become the treatment of choice.[115] These agents are generally used in patients with symptomatic Paget's disease, but their role in asymptomatic individuals is unclear.

Calcitonin

Calcitonin has a direct, receptor-mediated action on osteoclast function. In vivo studies show that within 30 minutes of calcitonin administration, osteoclasts cease synthetic activity and begin to detach from bone. Recruitment of osteoclasts and fusion of precursor cells is also halted, resulting in a rapid reduction in bone resorption. Calcitonin has a short half-life, so osteoclast activation recommences as soon as local concentrations return to basal levels. Nevertheless, calcitonin has proved to be useful in the management of Paget's disease, where it decreases bone pain and reduces the biochemical markers of bone turnover.[122] Salmon and porcine preparations of calcitonin are weakly antigenic, and neutralizing antibodies are formed during treatment by some patients, which may limit their long-term efficacy. Calcitonin may be given by subcutaneous injection or by intranasal administration, although the latter is not available throughout the world.

Bisphosphonates

Oral antiresorptive therapy for Paget's disease became practical for the first time with the introduction of etidronate in the late 1970s.[123] Disodium etidronate 400 mg daily decreases the biochemical markers of bone turnover by 40 to 60 percent.[115] Unfortunately, prolonged therapy with disodium etidronate may lead to impaired mineralization,[124] so courses of treatment should not exceed 6 months. Intravenous infusions of pamidronate decrease the biochemical markers of bone turnover by 60 to 70 percent, resulting in prolonged remission in many patients with Paget's disease.[115] Pamidronate may be given by weekly infusion of 30 mg for 6 weeks, or by three fortnightly infusions of 60 mg.[125] A 3-month course of oral tiludronate 400 mg daily decreases the biochemical markers of bone turnover by at least 50 percent in 70 percent of patients.[126] This may avoid the need for further treatment for at least 18 months.[126]

Fractures in the Elderly

The mechanical properties of an individual bone are determined by the amount of bone present, skeletal architecture, and bone quality. Aging is associated with a reduction in bone mass, disruption of trabecular architecture, and an increased prevalence of disorders such as osteomalacia and Paget's disease that adversely affect the quality of bone. Nevertheless, the risk of fracture is determined not only by skeletal factors, but also by the incidence of falls and by the presence or absence of protective mechanisms such as extending the arm on falling.[127] It is therefore not surprising that the incidence of fractures increases with advancing age. Although fractures in young adults usually occur after extensive trauma, fractures in the elderly may result from minimal trauma, such as falling from standing height. The major fractures occurring in the elderly are those of the forearm, vertebral body, humerus, pelvis, and femoral neck.[3,128] The incidence of these fractures increases with advancing age and is higher in women than men, because of their lower peak bone mass, more rapid bone loss, and greater risk of falls. There is considerable geographic variation in fracture incidence around the world,[128] which may reflect differences in bone mass due to race, smoking, alcohol consumption, and physical activity. The absolute number of fractures in the elderly is rising rapidly, due in part to the increasing numbers of elderly people and a rising age-specific incidence of fractures.[129–132] If present demographic trends continue in the United Kingdom, the number of young elderly people will remain reasonably constant over the next few decades, whereas the number of people over the age of 85 years will increase considerably.[130] Many of these elderly people will be frail, and therefore particularly at risk of fractures. There is also evidence of a rising age-specific incidence of fractures of the forearm, vertebral body, humerus, and femur, which has been attributed to the increased survival of frail individuals and secular changes in smoking, alcohol consumption, diet, and physical activity.[131,132]

Femoral Fractures

Femoral fracture is the most important fracture in elderly people because it causes greater mortality, higher morbidity, and more expenditure than all other fractures combined.[128] The incidence of this fracture rises steeply with age in both sexes, although it is considerably higher in women than men.[131] Using current age-specific incidence rates for England and Wales, it has been estimated that 12 percent of women and 5 percent of men will have sustained a femoral fracture by the age of 85.[133] Several risks factors have been identified for femoral fractures, including reduced bone mass, falls, low body weight, physical inactivity, muscle weakness, and the presence of osteomalacia.[1,25,35,58,113]

Femoral fractures are associated with a considerable mortality, particularly in older, more dependent individuals.[58] This excess mortality following femoral neck fractures has been reported to be about 17 percent over 5 years, although most deaths occur within 6 months of fracture.[58]

In addition to the excess mortality, femoral fractures are associated with considerable morbidity, with many patients becoming more immobile and more dependent. Between 25 and 50 percent of individuals are more dependent after fracture, with deterioration occurring more often in women over the age of 75 years, those with a poor clinical result, and those who were already dependent before fracture.[134–136]

There are few estimates of the total cost of femoral fracture, although it was suggested that the hospital costs alone of this fracture in England and Wales exceeded £165 million/year in 1987.[129] This figure takes no account of the cost of general practitioner or district nursing services, the expenses incurred by social service departments in providing home aides and places in day centers and residential homes, or the cost to the Department of Social Security of attendance allowance, invalid care allowance, and benefit payments to support private nursing home placement.

Forearm Fractures

Forearm fractures are the most common fractures before the age of 75 years.[128] The incidence rises steeply at the menopause in women and then plateaus above the age of 65 years, whereas the incidence changes little with age in men.[137] It has been suggested that the rise in incidence at the menopause is due to an increase in postural instability and therefore falls in women at this age,[137,138] and the absence of a further increase in incidence of forearm fractures after the age of 65 years may be due to the fact that the arm is less likely to be used to break a fall in elderly people.

Vertebral Fractures

The incidence and prevalence of vertebral fractures is difficult to quantify, as many patients with this fracture do not seek medical attention.[58] A Swedish study suggests that the prevalence of vertebral crush fractures in women is 1 percent in the seventh decade, 4 percent in the eighth decade, and 13 percent in the ninth decade, whereas the prevalence in men is 4 percent in the eighth decade and 7 percent in the ninth decade.[132] Nevertheless, data from the European Vertebral Osteoporosis Study (EVOS)[139] suggest that the prevalence of vertebral deformity may be higher in men than women, possibly due to trauma earlier in life. There is also a large variation in the incidence of vertebral fractures across Europe,[139] which may reflect differences in physical activity and other lifestyle factors.

In addition to back pain, loss of height, and kyphosis, vertebral fractures may also result in loss of energy, emotional problems, sleep disturbance, social isolation, and reduced mobility.[140] There is also an increased mortality associated with vertebral crush fractures of about 18 percent at 5 years, but this may be due to coexisting conditions associated with osteoporosis, rather than the fracture itself.[58]

References

1. Riggs BL, Melton LJ III: Involutional osteoporosis. N Engl J Med 1986;314:1676–1686
2. Francis RM: The pathogenesis of osteoporosis. pp. 51–80. In Francis RM (ed). Osteoporosis: pathogenesis and management. Kluwer, Lancaster, 1990
3. Francis RM, Sutcliffe A: Implications of osteoporotic fractures in the elderly. pp.87–93. In Drife JO, Studd JWW (eds): Hormone replacement therapy and osteoporosis. Proceedings of the 22nd Study Group of the Royal College of Obstetricians and Gynaecologists. Springer-Verlag, Berlin, 1990
4. Ross PD, Davis JW, Epstein RS, Wasnich RD: Pre-existing fractures and bone mass predict vertebral fracture incidence in women. Ann Intern Med 1991;114:919–923
5. Black DM, Cummings SR, Genant HK et al: Axial and appen-

dicular bone density predict fractures in older women. J Bone Miner Res 1992;7:633–638
6. World Health Organization: Assessment of fracture risk and its application to screening for postmenopausal osteoporosis. Report of a WHO Study Group. World Health Organization, Geneva, 1994
7. Melton LJ, Chrischilles EA, Cooper C et al: Perspective: how many women have osteoporosis? J Bone Miner Res 1992;7: 1005–1010
8. Slemenda CW, Christian JC, Williams CJ et al: Genetic determinants of bone mass in adult women: a reevaluation of the twin model and the potential importance of gene interaction on heritability estimates. J Bone Miner Res 1991;6:561–567
9. Cohn SH, Abesamis C, Yasumura S et al: Comparative skeletal mass and radial bone mineral content in black and white women. Metabolism 1977;26:171–178
10. Mazess RB: On aging bone loss. Clin Orthop 1982;165: 239–252
11. Smith DM, Nance WE, Kang KW et al: Genetic factors in determining bone mass. J Clin Invest 1973;52:2800–2808
12. Seeman E, Hopper JL, Bach LA et al: Reduced bone mass in daughters of women with osteoporosis. N Engl J Med 1989;320: 554–558
13. Morrison NA, Qi JC, Tokita A et al: Prediction of bone density from vitamin D receptor alleles. Nature 1994;367:284–287
14. Nilson BE, Westlin NE: Bone density in athletes. Clin Orthop 1972;77:179–182
15. Kanders B, Dempster DW, Lindsay R: Interaction of calcium nutrition and physical activity on bone mass in young women. J Bone Miner Res 1988;3:145–149
16. Sandler RB, Slemenda CW, LaPorte RE et al: Postmenopausal bone density and milk consumption in childhood and adolescence. Am J Clin Nutr 1985;42:270–274
17. Johnston CC Jr, Miller JZ, Slemenda CW et al: Calcium supplementation and increases in bone mineral density in children. N Engl J Med 1992;327:82–87
18. Stevenson JC, Lees B, Devenport M et al: Determinants of bone density in normal women: risk factors for future osteoporosis. BMJ 1989;298:924–928
19. Goldsmith NF, Johnston JO: Bone mineral: effects of oral contraceptives, pregnancy and lactation. J Bone Joint Surg 1975; 57A:657–668
20. Eisman JA, Kelly PJ, Morrison NA et al: Genetic and environmental interactions on bone mass, abstracted. Bone Miner 1992; 17(suppl 1):72
21. Peacock M, Johnston CC Jr, Christian J: Inheritance of calcium absorption, abstracted. Bone Miner 1992;17(suppl 1):92
22. Compston JE: Risk factors for osteoporosis. Clin Endocrinol 1992;36:223–224
23. Scane AC, Francis RM: Risk factors for osteoporosis in men. Clin Endocrinol 1993;38:15–16
24. Christiansen C, Riis BJ, Rodbro P: Predictions of rapid bone loss in postmenopausal women. Lancet 1987;1:1105–1108
25. Davidson BJ, Ross RK, Paganini-Hill A et al: Total and free estrogens and androgens in postmenopausal women with hip fractures. J Clin Endocrinol Metab 1982;54:115–120
26. Jick H, Porter J, Morrison AS: Relation between smoking and the age of natural menopause. Lancet 1977;1:1354–1355
27. Jensen J, Christiansen C, Rodbro P: Cigarette smoking, serum estrogens and bone loss during hormone-replacement therapy early after menopause. N Engl J Med 1985;313:973–975
28. De Vernejoul MC, Bielakoff J, Herve M et al: Evidence for defective osteoblastic function. A role for alcohol and tobacco consumption in osteoporosis in middle-age men. Clin Orthop 1983;179:107–115
29. Saville PD: Changes in bone mass with age and alcoholism. J Bone Joint Surg 1965;47B:492–499
30. Holbrook TL, Barrett-Connor E: A prospective study of alcohol consumption and bone mineral density. BMJ 1993;306: 1506–1509
31. Krolner B, Toft B, Pors Nielsen S, Tondevold E: Physical exercise as prophylaxis against involutional bone loss: a controlled trial. Clin Sci 1983;64:541–546
32. Krolner B, Toft B: Vertebral bone loss: an unheeded effect of therapeutic bed rest. Clin Sci 1983;64:537–540
33. Cooper C, Barker DJP, Wickham C: Physical activity, muscle strength, and calcium intake in fracture of the proximal femur in Britain. BMJ 1988;297:1443–1446
34. Lau E, Donnan S, Barker DJP, Cooper C: Physical activity and calcium intake in fracture of the proximal femur in Hong Kong. BMJ 1988;297:1441–1443
35. Boyce WJ, Vessey MP: Habitual physical inertia and other factors in relation to risk of fracture of the proximal femur. Age Ageing 1988;17:319–327
36. Riggs BL, Wahner HW, Melton LJ III et al: Dietary calcium intake and rates of bone loss in women. J Clin Invest 1987;80: 979–982
37. Stevenson JC, Whitehead MI, Padwick M et al: Dietary intake of calcium and postmenopausal bone loss. BMJ 1988;297:15–17
38. Parfitt AM: Dietary risks factors for age-related bone loss and fractures. Lancet 1983;2:1181–1185
39. Baker MR, Peacock M, Nordin BEC: The decline in vitamin D status with age. Age Ageing 1980;9:249–252
40. Gallagher JC, Riggs BL, Eisman J et al: Intestinal calcium absorption and serum vitamin D metabolites in normal subjects and osteoporotic patients: effect of age and dietary calcium. J Clin Invest 1979;64:729–736
41. Bullamore JR, Gallagher JC, Wilkinson R et al: Effect of age on calcium absorption. Lancet 1970;2:535–537
42. Endres DB, Morgan CH, Garry PJ et al: Age-related changes in serum immunoreactive parathyroid hormone and its biological action in healthy men and women. J Clin Endocrinol Metab 1987;65:724–731
43. Khaw KT, Sneyd MJ, Compston J: Bone density parathyroid hormone and 25-hydroxyvitamin D concentrations in middle aged women. BMJ 1992;305:273–277
44. Dawson-Hughes B, Dallal GE, Krall EA et al: Effect of vitamin D supplementation on wintertime and overall bone loss in healthy postmenopausal women. Ann Intern Med 1991;115: 505–512
45. Caplan GA, Scane AC, Francis RM: Pathogenesis of vertebral crush fractures in women. J R Soc Med 1994;87:200–202
46. Baillie SP, Davison CE, Johnson FJ, Francis RM: Pathogenesis of vertebral crush fractures in men. Age Ageing 1992;21: 139–141

47. Riggs BL, Melton LJ III: Evidence for two distinct syndromes of involutional osteoporosis. Am J Med 1983;75:899–901
48. Reid DM: Corticosteroid osteoporosis. pp. 103–144. In Francis RM (ed): Osteoporosis: Pathogenesis and Management. Kluwer, Lancaster, 1990
49. Bar-Shavit Z, Kahn AJ, Pegg LE et al: Glucocorticoids modulate macrophage surface oligosaccharides and their bone binding activity. J Clin Invest 1984;73:1277–1283
50. Smith R: Corticosteroids and osteoporosis. Thorax 1990;45: 573–578
51. Bataille R: Management of myeloma with bisphosphonates. N Engl J Med 1996;334:529–530
52. Krane SM, Schiller AL: Hyperostosis, neoplasms, and other disorders of bone and cartilage. pp. 1902–1910. In Braunwald E, Isselbacher KJ, Petersdorf RG et al (eds): Harrison's Principles of Internal Medicine. 11th Ed. McGraw-Hill, New York, 1987
53. Hahn TJ: Drug-induced disorders of vitamin D and mineral metabolism. Clin Endocrinol Metab 1980;9:107–129
54. Francis RM, Peacock M, Marshall DH et al: Spinal osteoporosis in men. Bone Miner 1989;5:347–357
55. Adams PH, Jowsey J, Kelly PJ et al: Effect of hyperthyroidism on bone and mineral metabolism. Q J Med 1987;36:1–15
56. Minnaire P, Meunier P, Edouard C et al: Quantitative histological data on disuse osteoporosis. Calcif Tiss Res 1974;17:57–73
57. Anon: Osteoporosis and activity. Lancet 1983;1:1365–1366
58. Cooper C: Epidemiology and public health impact of osteoporosis. pp. 459–477. In Reid DM (ed): Bailliere's Clinical Rheumatology—Osteoporosis. Bailliere Tindall, London, 1993
59. Scane AC, Masud T, Johnson FJ, Francis RM: The reliability of diagnosing osteoporosis from spinal radiographs. Age Ageing 1994;23:283–286
60. Saville PD, Nilsson BER: Height and weight in symptomatic postmenopausal osteoporosis. Clin Orthop 1966;45:49–54
61. Drinkwater BL, Nilson K, Chesnut CH III et al: Bone mineral content of amenorrheic and eumenorrheic athletes. N Engl J Med 1984;311:277–281
62. Cann CE, Martin MC, Genant HK, Jaffe RB: Decreased spinal mineral content in amenorrheic women. JAMA 1984;251: 626–629
63. Riggs BL, Melton LJ III: The prevention and treatment of osteoporosis. N Engl J Med 1992;327:620–627
64. Lindsay R: Prevention and treatment of osteoporosis. Lancet 1993;341:801–805
65. Stevenson JC, Cust MP, Gangar KF et al: Effects of transdermal versus oral hormone replacement therapy on bone density in spine and proximal femur in postmenopausal women. Lancet 1990;336:265–269
66. Felson DT, Zhang Y, Hannan MT et al: The effect of postmenopausal estrogen therapy on bone density in elderly women. N Engl J Med 1993;329:1141–1146
67. Stampfer MJ, Colditz GA: Estrogen replacement therapy and coronary heart disease: a quantitative assessment of the epidemiological evidence. Prev Med 1991;20:47–63
68. Hunt K, Vessey M, McPherson K, Coleman M: Long term surveillance of mortality and cancer incidence in women receiving hormone replacement therapy. Br J Obstet Gynaecol 1987;94: 620–635
69. Whitehead MI, Townsend PT, Pryse-Davies J: Effects of estrogens and progestins on the biochemistry and morphology of the postmenopausal endometrium. N Engl J Med 1981;305: 1599–1605
70. Bergkvist L, Adami HO, Persson I et al: Risks of breast cancer after estrogen and estrogen-progestin replacement. N Engl J Med 1989;321:293–297
71. Pike MC, Bernstein L, Ross RK: Breast cancer and hormone replacement therapy. Lancet 1990;335:297
72. Jones MM, Francis RM, Nordin BEC: Five year follow up of oestrogen therapy in 94 women. Maturitas 1982;4:123–130
73. Francis RM, Selby PL, Rodgers A, Davison CE: The management of osteoporosis. pp. 145–179. In Francis RM (ed): Osteoporosis: pathogenesis and management. Kluwer, Lancaster, 1990
74. Pors Nielsen S, Barenholdt O, Hermansen F, Munk-Jensen N: Magnitude and pattern of skeletal response to long term continuous and cyclic sequential oestrogen/progestin treatment. Br J Obstet Gynaecol 1994;101:319–324
75. Heaney RP, Recker RR, Saville PD: Menopausal changes in calcium balance performance. J Lab Clin Med 1978;92: 953–993
76. Lindsay R, Tohme J: Estrogen treatment of patients with established postmenopausal osteoporosis. Obstet Gynecol 1990;76: 1–6
77. Lufkin EG, Wahner HW, O'Fallon WM et al: Treatment of postmenopausal osteoporosis with transdermal estrogen. Ann Intern Med 1992;117:1–9
78. Selby PL, Horsman A, Peacock M: Norethisterone as an alternative to oestrogen in the management of postmenopausal osteoporosis. pp. 555–556. In Christiansen J, Johansen JS, Riis BJ (eds): Osteoporosis 1987. Osteopress ApS, Copenhagen, 1987
79. Lindsay R, Hart DM, Kraszewski A: Prospective double-blind trial of synthetic steroid Org OD 14 for preventing postmenopausal osteoporosis. BMJ 1980;280:1207–1209
80. Love RR, Mazess RB, Barden HS et al: Effects of tamoxifen on bone mineral density in postmenopausal women with breast cancer. N Engl J Med 1992;326:852–856
81. Francis RM: Oral bisphosphonates in the treatment of osteoporosis: a review. Curr Ther Res 1995;56:831–851
82. Storm T, Thamsborg G, Steinich T et al: Effect of intermittent cyclical etidronate therapy on bone mass and fracture rate in women with postmenopausal osteoporosis. N Engl J Med 1990; 322:1265–1271
83. Watts NB, Harris ST, Genant HK et al: Intermittent cyclical etidronate treatment of postmenopausal osteoporosis. N Engl J Med 1990;323:73–79
84. Harris ST, Watts NB, Jackson RD et al: Four-year study of intermittent cyclic etidronate treatment of postmenopausal osteoporosis: three years of blinded therapy followed by one year of open therapy. Am J Med 1993;95:557–567
85. Liberman UA, Weiss SR, Broll J et al: Effect of oral alendronate on bone mineral density and the incidence of fractures in postmenopausal osteoporosis. N Engl J Med 1995;333:1437–1443
86. Overgaard K, Hansen MA, Jensen SB, Christiansen C: Effect

of Salcatonin given intranasally on bone mass and fracture rates in established osteoporosis: a dose-response study. BMJ 1992; 305:556–561

87. Rico H, Henandez ER, Revilla M, Gomez-Castresana F: Salmon calcitonin reduces vertebral fracture rate in postmenopausal crush fracture syndrome. Bone Miner 1992;16:131–138

88. Prince RL, Smith M, Dick IM et al: Prevention of postmenopausal osteoporosis. A comparative study of exercise, calcium supplementation and hormone-replacement therapy. N Engl J Med 1991;325:1189–1195

89. Reid IR, Ames RW, Evans MC et al: Effect of calcium supplementation on bone loss in postmenopausal women. N Engl J Med 1993;328:460–464

90. Chapuy MC, Arlot ME, Duboeuf F et al: Vitamin D_3 and calcium to prevent hip fractures in elderly women. N Engl J Med 1992; 327:1637–1642

91. Heikinheimo RJ, Inkovaara JA, Harju EJ et al: Annual injection of vitamin D and fractures of aged bones. Calcif Tissue Int 1992;51:105–110

92. Francis RM, Boyle IT, Moniz C et al: A comparison of the effects of alfacalcidol treatment and vitamin D_2 supplementation on calcium absorption in elderly women with vertebral fractures. Osteoporosis Int 1996;6:284–290

93. Tilyard MW, Spears GFS, Thompson J, Dovey S: Treatment of postmenopausal osteoporosis with calcitriol or calcium. N Engl J Med 1992;326:357–362

94. Riggs BL, Hodgson SF, O'Fallon WM et al: Effect of fluoride treatment on the fracture rate in postmenopausal women with osteoporosis. N Engl J Med 1990;322:802–809

95. Kleerekoper M, Peterson EL, Nelson DA et al: A randomized trial of sodium fluoride as a treatment for postmenopausal osteoporosis. Osteoporosis Int 1991;1:155–161

96. Pak CYC, Sakhaee K, Adams-Huet B et al: Treatment of postmenopausal osteoporosis with slow release sodium fluoride. Ann Int Med 1995;123:401–408

97. Chesnut CH, Ivey JL, Gruber HE et al: Stanozolol in postmenopausal osteoporosis: therapeutic efficacy and possible mechanisms of action. Metabolism 1983;32:571–580

98. Need AG, Chatterton BE, Walker CJ et al: Comparison of calcium, calcitriol, ovarian hormones and nandrolone in the treatment of osteoporosis. Maturitas 1986;8:275–280

99. Peacock M: Osteomalacia. pp. 72–111. In Nordin beC (ed): Metabolic Bone and Stone Disease. 2nd Ed. Churchill Livingstone, Edinburgh, 1984

100. Nordin BEC, Peacock M, Aaron JE et al: Osteoporosis and osteomalacia. Clin Endocrinol Metab 1980;9:177–205

101. Haussler MR, McCain TA: Basic and clinical concepts related to vitamin D metabolism and action. N Engl J Med 1977;297: 974–983, 1041–1050

102. Poskitt EME, Cole TJ, Lawson DEM: Diet, sunlight and 25 hydroxyvitamin D in healthy children and adults. BMJ 1979; 1:221–223

103. Lawson DEM, Paul AA, Black AE et al: Relative contributions of diet and sunlight to vitamin D state in the elderly. BMJ 1979; 2:303–305

104. Fraser DR, Kodicek E: Unique biosynthesis by kidney of biologically active vitamin D metabolite. Nature 1970;228:764–766

105. Kodicek E, Lawson DEM, Wilson PW: Biological activity of polar metabolite of vitamin D_3. Nature 1970;228:763–764

106. Barragry JM, France MW, Corless D et al: Intestinal cholecalciferol absorption in the elderly and in younger adults. Clin Sci 1989;55:213–220

107. Skinner RK: 25 hydroxylation of vitamin D in the elderly. pp. 1011–1013. In Norman AW, Schaefer K, Herrath DV et al (eds): Vitamin D, basic research and its clinical application. Walter de Gruyter, Berlin, 1979

108. Dunnigan MG, McIntosh WB, Ford JA, Robertson I: Acquired disorders of vitamin D metabolism. pp. 125–150. In Heath DA, Marx SJ (eds): Clinical Endocrinology. 2: calcium disorders. Butterworths, London, 1982

109. Corless D, Beer M, Boucher BJ et al: Vitamin D status in long stay geriatric patients. Lancet 1975;2:1404–1406

110. Francis RM, Peacock M, Barkworth SA: Renal impairment and its effects on calcium metabolism in elderly women. Age Ageing 1984;13:14–20

111. Anderson I, Campbell AER, Dunn A, Runciman JBM: Osteomalacia in elderly women. Scott Med J 1966;2:429–436

112. Campbell GA, Kemm JR, Hosking DJ, Boyd RV: How common is osteomalacia in the elderly? Lancet 1984;2:386–388

113. Aaron JE, Gallagher JC, Anderson J et al: Frequency of osteomalacia and osteoporosis in fractures of the proximal femur. Lancet 1974;1:229–223

114. Campbell GA, Hosking DJ, Kemm JR, Boyd RV: Timing of screening for osteomalacia in the acutely ill elderly. Age Ageing 1986;15:156–164

115. Hosking D, Meunier PJ, Ringe JD et al: Paget's disease of bone: diagnosis and management. BMJ 1996;312:491–494

116. Siris ES: Paget's disease of bone. pp. 253–259. In Favus MJ (ed): Primer on the metabolic bone diseases and disorders of mineral metabolism. American Society for Bone and Mineral Research, Kelseyville, CA, 1990

117. Barker DJP, Clough PW, Guyer PB, Gardner MJ: Paget's disease of bone in 14 British towns. BMJ 1977;1:1181–1183

118. O'Driscoll JB, Anderson DC: Past pets and Paget's disease. Lancet 1985;2:919–921

119. Gordon MT, Anderson DC, Sharpe PT: Canine distemper virus localised in bone cells of patients with Paget's disease. Bone 1991;12:195–201

120. Kanis JA: Pathophysiology and Treatment of Paget's Disease of Bone Martin Dunitz, London, 1991

121. Frassica FJ, Tiegs RD, Unni KK, Sim FH: Paget's sarcoma of bone: clinicopathologic features and treatment in 51 cases. First International Symposium on Paget's Disease of Bone p. 25. Paget's Disease Foundation, New York, 1992

122. Cantrill JA, Anderson DC: Treatment of Paget's disease of bone. Clin Endocrinol 1990;32:507–518

123. Khairi MRA, Johnston CC, Altman RD et al: Treatment of Paget's disease of bone (osteitis deformans). Results of a one-year study with sodium etidronate. JAMA 1977;230:561–567

124. Gray RES, Yates AJP, Preston CJ et al: Duration of effect of oral diphosphonate therapy in Paget's disease of bone. Q J Med 1987;64:755–767

125. Richardson PC, Cantrill JA, Anderson DC: Experience of treating 218 patients with Paget's disease of bone using intravenous

3-amino-hydroxypropylidene-1-1-bisphosphonate (APD), abstracted J Bone Miner Res 1989;4 (suppl 1):S198

126. Fraser WD, Stamp TC, Creek RA et al: A double-blind, multicentre, comparative study of tiludronate and placebo in Paget's disease of bone. Postgrad Med J 1997;73:496–502
127. Cooper C, Barker DJP, Morris J, Briggs RSJ: Osteoporosis, falls and age in fracture of the proximal femur. BMJ 1987;295:13–15
128. Cummings SR, Kelsey JL, Nevitt MC, O'Dowd KJ: Epidemiology of osteoporosis and osteoporotic fractures. Epidemiol Rev 1985;7:178–208
129. Wallace WA: The scale and financial implications of osteoporosis. Int Med 1987;(suppl 12):3–4
130. Central Statistical Office: Social Trends No. 17. HMSO, London, 1987
131. Boyce WJ, Vessey MP: Rising incidence of fracture of the proximal femur. Lancet 1985;1:150–151
132. Obrant KJ, Bengner U, Johnell O et al: Increasing age-adjusted risks of fragility fractures: a sign of increasing osteoporosis in successive generations? Calcif Tissue Int 1989;44:157–167
133. Royal College of Physicians: Fractured neck of femur. Royal College of Physicians, London, 1989
134. Jensen JS, Bagger J: Long-term social prognosis after hip fractures. Acta Orthop Scand 1982;53:97–101
135. Thomas TG, Stevens RS: Social effects of fractures of the neck of femur. BMJ 1974;3:456–458
136. Beals RK: Survival following hip fracture—long follow up of 607 patients. J Chron Dis 1972;25:235–244
137. Winner SJ, Morgan CA, Evans JG: Perimenopausal risk of falling and incidence of distal forearm fracture. BMJ 1989;298: 1486–1488
138. Crilly RG, Richardson LD, Roth JH et al: Postural stability and Colles fractures. Age Ageing 1987;16:133–138
139. Silman AJ: The epidemiology of vertebral fractures. Osteoporosis Int 1996;6(suppl 1):86
140. Scane AC, Sutcliffe AM, Francis RM: The sequelae of vertebral crush fractures in men. Osteoporosis Int 1994;4:89–92

CHAPTER 82

Arthritis in the Elderly

DAVID L. SCOTT

Rheumatic diseases are common in elderly people and are often undiagnosed or undertreated. In general elderly patients have the same types of musculoskeletal disorders as younger age groups. However, there are differences in the pattern, severity, and effect of these diseases and variations in their optimal treatment. A few disorders such as polymyalgia rheumatica are far more common in elderly people.

Special problems in elderly patients with arthritis include the insidious nature of musculoskeletal symptoms, associated comorbidity and muscle weakness, slow response to treatment, poorer outcome, and greater propensity to adverse drug reactions. The main rheumatic diseases of the elderly, summarized in Table 82-1, include inflammatory arthritis, degenerative arthritis, connective tissue diseases, soft tissue rheumatism, and back pain.

Arthritis is the most common cause of disability in people aged over 75 years.[1] The most common cause of terminal dependency due to loss of mobility, confinement in bed or in the house, is also arthritis and rheumatism. One hospital-based survey in London showed that 76 percent of patients admitted to an acute elderly unit had peripheral arthritis, 48 percent had arthritis directly contributing to their functional disability, and 19 percent did not volunteer information about their joint disease.[2]

Zeidler[3] reviewed geriatric rheumatology and the epidemiology of musculoskeletal diseases in elderly patients. Although difficult to estimate, he noted that the prevalence rate of disabling joint diseases increases as people age. Osteoarthritis is the most common type of joint disease in geriatric patients. Symptomatic osteoarthritis has a much lower prevalence rate than does radiographic osteoarthritis. However, symptomatic disease is important in that it may motivate a patient to seek medical attention. The prevalence of rheumatoid arthritis (RA) also increases with advancing age. The onset of RA in both large and small joints in patients older than 60 years is more frequent and begins with greater disease activity as compared with patients younger than 60 years, RA runs a more severe course in older than in younger patients. Epidemiologic data suggest that elderly individuals are the major consumers of anti-inflammatory drugs. The prevalence of these disorders increases with advancing age and, coupled with increasing longevity, poses a growing challenge to practicing clinicians.

Disease Mechanisms

The Pathologic Changes of Arthritis

The pathologic changes seen in arthritis comprise increased number of cells on the surface of the synovium, moderate numbers of lymphocytes in perivascular areas, aggregates of lymphocytes and plasma cells in the subintimal synovium, prominent new vessel formation, and an increased connective tissue matrix into which the inflammatory cells have migrated. There are often considerable amounts of fibrin superficially within the synovium. The changes are nonspecific and are similar in RA and other inflammatory arthropathies.[4]

The synovial lining cells are derived from macrophages and fibroblasts. They show a variable increased number in rheumatoid synovia resulting from local proliferation and recruitment of macrophage-like cells. Underlying the lining cell layer is a variable subintimal layer and beneath that a more dense fibrotic collagenous layer. The subintimal synovium contains many blood vessels, reticular connective tissue components, tissue macrophages and occasional giant cells, and a variable lymphocytic and plasma cell infiltrate. Lymphocytes often form follicular aggregates. There is some fibrosis, although this is inconsistent. At the margins of the synovium is the pannus, which overlies the articular cartilage. It is often difficult to define a lining cell layer in the pannus and a continuous mass of cells is seen adjacent to the cartilage margins, which extends into the deeper tissues. Most cells of the pannus are large and mononuclear. Many have a fibroblastic appearance.

The main features of rheumatoid synovitis are summarized in Table 82-2. None is specific for RA. In osteoarthritis there is more fibrosis. In other forms of inflammatory synovitis there is less lymphocyte infiltration.

Cells Involved

Arthritis involves T and B lymphocytes, macrophages, synovial lining cells (a mixture of fibroblasts and macrophages), endothelial cells, and polymorphs. The polymorphs are found in high concentrations in synovial fluid but are rarely seen in the synovium itself.

The pathogenesis of arthritis involves cell adhesion and migration, T- and B-cell activation, cytokine release, and joint destruction. Many of the molecules that participate in these complex interactions, especially the various cytokines, have been cloned and sequenced and the function of their products

Table 82-1 The main musculoskeletal disorders of the elderly

Type of Disorder	Examples
Inflammatory synovitis	Rheumatoid arthritis Gout Pseudogout Septic arthritis
Degenerative arthritis	Osteoarthritis
Vasculitis and connective tissue diseases	Polymyalgia rheumatica Temporal arteritis Systemic lupus erythematosus
Soft tissue rheumatism	Rotator cuff shoulder lesions Frozen shoulder
Back pain	Mechanical back pain Lumbar spondylosis and spondylolisthesis Spinal stenosis Osteoporotic vertebral fracture Spinal malignancy

studied intensively. Despite such knowledge gathered from this reductionist approach we still do not understand fully the pathogenesis of the disease.[5] Synovitis is taking place within an individual in whom many other complex systems are interacting with the immune system. An example is the neuroendocrine system, which can down-regulate inflammation through the secretion of cortisol. Study of the hypothalamic-pituitary-adrenal axis in patients with RA has shown, for example, that it responds poorly to inflammatory stimuli. This defect may not only be an important factor in determining the severity of joint inflammation but could be an important early event in the switch from acute to chronic inflammation. It shows the need to have a view of the whole patient as well as a good knowledge of the individual components of joint inflammation.

T lymphocytes are generally thought to have a central pathologic role in inflammatory synovitis and especially in RA, although there is some debate as to whether or not they are of primary importance. The basic idea of a pathologic T-cell response in RA is supported by the demonstration that removing T cells by thoracic duct drainage, lymphapheresis, or total lymphoid irradiation ameliorates arthritis. On the other hand, the infiltrating T cells seem to be remarkably inactive and as a population to lack specificity for any particular antigen, leading some to conclude that their role is either passive or irrelevant.[6] Studies of T-cell receptor usage of individual T cells may give important insight into the pathogenesis of arthritis. Germline T-cell receptor complex polymorphisms may contribute to genetic susceptibility to arthritis.[7]

Synovial lining cell hyperplasia and mononuclear cell infiltration are conspicuous in the earliest stages of synovitis.[8] The changes in RA are indistinguishable from those of other inflammatory joint disease. T-cell distribution is similar in early and late synovitis and mature CD4+ lymphocytes are the predominant cells in both situations. The relationship of lining cell hyperplasia to subintimal cell infiltration is unknown; whether they develop simultaneously or one precedes the other is an important unanswered question. Production of enzymes such as metalloproteinases believed to be important in extracellular matrix destruction is an early event.

Macrophage-like synoviocytes originate in the bone marrow, like other mononuclear phagocytes, and are constantly replaced via the circulation.[9] In the rheumatoid synovium about 80 percent of the lining cells are macrophage-like cells functioning as antigen-processing and antigen-presenting cells to T lymphocytes. Monocyte and lymphocyte traffic into the RA synovium is mediated by adhesion molecules.

Signaling Between Cells: Cytokines and Growth Factors

Cytokines, cytokine inhibitors, and growth factors are recognized as important mediators of inflammation and joint destruction in arthritis.[10] Several classes of peptides are involved including interleukins, tumor necrosis factors, interferons, and a variety of peptide regulatory factors. These are summarized in Table 82-3.

Interleukin-1 (IL-1) is a small protein produced by monocytes and macrophages.[11] Two forms exist (α and β) with amino acid sequence homology of about 26 percent. IL-1β is the predominant form synthesized by human monocytes. Both forms bind to the same cell surface receptor. The systemic effects of IL-1 include fever, decreased appetite, and the induction of metabolic changes. In arthritis the local effects of IL-1 may be more important. These local effects include augmentation of T- and B-lymphocyte function; chemotaxis of neutrophils and other cells; proliferation of fibroblasts; and the

Table 82-2 The main pathologic features of rheumatoid arthritis

Synovial lining cell hyperplasia
Superficial fibrin deposition
Vascular proliferation
Lymphocytic infiltration and variable lymphocytic aggregation
Macrophages and plasma cells in subintimal synovium
Variable synovial fibrosis
Marginal pannus over articular cartilage
Destruction of adjacent articular cartilage and bone

Table 82-3 Cytokines and growth factors involved in arthritis

Cytokines Influencing Synovial Cells	Cytokines Influencing Neutrophils	Growth Factor Influencing Synovial Cells
Interleukin-1	Interleukin-8	Platelet derived growth factor
Interleukin-6		Insulin-like growth factor
Tumor necrosis factor-α		Fibroblast growth factor
		Transforming growth factor β

production of prostaglandin E_2 and collagenase by fibroblasts and chondrocytes. IL-1 may contribute to joint scarring and fibrosis by stimulating fibroblast proliferation either directly or indirectly through the induction of platelet-derived growth factor and other peptide regulatory factors. A variety of natural IL-1 inhibitors have been identified in cell supernatants and in human urine.[12] The term *IL-1 inhibitor* is a general one, and such substances could potentially act at many different levels in specific or nonspecific ways, such as reducing IL-1 synthesis, binding to IL-1, blocking IL-1 receptors, and interfering with the postreceptor effects of IL-1.

Tumor necrosis factor-α (TNFα) is another small peptide produced by monocytes and macrophages. It is usually secreted together with IL-1, although production of these two proteins is apparently regulated and controlled independently. As monocytes mature into macrophages their ability to produce IL-1 decreases while TNFα production is relatively unaffected. TNFα binds to separate receptors on target cells, although it has similar biological functions to IL-1; for example it also stimulates PGE_2 and collagenase production by synovial cells cultured in vitro. TNFα is present in synovial fluid and is synthesized by synovial tissue.[13] Similar to IL-1 the local effects of TNFα may be counteracted by regulatory or inhibitory proteins.

Interleukin-6 (IL-6) is a further small polypeptide produced by monocytes, T lymphocytes, and fibroblasts.[14] Both IL-1 and TNFα induce the synthesis and secretion of IL-6. Although IL-6 has similar actions to IL-1, it is a more potent inducer of hepatic synthesis of acute phase proteins and of immunoglobulin production by B lymphocytes. High levels of IL-6 are present in arthritic synovial fluids. IL-6 may both amplify some of the effects of IL-1 and TNFα and also induce the synthesis of acute phase proteins and rheumatoid factors.

Interleukin-8 (IL-8) is a different cytokine that activates neutrophils. It is also known as neutrophil-activating peptide-1.[15] It induces a range of responses in neutrophils including the expression of surface adhesion molecules and the production of reactive oxygen metabolites. IL-8 is a product of mononuclear phagocytes and also fibroblasts and other cells. In arthritis IL-8 could bring about the accumulation of neutrophils that are considered a major source of cartilage degrading enzymes. IL-8 levels are high in synovial fluids from patients with RA.[16]

How are the large number of different cytokines in the inflamed synovium regulated? Studies on synovial biopsies show persistent expression of mRNA to IL-1, TNFα, IL-6, and other cytokines. This stability and persistence of cytokine production suggests it plays an important role in the pathogenesis of the chronicity of synovitis in rheumatoid disease. There is evidence that TNFα is the dominant signal regulating IL-1 production,[17] although other noncytokine signals such as immune complexes may also be of significance.

Fibroblast growth factors (FGFs) are a family of related proteins including acidic and basic FGFs. They have some homology with IL-1. Basic FGF, the first to be isolated and biologically characterized, provides an example for the group. It increases DNA synthesis and cell division, effects angiogenesis, and is an intracrine growth factor.[18]

Cultured rheumatoid synovial cells express the gene for basic FGF, secrete the protein, and also proliferate in response to basic FGF.[19] Synovial cells may thus stimulate their own proliferation in an autocrine manner through modulators like basic FGF.

Transforming growth factor β (TGF-β) is present in lymphocytes and macrophages and has potent immunomodulatory effects.[20] There are five forms of TGF-β but only TGF-β1 and TGF-β2 seem important in arthritis.[21] TGF-β influences fibroblastic cell growth and facilitation of extracellular matrix remodeling.[22] TGF-β inhibits IL-1-induced lymphocytic proliferation and promotes synovial fibroblast hyperplasia.

Platelet-derived growth factor (PDGF) is released from the α granules of platelets during blood clotting.[23] PDGF-like polypeptides are also released from macrophages.[24] Biologically active PDGF, which comprises two subunits, is mitogenic for fibroblasts and chondrocytes.

Neuroendocrine Signaling

Renewed interest in the role of neuroendocrine factors in arthritis follows from studies of experimental arthritis, in particular the streptococcal cell wall model by Wilder and Sternberg.[25] In this model one inbred strain, Lewis female rats, are highly susceptible to developing severe T-lymphocyte-dependent proliferative and erosive arthritis after intraperitoneal injection of streptococcal cell walls. Conversely, another strain, Fischer female rats develop only a minimal, transient arthritis following an identical injection of cell walls. Studies with this model by Sternberg and others[26] have shown that Lewis rats have a very poor response from their hypothalamic-pituitary-adrenal axis to the stress of intraperitoneal injections of streptococcal cell walls. In comparison Fischer rats show a good stress response with rapid increases in serum adreno corticotsogic hormone (ACTH) and corticosteroid levels as well as increased hypothalamic release and synthesis of corticotropin-releasing hormone. Giving the Lewis rats physiologic levels of corticosteroids inhibits the development of arthritis. By contrast blocking the effects of corticosteroids in Fischer rats using a corticosteroid receptor antagonist leads to the development of severe arthritis in response to streptococcal cell walls. These results show the potential importance of the hypothalamic-pituitary-adrenal axis in the development of arthritis. In 1984 Munck et al.[27] suggested that the production of corticosteroids in the stress response of the hypothalamic-pituitary-adrenal axis was counter-regulatory and suppressed inflammation mediated by the immune system. The experiments with Lewis rats supports this concept. The implication is that a relative deficiency of corticosteroids may allow the development of unchecked immune activation and the persistence of arthritis in the Lewis rats. The case for using corticosteroids therapeutically is greatly strengthened.

Adhesion Molecules

Adhesion molecules are involved in cell-cell adhesion, antigen recognition, lymphocyte activation, and cell trafficking. There are three main groups of adhesion molecules each binding to different ligands[28]: molecules of the immunoglobulin supergene family, the integrins, and the selectins (Table 82-4).

Adhesion molecules from the immunoglobulin supergene family include receptors that react with antigens and antigen-independent receptors. Examples of the former group are the T-cell receptor/CD3 and surface immunoglobulin. An example of the latter group is the CD2 receptor, which reacts with the ligand lymphocyte function associated molecule-3 (LFA-3).

The integrins are a different family of adhesion molecules. They are transmembrane glycoproteins with an α/β heterodimer structure. The β_1 integrins, also called the VLA (very late activation) subfamily, has six members termed VLA 1–6. These are widely distributed and interact with extracellular matrix components such as fibronectin, laminin, and collagen. They are important in wound healing and cell migration in tissue remodeling and repair. The β_2 subfamily is also known as the leukocyte integrins and has three members. These are LFA-1, which binds to the ligands ICAM-1 (intercellular adhesion molecule-1) and ICAM-2; Mac-1, which binds to the ligand iC3b; and p150,95, which also binds to the ligand iC3b. Leukocyte integrins are exclusively expressed on leukocytes and are predominantly involved in immune adherence; they all belong to the CD11/CD18 heterodimer complex. The final class of β_3 integrins are expressed on endothelial cells and platelets, respectively. The name integrin was introduced to signify the role of these proteins in integrating the intracellular cytoskeleton with the extracellular matrix.[29]

The final group of adhesion proteins are the selectins. They are expressed on leukocytes and endothelial cells and are involved in leukocyte adhesion to endothelium in acute inflammation. There are three members of this group: endothelial cell adhesion molecule-1 (ELAM-1); leukocyte adhesion molecule-1 (LAM-1); and platelet-activation-dependent granule-external membrane (PADG-EM) protein.

Table 82-4 Classification of adhesion molecules

Families	Subfamilies	Examples
Immunoglobulin	T-cell receptor/CD3	
Supergene	CD2 receptor/LFA3	
Integrins	β_1 integrins	VLA 1–6
	β_2 integrins	LFA1 Mac-1 p150,95
	β_3 integrins	Vitronectin receptor Platelet glycoprotein IIб/IIIa
Selectins	ELAM-1 LAM-1 PADG-EM	

Table 82-5 Main components of the extracellular matrix

Type of Component	Examples	Distribution
Collagen	Collagen I and III Collagen II Collagen IV Collagen V	Interstitial connective tissues Cartilage Basement membranes Pericellular extracellular matrix
Noncollagenous structural glycoproteins	Fibronectin Laminin Vitronectin	Widely distributed in connective tissue Basement membrane component More limited pericellular distribution
Proteoglycans and glycosaminoglycans	Hyaluronic acid Heparan sulfate Keratan sulfate	Widely distributed Basement membranes proteoglycan Cartilage

A variety of extracellular and intracellular factors modify the expression of adhesion molecules.[30] Factors that up-regulate the expression and/or adhesiveness of these molecules include exposure to cytokines,[31] adhesion to extracellular matrix proteins,[32] and lymphocyte activation. They are widely distributed in the inflamed synovium. Adhesion molecules are also involved in lymphocyte recalculation and localization.

The Extracellular Matrix

The cells of the synovium interact closely with their surrounding extracellular matrix, which acts as a scaffolding and also controls a number of cellular activities including cell shape, cell migration, cell division, and differentiation.[33] Components of the matrix can also trap autoantigens and thus also may contribute toward disease pathology.[34] The main components of the extracellular matrix are summarized in Table 82-5.

Collagen is a ubiquitous protein found in a variety of forms in all body tissues. The main forms of collagen in connective tissues are collagens I, II, and III. They are fiber-forming collagens with a triple helical structure. Collagens I and III are found in the synovium and associated fibrous structures. Collagen II is the main collagen of cartilage. Collagen molecules can be classified into three groups: group 1 have continuous uninterrupted helical domains (types I, II, III, V, and XI); group 2 have interrupted helical domains (types IV and VII); and group 3 have short α-chains (types VI, IX, and X).[35] Collagen and its breakdown products are implicated in the process of inflammation; they are directly chemotactic for monocytes and fibroblasts to sites of injury and tissue damage in the early phases of the inflammatory process.

Immunohistochemical studies have localized the various collagens in normal and inflamed synovia from RA and other arthropathies.[36,37] Collagens III and VI are present in small amounts; collagen IV is present in the basement membrane of blood vessels in the synovium. Collagen IV is present around synovial lining cells. Collagen II is present only in the articular cartilage of the joint. However, degradation of the collagen is a major factor in cartilage damage caused by rheumatoid synovitis. Collagen type II is present in synovial phagocytes from patients with rheumatoid synovial fluids.[38] This is a potential sensitive immunohistochemical marker of cartilage erosion in rheumatoid disease and shows the potential importance of phagocytic cells in joint damage.

In arthritis the proliferation of the synovium leads to an increase in the amount of collagen within the joint and also to a change in its distribution, with increasing amounts of collagen III in the synovial lining cell layer and subintimal layer. Degradation of collagen and its associated components of the extracellular matrix is accomplished by proteolytic enzymes. The degradation products of collagen may have complex effects on cells and may play a role in signaling between cells.

Glycosaminoglycans include hyaluronic acid, chondroitin sulfate, dermatan sulfate, keratan sulfate and associated molecules, and heparan sulfate proteoglycan. Hyaluronate is responsible for many of the viscous properties of synovial fluid, but is also involved in many reactions in the tissues and is involved with a specific cell adhesion molecule.[39] The interaction between hyaluronate, its cell surface receptor, and the cell cytoskeleton may have important pathogenic roles in determining the chronic inflammatory response.[40] There is a marked increase in hyaluronate with free binding sites for its associated link protein in the rheumatoid synovium.[41] Hyaluronic acid is also present in the serum and its levels are high in rheumatoid disease. Proteoglycans such as chondroitin sulfate and keratan sulfate are major cartilage constituents. There is also evidence they are involved in the synovium.

The final group are the structural glycoproteins, a heterogeneous group of proteins that includes fibronectin, laminin, chondronectin, vitronectin, and possibly associated proteins such as tissue P component. This diverse group of large proteins may also modulate the pathogenesis of synovitis.

Proteolytic Enzymes

The resorption of the connective tissues of the joint seen in joint destruction in arthritis is a process similar to that at other sites of the body in normal events such as cell migration and tissue morphogenesis. Cell-cell and cell-matrix interactions are important in controlling the process, but the main factors involved are the production of proteolytic enzymes, activators, and inhibitors. The initial step is the extracellular degradation of connective tissues involving secreted matrix metalloproteinases and in inflammatory systems serine proteases are released by invading cells. Mechanical disruption and free radicals can augment the enzymic processes.

Collagenase is the most specific metalloproteinase (Table 82-6). Human fibroblast collagenase in its latent form is a 55-kd protein with a minor glycosylated form of 59 kd; on activation these sizes are reduced to 43 kd and 48 kd respectively.[42] The enzyme's activity for the different types of collagen is in the order III>I>II. Stromelysin is a metalloproteinase that degrades the protein core of proteoglycans causing the release of soluble glycosaminoglycans. It also degrades laminin, fibronectin, and type IV collagen.[43] The final enzyme in this family is gelatinase. It has a latent molecular weight of 72 kd.[44] On activation it degrades gelatin, which is itself degraded collagen, and also collagens type IV and V.[45] The properties of gelatinase suggest two roles in vivo. First, it further degrades small fragments of collagen released by the action of collagenase. Second, its ability to degrade native type IV collagen, which is a major constituent of basement membranes, indicates it may have a role during the invasion of this membrane by proliferating cells.

The connective tissue metalloproteinases are all specifically inhibited by a tissue inhibitor of metalloproteinase (TIMP). This is a heavily glycosylated protein of low molecular weight.[46] TIMP is present in connective tissues, and has also been identified in the culture media of many connective tissue cells and in synovial fluid. Metalloproteinases are inhibited by various proteins in addition to TIMP; α_2-macroglobulin is one of these and is especially important. Binding studies have shown that TIMP is unable to displace α_2-macroglobulin once a metalloproteinase is bound.[47] In the inflammatory response of RA, α_2-macroglobulin concentrations rise in plasma and there is greater capillary permeability, allowing it to reach sites such as synovial tissues. These circumstances may make α_2-macroglobulin a more effective metalloproteinase inhibitor.

The metalloproteinases are controlled in several ways: by the synthesis of the latent enzyme; by the need for an activation mechanism; and by the presence of inhibitory TIMPs. Expression of metalloproteinase and TIMP by cultured connective tissue cells is regulated by a number of cytokines, growth fac-

Table 82-6 Metalloproteinase enzymes of human connective tissue

Enzyme	Size (Latent), kd	Size (Active), kd	Substrates
Collagenase	55	43	Collagens I, II, and III
Stromelysin	57	48	Proteoglycan core protein Collagen IV Fibronectin Laminin Elastin Denatured collagens
Gelatinase	72	66	Denatured collagens Collagens IV, V, VII

tors, and hormones. The activity of metalloproteinases can also be influenced by their extracellular activation. The prometalloproteinases undergo a conformational change with the loss of about 80 N-terminal amino acids.[48,49] Proteolytic cleavage with trypsin, plasmin, or similar enzymes causes activation, although a final self-cleavage event occurs. The presence of stromelysin during collagenase activation causes a marked potentiation of over 10-fold in collagenase activity.

Free Radicals and Tissue Damage

A free radical is a molecule with one or more unpaired electrons; examples include the oxygen molecule, the hydrogen atom, and most transition metals. The unpaired electron(s) characteristic of an oxygen-derived free radical may confer a high level of instability and thus chemical reactivity of the molecule. Consequently, oxygen free radicals are often tissue damaging and usually only exist at low steady state concentrations in vivo.[50] When polymorphonuclear leukocytes engulf microbes they rapidly consume oxygen. This is termed the *respiratory burst*. The oxygen consumption is utilized to produce reactive, oxygen-derived species that are responsible for killing microbial pathogens.

A consequence of uncontrolled production of free radicals is damage to biomolecules leading to altered function and disease. There is much direct and indirect evidence implicating radicals in the pathogenesis of rheumatoid synovitis. Many cells involved in the inflamed synovium, such as macrophages, neutrophils, lymphocytes, and endothelial cells, have the capacity when isolated and stimulated to produce free radicals. When stimulated in the environment of critical biomolecules such as lipids, proteins, DNA, and glycosaminoglycans, they promote oxidative damage.

Interest in the tissue-destroying power of oxygen radicals was stimulated by the observation that they degrade hyaluronic acid, leading to a loss in its viscosity similar to that seen in rheumatoid synovitis.[51] This appeared to explain the paradox of low viscosity of rheumatoid synovial fluid in the absence of detectable hyaluronidase; however, it is now known that rheumatoid synovial lining cells secrete short chain hyaluronic acid polymers,[52] so it is not certain about the contribution of oxygen radicals toward the depolymerization process. Although there is ample evidence to implicate radicals in the pathogenesis of inflammatory synovitis, this requires an adequate supply of oxygen and the oxygen tension in inflamed synovial fluid is low.[53] There is a need to explain how, in the relatively hypoxic environment of the inflamed joint, free radicals are generated. This led Woodruff et al.[54] to propose that radicals are formed in synovitis by a hypoxic-reperfusion mechanism.

Ischemia-induced damage occurs in many disorders, such as coronary artery disease. Although ischemia itself can ultimately produce tissue death, in many clinical situations a substantial part of the injury is more properly termed reperfusion injury.[55] Much of the injury occurs when oxygen is reintroduced to the tissue by the restoration of the blood supply. When this happens free radicals are formed in abundance due to the uncoupling of a variety of intracellular redox systems, causing substantial microvascular and parenchymal damage. Several mechanisms can lead to hypoxic-reperfusion injury in rheumatoid joints. In the normal knee the intra-articular pressure is at or slightly below atmospheric pressure.[56] In normal knees contracting the quadriceps produces a subatmospheric pressure[57] whereas in rheumatoid patients, where there is a synovial effusion, quadriceps contraction produces high intra-articular pressures. This high pressure on exercise occludes the synovial capillary bed in arthritic patients with reperfusion injury.[58]

Age and Arthritis

Several features of old age are implicated in the etiology of arthritis. These include hormonal changes after the menopause in women and the loss of testicular function in men, the increased tissue damage from free radicals in later life and the gradual failure of antioxidant systems, the degenerative changes in articular cartilage and the reduced content of glycosaminoglycans in later years, the loss of bone in the elderly, the increase in muscle weakness, and a nonspecific decline in immune function together with an increased propensity to autoantibody production. Almost all arthropathies have an increased prevalence in old age. On the other hand, it is certainly a mistake to merely attribute a disease such as osteoarthritis to the aging process; it is far more of an active disorder with both genetic and environmental factors having a role in its etiology.

Symptoms and Signs of Arthritis

Local symptoms comprise pain, tenderness, swelling and stiffness in the joints, periarticular tissues, ligaments and tendons, and muscles. Pain is the predominant symptom. Usually persistent and moderately severe, it is often worse on movement and it invariably limits patients' lifestyles.

Stiffness is the most characteristic arthritic symptom. It comprises both early morning stiffness and postexercise stiffness. Morning stiffness points toward inflammatory arthritis or polymyalgia rheumatica. It usually lasts over 60 minutes and can be very prolonged. Postexercise stiffness points more toward osteoarthritis. Tenderness and swelling of the joints or tendons usually go together and indicate an inflammatory synovitis or tendonitis. They vary from very subtle to gross symptoms. Some elderly patients minimize the extent of their joint swelling, even though it is extensive on examination. Bony swelling of the joints usually indicates osteoarthritis.

Systemic symptoms vary. In rheumatoid arthritis or polymyalgia rheumatica they can be quite marked and include malaise, anorexia, weight loss, and depression. Low-grade fevers can occur, especially in connective tissue disorders.

The goal of the examination is to identify the presence and extent of joint swelling and tenderness, the numbers of joints

Table 82-7 Laboratory investigations

Class of Test	Category	Example of Abnormality
Haematology	Hemoglobin White cell count Platelet count ESR	Anemia in rheumatoid arthritis Leukocytosis in septic arthritis Thrombocytopenia in systemic lupus erythematosus Elevated in polymyalgia rheumatica
Biochemistry	Creatinine Uric acid CPK	High with involvement in systemic vasculitis Elevated in gout Elevated in polymyositis
Immunology	Rheumatoid factor Antinuclear antibody C-reactive protein Immunoglobulins Complement C_3 and C_4	Positive in rheumatoid arthritis Positive in systemic lupus erythematosus Elevated in rheumatoid arthritis Elevated in Sjögren's syndrome Low in active systemic lupus erythematosus
Synovial fluid microscopy	Crystals	Present in gout and pyrophosphate crystal deposition disease
Culture	Bacteria in septic arthritis	

or soft tissue structures involved, the distribution of joint inflammation, its severity, and the presence of effusions and deformities. Extra-articular features such as subcutaneous nodules should be sought. Regional problems such as back pain or shoulder problems require specific attention to those sites. Comorbidity is common in elderly patients with arthritis and general physical examination is essential.

Investigations

There are two reasons for investigating patients with arthritis: making or confirming the diagnosis and assessing disease severity or side effects to drugs. Investigations range from full blood counts and routine biochemistry to immunologic measures of rheumatoid factor and analysis of synovial fluid for crystals. The main tests are summarized in Table 82-7.

Rheumatoid Factor

Rheumatoid factor is an antibody against the Fc fragment of IgG. Rheumatoid factors react against different species of IgG including human and rabbit. Rheumatoid factors can involve different immunoglobulin classes giving IgM, IgG, and IgA rheumatoid factors. Different subclasses of antibody can also be involved, such as IgA_1 and IgA_2 rheumatoid factors. Most tests detect IgM rheumatoid factor. There is some evidence that IgA rheumatoid factor is more related to joint destruction. Rheumatoid factor positivity goes with worse disease and poorer outcome in rheumatoid arthritis and is associated with subcutaneous nodules, vasculitis, and other extra-articular features. Osteoarthritis, gout, and psoriatic arthritis should all be negative on tests for rheumatoid factor.

Other Immunologic Tests

Anti-nuclear antibodies are more important in connective tissue diseases, although rheumatoid arthritis is a common cause of low-titer positive anti-nuclear antibodies. There are many types of anti-nuclear antibodies and the less specific IgM subclass are more often seen in RA. Osteoarthritis, gout, and psoriatic arthritis should be negative for anti-nuclear antibodies.

The other main area of testing is for acute phase changes. An elevated C-reactive protein level, together with a high erythrocyte sedimentation rate (ESR) and changes in several serum proteins characterizes active RA. It is termed the *acute phase response*. It is mediated by the cytokine network, especially IL-1 and IL-6. The levels of these cytokines can be measured directly but they are labile and secreted in pulses and thus are poor measures of disease activity in many cases. The range of immunologic tests and methods are summarized in Tables 82-8 and 82-9.

Changes in Degenerative Arthritis

Osteoarthritis and inflammatory arthritis are characterized by cartilage damage and collagen turnover. Unfortunately the markers of this process are not ideal and at present no tests have a major role but investigations based on connective tissue biochemistry will be available in the future. They comprise measures of derivatives of collagen metabolism, cartilage breakdown products, and mediators of connective tissue turnover. Excluding crystal deposition disease by synovial fluid microscopy also helps in differential diagnosis.

Keratan sulfate has been most widely studied. It is a metabolite of cartilage degradation and can be measured in synovial fluid and blood. Serum levels of keratan sulfate may reflect proteoglycan metabolism. Its serum levels are elevated in some patients with osteoarthritis but it may merely reflect a negative acute phase reactant[59] and its levels may not always reflect cartilage damage. The measurement of other cartilage products, such as the expression of chrondroitin sulfate epitopes by monoclonal antibodies (e.g., 3B3 antibody) may be more helpful, but this work is at an early stage.

Collagen degradation leads to pyridinoline and deoxypyridinoline cross-link fragments in blood and urine, which can be measured in chromatographic or immunochemical assays. They are the most widely used markers in osteoarthritis[60] although they have not extended beyond clinical trials (Table 82-10).

These include measuring the products of cartilage damage such as keratan sulfate, which is a glycosaminoglycan in carti-

Table 82-8 Immunologic investigations

Acute Phase Changes	Immunoglobulins	Complement	Cytokines
ESR	IgG	C_3	TNF-α
C-reactive protein	IgA	C_4	IL-1
Serum amyloid A protein	IgM		IL-6

lage, and collagen turnover markers. The most well known of these are collagen propeptide fragments.

Imaging in Arthritis

Imaging arthritic joints has a variety of aims that depend on the specific circumstances. These include diagnosis, assessing progression and the effects of drugs, looking at early rapid changes in the extent of synovitis, and looking at joints at risk of progression and damage. The modalities of imaging are summarized in Table 82-11. Currently plain joint radiographs remain the most widely used method for determining the extent and nature of structural changes in arthritis. The main radiologic changes include periarticular osteoporosis and sclerosis, loss of joint space (reflecting cartilage damage), juxta-articular erosions, marginal osteophytes, joint destruction, and ankylosis.[61] Although joint radiographs are one of the most objective methods of assessing joint destruction many investigators have failed to demonstrate a significant correlation between the severity of radiographic findings on hand radiographs and functional status.[62]

Magnetic resonance imaging (MRI) gives the opportunity for far greater information to be gained from imaging joints. It will probably be the "gold standard" for evaluating the nature and extent of pathologic changes within the joints in future years. However, experience is still at an early stage. Essential information needs to be obtained before the place of MRI in the assessment of arthritis can be fully defined.[63,64]

Physiologic measurements and diagnostic assessments can both be achieved using nuclear medicine techniques and densitometry. The role of these alternative imaging procedures must not be overlooked. Most experience has been gained from using bone scans.[65] These examine a combination of bone blood flow and osteoblastic activity. Their resolution is poor and this is a limiting factor. The three-phase bone scan looks at initial uptake, the blood pool interval, and subsequent localization within the bones. The use of labeled white cells, such as indium-labeled leukocytes, allows the assessment of joint inflammation.[66] Labeled immunoglobulin may also be useful. The resolution of detectors allows better images of large joints such as the knee.

Densitometry has many advantages for assessing bone changes.[67] It can be either whole body densitometry or localized views of specific joints or regions. Until now it has mainly focused on assessing the effects of drugs on bone mineral density and the relation to fracture risk. The introduction of new systems may be more advantageous for looking at specific joints.

Drug Therapy

Conventionally anti-rheumatic drugs have been divided into nonsteroidal anti-inflammatory drugs (NSAIDs), slow-acting drugs, and steroids. Slow-acting drugs are often thought capable of modifying the course of RA and are sometimes termed "disease modifying" drugs. The belief that such drugs affect the course of RA is based on their effects on the radiologic progression of joint damage. There is evidence that some slow-acting drugs may reduce the rate of progression but the situation is not straightforward. Concerns have led to the suggestion that the classification of anti-rheumatic drugs should be changed and the concept of disease control introduced.[68]

Disease control implies a beneficial effect on inflammatory synovitis, leading to reduced anatomic damage, improved and maintained function, and an amelioration of systemic rheumatoid disease over a long period of time. Disease control must

Table 82-9 Immunologic methods

Method	Example of Use
Agglutination	IgM rheumatoid factor
Nephelometry	IgM rheumatoid factor
ELISA	IgA and IgG rheumatoid factors
Radial immunodiffusion	C-reactive protein
Immunodiffusion	ENA, e.g., Sm and RNP
Immunofluorescence	ANA, Crythidea
Radioimmunoassay	DNA binding

Table 82-10 Laboratory investigations in osteoarthritis

Type of test	Example
Synovial fluid analyses	Cell counts Crystals (in chondrocalcinosis) Cartilage damage markers (e.g., keratan sulfate)
Blood	Cartilage damage markers (e.g., keratan sulfate) Collagen turnover markers (e.g., collagen propeptides)
Urine	Collagen damage markers (e.g., pyridinium cross-links)

Table 82-11 Imaging methods

Modality	Example
Plain radiology	X-rays of hands in rheumatoid arthritis
Magnetic resonance imaging	Imaging of knee joint to show internal derangement
Computed tomography	Imaging of sacroiliac joint if infection suspected
Bone scan	Showing active joints in inflammatory synovitis
DEXA	Identifying osteoporosis with inflammatory synovitis

relate as much to an overall management strategy or drug combination as to a single drug.[69] Most anti-rheumatic drugs are symptomatically effective and this should be one determinant of their classification. If a drug or a therapeutic strategy then meets the criteria for disease control it can be reclassified accordingly. At least 12 months of disease-controlling activity is needed to predict improved long-term outcome.

Anti-Inflammatory Drugs

NSAIDs remain the central focus of antirheumatic therapy. They reduce the signs and symptoms of acute synovitis and relieve pain and are widely used in RA, osteoarthritis, gout, back pain, and soft tissue rheumatism. NSAIDs such as diclofenac, ibuprofen, and naproxen are well established and have been available for many years. New drug development has concentrated on reducing side effects while maintaining efficacy. The main NSAIDs are summarized in Table 82-12.

The concept that NSAIDs act by inhibiting prostaglandin biosynthesis has been a central tenet of antirheumatic drug development. Most of their effectiveness has been attributed to inhibition of the cyclo-oxygenase enzyme. We now know that this enzyme exists in two isoforms called COX-1 and COX-2.[70] They offer the possibility of producing a new generation of anti-inflammatory drugs that are less toxic. Although both enzymes are involved in the generation of prostaglandins, COX-1 is constitutively expressed whereas COX-2 is induced by inflammation. Almost all the current NSAIDs are COX-1 inhibitors and this may explain their gastrointestinal toxicity. The new generation of COX-2 inhibitors may reduce toxicity without affecting their anti-inflammatory effect.

Table 82-12 Commonly Used NSAIDs

Short Half-Life (Under 6 Hours)	Long Half-Life (Over 12 Hours)
Diclofenac	Azapropazone
Etodolac	Fenbufen
Ibuprofen	Nabumetone
Indomethacin	Naproxen
Ketoprofen	Piroxicam
Tiaprofenic acid	Sulindac

The main adverse effect of NSAIDs is their gastrointestinal toxicity, and their propensity to cause ulcers accounts for the peptic ulcers, bleeding, and perforations associated with their use. There is a significant morbidity and mortality. There are several strategies to reduce these adverse effects. The most widely used is coprescribing with misoprostol, a synthetic prostaglandin that reduces the gastrointestinal side effects of NSAIDs and both prevents and heals NSAID-associated ulcers.[71] It can be given by itself or in a combined fixed-dose combination with diclofenac (Arthrotec). Reducing gastric acid by H_2-antagonists such as ranitidine also heals NSAID-associated ulcers and has a role in their prevention. There is debate about whether all NSAIDs cause the same frequency of ulcers and the evidence suggests that some NSAIDs such as azapropazone may be more likely to result in gastrointestinal adverse effects. Newer NSAIDs have intrinsically less gastrointestinal adverse reactions. An example is a prodrug like nabumetone, which does not cause gastric damage itself.

NSAIDs cause many different adverse effects and these are summarized in Table 82-13. In addition to gastrointestinal problems renal and central nervous system reactions can be a special problem. The mild reactions of dizziness and confusion can be a particular difficulty in patients already taking many different medications and can lead to considerable disorientation.

The value of NSAIDs for symptomatic treatment in osteoarthritis is an area of controversy. Although most clinicians use

Table 82-13 Adverse effects of NSAIDs

Type of Adverse Reaction	Example
Gastrointestinal	Indigestion Erosions Peptic ulcer Hemorrhage and perforation Small bowel enteropathy
Hepatic	Hepatocellular damage Cholestasis
Renal	Acute renal failure Interstitial nephritis
Hematologic	Thrombocytopenia Neutropenia Hemolytic anemia
Skin	Photsensitivity Urticaria Erythema multiforme
Chest	Bronchospasm Pneumonitis
Central nervous system	Headache Dizziness Confusion

them, the supporting evidence is not strong. Dieppe et al.[72] highlighted the lack of randomized placebo-controlled trials of NSAIDs; the majority of trials in osteoarthritis compare one NSAID with another. One large study by Bradley et al.[73] compared ibuprofen against paracetamol in patients with osteoarthritis of the knee and suggested that there was no convincing evidence in favor of the NSAID. Brandt[74] has outlined in detail the deficiencies in the case for using NSAIDs in osteoarthritis. But the absence of good evidence for their use does not mean NSAIDs are ineffective, it merely indicates the inadequacy of randomized clinical trials in the area.

Disease-Controlling Drugs and Immunosuppression

Disease-controlling drugs and immunosuppression are mainly used to treat RA. The assessment of their effect includes clinical, laboratory, functional, and radiologic approaches. A central theme of therapy—disease control—is based on overcoming the inflammatory synovitis and thus reducing the progression of joint damage. The effects of generalized inflammation indicated by the acute phase response on the progression of RA are well known as is the association between radiologic progression and acute phase proteins such as C-reactive protein. Otterness[75] has shown that drugs that reduce C-reactive protein give the best outcomes. However, normalizing an elevated acute phase response may be insufficient, and only patients who consistently maintain low ESR and C-reactive protein levels have less radiologic progression. Further work is needed to define whether it is most important to control local or systemic inflammation in RA. Despite such uncertainties there is a clear need to control both symptoms of inflammatory synovitis and reduce the elevated acute phase response. Therapy with slow-acting drugs has this as a combined aim.

Aggressive RA or the early onset of erosions are indications for early treatment with a slow-acting drug. Most rheumatologists use sequential monotherapy, with one slow-acting drug following another in an attempt to control the disease without excessive side effects. The concurrent use of several second-line drugs is controversial. Wilke et al.[76] argued that as the long-term outcome of sequential monotherapy has been disappointing specific goals of treatment should be established and aggressive treatment given in a logical manner in early disease. As RA rarely remits, refractory disease is common and in this situation the therapeutic options include cyclosporine A, high-dose methotrexate, combination second-line agents, and tailored use of corticosteroids.

Gold, penicillamine, and sulfasalazine perform similarly, with about 60 percent of patients continuing to receive each drug for at least 1 year.[77] Patients with a longer disease duration showed a greater tendency to stop treatment. The median percentage improvement was 33 percent in pain score and 50 percent in ESR. Methotrexate has proved a major advance from the 1980s in the treatment of RA. Used initially in patients with psoriatic arthritis because of their skin disease, it induced improvement in synovitis. A subsequent placebo-controlled trial in RA confirmed its efficacy. Alarcon et al.[78] reviewed the clinical and radiologic effects of methotrexate questioned its effects on x-ray progression. They performed a meta-analysis of 353 methotrexate-treated subjects and 205 controls and computed a monthly rate of disease progression. The rates of disease progression were similar for methotrexate-treated cases and controls. A new agent for use in nonresponding RA is cyclosporine A, which controls the symptoms of early and late RA.[79] Cyclosporine A, slows radiologic progression in advanced disease.[80]

The use of several antirheumatic drugs concurrently is routine clinical practice. NSAIDs, slow-acting drugs, and steroids are often used together and may also include hormone replacement therapy. But the concept of combination therapy with two slow-acting drugs is more controversial. Tugwell et al.[81] have shown that the combination of cyclosporine A and methotrexate appear to be effective and this is an important focus of future therapy.

Steroids

In RA the efficacy of corticosteroids was demonstrated in early clinical trials. But their long-term side effects, particularly osteoporosis, have remained a substantial obstacle limiting their routine use. Short courses of oral prednisolone or a depot intramuscular injection are often used in active disease when commencing therapy with a slow-acting drug to control symptoms before the slow-acting drug has an appreciable effect.[82] Pulse therapy with intravenous steroids such as 0.5 to 1.0 g methylprednisolone has a rapid onset of action but its advantage is often not maintained and its use remains in some doubt.[83] The more prolonged use of oral steroids has been shown to be advantageous in early disease. Kirwan[84] showed that in early RA patients, low-dose prednisolone (7.5 mg/day) when used in conjunction with disease-modifying antirheumatic drugs reduced the progression of erosive disease. More studies are needed to establish the value and risks and benefits of steroids in this situation.

Hormone Replacement Therapy

The widespread use of hormone replacement therapy has been an important advance in the management of osteoporosis. There is evidence that hormone replacement therapy should be used as part of the integrated management of RA. Hall et al.[85] assessed the effect of hormone replacement therapy on bone mass in 200 postmenopausal female patients with RA treated with and without steroid therapy. They showed that hormone replacement therapy increases spinal bone mineral density and maintains femoral bone mineral density in postmenopausal RA. It is also effective in preserving bone mass in patients taking low-dose corticosteroids.

Supportive Nondrug Therapy

Physiotherapy, occupational therapy, supplying aids and appliances such as walking sticks, modifying footwear such as fitting insoles and providing surgical shoes, and chiropody all have important places. This is especially true in elderly patients with arthritis. Of equal importance is providing patient education and general advice about arthritis together where possible with simple exercise programs.

Rheumatoid Arthritis

RA is a chronic inflammatory synovitis of peripheral joints. It is usually polyarticular and symmetric in distribution. Many patients have radiologic evidence of juxta-articular erosions and are seropositive for rheumatoid factor. Extra-articular features such as subcutaneous nodules are common.

Epidemiology

RA is a common disorder. We know the incidence of new cases of rheumatoid arthritis from prospective studies such as the Norfolk Arthritis Register; there will be in the region of 50/100,000 new cases of inflammatory synovitis each year in the United Kingdom.[86] Most of these are due to RA. There is also a considerable amount of information about the prevalence of established RA; in Europe this varies from 0.5 percent to 2 percent or more depending on the exact population studied.[87] Some populations in North America have higher prevalence rates (Table 82-14).

The prevalence of RA increases with age. It is especially frequent in elderly women. A study from North America in the early 1960s showed that it was rare in men before the age of 45 years and in women before the age of 35 years. In the over 65 age group its prevalence increased to 1.8 percent males and 4.9 percent females.[88]

Disease Onset

The most common presentation is an insidious onset.[89,90] Up to three-quarters of cases start in this way. The characteristic features of an inflammatory synovitis are present including joint swelling, joint tenderness, and morning stiffness. These usually involve multiple sites in a symmetric distribution. There are often systemic features such as malaise and fatigue. A small number of cases, about 5 to 10 percent, have an acute onset with an "explosive" beginning and a rapid onset of symptoms over a few days or even less. Between these two extremes there is an intermediate onset of the symptoms over days and weeks. This is seen in nearly 20 percent of cases.

Early RA usually involves the proximal interphalangeal joints of the hands together with the wrists. The metatarsophalangeal joints of the feet are also commonly involved. A small number of patients have an atypical onset. These include intermittent episodes of arthritis termed *palindromic rheumatism*, polymyalgic and monoarticular onsets. Patients with a polymyalgic onset have predominant shoulder girdle symptoms with muscle pain and prolonged morning stiffness. Palindromic arthritis, which can develop into RA, is more a symptom complex than a disease entity.[91] Its features are transient synovial inflammation, involvement of different joints, and aysmptomatic periods without synovitis. When there is a monoarticular onset the knee is usually involved.

Table 82-14 Prevalence of rheumatoid arthritis in different populations

Population	Prevalence (%)
Europe	
United Kingdom	1.1
Netherlands	0.9
Finland	2.0
Denmark	0.8
North America	
US National Health Survey	1.0
Inuit Indians (Canada)	0.6
Pima Indians (United States)	5.3

Table 82-15 The course of rheumatoid arthritis

Disease Type	Frequency (%)	Description
Progressive course	70	Chronic disease with invariable progression and some fluctuations in severity
Intermittent course	25	Intermittent attacks of arthritis, often less than 1 year, and intermissions for variable periods of time
Brief remissions		Lasting less than 1 year in 10% of cases
Long remissions		Lasting over 1 year in 10% of cases
"Malignant" disease	Less than 5	Uncommon form of RA with severe extra-articular disease, especially vasculitis; often fatal.

Disease Course

RA is usually divided into progressive disease, an intermittent course, and cases with long clinical remissions, which form a variant of intermittent disease. A few patients with severe extra-articular disease can be described as having "malignant" RA. These different patterns are summarized in Table 82-15.

Clinical Features

Persistent joint inflammation is the central diagnostic feature of RA. The joints are swollen, tender, and stiff. Morning stiffness is prolonged and may last 60 minutes or longer. The joint involvement is symmetric and usually involves the hands (proximal interphalangeal and metacarpophalangeal joints), wrists, and feet (proximal interphalangeal and metatarsophalangeal joints). The elbows, knees, and ankles are often involved as well.

The synovitis is accompanied by systemic features of ill health with malaise, weight loss, occasional intermittent fever, and constitutional upset in many cases. As the arthritis progresses there are characteristic destructive changes, for example, ulnar deviation and the Swan neck and Boutonierre deformities of the fingers.

Extra-Articular Features

Subcutaneous nodules are the classic example. They are found on extensor surfaces such as the elbows or sites of pressure such as the lower back or in some parts of the hands. They occur in about 20 percent of cases. The other extra-articular features are summarized in Table 82-16.

The main clinical problems result from rheumatoid vasculitis. This is due to an inflammatory infiltration of small and medium-sized vessels. It usually occurs after 10 years or more of the disease in patients with high levels of rheumatoid factor and destructive disease.[92]

Clinical Assessments

The core data set, which has been agreed internationally,[93] is summarized in the accompanying box. The measures give a good overall picture of RA and permit assessment of progression and response to treatment.

Disease activity can be assessed by counting the number

Table 82-16 Extra-articular features of rheumatoid arthritis

Extra-Articular Feature	Specific Example
Subcutaneous nodules	Pressure area at elbow In wall of olecranon bursa At sacrum
Pulmonary	Pleural effusion Interstitial fibrosis
Cardiac	Pericarditis Valvular disease
Ocular	Keratoconjunctivitis sicca Episcleritis Scleritis
Neurologic	Carpal tunnel syndrome Mononeuritis multiplex Peripheral neuropathy Cervical myelopathy
Renal	Amyloidosis Drug toxicity
Vasculitis	Nail fold infarctions Leg ulcers Systemic vasculitis
Hematologic	Anemia Felty syndrome

Core data set in rheumatoid arthritis

Number of swollen joints
Number of tender joints
Pain assessed by the patient
Patient's global assessments of disease activity
Physician's global assessments of disease activity
Laboratory evaluation of an acute-phase reactant (ESR, C-reactive protein, or equivalent)
Self-administered functional assessment (such as the Health Assessment Questionnaire)

of active joints. The best joint count has been an area of recent investigation. Prevoo et al.[94] contrasted several available methods. The various indices had similar reliability and validity and no joint index was superior for measuring disease activity. The implication is that the simplest index, the 28 joint count, is best. Other studies have also concluded that the 28 joint count gives all the necessary information.

Patients can assess their disease activity in RA. A self-report measure of disease activity was developed by Stewart et al.[95] based on an articular index. The measure was sensitive to therapeutic change when completed by patients both before and after intra-articular corticosteroid injection. Although a self-report articular index has the potential to provide an inexpensive method for monitoring disease activity or treatment response in RA, it may be affected by confounding variables such as the patient's mood. Further work by Stucki et al.[96] has confirmed the value of patients' self-assessments.

Because RA is multidimensional its activity should be assessed in several areas or domains. There are apparent advantages in using a single index that pools several outcome measures to provide one overall measure. Examples include the disease activity index derived by van der Heijde et al.,[97] the Stoke index,[98] and the Mallya and Mace index.[99] Pooled indices may be difficult to calculate and interpreting their results may present problems.

Imaging

Joint imaging includes plain radiology, MRI, bone scans and isotope labeling methods, and DEXA scans for peri-articular osteoporosis. Conventional x-rays remain the gold standard for diagnosis and determining drug efficacy. MRI will be the future method of choice for defining cartilage and synovial changes in single joints. Isotope methods give the best indication of synovial inflammation.

Radiographs of the hands and feet can be scored by simple standardized methods. The most widely used methods are those of Sharp et al.[100] and Larsen et al.[101] Both methods are reproducible[102] and are composite indices combining joint space loss, erosions, and other changes. Their disadvantage is that they combine diverse changes in a single score and assign numerical values to qualitative changes. Radiographic changes in hands and wrists reflect changes in major joints. In early RA 70 percent of patients have radiographic damage at 3 years.[103] By 10 years X-ray progression is invariable in severe disease.[104]

Functional Assessments

The most familiar instruments used in RA are the Health Assessment Questionnaire (HAQ)[105] and the Arthritis Impact Measurement Scale (AIMS).[106] Both were developed specifically for RA. There are also several questionnaires designed to be relevant to a wide range of health problems, the so-called generic measures. A number of these generic instruments have been used to assess health status in RA,[107] including the Sickness Impact Profile, the Nottingham Health Profile (NHP), the Quality of Well-Being Scale, and the SF-36. The NHP and the Medical Outcome Study Short Form-36 (SF-36) have been widely used in RA.[108,109]

Laboratory Assessments

Rheumatoid factor levels assist in both diagnosis and assessment of severity. There are many different measures available including particle assays (e.g., latex test and RA particle agglutination), radioimmunoassays, enzyme-linked immunosorbent assays, and (ELISA). They use a variety of immunoglobulin sources including rabbit and human IgG and different classes of rheumatoid factors are measured. Traditional assays such as the latex test measure mainly IgM rheumatoid factor. ELISAs measure both IgG and IgA rheumatoid factor as well as IgM.

Rheumatoid factor status is an important prognostic indicator in all cases. When Isomaki[110] reviewed follow-up results of unselected adult arthritis cases he found outcome was worst in seropositive rheumatoid patients and best in seronegative oligoarthritis of unknown etiology. Increased rheumatoid factor levels in early RA, especially a high level of IgA rheumatoid factor within 3 years of the onset of symptoms, was prognostic for a more severe disease outcome 6 years after the onset of symptoms. The importance of rheumatoid factor status has been confirmed in many other studies.[111]

Single measures showing a high ESR or C-reactive protein level indicate a poor prognosis. A combination of measures or multiple values are better. Hassell et al.[112] evaluated disease activity annually over 7 years in 127 patients and found significant correlations between "areas under the curve" for the ESR and other disease activity measures and destructive RA.

General demographic features, predictive of a poor response in most disease, include age, gender, and disease duration. Kaarela[113] evaluated predictors of outcome in 442 patients with recent arthritis and compared 22 variables recorded at the onset of arthritis. Destructive RA was predicted by symmetric polyarthritis, female sex, and old age.

RA is related to HLA DR4 but there is debate about its value in predicting response. Some studies have shown little effect. Silman et al.[114] found no evidence that HLA DR4 was a useful indicator of subsequent outcome. But van der Heijde et al.[115] considered HLA typing to be useful in predicting the outcome in early RA. Emery[116] suggests that the combination of polyarthritis, high C-reactive protein levels, and genetic markers, especially DR4 status, will all help define the course of early disease.

Van Zeben et al.[117] looked at prognostic factors in early RA. A combination of three commonly available variables—number of swollen joints, IgM-rheumatoid factor, and the erosion score—predict outcome well. Corbett et al.[118] reported predictors of death, survival, and function after 15 years. Outcome could be correctly predicted in 73 percent of cases from a combination of early erosive change, seropositivity, poor grip strength, and cervical subluxation.

Clinical Outcomes

Studies of antirheumatic therapy tend to show that it is successful in the short term whereas there are poor results in the long-term outcome. This was first highlighted by Pincus.[119] Prospective long-term clinical studies show that most patients first seen as inpatients are moderately or severely impaired by 20 years and the average outpatient has a 30 percent chance of severe disability.[120]

Not all studies show that RA has a poor outcome. A review of 64 survivors from a prospective study of early RA found that after 15 years 60 percent of survivors had relatively normal function. In another study[121] 128 RA patients who developed the disease in 1985 were studied after 6 to 7 years: 32 percent had no articular swelling; 23 percent had normal x-rays and 31 percent had no erosions; and 31 percent had normal function. Rheumatoid factors and nodules were related to more severe outcomes.

RA leads to premature mortality. In hospitalized patients with RA nearly 20 percent of deaths are directly caused by RA. Wolfe et al.[122] reported results from a large study examining 922 deaths in 3,501 patients with RA. The standardized mortality ratio was 2.3. The causes of mortality in RA do not differ much from those in the normal population, although there is an increase in infection and lymphatic malignancies as a cause of death. The average shortening of life is not great and is in the region of 4 to 5 years. Patients with severe RA are most likely to die early.

Specific Problems in the Elderly

RA is increasingly becoming a disease of later life. The most common time for developing the disease is the sixth decade and as it lasts 10 to 20 years many patients with RA are over 65 years old. When its onset is in old age it is often overlooked or ignored by patients and physicians. It is difficult to manage complex RA in the elderly, especially if they have other problems with mobility. RA is frequently associated with other diseases and such comorbidity can be a serious clinical problem in the elderly. Finally they have increased risks of adverse effects with antirheumatic drugs such as nonsteroidal anti-inflammatory agents and this makes management more complex.

Osteoarthritis

Osteoarthritis is a heterogeneous condition with a variety of causes and patterns of expression. It is analogous to kidney or heart failure in which similar clinical and pathologic features develop irrespective of the underlying causes, and could be considered as "joint failure." Older age is the most significant factor in its development in a general population.[123] The joint most commonly affected is the knee, and osteoarthritis of the knee is one of the most common causes of pain and disability in the community. There is a rise in the annual consultation rate for osteoarthritis,[124] and this may reflect not only an increased incidence of disease but also decreased tolerance of joint problems.

Osteoarthritis can be considered as a synovial joint syndrome rather than a single disease. Pathologically it is characterized by a loss of and change in the composition of cartilage proteoglycans leading to failure of normal responses to stress. The results include cartilage fibrillation and loss, bone exposure, and a clinical syndrome of pain and disability. Rare forms of heritable chondrodysplasia lead to premature osteoarthritis but, in most instances, its cause is either excess, inappropriate, or insufficient mechanical demand, or traumatic, infective, inflammatory, endocrine, or metabolic disease. There remain idiopathic ("primary") cases in which no cause is demonstrable.[125]

Epidemiology

The prevalence of osteoarthritis rises steeply with age. Its frequency has been evaluated in both clinical and radiography studies. X-ray evidence of osteoarthritis exceeds its clinical frequency. In Europe and North America there is a similar prevalence rising from less than 1 percent of those aged under 35 years to over 30 percent of those aged over 75 years.[126,127] Both hand and knee osteoarthritis are more common in women than men. Hip osteoarthritis is less common and its prevalence rates in men and women appear to be more similar. The incidence of symptomatic osteoarthritis has been studied less often. One study from North America showed the incidence of knee and hip osteoarthritis was 200/100,000 person-years.[128] Felson et al.[129] evaluated 869 patients from the Framingham osteoarthritis study and found rates of incident disease were 1.7 times higher in women than in men, progressive disease occurred slightly more often in women, but rates did not vary by age. Among women, approximately 2 percent per year developed incident radiographic disease, 1 percent per year developed symptomatic knee osteoarthritis, and about 4 percent per year experienced progressive knee osteoarthritis.

Clinical Features

Osteoarthritis is characterized by articular pain, bony joint swelling, morning stiffness and inactivity stiffness, and associated functional disability and radiography changes (see accompanying box). Pain is the predominant symptom in osteoarthritis. It varies in severity and its exact nature both between patients and in individual cases over a period of time. Although pain is more marked in patients with severe joint destruction on x-rays, there is often no close relationship between pain and radiography abnormalities. Causes of pain in osteoarthritis include raised intraosseous pressure, inflammatory synovitis, periarticular problems, periosteal elevation, muscular changes, fibromyalgic amplification, and central neurogenic changes. There is often relatively little relationship between the severity and clinical importance of pain, stiffness, and physical function in patients with osteoarthritis.[130]

> ***Clinical features of osteoarthritis***
>
> Pain
> Stiffness
> Bony swelling and crepitus
> Loss of movement
> Instability
> Loss of function

Stiffness is experienced by most patients with osteoarthritis. "Stiffness" may refer to difficulty initiating movement, problems in completing a full range of movement, or the ache or pain of a joint on movement. It is often present first thing in the morning, but only lasts 10 to 25 minutes in many cases. More characteristically it comes on after inactivity, when it is frequently termed "gelling" of a joint.

Many patients have loss of movement or instability of one or more joints. Sometimes patients note that a joint will suddenly "give way." In some joints there is a sensation of inflammation due to an associated synovitis and the joint is swollen, tender, and warm.

On examination there is firm or bony swelling around the joint and crepitus on movement. The most characteristic bony swellings are the Heberden's and Bouchard's nodes of hand osteoarthritis. Coarse "crepitations" are usually felt on movement of the involved joint. In severe disease they can be audible. Effusions occur in some cases, especially in knee osteoarthritis. It is possible to use an articular index to standardize the clinical assessment of osteoarthritis and such an index was developed by Doyle et al.,[131] but assessment remains difficult to reproduce.

There are problems in diagnosing osteoarthritis. Although a set of clinical criteria has been developed,[132] these have been criticized for using rheumatoid patients who had not been age and sex matched as controls, using osteophytes as a feature of osteoarthritis, for circularity, and for inadequate validation.[133] Loss of cartilage on x-rays has been reported as the one feature present in all attempted definitions, but these are based on pathologic changes that are not often available to the clinician making the diagnosis.[134] Furthermore the relationship between the incidence of symptoms and the degree of radiologic change is not clear. Almost the entire population over the age of 65 years have at least one joint with evidence of radiographic osteoarthritis but the proportion with symptoms varies with joint, age, and sex.

Clinical Subgroups

Osteoarthritis includes several different subgroups that may all have different natural histories, patterns of joints affected, and different rates of disease progression. These include knee/hand osteoarthritis (often known as "generalized osteoarthritis"), inflammatory/erosive osteoarthritis, rapidly progressive osteoarthritis, secondary osteoarthritis, hypertrophic and atrophic osteoarthritis, and destructive osteoarthritis of the elderly. Set against the classification of osteoarthritis into such distinct subgroups are the findings of Cushnahan and Dieppe,[135] they found a strong relationship between age and the number of involved sites. This was thought to be due to the slow addition of new joint sites with age. However, there was no evidence of well-defined clinical subsets of patients.

Inflammatory osteoarthritis and destructive disease in the elderly deserve special consideration. Destructive osteoarthritis with radiographic findings of rapid severe joint destruction can be a diagnostic problem. The x-ray changes mimic septic arthritis, rheumatoid, and seronegative arthritis. Rapid progression of pain and disability are consistent clinical features. The condition mainly effects the shoulder, knee, and hip.[136] Progression to complete joint destruction takes only 1 to 2 years. Most patients are elderly women.

Laboratory Markers

Several biochemical markers such as keratan sulfate and pyridinoline have been investigated but there have been difficulties with all of these systems.[137] One of the major problems is that most of the body cartilage is in the intervertebral discs and costochondral junctions, and the joints that are affected by osteoarthritis form a small proportion of this total, and may develop only subtle biochemical changes in early disease. In addition, the concentration of cartilage degradation products depends on many factors, including rate of release of the compounds, diurnal variation, the route via which they reach the blood, and their distribution in the different body pools.

Imaging

X-rays are the main investigation in osteoarthritis (see accompanying box). Several changes are observed. The most important are loss of joint space, marginal osteophytes, subchondral sclerosis, cysts, tibial spiking (in the knees), and loss of alignment.

Radiologic features of osteoarthritis

Loss of joint space
Marginal osteophytes
Subchondral sclerosis
Tibial spiking
Loss of alignment

Several scoring systems quantify the radiographic changes in osteoarthritis. The first one, developed by Kellgren and Lawrence in 1957,[138] grades the disease on a scale of 0 to 4 in comparison to a set of standard films. Later methods of grading have paid less attention to osteophytosis, which may be related to normal aging. In 1987 the American Rheumatism Association reviewed the radiographic criteria commonly used in the assessment of progression in the hand, hip, and knee.[139] It showed that in knee osteoarthritis early joint space narrowing and changes in subchondral bone were more significant indicators of progression than a lone osteophyte.[140] Joint space narrowing appears to be the most reproducible feature of knee osteoarthritis.[141]

Polymyalgia Rheumatica and Giant Cell Arteritis

Polymyalgia rheumatica and giant cell arteritis, which is also known as temporal arteritis, are related diseases that form two ends of a single spectrum. They are both diseases of the elderly and their mean age of onset is 70 years, with a range from 50 to 90 years. Their onset is characteristically dramatic and many patients can give the exact date and hour of their first symptoms. Occasionally the onset is insidious and the symptoms may have been present for months or longer prior to the diagnosis.

Epidemiology

The diseases are relatively uncommon. One study from North America suggested the annual incidence of biopsy-proven giant cell arteritis between 1950 and 1985 in North America was 17 in 100,000 people aged over 50 years.[148] It was approximately three times more frequent in women. Studies from Europe suggest an incidence of 16.8 per 100,000.[149] In the United Kingdom the prevalence of polymyalgic symptoms in people over 65 years of age is approximately 330 per 100,000.[150]

Polymyalgia Rheumatica

The onset usually involves pain and stiffness in the muscles of the shoulder and neck. There is eventual involvement of the pelvic girdles in some patients. The symptoms are bilateral and symmetric. Stiffness is a predominant feature especially after rest or in the morning and usually lasts for longer than 1 hour. Muscle pain is diffuse, movement accentuates the pain, and it can be worse at night. Muscle strength is usually unimpaired although the pain makes testing difficult. There is often an associated synovitis especially of the knees, wrists, and small joints of the hands. It is usually transient and mild and erosive changes are unusual. The arthritis may overlap with rheumatoid disease in the elderly.

Giant Cell Arteritis

Headache is a predominant symptom and is present in a majority of cases (see Ch. 33). It often begins early in the course of the disease and may be a presenting symptom. Pain is severe and localized to the temple. There may be associated scalp tenderness. Visual disturbance is described in about one-quarter of the cases. Visual loss is less common and can involve 5 to 10 percent; blindness remains a significant risk. This is due to involvement of the ophthalmic artery, which is an end artery. Rare features of giant cell arteritis include hemiparesis, peripheral neuropathy, and deafness. Involvement of the coronary artery occasionally leads to myocardial infarction.

Constitutional Symptoms

Both polymyalgia rheumatica and giant cell arteritis are associated with fever, fatigue, anorexia, weight loss, and depression. Occasionally patients present with a fever.

Relationship Between Polymyalgia Rheumatica and Giant Cell Arteritis

Paulley and Hughes,[151] in 1962, were the first to link these two conditions, suggesting polymyalgia has many of the manifestations of temporal arteritis. Since then most authorities recognize the relationship between the two conditions.

Investigations

The ESR is usually but not always elevated and it is unusual to make the diagnosis in the presence of a normal ESR. There is often associated rise in the C-reactive protein levels and a mild anemia. Rheumatoid factor is usually negative. Biopsies of the temporal arteries should be undertaken in cases of giant cell arteritis and if there is diagnostic doubt. These will show the distinctive giant cell arteritis. However, skip lesions mean that a normal biopsy can occur despite the presence of the disease.

Treatment

Corticosteroids are the mainstay of therapy. A high dose of corticosteroids should be used in giant cell arteritis and 60 mg daily is a reasonable initial dose. A lower dose is used in patients with polymyalgia rheumatica of between 10 and 15 mg daily. In both diseases the steroids should be gradually withdrawn over a period of 12 to 18 months. Not all patients respond to steroids alone. Sometimes symptomatic treatment with an NSAID is needed and in some cases an additional disease-modifying drug such as azathioprine or methotrexate can be used. There is some evidence that intramuscular depomedrone may control symptoms with less risk of adverse reactions in polymyalgia rheumatica than conventional steroids and this is an area of ongoing research.

Gout

Gout is a syndrome caused by an inflammatory response to the formation of urate crystals. These crystals develop secondary to hyperuricemia. Gout can occur in both acute and chronic forms. The hyperuricemia may be due to environmental or genetic factors. Although it most frequently affects middle-aged males, there is an increasing frequency in elderly females taking diuretic tablets. The acute form is usually relapsing and self-limiting. The chronic form is associated with tophus formation and bone and joint destruction.

Epidemiology

Hyperuricemia has been investigated in many populations. In males the prevalence of hyperuricemia rises steeply after puberty and in females after the menopause although levels in women are usually lower than in men.[152] It is difficult to determine the precise incidence and prevalence of gout as it is a remitting and relapsing disease and patients frequently are misdiagnosed. It is rare in children and premenopausal women. It is uncommon in men under the age of 30. The peak onset in men is between 40 and 50 years. In women it occurs later. The epidemiology of gout is changing, with an increasing number of females having the disease. This is probably due to changes in lifestyle, drug therapy, and increased longevity. Gout remains the most common inflammatory arthritis in males over 40 years of age.[153] The prevalence of gout is between 5 and 28 per thousand males and 1 and 6 per thousand females. The annual incidence is between 1 and 3 per thousand males and 0.2 per thousand females. The plasma urate concentration is the most important determinant of the risk of developing gout.[154] An important identifiable cause is concomitant thiazide diuretic therapy.

Clinical Features

Asymptomatic hyperuricemia is far more frequent than gout. The risk of gout increases with a rising level of serum uric acid. However, many years of hyperuricemia may precede the onset of acute gout and many individuals with hyperuricemia do not develop the disease. When there is a severe acute overproduction of urate, as for example occurs with cytotoxic chemotherapy, there is a high risk of acute gout.

Acute gout is characterized by the rapid onset of pain, its exquisite nature, and the swelling and associated redness around the affected joint. The classic presentation is in the first metatarsophalangeal joint and in time this is affected in over 80 percent of patients with gout. Many joints may be involved. The lower limbs are involved more frequently than the upper limbs. Redness over the affected joints is a feature that sets gout apart from most other noninfective causes of arthritis. The swelling can be very marked over the entire region. The natural history of acute gout varies: mild attacks may resolve within 1 or 2 days. More severe attacks may last 1 or 2 weeks. Approximately 90 percent of initial attacks of gout are monoarticular. Concurrent features are mild or absent.[155]

Sometimes gout presents early in its course with polyarticular involvement and it can then be easily confused with other forms of arthritis. In the elderly, gout is often more indolent and is frequently mistaken for osteoarthritis, which results in a delay in diagnosis.[156] In elderly people polyarticular gout can be the presenting feature of an attack, especially in elderly women. Acute gout can be precipitated by a variety of factors including acute illness, trauma, surgery, and alcohol and drugs, which increase the uric acid concentration.

Incomplete resolution of acute gout normally indicates a concurrent arthropathy, especially osteoarthritis. However, a substantial proportion of patients with acute gout go on to develop a chronic phase of the disease. This is characterized by the formation of tophi. These are firm nodular or fusiform swellings that can occur at most sites of the body but are especially common on the hands and feet and around the ear. The inflammatory process in chronic gout is often mild although there can be supra added acute episodes. Most of the disability is due to the presence of tophi that can become ulcerated and infected. Long-term problems with chronic gout are usually due to the deposition of tophi in the kidney or other sites; allopurinol therapy (see below) has a role in preventing such renal involvement.

Associated Disorders

Gout is associated with obesity, hypertension with diuretic therapy, excess alcohol intake, hyperlipidemia, and other vascular disorders. There may also be an association with diabetes mellitus.

Investigations

The diagnosis of gout is based on identification of urate crystals in synovial fluid on polarizing light microscopy. This is usually undertaken on fresh synovial fluid. Occasionally material from a gouty tophus can be examined in a similar way.

Serum uric acid concentrations are usually elevated. It is very uncommon for acute gout to occur unless the uric acid level is high. On the other hand an elevated uric acid level does not necessarily mean the patient has gout.

There are often characteristic features on radiography. During an acute attack there may be soft tissue swelling or effusions. Most characteristic features are large erosions that are classically called "punched out" and are some distance from the joint surface. In late disease extensive erosive change may be difficult to differentiate from RA.

Treatment

Therapy in gout is directed toward controlling the symptoms in acute episodes and from preventing further attacks and complications in chronic gout.[157]

The acute episodes of gout normally respond to short-term treatment with relatively large doses of NSAIDs. An example of the dosage of NSAIDs used is to give indomethacin 50 mg qds. Occasionally colchicine is used. This is less satisfactory as it has a therapeutic dose relatively close to the toxic one. Normally 1 mg of colchicine is given initially followed by 0.5 mg every 2 to 3 hours until the attack tends to settle or diarrhea and vomiting occur. An alternative approach is to give intra-articular steroids, which can be very effective in the early stages of gout.

Preventing further episodes of gout is normally achieved by allopurinol. This inhibits the enzyme xanthine oxidase. The dosage varies from 100 to 600 mg daily. It is usual to start with a low dose and build up. The initiation of allopurinol may lead to an acute episode of gout and it is conventional to start allopurinol at the same time as giving NSAID therapy. Allopurinol may make an acute attack of gout worse so it is used subsequent to control of the joint inflammation with NSAIDs. Rarely patients develop hypersensitivity to allopurinol. In these circumstances a uricosuric drug can be used; for example, sulfapyrazone. Treatment in this situation is less satisfactory.

Calcium Pyrophosphate Crystal Deposition Disease

Calcium pyrophosphate crystal deposition disease is associated with calcium pyrophosphate dihydrate crystal deposition. Although it is usually sporadic, there are familial forms and it can be associated with other metabolic disturbances. It is predominantly a disease of the elderly and presents with an acute self-limiting arthritis that is termed *pseudogout*. There is a strong association and overlap with osteoarthritis. It mainly involves the large joints such as the knees and wrists. There is a spectrum of pathology; in some cases there is only chondrocalcinosis, which is the deposition of calcium in articular cartilage, and is usually asymptomatic. In other patients there is more widespread deposition of pyrophosphate crystal deposition disease and an associated synovitis develops. Thus although many patients with pseudogout have chondrocalcinosis, the latter can occur by itself and be asymptomatic or it may be seen against the background of osteoarthritis.

Epidemiology

Chondrocalcinosis has a female preponderance and is associated with aging. It is rare under the age of 50 years. In those aged between 65 to 75 years it affects 10 to 15 percent of the population and over the age of 85 years it affects up to 60 percent of the population.[158] The large population-based radiographic survey from Framingham,[159] which looked at a population ranging in age between 63 and 93 years, found an overall prevalence of 8 percent. No epidemiologic data exist for pyrophosphate arthropathy although it is generally thought to occur in the elderly with a female preponderance. Most studies show that the mean age of presentation is between 65 and 75 years. It is rare in younger cases although occasionally seen. There are many metabolic associations associated including diabetes, anemia, Paget's disease, and hypothyroidism. The strongest association is with hemochromatosis.[160]

Clinical Features

Pyrophosphate crystal deposition disease can occur as an acute synovitis, chronic arthritis, or as an incidental finding. The classic presentation is the acute synovitis of pseudogout, which is the most common cause of an acute monoarthritis in the elderly. The typical attack develops with severe pain, stiffness, and swelling maximal between 6 and 24 hours after the onset. The patient often describes the pain as very severe. There may be overlying erythema. Examination shows a tender joint with signs of marked synovitis such as warmth, a large intense effusion, joint line tenderness, and restriction of movement. Fever is common and this can be marked. Elderly patients often appear unwell and mildly confused. The acute attacks are self-limiting and usually resolve within 1 to 3 weeks.

Chronic pyrophosphate arthropathy is also predominantly found in elderly and female patients. It mainly involves the knees, wrists, and shoulder joints. Presentation is with chronic pain, early morning stiffness, inactivity stiffness, reduced movement, and functional impairment. Acute attacks may be superimposed upon this chronic history. Symptoms are often restricted to just a few joints. Occasionally, multiple joint involvement is seen. Affected joints usually reveal signs of osteoarthritis such as bony swelling, crepitus, and varying degrees of synovitis. Knee joints may be warm with some tenderness, effusion, and soft tissue thickening.

Examination may show more widespread evidence of osteoarthritis. There may also be occasionally more severe inflammatory features and the presentation may develop into pseudo RA, although the infrequency of tenosynovitis and the absence of extra-articular disease normally allows distinction.

Most patients present a benign course and a majority show stabilization of symptoms.[161] Occasionally, progressive severe destructive arthritis may occur, especially involving the knees, shoulders, or hips. This is almost entirely confined to elderly women, usually accompanied by severe night and rest pain and associated with a poor outcome.[162]

Atypical presentations include marked shoulder pain and stiffness that may cause confusion with polymyalgia rheumatica, severe spinal stiffness that may present with similarities to ankylosing spondylitis, tendonitis and tenosynovitis, bursitis, and even tophaceous or tumoral calcium pyrophosphate deposition.

Investigation

Aspiration of synovial fluid and identification of calcium pyrophosphate crystals on microscopy are the key to the diagnosis. The crystals can be difficult to see in some cases and it is usually best to examine fresh synovial fluid.

Standard radiographs show both the osteoarthritic pattern of joint destruction and calcification associated with crystal deposition disease. The latter occurs most commonly in fibrocartilage such as the knee menisci or triangular ligament of the wrist. It can also be seen in hyaline cartilage, particularly the knee and hip joints. Severe pseudogout can trigger a moderate acute phase response with elevation of the ESR and acute phase reactant such as C-reactive protein. The white cell count may also be elevated.

Management

The aspiration of synovial fluid in acute synovitis associated with calcium pyrophosphate crystal deposition disease can markedly improve the initially severe symptoms. Analgesics and NSAIDs are usually given and these also rapidly improve symptoms. Colchicine is effective but rarely warranted. For severe polyarticular attacks unresponsive to aspiration and injection, oral steroids may be considered although their efficacy is unproven. Once synovitis is settling active mobilization with attention to muscle training is worthwhile.

Unlike gout there is no specific therapy for chronic pyrophosphate arthropathy and treatment of the underlying metabolic disease has little effect on outcome. The main objective is to reduce symptoms, and maintain and improve function. Exercise programs, a reduction in obesity, and building up muscle strength are all immensely valuable. If osteoarthritic joint damage is a particular problem, surgical replacement must be considered.

Apatite Deposition Disease

Periarticular deposits of calcific material that are predominantly carbonated apatites or intra-articular deposits of a variety of basic calcium phosphates, also predominantly apatites, are seen in a variety of disease settings. Calcific periarthritis and the acute synovitis associated with apatite deposition have different etiologies and clinical courses but are united by the presence of calcium deposits in bone.

The presence of calcific periarthritis has been recognized for many years. However, the relationship between apatite deposition and joint diseases is more recent and was not described in detail until 1976.[163]

Epidemiology

Calcific periarthritis is relatively common. In one large study of office workers published in the 1940s there was a prevalence of 2.7 percent of shoulder calcification.[164] Subsequent studies have found relatively similar high levels of shoulder calcification. There have been few studies of the epidemiology of articular apatite deposition mainly because the relationship between pathologic and radiologic findings and symptoms of arthritis or the presence of an arthopathy or acute synovitis is uncertain. However, that apatite particles were found in 30 to 60 percent of osteoarthritic synovial fluids may be of some pathologic relevance.[165]

Clinical Features

Calcific deposits around the shoulder and elsewhere are often asymptomatic. They may be associated with a number of clinical syndromes. The most striking presentation is acute calcific periarthritis.[166] Over 70 percent of attacks occur around the shoulder although it may involve other sites. The episode may be preceded by mild trauma or illness but is often spontaneous. Patients present with a sudden onset of severe pain described as "acute hyperalgia." Within hours there is often associated swelling that might be hot and red. There is extreme local tenderness. Movement around the shoulder is very limited. The condition appears to be initiated by a rupture of the calcific deposit leading to crystals being shed into the adjacent periarticular tissues. Sites other than the shoulder that may be involved include the greater trochanter, the epicondyle, the wrist, and around the knee.[167]

Understanding the relationship between intra-articular apatite crystal and clinical symptoms is poor. It is possible that the deposition of apatite in aging articular cartilage is relatively common and usually benign. In some patients there may be an acute synovitis associated with the presence of apatite crystals and this may be a causal relationship. Chronic monoarthritis is also sometimes seen. More commonly apatite crystals are associated with osteoarthritis.[168]

The most important potential relationship is in large joint destructive arthropathies of the elderly. In 1981 McCarty and his colleagues[169] described this entity in some detail and used the term Milwaukee shoulder and suggested the apatite crystals were implicated in much of the damage. Others subsequently confirmed this finding and suggested apatite-associated destructive arthritis may be more descriptive. The clinical picture is characteristic.[170] Patients may or may not have a preceding history of chronic joint disease, they are usually over 70 years of age, and 90 percent are female. They present with a relatively short history over a few weeks and months of increasing pain, swelling, and loss of function of the affected joint which is usually a shoulder. Aspiration of the effusion reveals a large quantity of synovial fluid. It may be blood-stained and apatite crystals are found on evaluation.

Investigations

Plain joint radiology will show the presence of calcific periarthritis or associated changes within the joint. Aspiration and microscopy of the synovial fluid confirms the presence of apatite crystals. Other investigations add little, although alternative imaging modalities including MRI may be advantageous in due course.

Management

If calcific periarthritis or periarticular calcium deposits are found, asymptomatic individuals need no treatment. In an acute attack of calcific periarthritis, high doses of NSAIDs or even colchicine can be used initially. Local steroid injections also have a role although their exact place is controversial as they may increase calcification and make recurrent attacks more likely. Patients with chronic arthritis and osteoarthritis who have apatite deposition must be managed in the same way as the underlying condition. The destructive arthritis associated with Milwaukee shoulder is a difficult management problem. Anti-inflammatory drugs, analgesics, and local steroids have all been used but they are often ineffective. However, as symptoms do appear to be reduced in a majority of patients over a few months, conservative and simple symptomatic measures may eventually allow a resolution of the symptoms to occur as part of the natural history of the disease.

Diffuse Idiopathic Skeletal Hyperostosis

Diffuse idiopathic skeletal hyperostosis (DISH), also known as Forestier's disease, is a ubiquitous condition that predominantly affects the spine. It is a chronic age-related condition characterized by new bone growth. There may be a stiffening peripheral arthropathy. Growth factors, particularly insulin, are implicated in its pathogenesis. It is mainly identified on x-rays, which reveal hyperostosis and an increase in bone mass generally. It is associated with diabetes, gout, hypertension, obesity, and anemia.

Epidemiology

DISH is rare before the age of 45 years and is predominantly a disease of the elderly. In Scandinavia the incidence is estimated at 700 per 100,000 person-years with approximately half the risk in women.[171] Prevalence rates suggest it involves approximately 10 percent of males and 8 percent of females over the age of 65 years.

Clinical Features

DISH is diagnosed principally on radiologic findings. It is characterized by new bone formation with an increased amount of normal bone, heterotopic bone formation, and the presence of new bone growth into the entheses, where tendons, ligaments, joint capsules, and annulus fibrosus fibers insert into bone.[172] This is seen most commonly in the spine, especially the thoracolumbar spine. Other areas of the skeleton are also involved, including phalangeal tufting and increase in size of the sesamoid bones.[173]

The deposition of new bone in DISH is often asymptomatic apart from increased stiffness in the neck, back, and peripheral joints. Pain may be present when there is a peripheral enthesopathy such as a calcaneal spur. The relationship between the radiologic changes and the symptoms of pain is uncertain. DISH is often associated with degenerative hip disease and may modify the skeletal response to inflammatory and traumatic conditions.[174]

Investigations

DISH is diagnosed radiologically. Occasionally associated diseases may be diagnosed such as maturity onset diabetes or hyperlipidemia.

Management

In many cases no specific treatment is needed other than reassuring the patient. In patients where there is obesity or other problems, weight reduction may help. Local tender points can be treated by corticosteroid injections. This is especially true of patients with enthesopathies. Analgesics or anti-inflammatory drugs are of limited value.

Spondyloarthropathies

This group of diseases includes ankylosing spondylitis, reactive arthritis, the arthritis associated with Crohn's disease and ulcerative colitis, Reiter's syndrome, and psoriatic arthritis. These diseases principally involve young men and are rare in the elderly. They are characterized by sacroiliitis and inflammatory back disease and the presence of oligoarthritis involving large joints and occasionally with an enthesopathy.

There are extra-articular features such as uveitis or upper lobe pulmonary fibrosis in ankylosing spondylitis and conjunctivitis and urethritis in Reiter's syndrome. In the elderly some patients may have the end results of pre-existing ankylosing spondylitis but it is very unusual for the disease to present in old age.

Psoriatic arthritis is more frequently seen in the elderly but it still has a peak incidence under the age of 50 years. It is an inflammatory arthritis associated with psoriasis, has a variety of forms including a peripheral polyarthritis, which is a symmetric or inflammatory involvement of the distal phalangeal joints, and uncommonly a characteristic mutilating arthritis associated with telescoping of the fingers.

The treatment of seronegative spondyloarthropathies involves education and advice, analgesia, and anti-inflammatory medication, sulfasalazine and local steroid injections in some patients, and exercise programs in the majority of cases.

References

1. Abrahams M: Three Score Years and Ten. Age Concern, London, 1977
2. Jenkinson ML, Bliss MR, Brain AT, Scott DL: Peripheral arthritis in the elderly: a hospital study. Ann Rheum Dis 1989; 48:227–231
3. Zeidler H: Epidemiology of musculoskeletal conditions in the geriatric population. Eur J Rheumatol Inflamm 1994;14:3–6
4. Gardner DL: The Pathology of Rheumatoid Arthritis. Arnold, London, 1992
5. Panayi GS: The pathogenesis of rheumatoid arthritis: from molecules to the whole patient. Br J Rheumatol 1993;32: 533–536
6. Salmon M, Gaston JS: The role of T-lymphocytes in rheumatoid arthritis. Br Med Bull 1995;51:332–345
7. Bowness P, Bell J. T-cell receptors and rheumatic disease: approaches to repertoire analysis. Br J Rheumatol 1992;31: 3–8
8. Zvaifler NJ, Boyle D, Firestein GS: Early synovitis—synoviocytes and mononuclear cells. Sem Arthritis Rheum 1994; 23(suppl2):11–16
9. Cutolo M, Sulli A, Barone A et al: Macrophages, synovial tissue and rheumatoid arthritis. Clin Exp Rheumatol 1993; 11:331–339
10. Arend WP, Dayer J-M: Cytokines and cytokine inhibitors or antagonists in rheumatoid arthritis. Arthritis Rheum 1990;33: 305–315
11. Dinarello CA: Interleukin-1 and its biologically related cytokines. Adv Immunol 1989;44:153–205
12. Larrick JW: Native interleukin 1 inhibitors. Immunol Today 1989;10:61–66
13. Yocum DE, Esparza L, Dubry S et al: Characteristics of tumour necrosis factor production in rheumatoid arthritis. Cell Immunol 1989;122:131–145
14. Wong GG, Clark SC: Multiple actions of interleukin 6 within a cytokine network. Immunol Today 1988;9:137–139
15. Baggiolini M, Walx A, Kunkel SL: Neutrophil-activating peptide-1/interleukin 8, a novel cytokine which activates neutrophils. J Clin Invest 1989;84:1045–1049
16. Seitz M, Dewald B, Gerber N, Baggiolini M: Preferential production of interleukin-8 in rheumatoid arthritis. Clin Rheumatol 1990;9:569
17. Brennan FM, Field M, Chu CQ et al: Cytokine expression in rheumatoid arthritis. Br J Rheumatol 1991;30(suppl 1):76–80
18. Logan A: Intracrine regulation at the nucleus—a further mechanism of growth factor activity? J Endocrinol 1990;125: 339–343
19. Melnyk VO, Shipley GD, Sternfield MD et al: Synoviocytes synthesize, bind, and respond to fibroblast growth factor. Arthritis Rheum 1990;33:493–500
20. Wahl SM, McCartney-Francis N, Mergenhagen SE: Inflammatory and immunomodulatory roles of TGF-beta. Immunol Today 1989;10:258–261
21. Allen JB, Manthey CL, Hand AR et al: Rapid onset synovial inflammation and hyperplasia induced by transforming growth factor β. J Exp Med 1990;171:231–247
22. Keski-Oja J, Raghow R, Sawdey M et al: Regulation of mRNA's for type-1 plasminogen activator inhibitor, fibronectin, and type I procollagen by transforming growth factor-beta. Divergent responses in lung fibroblasts and carcinoma cells. J Biol Chem 1988;263:3111–3115
23. Deuel TF, Tong BD, Huang JS: Platelet-derived growth factor: structure, function and roles in normal and transformed cells. Curr Top Cell Regul 1985;26:51–64
24. Martinet Y, Bitterman PB, Mornex J-F et al: Activated human monocytes express the c-sis proto-oncogene and release a mediator showing PDGF-like activity. Nature 1986;319:158–160
25. Wilder RL, Sternberg EM: Neuroendocrine hormonal factors in rheumatoid arthritis and related conditions. Curr Opin Rheumatol 1990;2:436–440

26. Sternberg EM, Hill JM, Chrousos GP et al: Inflammatory mediator-induced hypothalamic-pituitary-adrenal axis activation is defective in streptococcal cell wall arthritis susceptible Lewis rats. Proc Natl Acad Sci USA 1989;86:2374–2378

27. Munck A, Guyre PM, Holbrook NJ: Physiological functions of glucocorticoids in stress and their relation to pharmacological actions. Endocrin Rev 1984;5:25–44

28. Springer TA: Adhesion molecules of the immune system. Nature 1990;346:425–434

29. Rouslahti E: Integrins. J Clin Invest 1991;87:1–5

30. Arnout MA: Leucocyte adhesion molecule deficiency: its structural basis, pathophysiology and implications for modulating the inflammatory response. Immunol Rev 1990;114: 145–180

31. Rothlein R, Czajkowski M, O'Niell MM et al: Induction of intercellular adhesion molecule-1 on primary and continuous cell lines by pro-inflammatory cytokines. J Immunol 1988; 141:1665–1669

32. Dougherty GJ, Murdoch S, Hogg N: The function of human intercellular adhesion molecule-1 (ICAM-1) in the generation of an immune response. Eur J Immunol 1988;18:35–40

33. Shimizu Y, Van Seventer GA, Horgan KJ, Shaw S: Role of adhesion molecules in T cell recognition—fundamental similarities between four integrins on resting human T cells (LFA-1, VLA-4, VLA-5, VLA-6) in expression, binding and costimulation. Immunol Rev 1990;114:109–143

34. Lake RA, Morgan A, Henderson B et al: A key role for fibronectin in the sequential binding of native dsDNA and monoclonal anti-DNA antibodies to components of the extracellular matrix: its possible significance in glomerulonephritis. Immunology 1985;54:389

35. Miller EJ: The structure of fibril forming collagens. Ann NY Acad Sci 1985; 460:1–13

36. Linck G, Stocker S, Grimaud J-A et al: Distribution of immunoreactive fibronectin and collagen (type I, II, IV) in mouse joints. Histochemistry 1983;77:323

37. Okada Y, Naka K, Minamoto T et al: R Localization of type VI collagen in the lining cell layer of normal and rheumatoid synovium. Lab Invest 1990;63:647–656

38. Moreland LW, Stewart T, Gay RE et al: Immunohistologic demonstration of type II collagen in synovial fluid phagocytes of osteoarthritis and rheumatoid arthritis patients. Arthritis Rheum 1989;32:1458–1464

39. Miyake K, Underhill CB, Lesley J, Kincade PW: Hyaluronate can function as a cell adhesion molecule and CD44 participates in hyaluronate recognition. J Exp Med 1990;172:69–75

40. Lacy BE, Underhill CB: The hyaluronate receptor is associated with actin filaments. J Cell Biol 1987;105:1395

41. Worrall JG, Bayliss MT, Edwards JCW: Distribution of hyaluronan in rheumatoid synovium. Br J Rheumatol 1989;28 (suppl 2):62

42. Doherty AJP, Murphy G: The metalloproteinase family and the inhibitor TIMP: a study using cDNAs and recombinant proteins. Ann Rheum Dis 1990;49:469–479

43. Okada Y, Nagase H, Harris ED: A metalloproteinase from human rheumatoid synovial fibroblasts that digests connective tissue matrix components. Purification and characterisation. J Biol Chem 1986;261:14245–14255

44. Sellers A, Reynolds JJ, Miekle MC: Neutral metalloproteinases of rabbit bone. Separation in latent forms of distinct enzymes that when activated degrade collagen, gelatin and proteoglycans. Biochem J 1978;171:493–496

45. Murphy G, McAlpine CG, Poll CT, Reynolds JJ: Purification and characterization of a bone metalloproteinase that degrades gelatin and types IV and V collagen. Biochim Biophys Acta 1985;831:49–58

46. Cawston TE: Protein inhibitors of metalloproteinases. pp. 589–610. In Barrett AJ, Salveson G (eds): Protein Inhibitors. Elsevier, Amsterdam, 1986

47. Cawston TE, Mercer E: Preferential binding of collagenase to alpha 2-macroglobulin in the presence of the tissue inhibitor of metalloproteinases. FEBS Lett 1986;209:9–12

48. Grant GA, Eisen AZ, Marmer BL et al: The activation of human skin fibroblast procollagenase. Sequence identification of the major conversion products. J Biol Chem 1987;262: 5886–5889

49. Nagase H, Enghild JJ, Suzuki K, Salvesen G: Stepwise activation mechanisms of the precursor of matrix metalloproteinase-3 (stromelysin) by proteinases and (4-aminophenyl)mercuric acetate. Biochemistry 1990;29:5783–5789

50. Blake DR, Allen R, Lunec J: Free radicals in biological systems—a review orientated to inflammatory processes Br Med Bull 1987;43:371–385

51. McCord JM: Free radicals and inflammation: protection of synovial fluid by superoxide dismutase. Science 1974;185: 529–531

52. Vuorio E, Einola S, Hakkarainen S, Penttinen R: Synthesis of underpolymerised hyaluronic acid by fibroblasts cultured from rheumatoid and non-rheumatoid synovitis. Rheumatol Int 1982;2:97–102

53. Lund-Oleson K: Oxygen tensions in synovial fluids. Arthritis Rheum 1990;13:769–776

54. Woodruff T, Blake DR, Freeman J et al: Is chronic synovitis an example of reperfusion injury? Ann Rheum Dis 1986;45: 608–611

55. McCord JM: Oxygen-derived free radicals in postischemic tissue injury. N Engl J Med 1985;312:159–163

56. Dixon AStJ, Hawkins C (eds): Raised Intra-Articular Pressure—Clinical Consequences. Bath Institute for Rheumatic Diseases, Bath, 1990

57. Jayson MIV, Dixon AStJ: Intra-articular pressure in rheumatoid arthritis of the knee. III. Pressure changes during joint use. Ann Rheum Dis 1970;29:401

58. Blake DR, Merry P, Unsworth J et al: Hypoxic-reperfusion injury in the inflamed human joint. Lancet 1989;1:289–293

59. Spector TD, Woodward L, Hall GM et al: Keratan sulphate in rheumatoid arthritis, osteoarthritis and inflammatory disorders. Ann Rheum Dis 1992;51:1134–1137

60. MacDonald AG, McHenry P, Robins SP, Rid DM: Relationship of urinary pyridinium crosslinks to disease extent and activity in osteoarthritis. Br J Rheumatol 1994;33:16–19

61. Scott DL, Adebajo AO, El-Badaway S et al: Disease controlling anti-rheumatic therapy: preventing or significantly decreasing the rate of progression of structural joint damage. J Rheumatol 1994;41:36–40

62. Regan-Smith MG, O'Connor GT, Kwoh CK et al: Lack of corre-

lation between the Steinbroker staging of hand radiographs and the functional health status of individuals with rheumatoid arthritis. Arthritis Rheum 1989;32:128–133

63. Yanagawa A, Takano K, Nishioka K et al: Clinical staging and gadolinium-DTPA enhanced images of the wrist in rheumatoid arthritis. J Rheumatol 1993;20:781–784
64. Jevtic V, Watt I, Rozman B et al: Precontrast and postcontrast (Gd-DTPA) magnetic resonance imaging of hand joints in patients with rheumatoid arthritis. Clin Radiol 1993;48: 176–181
65. al-Janabi MA: The role of bone scintigraphy and other imaging modalities in knee pain. Nucl Med Commun 1994;15: 991–996
66. Rydgren L, Wollmer P, Hultquist R, Gustafson T: 111-Indium-labelled leukocytes for measurement of inflammatory activity in arthritis. Scand J Rheumatol 1991;20:319–325
67. Deodhar AA, Brabyn J, Jones PW et al: Measurement of hand be one mineral content by dual energy x-ray absorptiometry: development of the method, and its application in normal volunteers and in patients with rheumatoid arthritis. Ann Rheum Dis 1994;53:685–690
68. Edmonds JP, Scott DL, Furst DE et al: Anti-rheumatic drugs: a proposed new classification. Arthritis Rheum 1993;36: 336–339
69. Edmonds JP, Scott DL, Furst DE, Paulus HE: New classification of anti-rheumatic drugs. The evolution of a concept. J Rheumatol 1993;20:585–587
70. Mitchell JA, Akarasereenont P, Theimermann C et al: Selectivity of nonsteroidal antiinflammatory drugs as inhibitors of constitutive and inducible cyclooxygenase. Proc Natl Acad Sci USA 1993;90:11693–11697
71. Ballinger A, Kumar P, Scott DL: Misoprostol and the prevention of gastroduodenal damage due to non-steroidal anti-inflammatory drugs. Ann Rheum Dis 1992;51:1089–1093
72. Dieppe PA, Frankel SJ, Toth B: Is research into the treatment of osteoarthritis with non-steroidal anti-inflammatory drugs misdirected? Lancet 1993;341:353–354
73. Bradley JD, Brandt KD, Katz BP et al: Comparison of an anti-inflammatory dose of ibuprofen, an analgesic dose of ibuprofen, and acetaminophen in the treatment of patients with osteoarthritis of the knee. N Engl J Med 1991;325:87–91
74. Brandt KD: Should nonsteroidal anti-inflammatory drugs be used to treat osteoarthritis? Rheum Dis Clin North Am 1993; 19:29–44
75. Otterness I: The value of C-reactive protein measurement in rheumatoid arthritis. Sem Arthritis Rheum 1994;24:91–103
76. Wilke WS, Sweeney TJ, Calabrese LH: Early, aggressive therapy for rheumatoid arthritis: concerns, descriptions, and estimate of outcome. Sem Arthritis Rheum 1993;23(suppl): 26–41
77. Capell HA, Porter DR, Madhok R, Hunter JA: Second line (disease modifying) treatment in rheumatoid arthritis: which drug for which patient? Ann Rheum Dis 1993;52:423–428
78. Alarcon GS, Lopez-Mendez A, Walter J et al: Radiographic evidence of disease progression in methotrexate treated and nonmethotrexate disease modifying antirheumatic drug treated rheumatoid arthritis patients: a meta-analysis. J Rheumatol 1992;19:1868–1873
79. Dougados M: Cyclosporin in rheumatoid arthritis. Clin Exp Rheumatol 1994;12(suppl 11):S75–78
80. Forre O, the Norwegian Arthritis Study Group: Radiologic evidence of disease modification in rheumatoid arthritis patients treated with cyclosporin: results of a 48-week multicentre study comparing low dose cyclosporin with placebo. Arthritis Rheum 1994;37:1506–1512
81. Tugwell P, Pincus T, Yocum D et al: Combination therapy with cyclosporin and methotrexate in severe rheumatoid arthritis. N Engl J Med 1995;333:137–141
82. Corkill MM, Kirkham BW, Chikanza IC et al: Intra-muscular depot methylprednisolone induction of chrysotherapy in rheumatoid arthritis: a 24 week randomised controlled trial. Br J Rheumatol 1990;29:274–279
83. Hansen TM, Kryger P, Elling H et al: Double blind placebo controlled trial of pulse treatment with methylprednisolone combined with disease modifying drugs in rheumatoid arthritis. BMJ 1990;301:268–270
84. Kirwan J: The effect of glucocorticoids on joint destruction in rheumatoid arthritis. N Engl J Med 1995;333:142–146
85. Hall GM, Daniels M, Doyle DV, Spector TD: Effect of hormone replacement therapy on bone mass in rheumatoid arthritis patients treated with and without steroids. Arthritis & Rheum 1994;37:1499–1505
86. Symmons DPM, Barrett EM, Bankhead CR et al: The incidence of rheumatoid arthritis in the United Kingdom: results from the Norfolk Arthritis Register. Br J Rheumatol 1994;33: 735–739
87. Silman AJ, Hochberg MC: Epidemiology of the Rheumatic Diseases. Oxford University Press, Oxford, 1994
88. Engel A, Roberts J, Burch TA: Rheumatoid arthritis in adults: United States, 1960–1962. Vital and Health Statistics, National Centre for Health Statistics, DHEW, Series 11, No 17, 1966
89. Fleming A, Crown JM, Corbett M: Early rheumatoid disease. I. Onset. Ann Rheum Dis 1976;35:357–360
90. Fleming A, Crown JM, Corbett M: Incidence of joint involvement in early rheumatoid arthritis. Rheumatol Rehab 1976; 15:92–96
91. Schumacher HR: Palindromic onset of rheumatoid arthritis. Arthritis Rheum 1982;25:361–369
92. Scott DGI, Bacon PA, Tribe CR: Systemic rheumatoid vasculitis: a clinical and laboratory study of 50 cases. Medicine 1981; 60:288–296
93. Felson DT, Andersen JJ, Boers M et al: The American College of Rheumatology preliminary core set of disease activity measures for rheumatoid arthritis clinical trials. Arthritis Rheum 1993;36:729–740
94. Prevoo ML, van Riel PL, van-'t HofMA et al: Validity and reliability of joint indices. A longitudinal study in patients with recent onset rheumatoid arthritis. Br J Rheumatol 1993; 32:589–594
95. Stewart MW, Palmer DG, Knight RG: A self-report articular index measure of arthritic activity; investigations of reliability, validity and sensitivity. J Rheumatol 1990;17:1011–1015
96. Stucki G, Stucki S, Bruhlmann P et al: Comparison of the validity of self-reported articular indices Br J Rheumatol 1995; 34:760–766

97. van der Heijde DMFM, van't HofMA, van Riel PLCM et al: Judging disease activity in clinical practice in rheumatoid arthritis: first step in the development of a disease activity score. Ann Rheum Dis 1990;49:916–920

98. Davis MJ, Dawes PT, Fowler PD et al: Comparison and evaluation of a disease activity index for use in patients with rheumatoid arthritis. Br J Rheumatol 1990;29:111–115

99. Mallya RAK, Mace BEW: The assessment of disease activity in rheumatoid patients using a multivariate analysis. Rheumatol Rehabil 1982;20:14–17

100. Sharp JT, Lidsky MD, Collins LC et al: Methods of scoring the progression of radiological changes in rheumatoid arthritis. Arthritis Rheum 1971;14:706–720

101. Larsen A, Dale K, Eek M: Radiographic evaluation of rheumatoid arthritis and related conditions by standard reference films, Acta Radiol (Diagn) 1977;18:481–491

102. Grindulis KA, Scott DL, Struthers GR: The assessment of radiological changes in the hands and wrists in rheumatoid arthritis. Rheumatol Int 1983;3:39–42

103. van der Heijde DM, van Leeuwen MA, van Riel PL et al: Biannual radiographic assessments of hands and feet in a three year follow up of patients with early rheumatoid arthritis, Arthritis Rheum 1992;35:26–34

104. Scott DL, Coulton BL, Popert AJ: Long term progression of joint damage in rheumatoid arthritis. Ann Rheum Dis 1986;45:373–378

105. Fries J, Spitz P, Young D: The dimensions of health outcomes: the Health Assessment Questionnaire disability and pain scales. J Rheumatol 1982;9:789–793

106. Meenan R, Gertman P, Mason J: Measuring health status in arthritis: the Arthritis Impact Measurement Scales, Arthritis Rheum 1980;23:146–152

107. Fitzpatrick R, Fletcher A, Gore S et al: Quality of life measures in health care: 1. Applications and issues in assessment BMJ 1992;305:1074–1077

108. Fitzpatrick R, Ziebland S, Jenkinson C et al: A comparison of the sensitivity to change of several health status instruments in rheumatoid arthritis. J Rheumatol 1993;20:429–936

109. Fitzpatrick R, Ziebland S, Jenkinson C et al: Transition questions to assess outcomes in rheumatoid arthritis. Br J Rheumatol 1993;32:807–811

110. Isomaki HA: An epidemiologically based follow-up study of recent arthritis. Incidence, outcome and classification. Clin Rheumatol 1987;6(suppl 2):53–59

111. van-Schaardenburg D, Hazes JM, de Boer A: Outcome of rheumatoid arthritis in relation to age and rheumatoid factor at diagnosis. J Rheumatol 1993;20:45–52

112. Hassell AB, Davis MJ, Fowler PD: The relationship between serial measures of disease activity and outcome in rheumatoid arthritis. QJ Med 1993;86:601–607

113. Kaarela K: Prognostic factors and diagnostic criteria in early rheumatoid arthritis. Scand J Rheumatol Suppl 1985;57:1–54

114. Silman AJ, Reeback J, Jaraquemada D: HLA-DR4 as a predictor of outcome three years after onset of rheumatoid arthritis, Rheumatol Int 1986;6:233–235

115. van der Heijde DM, van't HofMA, van Riel PL et al: Validity of single variables and composite indices for measuring disease activity in rheumatoid arthritis. Ann Rheum Dis 1992;51:177–181

116. Emery P: Assessment of rheumatoid arthritis—a clinician's viewpoint. J Rheumatol 1994;42(suppl):20–24

117. van Zeben D, Hazes JM, Zwinderman AH et al: Factors predicting outcome of rheumatoid arthritis: results of a follow-up study. J Rheumatol 1993;20:1288–1296

118. Corbett M, Dalton S, Young A et al: Factors predicting death, survival and functional outcome in a prospective study of early rheumatoid disease over fifteen years. Br J Rheumatol 1993;32:717–723

119. Pincus T: The paradox of effective therapies but poor long-term outcomes in rheumatoid arthritis. Sem Arthritis Rheum 1992;21(suppl 3):2–15

120. Scott DL, Symmons DPM, Coulton BL, Popert AJ: The long-term outcome of treating rheumatoid arthritis: results after 20 years. Lancet 1987;1:1108–1111

121. Suarez-Almazor ME, Soskolne CL, Saunders LD, Russell AS: Outcome in rheumatoid arthritis. A 1985 inception cohort study. J Rheumatol 1994;21:1438–1446

122. Wolfe F, Mitchell DM, Sibleg J et al: The mortality of 3501 persons with rheumatoid arthritis in the ARAMIS data banks. Arthritis Rheum 1991;34(suppl):D109

123. Acheson RM, Collart AB: New Haven survey of joint diseases. XVII. Relationship between some systemic characteristics and osteoarthrosis in a general population. Ann Rheum Dis 1975;34:379–387

124. Croft P: Osteoarthritis: review of UK data on the rheumatic diseases. Br J Rheumatol 1990;29:391–395

125. Gardner DL: Problems and paradigms in joint pathology, review. J Anat 1994;184(Pt 3):465–476

126. Van Saase JLCM, van Romunde LKJ, Cats A et al: Epidemiology of osteoarthritis: Zoetmeer survey. Comparison of radiological osteoarthritis in a Dutch population with that in 10 other populations. Ann Rheum Dis 1989;48:271–280

127. Felson DT: The epidemiology of osteoarthritis: results from the Framingham Osteoarthritis Study. Semin Arthritis Rheum 1990;20(suppl 1):42–50

128. Wilson MG, Michet CJ, Ilstrup DM, Melton LJ: Idiopathic symptomatic osteoarthritis of the hip and knee: a population-based incidence study. Mayo Clin Proc 1990;65:1214–1221

129. Felson DT, Zhang Y, Hannan MT et al: The incidence and natural history of knee osteoarthritis in the elderly. The Framingham Osteoarthritis Study. Arthritis Rheum 1995;38:1500–1505

130. Bellamy N, Wells G, Campbell J: Relationship between severity and clinical importance of symptoms in osteoarthritis. Clin Rheumatol 1991;10:138–143

131. Doyle DV, Dieppe PA, Scott J, Huskisson EC: An articular index for the assessment of osteoarthritis. Ann Rheum Dis 1981;40:75–78

132. Altman RD, Bloch DA, Bole Jr GG et al: Development of clinical criteria for osteoarthritis. J Rheumatol 1987;suppl 14:3–6

133. McAlindon T, Dieppe P: Osteoarthritis: definitions and criteria. Ann Rheum Dis 1989;48:531–532

134. McAlindon T, Dieppe P: The medical management of osteoar-

thritis of the knee: an inflammatory issue? Br J Rheumatol 1990;29:471–473

135. Cushnahan J, Dieppe PA: Study of 500 patients with limb joint osteoarthritis. I. Analysis by age, sex and distribution of symptomatic joint sites. Ann Rheum Dis 1991;50:8–13

136. Rosenberg ZS, Shankman S, Steiner GC et al: Rapid destructive osteoarthritis: clinical, radiographic, and pathologic features. Radiology 1992;182:213–216

137. Brandt KD: A pessimistic view of serologic markers for diagnosis and management of osteoarthritis. Biochemical immunologics and clinicopathologic barriers. J Rheumatol 1989;18: 39–42

138. Kellgren JH, Lawrence JS: Radiological assessment of osteoarthrosis. Ann Rheum Dis 1957;16:494–502

139. Altman R, Asch E, Bloch D et al: Development of criteria for the classification and reporting of osteoarthritis: classification of osteoarthritis of the knee. Arthritis Rheum 1986;29: 1039–1049

140. Altman RD, Fries JF, Bloch DA et al: Radiographic assessment of progression in osteoarthritis. Arthritis Rheum 1987; 30:1214–1225

141. Cooper C, Cushnaghan J, Kirwan J et al: Radiographic assessment of the knee joint in osteoarthritis. Br J Rheumatol 1990; 29:37

142. Voltanen EJ: Clinical comparison of triamcinolone hexacetonide and betamethasone in the treatment of osteoarthrosis of the knee joint. Scand J Rheumatol 1981;suppl 4:1–7

143. Chandler GN, Wright V: Deleterious effects of intra-articular hydrocortisone. Lancet 1958;2:661–663

144. Balch HW, Gibson JMC, El Ghobereg AF et al: Repeated corticosteriod injections into knee joints. Rheumatol Rehab 1977;16:137–140

145. Docherty M, Deippe PA: Effect of intra-articular Yttrium-90 (90Y) on chronic pyrophosphate arthropathy (CPA) of the knee. Ann Rheum Dis 1981;40:626

146. Dixon AS: Clinical trial of hyaluronate in patients with osteoarthritis of the knee. Curr Med Res Op 1988;11:205–213

147. Dawes PT, Kirlew C, Haslock I: Saline washout for knee OA: results of controlled study. Clin Rheumatol 1987;6:61–63

148. Machedo EBV, Michet CJ, Ballard DJ et al: Trends and incidence in clinical presentation of temporal arteritis. Olmsted Country, Minnesota 1950–85. Arthritis Rheum 1988;31: 745–749

149. Nordberg E, Bengtsson BA: Epidemiology of biopsy proven giant cell arteritis. J Intern Med 1990;227:233–236

150. Kyle V, Silverman B, Silman A et al: Polymyalgia rheumatica, giant cell arteritis and general practice. BJM 1985;13: 385–388

151. Paulley JW, Hughes JP: Giant cell arteritis or arthritis of the aged. BMJ 1962;15:62–67

152. Mikkelsen WM, Dodge HJ, Valkenburgh Hiems S: The distribution of serum uric acid value in a population unselected as to gout or hyperuricaemia. Ann J Med 1965;39:242–251

153. Rubenoff R: Gout and hyperuricaemia. Rheum Dis Clin North Am 1990;16:539–550

154. Campion VW, Glynn RG, DeLabre LO: Asymptomatic hyperuricaemia. Am J Med 1987;82:421–426

155. Lawry GV, Fan BT, Blueston ER: Polyarticular versus monoarticular gout; the prospective comparative analysis of clinical features. Medicine (Baltimore) 1988;67:335–343

156. Tear Borg EJ, Rasker JJ: Gout in the elderly: a separate entity? Ann Rheum Dis 1987;46:72–76

157. Wallace SL, Singer JZ: Therapy in gout. Rheum Dis Clin North Am 1988;14:441–447

158. Doherty M, Dieppe PA: Clinical aspects of calcium pyrophosphate dihydrate deposition. Rheum Dis Clin North Am 1988; 14:395–414

159. Felson DT, Anderson JJ, Naimarka Cannel W, Meenan RF: The prevalence of chondrocalcinosis in the elderly and its associations with knee osteoarthritis: the Framingham study. J Rheumatol 1989;16:1241–1245

160. Hamilton EBD: Diseases associated with CPPD deposition disease. Arthritis Rheum 1976;19:353–357

161. Mayer RA, Bush DC, Harrington TM: Acute calcific tendonitis of the hand and writs. J Rheumatol 1989;16:198–202

162. Pinals RS, Short CL: Calcific periarthritis involving multiple sites. Arthritis Rheum 1966;9:566–574

163. Dieppe PA, Huskisson EC, Crocker P, Willoughby DA: Appetite deposition disease: a new arthopathy. Lancet 1976;1: 266–269

164. Boswood BM: Calcium deposits in the shoulder and sub acromial bursitis. A survey of 12,222 shoulders. JAMA 1941;116: 2477–2482

165. Halverson P, McCarty DJ: Identification of hydroxy apatite crystals in synovial fluid arthritis. Arthritis Rheum 1979;22: 389–395

166. Swannel AJ, Underwood FA, Dixon AStJ: Periarticular calcific deposits mimicking acute arthritis. Ann Rheum Dis 1970;29: 380–385

167. Mayer RA, Bush DC, Harrington TM: Acute calcific tendonitis of the hands and wrists. J Rheumatol 1989;16:198–202

168. Deippe PA, Watt I: Crystal deposition in osteoarthritis. An opportunistic event. Clin Rheum Dis 1985;11:367–391

169. McCarty DJ, Halverson PB, Carrera GF et al: Milwaukee shoulder association of microsteroids containing hydroxyapaetite crystals, active collaginase and neutral protease with rotator cuff defects. Arthritis Rheum 1981;24:464–491

170. Campion GV, McCrae F, Alwan W et al: Idiopathic destructive arthritis of the shoulder. Semin Arthritis Rheum 1988;70: 232–245

171. Julkunen H, Heinoneno P, Knekt P, Maatela J: The epidemiology of hyperostosis of the spine together with its symptoms in related mortality in a general population. Scand J Rheumatol 1973;45:81–91

172. Littlejohn GO: More emphasis on the enthesis. J Rheumatol 1989;16:1020–1022

173. Littlejohn GO, Urowitz MB, Smythe HA, Keystone EC: Radiographic features of the hands in diffuse idiopathic skeletal hyperostosis (DISH): a comparative study with normals and acromegalics. Radiology 1981;140:623–629

174. Arlet J, Jacqueline F, Depeyre M et al: Le hanche dans l'hyperostose vertebrale. Rev Rheumal Osteoartic 1978;45:17–26

C H A P T E R 8 3

Connective Tissue Disease

A. J. FREEMONT

The term *connective tissues* encompasses a wide variety of different body materials, derived from mesoderm that support mammalian organs and tissues physically and chemically.[1] The majority consist of a matrix of insoluble complexed proteins,[2] the most abundant of which is collagen, in which are embedded cells. The main connective tissues are bone, cartilage, fibrous tissue, smooth and skeletal muscle, and fat. By and large the proportional volume of cells to matrix is less than 50 percent. The one major exception to these generalizations is adipose tissue in which the apparent matrix, fat, is intracellular.

The age-related changes in connective tissues have already been described (Chs. 7, 78, and 80). These changes clearly contribute to the pathology of the tissue, although there must always be debate as to the contribution of "age related",[3,4] and "non-age-related" phenomena to any perceived pathology, and, indeed, whether an appearance should be assessed as being "pathologic" relative to the "young normal" or "age-related normal".[5]

Diseases of three of the connective tissues, bone (Ch. 81), articular cartilage (Ch. 82), and skeletal muscle (Ch. 80) together with some of the consequences that result from alterations in the connective tissue components of elements of the cardiovascular system (Ch. 19) have already been described in detail and blood (Ch. 89) and skin (of which connective tissue is an important part, see Ch. 91) are discussed later. They will not be discussed here. This chapter concentrates on the common disorders of those connective tissues not already covered and their associations with aging.

There is a very marked relationship between certain types of connective tissue disease and age. Most of the disorders of connective tissues have their highest incidence in the young and middle-aged. If they are not the cause of significant mortality, these disorders can continue into the older age groups; however, these are not the diseases specific to old age. The number of connective tissue disorders, or their variants, that characteristically have an onset in the elderly age group rather than any other age groups is surprisingly small.

The reasons why certain connective tissue diseases arise in the elderly are not known. The discussion in Chapter 7 of the effects of aging on connective tissues may give some clues, but there are as many anomalies. Why, for instance, should one form of fibroblastic proliferation, Dupuytren's disease, be common in the elderly age group, when another, keloid, is not? Why does the incidence and range of malignant epithelial neoplasms increase in this age group whereas the diversity of malignant connective tissue neoplasms is so low?

In this chapter only those disorders characterized by a peak age of onset in the elderly age group are discussed. By necessity it cannot be exhaustive or comprehensive but highlights important issues and diseases affecting elderly people.

Nonmetabolic Diseases of Bone

The major nonmetabolic diseases of bone are fracture, osteomyelitis, Paget's disease, avascular bone necrosis, and bone neoplasms.

Fracture

There is a higher incidence of metastasizing neoplasms in the elderly. Such metastases often produce factors that stimulate osteoclasts leading to local osteopenia. This, together with the effects of osteoporosis, both in men and women, lead to a high incidence of pathologic fracture in this age group.[6] These disorders are dealt with in more detail elsewhere.

Osteomyelitis

With age, the decrease in native immunity increases the risk of developing infection. Osteomyelitis is an infection in bone marrow that usually reaches the bone by hematogenous spread from a primary site elsewhere.[7] In the elderly population, as in other age groups, the most common organism causing pyogenic osteomyelitis is *Staphylococcus aureus*. Mycobacterial infections, particularly of the spine, are increasingly common.

The inflammatory process is destructive, giving rise to loss of bone and increased risk of fracture. Inflammatory cells produce digestive enzymes that destroy bone directly and stimulate osteoclasts. If the inflammation breaks out of bone, non-osteoclast-mediated tissue degradation may result in damage to adjacent structures, such as the intervertebral discs in the spine, and articular structures in the synovial joints.

Paget's Disease

Paget's disease (see also Ch. 81) is a disorder of unknown etiology that causes an increase in the size of one or, rarely, more than one bone. Although sometimes classified with the metabolic bone disease, which are generalized skeletal disorders, it is this one characteristic of the disease that shows it as a separate entity. It is believed to develop slowly, manifesting itself predominantly in the elderly.[8] Initially, perhaps in every case, there is a decrease in bone mass, which is only later followed by an increase. Only in the late stages do clinical features usually manifest themselves. Even then probably as few as 10 percent of affected individuals present clinically.

Etiology and pathology

The incidence varies widely in Britain, being greatest in northwest England where at postmortem as many as 10 percent of individuals over 70 years of age show histologic changes of the disease. Histologically there is a generalized increase in bone cell activity that, in severe cases, leads to disruption of the normal lamellar structure of the collagen fiber arrays and uncoupling of osteoblastic and osteoclastic activity.[9] Together these two factors lead to the laying down of excessive quantities of weak bone. The bone marrow is very vascular and the normal hemopoietic marrow is replaced by fibrous tissue. By electron microscopy the osteoblasts are seen to contain viral particles, and modern research techniques, including immunohistochemistry and in situ hybridization, have shown that all bone cells are infected by a virus (Fig. 83-1 see also Plate 83-1). There is considerable controversy over the nature of this virus, which has been identified variously as measles, respiratory syncytial virus, and canine distemper virus.[10] Recent studies have shown that the viral infection causes profound changes in the function of osteoclasts and particularly their responsiveness to interleukin (IL)-6.[11] The implication of these findings indicates that the disease process is driven by inadequately controlled osteoclasts that are driving themselves through a viral-mediated novel autocrine loop.

Clinical features, diagnosis, and management

The abnormal bone matrix leads to weakness that manifests as bone pain and fracture.[12] The increased bone cell turnover, particularly of the osteoblast lineage, causes an increased risk of developing bone malignancies, most commonly osteosarcoma. The high vascularity within the affected bone or bones can, particularly in the elderly and others with poor cardiac function, lead to high output cardiac failure.[13]

The excessive bone cell activity causes an increase in the serum alkaline phosphatase and urinary collagen breakdown products. The bone itself is thicker, both clinically and radiologically, and the skin over the bone is warm to touch. As the disease is driven by the osteoclast, symptomatic relief can be obtained by the use of drugs that suppress osteoclast function, notably bisphosphonates and calcitonin.[14]

Avascular Bone Necrosis

With the exception of that form of avascular bone necrosis that follows fracture of the femoral neck or the carpal scaphoid there is no form of avascular bone necrosis that particularly affects the elderly population.[15]

Cartilage

Most cartilage is present within joints, either the articular surfaces of the synovial joints, or cartilaginous joints (e.g., the costosternal joints). The disease of these structures have been

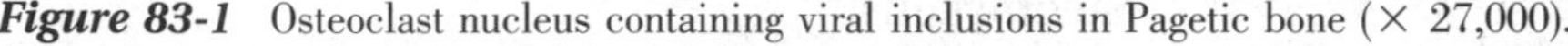

Figure 83-1 Osteoclast nucleus containing viral inclusions in Pagetic bone (× 27,000).

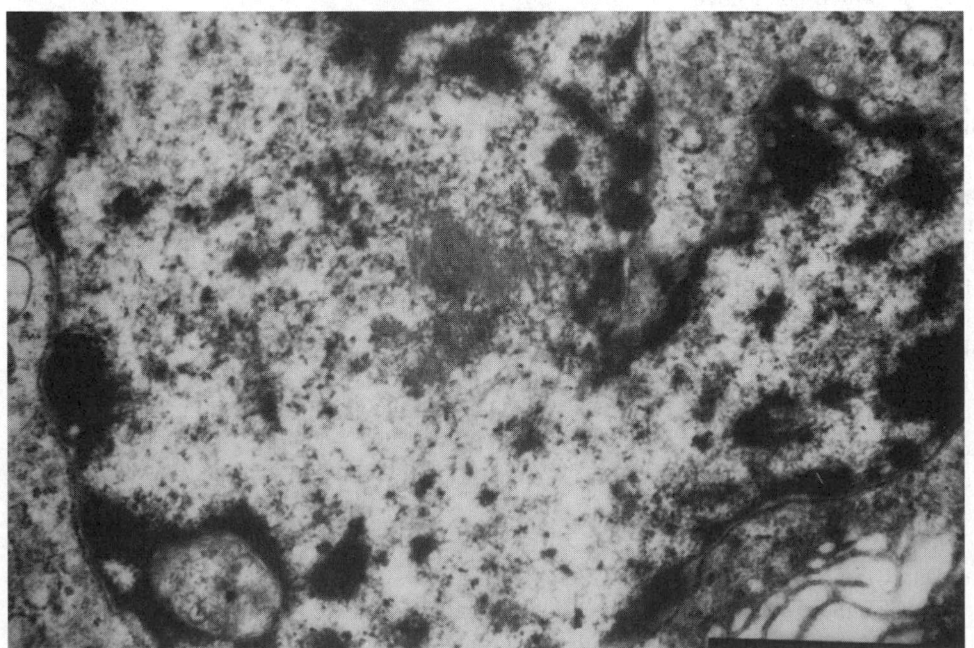

covered in the preceding chapter. Cartilage is present outside the joints mainly within the upper respiratory tract and the pinnae. There are few disorders of these cartilages and the most common, chondrosarcoma and relapsing polychondritis, are not disorders specifically of the elderly population.

The cartilage does, however, change its physical properties with age. As the water content increases so the compliance decreases.[16] In addition there is progressive dystrophic calcification and even ossification that can affect the function and load response characteristics of these tissues.[17] Finally crystals other than hydroxyapatite, such as monosodium urate and calcium pyrophosphate, can be deposited within this cartilage (see below).

Fibrous Tissue, Ligaments, and Tendons

Disorders of fibrous tissue, particularly the organized fibrous tissues of ligaments and tendons, are very common. They include proliferations such as keloid and the fibromatoses; trauma, either to the structure itself or to its insertion into bone (the enthesis); myxoid degeneration (ganglion formation); and metaplasia.

Keloid

Because of the changes that occur in fibroblast function with age, keloid[18] is rare in the elderly population, even in those ethnic groups in which it is most frequently encountered. The same applies to other fibrotic disorders such as Morton's metatarsalgia.

Dupuytren's Disease

Dupuytren's disease[19] is a disorder in which there is a nodular proliferation of fibroblasts within the palmar fascia and its digital extensions leading to dense collagen deposition, thickening and contracture within the fascia, and permanent deformity of the adjacent finger.[20]

Etiology and pathology

Many theories have been put forward to explain Dupuytren's disease. They include changes induced by mast cell and epidermal chemical mediators, alterations in the vasculature, and paraneoplastic changes in DNA. None has been unequivocally accepted.

Within the palmar fascia the fibroblastic proliferation is focal leading to small nodules of very active fibroblasts (Fig. 83-2; see also Plate 83-2). The nodular proliferation flits from area to area of the fascia resulting in a generalized increase in collagen deposition. As the collagen "matures," internal fiber cross-linking leads to an overall reduction in fiber length and consequent contracture.[21]

Clinical features, diagnosis, and management

The patient complains of a slowly progressive, painless nodule in the fascia that, as it worsens, shortens the affected ligament causing further thickening and fascial contracture. Each fascial slip is attached to a finger and the contracture leads to a permanent flexion deformity of the digit.

The clinical presentation is diagnostic, and so too are the biopsy appearances. Surgical excision is the treatment of choice, but the potential progression of the disease is not af-

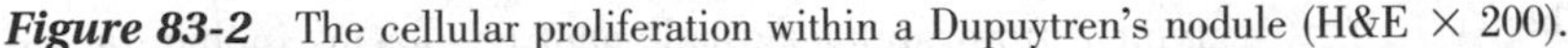

Figure 83-2 The cellular proliferation within a Dupuytren's nodule (H&E × 200).

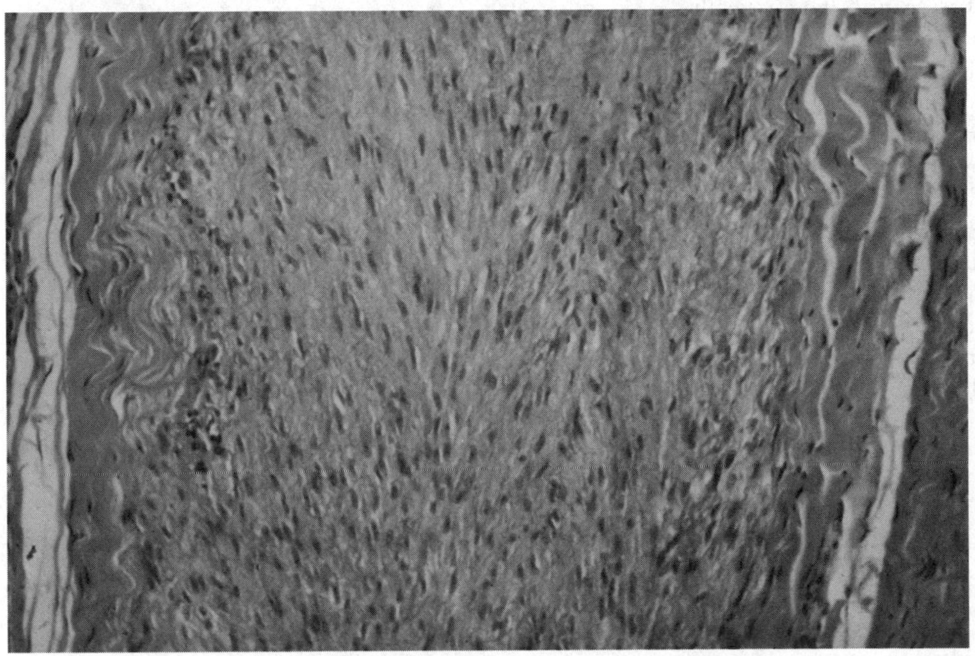

fected. The pathogenesis is unknown, indeed puzzling, as the fibroblast proliferation is difficult to reconcile with the behavior of skin fibroblasts from older people, which divide more slowly than those from younger individuals in vitro. There are other forms of non-neoplastic proliferation of fibroblasts within fascia, such as nodular fasciitis, proliferative fasciitis, and plantar fibromatosis (Lederhose's disease), but they all typically affect younger people.

Trauma

One consequence of alterations in fibroblast function with age is abnormal deposition and polymerization of collagen.[22] In addition, with increasing age, there is fatty infiltration of ligaments. Together these factors predispose elderly people to an increased risk of complete and partial ligamentous tears. The general decrease in excessive physical activity counters this risk to some extent as does the very high degree of cross-linking (and therefore increased strength) of the older collagen fibers.

Enthesopathies

Enthesopathy is the name given to a disparate group of disorders that occur at the entheses. The most striking of these are the inflammatory enthesopathies, seen in ankylosing spondylitis (AS)[23] and rheumatoid arthritis (RA).[24] Active enthesopathic AS is not a disease of elderly people and RA has been discussed previously. There are two other major causes of enthesopathy, hyperparathyroidism and trauma. Although the incidence of primary hyperparathyroidism peaks in elderly women, it is a mild form of the disease and the abnormal activity of the parathyroid glands is brought under control by an early resetting of the homeostatic mechanisms while the serum calcium is still within the normal range. There is therefore little of the bone erosion that is seen in the classically described histologic feature of the disease. In more severe disease hyperosteoclasis at the enthesis can weaken the insertion, leading to pain and ligament failure.

The changes in the collagen structure of the ligament/tendon and in the cartilage and bone at the enthesis make the incidence of partial or complete physical failure during exercise much higher in the increasingly fit elderly population.

Traumatic damage and even avulsion leads to a repair process with the development of bone outgrowths called traction spurs particularly at sites of maximum load, the insertion of the plantar fascia into the calcaneum, the insertion of the Achilles tendon, and the insertions of the long ligaments of the spine into the vertebral bodies.

Elastosis

An increase in elastic fibers is a common feature of the skin of elderly persons,[25] It happens in other connective tissues, notably cartilage. Its significance in disease terms is not known.

Adipose Tissue

The major disorders of fat, other than changes in its amount and distribution and the effects of trauma, are the inflammatory disorders, of fat itself and its septal known as panniculitis and neoplasms.[26] These are not disorders specifically of the elderly population.

Neoplasms of Connective Tissue

The most common neoplasms, generally, of the connective tissues[27,28] are secondary malignant tumors; as the incidence of primary malignancies increases with age, so too does the number of secondary neoplasms within connective tissues. The bone, or more accurately the bone marrow, is a common site of secondary epithelial malignancies, most commonly from primaries in the breast, bronchus, prostate, bowel, thyroid, and kidney.

Hemic neoplasms, leukemias, lymphomas, and myeloma also metastasize to or arise within bone marrow and other connective tissues, where they may mimic secondary carcinomas. In bone tumor, cell production of cytokines stimulates bone cells (most commonly osteoclasts, but more rarely osteoblasts[29]) leading to local changes in bone mass. Increased osteoclasis leads to local bone loss and increased risk of fracture.

Although many benign and malignant connective tissue neoplasms are seen in the elderly population, it is only very rare primary benign and malignant connective tissue neoplasms that have their peak incidence in this age group. Some, such as lipoma, persist if not treated, and therefore appear to increase in incidence with age, but there are others that are truly neoplasms of the elderly.[30] "Benign" neoplasms include atypical fibroxanthoma; malignant neoplasms include malignant fibrous histiocytoma, cutaneous angiosarcoma, and osteosarcoma arising in Paget's disease.

Atypical Fibroxanthoma

Atypical fibroxanthoma is a neoplasm that occurs principally on the actinic-damaged skin of the head and neck of elderly persons. It is not really correct to place it with benign neoplasms as its local behavior and histologic appearances are indistinguishable from malignant fibrous histiocytoma (see below). It responds exceptionally well to local excision.

Malignant Fibrous Histiocytoma

Malignant fibrous histiocytoma is the most common sarcoma of late adult life and is found predominantly in the skeletal muscle of the extremities or in the retroperitoneum.

Etiology and pathology

Malignant fibrous histiocytoma can be caused by radiation, but most cases are idiopathic. the tumor varies in size depending on site and growth rate. It is typically solitary and multilob-

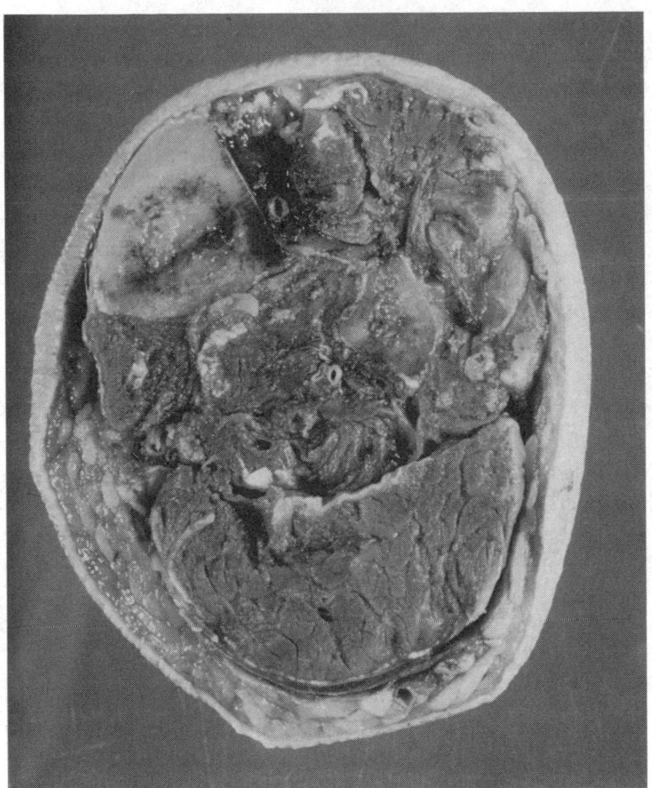

Figure 83-3 A macroscopic image of a malignant fibrous histiocytoma. Diameter approximately 5 cm.

ulated but may spread long distances along fascial planes (Fig. 83-3; see also plate 83-3). It may be firm or myxoid and contains areas of hemorrhage and necrosis. Histologically it consists of spindle-shaped cells arranged in a cartwheel or storiform pattern with scattered multinucleate cells. The spindle cells have an indeterminate phenotype whereas the multinucleate cells react with macrophage markers. The cell of origin of this neoplasm has yet to be determined. Malignant Fibrous histiocytoma metastasizes predominantly to the lungs (82 percent). The 2-year survival is 60 percent but of the survivors one-third will be expected to have a recurrence or metastasis.

Clinical features, diagnosis, and management

The patient usually presents with a painless swelling of a few months duration. The diagnosis is suggested by magnetic resonance imaging and made by biopsy. Wide local excision is the treatment of choice.

Cutaneous Angiosarcoma

Unlike other forms of angiosarcoma, cutaneous angiosarcoma primarily affects the elderly.

Etiology and pathology

The neoplasm arises on the head and neck, raising the possibility of sun exposure as a causative agent. The tumor consists of irregularly shaped vascular channels lined by atypical endothelial cells. About 40 percent of patients die of their disease. Metastasis is to the lung and liver.

Clinical features, diagnosis, and management

The neoplasm presents as small nodules resembling blood blisters or blue red macules. The lesions are often multiple and painless but may later ulcerate and bleed.

The tumors respond only poorly to radiotherapy, and wide local excision, the treatment of choice, is often very difficult on the face, head, and neck.

Paget's Sarcoma

Malignant change within a stem line occurs as a consequence of mutation within replicating DNA. The change of mutation is a function of the rate of replication of the stem cell line. In Paget's disease excessive production of cytokines induces rapid stem cell recruitment, particularly in the cells of the osteoblast lineage. As a consequence the opportunity for malignant transformation of osteoprogenitor stem cells is high. Approximately 1 in 40 of all patients with Paget's disease will develop a sarcoma within the affected bone and the overwhelming majority will be osteosarcomas.

Immune Mediated Connective Tissue Disorders

This group of clinicopathologic entities is characterized by an immune response against "self-antigens" leading to damage to "connective tissues" and blood vessels in multiple organs, notably joints, skin, glomeruli, and large and small blood vessels. Pathogenetically all these disorders exhibit immune complex deposition, and/or formation, within affected organs (usually on basement membranes) and consequent tissue damage. The intriguing thing about these disorders is that the balance of the organs affected by the disease process varies from condition to condition, so that in rheumatoid disease the joints are most commonly and severely affected, whereas in polyarteritis nodosa it is the blood vessels and in systemic lupus erythematosus, the skin and kidney.

Clinically all the "connective tissue diseases" are associated with nonspecific constitutional disturbances coupled with patterns of organ involvement and circulating antigens that determine the clinical designation. The major members of this group are rheumatoid disease, systemic lupus erythematosus, the vasculitides (including polyarteritis nodosa and giant cell arteritis), systemic sclerosis, and polymyositis.

Like all autoimmune diseases they most commonly present in young adult women. Some diseases, such as rheumatoid disease, which was discussed in Chapter (82), can present at any age and in the elderly may have a different presentation and course from that in the young. Others, notably giant cell arteritis and polymyalgia rheumatica, present in the elderly population and are truly disorders of this age group.

Systemic Lupus Erythematosus

Although the majority of cases of systemic lupus erythematosus,[31,32] occur in young adults, approximately 15 percent of cases present in those over the age of 60 years. The disease is characterized by the development of autoantibodies to nuclear antigens, especially double-stranded DNA and Sm. The antigens/antibody complexes form, or are deposited, on the basement membranes of the epidermis, joints, renal glomeruli, arteries, and the microvasculature in a variety of organs. Vascular injury and stimulation of the clotting mechanism lead to thrombosis and functional disturbances in the affected organ.

Disease starting in elderly patients is often insidious in onset and associated with a relatively high incidence of interstitial lung disease and a lower incidence of renal disease.

Vasculitides

The vasculitides are a group of disorders in which inflammation in the blood vessel wall leads to its damage, extravasation of vascular contents, and thrombosis. These disorders may be restricted to blood vessels or may be part of a broader spectrum of disease.[33] The vascular element may be classified in a number of ways but the simplest is on the basis (1) of the type of vessel involved (e.g., artery, microvasculature, etc.), and (2) by the nature of the inflammatory cell infiltrate (e.g., lymphocytic, granulocytic, etc.).

The inflammation is believed to be caused by immune complex deposition in the wall of the blood vessel but this is only infrequently possible to prove. Of the many types of vasculitis only one occurs specifically in the elderly: giant cell or temporal arteritis.

Giant Cell Arteritis and Polymyalgia Rheumatica

Giant cell arteritis (see also Ch. 34) is a relatively uncommon disorder (approximately 1:1,000 over 60 years) manifesting as an arterial vasculitis with a predilection for the arteries of the head,[34] particularly the external carotid and the retinal branch of the internal carotid arteries, in elderly women (F: M = 3:1).

Etiology and pathology

The American College of Rheumatology has proposed diagnostic criteria.[35] Early in the disorder there is a leukocytoclastic vasculitis, so called because the vessel wall contains viable polymorphs and polymorph debris, evidence of complement activation, and generation of toxic polymorph products. Not only do polymorphs perish in this environment but so too do the smooth muscle cells of the arterial wall, leading to segmented mural necrosis. Later the typical but rarely seen picture of chronic inflammation with giant cells within the wall of the vessel appears. The giant cells are of two types including (1) immune competent cells, primed to an unknown antigen, and (2) foreign body type cells that are phagocytosing the internal elastic lamina. Thrombosis is commonly seen. The disease has a focal distribution within the vessel and, in any one location, a short time course. After the inflammation has spontaneously settled the vessel wall undergoes fibrosis; if extensive this can indicate earlier destructive inflammation. The presence of fibrosis and loss of the internal elastic lamina cannot always be taken as evidence of previous inflammation, however, because fibrosis of arterial walls is a "normal" finding in the elderly population.

The etiology of the vasculitis is not known. There is familial aggregation[36] and association with HLA-DR4.[37] In the serum there are raised levels of IgG, total complement, C3, and C4 in the serum. Circulating immune complexes have been demonstrated in up to 90 percent of patients.[38] They have also been seen attached to the internal elastic lamina, perhaps by absorbence.

Clinical features, diagnosis, and management

Classically, but not universally, the patient complains of a severe headache, often in the temple. The external carotid artery is characteristically firm, tortuous, and pulseless (Fig. 83-4; see also Plate 83-4). The erythrocyte sedimentation rate (ESR) is elevated, arteriograms may be abnormal, and arterial biopsy sometimes shows the typical histologic appearances. Biopsy is less commonly performed nowadays because the focal nature of the disease and sometimes nonspecific features make the diagnostic yield low[39] and even if an abnormality is found there is poor correlation between the biopsy findings and disease activity.[40] Instead response to therapy is used as a diagnostic test. Steroids are the treatment of choice and the symptoms settle rapidly on adequately large doses. Early management is seen as essential if the most feared complication, retinal artery thrombosis and blindness, is to be prevented.

Polymyalgia Rheumatica

The local disorder giant cell arteritis is associated with a generalized condition known as polymyalgia rheumatica.[41] It is characterized by low-grade fever; weight loss; ill-defined pain and stiffness in the shoulder girdle, upper arms, and neck; malaise; and fatigue. Movement accentuates the pain, which is worst at night. Affected joints, particularly the knees and sternoclavicular joints, are actively inflamed. There is an increase in the number of cells within the synovial fluid and a normochromic, normocytic anemia. The ESR is very high but there is no leukocytosis. Tests for autoantibodies are negative. It also responds to steroids.

Metabolic Nutritional, and Endocrine Disorders

Metabolic (generalized) skeletal disorders have already been discussed, but similar disorders also affect other connective tissues. Prominent among these disorders are the crystal

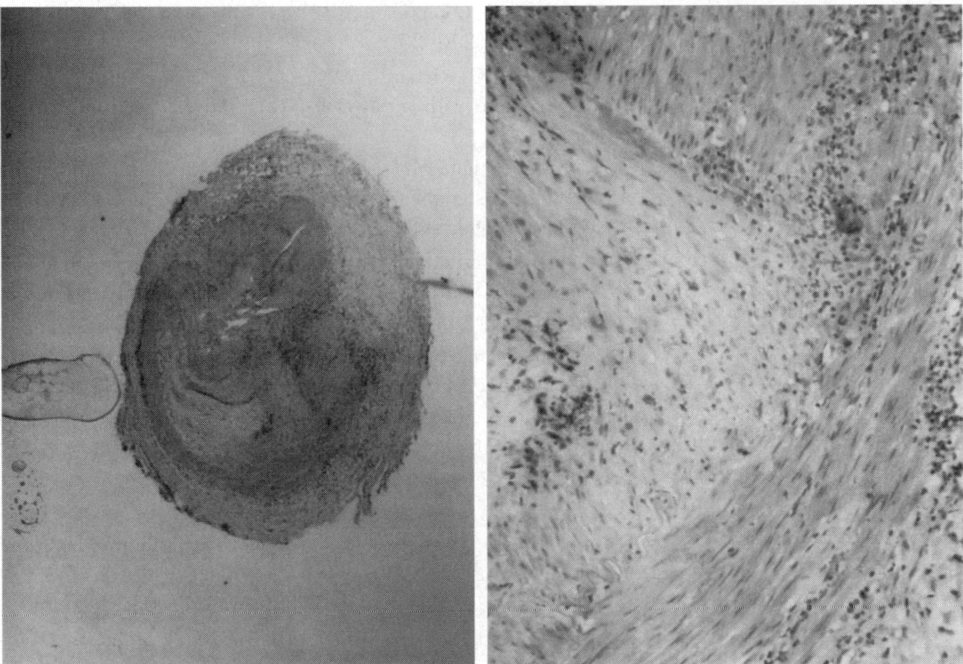

Figure 83-4 An artery from a patient with giant cell arteritis. (**A**) Virtual occlusion of the lumen. (H&E, × 10) (**B**) Inflammation including giant cells in the wall (H&E, × 150).

deposition diseases due to the accumulation within connective tissues of monosodium urate and calcium pyrophosphate. Other metabolic products can also accumulate in the connective tissues notably abnormal proteins such as glycosylated proteins in diabetes, and proteins with a β-pleated sheet molecular structure, the hallmark of amyloid.

Although there are many metabolic disorders, these are the most common in the elderly population.

Gout

Uric acid is a breakdown product of purine metabolism.[42] Most is excreted by the kidney.[43] Alteration in uric acid excretion either idiopathic or secondary to diuretic therapy leads to an increase in monosodium urate in the blood and extracellular fluid and its precipitation in the tissues. Cartilage, particularly articular fibrocartilage and nonarticular hyaline cartilage, and subcutaneous connective tissue are the most common sites of its accumulation. Here aggregates of the crystals induce a macrophage response. These "tophi" may ulcerate. In the elderly, tophaceous or nontophaceous gout occurs either due to an idiopathic decrease in urate secretion, generalized deterioration in renal function, or the use of certain diuretics.

Calcium Pyrophosphate Deposition Disease

Unlike monosodium urate deposition disease calcium pyrophosphate crystals precipitate out most commonly within joints, notably fibrocartilage.[44] Their anomalous activation of either macrophages and neutrophils, and the disease so caused,[45] were discussed in the chapter on joint disease (see Ch. 82).

Diabetes

Diabetes has been discussed at length. Its effects on connective tissues are much the same as those elsewhere. Both by nonenzymic glycosylation and alteration of intracellular metabolism diabetes results directly in the production and deposition of abnormal proteins. This is most prominent in bone in which structural and physicochemical changes in the matrix lead to deposition of an autofluorescent matrix. In addition, effects on the vasculature and nerves cause traumatic, infective, and infarctive events in connective tissues.

Amyloid

Normally proteins have a tertiary molecular structure in the form of an α-helix. In certain circumstances (including old age) the tertiary structure of a particular protein changes to a β-pleated sheet configuration.[46] In this form the protein is less readily degraded and therefore accumulates within the tissue. Certain proteins are more prone to undergoing β-pleated sheet configuration. Prominent among such proteins are immunoglobulin light chains, the acute phase protein, protein A, certain hormones (e.g., insulin and calcitonin), and, particularly in old age, a family of proteins similar to prealbumin and designated amyloid S (AS). These accumulate most commonly in the myocardium, synovium, cartilage, ligaments, menisci, and brain. These proteins accumulate preferentially within the walls of blood vessels, leading to poor perfusion, and in connective tissues such as fat, and articular cartilage. Their unique protein structure means they take up certain histologic dyes (such as Congo red) particularly well, and the parallel arrangement of these dye molecules attached to the β-pleated sheet makes the stained product birefringent.

The most common site for AS to assimilate in the elderly is in cartilage and synovium and there is a strong association between amyloid deposition and osteoarthritis.

Summary

The connective tissues are the most abundant in the whole body. Diseases of connective tissue can occur at any time of life and most present first during middle age. There are some that are specific to the elderly including Paget's disease of bone, Dupuytren's disease, malignant fibrous histocytoma, cutaneous angiosarcoma, giant cell arteritis and polymyalgia rheumatica and senile amyloid, discussed here, and osteoporosis and osteoarthritis, two of the most common noninfective diseases in the Western world, which are discussed in previous chapters. Many are significant causes of morbidity and even mortality.

References

1. Wainwright SA, Biggs WD, Currey JD, Gosline JM: Mechanical Design in Organisms. Edward Arnold, London, 1976
2. Hukins DSL, Weston SA, Humphries M, Freemont AJ: Extracellular matrix. pp. 181–230. In Bitter EE, Bitter N (eds): Principles of Medical Biology. JAI Press, Greenwich, CT, 1995
3. Rehman MTA, Hoyland JA, Denton J, Freemont AJ: Age related histomorphometric changes in bone in normal British men and women. J Clin Pathol 1994;47:529–534
4. Hoyland JA, Jayson MIV: Age related changes in the structures within and bordering the intervertebral foramen—associations with low back pain. pp. 94–110. In Hukins DW, Nelson MA (eds): The Ageing Spine. Manchester University Press, Manchester, 1987
5. Freemont AJ: Bone histomorphometry. pp. 77–90. In Tovey FI, Stamp T (eds): The Measurement of Metabolic Bone Disease. Parthenon Publishing Group, New York, 1995
6. Hall BK: Fracture repair and regeneration. In Hall BK (ed): Bone. Vol. 5. pp. 55–62. CRC Press, Boca Raton, FL, 1992
7. Freemont AJ: Inflammation. pp. 126–162. In Byers P, Salisbury J, Woods C (eds): Diseases of Bones and Joints. Chapman & Hall, London, 1994
8. Paget J: On a form of chronic inflammation of bones (osteitis deformans). Trans Med Chir Soc Lond 1877;60:37–63
9. Freemont AJ: The pathology of Paget's disease of bone. In Sharpe P (ed): The Molecular Biology of Paget's Disease. RC Landes & Co., 1996
10. Cartwright EJ, Gordon MT, Anderson DC, Sharpe PT. Paramyxovirus and Paget's disease. J Med Virol 1993;40:133–141
11. Hoyland JA, Freemont AJ, Sharpe P: Interleukin 6 (IL-6), IL-6 receptor and IL-6 nuclear factor gene expression in Paget's disease. J Bone Min Res 1994;9:75–80
12. Dalinka MK, Aronchick JM, Haddad JG: Paget's disease. Orthop Clin North Am 1983;4:3–19
13. Cawley MID: Complications of Paget's disease of bone. Gerontology 1983;29:276–287
14. Anderson DC, Richardson PC, Cantrill JC: Paget's disease and its treatment with intravenous APD. Adv Endocrinol 1986;6: 156–164
15. Catto M: Pathology of aseptic necrosis. pp. 417–442. In Harris NH (ed): Postgraduate Textbook of Clinical Orthopaedics. John Wright, Bristol, 1982
16. Venn MF. Variation of chemical composition with age in human femoral head cartilage. Ann Rheum Dis 1978;37:168–174
17. Middleton JF, Hunt S, Oates K: Electron probe X-ray microanalysis of the composition of hyaline articular and non-articular cartilage in young and aged rats. Cell Tissue Res 1988;253:469–475
18. Arnold H Jr, Grauer F: Keloids, etiology and management by excision and intensive prophylactic radiation. Arch Dermatol 1959;80:772
19. Dupuytren G, le baron: De la rétraction des doigts par suite d'une affection de l'aponeurose palmaire, opération chirurgicale qui convient dans ce cas. J Universal et Hebdomadaire de Médecine et de Chirurgie Pratiques 1831;5(2 ser):352–365
20. Mackenzie DH: The Differential Diagnosis of Fibroblastic Disorders. pp. 44–49. Blackwell Scientific Publications. Oxford 1970
21. Gabbiani C, Majno G: Dupuytren's contracture: fibroblast contraction? Am J Pathol 1972;66:131–146
22. Gardner DL: Pathological Basis of the Connective Tissue Diseases. Ch. 21. Edward Arnold, London, 1992
23. Freemont AJ: Pathology of ankylosing spondylitis. pp. 1–22. In Calabro DC, Carson DW (eds): New Clinical Applications—Rheumatology—Ankylosing Spondylitis. MTP Press, Lancaster, 1988
24. Freemont AJ: The Pathology of Rheumatoid Arthritis. pp. 83–114. In Henderson B, Pettifer R, Edwards J (eds): Mechanisms and Models in in Rheumatoid Arthritis. Academic Press, New York, 1995
25. Robert L, Jacob MP, Frances C et al: Interaction between elastin and elastases and its role in the aging of the arterial wall, skin and other connective tissues. A review. Mech Aging Dev 1984; 28:155–166
26. Lever WF, Shaumberg Lever G: Histopathology of the Skin Vol. 14. (6th Ed.) pp. 245–258. Lippincott-Raven, Philadelphia, 1984
27. Huvos AG: Bone Tumors, Diagnosis, Treatment and Prognosis. 2nd Ed. WB Saunders, Philadelphia, 1991
28. Enzinger FM, Weiss SW: Soft Tissue Tumors. CV Mosby, St Louis, 1983
29. McCullum P, Freemont AJ, Geary C, Liu Yin JA: A case of IgD myeloma presenting as diffuse osteosclerosis. J Clin Pathol 1988; 41:486–489
30. Hartley AL, Blair V, Harris M et al: Sarcomas in North West England: II Incidence. Br J Cancer 1991;64:1145–1150
31. Morgan SH, Hughes GRV: Connective tissue disorders. Med Int 1984;2:397–408
32. Wallace DJ, Dubois EL: Dubois' Lupus Erythematosus. 3rd Ed. Lea & Febiger, Philadelphia, 1987
33. McCluskey PT, Fienberg R: Vasculitis in primary vasculitides, granulomatoses and connective tissue diseases. Hum Pathol 1983;14:305–315

34. Horton BT, Magath BT, Brown GE: An undescribed form of arteritis of the temporal vessels. Arch Intern Med 1934;53:400–409

35. Hunder GG, Bloch DA, Michel BA et al: The American College of Rheumatology 1990 criteria for the classification of giant cell arteritis Arthritis Rheum 1990;33:1122–1128

36. Liang GC, Simkin PA, Hunder GG et al: Familial aggregation of polymyalgia rheumatica and giant cell arteritis. Arthritis Rheum 1975;17:19–24

37. Bignon JD, Barrier J, Soulillou JP et al: HLA DR4 and giant cell arteritis. Tissue Antigens 1984;24:60–62

38. Papaionnou CC, Gupta RC, Hunder GG, McDuffie FC: Circulating immune complexes in giant cell arteritis and polymyalgia rheumatica. Arthritis Rheum 1980;23:1021–1025

39. Mambo NC: Temporal (granulomatous) arteritis: a histopathological study of 32 cases. Histopathology 1970;3:209–221

40. Huston KA, Hunder GG, Lie JT et al: Temporal arteritis. A 25-year epidemiologic, clinical and pathologic study. Ann Intern Med 1978;88:162–167

41. Hunder GG, Allen GL: The relationship between polymyalgia rheumatica and temporal arteritis. Geriatrics 1973;28:134–142

42. Wyngaarden JB, Kelley WN: pp. 1043–1114. Gout. In Stanbury JB, Wyngaarden JB, Fredrickson DS et al (eds): The Metabolic Basis of Inherited Diseases. 5th Ed. McGraw Hill, New York, 1983

43. Levinson DJ: Clinical gout and the pathogenesis of hyperuricaemia. pp. 1645–1676. In McCarty DJ (ed): Arthritis and Allied Conditions: A Textbook of Rheumatology. (11th Ed. Lea & Febiger, Philadelphia, 1989

44. Brown WE, Gregory TM: Calcium pyrophosphate crystal chemistry. Arthritis Rheum 1976;19:446–463

45. Ryan LM, McCarty DJ: Calcium pyrophosphate crystal deposition disease; pseudogout; articular chondrocalcinosis. pp. 1711–1736. In McCarty DJ (ed): Arthritis and Allied Conditions: A Textbook of Rheumatology. 11th Ed. Lea & Febiger, Philadelphia. 1989

46. Isobe T, Araki S, Uchino F et al (eds): Amyloid and Amyloidosis. Plenum Press, New York, 1988

C H A P T E R 8 4

Orthopaedic Geriatrics

ELTON STRAUSS
CRAIG SCOTT BARTLETT III
ANDREW CASDEN
GIUSEPPE DIGIOVANNI
RICHARD A. FRIEDEN
MICHAEL HAHN
EVAN KARAS
ANN-MARIE PLATE
STEPHANIE SWEET

Trauma in the Geriatric Population: Surgical, Functional, and Social Aspects of Care

Physiologically, the elderly population presents a unique and complex picture that requires an understanding of the aging process and the effects of acquired diseases. With each passing year, individuals are living longer, healthier, and more active lives. These life-style changes are made possible by advances in the diagnosis and treatment of cardiovascular disease, diabetes, stroke, cancer, and arthritis. However, as their life spans increase and the scope of their activities broadens, elderly people are increasingly at risk for injury.

Trauma is now the fifth most common cause of mortality in people over the age of 65 years.[1–4] This age group accounts for 25 to 28 percent of accidental deaths, or approximately 28,000 cases per year.[1,3–9] Although engaged less often in the activities that place their younger counterparts at risk, the elderly are more susceptible and less tolerant of injury. In fact, the geriatric population has higher accident-related morbidity and mortality rates than any other age group.[2,4,5,8,10,11] Responsible for this are a reduction in physiologic reserve and complications arising from inadequacies in evaluation, monitoring, and treatment.[9–13] Three-quarters of trauma-related geriatric deaths have been reported to occur in the first 24 hours[14] with as many as one-third of these preventable.[9]

The cost of trauma care in the United States is overwhelming. More than $87 billion in direct medical expenditures and lost productivity is consumed annually,[15] with patients over 65 years of age accounting for nearly one-third of this.[1,8,11,16] Such an appropriation of a large portion of health care resources by a small segment of society prompts some of the most difficult ethical, sociologic, and therapeutic questions facing medicine.

Complicating the issue is the rapid growth of the geriatric population. In 1980, 11 percent of Americans—almost 26.5 million people—were over the age of 65 years. By 1990, this number had reached 30.9 million.[17] Present estimates indicate that this will swell to 51 million by the year 2020 and 68 million by 2040, then comprising 20 percent of our population. Those 85 years or older are growing at an even faster rate, expected to reach 6.7 million by 2020 and 12.2 million by 2040.[18]

Physiology of Aging

As aging progresses, there is an unavoidable decline of all organ systems that have a major impact on trauma in the elderly population.[3,19] Data from the National Health Survey[20] show that nearly 22 percent of all those over 65 years of age have a limiting heart condition, 4.7 percent have pulmonary disease, and 4 percent have diabetes. By age 70 years, as much as 70 percent of patients will have congestive heart failure, atrial fibrillation, leukemia, polycythemia, or diabetes.[2] Immunosenescence, an age-related and ill-defined decline in both cell- and humoral-mediated immunity, is responsible for decreased resistance to infection.[19]

Elderly patients generally have higher blood pressures than younger patients and progressive stiffening of the myocardium leads to reduced efficiency such that an 80-year-old has half the cardiac output of a 20-year-old.[21] The presence of atherosclerosis will further depress cardiac function by limiting coronary blood flow. Such changes can lead to conduction abnormalities, a decreased cardiac reserve, and a heart less sensitive to endogenous and exogenous catecholamines.[3,4] The normal compensatory response of tachycardia to hypovolemia, pain, and anxiety is often lacking. This response can also be blunted by medications (β- and calcium channel blockers) or intrinsic diseases (Lev's and Lenegre's).

With advancing age, pulmonary compliance decreases, total lung surface area diminishes, mucociliary clearance slows, and the oropharynx becomes colonized with gram-negative organisms.[4] In this setting, even a minor chest injury can be devastating. A decreased gag reflex, diminished respiratory muscle strength, and reduced lung capacity are in all likelihood responsible for the 40 percent complication rate in intubated geriatric patients.[22]

Renal mass declines progressively such that by age 65, there is a 30 to 40 percent loss of glomeruli.[4] The filtration rate is even further diminished due to degenerative changes in the tubules of the remaining glomeruli. Because they are less efficient in concentrating their urine and may be taking diuretics,[3] a normal serum creatinine may not represent normal renal function.

From age 30 years until menopause, bone is lost at 3 percent per decade in women, rising to 10 percent per decade after menopause.[3] This loss of bone mass predisposes the distal radius, proximal humerus, olecranon, hip, supracondylar femur, proximal and distal tibia, os calcis, and spine to fracture.[13] Approximately 80 percent of patients who sustain hip fractures have osteoporosis.[23]

Finally, subtle changes in cognitive ability, memory, and data acquisition are common in the elderly. Unfortunately, such findings may mask significant intracranial pathology.[4] Between the ages of 30 and 70 years, a progressively atrophic brain decreases in size by approximately 10 percent. The bridging veins become stretched, making them prone to significant bleeding even with minor trauma.[3] Should bleeding occur, dead space will permit an intracranial hematoma to expand more freely, leading to insidious development of symptoms.[21] Lastly, elderly patients have a decreased perception of pain, making them unaware of potential injuries.[3]

All of these physiologic changes with aging have an important impact on the occurrence, nature, and the outcome of trauma in the elderly.

Mechanisms of Injury

Motor vehicle accidents are the most common form of fatal accident for the elderly population through the age of 80 years, with falls a close second.[4,6,10,24] Only 13 percent of the 21.8 million licensed drivers in the United States are 65 years or older with one-third of these over the age of 75. Although only a small proportion of drivers, this group suffers from a crash rate second only to new drivers aged 16 through 25 years, and the highest rate of fatal crashes of any age group.[5] In 1985, persons over the age of 65 years accounted for 12.7 percent of all motor vehicle fatalities.[25] In contrast to younger drivers, elderly people are more likely to be involved in an accident during daylight hours, closer to home, and in good weather. However, alcohol use is less frequently involved.[25,26]

A combination of many factors explains the higher crash rates of the geriatric population. These include a diminution of cerebral and motor skills, alterations in visual or auditory acuity, pre-existing medical conditions, medications, and increased reliance on the motor vehicle as a primary source of transportation.[4] Cognitive defects in memory and judgment will often prevent the individual from recognizing and avoiding oncoming hazards.

Because they relate to postural stability, balance, motor strength, and coordination, the factors above also result in an increased risk of falling. After the age of 80 years, falls become the predominant mechanism of injury, probably due to changes in lifestyle and activity level. The older the individual, the more prone to tripping and less likely to stabilize oneself during a fall. Syncope can be caused by acute or chronic disease states that lead to a sudden decrease in cerebral blood flow (dysrhythmias, venous pooling, autonomic insufficiency) or metabolic derangement (hypoglycemia, hypoxia, anemia).[4] A sudden unexplained weakness of the lower extremities causing a fall (drop attacks) is common.

Although many falls occur on a level surface with only a limited amount of energy transfer, there is often significant morbidity and mortality. The incidence of fractures following a fall is reported to be between 8 and 40 percent.[27] Additionally, elderly people account for 70 percent of fall-related deaths[4,27] and of those hospitalized after falling, only 50 percent will be alive after 1 year.[28] Falling kills more individuals over 85 years of age than the number of motor vehicle fatalities among those aged 18 to 19.[3]

The third and most devastating mechanism of injury for the elderly involves the pedestrian motor vehicle accident (MVA). This comprises the majority of geriatric multiple trauma victims with the most commonly affected regions the head, chest, and tibia.[3] In addition to having the highest rate of pedestrian accidents,[29] those aged 65 years and older also have the highest population-based fatality rate of any age group.[25] This amounts to more than 22 percent of pedestrian MVA fatalities in the United States.[25] In Germany, 50 percent of all pedestrians killed in road traffic accidents are aged 65 years or older, and although amounting to only 16 percent of the population, the elderly population accounts for 27 percent of such fatalities in Sweden.[13]

It is interesting to note that the majority of MVAs involving elderly pedestrians occur at crosswalks[29] and that this age group represents 46 percent of crosswalk-associated fatalities.[25] Explaining this may be the fact that most traffic signals are set to allow a crossing rate of 4 feet per second. Such a brisk requirement will leave many older individuals trapped in the center of the roadway as the light changes. In addition, postural and sensory changes make it difficult to lift one's head to see signals or appreciate approaching danger.

Although falls and vehicular accidents constitute the majority of their serious injuries, elderly people are unfortunately often also the victims of violent crime. It is estimated that 800,000 members of this vulnerable population are presently the victims of physical abuse[30] with assaults accounting for 4 to 14 percent of their hospital admissions.[4,10,25,31,32]

Initial Evaluation and Treatment

Trauma care begins in the field. According to the American College of Surgeons, an age over 55 years should lower the threshold for triage to a trauma center.[11] Upon arrival at the hospital, it is important to obtain as rapid an assessment as possible. This includes a concise medical history, including details of the accident scene. One must not be misled by the appearance of a baseline senile dementia. It is often difficult to discern between this diagnosis and an intracranial hemorrhage or a transient ischemic attack.[11]

Because the states of the heart, lungs, and immunologic systems mainly determine the likelihood of survival,[19] they should receive particular attention. Thus, initial treatment priorities involve securing an airway, assessing cardiopulmonary function, providing humidified oxygen, controlling hemorrhage, and treating shock. Geriatric patients are much more likely to have dentures or other materials in their mouths that can lead to airway obstruction, the most rapidly fatal problem faced.[3] Military antishock trousers may be useful except in the setting of suspected head or chest trauma where they have the potential for increasing intracranial pressure.[3]

In those patients presenting with respiratory distress or in whom conservative methods of pulmonary support fail, early mechanical ventilation should be considered. Although this may lead to increased pulmonary infection rates, it is preferable to allowing the struggling patient to expend his or her limited supply of energy and become hypoxic.

Prudent administration of crystalloid is indicated, and the threshold for use of blood products should be low. However, elderly patients are as intolerant of over-resuscitation as they are of hypovolemia.[23] If the pressures stabilize after 1 L of crystalloid, then the patient in all likelihood has a volume deficit of less than 25 percent.[23] Should the patient fail to improve after hydration or an early response deteriorate, then blood products are indicated. Core body temperature must be monitored to avoid hypothermia from infusion fluids.

After the initial stabilization, a secondary survey is performed, including evaluation of the neurologic, cardiopulmonary, gastrointestinal, genitourinary, and musculoskeletal systems.

The cervical spine must be protected until properly evaluated. Bladder catheterization will allow fluid monitoring and potentially diagnose a genitourinary injury. A rectal exam is mandatory, particularly in men before catheterization. Detection of blood in the meatus or a high-riding boggy prostate may herald a urethral tear, usually secondary to a pelvic fracture. In this setting, a retrograde urethrogram is indicated.

If the patient has sustained chest trauma, fractured ribs, pneumothorax, hemothorax, cardiac contusion, and aortic injury should all be suspected. Although 80 to 90 percent of patients with an injured aorta are killed immediately, those that do survive must be diagnosed quickly because nearly one-half will die in the following 6 hours.[3] A cardiac contusion may lead to arrhythmias, congestive heart failure, and tamponade.[11] Although the electrocardiogram (ECG) has low sensitivity and specificity, it should be the initial study. Telemetry for 24 to 36 hours with serial ECGs and cardiac isozymes will help exclude contusion as a diagnosis.[3]

Abdominal visceral injuries are a serious problem, occurring in 35 percent of geriatric patients with multiple trauma.[8] Associated fractures are almost always present[8,11,33] and mortality rates can climb as high as 80 percent, nearly five times that of younger victims.[10] Also, the diagnosis of these injuries in the elderly patient can be difficult as the "gold standard" of diagnostic peritoneal lavage is rendered unreliable in the presence of previous abdominal surgery. In these cases, double-contrast computed tomography is a reasonable alternative as long as hydration is closely monitored.

The pelvis, entire spine, and all four extremities should be palpated, and if possible, joints moved and stressed. Unstable pelvic and femoral fractures play major roles in the development of shock due to massive blood loss.[8,13,33] Fractures must be immobilized and dislocations reduced.

A radiographic trauma series includes an anteroposterior (AP) chest, lateral cervical spine, and AP roentgenogram of the pelvis. Additionally, limbs in question require AP and lateral views. In the management of long bone fractures, it is mandatory that the two adjacent joints are included in the radiographs.

Once the geriatric trauma victim is deemed stable, or assessed as having only "minor injuries," it is important to guard against a false sense of security. Rapid deterioration is still a possibility[3,4,34] and, as discussed in the physiology section, heart rate, blood pressure, and urine output can be unreliable parameters in the elderly. After blood loss they cannot augment their cardiac output through increased contractility or heart rate. Thus, pressure is maintained by an increased systemic vascular resistance, which only further depresses output.[3]

Aggressive trauma care with invasive monitoring, especially of geriatric patients with an American Society of Anesthesiology class III or higher, can reduce mortality.[4,9,19,31,34] Utilizing this modality, Scalea et al.[34] found that some patients deemed "hemodynamically stable" actually had derangements in cardiac performance, vascular tone, and oxygen consumption. Cardiac outputs of less than 3.5 L/min or mixed venous oxygen saturations of less than 60 percent were indicative of inadequate oxygen delivery and a poor prognosis.[34] By improving oxygen consumption with accurate volume loading and inotropic support, they improved survival from 7 to 53 percent.

Surgical Considerations

Although they suffer from the same local complications as their younger counterparts,[13] geriatric patients have a mortality rate that is higher for nearly every type of surgery.[19,35] The greatest risks occur in the setting of trauma, where the victim's physiologic reserve is more easily surpassed. Thus, it is important that stabilization of major injuries be performed using the most effective but least invasive procedures. However, as modern surgical technique and equipment have improved, so have outcomes. Geriatric patients surviving surgery have displayed survival rates approaching age-matched controls.[19]

Although they are intolerant of exploratory laparotomy, elderly patients are even less tolerant of shock.[3] Thus, there is little margin for error. Treatment will often require compromise; for example, splenectomy may be preferable to salvage when the later will prolong surgery, increase bleeding, slow recovery, and potentially expose the patient to a second procedure.[3] Similarly, it may be prudent to perform an ileostomy rather than attempt a more lengthy anastomosis procedure.[3]

Although it is prudent to delay certain isolated fractures in medically stable geriatric patients,[11,36–38] the patient with polytrauma merits special consideration. Unstable pelvic and long bone fractures (especially the femur) are associated with increased risks of bleeding,[11,39] fat embolism,[40] and adult respiratory distress syndrome.[41] This last condition is the leading cause of death in the elderly trauma patient after 24 hours.[3] Thus, early stabilization within 24 hours is essential.[41] This will allow rapid mobilization of the patient, which optimizes respiratory function, the main source of morbidity and mortality in polytrauma.[8,12,13,41,42]

Open fractures in the elderly, occurring most commonly in the tibial region,[13] are treated with the same principles used for younger patients, including copious irrigation, adequate debridement, and stabilization of the fracture.[43–45]

Controlling pain in nonventilated patients will frequently ensure adequate pulmonary toilet. However, systemic analgesic therapy can lead to respiratory depression and must be used carefully. For this reason, regional therapy including epidural anesthesia, intrapleural catheterization, and intercostal nerve blocks is an attractive consideration.[11,13]

Maintenance of nutritional status is important as requirements significantly increase during the post-traumatic catabolic period.[11,31,46] Malnutrition, evident in 59 percent of elderly hip fracture patients, leads to immunocompetence, poor wound healing, decubitus ulcers, and subsequent wound infection or sepsis.[32] Also, hospital stays are longer, mortality greater, and patients less likely to return to their pre-injury level of function.[32] Thus, parenteral supplementation should be considered in a patient with hypoalbuminemia, negative nitrogen balance, and anergy.

General complications are related to immobilization with pneumonia, urinary tract infection, decubiti, thromboembolism, and pulmonary embolism being the most prevalent. The occurrence of these can lead to mortality with rates as high as 46 percent.[13] Thus, prophylaxis against deep venous thrombosis is recommended for all patients requiring bed rest. Strategies have included aspirin, warfarin, dextran, low-molecular-weight heparin, and intermittent external pneumatic compression. No one therapy has proven clearly superior.

Mortality

The overall mortality rate of hospitalized geriatric patients is reported to be in the range of 15 to 30 percent, far in excess of the 3 to 8 percent reported in younger patients with similar injuries.[6,8,10,14,21] Penning[13] noted that three-quarters of multiple trauma patients over age 75 years died, and in fact suggested that an increased likelihood of fatal outcome may exist after the age of 56. Although younger trauma patients typically succumb to irreversible brain damage,[10–12] the elderly are more likely to die of multiple organ failure and sepsis.[4] Still, severe brain trauma will lead to as high as a 90 percent mortality rate in this population, with survivors sustaining greater deficits and requiring longer hospitalization than younger victims.[3]

Finelli et al.[10] noted that mortality resulted singularly or in combination from pulmonary complications in 28 percent, infection in 27 percent, renal insufficiency in 71 percent, and cardiovascular collapse in 18 percent. However, Pennig[13] reported death due to head injury in 34 percent, hemorrhagic shock in 32 percent, and pulmonary complications in 24 percent. Also, Broos et al.[6] observed multiple system organ failure and head injury as the causes of death in 44 and 33 percent of cases, respectively. Furthermore, elderly patients with head trauma were nine times more likely to die than those with other injuries and two-thirds of those over 65 years of age arriving at the hospital unconscious died.

Specific factors correlated with death in elderly trauma patients include male sex; shock; bradycardia; burns; severe head, chest, or abdominal injuries; the need for ventilatory or inotropic support; age greater than 65 to 75 years; and the presence of infectious complications.[1,3,4,6,8,13,14,47–50] Elderly men were twice as likely to die as women and geriatric trauma victims with isolated chest injuries have a mortality rate two to three times that of their younger counterparts.[47] It is ironic that the stiffer rib cage of the elderly individual is protective against pulmonary contusion.[3]

Oreskovich et al.[8] noted that an elderly patient who requires prehospital intubation, displays hypovolemia in the field, has multiple injuries including a significant head injury, and requires pulmonary support for 5 days has virtually no chance for survival. However, they found the injury severity score (ISS) to be unreliable.

In contrast, other authors have shown that the ISS is a reasonable predictor of mortality.[1,4,10,14,50,51] Demaria et al.[12] using a modified ISS (Geriatric Trauma Survival Score), reported a 92 percent accuracy. Pellicane et al.[9] calculated a physiologic Trauma Score and while reporting that depressed scores predicted mortality in 90 percent of cases, noted that 52 percent of all deaths occurred in elderly patients with minimal impairment.

Although some authors have not noted a correlation with pre-existing cardiovascular disease, most have found this to increase a patient's risk of dying.[3,14,52] In addition, stroke has caused some postoperative deaths and postoperative delirium can interfere with physical therapy or lead to self-inflicted injury.[19] Other medical conditions that may be predictive of poor outcome include chronic renal insufficiency, cirrhosis, congenital coagulopathy, chronic obstructive pulmonary disease, and diabetes.[14,52] An elderly patient with one or more of these will often require a long period of hospitalization.[52,53]

Function

Although mortality rates are the most visible means of measuring outcome, functional status at the time of discharge and over the long term is of greater importance to patients and their families.[4] Oreskovich et al.[8] noted a poor long-term prognosis as only 8 percent of survivors returned to their previous level of independence. The remainder required some form of assistance at home or in a nursing facility. Even at 1 year after discharge, 72 percent were still in a nursing home.

In contrast, other authors have noted favorable functional results after multisystem trauma in elderly patients.[12,14,31,50] DeMaria and co-workers[31] reported that one-third of survivors were independent at discharge, one-third were dependent but living at home, and one-third required a nursing care facility. Eventually, 87 percent returned home and 57 percent were fully independent. Van-Aalst et al.[50] reported that two-thirds of surviving geriatric trauma victims regained a level of independence. However, only 49 percent of this group actually survived their initial injuries.

The Orthopaedic-Geriatric Unit

Modern management of geriatric fractures with collaboration by integrated teams of health care personnel was first promoted by Devas in 1977.[54] Since then, most studies have documented fewer complications, fewer transfers to intensive care units, improved ability to walk at time of discharge, and fewer discharges to nursing homes.[33,46,55–62] Reid et al.[60] noted that hospital stays were reduced by 41 percent and the percentage of those being discharged home increased from 10 to 32 percent. This was attributed to placement in the orthogeriatric unit within 1 day.

Generally, postoperative fracture patients fall into three groups: (1) those with little rehabilitation potential (severe dementia or long-term institutionalization), (2) those with a potential for rehabilitation, and (3) younger patients with no complications or comorbidities. The first group is best treated by transferral to an assessment and rehabilitation unit. The middle group is best served by placement in the orthogeriatric unit within 2 to 3 days of surgery. The third group usually does well regardless of placement and may remain on the orthopaedic unit until discharge home. Management without a designated unit is also possible[63] but more problematic.

Ogilvie-Harris et al.[64] have reported that a multidisciplinary approach using a care map will lead to decreased length of stay, decreased complications, and improved overall outcome. The tenets of this include appropriate consultations, laboratory tests, nursing care, diet, medications, activity, teaching, and discharge planning.

Preoperative anesthesiology and medical and gerontologic consultations will better prepare the patient for surgery. Early physiotherapy evaluation will mobilize the patient more quickly. Prompt attention to postoperative urologic problems will decrease the risk for infection.

Important aspects of nursing care include an egg-crate mattress and frequent turning every 2 to 3 hours to avoid decubiti, protection of the peroneal nerve, a trapeze, preoperative Buck's traction, and brief Foley catheterization. It is important to monitor input and output, mental status, respiration, and skin condition.

Appropriate analgesia must be given but not so great as to depress respiratory drive. Often, only simple analgesics are required. Iron supplements are often beneficial. In addition, stool softeners and a high-fiber diet will help avoid bowel dysfunction and its resultant lethargy, loss of appetite, and occasional irritable behavior. Laxatives, suppositories, and mild enemas are used as necessary.

A cornerstone of physiotherapy is early mobilization to avoid atelectasis. This begins by encouraging movement in bed, sitting on the side of the bed, and transferring to a standing position. As soon as patients can tolerate sitting, they should be out of bed to a chair, usually on the first postoperative day. Following this, transfer and gait training begin with the patient progressing to ambulation with a walker on the second day if possible. Preoperative instruction with regards to incentive spirometry and the early routines of mobilization will facilitate their use by the patient postoperatively. Occupational therapy for the patient's activities of daily living is also important.

During the postoperative phase, it is common to discover acute confusional states, anemia, malnutrition, hypothyroidism, osteomalacia, Parkinson's disease, strokes, cardiovascular malfunction, and infections. Each of these must be evaluated promptly and treated by the geriatric service, while the orthopaedic team follows fracture healing and prosthetic function.

Assessment of the patient's previous level of function, social supports, and present needs will improve the chances for discharge home or ease the transition from the hospital to another care facility.[13,64]

Socioeconomic Issues

Fitzgerald et al.[65] have reported that the diagnosis by related group (DRG)-based prospective payment system has decreased the average hospital stay after fracture of the hip from 16 to 10 days. A disturbing trend of poorer quality of care was also noted as rehabilitation sessions were decreased by 50 percent and the percentage of patients discharged to nursing homes doubled.

There is often no correlation between hospital cost and reimbursement as the system fails to adequately distinguish between different intensities and duration of treatment.[53] Several studies have reported grossly underestimated costs of patients with severe injuries, those with one or more complications, and those over 80 years of age.[4,10,14–16] Zietlow et al.[14] reported a reimbursement rate of only 66 percent in their study of geriatric trauma patients and Weingarten et al.[15] reported rates inversely proportional to age and length of stay.

Based on its present inadequacies, the DRG system appears to be incapable of supporting trauma care, especially that of the elderly. Because trauma centers are hospitals that specialize in high-severity high-cost patients, DRG payments will be routinely low. This can only lead to disproportionate financial losses and a discouragement of the regionalization of trauma care.[53]

Evaluation and Treatment of Hand, Wrist, and Elbow Problems in the Geriatric Population

History

The evaluation of the patient with hand, wrist, or elbow pain begins with a careful history. The location, nature, and duration of pain should be evaluated, as well as any alleviating or exacerbating symptoms. Exactly where the pain is located can be clarified by having the patient point with a single finger to the point of maximum tenderness. Radiation of pain can also be shown in this manner. Often the patient's use of anatomic terms is quite different from yours; misunderstanding is best prevented by having the patient simply point. The nature of the pain should also be described. Tingling, radiating, or burning pain is often due to nerve irritation, whereas a dull aching pain is more typical of tendinitis or osteoarthritis. Throbbing pain that wakens the patient at night is typical of infection if accompanied by erythema and swelling, whereas night pain in the absence of obvious infection can be due to a neoplastic process. The duration of the symptoms must also be carefully assessed, particularly in relation to any trauma or new activities. Although a recent fall is easily recognized as a cause for symptoms, less obvious are new exercise regimens, hobbies, or changes in lifestyle. An example is the wrist pain due to thumb extensor tendinitis often found in patients helping to care for infants. Activities that specifically worsen the pain should be described or demonstrated, as well as actions that help to relieve symptoms. The classic history of carpal tunnel syndrome is pain and numbness at night in the thumb, index, and middle finger relieved by shaking the hands. Pain unrelated to time of day or activities should heighten suspicion for malignancy, particularly of a severe nature. Inquiries should be made concerning the presence of similar symptoms in the past; patients will often surprisingly forget to mention that they had the exact problem 10 years ago, or more recently on the other side.

Physical Examination

The physical examination of the upper extremity is similar to a general physical examination in that a specific order should be followed. Establishing a routine makes an examination more efficient, and also prevents inadvertently forgetting portions. The abbreviation C-S-M for circulation, sensation, and motor is helpful in establishing a pattern. Circulation should be evaluated first. Unrecognized ischemia followed by necrosis makes the remainder of the evaluation a useless exercise. In addition, evaluation of circulation is the least invasive part of the examination. Evaluation should begin by examining the fingertips and assessing color and capillary refill. Capillary refill should be approximately 1 second; faster or slower are both bad and can indicate venous and arterial deficiency, respectively. The radial and ulnar arteries should also be palpated and an Allen's test performed. Checking the circulation is often forgotten; doing it first both prevents this, and also increases the patient's confidence in the examiner due to its pain-free nature in an already anxious setting.

Testing of sensation should also begin in the fingertips. It can be tested quickly in a gross fashion by gently stroking the patient's fingers and asking if it feels "normal" or "funny." It is often difficult for the patient to verbalize numbness or parasthesias more specifically. Responses of "funny" should be quantified by using two-point discrimination on both the radial and ulnar aspects of the finger pulp. Increased public awareness of carpal tunnel syndrome has given rise to a large number of patients who present with a "chief complaint" of carpal tunnel syndrome; this diagnosis should be called into question with the finding of an ulnar nerve deficit. Further neurologic testing, such as deep tendon reflexes, should also be done under the "S" portion of the examination.

The motor examination should measure individual muscle strength. Active and passive range of motion should also be performed. Finger flexion can be quickly recorded by measuring the distance from the fingertip to the distal palmar crease. When measuring range of motion of the wrist, one should remember to include supination and pronation in addition to flexion and extension. A passive range of motion greater than the active range of motion can indicate tendon rupture, whereas decrease in both active and passive range of motion is suggestive of contracture.

After the C-S-M portion of the examination, the physician should proceed with palpitation of painful areas. Here again the single finger method is useful. It forces the physician to be both accurate and gentle. Swelling or masses should also be looked for, and if found carefully described as to size, firmness, and mobility in relation to underlying structures.

A final aspect to consider is the presence of symptoms due to distant pathology. Pain in the hand or elbow can be associated with cervical spine or brachial plexus pathology.

Further Work-Up

After the history and physical examination, the diagnosis will be apparent in the majority of cases. Further studies may be necessary if the diagnosis remains unknown, or to assist in the planning of treatment. Radiographs are usually the first step in imaging. In cases of trauma with suspected fracture, radiographs are obviously indicated. Further studies, such as arthrograms, bone scans, computed tamography (CT), Magnetic resonance imaging (MRI), or electromyograms (EMGs), are more appropriately ordered by the specialist. Some of the more common uses of these studies are as follows:

- Arthrogram: assess ligamentous or triangular fibrocartilage complex of the wrist, usually with a triple injection technique (radiocarpal, distal radioulnar, and midcarpal joints).
- Bone scan: diagnosis of nondisplaced scaphoid fracture, avascular necrosis of the lunate, suspicion of metastatic disease (whole body bone scan).
- CT: occasionally for complex intra-articular distal radius fracture. Also for bony tumor.
- MRI: used increasingly for ligamentous and triangular fibrocartilage injuries of the wrist; also for soft tissue tumors.
- EMGs: commonly (perhaps unnecessarily) ordered to confirm carpal tunnel syndrome. Better reserved for atypical presentation.

Treatment

Although the treatment of hand, wrist, and elbow disorders are beyond the scope of this text, a description of the more commonly encountered problems will help to illustrate some of the options and dilemmas faced by the hand surgeon.

Fracture

Distal radius fractures are the most common upper extremity fracture in the elderly, with approximately 250,000 annually in the United States. These represent a pathologic fracture due to osteoporosis, which increases the difficulty of treating these injuries. Historically, treatment of distal radius fractures in the elderly consisted of closed reduction and casting, based on the belief that good clinical outcomes were obtained even with malunion. However, it is now recognized that the final outcome regarding pain, range of motion, and function are directly related to the adequacy of not initial, but final reduction. This point is critical, as almost all fractures can be temporarily reduced and placed in plaster. However, due to the compressive nature of the fracture, collapse in the cast is practically inevitable. Techniques now include percutaneous pinning, external fixation, open reduction and plating, and bone grafting. These can be used in almost any combination depending on the specific fracture pattern. More invasive techniques must be balanced against the risk of iatrogenically introduced stiffness. Although the current trend is toward more aggressive fixation, how much is too much is yet to be answered.

Osteoarthritis

The two most common sites of osteoarthritis in the upper extremity are the thumb carpometacarpal (CMC) or basal joint, and the distal interphalangeal (DIP) joints. They commonly present with pain with activity, and if present for a longer period, with deformity. Radiographs are diagnostic, with joint space narrowing and osteophytes. Initial treatment is symptomatic, with acetaminophen or nonsteroidal anti-inflammatory drugs (NSAIDs) and activity adjustment. Splints can be effective in basal joint arthritis. Treatment for failure of conservative therapy of the DIP joints usually consists of fusion. For the basal joint, partial or complete resection of the trapezium with ligament reconstruction and/or tendon interposition can be performed. Silicone implants have fallen out of favor in osteoarthritis, although they still play a role in rheumatoid arthritis. Osteoarthritis can also affect the elbow. The usual presenting symptoms are pain and flexion contracture.

Carpal Tunnel Syndrome

Carpal tunnel syndrome is due to compression of the median nerve in the carpal tunnel. Initial complaints include numbness and tingling in the thumb, index, and middle fingers, eventually with thenar muscle atrophy. Patients will often note dropping tea or coffee cups, due to the sensory and motor changes. Patients also typically have worsening of symptoms at nighttime. This is due to the usual flexed or extended position of the wrist while sleeping, both of which greatly increase carpal tunnel pressure. Initial treatment consists of NSAIDs to reduce presumed tenosynovitis, and nighttime wrist splints in a neutral position. Steroid injections have obtained mixed long-term results; however, most agree that a good short-term response to injection is an excellent prognostic indicator of surgical release. If there are signs of thenar atrophy at initial presentation, surgical release should not be delayed, as return in motor function is poor.

Tenosynovitis: Trigger Finger

Patients often present with a combination of carpal tunnel syndrome and trigger finger, as both are usually due to tenosynovitis. The trigger finger, a portion of the flexor tendon, becomes enlarged so that it barely fits through the A1 pulley located just proximal to the palmar-digital crease. The strong finger flexors are able to pull the tendon through the tight tunnel, but the weak extensor tendons cannot pull it back through, resulting in a finger stuck in flexion. Patient will report either strenuously extended the finger or having to open the finger with the other hand, usually with a painful popping sensation. Patients will sometimes only complain of pain in the region of the proximal interphalangeal joint; specific questions about triggering and palpating for a nodule over the A1 pulley can lead to the diagnosis. Permanent relief can be obtained with steroid injection; however, surgical release is sometimes necessary.

Tenosynovitis: De Quervain's

De Quervain's tenosynovitis affects the extensor tendon compartment, through which run the abductor pollices longus and the extensor pollices brevis. Patients present with pain over the distal lateral aspect of the radius, worsened by wrist extension and radial deviation. Treatment is analogous to the trigger finger, with initial conservative treatment followed by steroid injection and surgical release when necessary.

Dupuytren's Contracture

Dupuytren's contracture usually presents with painless progressive flexion contracture of the ring or small finger. Family history may be positive. A palpable nodule is often present, representing a thickening of the palmar fascia. Splinting is ineffective. Steroid injection can be used, but the standard treatment is surgical excision of the diseased fascia.

Rheumatoid Arthritis

Hand

Rheumatoid arthritis in the hand usually presents with involvement of the metacarpophalangeal (MCP) joints. Morning pain and stiffness is a common complaint. As the symptoms progress, there is a destruction of supporting ligaments and cartilage. Ulnar deviation of the digits at the MCP joints is the most common deformity. Patients also frequently develop swan neck of boutonniere deformities. Involvement of the thumb is particularly problematic; both the CMC and the MCP joints are commonly involved. Treatment of the deformities in the fingers and thumb is by a combination of fusion, occasional silicone arthroplasty, and ligament and tendon rebalancing.

Wrist

Rheumatoid arthritis in the wrist causes progressive deformity. Synovitis initially causes swelling, pain, and limitation of motion. As the rheumatoid synovium invades and destroys surrounding tendons, ligaments, cartilage, and bone, a pattern of deformity results. Surgical treatment is aimed at both preventing deformity and correcting deformity already present. The first procedures usually done involve the removal of synovium surrounding joints and tendons to alleviate pain and possibly prevent further destruction. Once tendon rupture occurs, surgery must be aimed at both reconstruction of the tendons and prevention of recurrent tendon damage. Usually by the time tendon rupture has occurred, synovial invasion has also caused significant ligament destruction and laxity, allowing the ulna and carpal bones to migrate. Thus, at this stage surgical intervention is also aimed at ligament reconstruction in order to restore the correct alignment of the bones. Tendons may also be transferred or tightened in order to provide additional and sometimes dynamic support to prevent recurrent bony migration. After bone and cartilage have been destroyed, surgical options consist of joint replacement or joint fusion.

Synovitis commonly is found around the extensor tendons on the dorsum of the wrist. Often, a transverse indentation in the swelling can be seen; this is due to the restraining effect of the dorsal retinaculum. Failure to control the synovitis with medical therapy over a period of 6 months is an indication of synovectomy; this is done in order to prevent rupture of the extensor tendons. A single extensor tendon rupture may present with only a mild extension lag due to the juncturae tendinea; however, subsequent ruptures will result in a more marked loss of range of motion and function. The extensor tendons are damaged both by direct invasion of the synovium and by fraying over the dorsally displaced ulna. This migration of the ulna occurs as synovium destroys ligaments that normally hold the distal radioulnar joint stable. As a result, the most common pattern of extensor tendon involvement is the small finger first, followed by the ring, middle, and index fingers. Extensor tendon rupture to just the small finger may be repaired with transfer of the distal stump to the ring finger extensor tendon; however, with multiple ruptures, simple transfer may not be possible, and the use of tendon transfers from the index finger, or even of the flexor tendons, may be necessary. In addition to being a more extensive procedure, the results of multiple extensor tendon reconstructions are not as predictable. Thus, it is preferable to perform synovectomy prior to tendon rupture. If dorsal migration of the ulna is present, this must also be addressed in order to prevent future tendon damage due to fraying. One method of returning the ulnar head to its normal position is to fuse it to the radius; this must be combined with a more proximal resection of a portion of the ulna in order to preserve pronation and supination. This preservation of the ulnar head is advocated by some to prevent future ulnar migration of the carpal bones. An approach more commonly used to address this displaced ulnar head is to remove it; this must be combined with a reconstruction of the ligaments in order to support the medial aspect of the wrist and prevent future dorsal migration of the remaining ulna.

Synovitis surrounding the flexor tendons presents with pain, symptoms of median nerve compression, and loss of motion. The swelling usually is not as prominent as on the dorsum of the wrist, and only a slight loss of the skin creases may be seen. Flexor tendon ruptures occur less commonly than extensor tendon ruptures; most often the thumb and index finger are involved due to fraying over a bony spur on the scaphoid. Treatment consists of synovectomy, tendon repair or transfer, and removal of any offending bony spurs.

Synovectomy of the wrist joints themselves remains somewhat more controversial. Although tenosynovectomy prevents tendon rupture, synovectomy of the wrist joints has not been firmly shown to prevent the progressive destruction of the joint, and has also been found by some to result in a loss of range of motion. However, it is generally agreed that for synovitis not responsive to medical treatment, in the presence of minimal cartilage and bone destruction, synovectomy will provide significant pain relief.

Once significant cartilage and bone destruction have occurred, surgical options include arthrodesis and arthroplasty, each of which has several variations with specific advantages and disadvantages. Although wrist fusion gives a stable and pain-free wrist, bilateral wrist fusions in the rheumatoid patient with bilateral disease cause significant difficulty with some activities of daily living. Partial fusions are another option. The pattern of joint destruction frequently shows severe radiocarpal disease with maintenance of the midcarpal joint. In such a patient, a fusion of just the radiocarpal joint leaving the midcarpal joint intact will relieve pain, yet retain 25 to 50 percent of wrist motion. Numerous other partial fusions may also be performed, the concept being to limit fusion to the diseased joints while preserving motion in the healthier joints.

Joint replacements have taken the form of either silicone or metal and plastic implants. While retaining motion, significant problems have been encountered. These include silicone synovitis, dislocation and breakage of the implants, progression of bone destruction, and infection. In addition, candidates must have adequate bone stock for the implant and functioning wrist extensors. High-demand patients also do more poorly after joint replacement. This must be kept in mind in a population that may require ambulatory aids. Silicone wrist implants have shown disappointing long-term results. Many surgeons now recommend their use only in very low-demand patients who specifically require wrist motion. Metal and plastic implants initially had problems with alignment of the center of rotation; newer designs appear to have solved this problem. The major remaining flaw seems to be loosening of the distal component. However, this has not prevented good long-term follow-up in properly selected patients. Although metal and plastic wrist arthroplasty show promise, their current use is primarily in rheumatoid patients who have bilateral wrist disease or significant loss of motion in their elbows and shoulders such that further loss of motion with wrist fusion would compromise function. In the patient with failed wrist arthroplasty, wrist fusion remains as a salvage procedure.

Elbow

The elbow is affected in 20 to 50 percent of patients with rheumatoid arthritis. Initial presentation is with synovitis causing pain, swelling, and loss of range of motion. Synovitis may cause so much swelling as to cause compression of surrounding structures, including the posterior interosseus and ulnar nerves. Synovectomy prior to evidence of bone and ligament involvement has shown good relief of pain for 3 years in about 90 percent of patients, and relief of pain for 5 years in 75 to 80 percent of patients. Some patients will also show some improvement in the range of motion. There is some controversy regarding the use of synovectomy in patients with joint destruction; however, although increases in the range of motion cannot be expected, many have reported significant pain relief in this group of patients. Radial head excision at the time of synovectomy is also a point of controversy. It is advocated by some, including us, to both improve exposure and to prevent future painful supination and pronation due to radiohumeral joint destruction. Others have proposed that removal of the radial head will destabilize the elbow, and with newer arthroscopic techniques, is unnecessary to facilitate adequate synovectomy. Patients with more severe joint destruction and instability or stiffness are candidates for one of the forms of arthroplasty.

Arthroplasty in the elbow can be performed using interposition of biologic material, nonconstrained metal components, or semiconstrained metal and plastic prostheses. A requirement for interpositional arthroplasty is adequate bone stock; this is often not present in the rheumatoid patient, and is more commonly used in patients with post-traumatic arthritis. The current selection of metal and plastic prostheses has evolved from earlier models with high failure rates. Early models with a simple hinge allowing only flexion and extension had unacceptably high rates of loosening, as any rotational or lateral forces were transferred directly to the prosthesis-bone interface. Newer designs have placed more reliance on muscles and ligaments for stability, thus protecting the bone-prosthesis interface. Nonconstrained or resurfacing models rely almost entirely on muscle and ligaments for stability; thus, they have the potential for dislocation. Semiconstrained models are interlocked "sloppy" hinges designed to have 7 to 10 degrees of toggle or play, thus having some inherent stability, but also relying on muscles and ligaments for stability. Theoretical benefits of the resurfacing models include less bone resection and lower loosening rates; benefits of the semiconstrained model include the use in previously unstable elbows and in revision surgery. Similar results have been reported in both types of prostheses. Relief of pain is noted in more than 90 percent of patients; a range of motion of 100 degrees in flexion and extension and 80 degrees in pronation and supination is also predictable, allowing most activities of daily living.

Complications of both resurfacing and semiconstrained elbow arthroplasty remain a concern. Although loosening rates have been decreased from 25 percent or more to 3 to 5 percent with newer designs, complications of infection, neuropraxia, and instability remain higher than for hip and knee arthroplasty. Infection rates of 3 to 11 percent are reported, due partly to the subcutaneous nature of the joint. Neuropraxias of the ulnar nerve are seen in about 7 percent of patients. Instability is found in 5 to 20 percent of patients. Revision options following failure include reimplantation of a semiconstrained prosthesis, interposition arthroplasty, and fusion. Because fusion causes severe limitations in activity, in addition to further stresses on often coexisting disease in the wrist and shoulder, it is considered by many surgeons only to be an option in cases of severe infection or where bone loss prohibits reimplantation. Recent reports show promising reductions in the rate of complications and need for revision surgery. For the properly selected patient, total elbow arthroplasty can be confidently predicted to provide relief of pain and a functional range of motion.

Degenerative Disorders of the Shoulder

This section discusses the relatively common degenerative conditions of osteoarthritis, rheumatoid arthritis, and rotator cuff disease in the geriatric population. Assessment of a patient with glenohumeral arthritis is similar to that of other joints. The history and physical examination strongly suggests the diagnosis and imaging studies are useful to confirm the clinical suspicion.

Pain is the chief complaint of almost all these patients, and is almost always associated with a functional deficit. The pain may radiate down the upper arm and forearm, or upward to the neck and trapezial area. In contrast, pain secondary to cervical spine pathology usually radiates to the superior or posterior aspect of the shoulder. A careful neurologic examination should help differentiate between these two causes of shoulder pain. Pain due to glenohumeral arthritis is usually worse at night, as it is exacerbated by use of the extremity and relieved with rest.

Inspection of the shoulder may reveal varying degrees of periscapular muscle atrophy. Pain upon palpation of the joint line as well as with shoulder motion is common. Tenderness upon palpation of the acromioclavicular joint should be assessed in all patients, as it is a very reliable indicator of acromioclavicular joint arthritis. Range of motion of the arthritic shoulder is painful and limited, and may be associated with palpable crepitus. Crepitus anteriorly and superiorly may indicate the presence of a massive rotator cuff tear with glenohumeral and humeroacromial arthritis (cuff tear arthropathy).[66] Strength of the shoulder musculature may be preserved (4/5 to 5/5) unless compromised by rotator cuff tear or pain.

Radiographic evaluation of the arthritic shoulder consists of true anteroposterior (AP) views of the shoulder in both internal and external rotation and an axillary view. The AP views are helpful to assess the degree of joint space narrowing and presence of osteophytes. The axillary view is used to assess posterior glenoid wear, which may alter the surgical technique. The radiographic pathoanatomy of osteoarthritis of the shoulder is similar to that of any disarthroid joint: narrowing of the joint space, subchondral sclerosis, peripheral osteophytes, and subchondral cyst formation. The largest osteophytes are usually located inferiorly. Osteophytes can enlarge the head of the humerus significantly and lead to a mechanical block to motion. Advanced cases are often associated with posterior glenoid wear from concomitant posterior shoulder instability.

Shoulder involvement in rheumatoid arthritis is common, affecting 50 to 60 percent of patients with the disease.[67,68] However, the course and severity of the disease varies greatly from individual to individual. All of the tissues about the shoulder are usually affected in rheumatoid arthritis. The subdeltoid-subacromial bursa can develop a painful bursitis that coexists with rotator cuff pathology. Attrition of the glenohumeral joint capsule and ligaments can lead to instability. The radiographic appearance of the proximal humerus and glenoid may appear normal or may demonstrate extensive erosions that parallel the degree of synovitis.

Conservative measures should be undertaken for initial treatment of mild to moderately severe shoulder arthritis. In addition, patients with severe disease who are poor surgical candidates because of medical comorbidities must also be managed nonoperatively. Physical therapy protocols designed to stretch and strengthen the rotator cuff and periscapular musculature are useful for increasing the range of motion and strength of the arthritic shoulder. Local modalities (e.g., heat, ice, ultrasound) and nonsteroidal anti-inflammatory medications may help to control swelling and pain.

Surgical treatment of the arthritic shoulder ranges from minimally invasive arthroscopic synovectomy to total shoulder replacement with glenoid and humeral prostheses. Arthroscopic synovectomy can provide pain relief for patients with rheumatoid arthritis, especially if attempted early in the course of their disease.[69–71] Prosthetic arthroplasty of the shoulder, if properly performed, provides predictable relief of pain with good or excellent functional results in more than 90 percent of patients.[72] Other surgical options with less predictable outcomes include capsular release, osteotomy, resection arthroplasty, and shoulder arthrodesis.

The rotator cuff consists of the tendinous insertions of the supraspinatus, infraspinatus, teres minor, and subscapularis muscles on the humeral head. It functions to both rotate the humeral head about its axis as well as to compress the humeral head into the concavity of the glenoid fossa, thus providing a fulcrum against which the powerful deltoid muscle can abduct, extend, and forward flex the humerus.[73] The rotator cuff is frequently involved in rheumatoid arthritis of the shoulder, but rarely involved in osteoarthritis.[74] The treatment of glenohumeral arthritis associated with rotator cuff tears is similar to that previously described. However, because of the biomechanical alteration of the joint kinematics, insertion of a glenoid component has been associated with a high rate of loosening and failure.[75] Therefore, hemiarthroplasty with a large-headed humeral component has become the accepted treatment for these patients.

Rotator cuff tears frequently present in the geriatric population without concomitant glenohumeral arthritis. The tendons of the rotator cuff are highly resistant to tearing in young patients, and full-thickness rotator cuff tears rarely occur in patients younger than 40 years of age. With increasing age and disuse, failure of the cuff tendons is more likely. The patient will typically present with the insidious onset of pain and weakness of shoulder abduction and external rotation. Complaints of inability to sleep on the affected side at night, placing the hand behind the head (e.g., combing hair), and placing objects on high shelves are common. Physical examination may reveal atrophy of the affected muscles in chronic cases. Occasionally, the cuff defect may be palpated by rotating the humeral head underneath the examiner's fingers. Strength in abduction and external rotation is decreased, and the patient may exhibit a positive "drop-arm" test (inability to maintain active shoulder abduction against manual downward pressure). The neck of a patient with a weak shoulder must also be examined to rule out cervical radiculopathy or branchial plexopathy as a cause of the patient's symptoms.

The radiographic analysis of patients with isolated rotator cuff tears is not as revealing as those associated with glenohumeral arthritis. Chronic tears may be associated with subacromial or treater tuberosity sclerosis or cyst formation. The coracoacromial ligament and/or cuff tendon insertion may be partially calcified. Arthrography, ultrasound, and magnetic resonance imaging are useful modalities to identify the presence and extent of the cuff pathology.

The treatment of a full-thickness rotator cuff tear must be tailored to the functional demands of the patient, the patient's symptoms, and the ability to achieve a durable repair. Low-demand patients with minimal symptoms may be treated nonoperatively with nonsteroidal anti-inflammatory medications and physical therapy modalities. Healthy patients with greater functional demands benefit significantly from surgical repair of the torn tendon edges to their anatomic insertion sites on the proximal humerus. As in any chronic condition, surgical repair is not an emergency and may be reserved for those patients who fail to respond favorably to nonoperative treatment.

Knee Problems in the Geriatric Patient

The importance of orthopaedic surgery in the geriatric population is to preserve independence. Although the musculoskeletal system at times does not take precedence in the treatment of the multitude of medical problems that elderly patients are faced with, the ability to get around as well as cognitive ability are the two most important factors in maintaining independence. The emergence of geriatrics as an increasingly important part of medicine in society has stressed the importance of orthopaedic surgery as a member of a multidisciplinary team in maintaining the independence and quality of life of elderly people.

Evidence suggests that older patients are weaker, have less endurance, and have smaller muscle fibers than do younger patients.[76] It is known that elderly people have fewer anterior horn cells.[77] However, part of their weakness is due to a lower level of condition, because older patients can increase both strength and endurance following training programs.[78,79]

In addition, the joint range of motion is diminished. The tendons, ligaments, and capsule surrounding joints lose elasticity as evidenced by the decrease in the joint range of motion and a sense of stiffness in older patients.[80] Stiffness following sleep, prolonged sitting, or exercise is more common and prolonged in older patients.

Rehabilitation is crucial after orthopaedic surgery and the physiatrists needs to take into consideration the special needs of the geriatric patient as discussed above. Also, the presence of osteoporosis should be determined before prescribing exercises that load the spine. Range of motion should be initiated slowly and not too vigorously. In principle the rehabilitation goals are to return each patient to the premorbid functional level of mobility and self-care, teach the exercises that are to be performed after hospital discharge, reduce the risk of falls, and ensure that the patient is discharged to a safe environment.

Background

Arthritis, joint, and musculoskeletal diseases commonly affect older patients. The knee is no exception, being affected by osteoarthritis, rheumatoid arthritis, pseudogout, polymyalgia-rheumatica, tumors, infection, and sports-related injuries. Certainly, degenerative joint disease (osteoarthritis) is by far the most common affliction of the knees in this population; knee osteoarthritis is more likely to result in disability than osteoarthritis of any other joint. Because of technology, an increased understanding of geriatric medicine, and the improved results obtained from total joint arthroplasty in the elderly population, orthopaedic surgeons are operating on increasing numbers of elderly patients with acute and chronic conditions of the knee that cause functional disability.

Osteoarthritis

Osteoarthritis is a slowly progressive monoarticular (or less commonly polyarticular) disorder of unknown cause and obscure pathogenesis. The condition occurs late in life, affecting principally the large weight-bearing joints, and is characterized clinically by pain, deformity, enlargement of the joint, and limitation of motion. For the elderly patient especially there is a rapid increasing limitation of motion that is more severe after a period of inactivity such as sitting in a chair or automobile or even after a night's sleep. For the knee, flexion is lost initially and later the patient develops an extensor lag (the inability to completely extend the knee). Deformity due to osteoarthritis is also troublesome causing an enlargement of the joint and in the knee a varus deformity (bowing) of the proximal tibia. Among the most bothersome symptoms for patients is their complaint of an abnormal gait. Even moderately severe osteoarthritis of a major joint (and especially in the weight-bearing area), causes dense sclerosis of the subchondral bone, cysts adjacent to the joint, and the presence of large marginal osteophytes. These radiographic findings are highly specific for osteoarthritis. Physicians treating the disease, therefore, rarely require other studies for substantiation of the disease.

Treatment

Treatment of osteoarthritis includes nonsteroidal anti-inflammatory drugs (NSAIDs) and joint injections.[81] Surgical treatments include joint replacement, osteotomy, and arthrodesis. In elderly patients arthrodesis is reserved mainly for failed total knee replacements. High tibial osteotomies are being performed in patients in their 60s and 70s who are active, which in the past has been reserved for younger patients. Rehabilitation techniques include decreasing weight-bearing on affected joints by the use of canes, crutches, walkers, and dieting. Exercise will increase the strength of muscles around involved joints, especially the knee extensors. Certainly, increasing the strength of these muscles by exercise will improve the muscular response after surgery.[82] Specific rehabilitation goals for total knee replacement are to regain full knee extension and at least 90 degrees of knee flexion as well as strengthening the quadriceps.

In the elderly population the choice to perform a total knee replacement is easier because age is not as great a consideration. In the younger patient who is active a total knee replacement might wear out and may not be the best choice. In the very aged (older than 80 years of age) with lower demands arthrodesis and osteotomy are not as indicated and total knee replacements become the procedure of choice. The elderly patient with pain in the knee significant enough to interfere with daily activities and with radiographic findings consistent with osteoarthritis are candidates for total knee replacements.

Total joint arthroplasty has proven to be a very successful procedure for older patients with severe osteoarthritis. However, most studies have focused on populations in their sixth and seventh decades of life. There is little literature published regarding total joint arthroplasty in the very aged (older than 80 years of age). Surgeons in the past have been reluctant to offer total joint replacements to patients in this age group for fear of subsequent mortality and morbidity. The results of total joint arthroplasty in patients in this age group have not been known until recently, with the surgery proving to be as beneficial and without significantly greater complications than in younger patients.[83–87] In the article by Tankersley et al.[86] 19 of 20 patients with a mean age of 87 years had good to excellent results with total knee replacements although most still used walking devices. Pain was the most common indication to perform the surgery and it seems that quality of life is much improved with the surgery. Good results has also been shown in performing total hip arthroplasty although there is a higher dislocation rate in patients greater than 80 years of age.[88–92]

Arthroscopy

There is much controversy and confusion regarding arthroscopic surgery in the elderly patient. Particularly in the geriatric knee with radiographic evidence of osteoarthritis, the orthopaedic surgeon has been reluctant to overuse arthroscopy for knee complaints. There are conditions afflicting the elderly in the knee that respond to arthroscopic surgery. Arthroscopic synovectomy in rheumatoid arthritis has shown beneficial effects.[93] Synovectomies in synovial chondromatosis and pigmented villonodular synovitis have also shown good results.

Unfortunately, the most common problem concerning the knee in the geriatric patient stems from the manifestations of chronic degenerative joint disease (i.e., loose fragments of articular cartilage, degenerative tears of the menisci, osteophyte formation). Arthroscopy has been used in the arthritic knee for joint debridements, miniscectomies, subchondral drillings, abrasion arthroplasties, and loose body removal.[80,94–97] Compared with resurfacing procedures (i.e., total joint replacements), however, arthroscopy should be considered a temporary measure and not a definitive operation. Success rates in terms of relief of pain and improvement in function do not compare favorably with those of arthroplasty. Certainly arthroscopy is preferable in patients whose poor medical conditions are contraindications to larger procedures and in those patients refusing the more drastic alternative.

Acute injuries also affect the geriatric knee. It was long believed that knee pain in the older patient who had minuscule tears was a result of the osteoarthritic changes seen in the radiograph. As a result, orthopaedic surgeons denied elderly patients with mechanical knee symptoms surgery because of the opinion that the result would not be satisfactory. Through the years, studies have shown that aging patients are prone to acute tears of the meniscus as well as degenerative tears.[98] The acute tear causing symptoms will do well with arthroscopic surgery and should not be denied to the elderly patient.

Rheumatoid Arthritis

Rheumatoid arthritis is less frequent than osteoarthritis and seems to be different in the elderly than in the younger person. The sex ratio is more equal, and the duration of the disease is shorter. The small joints of the hand are more frequently affected. Shoulder involvement is also striking and the synovitis seems more impressive. Knee involvement is less often seen. Radiographic findings are less severe. Despite the lack of radiographic findings, the disease is devastating to the function of the elderly person.

Fractures of the Lower Extremity in the Geriatric Population

The lower extremity comprises the bulk of major fractures in the elderly, is responsible for more than 90 percent of all fracture surgery, and presents unique treatment problems. Generally, there are two types of patients injured: an active younger group and a frail older one.[99] In the former, activities such as shopping, walking, or dancing often lead to falls or other trauma, whereas in the latter group, a fall indoors is the common mechanism of injury. Susceptibility to fracture is related to age, osteoporosis, sex, and geography.[100–105]

The large increase in fracture rate after the age of 60 years is mainly due to falls.[104] However, the absolute number of fractures in the elderly population is also rising rapidly, due in part to the advancing age of the geriatric population.[106–109] Another common factor is osteoporosis,[100,103,104] present in approximately 80 percent of hip fracture patients aged 80 years.[102] Women are more affected because of their lower peak bone mass, more rapid postmenopausal bone loss, and greater risk of falls. The association with geographic location is in all likelihood related to bone mass, which is in turn affected by race, smoking, alcohol consumption, and physical inactivity.[106,108,110]

Fractures in elderly patients unite over a similar period of time as in 30-year-olds.[111–113] The healing process per se does not therefore require any special treatment for the elderly patient and good alignment and early mobilization become the prime goals of management. Thus, treatment options do not differ greatly from those standard in younger patients. However, knowledge of comorbid conditions, the patient's physiologic age, and the quality of bone stock available is crucial to the decision-making process.

Significant displacement, an inability to obtain a closed reduction, and intra-articular fractures are often indicators for surgery. Good results can be obtained following open reduction and internal fixation if the proper patient is selected. However, in the lower extremity, it may be easier to treat a leg length discrepancy with a shoe lift rather than performing a bone graft with its weight-bearing delay and risk of nonunion.[113]

Fractures of the Pelvis and Acetabulum

Isolated fractures of the pubic ramus, pelvic insufficiency fractures, and small nondisplaced fractures involving the acetabulum or sacrum can be treated nonoperatively.[114,115] The patient is typically placed on a regimen of appropriate analgesics, limited abduction, and bed rest or restricted weight-bearing with a walking frame. However, this must not be prolonged because of the well-known risks of immobilization in the elderly. Typically, not more than 1 week is required for the bulk of these. For most acetabular fractures, a period of up to 8 weeks may be required.

The personality of the injury changes with the total disruption of the pelvic ring suffered by a pedestrian struck by a motor vehicle. Excessive blood loss from a bleeding pelvis venous plexus is among the most common causes of shock in the geriatric trauma patient.[116,117] Transfusion requirements averaged 29 units for closed and 763 units for open injuries in one series.[116] Major venous bleeding can often be controlled by placement of an external fixator, and arterial hemorrhage arrested by embolization in the angiography suite.[118] Unfortunately, external fixation can be tenuous in the brittle thin iliac bone of patient with osteoporosis.[113] Occasionally, an exploratory laparotomy is required to ligate the hypogastric vessels.

The overall rate of acute and delayed mortality from these fractures in the elderly population is 17 percent, approaching 90 percent with open injury.[116,119,120] Mortality rises from 3 percent in a normotensive patient to 38 percent in one with hypotension.[116]

Open reduction and internal fixation of selected displaced acetabular fractures in the elderly population has been shown to yield good results.[121] However, a high rate of failure of total hip arthroplasty performed after surgical stabilization of fractures has also been reported.[122] This may be due to excessive stripping of bone during the fracture fixation. Therefore, a primary total hip arthroplasty may be preferable to internal fixation in older patients and in those with signs of arthritis.

Fractures of the Proximal Femur

Fractures of the hip include those of the femoral neck and peritrochanteric region. Occurring with similar frequencies[123,124] and at an average age of 80 years,[118,125] these are associated with significant postoperative morbidity and mortality. They are the fourth largest cause of death in the elderly,[101,105] The pessimism permeating the medical community regarding their treatment is stated eloquently by DeLee[126] who writes: "We come into the world under the brim of the pelvis and go out through the neck of the femur."

As many as 300,000 Americans sustain hip fractures each year, comprising the majority of patients hospitalized with fractures.[127,128] Fractures of the proximal femur account for more than 70 percent of all operative procedures for fractures in patients over 70 years of age with the femur second at 16 percent.[113] This staggering number of injuries consumes a major portion of national health care resources estimated at $750 million each year,[105,129,130] an amount greater than that for all other fractures combined.[101]

More disturbing is that the number of fractures is increasing each year[105,131,132] and will probably double by 2050.[123] In England, by the age of 85 years, 12 percent of women and 5 percent of men will have sustained a hip fracture.[110] Gallagher et al.[133] noted that the rate of hip fracture doubled in each decade of life after age 50, and that by the age of 90, 32 percent of women and 17 percent of men had sustained a fracture.

Risk factors associated with fracture of the proximal femur include advancing age, female sex, falls, decreased bone mass, low body weight, physical inactivity, muscle weakness, and osteomalacia.[99,100,105,106,110,123,124,133–136] In elderly female patients, a fracture is nine times more likely to be the result of a fall than trauma.[137]

The magnitude and direction of applied forces as well as the degree of osteoporosis all contribute to variations in fracture pattern.[105,113,123] Direct forces include blows to the greater trochanter and impingement of the acetabular rim on the femoral neck (neck fractures). Indirect forces are primarily the pull of the abductors on the greater trochanter (intertrochanteric fractures).[123]

When an individual falls from a standing position, the energy sustained exceeds by many times that required to create a fracture of the femoral neck. The question then is why even more patients do not sustain fractures. Some of this potential energy is dissipated by use of the upper limbs to brace the fall and the elastic properties of soft tissues and other components of the skeleton.[105] Unfortunately, older, slower, weaker muscles cannot always contract enough to dissipate the energy of a fall.[123]

The postmenopausal loss of bone density that occurs in a majority of women not on hormone replacement therapy substantiates the 2:1 to 8:1 ratio of women to men found in most series of proximal femur fractures.[124] However, Stevens[105] noted in a large review that there is an uncertain relationship between osteoporosis and hip fracture and that after the age of 75 years protective neuromuscular responses may be more important.

Although neurologic conditions such as Parkinson's disease, stroke, and dementia will require special surgical considerations, they are not contraindications for either internal fixation or prosthetic replacement.[123,138]

The presence of osteoporosis also affects the choice of stabilization because fixation of the proximal fragment depends not just on the quality of reduction[139,140] but on the quality of cancellous bone present.[141] To this end, the Singh Index estimates the degree of osteoporosis by roentgenographic evaluation of trabecular patterns, grading them one through six.[142]

Evaluation and Initial Care

A rapid and concise evaluation is important for optimal treatment as noted in a recent report recommending that no patient spend greater than 1 hour in the emergency department.[110] Elderly patients living alone may lie undiscovered for hours or even days. These delays in medical treatment often leave the patient dehydrated and confused.

Displaced fractures will classically present with pain, shortening, external rotation, and an inability to stand or walk. Acutely, there may be swelling in the hip region, and later ecchymosis present over the greater trochanter. Neurovascular injury is rare.[123] With rotation of as much as 90 degrees, the findings associated with an intertrochanteric fracture are usually more obvious. Neck and nondisplaced fractures will often present without any clinical deformity.

Imaging studies include three radiographs. An anteroposterior radiograph of the affected hip taken in internal rotation will demonstrate the neck anatomy best. A similar view of the pelvis will allow comparison of the contralateral side. A cross-table lateral, better tolerated by a hip fracture patient, is important for evaluation of stability and displacement of the fracture.

Buck's traction is a light skin traction (up to 5 pounds) that provides some immobilization and maintenance of length of the extremity. However, it should be used carefully when peripheral vascular or sensory changes are present.

Occult Fractures

Occult fractures about the hip represent a difficult diagnostic and treatment problem. The patient often presents with a vague history of hip pain, minimal trauma, variable discomfort on motion, and an inability to bear weight.[143] In these cases, atraumatic diagnoses including arthritis, neoplasm, trochanteric bursitis, avascular necrosis, and spinal conditions are tempting. However, even with normal roentgenograms, a fracture should be considered. If suspicion is low or the patient not a candidate for further imaging studies, they can be made non-weight-bearing and repeat roentgenograms obtained in 1 week.

Otherwise, the traditional diagnostic procedure of choice has been technetium-99m bone scanning.[143,144] More recently however, magnetic resonance imaging (MRI) has become popular.[145] Its advantages include rapid procurement, greater specificity, an ability to delineate fracture lines, and few difficulties for a patient with renal or urinary tract problems. In addition, bone scanning may require postponement for several days to improve sensitivity,[118,146] thus increasing costs and delaying treatment.

Timing of Surgery

Historically, nonoperative management has resulted in nonunion or malunion, prolonged immobility, and very long hospital stays. These in turn have led to high rates of medical morbidity including contractures, decubiti, urinary tract and pulmonary infections, atelectasis, deep venous thrombosis, pulmonary emboli, and death.[105,118,123] Thus, surgery is almost always indicated.

In general, the shorter the interval between injury and surgery the fewer the complications. However, it is essential that all comorbid medical conditions be evaluated and treated promptly before surgery.[110,147–149] Del Guercio and Cohn[150] demonstrated that only 67 percent of elderly patients cleared for elective surgery had normal hemodynamic and respiratory function, and that 23 percent were in reality unacceptable surgical candidates, dying during subsequent procedures. Furthermore, perioperative physiologic monitoring using a Swan-Ganz catheter to assess optimum physiologic equilibrium has been reported to improve survival rates.[148,151,152]

Kenzora[147] reported that a delay of surgery less than 1 week was not associated with increased mortality. In fact, he noted that healthy patients operated on within 24 hours of injury had a 1 year mortality of 34 percent as opposed to 5.8 percent for those taken to the operating room after 2 to 5 days. In contrast, other authors have noted that those with two or fewer comorbid conditions have a higher rate of survival when operated on within 24 to 48 hours.[148,149] Thus, a guiding principle should be early intervention in healthy patients and initial medical optimization prior to surgery in those with multiple comorbidities.

For elderly patients with several risk factors for increased morbidity and mortality, surgery may not improve survival.[130,131,153–155] This has prompted some to recommend nonoperative management for these patients.[154] Although the risks of significant complications may be diminished by meticulous nursing care and early immobilization, this method must be chosen with caution.[130]

Fractures of the Femoral Neck

Fractures of the femoral neck are defined as intracapsular fractures beginning distal to the articular surface of the femoral head and ending just proximal to the intertrochanteric region. The presence of displacement often determines whether internal fixation or prosthetic replacement is to be performed.

Fracture displacement will disrupt the fragile blood supply coursing along the lateral capsule, leading to avascular necrosis of the femoral head. As the simple act of using a bedpan is sufficient to cause fracture displacement,[143] nondisplaced fractures should merit surgical consideration.[156] In addition, rigid fixation will avoid a poorly tolerated prolonged period of non-weight-bearing.[123]

The most accepted system for classification of this fracture is that of Garden:[157] A Garden type I is an incomplete and impacted fracture tilted into valgus; a type II is complete without displacement; a type III is partially displaced; and a type IV is completely displaced.

In general, nondisplaced fractures are treated with internal fixation, which usually involves the placement of three screws across the fracture site.[140] In those patients who are physiologically 75 years of age or younger, reduction and internal fixation for displaced fractures may be considered in the presence of good bone stock.[158,159]

Although nonunion (5 percent) and osteonecrosis (8 percent) are uncommon with nondisplaced fractures, their incidence rises to as high as 35 percent each in displaced fractures.[105,139,160,161] Rates are also typically higher in women[158] and in patients with advanced age.[162] In addition, one-third of patients with osteonecrosis and three-fourths with nonunion or early fixation failure will require additional surgery.[105,123,162]

Thus, prosthetic replacement in the form of cemented hemiarthroplasty is preferred for displaced fractures of the femoral neck.[105,123,159,163–165] Although not without its own problems of infection[164] and dislocation[126,163] this procedure avoids the morbidity and mortality associated with failure of internal fixation. Hemiarthroplasty is especially indicated for patients with a physiologic age over 65 years and in those whose medical condition is so tenuous that a second salvage for failure of primary fixation is not possible.[105,118] Also, patients over 75 years of age may benefit more with additional acetabular reconstruction, especially with pre-existing disease in this region (osteoarthritis, rheumatoid arthritis, Paget's disease).[105]

Other relative indications for prosthetic replacement include chronic renal disease, hyperparathyroidism, severe osteopenia (steroids, alcohol, malnutrition), and metastatic disease.[105,118,123] Internal fixation of fractures related to these conditions leads to high complication rates because of poor bone quality. A prosthesis may also be best for patients requiring a rapid return to ambulatory status because of other debilities such as blindness.

Fractures of the Intertrochanteric Region

Fractures of the intertrochanteric region are associated with significant morbidity and mortality.[166–168] They occur between the proximal tip of the greater trochanter and the distal aspect of the lesser trochanter. Because of their extracapsular nature and occurrence through well-perfused cancellous bone, healing is rarely a problem.[105,124]

Although many classification systems exist, the one of Evans[103] is perhaps the easiest to understand and use in clinical practice as it classifies fractures into stable (type I) and unstable (type II). The fracture may also be described in terms of the number of "parts," consisting of the proximal and distal fragments, and the two trochanters (i.e., two-, three-, and four-part fractures).

Surgical stabilization followed by early mobilization is preferred for both displaced and nondisplaced fractures. However, Hornby et al.[169] found no significant differences between patients treated surgically or conservatively for occult intertrochanteric fractures. But the latter group required hospitalization for an additional 26 days, leading to increased financial and social costs. Thus, nonoperative treatment may be suitable for only a small proportion of patients.

Although many implants have been used to treat intertrochanteric hip fractures, the method of choice is still fixation with a sliding hip screw device,[105,118,124,170–173] which has tolerated stress better than most static implants. Intramedullary devices may also have some applications.[113,124,171]

Unfortunately, complex unstable fractures can be associated with an 80 percent incidence of pain and collapse and poor bone quality can predispose to implant failure. To address these problems, osteotomies, bone cement, and hemiarthroplasty are occasionally required.[105,113,174–178]

The common finding of postoperative shortening can be partially overcome with a shoe lift, and reoperation in this frail group of patients is only required if the implant cuts out or causes severe pain.[105] In addition, angular and rotational deformities, osteonecrosis, implant failure, and screw migration are not uncommon.[114,124]

Pathologic Hip Fracture

Behr et al.[179] have noted that the most common primary tumor that metastasizes to the hip is that of the female breast. This tumor accounts for 45 percent of pathologic fractures, followed by 20 percent with myeloma, and 11 percent due to bronchial tumors.[179] Similar figures have been published by Haberman et al.[180] with the finding of a 59 percent 6-month and a 48 percent 1-year survival rate.

The goals of surgery should be to decrease pain, increase function, and to mobilize and discharge the patient home or to an alternative care facility as soon as possible.[118] Survival of pathologic long bone fractures has improved from 7.2 months in the 1960s to 18.8 months leading into the 1980s.[118] This later figure includes a 3.6-month survival for metastatic lung and 22.6-month survival for metastatic breast disease.

Although treatment principles are similar to non-neoplastic fracture treatment, hemiarthroplasty and the use of bone cement[118] is more common due to poor bone quality. Also, it is important to identify any other lesions, especially those in the femoral shaft, as these will also require surgical consideration.

Postoperative Care

Postoperative care should be directed toward early mobilization to avoid the complications of recumbency. Decubiti occur in up to one-third of patients with hip fractures within 2 weeks of admission.[181] Although troublesome, they are easily prevented by turning the patient every 2 hours. A manifestation of ischemia of the local skin and subcutaneous tissues, they occur most commonly at the sacrum, heels, and buttocks.[105]

Weight-bearing status remains an area of controversy. Although some have recommended restricted weight-bearing until healing, others have documented the use of unrestricted weight-bearing without deleterious effects.[123,124] In reality, there is little difference between the different weight-bearing statuses.[105,118]

Prohibiting weight-bearing does not lessen the muscle forces across the hip, which rise from one to 2.5 times body weight by simply raising one's leg in bed or turning over onto a bedpan.[118] Thus, full weight-bearing should begin immediately for patients with stable reductions. Treatment of nonsurgical candidates should consist of partial weight-bearing and mobilization as soon as pain permits.

After hemiarthroplasty by a posterior surgical approach, dislocation precautions are important. These include high chairs and toilets, and an abduction pillow, which avoid flexion and adduction—the position of least stability. For added security, a knee immobilizer that also limits flexion and adduction can be used.

Thromboembolism

The use of some form of therapy for prophylaxis against deep venous thrombosis is recommended. Strategies have included aspirin, warfarin, dextran, low-molecular-weight heparin, and intermittent external pneumatic compression. No one therapy has proven clearly superior. Warfarin is effective but carries increased risks of bleeding problems. Aspirin is effective and inexpensive; however, its effectiveness has been demonstrated primarily in men.[182] Low-molecular-weight heparin has been reported to be effective for patients undergoing hip fracture surgery.[183] External compression although effective and with a limited downside is costly.

By far, the most common postoperative complication, demonstrated in as much as 50 percent of patients by venography, is deep venous thrombosis.[105] Proximal thrombi are the most dangerous, leading to pulmonary emboli in 3 percent of patients and death in 1 percent.[105] However, it is the preference of many authors to avoid prophylactic anticoagulation because its benefits are often outdone by complications due to an increased bleeding tendency.[105,148] Once there is a clinical suggestion of thrombosis, evaluation and treatment must be aggressive. After the diagnosis has been confirmed using ultrasonography or ventilation-perfusion scans, treatment with heparin and subsequently warfarin is indicated.

Although some have described continuing warfarin for as little as 3 months, others have suggested a lifetime of prophylaxis. Stevens[105] suggests 3 to 6 months.

Morbidity and Mortality

Until the 1940s, in-hospital mortality rates after a fracture of the proximal femur were as high as 50 percent. However, since the 1960s, advancements in surgical treatment and hospital management have significantly reduced mortality[184–187] to approximately 10 percent today.[118] The greatest risk of death appears to exist during the first 4 to 6 months with a rate of 30 percent. This ranges from 14 to 50 percent during the year after injury, at which time mortality begins to resemble those of age- and sex-matched controls.[105,114,124,130,147,148,169,184–196]

Important variables adversely affecting morbidity and mortality include psychiatric or other central nervous system disease; multiple pre-existing and poorly controlled medical conditions including cardiac impairment, diabetes, chronic obstructive pulmonary disease, and rheumatoid arthritis; low weight; environment; immobilization; and poor previous level of function. Wood[197] noted that the most discriminating of these were dementia, postoperative chest or wound infection, neoplasia, and advanced age. Within 6 months, 74 percent of demented patients over the age of 85 years were dead.

Kenzora et al.[147] noted that mortality by 1 year was 11 percent for those with zero to three medical comorbidities and 25 percent for those with four or more. Sexson and Lehner[148] noted similar statistics for zero to two, and three or more comorbidities. The mortality rates for patients with cardiac disease, pulmonary disease, and diabetes were, respectively, 25, 32, and 9 percent at 1 year.

White et al.[196] noted a high degree of correlation with the grading system used by the American Society of Anesthesiologists. Those patients classified as grade I or II (healthy or mild systemic disease) had a 1 year mortality of 8 percent whereas those classified as III or IV (severe or incapacitating systemic disease) had a rate of 49 percent.

Although many investigators have found that advancing age is associated with increased mortality after fracture of the hip, others have challenged this view.[147,196] Controversy also exists over sex, with most authors noting increased mortality in males.[130,158,162,188,192,195] However, when other risk factors are controlled, this belief has been questioned.[130,137,147,148,198]

Postoperative complications have been consistently associated with an increased morbidity and mortality. In one study, the mortality rate associated with urinary tract infection, which occurred in as many as 30 percent of patients, was 24 percent.[199] Malnutrition, decubiti, and postoperative confusion have also been associated with an increased mortality rate after surgery.[130] Patients with decubiti also remain in the hospital longer than those without.[105]

A prolonged time under anesthesia and the type of anesthesia have not been consistently associated with increased mortality.[130,196,200] One study noted that early deaths were less likely with regional anesthesia (probably due to reduced thromboembolism); however, mortality rates did not differ by 8 weeks.[201]

There is evidence that proper coordination of health care services will improve outcomes[125,130,202–204] (also see Trauma in the Geriatric Population). The "orthogeriatric service" will improve rehabilitation. This is important as a significant relationship exists between discharge ambulatory status and mortality. Patients using a walker have a mortality rate of 7 percent compared with 26 percent for those using a wheelchair and 69 percent for those confined to bed.[148]

Function

A significant proportion of patients, ranging from 3 to 59 percent, do not regain the ability to walk after a fracture of the hip.[130,195,198,205] Some authors have noted that intertrochanteric fractures, particularly unstable ones, are more likely to impede walking[130,206] whereas others have noted no difference between these and neck fractures.[162,195,198,207,208]

A substantial number of elderly patients do not regain their preinjury ability to perform either basic (feeding, bathing, dressing, toileting) or instrumental (shopping, cooking, housework, using public transportation) activities of daily living (ADLs). The greatest degree of recovery occurs over the first 6 months with 33 to 40 percent of patients becoming independent with basic activities and 14 to 21 percent with instrumental activities by 1 year.[198,208]

Because of inability to ambulate and a deterioration of function, approximately 40 to 60 percent of patients will not return home directly after discharge.[129,130,208,209] Risk factors associated with a requirement for prolonged care include age greater than 60 to 80 years, female sex, poor general medical condition, cognitive deficits, limb contractures, poor abductor muscle function, lack of postoperative walking ability before 2 weeks, the need for assistance with ADLs, rehospitalization, a lack of social contacts, and prior dependency.[114,125,130,184,187,193,195,206,207,209–212]

Fractures of the Femur

The prevalence of proximal femur fractures is increasing as the average age of the population increases. The actual number of fractures has doubled in the past 20 years.[173] Approximately 250,000 proximal femur fractures occur in the United States each year and this number is predicted to triple by the year 2050.[213] These fractures occur predominantly in the elderly as low-energy injuries, such as a simple fall. These falls may be related to numerous factors including impaired vision, necrologic impairment, poor balance, altered reflexes, and muscular weakness. However, Firooznia et al.[214] demonstrated that those patients who developed proximal femur fractures do not have a higher rate of osteoporosis than their age-matched controls. Overall, the incidence is greatest for white women followed by white men, black women, and then black men. These rates are thought to reflect a difference in bone density between white and black people.[215] Prevention of these injuries lies in prevention of falls. Changes in daily activities or home life can help, such as eliminating throw rugs that may cause tripping, improved lighting, and slippers with a rubber or nonskid sole.

Subtrochanteric fractures refer to the region of the femur just below the lesser trochanter and up to 5 cm distal. These fractures account for 10 to 15 percent of all hip fractures and are among the most difficult to treat because this is the most stressed portion of the skeleton. It has been demonstrated that forces equivalent to six times body weight occur across this region.[216] In addition, it is encased by the quadriceps and hamstring muscles leading to various muscular forces that displace the fracture fragments. The proximal fragment is abducted by the illiopsoas and externally rotated by the short external rotators—piriformis, superior and inferior gemelli—while the distal fragment falls into varus due to the adductors.

In 1891, Allis described traction as a method of treatment but this led to high rates of varus deformity and nonunion, as well as pneumonia and pressure ulcers from sustained bed rest.[216] Therefore, internal fixation is the preferred treatment if the patient is medically stable. Specific treatment options vary from an intramedullary femoral nail to a dynamic hip screw to a dynamic condylar screw and plate. Regardless of the actual implant chosen, the aim is to form a stable construct so as to expedite the patient's return to ambulation, reduce pain, and restore anatomic and biomechanical function. The implant used, then, must endure the muscular forces and the weight-bearing forces described earlier. This explains the high rate of implant failure.

Fractures of the femoral midshaft, like those of the proximal femur, can be a major source of morbidity. Midshaft femur fractures require excessive forces, excluding pathologic fractures. The associated acute complications include extensive hematoma with blood loss, fat embolism, or adult respiratory distress syndrome. Future problems arise as a result of fracture shortening or malalignment causing a limp and post-traumatic arthritis.

A quick review of the anatomy will aid in a better understanding of the difficulty of femur fractures. The femur can be thought of as a tubular structure that widens distally for the condyles. It also has an anterior bow, thereby requiring any form of fixation to also have a "bow" or be prebent. The "tube" is surrounded by an envelope of muscle that aids in blood supply, but also causes deforming forces on the fracture fragments.

Treatment modalities include skeletal traction usually performed with a proximal tibial pin and approximately one-sixth body weight in traction weights. Often a short leg cast, called a Charnley boot, is placed that incorporates the tibial pin to reinforce it. Skeletal traction has been associated with a higher rate of knee stiffness and control of limb length is difficult with frequent shortening of 1.0 to 3.0 cm reported.[217] In addition, there is morbidity associated with prolonged bed rest, such as DVT, PE, and decubiti. It also requires an in-hospital stay of 6 weeks for traction followed by a unilateral spica cast or cast brace for 3 to 6 months.

Favor has shifted to an operative approach with early stabilization and ambulation. However, skeletal traction may still be used for stabilization prior to surgery or if a patient is unable to withstand an operative procedure. Surgical treatment frequently involves an intramedullary nail and only occasionally a plate and screws. The fixation chosen can be performed with spinal anesthetic, thereby eliminating the difficulty elderly patients have with general anesthesia. Studies comparing the results of intramedullary nailing with nonoperative treatment have repeatedly demonstrated the superiority of internal fixation, with fewer malunions, shorter hospitalization, less shortening, and increased healing times.[217] In addition, internal fixation allows for prompt mobilization of the patient, which improves pulmonary function and aids in the prevention of DVTs. The patient is mobilized out of bed as promptly as the next day after surgery and is relatively pain-free. Physical therapy begins postoperative day one with instruction in quadriceps strengthening exercises and progressive weight-bearing. As with hip fractures, patients are taught to ambulate with a walker until healing is complete.

Fractures of the Patella

A short discussion of patella fractures is also warranted in the elderly population. The patella is the largest sesamoid bone in the body and functions to increase the mechanical advantage of the quadriceps muscle. Patellar fractures result from direct injury such as a fall on the knee or striking the knee against the dashboard of an automobile during a vehicular accident. At presentation, the patient may have an abrasion or laceration over the patella. A palpable defect or separation of fragments is often present due to the subcutaneous location of the patella. Treatment is determined by the amount of displacement of the fragments and by the patient's ability or inability to extend the knee against gravity. If the patient is able to extend the knee, then there is little damage to the retinaculum and surgery is not indicated in minimally displaced fractures. The patient may be treated by immobilizing the knee in extension with a cylinder cast or brace for 6 weeks. The patient is weight-bearing as tolerated while the fracture is immobilized. For those without an intact extensor mechanism or with displacement of the fracture, surgical fixation is necessary. If the fracture involves only the distal pole and is commuted, a partial patellectomy is performed (excision of the fragment).[217] Otherwise, internal fixation with screws and wires is required. The exact hardware used will depend on the patient's bone quality and fracture pattern. Knee motion is usually begun within the first few weeks. Prognosis is good with return of normal knee motion; however, the articular cartilage destruction will lead to arthritis in the patella-femoral joint.

Fractures of the Tibia

Fractures of the tibia can be classified as proximal, shaft, and distal. The initial physical examination should be directed at the neurovascular status of the limb. Compartment syndrome must not be overlooked. After the initial evaluation, the limb should be splinted, elevated, and applications of ice can be intermittently used. Proximal intra-articular (plateau) and distal intra-articular (pilon) fractures present particularly difficult challenges in regards to evaluation and treatment. Ligamentous injury is often associated with plateau fractures, and soft tissue damage with pilon injuries. In the absence of contraindications for surgery, open reduction and internal fixation should be considered for unstable and displaced plateau[218] and pilon fractures. In some cases, percutaneous screw fixation alone may be possible for both plateau[219] and pilon fractures. Osteoporosis affects outcomes adversely.[218] Patients with osteoporosis have poor bone quality, making it difficult to obtain good purchase with screws and other implants.

The treatment of proximal tibia fractures is particularly troublesome because they involve the knee mechanism and any alteration in the anatomy can result in impaired function. Fractures of the tibial plateau make up 8 percent of fractures in the elderly popuhtim. These may involve the medial (10 to 23 percent), lateral (55 to 70 percent), or both plateaus (11 to 31 percent).[217] The mechanism of injury is a strong valgus or varus force with axial loading. Many occur as a result of a pedestrian being struck by the fender of an automobile (40 to 60 percent), hence the nickname fender fractures.[217]

The patient will present with complaints of pain and swelling of the knee. A valgus or varus deformity may be visible. Stressing the knee with a valgus or varus force will demonstrate whether the knee is stable, first in extension, then in 30 degrees of flexion. If the knee "opens" with stress (the examiner is able to cause a valgus or varus deformity of the knee) in full extension, then there is bony injury. However, if the knee opens in flexion only, then there is ligaments injury, such as a torn MCL or LCL. A hemarthrosis may be present causing a painful, tense knee and should be aspirated. The presence of fat in the aspirate is an indication of bony fracture.[217] Radiographs are warranted and should in the very least include an anteroposterior and lateral views. If a fracture is suspected but not observed then additional oblique views are necessary. Further, it may be necessary to obtain a computed tomography (CT) scan to evaluate the amount of articular fracture depression and to help with preoperative planning.

Treatment varies with the extent and severity of the fracture. If the fracture fragment is depressed this will lead to depression of the articular surface and cause long-term pain, instability, and arthritis. Nonoperative treatment is usually the course for those fractures that are not or minimally depressed. The most important determinant in the treatment of minimally displaced fractures is knee stability.[217] If the knee is unstable to valgus or varus stress, percutaneous pinning or even an open reduction may be necessary. Otherwise, a splint, cylinder cast, or fracture brace may be employed, but the patient remains non-weight-bearing on the affected extremity until healing has occurred, usually 6 to 8 weeks. The functional results for minimally displaced plateau fractures are good. Almost all will have a return to prefracture strength and motion.[217]

For those fractures that are displaced, indication for operative fixation is determined by the amount of depression, which is assessed by a CT scan. Treatment will also be dictated by the patient's ambulatory status. For example, a patient that is bed or wheelchair bound would probably not benefit from an operative procedure unless there was vascular or peripheral nerve damage secondary to the fracture. Most surgeons will not recommend operative treatment unless the depression is greater than 1 cm.[217] Operative fixation may vary from a couple of screws to a plate and bone graft. This is followed by a functional brace for about 6 to 8 weeks and non-weight-bearing for a total of 12 weeks.

Closed tibial shaft fractures are treated effectively with closed reduction and placement in a long leg cast for approximately 8 weeks. Elderly patients do not do well with crutches and are therefore given a walker for non- or full weight-bearing depending on the fracture pattern. However, unstable fractures or fractures that cannot be reduced require intramedullary nailing. Again, surgery is performed with a spinal or epidural anesthetic to reduce the risk of anesthesia. The patient is mobilized immediately after surgery to reduce the risk of DVT and to improve pulmonary function. The patient's weight-bearing status is dependent on the amount of fracture comminution and will range from non- to full weight-bearing immediately.

External fixation is often indicated with open fractures, poor soft tissue conditions, and periarticular fractures.[220] As with all open fractures, the incidence of infection increases. This is counteracted with perioperative antibiotics and thorough irrigation and debridement in the operating room. A patient is ambulatory with an external fixator the same as if he or she had a cast. There is a slight risk of pin tract infection, but this can be prevented with proper cleansing of the pins by the patient at home with hydrogen peroxide.

Fractures of the distal tibia extending into the ankle joint are known as pilon fractures. Osteoporotic bone is prone to this injury and makes internal fixation difficult because of the poor bone quality. The soft tissue envelope around the tibia is thin and therefore the soft tissues may be compromised. The fracture may be open or skin slough may occur even in closed fractures if the skin is markedly bruised or stretched.[217] Vascular compromise is rare, but dorsalis pedis and posterior tibial pulses should be monitored.

Treatment is dictated by the severity of comminution and joint incongruity.[217] Those without significant articular displacement can be treated nonoperatively with a gentle closed reduction and long leg cast. The patient is non-weight-bearing for 6 to 12 weeks. If there is joint incongruity or comminution, and a closed reduction is unsuccessful, an open reduction is mandated. Bone quality will determine the type of fixation. Internal fixation with a plate and screws provides the most stable fixation but requires good bone quality. An external fixator is often used with good results and the patient can be non-weight-bearing at home for 8 to 12 weeks. Early ankle motion is encouraged.[217] DVT prophylaxis is not necessary as long as the patient is ambulatory.

Fractures of the Ankle

Ankle fractures in the elderly can occur with great frequency due to osteoporosis. The same twisting injury that causes an ankle sprain in the young patient can cause a comminuted bimalleolar fracture in the elderly patient. The fracture is caused by the rotation of the leg on a stationary foot. The position of the foot (supinated versus pronated) and the deforming force (external, internal, abduction, adduction) on the leg will determine the fracture pattern. During this initial period, it is important to keep the leg elevated and iced to minimize the amount of swelling. Swelling will hinder an attempt at closed reduction and prevent the placement of a form-fitting cast.

Like all injuries, the initial evaluation begins with a neurovascular examination and an assessment of points of tenderness. Radiographs are a must in the elderly population as they rarely sprain their ankle. Radiographs must include anteroposterior, lateral, and mortise views of the ankle. It is also necessary to obtain full-length anteroposterior and lateral fibula views because the force of the fracture can propagate along the syndesmosis and exit proximally as a proximal fibula fracture. Without full-length films, this fracture is often missed. The mortise view (leg internally rotated 20 degrees) is extremely important in determining treatment. It allows for visualization of the clear space formed by the talus and the tibia and fibula, which is symmetric in the uninjured ankle. Any increased widening in the clear space must be reduced. The anteroposterior view is necessary to evaluate the integrity of the syndesmotic ligaments. Overlap of the lateral tibia and medial fibula of less than 10 mm on the anteroposterior is abnormal and indicates a disruption of the syndesmosis.[217] Injury to the syndesmotic ligaments should be suspected when the fibula is fractured at or above the level of the syndesmosis. This is important, as these fractures require surgical intervention with a syndesmotic screw.

The goals of treatment are to obtain an anatomic reduction and maintain this reduction until healing has occurred. Similar results are reported with nonoperative and operative treatment as long as the reduction is obtained and maintained throughout treatment. A closed reduction is attempted with all closed ankle fractures, except those with syndesmotic rupture, and immobilized in either a short or a long leg cast depending on the stability of the fracture. The patient remains non-weight-bearing for 6 weeks and is closely followed with weekly radiographs to ensure the reduction has not slipped. If a reduction cannot be achieved or maintained, or there is disruption of the syndesmotic ligaments, surgical intervention is warranted. Operative management involves internal fixation with screws and plates, which can remain idefinitely. The patient may still require postsurgical immobilization of the ankle especially in osteoporotic bone. Operative treatment of ankle fractures is performed to stabilize the fracture, not to allow earlier weight-bearing. All patients must remain non-weight-bearing for 6 weeks.

Fractures of the Foot

Foot fractures in the elderly are just as difficult to care for as those in younger adults. Fractures of the phalanxes and metatarsals are often easily underestimated. Tarsal bones are small bones with complex shapes, restricted motion, and multiple articulations.

Although anterioposterior and lateral roentgenograms should be obtained, certain views are additionally important to evaluate fractures of the foot. These include axial views for fractures of the calcaneus. If the diagnosis is in question, or surgery is planned, a CT scan is performed.

Regardless of treatment, splinting, elevation, and intermittent application of ice are important early treatment considerations.

Generally, closed reduction of phalangeal and metatarsal fractures followed by a cast or use of a hard shoe is effective. However, a malunion can conceivably lead to ill-fitting shoes and callosities. A common problem is nonunion of a fracture of the base of the fifth metatarsal (Jones fracture). This may require internal fixation.

Severe injury of the tarsi often leads to painful degenerative joint disease, which may ultimately require fusion. In order to lessen the likelihood of this problem, open reduction should be considered in the absence of factors mitigating against surgery.

Special Considerations: Spine Pathology in the Geriatric Population

Osteoporosis is the most common skeletal disorder in the world and is the second leading cause of musculoskeletal morbidity in the elderly population. More than 50 percent of all women aged 60 years have radiographic evidence of osteoporosis. By age 75 years approximately 90 percent are affected. The total cost of spinal fractures in the elderly population is approximately 6 billion dollars. Preventative measures for osteoporosis, medical management, and bracing principles have become increasingly important considerations in the geriatric population.

Osteoporotic fractures in general are associated with less severe trauma than fractures seen in patients with normal bone. It is known that rates of fracture directly increase with age and are higher in the female population. Most vertebral fractures in the elderly population are associated with bending or lifting. Sometimes these fractures have no clear precipitating cause. Falls are not as commonly associated with vertebral fractures; rather, they are mostly responsible for hip fractures and other long bone fractures. Vertebral fractures in patients between the ages of 50 and 75 years are most often related to acute compression and result in severe pain, whereas spinal fractures in patients over 75 years of age are often insidious in onset and are less painful.

By the age of 70 years, women have a 20 percent annual incidence of vertebral fractures, and by age 85 years the prevalence is 50 percent. The major differential diagnoses in spinal osteopenia include osteoporosis, osteomalacia, primary (myeloma) and metastatic malignancy, and marrow hyperplasia. Other causes of spinal problems in the elderly include Paget's disease, osteoarthritis, discogenic disease, and spinal stenosis.

Early recognition of osteopenia can play a large role in the prevention of future structural problems in the spine. A complete history and physical and work-up is essential, including bone densitometry if clinically indicated.

There are two basic principles in the management of spinal osteopenia in the elderly. The first is to prevent osteoporosis by early diagnosis. The second is to treat the acute and chronic sequelae of such osteopenia. The treatment of an acute compression fracture includes short-term bed rest, pain medication, heat, and possibly an orthotic. A home health aide and physical therapist may also be beneficial. The chronic component of this disease includes identifying those at high risk for fracture and treating this group. The high-risk group includes those patients with a family history; the postmenopausal female; white or Asian race; short stature with small bones; ectomorph; early menopause; nulliparity; low dietary calcium; low exercise level; excessive nicotine, caffeine, or alcohol; and steroid use. The high-risk group must be treated, for example, with calcium and possibly estrogen therapy or other modalities currently available.

Having recognized the cause and employed the treatment of osteoporotic compression fractures, the orthopaedic surgeon is now faced with a common and difficult problem. The patient continues to have pain, increasing deformity, and loss of height. Most of the loss of height comes from disc narrowing but a significant component is wedging and loss of vertebral height. Late neurologic abnormalities can be a problem and this is mostly related to the progressive onset of spinal stenosis secondary to progression of an angular deformity at the fracture site. The most common radiographic pattern includes a wedge-shaped deformity with loss of anterior vertebral height. Biconcave and flat (vertebra plana) patterns are also found. The clinical deformity is of two types: (1) generalized roundback, the most common type, and (2) acute angular localized deformity. Also, with lumbar fractures, loss of the normal lumbar lordosis is often seen. The degenerative scoliosis seen late in life is due to disc collapse and asymmetric facet loading, which is worsened by coexisting osteopenia.

The indications for surgery in the geriatric patient as related to osteoporotic back problems include (1) progressive deformity with significant pain in a scoliotic or kyphotic patient, (2) acute fractures with neurologic problems (very rare), and (3) osteoporosis in conjunction with spinal instability, usually associated with spinal stenosis.

There are several surgical problems encountered in the elderly patient with osteoporosis. The first is the often severely diminished mechanical properties of the bone, which makes internal fixation more difficult. The second is the difficulty in assessing the fusion mass postoperatively. The third is that many of these patients have coexisting disease. Spinal surgery, however, should be a consideration in the judiciously chosen geriatric patient. The development of better methods of internal fixation, better pre- and postoperative care, and the use of methylmethacrylate have made significant contributions to the success rate of these operations in the elderly population. We look toward future technological advances in order to make the formidable task of spinal surgery in the elderly even more successful.

Rehabilitation in the Orthopaedic Geriatric Patient

General Concepts

It is estimated that 30 percent of geriatric patients consult their physicians because of musculoskeletal problems such as backache, joint pain, and gait disturbances.[225] The following section describes the application of rehabilitation medicine concepts in the treatment of these patients.

General Principles of Rehabilitation Medicine

The main goal of rehabilitation medicine is the restoration of function. This begins with the classification of *impairment* (anatomic disturbance or deficit), *disability* (functional restriction), and *handicap* (environmental and societal barriers to optimum function). This is a multifaceted problem, because a focal process can cause restriction of many activities. It also means that addressing one area (e.g., the achievement of independent ambulation) does not guarantee restoration of independence in activities of daily living (ADLs), and vice versa.

The overall method used to achieve functional goals is the application of the interdisciplinary team. This approach coordinates the care of the multiple problems of elderly patients. It allows various clinicians to blend techniques, share ideas, and pool resources. The regular evaluation conferences with physicians, physical therapists, occupational therapists, nurses, vocational counselors, psychologists, and social workers provide individual patients with one plan of action suited to their needs.

The Need for Geriatric Rehabilitation

Normal aging causes a gradual reduction in activity and function. The observed reduction in exercise tolerance is more often related to changes in body composition, rather than to deterioration in cardiac function. Aging muscle uses oxygen less efficiently. This metabolic change responds favorably to training, just as it does for the younger population.

Aging brings stiffening of tendons and ligaments and loss of strength of cartilage. The posture changes in response to gravity. Changes in vision, hearing, joint position sense, and equilibrium have been documented. Gait deviations develop, other functional impairments become evident, and the older person's lifestyle becomes progressively constricted. For example, joint impairment and quadriceps weakness have been associated with declining walking velocity.[226]

There are increasing efforts to promote fitness and strength training in the geriatric population,[227] whether at home[228–230] or in an institution.[231] Biochemical and histologic studies of older participants have shown that their skeletal muscles respond vigorously to exercise.[229,232,233] Gymnastic facilities and personal trainers are adjusting fitness programs to meet the needs of the elderly. However, improvements in general fitness do not necessarily lead to improvements in function. The best way to improve an ambulatory skill or an ADL is by training specifically for that function. For example, a walking program increases the endurance for that activity but does not affect other functions.[234]

As increasing numbers of patients with orthopaedic and neurologic impairments survive into old age, they face additional challenges. One example is the population surviving and aging with spinal cord injuries.[235,236] Physical strain has been measured among persons with spinal cord injuries. Recommendations have been made for physical training to reduce the effort of ADLs.[237]

There are two areas in which osteoarthritis (OA)—or degenerative joint disease (DJD)—arises as a late complication from disorders acquired during youth. These are postpolio syndrome[238] and post-traumatic paraplegia. They both can lead to increased reliance on the shoulders and arms for mobility and weight-bearing. This causes increased joint stress and increased risk of OA.

There are also some conditions that may continue to evolve over time, such as recovery from stroke. One should remember that patients so affected require periodic monitoring and occasional intervention.

Conservative Interventions

The rehabilitation approach to the elderly patient with an orthopaedic problem (or any other disorder) starts with the initial assessment. This includes the following areas:

- Physical—range of motion (ROM), balance, coordination, strength, exercise tolerance
- Sensory—vision, hearing, joint and body position senses
- Cognitive—orientation, memory, language skills, judgment, abstract thinking, social interaction
- ADLs and instrumental ADLs—bathing, grooming, dressing, toileting, eating, shopping, meal preparation, etc.
- Environmental—positioning of carpeting, rugs, furniture, lights, stairs, thresholds, etc.

Patient evaluation starts with taking the history. A detailed personal and family history is usually the key to diagnostic evaluation. However, the functional status must be explored in depth, including self-care abilities, social supports, work skills and recreational pursuits, to estimate the degree of impairment of these tasks.

Pain reduction must be addressed before any remobilization or functional activity can be instituted. Pain is a complex psychophysiologic experience, consisting of the perception of noxious stimuli, the interpretation of those stimuli as painful, the creation of suffering, and the behaviors manifested by that suffering. Patient and family education regarding the nature and treatment of pain and use of behavioral modification and biofeedback relaxation techniques are part of the multifaceted approach to pain management. Pain is more debilitating for elderly patients than for the young.[239]

The physical examination includes specific aspects relevant to pain management. *Inspection* includes observation of patients as they enter the office, sit in a chair, and cooperate with the examiner. This demonstrates the gait pattern and ease of movement.

Palpation reveals the presence of tender and warm joints, tender muscle groups, and the quality of edematous areas.

The *motor* examination is often limited by pain itself. The presence of proximal weakness may be due to an inflammatory process, the use of steroid medications, or deconditioning.

The *sensory* examination can be influenced by medications, inflammatory conditions with nerve compression, or some systemic disorders with neurovascular sequelae, such as diabetes mellitus. Static (sessile) and dynamic (mobile) balance in sitting, standing, and walking should be included. The peripheral circulation must also be examined.

The first principle of pain treatment in the elderly is limitation of bed rest and instruction in bed mobility to avoid complications such as skin breakdown and pneumonia. Deconditioning can occur rapidly, so the situation must be monitored carefully.

Next, medication issues should be explored. One must avoid polypharmacy, be wary of medications that have central nervous system side effects, anticipate constipation from narcotic medications, and remember that there is a higher incidence of gastrointestinal bleeding from the use of many nonsteroidal anti-inflammatory drugs (NSAIDs) by elderly patients. Pain medications should be given on a regular schedule, not prn, so as to build and maintain a therapeutic blood level.

The "physical" part of physical medicine refers to the use of physical agents, or *modalities*, to decrease pain, reduce swelling, and increase distensibility of tissues. These modalities harness the energies of cold, heat, sound, light, and electricity.[240]

Cold is generally used for acute pain. Heat is useful for subacute or chronic situations. Combinations of heat and cold are used to reduce pain, decrease muscle spasms, and help prepare for exercise. Cold is usually delivered superficially by use of gel packs, brief applications of ice, or cold sprays such as ethyl chloride or fluorimethane. It may have a longer lasting effect on pain relief than heat, but it will not relieve stiffness.

Heat can be delivered superficially by heat lamps (infrared or ultraviolet), gel or hydrocollator packs, paraffin or whirlpool baths, or fluidotherapy (warm air blown through corn husks). Deeper heating is delivered by ultrasound, short-wave diathermy, or by electrical stimulation. Heat must be used cautiously, to avoid thermal burns, and should be avoided during acute inflammation. Each modality has its own advantages and shortcomings, and one must be aware of those facts when considering treatment.

Because the elderly do not tolerate temperature changes well, physical modalities that rely on extremes of heat and cold are used sparingly, with a tendency toward warmth.

Transcutaneous electrical nerve stimulation stimulates cutaneous nerve endings. It thus has an analgesic effect, thought to arise by blocking the signals from the noxious stimulus from reaching the spinal cord. It has only temporary effect and works best if an involved dermatome can be identified. Use of the device and selection of sites of application require review and supervision.

Due to the reported risk from using electrical stimulation

in patients with cardiac arrhythmias and those who rely on pacemakers, it is prudent to use modalities other than electricity for these patients.

Although acupuncture is neither part of Western medicine nor the classic rehabilitation armamentarium, it has been shown to decrease pain when used in certain ways. It has not been shown to modify the disease process.

Other treatments that have varying degrees of support among clinicians to reduce pain and encourage movement are biofeedback[241] and music therapy.[242]

Once patients have experienced reduced discomfort, *muscle strengthening* can begin. However, before embarking on a course of physical therapy (PT), patients should be confident that their doctor has examined, tested, and explained fully the condition and the plan of treatment. If patients are apprehensive or mistrusting, PT will not work. The goals are to control symptoms, increase function, and improve quality of life—not to provide a cure. Patients should be warned that they may experience muscle soreness after the first few sessions of PT. In fact, pain medications may be given before PT sessions to reduce the postexercise discomfort.

Therapeutic exercises serve to improve local muscle circulation, increase strength, increase mobility and flexibility, provide patients with tangible results, and build patient confidence. Exercises vary with the condition being treated. The therapist may modify the exercise program after the initial assessment. Patients should be warned not to hold their breath during exercises and to allow adequate time for repetitions.

Stretching exercises are important to maintain tensile properties of connective tissue and muscles, as well as to preserve joint ROM. Muscles must be strengthened in a coordinated fashion. These exercises start with gravity eliminated, such as when lying supine or with an assistant positioning the joint in this manner. Then, patients are taught to use the weight of the body part distal to the joint as the resistance to the exercise.

Very few devices are needed for an exercise program. Putty of various densities can be used to strengthen the hands. There are elastic bands that are color-coded in various resistances and are used to increase the work accomplished over small arcs of joint motion. Overhead pulleys can be used to preserve ROM, especially at the shoulders.

For patients with multiple limb involvement, swimming or taking a movement class in a warm pool can provide needed exercise. Dance-based aerobic exercise is being used in many university settings. Clinicians are finding reduced joint pain and swelling, decreased depression, and improved self-image and quality of life among patients participating in these projects. Recreational exercise serves not only as an emotional boost, but also as a means of maintaining mobility.[243,244]

Massage can reduce muscle tension, improve soft tissue distensibility, and improve circulation to muscles. It thus can reduce pain and prepare patients for exercise. It can be used as part of a relaxation technique or in the search for trigger points.

Fatigue or lack of endurance is common in pain patients. It can be attributed to a combination of muscle weakness from inactivity, effects of inflammation, side effects of medications (such as muscle relaxants and NSAIDs), sleep disruption, and deconditioning.

Passive exercise, that is, having another person perform the motions without patients' voluntary muscle action, can help preserve joint ROM. In the acute phase, passive ROM is needed. As the pain subsides, active assisted exercises will encourage patients to use muscle power for joint action. This is needed to preserve joint nutrition, muscle fiber nutrition, and bone mineralization. The term *active assisted* means that patients initiate the motion, and the assistant completes the range that patients cannot finish, due to either pain or muscle weakness.

The overall effects of active exercise are to increase the capacity of skeletal and cardiac muscle to do work. The metabolic and circulatory stress of exercise results in increased endurance.

Exercise should be task-specific, that is, geared to the functional aspects with which the patient has the most difficulty. Furthermore, people should exercise to goals that are not determined by pain. This is necessary because pain has lost its protective value. For example, one could exercise to a limited point, then stop to rest *before the pain starts*. This shows patients that it is possible to be active without pain.

After pain is controlled and strength is being built, mobility may still be impaired by a lack of *support and balance*. Gait deviations have many sources. The so-called antalgic gait pattern, or limp, results from pain (or the anticipation of pain) caused by bearing weight on the injured limb. Other changes in walking patterns are caused by muscle weakness, joint deformity, and balance disorders.

Kinesophobia, or fear of movement, is more pronounced in the elderly. Many patients will avoid moving certain ways for fear of triggering the pain. A problem-solving approach usually works for such a person. However, some elderly patients may refuse to get out of bed. In this situation, the patients may be suffering from "fall-o-phobia," that is, fear of the pain and instability causing falling and injury. These people require gentle coaxing, positioning to reduce discomfort, and a more gradual approach, often involving walking with the assistance of a person.

The use of a cane for added balance and to permit forward flexion may be initially difficult for some patients to accept, because it carries the societal stigma of infirmity. However, it could be presented as an aid to better endurance and further distance in walking. It is also not a substitute for having someone nearby if patients are fearful.

The patient may use a wooden or aluminum cane to assist balance and reduce pressure on affected leg joints. The cane should have one foot, a wide rubber tip, a built-up or pistol grip, and an angled or "ortho" handle to provide stability. Quadruped canes may appear to be more stable, but few patients will place all four feet on the ground at the same time. Therefore, not only are all four feet unavailable for stability, but the "airborne" feet can become tangled in furniture.

A walker is best for patients with bilateral leg problems, or if one wishes to transmit body weight through the arms instead of a painful spine. If patients have balance problems, it is best to use walkers with spring-loaded front wheels to reduce the effort of propulsion. Bearing weight on these walkers makes the front feet contact the floor, so the walker becomes stable. Patients whose grasp is ineffective due to weakness or arthritis can lean on a platform walker with their forearms.

More detailed descriptions of assistive devices for ambulation[245] and gait training[246] can be found elsewhere.

Back Pain

The differential diagnosis of back pain is broad. It includes visceral, neoplastic, metabolic, inflammatory, infectious, mechanical, and developmental disorders. One can usually rule out the majority of systemic illnesses that may refer pain to the back by the history and physical examination.

"Local" causes of back pain include degenerative joint disease (including facet joint changes), trauma, muscle strain, and disc degeneration. The presence of a disc bulge may be an incidental finding on an imaging study and may not correlate with the patient's complaints and examination.

In a recent study of spinal motion in asymptomatic elderly patients, it was found that degenerative disc changes correlated with limited spinal mobility more often than did degenerative facet joint changes.[247]

The importance of good posture cannot be overlooked, because it is known that body mechanics plays an important role in many spine conditions. An exaggerated thoracic kyphosis can be caused by osteoporosis in women and by Parkinson's disease in both men and women. Postural changes can also be associated with a lifetime of working at a desk or bent over a machine. Poor eyesight and/or hearing can cause patients to tilt the head to one side for better focus of sensory inputs. This can lead to neck and upper back strain. Scoliosis causes shifting of the center of gravity and increased back pain by muscle tension as well as ligamentous strain. There are many methods for analyzing postural control.[248]

Poliomyelitis and hemiparesis can produce long-term gait disturbances that can contribute to the development of back pain. Amputation of an arm or leg creates trunk imbalances and gait disturbances that can lead to back pain.

Obesity is a highly prevalent problem. Just as a strong abdominal wall is felt to be the "buttress" of the lumbar spine, excessive weight anteriorly can be the ballast that drags on the lumbar spine and creates increased postural deviations and pain.

Management of back pain employs many of the techniques mentioned in the first part of this section, including modalities to reduce pain and increase the ability to perform exercises. Judicious use of rest and exercise means enforcing the need for the patient to achieve adequate rest to avoid the fatigue that accompanies many conditions. Many patients require rest breaks during the day, especially if this means sitting for brief periods in a chair that provides adequate support. Pacing of work and alternation of activities are also included in this area of consideration.

Bracing of the trunk is occasionally required for severe back pain due to osteoporotic vertebral fractures. Clavicle or "figure-of-eight" straps can help remind patients to seek postural correction, usually by "squaring" the shoulders. However, reduction of a kyphosis due to osteoporotic vertebral collapse or arthritic facet joint deformity is not a feasible goal. Use of an abdominal binder or a girdle is better tolerated than a plastic body jacket or a device with rigid stays. It has been postulated that reliance on a thoracolumbar spinal orthosis (TLSO) may lead to further weakening of trunk and back muscles, with increased risk of re-injury. Patients who wear a TLSO must be encouraged to continue exercises unless contraindicated.

A corset may be a temporary support method. Patients can be weaned off the corset if they are first taught exercises to strengthen the abdominal muscles for back support, then started on a schedule of reduced wearing in the mornings.

In general, external supports are poorly tolerated by the elderly. There is an inverse correlation between the degree of support and the degree of comfort.

Exercise vary with the condition being treated. There has been a long-standing controversy over using strict flexion exercises (Williams) versus starting with extension and gradual inclusion of other positions (McKenzie). Although Williams flexion exercises can strengthen abdominal muscles, stretch back muscles and soft tissues, and open intervertebral foramina, they can raise intradisc pressure. Therefore, Williams exercises are not recommended for suspected disc disorders.

Although McKenzie exercises are usually thought of as consisting primarily of extension exercises, they are actually part of an approach to back pain. Patients are encouraged to seek positions that reduce the pain, centralize it (eliminate pain from the legs), and then abolish the pain altogether. This usually begins with extension but may be expanded to include other types of movements.

There are several sets of postural and balance exercises available.[245,249,250]

A positive correlation has been noted between back extensor muscle strength and vertebral bone mineral density.[251] Therefore, an exercise program designed to strengthen these muscles may have a beneficial effect. In addition, a flexion exercise program may cause more vertebral compression fractures than an extension exercise program.[252]

Joint Problems

Osteoarthritis

OA is the most common orthopaedic pathology in the elderly. It affects mainly the large weight-bearing joints and is associated with repeated minor trauma and obesity.[250] Although it is not an inflammatory process, OA can mimic inflammatory joint diseases. Gout, septic arthritis, multiple myeloma, neoplasms, or rheumatoid arthritis can all present with combinations of symptoms and signs that mimic OA.[253]

Another condition that can mimic the pain of OA is bursitis, which also causes pain around the hip (especially the trochanteric variety).[254] Ischial bursitis can cause buttock pain that may mimic sciatica. Iliopsoas bursitis causes anteromedial thigh pain. Bursitis is managed initially by applying physical agents, NSAIDs, and injections of local anesthetic-steroid combination.[255] Patients should be instructed to avoid painful positions, to use seating cushions, and to apply gentle stretch to the involved areas.[254,256]

Clinical manifestations of inflammatory arthritis or OA may begin with fatigue or lack of endurance. Morning stiffness and decreased ADLs are common complaints.[254] Muscle weakness can affect the lower extremities first, leading to difficulty climbing stairs, rising out of chairs, or getting into and out of the bathtub. Later, the upper extremities may become involved, leading to difficulty dressing, feeding, and bathing.

There may be progressive loss of spine mobility, leading to transfer of motion to available spinal segments. The excessive mobility at these levels can lead to back pain, disc disorders, and further degeneration.

The first technique of joint preservation is *splinting*. Provision of an external splint (orthosis) during an acute inflammatory episode can rest both the affected joint and the surrounding muscles. It can reduce pain and swelling that may be exacerbated by motion. Care must be taken not to encourage the development of contractures in other joints due to prolonged immobilization. Positioning in bed can help reduce the risk of contractures.

Upper limb orthoses are used to prevent deformity, reduced wrist pressure in carpal tunnel syndrome, or can be custom-made to provide substitute power to weak fingers. They must be as unobtrusive as possible, to permit maximal manipulation of the environment.

Lower limb orthoses provide support, reduce deformity, and make a small contribution to forward momentum during ambulation. The brace applies forces that act on the limb during weight-bearing. The added weight of an orthosis may impede mobility. Skin breakdown and nerve compression are potential risks of orthoses.

Many patients are advised to use *adapted equipment* (e.g., reachers, built-up handles). These can make daily life tasks easier, especially for patients with hand deformities or weakness. Cane use and weight loss can decrease the pressure on a painful hip.[254]

Anti-inflammatory drugs and joint injections are available medication options.[257]

Exercise protocols for arthritic joints begin with reducing pain and swelling by cold or hot packs or other modalities. When the pain is under control, passive movements are performed. These motions decrease stiffness and increase ROM. Increased pain is an indicator that the program is too aggressive. Strengthening exercises are necessary, because muscle wasting can occur as a response to joint inflammation. Muscle weakness leads to increased joint instability. It should be noted that a closely monitored, moderate intensity stationary cycling and vigorous intensity strength-training program has not been shown to increase joint discomforts in older adults with arthritis.[258]

Rehabilitation After Joint Surgery

When conservative methods no longer suffice to maintain functional independence, surgery offers renewed hope to the patient with arthritis. Surgical approaches to the arthritic joint include arthrodesis, or fusion, and arthroplasty, or replacement. One must remember that, in addition to the usual risks of surgical intervention, including that of general anesthesia, there is the potential to lose function while reducing pain.

Arthrodesis, for example, results in an immobile joint. The stresses formerly taken by that joint are then transmitted to joints proximal and distal to it. These structures can become painful.

Arthroplasty is the most common surgical intervention for arthritis in the elderly.[259] It results in loss of at least one grade in muscle power. Because stability of the new joint depends on the strength of the surrounding muscles, postoperative rehabilitation is needed before the patient can resume usual activities.

The postoperative course usually consists of education, practicing gait with assistive devices, gradual strengthening exercises, and review of self-care skills. Patients who receive cemented prostheses can start weight-bearing as tolerated, but use an assistive device (walker or crutches, depending on equilibrium) for approximately 6 weeks. Patients who receive noncemented prostheses start with toe-touch weight-bearing and must continue this way for 6 weeks. After that, gradual increases in the amount of partial weight-bearing occur every 2 weeks. Cane use may continue beyond the 12-week course.[259,260]

Although noncemented endoprostheses last longer than cemented devices, the energy expenditure for the initial non-weight-bearing period may exceed the ability of many older, medically complex patients.[261]

During the above course, patients are also being taught exercises to strengthen the muscles around the hip. They start with isometrics to maintain muscle tone and increase circulation. They learn to avoid certain motions that might contribute to dislocation of the endoprosthesis.[256,259] Position and bed mobility are also important.[254]

Select patients may benefit from a home exercise program with monitoring every 2 weeks.[262]

OA of the knee can cause reflex inhibition of the quadriceps. Patients may present initially not with pain but with subjective weakness ("giving way"). Pain and edema reduction are necessary prior to beginning a strengthening program. Muscle strengthening might protect the joint. Weight loss and cane use can decrease the pressure on the knee.

The postoperative rehabilitation protocol for knee replacement is similar to that for hip replacement. It also includes education to avoid complications, gait review with assistive devices, and Rom and strengthening exercises.[250,263–265] The use of passive motion (CPM) machines requires education and monitoring.[259,266] CPM machines may have little long-term effect on knee ROM.[267]

Trauma and Fractures

Etiology and Prevention

There are many patient (intrinsic) and environmental (extrinsic) factors that contribute to falls and injury.[268–270] Analysis of this problem usually begins with the patient, often after multiple falls and injuries have occurred.[271]

Analysis has not revealed significant differences in gait characteristics between healthy elderly individuals with a history of falling and those with no history of falling.[272] However, static balance, lower extremity strength, and ankle and hip flexibility may contribute to falls.[273,274]

Two important patient factors are disturbed balance and mobility.[275] Body weight during quiet standing is distributed between both legs (double support). The sensation of joint position is carried from the legs along the dorsal columns of the spinal cord to the brain. The cerebellum uses this information to coordinate the muscle contractions needed to maintain the standing posture. Adequate muscle strength is necessary to complete the task. Thus, both peripheral and central mechanisms are required.

The sense of balance may be disturbed at many levels.[276] Inadequate peripheral nerve sensory feedback (such as with diabetic neuropathy) can lead to difficulty standing with the feet together and the eyes closed. This removes an alternative means of feedback. Vestibular degenerative changes also deprive the patient of input. Cerebellar injury can cause problems during standing with the eyes open, as well as during ambulation. Thus, at a time when patients need maximum feedback to compensate for disturbed central mechanisms, their peripheral systems are also deteriorating.[277]

Postural disturbances affect balance and become more difficult to correct with aging. The head is held in a forward position, the shoulders are rounded, hip and knee flexion increase, and the lumbar lordosis changes (either flatter or more curved).[278] Trunk control decreases with age.[279]

Reduced muscle strength, slower reaction times, stiffer connective tissue, and less dense bones are other patient factors contributing to falls and injury.[280] For example, hip abductors keep the pelvis level during single-support weight-bearing. If one set is weak, the pelvis might drop away from that side, causing the trunk to follow (Trendelenburg sign). The compensatory action, which is elicited during gait, is to lean the trunk over the weight-bearing leg to keep the pelvis level (compensated Trendelenburg sign).[254] Strengthening the hip abductors and the calf muscles is critical for reduction of falls risk.

Slower reaction times contribute to falls because they signify an impaired ability to restore disturbed equilibrium. Reaction time can be prolonged by neurologic changes, medication, or fatigue.[281] This is especially hazardous when combined with rigidity, as in Parkinson's disease. Falls while turning are more likely to lead to a hip fracture than falls sustained while walking in one direction.[282]

It is known that exercise can increase strength and improve balance. In addition, more active people may be less likely to experience falls and fractures than do sedentary people.[283] However, resistive and balance training may not result in faster walking speed or more rapid ability to stand from sitting.[284,285]

The other main area of concern in preventing falls and injury is systematic environmental assessment. Much can be done to maximize safety and independence, whether clients reside in nursing homes, chronic care facilities, or in private homes. This includes the presence of alarms, adequate lighting, and adaptive equipment (e.g., grab bars, bath equipment). Special attention is paid to coordination of furniture dimensions and functions.[286] Rugs and room thresholds are potential hazards for ambulatory patients. The environmental assessment should be incorporated into the home visit protocol.[287]

Dependence in ADLs is associated with increased falls risk.[288] For example, transfer activities are essential for safe mobility of the dependent, nonambulatory patient.[289] Particular attention must be directed toward furniture positioning, appropriate footwear, clear instructions to the patient, and good body mechanics on the part of the caregiver. Transfer activities must be modified after lower extremity surgery, especially to avoid dislocation of a hip arthroplasty. Descriptions of transfer techniques can be found in textbooks of physical therapy.[290]

Rehabilitation After Lower Extremity Trauma or Fracture

Rehabilitation after fractures starts with assessment of patient function and the condition of the fractured limb. The latter includes measurement of pain, swelling, joint ROM, and muscle strength. Comparison is made between the fractured extremity and its contralateral partner.[291]

Patient confidence is vital to rapid remobilization. It is necessary to reassure the patient that the repair is solid and that the leg will provide support.[261] Confidence in the rehabilitation process is built by offering clear explanations, by setting goals based on the patient's individual needs and abilities, and by providing encouragement from both family and team members.

The success of fracture rehabilitation is judged by measuring increases in strength, muscle bulk, ROM, and endurance, and by checking for decreases in pain and swelling. Predictors of success also include assessment of balance, sitting and standing ability, and gait.[292] Repeated assessment is needed to monitor those patients at risk of long-term functional decline.[293]

The majority of femoral fractures in the elderly occur at the femoral neck or at the intertrochanteric (IT) area.[254] Conservative nonoperative management of femoral fractures is associated with the complications of prolonged immobilization.[256] If patients cannot tolerate surgery or are not expected to be ambulatory, pain control, closed reduction, splinting, and prevention of complications may be sufficient. Patients must be able to withstand not only the stresses of general anesthesia and surgical intervention, but also a postoperative course of rehabilitation.

Operative choices for femoral neck fractures include internal fixation and endoprosthetic replacement. Because the IT area is better vascularized than the femoral neck, internal fixation is the option of choice for IT fractures. Internal fixation with good reduction allows early mobilization, which is critical for older patients, especially those with concurrent neurologic conditions.[255]

Depending on the device used, patients start bed mobility and transfer training the first day after surgery. Patients may start partial weight-bearing by the second postoperative day. Standing and weight-shifting skills and ambulation with assistive devices should progress during the ensuing weeks.[260]

Pain with weight-bearing (after the initial postoperative period) should raise suspicions as to the status of the fixation. Electromagnetic fields and low-power ultrasound have been used to promote healing of nonunion of fractures.

Other problems that may arise after surgery include anemia, malnutrition, deep vein thrombosis, mental status changes, dehydration, and complications of immobility. These must by identified and treated quickly to optimize the patients' rehabilitation potential. If there is a limb length discrepancy, a shoe lift can be provided. Toilet seats and chairs should be raised for easier mobility.

Elderly patients with osteoporosis may present with pelvic fractures. Although they can cause pain referred to the hip area, these fractures are often not seen on standard radiographs. A bone scan is necessary if standard films are negative. Pain management and early mobilization are needed.[255]

Fractures distal to the hip generally require a higher velocity than that achieved in the usual falling episode. Thus, fractures around the knee are uncommon in the older population.

Lower limb deformities that occurred during youth may lead to joint problems in later life. DJD may cause either genu valgum ("knock-knees") or genu varum ("bow-legs"). Patients with either condition may be more vulnerable to ligament and meniscus injury during a fall.

Patients presenting with knee instability and pain require specific questions in the history part of the office visit to determine the mechanism of injury. A careful examination of the painful limb can reveal the structural damage.[265,294–297] Arthroscopy may be needed if the physical examination is inconclusive.[298]

Traumatic synovitis of the knee is seen in physical laborers, both during and after employment. Cold compresses for the first 24 to 48 hours are followed by gentle massage and mild heating, as well as immobilization to support weight-bearing. Isometric exercises are needed to prevent atrophy of the quadriceps femoris muscle. Bracing or taping is removed periodically to permit active assisted exercise. Prompt resumption of ambulation is critical to prevent deconditioning. More aggressive exercises can be pursued after the pain has subsided.[250]

Occasionally, a patient may complain of swelling and pain in a single joint (especially the knee), but does not recall a history of trauma, overuse, or migratory joint pain. This should not be dismissed as "arthritis" until a full diagnostic work-up has been performed, including the possibility of neoplasm.

Foot and ankle disorders are common in the older population.[281] Many are not recognized until the later stages of deformity because of lack of sensation, such as the neuropathic ("Charcot") foot associated with diabetes mellitus.

Examination of the foot/ankle complex is described elsewhere.[260,299,300] It should be remembered that the shape and position of the foot in quiet standing are different from those in the dynamic state. Therefore, examination of the patient requires analysis of both conditions, as well as non-weight-bearing. The shoes and any current orthotic devices must be checked for adequacy of fit, utility during gait, and asymmetric wear patterns reflecting uneven use.

A number of female patients have worn high heels for many years. This habit can cause tightening and shortening of the Achilles' tendons, which makes patients fall backward when they try to walk with a lower heel or go barefoot. Another factor contributing to falling and injury is the combination of high heels with the decline in sensory feedback, plantarflexion strength, and balance that occurs with aging.

Ankle sprains are treated initially by cold applications, rest, elevation of the leg, and wrapping with a compression bandage. After the first 24 to 48 hours, treatment includes daily use of heat (if the swelling and warmth have begun to recede), massage, and elastic bandages. Direct (galvanic) current has been used as a physical therapy modality for ankle sprains and edema.[250] Crutches and non-weight-bearing gait are encouraged.

Within 2 weeks, stretching and weight-bearing can begin. The patient should be pain-free before starting resistive exercises. External ankle support, which is helpful for compression and protection, is used for approximately 4 weeks. Gradually, the degree of exercise and functional activity is increased. Finally, education regarding footwear and exercises can help prevent further problems.[300,301]

Some patients have a history of chronic ankle sprains. This may be due to a combination of muscle weakness (especially the peroneal muscles) and impaired balance (proprioceptive loss). These patients are treated with strengthening exercises and balance training.[300]

Older patients with osteopenia are at risk for ankle fractures, usually due to forces transmitted from the feet. Treatment depends on classification and surgical intervention.[300,302]

The less flexible feet of older people are at increased risk for stress fractures. Most commonly, the metatarsals are involved. Fractures of the first four metatarsals are usually treated by limited activity for 4 to 12 weeks. Because fractures of the fifth metatarsal are prone to delayed or nonunion, they may require surgical fixation.[300]

Patients complaining of heel pain and/or pain along the sole of the foot with toe extension may have plantar fasciitis. The differential diagnosis is broad. Older, overweight, sedentary individuals are at increased risk of developing plantar fasciitis. Prolonged weight-bearing on hard surfaces, repeated trauma with heel strike, and fat pad atrophy are possible contributing factors. Treatment includes injection of steroid and long-acting anesthetic into the insertion of the plantar fascia, use of soft heel cups, and splinting to support the foot. Orthotics may be needed for dynamic correction for active people. Plantar fascia and Achilles tendon stretching are taught.[303–305]

Summary

A comprehensive rehabilitation evaluation includes muscle testing, joint ROM and notation of deformity, assessment of pain by a visual analog scale, and functional assessment combining self-care, vocational, and avocational activities. Rehabilitation intervention consists of judicious use of rest, exercise, splinting, thermal agents, other physical modalities, and education. Patients should be encouraged to seek adequate rest and accurate information.

Improvement in self-care and walking skills, decreased reliance on caregivers, and increased comfort are achievable goals for elderly patients. Important factors are age, physical condition, psychological condition, and social resources. Goals may be modified and the tempo may be changed to accommodate the patient.

In conclusion, successful orthopedic rehabilitation of the geriatric patient requires an interdisciplinary approach, an informed patient and family, and an individualized and carefully monitored treatment program.

References

1. Knudson MM, Lieberman J, Morris JA et al: Mortality factors in geriatric blunt trauma patients. Arch Surg 1994;129: 448–453
2. Laur AR: Age and sex relation to accidents. Traffic Safety Research Review 1959;3:21
3. Levy DB, Hanlon DP, Townsend RN: Geriatric trauma. Clin Geriatr Med 1993;9:601–620
4. Schwab CW, Kauder DR: Trauma in the geriatric patient. Arch Surg 1992;127:701–706
5. Accident Facts 1991 Ed National Safety Council, Chicago 1991
6. Broos PL, Stappaerts KH, Luiten EJ, Gruwez JA: Home-going: prognostic factors concerning the major goal in treatment of elderly hip fracture-patients. Int Surg 1988;73:148–150
7. Champion HR, Copes WS, Buyer D et al: Major trauma in geriatric patients. Am J Public Health 1989;79:1278–1282
8. Oreskovich MR, Howard JD, Copass MK, Carrico CJ: Geriatric trauma: injury patterns and outcomes. J Trauma 1984;24: 565–572
9. Pellicane JV, Byrne K, DeMaria EJ: Preventable complications and death from multiple organ failure among geriatric trauma victims. J Trauma 1992;33:440–444
10. Finelli FC, Jonsson J, Champion HR et al: A case control study for major trauma in geriatric patients. J Trauma 1989; 29:541–548
11. Lonner JH, Koval KJ: Polytrauma in the elderly. Clin Orthop 1995;318:136–143
12. DeMaria EJ, Kenny PR, Merriam MA et al: Survival after trauma in geriatric patients. Ann Surg 1987;206:738–743
13. Pennig D: Principles of fracture management in elderly patients. pp.120–137. In Newman RJ (ed): Orthogeriatrics: Comprehensive Orthopaedic Care for the Elderly Patient. Butterworth-Heinemann, Oxford, 1992
14. Zietlow SP, Capizzi PJ, Bannon MP, Farnell MB: Multisystem geriatric trauma. J Trauma 1994;37:985–988
15. Weingarten MD et al: Trauma and aging effects on hospital costs and length of stay. Ann Emerg Med 1988;17:10–14
16. DeMaria EJ, Merriam MA, Casanova LA et al: Do DRG payments adequately reimburse the costs of trauma care in geriatric patients. J Trauma 1988;28:1244–1249
17. US Bureau of the Census: Current population reports series P-25, No. 952: Projections of the population of the United States by age, sex, and race, 1883 to 2080. US Government Printing Office, Washington DC, 1984
18. Spencer G: Projections of the population of the United States by age, sex, and race: 1988 to 2080. US Bureau of the Census, Washington, DC, 1989. Current Population Reports, Ser. P-25, No. 1018
19. Keating HJ: Preoperative considerations in the geriatric patient. Med Clin North Am 1987;71:569–583
20. US Dept of Health, Education, and Welfare: Vital Health Statistics, Series 10, Number G-1, 1991
21. Kauder DR, Schwab CW: Comorbidity in geriatric patients. pp. 215–230. In Maull K, Cleveland H, Strauch G, Wolferth C (eds): Advances in Trauma. Mosby-Year Book, St. Louis, 1990
22. Seymour DG, Pringle R: Postoperative complication in the elderly surgical patient. Gerontology 1983;29:262–270
23. Demarest GB, Osler TM, Clevenger FW: Injuries in the elderly: evaluation and intial response. Geriatrics 1990;45: 36–42
24. Osler T, Hales K, Baack B et al: Trauma in the elderly. Am J Surg 1988;156:537–543
25. US Dept of Transportation Publication HS 807071: A Decade of Progress: Fatal Accident Reporting System, 1989. National Highway Traffic Safety Administration, Washington, DC, 1991
26. Waller JA, Goo JT: Highway crash and citation patterns and chronic medical conditions. J Safety Res 1969;1:13–18
27. Perry BC: Falls among the elderly: a review of the methods and conclusions of epidemiologic studies. J Am Geriatr Soc 1982;30:367–371
28. Rubenstein LZ: Falls in the elderly: a clinical approach. West J Med 1983;138:273–275
29. Rivera FB, Bergman AB: Factors associated with pedestrian vehicle collision injuries and fatalities. West J Med 1987;146: 243–245
30. Jones J, Dougherty J: Emergency department protocol for diagnosis and evaluation of geriatric abuse. Ann Emerg Med 1988; 17:1006–1015
31. DeMaria EJ, Kenny PR, Merriam MA et al: Aggressive trauma care benefits the elderly. J Trauma 1987;27:1200–1206
32. Patterson BM, Cornell CN, Carbone B et al: Protein depletion

and metabolic stress in elderly patients who have fracture of the hip. J Bone J Surg 1992;74A:251–260

33. Naam NH, Brown WH: Major pelvic fracture. Arch Surg 1983; 16:610–615
34. Scalea TM, Simon HM, Duncan AO et al: Geriatric blunt multiple trauma: improved survival with early invasive monitoring. J Trauma 1990;30:129–134
35. Boucher CA, Brewster DC, Darling RC et al: Determination of cardiac risk by dipyridamole-thallium imaging before peripheral vascular surgery. N Engl J Med 1985;312:389
36. Kenzora JE, McCarthy RE, Lowell JD et al: Hip fracture mortality. Clin Orthop 1984;186:45–56
37. Sexson SB, Lehner JT: Factors affecting hip fracture mortality. J Orthop Trauma 1987;1:298–305
38. Zuckerman JD, Skovron ML, Fessel K et al: The role of surgical delay in the long-term outcome of hip fractures in geriatric patients. Orthop Trans 1992–1993;16:750
39. Martin RE, Teberian G: Multiple trauma and the elderly patient. Emerg Med Clin North Am 1990;8:411–420
40. Riska EB, Bonsdorff H, Hakkinen S et al: Fat embolism in patients with multiple injuries. J Trauma 1982;22:891–894
41. Johnson KD, Cadambi A, Seibert GB: Incidence of adult respiratory distress syndrome in patients with multiple musculoskeletal injuries: effect of early operative stabilization of fractures. J Trauma 1985;25:375–384
42. Hardin GT: Timing of fracture fixation: a review. Orthop Rev 1990;19:861–867
43. Gustilo RB, Merkow RL, Templeman D: The management of open fractures. J Bone Joint Surg 1990;72A:299–304
44. Gustilo RB, Mendoza RM, Williams DN: Problems in the management of type III (severe) open fractures: a new classification of type III open fractures. J Trauma 1984;24:742–746
45. Gustilo RB, Anderson JT: Prevention of infection of one thousand and twenty-five open fractures of long bones. J Bone Joint Surg 1976;58A:453–458
46. Koval KJ, Zuckerman JD: Functional recovery after fracture of the hip. J Bone Joint Surg 1994;76A:751–758
47. Kulshrestha P, Iyer KS: Chest injuries: a clinical and autopsy profile. J Trauma 1988;28:844–847
48. Murphy PJ, Rai GS, Lowy M, Bielawska C: The beneficial effects of joint orthopaedic-geriatric rehabilitation. Age Ageing 1987;16:273–278
49. Santos AL, Gelperin A: Surgical mortality in the elderly. J Am Geriatr Soc 1975;28:42
50. Van-Aalst JA, Morris JA Jr, Yates HK et al: Severely injured geriatric patients return to independent living: a study of factors influencing function and independence. J Trauma 1991; 31:1096–1102
51. Baker SP, O'Neil B, Haddon E, Long WB: The injury severity score: a method for describing patients with multiple injuries and evaluating emergency care. J Trauma 1974;14:187–196
52. Morris JA, MacKenzie EJ, Edelstein SL: The effect of preexisting conditions on mortality in trauma patients. JAMA 1990; 263:1942–1946
53. MacKenzie EF, Morris JA, Edelstein SL: Effect of preexisting disease on length of hospital stay in trauma patients. J Trauma 1989;29:757–765
54. Devas MB: Geriatric Orthopaedics. Academic Press, London, 1977
55. Boyd RV, Hawthorne J, Wallace WA et al: The Nottingham orthogeriatric unit after 1000 admissions. Injury 1983;15: 193–196
56. Ceder L, Thorngren KG, Wallden B: Prognostic indicators and early home rehabilitation in elderly patients with hip fractures. Clin Orthop 1980;152:173–184
57. Gilchrist WJ, Newman RJ, Hamblen DL, Williams BO: Prospective randomized study of an orthopaedic geriatric inpatient service. BMJ 1988;297:1116–1118
58. Incalzi RA, Bernabei R, Carbonin P: The orthopedic-geriatric unit: a new model of hospital care [Italian]. Ann Ital Med Int 1995;10:49–52
59. Radke MS, Flynn JP, Smith M et al: Functional improvement in geriatric trauma patients admitted to a dedicated rehabilitation hospital. Md Med J 1992;41:981–987
60. Reid J, Kennie DC: Geriatric rehabilitation care after fractures of the proximal femur: one year follow up of a randomized clinical trial. BMJ 1989;299:25–26
61. Sainsbury R, Gillespie WJ, Armour PC, Newman EF: An orthopaedic geriatric rehabilitation unit: the first two years experience. NZ Med J 1986;99:583–585
62. Zuckerman JD, Sakales SR, Fabian DR, Frankel VH: Hip fractures in geriatric patients. Results of an interdisciplinary hospital care program. Clin Orthop 1992;274:213–225
63. Harrington MR, Brennant M, Hodkinson HM: The first year of a geriatric-orthopaedic liaison service: an alternative to "orthogeriatric" units? Age Ageing 1988;17:129–133
64. Ogilvie-Harris, Botsford DJ, Hawker RW: Elderly patients with hip fractures: improved outcome with the use of care maps with high-quality medical and nursing protocols. J Orthop Trauma 1993;7:428–437
65. Fitzgerald JF, Moore PS, Dittus RS: The care of elderly patients with hip fracture. Changes since implementation of the prospective payment system. N Engl J Med 1988;319: 1392–1397
66. Neer CS II, Craig EV, Fukuda, H: Cuff tear arthropathy. J Bone Joint Surg 1983;65A:1232–1244
67. Peterson CJ: Painful shoulders inpatients with rheumatoid arthritis. Scand J Rheum 1986;15:275–279
68. Crossan JF, Vallance R: The shoulder joint in rheumatoid arthritis. pp. 131–143. In Bayley I, Kessel L (eds): Shoulder Surgery. Springer-Verlag, New York, 1982
69. Pahle J: The shoulder in rheumatoid arthritis: synovectomy. Reconstruct Surg Traumatol 1981;18:33–47
70. Ogilvie-Harris D, D'Angelo G: Arthroscopic surgery of the shoulder. Sports Med 1990;9:120–128
71. Naranja RJ, Iannotti JP: Surgical options in the treatment of arthritis of the shoulder: alternatives to prosthetic arthroplasty. Sem Arthroplasty 1995;6:204–213
72. Cofield RH, Edgerton BC: Total shoulder arthroplasty. Complications and revision surgery. Instr Course Lect 1990;39: 449–462
73. Morrey BF, An K-H: Biomechanics of the shoulder. pp. 208–245. In Rockwood CA, Matsen FA II (eds): The shoulder, WB Saunders, Philadelphia, 1990

74. Nicholson GP, Misamore GW: Rotator cuff insufficiency in the arthritic shoulder: treatment alternatives. Sem Arthroplasty 1995;6:273–279
75. Franklin JL, Barrett WP, Jackins SE et al: Glenoid loosening in total shoulder arthroplasty. Association with rotator cuff deficiency. J Arthroplasty 1988;3:39–46
76. Shepard RJ: Physiology and Biochemistry of Exercise. Praeger, New York, 1982
77. Howard JE, McGill KC, Dorfman LJ: Age effects on properties of motor units action potentials: ADEMG Analysis. Ann Neurol 1988;24:207–212
78. Fiatrone MA, Marks EC, Ryan ND et al: High intensity strength training in nonagenarians, effects of skeletal muscle. JAMA 1990;263:3029–3034
79. Sidney KH, Shepard RT: Frequency and intensity of exercise training for elderly subjects. Med Sci Sports 1978;10: 125–131
80. Burks RT: Arthroscopy and degenerative arthritis of the knee: a review of the literature. Arthroscopy 1990;6:43–47
81. Wigley FM: Osteoarthritis: practical management in older patients. Geriatrics 1984;39:101–120
82. Flanagan SR, Ragnarsson KT, Ross MK, Wong DK: Rehabilitation of the geriatric orthopaedic patient. Clin Orthop 1995; 316:80–92
83. Cohr BT, Krackow KA, Hungerford DS et al: The results of total knee arthroplasty in patients eighty years and older. Orthop Rev 1990;19:451–460
84. L'Insalata MD, Stern SH, Insall JN: Total knee arthroplasty in elderly patients. J Arthroplasty 1992;7:261–266
85. Pritchard RW: Total knee replacements in the elderly. J Maine Med Assoc 1980;71:378–379
86. Tankersley SW, Hungerford DS: Total knee arthroplasty in the very aged. Clin Orthop 1995;316:45–49
87. Zicat B, Rorabeck CH, Bourne RB et al: Total knee arthroplasty in the octogenarian. J Arthroplasty 1993;8: 395–400
88. Ekelund A, Rydell N, Nilsson OS: Total hip arthroplasty in patients 80 years of age and older. Clin Orthop 1990;281: 101–106
89. Levy RN, Levy CM, Snyder J, DiGiovanni J: Outcome and long-term results following total hip replacement in elderly patients. Clin Orthop 1995;316:25–30
90. Newington DP, Bannister GC, Fordyce M: Primary total hip replacement in patients over 80 years of age. J Bone Joint Surg 1990;72B:450–452
91. Peterson VS, Solgard S, Simonsen B: Total hip replacement in patients aged 80 years and older. J Am Geriatri Soc 1989; 37:218–222
92. Phillips TW, Grainger RW, Cameron HAS, Bruce L: Risks and benefits of elective hip replacement in the octogenarian. Can Med Assoc J 1987;137:497–500
93. Altman RD, Gary R: Diagnostic and therapeutic uses of the arthroscope in rheumatoid arthritis and osteoarthritis. Am J Med 1983;31:50–55
94. Casscells SW: What, if any, are the indications for arthroscopic debridement of the osteoarthritic knee? Arthroscopy 1990;6: 169–170
95. Chang RW, Falconer J, Stulberg SD et al: A randomized, controlled trial of arthroscopic surgery versus closed-needle joint lavage for patients with osteoarthritis of the knee. Arthritis Rheum 1993;36:289–296
96. Jackson RW: The role of arthroscopy in the management of the arthritic knee. Clin Orthop 1974;101:28–35
97. Yang SS, Nisonson B: Arthroscopic surgery of the knee in the geriatric patient. Clin Orthop 1995;316:50–58
98. Eichenholtz SN, Jacobs B, Patterson RL: Meniscus injuries of the knee in the elderly. J Am Geriatr Soc 1968;16:281–289
99. Aaron JE, Gallagher JC, Anderson J et al: Frequency of osteomalacia and osteoporosis in fractures of the proximal femur. Lancet 1974;1:229–233
100. Cooper C, Barker DJP, Morris J, Briggs RSJ: Osteoporosis, falls and age in fracture of the proximal femur. BMJ 1987; 295:13–15
101. Cummings SR, Kelsey JL, Nevitt MC, O'Dowd KJ: Epidemiology of osteoporosis and osteoporotic fractures. Epidemiol Rev 1985;7:178–208
102. Demarest GB, Osler TM, Clevenger FW: Injuries in the elderly: evaluation and initial response. Geriatrics 1990;45: 36–42
103. Evans EM: The treatment of trochanteric fractures of the femur. J Bone Joint Surg 1949;31:190–203
104. Michel BA, Bloch DA, Fries JF: Physical activity and fractures over the age of fifty years. Int Orthop 1992;16:87–91
105. Stevens J: Fractures of the femoral neck. Hook-pin fixation in femoral neck fractures: a two-year follow-up study of 300 cases. Clin Orthop 1987;218:58–62
106. Boyce WJ, Vessey MP: Rising incidence of fracture of the proximal femur. Lancet 1985;1:150–151
107. Central Statistical Office: Social Trends, No. 17. HMSO, London, 1987
108. Obrant KJ, Bengner U, Johnell O et al: Increasing age-adjusted risks of fragility fractures: a sign of increasing osteoporosis in successive generations? Calcif Tissue Int 1989;44:157–167
109. Wallace WA: The scale and financial implications of osteoporosis. Int Med 1987;(suppl 12):3–4
110. Royal College of Physicians: Fractured neck of the femur, prevention and management. J R Coll Phys Lond 1989;23: 8–12
111. Devas MB: Geriatric Orthopaedics. Academic Press, London, 1977
112. Moran CG, Gibson MJ, Cross AT: Intramedullary locking nails for femoral shaft fractures in elderly patients. J Bone Joint Surg 1990;72B:19–22
113. Pennig D: Principles of Fracture Management in Elderly Patients. pp. 420–435. In Newman RJ (ed): Orthogeriatrics: Comprehensive Orthopaedic Care for the Elderly Patient. Butterworth-Heinemann, Oxford, 1992
114. Jensen JS: Determining factors for the mortality following hip fractures. Injury 1984;15:411
115. Tile M: Fractures of the Pelvis and Acetabulum. Williams & Wilkins, Baltimore, 1995
116. Naam NH, Brown WH: Major pelvic fracture. Arch Surg 1983; 16:610–615
117. Oreskovich MR, Howard JD, Copass MK, Carrico CJ: Geriatric

trauma: injury patterns and outcomes. J Trauma 1984;24: 565–572

118. Lyden JP: Fracture management of the elderly patient. pp. 269–287. In Sculco TP (ed): Orthopaedic Care of the Geriatric Patient. CV Mosby, St. Louis, 1985
119. Levy DB, Hanlon DP, Townsend RN: Geriatric trauma. Clin Geriatr Med 1993;9:601–620
120. Martin RE, Teberian G: Multiple trauma and the elderly patient. Emerg Med Clin North Am 1990;8:411–420
121. Helfet DL, Borrelli JB, DiPasquale T, Sanders R: Stabilization of acetabular fractures in elderly patients. J Bone Joint Surg 1992;74A:753–765
122. Karpik KD, Mears DC, Hardy SL: Total hip arthroplasty for post-traumatic arthritis following acetabular fractures. Presented at the Orthopaedic Trauma Association Specialty Day Symposium at The 63rd Annual Meeting of the American Academy of Orthopaedic Surgeons, Atlanta, February 25, 1995
123. Koval KJ, Zuckerman JD: Hip Fractures: I. Overview and evaluation and treatment of femoral neck fractures. J Am Acad Orthop Surg 1994;2:141–149
124. Koval KJ, Zuckerman JD: Hip Fractures: II. Evaluation and treatment of intertrochanteric fractures. J Am Acad Orthop Surg 1994;2:150–156
125. Ceder L, Thorngren KG, Wallden B: Prognostic indicators and early home rehabilitation in elderly patients with hip fractures. Clin Orthop 1980;152:173–184
126. DeLee JC: Fractures and dislocations of the hip. pp. 1211–1356. In Rockwood CA, Green DP (eds): Fractures in Adults. vol. 2. Lipincott, London, 1984
127. Barr JS: Trauma (Hip and Femur). p. 288. In Orthopaedic Knowledge Update I: Home Study Syllabus. American Academy of Orthopaedic Surgeons, Chicago, 1984
128. National Health Center for Health Statistics: Advance Data From Vitaland Health Statistics: 1985 Summary: Nutritional Hospital Discharge Summary. Public Health Service, Hyattsville, MD, 1986
129. Fitzgerald JF, Moore PS, Dittus RS: The care of elderly patients with hip fracture. Changes since implementation of the prospective payment system. N Engl J Med 1988;319: 1392–1397
130. Koval KJ, Zuckerman JD: Functional recovery after fracture of the hip. J Bone Joint Surg 1994;76A:751–758
131. Hedlund R, Lindgren U, Ahlbom A: Age- and sex-specific incidence of femoral neck and trochanteric fractures. An analysis based on 20,538 fractures in Stockholm County, Sweden, 1972–1981. Clin Orthop 1987;222:132–139
132. Ogilvie-Harris, Botsford DJ, Hawker RW: Elderly patients with hip fractures: improved outcome with the use of care maps with high-quality medical and nursing protocols. J Orthop Trauma 1993;7:428–437
133. Gallagher JC, Melton RJ, Riggs BL, Bergstrath E: Epidemiology of fractures of the proximal femur in Rochester, Minnesota. Clin Orthop 1980;150:163–171
134. Boyce WJ, Vessey MP: Habitual physical inertia and other factors in relation to risk of fracture of the proximal femur. Age Ageing 1988;17:319–327
135. Davidson BJ, Ross RK, Paganini-Hill A et al: Total and free estrogens and androgens in postmenopausal women with hip fractures. J Clin Endocrinol Metab 1982;54:115–120
136. Riggs BL, Melton LJ: Involutional osteoporosis. N Engl J Med 1986;314:1676–1686
137. Alffram PPA: An epidemiologic study of cervical and trochanteric fractures of the femur in an urban population. Analysis of 1,664 cases with special references to etiologic factors. Acta Orthop Scand Suppl 65, 1964
138. Coughlin L, Templeton J: Hip fractures in patients with Parkinson's disease. Clin Orthop 1980;148:192–195
139. Garden RS: Stability and union in subcapital fractures of the femur. J Bone Joint Surg 1971;53B:183–197
140. Stappaerts KH, Broos PLO: Internal fixation of femoral neck fractures: a follow-up study of 118 cases. Acta Chir Belg 1987; 87:247–251
141. Arnold WD: The effect of early weight-bearing on the stability of femoral neck fractures treated with Knowle's pins. J Bone Joint Surg 1984;66A:847
142. Singh M, Nagrath AR, Maini PS: Changes in trabecular pattern of the upper end of the femur as an index of osteoporosis. J Bone Joint Surg 1970;52A:457–467
143. Rizzo PF, Lynden JP, Schneider RN: Occult hip fractures: diagnosis and treatment. Contemp Orthop 1993;27:339–345
144. Fairclough J, Colhoun E, Johnston D, Williams LA: Bone scanning for suspected hip fractures: a prospective study in elderly patients. J Bone Joint Surg 1987;69B:251–253
145. Yao L, Lee JK: Occult intraosseous fracture: detection with magnetic resonance imaging. Radiology 1988;167:749–751
146. Geslien GE, Thrall JH, Espinosa JL, Older RA: Early detection of stress fractures using 99mTc polyphosphate. Radiology 1976;1121:683–687
147. Kenzora JE, McCarthy RE, Lowell JD et al: Hip fracture mortality. Clin Orthop 1984;186:45–56
148. Sexson SB, Lehner JT: Factors affecting hip fracture mortality. J Orthop Trauma 1987;1:298–305
149. Zuckerman JD, Skovron ML, Fessel K et al: The role of surgical delay in the long-term outcome of hip fractures in geriatric patients. Orthop Trans 1992–1993;16:750
150. Del Guercio LRM, Cohn JD: Monitoring operative risk in the elderly. JAMA 1980;243:1350–1355
151. Scalea TM, Simon HM, Duncan AO et al: Geriatric blunt multiple trauma: improved survival with early invasive monitoring. J Trauma 1990;30:129–134
152. Shultz RJ, Whitfield GF, LaMura JJ et al: The role of physiologic monitoring in patients with fracture of the hip. J Trauma 1985;25:309–316
153. Frew JFM: Conservative treatment of intertrochanteric fractures. In Proceedings of the British Orthopaedic Association. J Bone Joint Surg 1972;54B:748–749
154. Lyon LJ, Nevins MA: Management of hip fractures in nursing home patients: to treat or not to treat? J Am Geriatr Soc 1984; 32:391–395
155. Sherk HH, Snape WJ, Loprete FL: Internal fixation versus nontreatment of hip fractures in senile patients. Clin Orthop 1979; 141:196–198
156. Bently G: Treatment of nondisplaced fractures of the femoral neck. Clin Orthop 1980;152:93

157. Garden RS: Reduction and fixation of subcapital fractures of the femur. Orthop Clin N Am 1974;5:683–712
158. Asnis SE, Wanek-Sgaglione L: Intracapsular fractures of the femoral neck. J Bone Joint Surg 1994;76A:1793–1803
159. Swiontkowski MF: Current concepts review: intracapsular fractures of the hip. J Bone Joint Surg 1994;76A:129–138
160. Cobb AG, Gibson PH: Screw fixation of subcapital fractures of the femur: a better method of treatment? Injury 1986;17: 259–264
161. Lu-Yao GL, Keller RB, Littenberg B, Wennberg JE: Outcomes after displaced fractures of the femoral neck. J Bone Joint Surg 1994;76A:15–25
162. Barnes JT, Brown JT, Garden RS, Nicoll EA: Subcapital fractures of the femur; a prospective review. J Bone Joint Surg 1976;58B:2–24
163. Bochner RM, Pellicci PM, Lynden JP: Bipolar hemiarthroplasty for fracture of the femoral neck: clinical review with special emphasis on prosthetic motion. J Bone Joint Surg 1988;70A:1001–1010
164. Bray TJ, Smith-Hoefer E, Hooper A et al: The displaced femoral neck fracture: internal fixation versus bipolar endoprosthesis—results of a prospective, randomized comparison. Clin Orthop 1988;230:127–140
165. Robinson CM, Saran D, Annan IH: Intracapsular hip fractures. Results of management adopting a treatment protocol. Clin Orthop 1994;302:83–91
166. Ahman LA, Eckhoff DG, Kramer AM: Outcome studies of hip fractures: a functional viewpoint. Orthop Rev 1994;23:19–24
167. Haentjens P, Casteleyn PP, DeBoeck H et al: Treatment of unstable intertrochanteric and subtrochanteric fractures in elderly patients. J Bone Joint Surg 1989;71A:1214–1225
168. Laskin RS, Gruber MA, Zimmerman AJ: Intertrochanteric fractures of the hip in the elderly. Clin Orthop 1979;141: 188–195
169. Hornby R, Evans JG, Vardon V: Operative or conservative treatment for trochanteric fractures of the femur. J Bone Joint Surg 1989;71B:619–623
170. Bonamo JJ, Acettolo AB: Treatment of intertrochanteric fractures with a sliding nail-plate. J Trauma 1982;114:797–811
171. Goldhagen PR, Oconor DR, Schwarze D, Schwartz E: A prospective comparative study of the compression hip screw and the gamma nail. J Orthop Trauma 1994;8:367–372
172. Jensen JS, Sonne-Holm S, Tondevold E: Unstable trochanteric fractures. A comparative analysis of four methods of internal fixation. Acta Orthop Scand 1980;51:949–962
173. Kyle RF, Gustilo RB, Premer RF: Analysis of six hundred and twenty two intertrochanteric fractures. A retrospective and prospective study. J Bone Joint Surg 1979;61A:219–221
174. Broos PL, Rommens PM, Deleyn PRJ et al: Pertrochanteric fractures in the elderly: are there indications for primary prosthetic replacement? J Orthop Traum 1991;5:446–451
175. Chow SP, Tang SC, Pun WK et al: Treatment of unstable trochanteric fractures with Dimon-Hughston osteotomy displacement fixation and acrylic cement. Injury 1987;18: 123–127
176. Dimon JH, Hughston JC: Unstable intertrochanteric fractures of the hip. J Bone Joint Surg 1967;49A:440–450
177. Muhr G, Tscherne H, Thomas R: Comminuted trochanteric femoral fractures in geriatric patients. The results of 321 cases treated with internal fixation and acrylic cement. Clin Orthop 1979;138:41–44
178. Sarmiento A, Williams EM: The unstable intertrochanteric fracture. Treatment with a valgus osteotomy and I beam nail-plate. J Bone Joint Surg 1970;52A:1309–1310
179. Behr JT, Dobozi WR, Badrinath K: The treatment of pathological and impending pathological fractures of the proximal femur in the elderly. Clin Orthop 1985;198:173–178
180. Haberman EJ, Sachs R, Stern RE et al: The pathology and treatment of metastatic disease of the femur. Clin Orthop 1982; 169:70–82
181. Verluysen M: Pressure sores in elderly patients. The epidemiology related to hip operations. J Bone Joint Surg 1985; 67B:10–13
182. Feldman DS, Zuckerman JD, Walters J et al: Clinical efficacy of aspirin and dextran for thromboprophylaxis in geriatric hip fracture patients. J Orthop Trauma 1993;7:1–5
183. Gerhart TN, Yett HS, Robertson LK et al: Low-molecular weight heparinoid compared with warfarin for prophylaxis of deep-vein thrombosis in patients who are operated on for fracture of the hip: a prospective, randomized trial. J Bone Joint Surg 1991;73A:494–502
184. Beals RK: Survival following hip fracture—long term follow up of 607 patients. J Chron Dis 1972;25:235–244
185. Evans JG: Epidemiology of osteoporosis and fractures of the femoral neck. Int Med 1987;(suppl 12):4–6
186. Greatorex IF: Femoral neck fractures—improving efficiency in the case of elderly women. Commun Med 1986;8:185–190
187. Thomas TG, Stevens RS: Social effects of fractures of the neck of the femur. BMJ 1974;3:456–458
188. Dahl E: Mortality and life expectancy after hip fracture. Acta Orthop Scand 1980;51:163–170
189. Elmerson S, Zetterburg C, Andersson BJ: Ten-year survival after fractures of the proximal end of the femur. Gerontology 1988;34:186–191
190. Gilchrist WJ, Newman RJ, Hamblen DL, Williams BO: Prospective randomized study of an orthopaedic geriatric inpatient service. BMJ 1988;297:1116–1118
191. Goucke CR: Mortality following surgery for fractures of the neck of the femur. Anaesthesia 1985;40:578–583
192. Holmberg S, Conradi P, Kalen R, Thorngren KG: Mortality after cervical hip fracture. 3002 patients followed for six years. Acta Orthop Scand 1986;57:8–11
193. Ions GK, Stevens J: Prediction of survival in patients with femoral neck fractures. J Bone Joint Surg 1987;69B:384
194. Magaziner J, Simonsick EM, Kashner TM et al: Survival experience of aged hip fracture patients. Am J Pub Health 1989; 79:274–278
195. Miller CW: Survival and ambulation following hip fracture. J Bone Joint Surg 1978;60A:930
196. White BL, Fisher WD, Laurin CA: Rate of mortality for elderly patients after fracture of the hip in the 1980's. J Bone Joint Surg 1987;69A:1335
197. Wood D: MS Thesis. University of London, 1990
198. Jette AM, Harris BA, Cleary PD, Campion EW: Functional

recovery after hip fracture. Arch Phys Med Rehab 1987;68: 735–740

199. Craxford AD, Stevens J: Proximal femoral fractures in psychiatric patients. Injury 1979;11:19–22
200. Davis FM, Woolner DF, Frampton C et al: Prospective multicentre trial of mortality following general or spinal anesthesia for hip fracture surgery in the elderly. Br J Anaesth 1987;59: 1080–1088
201. McKenzie PJ, Wishart HY, Smith G: Long-term outcome after repair of fractured neck of the femur. Comparison of subarachnoid and general anaesthesia. Br J Anaesth 1984;56:581–584
202. Harrington MR, Brennant M, Hodkinson HM: The first year of a geriatric-orthopaedic liaison service: an alternative to "orthogeriatric" units? Age Ageing 1988;17:129–133
203. Reid J, Kennie DC: Geriatric rehabilitation care after fractures of the proximal femur: one year follow up of a randomized clinical trial. BMJ 1989;299:25–26
204. Zuckerman JD, Sakales SR, Fabian DR, Frankel VH: Hip fractures in geriatric patients. Results of an interdisciplinary hospital care program. Clin Orthop 1992;274:213–225
205. Niemann KMW, Mankin HJ: Fractures about the hip in an institutionalized patient population. II. Survival and ability to walk again. J Bone Joint Surg 1968;50A:1327–1340
206. Cummings SR, Phillips SL, Wheat ME et al: Recovery of function after hip fracture. The role of social supports. J Am Geriatr Soc 1988;36:801–806
207. Barnes B, Donovan K: Functional outcomes after hip fracture. Phys Ther 1987;67:1675–1679
208. Magaziner J, Simonsick EM, Kashner TM et al: Predictors of functional recovery one year following hospital discharge for hip fracture: a prospective study. J Gerontol 1990;45: 101–107
209. Broos PL, Stappaerts KH, Luiten EJ, Gruwez JA: Home-going: prognostic factors concerning the major goal in treatment of elderly hip fracture-patients. Int Surg 1988;73:148–150
210. Bonar SK, Tinetti ME, Speechley M, Cooney LM: Factors associated with short-versus long-term skilled nursing facility placement among community-living hip fracture patients. J Am Geriatr Soc 1990;38:1139–1144
211. Jensen JS, Bagger J: Long-term social prognosis after hip fractures. Acta Orthop Scand 1982;53:97–101
212. Mullen JO, Mullen NL: Hip fracture mortality: a prospective, multifactorial study to predict and minimize death risk. Clin Orthop 1992;280:214–222
213. Frandsen PA, Kruse T: Hip fracture in the county of Funen, Denmark. Implication of demographic aging and changes in incidence rates. Acta Orthop Scand 1983;54:681–686
214. Firooznia H, Rafii M, Golimbu C et al: Trabecular mineral content of the spine in women with hip fracture: CT measurement. Radiology 1986;159:737–740
215. Hinton RY, Smith GS: The association of age, race, and sex with the location of proximal femur fractures in the elderly. J Bone Joint Surg 1993;75A:752–759
216. Koch JC: The laws of bone architecture. Am J Anat 1917;21: 177–298
217. Rockwood C, Green D, Bucholz R: Rockwood and Green's Fractures in Adults. 3rd Ed. Lippincott-Raven, Philadelphia, 1991
218. Schatzker J, McBroom R, Bruce D: The tibial plateau fracture: the Toronto experience 1968–1975. Clin Orthop 1979;138: 94–104
219. Koval KJ, Sanders R, Borrelli J et al: Indirect reduction and percutaneous screw fixation of displaced tibial plateau fractures. J Orthop Trauma 1992;6:340–346
220. Yang EC, Weiner L, Strauss E et al: Metaphyseal dissociation fractures of the proximal tibia. Am J Orthop 1995;(Sept): 695–704
221. Grazier KL, Holbrook TL, Kelsey JL, Stauffer RN: The Frequency of Occurrence, Impact and Cost of Musculoskeletal Conditions in the U.S. AAOS, Chicago, 1984
222. Kostuik, JP. Compression fractures and surgery in the osteoporotic patient. In Frymoyer JW (ed): The Adult Spine. Principles and Practice. Lippincotts-Raven, Philadelphia, 1991
223. Kane WJ: Osteoporosis, osteomalacia and Pagets disease. In Frymoyer JW (ed): The Adult Spine. Principles and Practice. Lippincott-Raven, Philadelphia, 1991
224. Barth RW, Lane JM: Osteoporosis. Orthop Clin North Am 1988;19:845–858
225. Steinberg FU: Principles of geriatric rehabilitation. Arch Phys Med Rehabil 1989;70:67–68
226. Gibbs J, Hughes S, Dunlop D et al: Predictors of change in walking velocity in older adults. J Am Geriatr Soc 1996;44: 126–132
227. Frontera WR, Meredith CN: Exercise in the rehabilitation of the elderly. pp. 35–46. In Felsenthal G, Garrison SJ, Steinberg FU (eds): Rehabilitation of the Aging and Elderly Patient. Williams & Wilkins, Baltimore, 1994
228. Agre JC, Pierce LE, Raab DM et al: Light resistance and stretching exercise in elderly women: effect upon strength. Arch Phys Med Rehabil 1988;69:273–276
229. Aniansson A, Ljungberg P, Rundgren A, Wetterqvist H: Effect of a training programme for pensioners on condition and muscular strength. Arch Gerontol Geriatr 1984;3:229–241
230. King AC, Haskell WL, Taylor B et al: Group-vs home-based exercise training in healthy older men and women. JAMA 1991;266:1535–1542
231. Fisher NM, Pendergast DR, Calkins E: Muscle rehabilitation in impaired elderly nursing home residents. Arch Phys Med Rehabil 1991;72:181–185
232. Frontera WR, Meredith CN, O'Reilly KP et al: Strength conditioning in older men: skeletal muscle hypertrophy and improved function. J Appl Physiol 1988;64:1038–1044
233. Thompson LDV: Effects of age and training on skeletal muscle physiology and performance. Phys Ther 1994;74:71–81
234. MacRae PG, Asplund LA, Schnelle JF et al: A walking program for nursing home residents: effects on walk endurance, physical activity, mobility, and quality of life. J Am Geriatr Soc 1996;44:175–180
235. Eisenberg MG, Tierney DO: Changing demographic profile of the spinal cord injury population: implications for health care support systems. Paraplegia 1985;23:335–343
236. Yarkony GM: Aging after traumatic spinal cord injury. pp. 391–396. In Felsenthal G, Garrison SJ, Steinberg FU (eds): Rehabilitation of the Aging and Elderly Patient. Williams & Wilkins, Baltimore, 1994

237. Janssen TWJ, Van Oers CAJM, Van Der Woude LHV, Hollander AP: Physical strain in daily life of wheelchair users with spinal cord injuries. Med Sci Sports Exerc 1994;26:661–670

238. Halstead LS: Poliomyelitis. pp. 415–425. In Felsenthal G, Garrison SJ, Steinberg FU (eds): Rehabilitation of the Aging and Elderly Patient. Williams & Wilkins, Baltimore, 1994

239. Cutler RB, Fishbain DA, Rosomoff RS, Rosomoff HL: Outcomes in treatment of pain in geriatric and younger age groups. Arch Phys Med Rehabil 1994;75:457–464

240. Santiesteban AJ: Physical agents and musculoskeletal pain. pp. 181–193. In Gould JA (ed): Orthopaedic and Sports Physical Therapy. 2nd Ed. CV Mosby, St. Louis, 1990

241. Wagstaff P, Coakley D: The management of stroke. p. 17. In Physiotherapy and the Elderly Patient. MD, Aspen, Rockville, 1988

242. Wagstaff P, Coakley D: Music, leisure and exercise. pp. 173–180. In Physiotherapy and the Elderly Patient. MD, Aspen, Rockville, 1988

243. Hanser S: Music therapy with depressed older adults. pp. 222–231. In Spintge R, Droh R (eds): MusicMedicine. MMB Music, St. Louis, 1992

244. Turner SS: Expression through dance for the well-elderly. pp. 218–221. In Spintge R, Droh R (eds): MusicMedicine. MMB Music, St. Louis, 1992

245. Pierson FM: Ambulation aids, patterns, and activities. pp. 99–148. In Principles and Techniques of Patient Care. WB Saunders, Philadelphia, 1994

246. Epler M: Gait. pp. 602–625. In Richardson JK, lglarsh ZA (eds): Clinical Orthopaedic Physical Therapy. WB Saunders, Philadelphia, 1994

247. Weiner DK, Distell B, Studenski S et al: Does radiographic osteoarthritis correlate with flexibility of the lumbar spine? J Am Geriatr Soc 1994;42:257–263

248. Alexander NB: Postural control in older adults. J Am Geriatr Soc 1994;42:93–108

249. Johnson GW: Progressive exercise program: a model approach for working with elderly patients. pp. 197–210. In Jackson OL (ed): Therapeutic Considerations for the Elderly. Churchill Livingstone, New York, 1987

250. Shestak R: Handbook of Physical Therapy. Springer, New York, 1977

251. Sinaki M, McPhee MC, Hodgson SF et al: Relationship between bone mineral density of spine and strength of back extensors in healthy postmenopausal women. Mayo Clin Proc 1986;61:116–122

252. Sinaki M, Mikkelsen BA: Postmenopausal spinal osteoporosis: flexion versus extension exercises. Arch Phys Med Rehabil 1984;65:593–596

253. Karten I: Osteoarthritis in the elderly. Pract Gastroenterol 1986;10:34–38

254. Saudek CE: The hip. pp. 347–394. In Gould JA (ed): Orthopaedic and Sports Physical Therapy. 2nd Ed. CV Mosby, St. Louis, 1990

255. Ben-Yishay A, Zuckerman JD: Hip injuries: an orthopedic perspective. pp. 217–241. In Lewis CB, Knortz KA (eds): Orthopedic assessment and treatment of the geriatric patient. Mosby-Year Book, St. Louis, 1993

256. LeVeau B: Hip. pp. 333–398. In Richardson JK, Iglarsh ZA (eds): Clinical Orthopaedic Physical Therapy. WB Saunders, Philadelphia, 1994

257. Convery FR, Convery MM: Post-traumatic and degenerative arthritis. pp. 571–582. In Nickel VL, Botte MI (eds): Orthopaedic Rehabilitation. 2nd Ed. Churchill Livingstone, New York, 1992

258. Coleman EA, Buchner DM, Cress ME et al: The relationship of joint symptoms with exercise performance in older adults. J Am Geriatr Soc 1996;44:14–21

259. Nicholas II, Rosenberg AN: Arthritis and arthroplasties. pp. 97–106. In Felsenthal G, Garrison SJ, Steinberg FU (eds): Rehabilitation of the Aging and Elderly Patient. Williams & Wilkins, Baltimore, 1994

260. Lewis CB, Bottomley JM: Orthopedic treatment considerations. pp. 327–352. In Geriatric Physical Therapy: A Clinical Approach. Appleton & Lange, Norwalk, CT, 1994

261. Kampa K: Hip injuries: a rehabilitation perspective. pp. 243–262. In Lewis CB, Knortz KA (eds): Orthopedic Assessment and Treatment of the Geriatric Patient. Mosby-Year Book, St. Louis, 1993

262. Sashika H, Matsuba Y, Watanabe Y: Home program of physical therapy: effect on disabilities of patients with total hip arthroplasty. Arch Phys Med Rehabil. 1996;77:273–277

263. Cameron HU, Brotzman SB, Boolos M: Rehabilitation after total joint arthroplasty. pp. 283–311. In Brotzman SB (eds): Clinical Orthopaedic Rehabilitation. Mosby, St. Louis, 1996

264. Huo MH, Sculco TP: Complications in primary total knee arthroplasty. Orthop Rev 1990;19:781–788

265. Knortz KA: Knee injuries: a rehabilitation perspective. pp. 301–322. In Lewis CB, Knortz KA (eds): Orthopedic Assessment and Treatment of the Geriatric Patient. Mosby-Year Book, St. Louis, 1993

266. Mooney V, Becker S: Major fractures. pp. 601–610. In Nickel VL, Botte Mi (eds): Orthopaedic Rehabilitation. 2nd Ed. Churchill Livingstone, New York, 1992

267. Wasilewski SA, Woods LC, Torgerson WR, Healy WL: Value of continuous passive motion in total knee arthroplasty. Orthopedics 1990;13:291–295

268. Lewis CB, Bottomley JM: Principles and practice in geriatric rehabilitation. pp. 276–282. In Geriatric Physical Therapy: A Clinical Approach. Appleton & Lange, Norwalk, CT, 1994

269. Nyberg L, Gustafson Y, Berggren D et al: Falls leading to femoral neck fractures in lucid older people. J Am Geriatr Soc 1996;44:156–160

270. Stein BD, Felsenthal G: Rehabilitation of fractures in the geriatric population. pp. 123–139. In Felsenthal G, Garrison SI, Steinberg FU (eds): Rehabilitation of the Aging and Elderly Patient. Williams & Wilkins, Baltimore, 1994

271. Alexander NB: Gait disorders in older adults. J Am Geriatr Soc 1996;44:434–451

272. Gehlsen GM, Whaley MH: Falls in the elderly: Part I, gait. Arch Phys Med Rehabil 1990;71:735–738

273. Gehlsen GM, Whaley MH: Falls in the elderly: Part II, balance, strength, and flexibility. Arch Phys Med Rehabil 1990; 71:739–741

274. MacRae PG, Lacourse M, Moldavon R: Physical performance

measures that predict faller status in community-dwelling older adults. J Sports Phys Ther 1992;16:123–128

275. Steinberg FU: Disorders of mobility, balance, and gait. pp. 243–252. In Felsenthal G, Garrison SJ, Steinberg FU (eds): Rehabilitation of the aging and elderly patient. Williams & Wilkins, Baltimore, 1994

276. Lewis CB, Bottomley JM: Pathological manifestations of aging. pp. 111–122. In Geriatric Physical Therapy: A Clinical Approach. Appleton & Lange, Norwalk, CT, 1994

277. Sudarsky L: Geriatrics: gait disorders in the elderly. N Engl J Med 1990;322:1441–1446

278. Lewis CB, Bottomley JM: Assessment instruments. pp. 168–173. In Geriatric Physical Therapy: A Clinical Approach. Appleton & Lange, Norwalk, CT, 1994

279. Alexander NB, Fry-Welch DK, Marshall LM et al: Healthy young and old women differ in their trunk elevation and hip pivot motions when rising from supine to sitting. J Am Geriatr Soc 1995;43:338–343

280. Perry J: Gait characteristics. pp. 113–123. In Jackson OL (ed): Therapeutic Considerations for the Elderly. Churchill Livingstone, New York, 1987

281. Wagstaff P, Coakley D: Treatment of musculo-skeletal disorders. pp. 83–115. In Physiotherapy and the Elderly Patient. Aspen Rockville, MD, 1988

282. Cumining RG, Klineberg RJ: Fall frequency and characteristics and the risk of hip fractures. J Am Geriatr Soc 1994;42: 774–778

283. Smith EL, Gilligan C, Kwiatkowski BS: Osteoporosis: background and management. pp. 399–407. In Lewis CB, Knortz KA (eds): Orthopedic Assessment and Treatment of the Geriatric Patient. Mosby-Year Book, St. Louis, 1993

284. Hunter GR, Treuth MS, Weinsier RL et al: The effects of strength conditioning on older women's ability to perform daily tasks. J Am Geriatr Soc 1995;43:756–760

285. Judge JO, Whipple RH, Wolfson LI: Effects of resistive and balance exercises on isokinetic strength in older persons. J Am Geriatr Soc 1994;42:937–946

286. Karlqvist L: Environmental assessment: adaptations for maximal independence. pp. 155–171. In Jackson OL (ed): Therapeutic Considerations for the Elderly. Churchill Livingstone New York, 1987

287. Fabacher D, Josephson K, Pietruszka F et al: An in-home preventive assessment program for independent older adults: a randomized controlled trial. J Am Geriatr Soc 1994;42: 630–638

288. Langlois JA, Smith GS, Nelson DE et al: Dependence in adctivities of daily living as a risk factor for fall injury events among older people living in the community. J Am Geriatr Soc 1995;43:275–278

289. Thapa PB, Brockman KG, Gideon P et al: Injurious falls in nonambulatory nursing home residents: a comparative study of circumstances, incidence, and risk factors. J Am Geriatr Soc 1996;44:273–278

290. Pierson FM: Transfer activities. pp. 63–98. In Principles and Techniques of Patient Care. WB Saunders, Philadelphia, 1994

291. Gradisar IA: Fracture stabilization and healing. pp. 130–135. In Gould JA (ed): Orthopaedic and Sports Physical Therapy 2nd Ed. CV Mosby, St. Louis, 1990

292. Fox KM, Felsenthal G, Hebel JR et al: A portable neuromuscular function assessment for studying recovery from hip fracture. Arch Phys Med Rehabit 1996;77:171–176

293. Fox KM, Hawkes WG, Magaziner J et al: Markers of failure to thrive among older hip fracture patients. J Am Geriatr Soc 1996;44:371–376

294. Shoemaker SC, Skyhar MJ, Simmons TC: Rehabilitation of the knee. In Nickel VL, Botte MI (eds): Orthopaedic Rehabilitation. 2nd Ed. Churchill Livingstone, New York, 1992

295. Smith S: Knee injuries: an orthopedic perspective. pp. 263–299. In Lewis CB, Knortz KA (eds): Orthopedic Assessment and Treatment of the Geriatric Patient. Mosby-Year Book, St. Louis, 1993

296. Timm KE: Knee. pp. 399–482. In Richardson JK, lglarsh ZA (eds): Clinical Orthopaedic Physical Therapy. WB Saunders, Philadelphia, 1994

297. Wallace LA, Mangine RE, Malone TR: The knee. pp. 334–337. In Gould JA (ed): Orthopaedic and Sports Physical Therapy. 2nd Ed. CV Mosby, St. Louis, 1990

298. Keene JS: Ligament and muscle-tendon unit injuries. pp. 137–165. In Gould JA (ed): Orthopaedic and Sports Physical Therapy. 2nd Ed. CV Mosby, St. Louis, 1990

299. McPoil TG, Brocato RS: The foot and ankle: biomechanical evaluation and treatment. pp. 293–321. In Gould JA (ed): Orthopaedic and Sports Physical Therapy. 2nd Ed. CV Mosby, St. Louis, 1990

300. Riddle DL: Foot and ankle. pp. 483–562. In Richardson JK, lglarsh ZA (eds): Clinical Orthopaedic Physical Therapy. WB Saunders, Philadelphia, 1994

301. Esterson PS, Meadows MO: Leg and ankle injuries: a rehabilitation perspective. pp. 329–343. In Lewis CB, Knortz KA (eds): Orthopedic Assessment and Treatment of the Geriatric Patient. Mosby-Year Book, St. Louis, 1993

302. Karpman R: Leg and ankle injuries: an orthopedic perspective. pp. 323–327. In Lewis CB, Knortz KA (eds): Orthopedic Assessment and Treatment of the Geriatric Patient. Mosby-Year Book, St. Louis, 1993

303. Bistevins R: Footwear and footwear modifications. pp. 967–975. In Kottke FJ, Lehmann JF (eds): Krusen's Handbook of Physical Medicine and Rehabilitation. WB Saunders, Philadelphia 1990

304. Bottomley JM, Herman H: Foot injuries: a rehabilitation perspective. pp. 349–377. In Lewis CB, Knortz KA (eds): Orthopedic Assessment and Treatment of the Geriatric Patient. Mosby-Year Book, St. Louis, 1993

305. Brotzman SB, Brasel J: Foot and ankle rehabilitation. pp. 245–281. In Brotzman SB (ed): Clinical Orthopaedic Rehabilitation. Mosby, St. Louis, 1996

CHAPTER 85

Orthogeriatrics

MICHAEL A. HORAN
JOHN E. CLAGUE

What is Orthogeriatrics?

Geriatric medicine, unlike traditional organ-based medical specialties, emphasizes the context in which new problems arise. These problems are superimposed on underlying aging processes, on the accumulated deficits of a long life and, frequently, on coexisting chronic disorders. Modern geriatric medicine has acquired a corpus of knowledge and expertise that should ensure optimal management for such patients. However, these patients do not present only to geriatricians but to almost all other departments in a hospital. Thus, geriatric medicine might best be viewed as a dimension of medicine rather than as simply a subspecialty of general internal medicine. One service that deals with large numbers of these older patients is orthopaedic surgery. Orthopaedic surgeons are usually well aware of the problems and have often collaborated in schemes to ensure that the skills of geriatricians are routinely available for their patients. The term *orthogeriatrics* is generally used to denote any of a variety of such schemes.

How is Orthogeriatrics Organized?

Orthogeriatrics Units

Probably the first reported orthopaedics-geriatrics liaison for hip fractures was established in Hastings in 1962.[1] Orthopaedic surgeons would select patients for transfer to a dedicated orthogeriatrics ward and would share responsibility for them with geriatricians. Day-to-day care would be provided by staff from the geriatrics service and a multidisciplinary ward round would take place each week to review progress, to agree on rehabilitation goals, and to set up arrangements for discharge from the hospital. Generally, patients would remain in the orthogeriatrics unit for a finite time (maximum 6 weeks) and when the fracture ceased to be the main barrier to discharge, the patient would be transferred to a more appropriate ward.

Many orthogeriatrics units have now been established and tend to operate along similar lines, although the precise organization of the service has had to adapt to local circumstances. A survey of 289 departments of geriatric medicine in 1985[2] reported that 20 percent of them provided some kind of special unit for hip fracture patients. Furthermore, two influential reports[3,4] have suggested the Hastings system as a valuable model for other units.

Liaison Services

One concern about establishing special units is the associated, additional resource use, although the true costs of such schemes as those referred to above are not known. Some schemes have been established that seek to minimize use of resources. A nurse-based liaison service has been described.[5] A senior nurse with orthopaedic and geriatric experience liaised between a geriatric unit and the orthopaedic ward and was able to provide advice on rehabilitation, common medical problems, and the availability of community care. Although backup was available from the geriatricians only a few patients per month required transfer to the geriatric unit. A junior-doctor-led liaison service requiring no more than 3 hours per week input was reported by Harrington et al.[6] A multidisciplinary ward round was the mainstay of the service. Advice on symptoms management, holistic care, investigation of laboratory abnormalities, rehabilitation, and discharge goals were seen as the main input. Improvement in the quality of care and a reduced number of patients transferred for rehabilitation were seen as the main advantages of the system.

The Rapid Transit System

The rapid transit system is based on the ideas of Ceder et al.[7,8] and was popularized by Sikorski and colleagues[9] in Australia. It is based on reducing the time spent in the hospital to a minimum (as little as 5 days). Only essential investigations are done, narcotic and sedative drugs are not used, and general anesthesia is avoided. Surgery is done early, often after transfer to the operating room directly from the accident and emergency department. Full weight-bearing is encouraged within hours of surgery. Discharge planning starts the day after surgery and patients are discharged when they can move about the bed, achieve reasonable safety with transfers, and walk a few steps with or without aids. High levels of support are provided at discharge but this is reduced over 2 to 3 weeks toward prefracture levels.

Hospital-at-Home

Hospital-at-home (HAH) was established on a pre-existing, general practice-based, community nursing service in Peterborough. The aim is immediate rehabilitation and discharge planning by a team that oversees both in-hospital and postdischarge management. Intensive home nursing (24 hours/day, if needed) is provided, plus occupational therapists and physiotherapists. It is reported that up to 50 percent of hip fracture patients are suitable for this kind of management.[10,11]

Does Orthogeriatrics Work?

It is difficult to evaluate the effectiveness of orthogeriatrics care and most reported studies of orthogeriatrics units are intrinsically flawed in their design. The main outcome measure has been length of hospital stay, which can easily be reduced at the price of inappropriate admissions to continuing care.[12] Some studies have reported not only reduced length of stay but also better functional outcomes[13] and reduced cost.[14] Rapid transit has been reported to achieve reduced length of stay without jeopardizing functional outcome.[15] The HAH scheme has also been reported to be less expensive than conventional care[16] with only modestly increased readmission rates. However, accounting studies in this area are in their infancy and the overall cost will depend not only on the costs of acute and postacute care, but also on the ongoing care costs. No formal comparisons between liaison services and other models of orthogeriatric care have been made.

One major problem in comparing accelerated discharge schemes with hospital-based rehabilitation is that we do not yet know what constitutes optimal rehabilitation strategies for hip fracture patients. It seems likely that the amounts of physiotherapy time available in most geriatrics units is inadequate and most patients do not even get the prescribed level of treatment.[17]

What Should Be The Aims of an Orthogeriatrics Service?

The principal aims of orthogeriatrics should be to optimize management so that unnecessary deaths are avoided, inappropriate treatments are withheld or withdrawn, complications are prevented, predisposing factors are detected and treated, functional outcome is enhanced, and effective discharge procedures are implemented without undue delays. Most schemes have concentrated on patients with hip fractures but serious consideration should be given to the inclusion of patients with multiple injuries and fractures of the distal radius, proximal humerus, and pelvis.

In our hospital, we believe the best way to achieve these aims is to have a consultant geriatrician dedicated to the orthopaedics service who shares patient care with the orthopaedic surgeons. Primary responsibility often changes over time and is assumed by the consultant whose skills are most relevant for the dominant problem. The geriatrician visits the wards daily to assess all new admissions, to advise on fitness for surgery, to provide ongoing medical supervision, to select patients most likely to benefit from transfer to our orthogeriatrics rehabilitation unit, and to identify those who will require placement in continuing care. He also supervises the care of those transferred to the specialist unit. This approach should improve the quality of medical care, not only by the prompt recognition and treatment of coexisting medical and psychiatric conditions, but also by changing the mindset of the staff in the orthopaedic wards so that they become more attuned to the particular problems of older patients.

References

1. Devas MB, Irvine RE: The geriatric orthopaedic unit. J Bone Joint Surg 1963;46B:630–634
2. Brocklehurst JC, Andrews K: Geriatric medicine—the style of practice. Age Ageing 1985;14:1–7
3. Department of Health and Social Security: Report of a working party. Orthopaedic services: waiting time for out-patient and in-patient treatment (Chairman, Prof. R.B. Duthie). HMSO, London, 1981
4. Royal College of Physicians of London: Fractured neck of femur. Prevention and management. Report. 1989
5. Blacklock C, Woodhouse KW: Orthogeriatric liaison. Lancet 1988;1:999
6. Harrington MG, Brennant M, Hodkinson HM: The first year of a geriatric-orthopaedic liaision service: an alternative to orthogeriatric units? Age Ageing 1988;17:129–133
7. Ceder L, Lindberg L, Odberg E: Differentiated care of hip fracture in the elderly. Mean hospital days and results of rehabilitation. Acta Orthop Scand 1980;51:157–162
8. Ceder L, Stromqvist B, Hansson LI: Effects of strategy changes in the treatment of femoral neck fractures during a 17-year period. Clin Orthop 1987;218:53–57
9. Sikorski JM, Davis NJ, Senior J: The rapid transit system for patients with fractures of the proximal femur. BMJ 1985;290: 439–443
10. Mowat IG, Morgan RTT: Peterborough hospital at home scheme. BMJ 1982; 284:641–643
11. Meeds B, Pryor GA: Early home rehabilitation for the elderly patient with hip fracture. The Peterborough hip fracture scheme. Physiotherapy 1990;76:75–77
12. Fitzgerald JF, Fagan LF, Tierney W, Dittus RS: Changing patterns of hip fracture care before and after implementation of the prospective payment system. JAMA 1987;25:218–221
13. Reid J, Kennie DC: Geriatric rehabilitative care after fractures of the proximal femur: one year follow up of a randomized clinical trial. BMJ 1989; 299:25–26
14. Elliot JR, Wilkinson TJ, Hanger HC et al: The added effectiveness of early geriatrician involvement on acute orthopaedic wards to orthogeriatric rehabilitation. NZ Med J 1996;109: 72–73
15. Cameron ID, Lyle DM, Quine S: Accelerated rehabilitation after proximal femoral fracture: a randomized controlled trial. Disabil Rehabil 1993;15:29–34
16. Hollingworth W, Todd CJ, Parker MJ et al: A cost analysis of discharge policies after hip fracture. BMJ 307:903–906
17. Hanspal R, Wright M, Proctor D et al: Failure to deliver the formal therapy prescribed in an NHS rehabilitation unit. Clin Rehabil 1994;8:161–165

CHAPTER 86

Injury in the Aging

MICHAEL A. HORAN

The assertion that trauma is a disease of the young is wrong. Although injuries are certainly more common in younger people than in the older population, older people are much more likely to die as a result of their injuries, virtually regardless of injury severity.[1–8] People aged over 65 years account for about 28 percent of all fatal injuries, despite constituting only about 12 percent of the total population.[9] Falls are the cause of the majority of injuries in older people[10] but falls are common in all age groups. In one study, older people accounted for only about 14 percent of fall-related injuries but for about 50 percent of fall-related deaths.[11] Road traffic accidents account for the majority of multiple injuries.[10,12] American figures for 1986 report that 38 percent of hospital bed-days for all patients in whom injury was the primary reason for hospital admission were accounted for by those over the age of 65 years.[5] Using 1986 average daily costs in the hospital ($500) and in intensive care units ($1,200 to $2,000), their hospital expenses were estimated to exceed $4.4 billion. Despite these huge resource implications, most research has focused on younger victims of trauma.

Defining and Measuring Injury

The transfer of energy at rates and in amounts above the tolerance of tissues is the necessary and specific cause of injury. The amount of energy concentration outside the limits of tissue tolerance determines the severity of injury. Thus, injury generally refers to the damage to cells, tissues, and organs but may also include the nature and magnitude of the various physiologic responses in the recipient of the injury.

The measurement of injury is as important for planning management and studying outcomes as is measurement in any other disease where a variety of grading and staging systems may be used. The systems used for injury utilize either the anatomic extent of the injury, the (patho)physiologic responses of the recipient of the injury, or some hybrid of these two.

Anatomic indexes (e.g., Abbreviated Injury Scale, Injury Severity Score, Anatomic Profile), which require complete and accurate diagnosis, are of only limited use in the immediate management of an injured patient because full information is rarely available until much later. However, they are very useful in evaluating trauma systems and outcome assessment Scoring systems based on the response of the injured individual (e.g., Glasgow Coma Scale, Revised Trauma Score, Simplified Acute Physiology Score, APACHE) are particularly useful for triage and/or patient management. The most commonly used hybrids are the TRISS (Revised Trauma Score + Injury Severity Score) and ASCOT (A Severity Characterization of Trauma), the latter having been developed in response to the limitations of the anatomic component of TRISS and which appears to be a much better predictor of survival. None of the available systems is entirely satisfactory for all purposes, particularly for the prediction of outcomes other than death.[5,13]

The data used to derive most of these scoring systems come mainly from injured younger people and the systems may not perform well for old people.[6,14,15] Possible reasons for this are discussed by Horan et al.[16] Because old bones are weaker than young ones, less energy will be needed to exceed breaking tolerance and the associated soft tissue damage is likely to be less extensive, and thus anatomic scoring systems tend to overestimate the anatomic severity of injury. However, any age-related attenuation of the physiologic responses of the recipient of the injury would tend to underestimate the severity of the injury. This seems to be of only theoretical importance because old people tend to present greater physiologic perturbations (SAPS) for all but the most extreme anatomic injury severity scores (ISS).[17] Once age groups are stratified for SAPS score, age ceases to be an important outcome predictor, provided equivalent treatments are employed. A similar conclusion was reached in a study designed to validate the APACHE III scoring system, which showed that age alone accounted for very little of the variation of outcome; physiologic derangements and comorbid factors were much more important.[18]

Although well recognized, the deficiencies of the generally used scoring systems when applied to the elderly have not been adequately addressed. DeMaria et al.[15] devised a Geriatric Trauma Survival Score that was 92 percent accurate in predicting survival. This system is based on the ISS plus cardiac and infective complications as well as ventilator dependence. Other studies to address the utility of this scoring system seem not to have been done and it is not widely used.

Injuries at Specific Sites

Head Injuries

As the brain ages, its dura becomes tightly adherent to the skull, which makes epidural hematomas uncommon. A progressive loss of brain volume leads to an increase in the space around the brain that is thought to protect it against contusions, but makes subdural hematomas more likely. Intraparenchymal hemorrhage is also more common in elderly people. The epidemiology of head injuries has been reviewed recently.[19] Two aspects are particularly worthy of note: First, there is a modest increase in incidence rates after the age of about 60 years and, second, head injuries are more common in men than in women, even in extreme old age. Thus, crude figures, unadjusted for sex, may underestimate the importance of head injuries among older people owing to the preponderance of women in older age groups.

Head injuries in older people can be devastating. Severe injuries (Glasgow Coma Scale less than 8) have a fatality rate of about 90 percent.[20] Those who survive the initial injury have long hospital stays and more severe residual neurologic deficits. In a study comparing 33 younger patients with acute subdural hematomas with 34 older patients with similar lesions, none of the older patients with a GCS less than 13 made a functional recovery. It is widely believed that elderly people also have poorer outcomes after minor head injuries (GCS 13 or greater on presentation) but there is little published evidence to support this conclusion.

It is not clear why older people have such poor outcomes after head injuries. It is likely that comorbid factors, suboptimal management, and a predisposition to systemic complications play important roles, although a recent study suggests that there is a reduced capacity of the aging brain to recover from injuries.[21]

Thoracic Trauma

Older people with isolated chest injuries have a two to three times greater risk of death than similarly injured younger people.[2,22,23] Rib fractures often complicate even mild blunt trauma to the chest in older people. Similarly, insignificant falls or blows to the chest may cause occult pneumothorax or hemothorax and pulmonary contusions often accompany even mild thoracic injuries. Prompt mechanical ventilation is warranted in older patients showing signs of respiratory distress in any of these circumstances. A history of rapid deceleration should alert one to the possibility of traumatic rupture of the aorta in all older patients. Mediastinal widening or an ill-defined aortic knuckle are characteristic radiographic appearances. Although more than 80 percent of those with this complication die at the accident scene, the remainder may be hemodynamically stable on presentation.

Abdominal Trauma

The death rate in older patients with visceral injuries is about 80 percent.[6] The principles of management of abdominal injuries change little with age. However, it should be borne in mind that the old are intolerant of both shock and unnecessary laparotomy and their management demands a sense of urgency and a high degree of clinical acumen. Those with a history of previous significant abdominal surgery, young or old, should have either a computed tomography scan or ultrasound scan rather than diagnostic peritoneal lavage.

Fall-Related Fractures

The nature of the fall dictates the nature of the fracture. Fractures of the wrist and proximal humerus are believed to be associated with falls on an outstretched arm, implying that the person was moving reasonably fast at the time of the fall. Falls from a stationary position or during slow locomotion are generally considered most likely to result in proximal femoral fractures and it is these that account for most of the old-age peak in trauma deaths.[24] Falls also account for the majority of cervical spine fractures in older people.[25] Frail older people may sustain long bone fractures without a clear history of injury or falls.[26] These have been termed *minimal trauma fractures* and the only precipitating factor clearly identified is severely impaired mobility.

Falls have four distinct phases:(1) loss of balance, (2) a phase of descent, (3) an impact phase, and (4) a postimpact phase during which the faller eventually comes to rest.[27] Most work on falls and fall prevention has concentrated on the first of these (why people fall) and the results emphasize the importance of gait disorders, dementia, visual impairment, neurologic and musculoskeletal disorders, orthostatic hypotension, drugs, and environmental hazards. By contrast, little is known about the other three phases (how people fall) and how this relates to the risk of fracture. Cummings and Nevitt[28] consider that for a hip fracture to occur, there must be (1) impact near the hip, (2) failure of active protective mechanisms, and (3) insufficient passive energy absorption by local soft tissues. Under these conditions they suggest that sufficient force can be transmitted to the proximal femur to exceed its fracture load. Others have reported that in a typical fall, more than enough energy will be available to fracture an elderly hip.[29,30]

Experimental systems have been developed to get more precise measurements of the forces involved in falls under different experimental conditions. It was shown that impact in a state of muscle contraction (mainly trunk and back muscles) considerably increases impact force.[31] However, more physiologic studies on experimental falls suggest that eccentric contractions of these muscle groups can dissipate up to two-thirds of the available potential energy with further contributions from stiffness and damping in the hip and knee.[32] Thus, although falls among elderly subjects are associated with available potential energies between 400 J and 700 J, the actual energy available at impact could be only about one-third of these values. The strength of the proximal femur has been measured in cadaveric specimens tested in a loading configuration that simulated a fall with impact on the greater trochanter. It was found that fracture load is linearly related to bone mineral density.[33]

Nevitt and Cummings[34] compared fallers sustaining fractures and those who did not. Those who sustained fractures were more likely to have fallen sideways or straight down (odds ratio 3.3) and to have landed on or near the hip (odds ratio

32.5). For those who fell on their hip, the risk of fracture approximately doubled for every standard deviation decrease in bone mineral density at the hip. Similarly, Greenspan et al.[35] found that falling to the side increased fracture risk sixfold; increasing the potential energy of the fall by one standard deviation increased the risk threefold; and a reduction of body mass index by one standard deviation increased fracture risk twofold. A decrease in bone mineral density by one standard deviation increased fracture risk threefold.

The combined data from the above studies show an average impact force of about 5,600 N[32] and an average fracture load of about 4,170 N. Thus, those who do not sustain fractures under these conditions *must* employ energy absorbing/dissipating mechanisms to reduce the force delivered to the femur: eccentric contraction of large muscles, use of the outstretched hand, and energy absorption by soft tissues. These studies also suggest that pharmacologic interventions to increase proximal femur bone mineral density would have to show substantial effects in order to increase fracture load above the likely impact forces and interventions to prevent falls would probably have a much greater impact on fracture incidence.

Multiple Injuries

Visceral injuries in the absence of fractures are very rare in older trauma victims.[1] The bony injuries that present the most immediate threats to life are skull fractures (with underlying brain injury) and fractures of the pelvis. The main problem with pelvic fractures is massive bleeding from lacerations to the pelvic venous plexus, but this can generally be controlled by external fixators. About 15 percent of older people with closed pelvic fractures die, whereas for open fractures the death rate is approximately 80 percent.[36] Long bone fractures, especially the tibia, are common and must be stabilized early to control blood loss, reduce the risk of fat embolism, and enable early mobilization. Older people do not tolerate delays before surgical stabilization well,[37] even after isolated hip fractures.[38,39]

Responses to Injury

The Ebb and Flow Phases

The general response to physical injury is complex and is conventionally divided into two phases: the ebb phase and the flow phase.[40] In general, the ebb phase is one of increased fuel production and reduced metabolic rate whereas the flow phase is characterized by increased metabolic rate, catabolism, and fuel utilization. Because responses to injury in older people have not been systematically studied, it is impossible to give a complete account and so I will concentrate on those aspects that are best understood and those that seem of particular clinical importance.

The Hypothalamic-Pituitary-Adrenal Axis

One of the most rapid effects of injury is to provoke well-known neuroendocrine responses. The activity of the sympathoadrenal system and the hypothalamic-pituitary-adrenal (HPA) axis, and the secretion of a number of other hormones (growth hormone, prolactin, vasopressin, aldosterone, and glucagon), are increased. In some systems, such as the sympathoadrenal, the magnitude of the initial response increases with injury severity and may not be detectable at all with minor injuries. For other systems, such as the HPA axis, it is the duration of the response that increases with injury severity. Aging does not appear to impair these early neuroendocrine responses.

It has been repeatedly shown that the plasma cortisol concentration remains elevated at 2 weeks after proximal femur fracture, by which time it has returned to normal in younger patients with injuries of similar, and even greater, severity[41] and the difference from healthy or bed-ridden elderly control subjects can persist for at least 8 weeks.[42] Compared with healthy elderly women, patients 2 weeks after hip fracture have increased rates of cortisol production and urinary free cortisol excretion.[43]

The reason for the continued cortisol production is unclear. The early HPA response to injury may be provoked by a number of signals (volume depletion, hypotension, nociception, hypoxia, circulating cytokines), the relative importance of which will depend on the nature and severity of the injury. In patients with simple fractures, such stimuli should soon cease as appropriate treatments are instituted and this is consistent with the short-lived cortisol response in younger patients. We believe that older people have an impaired ability to down-regulate the response after resolution of the stimulus rather than a more persistent stimulus. Such a defect is observed in old rats and results from loss of corticosteroid receptors in the hippocampus, which play a role in feedback inhibition.[44] Evidence for the same process in humans comes from patients with Alzheimer's dementia, who have extensive hippocampal neuron loss and show impaired feedback inhibition of the HPA axis as measured by the dexamethasone suppression test. Resistance to dexamethasone suppression in depression is more common among elderly than among young patients and is associated with cognitive impairment.[44] We have found marked resistance to dexamethasone suppression in elderly patients with hip fracture[42,45] suggesting that their hypercortisolemia may also be due to degenerative changes in the hippocampus. Whether or not some older people are particularly predisposed to a prolonged cortisol response to stress is not known. Genetic factors have not been sought but early life events might dictate responses in later life. Recently, Barker[46] has drawn attention to the importance of perinatal events and the development of disease in later life. Levitt et al.[47] have shown that administration of glucocorticoids to rats in the last week of pregnancy leads to reduced numbers of hippocampal glucocorticoid receptors and the development of hypertension when the offspring reach adulthood. Likewise, their administration in the first week of life leads to similarly reduced numbers of hippocampal glucocorticoid receptors in adulthood.

It is still not known whether the persistent hypercortisolemia is maladaptive or a necessary adaptive response, but if the cause(s) is essentially pathologic, the former possibility is the more likely. The acute adrenocortical response helps protect against the effects of hypovolemia by increasing blood glucose and promoting compensatory fluid movement.[48] However, once fluid loss has been corrected, there is little evidence that a sustained elevation in cortisol concentration (as opposed to basal levels, which are known to protect against circulatory collapse) is required to maintain cardiovascular integrity.

If the response is a beneficial adaptation it might be expected that there would be evidence of acquired resistance to glucocorticoid effects, which has already been described in Alzheimer's disease[49] and as a transient phenomenon in depression, septic shock, and acquired immunodeficiency syndrome as well as in corticosteroid-resistant asthma, colitis, and rheumatoid disease.[50] Our own unpublished work has shown no evidence of resistance to glucocorticoid effects in circulating lymphocytes or polymorphonuclear leukocytes.

If it is a maladaptive response, we would expect to see evidence of its effects in the form of insulin resistance, muscle proteolysis, immune suppression, impaired wound healing, etc. Such effects are well known in patients with Cushing's disease and are found also in patients with major depression.[51] Animal experiments with glucocorticoid antagonists have shown that endogenous glucocorticoids have protein-catabolic and immunosuppressive effects soon after injury, when their concentrations are elevated.[52,53]

Metabolic Changes

Like the early neuroendocrine responses, the early metabolic changes after injury are not attenuated with aging. Plasma glucose concentrations rise with injury severity but plasma insulin fails to rise commensurately owing to suppression of insulin secretion by circulating catecholamines. Concentrations of lipid metabolites and lactate are also similar in young and old people after injury, although there is evidence that older people have higher rates of lipolysis and re-esterification of free fatty acids within adipose tissue for reasons that are not clear.

The flow phase is associated with elevations in metabolic rate and urinary nitrogen excretion caused by muscle protein catabolism. Older hip fracture patients show the expected rise in metabolic rate and nitrogen excretion.[54–56] The patients in these studies accumulated an energy and nitrogen deficit over about a week that was estimated to be preventable in most patients by dietary supplementation of about 300 kcal/day energy and 20 g/day protein. Those patients with a more marked protein deficiency had a reduced probability of survival.[55]

The flow phase also affects carbohydrate and fat metabolism. There is a shift from carbohydrate to fat as the preferred fuel and patients are resistant to the effects of insulin. The magnitude of insulin resistance in the injured elderly is reported to be significantly greater than in the young.[57] The cause of this exaggerated insulin resistance is unknown but it seems highly likely that the high cortisol concentrations are at least partly responsible.

Recovery Following Injury

Recovery following injury has at least three components: (1) resolution of the catabolic flow phase and restoration of the energy and protein deficits, (2) return of function of injured body parts, and (3) the psychosocial adjustment of the injured patient.

The Phase of Anabolism

It is not known whether the catabolic flow phase gives way to the phase of anabolism and recovery occurs simply by the passive termination of the signals that maintain the flow phase or whether it is actively driven by positive signals. Moore,[58] studying recovery from major surgery in younger patients, considered that the anabolic phase could not occur without the resumption of feeding but that this is not the signal that initiates it. He also thought that protein synthesis proceeds at its maximum rate and could not be increased further by endocrine manipulations or forced feeding. Only after the nitrogen debt is repaid and lean body mass is restored is fat deposited. Failure to increase dietary intake results in a failure to gain weight and recovery becomes stalled. Interestingly, even healthy older women fed an energy-replete but marginally protein-deficient diet over 9 weeks developed significant losses of lean body mass, muscle strength, and immune functions.[59]

The studies of Moore have not been confirmed. Indeed, it is surprising how little work has been done in this important area in patients of any age. Humberstone and Shaw[60] studied glucose and protein kinetics in eight patients aged 56 to 79 years following major surgery and showed that these patients were unable completely to oxidize glucose to carbon dioxide and there was increased glucose recycling to lactate. Glucose oxidation was reduced by about 40 percent. Glucose production was increased and this was not suppressed normally by the infusion of glucose. Basal insulin concentrations were elevated with a reduced response to glucose infusion.

The only other aspect of the whole body response to injury studied beyond the flow phase is fatigue.[61] Although there are modest reductions in isokinetic endurance and isometric strength of skeletal muscles during convalescence from moderate surgery, a sensation of fatigue is a very prominent symptom that persists for a month or more, at least in younger patients. Its cause is not known and the phenomenon has not been studied specifically in older trauma patients or patients undergoing elective surgery.

The importance of proper nutrition for older people, the high prevalence of undernutrition in older people in the hospital, and the severe morbidity and mortality associated with undernutrition are all well known, and yet undernutrition continues to be overlooked.[62] Many older people admitted with hip fractures already have evidence of undernutrition at the time of presentation[63,64] and it has been suggested that thinness[47] and weight loss after age 50 years[65] increase fracture risk through poorly understood mechanisms that presumably include a reduced ability to dissipate energy on impact.[28,35]

Surprisingly, it has been reported that one-third of orthopaedic surgeons in the north of England did not feel that malnutrition was an important problem in their patients with hip fractures.[66]

People presenting with hip fractures who are already undernourished fare worse than their well-nourished counterparts[64] and nutritional support improves their condition.[67,68] Bastow et al.[67] used overnight nasogastric feeding and Delmi et al.[68] claim impressive results with oral supplements, although oral supplements in large quantities are not well tolerated by older patients with hip fracture.[69] Although the concept of nutritional support for patients with hip fractures is well established, we do not know how best to tailor it to the needs of individual patients.

Return of Function

Recent studies have shown that only about 40 percent of patients with hip fractures who were ambulant without a walking aid before the injury returned to that state.[70,71] Lamb et al.[72] studied previously healthy patients with hip fractures and showed that extensor muscle power in the fractured leg was the most important determinant of walking speed and stair-climbing time and that the most important determinant of leg extensor power was pain. Other factors are also important. Comorbid conditions including depression and dementia, malnutrition, social supports, and prefracture functional abilities and fitness predict eventual functional recovery.[64,73–81]

Although many of the factors mentioned above are ameliorable, the only intervention that has actually been shown to modify recovery is nutrition. We, and others, are interested in the use of anabolic agents and other pharmacologic interventions, but none has been properly studied in the injured elderly population. Nevertheless, it would seem prudent to optimize management of comorbid conditions and take steps to prevent complications, for example by heparin prophylaxis for venous thromboembolism, perioperative antibiotics and competent fluid resuscitation. Early mobilization is also to be encouraged as immobilization results in further deconditioning,[82] muscle wasting, body fluid shifts, and in increased risk of venous thrombosis and decubitus ulcers. Some orthopaedic surgeons delay weight-bearing after insertion of a rigid fixation device. Such devices maintain good reduction of the fracture but reduce the callus response and slow fracture healing with the attendant risk of fixation failure. However, at least for hip fractures, this may not be a very important consideration. A recent study has shown that early, complete weight-bearing is not associated with a high risk of failure of fixation, nonunion, osteonecrosis, or prosthetic dislocation.[76]

Psychosocial Adjustment

The importance of psychological factors on recovery from illness and surgery has recently been stressed[83] but little is known about this in older people in any clinical setting. Only depression has been addressed in any detail.[75,84,85] It is common, often undiagnosed, and contributes to the syndrome of "failure to thrive."[86] Adequate screening instruments and effective treatments for depression are readily available.

Conclusion

Injuries are common in older people and poorly tolerated. There is evidence that, because of the greater physiologic disturbances induced by the injuries and because older patients (age greater than 50 years) are particularly predisposed to develop multiple organ failure,[87] a lower threshold for invasive monitoring will enhance survival. Indeed, aggressive treatment with early invasive monitoring has already been reported to be beneficial for outcome.[17,87,88] There is also evidence that some aspects of the endocrine-metabolic response may be maladaptive and may be amenable to therapeutic interventions (e.g., by controlled inhibition of glucocorticoid synthesis). Other factors that predispose to suboptimal outcomes are also known and are more readily amenable to modification (e.g., nutritional support, antidepressants, prevention of complications, treatment of comorbid conditions), although the ultimate benefits that might result have only been demonstrated for nutritional interventions. Early mobilization should also be done because the theoretical objections have been shown to be of little importance. However, we do not yet know what constitutes an optimal rehabilitation strategy after hip fracture, let alone after other injuries in the elderly population. Even if we did know what should be done, could we deliver?[89]

References

1. Oreskovich MR, Howard JD, Copass MK, Carrico CJ: Geriatric trauma: injury patterns and outcome. J Trauma 1984;24:565–572
2. Allen JE, Schwab CW: Blunt chest trauma in the elderly. Am Surg 1985;51:697–700
3. Evans JG: Falls and fractures. Age Ageing 1988;17:361–364
4. Osler T, Hales K, Baack B et al: Trauma in the elderly. Am J Surg 1988;156:537–543
5. Champion H, Copes W, Buyer D et al: Major trauma in geriatric patients. Am J Public Health 1989;79:1278–1282
6. Finelli FC, Jonsson J, Champion H et al: A case control study for major trauma in geriatric patients. J Trauma 1989;29:541–548
7. McCoy GF, Johnstone RA: Injury to the elderly in road traffic accidents. J Trauma 1989;29:494–497
8. Sklar DP, Demarest GB, McFeeley P: Increased pedestrian mortality among the elderly. Am J Emerg Med 1989;7:387–390
9. Lonner JH, Koval KJ: Polytrauma in the elderly. Clin Orthop Rel Res 1995;318:136–143
10. Zietlow SD, Capizzi PJ, Bannon MP, Farnell MB: Multisystem geriatric trauma. J Trauma 1994;37:985–988
11. Mosenthal AC, Livingston DH, Elcavage J et al: Falls: epidemiology and strategies for prevention. J Trauma 1995;38:753–756
12. van der Sluis CK, Klasen HJ, Eisma WH, ten Duis HJ: Major trauma in young and old: what is the difference? J Trauma 1996;40:78–82

13. Champion HR, Sacco WJ, Copes WS: Injury severity scoring again. J Trauma 1995;40:78–82
14. Horst HM, Obeid FN, Sorensen UJ, Bivins BA: Factors influencing survival of elderly trauma patients. Crit Care Med 1986; 14:681–684
15. DeMaria EJ, Kenney P, Merrian MA et al: Survival after trauma in geriatric patients. Ann Surg 1987;206:738–743
16. Horan MA, Barton RN, Little RA: Ageing and the response to injury. pp. 101–135. In Evans JG, Caird FI (eds): Advanced Geriatric Medicine 7. Wright, Bristol, 1988
17. Shabot MM, Johnson CL: Outcome from critical care in the "oldest old" trauma patients. J Trauma 1995;39:254–259
18. Knaus WA, Wagner DP, Draper EA et al: The APACHE III prognostic system: risk prediction of hospital mortality for critically ill hospitalized adults. Chest 1991;100:1619–1636
19. Jennett B: Epidemiology of head injury. J Neurol Neurosurg Psychiatr 1996;60:362–369
20. Amacher AL, Bybee DE: Tolerance of head injury by the elderly. Neurosurgery 1987;20:954–958
21. Vollmer DG, Torner JC, Jane JA et al: Age and outcome following traumatic coma: why older patients fare worse. J Neurosurg 1991;75:S37–S49
22. Kulshrestha P, Iyer KS: Chest injuries: a clinical and autopsy profile. J Trauma 1988;28:844–847
23. Shorr RM, Rodriguez A, Indeck MC et al: Blunt chest trauma in the elderly. J Trauma 1989;29:234–237
24. Tubbs N: A comparison of deaths from injury: 1947–56 compared with 1962–71. Injury 1976;7:233–241
25. Lieberman IH, Webb JK: Cervical spine injuries in the elderly. J Bone Joint Surg 1994;76B:877–881
26. Kane RS, Burns EA, Goodwin JS: Minimal trauma fractures in older nursing home residents: the interaction of functional status, trauma, and site of fracture. J Am Geriatr Soc 1995;43: 891–894
27. Hayes WC, Myers ER, Morris JN et al: Impact near the hip dominates fracture risk in elderly nursing home residents who fall. Calcif Tissue Int 1993;52:192–198
28. Cummings SR, Nevitt MC: A hypothesis: the causes of hip fracture. J Gerontol 1989;44:M107–M111
29. Frankel VH, Burstein AH: Orthopaedic Biomechanics. Lea & Febiger, Philadelphia, 1970
30. Muckle DS, Bentley G, Deane G, Kemp FH: Basic science of the hip. pp. 53–58. In Muckle DS (ed): Femoral Neck Fractures and Hip Joint Injuries. Wiley, New York, 1978
31. Robinovitch SN, Hayes WC, McMahon TA: Prediction of femoral impact forces in falls on the hip. J Biomech Eng 1991;113: 366–374
32. Hayes WC, Myers ER: Biomechanics of fractures. pp. 93–114. Riggs BL, Melton L (eds): In Osteoporosis— etiology, Diagnosis and Management. Lippincott-Raven, Philadelphia, 1995
33. Courtney AC, Wachtel EF, Myers ER, Hayes WC: Effects of loading rate on strength of the proximal femur. Calcif Tissue Int 1994;55:53–58
34. Nevitt MC, Cummings SR: Type of fall and risk of hip and wrist fractures: the study of osteoporotic fractures. J Am Geriatr Soc 1993;41:1226–1234
35. Greenspan SL, Myers ER, Maitland LA et al: Fall severity and bone mineral density as risk factors for hip fracture in ambulatory elderly. JAMA 1994;324:1326–1331
36. Martin RE, Teberian G: Multiple trauma and the elderly patient. Emerg Med Clin North Am 1990;8:411–420
37. Riska EB, Myllynen P: Fat embolism in patients with multiple injuries. J Trauma 1982;22:891–894
38. Rogers FB, Shackford SR, Keller MS: Early fixation reduces morbidity and mortality in elderly patients with hip fractures from low-impact falls. J Trauma 1995;39:261–265
39. Zuckerman JD, Skovron ML, Koval KJ et al: Postoperative complications and mortality associated with operative delay in older patients who have a fracture of the hip. J Bone Joint Surg 1995; 77A:1551–1556
40. Cuthbertson DP: Observations on disturbance of metabolism produced by injury to the limbs. Q J Med 1932;25:233–246
41. Frayn KN, Stoner HB, Barton RN, Heath DF: Persistence of high plasma glucose, insulin and cortisol concentrations in elderly patients with proximal femoral fractures. Age Ageing 1983;12:70–76
42. Roberts NA, Barton RN, Horan MA, White A: Adrenal function after upper femoral fracture in elderly people: persistence of stimulation and the roles of adrenocorticotrophic hormone and immobility. Age Ageing 1990;12:70–76
43. Barton RN, Weijers JWM, Horan MA: Increased rates of cortisol production and urinary free cortisol excretion in elderly women 2 weeks after proximal femur fracture. Eur J Clin Invest 1993; 23:171–176
44. Seeman TE, Robbins RJ: Aging and hypothalamic-pituitary-adrenal response to challenge in humans. Endocr Rev 1994; 15:233–259
45. Doncaster HD, Barton RN, Horan MA, Roberts NA: Factors influencing cortisol-adrenocorticotrophin relationships in elderly women with upper femur fractures. J Trauma 1993;34: 49–55
46. Barker DJP: Mothers, Babies and Disease in Later Life BMJ Publishing Group, London, 1994
47. Levitt NS, Lindsey RS, Holmes MC, Seckl JR: Dexamethasone in the last week of pregnancy attenuates hippocampal glucocorticoid receptor gene expression and elevates blood pressure in the adult offspring in the rat. Neuroendocrinology 1996;64: 412–418
48. Drucker WR, Chadwick CD, Gann DS: Transcapillary refill in haemorrhage and shock. Arch Surg 1981;116:1344–1353
49. Linder J, Nolgård P, Näsman B et al: Decreased peripheral glucocorticoid sensitivity in Alzheimer's disease. Gerontology 1993;39:200–206
50. Brönegård M, Stierna P, Marcus C: Glucocorticoid resistant syndromes—molecular basis and clinical presentations. J Neuroendocrinol 1996;8:405–415
51. Sternberg EM, Chroussos GP, Wilder RL, Gold PW: The stress response and the regulation of inflammatory disease. Ann Intern Med 1992;117:854–866
52. Hall-Angerås M, Angerås U, Zamir O et al: Effect of the glucocorticoid receptor antagonist RU38486 on muscle protein breakdown in sepsis. Surgery 1991;109:468–473
53. Cech AC, Shore J, Gallagher H, Daly JM: Glucocorticoid receptor blockade reverses post-injury macrophage suppression. Arch Surg 1994;129:1227–1232

54. Jallut D, Tappy L, Kohut M et al: Energy balance in elderly patients after surgery for a femoral neck fracture. JPEN 1990; 14:563–568
55. Patterson BM, Cornell CN, Carbone B et al: Protein depletion and metabolic stress in elderly patients who have a fracture of the hip. J Bone Joint Surg 1992;74A:251–260
56. Nelson KM, Richards EW, Long CL et al: Protein and energy balance following femoral neck fracture in geriatric patients. Metabolism 1995;44:59–66
57. Watters JM, Moulton SB, Clancey SM et al: Aging exaggerates glucose intolerance following injury. J Trauma 1994;37: 786–791
58. Moore FD: Bodily changes in surgical convalescence 1. The normal sequence: observations and interpretations. Ann Surg 1953;137:289–315
59. Castaneda C, Charnley JM, Evans WJ, Crim ML: Elderly women accomodate to a low-protein diet with losses of body cell mass, muscle function, and immune response. Am J Clin Nutr 1995; 62:30–39
60. Humberstone DA, Shaw JH: Isotopic studies during surgical convalescence. Br J Surg 1989;76:154–158
61. Christiansen T, Kehlet H: Postoperative fatigue. World J Surg 1993;17:220–225
62. Cedersholm T, Jägrén C, Hellström K: Outcome of protein-energy malnutrition in elderly medical patients. Am J Med 1995;98:67–74
63. Older MWJ, Delyth E, Dickenson JWT: A nutrient survey in elderly women with femoral neck fracture. Br J Surg 1980;67: 884–886
64. Bastow MD, Rawlings J, Allison SP: Undernutrition, hypothermia and injury in elderly women with fractured femur: an injury response to altered metabolism? Lancet 1983;1:143–145
65. Langlois JA, Harris T, Looker AC, Madans J: Weight change between age 50 years and old age is associated with risk of hip fracture in white women aged 67 years and older. Arch Intern Med 1996;156:989–994
66. Hussein A, Barer D: Nutritional assessment in patients admitted with proximal femoral fractures. Gerontology 1994;40:289
67. Bastow MD, Rawlings J, Allison SP: Benefits of supplementary tube feeding after fractured neck of femur: a randomised controlled trial. BMJ 1983;287:1589–1592
68. Delmi M, Rapin C-H, Bengoa J-M et al: Dietary supplementation in elderly patients with fractured neck of the femur. Lancet 1990;335:1013–1016
69. Stableforth PG: Supplementary feeds and nitrogen and calorie balance following femoral neck fracture. Br J Surg 1986;73: 651–655
70. Keene GS, Parker MJ, Pryor GA: Mortality and morbidity after hip fractures. BMJ 1993;307:1248–1251
71. Marottoli RA, Berkman LF, Cooney LM: Decline in physical function following hip fracture. J Am Geriatr Soc 1992;40: 861–866
72. Lamb SE, Morse RE, Evans JG: Mobility after proximal femoral fracture: the relevance of leg extensor power, postural sway and other factors. Age Ageing 1995;24:308–314
73. Ions GK, Stevens J: Prediction of survival in patients with femoral neck fractures. J Bone Joint Surg 1987;69B:384–387
74. Jette AM, Harris A, Cleary PD, Campion EW: Functional recovery after hip fracture. Arch Phys Med Rehabil 1987;68: 735–740
75. Mossey JM, Mutran E, Knott K, Craik R: Determinants of recovery 12 months after hip fracture: the importance of psychosocial factors. Am J Public Health 1989;79:279–286
76. Koval KJ, Skovron ML, Polatsch D et al: Dependency after hip fracture in geriatric patients: a study of predictive factors. J Orthop Trauma 1996;8:531–535
77. Mossey JM, Knott K, Craik R: The effects of persistent depressive symptoms on hip fracture recovery. J Gerontol 1990;45: M163–M168
78. Bernardini B, Meinecke C, Pagani M et al: Comorbidity and adverse clinical events in the rehabilitation of older adults after hip fracture. J Am Geriatr Soc 1995;41:894–898
79. Svensson O, Strömberg L, Öhlén G, Lindgren U: Prediction of the outcome after hip fracture in elderly patients. J Bone Joint Surg 1996;78B:115–118
80. Myers AH, Palmer MH, Engel BT et al: Mobility in older patients with hip fractures: examining prefracture status, complications, and outcomes from the acute-care hospital. J Orthop Trauma 1996;10:99–107
81. Ponzer S, Bergman B, Brismar B, Johansson LM: A study of patient-related characteristics and outcome after moderate injury. Injury 1996;27:549–555
82. Shahar A, Powers KA, Black JS: The risk of postoperative deconditioning in older adults. J Am Geriatr Soc 1996;44:471
83. Johnston M: Psychological factors in recovery from illness and from surgery. Proc R Coll Physicians Edinb 1996;26:451–460
84. Billig N, Ahmed SW, Kenmore P et al: Assessment of depression and cognitive impairment after hip fracture. J Am Geriatr Soc 1986;34:499–503
85. Fox KM, Hawkes WG, Magaziner J et al: Markers of failure to thrive among older hip fracture patients. J Am Geriatr Soc 1996; 44:371–376
86. Sarkisian CA, Lachs MS: "Failure to thrive" in older adults. Ann Intern Med 1996;124:1072–1078
87. DeMaria EJ, Kenney PR, Merrian MA et al: Aggressive trauma care benefits the elderly. J Trauma 1987;27:1200–1205
88. Scalea TM, Simm HM, Duncan AO: Geriatric blunt trauma: improved survival with early invasive monitoring. J Trauma 1990;30:29–34
89. Hanspal R, Wright M, Proctor D et al: Failure to deliver the formal therapy prescribed in an NHS rehabilitation unit. Clin Rehab 1994;8:161–165

CHAPTER 87

Podiatry

KATHERINE WARD

MARK KOSINSKI

As the next century brings a population explosion of older people, particular attention must be paid to the multiple and complex disorders that impair functional independence and compromise quality of life. One of the most important and sometimes overlooked topics is that of proper foot care and function. It has been estimated that 70 percent of the population over 65 years of age suffers from a foot problem.[1] Foot pain can easily jeopardize an individual's ability to perform many of the important instrumental activities of daily living including cooking, shopping, housekeeping, doing laundry, and using transportation.

Foot pain in the elderly may be caused by changes in gait, past foot care and management, hereditary problems, previous foot conditions that were not treated, changes in mental status, nutritional abnormalities, systemic and local disease, hospitalization and confinement to bed, and various medications. These factors are further compounded by the elderly person's increased susceptibility to infection, diabetes mellitus, other types of neurovascular impairment, and atrophy associated with degeneration of neuromuscular and musculoskeletal diseases.

This myriad of changes associated with aging results in a diminished homeostatic reserve, commonly manifested with loss of ambulation. The loss of ambulatory ability can be devastating to an older person. The change magnifies dependence on others, as well as increasing the risk of falls. For those without a family or social support network, loss of ambulation usually precedes admission into an institutionalized facility.

Proper foot care must be provided for elderly patients in an attempt to promote pain-free ambulation. The dire consequences of immobility in this age group certainly underscores this point. Podiatric problems are often preventable or readily treatable. Physical examination of the feet (combined with a comprehensive physical examination) is an important part of the geriatric assessment. The interdisciplinary team approach certainly benefits the older person with interrelated problems. Foot care is often complicated by cognitive, visual, and sensory impairment that requires contributions from a host of specialists. In this chapter, the diagnosis, treatment, and prevention of common pedal problems are discussed in an effort to promote health maintenance in the older population.

Orthopaedic/ Biomechanical Disorders

The foot and ankle may demonstrate the ravage of time like no other bones or muscles of the musculoskeletal system.[2] Lower extremity joint impairment and painful foot disorders also represent major causes of treatable gait disturbances. Heel pain is a common complaint of older individuals. Recent weight gain, increased walking or standing activities, hard floors or surfaces, and biomechanical abnormalities are the factors that predispose to the development of plantar calcaneal pain. Plantar calcaneal spurs (diagnosed by a lateral radiograph of the foot) are often aggravated by an atrophied fat pad. Conservative treatment includes rest, nonsteroidal anti-inflammatory drugs (NSAIDs), and accommodative shoes, such as a sneaker or running shoe, with a thick shock-absorbing insole. Viscoelastic heel cushions or heel cups (available commercially) can be inserted into existing shoes to provide additional cushioning. Prescription custom-made orthoses may be indicated to support the arch and to reduce traction of the plantar fascia from its origin on the calcaneus. To prevent recurrence, shoe modifications should be worn indefinitely. Another important treatment is stretching of the Achilles tendon and plantar fascia of the affected foot. Recalcitrant cases may require a series of local injections (local anesthetic combined with a corticosteroid) into the area of maximum tenderness (usually the anteromedial tubercle of the calcaneus). If not diagnosed and treated in a timely fashion, acute plantar heel pain can become a chronic condition, especially in patients who are overweight or have bilateral symptoms.[3]

When appropriate therapy fails to achieve expected results, one must consider systemic disease as a possible etiology of heel pain. Although the majority of heel pain is of biomechanical etiology, diseases such as rheumatoid arthritis, ankylosing spondylitis, psoriatic arthritis, and Reiter syndrome can also cause heel pain.

The joints of the feet such as first metatarsophalangeal joint, ankle, and midtarsal joints are also prone to osteoarthritis. Diagnosed by limited and painful range of motion as well as narrowed joint space on radiographs, this condition usually responds well to conservative measures. Shoe modifications such as balanced inlay orthoses and a forefoot rocker sole angled to follow the progression of gait provide good local treatment. Topical medications such as capsaicin (Zostrix) have been shown to relieve pain caused by degenerative joint disease, whereas systemic medications such as NSAIDs are also indicated.

Joint pains from bunions, hallux valgus, hammer toes, and mallet toes are also common lower extremity problems in elderly people. If the above-mentioned conservative measures fail to alleviate the pain, surgical correction may be considered. Foot surgery can provide improvement of function and quality of life, even in the presence of chronic illnesses. Of course, a prudent comprehensive surgical work-up in conjunction with the primary care physician, as well as an anesthesiologist, would be obligatory.

Because studies suggest an increased morbidity and mortality in patients over age 70 years related to elective surgeries,[2] the decision to perform a procedure should not be taken lightly. Preoperative concerns include diminished cardiac and pulmonary reserve, and coexisting chronic illnesses; postoperative concerns include altered response to infection, postoperative confusion, constipation, and urinary incontinence.

Gait disturbances are a common sequela of age-related changes in the central and peripheral nervous systems. Senile ataxia is a gait pattern characterized by a flexed posture with wide-based gait in men, and a waddling, narrow-based gait in women.[4] This is seen in neurologically healthy individuals and has no known etiology.

Features of pathologically induced gait disturbances are frequently nonspecific and overlap with those of senile ataxia, giving little clue as to the primary pathology. In Parkinson's disease and cerebellar atrophy, gait characteristics are specifically helpful in establishing the diagnosis. Shuffling and abducted gaits also produce increased stress and pressure on the soft tissues leading to dermal lesions (see dermatology section below).

It is important to search for an underlying etiology in the physical assessment, as approximately 25 percent of geriatric gait disturbances do have a treatable cause.[5] Frequently there is an underlying neurologic, endocrine, musculoskeletal, or psychological disorder. Other contributing factors include cardiovascular disease and impairment of equilibrium.

A complete evaluation, including a fall history and gait analysis, may provide some information regarding the extent and location of the underlying pathology. Demonstration of poor gait, difficulty with chair transfer, and a loss of balance when standing on tip-toe suggests an underlying neurologic or musculoskeletal disorder.[6]

Serum studies may reveal vitamin B_{12} deficiency, hypothyroidism, osteomalacia, or drug toxicity. Radiographic studies assist in excluding bone disease. Remember that stress fractures may not be evident at the time of injury. If signs and symptoms are consistent with fracture, treat as such and repeat the radiograph in 10 to 14 days. Computed tomography, magnetic resonance imaging, myelography, and electrophysiologic studies may offer a definitive diagnosis in cases of primary central nervous system pathology. Common etiologies of gait disorders include neurologic (cerebrovascular accident, dementia, Parkinson's disease, etc.), musculoskeletal (arthritis, osteoporosis, myopathy, etc.), endocrine (hypothyroidism, diabetes), psychological (depression, fear of falling), as well as medications.

Dermatologic Disorders

Hyperkeratotic lesions (corns and calluses and other keratotic lesions) are the most common podiatric complaints of the elderly. They frequently arise in areas of increased pressure or friction and over bony prominences. Although these conditions are common among all age groups, degenerative joint disease, atrophy of the plantar fat pad, and decreased pain threshold predispose the elderly to increased frequency of complaints. Depending on their depth and severity, there may be an associated adventitious bursa formation. Treatment consists of aseptic debridement and weight or pressure dispersion. Lesions on the plantar aspect of the foot should also be treated with a shock-absorbing insert to disperse the weight-bearing forces and implement an atrophic or displaced plantar fat pad. Injection of a small amount of soluble corticosteroid (e.g., dexamethasone sodium phosphate, 1 to 2 mg) may provide relief from the painful inflammation associated with an adventitial bursa.

It is especially important to debride chronic hyperkeratotic lesions in patients with vascular or neurologic impairment, as deep-seated lesions may give rise to soft tissue breakdown, ulcerations, and bone infection.

As noted earlier in this chapter, sneakers or running shoes are ideal footgear for biomechanical as well as dermatologic problems. A wide toe box is important for preventing pressure on the digits, and abundant cushioning on the sole of the foot is required to mitigate the excessive plantar pressures that cause the hyperkeratotic lesions.

Well-cushioned shoegear is often required to mitigate the consequences of atrophied subcalcaneal or submetatarsal fat pads. When the natural fat found on the plantar aspect of the feet atrophies, the underlying bony structures become more prominent and cause pain. When such pain occurs under the plantar aspect of the metatarsal head, it is called metatarsalgia. The complaint is frequently a callus or inflammation of the area (bursitis). Diagnosis can be made by clinical examination, and radiographs may reveal underlying bone pathology. Treatment consists of debridement of hyperkeratotic lesions with padding to disperse the weight. Long-term treatment includes the use of soft tissue supplements such as plastizote, which can be added to foot orthotics or inserted directly into the shoe.

Expensive custom-molded shoes are often unnecessary for all but the most severe foot deformities. If they are indeed indicated, they should include a high, wide toe box, a bunion last, and an extra depth feature to accommodate weight-dispersive orthoses. Surgical correction should always be considered as the last resort, after all conservative measures have failed. As mentioned previously, surgery must be weighed against the potential local risks (infection, prolonged swelling and pain, etc.) as well as its impact on the overall health of the patient.

Maceration and fissuring of the interspaces is another common dermatologic finding in the elderly population. Vision and dexterity loss make it difficult to examine and care for the feet, and digital deformities precipitate moisture accumulation between the toes. The dark and moist environment between the toes predisposes the area to fungal and bacterial infection. A Wood's light can be used to detect coral red fluorescence suggestive of *Corynebacterium minutissimum*, which is usually treated with topical erythromycin. A negative Wood's light is implicative of a fungal or yeast infection that can be treated with clotrimazole solution (Lotrimin, Mycelex) applied interdigitally twice daily for 2 to 4 weeks. Of course, meticulous cleaning and drying of the area while bathing is also necessary. In more severe cases, wet-to-dry gauntlet dressings using Burow's solution may be used. However, if lamb's wool or gauze is used to separate the toes, never encircle a digit. Such dressings may become constrictive and severely compromise the circulation.

In contrast, there is also a decrease in skin hydration as aging progresses. Combined with diminished sebaceous and eccrine activity, dry and scaly skin often results. Bathing followed by the use of a topical emollient can retard water loss, relieving pruritus and preventing fissuring that can lead to infection. If infection does develop, elderly people are less able to fight it.

Ulcerations of the leg, feet, and toes are also seen frequently in the geriatric population. The differential diagnosis of pedal ulcers includes arteriosclerosis obliterans, neurotrophic, chronic pernio, gout, mycobacterium tuberculosis, Raynaud's disease/phenomenon, scleroderma, and neoplasms, in addition to those caused by biomechanic, iatrogenic, or patient-induced diseases.[7]

Ischemic ulcers typically occur on the distal and dorsal digits, as well as the dorsal foot and lateral malleolar area. Symptoms include severe pain, worse at night and relieved by dependency. They are characterized by trophic skin changes, poor granulation tissue, poor color of tissue (cyanotic, gray, or black), and poor bleeding upon stimulation.

Neurotrophic ulcers commonly occur beneath pressure points or hyperkeratotic lesions (submetatarsal heads 1,5, lateral fifth metatarsal base, and dorsomedial navicular). There is usually no pain, as the patient is typically neuropathic. The ulcers are characterized by punched-out lesions with a red base and white rim, with excellent bleeding. Due to the high incidence of diabetic ulcers and their coexisting morbidity, this topic will be discussed thoroughly in a separate section within this chapter.

Decubitus ulceration is another common problem, clearly related to chronic skin changes in the elderly. It is often the result of chronic stasis dermatitis, secondary to altered venous circulation in the leg. The skin (typically around the medial malleolus) becomes pigmented as fragile venules leak hemosiderin. Edema and fibrosis contribute to damage of the local tissue. Poor circulation is an added risk factor that will impair healing and increase the chance of infection.

Treatment of these ulcers must address their etiology, and therefore requires a multidisciplinary approach. Edema can be reduced with elevation of the foot (above heart level), as well as with compressive boots and stockings. Individuals with a history of venous stasis ulcers shuld wear elastic supports daily. Wound care must be performed regularly to ensure a clean, moist granular bed of the ulcer. Aerobic and anaerobic cultures must be performed if infection is suspected, followed by the appropriate antibiotic coverage.

Lower extremity edema may also lead to discomfort in shoegear and alteration in gait patterns and mobility. Addressing the etiology of the pedal edema (whether it be cardiac, renal, hepatic, or vascular) in conjunction with elevation and support hose, should help to relieve symptoms.

It is important to keep in mind that a chronic ulceration, especially if it is not responding to appropriate therapy, has the potential for malignant degeneration. This is especially true for the common venous stasis ulcer. Any suspicious ulcer should be biopsied to include the most ominous border, along with normal skin for comparison. It is recommended to biopsy of the leading edge of ulcers, as the ulcer base is typically just granulation tissue. Multiple biopsies are certainly acceptable should there be several suspicious areas.

Nail Disorders

Toenail problems are also a common complaint within the geriatric population. Hypertrophy (thickening and hardening of the toenails) frequently occurs in patients with systemic disease, impaired vision, obesity, inability to bend, and/or loss of manual dexterity. This condition is caused primarily by onychomycosis impaired circulation, or repeated microtrauma over time. Mycotic nail infections respond poorly to topical therapy. The recent advent of safer oral agents such as Sporanox (itraconazole, Janssen Pharmaceutica) may help to achieve a cure in some patients. It was recently approved by the Food and Drug Administration for treatment of onychomycosis and is effective against dermatophytes, yeasts, and molds. However, older patients usually do best with serial nail debridement, which not only maintains comfort but decreases the chance of soft tissue infection, infected ingrown toenails, and subungual corns or ulceration.

It is important to differentiate mycotic nail infections from nail dystrophies secondary to systemic disease, vascular insufficiency, and trauma. For example, poor nutritional status can lead to toenails that are atrophic, thin, brittle, and lackluster, with possible longitudinal ridges. Other systemic diseases associated with common nail dystrophies include diabetes mellitus, syphilis, psoriasis, Reiter syndrome, ischemia, gout, rheumatoid arthritis, and systemic lupus erythematosus.

Although patients invariably attribute periungual pain as being secondary to an ingrown or incurvated nail, it is important to rule out ischemia as the etiology of the nail pain. Ischemic changes of the digit can often mimic nail pain and mislead both patient and physician.

Infected paronychias often exhibit adjacent chronic granulation tissue. It is incumbent that the physician biopsy all such lesions. We are too familiar with patients in whom Kaposi's sarcoma, amelanotic melanoma, and squamous cell carcinoma of the nail groove have given the appearance of a pyogenic granuloma.

Subungual hematomas are not uncommon in older individuals, usually from microtrauma secondary to shoegear. However, it is prudent to consider any subungual hyperpigmented lesion a melanoma until proven otherwise. To rule out melanoma, debride the nail plate as proximal as possible. Many times part of the nail can be removed easily to reveal subungual debris consistent with previous hemorrhage or fungal infection. If this is not the case, however, suspicious hyperpigmented lesions of the nail bed must be biopsied.

Foot Problems in Patients With Diabetes

Neuropathy, peripheral vascular disease, and immunopathy all play a role in the development of foot pathology in patients with diabetes. These three factors, combined with the reduced vision and mobility that impair the ability of older patients to inspect and care for their feet, can have disastrous consequences. When left unrecognized and therefore untreated, many minor foot problems (such as corns and calluses) progress to ulcerations and infections, producing the well-known morbidity associated with diabetes. Risk factors for diabetic foot ulcers include sensorimotor and autonomic neuropathy, peripheral vascular disease, limited joint mobility, high plantar pressures, bony deformities, history of previous ulceration, and visual or functional impairment.

Chronic sensory neuropathy is one of the most common long-term complications of diabetes mellitus. Symptoms frequently include numbness, dysesthesia, lancinating pain, burning, and hypersensitivity. Sensory loss is typically in a stocking-glove distribution and is often of insidious onset. In its early stages, patients may be unaware that a decrease in sensorium even exists. In those patients without diabetes, pedal neuropathy may be secondary to alcoholism, a herniated nucleus pulposus, heavy metals, vitamin deficiencies, and collagen diseases, among other systemic conditions.

Sensory neuropathy is often accompanied by a motor component. In the foot of a patient with diabetes, loss of motor fibers may lead to intrinsic muscle atrophy and imbalance between flexor and extensor muscles. Clawing of the toes, prominent metatarsal heads, and anterior displacement of an already atrophied plantar fat pad may increase the patient's risk for pressure-induced lesions.[8,9] Glycation of collagen leads to thickening and increased cross-linking of collagen bundles, resulting in thin, tight, and waxy skin and further restriction of joint movement.[10] Dry and atrophic skin is also caused by the autonomic neuropathy, which leads to denervation of the sweat glands. Cracks and fissures violate the skin defenses, leaving the patient vulnerable to bacterial infection.

Ulcerations may be caused by an acute event or repetitive minor trauma. It has been shown that constant pressure of 5 to 7 pounds per square inch over a bony prominence can cause ischemic necrosis in less than 7 hours.[11] If an ulcer is indeed caused by pressure or a biomechanical problem, it will never resolve if weight is not dispersed from the affected area, regardless of how much debridement of local wound care is given.

Peripheral vascular disease is 20 times more common in patients with diabetes than in nondiabetic individuals.[12] Micro- and macrovascular disease puts the patient at risk for gangrene and ulceration by reducing the perfusion pressure where tissue ischemia occurs. Diabetic occlusive disease has a predilection for the tibial and peroneal arteries, and tends to be bilateral and multisegmental.

Medial arterial calcification is a common finding in patients with diabetes and can be recognized on radiographs by its pipe-stem appearance. When present, it can alter the pulse wave form and falsely elevate ankle pressure. Ankle/brachial index and pulse volume recordings may therefore be of questionable value in assessing peripheral circulation in patients with diabetes, but they are useful if they are low.[10] In general, be suspicious if the ankle/brachial index is greater than 1.0. A reading of less than 0.5 indicates serious arterial compromise and poor healing potential.

The best treatment for the foot of a patient with diabetes is patient education and thorough, frequent foot examinations. The foot examination should be a regular part of each office visit. Both shoes and socks should be removed and the feet should be checked for trophic and pretrophic skin changes, thickened or incurvated nails, and hyperkeratosis. Hemorrhage within a callus may be suggestive of ulcer formation. The interspaces should be carefully inspected for maceration or fissuring.

The neurologic examination should include evaluation of deep tendon reflexes, sharp/dull discrimination, light touch, proprioception, and vibratory sensation using a 128-Hz tuning fork. Vibratory sensation and proprioception, both carried by the posterior columns, are the first to be affected by diabetic neuropathy. Keep in mind that decreased vibratory sensation may also occur as part of normal aging. Diminished or absent knee and ankle jerk reflexes are also common with aging, and in the absence of other pathology do not require further evaluation. Autonomic neuropathy can be recognized clinically by the absence of sweating, a relatively fixed heart rate, and postural hypotension.

A palpable popliteal pulse may be an unreliable indicator of circulation in the lower extremity, as 40 percent of patients with diabetes presenting with distal gangrene have a popliteal pulse.[13] Similarly, a palpable dorsalis pedis or posterior tibial pulse is an unreliable indication of circulation in the toes. Twenty percent of patients with diabetes with palpable pedal pulses have significant small vessel disease. Temperature gradient, capillary filling time, rubor on dependency, and pallor on elevation are useful adjunctive tests for assessing distal lower extremity circulation.

When evidence points to arterial insufficiency, a vascular referral is indicated with possible arterial reconstruction when appropriate. Unfortunately, due to the characteristics of diabetic angiopathy, surgery may not always be feasible.

The pain of diabetic neuropathy is another common complaint of patients with diabetes. It is difficult to control, especially in patients with poor glucose control. Topical capsaicin (Zostrix) applied 2 or 3 times a day may provide some relief. Tricyclic antidepressants may also prove advantageous.

It is important to counsel patients with diabetes regarding their shoegear. Those with neuropathy should wear shoes with laces or straps. Laced shoes are also preferred to loafers because they allow for swelling. "Slip-on" shoes cannot grip the midfoot and do not prevent forward migration of the foot during ambulation. Patients with neuropathy often purchase shoes that are too tight or pull their laces too tight because they cannot feel the reassuring snugness of a proper fit. Sneakers or running shoes provide a soft, wide toe box and sufficient plantar soft tissue supplementation. Patients with diabetes should always allow a slow break-in period for new shoes, with periodic self-inspection for any signs of irritation or blistering.

In addition to the proper shoegear, socks should be made of cotton or wool, rather than synthetic fibers. The use of mended stockings or stockings with seams should be discouraged. Patients with diabetes should not walk barefooted. Sandals, especially those with thongs between the toes, are to be avoided. Lotions containing ammonium lactate are useful in treating xerotic skin and preventing heel fissures. Conversely, web spaces should be kept dry.

Patients play an important role in preventing their foot problems. The following recommendations should be made at each office visit: stop smoking, inspect feet daily for cuts and blisters, inspect the inside and outside of shoes for foreign objects, do not walk barefooted, cut toenails straight across, avoid temperature extremes on the feet, and notify a physician of any problems immediately.

Ulcer Management

Despite our best efforts at preventing skin breakdown, ulcerations frequently occur. The mainstays of ulcer management are weight dispersion, debridement of devitalized tissue, and use of antibiotics when appropriate. Dressings should conform to the cavity left by an ulcer, and every effort should be made to maintain a moist wound environment that encourages growth of granulation tissue. Treatment of deep ulcers with osseous involvement may require surgical intervention. If bone is exposed in an ulceration, it is considered to be infected. Nutritional and glycemic control should be optimized during ulcer therapy, because low albumin and hyperglycemia may impair wound healing.

Ulcer treatment also requires the use of specialized shoegear to limit the propulsive period of gait as well as to decrease the pressure and friction of regular shoes. Recce-type surgical shoes are very useful in this regard. Their open-toe design accomodates digital lesions, and they can be modified with weight-dispersive materials for treating plantar lesions. There are also several commercially available enclosed convalescent shoes that provide a wide, high toe box and an extra-depth sole. A removable plastizote insole is usually provided on which weight-dispersive modifications can be made.

Management of diabetic infections may prove challenging, as they are often deep ulcers with polymicrobial growth. Correct culturing technique is imperative for obtaining accurate results. Prior to the culturing, a vigorous saline scrub of the ulcer surface, followed by deep curettage of the ulcer base is recommended. When culturing wounds, similarly prepare the site by cleansing the wound surface and surrounding skin with an antibacterial solution, followed by a sterile saline rinse. Be sure to take a deep culture. Pus contains phagocytized bacteria and therefore does not represent the best culture material. Use a sterile instrument to gently probe wounds and ulcers for sinus tracts. Be sure the culturette is capable of supporting both aerobic and anaerobic bacteria, and transport the specimen rapidly to the lab. Serial radiographs are recommended for deep ulcers to rule out osteomyelitis.

Diabetic infections are polymicrobial, with *Bacteroides fragilis* being one of the most common anaerobic isolates. Empiric antibiotic therapy for mild diabetic foot infections may include amoxicillin/clavulanate, cephalexin, or clindamycin. Moderate to severe infections mandate treatment with ciprofloxacin plus clindamycin, ticarcillin/clavulanate, mefoxin, or unasyn. The patient's renal status and general health must be considered prior to prescribing any of these medications. Consultation with an infectious disease specialist may also be necessary.

It must not be assumed that all chronic ulcers are infected: Positive cultures may reflect bacterial colonization, rather than actual infection. Clean, granulating ulcers that do not appear clinically infected do not need to be cultured. Antibiotic therapy is necessary only when skin and bone infection exist. Clean wounds may be treated with local wound care and weight dispersion alone.

It is also important to never become complacent when dealing with a wound in a patient with diabetes, even when response to treatment appears to be adequate. Consider hospitalization if any of the following are present: fever with ascending cellulitis, lymphangitis or lymphadenopathy, nonpalpable pedal pulses, need for surgical intervention (revascularization, amputation, or radical debridement), deep plantar space infection, malodorous drainage suggestive of an anaerobic infection, medical conditions requiring stabilization, failure to improve within 48 to 72 hours of outpatient therapy, and noncompliance with outpatient treatment. A team approach that includes the primary care physician, vascular surgeon, and podiatrist is often the most rational course for managing patients who require hospitalization.

Summary

The podiatrist can be a valuable team member in the multidisciplinary approach of geriatric assessment: Physical examination and functional health are addressed to promote quality of life. The physical, pharmacologic, and physiologic changes that accompany aging can result in an increased risk of loss of life or limb after podiatric problems develop in elderly patients. It is therefore necessary to prevent and treat the pedal manifestations of vascular, neurologic, musculoskeletal, and metabolic disorders in order to improve quality of life and ambulatory ability, while reducing pain and foot morbidity.

References

1. DellaCorte MP, Tsouris J, Buffone WF: Geriatrics. p. 73. In Birrer RB, DellaCorte MP, Grisafi PJ (eds): Common Foot Problems in Primary Care. Hanley & Belfus, Philadelphia, 1992

2. Luxenberg J: Geriatrics. pp. 534, 540. In Zier BG (ed): Essentials of Internal Medicine in Clinical Podiatry. WB Saunders, Philadelphia, 1990
3. Wolgin M, Cook C, Graham C, Mauldin D: Conservative treatment of plantar heel pain: long-term follow up. Foot Ankle 1995; 15:97–102
4. Rubine FA: Gait disorders in the elderly. Postgrad Med 1993; 94:185–190
5. Sudarsky L, Ronthal M: Gait disorders among elderly patients: a survey of 50 patients. Arch Neurol 1983;40:740–743
6. Tideiksaar R: Geriatric falls: assessing the cause, preventing recurrence. Geriatrics 1989;44:57–64
7. Kosinski M, Ramcharitar S: In-office management of common geriatric foot problems. Geriatrics 1994;49:43–47
8. Cavanaugh PR, Derr JA, Ulbrecht JS et al: Correlates of structure and function in the diabetic foot. Diabetologia 1991; 34(suppl 2):A39
9. Boulton AM: The diabetic foot. Med Clin North Am 1988;72: 1513–1530
10. Goodfield MJB, Millard LG: The skin in diabetes mellitus. Diabetologia 1988; 31:567–575
11. Sage R: Diabetic ulcers: evaluation and management. Clin Podiatr Med Surg 1987; 4:383–393
12. Gibbons GW, Freeman D: Vascular evaluation and treatment of the diabetic. Clin Podiatr Med Surg 1987;4:377–381
13. Bulat T, Kosinski M: Diabetic foot: strategies to prevent and treat common problems. Geriatrics 1995;50:46–55

CHAPTER 88

Aging and the Blood

MARIA H. GILLEECE
T. MICHAEL DEXTER

Peripheral blood cells play vital roles in an array of diverse function—they ensure tissue oxygenation, participate in tissue repair and hemostasis, and are major components of the immune response. The required heterogeneity of cell type and function is generated by the proliferation and differentiation of a small pool of multipotential hemopoietic stem cells. These cells initially seed the yolk sac during embryonic development, then the liver and spleen, and finally the bone marrow which is the main source of circulating blood cells by the time of birth. In the case of T lymphocytes, pre-T cells emanate from the bone marrow and pass through the thymus where they undergo further development before reaching maturity and then, like B lymphocytes, disseminate throughout the blood and lymphoid tissue.

Peripheral Blood

Early studies on red cell indexes in aging populations suggested that a fall in hemoglobin and a decrease in red cell mass were age-related changes,[1–4] and it was hypothesized that they might be secondary to the reduced oxygen demand associated with a sedentary lifestyle.[5] The confounding effects of intercurrent illness on red cell parameters were not fully appreciated until 1984 when agreement was reached regarding a definition of the healthy elderly population provided by the Senieur guidelines.[6] Even these suggested the use of a hemoglobin range lower than that applied to the rest of the adult population, based on an earlier study by Landahl et al.[7] Recent studies using the clinical recommendations of the Senieur protocol indicate that red cell indexes are well preserved even in centenarians.[8,9] However, peripheral blood lymphocyte populations do seem to show a significant change in age, with a fall in total numbers. $CD4^+$ T-helper cells, responsible for major histocompatibility complex class II restricted recognition of foreign antigen and subsequent activation of CD8+ T-suppressor, B-lymphocyte, and granulocyte effector cells of the immune response, show an overall decline with age[10,11] accompanied by a reduction in capacity to produce virgin $CD4^+CD45RA$ T cells.[12] The latter changes may be a consequence of stem cell exhaustion (considered unlikely in view of the apparently normal myelopoiesis occurring in these patients) or a defect in the ability of the stem cells to undergo differentiation to produce pre-T cells or the absence of a thymus or thymus-like microenvironment. Sansoni et al.[9] made a careful study of lymphocyte subsets and natural killer (NK) activity in the healthy elderly and showed that while the number of $CD4^+$ and $CD8^+$ T cells fell with age, there was a rise in the number of activated T cells of CD3 + HLA-DR + phenotype and a rise in the number of functional NK $CD16^+CD57^-$ and $CD16^-CD57^+$ cells in healthy centenarians. Curiously, a control group of middle-aged subjects (range 50 to 68 years) had relatively low NK activity compared to that of the centenarians and young subjects (range 19 to 30 years), and this has prompted speculation that maintenance of NK activity may be related to a "longevity phenotype."[9] B-lymphocyte numbers in peripheral blood decline with age,[9] but this may represent a redistribution of cells into lymphoid follicles[13] since immunoglobulins and IgG subclasses rise with age in the absence of malignancy.[14–16]

Bone Marrow

At birth all marrow is red hemopoietically active tissue, but then there is an orderly retreat of this tissue and replacement by yellow, hemopoietically inactive adipose marrow, beginning in the diaphysis and continuing in the distal metaphysis of each long bone and then in the proximal metaphysis.[17,18] These reversible changes can be triggered by decreased temperature and perfusion.[19,20] By early adulthood red marrow predominates only in the flat bones and vertebral bodies, with remnants in the proximal humeral and femoral bones. Gradual involution of red marrow continues but is especially marked after the age of 70 years when iliac crest marrow cellularity is reduced to about 30 percent of that found in young adults.[13,21–23] Nuclear magnetic resonance[19] is more sensitive to changes in cellularity than conventional microscopy and suggests that mechanical stress at the cervical and lumbar spine vertebral body endplates and medial portion of the femoral neck accelerates this conversion. At the same time, there is an increase in marrow necrosis and fibrosis, loss of bone substance which allows further expansion of adipose tissue with age, an increase in bone marrow iron stores,[24] a fall in the number of normoblasts,[25] and an accumulation of benign lymphoid aggregates.[13]

Stem Cells

Our present understanding of hemopoiesis derives from experimental and clinical observations of three interacting entities—the multipotent hemopoietic stem cells and their progeny, the stromal microenvironment, and growth factor molecules. During early hemopoietic development the stem cells retain the capacity to undergo self-renewal but can also, following appropriate stimuli, undergo successive cycles of proliferation and differentiation, a process known as lineage committment. Experimental evidence supports the notion that a single multipotential stem cell can, in an appropriate environment, give rise to a variety of more developmentally restricted and lineage-restricted progenitor cells capable of producing cells of different mature hemopoietic cell types.[26] Hemopoiesis is polyclonal in healthy young adults,[27–29] indicating that more than one stem cell clone contributes to the production of mature cells from the marrow at any one time. However, the short life span of many peripheral blood cells, 8 hours in the case of neutrophils, imposes a massive proliferative demand on the pool of hemopoietic stem and progenitor cells which must produce more than 10^{11} new cells each day in order to maintain the status quo. While maturation of some cells such as T lymphocytes and monocytes may occur outside the bone marrow, the process of stem cell renewal and lineage commitment appears to be almost entirely confined to the bone marrow.

The Marrow Environment

The stromal microenvironment of the bone marrow includes fibroblasts, adipose cells, macrophages, reticular cells, and endothelial cells and is essential for maintenance of hemopoiesis.[30] Bone marrow trephine histology[31] reveals the orderly arrangement of the developing cells in which early granulocytic cells can be found along the trabecular margins, while erythroid islands, megakaryocytes, and occasional lymphoid nodules are positioned in the intertrabecular spaces. These features suggest that within the stroma there are "niches" where particular developmental events are favored by the local arrangement of stromal cells, growth factors, and hemopoietic progenitor cells.

Self-renewal and Differentiation of Stem Cells

Although theoretical models have been proposed[32,33] to explain the hierarchy of mechanisms by which stem cells reenter the cell cycle to self-renew *or* to differentiate and undergo eventual clonal extinction, how the environmental factors discussed above work together to regulate self-renewal and differentiation of stem cells remains an enigma. Recent data[34] tend to favor a stochastic[35] over a deterministic[36] pattern. However, the contribution made by individual stem cells throughout an entire life span and the self-renewal capacity of the stem cell pool at a given point during that life span remain the focus of considerable debate. Some data suggest that stem cells have a finite proliferative capacity that falls progressively with age and can be accelerated by damage—a model that would explain the permanent reduction in marrow reserve caused by busulphan[37] and the limited capacity for repopulation in serial bone marrow transplantation.[38] More compelling data, however, support the idea that for all practical purposes stem cells have an indefinite capacity for self-renewal.[39–43] There is little evidence one way or the other indicating that there is a decline in the self-renewal or differentiating capacity of hemopoietic stem cells with age in humans. In mice, however, careful studies have shown that there is no decline in stem cells or their ability to regenerate hemopoiesis with age.[40,44]

Senescence and the Hemopoietic Stem Cell

Although stem cells probably constitute less than 0.01 percent of bone marrow mononuclear cells, they can be partly enriched using positive and negative selection ($CD34^+$ $Thy\text{-}1^{lo}$ $CD38^{lo}$ $CD45RA^{lo}$ $CD71^{lo}$).[45–49] Recent observations of the ribonucleoprotein telomerase activity in these cells suggest that there is a loss of proliferative capacity of stem cells with age. Telomeres, the ends of chromosomes, bear multiple tandem repeats of the nucleotide sequence TTAGGG, some of which are lost with each round of mitotic activity. This is because DNA polymerase uses only one primer and DNA is replicated in the $5' \rightarrow 3'$ direction, leading to progressive shortening of chromosomes with each cell division. Telomere shortening leads inexorably to chromosomal shrinkage and cell death, but cells that express telomerase are able to synthesize more TTAGGG repeats and extend the proliferative capacity of the cell. In addition to being an important part of tumor cell proliferative capacity, there is evidence that this is an important mechanism in normal proliferating cells. Vaziri et al.[50] have examined telomerase activity indirectly using chromosome terminal restriction fragment lengths and have demonstrated that candidate hemopoietic stem cells of the $CD34^+$ $CD45RA^{lo}$ $CD71^{lo}$ phenotype have longer TTAGGG repeat sequences than their progeny and that terminal differentiation of committed progenitor cells is associated with telomeric loss. They have also shown that stem cells from fetal liver have longer telomeres than those found in cord blood and that in the adult there appears to be a loss of stem cell telomere length with age. In other words if the self-renewal and/or proliferative capacity of the stem cell pool does decrease with age, this decline may be associated with a reduction in telomere length.

The Role of Lineage-Restricted Progenitor Cells

Stem cells are relatively few in number (perhaps 1 in 50,000 bone marrow cells),[51] and adequate production of mature cells is met by amplification and development of the more developmentally restricted progeny of the stem cells. Much more is known about the regulation of growth and development of these progenitor cells (colony forming unit-granulocyte erythroid monocyte macrophage [CFU-GEMM], granulocyte macrophage-colony forming cell [GM-CFC], macrophage-colony forming cell [M-CFC], granulocyte-colony forming cell [G-CFC], burst forming unit-erythroid [BFU-E], and colony forming unit-erythroid [CFU-E] than of the stem cells. Some of these progenitors retain the ability to produce multiple cell lineages (CFU-GEMM and GM-CFC), while others are committed to differentiation along only one cell lineage.

All these progenitor cells can be cultured in vitro using liquid medium containing essential growth factors.[51] Under these conditions they undergo clonal extinction associated with further proliferation and differentiation to produce mature blood cells. The requirement of these cells for growth factors is absolute, and in the absence of appropriate growth factors these progenitors die by apoptosis (programmed cell death).[52] It has been reported that in vitro colony formation from bone marrow derived from an aged population was inversely proportional to marrow cellularity.[53] These data suggest the possibility that as mitotic capacity of the hemopoietic stem cell population diminishes with age, equilibrium between renewal and differentiation shifts away from self-renewal in order to preserve peripheral blood function. This tends to predict the emergence of monoclonal hemopoiesis in the elderly, and this has in fact been described recently.[54]

More primitive progenitors can be grown in long-term bone marrow cultures (LTBMC)[55] when cultured in association with stromal cells. These stromal cells support the survival and development of the hemopoietic progenitor cells forming the characteristic "cobblestone" areas of hemopoietic foci within the stroma. The primitive cells that initiate hemopoiesis in LTBMC, the long-term culture initiating cells (LTCIC), are multipotential and have at least a limited self-renewal capacity allowing them to generate CFU-GEMM, GM-CFC, G-CFC, M-CFC, BFU-E, and CFU-E for periods extending to several months. In other words, the LTCIC have many characteristics in common with stem cells, and because of this the LTBMC system has been used to assess the function of the stromal layer and its interaction with primitive hemopoietic cells and their progeny and to measure the responses of hemopoietic cells to growth factors. In appropriate circumstances, however, the stromal cells can support the proliferation of "nonself" hemopoietic cells, and these secondary cultures have proved to be useful models for detecting possible age-related changes in model systems.[40,44,56–59] As yet, however, such cultures have not been used for a thorough analysis of possible loss of stromal function or hemopoietic response in elderly subjects.

Growth Factors in Hemopoiesis

Growth inhibitory and stimulatory molecules are produced or sequestered by the stromal cells and hemopoietic cells within the bone marrow, and such factors clearly play an important role in hemopoietic cell development.[51] Receptors with a high affinity for these growth factors are expressed by hemopoietic cells and transduce signals which can influence the cell cycle status and/or induce or facilitate differentiation and activation of mature cells. The type of growth factor, its concentration, the presence or absence of the appropriate receptor, the differentiation status of the cell, and the presence of other costimulatory or inhibitory growth factors are all important in determining the response of the target cells, that is, whether or not to enter the cell cycle, to self-renew, or to differentiate.[51] Furthermore, it is also now known that a major role of growth factors is to suppress apoptosis; indeed this may be one of the primary mechanisms that regulate normal levels of cell proliferation in the bone marrow and that is responsible for greater or fewer cells being released into the circulation.

In studies designed to investigate whether or not the response of hemopoietic cells to growth factors undergoes age-related changes,[60] it was found that in elderly patients (who had a hematologic malignancy or chronic disease or had received myelotoxic drugs), the hemopoietic response in vivo to recombinant hemopoietic growth factors was well conserved compared to that in young patients. However, an in vitro study of bone marrow from healthy elderly (70 to 80 years old) and healthy young (20 to 30 years old) volunteers revealed a decline in the proliferative response to G-CSF in the elderly group.[61] Another in vitro study has shown that stromal cells from healthy elderly subjects are less responsive to interleukin-1-induced expression of GM-CSF or G-CSF genes than younger subjects.[62] Apart from impaired responses due to aging, however, there may be changes in the relative importance of growth factors during a normal life span—it is known, for example, that interleukin-9[63] and interleukin-11[64] are of more importance in fetal than in adult hemopoiesis.

Conclusion

Animal studies have contributed relatively little to our understanding of how the aging process affects hemopoiesis in the human. However, various in vitro assay systems are now available to assess the function of both the stromal microenvironment and the hemopoietic stem and progenitor cells, and use of these systems should provide major insights into the mechanisms underlying defective hemopoiesis seen in elderly patients, as well as changes associated purely with senescence.

References

1. McLennan WJ, Andrews GR, Macleod C et al: Anaemia in the elderly. Q J Med 1973;42:1–13
2. Hill RD: The prevalence of anemia in the over-65s in a rural practice. Practitioner 1967;217:961–963
3. Myers MA, Saunders CRG, Chalmers DG: The hemoglobin level of fit elderly people. Lancet 1968;ii:261–263
4. Piomelli S, Nathan DG, Cummins JF et al: The relationship of total red cell volume to total body water in octogenarian males. Blood 1962;19:89–92

5. Besa EC: Approach to mild anemia in the elderly. Clin Geriatr Med 1988;4:43–55
6. Ligthart GJ, Corberand JX, Fournier C et al: Admission criteria for immunogerontological studies in man: the Senieur protocol. Mech Age Dev 1984;28:47–55
7. Landahl S, Jagenburg R, Svanburg A: Blood components in a 70 year old population. Clin Chem Acta 1981;112:301–314
8. Baldwin JJ: True anemia: incidence and significance in the elderly. Geriatrics 1989;44:33–36
9. Sansoni P, Cossarizza A, Brianti V et al: Lymphocyte subsets and natural killer cell activity in healthy old people and centenarians. Blood 1993;82:2767–2773
10. Roberts-Thompson IC, Whittingham S, Youngchaiyud U, Mackay IR: Ageing, immune response and mortality. Lancet 1974;ii:368–370
11. Weinberg K, Parkman R: Age, the thymus and T lymphocytes. N Engl J Med 1995;332:182–183
12. Mackall CL, Fleisher TA, Brown MR et al: Age, thymopoiesis, and $CD4^+$ T-lymphocyte regeneration after intensive chemotherapy. N Engl J Med 1995;332:143–149
13. Liu PI, Takanari H, Yatani R, Nelson G: Comparative studies of bone marrow from the United States and Japan. Ann Clin Lab Sci 1989;19:345–351
14. Radl J, Sepers JM, Skvaril F et al: Immunoglobulin patterns in humans over 95 years of age. Clin Exp Immunol 1975;22:84–90
15. Radl J: Effects of ageing on immunoglobulins. pp. 52–69. In Ritzmann S (ed): Pathology of Immunoglobulins. Alan R Liss, New York, 1982
16. Paganelli R, Quinti I, Fagiolo U et al: Changes in circulating B cells and immunoglobulin classes and subclasses in a healthy aged population. Clin Exp Immunol 1992;90:351–354
17. Kricun ME: Red-yellow marrow conversion: its effect on the location of some solitary bone lesions. Skeletal Radiol 1985; 14:10–19
18. Moore SG, Dawson KL: Red and yellow marrow in the femur: age-related changes in appearance at MR imaging. Radiology 1990;175:219–223
19. Ricci C, Cova M, Kang YS et al: Normal age-related patterns of cellular and fatty bone marrow distribution in the axial skeleton: MR imaging study. Radiology 1990;177:83–88
20. Kita K, Kawai K, Hirohata K: Changes in bone marrow blood flow with aging. J Orthop Res 1987;5:569–575
21. Meunier P, Aaron J, Edouard C, Vignon G: Osteoporosis and the replacement of cell populations of the marrow by adipose tissue. Clin Orthopaed 1971;80:147–154
22. Hartsock RJ, Smith EB, Petty CS: Normal variations with ageing of the amount of hematopoietic tissue in bone marrow from the anterior iliac crest: a study made from 177 cases of sudden death examined by necropsy. Am J Clin Pathol 1965;43: 326–331
23. Frisch B, Lewis SM, Burkhadt R, Bartl R: Biopsy Pathology of Bone and Marrow. Chapman and Hall, London, 1985
24. Yip R, Johnson C, Dallman PR: Age-related changes in laboratory values used in the diagnosis of an anaemia and iron deficiency. Am J Clin Nutr 1984;39:427–436
25. Lipschitz DA, Udupa KB, Milton KY, Thompson CO: Effects of age on hematopoiesis in man. Blood 1984;63:502–509
26. Dexter TM: Growth and differentiation in the haemopoietic system. Biochem Soc Trans 1991;19:303–306
27. Fialkow P: Primordial cell pool size and lineage relationships of five human cell types. Ann Hum Genet 1973;37:39–48
28. Vogelstein B, Fearon ER, Hamilton SR et al: Clonal analysis using recombinant DNA probes from the X-chromosome. Cancer Res 1987;47:4806–4813
29. Gale RE, Wheadon H, Linch DC: X-chromosome inactivation patterns using HPRT and PGK polymorphisms in haematologically normal and post-chemotherapy females. Br J Haematol 1991;79:193–197
30. Dexter TM, Moore MAS: In vitro duplication and "cure" of haemopoietic defects in genetically anaemic mice. Nature 1977; 269:412–414
31. Bain B, Clark D, Lampert IA: Bone Marrow Pathology. Blackwell Scientific Publications, Oxford, 1992
32. Brown G, Jones NA, Bunce CM et al: Haemopoiesis: a lottery or determinism. Br J Haematol 1991;79:527–529
33. Dexter TM, Spooncer ES: Growth and differentiation in the haemopoietic system. Ann Rev Cell Biol 1987;3:423–441
34. Fairbairn LJ, Cowling GJ, Reipert BM, Dexter TM: Suppression of apoptosis allows differentiation and development of a multipotent hemopoietic cell line in the absence of added growth factors. Cell 1993;74:823–832
35. Till JE, McCulloch EA, Siminovitch L: A stochastic model of stem cell proliferation based on the growth of spleen colony forming cells. Proc Natl Acad Sci U S A 1964;51:29–36
36. Curry JL, Trentin JJ: Haemopoietic spleen colony stimulating factors. Science 1967;236:1229–1237
37. Hellman S, Botnick LE: Stem cell depletion: an explanation of the late effects of cytotoxins. Int J Radiat Oncol 1977;2: 181–184
38. Ogden DA, Micklem HS: The fate of serially transplanted bone marrow cell populations from young and old donors. Transplantation 1976;22:287–290
39. Lajtha LG, Schofield R: Regulation of stem cell renewal and differentiation: possible significance in ageing. pp. 131–146. In Streliler BL (ed): Advances in Gerontological Research. Academic Press, New York, 1971
40. Schofield R, Dexter TM, Lord BI, Testa NG: Comparison of haemopoiesis in young and old mice. Mech Age Dev 1986;34: 1–12
41. Schofield R, Lord BI, Kyffin S et al: Self maintenance capacity of CFU-s. J Cell Physiol 1980;103:355–362
42. Harrison DE, Astle CM: Loss of stem cell repopulating ability upon transplantation. J Exp Med 1982;156:1767–1779
43. Jordan CT, Lemischka IR: Clonal and systemic analysis of long term hematopoiesis in the mouse. Genes Dev 1990;4:220–232
44. Tejero C, Testa NG, Hendry JH: Decline in cycling of granulocyte-macrophage colony-forming cells with increasing age in mice. Exp Hematol 1989;17:66–67
45. Lansdorp PM, Dragowska W: Long-term erythropoiesis from constant numbers of $CD34^+$ cells in serum-free cultures initiated with highly purified progenitor cells from human bone marrow. J Exp Med 1992;175:1501–1509
46. Civin CI, Strauss LC, Brovall C et al: Antigenic analysis of hematopoiesis. III. A hematopoietic progenitor cell surface anti-

gen defined by a monoclonal antibody raised against KG-1a cells. J Immunol 1984;133:157–165

47. Baum CM, Weissman IL, Tsukamoto AS et al: Isolation of a candidate human hematopoietic stem-cell population. Proc Natl Acad Sci U S A 1992;89:2804–2808
48. Craig W, Kay R, Cutler RL, Lansdorp PM: Expression of Thy-1 on human hematopoietic progenitor cells. J Exp Med 1993; 177:1331–1342
49. Terstappen LW, Huang S, Safford M et al: Sequential generations of hematopoietic colonies derived from single nonlineage-committed $CD34^+$ $CD38^-$ progenitor cells. Blood 1991;77: 1218–1227
50. Vaziri H, Dragowska W, Allsopp RC et al: Evidence for a mitotic clock in human hematopoietic stem cells: loss of telomeric DNA with age. Proc Natl Acad Sci U S A 1994;91:9857–9860
51. Metcalf D: The Colony Stimulating Factors. Elsevier, Amsterdam, 1984
52. Williams GT, Smith GT, Spooncer E et al: Haemopoietic colony stimulating factors promote cell survival by suppressing apoptosis. Nature 1990;343:76–79
53. Resnitzky P, Segal M, Barak Y, Dassa C: Granulopoiesis in aged people: inverse correlation between bone marrow cellularity and myeloid progenitor cell numbers. Gerontology 1987;33: 109–114
54. Fielding A, Gale RE, Linch DC: Analysis of X chromosome inactivation patterns in the elderly: implications for stem cell usage. p. 590A. In Griffin JD (ed): American Society of Haematology Thirty-Seventh Meeting, Seattle, Washington. WB Saunders, Philadelphia, 1995
55. Dexter TM, Allen TP, Lajtha L: Conditions controlling the proliferation of haemopoietic cells in vitro. J Cell Physiol 1977; 91:335–344
56. Boggs D, Patrene K: Hematopoiesis and aging. III. Anemia and a blunted erythropoietic response to hemorrhage in aged mice. Am J Hematol 1985;19:327–338
57. Mauch P, Botnick LE, Hannon EC et al: Decline in bone marrow proliferative capacity as a function of age. Blood 1982;60: 245–252
58. Inoue T, Cronkite EP: The influence of in vivo incubation of aged murine spleen colony-forming units on their proliferative capacity. Mech Ageing Dev 1983;23:177–190
59. Lipschitz DA, Udupa KB: Age and the haemopoietic system. Geriatr Biosci 1986;34:448–454
60. Shank WJ, Balducci L: Recombinant hemopoietic growth factors: comparative hemopoietic response in younger and older subjects. J Am Geriatr Soc 1992;40:151–154
61. Chatta GS, Andrews RG, Rodger E et al: Hematopoietic progenitors and aging: alterations in granulocytic precursors and responsiveness to recombinant human G-CSF, GM-CSF, and IL-3. J Gerontol 1993;48:207–212
62. Lee MA, Segal GM, Bagby GC: The hematopoietic microenvironment in the elderly: defects in IL-1-induced CSF expression in vitro. Exp Hematol 1989;17:952–956
63. Holbrook ST, Ohls RK, Schibler KR et al: Effect of interleukin-9 on clonogenic maturation and cell-cycle status of fetal and adult hematopoietic progenitors. Blood 1991;77:2129–2134
64. Schibler KR, Yang YC, Christensen RD: Effect of interleukin-11 on cycling status and clonogenic. Blood 1992;80:900–903

CHAPTER 89

Blood Disorders and Their Management in Old Age

MICHAEL L. FREEDMAN
DAVID G. SUTIN

Diseases of the Red Blood Cells

Anemia

Anemia can be defined as a reduction in the number of circulating red cells below the normal range. A U.S. national health and nutrition study defined the normal range of hemoglobin to be 13.3 to 17.7 g/dl for men and 11.7 to 15.7 g/dl for women[1,2] in the United States. The World Health Organization criteria for diagnosing anemia are a hemoglobin level of less than 14 g/dl in men and 12 g/dl in women.[3] A subsequent report[4] recommended that for males the critical hemoglobin level be reduced to 13 g/dl. In recent years, there has been considerable controversy regarding whether an "anemia of senescence"[2–15] exists. In order to examine this controversy, the physiologic variables affecting blood count in humans must be considered.

The normal red cell number, hematocrit, and hemoglobin levels can be raised by smoking, obesity, altitude, exertion, and stress.[16–20] Most normal men living at or near sea level whose red cell counts are above $6.0 \times 10^6/\mu l$ are smokers. This rise in red cells may be largely attributed to elevated carboxyhemoglobin[20] and chronic pulmonary disease.

The use of hematocrit and hemoglobin concentration to define anemia may be very misleading. When the peripheral blood is examined, it is assumed that the plasma volume remains constant; however, the plasma volume is the most variable portion of the whole blood (Table 89-1).[21–23]

Changes in plasma volume occur throughout the day and are dependent on daily activities. Exercise and activity tend to lower plasma volume and raise hematocrit and hemoglobin levels. The lack of exercise in the elderly tends to raise the plasma volume and therefore lower hemoglobin levels. Bed rest has a dual effect on hemoglobin levels. At first, there is a fall in plasma volume (an increase in hemoglobin due to an initial diuresis resulting from a decrease in antidiuretic hormone [ADH] secretion).[24] This is caused by an increase in thoracic blood volume which is followed by a decrease in extravascular (lymphatic) return of proteins and a further reduction in plasma volume and a rise in hemoglobin. Prolonged bed rest eventually, however, leads to a decrease in erythropoiesis and a lower red cell mass, as there is a decrease in oxygen demand.[25] Thus, after prolonged bed rest a person eventually develops an anemia.

When a young person stands up after being recumbent overnight, the plasma volume falls by about 300 ml.[26] This response is blunted in the normal elderly, presumably because of a defect in the afferent arm of the baroreceptor reflex arc distal to the vasomotor center.[27]

The elderly also do not respond in the same way as the young when exposed to high-altitude hypoxia. When a young person is exposed to high-altitude hypoxia, in the first 24 to 48 hours there is an increase in hemoglobin concentration due to a decrease in plasma volume,[28] an increase in 2,3-diphosphoglycreate (2, 3-DPC),[29] and an elevation of serum erythropoietin.[30] These changes result in a rapid increase in the oxygen delivery capabilities of the blood which is followed by an erythropoietin-stimulated increase in bone marrow and eventually in a polycythemic state.[31]

The decrease in plasma volume probably reflects a shift in intravascular fluid from blood to intracellular or extravascular spaces caused by vasoconstriction resulting from increased venomotor tone.[32] The increased venomotor tone in young people can be relieved by breathing 100 percent oxygen.[33] This hemoconcentration in young people is delayed in older people, and is possibly associated with an impairment in aldosterone release, also found in the elderly, at high altitudes.[34,35]

When measuring the red cell parameters in older people, all the variables must be taken into account. Very few studies have controlled for bed rest, exercise, altitude, time of day, fluid intake, salt intake, or plasma proteins. In addition, many drugs, particularly diuretics and antihypertensives can theoretically alter plasma volume and erythropoiesis.[32] Any antihypertensive medication that blocks the autonomic nervous system can decrease venomotor tone and therefore raise plasma volume (lower hemoglobin levels). Diuretics lower plasma volume but in renal failure may have the opposite effect. The chronic effect of any drug on erythropoiesis has not been carefully studied. Thus, any measurement of red cell parameters with age must control for medications, which has not been done.

Table 89-1 Factors affecting plasma volume and red cell parameters

Increased Physiologic Factor	Plasma Volume	Red Cell Parameters[a]
Capillary permeability	Decrease	Increase
Hormones		
Antidiuretic hormone	Increase	Decrease
Aldosterone	Increase	Decrease
Osmotic pressure (plasma protein)	Increase	Decrease
Venomotor tone		
Exercise	Decrease	Increase
Bed rest (prolonged)	Increased	Decrease

[a] *Red cell parameter = red blood cell, hemoglobin, or hemocrit.*

Aging does have an effect on blood production. There is evidence from both animal and human studies for the following age-related changes in bone marrow function.

1. The ratio of bone marrow cells to marrow fat decreases in the elderly,[36] although marrow from older people can be maintained by serial transplantation in tissue culture just as long as marrow from younger people; the number of normoblasts and committed erythroid stem cells (CFU-E) is lower, however. The number of earlier stem cells (BFU-E) was normal in the elderly.[37–39]
2. Iron incorporation into bone marrow cells from older people in vitro is the same as that from younger people. When stimulated with erythropoietin, an older person's marrow increases its iron incorporation to a lesser degree.[40]
3. Older animals do not respond to bleeding or hypoxia with increased erythropoiesis as well as younger animals.[41–42] It is not clear if the defect is in the hematopoietic elements themselves or is due to age-related changes in the marrow environment.
4. In humans, even though iron absorption from the gut is normal, an increase in ineffective erythropoiesis results in impaired incorporation of iron into heme in red cell precursors.[43]

There does seem to be a slightly lower red cell mass in the very elderly.[44] Red cell mass correlates best with lean body mass. It seems that the main determinant of red cell mass in the young is tissue oxygen requirements. Therefore, the decline in lean body mass and tissue oxygen requirements may explain at least part of the fall in red blood cell mass. However, the correlation between lean body mass and red cell mass also decreases with age.[44]

Elderly people respond to testosterone in pharmacologic doses, indicating that marrow function is preserved;[45] responsiveness to the hormone is not decreased. Red cell 2,3-DPG has been shown to decrease in aging men, indicating a decrease in the oxygen demand of the tissues.[29] It has been postulated that the "thermostat" for red cell production is set at a lower level, thus lowering the level at which red cell production is turned on. Red blood cell survival remains normal with advancing age.[46]

Normal, healthy young men have a hematocrit[13–15] of about 46 percent and a hemoglobin level of about 15.6 g/dl. By age 60, the normal hemoglobin has slipped approximately 1 g/dl and in subsequent years may fall as much as 1 g per decade. The decline for black men is even steeper than that for white men. The opposite is seen in women. Between age 30 and 60 women show an increase in hemoglobin level of 0.6 g/dl/decade.[47–49] After age 60, their red cell parameters decline in parallel to those of men. Black women at any age have red cell levels about 2 percent lower than those of white women. The difference between whites and blacks may represent nutritional differences or indicate thalassemia minor.[50]

In spite of these changes, most older people still have normal red cell counts, hemoglobin levels, and hematocrits.[13–15] Certainly, if older patients with hemoglobin levels less than 12 g/dl or hematocrits less than 36 percent are investigated, an underlying cause of the anemia is usually discovered.[10] The diagnostic workup for a mild anemia includes checking for blood loss, hemolysis, nutritional deficiencies, malignancy, infection, renal disease, any chronic disease, and any cause of an increase in plasma volume. Since all these factors are considered as part of a comprehensive geriatric assessment, the physician must always think in terms of what is causing the anemia. Even though there may be some very elderly people who have an anemia due to aging alone, most anemic elderly people have an underlying illness.

Classification of anemia in the elderly

Anemia can be classified either by morphology (Table 89-2) or by etiology (Table 89-3). However, in geriatric clinical practice, these two groups must be allowed to overlap to be of practical value. As discussed below, early in certain anemias, the morphology may be normocytic. For example, the microcytosis of iron deficiency is a late finding, as in the macrocytosis of vitamin B_{12} or folate deficiency. It is possible to diagnose these anemias long before morphologic changes appear in the blood smear or the rbc indices become abnormal.

Clinical features of anemia in the elderly

The symptoms and signs of anemia are the same in the elderly as in younger people, but the emphasis differs. Cardiovascular and cerebral features predominate, although many anemic patients have no complaints. Breathlessness and ankle edema are common manifestations and may be due to frank congestive cardiac failure. Left ventricle failure may occur, but angina is rare. Dizziness is common, and mental changes are important but are nonspecific. Apart from confusion there may be apathy and depression, leading to self-neglect or agitation, even with delusions and hallucinations.

The tongue is often smooth and pale, and the patient may complain of a burning sensation on the tongue; but a sore

Table 89-2 Morphologic classification of anemia

Microcytic
1. Iron deficiency
2. Anemia of chronic disease (often normocytic)
3. Sideroblastic anemia (often normocytic or macrocytic)
4. Thalassemia

Macrocytic
1. Megaloblastic
   a. Vitamin B_{12} deficiency
   b. Folic acid deficiency
   c. Myelodysplasia
2. Normoblastic
   a. Chronic liver disease
   b. Alcoholism
   c. Hypothyroidism
   d. Leukemia and myelodysplasia
   e. Aplastic anemia
   f. Increased reticulocytes

Normocytic
1. Blood loss
2. Hemolysis
3. Early-stage iron deficiency or megaloblastic anemia
4. Anemia of chronic disease
5. Anemia of renal disease
6. Anemia of liver disease
7. Anemia of endocrine disorders
8. Scurvy
9. Collagen-vascular disease
10. Bone marrow infiltration

tongue may be due to associated nutritional deficiencies rather than to the anemia itself. In such cases, there may be angular stomatitis or cheilosis. However, wearing an upper denture may produce lesions indistinguishable from angular stomatitis which may be misleading.

Pallor, especially if recent, is important but is rarely offered as a symptom. The skin of the elderly may be very difficult to assess, and attention should be paid to the color of the buccal and lingual mucosae and the nailbeds. Changes in the nails are rarely of help.

Table 89-3 Etiologic classification of anemia

Blood loss (acute or chronic)

Excessive red cell destruction (hemolytic anemia)

Impaired red cell formation
1. Deficiency of substances essential for erythropoiesis
   a. Iron deficiency
   b. Vitamin B_{12} deficiency
   c. Folic acid deficiency
   d. Vitamin C deficiency
   e. Protein malnutrition
   f. Heme deficiency
2. Disturbance of marrow function
   a. Aplastic anemia
   b. Myelophthisis
   c. Myelodysplasia

A spleen tip may be felt in severe long-standing anemia, but other causes must be excluded. Associated features should be sought, for example, bone tenderness, abdominal mass, lymphadenopathy, signs of neuropathy, or spinal cord lesions.

The essential feature of the chronic anemias—which are those most commonly seen in old age—is the insidious onset of symptoms and signs. Physiologic changes can compensate to some extent for the reduction in hemoglobin (e.g., an altered oxygen dissociation curve of hemoglobin to the right), allowing increased availability of oxygen to the tissues.[51–54] This allows the anemia to become marked before symptoms become troublesome. Furthermore, many old people are adverse to seeking medical (or other) help and may endure various symptoms without complaining. Thus, by the time an anemia is actually diagnosed in the elderly, the patient may in fact be very ill. In milder cases, untoward symptoms or failing general health may be accepted philosophically as part of "the burden of old age."

Investigation of anemia

A full blood count is a valuable routine investigation in all elderly patients. If anemia is found, it must be investigated before any attempt at treatment is made. Indiscriminate use of hematinics before investigation can cause further morbidity and make accurate diagnosis extremely difficult or delayed.

It is necessary to determine the type and cause of the anemia. Examination of the peripheral blood film may suggest the likely cause and indicate the type of anemia present. The cause is finally determined by careful history and examination, blood findings, and further investigations as required. Every initial geriatric assessment should include a complete blood count (CBC), and some authors advocate yearly testing. A healthy hemoglobin provides a basis for reassurance in a health-conscious population, whereas a hemoglobin in the anemic range (less than 12 g/dl in women and 13.5 g/dl in men is often used) alerts the physician to the potential presence of a disease process requiring early intervention.[55]

Once an anemia has been identified, the next step is to further characterize it utilizing the information already available from the CBC. An anemia accompanied by abnormalities in white blood cell and platelet counts suggests a primary marrow production problem, including aplastic anemia, marrow filled with tumor or infection, drug- or toxin-suppressed marrow, or nutrient-deprived marrow. The mean corpuscular volume (MCV) provides a clue to the red blood cell size, an important feature in classifying anemias. An MCV above 100 fl is considered macrocytic, an MCV less than 80 fl microcytic, and one 80 to 100 fl is normocytic. However, one should never rely entirely on the MCV or defining cell size. Examination of the peripheral blood smear is necessary to confirm automated counter measurements; what the counter identifies as macrocytic may actually be an abundance of reticulocytes with a typical polychromatophilic appearance on visual inspection. Likewise, a mixed population of macrocytes and microcytes might yield a MCV calculated in the normocytic range by the counter.[55] Red cell diameter width (RDW), a measure of anisocytosis, is often unreliable in the elderly.[56–57]

Examination of the peripheral blood smear is essential in establishing red cell morphology. With the aid of an atlas, even a nonhematologist can identify pathologic shapes such as teardrops, schistocytes, ovalocytes, poikilocytes, and burr cells—crucial clues to the pathogenesis of the anemia. Cell color (hypo- or normochromic) reflects the hemoglobin concentration and thereby also distinguishes the type of anemia.[55]

After review of the CBC and inspection of the peripheral smear, one additional useful test involves special staining of the peripheral blood cells for a reticulocyte count. Reticulocytes, or young erythrocytes, should be abundantly produced and released in situations of blood loss, such as bleeding or hemolysis, but are scarce in situations in which anemia is due to inadequate marrow production. A low reticulocyte count may be misleading in situations where blood loss has outstripped the supply of nutrients in the marrow, resulting in secondary marrow failure. Reticulocyte count norms are relative to the degree of anemia: the more anemic, the greater the reticulocyte count. The absolute reticulocyte count, corrected reticulocyte count, and reticulocyte production index (RPI) help one to assess the adequacy of the bone marrow response in the face of anemia. The RPI can be calculated in anemic patients in the following way.

$$\text{RPI} = \frac{\text{corrected reticulocyte count}}{2}$$

$$\text{Corrected reticulocyte count} = \text{reticulocytes (\%)} \times \frac{\text{patient hematocrit}}{\text{normal hematocrit}}$$

The usual normal hematocrit used is 0.45 L/L. The factor 2 in the denominator is used in anemic patients to take account of shift reticulocytes, prematurely released reticulocytes that take longer to lose their reticulin than normal reticulocytes. An adequate bone marrow response is usually indicated by an RPI greater than 3, and an inadequate one by an RPI less than 2.[58]

With the data accrued from one tube of blood (CBC, MCV, smear, and reticulocyte count), the anemia can usually be characterized.[55]

A bone marrow examination is rarely necessary in the initial evaluation of anemia in older patients. The vast majority of uncomplicated anemias can be diagnosed without a bone marrow examination. However, this procedure should be performed when the anemia is accompanied by abnormalities in white blood cells or platelets or when marrow infiltration is suspected. The examination is no more dangerous or painful in older people than in younger people.

Treatment of anemia—general principles

The first step is to identify and treat the underlying cause of the anemia. For example, in iron deficiency, the source of blood loss must be found and the bleeding stopped. After the cause of the anemia is found, a specific hematinic may be prescribed. If a rapid correction of the anemia is required, a red cell transfusion must be given after diagnostic blood tests have been performed.

Specific hematinics are iron, vitamin B_{12}, folic acid, and perhaps ascorbic acid and pyridoxine. Nonspecific hematinics include hormones such as androgens and growth factors such as erythropoietin and colony stimulating factors.

Following an accurate diagnosis the specific hematinic required should be used alone whenever possible, and the response to full doses assessed. This helps in confirming the diagnosis and simplifies the treatment. Combination preparations or hematinic "cocktails" are to be avoided, as they obscure the diagnosis.

The main indications for blood transfusion are when hematinic therapy will be ineffectual or inappropriate, when the gravity of the patient's condition precludes undue delay, or prior to surgery. Usually when the hematocrit is less than 25 percent or the hemoglobin concentration is below 8 g/dl, transfusion is necessary in patients over the age of 65. When transfusion becomes necessary in the elderly, every attempt must be made to avoid overloading the circulation. This is accomplished by using packed red cells in small volumes at a slow rate (e.g., 0.5 L in 6 to 8 hours), often adding a diuretic, and by careful clinical observation to avoid pulmonary congestion and a rise in venous pressure.

Microcytic Anemias

Iron deficiency anemia

A microcytic (MCV less than 80 fl) hypochromic anemia in an elderly individual means iron deficiency due to blood loss until proven otherwise. The current recommended dietary allowance for iron in elderly patients in the United States is 10 mg.[59] The most common anemia in the elderly is rarely due to dietary deficiency in industrialized nations because of the prevalence of iron fortification in wheat as well as a diet heavy in meat containing heme iron.[60] According to the Second National Health and Nutrition Examination Survey, 1976 to 1980, carried out by the U.S. National Center for Health Statistics, mean iron intake was 13 mg/d for men and 10 mg/d for women over 70 years of age.[61] In fact, since the body salvages and recycles heme iron and stores absorbed dietary iron, the elderly usually have accumulated ample stockpiles of iron over their lifetime. In addition, about one-third of the absorbed iron in the elderly is not utilized for erythropoiesis but is deposited in nonerythroid tissues, predisposing them to iron overload. Therefore, the only rationale for the use of iron supplements in the aged individual is for replacement therapy after a diagnosis of iron deficiency has been appropriately made or for dietary supplementation in an individual with low iron stores who malabsorbs dietary iron (e.g., status postgastrectomy).

Stages of iron deficiency There are four well-described stages of iron deficiency (Table 89-4), only the last two of which are reflected in the red blood cell indexes.[60,62]

Table 89-4 Four stages of iron deficiency

Stage	Bone Marrow Iron	Serum Ferritin	Serum Fe/TIBC	Erythrocyte Protoporphyrin	Red Blood Cell Morphology
Iron depletion	Low	Low	Normal	Normal	Normal
Iron deficiency without anemia	Low/absent	Low	Normal or low	Normal	Normal
Early iron deficiency anemia	Absent	Low	Low	High	Normal or slightly microcytic
Late iron deficiency anemia	Absent	Low	Low	High	Microcytic, hypochromic

Abbreviation: TIBC, total iron binding capacity.

Before the overt hematologic effects of iron deficiency manifest themselves, only bone marrow stains for iron or serum ferritin can be used to detect the two earlier stages reliably. In the first stage, known as iron depletion, serum ferritin is the most useful indicator because it is not practical to use bone marrow aspiration as a screening test. As iron deficiency progresses, bone marrow remains reduced or absent and serum ferritin remains low while other biochemical and hematologic changes occur. In the second stage, iron deficiency without anemia, there is a fall in serum iron with a corresponding rise in transferrin. In early iron deficiency anemia, the third stage, bone marrow iron is absent but red blood cells are usually still normocytic and normochromic. Additionally, the supply of transport iron for heme synthesis becomes limited and erythrocyte protoporphyrin is elevated. In the fourth and final stage of iron deficiency, the classic hematologic findings of microcytic, hypochromic anemia are seen.[60,62]

Diagnosis of iron deficiency Tests used to detect iron deficiency have various levels of diagnostic accuracy (Table 89-5),[62] and the limitations of each measurement must be kept in mind. Using anemia as a screening test for iron deficiency is limited because it is a late finding and does not distinguish it from other causes of anemia. Decreased MCV is also a relatively late finding. Additionally, other anemias that may be microcytic and difficult to distinguish from iron deficiency based on MCV alone are thalassemia minor, anemia of chronic disease (ACD), and sideroblastic anemia.

Other tests useful in detecting iron deficiency before overt anemia develops can present several problems from the standpoint of diagnostic accuracy. Whereas a low serum ferritin level always indicates iron deficiency, a normal level does not ensure adequate iron stores, as serum ferritin is often elevated into the normal range in the presence of chronic inflammation and liver disease. In a study by Guyatt et al.[63] on anemic patients over 65 years of age, a ferritin level less than or equal to 18 μg/L had a likelihood ratio of 41 for iron deficiency, and a level of 19 to 45 μg/L had a likelihood ratio of 3. Low transferrin saturation is unreliable because iron and serum transferrin levels are often decreased in the elderly as well as in those with chronic disease. Serum iron may be inaccurate because it can fluctuate depending on the time of day. Free erythrocyte protoporphyrin level increases at about the same time that microcytosis develops and is therefore a relatively late finding. Additionally, high levels of erythrocyte protoporphyrin may not distinguish iron deficiency from lead poisoning.

Thompson et al.[56] have evaluated the accuracy of RDW, MCV, and transferrin saturation in the diagnosis of iron deficiency in hospitalized patients. RDW measures the variability in red cell size (anisocytosis). In contrast to previous reports, the authors found that none of these tests were sensitive or specific enough to be considered an accurate screening test for the diagnosis of iron deficiency anemia in hospitalized patients and the elderly.

In cases where the diagnosis is in doubt, a bone marrow biopsy showing depletion of iron stores is diagnostic, and in the occasional patient who refuses a bone marrow biopsy, a trial of iron therapy for 1 month can be used.

Table 89-5 Limitations of tests used to diagnose iron deficiency

Test	Limitation
Hemoglobin/hematocrit	Anemia is a late finding, not specific
Microcytosis (MCV)	Late finding, not specific
Serum ferritin	Normal level not accurate with concurrent chronic disease or liver disease
Transferrin saturation	Low transferrin also found in the elderly and those with chronic disease
Serum iron	Levels may fluctuate during the day
Free erythrocyte protoporphyrin	Late finding, not specific
Red cell distribution width	Not sensitive or specific enough for screening

Abbreviation: MCV, mean corpuscular volume.

Metabolic role of iron Iron is essential by itself and as a portion of the heme molecule in many metabolic processes. Iron is present at the subcellular level, both by itself and in heme, where it functions as a component of various enzymes. The presence of iron is essential in mitochondria for generation of energy in the form of adenosine triphosphate (ATP) by oxidative phosphorylation. Several enzyme components of the respiratory electron transport chain contain iron, including cytochrome oxidase (containing two heme groups), succinate dehydrogenase (an iron flavoprotein), and other non-heme-containing compounds.[64] By itself, iron exerts a controlling effect on protein synthesis in the mitochondrion and may help maintain the integrity of the organelle.[65–67]

The cytoplasmic concentration of heme exerts crucial control of protein synthesis initiation and polyribosome formation in immature red cells,[68] and probably in all cells.[69–73] As heme concentration falls below a critical level, a translational repressor of initiation forms (the heme-controlled repressor [HCR_A]) from a noninhibitory form of the same protein (HCR_I) and stops the initiation of cytoplasmic protein synthesis.[74]

In sufficient amounts, heme can inhibit the formation of this repressor and reverse its activity. HCR_A has also been found in mature human and rabbit erythrocytes, while in reticulocytes that are actively synthesizing protein it is found in its inactive or HCR_I form. This is evidence that HCR plays a physiologic role in the maturation and cessation of protein synthesis in erythroid cells.[75]

HCR_A is a cyclic adenosine monophosphate (AMP)-independent protein kinase[76] which appears to act by phosphorylating and inactivating the initiation factor eIF-2 that mediates the binding of met-tRNAf to the 40S ribosomal subunit.[77–79] Even though HCR_A does not require cyclic AMP, mitochondrial γ-aminolevulinic acid (ALA-S) activity seems dependent on it.[80]

Freedman and Rosman[74] have proposed a working model for heme control of red cell hemoglobin synthesis. A decrease in heme concentration, such as in iron deficiency, ACD, or sideroblastic anemia, results in activation of HCR_A and diminished hemoglobin synthesis. Heme synthesis is also partially regulated by end product inhibition (by heme) of the rate-limiting enzyme ALA-S.[81] Consequently, when heme accumulates, ALA-S is inhibited and further heme synthesis stops.

This model of heme control of protein synthesis helps explain the balanced heme and globin synthesis seen in erythroid and other cells and is consistent with other strong evidence that heme synthesis is essential in erythropoiesis. Erythropoietin has been shown to first stimulate ALA-S and heme synthesis before affecting globin synthesis.[82] Using a system of bone marrow precursors in tissue culture, it has been shown that heme synthesis is maximal in the earliest precursor cells and decreases with cell maturity. This is consistent with the theory that in erythrocytes there must be sufficient intracellular heme to convert HCR from an inhibitory to a noninhibitory state before protein synthesis can proceed.[74]

In recent years, it has been shown that iron, independent of heme, is required for maximal mitochondrial protein synthesis.[61] Iron deficiency exerts a negative effect on mitochondrial protein synthesis, and there is decreased synthesis of the inner mitochondrial membrane. This results in decreased heme synthesis, a fall in cellular heme concentrations, and activation of HCR_A. Consequently, cytoplasmic protein synthesis is decreased, which in turn results in a decline in cytoplasmically synthesized mitochondrial proteins. This ensures a balance between cytoplasmic and mitochondrial protein synthesis.

In a situation where there is primary inhibition of cytoplasmic protein synthesis, free heme levels rise and decrease mitochondrial protein synthesis and feedback-inhibit ALA-S. Thus the effect of elevated heme levels on mitochondrial protein synthesis and ALA-S is another way the cell ultimately controls heme synthesis and integrates mitochondrial and cytoplasmic protein synthesis.[67]

Drug metabolism and iron Cytochrome P450 is another heme protein and is an important component of the hepatic drug metabolizing enzyme system which usually stays normal with aging. Heme production is regulated in hepatocytes by the balance between heme synthesis, controlled by ALA-S, and heme degradation, controlled by microsomal heme oxygenase. In aged rats, there is decreased hepatic heme synthesis caused by a decrease in ALA-S.[83] In addition, there is an increase in heme oxygenase and heme degradation.[84] In spite of this, heme levels and cytochrome P450 levels stay normal,[84,85] suggesting that an alternate pool of heme exists (such as tryptophan, pyrrolase, or hemopexin) which is increasingly used with age.[84,85] The net result is that with aging, cytochrome P450 is maintained by utilizing dietary heme. However, with iron deficiency, clearly cytochrome P450 is ultimately decreased.[85]

Iron overload also induces heme oxygenase and degrades heme,[86] leading to a decrease of cytochrome P450.[87] Since there is a degree of iron overload with aging, this may explain why in some elderly individuals there are problems in handling medications metabolized by cytochrome P450.[85]

Tissue iron deficiency In iron deficiency, it also has been shown that there is decreased activity of cytochrome c, cytochrome oxidase, succinic dehydrogenase, aconitase, xanthine oxidase, myoglobin, and other enzymes, including ribonucleotide reductase necessary for DNA synthesis.[60,88–94] Iron deficiency, therefore, is not manifested just as an anemia. In addition to its contributions to red blood cell production, iron is an important regulator of many cellular functions, including protein synthesis and energy production in all cells. Because of iron's ubiquitous involvement in many aspects of cell metabolism, its deficiency results in alterations in many tissues, as summarized in Table 89-6.

A lack of tissue iron seems to have a profound effect on various mucosal surfaces, resulting in several clinical entities. The mouth has been found to be affected by iron deficiency in a number of ways, including glossitis and angular stomatitis.[95] Additionally, several reports have described altered histology in the buccal mucosa of iron-deficient patients.[96–97]

The effects of iron deficiency on the esophagus have received much attention, beginning with the reports of Paterson, Kelly, and Vinson.[98–100] Sideropenic dysphagia, also known as Patterson-Kelly-Vinson syndrome, is characteristically associated with a mucosal web found in the postcricoid region of the hypopharynx. Although in most cases the web is found to consist of normal epithelium, carcinoma in situ is occasionally demonstrated.[101] Several investigators consider the postcricoid obstruction of Patterson-Kelly-Vinson syndrome to be a prema-

Table 89-6 Consequences of tissue iron deficiency

Tissue	Defect
Mouth	Glossitis, angular stomatitis, altered histology
Esophagus	Premalignant webs
Stomach	Atrophic gastritis
Small intestine	Malabsorption
Fingernails	Koilonychia
Lymphocytes	Poor function, leading to immunodeficiency
Heart	Hypertrophy
Muscle	Impaired endurance and ability to exercise
Brain	Decreased mentation
Catecholamine metabolism	Hypothermia

lignant lesion.[97,102–103] This syndrome has also been found to be associated with a variety of autoimmune disorders, including Sjögren's syndrome, Hashimoto's thyroiditis, and pernicious anemia, all of which are common in the elderly.[104–106] Patients may develop pagophagia,[107–108] or ice and starch eating, presumably as a mechanism for soothing irritated mucosal surfaces.[107–108]

The integrity of the gastric mucosa is affected adversely by a lack of iron. Iron deficiency is associated with a high frequency of atrophic gastritis. The loss of normal acid production in iron-deficient subjects may be secondary to the development of autoantibodies to gastric parietal cells.[104,109] Atrophic gastritis and achlorhydria seem to be reversible when iron is replaced before the age of 30, but the changes appear to be permanent when treatment occurs after that age.[110–111] Iron deficiency may also affect the mucosa of the small intestine; mucosal changes similar to those seen in sprue have been observed in children with iron deficiency anemia, however, the mucosa can revert to normal following iron replacement.[112]

There is evidence that adequate tissue levels of iron are necessary for normal growth and skeletal development. Iron-deficient children have been shown to be significantly underweight, and when iron was replaced, weight gain occurred.[113]

As previously mentioned, iron appears to be necessary to maintain the normal integrity of mitochondria, and when iron is deficient, gross abnormalities of mitochondrial structure are seen.[114,115] Mitochondria are found to be enlarged and to have cristae that are sparse, broken, deformed, and swollen. Inadequate tissue iron levels seem to be responsible for structural abnormalities of lymphocytes and may explain susceptibility to infection.[112]

Functional effects of iron deficiency Iron deficiency results in a decrease in work capacity out of proportion to the degree of anemia. The anemia compromises cardiovascular function by impairing the capacity to perform brief, intense forms of exercise as reflected by the VO_2max. Loss of iron at the cellular level results in a reduction in levels of muscle oxidative enzymes, resulting in impairment in the performance of endurance-type exercises.[116–124] Studies have shown that iron-deficient rats have impaired work performance even when the anemia is corrected by exchange transfusion. During exercise, possibly as a result of depletion in iron-containing mitochondrial enzymes (e.g., α-glycerophosphate oxidase), they accumulate excessive lactate which seems to impair physical activity.[125]

Iron deficiency predisposes individuals to certain infections. Decreases in both cellular immunity[126–130] and neutrophil function have been reported.[130–132]

In contrast to the evidence linking iron deficiency with a predisposition to infection, there are data suggesting that rapid correction of iron deficiency may promote certain bacterial and parasitic infections, particularly if iron-dextran[62,130,133–140] is used. In the tropics, where iron deficiency is widespread and life-threatening, it has been suggested that severely anemic patients be protected against malaria while they are being created with iron. In addition, such patients must be watched carefully for bacterial infections and treated aggressively if they occur. In otherwise healthy populations, there does not seem to be any reason to withhold iron therapy. However, in the very sick elderly, it is advisable to closely monitor for infection during treatment for iron deficiency. In those with active infections, it seems prudent to treat the infection first and to limit the use of parenteral iron-dextran.

There is considerable evidence linking iron deficiency to central nervous system (CNS) dysfunction in animals and humans.[60,62,141–162] Studies have been performed on younger people and animals, but to date there have been no studies on the elderly. Certainly iron deficiency should be treated in the elderly and should be tested for as part of the evaluation of a dementia or altered mental status.

Abnormalities in catecholamine metabolism and thermogenesis have been found in iron-deficient humans.[60,62,163–168] Elevated catecholamine levels have been reported in iron-deficient humans even in the absence of anemia. Additionally, impaired temperature maintenance has been demonstrated in iron-deficient individuals exposed to mild hypothermia.

Absorption of iron Normally, iron is absorbed by specific mucosal receptors located in the duodenum and upper jejunum. To be absorbed, iron must be in the form of heme, soluble ferrous salts, or ferric chelates.[60]

Heme is released by hydrolysis from food hemoglobin or myoglobin by HCl and intramural proteases. The heme is then auto-oxidized to hemin (ferri heme). Hemin enters upper mucosal cells intact, after which heme oxygenase releases the iron for entry into the bloodstream where it is bound to transferrin. Small amounts of heme may be carried by hemopexin directly to the bone marrow[169] (the alternate pool). With age the absorption of heme becomes increasingly important, emphasizing the need for heme-containing foods such as meat in the diet.[170–175]

Most food iron is in the form of ferric iron. For it to remain soluble and absorbable, HCl, reducing agents and low molecular weight weak chelates (such as sugars and amino acids) must be present.[176–179] In the absence of these factors, ferric hydroxide or insoluble complexes with phosphates and phytates form. Ferrous iron is actively transported into mucosal brush border cells by receptor-mediated endocytosis. Virtually no food iron is in the ferrous form, although medicinal iron is. Thus in achlorhydric older patients, there may be difficulty in absorbing food iron but not medicinal iron. Ascorbic acid has been shown to increase inorganic iron absorption in persons with iron deficiency,[180] and tea, coffee, pyhtates, and possibly calcium to reduce it. In the healthy elderly, iron absorption seems normal.[43,60]

Body iron is regulated within very narrow limits through iron absorption. It is hypothesized that an exchange equilibrium between transferrin iron and the iron content of mucosal cells regulates total body iron content.[80] Total body iron appears to rise modestly with increasing age. The average diet has 10 to 15 mg of iron, of which approximately 8 percent is absorbed.[61] A dietary deficiency of iron is extremely rare in the elderly, and takes 3 to 7 years to develop.[60,181]

Causes of iron deficiency in the elderly The diagnosis of iron deficiency in the absence of any history of hemorrhage should be taken as evidence of occult gastrointestinal bleeding, and gastrointestinal tract evaluations should be performed. Any hemorrhagic lesion of the gastrointestinal tract may be responsible. In a recent study by Rockey and Cello,[182] on 100 patients with iron deficiency anemia who underwent gastrointestinal examinations, an upper gastrointestinal tract bleeding source was found in 37 patients, 19 of which were peptic ulcers; colonoscopic lesions were found in 26, 11 of which were cancers.[182] There is some evidence that low serum ferritin, even in the absence of anemia, may be a useful aid in detecting patients harboring occult gastrointestinal tract lesions[183,184] and therefore might have some utility as a screening test for these lesions. In selected patients other sites of bleeding or malabsorption should be considered.

Treatment of iron deficiency anemia The first step is to find and to stop the source of bleeding. The iron deficiency is usually treated with oral ferrous iron.[55] Salts and enteric-coated or sustained-release preparations should be avoided, as they are not well absorbed. The simplest oral preparation is ferrous sulfate, 300 mg, which contains 60 mg of iron per tablet. One tablet taken three times a day, 1 hour before meals, supplies 180 mg of iron. As this preparation may cause constipation and gastric irritation, it is sometimes wise to begin with one tablet per day and increase the dose gradually over 1 to 2 weeks. Patients who are unable to tolerate ferrous sulfate because of gastrointestinal side effects may tolerate the iron polysaccharide complex (e.g., Niferex). Liquid preparations are available for those who are unable to swallow pills. It is important to appreciate that iron therapy may reduce the absorption of a wide variety of other drugs the patient may be taking, including L-dopa, ciprofloxacin, and thyroxine.[185,186] Response to treatment is monitored by hemoglobin, hematocrit, and ferritin levels, and it usually requires 6 months or more to replenish iron stores if bleeding has stopped (to restore the ferritin to normal). Hemoglobin and hematocrit levels can be raised to their normal levels in 2 months. In the patient who has severe malabsorption, who cannot tolerate oral iron, whose iron stores need rapid replenishing, or who has active bleeding, parenteral iron may be best.[55] Parenteral iron is available as iron-dextran and can be given intravenously or by deep intramuscular injection. This therapy has been associated with anaphylactic shock, and a test dose of 0.5 ml should be given before treatment begins. The maximum recommended dose is 2.0 ml per day (intravenously), which delivers 100 mg of iron (using IV Fed, as available in the US). Intravenous infusion should proceed no faster than at a rate of 1 ml/min. Side effects of iron-dextran include pain at the injection site, fever, and arthralgias. Intramuscular injections have been found under experimental conditions to produce sarcomas in various animals. The most expensive and potentially hazardous way to replete iron, of course, is by transfusion. Each milliliter of transfused red blood cells delivers 1 mg of iron.

Other causes of microcytic anemia

Anemias caused by abnormal hemoglobins (e.g., sickle cell anemia) are usually not first diagnosed in old age but obviously may be. Thalassemia minor, since it is asymptomatic, may first be found in old age. Thalassemia minor occurs in individuals who are heterozygous for genes that produce none or very little of the α- or β-hemoglobin chain. These conditions result in either microcytosis without anemia or a mild microcytic anemia with hypochromia, target cells, anisocytosis, poikilocytosis, polychromatophilia, and basophilic stippling of red blood cells on the peripheral blood smear. There is no reticulocytosis, and serum iron, TIBC, and ferritin are all normal. Hemoglobin electrophoresis may reveal an increase in the minor hemoglobins, A_2 and F, and in β-thalassemia, but in α-thalassemia no increase in these hemoglobins is seen. No treatment is usually required for these conditions. Iron therapy is contraindicated as it may produce iron overload.[58]

The anemia of chronic disease may be microcytic, but it is more commonly normocytic and will be discussed along with the normocytic anemias. Sideroblastic anemia may be microcytic, normocytic, or even macrocytic and will be discussed in the section on myelodysplastic syndromes.

Normocytic Anemias

Anemia of chronic disease

The most common normocytic (MCV 80 to 100 fl) anemia in the elderly is the anemia secondary to other chronic diseases. The anemia is mild to moderate, with variable hypochromia and hypoferremia despite abundant stores of iron in the body.[187] Approximately one-half of these anemias are caused by chronic inflammatory disorders such as infection, and the other half are caused by neoplasms. ACD is about 40 percent as common as iron deficiency anemia in people of European extraction of all ages.[188] It is probably more common in older people, as they have more chronic diseases.

Within 1 to 2 months of onset of a chronic inflammation or neoplasm, a modest anemia develops which tends to correlate in severity with the underlying disease but never progresses to severe anemia. Typically, hematocrit levels decline to about 30 to 40 percent (average about 34 percent).[189] The anemia is usually normocytic and in more than 50 percent of cases is hypochromic. Occasionally microcytosis is seen. The most characteristic pathogenic change is impairment of iron flow from the macrophage to the plasma.

In ACD, apoferritin synthesis by mononuclear phagocytes is increased by a cytokine (probably interleukin-1 [IL-1]).[190–192] This excess apoferritin directs newly mobilized iron to the storage pool, thereby blocking its release from the macrophage. The red cell precursors are then prevented from obtaining the iron necessary to form heme and hemoglobin. In addition, lactoferrin is released into the plasma from neutrophils during inflammation. Plasma lactoferrin binds to specific receptors on macrophages and competes with transferrin for iron,[193] which certainly contributes to the movement of iron away from the bone marrow and into storage in macrophages of the reticuloendothelial system.[194] This shifting of iron into storage is thought to represent a primitive immune mechanism for starving pathogens of necessary iron.[190–195]

Another factor that plays a role in the pathogenesis of ACD includes a modest reduction of erythrocyte survival without an adequate compensatory increase in the rate of red cell production. The reduced red blood cell survival is probably related to an increase in phagocytic activity by activated macrophages. IL-1 (which is increased in many chronic conditions) is also believed to act on T lymphocytes to produce γ-interferon which is believed to directly inhibit erythroid colony forming units.[196] Tumor necrosis factor is likewise felt to inhibit erythroid colony forming units in some cases. Erythropoietin secretion often appears to be less than optimal, and administration of this hormone results in an increasing hematocrit in certain individuals.[196]

Diagnosis of ACD In addition to the mild anemia and hypochromia, the reticulocyte count is also low. Serum iron is low, and in contrast to the situation in iron deficiency, so is iron binding capacity (transferrin levels). Serum ferritin is elevated, and bone marrow shows abundant iron.

Treatment of ACD Since the anemia is usually mild to moderate, no treatment is necessary in most instances. Occasionally blood transfusion may hasten the healing of wounds and stubborn infections. As a rule, however, the hazards of transfusion outweigh any potential benefits. Certain groups of patients for example, HIV-infected patients with severe anemia on zidovudine and with erythropoetin levels less than 500 mUnits/ml may respond to erythropoetin.[196] Unless the underlying disease is accompanied by iron deficiency, the administration of oral iron or parenteral iron is contraindicated. Hypoferremia does not appear to be dangerous and may represent a beneficial response on the body's part to protect against infection.[60,62,190,195] The only therapy usually necessary is treating the underlying inflammation or neoplasm.

Anemia of renal disease

In renal insufficiency a normochromic anemia develops which is very similar to ACD. In this condition there is a deficiency of erythropoietin production,[197] and there is evidence that the administration of erythropoietin, when the anemia is severe, can partially improve the condition. Improvement is usually not complete, as nonspecific substances accumulate in renal insufficiency that suppress hematopoiesis.[198,199] In addition, specific inhibitors may accumulate in uremia.[200,201] However, in patients on hemodialysis, erythropoietin is very effective in correcting the anemia, as these inhibitors are removed. It is important to correct any concomitant nutritional deficiencies such as those involving iron or folic acid, which are common in renal disease. In rare cases blood transfusions may be necessary to protect the patient's cardiovascular status.

Anemia of liver disease

In liver diseases a normocytic or macrocytic anemia develops. There are many causes of anemia in liver disease, including bleeding, iron deficiency, folate deficiency, hypersplenism, and sideroblastic anemia. Even when these are excluded, anemia is often present that is similar to ACD. In liver disease, however, serum iron is increased and there is an increase in transferrin saturation. Serum ferritin is also increased and often reflects total body iron overload.[202]

Anemia of endocrine disorders

Endocrine disorders that commonly produce anemia are hypothyroidism, hypopituitarism, and adrenal insufficiency. In all three cases the anemia is normocytic and normochromic but may be macrocytic. Hypothyroidism is commonly complicated by iron deficiency,[203] resulting in microcytosis and hypochromia, or by associated megaloblastic anemia,[204] in which the cells are macrocytic and normochromic. Unless a specific deficiency of iron, vitamin B_{12}, or folate is identified, the therapy for the anemia is again that for the underlying disorder.

Anemia of scurvy

Most scorbutic patients are anemic, and the anemia is usually normocytic and normochromic. Hypochromic microcytic anemia may also occur as a result of associated iron deficiency and blood loss. The bone marrow is normoblastic and hyperplastic. In rare cases, it is megaloblastic and the peripheral cells are macrocytic as a result of associated folate deficiency (malnutrition).

The anemia is due to impaired erythropoiesis but shortened red cell life span, and blood loss perhaps contributes. Ascorbic acid therapy produces a reticulocytosis and corrects the anemia. In some patients, there is also an associated iron deficiency, and these individuals should be treated with iron and ascorbic acid given simultaneously. If folate deficiency is present, folate should be added.

Protein malnutrition

Protein deficiency alone does not usually cause anemia but may be one factor in a situation predisposing to anemia (e.g., renal disease or cirrhosis).

Anemia of collagen-vascular diseases

ACD appears in collagen vascular diseases such as rheumatoid arthritis, polyarteritis, dermatomyositis, systemic lupus erythematosus, and temporal arteritis (including polymyalgia rheumatica). The latter is essentially a disease of geriatric patients. The anemia responds to steroid treatment as well as the entire symptom complex does.

"Unexplained anemia" of the elderly

A mild, normochromic, normocytic anemia with a hemoglobin concentration usually between 11 and 12 g/dl has been reported in people over the age of 70. This anemia cannot be accounted for by any underlying disease or deficiency, and the bone marrow does not contain ringed sideroblasts. This unexplained anemia is said to account for over 30 percent of the anemias in this age group.[126] It is associated with low neutrophil, lymphocyte, and platelet counts, and there is an increased red blood cell 2,3-DPG level, implying that this condition is not merely a normal age-related variant. The significance of this type of anemia is presently unknown, but it is probably a myelodysplastic syndrome.

Hemolytic Anemias

Frank hemolytic anemias are not common in the elderly, even though a shortened red cell survival is found in various types of anemia. The hereditary forms of hemolytic anemias are usually diagnosed in childhood or in early adolescence and are discussed in any standard textbook of hematology.

Acquired hemolytic anemia (i.e., hemolysis not due to congenital abnormalities of the red blood cell) is a normochromic, normocytic anemia which can occur at any age. The incidence of this disorder increases with advancing age. Peripheral destruction of red cells results in increased production of young red cells by the bone marrow, resulting in an increased reticulocyte count and polychromatophilia on the peripheral blood smear. As reticulocytes are larger than mature red cells, if the reticulocytosis is brisk enough, the indexes may become macrocytic. Red cell destruction results in increased serum unconjugated bilirubin, serum glutamic oxaloacetic transaminase (SGOT), and lactate dehydrogenase (LDH) decreased serum haptoglobin, and increased urine urobilinogen. If the hemolysis is intravascular, urine hemosiderin is increased as well. The direct antiglobulin test (Coombs' test) is used to detect antibody and/or complement on the red blood cell, and it can also identify the antigen to which the antibody is reacting.[205]

Causes of acquired hemolytic anemia

Idiopathic autoimmune hemolysis may be a result of warm-reaction antibodies of the IgG class or cold agglutinins which are usually of the IgM class. Idiopathic cold agglutinin disease is primarily a disease of old age. At times the cold agglutinin may be of the IgG class, or a nonagglutinin may be found.

Immune hemolysis may also be secondary to a variety of other illnesses. Approximately 30 percent of secondary immune hemolytic anemias are caused by lymphoproliferative diseases, including chronic lymphocytic leukemia, non-Hodgkin's lymphoma, Hodgkin's disease, and multiple myeloma. Agnogenic myeloid metaplasia, systemic lupus erythematosus, viral infections, mycoplasma pneumoniae infection, syphilis, and various nonhematologic malignancies are also associated with immune hemolytic anemia. This condition is more common in women, and the incidence of the secondary varieties rises with age.[206]

Another major cause of hemolytic anemia is a drug reaction. The elderly are more prone to develop this problem simply because they generally take more medications than younger individuals. Several types of drug-induced hemolysis have been described.[207–208]

Methyldopa causes autoantibody formation with antibodies directed against normal red blood cell antigens (usually Rh antigens) and is reported to occur in 10 to 40 percent of people taking the drug. These antibodies attach to the red blood cell, resulting in a positive direct Coombs' test against IgG. Less than 1 percent of these people actually develop hemolysis, however.[207,208] Discontinuation of the drug usually results in correction of the anemia, but autoantibodies may persist for months to years. Other drugs that in rare cases produce autoimmune hemolysis include ibuprofen, L-dopa, and procainamide. It is known that methyldopa inhibits T-suppressor cells both in vitro and in vivo.[209] The drug apparently causes a rise in lymphocyte cyclic AMP, which is believed to then cause the T-cell abnormality. This decrease in T-suppressor cells is thought to result in unregulated autoantibody production by a subset of B cells in some individuals. Those with HLA-B_7 seem to be at greatest risk. Total T-cells decrease in patients who have this positive antibody test.

A second type of drug-induced hemolytic anemia results when the drug binds to the surface of the red cell, acting as a hapten and eliciting an immune response. Antibodies, usually IgG, are made against the drug-red blood cell complex.[208] The direct Coomb's test is positive, and the indirect Coombs' test is positive as well. The most common drugs producing this problem are penicillin and the cephalosporins. The anemia clears when the drug is discontinued.

The third type of drug-induced immune hemolytic anemia occurs when a drug, either alone or bound to a plasma protein, stimulates the production of antibodies to the drug.[210] Drug antibody immune complexes form in the circulation and bind to the red blood cell. Intravascular hemolysis occurs because the complex activates on the red blood cell surface. The Coombs' test is positive for complement but not for IgG. The drugs most commonly associated with this type of hemolysis are sulfonamides, quinidine, quinine, and insulin, although many medications can produce this phenomenon. Again, hemolysis stops when the drug is discontinued.

Treatment of autoimmune hemolytic anemia

Idiopathic autoimmune hemolysis secondary to warm-reaction antibodies of the IgG class responds to steroid therapy approximately 75 percent of the time.[211] Prednisone in a dose of 60 mg/d in divided doses is the initial treatment, although occasionally 100 mg is needed. A rise in the hemoglobin and hematocrit and a drop in the reticulocyte count usually occur in the first 3 to 14 days, but the response may be delayed by as much as 8 weeks. Once remission occurs, steroids may be tapered by 5 mg/wk, but relapse requires increasing the dose by 15 to 20 mg followed by a more gradual taper in dose. Some patients continue to require a small daily dose or alternate – day therapy for long periods of time. If there is no response to 60 mg of prednisone per day after 4 to 8 weeks, higher doses may be tried or the blocked androgen, danazol, may be added at a dose of 200 mg two to four times a day.[212–214] If therapy still fails, the next step is usually splenectomy, which results in long-term remission in 50 to 75 percent of cases.[214] For patients who either do not respond to the above measures or are poor surgical candidates, immunosuppressive agents cyclo phosphamide or azathioprine may be useful.[215] Most patients with warm antibody immune hemolysis do not require transfusion, but for those who are extremely symptomatic because of their anemia, transfusion can be considered. Cross-matching blood is problematic, and the autoantibodies of course reduce the survival of the transfused red blood cells. Plasmapheresis is usually not successful, as IgG has a very large distribution in the body, but has been reported to work sometimes.

Idiopathic cold agglutinin disease due to IgM requires avoidance of exposure to the cold. Steroids and splenectomy are usually not useful, although they have been used with some success in small numbers of patients with disease due to either low-titer IgM or to IgG.[205,214] Plasmapheresis may provide temporary improvement, as the IgM is confined to the intravascular space.[216,217] Disease caused by cold-activated IgG hemolysin is also treated by avoiding exposure to the cold. In both diseases, transfusion should be done with washed red blood cells that have been warmed. Immune hemolytic anemia secondary to other diseases usually improves only with treatment of the underlying disease. If this strategy is not possible, therapy may be tried as described above, but success is less likely than in idiopathic disease.

As stated previously, treatment of drug-induced hemolytic anemia usually consists of simply discontinuing the responsible medication. In rare instances, methyldopa autoimmune hemolysis continues long enough to require a course of steroids as described above.

Occasionally intravascular hemolysis may be due to trauma, such as in patients with prosthetic heart valves or prolonged marching, and treatment in these patients should focus on the etiology.

Macrocytic Anemias

Macrocytic anemia is described as an anemia in which the MCV is greater than 100 fl. MCV increases slightly with increasing age but usually not enough to produce significant macrocytosis.[10] Relatively few disorders routinely result in macrocytic anemia (Table 89-2). The two common disorders that produce macrocytosis are megaloblastic anemias due to either vitamin B_{12} or folate deficiency.

Vitamin B_{12} deficiency

Vitamin B_{12} (also known as cobalamin) deficiency, has been reported to account for up to 9 percent of anemias in elderly populations. Vitamin B_{12} is found in most animal tissues but not in plants. A normal diet contains up to 5 to 30 μg/d. Vitamin B_{12} is stable in normal cooking and most of it is available from absorption, but only 2 μg can be absorbed from a single meal, as this is the limit for the ileal receptors.[218] B_{12} loss from the body is very small, being only about 0.1 to 0.2 percent of the total B_{12} pool daily regardless of the size of the pool.[219] Once absorbed, B_{12} is stored in the liver, which normally contains over 1 mg of the vitamin. Other organs also store this vitamin, so that total body B_{12} is 2 to 5 mg.[220,221] As a person becomes B_{12}-deficient, less B_{12} is lost than in normal people and less is required to maintain the steady state. This may explain why in latent B_{12} deficiency (B_{12} depletion) with mild malabsorption of B_{12}, an overt megaloblastic anemia may not occur (see below).

Vitamin B_{12} is usually absorbed by active transport with intrinsic factor (IF). Vitamin B_{12} in nature is always bound to R proteins (cobalophilin), which are present in virtually all body secretions as well as in food. R proteins are so named because they have rapid electrophoretic mobility, as contrasted to IF which has slow (S) mobility.

The cobalamin R complex is degraded partially in the stomach by acid peptic digestion and partially in the upper small intestine by pancreatic enzymes,[222] thus allowing formation of the cobalamin-IF complex. IF, a glycoprotein of 50,000 molecular weight, is secreted by the gastric parietal cells and binds cobalamin after it has been released from its R binder by digestive action. Once IF binds cobalamin, the IF-cobalamin complex travels to the terminal ileum where there are specific receptor binding sites for IF.[223,224] As the cobalamin-IF complex crosses the intestinal mucosa, IF is lost and cobalamin is transferred to the cellular R proteins.[224]

The second mechanism available for the absorption of cobalamin involves simple diffusion of the vitamin within the lumen of the gut. This process accounts for only 1 to 3 percent of the absorption of cobalamin under normal circumstances but may increase in significance when larger amounts of free vitamin are ingested. This situation might occur when pharmacologic, not physiologic, doses of vitamin B_{12} are being ingested. However, with usual dietary intake, if IF is absent, a deficiency of B_{12} eventually occurs.

Even though only 2 to 5 μg of cobalamin is absorbed daily, because of an extremely efficient enterohepatic circulation which recycles vitamin B_{12} from bile and other intestinal secretions,[225,226] the daily loss is only about 1 to 2 μg/d (half-life of cobalamin in the body is about 1,360 days). In fact, in cases of pure IF deficiency, such as after total gastrectomy, it may take up to 3 to 5 years to become overtly B_{12}-deficient.

TCII is the dominant carrier of vitamin B_{12} immediately after its absorption and separation from IF.[227–229] The complex is rapidly cleared from the plasma and taken up by the tissues. TCI and TCIII are thought to be the storage proteins. The physiologic transporter TCII is responsible for about 25 percent of the cobalamin circulating in plasma, and the rest is on other transcobalamins.[230–232] Once inside the cell, B_{12} is converted to methylcobalamin and adenosylcobalamin.[223] Adenosylcobalamin is the coenzyme of L-methylmalonyl-CoA mutase, an enzyme catalyzing the first step in the pathway of propionic acid metabolism, in which methylmalonyl-CoA is converted to succinyl-CoA. Thus, B_{12} deficiency leads to an increase in methylmalonic acid. Methylcobalamin is the coenzyme for methionine synthase needed to convert homocysteine to methionine. In the absence of B_{12}, homocysteine levels also increase. It is unclear whether deficient activity in one or both of these enzyme systems results in the neurologic abnormalities seen in B_{12} deficiency. The conversion of 5-methyltetrahydrofolate (which is how folate is stored in the body) to tetrahydrofolate is coupled to B_{12}, requiring conversion of homocysteine to methionine. Tetrahydrofolate is then converted to 5,10-methylene tetrahydrofolate which is necessary for thymidylate and DNA synthesis. Thus, a deficiency of either B_{12} or folate leads to deficient DNA synthesis and to subsequent hematologic manifestation of megaloblastosis.[233]

Vitamin B_{12} is stored in the liver in large quantities, so that after a lesion occurs that prevents B_{12} absorption, it takes many years to develop a B_{12} deficiency. For this reason, patients who are B_{12}-deficient may present with profound anemias which are well tolerated, with no volume depletion or orthostatic hypotension. In fact, these patients will be at risk for the development of congestive heart failure if they are transfused.

Etiology of vitamin B_{12} deficiency

PERNICIOUS ANEMIA (AUTOIMMUNE DISEASE) This anemia is the classically described cause of cobalamin deficiency. There is an overall prevalence of 1 percent occurring equally in men and women. It is more common in Scandinavians but can be found in any ethnic or racial group; it is usually diagnosed in people aged 60 or over.

Pernicious anemia appears to be an autoimmune disease with production of antibodies directed against gastric parietal cells and IF. It occurs more frequently in people who have another autoimmune disease, such as hypothyroidism, Graves' disease, Addison's disease, vitiligo, or hypoparathyroidism. Symptoms of pernicious anemia may be no more specific than fatigue due to profound anemia. Characteristically, however, patients develop glossitis with a smooth red tongue, mild jaundice, and neurologic changes. The neurologic findings include paresthesias, abnormal position and vibration sensation, gait ataxia due to degeneration of the posterolateral columns of the spinal cord, and various psychiatric disorders. These neurologic changes are not always corrected when the deficiency is treated.[50]

Laboratory abnormalities accompanying pernicious anemia include macrocytosis and hypersegmented polymorphonuclear leukocytes on the peripheral blood smear and increased serum bilirubin and LDH due to ineffective erythropoiesis. The platelet count and white blood cell count may be reduced, and the serum vitamin B_{12} level is low. Approximately 30 percent of patients with B_{12} deficiency have elevated serum folate levels. The bone marrow, if examined, will show characteristic megaloblastic changes.[233]

In pernicious anemia, there is a deficiency of IF produced in the stomach, resulting in malabsorption of cobalamin. The Schilling test,[50] which measures the oral absorption of radiolabeled vitamin B_{12} with and without the addition of oral IF, differentiates between pernicious anemia and other causes of B_{12} deficiency such as malabsorption and bacterial intestinal overgrowth. In pernicious anemia, the absorption of oral B_{12} alone is abnormal but can be corrected with IF. If absorption is not corrected with IF, the patient is treated for a few weeks with a broad-spectrum antibiotic and the test is then repeated. If absorption becomes normal, the problem is bacterial overgrowth. If the patient really has pernicious anemia and has been B_{12}-deficient for some time, however, they may malabsorb B_{12} because of malfunction of the small intestine as a result of B_{12} deficiency. To test this possibility, the patient should have the Schilling test repeated after a few months of B_{12}

Neuropsychiatric manifestations usually found in vitamin B_{12} deficiency

- Myelopathy
  - Posterior column disease
    - Acroparesthesias and other sensory disturbances
    - Poor coordination
    - Diminished vibration and/or position sense
    - Ataxia
    - Diminished deep tendon reflexes
  - Lateral column disease
    - Weakness
  - Spinothalamic tract
    - Nocturnal cramping in arms and legs
- Brain
  - Dementia
  - Personality changes (apathy, irritability, emotional instability)
  - Depression
  - Disturbances in taste and smell

supplementation. If it is still abnormal, the patient has intestinal malabsorption.[50] Treatment of B_{12} deficiency often requires lifetime parenteral B_{12} administration. Although 100 μg intramuscularly daily for the first 5 days is sufficient, it is usually more convenient to give 1,000 μg daily for the first week, then weekly for 4 weeks or until the hemocrit is normal, and then monthly for life. There is some evidence that daily doses of vitamin B_{12} (1,000 μg) per day orally may be sufficient therapy, with enough B_{12} being absorbed even in the absence of IF.[234] The response to treatment is usually evidenced by a brisk reticulocytosis within 1 week. While the anemia should be corrected within 1 month, peripheral blood smear abnormalities, particularly hypersegmented neutrophils, may persist for 1 year. Hypokalemia and hypophosphatemia may occur early in therapy, and serum phosphate and potassium should be monitored and supplementation given if necessary. Transfusion may produce volume overload, and if necessary, should be given slowly with careful monitoring of the patient. It should also be noted that misdiagnosis of B_{12} deficiency as folate deficiency and consequent treatment with folate alone may improve the hematologic disorder but does not treat the neurologic changes of B_{12} deficiency. It is, therefore, to be avoided at all costs.

Patients with pernicious anemia have been shown to be at increased risk of cancer of the stomach (2.9 standardized incidence ratio in a recent Swedish study), gastric carcinoids, and possibly other cancers as well.[235] Surveillance upper endoscopy can help locate tumors while they are still curable: two small gastric adenocarcinomas as well as two gastric carcinoids were found in 56 patients undergoing gastroscopy in a Finnish study.[236] The role, frequency, and cost of routine endoscopy is still being debated; however, all patients should clearly receive stool occult blood testing and endoscopy for any gastrointestinal symptoms.

Another frequent cause of vitamin B_{12} deficiency in the elderly is an inability to free B_{12} from its binding to dietary proteins. HCl and pepsin contribute to the release of cobalmin from dietary proteins so that B_{12} can bind to IF and thus be available for absorption. If there is a lack of either HCl or pepsin, B_{12} is not liberated from the protein and therefore not bound to IF. These patients have a normal Schilling test, as the B_{12} in the test is free and not bound to protein. It has been shown that Omeprazole, a potent inhibitor of gastric acid secretion, decreases B_{12} absorption.[237] It has also been demonstrated that about 30 percent of patients with a history of gastric surgery will become B_{12}-deficient.[238] Patients with B_{12} deficiency due to a lack of HCl can be treated with oral vitamin B_{12} pills on an empty stomach, as the B_{12} is free and not bound and therefore will be available to bind with IF.

Other causes of B_{12} deficiency such as such bacterial overgrowth and ileal diseases may occur as well and have been alluded to above.

Low serum B_{12} levels in the elderly–relationship to dementia The dementia of vitamin B_{12} deficiency can be identical to that of Alzheimer's disease. The most important unanswered questions in vitamin B_{12} research concern the frequency of dementia induced by cobalamin deficiency and how often neuropsychiatric changes occur in the absence of any hematologic abnormalities. These questions are still incompletely answered, but recent work has shown that 30 percent or more of patients with B_{12} deficiency and neuropsychiatric abnormalities that respond to B_{12} therapy have normal hemoglobin levels and MCVs.[239,240] It has also been suggested that patients whose duration of symptoms is less than 1 year have better responses to therapy than those whose cognitive deficits have lasted more than 1 year, suggesting a possible time-limited window of opportunity for maximum effect of therapy.[239]

It is generally agreed that patients with organic brain syndrome, unexplained psychosis, unexplained peripheral neuropathy, prior gastrectomy, hypersegmentation of the neutrophils on the peripheral blood smear, or unexplained macrocytosis should be tested for vitamin B_{12} deficiency. It has been demonstrated that sole reliance on these criteria may result in cases of B_{12} deficiency being missed.[241] The absence of an elevated MCV, which was previously felt to be a hallmark of B_{12} deficiency, has now been described by a number of authors.[239,240,242–245] RDW has been proposed as a useful screening test for B_{12} deficiency[246–247]; however, this deficiency does occur in patients with normal RDWs.[248] Hypersegmentation on the blood smear is more useful than either MCV or RDW as a screen for B_{12} deficiency.[243,248]

About 8 percent of patients hospitalized on an inpatient medical service had low serum vitamin B_{12} levels.[242,249,250] This included people who were elderly, but also younger people, particularly those with acquired immunodeficiency syndrome (AIDS).[241]

In an ambulatory elderly population, low serum vitamin B_{12} is found in 3 to 21 percent of those tested. In two studies, a 3 percent incidence was reported.[251,252] Other studies found the incidence to be about 7 percent.[253–255] Even higher incidences have been reported,[256–260] including 21.3 percent in people with early signs and symptoms of dementia.[261] The observation that holotranscobalamin II levels decline with age and that the percentage of vitamin B_{12} binding to transcobalamin II is less suggests that low serum B_{12} truly represents a body deficiency of cobalamin.[253] Demonstrations that B_{12} levels, holotranscobalamin II, and binding of B_{12} to transcobalamin II are lower in some people with dementia,[261,262] and that in these patients an abnormal deoxyuridine suppression test[250] or elevated methylmalonic acid and homocysteine levels[243] are found, and most importantly that some patients with cobalamin deficiency, neuropychiatric abnormalities, normal hemoglobin, and mean red cell volumes improved with cobalamin replacement[239,240] are strong evidence that in some people the symptoms of B_{12} deficiency are neuropsychiatric rather than hematologic.[261]

Evaluation of a low serum vitamin B_{12} level Low serum vitamin B_{12} levels are frequently not investigated.[242,263] As the consequences of B_{12} deficiency can be devastating, all low serum cobalamin levels should be further evaluated.

Gallium scans, red cell mass tests, thyroid scans, ^{32}P treatment, and bone scans can falsely elevate the radioactivity count and produce a falsely low B_{12} value. Other causes of falsely low B_{12} levels include pregnancy, folate deficiency, ingestion of high doses of absorbic acid, and multiple myeloma.[264,265] Numerous tests have been proposed to investigate low B_{12} levels, including Schilling and food Schilling tests, serum methylmalonic acid and homocysteine levels, deoxyuridine suppression testing of bone marrow, tests for anti-IF antibody assays, and holotranscobalamin II and transcobalamin II saturation with B_{12}.

Schilling tests are frequently used to evaluate low serum vitamin B_{12} levels. The two-stage Schilling test is superior to the one-stage test.[266] Carmel et al.[267] have recently shown that the food Schilling test is frequently abnormal in patients with a low B_{12} level and a normal fasting Schilling test. It appears that many elderly patients are unable to split off B_{12} from the R proteins in food because of either hypochlorhydria or pancreatic insufficiency. One of the biggest problems with Schilling tests is accurate collection of 24-hour urine specimens. This is especially problematic in geriatric patients who may experience urinary incontinence or have cognitive difficulties.

Both methylmalonic acid and homocysteine serum levels increase with vitamin B_{12} deficiency.[243] In a study by Savage et al.[268] only 1 patient out of over 400 patients with cobalamin deficiency had normal levels of both metabolites, 98 percent had elevation of methylmalonic acid levels, and 96 percent had elevated homocysteine levels. In a study by Stabler et al.[240] only 5 patients out of 86 who responded to cobalamin therapy did not have an elevated level of one of these metabolites, and these patients had an improvement in only one out of four parameters assessed.[240] Testing for these metabolite levels has therefore become very valuable in assessing patients' cobalamin status. Methylmalonic acid levels may also be elevated in renal insufficiency. Homocysteine levels may be increased in folate deficiency, pyridoxine deficiency, or renal insufficiency[269] or because of a variety of genetic defects.

The deoxyuridine suppression test of bone marrow DNA synthesis is felt to be a reliable measure of vitamin B_{12} status.[270,271] Carmel et al.[267] described 18 patients with abnormal deoxyuridine suppression levels, all of whom had normal levels of methylmalonic acid and homocysteine in their urine and only one of whom had a hypersegmented blood smear. Some patients had abnormal Schilling tests, and abnormal food Schilling tests were even more common. Two patients with normal test results had abnormal results 1 year later. Thus, deoxyuridine suppression tests appear to be useful in diagnosing metabolic abnormalities early in the course of B_{12} deficiency. The main disadvantage of the test is that it requires a bone marrow examination and is still restricted to special laboratories. If developed commercially, it is likely to be more expensive than serum measurement of methylmalonic acid or homocysteine. The specificity of the test seems to be excellent,[272] although there is some suggestion that malnutrition and certain drugs may cause false positive results.[273,274]

Antibodies to gastric parietal cells and to IF are common in classic autoimmune pernicious anemia. Parietal cell antibodies lack sufficient specificity to be useful; antibodies to IF are quite specific for pernicious anemia but have a sensitivity of only about 50 percent.[275] A positive test is very helpful, but a negative test should prompt further investigation. It is not known how many patients with low vitamin B_{12} levels have early autoimmune pernicious anemia. Many of these elderly people may not be able to absorb food B_{12} secondary to hypochlorhydria or a decrease in pancreatic enzymes and may never show anti-IF antibodies.

The stages of vitamin B_{12} deficiency One of the most intriguing developments in the study of vitamin B_{12} deficiency has been the recent model presented by Herbert.[276] It is proposed that there are four stages in the development of B_{12} deficiency: negative B_{12} balance,[277,278] B_{12} depletion, B_{12}-deficient erythropoiesis, and B_{12} deficiency anemia (Table 89-7). The first two stages are characterized by reduced holotranscobalamin II and decreased transcobalamin II saturation. The deoxyuridine suppression test is said to be normal, there is no hypersegmentation, and the methylmalonic acid level is normal. In the stage of B_{12}-deficient erythropoiesis, hypersegmentation of neutrophils occurs and the deoxyuridine suppression test becomes abnormal. Holotranscobalamin II and transcobalamin II saturation fall further. The patient's hemoglobin and MCV are still normal, and methylmalonic acid may or may not be increased. Only in the final stage does the patient become anemic and develop an elevated MCV. The model makes intuitive sense and has received some preliminary support, but as the authors acknowledge, it remains to be tested in a sufficiently large patient group.[276–278]

One of the most important questions related to this model concerns the stage at which myelin and brain damage occur. If it can occur prior to the development of hypersegmentation and methylmalonic acid elevation, this strongly argues for screening all elderly for B_{12} levels and ordering holotranscobalamin II levels and transcobalamin II saturations for all those with low or borderline results. Another important question is whether all patients who are in negative B_{12} balance or in the stage of B_{12} depletion will proceed to B_{12}-deficient erythropoiesis, neurologic damage, and dementia if untreated. This is an especially important question in regard to the elderly, as transcobalamin II saturation is low in many patients, even those with normal B_{12} levels.[253]

Elevated homocysteine levels have been associated with both arterial[279–281] and venous[280,282] occlusive disease. Naurath et al.[283] have shown that treating patients with elevated homocysteine levels with a mixture of vitamin B_{12}, folate, and pyridoxine, even in the absence of lowered pretreatment values of these vitamins, often lowers the homocysteine level. The question of routine screening of the elderly for elevated homocysteine levels must therefore be raised.

Current recommendations

1. We recommend screening all older adults for vitamin B_{12} deficiency. Many patients with this deficiency have normal

Table 89-7 Proposed four stages of vitamin B_{12} deficiency

Stage	Vitamin B_{12} Level	Holo-transcobalamin Levels	Transcobalamin II-B_{12} Binding	Methylmalonic Acid and Homocysteine Levels	Hypersegmented Neutrophils	Thymidine Uptake in DUST	Schilling Test	Mean Cell Volume	Hemoglobin
1. Negative vitamin B_{12} balance	Low normal	Normal	Normal	Normal	None	Normal	Normal	Normal	Normal
2. Vitamin B_{12} depletion	Low	Low	Low	Normal	None	Normal	Normal	Normal	Normal
3. Vitamin B_{12}-deficient hematopoiesis	Low	Low	Low	High	Few	High	Normal	Normal	Normal
4. Vitamin B_{12} deficiency anemia	Low	Low	Low	High	Many	High	Abnormal	High	Low

Abbreviation: DUST, deoxyuridine suppression test.

hemoglobin and MCVs, and the cognitive dysfunction associated with B_{12} deficiency may have only a short, time-limited window of opportunity for optimal response to therapy.[239] Elevated homocysteine levels, often found in B_{12} deficiency, have been associated with both arterial[279–201] and venous[280,282] occlusive disease. Patients with low B_{12} levels have been shown to have impaired antibody response to pneumococcal vaccine.[284] The above data suggest that all older patients may benefit from screening.

2. Serum vitamin B_{12} levels should be used in routine screening of elderly patients. A B_{12} of less than 350 pg/ml should be taken as evidence that further screening is required.[269] A study by Pennypacker et al.[285] in an outpatient geriatric clinic found elevated methylmalonic acid or homocysteine levels in 56 percent of patients with B_{12} levels from 201 to 300 pg/ml, compared to 62 percent of patients with lower serum cobalamin levels (less than or equal to 200 pg/ml),[285] suggesting that the higher level should be used as the cutoff value for patients requiring further screening.
3. These patients with B_{12} levels less than 350 pg/ml should then have their serum methylmalonic acid and homocysteine levels measured. An elevation to greater than three standard deviations above the mean in normal subjects is highly suspicious for vitamin B_{12} deficiency.[268]
4. Some patients have elevated metabolite levels due to other causes. Methylmalonic acid levels may be elevated in renal insufficiency, and homocysteine levels may be increased in folate deficiency, pyridoxine deficiency, renal insufficiency,[269] and a variety of genetic defects; therefore in the appropriate context these causes should be sought. A reduction to normal or to less than 50 percent of the pretreatment value of the metabolites is usually found in cobalamin-responsive patients.[240]
5. The use of further testing such as a Schilling test or determining anti-IF antibodies should be determined on an individual basis.

Issues that require further information include the following:

1. Some patients with vitamin B_{12} levels greater than 300 pg/ml have elevated methylmalonic acid and homocysteine levels. In the study by Pennypacker et al.[285] seven subjects who met these criteria and were treated with B_{12} had decreases in their metabolite levels.[285] Whether patients with these metabolite levels should be screened and their responses to therapy routinely monitored is an important issue.
2. Many patients with vitamin B_{12} levels less than 200 pg/ml have normal serum metabolites, for example, 38 percent in the study by Pennypacker et al.[285] In rare cases patients with low B_{12} levels and normal serum metabolites seem to respond to B_{12} therapy (see section on evaluation above). It is not clear what the best test is for detecting these occasional patients. Perhaps they should be tested with a peripheral blood smear looking for hypersegmented polymorphonuclear leukocytes and macrovalocytes, bone marrow biopsy, or trial of therapy, or perhaps they do not warrant any further tests for B_{12} deficiency as long as no other strong indicators of underlying B_{12} deficiency are present. It is not known whether the response of these rare patients was just due to random variations in test results and was not a true response, as might be suggested by the fact that the five cobalamin-responsive patients who had normal metabolite levels studied by Stabler et al.[240] had a response in only one out of four parameters assessed. Patients with B_{12} depletion and no deficiency can usually be treated with oral B_{12} initially and their responses closely monitored.
3. The cost-effectiveness of different screening strategies, as compared to routine oral vitamin B_{12} supplementation needs to be assessed.

4. The role of gastroscopic surveillance in detecting early neoplasms needs to be clarified.

Folate deficiency

Folic acid deficiency produces changes on the peripheral blood smear and in the bone marrow that are indistinguishable from those due to vitamin B_{12} deficiency. There is controversy concerning the incidence of folate deficiency in the elderly, partly because different groups define the lower limits of normal differently and because there are several different ways to determine folate levels.[286–295] Serum folate levels fluctuate rapidly and do not necessarily reflect body stores. Red blood cell folate levels are more reliable, but both radioimmunoassay and microbiologic methods are available for measuring both red blood cells and serum folate and there is frequently a discrepancy between the results from these methods.[295] Normal body stores of folate can be depleted in less than 6 months, and several conditions can cause folate deficiency to occur rapidly. These include malabsorption, poor nutrition, alcoholism, and states of increased folate utilization such as hemolytic anemia and neoplasia. Furthermore, drugs can cause folate deficiency, including anticonvulsants, antineoplastic drugs, trimethoprim, and nitrofurantoin. Many older people with psychiatric illnesses become folate-deficient because they do not eat. If the above-mentioned conditions are excluded, the vast majority of community-dwelling elderly are folate-replete.[295] Age does not predispose one to folate deficiency; disease states and medications are the reasons people become deficient. Certainly, if people do not eat, they become folate-deficient rapidly. However, even the poor elderly in the United States seem to have diets with sufficient amounts of this vitamin.[295]

Folate deficiency may result in neurologic changes which are virtually indistinguishable from those produced by vitamin B_{12} deficiency.[295] Included among the neuropsychiatric problems of folate-deficient individuals are intellectual impairment, confusion, psychosis, depression, stupor, coma, cerebral ischemia, and paraplegia.[295–317] Diagnosis of anemia due to folate deficiency rests on a peripheral blood smear with macrocytic red blood cells and hypersegmented neutrophils, a normal serum B_{12} level, and low serum folate and/or red blood cell folate. These values are frequently defined as below 2 μg/ml and below 100 μg/ml, respectively. Serum homocysteine levels are elevated in 90 percent of patients with folate deficiency, but methylmalonic acid levels are normal.[268] If methylmalonic acid levels are high, coexisting B_{12} deficiency must be considered. Bone marrow, if examined, will be indistinguishable from that seen in B_{12} deficiency. Treatment of folate deficiency consists of 1 mg of folic acid orally, and a parenteral form is available for patients with severe malabsorption. Again, it should be noted that treatment of a patient with megaloblastic anemia secondary to B_{12} deficiency with folate alone may correct the anemia but does not reverse the neurologic damage.

Macrocytosis can also be found in a number of other conditions, such as artifactual macrocytosis due to cold agglutinins; reticulocytosis may cause macrocytosis because these cells are larger than older red cells. A variety of medications such as hydroxyurea and zidovudine, myelodysplastic syndromes, alcoholism, liver disease, and hypothyroidism are all associated with macrocytosis as well.[318]

Diseases of White Blood Cells and the Reticuloendothelial System

Leukopenia and Agranulocytosis

The causes of a decrease in white cells are similar in any age group. In older people any severe infection may cause leukopenia, while in the young it is usually due to a viral illness. Psychotropic, cardiovascular, and antibiotic drugs are the drugs that most commonly cause a decrease in white cells in the elderly. Since the elderly take multiple medications, they are at greater risk for developing leukopenia.

Acute Leukemia

Acute leukemia is an accumulation of immature lymphoid or myeloid cells in the bone marrow and peripheral blood, tissue invasion by these cells, and associated bone marrow failure. Untreated, median survival is 3 months.

Acute leukemias are classified grossly as either acute lymphocytic leukemia (ALL) or acute nonlymphocytic leukemia based on the morphology of the cells in the peripheral blood and bone marrow smears, histochemical staining, and immunologic markers. The French-American-British Cooperative Group (FAB) classification of acute leukemias is the system most widely used to facilitate clinical studies and allows for some degree of prognostication.[319] This classification is shown in Table 89-8.

Incidence

Acute leukemia is primarily a disease of the elderly.[320] While there have been dramatic improvements in the treatment and survival of patients with leukemia, most of the dramatic results have been in the young. Leukemia has an incidence of about 15 per 100,000 in all age groups. However, the incidence begins to rise at age 40 and by age 80 is approximately 160 per 100,000. Eighty percent of adults with acute leukemia have acute nonlymphocytic leukemia, whereas 80 percent of all children with acute leukemia have lymphocytic leukemia. In spite of this, the incidence of ALL is four times higher in the elderly than in children.

Etiology

It is not clear what the etiology is in most cases of acute leukemia. Radiation exposure has been implicated as the cause in at least some cases. Data on atomic bomb survivors from Hiroshima and Nagasaki show a 10 to 20 percent increased incidence of acute nonlymphocytic leukemia. Likewise, diagnostic radiologists and patients who received radia-

Table 89-8 French-American-British classification of acute leukemias and myelodysplasia

A. Acute nonlymphocytic leukemia
   1. M1: myeloblastic without maturation
   2. M2: myeloblastic with maturation
   3. M3: promyelocytic
   4. M4: myelomonocytic
   5. M5: monocytic
      M5a: poorly differentiated (monoblastic)
      M5b: monocytic
   6. M6: erythroleukemia
   7. Other (megakaryoblastic, basophilic, eosinophilic)

B. Acute lymphoblastic leukemia
   1. L1: small cells predominate
   2. L2: large heterogeneous cells
   3. L3: large homogeneous cells (Burkitt's type)

C. Myelodysplasia syndrome
   1. Refractory anemia
   2. Refractory anemia with ringed sideroblasts (>15% ringed forms in the marrow)
   3. RAEB (5–20% blasts in the marrow, <5% circulating blasts)
   4. Chronic myelomonocytic leukemia (monocytosis ≥1,000/mm^2 in association with RAEB)
   5. RAEB in transformation (20–30% blasts in marrow, ≥5% circulating blasts)

Abbreviation: RAEB, refractory anemia with excess blasts.

tion therapy for ankylosing spondylitis in the earlier part of this century had a 2.5- and 14-fold increased risk, respectively, of developing acute nonlymphocytic leukemia. High-level benzene exposure in the workplace has been strongly implicated as increasing the risk of developing this type of acute leukemia.[321] It is now well established that long-term, low-dose therapy with virtually any type of chemotherapeutic alkylating agent can cause acute leukemia, mostly acute nonlymphocytic leukemia.[322] The combination of chemotherapeutic drugs and radiation increases the risk of developing leukemia. Chronic bone marrow disorders such as myelodysplastic syndromes, polycythemia vera, paroxysmal nocturnal hemoglobinuria, and aplastic anemia are sometimes followed by a rapidly progressive leukemic phase.[320] Viruses have long been suspected to be the cause of at least some acute leukemias.[323] Recent molecular genetic studies have demonstrated that oncogenes, the cellular homologs of retroviral transforming genes, appear to have a role in the induction and maintenance of the malignant state. Cytogenetic and molecular biologic techniques have shown that specific oncogenes are involved in nonrandom chromosome translocations or are found on deleted or reduplicated chromosomes.[324–326]

Pathophysiology and signs and symptoms

Primitive white blood cells accumulate rapidly in the bone marrow and invade many tissues including the liver, spleen, lymph nodes, and CNS. Normal bone marrow is replaced by these blasts, which results in severe anemia and thrombocytopenia with marked bleeding. Normal leukocytes are replaced by these primitive cells, which results in the patient developing infections.

Acute leukemia frequently presents as an apparent infection with an acute onset and high fever. Because of the thrombocytopenia, there are usually petechiae and ecchymoses as well as bleeding from the nose, mouth, and gastrointestinal and genitourinary tracts. There is often enlargement of the liver, spleen, and lymph nodes, but this is not always present. In the elderly, the disease can develop insidiously, with progressive weakness, pallor, a change in the sense of well-being, and delirium.[327]

Laboratory data and diagnosis

The total white blood count may be low, normal, or elevated. Blast forms are usually seen in the peripheral blood smear, but a bone marrow aspiration should always be performed to confirm the diagnosis. The bone marrow shows an excess of blast cells, with decreased or absent normal erythroid, granulocytic, and megarocytic cells. Histochemical stains and surface antigen markers help identify the type of acute leukemia. Cytogenetic markers are also useful to prognosticate the cause of the leukemia and to choose therapy.

Prognosis

The average patient will die within 4 to 6 months from clinical onset unless he is treated. Some patients die within days of the onset of the illness. Infection, bleeding, advanced age, high blast counts, and chromosomal abnormalities have all been proposed as poor prognostic indicators, while the presence of Auer rods (in acute myelogenous leukemia) and the development of hepatitis have been reported to be advantageous. Recent work has tried to define morphologic cytogenetic and in vitro growth characteristics as prognosticators. However, the literature is very controversial regarding all the prognostic signs.[320,327]

Advanced age has typically been considered a bad sign (advanced age in most series is defined as over 50 or 60 years). Much of the problem in treating the elderly seems to be their inability to tolerate the prolonged pancytopenia that accompanies aggressive induction chemotherapy regimens.

The elderly also have more complex karyotype abnormalities than younger patients,[320,328] and more of them have underlying primary marrow disorders such as myelodysplasia.[320] The presence of a prior hematologic marrow disorder (e.g., myelodysplasia or polycythemia vera) or a leukemia that is secondary to prior alkylating agent therapy seems to be a poor prognostic sign.[329,330]

Treatment

Older patients with ALL have an overall poor long-term survival compared to children, who have an excellent prognosis. The older patient with ALL usually is defined as high risk and often has a white blood cell count of more than 20,000/mm^3, a mediastinal mass, L2/L3 morphology, T-cell or B-cell leukemia, and meningitis. Therapy usually consists of a combination of drugs including vincristine, prednisone, and additional drugs that may include, among others, doxorubicin, cyclophosphamide, and L-asparaginase.[331] Most older people relapse within the first year of treatment. At the present time, therefore, there is no standard combination therapy.[320,327]

In acute nonlymphocytic leukemia, complete remission must first be obtained. The induction phase is the most crucial time because the patient is often infected and bleeding, and has a large tumor burden with little normal hematopoiesis. Complete remission is defined as the reduction of leukemic blasts to an undetectable level in the bone marrow (fewer than 5 percent blasts). Many induction regimens are currently being studied; the standard combination is cytarabine at 100 to 200 mg/m^2/d as a continuous intravenous infusion for 7 days and daunorubicin 45 mg/m^2 intravenously for the first 3 days.[331] By supporting the patient with platelets, red blood cells, and antibiotics, the current complete remission rate in people over age 60 is reported to be 40 to 76 percent.[320] The median survival is 1 to 2 years. New protocols are studying the value of different maintenance and consolidation chemotherapeutic regimens.[329,330,332]

Infections are the major cause of mortality and morbidity in acute leukemias because of the severe leukopenia and the destruction of normal cutaneous and mucosal barriers. Approximately 500 to 1,000 polymorphonuclear leukocytes per cubic millimeter are necessary for protection against infection. In many patients the endogenous bowel flora is the source of the infection. The pharynx, lungs, perirectal areas, and skin are also common sites of infection. The genitourinary tract and meninges are less common sites. Since the source of the infection is endogenous organisms, reverse isolation is of limited value. Viruses, protozoa, and anaerobic bacteria are uncommon pathogens early in therapy. Fungal infections usually occur after 7 to 14 days of antibiotic therapy in neutropenic patients.[333] The choice of antibiotic depends on the predominant organisms causing infection in a given hospital. Usually an aminoglycoside and a semisynthetic penicillin or cephalosporin are the drugs of choice, as the most common organisms in most hospitals are *Pseudomonas* and *Escherichia coli*. Recently, trimethoprim-sulfamethoxazole as prophylaxis has been suggested, particularly in patients who have had frequent admissions with fever and neutropenia.[334]

Metabolic problems are quite common during induction therapy. Hyperuricemia from the release of uric acid from the dead blasts should be treated prophylactically with allopurinol 300 mg/d. Hypokalemia can occur as a result of natriuresis and/or proximal renal tubular dysfunction. A renal tubular acidosis-like syndrome with hypokalemia, amino aciduria, and hyperphosphaturia occurs but is probably not related to lysozyme. Metabolic alkalosis, metabolic acidosis, hypocalcemia, and hyperphosphatemia are all common complications. Patients should be treated routinely with vigorous hydration, alkalinization of the urine, and allopurinol.[335,336]

Aggregates of blasts and thrombi may occlude small blood vessels throughout the body, particularly in the brain and lungs. Therapy revolves around hydration and rapid reduction of the blast count, usually with prompt treatment with a chemotherapeutic agent such as hydroxyurea, which rapidly lowers the white cell count.[337] Leukopheresis and cranial irradiation may be temporizing measures.[338,339]

The CNS is the most common site of extramedullary relapse in acute leukemia. The need for prophylactic meningeal therapy with cranial irradiation and intrathecal methotrexate or cystosine arabinoside has not yet been formally addressed in the elderly. Therefore, these methods must be used with extreme caution at the present time. Spinal cord compression, when it occurs, is usually responsive to local radiation. T-cell acute lymphocytic leukemias are most likely to cause either CNS or gonadal invasion. However, the role of prophylactic testicular radiation is currently unclear in the elderly.[320,326]

Disseminated intravascular coagulation is an uncommon complication and is mainly seen in M3 (promyelocytic leukemia). In general, it is self-limited and is most problematic during the rapid cell lysis of induction chemotherapy. The use of prophylactic heparin continues to be controversial.

Bone marrow transplant is rarely used in individuals over the age of 35. At present, this technique is not used in elderly patients.

Chronic Leukemias

Chronic leukemia is a neoplastic accumulation of mature lymphoid or myeloid elements of the blood which usually progresses more slowly than an acute leukemia. If lymphoid cells are the neoplastic type, the disease is called chronic lymphocytic leukemia. If myeloid cells are involved, it is termed chronic myeloid leukemia. Chronic myeloid leukemia will be discussed in the section on myeloproliferative disorders.

Chronic lymphocytic leukemia is primarily a disease of the elderly, while chronic myeloid leukemia usually occurs in the thirties and fourties, as well as in old age. In more than 95 percent of all cases chronic lymphocytic leukemia involves neoplastic proliferation of B cells.[340]

Incidence

Chronic lymphocytic leukemia is the most common leukemia in western society, accounting for 25 to 40 percent of all leukemias. Ninety percent of all patients are over the age of 50, with the vast majority being over age 60. Men are affected twice as often as women.[340]

Etiology

In contrast to the situation for chronic myelogenous leukemia, ionizing radiation plays no part in the etiology of chronic lymphocytic leukemia. There seems to be a genetic component, as the illness is more common in certain families, and in some of these families, there are immunologic abnormalities. Chronic viral infections (retroviruses) have been suggested as possible candidates.[341]

Pathophysiology and signs and symptoms

In this disorder there is an accumulation of monoclonal lymphocytes in peripheral blood, bone marrow, lymphoid tissue, and sometimes other organs. The cells appear morphologically mature, but the presence of receptors for mouse erythrocytes, HLA-DR antigens, and a small amount of surface immunoglobin suggests some degree of immaturity. Trisomy 12 has been described as a chromosomal abnormality in some cases (25 percent), and abnormalities of other chromosomes including 6, 11, and 13 have been described as well.[342] Infiltration of the bone marrow may eventually result in pancytopenia. Normal B cells are not present in adequate numbers, which often leads to bacterial infection. Transformation into diffuse large cell lymphoma (Richter's syndrome) or prolymphocytic leukemia may occur as a terminal event.[327,340]

The presentation is highly variable. Over 25 percent of patients have asymptomatic disease that is discovered on routine physical examination or blood analysis. The most common initial symptoms are fatigue, malaise, and decreased exercise tolerance. In many older people, exacerbation of coronary artery or cerebrovascular disease may be the initial manifestation.

Some patients report enlarged lymph nodes or complain of abdominal pain or early satiety due to splenomegaly. Lymphadenopathy is commonly found in the cervical, axillary, and supraclavicular areas, while inguinal adenopathy is rare. Splenomegaly is found in 50 percent of patients at presentation, and hepatomegaly may develop as the disease progresses. Lymphocyte infiltration can occur in any organ. Jaundice usually suggests hemolysis even though periportal lymph node enlargement with biliary tract obstruction can occur. In late-stage disease ecchymoses and petechiae from thrombocytopenia may be seen. Fever is usually secondary to infection, but late in the disease the possibility of transformation in to acute prolymphocytic leukemia or aggressive lymphoma should be considered. Clinical hyperviscosity is rare and occurs only when the white blood cell count is 800,000/mm^3 or greater.[327,340]

Laboratory data and diagnosis

The diagnosis of chronic lymphocytic leukemia requires the demonstration of sustained lymphocytosis and bone marrow lymphocyte infiltration in the absence of other causes. The absolute lymphocyte count is generally above 15,000/mm^3. Cells are mature in appearance, and there is a tendency for these lymphocytes to smudge on preparation of the blood smear. In B-cell chronic lymphocytic leukemia, the T and B cells are both increased in absolute number. However, B cells are preferentially increased and make up 40 to 90 percent of all lymphocytes. The B cells form rosettes with mouse erythrocytes; they are of monoclonal origin and express surface immunoglobins of one light-chain class. The surface immunoglobin is usually IgM but less commonly is IgD. Immunophenotypically they also express the cell markers CD5$^+$, CD19+, CD20+, CD23+, FMC7−/+ and CD22−/+.[342] In B-cell chronic lymphocytic leukemia, the ratio of helper to suppressor T cells is reversed because of an increase in the number of suppressor cells. This is thought to account for development of the pure red cell aplasia described in a few patients.[343]

Approximately 1 percent of patients have lymphocytes that form rosettes with sheep red blood cells, and their disease is classified as T-cell chronic lymphocytic leukemia. Both helper (T4$^+$) and suppressor (T8$^+$) forms are seen. The lymphocytes often demonstrate cytoplasmic azurophilic granules. Massive splenomegaly, marked neutropenia, skin infiltration, modest bone marrow infiltration, and a rapid clinical course leading to death are seen in less than one-half of these patients.[344] There is a high concurrence with rheumatoid arthritis.[344] Most cases, however, have indolent courses.[345]

Red blood cell morphology is usually normal. Anemia is found in 10 to 20 percent of all patients and is most often normochromic and normocytic. The anemia may be due to marrow replacement, hypersplenism, or suppressor mechanisms. The Coombs' test reveals IgG coating of red blood cells in about 20 percent of cases; however, immune hemolytic anemia is seen only 8 percent of the time. Thrombocytopenia is found in 10 to 20 percent of cases and may be due to marrow replacement, hypersplenism, or antiplatelet antibodies. Autoimmune thrombyctopenia occurs in about 5 percent of patients.[346] Bone marrow morphology shows interstitial or nodular infiltration in early disease and diffuse infiltration in advanced stages.[347,348]

In about 5 percent of cases, immunoglobin found on the cell surface is the same as that found in the serum as a monoclonal protein. About 50 to 75 percent of patients are hypo- or agammaglobulinemic.

Prognosis

On the basis of physical examination and a CBC, the patient can be staged clinically (Table 89-9).[349] Group A patients have fewer than three areas of lymphoid enlargement, including cervical, axillary, supraclavicular, or inguinal lymph nodes or liver or spleen. Generally, disease progression follows a stepwise pattern from mild to more severe illness. Patients in group C with anemia (less than 10 g/dl) or thrombocytopenia (less than 100,000/mm^3) usually survive less than 2 years.

Other poor prognostic signs include diffuse replacement of

Table 89-9 International workshop on staging of chronic lymphocytic leukemia

Stage	Definition
A	No anemia or thrombocytopenia and fewer than three areas of lymphoid enlargement, median survival >7 years
B	No anemia or thrombocytopenia with three or more involved areas, median survival <5 years
C	Anemia (hemoglobin <10 g/dl) and or thrombocytopenia (<100,000/μl) regardless of the number of areas of lymphoid enlargement, median survival <2 years

bone marrow, presence of trisomy 12[350] with other chromosomal abnormalities, IgM surface immunoglobin rather than IgD,[351] and a lymphocyte doubling time of under 12 months.

Although survival in chronic lymphocytic leukemia is often prolonged, the overall 5-year survival is only about 50 percent.

Treatment

Patients in group A usually do not require any treatment until their disease progresses. This approach is usually extended to individuals in group B, as the complications of chemotherapy such as infection or development of acute nonlymphocytic leukemia may be more deleterious than the chronic lymphocytic leukemia.[352]

In stage C,[340] chlorambucil is the agent most often used. It can be given daily (often at doses of 6 to 8 mg orally) or every 2 weeks (0.4 to 0.8 mg/kg body weight): resposes rates range from 40 to 70 percent, but complete responses are rare.[342] Patients who fail to respond can be given other chemotherapy (e.g., fludarabine).[342] Maintenance therapy is not usually employed. Steroids are often used for the treatment of patients with autoimmune hemolytic anemia or thrombocytopenia, and radiation therapy is used to reduce local bulky disease, vital organ compromise, or painful bone lesions.

The most common complications of chronic lymphocytic leukemia are bacterial infections, with pneumonia and urinary tract infections occurring most frequently. Gram-positive cocci, gram-negative rods, *Listeria*, fungi, and *Pneumocystis carinii* infection all occur. In addition to the appropriate antibiotics, some patients with hypogammaglobulinemia may benefit from regular infusions of immune globulin; however, the cost of this therapy is very high.[353] Patients with chronic lymphocytic leukemia have at least a fourfold risk of developing a carcinoma.

When transformation into either a prolymphocytic leukemia or into an aggressive lymphoma occurs, there is generally a poor response to chemotherapy or radiation.

Multiple Myeloma

Multiple myeloma is a neoplastic disorder resulting from the proliferation and accumulation of immature plasma cells in the bone marrow. Its major manifestations, which ultimately lead to death, result from both the direct effect of these cells and the characteristic proteins produced by them, as well as their secondary effects on other organ systems.[354–356]

The neoplastic plasma cells almost always synthesize abnormal amounts of monoclonal immunoglobulin (IgG, IgA, IgD, or IgE) κ or λ light chains. They are, therefore, usually classified by their immunoglobulin class. Rarely, there are cases in which there is no detectable secretion of immunoglobulin.[356]

Incidence

The annual incidence of multiple myeloma is approximately 3 per 100,000. However, at age 80, the incidence rises to 37 per 100,000. The disease is more common in blacks than in whites, and the incidence is slightly greater in men. Multiple myeloma usually occurs in people over the age of 50 and the incidence increases progressively with age.[354–356]

Etiology

There is an increased incidence of myeloma in first-degree relatives. This together with the higher frequency of the 4C complex of HLA antigens in myeloma patients and the increased incidence in blacks suggests that genetic factors play a role.[357–360]

There seems to be an enhanced risk of developing myeloma after high radiation exposure, as shown in Hiroshima and Nagasaki atomic bomb survivors.[361] Other etiologic possibilities suggested have included chronic antigenic stimulation such as cholecystitis, osteomyelitis, repeated allergen injections, rheumatoid arthritis, hereditary spherocytosis, and Gaucher's disease.[362–375] Asbestos and viral illnesses such as Aleutian mink disease have also been implicated.[376–381]

Since myeloma is also age-related, one possible influence might be the decrease in the T-lymphoid arm of the immune system. As T cells decrease, B-cell clones may proliferate excessively. Because of such monoclonal expansions, there may then be a higher probability of either spontaneous or externally induced genetic alteration of one such clone, allowing it to proliferate and secrete its immunoglobulin. This activity would still remain under control of the immune system and thus would be considered "benign monoclonal gammopathy." Finally, a second external oncogenic event could result in uncontrolled proliferation of these cells, and multiple myeloma would ensue.[382]

Much interest has recently been focused on a number of cytokines that may play a role in multiple myeloma. IL-6 has been suggested to be a myeloma cell growth factor, and high levels of IL-6 have been associated with a poor outcome in some studies on multiple myeloma.[383]

Pathophysiology and signs and symptoms

The consequences of abnormal plasma cell growth cell tumors include osteolysis, hematopoietic suppression, hypogammaglobulinemia, paraproteinemia, paraproteinuria, and renal disease.[354–356]

Plasma cell tumors usually develop in areas of hematopoietically active bone marrow. They can be seen in virtually any bone and rarely in extraskeletal sites. In most instances, even plasmacytomas that seem solitary eventually become generalized.

Osteolytic lesions are very common and are thought to result from the release of osteoclast activating factor (possibly IL-6) from the neoplastic plasma cell,[384] which stimulates osteoclasts to resorb bone.

Marrow function is impaired in proportion to the number of plasma cells in the bone marrow. Anemia is most common, but neutropenia and thrombocytopenia also occur.

In multiple myeloma, the single species of abnormal plasma cells produces a single type of immunoglobulin or portion of the immunoglobulin molecule in excess. There is concomitant suppression of the other classes of normal immunoglobulin, resulting in actual or functional hypogammaglobulinemia. In over 50 percent of patients, the monoclonal protein is an IgG, in 20 percent IgA, and 12 percent IgM (macroglobulinemia). IgD is found in about 2 percent of cases, and IgE is very rare. About 10 percent of patients produce only light chains, and less than 1 percent produce only heavy chains. In rarer cases patients produce two or more monoclonal proteins, and about 1 percent of patient do not have any monoclonal protein in their serum or urine.[354–356]

About one-half of patients with multiple myeloma have renal disease. Urinary tract infections, glomerular deposits of amyloid, stones from hypercalcemia and hyperuricemia, and plasma cell infiltration of the kidney all may occur. However, the major cause of renal failure is tubular damage associated with the excretion of light-chain proteins. Not all these proteins are nephrotoxic, and some patients may excrete large amounts of them for years without developing renal failure. Patients excreting λ light chains are at greater risk than those excreting κ light chains.[354–356]

Multiple myeloma is usually a progressive disease. The doubling time of the abnormal plasma cells has been estimated to be 3 to 10 months. In rare cases, however, the preclinical stage may have a duration of years.[354–356]

The most frequent symptom of multiple myeloma is bone pain which occurs in about 70 percent of patients. Pain is often in the lower back or ribs and gradually increases in intensity. Sudden onset of pain often means that a vertebra has collapsed or there has been a spontaneous fracture through an involved area such as the shaft of a long bone, the pelvis, a rib, or a clavicle.

Systemic signs and symptoms include pallor, weakness, fatigue, dyspnea on exertion, and palpitations. These all result from the anemia present in about 70 percent of patients at the time of diagnosis. Signs of thrombocytopenia are common, such as ecchymoses, purpura, epistaxis, or excessive bleeding from trauma. Signs of infection also occur frequently as a result of neutropenia and immunoglobulin deficiency, and the patient may present with pneumonia, pyoderma, or pyelonephritis. Cold insensitivity and urticaria may result from cryoglobulinemia. Nephrotic syndrome is a rare presentation.

Hypercalcemia is very common in patients with destructive bone lesions and may result in anorexia, nausea, vomiting, polyuria, polydipsia, constipation, and dehydration. Particularly in the elderly, drowsiness, confusion, and coma can result from hypercalcemia.[354–356]

Acute renal failure may also develop in patients who have azotemia and who receive hypertonic contrast media during the performance of a diagnostic procedure. In patients with multiple myeloma, procedures such as intravenous or retrograde pyelograms or open bone biopsies should not be performed unless there is ample urine flow and hypercalcemia and hyperuricemia have been corrected.

Hyperviscosity syndrome occurs about 50 percent of the time if the monoclonal immunoglobulin is IgM (macroglobulinemia). It is uncommon in multiple myeloma with another monoclonal protein. Purpura, ecchymoses, epistaxis, gastrointestinal bleeding; blurred vision (associated with venous congestion, hemorrhages, and exudates), and ischemic neurologic symptoms are common signs of hyperviscosity.[354–356]

Neurologic signs and symptoms include mental confusion due to hypercalcemia, spinal cord and nerve root compression, myelomatous meningitis, carpal tunnel syndrome (due to deposition of amyloid), and sensorimotor polyneuropathy not due to amyloid or infiltration with plasma cells. Rarer CNS symptoms include intracerebral plasmacytomas, herpes zoster, and multifocal leukoencephalopathy.[354–356]

Laboratory data and diagnosis

The order of evaluation depends on the mode of presentation. If a monoclonal serum component is found in an otherwise asymptomatic patient, the skeleton should be x-rayed and a bone marrow aspiration should be performed. The absence of both lytic bone lesions and plasma cell infiltration makes a diagnosis of benign monoclonal gammopathy likely. Confirmatory tests for this diagnosis include absence of significant (less than 60 mg/24 h) amounts of a single type of light chain (Bence-Jones protein) in the urine and a serum monoclonal gammopathy of less than 2 g/dl. The presence in the bone marrow of more than 10 percent mature and immature plasma cells, osteolytic bone lesions, and a serum monoclonal protein is diagnostic of multiple myeloma. Excretion of light chains of more than 60 mg/24 h and of a monoclonal protein of greater than 2 g/dl (although it is usually greater than 3 g/dl) is very suggestive of multiple myeloma. If bone marrow plasmacytosis is not demonstrated, a repeat bone marrow aspiration and a search for an extraskeletal plasma cell tumor should be undertaken. Finally, one must keep in mind that idiopathic monoclonal components are sometimes seen with other cancers.[354–356]

Prognosis

The only way to differentiate between some cases of early multiple myeloma and benign monoclonal gammopathy is observation over time. In a long-term follow-up study (median 22 years) in patients at the Mayo clinic with apparently benign monoclonal gammopathy, 19 percent had benign monoclonal gammopathy, 10 percent had a serum monoclonal protein value of 3 g/dl or more but did not require chemotherapy, 47 percent had died without evidence of myeloma, and 24 percent had multiple myeloma (66 percent of this group), systemic amyloidosis, macroglobulinemia, or malignant lymphoproliferative disease. In patients who developed multiple myeloma this was diagnosed a median of 10 years after the monoclonal protein was found, emphasizing the need for long term follow-up.[385]

Once a diagnosis of multiple myeloma is made, the patient can be classified as a good or a poor risk. A good risk is defined as a hemoglobin of 9.0 g/dl or greater, a blood urea nitrogen of 30 mg/dl or less, and a serum calcium level of 12 mg/dl or less after hydration. The poor-risk group consists of patients who fail to meet these criteria.[354] With therapy, the good-risk group has a median survival of 42 months and the poor-risk group has only a 21-month survival. Both groups respond equally well to initial therapy. Besides clinical status, other important prognostic features are the β_2-microglobulin level which is an indicator of tumor mass,[386] the plasma cell labeling index which measures the proliferative rate of the plasma cells,[386] and possibly the IL-6 level.[383,386]

In some elderly people who fulfill the good-risk diagnostic criteria for multiple myeloma the disease progresses very slowly. If the patient is asymptomatic or only mildly symptomatic and is not at risk of developing a complication, he can be followed over time to determine the pace of the illness. In addition, occasionally there are elderly patients with advanced-stage myeloma with a good prognosis. As a general rule, if an elderly patient is feeling well, one should wait until the pace of the illness is determined.

Treatment

Since multiple myeloma is a neoplastic disorder, the mainstay of treatment is chemotherapy. Radiation is reserved for localized lesions and is most helpful in relieving back pain from osteolytic lesions. However, if extensive bone demineralization is causing the back pain, radiation is usually not palliative and chemotherapy should be used.[354–356]

All patients should be encouraged to keep active to prevent further bone demineralization. Lumbar corsets and braces may help to relieve pain and prevent further damage. Large osteolytic lesions should be irradiated before fractures occur. Actual fracture through a lytic lesion requires an intramedullary pin and radiation.

Patients must drink 2 to 3 L of fluid per day to maintain increased urine output to allow excretion of light chains, calcium, uric acid, and other metabolites. All infections must be treated promptly. Hyperuricemia should be treated with allopurinol. Hypercalcemia is usually treated with hydration and prednisone until serum calcium returns to normal (usually 1 to 5 days). Calcitonin or a bisphosphonate may be used if the above therapy does not work but usually is not needed.[387] Daily oral therapy with sodium or potassium phosphate may also be helpful in some patients with moderate hypercalcemia.

Many chemotherapeutic regimens are currently in use for multiple myeloma. In the elderly with decreased bone marrow reserve, the most common regimen is intermittent melphalan and prednisone. The two drugs are given daily for 4 days, and treatment is repeated at intervals of 4 to 6 weeks for at least three courses before remission or resistance is confirmed.[387] In approximately 40 percent of patients remission is induced with the above therapy. The median duration of remission is about 2 years, and median survival about 3 years.[387] For patients who do not respond to the aforementioned regimen a wide variety of other options (e.g., vincristine, doxorubicin, and dexamethasone) are available.[387] Several maintenance therapies including continued melphalan and prednisone have been used,[387] and some success with increased remission duration has recently been reported with α-interferon.[388] Which maintenance therapies, if any (most studies do not show increased survival), to use are determined on an individual basis.

Hyperviscosity can be treated effectively in the short term by plasmapheresis.

Lymphoma

Lymphomas are primary malignancies of the lymph nodes and include Hodgkin's disease and non-Hodgkin's lymphoma. They are distinct entities characterized by different patterns of spread, clinical behaviors, and cell of origin. Hodgkin's disease usually has a predictable pattern of spread to contiguous lymph node areas, while non-Hodgkin's lymphoma is usually widespread at diagnosis. Non-Hodgkin's lymphoma is more likely to have extranodal involvement. Both can be divided into subsets based on the histologic appearance of the lymph nodes.[320,389,390]

The diagnosis of Hodgkin's disease depends on histologic finding in the lymph node of the Reed-Sternberg cell, a giant cell with twin nuclei that give the cell the appearance of "owl's eyes." The Reed-Sternberg cell is probably the malignant cell, and the other cells surrounding it probably represent tissue reaction.[320,389,390]

Histologically, Hodgkin's disease is subdivided into the following four major types.

1. *Lymphocyte predominant*: mainly adult lymphocytes with few Reed-Sternberg cells
2. *Mixed cellularity*: a cellular response of mature lymphoid cells, plasma cells, eosinophils, and Reed-Sternberg cells
3. *Lymphocyte-depleted*: a paucity of lymphoid cells with a majority of histiocytes, fibrotic reaction, and Reed-Sternberg cells
4. *Nodular sclerosis*: effacement of lymphoid tissue by nodular aggregates of mature lymphoid cells and "lacunar" variants of Reed-Sternberg cells separated by bands of adult collagen.

Before modern therapies became available, it was noted that lymphocyte predominant and nodular sclerosis types carried a better prognosis.[320,389,390]

Systematic clinical staging is extremely important in the management of Hodgkin's disease. The currently accepted clinical stages are listed in Table 89-10.

Non-Hodgkin's lymphomas are a heterogeneous group of lymphoid malignancies which have some common but many different features. The classification of non-Hodgkin's lymphomas has been a controversial subject and is undergoing revision. There are currently two complementary approaches to classifying these illnesses: classic description of architecture and histology and use of immunologic markers. Table 89-11 shows the histologic classification of Rappaport[391] and the international panel working formulation[392] based on the type of lymphocyte seen. Recently a new classification has been suggested by the International Lymphoma Study Group. It di-

Table 89-10 Clinical staging of Hodgkin's disease[a]

Stage	Definition
I	Disease limited to one anatomic region
II	Disease in two or more anatomic regions on the same side of the diaphragm
III	Disease on both sides of the diaphragm but limited to lymph nodes, spleen, and/or Waldeyer's ring
III_1	Involvement limited to spleen, splenic nodes, and celiac and/or portal nodes
III_2	Involvement of para-aortic, pelvic, and iliac nodes
IV	Extranodal disease not directly contiguous with a nodal area (i.e., bone marrow, lung, pleura, liver)

[a] *All stages are subclassified into A and B; A, no systematic symptoms; B, any one symptom of unexplained fever, or night sweats, or 10% or more loss of body weight.*

Table 89-11 Histologic classification of the non-Hodgkin's lymphomas

Working Classification	Rappaport's Classification
Low grade	
Small lymphocytic	Well-differentiated lymphocytic lymphoma (WDL)
Follicular small cleaved lymphocytic	Nodular poorly differentiated lymphocytic (NPDL)
Mixed follicular small cleaved cell and large cell	Nodular mixed lymphoma (NM)
Intermediate grade	
Follicular, predominantly large cell	Nodular histiocytic lymphoma (NHL)
Diffuse small cleaved cell	Diffuse poorly differentiated lymphocytic lymphoma (DPDL)
Diffuse large cell (cleaved or uncleaved)	Diffuse histiocytic lymphoma (DHL)
High grade	
Diffuse large cell immunoblastic	Diffuse histiocytic lymphoma (DHL)
B cell	
T cell	
Polymorphous	
Epithelial cell component	
Lymphoblastic	Lymphoblastic lymphoma
Convoluted	
Nonconvoluted	
Small noncleaved	Diffuse undifferentiated lymphoma (DUL)
Burkitt's	
Non-Burkitt's	

vides lymphoid neoplasms into B-cell neoplasms, T-cell neoplasms, and Hodgkin's disease and also lists classes not previously well defined such as mantle cell lymphoma and marginal zone B-cell lymphoma, which includes the mucosa-associated lymphoid tissue (MALT) type.[393]

Clinical staging is similar to that for Hodgkin's disease. However, over 90 percent of patients have stage III or IV disease at the time of presentation.

Incidence

The incidence of Hodgkin's disease is 2 per 100,000 per year in the United States, and there is a bimodal distribution as a function of age. There is an initial peak between 15 and 35 and a subsequent peak at age 50 to 80. At age 25, the incidence is approximately 5 per 100,000 per year, and at age 75 it is 7 per 100,000. The incidence is slightly greater for men.

The age-adjusted incidence of non-Hodgkin's lymphoma is 2.6 to 5.8 per 100,000 per year. There is a progressive increase in incidence with age similar to that seen in acute leukemia. At age 80, the incidence is approximately 40 per 100,000 per year.[320,389,390]

Etiology

The etiology of Hodgkin's disease remains unknown. However, based on seroepidemiologic studies, there has been interest in the Epstein-Barr virus and other oncogenic viruses in relation to this disease. Patients with immunodeficiencies and autoimmune disease are at increased risk, which suggests that the immune system plays a role in the etiology. There are some suggestions that in the young, Hodgkin's disease may be an infectious disease, while in the elderly it is more likely a conventional malignancy.[394]

The etiology of most non-Hodgkin's lymphomas is also unknown. However, immunosuppressed patients (e.g., renal transplant recipients) and those with excessive function of the immune system (e.g., with Sjögren's syndrome) are at greater risk.[395] Viral etiologies are involved in at least some non-Hodgkin's lymphomas. African Burkitt's lymphoma is associated with Epstein-Barr virus infection,[395] and an aggressive T-cell leukemia or lymphoma is associated with HTLV-I infection in Japan and the Caribbean. Similarly, patients with human immunodeficiency virus (HIV) infection often develop aggressive non-Hodgkin's lymphoma and sometimes Hodgkin's disease.[396–399] It has been postulated that in acquired immunodeficiency syndrome (AIDS), lymphomas are secondary to Epstein-Barr virus activation of oncogene expression.[400] There is also some evidence that some early MALT-type tumors are antigen-responsive, and therapy directed against the antigen may result in regression of early lesions (*Helicobacter pylori* in gastric lymphoma).[401,402]

Chromosomal abnormalities are frequent in patients with lymphoma, and several abnormalities are often found simultaneously.[403] Translocations involving chromosomes 14 and 18 are the most common abnormalities found in non-Hodgkin's lymphoma. An oncogene *bcl-2* has been cloned from the region involved on chromosome 18 and has been shown to be activated through juxtaposition with the immunoglobulin heavy-chain locus.[403] The gene *bcl-2* produces a protein that helps block programmed cell death of B lymphocytes, possibly resulting in extended survival of cells carrying this translocation.[403]

Pathophysiology and signs and symptoms

In Hodgkin's disease normal lymphoid tissue is replaced by the malignant lymphoma, which can result in immunodeficiency and infections. The bone marrow may be replaced, resulting in pancytopenia and subsequent anemia, bleeding, and infection. The tumor bulk may obstruct vital organs and ultimately invade vital organs and cause death.

Patients with Hodgkin's disease usually have enlarged lymph nodes in the neck on presentation. Although any nodal group can be involved, the cervical or axillary lymph nodes are the most common. The patient may be asymptomatic, or the onset of symptoms may be marked by the B symptoms of fever, night sweats, or weight loss of greater than 10 percent of normal body weight. Pruritus may be present, but it is no longer considered diagnostic of a B classification. These constitutional symptoms are often associated with extensive disease. Patients may also present with advanced disease consisting of diffuse adenopathy and involvement of the spleen, liver, bone marrow, or lung. The elderly are more likely to present with B symptoms and advanced disease.[404]

Non-Hodgkin's lymphomas at all ages appear to be multicentric in origin and have a tendency to spread widely during the course of the disease. A peripheral blood leukemic phase is not uncommon. Most patients seek medical care because of neck or inguinal node enlargement. However, skin, gastrointestinal tract, bone, liver, and CNS lymphomas make up about 10 to 20 percent of the primary sites at presentation. Splenomegaly, bone marrow failure, autoimmune hemolytic anemia, and autoimmune thrombocytopenia are occasional presenting features. Systemic B symptoms are not as common as in Hodgkin's disease. Waldeyer's ring involvement is strongly associated with gastrointestinal lesions. Hypercalcemia is a prominent feature in HTLV-I-related non-Hodgkin's lymphoma but it is rare in other lymphomas. Hypogammaglobulinemia may be present, but patients occasionally have a monoclonal serum M component.[320,389]

Laboratory data and diagnosis

The diagnosis is made based on biopsy and the histologic picture of malignant lymphoma.

In Hodgkin's disease clinical staging is extremely important to determine treatment, and systemic staging includes the following.

1. Complete physical examination with careful attention to all lymph node areas.
2. Routine chemistry profile and CBC.
3. Computerized tomography scans of the abdomen, pelvis, and in some cases, the chest.
4. Lymphangiography via the pedal lymphatics to outline the femoral, inguinal, pelvic, and para-aortic nodes.
5. In cases in which the clinical stage may change the treatment modality, laparotomy (sometimes including splenectomy), liver biopsies, and sampling of suspicious nodes should be performed. A bone marrow biopsy is also required if it will change treatment. Up to 30 percent of patients have different clinical and pathologic stages. In the elderly, however, Hodgkin's disease is more likely to be manifested as advanced disease (stage III or IV). It has been suggested that patients past the age of 40, particularly those with mixed cellularity or lymphocyte depletion histologies, may not benefit from laparotomy.[320,389]

In non-Hodgkin's lymphoma systemic staging is rarely required. After a complete physical examination, CBC, chemistry profile, bone marrow aspirate and biopsy, chest x-ray, and abdominal computerized tomography, about 90 percent of all patients are shown to have advanced-stage disease. Staging laparotomy is usually not required. Other studies such as serum protein electrophoresis, skeletal x-rays, and intravenous urography are sometimes useful.[320,389]

Prognosis

In Hodgkin's disease, the elderly with advanced stages do not do as well as young people since they are unable to tolerate maximal radiation and chemotherapy doses.[405] In non-Hodgkin's lymphoma, the prognosis relates to both age and factors that are intrinsic to the disease. Good prognostic indicators are nodular histology, limited stage, and young age. Marrow involvement is a poor prognostic sign in unfavorable histologies but not in favorable or intermediate histologies. Other poor prognostic signs are bulky abdominal disease, hemoglobin less than 12 g/dl, and serum LDH greater than 250 units/L.[395] Based on five clinical factors—age, tumor stage, serum LDH, performance status, and number of extranodal disease sites—some physicians categorize patients into four groups which help to predict complete response rates and survival.[406]

Treatment

In Hodgkin's disease, the primary therapeutic maneuver is the treatment of known disease and the next potential site of involvement. In general, limited radiation therapy is used for stages I and II (many institutions use chemotherapy and radiation therapy for stages IB and IIB), and combination chemotherapy with or without radiation is recommended for stages III and IV. The current recommendations are shown in Table 89-12.[320,389] However, it must be kept in mind that regeneration of the bone marrow after radiation or chemotherapy is markedly diminished in patients past the age of 40, and gastrointestinal side effects are much more severe. Thus, one must consider limiting the usual mantle field in elderly patients with early-stage disease. Similarly, it may be impossible to give optimal chemotherapy to elderly patients, even though the ben-

Table 89-12 Treatment of patients with Hodgkin's disease

Stage	Therapy	Five-Year Disease-Free Survival (%)
IA, IIA	Mantle and para-aortic irradiation[a]	90
$IIIA_1$	Total nodal irradiation	50
	Chemotherapy and extended field irradiation	85
IB and IIB	Similar to IA and IIA[b]	80–90
$IIIA_2$ and IIIB	Chemotherapy and involved field irradiation[c]	80–85
IVA and IVB	Chemotherapy with or without irradiation of bulk disease	25–40

[a] *If the mediastinal mass is more than one-third the diameter of the chest, combined modality therapy consisting of chemotherapy and mantle irradiation is preferable to radiation alone.*

[b] *Many institutions give chemotherapy as well.*

[c] *Radiation therapy used only in certain cases.*

efits of aggressive chemotherapy outweigh the risks. The survival of patients given palliative treatment rather than aggressive therapy is dramatically less. Many elderly patients can tolerate only 30 to 50 percent of the optimal dose of chemotherapy.[405] The duration of chemotherapy is 6 to 12 months or at least 2 months following attainment of complete remission. There is an increased incidence of a second malignancy in patients with Hodgkin's disease receiving therapy.[407,408] In a study at Stanford University acute leukemia developed in about 4 percent of patients. However, the risk appeared to level off after 10 years,[408] and it was believed that risks were largely due to the chemotherapy. About 20 percent of patients developed solid tumors by 20 years after treatment, and these were believed to be primarily irradiation-induced.[408] In the aforementioned study, by 18 years after treatment, about 5 percent of patients had developed non-Hodgkin's lymphoma.

In non-Hodgkin's lymphoma, there are marked differences in prognosis based on pathologic classification. Very few cases are stage I, and therefore curative radiation is rarely possible. Most patients have advanced-stage disease and require chemotherapy. Chemotherapeutic "cures" in non-Hodgkin's lymphoma paradoxically tend to occur only in patients with intermediate and unfavorable prognosis histologies. In contrast, in lymphomas with a favorable prognosis, while they are extremely sensitive to chemotherapy, aggressive therapy does not seem to prolong survival. For these reasons, therapy is minimal in cases with a favorable prognosis and aggressive in those with unfavorable pathology.[320,389,395]

Favorable prognosis histology in non-Hodgkin's lymphoma Regional radiation is used in what appears to be disease of stage I or II, if any therapy is given. However, most patients relapse either because they were not truly in an early stage or because the disease is so indolent that recurrence may not occur for 5 to 10 years. Chemotherapy is rarely indicated in stage I or II and often no therapy is needed. Particularly in the elderly, close follow-up without treatment until problems develop is often a practical approach.[320,389]

In stages III and IV, the disease is still very indolent. Most patients respond to chemotherapy, but the relapse rate is 10 to 20 percent per year. Even though 80 to 90 percent with favorable prognosis histology achieve complete remission, at the 10-year mark only 10 to 20 percent will be without disease. Consequently, it is often wise to avoid both the serious systemic toxicity inherent in aggressive combination therapy and the potential risk of acute nonlymphocytic leukemia associated with chronic low-dose alkylating agents.[409] If treatment is necessary, chlorambucil is often used. Newer protocols involving different agents that have shown some promise in indolent lymphoma, such as fludarabine, are currently underway.[402]

Intermediate and unfavorable prognosis histology in non-Hodgkin's lymphoma These aggressive non-Hodgkin's lymphomas are rapidly growing tumors with a short natural history. For this reason patients are generally treated with combination chemotherapy. Some patients with localized disease are, however, treated with combined limited-term chemotherapy and radiation therapy.[402] Regimens that might offer better tolerability in the elderly than older ones are being developed.[406]

Waldenstrom's Macroglobulinemia

Waldenstrom's macroglobulinemia[355] is a lymphoproliferative disorder of the elderly associated with the production of monoclonal IgM greater than 2 g/L. It is usually found in men past the age of 50. The illness is insidious, with fatigue and weight loss being the predominant clinical findings. As the level of IgM monoclonal protein rises, hyperviscosity syndrome ensues with visual disturbances, lethargy, confusion, muscle weakness, neurologic findings, and sometimes congestive heart failure. If the macroglobulins are cryoglobulins, Raynaud's phenomenon may occur. Tissue deposition of the macroglobulin may result in peripheral neuropathy, renal disease (although this is less common and usually less severe than in multiple myeloma), or amyloidosis.[410]

Physical examination shows retinal changes with engorged veins, hemorrhages, exudates, and blurred disk margins. Bleeding manifestations may occur as a result of interaction of the macroglobulin with platelets and coagulation factors. There is often anemia, but it may be artificially low because IgM causes expansion of the plasma volume. There is usually moderate lymphadenopathy and hepatosplenomegaly. Bence-Jones proteinuria may also be observed.[410]

The diagnosis is made by demonstrating an IgM monoclonal spike in serum protein electrophoresis. Immunoelectrophoresis confirms that there is a monoclonal IgM. A bone marrow examination reveals infiltration by lymphocytes, plasma cells, and plasmacytoid lymphocytes with immature forms. The peripheral blood smear often shows a mild lymphocytosis with plasmacytoid lymphocytes. When the disease is advanced, the organs are infiltrated with these cells. Treatment is necessary when there is anemia, bleeding, organomegaly, or hyperviscosity symptoms. In its early stages Waldenstrom's disease does not require therapy. Treatment usually involves chemotherapy with an alkylating agent (traditionally chlorambucil), often together with prednisone. Other therapies, involving agents such as α-interferon or fludarabine, are sometimes tried.[410] Hyperviscosity is controlled with plasmapharesis.[355]

Hairy Cell Leukemia

Hairy cell leukemia (leukemic reticuloendotheliosis) is an uncommon chronic lymphoproliferative disease originating usually as a lymphoma of splenic B cells (rarely T cells) which eventually results in splenomegaly, pancytopenia, and the presence of "hairy" lymphocytes in the blood and bone marrow. These hairy lymphocytes are unique in that they contain tartrate-resistant isozyme 5 of acid phosphatase, ribosomal lamellar aggregates in the cytoplasm seen on electron microscopy, receptors for C3b, on their surface receptors for the Fc portion of IgG (Fc R), and frequent expression of monoclonal S IgG.[360,361]

Hairy cell leukemia usually appears at an earlier age, the median age being 53; the male/female ratio is more than 5:1. Hairy cell leukemia is a chronic disease, with most patients surviving for more than 5 years. Initial presentation includes fatigue, weight loss, and weakness. The most prominent clinical finding is splenomomegaly. The massive splenomegaly is responsible for symptoms and for the hematologic picture of hypersplenism.

At diagnosis, most patients are pancytopenic, and the characteristic hairy cells are seen on the peripheral blood smear. Bone marrow aspirate is usually unsuccessful, and a biopsy is necessary to demonstrate marrow infiltration. Less common findings include osteolytic bone lesions, paraproteinemia, and skin involvement. Death is usually a result of infection and, less commonly, second malignancies.[411]

Therapy for hairy cell leukemia has been very satisfactory. At the present time, when treatment is required, the choices include splenectomy, α-interferon, deoxycoformycin (pentostatin), and 2-chlorodeoxyadenosine.[412]

Angioimmunoblastic Lymphadenopathy

Angioimmunoblastic lymphadenopathy is a systemic benign-appearing largely T-cell lymphoproliferative disorder with about a 20 percent prediliction for transformation into lymphoma.[413] This is a disorder of late midlife (median age 60). Patients present with fever, night sweats, weight loss, pruritus, abdominal pain, painful cervical or generalized adenopathy, erythematous maculopapular rashes, and hepatosplenomegaly.[414] Frequently an anemia (often Coombs-positive) and polyclonal hypergammaglobulinemia are also found.[415] The clinical course is usually aggressive, with median survival of between 11 and 30 months, though some patients may experience spontaneous remission.[415] The major cause of mortality is infection or transformation into lymphoma, usually large cell immunoblastic lymphoma, periphereal T-cell lymphoma, or Hodgkin's disease.[415] Treatment is usually combination chemotherapy that includes prednisone.

Myeloproliferative Diseases

Myeloproliferative disorders share a common origin in that they arise from monoclonal proliferation of the hematopoietic pluripotent precursor cell. In this respect, these illnesses can all be classified as malignancies. However, since in most myeloproliferative diseases the pluripotential precursor cells retain the ability to differentiate and mature into functional cells, they are usually fairly benign and chronic.[416,417]

Classification

Myeloproliferative diseases can be classified by their degree of maturation. Thus, they range from benign to dysplastic to malignant. The hyperplastic syndromes are polycythemia vera and essential thrombocythemia. Myeloid metaplasia is the dysplastic phase, and acute myelosclerosis, paroxysmal nocturnal hemoglobulinuria, aplastic anemia, and leukemia are malignant. This classification allows for the degree of overlap between the syndromes and the transition from one stage to the other (from more benign to more malignant). In these disorders, there is also a variable amount of fibrosis in the bone marrow.[416] Fibroblastic proliferation in myeloproliferative disease is of polyclonal origin and is a reactive phenomenon.[418]

The most benign proliferative states are characterized by panmyelosis of the central skeletal marrow with intact maturation of the red cells, white cells, and platelets (polycythemia vera and essential thrombocythemia). Dysplastic syndromes are characterized by reversion to a fetal distribution of the hematopoietic organ involving centrifugal expansion of the bone marrow from the axial skeleton to the long bones and reactivation of extramedullary hematopoiesis in the spleen and liver (myeloid metaplasia). This occurs in agnogenic myeloid metaplasia, polycythemia vera with myeloid metaplasia, and postpolycythemic myeloid metaplasia. Further malignant deterioration in myeloproliferative disease is characterized by ineffective erythropoiesis and a decrease in peripheral blood counts. Normal maturation is overcome by the production of abnormal cells. During this phase, hematopoiesis may develop into aplastic anemia, a myelodysplastic syndrome, or paroxysmal nocturnal hemoglobinuria. Final malignant deterioration is seen as acute nonlymphocytic or lymphocytic leukemia.[416]

Chronic myelogenous leukemia is also a clonal myeloproliferative disorder originating from a neoplastic transformation at the level of multipotential stem cells and is characterized by massive overproduction of slightly defective granulocytes. This illness does not arise from the other more benign myeloproliferative disorders but terminates with further deterioration to acute leukemia.[419–421]

Incidence

Accurate information on the incidence of myeloproliferative disorders is not available. These disorders are observed during the middle and later years of life and are rare in the young. Males are afflicted slightly more frequently than females. It has been suggested that there is an increased incidence in Ashkenazi Jews, but this is debatable.[416]

Etiology

Rare cases with a familial incidence or a history of exposure to mutagens or bone marrow toxins (benzene, radiation) suggest that there may be a chromosomal abnormality. However, this idea remains very speculative, except for chronic myelogenous leukemias.[421] At the present time, the etiology of these illnesses is still unknown.

Pathophysiology and signs and symptoms

Uncontrolled production of mature red blood cells is the predominant proliferative feature of polycythemia vera. This activity must be distinguished from other causes of erythrocytosis by the presence of an elevated red cell mass, normal oxygen saturation in the blood, normal p50 of the hemoglobin, and normal renal ultrasound (in selected patients abdominal and brain imaging studies to exclude certain specific diseases associated with erythrocytosis may also need to be performed). The erythropoiltin level is low. A bone marrow biopsy shows hypercellularity, with most patients having trilinear hyperplasia. The leukocyte and platelet counts are usually elevated, and high leukocyte alkaline phosphatase and vitamin B_{12} levels are also often found. The increased blood volume and increased circulatory red cell mass lead to the complications of thrombosis and bleeding. Thrombosis may be arterial (coronary, cerebral, or peripheral vascular) or venous (peripheral, hepatic, or portal). Elderly patients are at increased risk for thrombotic events.[422,423] Small vessel insufficiency produces cyanosis, erythromelalgia, or even frank gangrene of the fingers and toes. Mild hemorrhagic tendencies such as epistaxis, bruising, and gingival bleeding are common, while severe gastrointestinal, genitourinary, or pulmonary bleeding occurs in about 10 percent of patients. The major causes of mortality in untreated patients are thrombosis and hemorrhage.[416,417]

In essential thrombocythemia there is also hemorrhage and microvascular occlusions. However, there is generally a poor correlation between the occurrence of hemorrhagic phenomena and the platelet count or the presence of in vitro platelet function abnormalities. It seems that the combination of erythrocytosis and thrombocytosis predisposes to large vessel thrombosis. Thrombocythemia in the absence of an elevated red cell mass does not lead to large vessel thrombosis. However, microvascular occlusion occurs very frequently, as does bleeding.[416,417]

In myeloid metaplasia, the degree of splenic involvement by extramedullary hematopoiesis is independent of the degree of marrow fibrosis. The dissociation invalidates the idea that myeloid metaplasia is compensatory to diminished bone marrow function.[416,417] The finding of increased numbers of granulocytic stem cells in the peripheral blood that show fetal characteristics suggests that it is possible that myeloid metaplasia arises from a homing of these cells to a favorable environment in the spleen and liver. When myeloid metaplasia occurs de novo, it is referred to as agnogenic myeloid metaplasia. The most common symptoms of agnogenic myeloid metaplasia are due to anemia or splenomegaly; half of patients have leukocytosis, and half have either thrombocytosis or thrombocytopenia.[424] In 12 percent of patients with polycythemia vera, about 10 years after diagnosis there is evolution into a picture indistinguishable from that of myeloid metaplasia. This may occur more frequently after ^{32}P treatment. Myeloid metaplasia may also occur early in the course of polycythemia vera. It is far less common to see myeloid metaplasia in the course of essential thrombocythemia.[416,417]

Patients with polycythemia and agnogenic myeloid metaplasia are at greater risk for developing acute leukemia. The leukemia may be acute lymphocytic, acute nonlymphocytic, or biphenotypic and is characteristically resistant to chemotherapy. Transformation into acute leukemia is an expression of myelodysplasia and occurs in both treated and untreated patients, even though it is more common in those who have received alkylating agents and radiation.

In chronic myelogenous leukemia over 90 percent of patients have the Ph^1 (Philadelphia) chromosome: this abnormality results from a T (9;22) translocation. The presence of this marker forecasts both a better prognosis and a better response to therapy.[421]

Patients with chronic myelogenous leukemia may present with almost identical physical and peripheral blood counts as myeloid metaplasia. However, in chronic myelogenous leukemia leukocytosis is usually more prominent, teardrop cell forms are absent, and fibrosis of the bone marrow is uncommon. The differentiating features of chronic myelogenous leukemia are the presence of the Ph^1 chromosome, low or absent neutrophil alkaline phosphatase activity, and a high vitamin B_{12} serum level with a very high unsaturated binding capacity due to an increase in transcobalamin I.[416,417]

In other myeloproliferative disorders, the Ph^1 chromosome is not found, the neutrophil alkaline phosphate activity is normal or high, and serum vitamin B_{12} is only slightly elevated. In these other conditions, elevation is due to the elaboration of transcobalamin III. There is considerable elevation of the unsaturated B_{12} binding capacity.[416,417]

Early in the course of chronic myelogenous leukemia, the illness may be mistaken for another myeloproliferative disorder. It is important to distinguish it, as the prognosis and the treatment will be very different.

Prognosis

The median survival of patients with polycythemia vera who are treated is approximately 10 to 15 years.[425] In primary thrombocythemia, the median survival is about 5 years. Myeloid metaplasia patients have a 60 percent decrease in 5-year survival as compared to controls matched for age and gender.[419,420] Acute leukemias and myelosclerosis are usually rapidly fatal within months. Chronic myelocytic leukemia patients treated with conventional chemotherapy have a median survival of 47 months, and in rare cases patients survive for decades.

Treatment

In polycythemia, restoration of a normal blood volume and hematocrit markedly reduces the incidence of complications.[425] At diagnosis the patient should undergo a series of phlebotomies of 250 to 500 ml every second or third day. If hydration is maintained, there is no need to readminister the patient's plasma. In patients with cardiovascular disease and in people over 75 years of age, it is usually prudent to phlebotomize only about 250 to 350 ml each time. Once the hematocrit is reduced to below 42 percent, the phlebotomy should be repeated as required to maintain the hematocrit at the desired level, at about 40 to 44 percent. Phlebotomy inevitably results in iron deficiency which serves to limit erythropoiesis. The phlebotomy requirement in iron deficiency should be less than 8 units per year. If an electronically derived hematocrit is used, it should be recognized that in the face of microcytosis the electronic cell counter underestimates the hematocrit up to 7 percent. Iron should not be given to correct the iron deficiency, as it will stimulate erythropoiesis.[425]

Occasionally a patient cannot tolerate phlebotomies or finds the symptoms of iron deficiency very troublesome. There are also certain subgroups of patients who are at especially high risk for thrombosis: patients older than 70 years of age, patients in whom erythropoiesis is so active that they have a high frequency of phlebotomy, and patients with a prior history of thrombosis.[423] In these individuals it is necessary to consider the use of myelosuppressive therapy. However, in patients treated with ^{32}P or chlorambucil, there is a danger of inducing leukemia or a second malignancy,[425] and the overall benefit of aggressive therapy has been questioned.[422] In a recent study in Italy four times as many patients who had previously received radiophosphorous alkylating or nonalkylating myelosuppressive agents died of cancer compared with patients who received phlebotomy or other pharmacologic treatments.[422] At the present time, when myelosuppression is necessary, hydroxyurea is often used, although the previously believed safety of this agent in terms of mutagenicity has also recently been questioned.[423] Pruritus does not respond to phlebotomy and requires myelosuppression. Interferon is being used experimentally with some success in treating this disease.[423]

In essential thrombocythemia, myelosuppression is indicated in patients past the age of 60 who have marked thrombocythemia (platelet counts consistently over $1 \times 10^6/\text{mm}^3$) or a lower thrombocythemia with a past history of thrombosis or hemorrhage or a coexisting condition that places them at increased risk of these complications. Myelosuppression is usually achieved with hydroxyurea used in the same manner as in polycythemia vera.[426] The platelet count is usually reduced to a level of $500{,}000/\text{mm}^3$. If surgery is necessary, the platelet count should be reduced to less than $500{,}000/\text{mm}^3$. Postoperative bleeding should be managed with transfusion of normal platelets regardless of the platelet count. If a patient with thrombocythemia is bleeding or has active thrombosis, the platelet count should be reduced rapidly with plateletpheresis and hydroxyurea.[426] In any myeloproliferative disorder, the platelet count and red cell count must be normal before any surgery is performed. Newer approaches involving therapy with anagrelide, an agent believed to impair megakaryocytic maturation, is being evaluated with some success in patients with this disorder.[427]

In the asymptomatic phase of myeloid metaplasia no therapy is necessary unless the patient has thrombocythemia and is being prepared for surgery.[418] In myeloid metaplasia splenomegaly is usually responsible for the major complications of the illness. Splenomegaly in myeloid metaplasia usually responds to myelosuppression. Hydroxyurea in doses of 1.0 g/d orally usually reduces the size of the spleen without achieving a significant decrease in marrow function. Anemia is not a contraindication to the use of myelosuppression, as transfusion may be given.[416]

Myelosuppressive therapy, however, cannot be used in the setting of neutropenia and thrombocytopenia because of hypoplasia or fibrosis of the bone marrow. Splenic irradiation has been tried, but even localized therapy is myelosuppressive. Therefore, splenic irradiation must be used sparingly and with extreme caution.[416–418] Splenectomy is used in some patients, but there is significant mortality and morbidity in elderly patients with myeloid metaplasia. Embolism via an arterial catheter has been proposed for use in the elderly as an alternate safer method of infarcting the spleen.[418] Indications for splenectomy may include symptomatic splenomegaly, refractory thrombocytopenia, refractory hemolytic anemia, and portal hypertension due to splenomegaly.[424] Early splenectomy (at the point at which significant pancytopenia is present) in the elderly has been advocated before cardiovascular complications occur.[416] Splenectomy is contraindicated if diffuse intravascular coagulation is found on laboratory testing (12 percent of patients have this condition without clinical bleeding). Thrombocythemia should be treated with hydroxyurea prior to splenectomy. Surgery is palliative therapy and usually should not be performed if there is high serum alkaline phosphatase, anemia with a spleen estimated to be greater than 3 kg, or anemia with a spleen estimated to be less than 1 kg.[416] Measurement of red cell production, survival, and splenic sequestration are not predictive of the effect of splenectomy on the anemia. The anemia should be evaluated to be sure that deficiencies are not present, such as iron, folate, or vitamin B_{12}. Hemolysis may respond to the use of corticosteroids and should be evaluated with chromium red blood survival. If ineffective erythropoiesis is present (shown by ferrokinetics), pyridoxine and androgens may be tried.[416–418,424]

The malignant phases of myeloproliferative disorders are

notoriously resistant to therapy. However, treatment is similar to that described in previous sections.

In all myeloproliferative disorders hyperuricemia is treated with allopurinol. Hydration should be maintained, and hypertonic solutions for diagnostic purposes should be avoided as much as possible. Histamine symptoms (itching and pruritus after baths) may be relieved by use of the potent antihistamine agent cyproheptadine, 4 mg orally; other antihistaminics are usually not successful. Symptoms of gastrointestinal hyperacidity may be controlled with H2 blockers and/or antacids.[416]

Chronic myelocytic leukemia used to be controlled with oral busulfan or hydroxyurea. The current therapy for chronic myelocytic leukemia is evolving, however, and some studies have suggested that α-interferon prolongs survival and delays progression to the blastic phase when compared to therapy with hydroxyurea or busulfan.[428] Therefore interferon-based regimens are being recommended more often. Bone marrow transplantation, which has met with some success in younger patients, is rarely used in the elderly because of the high mortality associated with this procedure.[428]

Myelodysplastic Syndromes

Myelodysplastic syndromes are a heterogeneous group of disorders in which the hematopoietic precursors are abundant but morphologically abnormal. There is ineffective hematopoiesis, and normal numbers of mature peripheral blood cells are not produced. If only the red cell line is affected, the term *refractory anemia* is used. There is often a progression from refractory anemia to a more serious myelodysplastic syndrome involving white cells and platelets.[429]

Morphologic criteria are still the basis on which these myelodysplastic syndromes are classified (Table 89-8). If only the red cell line is involved and there are no ringed sideroblasts, the disorder is called refractory anemia. If there are more than 15 percent ringed sideroblasts, the diagnosis is refractory anemia with ringed sideroblasts. When there are excess blasts in the marrow but not in the peripheral blood, refractory anemia with excess blasts (RAEB) is the diagnosis. When RAEB is accompanied by peripheral blood monocytosis (1,000/mm^3 or greater), the illness is called chronic myelomonocytic leukemia. Finally, when there are 5 percent or more peripheral blood blasts, the illness is called RAEB in transformation. There terms have for the most part replaced the old term *preleukemia*, as only about 10 to 30 percent of patients with a myelodysplastic syndrome go on to develop acute leukemia.[320,429]

Incidence

The exact incidence is not known, but these syndromes are fairly common in elderly people. Ineffective erythropoiesis increases with the age of a population and in some studies on the elderly up to 20 percent had unexplained refractory anemia. These syndromes are more common in men than in women and are extremely rare under the age of 40. The older one gets, the more likely one is to develop these disorders (see the section on etiology). A history of exposure to radiation and/or chemical leukemogens is common.[430]

Etiology

While the etiology in most patients is unknown, it has become clear that treatment with prolonged courses of alkylating agents is associated with an increased risk of myelodysplastic syndromes and acute nonlymphocytic leukemia. Long courses of phenylalanine mustard for treatment of multiple myeloma or ovarian carcinoma, or of chlorambucil or nitrogen mustard plus radiation therapy for Hodgkin's disease, result in an incidence of acute nonlymphocytic leukemia of 2 to 7 percent. Anemia or pancytopenia associated with changes in the bone marrow and peripheral blood identical to those in myelodysplastic syndromes develops 2 to 10 years after therapy.[431] The acute nonlymphocytic leukemia that may result is invariably fatal. It is very likely that this long-term complication of successful chemotherapy will become more prevalent, especially in an aging population, as the survival of patients with cancer continues to improve. Chemotherapeutic drugs that are not alkylating agents, such as methotrexate, do not seem to be associated with this danger.

Other etiologic possibilities include RNA viruses, somatic mutations, radiation, and environmental toxins. Aging seems critical, and this has been interpreted as being related to the multi-hit theory of carcinogenesis.[432] Drugs and various illnesses can cause sideroblastic anemia. In these conditions, the inhibition of mitochondrial and heme synthesis and accumulation of the heme-controlled suppressor seems to be the pathogenic event.[15,67,74,85,433]

Pathophysiology and signs and symptoms

Most of these syndromes are thought to arise from a lesion in the pluripotential hematopoietic stem cell pool and to evolve from clonal expansion of a single stem cell or a very small number of such cells. Deletion of a major portion of the long arm of chromosome 5[59] is encountered in a wide spectrum of acquired hematologic disease, including refractory anemias, acute nonlymphocytic leukemias, myeloproliferative diseases, lymphomas, and occasional solid tumors.[434] About 50 percent of patients with myelodysplastic syndrome have chromosomal abnormalities, and abnormalities of chromosomes 7, 8, 11, 12, and 20 have also been described in addition to the abnormalities on chromosome 5.[435] The major specific pathophysiologic mechanism is ineffective hematopoiesis, the defective maturation of marrow precursor cells. Proliferation of progenitor and early precursor cells is usually normal or enhanced, producing a hypercellular marrow, but there is a deficiency of the circulating fully mature cells. There is also a mild decrease in the cells' life span which contributes to the cytopenias.[320,429]

There are rare instances of such myelodysplastic syndromes in families. A protracted myelodysplastic syndrome lasting for 1 to 20 years occurs in about 5 to 10 percent of all cases of acute nonlymphatic leukemia.[320,429] The patient generally seeks medical care for symptoms of anemia, thrombocytopenia, or leukopenia. Thus, fatigue, decrease in exercise tolerance, purpura, fever, and infections are the common presenting problems. The male/female ratio is 2:1; and the patient is usually elderly. Hepatomegaly is present in about 5 percent of cases, while splenomegaly is present in about 10 percent. Pallor is found in about 50 percent of cases. Often the patient complains of arthralgias. Because development of the cytopenias is slow, many patients are asymptomatic and the diagnosis is made incidentally or the anemia is falsely attributed to aging.[429]

Laboratory data and diagnosis

The hallmark of the illness is anemia with reticulocytopenia, and red cell morphology is usually abnormal. A dimorphic population of red cells is usually present; some cells are microcytic and hypochromic, and others are normochromic and normocytic or macrocytic. Basophilic stippling, target cells, schistocytes, and nucleated red blood cells are often seen.[320]

Leukopenia is moderate in the white blood cell range of 1,000 to 4,000/mm^3, with neutropenia being more pronounced than lymphopenia. Neutrophils are frequently poorly granulated, neutrophil alkaline phosphatase may be low, and acquired pseudo-Pelger-Huet anomaly (hypolobulation of the nuclei of the mature neutrophil) may be present. Granulocytes often have abnormal function, which further adds to the increased susceptibility to infection. Monocytosis is present in 30 percent of patients, and thus serum and urinary lysozyme may be elevated. Immature myeloid cells may seem to be present in the peripheral blood smear.[320]

Thrombocytopenia is common, even though patients occasionally have thrombocytosis. Platelets may have functional defects.

The bone marrow is diagnostic of myelodysplastic syndromes.[320] Erythroblasts may have double or fragmented nuclei or intranuclear bridging and budding. Ringed sideroblasts (excess iron in mitochondria) may be prominent and are usually found in patients with primarily abnormalities in red cell precursors. With mainly erythroid dysplasia, the ratio of myeloid to erythroid precursors (M/E ratio) is 1:1 to 1:10. There is an increase in reticuloendothelial iron, and serum iron and ferritin levels in plasma are elevated. Dyserythropoiesis results in moderate elevation of serum LDH and indirect bilirubin. Iron turnover studies reveal the ineffective erythropoiesis; there is an increase in the iron turnover rate but decreased incorporation of iron into circulating erythrocytes.[320]

Marrow myeloid cells may show poor maturation to mature neutrophils and have the acquired pseudo-Pelger-Huet anomaly. They are often poorly granulated. Eosinophils and basophils may also be dysplastic. In patients with mainly myeloid dysplasia, the M/E ratio is 3:1 to 10 to 20:1. Megakarocytes may be immature and dysplastic as well.[320]

Most patients have increased iron stores, and many show clinical hemochromatosis with diabetes, cirrhosis, infiltrative heart disease, and pituitary dysfunction.[320]

Prognosis

Prognosis is variable, with survival of a few months to 10 to 15 years. Median survival ranges from 6 years for patients with refractory anemia with ringed sideroblasts to 5 months for those with refractory anemia with excess blasts in transformation.[435] The proportion of patients whose disease transforms into acute nonlymphocytic leukemia varies in the different subgroups, being about 50 percent in refractory anemia with excess blasts in transformation, 40 percent in refractory anemia with excess blasts, 35 percent in CMML, 15 percent in refractory anemia, and 5 percent in refractory anemia with ringed sideroblasts.[435] In a recent study from Australia on patients with myelodysplastic syndrome, the causes of death were infection (37 percent), acute leukemia (20 percent), bleeding (11 percent), and causes unrelated to myelodysplasia (37 percent). In 9 percent the cause of death was not recorded.[436]

Treatment

Transfusion of blood products is the mainstay of treatment[320]; however, this should be limited as much as possible. Transfusion of packed red cells entails the risk of iron overload, alloimmunization to red cell, white cell, and platelet antigens, and transmission of a variety of infections. Washed red blood cells may slow the development of alloimmunization. Platelet transfusions should be used if the patient is thrombocytopenic and there is bleeding or if surgery is necessary. Granulocyte transfusions should be used only in neutropenic patients with documented gram-negative infections who do not respond to antibiotics alone.[437] Colony stimulating factors are often used to try to improve peripheral cell counts to avoid transfusions. Erythropoetin is frequently used to try to raise the hematocrit. About 20 percent of patients show a significant response,[438,439] and there is some evidence that those with lower erythropoetin levels are more likely to respond.[439] GM-CSF and G-CSF regularly correct neutropenia but have not been shown to increase survival.[438]

Occasionally patients with ringed sideroblasts respond to pharmacologic doses of oral pyridoxine, 100 to 300 mg/d.[320] The response is only partial, and abnormal red cell morphology usually persists. Androgens and corticosteroids have usually been of little benefit.[437] Consideration should be given to the use of desferrioxamine when the total number of transfused units of red cells approaches 100.

Early treatment of myelodysplasia with excess blasts using chemotherapy has not shown any benefit on survival. The use of low-dose cytosine arabinoside to induce differentiation of blasts has been very controversial.[320,437] When the patient develops acute nonlymphocytic leukemia, the remission rate is even less than in cases of nonlymphocytic leukemia where patients did not have prior myelodysplasia. Individuals with this secondary form of nonlymphocytic leukemia have prolonged marrow aplasia after chemotherapy. Recent approaches in the elderly have involved supportive care with blood products and an attempt to keep the white blood cell count below

50,000/mm^3 with oral hydroxyurea.[320] Bone marrow transplantation, which is sometimes used in younger patients with myelodysplastic syndromes, is seldom used in older adults because of poor tolerability and survival.

Disorders of Hemostasis

Hemostasis is maintained by a mechanism involving vascular, platelet, and coagulation components. A tendency to bleed may result from a disorder of one or more of these components. As a general rule, coagulation defects in the elderly may be treated as they are in other age groups. Purpura may occur with or without demonstrable platelet abnormalities. The most common purpura in the elderly are nonthrombocytopenic.

Nonthrombocytopenic Purpuras

This condition has a different significance in the elderly than in the young. Anaphylactoid purpura is rare in old age, whereas senile purpura is very common.

Senile purpura

Senile purpura[440–442] occurs mainly on the extensor surfaces of the forearms and hands and may be seen in many otherwise normal old people. Loss of subcutaneous fat and changes in aging connective tissue permit undue mobility of an old person's skin, and the resulting shearing forces allow rupture of small vessels. The extravasated blood tracks widely, and the tissues' reaction to it is impaired. No history of trauma is usually obtained. In senile purpura individual lesions last longer than other types of purpura (from 1 to 3 weeks) and do not undergo the typical color changes as they resolve because of the poor phagocytic response to the extravasated blood. Senile purpura is more common in women. Platelets are normal both qualitatively and quantitatively in patients with senile purpura, and no correlation has been shown with ascorbic acid deficiency.

Scurvy

Scurvy is associated with purpura and more widespread bleeding from body surfaces, under the periosteum, or in the viscera. This hemorrhagic tendency has for a long time been attributed to disturbed collagen synthesis and an endothelial defect in the capillaries. In recent years, it has been demonstrated that impaired platelet function is also a feature of scurvy.[443] Dysproteinemias, infections, hypothermia, neoplasia, and drugs, have been implicated as causes of nonthrombocytopenic purpura.

Purpura Due to Platelet Defects

Thrombocytopenia may occur as a primary (idiopathic) disorder or a secondary phenomenon (drug-induced or associated with other blood diseases, infections, neoplasia, or various other conditions). Occasionally thrombocythemia, thrombasthenia, or combined defects may be present.

Autoimmune (idiopathic) thrombocytopenic purpura

IgG autoantibodies against platelets can sensitize the platelets for destruction.[444] The structure of the antigens involved is unknown, but the antigens are present in the platelets in most people. Platelet autoantibodies may be a primary or secondary phenomenon. If they are secondary, they usually arise in the setting of systemic lupus erythematosus, immunodeficiency disorders, or B-cell lymphoproliferative syndromes (e.g., chronic lymphoytic leukemia).[444–445] Autoimmune thrombocytopenia may be the first sign of HIV infection and is found in about 10 percent of patients with AIDS. In children, acute autoimmune thrombocytopenia often follows a viral infection and remits spontaneously. In older people the onset is usually insidious and is not clearly related to another illness. The course is usually chronic and intermittent.[444–445]

Autoimmune platelet destruction results in thrombocytopenia and manifestations of hemorrhage in the patient. Unless severe acute or chronic bleeding has occurred or the patient has Evan's syndrome (immune hemolytic anemia and thrombocytopenia), the red and white cell counts are normal. Few platelets are seen in the peripheral blood smear, and those that are present are large ("megathrombocytes").[444] The bone marrow shows an increase in megakaryocytes. There is usually no splenomegaly. In the serum, there are antibodies of the IgG class, and the few circulating platelets can be shown to be coated with antiplatelet IgG, C3, or both.[444,445] Testing for the presence of antibodies on platelet surfaces is, however, associated with many false positive results. Antibodies to specific platelet antigens (e.g, IIb/IIIa or Ib/IX complex) have been found in many patients with autoimmune thrombocytopenia, but tests for these are not available in most hospitals.[446] Treatment is usually initiated for bleeding or very low platelet counts (usually less than 30,000/μl) or prior to surgery. Therapy usually involves corticosteroids (prednisone 1 to 2 mg/kg/d). About 80 percent of patients respond in about 3 to 28 days after treatment is started.[446] Once a response has occurred, steroids should be tapered over 4 to 8 weeks. Splenectomy is often recommended for patients who relapse or who require high doses of prednisone to keep the platelet count acceptable. In life-threatening situations, high-dose methylprednisolone or intravenous γ-globulin is useful.[446] Other methods of treatment, if corticosteroids fail, are plasmapharesis,[446] more potent immunosuppressive drugs such as vinca alkaloids, danazol, or a monoclonal anti-FCR III antibody.[396,445]

Secondary thrombocytopenia

Drugs are a very important cause of thrombocytopenia. They may be direct marrow toxins or cause idiosyncratic or hypersensitivity reactions. Any drug capable of producing aplastic anemia can reduce platelets, either selectively or as part of the aplastic picture. In addition, some drugs are known to cause selective thrombocytopenia only by decreasing megakarocytes. They are all low-risk drugs and include sedormid, quinidine, sulfonamides, penicillin, tetracycline, chloramphenicol, salicylates, barbiturates, desipramine, chlorothiazide, digitoxin, insulin, cimetidine, and myelosuppressive drugs used as chemotherapeutic agents.[447]

Medication can also induce immune-mediated platelet destruction. Penicillin, quinidine, and quinine elicit antibodies that cause reactions similar to the hemolytic disorders produced by these drugs.[448] Antibodies against the anticoagulant heparin may produce thrombocytopenia, possibly because the heparin-antibody complexes bind to the platelets and activate them by binding to the platelet Fc receptor.[449] At the same time that the patient is at risk of bleeding from the thrombocytopenia, they are thus also subject to arterial thrombosis. In some cases, switching from bovine to porcine heparin stops the thrombocytopenia. Although the incidence of this complication is low, the widespread use of heparin in clinical practice makes it a familiar problem.[449]

Secondary thrombocytopenia is seen in acute and chronic leukemias, lymphomas, infections, myelodysplastic syndromes and myeloproliferative disorders, neoplasms, collagen-vascular diseases, splenomegaly, paraproteinemia, cirrhosis of the liver, and hypersensitivity reactions. Ethanol use may also be associated with thrombocytopenia by direct suppression of platelet production, reduced survival, and secondary to the hypersplenism or folate deficiency that may be found in some alcoholics.

Transfusion thrombocytopenia

Antibodies directed against a platelet surface antigen (PL^{A1}), an epitope of platelet membrane glycoprotein IIb/IIIa, are very destructive to platelets.[447] However, the PL^{A1} antigen is present on platelets of more than 98 percent of persons. Therefore, antibodies against PL^{A1} antigens only rarely are a problem in platelet transfusion therapy. However, persons who lack the PL^{A1} antigen on their platelets and also receive transfusions of PL^{A1}-bearing platelets may develop a condition called post-transfusion purpura. The platelets contained in whole blood transfusions are sufficient to elicit this disorder. At some time following the transfusion, the patient generates anti-PL^{A1} antibodies. These antibodies are believed to bind PL^{A1} antigen released from the transfused platelets, and the antigen-antibody complex then binds to the patient's own PL^{A1}-negative platelet. The binding of these complexes causes the destruction of the patient's platelets. The disorder is self-limited and remits completely.[447]

Thrombocytopenia caused by bone marrow failure is a common problem in hematology. It is treated with supportive care with platelet transfusions. However, platelet surfaces have histocompatibility (HLA) antigens, and anti-HLA antibodies arise in many patients and become a limiting factor in the effectiveness of platelet support therapy. The time of detection of anti-HLA antibodies against infused platelets correlates with the onset of refractoriness to the hemostatic effectiveness of the transfusions; the platelet count in the recipient no longer rises in response to transfusions from the donor to whose platelet antigen the recipient is sensitized. Judicious HLA antigen matching of donors with recipients can prevent such isosensitization and eventually find platelets that can survive in such a sensitized recipient. Unfortunately, HLA matching is a somewhat laborious and expensive procedure.[447] Thrombopoietin, the hormone thought to stimulate megakaryocytes, has recently been purified and cloned.[450] This may in time lead to advances in the treatment of a wide range of conditions associated with reduced platelet production, such as is seen after chemotherapy. The safety of this hormone for use in human is currently being investigated.

Thrombotic thrombocytopenic purpura

Thrombotic thrombocytopenia purpura (TTP)[451] is a mysterious and deadly disease in which fibrin plugs appear in small blood vessels throughout the body, with little apparent activation of the clotting cascade or the fibrinolytic system. In some people the condition appears to be initiated by toxic endothelial damage: the toxin produced by *E coli* 0157:H7 and various drugs including mitomycin C and cyclosporin A have been implicated in some cases.[446] The disease has a rapid onset, with widespread manifestations appearing over the course of a day or two. In the classic case, fever, thrombocytopenia with bleeding, traumatic hemolytic anemia, acute renal failure, and CNS disturbances are seen. Laboratory findings are very helpful in confirming the diagnosis and especially in making the sometimes difficult distinction between TTP and disseminated intravascular coagulation. The changes of traumatic anemia are present, including a low hematocrit and fragmented red cells on the blood smear. The platelet count is low, but there are many megakaryocytes in the marrow, indicating that the reduction in platelets is attributable to increased consumption rather than decreased production. Other clotting studies are usually normal, fibrinogen levels are normal or increased, and split products are usually absent. The diagnosis often has to be made on clinical grounds, but it can sometimes be made by biopsy, usually of the gum. The diagnostic finding is an arteriole containing a mass of fibrin. There is no evidence of inflammation, immunoglobulin, or complement to be found. The finding of an arteriole filled with a fibrin plug is pathognomonic for TTP in this clinical setting.[451]

TTP is usually treated by large-volume plasma exchanges, usually in combination with steroids. This form of therapy has decreased the mortality rate of TTP from 90 percent to less than 50 percent; no one knows why. In patients with TTP who do not respond to plasma exchange, a combination of steroids, antiplatelet agents, and emergency splenectomy has been used with some success.

Thrombasthenia

This rare qualitative platelet defect affects platelet function and leads to a hemorrhagic tendency due to impaired platelet adhesiveness and a failure of clot retraction (despite a normal platelet count). Though mostly a hereditary disease, it is occasionally first diagnosed in older adults. It may also be secondary to scurvy, uremia, thrombocythemia, or macroglobulinemia.[448]

Drugs affecting platelet function

There has been much recent work on platelet function in the hope of ultimately influencing the natural history of thrombosis and atherosclerosis. Many drugs have been shown to have effects on platelet behavior (adhesiveness, aggregation, and release phenomenon). Aspirin is the drug most commonly used and may be important in preventing thrombosis in older people.[452–453]

Defects of Blood Coagulation

Survival with congenital coagulation disorders in later life is possible, especially in von Willebrand's disease. Acquired disorders include vitamin K deficiency, which leads to a reduction in prothrombin (factor II) and in factors VII, IX, and X. This condition may occur in malabsorption syndromes, liver disease, prolonged obstructive jaundice, and biliary fistula and with oral broad-spectrum antibiotic therapy.[448,454]

Anticoagulant therapy with warfarin reduces hepatic synthesis of the same four factors. Chronic liver disease may lead to reduction in the above factors and also in fibrinogen (factor I) and factor V, XI, XII, and XIII. Factor X deficiency occurs in amyloidosis.

Circulating anticoagulants

Circulating anticoagulants inhibit clotting factors, usually factor VIII. The presence of this anticoagulant often means that the patient has lupus, but in the elderly it is often observed as an isolated entity.[455,456] This anticoagulant rarely causes problems and usually proves to be the explanation for a prolonged partial thromboplastin time not corrected by normal plasma. Other acquired anticoagulants are seen when there is an elevation of fibrin, split products, and an anti-factor VIII antibody in hemophilia; when there are abnormal paraproteins; or if the patient is taking anticoagulant drugs.[448,454]

Fibrinogen deficiency

Fibrinogen deficiency may result from impaired formation (liver disease), intravascular clotting, or overactive fibrinolysis.[454]

Regulation of clotting

The clotting process is regulated by two general mechanisms: elimination of activated clotting factors and destruction of the fibrin clot (fibrinolysis). The activated clotting factors are removed by two circulating anticoagulant systems: the antithrombin III proteoglycan system and the protein C-protein S system.

Antithrombin III is a protease inhibitor which acts against all the proteolytic clotting factors except VIIa.[457–459] Antithrombin III binds to proteoglycans on the endothelial surfaces of blood vessels, thus layering them with an anticoagulant. Heparin works via its interaction with antithrombin III. An inherited deficiency of this molecule leaves the individual highly suspectible to venous thrombosis.[457–459]

Protein C is a vitamin K-dependent protease that neutralizes factors V and VIII and must be activated by thrombin to work. Thrombin in turn must be modulated by a protein, thrombomodulin, before it can become an activator of protein C. Activated protein C then destroys the activity of factors V and VIII. To work, activated protein C requires $Ca,^{2+}$ phospholipid, and another vitamin K-dependent protein, protein S (the accelerator). A deficiency in either protein C or S leads to a greatly increased risk of venous thrombosis.[459–460] Resistance to activated protein C has also been described as a major risk factor for thrombosis. In most cases it is the result of a single point mutation in the factor V gene, making factor V less sensitive to activated protein C-mediated inactivation.[461] Activated protein C resistance is found in about 4 percent of the population.[461] The presence of this abnormality may be especially important if the patient has other risk factors for thrombosis. High homocysteine levels have also been suggested as risk factors for thrombosis (see section on vitamin B_{12} deficiency), a recent study has suggested that patients with homocysteinuria and activated protein C resistance are at especially high risk for thrombosis.[462]

Fibrinolysis

Fibrinolysis is accomplished by a fibrin-splitting protease, plasmin. Plasmin is derived from its precursor, plasminogen.[463]

Disseminated intravascular coagulation

A syndrome of diffuse intravascular coagulation (DIC) may be seen in the elderly in an acute, subacute, or chronic form.[448–454] There is always a serious underlying disease process that leads to thromboplastic substances (from damaged or neoplastic tissues) entering the circulation and activating the extrinsic clotting system. The intrinsic clotting system may also be involved—endothelium may be damaged by endotoxins, which also induce platelet aggregation. Antigen-antibody reactions may also lead to platelet aggregation. Platelet factor III is released and participates in the coagulation process. Intravascular fibrin deposition follows, but fibrinolysis is activated simultaneously. The net result of these changes is bleeding, thromboses, shock, hemolysis, and renal failure.[448–454]

Criteria for diagnosis are not well defined; the most useful are a low platelet count, prolonged prothrombin time, and also often activated partial thromboplastin time, positive plasma protamine test for fibrin, monomer-fibrinogen complexes, D dimers, and levels of fibrinogen and fibrin degradation products related to the clinical condition. Therapy may include under certain circumstances, restoration of depleted blood components with platelet concentrates, cryoprecipitate, and fresh frozen plasma,[464] especially if the patient is bleeding. The most important therapy is to stop the triggering factors and the underlying disease (e.g., infection, neoplasia, or various forms of tissue damage from trauma, burns, heatstroke, surgery, antigen-antibody reactions, drugs, incompatible transfusion, anaphylactic shock, and intravascular hemolysis). Aortic aneurysms have been associated with extensive coagulation disorders. Liver disease, acute pancreatitis, and nonbacterial thrombotic endocarditis have also been shown to cause DIC.[448–454]

The use of heparin in the treatment of DIC is controversial.

It may have a place in chronic varieties with thrombotic manifestations and/or dermal necrosis. Replacement of hemostatic factors may require the "cover" of continuous heparin infusion, especially in complex situations such as promyelocytic leukemia, however, some physicians question the routine use of heparin in acute promyelocytic leukemia.[464] In most cases of DIC (about 95 percent), heparin has not proved to be of value and may sometimes be harmful. Heparin may itself cause thrombocytopenia and thrombosis.[448–454]

Primary fibrinogenolysis (fibrinolysis)

Primary fibrinogenolysis occurs when active plasmin is generated in the circulation at a time when the clotting cascade is not operating. It is very rare and occurs only occasionally in severe liver disease, cancer of the prostate and lung, or heatstroke.[465]

The illness is characterized by severe bleeding and must be differentiated from DIC. The two conditions are similar in that the partial thromboplastin time, prothrombin time, and thrombin time are prolonged. In addition, in both, fibrinogen levels are low and fibrin degradation products are seen in the plasma. Traumatic hemolytic anemia may also be present.[448,465]

To make a diagnosis of primary fibrinogenolysis, the platelet count must be normal (low in DIC). The euglobulin clot lysis time is shortened (normal in DIC), and fibrin degradation products are present when detected by immunologic or staphyloccal clumping assays but negative when detected by paracoagulation assays (ethanol or protamine). In contrast, in DIC these tests are both positive. The reason for this difference is that in DIC the plasma contains fibrin monomers that are unable to form a fibrin gel because they form complexes with degradation products. When ethanol or protamine is added to plasma, these complexes fall apart and the liberated fibrin monomers polymerize to form a gel. In fibrinogenolysis there are no fibrin monomers, and so a gel does not form. Assays for D dimers are also negative.[464]

It is important to make this distinction between DIC and fibrinogenolysis, as the latter can be treated with ϵ-aminocaproic acid, which inhibits both plasmin and plasminogen. If this drug is used in DIC, it will be very dangerous and thrombosis will be enhanced.

Biologic Therapy in Hematology

A new era is dawning in that biologic materials derived from humans are being used to treat deficiencies of blood cells and hematologic malignancies. The availability today of erythropoietin, granulocyte or granulyte-macrophage colony stimulating factors (G-CSF and GM-CSF) offer a potential for treating these specific anemias or leukopenias without resorting to transfusions.[466] Bone marrow transplantation is invaluable in treating young people with hematologic malignancy or aplastic anemia. While we do not yet know the efficacy of these treatments in the elderly, it is hoped that over the next few years we will see research in this area.[467]

Other biologicals are being developed to treat malignancies, including agents that boost host deficiencies, agents that kill tumors directly, and agents that alter tumor biology. The first class of agents (active immunotherapy) includes tumor-specific (tumor cell vaccines) and nonspecific agents (lymphokines, such as IL-2). The second category, immunotherapy, also includes tumor-specific (antitumor monoclonal antibodies) and nonspecific agents (tumor necrosis factor). Interferon has several modes of action in this category. The final category includes any agent that interferes with tumor biology and includes differentiating agents (retinoids), agents that block tumor growth (antibodies to growth receptors), and agents that alter the process of metastasis (laminine fragments).[468] Ultimately, it may be possible to alter the DNA of the tumor cell and thereby cure malignancy.[469]

At the present time, we have to combine biologic therapy with traditional radiation and chemotherapy in treating hematologic malignancies. Certainly growth factors such as GM-CSF may make it possible to deliver higher levels of chemotherapy which hopefully will prove to be beneficial in treating the elderly. All these new developments in biologic therapy should prove to be invaluable resources in geriatric medicine.

References

1. Department of Health, Education, and Welfare: The First Health and Nutrition Examination Survey. DHEW (HSM), Washington, DC, 1971–1972
2. Yip R, Johnson C, Dallman PR: Age-related changes in laboratory values in the diagnosis of an anemia and iron deficiency. Am J Clin Nutr 1984;39:427–436
3. World Health Organization: Iron Deficiency Anemia. Report of a Study Group. p. 4. WHO Technical Reports Series 182. World Health Organization, Geneva, 1959
4. World Health Organization: Nutritional Anemias. Report of a WHO Scientific Group. WHO Technical Reports Series 405. World Health Organization, Geneva, 1968
5. Hill RD: The prevalence of anemia in the over 65s in a rural practice. Practitioner 1967;217:963–965
6. Myers MA, Saunders CRG, Chalmers DG: The hemoglobin level of fit elderly people. Lancet 1968;ii:261
7. Milner JS, Williamson J: Hemoglobin, hematocrit, leukocyte count and blood grouping in older people. Geriatrics 1972; 27:118–126
8. Department of Health and Social Security: A nutritional survey of the elderly. p. 57. Report on Health and Human Subjects 3. HMSO, London, 1972
9. Brocklehurst JC, Leeming JG, Carty MH, Robinson JM: Medical screening of old people accepted for residential care. Lancet 1978;ii:141–143
10. Htoo MS, Kofkoff RL, Freedman ML: Erythrocyte parameters in the elderly: an argument against new geriatric normal values. J Am Geriatr Soc 1978;27:547–555
11. Williams WJ: The effect of aging on the blood count. Compr Ther 1960;6:7–9

12. Lipshitz DA, Mitchell CO, Thompson C: The anemia of senescence. Am J Hematol 1981;11:47–54
13. Freedman ML, Marcus DL: Anemia and the elderly: is it physiology or pathology? Am J Med Sci 1980;280:81–85
14. Freedman ML: Anemias in the elderly. Compr Ther 1983;i:45–53
15. Babitz L, Freedman ML: Anemia and the elderly patient. Compr Ther 1988;14:55–64
16. Tibblin E, Bengtsson C, Hallberg L, Lennartsson J: Hemoglobin concentration and peripheral blood counts in women. Scand J Haematol 1979;22:5–16
17. Eisen ME, Hammond EC: The effect of smoking on packed cell volume, red cell counts, haemoglobin and platelet counts. Can Med Assoc J 1956;75:520–523
18. Isager H, Hagerup L: Relationship between cigarette smoking and high packed cell volumes and haemoglobin level. Scand J Haematol 1971;8:241–244
19. Sagone AL Jr, Bakcerzak SP: Smoking as a cause of erythrocytosis. Ann Intern Med 1975;82:512–515
20. Vaisrub S On the fringes of smoke rings. JAMA 1976;234:520
21. Albert SN: Blood Volume. p. 24. Charles C Thomas, Springfield, Il, 1963
22. Besa EC, Gorshein D, Gardner FH: Androgens and human blood volume changes. Arch Intern Med 1974;133:418–425
23. Besa EC: Physiological changes in blood volume. Crit Rev Clin Lab Sci 1975;6:67–79
24. Beaumont WV, Greenleaf JE, Juhos L: Disproportional changes in hematocrit, plasma volume and proteins during exercise and bed rest. J Appl Physiol 1972;33:55–61
25. Taylor HL, Ericson L, Hemschel A, Keys A: The effect of bed rest on the blood volume of normal men. Am J Physiol 1945;144:227–232
26. Fawcett JK, Wynn V: Effects of posture on plasma volume and some blood constituents. J Clin Pathol 1960;13:304–310
27. Rowe JW, Minaker KL, Sparrow D, Robertson GL: Age related failure of volume-pressure-mediated vasopressin release. J Clin Endocrinol Metab 1982;54:661–664
28. Sanchez C, Merino C, Figallo M: Simultaneous measurement of plasma volume and cell mass in polycythemia of high altitude. J Appl Physiol 1970;28:775–778
29. Purcell H, Brozovic B: Red cell 2,3-diphosphoglycerate concentration in man decreases with age. Nature 1974;251:511–512
30. Miller ME, Rorth M, Parving HH et al: pH effects on erythropoietin response to hypoxia. N Engl J Med 1973;288:706
31. Rorth M: Hypoxia, red cell oxygen affinity and erythropoietin production. Clin Haematol 1974;3:595–3607
32. Besa EC: Approach to mild anemia in the elderly. Clin Geriatr 1988;4.1:43–55
33. Woo JE, Roy SB: The relationship of peripheral venomotor response to high altitude pulmonary edema in man. Am J Med Sci 1980;259:56–65
34. Dill BD, Horvath SM, Dahms TE et al: Hemoconcentration at altitude. J Appl Physiol 1969;27:514–518
35. Jung RC, Dill DB, Horton R, Hovarth SM: Effects of age on plasma aldosterone levels and hemoconcentration at altitude. J Appl Physiol 1971;31:593–597
36. Hartsock RJ, Smith EB, Petty CS: Normal variations with aging in the amount of hematopoietic tissue in bone marrow from the anterior iliac crest. J Am Clin Pathol 1965;43:326–331
37. Lipshitz DA, Udupa KB, Milton KY, Thompson CO: Effects of age on hematopoiesis in man. Blood 1984;63:502–509
38. Chen MG: Age related changes in hematopoietic stem cell populations of long lived hybrid mouse. J Cell Physiol 1971;78:225–232
39. Harrison DE: Normal function of transplanted marrow cell lines from aged mice. J Gerontol 1975;30:279–285
40. Freedman ML: Heme and iron metabolism in aging. Blood Cells 1987;13:234–241
41. Refino CJ, Dallman PR: Rate of repair of iron deficiency anemia and blood loss anemia in young and mature rats. Am J Clin Nutr 1983;37:904–909
42. Boggs DR, Patrene KD: Hematopoiesis and aging III: anemia and a blunted erythropoietic response to hemorrhage in aged mice. Am J Hematol 1985;19:327–328
43. Marx JJM: Normal iron absorption and decreased red cell iron uptake in the aged. Blood 1979;53:204–211
44. Piomelli S, Nathan DG, Cummins JF, Gardner F: The relationship of total red cell volume to total body water in octogenarian males. Blood 1962;19:89–98
45. Nathan DG, Piomelli S, Gardner F, Limauro AL: The effects of androgen on some aspects of body composition and erythropoiesis in octogenarian males. Ann N Y Acad Sci 1967;110:965–977
46. Hurdle ADF, Rosin AJ: Red cell volume and red cell survival in normal aged people. J Clin Pathol 1962;15:343–345
47. Myers AM, Saunders CR, Chalmers DG: The haemoglobin level of fit elderly people. Lancet 1968;ii:261–263
48. Smith JS, Whitelaw DM: Hemoglobin values in aged men. Can Med Assoc J 1971;105:816–818
49. McLennan WJ, Andrews GR, Macleod C, Caird FI: Anemia in the elderly. Q J Med 1973;42:1–13
50. Jandl JH: Blood: Textbook of Hematology. Little Brown, Boston, 1987
51. Huehns ER: Control of red cell oxygen affinity by 2,3-DPG in disease. pp. 38–55. In Huntsman RG, Jenkins GC (eds): Advanced Haemotology. Butterworth, London, 1974
52. Huehns ER: The structure and function of haemoglobin: clinical disorders due to abnormal haemoglobin structure. pp. 526–629e. In Hardisty RM, Weatherall DU (eds): Blood and Its Disorders. Blackwell, Oxford, 1974
53. Brewer GJ: Red cell metabolism and function pp. 473–508. In Surgenor DN (ed): The Red Blood Cell. 2nd Ed. Academic Press, New York, 1974
54. Thomas HM, Lefrak S, Irwin RS et al: The oxyhemoglobin disassociation curve in health and disease. Am J Med 1974;57:331–348
55. Weintraub NT, Freedman ML: Anemias. pp. 643–684. In Abrams WB, Berkow R (eds): The Merck Manual of Geriatrics. Merck, Sharp & Dohme, Whitehouse Station, NJ, 1990
56. Thompson W, Meola T, Lipkin M Jr, Freedman ML: The utility of the RDW, MCV and transferrin saturation in the diagnosis

of iron deficiency anemia. Arch Intern Med 1988;148: 2128–2130

57. Thompson WG, Cassino C, Babitz L et al: Hypersegmented neutrophils and vitamin B_{12} deficiency. Acta Haemotol 1989; 81:186–191
58. Coates CA: Routine testing in hematology. pp. 127–144. In Rodak BF: Diagnostic Hematology. WB Saunders, Philadelphia, 1995
59. The Editors. Tenth Edition of the RDA. Nutr Rev 1990;48: 28–29
60. Marcus DL, Freedman ML: Clinical disorders of iron metabolism in the elderly. Clin Geriatr Med 1985;1:729–745
61. Assessment of Iron Nutriture. pp. 129–151. In DHSS Publication 89–1255, National Center for Health Statistics.
62. Schultz BM, Freedman ML: Iron deficiency in the elderly. pp. 291–313. Bailliere's Clinical Haematology 1.
63. Guyatt GH, Patterson C, Ali M et al: Diagnosis of iron deficiency in the elderly. Am J Med 1990;88:205–209
64. Jacobs A: Non-haematologic effects of iron deficiency. Clin Haematol 1982;11:353–365
65. Marcus DL, Ibrahim NG, Gruenspecht N, Freedman ML: Iron requirement for isolated rat liver mitochondrial protein synthesis. Biochim Biophys Acta 1982;607:136–143
66. Marcus DL, Ibrahim NG, Freedman ML: Age-related decline in the biosynthesis of mitochondrial inner membrane proteins. Exp Gerontol 1980;17:333–341
67. Marcus DL, Freedman ML: Role of heme and iron metabolism in controlling protein synthesis. J Am Geriatr Soc 1986;34: 593–600
68. Rabinovitz M, Freeman ML, Fisher JM, Maxwell CR: Translational control in hemoglobin synthesis. Symp Quant Biol 1969; 34:567–568
69. Gross M, Rabinovitz M: 1972 Control of globin synthesis by hemin: factors influencing formation of an inhibitor of globin chain. initiation in reticulocyte lysates. Biochim Biophys Acta 1972;287:340–352
70. Rhoads RE, McNight GS, Schimke RT: Quantitative measurement of ovalbumin messenger ribonucleic activity: localization in polysomes, induction by estrogen, and effect of actinomycin D. J Biol Chem 1973;248:2031–2037
71. Freedman ML, Karpatkin S: Requirement of iron for platelet protein synthesis. Biochem Biophys Res Commun 1973;54: 475–481
72. Lodish HF, Desalu O: Regulation of synthesis of nonglobin proteins in cell-free extracts of rabbit reticulocytes. J Biol Chem 1973;248:3420–3428
73. Lodish HF: Model for the regulation of mRNA translation applied to haemoglobin synthesis. Nature 1974;251:385–392
74. Freedman ML, Rosman J: A rabbit reticulocyte model for the role of hemin-controlled repressor in hypochromic anemias. J Clin Invest 1976;57:594–603
75. Freedman ML, Geraghty M, Rosman J: Hemin control of globin synthesis: isolation of a hemin-reversible translational repressor from human nature erythrocytes. J Biol Chem 1974;240: 7290–7302,
76. Freedman ML, Spieler PJ, Rosman J, Wildman J: Cyclic AMP maintenance of rabbit reticulocyte haem and protein synthesis in the presence of ethanol and benzene. Br J Haematol 1977; 37:179–185
77. Ranu RS, London IM: Regulation of protein synthesis in rabbit reticulocyte lysates: purification and initial characterization of the cyclic 3′:5′-AMP independent protein kinase of the hemeregulated translational inhibitor. Proc Natl Acad Sci U S A 1976;73:4349–4355
78. Trachsel H, Staehelin T: Binding and release of eukaryotic initiation factor of eIF-2 and GTP during protein synthesis initiation. Proc Natl Acad Sci U S A 1978;75:204–211
79. deHaro C, Datta A, Ochoa S: Mode of action of the hemin controlled inhibitor of protein synthesis. Proc Natl Acad Sci U S A 1978;75:243–252
80. Ibrahim NG, Spieler PJ, Freedman ML: Ethanol inhibition of rabbit reticulocytes at the level of delta-aminolevulinic acid synthase. Br J Haematol 1979;41:235–241
81. Irbahim NG, Gruenspecht NR, Freedman ML: Feedback inhitition rat reticulocyte delta at the level of delta aminolevulinic acid synthase. Biophys Res Commun 1978;80:722–730
82. Beuzard Y, Rodvien R, London IM: Effect of hemin on the synthesis of hemoglobin and other proteins in mammalian cells. Proc Natl Acad Sci U S A 1973;70:1022–1031
83. Ibrahim NG, Marcus DL, Freedman ML: Maintenance of cytochrome P-450 content in old rat livers in spite of decreased mitochondrial protein synthesis. J Clin Exp Gerontol 1981;3: 327–337
84. Ibrahim NG, Levere RD, Freedman ML: Effect of age on rat liver heme and drug metabolism. Exp Gerontol 1985;20: 277–284
85. Freedman ML: Heme and iron metabolism in aging. Blood Cells 1987;13:234–241
86. Ibrahim NG, Hoffstein ST: Induction of liver cell haem oxyganese in iron overloaded rats. Biochem J 1979;180:257–263
87. Marcus DL, Lew G, Freedman ML: Increased inactivation of cytochrome P-450 in iron overloaded rats. J Clin Exp Gerontol 1985;7:257–270
88. Gubler CJ, Cartwright GE, Wintrobe MM: Studies on copper metabolism. XX. enzyme activities and iron metabolism in copper and iron deficiencies. J Biol Chem 1957;224:533–546
89. Beutler E: Iron enzymes in iron deficiency. I. cytochrome c. Am J Med Sci 1968;234:517–527
90. Beutler E: Iron enzymes in iron deficiency. IV. cytochrome oxidase in rat kidney and heart. Acta Haematol 1959;21: 371–377
91. Beutler E, Blaisdell RK: Iron enzymes in iron deficiency. V. succinic dehydrogenase in rat liver, kidney and heart. Blood 1960;15:30–35
92. Masuya T: Pathophysiological studies in sideropenic symptoms: biochemical considerations. Isr J Med Sci 1965;1: 733–734
93. Srivastava SK, Sanwal GG, Tewari KK: Biochemical alterations in rat tissue in iron deficiency and repletion. Indian J Biochem 1965;2:257–263
94. Dagg JH, Jackson JM, Curry B, Goldberg A: Cytochrome oxidase in latent iron deficiency (sideropenia). Br J Haematol 1966;12:331–333
95. Beveridge BR, Bannerman RM, Evanson JM, Witts L: Hypochromic anemia: a retrospective study and follow-up of 378 in-patients. Q J Med 1965;34:145–153

96. Jacobs A: Oral cornification in anaemic patients. J Clin Pathol 1959;12:235–241
97. Jacobs A: The buccal mucosa in anaemia. J Clin Pathol 1960; 13:463–470
98. Paterson DR: A clinical type of dysphagia. J Laryngol Rhinol Otol 1919;34:289–295
99. Kelly AB: Spasm at the entrance to the oesophagus. J Laryngol Rhinol Otol 1919;34:285–289
100. Vinson PP: Hysterical dysphagia. Minnesota Med 1922;5: 107–111
101. Entwistle CC, Jacobs A: Histological findings in the Patterson-Kelly syndrome. J Clin Pathol 1965;18:408–413
102. Ahlbom HE: Simple achlorhydric anemia, Plummer-Vinson syndrome and carcinoma of the mouth, pharynx, and esophagus in women. BMJ 1936;ii:331–336
103. Wynder EL, Hultberg S, Jacobsson F, Bross IJ: Environmental factors in cancer of the upper alimentary tract. Cancer 1957; 10:470–475
104. Dagg JH, Goldberg A, Anderson JM et al: Autoimmunity in iron deficiency anemia. BMJ 1964;i:1349–1355
105. Chisholm M, Ardran GM, Callender ST, Wright R: A follow up study of patients with postcricoid webs. Q J Med 1971;40: 409–420
106. Chisholm M, Ardran GM, Callender ST, Wright R: Iron deficiency and autoimmunity in postcricoid webs. Q J Med 1971; 40:421–433
107. Coltman CA Jr: Pagophagia and iron lack. JAMA 1969;207: 513–521
108. Sayers G, Lipschitz DA, Sayers M: The relationship between pica and iron nutrition in Johannesburg Bantu adults. South C J Nutr 1974;48:53–60
109. Markson JL, Moore JM: Autoimmunity in pernicious anaemia and iron deficiency anaemia. Lancet 1962;ii:1240
110. Jacobs A, Lawrie JH, Entwistle QC, Campbell H: Gastric acid secretion in chronic iron deficiency anaemia. Lancet 1966;ii: 190–196
111. Stone WD: Gastric secretory response to iron therapy. Gut 1968;9:99–104
112. Jacobs A: Non-haematologic effects of iron deficiency. Clin Haematol 1982;ii:353–365
113. Judish JM, Naiman JL, Oski FA: The fallacy of the fat iron deficient child. Pediatrics 1965;37:987–993
114. Dallman PR: Tissue effects of iron deficiency. pp. 437–475. In Jacobs A, Worwood M (eds): Iron in Biochemistry and Medicine. Academic Press, London, 1974
115. Hood DA, Kelton R, Nishio ML: Mitochondrial adaptations to chronic muscle use: effect of iron deficiency. Comp Biochem Physiol 1992;101A:597–605
116. Holloszy JO: Biochemical adaptations in muscle: effects of exercise on mitochondrial oxygen uptake and respiratory enzyme activity in skeletal muscle. J Bio Chem 1967;242: 2278–2282
117. Ekblom B, Goldbarg AN, Gullbring B: Response to exercise after blood loss and reinfusion. J Appl Physiol 1972;33: 175–180
118. Viteri FE, Torun B: Anaemia and physical work capacity. Clin Haematol 1974;3:609–617
119. Finch CA, Miller LR, Inamdar AR et al: Iron deficiency in the rat: physiological and biochemical studies of muscle dysfunction. J Clin Invest 1976;58:447–453
120. Gardner GW, Edgarton VR, Senewiratne B et al: Physical work capacity and metabolic stress in subjects with iron deficiency anemia. Am J Clin Nutr 1977;30: 910–917
121. Basta SS, Soekirman MS, Karydi D, Scrimshaw NS: Iron deficiency anemia and the productivity of adult males in Indonesia. Am J Nutr 1979;32:916–922
122. Edgerton VR, Gardner GW, Ohira Y et al: Iron deficiency anaemia and its effect on worker productivity and activity patterns. BMJ 1979;2:1546–1549
123. Davies KJA, Packer L, Brooks GA: Biochemical adaptation of mitochondria muscle, and whole animal respiration to endurance training. Arch Biochem Biophys 1981;209:538–553
124. Dallman PR: Manifestations of iron deficiency. Semin Hematol 1982;19:19–30
125. Finch CA, Gollnick PD, Hlastala MP et al: Lactic acidosis as a result of iron deficiency. J Clin Invest 1979;64:129–137
126. Chandra RK, Saraya AK: Impaired immunocompetence associated with iron deficiency. J Pediatr 1975;86:899–909
127. Joynson DHM, Jacobs A, Walker DM, Dolby AE: Defect of cell mediated immunity in patients with iron deficiency anaemia. Lancet 1972;ii:1058–1059
128. Higgs JM, Wells RS: Chronic mucocutaneous candidiasis: associated abnormalities of iron metabolism. Br J Dermatol 1973;86(suppl 8):88–93
129. Macdougal LG, Anderson R, McNab GM, Katz J: The immune response in iron deficient children: impaired cellular defence mechanisms with altered humoral components. J Pediatr 1975; 86:833–840
130. Cook JD, Lynch SR: The liabilities of iron deficiency. Blood 1986;68:803–809
131. Chandra RK: Reduced bacterial capacity of polymorphs in iron deficiency. Arch Dis Childhood 1973;48:864–870
132. Sagone AL, Balcerzak SP: Activity of iron containing enzymes in erythrocytes and granulocytes in thalassemia and iron deficiency. Am J Med Sci 1970;259:350–355
133. Sussman M: Iron and infection. pp. 664–679. In Jacobs A, Woorwood M (eds): Iron in Biochemistry and Medicine. Academic Press, London, 1974
134. Masawe AEJ, Muindi JM, Swai GRB: Infections in iron deficiency and other types of anaemia in the tropics. Lancet 1974; ii:314–320
135. Barry DMJ, Reeve AW: Increased incidence of gram negative sepsis with intramuscular iron administration. Pediatrics 1977;60:908–913
136. Murray MJ, Murray AB, Murray MB, Murray CJ: The adverse effect of iron repletion on the course of certain infections. BMJ 1978;ii:1113–1121
137. Payne SM, Finkelstein RA: The critical role of iron in host-bacterial interactions. J Clin Invest 1978;61:1428–1435
138. Bullen JJ, Rogers HJ, Griffiths J: Role of iron in bacterial infection. Curr Topics Microbiol Immunol 1978;80:1–12
139. Fleming AF: Iron deficiency in the tropics. Clin Haematol 1982;11:365–371
140. Weinberg ED: Iron withholding: a defence against infection and neoplasia. Physiol Rev 1984;64:65–72

141. Glover J, Jacobs A: Activity pattern of iron deficient rats. BMJ 1972;ii:627–633
142. Webb TE, Oski FA: Iron deficiency anemia and scholastic achievement in young adolescents. J Pediatr 1973;82: 827–833
143. Webb TE, Oski FA: Behavioral status of young adolescents with iron deficiency status. J Spec Educ 1974;8:153–160
144. Pollitt E, Leibel RL: Iron deficiency and behavior. J Pediatr 1976;88:372–381
145. Tamir H, Klein A, Rapport MM: Serotonin-binding protein: enhancement of binding by Fe^{2+} and inhibition of binding by drugs. J Neurochem 1976;26:871–878
146. Youdim MBH, Green AR: Biogenic monoamine metabolism and functional activity in iron deficient rats: behavioral correlates. pp. 201–221. In Porter R, Fitzsimons DW (eds): Iron Metabolism. Elsevier/North Holland, Amsterdam, 1977
147. Oski FA, Honig AS: The effects of therapy on the developmental scores of iron-deficient infants. J Pediatr 1978;92: 21–28
148. Bothwell TH, Carlton RW, Cook JD, Finch CA: Iron Metabolism in Man. Blackwell, Oxford, 1979
149. Weinberg J, Dallman PR, Levine S: Iron deficiency during early development in the rat: behavioral and physiological consequences. Pharmacol Biochem Behav 1980;12:493–502
150. Williamson AM, Ng KT: Activity and T-maze performance in iron deficient rats. Physiol Behav 1980;24:1157–1162
151. Youdim MBH, Green AR, Bloomfield MR: The effects of iron deficiency on brain biogenic monoamine biochemistry and function in rats. Neuropharmacology 1980;19:259–267
152. Deinard A, Gilbert A, Dodds M, Egeland B: Iron deficiency and behavioral defects. Pediatrics 1981;68:828–833
153. Sourkes TL: Transition elements and the nervous system. pp. 1–29. In Pollitt E, Leibel AL (eds): Iron Deficiency and Behavior. Raven Press, New York
154. Youdim MBH, Yehuda S, Ben-Shachar D: Behavioral and brain biochemical changes in iron deficient rats: the involvement of iron in dopamine receptor function. pp. 39–56. In Pollit E, Leibel R (eds): Iron Deficiency: Brain Biochemistry and Behavior. Raven Press, New York, 1982
155. Lotzoff B, Brittenham GM, Viteri FE et al: Developmental deficits in iron-deficient infants: effects of age and severity of iron lack. J Pediatr 1982;101:948–956
156. Mackler B, Finch C: Iron in central nervous system oxidative metabolism. pp. 31–38. In Pollitt E, Leibel RL (eds): Iron Deficiency: Brain Biochemistry and Behavior. Raven Press, New York, 1982
157. Walter T, Kovalskys J, Stekel A: Effect of iron deficiency on infant mental development. J Pediatr 1983;10:519–525
158. Pollitt E, Leibel RL, Greenfield DB: Iron deficiency and cognitive test performance in preschool children. Nutr Behav 1983; 1:137–142
159. Schoene RB, Escourrou P, Robertson HT et al: Iron depletion decreases maximal exercise lactate concentrations in female athletes with minimal iron deficiency anemia. J Lab Clin Med 1983;102:306–311
160. Vyas D, Chandra RK: Functional implications of iron deficiency. pp. 45–59. In Stekel A (ed): Iron Nutrition in Infancy and Childhood. Raven Press, New York, 1984
161. Tucker DH, Sanstead HH, Penland JG et al: Iron status and brain function: serum ferritin level associated with asymmetries of cortical electrophysiology and cognitive performance. Am J Clin Nutr 1984;39:105–112
162. Soemantri AG, Pollitt E, Kim I: Iron deficiency and education achievement. Am J Clin Nutr 1985;42:1221–1227
163. Symes AL, Missala K, Sourkes TL: Iron- and riboflavin dependent metabolism of a monoamine in the rat in vivo. Science 1981;74:153–155
164. Voorhess ML, Stuart MJ, Stockman JA, Oski FA: Iron deficiency anemia and increased urinary epinephrine excretion. J Pediatr 1975;86:542–547
165. Youdim MBH, Woods HF, Mitchell B, Boudin D: Human platelet monoamine oxidase activity in iron-deficiency anaemia. Clin Sci Mol Med 1976;48:289–295
166. Woods HF, Youdim MBH, Boudin D, Mitchell B: Monoamine metabolism and platelet function in iron-deficiency anaemia. Ciba Found Symp 1977;51:227–248
167. Dillman E, Johnson DG, Martin J et al: Catecholamine elevation in iron deficiency. Am J Physiol 1979;237:R297–R300
168. Dillman E, Mackler B, Johnson D et al: Effect of iron deficiency on catecholamine metabolism and body temperature regulation. pp. 57–62. In Pollitt E, Leibel RL (eds): Iron Deficiency: Brain Biochemistry and Behavior. Raven Press, New York, 1982
169. Davies DM, Smith A, Muller-Eberhard U, Margan WR: Hepatic-subcellular metabolism of heme from hemopexin: incorporation of iron into ferritin. Biochem Biophys Res Commun 1979;91:1504–1511
170. Callender ST, Mallet BJ, Smith MD: Absorption of hemoglobin iron. Br J Haematol 1957;3:186–192
171. Hussain R, Walker RB, Layrrise M et al: Nutritive value of food iron. Am J Clin Nutr 1965;16:464–471
172. Hallberg L, Solvell L: Absorption of hemoglobin iron in man. Acta Med Scand 1965;181:335–354
173. Conrad ME, Benjamin BI, Williams HL, Foy AL: Human absorption of hemoglobin iron. Gastroenterology 1967;53:5–10
174. Weintraub LR, Weinstein MB, Huser HJ, Rafal S: Absorption of hemoglobin iron: the role of a heme-splitting substance in the intestinal mucosa. J Clin Invest 1968;47:531–539
175. Raffin SB, Woo CH, Roost KT, Schmid R: Intestinal absorption of hemoglobin iron-heme cleavage by mucosal heme oxygenase. J Clin Invest 1974;54:1344–1352
176. Brown ER Jr, Justus BW: In vitro absorption of radioiron by everted pouches of rat intestine. Am J Physiol 1958;194: 319–326
177. Beutler E, Kelly BM, Beutler F: The regulation of iron absorption. II. the relationship between iron dosage and iron absorption. Am J Clin Nutr 1962;11:559–567
178. Pollack S, Kaufman RM, Crosby WH: Iron absorption: effects of sugars and reducing agents. Blood 1964;24:577–581
179. Rhodes J, Beton D, Brown DA: Absorption of iron instilled into the stomach, duodenum and jejunum. Gut 1968;9:323–324
180. Bendrich A, Cohen M: Ascorbic acid safety: analysis of factors affecting iron absorption. Toxicol Lett 1990;51:189–201
181. Lynch SR, Finch CA, Monsen ER, Cook JD: Iron status of elderly Americans. Am J Clin Nutr 1982;36:1032–1045

182. Rockey DC, Cello JP: Evaluation of the gastrointestinal tract in patients with iron-deficiency anemia. N Engl J Med 1993; 329:1691–1695

183. Joosten E, Dereymaeker L, Perelmans W, Hiele M: Significance of a low serum ferritin level in elderly in-patients. Postgrad Med J 1993;69:397–400

184. Griffiths EK, Schapira DV: Serum ferritin and stool occult blood and colon cancer screening: cancer detection and prevention. 1991;15:303–305

185. Campbell NRC, Hasinoff BB: Iron supplements: a common cause of drug interactions. Br J Clin Pharmacol 1991;31: 251–255

186. Campbell NRC, Hasinoff BB, Stalts H et al: Ferrous sulfate reduces thyroxine efficacy in patients with hypothroidism. Ann Intern Med 1992;117;1010–1013

187. Cartwright GE, Lee GR: The anaemia of chronic disorders. Br J Haematol 1971;21:147–152

188. Frey R, Grimm J, Trachsler M, Rhyner K: Die wertigkeit von serum-ferritin, serumeisen and eisenbindungskapazitat in der differential diagnose der mikrozytarenhypochromen anamie. Schewiz Med Wochenschr 1982;112:13–17

189. Cartwright GE: The anaemia of chronic disorders. Semin Hematol 1996;3:351

190. Kluger MJ, Rothenburg BA: Fever and reduced iron: their interaction as a host defense response to bacterial infection. Science 1979;203:374–376

191. Pekarek RS: The effect of leukocytic endogenous mediator (LEM) on the tissue distribution of zinc and iron. Proc Soc Exp Biol Med 1972;140:684–686

192. Karle H, Hansen NE, Malmquist J et al: Turnover of human lactoferrin in the rabbit. Scand J Haematol 1979;23:303–312

193. Van Snick L, Masson PL: The binding of human lactoferrin to mouse peritoneal cells. J Exp Med 1976;144:1568–1580

194. Van Snick L: The ingestion and digestion of human lactoferrin by mouse peritoneal macrophages and the transfer of its iron into ferritin. J Exp Med 1977;146:817

195. Weinberg J: Iron and infection. Microbiol Rev 1978;42:45–66

196. Krantz SB: Pathogenesis and treatment of the anemia of chronic disease Am J Med Sci 1994;307:353–359

197. Radtke HW, Claussner HW, Erbes PM et al: Serum erythropoietin concentration in chronic renal failure: relationship to degree in anemia and excretory renal function. Blood 1979; 54:877–884

198. Bozzini CE, DeVoto FEH, Tomio JM: Decreased responsiveness of hematopoietic tissue to erythropoietin in acutely uremic rats. J Lab Clin Med 1966;68:411–417

199. Van Dyke D, Keighley G, Lawrence J: Decreased responsiveness to erythropoietin in a patient with anemia secondary to chronic uremia. Blood 1963;22:838

200. Urabe A, Chiba S, Kosaka K, Takaku F: Response of uraemic bone marrow cells to erythropoietin in vitro. Scand J Haematol 1976;17:335–340

201. Wallner SF, Vautrin RM: The anemia of chronic renal failure: studies of the effect of organic solvent extraction of serum. J Lab Clin Med 1978;92:363–369

202. Pricto J, Barry M, Sherlock S: Serum ferritin in patients with iron overload and acute and chronic liver disease. Gastroenterology 1975;68:533–535

203. Larsson SD: Anemia and iron metabolism in hypothyroidism. Acta Med Scand 1967;157:349–363

204. Tudhope GR, Wilson GM: Anemia in hypothyroidism: incidence pathogenesis and response to treatment. J Med 1960; 29:513–537

205. Freedman ML: pp. 109–131. In Denham MJ, Chanorin I (eds): Haemolytic Disease, in Blood Disorders in the Elderly. Churchill Livingstone, London, 1985

206. Dacie JV, Worlledge S: Autoimmune hemolytic anemias. Prog Hematol 1969;6:82–120

207. Worlledge S: Immune drug-induced hemolytic anemias. Semin Hematol 1969;6:181–200

208. Petz LD: Drug-induced immune hemolytic anemia. Clin Haematol 1980;4:181–197

209. Kirtland HH III, Mohler DN, Horowitz DA: Methyldopa inhibition of suppressor-lymphocyte function: a proposed cause of autoimmune hemolytic anemia. N Engl J Med 1980;30: 825–832

210. Petz LD, Garratty G: Drug-induced haemolytic anaemia. Clin Haematol 1975;4:181–197

211. Pirofsky B: Autoimmunization and the Autoimmune Hemolytic Anemias. Churchill Livingstone, London, 1980

212. Madanes AE: Danazol. Ann Intern Med 1982;96:625–630

213. Ahn YS, Harrington WJ, Mylvaganam R: Danazol therapy in autoimmune hemolytic anemia. Blood 1983;62(suppl):102a

214. Jayid J: Immune hemolytic anemia in the aged. Clin Geriatr Med 1985;1:747–772

215. Allgood JW, Chaplin A Jr: Idiopathic acquired hemolytic anemia: a review of forty-seven cases treated from 1955 through 1965. Am J Med 1967;43:254–273

216. Kutti N, Wadenvik H, Safai-Kutti S et al: Successful treatment of refractory autoimmune hemolytic anaemia by plasmapheresis. Scand J Haematol 1984;32:149–152

217. Murphy S, LoBuglio AP: Drug therapy in autoimmune hemolytic anemia. Semin Hematol 1976;13:323–334

218. Heyssel RM, Bozian RC, Darby WJ, Bell MC: Vitamin B_{12} turnover in man: the assimilation of vitamin B_{12} from natural foodstuffs by man and estimates of minimal daily requirements. Am J Clin Nutr 1966;18:176–184

219. Hall CA: Long-term excretion of Co-57 B_{12} and turnover within the plasma. J Clin Nutr 1964;14:156–162

220. Adams JF: Considerations governing the maintenance treatment of patients with pernicious anemia. In Heinrich HC (ed): Vitamin B_{12} and Intrinsic Factor. Second European Symposium. Enke, Stuttgart, 1962

221. Grasbech R: Calculations on vitamin B_{12} turnover in man. Scand J Clin Lab Invest 1959;11:250–258

222. Beck WS: Metabolic aspects of vitamin B_{12} and folic acid. pp. 311–331. In Williams WJ, Beutler E, Erislev AJ, Lichtman MA (eds): McGraw-Hill, New York, 1983

223. Herbert V, Castle WB: Divalent cation and pH dependence of rat intrinsic factor action in everted sacs and mucosal homogenates of rat small intestine. J Clin Invest 1961;40: 1978–1983

224. Grasbeck R: Soluble and membrane-bound vitamin B_{12} transport proteins. p. 743. In Zagalak B, Freidrich W (ed): Vitamin

B_{12} Proceedings of the Third European Symposium on Vitamin B_{12} and Intrinsic Factor. Walter de Gruyter, New York, 1979

225. Grasbeck R, Nyberg W, Reizenstein PG: Biliary and fecal vitamin B_{12} excretion in man: an isotope study. Proc Soc Exp Biol Med 1958;97:780–784
226. Reizenstein PG: Excretion of non-labelled vitamin B_{12} in man. Acta Med Scand 1959;165:313–319
227. Benson RE, Rappazzo ME, Hall CA: Late transport of vitamin B_{12} by transcobalamin II. J Lab Clin Med 1972;80:488–495
228. Gizis EJ, Arkun SN, Miller IF et al: Plasma clearance of transcobalamin I- and transcobalamin II-bound Co vitamin B_{12}. J L Clin Med 1969;74:574–580
229. Finkler AE, Hall CA: Nature of the relationship between vitamin B_{12} binding and cell uptake. Arch Biochem Biophys 1967; 120:79–85
230. Carmel R, Herbert V: Deficiency of vitamin B_{12} binding alpha globulin in two brothers. Blood 1969;33:1–12
231. Hakami N, Neiman PE, Canellos GP, Lazerson: Neonatal megoblastic anemia due to inherited transcobalamin II deficiency in two siblings. N Eng J Med 1971;285:1163–1170
232. Allen RH: The plasma transport of vitamin B_{12}. Br J Haematol 1976;33:161–167
233. Herbert V: Megaloblastic anemias. Lab Invest 1985;52:3–19
234. Lederle FA: Oral cobalamin for pernicious anemia: medicine's best kept secret. JAMA 1991;265:94–95
235. Hsing AW, Hansson L, McLaughlin JK et al: Pernicious anemia and subsequent cancer: a population based cohort study. Cancer 1993;71:745–750
236. Sjoblom SM, Sipponen P, Jarvinen H: Gastroscopic follow up of pernicious anemia patients. Gut 1993;34:28–32
237. Marcaurd SP, Albernaz L, Khazanie PG: Omeprazole therapy causes malabsoption of cyanocobalmin. Ann Intern Med 1994; 120:211–215
238. Sumner AE, Chin MM, Abrahm JL et al: elevated methymalonic acid and total homocysteine levels show high prevalence of vitamin B_{12} deficiency after gastric surgery. Ann Intern Med 1996;124:469–476
239. Martin DC, Francis J, Protetch J, Huff JF: Time dependency of cognitive recovery with cobalamin replacement: report of a pilot study. J Am Geriatr Soc 1992;40:168–172
240. Stabler SP, Allen RH, Savage DG, Lindenbaum J: Clinical spectrum and diagnosis of cobalmin deficiency. Blood 1990; 76:871–881
241. Babior BM, Buhn HG: Megaloblastic anemias. p. 1503. In Braunwald E, Isselbacher KJ, Petersdorf RG et al (eds): Harrison's Principles of Internal Medicine. McGraw-Hill, New York, 1987.
242. Thompson WG, Babitz L, Cassino C et al: Evaluation of current criteria used to order vitamin B_{12} levels. Am J Med 1987;82: 291–294
243. Lindenbaum J, Healton EB, Savage DG et al: Neuropsychiatric disorders caused by cobalamin deficiency in the absence of anemia or macrocytosis. N Engl J Med 1988;318:1720–1728
244. Carmel R: Pernicious anemia: the expected findings of very low serum cobalamin levels, anemia, and macrocytosis are often lacking. Arch Intern Med 1988;148:1712–1714
245. Spivack JL: Masked megaloblastic anemia. Arch Intern Med 1982;142:2111–2114
246. Bessman JD, Gilmer PR Jr, Gardner FH: Improved classification of anemias by MCV and RDW. Am J Clin Pathol 1983; 80:322–326
247. Bergia JJ: Evaluation of anemia. Postgrad Med 1985;77: 253–269
248. Thompson WG, Cassino C, Babitz L et al: Hypersegmented neutrophils and vitamin B_{12} deficiency. Acta Haematol 1989; 81:186–191
249. Cooper BA, Fehedy V, Blanshay P: Recognition of deficiency of vitamin B_{12} using measurement of serum concentration. J Clin Lab Med 1986;107:447–452
250. Karnaze DS, Carmel R: Low serum cobalamin levels in primary degenerative dementia: do some patients harbor atypical cobalamin deficiency states? Arch Intern Med 1987;147:429–431
251. Grinblat J, Marcus DL, Hernandez F, Freedman ML: Folate and vitamin B_{12} levels in an urban elderly population with chronic disease: assessment of two laboratory folate assays: microbiologic and radioassay. J Am Geriatr Soc 1986;34: 627–632
252. Garry PJ, Goodwin JS, Hunt WC: Folate and vitamin B_{12} status in a healthy elderly population. J Am Geriatr Soc 1984;32: 719–726
253. Marcus DL, Shadick N, Grantz J, Freedman ML: Low serum B_{12} levels in a hematologically normal elderly subpopulation. J Am Geriatr Soc 1987;35:635–638
254. Norman EJ: Gas chromatography mass spectrometry screening of urinary methylmalonic acid: early detection of vitamin B_{12} deficiency to prevent permanent neurologic disability. Gas Chromatogr Mass Spectrum News 1984;12:120–129
255. Weiland RG: Vitamin B_{12} deficiency in non-anemic elderly. J Am Geriatr Soc 1986;34:618
256. Kilpatrick GS, Withey JL: The serum vitamin B_{12} concentration in the general population. Scand J Haematol 1965;2: 220–229
257. Elsborg L, Lund V, Bastrup MP: Serum B_{12} levels in the aged. Acta Med Scand 1976;200:309–314
258. Matchar DB, Feussner JR, Watson DJ et al: Significance of low serum B_{12} levels in the elderly. J Am Geriatr Soc 1985; 34:680A–681A
259. Blundell EL, Matthews JH, Allen SM et al: Importance of low serum vitamin B_{12} and red cell folate concentrations in elderly hospital inpatients. J Clin Pathol 1985;38:1179–1184
260. Elwood PC, Shinton NK, Wilson CID et al: Haemoglobin, vitamin B_{12} and folate levels in the elderly. Br J Haematol 1971; 21:557–563
261. Freedman ML: Status of vitamin B_{12} and folic acid in the elderly in the United States. pp. 25–31. In The Role of Folate and Vitamin B_{12} in Neurotransmitter Metabolism and Degenerative Neurological Changes Associated with Aging. NIA, NIDDKD Publication. Federation of American Societies for Experimental Biology, Bethesda, MD, 1989
262. Cole MG, Prichal JF: Low serum B_{12} in Alzheimer-type dementia. Age Ageing 1984;13:101–105
263. Carmel R, Karnaze DS: Physician response to low serum cobalamin levels. Arch Intern Med 1986;146:1161–1165
264. Lindenbaum J: Status of laboratory testing in the diagnosis of megaloblastic anemia. Blood 1983;61:624–627

265. Carethers M: Diagnosing vitamin B_{12} deficiency, a common geriatric disorder. Geriatrics 1988;43:89–112

266. Fairbanks VF: Test for pernicious anemia: the "Schilling test." Mayo Clin Proc 1983;58:541–544

267. Carmel R, Sinow RM, Siegel ME, Samloff M: Food cobalamin malabsorption occurs frequently in patients with unexplained low serum cobalamin levels. Arch Intern Med 1988;148: 1715–1719

268. Savage DG, Lindenbaum J, Stabler SP, Allen RH: Sensitivity of serum methylmalonic acid and total homocysteine determinations for diagnosing cobalamin and folate deficiencies. Am J Med 1994;96:239–246

269. Stabler SP: Screening the older population for cobalamin deficiency. J Am Geriatr Soc 1995;43:1290–1297

270. Metz J, Kelly A, Swett VC et al: Deranged DNA synthesis by bone marrow from vitamin B_{12}-deficient humans. Br J Haematol 1968;14:575–592

271. Lindenbaum J: Status of laboratory testing in the diagnosis of megaloblastic anemia. Blood 1983;61:624–627

272. Metz J: The deoxyuridine suppression test: a review of its clinical and research applications. Crit Rev Lab Sci 1984;20: 205–241

273. Wickramasinghe SN: The deoxyuridine suppression test: a review of its clinical and research applications. Clin Lab Haematol 1981;3:1–18

274. Wickramasinghe SN, Akinyanju OO, Grange A, Litwinczuk RAG: Folate levels and deoxyuridine levels in protein-energy malnutrition. Br J Haematol 1983;53:135–143

275. Fairbanks VF, Lennon VA, Kokmen E, Howard FM: Test for pernicious anemia: serum intrinsic factor blocking antibody. Mayo Clin Proc 1983;58:203–204

276. Herbert V: Don't ignore low serum cobalamin (vitamin B_{12}) levels. Arch Intern Med 1988;148:1705–1707

277. Herbert V, Herzlich B: A proposed model of sequential stages in the development of vitamin B_{12} deficiency, abstracted. Blood 1985;66(suppl 1):54a

278. Herzlich B, Herbert V: Depletion of serum holotranscobalamin II: an early sign of negative vitamin B_{12} balance. Lab Invest 1988;58:332–337

279. Perry IJ, Refsum H, Morris RW et al: Prospective study of serum total homocysteine concentration and risk of stroke in middle-aged British men. Lancet 1995;346:1395–1398

280. Fermo I, Vigano D'Angelo S, Paroni R et al: Prevalence of moderate hyperhomocysteinemia in patients with early onset venous and arterial occlusive disease. Ann Intern Med 1995; 123:747–753

281. Stampfer MJ, Malinow R, Willet WC et al: Prospective study of plasma homocysteine and risk of myocardial infarction in U.S. Physicians. JAMA 1992;268:877–881

282. Den Heijer M, Koster T, Blom HK et al: Hyperhomocysteinemia as a risk factor for deep vein thrombosis. N Engl J Med 1996;334:759–762

283. Naurath HJ, Joosten E, Riezler R et al: Effect of vitamin B_{12} folate, and vitamin B_6 supplements in elderly people with normal serum vitamin concentrations. Lancet 1995;346:85–89

284. Fata FT, Herzlich BC, Schiffman G, Ast AL: Impaired antibody responses to pneumococcal polysaccharide in elderly patients with low serum vitamin B_{12} levels. Ann Intern Med 1996;124: 299–304

285. Pennypacker LC, Allen RH, Kelly JP et al: High prevalence of cobalamin deficiency in elderly outpatients. J Am Geriatr Soc 1992;40:1197–1204

286. Read AE, Gough GH, Pardoe LJ, Nicholas A: Nutritional studies on the entrants to an old people's home with particular reference to folic acid deficiency. BMJ 1965;ii:843–848

287. Batata M, Spray GH, Bottom FG et al: Blood and bone marrow changes in elderly patients with special reference to folic acid, vitamin B_{12}, iron and ascorbic acid. BMJ 1967;ii:667–669

288. Girdwood RH, Thompson AD, Williamson J: Folate status in the elderly. BMJ 1967;ii:670–672

289. Bailey LB, Wagner PA, Christakis GH et al: Folacin and iron status and hematological findings in predominately black persons from urban low-income households. Am J Clin Nutr 1979; 32:2346–2353

290. Rosenberg IH, Bowman BB, Cooper BA et al: Folate nutrition in the elderly. Am J Clin Nutr 1982;16:1060–1066

291. Wagner PA, Bailey LB, Krista ML et al: Comparison of zinc and folacin status in elderly women from differing socioeconomic backgrounds. Nutr Res 1971;1:565–569

292. Baker H, Frank O, Thind IS et al: Vitamin profiles in elderly persons living at home or in nursing homes versus profile in healthy young subjects. J Am Geriatr Soc 1979;27:444–450

293. Hayes AN, Willans DJ, Skelton D: Vitamin B_{12} (cobalamin) and folate blood levels in geriatric reference group as measured by two kits. Clin Biochem 1985;18:56–61

294. Garry PJ, Goodwin JS, Hunt WC: Folate and vitamin B_{12} status in a healthy elderly population. J Am Geriatr Soc 1984;32: 719–726

295. Grinblat J, Marcus DL, Hernandez F et al: Folate and vitamin B_{12} levels in an urban elderly population with chronic diseases. J Am Geriatr Soc 1986;34:627–632

296. Marcus DL, Freedman ML: Folic acid deficiency in the elderly. J Am Geriatr Soc 1985;33:552–558

297. Botez MI, Young SN, Bachevalier J, Gauthier S: Effect of folic acid and vitamin B_{12} deficiencies in 5-hydroxyindoleacetic acid in human cerebrospinal fluid. Ann Neurol 1982;12: 479–484

298. Reynolds EH, Mattson RH, Gallagher BB: Relationships between serum cerebrospinal fluid anticonvulsant drug and concentrations in epileptic patients. Neurology 1972;22:841–844

299. Lanzkowsky P, Erlandson ME, Bezan AI: Isolated defects of folic acid absorption associated with mental retardation and cerebral calcification. Blood 1969;34:452–465

300. Coleman N: Folate deficiency in humans. p. 80. In Draper HH (ed): Advances in Nutritional Research. Vol. 1. Plenum, New York, 1977

301. Herbert V: Experimental nutritional folate deficiency in man. Trans Assoc Am Phys 1962;75:307–320

302. Reynolds FH, Rothfield P, Pincus JH: Neurological disease associated with folate deficiency. BMJ 1973;ii:398–400

303. Runcie J: Folate deficiency in the elderly. pp. 493–595. In Boetz M, Reynolds EH (eds): Folic Acid in Neurology, Psychiatry and Internal Medicine. Raven Press, New York, 1979

304. Shulman R: An overview of folic acid deficiency and psychiat-

ric illnesses. pp. 463–474. In Botez MI, Reynolds EH (eds): Folic Acid in Neurology, Psychiatry and Internal Medicine. Raven Press, New York, 1979

305. Carney MWP: Psychiatric aspects of folate deficiency. pp. 475–492. In Botez MI, Reynolds EH (eds): Folic Acid in Neurology, Psychiatry and Internal Medicine. Raven Press, New York, 1979
306. Botez MI, Botez T, Leville J et al: Neuropsychological correlates of folic acid deficiency: facts and hypotheses. pp. 435–462. In Folic Acid in Neurology, Psychiatry and Internal medicine. Raven Press, New York, 1979
307. Rosenberg IH, Bowman BB, Cooper BA et al: Folate nutrition in the elderly. Am J Clin Nutr 1982;36:1060–1066
308. Reynolds EH: Neurological aspects of folate and vitamin B_{12} metabolism. Clin Haematol 1976;5:661–696
309. Botez MI, Bachevalier J: The blood brain barrier and folate deficiency. Am J Clin Nutr 1981;34:1725–1730
310. Coleman N, Herbert V: Folate metabolism in brain. p. 103. In Kumar E (ed): Biochemistry of the Brain. Pergamon Press, Oxford, 1979
311. Sneath RW, Chanarin I, Hodkinson HM et al: Folate status in a geriatric population and its relation to dementia. Age Ageing 1973;2:177–182
312. Melamed E, Reches A, Hershko C: Reversible central nervous system dysfunction in folate deficiency. J Neurol Sci 1975; 25:93–98
313. Strachan RW, Henderson JG: Dementia and folate deficiency. J Med 1967;36:189–204
314. Hurdle ADF, Picton-Williams TC: Folic acid deficiency in elderly patients admitted to hospital. BMJ 1966;ii:202–207
315. Shulman R: An overview of folic acid deficiency and psychiatric illness. p. 463. In Botez MI, Reynolds EH (eds): Folic Acid in Neurology, Psychiatry and Internal Medicine. Raven Press, New York, 1979
316. Ten-State Nutrition Survey 1968–1970 (1970) IV DHEW Publication No. (HSM) US Department of Health, Education and Welfare, Communicable Disease Center IV: 72
317. Carney MWP: Serum folate values in 423 psychiatric patients. BMJ 1967;4:512–516
318. Brigden ML: A systematic approach to macrocytosis: sorting out the causes. Postgrad Med 1995;97:171–186
319. Bennett JM, Catovsky D, Daniel MT: Proposals for the classification of the acute leukaemias. Br J Haematol 1976;33: 451–458
320. Antin JH, Rosenthal DS: Acute leukemias, myeloplasia and lymphomas. Clin Geriatr Med 1985;1:795–826
321. Cohen HS, Freedman ML, Goldstein BD: The problem of benzene in our environment: critical and molecular considerations. Am J Med Sci 1978;275:124–136
322. Kyle RA: Second malignancies associated with chemotherapeutic agents. Semin Oncol 1982;9:131–142
323. Blayney W, Jaffe ES, Fisher RI et al: The human T-cell leukemia/lymphoma virus, lymphoma, lytic lesions and hypercalcemia. Ann Intern Med 1983;98:144–151
324. Chaganti RSK: The significance of chromosome change to hematopoietic neoplasms. Blood 1983;62:515–524
325. Bishop JM: The molecular genetics of cancer. Science 1987; 235:305–311
326. Holt JT, Morton CC, Neinhuis AW, Leder P: Molecular mechanisms of hematological neoplasms. pp. 347–376. In Stamatoyannopoulos G, Neinhuis AW, Leder P, Majerus PW (eds): The molecular basis of blood diseases. WB Saunders, Philadelphia, 1987
327. Hayhoe FGJ, Rees J: The leukemias. pp. 188–207. In Denham MJM, Chanarin I (eds): Blood Disorders in the Elderly. Churchill Livingstone, London, 1985
328. Yunis JJ, Brunning RD, Howe RB, Lobell M: High-resolution chromosome as an independent prognostic indicator in adult acute non-lymphocytic leukemia. N Engl J Med 1984;311: 812–818
329. Bloomfield CD: Acute myeloid leukemia. Semin Oncol 1987; 14:357–471
330. Koeffler HP: Syndromes of acute non-lymphocytic leukemia. Ann Intern Med 1987;107:74–75
331. Devine SM, Larson RA: Acute leukemia in adults: recent developments in diagnosis and treatment. CA Cancer J Clin 1994;44:326–352
332. Champlin R, Gale RP: Acute myelogenous leukemia: recent advances in therapy. Blood 1987;69:1551–1562
333. Bodey GP, Bolivar R, Fainstein V: Infectious complications in leukemic patients. Semin Hematol 1982;19:193–236
334. Weiser B, Lange M, Fialk MA et al: Prophylactic trimethoprim sulfamethoxazole during consolidation chemotherapy for acute leukemia: a controlled trial. Ann Intern Med 1981;95: 436–438
335. Mir MA, Delamore IW: Metabolic disorders in acute myeloid leukemia. Br J Haematol 1978;40:79–92
336. O'Regan S, Carson S, Chesney RW, Drummond KN: Electrolyte and acid base disturbances in the management of leukemia. Blood 1977;49:345–353
337. Grund FM, Armitage JO, Burns CP: Hydroxyurea in the prevention of the effects of leukostasis in acute leukemia. Arch Intern Med 1977;137:1246–1247
338. McKee I, Collins RD: Intravascular leukocyte thrombi and aggregates as a cause of morbidity and mortality in leukemia. Medicine 1974;53:462–478
339. Littman MA, Rowe JM: Hyperleukocytic leukemia: rheological, clinical and therapeutic considerations. Blood 1982;60: 279–283
340. Stahl R, Silber R: Chronic lymphocytic leukemia. Clin Geriatr Med 1985;1:857–867
341. Mann DL, DeSantis PM, Mark G et al: HLTV-1 associated B-cell CLL: indirect role for retrovirus in leukemogenesis. Science 1987;236:1103–1106
342. Rozmin C, Montserrat E: Chronic lymphocytic leukemia. N Engl J Med 1995;333:1052–1057
343. Mangan KF, Chikkappa G, Farley PC: T gamma cells suppress growth of erythroid colony-forming units in vitro in the pure red cell aplasia of B-cell CLL. J Clin Invest 1982;70:1148–1156
344. Brouet JC, Flandrin G, Sasportes M et al: CLL of T cell origin: immunologic and clinical evaluation in 11 patients. Lancet 1975;ii:890–893
345. Newland AC, Catovsky D, Lynch D et al: Chronic T cell lymphocytosis: a review of 21 cases. Br J Haematol 1984;58: 433–466

346. Rai KR, Sawitsky A: Studies in clinical staging, lymphocyte function, and markers as an approach to the treatment of CLL. In Silber RL, Gordon AS, Lobue J et al (eds): Contemporary Hematology Oncology. Vol 2. Plenum, New York, 1981
347. Carbone A, Santoro A, Pilotti S, Rilke F: Bone marrow patterns and clinical staging in CLL. Lancet 1978;i:606
348. Charron D, Dighiero G, Raphael M, Binet JL: Bone marrow patterns and clinical staging in CLL. Lancet 1977;ii:819
349. Binet JL, Catovsky D, Chandra P et al: CLL: proposals for a revised prognostic staging system. Br J Haematol 1981;48: 365–367
350. Han T, Ozer H, Sadamori N et al: Prognostic importance of cytogenetic abnormalities in patients with CLL. N Engl J Med 1989;310:288–292
351. Ligler FS, Kettman JR, Smith G, Frenkel EP: Immunoglobin phenotype on B cells correlates with clinical stage CLL. Blood 1983;62:256–263
352. Lee JS, Dixon DO, Kantarjian HM et al: Prognosis of chronic lymphocytic leukemia: a multivariate regression analysis of 325 untreated patients. Blood 1987;69:929–936
353. Weeks JC, Tierney MR, Weinstein MC: Cost effectiveness of prophylactic intravenous immune globulin in chronic lymphocytic leukemia. N Engl J Med 1991;325:81–86
354. Cohen HJ: Multiple myeloma in the elderly. Clin Geriatr Med 1985;1.4:827–855
355. Reid CDL: Plasma cell disorders. In Denham MJ, Chanarin I (eds): Blood Disorders in the Elderly. Churchill Livingstone, London, 1985
356. Farhangi M (ed): Plasma cell myeloma and myeloma proteins. Semin Oncol 1986;13:1–382
357. Maldonado JE, Kyle RA: Familial myeloma: report of eight families and a study of serum proteins in their relatives. Am J Med 1976;57:875–884
358. McPhedran P, Health CW Jr, Garcia J: Multiple myeloma incidence in metropolitan Atlanta, Georgia: racial and seasonal variations. Blood 1972;39:866–873
359. Bertrams J, Kuwert E, Bohmeu U et al: HLA-antigens in Hodgkin's disease and multiple myeloma. Tissue Antigens 1972; 2:41–46
360. Smith G, Wolford RL, Fishkin B et al: HLA phenotypes, immunoglobins and K and L chains in multiple myeloma. Tissue Antigens 1976;4:374–377
361. Ishimaru M, Ishimaru T, Mikamin M, Matsunaga M: Multiple myeloma among atomic bomb survivors, Hiroshima and Nagasaki, 1950–1976. Radiation Effects Research Foundation, Technical Report 9-79. Radiation Effects Research Foundation, Hiroshima, 1976
362. Isobe T, Osserman EF Pathologic conditions associated with plasma cell dyscrasias: a study of 806 cases. Ann N Y Acad Sci 1971;190:507–516
363. Osserman EF, Takatsuki K: Considerations regarding the pathogenesis of the plasmacytic dyscrasias. Ser Haematol 1965;4:28–49
364. Schafer AI, Miller JB: Association of IgA multiple myeloma with a preexisting disease. Br J Haematol 1979;41:19–24
365. Wohlenberg H: Osteomyelitis and plasmacytoma. N Engl J Med 1979;283:822–823
366. Penny R, Hughes S: Repeated stimulation of the reticuloendothelial system and the development of plasma cell dyscrasias. Lancet 1970;i:77–78
367. Rosenblatt J, Hall AC: Plasma-cell dyscrasias following prolonged stimulation of reticuloendothelial system. Lancet 1970; i:301–302
368. Goldenberg GJ, Paraskevas F, Israels LG: The association of rheumatoid arthritis with plasma cell and lymphocytic neoplasms. Arthritis Rheum 1969;12:569–579
369. Wegelius O, Skrifvars B: Rheumatoid arthritis terminating in plasmacytoma. Acta Med Scand 1970;187:133–138
370. Isomaki HA, Hakulmen T, Joustenlahti U: Excess risk of lymphomas, leukemias and myeloma in patients with rheumatoid arthritis. J Chron Dis 1978;31:691–696
371. Schaefer AI, Miller JB, Lester EP et al: Monoclonal gammopathy in heredity spherocytosis: a possible pathogenetic relation. Ann Intern Med 1978;88:45–46
372. Pratt PW, Estren S, Kochwa S: Immunoglobulin abnormalities in Gaucher's disease: report of 16 cases. Blood 1968;31: 633–640
373. Wolf P: Monoclonal gammopathy in Gaucher's disease. Lab Med 1973;4:28
374. Turesson I, Rausing A: Gaucher's disease and benign monoclonal gammopathy. Acta Med Scand 1975;197:507–512
375. Macdonald M, McCathie M, Faed MJ: Gaucher's disease with biclonal gammopathy. J Clin Pathol 1975;28:757
376. Gerber MA: Asbestosis and neoplastic disorders of the hematopoietic system. Am J Clin Pathol 1970;53:204–208
377. Kagan E, Jacobson RJ, Yeung KY et al: Asbestos associated neoplasm of B cell lineage. Am J Med 1979;67:325–330
378. Porter DD, Dixon FJ, Larson AE: The development of a myeloma-like condition in mink with Aleutian disease. Blood 1965;25:736–742
379. Chapman I, Jimenez FA: Aleutian mink disease in man. N Engl J Med 1963;269:1171–1174
380. Helmboldt CR, Kenyon AJ, Dessel BH: The comparative aspects of Aleutian disease. pp. 315–319. In Slow, Latent and Temperate Virus Infections. NINBD Monograph 2. National Institute of Health, Bethesda, MD, 1964
381. Henry LW: Multiple myeloma in a mink handler following exposure to Aleutian disease. Cancer 1979;44:273–275
382. Radl J: Benign monoclonal immunopathy (idiopathic paraproteinemia). Am J Pathol 1981;104:91–93
383. Klein B: Cytokine, cytokine receptors, transduction signals and oncogenes in human multiple myeloma. Semin Hematol, 1995;32:4–19
384. Durie BG, Salmon SE, Mundy GR: Relation of osteoclast activating factor production to extent of bone marrow disease in multiple myeloma. Br J Haematol 1981;47:21–30
385. Kyle RA: Benign monoclonal gammopathy—after 20 to 35 years of follow-up. Mayo Clin Proc 1993;68:26–36
386. Kyle RA: Why better prognostic factors for multiple myeloma are needed. Blood 1994;83:1713–1716
387. Alexian R, Dimopoulous M: The treatment of multiple myeloma. N Engl J Med 1994;330:484–489
388. Nordic Myeloma Study Group: Interferon-a2b added to mel-

phalan-prednisone for initial and maintanance therapy in multiple myeloma. Ann Intern Med 1996;124:212–222

389. Malpas JL: The lymphomas. pp. 264–265. In Denham MG, Chanarin I (eds): Blood Disorders in the Elderly. Churchill Livingstone, London, 1985

390. Koduru PR, Filippa DA, Richardson ME: Cytogenic and histological correlations in malignant lymphoma. Blood 1987;69: 97–102

391. Rappaport H: Tumors of the hematopoietic system. pp. 97–161. In Atlas of Tumor Pathology. Section III, Fascicle 8. Armed Forces Institute of Pathology, Washington, DC, 1966

392. Non-Hodgkins Lymphoma Pathologic Classification Project: National Cancer Institute sponsored study of classification of non-Hodgkin's lymphoma: summary and description of a working formulation for clinical usage, 1982

393. Harris NL, Jaffe ES, Stein H, Banks P et al: A revised European-American classification of lymphoid neoplasms: a proposal from the International Lymphoma Study Group. Blood 1994;84:1361–1385

394. MacMahon B: Epidemiology of Hodgkin's disease. Cancer Res 1966;26:1189–1200

395. Jandl J: Non-Hodgkin's lymphoma. pp. 891–964. In Blood: Textbook of Hematology. Little Brown, Boston, 1964

396. Baer DM, Anderson ET, Wilkinson LS: Acquired immune deficiency syndrome in homosexual men with Hodgkin's disease: three case reports. Am J Med 1986;80:738–740

397. Ioachim HL, Cooper MC, Hellman GL: Lymphomas in men at high risk for acquired immune deficiency syndrome (AIDS): a study of 21 cases. Cancer 1985;56:2381–2842

398. Levine AM, Gill PS, Meyer PR et al: Retrovirus and malignant lymphomas in homosexual men. JAMA 1985;254:1921–1925

399. Ioachim HL, Cooper MC: Lymphomas of AIDS. Lancet 1986; i:96

400. Groopman JE, Sullivan JL, Mulder C et al: Pathogenesis of B cell lymphoma in a patient with AIDS. Blood 1986;67: 612–625

401. Wotherspoon AC, Doglioni C, Diss TC et al: Regression of primary low grade B-cell gastric lymphoma of mucosa-associated lymphoid tissue type after eradication of *Helicobacter pylori*. Lancet 1993;342:575–577

402. Cavelli F: Recent advances in the management of lymphoma. Eur J Cancer 1995;31A:841–844

403. Mrozek K, Bloomfield CD: Cytogenetics of indolent lymphomas. Semin Oncol 1993;20(suppl 5):47–57

404. Lokich JJ, Pinkus CG, Moloney WC: Hodgkin's disease in the elderly. Oncology 1974;29:484–500

405. Eghbali H, Hoerni-Simon G, deMascarel I et al: Hodgkin's disease in the elderly: a series of 30 patients older than 70 years. Cancer 1984;53:2191–2193

406. Lichtman SM: Lymphoma in the older patient. Semin Oncol 1995;22(suppl 1):25–28

407. Boivin JF, Hutchinson GB: Second cancers after treatment for Hodgkin's disease: a review. In Boice JD, Fraumene JF Jr (eds): Radiation Carcinogens: Epidemiology and Biological Significance. Raven Press, New York, 1984

408. Rosenberg SA: The treatment of Hodgkin's disease. Ann Oncol 1994;5(suppl 2):17–21

409. Portlock CS: Management of the indolent non-Hodgkins lymphomas. Semin Oncol 1980;3:292–301

410. Dimopoulos MA, Alexian R: Waldenstrom's macroglobulinemia. Blood 1994;83:1452–1459

411. Westbrook CA, Groopman JE, Golde DW: Hairy cell leukemias: disease pattern and prognosis. Cancer 1984;59: 500–506

412. Morrison VA: Chronic leukemia. CA Cancer J Clin 1994;44: 353–377

413. Weiss LM, Strickler JG, Dorfman RF et al: Clonal T-cell populations in angioimmunoblastic lymphadenopathy and angioimmunoblastic lymphadenopathy-like lymphoma. Am J Pathol 1986;122:392–397

414. Lukes RJ, Tindle BH: Immunoblastic lymphadenopathy: a hyperimmune entity resembling Hodgkin's disease. N Engl J Med 1975;292:1–8

415. Freter CE, Cossman J: Angioimmunoblastic lymphadenopathy with dysproteinemia. Semin Oncol 1993;20:627–635

416. Gilbert HS: Myeloproliferative disorders. Clin Geriatr Med 1985;1:773–793

417. Middleton AM: Polycythemia and myelofibrosis. pp. 234–244. In Denham MJ, Chanarin I (eds): Blood Disorders in the Elderly. Churchill Livingstone, London, 1985

418. Gilbert HS: Myelofibrosis revisited: characterization and classification of myelofibrosis in the setting of myeloproliferative disease. pp. 3–18. In Berk PD, Castro-Malaspina H, Wasserman LR (eds): Myelofibrosis and the Biology of Connective Tissue. Alan R Liss, New York, 1984

419. Champlen RE, Golde DW: Chronic myelogenous leukemia: recent advances. Blood 1985;65:1039–1047

420. Sokol JE, Baccarani M, Russo D, Tura S: Staging and prognosis in chronic myelogenous leukemia. Semin Hematol 1988;25: 49–61

421. Cannistraa SA Chronic myelogenous leukemia as a model for the genetic basis of cancer. Hematol Oncol Clin North Am 1990;4:337–357

422. Gruppo Italiano Studio Policitemia: Polycythemia vera: the natural history of 1213 patients followed for 20 years. Ann Inter Med 1995;123:656–664

423. Bilgrami S, Greenberg BR; Polycythemia rubra vera. Semin Oncol 1995;22:307–326

424. Tefferi A, Silverstein MN, Noel P: Agnogenic myeloid metaplasia. Semin Oncol 1995;22:327–333

425. Berk PD, Goldberg JD, Donovan PD et al: Therapeutic recommendations in polycythemia vera based on Polycythemia Vera Study Group protocols. Semin Hematol 1986;23:132–143

426. Mitus AJ, Schafer AI: Thrombocytosis and thrombocythemia. Hematol Oncol Clin North Am 1990;4:157–178

427. Tefferi A, Silverstein MN, Hoagland CH: Primary thrombocythemia. Semin Oncol 1995;22:334–340

428. Giralt S, Kantarjian H, Talpazn M: Treatment of chronic myelogenous leukemia. Semin Oncol 1995;22:396–404

429. Griffin JD: Myelodysplasias. Clin Hematol 1986;15:909–1111

430. Brandt L: Environmental factors and leukemia. Med Oncol Tumor Pharmacother 1985;2:7–10

431. Zarrabi MH, Rosner F: Second neoplasms in Hodgkin's disease: current controversies. Hematol Oncol Clin North Am 1989;3:303–318
432. Jacobs A, Clark RE: Pathogenesis and clinical variations in the myelodysplastic syndromes. Clin Hematol 1986;15:925–951
433. Freedman ML: Hemoglobin synthesis in normal and abnormal states. pp. 47–101. In Gordon AS, Silber R, LoBue J (eds): The Year in Hematology 1977. Plenum, New York, 1977
434. Bunn HF: 5Q and disordered hematopoiesis. Clin Hematol 1986;15:1023–1035
435. Greenberg PL: Myelodysplastic syndrome. pp. 1098–1142. In Hoffman R, Benz E, Shattil S et al (eds): Hematology: Principles and Practice. 2nd Ed. Churchill Livingstone New York 1995
436. Cunningham I, MacCallum SJ, Byth K et al: The myelodysplastic syndromes: an analysis of prognostic factors in 226 cases from a single institution. Br J Haematol 1995;90:602–606
437. Spriggs DR, Stone RM, Kufe DW: The treatment of myelodysplastic syndromes. Clin Hematol 1986;15:1081–1107
438. Estey EH: Treatment of acute myelogenous leukemia and myelodysplastic syndromes. Semin Hematol 1995;32:132–151
439. Hellstrom-Lindberg E: Efficacy of erythropoietin in the myelodysplastic syndromes: a meta-analysis of 205 patients from 17 studies. Br J Haematol 1994;89:67–71
440. Shuster S, Scarborough H: Senile pupura. Q J Med 1961;30: 33–41
441. Shuster S, Black MM, McVitie E: The influence of age and sex on skin thickness, skin collagen, and density. Br J Dermatol 1975;93:639–643
442. Fritsch WC: Managing age-related vascular skin lesions. Geriatrics 1975;30:45–48
443. Jandl J: Blood: Textbook of Hematology. pp. 1019–1039. Little Brown, Boston, 1987
444. Karpatkin S: Autoimmune thrombocytopenia purpura. Semin Hematol 1985;22:260–280
445. Bussel JB: Autoimmune thrombocytopenia purpura. Hematol Oncol Clin North Am 1990;4:179–191
446. Rutherford CJ, Frenkel EP: Thrombocytopenia issues in diagnosis and therapy. Med Clin North Am 1994;78:555–574
447. Jandl J: Disorders of platelets. pp. 1041–1094. In Blood: Textbook of Hematology. Little Brown, Boston, 1987
448. Machin SJ: Bleeding and coagulation disorders. pp. 132–156. In Denham MJ, Chanarin I (eds): Blood Disorders in the Elderly. Churchill Livingstone, London 1985
449. Warkentin TE, Kelton JG: Heparin and platelets. Hematol Oncol Clin North Am 1990;4:243–264
450. Shick BP: Hope for treatment of thrombocytopenia. N Engl J Med 1994;331:875–876
451. Ruggenenti P, Remuzzi G: Thrombotic thrombocytopenic purpura and related disorders. Hematol Oncol Clin North Am 1990;4:219–241
452. Webster MWI, Chesboro JH, Foster V: Platelet inhibitor therapy. Hematol Oncol Clin North Am 1990;4:265–289
453. Smith T, Viverette F, Adelman B: The use of antithrombotic therapy in the elderly. Clin Geriatr Med 1985;1:887–897
454. Stemerman MB: Coagulation in the elderly. Clin Geriatr Med 1985;1:869–885
455. Schleider MA, Nachman RL, Jaffe EA, Coleman M: A clinical study of the lupus anticoagulant. Blood 1976;48:499–509
456. Shapiro SS, Thiagarjian P: Lupus anticoagulants. Prog Hemost Thromb 1982;6:263–285
457. Chan TIC, Chan V: Antithrombin III, the major modulator of intravascular coagulation, is synthesized by human endothelial cells. Thromb Haemost 1981;46:504–506
458. Wunderwald P, Schrenk WJ, Port H: Antithrombin from human plasma: an antithrombin binding moderately to heparin. Thromb Res 1986;25:177–191
459. Furie B, Furie BC: The molecular basis of blood coagulation. Cell 1988;53:505–518
460. Clouse LH, Comp PC: The regulation of hemostasis: the protein C system. N Engl J Med 1986;314:1298–1304
461. Dahlback B: Inherited thrombophilia: resistance to activated protein C as a pathogenic factor of venous thromboembolism. Blood 1995;85:607–614
462. Mandel H, Brenner B, Berant M et al: Coexistence of hereditary homocysteinuria and factor Vleiden effect on thrombosis. N Engl J Med 1996;334:763–768
463. Kaplan AP: Initiation of the intrinsic coagulation and fibrinolytic pathway of man. Prog Hemost Thromb 1978;4:127–175
464. Seligsohn U: Disseminated intravascular coagulation. pp. 1289–1317. In Hardin RI, Lux SE, Stossel TP (eds): Blood: Principles and Practice of Hematology: JB Lippincott, Philadelphia 1995
465. Barbior BM, Stossel TP: Hematology: A Pathophysiological Approach. 2nd ed. Churchill Livingstone, London 1990, pp. 221–229
466. Golde DW (ed): Hematopoietic growth factors. Hematol Oncol Clin North Am 1989;3:369–554
467. Goldstone AH (ed): Autologous bone marrow transplantation. Clin Haematol 1986;15:1–267
468. Longo DL: Principles of cancer treatment. pp. 1214–1228. In Kelley WN (ed): Textbook of Internal Medicine. JB Lippincott, Philadelphia, 1989
469. Deisseroth AB: Molecular approaches to the management of malignant disease. pp. 1228–1232. In Kelley WN (ed): Textbook of Internal Medicine. JB Lippincott, Philadelphia, 1989

CHAPTER 90

Aging of the Skin

CHRISTOPHER E. M. GRIFFITHS

The most immediate, and perhaps most telling, evidence of an individual's age is the appearance of his or her skin, hair, and nails. After all, the most that the outside world sees of us are our faces and hands and as both of these are sun-exposed sites this introduces a superimposed complexity almost unique to skin aging namely the role of environmental factors (i.e., sun exposure). It is only in the past 15 years that researchers have become aware of the distinction between intrinsic, chronologic aging of the skin—which exists in its purest form in non-sun-exposed (photoprotected) body sites such as the buttocks—and extrinsic aging due to habitual sun exposure, most evident on face and hands. Extrinsic aging is never a pure phenomenon as it is inevitably superimposed on some degree of chronologic aging, thus the term *photoaging*. However, as elucidated in this chapter, the changes that sunlight wreaks upon the skin are more pronounced than those produced by longevity alone. It is this inability to distinguish extrinsic from intrinsic skin aging that has eventuated in erroneous beliefs regarding wrinkles and age or liver spots: these clinical features, so often synonymous with old age, are merely the consequence of cumulative sun exposure. Proof of this is the paucity of wrinkling in black skin (markedly sun protected by virtue of melanin) unless greatly sun exposed. This confusion has led to use of inappropriate terms such as premature or accelerated aging occurring in response to chronic sun exposure. This chapter serves to dispel these myths and helps distinguish between intrinsic and extrinsic aging (photoaging), and illustrates how little is known about the processes that underlie intrinsic skin aging.

An anatomic approach to the epidermis and dermis and the cell types contained therein has been adopted and the clinical and histologic features of intrinsic and photoaged skin compared and contrasted. The psychological effects of skin senescence probably outweigh the physiologic effects and on these grounds alone there is an increasing need for prevention and/or treatment. On this basis the chapter closes with a brief discussion of the nonsurgical approaches under investigation for treatment of aged skin.

Epidermis

The epidermis is composed of a nonviable stratum corneum composed of enucleated squames and keratin and a viable cellular layer composed of keratinocytes, Langerhans cells, and melanocytes.

Stratum Corneum

The stratum corneum supplies a barrier function to skin and it appears that this integral role is not appreciably affected by age.[1] Stratum corneal thickness is unchanged in the elderly[2] although its moisture content and cohesiveness are reduced coupled with an increase in renewal time of damaged stratum corneum.[3] These changes are manifest clinically as dry, rough skin—so often the bane of elderly people—and enhanced susceptibility to irritants with consequent pruritus. Self-evidently such xerosis-induced pruritus is best treated with emollients as opposed to antihistamines and sedatives.

Keratinocytes

Epidermal thickness decreases slightly[4] with age; in men this is a gradual process beginning between 20 and 30 years of age,[5] and in women a reduction in epidermal thickness is apparent only after the menopause.[5] There is some evidence that estrogen replacement can slow or prevent this epidermal atrophy in women.

Photoaged epidermis is initially thickened but eventually atrophies.[6] Human epidermis is highly proliferative but in a steady-state condition dependent, as are other self-renewing structures, on slowly cycling, undifferentiated stem cells.[7] These stem cells are located within the basal compartment of the epidermis—the nonserrated keratinocytes at the tips of the epidermal rete ridges.[8] Loss of rete ridges and consequent flattening of the dermal-epidermal junction is a hallmark of intrinsically aged skin.[9] Such flattening results in a reduction in mean surface area of the dermal-epidermal junction. One study has estimated a reduction in mean area of dermal-epidermal junction/mm^2 from 2.6 at age 21 to 40 years to 1.9 at age 61 to 80 years.[10] These changes are accompanied by a reduction in microvilli[11]—cytoplasmic projections from basal keratinocytes into the dermis. This overall loss of integrity between epidermis and dermis manifests as an enhanced susceptibility of aged skin to simple trauma and shearing forces. This is demonstrated by the ease with which suction blisters can be raised on aged as opposed to young skin.[1] Photoaged skin has even greater fragility mainly because structures tethering epidermis to dermis, namely collagen VII-containing anchoring fibrils[12] and fibrillin fibers,[13] are greatly reduced in number in sun-exposed sites. The rate of epidermal renewal is reduced in the skin of individuals aged 60 years or greater.[14] Aging as a single factor reduces the ability of keratinocytes to proliferate in vitro.[15] This observation is in keeping with the Hayflick hypothesis of reduced numbers of cellular doublings with longevity.[16] Gilchrest et al.[17] have shown that the interleukin-1 receptor antagonist gene is increased in aged but decreased in photoaged epidermal keratinocytes. Furthermore, levels of interleukin-1 in keratinocytes are not affected by intrinsic aging.[17] The ability of epidermal growth factor (EGF) to bind to its receptor is compromised in intrinsically aged skin and subsequently this may impair epidermal keratinocyte proliferation.

There is little difference in keratinocyte differentiation between photoaged, aged, and young epidermis although there is marked heterogeneity of keratinocyte size and shape in intrinsically aged skin.[18] Melanin is uniformly distributed within aged keratinocytes but shows characteristic irregular clumping in photoaged epidermal keratinocytes.

Melanocytes

Melanocytes are decreased in number in intrinsically aged epidermis, although the estimates of this decrease vary from study to study according to the methodologies used to quantitate melanocyte numbers. This said, the reduction is in the order of 8 to 20 percent per decade compared to young adult skin.[19,20] By marked contrast, in chronically sun-exposed, photoaged skin there is an increase in numbers of melanocytes.[20] In addition to a reduction in melanocyte numbers there is loss of melanocyte function eventuating in reduced tanning ability of intrinsically aged skin in response to ultraviolet radiation. The serious sequel to loss of melanocyte number and function in elderly skin is loss of photoprotection leading to an increased risk of skin cancer. Age or "liver" spots are more correctly known as *actinic lentigines*; these lesions are observed only on chronically sun-exposed sites, most particularly the dorsa of the hands. Their popular names, which include "autumn leaves" and "coffin spots" connote impending senility; however they are more common in the elderly only because cumulative sun exposure is necessarily greater in this group. Histologically, actinic lentigines are characterized by clusters of large, dendritic melanocytes within the basal layer of epidermis.

Langerhans Cells

The furthermost outposts of the body's immune system, epidermal Langerhans cells, are bone-marrow-derived cells that function as antigen-presenting cells integrally involved in immune surveillance. The number of Langerhans cells is reduced in intrinsically aged epidermis,[21] a decrease that is compounded in photoaging.[22] Gilchrest et al.[21] demonstrated that subjects aged 62 to 86 years had a 42 percent reduction in the number of Langerhans cells in sun-protected skin as compared to young subjects aged 22 to 26 years. A reduction in Langerhans cell number equates to a loss of immune surveillance and consequent increased risk of skin cancer and may help explain the difficulty in sensitizing aged skin to contact allergens.

Dermis

Human dermis is divided into two components: a superficial, immediately subepidermal papillary dermis and the deeper reticular dermis. Although in comparison to epidermis the dermis is relatively hypocellular and has a longer cell turnover time, the changes wrought on it by chronologic aging and photoaging are far more evident. Indeed it is dermal change that causes some of the more characteristic features of cumulative sun exposure, namely wrinkles and elastosis (Fig. 90-1). Dermal changes also provide the most striking differences between the effects of chronologic aging and photoaging, namely atrophy and hypertrophy, respectively. Sex differences are also apparent within the dermis in that it is generally thicker in males than in females, especially postmenopause.[1] The principal cells within the dermis are fibroblasts although endothelial cells and mast cells are also affected by aging.

Fibroblasts

Numbers of dermal fibroblasts decrease with age associated with a reduction in fibroblast size and impaired capacity to produce extracellular matrix components, namely collagen, elastin, and glycosaminoglycans.[23] Collagen I is the predominant constituent of extracellular matrix and collagen in total accounts for 70 percent dry weight of dermal tissue. Collagen provides skin with its tensile strength. Thus any loss in collagen imbues skin with a susceptibility to shearing force trauma. Age- related reduction in collagen is a subtle process, difficult to ascertain, whereas photoaging produces marked loss of collagen. Loss of collagen due to photoaging is a bipartite process resulting from decreased synthesis[24] coupled with increased breakdown by matrix metalloproteinases.[25] In photoaged skin the papillary dermis is almost devoid of collagen synthesis[26] and collagen VII-containing anchoring fibrils, which tether epidermis to dermis, are significantly reduced in number.[12] Wound healing is impaired in intrinsically aged as compared to young skin in that rate of healing is appreciably slower but paradoxically the resultant scar is usually more cosmetically acceptable.

Loss of papillary dermal collagen and related structures most likely account for wrinkling due to photoaging. Sunlight is not the only extrinsic function that causes skin wrinkling. Several studies[27,28] have confirmed that smoking is an independent causative factor of facial wrinkles, possibly as a result of metalloproteinase activation.

Dermal glycosaminoglycans, especially dermatan sulfate and hyaluronic acid, are diminished with age and this may contribute to loss of dermal thickness and skin suppleness. By comparison photoaging greatly increases dermal content of glycosaminoglycans;[29] however, little is known about the nature of these glycosaminoglycans and whether or not they are functional.

One of the features of early, evolving photoaging is the presence of a periadnexal inflammatory infiltrate, consisting of macrophages and neutrophils.[30] It is postulated that en-

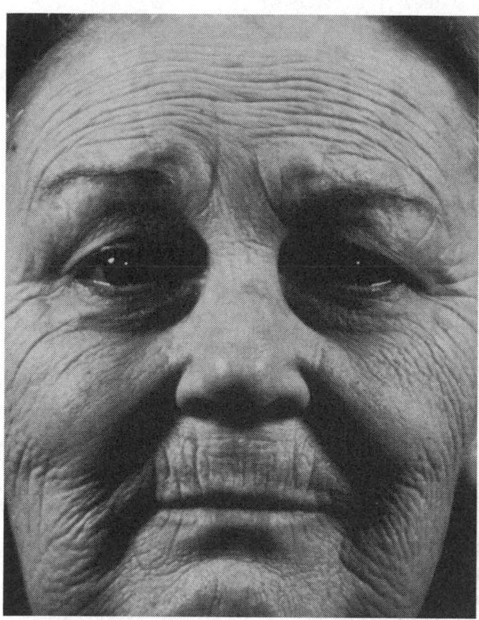
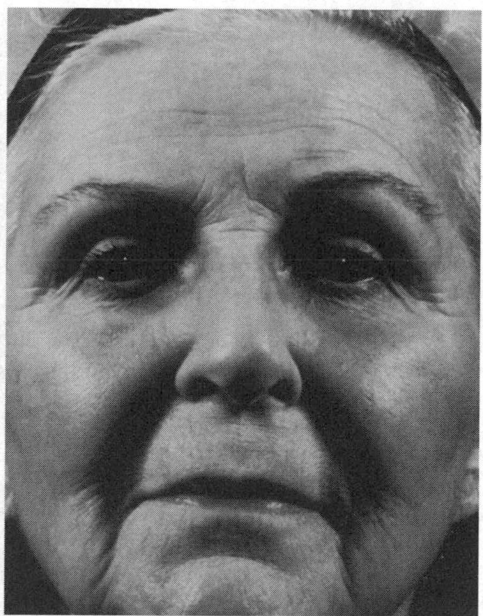

Figure 90-1 Faces of two 71-year-old women. The woman on the right has avoided sun exposure for most of her life and the changes are mostly those of intrinsic, chronologic aging. The woman on the left has suffered a great deal of sun exposure and the wrinkles and thickened skin are evidence of photoaging. To the untrained observer the woman on the left appears older than her stated age.

zymes and/or cytokines produced by this inflammatory infiltrate are responsible for the gross disruption of extracellular matrix observed in photoaged skin. No inflammation is seen in normal, intrinsically aged skin.

Fibroblasts also produce elastin, a protein that provides skin with its elasticity. Elastin content of intrinsically aged and photoaged skin is very different (Fig. 90-2). Intrinsically aged skin displays a reduction in elastic tissue, particularly the finer fibers in the vicinity of the dermal-epidermal junction. Thicker elastin fibers deeper in the reticular dermis are disorganized, frayed, and contain cystic spaces.[11,31] These changes are most probably a combination of reduced synthesis and/or elastolysis. Photoaging markedly increases elastotic material within the dermis, so much so that the relatively subtle changes produced by intrinsic aging are over-shadowed. Clumps of truncated, disorganized elastotic material are observed throughout the reticular dermis of photoaged skin. Chronic sun exposure has a hypertrophic effect on elastic tissue. The mechanisms underlying this change are not fully understood. The elastotic material manifests clinically as yellow, pebbled, elastosis most easily observed on the temples of chronically sun-exposed individuals.

Endothelium

Aged skin is relatively hypovascular, particularly due to loss of small capillaries that run perpendicular to the dermal-epidermal junction and form capillary loops.[32] This loss is concomitant with the loss of epidermal rete ridges.[33,34] Blood vessels within the reticular dermis are reduced in number and their walls are thinned. The consequent compromised blood flow is manifest physiologically as pale skin and an impaired capacity to thermoregulate[1,35]—possibly a contributing factor in the increased susceptibility of elderly individuals to hypo- and hyperthermia.

Likewise photoaged skin is depleted of blood vessels but those remaining are tortuous, dilated, and telangiectatic,[1,6,34] resulting in venous lakes seen on the faces of photoaged individuals. The vessel walls are often thickened and rigid and this, coupled with loss of the buffer effect of perivascular collagen in sun damage, makes such blood vessels more susceptible to trauma resulting in Bateman's or senile purpura on sun-exposed sites.

Mast Cells

There is an approximate 50 percent reduction in numbers of mast cells in intrinsically aged skin.[36] Such a reduction may explain the relative rarity of urticaria in the elderly population.

Appendages

Sweat Glands

Eccrine glands are reduced in number and function in aged skin.[1,18] Impairment of sweating, as with loss of microcirculation, negatively affects the thermoregulatory capacity of chronologically aged skin. Eccrine gland response to thermal and chemical (acetylcholine) stimuli is impaired. Apocrine gland

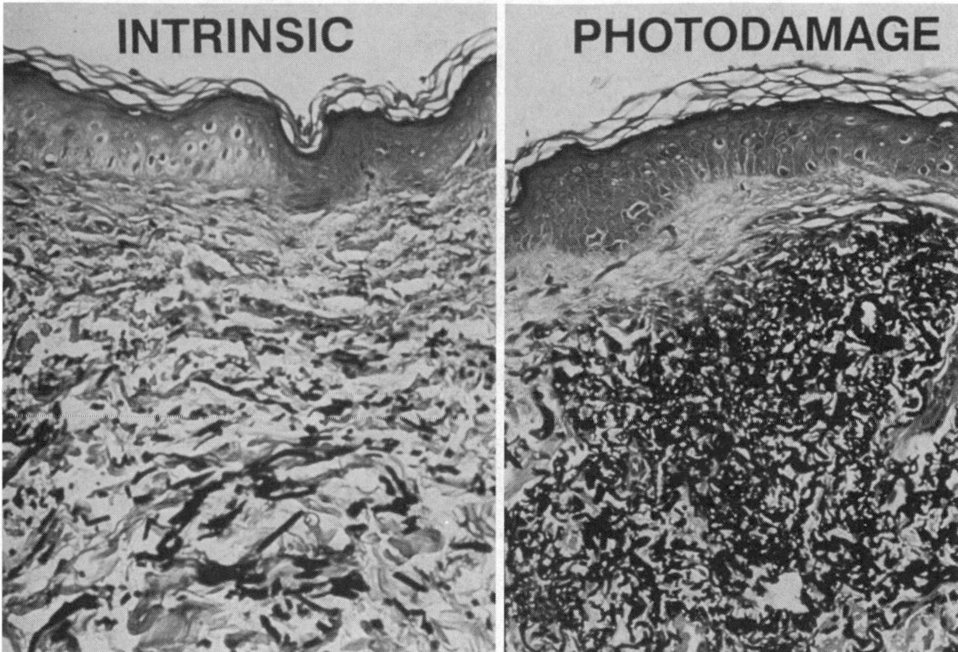

Figure 90-2 Photomicrographs of histologic sections of intrinsically and extrinsically aged skin stained with Verhoeff van Giesen stain for elastin. The salient difference is the gross increase in black-staining, elastotic material in the reticular dermis of extrinsic, photoaged skin. (×40.)

activity is diminished, probably as a consequence of declining testosterone levels, leading to a reduction in pheromone secretion and body odor.[37] Both apocrine[18] and eccrine glands[38] in aged skin contain deposits of lipofuscin.

Sebaceous Glands

Age does not alter the number of sebaceous glands although they become hyperplastic and larger[39]: mean sebaceous gland size increases from 0.22 mm^2 in young adults to 0.4 mm^2 in the elderly. Although aged sebaceous glands are increased in size they produce 50 percent less sebum than their younger counterparts.[40] The constituency of aged sebum is altered in that it contains less free cholesterol but more squalene.[41] Sebaceous gland hyperplasia presents clinically as giant comedones. Such hyperplasia is greatly exaggerated in photoaging especially on the face. Some investigators believe that the reduction in sebum production that occurs with age, and contributes to xerosis of aged skin, is a reflection of reduced testosterone[42] although this does not explain the hyperplasia.

Nerves

Skin is richly supplied by sensory receptors and free nerve endings that may permeate the epidermis and interact with Langerhans cells.[43] Age probably reduces and disorganizes the nerve supply of the skin; indeed there is an approximate two-thirds reduction in numbers of Pacinian and Meissner's corpuscles with age.[44] Partly as a consequence of these anatomic changes there is an increased threshold to pain in aged skin.[45]

Hair

Graying of scalp and beard hair is due to reduction (gray hair) or loss (white hair) of melanin from hair follicles and is an unambiguous manifestation of advancing years.[46] Hair, particularly scalp hair, is lost with age in both sexes[47] and is associated with transition of terminal to vellus hairs. An Australian study reported that gray hair was found in only 22 percent of men aged 25 to 34 years as opposed to 95 percent of men over the age of 55 years.[1] Patterned, androgenetic alopecia is a genetically predetermined condition arising from increased sensitivity of hair follicles to the effects of dihydrotestosterone produced by breakdown of free testosterone by the enzyme 5α reductase. In some studies the prevalence of significant scalp hair loss approaches 70 percent in men over the age of 50 years.[46] The rate of hair growth decreases with age. Hair is not universally lost in that men in particular have an associated increase in hair growth in the nostrils, eyebrows, and on the ears. Elderly women often display conversion of vellus to terminal hairs on the chin and moustache areas.

Nails

Nails grow more slowly in the elderly and are characterized by brittleness and longitudinal, beaded ridging—so-called sausage links.

Psychological Effects

Although nobody has died as a result of cutaneous senescence (skin does not totally fail) the detrimental consequences of cutaneous aging, whether it be intrinsic or extrinsic, are not merely physiologic. Skin represents our appearance to others and wrinkled, blemished, sagging skin is often as repugnant to the elderly as to the young. In modern day youth-driven society the search for preservation of youthful appearance has never been so important. Attractiveness induces feeling of self-worth and is strongly related to how favorably others perceive us. Furthermore, there is evidence that physically attractive individuals may live longer.[48] Men who looked "young for their age" lived longer than men who appeared older than their stated age.[48]

Treatment

Most of the cutaneous features erroneously associated with aging are merely a result of chronic sun exposure. One strategy, although very long term, is to prevent the ravages of excess sun exposure by educating young people about the dangers of ultraviolet irradiation and encouraging them to practice sun avoidance and use of sunblocks. It is estimated that 50 percent of sun exposure occurs before the age of 20 years; thus if you want to look good as a grandparent begin while your grandparents are still alive!

The "fountain of youth" is a mythical prize but nowadays may be more attainable than Ponce de Leon ever thought possible. Nonsurgical manipulation of aged and photoaged skin is feasible. In this regard, attention has been focused on the steroid hormone receptor superfamily that contains the receptors for retinoic acid, vitamin D, thyroid hormone, and glucocorticoids, among others.[49] Topical retinoids, particularly all-*trans* retinoic acid, a metabolite of vitamin A, may improve clinical features of photoaged[50,51] and possibly intrinsically aged skin[49]. Retinoic acid effaces wrinkles by inducing synthesis of collagen I within the papillary dermis[26] both directly by stimulating fibroblasts[53] and indirectly by inducing transforming growth factor-β,[54] which in turn stimulates fibroblast production of collagen. Topical retinoid use also increases anchoring fibril numbers at the dermal-epidermal junction of photoaged skin.[55] Recent work has demonstrated that topical retinoids may inhibit the induction of matrix metalloproteinases by ultraviolet irradiation,[25] thereby preventing collagen breakdown. α-Hydroxy and glycolic acids may also have a reparative effect on photoaged and perhaps aged skin,[56] but there is a marked scarcity of data to support such claims.

Although the effects of topical retinoids on intrinsically aged skin are more difficult to address it appears that there may be an enhanced sensitivity of intrinsically aged skin to the reparative mechanisms of topical retinoids. Aged skin, as compared to young skin, appears to have less retinoid activity.[57] It may be that a feature of cutaneous aging is gradual loss of steroid superfamily activity: testosterone and estrogen are reduced as is vitamin D synthesis.

Conclusions

Aging of the skin is, as with other organs, a highly complex process and intrinsic aging must be separated from the effects of environmental factors. The study of aging skin particularly as a consequence of the ready accessibility of cutaneous tissue is one that presents a paradigm for aging of other organs. With the exponential rise in numbers of old and very old individuals coupled with the ever-increasing emphasis on youth, the search for the "foundation of youth" will be redoubled as we approach the penumbra of the 21st century.

References

1. Balin AK, Pratt LA: Physiological consequences of human skin aging. Cutis 1989;43:431–436
2. Lavker RM: Structural alterations in exposed and unexposed aged skin. J Invest Dermatol 1979;73:59–66
3. Potts RO, Buras EM, Chrisman DA: Changes with age in the moisture content of human skin. J Invest Dermatol 1984;82: 97–100
4. West MD: The cellular and molecular biology of skin aging. Arch Dermatol 1994;130:87–95
5. Branchet MC, Boisnic S, Frances C, Robert AM: Skin thickness changes in normal aging skin. Gerontology 1990;36:28–35
6. Lober CW, Finske NA: Photoaging and the skin: differentiation and clinical response. Geriatrics 1990;45:36–42
7. Miller SJ, Lavker RM, Sun TT: Keratinocyte stem cells of cornea, skin and hair follicle: common and distinguishing features. Dev Biol 1993;4:217–240
8. Lavker RM, Sun TT: Heterogenicity in epidermal basal keratinocytes: morphological and functional correlations. Science 1982; 215:1239–1241
9. Hill WR, Montgomery H: Regional changes and changes caused by age in the normal skin. J Invest Dermatol 1940;3:321–345
10. Katzberg AA: The area of the dermal-epidermal junction in human skin. Anat Rec 1958;131:717–723
11. Lavker RM, Zheng PO, Dong G: Aged skin: a study by light transmission electron and scanning electron microscopy. J Invest Dermatol 1987;88:44S–51S
12. Craven NM, Watson REB, Jones C et al: Collagen VII in photoaged skin abstracted. J Invest Dermatol 1995;105:488
13. Watson REB, Craven NM, Shuttleworth CA et al: Fibrillin in photoaged skin, abstracted. Br J Dermatol 1996;134:573
14. Grove GL: Age-associated changes in human epidermal cell renewal and repair. pp. 193–204. In Balin AK, Kligman AM (eds): Aging and the Skin. Lippincott-Raven, Philadelphia, 1989
15. Gilchrest BA: In vitro assessment of keratinocyte aging. J Invest Dermatol 1983;81:184S–189S
16. Hayflick L: The cellular basis for biological ageing. In Finch CE, Hayflick L (eds): Handbook of the Biology of Aging. Van Nostrand Reinhold, New York, 1977
17. Gilchrest BA, Garmyn M, Yaar M: Aging and photoaging affect gene expression in cultured human keratinocytes. Arch Dermatol 1994;130:82–86
18. Montagna W: Morphology of the ageing skin: the cutaneous appendages. pp. 1–16. In Montagna W (ed): Advances in Biology of the Skin. Vol. 6. Pergamon Press, Oxford, England, 1965
19. Quevedo WC, Szabo G, Virks J: Influence of age and UV on the populations of dopa-positive melanocytes in human skin. J Invest Dermatol 1969;52:287–290
20. Gilchrest BA, Blog F, Szabo G: Effect of aging and chronic sun-

exposure on melanocytes in human skin. J Invest Dermatol 1979; 73:141–143

21. Gilchrest BA, Murphy GF, Soter NA: Effect of chronologic aging and ultraviolet irradiation on Langerhans' cells in human epidermis. J Invest Dermatol 1982;79:85–88
22. Gilchrest BA, Szabo G, Flynn E et al: Chronologic and actinically induced aging in human facial skin. J Invest Dermatol 1983;80: 81S–85S
23. Andrew W, Behnke R, Sato T: Changes with advancing age in the cell population of human dermis. Gerontologica 1964;10: 1–19
24. Talwar HS, Griffiths CEM, Fisher GJ et al: Reduced type I and type III procollagens in photodamaged adult human skin. J Invest Dermatol 1995;105:285–290
25. Fisher GJ, Datta SC, Talwar HS et al: Molecular basis of sun-induced premature skin ageing and retinoid antagonism. Nature 1996;379:335–339
26. Griffiths CEM, Russman AN, Majmudar G et al: Restoration of collagen formation in photodamaged human skin by tretinoin (retinoic acid). N Engl J Med 1993;329:530–535
27. Daniell H: Smoker's wrinkles. A study in the epidemiology of "Crow's feet". Ann Intern Med 1971;75:873–880
28. Kadunce DP, Burr R, Gress R et al: Cigarette smoking: a risk factor for premature facial wrinkling. Ann Intern Med 1991;114: 840–844
29. Smith JG, Davidson EA, Sams WM et al: Alterations in human dermal connective tissue with age and chronic sun damage. J Invest Dermatol 1962;37:447–452
30. Lavker RM, Kligman AM: Chronic heliodermatitis: a morphologic evaluation of chronic actinic damage with emphasis on the role of mast cells. J Invest Dermatol 1988;90:325–330
31. Braverman IM, Fonferko E: Studies in cutaneous aging, I: the elastic fiber network. J Invest Dermatol 1982;78:434–443
32. Montagna W, Carlisle K: Structural changes in aging human skin. J Invest Dermatol 1979;73:47–53
33. Braverman IM, Fonferko E: Studies in cutaneous ageing, II: the microvasculature. J Invest Dermatol 1982;78:444–448
34. Kligman AM: Perspectives and problems in cutaneous gerontology. J Invest Dermatol 1979;73:39–46
35. Howell TH: Skin temperature gradient in the lower limbs of old women. Exp Gerontol 1982;17:65–67
36. Gilchrest BA, Stoff J, Soter NA: Chronologic aging alters the response to ultraviolet-induced inflammation in human skin. J Invest Dermatol 1982;79:47–53
37. Hurley JH, Shelley WB: The Apocrine Sweat Gland in Health and Disease. Charles C Thomas, Springfield, IL, 1960
38. Cawley E, Hsu YT, Sturgill BC, Harman LE: Lipofuscin (wear-and-tear pigment) in human sweat glands. J Invest Dermatol 1973;61:105–107
39. Plewig G, Kligman AM: Proliferative activity of the sebaceous glands of the aged. J Invest Dermatol 1978;70:314–317
40. Pochi PE, Strauss JJ, Downing DT: Age-related changes in sebaceous gland activity. J Invest Dermatol 1979;73:108–111
41. Smith L: Histopathologic characteristics and ultrastructure of aging skin. Cutis 1989;43:414–424
42. Gilchrest BA: Aging. J Am Acad Dermatol 1984;11:955–997
43. Hosoi J, Murphy GF, Egan CL et al: Regulation of Langerhans cell function by nerves containing calcitonin gene-related peptide. Nature 1993;363:159–163
44. Schludermann E, Zubeck JP: Effects of age on pain sensibility. Percept Motor Skills Res Exchange 1962;14:295–301
45. Grove GL, Duncan S, Kligman AM: Effect of ageing on the blistering of human skin with ammonium hydroxide. Br J Dermatol 1982;107:393–400
46. Burch PRJ, Murray JJ, Jackson D: The age prevalence of arcus senilis, greying of hair and baldness; etiological considerations. J Gerontol 1971;26:364–372
47. Barman JM, Astore I, Percorara V: The normal trichogram of the adult. J Invest Dermatol 1965;44:233–236
48. Borkan GA, Norris AH: Assessment of biologic age using a profile of physical parameters. J Gerontol 1980;35:177–184
49. Evans RM: The steroid and thyroid hormone receptor superfamily. Science 1988;240:889–895
50. Kligman AM, Grove GL, Hirose R et al: Topical tretinoin for photoaged skin. J Am Acad Dermatol 1986;15:836–859
51. Weiss JS, Ellis CN, Headington JT et al: Topical tretinoin improves photoaged skin: a double-blind, vehicle-controlled study. JAMA 1988;259:527–532
52. Kligman AM, Dugadkina D, Lavker RM: Effects of topical tretinoin on non-sun-exposed skin of the elderly. J Am Acad Dermatol 1993;29:25–33
53. Federspiel SJ, DiMari SJ, Howe AM et al: Extracellular matrix biosynthesis by cultured fetal rat lung epithelial cells IV. Effects of chronic exposure to retinoic acid on growth, differentiation and collagen biosynthesis. Lab Invest 1991;65:441–450
54. Glick AB, Flanders KC, Danielpour D et al: Retinoic acid induced transforming growth factor-β_2 in cultured keratinocytes and mouse epidermis. Cell Regul 1989;1:87–97
55. Woodley DT, Zelickson AS, Briggaman RA et al: Treatment of photoaged skin with topical tretinoin increases dermal-epidermal anchoring fibrils: a preliminary report. JAMA 1990;263: 3057–3059
56. Ditre CM, Griffin TD, Murphy GF et al: Effects of α-hydroxy acids on photoaged skin: a pilot clinical, histologic and ultrastructural study. J Am Acad Dermatol 1996;34:187–195
57. Varani J, Perone P, Griffiths CEM et al: *All-trans* retinoic acid (RA) stimulates events in organ-cultured human skin that underlie repair. J Clin Invest 1994;94:1747–1756

CHAPTER 91

Skin Diseases and Old Age

BARBARA A. GILCHREST

Demographic and Epidemiologic Considerations

Skin disease and symptoms referable to the skin are exceedingly common among the elderly. In the United States, nearly 20 percent of all outpatient visits to physicians by patients aged 65 years or older are motivated at least in part by a skin complaint[1]; approximately two-thirds of ambulatory older persons examined in survey studies have one or more dermatologic disorders.[1–3] Including the cosmetically distressing and often anxiety-provoking benign neoplasms and other skin changes associated with aging, the percentage of the elderly population affected by abnormalities of the skin increases to 100 percent. Although these disorders are only rarely life threatening, they detract substantially from the quality of life and often lower self-esteem and psychosocial well-being.[4] The following sections seek to explain this high prevalence of skin disease and discuss the pathophysiology, diagnosis, and management of the more common disorders encountered in a geriatric practice.

Factors Predisposing to Skin Disease in the Elderly

Skin is the principal barrier between the body and its external environment. Thus, over many decades, the skin is modified not only by intrinsic aging processes, as are all tissues in the body, but also by cumulative environmental impacts. The relative contributions of these intrinsic and extrinsic processes on age-associated predisposition to injury and disease varies dramatically among individuals and from site to site on the skin surface. For most individuals, particularly fair-skinned Caucasians, the major life-long environmental impact on skin is sun exposure. *Photoaging*, discussed separately below, is the term used to describe this superposition of cumulative sun damage on intrinsic aging.

Intrinsic aging processes have been shown to decrease maximum function and reserve capacity in skin as assessed in a variety of assays.[5,6] These age-associated functional decrements are widely and reasonably presumed to contribute to clinical skin disease, as well as to contribute to systemic health problems of the elderly. Of note, however, these decrements have relatively minor impact on the appearance of skin either clinically or histologically.[5,6] Photoaging exaggerates most of the functional losses observed in sun-protected old skin and greatly increases the risk of carcinogenesis.[7] In addition, photoaging is responsible for the great majority of age-associated changes in the skin's appearance.[7] Understanding this duality of aging processes in the skin is important not only in preventing and managing geriatric skin disease, but serves as well as an important reminder that the apparent aging of all organ systems is the combined result of innate aging and environmental influences.

Approach to Dermatologic Disease in Older Patients

Proper evaluation of a dermatologic complaint entails at a minimum a pertinent medical history and skin examination. Patients with evidence of sun damage, particularly those with actinic keratoses (see below), should have a full skin examination at least annually, whether or not they have symptoms referable to the skin, in order to detect lesions suspicious for skin cancer. It is also important to inquire regarding topical and systemic treatments, either prescribed or self-determined. Over-the-counter topical remedies, cosmetics, bathing habits, and exposure to harsh detergents or inappropriate cleansers such as isopropyl alcohol, for example, often exacerbate skin conditions. The duration of a complaint, response to previous treatments, presence of similar condition in close contacts, and the patient's own opinions regarding etiology are among the information items to be elicited.

Often important physical findings are found in areas other than those mentioned by the patient. For example, the patient may not necessarily complain of genital lesions or may be unaware of cutaneous malignancies or other significant conditions unrelated to the chief complaint. Finally, age-associated blunting of vascular and immune responses may make skin findings more subtle in elderly patients than in younger patients with similar disorders, complicating diagnosis.

The older patient often has difficulty complying with topical treatment. He or she may not be able to reach the feet or back; may not be able to bathe, shower, or shampoo without assistance; and, as with oral medications, may become confused by complex regimens. Patient comprehension, mobility, and home situation should be carefully assessed initially and at the time of follow-up visits, particularly in the event of treatment failure.

Selected Skin Diseases

Numerous skin diseases affect the elderly.[8] Those covered in the following sections are highly prevalent and/or highly symptomatic, mandating a geriatrician's familiarity with their pathogenesis, diagnosis, and treatment.

Herpes Zoster

Herpes Zoster (HZ), or "shingles," is due to reactivation of a latent varicella virus infection. Following a primary varicella infection, usually in childhood, the virus may remain dormant in dorsal sensory root ganglia and reactivate decades later at times of physical stress or reduced immunosurveillance. The annual incidence of HZ in apparently healthy person ranges from approximately 1 to 2 cases per thousand in adolescents and young adults to 10 times this incidence in those aged 80 years and older.[9] The incidence of HZ in individuals with additional age-associated predisposing factors such as cancer, immunosuppressive therapy, and surgery is considerably higher. The lifetime risk of HZ is approximately 50 percent, with 10 percent of individuals experiencing at least two episodes,[9] making HZ a statistically likely event in the later decades of life.

HZ classically presents as paresthesia and/or dysesthesia affecting a single dermatome. These symptoms usually persist for several days, rarely more than a week, before skin lesions appear. The eruption of HZ is virtually pathognomonic. Clusters of vesicles, usually superimposed on erythematous plaques, erupt in a dermatomal distribution. In 98 percent of patients, the eruption is unilateral and lesions do not cross the midline, although occasional individual vesicles can be found outside the affected dermatome. The diagnosis of herpes virus infection may be confirmed by a Tzanck test of material scraped from the base of an intact vesicle. A positive test is indicated by the appearance of multinucleated giant cells characteristic of herpetic infection, although this test cannot distinguish herpes simplex from herpes zoster. The initially clear vesicles may become pustular or, especially in the elderly, hemorrhagic within a few days. New lesions continue to appear for several days, often progressing distally along the dermatome. Widespread dissemination, if it is to occur, usually does so during this period. Pain and hyperesthesia are frequently prominent during the first days of the eruption. Vesicles usually begin to crust in the second week and resolve within 4 weeks in most patients; the eruption tends to persist longer and to be more severe in the elderly than in younger adults. Permanent dyspigmentation or even hypertrophic scarring may occur in lesional skin.

Vesicle fluid is contagious, but the attack rate (cases of varicella) in susceptible household contacts is much less than for chickenpox (primary varicella infection). The course of HZ infection in young and old adults differs primarily in the incidence and severity of postherpetic neuralgia, variably defined as pain persisting after healing of skin lesions or pain of greater than 1 to 3, or 6 months duration. This problem occurs in approximately 10 percent of HZ cases overall, but although postherpetic neuralgia is uncommon in patients less than 40 years of age, it occurs in over one-half of patients aged 60 years and in over three-quarters of patients aged 70 years.[10] With age, the increase in severity and duration of postherpetic neuralgia is even more marked than the increase in incidence. Persistent pain is especially common in those patients with trigeminal involvement (10 to 15 percent of reported cases). The basis of the increased risk of postherpetic neuralgia in the elderly is unclear, but may be the consequence of less successful healing, with a greater tendency to perineural fibrosis and/or failure of involved neurons to re-establish normal signal transduction thresholds after the acute viral infection.

At this time, there is no effective means of preventing HZ infection. Therapies are directed at reducing discomfort during the acute eruption and preventing or ameliorating postherpetic neuralgia.

During the acute phase of HZ infection, some patients require narcotic analgesics for adequate relief of pain. These agents should be prescribed cautiously in the elderly to avoid overmedication and adverse systemic effects. Early skin lesions are best treated with local compresses of Burow's solution (1:20 in cool water) or other hypertonic soaks for 10 minutes, three to four times daily, followed by gentle washing with Hibiclens or other antibacterial soap to hasten drying and prevent bacterial superinfection. A topical antibiotic alone, such as mupirocin ointment, should be applied two to three times daily to already crusted lesions. Systemic treatment is optimal in the immunocompetent host but studies have shown that patients who receive antiviral therapy experience faster healing, a shortened duration of viral shedding, and a decrease in the severity and duration of acute pain.[11] Treatment should be started within 72 hours of the onset of symptoms to be effective. Currently there are three antiviral drugs approved for the treatment of HZ: acyclovir 800 mg five times a day for 7 to 10 days, its analog famcyclovir 500 mg three times a day for 7 days, and its prodrug valacyclovir 1,000 mg three times a day for 7 days.[9]

Although antiviral therapy has definite proven benefit for the treatment of acute zoster, its role in the prevention of postherpetic neuralgia is less definite.[9] Whereas some studies conclude that treatment of acute HZ does not affect the outcome of postherpetic neuralgia, others have shown benefit. In one study acyclovir 800 mg five times a day for 10 days decreased the incidence of postherpetic neuralgia from 16.7 percent in the placebo group to 4.2 percent in the treated group during the first 3 months.[11] From 4 to 6 months, the groups did not differ statistically in neuralgia prevalence. These patient groups averaged 55 and 59 years of age, respectively, with more than 70 persons aged 50 years or older in each group, but data for the more elderly cohorts were not analyzed separately. However, no reduction in postherpetic neuralgia was detected in a second study of 364 patients aged 60 years or older,[12] using a very similar design in which acyclovir was administered for only 7 days. Neither study found medically significant side effects of acyclovir. In a separate double-blind controlled study of HZ ophthalmicus, acyclovir 600 mg five times a day for 10 days was found to reduce the rate of ocular complications such as keratitis and uveitis when treatment was initiated as late as 7 days after the appearance of lesions.[13]

Treatment with systemic corticosteroids is likewise controversial. A randomized, controlled study of 349 subjects comparing 7- and 21-day treatments of acyclovir alone or in addition to prednisolone revealed that a longer course of acyclovir or the addition of steroids offered only minimal benefit, although an increase in adverse events was reported in the group treated with steroids.[14] These data contrast with earlier controlled trials examining the efficacy of oral corticosteroids in HZ management that reported a reduction in pain during the acute episode in all four of the five trials in which this variable was assessed.[9] All studies employed a dose of prednisone or its equivalent at a dose of 40 to 60 mg/day tapered over 21 to 28 days, and none found an increase in HZ complications or steroid-associated side effects in treated patients. Two of the five trials found that corticosteroid therapy during the acute episode reduced the prevalence or severity of postherpetic neuralgia. Whether these discrepant results are the result of different selection criteria and patient age or borderline effectiveness of the intervention is unclear.

Treatment of already established postherpetic neuralgia can be frustrating. Often topical therapy is initiated as first-line treatment owing to its safety as compared with other modalities. Capsaicin, which exerts its effects via the local depletion of substance P and other neuropeptides, applied as a 0.75 percent cream three to four times a day for 6 weeks decreased the pain of postherpetic neuralgia by at least 40 percent within 6 weeks of therapy in the majority of patients, as compared to only 6 percent of patients treated with vehicle control.[15] A 0.25 percent capsaicin cream is presently the only FDA-approved topical treatment for this neuralgia. However, transient stinging and burning at the time of application, incomplete pain relief, and the requirement for frequent, indefinite treatment greatly decrease patient satisfaction with this modality. Other topical treatments include topical anti-inflammatory agents, such as formulations containing aspirin or indomethacin, and topical anesthetics, such as EMLA (eutectic mixture of local anesthetics). This cream is most effective if applied under plastic wrap occlusion for a minimum of 1 hour, on a schedule dictated by patient symptoms. Data on the long-term efficacy of these agents are very limited.[10]

Despite trials and anecdotal use of numerous systemic agents for the treatment of postherpetic neuralgia, antidepressants such as amitriptyline remain the most consistently effective.[9,16] These drugs appear to act by blocking uptake of norepinephrine and serotonin by spinal neurons involved in pain perception, and often doses lower than those needed for antidepressant action are effective. Patients may begin with 12.5 to 25 mg at bedtime, increasing until the pain is controlled or unacceptable side effects are encountered. Typical effective and well-tolerated doses are 75 to 150 mg/day. Particularly in patients with lancinating pain, carbamazepine 160 mg/day, increasing cautiously as necessary, may prove to be an effective alternative. A variety of nonmedical therapies, such as nerve blocks, transcutaneous electrical nerve stimulation, and deep brain stimulation have also been employed.

Pruritus

Elderly people often experience localized or generalized pruritus. Depending on the population surveyed and the criteria employed, up to two-thirds report frequent bothersome itching.[1] For some, it is a minor annoyance; for others the pruritus leads to extensive, slow-healing excoriations or loss of sleep with associated irritability and impaired mental function.

Many patients presenting to the physician because of pruritus in fact have an eruption that is responsible for the symptom,[17] although its other manifestations may be so subtle that the patient or even the physician does not notice the rash. Because inflammatory responses may be muted in the elderly, a careful history and physical examination are necessary before excluding primary disorders of the skin such as eczema, early bullous pemphigoid, urticaria, scabies, or pediculosis. Proper identification of a causative dermatosis leads to effective treatment in most patients and enables the patient to avoid the hematologic, radiographic, and other laboratory procedures that constitute the work-up for unexplained generalized pruritus.

Among all patients seeking medical attention for pruritus, the prevalence of underlying systemic disease has been reported as 10 to 50 percent,[18] the percentage depending on patient selection, diagnostic evaluation, and period of follow-up. Many authorities, however, believe the statistical association is far less strong among unselected older persons presenting to physicians with this symptom.

Numerically, perhaps the most important known cause of persistent generalized pruritus is chronic renal failure. However, the degree of renal failure necessary to cause pruritus is unknown, complicating interpretation of this symptom in the elderly patient with mild to moderate renal insufficiency. From a practical viewpoint, it is probably unwise to attribute pruritus to otherwise asymptomatic renal failure, or to renal insufficiency not requiring specific therapy for metabolic imbalance.

Pruritus is probably the most distressing and consistent symptom of chronic cholestasis, which underlies all the hepatic disorders associated with pruritus. Overall, pruritus occurs in approximately 20 to 25 percent of jaundiced patients, but it is rare in those with hepatic disease lacking cholestasis. Drugs that can cause pruritus by inducing cholestasis include phenothiazines, tolbutamide, erythromycin estolate, anabolic hormones, estrogens, and progestins. Opiates are perhaps the most common drugs to cause non-immunologically-mediated pruritus without cholestasis.

Approximately 30 to 50 percent of patients with polycythemia vera and up to 20 percent of patients with Hodgkin's disease experience pruritus. The incidence and significance of pruritus in other lymphomas and leukemias are unknown, but the occasional association cannot be disputed. Generalized pruritus has been reported as an initial symptom in patients with multiple myeloma, Waldenström's macroglobulinemia, and benign gammopathies. Iron deficiency anemia has been reported as the cause of generalized pruritus in more than 50 patients,[19] including 6 with polycythemia,[20] although this association is apparently rare. Pruritus attributable to endocrine or specific "miscellaneous" causes is rare.

Most elderly people experience extensive or generalized pruritus for which there is no apparent explanation. Hence, one must either accept a higher incidence of idiopathic pruritus with advancing age or infer the existence of "senile pruritus." Physiologic factors that may contribute to this hypothetical entity include age-associated alterations in the skin, peripheral nerve endings, and dermal neuropeptide release.

Alterations in the barrier function of the skin, possibly facilitating low-grade irritant dermatitis, include decreased keratohyalin granule formation in the epidermis, decreased skin surface hydration, diminished stratum corneum lipids, and a slower rate of stratum corneum barrier repair.[21,22] In addition, altered sensory thresholds of C-fiber neurons as well as modifications in the synthesis, release, and clearance of dermal neuropeptides, such as substance P, histamine, neurokinin A, calcitonin generelated peptide, and other mediators with opiate activity may also play a role.[22]

The appropriate laboratory evaluation for the patient with unexplained generalized pruritus remains a matter of opinion, as cost/benefit ratios for individual procedures have not been determined. Measurement of serum creatinine, blood urea nitrogen, bilirubin, hepatic enzymes, and a complete blood count seem to constitute a reasonable survey; a chest x-ray may also be justified as a screening for malignancy. Appropriate physical examination includes examination of the thyroid gland, lymph nodes, liver, and spleen. Additional tests may be suggested by history, review of systems, or physical examination.

The pathophysiology of pruritus associated with systemic disease is incompletely understood, and the optimal therapy is that for the underlying disease whenever possible. Specific approaches to the treatment of the pruritus itself are available in a few instances, but for most patients, nonspecific therapies must be employed.[22,23] Often it is worthwhile to prescribe an emollient, even in the absence of clinical xerosis, because minimal or intermittent "dryness," present in virtually all elderly individuals, may notably exacerbate pruritus of another cause. Patients should be cautioned specifically against topical application of alcohol or hot water (both of which may temporarily relieve but ultimately exacerbate pruritus) or excessive washing, especially with soap. Topical application of menthol and camphor in an emollient base, such as in Sarna lotion, may provide considerable temporary relief; other topical anesthetics can be used only at the risk of allergic sensitization. Oral antihistamines are widely prescribed for pruritus of all causes, although their efficacy is slight in most instances, even when combinations of H_1 and H_2 blockers are used. The use of antihistamines by the elderly may result in the additional problems of urinary retention, paradoxic restlessness, or significantly impaired psychomotor function. Newer nonsedating antihistamines have fewer neurologic side effects, but care must still be taken to avoid potential drug interactions.

Xerosis

Xerosis is the term used to describe the "dry" or rough quality of skin that is almost universal among the elderly. The condition may be generalized but is especially prominent on the lower legs and is exacerbated by low humidity environments classically found in overheated rooms during cold weather. "Xerosis" is a misnomer; the initial assumption that the disorder resulted from a lack of water in the skin overall has been disproved.[24] In vivo and in vitro measurements demonstrate diminished hydration of the superficial portion of the stratum corneum only, with the deeper portion maintaining normal hydration.[25] The occasional classification of xerosis as a disorder of sebaceous (oil) glands is similarly without experimental basis. Xerosis probably reflects minor abnormalities in epidermal maturation that, in turn, result in an irregular surface and altered composition of the stratum corneum. Xerotic skin in the elderly is often pruritic and may show evidence of inflammation, probably due to defects in the stratum corneum, with secondary entry of irritating substances into the dermis. The resulting inflammatory conditions, including *erythema craquele* or *winter eczema*, respond promptly to topical corticosteroid ointment and/or emollients, although these preparations do not correct the xerosis itself.

Frequent, regular use of a topical emollient makes dry skin more attractive and more comfortable and prevents the complications discussed previously. Emollients are most effective when applied to already moistened skin (e.g., immediately after the bath or shower). "Heavy," frankly greasy emollients are sometimes appealing to the elderly. They are often inexpensive and have the additional property of perceptibly coating the skin, producing a smooth surface film, and they are usually good barriers against evaporation. Preparations containing ammonium lactate[36] or other α-hydroxy acids are more cosmetically elegant and often provide longer lasting improvements in skin barrier function and xerosis. Finally, it should be noted that emollients applied to the skin immediately after bathing retain water more effectively than gels or oils added to the bath water. As well, bath oils coat the bathtub as well as the skin, producing a dangerously slippery surface that is difficult to clean.

Seborrheic Dermatitis

Seborrheic dermatitis is a very common dermatologic condition in the geriatric population.[1,2] Clinically, it presents as erythema and greasy-appearing scales in what is referred to as a *seborrheic distribution*, namely the scalp; postauricular folds; central face, particularly the eyebrows, glabella, perinasal, nasolabial folds, and beard area; and the central chest and interscapular areas. On the scalp, it is referred to in lay terms as dandruff. Seborrheic dermatitis is found with greater frequency among patients with underlying neurologic conditions, such as Parkinson's disease, facial nerve injury, spinal cord injury, poliomyelitis, and syringomyelia, as well as in patients taking neuroleptic medications with parkinsonian side effects. Human immunodeficiency virus infection has also been associated with severe seborrheic dermatitis.

The role of resident lipophilic yeast, *Pityrosporum ovale*, is controversial, although studies have shown the organism to be present in greater numbers in patients with seborrheic dermatitis. Treatment is directed at either killing the yeast with topical antifungal preparations or directly suppressing inflammation via low-potency topical steroids. It should be noted that the antifungal agent ketoconazole also has some anti-inflammatory properties. In a double-blind study comparing 2 percent ketoconazole cream to 1 percent hydrocortisone cream, therapeutic response was noted in 80.5 percent of subjects using ketoconazole and 94.4 percent of those using hydrocortisone, demonstrating a somewhat higher efficacy of hydrocortisone, although establishing ketoconazole as an effective, steroid-sparing alternative.[40] For hair-bearing regions, shampoos containing ketoconazole, selenium sulfide, salicylic acid, zinc pyrithione, or tar are effective; for severe cases, a steroid-containing solution can be applied to the scalp after shampooing.

Rosacea

Also called acne rosacea, this is an idiopathic facial disorder of middle-aged and elderly fair-skinned persons consisting of inflammatory papules and pustules, telangiectasia, and easy sometimes florid flushing. The relative severity of these components varies markedly among patients; some, particularly men, may also develop marked coarsening and hypertrophy of the nasal skin, so-called rhinophyma.

The acneiform lesions usually respond dramatically to low-dose tetracycline (e.g., 250 to 500 mg twice daily) or other broad-spectrum antibiotics. Many patients can be maintained on even lower doses, and perhaps one-third have long-term remissions after a single 2- to 3-month antibiotic course. Topical antibiotics, particularly metronidazole, may also provide good to excellent control of the lesions. The mechanism of action of these agents is unknown, but their anti-inflammatory properties are suspected to play a role.

Management of the vascular component of rosacea is more difficult. The above antibiotics are claimed to reduce both telangiectasia and flushing, but the evidence for this benefit is slight. Patients should be advised to avoid known precipitants of flushing, such as alcohol, hot or spicy food, intense exercise, and emotional stress, but many are unable or unwilling to do so. Electrocautery and, more safely and reliably, pulsed dye laser therapy can eradicate individual dilated vessels; in extreme cases, laser treatment of the entire facial area subject to flushing can be performed and is reported to decrease the severity of vasodilation after challenge.

Reshaping of the rhinophymatous nose with removal of excess thickened skin can be accomplished by conventional surgery or use of the CO_2 laser.

Scabies

Scabies is a severely pruritic infestation by the *Sarcoptes scabiei* mite. Symptoms are due to a hypersensitivity reaction to the mite, explaining why pruritus can persist for days to weeks following adequate treatment and conversely why infested persons may be asymptomatic for days to weeks. While the male mite remains on the surface of the skin, the female burrows through the stratum corneum to lay her eggs. In an average infested host, only 10 to 12 live female mites are present at one time. Transmission is through person-to-person contact, and epidemics can arise among institutionalized or nursing home patients, necessitating widespread treatment of patients, staff, and visitors.

The hallmark lesion of scabies is the burrow, a linear ridge often ending with a tiny vesicle. Other cutaneous manifestations are papules, vesicles, nodules, and excoriations. Lesions are concentrated in the interdigital web spaces, axillae, umbilicus, and on the volar wrists and genitalia. Diagnosis is confirmed by scraping the contents of the burrow onto a slide with mineral oil and examining it microscopically. The presence of a mite, eggs, or feces confirms the diagnosis, but this evidence is not essential to making the diagnosis if clinical suspicion is high. Immunocompromised patients or those who have an impaired ability to scratch may have an extensive hyperkeratotic and highly contagious eruption harboring thousands of mites.[26]

The two most widely used treatments are topical lindane and permethrin. Permethrin lacks the neurologic toxicity sometimes seen with lindane, and it has the advantage of being able to kill the scabies eggs as well as mites; thus, in theory only one application is necessary. For successful treatment, all household members and other close contacts must be treated at the same time as the affected patient even if asymptomatic, because newly infested individuals develop pruritus only when allergically sensitized, often after a delay of 2 weeks or more. The medication is applied from the neck down, with particular attention to the subungual area and lesion-bearing sites including the genitalia, then washed off after 8 hours. At that time all clothing and linens should be washed in hot water, and dry cleaned, or placed in a hot dryer. One week later, the entire process is repeated to kill any larvae that have hatched since the first treatment. It is essential to avoid application of lindane immediately following a hot bath, as increased absorption has been reported to cause seizures in some elderly individuals. Oral ivermectin has been reported to be as effective as topical lindane or permethrin in curing scabies,[27] but is not approved for this indication. Residual pruritus can be managed with topical steroids or antihistamines. However, if pruritus continues beyond a few weeks or if new lesions appear, treatment failure, reinfestation, or misdiagnosis should be considered.

Drug Eruptions

Adverse cutaneous reactions to medications include expected, usually dose-related side effects, such as an acneiform eruption following corticosteroid administration or xerosis from retinoids, and unexpected, immune-mediated, allergic reactions. These latter reactions typically occur within 3 days to 2 weeks of challenge and persist up to 2 weeks after the drug is discontinued. Rechallenge results in a more rapid onset of the eruption. Less commonly, a patient may have an adverse reaction to a medication after weeks, months, or rarely years of use.

Any medication can cause a drug eruption, but certain medications are statistically more likely to do so. In two separate survey studies of over 22,000 and 15,000 inpatients, respectively, the Boston Collaborative Drug Surveillance Program[28] identified the following as most likely to cause a drug eruption: amoxicillin, ampicillin, penicillin, semisynthetic penicillins, trimethoprim-sulfamethoxazole, transfused blood, cephalosporins, gentamycin sulfate, acetylcysteine, allopurinol, quinidine, and dipyrone. Conversely, digoxin, antacids, meperidine, promethazine, and acetaminophen were among those medications administered to more than 1,000 patients with no reported cutaneous eruptions.

Central to management of a drug eruption is discontinuation of the culprit medication. In a patient ingesting multiple medications, it is prudent to discontinue or replace with a non-cross-reacting alternative all but those essential to his or her survival. This is particularly essential in the more serious and potentially life-threatening reactions. Failure to remove the immunologic challenge may lead to a progressively more severe eruption. Midpotency topical steroids, antihistamines, and antipruritic lotions provide symptomatic relief during the period of resolution, after withdrawal of the suspected offending agent(s). Oral corticosteroids are not indicated in the management of drug eruptions, with the possible and controversial exception of those that are life threatening.

The most common form of drug eruption is the morbilliform or exanthematous eruption. Sometimes referred to as a "maculopapular" eruption, it is characterized by discrete and coalescing erythematous macules and papules symmetrically distributed on the trunk and extremities. The most common causative agents are those listed above. Morbilliform eruptions typically begin within 1 week of exposure, except in the case of penicillins when they may occur 2 weeks or longer after the initial exposure.[29]

Other forms of drug eruption include photosensitivity, as is seen with doxycycline or thiazides; a lichenoid or lichen planus-like eruption, seen with gold and phenothiazines; and urticaria, often associated with penicillin or iodine-containing contrast media. Fixed drug eruption is manifest by one or few red to violaceous, round plaques that recur in the identical location if the patient is rechallenged. These lesions resolve with hyperpigmentation, which becomes more pronounced with each episode. Causes of fixed drug eruption include tetracyclines and nonsteroidal anti-inflammatory drugs.[30] Vasculitis, presenting as palpable purpura, can occur as the result of medication hypersensitivity, among many other possible causes. Immune complex formation can lead to a serum sickness reaction, characterized by an urticarial eruption, fever, arthritis, nephritis, and sometimes neurologic symptoms. Penicillins, sulfonamides, and streptomycin are among the causative agents.[29]

Some uncommon drug reactions are important due to their life-threatening nature. These include hypersensitivity reaction, anaphylaxis, exfoliative erythroderma, erythema multiforme major (Stevens-Johnson syndrome), and toxic epidermal necrolysis (TEN). These conditions often require hospitalization with intensive supportive care, as well as discontinuation of the causative agent.

Hypersensitivity reaction was first described with phenytoin, and is now recognized with drugs other than anticonvulsants, particularly sulfonamides. It is a multisystem response manifest by a cutaneous eruption, which may be of any type, in conjunction with fever, adenopathy, hematologic abnormalities, and hepatitis.[3] It should be noted that phenytoin, carbamazepine, and phenobarbital cross-react with each other, so that all three agents are contraindicated in patients sensitive to any of them.

Anaphylaxis occurs on a spectrum of IgE-dependent reactions including urticaria, bronchospasm, laryngeal edema, and hypotension. Penicillins are the drugs most commonly associated with anaphylaxis, and the reaction is more likely to occur with intravenous administration.[29] Exfoliative erythroderma presents as diffuse erythema and scaling. Temperature, fluids, electrolytes, and nutrition must be carefully monitored. Erythema multiforme is recognized by pathognomonic target lesions: a dusky center that sometimes progresses to a central blister or erosion, surrounded by pale edematous skin, with a macular erythematous perimeter. When mucous membranes are involved the eruption is classified as Stevens-Johnson syndrome. Large areas of sloughed skin are the hallmark of (TEN); TEN is characterized by skin tenderness and a positive Nikolsky sign, the shearing off of the epidermis with lateral force. TEN may appear de novo or may evolve from severe erythema multiforme. Again, fluid and electrolyte management and the avoidance of sepsis are crucial. Reported mortality rates for TEN are 30 to 50 percent and patients are best managed in a burn unit.[32]

Skin Cancer

Malignant neoplasms are strongly age-associated in most organ systems, including the skin. The most common cutaneous malignancies, basal cell carcinoma (BCC), squamous cell carcinoma (SCC), and malignant melanoma, account for perhaps one-half of all human malignancies and are rapidly increasing in incidence, to 800,000 to 1,200,000 cases per year as compared with half that number two decades ago.[33,34] Understandably, many authorities describe skin cancer as an epidemic, particularly affecting the elderly.

Ultraviolet irradiation, particularly ultraviolet B (290 to 320 nm, sunburn spectrum) is the major causative agent of skin cancer. The incidence of BCC and SCC rises with increased cumulative ultraviolet exposure, as assessed by lifelong geographic residence, employment, and recreational histories. Melanoma is better correlated with intense intermittent exposures, such as those causing blistering sunburns.[35] Other risk factors include male gender and the interrelated features of fair skin, freckling, blue or light colored eyes, red or blond hair, and a tendency to sunburn rather than tan.[36] Cigarette smoking is also statistically associated with increased skin cancer risk.[37]

Unlike most malignancies, virtually all skin cancers can be recognized early in their course due to their visibility on the skin's surface. Cutaneous malignancies detected and treated at an early stage are nearly always curable, particularly in the case of nonmelanoma skin cancer, whereas malignancies left untreated have a greater risk of cosmetic disfigurement, functional impairment, metastasis, and fatal outcome.

Basal Cell Carcinomas

Approximately three-fourths of skin cancers are BCCs. Typical early lesions are asymptomatic, firm, opalescent or "pearly" papules, with fine surface telangiectases. Ninety percent occur on the face and neck. BCCs enlarge very slowly, and patients frequently insist that 4-mm lesions have been present for years. The classic, neglected "rodent ulcer" is uncommon today but can still be identified by its firm, opalescent, telangiectatic, rolled border. Differential diagnosis of BCC includes dermal nevi, which are flesh-colored but not as firm, and sebaceous hyperplasia, which is also less firm and is characterized by a slightly yellow color and a central punctum, the sebaceous orifice. Subtypes include nodular BCC, described above; superficial or multicentric BCC, which presents as a scaly red macule; morpheiform BCC, which appears waxy and scar-like and can often extend far beyond its clinically apparent borders; and pigmented BCC with black, brown, and gray pigmentation, often mistaken for a melanoma or seborrheic keratosis.[36]

BCCs have an extremely low incidence of metastasis, and thus mortality is low. However, if the lesion is untreated it may erode into adjacent structures and cause considerable local destruction.

A variety of treatment modalities exist. These include simple excision, micrographic surgery, electrodesiccation and curettage, cryotherapy, and X-irradiation, all of which have 5-year recurrence rates between 1 and 10 percent.[38] The appropriate choice of treatment depends on numerous factors, such as the location, histologic variant, size, and primary or recurrent status of the BCC, and the general health and cosmetic concerns of the patient.

Squamous Cell Carcinomas

SCCs occur in the same fair-skinned patient population, primarily in habitually sun-exposed areas, such as the head, neck, and upper extremities, but occasionally in sites of chronic ulceration or other skin damage. Early lesions are asymptomatic, firm red papules or plaques, usually with scale; more advanced lesions tend to ulcerate. Differential diagnosis includes premalignant actinic keratoses and, in the case of verrucous lesions, viral warts. Biopsy of suspect lesions is always indicated.

Like BCC, most SCCs are only locally invasive, but 2 to 10 percent metastasize.[36,39] Factors predisposing to metastasis are location on the lip or in areas of chronic inflammation, scarring or sites of prior ionizing irradiation, size greater than 1 cm in diameter and greater than 4 mm in thickness, and immunosuppression.[36] Treatment is usually simple excision or micrographic surgery.

Actinic Keratoses

Actinic keratoses (AKs) are SCC precursor lesions. They occur in the same distribution, namely the head, neck, dorsal hands, and arms. Clinically, they appear as rough, scaly, pink-red, poorly circumscribed macules. Identification is sometimes easier by palpation than by visualization. Induration may be a sign of progression to SCC or simply a manifestation of inflammation, and such lesions require biopsy to exclude malignancy. Multiple lesions are common. The rate of malignant transformation for individual AKs is difficult to ascertain, and estimates range from less than 1 per 1,000 per year to 20 percent although the true rate is probably closer to the former. An estimated 10 to 36 percent regress spontaneously.[40] particularly with sun avoidance.[41] Lesions are usually spot-treated with cryotherapy or topical fluorouracil or masoprocol cream, but recurrences are common. Several studies have shown that sun avoidance and observation alone are acceptable alternatives unless lesions are advanced (indurated). Nevertheless, all patients with multiple AKs should be monitored at least annually because of their high statistical risk of skin cancer of all types.

Malignant Melanoma

Malignant melanoma is rare in comparison with nonmelanoma skin cancer, but in the United States it is now more common than Hodgkin's disease or thyroid carcinoma,[33] and incidence is increasing faster than for any other cancer.[42] Age-specific incidence increases throughout life, with statistically excess mortality among older men.[43] Even more than with other cutaneous malignancies, successful treatment depends on early recognition.

Clinical criteria for the diagnosis of melanoma have been extensively reviewed.[44] Signs include diameter greater than 6 mm, variation in color (red, white, and blue areas within a brown-black lesion), irregular border, and irregular surface topography. Bleeding and pain are late findings. The extremely common seborrheic or senile keratoses can usually be differentiated by their "stuck on" quality, even brown pigmentation, and "regularly irregular" surface. Any change or rapid growth of an existing nevus or new pigmented lesion arising in an elderly individual is suspect, however.

As is the case with BCCs, there are several clinical subtypes of melanoma. The most common type is superficial spreading melanoma, accounting for approximately 70 percent of cases. Lentigo maligna melanoma, arising from its slow growing precursor, lentigo maligna, is often a large lesion with varied pigmentation, and occurs on sun-exposed surfaces, usually the face. Nodular melanomas are rapidly growing lesions that tend to invade deeply early in their course, with a resultant poor prognosis. Acrolentigenous melanoma, by definition a lesion of the hands and feet, often periungual, is the most common form of melanoma in blacks and Asians. A variant of this type of melanoma occurs on mucosal surfaces. Amelanotic melanoma accounts for less than 1 percent of all subtypes and poses a particular diagnostic challenge, owing to its lack of pigmentation.

The most important prognostic indicator in melanoma is the Breslow tumor thickness, the depth of malignant cell invasion as determined histologically. Five-year survival for lesions less than 0.76 mm thick is 96 percent, and for lesions between 0.76 and 1.49 mm 87 percent, whereas survival falls to 75, 66, and 47 percent for lesions 1.5 to 2.49 mm, 2.5 to 3.99 mm, and greater than 4 mm thick, respectively. In general, older patients have a worse prognosis than younger ones.[44]

Surgical excision is the mainstay of treatment, and recommended margins of excision increase with tumor thickness. The benefit of elective lymph node dissection and/or adjuvant therapy in medium to thick melanomas is controversial,[45] although recently α-interferon therapy after definitive surgical excision has been shown to improve survival.[45] Patients diagnosed with melanoma must be closely monitored for local recurrence, metastasis, or development of a second primary melanoma, for which they are at increased risk. Such follow-up is best done by a physician with extensive experience in this field.

Photoaging

Many older persons are distressed by the appearance of their skin. Treatment of the changes due to life-long sun exposure may provide a substantial morale boost; as well, participation in a comprehensive treatment regimen expected to improve their appearance may motivate otherwise noncompliant patients to avoid further sun exposure and thus reduce their skin cancer risk (see above).

It is now well established that sun avoidance and regular sunscreen use for periods as brief as 6 to 7 months can improve the skin's appearance[46–48] and permit regression of AKs.[41] Daily application of tretinoin 0.05 to 0.1 percent for 4 to 6 months in the context of such a regimen gives further improvement, with decreases in roughness, fine wrinkling, and mottled hyperpigmentation in 60 to 80 percent of patients[46–48] and an approximately 60 percent reduction in size and number of AKs. Histologic studies have established that tretinoin therapy reduces and redistributes epidermal melanin[50,51] and increases collagen deposition in the superficial dermis,[52] leading to lighter, more even skin color and decreased wrinkling, respectively. The mechanism of tretinoin's effect on AK regression is not known, but is presumably the same as for other retinoid compounds' anti-neoplastic effects.[53]

Tretinoin 0.05 percent emollient cream, recently approved for the indication of photoaging in the United Kingdom as Retinova and in the United States as Renova, is customarily applied at bedtime to the face, dorsa of the hands, and other target areas. Moisturizer and sunscreen are applied in the morning. During the first weeks of treatment, nearly all patients experience retinoid dermatitis, consisting of erythema scaling, and itching or burning.[46–49] For most, symptoms are mild, peak at approximately 2 weeks, and then abate. Patients should be instructed to skip occasional days of application as necessary until their skin accommodates. As during other forms of topical chemotherapy, AKs may "light up," becoming more apparent during the early weeks of therapy. Treatment may be continued indefinitely, although improvement in appearance may plateau after 6 to 12 months. Less frequent tretinoin applications may then permit prior benefit to be retained in many patients.

Preparations containing α-hydroxyacids (AHAs) such as lactic acid or glycolic acid also improve the appearance of photodamaged skin when applied daily for several months[54,55] and may be less irritating than tretinoin, although in general less information is available regarding their effects. AHA-containing moisturizers are also highly effective in removing the hyperkeratosis (retained scale) often present on the extremities of older patients, as well as in areas of photodamage.

Bullous Pemphigoid

Bullous pemphigoid (BP) is an idiopathic, antibody-mediated disease, which can be differentiated clinically, histologically, and immunologically from the much less common pemphigus vulgaris. The elderly are affected far more commonly than young adults, and BP is the most common immune-mediated blistering disease affecting older patients. The disease is self-limited, lasting months to years, with recurrences following disease-free periods in a minority of patients.[56] Untreated, it ranges in severity from mild to disabling, and the resulting prolonged loss of an effective cutaneous barrier may be fatal.

BP is characterized clinically by tense bullae arising on either erythematous or normal-appearing skin. Preceding or accompanying pruritus is common and may be intense. Crusted erosions and urticarial wheals may coexist with intact bullae, and hemorrhagic bullae are not unusual. Lesions occur most often on the trunk and proximal extremities, with a predilection for flexural surfaces. Approximately one-third of patients have oral blisters, although, unlike pemphigus vulgaris, the mouth is rarely the initial site of involvement. In some patients, bullae remain localized to one area for several months, and in a few, the lesions never become widespread.

Diagnosis is confirmed by skin biopsy. Immunofluorescent staining of perilesional skin is virtually pathognomonic, showing linear deposition along the basement membrane zone of C_3 (third component of complement) in all patients and of IgG in most. Indirect immunofluorescent studies demonstrate anti-basement-membrane zone antibodies of the IgG class in approximately 70 percent of patients.[56]

The two recognized autoantibodies in BP are components of the hemidesmosome,[57] a structure that attaches the basal keratinocyte to the basement membrane. Immune-mediated disruption of this attachment leads to dermoepidermal separation and blister formation.

Corticosteroids are the first line of therapy. In mild or localized cases, topical or intralesional steroid application may control the lesions, but almost all patients require systemic treatment at least initially. Patients with extensive or rapidly progressive, disabling disease should begin therapy with prednisone, 60 to 100 mg daily (some authors recommend two to three times this dose). Patients should be re-evaluated at weekly intervals and the prednisone dose slowly and progressively reduced once new blisters cease forming and clinical remission is achieved. An immunosuppressant such as azathioprine, cyclophosphamide, or methotrexate may be added to the regimen initially or at the time of remission in order to reduce the prednisone requirement.[56,58,59] Six to 8 weeks are required for full expression of the steroid-sparing effect. Patients with less severe disease may initiate therapy with 40 to 60 mg of prednisone on alternate days and/or an immunosuppressant. In all patients, drug dosages are decreased gradually to zero over many months, provided the disease remains in remission. Recently, successful therapy with tetracycline (500 mg four times a day) and nicotinamide (500 mg three times a day) has been suggested as an alternative to prednisone.[60] Sulfapyridine or sulfones are also alternative therapies for patients with major contraindications to systemic steroids. Most patients achieve prolonged remissions and can ultimately discontinue treatment without recurrence of lesions. However, the possibility of disease exacerbation and the potential complications of therapy require close, expert monitoring of all patients throughout the course of their disease.

References

1. Fleischer Jr AB, McFarlane M, Hinds MA, Mittelmark MB: Skin conditions and symptoms are common in the elderly: the prevalence of skin symptoms and conditions in an elderly population. J Geriatr Dermatol 1996;4:78–87
2. Beauregard S, Gilchrest BA: A survey of skin problems and skin care regimens in the elderly. Arch Dermatol 1987;123: 1638–1643
3. Tindal JP: Skin changes and lesions in our senior citizens: incidences. Cutis 1976;18:359–362
4. Lutsky NS: Attitudes toward old age and elderly persons. pp. 287–336. In Eisdorfer C (ed): Annual Review of Gerontology and Geriatrics. Springer, New York, 1980
5. Gilchrest BAI: Skin and Aging Processes. CRC Press, Boca Raton, FL, 1984
6. Gilchrest BA: Age-associated changes in the skin. J Am Geriatr Soc 1982;30:139–143
7. Gilchrest BA: Photodamage. Blackwell Science, Cambridge, MA, 1995
8. Woodwell DA, Schappert SM: National Ambulatory Medical Care Survey: 1993 Summary. Advance Data from Vital and Health Statistics Number 40. National Center for Health Statistics, Hyattsville, 1995
9. Kost RG, Straus SE: Postherpetic neuralgia—pathogenesis, treatment, and prevention. N Engl J Med 1996;335:32–42
10. Lee JJ, Gauci CAG: Postherpetic neuralgia: current concepts and management. Br J Hosp Med 1994;52:565–570
11. Huff JC, Bean B, Balfour HH et al: Therapy of herpes zoster with oral acyclovir. Am J Med 1988;85(suppl 2A):84–89
12. Wood MJ, Ogan PH, McKendrick MW et al: Efficacy of oral acyclovir treatment of acute herpes zoster. Am J Med 1988; 85(suppl 2A):79–83
13. Cobo M: Reduction of the ocular complications of herpes zoster ophthalmicus by oral acyclovir. Am J Med 1988;85(suppl 2A): 90–93
14. Wood MJ, Johnson RW, McKendrick MW et al: A randomized trial of acyclovir for 7 days or 21 days with and without prednisolone for treatment of acute herpes zoster. N Engl J Med 1994; 330:896–900
15. Bernstein JE, Korman NJ, Bickers DR et al: Topical capsaicin treatment of chronic postherpetic neuralgia. J Am Acad Dermatol 1989;21:265–270
16. Rowbotham MC: Treatment of postherpetic neuralgia. Semin Dermatol 1992;11:218–225
17. Klecz RJ, Schwartz RA: Pruritus. Am Fam Physician 1992;45: 2681–2686
18. Gilchrest BA: Pruritus: pathogenesis, therapy and significance in systemic disease states. Arch Intern Med. 1982;142: 101–105
19. Lewiecki MEM, Rahman F: Pruritus: a manifestation of iron deficiency. JAMA 1976;236:2319–2320
20. Salem HH, van der Weyden MB, Young IF, Wiley JS: Pruritus and severe iron deficiency in polycythemia vera. BMJ 1982; 285:91–92
21. Ghadially R, Brown BE, Sequeira-Martin SM et al: The aged epidermal permeability barrier: structural, functional, and lipid biochemical abnormalities in humans and a senescent murine model. J Clin Invest 1995;95:2281–2290
22. Gilchrest BA: Pruritus in the elderly. Semin Dermatol 1995; 14:317–319
23. Fleischer AB: Pruritus in the elderly: management by senior dermatologists. J Am Acad Dermatol 1993;28:603–609
24. Kligman AM: Perspectives and problems in cutaneous gerontology. J Invest Dermatol 1979;73:39–46
25. Tagami H: Quantitative measurements of water concentration of the stratum corneum *in vivo* by high-frequency current. Acta Derm Venereol 1994;185:29–33
26. Estes SA, Estes J: Therapy of scabies: nursing homes, hospitals, and the homeless. Semin Dermatol 1993;12:26–33
27. Meinking TL, Taplin D, Herminda JL et al: The treatment of scabies with invermectin. N Engl J Med 1995;333:26–30
28. Arndt KA, Jick H: Rates of cutaneous reactions to drugs: a report from the Boston Collaborative Drug Surveillance Program. JAMA 1976;235:918–922; Bigby M, Jick S, Jick H,

Arndt K: Drug-induced cutaneous reactions: a report from the Boston Collaborative Drug Surveillance Program on 15,438 consecutive inpatients, 1975 to 1982. JAMA. 1986;256: 3358–3363
29. Wintroub BU, Stern R: Cutaneous drug reactions: pathogenesis and clinical classification. J Am Acad Dermatol 1985;13: 167–179
30. Goldstein SM, Wintroub BU: A Physician's Guide—Adverse Cutaneous Reactions to Medication. CoMedia Inc, New York, 1994
31. Shear NH, Spielberg SP: Anticonvulsant hypersensitivity syndrome: in vitro assessment of risk. J Clin Invest 1988;82: 1826–1832
32. Roujeau JC, Stern RS: Severe adverse cutaneous reactions to drugs. N Engl J Med 1994;331:1272–1285
33. Parker SL, Tong T, Bolden S, Wingo PA: Cancer statistics, 1996. CA Cancer J Clin 1996;46:5–27
34. Miller DL, Weinstock MA: Nonmelanoma skin cancer in the United States: incidence. J Am Acad Dermatol 1994;30: 774–778
35. Elmets CA, Mukhtar H: Ultraviolet radiation and skin cancer: progress in pathophysiologic mechanisms. Prog Dermatol 1995; 30:1–16
36. Preston DS, Stern RS: Nonmelanoma cancers of the skin. N Engl J Med 1992;327:1649–1662
37. Karagas MR, Stukel TA, Greenberg ER et al: Risk of subsequent basal cell carcinoma and squamous cell carcinoma of the skin among patients with prior skin cancer. JAMA 1992;267: 3305–3310
38. Rowe DE, Carroll RJ, Day CL: Long-term recurrence rates in previously untreated (primary) basal cell carcinoma: implications for patient follow-up. J Dermatol Surg Oncol 1989;15: 315–328
39. Salasche SJ, Cheney ML, Varvares MA: Recognition and management of the high-risk cutaneous squamous cell carcinoma. Curr Probl Dermatol 1993;5:141–192
40. Frost CA, Green AC. Epidemiology of solar keratoses. Br J Dermatol 1994;131:455–464
41. Thompson SC, Jolley D, Marks R: Reduction of solar keratoses by regular sunscreen use. N Engl J Med 1993;329:1147–1151
42. Ries LAG, Miller BA, Hankey BF et al (eds): SEER Cancer Statistics Review, 1973–1991: Tables and Graphs, National Cancer Institute. NIH Pub. No. 94-2789. pp.287–299. Bethesda, MD, 1994
43. Geller AC, Koh HK, Miller DR et al: Death rates of malignant melanoma among white men: United States, 1973–1988. MMWR 1992;41:20–21, 27
44. Koh HK: Cutaneous melanoma. N Engl J Med 1991;325: 171–182
45. Johnson TM, Smith JW, Nelson BR, Chang A: Current therapy for cutaneous melanoma. J Am Acad Dermatol 1995;32: 689–707
46. Weinstein GD, Nigra TP, Pochi PE et al: Topical tretinoin for treatment of photodamaged skin: a multicenter study. Arch Dermatol 1991;127:659–665
47. Olsen EA, Katz HI, Levine N et al: Tretinoin emollient cream: a new therapy for photodamaged skin. J Am Acad Dermatol 1992;26:215–224
48. Gilchrest BA: A review of skin ageing and its medical therapy. Br J Dermatol 1996;135:867–875
49. Kligman AM, Thorne EG: Topical therapy of actinic keratoses with tretinoin. pp.66–73. In Marks R (ed): Retinoids in Cutaneous Malignancy. Blackwell Scientific, Oxford 1991
50. Bhawan J, Gonzalez-Serva A, Nehal K et al: Effects of tretinoin on photodamaged skin: a histologic study. Arch Dermatol 1991; 127:666–672
51. Rafal ES, Griffiths CEM, Ditre CM et al: Topical tretinoin (retinoic acid) treatment for liver spots associated with photodamage. N Engl J Med 1992;326:368–374
52. Griffiths CEM, Russman AN, Majmudar G et al: Restoration of collagen formation in photodamaged human skin by tretinoin (retinoic acid). N Engl J Med 1993;329:530–535
53. Moon RC, Itri LM: Retinoids and cancer. pp. 327–372. In Sporn MB, Roberts AB, Goodman DS (eds): The Retinoids. Vol.2 Academic Press, New York, 1984
54. Ditre CM, Griffin TD, Murphy GF et al: Effects of alpha hydroxy acids on photoaged skin: a pilot clinical, histologic, and ultrastructural study. J Am Acad Dermatol 1996;34:187–195
55. Stiller MJ, Bartalone J, Stern R et al: Topical 8% glycolic acid and 8% L-lactic lactic acid creams for the treatment of photodamaged skin. Arch Dermatol 1996;132:631–636
56. Mutasim DF: Bullous pemphigoid: review and update. J Geriatr Dermatol 1993;1:62–71
57. Ishiko A, Shimizu H, Kikuchi A et al: Human autoantibodies against the 230-kD bullous pemphigoid antigen (BPAG1) bind only to the intracellular domain of the hemidesmosome, whereas those against the 180-kD bullous pemphigoid antigen (BPAG2) bind along the plasma membrane of the hemidesmosome in normal human and swine skin. J Clin Invest 1993;91: 1608–1615
58. Fine JD: Management of acquired bullous skin diseases. N Engl J Med 1995;333:1475–1484
59. Paul MA, Jorizzo JL, Fleischer AB, White WL: Low-dose methotrexate treatment in elderly patients with bullous pemphigoid. J Am Acad Dermatol 1994;31:620–625
60. Fivenson DP, Breneman DL, Rosen GB et al: Nicotinamide and tetracycline therapy of bullous pemphigoid. Arch Dermatol 1994;130:753–758

CHAPTER 92

Drug Safety and Effectiveness in the Elderly

C. G. SWIFT

The principles of pharmacology in old age and their implications for prescribing are dealt with in Chapter 11 of this volume, including nondrug options, the principles of dosage, and the need for strategies to achieve satisfactory drug compliance. The purpose of this chapter is to examine the issues concerned with the overall safety and effectiveness of drug therapy in the older population (as distinct from variability in individual drug response), and the measures required to optimize the results of drug therapy in this age group.

The background to this is the historic association of major expenditure with what appear to be rather poor results. Evidence of clear benefit for older recipients has often been lacking, whereas the frequency of adverse drug reactions (ADRs) has appeared disproportionately high, suggesting a picture of escalating drug utilization of questionable appropriateness. It is therefore important to appraise the evidence for both the scale of iatrogenic disease and the efficacy and effectiveness of therapeutic regimens. The now legendary distinction between efficacy and effectiveness is expounded in the classic articles of Cochrane.[1] These concepts underlie current interest in "evidence-based medicine" and are clearly appropriate to consideration of drug utilization in the older population.

Evidence for Adverse Drug Reaction Susceptibility

Anecdotal reports of older patients being less well able to tolerate drugs have become almost part of the language of geriatric medicine. The vignette of the geriatrician drawing a straight line through the prescribing sheet followed by the reportedly dramatic recovery of the patient is a familiar one. Such reports have suggested culpability (with variable justification) on the part of (1) the prescribers, (2) the drugs themselves, and (3) the aging process, and have added some impetus toward acquiring more scientific evidence. They may also have promoted inappropriately negative attitudes about the benefits of drug therapy for older people.

More concrete links between drug toxicity and advancing age have emerged from organized methods of drug surveillance (pharmacovigilance).[2] These have included (1) observational cohort studies using detection methods of greater or less sensitivity, (2) formal prospective ADR surveillance initiatives, (3) spontaneous reporting systems, (4) record linkage studies, (5) case cohort studies, and (6) case control studies.

In one of the earliest prospective observational cohort studies,[3] 15.3 percent of prescribed drug takers admitted to departments of geriatric medicine in the United Kingdom were found to have ADRs, which in most cases were judged to have contributed to the need for admission. The frequency of ADR was also related to the number of prescribed drugs (Fig. 92-1). Although in theory subject to observer bias, this was one of the first reports to move the epidemiology beyond anecdote. Subsequent studies of this type with broadly similar findings have been undertaken with other selected populations, such as nursing home occupants,[4] outpatients,[5,6] or patients requiring hospital readmission.[7]

Early prospective small-scale surveillance studies[8] and larger scale ADR detection studies[9,10] showed an increased frequency of unwanted drug effects with increasing age in hospital patients. The former focused on drugs in general, whereas the latter sought to single out specific drug groups.

Spontaneous reporting system (e.g., the U.K. yellow card system) have shown both an increased preponderance of ADRs in general in older age groups and also increased susceptibility to drug-specific ADRs, such as nonsteroidal induced gastrointestinal bleeding.[11] Both record linkage and case cohort studies of nonsteroidal anti-inflammatory drug (NSAID) use have shown age to be a defined determinant of ADRs.[12,13]

Interpretation of these data presents a number of difficulties in the following areas:

1. *Clinical significance*. The distinction between relatively trivial and very important ADRs is often unclear from broadly based pharmacovigilance data, although often explored in studies of specific drug classes, such as NSAIDs, where age predisposes to serious adverse events independently of prescription rate.[11]
2. *The distinction between adverse events and ADRs*. Many reported adverse events are in categories that exhibit an increasing incidence with age, irrespective of drug therapy. Thus the risks attributable to drugs in such reports may be overestimated unless the occurrence of non-drug-related events can be identified and allowed for. This is one of the arguments in support of record linkage systems and of case control studies.[12,14] Measures to improve the sensitivity of ADR diagnosis in observational studies have included the use of algorithms (e.g., the Adverse Drug Reaction Probability Scale) and Bayesian probability calculations.[15,16]
3. *Reporting biases*. Apart from the well-known tendency of

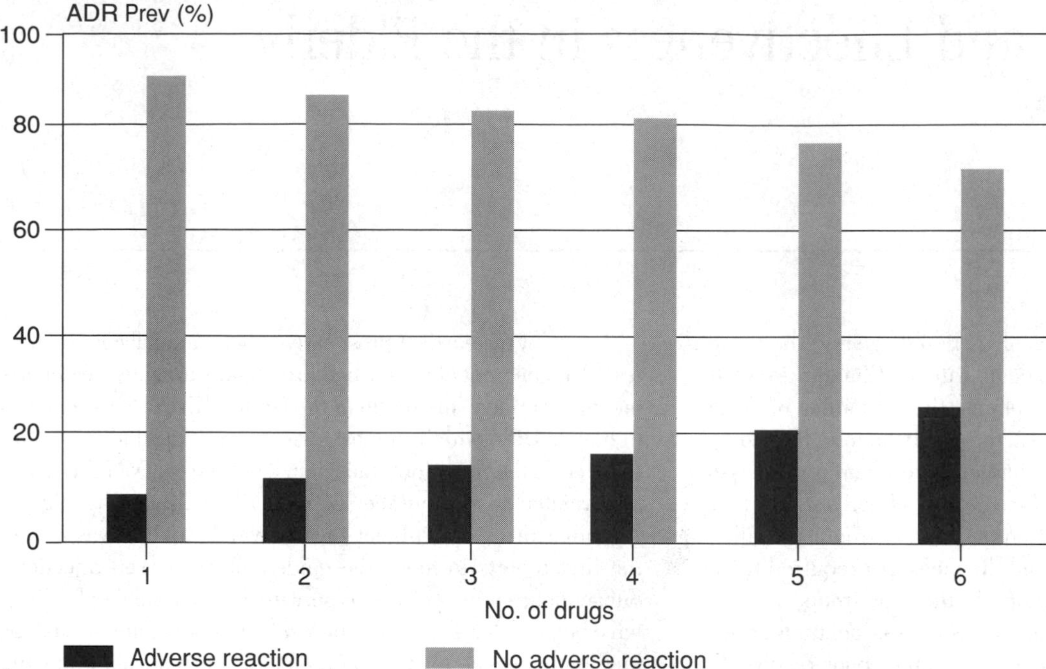

Figure 92-1 Relationship between number of prescribed drugs and adverse drug reactions in an observational cohort study. (From Williamson and Chopin,[3] with permission.)

spontaneous reporting systems to attract only a fraction of legitimately notifiable events, their focus tends to be on serious and unexpected problems. Thus, type A ADRs (dose-related, predictable, and an accentuation of a drug's known pharmacologic action) are likely to be under-represented by comparison with type B (idiosyncratic, unpredictable, and largely unrelated to a drug's main pharmacologic action). Unfortunately, most drug-related morbidity among older people is probably due to type A reactions, many of which are not judged to be severe enough to prompt a spontaneous report. Studies based on self-reporting indicate it to be almost certainly the least reliable method,[5,17] possibly because of a reduced awareness or appreciation of some symptoms with increasing age.

4. *Different study populations*. Although hospital inpatient data more consistently (although not invariably) have shown an age-dependent increase in susceptibility,[9,18–20] less consistent findings have been reported in other groups, such as outpatients.[6,21]

Taken overall, the cumulative evidence points convincingly to an increase in susceptibility to ADRs with increasing age, although in discriminant analysis age-associated contributory variables often appear to predominate over any independent effect of age itself.[19] Major factors commonly implicated in this problem include the following:

1. *Excessive prescribing (number and duration)*. Drug utilization in developed populations is disproportionately high among older people and there is a continuing upward trend.[22] This raises concerns about both cost and morbidity. A positive correlation between total numbers of prescriptions and ADR frequency is to some extent predictable and has been demonstrated in several studies.[3,11] Whether or not prescribing is excessive is difficult to establish without detailed assessment of appropriateness.

2. *Inappropriate prescribing*. There is still a paucity of evidence about the benefit-risk ratio of many drugs in this age group (especially large-scale studies incorporating valid clinical outcome measures). Some drug use is, however, generally agreed to be higher than desirable (e.g., neuroleptic use in dementia) and one approach to the assessment of appropriateness is the development and application of consensus criteria.[23, 24] A problem with this approach, if directly applied, is its relative inflexibility to individual variation in usage and indication (i.e., case mix).

Recent work has explored both the practicability and the reliability of a set of indicators of overall prescribing quality in older patients, based on (1) purely descriptive data (e.g., number of prescribed items per patient), (2) evidence of unnecessary or harmful prescribing (e.g., duplication), or (3) the appropriateness of use of individual drugs or combinations (e.g., inhaled steroids with β-2 agonists).[25] Figure 92-2 shows the algorithm used for assessing the appropriateness of co-prescription (when observed) of an angiotensin-converting enzyme (ACE) inhibitor and a potassium-sparing diuretic. It will be seen that this method, using largely drug-chart-based information supplemented by objective clinical evidence where required, enables the assessment of prescribing quality while also accounting for variation due to case mix.

The emergence of better audit tools is welcome and should

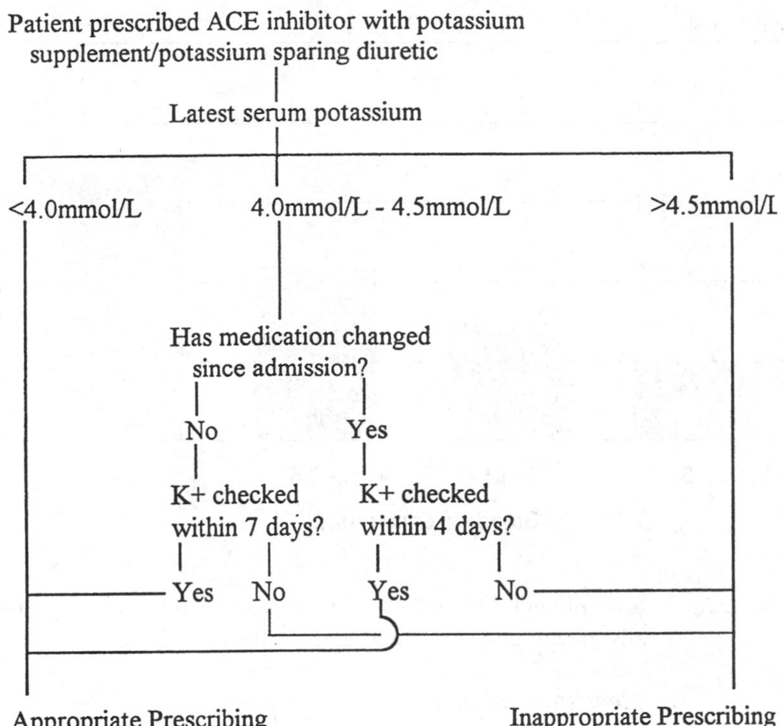

Figure 92-2 Algorithm used for assessing the appropriateness of co-prescription of an ACE inhibitor and a potassium-sparing diuretic. One of a set of prescribing indicators. (From Oborne et al.,[25] with permission.)

result in a clearer assessment of prescribing quality (alongside existing measures of quantity) for the future. It is, however, difficult to criticize poorly rationalized prescribing where the hard data required are unavailable (e.g., because of the historic exclusion of older people in clinical trials). Thankfully, this situation has begun to improve (see below) although direct evidence in very old and sick patients still presents particular difficulties, leaving the clinician dependent on cautious extrapolation from controlled studies of less complex individuals fulfilling trials criteria.

3. *Unsatisfactory "medication management" (noncompliance)*. The contribution of problems of medication management to ADR is generally considered to be small. There is no evidence that age per se is predictive of poor drug compliance, although some of the associated factors, such as social isolation and illness of long duration, may be implicated. Problems of compliance are, however, directly proportional to the number and complexity of prescriptions.[26,27] Poor professional communication[28] and unsatisfactory presentation of drugs (e.g., childproof containers)[29] have also been found to contribute. As a general rule there is little point in issuing a prescription to an individual with impaired cognition unless the assistance of a caregiver or other third party can be assured. The principal consequence of poor compliance appears to be failure of therapeutic outcome rather than drug toxicity.

4. *Altered dose-related aspects of drug handling and response (due to the combined or separate effects of aging and disease states)*. Several studies have shown a clear effect of both age and dose on the occurrence of ADRs, strongly suggesting a key contribution of altered pharmacokinetics or pharmacodynamics to type A reactions in the older population. The biologic mechanisms are outlined in Chapter 11. Figure 92-3 shows the effect of dose on the relative risk of upper gastrointestinal ADRs in a case cohort study of older NSAID consumers.[13] The dose-dependent mechanisms involved here are not entirely understood, but might relate to a reduction with increasing age in mucosal prostaglandin content. Another example is the age-related incidence of unwanted sedation from benzodiazepines, which is also dose dependent, and is probably due to enhanced central nervous system "sensitivity".[30]

In summary, the measures required to improve drug safety in older recipients comprise (1) the development of drugs with safer pharmacologic actions, (2) the on-going and systematic investigation of dose-response relationships in this age group, both for drug classes and individual compounds, and (3) the continued improvement and application of pharmacovigilance methods to quantify safety in relation to efficacy. These in turn will provide the necessary information with which (4) to influence and modify prescribing practice. A useful vehicle for dissemination may well be the preparation of consensus statements, such as that published by the U.K. Royal College of Physicians.[31] Other more explicitly audit-driven initiatives, such as implementation of the Omnibus Budgetary Reconciliation Act of 1987 (OBRA-87) (designed to reduce unnecessary drug use, including the inappropriate prescription of neuroleptic drugs in nursing homes, in the United States)[32] and training programs[33] may also have a place, provided that the impetus is driven by sound science and not just economic imperatives. Measures to improve medication management probably have more to do with ensuring efficacy than with drug safety, although gross instances of poor compliance will, of course, carry risks.

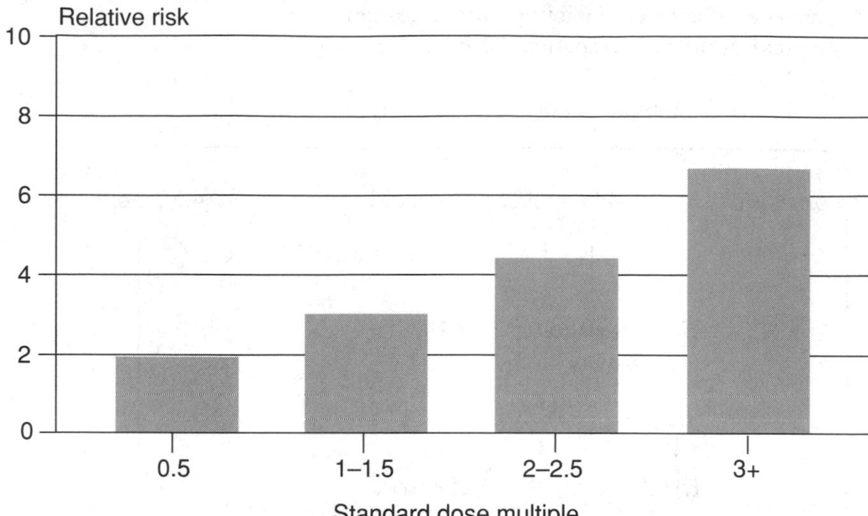

Figure 92-3 The effect of dose on the relative risk of upper gastrointestinal adverse drug reactions in a case cohort study of older nonsteroidal anti-inflammatory drug consumers. From Griffin et al.,[13] with permission.)

The reader is referred to other reviews dealing with aging and adverse drug reactions.[34,35]

Evidence for Drug Efficacy

The relative paucity of good clinical trials information underpinning drug therapy in this age group has already been mentioned. The organized participation of older patients in such trials is still a comparatively recent phenomenon. It has been largely driven by an increased awareness of the special problems of safety and the resulting emergence of defined regulatory requirements for drug development. As a result, the situation has improved, bringing with it (1) greater experience of the special considerations involved in conducting such experiments and (2) confirmation of the possibility of gratifying results from carefully managed drug treatment, even in patients of very advanced years. The availability of such information is vital, not least because many of the conditions concerned are of the "long-term limiting" variety and therefore necessitate protracted or permanent administration of drugs. The resulting costs in terms of expense, inconvenience, and possible side effects are potentially so considerable that there can be little justification for embarking on the use of such medication unless the evidence of genuine benefit is clear.

Conduct of Clinical Trials

The particular constraints facing clinical investigators working with older subjects are as follows:

Heterogeneity

It is well recognized that the heterogeneity of human population samples increases with age. As a result, larger numbers of trial subjects may be required to produce trials of adequate power, while at the same time the practical recruitment of large numbers of older participants tends to be more, rather than less, difficult. The net effects in completing the study are usually greater cost, time, and organizational difficulty.

Measurement error

Measurement error is a further potential consequence of heterogeneity. Many clinical and biological measurements lose sensitivity if intersubject variability is high, but it may be logistically, economically, or scientifically impractical to utilize the most sensitive and specific methods in large population samples or away from tightly controlled environments. Under these circumstances the investigator may have to accept a compromise between the method of choice on the one hand and the applicability of the findings to the broad elderly population on the other. The decision will depend on a definition of the precise question.

Ethical issues

Justification The justification (see also Ch. 46) for undertaking clinical experimentation involving older subjects and the ethical concerns may be summarized as follows: (1) It is arguably unethical not to conduct such research because of the potential risk to much larger numbers of older patients if the required hard information on efficacy and safety is lacking; (2) there is no valid scientific alternative to properly designed and conducted clinical trials; (3) the issue then becomes that of balancing the risks undertaken by consenting individuals in clinical trials against the wider common good. The imperative to undertake the necessary research is counterbalanced by the proportionately greater responsibility of the research community to safeguard the interests of older participants in trials. The underlying ethical principles are the same as for all trial subjects, only more so.

Safety Clinical trials in general have an excellent safety record. Most studies of large numbers of trial subjects both in Britain and the United States have reported no deaths, very low levels of suspected serious reactions, and levels of minor suspected drug-related events of the older of 2 to 6 percent.[36–38] The safety data specifically in older trial participants remain to be adequately studied, but there is to date no indication that these differ. The existence of increased background morbidity in older patient groups is inevitable, however, and the possibility of higher risk to older individuals is significant. These important issues require careful consideration when deciding how, when, where, and by whom clinical studies should be undertaken. Heightened awareness and greater care are required, and there are strong arguments for basing such work more or less exclusively in centers with demonstrable and predominant specialist expertise in clinical research in older human subjects.

Scientific validity Because of the above factors the temptation to make scientific compromises for reasons of time, convenience, or cost is pressing. To do so, however, may be to expose older subjects to the risks of a clinical trial from which no valid conclusions can be drawn. There are many such studies in the published literature. Bad studies and pseudoscience should be regarded as unethical. It is probably right that an increased role for ethics committees in scientific scrutiny is currently gaining ground.

Information handling Advanced age per se in no way results in the loss of ability to give or withhold informed consent. It may be appropriate, however, to build in additional safeguards with some older participants, particularly patients or those in institutional settings. All concerned, including the local Ethics Committee, should be satisfied that information is presented in a way that is operationally meaningful (i.e., in terms sufficiently nontechnical to convey a faithful account to the participant of the content, purpose, and risks of the proposed study).

Particular care is necessary at all times to safeguard the autonomy of trial participants. The reasons why older people take part have been found to differ from those influencing the standard young healthy volunteer (in whom the motivation is with few exceptions overwhelmingly financial). There is usually a clearly stated wish to be of help to others, there is an increased likelihood that previous treatment will have been beneficial, and because many disorders are age-related, there is a sense of moral duty on the part of older people to offer help.[39]

These issues require sensitive and professional handling. A common additional practice in the consent procedure, particularly with vulnerable groups (see below) is to involve an independent but sympathetic observer (e.g., senior nurse) who should establish and confirm his or her satisfaction about the presentation of information and the understanding and consent or refusal of the intended participant. The informal involvement of relatives or principal caregivers should, when possible, be encouraged, although there needs to be an awareness of the occasional possibility of inappropriate pressures from these sources. Written consent alone has commonly been found to be an inadequate safeguard in circumstances where the absolute autonomy of the intended participant is in doubt to any degree.

Vulnerable groups Special protective strategies are appropriate for certain groups of older subjects where clinical trial participation is potentially associated with greater psychological pressure or actual risk. These groups may include (1) those with impaired cognition, (2) those with intractable conditions unresponsive to previous treatment, (3) those living in institutional surroundings, (4) those on their own without the support of family or other advocates, and (5) those (in some health care systems) living in circumstances of poverty.

Evidence From Controlled Clinical Studies

Clinical trials within the framework of drug development are usually categorized into phases I to IV.

Phase I studies

Phase I studies (in the usually defined sense of a drug's first introduction to human following preclinical evaluation) have seldom involved older individuals. The objectives are to define and measure the effects of a range of doses in healthy adult human volunteers, to ascertain the dose range of tolerability, and to investigate the human pharmacokinetics and pharmacodynamics in order to arrive at a projected estimate of the likely therapeutic dose.

In recent years, age changes in pharmacokinetics and pharmacodynamics have been characterized in many studies of "phase I" type in older human subjects (including healthy volunteers) (see Ch. 11) as a means of quantifying such effects and making informed recommendations on dosage for subsequent trials and for clinical use in older patients.

Phase II studies

The extent to which phase II studies involve older individuals has depended historically on the perceived particular importance of the target condition in older patients. There has in general been inadequate representation. Sound phase II studies are characterized by tight control, small numbers, rigid design, close monitoring, and the most sensitive possible quantification of response. They are intended to confirm the estimated effective dose, the drug effect and tolerability in patients, and the therapeutic ratio and to predict the likely value of the treatment in a broader range of patients. It may be necessary for surrogate rather than generalizable endpoints to be utilized.

A phase II study of tacrine hydrochloride[40] illustrates the value of this approach in the difficult area of dementia of Alzheimer type and has provided the basic model for most subsequent studies of cholinesterase inhibitors in this field. The study was of careful randomized controlled design with closely defined subject selection criteria, accepted objective measures of impaired cognition, and exclusion on the basis of concurrent illness or medication, or the absence of a reliable caregiver to ensure compliance with the protocol. This rigorous approach resulted in a 50 percent exclusion of patients assessed for entry, in addition to which some 27 percent of subjects were

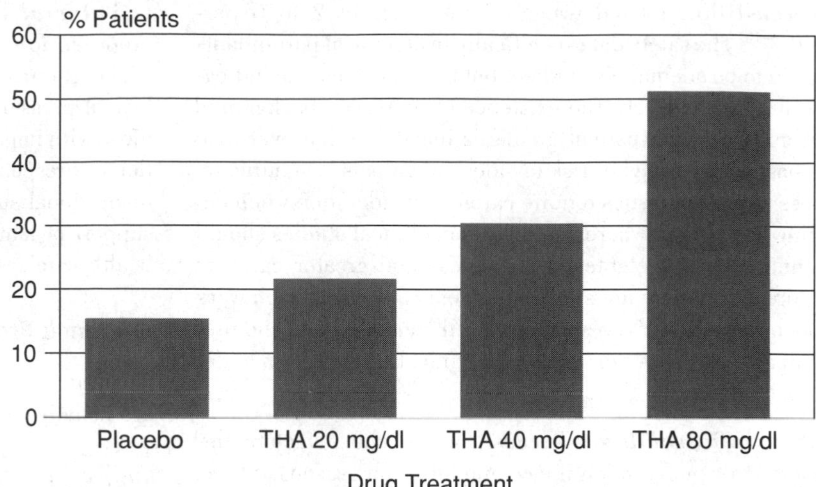

Figure 92-4 Percentage of patients with a four-point improvement on the Alzheimer's Disease Assessment Scale cognitive subscale after 12 weeks of treatment in a controlled trial. (From Farlow et al.,[41] with permission.)

withdrawn after entering the study. The largely surrogate measures of outcome used (e.g., changes in Mini Mental Status Examination score and the neuropsychological variables of the CAMCOG test battery) were selected primarily because of their anticipated sensitivity as measures of change rather than their criterion validity. As a result of the care in design and execution, this was one of the first studies to demonstrate convincingly the dose-dependent efficacy of any compound in treating this condition. It was left to studies with larger numbers to provide further evidence of efficacy by reproducing the findings[41] (Fig. 92-4) and in addition showing benefit on the more "real" (but less sensitive) endpoints, such as caregiver ratings. The wider effectiveness and safety of cholinesterase inhibitors remain to be established by means of extended phase III and IV studies. In the absence of phase II data, however, such studies would probably not have been justifiable, nor their design informed.

Phase III and large-scale intervention studies

There has been a welcome growth in the involvement of older patients in phase III and large-scale intervention studies. Well-known examples include the European Working Party and other major studies in hypertension,[42–45] several of the international studies of thrombolysis and secondary prevention in myocardial infarction[46–49] and of ACE inhibition in systolic heart failure and left ventricular dysfunction,[50] the Scandinavian Simvastatin Study (4S) of cholesterol reduction,[51,52] and the studies of antithrombotic agents in atrial fibrillation[53–55] and established stroke.[56] The evidence of benefit irrespective of advanced age has been a feature of many of the findings, in some cases showing an apparently preferential benefit with increasing age, even with correction of the data for the higher baseline incidence of the target endpoints in older subjects. Figure 92-5, for example, shows the effect of the combination of streptokinase and aspirin on 5-week percentage mortality in the ISIS-2 study with the data also expressed as the reduction in deaths per thousand patients.[47] The beneficial effects on mortality and symptoms of long-term ACE inhibition after myocardial infarction with left ventricular dysfunction have been shown clearly in older as well as younger patients.[50]

We are thus entering a period where the benefits of both acute and long-term drug interventions are becoming more clearly demonstrated in older populations of patients than ever before. This has profound implications for the provision of health care, but also necessitates an urgent review of the approach to medication management, particular for long-term medication, because the benefits demonstrated in large-scale trials generally relate to defined dose regimens administered under close scrutiny. The long-term co-administration to patients with ischemic heart disease of a diuretic, an anticoagulant or aspirin, an ACE inhibitor, an antiarrhythmic, a calcium channel blocker, and a lipid-lowering agent might now be argued to be justified by the evidence of benefit. Suboptimal compliance with such a complex regimen would, however, negate the benefits of all these preparations and hence the cost effectiveness of the entire exercise. For these reasons, the need to assist with medication management where necessary appears more than ever important and a challenge to interprofessional practice involving especially doctors, nurses, and pharmacists.

Drug Regulation

Where drug regulatory procedures have become well established, the requirement of pharmaceutical companies to submit information on the clinical pharmacokinetics, dose requirements, efficacy, and safety of any new compound with respect to older recipients as part of the premarketing dossier and product licence application has now been an accepted element of drug development for about the last two decades. This has undoubtedly contributed to a wider awareness among both manufactures and prescribers of the importance of advanced age as a risk factor for ADR. Sporadic instances where drugs have been withdrawn or restrictions imposed on their use because of an apparently age-defined incidence of reports to the regulatory bodies (e.g., terodiline, mianserin) have also served to highlight the issues. An optimistic view that both care in prescribing and drug safety in the older population as a whole have improved as a result might be justified, although there is as yet no hard evidence. The need for a shift in clinicians' thinking in the direction of maximizing the effectiveness of drug treatment (rather than simply avoiding its dangers) is now supported by the evidence.

Initiatives have been taken to harmonize internationally the regulatory requirements for new drug evaluation in the older population. The recommendations of the International Committee on Harmonization[57] are encapsulated in abbreviated form in Table 92-1. Although deliberately amenable in part to interpretation, these guidelines provide a framework (built on experience and capable of further fine tuning) for future care both in the development of new drugs and in the conduct of the phases of clinical trials. A minor risk is that mechanical repetition of a prescribed set of criteria may result in spurious work that misses the key questions relevant to individual drugs. At present, however, the interface between specialists in clinical age research and industry looks sufficiently healthy to safeguard against this and the regulatory bodies themselves are developing a more interactive role with companies in the compilation of product licence applications. All of these developments are welcome contributions to the well-being of older medication consumers.

Table 92-1 International Committee on Harmonization Guidelines for drug development research in older people—rationale and content

Scope
Significant use due to prevalence or age-associated condition
New entities
New formulations/combinations
New uses
Pharmacokinetic studies
Formal studies as a rule
Volunteers or patients
Single/multiple dose
Pharmacokinetic screening under certain circumstances
Renal/hepatic impairment
Pharmacodynamic studies
Drugs that sedate
Unexplained response differences
Phase II/III
Meaningful numbers to permit comparison (e.g., minimum 100: higher % for Alzheimer's disease)
Further studies if indicated by findings
Combined or separate (age-specific) studies
Interaction studies
Digoxin
Oral anticoagulants
Enzyme induction
Enzyme inhibition
Likely concomitant drugs

(From Food and Drug Administration,[57] with permission.)

Conclusions

The available information indicates that advancing age is associated with both an increase in susceptibility to ADR and a growing potential to benefit from effective modern drug therapy. Greater safety may be achieved by the development of better, more specific drugs, clearer delineation of age changes in dose-response relationships and the factors underlying

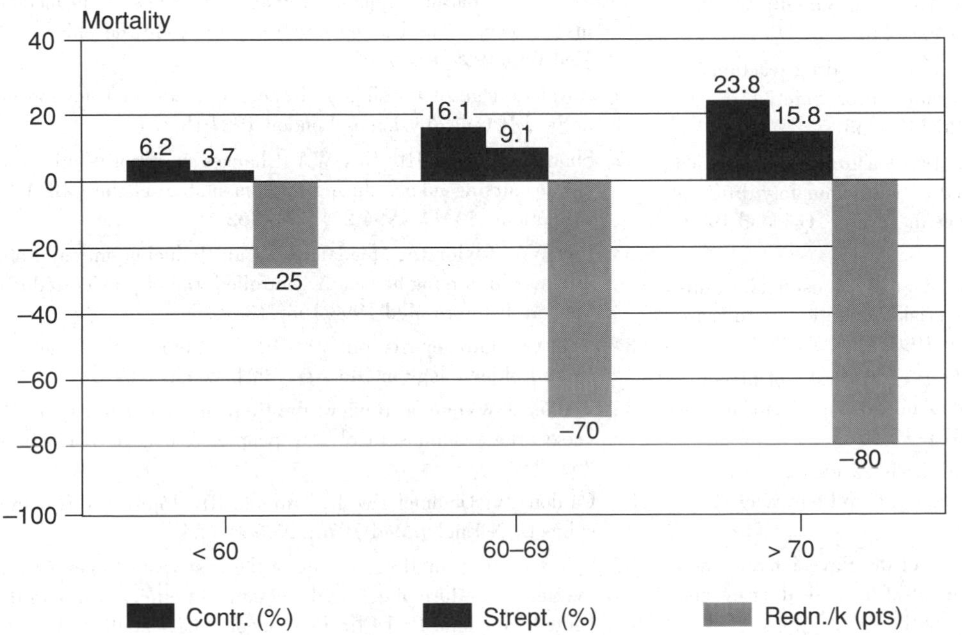

Figure 92-5 Effect of streptokinase plus aspirin on 5-week mortality by age in the ISIS-2 trial. (From ISIS-2 Collaborative Group,[47] with permission.)

them, and more circumspect, better informed prescribing. The promise of more effective drug therapy has increased dramatically in recent years and may be realized by proper measurement of efficacy in carefully designed and executed clinical trials in the age group, together with improved communication about the risks and benefits of drugs and serious, preferably interdisciplinary, strategies to ensure access and promote optimal medication management. These are exciting challenges for both scientists and the health care professions.

References

1. Cochrane AL: Archie Cochrane in his own words. Selections arranged from his 1972 introduction to "Effectiveness and Efficiency: Random Reflections on the Health Services" 1972 [classical article]. Controlled Clin Trials 1989;10:428–433
2. Rawlins MD: Pharmacovigilance: paradise lost, regained or postponed? J R Coll Phys 1995;29:40–49
3. Williamson J, Chopin JM: Adverse reactions to prescribed drugs in the elderly: a multicentre investigation. Age Ageing 1980;9:73–80
4. Cooper JW: Probable adverse drug reactions in a rural geriatric nursing home population: a four-year study. J Am Geriatr Soc 1996;44:194–197
5. Klein LE, German PS, Levine DM et al: Medication problems among outpatients. Arch Intern Med 1984;144:1185–1188
6. Schneider JK, Mion LC, Frengley JD: Adverse drug reactions in an elderly outpatient population. Am J Hosp Pharm 1992;49:90–96
7. Bero LA, Lipton HL, Bird JA: Characterization of geriatric drug-related hospital readmissions. Med Care 1991;29:989–1003
8. Hurwitz N: Predisposing factors in adverse reactions to drugs. BMJ 1969;1:536–539
9. Greenblatt DJ, Allen MD, Shader RI: Toxicity of high-dose flurazepam in the elderly. Clin Pharmacol Ther 1977;21:355–361
10. Greenblatt DJ, Allen MD: Toxicity of nitrazepam in the elderly: a report from the Boston Collaborative Drug Surveillance Program. Br J Clin Pharmacol 1978;5:407–413
11. Castleden CM, Pickles H: Suspected adverse drug reactions in elderly patients reported to the Committee on Safety of Medicines. Br J Clin Pharmacol 1988;26:347–353
12. Beardon PH, Brown SV, McDevitt DG: Gastrointestinal events in patients prescribed non-steroidal anti-inflammatory drugs: a controlled study using record linkage in Tayside. Q J Med 1989;71:497–505
13. Griffin MR, Piper JM, Daugherty JR et al: Nonsteroidal anti-inflammatory drug use and increased risk for peptic ulcer disease in elderly persons. Ann Intern Med 1991;114:257–263
14. Langman MJS, Weil J, Wainwright P et al: Risks of bleeding peptic ulcer associated with individual non-steroidal anti-inflammatory drugs. Lancet 1994;343:1075–1078
15. Lanctot KL, Naranjo CA: Computer-assisted evaluation of adverse events using a Bayesian approach. J Clin Pharmacol 1994;34:142–147
16. Lanctot KL, Naranjo CA: Comparison of the Bayesian approach and a simple algorithm for assessment of adverse drug events. Clin Pharmacol Ther 1995;58:692–698
17. Kellaway GSM, McCrae E: Intensive monitoring of adverse drug effects in patients discharged from acute medical wards. N Z Med J 1973;78:525–528
18. Classen DC, Pestotnik SL, Evans RS, Burke JP: Computerised surveillance of adverse drug events in hospital patients. JAMA 1991;266:2847–2851
19. Carbonin P: Is age and independent risk factor of ADRs in hospitalised medical patients. J Am Geriatr Soc 1991;39:1093–1099
20. Ogilvie RI, Ruedy J: Adverse drug reactions during hospitalisation. Can Med Assoc J 1967;97:1450–1457
21. Hutchinson TA, Flegel KM, Kramer MS et al: Frequency, severity and risk factors for adverse drug reactions in adult populations: a prospective study. J Chron Dis 1986;39:533–542
22. Griffin JP, Chew R: Trends in usage of prescription medicines by the elderly and very elderly between 1977 and 1988. In: The Challenges of Ageing. ABPI, London, 1990
23. Beers MH, Ouslander JG, Rollingher I et al: Explicit criteria for determining inappropriate medication use in nursing homes. Arch Intern Med 1991;151:1825–1832
24. Beers MH, Ouslander JG, Fingold SF et al: Inappropriate medication prescribing in skilled-nursing facilities. Ann Intern Med 1992;117:684–689
25. Oborne CA, Batty GM, Maskrey V et al: Development of prescribing indicators for elderly medical inpatients. Br J Clin Pharmacol (in press)
26. Hulka BS, Kupper LL, Cassel JC, Efird RL: Medication use and misuse: physician-patient discrepancies. J Chronic Dis 1975;28:7–21
27. Clinite JC, Kabat HF: Prescribed drugs: errors during self administration. J Am Pharm Assoc 1969;9:450–452
28. Cartwright A: Medicine taken by people aged 65 or more. Br Med Bull 1990;1:63–76
29. Atkinson L, Gibson I, Andrews J: An investigation into the ability of elderly patients continuing to take prescribed drugs after discharge from hospital and recommendations concerning improving the situation. Gerontology 1978;24:225–234
30. Swift CG: Pharmacodynamics: changes in homeostatic mechanisms, receptor and target organ sensitivity in the elderly. Br Med Bull 1990;46:36–52
31. Royal College of Physicians: Report on medication for the elderly. J R Coll Physicians London 1984;18:7–17
32. Shorr RI, Fought RL, Ray-WA: Changes in antipsychotic drug use in nursing homes during implementation of the OBRA-87 regulations. JAMA 1994;271:358–362
33. Ray WA, Taylor JA, Meador KG et al: Reducing antipsychotic drug use in nursing homes. A controlled trial of provider education. Arch Intern Med 1993;153:713–721
34. Swift CG: Iatrogenesis. pp. 398–407. In Ebrahim S, Kalache A (eds): Epidemiology in Old Age. BMJ, London, 1996
35. Walker J, Wynne H: Review: the frequency and severity of adverse drug reactions in elderly people. Age Ageing 1994;23:255–259
36. Cardon PV, Dommel FW Jr, Trumble RR: Injuries to research subjects. N Engl J Med 1976;295:650–654
37. Spiers CJ, Griffin JP: A survey of the first year of operation of the new procedure affecting the conduct of clinical trials in the United Kingdom. Br J Clin Pharmacol 1983;15:649–651

38. Royle JM, Snell ES: Medical research on normal volunteers. Br J Clin Pharmacol 1986;21:548–551
39. Kinirons MT, Maskrey V, Swift CG, Jackson SHD: Elderly volunteers' opinion and attitudes to clinical research Age Ageing 1995; 24(S2):6
40. Eagger SA, Levy R, Sahakian BJ: Tacrine in Alzheimer's disease. Lancet 1991;337:989–992
41. Farlow M, Stephen I, Gracon DVM et al: A controlled trial of tacrine in Alzheimer's disease. JAMA 1992;268:2523–2529
42. SHEP Cooperative Research Group: Prevention of stroke by antihypertensive drug treatment in older persons with isolated systolic hypertension. Final results of the Systolic Hypertension in the Elderly Program (SHEP). JAMA 1991;265:3255–3264
43. Amery A, Birkenhager W, Brixko P et al: Influence of antihypertensive drug treatment on morbidity and mortality in patients over the age of 60 years. European Working Party on High blood pressure in the Elderly (EWPHE) results: sub-group analysis on entry stratification. J Hypertens Suppl 1986;4:S642–647
44. Lever AF, Brennan PJ: MRC trial of treatment in elderly hypertensives. Clin Exp Hypertens 1993;15:941–952
45. Ekbom T, Dahlof B, Hansson L et al: Antihypertensive efficacy and side effects of three beta-blockers and a diuretic in elderly hypertensives: a report from the STOP-Hypertension study. J Hypertens 10:1525–1530
46. Gruppo Italiano per lo Studio della Sopravvivenza nell'Infarto Miocardico: GISSI-2: a factorial randomised trial of alteplase versus streptokinase and heparin versus no heparin among 12,490 patients with acute myocardial infarction. Lancet 1990; 336:65–71
47. ISIS-2 (Second International Study of Infarct Survival) Collaborative Group: Randomised trial of intravenous streptokinase, oral aspirin, both, or neither among 17,187 cases of suspected acute myocardial infarction: ISIS-2. Lancet 1988;2:349–360
48. ISIS-3 (Third International Study of Infarct Survival) Collaborative Group: ISIS-3: a randomised comparison of streptokinase vs tissue plasminogen activator vs anistreplase and of aspirin plus heparin vs aspirin alone among 41,299 cases of suspected acute myocardial infarction. Lancet 1992;339:753–770
49. The GUSTO Angiographic Investigators: The effects of tissue plasminogen activator, streptokinase, or both on coronary-artery patency, ventricular function, and survival after acute myocardial infarction. N Engl J Med 1993;329:1615–1622
50. ISIS-4 (Fourth International Study of Infarct Survival) Collaborative Group: ISIS-4: a randomised factorial trial assessing early oral captopril, oral mononitrate, and intravenous magnesium sulphate in 58,050 patients with suspected acute myocardial infarction. Lancet 1995;345:669–685
51. Scandinavian Simvastatin Survival Study (4S): Randomised trial of cholesterol lowering in 4444 patients with coronary heart disease. Lancet 1994;344:1383–1389
52. Glasser SP, DiBianco R, Effron BA et al: The efficacy and safety of pravastatin in patients aged 60 to 85 years with low-density lipoprotein cholesterol > 160 mg/dl. Am J Cardiol 1996;77: 83–85
53. Ezekowitz MD, Bridgers SL, James KE et al: Warfarin in the prevention of stroke associated with nonrheumatic atrial fibrillation. Veterans Affairs Stroke Prevention in Nonrheumatic Atrial Fibrillation Investigators. N Engl J Med 327:1406–1412
54. Stroke Prevention in Atrial Fibrillation Study: Final results. Circulation 1991;84:527–539
55. Connolly SJ, Laupacis A, Gent M et al: Canadian Atrial Fibrillation Anticoagulation (CAFA) Study. J Am Coll Cardiol 1991;18: 349–355
56. International Stroke Trial (in press)
57. Food and Drug Administration, Department of Health and Human Services (USA): International Conference on Harmonization; Guideline on Studies in Support of Special Populations: Geriatrics; Availability. Fed Reg 1994;59:33398–33400

C H A P T E R 93

Geriatric Oncology

MARGOT GOSNEY

Cancer is a major cause of death and morbidity in elderly patients with over 50 percent of new cases occurring in those aged 70 years or older. Cancer death rates in older people have increased by 17 percent despite a 23 percent decrease in the cancer death rate in those aged 65 years or less.[1] As the incidence and prevalence of cancer increases, coupled with improved diagnostic certainty and life expectancy, many doctors will be faced with caring for elderly patients with cancer. It is estimated that 6 percent of NHS expenditure is used in cancer care with elderly patients responsible for a large proportion of this expenditure. Although cancer was chosen as a key area in the "Health of the Nation" document,[2] elderly people were not specifically targeted and in the Department of Health document, "A Policy Framework for Commissioning Cancer Services,"[3] which provides guidance for purchasers and providers of cancer services, there is no mention of involvement of geriatricians in the acute care or rehabilitation of elderly patients with cancer. The true impact of cancer in older people is unknown because of poor histologic verification; often the first registration of cancer is at death certification. In the US, in an attempt to focus attention on geriatric oncology, the American Cancer Society, the American Society of Clinical Oncology, and other research groups have formed subgroups specifically to deal with the problem of geriatric oncology. However, less interest in this subspeciality of geriatric medicine has been seen in the UK despite a clear need for geriatricians to be involved in the diagnosis of cancer and the planning of subsequent therapy.

Cancer and Aging

There is no doubt that older people are more likely to develop cancer and differences in tumor growth and spread occur as a result of aging. The relationship between cancer and aging is complex, and various factors including changes in host tumor defenses, and exposure to carcinogens, have roles to play in the etiology of tumors. Although there are several distinct theories of cancer causation in older people, including decreased ability to repair DNA, oncogene activation or amplification, tumor suppressor gene loss, decreased immune surveillance, prolonged duration of carcinogenic exposure, or increase susceptibility of aged cells to carcinogens, no one theory has universal backing.[4]

There is debate as to whether carcinogenesis and aging are related phenomena. Many believe such a relationship exists[5,6] with some postulating that cancer develops due to normal processes occurring during aging[7] and others favoring a common etiological origin for both cancer and aging.[8] There is a relationship between chromosomal alterations and malignancy.[9] Several inherited disorders, featuring both chromosomal breakage and an increased frequency of malignant disease, show abnormalities of DNA repair or recombination[10] and many genetically determined syndromes have both an accelerated progression of biologic aging and a high frequency of malignant disease.[11]

In 1858, Virchow[12] stated that each tissue present in the body has a limited response to injury. Since then, further work has described how various tissues of the body respond to damage. Those tissues having continuously mitotic cells, such as the gut and marrow, develop tumors while those with intermittently mitotic cells, such as endothelial or smooth muscle, develop degenerative diseases such as atherosclerosis, but only rarely malignant change. Nonmitotic cells such as the neurone, virtually never develop tumors, but are associated with disorders such as Alzheimer's or Parkinson's disease, illustrating that frequent cell turnover is required for tumor development.[13]

A reduction in DNA methylation in some genes is more common in older subjects and results in an increase in cancer,[14,15] although this is not a consistent finding in all genes.[16] The formation of DNA adducts in a variety of tissues is seen in chemical carcinogenesis[17] and, in certain animal models, adduct-like compounds (I-compounds) accumulate with age.[18] Whether the I-compounds are responsible for tumor development or are merely markers of the aging process is debatable,[19] but they do have the capability to carry mutations, DNA chain breaks, and gene rearrangements.[18] Further evidence for the role of altered DNA repair in cancer causation is provided by the increased susceptibility of cells from older persons to chromosomal damage by ^{3}H-thymidine and to the toxic consequences of irradiation.[20]

In considering cancer in elderly people, the role of factors that increase life span (geroprotectors) and their effects on tumor development must be noted. Geroprotectors are of three types. First, those that decrease the mortality of a long-living subpopulation, are effective in inhibiting carcinogenesis, prolong tumor latency, and decrease the incidence of cancers (e.g., calorie restricted diet). Second, those that increase the survival in a short-living subpopulation without a change in the maximum life span and may increase tumor incidence in an exposed population (e.g., tocopherol). Finally, geroprotectors that prolong the life span equally in all members of the population, postpone the beginning of population aging, and in general do not influence the incidence of tumors, but do prolong tumor latency (e.g., 2-mecaptoethylamin).[21]

A large literature describes the gradual alteration of immune function that occurs with advancing age and that may contribute to the increase in malignancy. Many of these changes occur with the onset of thymic involution, which begins at puberty and results in only 10 percent of thymic function remaining by the age of 45. Although the total population of T lymphocytes does not decline, the number of suppressor and killer cells decreases, the helper-suppressor ratio reverses, and there is an increase in the number of immature lymphocytes in the peripheral blood. Immune surveillance depends on the integrity of lymphocytes, and thymic function is critical for monitoring and disposing of cells that harbor replicative aggregations. Thymic hormones not only decline with age, but have also been shown to be significantly lower in age-matched patients with malignant disease.[22] Although reduction in immune surveillance may play a role in the development of cancer in older people, if it were to result in tumor development as seen in immunosuppressed patients, a lack of tumor diversity would be expected, which is not the case.[23]

Administration of L-argenine acts directly on the pituitary to increases thymulin levels and thus, the number of lymphocyte peripheral subsets.[22] However, there are no data on the use of L-argenine in immune activation in elderly patients with cancer.

There is conflicting opinion regarding the growth and spread of cancer in older patients, and although some evidence shows death to be earlier in older subjects, coexisting diseases have obvious effects on morbidity and mortality. Some experimental work has demonstrated slower tumor growth, fewer metastases, and longer survival in older rodents and others have shown decreased tumor growth associated with impaired T-cell function.[24] Cultures from melanoma cell lines have demonstrated that T cells from young, but not old, donors stimulate the growth of tumor cells, and T cells from young, but not old, mice produce angiogenic factors resulting in a richer vascular supply that may be responsible for increased growth and metastases. The therapeutic implications of angiogenic factors produced by T cells has yet to be explored. Additionally, a relationship between anergy and cancer mortality, although not statistically significant, has been noted in older patients.[25]

Many elderly subjects have been exposed to carcinogenic agents as a result of their occupation (asbestos; inorganic chemicals such as arsenic or nickel; and plant products such as aflatoxin, polycyclic hydrocarbons, and dyes). Lifestyle and diet is dominated in older subjects by tobacco consumption and atmospheric pollution and although studies have shown an increased incidence of cancer of the endometrium and breast associated with diet, other dietary factors such as fiber may protect against the development of carcinoma of the bowel.

The relationship between cancer and aging is clearly complex and various factors, including exposure to carcinogens and changes in the host defence, have roles to play in the etiology of tumors. With further understanding of normal aging its relationship to carcinogenesis should be further understood.

Cancer Prevention

There are two main approaches to cancer prevention: *primary prevention*, which may be less applicable to older people, relates to changes in lifestyle, exercise, and diet to preclude the development of cancer; and *secondary prevention*, which involves screening tests and examinations to aid early detection of tumors, thereby decreasing morbidity and mortality, increasing the chance of cure, and prolonging disease-free interval following therapy.

Cancer becomes 100 times more common in men and 30 times more common in women between the ages of 25 and 75 years,[26] and therefore, secondary prevention should perhaps be targeted at older people rather than in the young.[27]

Screening

For screening to be applicable, a disease must be common, curable if diagnosed early, and the test involved must be highly sensitive. Screening in the UK is almost exclusively for tumors of the breast and cervix and is uncommonly performed in older people. The approach to screening varies, the US performing screening tests until studies show them to be ineffective, while in many areas of Europe screening is not carried out until shown to be effective. Older subjects are less likely than younger age groups to participate in screening and cancer detection behaviors[28,29] and this may be due to inadequate knowledge about cancer,[30] lower educational level, or being unaware of an increased risk.[31] Other factors such as fear of cancer and its treatment, difficulty differentiating between normal physiologic changes and early symptoms or signs of cancer,[32] and fatalism[33] have also been implicated. Men participate less than women in screening procedures[34,35] and it has been found that elderly people who scored highly in a health perception questionnaire, which measured current health, prior health, health outlook, health worry/concern, resistance or susceptibility to illness, and rejection of the sick role, were also more likely to have participated in cancer screening programs.[35] This perception of health by older people playing an important role in cancer prevention has been reported by others.[36–39]

If screening in older subjects increases, the involvement of nurses will be important, although evidence suggests that patients perceive nurses not to focus on health promotion activities and to be more likely to perform examination themselves, rather than teaching elderly women to examine their own breasts.[40]

In order to improve the early detection of cancer, several questions including the attitudes of older people towards screening, and the barriers perceived by the patient especially for skin, breast, and cervical cancer need to be explored.[41–43]

Elderly people must be taught to differentiate symptoms and signs of aging from those of cancer, and the reasons for delay in seeking a medical opinion must be sought.

Breast cancer studies have shown a positive relationship between stage of disease and age at diagnosis.[28] However, older women are less likely to participate in screening programs for breast cancer than younger women.[29,44] In the UK screening by mammography for women aged 50 to 64 on a triennial basis was recommended by the Forrest Report, and although women aged 65 years or older may attend for routine mammography, they are not invited to do so. Mammography reveals more tumors in older patients than in younger subjects[45] and despite early detection resulting in reduced mortality[46] and mammography increasing the proportion of early cancers[47] and thereby reducing mortality,[48,49] only 16 percent of all those performed are on women aged over 60 years.[31] Hobbs et al.[50] found that less women aged 65 to 79 (61 percent) than aged 50 to 64 years (77 percent) attended mammography after invitation, although the "pick up" rate was three times greater in the older group. Factors that may reduce the number of elderly women attending for mammography are that they consider themselves less at risk for developing breast cancer than younger women[51] and consider self-examination to be adequate. Older women are less likely to have breast examinations performed by their doctors[52] despite this having been shown to result in less advanced disease at presentation[53] and physicians are less likely to send older people for screening.[54] Although it has been suggested that elderly subjects refuse to attend for screening, there is little evidence to support this.

If the percentage of older women who receive mammograms and breast examinations increased to 80 percent, mortality in this age group would fall by 30 percent[55] and data obtained from the SEER program showed a life extension of 178 days for those over 85 years and 617 days for those aged 65 to 69[56] if screening was extended. If quality of life is good following the diagnosis of cancer, the benefits of screening outweigh any anxiety generated by the procedures. There is no data to exclude women from breast cancer screening on an age basis alone.[57]

Colorectal screening using fecal occult blood, digital rectal examination, and sigmoidoscopy, although well-accepted in the US, is not commonly performed in the UK.[58,59] Colon cancer is related to the presence of premalignant adenomas, which are more common in elderly people,[60,61] and although the life expectancy of many elderly patients with colorectal cancer is short, if early detection results in a reduction in the number of older people presenting with inoperable bowel obstruction secondary to advanced tumors, it should be considered. Although some studies have shown no increased survival following screening,[62] there is controversy surrounding patient numbers.[63]

Screening for prostatic cancer using digital rectal examination is controversial,[57,64,65] as autopsy studies have shown that foci of adenocarcinoma in the prostate are almost universal in elderly men dying from unrelated causes. The presence of prostatic cancer does not equate with significant disease and the tumor may remain latent for some time. Prostatic symptoms are common in older men and if rectal examination were to reveal a tumor in an otherwise asymptomatic patient, there is debate as to the best therapeutic intervention.

Although lung cancer is common, survival is not improved by screening programs[57] and many physicians consider that older subjects have little or no benefit from smoking cessation despite a lack of evidence that ability to stop alters with age.[66] Immediately after cessation of smoking, a decline in the risk of developing lung cancer is seen such that 5 to 9 years after stopping, the risk is half, and by 15 years the risk is that of a lifelong nonsmoker.[67] Therefore, this, together with the life expectancy of patients aged 65 years being as great as 17 years, indicates that smoking cessation clearly has benefits.

Cervical screening has been aimed at young women, with over one-half the women aged 65 years or older not having had a Papanicolaou screen in the previous 3 years.[68] As the incidence of cervical cancer continues to increase in older women, a 63 percent improvement in mortality could result from routine screening of those over age 65.[69] Various methods of improving participation in cervical screening, including the availability of testing in older persons accommodation, has been suggested.[70]

Incidence

Malignant disease has a rising incidence with age, particularly for tumors of the prostate, stomach, colorectum, pancreas, and esophagus. In the case of primary lung and breast tumors, although there is a similar rise, this falls away in the older age groups, which may be due to poorer standards of diagnosis and certification or due to an increase in deaths from other causes. Smith[71] found that although mortality rates increase with age, the relative frequency of cancer deaths declined. Almost 40 percent of all deaths between the ages of 50 and 69 years, but only 4 percent of deaths in those aged 100 years or older, were due to malignant disease. Of the 524 patients aged 100 years or older who died from malignant disease in the US in 1990, the most common single site was the breast in 70 women, with 45 men dying of carcinoma of the prostate.[71] Similar studies in England and Wales looking at patients aged over 100 at the time of death showed a decreased mortality rate for males but a slow nonexponential increasing mortality rate in females.[72]

Diagnosis

There is evidence that stage of disease varies in older subject at presentation. In breast cancer, it has been found to be earlier in these subjects when screening is utilized.[45] However, many older patients delay seeking medical advice and this may result in cancer being diagnosed at an advanced stage. The delay in diagnosis may have the same cause as the failure to participate in screening, namely a general lack of awareness of possible signs and symptoms of malignancy. Older people may still view cancer to be untreatable and to be invariably fatal. Some studies have found that elderly patients may have difficulty accessing diagnostic interventions.[73,74] When the stage of disease at diagnosis is considered, there is a clear relationship not only between age and stage at diagnosis, but also between age at diagnosis and treatment received by the patient with cancer.[75–77] The relative lack of investigations that are undertaken on an elderly person is partly due to the oncologist's lack of understanding normal aging. Geriatricians are experienced in assessing pre-existing disability and concurrent disease, understanding functional status, level of dependency, and psychological adjustment. This enables joint decisions with regard to further therapy prior to the rehabilitation and, hopefully, recovery of the elderly patient with cancer.[78]

Treatment

Elderly patients should receive therapy comparable to their younger counterparts, although this is often not the case. Older patients with cancer are less likely to receive definitive treatment than younger people after the diagnosis of cancer.[76,79–82] When a comparison of the 1990 incidence data from the NCI Surveillance, Epidemiology and End Results (SEER) program[83] was made to the National Cancer Institute (NCI) Treatment Trials, which included more than 8,000 elderly patients, a significant discrepancy between the incidence of cancer and participation in cancer treatment protocols was found. Only 39 percent of males and 25.9 percent of the women involved in the trials were 65 years or older and as a result of this the US, under the auspices of the NCI, have sponsored a number of trials specifically targeting older patients. Data published by Trimble et al.[84] showed the mean age of those receiving chemotherapy to be significantly younger than the mean age of those registered as incidence cases of cancer by SEER and Mor et al.[75] showed that age was related inversely to subsequently receiving either chemotherapy or radiotherapy after controlling for the stage of disease and comorbidity. Patients with breast cancer aged 75 years or older were twice as likely as patients aged 45 years to undergo surgery as sole treatment and 60 percent of patients under 45 years with regional node involvement received adjuvant chemotherapy compared to just 27 percent of those 65 years or older.[85]

The reasons behind the under-representation of older subjects in treatment figures are complex. The patient may not have full investigation and staging, and therefore, not be eligible to enter into a trial. Some argue that older patients are more likely to suffer from toxicity with chemotherapy,[86] and although an increase in hematological toxicity with methotrexate and methyl-CCNU has been reported,[87] this may in part be due to aging changes present in the bone marrow and its response to growth factors.[88,89] Other authors[90] have found no increase in nephrotoxicity in elderly subjects despite clear pharmacologic reasons why they may occur.

Data from chemotherapeutic studies have shown that attempts at curative cancer therapy decline in proportion to the age of the patient[76] and although the risk of adverse drug reactions may increase sevenfold in patients older than 70 years of age when compared with younger adults, most elderly patients benefit from anticancer therapy even when the therapeutic index is reduced.[91]

When side effects of chemotherapeutic agents are considered, studies have documented that younger patients report more nausea, fatigue, and vomiting than their older counterparts,[92,93] and one possible explanation for the reduction in nausea and vomiting in older people is that younger patients have higher anxiety levels and greater expectation of being sick.[94]

Putative problems with compliance in older people has been cited as a reason for their nontreatment and elderly women with breast cancer have been found not to follow the prescribed adjuvant chemotherapy, although the reasons for this were not clear.[95] Further planning with regard to patient education is required as more elderly people undergo complex oral chemotherapeutic regimes at home. Other studies have shown, in contrast, that older patients are more compliant with therapeutic regimens than younger patients.[96]

Other reasons given for the nontreatment of elderly subjects with cancer have included the advanced stage of the disease at presentation, and although there is evidence that patients over 55 years of age have more advanced disease, at presentation this is not universal.[28,75,77,85,97,98]

Some doctors caring for elderly patients with cancer consider that they are less likely to wish to receive treatment than their younger counterparts. This was not the finding of Yellen et al.,[99] who used structured scenarios to assess patients' willingness to accept toxic chemotherapy to enhance survival, and found that older patients were as willing to choose chemotherapy as younger patients, though the former required a greater survival advantage before they would choose a toxic regime over a less toxic alternative.

Poor life expectancy in elderly subjects has been cited as a further reason for nontreatment, however, it must be remembered that a 90-year-old has a life expectancy of 5 years, an 80-year-old of 8 years, and a 70-year-old of 15 years—age alone should not be used to discriminate against treatment.[100]

Greenfield et al.[79] found that the presence of comorbidity was associated with less treatment for breast cancer in older women, but even when controlled for comorbidity, there were substantial age effects on treatment decisions. Following an interview of 800 patients aged 65 years or older with newly diagnosed cancer of the breast, prostate, colon or rectum, logistic regression was used to assess factors potentially influencing the receipt of definitive treatment to each individual. The study showed that for breast and prostate cancer there was a clear increase in the percent of patients not receiving definitive treatment with increasing age,[101] and in colorectal cancer, men were more likely to receive definitive therapy than women.[101] This latter finding is in contrast to previous studies that have shown no effect of sex on treatment for colon cancer.[76] Other studies have found factors determining nontreatment with chemotherapy to include impaired ability to perform ADL, access to transportation, being unmarried, low income, and low educational achievement.[101] Surprisingly, the presence of other medical disorders, although reducing definitive treatment, was not statistically significant in the analysis. In contrast, advanced age, impaired access to transportation, and poor functional and cognitive status showed little influence on receipt of surgical therapy.

Drug Therapy

The normal physiologic changes of aging affect drug absorption, distribution, metabolism and elimination and thus, when prescribing any drug for an elderly person, drug pharmacokinetics must be considered. Elderly patients with cancer may receive a wide range of drugs including chemotherapeutic agents, analgesics, antiemetics, antibiotics, and others, in addition to drug therapy that has previously been prescribed for coexisting medical disorders.

While there is evidence that drug absorption is not significantly altered by age per se,[102] some normal changes of aging do affect drug absorption. Oral drugs are modified by gastric motility and emptying time while the absorption of parenterally administered drugs is dependent on local blood flow in muscles and fatty tissue. Drug distribution is affected by the decrease in total body water and albumin and the change in the ratio of lean body weight to fat. The reduction in albumin results in a greater concentration of unbound drugs in the circulation able to exert their effects, such as the highly lipophilic agents, CCNU and procarbazine.

Drug metabolism is affected by decreased liver mass and hepatic blood flow as well as decreased microsomal enzymatic activity in the liver and effects drugs such as adriamycin, which is degraded by a mixed-function oxidase system.[103] Elimination is affected by the reduction in glomerular filtration rate, decreased renal blood flow, and renal tubular function, and is particularly important with cyclophosphamide and methotrexate, which are both renally excreted.

Chemotherapy

Older patients are less likely to receive chemotherapy, and if treated, it is more likely to be outside a clinical trial. This is due partly to age restrictions on trial entry, and partly to clinicians without clinical evidence, feeling the need to reduce drug dosages in such patients. All drug therapy in elderly people is effected by altered pharmacokinetics and pharmacodynamics and some chemotherapeutic agents pose special problems.[86,104,105] Reduction of chemotherapeutic drug dosages may reduce both toxicity and response rates,[106] lower response rate without effect on toxicity, or result in better tolerance, but provide no survival advantage.[97,107,108]

Other researchers have found that elderly subjects, when receiving drug dosages similar to their younger counterparts, have similar toxicity rates although some trials do not clearly define how the patients aged over 70 years were selected.[86,87,109]

In order to avoid unnecessary toxicity, a decision regarding dose reduction should be made on the onset of treatment, because if dose reductions vary from cycle to cycle of therapy, although tailored for individual patients, little evidence is accrued with regard to toxicity and efficacy.

There is an age dependent decrease in bone marrow stem cells, which result in increased liability to neutropenic episodes. Both granulocyte macrophage-colony stimulating factor (GM-CSF) and granulocyte-colony stimulating factor (G-CSF) reduce the duration of severe neutropenia and accelerate neutrophil recovery following chemotherapy. There is no evidence that older people respond differently from younger patients to such agents,[110] and in patients aged between 60 and 70 years being treated with aggressive chemotherapy for non-Hodgkins lymphoma, the addition of G-CSF reduced the number of chemotherapy courses that were delayed, the mean duration of delay, the incidence of severe infections, and hospitalization. Additionally, G-CSF was found to be cost-effective in this group of older people.[111]

The following are some of the drugs that are commonly used in older subjects with particular problems in this age group highlighted.

Cyclophosphamide is a stable inactive compound that is activated in the liver via the cytochrome-P450 system and that is well-absorbed when taken orally. It is used in solid tumors such as small cell lung cancer, lymphomas, and breast or ovarian cancer. The side effect profile includes nausea and vomiting, hematological toxicity, pulmonary fibrosis, and hemorrhagic cystitis.

Chlorambucil is an oral-alkylating agent with a myelosuppressive effect that is gradual in onset. It is used in the palliative treatment of ovarian cancer and in low-grade lymphomas.

Methotrexate is a folic acid antagonist that can be administered orally, intravenously, or intrathecally. Toxicity is usually to the gastrointestinal tract, mucous membranes, and bone marrow and if ascites or a pleural effusion are present, methotrexate may accumulate in these sites to be later released and result in toxicity. The drug is 50 percent bound to albumin and can be displaced by drugs such as salicylates and phenytoin. Its excretion is mainly unchanged in the urine and is affected by glomerular and tubular alterations in older subjects. It is widely used in ovarian and breast carcinoma, as well as lymphomas and leukemia.

5-Fluorouracil is an agent that interferes with nucleic acid synthesis and is widely used for colorectal metastases, although also having activity in breast and ovarian tumors. It is well tolerated both orally and intravenously, but may cause nausea, diarrhea, myelosuppression, and cardiac disturbances.

Vincristine is an alkaloid that is administered intravenously in the treatment of lymphomas, small cell carcinoma, and tumors of the breast. Its toxicity is mainly neurologic with peripheral neuropathy occurring especially in older people and in those with hepatic impairment. The neuropathy is characterized by early loss of reflexes and paresthesia, with motor weakness and peripheral sensory signs at a later stage. Although nerve conduction is usually preserved, the EMG shows denervation and in elderly patients an autonomic neuropathy may result in constipation and ileus.

Etoposide is one of the most widely used chemotherapeutic drugs in elderly patients and may be administered orally or intravenously. Its main role is in the palliative treatment of small cell lung cancer, although it has been widely used in lymphomas in older patients. Its main toxic effects are nausea, vomiting, and neutropenia.

Cisplatin is a platinum complex used primarily in carcinoma of the ovary, although it has a role in the management of lymphomas and small cell carcinoma of the bronchus. It is highly nephrotoxic and a high urine flow must be obtained prior to drug administration. Even when there is adequate hydration and diuresis, renal function usually worsens during repeated cycles of therapy and repeated creatinine clearance estimations are mandatory. Nausea and vomiting, ototoxicity that may be irreversible, peripheral neuropathy, and biochemical abnormalities of potassium, magnesium, and calcium are common documented side effects.

Adriamycin is an anthracycline antibiotic that is given intravenously and because of hepatic metabolization may result in toxicity in older patients with impaired liver function. Its main side effects are bone marrow depression, nausea, vomiting, and alopecia. Cardiotoxicity may result in arrhythmias or cardiac failure and is related to the total dose administered. The main roles for adriamycin are in the management of lymphomas, small cell carcinoma, and adenocarcinoma of the breast, ovary, and stomach.

Hormonal Therapies

Hormonal therapies may provide a benefit to elderly patients with advanced cancer of the breast, prostate, and endometrium. In the management of metastatic breast cancer, the beneficial effects of estrogen therapy increase steadily with age in all postmenopausal women probably due to the increased incidence of estrogen-receptor positive tumors in older women that result in an increased response rate to such therapy.

Radiotherapy

Little is known about organ-specific tolerance to radiation in relation to aging, although there is evidence that tolerance of normal tissues to radiation therapy is 10 to 15 percent less in the very old. Additionally, lymphocytes from both elderly experimental animals and man are more susceptible to damage induced by ionizing radiation. Because most radiotherapy in elderly patients is palliative in intent, it is important that minimal toxicity is experienced.

Myelosuppression may be problematic as elderly patients have less functional bone marrow and a slowed recovery of normal tissue. Fatigue may result in compliance problems and radiation may result in dry skin that is more susceptible to infection.[112] The normal aging of the gastrointestinal tract may result in increased susceptibility to anorexia and stomatitis following radiotherapy.[113]

The more commonly seen radiation side effects that occur in elderly subjects are predicated on pre-existing conditions; thus radiation to emphysematous lungs will increase dyspnea and irradiation of the mediastinum will impair declining left ventricular function. Compliance with radiotherapy in elderly subjects is additionally hampered by multiple visits and traveling. The use of split fractions does, however, reduce toxicity and is essential in the treatment of many tumors in older patients.

Nursing Care

Nursing research dealing with older subjects is limited, and where it does exist is most often related to the elderly people in nursing homes or long-term care. In 1986, Adams[114] reviewed 154 studies, and although the studies covered hypertension, medication, and chronic illness in older people, none dealt with cancer. In a similar fashion to medical papers on older people, most nursing research describes elderly subjects to be "65 years of age or over," which means that their findings may not be applicable to those patients usually seen in geriatric medicine practice who are frequently over 80 years.[41]

Agism is an important adverse influence on the prevention and diagnosis of cancer, but also in the nursing care of elderly patients with cancer, and nurses are just as likely as others to be biased by agism.[115] This may be due to the inadequate preparation of nurses[116] or to a perceived lack of attractiveness of a gerontological career.[117] The nurse may view cancer prevention to be unnecessary, may promote dependency and learned helplessness, and minimize the need for referral to clinicians or community resources.[116]

The experience of cancer for both the patient and family is stressful, and although many treatments for cancer can be given on an outpatient basis, many require prolonged hospitalization. Upon discharge to the community, much of the physical and psychological care of the patients is placed on the family. This puts an enormous stress on elderly patients and their care givers. Not surprisingly, there is a high correlation between severity of symptoms and impact on activities of daily living.[118] Additionally, there is evidence that many patients with cancer have depressive symptoms[119] and there is a positive correlation between patients' selfcare needs and mood.[120] Kurtz et al.[121] assessed the mental health of patients and family members and found of the 208 patients in the study, in 83 of whom were aged 65 years or older; the most common five symptoms were fatigue, pain, nausea, poor appetite, and constipation. In this study there was no relationship between age and level of symptoms, although older people tend to under-report and this may counteract a genuine age-related increase in symptoms. Caregivers are more likely to be wives than husbands and to care single-handedly. Wives provide twice the hours of care that husbands provide, although this is compensated by female patients having more outside care than males.[122] When the patient was younger, the caregivers tended to be more depressed, and caring had a greater impact on the caregiver's schedule; friends did provide more support to the caregiver. In 82 percent of cases, the caregivers were spouses of the patients and it is likely, therefore, that elderly spouses will be solitary caregivers and have little support from other friends and relatives.[121] Elderly caregivers require counseling, but this may present logistic difficulties. The use of telephone counseling is of potential value and removes the need for transport and alternative care arrangements.[123]

Rehabilitation

Where data are available on elderly patients following treatment for cancer, functional status assessment is usually via the Karnofsky performance status. This however, is not specific to older subjects and ignores many of the more important activities of daily living that are included in well-validated rating schemes used frequently by geriatricians. When geriatricians and oncologists work together in the assessment of elderly patients, a functional assessment that is familiar to both is mandatory.

Survival

Relative survival is lower among older people with cancer than among their younger counterparts. There are many possible explanations for these differences and these include tendency for cancer to be diagnosed at a later stage in older subjects, and differences in the treatments received by elderly patients. Other age-related factors, such as comorbidity, obviously alter outcome.[28,75,77,124]

References

1. Byrne A, Carney DN: Cancer in the elderly. Curr Prob Cancer 1993;17:145–218
2. Paine C: The Health of the Nation. HMSO, Department of Health, London, 1992
3. Calman K: A Policy Framework for Commisioning Cancer Services. HMSO, Department of Health, 1995
4. Cohen HJ: Biology of aging as related to cancer. Cancer 1994; 74(suppl 7):2092–2100
5. Dix D, Cohen P, Flannery J: On the role of aging in cancer incidence. J Theor Biol 1980;83:163–173
6. Ebbesen P: Cancer and normal aging. Mech Ageing Dev 1984; 25:269–283
7. Dilman VM: Aging and cancer in the light of ontogenetic "model of medicine". pp. 21–23. In Likhachev A, Anisimov V, Montesano R (eds): Age Related Factors in Carcinogenesis. IARC Science, Lyons, 1985
8. Cutler RG, Semsei I: Development, cancer and ageing: possible common mechanisms of action and regulation. J Gerontol A: Biol Sci Med Sci 1989;44:25–34
9. Yunis JJ: The chromosomal basis of human neoplasia. Science 1983;221:227–236
10. Setlow RB: Repair deficient human disorders and cancer. Nature 1978;271:713–717
11. Goldstein S: Human genetic disorders which feature accelerated aging. pp. 171–224. In Schneider EL: The Genetics of Aging. Plenum, New York, 1978
12. Virchow RLK: Cellular Pathology as Based Upon Physiological and Pathological Histology. A Hirschwald, Berlin, 1858
13. Lipschitz DA, Goldstein S, Reis R et al: Cancer in the elderly: basic science and clinical aspects. Ann Intern Med 1985;102: 218–228
14. Ono T, Takahashi N, Okada S: Age-associated changes in DNA methylation and mRNA level of the *c-myc* gene in spleen and liver of mice. Mutat Res 1989;219:39–50
15. Mays-Hoopes LL: Age-related changes in DNA methylation: do they represent continued developmental changes? Int Rev Cytol 1989;114:181–220
16. Ono T: Changes of DNA methylation in aging and carcinogenesis. Cancer Res Clin Oncol 1990;116(suppl):1056
17. Singer B, Gruneberger D: Molecular Biology of Mutagens and Carcinogens. Plenum, New York, 1983
18. Randerath K, Liehr JG, Gladek A, Randerath E: Age-dependent covalent DNA alterations (I-compounds) in rodent tissues: species, tissue and sex specification. Mutat Res 1989; 219:121–133
19. Warner HR, Price AR: Involvement of DNA repair in cancer and aging. J Gerontol A: Biol Sci Med Sci 1989;44:45–54
20. Staiano-Coico L, Darzynkiewics Z, Melamed MR, Weksler ME: Changes in DNA content of human blood mononuclear cells with senescence. Cytometry 1982;3:79–83
21. Anisimov VN: Carcinogenesis and Aging. Vol. 1 and 2. Boca CRC Press, Boca Raton, FL, 1987
22. Mocchegiani E, Cacciatore L, Talarico M et al: Recovery of low thymic hormone levels in cancer patients by lysine-arginine combination. Int J Immunopharmacol 1990;12:365–371
23. Ershler WB: Geriatric correlates of experimental tumor biology. Oncology Huntingt 1992;6(suppl 2):58–61
24. Weksler ME, Tsuda T, Kim YT, Siskind GW: Immunobiology of aging and cancer. Cancer Detect Prev 1990;14:609–611
25. Wayne SJ, Rhyne RL, Garry PJ, Goodwin JS: Cell-mediated immunity as a predictor of morbidity and mortality in subjects over 60. J Gerontol 1990;45:M45–48
26. Brownson RC, Reif JS, Alavanja MCR, Bal DG: Cancer. pp. 137–167. In Brownson RC, Remington PW, Davis JR (eds): Chronic Disease, Epidemiology and Control. American Public Health Association, Washington DC, 1993
27. Bal DG, Lloyd J: Advocacy and government action for cancer prevention in older persons. Cancer 1994;74:2067–2070
28. Holmes F, Hearne E: Cancer stage-to-age relationship: implications of cancer screening in the elderly. J Am Geriatr Soc 1981;19:55–57
29. Costanza ME: The extent of breast cancer screening in older women. Cancer 1994;74(suppl 7):2046–2050
30. Weinrich SP, Weinrich MC: Cancer knowledge among elderly individuals. Cancer Nurs 1986;9:301–307

31. Robie PW: Cancer screening in the elderly. J Am Geriatr Soc 1989;37:888–893
32. Frank-Stromborg M: The role of the nurse in early detection of cancer: population sixty-six years of age and older. Oncol Nurs Forum 1986;13:66–74
33. Powe BD: Fatalism among elderly African Americans. Effects on colorectal cancer screening. Cancer Nurs 1995;18: 385–392
34. Warren B, Pohl JM: Cancer screening practices of nursing practitioners. Cancer Nurs 1990;3:143–151
35. Zabalegui A: Secondary cancer prevention in the elderly. Cancer Nurs 1994;17:215–222
36. Yoder LE, Jones SC, Jones PK: The association between health care behaviors and attitudes. Health Values 1985;9:24–31
37. Speake DL: Health promotion and activity in the well elderly. Health Values 1987;11:25–30
38. Speake DL, Cowart ME, Pellet K: Health perceptions and lifestyles of the elderly. Res Nurs Health 1989;12:93–100
39. Barnes S, Thomas A: A modified cancer education program. Effect on cancer knowledge and beliefs of the elderly. Cancer Nurs 1990;13:48–55
40. Ludwick R: Registered nurses' knowledge and practices of teaching and performing breast exams among elderly women. Cancer Nurs 1992;15:61–67
41. Given B, Given CW: Cancer nursing for the elderly: a target for research. Cancer Nurs 1989;12:71–77
42. Rubenstein L: Strategies to overcome barriers to early detection of cancer among older adults. Cancer 1994;74(suppl 7): 2190–2193
43. Roetzheim RG, Van-Durme DJ, Brownlee HJ et al: Barriers to screening among participants of a media-promoted breast cancer screening project. Cancer Detect Prev 1993;17: 367–377
44. Foster RS, Long SP, Costanza MC et al: Breast self-examination practices and breast cancer stage. N Engl J Med 1978; 299:265–270
45. Faulk RM, Sickles EA, Sollitto RA et al: Clinical efficacy of mammographic screening in the elderly. Radiology 1995;194: 193–197
46. Collette DJA, Day NE, Rombach JJ, de Waard F: Evaluation of screening for breast cancer in a non-randomized study (the Dom project) by means of a case-control study. Lancet 1984; i:1224–1226
47. Tabar L, Fagerberg G, Day NE et al: Breast cancer treatment and natural history: new insights from results of screening. Lancet 1992;339:412–414
48. Morrow M: Breast disease in elderly women. Surg Clin North Am 1994;74:145–161
49. Chen HH, Tabar L, Fagerberg G, Duffy SW: Effect of breast cancer screening after age 65. J Med Screen 1995;2:10–14
50. Hobbs P, Kay C, Friedman EHI et al: Response by women aged 65–79 to invitation for screening for breast cancer by mammography: a pilot study. Br Med J 301:1314–1316
51. Harris RP, Fletcher SW, Gonzalez JJ et al: Mammography and age: are we targeting the wrong women? A community survey of women and physicians. Cancer 1991;67:2010–2014
52. King ES, Resch N, Rimer B et al: Breast cancer screening practices among retirement community women. Prev Med 1993;22:1–19
53. Samet JM, Hunt WC, Goodwin JS: Determinants of cancer stage. A population-based study of elderly New Mexicans. Cancer 1990;66:1302–1307
54. Weinberger M, Saunders AF, Samsa GP et al: Breast cancer screening in older women: practices and barriers reported by primary care physicians. J Am Geriatr Soc 1991;39:22–29
55. Albert M: Health screening to promote health for the elderly. Nurse Pract 1987;12:42–58
56. Mandelblatt JS, Wheat ME, Monane M et al: Breast cancer screening for elderly women with and without comorbid conditions. A decision analysis model. Ann Intern Med 1992;116: 722–730
57. Oddone EZ, Feussner JR, Cohen HJ: Can screening older patients for cancer save lives? Clin Geriatr Med 1992;8:51–67
58. Weinrich SP, Weinrich MC, Stromborg MF et al: Using elderly educators to increase colorectal cancer screening. Gerontologist 1993;33:491–496
59. Wagner JL, Herdman RC, Wadhwa S: Cost effectiveness of colorectal cancer screening in the elderly. Ann Intern Med 1991;115:807–817
60. Rex DK, Lehman GA, Ulbright TM et al: Colonic neoplasia in asymptomatic persons with negative fecal occult blood tests: influence of age, gender, and family history. Am J Gastroenterol 1993;88:825–831
61. DiSario JA, Foutch PG, Mai HD et al: Prevalence and malignant potential of colorectal polyps in asymptomatic, average-risk men. Am J Gastroenterol 1991;86:941–945
62. Kronberg O, Fenger C, Olsen J et al: Repeated screening for colorectal cancer with faecal occult blood test. Scand J Gastroenterol 1989;24:599–606
63. Moss S, Draper GJ, Hardcastle JD, Chamberlain J: Calculation of sample size in trials for early diagnosis of disease. Int J Epidemiol 1987;16:104–110
64. Optenberg SA, Thompson IM: Economics of screening for carcinoma of the prostate. Urol Clin North Am 1990;17:719–737
65. Gerber FS, Chodak GW: Routine screening for cancer of the prostate. J Nat Cancer Inst 1991;83:329–335
66. Pederson LL: Compliance with physician advice to quit smoking. A review of the literature. Prev Med 1982;11:71–84
67. Holbrook J: Tobacco smoking. pp. 1302–1305. In Petersdorf, Adams, Braunwald et al. (eds): Harrison's Principles of Internal Medicine. 10th Ed. McGraw-Hill, New York, 1983
68. Power EJ: Cervical cancer screening in elderly women: Congressional Office of Technology Assessment. JAMA 1990;263: 2996
69. Fletcher A: Screening for cancer of the cervix in elderly women. Lancet 1990;335:97–99
70. White JE, Begg L, Fishman NW et al: Increasing cervical cancer screening among minority elderly. Education and on-site services increase screening. J Gerontol Nurs 1993;19: 28–34
71. Smith EWE: Cancer mortality at very old ages. Cancer 1996; 77:1367–1372
72. Barrett JC: The mortality of centenarians in England and Wales. Arch Gerontol Geriatr 1985;4:211–218

73. Mor V, Guadagnoli E, Weitberg A et al: Influence of old age, performance status medical, and psycholsocial status on management of cancer patients. pp. 127–146. In Yancik R, Yates J (eds): Cancer in the Elderly. Springer Publishing, New York, 1989
74. Bennett C, Greenfield S, Avonow H et al: Patterns of care related to age of men with prostate cancer. Cancer 1991;67: 2633–2641
75. Mor V, Masterson-Allen S, Goldberg R, et al: Relationship between age diagnosis and treatments received by cancer patients. J Am Gerontol Soc 1985;33:585–589
76. Samet JM, Hunt WC, Key CR et al: Choice of cancer therapy varies with age of patient. JAMA 1986;255:3385–3390
77. Goodwin J, Sament J, Key C et al: Stage at diagnosis of cancer varies with age of the patient. J Am Geriatr Soc 1986;34: 20–26
78. Corner J: Some reflections on frailty in elderly patients with cancer. Eur J Cancer Care 1993;2:5–9
79. Greenfield S, Blanco VM, Elashoff RM, Ganz PA: Patterns of care related to age of breast cancer patients. JAMA 1987;257: 2766–2770
80. Silliman RA, Guadagnoli E, Weitgerg AB, Mor V: Age as a predictor of diagnostic and initial treatment intensity in newly diagnosed breast cancer patients. J Gerontol 1989;44:46–50
81. Bergman L, Dekker G, van Leeuwen FE et al: The effect of age on treatment choice and survival in elderly breast cancer patients. Cancer 1991;67:2227–2234
82. Markman M, Lewis JL, Saijo P et al: Epithelial ovarian cancer in the elderly: the Memorial Sloan-Kettering Cancer Center experience. Cancer 1993;71:634–637
83. McBean AM, Warren JL, Babish JD: Measuring the incidence of cancer in elderly Americans using Medicare claims data. Cancer 1994;73:2417–2425
84. Trimble EL, Carter CL, Cain D et al: Representation of older patients in cancer treatment trials. Cancer 1994;74(suppl 7): 2208–2214
85. Allen C, Cox E, Manton R, Cohen H: Breast cancer in the elderly. Current patterns of care. J Am Geriatr Soc 1986;34: 637–642
86. Begg CB, Cohen JL, Ellerton J: Are the elderly predisposed to toxicity from cancer chemotherapy? An investigation using data from the Eastern Cooperative Oncology Group. Cancer Clin Trials 1980;3:369–374
87. Begg CB, Carbone PP: Clinical trials and drug toxicity in the elderly. Cancer 1983;52:1986–1992
88. Chatta GS, Andrews RG, Rodger E et al: Hematopoietic progenitors and aging: alterations in granulocytic precursors and responsiveness to recombinant human G-CSF, GM-CSF, and IL-3. J Gerontol 1993;48:M207–12
89. Chatta GS, Price TH, Stratton JR, Dale DC: Aging and marrow neutrophil reserves. J Am Geriatr Soc 1994;42:77–81
90. Hrushesky WJM, Shimp W, Kennedy BJ: Lack of age-dependent crisplatin nephrotoxicity. Am J Med 1984;76:579–584
91. Balducci L, Mowry K: Pharmacology and organ toxicity of chemotherapy in older patients. Oncology 1992;6:62–68
92. Nerenz D, Leventhal H, Easterlin DV, Love RR: Psychosocial consequences of cancer chemotherapy for elderly patients. Health Serv Res 1986;20:961–976
93. Dodd MJ, Onishi K, Dibble SL, Larson PJ: Difference in nausea, vomiting and retching between younger and old out-patients receiving cancer chemotherapy. Cancer Nurs 1996;19: 155–161
94. Fallowfield LJ: Behavioral interventions and psychological aspects of care during chemotherapy. Eur J Cancer 1992;28a: S39–41
95. Bonnadonna G, Valagussa P: Dose-response effect of chemotherapy in breast cancer. N Engl J Med 1981;304:10
96. Holland JC, Massie MJ: Psychosocial aspects of cancer in the elderly. Clin Geriatr Med 1987;3:2766–2770
97. Cohen H, Silberman H, Forman W et al: Affect of age on response to treatment and survival of patients with multiple myeloma. J Am Geriatr Soc 1983;31:372–377
98. Warnecke RB: The elderly as a target group for prevention and early detection of cancer. pp. 3–14. In Yancik R, Yates JW (ed): Cancer in the Elderly: Approaches to Early Detection and Treatment. Springer Publishing, New York, 1989
99. Yellen SB, Cella DF, Leslie WT: Age and clinical decision making in oncology patients. J Natl Cancer Inst 1994;86: 1766–1770
100. Ganz PA: Does (or should) chronologic age influence the choice of cancer treatment? Oncology Huntingt 1992;6(suppl 2):45–49
101. Goodwin JS, Hunt WC, Samet JM: Determinants of cancer therapy in elderly patients. Cancer 1993;72:594–601
102. Lamy P: Comparative pharmacokinetic changes and drug therapy in an older population. J Am Geriatr Soc 1982;30:S11–19
103. Robert J, Hoerni B: Age dependence of the early phase pharmacokinetics of doxorubicin. Cancer Res Clin Oncol 1983; 43:4467–4469
104. Hansen HH, Selawry OS, Holland JF, McCall CB: The variability of individual tolerance to methotrexate in cancer patients. Br J Cancer 1971;25:298–305
105. Haas CD, Coltman CA, Gottlieb AJ: Phase II evaluation of bleomycin: a Southwest Oncology Group study. Cancer 1976; 38:8–12
106. Frei E, Canellos GP: Dose: a critical factor in cancer chemotherapy. Am J Med 1980;69:585–594
107. Bonadonna G, Valagussa P: Dose response effects of adjuvant chemotherapy in breast cancer. N Engl J Med 1981;304: 10–15
108. Gelman R, Taylor SG: Cyclophosphamide, methotrexate and 5-fluorouracil chemotherapy in women more than 65 years old with advanced breast cancer: the elimination of age trends in toxicity by using doses based on creatinine clearance. J Clin Oncol 1984;2:1404–1403
109. Leslie WT: Chemotherapy in older cancer patients. Oncology Huntingt 1992;6(suppl 2):74–80
110. Shank W, Balducci L: Recombinant hemopoietic growth factors may protect older patients from chemotherapy myelodepression. Proc Am Soc Clin Oncol 1991;10:326
111. Kayahara M, Nagakawa T, Ueno K et al: Pancreatic resection for periampullary carcinoma in the elderly. Surg Today 1994; 24:229–233
112. Hilderley L: Clinical reviews: skin care in radiation therapy: a review of the literature. Oncol Nurs Forum 1983;10:51–56

113. Gunn W: Radiation therapy for the aging patient. Cancer 1980; 30:337–347

114. Adams M: Aging: gerontological nursing research. Annu Rev Nurs Res 1986;4:77–103

115. Chandler JT, Rachal JR, Kazelskis R: Attitudes of long term care nursing personnel towards the elderly. Gerontologist 1986;26:551–555

116. Boyle DM, Engelking C, Blesch KS et al: Oncology nursing society position paper on cancer and aging: the mandate for oncology nursing. Oncol Nurs Forum 1992;19:913–933

117. Siu AL: The quality of medical care received by older persons. J Am Geriatr Soc 1987;35:1084–1091

118. Holmes S, Dickerson J: The quality of life: design and evaluation of self-assessment instrument for use with cancer patients. Int J Nurs Stud 1987;24:15–24

119. Derogatis LR, Morrow G, Fettig J et al: The prevalence of psychiatric disorders among cancer patients. JAMA 1983;249: 751–757

120. McCorkle R, Quint-Benoleil J: Symptoms distress, current concerns and mood disturbance after diagnosis of life-threatening illness. Soc Sci Med 1983;17:431–438

121. Kurtz ME, Given B, Kurtz JC, Given CW: The interaction of age, symptoms and survival status on physical and mental health of patients with cancer and their families. Cancer 1994; 74:2071–2078

122. Allen SM: Gender differences in spousal caregiving and unmet need for care. J Gerontol 1994;49:S187–195

123. Skipwith DH: Telephone counseling interventions with caregivers of elders. J Psychosoc Nurs Ment Health Serv 1994; 32:7–12

124. Fentiman IS, Tirelli U, Monfardini S et al: Cancer in the elderly: why so badly treated? Lancet 1990;335:1020–1022

CHAPTER 94

Constipation and Fecal Incontinence in Old Age

J. C. BROCKLEHURST

The knowledge base relating to constipation and fecal incontinence has grown considerably in the past 10 years as a result of a burst of research activity in this field. Almost all of this work, however, has been with subjects under the age of 65 and much of it awaits validation in people aged 70 and above. In particular, the effects of aging, immobility, and mental impairment may strikingly alter the causes and management of these conditions in elderly people. This chapter will review contemporary understanding of colorectal motility and defecation before considering how these factors relate to continence and fecal incontinence in old age.

Investigations

The main methods of investigation used in both research and practice include transit time; colonic, rectal, and anal manometry; defecography; anal endosonography; and electromyography (EMG). These techniques are briefly reviewed here. For more detailed consideration the reader is referred to the monograph by Barratt.[1]

Transit Time

The measurement of transit time—the time it takes for markers that are swallowed to appear in the stool—is now a well-established method of investigating bowel function. Radio-opaque markers (usually 20 markers 1 to 2 mm long cut from radio-opaque tubing with an external diameter of 3 mm and contained in two gelatin capsules) are swallowed, and the length of time required for them to be passed is monitored by x-ray. This can be done either by x-raying the abdomen (usually on days 3, 5, 7, and if necessary 14) or, if it is possible to collect the stool, x-raying the stools as each day. The time taken for 80 percent of the markers (i.e., 16) to be passed is the measurement usually recorded and is called the 80 percent transit time. The upper limit of normal 80 percent transit time is generally regarded as 5 days.[2,3]

Variations of this method have been developed—employing shaped markers on three consecutive days[4] or using isotope markers.[5,6] That transit time is strongly dependent on intake of dietary fiber has been well demonstrated by the work of Birkett and colleagues.[7] The relationship among transit time, stool weight, and dietary fiber has been demonstrated on a number of occasions.[8]

Manometry

Motility within the colon has been investigated by using balloons and open-ended tubes inserted through the anus or through a colostomy opening; pressure telemetering capsules that can be swallowed are also employed. Since the colon is an open-ended cylinder, the recording of pressure changes within it presents a more difficult problem than in a closed organ such as the urinary bladder. While balloons record isotonic contraction and open-ended tubes record isometric contraction, neither one alone can adequately record both types.[9]

One shortcoming of recording colonic motility is its unpredictable nature and the fact that motility patterns are not necessarily reproducible in one individual throughout subsequent periods. To overcome this problem, maximum stimulation of colonic motility by injection of neostigmine (prostigmine)[10] or by ingestion of a meal[11] is used. The most satisfactory formula for interpretating such data can be obtained with the motility index.[12]

Anal manometry uses similar techniques or a solid-state strain gauge system.[13] Anal manometric measures are usually taken in a resting state, regarded as a measure of internal sphincter function, and also at maximum voluntary squeeze, indicating external sphincter function.

Electromyography

EMG measures anal sphincter electromyographic frequency (and thus internal sphincter pressure).[14] Single-fiber EMG measures single-fiber nerve density as an expression of motor denervation (e.g., in the pudendal nerve).[15,16]

Pudendal nerve terminal motor latency is the response time of the external sphincter to transrectal stimulation of the pudendal nerve[17] and is a measure of pudendal nerve atrophy.

Imaging

Defecography demonstrates perineal descent, rectocele, and intussusception. Endosonography is now the method of choice in demonstrating sphincter deficits.[18]

Sensation

Intrarectal sensation is usually measured by gradual distention of a water-filled balloon[19] or by a bipolar ring electrode in contact with the rectal wall producing a sensation of tingling or throbbing when the sensory threshold is reached.[20]

Physiology

Colorectal Motility

It is generally agreed that there are two main types of colonic motility, namely, segmental or "shuttling" motility and mass peristalsis. A study on healthy young volunteers involving open-ended catheters placed in the transverse, descending, and sigmoid colons and maintained for 24 hours demonstrated these well.[21] The first (Fig. 94-1A) consisted of bursts of nonprogressive low-amplitude contractions which were least frequent during the night, were most frequent after waking and breakfast, and showed additional increases after lunch and dinner. The second, mass peristalsis (Fig. 94-1B) consisted of very high-amplitude contractions, occurring on average 4.4 times in 24 hours and moving sequentially through the three sites in an anal direction and occasionally followed 1 or 2 minutes later by a second and indeed a third high-amplitude contraction. These seemed to originate in the transverse colon. Twenty-five percent were felt as an urge to defecate, and in two of the seven subjects defecation followed immediately. The propagation velocity was 1 cm/s.

It has been claimed that the gradient of segmental motility is such as to prevent propulsion away from the mouth.[22]

Major propulsive movements start at the transverse colon and are likely to follow a main meal,[23] the so-called gastrocolic reflex. Connell[24] suggested that this reflex was incorrectly named since it is humoral rather than nervous and occurs in paraplegic patients and in those who have had a gastrectomy or a vagotomy. The injection of gastrin, for instance, causes colonic motility similar to that initiated by a meal. However, the postprandial increase in motility is probably not mediated

Figure 94-1 Tracings of (**A**) shuttling motility and (**B**) mass peristalsis recorded from four balloons in situ as shown in diagram. (From Narducci et al.[21] with permission.)

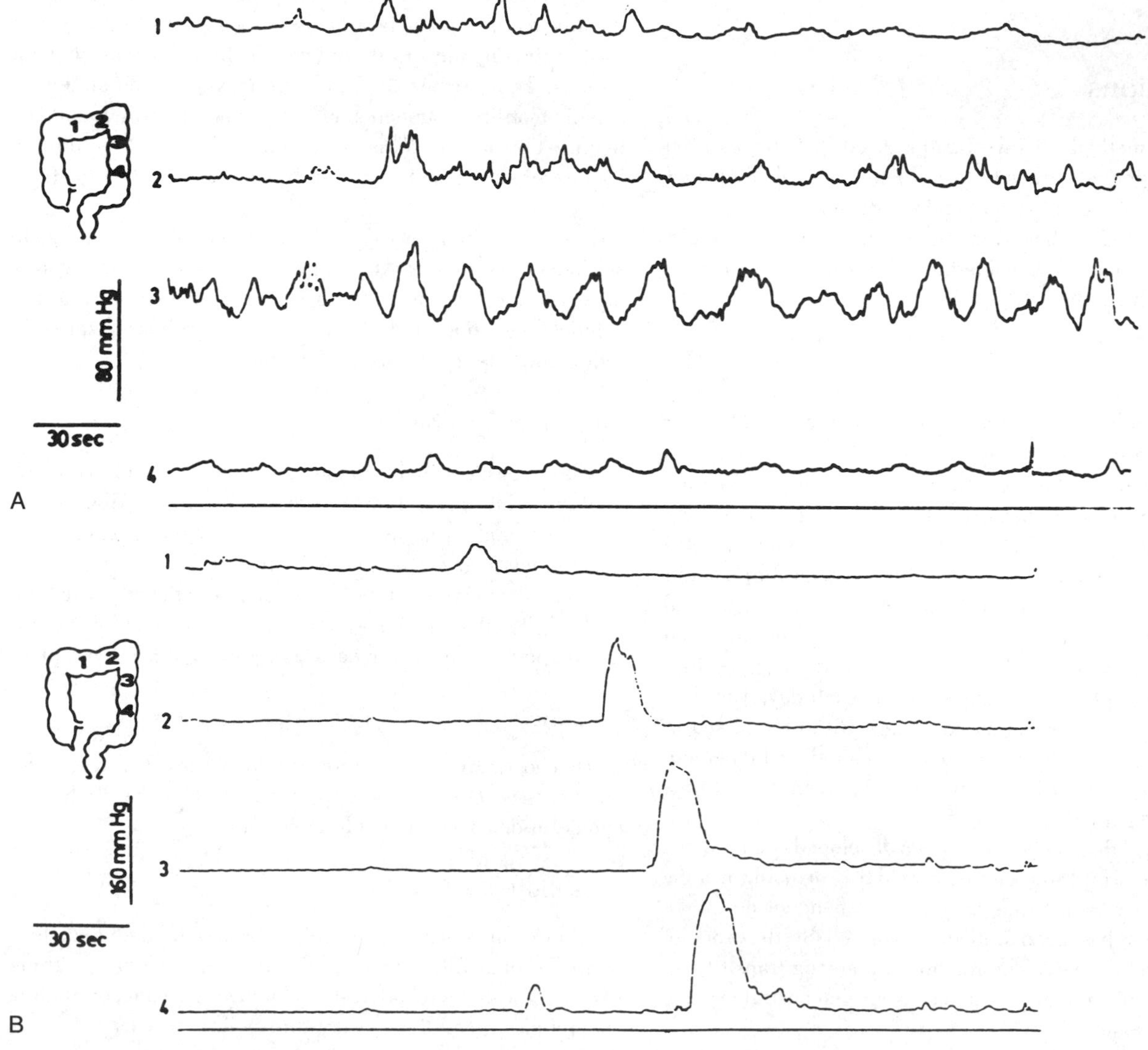

by gastrin since it is observed in patients who have been gastrectomized.[25] It is more probably due to the enzyme cholecystokinin or other intestinal peptides.[26]

Essential for social functioning is the ability to distinguish among fluid, flatus, and feces.[27] The presence of a sensory zone at the upper end of the anal canal allowing this discrimination has been disputed.[28]

Physical activity contributes to mass peristalsis,[29] and the gastrocolic reflex was rarely found to be associated with propulsive activity in resting patients. This observation is clearly important in regard to disabled elderly people who are generally immobile.

Most studies on motility have been carried out on healthy and relatively young subjects, however, one study compared healthy elderly (mean age 72) subjects with healthy younger (mean age 29) subjects.[30] No difference was found between old and young in the amplitude or duration of contractions during fasting, during consumption of a meal, or after a meal.

The incidence of mass peristaltic waves is significantly increased by administration of a contact laxative (e.g., bisacodyl).[31]

Motility in the rectum is different from that in the colon, and indeed a functional rectosigmoid sphincter may result from shuttling motility at this point moving the fecal bolus proximally. Certainly, there seems to be an alteration in the pattern of myoelectrical activity at this point.[32,33] Slow waves of contraction appear to be present in the rectum more continuously than elsewhere in the colon.[34,35] The increase in segmental activity at the lower end of the sigmoid may be an important factor in the development of colonic diverticula and the reason why these commonly start in the sigmoid colon (see Ch. 62), and when the rectum is distended, phasic contractions develop in most subjects,[36] more commonly in old people with chronic brain failure than in those without.[37]

Normally the resting rectum is not necessarily empty[38]—feces may be present without an urge to defecate.[39] Feces can return from the rectum to the sigmoid colon.[39]

Sensation

The only conscious sensation normally arising from the large bowel is that of rectal distension producing a sensation of fullness and a desire to defecate. This sensation may be diminished in elderly people.[40–42]

The volume required to produce an urge to defecate and pain is diminished after a meal.[43] Stress increases the sensitivity of the rectum to distention[44] and so does hysterectomy.[45] It is suggested that the sensation of fullness and impending defecation arises from nerve receptors not in the rectum itself but rather in the muscles of the pelvic floor,[46] but this is disputed. This sensation is absent in patients with spinal cord lesions from the fifth cervical to the tenth thoracic level.[47]

The anal canal is sensitive to light touch, pressure, pain, and temperature.

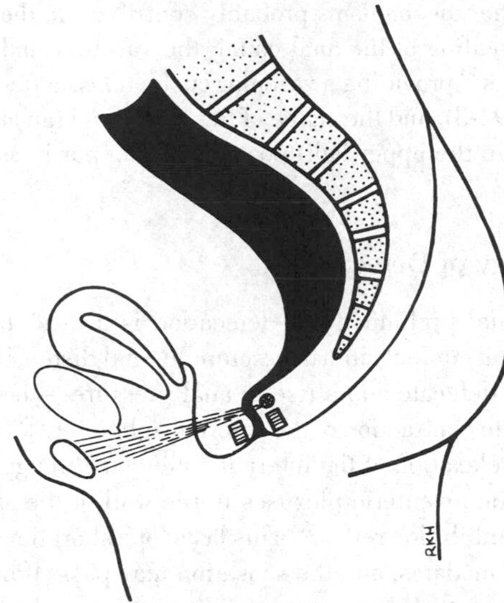

Figure 94-2 The anorectal angle, maintained by puborectalis sling.

Continence Mechanisms

Anal continence is maintained by a number of separate and important mechanisms. One is the anorectal angle maintained principally by the puborectalis sling (Fig. 94-2). The puborectalis arises from the posterior surface of the symphysis pubis and is inserted into a raphe on the posterior surface of the anorectal junction. There is some evidence that, unlike the other pelvic floor muscles, which are supplied by the external pudendal nerve, it may be innervated by a direct branch from spinal segments S3 to S4.[48]

The internal anal sphincter is a continuation of the circular smooth muscle of the rectum (Fig. 94-3) which provides 75 to 80 percent of the anal closing pressure at rest.[49] The external sphincter is a striated muscle in close proximity to the puborectalis and is innervated by the external pudendal nerve. It is under voluntary control and in the resting state contributes only a small amount to anal pressure. When the rectum is distended, this muscle contracts reflexly and, after sudden substantial distension, contributes about 60 percent of the closing pressure.[49]

Figure 94-3 Muscles involved in anal continence.

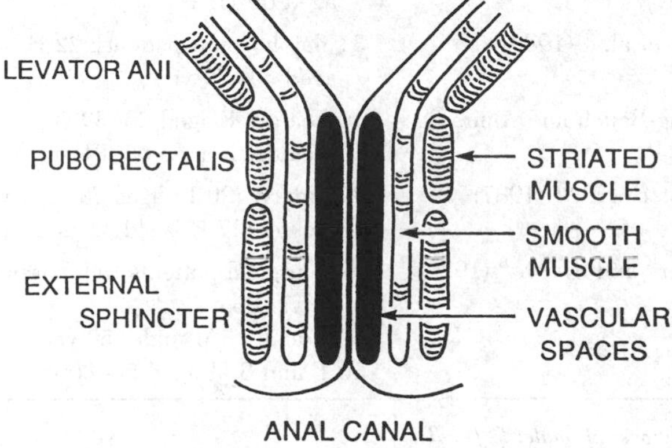

Two other mechanisms probably contribute to the fine closure and sealing of the anal canal: the vascular and mucosal components[50] providing a vascular cushion and a fine mucosal seal (Fig. 94-3), and the shape of the anal canal (an anteroposterior slit in the upper half) possibly acting partly as a flutter valve.[51]

Physiology of Defecation

The usual preliminary to defecation is a mass peristalsis moving fecal contents into the rectum. Rectal distension causes an urge to defecate and a rise in anal pressure—the inflation reflex due to contraction of the external sphincter.[52] This is followed by relaxation of the internal sphincter through local reflexes in the myenteric plexuses in the wall of the anorectum called the inhibition reflex.[53] This lasts for a short time, the rectum accommodates, and the sensation may pass. If defecation is to proceed, the appropriate position is assumed, abdominal pressure is raised, the puborectalis and anal sphincters relax, the anorectal angle is widened, the rectum and anus assume a funnel shape, and the contents are expelled. At the end of defecation the external sphincter contracts momentarily (the closing reflex), and the internal sphincter resumes its contraction.[54] The external sphincter, of course, contracts reflexly during coughs and sneezes or other events that lead to a sudden rise in intra-abdominal pressure, and it is also under voluntary control.

Age Changes

Age changes in both morphology and function have been recently reviewed.[55] Gender differences are to be expected since childbearing has been shown to affect the pudendal nerve, leading to a loss of cells in the external sphincter and puberectalis muscle.[48,56,57] Similar pudendal neuropathy may be caused by the "descending perineum" secondary to long, continued straining in defecation [58–60] and in diabetes.[61] However, pudendal neuropathy occurs as an age-associated change, especially in those above 70 in both sexes,[62] and progresses with time.[63]

A diminution in squeeze (external sphincter) pressure with age has been shown by many workers (Table 94-1). There is less unanimity about changes in resting (internal sphincter) pressure with age (Table 93-1). Decreased anal sphincter pressure has also been demonstrated in Parkinson's disease.[69]

Morphometric changes in the internal sphincter include an increased amount of collagen between small muscle cells[70,71] reflected in thickening shown on endosonography.[72]

External sphincter function is affected by the selected loss of type I (slow) fibers with age, especially after 80 years.[73]

Transit time is not affected by age,[74] but it is prolonged in hypothyroidism[75] and in Parkinson's disease.[69] However, several studies have shown that in geriatric long-stay patients—who are mainly bed ridden or chairfast and most of whom suffer from disabling neurologic disease—80 percent transit time is much prolonged and in some case may exceed 14 days.[76] The delay occurs largely in the rectosigmoid area—a situation that has been described as terminal reservoir syndrome.

No difference in the volume or pressure of rectal distension needed to produce first sensation in old and young subjects has been seen.[67] For the old, however, a smaller volume of rectal distension was needed to trigger the desire to defecate but was not related to pressure. The maximum tolerable volume

Table 94-1 Effect of aging on internal and external sphincter pressures—results from various studies

Study	Subjects	In Elderly Group	
		Anal Resting Pressure (Internal Sphincter)	**Anal Maximum Squeeze Pressure (External Sphincter)**
McHugh and Diamant[64] (1987)	157 healthy M and F volunteers aged 20–89 yr	Decreased	Decreased (F only)
Mattheson and Keighley[65] (1981)	125 surgical patients; 46 M and F aged 60 yr +	Decreased (over 70)	Decreased (F over 70 only)
Barrett et al.[37] (1989)	31 day-hospital patients; 22 F aged 74–79 yr	No significant difference	Decreased
Loening-Bauch and Anuras[66] (1984)	10 healthy F aged 23–39 yr 10 healthy F aged 65–81 yr	No significant difference	No significant difference
Bannister et al.[67] (1987)	37 elderly (20 F) aged 78 ± 1 yr 48 young (27 F) aged 32 ± 2 yr	Decreased	Decreased
Laurberg and Swash[68] (1989)	121 surgical patients with normal pelvic floor 52 F and 11 M under 50 yr 50 F and 8 M aged 50–80 yr	No significant difference	Decreased (F only)

Abbreviations: M, male; F, female.

was also decreased. Old people were less able to expel a simulated stool within a short period of time (20 seconds), although by 5 minutes there was no difference. There was no difference between the anorectal angle in old and young. Rectal pressure rose more rapidly for lower volumes in elderly women. These measurements, however, have been shown to be subject to considerable day-to-day variation.[77]

Bowel Habits

Reports on the bowel habits of old people are conflicting. Two showed no difference between old and young, though laxative consumption was greater in the old.[78,79] A third[80] showed that five or fewer bowel movements weekly were twice as common in those older than 50 compared with younger people, and a fourth[81] reported an increase in bowel movements among the older. A study on self-reported constipation among elderly people living at home[82] indicated a prevalence of 30 percent—although only 3 percent of these individuals had fewer than three bowel movements a week.

The need for regular purgation even if bowel function is quite regular is apparently a strongly held belief among 25 percent of the population of the United Kingdom, no matter what their age.[82] Indeed, many of these people thought it harmful if the bowels were not opened every day. Clearly there is a good deal of confusion in the public mind about bowel habits, constipation, and the need for laxatives, and this may be an inheritance from the early part of the twentieth century when the theory of autointoxication from the colon was firmly held by the medical profession, regular purgation and even colectomy[83] being widely recommended.

Constipation

Constipation is a symptom and as such may mean different things to different individuals. It may signify bowel movements that are less frequent than they used to be or that are more difficult to pass. On the other hand, it may simply mean that bowel movements are less frequent than the person thinks they ought to be. Constipation may be a symptom of diseases such as hypothyroidism, depression, and states causing hypercalcemia. It may be associated with neurologic disease such as paraparesis, or it may reflect pathology in the large bowel such as cancer or aganglionosis. It may be associated with certain drugs or a poor (generally low-residue) diet, or it may be a primary condition often considered idiopathic.

Primary or idiopathic constipation has been studied mainly in younger adults and with conflicting conclusions. It has been categorized in various ways. For instance, Lanfranchi and colleagues[84] classified it as either painful or painless, with differences in transit time, anal resting pressure, threshold for rectal sensation, and inhibition reflex. They suggested that the painful type was a form of spastic constipation which may be associated with irritable bowel syndrome, whereas the painless type may be a form of atonic constipation possibly associated with reduced motor activity or reduced colonic wall sensitivity. Another study on 39 chronically constipated younger adults divided them into three types—slow transit, normal transit, and megarectum. None of those in the last mentioned group were able to expel a water-filled balloon, and this could be done by only a quarter of those with slow transit and by only half of those in the normal transit group.[85]

Constipation with slow transit time and no response to the introduction of bisacodyl into the lower rectum (normally a contact effect) was thought to be due to impairment of the myenteric plexuses,[86,87] a theory upheld by other investigators.[88]

Slow-transit constipation may also be due to outlet obstruction which may be caused by paradoxical puborectalis contraction (i.e., absence of relaxation of the muscle on attempted defecation),[89–91] although this is apparently common in nonconstipated individuals and may occur in spinal cord disorder.

Thus constipated patients may show one or more of the following:

- Failure to widen the anorectal angle on attempted defecation
- Failure to inhibit the external sphincter on attempted defecation
- Higher rectal volume to induce desire to defecate
- Higher rectal volume to stimulate rectal contractions
- More difficulty in passing simulated stools
- Prolonged transit time

These findings indicate impairment of the innervation and reflexes involved in defecation. Possible causes include very long-term use of irritant laxatives[92] and Parkinsonism.[93] While several of these factors may be operating in constipation in old age, immobility may be another important factor. An interesting comparison of defecation patterns in normal and active elderly people and in those more disabled and immobile was described by Donald and colleagues,[94] comparing 111 patients randomly drawn from a general practice list with 90 patients attending a geriatric day hospital. The findings (Table 94-2) show striking differences, between the two groups in mobility, depression, and arthritis. In the day hospital group only, there was also a correlation between feces in the rectum and constipation. The association between physical mobility and defecation has already been noted and moderate exercise has been shown to decrease transit time.[95]

Diagnosis

While constipation should be considered when bowel habits change, when bowel movements occur less than three times weekly, and when colic, paradoxical diarrhea, or fecal incontinence is present, there are few other specific symptoms. Urinary frequency, incontinence or retention, and mental confusion may be associated symptoms.

Table 94-2 Comparison of elderly people attending a day hospital with matched group selected randomly from general practice lists[a]

	General Practice List ($n = 111$)	Day Hospital Attenders, ($n = 90$)
Bowel motion ≥ 3 times weekly	95	85
Reported constipation	23	55
Laxatives ≥ once weekly	15	22
Reported straining	25	53
Large amount of feces on rectal examination	27	40
Homebound	9	69
Depressed	20	50
Arthritis	22	47

[a] *Figures are percentages.*
(From Donald and Smith,[94] with permission.)

Abdominal distention, pain, tenderness, or a palpable fecal mass may be present. Rectal examination may have a low sensitivity in the diagnosis of constipation. Cox and colleagues[96] carried out rectal examinations in 220 patients newly admitted to a geriatric unit, all aged over 75 (mean age 82). Twenty-five percent of those who said their bowel habits were regular were found to be impacted. Those impacted were more likely to be confused and to have perineal fecal staining. Abdominal x-ray evidence of constipation (visible feces throughout the colon with heavy loading at one site) correlated significantly with the complaint of constipation with pain and straining and laxative use. Smith and Lewis[97] showed no correlation between rectal examination and abdominal x-ray findings, and 30 percent of subjects with an empty rectum had a large amount of feces in the rectosigmoid areas. Straight abdominal x-rays in 66 newly admitted geriatric patients (mean age 79)[98] found 43 with a feces-filled cecum and 23 with a gas-filled cecum. There was no difference between the two types in overall transit time, but the distribution of the pellets showed a larger number in the descending colon and rectum in association with the gas-filled cecum, which seems to correlate with terminal reservoir syndrome.

In summary then, it is clear that in old age constipation may be a symptom of underlying general disease, a symptom of disease of the colon or rectum, an effect of diet or of drugs, or alternatively more akin to the idiopathic constipation of younger people, possibly consisting of two types based on normal or prolonged transit time and major delay in the right or left side of the colon. In the latter case the disorder is associated particularly with immobility and mental confusion.

Treatment

It is clear from the considerable literature on the use of laxatives in old people, both at home and in institutions, that a very large number are taken unnecessarily. Laxative use can be strikingly diminished by adding fiber or bran to the diet[99] and by regular exercise in the case of long-stay patients.[100] Dietary fiber or bran is contraindicated in immobile old people and should not be used in impacted subjects until the impaction has been relieved. Laxatives given to patients with terminal reservoir syndrome are likely to produce fecal incontinence, and their use should therefore be limited to occasional symptomatic relief of constipation in mobile elderly people. Some laxatives in regular use are contraindicated, for instance, liquid paraffin (mineral oil) may predispose to inhalation pneumonia, deficiency of fat-soluble vitamins, fecal incontinence, and possibly colorectal cancer. Those that can be recommended are the following:

- *Standardized senna*: an anthroquinone preparation thought to stimulate Auerbach's plexus and increase the bulk and softness of the stool by inhibiting water absorption[101]
- *Bisacodyl*: a diphenylmethane which stimulates propulsive motility in the colon by action on the sensory nerves that is possibly associated with diminished water absorption[101]
- *Lactulose*: a synthetic disaccharide not significantly digested or absorbed; exerts an osmotic effect in the small intestine and thereby increases fecal weight, volume, and water content[102]
- *Ispaghula and other natural gums*: substances that absorb water and are effective as bulk laxatives (swallowed with a large draft of water lest the granules lodge at the lower end of the esophagus); regarded as being as effective as bran, more palatable, and more acceptable to the elderly[103]
- *Dioctyl sodium sulfasucconate*: a "stool softener" with a detergent effect which allows water to penetrate hard feces

If the stool is soft, senna or bisocodyl should be the first choice, and if it is hard, lactulose. More drastic purgatives are available but must be used with care in the old, starting with less than the recommended dosage. These include the following:

- *Sodium picosulfate with magnesium citrate (Picolax)*: a combined irritant purgative with a fairly rapid effect (2 to 4 hours)
- *Magnesium sulfate (Epsom salts) and magnesium citrate*: both osmotic laxatives

A recent development has been the use of Misoprostol, a synthetic prostaglandin E analog, in chronic constipation,[104] and further study is awaited.

Immobile patients with terminal reservoir syndrome are generally best treated from below with enemas (e.g., 128 ml disposable phosphate enema) or suppositories (bisacodyl or glycerin). To be effective, these treatments must be given every day, sometimes for 7 to 10 days. Rectal necrosis with phosphate enemas has been reported,[105] and users should be instructed to angle the nozzle posteriorly after passing it through the anal canal. Alternative methods of emptying the impacted rectum and descending colon are by using mannitol (1 L 10% iced mannitol with fruit juice, taken over 30 minutes and followed by fluids ad lib).[106] Another regimen involves using Golytely (polyethylene glycol 80 ml/L in a balanced electrolyte solution), 2 L/d of which should be taken for 2 days.[107]

Occasionally, manual evacuation is required for disimpaction of hard fecal matter. This is a procedure that should generally be performed by a medical practitioner or a qualified nurse with special training.

Once the impacted feces have been fully removed, it is equally important to ensure that impaction does not occur again; the condition will certainly recur if the patient remains as before. Bran, fiber, and bulk laxatives should not be used before disimpaction but in mobile patients may be carefully introduced thereafter.[108] In general, however, it is probably best to ensure nonrecurrence by using an enema or suppositories twice weekly, although in some cases a laxative given twice weekly may be successful without causing fecal incontinence. Whenever possible, physical mobility should be increased. Daily exercise in bed and the use of abdominal massage have been shown to reduce laxative and enema use and fecal incontinence in chairfast geriatric long-stay patients—although they did not affect transit time.[100]

Other treatment modalities include digital stimulation and biofeedback. Digital stimulation (or digitation) with or without mild laxatives was studied in a group of 48 stroke patients. Circular motion of the finger within the anus for 30 seconds was claimed to induce peristalsis and relax the anal sphincter. Regular bowel habits were established in 24 of 25 patients receiving this daily regimen.[109] Visual feedback with EMG display has been shown to be no more effective than muscle training without feedback in 59 patients with idiopathic constipation.[110]

Complications

Megacolon and Megarectum

One of the complications of constipation in elderly people is idiopathic megacolon and megarectum. In *rare* cases this condition may be associated with adult Hirschsprung's disease (absence of anal inhibition on rectal distension), which may be amenable to surgery.[111] Other forms may or may not be accompanied by increased anal pressure. The disorder has also been described in association with Parkinsonism.[112]

Idiopathic megacolon in old people is manifested as gross tympanitic abdominal distension usually associated with diarrhea and fecal incontinence. The diagnosis is easily made from an x-ray, and manometric findings have also been described.[113] Diarrhea due to anaerobic bacterial colonization may be superimposed and require treatment with metronidazole. The main danger of idiopathic megacolon is the development of volvulus of the sigmoid. Treatment is similar to that for terminal reservoir syndrome and is often unsatisfactory. Colectomy may be the ultimate answer.

Figure 94-4 (**A**) Anteroposterior and (**B**) lateral radiographic views of volvulus sigmoid colon.

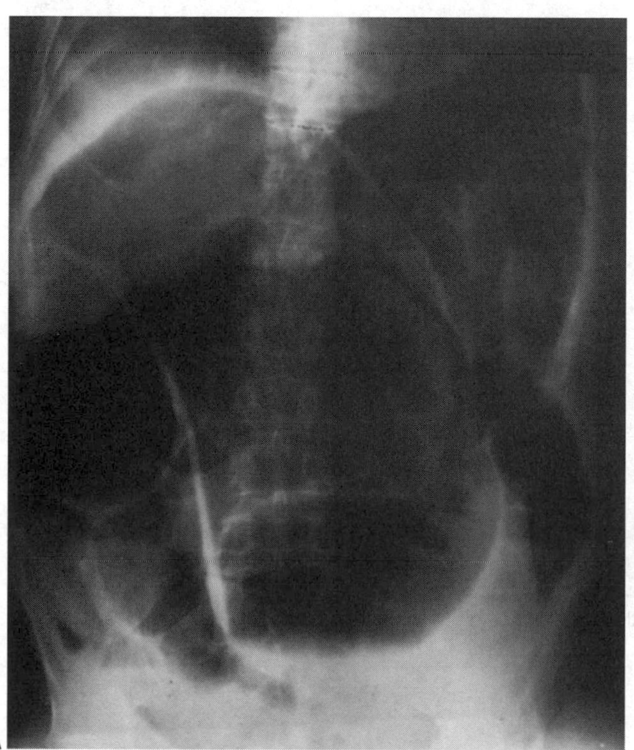

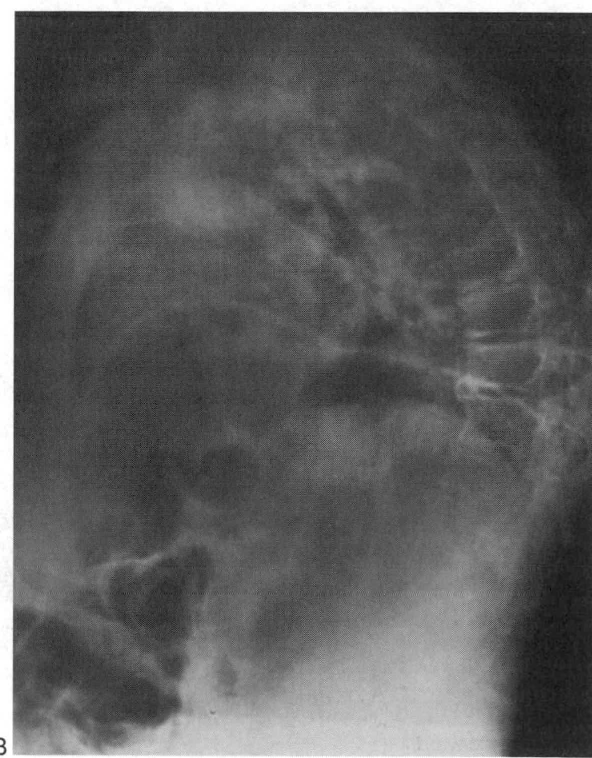

Volvulus

Volvulus of the sigmoid colon (Fig. 94-4) is a disorder occurring particularly in institutionalized and immobile patients.[114] The early diagnosis requires a high index of suspicion since the symptoms are nonspecific. They may include abdominal distension, which may be minor, or considerable cramping, abdominal pain, and constipation. Hypercalcemia, a high-residue diet, and explosive treatment of constipation have also been suggested as possible associated factors. The mortality is high, and this is no doubt in part due to slowness in making the diagnosis. Sigmoidoscopy itself is sometimes all that is required to reduce the volvulus, but over 50 percent of cases require surgical intervention.[114]

Other complications seen on defecography include intussusception, enterocele,[115] sigmoidocele,[116] and rectocele.[117]

Hemorrhoids are not caused by constipation in younger people, but there appears to be a direct association between the two in elderly people. They may block defecation by causing abnormally high pressure in the anal canal on straining.[118,119]

Fecal Incontinence

The prevalence of fecal incontinence may be gauged from a limited number of studies showing reasonable concordance. These are illustrated in Figure 94-5 which shows a slight increase in people above the age of 65 living in their own homes—most marked in the very old—but escalation of the problem in various institutional settings involving increasing levels of physical and mental dependency. The definition of fecal incontinence used in these studies varies both as to frequency (e.g., more or less than once weekly) and extent (e.g., inclusion or exclusion of staining). Incontinence of flatus is not reported in these studies although it probably also increased with age. In institutions, of course, the prevalence rate depends on management policies and the success with which they are carried out.

Definition

Fecal incontinence can be defined as the involuntary or inappropriate passage of feces. Anal incontinence also includes the involuntary passage of flatus.[120]

Causes of Fecal Incontinence

In adults of all ages fecal incontinence may be a symptom of many different pathologic processes or may be associated with drugs, diet, or disabilities impairing access to toilets. Of particular importance in women are the effects of childbirth, both in causing sphincter disruption and pudendal nerve atrophy. It has been estimated that 35 percent of primipara developed a sphincter defect after vaginal delivery and 6 percent had a disturbance of anal continence.[121] The primary repair of third-degree tears following childbirth leaves many women with sphincter damage. In the very old and those in institutions, however, the emphasis is different, with overflow incontinence

Figure 94-5 Prevalence of fecal incontinence in various settings. (From Ref. 120, with permission.)

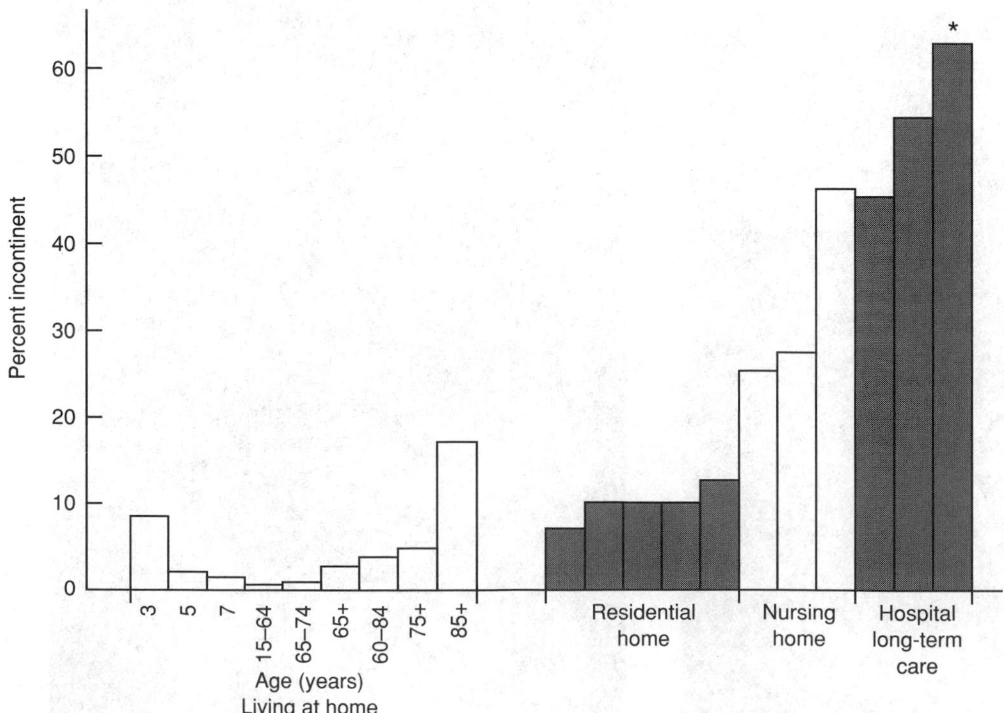

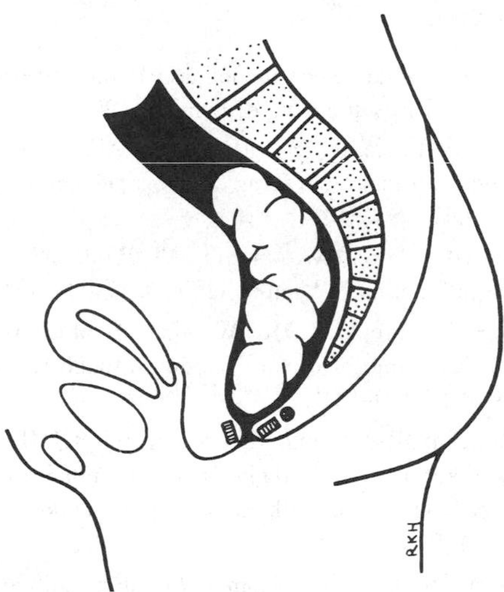

Figure 94-6 Anorectal angle in terminal reservoir syndrome (fecal impaction of rectum).

resulting from fecal impaction and incontinence due to dementia and confusion being the main causes.

Overflow Incontinence and Fecal Impaction

The relationship between fecal impaction and incontinence lies in the obtuseness of the anorectal angle (Fig. 94-6) and the continual presence of an impacting fecal mass in the rectum, leading to a blunting of rectal sensation and also of the anorectal reflexes with a consequent diminution in resting anal pressure.[122] An old person with fecal impaction is likely to feel constantly uncomfortable, unsure as to whether the discomfort is due to gas or solid, and have laxity of the anal sphincters. Leakage of feces occurs, and the clinical characteristic of fecal incontinence secondary to impaction is soiling by liquid or semisolid feces many times a day.

Uninhibited Incontinence

A second major cause of fecal incontinence in elderly people is that which is regarded as uninhibited (formerly called neurogenic) in as much as it is associated with global cerebral disease, particularly senile dementia. When the gastrocolic reflex occurs and feces enter and distend the rectum, feces are passed, possibly because of an abnormal sphincter response or possibly because the patient, being disoriented, allows the formed stool to be passed inappropriately. Clinically this form of incontinence is characterized by a formed stool once or twice a day, which usually distinguishes it from that due to fecal impaction. An analogy may be with the uninhibited neurogenic bladder in patients with dementia, and some similarities have been drawn between the cystometrogram and the proctometrogram.[123] However, there has been very little research on this condition. Barrett and colleagues[124] showed a significantly larger number of intrinsic rectal contractions following rectal distension in patients with low mental test scores, compared with others.

Symptomatic Incontinence

The third and perhaps most critical cause of fecal incontinence in elderly people is secondary to organic disease of the colon or rectum. The differential diagnosis, therefore, must include colorectal cancer, diverticular disease, inflammatory bowel disease, diabetic autonomic neuropathy, and so on. Inappropriate use of laxatives may also cause secondary fecal incontinence.

Anorectal Incontinence

A fourth type of fecal incontinence is anorectal fecal incontinence syndrome (also known as idiopathic fecal incontinence and neurogenic fecal incontinence). This concept was introduced by Parks and associates[56] who described it as a form of fecal incontinence not caused by systemic neurologic disorder. This condition is characterized by a disturbance of anorectal sensation (inability to differentiate flatus from feces), a patulous anus, absence of the anal reflex, and widening of the anorectal angle, possibly associated with degrees of rectal prolapse. It is associated with histologic evidence of denervation in the pelvic musculature, most prominent in the external anal sphincter and least prominent in the levator ani, which could follow entrapment or stretch injury to the pudendal or perineal nerves either as a consequence of repeated straining at defecation or attempted defecation or of childbirth injuries.[125] Similar changes in elderly nonincontinent subjects were less pronounced than in some elderly incontinent patients.[126] More recently, concomitant damage to the internal sphincter has also been described in anorectal incontinence.[127,128]

Allied with anorectal incontinence is the fecal incontinence associated with diabetic autonomic neuropathy and intermittent diarrhea. The average duration of diabetes in one study was 15 years, and patients had a lower resting anal pressure than a series of controls.[80,129] Somatic peripheral neuropathy may also be associated with fecal incontinence and prolonged pudendal nerve terminal motor latency.[61]

Management

The approach to fecal incontinence in elderly patients generally depends on whether the patient is in long-term care or very immobile at home on the one hand or is an otherwise moderately active person on the other. In the latter case the diagnosis of sphincter disruption due to childbirth or prolonged straining at defacation (idiopathic incontinence) requires early exclusion, as does the possibility of colorectal cancer. In the case fecal impaction or uninhibited (neurogenic) former incontinence is more likely.

Duration of incontinence, its frequency, and the nature of the stool must be determined. Fecal incontinence of recent onset suggests that the symptom is secondary to colorectal disease. If the patient is constipated, this problem should be dealt with first as outlined above. As soon as the colon and rectum have been emptied, the incontinence will disappear if it was due simply to fecal impaction but will otherwise persist, and lower bowel investigation is required which may include one or more of the investigations described above.

If incontinence is of long duration with one or two formed stools a day, it is likely to be uninhibited incontinence; frequent soiling with soft stool suggests fecal impaction. In any case, impaction first requires treating, and once it clears up, steps must be taken to ensure that it does not recur. Uninhibited incontinence can be managed by a regimen that diminishes mass peristalsis, producing a degree of constipation, and then superimposes evacuations at preplanned intervals—usually twice a week. Constipating drugs such as loperamide or codeine phosphate should be given daily, and enemas or suppositories twice a week. Alternatively, a laxative such as senna at night to produce a controlled bowel motion first thing in the morning and then codeine phosphate for the rest of the day may be used.[130] Attempts to improve the mobility of patients using a planned exercise regimen have been shown to be effective in diminishing laxative consumption and fecal incontinence.[100]

Idiopathic Incontinence

Treatment involves either pelvic floor muscle re-education (with or without biofeedback) or surgery. Exercises for the pelvic floor are as for urinary incontinence and should generally be supervised by a physiotherapist. Biofeedback addition to exercise has had reported success in the elderly[131] as well as in younger subjects.[132]

Many elderly people have difficulty cooperating with such biofeedback and exercise regimens. For them and for others with anorectal incontinence in whom pelvic floor re-education is unsuccessful, surgical correction is needed. The favored operation is postanal repair[133] which is not a prolonged or difficult procedure. Reported results of postanal repair, however, are equivocal.[134]

Fecal incontinence is all too often regarded as an inevitable concomitant of long-term care of old people in institutions. This point of view is totally unacceptable. One study[135] has shown that the 10 percent fecal incontinence among residents of old peoples' homes could be reduced by 87 percent using appropriate medical and nursing intervention. A clinical diagnosis of the cause of incontinence was made, treatment was ordered as outlined above, and, where this was conscientiously carried out by general practitioners and nurses, by 2 months after the instigation of treatment, there was an 87 percent cure rate compared with 32 percent in the control group. Incidentally, less than 4 percent of the residents with fecal incontinence had been referred to their general practitioner for this condition and yet 73 percent had suffered from incontinence for over a year.

Audit

Clinical audit schemes for providing high-quality care in the promotion of fecal continence in long-term care[136] and for the management of fecal incontinence[137] are published by the Royal College of Physicians of London.

References

1. Barrett JA: Faecal Incontinence and Related Problems in the Older Adult. Edward Arnold, London, 1993
2. Hinton JM, Lennard-Jones JE, Young AC: A new method of studying gut transit time using radioopaque markers. Gut 1969; 10:842–847
3. Wyman JB, Heaton KW, Manning AT, Wicks ACB: Variability of colonic function in healthy subjects. Gut 1978;19:146–150
4. Cummings JH, Jenkins DJA, Wiggins HS: Measurement of the mean transit time of dietary residue through the human gut. Gut 1976;17:210–218
5. Van der Sijp JRM, Camm MA, Nightingale GJMD et al: Radio isotope determination of regional colonic transit in severe constipation: comparison with radio isotope markers. Gut 1993; 34:402–408
6. Notghi A, Hutchinson R, Kumar D et al: Simpified method for measurement of segmental colonic transit time. Gut 1994;35: 976–981
7. Burkitt DP, Walker ARP, Painter NS: Effect of dietary fibre on stools and the transit time and its role in the causation of disease. Lancet 1972;ii:1408
8. Paylor DK, Pomare EW, Heaton KW, Harvey RF: The effect of wheat bran on intestinal transit. Gut 1975;16:209–213
9. Ritchie GM, Ardran MD, Truelove S: Motor activity of the sigmoid colon of humans. Gastroenterology 1962;43:642–668
10. Misiewicz JJ, Connell AM, Pontes FA: Comparison of the effect of meals and prostigmine on the proximal and distal colon in patients with or without diarrhoea. Gut 1966;7:468–473
11. Meunier P, Rochas A, Lambert R: Motor activity of the sigmoid colon in chronic constipation: a comparative study with normal subjects. Gut 1979;20:1095–1101
12. Rogers J, Misiewicz JJ: Fully automated computer analysis of intracolonic pressures. Gut 1989;30:642–649
13. Kamm MA: Pelvic floor tests in constipation. pp. 145–156. In Kamm MA, Lennard-Jones JE (eds): Wrightson Biomedical Publishing, Petersfield, 1994
14. Farouk R, Duffy GS, MacGregor AB, Bartolo DC: Evidence of electromechanical dissociation of the internal anal sphincter in idiopathic faecal incontinence diseases. Colon Rectum 1994; 37:595–601
15. Aanestad O, Flink R: Interference pattern in perineal muscles: a quantitative electromyographic study in patients with faecal incontinence. Eur J Surg 1994;1060:111–118
16. Neill ME, Swash M: Increase motor unit fibre density in the external anal sphincter in ano-rectal incontinence: a single fibre EMG study. J Neurol Neurosurg Psychiatry 1980;43:343–347
17. Swash M, Snooks ST: Motor nerve conduction studies of the pelvic floor innervation. pp. 196–206. In Henry MM, Swash M (eds): Coloproctology and the Pelvic Floor. 2nd Ed. Butterworths, London, 1992
18. Law PJ, Bartram CI: Anal endosonography—technique, normal anatomy. Gastrointest Radiol 1989;14:349–353
19. Broens PM, Penninck FM, Lestar B, Kerrimans RP: The trigger for rectal filling. Int J Colorect Dis 1994;9:1–4
20. Kamm MA, Jones JE: Rectal mucosal electro sensitivity testing: evidence for a sensory neuropathy in severe constipation. Colon Rectum 1990;33:419–423

21. Narducci F, Bassotti G, Gaburri M, Morelli A: Twenty four hour manometric recording of colonic motor activity in healthy man. Gut 1987;28:17–25
22. Chauve A, Devroede G, Bastin E: Intraluminal pressures during perfusion of the human colon in situ. Gastroenterology 1976; 70:336–340
23. Schang JC, Devroede G: Fasting and postprandial myoelectric spiking activity in the human sigmoid colon. Gastroenterology 1983;85:1048–1053
24. Connell AM: Motor activity of the large bowel. pp. 2075–2091. Handbook of Physiology. Section 6, Vol. IV. American Physiological Society, Bethesda, MD, 1968
25. Holdstock DJ, Misiewicz JJ: Factors controlling colonic motility: colonic pressures and transit after meals in patients with total gastrectomy, pernicious anaemia or duodenal ulcer. Gut 1970;11:100–110
26. Akkermans LMA, Van Der Heide D: Metabolic and endocrine factors in constipation. pp. 60–61. In Kamm MA, Lennard-Jones J E (eds): Wrightson Biomedical Publishing, Petersfield, 1994
27. Duthie HL, Bennett RC: The relation of sensation in the anal canal to the functional anal sphincter: a possible factor in anal incontinence. Gut 1963;5:179–182
28. Read MG, Read NW: Role of ano-rectal sensation in preserving continence. Gut 1982;23:345–347
29. Holstock DJ, Misiewicz T, Smith T, Rowlands EN: Propulsion (mass movements) in the human colon and its relationship to meals and somatic activity. Gut 1970;11:91–99
30. Loening-Baucke V, Anuras S: Sigmoidal and rectal motility in healthy elderly. J Am Geriatr Soc 1984;32:887–891
31. Karaus M, Sarna S, Ammon HV, Weinbeck M: Effect of oral laxatives on colonic motor complexes in dogs. Gut 1987;28: 1112–1110
32. Taylor I, Duthie HL, Smallwood R, Lingens D: Large bowel myoelectric activity in man. Gut 1975;16:808–814
33. Prior A, Fearn US, Read NW: Intermittent rectal motor activity: a rectal motor complex? Gut 1991;32:1360–1363
34. Daniel EE: Electrophysiology of the colon. Gut 1975;16: 298–329
35. Kumar D, Williams NS, Waldron D, Wingate DL: Prolonged manometric recording of anorectal motor activity in ambulant human subjects: evidence of periodic activity. Gut 1989;30: 1007–1011
36. Read NW, Haynes WG, Bartow DW et al: Use of ano rectal manometry during rectal infusion of saline to investigate sphincter function in incontinent patients. Gastroenterology 1983;85: 105–113
37. Barrett JA, Brocklehurst JC, Kiff ES et al: Anal function in geriatric patients with faecal incontinence. Gut 1986;30: 1244–1251
38. Donald IP, Smith RG, Cruikshank JG, Elton RA: A study of constipation in the elderly living at home. Gerontology 1985; 31:112–118
39. Halls J: Bowel contents shift during normal defaecation. Proc R Soc Med 1965;58:859–860
40. Newman HF, Freeman J: Physiological factors affecting defecatory sensation: relation to aging. J Am Geriatr Soc 1974;22: 553–554
41. Loeining-Baucke V, Anuras S: Anorectal manometry in healthy elderly subjects. J Am Geriatr Soc 1984;32:636–639
42. Read NW: Ano-rectal sensation. pp. 88–89. In Kamm MA, Jones JE (eds): Constipation. Wrightson Biomedical Publishing, Petersfield, 1994
43. Musial F, Crowell MD, Kalveram KT, Enck P: Nutrients ingestion increases rectal sensitivity in humans. Physiol Behav 1994; 55:953–956
44. Erchenbrecht JF: Noise and intestinal motor alterations. pp. 93–96. In Bueno L, Collins S, Junien JL (eds): Stress and Digestive Motility. John Libbey, Paris, 1989
45. Prior A, Stanley K, Smith ARB, Read NW: Effect of hysterectomy on ano-rectal and urethral visceral physiology. Gut 1992; 3:264–267
46. Lane RHS, Parkes HE: Function of the anal sphincters following colo-anal anastomosis. Br J Surg 1977;64:569–599
47. Wheatley IC, Hardy KJ, Dent J: Anal pressure studies in spinal patients. Gut 1977;18:488–490
48. Percy JP, Swash M, Neill ME, Parks AG: Electrophysiological study of motor nerve supply of pelvic floor. Lancet 1980;i: 16–17
49. Schweiger M: Method for determining individual contributions of voluntary and involuntary anal sphincters to resting tone. Dis Colon Rectum 1979;22:415–416
50. Gibbons CP, Trowbridge EA, Bannister JJ, Read NW: Role of the anal cushions in maintaining continence. Lancet 1986;i: 886–888
51. Phillips SF, Edwards AW: Some aspects of anal incontinence and defaecation. Gut 1965;6:396–405
52. Kerremans R: Morphological and Physiological Aspects of Anal Acute Continence and Defaecation. Presses Academiques Europeennes, Brussels, 1965
53. Lubowski DZ, Nicholls RJ, Swash M, Jordan MJ: Neurological control of internal anal sphincter function. Br J Surg 1987;74: 668–670
54. Shorovon PJ, McHugh SM, Diamont NE et al: Defaecography in normal volunteers: results and implications. Gut 1989;30: 1737–1749
55. Lovat LB: Age related changes in gut physiology and nutritive status. Gut 1996;38:306–309
56. Parks AG, Swash M, Urich H: Sphincter denervation in anorectal incontinence and rectal prolapse. Gut 1977;18:656–665
57. Henry MM, Parks AG, Swash M: The anal reflex in idiopathic faecal incontinence in an electro-physiological study. Br J Surg 1980;67:781–783
58. Engel AF, Kamm MA: The acute effect of straining on pelvic floor neorological function. Int J Colorect Dis 1994;9:8–12
59. Kiff ES, Barnes PRH, Swash M: Evidence of pudendal neuropathy in patients with perineal descent and chronic straining stool. Gut 1984;25:1279–1282
60. Engel AF, Kamm MA: The acute effect of straining on pelvic floor and neurological function. Int J Colorect Dis 1994;9:8–12
61. Pinna-Pintour M, Zara GP, Falletto E et al: Pudendal neuropathy in diabetic patients with faecal incontinence. Int J Colorect Dis 1994;9:105–109
62. Vaccaro CA, Cheong DMO, Wexner SD et al: Pudendal neuropathy in evacuatory disorders. Dis Colon Rect 1995;38:166–171

63. Hill T, Muratay A, Kiff ES: Pudendal neuropathy in patients with idiopathic faecal incontinence progresses with time. Br J Surg 1994;81:1494–1495
64. McHugh SM, Diamont NE: Effect of age, gender and parity on anal canal pressures: contribution of impaired anal sphincter function to faecal incontinence. Dig Dis Sci 1987;32:726–736
65. Mattheson DM, Keighley MRB: Manometric evaluation of rectal prolapse and faecal incontinence. Gut 1981;22:126–129
66. Loening-Baucke, Anuras S: Anorectal manometry in healthy elderly subjects. J Am Geriatr Soc 1989;32:636–639
67. Bannister JJ, Abouzekry I, Read NW: Effect of aging on anorectal function. Gut 1987;28:353–357
68. Laurberg S, Swash M: Effects of aging on the anorectal sphincters and their innervation. Dis Colon Rectum 1989;32:737–742
69. Edwards LL, Quigley EM, Harned RK et al: Characterisation of swallowing and defaecation in Parkinson's disease. Am J Gastroenterol 1994;89:15–25
70. Swash M, Gray A, Lubowski DZ, Nicholls RJ: Ultrastructural changes in internal anal sphincter in neurogenic faecal incontinence. Gut 1988;29:1692–1698
71. Speakman CT, Hoyle CH, Kamm MA et al: Abnormal internal anal sphincter fibrosis and elasticity in faecal incontinence. Disease Colon Rectum 1995;38:407–410
72. Burnett SJ, Bartram CI: Endosonographic variations in normal internal anal sphincter. Int J Colorectal Dis 1991;6:2–4
73. Lierse W, Holschneider AM, Steinfeld J: The relative proportions of type I and type II muscle fibres in the external sphincter ani muscle at different ages and stages of development: observations on the development of continence. Eur J Paediatr Surg 1993;3:28–32
74. Melkersson M, Andersson H, Bosaeus I, Falkheaden T: Intestinal transit time in constipated and non-constipated geriatric patients. Scand J Gastroenterol 1983;18:593–597
75. Rahman Q, Haboubi NY, Hudson PR et al: The effect of thyroxine on small intestinal motility in the elderly. Clin Endocrinol 1991;35:443–446
76. Brocklehurst JC, Kirkland JL, Martin J, Ashford J: Constipation in long stay elderly patients: its treatment and prevention by lactulose, poloxalkol dihydroxyanthroquinolone and phosphate enemas. Gerontology 1983;29:181–184
77. Goke M, Donner K, Meyer-Zym-Buschenfelde KH: Intra-individual variability of ano-rectal manometry parameters. Gastroenterology 1992;30:243–246
78. Connell AM, Hilton C, Irvine C et al: Variations in bowel habit in two population samples. BMJ 1965;2:1095–1099
79. Milne JS, Williamson J: Bowel habit in older people. Gerontol Clin 1972;14:56–60
80. Levi N, Stermer E, Steiner Z et al: Bowel habits in Israel: a cohort study. J Clin Gastroenterol 1993;16:295–299
81. Longsteth GF: Bowel patterns and anxiety: demographic factors. J Clin Gastroenterol 1993;17:128–132
82. Moore-Gillon V: Constipation—what does the patient mean? J R Soc Med 1984;77:108–110
83. Lane WA. The Operative Treatment of Chronic Intestinal Stasis. Nisbet, London, 1915
84. Lanfranchi GA, Bazzocchi G, Brignola C et al: Different patterns of intestinal transit time and anorectal motility in painful and painless chronic constipation. Gut 1984;25:1352–1357
85. Barnes PRH, Lennard-Jones JE: Balloon expulsion from the rectum in constipation of different types. Gut 1985;26: 1049–1052
86. Preston DM, Lennard-Jones JE: Anismus in chronic constipation. Dig Dis Sci 1985;30:413–418
87. Preston DM, Lennard-Jones JE: Pelvic motility and response to intraluminal bisacodyl in slow-transit constipation. Dig Dis Sci 1985;30:289–294
88. Krishnamurthy S, Schuffler MD, Rohrmann CA, Pope CE: Severe idiopathic constipation is associated with a distinctive abnormality of the colonic myenteric plexus. Gastroenterology 1985;88:26–34
89. Karbon U, Pöhlman L, Nilsson S, Graf W: Relationship between defaecographic findings, rectal emptying and colonic transit time in constipated patients. Gut 1995;36:907–912
90. Lubovski DZ, King DW, Finlay IG: Electromyography of the pubococcygeus muscle in patients with obstructed defaecation. Int J Colorectal Dis 1992;184–187
91. Herbaut AG, Van De Stadt J, Panzer JM et al: Paradoxical contraction of pelvic floor muscles: clinical significance. Acta Gastroenterol Belg 1994;57:13–18
92. Smith B: The effect of irritant purgatives on the myenteric plexus in man and mouse. Gut 1968;9:139–143
93. Singaram C, Ashref W, Gaummitz A et al: Dopaminergic defects of enteric nervous system in Parkinson's disease patients with chronic constipation. Lancet 1995;346:861–864
94. Donald IP, Smith RG, Cruikshank JG, Elton RA: A study of constipation in the elderly living at home. Gerontology 1985; 31:112–118
95. Oettlés SJ: The effect of moderate exercise on bowel habit. Gut 1991;32:941–944
96. Cox J, Chittenden J, Heaton G et al: Rectal examination revealing the presence of faecal impaction. Geriatr Med 1989;Jan: 22–23
97. Smith RG, Lewis S: The relationship between digital examination and abdominal radiographs in elderly patients. Age Ageing 1990;19:142–143
98. McKay LF, Smith RG, Eastwood MA et al: An investigation of colonic function in the elderly. Age Ageing 1983;12:105–110
99. Sandman RN, Adolfsson R, Hallmans G et al: Treatment of constipation with high bran bread in long term care of severely demented elderly patients. J Am Geriatr Soc 1983;31:289–293
100. Resende TL, Brocklehurst JC, O'Neill PA: A pilot study on the effect of exercise and abdominal massage on bowel habit in continuing care patients. Clin Rehabil 1993;7:204–209
101. Bennett A: Pharmacology of colonic muscle. Gut 1975;16: 307–314
102. Bass P, Dennis S: The laxative effects of lactulose in normal and constipated subjects. J Clin Gastroenterol 1981;3(suppl 1): 23–28
103. Eastwood MA, Passmore R: Dietary fibre. Lancet 1983;ii: 202–206
104. Soffer EE, Metcalfe A, Launspach J: Misoprostol is effective treatment for patients with severe constipation. Science 1994; 39:929–933

105. Smith I, Carr N, Corrado OJ, Young A: Rectal necrosis after a phosphate enema. Age Ageing 1987;16:328–330
106. Palmer KR, Khan AN: Oral mannitol: a simple and effective bowel preparation for barium enema. BMJ 1979;2:1038
107. Puxty JAH, Fox RA: Golytely—a new approach to faecal impaction in old age. Age Ageing 1986;15:182–184
108. Grecors HC, Brooks J: Alleviation of constipation in the elderly by dietary fibre supplementation. J Am Geriatr Soc 1980;28: 410–414
109. Munchiando JF, Kendall F: Comparison of effectiveness of two bowel programmes for CVA patients. Rehabil Nurs 1993;18: 168–172
110. Koutsomaris D, Lennard Jones JE, Rox AS, Kanis MA: Controlled randomised trial of visual feedback versus muscle training without a visual display for intractible constipation. Gut 1995;37:95–99
111. Taylor I, Hammond P, Darby C: An assessment of anorectal motility in the management of adult megacolon. Br J Surg 1980; 67:754–756
112. Rosenthal M, Marshall CE: Sigmoid volvulus in association with Parkinsonism—report of four cases. J Am Geriatr Soc 1987; 35:683–684
113. Chiarioni G, Bassotti G, Germani U et al: Idiopathic megarectum in adults: an assessment of manometric and radiological variables. Dig Dis Sci 1995;10:2286–2292
114. Arnold GJ, Nance FC: Volvulus of the sigmoid colon. Ann Surg 1973;177:527–537
115. Karboun U, Pahlman L, Nilsson TT, Graf W: Relationship between defaecographic findings, rectal emptying and colonic transit time in constipated patients. Gut 1995;36:907–912
116. Jorge JM, Yang YK, Wexner SD: Incidence and clinical significance of sigmoidoceles as determined by a new classification system. Dis Colon Rectum 1994;37:1112–1117
117. Karaskick S, Ehrlich SM: Is constipation a disorder of defaecation or impaired mobility? distinction based on defaecography and colic transit studies. Am J Roentogenol 1996;166:63–66
118. Johanson JF, Sonenberg A: The prevalence of haemorrhoids and chronic constipation: an epidemiological study. Gastroenterology 1990;98:380–386
119. Sum WM, Read NW, Shorthouse AJ. Hypertensive anal cushions as a cause of the high anal canal pressure in patients with haemorrhoids. Br J Surg 1990;77:458–462
120. Incontinence: Causes, Management and Provision of Services. Royal College of Physicians, London, 1995
121. Bartram CI, Sultan AH: Anal ultra-sonography in faecal incontinence. Gut 1995;37:4–6
122. Read NW, Abouzekry L: Why do patients with faecal impaction have faecal incontinence? Gut 1986;27:283–287
123. Godec CJ, Cass AS: A comparison of pressure measurements in the lower urinary and lower faecal pathways. J Urol 1980; 123:58–60
124. Barrett JA, Brocklehurst JC, Kiff, ES et al: Rectal motility studies in geriatric patients with faecal incontinence. Age Ageing 1990;19:311–317
125. Swash M, Gray A, Lubowski DZ, Nicholls RJ: Ultrastructural changes in internal anal sphincter in neurogenic faecal incontinence. Gut 1988;29:1692–1698
126. Percy JP, Neill ME, Kandiah TK, Swash M: A neurogenic factor in faecal in continence in the elderly. Age Ageing 1982;11: 175–179
127. Lubowski DZ, Nicholls RJ, Burleigh DE, Swash M: Internal anal sphincter in neurogenic faecal incontinence. Gastroenterology 1988;95:997–1002
128. Farouk R, Duffy GS, Pryde A et al: Internal anal sphincter disfunction in neurogenic faecal incontinence. Br J Surg 1993; 80:259–261
129. Schiller LR, Santa Ana CA, Schmulen AC et al: Pathogenesis of faecal incontinence in diabetes mellitus. N Engl J Med 1982; 307:1666–1671
130. Jarret AS, Exton-Smith AN: Treatment of faecal incontinence. Lancet 1960;i:925
131. Whitehead WE, Burgio KL, Engel BT: Biofeedback treatment of faecal incontinence in geriatric patients. J Am Geriatr Soc 1985,33.320–324
132. Chiarioni G, Scatoloni C, Bonfante F, Van Tini I: Liquid stool incontinence with severe urgency: anorectal function and effective biofeedback treatment. Gut 1993;34:1576–1580
133. Browning GGP, Parks AG: Post anal repair for neuropathic faecal incontinence in correlation of clinical results and anal canal pressures. Br J Surg 1983;70:101–104
134. Jameson JS, Speakman CT, Darzi A et al: Audit of postanal repair in the treatment of faecal incontinence. Dis Colon Rectum 1994;37:369–372
135. Tobin GW, Brocklehurst JC: Faecal incontinence in residential homes for the elderly: prevalence, aetiology and management. Age Ageing 1986;15:41–46
136. Hopkins A, Brocklehurst JC, Dickinson E: The CARE Scheme: Clinical Audit of Long Term Care in Elderly People. 2nd Ed. Royal College of Physicians of London, 1997
137. Brocklehurst JC: Clinical Audit Scheme for Urinary and Faecal Incontinence. Royal College of Physicians of London, London, 1997

CHAPTER 95

Urinary Incontinence

JAMES MALONE-LEE

Developments in the sciences concerned with the lower urinary tract make incontinence an extremely interesting subject which is varied and clinically very rewarding. It is now difficult to support the view that incontinence is a "Cinderella" subject, not taken sufficiently seriously by a majority of clinical staff. However, there remains a shortage of centers that can provide training in the clinical skills needed for this subject, and people new to the speciality are advised to make early arrangements for training.

In the United Kingdom the prevalence of urinary incontinence increases from 2 percent of men and 9 percent of women aged 15 to 64 to 7 percent of men and 12 percent of women aged 65 and older.[1] A more recent survey has supported these observations.[2] The increased prevalence of incontinence in late life reflects functional deterioration and coincidental disability, the two working additively,[3] as would be expected intuitively.

Anatomy and Physiology

The smooth muscle fibers of the bladder, termed the detrusor, funnel at the bladder neck and continue into the urethra as longitudinal fibers forming a tube. In the male these fibers are inserted into the verumontanum, but in the female they terminate in the distal urethra. Contraction of the detrusor results in a rise in bladder pressure associated with shortening of the urethra. The trigone forms a triangular base plate with its apex at the bladder neck and its base running between both ureters. Contraction of the muscle of the trigone results in funneling of the bladder neck. Some fibers inserted into the external surface of the trigone distally pull the distal margins of the trigone apart, thus opening the bladder neck.

The detrusor has the ability to stretch considerably without developing an increase in tension. This means that it is normal for a bladder to be filled to 500 ml or more without an increase in intravesical pressure other than the pressure head resulting from the height of the fluid in the bladder, which is approximately 8 cmH_2O at 500 ml. If, during the filling phase of a urodynamic study, the detrusor contracts spontaneously, despite attempts to inhibit this, and thereby increases the pressure in the bladder, the detrusor is said to be unstable. If the tension on the detrusor increases in association with filling, irrespective of any contractions, the bladder is said to lack compliance. Low compliance may result from fibrosis, detrusor hypertrophy, or increased resting tone secondary to reduced neural inhibition.[4] The terminology is a little unsatisfactory. True compliance is a static measure obtained from a length-versus-tension curve in which each pair of measures are taken at steady state. Many urodynamicists measure compliance from filling urodynamic studies during which bladder volume changes continuously. This means that the measurements are the sum of compliance and tissue viscosity.

The normal mechanism for activating contraction of the detrusor is the release of acetylcholine from parasympathetic nerves, stimulated by the spinobulbospinal micturition reflex, the main micturition reflex. Tension receptors in the detrusor activate afferents traveling in the pelvic nerves, and these afferents pass through the lumbosacral dorsal roots to ascending tracts up to the pons. At this level the pontine micturition center provides the site where connections are made with descending motor tracts destined for the sacral parasympathetic nuclei. Preganglionic sacral parasympathetic axons originate in the sacral parasympathetic nuclei, leave the spinal cord through ventral roots, and travel in the pelvic nerves to ganglia in the pelvic plexus.[5,6]

While much of the functional neuroanatomy of the lower urinary tract has been explored by experiments conducted on cats, the advent of positron emission tomography has allowed some impressive studies on humans. These have shown that humans and cats have remarkably similar arrangements. They can show that micturition is associated with activity in the hypothalamus, periaqueductal gray matter, right prefrontal cortex, anterior cingulate gyrus, and dorsomedial pontine tegmentum. It seems that all these functional areas are found exclusively on the right side.[7]

Since higher cerebral centers tend to inhibit the pontine micturition center, lesions above this are associated with detrusor overactivity. Subpontine lesions are more complex. Some spinal micturition reflexes are located below the pons which are weak in the adult and probably inactive in health. Therefore, lesions of the spinal cord below the pons, but rostral to the sacral nuclei, result in bladder areflexia initially. Subsequent to the injury, over weeks or months, reflex mechanisms in the spinal cord become active, resulting in some uncoordinated and poorly sustained reflex bladder activity. However, if a spinal lesion involves complete destruction of the sacral nuclei, bladder areflexia will be permanent.[5,6]

The internal urethral sphincter is present only in the male, forming a circular collar continuous with the smooth muscle of the prostate. This sphincter is not part of the continence mechanism but contracts during ejaculation to prevent retrograde flow of semen into the bladder. Failure of this sphincter leads to infertility, dry ejaculation, and seminuria. The internal sphincter is cut during transurethral resection of the prostate, however, continence is maintained.[5,6,8]

The external urethral sphincter is the principal mechanism for maintaining urethral continence in both sexes. The circularly arranged muscle fibers are striated and predominantly slow twitch. The striated muscles of the pelvic floor and the external sphincter are supplied by somatic efferents originating in the anterior horns of sacral cord segments S2 to S4. The motor neurons are grouped in a specific region called Onuf's nucleus. This nucleus differs from other somatic motor nuclei with histochemical appearances similar to sacral parasympathetic nuclei along with evidence of adrenergic innervation. The axons originating from Onuf's nucleus pass to the periphery through the pudendal nerve and the pelvic nerves. External sphincter activity is supported by the adrenergic smooth muscle of the urethra.[5,6,8]

Sympathetic innervation for the lower urinary tract comes from postganglionic nerves traveling in the hypogastric plexus, pelvic nerves, and pudendal nerves. The sympathetic innervation inhibits the detrusor and stimulates the urethral smooth muscle and the sphincters. The stimulatory receptors on the urethra, sphincter myocytes, and prostatic smooth muscle are predominantly α_{1A} (sometimes termed α_{1C}) with some contribution from α_{1L} receptors.[9,10] The inhibitory noradrenergic receptors on detrusor cells are sparse and are of the β_2 type. The stimulatory action of noradrenaline on the smooth muscle of the prostate has precipitated an interest in selective α_{1A} receptor antagonists in the treatment of prostatism.[5,6]

Acetylcholine acts on muscarinic receptors which when stimulated activate second messengers, causing release of Ca^{2+} ions from intracellular stores in the sarcoplasmic reticulum. The rise in intracellular Ca^{2+} ion concentration activates the actin and myosin, thereby promoting contraction. We know that the detrusor cell can depolarize with the inward current consisting of Ca^{2+} ions passing through L-type channels in sufficient magnitude to support depolarization.[11] The calcium influx can then trigger further intracellular Ca^{2+} ion release. However, acetylcholine does not cause depolarization, and the role of detrusor depolarization is unexplained. It may be that its limited influence explains the lack of efficacy of calcium channel blockers in the treatment of detrusor instability.[11–13]

The muscarinic receptor itself is the focus of much current interest. Molecular biologic studies have identified five subtypes of muscarinic receptors (m1 to m5) which are distributed throughout the central nervous system and in the periphery. Selective agonists and antagonists have identified three pharmacologic subtypes (M1 to M3) which correspond to the cloned m1 to m3 receptors. M1 activity is detected in the autonomic ganglia and central nervous system, M2 activity is found predominantly in the heart, and M3 activity is observed in glandular tissue and smooth muscle. mRNA activity for m4 receptors has been identified in rat striatum and rabbit lung. We know nothing about the role of m5 receptors.

Ligand studies on M2 and M3 receptors have shown that in the bladder the greater proportion (85 percent) are M2 receptors, only 20 percent being M3. It was thought that M2 receptors were largely redundant and that all the contractile activity could be attributed to the M3 receptor, however, recent studies suggest that the M2 receptor may be active after all.[14] In other smooth muscles the M2 receptor, on stimulation, inhibits adenylate cyclase which is activated by adrenoceptors. It is not known whether this system is active in the human bladder,[15] but it has been found that some muscarinic antagonists prove highly selective for the bladder, and this tissue specificity seems to be associated with either M2 selectivity or lack of M3 selectivity.[16–18]

It is now known that acetylcholine and noradrenaline are not the only significant neurotransmitters in the lower urinary tract. Nonadrenergic noncholinergic (NANC) neurotransmitters are neuropeptides that modulate the actions of the classic transmitters and may act as transmitters themselves. Neuropeptide Y (NPY) and vasoactive intestinal polypeptide (VIP) are important neuromodulators which are released at neuromuscular junctions to influence the release and uptake of acetylcholine and noradrenaline. Adenosine triphosphate (ATP) is thought to be an important neurotransmitter and is known to cause depolarization of the detrusor. While ATP is not important in the normal human bladder, there is evidence that in diseased states the activating mechanisms of the detrusor change and NANC transmitters exert a much greater influence on the bladder.[16–18] There is also a growing interest in the activity of calcitonin-gene-related peptide (CGRP) as an afferent pathway stimulant since inhibition of this substance might be used to treat detrusor instability.[19]

Presentation

It is frequently stated that the bladder is an unreliable witness and that the symptoms a patient describes do not point to the true pathology.[20] This belief has arisen from the dubious assumption that patients can be fitted into distinct diagnostic categories and that meaningful symptoms are unique to the diagnostic groups. In truth, it seems that our diagnostic categories form intersecting continua which share some symptoms. This is important because erroneous faith in diagnostic absolutes leads to dismissal of the significance of symptoms, which are patients' experience of disease. I believe that the majority of symptoms can be explained by the physiologic and mechanical principles governing the lower urinary tract and that what patients say usually makes sense. To date, experimental data have supported this thesis, but rigor demands that we explore the subject much further. However, I will discuss critically the nature of symptoms because fluency in this subject is important for doctor-patient relationships.

Frequency, urgency, urge incontinence and nocturnal enuresis are symptoms associated with unstable contractions of the bladder and have been shown to be present during unstable bladder activity[21] and to be reduced with documented resolution of the instability.[22,23] Frequency and urgency may be more noticeable when a person is going out or while opening the door on returning home and are subject to diurnal and seasonal variation. Intercurrent illness, particularly urinary infection, exacerbates instability. Urgency may vary as an experience among individuals. Some describe the idea of a growing potential for loss of bladder control, whereas others tell of a wholly physical sense of near incontinence.

Stress incontinence is the experience of incontinence associated with coughing, sneezing, and other physical activity. It is associated with avoidance behavior prior to coughing. The term *genuine stress incontinence* is used to describe stress incontinence caused by an incompetent urethral sphincter. This terminology arose because it was noted that some women with symptomatic stress incontinence had unstable bladders, and it was believed that coughing induced unstable contractions which led to incontinence. It was proposed that instability could masquerade as stress incontinence. In fact, there are degrees of sphincter incompetence which can coexist with degrees of detrusor instability, and the two may interact.[24] We now know that the symptom of stress incontinence, with or without instability, is clearly associated with reduced sphincter function.[24,25] Where detrusor instability coexists, treatment of the instability may result in resolution of both symptom groups. This should be expected if the two pathologies work synergistically. Response to treatment of one pathology does not exclude the presence of the other.[26] Based on current evidence, if a woman describes stress incontinence, there is a probability of some degree of sphincter dysfunction.

Sphincter dysfunction results in a reduction in the maximum closing pressure that can be generated in the urethra. For continence this closing pressure must exceed the pressure of urine at the bladder neck. As the bladder fills, pressure develops equal to the hydrostatic pressure of urine in the bladder plus the weight of any viscera pressing on the bladder. The hydrostatic pressure at 400-ml capacity is about 7 cmH_2O. If the maximum closure pressure is reduced below 10 cmH_2O, the woman will develop a sense of pending incontinence as the hydrostatic pressure rises toward the urethral threshold, and minor positional changes may exacerbate this sensation. The woman will be forced to maintain a bladder capacity with a hydrostatic pressure below the threshold. The symptoms of frequency, urgency, and urge incontinence may all therefore be induced by an incompetent urethral sphincter. Additionally, rising during or at the end of the night with a full bladder and suddenly applying increased hydrostatic pressure to the faulty sphincter can lead to very severe urgency and precipitancy.

Hesitancy, a reduced stream, intermittency of stream, straining to void, manual abdominal compression during voiding, terminal dribbling, postmicturition dribbling and incomplete emptying are recognized symptoms of a voiding problem, be it obstructive or due to failure of detrusor emptying function. Their presence correctly points to a need to check voiding efficiency. However, the physiology of micturition indicates that high frequency of voiding leads to similar symptoms. The bladder empties more efficiently from a higher capacity[27] when the hydrostatic pressure is greater, helping to open the urethra. Elongation of the detrusor fibers in response to filling promotes optimum contact between the actin and myosin so that better contraction can be obtained.[28] Flow rates are well known to be related to the voiding bladder volume.[27] People with frequency therefore commonly describe symptoms of poor voiding in the absence of detrusor underactivity or obstruction.

Dysuria is the experience of pain in association with micturition. The classic symptom of burning in the urethra during voiding, caused by infection, is well known. Less appreciated is the external dysuria experienced by women with vaginitis when urine passes over the labia.[28] A persistent low abdominal pain, partially relieved by micturition, is a feature of chronic cystitis, particularly interstitial cystitis.[29,30] Instability may also cause poorly localized pain associated with unstable activity, which is particularly marked on rising in the morning. Very high frequencies may also result in lower urinary tract discomfort, which tends to fan the flames of frequency.

A variety of factors unrelated to bladder physiology should be explored at the time of presentation. These commonly interact with a greater propensity for incontinence so as to cause it, and so correction leads to continence. The possibility of adverse drug reactions, especially those caused by diuretics, sedatives, and α-receptor antagonists, should be investigated. Diabetes can certainly manifest itself as urinary incontinence. Toxic confusional states and intercurrent illness can precipitate the problem, as can postoperative urinary retention, particularly in an orthopedic unit. It is often stated that fecal impaction causes urinary incontinence. While it certainly causes fecal incontinence and may cause urinary retention, I am less certain of a valid relation with urinary incontinence. Physical problems regarding access to lavatory facilities also need to be considered.

Urodynamics

A urodynamic study has been the principal method used to explore the physiologic changes particularly associated with the elderly. This study is not necessary for the primary treatment of anyone presenting with urinary incontinence, be they young or old, and age does not contribute to the decision to make the investigation. However, an understanding of the test is certainly worthwhile.

A urodynamic study describes a number of aspects of lower urinary tract function extremely accurately,[31] particularly if proper attention is given to the laws of mechanics and physiology governing the process. Investigators err when they assume that their theoretical beliefs will be supported by the results of the study. For example, a urodynamic study measures urinary outflow obstruction precisely.[31] It has been found that urologists operate on the basis of symptoms rather than on the physical demonstration of obstruction.[32] Because similar symptoms are found in urodynamically obstructed and unobstructed men, it is inevitable that a clinical syndrome bearing the name *obstruction* is divorced from the urodynamic measure. Similarly, according to the definition of detrusor instability given here, patients with urge incontinence may prove to have stable bladders. The problem is not with the measure but with our theories about the nature of the clinical problem. With that said, I will describe the test process.[31,33]

On presentation, patients are asked to empty their bladders while the urine flow rate is measured by means of a flow meter positioned in an adapted commode. A Jaques catheter (French gauge 10) and a nylon catheter (16G) are placed in the bladder via the urethra, which is anesthetized with 2 percent lignocaine gel. The postmicturition residual urine is drained off and measured. Another catheter (French gauge 10) tipped with a perforated latex sheath, to avoid fecal plugging, is introduced into the rectum. The smaller bladder catheter and the rectal catheter are filled with normal saline and then connected to force displacement transducers mounted at the level of the superior ramus of the pubic bone. This reference point is used to establish atmospheric pressure. The detrusor pressure, generated by the walls of the bladder, is calculated by subtracting the intra-abdominal pressure (measured via the rectal catheter) from the intravesical pressure (measured via the epidural catheter). The bladder is filled with a fluid (usually normal saline at 20°C) at a rate of between 50 and 100 ml/min. Unfortunately, the filling rate, fluid temperature, and content are not standardized and vary with department preference.

The analog data obtained from the transducers can be digitized and collected on a magnetic disk. The bladder is filled until either a maximum of 500 ml has been infused, until unstable detrusor activity prohibits further filling, or until the patient is unable to tolerate any further infusion. On completion of the filling study, the Jaques catheter, which was used for filling, is withdrawn from the bladder, leaving the pressure measuring catheter in situ. The patient is then asked to void to completion. During voiding the bladder and rectal pressure and the flow rate are recorded simultaneously.

During normal filling to 500 ml the detrusor pressure rises to about 8 cmH_2O consequent on the pressure head of infused fluid and relaxation of the detrusor in response to filling (Fig. 95-1). If the detrusor contracts while the patient is attempting to inhibit micturition, an unstable bladder or detrusor instability is diagnosed. If this condition coexists with neurologic disease, detrusor hyper-reflexia is diagnosed. This nomenclature is based on assumptions about pathophysiology and not on observed differences in behavior,[34] although recent work supports such a distinction.[35]

This basic test can be supplemented by fluoroscopic radiography and a number of other embellishments, although the value of these additions lacks evidence.[36]

Age-related Pathophysiology

Early studies on age-related urodynamic findings were conducted on samples from elderly populations without comparisons from younger groups.[37–39] More recently studies have compared people with lower urinary tract symptoms across all age groups.[24,40–42] In 1995 data were published on normal asymptomatic elderly people but without comparative controls.[43]

Urge incontinence is the more common cause of urinary incontinence in the elderly and is due chiefly to detrusor insta-

Figure 95-1 Detrusor pressure against infusion volume. Record obtained from a normal woman with a stable bladder.

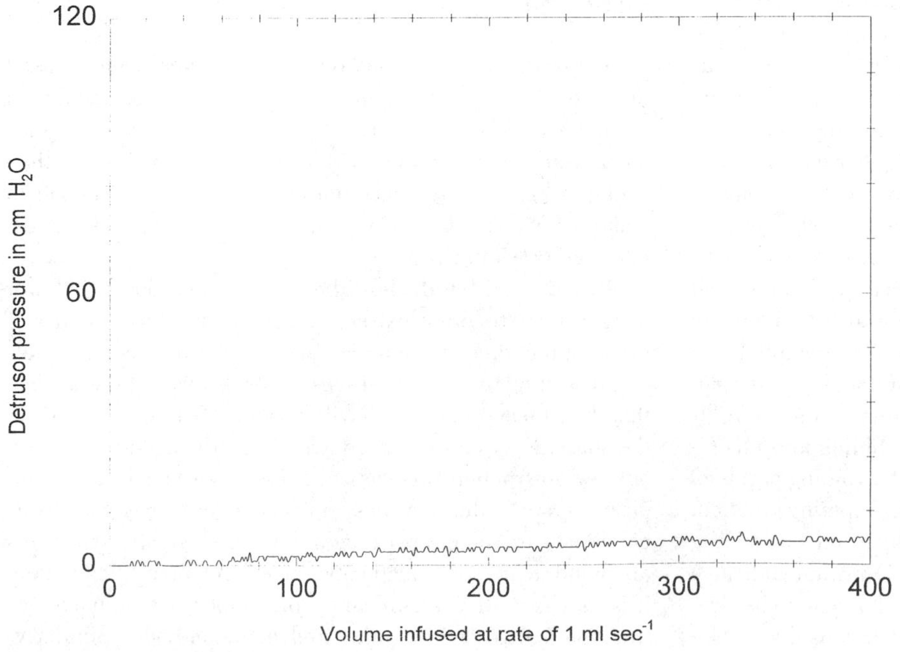

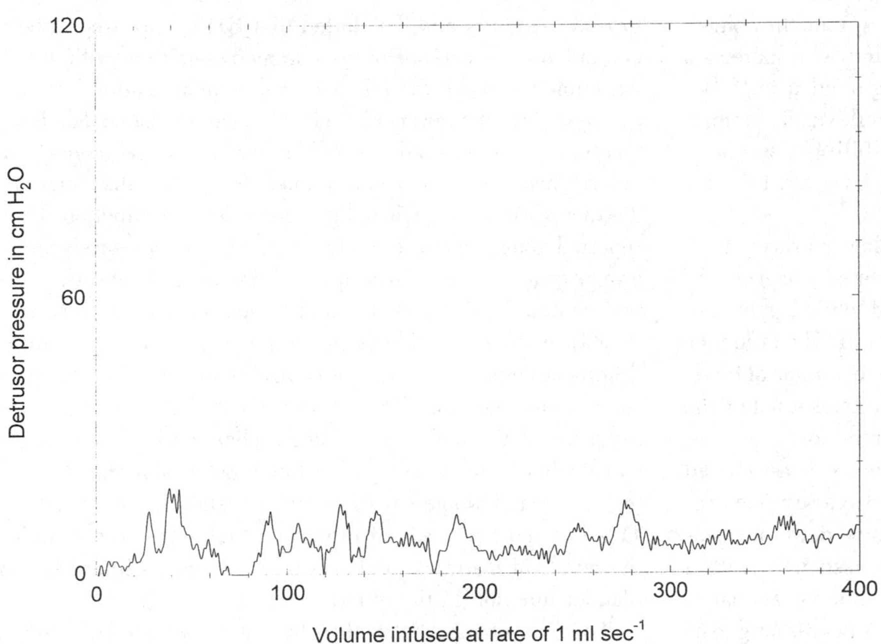

Figure 95-2 Detrusor pressure against infusion volume. Record obtained from a patient with instability.

bility. This is particularly the case in elderly people living in institutions.[44,45] Among outpatients with lower urinary tract symptoms, between 75 and 85 percent of women aged 75 and older and 85 and 95 percent of similarly aged men are found to have detrusor instability.[46]

Figures 95-2 and 95-3 are recordings obtained from women with detrusor instability and hyper-reflexia (detrusor instability with neurologic disease). There are differences in the patterns of detrusor instability between men and women. In addition, among women, contractions differ in relation to age and neuropathologic state. Hyper-reflexic contractions occur against a background of poor compliance, caused by persistent muscle tone, and tend to summate. This pattern differs from that seen in detrusor instability where the contractions are less

Figure 95-3 Detrusor pressure against infusion volume. Record obtained from a patient with multiple sclerosis. A hyper-reflexic bladder.

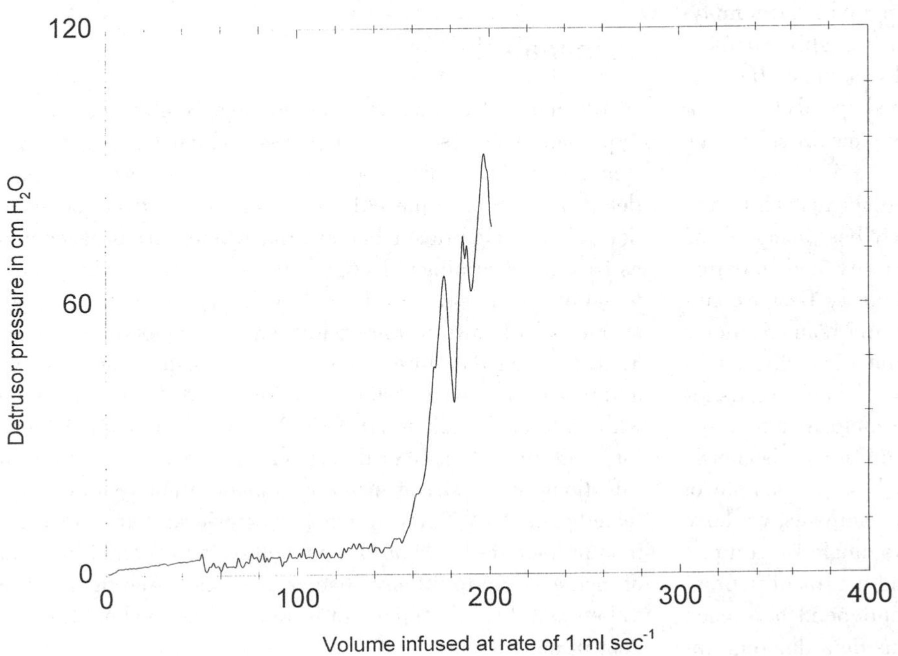

consistent against a background of persistent tone. In women, with aging, detrusor instability is associated with increased excitability and similarly increased background tone.[42] Because of the similarities to detrusor hyper-reflexia, it is tempting to suspect that, in late life, detrusor instability is associated with age-related neurologic degeneration, however, this has yet to be explored.

It is interesting to note that men with lower urinary tract symptoms do not demonstrate the age-related changes observed in women.[41] This probably is related to the higher urethral resistance provided by the prostate gland. The influence of this "obstructive" organ may dominate the evolution of bladder physiology. A recent publication comparing obstructed and unobstructed elderly men supports this contention.[47]

Detrusor instability in both men and women is associated with lower bladder capacity in the elderly.[41] Contrary to expectation, lower bladder capacity, more aggressive detrusor instability,[42] and older age do not appear to be associated with a poorer therapeutic prognosis.[46] In fact, there do not appear to be any urodynamic variables indicative of a poorer prognosis for treatment of detrusor instability.[48] It is not appropriate therefore to talk of severity of detrusor instability.

In women there are some interesting age-related changes involving bladder sensation. It has been found that appreciation of bladder filling is reduced with aging and that this change in perception is much more marked in women with detrusor instability and/or genuine stress incontinence.[40] This finding is unexpected since lower bladder capacities seem to favor a contrary experience. Studies on bladder sensation combined with tests of cortical perfusion and cognition have shown that reduced bladder sensation in the elderly is associated with impaired cognition and reduced perfusion of specific parts of the cortex.[49,50]

Both men and women void less successfully in late life, and voiding is associated with higher residual urine volumes and a higher proportion of patients with incomplete bladder emptying.[39,41,45] The explanations for this are probably complex. Obstruction plays a part in men, but it is by no means the only explanation. There is evidence for a reduced speed of detrusor shortening in late life,[41] as well as problems in sustaining adequate voiding contractions.[39,41,45]

Observation of the combination of detrusor instability and incomplete bladder emptying in the elderly has prompted the controversial notion of detrusor hyperactivity and impaired contractility (DHIC)[39] which was described by Resnick and Yalla[39] when reporting on 32 elderly nursing home residents in 1987.[39] They identified a specific physiologic entity, a subset of detrusor hyper-reflexia in the elderly. The characteristics were unstable detrusor contractions, postmicturition residual urine volume, and reduced speed and amplitude of isometric detrusor contractions. In studying a much larger sample of elderly people, as compared with younger subjects, we have been unable to detect such a distinct physiologic subgroup.[41] Voiding problems, detrusor instability, and contractility problems exist in the elderly but seem to be independent of each other. Griffiths also examined this issue using a different approach than ours and concluded that DHIC appeared to be a coincidental occurrence of two common conditions with different etiologies (Griffiths DJ, personal communication, 1996).

However, Elbadawi et al.[51] (1993) have published data from electron microscopy studies on bladder biopsy specimens from elderly men ($n = 11$) and women ($n = 24$) that support distinct pathophysiologic subgroups of detrusor function. They reported four structural patterns matching four urodynamic groups exactly with no overlap. Additionally two subsets, "normal contractility" ($n = 11$) and "impaired contractility" ($n = 24$), matched histologic subsets exactly. These findings, despite attempts, have not been corroborated (Gosling JA, personal communication, 1996). Carey et al.[52] have reported finding some of the defining histologic characteristics described by Elbadawi et al.[51] evenly distributed between normal women ($n = 15$) and women with detrusor instability ($n = 22$).[52] This is a most interesting problem which currently occupies the minds of many clinical and basic scientists interested in bladder function in the elderly.

There are changes in urethral function associated with aging in women. Figure 95-4 demonstrates a plot of voiding detrusor pressure against flow rate recorded in a urodynamic study. The pressure-versus-flow plot is extremely important in urodynamic analysis, and its properties have been well reviewed elsewhere.[31,53] It has been demonstrated that the two pressure intercepts shown, $p_{det.close}$ and $p_{det.open}$, are invariably elevated in the presence of detrusor instability and lowered in the presence of genuine stress incontinence. Where both conditions exist, the values take the middle ground. The highest values are seen in neurologic diseases such as multiple sclerosis (Fig. 95-5). It has been shown that greater age in women is associated with lower values of both $p_{det.close}$ and $p_{det.open}$, even in the presence of detrusor instability (Fig. 95-6).[24] Thus aging in women is associated with a loss of urethral competence.

Urinanalysis

Biochemical testing and microbiologic culture of urine is important in the assessment of patients with lower urinary tract symptoms. This subject has been recently reviewed in some detail in relation to the elderly.[54] Confusion exists about the definition of significant bacteriuria, which may be accepted as 10^5 colony forming units (CFU) of a single species in asymptomatic women but may be as low as 10^2 CFU of a single species of a known urinary pathogen in symptomatic women. Many automated culture systems have a sensitivity of 10^4 CFU, and urinary leukocyte esterase and nitrite tests correlate only with cultures as high as 10^5 CFU.[55] In addition, many laboratory culture systems can detect only just over 50 percent of infections in midstream urine specimens from genuinely infected patients.[55,56] Asymptomatic bacteriuria is far more common in the elderly. About 20 percent of women and 3 percent of men aged 65 to 70 have bacteriuria, and these figures rise to between 20 and 50 percent in women and to about 20 percent in men aged over 80.[54]

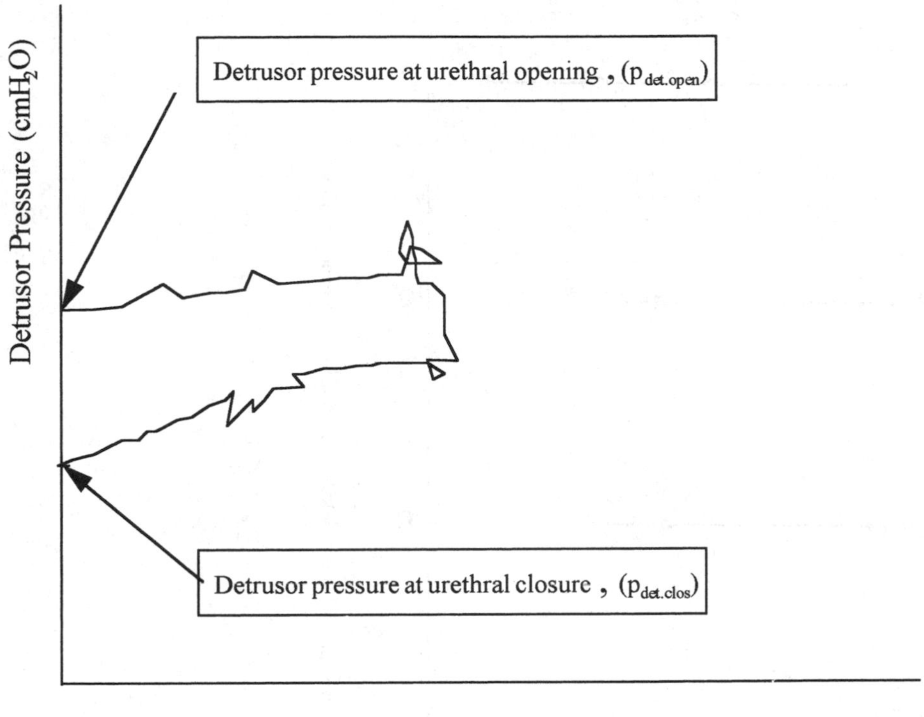

Figure 95-4 The pressure-flow plot.

Figure 95-5 Detrusor pressures at urethral opening and closure for women with lower urinary tract symptoms.

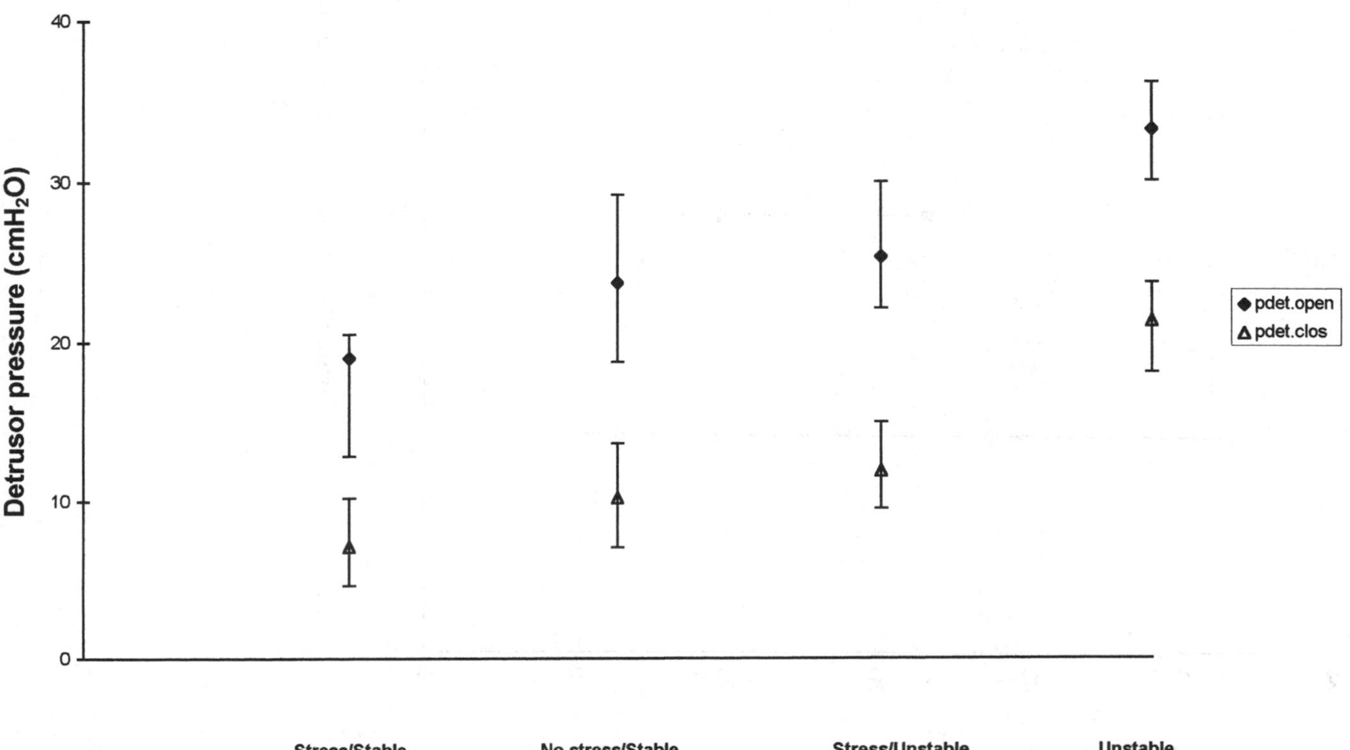

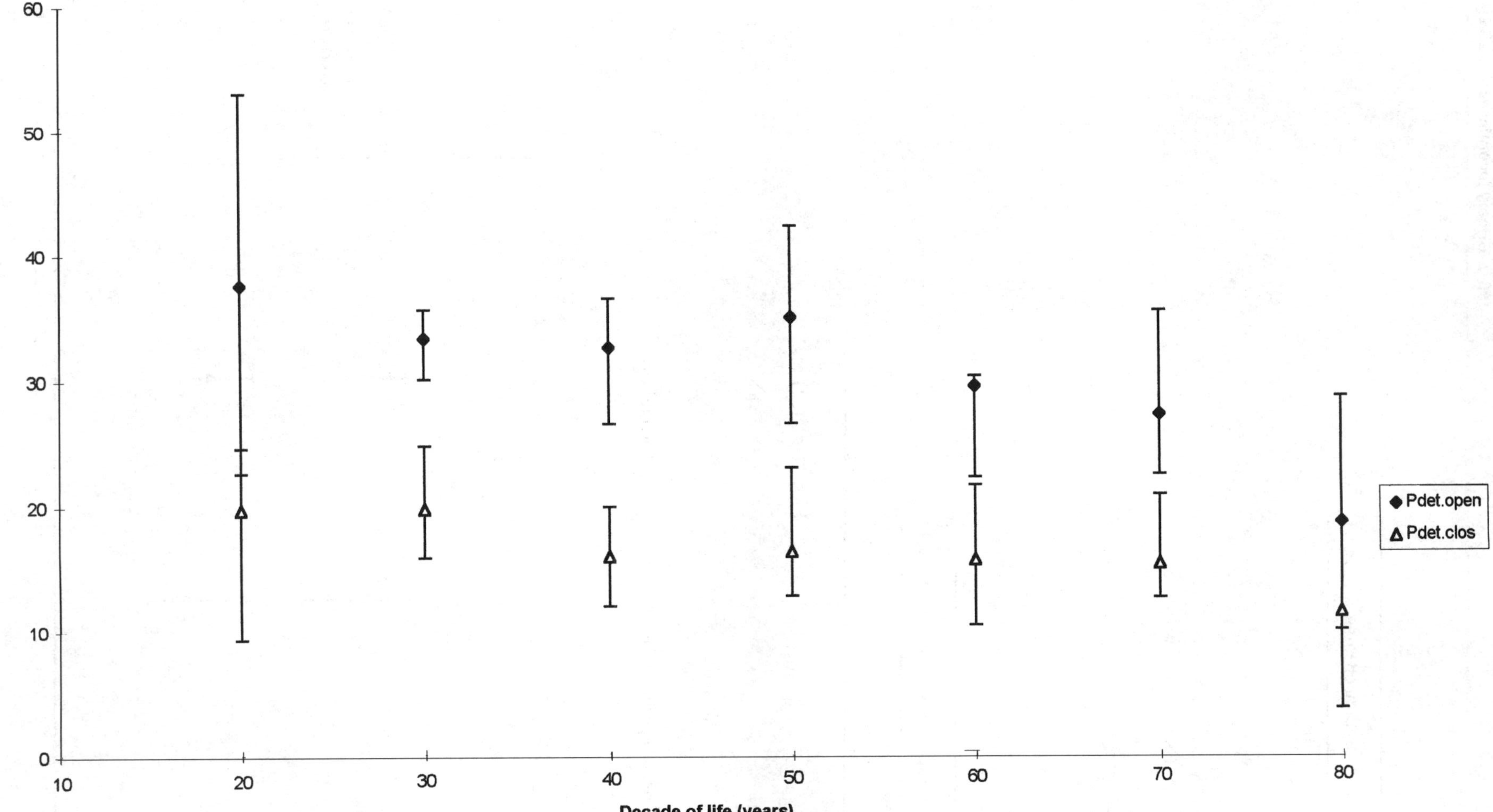

Figure 95-6 Detrusor pressures at urethral opening and closure for women with pure detrusor, instability by decade of life.

Greater morbidity has been associated with bacteriuria in the elderly,[57] but this may only be a reflection of susceptibility since there are no data indicating that treating asymptomatic bacteriuria influences the general health state.[54,58,59] Similarly, no data are available justifying the treatment of nonacute dysuric bacteriuria in the incontinent elderly. It has been found that detection of "asymptomatic" bacteriuria in the elderly at the time of urodynamic assessment does not seem to be related to the course of events following investigation.[60]

The Treatment of Urinary Incontinence

Treatment of urinary incontinence is likely to be directed toward one or all of the following goals: (1) reduction of bladder sensitivity, (2) stabilization of the detrusor (3) promotion of adequate bladder emptying during voiding, and (4) restoring competence of the urethral sphincter. Since several therapeutic options can promote more than one of these objectives, it is easier to consider treatment modalities individually.

Bladder Retraining

This pragmatic technique uses a protocol designed to encourage the patient to reduce the frequency of micturition. Several methods have been proposed, and none has been shown to be any better than the others. The patient uses a chart to keep a record of episodes of micturition. During this time efforts are made to delay micturition long after the urge to urinate is experienced. It has been found that while practicing this technique the frequency of micturition tends to decrease.[61–63] In a recent randomized controlled trial[64] which included bladder retraining, we found that in patients who responded, the period of change, lasted about 3 weeks.

Patients with sensory urgency who experience an inappropriate desire to micturate at low bladder capacities in the absence of detrusor activity, can use bladder retraining to reduce their frequency. However, retraining is not necessarily easy, and the patient should be warned of this and persuaded of the great importance of compliance if there is to be any hope of recovery.

An unstable bladder tends to become less reactive if stretched by higher bladder volumes. This principle is used to treat detrusor instability where frequency itself promotes very low bladder capacities. Some patients with detrusor instability experience pain while delaying micturition, and there is a real possibility of urge incontinence while working with the regimen. Because the goal is to stretch the bladder, the process can be augmented by encouraging higher fluid intakes while the patient is at home and not exposed to public scrutiny should an episode of incontinence occur.

As previously stated, if the urethral sphincter is incompetent, the greater pressure head applied to the bladder neck by larger bladder volumes will result in a strong sense of pending incontinence. This results in frequency being a feature of sphincter incompetence. For this reason it is appropriate to use a bladder retraining regimen as part of the treatment of genuine stress incontinence, provided of course that attention is also applied to the sphincter lesion.

Because a bladder always empties more efficiently from a higher capacity, it is logical to use a bladder retraining regimen to treat voiding problems secondary to detrusor muscle lesions. A proviso is to avoid excessive delay such that the bladder capacity rises substantially above 500 ml when there will be a danger of reducing detrusor power by overextension of the detrusor muscle fibers.

Stabilization of the Bladder

Attempts to prevent unstable bladder contractions are the main focus of much of our pharmacologic effort. It is very probable that the most immediate precipitant of unstable detrusor contractions is the action of acetylcholine on the M3 muscarinic receptor on the detrusor membrane. None of the drugs currently available for treating detrusor instability were developed with the bladder in mind, and we have been dependent on the accident of side effects for a very long time. However, two new antimuscarinic agents, Tolterodine and Darifenacin,[14,23,65] are subjects of phase 3 studies, and both these molecules have been developed specifically for the bladder.

Oxybutynin hydrochloride (Ditropan, Cystrin) seems to be the drug of first choice in treatment of the unstable bladder at most centers.[64,66–70] It is a tertiary amine with powerful anticholinergic, local anesthetic, and papaverine-like properties. It is very well absorbed from the gastrointestinal tract, reaching maximum plasma concentration 30 minutes after ingestion. It is excreted by the kidneys and has a plasma half-life of about 3 hours which is very slightly increased in the elderly. The side effects involve dry mouth, constipation, reflux esophagitis (the usual reason for withdrawal of this medication), dry skin, visual accommodation problems, and minor ankle swelling. Recent work has supported doses lower than those recommended on the data sheets for all age groups. We start all patients on 2.5 mg (or 3 mg) bid and titrate the dose in response to efficacy and side effects.[70] It is probably best to wait 4 weeks between dose alterations, as the dynamics of the drug seem to be slower than the kinetics suggest.[64,71]

The tricyclic antidepressant imipramine (Tofranil) has anticholinergic, α-agonistic, antihistaminic, and anti-5-hydroxytryptamine properties.[72–76] Most patients respond to a single dose of between 10 and 25 mg at night, but some individuals with troublesome daytime symptoms require an extra dose in the morning. The side effects are similar to those of oxybutynin but are milder; in addition, postural instability and drowsiness are problems experienced by the elderly. Imipramine is probably not as effective as oxybutynin, but there are a number of references in the literature reporting anecdotal observations of synergism in combination with oxybutynin (both drugs being administered in low dose) when treating particularly resistant patients.[77–79]

The quaternary ammonium compound propantheline (Probanthine), is recommended by some clinicians. It is not well absorbed from the gastrointestinal tract, and therapeutic levels are difficult to achieve. Evidence of efficacy in published works is not convincing and is based on within-group analysis of negative comparative studies. Doubt exists as to what dose should be used, and it is probable that a dose higher than that recommended on the data sheet would be required to achieve a response.[80–83] Emepromium bromide (Cetiprin), another quaternary ammonium compound, is no longer available in the United Kingdom but is available elsewhere.[84–87] There are considerable doubts about its efficacy, gastrointestinal absorption is not good, and it has a reputation for causing esophageal ulceration.

Interest has been shown in calcium channel blocking drugs for use in the treatment of detrusor instability. Terodiline (Micturin) was the most well known of this group[88–90] but was withdrawn from the market in 1991 following reports of serious adverse cardiac events, in particular arrythmia of torsades de points.[91–93] Terodiline has anticholinergic properties as well, but it is highly likely that the cardiac effects were caused by the calcium channel blocking properties. Other anticholinergics used to treat the unstable bladder have not been linked to this problem. In a small study on the elderly, which lacked power, no difference in symptom change was detected in a control group on placebo bladder retraining.[89]

Flavoxate hydrochloride (Urispas) is a drug with papaverine-like properties. At one time it was used extensively for treating the unstable bladder, but doubts arose as to its efficacy and these were confirmed by data from controlled clinical trials. It is no longer considered an effective drug for treating this condition.[94,95]

Surgery for Detrusor Instability and Hyperreflexia

Three surgical procedures should be mentioned. Cystodistension, by inflating a balloon in the bladder under an anesthetic, produces a transient and unhelpful benefit.[96] Subtrigonal phenol injection was advocated for a while but has not stood the test of time.[97] "Clam" cystoplasty has proved to be a most important operative intervention for resistant patients.[98,99] There are some doubts about its applicability in late life since the procedure makes voluntary bladder emptying ineffective, and so voiding difficulties are inevitable. Patients therefore require clean, intermittent self-catheterization to empty their bladders. This is particularly important when the procedure has been performed for detrusor hyper-reflexia.[100] Some elderly patients can cope with intermittent self-catheterization, but the prevalence of multiple disabilities in late life demand some circumspection regarding the use of this technique.

Correcting Sphincter Incompetence

Pelvic floor exercises are a popular means of offering nonsurgical therapy to patients with urethral sphincter incompetence.[101] The evidence for their efficacy is far from established and is based on data from open studies or within-group analyses of comparative trial data.[102–104] These exercises have not been found to be superior to surgery. There is little consistency in the techniques adopted by different centers.[101] While they have been advocated for the treatment of stress incontinence in older women,[105,106] there is no evidence supporting any specific effectiveness in the elderly. Regrettably no large-scale studies of efficacy that include age comparisons have been conducted, and so doubt hangs over the usefulness of these exercises.

The most widely accepted surgical approach is colposuspension, which seems to achieve the most consistent success at a wide variety of centers.[107,108] Some less invasive techniques are currently being studied, in particular, modifications of Stamey endoscopic bladder neck suspension[109,110] and of injection of paraurethral tissues.[111] Unfortunately, the results of these procedures are rather disappointing, and that in itself is a good argument for using colposuspension as a first choice.

The AS artificial urinary sphincter is an option for the management of urethral sphincter failure in both men and women. It is best suited to people who do not have unstable bladders. The operation involves insertion of a cuff around the urethra which is passively inflated from a reservoir of fluid placed in the pelvis. The cuff can be deflated, so as to allow voiding, by activating a pump placed in the scrotum or labia major; after voiding, the cuff reinflates spontaneously. Complications include infection, displacement of the device, and mechanical failure, and some manual dexterity is required. These devices have been in use since 1972, and there is considerable experience and development favoring success. In correctly selected patients this prosthetic sphincter is highly effective.[112–114]

Treating Voiding Disorders

Intermittent self-catheterization has gained general acceptance in the management of voiding disorders associated with neurologic disease.[115–117] Both elderly men and elderly women have an increased tendency toward incomplete bladder emptying, and this frequently coexists with detrusor instability. Voiding disorders in the elderly may occur in the absence of symptoms,[118] and treating detrusor instability in the presence of a voiding disorder may exacerbate incomplete bladder emptying. The latter can be managed by intermittent catheterization, although at this stage little is known about the efficacy of this technique in the elderly. In addition, it is unclear which patients with voiding disorders can be safely left unattended.

The policy in my department is to identify patients with voiding disorders by including determination of the postmicturition residual urine volume as part of our standard assessment protocol. When we discover a significant problem, which we define as a residual of 150 ml or more, we institute a temporary, once-daily intermittent catheterization program. If this results in a rapid, significant improvement in symptoms, we establish a more permanent regimen; otherwise we take no further action.

There are practical difficulties in using this technique because of cognitive impairment and lack of manual dexterity. It is more usual to enlist the services of a spouse or partner to administer the procedure, although a number of elderly people can self-catheterize. We have found that the fluid output in elderly people tends to be lower, and so a less frequent regimen of daily or twice daily catheterization may prove adequate. Complications in our selected elderly patients do not seem to be greater than among the young. Some older women with delicate atrophic urethras appear to be able to reduce urethral trauma by taking oral estrogen replacement therapy.

Estrogen Replacement Therapy

The role of estrogen replacement therapy in the treatment of urinary incontinence remains unclear. Studies do not supported its efficacy, despite widespread advocacy based on anecdotal reports.[119–121] Estrogen may, however, have a role in the management of recurrent urinary infection.[119,122] Estrogen withdrawal is associated with a fall in the level of intravaginal glycogen on which lactobacilli depend. These bacteria cease to colonize the vagina, which then becomes occupied by colonic organisms that thrive at the lower pH associated with this change. Atrophy of the urothelium encourages colonization by gram-negative fecal organisms, and the urothelium becomes more adherent for these bacteria. There is some slim evidence that estrogen replacement therapy can reverse this process and give protection to elderly women with recurrent urinary tract infections.[119,121]

The primary concern in relation to hormone replacement therapy is the risk of stimulating carcinoma of the uterus. This can be countered by using cyclic progestogen, which means that in women with a uterus, combined cyclic estrogen and progestogen therapy should be used. There may be a very slightly increased risk of breast carcinoma associated with the use of hormone replacement therapy over a long period of time, but this may be offset by the reduced risk of osteoporosis, stroke, and cardiac infarction.[119,123]

A disadvantage of cyclic combined therapy is bleeding, which is not popular among elderly women. Estriol (Ovestin) may be useful in avoiding this problem. There are no endometrial receptors, and so there is no risk of stimulating endometrial carcinoma. It can therefore be used continuously without progestogen in women who have not had a hysterectomy. The receptors for estriol are primarily found in the vagina and lower urinary tract. Estriol does not affect bone, and so it is not possible to achieve an osteoporosis sparing effect with this drug.[124]

Treating Urinary Infection

Urinary infections should be treated with drugs that are well absorbed from the gastrointestinal tract and therefore do not accumulate in the colon, are excreted in the urine rapidly, are not associated with high resistance rates, and are inexpensive. Nitrofurantoin (Furadantin) meets these criteria. Some patients experience nausea when using this drug, and under these circumstance the macrocrystals (Macrodantin) prove useful. Trimethoprim (Monotrim) is a useful urinary antibiotic provided there is not a great deal of local resistance. Amoxycillin (Amoxil) continues to be recommended for urinary infections; it is effective but is particularly associated with the development of vaginal thrush infections. These occur in 25 percent of women prescribed Amoxicillin. Nalidixic acid (Negram) is also a useful urinary antibiotic worth considering as a nontoxic first-line treatment. The newer quinolones such as ciprofloxacin (Ciproxin) should really be used as second-line therapy for resistant infections.[54,56]

The dose and duration of a therapy should be designed to limit the period of treatment. Clinical trials have shown that uncomplicated cystitis usually responds to a single dose of 3 g of Amoxicillin or 400 mg of trimethoprim. Recurrent postcoital cystitis usually responds to 100 mg nitrofurantoin immediately after intercourse. If the bladder is abnormal, this may be less efficacious. The antibiotic should be prescribed in a generous dose to be taken every 12 hours from the first hint of symptoms until the symptoms have cleared. This is an easy protocol for patients to follow and results in short courses of about 2 days.[125] Our preference is for nitrofurantoin as first-line therapy and ciprofloxacin as second-line treatment if a urine culture has not provided sensitivity data. In rare situations where prophylactic therapy is used in a patient with recurrent urinary infections, this is given as nitrofurantoin 50 mg at night for 3 months. Long-term use of this drug may, very rarely, cause peripheral neuropathy and pulmonary fibrosis. Since the action of nitrofurantoin depends on rapid renal excretion, it is of no great use in renal impairment.[54,56]

Devices

Incontinence pads continue to play an important role in the management of uncontrolled urinary or fecal incontinence. They are best suited to patients with dementia and severe progressive disability. However, ambulant patients may need to use these devices while awaiting a permanent cure. The design, technology, function, and performance of incontinence pads have been reviewed with meticulous detail elsewhere.[126,127] Currently there are some very effective products available, but care should be taken when choosing a suitable pad. There are now considerable data on which to base an informed judgment. It is worth auditing the criteria adopted by local organizations when purchasing incontinence aids.[126–128]

Permanent indwelling catheters have a role in the management of some patients. They are not suitable for people with uncontrolled instability or hyper-reflexia since they cause pain and bypassing. They are best reserved for people with voiding problems, with or without controllable instability, who are unable to manage intermittent self-catheterization. A suprapubic catheter is by far the better option. It is easier to maintain and does not traumatize the urethra. Urethral catheters in women may induce a vesico-vaginal fistula. If the bladder is impalpable, the suprapubic catheter must be inserted under cystoscopic scrutiny.

Recurrent blocking and infections are complications of permanent catheterization. Anecdotal reports favor the use of vitamin C 1 g qds and cranberry juice to combat blockage and infection, but there are no clinical trial data supporting this remedy although cranberry juice seems to have urinary antiseptic properties.[129] The former acidifies the urine and the latter reduces the tenacity of bacterial adhesion. Suby G bladder washouts protect against blocking. A successful indwelling catheter must be changed only once every 3 months. Asymptomatic bacteriuria should be left untreated.[130–133]

External sheath drainage is an option in some men. The old, cumbersome latex contraptions have given way to penile sheaths, developed from the condom, which are fixed to the penis using adhesives specifically developed for this purpose. The urine drains from a tube connected at the apex of the sheath. The main problem is difficulty in fixation caused by penile retraction. Additionally, some patients have problems with displacement in response to the physical stresses of movement. There is an increased incidence of urinary infection from organisms ascending in the urinary column. While skin ulceration has been reduced with the advent of better adhesives, it remains a complication. A retractile penis can be splinted internally by implanting the Small Carrion prosthesis normally used for managing erectile failure.[134]

References

1. Thomas TM, Plymat KR, Blannin J, Meade TW: The prevalence of urinary incontinence. BMJ 1980;281:1243–1245
2. Brocklehurst JC: Urinary incontinence in the community—analysis of a MORI poll. BMJ 1993;306:832–834
3. Ding YY, Lieu PK, Choo PWJ, Tjia TTL: Urinary incontinence after ischaemic stroke—predictive factors for is prevalence. Neurourol Urodyn 1996;15:262–264
4. Brading AF, Turner WH: The unstable bladder: towards a common mechanism, abstract ed. Br J Urol 1994;73:3–8
5. Hoyle CHV, Lincoln J, Burnstock G: Neural control of pelvic organs. pp. 1–54. In Rushton DN (ed): Handbook of Neuro-Urology. Marcel Dekker, New York, 1994
6. De Groat WC: Neurophysiology of the pelvic organs. pp. 55–93. In Rushton DN (ed): Handbook of Neuro-Urology. Marcel Dekker, New York,1995
7. Blok BFM, Holstege G: The human brain in the control of micturition and urine storage: a positron emission tomography study. Neurourol Urodyn 1996;15:261–262
8. Myers RP: Male urethral sphincteric anatomy and radical prostatectomy. Urol Clin North Am 1991;18:211–227
9. Marshall I, Burt RP, Green M et al: RS 17053 distinguishes between alpha-1A adrenoceptors in human prostate and the alpha-1a sybtype clone. Neurourol Urodyn 1996;15:343–344
10. Testa R, Hieble PJ, Guarneri L et al: The potency of alpha-1 adrenoceptor antagonists for lower urinary tract tissues is related to their affinity for the alpha-1L adrenoceptor subtype. Neurourol Urodyn 1996;14:346–347
11. Montgomery BSI, Fry C: The action potential and net membrane currents in isolated human detrusor smooth muscle cells, abstracted. J Urol 1992;147:176–184
12. Palfrey ELH, Fry CH, Shuttleworth KED: A new in vitro perfusion technique for the investigation of human detrusor muscle. Br J Urol 1984;56:635–640
13. Wu CU, Kentish KJ, Fry CH: The effects of pH on Ca^{2+} activated force in α-toxin permealised detrusor smooth muscle isolated from guinea-pig bladder. J Physiol 1994;477:42
14. Nilvebrant L, Sundquist S, Gillberg PG: Tolterodine is not subtype (m1–m5) selective but exhibits functional bladder selectivity in vivo. Neurourol Urodyn 1996;15:310–311
15. Shishido K, Yamaguchi O, Yokota T: Muscarinic receptor subtypes and their functional roles in rat detrusor muscle. Neurourol Urodyn 1996;15:313–314
16. Jurgen W: Molecular basis of muscarinic acetylcholine receptor function, abstracted. Trends Pharmacol Sci 1993;14:308–313
17. Eglen RM, Reddy H, Watson N, Challis JRA: Muscarinic acetylcholine receptor subtypes in smooth muscle, abstracted. Trends Pharmacol Sci 1994;15:114–119
18. Andersson K-E, Holmquist F, Fovaeus M et al: Muscarinic receptor stimulation of phosphoinositide hydrolysis in the human isolated urinary bladder, abstracted. J Urol 1991;146: 1156–1159
19. Vale P, Barroso C, Afonso F et al: Peptidergic innervation of the human urinary bladder. Neurourol Urodyn 1996;15:372–373
20. Blaivas JG. The bladder as an unreliable witness. Neurourol Urodyn 1996;15:443–445
21. van Waalwijk, van Doorn ES, Remmers A, Janknegt RA: Extramural ambulatory urodynamic monitoring during natural filling and normal daily activities: evaluation of 100 patients. J Urol 1991;146:124–131
22. Tapp JS, Cardozo LD, Versi E, Cooper D: The treatment of detrusor instability in post-menopausal women with oxybutynin chloride: a double-blind placebo-controlled study. Br J Obs Gynaecol 1990;97:521–526
23. Naerger H, Fry CH, Nilvebrant L: Effect of Tolterodine on electrically induced contractions of isolated human detrusor muscle from stable and unstable bladders. Neurourol Urodyn 1995;14: 76–77
24. Wagg AS, Lieu PK, Ding YY, Malone Lee JG: Age-related changes in female urethral function in association with detrusor instability. J Urol 1996;156:1984–1988
25. Lieu PK, Ng KJ, Malone-Lee JG: The voiding/pressure flow plot in the water cystometrogram is useful in inferring the possible existence of urethral sphincter incompetence in women. Neurourol Urodyn 1993;12:308–310
26. Wagg AS, Malone Lee JG: Pressure-flow plot analysis in women with detrusor instability and stress incontinence. Neurourol Urodyn 1995;14:439–440

27. Haylen BT, Parys BT, Anyaegbunam WI et al: Urine flow rates in male and female urodynamic patients compared with the Liverpool nomograms. Br J Urol 1990;65:483–487
28. Hill AV: The heat of shortening and the dynamic constants of muscle. Proc Roy Soc 1938;126:136–195
29. Karram MM: The painful bladder: urethral syndrome and interstitial cystitis. Curr Opin Obstet Gynecol 1990;2:605–611
30. Frazer MI: Idiopathic sensory urgency and early interstitial cystitis. Int Urogynecol J 1993;4:43–49
31. Schafer W: Principles and clinical application of advanced urodynamic analysis of voiding function. Urol Clin North Am 1992; 17:553–566
32. Cannon A, Chambers L, Bartlett E et al: The natural history of bladder outlet obstruction and the long-term follow up of transurethral resection of the prostate. Neurourol Urodyn 1996; 15:381–382
33. Griffiths DJ: Urodynamic assessment of bladder function. Br J Urol 1977;49:29–36
34. International Continence Society: Standardisation of terminology of lower urinary tract function. Neurourol Urodyn 1988;7: 403–426
35. Malone-Lee JG, Wagg A, Mundy A et al: Science of urinary incontinence. Lancet 1994;344:311–315
36. Mundy AR, Stephenson TP, Wein AJ (eds): Urodynamics: Principles, Practice and Application. pp. 89–211. Churchill Livingstone, London, 1994
37. Castleden CM, Duffin HM, Asher MJ: Clinical and urodynamic studies in 100 elderly incontinent patients. BMJ 1981;282: 1103–1105
38. Hilton P, Stanton SL: Algorithmic method of assessing urinary incontinence in elderly women. BMJ 1981;282:940–942
39. Resnick NM, Yalla SV: Detrusor hyperactivity with impaired contractile function: an unrecognised but common cause of incontinence in elderly patients. JAMA 1987;257:3076–3081
40. Collas DM, Malone-Lee JG: Age associated changes in detrusor sensory function in patients with lower urinary tract symptoms. Int Urogynecol J 1996;7:24–29
41. Malone-Lee JG, Wahedna I: Characterisation of detrusor contractile function in relation to Old-Age. Br J Urol 1993;72: 873–880
42. Malone-Lee JG, Orugon O: A data reduction technique for describing and quantifying detrusor instability. Int Urogynecol J 1993;4:204–211
43. Resnick NM, Elbadawi A, Yalla SV: Age and the lower urinary tract: what is normal? Neurourol Urodyn 1995;14:577–579
44. Resnick NM, Yalla SV, Laurino E: The pathophysiology of urinary incontinence among institionalized elderly persons. N Engl J Med 1989;320:1–7
45. Griffiths DJ, McCracken PN, Harrison GM, Gormley EA: Characteristics of urinary incontinence in elderly patients by 24-hour monitoring and urodynamic testing. Age Ageing 1992;21: 194–201
46. Malone-Lee JG. Incontinence. Rev Clin Gerontol 1992;2: 45–61
47. Lieu PK, Ding YY, Choo PWJ: Distinguishing unstable detrusor contractions of bladder outlet obstruction and cerebral disease. Neurourol Urodyn 1996;15:262–263
48. Wagg AS, Bayliss M, Arnold KG, Malone-Lee JG: Urodynamic prognosticators in detrusor instability. Neurourol Urodyn 1996; 15:279–280
49. Griffiths DJ, McCracken PN, Harrison GM et al: Cerebral aetiology of urinary urge incontinence in elderly people. Age Ageing 1994;23:246–250
50. Griffiths DJ, McCracken PN, Harrison GM, Moore KN: Urinary incontinence in the elderly: the brain factor. Scand J Urol Nephrol 1994;157:83–88
51. Elbadawi A, Yalla SV, Resnick NM: Structural basis of geriatric voiding dysfunction. I. methods of a prospective ultrastructural/urodynamic study and an overview of the findings. J Urol 1993; 150:1650–1656
52. Carey M, Sapountzis K, Friedhuber A et al: Electron microscopy study of detrusor muscle cell junctions in women with detrusor instability and controls. Neurourol Urodyn 1996;15:431–432
53. Griffiths DJ: Urodynamics: The Mechanics and Hydrodynamics of the Lower Urinary Tract. Adam Hilger, Bristol, 1980
54. Gray RP, Malone-Lee J: Urinary tract infection in elderly people—time to review management? Age Ageing 1995;24: 341–345
55. Pappas PG: Laboratory in the diagnosis and management of urinary tract infections. Med Clin North Am 1991;75:313–325
56. Hooton TM, Stam WE: Management of acute uncomplicated urinary tract infection in adults. Med Clin North Am 1991;75: 339–357
57. Nicolle LE, Henderson E, Bjornson J et al: The association of bacteriuria with resident characteristics and survival in elderly institutionalized men. Ann Intern Med 1987;106:682–686
58. Nicolle LE, Mayhew JW, Bryan L: Prospective randomised comparison of therapy and no therapy for asymptomatic bacteriuria in institutionalised women. A J Med 1987;83:27–33
59. Orr PH, Nicolle LE, Duckworth H et al: Febrile urinary infection in the institutionalized elderly. A J Med 1996;100:71–77
60. Harari D, Malone-Lee JG, Ridgway GL: An age related investigation of urinary tract symptoms and infection following urodynamic studies. Age Ageing 1994;23:62–64
61. Frewen WK: A reassessment of bladder training in detrusor dysfunction in the female. Br J Urol 1982;54:372–373
62. Jarvis GJ, Millar DR: Controlled trial of bladder drill for detrusor instability. BMJ 1980;281:1322–1323
63. Jarvis GJ, Miller DR: Controlled trial of bladder drill for detrusor instability. BMJ 1980;281:1322–1323
64. Szonyi G, Collas DM, Ding YY, Malone-Lee JG: Oxybutynin with bladder retraining for detrusor instability in elderly people: a randomized controlled trial. Age Ageing 1995;24:287–291
65. Nilvebrant L, Stahl M, Andersson KE: Interaction of Tolterodine with cholinergic muscarinic receptors in human detrusor. Neurourol Urodyn 1995;14:75–76
66. Malone-Lee JG: The clinical efficacy of oxybutynin. Rev Contemp Pharmacother 1995;5:195–202
67. Ouslander JG, Schnelle JF, Uman G et al: Does oxybutynin add to the effectiveness of prompted voiding for urinary incontinence among nursing home residents? a placebo-controlled trial. J Am Geriatr Soc 1995;43:610–617
68. Yarker YE, Goa KL, Fitton A: Oxybutynin: a review of its pharmacodynamic and pharmacokinetic properties, and its therapeutic use in detrusor instability. Drugs Aging 1995;6:243–262

69. Hughes KM, Lang JCT, Lazare R et al: The measurement of oxybutynin and its *N*-desethyl metabolite in plasma and its application to pharmacokinetic studies in young volunteers and elderly and frail elderly volunteers. Xenobiotica 1992;22: 859–864

70. Malone-Lee JG, Lubel D, Szonyi G: Low dose oxybutynin for the unstable bladder. BMJ 1992;304:1053

71. Yarker YE, Goa KL, Fitton A: Oxybutynin: a review of its pharmacodynamic and pharmacokinetic properties, and its therapeutic use in detrusor instability. Drugs Aging 1995;6:243–262

72. Hindmarch I, Alfford C, Barwell F, Kerr JS: Measuring the side effects of psychotropics: the behavioural toxicity of antidepressants. J Psychopharmacol 1992;6:167–173

73. Peterson JS, Patton AJ, Noronha-Blob L: Mini-pig urinary bladder function: comparisons of in vitro anticholinergic responses and in vivo cystometry with drugs indicated for urinary incontinence. J Auton Pharmacol 1990;10:65–73

74. Barker G, Glenning PP: Treatment of the unstable bladder with propantheline and imipramine. Aust N Z J Obstet Gynaecol 1987;27:152–154

75. Castleden CM, Duffin HM, Gulati RS: Double-blind study of imipramine and placebo for incontinence due to bladder instability. Age Ageing 1986;15:299–303

76. Jarvis GJ: A controlled trial of bladder drill and drug therapy in the management of detrusor instability. Br J Urol 1981;53: 565–566

77. Karram MM, Bhatia NN: Management of coexistent stress and urge urinary incontinence. Obstet Gynecol 1989;73:4–7

78. Wall LL: The management of detrusor instability. Clin Obstet Gynecol 1990;33:367–377

79. Bent AE: Etiology and management of detrusor instability and mixed incontinence. Obstet Gynecol Clin North Am 1989;16: 853–868

80. Holmes DM, Montz FJ, Stanton SL: Oxybutinin versus propantheline in the management of detrusor instability: patient-regulated variable dose trial. Br J Obstet Gynaecol 1989;96: 607–612

81. Thuroff JW, Bunke B, Ebner A et al: Randomized, double-blind, multicentre trial on treatment of frequency, urgency and incontinence related to detrusor hyperactivity: oxybutynin versus propantheline versus placebo. J Urol 1991;145:813–817

82. Zorzitto ML, Jewett MAS, Fernie GR et al: Effectiveness of propantheline bromide in the management of geriatric patients with detrusor instability. Neurourol Urodyn 1986;5:133

83. Blaivas JG, Labib KB, Michalik SJ, Zayed AA: Cystometric response to propantheline in detrusor hyperreflexia: therapeutic implications. J Urol 1980;124:259–262

84. Sole GM, Arkell DG: A symptomatic and cystometric comparison of terodiline with emepronium in the treatment of women with frequency, urgency and incontinence. Scand J Urol Nephrol Suppl 1984;87:55–57

85. Perera GL, Ritch AE, Hall MR: The lack of effect of intramuscular emepronium bromide for urinary incontinence. Br J Urol 1982;54:259–260

86. Walter S, Hansen J, Hansen L et al: Urinary incontinence in old age: a controlled clinical trial of emepronium bromide. Br J Urol 1982;54:249–251

87. Williams AJ, Prematalake JK, Palmer RL: A trial of emepronium bromide for the treatment of urinary incontinence in the elderly mentally ill. Pharmatherapeutica 1981;2:539–542

88. Norton P, Karram M, Wall LL et al: Randomized double-blind trial of terodiline in the treatment of urge incontinence in women. Obstetr Gynecol 1994;84:386–391

89. Wiseman PA, Malone Lee J, Rai GS: Terodiline with bladder retraining for treating detrusor instability in elderly people. BMJ 1991;302:994–996

90. Langtry HD, McTavish D: Terodiline: a review of its pharmacological properties and therapeutic use in the treatment of urinary incontinence. Drugs 1990;40:748–761

91. Thomas SH, Higham PD, Hartigan-Go K et al: Concentration dependent cardiotoxicity of terodiline in patients treated for urinary incontinence. Br Heart J 1995;74:53–56

92. van der Klauw MM, van Rey FJ, Stricker BH: Polymorph ventricular tachycardia with torsades de pointes caused by administration of terodiline (Mictrol). Ned Tijdschr Geneeskd 1992; 136:91–93

93. Anonymous: Terodiline and torsades de pointes. BMJ 1991; 303:519–520

94. Ruffmann R: A review of flavoxate hydrochloride in the treatment of urge incontinence. J Intern Med Res 1988;16:317–330

95. Robinson JM, Brocklehurst JC: Emepronium bromide and flavoxate hydrochloride in the treatment of urinary incontinence associated with detrusor instability in elderly women. Br J Urol 1983;55:371–376

96. Lasanen LT, Tammela TL, Kallioinen M, Waris T: Effect of acute distension on cholinergic innervation of the rat urinary bladder. Urol Res 1992;20:59–62

97. Chapple CR, Hampson SJ, Turner Warwick RT, Worth PH: Subtrigonal phenol injection: how safe and effective is it? Br J Urol 1991;68:483–486

98. Flood HD, Malhotra SJ, O'Connell HE, Ritchey MJ et al: Long-term results and complications using augmentation cystoplasty in reconstructive urology. Neurourol Urodyn 1995;14:297–309

99. George VK, Russell GL, Shutt A et al: Clam ileocystoplasty. Br J Urol 1991;68:487–489

100. Singh G, Thomas DG: Intermittent catheterization following enterocystoplasty. Br J Urol 1995;76:175–178

101. Mantle J, Versi E: Physiotherapy for stress urinary incontinence: a national survey. BMJ 1991;302:753–755

102. Mouritsen L, Frimodt Moller C, Moller M: Long-term effect of pelvic floor exercises on female urinary incontinence. Br J Urol 1991;68:32–37

103. Ferguson KL, McKey PL, Bishop KR et al: Stress urinary incontinence: effect of pelvic muscle exercise. Obstet Gynecol 1990; 75:671–675

104. Wilson PD: Conservative management of urethral sphincter incompetence. Clin Obstet Gynecol 1990;33:330–345

105. Herzog AR, Fultz NH, Normolle DP et al: Methods used to manage urinary incontinence by older adults in the community. J Am Geriatr Soc 1989;37:339–347

106. Keating JC Jr, Schulte EA, Miller E: Conservative care of urinary incontinence in the elderly. J Manipulative Physiol Ther 1988;11:300–308

107. Alcalay M, Monga A, Stanton SL: Burch colposuspension: a 10–20 year follow up. Br J Obstet Gynaecol 1995;102:740–745

108. Jarvis GJ: Surgery for genuine stress inconitnence. Br J Obstet Gynaecol 1994;101:371–374
109. Ganabathi K, Abrams P, Mundy AR et al: Stamey-Martius procedure for severe genuine stress incontinence. Br J Urol 1992; 69:34–37
110. Hilton P, Mayne CJ: The Stamey endoscopic bladder neck suspension: a clinical and urodynamic investigation, including actuarial follow-up over four years. Br J Obstet Gynaecol 1991; 98:1141–1149
111. Shortliffe LM, Freiha FS, Kessler R et al: Treatment of urinary incontinence by the periurethral implantation of glutaraldehyde cross-linked collagen. J Urol 1989;141:538–541
112. Mundy AR: Artificial sphincters. Br J Urol 1991;67:225–229
113. Wang Y, Hadley HR: Management of persistent or recurrent urinary incontinence after placement of artificial urinary sphincter. J Urol 1991;146:1005–1006
114. Mundy AR: Artificial sphincters. Br J Urol 1991;67:225–229
115. Hunt GM, Oakeshott P, Whitaker RH: Intermittent catheterisation: simple, safe, and effective but underused. BMJ 1996;312: 103–107
116. Wyndaele JJ, Maes D: Clean intermittent self-catheterization: a 12-year followup. J Urol 1990;143:906–908
117. Klauber GT, Sant GR: Complications of intermittent catheterization. Urol Clin North Am 1983;10:557–562
118. Smith NKG, Morrant JD: Post-operative urinary retention in women: management of intermittent catheterization. Age Ageing 1990;19:337–340
119. Cardozo LD, Kelleher CJ: Sex hormones, the menopause and urinary problems. Gynecol Endocrinol 1995;9:75–84
120. Ouslander JG: Geriatric urinary incontinence. Dis Mon 1992; 38:65–149
121. Cardozo L: Role of estrogens in the treatment of female urinary incontinence. J Am Geriatr Soc 1990;38:326–328
122. Nygaard IE, Johnson JM: Urinary tract infections in elderly women. Am Fam Physician 1996;53:175–182
123. Levin RM: Osteoporosis: prevention is key to management. Geriatrics 1993;48(suppl 1):18–24
124. Molander U, Milsom I, Ekelund P et al: A health care program for the investigation and treatment of elderly women with urinary incontinence and related urogenital symptoms. Acta Obstet Gynecol Scand 1991;70:137–142
125. Stamey A: Recurrent urinary tract infections in female patients: an overview of management and treatment. Rev Infect Dis 1987; 9:S195–S208
126. Cottenden AM, Fader MJ, Barnes KE et al: The clinical performance of incontinence products in relation to technical testing. Proc INSIGHT 1987;2:1–30
127. Cottenden AN, Malone-Lee JG, Butchers D: Technical testing and user requirements for adult incontinence products. Proc INSIGHT 1988;1:1–16
128. Cottenden AM, Fader MJ, Barnes KE et al: The clinical performance of incontinence pads in relation to their design and constitutent materials. Proc TAPPI 1987;1:155–168
129. Avorn J, Monane M, Gurwitz JJ et al: Reduction of bacteriuria and pyuria after ingestion of cranberry juice. JAMA 1994;271: 751–754
130. Abrutyn E, Berlin J, Mossey J et al: Does treatment of asymptomatic bacteriuria in older ambulatory women reduce subsequent symptoms of urinary tract infection? J Am Geriatr Soc 1996;44:293–295
131. Jain P, Parada JP, David A, Smith LG: Overuse of the indwelling urinary tract catheter in hospitalized medical patients. Arch Intern Med 1995;155:1425–1429
132. Sandock DS, Gothe BG, Bodner DR: Trimethoprim-sulfamethoxazole prophylaxis against urinary tract infection in the chronic spinal cord injury patient. Paraplegia 1995;33:156–160
133. Stamm WE: Catheter-associated urinary tract infections: epidemiology, pathogenesis, and prevention. Am J Med 1991;91: 65S–71S
134. Pryor JP: Penile prostheses. pp. 365–372. In Gingell C, Abrams P, (eds): Controversies and Innovations in Urological Surgery. Springer-Verlag, London, 1988

CHAPTER 96

Falls

JOANNA DOWNTON

Falls and their consequences occur at all stages of life but are rightly seen as a particular problem for old people. Falls occur much more commonly in old age, and the elderly are more likely to injure themselves when they do fall. Most deaths due to falls occur in the elderly. The psychological impact of falls on old people is less immediately apparent but equally important. But the very frequency with which falls occur and the wide range of factors that may predispose elderly people to balance problems create difficulties in managing fallers and identifying why falls happen. The problems causing falls may be very specific or completely nonspecific, and a fall may be due to a single cause or, more commonly, to multiple problems. However, by systematically studying falls and incorporating information from the many studies that have been performed, it is possible to devise a logical and helpful way to approach the problem.

Epidemiology of Falls

The epidemiology of falls has been studied extensively over the last 30 years; however, estimates of the prevalence of falling vary widely. There may be genuine large differences in likelihood of falling between and within populations, but the ways in which research has been performed may explain some of the inconsistencies.[1] Studies have used different ways of selecting populations, definitions of falls have varied, and not all studies have taken account of the likelihood that fallers forget or do not report their falls. However, several large, well-designed population studies on elderly people have now been reported, allowing a reliable estimate of the prevalence of falls in community-dwelling older people. These methodologically sound epidemiologic studies on falls indicate an incidence of 28 to 35 percent in those aged 65+,[2–5] 35 percent in those aged 70+,[5,6] and 32 to 42 percent in those aged 75+.[7,8] The healthy elderly fall less frequently—only about 15 percent of a group of fit elderly fell over the course of a year.[9] Those who have already had a fall have a higher rate of falling (60 to 70 percent) in the subsequent year.[10] It is difficult to draw conclusions about the prevalence of falls in the elderly in institutional care, though it is certainly higher. It is estimated that at least 50 percent of elderly people in institutional care are subject to falls.[11]

Complications of Falling (See Also Chs. 44, 85, and 86)

Death

The majority of deaths due to falls occur in those older than 65,[12] and complications caused by falls are the leading cause of death from injury in people older than 65.[13] Death directly as a result of a fall occurs in approximately 2 per 1,000 of the population older than 65 per year, with a higher risk in men than in women and a tendency for risk to increase with age.[14] Almost half of all deaths follow a hip fracture. Falls can also be a marker of increased risk of dying. They were found to be one of a number of predictors of subsequent death in a community study in New Zealand,[15] and fallers had more than double the death rate over 2 years compared to a matched group of nonfallers.[16]

Injury

Injuries following falls are common, occurring in one-third to three-quarters of falls, though most injuries are relatively trivial[10,17,18] and more than half of fallers do not seek medical attention.[8] Most serious injuries and most fractures in the elderly are caused by falling,[19,20] though fractures occur in less than 10 percent of falls.[8,14] There seems to be a higher risk of injury for those individuals who fall away from their home, perhaps because they tend to be members of a healthier, more active group who are likely to suffer more violent falls.[21] The incidence of femoral neck fracture is reported to be approximately 5 per 1,000 population older than 65 per year[22] but varies in different parts of the world.[23] The rate of injury is substantially higher in institutionalized elderly than in those living independently.[24]

Fear of falling

Fear of falling is reported to be at least as common as falls themselves,[7,10,25,26] and although there is a strong association between the two factors, a third of those who had not had a fall the previous year reported that they limited their activity because of fear of falling.[27] In some cases, such fear can have catastrophic effects on mobility and independence.[28] There is some evidence that falls produce symptoms of anxiety and depression,[27,29] and depressive symptoms are common in patients following hip fracture.[30] Falls can have major effects on relatives and caregivers because of implications concerning the need to provide care for the elderly person and the restrictions this may involve. These issues may bring to light problems in the relationship between caregiver and faller.

"Long lie"

Although they may be uninjured, a proportion of elderly fallers are unable to get up without assistance after a fall and may suffer a "long lie." The proportion unable to get up alone has been reported to be as high as 50 percent.[31] A large prospective study of community-living fallers found that 14 percent were unable to get up for at least 5 minutes and 3 percent remained on the floor for more than 20 minutes.[17] Those who are unable to get up are at risk of dehydration, pneumonia, pressure sores, and rhabdomyolysis[32,33] and are older and frailer than those who can get up unaided.[31] They also have a higher risk of death, decline in independence, and requirement for institutional care.[31]

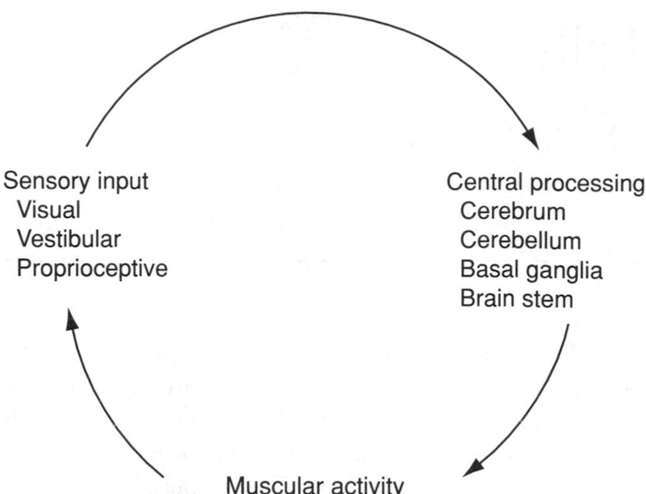

Figure 96-1 Control of balance.

Reduction in activity and independence

Falls lead to old people restricting their activity,[34,35] sometimes because they are advised to by health care workers[17] and sometimes because of continuing pain or disability from injury.[25] Femoral neck is recognized to result in a decline in functional abilities compared with the prefracture state,[36] and there is also evidence that other types of fractures have a significant effect on independence.[37] Those who are frailer and more dependent prior to their injury have worse outcomes, though this can be mitigated by thorough assessment and rehabilitation.[38] Fallers, particularly those who fall repeatedly, are more likely to require institutional care.[39,40]

Balance, Gait, Aging and Falls

Disturbances of gait and balance are covered in detail in Chapter 39 but will be discussed here briefly to aid in understanding some of the factors that predispose the elderly to falling. The upright human is basically unstable, with a small base of support, a high center of mass, and a tendency for any activity to lead to the center of mass being outside the base of support. Any activity increases this imbalance, and a complex neuromuscular system has therefore evolved to maintain balance during all the varied activities associated with everyday life. In simple terms this is a feedback loop (Fig. 96-1) with sensory input from vision, proprioception, and the vestibular apparatus of the inner ear. Many parts of the brain are involved in processing this information, and muscular contractions to adjust balance occur in response to neural impulses from the central control areas. As well as reactive responses to changes in position and balance stresses, there are also anticipatory reflexes with stabilization of the body position before planned movements. These various reactions and reflexes occur in consistent patterns, as in the long-latency postural response producing distal-to-proximal lower limb muscle activation in response to movement of a supporting surface.[41,42]

The sensory input for the balance system provides considerably more information than is normally required. This redundancy of input means that balance can normally be maintained in the absence of some information (e.g., when the eyes are closed), though it may be less finely tuned in these situations. Vision provides the most important sensory information and can normally compensate for the absence or unreliability of other sensory input. Vestibular input is less crucial, being more concerned with visual fixation via the vestibulo-ocular reflex. Proprioceptive input comes from the soles of the feet, the lower limb muscle spindles and joints, and the very rich sensory supply to the cervical spine mechanoreceptors. It is prone to distortion if joints are damaged by arthritis, resulting in sensory conflict which may lead to imbalance and unsteadiness. In young, healthy subjects, infiltration of the cervical spine facet joints with local anesthetic produces vague symptoms of dizziness and unsteadiness similar to those many elderly people complain of.[43,44]

Balance control is thought to be organized on several levels. At the lowest level are the sensory and musculoskeletal systems; the middle level consists of the central processing areas such as the cerebellum, the brain stem, and the motor and sensory cortexes; and the highest level of control resides in the motor planning areas including the frontal lobes. This classification allows gait and balance abnormalities to be described and understood in a way that makes sense of clinical observations.[45]

One of the problems of investigating changes in balance and gait with aging is separating age-related changes from those due to disease since many elderly have accumulated a number of pathologic conditions that may affect balance. Consistent findings in normal elderly subjects are that they demonstrate a small increase in onset latency of long-latency postural reflexes and tend to show reversal of the distal-to-proximal pattern of muscle activation in response to movement of the supporting surface.[42] Studies on responses to perturbations show that the elderly are more likely to use the hip strategy (a proximal-to-distal activation of muscle contraction) which results in more loss of balance.[46]

Healthy elderly tend to walk more slowly than younger adults, with a corresponding reduction in stride length, but have no difficulty initiating walking, no shuffling, and only mild imbalance. It has been suggested that this is better termed a cautious gait[45] than a senile gait[47] since younger people adopt a similar pattern when walking slowly. Factors other than gait and balance problems can affect walking speed, such as cardiovascular fitness,[48] confidence, usual level of activity,[49] and other diseases such as arthritis or other musculoskeletal problems.

Classification of Fallers

There have been several attempts to classify falls and fallers in an effort to detect patterns that will aid in diagnosis and management. The simplest division is between fallers and nonfallers, though some workers have suggested that nonfallers should include those falling less than twice a year.[50,51] There is evidence that these two groups describe two separate populations with substantially different risks of falling.[50] Falls are commonly divided into external or internal types,[5] that is, whether the loss of balance is primarily due to an internal or intrinsic liability to fall or to an extrinsic stress (a trip or a slip). This is complicated by the fact that simple trips and slips, as well as internal falls, are also common in the balance-impaired elderly. However, it seems appropriate that nontrip falls should stimulate a more thorough search for health problems underlying the fall.

Factors Associated with Falls

It is possible to find studies showing an association between practically any factor and falls and almost as many showing that such factors are not associated. It is not clear whether falls are random, unpredictable accidents or whether it is possible to pick out those who will fall from those who will not. Many factors are implicated, and it seems likely that combinations of factors are more important than single problems. Many factors are interdependent, for example, age and cognitive function, confusion and dependency, and neurologic disease and abnormal gait, and therefore multivariate analysis is required to determine independent associations. This has rarely been done, and therefore the relative risk of any particular factor cannot be estimated. Studies using multivariate analysis have shown limited ability to predict who would be classified as a faller or a nonfaller even when used retrospectively on the population from which the factors were derived.[2,4]

Virtually all studies have shown increasing risk of falling with increasing age, and most have shown women to be more likely to fall than men, though the reverse may be true in hospital populations.[52] In some studies the very elderly have a lower prevalence, perhaps because of selective survival of a particularly fit cohort.[3,53] Among those in institutional care, the young elderly (those under 75 years old) seem to be more prone to falling.[54,55] The presence of multiple illnesses also seems to predispose to falls.[56,57] Living alone,[2,3,10] spending the greater part of the day alone,[10] and living in specialized housing for the elderly[11] have been identified as risk factors for falls, though it is likely that they are merely markers for physical or other problems increasing the risk of falling.

Psychological factors may increase an individual's risk of falling. Cognitive impairment may cause lack of insight into problems, leading to poor compliance with medical treatment or advice; depression can result in poor concentration and failure to appreciate risks; and occasionally falls may be a manifestation of attention-seeking behavior.[58] Fear of falling may lead to extensive restriction of activity, which can increase the risk of falling because of the deconditioning effect of lack of activity.[59,60] Several studies have shown anxiety and/or depression to be risk factors for falling.[2,9,11,57]

Causes of Falls

Age-related Factors

It is difficult to separate the changes in gait and postural stability due to age alone from those caused by pathology. However, a proportion of the very elderly appear to retain normal balance and gait.[61] One of the important age-related changes that may predispose older people to falling is the tendency toward slowing of central integrative mechanisms important for postural reflexes.[62,63] Aging seems to reduce processing capacity and impair the ability to divide attention. Thus the appropriate allocation of central processing resources among concurrent tasks is upset.[62] If concentration is distracted, for example, by another cognitive task, there is slower recovery from postural perturbation.[64] Objective measurement has shown some association between impaired gait and balance and risk of falling,[65] though this has not always been useful in predicting who will fall.[66]

Specific Diseases

1. *Epilepsy*: Epilepsy increases in prevalence with increasing age and is often associated with loss of consciousness; thus it may be a cause of falls. Without a description from a reliable witness, diagnosis can be difficult. Epilepsy is discussed in Chapter 31.

2. *Parkinson's disease*: Parkinson's disease has long been recognized as a potent cause of falls.[67,68] Disturbance of posture and equilibrium is one of the cardinal signs of the disease, and a number of gait abnormalities are common.[69] Parkinson's disease is discussed in Chapter 38.

3. *Myopathies and peripheral neuropathies*: Lower limb weak-

ness has been shown to be a risk factor for falling.[70,71]; thus myopathies and motor neuropathies, especially those affecting the lower limbs, may result in falls. Sensory neuropathies can contribute to falls because of degradation of postural sensory information.

4. *Cardiogenic syncope*: Cardiac arrhythmias have been shown in some studies to be associated with a higher risk of falls[72] and fractures,[73] though this connection has been disputed.[74] Recent work suggests that a significant number of fallers may have cardiac arrhythmias precipitated by carotid sinus hypersensitivity.[75,76] This topic is discussed in Chapters 26 and 32.

5. *Cervical spondylosis*: There are two ways in which this condition may predispose a person to falling. Impairment of proprioceptive input from the cervical spine mechanoreceptors is a source of symptoms of vague dizziness and imbalance in elderly sufferers,[44] and cervical myelopathy with associated lower limb spasticity may affect gait adversely, particularly producing a tendency to trip.

6. *Normal pressure hydrocephalus*: The hallmark of this disorder is an abnormality of gait together with cognitive impairment and urinary incontinence.[77,78] Both the gait abnormality and the cognitive impairment predispose to falling, and as the condition progresses, a "frontal gait disorder" develops (see below).

7. *Dementia*: Demented subjects are at high risk of falling. Impairment on simple mental test scores has been shown in fallers compared with nonfallers.[2,3] A case-control study found three times as many falls in a demented group as in controls.[79] Lack of insight into their limitations is almost universal in such individuals and creates significant problems in independent living. It is possible that impaired balance mechanisms occur as part of the neurologic deterioration associated with dementia.[80] Dementia sufferers are at significantly higher risk of fracturing a hip than those with normal cognitive function.[81]

8. *Autonomic dysfunction or postural hypotension*: Autonomic dysfunction is not very common in healthy community-dwelling elderly but can be a potent cause of falls because of postural hypotension.[82] Autonomic failure is discussed in Chapter 37. Postural hypotension without autonomic failure seems to be more common and can be precipitated by drugs, fluid depletion, or immobilization.

Falling syndromes

1. *Multiple sensory deficits*: It is likely that some of the symptoms of dizziness, imbalance, and falls in the frailer elderly are related to multiple, sometimes relatively minor, deficits in a number of sensory systems.[42] Individual deficits increase the likelihood of falling, but combinations of deficits can compound the problem.

2. *Cerebrovascular disease*: This condition can produce a variety of disorders associated with a high risk of falling. Multi-infarct dementia commonly results in gait disorder as well as cognitive impairment, both of which predispose to falling. Stroke itself significantly increases the risk of falling.[83] Fallers are much more likely to show white matter hypodensity on a computed tomography scan than nonfallers, and much of it is due to vascular ischemic damage.[84]

3. *Frontal lobe gait and balance disorders*: A variety of these have been described, and the terminology is not always used consistently. A recent review has produced a more systematic classification, though there seems to be some overlap between the categories.[45] These disorders are often associated with falls, and a simple clinical assessment of gait and balance (see below) can demonstrate difficulties in gait ignition, unsteadiness on turning, irregularity of gait cadence, and/or shuffling gait.

4. *Drop attacks*: These attacks have been recognized for many years[85] but are not well understood. The term tends to be used as a convenient description for any sudden falling attack, but idiopathic drop attacks need to be distinguished from symptomatic drop attacks due to such conditions as epilepsy, cataplexy, and focal structural central nervous system lesions.[86] Idiopathic drop attacks have been defined as "falling without warning, not associated with loss of consciousness, not apparently due to any malfunction of legs, not induced by changes of posture or movement of the head, and not accompanied by vertigo or other cephalic sensation, not associated with myoclonic jerks."[87] It is difficult to be certain about the etiology since studies on the phenomenon have rarely been rigorous in excluding symptomatic drop attacks. The main theories are that they are due to abnormalities in postural function or to transient dysfunction of the brain stem centers in the reticular formation controlling tone in the antigravity muscles.[88] True idiopathic drop attacks appear to have a good prognosis[89] other than the risk of injury sustained during the fall.

Drugs

It is difficult to separate the effects of drugs from the effects of the diseases for which they are prescribed, but it seems that consumption of any drug is associated with an increase in the likelihood of falling.[3] Drugs may have an effect on postural stability because of their central depressant effect (e.g., minor tranquillizers, sedatives, hypnotics), because they may cause postural hypotension (e.g., antihypertensives, anti-Parkinsonian drugs), or both (e.g., tricyclic antidepressants, major tranquillizers). In each of these cases, an association has been found between consumption of the drug and either falling or fractures secondary to falls.[2,4,7,90,91] Drugs for which there is most compelling evidence that they increase the likelihood of falling are benzodiazepines and tricyclic antidepressants. In the case of benzodiazepines the argument for limiting new prescriptions and withdrawing the drug from long-term users to prevent falls and fractures is strong.[90] There may also be risks with other drugs, for example, nonsteroidal anti-inflammatory drugs which can produce symptoms of dizziness in elderly people.[92]

The evidence concerning diuretics is conflicting. Some investigators claim that thiazides protect against fracture because of their hypocalciuric effect[93] despite being associated with a high incidence of symptoms of dizziness, fainting, and blacking out,[94] while others have found an association between thiazide intake and femoral fracture.[95] The relationship between alcohol consumption and falls, particularly in the elderly, has been little studied.[96] It seems likely, however, that alcohol increases the risk of falling since it tends to increase postural instability.[97] No association was found between fall injury events and self-reported alcohol use,[98] though it is a significant risk factor for head injury.[99] A study measuring breath or blood alcohol in elderly fallers admitted to an emergency room found that only 6 percent had any evidence of recent alcohol ingestion.[100]

Environmental Factors

Environmental factors are recognized to be important in the causation of falls,[101] though separating intrinsic and extrinsic causes is difficult. It seems that environmental factors predominate in about a third of falls,[102] though the proportion is less in the very elderly.[103] The environment can combine with intrinsic factors to increase the risk of falling. Studies on the interaction of vision and surroundings demonstrate the problems that elderly people may have negotiating stairs if their vision is impaired or lighting levels are low.[104,105]

In hospitals and institutions higher staffing levels may reduce fall frequency.[106] However, very low staffing levels may be associated with fewer falls because activity is discouraged.[107] There is a suggestion that environmental temperature affects the risk of falling, at least in women,[108] though this may occur only in thin or undernourished women, perhaps because of a relationship between nutritional state and thermoregulation.[109]

Acute Ill Health

Falling is one of the "geriatric giants," being one of the common ways in which acute ill health may be manifested nonspecifically in the elderly. One reason for this may be that in the frail elderly person, cerebral perfusion may normally be impaired by an accumulation of chronic health problems such as heart failure, cerebrovascular disease, lung disease, and so on, so that even when the person is relatively well cerebral perfusion is only just above the level required for maintenance of consciousness.[110] Any acute illness can cause a transient drop in cerebral perfusion (e.g., because of hypotension) sufficient to result in transient impairment of consciousness and a fall. It is therefore important to consider the possibility of acute ill health in any older person who has fallen.

Clinical Management of Fallers

There is always a reason why someone falls. It is usually possible to determine at least some of the factors that have caused the fall, and it is often possible to do something about some or all of them to reduce the risk of further falls.[111] Any fall is the result of an interaction of a number of factors. The question that needs to be answered is why a particular person

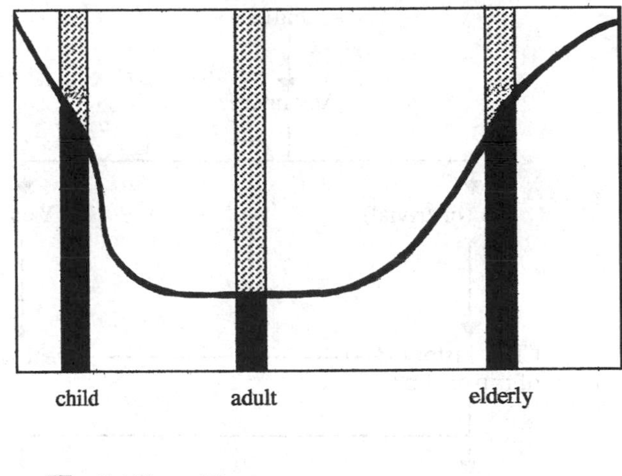

Figure 96-2 Liability versus opportunity to fall at different ages.

fell at a particular time in a particular place. This implies that there are internal and external (environmental) factors, both of which may be fixed or variable with time. For a fall to occur, there must be an opportunity as well as a liability to fall. The relative contributions of liability and opportunity vary at different ages (Fig. 96-2) and contribute to the different rates of falling with age. They also vary in an individual from moment to moment depending on tiredness, concentration, health factors, and so on. Almost any medical condition can increase an elderly person's risk of falling; conversely, not everyone with a particular problem suffers falls.

There are two main elements in the management of falls. First, there is assessment and management of the faller once a fall has taken place, and second, there is a general evaluation of both the elderly person and their environment to look for factors increasing the risk of falls and injury. Assessment of fallers, particularly at the time of or shortly after the fall, is obviously necessary to detect any injury, but it is also often possible to detect potentially treatable causes or predisposing factors for falls (Fig. 96-3).

Clearly, the first priority is to deal with any injury sustained. Once the patient's condition is stabilized, the question of what caused the fall can be addressed. A proportion of falls at any age occur for predominantly external reasons—so-called trips or slips. Changes with aging may make trips or slips more likely because of changes in gait and postural reflexes, and they may make falls more likely if trips or slips occur because of slowed reactions and impaired righting reflexes. A note of caution is needed here—there is often an element of rationalization: "I fell. People fall because they trip. Therefore I must have tripped." If the patient says, "I *must have* tripped," then it is very likely that they did not trip. If, however, they are able to describe clearly the cause of the fall and the circumstances leading up to it (e.g., tripping over uneven paving stones, slipping on a patch of ice), then the fall can more confidently be

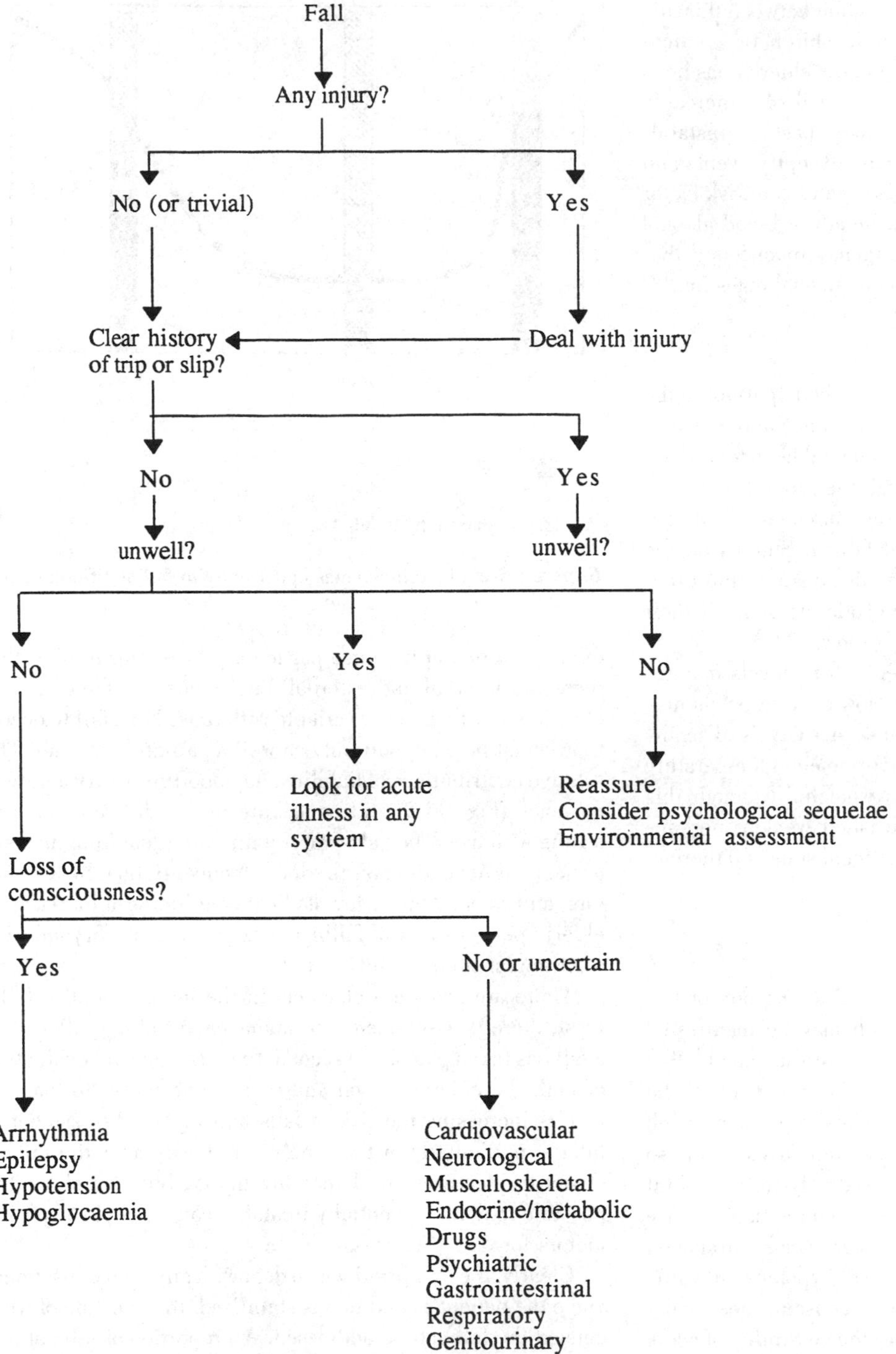

Figure 96-3 Management of a faller.

ascribed to a trip or a slip. Another caution is that ill health may mean that an elderly person is more likely to trip, as well as to suffer a nontrip fall, and it is therefore important that the possibility of an underlying illness be considered even if the fall was clearly due to a simple trip. If the fall is of a nonspecific or nontrip type, the next question to consider is whether it was the manifestation of an acute illness of any type. If this does not seem to be the case, then the wide range of potential causative or contributory factors should be considered.

History

An elderly person who has had a fall should be asked to describe what happened. A general question such as "Why did you fall?" or "What caused your fall?" may not provide much helpful information, though people who have had a straightforward trip or slip are likely to be able to describe the circumstances of their fall in response to such questions. More useful questions include the following:

- What were you doing at the time of your fall (e.g., walking, standing still, getting up from a chair, etc.)?
- Were you feeling quite well before you fell?
- Did you notice any symptoms (e.g., dizziness, palpitation, chest pain, visual disturbance) prior to or following your fall?
- Did you black out or lose consciousness when you fell?

Terms such as *dizziness* or *palpitations* need to be carefully defined, as they may be used to describe a number of different sensations.

The description of the fall obtained from the faller may be very vague or even nonexistent, and in the absence of a witness it is often difficult to know how much reliance to place on it, particularly if there is any cognitive impairment. Loss of consciousness may not be remembered.[76] If witnesses are available, particularly if it is possible to interview them shortly after the fall, as much information as possible should be obtained about the circumstances of the fall, the appearance of the faller, whether there was any loss of consciousness, and so on, and whether there have been previous similar episodes.

An inquiry about the faller's normal functional status is helpful. The likely causes of a fall in someone who is normally poorly mobile and very dependent may well be different from those in a healthy, independent elderly person. Because of the wide range of potential causes of falls and the fact that various factors may interact to produce an increased risk of falling, a thorough medical history is usually necessary. Drug treatment has been clearly implicated in causing some falls, and so medication must be reviewed.

Examination

In many cases a full medical examination is appropriate, particularly if the fall seems to be due to acute illness, which may be of any type. It is also often appropriate in the assessment of someone having recurrent falls, where again the problem or problems may be in any body system. Special attention should be paid to the cardiovascular, neurologic, and musculoskeletal systems. Specific factors that may be useful in the examination of someone who has fallen are shown in the accompanying boxed list.

Assessment of balance, gait, and mobility in the elderly has been studied extensively.[112] Many of the assessments devised are complex and time-consuming and, although very thorough, are unsuitable for day-to-day use in clinical assessment. There are, however, a number of simple balance and gait assessments suitable for use in clinical situations, and some of them can be carried out routinely in the assessment of elderly fallers. The simplest test is the Romberg test, which demonstrates stability on standing with the feet together, with eyes open and closed. There is normally more sway with closed eyes, but loss of balance when the eyes are closed suggests vestibular and/or proprioceptive impairment with over-reliance on vision to maintain static posture. Stability can be stressed by a gentle push on the sternum,[113] and the patient's response to this indicates the state of the postural and protective responses. Dynamic postural control can be tested using "functional reach," where the subject stands still and reaches forward as far as possible along a fixed rule.[114] This has been shown to correlate with other measures of mobility and balance and with risk of falling.[115] A simple assessment of gait and mobility is the timed walk, recording either the time taken to complete a given distance or the distance walked in a given time.[116,117] This test can be used to monitor response to treatment. A composite measure of balance and gait can be made using the "get up and go" test[118] with the more refined "timed up and go" test[119] if serial measures are needed to monitor response to treatment. Simple measures of balance, gait, and mobility should be part of the assessment of all elderly fallers.

Examination of a faller–specific factors

Pulse rate and rhythm
Supine and standing blood pressure
Mental status
Visual acuity and visual fields
Muscle power, especially in lower limbs
Neck movements (limitation, precipitating dizziness)
Knee joint stability
Foot deformities
Romberg test
"Get up and go" test (see text)

Management of Fallers

Treatment

Once any injury has been dealt with, treatment of a faller is dictated by the assessment of the cause of the fall. Identification of specific medical factors as probable causes should lead to these factors being improved by appropriate intervention, such as discontinuing an offending drug. In situations where the cause seems predominantly external, environmental assessment by an occupational therapist may be useful to identify potential risks, though people are often reluctant to make adaptations to their surroundings. It is impossible to get rid of all risks, and attempts to do so may lead to unacceptable restrictions on the autonomy of elderly people.

Gait assessment and retraining by a physiotherapist may be helpful, though the only reported study on physiotherapy for fallers failed to show a clear benefit.[120] Teaching someone how to get up after a fall may avoid the potentially dangerous "long lie" if further falls occur and is often of psychological benefit to the faller, though either the faller or the therapist may be reluctant to undertake this type of training.[121] Providing some sort of alarm device, particularly a body-worn one, may also help to prevent debilitating fear of future falls and reassure the faller and their relatives or caregivers that help will be summoned if a fall occurs.

Rehabilitation

Rehabilitation of fallers needs to be adapted to individuals and the specific problems they have. This implies that the first step is full assessment of the causes of the fall and the particular medical and functional difficulties of the individual. There also should be an awareness of the effects (both physical and psychological) of the fall. One of the most difficult problems is that fallers may have a degree of cognitive impairment and thus may not fully appreciate their limitations. Since there are many potential reasons for falling, no general recommendations can be made. Many fallers have abnormalities of balance or gait, and input from a physiotherapist along with graded balance and mobility exercises may be helpful.[122] It is often useful to visit the home of the faller to assess whether there are any alterable risk factors in their environment, though recent work suggests that the approach of reducing home hazards has been over-rated.[123,124]

Prevention of Falls

Because of the frequency of falls and their complications in older people, the prevention of falls is an important public health issue. Primary prevention may be possible in some circumstances. For example, elderly people in institutional care seem to be at particular risk of falling. Assessment of such populations and of their environment may yield remediable factors that affect accident risk. Such assessment should occur when someone first enters institutional care and should also be part of the regular monitoring of all residents. The value of this procedure is suggested by a study on institutionalized subjects with Alzheimer's disease in whom a changing level of dependency was a clear risk factor for falls.[125] It is possible that determining "risk scores" might be useful in detecting those who are likely to fall,[126] though it is probable that large proportions would be classified as high risk.[127] Both falls and fractures can probably be reduced by a healthier diet and lifestyle during youth and middle age since this would result in higher bone mass and better balance and postural reflexes.

For the elderly population as a whole, general strategies in primary prevention may reap benefits. Maintaining physical fitness as far as possible by regular exercise sessions can reduce risk of falling and injury by improving muscular function,[128] limiting osteoporosis, and possibly maintaining cognitive function.[129]

Secondary prevention is perhaps a more useful strategy. People who have actually suffered a fall have demonstrated an increased tendency to fall, and it is usually possible to identify one or more factors that increase their risk of falling. Much secondary prevention could take place on an opportunistic or case-finding basis, as many elderly people are in contact with their general practitioners. Elderly people who visit emergency rooms following a fall also comprise a high-risk group that merits attention.

There is now valid, research-based advice available on how to prevent falls in the elderly population. There is evidence that those at higher risk of falling can be identified by a simple assessment of risk factors.[17,126,130–132] Multifactorial assessment and intervention seem to benefit the frailer elderly,[16] and the fitter elderly seem to benefit from exercise that includes a balance component.[133,134]

In 1990 a large multicenter set of studies was set up in the United States to investigate a number of issues relating to falls and fall-related injuries in older people. The Frailty and Injuries Cooperative Study of Intervention Techniques (FICSIT) was an ambitious attempt to answer some of the questions relating to treatment and prevention of frailty, falls, and injuries in the elderly.[135] In total, over 2,300 subjects were enrolled in nine studies examining various types of assessment and intervention in both healthy and frail subjects. Each study had a specific focus, and most had primary outcome measures relating to balance, falls, and injuries. A planned meta-analysis was carried out to try to answer questions about the prevention and treatment of falls.[133]

Results from some of the FICSIT studies suggest that a number of interventions are useful in preventing falls in various groups of older people. In community-living elderly, multiple risk factor intervention (e.g., adjustment in medication, behavioral instructions, exercise programs, correction of visual and hearing impairment, identification of environmental hazards) intended to reduce any risk factors identified has been shown to be effective in significantly reducing the risk of falling.[136–138] Exercises of various types can improve lower limb strength, reaction time, neuromuscular control, amount of sway, gait velocity, and overall levels of physical activity both in frail institutionalized elderly[139] and in healthy community-living elderly.[134] Exercise programs can also improve the ability to perform daily tasks.[140] However, the effect on falling is small, with significant reductions in only specific types of falls such as nonaccidental falls, falls due to loss of balance, and multiple falls.[134] Exercises including a balance component (e.g., tai chi) seem particularly useful in preventing falls.[133] As secondary prevention, a postfall assessment with intervention to deal with risk factors for falling and any underlying health problems can have a significant effect on the need for subsequent hospitalization and a small effect on the risk of further falls.[16]

Assessment of the home to detect hazardous factors is probably not a particularly useful element in the prevention of falls since falls are not strongly associated with the presence of home hazards,[123,124] except in the vigorous elderly whose risk of falling is otherwise fairly low.[123] If one accepts that it is not possible to prevent all falls, it may be worthwhile considering what can be done to prevent or reduce injury due to falls. Simple hip protectors have been shown to reduce the incidence of hip fractures in an institutional group at high risk of falling[141] though more work is needed to make the devices more acceptable to frail elderly.[142] It is also useful to look at floor coverings, as the surface on which someone falls affects the likelihood of injury. There is still much to be done in the area of fall prevention.[143]

It is important to remember that although much can be done to reduce the risk of falling in populations and in individuals, it is not possible to prevent all falls and that unrealistic attempts to do so may have a detrimental effect on quality of life in the frailer elderly. It is important to remain realistic and accept that some risk is unavoidable if life is to remain worth living.[144]

References

1. Downton J: The problems of epidemiological studies of falls. Clin Rehabil 1987;1:243–246
2. Campbell AJ, Reinken J, Allan BC, Martinez GS: Falls in old age: a study of frequency and related clinical factors. Age Ageing 1981;10:264–270
3. Prudham D, Evans JG: Factors associated with falls in the elderly: a community study. Age Ageing 1981;10:141–146
4. Blake AJ, Morgan K, Bendall MJ et al: Falls by elderly people at home: prevalence and associated factors. Age Ageing 1988; 17:365–372
5. Campbell AJ, Borrie MJ, Spears GF et al: Circumstances and consequences of falls experienced by a community population 70 years and over during a prospective study. Age Ageing 1990; 19:136–141
6. Campbell AJ, Borrie MJ, Spears GF: Risk factors for falls in a community-based prospective study of people 70 years and older. J Gerontol 1989;44:M112–117
7. Tinetti ME, Speechley M, Ginter SF: Risk factors for falls among elderly persons living in the community. N Engl J Med 1988; 319:1701–1707
8. Downton JH, Andrews K: Prevalence, characteristics and factors associated with falls among the elderly living at home. Aging 1991;3:219–228
9. Gabell A, Simons MA, Nayak USL: Falls in the healthy elderly: predisposing causes. Ergonomics 1985;28:965–975
10. Nevitt MC, Cummings SR, Kidd S, Black D: Risk factors for recurrent non-syncopal falls: a prospective study. JAMA 1989; 261:2663–2668
11. Tinetti ME, Speechley M: Prevention of falls amongst the elderly. N Engl J Med 1989;320:1055–1059
12. Waller JA: Injury in aged: clinical and epidemiological implications. N Y State J Med 1974;74:2200–2208
13. Sattin RW: Falls among older persons: a public health perspective. Ann Rev Public Health 1992;13:489–508
14. Sattin RW, Lambert Huber DA, DeVito CA et al: The incidence of fall injury events among the elderly in a defined population. Am J Epidemiol 1990;131:1028–1037
15. Campbell AJ, Diep C, Reinken J, McCosh L: Factors predicting mortality in a total population sample of the elderly. J Epidemiol Community Health 1985;39:337–342
16. Rubenstein LZ, Robbins AS, Josephson KR et al: The value of assessing falls in an elderly population: a randomized clinical trial. Ann Intern Med 1990;113:308–316
17. Nevitt MC, Cummings SR, Hudes ES: Risk factors for injurious falls: a prospective study. J Gerontol 1991;46:M164–M170
18. O'Loughlin JL, Robitaille Y, Boivin JF, Suissa S: Incidence of and risk factors for falls and injurious falls among the community-dwelling elderly. Am J Epidemiol 1993;137:342–354
19. Oreskovich MR, Howard JD, Copass MK, Carrico CJ: Geriatric trauma: injury patterns and outcome. J Trauma 1984;24: 565–572
20. Melton LJ III, Riggs BL: Epidemiology of age-related fractures. pp. 1–30. In LV Alvioli (ed): The Osteoporotic Syndrome. Grune & Stratton, New York, 1987
21. Speechley M, Tinetti M: Falls and injuries in frail and vigorous community elderly persons. J Am Geriatr Soc 1991;39:46–52
22. Evans JG, Prudham D, Wandless I: A prospective study of fractured proximal femur: incidence and outcome. Public Health 1979;93:235–241
23. Lewinnek GE, Kelsey J, White AA, Kreiger NJ: The significance and a comparative analysis of the epidemiology of hip fractures. Clin Orthop 1980;152:35–43
24. Luukinen H, Koski K, Honkanen R, and Kivela SL: Incidence of injury-causing falls among older adults by place of residence: a population-based study. J Am Geriatr Soc 1995;43:871–876
25. Grisso JA, Schwarz DF, Wolfson V et al: The impact of falls in an inner-city elderly African-American population. J Am Geriatr Soc 1992;40:673–678
26. Maki BE, Holiday PJ, Topper AK: Fear of falling and postural performance in the elderly. J Gerontol 1991;46:M123–M131
27. Downton JH, Andrews K: Postural disturbance and psychological symptoms amongst elderly people living at home. Int J Geriatr Psychiatry 1990;5:93–98
28. Murphy J, Isaacs B: The post-fall syndrome: a study of 36 elderly patients. Gerontology 1982;28:265–270
29. Vetter NJ, Ford D: Anxiety and depression scores in elderly fallers. Int J Geriatr Psychiatry 1989;4:159–163
30. Billig N, Ahmed SW, Kenmore P et al: Assessment of depression and cognitive impairment after hip fracture. J Am Geriatr Soc 1986;34:499–503
31. Tinetti ME, Liu WL, Claus EB: Predictors and prognosis of inability to get up after falls among elderly persons. JAMA 1993; 269:65–70
32. Wild D, Nayak USL, Isaacs B: How dangerous are falls in old people at home? BMJ 1981;282:266–268
33. Mallinson WJW, Green MF: Covert muscle injury in aged patients admitted to hospital following falls. Age Ageing 1985; 14:174–178
34. Vellas B, Cayla F, Bocquet H et al: Prospective study of restriction of activity in old people after falls. Age Ageing 1987;16: 189–193
35. Kosorok MR, Omenn GS, Diehr P et al: Restricted activity days among older adults. Am J Public Health 1992;82:1263–1267
36. Marotolli RA, Berkman LF, Cooney LM: Decline in physical function following hip fracture. J Am Geriatr Soc 1992;40: 861–866
37. Greendale GA, Barrett-Connor E, Ingles S, Haile R: Late physi-

cal and functional effects of osteoporotic fracture in women: the Rancho Bernardo study. J Am Geriatr Soc 1995;43:955–961

38. Bernardini B, Meinecke C, Pagani M et al: Comorbidity and adverse clinical events in the rehabilitation of older adults after hip fracture. J Am Geriatr Soc 1995;43:894–898
39. Baker SP, Harvey AH: Fall injuries in the elderly. Clin Geriatr Med 1985;1:501–508
40. Dunn JE, Furner SE, Miles TP: Do falls predict institutionalization in older persons? J Aging Health 1993;5:194–207
41. Woollacott MH, Shumway-Cook A, Nashner LM: Aging and posture control: changes in sensory organization and muscular coordination. Int J Aging Hum Dev 1986;23:97–114
42. Manchester D, Woollacott M, Zederbauer-Hylton N, Marin O: Visual, vestibular and somatosensory contributions to balance control in the older adult. J Gerontol 1989;44:M118–M127
43. de Jong PTVM, de Jong JMBV, Cohen B, Jongkees LBW: Ataxia and nystagmus induced by injection of local anaesthetics in the neck. Ann Neurol 1977;1:240–246
44. de Jong JMBV, Bles W: Cervical dizziness and ataxia. In Bles W, Brandt T (eds): Disorders of Posture and Gait. Elsevier Science Publishers, Amsterdam, 1986
45. Nutt JG, Marsden CD, Thompson PD: Human walking and higher-level gait disorders, particularly in the elderly. Neurology 1993;43:268–279
46. Horak FB, Shupert CL, Mirka A: Components of postural dyscontrol in the elderly: a review. Neurobiol Aging 1989;10: 727–738
47. Koller WC, Glatt SL, Fox JH: Senile gait: a distinct neurological entity. Clin Geriatr Med 1985;1:661–668
48. Cunningham DA, Rechnitzer PA, Pearce ME, Donner AP: Determinants of self-selected walking pace across ages 19–66. J Gerontol 1982;37:560–564
49. Imms FJ, Edholm OG: Studies of gait and mobility in the elderly. Age Ageing 1981;10:147–156
50. Campbell AJ, Spears GF: Fallers and non-fallers. Age Ageing 1990;19:345–346
51. Evans JG: Fallers, non-fallers and Poisson. Age Ageing 1990; 19:268–269
52. Berry G, Fisher RH, Lang S: Detrimental incidents, including falls, in an elderly institutional population. J Am Geriatr Soc 1981;29:322–324
53. Woodhouse PR, Briggs RS, Ward D: Falls and disability in old people's homes. J Clin Exp Gerontol 1983;5:309–321
54. Gryfe CI, Amies A, Ashley MJ: A longitudinal study of falls in an elderly population. I. incidence and morbidity. Age Ageing 1977;6:201–210
55. Haga H, Shibata H, Shichita K et al: Falls in the institutionalised elderly in Japan. Arch Gerontol Geriatr 1986;5:1–9
56. Morse JM, Tylko SJ, Dixon HA: Characteristics of the fall-prone patient. Gerontologist 1987;27:516–522
57. Granek E, Baker SP, Abbey H et al: Medications and diagnoses in relation to falls in a long-term care facility. J Am Geriatr Soc 1987;35:503–511
58. Belfield PW, Young JB, Bagnall WE, Mulley GP: Deliberate falls in the elderly. Age Ageing 1987;16:123–124
59. Harper CM, Lyles YM: Physiology and complications of bed rest. J Am Geriatr Soc 1988;36:1047–1054
60. Creditor MC: Hazards of hospitalization of the elderly. Ann Intern Med 1993;118:219–223
61. Bloem BR, Haan J, Lagaay AM et al: Investigation of gait in elderly subjects over 88 years of age. J Geriatr Psychiatry Neurol 1992;5:78–84
62. Teasdale N, Stelmach GE, Bard C, Fleury M: Posture and elderly persons: deficits in the central integrative mechanisms. In Woollacott M, Horak F (eds): Posture and Gait: Control Mechanisms. University of Oregon, Portland, 1992
63. Stelmach GE, Worringham CJ: Sensorimotor deficits related to postural stability: implications for falling in the elderly. Clin Geriatr Med 1985;1:679–694
64. Stelmach GE, Zelaznik HN, Lowe D: The influence of aging and attentional demands on recovery from postural instability. Aging 1990;2:155–161
65. Maki BE, Holliday PJ, Topper AK: A prospective study of postural balance and risk of falling in an ambulatory and independent elderly population. J Gerontol 1994;49:M72–M84
66. Fernie GR, Gryfe CI, Holliday PJ, Llewellyn A: The relationship of postural sway in standing to the incidence of falls in geriatric subjects. Age Ageing 1982;11:11–16
67. Klawans HL, Topel JL: Parkinsonism as a falling sickness. JAMA 1974;230:1555–1557
68. Bloem BR: Postural instability in Parkinson's disease. Clin Neurol Neurosurg 1992;94(suppl):S41–S45
69. Brown P, Steiger MJ: Basal ganglia gait disorders. In Bronstein AM, Brandt T, Woollacott M (eds): Clinical disorders of Balance, Posture and Gait. Edward Arnold, London, 1996
70. Tinetti ME: Factors associated with serious injury during falls by ambulatory nursing home residents. J Am Geriatr Soc 1987; 35:644–648
71. Whipple RH, Wolfson LI, Amerman PM: The relationship of knee and ankle weakness to falls in nursing home residents: an isokinetic study. J Am Geriatr Soc 1987;35:13–20
72. Gordon M: Occult cardiac arrhythmias associated with falls and dizziness in the elderly: detection by Holter monitoring. J Am Geriatr Soc 1978;26:418–423
73. Abdon NJ, Nilsson BE: Episodic cardiac arrhythmia and femoral neck fracture. Acta Med Scand 1980;208:73–76
74. Clarke PI, Glasser SP, Spoto E: Arrhythmias detected by ambulatory monitoring: lack of correlation with symptoms of dizziness and syncope. Chest 1980;77:722–725
75. Kenny RA, Traynor G: Carotid sinus syndrome—clinical characteristics in elderly patients. Age Ageing 1991;20:449–454
76. McIntosh SJ, Lawson J, Kenny RA: Clinical characteristics of vasodepressor, cardioinhibitory, and mixed carotid sinus syndrome in the elderly. Am J Med 1993;95:203–208
77. Knutsson E, Lying-Tunell U: Gait apraxia in normal pressure hydrocephalus: patterns of movement and muscle activation. Neurology 1985;35:155–160
78. Sorensen PS, Jansen EC, Gjerris F: Motor disturbances in normal pressure hydrocephalus: special reference to stance and gait. Arch Neurol 1986;43:34–38
79. Morris JC, Rubin EH, Morris EJ, Mandel SA: Senile dementia of the Alzheimer's type: an important risk factor for serious falls. J Gerontol 1987;42:412–417
80. Visser H: Gait and balance in senile dementia of Alzheimer's type. Age Ageing 1983;12:296–301

81. Melton LJ, Beard CM, Kokmen E et al: Fracture risk in patients with Alzheimer's disease. J Am Geriatr Soc 1994;42:614–619
82. Mader SL, Josephson KR, Rubenstein LZ: Low prevalence of postural hypotension among community dwelling elderly. JAMA 1987;258:1511–1514
83. Forster A, Young J: Incidence and consequences of falls due to stroke: a systemataic inquiry. BMJ 1995;311:83–86
84. Masdeu JC, Wolfson L, Lantos G et al: Brain white matter changes in the elderly prone to falling. Arch Neurol 1989;46: 1292–1296
85. Sheldon JH: The Social Medicine of Old Age: Report of an Inquiry in Wolverhampton. Oxford University Press, London, 1948
86. Lee MS, Marsden D: Drop attacks. pp. 177–187. In Bronstein AM, Brandt T, Woollacott M (eds): Clinical Disorders of Balance, Posture and Gait. Edward Arnold, London, 1996
87. Stevens DL, Matthews WB: Cryptogenic drop attacks: an affliction of women. BMJ 1973;1:439–442
88. Overstall P: Drop attacks. pp. 299–308. In Kenny RA (ed): Syncope in the Older Patient. Chapman & Hall Medical, London, 1996
89. Meissner I, Wiebers DO, Swanson JW, O'Fallon WM: The natural history of drop attacks. Neurology 1986;36:1029–1034
90. Myers AH, Baker SP, Van Natta ML et al: Risk factors associated with falls and injuries among elderly institutionalized persons. Am J Epidemiol 1991;133:1179–1190
91. Ray WA, Griffin MR, Malcolm E: Cyclic antidepressants and the risk of hip fracture. Arch Med 1991;151:754–756
92. Goodwin JS, Regan M: Cognitive dysfunction associated with naproxen and ibuprofen in the elderly. Arthritis Rheum 1982; 25:1013–1014
93. Rashiq S, Logan RFA: Role of drugs in fractures of the femoral neck. BMJ 1986;292:861–863
94. Hale WE, Stewart RB, Marks RG: Central nervous system symptoms of elderly subjects using antihypertensive drugs. J Am Geriatr Soc 1984;32:5–10
95. Heidrich FE, Stergachis A, Gross KM: Diuretic drug use and the risk for hip fracture. Ann Intern Med 1991;115:1–6
96. Hingson R, Howland J: Alcohol as a risk factor for injury or death resulting from accidental falls: a review of the literature. J Stud Alcohol 1987;48:212–219
97. Jansen EC, Thyssen HH, Brynskov J: Gait analysis after intake of increasing amounts of alcohol. Z Rechtsmed 1985;94: 103–107
98. Nelson DE, Sattin RW, Langlois JA et al: Alcohol as a risk factor for fall injury events among elderly persons living in the community. J Am Geriatr Soc 1992;40:658–661
99. Pentland B, Jones PA, Roy CW, Miller JD: Head injury in the elderly. Age Ageing 1986;15:193–202
100. Turner GF, Wilson P, Ward G et al: What proportion of falls in elderly people who present to hospital are related to alcohol drinking? 1990;2:413–414
101. Gibson MJ: The prevention of falls in later life: a report of the Kellogg International Workgroup on the Prevention of Falls by the Elderly. Dan Med Bull suppl 1987;4:1–24
102. Citron N: Femoral neck fractures: are some preventable? Ergonomics 1985;28:993–997
103. Morfitt JM: Falls in old people at home: intrinsic versus environmental factors in causation. Public Health 1983;97:115–120
104. Cohn TE, Lasley DJ: Visual depth illusion and falls in the elderly. Clin Geriatr Med 1985;1:601–615
105. Archea JC: Environmental factors associated with stair accidents by the elderly. Clin Geriatr Med 1985;1:555–568
106. Blake C, Morfitt JM: Falls and staffing in a residential home for elderly people. Public Health 1986;100:385–391
107. Morris EV, Isaacs B: The prevention of falls in a geriatric hospital. Age Ageing 1980;9:181–185
108. Campbell AJ, Spears GFS, Borrie MJ, Fitzgerald JL: Falls, elderly women and the cold. Gerontology 1988;34:205–208
109. Bastow MD, Rawlings J, Allison SP: Undernutrition, hypothermia, and injury in elderly women with fractured femur: an injury response to altered metabolism? Lancet 1983;1:143–146
110. Lipsitz LA: Syncope in the elderly. Ann Intern Med 1983;99: 92–105
111. Rubenstein LZ, Robbins AS, Schulman BL et al: Falls and instability in the elderly. J Am Geriatr Soc 1988;36:266–278
112. MacKnight C, Rockwood K: Assessing mobility in elderly people: a review of performance-based measures of balance, gait and mobility for beside use. Rev Clin Gerontol 1995;5:464–486
113. Weiner WJ, Nora LM, Glantz RH: Elderly in-patients: postural reflex impairment. Neurology 1984;34:945–947
114. Weiner DK, Duncan PW, Chandler J, Studenski SA: Functional reach: a marker of physical frailty. J Am Geriatr Soc 1992;40: 203–207
115. Studenski S, Duncan PW, Chandler J et al: Predicting falls: the role of mobility and nonphysical factors. J Am Geriatr Soc 1994;42:297–302
116. Lipsitz LA, Jonsson PV, Kelley MM, Koestner JS: Causes and correlates of recurrent falls in ambulatory frail elderly. J Gerontol 1991;46:M114–M122
117. Thapa PB, Gideon P, Fought RL et al: Comparison of clinical and biomechanical measures of balance and mobility in elderly nursing home residents. J Am Geriatr Soc 1994;42:493–500
118. Mathias S, Nayak USL, Isaacs B: Balance in elderly patients: the "get up and go" test. Arch Phys Med Rehabil 1986;67: 387–389
119. Podsiadlo D, Richardson S: The timed "up & go": a test of basic functional mobility for frail elderly persons. J Am Geriatr Soc 1991;39:142–148
120. Obonyo T, Drummond M, Isaacs B: Domiciliary physiotherapy for old people who have fallen. Int Rehabil Med 1983;5: 157–160
121. Simpson JM, Salkin S: Are elderly people at risk of falling taught how to get up again? Age Ageing 1993;22:294–296
122. Hogan DB, Berman P, Fox RA, Hubley-Kozey CL et al: Idiopathic gait disorders in the elderly. Clin Rehabil 1987;1:17–22
123. Northridge ME, Nevitt MC, Kelsey JL, Link B: Home hazards and falls in the elderly: the role of health and functional status. Am J Public Health 1995;85:509–515
124. Clemson L, Cumming RG, Roland M: Case-control study of hazards in the home and risk of falls and hip fractures. Age Ageing 1996;25:97–101
125. Brody EM, Kleban MH, Moss MS, Kleban F: Predictors of falls

among institutionalised women with Alzheimer's disease. J Am Geriatr Soc 1984;32:877–882

126. Tinetti ME, Williams TF, Mayewski R: Fall risk index for elderly patients based on number of chronic disabilities. Am J Med 1986;80:429–434
127. Fife DD, Solomon P, Stanton M: A risk/falls program: code orange for success. Nurs Management 1984;15:50–53
128. Rickli R, Busch S: Motor performance of women as a function of age and physical activity level. J Gerontol 1986;41:645–649
129. Molloy DW, Richardson LD, Grilly RG: The effects of a three-month exercise programme on neuropsychological function in elderly institutionalized women: a randomized controlled trial. Age Ageing 1988;17:303–310
130. Tinetti ME, Doucette JT, Claus EB: The contribution of predisposing and situational risk factors to serious fall injuries. J Am Geriatr Soc 1995;43:1207–1213
131. Tinetti ME, Doucette JT, Claus E, Marottoli R: Risk factors for serious injury during falls by older persons in the community. J Am Geriatr Soc 1995;43:1214–1221
132. Tinetti ME, Inouye SK, Gill TM, Doucette JT: Shared risk factors for falls, incontinence, and functional dependence: unifying the approach to geriatric syndromes. JAMA 1995;273:1348–1353
133. Province MA, Hadley EC, Hornbrook MC et al: The effects of exercise on falls in elderly patients: a preplanned meta-analysis of the FICSIT trials. JAMA 1995;273:1341–1344
134. Lord SR, Ward JA, Williams P, Strudwick M: The effect of a 12-month exercise trial on balance, strength, and falls in older women: a randomized controlled trial. J Am Geriatr Soc 1995; 43:1198–1206
135. Ory MG, Schechtman KB, Miller JP et al: Frailty and injuries in later life: the FICSIT trials. J Am Geriatr Soc 1993;41:283–296
136. Tinetti ME, Baker DI, McAvay G et al: A multifactorial intervention to reduce the risk of falling among elderly people living in the community. N Engl J Med 1994;331:821–827
137. Wagner EH, Lacriox AZ, Grothaus L et al: Preventing disability and falls in older adults: a population-based randomized trial. Am J Public Health 1994;84:1800–1806
138. Hornbrook MC, Stevens VJ, Wingfield DJ et al: Preventing falls among community-dwelling older persons: results from a randomized trial. Gerontologist 1994;34:16–23
139. Fiatarone MA, O'Neill EF, Ryan ND et al: Exercise training and nutritional supplementation for physical frailty in very elderly people. N Engl J Med 1994;330:1769–1775
140. Hunter GR, Treuth MS, Weinsier RL et al: The effects of strength conditioning on older women's ability to perform daily tasks. J Am Geriatr Soc 1995;43:756–760
141. Lauritzen JB, Petersen MM, Lund B: Effect of external hip protectors on hip fractures. Lancet 1993;341:11–13
142. Wallace RB, Ross JE, Huston JC et al: Iowa FICSIT trial: the feasibility of elderly wearing a hip joint protective garment to reduce hip fractures. J Am Geriatr Soc 1993;41:338–340
143. Tinetti ME: Prevention of falls and fall injuries in elderly persons: a research agenda. Prev Med 1994;23:756–762
144. Wynne-Harley D: Living dangerously: risk-taking, safety and older people. Centre for Policy on Ageing, Report 16, London, 1991

C H A P T E R 97

Pressure Sores: Etiology and Prevalence

GERALD C. J. BENNETT
MARY R. BLISS

History

The current renaissance in the scientific study of pressure sores has brought this important topic into the mainstream of clinical research for many groups of health care professionals. Pressure sores as a clinical problem and theories regarding their causation, management, and prevention have interested doctors and nurses throughout history, however.

When the mummified body of an Egyptian priestess of Amen (Twenty-first Dynasty) was unwrapped in the British Museum,[1] she was found to have pressure sores over her buttocks and shoulders. Indeed, her Egyptian embalmers had performed the first known skin graft by placing gazelle skin over the sores in an effort to restore her prior to her journey to the afterlife. There are apparent biblical references to pressure sores, and they are mentioned in the writings of Moses Maimonides.[2,3] Four hundred years ago Fabricius[4] speculated on their causation, blaming "pneums" resulting from nerve severance and (importantly) loss of blood supply. In 1749 Quesnay[5] classified sores as those caused by pressure and those due to other diseases. By 1852 Brown-Sequard[6] (still a respected physician before his "elixir of youth" foray) confidently concluded that skin pressure and moisture were the two most important etiologic factors. He based this theory on experiments in which he failed to produce ulcers or sores in cord-transected animals if the skin was kept dry. In 1873 Paget[7] wrote, "Bedsores may be defined as the sloughing and mortification or death of a part produced by pressure."

Progress was halted, however, by the intervention of Charcot[8] (probably the most powerful voice in medicine at the time) who in 1879 published a theory on the causation of pressure sores stating that nerve injury released a neurotrophic factor resulting in tissue necrosis. So influential were his opinions that, despite any evidence backing his ideas, the scientific study of pressure sores became redundant. In 1874 Leyden[9] had already claimed that pressure sores were inevitable in desensitized skin. This powerful pessimism, especially in the field of paraplegia, held sway and was still being advocated in 1940 when Munro[10] opposed surgical treatment for patients with paraplegia because it was proposed that following spinal cord injury, a disturbed autonomic nervous system altered skin reflexes and inevitably predisposed the patient to ulceration.

During this dark era others reported their work but failed to receive recognition. In 1908 Van Gehuchten[11] discussed the etiologic factors in muscle wasting leading to sore formation, while Kuster[12] focused attention on bacterial infection in acute sores. World War I casualties enabled Marie and Roussy[13] to assert that not only paraplegics but also debilitated patients developed pressure sores and that, more importantly, both prevention and treatment were possible. World War II focused attention on this topic again, in no small part as a response to the large numbers of young paraplegics and debilitated people developing pressure sores and requiring treatment. This led to a resurgence of interest in surgical intervention, beginning with the work of Davis[14] who had in 1938 first used pedicle flaps to close wounds. By 1944 Scoville[15] and Lamon and Alexander[16] had reported the first successful excision of a sacral ulcer by primary closure in patients protected by parenteral administration of penicillin.

The postwar era has been dominated by the billion dollar wound healing product industry, obscuring somewhat the important work in physiology and biomechanics as well as in prevention. We are entering a time of medical and nursing liaison involving prevention, management, and treatment procedures using the exciting new information available from scientific research into the etiology and pathophysiology of pressure sores.

Etiology

To prevent and treat pressure sores it is essential to understand that it is peripheral circulatory failure and not nursing neglect that is the primary etiologic factor. The condition may be due to a variety of intrinsic and extrinsic causes, as indicated in the accompanying box.

Intrinsic Causes

Acute Illness

Pressure sores are an aspect of the multiorgan failure that may occur in acute illness or trauma.[17] Changes in blood flow in organs, including muscle and skin, occur in patients with septicemia.[18–20] Failure of reactive hyperemia and decreased oxygen uptake further reduce the ability of tissues to withstand ischemia.[21–23] Similar pathophysiologic changes occur in patients without apparent sepsis.[17] It has been observed that pressure sores accompany relapses in multiple sclerosis and in a wide variety of acute and chronic illnesses associated with low plasma albumin.[24–25] Myopathy and neuropathy amount-

Intrinsic and extrinsic causes of pressure sores

Intrinsic
- Acute illness
- Neurologic disease
- Peripheral vascular disease
- Pain
- Drugs
- Incontinence
- Nutrition
- Age

Extrinsic
- Pressure and shearing forces
- Macerated skin

ing to quadriplegia have been shown to occur in critically ill patients with and without sepsis.[26] Barton[27] thought that bacteremia and endotoxemia were the most important causes of deep sores but that they could also result from metabolic acidosis, dehydration, burns, tissue trauma, hypoxia, circulatory stasis, and "reticuloendothelial depression." Common factors are likely to be the interaction of various mediator systems, including interleukin-1 and interleukin-6, tumor necrosis factor (TNF), and platelet activating factor, and their effects on the vascular endothelium.[17] Leukocyte and platelet aggregation with increased vascular permeability causes microthrombi and interstitial edema[17] which have also been shown to occur in pressure sores.[27]

The importance of illness in the etiology of pressure sores is emphasized by the fact that they occur in dying patients of all ages. In one study 64 percent of pressure sores in hospice patients occurred within 2 weeks of death.[28] Up to 50 percent of elderly patients who develop pressure sores die within 4 months, and this increases to 90 percent of patients with interstitial or deep sores.[29] Necrosis of peripheral tissue with pressure may occur in any acutely ill person but is more common, and is associated with apparently less severe illness, in patients with neurologic and vascular disease.

Neurologic disease

Normally pressure sores are prevented by ischemic discomfort which stimulates movement; indeed, a sleeping adult moves about once every 10 minutes and completes up to 40 full turns in an 8-hour night.[30–32] Elderly patients make fewer movements than younger ones, and people with Parkinson's disease and dementia fewer still.[33,34] It was shown that decreased movement in elderly patients in bed was highly correlated with the development of pressure sores.[35] The critical period during which tissues can experience ischemia and recover depends on the type of pressure and the physical condition of the person. Patients with new spinal cord injury require turning onto their sides for 1 minute every half-hour to prevent tissue necrosis, but healthy para- and quadriplegic patients with healed lesions may be able to lie in one position for 4 hours or more.[36] The supporting surface and the patient's posture are also important. Normal young adults lying in a hospital bed in a lateral position (the site of highest pressure) developed persistent erythema over the greater trochanter after 90 minutes.[37] Patients with spinal cord injury and other neurologic illnesses may also have damaged impaired vasomotor reflexes.[25] There is reduced reactive hyperemia following local pressure in patients with spinal cord injury, most marked in those with sensory impairment.[38] Bader and Gent[23] found that normal young adults had adaptive responses with improved transcutaneous oxygen tensions after repeated tissue loading, compared with "elderly, immobile, and insensitive patients" at risk of pressure sores who tended to have reduced levels.[23]

Peripheral vascular disease

Microvascular disease (seen in diabetes, smoking, hypertension) reduces the ability of the arteries and capillaries to respond to pressure ischemia. Impaired red cell and leukocyte deformability and increased packed cell volume, fibrinogen levels, and platelet aggregability allow vascular obstruction and thrombosis to occur with minor pressure.[39] Further injury caused by neutrophils and free radicals may increase the extent of tissue damage.[40] Heel sores are common in patients with strokes and are four times more common in smokers than in nonsmokers.[41] Virtually all diabetic foot sores are pressure sores due to sensory neuropathy and abnormal vascular responses to trauma.[42] Following minor pressure, patients with vasculitis due to rheumatoid arthritis also frequently develop sores which are slow to heal.[43]

Pain

Pain is associated with an increased risk of pressure sores,[44] partly because of the connection with acute illness and trauma but also because pain inhibits movement. When pain is due to pressure sores, a vicious cycle is established. Severe pain also raises oxygen demand because of increased skeletal muscle activity.[45]

Drugs

Sedatives, including excessive doses of opiate analgesics, exacerbate peripheral tissue ischemia by causing drowsiness and reducing appreciation of pressure pain. High doses of phenothiazines and butyrophenones can cause hypotension, dehydration, and reduced mobility due to Parkinsonism and may have a particular tendency to precipitate deep pressure necrosis in elderly patients with dementia. Nonsteroidal anti-inflammatory drugs depress reactive hyperemia and impair healing.[41,46] β-Adrenoceptor blocking drugs increase susceptibility to tissue necrosis by causing hypotension and peripheral vasoconstriction. Inotropes used to support the systemic circulation in critically ill patients may cause peripheral gangrene without pressure.[47] Many other drugs increase susceptibility to pressure necrosis in older people by causing nausea or diarrhea (e.g., antibiotics), constipation, hypotension, or a confusional state.

Incontinence

The importance of incontinence as a risk factor is in part due to its association with neurologic disease and acute illness. Urinary incontinence is less significant than double incontinence which tends to occur in more advanced disease, and catheterized and noncatheterized patients have been shown to be equally susceptible.[48] Fecal incontinence due to severe constipation (even causing subacute obstruction) is also common in patients with pressure sores.

Nutrition

Malnutrition is often cited as a cause of pressure sores.[49] Using B-mode ultrasound, Clark et al.[50] showed that elderly hospital patients with pressure sores tended to have less soft tissue over the sacrum than controls. This was significant, however, only in patients with incontinence, and thus malnutrition alone has not been shown to be an independent risk factor.[51] Low plasma albumin, the only hematologic or biochemical factor correlated with the development of pressures sores, is probably more important as an indicator of illness than of malnutrition.[52]

Age

Approximately 70 percent of patients with pressure sores are past the age of 70, but age alone has not been shown to be significant.[53] The high incidence in old age is likely due to the increased prevalence of neurologic and vascular disease and of acute and terminal illness rather than to age itself. Elderly hospital patients have been shown to have reduced hyperemic responses, but this is less marked in healthy old people living at home.[54] Aging skin has relatively well-preserved skin blood flow and healing ability.[55–57]

Extrinsic Causes

Numerous authors have stressed the fact that pressure per se is one of the main determinants in pressure sore formation.[35,58–61] The skin breaks down when sufficient pressure is applied to overcome the capillary pressure of 32 mmHg at the arterial end, especially over a bony prominence.[62] There is, however, debate as to what constitutes normal capillary pressure in a frail elderly person.[63] Pressure in excess of capillary pressure results in anoxia and cellular death, leading to abnormal metabolic processes resulting in inflammation.[64–66] If pressure is removed in the early stages, some of this damage is initially reversed (normal reactive hyperemia results from a vasodilation response to ischemia).[67]

Pressure on peripheral tissue has two sources, external pressure on skin and internal pressure due to bony prominences causing superficial and deep sores, respectively (Figs. 97-1 and 97-2; see also Plates 97-1 and 97-2). The tissues are trapped in between these two sources of pressure, resulting in a pressure gradient which is highest over the bone and decreases toward the surface (Fig. 97-3). A clinically important study showed that altering or relieving pressure for as little as 5 minutes may allow tissue to withstand higher pressures for longer periods of time.[68]

It is apparent, however, from Kosiak's[65] experiments on dogs that the "pressure-ischemia" explanation for the pathogenesis of pressure sores is not complete in that some of his animals were exposed to continuous cutaneous pressures of 100 mmHg for periods of up to 12 hours (and 150 mmHg for 11 hours) without developing sores. Dinsdale[69,70] added friction to the pathogenesis argument following his research using pig skin: "The different pressures required to produce skin necrosis do not correlate closely with the pressure exerted on the human skin during normal activities of daily living."

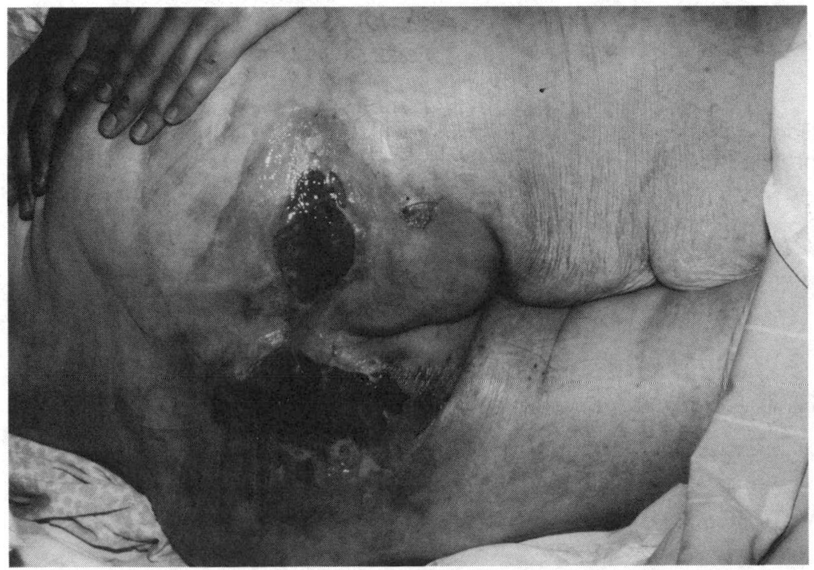

Figure 97-1 Superficial sore.

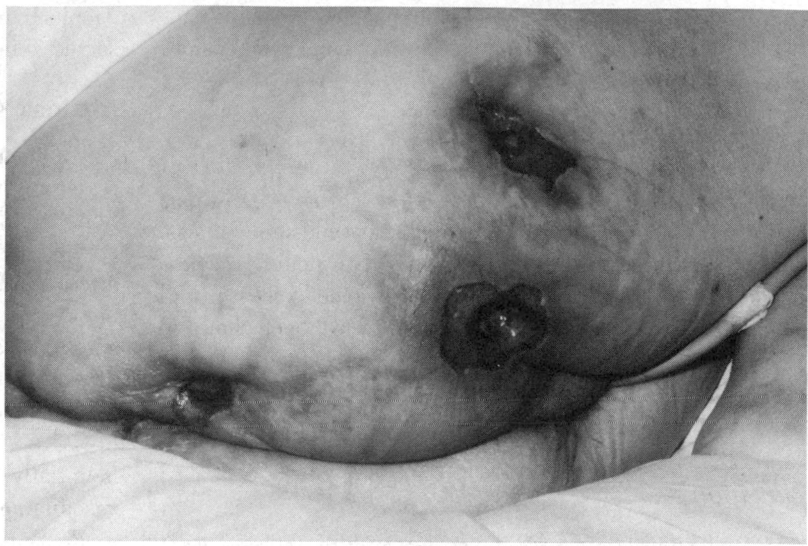

Figure 97-2 Deep interstitial sore.

There are, according to Barton and Barton,[41] two coexisting processes that cause reduced tissue perfusion and eventually result in anoxic necrosis of the skin:

1. Exclusion of blood from the skin by the application of sustained pressure in excess of mean capillary pressure
2. Thrombosis of the microcirculation caused by the application of disruptive and shearing forces

Extrinsic pressures causing sores are higher than those elderly people normally experience or are pressures for which they have reduced physiologic tolerance because of their physical condition. The effect of illness must be taken into account when considering "occlusion pressures" and so-called safe interface pressures measured in healthy subjects.[71] Common sites of sores are shown in the accompanying box.[72]

Most sores occur over the sacrum, the area carrying the most weight in a recumbent sick person (Fig. 97-4; see also Plate 97-3). It has been shown that shocked and dehydrated patients with femoral neck fractures can spend 12 hours (with

Figure 97-3 Possible etiologic model for a pressure sore (Bliss). In general, the higher the pressure, the shorter the time required to cause a sore, but it is important to note that low pressure sustained for long periods is as damaging as high pressure for short periods. Deep pressure in the subcutaneous tissues and muscle next to bone may be considerably higher than the pressure measured on the skin, and the body is probably better adapted physiologically to deal with short periods of high pressure than with prolonged low pressure.

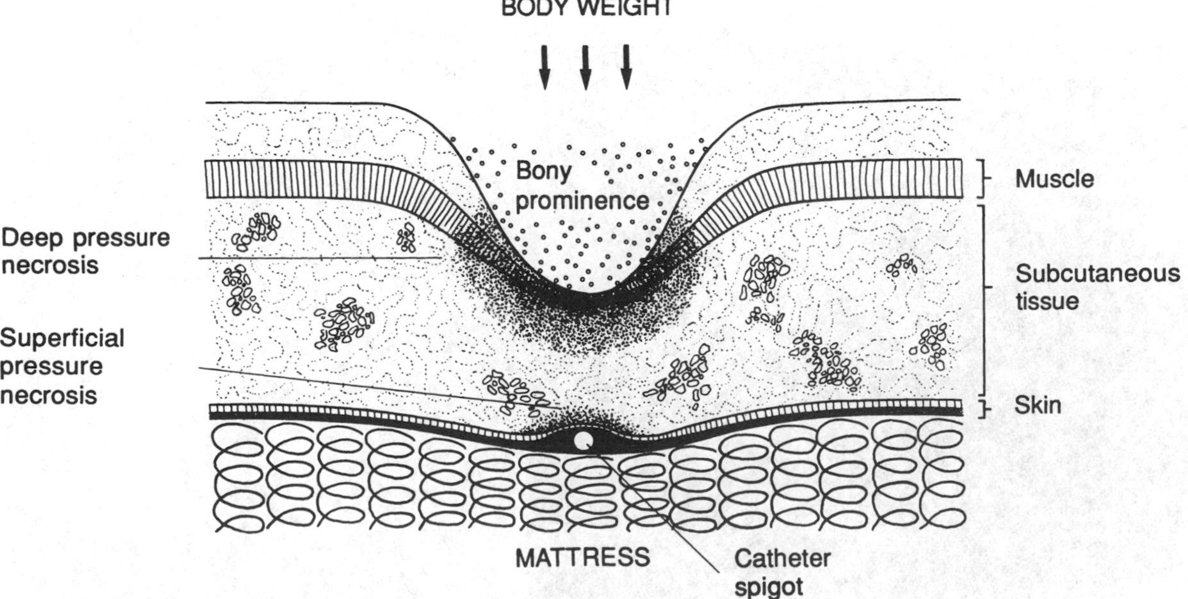

Sites of pressure sores in elderly patients

Sacrum
Ischial tuberosities
Hip
Heel
Elbow
Knee
Ankle
Occiput

sacral pressures up to 60 mmHg) lying on an unprotected gurney in an emergency room.[73] Elderly patients should spend as short a period of time as possible in the emergency room, preferably not more than an hour. However, this is not always practicable, and emergency pressure relief needs to be provided from the time of arrival until transfer to a hospital room. If a patient has to spend a long time on an x-ray table, it should be padded and, if necessary, the plates inserted between the padding and the patient. Similar pressures occur in patients admitted on worn mattresses (fire-retardant agents decrease the life of mattresses). Greater trochanter sores (Fig. 97-5; see also Plate 97-4) can be provoked by poorly fitting mattress covers or by sheets causing a "hammocky" effect, while sitting a patient up in bed can cause shear stresses over the sacrum, increasing capillary distortion and occlusion and the likelihood of deep tissue necrosis. Heels (Fig. 97-6; see also Plate 96-5) are sensitive sites for the development of sores because of the junction between two different skin types (thick plantar and thin posterior heel), and sores can be caused by tightly tucked-in sheets and quilts and by sitting patients up, which increases pressure on the heels. Nursing sick elderly patients in chairs can result in the formation of additional sores over the ischial tuberosities. Pressure is more difficult to relieve in a chair than in bed, and many studies have shown that patients nursed in chairs are liable to have more sores and more severe sores than patients who are nursed predominantly in bed (Fig. 97-7; see also Plate 97-6).[53,74,75]

Pressure sores at less common sites may be caused by traction apparatus, casts, prostheses, shoes, condom devices, catheters, nasal tubes, and so on. Bandages are a common, usually unrecognized, cause of necrotic pressure sores of the legs and feet in patients with vascular disease (Fig. 97-8; see also Plate 97-7)

Physiologic Measurement

Pressure

The accuracy of interface pressure measuring systems has been investigated by Allen et al.[76] Their study indicated that different interfaces affected accuracy markedly and that repeatability was affected when a nonhomogenized interface was used. It also showed that errors associated with interface pressure measurement systems could be substantial and vary from one system to another. The role of pressure measurement in pressure sore research has been pioneered by Bader and Hawker[77–79] with special reference to the spinal cord injury patient. Pressure measurement has also been used to evaluate specialized support surfaces.[80]

Microcirculation

The regulation of blood flow in the microvasculature is affected mainly by the smooth muscle cells surrounding the venous and arterial vessels. These cells are either controlled by nerve fibers (multiunit type) or possess internal activity (unitary type).[81] The latter type is most common in the smallest branches of the vascular tree and is believed to give rise to the rhythmic variations in microvascular blood flow.[82] These variations in blood flow, which can be recorded by laser Doppler flowmetry, are assumed to reflect the varying pressure recorded in the capillaries.[83] Laser Doppler flowmeters have

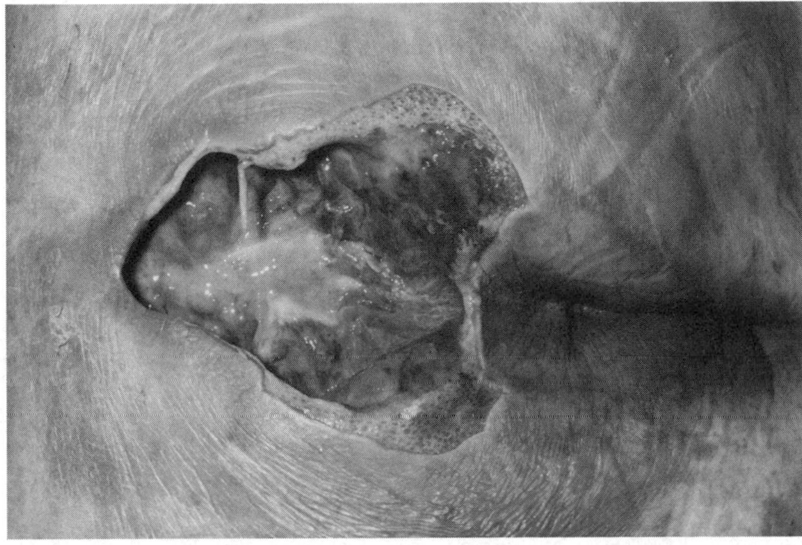

Figure 97-4 Sacral sore.

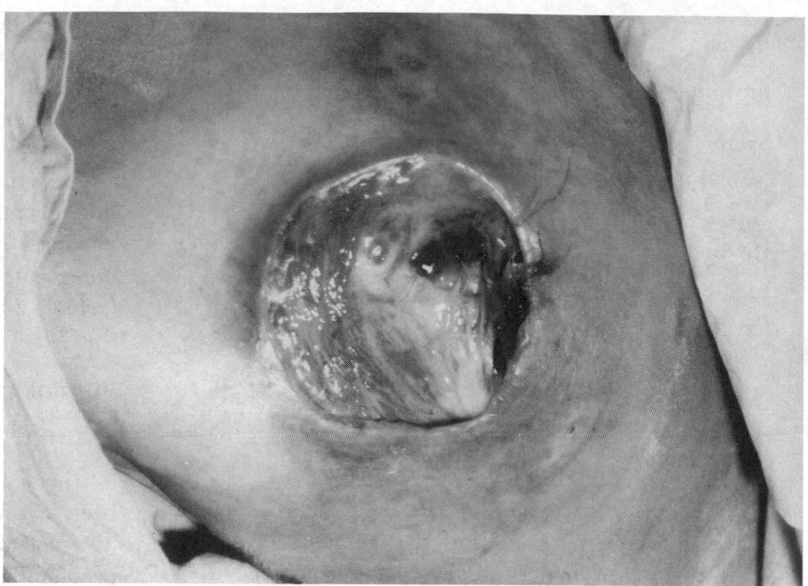

Figure 97-5 Grade 4 sore over the greater trochanter.

been extensively used in studying the etiology of pressure sores by virtue of their measurement of cutaneous skin flow.[84–86]

Schubert et al.[87] compared skin microcirculation over a damaged risk area, the sacrum, with that over an area of undamaged skin in the gluteal region using laser Doppler fluxometry. This study also examined nutritive transport using fluoroscan flowmetry and skin temperature. There was increased skin microcirculation in the early stage of pressure sore formation but no increase in skin temperature. The increase in blood flow in subpapillary tissue layers effectively dissipated the heat generated by the damage and the increased metabolic activity.[87] The heel has been shown to be vulnerable to compression using laser Doppler fluxometry.[88]

Transcutaneous gas tension

The measurement of skin or cutaneous "respiration" began in 1851 when Von Gerlach[89] studied oxygen diffusion through human skin. The use of skin measurement to determine arterial oxygen pressure (PaO_2) was pioneered by Baumberger and Goodfriend[90] in 1951, and the method validated by Roth et al.[91] in 1957. In 1969 Huch et al.[92] reported PaO_2 measurements by employing surface sensors on the scalp of normal newborns using a nicotinic acid derivative as a vasodilating agent. This study showed that PaO_2 values relatively close to arterial ones could be obtained. A technical advance occurred with the work of Eberhard[93] and Huch[94] who proposed that the sensor be heated to temperatures between 42°C and 45°C.

This method was applied in investigating the effect of external pressure on the skin,[23,95,96] especially in patients with spinal cord injuries.[97–99] The susceptibility to pressure sores in this group may be due to the interactive effects of prolonged immobilization and injury-related autonomic dysfunction associated with reduced tissue perfusion. Transcutaneous gas tension measurement has also been used to assess the effect on tissue oxygenation of specialized versus conventional hospital support surfaces (Fig. 97-9; see also Plate 97-8).[100–102]

Figure 97-6 Heel sore.

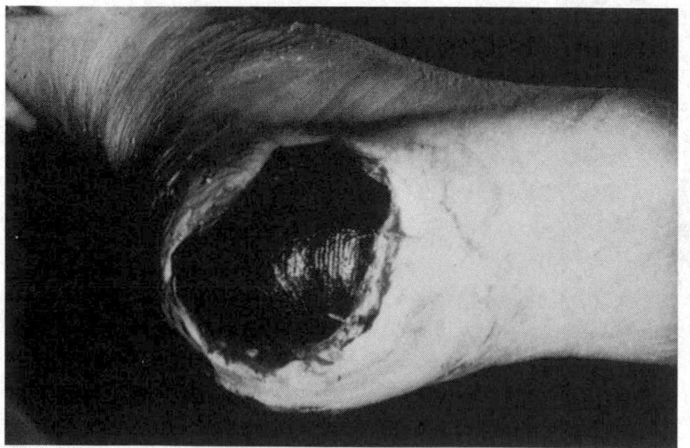

Figure 97-7 Chair sores.

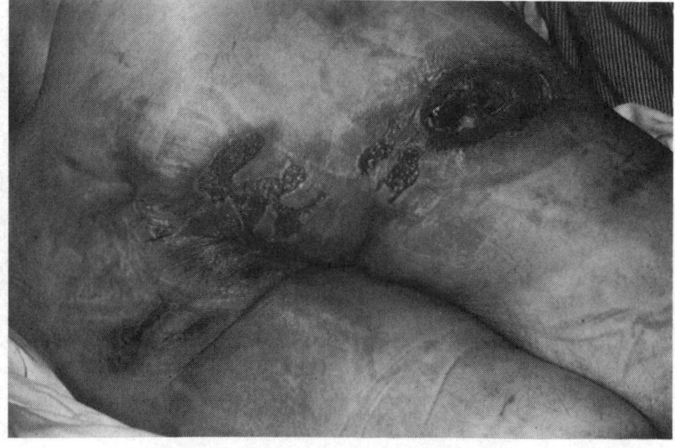

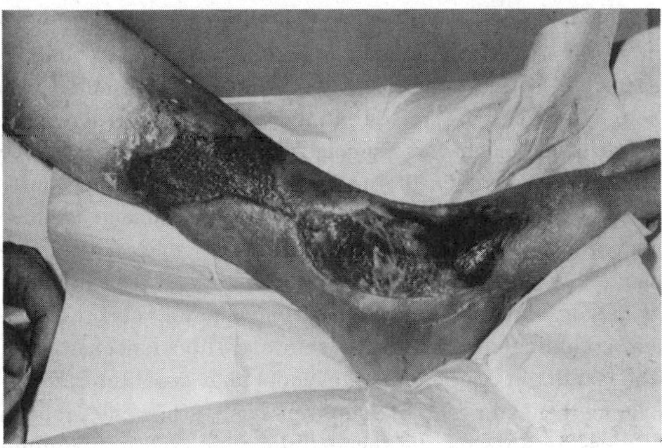

Figure 97-8 Pressure sore caused by a bandage. Note characteristic deep necrosis over the instep.

Pathology

Tissue damage due to pressure is always strictly confined to the area of the original ischemia so that pressure sores, like burns with which they are often confused, are clear-cut wounds occurring in usually normal skin. Contrary to common belief, they never extend to involve surrounding tissues, and new necrosis is always an indication of continuing pressure.

There are two pathophysiologic types of pressure sores: superficial, confined to the epidermis and dermis; and deep, involving periosteum, muscle, subcutaneous fat, and associated structures. However, for the purposes of audit and research, they are conventionally divided into four grades. The accompanying box shows a modification of the system used by the U.S. National Pressure Ulcer Advisory Panel.[103] The principal difference in this classification is the inclusion of only *colorless* blisters, indicating damage limited to the epidermis, in grade 2. Blue or black discoloration, or edema, always denotes involvement of at least dermal or subdermal tissue, and so all discolored or edematous sores are included in grade 3 or 4. Other workers have suggested five grades, including blanching erythema as grade 1.[104] The actual extent of damage often cannot be confirmed until the necrotic tissue breaks down.

Figure 97-9 Measurement of transcutaneous gas tension.

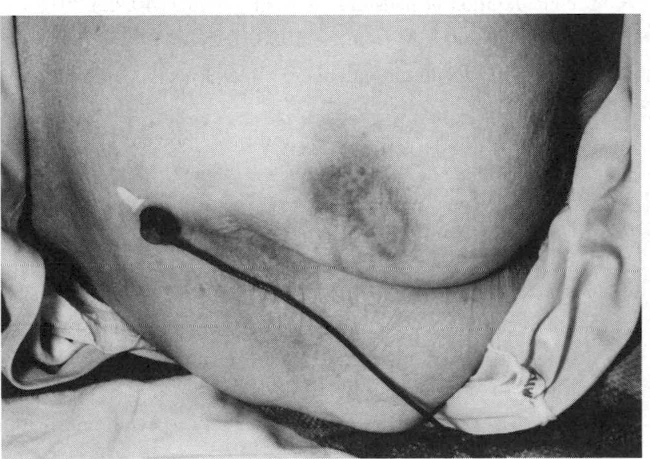

Prevalence

A 1971 study in Denmark showed that 3 percent of all hospital patients studied had a pressure sore, the minimum inclusion being "at least an epithelial defect."[105] The two large-scale U.K. surveys were performed in the greater Glasgow[106] and Borders[107] health board areas in 1976. These prevalence surveys were completed on a single day using a questionnaire completed by staff for hospital patients, excluding maternity, psychiatry, and learning disability but not psychiatry of old age patients. Those in the community were included if they received a district nurse visit that day.

The greater Glasgow survey contained data on 10,751 patients. The sore prevalence rate was 8.8 percent, 1.5 percent of the patient population having a sore in the most severe category. Only established sores were included, not incipient sores or early tissue damage. The Borders survey covered a much smaller population in which the overall sore prevalence rate was 9.4 percent, with 2.1 percent having a severe sore. Subanalysis involving community and hospital patients revealed a sore prevalence rate of 4.8 percent for patients nursed

Staging of pressure sores

Stage I

Nonblanchable erythema of intact skin, the heralding lesion of skin ulceration. In individuals with darker skin, discoloration of the skin, warmth, edema, induration, or hardness may also be indicators.

Stage II

Colorless blisters indicating damage limited to the epidermis.

Stage III

Full-thickness skin loss involving damage to or necrosis of subcutaneous tissue that may extend down to, but not through, underlying fascia. The ulcer presents clinically as a deeper crater with or without undermining of adjacent tissue.

Stage IV

Full-thickness skin loss with extensive destruction, tissue necrosis, or damage to muscle, bone, or supporting structures (e.g., tendon, joint capsule). Undermining and sinus tracts also may be associated with stage IV pressure ulcers.

(From Macklebust,[103] with permission.)

at home versus 11.7 percent for those nursed in a hospital. However, if patients of similar disability are compared, the difference disappears. The survey findings in Denmark and Scotland were analyzed by Barbanel et al.[108] who felt that, despite differences in the nature and composition of the survey population, the differences in the sore prevalence rate were real.

Prevalence rates within four European countries have been documented, as well as prevalence rates in hospitals in the greater Paris region.[109,110] There are very few data on the nursing or residential home population in the United Kingdom. Reports in the United States indicate that between 20 and 35 percent of elderly people have pressure sores at the time of admission to a nursing home.[111–112] Most prevalence studies in the United Kingdom indicate that between 8 and 20 percent of people in the hospital sector have pressure sores.[113–115] Similar figures are found in the U.S. in patient population,[116–117] however, lower prevalence rates have been reported in the United Kingdom,[118] especially in units with a specialized interest. Some units have been estimated to have 30 to 50 percent of patients affected by pressure sores.[41] There is confusion concerning the correct use of the terms *prevalence* and *incidence*.[119] Interpretation of results is also complicated by the use of a variety of populations within a variety of settings, including continuing care.[120–123] Incidence rates have been reported as either percentages of subjects[123] or as a number or range per 1,000 patient-days (e.g., 0.20 to 0.56 per 1,000 patient-days).[124,125] In a 2-week prospective cohort study of elderly patients at risk (less than 17 on the Braden scale), the incidence of pressure ulcers was 14 per 1,000 patient-days.[126]

Medical responsibility and medical education

The essential feature of pressure sore management is prevention, and to be successful, prevention must form part of the emergency care of susceptible patients. Doctors need to accept responsibility for maintaining the peripheral circulation as well as that of the heart or kidneys or any other organ. Pressure sores are a common, severe complication of illness in elderly patients and cause great pain and suffering. They delay recovery and may result in permanent disability or even death.[127,128] Ninety-five percent are probably preventable with proper early management,[129] and so they are likely to be an increasing basis of claims for compensation[130] and an important parameter in clinical audit or in quality of care.[116,131]

Preventing pressure necrosis requires a thorough understanding of the etiology and pathology of peripheral circulatory failure and skilled clinical judgment which should not be delegated to nurses alone. Patients at risk are found in almost every branch of medical practice, and clinicians and acute services care managers need to ensure that all health workers are trained to recognize susceptible patients and know how to provide appropriate treatment. Pressure care nurse specialists should be appointed in every health district. They should liaise with supplies officers and manufacturers to ensure that cost-effective, up-to-date pressure-relieving equipment is available in hospitals and in the community 24 hours a day[132] and responsible for servicing and redistribution. They should also help to organize in-service training sessions on pressure care. However, although nurse specialists may give general advice about pressure relief, the decision to use specialized equipment should be a joint responsibility of the physician and nurse and form part of the general medical and nursing plan of treatment.[128]

History and examination should encompass every organ system including at-risk areas of skin and subcutaneous tissue. The fact that pressure relief prevention may constitute a medical emergency in at-risk groups emphasizes how the problem of pressure sores can be successfully addressed in the future only if pressure relief is accepted as an essential part of medical student training. A survey of medical schools and colleges in the United Kingdom indicated that medical education in wound care was inadequate for their clinical and medicolegal needs.[133]

References

1. Thompson RJ: Pathological changes in mummies. Proc R Soc Med 1961;54:409–415
2. Daniel RJ, Hall EJ, Macleod MK: Pressure sores—a reappraisal. Ann Plast Surg 3:53–63
3. Maimonides M: The Medical Aphorisms of Moses Maimonides. Vols. 1 and 2. RF Bloch (trans and ed).
4. Fabricius H: De Gangrene et Sphacelo Tractatus Methodicus. 10th Ed. JT de Bry, Leyden, 1593
5. Quesnay M: Trite de Gangrene. pp. 319–353. Paris, 1749
6. Brown-Sequard E: Experimental Researches Applied to Physiology and Pathology. H Bailliere, New York, 1853
7. Paget J: Clinical lectures on bedsores. Students J Hosp Gaz London 1873;1:144
8. Charcot JM: Lectures on the Diseases of the Nervous System. Delivered at La Saltpetriere. 2nd Ed. Sigerson G, Henry C Lea, Philadelphia, 1879
9. Leyden E: Klinik de Ruckenmarks—Kraukheiten. p. 156. Vol. 1. A Hirchwald, Berlin, 1874
10. Munro D: Care of the back following spinal cord injuries: consideration of bedsores. N Engl J Med 1940;223:391
11. Van Gehuchten A: Neuraxe 1908;10:298
12. Kuster I: Decubitus eulenberg. Real Encyclopadie 1908;3:671
13. Marie P, Roussy G: Sur la possibilitie de prevenir la formation des escarres dans les traumatismes de guerre. Bull Acad Med Paris 1915;73:602
14. Davis JS: Operative treatment of scars following bedsores. Surgery 1938;3:1
15. Scoville WB: Cited by Bailey BN in Bedsores. Edward Arnold, London, 1967
16. Lamon JC, Alexander E: Secondary closure of decubitus ulcers with the aid of penicillin. JAMA 1945;127:396
17. Beal AL, Cerra FB Multiple organ failure syndrome in the 1990's. JAMA 1994;271:226–233

18. Wyler F, Neutze JM, Rudolph AM: Effects of endotoxin on distribution of cardiac output in unanaesthetised rabbits. Am J Physiol 1970;219:246–251
19. Berstein A, Sibbald WJ: Circulatory disturbances in multiple system organ failure. Crit Care Clin 1989;5:233–254
20. Naumann CP, Ruetsch YA, Fleckenstein W et al: PO_2 profiles in human muscle tissue as indication of therapeutical effects in septic shock patients. Adv Exp Biol 1992;317:869–877
21. Sibbald WJ, Lam C, Tyme K, Rantin C: Microvascular perfusion is impaired in rat model of normotensive sepsis. J Clin Invest 1994;94:2077–2083
22. Bernandi L, Radaelli A, Solda PL et al: Autonomic control of skin microvessels: assessment by power spectrum of photoplethysmographic waves. Clin Sci 1996;90:345–355
23. Bader DL, Gent CA: Changes in transcutaneous oxygen tension as a result of prolonged pressures at the sacrum. Clin Physiol Meas 1988;9:33–40.
24. Loeper J, Rameix P: Le problem des escarres et leur traitment chez le sujet age. Semaine Hopitaux Paris 1960;10:635–638
25. Bliss MR: Aetiology of pressure sores. Rev Clin Gerontol 1993;3:379–397
26. Latronico N, Fenzi F, Recupero D et al: Critical illness myopathy and neuropathy. Lancet 1996;347:1579–1582
27. Barton AA: Pressure sores. pp. 53–57. In Barbanel JC, Forbes CD, Lowe G (eds): Pressure Sores. Macmillan, London, 1993
28. Hanson D, Langermo DK, Olson B et al: The prevalence and incidence of pressure ulcers in the hospice setting: analysis of two methodologies. Am J Hosp Palliative Care 1991;5:18–22
29. Bliss MR, Silver JR: Pressure sores. pp. 97–112. In Mark BE, Graham-Brown RAC, Sarkang I (eds): Skin Disorders in the Elderly. Blackwell Scientific Publications, Oxford, 1988
30. Keane F: The minimum physiological mobility requirement of man supported on a soft surface. Paraplegia 1979;16:383–389
31. Johnson HM, Swan TH, Weigand GE: In what positions do healthy people sleep? JAMA 1930;94:2058–2062
32. Barbanel JC: Movement studies during sleep. pp. 249–260. In Bader DL (ed): Pressure Sores: Clinical Practice and Scientific Approach. Macmillan, Basingstoke, UK, 1990
33. Bar CA, Lloyd S, Pathy MS, Chawla JC: A system to monitor gross positional changes in recumbent parts. Care Sci Pract 1983;2:4–7
34. Nicholson PW, Leeman AL, O'Neill CJA et al: Pressure sores: effect of Parkinson's disease and cognitive function on spontaneous movement in bed. Age Ageing 1988;17:111–115
35. Exton-Smith AN, Sherwin RW: The prevention of pressure sores: significance of spontaneous bodily movements. Lancet 1961;ii:1124–1126
36. Cönnewicht BR: Pressure sores and spinal cord injury. J Wound Care 1996;5:114
37. Barnett RI, Ablarde JA: Skin vascular reaction to standard patients persisting on a hospital mattress. Adv Wound Care 1994;7:58–65
38. Schubert V, Fagnell B: Post occlusive reactive hyperaemia and thermal response in the skin micro-circulation of subjects with spinal cord injury. Scan J Rehabil Med 1991;23:33–40
39. Walmsley D, Wiles PG: Impaired hyperaemic response to skin microtrauma in diabetes is associated with retinopathy. Clin Sci 1988;74(suppl 18):24–25
40. Brady AJ, Williams FM, Williams TJ: Inflammatory injury in myocardial ischaemia. Clin Sci 1992;83:511–518
41. Barton A, Barton M: The Management and Prevention of Pressure Sores. Faber and Faber, London, 1981
42. Rayman G, Malik RA, Sharma AK, Day JL: Microvascular response to tissue injury and capillary ultrastructure in the foot skin of type 1 diabetic patients. Clin Sci 1995;89:467–474
43. Salaman RA: The aetiology and healing rates of chronic leg ulcers. J Wound Care 1995;7:320–323
44. Barnet E: A review of risk assessment methods. Care Sci Pract 1988;6:49–52
45. Anderson WG: Anaesthesia for patients with cardiac disease: post operative care. Br J Hosp Med 1987;37:411–418
46. Koller A, Kaley G: Role of endothelium in reactive dilatation of skeletal muscle arterioles. Am J Physiol 1990;259: 1313–1316
47. Hayes MA, Yau EHS, Hinds CJ, Watson JD: Symmetrical peripheral gangrene with noradrenaline administration. Int Care Med 1992;18:433–436
48. Piloian BB. Defining characteristics of the nursing diagnosis "high risk for impaired skin integrity." Decubitus 1992;5: 32–47
49. Perkash A, Brown M: Anaemia in patients with traumatic spinal cord injury. Paraplegia 1982;20:235–236
50. Clark M, Rowland LB, Wood HA, Crow RA: Comparison of contact pressures measured at the sacrum of young and elderly subjects. J Biomed Eng 1989;11:200–202
51. Finucane TE: Malnutrition, tube-feeding and pressure sores: data are incomplete. J Am Geriatr Soc 1995;43:447–451
52. Lehmann AS: Nutrition in old age: an update and questions for future research. 1. Reviews in Clin Gerontol 1991;1:135–145
53. Barbanel JC, Jordan MM, Nicol SM, Clark MO: Incidence of pressure sores in the greater Glasgow health board area. Lancet 1977;ii:548–550
54. Ek AC, Lewis DH, Zetterqvist H, Svensson PG: Skin blood flow in an area of risk for pressure sores. Scand J Rehabil Med 1984;16:85–89
55. Schubert V, Fagnell B: Local skin pressure and its effects on skin microcirculation as evaluated by laser-Doppler fluometry. Clin Physiol 1989;9:535–545
56. Henderson HP: Plastic and reconstructive surgery. pp. 303–329. In Mark BE, Graham Brown RAC, Sarkany I (eds): Skin Disorders in the Elderly. Blackwell Scientific Publications, Oxford, 1988
57. Ashcroft GS, Horan MA, Ferguson MWJ: The effect of ageing on cutaneous wound healing. Clin Sci 1995;89:43–44
58. Walden RH: Inoperable pressure sores: prevention and management. N Y State J Med 71:657
59. Guttman L: The problem of treatment of pressure sores in spinal paraplegics. Br J Plast Surg 1955;8:196
60. Kosiak M: Evaluation of pressure as a factor in the production of ischial ulcers Arch Phys Med Rehabil 1958;39:623
61. Reswick JB, Simoes N: Application of engineering principles in the management of spinal cord injured patients. Clin Orthop 1975;112:124

62. Landis EM: Microinjection studies of capillary blood pressure in human skin. Heart 1930;15:209–228
63. Rithalia SVS: Comparison of pressure distribution in wheelchair seat cushions. Care Sci Pract 1989;7:87–89
64. Hussain T: An experimental study of some pressure effects on tissues with reference to the bedsore problem. J Pathol Bacteriol 1953;66:347
65. Kosiak M: Etiology and pathology of decubitus ulcers. Arch Phys Med 1959;40:62
66. Kosiak M: Etiology of decubitus ulcers. Arch Phys Med 1961; 42:19
67. Lewis T, Gant RT: Observations upon reactive hyperaemia in man. Heart 1925;12:73
68. Lindon O: Pressure distribution on the surface of the human body. Arch Phys Med 1965;46:378
69. Dinsdale SM: Decubitus ulcers in swine: light and electron microscopy study of pathogenesis. Arch Phys Med Rehabil 1973;54:51–56
70. Dinsdale SM: Decubitus ulcers: role of pressure and friction in causation. Arch Phys Med Rehabil 1974;55:147–153
71. Reswich JB, Rogers JE: Skin surface PO_2 and blood flow measurements over the ischial tuberosity. Arch Phys Med Rehabil 1982;63:553–556
72. Jordan MM: Report on Pressure Sores in the Elderly. Bioengineering Unit, University of Strathclyde, Glasgow, 1976
73. Versluysen M: How elderly patients with femoral fracture develop pressure sores in hospital. BMJ 1986;292:1311–1313
74. David J: The size of the problem of pressure sores. Care Sci Pract 1981;1:10–13
75. Nyquist R, Hawthorn PJ: The prevalence of pressure sores within an area health authority. Nursing 1987;12:183–187
76. Allen V, Ryan DW, Loman N, Murray A: Accuracy of interface pressure measurement systems. J Biomed Eng 1993;15: 344–348
77. Bader DL, Hawker MB: Pressure distribution under the ischium of normal subjects. J Biomed Eng 1986;8:353–357
78. Bader DL: The recovery characteristics of soft tissues following repeated loading. J Rehabil Res Dev 1990;27:141–150
79. Bader DL: Effect of compressive loading regimes on tissue viability. pp. 191–201. In Bader DL (ed): Pressure Sores—Clinical Practice and Scientific Approach. Macmillan, Basingstoke, UK, 1990
80. Patel UH, Jones JT, Babbs CF et al: The evaluation of five specialised support surfaces by use of a pressure sensitive mat. Decubitus 1993;6:28–31,34,36–7
81. Ottosan D: Nervsystemets Fysiologi. Natur Och Kulhur, Stockholm, 1970
82. Wiedeman MP, Tuma RF, Mayrovitz HN: An Introduction to Microcirculation. Academic Press, London, 1981
83. Mahler F: Blood pressure fluctuations in human nailfold capillaries. Am J Physiol 1979;263:888–893
84. Holloway G, Watkins D: Laser-Doppler measurement of cutaneous blood flow. J Invest Dermatol 1977;3:69:306–309
85. Nilsson G: Evaluation of a laser-Doppler flowmeter for measurement of tissue blood flow. Trans Biomed Eng 1980;27: 10:597–604
86. Powers E, Frayer W: Laser-Doppler measurement of blood flow in the microcirculation. Plast Reconstr Surg 1978;61:2: 250–255
87. Schubert V, Perbeck L, Schubert PA: Skin microcirculatory and thermal changes in elderly subjects with early stage pressure sores. Clin Physiol 1994;14:1–13
88. Abu-Own A, Sommerville K, Scur JH, Coleridge-Smith PD: Effects of compression and type of bed surface on the microcirculation of the heel. Eur J Vasc Endovasc Surg 1995;9: 327–334
89. Von Gerlach: Uber das hautatmen. Arch Anat Physiol 1851; 431–479
90. Baumberger J, Goodfriend R: Determinatin of arterial oxygen tension in man by equilibration through intact skin. FASEB J 1951;10:10–11
91. Roth G, Sjostedt S, Caligara F: Bloodless determination of oxygen tension by polarography. Sci Tools LKW Instrum J 1957;4:37–45
92. Huch A, Huch R, Lubbers D: 1969. Quantitative polargraphische sauerstoffdruck messing auf der kopfhaut des neugeborenen. Arch Gynaetol 1969;207:443–451
93. Eberhard P: Perkutane Messing des Sauerstoffpartialdrukkes Methodik und Anwendungen. Proc Medizin-Technik 1972, Stuttgart 26, 1972
94. Huch A: Eine schnelle beheizte Pt-Oberflachen Electrode zur kontinuierlichen Uberwachung des PO_2 bein Menschen Elektrodenauf bau und Eigenschaften. Proc Medizin-Technik 1972, Stuttgart 26, 1972
95. Newson T, Percy M: Skin surface PO_2 measurement and the effect of externally applied pressure. Arch Phys Med Rehabil 1981;62:390–392
96. Seiler WO, Stahelin HB: Skin oxygen tension as a function of imposed skin pressure: implications for decubitus ulcer formation. J Am Geriatr Soc 1979;27:298–301
97. Bogie KM, Nuseibeh I, Bader DL: Transcutaneous gas tensions in the sacrum during acute phase of spinal cord injury. Proc Inst Mech Eng Part H J Eng Med 1992;206(1):1–6
98. Mawson AR, Siddiqui FH, Connolly BJ et al: Sacral transcutaneous oxygen tension levels in the spinal cord injured: risk factors for pressure ulcers. Arch Phys Med Rehabil 1993;74: 745–751
99. Bogie KM, Nuseibeh I, Bader DL: Early programme changes in tissue viability in the seated spinal cord injured subject. Paraplegia 1995;33:141–147
100. Feldman DL, Sepka RS, Klitzman B: Tissue oxygenation and blood flow on specialised and conventional hospital beds. Ann Plast Surg 1993;30:441–444
101. Jakobsen J, Christensen KS: Transcutaneous oxygen tension measurement over the sacrum on various antidecubitus mattresses. Dan Med Bull 1987;34:300–331
102. Neander KN, Birkenfeld R: The influence of various support systems for decubitus ulcer prevention on contact care and percutaneous oxygen pressure. Int Care Nurs 1991;7:120–127
103. Maklebust JA: Pressure ulcer staging systems. Adv Wound Care 1995;8:2811–2814
104. Torrance C: Pressure sores: aetiology, treatment and prevention. Groom Helm, London, 1983:11–20

105. Petersen NC, Bittman S: The epidemiology of pressure sores. Scand J Reconstr Surg 1971;5:62
106. Jordan MM, Clark MO: Report on the Incidence of Pressure Sores in the Patient Community of the Greater Glasgow Health Board Area on Jan 1st 1976. University of Strathclyde, Glasgow, 1976
107. Jordan MM, Nichol SM, Melrose AL: Report on the Incidence of Pressure Sores in the Patient Community of the Borders Health Board Area on 13th October 1976. University of Strathclyde, Glasgow,
108. Barbanel JC, Jordan MM, Nichol SM, Clark ML: Incidence of pressure sores in the Greater Glasgow Health Board Area. Lancet 1977;ii;548–550
109. O'Dea K: The prevalence of pressure sores in four European countries. J Wound Care 1995;4(5):234–236
110. Barrois B, Allaert FA, Colin D: A survey of pressure sore prevalence in hospitals in the greater Pans region. J Wound Care 1995;4:234–236
111. Shaughnessy PW, Kramer AM: Increased needs of patients in nursing homes and patients receiving home health care. N Engl J Med 1990;332:21–27
112. Sternberg J, Spector WD, Kapp MC, Tucker RJ: Decubitus ulcers on admission to nursing homes: prevalence and residents characteristics. Decubitus 1988;1:14–20
113. Lowthian P: Pressure sore prevalence. Nurs Times 1979;75: 358–360
114. Nyquist R, Hawthorn PJ: The prevalence of pressure sores within an area health authority. Nursing 1987;12:183–187
115. O'Dea K: Prevalence of pressure damage in hospital patients in the UK. J Wound Care 1993;2:221–225
116. Allman RM: Pressure ulcers among the elderly. N Eng J Med 1989;320:850–853
117. Meehan M: National Pressure Ulcer Prevalence Survey. Adv Wound Care 1994;7:27–38
118. Hibbs P: Pressure Area Care for the City & Hackney Health Authority. City & Hackney Health Authority, London, 1988
119. Dealey C: Measuring the prevalence and incidence of pressure sores. Br J Nurs 1993;2:998–1000,1002–1006
120. Dealy C: The size of the pressure-sore problem in a teaching hospital. J Adv Nurs 1991;16:663–670
121. Allcock N, Wharrad H, Nicolson A: Interpretation of pressure sore prevalence. J Adv Nurs 1994;20:37–45
122. Clark M, Watts S: The incidence of pressure sores within a National Health Services Trust hospital during 1994. J Adv Nurs 1994;20:33–36
123. Martin BJ: Incidence of pressure sores in geriatric long-term hospital care 1995. J Tissue Viability 1995;5:83–87
124. Brandeis GH, Ooi WL, Hossain M et al: A longitudinal study of risk factors associated with the formation of pressure ulcers in nursing homes. J Am Geriatr Soc 1994;42:388–393
125. Rudman D, Mattson DE, Alvemo L et al: Comparison of clinical indicators in two nursing homes. J Am Geriatr Soc 1993; 41:1317–1325
126. Bergstrom N, Braden B: A prospective study of pressure sore risk among institutional elderly. J Am Geriatr Soc 1992;40: 747–758
127. Baker JHE, Silver JR, Tudway AJC: Late complications of pressure sores, Care Sci Pract 1984;3:56–59
128. Andrews J, Balai R: The prevention and treatment of pressure sores by use of pressure distributing mattresses. Decubitus 1988;1:4–21
129. Hibbs PJ: Prevention: Can We Afford It? The Third Pressure Sore Symposium, Bath, 11–12 March, 1987
130. Editorial: Care Sci Prac 1987;5:2
131. Barton AA, Barton M, Crow M: Mortality, morbidity and resource allocation. BMJ 1981;282:484
132. Hibbs PJ: Pressure sores: a system of prevention. Nurs Mirror 155:25–29
133. Bennett GCJ: Teaching of wound care to medical undergraduates (results from a U.K. national survey). J Tissue Viability 1992;2:50–51

CHAPTER 98

Pressure Sore Prevention and Management

MARY R. BLISS

GERALD C. J. BENNETT

Prevention

Identifying Patients at Risk

One of the chief difficulties in preventing pressure sores (decubitus ulcers) in elderly patients is deciding which patients are susceptible before signs of tissue damage occur. Unlike intensive care or spinal injury patients, almost 100 percent of whom are at risk, risk in elderly patients varies according to the presence or absence of neurologic and vascular disease and the degree of acute illness. Numerous prediction scores have been developed to try to help nurses decide which patients need pressure relief.[1] Most have been based on the Norton score (Table 98-1) originally devised for geriatric patients.[2] Subsequent modifications have mainly tried to improve its specificity and to increase its applicability to other patient groups.[1,3] However, it is impossible to test the validity of prediction scores in practice,[4] and the method has many disadvantages: some scores such as the Norton score, which gives as much weight to disability and nursing procedure as to illness, have a high sensitivity but a low specificity, thus encouraging overuse of scarce resources[1]; there is controversy about which is the most appropriate score for different types of patients, with the result that many different systems are in use, making comparisons between studies difficult; some scores are time-consuming (taking up to 10 minutes to estimate) and require prior knowledge of the patient[5]; it is uncertain how often patients need to be rescored—only once is clearly insufficient for patients whose condition may change hourly[6]; there is a tendency for scores to be simply repeated, over looking significant changes in a patient's condition; and a not-at-risk score may provide a false sense of security.

The simplest score, devised by Andersen et al.[7] in which 2 or higher indicates the need for pressure relief, has been shown to have as high a sensitivity and specifity for grade 2 scores as more complicated systems.[1] In this score unconsciousness, dehydration, and paralysis are absolute risk factors (score 2), and age over 70 years, reduced mobility, incontinence, pronounced emaciation, and redness over bony prominences are relative risk factors (score 1). Including the condition of the skin over the pressure areas as a risk factor has the merit of ensuring that patients are examined and that those with early tissue damage are likely to be treated.

However, if the importance of illness in the development of peripheral tissue necrosis is appreciated, all scoring systems are probably unnecessary and potentially misleading. A dehydrated patient admitted to a hospital is given intravenous fluids for the first 2 or 3 days as part of his general medical care without the need to calculate a clinical score. Similarly, all patients in high-risk groups, (i.e., those with spinal cord injury, neurologic disease, or cardiovascular disease, or who are more than 70 years old) should be considered as being likely to require pressure care from the moment of onset of an acute illness however trivial. It is important to remember that manifestation of illness in elderly patients is often nonspecific and that a fall, acute confusion, loss of appetite, dehydration, new incontinence, or constipation may signify an infection. Acute trauma (including surgery) is an indication of the need for pressure care in an old person. The pressure areas (sacrum, hips, heels) must be examined. An area of erythema that does not blanch on pressure or persists for longer than 30 minutes should be assumed to be a grade 1 pressure sore (Fig. 98-1; see also Plate 98-1) and an indication for immediate action to prevent further tissue damage.

Pressure relief should be continued until the patient's general condition and mobility show that there is no longer a risk of tissue necrosis. For many, it will be obvious almost immediately from their mental acuity or mobility that pressure-relieving measures are unnecessary; however, many others will prove to be more ill than had originally been suspected, and for them it is essential that pressure relief be instituted early before, not after, tissue death occurs. When the patient has recovered and is able to spend more than 6 hours out of bed daily without developing pressure marks on the skin (normally within 2 weeks) pressure-relieving aids can usually be safely removed. However, the pressure areas should continue to be examined daily, and if they show evidence of deterioration, pressure relief must be restored immediately.

Whenever possible, pressure care should begin in the community. General practitioners and community nurses, as well as hospital staff, need to learn to recognize susceptible patients, know how to prevent pressure necrosis, and know where to obtain necessary equipment.

General Measures

The cause of the acute illness must be diagnosed and, if possible, treated. Pain should be relieved early (e.g., in the emergency room) with opiates, if necessary, and by careful support, warmth, and blankets. Decisions about the need for an operation or other contraindications to oral fluids should be made as soon as possible so that appropriate patients may be offered hot drinks and food.

Table 98-1 Norton pressure sore prediction score[a]

Physical Condition	Mental State	Activity	Mobility	Incontinence
4 Good	4 Alert	4 Ambulent	4 Full	4 Not
3 Fair	3 Confused	3 Walks with help	3 Limited	3 Occasional
2 Poor	2 Apathetic	2 Chairbound	2 Very limited	2 Usually urine
1 Bad	1 Stuporose	1 In bed	1 Immobile	1 Doubly incontinent

[a] *Patients with a score of 14 or lower are liable to develop pressure sores.*

In the hospital room, the patient must be given adequate fluids, including frequent drinks if possible. Oral hygiene is very important. Monilial infection is common in elderly patients at risk of pressure sores and exacerbates dehydration and poor nutrition by preventing drinking and eating. The mouth should be examined daily and treated with fungicides if necessary. Where possible, patients should be fed orally with suitably prepared nutritious meals. The need for artificial feeding depends on the cause of the patient's illness and general condition, but enterostomal feeding has not been shown to prevent pressure sores.[8]

Incontinent patients should be changed frequently. Condom urine drainage can be used for men, with care to avoid tension on sensitive skin. Both sexes may benefit from a temporary indwelling catheter. Urine drainage bags must be well supported by clipping them to the side of the bed or by waist suspension so as to avoid the risk of traction on the balloon causing pressure on the trigone[9] or penis. Leg bags are not suitable for ambulant old people, as they slip when full. Constipation, which is almost invariably present in patients ill enough to be susceptible to pressure sores, must be vigorously treated.

Skin Hygiene

The skin should be kept clean and dry and exposed to the air as much as possible by regular repositioning. Barrier creams do not prevent pressure sores. In the past, skin "hardeners" (e.g., soap, alcohol, witch hazel) were often advocated in the mistaken belief that sores were caused by the effects of pressure on the skin rather than on the underlying blood supply. Many were potentially damaging, causing dryness or vasoconstriction in already, ischemic areas. However, massaging of the skin of the pressure areas every 2 to 4 hours which has also been condemned by some authorities,[10] has been found to be effective for preventing sores in spinal injury patients,[11] probably mainly because it allowed periodic pressure relief if only for short periods.

Bed Rest

Patients at risk of pressure sores should be nursed mainly or wholly in bed. Those with a new spinal cord injury are confined to bed until their spinal lesion has stabilized (in 2 to 3 months).[12] They are then allowed out of bed for gradually increasing periods of time. The pressure areas are examined daily, and if a patch of persistent erythema indicating excessive pressure is found, the patient is returned to bed until it is healed.[12,13] A similar but faster approach should be adopted for elderly patients. As soon as they are fit, they should be allowed out of bed for physiotherapy and to walk to the toilet, but they should not sit in a chair for longer than 1 to 2 hours daily until they are able to do so comfortably and willingly without developing significant dependent edema or pressure marks on the skin. In a crossover study, Gebhardt and Bliss[14] showed a significantly reduced incidence of pressure sores in

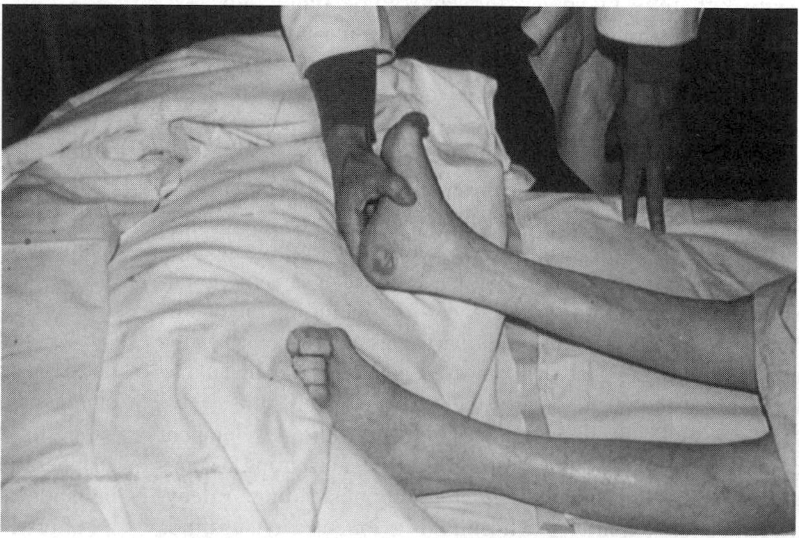

Figure 98-1 Persistent erythema—grade 1 pressure sore.

elderly orthopedic patients for whom chair nursing was limited to 2 hours per session compared with unlimited chair nursing (median 6 hours). Patients should be encouraged to get on and off their beds as often as they wish and to have a siesta for rest and a complete change of position after meals.

Acute spinal injury patients are normally treated with anticoagulants, but this is probably necessary only in elderly patients who have suffered recent trauma (e.g., femoral neck fracture) or who have known thromboembolic disease. Other patients do not have an increased risk of venous thrombosis, and the velocity of blood flow in the legs is increased up to 20-fold in the horizontal position compared with the sitting position.[15] Chest infection, another commonly cited complication of bed rest,[16] was found by Gebhardt and Bliss[14] to be reduced rather than increased by increased bed rest, while diminished exercise tolerance, muscle and bone atrophy, and joint contracture are irrelevant for the brief period of pressure relief required during an acute illness; any disadvantage is more than outweighed by the benefits of faster recovery and freedom from pressure sores. Urinary incontinence may be increased by bed rest, because of the resorption of edema and diuresis that occurs in sick old people in the horizontal position,[17] but usually improves as the patient gets better.

In bed, the patient should be laid as flat as possible. However, many old people need to be nursed sitting up. The backrest and pillows should be positioned so as to give firm support to the lower back and spine, with a triangular arrangement to prevent pressure over prominent dorsal vertebrae if necessary and a pillow under the head. The sheets should be smooth and dry. A bed cradle should be provided, or a pleat made in the sheet and coverlet over the feet to relieve pressure on the heels. A duvet may be used instead, but care should be taken that duvets and blankets are not left folded over the feet when not in use. Patients with peripheral vascular disease, or with rough, sore heels but no localized necrosis, may benefit from a good-quality nursing fleece placed over the whole of the lower third of the bed. This helps to prevent ankle and heel sores and is more comfortable and less restrictive than bootees.

Pressure Relief

Traditionally, nurses have tried to prevent pressure sores in patients in bed by regular turning or repositioning. The method was first established in the 1940s in early spinal injury units and is still the principal system used for paraplegic patients today.[18] Patients are nursed on pressure relieving foam mattresses[9] or pillow packs[13] and are log-rolled between three and four positions throughout the 24 hours according to personalized turning plans[9] (Fig. 98-2). If one area shows a patch of nonfading erythema, that area is omitted from the turning plan until it is completely healed. In this way more than 80 percent of these highly vulnerable patients can be kept free of sores. However, the system is generally impracticable for the elderly. Many old people need to be nursed in the sitting position because of heart or lung disease. Patients requiring intensive care also frequently cannot be repositioned because of the presence of life support equipment or of unstable heart rhythms.[19] In addition, most elderly patients, particularly those with cerebrovascular disease and at high risk of pressure sores, dislike laying on their side and often scream when turned or more out of position. Successful repositioning requires meticulous care and a high staff/patient ratio, which is rarely available in general and geriatric units or in the community. As a result, patients are frequently merely turned from one hip to the other

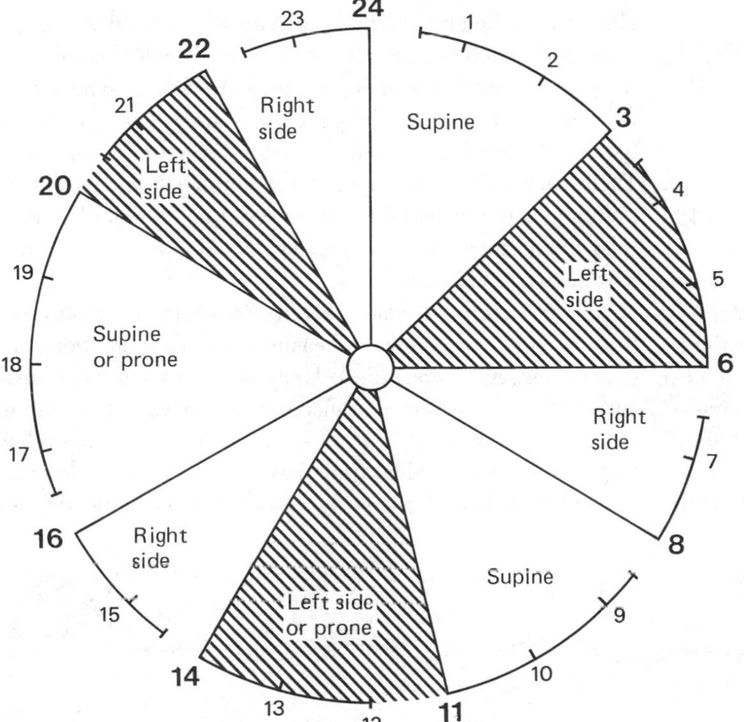

Figure 98-2 Twenty-four hour turning clock. (Courtesy of P. Lowthian.)

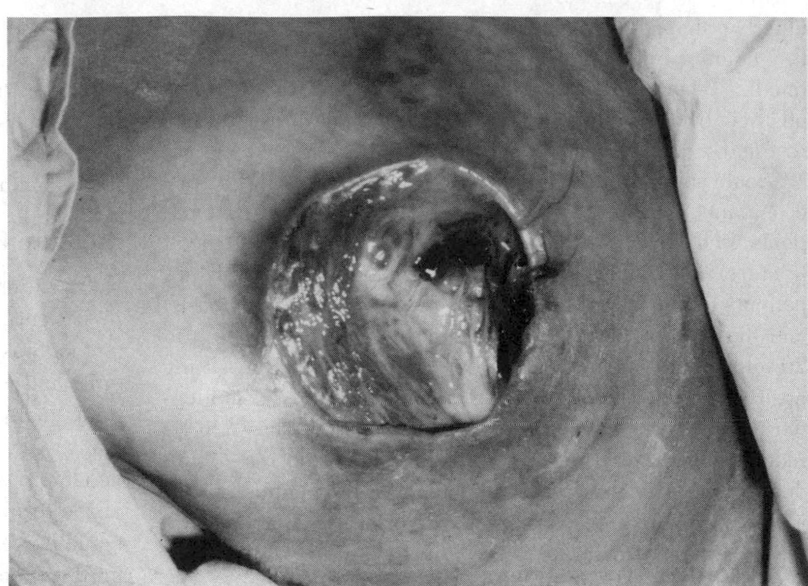

Figure 98-3 Grade 4 sore over the greater trochanter.

on a normal hospital mattress, throwing excessive pressure onto the greater trochanters with often disastrous results (Fig. 98-3). Tilting regimens may be less damaging[18] but are no better liked by elderly patients. Pressure relieving beds or mattresses that reduce or avoid the need for regular repositioning except for comfort are therefore very important.

Pressure-Relieving Supports

Pressure relieving supports fall into three categories: turning beds, constant low-pressure mattresses and beds, and alternating-pressure mattresses.

Turning beds

Turning beds are used in spinal injury units to assist turning but are unsuitable for elderly patients and so will not be discussed here.

Constant low-pressure supports

These are soft or flotation mattresses and beds (Fig. 98-4) which aim to distribute the body weight as widely as possible so as to reduce localized areas of high pressure over bony prominences which causes tissue distortion and ischemia. Flotation water beds have been used since the early 1800s.[20] The patient lies in a bath of water on a very loose waterproof sheet which allows the body to sink into it as if floating. This provides multiaxial support to the body which prevents capillary distortion and occlusion. Deep water beds prevent sores[7] but have many disadvantages: they are very heavy and difficult to install, and so they cannot be used for emergency prevention; they increase dependency; they make some patients feel seasick; they are unsuitable for many patients (e.g., heavy patients, those who need to sit up, patients with unstable fractures, patients likely to require resuscitation, or those undergoing rehabilitation); and they make nursing difficult (e.g., washing, feeding, toileting, and especially getting patients in and out of bed).

In an attempt to overcome some of these problems, flotation air beds, such as low air loss[21] and air-fluidized beads beds,[22] have been developed in which the floating action can be temporarily suspended to provide a stable surface for nursing procedures. A low air loss bed has been shown in a randomized controlled trial to prevent sores in intensive care patients.[21] However, air flotation beds share many of the disadvantages of water beds, such as difficulty of installation and of getting patients in and out,[22] and of dependency. Air-fluidized beds have been reported to cause dehydration[23] and electrolyte disturbances.[24] Flotation air beds generally are also expensive.[21] Their use has therefore largely been confined to intensive care units and to treatment rather than prevention. Low air loss mattress replacements are less expensive and more practical and may be just as effective.[1]

Efforts have been made to develop static soft mattresses that are more economical and easier to use than flotation beds (e.g., of air, gel, foam, fiber). Many show low interface pressures[25–27] and sustained transcutaneous oxygen tensions in studies in volunteers,[28] but these observations may not relate to practice[29] and clinical trials have proved difficult to carry out and to evaluate.[1] Sideranko et al.[30] found a static air mat-

Figure 98-4 Mechanism of action of constant low-pressure supports such as air or foam overlays, low air loss or air-fluidized bead beds.

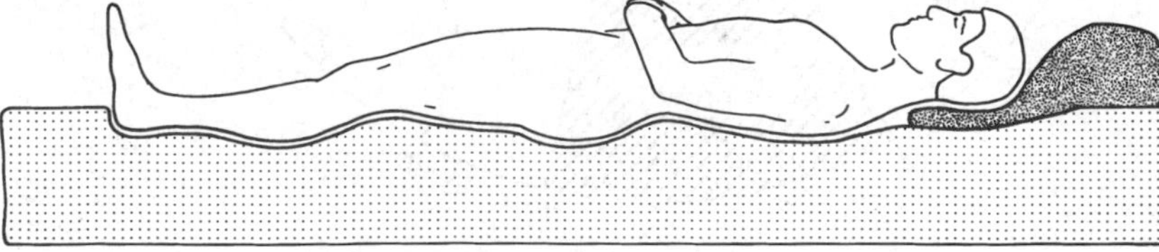

tress to be effective in a surgical intensive care unit with only a 5 percent incidence of sores compared with 12 percent with a water mattress and 25 percent with a small-cell alternating-pressure mattress. Sylvia[31] noted that the incidence of sores in a university teaching hospital increased when static air overlays were discontinued and improved when they were reintroduced. However, in elderly private nursing home residents, Lazzara and Buschmann[32] did not find any difference in the incidence of sores (about 15 percent) on air and gel overlays, noting that the former were difficult to maintain correctly inflated and easily punctured and that the latter were heavy. In a study of elderly patients with femoral neck fracture, a bead support system[33] consisting of individual cushions was shown to be effective in preventing sores compared with standard surfaces (16 percent and 49 percent incidence, respectively) but has since been discontinued probably because of practical difficulties. Conine et al.[34] found a 59 percent incidence of sores in chronic neurologic patients on a fiberfill overlay; patients also complained that it restricted movement and stability and developed an unpleasant odor. Kemp et al.[35] reported a greater incidence of sores in geriatric patients on a convoluted overlay (47 percent) than on a solid foam overlay (31 percent). However, compared with ordinary hospital mattresses, a slit foam mattress[36] and a variety of other specialized foam mattresses[1] have been shown to have significant benefit in preventing sores in orthopedic patients. In a randomized trial in long-stay geriatric patients (only about 40 percent of whom were scheduled for 4-hour turning), Bliss[37] found that significantly fewer patients with grade 1 and 2 sores deteriorated on three slit foam mattress overlays (about 35 percent) compared with a water overlay (47 percent) and two fiberfill overlays (about 52 percent); however, only 13 percent deteriorated on a large-cell alternating-pressure mattress. Gebhardt et al.[38] found that 40 percent of intensive care patients developed pressure sores on a variety of constant low-pressure mattresses and overlays, compared with none on large-cell alternating-pressure mattresses.

The results of these trials suggest that static air overlays and slit foam mattresses are probably the most useful nonflotation low-pressure supports but that neither can be relied on to prevent sores without regular repositioning.

Alternating-pressure supports

Alternating-pressure mattresses and overlays work on a different principle than constant low-pressure supports. They do not aim solely to reduce pressure but to reproduce the alternation of high and low pressure in the weight-bearing areas that occurs in normal people as a result of postural changes in response to pressure pain. The repeated movement in the tissues allows reopening of capillary beds and reactive hyperemia which prevents prolonged ischemia and cell death.

Alternating-pressure mattresses consist of two alternating systems of air cells which inflate and deflate reciprocally over a 5- to 10-minute cycle underneath the recumbent body, thus continually changing the areas of support (Fig. 98-5). The cells

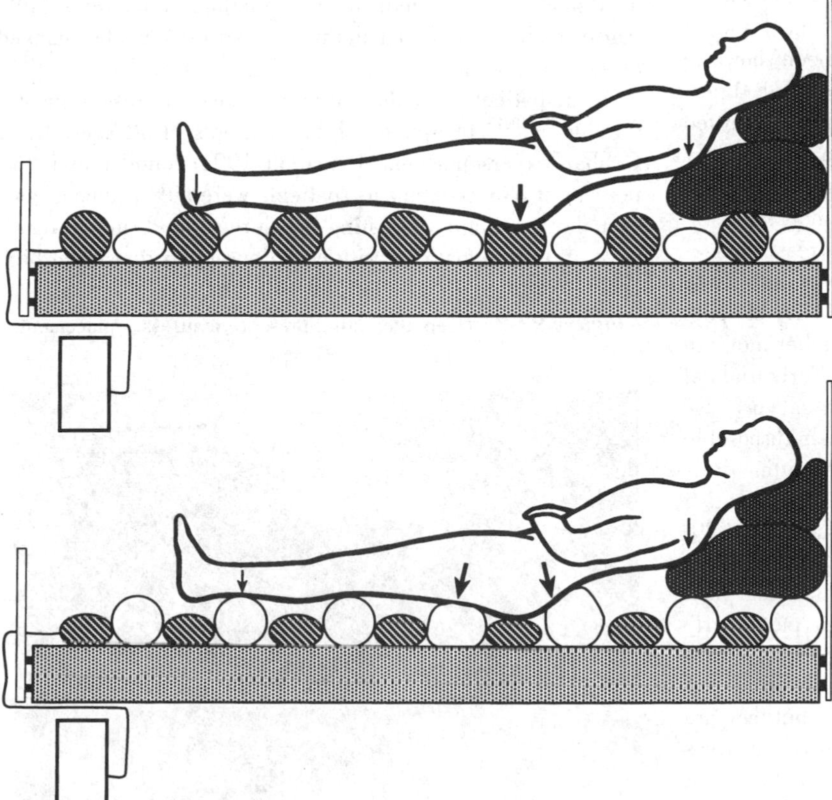

Figure 98-5 Mechanism of action of alternating-pressure supports.

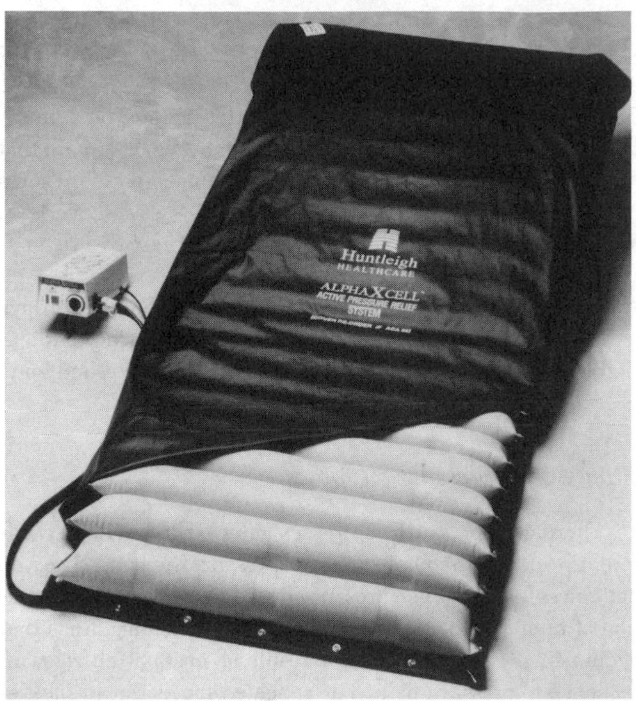

Figure 98-6 Large-cell alternating-pressure overlay.

must have adequate diameter to lift the body sufficiently clear of the underlying mattress or bed to allow restoration of the blood supply. A randomized controlled trial in acute geriatric patients indicated that large-cell mattresses with cells 15 cm in diameter were more effective at preventing pressure sores than small-cell mattresses with cells less than 5 cm in diameter.[1,39] Twenty five percent of intensive care patients[30] and 54 percent of chronic neurologic patients[34] have been shown to develop sores on small-cell mattresses compared with 0 percent of intensive care patients,[38] 4 percent of newly admitted general hospital patients,[7] and 13 percent of long-stay elderly patients[37] on medium-depth large-cell (10 cm) mattresses (Fig. 98-6 see also Plate 98-2). Deeper (about 15 cm), more sophisticated, and expensive alternating-pressure mattress replacements with double layers of cells[40] (Fig. 98-7; see also Plate 98-3) or rectangular cells[41] are often used for heavy patients or for treating sores,[42] but it is not known whether they are more effective than medium-depth mattresses. Early trials of alternating-pressure supports are difficult to evaluate because demand was mainly for small-cell inexpensive, semidisposable machines which constantly broke down, thus permitting pressure sores to occur.[34,40,43–45] Following publication of a British standard for alternating-pressure air mattresses in 1989, stronger models have become available. Alternating-pressure supports are now widely used in British hospitals and hospices,[46] with a reduction in the incidence of sores, particularly of deep sores.[47]

Large-cell alternating-pressure overlays have the disadvantage of requiring a motor which may be noisy,[34] but they are generally more portable and easier to install on the mattress of a patient's bed in the hospital or in the community than most low-pressure overlays. Patients can be nursed on them as on an ordinary mattress, including sitting up with a backrest if necessary. Regular repositioning is not essential, but patients can be turned if required.

Careful training of doctors and nurses in the use of alternating-pressure mattresses is essential. The mattress must be correctly anchored on the bed, the tube attachments secured, the pressure dial adjusted for the patient's weight if required, and the motor plugged in and switched on. Special care must be taken to ensure that the air tubes connecting the mattress and motor are not kinked by being tucked under the mattress of the bed. Backrests should normally be placed on top of the overlay, but some alternating-pressure mattresses can be used over a backrest or on a gatched bed to protect the back and shoulders. A blanket or similar flexible insulating material may be placed over the mattress under the bottom sheet to reduce humidity and improve comfort.[48] The original Airwave mattress[40] had a full-length nursing fleece which did not impair its performance and which may have helped to prevent superficial sores. Thick foam overlays, incontinence pads, pillows, bootees, and so on, must not, however, be placed between the patient and the support.

Most modern alternating-pressure mattresses have devices enabling them to remain inflated while patients are being transported to the operating room. They can then be reconnected to an electrical outlet in the recovery room ready to receive them following the operation. Most also have emergency deflation devices for cardiac resuscitation although it is uncertain whether these are essential and they clearly add to the hazards of misuse. Mattresses must be checked daily to ensure that they are correctly inflated. Most are fitted with audible as well as visual alarms to indicate malfunction. If no remediable cause can be found for an alarm, the mattress must be changed as soon as possible.

Some patients find alternating-pressure mattresses uncomfortable.[34,38,45] In a study of 115 patients of all ages, K. S. Gebhardt (personal communication 1996) found that in 65 percent of 593 assessments, patients were either unconscious or unaware of their alternating-pressure support (including almost all elderly patients with cerebrovascular disease at high

Figure 98-7 Deep alternating-pressure mattress replacement.

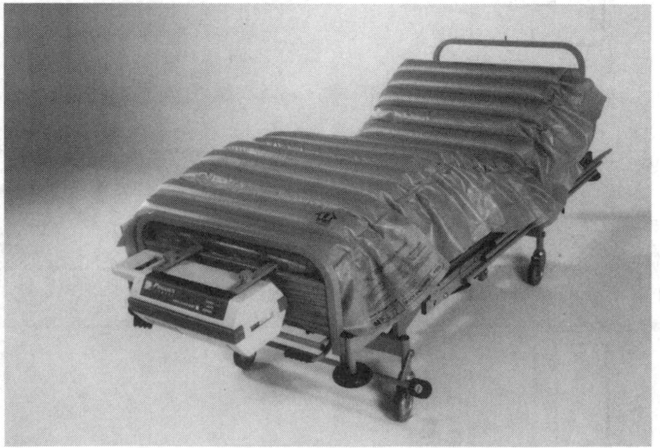

risk of pressure sores); 17 percent said it was comfortable; 15 percent found that it was tolerable; and 3 percent reported that it was uncomfortable. Eight patients asked to have their mattress removed. Patients with painful illnesses such as cancer are particularly likely to find them upsetting. For these individuals, a static air overlay[31,49] may be useful, but care must be taken to ensure that it is properly inflated. Alternatively, a low air loss overlay may be tried.[1] However, many patients who complain about the discomfort of an alternating-pressure mattress are sufficiently alert and responsive to no longer be in need of special support.

Pressure-relieving cushions

Pressure-relieving cushions are seldom indicated for elderly patients. Those ill enough to be at risk of pressure sores are usually too weak to be nursed out of bed for more than 2 hours at a time, during which they can safely sit in an ordinary armchair with the knees well supported at a right angle to ensure optimum distribution of pressure over the ischial tuberosities and thighs. Pressure-relieving cushions are less effective than pressure-relieving mattresses,[50] and seat cushions hinder patients' mobility and efforts to relieve their own pressure areas. Immobile old people living at home who insist on spending most of their days—and often nights—in a chair may occasionally benefit from a special cushion, but this is unlikely to prevent tissue breakdown as they become more ill. Pressure-relieving cushions for healthy wheelchair-bound patients are, however, essential[51] and need to be chosen with the help of an occupational therapist. Comfort, stability, ease of transfer, cleaning, durability, and cost are as important as pressure relief.[52] A simple 4-inch foam cushion which is replaced every 6 months may be more suitable than an expensive cushion, for example, a Roho air cushion[53] (Fig. 98-8; see also Plate 98-4) which gives good pressure distribution but is difficult to keep correctly inflated and hinders transfers, or a gel cushion[54] which is heavy. Alternating-pressure cushions are available[55] but are less effective than mattresses.

Gurneys and x-ray and operating tables

Elderly patients should spend as little time as possible in the emergency room, preferably not more than an hour.[56] However, this is not always practicable, and emergency pressure relief needs to be provided from the time of arrival until transfer to a hospital room. It is difficult to reposition ill or traumatized patients on a narrow gurney,[57] and large-cell alternating-pressure pads are unsuitable for patients who have to be moved frequently. Static air mattresses are also difficult to maintain correctly inflated. A good-quality slit foam pad is probably the most practical and most likely to provide adequate pressure relief for a short period. Patients with paralyzed legs (e.g., due to a femoral neck fracture or stroke) should have a pillow or foam gutter placed under the calf so that the heel hangs free of pressure.

If a patient has to spend a long time on an X-ray table, it should be padded and, if necessary, the plates inserted between the padding and the patient.

Bead,[33] gel,[58] foam,[57,59] air,[59] liquid replacement,[60] and small-cell alternating-pressure pads and pillows have been used to relieve pressure on operating tables, but none has proved wholly satisfactory. Stability, durability, ease of use and of cleaning and sterilizing, and antistatic properties are as important as the ability to relieve pressure and capital cost.[58] If no special support is available, very high-risk patients such as spinal injury patients and those undergoing cardiovascular operations, should be carefully positioned with pillows under the lumbar area and thighs to relieve pressure over the sacrum, and under the calves to protect the heels. A channeled pillow may be used under the head to relieve pressure on the occiput.[59] If possible, the patient should be moved or lifted at intervals to allow restoration of the peripheral circulation to all parts of the body.

Discontinuing pressure relief

Most elderly patients with acute illness require pressure relief for only about 1 or 2 weeks. As soon as they are able to sit up out of bed comfortably for more than 6 hours and do not have sores, special supports should be removed. Pressure-relieving mattresses are bulky and unstable and hinder rehabilitation by making it difficult for patients to move and to get on and off their beds unaided. They should always be removed for at least a few days before discharge from the hospital to ensure that the patient is safe without a special support before returning home or to a nursing home. A few chronically ill patients may need to continue to be nursed on special supports

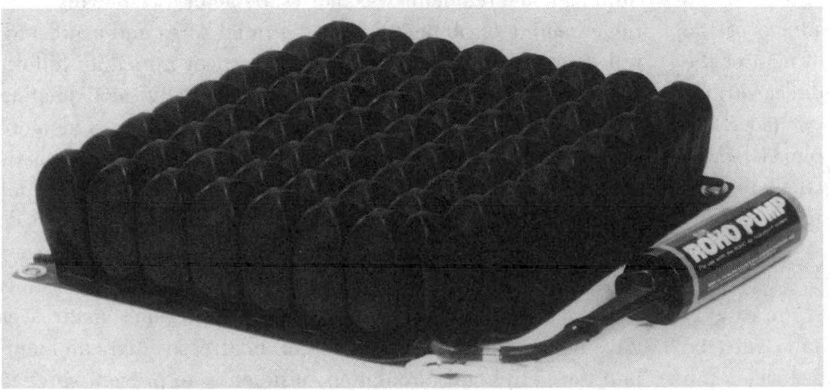

Figure 98-8 Roho cushion.

in the community to prevent tissue breakdown, and this arrangement should be before discharge.

Supply of pressure-relieving supports

In the United Kingdom tissue viability nurse specialists are increasingly being appointed with joint responsibilities in hospitals and in the community[61] to advise about pressure care and to ensure that equipment such as alternating-pressure overlays is available wherever it is needed. They are also responsible for retrieving units no longer needed so that they can be cleaned and serviced before reuse. Most pressure-relieving mattress replacements and overlays, including alternating-pressure mattresses, can be cleaned by sponging with hot water and an antiseptic according to the manufacturer's instructions. Supports used for patients requiring barrier nursing (e.g., for methicillin-resistant *Staphylococcus aureus*) need to be cleaned by a gas cleaner or Formalin spray (including the motor). All pressure-relieving supports used in hospitals should be serviced and sterilized every 3 months.[62]

Healing Pressure Sores

Pressure sores are acute wounds consisting of discrete areas of dead tissue caused by ischemia due to pressure. Except in patients with peripheral vascular disease, the surrounding tissues are usually healthy so that, providing pressure can be relieved and the blood supply restored, healing takes place rapidly. The idea that pressure sores are chronic[63] is almost entirely due to the inadequacy of pressure relief. Even pressure sores of the legs and feet in patients with peripheral vascular disease usually heal steadily with pressure relief and bed rest to maximize circulation. Local treatment is of minimal importance and should be as simple as possible, avoiding injurious agents that delay natural healing.

Healing of a traumatic wound such as a pressure sore takes place in four stages: debridement, granulation and contraction, re-epithelialization, and remodeling. With restoration of the blood supply, eicosanoids and free radicals[64] released from the dead cells attract inflammatory cells which phagocytose the dead tissue and liberate proteolytic enzymes which liquify it and allow it to be discharged.[65] They also secrete cytokines which promote the growth of granulation tissue by stimulating angiogenesis and recruiting fibroblasts and myofibroblasts. When the slough has separated in about 2 to 4 weeks, the latter contract,[66] causing a reduction in the volume of the sore to about half its original size with closure of most of the sinuses. Epithelial cells then migrate over the reduced surface area by binding to macromolecules to close the wound.[64] Finally the highly cellular granulation tissue is remodeled by further deposition of collagen and apoptosis over the following year to form a strong but relatively acellular scar.

Pressure relief

Measures for relieving pressure to heal sores are exactly the same as for prevention except that they usually must be continued for much longer. This depends on the size and depth of the original wound; small, superficial sores may heal within 1 week, but a large, full-thickness sore may take 6 months or more. Very extensive areas of tissue loss may never heal satisfactorily without plastic surgery.

Bed rest

Bed rest is essential for healing almost all pressure sores. A patient with a new necrotic sore is invariably ill, and so bed rest is a necessary part of his general medical treatment. It becomes more difficult to enforce with both the patient and the nurses as recovery is made. The belief that nursing patients out of bed is good for "bedsores" persists and is still often taught to nurses and medical students. However, healing is inevitably delayed or prevented if a sore is deprived of a blood supply by sitting in a chair for the greater part of the day. Pressure-relieving cushions do not allow adequate circulation to permit healing, and pressure in the seated posture risks causing new necrosis. Patients should therefore spend as much time as possible on a pressure-relieving mattress on their bed. Where practicable, the injured area should be kept free of pressure by careful repositioning. Sleep is important for healing[67] and may be encouraged during the day as well as at night. As the patient's condition improves, they may be dressed and allowed to get up for physiotherapy and for meals and to walk to the toilet but should return to rest on their bed at all other times.

Pressure-relieving supports

The results of trials of pressure-relieving supports for healing sores are similar to those for prevention. Five randomized trials of flotation beds for healing have been carried out, three on an air-fluidized bead bed,[22,68,69] and two on low air loss flotation beds.[1,70] They included a variety of different types of patients with pressure ulcers ranging from grade 2 to 4 (see Ch. 96). Not surprisingly all showed beneficial results compared with the control regimens: turning every 2 hours on a hospital bed, sheepskins, gel pads, convoluted foam mattresses, and small-cell alternating-pressure pads. However, two of the trials of the air-fluidized bead bed were limited to periods of about 2 weeks because of the expense, and 50 percent of patients in the third trial were withdrawn over the 36-week trial period.[1] A trial of a low air loss bed for elderly nursing home residents was more satisfactory,[70] showing complete healing of 60 percent of superficial sores and a substantial decrease in the size of deep sores over a median follow-up period of 37.5 days. Caley[1] found equally good healing rates over 24 days in patients on less expensive and more practical low air loss overlays. However, all air flotation beds and overlays are bulky and unstable, making it difficult for patients undergoing rehabilitation to get on and off their beds easily and to help themselves. Static soft mattresses and overlays are more practical but less effective.[37,68,70]

Few trials of healing on alternating-pressure mattresses have been attempted, but large-cell mattresses that can maintain the peripheral circulation sufficiently to prevent sores in intensive care patients[38] are also likely to permit healing. Bliss[37] found that 45 percent of grade 2 sores healed in 18 days on medium-depth large-cell alternating-pressure mattresses compared with 37 percent on slit foam and 24 percent and 20 percent on water and fiberfill overlays, respectively. Devine[42] showed, a similar reduction in the size and healing of grades 2 to 5 sores in 4 weeks on two types of deep alternating-pressure mattresses. Results on small-cell mattresses have been less successful[22,70] but are difficult to evaluate because of the use of foam sheets, fleeces, bootees, and so on, in addition to alternating pressure.

Alternating-pressure mattresses provide a more stable surface than flotation supports and are therefore more suitable for long-term use for healing sores in patients undergoing rehabilitation. They are also usually less expensive. They are relatively easy to install in a patient's home so that healing can be continued in the community if necessary. A patient with a sacral lesion can be nursed on alternate sides without danger of developing sores over the greater trochanters, but a pillow should be placed between the legs to prevent the formation of sores over the knees.

Heel sores

Bed rest is important in healing heel sores. The purpose is not to relieve pressure on the heels, which is more difficult in bed than in a chair, but to optimize the circulation. Arterial blood flow is increased by dependency, but venous return is greatly reduced in the sitting position compared with the horizontal position.[15] This results in capillary stasis and edema which slows healing and exacerbates infection. Diuretics alone are ineffective in reducing edema in the dependent leg, and elevation on a footstool causes intolerable pressure on the heels and ischial tuberosities. Rest in the horizontal or semirecumbent position on a bed or on a chaise lounge, with or without diuretics, produces an immediate reduction in the venocapillary pressure with improvement in the circulation, resolution of edema, and the beginning of healing, usually within 2 days. In elderly patients, the leg should not be raised above the horizontal because of the risk of causing arterial insufficiency. A pillow or foam wedge may be placed under the calves to relieve pressure on the heels, but care should be taken to ensure that it is *not placed under the heels themselves*. There is no evidence that the increased pressure on the calves causes deep vein thrombosis. If possible, the patient should be nursed on a large-cell alternating-pressure mattress. As the sore heals and mobility improves, the patient can cautiously sit up out of bed for longer periods, providing edema does not recur. The legs should be dependent while sitting in a chair, as this provides optimum pressure relief and is usually most comfortable; but the patient should return to rest on the pressure-relieving mattress on their bed at frequent intervals until the sore is healed.

Pain

Both superficial and deep pressure sores in elderly patients are usually very painful. Pain limits mobility, impairs sleep and appetite, and has a deleterious effect on healing.[7] Measures to relieve pain must be started as soon as possible. For superficial sores, careful positioning with pillows to avoid pressure on the sore area, a pressure-relieving mattress, and an occlusive dressing, if appropriate, may be adequate. Analgesics such as paracetamol or co-proxamol are ineffective. A patient with a new deep sore is usually toxic and shocked as well as in severe pain. The presence of a large amount of necrotic tissue initiates the systemic inflammatory response syndrome,[72] causing pyrexia, tachycardia, and leukocytosis without infection. Surgical debridement and packing the wound greatly exacerbate pain[73] without speeding healing and should be avoided. The patient should be treated with bed rest, fluids, and analgesics. Nonsteroidal anti-inflammatory drugs may relieve traumatic pain[71] but delay healing and increase susceptability to further tissue damage.[74] Systemic opiates are usually necessary. Short-acting drugs such as pethidine are not appropriate. Diamorphine 2.5 to 5 mg or morphine 5 to 10 mg should be given every 4 hours orally, or via a subcutaneous pump, until the sloughs have separated and the sore has begun to granulate, usually in 2 to 4 weeks. In elderly patients these small doses rarely cause nausea, and so antiemetics are unnecessary. They can also safely be given to patients with respiratory disease. Long-acting preparations are less effective and more likely to cause drowsiness and confusion. Excessive drowsiness is usually due to an unnecessarily high dosage, but it is important to remember that sleep promotes healing and that in some dying patients a drowsy state is preferable. Effective pain relief with opiates can also delay death in terminally ill patients by improving rest, appetite, and a feeling of well-being. The most important side effect is constipation. Regular enemas and stimulant laxatives are required for almost all patients with pressure sores.

Nutrition

Good hydration and nutrition are important for optimal healing, but decisions about artificial feeding for old people who cannot be fed orally should depend on their prognosis and the wishes of patients and their families. In a study of long-term care, prolonged tube feeding of patients did not prevent sores or facilitate healing.[75]

With an intact blood supply, the early processes of repair take place even in a catabolic dying patient, but it has been calculated that twice the normal daily protein intake is required as for complete healing of a full-thickness sore in a young person.[66] A high-protein diet is therefore important. Carbohydrate is also required to provide fuel for cellular metabolism.[76] Vitamin C is important, both because of its role in the synthesis of hydroxyproline and hydroxylysine (constituents of collagen) and as a scavenger of free radicals.[76] However, supplements have not been shown to accelerate healing,[77] and megadoses have been reported to cause tissue breakdown if they are suddenly stopped.[78] Zinc is also important for collagen syntheses, but systemic and topical supplements have not been shown to promote healing and may retard it by upsetting calcium concentration.[79] Iron is a cofactor for the hydroxylation of lysine and proline[78] and so is essential for collagen synthesis as well as for maintaining the hemoglobin level and oxygen-carrying capacity of blood. Hemoglobin and iron status should be checked, and supplements given if necessary. Very debilitated patients with anemia of chronic disease may be helped by an initial blood transfusion. Copper, manganese, and calcium are also involved in collagen synthesis, but supplements are rarely required. Many nutritional parameters are altered by illness and age[80] and do not necessarily reflect intake or whole body balance. Anabolic steroids,[81] insulin,[82] and more recently growth hormone[83] have been used in attempts to improve nutrition, but without success. However, in most patients, appetite improves when pressure is relieved and pain and further tissue necrosis is prevented, so that nutritional supplements and drug therapy are unnecessary.

Infection

Cellulitis, edema, pyrexia, and leutoctytosis in a patient with a new pressure sore are a normal reaction to the presence of dead tissue and do not indicate infection or the need for antibiotics. It is also important to realize that the subsequent liquification and discharge of dead tissue as a foul-smelling exudate with apparent enlargement of the sore is the first stage of healing and not a sign of worsening infection.[84] Although a discharging sore is always heavily colonized with local bacteria, including pathogens, these seldom cause clinically significant infection[85] and may even help to liquify the sloughs.[86] Galpin et al.[87] found bacteremia in 76 percent of of patients with deep sores, but half of these individuals died despite being given antibiotics, suggesting that they were very ill and that pressure relief was inadequate.

Unnecessary treatment with antibiotics is merely likely to impair appetite or to cause diarrhea and to encourage the growth of resistant organisms. A pressure sore needs to be swabbed only if following debridement it develops a secondary infection and cellulitis or if the patient shows new signs of systemic toxicity. An infected sore is usually painful, glistening, friable, and bright red and may have a characteristic odor, in contrast to healthy granulation tissue which is relatively painless, dull pink, and nonfriable with little or no discharge. Most patients who require antibiotics for a secondary infection are diabetics. Gram-negative organisms, coliforms, proteus, and pseudomonas predominate, but group A streptococci and *Staphylococcus aureus*, including methicillin-resistant strains, and anaerobes are common. Infections are not usually considered clinically significant unless there are more than 10^5 organisms per gram of tissue.[66] Some authorities recommend wound biopsy as a more reliable means of identifying the responsible organism,[88] but this is rarely necessary. If antibiotics are required, they should be given systemically.

Local Treatment

Debridement

Surgical debridement of pressure sores in elderly patients is rarely indicated. The sores are less extensive than those in spinal injury patients and hardly ever extend into joints or bone. Surgery merely introduces the hazards of an anesthetic and of new pressure trauma in a sick patient. Providing pressure is relieved, the sloughs separate naturally within 1 to 4 weeks with or without the help of hydrolyzing agents (Fig. 98-9; see also Plate 98-5). As they loosen, they can be snipped free with scissors and the cavities washed out twice daily with normal saline or tap water.[84] In the rare cases in which the sloughs do not separate spontaneously, the patient is usually dying.[74]

Wound healing agents

Antiseptics such as Eusol and povidone iodine are toxic to granulation tissue[84,89,90] and prevent epithelialization.[91] They are thus likely to delay rather than to accelerate healing and should not used. Topical antibiotics should similarly be avoided, as they are liable to cause sensitivity reactions and to encourage the growth of resistant organisms. Pierce et al.[92] reported accelerated healing of "chronic" pressure ulcers in elderly nursing home residents with the use of platelet-derived

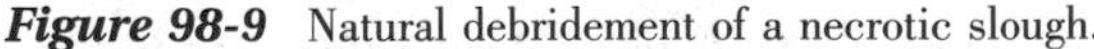

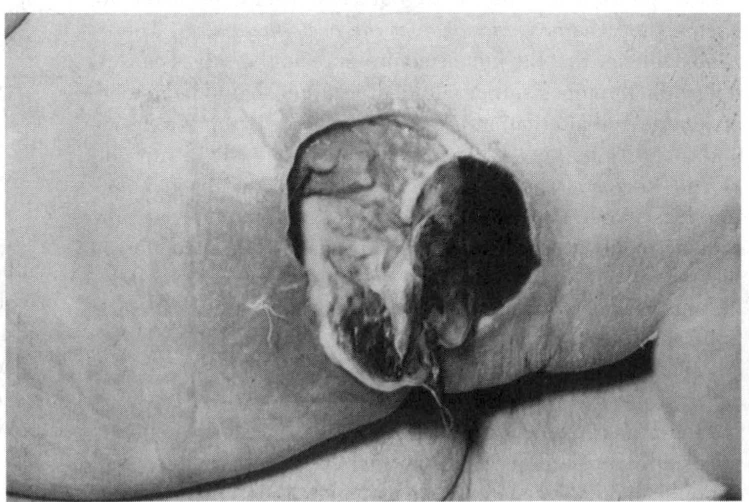

Figure 98-9 Natural debridement of a necrotic slough.

growth factor, as shown by reduction in the volume of the wound and by tissue biopsy over 28 days, but no information is given about concurrent pressure relief. Similarly, studies on low-frequency[93] and high-frequency[94] electromagnetic energy, laser therapy,[95] ultrasound,[96] and hyperbaric oxygen[97] purported to show benefits for chronic wound healing, have either been poorly controlled and not included pressure relief or have been carried out on different types of wounds (e.g., venous or arterial ulcers and diabetic foot sores).

Dressings

In experimental animals[98,99] and in humans,[100] healing has been shown to proceed more rapidly in a moist than in a dry environment, but there has been a lack of clinical trials, and many health care workers still prefer dry healing for some types of wounds.[84] Dry dressings, including "nonadhesives," tend to become incorporated into slough and developing granulation tissue so that the wound is retraumatized each time they are changed.[84] Occlusive and semiocclusive dressings (which allow passage of water vapor and oxygen but not of water and bacteria) reduce pain[101] and prevent drying and scab formation, thus permitting faster resolution of the sloughs and epithelialization.[84] Hydrocolloid dressings also reduce infection[102] by providing a partially self-sterilizing fluid medium.[84] However, the presence of microorganisms does not necessarily affect healing rates,[85,86,103] and different types of dressings may be needed in different situations. Bio-occlusive and hydrocolloid dressings are useful for treating sores on nonpressurized skin (e.g., over the greater trochanters or malleoli), but in pressure areas such as the sacrum and heel they tend to rumple or harden and to pull on the skin, causing further pressure and tissue damage. They are also unsuitable for necrotic sores with a heavy exudate.

Packing

Deep pressure sores do not need to be packed. Packing is unnecessary to prevent loculation of infected material, as this never occurs in pressure sores in elderly patients. Packing with solid substances such as gauze obstructs discharge of necrotic material, prevents contraction by damaging granulation tissue, and is very painful.[73] Alginates or foam are less damaging, but all packing agents require a secondary dressing to keep them in place, which is liable to cause dermatitis on the margin of the wound.[84] Nonirritant substances such as honey, which has antibacterial properties,[104] or hydrogels,[105] which help to hydrolyze slough, can be placed in the cavity, but there is no research evidence that they have any advantage over leaving it empty. Deep pressure sores usually heal rapidly if they are simply dressed with sheets of absorbent material secured across the mouth of the wound and changed as often as possible. Superficial and deep sacral sores near the anus cannot be dressed effectively but heal well if they are simply kept clean with frequent changes of underpad. Open wounds are undesirable in institutions where they may act as a source of infection but cause little or no harm to the patient and may be unavoidable.

A hydrogel may be combined with metronidazole powder to reduce odor in a necrotic wound.[105] Activated charcoal dressings should be avoided as they are costly, are ineffective when saturated, and may interfere with the growth of fibroblasts.[105] It is also important to realize that, unlike that in fungating cancers, odor in a pressure sore subsides spontaneously within 1 or 2 weeks following separation of the sloughs.

Heel sores

Superficial and deep heel sores are usually best treated, at least initially, by being exposed and allowed to dry. Heal sores heal slowly, partly because of scanty subcutaneous tissue which limits contraction and partly because of the frequent presence of peripheral vascular disease. Attempts to keep the area moist to promote early debridement often merely increase maceration and pain and hinder mobility. If the sore is allowed to dry and surrounding inflammation to subside, with bed rest to maximize the circulation, pain usually improves so that the patient can begin to walk about. Superficial transparent or black dried blisters can be ignored and soon detach themselves. Full-thickness eschars also often cause little inconvenience, but if required, final debridement can be expedited by applying a small hydrogel or hydrocolloid dressing. An enzyme preparation can also be used but is expensive and must be applied twice daily.[84] Injecting enzymes under an eschar or debriding with a scalpel is painful and injurious and is not recommended. If a bandage is necessary, it should be applied loosely in order to avoid causing a new pressure injury on the foot.

Plastic surgery

Surgery is seldom required to heal pressure sores in elderly patients. Most sores heal steadily with relief of pressure, and in the rare exception the patient is usually too ill for surgery or is dying. Elderly patients who have developed deep pressure sores often need long-term nursing with continuous pressure relief, and so the protracted healing of the sores themselves causes little extra inconvenience.

However, with modern anesthetic techniques age itself is no bar to surgery, and an alert, active patient who has suffered a deep pressure sore preventing them from achieving full mobility or discharge from the hospital should be considered for plastic surgery. Split skin or pinch grafts are usually unhelpful and cause an additional lesion in the donor area. Simple suturing is also seldom satisfactory, and a full-thickness skin flap is usually required.[106] The patient should be rendered as fit as possible by physiotherapy, a high-protein diet, and a blood transfusion and/or antibiotics if indicated. The wound is sterilized preoperatively by using packs soaked in a strong antiseptic such as Eusol or silver sulfadiazine. This is the only situation in which the use of an antiseptic may be justified. The whole sore is then excised, together with any associated bursae, followed by removal of underlying prominences. The tissue defect is closed by direct suture or a local skin flap. In spinal injury patients myocutaneous flaps can be used to increase tissue bulk over bony prominences. Scrupulous pressure relief in the perioperative period is essential. If a suitable pressure-relieving support (e.g. an alternating-pressure or low air loss overlay) is not available, a careful repositioning schedule will be necessary. In very debilitated elderly patients pressure relief may have to be continued indefinitely.

Methicillin-resistant Staphylococcus aureus

Many elderly patients are contaminated with methicillin-resistant *S. ureus* (MRSA), and their pressure sores soon become colonized. However, this rarely affects healing which depends primarily on pressure relief. The main danger is of cross-infection in hospitals where isolation, barrier nursing, and eradication therapy are usually required. The patient should be discharged as soon as possible. In the community, colonization with MRSA poses little threat and should not constitute a reason for refusing admission to a residential or nursing home.[107] Affected residents should be given a single room if available but may share a room with another resident who does not have an open skin lesion if necessary. They should not be isolated from other residents. Their wound should be covered by a dressing, preferably impermeable, but no precautions are necessary with other items touched or handled by them. Staff should use disposable gloves and aprons when dressing the wound, performing catheter care, or dealing with soiled bedding, but thorough hand washing by both the resident and staff members after other activities is sufficient. Clothes and bedding should be machine-washed, preferably at a hot setting, or dry cleaned if unsuitable for machine washing.

Cost

In the United Kingdom pressure-relieving mattress overlays and replacements are normally purchased by health authorities so that they are readily available for prevention. Single-layer large-cell alternating-pressure overlays cost between £700 ($1,052) and £900 ($1,353) and with proper servicing should last for 5 years. Deep alternating-pressure-large-cell mattress replacements cost about £2,000 ($3,006) and £4,000 ($6,012) and have a similar working life. Thrice monthly servicing and sterilization cost about (£30 ($45). In the United States, supports are usually hired by the day at about $15 to $25 (£9.4 to £15.6) for a medium-depth large-cell alternating-pressure mattress overlay and $25 to $60 (£15.6 to £37.5) for a deep mattress replacement and are more likely to be used for treatment than for prevention.

In their report to the U.K. Department of Health in 1993, Touche Ross[108] estimated that, ignoring pain and suffering (and possible litigation), it was less expensive to treat sores allowed to develop than to prevent them, despite the expense of dressings and surgery and considerable opportunity costs due to the prolonged hospital stay of patients with sores. This was mainly because of the large number of at-risk patients requiring special treatment (e.g., regular turning) to prevent sores compared with the relatively small number whom it was estimated would actually develop them without this preventive treatment and the very high cost of staff time involved—£510,000 to £2,399,000 ($766,530 to $3,605,697) per annum for a 600-bed district general hospital, compared with £185,000 to £443,000 ($278,055 to $665,829) for treatment. But if obligatory turning, which in any case is seldom effective for elderly patients, can be avoided and the majority of pressure sores occurring in a hospital prevented by the routine use of single-layer large-cell alternating-pressure overlays for about the first 2 weeks of admission for patients at risk (i.e., those requiring intensive care, acutely ill or traumatized elderly patients, and patients with neurologic disease), the costs of both prevention and treatment are likely to be very much less—and pain and suffering can be avoided. Effective prevention of pressure sores during the period of acute illness is also likely to facilitate rehabilitation and permit earlier discharge. However, in the long term, like all resuscitative treatments for frail patients, it may contribute to greater overall costs by increasing longevity.

REFERENCES

1. The Prevention and Treatment of Pressure Sores. Effective Health Care. Nuffield Institute of Health, University of Leeds, 1995
2. Norton D, McLaren R, Exton Smith AN: An investigation of geriatric nursing problems in hospital. Churchill Livingstone, Edinburgh, 1975
3. Hitch S: NHS Executive Nursing Directorate: strategy for major clinical quidelines— prevention and management of pressure sores, a literature review. J Tissue Viability 1995;5: 3–24
4. Jones R. Scoring the risk scores. J Tissue Viability 1994;4: 65–67
5. Gosnell DJ: Pressure sore risk assessment: a critique. 1. the Gosnell scale. Decubitus 1989;2:32–38
6. Hibbs P: The economics of pressure sore prevention. pp. 35–42. In Bader DL (ed): Pressure Sores: clinical Practice and Scientific Approach. Macmillan, Basingstoke, England, 1990
7. Andersen KE, Jensen O, Kvorning SA, Bach E: Decubitus prophylaxis: a prospective trial of the efficiency of alternating pressure air mattresses and water mattresses. Acta Dermatovener (Stockholm) 1982;63:227–230
8. Finucane TE: Malnutrition, tube feeding and pressure sores: data are incomplete. J Am Geriatr Soc 1995;43:447–451
9. Lowthian P: Preventing pressure sores. Nurs Mirror 1985;160: 18–20
10. Olson B: Effects of massage for prevention of decubitus ulcers. Decubitus 1990;2:32–37
11. Vilain R: Five years of prevention: why are there still decubitus ulcers? Semaines Hopitaux Paris 1960;36:3296–3300 (suppl 594–596)
12. Watson N: Spinal shock in paraplegia—early skin care. pp.

91–94. In Barbenel JC, Forbes CD, Lowe GDO (eds): Pressure Sores. Macmillan, London, 1983

13. Rogers MA: Living with paraplegia. pp. 46–63. Faber and Faber, London, 1986
14. Gebhardt KS, Bliss MR: Preventing pressure sores in orthopaedic patients. J Tissue Viability 1994;4:51–54
15. Ashby EC, Ashford NS, Campbell MJ: Posture, blood velocity in common femoral vein, and prophylaxis of venous thromboembolism. Lancet 1995;345:419–421
16. Harper CM, Lyles YM: Physiology and complications of bedrest. J Am Geriatr Soc 1988;36:1047–1054
17. Guite GH, Bliss MR, Mainwaring-Burton RW et al: Hypothesis: posture is one of the determinants of the circadian rhythm of urine flow and electrolyte excretion in elderly female patients. Age Ageing 1988;17:241–248
18. Gunnewicht BR: Management of pressure sores in a spinal injury unit. J Wound Care 1995;5:36–39
19. Malone C: Intensive pressures. Nurs Times 1992;88;57–64
20. Editorial: Hydrostatic bed for invalids. London Med Gaz 1832; 10:712–714
21. Inman KJ, Sibbald WJ, Rutledge FS, Clark BJ: Clinical utility and cost effectiveness of an air suspension bed in the prevention of pressure sores. JAMA 1993;269:1139–1143
22. Allman RM, Walker JM, Hart MK. et al: Airfluidised beds or conventional therapy for pressure sores—a randomised controlled trial. Ann Intern Med 1987;107:641–648
23. Breslaw RA: Nutrition and air fluidised beds: a literature review. Adv Wound Care 1994;7:57–62
24. Micheels J, Sorensen B: Water and sodium balance: the effect of an airfluidised bed on burned patients. Burns 1983;9: 305–311
25. Clark M, Rowland LB: Preventing pressure sores: matching patient and mattress using interface pressure measurements. Decubitus 1989;2:34–39
26. Petrie LA, Hummel RS III: A study of interface pressure for pressure reduction and relief mattresses. J Enterostomal Ther 1990;17:212–216
27. Swain I: PSI Evaluation: Foam Mattresses. Her Majesty's Stationary Office, London, 1993
28. Jakobsen J, Stenild CK: Transcutaneous oxygen tension measurement over the sacrum on various anti-decubitus mattresses. Dan Med Bull 1987;34:330–331
29. Krouskop TA, Garber SL: Interface pressure confusion. Decubitus 1989;2:8
30. Sideranko S, Quinn A, Burns K, Froman RD: Effects of position and mattress overlay on sacral and heel pressures in a clinical population. Res Nurs Health 1992;15:245–251
31. Sylvia CJ: Determining the right mix of support surfaces to minimize hospital aquired pressure ulcers. Ostomy Wound Management 1993;39:12–16
32. Lazzara DJ, Buschmann MBT: Prevention of pressure ulcers in elderly nursing home residents: are support surfaces the answer? Decubitus 1991;4:42–48
33. Goldstone LA, Norris M, O'Reilly M, White JA: Clinical trial of a bead bed system for the prevention of pressure sores in elderly orthopaedic patients. J Ad Nurs 1982;7:545–548
34. Conine JA, Daechsel D, Laus MS: The role of alternating air and silicone overlays in preventing decubitus ulcers. Int J Rehabil Res 1990;13:57–65
35. Kemp MG, Kopanke D, Tordecilla L et al: The role of support surfaces and patient attributes in preventing pressure ulcers in elderly patients. Res Nurs Health 1993;16:89–96
36. Hofman A, Geelkerken RH, Hamming JJ et al: Pressure sores and pressure decreasing mattresses: controlled clinical trial. Lancet 1994;343:568–571
37. Bliss MR: Preventing pressure sores in elderly patients: a comparison of seven mattress overlays. Age Ageing 1995;24: 297–302
38. Gebhardt KS, Bliss MR, Winwright PL, Thomas JM: Pressure relieving supports in an ICU. J Wound Care 1996;5:116–121
39. Bliss MR, McLaren R, Exton Smith AN: Mattresses for preventing pressure sores in geriatric patients. Med Bull Ministry Health 1966;25:238–267
40. Exton Smith AN, Overstall PW, Wedgewood J, Wallace G: Use of the "Airwave system" to prevent pressure sores in hospital. Lancet 1982;ii:1288–1290
41. Dunsford C: A clinical evaluation of the Nimbus Dynamic Flotation System. J Tissue Viability 1991;1:75–78
42. Devine B: Alternating pressure air mattresses in the management of established pressure sores. J Tissue Viability 1995; 5:94–98
43. Bedford PD, Cosin LZ, McCarthy TF, Scott BO: The alternating pressure mattress. Gerontol Clin 1961;3:79–82
44. Bliss MR: The use of Ripplebeds in hospitals: Hosp Health Ser Rev 1979;74:190–193
45. Stapleton M: Preventing pressure—an evaluation of three products. J Br Geriatr Nursing 1986;6:23–25
46. Bale S: Pressure sore prevention in a hospice. J Wound Care 1995;4:465–468
47. James HM, Fong A: Implementing and evaluating a pressure sore policy. J Tissue Viability 1996;6:43–45
48. Clark M: Pegasus Airwave and fleeces. J Tissue Viability 1996;6:62
49. Ecomomides NG, Skoutakis VA, Carter CA, Smith VH: Evaluation of the effectiveness of two support surfaces following myocutaneous flap surgery. Adv Wound Care 1995;8:49–53
50. Bader DL, Hawken MB: Ischial pressure distribution under the seated person. pp. 223–233. In Bader DL (ed): Pressure Sores: Clinical Practice and Scientific Approach. Macmillan, Basingstoke, England, 1990
51. Rithalia SVS: Comparison of pressure distribution in wheelchair seat cushions. Care Sci Pract 1989;7:87–89
52. Wilson J: Wheelchair cushioning. Spinal Injuries Assoc Newslett 1992;65:25
53. Cheshire L: A survey of Roho cushion users (1986). Care Sci Pract 1987;5:8–14
54. Conine TA, Hershler C, Daeschel D et al: Pressure ulcer prophylaxis in elderly patients using polurethane foam or Jay wheelchair cushions. J Int Rehabil Res 1994;17:123–137
55. Rithalia S, Altard J, Kulkarni J: Interface pressure and cycle time characteristics in alternating pressure air cushions. J Tissue Viability 1995;5:107
56. Editorial: Fractured neck of femur: prevention and management. Summary and recommendations of a report of the Royal

College of Physicians. J R College Physicians London 1989; 23:8–12

57. Bulstrode C: Orthopaedics. pp. 55–64. In Bader DL (ed): Pressure Sores: Clinical Practice and Scientific Approach. Macmillan, Basingstoke, 1990
58. Neander KD, Birkenfeld R: Decubitus prophylaxis in the operating theatre. J Tissue Viability 1991;1:71–74
59. Lowthian P: Pressure sore prevention. Nursing 1989;3:17–23
60. Moore E, Rithalia S, Gonsalkorale M: Assessment of the Charnwood operating table and hospital trolley mattresses. J Tissue Viability 1992;2:71–72
61. Malone C: Uniting services in tissue viability care. Nurs Standard 1995;9:39–42
62. Hookway J: A pressure relieving equipment manager. J Tissue Viability 1996;6:45
63. Gebhardt KS: Editorial. Tissue Viability 1996;6:34–35
64. Van de Kerkhof PCM: Inflammation versus reepithelialisation during wound healing. Wound Management 1996;1:1
65. Rodeheaver G, Baharestani MM, Brabec ME et al: Wound healing and wound management: focus on debridement. Adv Wound Care 1994;7:22–39
66. Constantian MB, Jackson HS: Biology and care of the pressure ulcer wound. pp. 69–100. In Constantian MB (ed): Pressure Ulcers: Principles and Techniques of Management. Little, Brown, Boston, 1980
67. Adam K, Oswald I: Sleep helps healing. BMJ 1984;289: 1400–1401
68. Munro BH, Brown L, Heitman BB: Pressure ulcers: one bed or another. Geriatr Nurs 1989;10:190–192
69. Strauss MJ, Gong J, Gary BD et al: The cost of home air fluidised therapy for pressure sores. J Fam Pract 1991;33: 52–57
70. Ferrell BA, Osterweil D, Christensen P: A randomised trial of low air loss beds for treatment of pressure ulcers. JAMA 1993; 269;494–497
71. Rice ASC: Pain, inflammation and wound healing. J Wound Care 1994;3:246–248
72. Beal AL, Cerra FB: Multiple organ failure syndrome in the 1990s. JAMA 1994;271:226–233
73. Williams C: Painful dressings. J Tissue Viability 1996;6:57
74. Barton A, Barton M: The Management and Prevention of Pressure sores. London, Faber and Faber, London, 1981
75. Henderson CT, Trumbore LS, Morharban S et al: Prolonged tube feeding in longterm care: nutritional status and clinical outcomes. J Am College Nutrition 1992;11:309–325
76. Lewis BK, Harding KG: Nutritional intake and wound healing in elderly people. J Wound Care 1993;2:227–229
77. Reit G, Kessels AG, Knipchild PG: Randomised clinical trial of ascorbic acid in the treatment of pressure ulcers. J Clin Epidemiol 1995;48:1453–1460
78. Tyrrell DAJ: Vitamin C and the common cold. Prescribers J 1988;14:21–24
79. Lansdowne ABG: Zinc in the healing wound. Lancet 1996; 347:706–707
80. Lehman AB: Nutrition in old age: an update and questions for future research. 1. Rev Clin Gerontol 1991;1:135–145
81. Irvine RE, Memon AH, Shera AS: Norethandrolone and prevention of decubitus ulcers. Lancet 1961;ii:1333–1334
82. Joseph B: Insulin in the treatment of non diabetic bedsores. Ann Surg 1930;92:318
83. Rudman D, Feller AG, Nagraj HS et al: Effects of growth hormone in men over 60 years old. N Engl J Med 1990;323: 1–6
84. Miller M, Dyson M: Principles of wound care. Macmillan, London, 1996
85. Bowler PG: The role of occlusive dressings in infection control. Wound Management 1996;1:5–6
86. Hutchinson JJ, Lawrence JC: Wound infection under occlusive dressings. J Hosp Infect 1991;17:83–94
87. Calpin JE, Chow AW, Bayer AS, Guze LB: Sepsis associated with decubitus ulcers. Am J Med 1976;61:346–350
88. Stotts NA: Determination of bacterial burden in wounds. Adv Wound Care 1995;8:28/46–28/52
89. Cameron S, Leaper D: Antiseptic toxicity in open wounds. Nurs Times 1988; 84:77–78
90. Tatnall FM, Leigh IM, Gibson JR: Comparative study of antiseptic toxicity on basal keratinocytes, transformed keratinocytes and fibroblasts. Skin Pharmacol 1990;3:157–163
91. Barnett SE: Histology of the human pressure sore. Care Sci Pract 1987;5:13–18
92. Pierce GF, Torpley JE, Allman RA et al: Tissue repair processes in healing chronic pressure ulcers treated with recombinant platelet-derived growth factor BB. Am J Pathol 1994; 145:1399–1410
93. Stefanovska A, Vodovnik L, Benko H, Turk R: Treatment of chronic wounds by electric and electromagnetic fields. 2. value of FES parameters for pressure sore treatment. Med Biol Eng Comput 1993;31:213–220
94. Eason A, Lee MHM, Folk FS: Accelerated wound healing of pressure ulcers by pulsed high peak power electromagnetic energy (Diapulse). Decubitus 1991;4:24–34
95. Mester AF, Mester A: Wound healing. Laser Ther 1989;1: 7–15
96. Dyson M, Franks C, Suckling J: Stimulation of healing of varicose ulcers by ultrasound. Ultrasonics 1976;14:232–236
97. Upson AV: Topical hyperbaric oxygen in the treatment of recalcitrant open wounds. Practice 1986;66:1408–1412
98. Winter GD: Formation of the scab and the rate of epithelialisation of superficial wounds of the skin of the young domestic pig. Nature 1962;193:293–294
99. Dyson M, Young S, Pendle CL et al: Comparison of the effects of moist and dry conditions on dermal repair. J Invest Dermatol 1988;91:434–449
100. Hinman CD, Cameron D, Maibach H: Effect of air exposure and occlusion on experimental human skin wounds. Nature 1963;200:377–379
101. Field FK, Kerstein MD: Overview of wound healing in a moist environment. Am J Surg 1994;167:2S–6S
102. Mertz PM, Marshall PA, Eaglstein WH: Occlusive wound dressings to prevent bacterial invasion and wound infection. J Am Acad Dermatol 1985;12:662–668
103. Katz S, McGinley K, Leyden JJ: Semipermeable occlusive dressings: effects on growth of pathogenic bacteria and reepi-

thelialisation of superficial wounds. Arch Dermatol 1986;122: 58–62

104. Greenwood D: Honey for superficial wounds and ulcers. Lancet 1993;341:90–91

105. Thomas S: Wound management and dressings. Pharmaceutical Press, London, 1990

106. Constantian MB, Jackson HS: The sacral ulcer, the trochanteric ulcer, the ischial ulcer: ulcers in less common sites. pp. 149–258. In Constantian MB (ed): Pressure ulcers: Principles and Techniques of Management. Little Brown, Boston, 1980

107. Working Party Report. Guidelines on the control of methicillin resistant *Staphylococcus aureus* in the community. J Hosp Infect 1995;31:1–12

108. Touche Ross and Company: The Costs of Pressure Sores. Report to the Department of Health December, 1993

CHAPTER 99

Sleep and Insomnia in Later Life

KEVIN MORGAN

Changes in the structure and quality of sleep have long been recognized as a feature of the aging process. Writing in *The Lancet* more than 150 years ago, for example, Dr. George Sigmond observed that, "The duration of sleep should be, in manhood, about the fourth or the sixth of the 24 hours; children, the younger they are the more sleep they require; in advanced age there is more watchfulness."[1] Similar associations between "watchfulness" and age were noted by Herman Melville who, in his novel *Moby Dick* commented, "Old age is always wakeful; as if, the longer linked with life, the less man has to do with aught that looks like death."[2] Developments in research methodology, particularly polysomnography, have since confirmed these changes in sleep structure that accompany advancing age,[3] while epidemiologic studies have clearly described the age-related increase in complaints of insomnia.[4] Sleep disorders in later life are now widely regarded as a significant policy issue[5] and an important focus for clinical[3] and economic[6,7] concern. This chapter focuses mainly on insomnia, and aims to provide the background to this concern, and introduce the basis for clinical assessment and management. Because advances in sleep research have engendered an increasingly sophisticated taxonomy of sleep disorders, some familiarity with currently used diagnostic and classificatory systems is essential.

Presentation and Classification of Insomnia

Broadly, complaints of disturbed sleep may be divided into sleep onset problems (trouble getting to sleep), sleep maintenance problems (trouble staying asleep), and early morning awakening. These symptoms may occur singly or in combination, and may be transient or long-term. Disturbed sleep may also present, not as a complaint of sleeplessness, but rather as a report of excessive daytime sleepiness (hypersomnia). Building on these rather straightforward subjective reports, insomnia is now explicitly defined in three diagnostic systems: the ICD–10 Classification of Mental and Behavioral Disorders[8]; the Diagnostic and Statistical Manual of Mental Disorders (DSM-IV)[9], and the International Classification of Sleep Disorders (ICSD).[10] While all three classifications largely agree on the symptoms of insomnia, there are important differences both in terminology and emphasis.

Insomnia: International Classification of Mental and Behavioral Disorders-10

The ICD-10 broadly divides sleep disorders into organic and nonorganic, with the latter category further subdivided into dyssomnias (disturbances of the amount, quality, or timing of sleep) and parasomnias (abnormal episodic events occurring during sleep, for example sleepwalking, nightmares, etc.). In this system, "nonorganic insomnia" is a dyssomnia characterized by persistent (i.e., at least 3 times a week for at least 1 month) difficulty in getting to sleep or staying asleep (or poor quality sleep), which causes the individual concern, and markedly interferes with social or occupational functioning. The ICD-10 does not explicitly discriminate between primary insomnia (where the sleep disturbance may be the presenting condition) and secondary insomnia (where the sleep disturbance accompanies other physical or mental disorders).

Insomnia: Diagnostic and Statistical Manual of Mental Disorders-IV

DSM-IV uses a broader classification that recognizes four main types of sleep disorder: sleep disorders related to another mental disorder, sleep disorders due to a general medical condition, substance-induced sleep disorders, and primary sleep disorders (i.e., those not associated with a psychiatric, medical, or pharmacologic cause). *Primary sleep disorders* in DSM-IV are analogous to the *nonorganic sleep disorders* of ICD-10, and are similarly divided into dyssomonias and parasomnias, with insomnia (as "primary insomnia") again subsumed within the dyssomnias. In DSM-IV the diagnostic features of primary insomnia are also similar to those described in ICD-10 and include a persistent (i.e., for at least 1 month) complaint of difficulty initiating or maintaining sleep (or of nonrestorative sleep), which causes the individual "significant" distress and is associated with impaired social or occupational functioning. Unlike ICD-10, however, DSM-IV taxonomically separates primary insomnia from those secondary insomnias associated with other disorders. Nevertheless, the system does recognize that, under some circumstances, distinguishing *primary insomnia* from *insomnia related to another mental disorder* ". . . can be especially difficult," and that *sleep disorders due to general medical conditions* are ". . . characterized by symptoms similar to those in primary sleep disorders."

Insomnia: International Classification of Sleep Disorders

The most detailed classification of sleep disorders is that provided by the ICSD, which defines 12 subtypes of "insomnia disorder" (i.e., disorders of initiating or maintaining sleep), and more than 50 different insomnia syndromes. Because many of these diagnoses require specialized instrumental monitoring (often laboratory-based polysomnography) the value of the ICSD in everyday practice is probably limited. The most common forms of insomnia recognized by this classification (and those closest to the "nonorganic" and "primary" insomnias of ICD-10 and DSM-IV) include *psychophysiologic insomnia* (characterized by psychosomatic arousal, excessive concern about sleep adequacy, and somatisized tension) *inadequate sleep hygiene* (where the sleep problem appears to be caused or maintained by maladaptive practices), and so-called *sleep-state misperception* (where the chronic complaint of insomnia is not "corroborated" by polysomnographic findings). Though relatively rare, the ICSD diagnosis of *idiopathic insomnia* (a near lifelong constitutional predisposition to poor quality sleep) may also be regarded as a "classic" insomnia.

Overall, then, ICD-10, DSM-IV, and ICSD show widespread consensus as to what constitutes insomnia, with many apparent differences being terminologic rather than fundamental (in each system, for example, the same clinical presentation could attract the diagnosis of "organic insomnia," "primary insomnia," or "psychophysiologic insomnia," respectively). In clinical field studies where all three systems have been used, diagnoses have been found to logically inter-relate.[11] Nevertheless, there remain important areas of disagreement. The rather judgmental ICSD label of *sleep-state misperception*, for example, has met with criticism, being described as an unhelpful pseudodiagnosis.[12]

Insomnia and Aging

While formal diagnostic classification is increasingly being used in epidemiologic studies of insomnia,[13,14] such categorization remains the exception. Nevertheless, since the seminal studies of McGhie and Russell[16] in the UK, and Karacan et al.[17] in the US, community surveys have been remarkably consistent in describing the prevalence and natural history of poor sleep quality.

Descriptive Epidemiology

The prevalence of insomnia increases steadily with age,[15–21] and is commonly reported by up to one in three people aged 65 and over[14,15,18,22] (see Table 99-1). Epidemiologic studies have also consistently shown that dissatisfaction with sleep is more common among elderly women than among elderly men (Table 99-1),[13,14,15,22] and is higher among lower income and lower educational attainment groups.[13,15,23–25] Evidence from the US[24] also shows clear racial differences in levels of insomnia, with older African Americans reporting significantly fewer sleep complaints than their white contemporaries. However, whether these latter findings reflect differences in the propensity to express complaints, or fundamental differences in the sleep experience, remains unclear.

In contrast to the abundance of prevalence data, information on the *incidence* of insomnia (i.e., the rate at which new cases come into existence) is scarce. Nevertheless, in one of the few studies to examine this issue, a clear, though modest, age gradient in the 1-year incidence of insomnia was present, with incident complaints rising from 5.7 percent among those aged 18 to 25, to 7.3 percent among those aged 65 and over.[13]

Increasing age is also associated with changes both in the nature and the duration of sleep complaints. Problems in getting to sleep (sleep onset problems) tend to predominate in younger insomniacs, while problems *staying* asleep (sleep maintenance problems) become increasingly common in later life.[14,19] Complaints of early-morning awakening (EMA) also increase with age,[26] but remain less common than sleep maintenance problems in elderly populations (Table 99-2). Several epidemiologic studies report data that indicate that symptoms of disturbed sleep are more persistent in older age groups.[18,27] When asked to quantify the severity of insomnia, for example, older respondents are more likely to report that the problem occurs "often or all the time"[17] or "a lot."[18] In a longitudinal follow-up, Morgan and colleagues[28] found that of 82 insomniacs aged 65 to 74, 69 (84 percent) continued to complain of poor sleep when interviewed 18 to 24 months later.

The extent to which reported dissatisfaction with sleep among elderly people (as measured in community surveys) translates into complaints of poor sleep (in primary care settings) has only recently attracted research attention. The evidence clearly shows, however, that insomnia remains both widely reported,[20,27,29] and widely treated in general practice settings. In addition, those reporting sleep problems tend to show significantly higher general practice consultation rates than those who do not.[20,21]

Structural Changes in Sleep

Since the discovery of rapid eye movement (REM) sleep,[30] and the subsequent upsurge of interest in all-night polysomnography, numerous EEG studies have reported age-related changes in the continuity, duration, and depth of sleep. Each of these changes has profound implications for subjective sleep quality as reported in population surveys, and each will be considered in turn.

Continuity of Sleep

Relative to that of the young, the sleep of elderly people is characterized by more frequent "shifts" from one sleep stage to another, and more frequent episodes of intervening wakefulness during the night (Fig. 99-1). Both events result in sleep that is more broken, and more likely to be rated as poor in quality.[31] Brief periods of EEG wakefulness (alpha activity)

Table 99-1 Prevalence of insomnia (variously defined) among older people living in the community

Location	Age	No. of Older Respondents	Prevalence (%) Overall	Women	Men
Florida (US)	60–69	NR	20.9[a]	22.6	18.3
	70+	NR	25.9[a]	29.4	20.0
National Sample (US)	65–79	798	25.0[b]	NR	NR
Nottingham (UK)	65+	1,023	22.5[c]	27.7	14.6
			16.0[d]	19.0	11.6
NIMH Catchment Area (US)	65+	1,801	12.0[e]	NR	NR
Paris (France)	55+[k]	758	31.0[f]	42.5	22.5
Mannheim (Germany)	66–92	330	23.0[g]	29.1	7.9
			17.0[h]	17.5	16.9
National sample (France)[15]	65+	NR	NR	37.3[i]	28.7[i]
East Boston (US)[14]	65+	3,537	33.7[j]	36.4	29.4
New Haven, Connecticut, (US)[14]	65+	2,717	27.5[j]	31.1	21.2
Iowa (US)[14]	65+	3,028	23.2[j]	25.4	19.5

Abbreviation: NR, data not reported. Insomnia defined as follows:
[a] *Trouble sleeping "often/all the time."*
[b] *"... had trouble and was bothered a lot" by "trouble falling asleep or staying asleep."*
[c] *Problems sleeping "often/all the time."*
[d] *Problems sleeping "sometimes."*
[e] *"... had trouble falling asleep, staying asleep, or waking too early" for a period of 2 weeks or more, and consulted a professional about it, took medication for it, or stated that it interfered with life a lot, and "... if it was not always the result of physical illness."*
[f] *Reported "sleep disturbances."*
[g] *DSM-III-R criteria for severe insomnia.*
[h] *DSM-III-R criteria for severe insomnia but* without *daytime impairment.*
[i] *"... unsatisfied with sleep* or *taking medication for sleeping difficulties or anxiety with sleeping difficulties."*
[j] *"... trouble falling asleep and/or waking up too early and not being able to fall asleep again most of the time."*
[k] *Age range = 55 to unspecified retirement (sample comprised wage-earners only).*

during the sleep period are normal at any age, but tend to become more frequent[32,33] in later life. Throughout adult life these "spontaneous" nocturnal awakenings tend to be more common among men, a finding possibly related to the disturbing effects of nocturnal penile tumescence (NPT), which occurs quite mechanically during REM sleep in sexually nondysfunctional men of all ages.[34–36]

In addition to the more conventionally recorded EEG awakenings (which can last for several minutes) "transient arousals" (2 to 15 second bursts of alpha activity) have also been observed in the sleeping EEG of elderly subjects.[37] While unrelated to behavioral awakenings, these brief episodes of α activity, indicative of sleep fragmentation, are positively related to daytime sleepiness (as measured by the multiple sleep latency test).[37]

Duration of Sleep

As periods of intervening wakefulness increase with age in both frequency and duration, the total time spent asleep at night shows a reciprocal decrease. As a result, sleep efficiency (time spent asleep divided by time spent in bed) also tends to decrease.[3] One of the most consistently reported age-related structural changes within non-REM (NREM) sleep is the progressive reduction in EEG slow waves (those associated with stages 3 and 4 or slow-wave sleep)[38] and, for many people, the virtual disappearance of stage 4 altogether (Fig. 99-1).

Depth of Sleep

With advancing age, depth of sleep appears to be affected both quantitatively and qualitatively. Changes in the architecture of sleep so far considered result in a diminution of deeper slow-wave sleep (SWS), and a reciprocal increase in stages 2 (light sleep) and 1 (drowsiness). The sleep of the elderly is, therefore, *structurally* lighter. In addition, studies of auditory awakening thresholds (the minimum amount of noise required to wake a sleeping person) show qualitative changes in the depth of individual sleep stages. It has been shown, for example, that during stages 2, 4, and REM, older people are more easily awakened by noise (i.e., have lower auditory awakening thresholds) than are younger people (this despite reductions

Table 99-2 Distribution of sleep complaints among older people living in the community

Place	Age	Reported Sleep Problems (%)[a]		
		Onset	Maintenance	EMA
Florida (US)[17]	60–69[b]	58.1	20.2	4.0
	70+[b]	53.8	20.9	3.3
Nottingham (UK)[22]	65+[b]	70.6	63.2	33.6
Uppsala (Sweden)[19]	60–69[c]	21.8	31.5	NR
East Boston (US)[14]	65+(W)[c]	25.0	32.0	26.0
	65+(M)[c]	19.0	28.0	19.0
New Haven, Connecticut (US)[14]	65+(W)[c]	23.0	26.0	19.0
	65+(M)[c]	14.0	18.0	13.0
Iowa (US)[14]	65+(W)[c]	16.0	34.0	15.0
	65+(M)[c]	10.0	34.0	12.0

Definitions: Onset, problems getting to sleep; maintenance, problems staying asleep; EMA, early morning awakening; NR, data not reported; W, women; M, men.
[a] *Categories not mutually exclusive.*
[b] *Base = total insomniacs in study.*
[c] *Base = total respondents in study.*

in the hearing sensitivity of older subjects).[39] Age-related differences in auditory awakening thresholds have also been observed in comparisons of pre- and postadolescent males (with older subjects again showing lower awakening thresholds).[40] Taken together, then, the evidence suggests a near lifelong modification of processes underlying arousal from sleep. It is relevant to note, however, that *outside* the laboratory, auditory awakening thresholds may not be the best predictor of a given individual's response to nocturnal sound. In an extensive field study of the effects of aircraft noise on the sleep of people living near Heathrow Airport, London, Horne et al.[41] found that sleep disturbances did not increase with age. Rather, the behavior of bed partners and others living in the household appeared to be a more influential factor than aging in determining intrasleep arousals.

Figure 99-1 Shifts of sleep stage in the elderly.

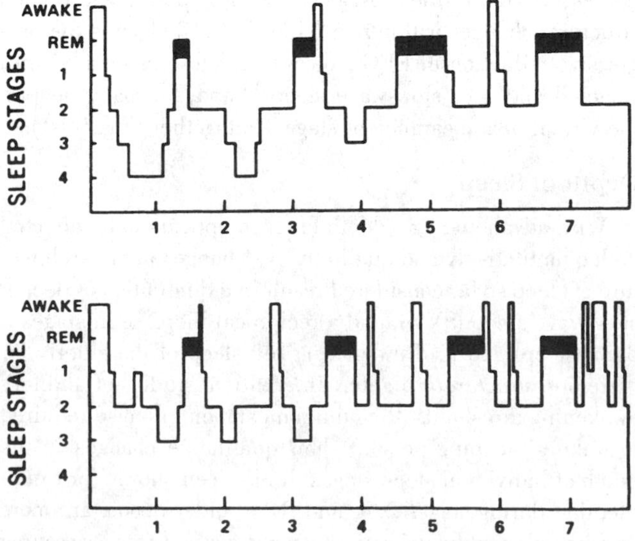

Gender Differences in Sleep Quality

Collectively, then, these structural changes in sleep are broadly consistent with the subjective reports from community surveys. It is interesting to note, however, that while epidemiologic studies tend to show that women are more likely to report sleep difficulties in old age, the EEG studies[33] indicate that it is men who experience the greater deterioration in their sleep architecture.[42] The reasons for this discrepancy are not clearly understood, but possibly reflect cultural influences on the willingness of men and women to disclose symptoms and problems.

The Aging Circadian Rhythm

In addition to changes in the architecture and depth of (usually night time) sleep, the circadian rhythm itself also shows evidence of age-related decay, with sleep becoming desynchronized and more likely to encroach on daytime activities. Disturbances of the sleep-wake cycle, such as those which result from transmeridian travel,[43] shift work,[44] or sleep deprevation[45] are also less well tolerated by older people.

Evidence that the strength of the circadian rhythm is strongly influenced by age-related changes in melatonin secretion has accumulated in recent years.[46,47] In clinical trials among elderly people it has been shown that controlled-release melatonin replacement therapy can significantly improve both sleep efficiency[48,49] and sleep onset.[49] Nevertheless, psychological contributions to circadian synchronization, such as the ability to perceive and respond to social zeitgebers (time cues), and the importance of maintaining regular social habits, should not be overlooked.[50,51]

Structural Changes in Sleep

While contemporary sleep research has yielded several well-argued and scientifically profitable "global" theories,[52,53] there exists no overall consensus regarding either the functions of sleep, or the specific relevance of age-related change in sleep architecture. Recent debate, however, has increasingly focused on whether such change is normal or pathologic.[3,54] Ostensibly measured in healthy subjects, it has long been assumed that many of the age-related structural changes recorded in EEG laboratories reflected aspects of normal ontogenetic change. However, the possibility has now arisen that some of these apparently normal changes may be related to sleep-related respiratory disturbance (SRRD) or period leg movements (PLM), awareness of which has grown rapidly in the past 10 years. Both SRRD and PLM are extremely prevalent in later life,[55–57] and are known to be disruptive of sleep continuity and quality. Whether, and to what extent, these conditions have "contaminated" earlier normative studies of human sleep, or whether structural changes in sleep predispose the individual to SRRD and PLM (or vice versa), remains unknown. Issues relating to SRRD are more fully discussed below.

The Origins of Insomnia

Given that in old age structural changes in sleep are experienced by the majority, while complaints of unsatisfactory sleep quality are expressed by the minority, it is reasonable to conclude that age-related change, per se, is not a sufficient condition for the development of insomnia. Rather, the experimental and epidemiologic evidence clearly points to the existence of health, situational, and psychological factors that are strongly associated with the onset and/or the maintenance of disturbed sleep. Because these factors may occur in combination, and are often superimposed upon sleep already compromised by ontogenetic change, it follows that sleep problems in later life are frequently multifactorial in origin. Some of the more important factors known to influence sleep quality in later life have been selected here for discussion.

Mental and Physical Health Status

As a correlate of psychological well-being, insomnia continues to be regarded as a useful indicant of mental ill health, appearing as a prominent diagnostic feature in both ICD-10[8] and DSM-IV.[9] The symptom of disturbed sleep is also included in most of the available schedules for assessing the mental health of elderly people, including the Geriatric Mental State Schedule (GMS),[58] the Cambridge Mental Disorders of the Elderly Examination (CAMDEX),[59] and the Comprehensive Assessment and Referral Evaluation (CARE).[60] It is likely, however, that the specificity of insomnia as a symptom of mental ill health is lowest in later life. Thus, while complaints of insomnia steadily increase from early adulthood to at least the sixth or seventh decade of life,[15,18–21] the prevalence of those mental health problems most closely associated with insomnia, depression, and anxiety, appears to peak in earlier adulthood, and decline thereafter.[61–64]

The relative contributions of mental and physical health factors to late-life insomnia can be more directly assessed from the existing literature. Comparing the performance of various CARE indicator scales, Golden and associates[60] found high correlations not only between the sleep disorder and depression scales (r = 0.55), but also between sleep disorders and somatic symptoms (r = 47), arthritis (r = 0.36), and leg swelling (r = 0.36) scales. Similar associations are reported by Habte-Gabr et al.[23] for 3,097 elderly people living in rural Iowa, US. In this extensive survey of health and disturbed sleep, recent hospitalization, limitations of physical function, self-perceptions of health, joint pain and stiffness, emphysema, a history of stroke or heart disease, and depressive symptoms were all significantly associated with poor quality, unrefreshing sleep.

Similarly, Gislason and Almqvist,[19] in their extensive postal survey among a random sample of Swedish men of all ages, conclude, "Complaints of DMS [difficulty maintaining sleep] increased with increasing age . . . multiple regression clarified that the increase was related to reporting of somatic diseases and overweight". From the same study its was also found that sleep complaints, ". . . were almost twice as common among men attending regular medical check-ups for somatic diseases . . .". Mental health problems (particularly depression and anxiety) are nevertheless, prevalent among older insomniacs, and in a recent review of community studies, were found to be associated with more than 30 percent of later life sleep complaints within random samples.[26] It is likely, however, that much higher levels of psychiatric comorbidity would be found among clinic populations and general practice attenders.[65]

Factors influencing sleep quality in later life

- Age-related changes in sleep structure[33]
- Age-related changes in sleep depth[39]
- Mental health status
  - Depression[13]
  - Dementia[66]
- Physical health status
  - General symptoms[23]
  - Sleep-related respiratory disturbance[110]
  - Periodic leg movements (nocturnal myoclonus)[121]
- Institutionalization[78]
- Poor sleep hygiene[98]
- Personality factors[28]
- Loss of stimulus control[74]

Dementia

Dementia presents a special area of concern in late-life sleep disturbance, because many of the polygraphic sleep changes seen in normal aged individuals, and described above, are amplified in dementing illness. Relative to age-matched controls, demented individuals take longer to get to sleep,[66] wake up more frequently during the night,[66,67] stay awake longer when disturbed,[67] tend to be more active during periods of wakefulness,[66] and in one study were found to be up to 20 times more likely to fall asleep during the day.[67] Changes in the circadian organization of *total* sleep have also been reported. In a detailed comparison of demented and non-demented inpatients Allen et al.[66] found that patients with dementia not only slept more during the day, but that some (10 percent) actually slept more during the day than during the night (so called day-night reversal).

These changes in the architecture and circadian timing of

sleep, often accompanied by episodes of night-time agitation and wandering (or "sundowning"),[3] contribute substantially to the demands of caring and are among the most frequently cited reasons for the breakdown of caregiving in the community.[68–70] Evidence linking the severity of cognitive impairment, as indexed by psychometric ratings, with the degree of sleep disturbance[38] highlights the role of neuronal degeneration in explaining dementia-related sleep disorders. However, the existence of wide individual differences in the degree of sleep disturbance among similarly impaired individuals,[71] and the failure of sleep disturbance indicators reliably to discriminate between mildly demented patients and nondemented controls[72] suggest that etiological factors are not alone in determining sleep disruptions in dementia. This conclusion is supported by the findings of Meguro et al.[73] who report that dementia severity (as indexed by the extent of white matter lesions) and lowered activity levels (as measured by ADL scores) interact to increase sleep fragmentation.

Whatever the organic origin, it is likely that the disruption of sleep in dementia is exacerbated by behavioral factors. The research evidence clearly indicates that regularizing daytime and night-time activities, optimizing daytime stimulation, minimizing daytime naps, and maximizing the psychological association between the bedroom and sleep, all make significant contributions to the maintenance of satisfactory sleep-wake cycles in nondemented insomniacs.[74] In dementing illness, however, the influence of these and other factors may be greatly diminished or lost. For example, a demented patient with severely disturbed night-time sleep may be left to nap ad lib during the day by an exhausted relative. As a result, the patient may be less tired and less likely to sleep during the night, which in turn can lead to sleepiness and excess napping the following day, and so on. Support for the general proposition that behavioral factors exacerbate sleep fragmentation in dementia can be found in the clinical literature. Hinchcliffe et al.[75] for example, describe the successful management of dementia-related night-time sleeplessness and wandering through stimulating daytime "distractions," which prevented excessive napping.

Institutionalization

Relationships between institutionalization and disturbed sleep are strongly suggested by the high levels of hypnotic drug consumption that have consistently been found in hospitals and rest, residential, and nursing homes.[76–80] Within each of these settings sleep disturbance can be related to the act of admission itself, the personal circumstances necessitating admission, or to the institutional environment. Each of these factors will be considered in turn.

The act of admission

It is well recognized in contemporary sleep research that environmental novelty (such as the first night in the EEG laboratory) results in sleep which is shorter, lighter, and more broken; a phenomenon originally described as the "first night effect"[81,82] and observed in laboratory studies of older subjects.[33] After a brief period of adaptation (1 to 2 nights), however, sleep returns to its more "normal" structure.[33] There is no reason to suppose that such phenomena do not accompany institutional admissions. There are, however, very good reasons to suppose that such sleeplessness may be interpreted as a clinical event, and inappropriately treated with hypnotic drugs.[83]

Reason for admission

Institutionalization is often accompanied by events that in themselves can be expected to disturb sleep—anxiety, discomfort, pain, bereavement, etc. In hospital settings it is also becoming increasingly apparent that many surgical and medical procedures have a detrimental effect on sleep continuity.[84,85]

The institutional environment

Undoubtedly, one of the most significant environmental factors that has been shown to influence sleep quality in institutional settings is noise.[86–88] Thus, despite the theoretical importance of sleep in healing and tissue restoration,[89] hospitalization remains a major cause of insomnia.[90] A particularly interesting research finding that may help to explain this state of affairs concerns the discrepancy between sleep parameters as measured by the EEG, and sleep parameters as judged by observers. It has been shown in several studies that, when compared with EEG measures recorded over the same period, nurse ratings consistently overestimate the sleep of hospital patients,[91,92] even in intensive care units where patients are continuously observed.[84] Indeed, in a comparison of 26 studies in which the sleep of elderly people had been either observed or polygraphically recorded, direct observations were found to yield the highest estimates of total sleep time.[71]

The research evidence also suggests that institutional *regimes* can adversely affect sleep quality in old age. Again, while days lacking in structure and stimulation can disturb sleep at almost any age, elderly people do appear to be most at risk. In nursing home residents, for example, disturbed night-time sleep has been associated with excessive periods in bed. Using wrist actigraphy[93] to monitor sleep and waking, Ancoli-Israel et al.[94] recorded up to 5 episodes of sleep during the day, and up to 32 episodes of wakefulness during the night in nursing home residents. These investigators concluded that residents had, ". . . very little sustained wakefulness and very little sustained sleep." Physical activity levels have also been implicated as a factor contributing to poor sleep in nursing home residents, though the evidence cautions against a simple cause-effect explanation. Thus, while lower activity levels have been significantly associated with sleep fragmentation in elderly nursing home residents,[73] structured activity programs appear to have little impact on the sleep quality of elderly people who are similarly institutionalized.[95]

Lifestyle

In recent years the clinical and research literature has established clear links between aspects of lifestyle (e.g., diet, exercise, sleeping habits, etc.) and sleep quality. Thus, degraded sleep quality in later life has been associated with tea consumption,[28] excessive daytime napping,[94] excessive time spent in bed,[94] and by unaccustomed night-time food and drinks.[96] Furthermore, in middle-aged people, body weight has also been shown to influence total and percentage REM sleep.[97] Improvements in "sleep hygiene," on the other hand, have been associated with significant and sustained improvements in sleep quality, particularly when combined with psychological therapies.[98] Certainly, regularizing daytime and night time activities, optimizing daytime stimulation, minimizing daytime naps, and maximizing the psychological association between the bedroom and sleep all make a significant contribution to the maintenance of satisfactory sleep-wake cycles in both elderly[99] and young[100] insomniacs.

Personality Factors

Studies comparing the personality profiles of otherwise healthy good and poor sleepers have found consistent differences in young,[101] middle-aged,[102] and elderly[28] subjects. In all cases, poor sleepers have shown significantly elevated levels of anxiety and neuroticism as measured by the Minnesota Multiphasic Personality Inventory (MMPI),[101] the Taylor Manifest Anxiety Inventory,[102] the Spielberger State-Trait Anxiety Inventory, and the Eysenck Personality Questionnaire.[28] Similar relationships between insomnia and anxiety/neuroticism have also been found in sleep clinic patients[103] and representative survey populations.[104] Given that many of these instruments reflect what are presumed to be enduring traits, such characteristics may act as risk factors for insomnia either directly, by contributing to levels of emotional arousal, or indirectly by lowering the threshold at which sleep is perceived to be a problem. That sleep quality is significantly influenced by constitutional factors is also strongly supported by evidence on heriditary predispositions. In a study of over 10,000 elderly people in Sweden, levels of insomnia were found to be significantly higher among those of which both parents were also poor sleepers.[105]

Learning and Stimulus Control

Stimulus control theory[106] presumes the influence of both operant and classical learning in the onset and maintenance of insomnia. As an operant behavior reinforced by sleep itself, sleep *onset* becomes associated with a number of factors (getting into bed, switching off the light, settling down to sleep), which ultimately become discriminative stimuli for reinforcement (in the presence of which sleep onset becomes more probable). In chronic insomnia, however (whatever the cause), where long periods in bed are increasingly associated with wakefulness, connections between these stimuli and sleep onset can be significantly weakened. Furthermore, through the repeated pairing of bedroom cues with the frustration of sleeplessness, these same stimuli can now, through the mechanisms of classical conditioning, become conditioned stimuli for negative emotional responses that antagonize and sustain episodes of insomnia. Thus, factors that initiate insomnia may differ from those factors which maintain insomnia. Treatment, therefore, aims to maximize the stimulus control properties of the bedroom and recondition the environmental cues.[106]

Sleep-Related Respiratory Disturbance

Classified within the ICSD[10] as a dyssomnia giving rise to either insomnia disorders or to disorders of excessive sleepiness, sleep-related respiratory disturbances (SRRD) refer to episodes of apnea and hypopnea which, in affected individuals, suppress the deeper stages of sleep. While criteria and terminology used to describe SRRD varied considerably in earlier studies,[107] the use of the respiratory disturbance index (RDI) has now been widely adopted for clinical and research purposes. Defined as the average number of apneic plus hypopneic episodes per hour of sleep, an RDI of greater than or equal to 5 was originally considered pathognomonic of sleep apnea syndrome (SAS).[108] In recent years, however, higher RDI levels (e.g., RDI greater than or equal to 15) have been found to offer a more realistic criterion for SAS.[109]

The prevalence of SRRD increases significantly with age,[110] with additional risk factors including being male, snoring, and obesity.[111] Indeed, associations with daytime sleepiness and snoring have proved so robust that these two factors have been described as the "cardinal symptoms" of SAS.[3] The clinical relevance of SRRD in the absence of daytime symptoms, however, remains unclear. Community-based studies have shown that low levels of SDB (RDI greater than or equal to 5) are relatively common among noncomplaining older people, affecting approximately 24 percent of asymptomatic Americans aged 65 and over.[112] In studies that have found similar levels of SRRD among healthy elderly volunteers, no relationships were found between SRRD and measures of daytime sleepiness,[113,114] sleep-wake complaints,[55] cognitive performance, personality, or health status.[114]

Using the more stringent criterion of RDI greater than or equal to 15, however, there appears to be general agreement that SRRD is a major cause of reported sleep disturbance and excessive daytime somnolence in older people.[110] Nevertheless, though associated with significant levels of morbidity in younger age groups, these higher RDI levels do not emerge as independent predictors of mortality (when chronologic age and comorbidity are controlled) in elderly samples.[115,116]

While high in normal aged populations, levels of SRRD appear to be even higher among the demented,[117] particularly demented women.[118] Within small groups of women selected from an Australian retirement village, for example, 72 percent of the demented, compared with 46 percent of controls, were found to have RDIs of greater than or equal to 5.[119] Again, the precise clinical relevance of these events is uncertain. It seems reasonable to assume that respiratory disturbances that can be accompanied by prolonged oxygen desaturation and hypoxemia may further compromise neuropsychological functioning in dementing illness. In mildly and moderately demented people, however, Hoch et al.[120] found no consistent correlations between RDIs, apneic events per hour, lowest oxyhemoglobin desaturation, and psychometric test performance.

Periodic Leg Movements

Also classified within the ICSD[10] as a cause of both insomnia and excessive daytime sleepiness, PLM is characterized by involuntary limb movements that can occur in all stages of sleep, but tend to predominate in the lighter stages (stages 1 and 2).[121] While movement and positional changes occur throughout normal sleep, four or more consecutive limb movements lasting 0.5 to 5 seconds (with an intermovement interval of 4 to 90 seconds) are regarded as PLM episodes.[122] More than five such episodes per night is considered pathologic.[122] As with SRRD, PLM also increases with age, with an estimated prevalence among elderly people living at home of about 45 percent.[56] Once again, however, not all those showing signs of PLM experience disturbed sleep. Thus, while undoubtedly a cause of disturbed sleep in later life, many of the links between PLM and sleep complaints remain to be explored.

Managing Insomnia

Advances in the understanding of factors that disturb sleep have, in recent years, been accompanied by substantial progress in the development of effective therapies and strategies for managing insomnia. These therapeutic options range from health education messages, through short-term drug management, to longer-term psychological therapies, and their deployment places particular demands on clinical assessment and resource targeting. Combining empirical research findings, authoritative clinical advice, and current prescribing recommendations, a schematic overview of management is presented in Figure 99-2, and elaborated below. The aim here is to de-

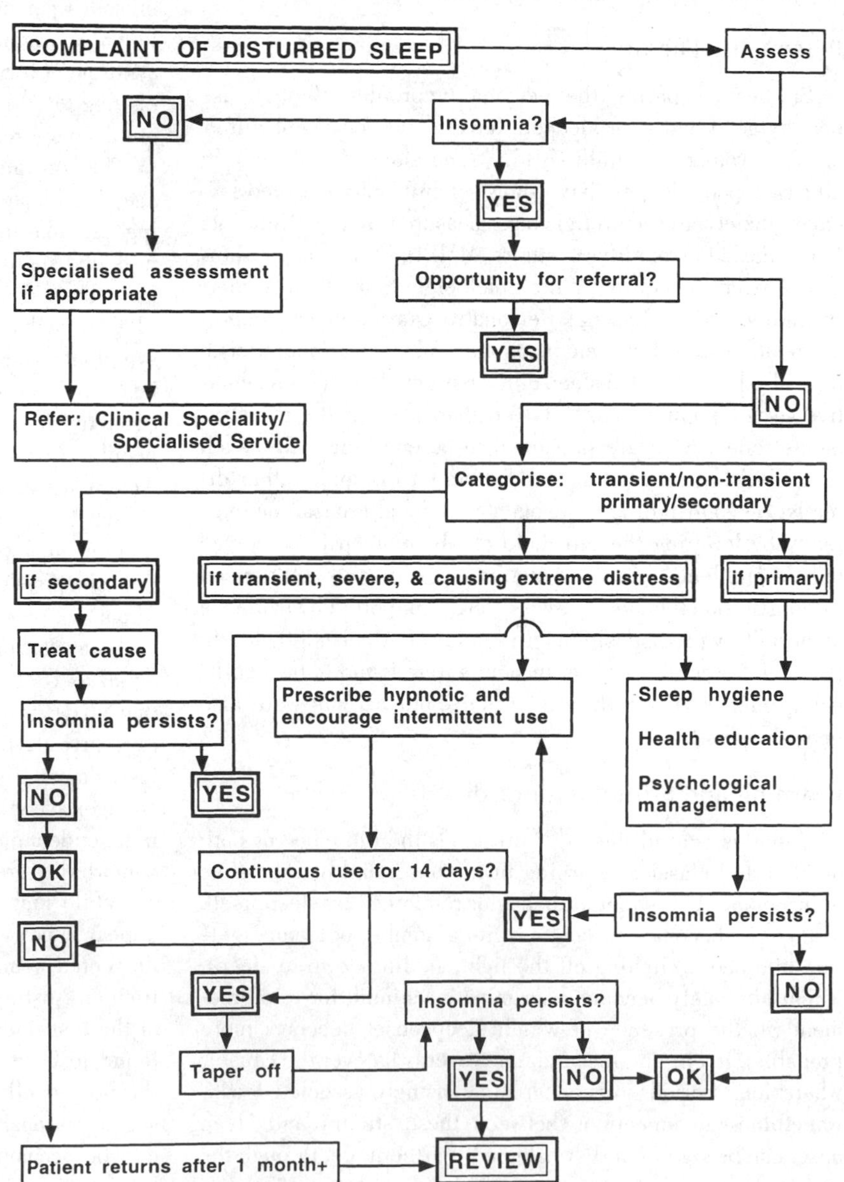

Figure 99-2 Schematic overview of the management of insomnia.

Sleep latency (minutes)	120+															
	60															
	50															
	40															
	30															
	20															
	10															
Total sleep (hours)	8+															
	7															
	6															
	5															
	4															
	3															
	2															
	1															
Sleep quality	Very good															
	Good															
	Average															
	Poor															
	Very Poor															
Day		1	2	3	4	5	6	7	8	9	10	11	12	13	14	15
Start Date																

Figure 99-3 Daily sleep chart.

scribe the *structure* of management, and introduce the appropriate therapeutic concepts. Issues of therapeutic practice are dealt with in greater detail in the literature cited.

Assessment

Possibly one of the weakest components of contemporary insomnia management, assessment should aim to clarify the history and current dynamics of the presenting problem, and identify realistic targets for clinical intervention. Because sleep problems occur over time, serial assessment of sleep patterns, using self-completed daily ratings (Fig. 99-3) or daily sleep diaries (Fig. 99-4), is extremely useful. Such ratings, continued throughout treatment and follow-up periods, also provide valuable outcome information, and can therefore be used to monitor and adjust management. Assessment should also cover relevant aspects of general health, the patient's sleep history and sleep hygiene, and their current expectations and understanding of sleep.

While assessment methods can vary from formal questionnaire procedures,[74,123] to less structured clinical consultations, it is worth emphasizing here two assessment-related principles that emerge clearly from the scientific evidence reviewed above. First, because many patients enter middle and later life with pre-existing sleep problems, it should be recognized that sleep disturbances that are reported in old age are not necessarily due to old age. And second, given the operation of stimulus control influences, it should be remembered that factors which originally caused a sleep problem (e.g., acute trauma) may be less important than those behavioral factors that can maintain a sleep problem (e.g., the acquisition of maladaptive sleep habits).

Following assessment, onward referral may be considered

Figure 99-4 Daily sleep diary.

Name	Date	
1	At what time did you go to bed last night?	
2	At what time did you settle down to sleep?	
3	How long did it take you to fall asleep?	
4	How many times did you wake up?	
5	What woke you up?	
6	For how long do you think you were awake on each of these occasions?	
7	At what time did you finally wake up?	
8	How did you feel when you woke up this morning? (tick one)	Refreshed and alert ☐ Alert but not at peak ☐ Tired ☐ Absolutely shattered ☐
9	At what time did you get up?	
10	How would you rate last night's sleep? (tick one)	Very Good ☐ Good ☐ Average ☐ Poor ☐ Very Poor ☐
11	What medicines did you take yesterday?	
12	How much alcohol did you drink yesterday?	

depending on local resources (e.g., the existence of a specialized service for insomnia or sleep apnea). If referral is not considered, then treatment may be delivered on the basis of triage, as shown in Figure 99-2. Where insomnia is secondary (as, for example, in depression or arthritis) treatment, or a review of treatment, of the underlying cause may prove sufficient. Alternatively (or additionally), insomnia may be treated with one or more specific options as indicated in Figure 99-2.

Treatment Options

Having assessed the patient's understanding and management of their own sleep, information and sleep hygiene advice are appropriately offered. The remaining treatments can broadly be divided into: drug management, stimulus control approaches, relaxation-based approaches, and cognitive approaches[74,123,124] (with the latter three collectively referred to as "psychological management" in Figure 99-2).

Drug management

There is now widespread agreement that, "... hypnotic medication should not be the mainstay of management for most of the causes of disturbed sleep."[5] Nevertheless, hypnotics appear to have an important role in the management of *short-term* insomnias where the daytime consequences of such disturbance are, "severe, disabling, or subjecting the individual to extreme distress."[125] From both a pharmacologic and psychological perspective, great caution is required in the drug management of late-life insomnia, with hypnotics avoided if at all possible. Where drug management is unavoidable, shorter half-life drugs (at the lowest possible dose) are clearly preferable,[126] with intermittent use encouraged, and a limited "course" of drugs prescribed. Because even brief periods of hypnotic drug consumption may be accompanied by tolerance, products which minimize withdrawal effects should also be preferred, and abrupt discontinuation of the drug avoided.

Stimulus control procedures

One of the most successful psychological methods for treating insomnia, stimulus control includes a variety of strategies for strengthening and maintaining associations between bedroom and sleep onset (see above). These include going to bed only when tired, using the bedroom only for sleep and sex, leaving the bedroom if sleep onset does not occur within 15 to 20 minutes (following either "lights-out," or a nocturnal awakening), and arising at a preset time irrespective of the amount slept. While shown to be effective in the management of late-life insomnias,[26] the standard stimulus control instructions (arising from bed in the night, for example) may not be appropriate for all elderly patients.

Relaxation-based treatments

Progressive relaxation, autogenic training, and electromyographic feedback techniques for reducing somatic tension have all been found effective in the management of sleep-onset insomnia, with long-term benefits apparent at follow-up.[74] Evaluation studies among elderly people, however, remain rare. Nevertheless, it is reasonable to suggest that, under some circumstances (e.g., coexisting arthritis) progressive relaxation, with its emphasis on muscle tension, may be inappropriate.

Cognitive treatments

Cognitive therapies have been found effective in the treatment of older insomniacs,[127] chronic insomniacs,[128] and clinically heterogeneous insomniac groups.[129] Aimed primarily at reducing cognitive arousal and focusing presleep mentation, therapeutic strategies vary from imagery training to paradoxical intention (i.e., instructing the patient to remain awake, and thereby reducing anxieties about getting to sleep[74]). While effective both alone, and in combination with relaxation therapies, the evidence does suggest that the benefits from some cognitive approaches may be less robust, and more variable than others.[130]

Review

While the postassessment triage in Figure 99-2 suggests clear boundaries between diagnostic categories, the "Review" box acknowledges that not all the treatment options indicated will benefit all the patients. Review, therefore, presents an opportunity to consolidate experience gained, and consider remaining options. Persistent insomnias at first assumed to be transient, those who show poor compliance with psychological treatments, patients with complex sleep problems who may otherwise become chronic drug users, and secondary insomnias where the underlying condition, and hence, the insomnia, vary in severity may all require reconsideration at this point.

Conclusions

In addition to senescent changes that directly influence the structure and quality of sleep, advancing age is also associated with an increasing number of events that can influence and disturb sleep indirectly. As a result, sleep problems in old age are both prevalent and complex. Academic and clinical sleep research has, in recent years, made considerable progress in identifying and clarifying some of the specific causes and correlates of disturbed sleep in later life. It is now clear that such problems, often multifactorial in origin, require a broad and flexible clinical response. Consonant with this growth in research knowledge, treatment approaches have become increasingly systematized in recent years, with due emphasis given to sleep assessments, health education, and sleep hygiene, and the appropriate deployment of both pharmacologic and psychological therapies. In this respect, it is relevant to note that nonpharmacological treatments may often be more acceptable to patients.[131] The evidence also suggests, however, that there are many situations where, as elsewhere, prevention is better than cure.

References

1. Sigmond GG: Lectures on materia medica and therapeutics. Lancet 1836;37:214–220
2. Melville H: Moby Dick. p. 29. First published 1851. Penguin popular classics 1994. Penguin, Harmonsworth, U.K. p. 132
3. Bliwise D: Sleep in normal aging and dementia. Sleep 1993; 16:40–81
4. Partininen M: Epidemiology of sleep disorders. pp. 437–452. In Roth T, Dement WC (ed): Principles and Practice of Sleep Medicine. WB Saunders, Philadelphia, 1994
5. National Institutes of Health: Consensus development conference statement: the treatment of sleep disorders of older people. Sleep 1991;14:169–177
6. Leger D: The cost of sleep related road accidents: a report for the National Commission on Sleep Disorders Research. Sleep 1994;17:84–93
7. Leger D: The cost of sleepiness: a response to comments. Sleep 1995;18:281–284
8. World Health Organization: The ICD-10 Classification of Mental and Behavioural Disorders. World Health Organization, Geneva, 1993
9. American Psychiatric Association: Diagnostic and Statistical Manual of Mental Disorders: DSM-IV. American Psychiatric Association, Washington, DC, 1994
10. American Sleep Disorders Association: The International Classification of Sleep Disorders: Diagnostic and Coding Manual. American Sleep Disorders Association, Rochester, Minnesota, 1990
11. Buysse DJ, Reynolds CF, Kupfer DJ et al: Clinical diagnoses in 216 insomnia patients using the International Classification of Sleep Disorders (ICSD), DSM-IV and ICD-10 categories. A report from the APA/NIMH DSM- IV field trial. Sleep 1994; 17:630–637
12. Trinder J: Subjective insomnia without objective findings: a pseudodiagnostic classification? Psych Bull 1988;103:87–94
13. Ford DE, Kamerow DB: Epidemiologic study of sleep disturbances and psychiatric disorders. J Am Med Assoc 1989;262: 1479–1484
14. Foley DJ, Monjan AA, Brown SL et al: Sleep complaints among elderly persons: an epidemiologic study of three communities. Sleep 1995;18:425–432
15. Ohayon M: Epidemiologic-study on insomnia in the general-population. Sleep 1996;19:S7–S15
16. McGhie A, Russell SM: The subjective assessment of normal sleep patterns. J Ment Sci 1962;108:642–654
17. Karacan I, Thornby JI, Anch H et al: The prevalence of sleep disturbance in a primarily urban Florida county. Soc Sci Med 1976;10:239–244
18. Mellinger GD, Balter MB, Uhlenhuth EH: Insomnia and its treatment. Arch Gen Psych 1985;42:225–232
19. Gislason T, Almqvist M: Somatic disease and sleep complaints. Acta Med Scand 1987;221:475–481
20. Weyerer S, Dilling H: Prevalence and treatment of insomnia in the community: results from the upper Bavarian field-study. Sleep 1991;14:392–398
21. Jacquinet-Salord MC, Lang T, Fouriaud C et al: Sleeping tablet consumption, self reported quality of sleep, and working conditions. J Epidemiol Comm Health 1993;47:64–68
22. Morgan K, Dallosso H, Ebrahim S et al: Characteristics of subjective insomnia among the elderly living at home. Age Ageing 1988;17:1–7
23. Habte-Gabr E, Wallace RB, Colsher PL et al: Sleep patterns in rural elders: demographic, health, and psychobehavioral correlates. J Clin Epidemiol 1991;44:5–13
24. Blazer DG, Hays JC, Foley DJ: Sleep complaints in older adults: a racial comparison. J Geronotol 1995;50A: M280–M284
25. Geroldi C, Frisoni GB, Rozzini R et al: Principal lifetime occupation and sleep quality in the elderly. Gerontology 1996; 42:163–169
26. Morgan K: Mental health factors in late-life insomnia. Rev Clin Gerontol 1996;6:75–83
27. Hohagen F, Käppler C, Schramm E et al: Prevalence of insomnia in general practice attenders and the current treatment modalities. Acta Psych Scand 1994;90:102–108
28. Morgan K, Healey DW, Healey PJ: Factors influencing persistent subjective insomnia in old age: a follow-up study of good and poor sleepers aged 65–74. Age Ageing 1989;18:117–122
29. Pharoah PDP, Melzer D: Variations in prescribing of hypnotics, anxiolytics and antidepressants between 61 general practices. Br J Gen Prac 1995;45:595–599
30. Aserinsky E, Kleitman N: Regularly occurring periods of eye motility, and concomitant phenomena during sleep. Science 1953;118:273–274
31. Oswald I: Sleep studies in clinical pharmacology. Br J Clin Pharmacol 1980;10:317–326
32. Webb WB: Sleep in older persons: sleep structures in 50- to 60-year-old men and women. J Gerontol 1982;37:581–586
33. Reynolds CF, Kupfer DJ, Taska LS et al: Sleep of healthy seniors: a revisit. Sleep 1985;8:20–29
34. Karacan I, Williams RL, Thornby JI, Salis PJ: Sleep-related tumescence as a function of age. Am J Psych 1975;132: 932–937
35. Schiavi RC, Schreiner-Engel P: Nocturnal penile tumescence in healthy aging men. J Gerontol (Med Sci) 1988;43: M146–150
36. Gheorghiu S, Mulligan T, Veldhuis JD: Lack of temporal association among REM sleep, LH secretion, testosterone secretion, and nocturnal penile tumescence (NPT) in healthy aged men. J Am Geriatr Soc 1995;43:SA81
37. Carskadon MA, Brown ED, Dement WC: Sleep fragmentation in the elderly: relationship to daytime sleep tendency. Neurobiol Aging 1982;3:321–327
38. Prinz PN, Vitaliano PP, Vitiello MV et al: Sleep, EEG and mental function changes in senile dementia of the Alzheimer's type. Neurobiol Aging 1982;3:361–370
39. Zepelin H, McDonald CS, Zammit GK: Effects of age on auditory awakening thresholds. J Gerontol 1984;39:294–300
40. Busby KA, Mercier L, Pivik RT: Ontogenic variations in auditory arousal threshold during sleep. Psychophysiology 1994; 31:182–188
41. Horne JA, Pankhurst FL, Reyner LA et al: A field study of sleep disturbance: effects of aircraft noise and other factors

on 5,742 nights of actimetrically monitored sleep in a large subject sample. Sleep 1994;17:146–159

42. Rediehs MH, Reis JS, Creason NS: Sleep in old age: focus on gender differences. Sleep 1990;13:410–424
43. Dement WC, Seidel WF, Cohen SA et al: Sleep and wakefulness in aircrew before and after transoceanic flights. Aviat Space Environ Med 1986;(suppl 12):B14–B28
44. Monk TH: Shift work. pp. 471–481. In Kryger MH, Roth T, and Dement WC, (eds): Principles and Practice of Sleep Medicine. WB Saunders, Philadelphia, 1994
45. Webb WB: Sleep stage responses of older and younger subjects after sleep deprivation. Electroenceph Clin Neurophysiol 1981;52:368–371
46. Short RV: Melatonin: hormone of darkness. Br Med J 1993; 307:952–953
47. Haimov I, Laudon M, Zisapel N et al: Sleep disorders and melotonin rhythms in elderly people. Br Med J 1994;309:167
48. Garfinkel D, Laudon M, Nof D, Zisapel N: Improvement of sleep quality in elderly people by controlled-release melatonin. Lancet 1995;346:541–544
49. Haimov I, Lavie P, Laudon M et al: Melatonin replacement therapy of elderly insomniacs. Sleep 1995;18:598–603
50. Minors DS, Rabbitt PMA, Worthington H: Variation in meals and sleep-activity patterns in aged subjects: its relevance to circadian rhythm studies. Chronobiol Int 1989;6:139–146
51. Monk TH, Reynolds CF, Machen MA, Kupfer DJ: Daily social rhythms in the elderly and their relationship to objectively recorded sleep. Sleep 1992;15:322–329
52. Adam K, Oswald I: Protein synthesis, bodily renewal and the sleep-wake cycle. Clin Sci 1983;65:561–567
53. Horne J: Why We Sleep: The Functions of Sleep in Humans and Other Mammals. Oxford University Press, Oxford, 1988
54. Bliwise DL: Normal aging. Principles and Practice of Sleep Medicine. 2nd Ed. WB Saunders, Philadelphia, 1994
55. Mosko SS, Dickel MJ, Paul T et al: Sleep apnea and sleep-related periodic leg movements in community resident seniors. J Am Geriatr Soc 1988;36:502–508
56. Ancoli-Israel S, Kripke DF, Klauber MR et al: Periodic limb movements in sleep in community dwelling elderly. Sleep 1991;14:496–500
57. Ancoli-Israel S, Kripke DF, Klauber MR et al: Sleep disordered breathing in community dwelling elderly. Sleep 1991; 14:486–495
58. Copeland JRM, Kelleher MJ, Kellett JM et al: A semi-structured clinical interview for the assessment of diagnosis and mental state in the elderly. The Geriatric Mental State Schedule. 1. Development and reliability. Psychol Med 1976;6: 439–449
59. Roth M, Tym E, Mountjoy CQ et al: CAMDEX: a standardised instrument for the diagnosis of mental disorder in the elderly with special reference to the early detection of dementia. B J Psych 1986;149:698–709
60. Golden RR, Teresi JA, Gurland BJ: Development of indicator scales for the Comprehensive Assessment and Referral Evaluation (CARE) interview schedule. J Gerontol 1984;39: 138–146
61. Myers JK, Weissman MM, Tischler GL et al: Six-month prevalence of psychiatric disorders in three communities: 1980–1982. Arch Gen Psych 1984;41:959–967
62. Blazer D, Hughes DC, George LK: The epidemiology of depression in an elderly community population. Gerontologist 1987;27:281–287
63. Kay DWK: Anxiety in the elderly. pp. 289–310. In Noyes R, Roth M, Burrows GD (eds): Handbook of Anxiety. Vol 2. Classification, Etiological Factors and Associated Disturbances. Elsevier Science Publishings, Amsterdam, 1988
64. Robins LN, Helzer JE, Weissman MM et al: Lifetime prevalence of specific psychiatric disorders in three sites. Arch Gen Psych 1984;41:949–958
65. Schramm E, Hohagen F, Kappler C et al: Mental comorbidity of chronic insomnia in general practice attenders using DMS-III-R. Acta Psych Scand 1994;91:10–17
66. Allen SR, Seiler WO, Stähelen HB, Speigel R: Seventy two hour polygraphic and behavioral recordings of wakefulness and sleep in a hospital geriatric unit: comparison between demented and nondemented patients. Sleep 1987;10: 143–159
67. Prinz PN, Peskind ER, Vitaliano PP et al: Changes in the sleep and waking EEGs of nondemented and demented elderly subjects. J Am Geriatr Soc 1982;30:86–93
68. Gilhooly M: the social dimensions of senile dementia. pp. 88–135. In Hanley I, Hodge J (eds): Psychological Approaches to the Care of the Elderly. Croom Helm, London, 1984
69. Gilleard CJ: Living with Dementia. Croom Helm, London, 1986
70. Pollak CP, Perlick D: Sleep problems and institutionalization of the elderly. J Geriatr Psych Neurol 1991;15:123–135
71. Regestein QR, Morris J: Daily sleep patterns observed among institutionalized elderly residents. J Am Geriatr Soc 1987;35: 767–772
72. Vitiello M, Prinz, PN, Williams DE et al: Sleep disturbances in patients with mild-stage Alzheimer's disease. J Gerontol 1990;45:M131–138
73. Meguro K, Ueda M, Kobayashi I et al: Sleep disturbance in elderly patients with cognitive impairment, decreased daily activity and periventricular white matter lesions. Sleep 1995; 18:109–114
74. Espie CA: The Psychological Treatment of Insomnia. Wiley, Chichester, 1991
75. Hinchcliffe AC, Hyman I, Blizard B, Livingston G: The impact on carers of behavioural difficulties in dementia: a pilot study on management. Int J Geriat Psychiatry 1991;7:579–583
76. Buck JA: Psychotropic drug practice in nursing homes. J Am Geriatr Soc 1988;36:409–418
77. Seppala M, Rajala T, Sourander L: Subjective evaluation of sleep and the use of hypnotics in nursing-homes. Aging Clin Exp Res 1993;5:199–205
78. Middelkoop HAM, Kerkhof GA, Smilde-Van Den Doel DA et al: Sleep and ageing: the effects of institutionalisation on subjective and objective characteristics of sleep. Age Ageing 1994;23:411–417
79. Snowdon J, Vaughan R, Miller R et al: Psychotropic-drug use in Sydney nursing-homes. Med J Austr 1995;163:70–72

80. Alessi CA, Schnelle JF, Traub S, Ouslander JG: Psychotropic medications in incontinent nursing home residents: association with sleep and bed mobility. J Am Geriatr Soc 1995;43:789–792

81. Agnew HW, Webb WB, Williams RL: The first night effect: an EEG study of sleep. Psychophysiology 1966;12:412–415

82. Scharf MB, Kales A, Bixler EO: Readaptation to the sleep laboratory in insomniac subjects. Psychophysiology 1975;12:412–415

83. Dement WC, Miles LE, Carskadon MA: "White paper" on sleep and aging. J Am Geriatr Soc 1982;30:25–50

84. Aureff J, Elmqvist D: Sleep in the surgical intensive care unit: continuous polygraphic recording of sleep in nine patients receiving postoperative care. Br Med J 1985;290:1029–1032

85. Meyer TJ, Eveloff SE, Bauer MS et al: Adverse environmental-conditions in the respiratory and medical ICU settings. Chest 1994;105:1211–1216

86. Hilton BA: Noise in acute patient care areas. Res Nursing Health 1985;8:283–291

87. Soutar RL, Wilson JA: Does hospital noise disturb patients? Br Med J 1986;292:305

88. Yinnon AM, Ilan Y, Tadmor B et al: Quality of sleep in the medical department. Br J Clin Pract 1992;46:88–91

89. Adam K, Oswald I: Sleep helps healing. Br Med J 1984;289:1400–1410

90. Closs J: Patients' sleep-wake rhythms in hospital. Nursing Times 1988;84:48–50, 84:54–55

91. Kupfer DJ, Wyatt RJ, Snyder F: Comparison between electroencephalographic and systematic nursing observations of sleep in psychiatric patients. J Nerv Ment Dis 1970;151:361–368

92. Weiss BL, McPartland RL, Kupfer DL: Once more: the inaccuracy of non-EEG estimates of sleep. Am J Psych 1973;130:1282–1285

93. Sadeh A, Hauri P, Kripke DF, Lavie P: The role of actigraphy in the evaluation of sleep disorders. Sleep 1995;18:288–302

94. Ancoli-Israel S, Parker L, Sinaee R et al: Sleep fragmentation in patients from a nursing home. J Gerontol: Med Sci 1989;44:M18–21

95. Alessi CA, Schnelle JF, MacRae PG et al: Does physical activity improve sleep in impaired nursing home residents? J Am Geriatr Soc 1995;43:1098–1102

96. Adam K: Dietary habits and sleep after bedtime food drinks. Sleep 1980;3:47–58

97. Adam K: Total and percentage REM sleep correlate with body weight in 36 middle-aged people. Sleep 1987;10:69–77

98. Schoicket SA, Bertelson AD, Lacks P: Is sleep hygiene a sufficient treatment for sleep-maintenance insomnia. Behav Ther 1988;19:183–190

99. Morin CM, Azrin NH: Behavioral and cognitive treatments of geriatric insomnia. J Consul Clin Psych 1988;56:748–753

100. Lacks P, Morin CM: Recent advances in the assessment and treatment of insomnia. J Consult Clin Psych 1992;60:586–594

101. Monroe LJ: Psychological and physiological differences between good and poor sleepers. J Abnor Psych 1967;72:255–264

102. Adam K, Tomeny M, Oswald I: Physiological and psychological differences between good and poor sleepers. J Psych Res 1986;20:301–316

103. Kales A, Caldwell AB, Soldatos CR et al: Biopsychobehavioral correlates of insomnia. II: Pattern specificity and consistency with MMPI. Psychosom Med 1983;45:341–356

104. Hyyppa MT, Kronholm E, Mattlar CE: Mental well-being of good sleepers in a random population sample. Br J Med Psych 1991;64:25–34

105. Asplund R: Are sleep disorders hereditary? A questionnaire survey of persons about themselves and their parents. Arch Gerontol Geriat 1995;21:231

106. Bootzin RR, Epstein D, Wood JM: Stimulus control instructions. pp. 19–28. In Hauri P (ed): Case Studies in Insomnia. Plenum, New York, 1991

107. Berry DTR, Phillips BA: Sleep disordered breathing in the elderly: review and methodological comment. Clin Psych Rev 1988;8:101–120

108. Guilleminault C, van den Hoed J, Mitler M: Clinical overview of the sleep apnea syndromes. pp. 1–11. In Guilleminault C, Dement W (eds): Sleep Apnea Syndromes. Alan R Liss, New York, 1979

109. Gould GA, Whyte KF, Rhind GB et al: The sleep hypopnea syndrome. Am Rev Respir Dis 1988;137:895–898

110. Ancoli-Israel S, Coy T: Are breathing disturbances in elderly equivalent to sleep apnea syndrome? Sleep 1994;17:77–83

111. Bliwise DL, Feldman DE, Bliwise NG et al: Risk factors for sleep disordered breathing in heterogeneous geriatric populations. J Am Geriatr Soc 1987;35:132–141

112. Ancoli-Israel S, Kripke DF, Mason WJ et al: Sleep apnea and PMS in a randomly selected elderly population: final prevalence results. Sleep Res 1986;15(abstr.):101

113. Carskadon MA, Brown ED, Dement WC: Sleep fragmentation in the elderly: relationship to daytime sleep tendency. Neurobiol Aging 1982;3:321–327

114. Berry DTR, Phillips BA, Cook YR et al: Sleep-disordered breathing in healthy aged persons: possible daytime sequelae. J Gerontol 1987;42:620–626

115. Mant A, King M, Saunders NA et al: Four-year follow-up of mortality and sleep-related respiratory disturbance in non-demented seniors. Sleep 1995;18:433–438

116. Ancoli-Israel S, Kripke DF, Klauber MR et al: Morbidity, mortality and sleep-disordered breathing in community dwelling elderly. Sleep 1996;19:277–282

117. Erkinjuntti T, Partinen M, Sulkava R et al: Sleep apnea in multi-infarct dementia and Alzheimer's disease. Sleep 1987;10:419–425

118. Frommlet M, Prinz P, Vitiello MV et al: Sleep hypoxemia and apnea are elevated in females with mild Alzheimer's disease. Sleep Res 1986;15(abstr.):189

119. Mant A, Saunders NA, Eyland AE et al: Sleep-related respiratory disturbance and dementia in elderly females. J Gerontol (Med Sci) 1988;43:M140–144

120. Hoch CC, Reynolds CF III, Nebes RD et al: Clinical significance of sleep-disordered breathing in Alzheimer's disease: preliminary data. J Am Geriatr Soc 1989;37:138–144

121. Montplaisir J, Godbout R, Pelletier G, Warnes H: Restless legs syndrome and periodic movements during sleep. pp.

589–597. In Kryger MH, Roth T, Dement WC (eds): Principles and Practice of Sleep Medicine. WB Saunders, Philadelphia, 1994

122. Coleman RM: Periodic movements in sleep (nocturnal myoclonus) and restless legs syndrome. pp. 265–295. In Guilleminault C (ed): Sleeping and Waking Disorders: Indications and Techniques. Addison-Wesley Publishing, Menlo Park, California, 1982
123. Morin CM: Insomnia: Psychological Assessment and Management. The Guildford Press, New York, 1993
124. Kryger MH, Roth T, Dement WC (eds): Principles and Practice of Sleep Medicine. WB Saunders, Philadelphia, 1994
125. Committee on Safety of Medicines: Benzodiazepine dependence and withdrawal. Curr Prob 1988;21:1–2
126. Morgan K: Hypnotic drugs, psychomotor performance and ageing. J Sleep Res 1994;3:1–15
127. Morin CM, Azrin NH: Behavioral and cognitive treatments of geriatric insomnia. J Consult Clin Psych 1988;56:748–753
128. Espie CA, Lindsay WR, Brooks DN et al: A controlled comparative investigation of psychological treatments for chronic sleep-onset insomnia. Behav Res Ther 1989;27:79–88
129. Morin CM, Culbert JP, Schwartz SM: Nonpharmacological interventions for insomnia: a meta analysis of treatment efficacy. Am J Psych 1994;151:1172–1180
130. Lacks P, Morin CM: Recent advances in the assessment and treatment of insomnia. J Consult Clin Psych 1992;60:586–594
131. Morin CM, Gaulier B, Barry T, Kowatch RA: Patients' acceptance of psychological and pharmacological therapies for insomnia. Sleep 1992;15:302–305

CHAPTER 100

Eating Disorders

GERALD BLANDFORD

All living things must receive adequate nutrition to survive. In both animals and man the acts of food gathering and eating are innate and failure results in malnutrition, morbidity, and death. However, in man the acts and processes of food acquisition and preparation that precede eating are much more complicated than in other species. For the elderly, eating is a task that is not only complex, but often lonely and onerous, and hindered by multiple factors. These include the effects of aging, economic deprivation, poor social support, physical disability, acute and chronic disease states, and medication usage. As a consequence, the process of eating for the elderly is highly susceptible to failure, with subsequent inanition and its outcomes.[1] These consequences form the imperative for this chapter, which will review the underlying causes, and diagnostic and management strategies for impaired eating in old age.

Epidemiology

The principle indicator for the presence of disordered eating in aging is malnutrition. The measurement of nutritional status is relatively imprecise and the prevalence of malnutrition varies based on the methods used and the population studied.[2–4] Most geriatric studies have concentrated on protein calorie malnutrition. The prevalence of malnutrition in the elderly is variously estimated at 10 to 25 percent for those in the community over 65 years,[5–6] 30 to 61 percent for hospital patients,[5,7] and 17 to 85 percent for nursing home residents.[2,5,8] Any clinical condition with such serious consequences and such high prevalence must be taken seriously. Potential underlying causes require rigorous investigation.

Aging and the Process of Eating

The requirements for eating are listed in Table 100-1. Eating and drinking are driven by hunger or thirst, habit, or a deliberate wish to eat. Food must be acquired, prepared, and presented for eating, and the individual must be able to get the food from plate to mouth. There follows the complex neuromuscular processes of mastication, bolus preparation, and swallowing. Every part of this process may be impacted by some of the losses and problems of aging, whether physiologic, pathologic, iatrogenic, functional, psychological, or sociologic.

Motivation

The motivation to eat and drink may be voluntary or involuntary. Humans may eat because they wish to, whether hungry or not, or whether it is good for them or not. The choice is a cognitive process that may become a bad habit or idiosyncrasy carried into old age with resultant over- or undernutrition, and vitamin or mineral deficiencies. Because choice significantly affects dietary intake, cognitive impairment may also significantly alter the quality or quantity of what is eaten. In late Alzheimer's disease, however, and probably other progressive dementias, agnosias occur, with a failure to recognize the need to eat or the nature of food, and patients may therefore ignore food or eat nonedibles.[9–13] Further, when attempts are made to spoon-feed such patients they may exhibit resistive aversive feeding behaviors such as biting, pushing away the hand that feeds, or striking out,[9–13] which further compromise food intake.

Appetite

Hunger is the involuntary drive to eat. It is regulated by various chemical mediators including hormones (e.g., insulin, corticosteroids, growth and thyroid hormones) and various cytokines (e.g., cholecystokinin,[14] serotonin,[15] interleukin-1-β (IL-1-β), tumor necrosis factor-α (TNF-α),[16] neuropeptide Y[17]), acting directly or indirectly through the hypothalamus and basal brain. Some increase in aging resulting in early satiety (e.g., cholecystokinin), some rise in response to stress or depression (e.g., serotonin), and others are produced in response to common disease processes in aging such as infection, inflammation, or cancer (e.g., TNF-α, IL-1-β). Endocrine diseases such as thyrotoxicosis or myxedema and diabetes produce their effects on nutritional status and eating by altering the body's metabolism. The metabolic rate is often reduced in aging because of an increasingly sedentary existence brought about by disease, disability, or various psychosocial factors. In addition, various chemical mediators, be they hormones, cytokines, or drugs, may have their effects on appetite altered because of changes in receptor status that accompany old age (e.g., decreased opiod and insulin receptors).

Thirst

Body fluid homeostasis is frequently impaired in aging with potentially lethal consequences if the body is subject to certain stresses (e.g., increased ambient temperature, fever, vomiting).

Table 100-1 The requirements for eating

Motivation
Involuntary drives
Hunger
Thirst
Voluntary drives
Recognition of the need to eat or drink
Acquired habits
Eccentricity
Functional resources
Cognitive function
Prepare shopping list
Obtain food
Prepare a meal
Recognize the need to eat
General physical function
Ability to shop (transportation, ambulation)
Food preparation
Ability to get food to mouth
Social support system
Family or other care provider
Societal resources
Economic resources
Transportation
Senior/community center
Meals-on-wheels
Home care
The act of eating
Ability to suck, moisten, chew
Prepare bolus
Progress bolus through oropharyngeal and esophageal phases of swallowing

Changes occur in fluid ingestion in aging.[18] Thirst may be diminished by failure of osmotic regulation, by inappropriate antidiuretic hormone secretion or by changes in the basal brain. In addition, changes in renal function may impair the glomerular filtration rate, and electrolyte and water handling. In healthy elderly persons the nonstressed water deficits are generally made up by coingestion of water with solids.[18] However, this compensatory mechanism is not adequate if solid food ingestion is diminished from any cause, resulting in dehydration and its significant morbidity and mortality.

Many medications are anorexogenic or have a direct effect on fluid or electrolyte balance and may, therefore, contribute significantly to reduced nutritional intake, dehydration, or water overload. The multiple medications used in the management of various clinical problems of the elderly are a major cause of anorexia and impaired fluid homeostasis.

Food Acquisition

Food gathering for man is a highly complex activity. It requires cognitive input—acknowledgement of the need to obtain food; ability to identify the food required; knowing where it can be acquired; having the necessary fiscal resources; and having the physical ability or the cognitive, financial, or social resources to acquire it and bring it home. Food then needs to be prepared, which requires cognitive input, a certain level of physical functioning (e.g., vision, upper extremity dexterity), and certain domestic resources (e.g., stove, microwave, a power supply). It is, therefore, apparent that depression, dementia, many different kinds of physical disability, poverty, lack of transportation, or an inadequate social support system, can all prejudice the food supply. The last step in food acquisition is the ability to get prepared food from table to mouth. Again, impaired vision and upper limb weakness, incoordination, or tremor may be causative factors.

The Act of Eating

Before the benefits of acquired nutrition and hydration can be realized, food and water must reach the absorptive surfaces of the gastrointestinal tract below the esophagus. The processes required to achieve this task are highly sophisticated and delicately organized.

The oropharynx is the locus for the sensations of taste and smell, which affect what is eaten. The teeth, dental prosthesis, mucus membranes, and saliva are involved in mastication and bolus formation. The tongue and neuromusculature of the oropharynx transfer the bolus to the posterior pharynx where closure of the airways and opening of the upper esophageal sphincter are orchestrated. This sequence involves sensory nerve endings, motor nerves, voluntary and involuntary striated muscle, teeth, salivary glands, articular cartilage, joints, and the swallowing center in the basal brain. All may be affected by aging, disease, or by various therapeutic interventions.

Chemosensory Changes, Oral Health, and Eating

The changes in taste and smell associated with aging, the effect these changes have on food intake, and the changes in mastication caused by dental problems, altered salivation, and oral motor performance in aging have been the subject of an excellent detailed review.[19]

Healthy older persons' ability to taste, food enjoyment, and salivary output are essentially unaffected, while chewing efficiency and swallowing are slightly diminished and smell is significantly diminished. In contrast, all are significantly diminished in medically compromised patients. The oral and systemic etiologies of gustatory and olfactory dysfunction, food selection, and chewing and swallowing problems in the geriatric population are summarized in Tables 100-2 and 100-3. They may lead to anorexia, oral pain, less enjoyment of eating, and selective, though often unconscious, changes in food consistency or avoidance of certain foods. Smaller meals and smaller mouthfuls are taken, and the whole process of eating is slowed. These changes may also impair social interactions

Table 100-2 Oral etiologies of gustatory and olfactory dysfunction, food selection, chewing, and swallowing problems

Etiology	Smell and Taste Problem	Food Selection and Chewing Problem	Swallowing Problem
Oral trauma			
Burns, lacerations, chemical damage	x	x	x
Anesthetic, surgical	x	x	
Removable prosthetic appliance	x	x	x
Oral diseases and problems			
Periodontal diseases	x	x	
Dental-alveolar and other infections	x	x	
Soft tissue lesions/oral tumors	x	x	x
Candidiasis, denture stomatitis	x	x	
Burning mouth syndrome	x	x	
Salivary dysfunction	x	x	x
Tooth loss		x	x
Diminished activity of masticatory muscles		x	x
Impaired chewing	x	x	x
Velopharyngeal incompetence			x
Oral pain		x	
Treatment of oral diseases			
Oral mouth rinses, gels, and dentifrices	x		
Removable prosthetic appliances	x	x	x
Drugs in saliva	x		
Dental material interactions, galvanism	x		
Poor dental restorations		x	
Chemosensory problems			
Dysosmia	x	x	
Dysgeusia	x	x	
Halitosis	x	x	

(From Ship et al.,[19] with permission.)

because of the particular food requirements and perceptions that certain changes in eating habits may be socially unacceptable.

Swallowing

The swallowing process[20] and its changes in aging[21–23] have been well-reviewed. The conscious awareness of eating stops when the act of swallowing begins. The movement of the bolus is automatic through the oral cavity, pharynx, and esophagus. The swallowing reflex requires an intact medullary swallowing center, healthy striated muscle, sensory input from the V, X, and XI cranial nerves, and motor input from cranial nerves V, VII, IX, and XII. Respiration ceases, and an invariable sequence of events occurs. There is closure of the airways, velar elevation, laryngeal elevation, pharyngeal shortening, opening of the upper esophageal sphincter, and pharyngeal contraction. This takes normally less than 1 second. The bolus falls into the esophagus and is propelled into the stomach by smooth muscle peristalsis. When the bolus approaches the stomach, the lower esophageal sphincter relaxes. The process takes about 8 seconds for solids and 3 seconds for liquids.

Normal aging is associated with frequent, though clinically insignificant, delay in initiating the swallow. Increased laryngeal penetration has been reported in one study[24] but not in another.[25] However, the occurrence of aspiration in healthy old age has not been reported. Esophageal motility declines with age with increased transit times and less efficient peristalsis[26] and gastroesophageal reflux occurs with greater frequency[27] but neither have been associated with dysphagia.[28]

Oropharygeal and pharyngoesophageal dysphagia occur

Table 100-3 Systemic etiologies of gustatory and olfactory dysfunction, food selection, chewing, and swallowing problems

Etiology	Smell and Taste Problem	Food Selection and Chewing Problem	Swallowing Problem
Upper respiratory tract problems			
Lesions of the nose/airways	x		
Viral and bacterial infections	x		
Exposure to toxic airborne contaminants	x		
Peripheral or central nervous system pathologies			
Head and neck trauma	x	x	x
Tumors, lesions	x		x
Neurological diseases (e.g., Alzheimer's)	x	x	x
Systemic diseases			
Systemic conditions			
Cerebrovascular diseases	x	x	x
Head and neck cancers	x	x	x
Arthritides		x	x
Psychiatric disorders	x	x	
Endocrinopathies (e.g., diabetes)	x	x	x
Pulmonary diseases			x
Gastrointestinal disorders	x	x	x
Swallowing disorders		x	x
Sjögren's syndrome	x	x	x
Treatment of systemic conditions			
Prescription and nonprescription drugs	x		x
Head and neck irradiation	x	x	x
Chemotherapy	x	x	x
Head and neck surgery	x	x	x
Gastrointestinal surgery			x
Nutritional and dietary problems			
Inappropriately restricted diet		x	
Monotonous diet, poor texture and color		x	
Insufficient smell/taste cues to initiate eating		x	
Nutritional deficiencies	x	x	x
Psychosocial problems			
Eating alone		x	
Perceived chewing and eating problems		x	
Low socioeconomic status		x	
Others			
Aging	x	x	x
Circadian variation	x		
Functional problems (ADL, IADL)		x	

(Modified from Ship et al.,[19] with permission.)

commonly after cerebrovascular accidents and in various neurologic disorders, particularly Alzheimer's disease and Parkinson's disease, in various systemic diseases, as with cervical osteophytes, is a matter of course with head and neck cancers, and following the surgical or radiation treatments used for these conditions. Dental problems and dentures may cause oropharyngeal dysphagia. In the latter case, impaired oral sensation, oral stereognosis, and taste are suggested causes although clinical significance has not yet been proved.[29] Salivary gland dysfunction and xerostomia caused by medications and Sjögren's syndrome may also cause delay in the initiation of swallowing and complaints of dysphagia.[30,31]

Other Functional Impairments

The common end point of all functional impairment is dependency for the task impaired. Thus, when a person has impaired vision, hearing, ambulation, toileting, bathing, or eating, they become more or less dependent for that task. We have seen that in the community, eating requires cognition, vision, ambulation and/or transportation, economic resources, social supports, manual dexterity, and the ability to eat safely. There are, therefore, many points at which the individual is potentially dependent and, if these dependencies are not adequately addressed then the food supply will be compromised and nutritional intake will decline resulting in morbidity and mortality. It is, therefore, essential when working up a patient for malnutrition to investigate the whole of the community support system and to ensure that it is included in developing care plans and in monitoring progress.

Sadly, even in professional care settings such as hospitals and nursing homes, where care for dependent persons should be optimal, feeding patients is critically wanting. Butterworth[32] in 1974 declared that malnutrition was the skeleton in the acute care hospital closet. There is still inadequate flesh on those bones[7] and nursing home closets contain the same skeletons.[8,9,33,34] The main causes for this problem have been known for more than 20 years,[35,36] yet the problem remains. The causes are itemized in the accompanying boxed list, "Causes of Continued Malnutrition in Institutional Settings." As can be seen, the problems identified indicate that interdisciplinary care is required. The services of the dietitian, nursing staff, nursing attendants, physicians, and administration are needed to provide corrective action. Absent any other leader, the geriatrician should be the captain of this team and vigorously address all of the eating problems with the patient and the care team.

"Failure to Thrive"

The most frequent presentation of an eating problem is either an older person brought to the office for increasing dependency or vague weight loss, or an incidental finding of malnutrition in the office, at the hospital, or in the nursing home. Typical of geriatric medicine, this problem is a vague clinical syndrome without a single, potentially preventable, treatable, or identifiable pathogenesis. It is most frequently termed "failure to thrive" (FTT), although many other terms have been applied.[37,38] Failure to thrive was given its own International Classification of Diseases, Ninth Revision (ICD-9) code in 1979, even though it does not fulfill the criteria for a specific disease entity. It has been defined by the National Institute on Aging as, "a syndrome of weight loss, decreased appetite, poor nutrition, and inactivity, often accompanied by dehydration, depressive symptoms, impaired immune function, and low cholesterol".[39] But this definition fails to include an important common association, namely cognitive impairment. All conditions associated with impaired eating cause FTT if present for long enough. An historic perspective, review of the syndrome, and a logical approach to its evaluation has been offered.[36] Evaluation begins with a nutritional assessment.

Causes of continued malnutrition in institutional settings

- Failure to set up food trays properly
- Failure to provide needed assistance with feeding
- Failure to comply with patient food preferences
- Providing food of the wrong consistency
- Inducing nausea and anorexia by giving medications before meals when this is not necessary or when less anorexogenic medications are available
- Failure to provide multiple small feedings when this would be helpful
- Failure to provide a comfortable setting conducive to eating
- Inducing confusion by frequent room changes or medications

(Adapted from Sullivan,[2] with permission.)

Nutritional Assessment

Many instruments have been developed to detect risk for malnutrition at various steps along the pathway to malnutrition from "at risk" to severely malnourished. Nutritional screening methods, which could be used for assessment as a part of a multidimensional geriatric assessment in older persons in various settings, have been the subject of an excellent review.[40] A screening instrument should be cheap, sensitive, specific, and have some predictive value. In general, specificity is sacrificed to sensitivity with the expectation that the presence of malnutrition will lead to more specific investigations. There needs to be both good inter-rater and test-retest reliability. Finally, a screening test should lead to findings for which there are effective and affordable therapeutic interventions. The ability of the available instruments to detect risk varies between 36 percent to 93 percent for sensitivity and from 44 to 85 percent for specificity. Three instruments, designed for use in the hospital setting (Subjective Global Assessment,[41] Prognostic Nutritional Index [PNI],[42] and Nutritional Risk Index[41]), have been shown to be valid predictors for potential improvement with a nutritional intervention, and one of these (PNI) has been effective when used in ambulatory and nursing home patients. A new and promising internationally developed instrument, the Mini Nutritional Assessment, has been developed as a rapid and simple evaluation for the at risk elderly and has been cross-validated in elderly populations from the very frail to the healthy.[43] An assessment instrument for aversive feeding behavior in dementia has been developed[44] and is currently being tested.[13] Results on the therapeutic usefulness of these instruments are pending. There are no data on the cost/benefit of using any of these instruments.

On examination, low body weight, muscle wasting, absence of subcutaneous fat, sometimes clinical features of specific vitamin deficiencies (particularly vitamin C, thiamine, and B_{12}), various anthropomorphic measurements, the presence of a low serum albumin, low cholesterol, low levels of vital nutrients (e.g., iron, zinc), and various vitamins can confirm the diagnosis of malnutrition and provide clinical parameters to follow progress.

Once a diagnosis of malnutrition has been made, then the

usual diagnostic protocols are applied to identify specific treatable conditions (e.g., cancer, malabsorption, chronic inflammatory diseases, or endocrine abnormalities) and at the same time consideration must be given to the multiple functional and psychosocial factors that contribute to disordered eating and which are outlined in Table 100-1.

Diagnosing Dysphagia

After malnutrition and dental problems, the most frequent diagnosis made regarding eating disorders is that of "dysphagia." The word is derived from the Greek and means "difficulty eating." Specialists divide dysphagia symptomatically into oropharyngeal, pharyngoesophageal and esophageal types; however, common usage in medical practice has tended to limit it to describing only the involuntary, pharyngoesophageal and esophageal phases of swallowing. These are characterized by coughing, choking, nasal regurgitation, or food "sticking" somewhere behind the sternum. A threat of aspiration is present when the voice is wet or gurgling in quality. The causes of esophageal dysphagia are presented in the accompanying boxed list.

Difficulty in the earlier, voluntary, oropharyngeal phase of eating, which includes mastication, bolus preparation, and initiating the swallow, should also be called dysphagia, but it is diagnosed and even more rarely recognized in the one circumstance where it may be most frequent, namely late-stage dementia. The signs include failure to open the mouth, dysarthria, tongue movement abnormalities, food residues remaining between cheek and gum or under the tongue, or inability to transfer ("swallow") the bolus to the posterior pharynx. The causes of oropharyngeal dysphagia are listed in Table 100-4.

The symptoms of oropharyngeal dysphagia can usually be accurately described by the cognitively unimpaired. A simple physical examination frequently identifies the cause of the problem (e.g., tumors, stroke, pseudobulbar palsy, Parkinson's disease, cranial nerve lesions) and the word "dysphagia" may never appear in their diagnosis.

In contrast, late-stage dementia patients, who may all ultimately develop this problem,[9,13] are generally unable to speak or express themselves. They usually reside at home or in a nursing home and their problem is described to the primary physician by feeders as difficulty swallowing, "dysphagia", or "refusal" to eat or swallow. This frequently results in tube feeding or the use of sedatives without further work-up. Careful observation of these patients, however, reveals a pattern of aversive feeding behaviors that hinder or prevent effective oral feeding, which may be managed without tube feeding.[9–13,44] Among them are a group of oral feeding dyspraxias (e.g., pursing of the lips instead of opening the mouth; failure to suck, chew, or swallow; pocketing of food; pushing food out of the mouth).[9,13] These are the last aversive feeding behaviors to appear and occur almost exclusively in bed-bound, incontinent, noncommunicative, end stage patients incapable of any voluntary activity.[13] All imply a severe degree of incoordination of the oropharyngeal phase of eating and, if they fail to remit, which is usually the case, they further imply the presence of a terminal state because the patient will die unless provided with life-sustaining nutrition by artificial means. Management of these patients then requires a much more careful analysis than simply placing a feeding tube. This should

Causes of esophageal dysphagia

- Achalasia
- Diffuse esophageal spasms
- Carcinoma
- Strictures
- Webs
- Rings
- Medication (chemical) injuries to gastric lining

Table 100-4 Causes of oropharyngeal dysphagia

Neuromuscular
Stroke
Parkinson's disease
Brain stem tumors
Multiple sclerosis
Amytrophic lateral sclerosis
Mononeuritis multiplex
Skeletal muscle disorders
Inflammatory myopathies
Polymyosistis
Dermatomyositis
Muscular dystrophies
Myotonic dystrophy
Oculopharyngeal dystrophy
Myasthenia gravis
Metabolic myopathies
Hyperthyroidism
Hypothyroidism
Steroid myopathy
Mechanical obstruction
Inflammatory conditions
Extrinsic compression (thyromegaly, cervical hyperostosis, lymphadenopathy)
Postsurgical changes
Radiation scarring
Motility disorders
Zenker's diverticulum
Cricopharyngeal bar
Salivary problems
Medications
Sjögren's syndrome
Postradiation
Cognitive dysfunction
Alzheimer's disease
Parkinson's disease

include consideration of the benefits and burdens of artificial feeding and hydration, the patient's prior wishes regarding tube feeding, and the ethical and legal standards that have been set for medical practice in these patients.

Barium radiographic studies are the most useful tests for defining dysphagia. They should include anteroposterior and lateral projection videoradiography to properly elucidate mechanisms, and a solid bolus (cookie swallow) to identify obstructive lesions. An obstructive lesion may require endoscopy and biopsy. Motility disorders can be further elucidated with manometric studies. Sophisticated manometric studies help elucidate physiologic mechanisms, but at present are of little practical help. In contrast, video-radiography can define strategies to improve feeding by identifying positional changes that circumvent the hazards of pharyngeal penetration. Unfortunately, most late-stage dementia patients are unable to cooperate sufficiently for these studies to be clinically useful.

Management of Eating Disorders

Throughout the foregoing, the need for an interdisciplinary approach has been emphasized. The social, economic, ADL, IADL, medical, psychological, and iatrogenic causes must be elucidated and comprehensively addressed. Clearly, this requires a great deal of professional time and expertise, and substantial and varied resources. The expense is considerable and pragmatism is necessary in determining what is reasonable and what is not. Correctable medical problems should obviously be addressed. Unfortunately, data on cost-effectiveness on most aspects of assessing nutritional impairment is absent.[40] The available data on replenishing and preventing nutritional deficits, with few exceptions, lack scientific support for their effectiveness.[2,38,40] Nevertheless, it is reasonable, humane, and civilized to try to ensure that individuals receive adequate nutrition and social supports. This may at least improve the quality of life.

Management of Dysphagia

Treatment depends upon underlying causes and the nature of the problem. Appropriate treatment for malignancies and diseases such as polymyositis, Parkinson's disease, thyroid dysfunction, or myasthenia gravis, may result in significant improvement in swallowing. The more permanent problems that follow a stroke, head and neck surgery, radiation or trauma, or degenerative neurologic diseases, such as Alzheimer's disease or motor neurone disease, can be managed or improved to some extent by mechanical strategies and behavior modification.[45] Strategies that minimize laryngeal penetration include changes in food consistency and volume of feedings, postural modifications, instruction on certain physical maneuvers, and dental, prosthetic, or surgical interventions.[46] A speech therapist can be invaluable in assisting the care team identify the appropriate treatment. If these strategies are ineffective then enteral feeding should be considered.

Tube Feeding

The principle mode of ensuring increased or sufficient nutritional intake in patients who are unable to eat is tube feeding. In this invasive procedure (which should therefore require the patient's consent) a tube is inserted into the stomach through the nose (nasogastric [NG] tube), through an abdominal incision into the stomach (percutaneous endoscopic gastrostomy [PEG] or the jejunem (percutaneous endoscopic jejunostomy [PEJ]) through which nutrition, hydration, and medications can be passed. It is clearly indicated to provide nutrition and hydration to patients with serious acute illness where there is expectation of recovery of the ability to eat. It is also appropriate to supplement feeding in the short-term for patients unable to eat or drink sufficient amounts, to preserve or restore their fluid and nutritional balance while recovering from some temporary disability. In incurable illness, tube feeding may be palliative, relieving hunger or thirst such as frequently occurs with head and neck tumors, postsurgery and/or radiation, or in treating the wasting syndromes of AIDS and cancer patients, if some improvement in there condition or function can be reasonably expected. However, there is no evidence that prolonged tube feeding patients with advanced dementia is either palliative or therapeutic. These patients fail to exhibit symptoms of hunger or thirst that might be relieved, and the primary underlying brain pathology is neither arrested nor reversed.

Four myths concerning tube feeding have been promulgated over time.[47] They are (1) that it is ordinary care analogous to spoon feeding, (2) that it prevents aspiration pneumonia, (3) that swallowing evaluations identify patients who should receive tube feeding, and (4) that withholding or withdrawing tube feeding leads to a painful death. All of these myths can be substantially refuted.

First, tube feeding provides only chemical nutrition not food, and it is a potentially harmful and even a life-threatening procedure (see accompanying boxed lists on enteral tube feeding and gastronomy and jejunostomy tube feeding). Second, the literature on aspiration pneumonia is confounded by the inconsistent definitions of the syndrome, and by the fact that the syndrome continues to occur in many tube-fed patients regardless of whether it is an NG, PEG, or JEG. This may be due to aspiration of saliva or oral bacteria, by NG tubes causing incompetence of the gastroesophageal sphincter, by PEG tubes increasing gastroesophageal reflux, or by regurgitation from an over-full stomach. These problems may be minimized by keeping the patient at 30 to 35 degrees when in bed, by monitoring gastric residual before each feeding, and by ensuring that tube placement is correct. Third, the diagnostic procedures for dysphagia, briefly described above, may clearly characterize abnormalities of the process of swallowing, but the clinical significance of the very subtle changes that can be identified requires careful consideration. Significant clinical judgment is required, taking into account both the severity of symptoms and the nature of the underlying disease. An abnormal result from a swallowing evaluation is not a categorical requirement to tube feed. Finally, the cruel and painful death

Complications of enteral tube feeding

- Discomfort
- Self-extubation
- Dislodgement
- Incorrect placement
- Tube trauma
- Erosions of nasal septum and passages
- Bleeding
- Tracheal perforation
- Pneumothorax
- Electrolyte disturbance
- Bloating
- Regurgitation
- Diarrhea
- Aspiration pneumonia
- Anxiety
- Imposition of chemical or mechanical restraints

by starvation claimed by some to occur when tube feeding is not provided has no scientific foundation.[48]

Summary

Malnutrition is common in aging and has multiple causes. Its presence indicates some disorder of eating. The common causes are anorexia, physical difficulty with eating, and failure to acquire or prepare food or to eat food provided. The great variety of causes for the syndrome is only exceeded by the heterogeneity of the elderly population.

The approach to identifying causes and developing appropriate care plans include multidimensional assessment, nutritional status evaluation, and studies of the physiologic processes of eating.

Management strategies focus first on treating underlying causes. In spite of the fact that supplemental feedings have rarely been satisfactorily proven to be of significant benefit in most circumstances, strategies to enhance and restore nutritional status should be developed and implemented. Enteral feeding should be used with discretion, especially in late-stage dementia.

Further research into this clinically problematic area of geriatric medicine is urgently needed. The elderly population in general, and of those who will suffer from disordered eating in particular, is growing faster than most other population groups in society. The methods for nutritional status evaluation and the results of nutritional interventions require further validation, and society will require that their respective cost/benefit ratio be favorable.

Complications of gastrostomy and jejunostomy tube feeding

- All the complications of enteral tube feeding
- Peristomal discomfort
- Abdomonal wall cellulitis
- Peritonitis
- Gastrointestinal bleeding
- Leakage
- Ileus
- Bowel obstruction
- Small bowel perforation and death
- Anesthetic problems (e.g., cardiopulmonary arrest)

References

1. Sullivan DH: The role of nutrition in increased morbidity and mortality. Clin Geriatr Med 1995;11:661–673
2. Sullivan DH: Impact of nutritional status on health outcomes of nursing home residents. J Am Geriatr Soc 1995;43:195–196
3. Reuben DB, Greendale GA, Harrison GG: Nutrition screening in older persons. J Am Geriatr Soc 1995;43:415–425
4. Guigoz Y, Vellas B, Garry PJ: Assessing the nutritional status of the elderly: the Mini Nutritional Assessment as a part of geriatric evaluation. Nutr Rev 1996;54:S59–S65
5. Verdery RB: Failure to thrive in the elderly. Clin Geriatr Med 1995;11:653–659
6. Wallace JI, Schwartz RS, LaCroix AZ et al: Involuntary weight loss in older outpatients: incidence and clinical significance. J Am Geriatr Soc 1995;43:329–337
7. Mowe M, Bohmer T: The prevalence of undiagnosed protein-calorie undernutrition in a population of hospitalized elderly patients. J Am Geriatr Soc 1993;41:283–296
8. Morley JE, Silver AJ: Nutritional issues in nursing home care. Ann Intern Med 1995;123:850–859
9. Siebens H, Trupe E, Siebens A et al: Correlates and consequences of eating dependency in institutionalized elderly. J Am Geriatr Soc 1986;34:192–198
10. Norberg A, Athlin E: Eating problems in severely demented patients. Issues and ethical dilemmas. Nurs Clin North Am 1989;24:781–787
11. Volicer L, Seltzer B, Rheaume Y et al: Eating difficulties in patients with probable dementia of the Alzheimer type. J Geriatr Psych Neurol 1989;2:188–194
12. Watkins LB, Blandford G: Aversive feeding behavior in dementia. J Am Geriatr Soc 1994;43:32
13. Blandford G, Watkins LB, Mulvihill MN et al: Assessing abnormal feeding behavior in dementia: a taxonomy and initial findings. Research and Practice in Alzheimer's Disease. Springer Publishing, New York, 1997 (in press.)
14. Morley JE, Silver AJ: Anorexia in the elderly. Neurobiol Aging 1984;9:9

15. Wallin MS, Rissanen AM: Food and mood: relationship between food, serotonin and affective disorders. Acta Psych Scand 1994; 377(suppl):36–40

16. Martinez M, Arnalich F, Hernanz A: Alterations in anorectic cytokines levels from plasma and cerebrospinal fluid in idiopathic senile anorexia. Mech Aging Dev 1993;72:145–153

17. Leibowitz SF: Brain neuropeptide Y: an integrator of endocrine, metabolic and behavioral processes. Brain Res Bull 1991;27: 333–337

18. de Castro JM: Age-related changes in natural spontaneous fluid ingestion and thirst in humans. J Gerontol 1992;47:P321–P330

19. Ship JA, Duffry V, Jones JA, Langmore S: Geriatric oral health and its impact on eating. J Am Geriatr Soc 1996;44:456–464

20. Grohan ME: Dysphagia: diagnosis and management. 3rd Ed., Butterworth-Heinemann, Boston, 1997

21. Castell JA, Castell DO. Upper esophageal sphincter and pharyngeal function and oropharyngeal (transfer) dysphagia. Gastroenterol Clin North Am 1996;25:35–50

22. Sonies BC: Oropharyngeal dysphagia in the elderly. Clin Geriatr Med 1992;8:569–577

23. Schroeder PL, Richter JE: Swallowing disorders in the elderly. Semin Gastrointest Dis 1994;5:154–165

24. Robbins J, Hamilton JW, Lof GL, Kempster GB: Oropharyngeal swallowing in normal adults of different ages. Gastroenterology 1992;103:823–829

25. Tracy JF, Logemann JA, Kahrilas PJ et al: Preliminary observations on the effects of age on oropharyngeal deglutition. Dysphagia 1989;4:90–94

26. Mandelstam P, Lieber A: Cineradiographic evaluation of the esophagus in normal adults. Gastroenterology 1970;58:32–38

27. Dodds WJ, Hogan WJ, Helm JF, Dent J: Pathogenesis of reflux esophagitis. Gastroenterology 1981;81:376–394

28. Ergun GA, Miskovitz PF: Aging and the esophagus: common pathologic conditions and their effect upon swallowing in the geriatric population. Dysphagia 1992;7:58–63

29. Tallgren A, Tryde G. Chewing and swallowing activity of masticatory muscles in patients with complete upper and lower partial denture. J Oral Rehab 1991;18:285–299

30. Loesche WJ, Bromberg J, Terpenning MS et al: Xerostomia, xerogenic medications and food avoidances in selected geriatric populations. J Am Geriatr Soc 1995;43:401–407

31. Caruso AJ, Sonies BC, Atkinson JC, Fox PC: Objective measures of swallowing in patients with primary Sjogren's syndrome. Dysphagia 1989;4:101–105

32. Butterworth CE: The skeleton in the hospital closet. Nutrition Today 1974;March/April:4–8

33. Shaver HJ, Loper JA, Lutes N: Nutritional status of nursing home patients. J Parent Enteral Nutr 1980;4:367–370

34. Rudman D, Mattson DE, Nagmraj HS et al: Antecedents of death in men of a Veterans Administration nursing home. J Am Geriatr Soc 1987;35:496–502

35. MacLennan WJ, Martin P, Mason BJ: Causes for reduced dietary intake in a long-stay hospital. Age Aging 1975;4:175–180

36. Edwards KA: Dining experience in the institutional setting. Nursing Homes 1979; March/April:6–17

37. Sarkisian CA, Lachs MS: "Failure to thrive" in older adults. Ann Intern Med 1996; 124:1072–1078

38. Verdery RB: Failure to thrive in older people. J Am Geriatr Soc 1996;44:465–466

39. Lonergan ET (ed): Extending Life, Enhancing Life: A National Research Agenda. National Academy Pr, Washington, DC, 1991

40. Reuben DB, Greendale GA, Harrison GG: Nutrition screening in older persons. J Am Geriatr Soc 1995;43:415–425

41. Veterans Affairs Total Parenteral Nutrition Cooperative Study Group: Perioperative total parenteral nutrition in surgical patients. N Engl J Med 1991;325:525–532

42. Dempsey DT, Mullen JL: Prognostic value of nutritional indices. JPEN 1987;11:109–114S

43. Guigoz Y, Vellas B, Garry PJ: Mini Nutritional assessment: a practical assessment tool for grading the nutritional state of elderly patients. Facts Res Gerontol 1994;(suppl. 2):15–59

44. Blandford G, Watkins L, Mulvihill M, Taylor B: Feeding Alzheimer's patients. Facts Res Gerontol Newsletter 1995;4:5–8

45. Linden P: Treatment strategies for adult neurogenic dysphagia. p.255. In Sonies B (eds): Seminars in Speech and Language. Thieme, New York, 1991

46. Logemann J: Evaluation and Treatment of Swallowing Disorders. College Hill Press, San Diego, 1993

47. Ahronheim JC: Nutrition and hydration in the terminal patient. Clin Geriatr Med 1996;12:379–391

48. Ahronheim JC, Gasner MR: The sloganism of starvation. Lancet 1990;1:278–279

CHAPTER 101

Pain Problems in Old Age

BENNY KATZ

ROBERT D. HELME

The optimal approach to the management of pain is to treat the underlying cause of disease. As the disease resolves, by natural healing or in response to intervention, pain usually subsides and short-term symptomatic treatment may be all that is required. In older people there is an increased prevalence of chronic pain, often because the general health status of the patient or the nature of the underlying condition causing the pain precludes definitive treatment. Regardless of etiology, chronic pain interferes with enjoyment of life, has deleterious effects on mood, social interaction, function, mobility, and independence. Despite an age-related increase in prevalence, chronic pain should not be regarded as a normal consequence of the aging process. Pain is always due to pathology, either physical or psychological. When pain persists, and the underlying cause cannot be eradicated, the pain rather than disease becomes the major problem and is the focus of therapy.

Chronic pain is not merely acute pain that has persisted, it is not solely a sensory phenomenon. Emotional responses often determine whether a sensation is pleasant or unpleasant, and whether an acute pain becomes chronic. The International Society for the Study of pain has defined pain as "an unpleasant sensory and emotional experience associated with actual or potential tissue damage or described in terms of such damage".[1] Failure to recognize the complex interaction between pain and suffering may lead to inappropriate interventions. An individual who has persistent pain despite what appears to be conventional therapy should be carefully reassessed to determine why there has been a failure of response to treatment. Merely increasing the dose of an ineffective medication is futile, placing the individual at increased risk of adverse effects, and leading to frustration, despair, depression, or other psychological consequences. Addressing the pain from a pathophysiologic perspective assists in the selection of appropriate treatment modalities and in determining prognosis.

Types of Pain

Acute pain usually has an identifiable temporal relationship with an injury or disease. In this setting, pain may be seen to serve a useful role in drawing attention to injured tissues, altering behavior, and hence, preventing further tissue damage. Autonomic overactivity such as diaphoresis and tachycardia may be present. There is little data to suggest that the overall prevalence of acute pain is influenced by aging. Crook and colleagues[2] reported a prevalence of approximately 5 percent for acute pain across all age groups. Pain in older people may not be the cardinal symptom of disease as it is in a younger population. Approximately one-third of myocardial infarctions are silent. The incidence of silent myocardial infarction is strongly influenced by age with 47 percent being unrecognized between the ages of 75 and 79 years.[3] In a retrospective study of elderly patients with peritonitis, abdominal pain was absent in nearly one-half of the cases.[4] There is no clear explanation why the elderly are more likely to have painless presentations of typically painful diseases.[5]

In contrast, *chronic pain* persists beyond the normal duration of injury or tissue damage. The time frame for the transition from acute to chronic pain is somewhat arbitrary, often determined by the underlying pathology, and not necessarily characterized by a change in quality or severity of symptoms. Psychological and functional consequences are often apparent in chronic pain and autonomic overactivity is not a feature. There may be no identifiable pathology to account for the pain. Once reversible factors have been excluded, the pain rather than the pathology is considered the major problem. The goals of treatment shifts from a disease eradication approach to improving function and decreasing suffering.

The prevalence rates of chronic pain vary widely among studies, related to difference in the populations sampled and the methodologies of the studies.[6–8] Crook and colleagues[2] reported age-specific rates of persistent pain of 7.6 percent in subjects aged 18 to 30 years, increasing in each progressive age cohort to 29 percent for those aged between 71 and 80 years. An age-associated increase in prevalence of chronic pain is a consistent finding up to age 65 years, although some studies have reported an attenuation in the prevalence of pain report in the over-85-year age group.[9–11] Reasons that might contribute to this include survivor effects, poor response rates in surveys, and sequestration of the sickest old in institutions. There is some consensus from epidemiologic studies that pain affecting joints, the feet, and legs is increased with age, that pain in the head, abdomen, and chest is reduced, and that back pain report is widely variable.[10–12] Chronic pain has a deleterious effect on function and mood[9,12] and is an important symptom in the final stage of life. Studies undertaken in residential care settings for the elderly have shown prevalence rates of chronic pain between 66 and 80 percent,[13,15] with low back pain reported in 40 percent, arthritis of appendicular joints 24 percent, followed by old fracture site pain and painful neuropathies.[15] Moss and colleagues[17] reported that during the last year of life 66 percent of individuals had frequent or continuous severe pain.

As women represent a higher proportion of the older population, the impact of the trend for a higher prevalence of pain in women in a several of epidemiologic studies should not be underestimated.[9,10,12,17] Disease presentation is influenced by gender, for instance rheumatoid arthritis, fibromyalgia, and migraine headaches are more prevalent in women, whereas gout, ankylosing spondylitis, and coronary artery disease are more prevalent in men. Hormonal factors may also play a role in pain perception. Lifestyle factors and preparedness to report pain are relevant, but are unlikely to be the whole explanation.[17–19] Literature on gender differences in pain perception beyond the reproductive years is scarce, and further research in this area is required.

Age-Related Changes in Pain Perception

The way an individual perceives a sensory stimulus influences the response to that stimulus. There are widespread morphologic, electrophysiologic, neurochemical, and functional changes within the sensory pathways, and psychological factors that may alter the experience of pain in the elderly.[6] Attempts to experimentally measure the effects of age on pain perception have resulted in contradictory results. Whether or not age affects the level of discomfort and suffering associated with clinical pain is uncertain.[20] Some areas of pain perception and report are modified by the aging process, which may make it easier for the elderly to deal with minor degrees of pathology, however when pain is perceived the experience is the same. There is a change is in threshold of pain report, rather than actual experience of pain itself.[6] Clinicians should not underestimate the potential seriousness of underlying pathology when minimal pain is reported by older people.

Pathophysiologic Perspective

Pain may be considered from a number of perspectives. Usually the onset, quality, site, and etiology of pain are considered in determining a management strategy. Chronic pain may be subdivided into three subtypes based on pathophysiologic criteria. An understanding of the pathophysiologic basis of the pain may assist in selection of therapy and in determining prognosis. Pain that arises from noxious stimulation of specific peripheral or visceral nociceptors is termed *nociceptive pain*. Examples include pain arising from osteoarthritis and soft tissue injuries. When pain arises from pathology of the peripheral nerves or within the central nervous system it is termed *neuropathic pain*. Examples include painful peripheral neuropathies, phantom limb pains, postherpetic neuralgia, trigeminal neuralgia, and central post-stroke pain. When psychological or psychiatric factors are dominant, the pain is termed *psychogenic pain*. In the Diagnostic and Statistical Manual of Mental Disorders-IV (DSM-IV) of the American Psychiatric Association,[21] this entity is referred to as "Pain Disorder" and is diagnosed when psychological factors are judged to have the major role in the onset, severity, exacerbation, or maintenance of the pain. Pain disorder is not diagnosed if pain is better accounted for by a mood, anxiety, or psychotic disorder. There may or may not be an associated medical condition. The absence of obvious pathology to account for the pain should not lead to the assumption that the pain is of psychogenic origin. The diagnosis of psychogenic pain should only be made in the setting of psychopathology. Previously, this entity was called *somatoform pain disorder*.

It is not unusual for an older individual to have multiple mechanisms to account for their pain. Specifically, chronic pain regardless of etiology is often associated with deleterious effects on mood, such as depression, anxiety, or anger. Pains associated with cancer often have features of acute and chronic pain, with different pathophysiologic factors contributing to a variable extent at different times.

Evaluation of the Patient with a Persistent Pain Problem

The assessment of a patient with a complex pain problem may need to take place over several consultations. The history should focus on the onset and temporal pattern of the symptoms, site and quality of the pain, aggravating and relieving factors, and the impact that pain is having on the patient's lifestyle. The reliability of the history may be affected by the chronicity of the pain, past interventions, and cognitive impairment. One must be vigilant not to falsely attribute drug side effects to the underlying pathology. Physical examination should place special emphasis on the musculoskeletal and neurologic examinations because of their importance in the genesis of pain in the elderly. Abnormalities on sensory examination should be demonstrable in neurogenic pain disorders. The assessment should include functional and psychological aspects. Where possible, the individual should be assessed within their own environment. The open ended question, "What would you do if you no longer had pain?" often reveals valuable information regarding mood state, attitudes, and disability.

There are a number of validated instruments available to quantify and communicate the patient's pain experience. The McGill Pain Questionnaire[22] is a widely used measure consisting of 78 adjectives describing emotional, sensory, and evaluative dimensions of the pain experience. Words such as throbbing, sharp, cramping, burning, and aching describe a sensory dimension, whereas tiring, exhausting, cruel, punishing, fearful, and sickening describe an affective component. Among simpler instruments are the Visual Analog Scales for pain and unpleasantness and the Present Pain Intensity Scale of the McGill Pain Questionnaire. A Visual Analog Scale is a 100mm line, marked at one end with words such as "No Pain" and at the other "Worst Possible Pain". The patient places a mark along the line to indicate the severity of the pain. The Present Pain Intensity Scale is a word descriptor; the patients chooses the most appropriate adjective: "No Pain, Mild, Discomforting, Distressing, Horrible, Excruciating". Pain scales are usually combined with other psychometric instruments to describe the broader dimensions of the pain experience. These may include measures of depression, anxiety, pain impact, and activities of daily living.

The vagaries of the history and physical examination in the older patient places increased emphasis on the use of investigative procedures to establish a diagnosis and exclude more serious pathology. However, a high frequency of abnormal laboratory or radiologic findings in asymptomatic individuals may lead to false attribution of the cause of the symptoms. For example, computed tomography[23] and magnetic resonance imaging (MRI) studies[24] of the lumbar spine in asymptomatic individuals over 60 years of age reveal more than 80 percent with abnormal findings, and 21 percent with spinal canal stenosis.[25] Even after thorough assessment a definitive cause of low back pain cannot be established in 85 percent of cases.[26] Thus, the identification of pathology on diagnostic investigations does not necessarily indicate causality; abnormal findings must be interpreted in light of the clinical setting.

Psychological Assessment

A comprehensive psychological assessment is not usually required in the setting of acute pain. However, chronic pain may have profound effects on mood, interpersonal relationships, and activity level. It is often difficult to ascertain which is cause and which is effect. Psychological evaluation is indicated when medical evaluation fails to adequately explain the degree of pain behavior. Psychological evaluation can also be valuable when the pain causes severe distress, results in excessive health service utilization, or interferes with normal activities or interpersonal relationships. Chronic pain patients are often resistant to psychological evaluation, considering this an inference that the pain is "in the head" rather than a physical problem. Patients often require careful explanation regarding the complex interaction between mind and body, which often influences pain, suffering, and disability.[27] Acknowledging that the pain is real preserves the patient's sense of legitimacy and allows for a more complete evaluation of the psychological factors contributing to the maintenance of pain.

It is important to evaluate how the patient and their relatives conceptualize the pain and goals of treatment. It is often the case that they believe that the pain has persisted because the medical workup has been inadequate or specific interventions denied. Each time a new intervention is tried and fails the psychological distress is reinforced. Psychological strategies are not likely to be effective in teaching the patient how to manage with ongoing pain while the patient remains focused on seeking a cure. Pain behaviors such as limping, grimacing, inactivity, and verbalizing of pain complaints may be reinforced by social influences such as gaining attention, sympathy, or the ability to avoid unpleasant responsibilities. Fear of causing further pain or injury may lead to avoidance of activity. Attempts at management with medications and physical therapies, without addressing psychological factors are often unsuccessful.

Assessment of Pain in the Presence of Dementia

The prevalence of cognitive impairment rises sharply with advancing age with rates in excess of 30 percent after the age of 80 years. Significant cognitive impairment should be screened using a standard instrument such as the Mini-Mental Status Examination of Folstein.[28] Dementia represents a major impediment to the evaluation and management of pain. Report of pain in demented individuals may be affected by memory impairment or communication disturbances common in dementing illnesses. A corroborative history from relatives or previous therapists is often required.

Cognitive impairment may be aggravated by pain or medications used to treat the pain.[29] There is no convincing evidence of enhancement of pain by dementia. In fact, Parmalee and colleagues[15] found a small negative relationship between pain intensity and cognitive impairment in a sample of 758 elderly institutionalized residents. Individuals with marked cognitive impairment were less likely to report pain in the back and joints. However, when pain was reported there was no difference in the presence or absence of a likely physical cause. In a sample of 325 nursing home residents, Ferrell and colleagues[30] reported that elderly subjects with mild to moderate cognitive impairment often require more time to assimilate and respond to questions regarding pain, but of the 62 percent reporting pain complaints 83 percent were able to complete a unidimensional pain-intensity scale, with the Present Pain Intensity Scale of the McGill Pain Questionnaire having the highest completion rate of 65 percent. Pain report should not be disregarded because the individual has cognitive impairment.

Define the Goals of Therapy

Prior to embarking upon a treatment program, the patient and the clinician should agree on the goals of therapy, particularly when pain eradication is not feasible. A frank discussion about the prognosis and therapeutic options is often accepted with gratitude. Even if the sensory component of pain cannot be eliminated, improved outcomes can be achieved by addressing factors such as disability and mood disturbance. Disability may be more important to the patient than the pain. Medication side effects may be more troublesome than the condition for which they were prescribed. Pain management programs combine cognitive and rehabilitative approaches to enhance coping strategies and minimize the impact that persistent pain has on the individual. A marginal improvement may make the difference between coping and not coping at home.

Management

Most pain encountered in clinical practice is associated with stimulation of peripheral nociceptors. Nociceptive pains are usually well-localized and described in terms such as aching, heaviness, sharp, or throbbing. Nociceptive pains tend to respond to analgesic medications and physical therapies. Pain of neuropathic origin is often associated with abnormal and unpleasant sensations (dysasthesia) and have a burning or shooting quality. Mild normally non-noxious stimuli in the affected region may cause pain (allodynia), and repetitive stimulation results in summation and after-pain (hyperpathia). There may be a delay between the precipitating injury and the onset of pain[31] and pain often persists in the absence of ongoing tissue damage. Neuropathic pain is difficult to eradicate and is typically insensitive to usual doses of simple and opioid analgesic medications.[32]

Medications

Pharmacological approaches with simple analgesics and nonsteroidal anti-inflammatory drugs (NSAIDs) are the mainstay of most interventions for pain, whether self-initiated or prescribed by the doctor. This is often the most convenient and cost-effective approach. Selection of appropriate drug therapy for the older patient requires an understanding of age-related pharmacokinetic and pharmacodynamic changes, and also needs to take into account any coexisting diseases, which may be adversely affected by the new treatment. In general, drugs with shorter half-lives are preferable, commenced at low doses and titrated upward. Concern regarding potential adverse effects of medications should not result in the patient suffering unnecessarily.

Simple analgesics

Simple, nonopioid analgesics include paracetamol (acetaminophen), aspirin, and the NSAIDs. Paracetamol is the preferred analgesic for the elderly, particularly in noninflammatory musculoskeletal conditions as it has relatively few side effects in standard doses, and no dose adjustment is required.[29] Aspirin is less well-tolerated for rheumatologic conditions than NSAIDs.

The trend toward the earlier use of disease-modifying agents in rheumatoid arthritis may decrease the requirement for NSAIDs. More than one half the prescriptions for NSAIDs are for osteoathritis.[33] They have proved efficacious for short-term use in musculoskeletal back pain and osteoarthritis, but their value over long periods is uncertain.[33] The side effect and drug interaction profile of NSAIDs is of particular concern. Gastrointestinal side effects occur in 10 to 60 percent of NSAIDs users, with symptomatic and potentially life-threatening ulcer complications reported in 2 to 4 percent of patients taking NSAIDs for a year. Risk factors for serious upper gastrointestinal hemorrhage include age greater than 75 years, history of peptic ulcer or bleeding, and cardiovascular disease. Patients with rheumatoid arthritis with these risk factors have a 9 percent risk of a major complication in 6 months.[34] Many patients taking NSAIDs for osteoarthritis can achieve equivalent symptom control with paracetamol.[35] If a NSAIDs cannot be discontinued in an older patient who has other risk factors, consideration should be given to the prophylactic use of the prostaglandin E_1 analog misoprostol, which can reduce serious NSAIDs upper gastrointestinal complications by 40 percent.[34] Other antiulcer treatments may be better tolerated than misoprostol, but as yet evidence of their comparative efficacy is not available. Other important side effects of NSAIDs include aggravation of renal impairment, cardiac failure, and hypertension, as well as dermatologic complications, headaches, and confusional states.

The vast majority of patients will respond to a NSAID in 10 to 14 days. If this does not occur, the NSAID should be ceased, and if appropriate another tried of a different chemical class. The basis for these individual difference in response to different NSAIDs is not clear.[35] Most NSAIDs have a dose-response relationship and a ceiling effect, whereby increasing the dose above a certain level does not impart any greater analgesia, but increases the likelihood of drug toxicity. There is no evidence that the combined use of two NSAIDs provides superior analgesia to a single NSAID, but rather it may place the patient at increased risk of adverse effects.

Opioid analgesics

Opioid analgesics may be divided into weak and strong categories according to their potency. All opioid analgesics have the potential to cause sedation, respiratory depression, and impair mental abilities. They are reserved for moderate or severe pain. The elderly tend to be more sensitive to equivalent doses and blood levels of opioids, receiving greater and more prolonged pain relief.[29,36] Codeine (methylmorphine), the parent compound of the weak opioid analgesic group, may exert its moderate analgesic effect through its partial biotransformation to morphine by the liver. It has frequent side effects in the elderly, particularly constipation, nausea, and confusion. Other weak opioids include oxycodone and propoxyphene. Oxycodone is classified as a weak opioid by virtue of the small content in proprietary compounds, although pharmacologically it is a strong opioid. Propoxyphene should be used with caution in the elderly because of the long half-life of its major metabolite and potential for CNS side effects including hallucinations and seizures. Combinations of nonopioids with weak opioids such as aspirin or paracetamol with codeine offer enhanced analgesia. The combined medications may result in a lower incidence of side effects as each analgesic can be used at a lower dose. The weak opioids have a ceiling effect for analgesia, if adequate pain relief is not obtained at optimal doses, change to a strong opioid should be considered.

Morphine is the parent compound of the strong opioid group. The analgesic properties of morphine are not limited by a ceiling effect, however, side effects are common, including nausea, vomiting, constipation, respiratory depression, and cognitive dysfunction. Delayed-release morphine preparations may be used in the elderly, but care must be taken to prevent accumulation of the drug. Constipation secondary to opioids should be managed concurrently with bowel stimulants. Tolerance to other side effects develops more rapidly than tolerance to analgesic effects. Other strong opioids include methadone, pethidine (meperidine), and fentanyl. Pethidine is not appropriate for long-term use because of the risk of accumulation of its metabolite, norpethidine, resulting in CNS excitation, tremors, and seizures.[37] Methadone must be used with caution because it has a long half-life up to 2 or 3 days,[37] resulting in accumulation in the elderly.

Tolerance may develop with repeated administration of all opioids whereby higher doses are required to maintain equivalent analgesic effects. The rate of development of tolerance varies greatly. To overcome tolerance, the dose or frequency of dosing may be increased. Cross-tolerance with other opioids is not complete and it is often advisable to try a another oral opioid, at one-half of the equianalgesic dose.[38] When a patient is unable to tolerate oral opioids, or has refractory pain, parenteral analgesia by the subcutaneous, venous, or epidural route should be considered.

Adjuvant analgesics

Some medications that do not have primary analgesic properties have been shown to have analgesic properties in addition to their primary action. They often enhance the response of known analgesics. The major groups in this category are tricyclic antidepressants and anticonvulsants, although antipsychotic medications and local anesthetics may be used for this indication. Controlled trials have demonstrated response to tricyclics in a variety of painful disorders, including postherpetic neuralgia, diabetic neuropathy, tension and migraine headache, atypical facial pain, rheumatoid arthritis, chronic low back pain, and cancer.[31,39] Watson and colleagues[40] reported that more than 60 percent of patients with postherpetic neuralgia achieved good results with amitriptyline or nortriptyline, at a median dose of 50 to 70 mg daily. A recent meta-analysis of 39 placebo-controlled trials reported a statistical difference between the analgesic effect of tricyclic antidepressants and placebo in 28 of the studies, with a median of 58 percent of patients reporting at least 50 percent pain reduction.[39] Only four studies had a negative mean effect. When comparisons have been undertaken, no antidepressant has been found to be as consistently effective as amitriptyline, although other agents may be better tolerated. The analgesic effects of tricyclic antidepressants are independent of the antidepressant effects, and occur more rapidly and at a lower dose than used in depression. The sedating side effects may be used to advantage for individuals with pain-related insomnia. Older patients are prone to postural hypotension, falls, and urinary retention induced by these agents,[29] hence a low starting dose is recommended.

Carbemazepine is the drug of choice in trigeminal neuralgia, pain control is achieved in about 75 percent of patients.[41] It may be valuable in other neuropathic pains, which have a lancinating component such as phantom limb pain and central poststroke pain.[32] Its effectiveness in older patients is often limited by side effects, particularly sedation, confusion, and ataxia. Other anticonvulsants such as gabapentin, sodium valproate, phenytoin, and clonazepam may be trialed to obtain the best balance of analgesia and side effects. The cautious use of an anticonvulsant in combination with a tricyclic antidepressant may be indicated for use in patients troubled by refractory neurogenic pains not responsive to single therapy. The use of antipsychotic agents as adjuvant analgesics in the elderly is not recommended because of low efficacy and high potential for adverse side effects.[32] Mexilitene and baclofen may have a role in the management of refractory neurogenic pains not responding to antidepressant or anticonvulsant medications.[41] Treating symptoms such as insomnia, nausea, and constipation may assist the patient to cope better with pain.

Physical Therapies

Individuals with chronic pain are often physically deconditioned. The elderly are more likely to have pathologies additional to those causing the pain, compounding the tendency to physical inactivity and deconditioning. Regular physical activity increases fitness, enhances feeling of well-being and confidence, and may have a beneficial effect on reducing the impact of pain. There is accumulating evidence that even frail, chronically ill older people are able to exercise and improve their physical fitness.[42,43]

The combination of pharmacologic and physical therapies often provides superior relief to individual therapies. Simple adjustments in posture and daily routines, such as preparing meals in a seated position, breaking up the housework, or the provision of a walking aid can reduce the impact of pain on daily life. The use of a walking frame, which causes a mild degree of lumbar flexion, will ease the pain of lumbar canal stenosis. Attention to posture may improve back and neck pains. Hydrotherapy should be considered when weight-bearing exercises aggravate pain. The buoyancy effect of water reduces the weight of the body, allowing joints to be moved with minimal friction through a full range of movements. The warmth of the water decreases pain and muscle spasm. Hydrotherapy programs also have a beneficial socializing aspect.

Transcutaneous electric nerve stimulation (TENS) is a popular method of symptom relief for a wide range of painful conditions in the elderly such as low back pain, osteoarthritis, and postherpetic neuralgia. The response to TENS is unpredictable, but some individuals appear to obtain great benefit. Others who have previously been classed as nonresponders to TENS can obtain benefit when the settings are altered or the unit is worn longer, up to several hours per day. Transcutaneous electric nerve stimulation has the benefit of being portable, safe, and inexpensive. It may offer pain relief and reduce the need for medication. The effectiveness of TENS has been questioned by inconsistent findings in placebo-controlled trials,[44,45] nevertheless it is worth considering for patients of all ages with chronic pain. Other physical therapies including massage, cold and heat treatments, acupuncture, and electrical stimulation are used for a wide range of painful conditions.

Psychological Approaches

Psychological factors may contribute to the maintenance of pain, or be causally related. Regardless of the pathophysiologic basis of chronic pain, psychological strategies have a role in management. The essence of management is to establish appropriate pain-coping strategies and discourage behaviors that may perpetuate the pain syndrome. Usually a combination of behavioral and cognitive strategies are employed. Cognitive strategies are aimed at modifying belief structures, attitudes, and thoughts in order to modify the experience of pain and suffering. These include distraction therapy, relaxation, biofeedback, and hypnosis. The patient is encouraged to take an active role and accept responsibility for pain management, rather than being a passive victim.

Cognitive strategies are usually combined with a behavioral approach. Respondent behavior refers to the responses elicited by a noxious stimulus, while operant behavior is that which becomes reinforced by subsequent environmental, social, and interpersonal influences. In the elderly these behaviors may become reinforced through gaining attention, concern, and social contact, which may not have otherwise been available. Invalidism and abnormal pain behavior may persist even in the absence of continuing noxious stimulation. Behavioral operant conditioning discourages pain behaviors such as limping, grimacing, inactivity, and verbalizing of pain complaints. Usually, in conjunction with the patient's relatives, positive reinforcement is provided for behavior unrelated to pain and for successfully achieving preset goals. All other pain behaviors, such as moaning are ignored. A number of studies have demonstrated increased activity, reduced analgesic consumption, and improved mood in middle-aged adults, with some reporting benefit for elderly patients with chronic pain.[46,47] Supportive psychotherapy and pharmacologic approaches may be of benefit in the management of somatoform pain disorders and depression. Pilowsky and Barrow[48] evaluated the management of somatoform pain disorder with amitriptyline and psychotherapy, individually and in combination. Amitriptyline reduced pain intensity and increased activity level. Psychotherapy was more effective than supportive counseling. There was a complex interaction between amitriptyline and psychotherapy, which favors the use of combination therapy in this setting.

Pain and Cancer

Half of all cancers occur in the population over 65 years of age.[49] In the advanced stages of cancer 70 percent experience pain, of which 80 percent is severe and persistent.[50] In up to 90 percent of cases cancer pain can be managed by relatively simple means.[51] The World Health Organization (WHO) has developed the Cancer Pain Relief Program to offer adequate pain relief to all cancer patients in the world, through the existing health system.[50]

The WHO method for relief of cancer pain centers around a three-step approach to the use of analgesia. The first step of the WHO analgesic ladder is the nonopioid analgesics, the second step is the weak opioids, and the third step is the strong opioid group. Nonopioid analgesics are usually combined with an opioid in steps two and three to give additive analgesia. At each stage, adjuvant analgesic drugs such as antidepressants and anticonvulsants should be added when there is a specific indication. Symptoms such as insomnia, nausea, vomiting, and constipation should be treated aggressively. To maintain effective blood levels, analgesics should be given on a regular basis. Additional doses may be required for "breakthrough pain", such as prior to dressings or activity. Whenever possible, analgesia should be given orally, by "the ladder", and with frequent re-evaluation. The parenteral route of administration should be considered if medications are not tolerated orally. Excellent pain relief is not always achievable, in which case a specific set of aims is useful; initially aimed to increase hours of pain-free sleep, then to relieve the pain while at rest, followed by pain relief while standing or during activity. The use of the WHO analgesic ladder and careful dose titration allow the correct choice of drug in the shortest possible time period.

Zech and colleagues[52] reported nearly 90 percent of 2,118 palliative care patients were able to obtain satisfactory pain control on this regimen up to the time of death. Patients with residual pain were often content with the balance of analgesic efficacy and troublesome side effects. Emotional, spiritual, and functional aspects should not be neglected. Despite the widespread dissemination of the WHO ladder, most cancer pain patients around the world still appear to have inadequate analgesia.[53]

The principles of the WHO method for relief of cancer pain offers a rational approach to the pharmacologic management of chronic nonmalignant pain. Patients with pain of nonmalignant pain origin are less likely to accept medication side effects that interfere with daily activity more than the pain or disease. Physical and psychological interventions should be introduced early to reduce dependence on pharmacologic approaches.

The Use of Opioids in Chronic Nonmalignant Pain

There is clear consensus about the use of opioids in severe malignant pain, however the role of opioid therapy for the management of chronic pain of nonmalignant origin remains controversial.[54] Clinical experience demonstrates that selected patients obtain considerable benefit.[55] Exaggerated fear of adverse effects should not prevent a trial of opioid therapy in appropriately selected individuals who have not responded to other therapies. Opioid tolerance is rarely a major problem in the older age groups. It can be managed with dose adjustment or chemical substitution. Physical or psychological dependence are rarely significant issues in elderly patients.

Maintenance opioid therapy for chronic pain of nonmalignant origin should not be considered until the patient has been thoroughly evaluated and has not responded to other conventional therapies. There is an increased onus on the clinician to ensure the patient understands the risks and benefits of this therapy. The more serious the risk, the more important it is for the physician to outline such risk, even if the probability of it eventuating is small. The patient must understand the potential for dependence and withdrawal symptoms. The physician must be familiar with and observe statutory requirements regarding the supply of opioids.[54] Both parties must agree to close supervision for the duration of therapy. The aims of treatment should be explicit, often aimed at easing the pain rather than total eradication. Total eradication of pain may occur at the expense of intolerable side effects. Four factors should be regularly monitored; the dose of opioid, pain relief, side effects, and overall functional status. The dose may be increased to obtain better pain control or functional status. If, however, the opioid dose is escalating at a time when pain control or functional status is declining, management should be reviewed.[56] Episodes of increased pain are more likely related to progression of the underlying disease than the development of opioid tolerance.

Concluding Remarks

Advancing age is associated with an increased prevalence of chronic pain. Various factors may preclude the older patient from the benefit of definitive therapy to eradicate pain and under these circumstances symptom management is indicated. The persistence of pain, despite apparently appropriate therapy, raises the possibility of unrecognized mood disturbance, pain of neurogenic origin, or advancing pathology. Overemphasis on pharmacologic approaches, ignores the potential benefits of physical and cognitive-behavioral strategies. The patient should never be described as having failed to respond to therapy, a failure of response reflects inappropriate therapy. A multidisciplinary pain management approach involving medical, physical, and psychologic therapeutic modalities is often more effective than a single disciplinary approach.[57] The proliferation of multidisciplinary pain management clinics over the past 30 years offers greater access to individuals with chronic pain, yet few have expertise or interest in geriatric medicine.[58] Age should not, however, be regarded as a barrier to successful outcomes from multidisciplinary management of pain problems in older people.

References

1. Merksey H: Classification of chronic pain: description of chronic pain syndromes and definition of pain terms. Pain 1986; (suppl 3):1
2. Crook J, Rideout E, Browne G: The prevalence of pain complaints in a general population. Pain 1984;18:299–314
3. Sigurdsson E, Thorgeirsson G, Sigvaldason H, Sigfusson N: Unrecognized myocardial infarction: epidemiology, clinical characteristics, and the prognostic role of angina pectoris. The Reykjavik Study. Ann Intern Med 1995;122:96–102
4. Wroblewski M, Mikulowski P: Peritonitis in geriatric inpatients. Age Ageing 1991;20: 90–94
5. Ambepitiya GB, Iyengar EN, Roberts ME: Review: silent exertional myocardial ischaemia and perception of angina in elderly people. Age Ageing 1993;22:302–307
6. Gibson SJ, Helme RD: Age differences in pain perception and report: a review of physiological, psychological, laboratory and clinical studies. Pain Rev 1995;2:111–137
7. Ruiz-Lopez R: The epidemiology of chronic pain. Pain Digest 1995;5:67–68
8. Crombie IK, Davies HTO, Macrae WA: The epidemiology of chronic pain: time for new directions. Pain 1994;57:1–3
9. Mobily PR, Herr KA, Clark MK, Wallace RB: An epidemiologic analysis of pain in the elderly. J Ageing Health 1994;6: 139–154
10. Andersson HI, Ejlertsson G, Leden I, Rosenberg C: Chronic pain in geographically defined general population: studies of different age, gender, social class, and pain localization. Clin J Pain 1993;9:174–182
11. Brattberg G, Thorslund M, Wilkman A: The prevalence of pain in a general population. The results of a postal survey in country Sweden. Pain 1989;37:215–222
12. Von Korff M, Dworkin SF, Resche L, Kruger A: An epidemiologic comparison of pain complaints. Pain 1988;32:173–183
13. Sengstaken EA, King SA: The problems of pain and its detection among geriatric nursing home residents. J Am Geriatr Soc 1993; 41:541–544
14. Ferrell BA, Ferrell BR Osterweil D: Pain in the nursing home. J Am Geriatr Soc 1990;38:409–414
15. Parmalee PA, Smith B, Katz IR: Pain complaints and cognitive status among elderly institution residents. J Am Geriatr Soc 1993;41:517–522
16. Moss MS, Lawton MP, Glicksman A: The role of pain in the last year of life of older persons. J Gerontol 1991;46:51–57
17. Tibblin G, Bengtsson C, Furunes B, Lapidus L: Symptoms by age and sex. Scand J Prim Health Care 1990;8:9–17
18. Berkley KJ: Sex and chronobiology: opportunities for focus on the positive. Newsletter of the International Society for the Study of Pain, January 1993
19. Ruda MA: Gender and pain. Pain 1993;53:1–2
20. Harkins SW, Price DD, Bush FM, Small RE. Geriatric pain. pp. 769–784. In: Wall PD, Melzack R (eds): Textbook of Pain. 3rd Ed. Churchill Livingstone, New York, 1994
21. American Psychiatric Association: Diagnostic and Statistical Manual of Mental Disorders. 4th Ed. American Psychiatric Association, Washington, DC, 1994
22. Melzack R: The McGill Pain Questionnarie: major properties and scoring methods. Pain 1975;1:275–297
23. Wiesel SW, Tsourmas N, Feffer HL et al. The incidence of positive CAT scans in an asymptomatic group of patients. Spine 1984;9:549–551
24. Jensen M, Brant-Zawadzki MN, Obuchowski N et al: Magnetic resonance imaging of the lumbar spine in people without back pain. N Engl J Med 1994;331:69–93
25. Boden SD, Davis DO, Dina TS et al: Abnormal magnetic-resonance scans of the lumbar spine in asymptomatic subjects. J Bone Joint Surg 1990;72A:403–408
26. Deyo RA: Magnetic resonance imaging of the lumbar spine. N Engl J Med 1994;331:115–116

27. Turner JA, Romano JM: Psychological and psychosocial evaluation. In Bonica JJ (ed): The Management of Pain. 2nd Ed. Philadelphia: Lea & Febiger, 1990
28. Folstein MF, Folstein SE, McHugh P: "Mini-mental state": a practical method for grading the cognitive state of patients for the clinician. J Psychiatr Res 1975; 21:189–198
29. Montamat SC, Cusack BJ, Vestal RE: Management of drug therapy in the elderly. N Engl J Med 1989;321:303–309
30. Ferrell BA, Ferrell BR, Rivera L: Pain in cognitively impaired nursing home patients. J Pain Symptom Manage 1995;10: 591–598
31. Andersen G, Vestergaard K, Ingeman-Nielsen M, Jansen TS: Incidence of central post-strokc pain. Pain 1995;61:187–193
32. Fields HL: Pain. New York, McGraw-Hill, New York, 1987
33. Brooks PM, Day RO: Nonsteroidal antiinflammatory drugs: differences and similarities. N Engl J Med 1991;324:1716–1725
34. Silverstein FE, Graham DY, Senior JR et al: Misoprostol reduce serious gastrointestinal complications in patients with rheumatoid arthritis receiving nonsteroidal anti-inflammatory drugs. Ann Intern Med 1995;123:241–249
35. Brooks PM, March LM: New insights into osteoarthritis. Med J Aust 1995;163:367–369
36. Bellville JW, Forrest WH, Miller E, Brown BW: Influence of age on pain relief from analgesics. JAMA 1971;217:1835–1841
37. Twycross RG: Opioids. pp 943–960. In Wall PD, Melzack R (eds): Textbook of Pain. 3rd Ed. Churchill Livingstone, Edinburgh, 1994
38. Wall RT: Use of analgesic drugs in the elderly. Clin Geriatr Med 1990;6:345–363
39. Onghena P, Van Houdenhove B: Anti-depressant induced analgesia in chronic non-malignant pain: a meta-analysis of 39 placebo-controlled studies. Pain 1992;49:205–220
40. Watson CPN, Evans RJ, Watt VR, Birkett N: Post-herpetic neuralgia: 208 cases. Pain 1988;35:289–297
41. Fields HL: Treatment of trigeminal neuralgia. N Engl J Med 1996;334:1125–1126
42. Fiatarone MA, O'Neill EF, Ryan ND et al: Exercise training and nutritional supplimentation for physical frality in very elderly people. N Engl J Med 1994;330: 1769–1775
43. Ettinger WH: Physical activity and older people: a walk a day keeps the doctor away. J Am Geriatr Soc 1996;44:207–208
44. Deyo RA, Walsh NE, Martin DC et al: A controlled trial of Transcutaneous Electrical Nerve Stimulation (TENS) and exercise for chronic back pain. N Engl J Med 1990;322:1627–1634
45. Marchand S, Charest J, Li J, Chenard J-R et al: Is TENS purely a placebo effect? A controlled study on chronic low back pain. Pain 1993;54:99–106
46. Gibson SJ, Katz B, Corran TM et al: Pain in older persons. Disabil Rehab 1994;16:127–139
47. Puder RS: Age analysis of cognitive-behavioural group therapy for chronic pain outpatients. Psychol Ageing 1988;3:204–207
48. Pilowsky I, Barrow CG: A controlled study of psychotherapy and amitriptyline used individually and in combination in the treatment of chronic intractable, "psychogenic" pain. Pain 1990;40:3–19
49. Cohen HJ: Oncology and aging: general principles of cancer in the elderly. pp 77–105. In Hazzard WR, Bierman EL, Blass JP, et al (eds): Principles of Geriatric Medicine and Gerontology. 3rd Ed. McGraw-Hill, New York, 1994
50. Tadeka F: WHO cancer pain relief programme. pp. 467–474. In Bond MR, Charlton JE, Woolf CJ (eds): Proceedings of the VIth World Congress on Pain. Elsevier, Amsterdam, 1991
51. Jacox A, Carr DB, Payne R: New clinical-practice guidelines for the management of pain in patients with cancer. N Engl J Med 1994;302:651–655
52. Zech DFJ, Grond S, Lynch J et al: Validation of World Health Organization guidelines for cancer pain relief: a 10 year prospective study. Pain 1995:63:65–76
53. Jadad AR, Browman GP: The WHO Analgesia Ladder for cancer pain management. JAMA 1995;274:1870–1878
54. Mendelson G, Mendelson D: Legal aspects of the management of chronic pain. Med J Aust 1991;155:640–643
55. Zenz M, Strumpf M, Tryba M: Long term oral opioid therapy in patients with chronic nonmalignant pain. J Pain Symptom Manage 1992;7:69–77
56. Schug SA, Large RG: Opioids for chronic noncancer pain. Clinical Updates. International Association for the Study of Pain, Seattle, 1995
57. Flor H, Fydrich T, Turk DC: Efficacy of multidisciplinary pain treatment centres: a meta-analytic review. Pain 1992;49: 221–230
58. Harkins SW, Price DD: Assessment of pain in the elderly. pp. 315–331. In Turk DC, Melzack R (eds): Handbook of Pain Assessment. The Guilford Press, New York, 1992

CHAPTER 102

Elder Abuse

ANTHEA TINKER
CLAUDINE McCREADIE

Most medical practitioners are well aware of child abuse,[1] as are other health and social services professionals. Much research, both medical and social, has been carried out on this topic.[2–4] What is much less clear, however, is knowledge by professionals about elder abuse. Even more fundamental is the lack of knowledge and research in the UK about it as a problem, and how it should be dealt with. In this chapter, we first examine the historic development of concern, definitions, prevalence, and risk factors. We then discuss ways in which elder abuse may be identified and consider prevention, treatment, and management. We write from the perspective of developments in the UK, themselves substantially influenced by experience in North America.[5–8] In particular, the paucity of research in the UK has meant that much understanding of the issue has come from the extensive North American research.[9] There is scope for continuing to draw lessons from crossnational perspectives on the problem, along with due recognition of differences in service provisions and the legal position between countries. Throughout we are concerned that simplistic parallels might be drawn with child abuse.

Historic Development

In the UK, there are a number of strands in the development of concern about the problem of elder abuse. The earliest saw a parallel with child abuse and placed the issue in the wider context of the care of older people both in their own homes and in institutions, emphasizing both the importance of awareness by doctors and of good geriatric practice.[10,11] Little was done to follow-up this early recognition of the problem and, most crucially, virtually no research was undertaken in the UK until 1990.[12] In its absence, abuse was linked to concerns about family caregivers and the stress placed on them by the care of older people, particularly those with dementia.[13] There was concern with the appropriateness of applying contemporary law to situations involving older people with dementia and situations involving risk of harm to all "vulnerable" adults, including those with learning disabilities and severe mental illness. This resulted in a major review of law involving extensive proposals for change.[14] Finally, in England from 1990 on, the Department of Health's Social Services Inspectorate, responsible for professional and policy development in social care, has been in the forefront of developing policy and practice guidance on elder abuse.[15,16] Increasingly, there is a realization of the importance of drawing constructive lessons from the child protection experience.[17]

In contrast, in the US, the role of government, notably at the state level, has been more proactive and a significant benefit of this is that a substantial amount of research has taken place. Most interestingly, from the British point of view, where the focus for many years was on abuse by caregivers, much of this research took place from a perspective of family violence[18] as did a major research initiative funded by the Canadian Federal Government in 1991.[19]

Definition

Elder abuse refers to the ill-treatment of an older person (usually defined as over age 65). Abuse may occur both in domestic settings—the older person's own home, a relatives home, in sheltered housing or in institutions—day care, residential care, nursing homes, and hospitals. Some kinds of behavior defined as abuse are criminal acts, such as assault and theft; other, such as verbal abuse, or the restraint of someone who is aggressive, may seem much more contingent upon particular circumstances.

The Importance of Relationship to the Concept of Abuse

Where protection of the older person has dominated policy development, as in the US, self-neglect is invariably included as part of the definition, and accounts for substantial numbers of reports of abuse.[20,21] However, there is a strong argument for treating self-neglect as a problem in its own right, because it will almost certainly have a different set of explanations to the problem of abuse by others and require different interventions.[7,22] In this chapter, therefore, abuse refers to behavior within a relationship connoting trust. This distinguishes actions by those closely linked to the older person—family members or others in positions of responsibility for their care—from actions by strangers.

Different Types of Abuse

A recent review of the research on elder abuse suggests that under the "umbrella" heading of elder abuse there is a diversity of problems and that it is of fundamental importance to distinguish these.[23] There is now widespread agreement about five categories of abuse: physical violence; psychological abuse, often measured by persistent verbal aggression; financial abuse; sexual abuse; and neglect.[24,25] Although sexual abuse is sometimes subsumed under physical abuse, it has been increasingly recognized as a form of abuse in its own right.[26] There is still very limited information on how far these types of abuse occur together and how far they are separate phenomena, but the research suggests that they both occur singly *and* in combination, and that where they are occurring singly, the explanations for the abuse, and therefore the factors relevant to risk, may vary between the different types.

Severity of Abuse

The greater the violation of an individual, the more severe the harm to the person and the more distressed they may be.[27] Considering the degree of severity of effect of the abuse, its frequency, how long it has been going on, and the intentions of the abuser should help practitioners to judge the case for intervention and the kind of intervention that may be appropriate.[7] Table 102-1 provides standard definitions and gives examples of both behavior and effect.

Prevalence

There have been two major studies of community prevalence in North America.[32,33] These used the same definitions, and were based on telephone interviews. The only survey in Great Britain[34] employed broader definitions, and the different levels of abuse reported are more likely to reflect the questions asked rather than the actual levels of abuse in the community. The studies also need to be related to their own social and cultural context. One particular difficulty for prevalence studies using the general population is that people who are highly dependent on another person, and particularly people who have significant mental impairment, are unable to participate, except by proxy. Yet it is precisely these people whom practitioners would identify as most at risk.[8] In Australia, the medical records of all patients over the age of 65 referred to an area-based geriatric and rehabilitation service were examined over a 1-year period using similar definitions to the two North American studies.[35] Higher rates of prevalence have been recorded by interviewing carers of older people with substantial disabilities including dementia.[12,36,37] Table 102-2 shows prevalence of elder abuse in North America, the UK, and Australia.

Risk Factors

Risk needs to be related both to the different types of abuse, and to the different settings in which it may occur. Some of these areas remain almost completely unresearched, so little can be said about them.

Table 102-1 Definitions of types of abuse, with examples of behaviour and effects

Physical abuse: "The non-accidental infliction of physical force that results in bodily injury, pain or impairment".[28,29]

Examples of behavior: hitting, slapping, pushing, burning, physical restraint

Examples of effects: bruises, fractures, burns, broken teeth, sprains, cuts, hair loss, bleeding from scalp, fear, anxiety, depression

Psychological abuse: The persistent use of threats, humiliation, bullying, swearing and other verbal conduct, and/or of any other form of mental cruelty, that results in mental or physical distress.[18]

Examples of behavior: treating elder as a child, blaming, swearing, intimidating, name-calling, threatening violence, isolating elder

Examples of effect: fear, depression, confusion, loss of sleep, loss of appetite

Financial abuse: "The unauthorized and improper use of funds, property or any resources of an older person".[28]

Examples of behavior: misappropriating money, valuables, or property; forcing changes to will; denying elder right to access personal funds

Examples of effect: loss of money, etc., inability to pay bills, deterioration in health or standard of living, lack of amenities, unusual activity in bank accounts, signatures on documents uncertain, lack of solid arrangements for financial management, eviction or house sale notices

Sexual abuse: Direct or indirect involvement in sexual activity without consent.

Examples of behavior–non-contact: looking, photography, indecent exposure, harassment, serious teasing or innuendo, pornography. *Contact:* touching breast, genitals, anus, mouth; masturbation of either or both persons; penetration or attempted penetration of vagina, anus, mouth, with or by penis, fingers, other objects.[26,30]

Examples of effect: difficulty in walking or sitting, bruises, bleeding, venereal disease, psychological trauma

Neglect: "The repeated deprivation of some assistance that the older person needs for important activities of daily living".[31]

Examples of behavior: failure to provide food, shelter, clothing, medical care, hygiene, personal care; inappropriate use of medication or over medication.

Examples of effect: malnutrition, pressure sores, oversedation; untreated medical problems, depression, confusion

Physical and Verbal Abuse: Domestic Settings

This has been the most thoroughly researched area of elder abuse. The key conclusions are.

1. Risk is higher for older people who live with someone.[32,33,38] The majority of men of all ages in Great Britain live with a partner, but for women the pattern changes with age.[39] In Britain, two-thirds of women over the age of 80 live on their own.[39] Older people may be abused by their partners, and by other relations including their adult children.
2. Some abuse is long-standing—Homer and Gilleard[12] refer to the "elderly graduates of domestic violence."
3. Dependency in the abused person, measured in terms of

Table 102-2 Prevalence of elder abuse in Boston, US, 1986, Canada, 1990, Great Britain, 1992 and Australia, 1990–1991

Type of Abuse	Boston, US 1986 Rate per 1,000 Elderly	Canada, 1990 Rate per 1,000 Elderly	Great Britain, 1992 Rate per 1,000 Elderly	Australia, 1990–1991 Rate per 1,000 of Geriatric and Rehabilitation Service Community Patient Population
Physical	20	5	15	21
Psychological[a]	11	11	54	25
Financial	Not in study	25	15	11
Neglect	4	4	Not in study	14
Multiple	Not in study	8	Not in study	18
Sample size	2,020	2,008	593	1,176

[a] *Persistent verbal abuse.*
(Data from Pillemer and Finkelhor,[32] Podnieks,[33] Ogg and Bennett,[34] and Kurrle and associates.[35])

their need for help with activities of daily living, has not been found to be a significant risk factor.[32,33,40,41] Dependent older people may, however, be most at risk in the sense of actually being harmed since those who are most impaired both physically and mentally are least able to protect themselves.[18]

4. There is little evidence that the stress of caring for a dependent elder is on its own a cause of abuse.[35,37,38,42,43] Large numbers of carers of are "under stress", but do not abuse their relative. The crucial issue is to try and discriminate between abusing and nonabusing situations.[44]
5. Risk appears to depend more on characteristics associated with the abuser—particularly their physical and mental health and notably, in many studies, their consumption of alcohol.[12,33,42,45–49]
6. Studies specifically of patients with dementia indicate that the patient may be violent, and that their aggression may be associated with aggressive behavior in the person caring for them.[12,50–54]

Physical and Verbal Abuse: Institutional Settings

There is very little research about abuse occurring in institutions.[55] Although the definitions used in the domestic setting apply to the communal one, methods of caring assume significance, particularly as the prevalence of physical and mental disability is generally so high among older people in communal settings.[56] Numerous inquiries in Britain into grave deficiencies in various areas of institutional care for all age groups have shown that abuse flourishes within a culture that allows it to be acceptable.[57] Research in 57 residential and nursing homes in the USA found that 10 percent of staff admitted to at least one act of physical abuse in the preceding year; excessive restraint was the most frequently recorded form. Thirty-six percent of respondents had observed at least one act of physical abuse by others in the preceding year; restraint accounted for around two-thirds of reports.[58] Staff reported a very much higher rate of verbal than of physical abuse. Significant factors in explaining both kinds of abuse were staff burnout, patient aggression, and staff/patient conflict.[59]

Sexual Abuse

This type of abuse has been little researched, but such work as there is suggests that the victims are overwhelmingly female, and dependent on others for their care.[60,61] Dementia may be an important risk factor.[26,51] It has been suggested that greater attention should be paid to the risk of sexual abuse in residential and nursing home settings.[62]

Financial Abuse

While nearly all definitions of elder abuse include financial abuse, there has been little research into financial abuse in its own right. It has been stressed recently that there is a gray area between the financial mismanagement of people's affairs when they grow older and actual abuse.[63] The financial affairs of older people with dementia appear invariably to be incorrectly ordered, thus increasing the risk of financial abuse.[64,65] In contrast to physical and verbal abuse, the risk of abuse to older people in the community may be greater when they are living on their own.[33] This may in turn link to age,[38] to gender (the substantially higher numbers of older women on their own) and to mental incapacity.[66] There is some evidence that financial abuse is more likely to be perpetrated by not-so-close relations.[33,40] Within institutional settings, very little is known. Again, there is an important issue over whether the appropriate arrangements for handling people's financial affairs are in place and whether there is someone responsible for seeing that these protect them from financial exploitation.[63]

Neglect

Although research suggests that neglect is the least prevalent of the different types of abuse, it is the type, apart from sexual abuse, that most nearly fits what has been the popular picture of abuse. Neglected older people are invariably in poor health, dependent on a caregiver, and may be mentally frail.[33,40]

Identification

The majority of cases, whether in domestic or instititutional settings, are likely to arise in either primary or secondary care as part of some other presenting problem. Identification depends on a high index of suspicion.[7,67] Abuse is frequently denied.[68] Physical symptoms may be common to frail older people suffering from chronic disease and be unreliable indicators.[6,12,67,69] When prevalence is relatively low, accurate diagnosis assumes great importance.[68,69] Incorrect diagnosis followed by misplaced interventions may damage all those concerned. Apart from increased sensitivity and awareness of the possibility of abuse, the first general principle, common to all good practice in geriatric medicine[70] and old age psychiatry[7] is that assessment, "must be as holistic as possible".[6] This may be time-consuming and it has been recognized that some doctors may, under pressures of time and shortage of resources, be particularly unwilling to address issues of family violence.[1] However, it is fundamental to view the patient in the context of their lifestyle and family or institutional environment.[69] While current research findings are limited, their logic is that the suspected perpetrator should be assessed as thoroughly as the victim of abuse. In the UK, existing law lends itself to an approach that sets suspected abuse in the context of assessment of needs for service provision embracing social care, health care, and housing.[16,23] Caregivers who provide a substantial amount of care on a regular basis also have the right to request their local authority for an assessment when the needs of the person for whom they are caring are being assessed, and the results of this assessment must be taken into account when making decisions about any services to be provided.

In the USA, where the law requires mandatory reporting of abuse cases, it is recommended that routine questioning should be built into daily practice and that in every clinical setting there should be a protocol for the detection and assessment of elder abuse.[71] However, in a different legal context, it has been concluded, that while doctors need to be alert to the possibility of abuse, there is currently insufficient evidence either for including or excluding case finding for elder abuse as a matter of routine.[25]

The issue of financial abuse is one that doctors may well encounter in various ways. The *scope* for financial abuse among older people with dementia begins with the management of their finances, if they are no longer able to manage them themselves. Doctors may be approached to advise on this[65] and need to know to whom to refer people for appropriate guidance. However, they may also come across actual abuse in the course of patient contact and it is then necessary for them to know to whom the older person is most appropriately referred.

Prevention, Treatment, and Management

The key objectives are the prevention of abuse and the promotion of the older person's autonomy.[7,18,25] At the level of policy and guidance, it is essential that the medical profession is properly represented where any professional or local initiatives are taking place to develop a response to abuse. In the context of patient care, doctors need to be sensitive to the appropriateness of arrangements for an older person's care—an issue raised directly in considering discharge arrangements—particularly from an accident or emergency department. The same considerations apply when considering the discharge of patients with challenging or aggressive behavior to an older person household: are those caring for them able and equipped to provide appropriate care? Two further general principles are "meticulous documentation"[69,71] and consultation with other professionals, both within and outside medicine.[18,69] The need to consult raises difficult ethical questions in terms of confidentiality of the doctor-patient relationship, should the older person request the doctor to "do nothing". The older person's rights to autonomy have to be balanced with the need for protection[25] and the possible danger in which they might be placed by misplaced intervention. The assessment of mental capacity, therefore, is of crucial importance and helps direct physicians to the options for intervention if the older person is unwilling to accept any help.

Figure 102-1, interpreted in relation to the relevant type of abuse and to the legal and service provision context in which medical practitioners are working, gives general guidance. In the UK, the number of laws that potentially bear on abuse are considerable, and legal advice may be needed, because the issues around mental capacity are particularly difficult.[72] In the event of an emergency, the medical practitioner needs to make immediate contact with other responsible agencies, notably the police and social services in the UK, adult protection services in the USA, and act to protect the older person from any further harm. While safety of the victim is the first priority, situations arising are such that it is also essential to pay attention to the physical and psychological health of the suspected abuser, who themselves may be vulnerable.[7]

Conclusion

Elder abuse "appears in many forms and for many reasons".[7] It encompasses domestic violence and harms inflicted on vulnerable adults. Overall, the primary aim should be to prevent it from occurring. There would appear to be four planks in prevention. The first is the provision of effective health and welfare services for older people, including pension and housing provision.[68,73] The second is awareness among a wide range of professionals, of whom the medical profession are crucial, that abuse can and does exist and requires a response.[1,19,74,75] The third, particularly in the context of the policy emphasis on care in the community, is recognition and

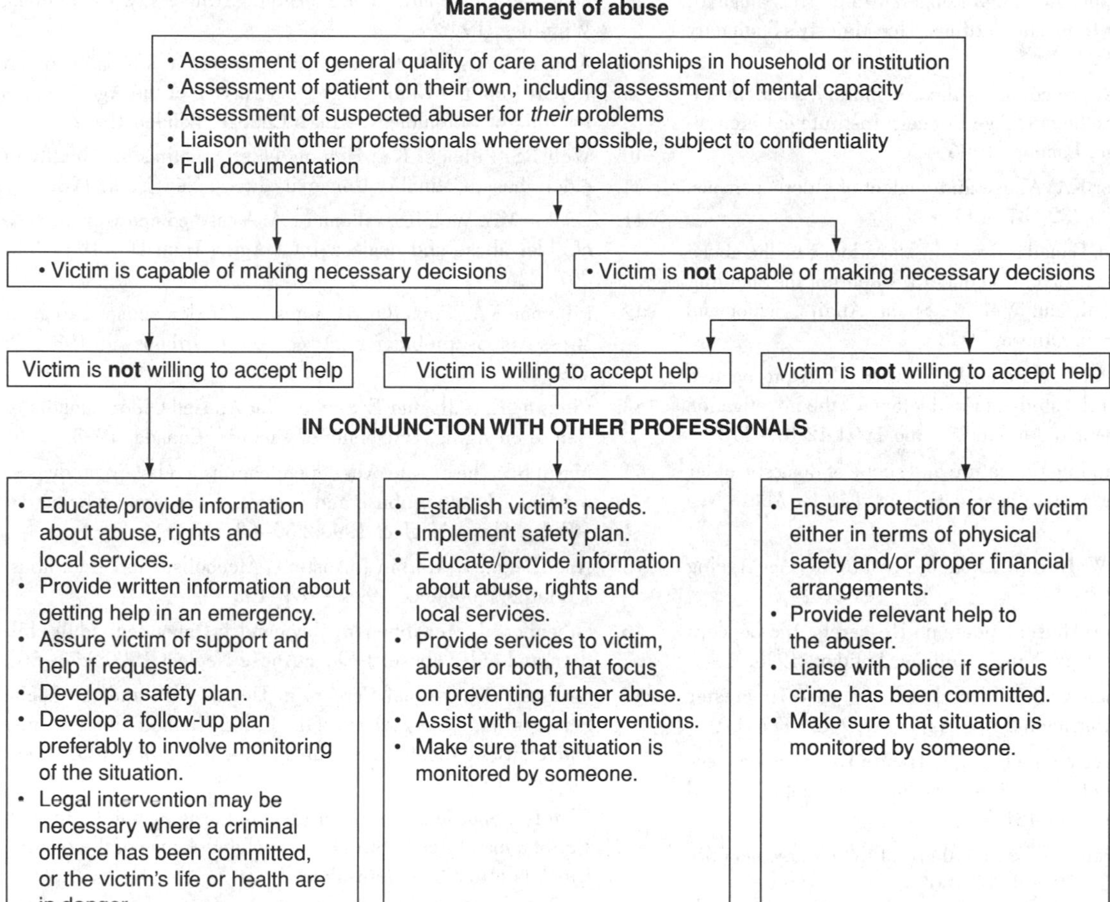

Figure 102-1 Management of abuse. (Data from Fisk,[7] Lachs and Pillemer,[18] Kurrle,[67] and American Medical Association.[71])

action around caregivers, who may be both abuser and/or abused, older or younger themselves, and in their own right suffering from physical or mental illness.[76] Finally, in the context of institutional care, it is essential that all requirements within a nation for the monitoring or regulation of the quality of care are met, and that there is a general imperative to provide quality care to older people.[77] It is the worst of all possible worlds, as older people themselves are only too aware, to move an older victim to an institution only for them to suffer abuse there. In summary, "the challenge is to make sure that efforts on behalf of mistreated older persons do more good than harm and do not lead to the neglect of other societal needs".[78]

References

1. Lachs MS: Preaching to the unconverted: educating physicians about elder abuse. J Elder Abuse Neglect 1995;4:1–12
2. Bullock R, Little M, Millham S, Mount K: Child Protection: Messages from Research. Department of Health, London, 1995
3. Gough D: Child Abuse Interventions: A Review of the Research Literature. Department of Health, London, 1993
4. National Research Council: Understanding Child Abuse and Neglect. National Academy Press, Washington, DC, 1993
5. McCreadie C, Tinker A: Review: abuse of elderly people in the domestic setting: a UK perspective. Age Ageing 1993;22:65–69
6. Bennett GCJ, Kingston P: Elder abuse: concepts theories and interventions. Chapman and Hall, London, 1993
7. Fisk J: Abuse of the elderly. pp. 901–914. In Jacoby R, Oppenheimer C (eds): Psychiatry in the Elderly. Oxford University Press, Oxford, 1992
8. Decalmer P, Glendenning F (eds): The Mistreatment of Elderly People. Sage, London, 1993
9. McCreadie C: A Guide to Research on Elder Abuse in the U.K. Action on Elder Abuse, London, 1995
10. Baker AA: "Granny-battering". Mod Geriatr 1975;8:20–24
11. Burston GR: Do your elderly patients live in fear of being battered? Mod Geriatr 1977;5:54–55
12. Homer A, Gilleard CJ: Abuse of elderly people by their carers. Br Med J 1990;301:1359–1362
13. Tomlin S: Abuse of Elderly People: An Unnecessary and Preventable Problem. British Geriatrics Society, London, 1989
14. Law Commission: Mental Incapacity. (Law Com. No. 231) Her Majesty's Stationary Office, London, 1995
15. Social Services Inspectorate: Confronting Elder Abuse. Her Majesty's Stationary Office, London, 1992

16. Social Services Inspectorate. No Longer Afraid: The Safeguard of Older People in Domestic Settings. Her Majesty's Stationary Office, London, 1993
17. Stevenson O: Elder protection in the community: what can we learn from child protection? Age Concern Institute of Gerontology, King's College, London, 1996
18. Lachs MS, Pillemer KA: Abuse and neglect of elderly persons. N Engl J Med 1995;332:437–443
19. House of Commons, Canada: Breaking the silence on the abuse of older Canadians: everyone's concern. Report of the Standing Committee on Health and Welfare, Social Affairs, Senior and the Status of Women, Ottawa, 1993
20. Lachs MS, Berkman L, Fulmer T, Horwitz RI: A prospective community-based pilot study of risk factors for the investigation of elder mistreatment. J Am Geriatr Soc 1994;42:169–173
21. Tatara T: Understanding the nature and scope of domestic elder abuse with the use of state aggregate data. J Elder Abuse Neg 1994;4:35–58
22. Cooney C, Hamid W: Review: Diogenes Syndrome. Age Ageing 1995;24:451–453
23. McCreadie C: Elder Abuse: Update on Research. Age Concern Institute of Gerontology, King's College, London, 1996.
24. Vernon MJ, Bennett GCJ: Elder abuse: the case for greater involvement of geriatricians. Age Ageing 1995;24:177–179
25. Canadian Task Force on the Periodic Health Examination: Secondary prevention of elder abuse and mistreatment. Can Med Assoc J 1994;10:1413–1421
26. Benbow SM, Haddad PM: Sexual abuse of the elderly mentally ill. Postgrad Med J 1993;69:803–807
27. Johns S, Hydle I, Aschjem O: The act of abuse: a two-headed monster of injury and offense. J Elder Abuse Neglect 1991;1: 53–64
28. Stein KF: A national agenda for elder abuse and neglect research: issues and recommendations. J Elder Abuse Neglect 1991;3:91–108
29. McCreadie C: Introduction: the issues, practice and policy. pp. 3–22. In Eastman M (ed): Old Age Abuse. 2nd Ed. Age Concern England/Chapman and Hall, London, 1994
30. Brown H, Turk V: Defining sexual abuse as it affects adults with learning disabilities. Mental Handicap 1992;20:44–55
31. Clarke M and Ogg J: Identifying the elderly at risk J Comm Nursing 1994;8:4–9
32. Pillemer KA, Finkelhor D: The prevalence of elder abuse: a random sample survey. Gerontologist 1988;28:51–57
33. Podnieks E: National Survey on Abuse of the Elderly in Canada. Ryerson Polytechnical Institute, Toronto, 1990
34. Ogg J, Bennett GCJ: Elder abuse in Britain. Br Med J 1992; 305:998–999
35. Kurrle SE, Sadler PM, Cameron ID: Patterns of elder abuse. Med J Australia 1992;157:673–676
36. Compton S: The Prevalence and Antecedents of Elder Abuse in People with Dementia. Bulletin 15, Action on Elder Abuse, London, 1996
37. Cooney C, Mortimer A: Elder abuse and dementia: a pilot study. Int J Soc Psych 1995;41:276–283
38. Penning MJ: Elder Abuse Resource Centre. Research component—Final Report. Centre on Aging. University of Manitoba, Winnipeg, 1992
39. Askham J, Grundy E, Hancock R, Tinker A: Life after 60. A Report from the Gerontology Data Service of the Age Concern Institute of Gerontology, King's College, London, 1992
40. Wolf RS, Pillemer KA: Helping elderly victims: the reality of elder abuse. Columbia University Press, New York, 1989
41. Godkin MA, Wolf RS, Pillemer KA: A case-comparison analysis of elder abuse and neglect. Int J Aging Hum Dev 1989;288: 207–225
42. Pillemer KA, Finkelhor D: Causes of elder abuse: caregiver stress versus problem relatives Am J Orthopsych 1989;59: 179–187
43. Pittaway E, Gallagher E: Services for Abused Older Canadians. Centre on Aging, University of Victoria, Canada, 1995
44. Marin RS: The debate over dependency as a relevant predisposing factor in elder abuse and neglect. A research perspective. J Elder Abuse Neglect 1990;2:59–63
45. Anetzberger G, Korbin J, Austin C Alcoholism and elder abuse J Interpers Violence 1994;9:184–193
46. Greenberg J, McKibben M, Raymond J: Dependent adult children and elder abuse. J Elder Abuse Neglect 1990;2:73–86
47. Saveman B-I: Formal Careers in Health Care and the Social Services Witnessing Abuse of the Elderly in their Homes. Umea University Medical Dissertations, New Series no. 403, Umea, Sweden, 1994
48. Wolf RS: Spouse abuse and neglect in the aging family. In Wolf RS, bergman S (eds): Stress, Conflict and Abuse of the elderly. Brookdale Institute, Jerusalem, 1989
49. Bristowe E, Collins JB: Family mediated abuse of non-institutionalized frail elderly men and women living in British Columbia. J Elder Abuse Neglect 1989;1:45–64
50. Levin E, Sinclair I, Gorbach P: Families, Services and Confusion in old age. Gower Publishing Company, Avebury, Aldershot, 1989
51. Paveza GJ, Cohen D, Eisdorfer C et al: Severe family violence and Alzheimer's Disease: prevalence and risk factors. Gerontologist 1992;32:493–497
52. Pillemer KA, Suitor JJ: Violence and violent feelings: what causes them among family caregivers? J Gerontol 1992;47: S165–S172
53. Coyne A, Reichman WE, Berbig LJ: The relationship between dementia and elder abuse. Am J Psych 1993; 150:643–646
54. Cahill S, Shapiro M: "I think he might have hit me once": aggression towards caregivers in dementia care. Austr J Ageing 1993;4:10–15
55. Gilleard C: Physical abuse in homes and hospitals. pp. 93–110. In Eastman M (ed): Old Age Abuse. 2nd ed. Age Concern England/Chapman and Hall, London, 1994
56. Martin J, Meltzer H, Elliot D: The Prevalence of Disability Among Adults. OPCS Surveys of Disability in Great Britain. Report 1. London, Her Majesty's Stationary office, 1988
57. Clough R: Scandals in residential care: report to the independent review of residential care. (Chair: G Wagner). National Institute for Social Work, London, 1988
58. Pillemer KA, Moore D: Abuse of patient in nursing homes: findings from a survey of staff. Gerontologist 1989;3:314–320

59. Pillemer KA, Bachman-Prehn R: Helping and hurting: predictors of maltreatment of patients in nursing homes. *Res Aging* 1991;1:74–95

60. Ramsey-Klawsnik H: Elder sexual abuse: preliminary findings. J Elder Abuse Neglect 1991;3:73–90

61. Holt M: Elder sexual abuse in Britain; preliminary findings. J Elder Abuse Neglect 1993;2:63–73

62. Sengstock M, McFarland MR, Hwalek M: Identification of elder abuse in institutional settings. J Elder Abuse Neglect 1991;1: 31–50

63. Langan J, Means R: Financial management and elderly people with dementia in the UK: as much a question of confusion as abuse? Ageing Soc 1996;16:287–314

64. Langan J, Means R: Personal finances, elderly people with dementia and the "new" community care. Anchor Res. Rep. 8. Anchor Housing Association, Oxfordshire, 1995

65. Rowe J, Davies KN, Baburaj V, Sinha RN: F.A.D.E. A.W.A.Y.: The Financial Affairs of Dementing Elders and Who Is the Attorney? J Elder Abuse Neglect 1993;2:73–79

66. Blunt AP: Financial exploitation of the incapacitated: investigation and remedies. J Elder Abuse Neglect 1993;1:19–32

67. Kurrle S: Elder abuse: a hidden problem. Mod Med Austr 1993; 9:58–72

68. McCallum J: Elder abuse: the "new" social problem? Mod Med Austr 1993;9:74–83

69. Lachs M, Fulmer T. Recognising elder abuse and neglect. Clin Geriatr Med 1993;3:665–679

70. Rubenstein LZ, Rubenstein LV: Multidimensional geriatric assessment. In Brockelhurst JC, Tallis RC, Fillit HM (eds): Textbook of Geriatric Medicine and Gerontology. 4th Ed. Churchill Livingstone, New York, 1992

71. American Medical Association: Diagnostic and Treatment Guidelines on Elder Abuse and Neglect. American Medical Association, Chicago, 1992

72. British Medical Association: Assessment of Mental Capacity: Guidance for Doctors and Lawyers. Joint Report of the BMA and the Law Society. British Medical Association, London, 1996

73. Callahan JJ: Elder abuse: some questions for policymakers. Gerontologist 1988;4:453–458

74. Blakely BE, Dolon R: Area agencies on aging and the prevention of elder abuse: the results of a national study. J Elder Abuse Neglect 1991;2:21–40

75. Wolf RS: Testimony on behalf of the National Committee for the Prevention of Elder Abuse before the U.S. House Select Committee on Aging, Subcommittee on Human Services. J Elder Abuse Neglect 1991;4:87–99

76. Homer A: Prevalence and prevention of elder abuse. pp. 31–50. In Eastman M (ed): Old Age Abuse. 2nd Ed. Age Concern England/Chapman and Hall, London, 1994

77. Royal College of Physicians: High quality long-term care for elderly people: guidelines and audit measures. Report, Royal College of Physicians, British Geriatrics Society. Royal College of Physicians, London, 1992

78. Wolf RS: Making an issue of elder abuse. Gerontologist 1992; 3:427–429

CHAPTER 103

Sexuality in Old Age

ROBERT N. BUTLER
MYRNA I. LEWIS

Misinformation, Myths, and Prejudices About Sexuality in the Later Years

Older patients' sexuality is frequently overlooked by physicians during the typical medical examination and evaluation. As a result, physicians may miss the opportunity to offer their older patients reassurance about the normal changes in sexuality that may be troubling them; they may not advise these patients about the side effects of medications that can impact adversely on continuing sexual activity; and they may fail to diagnose sexual dysfunction and recommend treatment possibilities.[1]

Lack of public and professional medical education is partially to blame for this neglect of late-life sexuality in the medical encounter. Centuries of myths about aging, as well as prudery and ignorance, have helped close the minds of laypeople and professionals alike to the fact that many older people wish to and do continue expressing their sexuality until the end of their lives. Because few studies have been conducted on sexuality in general, and on late-life sexuality in particular, there have been scant data about the nature and frequency of sexual activity among older persons. However, self-reports from surveys of older people have demonstrated that for many, sexual desire and satisfaction remain important aspects of their lives. The main barriers to sexual expression in late life are medical and psychological problems and social obstacles. A problematic marital relationship or lack of a partner due to the death of a spouse or companion may also interfere.[1]

Normal Aging and Changes in Sexuality

Many older people maintain desire (libido) and sexual capacity and satisfaction so long as they have their health, a healthy partner, and a good relationship with that partner. They experience the same four stages of the sexual act as younger people: desire, arousal, climax, and recovery. Sexual expression remains a highly complex process in old age, comprising fantasy, the central nervous and peripheral nervous systems, the circulatory system, and all six senses. The capacity for fantasy may, however, decline for older men, according to the National Institute on Aging's Baltimore Longitudinal Study on Aging. We do not know if this is equally true for women because sexual fantasy in women was not documented in this study.

Normal change in sexual functioning is usually manifested as a gradual slowing, that is more time is needed for arousal (erection in men; lubrication in women) and reaching a climax. Unlike women, healthy men can remain fertile until the end of life. There is no discrete climacteric for men, but rather a gradual decline of testosterone levels after age 30 that usually do not fall below normal. Testosterone levels in 70 percent of healthy older men are in the same range as those of younger men. With aging, the testes may become smaller and penile flaccidity greater. More direct stimulation of the penis may be necessary to reach engorgement and erection. For some older men, orgasm may last a shorter time than it did when they were younger. The force of ejaculation and the volume of ejaculate decrease. A great concern for older men (and for younger men as well) is their ability to maintain sexual potency. Impotence is often automatically and inaccurately attributed to increasing age. It can, in fact, occur at any age for a variety of reasons, and once it is properly diagnosed, it is often treatable[1,2] (see Impotence below).

Older women are less concerned about sexual performance than are men, but may be more concerned than men about appearance and their desirability. Those women who are healthy can usually continue earlier patterns of sexual functioning. Women's multiorgasmic capacity remains throughout life. For some women, sexual interest may increase after the menopause because they no longer experience concern about becoming pregnant. However, reduced estrogen production due to the menopause may present both physical and emotional problems to some older women. Physical problems include a change in vaginal shape, vaginal dryness, and thinning of the vaginal walls, which may lead to pain and bleeding during coitus and a less well-protected bladder and urethra, with recurrent cystitis as a result. Less acidic vaginal secretions may lead to greater incidence of vaginal infections. Emotional problems accompanying menopause include increased irritability and lability often due to sleep deprivation, which is itself a menopausal symptom. Some peri- and postmenopausal women experience anxiety over whether to initiate estrogen replacement therapy, which has been shown to help relieve symptoms and protect older women from heart disease and osteoporosis. Extensive studies over the next decade at the National Institutes of Health may help clarify indications, contraindications, and risks of hormone replacement therapy. Women who cannot or will not take replacement estrogen can often find relief for vaginal dryness and irritation during intercourse with water-based vaginal lubricants.[1,2]

Women who wish to remain sexually active in later life may face barriers that have nothing to do with physical symptoms. Because women live nearly 7 years longer than men and tend to marry men 3 or more years older than they are, they have a much greater chance of surviving their male partners. About 60 percent of older women are without a spouse, as opposed to 20 percent of men, and many others may be living with a disabled spouse who cannot be a sexual partner. As they grow older, the ratio of women to men increases greatly, and the chances of finding another partner are greatly reduced. There are approximately 150 women to 100 men over the age of 65, and 250 women to 100 men over the age of 85.

It has been estimated that up to 10 percent of the general population is homosexual, although the exact number is unknown. Similar to the older heterosexual population, many lesbians and gay men have long-term relationships and are emotionally stable, successful, and happy in their later years. When sexual difficulties occur for lesbian or gay male couples, they involve many of the same interpersonal, physical, social, and psychological problems faced by heterosexual couples. Physicians need to be as sensitive to and accepting of gay lifestyles as they are of heterosexual ones.[3]

Examination and Evaluation of the Patient

The general medical evaluation of an older person should include a thorough sexual history, current sexual function, and a careful physical examination. The physician should initiate questions in these areas because older patients may not volunteer sexual information about themselves. Questions should be asked in an unintimidating and unembarrassing fashion. During the examination, the physician should pay special attention to the neurologic, circulatory, and endocrine systems. Because some medical conditions, surgical procedures, and medications can affect sexual functioning, the physician should be sure to include a discussion of sexuality when treating disease or prescribing medication in patients for whom continuing sexual activity is important.

The physician should be aware of the fact that sexually transmitted diseases (STDs) occur in old as well as young persons. People of all ages should practice "safe sex." Ten percent of all AIDS patients in the US are over 55 years of age, and not all of them contracted HIV through blood transfusions. Hepatitis B is the only sexually transmitted virus preventable by vaccine.[3]

Effects of Medical Problems, Surgery, and Medications

Sexual interest and capacity wane in the presence of illness, and some diseases have a much more powerful effect upon sexuality in the later years because of their frequency and character. Heart disease is three times more common in men than in women probably because of the protection afforded by estrogen in premenopausal women. However, after the menopause the incidence of heart disease in women begins to rise and eventually reaches that of men. Heart disease is a source of considerable concern to sexually active older people because sexual activity increases the heart rate. Many who have had angina or a heart attack become anxious about future sexual encounters. The fear of dying during intercourse may also compound depression that is already present in response to the heart disease itself. Physicians should point out to their concerned patients that, in fact, oxygen usage or "debt" in a sexual encounter is the rough equivalent of walking up one or two flights of stairs. Physicians should reassure their patients that anyone who can carry out usual daily activities is able to engage in sexual activity. A large Japanese study showed that the rare occasions of death following orgasm occurred in individuals who were involved in extramarital sexual encounters, under stress, and following heavy meals and considerable alcohol intake.[4]

Patients are often uneasy about recommencing their sex lives following coronary bypass surgery. Some 4 weeks or more of abstinence is recommended before resuming sexual activity to allow full healing to occur.

Other medical conditions that can impact significantly on sexuality are stroke, diabetes, chronic prostatitis in men and stress incontinence in women, osteoarthritis and rheumatoid arthritis, backache, Parkinson's disease, and chronic emphysema and bronchitis. The effects on sexuality of these diseases and their treatment are summarized in Table 103-1.

Surgery can significantly impair sexual functioning as well. Common surgical procedures and their effects on sexuality are outlined in Table 103-2. Embarrassment or discomfiture from surgical procedures such as mastectomies or ostomies can inhibit sexual drive and performance. Prostate surgery is discussed in the section on impotence below.

Medications are among the most common causes of sexual dysfunction, especially in men, but in women as well. Commonly prescribed medications that adversely affect sexuality are listed in Table 103-3. Physicians should familiarize themselves with medications that have less toxic effects on sexual function and prescribe them whenever possible. For example, angiotensin-converting enzyme (ACE) inhibitors taken for hypertension are less apt to cause sexual dysfunction than methyldopa. In addition, it is possible to reduce the dosage of some drugs to avoid adverse sexual and other effects without reducing the benefits of the drugs to the patient. In certain cases, brief "drug holidays" may improve sexual function, but this requires discussion with one's physician.

Table 103-1 Effects of medical conditions on sexuality

Medical Condition	Effect on Sexuality	Treatment
Arthritis	Sexual desire is usually unaffected, but disability due to osteoarthritis and rheumatoid arthritis may interfere with performance	Trying sexual positions that do not aggrevate joint pain; planning sexual activity for times of day when pain and stiffness are diminished
Chronic emphysema and bronchitis	Shortness of breath hinders physical activity, including sex	Rest; supplemental oxygen
Chronic prostatitis	Pain may diminish sexual desire	Antibiotics; warm sitz baths, prostatic massage; Kegel exercises
Chronic renal disease	Impotence, possibly with anxiety and depression	Dialysis; psychotherapy for underlying emotional problems; kidney transplantation may restore sexual capacity
Diabetes mellitus	Impotence is common	Very tight control of diabetes may restore potency
Heart and vascular disease		
Myocardial infarction	8–14 week recuperation period recommended before resuming sexual intercourse; depression and antidepressant drugs may reduce libido and capacity; fear of bringing on another heart attack if patient resumes sexual activity	Reassurance from the M.D. about safety of sexual activity; exercise programs to improve cardiac function
Heart failure	Sexual dysfunction due to physical symptoms or medications; a 2–3 week recovery period is advised before resuming sex in cases of pulmonary edema	Reassurance from MD about safety of sexual activity for patients with effectively managed heart failure; exercise programs to improve cardiac function
Coronary bypass surgery	4 weeks or more of abstinence is recommended before resuming sexual intercourse	Alternatives such as self-stimulation or masturbation can usually be started earlier in the recovery period; exercise programs to improve cardiac function
Pelvic steal syndrome	Example of vascular impotence—male loses erection as soon as he enters his partner and begins pelvic thrusting due to gravity's redirecting blood supply away from the pelvis	Changing position may help (man should lie on his back or side)
Hypertension	Incidence of impotence in untreated male hypertensive patients is about 15%; effects on women not established	Choose hypertensive drugs that do not impair sexual response
Parkinson's disease	Lack of sexual desire in both men and women; impotence in men	Levodopa can improve sex drive and performance in some men for a limited period
Peyronie's disease	Intercourse is painful for many men with the disease; penetration may be difficult or impossible when penis is angled too sharply	Psychotherapy to help patient adjust to changes in the penis; symptoms occasionally disappear spontaneously; surgery helps in some cases
Stress incontinence	Sexual dysfunction has been reported in up to 50% of women with this condition	Solving the underlying problem may help; Kegel exercises to strengthen muscles supporting bladder; estrogen taken orally or locally to firm up vaginal lining; biofeedback training
Stroke	Sexual desire may not be impaired, but sexual performance likely to be affected (e.g., male erectile dysfunction either due to physical or psychological reasons, anesthetic areas, and/or physical limitations due to paralysis)	Mechanical adjustments to assist positioning necessary for sexual activities; treatments for impotence

(Data from Butler and Lewis.[1,3]*)*

Table 103-2 Effects of surgery on sexuality

Surgical Procedure	Effect on Sexuality
Hysterectomy	Need to refrain from sexual activity during healing (6–8 weeks after surgery); depression; possible reduction in sensation during orgasm
Mastectomy	Emotional reactions such as depression; loss of sexual desire due to emotional reactions of patient and partner
Prostatectomy	Need to refrain from sexual activity during healing (6 weeks); possible impotence due to surgery (nerve-sparing techniques help avoid this effect in some cases); possible psychogenic impotence
Orchiectomy	Impotence is common
Colostomy and ileostomy	Emotional reactions that can affect desire and potency (participation in ostomy clubs is recommended)
Rectal cancer surgery	Impotence is common

(Data from Butler and Lewis.[1,3]*)*

Addiction to substances such as alcohol and tobacco also impairs sexuality (see Table 100-3). Alcohol may increase desire, but decrease performance. Tobacco adversely affects male sexuality and causes wrinkles in both men and women.

Impotence (Erectile Dysfunction)

Because even occasional impotence can have significant emotional consequences for many men, which can, in turn, exacerbate physical problems, diagnosis should be made carefully. Impotence should only be diagnosed when failure in sexual encounters occurs in at least one-fourth of all attempts.

It is estimated that from 10 to 20 million men in the US experience some degree of impotence. Although impotence affects men of all ages, it tends to increase progressively with age because of the greater likelihood of accompanying medical conditions. Relatively few men seek help for impotence from their doctors, however.

It is estimated that 90 percent of impotence cases are due to physical causes, including vascular disorders such as atherosclerosis and pelvic steal syndrome (Table 103-1); neurologic disorders such as trauma (e.g., sports injuries) and diabetic neuropathy; and endocrine disorders, such as thyroid disease, diabetes, and low testosterone levels, although low testosterone affects only about 4 percent of men. Radiation and chemotherapy for cancer may destroy testicular function. In men with heart disease, fear that sex will cause a heart attack can cause impotence.

Table 103-3 Selected medications and substances that may adversely affect sexual functioning

Psychotropics
- Tricyclic antidepressants
  - Clomipramine
  - Amitriptyline
  - Doxepin
  - Imipramine
  - Nortriptyline[a]
  - Desipramine[a]
- Monoamine oxidase inhibitors
  - Isocarboxazid
  - Phenelzine
  - Tranylcypromine[a]
- Serotonin reuptake inhibitors
  - Fluoxetine
  - Paroxetine
  - Sertraline
  - Fluvoxamine
  - Venlafaxine
- Mood stabilizers/anticonvulsants
  - Lithium[b]
  - Valproate[a]
  - Carbamazepine
  - Phenytoin
  - Phenobarbitol

Antipsychotics/neuroleptics
- Phenothiazines
  - Chlorpromazine
  - Fluphenazine[a]
  - Perphenazine
  - Thioridazine
- Other
  - Haloperidol
  - Thiothixene
  - Risperidone

Antianxiety agents/tranquilizers
- Benzodiazepines

Diuretics
- Thiazide-type
  - Chlorthalidone
  - Hydrochlorothiazide
  - Indapamide[a]
- Loop diuretics
  - Furosemide[a]
- Potassium-sparing
  - Spironolactone

Antihypertensives
- Reserpine
- Methyldopa
- Guanethidine
- β-Blockers
  - Propanolol
  - Atenolol
  - Metoprolol
  - Bisoprolol
  - Timolol
  - Betaxolol
- α_1-Blockers
  - Prazosin[a]
  - Doxazosin[a]
- α_2-Agonists
  - Clonidine
  - Guanfacine
- ACE inhibitors[c]
  - Captopril[a]
  - Enalapril
- Calcium-channel blockers
  - Amlodipine
  - Verapamil
  - Diltiazem

Anticancer drugs
- Vinblastine
- 5-Fluorouracil
- Tamoxifen

Cold/allergy medications
- Chlorpheniramine
- Diphenhydramine hydrochloride
- Pseudoephedrine

Antiulcer medications
- Cimetidine
- Famotidine[a]
- Nizatidine[a]
- Ranitidine[a]

Stimulants/anorectics
- Phentermine
- Fenfluramine
- Phenylpropanolamine
- Diethylpropion
- Mazindol

Commonly abused substances
- Alcohol
- Barbiturates
- Cannabis
- Cocaine
- Opioids
- Methylphenidate
- Amphetamine
- Nicotine

Hormones
- Progesterone
- Cortisol

[a] *Studies indicate that these drugs may have fewer sexual side effects than others in their class.*

[b] *Direct sexual side affects of lithium are only confirmed when taken in conjunction with benzodiazepines.*

[c] *ACE inhibitors have fewer sexual side effects than other classes of antihypertensives.*

(Data from Crenshaw and Goldberg.[7]*)*

Impotence may also be caused by structural abnormalities such as Peyronie's disease (Table 103-1). Prostatecomies often create sexual problems. In some cases, a man who has had prostate surgery and has lost interest in sex may use the surgery as an excuse for avoiding sexual contact. Impotence may follow prostate surgery, but nerve-sparing surgical techniques, developed by Dr. Patrick Walsh of The Johns Hopkins University, are available and can help avoid erectile dysfunction in many cases.[5]

Certain drugs may also cause impotence, including antihypertensives, antidepressants, antipsychotics, and others (Table 103-3), as can overconsumption of alcohol.

Ten percent of impotence cases are due to psychological causes, including performance anxiety, stress, exhaustion, anger, and depression. Sexual problems can be both the origin of depression and symptomatic of it. Widowhood may be followed by grief, sometimes complicated by depression. It may lead to a kind of "enshrinement" of the lost partner. In such cases, "widower's guilt" may block the development of new relationships and cause erectile dysfunction when the man tries to engage in sexual intercourse with a new partner.[3]

Proper diagnosis of erectile dysfunction depends on taking a thorough history; asking questions about changes in libido, nocturnal erections, and problems with relationships; and a review of diseases and medication and alcohol use. This should be followed by a physical examination and laboratory evaluation, including a testosterone level. Erectile dysfunction during sleep can be checked by rigiscan, a means of measuring nocturnal tumescence associated with REM sleep. It should be noted, however, that this is an imperfect method for diagnosing impotence.

Impotence can often be successfully treated. For psychogenic cases, psychotherapy, marital therapy, group therapy, and sex therapy, which is based on Masters and Johnson's use of "sensate focusing," may be beneficial. These approaches are also useful when impotence is physical in origin because there are often associated or concommitant emotional reactions to impotence, and because such therapeutic approaches can help reassure the patient and his partner. For physically caused impotence, there are now four main treatment approaches:

- Treatment of the underlying cause, such as diabetes or reactions to medications.
- Pharmacotherapy, which involves self-injection directly into the corpus cavernosum with vasoactive compounds. Phentolamine, atropine, and prostaglandin-E have been shown to be effective given individually or together. Prostaglandin-E (Caverject) is the first FDA-approved prescription medication to treat impotence. Erection should occur within 5 to 10 minutes after injection, and the erection can last 30 minutes or more. Injection with these substances should not be done more than once every 24 hours and three times per week. Problems with this therapy include priapism (4 percent), which can be reversed with epinephrine or ephedrine; mild to moderate pain at the site of injection; and some scarring. Contraindications include presence of sickle-cell anemia, multiple myeloma, leukemia, anatomical deformities, and implants. The use of a tiny plunger or pill to overcome the necessity for injection is now in clinical trials. In a recent study, treatment of 1,511 men with erectile dysfunction, aged 27 to 88, with transurethral alprostadil (a synthetic compound identical to prostaglandin-E1) was shown to be effective in 66 percent of cases, regardless of age. A major advantage of this treatment is that the drug is delivered transurethrally via an applicator, rather than through injection.[6] Nitric oxide, a neurotransmitter that dilates the cavernosa, may help sustain erections and may one day be administered as a therapeutic modality.
- Vacuum therapy involves placing a cylinder over an unerect penis, sucking out air to produce an erection, and applying a wide rubber band at the base to maintain the erection. A third of individuals who try vacuum devices find them helpful. They should not be used by men taking anticoagulants or those who have low platelet levels.
- Implants (permanent penile prostheses) may help patients with otherwise untreatable impotence. These prostheses are irreversible and therefore should be used only as a last-resort therapy. Penile implants can be noninflatable (positionable or semirigid rod prosthesis) and inflatable. Inflatable implants include an inflate/deflate pump with the cylinder in the penis or placed below the skin in the scrotum. There is a reservoir in the scrotum. Cylinders are placed behind the abdominal muscles. Contraindications to this treatment include psychiatric problems such as psychosis and untreated depression.[3]

Revascularization surgery is still largely experimental. Some studies of the substance Yohimbine, which comes from the bark of an African tree, have shown that it has a positive effect on erection, probably because it acts on neurotransmitters such as acetylcholine and dopamine that are involved in the sexual response.

A self-help organization based in Washington DC, called Impotents Anonymous, provides valuable information and referral services.

In general, the old adage "use it or lose it" appears to be true. Erections bring oxygen-rich blood to the penis, which is contributory to continuing healthful functioning. Otherwise, damage to the lining of blood vessels can occur. Good health habits promote sexual capability. In addition to helping people stay healthy, a balanced diet, no tobacco, moderate consumption of alcohol, and exercise programs all help prevent sexual dysfunction as well.

The "Second Language of Sex"

Some older people are not interested in sex because they were never interested in it, or their sexual desire has decreased, or their opportunities for sexual activity are significantly diminished, or other reasons. Other older people *are* interested and want to continue to be sexually active. The point is, whatever the older patient's wishes are, they should be respected. Older people should not be stereotyped as being, on the one hand, loveless and sexless, and on the other, as sex-crazed "dirty old men" and "lascivious old women," undeserving of medical attention when they present sexual problems. There is a range of interest and degree of sexual activity among older people just as there is among other age groups, and treatment options can be as effective for them as for younger people.

The "first language" of sexuality, generally associated with youth, is biologic and intense. The "second language" of sexuality, broader than the first, may be better learned by experience over a lifetime. Of course, some younger people are naturally adept at expressing the second language of sexuality and, conversely, some older people never quite learn it. But for many people, focus on genital contact gives way over time to a more encompassing definition of sexuality, which includes intimacy, mutuality, trust, love, romance, friendship, and caring.[3]

It is not known if there is a clear association between sexual satisfaction and longevity, but there is evidence that married people survive the longest and that love and sex enhance the quality of life. Some of the greatest obstacles to successful, intimate relationships in later life are the negative attitudes and practices toward older persons found among health professionals and the public at large. Health professionals must realize that their older patients have sexual interest, capacities, and pleasures, and that we have the means to repair many of the physical, emotional, and social impediments to continuing sexuality in late life through education and other interventions.

References

1. Butler RN, Lewis MI: Sexuality. In pp. 827–839. Merck Manual of Geriatrics, 2nd Ed., Merck Research Laboratories, West Point, PA, 1995
2. Weg RB: Sexuality, sensuality and intimacy. pp. 479–488. In Enclyclopedia of Gerontology. Vol. 2. Academic Press, New York, 1996
3. Butler RN, Lewis ML: Love and Sex After 60. Ballantine Books, New York, 1993
4. Veno M: The so-called coital death. Jap J Legal Med 1963;17: 535
5. Walsh PC: The preservation of sexual function in the surgical treatment of prostatic cancer. An anatomical surgical approach. In Devica VT, Hellman S, Rosenberg SA (eds): Important Advances in Oncology. Lippincott-Raven, Philadephia, 1988
6. Padma-Nathan H, Hellstrom, WJG, Kaiser FE et al: Treatment of men with erectile dysfunction with transurethral alprostadil. N Engl J Med 1997;336:1–7
7. Crenshaw TL, Goldberg JP: Sexual Pharmacology: Drugs That Affect Sexual Functioning. WW Norton, New York, 1996

CHAPTER 104

The Elderly in Society: An International Perspective

ROBERT N. BUTLER
MIA OBERLINK
MALVIN SCHECHTER

The Longevity Revolution

Historical Perspective

With the Industrial Revolution in the 1800s came the development of scientific medicine and a transformation in understanding the causes and transmission of disease. New scientific understandings and public health efforts yielded dramatic reductions in maternal, infant, and child mortality rates in the 19th century. The 20th century reaped an unprecedented gain in life expectancy at birth; over 25 years throughout the industrialized world and more modest though significant increases in the developing world. This includes gains in late life, that is, reductions in deaths from heart disease and stroke after age 65. The goal of this chapter is to increase awareness of the worldwide phenomena of increased longevity and population aging, as well as approaches to geriatrics, productive aging, and long-term care policy. It presents selected international data pertaining to these topics in both developed and developing countries.

Japan has the highest life expectancy at birth of any nation: 76.5 years for men and 83.1 years for women (1993).[1] This compares with a 55-year life expectancy just prior to World War II. The speed of the aging of Japan's population is remarkable. It took 45 years for the 65 and over population of the UK to increase from 7 to 14 percent of its total population, Sweden required 85 years, and France 115 years. It took Japan only 26 years. The 65 and over population in the US will reach 14 percent in about 2012, or 68 years after it constituted only 7 percent of the total population.[2] This worldwide demographic revolution is a stunning social achievement. Yet, the consequences of longevity for family life, individual and social productivity, and the organization, delivery, and financing of health care, social services, and housing arrangements are not well understood. As the world faces larger numbers and proportions of older people, each nation will have to grapple with the impact of greater longevity on its people and institutions.

Organized and academic medicine have been slow to respond to population aging trends. Interdisciplinary geriatrics appeared first in Great Britain in the 1930s, stimulated by Dr. Marjorie Warren's efforts to reduce institutionalization of the elderly poor. The term "geriatrics" was coined in the US by Dr. Ignatz Nascher in 1909, but not until 1988 did American medicine establish a certificate of competency in geriatrics for physicians licensed in internal medicine and family practice. Geriatrics is growing as a specialty in some countries such as the Scandinavian nations and Japan.

Clinical practice, biomedical research, and professional medical training are being shaped by the forces of population aging. Knowledge about the role of aging in health and disease is critical to assuring a high quality of life for human beings across the life span, from early stages of development to old age. New knowledge may improve the effectiveness of care and preventive measures as well as economize on expenditures for later-life disabilities.

This chapter presents data on demographic trends, life expectancy, age- and sex-specific death rates for selected diseases, labor force participation rates, dependency ratios, and various economic indicators in selected countries. The statistics, while not exhaustive or entirely comparable nation-by-nation, are supplemented by some necessarily brief impressions of several countries. The authors offer reflections based on visits to the countries, the Almanac Project on Longevity and Society conducted by the International Longevity Center, and experience with international organizations studying aging.

Trends Among National Populations

Age Distributions

The demographic transition to an older population is a worldwide phenomenon. Currently, the world's elderly population is growing at an annual rate of 2.8 percent. That is much faster than the general rate of growth for the global population (1.6 percent).[3] Figure 104-1 shows the percentage increase in elderly populations from 1994 to 2025. Whole populations are

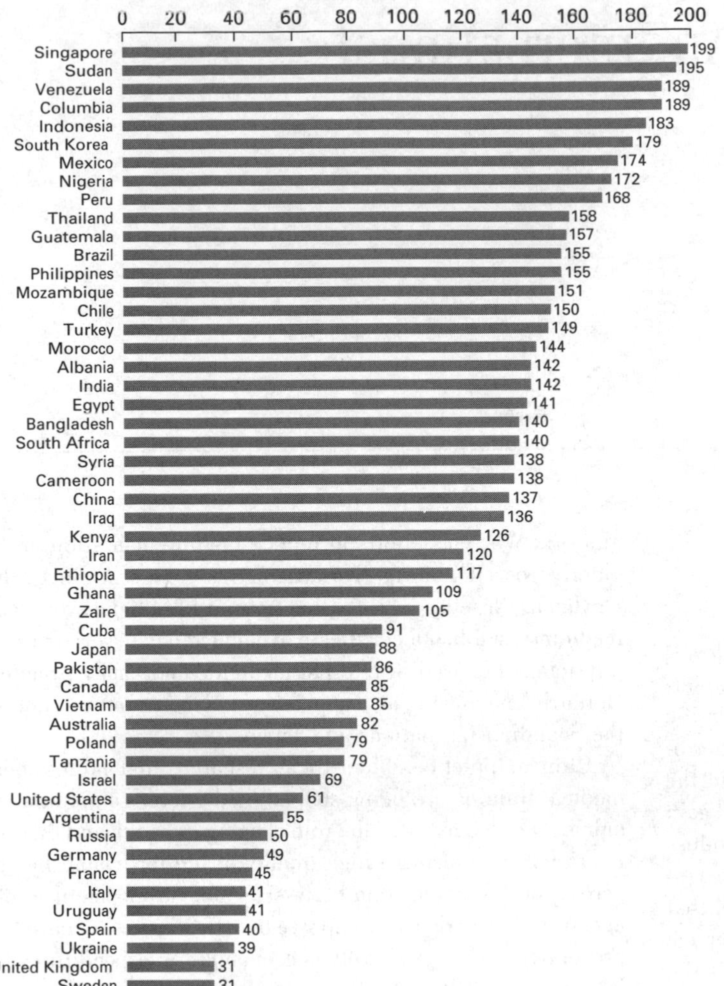

Figure 104-1 Projected percentage increase in population aged 65 and over, 1994–2020. (Adapted from Hobbs and Damon,[3] with permission.)

said to "age" when mortality and fertility rates fall and survival from birth through older ages increases. However, individual countries are at different stages of this transformation, with varying implications.

As the 20th century draws to a close, most of the developed world has at least 10 percent of its population aged 65 and over (Table 104-1). By the year 2000, about 418 million persons will be age 65 or over, with about 40 percent living in developed countries.[3] As the table indicates, Sweden's population has the highest proportion of elders: 17.5 percent.

In developed countries, increased life expectancy can put pressure on established security networks. For healthy older people who have both the desire and ability to work, problems arise from the maintenance of practices designed to remove them from the labor force and create opportunities for younger workers. High unemployment also results in fewer opportunities to work. These problems may be intensified when programs designed to provide for older people are strained by a growing older population. In addition, older people who are not healthy may place financial stress on medical systems that were designed for acute care rather than long-term care and do not adequately promote the prevention of disease associated with aging.[4]

By the year 2020, developing nations will have 65 percent of the world's population age 65 and over, up from 55 percent in 1994.[3] Despite a faster growth of their older population (see Figure 104-1), developing countries will continue, for the most part, to have smaller proportions of older people than developing countries. Table 104-2 lists developing countries which, in 1994, had less than 10 percent of their population age 65 and over. However, developing countries are experiencing the same strains due to increased longevity as developed countries, with added complications. They must struggle to achieve growth within the constraints of the world economy, while basic needs are not being met for the majority of their people. These hardships are compounded in countries where fertility rates have not fallen in pace with mortality rates, creating a growing number of children as well as older people.[4]

The absolute number of elders is quite large. In 1994, China, India, and the US each had more than 25 million resi-

Table 104-1 Aging countries: countries with at least 10 percent of population aged 65 and over in 1994

Country	Total Population (Thousands)	Percentage Aged 65 and Over
Western Europe		
France	57,840	15.4
Germany	81,088	15.4
Italy	58,138	15.9
Poland	38,655	10.9
Spain	39,303	14.7
Sweden	8,788	17.5
UK	58,135	15.8
Eastern Europe		
Russia	149,609	11.6
Ukraine	51,847	13.8
Asia		
Japan	125,107	13.7
Americas		
Canada	28,114	12.1
US	261,090	12.7
Uruguay	3,199	12.2
Middle East		
Israel	5,051	10.2
Oceania		
Australia	18,007	11.7

(From Hobbs and Damon,[3] with permission.)

dents aged 65 and over (Table 104-3). The People's Republic of China—the country with the greatest number of persons age 65 and over—had 71 million in 1994 and expects 168 million by 2020.[3]

The foregoing statistics cover the elderly within the broad category of "65 years and over." To help disaggregate the growth of elderly populations by size and age, Table 104-4 shows the number and proportion of persons in the age groups 60 to 69, 70 to 79, and 80 and over in 1994 for selected countries. Comparison with Table 104-5 provides the change in population age 60 and over between 1994 and 2020 for each of these countries.

Figure 104-2 illustrates the rapid growth of the "oldest old" population (those aged 80 and over) by showing their percentage of the total population in 1994 along with the projected growth rate for the year 2020. The growth of the "oldest old" population has important social implications. First, it implies a strain on current pension systems, as people survive well past the age limits on many pension programs. More older people depend on these programs for a longer period of time while increased costs result in pressures to reduce spending on these programs by both legislators and employers.

Table 104-2 Countries with less than 10 percent of population aged 65 and over in 1994

Country	Total Population (Thousands)	Percentage Aged 65 and Over
Asia		
Bangladesh	125,149	3
China	1,190,431	6
India	919,903	3.9
Indonesia	200,410	3.4
Iran	63,120	3.8
Pakistan	128,856	3.9
Singapore	2,859	6.5
South Korea	45,083	5.3
Thailand	59,510	4.7
Vietnam	73,104	4.9
Sub-Saharan Africa		
Cameroon	13,132	3.4
Ethlophla	54,253	2.7
Ghana	17,255	3
Kenya	28,241	2.3
Mozambique	17,346	2.5
Nigeria	98,091	2.9
South Africa	43,931	4
Sudan	29,420	2.2
Tanzania	27,986	2.8
Zaire	42,684	2.7
North Africa		
Egypt	60,765	3.4
Morocco	28,561	4.2
Middle East		
Iraq	19,890	3.1
Saudi Arabia	18,196	2.2
Syria	14,887	2.8
Turkey	62,154	5.1
Latin America		
Argentina	33,913	9.6
Brazil	158,739	4.5
Chile	13,951	6.5
Columbia	35,558	4.3
Cuba	11,064	9.2
Guatemala	10,721	3.4
Mexico	92,202	4.2
Peru	23,650	4
Venezuela	20,562	4.2
Eastern Europe		
Albania	3,374	5.7
Uzbekistan	22,609	4.6

(From Hobbs and Damon,[3] with permission.)

Table 104-3 Ten places with the largest number of persons 65 and over in 1994 (in thousands)

Country/Area	Population Aged 65 and Over
China	71,073
India	35,282
US	33,169
Russia	17,384
Japan	17,140
Germany	12,476
Italy	9,258
UK	9,175
France	8,924
Ukraine	7,155

(From Hobbs and Damon,[3] with permission.)

In addition, this growth of the "oldest old" population reflects a growing number of older people in need of medical care and/or help with daily living, because they tend to be sicker than the young old. These needs occur while many family members are themselves middle-aged or older and may have other obligations or medical conditions that prevent them from being caregivers.[4]

Life Expectancy

The high-life expectancies at birth shown in Figure 104-3 indicate a reduction in infant and childhood mortality due to improvements in health care, parenting, and living conditions. In virtually all societies, average life expectancy for females is longer than for males. The exact reasons for this phenomenon are still not known. These numbers are used to predict the number of older people in future years, but do not necessarily indicate a high quality of life for older people. Quality of life depends on the availability of sufficient income, access to housing and health care, and other factors that may vary from culture to culture.

Table 104-4 Population of people aged 60 and over by country in 1994

Country	Total Population (Thousands)	Total 60+ (Thousands)	60+ (%)	60–69 (Thousands)	60–69 (%)	70–79 (Thousands)	70–79 (%)	80+ (Thousands)	80+ (%)
Sweden	8,778	1,944	22.1	813	9.3	724	8.2	407	4.6
Italy	58,138	12,567	21.6	6,365	10.9	3,982	6.8	2,221	3.8
Germany	81,088	16,767	20.7	8,251	10.2	5,204	6.4	3,313	4.1
UK	58,135	11,979	20.6	5,458	9.4	4,179	7.2	2,342	4
France	57,840	11,862	20.5	5,673	9.8	3,626	6.3	2,563	4.4
Japan	125,107	24,403	19.5	13,344	10.7	7,462	6	3,597	2.9
US	261,091	43,503	16.7	20,473	7.8	15,270	5.8	7,760	3
Russia	149,609	24,768	16.6	14,863	9.9	6,588	4.4	3,317	2.2
Canada	28,114	4,579	16.3	2,252	8	1,550	5.5	777	2.8
Poland	38,655	6,064	15.7	3,449	8.9	1,761	4.6	854	2.2
Australia	18,077	2,825	15.7	1,407	7.8	982	5.4	438	2.4
Israel	2,051	6.85	13.6	332	6.6	240	4.8	113	2.2
Argentina	33,913	4,564	13.5	2,476	7.3	1,522	4.5	567	1.7
Chile	13,951	1,333	9.6	769	5.5	416	3	147	1.1
Singapore	2,859	276	9.6	161	5.6	82	2.9	33	1.1
China	1,190,431	109,199	9.2	67,326	5.7	32,864	2.8	9,010	0.8
Brazil	158,739	10,903	6.9	6,743	4.2	3,271	2.1	889	0.6
India	919,903	58,247	6.3	37,929	4.1	16,297	1.8	4,021	0.4
Mexico	92,202	5,766	6.3	3,306	3.6	1,713	1.9	745	0.8
Indonesia	200,410	11,866	5.9	8,272	4.1	2,985	1.5	609	0.3
Philippines	71,631	3,997	5.6	2,439	3.4	1,228	1.7	330	0.5
Egypt	60,765	3,414	5.6	2,276	3.7	934	1.5	204	0.3
Bangladesh	125,149	6,020	4.8	3,993	3.2	1,787	1.4	240	0.2
Nigeria	98,091	4,612	4.7	3,095	3.2	1,299	1.3	217	0.2

(From Hobbs and Damon,[3] with permission.)

Table 104-5 Projected population of people aged 60 years and over by country in 2020

Country	Total Population (Thousands)	Total 60+ (Thousands)	60+ (%)	60–69 (Thousands)	60–69 (%)	70–79 (Thousands)	70–79 (%)	80+ (Thousands)	80+ (%)
Japan	126,062	39,455	31.3	15,322	12.2	14,772	11.7	9,362	7.4
Germany	82,385	24,480	29.7	10,998	13.3	7,594	9.2	5,889	7.1
Italy	57,844	16,881	29.2	7,228	12.5	5,512	9.5	4,142	7.2
France	61,793	16,877	27.3	7,605	12.3	5,518	8.9	3,754	6.1
Sweden	9,469	2,572	27.2	1,083	11.4	947	10	542	5.7
UK	60,042	15,750	26.2	6,964	11.6	5,386	9	3,400	5.7
Canada	34,347	8,622	25.1	4,320	12.6	2,707	7.9	1,595	4.6
Poland	42,474	10,386	24.5	5,492	12.9	3,017	7.1	1,877	4.4
Singapore	3,335	819	24.5	472	14.1	238	7.1	109	3.3
Russia	159,263	36,823	23.1	19,925	12.5	9,707	6.1	7,191	4.5
Australia	22,724	5,249	23.1	2,602	11.4	1,723	7.6	925	4.1
US	326,322	73,905	22.6	37,919	11.6	22,980	7	13,007	4
Israel	6,935	1,183	17.1	606	8.7	366	5.3	210	3
China	1,424,725	241,594	17	142,233	10	70,624	5	28,737	2
Chile	19,225	3,246	16.9	1,730	9	1,036	5.4	480	2.5
Argentina	43,190	6,940	16.1	3,600	8.3	2,268	5.3	1,072	2.5
Brazil	197,466	26,679	13.5	15,392	7.8	8,156	4.1	3,132	1.6
Mexico	136,096	15,189	11.2	8,243	6.1	4,650	3.4	2,296	1.7
Indonesia	276,474	31,081	11.2	20,134	7.3	7,913	2.9	3,034	1.1
India	1,320,746	136,940	10.4	84,832	6.4	39,469	3	12,639	1
Philippines	115,988	10,213	8.8	6,335	5.5	2,948	2.5	930	0.8
Egypt	92,604	7,981	8.6	5,152	5.6	2,247	2.4	582	0.6
Bangladesh	210,428	14,407	6.9	9,482	4.5	4,227	2	697	0.3
Nigeria	215,893	11,549	5.3	6,951	3.2	3,699	1.7	900	0.4

(From Hobbs and Damon,[3] with permission.)

A country may have a low-life expectancy at birth, resulting in a smaller older population, but a high-life expectancy at age 65 and a high quality of life for older people. However, unlike life expectancy at birth, life expectancy at age 65 has not shown continued linear improvement in some countries (Fig. 104-4). In some Eastern European countries and India, there appears to have been a decline or, at least, stagnation in life expectancy at age 65. The reasons for this phenomenon appear to include alcoholism, cigarette smoking, excess fat consumption, and political destabilization. In the former USSR, national public health services have declined and diseases such as cholera and diphtheria have increased.

Causes of Death

The probability of eventually dying from specific causes is presented in Table 104-6. The country differences are starting points for epidemiologists in exploring the relationships between diseases and specific risk factors.

Of particular interest to the study of psychosocial factors in longevity is the phenomenon of relatively high rates of suicide among the aged in many countries (Table 104-7). For example, the male suicide rate in the US is nine times higher at age 75 than the female rate and also more than twice as high as the suicide rates for adult males through age 64.

Economic Indicators

Male labor force participation rates at various older ages are shown in Table 104-8. A fall in labor force participation usually occurs past age 65, and sometimes earlier, depending on factors such as retirement age and benefits. The trend toward earlier retirement, however, may be leveling off or reversing in some cases as older people begin to have more years of healthy productive living, especially among the "younger old" (age 65 to 74).

There are many economic variables that can indicate the well being of older people, most of which are not tabulated internationally. Table 104-9 shows some of these indicators for selected countries, including Gross Domestic Product (GDP),

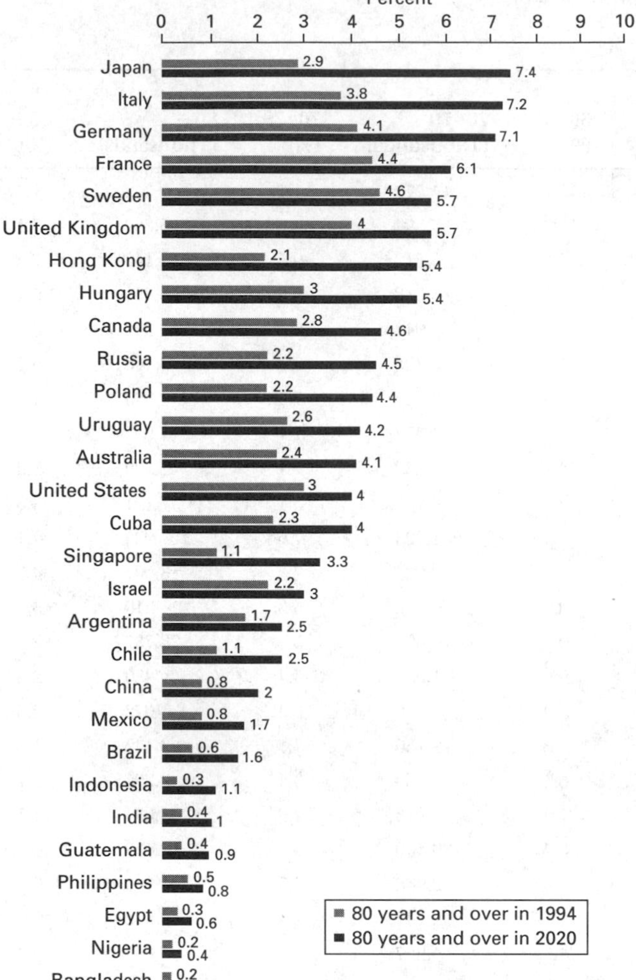

Figure 104-2 Percentage of population aged 80 and over, 1994 and 2020. (From Hobbs and Damon,[3] with permission.)

growth rates of GDP, central government expenditure on human services, and social security transfers to households as a percent of GDP. These figures, when compared with the size and growth of the older population, can help to indicate a government's commitment to its older population.

Social Responses to Longevity in Selected Countries

The Industrial Revolution increased the aggregate wealth of countries, but simultaneously produced mass urbanized poverty in Western nations. Among ameliorative efforts was the development of social security systems, originally focused on the problems of poverty in old age. Under Chancellor Otto Von Bismarck, pension legislation was enacted in 1889 in Germany.[5] Social security systems have played an increasingly important role since World War II. The number of countries with public pension systems has increased from 33 in 1940 to 155 in 1993.[6] Depending on the country, a social security program finances pensions only or includes medical care and such other benefits as disability and survivor coverage. The expanded systems recognize the relationship of poverty to sickness by incorporating both income-maintenance and health care financing.

One of the legacies of the early Industrial Revolution is the notion that workers are "used up" or useless in factories by their 40s.[7] Chronic illness and disability in old age prompted fears that the growing number of older persons would reduce the economic productivity of society, drain its resources, and create intergenerational conflict. In point of fact, the reduction of premature disease and death has enhanced societal productivity. There is a longer lifetime in which to produce wealth for self, family, and society. Only a minority, albeit a significant one, of a birth cohort in industrialized countries becomes disabled in old age or survives into late life with long-standing, progressive disabilities.

Although costs have been a concern in most European nations, Japan, and the US, most developed countries have been able to fund social security, private pensions, and health care programs. However, since 1990 the control of costs of "entitlements" has become a growing concern. The increased survivorship of older persons has enriched the life of the family and community, but this change has come about so dramatically and rapidly that social institutions and individuals are still adjusting to it.

National responsiveness to population aging has varied not only as a matter of industrial, scientific, and economic development but also as a matter of culture and history. Notable facts and responses to increased longevity in selected countries are briefly described below.

Japan

Japan has the world's longest life expectancy. Japan has put in place a health care financing system that gives essentially free care (only a 5 percent copayment is required) for all persons over age 70. Until recently, the system for delivering health care emphasized hospitalization; lengths of stay for elderly patients were much longer than in other countries. A "Golden Plan" was announced in 1990 for expanding home- and community-based services, particularly rehabilitation and adult day care.

Along with the US, Japan has endeavored to elevate the age of retirement. Although they are expected to retire from their full-time careers at age 60 for men and 56 for women, many retirees in Japan continue to work many years beyond these ages for financial and psychological reasons. In 1992 in Japan, 38.2 percent of men aged 65 and over and 16.7 percent of women that age were in the labor force[8] (compared with 16 percent and 7.4 percent, respectively, in the US).[7] Many more retire before or at age 60; however, this earlier retirement age coupled with a longer life expectancy make an extensive public pension system prohibitively expensive. In Japan, savings by individuals remain a major component

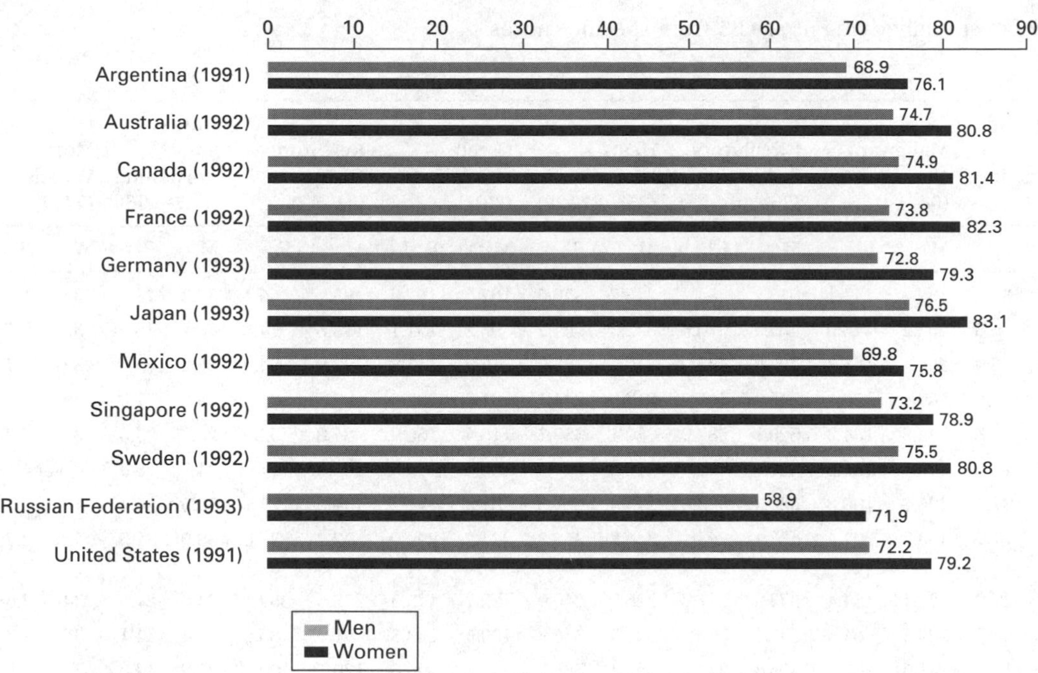

Figure 104-3 Average life expectancy in years at birth, by sex, for selected countries. (From World Health Organization,[1] with permission.)

of late-life resources. In the 1987 tax reform, incentives for individual savings were provided for.

Worry about the government's capacity to cope with a growing older population now and in the future was indicated in a book published in the early 1980s called *Japan in the Year 2000*.[9] This report by Japan's Long-Term Outlook Committee cited three major trends to be considered in national planning: (a) internationalization of the economy, (b) structural changes in the economy, and (c) population aging. Japan has recently created a national center on longevity science in Nagoya.

Figure 104-4 Average years of life remaining at age 65, by sex and country. (From World Health Organization,[1] with permission.)

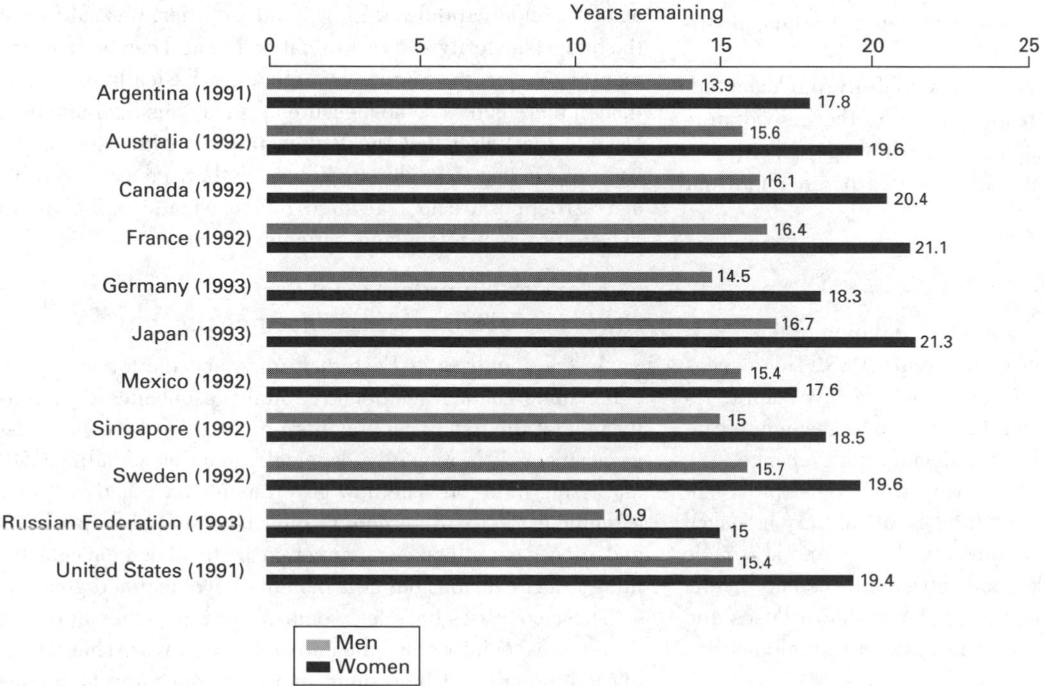

Table 104-6 Probability of eventually dying at age 65 from specific causes of death[a]

Country	Reported Year	Infectious and Parasitic (01–07)		Malignant Neoplasm (08–14)		Circulatory System (25–30)		Heart Disease (251, 27–28)		Cerebro-vascular (29)		Respiratory Disease (31–32)		Injury and Poisioning (E47–E56)		Motor Vehicle (E471)	
		M	F	M	F	M	F	M	F	M	F	M	F	M	F	M	F
Argentina	1991	29.5	31	186.4	141.1	515	584.1	345.2	370.6	107.6	127.8	83	66.4	30.3	21.7	3.9	1.9
Australia	1992	6.7	6.8	252.2	173.8	482.9	570.6	342.3	369.2	98.2	151.1	115.6	74.8	20.2	18.6	3.5	2.7
Canada	1992	6.2	6.9	264	195.3	433.9	487.9	316.7	325.9	76.3	113.8	122.9	94.9	25.2	25.6	3.6	2.7
France	1992	14	14.9	289	179	355.9	417.7	219.6	244.1	91.5	122.5	97.5	81.7	53.2	57.3	4.4	2.5
Germany	1993	6	5.8	242.5	184.2	520.1	587.9	350.1	359.1	116.4	156.9	86.8	52.9	25.2	25.5	3.1	1.8
Japan	1993	15.8	11.6	246.6	156.5	367.1	467	212.5	264.3	133.6	175.5	196.6	147	34.7	28.3	6.4	4
Mexico	1992	43.5	37.5	126.7	108.8	334.3	383.8	213.3	229.5	81.3	97	134.6	114.1	50.5	26.4	11	4.2
Russian Federation	1993	5	1.7	163.8	97.4	633.4	745.1	346.8	358.8	224.2	299.9	77.2	34.6	38.9	21.5	4.1	2.7
Singapore	1992	19.1	27.2	225.1	154.4	375.9	447.7	226.5	240.9	122.7	172.5	278.6	239	24.8	21.6	3.8	2.6
Sweden	1992	6.6	8.3	208.5	164.9	543.1	562	388.3	356.8	100.4	143.3	91.9	83.6	27.4	24.1	3.3	1.3
US	1991	12.6	14.5	241.6	180	475.6	534.1	368.4	388.3	67.3	96.5	120	100	25.9	17.8	5	3.2

Abbreviations: M, male; F, female.
[a] *All diseases are classified by ICD-9 Basic Tabulation List.*
(From World Health Organization,[1] with permission.)

The People's Republic of China

The People's Republic of China has the world's largest population. Even though life expectancy in China is lower than in the industrialized world 1 in 16 Chinese are elderly, for a total of 71 million. The village system provides roles for elders with the guiding concept of generations standing together. This and a Confucian background contribute to the people's high regard for elders. However, as in Japan, the extraordinary growth in the number of older people threatens traditional attitudes toward the elders.

The policy of one child per family, if fully implemented, would alter remarkably the responsibility of the individual to his or her parents and grandparents as they age; potentially, one child would bear responsibility for two parents and four grandparents.

Singapore

Twenty-six percent of Singapore's population of three million persons will be over 65 in the year 2035. This causes some anxiety in Singapore, because, having few natural resources, the country must depend on its human resources. Singapore is already planning for this demographic change.

Singapore is also noted for having the largest provident fund in the world. A provident fund is a publicly managed investment fund in which compulsory deductions are made from wages to be paid back upon retirement, usually in the form of a lump sum. Provident funds have shown losses and been abandoned in several countries, but Singapore has had positive results so far.[7]

The United Kingdom

The UK has been guided by the Beveridge Plan of the 1940s in developing a "cradle to grave" set of social entitlements akin to those of other Western European democracies. Generally, however, these countries are in the midst of retrenchment of entitlements in health and social services.

In the UK, geriatric medicine was incorporated into the postwar National Health Service. The Service, often criticized as being undercapitalized in hospital facilities, was subject to the budget austerity and re-evaluation by the Thatcher government. However, the Service has remained basically intact, although there is now some measure of private medical practice. Despite the belief that the British ration health care on the basis of age (for example, no dialysis authorized after age 55), age restrictions are not legislated, but are a matter of individual decision by physicians and patients.

The former Union of Soviet Socialist Republic (USSR) and east bloc nations

As the countries of Eastern Europe and the former Soviet Union undergo the transition to capitalist economies, the maintenance of the extensive benefits provided by the communist governments is in jeopardy, especially in a time of falling GDP and rising inflation. The new governments have had to spend as much as 10 to 13 percent of their GDP on public pensions and impose payroll taxes ranging from 35 to 50 percent contributing to tax evasion, but still benefits have declined greatly.[7]

These countries have lost years of life expectancy in recent decades, especially since the end of the Cold War. This probably is a function of high infant mortality rates and high con-

Table 104-7 Death by suicide and self-inflicted injury by age and sex (rates per 100,000 population)

Country	Sex	Total	5–14	15–25	25–34	35–44	45–54	55–64	65–74	75+
Argentina, 1991	M	9	0.8	6.5	9.4	9.7	12.9	17.3	26.8	46.5
	F	3	0.3	2.3	3.3	3.3	4	5.4	8.5	7.6
Australia, 1992	M	20.5	0.3	27.3	28.7	24.7	24.9	23.8	26.6	29.1
	F	5.3	0.2	5.6	6.8	6.3	6.3	7.4	7.4	9.1
Canada, 1992	M	20.7	1.3	24.7	28.8	27.3	24.7	26.2	20.5	27.2
	F	5.5	0.4	6	6.2	7.9	9.1	6.6	5.9	4.2
France, 1992	M	30.2	0.5	14	32.4	40.4	40.3	38.8	46.1	103.3
	F	10.9	0.1	4.3	8.9	12.6	16.4	16.9	17.4	24.3
Ireland, 1992	M	16.8	0.6	21.5	30.4	22	20.9	23.8	20	13.9
	F	3.3	*	2	5.2	2.5	5.7	7.1	6.1	5
Japan, 1993	M	22.3	0.4	10.1	18.1	24.5	36.1	37.8	31.7	51.8
	F	11.1	0.3	4.4	7.5	8.8	12.9	15.9	20.6	37
Germany, 1993	M	22.6	1	12.7	20	24.6	28.9	31.7	33.7	87.5
	F	8.9	0.3	3.4	5.5	6.8	12	12.6	15.2	24.4
Italy, 1991	M	11.5	0.2	5.7	10	10.5	12.5	18.3	23	41.9
	F	4.2	0.1	1.6	3.2	4	5	6.4	8.7	9.6
Mexico, 1992	M	4.3	0.4	5.7	7.1	6.4	6.7	7.6	9.8	18
	F	0.8	0.2	1.3	1.2	1	0.7	1	1.1	1.1
New Zealand, 1992	M	23.6	1.5	39.9	36.9	24.2	22.8	32.3	20.6	25.5
	F	5.5	0.4	6.2	5.4	5.6	11.4	11.5	4.9	6
Singapore, 1992	M	11.8	1	10.2	16.1	14	12.2	11.8	29.9	59.9
	F	9.3	0.5	6	11.5	9.7	6.5	11.7	29	56.4
Sweden, 1992	M	21.9	0.6	10	23	27.7	32.2	27.7	31.1	52.2
	F	9.6	*	6.7	8.4	10.4	14.8	13.6	15.9	13.3
US, 1991	M	20.1	1.1	21.9	25	23	23.7	25.3	30.7	56
	F	4.7	0.3	3.8	5.4	6.5	7.6	6.5	6	5.9
Russian Federation, 1993	M	66.2	2.8	41.7	82.1	99.4	118.2	100.7	80.7	103.8
	F	12.9	0.8	7.9	10.3	13.9	18.5	19	22.6	31.6

Abbreviations: M, male; F, female.
(From World Health Organization,[1] with permission.)

sumption of alcohol and tobacco. Remarkable longevity has been reported for the "long-lived" people of Soviet Georgia, but in truth no one has confirmed an age beyond 113. Nutrition, a strong role in family and community, and steady physical activity over the entire life cycle may contribute to the apparent increased survivorship in that region. The suggestion that such long-lived people existed in the Dark Ages may indicate a genetic component. The Ukraine had one of the first research institutes on aging.

Sweden

This country has long been acknowledged as being in the forefront of systematic development of social services, medical care, housing, and geriatric medicine. However, there have been cutbacks in these areas in the 1990s. With a sophisticated array of state-provided services, Sweden has the highest proportion of older persons in the world. The University of Göteborg has conducted longitudinal studies of older persons by 5-year birth cohorts and shown that socioeconomic improvement advances the health of older persons.[10,11]

Argentina

Argentina is the third richest country in Latin America, in which 8 percent of the world's elderly will be living in 2020. Yet despite rich natural and human resources, Argentina has been hit particularly hard by the debt crisis. The structural adjustment policies enforced by international creditors have resulted in inflation, shrinking state services, and conflict between workers and the state over the privatization of state-owned industries. Older persons have suffered because the values of their pensions have declined under the presidency of Carlos Saul Menem, who was elected in 1989.

Chile

Chile privatized its Social Security system in 1980, after a growing older population, high rates of tax evasion, and a stagnant economy resulted in a crisis of the public system. The

Table 104-8 Male labor force participation rates (percent economically active), by age

Country	Year	45–54 Years	55–59 Years	60–64 Years	65 Years and Over
Argentina	1990	93	79.4	56.1	50.9
Australia	1992	89	74.1	48.1	9.3
Canada	1992	90	62[a]		11
France	1992	93	68.7	19.2	3.5
Germany (Federal Republic)	1990	91.7	78.5	34.8	4.6
Japan[c]	1992	97.6	93.6	75	38.2
Mexico	1993	94.3	88.6	79.8	60.1
Russia[d]	1989	91.5[b]	78.8	35.3	13.5
Sweden	1992	93.1	84.9	60.9	13.7
UK	1992	91	78	52.9	8.7
US	1992	90.1	78.2	54.1	15.5

[a] *Refers to ages 55–84.*
[b] *Refers to ages 50–54.*
[c] *Data from U.S. Bureau of the Census, International Data Base.*[8]
[d] *Data from Velkof and Kinsella*[20] *U.S. Census Bureau, P95/93-1. Printing Office, Washington D.C.*

new system has been the focus of international attention. Workers are required to contribute 10 percent of their earnings to one of many competing private investment funds regulated by the government. Returns have fluctuated but remained positive so far, resulting in the privatization of pension funds by several countries. However, the question remains, will the Chilean system be able to weather the business cycle, particularly a deep economic recession?

Productive Aging and Long-Term Care

Two critical areas of needed societal adjustment to population aging are productive aging and long-term care. The former refers to the productive capabilities of older people—through paid employment, volunteering and other means—in meeting personal, family, and social needs. The other is organized long-term care in the home, community, and institution as part of comprehensive geriatrics, which includes prevention, acute care, and long-term care as well as end-of-life hospice care. An impediment to developing both areas is agism, or prejudice against older persons. They may be seen as unworthy to hold jobs and to receive medical care, personal care, and other services. Age-based rationing of health and social services and officially sanctioned limits on the productive social contributions of older people seem to be consequences of inadequate or irrational public policymaking.

Public Policy Implications

An astute public policy would recognize the value of maintaining older people in productive roles through conventional paid employment, volunteer service, and public-service occupations.[12] For many older persons, work contributes to physical, mental, and financial well-being. In serving families with youngsters while parents are off to work, elders may contribute to social productivity. Moreover, well elders may find esteem and income from serving frail elders in service programs. Whatever promotes life satisfaction and a sense of worth and usefulness may provide a potentially effective means of reducing costs of physical and mental illness in late life. The more self-reliant the elder population, the less need to spend on care. Productive aging, therefore, may be seen as a result of, as well as a stimulus for, comprehensive geriatrics. It may also help to reduce long-term care needs and to help finance them.

An astute public policy also recognizes long-term care benefits as supportive of the working family as well as of elders. For example, family members typically provide the lion's share of custodial care to the community-living elder. However, their abilities and energies may reach limits; without support, problems that could be dealt with at home with the help of medical and other professional persons must be transferred to institutions. Family burnout also may be a major factor in decisions to transfer the elder into a nursing home or other site of care. Furthermore, the burden of care falls mainly to women, more and more of whom are in the workforce away from home. The care duties become overwhelming without such aid as respite services, home-care and homemaking services, and adult day care. Thus, long-term care policy can promote individual productive aging and total social productivity. In the process, fears over national "bankruptcy" from expenses of disability in late life could be allayed.

With this background, we will consider some developments in productive aging and long-term care.

Productive Aging

The concept of productive aging offers a basis for personal and social strategies as populations age.[11] In more developed countries, notably the US, the age of retirement from the labor

Table 104-9 Summary of selected economic variables by country (recent period)

							Central Government Expenditure			Central Government Revenue			
Country	Year	Real GDP per Capita	Average Annual Growth Rate in Real GDP per Capita (Percent) (1980–1990)	Government Consumption Expenditure as a Percent of GDP	Real GDP per Worker	Percent Increase in Real GDP per Worker (1980–1990)	Year	Social Security Transfers to Households as a Percent of GDP	Human Services as a Percent of Central Government Expenditure	Year	Taxes as a Percent of GDP	Social Security Revenues as a Percent of Adjusted Tax Revenue	Percent of Total Population Age 65+[a]
Argentina	1990	4,095	2.1	3.5	10,009	−23	1989	4.7	53	1989	18.8	36.8	9.6
Australia	1990	17,144	6.2	10.4	30,019	9.2	1991	8.1	52	1991	30.7	—	11.7
Brazil	1990	4,588	4.5	13.8	10,871	−8.5	1990	8.7	26.4	1990	27	39.7	4.5
Canada	1990	20,694	6.9	10.1	34,864	20.5	1989	8	44.5	1989	35	15.3	12.1
Congo	1990	2,824	9.8	55.3	4,971	15.4	1989	2.1	—	1988	—	17.5	3.4
Egypt	1990	2,030	6.8	27.5	6,824	14.6	1989	0.9	27.8	1988	11.7	8.9	3.4
FR Germany	1990	18,122	6.9	11.2	29,831	14.2	1989	14.3	87.7	1991	47.1	53.9	15.5[b]
France	1990	16,881	6.4	12.1	30,423	13.1	1989	18.9	89.2	1991	45.9	47.8	15.4
India	1990	1,252	8.5	17.8	2,738	38	1990	0.2	10.9	1990	12.5	—	3.9
Indonesia	1990	2,234	10.1	12.2	4,942	47	1990	—	14	1990	18.8	—	3.4
Israel	1990	10,098	6.6	24.7	22,128	10	1990	10.8	41.4	1990	29.9	9.3	10.2
Italy	1990	15,082	7.2	9.9	30,967	14	1988	17.6	59.7	1991	41.5	29.6	14.9
Japan	1990	17,792	8.5	6.4	23,419	40.7	1989	0.5	53	1990	20.9	—	13.7
Mali	1990	598	5.5	15.4	1,096	−28.7	1988	0.9	27.8	1988	11.7	6.9	3.4
Mexico	1990	6,319	5.2	7.5	15,705	−11.8	1990	2.3	28.8	1990	6.7	12.3	4.2
Netherlands	1990	15,543	6.2	9.4	30,859	5.2	1991	20.5	65.8	1991	47.4	39.2	13.3
Pakistan	1990	1,599	7.4	17.4	4,525	24.1	1988	1.3	13.5	1991	24.8	—	3.9
Philippines	1990	2,080	4.5	13	4,752	−7.7	1991	0.5	32.5	1991	15.3	—	3.6
Singapore	1990	13,232	10.5	6.9	2,262	51.7	1990	0.5	33.9	1990	15.8	—	6.5
Spain	1990	11,653	7.2	10.4	26,588	22.2	1989	12.5	57.9	1990	33.7	39	14.7
Sweden	1990	17,320	6.5	18.4	27,876	13.6	1991	23	66.1	1989	51.8	37.2	17.5
UK	1990	15,374	7.3	13.8	26,454	26.2	1990	10.7	48.2	1990	35.9	17.9	15.8
US	1990	21,571	6.4	10.9	37,473	19.8	1991	6.6	44.5	1991	26.8	38.1	12.7

Abbreviation: GDP, gross domestic product.

[a] *Data from Hobb's and Damon.*[3]

[b] *Data from Germany.*

(Adapted from Muller,[4] *with permission.)*

force and the proportion of the life span spent at work have been dropping while average life expectancy has risen.

Because these added years are also years of higher use of health and long-term care services, doubts have grown about national economic capacity to maintain or improve pension and health benefits. Attention is gradually focusing on methods of prolonging the working life by retraining and improving job conditions and by efforts to encourage health promotion and disease prevention.

In the US, for example, mandatory retirement has been almost entirely prohibited by law as outlined in the Anti-Age Discrimination Act of 1967, which was amended in 1978 and 1986.[12] The Social Security system has been programmed for a higher age of retirement with full benefits; the age shift to 67 is phased-in gradually in 2003 to 2027.[13] Employers have begun to consider special programs to hire, keep, and retrain older workers. One insurance company found it profitable to hire its pensioners for limited service rather than to employ temporary workers unfamiliar with the company.[14] Recognizing productivity losses due to absenteeism and time spent in caring for a disabled family member, some large employers have begun to offer assistance to workers' families in locating social, counseling, health care, housing, and other services.

Taken as a measure of society's economic capacity to maintain a growing elder population are changes in demographic "support ratios" (Fig. 104-5). As seen in Table 104-5, the populations aged 20 to 64 will dwindle relative to the populations aged 65 and over during the period 1990 to 2025. This trend is interpreted to mean that there will be relatively fewer workers to support relatively more dependents. However, this is not necessarily true. Obviously, some people are still workers after age 65 just as some are dependents in the age range of 20 to 64. Early retirement has reduced the proportion economically active before 65. Other qualifications are in order. For example, there are also fewer children to care for in the population. Nonetheless, it is clear that factors excluding people from the workforce necessarily complicate problems of supporting dependents or dependent phases of one's own life.

An increasing number of older women in the labor force has resulted in less time and more stress connected with care at home. To preserve earnings, families have had to find paid caregivers for the homebound. The need to finance long-term care has prompted debate concerning roles for public and private insurance, the capacities of individuals and families to afford private policies, the adequacy of "affordable" insurance, and steps to organize and staff geriatrically oriented systems of care.

Japan has developed strategies for elevating the age of retirement from the 1950s into the 1960s. Its Silver Manpower Centers offer an avenue for the productive use of retired workers and the generation of needed retirement income. The enlarging older population may provide volunteered as well as paid services related to chronic disability, education of children and young workers, and support of maturing families. Labor shortages are seen in some countries where willing and able elders are available to work.

With the globalization of economies, each country's financial ability to provide for, and make use of, older people is

Figure 104-5 Support ratios, 1990 and 2025. (From Kinsella and Taeuber,[2] with permission.)

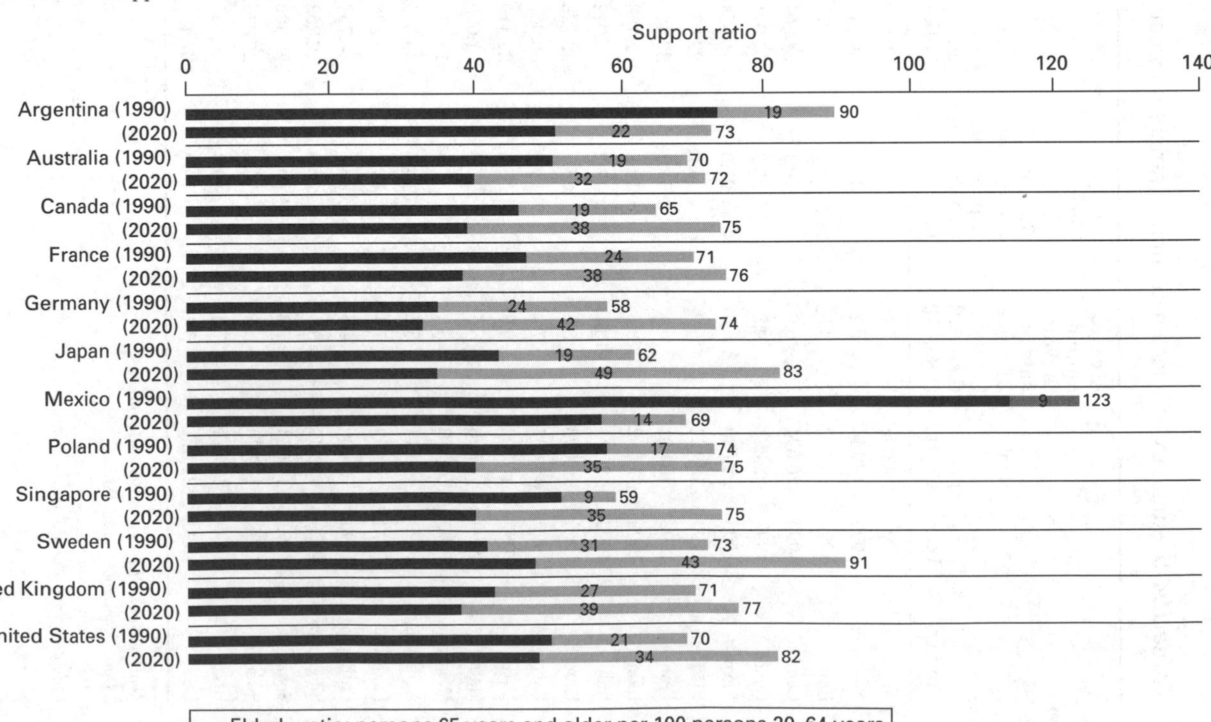

affected by conditions beyond its borders. The tendency of manufacturers to locate jobs where labor is cheap has strong implications for the financing of Social Security and other social welfare programs, including health services. Both the more developed and the less developed nations have a common stake in finding solutions to problems that come with the longevity revolution. Among other things, this common stake should promote sharing of information in gerontology and geriatrics, the effective and efficient development of health and social services (including supportive housing), and practical applications of productive-aging concepts to employment and community service.

As the less developed countries industrialize, internal migration affects elders in several ways. They are left behind as younger family members move to the cities. Rural villages become "settlements for the old and the very young," with consequent reduction in crop yields and the importing of food into previously self-sufficient areas. For elders moving to urban centers, the changes can be abrupt and radical. They may have less living space and experience isolation due to differences in language and customs, or the loss of roles.

Long-Term Care Systems

Provisions for long-term care are as diverse as the many countries that have them. Acute care services, principally in the hospital, tend to be more alike around the world because of the heavy reliance on modern technology. Long-term care, growing out of social patterns, cultural traditions, and housing or household patterns, is far more diverse.[15]

The rapid growth of old and very old populations has required linkages between acute and long-term care services, the combination representing pillars of comprehensive geriatrics. While caregiving is still carried out primarily by families, the structure of families and their capabilities as caregivers to elders have changed in response to modern conditions. There appears to be increasing reliance on publicly provided services to help elders who are alone and family caregivers.

Among goals commonly found in long-term care programs in industrialized countries is the prevention of impoverishment. A major exception is the US, where the only available public funding is part of public assistance for the poor (e.g., Medicaid). Most industrialized nations have publicly supported programs of social and personal care (e.g., respite care, home help, adult day care); services are allocated according to individual need, not ability to pay.

Expansion of hospital, nursing home, and community-based services as well as assisted-living housing (e.g., apartment houses with meal and other services for the frail and disabled) are recognized in most industrial countries as necessary adaptations to population aging.

Sweden has one of the most systematic approaches to long-term care. A continuum of services is available to elders, including nursing home care and housing. The costs are paid chiefly by taxpayers; out-of-pocket spending is limited. About one-third of gross national product goes for health and social security in Sweden. By contrast, about half of nursing home bills and even more of home-care bills in the US are paid privately and without insurance.

In Great Britain, commercialism in long-term care has burgeoned. In Australia, long-term care is mostly in the private sector, if one counts retirement villages, hostels, and nursing homes operated by voluntary agencies and private corporations. State governments provide a smaller portion of aggregate services.[16]

China's long-term care challenges derive in part from its birth control program of one child per family. Without siblings, adult children may find it more difficult to aid multiple elderly family members as the very old population increases in the future.[17]

In 1990, the Japanese government announced a 10-year Golden Plan for the Welfare of the Aged, in preparation for having a population of which 31.3 percent will be aged 60 and over in 2020, greater than the proportions expected in Sweden and West Germany. The comparable proportion expected in the US is 22.6 percent and in the UK is 26.2 percent.[4]

The Japanese plan is part of a general set of policies, including income security, employment, lifelong learning, and housing, as well as health services and welfare. A prominent feature is support of family caregivers, chiefly women, in a way that permits them to continue in paid employment away from home during working hours. The plan exemplifies attempts to systematize and balance the institutional and community-based aspects of comprehensive geriatrics, the social and medical components, and the housing and family considerations. Other distinctions include systematic development of personnel and facilities, particularly in the community, and a tripling of spending in the 1990's compared with the 1980's. Day care services, including functional training, will be provided in 10,000 centers in 1999 compared with 1,780 in 1990. The program will encourage the development of "domiciliary care support" centers, offering home visiting, counseling, and care coordination. In 1989 there were no centers. Today there are 300, and the plan calls for 10,000 in 1999.

The prevention and minimization of illness and disability are among the chief goals of the plan. It calls for primary prevention, rehabilitation, and prosthetics extending to housing and other environmental modifications to assist mobility and other functioning.

Other elements of the plan include measures to promote morale among elders ("provide the aged with something to live for"), through jobs, sports, and social activities. The plan provides for developing volunteers, and promoting gerontological research.

The US, where per capita health care expenditures are highest in the world, has a fragmented health care delivery system with little coordination between acute and long-term care. Furthermore, geriatrics and gerontology are underrepresented in biomedical and epidemiologic research and training of research personnel. At this writing, it is unclear how the burgeoning managed care industry in the US will affect both acute and long-term care delivery for older people. Currently, only

10 percent of Medicare beneficiaries are enrolled in managed care plans. That number is expected to grow rapidly in the next 5 to 10 years, however.

In the US, a novel approach to integrating services is the social and health maintenance organization, or SHMO, which are being tested at different sites and under different auspices. They combine the basic hospital and medical services of the health maintenance organization (HMO) with a limited set of custodial care benefits at home and in the nursing home. The key SHMO feature is "case management", or care coordination; this offers families advice and service up to a certain limit. The SHMO pools funds from Medicare (basically an acute-care program for virtually all elders) and Medicaid (acute- and long-term care for poor persons). For the long-term care benefits, the non-poor participants pay an amount above Medicare user fees. Because the geriatric advantages of the SHMOs cannot be widely understood without educational effort, and because of the need to compete with conventional commercial insurance plans (filling in the gaps in Medicare payments), SHMOs have achieved solvency with difficulty. They might thrive, however, under broad public insurance (e.g., expansions of Medicare, as some have advocated, into long-term care).

In 1990, a Congressional commission advocated a geriatrics-informed plan for universal coverage of long-term care through social insurance, with a supplementary role for private insurance. Some 1.5 million or more commercial insurance policies have been sold. These policies offer indemnity payments for individuals determined by physicians (who need not have any geriatrics expertise) to need nursing home care. An assessment of patient needs may be invoked by the commercial insurer as a check on physician judgment.

The features of long-term care programs in developed nations may not be useful in developing countries without extensive adjustment for the cultural and socioeconomic contexts. It could be argued that many of the difficulties of establishing sound patterns of family-based long-term care in developed countries could be avoided if developing nations guarded against undermining communities and families as they adapt to industrialization. Long-term care, rarely highly technical, may remain safely in trained, lay hands. Perhaps the best approach is to retain as much of long-term care as possible within existing family structures and communities.

International Aging Organizations

The Maltese ophthalmologist and politician, Vincent Tabone, observed the rising numbers and proportions of older persons and encouraged Malta to become a major proponent of discussion and action in the United Nations concerning population aging. Similar observations about the US were made by American legislators led by Senator Frank Church and Representative Claude Pepper in the 1970s. As a result of these and other efforts, the United Nations called a World Assembly on Aging (UNWAA) for 1982. This 2-week conclave of 123 nations authorized an International Plan of Action on Aging.[18]

Many persons have been disappointed by the lack of governmental or private sector response to the UNWAA and its plan. However, there have been some developments. One was the creation in Malta of the United Nations International Institute on Aging. The institute is directed to applied research and training, with emphasis on the Third World. Malta is well positioned to concern itself with the developing world. The southernmost point of Europe in the Mediterranean, Malta is 70 miles north of Africa. It also has cultural and historic ties to the Middle East.

Following the UNWAA, the World Health Organization began to strengthen its global program on aging, relocating its offices from Copenhagen to the WHO headquarters in Geneva. The US National Institute on Aging developed an international research effort. A private sector group, the American Association on International Aging, was created. Already on the scene was the International Federation on Aging spearheaded by Age Concern in Great Britain and partially financed by the American Association of Retired Persons. The International Association of Gerontology, meeting quadrennially, brings both research and policy concerns to its member societies. Among other nations showing great interest in population aging were the Dominican Republic and Costa Rica.

The care and financing of older populations are complex topics of study. Universities and other organizations in various parts of the world are engaged in biological, medical, and behavioral research on processes of aging and age-related diseases. The impact of population aging upon social institutions, on the one hand, and the impact of changing institutions on the lives of older people, on the other, are equally important concerns in the social sciences, public administration, economics, and public policy.

In 1990, the International Longevity Center (ILC) was founded with units in New York City and Japan. The ILC is the only nonpartisan, nonprofit organization devoted exclusively to the study of worldwide population aging and its impact on individuals, families, societies, and their institutions. As of this writing, there are three ILCs: ILC (US), ILC (Japan), and ILC (France) that work separately and collaboratively on a variety of projects in the areas of economics, medicine, ethics, and demography.

Conclusion

In meeting the challenges of health care and productive aging, roles must be played by the individual, family, community, employers, and government.[20] The individual has the responsibility to maintain good health habits, to develop and protect personal economic resources, and to contribute to the social and physical environment that all share. The family's role is to assist disabled family members of all ages. The community can help provide opportunities for productive expression and access to health and housing services of good quality.

Employers and unions have responsibilities for maintaining healthful working conditions and negotiating practical pension and health care arrangements for employees of all ages. And finally, government needs to assure a basic floor of economic security for all its citizens and provide opportunities for older people to remain contributing members of society for as long as possible.

Note: The authors are based in the International Longevity Center (US), Department of Geriatrics and Adult Development, Mount Sinai School of Medicine, New York.

References

1. World Health Organization. World Health Statistics Annual 1994. World Health Organization, Geneva, 1995
2. Kinsella K, Taeuber C: An Aging World II. U.S. Census Bureau, International Population Reports, P25, 92–93. Government Printing Office, Washington DC, 1993
3. Hobbs F, Damon B: 65 + in the United States. U.S. Census Bureau, Current Population Reports, P23, 190. Government Printing Office, Washington DC, 1996
4. Muller C: Social Adjustment to Longevity: The Search for Indicators (Almanac Phase II). International Longevity Center (U.S.), New York, 1996
5. Achenbaum WA: Social Security: Visions and Revisions. Cambridge University Press, Cambridge, 1986
6. Kinsella K, Gist Y: Older Workers Retirement, and Pensions: A Comparative International Chartbook. U.S. Census Bureau, IPC/95-2. Government Printing Office, Washington, DC, 1995
7. Crichton-Browne J: The Prevention of Senility. Macmillan, New York, 1905
8. U.S. Bureau of the Census, International Data Base.
9. Long-Term Outlook Committee, Economic Council, Economic Planning Agency: Japan in the Year 2000: Preparing Japan for an Age of Internationalization, the Aging Society, and Maturity. The Japan Times, Tokyo, 1983
10. Svanborg A: Environmental Influences on Aging. In Butler RN, Gleason HP (eds): Productive Aging: Enhancing Vitality in Later Life. Springer, New York, 1985
11. Butler RN, Schechter M, 1985 Oberlink M (eds): The Promise of Productive Aging. Springer, New York, 1990
12. National Institute on Aging: Toward an Independent Old Age: A National Plan for Research on Aging. NIA, Bethesda, MD, 1982
13. Schulz JH: The Economics of Aging, Sixth Ed. Auburn House, Dover, MA, 1995
14. U.S. Senate Special Committee on Aging: *Personnel Practices for an Aging Workforce: Private Sector Examples*. Washington, DC, 1985
15. Schwab T (ed): Caring for an Aging World: International Models for Long-Term Care, Financing and Delivery. McGraw-Hill, New York, 1989
16. Moss B: Long-term care for the elderly in Australia. p. 242. Schwab, Schwab T (ed): Caring for an Aging World: International Models for Long-term Care, Financing and Delivery. McGraw-Hill, New York, 1989
17. Liang J, Gu S: Long-term care for the elderly in China. pp. 284–285. In Schwab T (ed): Caring for an Aging World: International Models for Long-Term Care, Financing and Delivery. McGraw-Hill, New York, 1989
18. Oriol WE: Aging in All Nations: A Special Report on the United Nations World Assembly on Aging. Washington, DC, 1982
19. Butler RN, Kükuni K: Who is Responsible for My Old Age? Springer, New York, 1993
20. Velkoff V, Kinsella K: Aging in Eastern Europe and the Former Soviet Union. U.S. Census Bureau, P9S/93-1. Government Printing Office, Washington DC, 1993

CHAPTER 105

Health Promotion and Physical Activity

DAVID C. KENNIE
SUSIE DINAN
ARCHIE YOUNG

Health Promotion

Although there is significant overlap between the two concepts, health promotion and disease prevention are not synonymous. They have different goals and use different strategies to improve health. Traditional preventive care has taken place within health services and has concentrated on the primary and secondary prevention of disease. Health promotion, however, has a wider remit. Just as "health" is more than the mere absence of disease,[1] so "health promotion" is more than the prevention or avoidance of disease. Essentially, health promotion aims for the personal development of people toward a better understanding and control of their own health and positive well-being. Its strategies often focus on society and on the environment.[2–4]

This broad approach demands a multiagency, intersectoral approach with much activity outside the traditional health arena. Nevertheless, elderly people need both preventive care and health promotion. It is essential that the health professions become fully engaged in both. Indeed, if the medical profession were to adopt a truly holistic approach, the terms preventive medicine and health promotion would be seen as merely the ends of a spectrum of interventions. Such a unified approach would deliver the many benefits of appropriate medical care and would also recognize the value of the medical care process as a major channel for the delivery of certain aspects of health promotion.

Although this chapter concentrates on the health promotion end of that spectrum, the authors' intention is that it will be a step toward a broad-based, unified approach to the full spectrum of health promotion and disease prevention.

A Multidimensional Model

Health has been defined by the World Health Organization (WHO) as a "state of complete physical, mental and social wellbeing".[1] Taken to its extreme, however, this means that the giving of almost any physical goods could be justified as a health promotion strategy, provided it kept the recipient satisfied.

A more realistic model of health in old age says that it depends on a matrix of an intrinsic factor (the individual) and three interwoven extrinsic factors: freedom from disease, optimal functional status (physical, mental, and social), and an adequate system of social and environmental supports (Fig. 105-1).

It follows that health promotion strategies must be multidimensional. For freedom from disease, the fundamental requirement is equity of access to the full range of acute, rehabilitative, supportive, and preventive medical services. Because the diagnosis, treatment, and prevention of disease are addressed elsewhere, however, this chapter concentrates on the other areas, on examples of improving functional independence, maintaining social supports, and enabling the personal development of older people toward taking responsibility for the control of their own health and well-being.

Issues Relating to Functional Status

Poor Mobility and Falls

Safe mobility is the cornerstone of independent physical functioning and strategies to promote this are essential components of health promotion for an elderly population. Fall prevention is discussed in Chapter 95 and the functional benefits of physical activity are considered in more detail later in this chapter.

Impaired Social Functioning

Many older people experience a reduction in their level of social functioning. This occurs as a result of bereavement, weakness, fatigue, and the "ecological gap"[5] (i.e., the demands made by urban environments on a relatively disabled population, who may have difficulty walking distances, may no longer own a car, and may feel unsafe on the streets after dark). Local government must, therefore, support and promulgate models of urban planning that take into account the needs of older people and facilitate social integration.

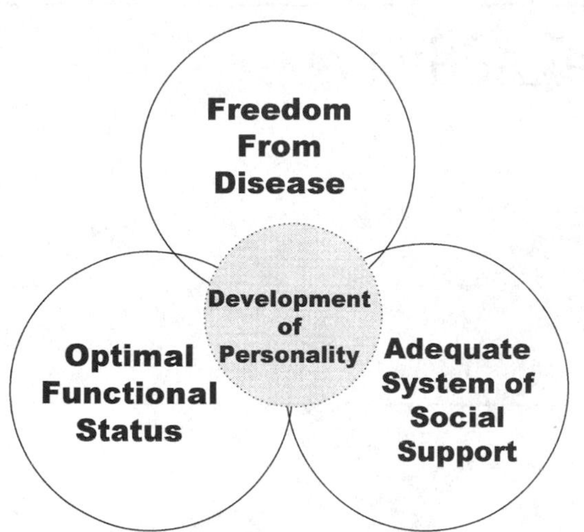

Figure 105-1 Matrix of domains determining health and well-being in old age.

The promotion of social functioning

A supportive environment
- Spaced out regular sitting areas
- Conveniently located public toilets
- Effective community policing
- Street lighting
- Home security and alarm provision
- Personal attack alarms
- Victim support schemes

Transport and access
- Traffic management for older pedestrians and drivers
- Access to public buildings
- Ramped curbs
- Convenient public transport
- Dial-a-lift services

Leisure
- Mobile library services
- Library services in long-term care
- Large print and audio books
- Information services relevant for elderly people
- Opportunities for physical recreation (see Box 5)

Continuing education
- Preretirement education courses
- Self-education groups
- Curriculum development for services to retired people
- University of the Third Age

Motoring Accidents

The rate of crashes, the severity of injuries and the mortality rates (standardized for distance driven) all rise dramatically after age 60, and especially after 75 years of age.[6] Visual, perceptual, and cognitive impairments are important factors.

Various targeting strategies have been employed to identify those at risk. These include self-reporting of illness, medical examination, simulated driving experiences, and traffic recognition tests. None, however, is as informative as testing driving ability on the road. While regular retesting of drivers after a specific age threshold would seem a sensible option, it raises important issues of civil liberty. It would also have an adverse effect on the barred drivers' level of social functioning. It is important, therefore, that it is not introduced without clear evidence of its effectiveness as a measure to reduce major trauma, especially as there is some Scandinavian evidence that it may merely result in an increased number of equally severe pedestrian-related car accidents.

Issues Relating to the Support System

Economic and Social Marginalization

Financial security is not only important in itself, it is also a prerequisite for access to healthy choices in lifestyle.[2] Older people make up the largest low income group in the UK, with one-half of all pensioner households depending on their state pension for 75 percent of their income.[7] This has serious implications for their health; poverty, or more precisely, relative poverty, shows a clear association not just with mortality in old age, but with increased morbidity in terms of chronic conditions and deteriorating functional status (Fig. 105-2).[8]

The traditional response has been to lobby government to ensure that elderly people are given an adequate basic pension and, if necessary, additional welfare benefits. This safety net is important, but cannot be relied upon for future generations of older people; such pensions threaten the fiscal integrity of most nations with an aging society. Social disadvantage may result from both the stigma of having left the workforce and constraints imposed by lack of money.

A task of health promotion may, therefore, be to educate middle-aged and elderly people into the techniques of once again generating their own income, probably not through employment, but perhaps through home-based businesses, made possible through technological improvements in communication. For this to be effective, however, some disincentives must be removed from the income tax structure. Alternatively, government might consider a greater financial acknowledgement of the role of older people as caregivers.

Social marginalization is also caused by geographic, cultural, and linguistic barriers and by ageism, which is pervasive within society. Health promotion measures to counteract agism within the health services include: professional education on the opportunities in caring for older people, legal action on

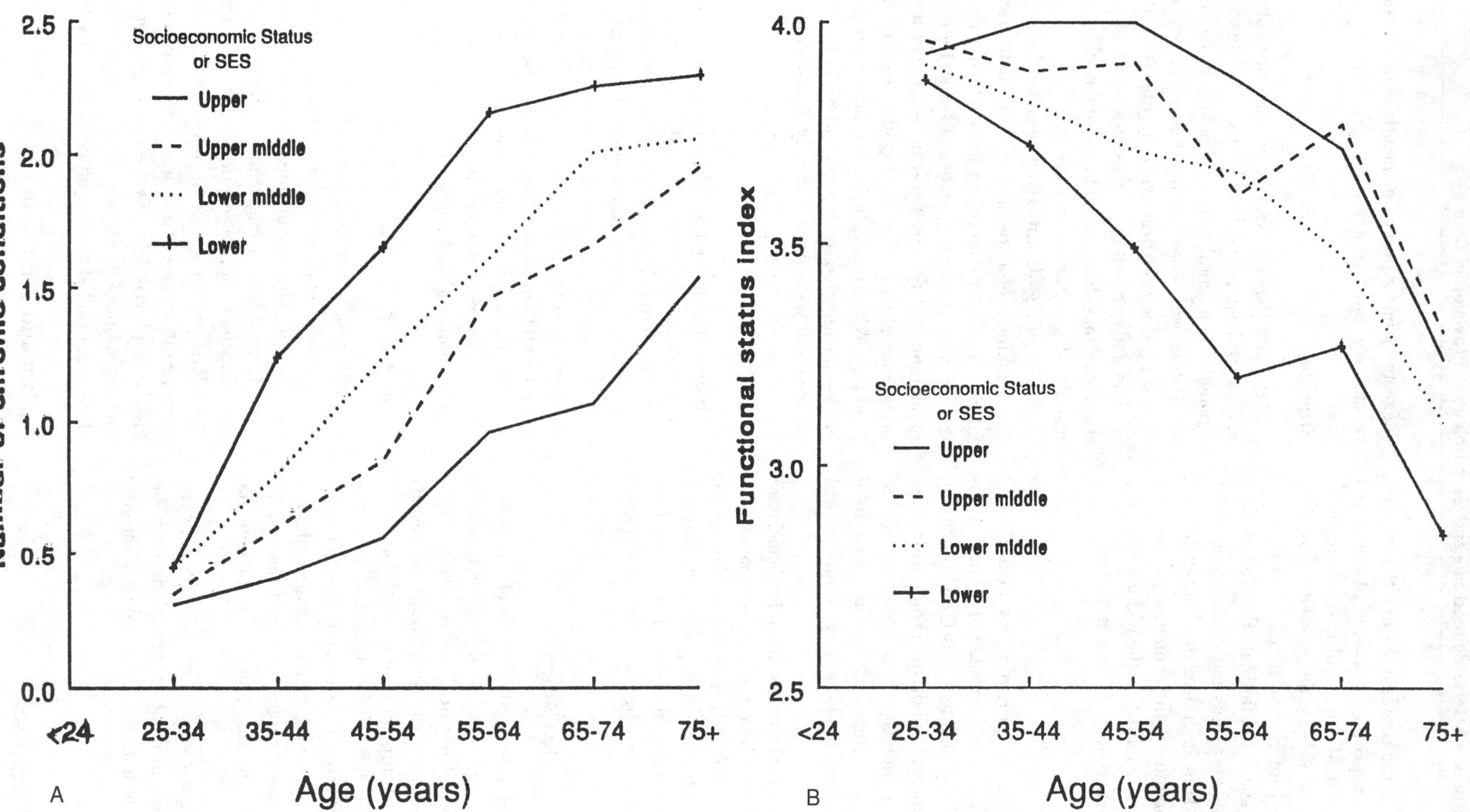

Figure 105-2 Relationship between socioeconomic status and health at different ages. **(A)** Chronic conditions; **(B)** functional status. (From House, et al.,[8] with permission.)

age-related discrimination in the provision of health care, and greater participation by older people in service planning and policy making. Initiatives outside the health sector include: positive media stereotypes of old people, a greater "political voice" for older people, and intergenerational projects.

Health promotion must strive to eliminate the marginalization of elderly people and foster their inclusion in the wider concept of "community". This includes: the household, the family, the institutional community, the community of interest, the community of faith, the neighborhood, the wider geographic community, and the political process of community.

Substandard Housing

Housing is a key element in providing for health, well-being, and independence, yet nearly one-half of all unfit properties are occupied by elderly people.[3] Substandard housing leads to: illness from dampness, hypothermia from inadequate heating and draughts, problems of access and being housebound from inadequate design, falls and accidents from problems of layout, and frustration and anxiety from the need for repair.

Effective health promotion strategies include: home care and repair schemes, gardening chore workers, heating and insulation strategies, and the installation of aids and adaptations. Strategies aimed at allowing the elderly inhabitant to stay put and avoid unnecessary moves are also effective and include the provision of personal and domestic care services and community alarm systems.

Stress and Burden on Family Caregivers

The impact of the caring role on the health of family and other informal caregivers can be considerable. Several studies attest to a significant degree of physical and psychological ill health. Caregiving also involves a degree of financial penalty and may place intolerable strains on family relationships.

Regrettably, the identification of the impact of the caring role on caregivers is a skill infrequently taught to health care professionals. Most rely on open-ended and unstructured interviews. Identification can, however, be enhanced through the use of validated measurement instruments for burden and stress.[9]

Health promotion strategies such as day and respite care, counseling, and skill training prolong the period of time informal caregivers are willing to undertake that role and improve caregivers' well-being.[10]

Issues Relating to Personal Development

Unhealthy Lifestyle Practices

In younger adults, there is a correlation between lifestyle and morbidity. In cross-sectional studies, this association is sometimes less clear for elderly people.[3] Nevertheless, considerable scientific evidence, including some prospective studies, suggests scope for promoting health by addressing key lifestyle practices in older people.

Smoking

Although the relative risk of total mortality from smoking may fall with age, considerable evidence attests to its still being a potentially harmful activity. Smoking has a well-documented correlation with coronary heart disease; peripheral vascular disease; chronic obstructive lung disease; lung, pancreatic, bladder and cervical cancer; osteoporosis; loss of body weight; decreased muscle strength; functional decline; skin wrinkling; macular degeneration; and fire risk.[3]

Although significant advantages can be achieved by quitting smoking even in old age, and although strategies of proven efficacy (such as counseling those at high risk coupled with the use of nicotine gum/patches) do exist, their use in this older population is still poor. Nevertheless, the cost-effectiveness of brief counseling advice on stopping smoking appears to be a good buy. When made during routine doctor-patient contact it has been estimated to be $950 and $1,411 per life-year saved for men and women, respectively, aged 65 to 69 years.[11]

Poor diet

Improved nutrition for older people continues to hold out much promise for improved health, but the reality from controlled trials has been more limited. For example, recent attempts at the primary prevention of various types of cancer with β carotene and antioxidants has been unimpressive. A different area of nutritional interest for promoting health of the older population is in those who are dependent for feeding (e.g., in nursing homes and hospitals) and around times of illness or surgical intervention.[12] Further discussion of nutrition is contained in Chapter 63.

Poor Health Literacy

Older people may lack the skills necessary to gain access to or to understand and use information in ways that promote good health. This might impair motivation to adopt healthy lifestyle practices or might impede the safe and effective use of medications. Improved esteem and self-worth can empower the elderly person to have the necessary confidence to become more health literate. Specific health education programs may also be employed, tailoring their messages for greatest impact. The promotion of health literacy also requires the development of personal and shared resources for self care.

Ageism and Self Worth

Many elderly people have a relatively low opinion of their value to society. Perhaps more than any, they hold ageist attitudes. These perceptions arise from many factors: their cultural inheritance, low income, social marginalization, boredom, and loneliness. These negative perceptions of self-worth delay self-referral for illness and disability, diminish advocacy and control, and reduce motivation to seek positive resources for health.

Many, very varied, factors can maintain self-esteem. They range from gainful and income-generating activity, through socialization, to a rewarding sex life. Participation on health planning and implementation groups can improve the sense of control. Elderly people also need more positive images of old age, providing a vision of what might be possible. Unless as a society we allow older people a dream of what old age can be like at its most favorable, we will continue with ageist stereotypes and with old people themselves assuming little responsibility or drive for their own future. Perhaps most of all, elderly people need positive affirmation by all sectors of society, from government to loved ones, of a belief in their value as human beings.

Adapting to Loss and Imminent Death

In the final analysis, every elderly person has to adapt to various sorts of loss and to the imminence of death. The ability to do this successfully and with dignity is the final life goal.[13] It largely depends on intrinsic coping skills acquired through life, but may be enhanced by open communication with loved ones and society at large and by freedom from pain and distress in the dying trajectory.

Tasks

If health promotion is to be effective for the elderly population, a large number of tasks need to be performed by many sectors of society, both individually and collectively (see accompanying box). Some tasks specific to the health services are considered further.

Tasks for Health Services

Public health professionals can assist purchasers of health care to buy an appropriate mix of health services that will have maximum impact on the health of an older population. Broad-based strategies that minimize the functional consequences of disease are as important as treatment modalities for specific disease processes. While many of these decisions will be evidence-based, it is important to realize that lack of evidence of efficacy is not the same as evidence of lack of efficacy and should not necessarily deter the adoption of a health promotion strategy that appears intuitively correct simply because sufficient research has, as yet, not been conducted on it.

Public health professionals, in the UK at least, have responsibility for assessing the local needs of their elderly communities. This presents the opportunity to develop a countrywide database on the current health, function, and social dependence of identifiable elderly populations, preferably using standardized measurement instruments and including sufficient data to permit the longitudinal measurement of disability-free life expectancy. In conjunction with local government, public health professionals might also produce a community health report that would include the current status of housing, transport, community security measures, leisure and sports activities, and continuing education for older residents.

Purchasers of health care can use the contracting process to ensure that effective medical services are available, accessible, and equitable. This applies to acute services, rehabilitation services, and also to primary care. They can use their financial leverage to promote a more holistic approach, for example by removing barriers between specialisms and between agencies.

Health purchasers should also review their relationships with nonhealth funding agencies. Barriers between funding agencies commonly result in perverse financial rulings that, overall, cost more money for the nation and are detrimental to the health of elderly people.

Health providers can assist in the promotion of health by adopting multidimensional, problem-orientated case records that take account not just of biomedical data, but of functional dependence and social support. The skills of staff, such as community nurses, should be expanded to include techniques to screen for visual and hearing impairment, physical functioning, cognitive status, depression, and caregiver burden and stress. Mouth care and foot care can be enhanced by developing a cadre of assistants for such purposes working as part of a team with the relevant fully trained professional. Bereavement counseling skills should be a required part of training for key personnel working in long-term care institutions. Health providers can collaborate with social services to ensure: an interagency policy on elder abuse, a comprehensive health assessment as part of more generalized assessment for long-term care (e.g., the US National Resident Assessment Instrument), the development of an agreed package of health promotional measures for implementation upon referral for social day care or on admission to long-term care.

The appointment of health promotion facilitators into community and primary care services specifically to educate and manage health promotion may also do much to advance the strategies adopted locally. This has certainly been the experience with traditional preventive care measures.[14]

Assessing Issues and Strategies

In order to safeguard essentially healthy people from unnecessary interference and disruption to lifestyle, to safeguard them from iatrogenic insult, and to prevent unnecessary costs to individuals and to society, health promotion strategies should be reviewed against the following criteria, originally evolved critically to examine the prevention of biomedical disorders,[15] but which have equal relevance to the broader aspects of health promotion.

Importance of the Problem

This needs to be considered first in terms of the older person's suffering, from functional disability, other morbidity, and mortality. The degree of burden that the problem imposes on caregivers and its impact on society in general are also important, because of their adverse effects both on society's views of elderly people, and also on the elderly individual's own sense of worth and well-being.

Detection of the Problem

Detection takes many forms. In primary and secondary prevention the priority issue is to refine the accuracy of identification of those individuals at risk of, or with, the particular health problem. For tertiary prevention, improved detection depends first on increasing the awareness of health care professionals that there might be a problem at all.

Effectiveness of Intervention

The Canadian Task Force on the Periodic Health Examination and the United States Preventive Services Task Force have scientifically scrutinized the effectiveness of many preventive care and health promotion strategies.[15] It is largely upon their criteria that evidence-based medicine is now founded.

Intervention in the Real World

Although a strategy may appear effective in a randomized controlled trial, it may not work in the real world. For it to be transportable out of the scientific setting, the populations under consideration must be similar, adequate resources must be available, compliance by elderly people and their caregivers must be likely, and ethical considerations in care should not be likely to bar progress.

Cost

Despite popular misconception, the scientific evidence suggests that the majority of health promotion strategies add to costs rather than create savings.[16,17] Wherever possible, therefore, the assessment of any health promotion strategy should include scrutiny of cost-effectiveness.

The Optimal Time for Implementation

Health promotion measures should be employed on a life-cycle approach optimizing their implementation to the time in life when most benefit can be achieved. The life-cycle idea is rooted in the concept that success or failure at previous life stages can play an important role in determining the probability of success in progressive life transitions.

Physical Function and Aging
Physical Activity as a Health Promotion Strategy

The decline in physical abilities with increasing age poses important challenges to older people and the ability to perform comfortably and safely everyday activities is central to well-being. This is partly through the aesthetic satisfaction of optimal physical function, but perhaps more through the importance of physical function for autonomous and wide-ranging social function. The adoption of a lifestyle that incorporates the necessary physical activities, therefore, is potentially a very important element of personal health promotion.[18] Its justification and requirements are now considered, along the lines suggested above.

Age-Related Changes in Physical Function

Strength

From middle age onward, there is a steady loss of muscle mass with increasing age. This results in a progressive and substantial loss of strength. Even in the absence of symptomatic or diagnosed disease, people aged 65 to 89 years show differences in strength consistent with the loss of strength at some 1 to 2 percent per year.[19] (See also Ch. 79).

The muscular cachexia (or "sarcopenia") of aging has sometimes been attributed to a reducing level of habitual physical activity with increasing age. This explanation is unconvincing, however, as it leaves unexplained the similar age-related decline in performance seen in elite, veteran sportsmen competing in strength events.

The loss of muscle is principally a reduction in the number of muscle fibers. This, in turn, is associated with a reduced number of motoneurones. It seems likely that the sarcopenia of aging is due to a slowly progressive denervation, incompletely compensated by an increase in the size of the remaining motor units.[20–22]

In addition to the reduction in the number of muscle fibers, there may also be a reduction in the size of the remaining muscle fibers, especially in the presence of pathology, following immobilization, and in advanced old age.[20–22] Unlike the reduction in the number of muscle fibers, this may be amenable to improvement by increased activity.[23,24]

Power

"Strength" and "power" are not synonymous. "Strength" refers to force (or torque). "Power," the rate of performing work, is calculated as the product of force and speed. Age-related differences in explosive power observed in healthy elderly subjects are equivalent to a loss of 3 to 4 percent per year.[19] Similarly, differences in power between healthy elderly people and patients of the same age are much greater than the differences in strength.

The weaker a muscle, the slower the contraction it must

make to overcome an unchanged external resistance. As a result, power is reduced not only to the same degree as strength, but also as a result of an enforced shift to a less favorable point on the power-velocity relationship. The greater the required force in relation to the muscle's maximal strength, the more pronounced is this "extra" deficit in power.[25]

Endurance

The ability to perform prolonged dynamic exercise without fatigue or discomfort depends on the percentage of the individual's maximal aerobic power (maximal oxygen uptake, or $\dot{V}O_2max$) required for the activity. $\dot{V}O_2max$ declines with increasing age, at approximately the same rate as, and perhaps partly because of, the loss of muscle mass.[26,27] The contribution of the gradual age-related reduction in maximal heart rate is still a matter for debate. The age-related decline in the performances of elite veteran endurance athletes indicates that the age-related decline in $\dot{V}O_2max$ cannot be explained as merely the result of habitual inactivity.

Functional Consequences

Strength and Power

A young person's strength includes a generous safety margin, but even healthy elderly people have strength (and power) below, or near to, functionally important thresholds and so have lost, or are in danger of losing, the ability to perform some important everyday tasks.[28–30] Women are weaker than men, both in absolute terms and also in relation to body weight. Their lower power:weight ratios mean that they are functionally vulnerable at least 10 years earlier than men. This helps explain the lower step heights achievable by healthy elderly women.[19,28] It may also contribute to the greater prevalence of disability and of falls among elderly women than among elderly men, and to the age-related decline in the percentage of elderly women using public transport on their own. There is a strong case, therefore, for ensuring that any interventions to improve muscle function are directed at least as strongly to women as to men.

The adverse effect of cooling on muscle power may be especially important in those elderly people who are immobile, thin, and living in poorly heated accommodation, perhaps contributing to the increased incidence of indoor falls and fractures in cold weather.

Endurance

The age-related decline in $\dot{V}O_2max$, especially when combined with the effects of disease, means that many elderly people need only a small further decline to render some everyday activities either impossible or so dependent on anaerobic metabolism as to be unpleasant to perform.[29]

The ability comfortably to sustain a walking speed of perhaps just 3 mph may be lost as a result of the age-related reduction in $\dot{V}O_2max$. This is especially true for women, as a result of their lower $\dot{V}O_2max$. For aerobic power, as for explosive power, a woman is functionally disadvantaged in weight-bearing activities (compared to a man of the same age) by her lower power:weight ratio. In very elderly female patients, even just sitting still may demand such a high proportion of $\dot{V}O_2max$ that this apparently trivial activity cannot be sustained for more than 2 to 3 hours at a time.[31]

Suppleness

In patients with arthritis, more than 120 degrees of shoulder abduction are necessary to wash hair without difficulty.[32] In the English National Fitness Survey (a representative sample of noninstitutionalized people), there was a gradual reduction in the mean range of shoulder abduction with increasing age, which was somewhat more pronounced in the women. More than a quarter of the men aged 75 and over and more than one-third of the women aged 75 and over had a range of shoulder abduction below this functional threshold.

Detecting the Need for Intervention

Although the benefits of physical training for the performance of everyday tasks do not become prominent until late middle age, increased physical activity brings other health benefits throughout life.[33] The promotion of physical activity is, therefore, a population-based intervention, from which older people must not be excluded. Population data on the strength, power, endurance, and suppleness of older people are invaluable, not so much to detect those who need the intervention, but to identify those who are likely to be most receptive to a promotional message based on the preservation of functional abilities.

Effectiveness of Physical Training

Psychosocial Impact

Physical activity relieves anxiety and mild depression, at least in younger adults. It can also improve short-term alertness.[34,35] Recreational exercise offers important opportunities for socialization and socially acceptable, nonclinical, physical contact.

Prevention of Disease

Habitual physical activity protects against conditions important in old age, notably osteoporosis, noninsulin-dependent diabetes mellitus (NIDDM), hypertension, ischemic heart disease, stroke, and probably also colonic cancer.[33,36–38]

Impact on Disability

Physical function depends on strength, power, endurance, coordination (including balance), and suppleness. Even in the absence of disease, these attributes are all eroded with increasing age, but all can be improved by appropriate physical training. Disability can even be ameliorated in the presence of established disease (e.g., in angina, claudication, airflow limitation).

Strength, power, and related functional ability

Training by maximal or near maximal muscle contractions produces improvements in strength and power. Typically, strength training might comprise 2 to 3 sets of 6 to 12 muscle contractions at perhaps greater than 70 percent of maximal strength, for each muscle group. The weakness of old age, however, means that this can be achieved with very little in the way of specialized equipment. Indeed, just body weight can be used to good effect.[30,40]

In randomized controlled trials, both healthy[39] and frail[41] elderly people (mean age 80 and over) following progressive-resistance, strength-training programs experienced improvements similar (in percentage terms) to those expected in much younger subjects. Unfortunately, there is no evidence that strength training halts the underlying loss of muscle fibers. Nevertheless, even if strength continues to be lost at some 1 to 2 percent per year, an improvement in isometric strength of, say, 20 to 25 percent is still equivalent to a substantial "rejuvenation" of strength.

Training-induced improvements in strength and power may result in improvement in selected functional abilities,[39,41] but functional gains are more likely if the performance of strengthening exercises is accompanied by practice of the specific functional skills.[42]

Endurance and related functional ability

Up to 70 years of age, it seems that a 10 to 20 percent improvement in $\dot{V}O_2max$ can be expected from endurance training.[43] New data suggest that even beyond 80 years of age, a meaningful reduction in the strain of submaximal exercise can be expected (Malbut-Shennan KE, Dinan SM, Verhaar H, Young A: personal communication, 1996). Functional benefit in everyday life, however, cannot be assumed, no matter how likely it seems. This is an important area for further research.

Balance

Evidence is now emerging that not only is balance improved by balance training,[44] but that it may even result in fewer falls.[45] Strength training may also contribute to improved balance.[46]

Promoting Physical Activity in the Real World

Merely advocating a nonspecific increase in habitual activity is unlikely to do much to encourage the patterns of exercise that might be expected to have substantial training effects. More specific advice is required, especially for strengthening exercise, and would be welcomed by older people themselves. A simple guide to strengthening exercise suitable for older people[47] distributed in the UK through the research charity "Research into Ageing" has uncovered a high level of demand.

The content of a fitness program suitable for older people includes all the elements common to any general fitness program, but with particular emphasis on the areas set out in the accompanying box and with appropriate adjustment of speed, intensity and content.

The widespread adoption of a combination of recreational brisk walking, swimming, and selected exercises (for flexibility and strengthening) would benefit most older people. There is also considerable scope for improving the independent use of recreational sports facilities. In addition, many seniors would welcome the opportunity to participate in a supervised exercise group, for guidance, for encouragement, and for socialization. The design and supervision of a seniors' exercise group are specialized skills. Efforts to increase the number of such groups, and to ensure enjoyment, effectiveness, and safety, should include insistence that group leaders hold an appropriate specialist qualification (see below).

Safety

Physical activity is not without its potential hazards. For most participants, the benefits greatly outweigh the hazards. Nevertheless, it is essential that everything possible is done to ensure the optimal balance between benefits and hazards

Principal components of a fitness program for seniors

As for any age group
- Progressive
- Regular
- Balanced
- Enjoyable
- Strength
- Endurance
- Flexibility
- Coordination
- All major muscle groups
- Full ranges of movement

Also, specifically for older people . . .
- Load the bones
- Target postural and pelvic floor muscles
- Target functional movements
- Develop body awareness and balance skills
- Cater for a wider range of
  - Initial activity levels
  - Disabilities and pathologies
  - Personal goals
- Injury prevention a higher priority

for each individual. This is especially true for those participants most at risk of adverse events. This requires the accurate identification of those for whom the standard exercise advice requires modification or who warrant some other precaution.

Safety also requires that the intensity of the activity can be accurately judged and controlled, ensuring an intensity high enough to produce benefit, but not so high as to be unduly hazardous.

Furthermore, it must be possible to meet both these requirements despite the considerable heterogeneity encountered in an unselected group of older people. The unfortunate, stereotyping effect of the expression "the elderly" encourages the assumption that all those aged over 65 are similar. On the contrary, the assessment of potential participants and of their responses to exercise must be able to take account of considerable diversity in age, initial fitness levels, and coincidental chronic diseases. An important priority should now be the development of evidence-based guidelines (or the validation of suitable existing guidelines) for a demedicalized approach to enjoyable, safe, and effective physical activity. In the meantime, in the absence of direct evidence, those responsible for giving exercise advice and for supervising exercise groups, as discussed below, must be more knowledgeable and more skilled than those working with younger groups.

Assessment of potential participants

Such guidelines as exist not only lack evidence of efficacy, but are also open to two other important criticisms. They were devised originally to have a high specificity for the identification of "safe" exercisers, but this is achieved only by excluding the majority of potential participants. What is actually required is an approach that excludes no one but, instead, indicates how each individual may enjoy effective exercise with the greatest safety.

Many existing guidelines identify those potential participants who supposedly should be advised to seek medical advice before increasing their habitual level of physical activity. The Canadian Physical Activity Readiness Questionnaire (PAR-Q) is often used in this way, although it was not devised for this purpose. Yet there is little to guide the doctor when faced with the potential exerciser. The Physical Activity Readiness Examination (PAR-X) was devised as an aide-memoir for primary care physicians confronted by people identified by the PAR-Q as requiring medical review before they would perform an unsupervised exercise test. For the moment, it would seem reasonable also to use it with those considering an increased level of habitual activity, but there is no evidence of its efficacy for this purpose, or even of the value of any medical involvement. Furthermore, if potentially important abnormalities are identified, what action should be taken? Whereas the exclusion of such an individual would have been a sufficient and appropriate response when the PAR-X was being used for its original purpose, this is not sufficient when the purpose of medical involvement is to enable participation. The doctor's role in assessment should be as an adviser (guiding the potential exerciser—see accompanying box) and not as a gatekeeper (barring the way to participation).

Ensuring safety–the doctor's responsibilities in fitness for seniors

- Able to recognize a well-run group
- Identify disorders that are present
- Ensure their accurate communication
  - To exerciser
  - By exerciser to others
- Educate exerciser
  - To recognize normal responses
  - To respect abnormal responses
  - About their medication

Assessment of exercise intensity

There is a "window" of exercise intensity for the optimal balance between benefit and hazard. As a result of the decline in maximal oxygen uptake with increasing age, the older the participants, the smaller the window and the more accurate the control of exercise intensity must be.

Pulse counting is still widely used in an attempt to monitor, and so control, the intensity of self-paced exercise. There are several reasons why this is usually futile. It is rarely accurate and the relationship between the "immediate" postexercise heart rate and the exercising heart rate is inconsistent.[48] Furthermore, even if pulse rate could be reliably monitored, the intensity rating still depends on knowing the individual's maximal heart rate. However, there is considerable interindividual variation in maximal heart rate among subjects of the same age. (For example, it ranged from 110 to 180 beats per minute in a small group of healthy 80-year-old men.[49]) A useful age-based prediction of maximal heart rate is not possible for an individual, and direct measurement in the laboratory for every potential participant would be completely impracticable. Finally, there is a further problem in the use of the heart rate if the participant is taking digoxin or a β-blocker.

The "talk test" has been suggested as an alternative. This ruled that the ability to converse during exercise indicated that the intensity was not excessive and was based on the supposition that speech during exercise would impose a concurrent additional demand for ventilation.[50] This is now known to be incorrect; speech during exercise is achieved by a temporary *reduction* in ventilation, in order to permit phonation.[51] Moreover, young subjects could still read a test passage even at nearly 90 percent of their predicted maximal heart rate.[51] The degree of respiratory embarrassment during simultaneous speech and exercise may yet provide an aid to the subjective assessment of exercise intensity, but the original concept of the "talk test" cannot be relied upon.

In the end, one must still rely on reasoned, sensible guidelines[52] and, where appropriate, the exercise teacher's observational skills. However, most important of all are the participant's subjective judgment and their ability to "listen to their body," learned during a very gradual increase in exercise intensity from a very low starting level over the first few months of an exercise program. This is not a matter for regret or apology as it is arguably preferable to a more medicalized approach based on pulse-counting. On the other hand, it is important that this approach and the guidelines used should be scientifically validated.

Injury avoidance

To maintain enjoyment and adherence, the avoidance of even minor soft-tissue injuries[53] and the recommendation of adequate rest between activity sessions should have high priority.

Assessment of teachers' competence and knowledge

An approach, such as that outlined above, which aims to exclude virtually no one and which depends on the use of the participant's own judgment for the assessment of exercise intensity, demands excellent communication between participants and their exercise advisors. It also demands that those working with older participants will be aware of the features of conditions likely to be present and of how to adapt their exercise advice accordingly. The coaching, teaching, and programming skills (see accompanying boxes) required to work effectively and safely with older participants are, in many ways, as specialized as those required to work with elite athletes. This has been recognized by some of the professional bodies concerned with physical training.[54]

On the other hand, a true population approach cannot depend upon exercise supervision by a relatively small group of specialist exercise teachers. There just cannot be enough of them. Older people are going to have to take responsibility for maintaining an increased level of habitual physical activity. The specialist teachers' role must evolve into "introduction to exercise" groups, the training of lay seniors as "peer mentors", and the supervision of very highly specialized groups for people with particularly severe disability or unstable disease.

Ensuring safe and successful fitness sessions for seniors–recommendations for teachers

- Emphasize posture and technique
- Give more teaching points and repeat more often
- Give more warning of directional and step changes
- Improve own body language and demonstration skills
- Improve own observation, monitoring, and correction skills
- Offer more choices
- Offer more information
- Be polished and punctual

(Adapted from Young and Dinan,[54] with permission.)

Ensuring successful fitness sessions for seniors–recommendations for programming

- Include older people
  - In planning and staffing
  - In evaluation
  - In promotional material
- First session is an individual assessment
- Progressive and multilevel program
- Mixture of activities
- Ensure essential facilities
- Appropriate scheduling and costing
- Include socialization time

(Adapted from Young & Dinan,[54] with permission.)

Changing Exercise Behavior

In an experimental setting, even a deeply engrained, multifactorial habit, such as customary physical activity, can be changed.[55] It is less clear if this holds true for older people in more realistic settings. There are a few promising early indications.[56–58] On the other hand, at least one study has shown that it cannot be assumed that the beneficial effects identified in tightly supervised research studies will be induced through sustainable, low-cost, "real life" interventions.[59]

Measuring changes in habitual physical activity

Adequate evaluation of strategies to promote physical activity requires a suitable method for the objective measurement of the duration and intensity of episodes of increased activity. Diaries and recall are insufficient. Movement monitors have been used, but may be insensitive to changes in the intensity of exercise. Twenty-four-hour recordings of heart rate have also been used, as a proxy for oxygen consumption, but it is not possible to identify which episodes of tachycardia are due to emotion or to intensive use of small muscle groups and which (the important ones) are due to the intensive use of large muscle groups. Perhaps a combination of the two approaches will prove suitable.

Cost

This chapter has recommended a demedicalized, population-based strategy for the promotion of physical activity, perhaps with an emphasis on walking as the core activity. This approach will have the added advantage of avoiding excessive costs. Nevertheless, adherence will depend on the individual participant finding the activity enjoyable. For many this will mean the use of leisure center facilities, at a cost. Those who wish to join an exercise group with a skilled teacher will have to pay. There may also be equipment and/or clothing costs. There may be medical costs associated with the management of soft tissue injuries.

On the benefit side of the balance, it is hard to know what value to put on subjective well-being, but reasoned estimates can be made of the savings to be expected from reductions in disease, disability, and dependence. Although the estimates are rather vague, exercise promotion among those below retirement age would seem to be a "good buy",[37,60–62] no matter what value is put on the gains in subjective well-being. The economic "bottom line" for encouraging physical activity among older people also seems encouraging[63] but is, as yet, even less securely documented.

The Optimal Time for Implementation

All the evidence to date is that the fitness of elderly people is just as trainable, in relative terms, as that of younger people. The message is simple: it's never too late for potentially beneficial physiologic adaptations in response to increased physical activity.

The crucial question is at what stage in life are people most open to advice about changes in exercise behavior? Unfortunately, little is known about the factors (such as beliefs, attitudes, expected benefits, self-efficacy, educational level) that might influence receptiveness of older people to such advice.[64] Nevertheless, it is appealing to suppose that future generations of seniors will find it easier to become, or remain, physically active in later life if they have been equipped with a suitably broad-based, multiactivity, physical "literacy" during childhood.

Acknowledgment

We are indebted to Tricia Labro for bibliographic assistance.

References

1. World Health Organization: Constitution of the World Health Organization: Annexe 1. The First Ten Years of the World Health Organization. WHO, Geneva, 1958
2. British Geriatrics Society: Health promotion in later life. Issue 1:4/93. In BGS Compendium. British Geriatrics Society, London, 1993
3. Kennie DC: Preventive Care for Elderly People. Cambridge University Press, Cambridge, 1993
4. Anonymous: Health and Well-being: A Guide for Older People. Department of Health, Leeds, 1995
5. Evans JG: A framework for promoting mobility and independence. pp. 1–9. In Towards a Framework for Promoting the Health of Older People. Four Perspectives of the Multiperspective Framework: Workshop Papers, Health Education Authority, London, 1996
6. Malfetti J: Drivers 55 Plus. AAA Foundation for Traffic Safety, Falls Church, Virginia, 1985
7. Teale C: Caring for older people: money problems and financial help. Br Med J 1996;313:288–289
8. House JS, Kessler RC, Herzog AR: Age, socioeconomic status and health. Milbank Q 1990;68:383–411
9. Vitaliano PP, Young HM, Russo J: A review of measures used among caregivers of individuals with dementia. Gerontologist 1991;31:67–75
10. Knight BG, Lutzky SM, Macofsy-Urban F: A meta-analytic review of interventions for caregiver distress: recommendations for future research. Gerontologist 1993;33:240–248
11. Cummings SR, Rubin SM, Oster G: The cost-effectiveness of counselling smokers to quit. J Am Med Assoc 1989;261:75–79
12. Sullivan DH: The role of nutrition in increased morbidity and mortality. In Lipschitz DA (ed): Nutrition, Aging and Age-Dependent Diseases, WB Saunders, Philadelphia, 1995
13. Christiansen D: Dignity in aging: notes on geriatric ethics. J Humanist Psych 1978;18:41–54
14. Dietrich AJ, O'Conner GT, Keliar A: Cancer: improving early detection and prevention. A community practice randomised trial. Br Med J 1992;304:687–691
15. Report of the US Preventive Services Task Force: Guide to Clinical Preventive Services. Williams & Wilkins, Baltimore, 1989
16. Russell LB: Is Prevention Better than Cure? Brookings Institution, Washington DC, 1986
17. Cohen DR, Henderson JB (eds): Health, Prevention and Economics: Oxford University Press, Oxford, 1988
18. Casperson CJ, Powell KE, Merritt RK: Measurement of health status and well-being. pp. 180–202. In Bouchard C, Shephard RJ, Stephens T (eds): Physical Activity, Fitness, and Health: International Proceedings and Consensus Statement. Human Kinetics, Champaign, IL, 1994
19. Skelton DA, Greig CA, Davies JM, Young A: Strength, power and related functional ability of healthy people aged 65–89 years. Age Ageing 1994;23:371–377
20. Young A: Muscle function in old age. New Issues Neurosci 1988;1:141–156
21. Faulkner JA, Brooks SV, Zerba E: Skeletal muscle weakness and fatigue in old age: underlying mechanisms. Annu Rev Gerontol Geriat 1990;10:147–166
22. Lexell J, Taylor CC: Variability in muscle fibre areas in whole human quadriceps muscle: effects of increasing age. J Anat 1991;174:239–249
23. Aniansson A, Grimby G, Hedberg M: Compensatory muscle fiber hypertrophy in elderly men. J Appl Physiol 1992;73: 812–816
24. Klitgaard H, Mantoni M, Schiafino S et al: Function, morphology and protein expression of ageing skeletal muscle: a cross-sectional study of elderly men with different training backgrounds. Acta Physiol Scand 1990;140:41–54

25. Harridge SDR, Young A: Skeletal muscle. In Pathy MSJ (ed): Principles and Practice of Geriatric Medicine. 3rd ed. John Wiley, London, 1997
26. Asmussen E: Aging and exercise. pp. 419–428. In Horvath SM, Yousef MK (eds): Environmental Physiology: Aging, Heat and Altitude. Elsevier North Holland, Amsterdan, 1980
27. Lakatta EG: Hemodynamic adaptations to stress with advancing age. Acta Med Scand 1986;(suppl 711):39–52
28. Levy DI, Young A, Skelton DA, Yeo A-L: Strength, power and functional ability. pp. 85–93. In Passeri M (ed): Geriatrics '94. CIC Edizioni Internazionali, Rome, 1994
29. Young A: Exercise physiology in geriatric practice. Acta Med Scand 1986; (suppl 711):227–232
30. Buchner DM, Larson EB, Wagner EH et al: Evidence for a nonlinear relationship between leg strength and gait speed. Age Ageing 1996;25:386–391
31. Young A: Exercise, fitness and recovery from surgery, disease, or infection. pp. 589–600. In Bouchard C, Shephard RJ, Stephens T et al (eds): Exercise, Fitness and Health: A Consensus of Current Knowledge. Human Kinetics, Champaign, IL, 1990
32. Badley EM, Wagstaff S, Wood PHN: Measures of functional ability (disability) in arthritis in relation to impairment of range of joint movement. Ann Rheum Dis 1984;43:563–569
33. Bouchard C, Shephard RJ, Stephens T (eds): Physical Activity, Fitness, and Health: International Proceedings and Consensus Statement. Human Kinetics, Champaign, Illinois, 1994
34. Chodzko-Zajko W, Moore KA: Physical fitness and cognitive functioning in aging. Exercise Sport Sci Rev 1994;22:195–220
35. Netz Y, Jacob T: Exercise and the psychological state of institutionalized elderly: a review. Percept Motor Skills 1994;79: 1107–1118
36. Powell KE, Blair SN: The public health burdens of sedentary living habits: theoretical but realistic estimates. Med Sci Sports Exerc 1994;26:851–856
37. Pate RR, Pratt M, Blair SN et al: Physical activity and public health. A recommendation from the Centers for Disease Control and Prevention and the American College of Sports Medicine. J Am Med Assoc 1995;273:402–407
38. Blair SN, Franks AL, Shelton et al (eds): Physical Activity and Health: A Report of the Surgeon General. US Department of Health and Human Services, Centers for Disease Control and Prevention, National Center for Chronic Disease Prevention and Health Promotion, Atlanta, 1996
39. Skelton DA, Young A, Greig CA, Malbut KE: Effects of resistance training on strength, power, and selected functional abilities of women aged 75 and older. J Am Geriatr Soc 1995;43: 1081–1087
40. Aniansson A, Gustafsson E: Physical training in elderly men with special reference to quadriceps muscle strength and morphology. Clin Physiol 1981;1:87–98
41. Fiatarone MA, O'Neill EF, Ryan ND et al: Exercise training and nutritional supplementation for physical frailty in very elderly people. N Engl J Med 1994;330:1769–1775
42. Skelton DA, McLaughlin AW: Training functional ability in old age. Physiotherapy 1996;82:159–167
43. Greig C, Young A: Aerobic exercise. pp. 601–604. In Evans JG, Williams TF (eds): Oxford Textbook of Geriatric Medicine. Oxford University Press, Oxford, 1992
44. Wolfson L, Whipple R, Derby C et al: Balance and strength training in older adults: intervention gains and tai chi maintenance. J Am Geriatr Soc 1996;44:498–506
45. Wolf SL, Barnhart HX, Kutner NG, et al: Reducing frailty and falls in older persons: an investigation of tai chi and computerized balance training. J Am Geriatr Soc 1996;44:489–497
46. Nelson ME, Fiatarone MA, Morganti CM et al: Effects of high-intensity strength training on multiple risk factors for osteoporotic fractures. J Am Med Assoc 1994;272:1909–1914
47. Skelton DA: Exercise for Healthy Ageing. Research into Ageing, London, 1994
48. Bell JM, Bassey EJ: Postexercise heart rates and pulse palpation as a means of determining exercising intensity in an aerobic dance class. Br J Sports Med 1996;30:48–52
49. Malbut KE, Dinan SM, Verhaar H, Young A: Maximal oxygen uptake in 80 year old men. Clin Sci 1995;89 (suppl. 33)(abstr.): 31P
50. Cotes JE: The ventilatory cost of activity. Br J Ind Med 1975; 32:220–223
51. Doust JH, Patrick JM: The limitation of exercise ventilation during speech. Resp Physiol 1981;46:137–147
52. Fentem PH, Bassey EJ: 50+ A Safe Approach for Leaders. Guidelines for Those in Charge of Activity Groups. Sports Council, London, 1993
53. Kallinen M, Markku A: Aging, physical activity and sports injuries. An overview of common sports injuries in the elderly. Sports Med 1995;20:41–52
54. Young A, Dinan S. Fitness for older people. Br Med J 1994; 309:331–334
55. Dishman RK, Buckworth J: Increasing physical activity: a quantitative synthesis. Med Sci Sports Exerc 1996;28:706–719
56. Frändin K, Johannesson K, Grimby G: Physical activity as part of an intervention program for elderly persons in Göteborg. Scand J Med Sci Sports 1992;2:218–224
57. Browne D: Encourage active community life. Br Med J 1994; 309:872
58. Hillsdon M, Thorogood M: A systematic review of physical activity promotion strategies. Br J Sports Med 1996;30:84–89
59. McMurdo MET, Johnstone R: A randomized controlled trial of a home exercise programme for elderly people with poor mobility. Age Ageing 1995;24:425–428
60. Morris JN: Exercise in the prevention of coronary heart disease: today's best buy in public health. Med Sci Sports Exerc 1994; 26:807–814
61. Kaman RL, Patton RW: Costs and benefits of an active versus an inactive society. pp. 134–144. In Bouchard C, Shephard RJ, Stephens T (eds): Physical Activity, Fitness, and Health. Human Kinetics, Champaign, Illinois, 1994
62. Shephard RJ: Costs and benefits of an exercising versus a non-exercising society. pp. 49–60. In Bouchard C, Shephard RJ, Stephens T et al: (eds): Exercise, Fitness, and Health. Human Kinetics, Champaign, Illinois, 1990
63. Shephard RJ: Aging, Physical Activity, and Health. pp. 370–373. Human Kinetics, Champaign, IL, 1997
64. Dishman RK: Motivating older adults to exercise. South Med J 1994;87:S79–S82

CHAPTER 106

Preventive and Anticipatory Care

IDRIS WILLIAMS

This chapter examines preventive and anticipatory care for older people in the community provided by a primary care service. Such an approach is, however, relevant to all those concerned with such care whatever the setting. The provision of comprehensive care for older people in the community inevitably includes health and social services working in close harmony. Not only does this concern the saving of lives and reduction of suffering, but also improvement in the quality of life. This means an integrated service that includes acute and continuing care as well as preventive care. These are closely linked; for example, a very important aspect of preventive care is good acute care.

The demographic changes experienced by both developed and developing countries mean increased proportions of older people in the population and especially of very old people with increased levels of high disability. The high cost of caring for this section of the community has led governments to look at ways of reducing the burden of disability. A preventive approach is attractive, and in the UK this has been introduced contractually. In the US, with its different system of health care, specialized geriatric assessment and treatment programs are increasing, based mainly on geriatric evaluation units, but they also take place in an ambulatory setting. These programs use a multi-dimensional, usually interdisciplinary, approach to evaluate an older individual's medical, physical, and functional capabilities and problems, with the intention of producing a comprehensive plan for therapy and long-term follow-up. Controlled trials have demonstrated that patients benefit significantly in several ways.[1] In Europe, many countries are examining their community and rehabilitation services and, in particular, discussing preventive approaches that could enhance functional health of older people.[2]

Objectives of Care of Old People in Primary Care

The UK has a well-developed system of primary care, multiprofessional in nature, but largely based on general practice. The principal aim is to keep an older person in as good effective health as possible in the environment of their choice. This is normally their own home, but an old person may want to be in more sheltered care and this should be recognized. Included in this aim are some specific objectives. These are detailed in Table 106-1.[3] These require a large number of services, but are largely fulfilled by the primary care system. In the past, preventive care was not provided very adequately, but has developed significantly in the past 25 years.

Development of Anticipatory Care

In most developed countries, medical care was traditionally initiated by a request from the patient for help at a consultation or home visit. The doctor's response was prompt and the objective was cure. Most general practitioner care was of this reactive type and still is. However, it was recognized that old people might also need some form of proactive care if only to keep an eye on long-term problems. Before the National Health Service, general practitioners in the UK pragmatically provided a primitive form of anticipatory care for their older patients by visiting them routinely. Unfortunately, those who really needed these visits rarely received them and the incentive for doctors was often the fee. Nevertheless, the idea persisted among old people that regular doctor visits were helpful.

In the UK the New Contract for General Practice was introduced in 1990[4] and included a requirement to undertake proactive annual health checks on patients aged 75 and over. This program is UK-specific, but the principle involved could have worldwide applicability. The method chosen for providing a preventive program is only one of several that have been developed and tested in the UK over the past 25 years; others may be more relevant to other countries. Screening clinics for the elderly were first developed in the UK by Cowan and Anderson.[5] They assessed patients referred to them by GPs, but the real incentive to the development of comprehensive screening of older people came from Willimason and his colleagues.[6] Disturbed by the people aged 65 and over arriving in the hospital with late-stage treatable illness, but who had not seen their GP for a considerable time, they studied a sample of over 65-year-old people at home and found a substantial amount of unreported need. This is often termed the "iceberg phenomenon," with reported needs only representing the tip of the iceberg. Most, but not all, subsequent studies have confirmed these findings.

Williamson's work stimulated interest among general practitioners in the UK who appreciated its relevance to their own work and experience. A need to discover illness at an early stage became the rationale behind early comprehensive screening activities. Important early screening was carried out by general practitioners.[7–11] It was realized that the age of 75 years was important, and that beyond this the real problems of old age became more common. The first community-based comprehensive assessment of all over 75-year-old patients in a practice was carried out by Williams and his colleagues[12] in 1970. Out of this study came some important concepts. It

Table 106-1 Objectives for health care of old people in primary care

1. To establish, when illness occurs, an accurate diagnosis on which logical treatment and accurate prognosis can be based: this implies good day-to-day care of older people and effective management of acute illness. Similarly, when social crises occur, effective assessment and response are needed. Often there are health and social components in an acute episode.
2. To identify the social environmental needs of older people and refer appropriately to social and environmental services.
3. To improve, and if this is not possible, to maintain, an older person's functional performance: cure may not always be possible, but an attempt should always be made to maximize effective health.
4. To provide effective continuing care for those needing long-term medical maintenance therapy, surveillance, and rehabilitation.
5. To provide adequate resettlement for patients who are discharged from hospital back into the community: proper reception of patients is crucial to their continuing care.
6. To provide adequate care for dying patients, especially when they wish to die at home.
7. To give support and relief to informal caregivers who are looking after older people.
8. To be prepared to be an older person's advocate in situations of difficulty.
9. To enable older people to be outward looking and to accept responsibility for caring for themselves: in this sense the provision of care itself is not the prime aim of the community worker; it is rather by education and encouragement, to facilitate self-care amongst older people.
10. To recognize "at risk" situations: examples of these are patients living alone, the housefast, the over 75-year-olds, the bereaved, and those recently discharged from hospital. Special care is needed for these people.
11. To provide information and education for older people in the neighborhood.
12. To foster a team approach to the provision of care: this should involve both health and social workers, who should form a community care team. It is no longer acceptable that a doctor should be involved solely in the medical aspects of old age, and a social worker only in the social care. Health and social problems are inevitably linked and both need attention if the overall situation is to be improved. This has long been a principle of care in the hospital where doctors, nurses and medical social workers worked in close cooperation. In the community such cooperation is no less essential.
13. To establish good relationships between the community care team for older patients and those providing care in hospitals or other institutions.
14. To provide a responsive service, both in social support and health care, with sufficient flexibility to provide high intensity care, where necessary, as in the "hospital at home" schemes.
15. To assess the needs of the older people in the local community, so that effective service can be provided.
16. To provide adequate education and training for health and social workers in matters relating to good primary care of older people.
17. To carry out medical audit on care programs for older people and be aware of quality control requirements.

was a *socio*medical study and showed the relationship between health and social ability. It confirmed unreported need, but showed that its importance was the effect it had on functional ability. The idea of effective health that judged a person's health mainly on functional grounds rather than freedom from disease was introduced. Much of this early screening work deepened understanding of the natural history of old age in the community, placing aging into a highly variable longitudinal perspective, which gave it a dimension that could be seen only from general practice. Other studies followed; not all, however, confirmed unreported need.[13–15]

Later, it became clear that full comprehensive screening was impracticable because of the workload on general practitioners and other members of the primary care team. Doubt was also cast on its value. Convincing evidence of health benefit measured by cure of illness did not appear to be demonstrated by follow-up studies in general practice.[16–18]

Despite this, the idea of tertiary screening continued to be developed. Based on the assumption that some elderly people needed such care more than others, a selective approach was adopted that led to schemes which examined subjects within certain "at risk" groups. The aim was to increase the yield of unreported illness.[19] On the other hand, Barber et al.[20] achieved a more selective cohort of patients by using a questionnaire to identify patients in need of screening. Pike[21] screened only those patients who were currently not on treatment. Again, clear health benefit was not demonstrated as a result of these selective methods.

By 1983, relatively few general practitioners were undertaking or interested in formal screening.[22] They asserted that most elderly patients were being seen anyway and that tertiary screening could be undertaken during normal consultation. This had been proposed by Van den Dool[23] in The Netherlands and in the UK was described by Stott and Davis,[24] who drew attention to the enormous potential of the consultation as an opportunity for preventive care, health promotion, and case finding. It involved expeditious, but careful, screening during normal contact between patient and health worker. It depended on a high proportion of elderly persons seeing their doctor regularly. At this time it was demonstrated that over 90 percent of the over 75-year-old population in a practice was seen at least once in a year by the general practitioner and that those not seen were in reasonably good health.[25,26] This was also found to be the most favored approach among general practitioners.[22]

Nevertheless, several options presented themselves. These included full comprehensive assessment for all, selective screening for specific groups, methods of identifying those with specific needs, for example, by postal questionnaire, case-finding visits, or opportunistic assessment at routine primary care contacts. Prior to 1990 in the UK, between 10 and 20 percent of GPs were doing formal geriatric assessments for their patients, with an unknown number doing them opportunistically.[22] As already noted, the 1990 Contract for GPs in the UK introduced a health check program for patients aged 75 years and over and this will be described later. The general conceptual background needs to be described first with a closer look at other options that may be more appropriate in different health care settings.

Definitions

Because there has been some confusion about the precise meaning of certain words, the terms used when describing anticipatory care need to be defined.[3]

- *Primary prevention:* stopping disease before it has had the chance to arise, e.g., immunization.
- *Secondary prevention:* the detection of disease when it is asymptomatic and often curable, e.g., cervical cytology.
- *Tertiary prevention:* early recognition and seeking out of established symptomatic disease or social detriment so that treatment and social support can be instituted to improve the quality of life and reduce the functional deficit present.
- *Anticipatory care:* this describes a program that looks ahead and aims to forestall any problems that may occur and thereby improve the quality of life. It includes all types of prevention and information about healthy lifestyle and avoidance of hazard.
- *Opportunistic anticipatory care:* this is the form of anticipatory care undertaken during normal contact with health workers, using, for instance, the opportunity presented by the patient/client seeking advice about other matters.
- *Case finding:* this is not easy to define and was coined to describe what happens when a health worker or social worker identifies a problem (or case) as part of a formal screening activity or when checked opportunistically. The problem could include physical, mental, social or family disease or dysfunction. It implies further assessment to work out solutions and formulate management plans.
- *Health check:* this is the first stage of the contractual obligation to examine old people and is a problem-identifying exercise that can lead to further assessment and management in primary care or, occasionally, full interdisciplinary assessments, often in secondary care facilities.
- *Assessment:* a broad term used when an old person is examined for specific purposes. For instance, to deal with incipient health or social breakdown; to deal with actual breakdown; when there is a change in circumstance, e.g., discharge from hospital, move to residential care; and, on an occasional basis, to monitor long-term care.
- *Effective health:* describes the health status of an old person, not by the presence or absence of disease, but on the basis of the ability to perform various activities of daily living.
- *World Health Organization Convention:* The convention of usage that is recommended by the World Health Organization[27] contains three definitions that are helpful when considering functional ability. The convention can be summarized as follows: impairment (the disease) gives rise to disability (the functional loss), which in turn gives rise to handicap (the effect on lifestyle).
    - *Impairment:* Any loss or abnormality of psychological, physiologic, or anatomic structure or function.
    - *Disability*: Any restriction or lack of ability (due to an impairment) to perform an activity in a manner or within the range considered normal for a person.
    - *Handicap*: A disadvantage resulting from an impairment or disability that limits or prevents the fulfilment of a role. (The role may be relative to age, sex, social, cultural, or economic factors.)

Preventive endeavors for older people are ultimately concerned with avoiding or reducing handicap.

Tertiary Prevention (Rationale)

Tertiary prevention is the basis of preventive activity among old people and the rationale for it needs to be clarified. There are two age-related factors that contribute: the tendency for older people to under-report medical and social problems and the almost universal presence of multiple pathology and morbidity. Added to this is the tendency for doctors to underdetect medical and social problems.

The main reason for unreported illness is patient inertia, which can be due to a number of causes, such as fear of hospitalization and unpleasant investigations, the risk of involuntary removal to residential care, lack of information, and imagining that symptoms are not amenable to treatment. Health workers tend to collude with a patient and compound the inertia; "it's your age" is a phrase often used, implying that nothing can be done.

Multiple pathology can be a major factor, though many of the problems may not be individually life-threatening or even disabling (e.g., hallux valgus, varicose ulcers, osteoarthritis, and obesity) the cumulative effect of several of these may be loss of function resulting in, for example, poor mobility.

An equation of diminishing function can, therefore, be written:

Unreported need
+ multiple pathology → Loss of function
and reduction in quality of life

Although the aging process is often invoked as a catalyst, other causal factors are more important; these include acute illness, injury, mental impairment, chronic disease, economic distress, loneliness, and social stress. Functional ability is the most important aspect of health in older age, especially beyond the age of 75.

Aim of Tertiary Prevention

The aim of tertiary prevention in older people is to identify and alleviate established disease at an early stage in order to improve or maintain functional status. Even if the impairment itself is not amenable to specific treatment, the preventive process is concerned with preventing disability and handicap, not impairment. This is the aim of the health check program for patients of 75 years and over.

Functional Ability

The rationale for tertiary prevention, therefore, depends upon the ability to prevent disability and handicap, but not necessarily the impairment itself. Ability to function is the measure of health in old age, not necessarily the absence of disease. In some situations the relationship between disease presence and functional decline is clear: for example, osteoarthritis of the hips causing a reduction in mobility. However, disease can be present without disability: for example, well-controlled diabetes mellitus. Such patients, although needing long-term continuing care, nevertheless remain functionally intact for a long period. Interestingly, diseases can seemingly be absent and yet functional loss exists. These situations are often seen in primary care. Causes can include situational factors such as isolation, inappropriate housing, and poverty; or personal factors such as poor motivation, psychological disturbance, and family upset. The ideal situation is disease absence and full functional ability—the classic definition of health. It is possible, however, that at least in advanced old age, most have some minor problem, though it may not be severe enough to impair function.

Functional ability is usually expressed through activities of daily living and a tertiary prevention program must take these into account. Observing changes in these indicate the need to search for possible causes that are amenable to being relieved.

The activities can be divided into three types:

- Sociable: how the person relates to the outside world in leisure and social activities (e.g., visiting friends, going to the cinema).
- Domestic: how the person keeps the household going (e.g., cooking, cleaning, laundering, attending to household repairs, keeping the house safe).
- Personal: how the person attends to personal needs (e.g., bathing, cutting toenails, dressing, toileting).

The convention is to use the term "activities of daily living" (ADLs) to cover personal tasks and "instrumental activities of daily living" (IADLs) to cover household tasks and sociability. Although it is possible to look separately at the three levels, and there is a dynamic link between them. They can be seen as three concentric rings surrounding the person—the outer ring representing sociability, the middle ring representing domestic tasks, and the inner ring representing personal tasks[28] (Fig. 106-1).

Functional decline, when it occurs, tends to start at the outer ring and progress inward to the other two levels. Thus, the first sign of breakdown usually happens in the outer ring: the old person ceases to go out to a place of worship, make visits to friends, or attend to hobbies. Signs of more serious decline occur at the next level and herald domestic deterioration: the house is uncleaned, repairs are not undertaken, and cooking becomes irregular. The final level of breakdown comes when personal activities are neglected: baths are not taken, toenails remain uncut. There may be gradual deterioration through the levels as time passes, often with intervening stable periods, but illness, either physical or mental, usually results in accelerated decline and a change in functional ability can take place within a very short time. Other catalysts also exist, some of which can be gathered together under the term *social detriment*. These include psychological factors, economic circumstances, the environment, loneliness, lack of privacy, opportunities to experience personal warmth, and a perceived loss of status. All of these can interfere with the psychological balance of an old person and affect the will to self-care, which results in functional loss.

Fortunately, decline is often reversible: appropriate treatment or social input can restore function and reinstate the integrity of the rings. A similar model can indicate the type of input necessary at each stage to achieve this, often complementing the medical treatment of the condition producing the deterioration[28] (Fig. 106-2).

The model has several uses: to provide three functional checklists when assessing old people; to take account of the timing of social deterioration; to highlight the place of physical and mental illness in causing accelerating functional decline; to place emphasis on early restoration of function, either by treatment or care input; to help caregivers to understand the significance of functional deterioration; and to help identify and manage problems earlier. It can also take account of caregiver intolerance. When deterioration reaches the inner level, caregivers begin to feel stressed and often cannot cope.[29] This needs to be recognized early so that relief is made available. In anticipatory care, an eye to function as measured by activities of daily living can alert the professional to hidden disabil-

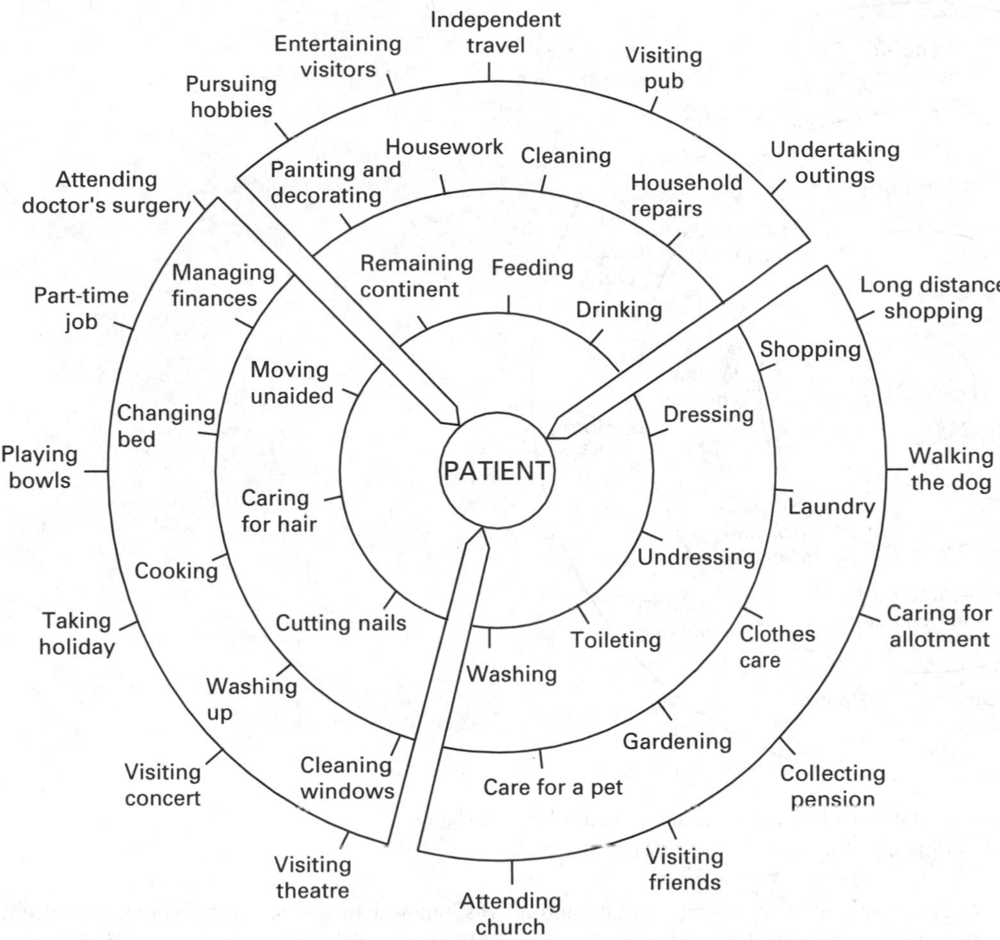

Figure 106-1 A model of social performance levels in older people. (From Williams EI: A Model to Describe Social Performance Levels in Elderly People. Br J Pract; 36:422–3.)

ity, and improvement can act as a measure of successful intervention.

Options for Tertiary Prevention

There has emerged over the past 20 years an understanding of the principle of tertiary prevention in old age and the availability of options for putting these into practice in primary care. Tertiary prevention should, of course, start at an early age. Most people in the 65 to 75 age group are in good functional health, and it is usual to start formal tertiary prevention checks from the age of 75 years. None of the options for undertaking tertiary prevention in the community have been totally satisfactory. With the introduction of contractual health checks in 1990, which is essentially a case-finding activity, other methods have been abandoned in the UK. The range, however, will be described briefly as the options may be more appropriate in other health care systems.

The options available are as follows:

1. To do nothing except to provide normal service or undertake a record review
2. To undertake a comprehensive screening of all 75 and over patients
3. To provide selective screening for specific "at risk" groups (e.g., those living alone, the recently bereaved, the very old)
4. To undertake a postal survey followed by full assessment of those found to be in need
5. To rely on health visitor or nurse case-finding visits, followed by a full assessment of those found to be in need
6. To carry out opportunistic case finding during doctor or health worker/patient contact, followed by full assessment of those found to be in need

The first option is to do nothing, and the argument for this is that the iceberg of illness is a myth and that unreported illness has not always been found or that the level may be overstated in the literature. The argument is tempered by the assertion that health care workers see most old people anyway and are likely to identify significant unreported illness. Nihilism does still exist, however, and an argument "to leave well alone," is still heard. Regular comprehensive screening of all old people at designated clinics has proved to be impractical. There is no evidence that unreported need is found only in

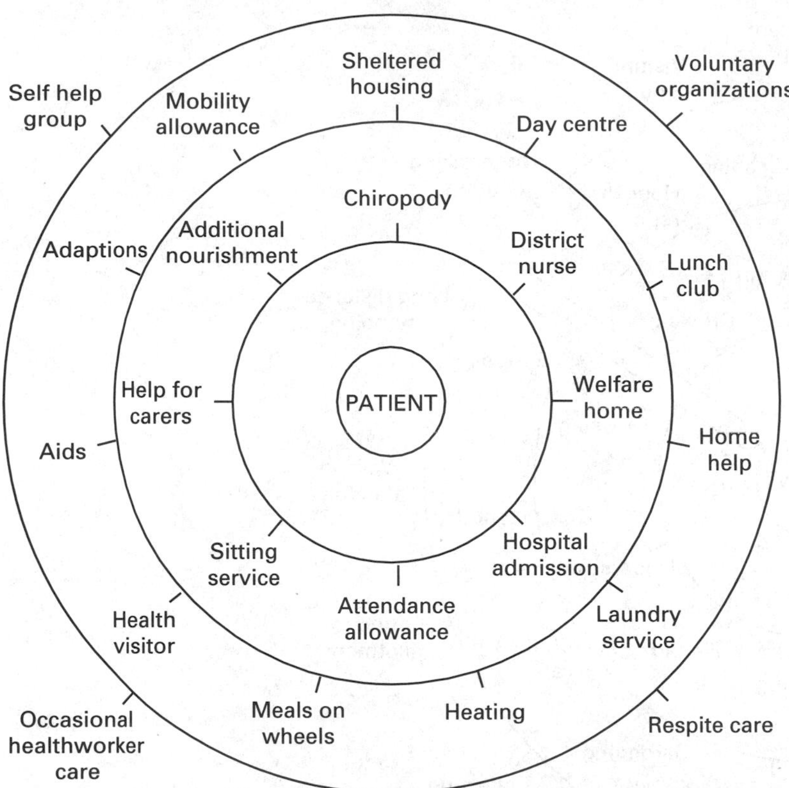

Figure 106-2 A model of services available to older people. (From Williams EI: A Model to Describe Social Performance Levels in Elderly People. Br J Pract; 36:422–3.)

"at risk" groups and this argues against selective screening. The last three options are basically case-finding exercises and depend upon a two-stage approach; initial surveillance with the aim of identifying problems, followed by further fuller assessment when this is indicated. Health worker initiated case-finding home visits and opportunistic case-finding at patient contact are the features of the contractual health check program. Postal screening is no longer carried out in the UK, but could have a place in other countries.

The postal questionnaire was developed by Barber and his colleagues[20] and contains nine questions requiring "yes" or "no" answers. These are as follows:

1. Do you live on your own?
2. Are you in a position to have no relative whom you can rely on for help?
3. Do you need help with housework or shopping?
4. Are there days when you are unable to prepare a hot meal for yourself?
5. Are you confined to your home through ill health?
6. Is there any difficulty or concern over your health you have still to see about?
7. Do you have any problem with eyes or eyesight?
8. Do you have any difficulty with hearing?
9. Have you been in hospital during the past year?

Each elderly patient was sent a letter, often on their birthday, and a "yes" answer to any of the questions or nonreply to the letter indicated that the patient was in need of comprehensive assessment by health visitor or doctor. The questionnaire was designed to cover known areas of risk to the patient's physical, mental, and social state. There are variations in both the way the questionnaire is set out and in the questions themselves. The method is designed to reduce workload by identifying groups of people which may have a high yield of unreported need. It is essentially a two-tier exercise. A full account of this program is set out in RCGP Occasional Papers Nos. 35 and 45.[30,31]

Evidence of Effectiveness

In the UK, early interest in assessment of older people was based on demonstrated unreported need. The aim was not necessarily to cure, but to alleviate the problem and reduce or prevent associated disability and handicap. Evidence for unreported need has consistently been recorded over the last 25 years and it would seem not to be merely a cohort effect.[32–36] Evidence of the effectiveness of a preventive assessment program has been harder to produce. Part of the reason for this has been a search for benefit in terms of clinical improvement, whereas the most likely benefit has turned out to be in such aspects as quality of life and a reduction in the need for institutional care.

Hendriksen[37] (1995) has analysed 10 randomized controlled studies published between 1984 and 1994 that looked at in-home preventive health checks using comprehensive geriatric assessment. The design and main results of these studies are summarized in Table 106-2.[15,34,36,38–44] The studies are different in many respects; for instance age range, the visitors, the content and the frequency of the visits. The results show, however, some remarkable similarities, and Hendriksen draws some tentative conclusions; for example one visit does not appear to be enough. In order to provide effective preventive prevention it seems necessary to develop a good rapport with the old person and formally follow-up an assessment. Professionals such as health visitors seem to get better results than volunteer visitors. Despite the problems of comparison, Hendricksen maintains that the predominant message from these preventive home assessment studies is very promising. He also puts forward interesting ideas about the causality of the favorable effects. For instance, at the completion of the Danish project[38] participants reported that the visitors had contributed to an increased feeling of confidence, and improved their contacts with other formal services. The result was higher self-esteem leading to better use of personal resources and maximizing support from family and friends. This allowed for improved self-care and also ability to cope with illness. This preserved or increased functional capacity and reduced the need for hospital and nursing home care.

Stuck et al.[45] (1993) published a detailed meta-analysis of controlled studies on the effects of comprehensive geriatric assessment on survival, residence, and function. The studies were from a variety of settings in different countries. Some were based on institutions, whereas others were not. Institutional-based studies included geriatric evaluation and management units; inpatient geriatric consultation services; and post-hospital services. Noninstitutional bases included home assessment services and outpatient assessment services. The overall results were encouraging, particularly for geriatric evaluation and management units. Stuck et al.[46] have taken this further and looked specifically at the seven home assessment studies included in the analysis. Overall, compared to controls, the odds of death were significantly reduced by about 15 percent for patients checked by home assessment services, and the odds of living at home significantly increased by more than 20 percent. The effect of (Home Assessment Services) (HAS) on the prevention of hospital admissions was heterogeneous, and thus not immediately interpretable. Examination of the study odds ratio/confidence bands reveal that two trials show statistically significant reductions in hospital use, while the

Table 106-2 A summary of the randomized controlled studies of preventive home visits

Authors/Country	Inclusion Criteria (years)	Number of Subjects	Visitor	Number of Visits	Results
Vetter,[15] UK	70+	I:577 C:571	Health visitor	3 in 2 years	Urban setting; lower mortality; higher quality of life
Hendricksen,[38] Denmark	75+	I:285 C:287	Nurses, physician	12 in 3 years	Lower mortality; reduction in hospital admissions and bed-days, fewer emergency medical calls
Sorenson,[39] Denmark	75, 80, 85	I:585 C:777	Social worker, physician	1 Visit	No differences
Carpenter,[40] UK	75+	I:272 C:267	Volunteers	6–12 in 3 years	Reduction in days spent in institutions
McEwan,[34] UK	75+	I:151 C:145	Nurse	1 Visit	No differences
Hall,[41] Canada	65+ and home care	I: 81 C: 86	Nurse	Depends on needs	More alive and living at home
Pathy,[36] UK	65+	I:369 C:356	Health visitors	Depends on needs	Lower mortality, shorter duration of stay in hospitals among 65–75 years superior self-rated health
Clarke,[42] Canada	75+	I:261 C:262	Layworker	3 in 2 years	Improved perceived health
Van Rossum,[43] Holland	75–85 without home nurse	I:292 C:288	Nurses	12 in 3 years	Subgroup rating their health as poor: lower mortality, reduced number of bad-days in hospital
Fabacher,[44] USA	70+; veterans	I:131 C:123	Nurse, volunteers	3 in 1 Year	Higher IADL scores

Abbreviations: C, control group; I, intervention group.

remaining trials had no such effects. Stuck concluded that in the ambulatory setting home-based comprehensive geriatric assessment appears to be the most efficacious format in that it optimizes comprehensive evaluation and close individual patient follow-up. He warned, however, about the variability of the methods of assessment and emphasized that studies have been restricted to those carried out in Europe with health care systems different from those in other countries. It is recommended that more research is needed to improve intervention methods and to address their impacts on the health care system.

The UK Health Check Program

The 1990 NHS Contract[4] obliged GPs to offer annual health checks to patients of 75 years and over who were registered with them. The importance of a domiciliary visit was stressed and the content of the assessment was to include, where appropriate, sensory functions, mobility, mental condition, physical condition including continence, social environment, and the use of medicine. Nothing is said in the Contract about the objectives or organization of such a program; it was presumably left to the professionals to determine these matters. The aim has been seen as providing a tertiary prevention program with the purpose of improving functional ability and quality of life.

Several other objectives have been added:

- To provide an opportunity for health promotion and health education
- To provide an opportunity for primary and secondary prevention
- To review the needs of caregivers
- To construct a database of relevant patient information

Problems that are identified in health checks need to be interpreted in terms of their effect on patients' function and ability to live independently. This is an important process that requires skill and experience. The health check should be seen as part of an overall program of care for older people. Time and energy should not be deflected from other effective ways of improving health and functional ability such as providing good acute care. Experience in practice has shown that the process has three stages (Fig. 106-3).[3]

Stage 1

This is the initial health check, the purpose of which is problem identification. It is essentially a structured conversation covering the following areas: social assessment, home assessment, mobility, general function (ADLs and IADLs), senses (vision and hearing), continence, medication, mental function, finances, and lifestyle. There is flexibility in the detail as to what is done at the initial health check. A full examination is rarely carried out, but selective examination is often performed: for instance blood pressure, urine test, sight and vision, and checks on aids and appliances. The importance of early recognition of atrial fibrillation means that it is increasingly recommended that examination of the pulse should take place. Some specific questions are also asked about falls, poor

Figure 106-3 The three stages of the health check.

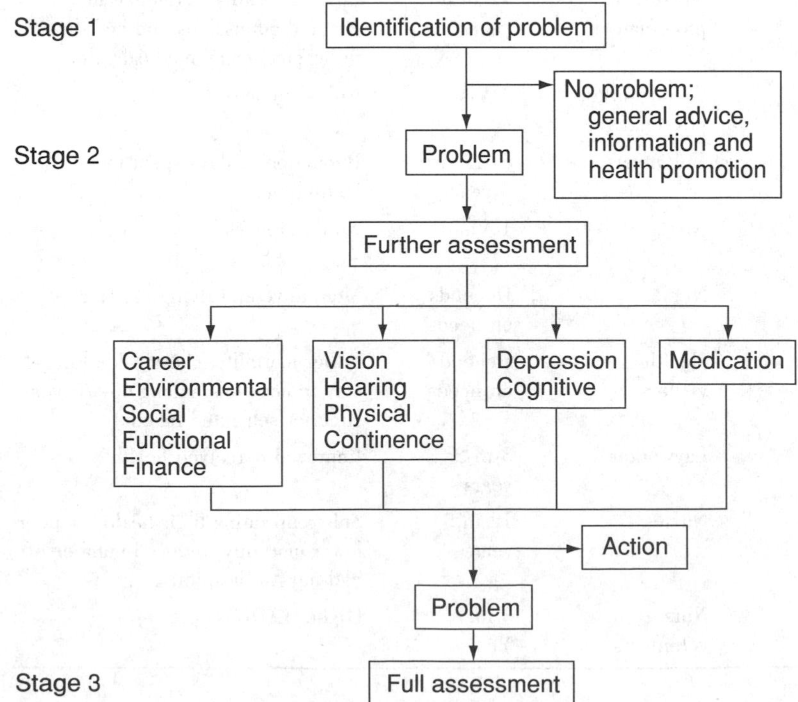

appetite, indigestion, dental problems, breathlessness, ankle swelling, unsteadiness, skin irritation, foot problems, hernia, and hemorrhoids. Sometimes quality-of-life questions are included.

There are many protocols/schedules that have been designed for use at stage 1. A useful one is included in RCGP Occasional Paper No. 59[47] and has the advantage of suggested questions that can trigger further examination at stage 2. Experience will allow more sensitive targeting of the trigger questions and possibly allow attention to focus on a group of old people with mild to moderate disability as well as those with severe degrees of frailty. Experience has shown that the first stage health check is undertaken both at home and at the surgery/office by either a nurse or doctor. There are situations where the check is carried out by specially trained link workers.[48] In the UK, about one-half the patients receiving a health check will be well and in good social circumstances; if problems exist they will be under active supervision.[49] For these patients the reassurance is helpful, but opportunities also exist for health promotion advice and information about existing available services.

Stage 2

Where problems have been identified, further assessment is needed. This usually takes place within the domain of primary care. This requires assessment related specifically to the problem identified. Most problems will be dealt with at this stage. The assessment will usually consist of a fuller history, some specific examinations, sometimes the completion of an assessment instrument and probably some other investigations. The RCGP Occasional Paper No. 59[47] contains appropriate guides to this further assessment. Specific standardized scales, for instance Barthel,[50] AMTS,[51] and GDS,[52] are recommended. If the health check is done initially by a GP, further management is along the usual clinical lines. Where the check is done by a nurse in the patient's home it is likely that most problems identified will be passed to the GP. Even so, many problems are dealt with by a nurse, health visitor, or social worker. Sometimes referral to specific specialists is needed, for example an eye surgeon or dermatologist; or to Social Services or Housing Agencies. A full description of the second stage review is found in "Caring for Older People in the Community" by E. I. Williams.[3]

Stage 3

Following health checks, full assessment is required when an identified problem cannot be successfully resolved in a primary care setting and help from secondary services is needed. Usually this means that there is a potential or actual breakdown in independent living or a serious medical problem has been found. It is not a common occurrence. The assessment needed is often led by a specialist in geriatric medicine, but is often multi-professional. It results in a detailed investigation of an individual's total situation including physical, mental, psychological, and functional state, together with an assessment of the support needed and the physical environment.

Effectiveness of the Health Check Program

The program of assessment of those aged 75 and over has now been in operation for over 5 years and an evaluation has been attempted. The imposition of a program that brought with it an additional workload was not favorably received by GPs and there was a feeling that there was not enough research evidence as to its value to justify its introduction. The result is that, despite the contractual need, assessments have only been patchily undertaken. Jill Tremellen[53] in a random sample of old people found 64 percent had accepted the assessment offer. Sixty-one percent of these were carried out at the patient's home with nurses doing most of the work. A sample of GPs were also interviewed and 68 percent of them thought assessments were unnecessary, but at similar interviews 52 percent of nurses thought them important. Ninety-three percent of the patients who were assessed found them to be useful. Doctors who undertook the assessments, mainly opportunistically, picked up few new problems. It was clear that nurses were much more enthusiastic, but required training to enable them to do home visits confidently.

Brown et al.[49] looked at what had happened in a structured random selection of 20 practices in a Health Authority area. These practices were visited to collect information on how assessments were organized and carried out. Three practices had performed no health checks. There was considerable variation in the way that assessments were organized and few of the practices had completed an assessment on all their patients during this time. Altogether, a total of 43 percent of patients assessed had a new problem that required action. It was concluded that the need for annual assessment should be kept under review and that adequate resources should be made available for the needs discovered. In this study, too, improved training for practice nurses was thought to be needed. The study reconfirmed the existence of unmet and unreported need. In a questionnaire to all practices in the same Health Authority, Brown and Groom[54] found that 99 percent of responding practices offered checks, but nearly one-quarter estimated that under 50 percent of their elderly population had actually received one. Practices with smaller numbers of elderly people were more likely to estimate high response rates to invitations and more likely to follow up those who did not respond. They indicated that it might be reasonable if more resources were not available to concentrate on assessing only those elderly people most at risk.

Chew et al.[55] reported on a study describing how the requirement to offer annual assessments had been implemented; what role was played by the Health Authority; how GPs and practice nurses viewed the assessment; and the experience and view of older people. Although only a small minority of GPs felt that the checks were of great value in improving the overall health of older people, most felt it was a useful way of providing advice and resources to a specific group of patients. More than two-thirds of the GPs would offer some selected groups of old people an assessment even if the requirement was removed, but only 28 percent would offer them to all older people. The majority of nurses, however, thought that routine assessments of those aged 75 and over were useful in many respects. Old people themselves were very positive and those who experienced them were equally positive about the reality.

Ongoing follow-up studies are being undertaken and the UK Medical Research Council has a multicenter trial that is looking at the best methods of undertaking home-based health checks in the very old. It will be some time before the results of these studies become available.

The Wider Concept of Anticipatory Care

The regular contact provided by the health check program between an old person and the health care services allows a range of other health promotion activities to be undertaken. Immunization against influenza for old people is recommended,[56] and it can be argued that maintenance of tetanus immunization is as necessary in older age as in young people. The age to which routine breast screening and cervical cytology should be available is debatable, but there are arguments that say that they should be available well beyond the age of 65 years.[57,58] The treatment of hypertension is recommended up to at least the age of 80 years and possibly beyond.[59]

There is also a valuable opportunity for health education. Older people should be encouraged to care for themselves, preserve autonomy, and maintain social contacts. Advice about not smoking, alcohol intake, diet, and avoidance of accidents are all important. Many problems suffered by older people arise because of lack of information. The opportunity presented by regular contact with them to give information about the practice, the services available in the community, financial services and social services should be used to the full.

Dangers

There are potential dangers with a health check program. Overtreatment is a temptation and old age may become overmedicalized. Expectations may be raised unrealistically and the offer of a regular check may reduce an old person's autonomy and the need to be responsible for their own health. Treatable illness may be missed. This is possible if untrained personnel are used for health checks and interventions are limited to only filling in a checklist. Ignoring other aspects of care is a risk if overemphasis is placed on a tertiary assessment program.

There are also ethical issues. Resources must be available to deal with positive findings. Confidentiality must be assured. Each team member must understand the boundaries of their own confidentiality and the patients need to know with whom information acquired during health checks is to be shared. An understanding of the mandate given by the patient needs to be clear. It is possible that the patient agrees to be examined, but not to the action indicated when problems are identified. It is necessary to look at the situation through the old person's eyes. Conditions that would be unacceptable to the interviewer may be seen as the norm to the patient. Unnecessary interference should, therefore, be avoided. A health promotion program for old people might be argued for on the grounds of equity alone. Such programs abound for well women and men at ages when the incidence of serious disease is trivial compared with those in their 70s and 80s.

Costs

Few attempts have been made to investigate the economic implication of health checks. McEwan and Foster[60] have undertaken a review of the costs of assessing old people in UK general practice. This has been difficult because of the lack of information in many of the published studies. Where information was available the cost was high. Additional costs to individual practices are calculable and include nurse time, traveling expenses, receptionist/secretarial time, doctor's time, telephone, postage, and stationery. An audit of the cost in a medium-sized practice revealed that the outlay amounted to around one-third of the capitation fees attracted by the patients in the practice who were 75 years and over.[61]

Vulnerable Groups of Old People

A comprehensive health check program will inevitably identify groups of old people with special problems. Examples would include those in residential care, those who either act as a caregiver or are dependent on a caregiver, membership of an ethnic minority, and those recently discharged from hospital. Caregivers have tolerance limits: some factors such as sleep disturbance, fecal incontinence, and mental illness in those being cared for are poorly tolerated and indicate that the provision of care is brittle and vulnerable to breakdown. If the caregiver themself is old, this needs to be recognized. Residents of residential homes and nursing homes should also receive health checks; maintenance of as good a functional status possible in these homes is no less vital.

An important subgroup of older old people are those belonging to the ethnic minorities. An increase in their number is predicted and little is known about their health needs. In the UK, a survey of older people born in India and Pakistan showed that over one-half those aged over 75 years were not fully independent in the basic activities of daily living.[62] Communication problems are likely to exist if the first language is not English, and this probably contributes to the underuse of services in this group.[63] Doctors will need to identify such patients on their list and liaise with community workers in meeting special needs, for instance, interpreters.

One advantage in undertaking health checks on old people is that it allows a health and social disability database to be completed for each patient. Such information is useful when patients move between care systems such as in and out of the hospital. Information about preadmission status is likely to be valuable to hospital clinicians, occupational therapists, and social workers. Communication of this information should be considered. Examples of basic data that could be available would include: caregiver availability, special "at risk" situations, existing medical problems, medication, services received before admission, activities of daily living, and reasons for a postdischarge visit.

Conclusions

The community care of older people is an issue that is important not only to industrialized countries, but also to developing countries, where often this group is the fastest growing section of the population. On any given date in the UK 95 percent of those aged 75 years and over are under the care of a GP and most older people never see a geriatrician throughout their lives.[64] A program of community-based anticipatory care, including tertiary prevention, with the aim of preserving functional activity and autonomy after the age of 75, has therefore, to be seriously considered. Equity demands that old people should have the same health promotion care as other sections of the community. Evidence of the effectiveness of comprehensive geriatric assessment is growing; in particular there are encouraging research findings that support their value in a community setting, especially when associated with good aftercare facilities. More flexible assessment instruments may be needed which allow better identification of those on the borderline of frailty for whom there is likelihood of real benefit. In the UK some progress has been made; implementation of evidence-based preventive screening in primary care will take time, but it will need professional attitude shifts if it is to be fully achieved.

References

1. Rubenstein L, Josephson K, Wieland D et al: Effectiveness of a geriatric evaluation unit: a randomised controlled trial. N Engl J Med 1984;310:1664–1670
2. Harmonizing Assessment of the Elderly in Europe: Gisela A. Fischer and Working Party. Department of General Practice and Family Medicine, Hannover, Germany, (research in Progress 1995–1997).
3. Williams EI: Caring for Older People in the Community. 3rd Ed. Radcliffe Medical Press, Oxford, 1995
4. National Health Service and Community Care Act 1990. Her Majesty's Stationary Office, London
5. Cowan NR, Anderson WF: Experiences of a consultative health centre for old people. Pub Health 1952;74:377–382
6. Williamson J, Stokoe IH, Gray S et al: Old people at home: their unreported needs. Lancet 1964;1:1117–1120
7. Thomas P: Experiences of two preventive clinics for the elderly. Br Med J 1968;2:357–360
8. Pike LA: A screening programme for the elderly in general practice. The Practitioner 1969;203:805–812
9. Hodes C: Geriatric screening and caring group practice. J Coll Gen Pract 1971;311,109:469–472
10. Irwin WG: Geriatric practice and the health centre. Mod Geriatr 1971;1:265
11. Dunn TB: The Red Bridge Scheme for routine medical examination of elderly patients. Mod Geriatr 1971;1:261–263
12. Williams EI, Bennett FM, Nixon J et al: Socio medical study of patients over 75 in general practice. Br Med J 1972;II:455–458
13. Currie G, McNeill RM, Walker JG et al: Medical and social screening of patients aged 70–72 by an urban general practice health team. Br Med J 1974;II:108–111
14. Freedman GR, Charlewood JE, Dodd PA: Screening the aged in general practice. J RCGP 1978;28:421–425
15. Vetter NJ, Jones DE, Victor CR: Effect of health visitors working with elderly patients in general practice: a randomised controlled trial. Br Med J 1984;288:369–372
16. Lowther CP, McLeod RDM, Williamson J: The evaluation of early diagnostic services for the elderly. Br Med J 1970;III: 275–277
17. Williams EI: A follow-up of geriatric patients: socio medical assessments. J Roy Coll Gen Pract 1974;24:341–346
18. Tulloch AG, Moore V: A randomised controlled trial of geriatric screening and surveillance in general practice. J Roy Coll Gen Pract 1979;29:730–733
19. Taylor R, Ford G, Barber H: Research perspective on ageing: The Elderly at Risk. Age Concern, London, 1983
20. Barber JH, Wallis JB, McKeating E: A postal screening questionnaire in preventive geriatric care. J Roy Coll Gen Pract 1980;30:49–51
21. Pike EA: Screening the elderly in general practice. J Roy Coll Gen Pract 1976;26:698–703
22. Williams EI: The general practitioner and the disabled. J Roy Coll Gen Pract 1983;33:296–299
23. Van den Dool CWA: Huisarts en Wetenschap 1970;13:3–59
24. Stott N, Davis, RH: The exceptional potential for prevention in the primary care consultation. J Roy Coll Gen Pract 1979;29: 201–205
25. Williams EI: Characteristics of patients over 75 not seen during one year in general practice. Br Med J 1984;288:119–121
26. Ebrahim S, Hedley R, Sheldon M: Low levels of ill-health among elderly non-consulters in general practice. Br Med J 1984;289: 1873–1875
27. World Health Organization: International Classification of Impairments, Disabilities and Handicaps. WHO, Geneva, 1980
28. Williams EI: A model to describe social performance levels in elderly people. J Roy Coll Gen Pract 1986;36:422–423
29. Sanford JRA: Tolerance of debility in elderly dependants by support at home: its significance for hospital practice. Br Med J 1975;3:471–473
30. Taylor RC, Buckley EG: Preventive care of the elderly: A Re-

view of Current Developments. Occasional Paper No. 35. Royal Coll of Gen Pract London, 1987

31. Williams EI, Buckley EG, Freer CB: Care of Old People: A Framework for Progress. Occasional Paper No. 45. Royal College of General Practitioners, London, 1990
32. Tobias B: Dental aspects of an elderly population: Age Ageing 1988;17:103–110
33. Mulley GP, White EG: Footcare for very elderly people: a community survey. Age Ageing 1989;18:275–278
34. McEwan RT, Davison N, Foster DP et al: Screening elderly people in primary care: a randomised controlled trial. Br J Gen Pract 1990;40:94–97
35. Iliffe S, Haines A, Gallivan S et al: Assessment of elderly people in general practice: 1. Social circumstances and mental state. Br J Gen Pract 1991;41:9–12
36. Pathy MSJ, Bayer A, Harding K et al: Randomised trial of case finding and surveillance of elderly people at home. Lancet 1992;340:890–893
37. Hendriksen C: Preventive home visits to elderly persons: status and perspectives. p. 231–239. In Rubenstein LZ, Wieland D, Bernabei R (eds): Geriatric Assessment Technology: The State of the Art. Editrice Kurtis, Milano, 1995
38. Hendriksen C, Lunde E, Stromgard E: Consequences of assessment and intervention among elderly people: a three year randomised controlled trial. Br Med J 1984;289:1522–1524
39. Sorensen KH: Follow-up three years after intervention to relieve unmet medical and social needs of old people. Compr Gerontol 1988;2:85–91
40. Carpenter GI, Demopoulos GR: Screening the elderly in the community: controlled trial of dependency surveillance using a questionnaire administered by volunteers. Br Med J 1990; 300:1253–1256
41. Hall N, De Beck P, Johnson D et al: Randomised trial of a health promotion programme for frail elderly. Can J Age 1992; 72:91–92
42. Clarke M, Clarke SJ, Jagger C: Social intervention and the elderly: a randomised controlled trial. Am J Epidemiol 1992;136: 1517–1523
43. Van Rossum E, Frederiks CMA, Philipsen H et al: Effects of preventive home visits for elderly people. Br Med J 1993;307: 27–32
44. Fabacher D, Josephson K, Pietruszka F et al: An in-home preventive assessment programme for independent older adults: a randomised controlled trial. J Am Geriatr Soc 1994;42: 630–638
45. Stuck AE, Siu AL, Wieland GD, et al: comprehensive geriatric assessment: a meta analysis of controlled trials. Lancet 1993; 342:1032–1036
46. Stuck AE, Wieland D, Rubenstein LZ et al: comprehensive geriatric assessment: meta analysis of main effects and element enhancing effectiveness. pp. 11–27. In Rubenstein LZ, Wieland D, Bernabei R (eds): Geriatric Assessment Technology: The State of the Art. Editrice Kurtis, Milano, 1995
47. Williams EI, Wallace P: Health Checks for People Aged 75 and Over. Occasional Paper No. 59 Royal College of General Practitioners, London, 1993
48. Wallace PG: Linking up with over 75s. Br J Gen Pract 1990; 40:267–269
49. Brown K, Williams EI, Groom L: Health checks on patients 75 years and over in Nottinghamshire after the new GP contract. Br Med J 1992;305:619–621
50. Wade DT, Colin C: The Barthel ADL Index: a standard measure of disability. Int Disabil Stud 1988;10:64–67
51. Hodkinson HM: Evaluation of a mental test score for assessment of mental impairment in the elderly. Age Aging 1972;1: 233–238
52. Sheik JI, Yesavage JA: Geriatric Depression Scale (GDS): recent evidence and development of a shorter version. In Brink TL (ed): Clinical Gerontology: A Guide to Assessment and Intervention. Howarth, New York, 1986
53. Tremellen J: Assessment of patients aged 75 and over in general practice. Br Med J 1992;305:621–624
54. Brown K, Groom L: General practice health checks and elderly people: a county wide survey. Health Trends 1995;27: 89–91
55. Chew CA, Wilkin D, Glendenning C: Annual assessments of patients aged 75 years and over: general practitioners and practice nurses views and experience. Br J Gen Pract 1994;44: 263–267
56. Chief Medical Officer: Letter to Family Practitioner Committees for Circulation to all General Practitioners, Regional Medical Officers and District Medical Officers. 19th September. PLCMO(89)C. Department of Health, London, 1989
57. Forrest P (Chairman): Breast Cancer Screening. Report to Health Ministers of England, Wales, Scotland and Northern Ireland by Working Group. Her Majesty's Stationary Office, London, 1986
58. Fletcher A: Screening for cancer of the cervix in elderly women. Lancet 1990;335:97–99
59. Beard K, Bulpitt C, Mascie-Taylor H et al: Management of elderly patients with sustained hypertension. Br Med J 1992; 304:412–416
60. McEwan RT, Forster DP: A review of the costs and effectiveness of assessing the elderly in general practice. Fam Pract 1993; 10:55–62
61. Williams EI: Audit of care of older people. p. 306–314. In: Caring for Older People in the Community. Third Ed. Radcliffe Medical Press, Oxford, 1995
62. Donaldson LJ: Health and social status of elderly Asians: a community service. Br Med J 1986;293:1079–1082
63. Kelsi N, Constantinides P: Working towards Racial Equality in Health Care: The Haringay Experience. King's Fund, London, 1989
64. Pereira Gray D: Health in old age. J Roy Soc Med 1994;87: 474–476

CHAPTER 107

Geriatric Medicine: History and Current Practice in Europe

J. C. BROCKLEHURST

J. L. DALL

The United Kingdom

For various historic reasons, specialist geriatric services have developed as an integral part of the National Health Service in the UK to a greater extent than in any other part of Europe. This chapter, therefore, deals principally with the evolution and present state of geriatric medicine in the UK. The second part deals more briefly with various aspects of geriatrics in a number of other European countries.

Geriatric medicine was established in the late 1930s by Margery Warren. Her message was the need for assessment and rehabilitation of elderly disabled people, education of medical students, and research into the problems of aging and old age.[1,2] This derived from her work in the workhouse infirmary associated with the West Middlesex Hospital in London—it is in the workhouse infirmary that the history of elder care ended and the modern era began.

Britain has been somewhat unique in the world inasmuch as care of old people has been a state responsibility for about 400 years. In 1533, King Henry VIII divorced his first wife, Catherine of Aragon (who had produced no heir) and married Anne Boleyn. Because the Pope would not sanction the divorce, Henry broke with the church of Rome and established the Church of England, of which he declared himself head. As an attempt to remove the influence of the Roman Church he systematically dissolved the monasteries throughout the land that had until then provided refuge for the aged and chronic sick. As a result the, "churches, streets and lanes of London became filled with sick and infirm poor men lying begging".[3] In 1552, a census—perhaps the first attempt ever to assess social need in England—was carried out by the citizens of London. It defined those in the city needing care as "fatherless children 300; children over burdening their parents 350; sick and lame persons 200; aged and infirm 400; poor householders 600; idle vagabonds 200". Christ's Hospital was to take care of the children, while Bridewell took charge of the idle, and Bedlam the insane. St. Bartholomew's and St. Thomas' Hospitals between them cared for the remainder, "curable and incurable alike".[3] However, the problems remained, and in 1601 the responsibility for care was devolved on the local parishes under the Poor Relief Act. They were to provide for

- the able bodied to work
- children to be bound apprentice
- the lame, impotent, old, and other persons unable to work to be relieved

Relief could be in kind, but an Act of Parliament (the Knatchbull Act of 1723) permitted parishes to set up poor houses providing indoor relief. Parishes gradually ceased paying outdoor relief, poor houses gradually became "workhouses", also known as houses of industry and houses of correction. Gilbert's Act of 1782 was intended to promote humane houses for the old and indigent, but few were created. Gilbert's Act also empowered parishes to join together in unions to build workhouses that gradually included infirmaries for the sick (the hospitals established at that time specifically excluding incurables). A Poor Law Commission was set up in 1832 and its report 2 years later (leading to the Poor Law Amendment Act of 1834) established the principle of less eligibility—that is life in the workhouse had to be less eligible (or more unpleasant) "than the situation of the independent labourer of the lowest class". The intention was to discourage all but the most desperate from entering the workhouse. Separation of the sexes was to be absolute, they were to "live, sleep and take their meals in totally different parts of the building each with its own enclosed yard". The work to be engaged in was "the hardest and most tedious labour human ingenuity could devise". Special treatment was to be provided for the "aged poor of good conduct", but this seldom occurred. As for those whose conduct was not regarded as good, the Minority Report had this to say, "For old men and women of this kind the general mixed workhouse with its stigma of pauperism, its dull routine its exaction of such work as its inmates can perform and its deterrent regulations seems a fitting place in which to end a misspent life".

Because national old age pensions were not introduced until 1908, most people surviving into old age and having no savings and impoverished families had no alternative but to enter the generally hated workhouse.

The Metropolitan Asylums Board established provision in 1867 for Poor Law infirmaries separate from workhouses in London. "Chronic sick wards" were later provided in municipal hospitals set up under the Public Health Act of 1878. General hospitals established at that time specifically excluded "incurables".

In 1929 the Local Government Act superceded the Boards of Guardians by local and county authorities and gradually there developed a series of general hospitals within whose walls many of the aged found refuge. A two-tiered hospital system resulted. The newly created municipal hospitals retained responsibility for those with chronic diseases (predominantly elderly people) whom the long established voluntary hospitals (the seat of all medical training and research) would not admit. Huge waiting lists developed for admission to this chronic sick hospital accommodation. It was in the workhouse infirmary and municipal hospitals that geriatrics was born. In 1935, Margery Warren (a medical officer at the West Middlesex Hospital[4]), took over care of 858 chronic patients (including 144 mentally ill) in the adjoining workhouse infirmary. Following medical examination, 200 of these could be transferred elsewhere, beds were removed, wards improved physically, and gradually the numbers were reduced to 400 beds.[2] Her methods—careful medical and social assessment, medical treatment and rehabilitation—were described in a series of publications.[1,2,4] Her general conclusion was that chronic sick patients should be treated in a special block in a general hospital because[1]

Geriatrics is a significant subject for the teaching of medical students. It should comprise an essential part of the training of student nurses. General hospital facilities are necessary for correct diagnosis and treatment. Research on disease in old age can only be undertaken with the full facilities of a general hospital.

These were visionary proposals in 1943.

The coming of the National Health Service (NHS) in 1948 marked the end of the Poor Law. It firmly divided responsibility for elderly people between local authorities and the newly established Regional Hospital Boards. At first many of the former workhouses in which there were both dormitory and hospital accommodation became joint-user establishments between the NHS and the local authorities. However, Part III of the National Assistance Act of 1948 required the local authorities to provide care and attention for those who could not look after themselves and many old people's homes were set up by these authorities as a result. Some were no more than old workhouses with slight modifications, others were large private houses or hotels that were especially adapted, and gradually the principle of purpose building of special residential accommodation for the elderly became established. There remained then under the Regional Hospital Boards a disparate collection of workhouse infirmaries, chronic sick wards in municipal hospitals and, as time went by, other hospitals whose use was changing (e.g., infectious diseases hospitals) into which elderly and infirm people were being admitted.

Throughout the 1940s a great deal of thought and discussion was given to the problems of the "chronic sick". Lord Amulree and Dr. E. C. Sturdee both at that time working in the Ministry of Health and having been involved with chronic sick patients who were evacuated during the war to sector hospitals under the emergency medical service, carried out surveys of hospitals in different parts of the country and gave an overview to the Parliamentary Medical Group (PMG) as reported in the *British Medical Journal*.[5] They indicated that not all the chronic sick were old (figures in 1943 showed 29 percent under 65), and many need not have been in hospital. They clarified the reasons as to how their status as "chronic sick" had come about:

". . . patients with diseases which have become chronic and difficult to treat because they have not been placed under childhood treatment early enough.
Patients with a disability taken into hospital only if their friends are unable to look after them.
Patients suffering from an illness which could have been prevented.
Patients admitted with so-called chronic diseases which under treatment have improved so that they could return home but they have nowhere to go."

These four categories encapsulated (perhaps unwittingly) the whole impetus for the emergence of geriatrics as a speciality.

Amulree and Sturdee suggested that 10 to 20 percent of beds in general hospitals should be allotted to this group of patients partly to counter the "present day tendency of giving priority to acute patients and leaving the others to shift for themselves" and to ensure accurate diagnosis and treatment. Their care should be "part of the duties of the more experienced medical staff."

They discussed accommodation for those no longer needing hospital care, recommending "hostels" run on the lines of boarding houses or hotels with special attention to the requirements of old people, some single rooms and no more than four in any room. They should have good lighting (including over bed lighting), "old people often like to read and knit in bed", good heating, nonslip floors, chairs easy to get out of, and so on. In some cases, the hostel may be part of a group of "cottage homes". For long-stay patients requiring nursing care, small units with a homely atmosphere was required and "everything should be done to remove the institutional stigma."

Early followers of Margery Warren were Dr. Lionel Cosin,[6] an orthopedic surgeon at Orsett Hospital, Essex, who promoted early rehabilitation, especially of fractured femur patients, Dr. Eric Brooke at St. Helier's Hospital, Carshalton, who had begun visiting waiting list patients in their own homes by a "geriatric social worker" and Dr. Trevor Howell at the Royal Hospital, Chelsea (for retired servicemen).[7]

Surveys of Need

The dawning recognition of the needs of old people in an aging society led to a number of major surveys being carried out, producing data for the planning of services. In 1945, Curran and colleagues[8] published figures about 1,001 males aged 65 and females aged 60 and over living in poorer areas of Glasgow, all of whom were visited at home. A social and medical survey of people aged 65 and over in England was set up by the Nuffield Foundation in 1943, the results of which were published in two reports—*Old People* (1947)[9] and the *Social Medicine of Old Age* (1948).[10] The former covered several localities, while the latter was a random sample of the inhabitants of the town of Wolverhampton, yielding 143 males and 334 females aged 65 and over each visited at home by Dr. Sheldon. Shortly afterward, a study of medical and social problems in old people in Northern Ireland was carried out by Adams and Cheeseman (1951).[11] This involved visits to 1,625 patients aged 60 and over in Northern Ireland hospitals, as well as a community survey in Belfast that included findings on medical examination. A further study in the UK was that of Hobson and Pemberton (1955).[12]

A more detailed study of disease and disability in 1,062 men aged 60 to 69 all on the lists of 11 general practitioners in Birmingham was reported by Brown et al.[13] in 1958, which showed a clear relationship between disease, disability, and social class. Nevertheless, 75 percent of men aged 66 and 50 percent aged 70 were still in full-time work.

In 1947, J.W. Affleck, a psychiatrist, published a survey of 788 chronic sick patients in five hospitals in Leeds[14] (all were cared for by general practitioners, 80 percent were over 65 and 35 percent suffered primarily from mental disorder). Affleck concluded "the study of disease of the aged would be greatly assisted if, as suggested, by Warren (1946) the 'geriatrics specialty' was developed in this country to the same extent as the paediatric to which it is analogous. It might develop into one of the most important services of the future anywhere."

In 1949, in his Lumleian Lectures to the Royal College of Physicians, A. P. Thompson[15] (Professor of Therapeutics at the University of Birmingham) described results of a survey of 50 institutions in Birmingham concerned with the reception of the aged and chronic sick—a total of 5,780 beds. These comprised 45 percent of all beds for general medicine and surgery in the region. For every 100 chronic sick beds there were 2 trained nurses, 21 assistant nurses, 22 domestic workers, and 5 administrators. In one hospital (Western Road Hospital) five full-time medical officers cared for 1,000 bedfast patients in addition to other responsibilities, including maternity beds and a venereal disease department. There was no physiotherapy, no attempt at rehabilitation, all day rooms were full of beds, and 97 percent of patients were bedfast, among whom one-half were incontinent. Thompson analyzed the reasons for this state of affairs in great detail. He concluded 100 days to be the critical period in hospital for elderly people—beyond that the expectation of discharge diminished as did visiting by relatives. At that time also all the hazards of the bedfast state—contractures, decubitus ulcers, incontinence, apathy, and acceptance became firmly established. Although he noted that in two hospitals where wards were reserved especially for patients over the age of 65 irrespective of the cause leading to admission treatment and discharge were better run, nevertheless, he did not support the concept of developing geriatrics as a specialty, but rather the establishment of wards in general hospitals, especially in teaching hospitals, where

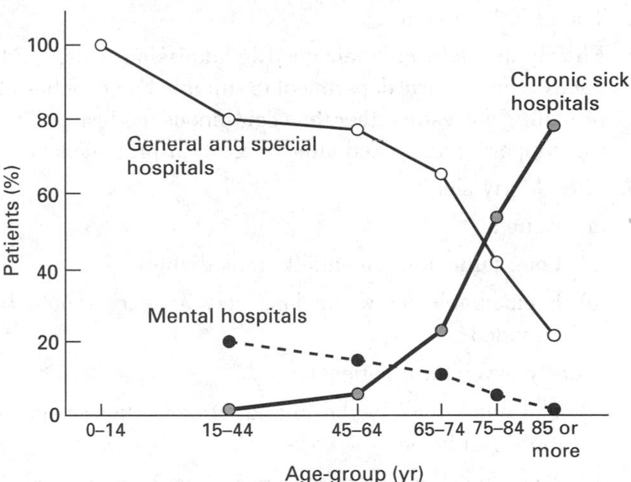

Figure 107-1 Age range of people treated in three different types of hospitals in Birmingham in 1960. (From Macintosh et al.[16] with permission.)

the aged and chronic sick would be cared for by general physicians.

In 1958 through 1959, a further study of hospital patients in all Birmingham general, special, and chronic hospitals was carried out by Thomas McKeown (Professor of Social Medicine) and his associates.[16] This involved 4,274 patients of whom in 4.7 percent it was considered that there were insufficient medical grounds for admission (11.8 percent in the chronic hospitals). The striking relationship of age with the type of hospital in which the patient was situated is shown in Figure 107-1. They concluded, "irrespective of their needs for care, physically ill patients are almost always in general and special hospitals if they are young and in chronic hospitals if they are old" and "the distribution of mentally disturbed patients who do not need the full services of a modern hospital between mental and chronic hospitals is sharply related to age and at ages 85 and over there are more of such patients in chronic than in mental hospitals".

The British Medical Association set up a Working Group in 1947 to review care of the elderly and infirm and make recommendations.[17] Of 21 members, 4 were active in the new specialty of geriatrics (Amulree, Brooke, Cousin, Warren). They noted that many elderly patients in institutions and hospitals for the chronic sick

> . . . drift into "infirmary decubitus" with avoidable contractures and deformities fixed and immobile, unable to feed themselves or sit up in bed. An atmosphere of hopelessness is shared by staff and patients alike. The situation can lead to wasteful use of nurses and hamper recruitment to an already depleted profession. Grave likelihood that hospitals throughout the country already handicapped by a shortage of beds due to insufficient nurses will be still further crippled.

The Report proposed a classification of the elderly as follows:

1. The elderly at home
2. Elderly and infirm; "their need is admission under guidance of the geriatric department to suitable homes or hostels providing domestic rather than continuous medical or nursing support" and looked after by general practitioners
3. The elderly sick
   (a) Acute:
   (b) Long-term sick (potentially remediable)
   (c) Irremediable for whom long stay annexes should be provided
4. Elderly psychiatric patients
   (a) Those not requiring hospital treatment who can stay in their own homes
   (b) Those needing custodial care in long stay annexes
   (c) Those in need of active psychiatric care or treatment in a mental hospital

They recommended the gradual establishment in general hospitals, including teaching hospitals, of special geriatric departments. A geriatric department was described as comprising wards in a general hospital reserved exclusively for elderly patients, all of whom are undergoing investigation or active treatment and rehabilitation so that in due course they may be discharged from such wards either to their own homes or after classification, to other appropriate accommodation. This included long-stay annexes which, under medical supervision of the geriatric department, would provide accommodation and nursing care for irremediable patients who after full investigation and treatment in the geriatric department show no promise of further improvement. Residential homes would each provide, in close association with the geriatric department, accommodation for 20 to 40 elderly people in need of residential, but not nursing care.

Admission to the geriatric department was to be directly from their own homes, or in some cases transfer from other hospital wards for rehabilitation and resettlement. It was hoped that, "this department will be able to absorb older patients from the acute medical wards and also relieve the surgical wards of their elderly patients after the post-operative phase and there must be sufficient beds in the long stay annexes to absorb the "20% residuum" which will be transferred to them from time to time".

The department should also have outpatient clinics, not only for consultation and investigation, but also for group exercises in which old people could benefit from the companionship of their fellows and from the stimulation of competition. Such an arrangement would, "facilitate discharge and prevent readmission" (a harbinger of the day hospital). Vehicles should be provided for this department so that it was not wholly dependent on ambulance service of the local authorities. Liaison with local authorities and other bodies public and voluntary, concerned with the problems of old age was regarded as of the highest importance.

This detailed account was published not only in the report of 1949—the Care and Treatment of the Elderly and Infirm—but in a supplement to the Report published in 1948, "The Right Patient in the Right Bed."[17]

Regarding the fourth category—elderly psychiatric patients—the report proposed observation wards within the geriatric department that would be used for assessment by a psychiatric consultant as to whether the patient should be sent to a long-stay annex as irremediable or to a mental hospital as likely to benefit from the advice and from the active treatment. It emphasized the importance of avoiding the stigma (for the family) of mental hospital admission for the "mental debility associated with old age".

In 1972, the Royal College of Physicians of London set up a Working Party whose membership consisted of 13 geriatricians and some college officers.[18] It pointed out the varying admission procedures that were developing at different geriatric departments (e.g., participating in general medical rotas; admitting all patients age 75 and over; only admitting patients referred from other clinicians). Regarding beds it reported, "most geriatric departments allot 30–40% of their beds for "continuing care", but it is obvious that the actual number of hospital beds for such patients with physical and mental infirmity must be increased during the next 30 years even if local authorities also expand their facility for the frail elderly (a prophecy which is being fulfilled in 1997 if "nursing home" is substituted for "hospital"). Problems of recruitment to the specialty were clearly indicated by the fact that there were 40 vacancies for consultant geriatricians at that time and the hope was expressed that the recently created academic departments would increase awareness of the role of geriatric medicine and the satisfaction this form of practice offers as a career. The need for specialist psychogeriatric services was also emphasized.

In 1976, yet another report of the British Medical Association was published.[19] Of a total working party membership of 17, 6 were consultant geriatricians (including 3 professors). A number of new developments were referred to, including assessment of unreported illness, good neighbor schemes, night sitters, soiled linen services, and admissions for respite care. Once again, staff shortages and inappropriate accommodation were emphasized. The importance of psychiatric assessment before the admission of mentally infirm elderly people to hospital, the involvement of health visitors in the early detection of unreported illness, and the recognition of one particular general practitioner as a visiting medical officer in a residential home with responsibility (in consultation with his colleagues) for contributing to medical policy within the home were all emphasized. Also, the importance of periodical review of medical and social needs of elderly people in residential homes and the possibilities for discharge.

The Structure of a Geriatric Service

In 1948, the year the National Health Service began, the first new appointment of a Consultant Geriatrician was made in Cornwall, Dr. Tom Wilson. This marked the recognition of a new specialty and one whose official status was the same as all other hospital specialties. By 1995, there were more than 600 consultant geriatricians in the UK. The first-generation geriatricians were each appointed to hospital management groups serving an average total population of between 200,000 and 250,000 people. The consultant was given responsibility for all the "chronic sick" beds usually in several hospitals and numbering between 200 and 400. There was generally a waiting list of similar proportions. The consultant's first clinical responsibility was to examine the patients occupying the beds, to make a diagnosis, and try to identify those who might respond to physical therapy and at least be able to be up and about and, in some cases, to move to residential homes or very occasionally, back home. At the same time, it was necessary to review those on the waiting list by visiting them at home or in the acute hospital beds that they occupied, attempting to decide some alternative to long-term care and to allot some order of priority, having in mind again those likely to respond to treatment once properly assessed. It was then necessary to decide which of the hospital wards should be used for admission and assessment and which might appropriately be used for long-term care. A number of documented accounts for this process are available.

In 1949, Exton-Smith and Crockett[20] described the initiation of a service at a London County Council Hospital (St. Pancras) after it had been taken over by a London teaching hospital (University College Hospital) under the care of a consultant, Lord Amulree. They described what they claimed was the first unit of its kind (being part of a teaching hospital) with facilities for investigation, treatment, and research. In 1949 also, Adams[21] described his work at the Belfast City Hospital, at one time the largest Poor Law Union Infirmary in the UK, but by then partly converted to a geriatric hospital with 500 to 600 of its 1,800 beds set aside for the chronic sick. Three hundred and fifty of these were in a "remote and antiquated brick building euphemistically named the 'convalescent buildings'." They comprised 60 bedded wards with "no lifts, narrow stairs and poor light". Patients were kept in bed all day to avoid falls because staff was minimal (at times, only one nurse and an orderly for 60 beds) and apathy was everywhere. This description echoes that of Marjory Warren and was repeated throughout the country where the first geriatric consultants were appointed—O. T. Brown in Glasgow, H. Droller in Leeds, J. Agate in Ipswich, T. Wilson in Truro, O. Olbrich in Sunderland, and so on.

The Style of Practice

Marjory Warren proposed that long-term care should be separate from other geriatric beds and most developments were along these lines.[22,23] Not all agreed however. Adams,[24] believed that all hospital wards should share the responsibility of care for long-stay patients and in designing new wards for his unit in Belfast, each L-shaped 40-bed ward included 16 long-stay beds in a separate area, but integral to the ward and cared for by the ward staff. Because most first-generation geriatricians were given beds in more than one hospital, it became effective to designate those at different sites for different purposes. Wards in a general hospital were best used for acute admissions (often called assessment wards) because of laboratory and radiologic facilities and easy access to other specialists. Other beds were often in former tuberculosis sanatoria or infectious diseases hospitals and might adapt well to rehabilitation with space for physiotherapy and occupational therapy. Later, day hospitals developed in association with many of these. So a system of "progressive patient care" developed in many departments (reviewed by Irvine in 1963).[25] A national survey of style of practice was carried out in 1984 by Andrews and Brocklehurst.[26,27] Two hundred and thirteen geriatric departments provided information as follows: in 38 percent acute and rehabilitation patients shared the same wards and long-stay patients were separate; 24 percent practiced complete progressive patient care with separate acute, rehabilitation, and long-stay wards; and 24 percent combined all forms of care in all wards. In 8 percent the acute assessment wards were separate and rehabilitation and long-term care combined.

The department at Hull was a leading proponent of managing all types of patients in all wards.[28] The department consisted of 433 beds in three different hospitals. An age-related admissions policy was developed (all medical emergencies aged over 75 being admitted to these beds). By 6 years after the inception of this policy, long-stay beds had been reduced to 20 percent, 5 to 6 percent of patients were transferred from other units and mean in-patient stay had been reduced to under 30 days (including long-stay patients).

The advantages of progressive patient care include better use of medical staff time—consultant ward rounds being daily or at least 2 to 3 times weekly in acute wards, once weekly in rehabilitation wards, and less frequently in long-stay wards.[27] The ward structure and process also fit the different types of patients—technical medical procedures in acute wards, all staff involved in promoting independence in rehabilitation wards, and a homely atmosphere and provision of recreational activities in long-stay wards. The disadvantage of progressive patient care was the need for patients to move between different wards and different nurses, although medical staff usually maintained continuity; also the need to maintain available beds in a number of different locations. A profile of a geriatric rehabilitation ward in 1985[29] indicated an average length of stay of 31 days for patients being discharged home, but more than twice that for patients awaiting placements in nursing homes or long-stay wards.

The concept of a "halfway house" for patients who had completed their medical care, but were not yet ready to live independently at home, was promoted by the National Corporation for the Care of Old People who set up a number of such units, usually in large houses outside hospital precincts.[30] In time, their short-stay function became lost and they added to long-stay beds. Most now have been closed or taken over as nursing homes by independent operators.

Coordination of Discharge

As the specialty developed, the need for coordination between the many agencies involved became apparent.[31] This applied not only within the hospital service, but also in the interface between primary care and hospital care and between geriaticians and psychiatrists.[32,33] The problems with aftercare led to increasing concern about discharge. While discharge planning was generally well-organized in departments of geriatric medicine, major problems remained in other hospital departments. In one study, 39 percent of the sample of people aged 65 and over were given less than 24 hours notice of discharge and less than 50 percent reported that a member of the hospital staff discussed their discharge with them while they were in hospital.[34] Lack of advice at the time of discharge was noted in 51 percent of elderly people readmitted within 28 days of discharge.[35] Another study[36] concluded that planned discharge for 650 patients aged 75 and over discharged over a period of 18 months from one hospital, could have saved 6,700 bed days by preventing a readmission. Detailed guidance for hospital discharge has recently been published.[37]

Integrated Services

An uneasy relationship between geriatric and general medicine was the constant background to the emergence of geriatrics as a specialty,[38,39] especially in two regards—the gatekeeper role of geriatrics for long-term care, which involved patients in general medical beds as well as the community; and increasing involvement of geriatricians in acute medicine of old age. Geriatricians relinquished care of patients under 65 with chronic illness as Young Disabled Units were established.[40] For those aged 65 and over, various admission policies were set up—some departments admitted according to need (i.e., those patients presenting with the "geriatric giants" or with mixed medical and social problems for which the geriatric department was specially adapted). Others were admitted on an age-related basis (varying from 65 and over to 85 and over).[41,42] These policies applied to emergency admissions while "cold" admissions referred by general practitioners through outpatients or domiciliary consultation usually included anyone 65 and over.[43] Most recently, a reintegration with general medicine for emergency admissions is gaining impetus[43–45] and now about one-fifth of geriatrics departments are integrated.[43] By this system, all emergency admissions over the age of 65 (which constitutes the majority of medical/geriatric in patients) are to joint acute wards staffed on a rota by general physicians and geriatricians. While dealing with acute problems of patients of all ages, geriatricians retain responsibilities for outpatient clinics, day hospitals, and rehabilitation of elderly people. The move towards integration has been partially driven by the need to reduce junior hospital doctors' hours of work and the problem of "outliers"—patients of one consultant being admitted to many different wards of the hospital when their wards are full. Accommodation to these difficulties acquired more rational and economic use of beds and staff. At present, age-related admission policies are dominant, but integrated services are progressively increasing.[43] Many geriatricians are concerned that these developments may foretell the end of the geriatric specialty to the disadvantage of older people. Already the geriatricians' involvement in long-term care is diminishing, and in some areas, has completely disappeared (see Ch. 111) and the role of day hospitals is coming under critical scrutiny.[46,47] (See Ch. 114.)

While most geriatricians are full-time specialists some have always had sessions in general medicine (joint appointments). These numbered 20 percent of geriatricians in 1988.[42] Half of these had five or more sessions devoted to general medicine (a full time National Health Service consultant contract is for 10 sessions a week). Specialism on a part-time basis within geriatric practice is also increasing. In 1988, 26 percent of full-time geriatricians and 48 percent of those with joint appointments practiced special interests.[42] Gastroenterology was the most frequent (24 percent) followed by cardiology (20 percent) and diabetes (16 percent).

Domiciliary Consultation

The practice of seeing the patients in their own homes was an essential part of geriatric practice in its early stages when consultants inherited large waiting lists. Such home visits were initiated by the hospital consultant, who usually carried out the visit, or sometimes by a social worker from the department.[48] Within the National Health Service they were part of the consultant's contract and called Assessment Visits.[49,50]

Apart from deciding priority for admission, or whether some alternative form of care was more appropriate, these visits had the advantage of establishing a personal rapport between doctor and patient and affording the doctor an insight into the social circumstances of his patients (and of the geographic catchement area). They allowed discussion with patients and relatives of the proposed line of action and often allowed direct contact between consultant and general practitioner.[51] They also came to have a role in the teaching of medical students.[51] Now most geriatrics departments are able to admit patients immediately on referral if they have acute problems or from outpatients or the day hospital if problems are less acute. However, a facility for consultants to offer advice to general practitioners on the diagnosis and management of patients at home remains and is allowed for within the National Health Service by a second type of home visit called a Domiciliary Consultation. This is initiated by the general practitioner and attracts a fee to the specialist. While the intention of such consultations was that the specialist and general practitioner should both be present, in fact this only happens in a minority of cases.[51] A review in 1991 suggested that a study was needed to identify the problems for which consultants and general practitioners thought domiciliary consultations might be useful (such as planning domiciliary palliative care).[52]

Special Units

Stroke units and orthogeriatric units have been developed in a number of geriatric departments (in 1985, stroke units in 11 percent and orthogeriatric units in 20 percent of departments[26]). These functioned with varying patterns—orthogeriatric wards having shared staffing with surgeons and geriatricians, stroke units usually being entirely staffed by geriatricians, but with specially trained physiotherapists, occupational therapists, and nurses. Early assessments of the effectiveness of some of these units was rather discouraging, but more recently have been very positive.[53,54] (See also Ch. 85.)

Prevention in Care of the Elderly

There are many reasons why elderly people may not consult their doctors with their symptoms—they regard them as inevitable accompaniments of aging, the doctor was regarded as too busy to be bothered by them, they have no telephone to make an appointment, or they have no transport to get to the general practitioner's surgery. The extent of unreported illness was investigated in Edinburgh in 1964 by Williamson and colleagues[55] who reported a considerable iceberg of morbidity. A clinic providing medical assessment associated with access to a health visitor (nurse), physiotherapist, chiropodist, and a voluntary welfare organizer was set up in 1952 in Rutherglen near Glasgow by Ferguson Anderson and Nairn Cowan.[56] Clients were referred by their general practitioners and findings on the first 500 were described in 1955.[56] Other schemes of screening or case finding have been published since then.[57–60] The responsibility for this service has been made a contractual obligation for general practitioners in the NHS and is now offered to all people aged 75 and over.

The Geriatric Day Hospital

Geriatric day hospitals were preceded in the UK by some patients attending in the daytime only at geriatric wards or rehabilitation units, coming from their own homes.[61] The first day hospitals described in the literature were in Oxford[62] and Leeds.[63] In 1958 through 1959 James Farndale[64] visited nine geriatric day hospitals, describing them as small and experimental. The first purpose-built day hospital was opened at Cowley Road Hospital, Oxford in 1958. The work of geriatric day hospitals was described in a number of publications in the early 1960's.[65–67] The first attempt to carry out a controlled trial of day hospital care was published by Woodford Williams and colleagues[68] in 1962. Further developments in geriatric day hospitals are described in Chapter 114.

Psychogeriatrics

The present structure and process of the specialty of psychogeriatrics is described by Arie (Ch. 42). The plight of mentally ill older people in general and chronic sick hospitals was highlighted in Thompson[15] in his report—indicating 25 percent of the 1,000 patients in the Western Road Infirmary in Birmingham in 1948 as being certifiably insane. Twenty-two years later, a further study of patients in hospital in Birmingham[16] showed the switch in the number of patients requiring some supervision because of their mental state between mental hospital and chronic sick hospitals as a function of advancing age (Fig. 107-1). The widespread mixing of patients with mental illness and physical disability in mental hospitals, geriatric wards and residential wards in Newcastle was highlighted by Kay and colleagues[69] in 1966 (Table 107-1). They advocated comprehensive psychogeriatric assessment units attached to general hospitals and staffed by geriatricians and psychiatrists. Developments in joint care between geriatrics and psychiatry by providing joint-assessment beds were demonstrated in Edinburgh in 1960,[70] in Nottingham in 1968,[71] and in Cornwall (together with a joint day hospital) in 1970.[72] Joint-assessment wards received encouragement from the Department of Health in 1970.[73] Specialist consultant psychogeriatricians began to be appointed in the National Health Service through the 1970's and the specialty received official recognition by the Department of Health in 1989.

Professional Training

In the UK, registration as a medical practitioner requires 5 years undergraduate study leading to the degree of Bachelor of Medicine and Bachelor of Surgeon (BMBS) followed by 1-year internship as a House Officer (6 months medicine and 6 months surgery). Thereafter, specialist training involves at least a further 7 years. Geriatric specialization is usually by dual accreditation in geriatric medicine and general internal medicine. This involves 3-years in general internal medicine and 4 years in geriatric medicine. The latter must include 2 years in posts involving clinical responsibilities for care of elderly patients in all relevant settings. The other 2 years provide for a number of options—for example, academic experience (research or postgraduate degree course); subspecialty within general internal medicine; related specialty, for example, public health medicine, general practice, rehabilitative/palliative medicine, or further experience in geriatric medicine including psychiatry of old age, stroke, etc. The diploma of membership of one of the Royal College of Physicians in the UK (MRCP) by written or clinical examination is essential, and is usually obtained within the first 2 years of training. For those intending to specialize within academic geriatrics, a doctors degree obtained by thesis (M.D. or Ph.D.) is also generally required.

Early Personalities and Publications

The British Geriatrics Society was formed as the Medical Society for the Care of the Elderly at a meeting convened by Dr. Trevor Howell in 1947. Those present included Lord

Table 107-1 Mental and physical status of aged patients in three types of institutions

	Mental Hospitals $n = 133$	Geriatric Wards $n = 50$	Welfare Homes $n = 73$
Mental			
Severe brain syndrome	49	42	29
Mild brain syndrome	0	18	11
Other mental syndrome	57	24	24
Physical			
Severe physical disability	28	48	12
Housebound (before admission)	34	30	40
Bedfast (before admission)	0	20	4
	Figures %		

(From Kay et al.,[69] with permission.)

Amulree, Dr. Sturdee, Dr. Marjory Warren, Dr. Eric Brooke, Mr. Lionel Cousin, Dr. Thomas Wilson, and Dr. Alfred Mitchum and Dr. Trevor Howell, who may be regarded as the founder members.[74]

In 1959, the name was changed to The British Geriatrics Society, and since then there have been episodic discussions about changing the name once more because of the fairly widespread use of the word *geriatric* in a pejorative manner (*"he's just an old geriatric"*), but this is largely a UK phenomenon, relating probably to the workhouse origin of the specialty, and Nascher's word, *geriatric*, remains paramount worldwide. In the UK, many departments now call themselves Care of the Elderly or some similar title, but the Society's name persists. Membership in 1995 numbers, 1770.

Marjory Warren, CBE (1897–1960) In 1936, Marjorie Warren became an Assistant Medical Officer at the West Middlesex County Hospital. Among her duties, she undertook more than 4,000 surgical operations. In 1935, the adjacent workhouse infirmary was annexed to the hospital and she took charge of it as described elsewhere. The reformed wards, with beds eventually diminished from 714 to 200, became a geriatric "Mecca" visited by physicians and others worldwide and inspiring the early pioneers to emulate her methods. She died prematurely in a car crash at the height of her career[75,76] (Fig. 107-2).

Lord Amulree, KBE (1900–1983) Lord Amulree was recruited to the Ministry of Health in 1933 with responsibilities among others for the Poor Law. At the time, due to wartime bombing of cities, many patients from chronic sick hospitals were transferred to temporary hospitals in the country, and Amulree, among others, became aware of the neglected state of these patients. Along with his senior colleague Sturdee, he brought this to the notice of the House of Lords[5] in 1946, and in 1949 he was appointed Consultant Physician in Geriatric Medicine at St. Pancras' Hospital annexed to University College Hospital. This was the first teaching hospital appointment in geriatrics. He was President of the British Geriatrics Society from its inception in 1946 for 25 years[77] (Fig. 107-3).

A. L. Sturdee After service in the Royal Navy in World War I, A. L. Sturdl joined the Minister of Health with responsibilities for the administration of the Poor Law. He presented

Figure 107-2 Dr. Marjory Warren–the founder of British geriatric medicine. (From Adams,[75] with permission.)

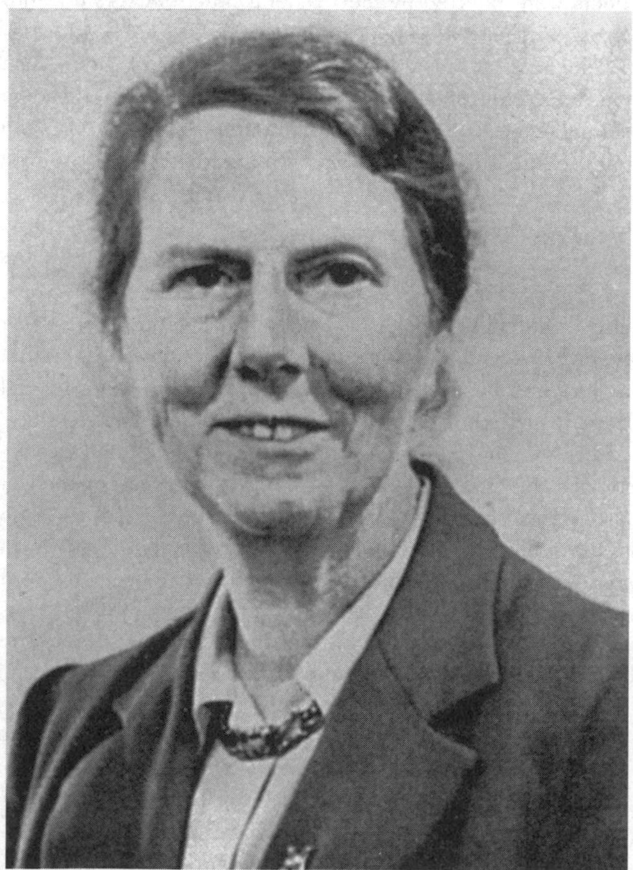

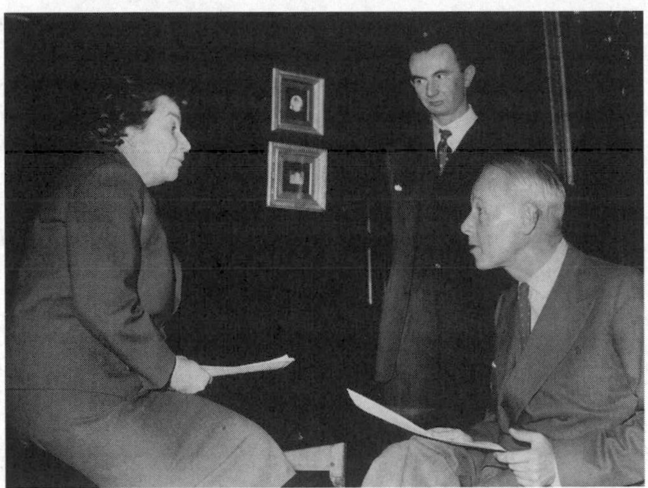

Figure 107-3 Lord Amulree (seated, right), first president and founding member of the Society for Care of the Elderly, later British Geriatrics Society (1948–1973); Professor Norman Exton-Smith (standing) first Joint Editor of both *Gerontolgia Clinica* and *Age and Ageing*, President of British Geriatrics Society (1978–1981); Professor Anna Aslan, Director, Institue of Gerontology, Bucharest, Romania.

the case for geriatrics in the House of Lords (with Amulree as assistant).[5]

Eric Brooke (1896–1956) Eric Brooke was Medical Superintendent of St. Helier's Hospital in Surrey like Marjory Warren and was confronted with a large number of chronic sick beds and a considerable waiting list. He decided to visit the patients at home accompanied by a social worker—this was regarded as the beginning of domiciliary assessment visits. He is also credited with the origins of the day hospital, bringing patients up to hospital wards for physiotherapy and preventing the need for admission.[78]

Lionel Cosin (1913–1944) Lionel Cosin was an orthopaedic surgeon who became Medical Superintendent of Orsett Hospital in Essex in 1937, and like Warren and Brooke, was confronted with the problem of the chronic sick. He developed a rehabilitation program and when he moved to Cowley Road Hospital in Oxford he established an early model geriatric unit, which became another focus for national and international visitors. He planned and developed the first purpose-built geriatric day hospital in 1958.[79]

Trevor Howell (1908–1988) Trevor Howell, the prime mover in creating the Medical Society for Care of the Elderly, was its first secretary. After a period in general practice he was posted during World War II as a Medical Officer to the Royal Hospital Chelsea—a large hospital for retired military personnel. His interest in clinical aspects of aging led to a research fellowship after the war followed by consultant appointment as a Physician in Geriatric Medicine at St. John's Hospital, Battersea, and subsequently at Queen's Hospital, Croydon.[80] He published widely in clinical medicine and medical history, including one of the early books (in 1946), *Old Age: Some Practical Points In Geriatrics*[81] (Fig. 107-4).

Thomas Wilson (1918–) After wartime service in the RAF, Thomas Wilson joined Trevor Howell at St. John's Hospital, and among other achievements, carried out the first series of cystometrograms in elderly people.[82] In 1948 he was appointed to the first advertised post of consultant geriatricians in the National Health Service, at Truro, Cornwall, where he developed early geriatric/psychogeriatric co-ordination.[82]

Dr. J. A. Sheldon, CBE (1893–1972) Dr. Sheldon, whose survey of aging in Wolverhampton has been referred to already[10], served as President of the Second International Congress of the International Association of Gerontology held in London in 1954. His researches included falls in old age and he developed what was probably the first measurement of sway.[83]

Sir Ronald Tonbridge (1906–1954) Sir Richard Tonbridge was Professor of Medicine at the University of Leeds in 1944, and promoted the cause of geriatrics being one of the two UK representatives at the formation of the International Association of Gerontology IGA (St. Louis, 1951) and Served as Chairman of the Second Congress of the IGA in 1954.

Figure 107-4 Dr. Trevor Howell—first secretary and founding member of the Medical Society for Care of the Elderly, later British Geriatrics Society.

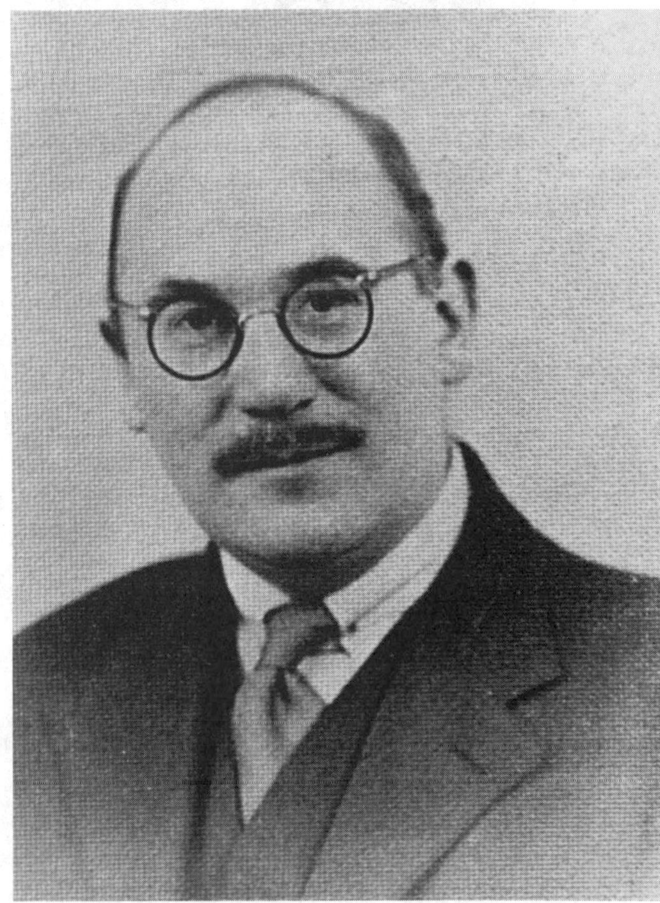

The individuals mentioned above were the early members of the British Geriatrics Society. Other early pioneers included Charles Andrews, who surveyed workhouses in Cornwall and recommended a countywide geriatric service headed by consultant geriatricians, which materialized in the appointment of Thomas Wilson. George Adams, CBE, whose study of the aged in community and hospitals in Northern Ireland has already been referred to,[21] attended the first meeting of the Medical Society for Care of the Elderly in 1948 and became second President of the British Geriatrics Society. He became consultant, and later Professor of Geriatric Medicine in Belfast. Sir Ferguson Anderson, appointed Coordinator of Geriatric Services in Glasgow subsequently occupied the first Chair of Geriatric Medicine in the UK. He became President of the Royal College of Physicians and Surgeons in Glasgow and the third President of the British Geriatrics Society (Fig. 107-5).

Publications

Among early British publications concerned with old age was "Records of Longevity" by Thomas Bailey (1857)—an essay on the history of longevity followed by notes on hundreds of individuals reputed to have lived 100 years or longer, and Charcot's lectures to the New Sydenham Society in 1881. In 1922, Sir Humphrey Rolleston developed his Linacre lectures into *Aspects of Old Age*, a well-documented book. His definition of old age as the *period at which man ceases to adjust himself to his environment* is not far from a modern definition of aging as a failure of homeostasis.

Figure 107-5 Professor Sir Ferguson Anderson—first professor of Geriatric Medicine in the UK President of the British Geriatrics Society (1975–1979).

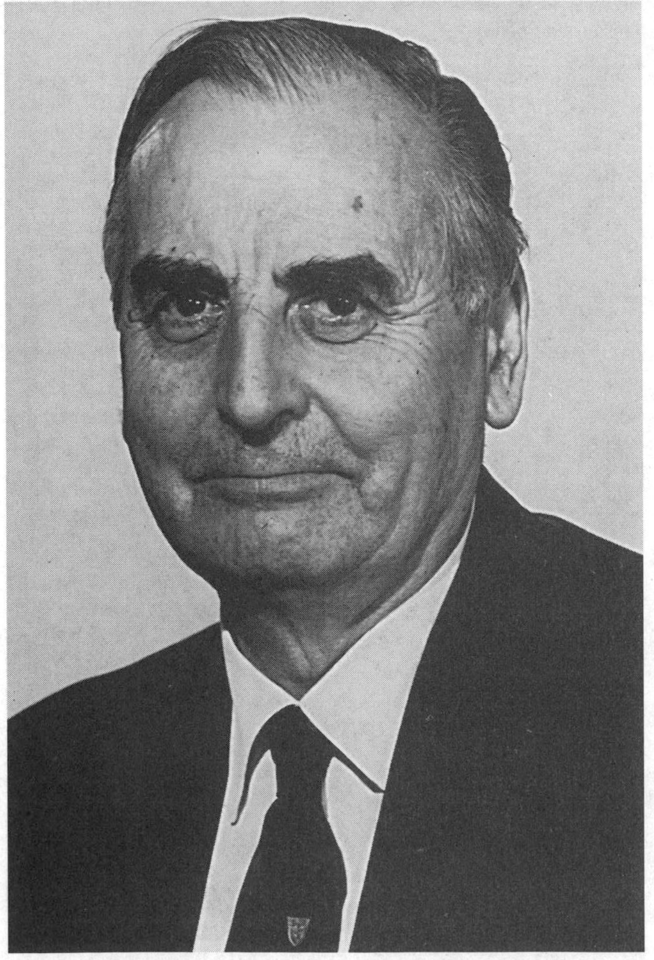

Books describing aspects of geriatric practice include, *Old Age—Some Practical Points in Geriatrics* (Howell, 1946), *Adding Life to Years* (Amulree, 1957), *Medical Problems of Old Age* (Exton-Smith, 1955), *Modern Trends in Geriatrics* (Hobson, 1956), *Rehabilitation of the Elderly Invalid at Home* (Adams, 1957), and *Social and Medical Problems of the Elderly* (Hazel, 1960).

The first large textbook was the First Edition of the present volume, *Geriatric Medicine and Gerontology*, Edited by J. C. Brocklehurst. It contained 760 pages contributed by 44 authors—modest numbers when compared with the present Fifth Edition.

Monographs include the two reports from the Nuffield Foundation already referred to—*Old People* (1947), and the *Social Medicine of Old Age* Sheldon (1948); *Incontinence and Old People* (Brocklehurst, 1951); which described cystometry and anoarectal manometry (using smoked drums and rubber tambours in the pretransducer era) and *Skill and Age* (Welford, 1951). Others include *The Biology of Senescence* (Comfort, 1956), *Family Life and Old People* (Townsend, 1957), *Physiological and Pathological Ageing* (Korenchevsky, 1958) and *Valvular Disease of the Heart in Old Age* (Bedford and Caird, 1960).

The first European journal, *Gerontologia Clinica*, edited by Woodford Williams and Exton-Smith and published by Karger became the official publication of the British Geriatrics Society (first published in 1956) until its own journal, *Age and Ageing*, was produced in 1971, edited by Exton-Smith and Hodkinson. *Gerontologia Clinica* continues as the European journal of gerontology.

Europe

It is still a minority of countries that have a nationally recognized specialty of geriatric medicine. Nevertheless, in most parts of Europe there are physicians who have been trained, or trained themselves, to develop a special interest in this field. Each country has developed in its own way, but an important catalyst has been the International Association of Gerontology (IAG). This organization was inaugurated at the first International Congress held in Liege in 1951 under the presidency of Professor Brull. Participants in the congress came from a wide range of experience and interest in aging in the domains of biology, social and behavioral science, and clinical medicine. An important purpose in setting up the IAG was to attract the attention of governments to the developing phenomenon of population aging and the rudimentary services and professional expertise that were available to meet this challenge.

A seminar was held in 1995[84] examining the arrangements for teaching of geriatric medicine throughout the European Union (EU). The report provided information about the geriatric services in the Union. Two streams were identified—specialist geriatricians working in hospitals, and general practitioners with specialist training working in long-term care institutions. An autonomous speciality in geriatric medicine was present in Belgium, Denmark, Finland, France, Germany, Italy, Ireland, The Netherlands, Norway, Spain, Sweden, Switzerland, and the UK, although in most cases this was not usually applied universally throughout the nation. In non-EU countries there is a specialty in several countries of the former USSR, notably Ukraine. Following are examples from a number of representative European countries, of their approach to medicine in old age.

The Netherlands

Much of the following information is derived from a paper by Dr. R. J. van Zonneveld.[85] From the 15th century, hovges (small courts) were created by employers for some of their former employees or servants and by churches and other charitable groups for the accommodation of elderly people. Special buildings, gasthhizen (guesthouses), were developed in the 16th and 17th centuries for the sick, the poor, the aged, and vagabonds, followed by poorhouses later becoming workhouses in the 18th century. While many ill elderly people were cared for in hospitals and asylums, nursing homes gradually developed in the 20th century—increasingly on a nonprofit basis, which from 1968 on (the General Special Sickness Expenses Insurance Act) were publicly funded. Gradually, a small number of specialists in geriatric medicine appeared, notably, Dr. I. T. H. Schreuder in Zonnestraal (a former diamond workers' sanitorium) in Hilversum where he developed in particular, a multiple disciplinary rehabilitation unit for stroke patients with an impetus on group work and with several novel developments, including the employment of pantomime actors to promote various methods of expression. Jaap Schouten developed a geriatric service in a teaching hospital in Amsterdam and others followed his example. The specialty of geriatrics is recognized, but not yet universally. The associated specialty of "Nursing Home Medicine" was pioneered in The Netherlands.

Sweden

As elsewhere, the aged and chronic sick in Sweden were cared for in a variety of institutions without any national planning until 1951, when the general wards for the chronically sick were recognized,[86] and a Hospital Act of 1959 made it possible to organize special units with their own consultants for long-term care within the framework of the general hospital. The specialty of "Long Term Care Medicine" became officially recognized in 1969. Long-term wards were established both in general hospitals and in separate hospitals with good resources for rehabilitation, the provision of day care, and outpatient consultation. There was a notable development in the city of Götenburg where the Department of Long Term Care

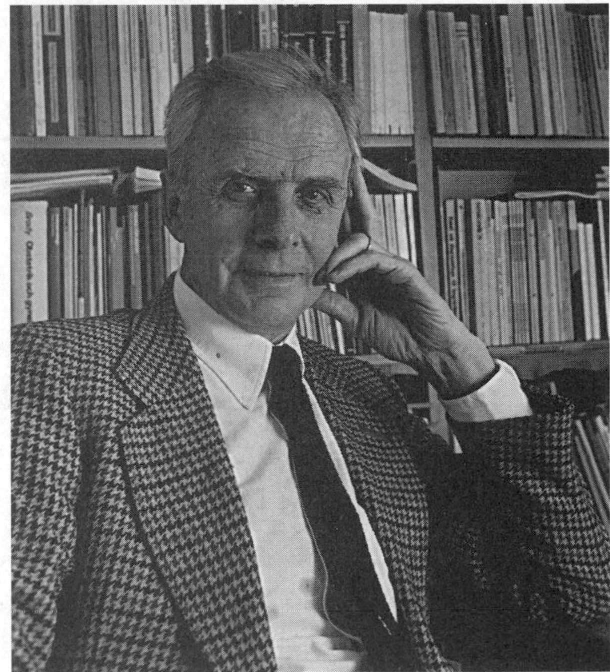

Figure 107-6 Professor Alvar Svanborg—Founder of geriatric medicine in Götenborg, Sweden and of the Göttenborg Longitudinal Study.

Medicine developed within the Vasa Hospital under the direction of Alvar Svanborg. (Fig. 107-6). Not only service and teaching were provided, but an ambitious and successful program of research, including one of the first, and probably the most comprehensive, longitudinal study of aging.[87]

Denmark

A different approach from Denmark was the development of an experimental unit for aged and chronically ill patients in Copenhagen. De Gamles By (Old Peoples Town) was where the Physician In-Chief Torben Geill was appointed in 1936 (Fig. 107-7). Thirty years later at the time of Geill's retirement in 1966, the "experiment" had grown to 1,500 hospital beds with 19 physicians' laboratories and rehabilitation services.[88]

Italy

Enrico Greppi, Professor in the Medical Clinic, University of Florence, (Fig. 107-8) developed an early interest in clinical problems of old age, leading to the formation of a Department of Gerontology in the university with colleagues F. M. Antonini and A. Zilli. An outpatient clinic, the Centro di Gerontologia e Geriatria, attached to the Department of Gerontology, in addition to its consultative role, developed a preventative program, examining groups of pensioners from the city and environs of Florence.

France

A prime mover in geriatric development in France was J. A. Huet, Professeur at L.'Ecole d'Anthropologie in Paris who had a special interest in difficulties found by retired employees

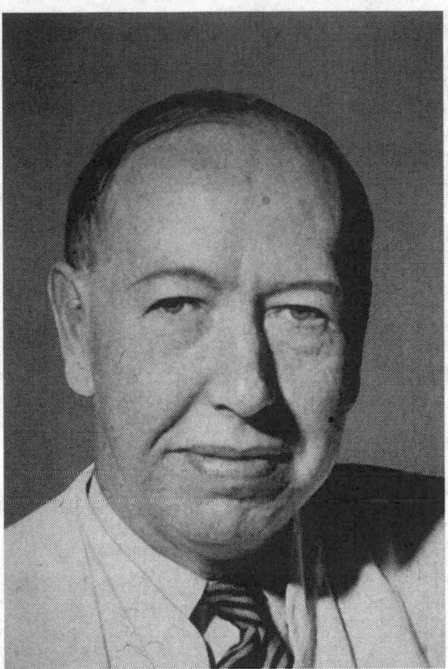

Figure 107-7 Dr. Torben Geill—founder of geriatrics in Denmark. Chief Physician De Gamles By (1936–1966). President IGA (1963–1966).

Figure 107-8 Professor Enrico Greppi—founding member of the International Association of Gerontology and President (1957–1959). President of Italian Society of Gerontology and Geriatrics (1950–1969).

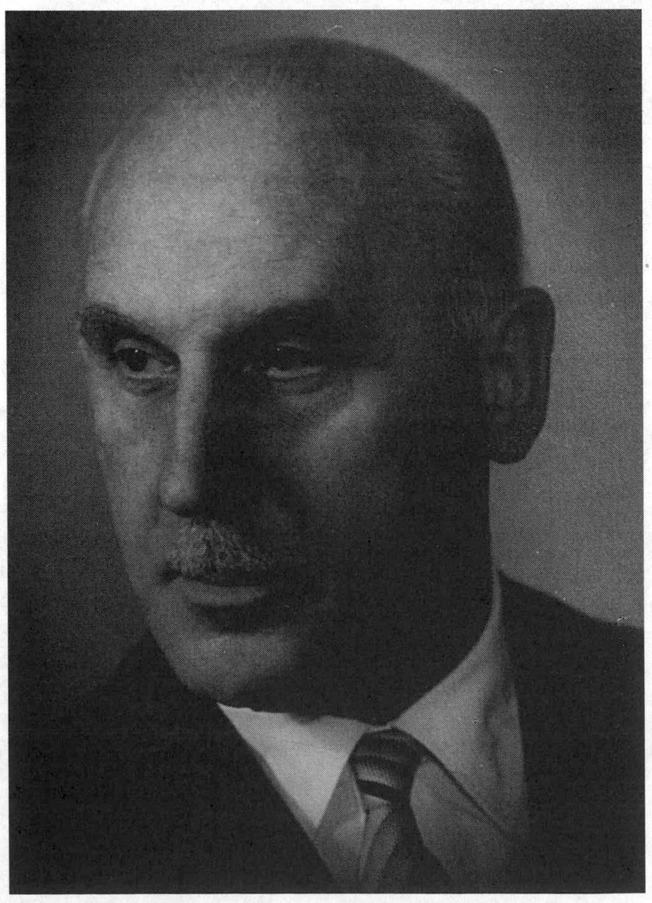

and was a founder of the IAG. A large chronic diseases hospital in Paris at Ivry Sur Seine became a focus of geriatric development under the guidance of Dr. Vignalou and Professor Berthaux. Other clinical departments were established in France (e.g., by Huganot in Grenoble, and Peters in Mulhouse). While the specialty of geriatrics is not universally recognized in France, much care of old people is centered in hospices that also provide care for mentally ill and mentally subnormal patients. Most medical schools provide some teaching on geriatrics and gerontology and there are training programs for specialists and general practitioners. One of the early European institutes of gerontology was established by Professor Bourliére in Paris who also published an early text, *Precis de Gerantologie* with L. Binet. In 554 pages it covers all major body systems, surgery, and psychiatry.

Germany

Developments have been predominant in psychogeriatrics in Germany. Hans Thomae, Professor of Psychology at the University of Bonne, pioneered a longitudinal study (Bonn Longitudinal Study of Ageing) with a special emphasis on personality, coping, and social interaction. Manfred Bergmann, Professor of Psychiatry at Heinrick Heine University, Düsseldorf, has been a pioneer in this field and was the first President of the International Psychogeriatric Association.

The specialty of geriatric medicine has had official recognition since 1996. Recognition is available to specialists in general medicine, neurology, and psychiatry. In some states an oral examination is mandatory, in others a 2-year residency in a geriatric department. Early hospital geriatric departments were developed in the 1970's by among others, Hartleb (Leverkusan-North Rhine Westphalia) and Martin (Duisberg). There are 32 day hospitals in the country with more planned, three Chairs of Geriatric Medicine (Universities of Berlin, Bochum, and Herdecke), and one Chair of Gerontology (Erlangan University).

Ukraine

In the former USSR, a notable institute of gerontology was established in Kiev (Institute of Gerontology of the USSR Acadamy of Medical Sciences) headed by Professor D. F. Chebotarev. A mass survey of 13,000 people aged 80 and over has been carried out, as well as studies on centenarians in Georgia. In Kiev also, a Chair of Geriatrics and Gerontology was established in 1970 in the Institute to further postgraduate training in problems of old age. Geriatrics polyclinics are found in centers throughout the former USSR.[89] There is particular emphasis on preventative aspects with a widespread system of Groups of Health—keep fit institutions for elderly people.

References

1. Warren MW: Care of chronic sick. A case for treating chronic sick in blocks in a general hospital. Br Med J 1943;ii:822–823
2. Warren MW: Care of the chronic aged sick. Lancet 1946;i: 841–843

3. Ives AGL: Responsibility for the "chronic" sick: the historical perspective. Lancet 1946;ii:915–916
4. Warren MW: The role of a geriatric unit in a general hospital. Ulster Med J 1949;(May) 3–12
5. Lord Amulree, Sturdee AL: Care of the chronic sick and of the aged. Br Med J 1946;617–619
6. Cosin L: A Statistical Analysis of Geriatric Care: Proceeding of the Royal Society of Medicine 1948;XLI:333–336
7. Howell T: Aspects of the history of geriatric medicine. Proc Roy Soc Med 1976;69:445–449
8. Curran M, Hamilton J, Orr JS et al: The care of the aged: observations based on experience in Glasgow Outdoor Medical Service. Lancet 1945;i:149–152
9. Nuffield Foundation: Old People. Oxford University Press, Oxford, 1947
10. Sheldon JH: The Social Medicine of Old Age. Oxford University Press, Oxford, 1948
11. Adams GF, Cheeseman EA: Old people in Northern Ireland; A Report to the Northern Ireland Hospital Authority on Medical and Social Problems of Old Age, 1951
12. Hobson W, Pemberton JA: The Health of the Elderly at Home. Butterworth, London, 1955
13. Brown RG, McKeown T, Whitfield AGM: Observations on the medical condition of men in the seventh decade. Br Med J 1958;555–562
14. Affleck JW: The chronic sick in hospital: a psychiatric approach. Lancet 1947;i:355–359
15. Thomson AP: Problems of ageing and chronic sickness. Br Med J 1949;i:243–249, 300–305
16. McKeown T, MacKintosh JM, Lowe CR: Influence of age on type of hospital to which patients are admitted. Lancet 1961; i:818–820
17. British Medical Association: The care and treatment of the elderly and infirm. Report of a Special Committee of the British Medical Association. British Medical Association, London, 1949; and The right patient in the right bed. Supplement to a Report of the British Medical Association Committee on the Care and Treatment of the Elderly and Infirm. British Medical Association, London, 1947
18. A Report of the College Committee on Geriatric Medicine. Royal College of Physicians of London, London, 1972
19. British Medical Association: Care of the Elderly. British Medical Association Board of Education Science. British Medical Association, London, 1976
20. Exton-Smith AN, Crockett GS: The chronic sick under new management: experiences in starting a geriatric unit. Lancet 1949;i:1016–1018
21. Adams, GF: Geriatrics in Northern Ireland. Lancet 1949;ii: 1095–1097
22. Lord Amulree, Exton-Smith AN, Crockett, GS: Proper use of the hospital in treatment of the aged sick. Lancet 1951;i:123–126
23. Exton-Smith AN: Progressive patient care in geriatrics. Lancet 1962;i:260–262
24. Adams GF: The third phase in geriatric medicine: design and purpose of a hospital geriatric department. Lancet 1960;i: 815–817
25. Irvine RE: Progressive patient care in the geriatric unit. Postgrad Med J 1963;39:401–407
26. Andrews K, Brocklehurst JC: Geriatric medicine: the style of practice. Age Ageing 1985;14:1–7
27. Andrews K, Brocklehurst JC: British Geriatric Medicine in the 1980's. King Edward's Hospital Fund for London, London, 1987
28. Bagnall WE, Datta SR, Knox J, Horrocks P: Geriatric medicine in Hull: a comprehensive service. Br Med J 1977;ii:102–104
29. Andrews K, Brocklehurst JC: A profile of geriatric rehabilitation units. J Roy Coll Phys London 1985;19:240–243
30. Adams GF: Betwixt and between: a recovery home for the old. Lancet 1954;ii:486–488
31. Brocklehurst JC: Co-ordination of care of the elderly. Lancet 1966;i:1363–1366
32. Brocklehurst JC, Shergold M: What happens when geriatric patients leave hospital. Lancet 1968;ii:1133–1135
33. Brocklehurst JC, Shergold M: Old people leaving hospital. Gerontol Clin 1969;11:115–126
34. Victor VR, Vetten MJ: Preparing the elderly for discharge from hospital: a neglected aspect of patient care. Age Ageing 1988; 17:155–163
35. Williams AEI, Fitton F: 1988 Factors affecting early unplanned re-admission of elderly patients to hospital. Br Med J 1988; 297:784–787
36. Townsend J, Piper M, Frank AO et al: Reduction in hospital in readmission stay of elderly patients by a community based hospital discharge scheme: a randomised control trial. Br Med J 1988;297:544–547
37. British Geriatrics Society: The discharge of elderly persons from hospital for community care. A Compendium Document. Section 7. British Geriatrics Society, London, 1995
38. Leonard JC: Can geriatrics survive? Br Med J 1976;i: 1335–1336
39. O'Brien TD, Joshi DM, Warren EW: No apology for geriatrics. Br Med J 1975;iv:277–280
40. Young Disabled Units: Chronically Sick and Disabled Persons Act 1970. Her Majesty's Stationary Office, London, 1970
41. Kafetz K, O'Farrell J, Parry A et al: Age related geriatric medicine: relevance of special skills of geriatric medicine to elderly people admitted to hospital as medical emergencies. J Roy Soc Med 1995;88:629–633
42. Brocklehurst JC, Davidson C: Interface between geriatric and general medicine. Health Trends 1989;21:48–50
43. British Geriatrics Society: Acute Medical Care of Elderly People. British Geriatrics Society Compendium Document: 12.2 Appendix 1. British Geriatrics Society, London, 1995
44. Grimley Evans J: Integration of geriatric with general medical services in Newcastle. Lancet 1983;i:1430–1433
45. Royal College of Physicians: Ensuring Equity and Quality of Care for Elderly People: The Interface between Geriatric Medicine and General (Internal) Medicine. Royal College of Physicians, London, 1994
46. National Audit Office: National Health Service Day Hospitals for Elderly People in England. Report by Comptroller and Auditor General. Her Majesty's Stationary Office, London, 1994
47. House of Commons Committee of Public Accounts: National

Health Service Day Hospitals for Elderly People in England. Her Majesty's Stationary Office, London, 1995

48. Care of the old in their homes. Lancet 1949;i:462
49. Arcand M and Williamson J: An evaluation of home visiting of patients by physicians in geriatric medicine. Br Med J 1981; 283:718–720
50. British Geriatrics Society: Assessment domiciliary visits. British Geriatrics Society Compendium Document. Section 22.1. British Geriatrics Society, London, 1995
51. Donaldson LJ, Hill PM: The domiciliary consultation service: time to take stock. Br Med J 1991;302:449–451
52. Forsythe M: Domiciliary visits: we need to identify the ones worth doing. Br Med J 1991;302:426–427
53. Gladman J, Barer D, Langhorne P: Specialist rehabilitation after stroke. Br Med J 1996;312:1623–1624
54. Hempsall VJ, Robertson DRC, Campbell MJ, Briggs RS: Orthopaedic Geriatric Care: is it defective? J Roy Coll Phys 1990; 24:47–50
55. Williamson J, Stokoe IH, Grey S et al: Old people at home: their unreported need. Lancet 1964;i:117–120
56. Anderson WF, Cowan NR: A consultative health centre for old people: the Rutherglen experiment. Lancet 1955;ii:239–240
57. Lowther CP, Macleod RDM, Williamson J. The evaluation of early diagnostic service for the elderly. Br Med J 1970;iii: 275–277
58. Williams EI: A follow-up of geriatric patients: socio-medial assessments. J Roy Coll Gen Pract 1974;24:341–346
59. Pike EA: Screening of the elderly in general practice. J Roy Coll Gen Pract 1976;26:698–703
60. Tulloch AJ, Moore V: A randomised controlled trial of geriatric screening and surveillance in general practice. J Roy Coll Gen Pract 1979;730–733
61. Brocklehurst JC: The geriatric day hospital. King Edward's Hospital Fund for London, London, 1970
62. Cosin L: The place of the day hospital in the geriatric unit. The Practitioner 1954;552–559
63. Droller H: A geriatric outpatient department. Lancet 1958;ii: 739–741
64. Farndale J: The day hospital movement in Great Britain. Pergammon Press, London, 1961
65. McComb SJ, Powell DJD: A geriatric day hospital. Gerontol Clin 1961;3:146–151
66. Fine W: Integration of a day hospital into a geriatric service. Geront Clin 1964;6:129–142
67. Brocklehurst JC: The work of a geriatric day hospital. Gerontol Clin 1964;6:151–166
68. Woodford Williams E, McKeown A, Trotter S: The day hospital in community care of the elderly. Gerontol Clin 1962;4: 241–256
69. Kay DW, Roth M, Hall MRP: Special problems of the aged and the organisation of hospital services. Br Med J 1966;ii:967–972
70. Fish F, Williamson J: A delirium unit in an acute geriatric hospital. Gerontol Clin 1964;6:71–80
71. Morton EVB, Barker ME, MacMillan D: The joint assessment and early treatment unit in psychogeriatric care. Gerontol Clin 1968;10:65–73
72. Wilson TS: A psychogeriatric service in Cornwall. Mod Geriatr 1970;Oct:29–39
73. DHSS Psychogeriatric Assessment Unit: Circular HM (70) 11. Her Majesty's Stationary Office, London, 1970
74. Howell T: Origins of the British Geriatrics Society. Age Ageing 1974;3:69–72
75. Adams GF: Margery Warren CBE 1897–1960. Gerontol Clin 1961;3:1–4
76. Matthews DA: Dr Margery Warren and the origin of British geriatrics. J Am Geriatr Soc 1984;32:253–258
77. Lord Amulree: Obituary; Munks Roll. Vol. VII. pp. 12–13. Royal College of Physicians, London, 1984
78. Brooke E: Obituary; Munks Roll. Vol. V. pp. 52–53. Royal College of Physicians, London, 1968
79. Cosin L: Obituary. British Geriatrics Society Newsletter, London, May 1994
80. Howell JH: Obituary. British Geriatrics Society Newsletter, London, July 1988
81. Howell TH: Old age: some practical points of geriatrics. Lewis, London, 1944
82. Wilson TS: Incontinence of urine in the aged. Lancet 1948;ii: 374–377
83. Sheldon JH: Natural history of falls in old age. Br Med J 1960; ii:1685–1690
84. Role of geriatrics/gerontology in the training and practice of physicians in Europe. Ministere du Travail et des Affaires Sociales, Paris, 1995
85. Van Zonneveld RJ: The Netherlands. In Geriatric Care in Advanced Society. Brocklehurst JC (ed): MTP, Lancaster, 1975
86. Svanborg A: Sweden. In Geriatric Care in Advanced Societies. Brocklehurst JC (ed): MTP, Lancaster, 1975
87. Rinder L, Rupe S, Steen B and Svanborg A: Seventy-year old people in Gottenburg: a population study in an industrialised Swedish study. Acta Med Scand 1975;198:397–407
88. Torben Geill on his seventieth birthday. Apolekerforensing, Copenhagen, 1966
89. Revutskya RG: USSR. In Geriatric Care in Advanced Societies. Brocklehurst JC (ed): Lancaster, MTP, 1975

CHAPTER 108

Geriatrics in North America

WILLIAM H. BARKER

The present and future status of geriatric medicine in North America reflects trends in demography and delivery of health services, as well as academic and practice initiatives within the medical profession. This contribution reviews these several elements in the development of geriatrics in the US and briefly considers and contrasts their counterparts in Canada.

Demography and Disability Trends

During the 20th century, the US has experienced a classic epidemiologic and demographic transition, from a society characterized by mortality caused by short-lived acute infectious diseases and an average life expectancy of 47 years of age in 1900, to one characterized by mortality from protracted chronic diseases with average life expectancy of over 75 years of age at the close of the century.[1] While increase in life expectancy (LE) during the first half of the century was almost entirely attributable to dramatic decline in infant mortality, during the final quarter of the century an unprecedented additional increase in LE has occurred among persons after attaining 65 years of age. While LE at age 65 increased by only 2 years, from 74 to 76 years, between 1900 and 1960, it increased by 3 more years to 79 years, between 1960 and 1990.[2] As a consequence of this extended average LE late in life, numerous studies have projected a disproportionately greater percentage growth in the population over 85 years of age in the first decades of the 21st century.[3]

Cross-sectional surveys conducted in the US in the 1980's document strong correlations between increasing age, prevalence of chronic medical conditions, and need for assistance with activities of daily living. While 35 percent of men and 45 percent of women between 60 and 69 years of age report two or more chronic conditions, these figures rise to 53 and 70 percent, respectively, over the age of 80. Need for assistance increases from 9 to 10 percent between 65 to 75 years of age to 45 percent at age 85 and above.[2] Recent studies of successive cohorts of aging persons in the US reported lessening degrees of disability in general, and specific conditions such as stroke during the 1980's.[4] In spite of such gratifying trends toward a healthier old age, the rapidly growing absolute numbers of very old persons portend a growing need for both acute and chronic care services.

Delivery Systems Trends

The evolution of financing and organization of acute and chronic care health services for older persons in the US in the 20th century has created dilemmas as well as opportunities for geriatric medicine. At the outset of the century, voluntary community hospitals, once equally open to young victims of accidents or infections and to aged persons with incurable and disabling chronic problems, began systematically to exclude the latter, leaving them to seek care in public almshouses or room and board homes. Despite compelling arguments in the pages of the forerunner of the *New England Journal of Medicine* and from the founder of Johns Hopkins Hospital, among others, exclusion of chronic care of older persons from the modern American hospital, and effectively from the study and practice of modern medicine, was a fait accompli in the US by early in the century. Hardships of the Great Depression in the 1930's led to two important developments that further promoted the pattern of separate acute and chronic care sectors. First was the introduction of the Blue Cross and Blue Shield programs of voluntary private health insurance, whereby subscribers protected themselves against costs of acute hospitalization and physician services. This ushered in the now widely prevalent convention of private health insurance to pay for discrete episodes of hospital and physician care, but explicitly excluding coverage for continuing chronic care in the community or in institutions. Fueled by health insurance financing along with the rapid growth of medical science following World War II, the modern acute care hospital and hospital-oriented subspecialty medicine came to dominate health care in the US.[5]

The second watershed event was the 1935 passage of the Social Security Act, which established a federally mandated payroll deduction to assure financial security in old age. Given the absence of dedicated funding or services for care of chronically ill older persons, the newly available pensions created a source of funds for privately operated rest homes. Thus was born the American private nursing home industry, which has flourished in parallel, but separately from, the acute care hospital industry.

The distinctly separate financing and development of the hospital and nursing home sectors, begun in the 1930s, was brought to fruition with passage of the landmark Medicare and Medicaid legislation in 1965. In this unprecedented legislation, the federal government expanded the Social Security payroll deduction to include a mandatory contribution to a trust fund (Medicare) to provide universal hospital insurance for retirees. Medicare includes limited coverage for posthospital,

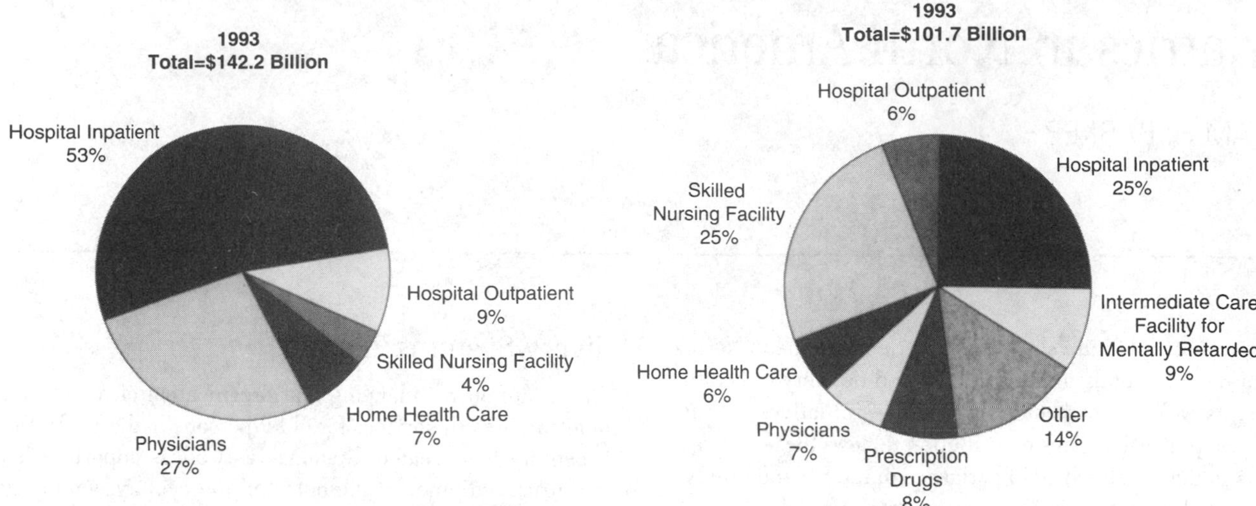

Figure 108-1 Distribution of Medicare (left) and Medicaid (right) dollars (Health Care Financing Administration).

short-term skilled home care or nursing home care. This "comprehensive health insurance" for the aged and disabled excludes coverage for chronic or long-term care, explicitly referred to as "custodial care". Enter Medicaid—this companion legislation is intended to provide comprehensive health insurance for the "medically indigent", primarily poor women and children; however, the program also covers the cost of custodial nursing home care, a benefit largely used by elderly persons who divest themselves of their capital ("spend down") in order to qualify.

From comparatively modest beginnings, these two major financing programs have grown astronomically—Medicare from some 19 million beneficiaries and $4 to 5 billion expenditures in 1966 to 38 million beneficiaries and over $160 billion in 1995; and Medicaid from a "means tested" recipient population of 18 million and annual expenditures of $12 billion in the early 1970s to 36 million recipients and over $100 billion expenditures in the early 1990s. The pie charts in Figure 108-1 show proportionately how the Medicare and Medicaid dollars are spent among hospital, nursing home, home health, physician, and other services. While Medicare dollars go primarily to hospital and physician services that meet the strict criterion of "medically indicated", the greatest single proportion (34 percent) of Medicaid dollars go to pay for chronic care for older persons in nursing facilities.[6]

Geriatric Medicine—Academic Evolution

Study of the aging process and the characteristics and care for disease in old age have been of some identified interest to medical practitioners and investigators in the US since the beginning of the century, long before the demographic transition to an "aging society". The seminal figure in this regard is Ignatz Leo Nascher (Fig. 108-2), a generalist physician, who devoted his career to studying, practicing, and promoting the medicine of old age—a field of work for which he first coined the now universal term, "geriatrics." Nascher vividly recalls an event that first kindled his lifelong interest during his medical school days in New York City in 1883[7]:

A section of the class was taken to the Almshouse by one of the instructors. An old woman hobbled up to him with some complaint. The instructor said she was suffering from old age. "And what could be done for it?" "Nothing." Was old age, then, a painful,

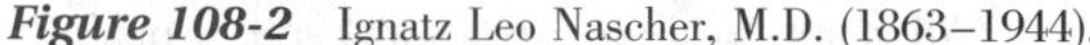

Figure 108-2 Ignatz Leo Nascher, M.D. (1863–1944).

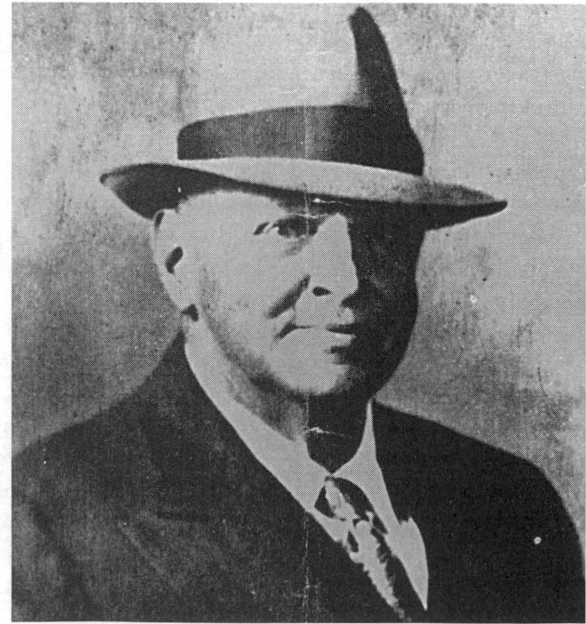

incurable disease from which those who reached advanced age must suffer and for which nothing could be done?[7]

Nascher thought otherwise, and devoted his career to refuting this conventional wisdom of the times. A prolific writer in professional and lay publications and author of a comprehensive text, *Geriatrics: The Diseases of Old Age and Their Treatment* (1914), he was convinced, partly through close collegial association with Dr. Abraham Jacobi, founder of the specialty of pediatrics, that geriatrics would become a thriving speciality. "There are hopeful signs that such interest is spreading, that the cardinal principles of Geriatrics are becoming recognized, and that Geriatrics will soon be taught and practiced as one of the major specialties of medicine."[7] Nascher's "prophetic words" fell on deaf ears and little formal attention to geriatrics as a specialty was heard for decades to follow.

In spite of the failure of geriatrics to receive the formal recognition forecast by Nascher, nonetheless, the challenges to study and treat medical problems of aging, which he articulated so well, received growing organized attention in other important ways. Beginning in the 1930s, the Josiah Macey Jr. Foundation sponsored a series of annual gerontology research conferences, each resulting in published proceedings, beginning with *The Problems of Aging* (1939), edited by the distinguished biologist, E.V. Cowdry. An outgrowth of the Macey Foundation's interest was establishment of the US Public Health Service Gerontology Research Center that has flourished to this day and has produced a formidable body of research on normal aging processes.[8] The 1940s saw the founding of the American Geriatrics Society (AGS) and the Gerontological Society of America (GSA), the former primarily representing practicing physicians, the latter primarily representing academicians from a number of disciplines concerned with biological, social, psychological, economic, and other dimensions of aging. At the public policy level, a series of White House Conferences on Aging, beginning in 1950, attended by scientists, consumers and policy makers, have crystallized and advanced major national initiatives to address medical and related problems of old age. The 1961 Conference was instrumental in promoting the subsequent 1965 enactment of the Medicare legislation, as well as the parallel Older Americans Act to support development of community social services.

American Geriatrics Society

The AGS was founded in 1942, through the spirited leadership of Dr. Malford Thewlis, a kindred spirit and longtime associate of Nascher's. From its original 30 physician members, the Society has burgeoned to a membership of some 6,000.[9]

At its 1952 meeting, the members voted to establish a peer-reviewed journal, and in January 1953, the *Journal of the American Geriatrics Society* was launched. In an inaugural essay, "Aging Comes of Age—The Modern Concept of Geriatrics," journal editor Willard Thompson, M.D., laid out the broad philosophy that characterizes this field of medical work[10]:

Geriatrics presents a great variety of problems and must be looked upon from the broadest possible point of view. The care of older people concerns physicians in practically every special field of medicine as well as the general practitioner who probably sees more older people than the specialist . . .. Studies of the causes of aging and attempts to improve the medical care of older people must be correlated with developments in all other fields which contribute to the welfare of the aging population.[10]

After Thompson's untimely death in 1954, Dr. Edward Henderson assumed editorship for the next 18 years, during which he also served as executive director of the AGS. The Society's highest lectureship award is named for Dr. Henderson.

The AGS has taken active positions on national public policy since the early 1960s, when, ironically, along with most of organized medicine, it testified against the forerunner to the Medicare legislation, being wary of the effect of a government health insurance program on the practice of medicine. Issues of note on which the AGS has subsequently developed more progressive positions and testified before the US Congress include nursing home standards and the concept of medical directors for nursing homes; patient and family rights to make decisions regarding life-sustaining interventions at the end of life; appropriate Medicare reimbursement for geriatric assessment, house calls, and nursing home visits; and financing for a continuum of long-term care services as part of national health care reform. Medical education has been a principal concern of the Society since its origin when one of two standing committees was established to aid medical societies in arranging geriatrics programs for practicing physicians. This focus has recently seen development of "The Geriatrics Review Syllabus," a self-administered core curriculum for physicians in training and in practice.

National Institute on Aging

The principal legacy of the 1971 White House Conference on Aging was the 1974 founding of the National Institute on Aging (NIA) as a component of the National Institutes of Health. The leadership at the NIA during its first decades reflects several distinctive perspectives on solving medical problems of old age. The founding director, Dr. Robert Butler (1974 to 1982), a psychiatrist, brought to the agency a broad background of teaching, research, and practice, with an emphasis on mental health. His Pulitzer prize-winning book, *Why Survive? Being Old in America*, published in 1975, brought to a wide professional and lay audience recognition of social and attitudinal ("agism") challenges as well as unmet chronic-care needs. Following his tenure at the NIA, he joined the Mt. Sinai Medical Center to be chairman of the first and only free-standing medical school geriatrics department in the US. The Institute's second director (1983 to 1991) was Dr. T. Franklin Williams, an internist with a strong background in chronic metabolic diseases. Prior to his appointment, he served as medical director of a 600-bed former county poor farm in Rochester, New York, which was transformed under his leadership into a nationally renowned university affiliated center (Monroe

Community Hospital) for treatment, teaching, and research related to chronic disease and disability of old age.[11] From this legacy he remains a tireless advocate for bringing geriatric assessment and rehabilitation to the mainstream of American medical education and practice. The third director of the NIA (1994 to the present), Dr. Richard Hodes, comes from a background in molecular biology research at the National Cancer Institute, and signals increasing focus on basic science as related to aging, while retaining the Institute's existing broad agenda of research.

In its first two decades, with an annual budget growing to over $400 million, the NIA has sponsored research on a number of long-neglected specific health problems associated with aging as well as investigating fundamental biomedical, sociobehavioral, epidemiologic, and health services problems. Exemplary large, multisite projects sponsored or cosponsored by the agency include:

- Established Populations for Epidemiologic Studies of the Elderly (EPESE): A longitudinal observational study of the natural history of many age-related problems, conducted in four different geographic sites and involving a combined cohort of some 10,000 subjects.
- The Teaching Nursing Home: A program devised to bridge the gap between acute medical and long-term care sectors by attracting medical school faculty and students to nursing homes for purposes of education, research, and practice.[12]
- Frailty and Injuries: Cooperative Studies of Intervention Techniques (FICSIT): A series of randomized clinical trials of various interventions to reduce musculoskeletal frailty and related injuries in later life, conducted at eight different sites.[13]
- Systolic Hypertension in the Elderly Program (SHEP): A randomized clinical trial of effectiveness of treating isolated systolic hypertension, conducted in collaboration with the National Heart, Lung, and Blood Institute, and involving some 4,800 subjects.[14]
- The Claude Pepper Older American Independence Centers: Named for a tireless congressional advocate in behalf of older people and based at a number of universities for the purpose of bringing together multidisciplinary research, training, and information dissemination on a variety of preventable or reversible causes of dependency.
- Alzheimer's Disease Centers: Based at 28 major medical institutions with the broad objective of conducting basic research on etiology, improving diagnosis and classification, evaluating clinical interventions, and disseminating information on Alzheimer's disease and related disorders.

Education and Training

In spite of long-standing recognition that the health problems of old age are important, both for research and as a focus of national academic societies and journals, fully a decade following passage of the Medicare legislation there was a remarkable dearth of physician practice or educational commitment to the field. The American Medical Association (AMA) physician master file for 1977 revealed that only 0.2 percent of physicians listed geriatrics as a principal area of practice.[15] Surveys of medical students and practicing physicians in the 1970's revealed little formal training and a generally negative attitude toward care of the elderly. The failure of the field to develop as a medical specialty, analogous to pediatrics, is attributed to a lack of certain critical historic elements. The field clearly did not fit neatly into either of the two dominant trends in medical career development of the post-World War II era: biomedical subspecialities, dominant from 1945 to 1970; and primary care specialities from 1955 to 1980.[16]

Facing this climate of medical noninvolvement, the US has witnessed a spate of initiatives to redress the gap in medical education and training in geriatrics. Foremost among these has been a series of three major reports issued by the National Academy of Science's Institute of Medicine (IOM), which advises the federal government on health policy matters. The first report (1978) under the leadership of Dr. Paul Beeson, a preeminent American Professor of Medicine and former Regius Professor of Medicine at Oxford, recommended that geriatrics be recognized as an academic discipline with a strong curricular presence in all medical schools. This would be accomplished by encouraging faculty to develop new courses or integrate pertinent material into existing courses. A variety of such undertakings ensued in response to state and federal grant support; however, relatively little substantial commitment to geriatrics was evident 5 years later. Re-evaluating the situation in 1985, Dr. Beeson indicated his disappointment with, "the half-way measures that we recommended" and cited certain more fundamental requirements for the success of geriatrics as a medical discipline. These included a tentative endorsement of the development of independent academic departments of geriatric medicine. Such departments would have their own faculty and required curriculum. He further pointed out the essential need for, "a change in our system of health care payments whereby cognitive work and time spent in the care of people with chronic multiple disabilities is rewarded in a manner comparable to the rewards that come from carrying out procedures."[17]

The second IOM report (1987) recognized modest but clearly insufficient development of formal geriatrics undergraduate and postgraduate education. About 75 percent of medical schools reported offering elective courses, but fewer than 4 percent of students had enrolled. Only 40 percent of medical residencies offered geriatrics rotations and few residents took them. More than 60 small 1- or 2-year geriatrics fellowship programs had developed, but over 25 percent of the approximately 200 positions were unfilled. A fundamental problem in attracting candidates to the field was the absence of a well-defined career ladder, something which by contrast was noted to be well-developed in Great Britain. Two critical steps toward defining career standards were recognized and applauded by the report. The first was a set of Guidelines for Fellowship Training Programs in Geriatric Medicine, developed and published in 1987 by the AGS.[18] The second was the joint development by the American Boards of Internal Medicine and Family Practice of an examination to award a Certificate of Added Qualifications (CAQ) in geriatric medicine. Candidates qualified for the exam based on several educational and practice pathways indicative of expertise and commitment to care of the elderly. Of 4,282 candidates who sat for the first exam in 1988, 2,398 (56 percent) passed and were awarded the CAQ.

With the forward-looking mission of defining and meeting needs for "Academic Geriatrics for the Year 2000", the 1987 IOM Report focused upon current versus projected numbers of faculty. Compared to a projected need for up to 1,600 faculty in geriatric medicine and 450 in geriatric psychiatry, as well as a complement of dedicated Ph.D. investigators, by the end of the century, it was noted that only 250 to 300 of all medical school faculty in the mid-1980's devoted substantial time to teaching aspects of geriatrics. To close this gap, the report emphasized the development of academic "centers of excellence" in geriatrics, analogous to cancer centers, which had greatly strengthened academic career development in the field of oncology. Each "center of excellence" would meet three central goals: (1) develop a geriatrics training program fulfilling the 1987 guidelines; (2) conduct a strong body of research and research training; and (3) provide clinical care in a variety of community and institutional settings. Existing Geriatric Research, Education and Clinical Centers (GRECCs) based at academically affiliated Veteran's Administration Hospitals were cited as models. It was recommended that funding for the proposed future "centers of excellence" come from a variety of sources, including the NIA, the National Institute for Mental Health, and other government agencies and private foundations.[19]

The third IOM report, "Strengthening Training in Geriatrics for Physicians," published in 1993, took stock of the progress to date and focused on future potentials as well as obstacles.[20] A background document, drawing on extensive survey research conducted at UCLA and the RAND Corporation in the late 1980's and early 1990's, addressed the persisting modest progress in development of careers and education in geriatrics in the US. As of 1992, 6,775 physicians from internal medicine, family medicine, and psychiatry, most of whom had not taken geriatric fellowships, had received certification in geriatrics. By 1994, there were 101 accredited geriatric medicine fellowship training programs with over 300 positions offered annually, but with fewer than 70 percent of positions filled. A high percentage of fellowship graduates were satisfied with their decision to pursue a career in geriatrics. A survey of residency programs found that 80 percent of family medicine programs, but only 36 percent of internal medicine programs reported required curriculum in geriatric medicine. Among 126 medical schools as of 1993, 14 taught geriatrics as a separate required course, while 102 taught geriatrics in the context of other required courses; only 2.9 percent of graduating students had taken an elective in geriatrics— essentially no change from 1987. With the exception of steady growth in the number and academic productivity of GRECCs in the VA system (a total of 16 sites with 284 completed traineeships and 617 total publications as of 1993), the development of centers of academic excellence was limited.

To explain the lack of greater progress, the 1993 IOM report noted the variable enthusiasm with which traditional leaders of academic medicine acknowledged the importance of geriatrics; the difficulty in finding stable funding to support both fellowships and centers of academic excellence; and, most fundamentally, the inadequate reimbursement provided by Medicare and other health insurers for the time-consuming, largely cognitive rather than procedure-governed work of those who would pursue a career in clinical geriatrics.

In an effort to awaken the academic establishment, the Association of Professors of Medicine convened a well-attended conference in 1993 on geriatrics curriculum. The conference was chaired by Dr. William Hazard, president of the AGS and Chairman of Internal Medicine at the Bowman Gray School of Medicine. Among highlights were presentations on the extensive geriatric training programs of the VA and innovative mid-career geriatrics training programs for internists as well as for physicians in other specialities (e.g., gynecology, urology, orthopedics) sponsored by the John A. Hartford Foundation. Of particular interest was the strong recommendation that geriatrics as practiced in the US should not be considered a subspecialty, but was rather more akin to primary care, a "supraspecialty" with added qualifications.[21] Bolstering this point of view was a survey of physicians who had taken the 1988 CAQ exam, which found that on average approximately 70 percent of their work represented primary care.[22] Others have made a persuasive argument, drawing comparisons to cardiology, rheumatology, and others, that the work pattern of the geriatrician more nearly fits that of a consulting subspecialty.[23] Depending on their work setting, geriatricians in the US will de facto serve in some instances more like primary care practitioners, in other instances more like subspecialists.

National attention was most recently drawn to the serious shortage of physicians with geriatric training by a widely publicized report from the Alliance for Aging Research submitted to the US Senate Committee on Aging in May 1996.[24]

Geriatric Medicine—Practice Evolution

By the mid-20th century as some members of the medical profession were becoming energized in Nascher's spirit, other professional and institutional associations were recognizing the implications of the trends in aging and chronic illness for organization and staffing of health services. In a joint report issued in 1947, addressed to the "general public as well as legislators and members of the health and welfare professions," the AMA, the American Hospital Association (AHA), the American Public Health Association, and the American Public Welfare Association made the following sweeping recommendations[25]:

- The care of the chronically ill should be inseparable from general medical care.
- Major emphasis should be placed on home and office care, with hospital care, convalescent care, and rehabilitation serving where possible to return the chronically ill to productive community life, and with nursing home facilities providing for those whose medical condition is such that they cannot remain in their home environment.
- Major emphasis must be given to coordination and integration of services. Because the medical condition of the chronically ill person is not static, but changes with time, it is essential to develop smoothly operating mechanisms for referral from one type of care to another.

When Medicare was legislated in 1965, as pointed out earlier, insurance coverage was restricted to physician, hospital, and post- hospital services for discrete illness episodes, explicitly excluding chronic care. The long-term care sector accordingly grew up separately from mainstream health service financing and delivery. By the 1980's, in the absence of a system for managing both acute and chronic care interchangeably, to wit, "smoothly operating mechanisms for referral from one type of care to another," a variety of inappropriate service utilization patterns emerged. Particularly conspicuous and costly among these were growing numbers of frail older patients "blocking beds" in acute care hospitals where restorative and health maintenance needs were neglected; and frequent disruptive transfers of nursing home residents to hospitals because of the failure to provide timely onsite care for acute medical problems. Recognizing the dilemmas caused by the lack of integrated services for chronically ill aged persons, many groups called for national health policy reform to address the situation. Exemplary of such efforts was a position paper on "Long-Term Care of the Elderly" issued by the American College of Physicians, which stated[26]:

> At present, there is not a comprehensive system of long-term care for the elderly in the United States. A confusing, fragmented, and expensive system exists that contains both gaps and duplication of services . . .. Reimbursement procedures, both public and private, tacitly recognize the existence of two separate systems of health care: one for acute care and another for long-term care . . .. A full array of services should be available through an integrated long-term care system. Such a continuum of care would better ensure that the elderly obtain appropriate services. The reimbursement system should foster, not impede, networking among hospitals and nursing homes.

In spite of a number of major health care reform proposals and legislative efforts in the late 1980s and early 1990s, most recently the thwarted effort of the Clinton Administration in 1994, national health care policy incorporating long-term care has not evolved and looks unlikely as the year 2000 approaches. Nonetheless, through public and privately funded demonstration projects, a variety of innovative health care strategies for meeting needs of frail older people have flourished during this time period. A selective review of such projects across the spectrum of care sites reveals the unmistakable strong presence of principles of geriatric medicine and leadership by trained geriatricians.

Hospitals

Largely emulating experiences pioneered in geriatric units in Great Britain, inpatient geriatric assessment services have been introduced in general hospitals in the US in several distinctly different ways, as shown in Figure 108-3. These include, as labeled: geriatric consultation services (C), geriatric

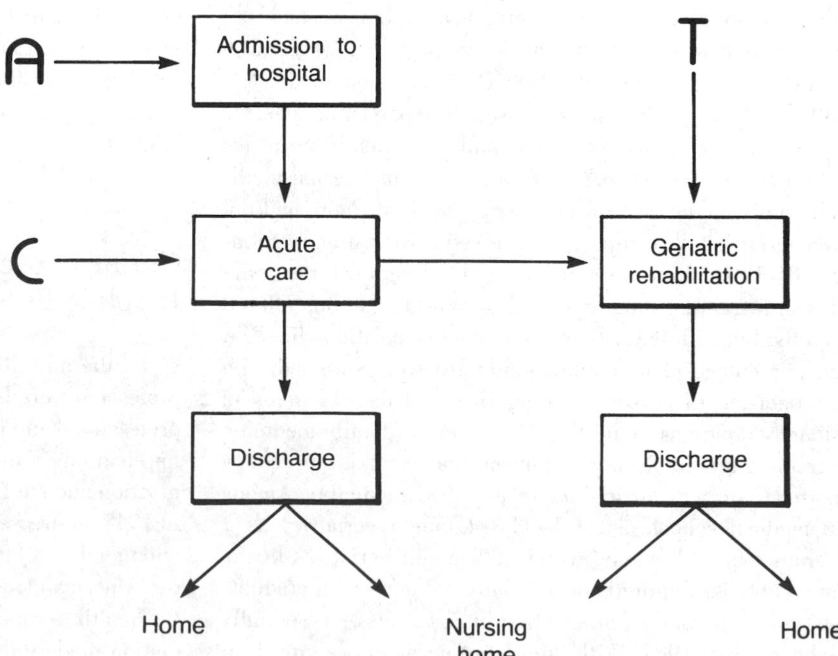

Figure 108-3 Potential intervention by special geriatric services in the course of acute hospital admission in the United States. A = Admit to acute geriatric service; C = geriatric consultation on acute medical and surgical services; and T = postacute transfer to special geriatric rehabilitation unit. (From Barker,[5] with permission.)

rehabilitation transfer units (T), and acute geriatric admission units (A).

Geriatric consultation services, being least obtrusive and demanding of hospital resources, represent the earliest and most widely implemented hospital-based geriatric strategy. Early observational studies reported extensive findings of unaddressed problems among older patients, but only limited evidence of significant impact on patient functional status, length of stay, or level of care at discharge. Two later randomized trials failed to find measurable differences between patients receiving geriatric consultation and controls.[27,28] In thoughtful commentary, Winograd and colleagues,[27] as well as others, have drawn the general conclusion that such consultation services have little measurable impact because of lack of control over clinical management for implementing their recommendations and indifferent attitudes of non-geriatric-trained hospital staff toward geriatric practices and patients.

Transfer units have been established and studied in a variety of hospital settings, including VA hospitals, academic medical centers, chronic disease hospitals, and rural community hospitals. The flagship example of this concept is the rigorously evaluated geriatric evaluation unit (GEU) developed at the Sepulveda VA Medical Center in Los Angeles. In a randomized clinical trial, Rubenstein and colleagues[29] reported that GEU patients, when compared with controls over a 1 year follow-up, experienced significantly lower mortality, reduced likelihood of nursing home admission, fewer overall acute hospital or nursing home days, greater improvement in functional status and morale, and lower average cost of care. A randomized trial of a unit developed and evaluated by Applegate and colleagues[30] in a large general hospital complex reported very similar findings.

Acute geriatric admission units have been introduced in relatively few US hospitals. One exemplary exception is the Acute Care for the Elderly (ACE) unit recently developed and carefully evaluated by Landefield and colleagues[31] at the Case Western Reserve Medical Center in Cleveland, Ohio. Designed to avoid the cascade of "hazards of hospitalization" for older patients,[32] the ACE unit incorporates a set of explicit geriatric care principles into routine acute care from the time of admission to hospital. These include environmental modification for safety and convenience; patient-centered care protocols dealing with potential problems with continence, mobility, skin integrity, mental health, etc.; and daily rounds by a multidisciplinary team led by medical and nursing directors. A randomized trial involving 651 patients showed significantly better functional status at discharge and lower rate of posthospital nursing home placement for the ACE unit patients, with comparable 7- to 8-day lengths of stay and hospital billing for intervention and control groups.

From their collective experience, hospital-based geriatric evaluation and management services (GEMs as they have come to be called), implemented in US general hospitals as inpatient and as outpatient modalities, appear to be both effective and efficient in influencing patient health status and health service utilization, particularly when they incorporate continuing care services.[33] Toward better defining the critical elements for successful GEM services and the generalizability of these services, further research was recommended at a national consensus conference among leaders in geriatric medicine in 1989.[34] As one outcome, a multisite randomized trial involving 10 VA medical centers and a target population of 1,400 patients was begun in 1995.

Nursing Homes

From the perspective of comprehensive medical services, perhaps the most costly and challenging problem among the 14,000 nursing homes in the US is the high rate of transfer of acutely ill, frail residents to short-term hospitals in lieu of managing their medical problems onsite. Multiple national and regional surveys have documented rates of 20 to 30 such hospitalizations per 100 nursing home beds per year, extrapolating to some 300 to 400,000 in the country annually.[35]

A number of practical care strategies have been shown to significantly reduce hospital transfer from nursing homes.[36] The introduction of geriatric nurse practitioners to deal with intercurrent acute medical problems, as well as ongoing health promotion, has been most widely studied and consistently shown to reduce hospital use by nursing home residents.[37] This effect is attributable to both earlier identification and management of potentially serious illness (e.g., urinary tract infections, poor control of diabetes) and to the clinical management of frankly serious illness onsite (e.g., pneumonia, congestive heart failure). A second strategy that has received limited formal evaluation consists of providing financial incentives to physicians, nursing homes, and ancillary services (e.g., laboratory, radiology) to care for serious acute illness episodes within the facility. A further dimension of geriatric care that has the potential to reduce hospitalization of nursing home residents is the growing use of advance directives to express patient or family preferences for receiving or withholding life-saving medical interventions, including hospitalizations. This ethical-legal strategy has been embodied in a variety of formal modalities, including "do not resuscitate" (DNR) orders, living wills, and health care proxies.[38]

Toward assuring quality care within nursing homes, ongoing monitoring with a uniform Resident Assessment Instrument was introduced in all US nursing homes in 1991 as a condition of participation in the Medicare and Medicaid programs. Details of this geriatric assessment and management strategy and its broadly positive effects in nursing homes are reported in the August 1997 issue of the *Journal of the American Geriatrics Society*.

Home and Community

In the US as elsewhere, more than 95 percent of persons over age 65, including most of those with chronic diseases and disabilities, live in the community. How best to anticipate and limit the impact of new intercurrent illness, prevent functional decline, and avoid admission to hospital and nursing homes among community-dwelling older persons has been the focus of extensive public policy experimentation in the past two decades and of targeted clinical geriatric strategies more recently.[39]

During the 1980's, more than two dozen largely government sponsored controlled studies of community-based long-term care (CBLTC) demonstrations emphasizing home care and day care social support modalities, were conducted. In a careful synthesis of results it was found, with rare exception, that there was no improvement in functional status or survival, nor cost savings among those receiving the interventions. Among major concerns noted was the failure to include a strong clinical geriatric medicine component to complement the social component of these projects.[40]

While national policy for CBLTC or "home care" remains a quandry, there has been very active expansion of provision of "home health care" alternatives to hospital care, largely under sponsorship of the Medicare program. The focus has been to avoid or shorten hospitalizations by providing high-tech and acute and subacute care services in the home (e.g., parenteral nutrition and antibiotics, respirators, etc.).[41]

Often missing from both the chronic social support "home care" and acute hospital alternative "home health" models are care modalities to meet the ongoing medical and medically related needs of vulnerable community-dwelling older persons. Strategies, remarkably similar to ones long practiced in Great Britain have recently been introduced in the US. First, is provision of annual in-home geriatric assessment by a geriatric nurse practitioner-geriatrician team. In a recently completed 3-year randomized trial,[42] those receiving this intervention experienced significantly less functional decline and permanent placement in nursing homes. In a variation on this strategy, a multisite demonstration supported by the Hartford Foundation has implemented practice models in which the ongoing care of frail older patients is shared by primary care physicians and geriatric nurse practitioners (GNPs). In this strategy, the patients are regularly seen at office visits by the physician and the GNP in tandem, while the GNP provides continuing care liaison. Geriatric nurse practitioner continuing care includes home visiting and telephone consultation with the objective of early detection and management of changes in mental or physical health as well as counsel on preventive health behaviors, etc. The next phase of this project focuses on developing techniques for training future physicians, nurses, and social workers to work effectively in such collaborative model (personal communication Donna Regenstreif, Ph.D.).

Managed Care Organizations

While, as evidenced above, there has been exciting progress with geriatric strategies at all levels of health care delivery, nonetheless, these specially funded "demonstrations" are the exception, not the rule, and will remain so as long as financing of health care is fragmented and fails to foster incorporation of such geriatric practices. Interestingly, as aspirations for comprehensive national health care reform have seriously waned since 1994, the dramatic surge of managed care organizations (MCOs) is providing, if not compelling, opportunities for the practice of geriatric medicine to flourish. In fact, the role of managed care organizations in care of older persons was the theme for special full-day workshops at the annual scientific meetings of both the AGS and the GSA in 1996 and 1997. The essence of MCOs is linking together a network of physician, hospital, home care, nursing home, and other service modalities to provide a defined scope of health care services for an enrolled population within a fixed budget, with considerable flexibility regarding the mix of service settings and personnel provided to meet the members' medical needs.

From the perspective of comprehensive services for older persons, three distinctly different variations on the MCO paradigm are briefly considered below: the Medicare Health Maintenance Organization (HMO), which provides a full complement of standard Medicare-coverable services, the Social Health Maintenance Organization (SHMO), and On Lok/Program of All-Inclusive Care for the Elderly (PACE), both of which represent models which also incorporate chronic care services.

Medicare health maintenance organization

As a potential cost-saving policy, the Medicare program was amended in the 1980's to encourage HMOs to enroll large populations of Medicare beneficiaries and provide their full range of benefits under capitated payment, representing approximately 95 percent of the average fee-for-service cost per member. By late 1996 more than 10 percent of Medicare's 33 million beneficiaries were enrolled in HMOs. Surveys in the early 1990's found that over one-half of the Medicare HMOs employed geriatricians and were supporting some form of organized geriatric practices. Practices given priority in a sample of plans include geriatric assessment and targeted case management for high-risk patients, subacute geriatric rehabilitation services, and utilization of geriatric nurse practitioners.[43]

An exemplary Medicare HMO, the Health Partners plan, located in the city of Minneapolis and caring for some 24,000 elderly persons (a subset of an all ages HMO enrollment of 265,000) is illustrated in Figure 108-4. Those members of the older population who are identified as "frail" based on medical-functional-social assessment, are tracked by trained geriatricians who provide both consultative services to other physicians, as well as some direct patient care service. Geriatric services, involving nurse practitioners and full multidisciplinary team care under geriatrician leadership, are provided respectively in the ambulatory setting emphasizing case management in the community; in the acute hospital emphasizing expeditious and safe discharge; in short-stay geriatric rehabilitation units located in skilled nursing homes; and in long-stay nursing homes, managing intercurrent illness episodes onsite in lieu of transfer to a hospital.[44]

Social health maintenance organization

While Medicare HMOs do not typically provide ongoing chronic, supportive care, a variant demonstration model sponsored by the Medicare program in the late 1980's, and known

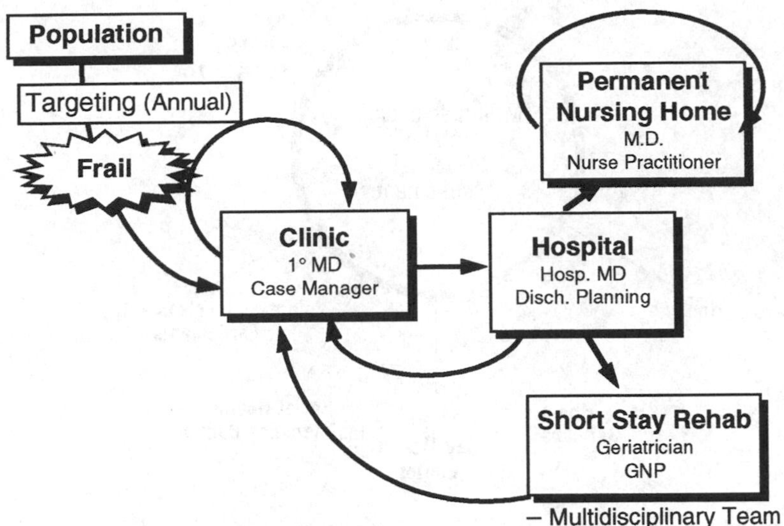

Figure 108-4 Network of services for Medicare patients enrolled in Health Partners health maintenance organization. (Courtesy of Thomas von Sternberg, M.D.)

appropriately as the SHMO, does, in fact, provide enrollees a limited amount of extended care service. The SHMO enrolls a relatively large population representing a cross-section of Medicare beneficiaries, all of whom agree to pay a supplemental premium into a fund that will finance a specified range of chronic social support services when, and if, needed. The chronic care benefits include case management, home nursing, homemaker services, day care, transportation, home-delivered meals, and limited amounts of skilled and custodial care in nursing homes.[45] While successful in many respects, the initial SHMO demonstration sites encountered difficulties in efficiently integrating traditional medical services with the supplemental chronic care services. In an effort to overcome these problems, a second-generation SHMO demonstration, launched at several sites in 1995, is designed to more explicitly incorporate "a geriatric style of practice," emphasing comprehensive assessment and rehabilitation and including pivotal roles for geriatricians in coordination of services.

On LOK/program of all-inclusive care for the elderly

The Program for All-Inclusive Care for the Elderly is a government-sponsored multisite demonstration designed to replicate the highly successful On Lok program, which integrates financing and delivery of a full range of acute and chronic care services for an enrolled population of several hundred disabled older people. The prototype program evolved from its origins as a multipurpose day care center in the Chinatown section of San Francisco to become a comprehensive system of medical and social services for functionally dependent elderly persons as illustrated in Figure 108-5. Combined Medicare-Medicaid funding provides coverage for all medical, rehabilitative, and long-term care services. The resulting comprehensive delivery of care that is provided by a multidisciplinary geriatric team and emphasizes noninstitutional modalities, has been achieved at per capita costs substantially lower than would be incurred under the traditional fragmented provision of acute and long-term care services.[46] On Lok/PACE replications are being conducted and evaluated in over 10 widely dispersed sites and the staff at these sites are frequently called upon to consult with other groups interested in implementing the model elsewhere in the US, as well as other countries.[47]

Canada

Canada shares with the US the 20th century demographic transition to an aging society with its attendant "geriatric imperative." Life expectancy increased from 49 to 70 years of age between 1900 and 1965 in Canada and has increased to over 76 as the century ends.

While sharing a common heritage of European conquest and colonization, Canada in contrast to its breakaway neighbor to the south, remained formally linked with Great Britain well into this century and has consequently retained certain distinctly European influences in both health service delivery and medical culture.

In the first instance, government financing of universal access to comprehensive health services, including substantial provision of chronic care, are fundamental principles of the Canada Health Act.[48] In the second instance, as in Great Britain, the roles of the medical profession are sharply divided between primary care and specialty medicine, the latter seeing patients on referral from the former.

Recognizing the need to address the health problems of increasing numbers of older Canadians, the Canadian Medical Association at its annual meeting in 1965 unanimously adopted a broad "Statement of Policy on Ageing."[49] Recommendations included placing greater emphasis on aging in medical school and resident training and in programs for practicing physicians; increasing numbers of medical and nonmedical professionals with primary interest in older people; increasing rehabilitation services, chronic hospitals, nursing homes, and community programs to serve frail older people; and targeting research on aging and chronic illness.

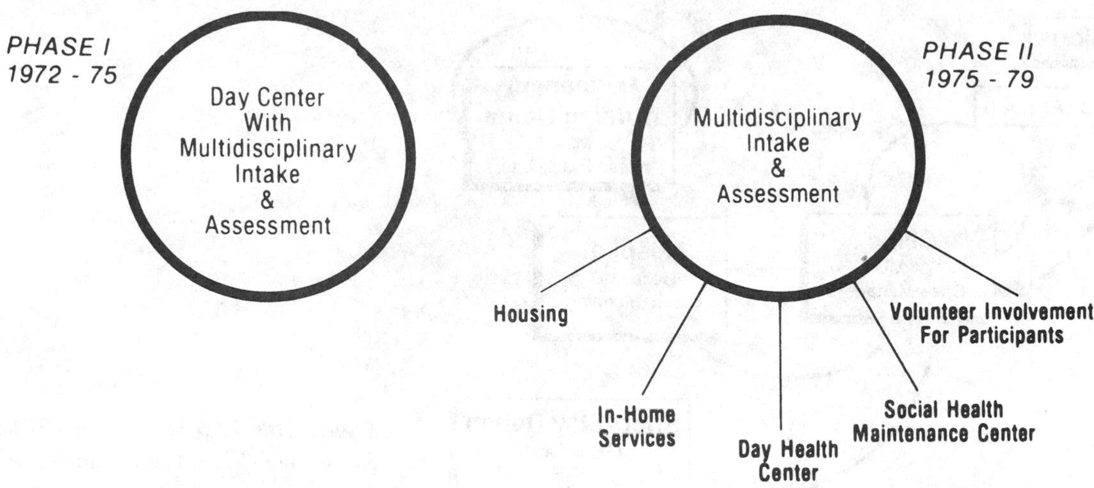

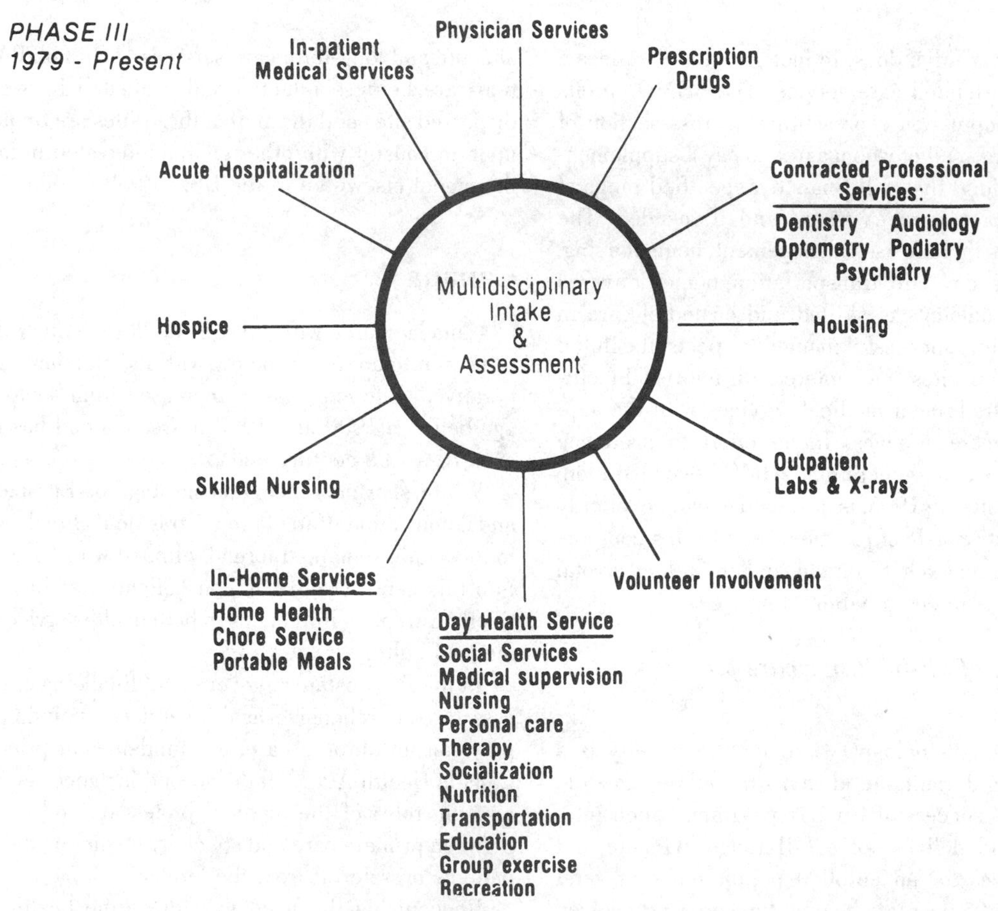

Figure 108-5 On Lok's health program development, 1972–1981. (From Barker,[5] with permission.)

In 1978, following several years of debate, the Canadian Royal College of Physicians and Surgeons voted to establish geriatric medicine as an academic and consultative subspecialty within internal medicine.[50] A set of requirements was developed to be used both for accrediting graduate training programs and for establishing eligibility of candidates to sit for the exam for the Certificate of Special Competence in Geriatric Medicine. Eligibility requirements included Royal College certification in internal medicine and completion of a 2-year program in geriatric medicine, which could be fulfilled through a variety of pathways. Importantly, in addition to acquiring attitudes, knowledge, and skills specific to medical problems of old age, trainees were to experience management of problems in inpatient and community settings, work with multidisciplinary health care teams, and learn to function primarily as a consultant, including planning for continuing care. In 1993, a revised specification of objectives for accredited training programs was issued by the Committee on Geriatric Medicine, again emphasizing the consultant role of the specialty.[51]

Within 5 years of the establishment of the specialty, accredited training programs were in place at 8 of Canada's 16 medical schools and 26 of 39 candidates had passed the certifying exam. The number of certified geriatricians increased to 42 in 1987 and 91 in 1994. Their roles have primarily consisted of developing and staffing academic programs in medical schools and geriatric consultative services in major population centers. A Royal College study in 1987 predicted the country would need between 500 and 700 geriatricians by the year 2000, a goal which like its US counterpart will be seriously underattained at current rates of growth of the field.[51] The Canadian Society of Geriatric Medicine was established in the early 1980's to serve the professional interests of the new specialty.

The response to the call for dedicated geriatric content in medical school curricula has been well-documented through a series of surveys completed by geriatric medicine training program directors. Mandatory geriatric curriculum time increased from averages of 10 hours in 1982 (range of 0 to 50 hours) and 31 hours in 1987 to 65 hours (range of 3 to 205 hours) in 1992. In most schools, the majority of the teaching occurs during clinical training. Electives in geriatrics are taken by less than 2 percent of students.[52] At the graduate level, increasing numbers of family medicine and internal medicine residencies require a month or more of geriatric training, and the College of Family Physicians has established an optional 6 to 12 month add-on period of training in health care for elderly.

Dedicated geriatrics services, while developed to varying degrees from province to province, are in principle fully covered as part of mainstream medical care under Canada's universal health system. As such, an older patient with acute and associated chronic care needs may be readily managed in a flexible continuing-care process under a global budget in Canada, in contrast to the fragmented approach to meeting (or possibly not meeting) the same care needs in mainstream medical services in the US.[53] Given the status of geriatricians as a recognized part of the nation's health system, Canadian geriatricians have implemented a variety of strategies and systems of care within the instititutional and community settings in which they work. In many instances they have emulated acute hospital-based units, day hospitals, and community outreach strategies developed in Great Britain or the US.

Of particular note are several exemplary initiatives in which geriatricians have organized consultative and/or direct care systems that span the continuum of acute and chronic care services.

The Ottawa Regional Geriatric Assessment Program, implemented in the 1980's, comprises a model network of inpatient, day hospital, and mobile geriatric assessment team services for meeting needs of community-dwelling frail older persons living within a defined area (personal communication, Dr. William Dalziel.) The Regional Geriatric Program of Metropolitan Toronto serves primarily as a clearinghouse for facilitating efficient referrals of older patients from general practitioners to specialized geriatric services within a very large metropolitan health care system (Personal communication, Dr. Duncan Robertson.) The Baycrest Centre for Geriatric Care, a microcosm of the Toronto metropolitan system, represents a model single institution providing a full spectrum of acute, short- and long-term rehabilitation, and chronic care services.[54] Seeking to provide similar comprehensive care services for community-dwelling populations of permanently disabled older persons, the Quebec Ministry of Health and Social Services has embarked on a planning grant to develop "Systems of Integrated Care for Dependent Elderly," drawing on approaches used in the US PACE model (personal communication, Dr. Howard Bergman.)

Development of the specialty of geriatric medicine in Canada has, from the beginning, received important contributions from British geriatricians, both as hosts to visitors in their home departments in Great Britain and as consultants onsite in Canada. Exemplary among these are Professor George Adams (Belfast) who during a sabbatical in Manitoba provided valued counsel on the decision in the 1970s to establish the specialty of geriatrics; Professor John Brocklehurst (Manchester) who planned and helped to implement Canada's first acute hospital-based geriatric service at the University of Saskatchewan; Professor James Williamson (Edinburgh) who consulted on geriatrics curriculum and service development at McMaster University and the University of British Columbia; and Dr. John Dall (Glasgow) who provided extensive consultation on the development of regional geriatrics services in Ottawa.

Summary

The need for geriatric medicine, as one response to the aging of society, has been well-articulated in both the US and Canada. With a legacy begun by Nascher, academic interest, particularly research in the medicine of old age, has flourished in the US. Medical training and professional certification have evolved to accommodate both primary care and consultant geriatirician roles without formally recognizing geriatrics as a subspecialty. Many innovative geriatric service modalities, including several managed care models have been introduced as demonstrations, but such services are not regularly covered under prevailing health care financing programs. In Canada, geriatric medicine has evolved as a medical subspecialty, complementary to, but distinct from, primary care. Within the context of comprehensive national health services, regional geriatric consultation and delivery systems are in place, or planned in many, but not all, parts of the country. Both countries approach the 21st century with a pressing challenge to overcome projected serious shortfalls in the supply of physicians trained in geriatrics to meet the needs of increasing numbers of older citizens.

Acknowledgments

A number of persons provided valuable resources and advice, in particular, Dr. T. Franklin Williams in the US and Dr. Howard Bergman in Canada.

References

1. Omran AR: Epidemiologic Transition in the United States: The Health Factor in Population Change. Population Bulletin Vol. 32, No. 2. Population Reference Bureau, Washington, D.C., 1980
2. U.S. Bureau of the Census: Current Population Reports, Special Studies, Sixty-Five Plus in America. U.S. Government Printing Office, Washington, D.C., 1992
3. Suzman RM, Willis DP, Manton KG: The Oldest Old. Oxford University Press, Oxford, 1992
4. Manton KG, Corder LS, Stallard E: Estimates of change in chronic disability and institutional incidence and prevalence rates in the U.S. elderly population from the 1982, 1984 and 1989 national long term care survey. J Gerontol 1993;48: Sl53–Sl66
5. Barker WH: U.S. Health services for the elderly to 1980. In Adding Life to Years. Organized Geriatrics Services in Great Britain and Implications for United States. Johns Hopkins University Press, Baltimore, 1987
6. DeLew N: The first 30 years of Medicare and Medicaid. JAMA 1995;274:262–267
7. Nascher IL: A history of geriatrics. Med Rev Rev 1926;32: 281–284
8. Schock NW, Gruelich RC, Andres R et al: Normal Human Aging: The Baltimore Longitudinal Study of Aging. NIH Publication No. 84-2450. National Institutes of Health, Bethesda, 1984
9. Thewlis MW: History of the American Geriatrics Society. J Am Geriatr Soc 1953;1:3–8
10. Thompson WO: Aging comes of age. J Am Geriatr Soc 1953; 1:1
11. Williams TF, Izzo AJ, Steel K: Innovations in teaching about chronic illness and aging in a chronic disease hospital. In Teaching of Chronic Illness and Aging, Clark DW, Williams TF (eds): DHEW Publication No. (NIH) 75–876. National Institutes of Health, Bethesda, 1975
12. Schneider EL, Wendland CJ, Zimmer AW et al: The Teaching Nursing Home. Raven Press, New York, 1985
13. Ory MG, Schechtman KB, Miller JP et al: Frailty and Injuries in later life: The FICSIT trials. J Am Geriatr Soc 1993;41: 283–343
14. SHEP Cooperative Research Group: Prevention of stroke by antihypertensive drug treatment in older persons with isolated systolic hypertension. JAMA 1991;265:3255–3264
15. Kane RL, Solomon D, Beck J et al: The future need for geriatric manpower in the United States. N Engl J Med 1980;302: 1327–1332
16. Maklan, C: Geriatric Specialization in the U.S.: Profile and Prospects. Ph.D. diss., University of Michigan. University Microfilms International, Ann Arbor, Michigan, 1984
17. Beeson, PB: The Institute of Medicine report in aging and medical education: 1984 update. Bull NY Acad Med 1985;61: 478–483
18. Guidelines for fellowship training programs in geriatric medicine. J Am Geriatr Soc 1987;35:792–795
19. Report of the Institute of Medicine: Academic geriatrics for the year 2000. J Am Geriatr Soc 1987;35:773–791
20. Institute of Medicine: Training Physicians to Care for Older Americans: Progress, Obstacles, and Future Directions. National Academy Press, Washington, D.C., 1994
21. Hazard WR (ed): Geriatrics curriculum development conference and initiative. Am J Med 1994;97:4AlS–59S
22. Reuben DB, Zwanziger J, Bradley TB et al: Is geriatrics a primary care or subspecialty discipline? J Am Geriatr Soc 1994; 42:363–367
23. Morley JE: Geriatric medicine: a true subspecialty. J Am Geriatr Soc 1993;41:1150–1154
24. Alliance for Aging Research: Will You Still Treat Me When I'm 65? The National Shortage of Geriatricians. Alliance for Aging Research, Washington, D.C., 1996
25. Special Article: Planning for the chronically ill. JAMA 1947: 343–347
26. American College of Physicians: Health and Public Policy Committee: long-term care of the elderly. Ann Intern Med 1984; 100:760–763
27. Winograd CH, Gerety MB, Lai NA: A negative trial of inpatient geriatric consultation. Lessons learned and recommendations for future research. Arch Intern Med 1993;153:2017–2023
28. Reuben DB, Borok GM, Wolde-Tsadik G et al: A randomized trial of comprehensive geriatric assessment in the care of hospitalized patients. N Engl J Med 1995;332:1345–1350
29. Reubenstein L, Josephson K, Wieland G et al: Effectiveness of a geriatric evaluation unit: A randomized clinical trial. N Engl J Med 1984;311:1664–1670
30. Applegate WB, Miller ST, Graney MJ et al: A randomized controlled trial of a geriatric assessment unit in a community rehabilitation hospital. N Engl J Med 1990;322:1572–1578
31. Landefield SC, Palmer RM, Kresevic DM et al: A randomized trial of care in a hospital medical unit especially designed to improve the functional outcomes of acutely ill older patients. N Engl J Med 1995;332:1338–1344
32. Creditor MC: Hazards of hospitalization of the elderly. Ann Intern Med 1993;118:219–223
33. Stuck AE, Siu AL, Wieland D et al: Comprehensive geriatric assessment a meta-analysis of controlled trials. Lancet 1993; 342:1032–1036
34. Jahnigen DW, Applegate WB, Cohen HJ: Working group on recommendations: research on content and efficacy of geriatric evaluation and management interventions. J Am Geriatr Soc 1991;39S:42S–44S
35. Barker WH, Zimmer JG, Hall WJ et al: Rates, patterns, causes, and costs of hospitalization of nursing home residents: a population-based study. Am J Pub Health 1994;84:1615–1620
36. Rubenstein LZ, Ouslander JG, Wieland D: Dynamics and clinical implications of the nursing home-hospital interface. Clin Geriatr Med 1988;4:471–491
37. Garrard J, Kane RL, Ratner ER, Buchanan JL: The impact of nurse practitioners on the care of nursing home residents. In

Katz PR et al (eds): Advances in Long-Term Care I. Springer Publishing Company, New York, 1991

38. Miller TE: Advance directives: moving from theory to practice. In Katz PR et al (eds): Quality Care in Geriatric Settings. Springer Publishing Company, New York, 1995
39. Campion EW: New hope for home care? N Engl J Med 1995; 333:1213–1214
40. Weissert WG, Hedrick SC: Lesson learned from research on effects of community-based long-term care. J Am Geriatr Soc 1994;42:348–353
41. Vladeck BC, Miller NA: The Medicare home health initiative. Health Care Financ Rev 1994;16:7–16
42. Stuck A, Aronow HV, Steiner A et al: A trial of in-home comprehensive geriatric assessments for elderly people living in the community. N Engl J Med 1995;333:1184–1189
43. Friedman B, Kane RL: HMO medical directors perceptions of geriatric practice in Medicare HMOs. J Am Geriatr Soc 1993; 41:1144–1149
44. von Sternberg T: Geriatrics as a value-added service within an HMO. Clin Geriatr 1995;3:42–45
45. Leutz WN, Greenberg J, and Abraham R et al: Changing Health Care for the Aging Society-Planning for the Social Health Maintenance Organization. D.C. Health, Lexington, 1985
46. Ansak M: The On Lok model: consolidating care and financing. Generations 1990;14:73–74
47. Kane RL, Illston LH, Miller NA: Qualitative analysis of the program of all-inclusive care for the elderly (PACE). Gerontologist 1992;32:771–780
48. Taylor MG: Insuring National Health Care. The Canadian Experience. University of North Carolina Press, Chapel Hill, 1990
49. Canadian Medical Association: Statement of policy on aging. Can Med Assoc J 1965;93:779
50. Cape RT, MacDonell JA: Integrated university training program in geriatric medicine accredited and evaluated by the Royal College of Physicians and Surgeons of Canada. J Am Geriatr Soc 1986;34:787–789
51. Hogan DB, Patterson C, Boustcha E et al: Writing terminal educational objectives for the Royal College of Physicians and Surgeons of Canada accredited training programs in geriatric medicine. Ann Roy Coll Phys Surg Can 1995;28:291–296
52. Dalziel WB, Man-Son-Hing M: Survey of geriatric content in Canadian undergraduate medial school curricula. Ann Roy Coll Phys Surg Can 1994;27:476–478
53. Bergman H, Clarfield AM, Ouslander J et al: Same patients, different systems: clinical implications for the care of the elderly. J Am Geriatr Soc 1992;40:1178–1182
54. Gordon M: Baycrest Centre for Geriatric Care: 75 years from clinical roots to academic present. Ann Roy Coll Phys Surg Can 1993;26:20–22

CHAPTER 109

Future Prospects for Geriatric Medicine in Developing Countries

ALEXANDRE KALACHE

This chapter addresses the rapidity of the aging process in the developing world, discusses the interrelated contributing demographic and socioeconomic factors, and examines its public health implications. This is followed by a discussion on the need for appropriate policies within a conceptual framework of health promotion and the strengthening of the primary care sector.

Rapid Aging in Developing Countries

In 1950 average life expectancy at birth in the developing world was around 40 years. By 1990 it had increased to 62 years and it is projected to reach 70 years within the next two decades.[1] Such rapid increases reflect sharp declines in mortality rates, particularly through the treatment and/or prevention of diseases commonly associated with premature death. Thus, the advent of specific treatment for a range of infectious diseases—for example, tuberculosis, respiratory infections, and gastroenteritis in childhood—associated with the prophylaxis of many others—such as diphtheria, poliomyelitis and measles—were the chief contributors to the survival of millions of children to adulthood throughout the developing world within the last 50 years. These adults are now aging.

In addition to these sharp declines in mortality, most of the developing world had experienced substantial decreases in fertility rates over a more recent past. For instance, in China, total fertility rates (TFR, that is the total number of children a woman in a given society expects to have at the end of her reproductive life) declined from 6.2 to 2.2 from 1970 to 1990. In Brazil, respective figures from 1976 to 1992 are 5.8 to 2.4.[2] As with the declines in mortality, fertility declines were made possible only through interventions based on medical technology. The availability of modern contraceptive methods has made it possible for such sharp declines in only a few years. In the same way that differences in life expectancy at birth in different regions of the world are rapidly disappearing, the large differentials between fertility rates are also decreasing. By the year 2025, TFRs for most of the developing world will be virtually the same as for industrialized countries.[3]

The combined effect of this shift from high to low mortality/fertility (commonly referred to as the demographic transition) is population aging: less children and more individuals surviving into old age.

The Contrast With Already Aged Societies

In the developed world, population aging also resulted from the demographic transition. However, the process took longer. For instance, in France it took 120 years for the proportion of elderly people to increase from 7 to 14 percent—achieved by 1952. Countries such as China, Malaysia, Jamaica, Brazil, and Thailand will replicate such doubling by the beginning of the century, in less than 30 years.[4]

The fundamental difference is due to the backgrounds in which the demographic transition took place in the past in the developed world and now in the developing world. In developed countries, the process followed the industrial revolution. Gradually, increasing segments of the population improved their living conditions by benefiting from rising socio-economic standards. They were better housed, better nourished, and enjoying healthier environments with improved working conditions. The contribution of medical technology was minimum. Tuberculosis, for example, was the leading cause of death in the US by 1900; 50 years later—that is, before the availability of specific treatment for the disease—mortality rates had declined to 10 percent of the 1900's level. Few of the "premature killers" could be prevented by immunization before the second World War—which also marks the advent of antibioticotherapy.

In contrast, the demographic transition in the developing world has been largely the result of medical intervention—effective treatment and vaccines for a wide range of infectious diseases. In spite of the poor—even miserable—conditions in which large proportions of the population in developing countries still live, survival into adulthood (and from there to old age) is increasingly becoming the norm rather than the exception.

Furthermore, in the past, high educational levels were a precondition for a woman to limit the size of her family. Today powerful contraceptive methods are effectively used throughout the world, irrespective of women's literacy.

Beyond 2000: The Old Age Century

Countries such as Indonesia, Kenya, Mexico, Taiwan, and Costa Rica will experience an increase of 300 percent or more in their elderly population from 1990 to 2025—far higher than the increase in the total population within the same period.[5] By early in the next century, 8 out of the 11 largest elderly populations will be in the developing world: China, India, Brazil, Indonesia, Pakistan, Mexico, Bangladesh, and Nigeria. By 2025 there will be 285 million people over the age of 60 years in China alone—more than the total present population of the US; in India the total will be close to 150 million; while Brazil and Indonesia, with 32 million each, will have elderly populations virtually as large as that of Japan.[1]

Figures 109-1 and 109-2 show the current age structure and that projected for the year 2025 for Asia and Latin America, respectively. The shift towards aging is quite evident in both these continents. However, it should be noted that the further aging of already aged societies will be a prominent feature of the coming century—as clearly shown through the age structures for Europe now and in 2025 (Figure 109-3).

Public Health Implications of Aging

Current WHO projections indicate that by the year 2020 over three-quarters of the deaths occurring in the developing world will be caused by noncommunicable disease (NCD)—a significant increase from current levels as shown in Figure 109-4. The contribution of communicable diseases will be reduced to around 12 percent of the deaths—the same as for those caused by injuries.[6] However, this reduction does not mean that communicable disease will have become less important as public health threats. In order to keep them at bay it will be necessary to invest considerable resources toward their prevention (e.g., comprehensive vaccination and sanitation campaigns) and treatment (a challenge in the face of the reemergence of epidemics from biopathogens increasingly resistant to available drugs).

This "double burden"—continuing public health problems related to infectious diseases coupled to the emergence of noncommunicable diseases—is already affecting many developing nations. In all probability, it will become a standard feature in most of the developing world for the foreseeable future.

The challenge for public health policymakers is huge: scarce resources will be increasingly required to deal with NCD, while the "old" diseases will continue to be prevalent. This is an unprecedented phenomenon closely linked to the aging process. Never before in the history of humankind it had been possible for societies to age—thus, changing disease patterns—in the context of poverty. It is also a paradox: aging also makes it imperative for society to redefine itself.

The very nature of the health problems associated with aging—long-term, treatable but not curable, often requiring life-long costly care, frequently disabling—highlight the importance of developing appropriate and cost-effective policies. In their absence, consequences for society could be devastating, eroding the very basis of overcoming underdevelopment.

Even the richest countries, which have taken much longer to age and to adapt to the new demographic order, are finding

Figure 109-1 Population pyramid—Asia (1995 and 2025).

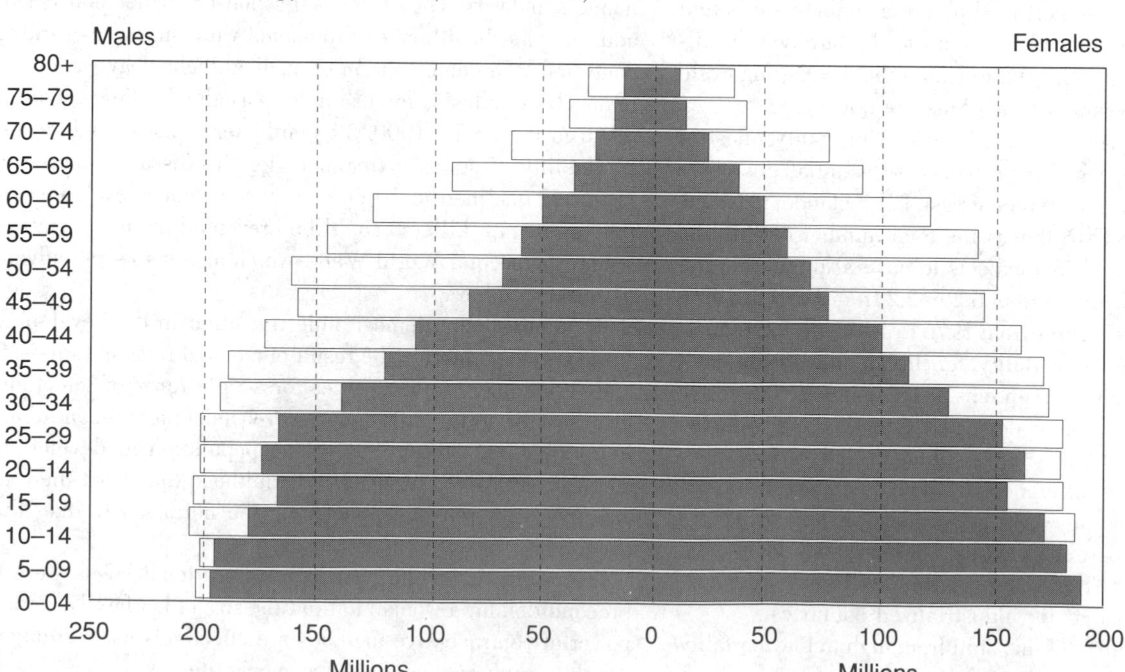

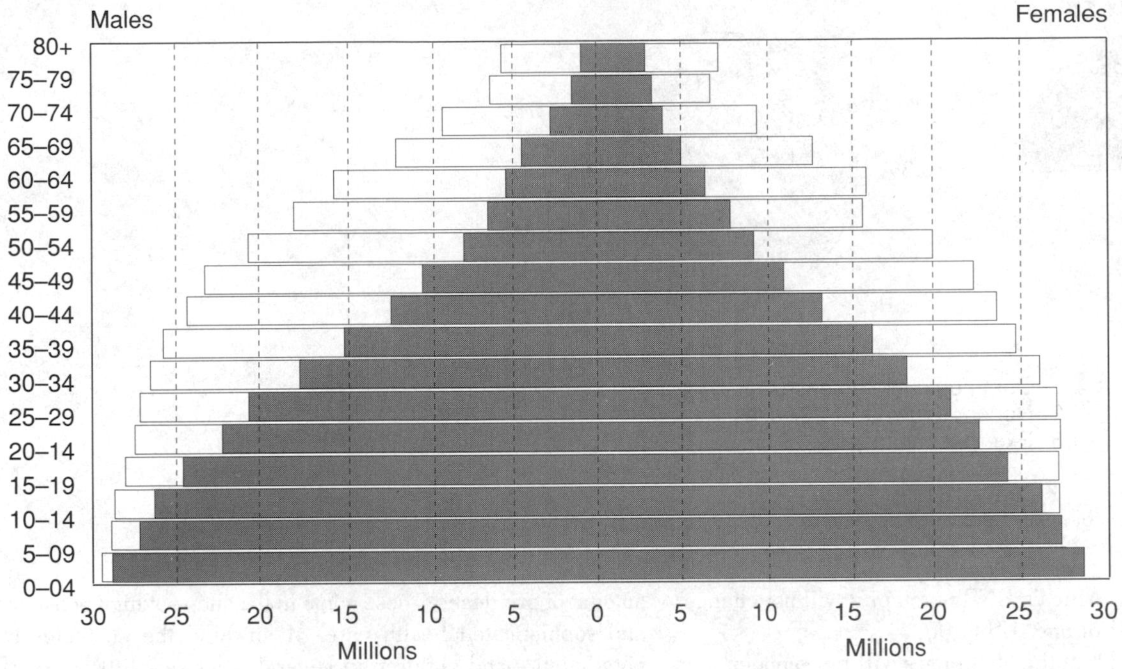

Figure 109-2 Population pyramid—Latin America (1995 and 2025).

it difficult to find solutions. The crisis of the welfare state throughout Europe is a clear example. Yet, World Bank figures indicate that in today's rich societies available resources are relatively much larger than those that will be at disposal of developing countries by the time they become as old as the developed world is today. According to the World Bank in 1992, the per capita income in OECD countries was around US $18,000 (projected to reach US $44,000 by 2030). Respective figures for Latin America are US $1,500 and US $6,000.[7] That means that by 2030, when the Latin American demographic structure will be very similar to that of the OECD countries today, there will be merely one-third of the resources to be shared by competing problems. By then, South Asian countries are expected to reach the current US $1,500 current Latin

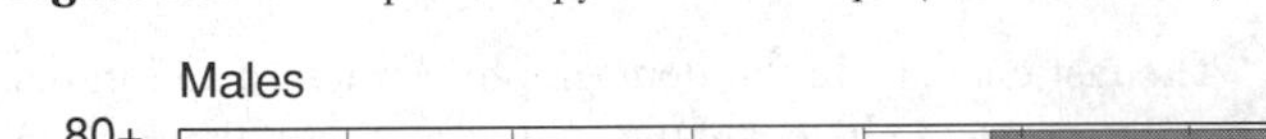

Figure 109-3 Population pyramid—Europe (1995 and 2025).

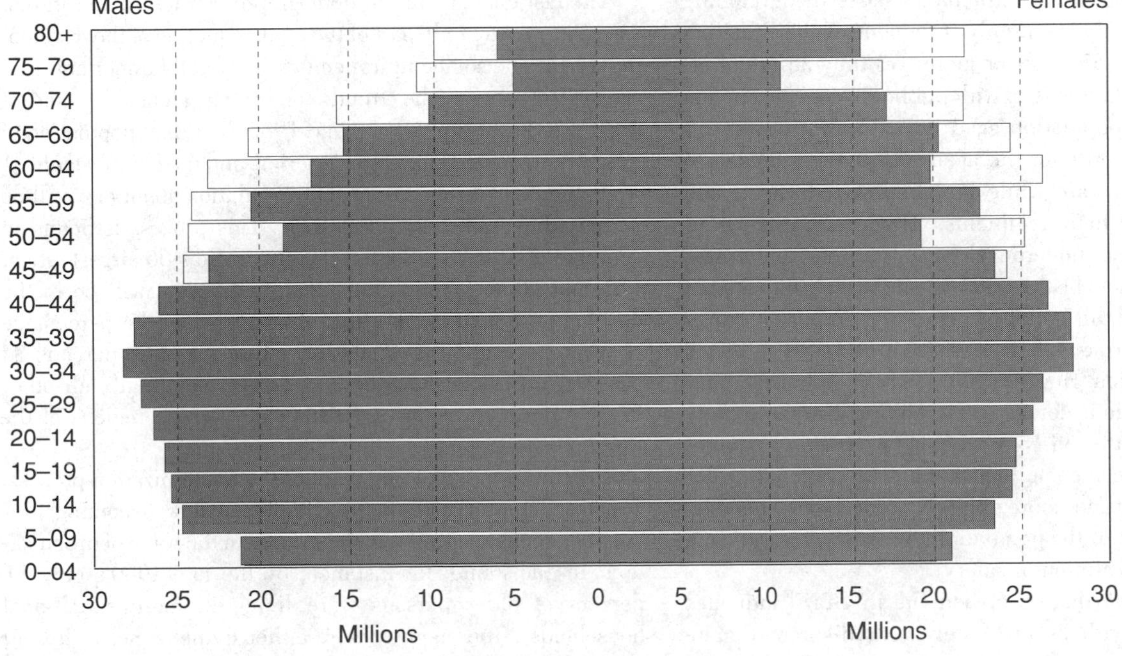

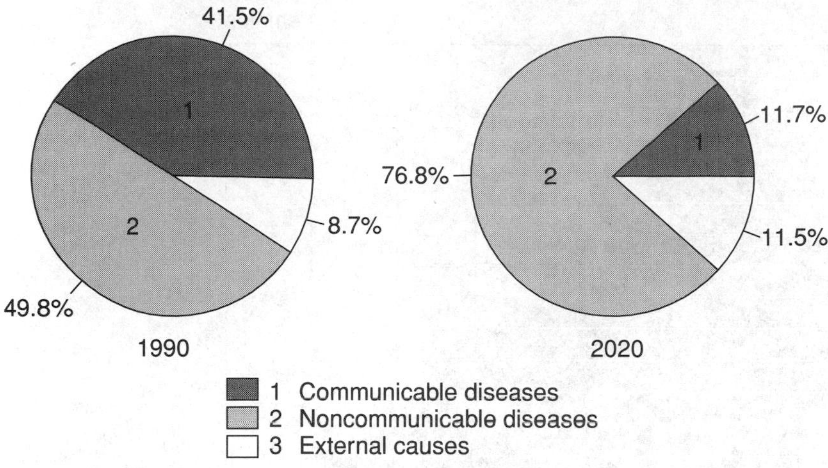

Figure 109-4 Causes of death in developing regions.

American level while Africa's GNP per capita will not change from the 1990's level of only US $300.

It should be added that the challenges will be compounded by the technological gap that will continue to grow separating rich and poor nations. The US $44,000 GNP per capita in the OECD countries will be translated into a level of technologic sophistication that is impossible to figure out today. This will put extra pressure on developing countries—where the elites will continue to expect the same level of sophisticated health care that their counterparts will be enjoying in the rich world.

Aging as a Development Issue

A study on public spending on social programs in the mid-1980's in Brazil illustrates the dilemmas faces by developing nations as they age. By then, only 9 percent of the Brazilian population was aged 55 years or more, yet they absorbed 48 percent of the benefits provided with public money. the respective figures for the population aged under 15 years were 34 and 28 percent. Benefits for the aged were mostly related to pensions and health care while for children education and health care were the main recipients.[8] Obviously, it is inconceivable to overcome underdevelopment unless tomorrow's adults will grow in good health and will attain high educational levels. Furthermore, the social fabric of any country requires intergenerational harmony. The tensions are clearly reflected in the Brazilian figures. However, they hide another basic prerequisite for harmonious development: equity. The same study indicated that the better-off 15 percent of the Brazilian population (with an average income higher than two minimum salaries) attracted seven times more publicly funded social benefits than the poorest fifth of the population (whose average income was less than half a minimum salary).

All in all, the distribution of benefits in Brazil indicates that older rich individuals are receiving a disproportionate amount of privileges. These come in the shape of high pensions and sophisticated health care. Meanwhile, the poor elderly population—and children in general—get very little in relative terms.

Aging-related policies in the developing world will have to take into account such inequities, because they could severely impair the capacity of societies to overcome underdevelopment. The models and practices from developed countries are of little relevance in this respect. Neither the resources they have available nor the pace of their aging process resemble what is now occurring in the developing world.

The Changing Sociocultural Context

The fast changes in the demographic structure and in disease patterns are only part of the aging equation of the developing world. The sociocultural context is equally important. Figure 109-5 shows the trends on aging alongside that of urbanization. Between 1950 and 1985 the urban population of most countries in Asia, Latin America, and the Pacific doubled, while the number of cities with a population about one million increased sixfold, from 34 to 213.[9] This process is bound to continue. By the year 2000, 50 of the world's 66 largest cities, with more than four million inhabitants each, will be in the developing world. By the turn of the century, the percentage of urban population in Argentina will be about 90 percent, 84 percent in Brazil, and over 75 percent in virtually all other Latin American countries.[10] Other developing regions of the world will follow suit.

Urbanization is but one mark of the modernization process. The trend toward the nuclear family is now becoming pronounced in many developing countries in the wake of urbanization. In São Paulo, for instance, by the late 1980's only 11 percent of older persons were living in multigenerational households—the majority were either living alone, with their

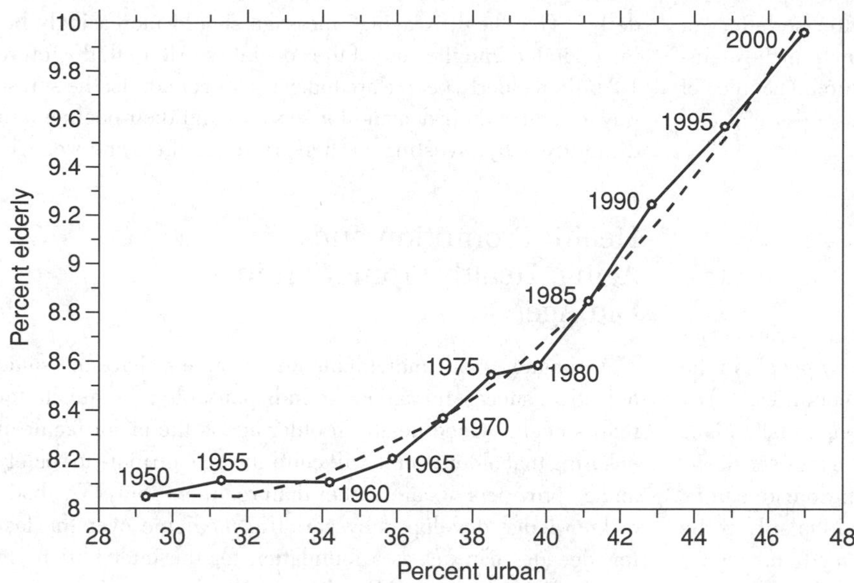

Figure 109-5 Population aging and urbanization, 1950 to 2000.

spouses only or in two-generation (nuclear family) households as shown in Table 109-1. This change in family structure—the social institution, which traditionally has cared for the aged—is not only in size, but also in its capacity to provide fully for its aging members. Constraints include crowded housing, limited financial resources, and the increasing employment of women—the traditional carers for the frail and dependent in any society.

In addition, urbanization entails two phenomena of large significance to population aging. On one hand, throughout the world, millions of previous rural migrants are now aging without having been fully assimilated into the mainstream of their new home environment. Figure 109-6 shows the situation in São Paulo. Among the more affluent elderly population, the proportion of individuals originally from a rural area was only 23 percent, while among the poor, the proportion grows to 72 percent.[12] On the other hand, those who migrate to urban areas are usually the young—leaving behind their elderly relatives without immediate support; unless they succeed in the city (a prospect often denied to unskilled workers) they will not be in a position to assist financially their now distant relations, whatever their intentions were at the point of departing.

Policymakers in developing countries are now starting to realize that unless family and community traditions of mutual aid are strengthened, a vast, yet unaffordable, service infrastructure would be required in coming decades to replace and expand previous informal caregiving.

It should also be noted that shifts from extended to nuclear families imply the loss of older persons roles as heads of families, and thus of their decision-making functions and financial responsibilities/privileges. Modernization undermines the status of older people by making their experience and attachment to tradition appear outmoded and irrelevant to technological progress. The socioeconomic changes that are now taking place

Table 109-1 Urban household composition of elderly population, by sex, in São Paulo, Brazil, (percentage) 1989

	São Paulo	
Household Type	**Male**	**Female**
One-person	16	32
Conjugal	21	17
2-generation (nuclear)	33	24
2–4 generation	11	11
Other	20	17

(Adapted from Hashimoto,[12] with permission.)

Figure 109-6 Older persons living in the community—rural vs. urban origin, São Paulo, Brazil, 1990. (From Ramos et al: Rev Sande Publica 1993;27(2):87–94.)

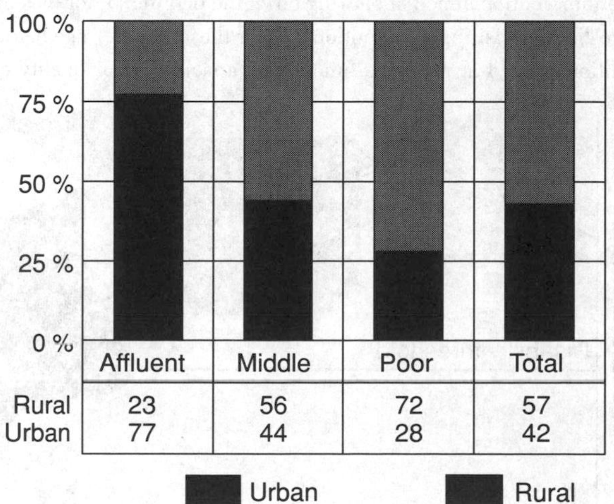

throughout the developing world often have the net effect of marginalizing the aged—that is, removing them from the mainstream of development, weakening their traditional sources of material support, and eliminating their purposeful social and economic role.

Geriatric Medicine at a Crossroad

By the year 2025—that is, less than 30 years from now—there will be more than 1.2 billion elderly people in the world, three-quarters of them in developing countries.[11] The context in which this fast aging process is going to take place has been outlined previously in this chapter. However desirable, it is inconceivable that specialized geriatric care can be provided for such vast numbers of aged individuals. Here lie the challenges and opportunities for geriatric medicine for the years to come. It will be necessary for the specialty to reinvent itself.

First, physicians in geriatric medicine will need to take the lead in disseminating their expertise and sharing their knowledge with other health professionals. This is easier said than done. Sharing knowledge is sharing power—an intrinsically difficult demand. Most of the problems presented by older people occur at community level where they will be expected to be solved—otherwise the costs will be prohibitive. Yet, primary health care workers are mostly ill-equipped to deal with the problems of old age. They need to be trained to acquire new knowledge and skills. The opportunities for geriatric medicine are immense. If the specialists seize these adopting active roles as trainers, disseminators of knowledge, advocates of change, and policy developers, a revived discipline will emerge.

Second, geriatric medicine in the developing world should expand to encompass aging rather than only "care of the elderly". The "healthy aging" message should increasingly be incorporated into the core of the speciality. After all, the future 1.2 billion elderly people are today's younger adults: the surest way to reduce their demand for services and their decline into disability is by investing on their health as they, and we, age.

Health Promotion and Aging: Health Promotion in Old Age

Ultimately, both individuals and societies share the same objective: successful aging. An indispensable prerequisite for that is health. Good health in older age is the major factor in ensuring that older people will continue to contribute to society and be providers of care, rather than recipients only. The body of knowledge developed by geriatric medicine over the last few decades can act as a foundation for the interventions to be widely implemented. For that, it will be necessary to adopt a life-course perspective. Good health in older age depends largely on interventions and behavior changes that took place much earlier in life. However, it is never too late to promote health, as evidence presented elsewhere in this book demonstrates clearly.

In this respect, the conceptual framework summarized in Figure 109-7 may be helpful. It refers to the disability threshold, the fitness gap,[13] and the interventions required throughout life to maintain and increase the level of functional capacity in later life. Physicians in geriatric medicine should increasingly become involved in determining which interventions early in life will ensure that most individuals reach the highest possible level of functional capacity in early adulthood. It is equally important to assist individuals throughout adulthood to slow down the pace of decline of different functional capacities—for example, encourage physical activity and avoidance of smoking to prevent a fast decline in ventilatory capacity.

Figure 109-7 Life-course perspective for maintenance of the highest possible level of functional capacity. 1. Early life interventions to ensure attainment of highest possible peak; 2. adult life intervention aimed at slowing down the decline; 3. for those in older age above the disability threshold, revisiting interventions; 4. for those in older age below the disability threshold, interventions aimed at restoring functional capacity and/or quality of life.

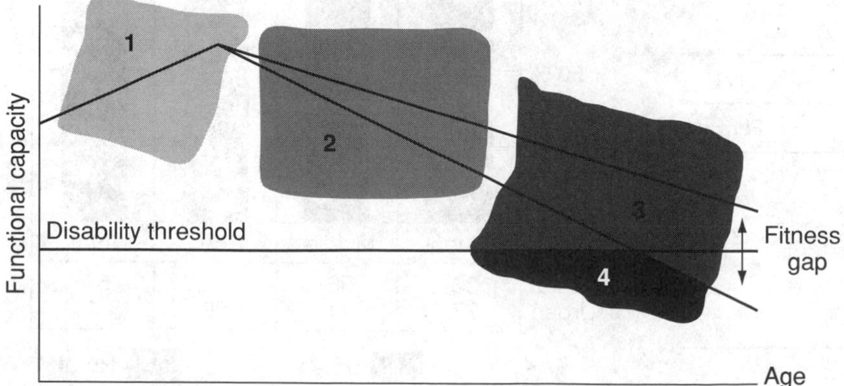

Later, in older age, the interventions previously implemented will need to be revisited and adapted: social and physiologic changes require a reassessment of strategies. For those who fall below the disability threshold, there are interventions that could restore function (e.g., cataract operations, hip replacements, hearing aids) or improve the quality of life (e.g., installation of assistive devices in the home or support for the informal caregiver).

Geriatric medicine in developing countries should avoid the limitations imposed by the adoption of a narrow disease-oriented model. Instead, it is health gains that should orient its development. This requires a combination of:

1. Clinical interventions with emphasis on community-based interventions; informing and supporting effective primary health care interventions.
2. Preventive interventions at primary, secondary, and tertiary levels.
3. Multisectoral actions, health, particularly in older age, depends on interventions from a wide range of sectors whose individual contributions and role need to be defined. Geriatric medicine specialists could play a critical role in acting as catalysts, mediators, facilitators, and advocates, as well as providers of services.

The WHO Ageing and Health Programme

Reflecting the above considerations and conceptual framework, and building on the achievements of its previous Health of the Elderly Programme, in April 1995 WHO launched the program on Ageing and Health, which incorporates the following perspectives: life course (elderly people not compartmentalized, but part of the life cycle as is any other age group); health promotion (with a focus on healthy aging/aging well); cultural (the settings in which individuals age will determine their health status in older age); gender (differences in both health and ways of living); intergenerational (with emphasis on strategies to maintain cohesion between generations); and ethical (multiple considerations emerge as populations age: e.g., undue hastening or delaying of death; human rights; long-term care; abuse).

The opportunity is timely. The World Health Organization is being required to provide worldwide leadership on the health dimension of what is increasingly becoming a dominant societal issue as the year 2000 approaches. Ageing and Health is essentially a horizontal program, acting as a catalyst for action among other WHO divisions, the Regional Offices, Member States, and other agencies. Collaborative work is being established with academic institutions and non-governmental organizations. Key program components are information base strengthening; policy development; advocacy; community-based programs; training; and research. A WHO global media strategy on healthy aging is to be established.

The purpose of the program is to promote health and well-being throughout the life span, thus ensuring the attainment of the highest possible level of quality of life for as long as possible, for the largest possible number of older people. For this to be achieved, WHO will be required to advance the state of knowledge about geriatrics and gerontology through special training and research efforts. These will give special emphasis to the unprecedentedly fast aging of developing country societies in a context of prevailing poverty and continuing demands arising from unsolved problems related to communicable diseases. Within this framework, aging is perceived by the Ageing and Health Programme as a developmental issue urgently requiring action and policies.

The challenge has been encapsulated in a Declaration launched at the end of an international conference on ageing in Brasilia, sponsored by the Brazilian Government and coordinated by the WHO Programme on Ageing and Health. (Brasilia Declaration on Ageing, Appendix 1).

References

1. Kalache A: Ageing in developing countries. pp. 1517–1528. In Pathy MSJ (ed): Principles and Practice of Geriatric Medicine. 2nd Ed. John Wiley & Sons, 1991
2. Population Ageing: a public health challenge, WHO fact sheet no. 135, October 1996
3. Stolnitz G (ed.): UN Demographic Causes and Economic Consequences of Population Ageing, Economic Studies No. 3, United Nation, New York, 1992
4. Kinsella K, Taeuber C: An Ageing World II. International Population Reports P95/92-3. U.S. Department of Commerce, Bureau of the Census, 1993
5. Global aging: comparative indicator and future trends, U.S. Department of Commerce, Bureau of Census, 1993
6. Murray C, Lopez A: Global Burden of Diseases, WHO, Harvard, 1996
7. World Bank, World Development Report, Washington, D.C., 1992
8. Brazil: Public Spending on Social Programs; Issues and Options, Report No. 7086-BR, World Bank, 1988
9. Macura M, Coleman D: International Migration: Regional Processes and Responses, Economic Studies No. 7, United Nations, New York, 1994
10. World Bank: World Development Report, 1993
11. WHO: 1995 World Health Statistics, Geneva, 1996
12. Hashimoto A: Aging and Urbanization, United Nations, New York, 1991
13. Muir-Grag JA: Social and community aspects of ageing. pp. 17–56. In Rathy MSJ (ed): Principles and Practice of Geriatric Medicine. John Wiley and Sons, New York, 1985

Brasilia Declaration on Ageing 1–3 July, 1996

Recognizing the importance of aging of the population, the Government of Brazil, in collaboration with the Program on Ageing and Health of the World Health Organization, convened an international meeting 1–3 July, 1996 to develop an agenda for the reminder of the 20th century and beyond. Attending the meeting was a multi-disciplinary group of experts—from all parts of Brazil, as well as from 21 countries including many from developing countries.

Aging is a development issue. Healthy older persons are a resource for their families, their communities and the economy. Their usually unpaid and unsung contributions are indispensable for development.

Aging is universal, affects every individual and family, community and society. The numbers of older persons are growing steadily. There are gender implications; older women are disproportionately represented among the oldest old and the most disadvantaged and they constitute the backbone of caregiving.

Aging is a normal dynamic process. It is not a disease. While aging is inevitable and irreversible, the chronic disabling conditions that often accompany ageing can be prevented or delayed, not only by medical but also by social, economic and environmental interventions. There are major inequities in ageing reflected in life expectancy, morbidity, premature mortality, disability and quality of life. The basic prerequisites of quality of life include adequate food, clean water, shelter, safety, basic economic security and access to primary health care.

This declaration takes into account the UN International Vienna Plan of Action on Aging, and it is consistent with conventions signed in Cairo, Copenhagen, and Beijing; with the Ottawa Charter on Health Promotion and with Habitat II.

The Conference recommends the following principles for action:

1. Addressing the needs of an ageing population must take place within the context of broader social policy and issues and take a life course perspective. Interventions should occur at the community level rather than focusing solely on the individual and should be culturally relevant.
2. All actions must be inter-sectoral and take into account the bio-physical, social, psychological, economic and environmental determinants of health. Policies across all sectors must be coordinated and harmonised.
3. Policies and practices should be developed to address ethical issues, including equal access to care and services and equitable distribution of resources.
4. To succeed, the approach must develop and build on partnerships between governments at all levels, non-governmental agencies, religious organisations, social movements and the private sector. It must also clearly include the active participation of those who benefit from policies and programmes.
5. Fiscally responsible action suggests a two-pronged approach that involves targeting the most vulnerable while at the same time engaging in disease prevention and health promotion.
6. Actions must promote and support family cohesion and intergenerational solidarity.
7. The multiple roles of ageing women and the impact of those roles on health and economic security must be recognised and supported by legislation, policy and programmes.
8. Education and training is needed at all levels and for all groups concerned with ageing. This includes education for seniors to enhance their capacity for self-help and mutual aid, advocacy and leadership; education of paraprofessional and professional health and social service providers that includes gerontology and geriatrics in the basic curriculum, as well as opportunities for specialisation and continuing education; practical training of family and social networks; and public education to dispel myths and stereotypes.
9. Research capacity must be developed in order to assess and define need, develop and evaluate models of intervention, disseminate best practices and inform policy. Training to utilise existing information and develop new databases is part of research capacity building. Longitudinal databases that facilitate the monitoring and determination of outcomes are a priority as is training in scientific research methods including quantitative, qualitative, participatory and action research methods. The emphasis should be on applied research.
10. To serve as a resource to support these recommendations, an international centre for ageing should be established in Brazil. This centre will serve as a clearing-house for best practice models, as a repository of comparative research data, and resource for education and training. This centre should also facilitate inter-country collaboration both between countries of the South as well as between North and South countries.

C H A P T E R 1 1 0

Rehabilitation

D. BARER

Although much has changed in both the theory and the practice of rehabilitation for elderly people in the last few years, advances in some areas have been mixed with muddle and frustration in others. Various factors, including scientific progress, political demographic and social change, and health service reorganization, are beginning to redefine the role and scope of rehabilitation.

The concepts of impairment, disability, and handicap are at last becoming common elements among clinicians, and this has focused attention on the broader, long-term aims of rehabilitation.[1] Its scope has been considerably widened by the increasing recognition of the psychosocial consequences of disease, but practical action is still often constrained by negative attitudes of society toward the role of elderly people, and sometimes by ambivalence in the expectations of elderly people themselves. These expectations are changing fast, and this process is likely to accelerate as the first postwar generations reach "old age."

The complexities of diagnosis and treatment in frail elderly people, with multiple pathology and reduced functional reserve, have forced us to reconsider our definitions of aging and disease and the boundary between them. These are increasingly seen as belonging on a continuum, with the universal and irreversible changes of aging at one extreme and the highly variable manifestations of acute curable illness at the other. Since the time of Marjorie Warren,[2] geriatric medicine has been pushing back the boundary, so that mental and physical disabilities that previously were considered inevitable consequences of aging have been shown to be remediable. Although the aging process has probably evolved entirely through the action on multiple gene complexes of selective pressures for survival and reproduction,[3] many of its deleterious effects on physical and mental function can clearly be mitigated by changes in environment and behavior.

If the "rehabilitation approach"—creating a stimulating environment and encouraging greater activity and autonomy—can hold back the juggernaut of age-related functional decline, its potential scope is widened enormously to include primary prevention of disability and disease. The aging of the human race is an unprecedented phenomenon, which is likely to prove the greatest world wide challenge of the next century.[4] Because evolution has ensured that the aging process involves an extremely complex series of interactions between multiple genes, affecting every system in the body in different and unpredictable ways, molecular biology is unlikely to provide a simple solution. The rehabilitation approach, on the other hand, is able to focus on whichever body systems are at greatest risk of failure, and thus offers a practical alternative that can be tailored to individual needs.

To meet this challenge effectively, however, the practice of rehabilitation will have to be based on much more secure scientific foundations. Not only must the mechanisms for the interactions between activity, environment, and physiologic change be established, but the yet more complex relationships between disability, social roles, and life satisfaction need to be explored. Progress in basic science has so far had only limited influence on everyday practice in rehabilitation, which remains an uneasy combination of art, magic, and applied commonsense. Until recently the empirical approach, based on methodologically sound clinical trials, has also had less success than might have been hoped. As we shall see, both of these deficiencies are now being corrected, and there is good reason to except rapid progress in the next few years, which should transform both practice and expectations.

In Britain, although geriatric medicine is well established as a specialty, there is still intense debate about the need for specific rehabilitation services for older people,[5] either within the "postacute care" sector of the reformed National Health Service or within the community at large. Care in the community for such people is still largely seen in terms of providing long-term support, rather than as a progressive, goal-directed process aimed at restoring greater health, dignity, and autonomy. If progress in rehabilitation achieves anywhere near its potential, the socioeconomic benefits will be enormous and attitudes to aging itself could be revolutionized.

Basic Concepts

Impairment, Disability, and Handicap

Many definitions of rehabilitation have been proposed but none has been able to capture all its aspects. The dictionary defines it in terms of restoration to "privileges, reputation, or proper condition," thus clearly emphasizing the social dimension (handicap), whereas most clinical (especially hospital-based) rehabilitation tends to focus on disability. Medical and surgical treatment, on the other hand, usually concentrates on reducing impairments, yet all three activities are essential components of the rehabilitation process.

The framework provided by the International Classification

of Impairments, Disabilities, and Handicaps[6] (see accompanying box) adopted by the World Health Organization (WHO) in 1980, has proved especially useful in clarifying these aims and sometimes in resolving conflicts over priorities. Thus the pain and stiffness (impairment) in an arthritic knee might be treated by replacing it with a prosthesis, whereas a course of physiotherapy with muscle strengthening exercises and provision of a walking aid might reduce the associated locomotor disability. Alternatively a move to a ground floor apartment or provision of appropriate transportation might do as much or more to restore self-sufficiency and improve the patient's quality of life. Which of these options, singly or in combination, is chosen depends on individual circumstances, associated pathology, the presence of other disabling conditions, and, above all, the patient's own priorities.

Knowledge of the underlying pathology and natural history is also essential in deciding the timing of various interventions. Thus in acute stroke the "ischemic cascade" (pathologic process) may develop over a few hours, leaving a short time period for treatment to reduce the infarct size.[7] The hemiparesis (impairment) may stabilize after a few days, after which treatment designed to promote neural plasticity or "repair" within the damaged brain areas is unlikely to work.[8] The resultant difficulty with walking (disability) may yet be substantially reduced in a few weeks of physiotherapy, focusing on motor relearning and compensatory strategies, and further "top-up" courses given at a later stage may help the patient regain any lost ground, although the benefits may only be temporary.[9]

Even if long-term disability can be minimized through a combination of these approaches, the stroke is still likely to have a major impact on the patient's psychological state, on his or her social life, on family relationships, and quite possibly on financial circumstances and housing. There are any number of strategies for reducing this social disadvantage (handicap), many of which go well beyond the traditional boundaries of "health care," but which must still be evaluated as part of the overall rehabilitation package.

Thus rehabilitation should be concerned not just with reablement, but also with resettlement, readjustment, role fulfillment, and the realization of potential in every sphere of life. These concepts can be applied in various ways in many different situations, ranging from physical medicine for war injuries, to behavioral therapy for drug dependency. The common principles include comprehensive (usually multidisciplinary) assessment, goal setting, and careful monitoring of progress with selective feedback of information to the patient to reinforce positive attitudes.

Definitions of impairment, disability, and handicap

Impairment: any loss or abnormality of psychological, physiological, or anatomic structure or function

Disability: any restriction or lack (due to an impairment) of the ability to perform an activity in the manner or within the range considered normal for a human being

Handicap: a disadvantage resulting from an impairment or disability, that limits or prevents the fulfillment of a role appropriate to a person's age, sex, social, and cultural circumstances

(From World Health Organization,[6] with permission.)

Assessment

Comprehensive clinical, functional, and psychosocial assessment has long been regarded as a cornerstone of geriatric medicine. In the face of frailty and multiple pathology, a full list, not only of the patient's problems but of strengths and resources, is required if appropriate care is to be planned. Strategies for reducing impairment, disability, and handicap should all be considered, and assessment must take place at all levels and must cover all aspects of the patient's current, former, and probable future situation.

Clinical practice often falls far short of the ideal, however, and many problems (and strengths) go undetected. The use of checklists and standardized assessment scales may certainly help, and enormous efforts have gone into developing a host of different instruments, both for everyday practice and research.[10] These cover every level from measurement of strength in a limb to grandiose concepts like "meaning in life,"[11] and range from simple checklists to sophisticated measures designed to simulate equal-interval scales, derived from mathematical modeling of large data sets.[12] There is much duplication and blurring of the boundaries among different domains of measurement, however.[10]

Although there is no doubt about the need to incorporate objective, scientific measurement into our everyday routine in rehabilitation, as much as in other areas of clinical practice,[13] this Babel-like proliferation of assessment scales can only hinder progress. Without standardization of basic measures the science of rehabilitation is like physics without a standard unit of distance or time. Some measures, such as the Barthel Index of activities of daily living (ADLs);[14,15] the Abbreviated Mental Test Score (AMT),[16,17] and the Geriatric Depression Scale[18] are so widely used, at least within Britain, that they are close to becoming part of the "common clinical language" for rehabilitation. As with ordinary language, however, local usage varies and changes over time, departing ever further from the original standard.

A Joint Working Party of the British Geriatrics Society (BGS) and the Royal College of Physicians of London (RCP) has recommended a set of "standardized clinical instruments and measurement scales (SCIMS)" for assessing basic ADLs, screening for visual, hearing and communication difficulties, cognitive impairment and depression, as well as assessing patients' social circumstances and subjective well-being (see Table 110-1).[19]

The use of SCIMS should enhance communication between those who care for elderly people in different settings, encour-

Table 110-1 Standardized clinical instruments and measurement scales for elderly people

Property Assessed	Recommended Scale	Domain of Interest	Comments
Basic activities of daily living	Barthel Index[13,14]	Disability	Informal observation of what patient *does* do 10 activities 1–3 points each giving maximum 20 points[14] Ceiling effect in outpatients
Vision, hearing, communication	Lambeth Disability Screening Questionnaire[15]	Disability	Originally postal questionnaire Not validated in hospitalized patients
Memory and cognitive function	Hodkinson Abbreviated Mental Test (AMT)[16]	Mental impairment	10 questions from longer Roth-Hopkins Test Can be shortened by dropping 3 of the 5 time-related questions[17]
Depression	Geriatric Depression Scale[18]	Depressive symptoms	Interview or self-administered screening test Standard 30-question form 15-question short form[19]
Subjective morale	Philadelphia Geriatric Center Morale Scale (Anglicized)[20]	Quality of life	Distinct from depression, though some overlap
Accommodation support, needs	Social Indicators Checklist[12]	Social circumstances	Checklist rather than measurement scale Useful as case mix indicator

(From Royal College of Physicians and British Geriatrics Society Joint Workshops,[19] with permission.)

aging the development of a common clinical language as well as comprehensive assessment software. For instance, it is recommended that the results of standardized assessments should accompany every communication between the hospital and primary care teams. The educational value of SCIMS is also emphasized: their use should "enhance the training of all professionals who come into contact with elderly people."[19]

The report also outlines a program for future development and research based on the use of these and other SCIMS, aimed at providing the information on which real advances in patient care[20] and efficient use of resources[21] can be based. Many difficulties remain, however, and much work needs to be done to assess the feasibility, advantages, and costs of translating these recommendations into routine clinical practice.

Whether or not standardized instruments are used, thorough multidisciplinary assessment is one of the cornerstones of geriatric medicine. Indeed in North America the process of "comprehensive geriatric assessment" is regarded as the defining feature of medical care for older people, the "new technology of geriatrics" by which the effectiveness of the whole specialty can be judged.[22] As we shall see, despite initial doubts,[22] evidence of its value is steadily accumulating.

The Aims of Rehabilitation

The ultimate aim of rehabilitation has been described as "to restore the individual to his or her fullest physical, mental and social capability."[23] This lofty view is useful in defining the overall scope of the enterprise but a more focused approach is needed in everyday practice.

One concept of particular relevance to elderly people is that of autonomy—the right to self-determination. Respect for autonomy is an ethical imperative in health care, and this means that the long-term aims should be those of the patient, rather than those of the staff or family.[24] Of course it is not always easy to ascertain the patient's true wishes, and even when they are clearly expressed they may appear totally unreasonable. Time and effort spent in trying to find out what each patient really wants to achieve and skill in resolving conflicting priorities are crucial to success.

Despite its importance there has been little systematic study of the aims and expectations of patients undergoing rehabilitation. Some studies have shown discrepancies in the values put on various daily living activities by patients and relatives,[25] and various systems have been devised to enable patients to set their own priorities.[26] These tend to be more appropriate to people of working age, however, and the agenda might be quite different for older people.

Many old people appear to value independence above all else and to wish only to return to a way of life that appears miserable or squalid to professional staff and to society in general. Restoring independence often involves taking calculated risks and it is essential that families and staff, who are both inclined to be overprotective, understand when this is being done according to the wishes and in the best interests of patients.

The idea of elderly patients as "consumers" or "customers" is beginning to take root but is still out of tune with the "we know best" attitude of many professionals. Indeed, traces of the workhouse origins of geriatric medicine in Britain can still occasionally be found in the authoritarian attitudes of some staff and the passive fatalism of many elderly patients. In general, however, expectations have changed a lot from the days of the Poor Law institutions and even frail old people have the right to choose their own lifestyle. The rights, wishes, and needs of caregivers must also be taken into account, however, and easing the physical and psychological burdens of care is one of the main aims of rehabilitation.

These general principles must be translated into specific overall aims in each individual case, involving the patient and family as much as possible. These long-term "aims" must then be broken down into a series of explicit intermediate steps (medium-term "objectives" and short-term "targets") and great efforts made to ensure that everyone involved with the patient's care is aware of and in agreement with them.[27] Rehabilitation is essentially a goal-driven process, and at every stage of every case, the short, medium-, and long-term goals should be clear.

Teamwork

Teamwork is the magic ingredient that makes rehabilitation work. It is difficult to overestimate the impact of a well-organized interdisciplinary team, applying their various skills in working toward common goals, in restoring morale and confidence in the face of illness and disability. Good teamwork multiplies the benefits of individual contributions, but by the same token poorly coordinated care, in which contradictory advice is given by different people and decisions are taken without reference to the team as a whole, can do great harm.

Just as accurate diagnosis is the basis for medical treatment, detailed assessment is needed before achievable goals can be set in rehabilitation. This assessment must be done by experts, but once the plans have been made it is the job of every member of the team to implement them. The scarcity of specialist therapists means that even in relatively well-resourced units only a tiny part of each patient's day is spent in individual therapy, so it is essential for others to contribute to the treatment program. In hospital the key workers are usually the nurses, who spend more time with the patient and have more influence on the overall environment than any other professional group. In the community it is the patient's family and informal caregivers who fulfill this role, so it is vital for them to be equipped with the necessary basic skills.

Thus the main contributions of specialist members of the team are in performing detailed assessments, helping in the process of goal setting and monitoring, and in teaching basic skills to enable others to implement the treatment plan, rather than in providing direct one-to-one treatment. This emphasis on collaboration toward a common purpose and skill sharing, together with a general air of efficiency, enthusiasm, and optimism, is the hallmark of good teamwork.

Motivation and Barriers to Recovery

The patient is always the most important member of the rehabilitation team, and the best efforts of the professionals are unlikely to succeed if the patient appears not to want to get better or not to understand what needs to be done to achieve this.

Apparent lack of motivation is all too often blamed on laziness, but in fact is usually due to a specific mental or physical disorder, one of the so-called barriers to rehabilitation. These may be due to the disease process itself (e.g., disordered perception after a stroke[28]), to complications (e.g., painful pressure areas, constipation), to comorbid conditions (e.g., unrecognized cardiac failure, thyroid disorders, drug side effects), to short-term psychological reactions (severe anxiety, subacute confusional states, embarrassment or fear of incontinence), or to more serious and chronic depression or dementia. One of the doctor's main roles is to detect and deal with these factors, but even so they are often missed.[29]

Sometimes there may be genuine hopelessness about the future because of bereavement, lack of social support or unsuitable housing, but even patients in apparently dreadful circumstances rarely "give up" in the absence of other, often remediable, factors.

Measurement of Effectiveness: The Rehabilitation "Black Box"

Rehabilitation is a complex process, often thought of in terms of a package or "black box," but surprisingly little work has been done to define its contents. This makes it difficult to apply objective findings obtained in one particular setting to clinical practice in another. Although differences in the structure and style of geriatric medical services have been fairly well documented,[30] very little is known about differences in the processes of care (including the overt and less overt means of patient selection), making it virtually impossible to make meaningful comparisons of outcome.[31]

In the accompanying box are listed some of the components of the rehabilitation packages, which highlight the emphasis on comprehensive assessment, communication, and exploitation of the patient's own skills and resources, rather than on providing "hands-on treatment." The time spent in talking to, listening to, understanding, and counseling patients and families has been termed *soft rehabilitation*[1] and is probably the most important part of the overall package.

By their nature these processes are difficult to quantify and, until they can be reliably measured (together with their individual effects on outcome) it will only be possible to make the most vague and general statements about the effectiveness of rehabilitation.

The Challenge of Rehabilitation in Old Age

The Scale of the Problem

There is nothing surprising in the fact that the prevalence of disability and dependency increases with age, but detailed information from epidemiologic surveys using standardized methods is vital in planning services.[32] The British National

Some components of the rehabilitation "black box"

Medical assessment (diagnosis, associated pathology, impairments)
Assessment of nursing needs (caring/encouraging)
Surveillance and preventative care (sores, contractures, bowel, bladder, DVT, anxiety, depression, etc.)
Assessment of impairments (physiotherapy, occupational and speech therapy)
Assessment of disabilities (physiotherapy, occupational and speech therapy)
Assessment of mental function and psychological state
Assessment of patient's strengths and resources
Assessment of patient's and family's priorities
Goal setting
Specific therapies
Progress monitoring
Discussion, explanation, and education of family/caregivers
Discharge planning
Long-term goal setting and review

Disability Survey, conducted by the OPCS in the mid-1980s, provided a wealth of such data, using strict definitions and a comprehensive measure of disability carefully developed for the purpose.[33]

Among its findings were that more than one-half of people aged over 75 years living in private households have some form of disability, most often due to musculoskeletal problems or sensory impairment.[33] The prevalence of severe disability increases particularly steeply with age, and nearly two-thirds of those in the most severe categories are aged over 70 years (40 percent are aged over 80 years).

Elderly women are much more likely to be disabled than men, and we know from other sources that although the "active life expectancy" of women is longer, the expected period of "terminal disability" and dependency is about twice that for men.[34] Despite its association with increased mortality at all ages, poverty is also a strong risk factor for disability in old age.

Commonly reported causes of severe disability among elderly people include arthritis, neurologic problems (probably stroke and Parkinson's disease), deafness, visual impairment, and cardiorespiratory disease. Mental disorders (depression and cognitive impairment), falls, painful feet, and incontinence of urine are also common but often underreported. Severe neurologic disability and dementia are very common in institutional care.[33]

Whatever happens to the incidence of these conditions in the next few years, demographic trends will ensure that numbers of very old people with severe disability will increase rapidly,[35] as will the need for rehabilitation services.[36] These will need to be planned on a community-wide or primary care basis,[37] with specialist hospital units focusing on common conditions such as stroke, where early intervention may reduce or prevent long-term dependency.[38]

In developing countries, where the rate of increase in the elderly population is even faster,[39] the need for cost-effective measures to control the burden of chronic illness and disability is yet more pressing.

Dependency and Institutionalization

Social, psychological, and economic factors make the difference between disability and dependency, and the relationship changes markedly with age. Perhaps the most striking finding is the speed with which dependency increases in older people, once illness and disability begin to appear. In a follow-up survey of people over 75 years of age living at home in the small town of Melton Mowbray, 82 percent of those survivors who were able to perform basic selfcare activities initially were still able to do so when contacted again after 5 years (one third had died).[40] When dependency was measured (in terms of the "interval of care need"[41]) rather than disability, however, only 22 percent of those survivors who had not required help initially remained fully independent 5 years later, and over one half needed help or supervision at frequent intervals.[42]

Numerous studies have shown that older people are much more likely to go into long-term institutional care than younger ones with equal disability. To a large extent this may be due to bereavement and social isolation, but attitudes of older people themselves, their families, and society in general undoubtedly play a major part.

Agism and Rationing

As a group, older people are heavy consumers of health care, and in an era of increasing pressure on budgets, there is a danger that they will be the target of cuts. Rationing decisions cannot be avoided, but they must be based on a clear assessment of how to maximize the "health gain" from finite resources, rather than on agist prejudice and "demographic panic."

Efforts to save money by cutting services for elderly people or denying them access to "high-tech" medical care are usually based on the misconception that the only purpose of treatment is to prolong life, and that old people are therefore less deserving or have less to gain than younger ones. In rehabilitation the aim is nearly always to increase the quality rather than the duration of life and, as we have seen, the needs and thus the potential benefits are greatest in the elderly population. Indeed effective rehabilitation for frail elderly people might reduce the need for enormously expensive long-term supportive care (both domiciliary and institutional), and thus save money overall.

These difficult resource use decisions must be based on sound evidence, and much more effort should go into research into the effectiveness of rehabilitation services and the correct balance between rehabilitation, social, and financial support.[43] There is already encouraging evidence that some forms of rehabilitation, such as stroke unit, care, may pay their way in terms of preventing long-term dependency.[38]

Attitudes and Expectations

Negative attitudes towards older people can be found at many levels and may influence all aspects of health care. A stereotyped, often strangely patronizing, view of elderly people, which takes no account of their rich and varied lifestyles, is common and may inhibit many patients from achieving their full potential. In extreme cases, deafness, communication difficulties, and bewilderment in the strange and often hostile surroundings of the acute hospital ward may be misinterpreted as dementia, with disastrous results. Cultural and educational differences can also be mistaken for stupidity, so that little effort is made to involve elderly patients in setting goals and establishing priorities, or to try out "high-tech" treatments or devices, which are often used in the rehabilitation of younger people.

The stoical attitudes ("I didn't want to bother the doctor") and low expectations ("what can I expected at my age?") of some older people themselves may be a further hindrance to successful rehabilitation, and may even reinforce agist prejudices.

Surveys confirm that many people regard functional limitations as a normal part of growing old. The proportion of people over 75 years of age who reported specific disabilities in the OPCS survey far exceeded the number who complained of "limiting longstanding disability" in the General Household Survey, done at about the same time.[33] Below the age of 75 years the proportions were reversed, indicating that younger people are more likely to feel restricted or handicapped by minor problems, whereas older people are often fatalistic even in the face of severe disability.

Caregivers

The vast majority of the burden of care for disabled elderly people is carried by their families and friends rather than by professionals or organized services. Caregivers are often elderly themselves and the mental, physical, and financial strains of caring can be enormous.[44] Far more practical help could and should be given to informal caregivers[45] and more research is needed into the savings that this might produce in preventing breakdown in their own health.

The moral support that can be provided by a good rehabilitation service should not be underestimated, however. As we shall see, the positive atmosphere of a well-organized unit, the enthusiasm of the staff for helping patients overcome their problems, and the high expectations generated, probably account for many of the undoubted benefits of the rehabilitation package. Families stand to gain almost as much as patients, especially by being involved in a progressive goal-setting process, which ensures that physical improvement or psychological readjustment continues long after the hospital phase of treatment. Indeed, improving the situation of caregivers should always be one of the main aims of rehabilitation.

As well as those providing day-to-day care, there are often other family members who are concerned about the patient's welfare but live too far away to provide much physical help. These "worried would-be caregivers" are often overprotective, sometimes through feelings of guilt, and may put pressure on professional staff to restrict the patient's independence or even to persuade them to go into a "home." This attitude can pose a serious threat to successful rehabilitation and can only be countered by trying to reach a consensus on overall goals. In some countries the threat of litigation has led to defensive and sometimes inhumane practices, such as the use of physical restraints in restless patients.[46] Staff and relatives should be reminded, however, that these not only eliminate the possibility of functional recovery, but may often cause more injuries than they prevent.[47,48]

Even when functional recovery is unlikely, caring has its positive side. Physical helplessness at the end of life may be a cruel caricature of that at its beginning, and the loss of dignity is often hard to bear, but occasionally the dependent role is accepted willingly, and in some families the process of terminal care may be the culmination of a lifelong loving relationship. Many older people would rather be looked after by their families than struggle to continue an independent but lonely life.

Serious difficulties are most likely to arise when previous family relationships have been bad, or when unpleasant personality traits are exaggerated by physical infirmity or senility. The term *elder abuse* originally applied mainly to extreme cases of physical violence, has been widened to include all forms of inadequate care or exploitation of frail, vulnerable people[49] and is probably more common than previously realized.[50] Although broadening the scope of the term will certainly improve recognition of the problem, a more flexible, nonconfrontational approach is needed to deal with minor cases.[50,51]

Frailty and Multiple Pathology

Frail people have reduced functional reserve, but may still be fully independent when well. When stressed by illness, injury, or sometimes by environmental factors, however, their ability to perform the basic tasks of everyday life starts to break down. Inactivity and immobility can also drastically impair muscle strength and stamina, as well as joint flexibility, balance, and reaction speed.[52] Under these circumstances even minor illness can have disastrous functional consequences.[53]

Thus in rehabilitating elderly patients after illness, enough time should be allowed to improve general fitness and functional capacity well above the threshold levels for performing everyday activities,[54] otherwise the discharge is likely to fail with the first minor setback. There is no doubt about the effectiveness of exercise training in improving fitness, muscle strength, flexibility, and mobility in very frail older people, especially those living in residential and nursing homes.[55–57]

Similar benefits can be achieved with slightly fitter elderly people living at home,[58] but it is more difficult to maintain long-term interest and motivation.[59,60] This is less likely to be a problem in the hospital rehabilitation setting, however.

As well as their general frailty, elderly patients often have multiple disease and impairments with which to contend. Diagnosis of these associated conditions and assessment of their contribution to overall disability is important, but treatment should not be overaggressive. Polypharmacy is the "partner in crime" of multiple pathology—the more dangerous partner—and the pros and cons of each treatment should be weighed in terms of its potential contribution to overall fitness. The need to avoid delays in mobilizing elderly patients and returning them to the community must also be borne in mind.

If patients with multiple pathology are to be rehabilitated successfully it is essential for one team to be in overall charge of their management. Fragmentation of care among multiple specialists, supervising different aspects of treatment, is not only expensive but extremely dangerous.

Acute Illness

Acute illness in a frail person often presents as a functional deterioration or as a social problem ("failure to cope"), and there is great danger that the first response may be to increase social support rather than to provide urgently needed medical treatment.[53] Once the need for medical treatment is recognized, rehabilitation must also start immediately, to avoid the disastrously rapid loss of functional reserve that illness and immobility bring about. It becomes vastly more difficult to mobilize elderly patients after even a few days of total inactivity, whether in bed or in a chair. Thus geriatric rehabilitation is essentially an "acute" specialty, whose place is more on the acute wards than in remote rehabilitation centers.

The Process of Rehabilitation

Rehabilitation is an iterative, learning-based, problem-solving process, whose main steps are assessment, goal setting, and monitoring of progress. The details may vary according to the setting but *comprehensive assessment* is always an essential first step. A list of problems should be complied, preferably using the framework of pathologies (medical diagnoses), impairments, and disabilities, and estimating the contribution of each of these to overall handicap. The relationships may not be simple and will undoubtedly vary over time, as some diseases abate while others progress remorselessly.

To be comprehensive, assessment needs to be multidisciplinary, because individual professionals are still poor at assessing problems outside their own area of expertise.[61] The use of SCIMS[19] as checklists may reduce the number of problems missed and can certainly help communication within the team,[62] but is no substitute for detailed evaluation by experts. Misconceptions and suspicions about the purpose of such SCIMS among some professional groups may account for some of the difficulty in introducing them into routine practice.[63]

Having catalogued the problems an *approximate prognosis* must be made, based on knowledge of the natural course of the conditions present and their likely response to treatment. This is never easy in older people because of their limitless diversity, the inevitable presence of multiple pathology, and the difficulty in predicting how they will respond to the "softer" components of the rehabilitation package.[37]

Wherever possible, predictions of the likely clinical course should be based on objective evidence from representative case series, so that *appropriate goals* can be set. These goals should be realistic but also ambitious, as there is evidence that aiming high tends to encourage greater engagement and better progress.[64] Most importantly, all goals should be understood and agreed by the patient, the family, and all other members of the rehabilitation team.

Although the principles of team care and goal setting are widely accepted in geriatric medicine, they are often difficult to follow in everyday practice. Patients are in fact rarely asked explicitly about their overall aims and there is still a tacit assumption that they share the same general priorities as professional staff. Even more problematic, in many hospitals there is little evidence of steps being taken to promote effective interdisciplinary communication and ensure that all members of the team are aware of the current goals, problems, and progress.[65,66] Efforts are being made in several units to remedy this by introducing goal-oriented, shared team notes, although this is often hampered by unjustified medicolegal concerns and by pressure from management to break down every activity of each profession into costed items of service.

Having agreed on explicit short-, medium-, and long-term goals, the patient's *rate of progress must be monitored* and compared with the predicted recovery curve. Here standardized clinical instruments are extremely useful, although simple disability measures such as the Barthel ADL Index may not be sensitive enough to register a change during some phases of rehabilitation, even though the patient is improving in other ways.

More sensitive (or "responsive") measures should focus on single activities, so that progress can be readily demonstrated to and understood by the patient and all members of the team. This *selective feedback* is essential for reinforcing positive attidues and maintaining morale. When functional recovery is likely to take weeks or months, as after a bad stroke for example, the patients should be encouraged to focus on the short term, taking things "one day at a time," and not to worry about the long-term future. This enhances the patient's sense of control and may help to reduce anxiety and avoid hopelessness and depression.

Slow progress should prompt a search for one of the barriers to rehabilitation discussed above, and functional deterioration should always raise suspicions of acute illness or adverse drug effects.

The Interdisciplinary Team

The most important members of the rehabilitation team are clearly the patients and other members of the family. Progress will be seriously hampered if they are not actively involved at every stage, and the business of the professional staff is to establish their priorities and then guide their efforts, reinforcing positive attitudes, boosting confidence, and making sure that progress is recognized and rewarded.

Having shared objectives is the cement that bonds the team together, but an organized structure and leadership are also needed. Traditionally, in Britain at least, the role of team leader has been assumed by the doctor. This is probably a reflection of historically unequal interprofessional (and gender) relationships, but change is slow and the system usually works well enough, provided leadership is not confused with autocracy. It is vital that initiative should not be suppressed and that all members of the team enjoy mutual respect and trust. The team leader is responsible for ensuring that consensus is reached on priorities and goals, that accurate information is given to patients and relatives and shared among the rest of the team, and that patient's autonomy, dignity, and confidentiality are protected.

Full team meetings should usually be held weekly to review each patient's progress, set new goals, and make discharge plans (the "social rounds" held on some acute care wards to discuss the latter are inadequate for complex interdisciplinary rehabilitation). Any major changes in the patient's condition, in treatment policy, or in discharge plans that occur between team meetings must be fully documented and communicated to the whole team.

The specialist roles of professional staff within the team are usually obvious but some points should be emphasized. Close medical attention is always needed to diagnose and treat the underlying disease, associated conditions, and the frequent episodes of acute illness that occur during the course of rehabilitation.

For physiotherapists the main focus is on improving mobility, balance, flexibility, strength, stamina, and respiratory function, by means of exercises and practice in everyday activities such as transferring, walking, and climbing stairs. They may also use a variety of physical treatments such as applied heat, cold, and transcutaneous electrical stimulation. The latter is mostly used for pain relief but "patterned neuromuscular stimulation" is now being increasingly used for improving musculoskeletal function.

Occupational therapists mostly concentrate on assessment and practice in performing ADLs, including provision of aids, but individual therapists may have specific expertise in assessment of perceptual disorders, driving, counseling, relaxation, and leisure therapy.

Speech therapists advise on both communication and swallowing problems and clinical psychologists can often help patients with cognitive and memory difficulties, emotional disorders, and dysfunctional or disturbed behavior. Both professions may work together with other therapists to overcome communication or psychological difficulties that may be hampering progress in other areas.

Social workers often have both a longer and a wider perspective than other members of the team, seeing their elderly clients in the context of their lives within the family and the community, rather than merely as patients with problem lists. They often take on a role as the patient's advocate, trying to establish their real wishes, protect their autonomy, and resist high-handed professional attitudes. Unfortunately nowadays their role as gatekeepers to community services exposes them to enormous financial pressures, and they are often forced to make compromises in trying to conserve scarce resources and resolve competing demands.

Nurses are the only professional group that is with the patient around the clock, and only they can transform the often confusing and frightening atmosphere of an acute hospital ward into a stimulating environment that encourages patients back to normal life. Simple things, like ensuring that patients look presentable in clothes and footwear that fit; that dentures, hearing aids, and spectacles are worn when necessary; and that catheter bags are strapped securely to the leg and out of sight, can make a huge difference. Good nursing is the key to creating a successful inpatient rehabilitation unit, and it is important that night staff feel as much part of the team as those working during the day, and that all work actively towards the same goals. Continence promotion, feeding, skin, bladder and bowel care, and dealing with day-to-day psychological needs are particular areas of expertise.

The need to promote independence may sometimes conflict with the nurse's traditional caring role, and nurses often feel that their training does not equip them to take the initiative in rehabilitation. This attitude can be a major problem because patients will not get better if the only time they do any "rehabilitation activity" is during their brief sessions with the physiotherapist, or if they have to wait a week for a speech therapist to review their swallowing before a more appetizing diet can be provided.

In practice, these difficulties can usually be overcome by setting up a ward-based "rehabilitation interest group" to discuss the role of each member of the team and to share basic knowledge and skills in their own fields of expertise. If well attended, such seminars can make a huge contribution to improving the morale and team spirit of a rehabilitation unit.

Even if they do not always initiate the rehabilitation plans, nurses should certainly play the key role in carrying them out. They can determine whether most activities that patients do on the ward (sitting, transferring, standing, using the toilet, washing, dressing, etc.) are performed in a way that encourages dependency or one that promotes recovery. The difference may be subtle but it is crucial and is mainly a question of attitude and confidence in basic skills. Patients should be expected to do things for themselves, even if it takes twice as long, and reasonable risk-taking should be encouraged, provided this serves to boost rather than undermine confidence. The vast majority of rehabilitation activity, including most physiotherapy sessions, should take place on the ward with the nurses present. In this way what is learned in the brief time with the specialist therapists can be practiced throughout the rest of the day.

In the community the key coordinating role is played by the patient's family or caregivers. Therapists, and especially those who are in short supply such as speech and language therapists, depend on such key workers and on lay and professional helpers to implement their treatment plans. The same principle applies to dieticians, hearing therapists, optometrists, chiropodists, and other professionals, who rarely pay more than occasional visits. Even physiotherapists often feel that they can achieve far more in a short time by teaching simple techniques to other staff and caregivers, than they can in several sessions with the patient alone. It is therefore unfortunate that professional policies tend to discourage skill sharing and aim to replace less skilled but more readily available helpers with highly trained, and much more expensive, therapists.[67]

Dealing With "Minor" Problems

When trying to restore function in a complex system, small things can make a big difference. Patients and relatives sometimes appear to worry more about a lost hearing aid than about the heart attack that has just been successfully treated, so paying attention to such minor problems (which are often easy to resolve) can do a lot to build up trust.

The first priority is to safeguard patients' basic dignity and comfort by ensuring that private parts and feet are covered, that they are seated in chairs that would not disgrace a living room, that possessions, books, and drinks are within reach, and if possible that they are not in perpetual terror of being incontinent.

Hearing aids, spectacles, and dentures are valuable possessions that must be treated with care and kept in working order. If they are not being used, it may be because they are not working or no longer adjusted to the patient's needs. Hearing aids may get clogged with wax (best dealt with by means of a paper clip), may fit poorly (often producing a loud positive feedback whistle), and the batteries frequently run out. Visual acuity for both near and distant vision should be tested with and without glasses. Ill-fitting dentures, common in patients with neuromuscular disease (especially stroke), can be embarrassing and painful. They affect both communication and feeding and can be an important cause of malnutrition, although minor problems can often be dealt with by using dental fixative.

Sensory impairments and communication difficulties are extremely common among patients on geriatric wards.[68] Surveys show that much more could be done, both to diagnose the causes,[68] and to promote rehabilitation by providing aids and by simple environmental improvements.[69] Every effort should be made to speak clearly, to reduce unnecessary noise from radios and televisions, to use communication aids or writing where appropriate, and to use large print for menus and large signs to help patients find their way around the ward.

Most patients require walking aids at some stage of rehabilitation and mobilization will be seriously hampered if these are mislaid or kept out of reach. Foot problems are very common and make a major contribution to overall disability.[70,71] Careful examination of each patient's feet is important and often gives valuable information about overall function and lifestyle. Providing basic foot care and ensuring that appropriate shoes or slippers are worn at all times is an essential part of rehabilitation practice.

Resettlement, Discharge Planning, and Support

Discharge planning should begin as soon as the patient's condition stabilizes and the likely functional outcome starts to become clear. The main factors determining whether or not the patient can return home are the amount of support available and the "interval of care."[41] The need for regular care at night, major difficulty with transfers, unpredictable changes in condition, and disruptive behavior are all serious obstacles. If it is clear that nursing home care will be needed, rehabilitation goals should refocus immediately on readjusting to disability and things that may improve the quality of life in institutional care (improving swallowing, comfortable positioning and seating, etc.). Long periods of hospital rehabilitation without clear goals (or with no hope of achieving them) can be extremely disillusioning and frustrating, and such patients should be resettled in a more home-like environment as soon as possible, and allowed to improve at their own pace.

If a return home is planned, the family can usually give detailed information about the home situation and support available, although a predischarge home visit is often necessary if the patient lives alone. Such visits can cause delay and anxiety and many patients perform well below their best with an audience of anxious relatives and professionals. They may also give an inadequate picture of the problems that are likely to occur, particularly at night. The recent practice of some social services departments of demanding occupational therapist home visits before domiciliary services can be arranged is merely a delaying tactic and to be deplored.

Full case conferences, involving representatives from the hospital, community, and primary health care and social services teams, as well as relatives and caregivers, are another time-consuming (and sometimes time wasting) maneuver. More efficient ways of communicating information about care needs and rehabilitation goals between teams are needed for all but a handful of cases.

For a frail person, discharge from the hospital, especially after a prolonged stay, can be a very stressful experience. Both the familiarity of the home environment, and its sudden strangeness to a newly disabled person, can be sources of danger. The lessons learned in rehabilitation, and even the disability itself, are forgotten as patients settle back into the old routine, until they realize with a shock the gap between their past and present capabilities. This realization often comes as a severe psychological blow, or often as a physical trauma (a fall), both of which can lead to disastrous loss of confidence, crisis reactions, abandonment of carefully nurtured rehabilitation plans, and despair.

The transition from hospital to home is often made more difficult by poor communication between hospital and community services.[72] Failure of promised services and aids to arrive, sometimes until long after they are needed, and the sudden withdrawal of contact with therapists, other staff, and patients, all add to the sense of abandonment. Despite this, most older people come through this traumatic period apparently unscathed, although it may have an effect on their long-term confidence.

The benefits of discharge liaison and support schemes are difficult to demonstrate in the short term, but may be important later. In a large trial in London, patients aged over 75 years and living alone were randomly allocated to receive either standard aftercare or support from a home care attendant scheme (practical care and help with rehabilitation) after discharge from the hospital.[73] After 3 months there were no significant differences in terms of mortality, physical independence, or morale. Over the next 18 months, however, hospital readmissions were significantly reduced in the intervention group, and the total number of days in the hospital were cut by nearly one-half, despite the fact that the extra support had been given for only 2 weeks after discharge.[73]

If these benefits are confirmed, with a policy of providing extra short-term home support to all patients over the age of 75 years discharged to live alone, an average health district with 250,000 people might expect to save about 23 hospital beds, more than paying for the cost of the service.

Audit and Effectiveness

Most patients get better with rehabilitation so it is always tempting to assume that they get better because of the rehabilitation. This simple fallacy often leads to another: that the quality of care provided can be judged by measuring patient outcomes. This false logic underpins the current political fashion for generating "league tables" of patient outcomes for comparing the performance of different units. Sophisticated methods have been developed for adjusting for differences in "case mix" in such comparisons, but these are almost certainly inadequate.[74,75]

This is not to belittle the importance of quality assurance and audit as part of the clinical routine, but it is far better to concentrate on assessing and improving the quality of care rather than measuring outcomes. Various methods for assessing the quality of notekeeping, interdisciplinary communication, goal setting, and monitoring of progress have been developed, and are being standardized. As an example, an Intercollegiate Working Group, representing the professional associations of all those working with stroke patients, has agreed on a comprehensive interdisciplinary audit package for stroke care. Analysis of cases where complications have occurred, or where outcome was worse than expected, can also be useful.

One approach, which involves a form of outcome measurement while still focusing on the process of rehabilitation, is "goal attainment scaling."[76] This assesses the extent to which goals set at the beginning of treatment are achieved. It is a useful way of analyzing the procedures used in setting goals and monitoring progress, but is too susceptible to observer bias to be an appropriate means of comparing different methods of treatment or different rehabilitation units.

Aids and Appliances

Aids and appliances can compensate for impairments and disabilities of various kinds, and may make the difference between independent life and institutional care for an elderly person. Although aids and devices are available to improve the quality of almost every aspect of life,[77] only a very limited selection tend to find their way into geriatric practice. Unfortunately even these are often underprovided (especially bath, kitchen, and toilet aids), underused, or faulty,[78] and delivery may be delayed until after the need for them has passed.[72]

This is probably largely due to lack of interest in or knowledge about this aspect of patient care among professionals, especially doctors. This deficiency has been substantially remedied by a host of excellent studies, articles, and lectures emanating from the Department of Medicine for the Elderly at Leeds. A very useful series of articles, published in the British Medical Journal, covering walking aids; wheelchairs; easy chairs; commodes; hoists; vision, hearing, and communication aids; toilet and bath aids; and devices to assist those with urinary incontinence, is now available in book form.[79] Illustrations are given of the types of aids available, when and where they might be useful, where to obtain them, and how to check that they are safe and in good working order. All members of the rehabilitation team should also know what resources there are locally and where to refer patients and relatives for expert advice.[80]

Many devices are available to help with higher level activities such as housework, gardening, driving, and a range of leisure activities, but probably much more could be done by applying modern technology to ease the restrictions in lifestyle imposed by aging and frailty.[81] The increasing numbers and political and economic power of older people should ensure that more attention will be paid in the future to their wishes and needs in the design and marketing of goods of all kinds. Thus the designed environment should gradually become more convenient and more enabling to elderly people with functional limitations.

Rehabilitation and the "Geriatric Giants"

The concept of the Geriatric Giants—immobility, instability, incontinence, and intellectual impairment—encapsulates the essence of geriatric practice as much today as when it was introduced by Isaacs 30 years ago.[82] All are multifactorial problems, resulting from a combination of reduced functional reserve and age-related disease, which may be acute or chronic. Whether they are the main problem needing rehabilitation or merely a complicating factor, they require careful assessment and a multidisciplinary approach to management, which can be surprisingly effective. In practice, however, assessment is often inadequate and management very poor.

Immobility

As always, assessment starts with a careful history and examination. Deteriorating mobility may be due to general or localized weakness, lack of energy or cardiorespiratory fitness, pain, sensory impairment, apraxia, loss of balance, or loss of confidence, and each of these may have many causes. As with all the Geriatric Giants "going off legs" may be a nonspecific presentation of acute illness, so delay in diagnosis and appropriate treatment can be disastrous.

Once the causes are established, the next priority is to measure the severity of the problem so that progress in rehabilitation can be monitored. Of the huge number of performance-based measures of mobility and balance available,[83] one simple, relevant, and practical example is the "Get Up and Go" test, devised by Isaacs and colleagues.[84] A more elaborate version, in which the patient is timed getting up from a chair, walking 3 meters, and sitting down again,[85] can easily discriminate among subjects using different walking aids. The average time to complete the test was 14 seconds for those requiring no aids, 20 seconds for those needing a stick, and 41 seconds for those using a walking frame.[86]

As well as measuring speed, the gait pattern should be assessed. Gait analysis can be complex but a useful classification of the common disorders found in elderly people, according to the "sensorimotor level" involved, has recently been developed.[87] Examples of highest-level gait disorders are the "overcautious gait," in which excessive time is spent in the support phase of walking, and "isolated gait ignition failure." The hemiplegic, cerebellar ataxic, and Parkinsonian gait patterns are classified as middle-level disorders, whereas examples of lowest level gait abnormalities include the patterns seen in people with severe arthritis, sensory loss, or visual impairment. In complex cases videotaping of the patient's gait can occasionally be useful.

The measures taken to improve mobility depend on the nature of the problem, but simple practical measures, including the use of aids, should always be considered.

Walking aids

Walking aids are among the most important tools for living. In a frail person, they may make the difference between independence and the need for constant supervision or even institutional care. On the other hand, if inappropriately selected or used, they may interfere with normal gait, increasing instability, damaging confidence, and eventually increasing dependency. As with all aids, expertise and care are needed in their selection and their use should be monitored to see that they are achieving the desired purpose. Many elderly people regard walking aids as a badge of frailty (and an invitation to muggers and thieves), and the use of sticks and frames as a capitulation to advancing age and infirmity. For this reason, many aids provided with good intent are discarded the minute the doctor or therapist is out of sight. Many a walking frame has been found on a domiciliary visit, doing sterling service as a clothes dryer.

Walking aids widen the base of support, but in doing so they may interfere with the normal bipedal gait pattern. Indeed a Zimmer frame replaces the normal reciprocal striding action with a halting, stepping motion, which has been described as more reptilian than human. The psychological effects of such a dramatic change in the speed and fluency of walking may be profound, leading to loss of dignity and self-esteem and even more serious consequences.

If aids are used they must be of the right type and size, correctly used, and properly maintained. For instance, Zimmer frames may be dangerous in "backward leaners" or a hindrance in patients with Parkinson's disease or those with "gait ignition failure." The handle of a walking stick should generally reach the level of the greater trochanter, or the distal wrist crease when the patient stands upright with arms hanging comfortably by the side. Someone with a bad hip should generally hold the stick in the opposite hand to support the hip abductors on the affected side. Zimmer frames should never be used to pull oneself up out of a chair and should not be carried up and down stairs (patients may need one frame for upstairs and another for down). Rubber ferrules should always be inspected for wear and to make sure that stones do not lodge in the grooves, making them slippery on contact with the ground.

Instability and Falls

Community surveys have shown that over one-third of people aged over 75 years fall in any given year,[88–91] and that around two-thirds of those who have already had one fall will have a recurrence in the following year.[92](see also Ch. 96). About one-half of these falls result in significant injury,[91] which can be rated serious in about 10 percent.[93] Traumatic injuries account for about one-half of all emergency department attendances by elderly people, and most of these are due to falls.[94]

Only a small minority of these falls can be blamed on environmental hazards; most are related to frailty, poor balance, impaired reflexes, and reduced functional reserve.[95,96] A fall in a frail person often marks the transition from independence to loss of confidence, "inability to cope," dependency, institutionalization[97] and terminal decline, so prevention and rehabilitation are both of the utmost importance.

Primary prevention

Attempts at primary prevention are feasible because falls are common and risk factors are fairly easy to identify. These include any kind of impairment of mobility or abnormality of gait, weakness or stiffness of limbs, foot problems, multiple medications (especially psychoactive or sedative drugs), postural hypotension, impaired vision, and poor balance.[98,101] In one study, 78 percent of those who had four or more of these risk factors fell, compared to only 8 percent of those with no risk factors.[98]

A multifactorial falls prevention program based on correction of risk factors has been developed in the United States and evaluated as part of the FICSIT (Frailty and Injuries: Cooperative Studies of Intervention Techniques) collaboration.[102] Men and women aged over 70 years, living in the community, were randomly allocated to receive either routine primary medical care or an individualized intervention package, including review of medications, full assessment, instructions and exercises from a physiotherapist, provision of aids, and removal of environmental hazards. Over the following year the risk of falling was reduced by nearly one-third (95 percent CI: 10 to 48 percent relative reduction) in the intervention group compared to those receiving routine care. Most of this benefit could be attributed to successful risk factor modification, but over one-third of those receiving the intervention package still fell. The cost of the program was about $2,000 per fall prevented, or $12,400 for each fall requiring urgent medical care.[102]

In another randomized trial involving a random sample of elderly people enrolled in an American health maintenance organization (HMO), those receiving a nurse assessment visit and follow-up interventions to reduce risk factors had a reduced risk of falls or functional decline over the next year, compared to those receiving usual care.[103] Although this was the larger trial, the HMO intervention appears to have been less comprehensive and less well targeted than that in the Tinetti et al. study,[102] and the benefits were more modest and had diminished by the end of the second year.[103]

These results are of great importance because they provide the first convincing demonstration that an appropriately targeted intervention can prevent potentially disastrous problems in elderly people who are frail yet still living independent lives. They will encourage further efforts to widen the scope of interdisciplinary, multifaceted geriatric rehabilitation to include primary preventative care and bring its benefits to the community at large.

Secondary prevention

In people who have already had a bad fall the same preventative principles apply, but the immediate consequences of the fall must first be addressed. Rehabilitation after fractures is discussed below, but whatever the injury the main aim is always to encourage early mobilization, as soon as pain and skeletal stability allow, partly to avoid the complications of immobility and partly to restore confidence as quickly as possible.

The psychological consequences of a fall can be at least as disabling as the physical effects, particularly if it is followed by a long lie on the floor. Fear of falling is such an important factor in rehabilitation that a specific measurement scale has been developed to help distinguish psychological reactions from purely physical disability.[104] Fear of falling affects balance performance and is associated with functional decline and restriction of activities,[105] although this effect may wear off in time if further falls are avoided.[106] Thus the aim must first be to mobilize the patient as soon as possible, in safe surroundings with full support, and then to take measures to improve balance, sharpen reflexes, and increase confidence.

Risk factors should be assessed as in primary prevention, but a much more detailed examination of muscle strength, joints, feet, eyesight, central and peripheral nervous system, and balance function is required. Muscular weakness, particularly in the knee extensors and the ankle dorsiflexors, is an important risk factor for recurrent falls, so particular care must be taken to examine quadriceps and tibialis anterior muscle strength in frail fallers.[101] Vision should also be carefully assessed, as both low-contrast visual acuity and difficulty adjusting to changes in lighting are associated with multiple falls.[101,107] The value of sensory testing is less clear-cut, with reduced vibration sense but not light touch being more common in fallers.[101]

Many complex laboratory-based tests of postural control and balance have been devised, but activity-based tests are more useful because the correspondence between functional ability and specific neuromuscular impairments is weak. Many subjects who perform poorly during everyday motor tasks such as standing up, sitting down, transferring, or turning have no obvious neuromuscular abnormalities.[108] Practice in such tasks, which often simulate the circumstances in which falls tend to occur, is also an important part of balance training.

Vestibular exercises

Although dizziness is a very common complaint among elderly people,[109] vestibular dysfunction is probably not a major cause of falls.[101,110–112] Nevertheless, "vestibular habituation exercises," in conjunction with balance retraining, may be useful in relieving symptoms and increasing confidence when vertigo is present.[113,114] In these exercises, various types of head motion that induce a sense of dizziness or instability are practiced for short periods each day.

Benign positional vertigo is not uncommon and can usually be diagnosed,[115] and sometimes successfully treated,[116] by simple head positioning maneuvers in the clinic. On the other hand, most reported symptoms of dizziness are not due to true vertigo and investigations rarely reveal a specific cause, although musculoskeletal and cardiovascular abnormalities are common.[117] Thus many of the risk factors for falls seem to be associated with dizziness as well, and a multimodal "fitness training" approach is needed to deal with them.

Balance training

Few patients receive specific balance training after a fall, and even when attempts are made they often consist of general exercises involving movement, stretching, and relaxation of major muscle groups, which are not very effective in improving balance.[118,119] On the other hand, intensive strength training can significantly improve balance in older people.[120] It is not entirely clear why progressive resistive exercises designed to strengthen muscles should improve balance, but in very frail people, especially those living in institutions, the proportional improvements in thigh muscle strength following this type of training can be enormous.[120] Discrepancies in the results of different trials of strength training in older people probably reflect differences in the intensity of the exercise regimens and the consequent improvement in muscle function.[121,122]

A reduced capacity for organizing and weighting different sensory inputs may be a more important cause of instability and falls than muscular weakness in older people.[123,124] Hu and Woollacott[125,126] have developed a system of progressive exercises that emphasize integration of different sensory stimuli with motor tasks. These exercises combine balance drills such as side stepping, bending to touch the knees, and reaching overhead, with "dynamic vestibular stimulation" by shaking and nodding the head while maintaining a fixed visual focus. Sensory balance training involves progressively reducing the normal sensory feedback used in maintaining upright stance by closing the eyes, tilting the head backward, or standing on a foam pad. After training an hour each day for 10 days, elderly subjects showed improved stability under changing sensory conditions as well as more rapid righting reactions. The tendency to fall was significantly reduced on balance platform tests[125,126] and investigations are under way to see whether this improvement can be carried over into everyday situations.

Weight-shifting exercises are an important component of balance training and can be practiced, in classes or alone, as part of a gentle aerobic exercise regime. Tai Chi Chuan is a form of slow weight-bearing exercise, appropriate for people with a wide range of locomotor abilities,[127] which can improve gait speed, strength and stability in elderly people when used in conjunction with resistance exercises.[128] Tai-Chi group work (twice weekly for 15 weeks) has been incorporated into an exercise program for frail people aged over 70 years in the United States, and evaluated as part of the multicenter FICSIT collaboration.[129] In a randomized study comparing different exercise regimens, those including Tai-Chi were associated with a reduced risk of falling, although no reduction in fall-related injuries has yet been demonstrated.[130]

Practical measures

Walking aids are mostly used to increase stability by widening the base of support, although they also may be useful in increasing sensory input. The main aim is to increase confidence, but if the speed and fluency of gait are severely hampered, the result may be a lowering of expectations with paradoxic worsening of instability and dependency. Thus selection of walking aids should not be based on theoretical principles alone but on careful assessment of the patient's actual performance with various types of aid. A systematic procedure has been developed in which patients are tested with various aids over an S-shaped course, using specific criteria to assess their stability, gait speed and ability to complete the course.[131] This "S-test" now needs to be validated by comparing the results with the patient's performance with the selected aid (and the incidence of falls) over a longer period of use.

In a recent survey of elderly people who fell, less than one-half were able to get up or summon help, yet only 13 out of 552 potential fallers had been taught how to get up off the floor.[132] When a training program was set up, however, only 63 percent of the 105 who were physically and mentally suitable for teaching were willing to learn. Of those who underwent the training, 44 percent were able to get up independently, 16 percent required some verbal assistance, and 40 percent required physical help to get up. Only 5 of the 15 people who claimed to have stood up independently after their last fall could do so in the test situation.[132]

Shoes that support the feet are at least as important as walking aids in promoting stability, and inspection of footwear is an essential part of both foot examination and gait assessment. Balance beam tests in elderly subjects wearing running shoes with soles of different thickness and hardness have been used in an attempt to make objective estimates of the contribution of footwear to dynamic balance.[133] From this point of view the best shoes were thin and hard and felt less comfortable. All shoes impaired foot position sense, however, to some extent offsetting the benefits of increased support.[134] Foam slippers, on the other hand, not only provide no support but seem designed to maximize the sensory deficit, and should be avoided wherever possible (if no suitable shoes or slippers are available, "grip-socks" are probably better).

Overall effectiveness of measures to prevent recurrent falls

As we have seen, primary preventative measures in elderly people living at home can be effective, provided they are appropriately targeted. It follows that the absolute benefits of such measures must be even greater in those who have already had a fall, as they are at higher risk. The results cannot necessarily be applied to very frail people in institutional care or sick elderly people in hospital, however, where different factors may have contributed to the cause of the fall and may affect the feasibility of rehabilitation.

Rubenstein and colleagues[135] organized a randomized controlled trial in 160 frail but ambulant residents (mean age 87 years) in an old people's home who had fallen within the past week. The intervention group received a package including full diagnostic and rehabilitation assessment, review of medication, physiotherapy, walking aids, removal of environmental hazards, or provision of new shoes when necessary, whereas the control group received normal medical care. About two-thirds of the primary care physicians followed the recommendations of the intervention team, and many remediable problems (weakness, orthostatic hypotension, drug side effects, gait dysfunction) were detected. At the 2-year follow-up, residents in the intervention group had fewer hospital admissions and spent significantly less time in the hospital. Although there were trends toward a reduction in falls and even in overall mortality, these did not reach the 5 percent significance level, suggesting that the effects of the intervention on general health were modest and not confined to the prevention of falls.[135]

Incontinence of Urine and Feces

Urinary incontinence

The normal pattern of bladder filling and voiding depends on a relatively delicate anatomic arrangement, with a complex reflex and voluntary neural control mechanism (see also Ch. 95). Various age-related changes may affect all parts of this system, so it is not surprising that it often breaks down during illness. Up to one-half of patients on elderly care wards are incontinent of urine (or catheterized) in any given day, and the proportion who suffer from at least one episode of wetting during their hospital stay is much higher.

During recovery from acute illness or disability, control of bowel and bladder function usually returns, but continual "accidents" not only cause distress but may well compromise overall functional recovery. Episodes of, and even fear of, incontinence are so damaging to dignity and self-esteem that restoration of continence may be a necessary precondition for improvement in other areas. After stroke, for instance, bladder control is such an important prognostic indicator that specific measures to restore continence in the early stages could well have a major impact on overall functional outcome.[136] This hypothesis is now being tested in controlled trials.

Effective management depends on establishing the pattern and likely cause of incontinence. Diagnosis is discussed in more detail elsewhere, but simple clinical assessment will almost always give a clear enough indication of the likely mechanism, at least to justify a trial of "behavioral treatment," and invasive urodynamic tests are rarely needed. Much more attention should be given to establishing the pattern of incontinence, sometimes in relation to fluid intake, by involving the patient in keeping a "frequency/volume" chart (the volume measurements only need be approximate).

Urgency of micturition with occasional flooding usually indicates either detrusor instability or "sensory urgency." In both cases the mainstay of treatment is habit retraining. The principle is to restore the patient to dryness by regular toileting (even if this means going every 10 minutes at first) and thus to establish confidence that the problem can be controlled. The interval between visits can then be gradually lengthened. In most cases, bladder capacity can be improved so that daily life is no longer dominated by the need to be within a few seconds of a toilet. Occasional accidents will still occur and the patient must be reassured that this does not indicate total failure (the continence chart should confirm this). This approach depends entirely on the active involvement of the patient, but when it is consistently followed, anticholinergic drugs and other measures are rarely necessary.

Symptoms of stress incontinence are almost always an indication to try pelvic floor exercises. These involve repeated contractions of the voluntary sphincter, as if to prevent soiling during a bad attack of diarrhea. Pelvic floor exercises are easy and unobtrusive to do, and effective if they are done properly, but they require motivation and persistence[137] and are difficult to monitor. Their effectiveness may sometimes be enhanced by biofeedback monitoring,[138] and myoelectrical stimulation has also been recommended, although the marked subjective benefits do not seem to be matched by objective cystometric evidence.[139] Pelvic floor exercises may also be helpful in the management of urgency and they are often combined with habit retraining in "behavioral" treatment of incontinence.[140]

Although direct comparative trials have not been done, there is little doubt that far more elderly patients could be helped by continence advisers using these simple "rehabilitation" approaches than by drug and surgical treatments. The main difficulty seems to be in convincing patients that effective help can be given to enable them to regain control through their own efforts. In a general practice-based trial, 197 (68 percent) of 292 women aged over 35 years with regular incontinence reported cure or improvement after a four-session course of pelvic floor exercises and bladder retraining, supervised by a nonspecialist nurse (who had had only 3 weeks of training), compared to 5 percent of controls.[141] Only one-half of the people found to have urinary incontinence in the initial survey had taken up the offer of treatment, however.[141]

These behavioral treatments encourage patients to establish control over their symptoms, thus overcoming the most demoralizing psychological consequences of incontinence. Success depends on active understanding and involvement on the part of the patient, however. The benefits of this approach certainly extend to elderly people with multiple medical problems, especially those with mixed incontinence, provided they are willing and able to play a full part in the process.[142]

Fecal incontinence

In elderly patients immobilized through sickness or disability, fecal incontinence is almost always associated with constipation and fecal impaction (see also Ch. 94). This can usually be confidently diagnosed by abdominal and, when necessary, rectal examination, although occasionally an abdominal x-ray is helpful, especially when the patient has "diarrhea."

Treatment with enemas and laxatives is often successful in restoring both fecal and urinary continence, although careful explanation must be given to the patient and family to make sure they understand the nature of the problem and what the treatment is trying to achieve. Constipation must then be prevented and continence maintained by encouraging suitable diet, activity, and where necessary abdominal massage.[143]

When incontinence is due to behavioral disturbance in the absence of constipation or diarrhea, treatment is based on "conditioning" principles: following a regular routine and providing cues for defecation at appropriate times. The effectiveness of these measures has been shown in several studies,[144] and fecal incontinence should therefore be regarded as a preventable problem, the control of which should be a quality standard for clinical audit.

"Intellectual Impairment"

Detailed discussion of the management and care of patients with cognitive impairment (see also Chs. 48 and 51) is beyond the scope of this chapter but certain principles can be outlined. First, dementia can be regarded as a terminal illness, so the long-term goals of rehabilitation should be seen in this light. Second, patients with severe impairment of memory, orientation, or concentration are unlikely to be able to participate actively in the rehabilitation process, let alone to lead it. Third, the learning process is likely to be severely damaged so there is often little carry over between therapy or practice sessions.

Dementia, therefore, affects every stage of the rehabilitation process and often constitutes an insuperable barrier to success. Nevertheless much can be done to improve the apparent quality of patients' lives and to overcome difficult or distressing behavior by providing a stimulating environment and a settled routine. In fact stability of environment and routine are so important that resettlement is nearly always the most urgent priority. Otherwise the benefits of prolonged hospital rehabilitation may be completely undone by a subsequent move into new surroundings.

Apparent mental confusion is not always due to dementia and, in rehabilitation as in other settings, it is essential to rule out alternative causes such as deafness, dysphasia, delirium, or depressive pseudodementia.

The Rehabilitation of Specific Conditions

Fractured Neck of Femur

Surveys in several countries indicate that the age-specific incidence of femoral neck fractures is continuing to rise.[145–148] By contrast there is little evidence of a similar rise in the rate of vertebral fractures,[149] so factors other than osteoporosis are probably involved.

Hip fractures commonly occur in active elderly people who may have accidental falls, often in icy weather, as well as in very frail older people with multiple pathology whose falls tend to occur indoors.[150] It is the latter group that is the main concern of the geriatrician, whose intervention may make the difference between a return to independent living and a lapse into dependency and terminal institutionalization.

The more fit patients can usually be dealt with quite adequately and speedily by most orthopaedic departments, but it is important to be clear about the case mix when interpreting "performance indicators" from any unit because small differences in the proportion of frail patients can make a big difference to the average outcome and length of stay in the hospital. When length of stay is arbitrarily constrained for financial reasons, the consequences may be disastrous for frail patients. This occurred in the United States when a diagnosis-related group payment system for hospital care was introduced, which took no account of age, illness severity, frailty, or other important indicators of case mix. The result was a reduction by over 40 percent in mean length of stay in the acute care hospital for patients with femoral neck fractures, but a more than 50 percent increase in the proportion discharged to nursing homes and a huge increase (from 9 to 33 percent) in the proportion who remained in institutional care 1 year later.[151]

The principles of "orthogeriatric" rehabilitation include good collaboration between orthopaedic surgeons and geriatricians, early surgical fixation, early mobilization, aggressive management of complications, and interdisciplinary team work with setting of time-limited but realistic goals. The geriatrician should therefore be familiar with the principles guiding the choice of operation and prosthesis[152] and the main complications associated with each one, as well as with appropriate policies for early weight-bearing and movement precautions to prevent dislocation.[153] In addition there should be agreed, evidence-based policies for pressure sore prevention, thromboprophylaxis, antibiotic use (bearing in mind the increasing menace of resistant organisms and *Clostridium difficile* diarrhea), use of bladder catheters, and nutritional support.

Ideally the geriatrician should be involved from the outset, performing preoperative assessments, making an approximate estimate of the likelihood of functional recovery, and anticipating likely postoperative problems in frailer patients. The concept of triage is useful: Patients in the fast stream can usually go home straight from the orthopaedic ward in a few days, provided there is extra community support for the first week or two,[154] whereas the chances of functional recovery in the middle group may depend critically on efficient inpatient rehabilitation. The most frail group is unlikely to recover independence, although as in the case of stroke, a trial period of active inpatient rehabilitation with modest initial goals should be planned, so that potential for unexpected functional recovery is not missed.

As always, simple measures can be important and it is likely that much of the difference between well-organized orthogeriatric rehabilitation and "routine" care is due to more careful and shorter term use of opioid analgesics and sedatives, greater attention to bowel and bladder care, and earlier provision of day clothes and appropriate footwear. Coordinated discharge planning is another common sense measure given insufficient attention on most acute units.

Other important simple measures, more often but by no means always remembered, include short-term use of in-dwelling catheters during the perioperative phase, prophylactic antibiotics for patients with arthroplasties, chest physiotherapy, adequate fluid intake, and early mobilization with use of stool softeners to prevent constipation. Delirium is common during the early postoperative phase, and should be managed by treating the underlying causes and aggravating factors as above, avoiding inappropriate medication, and providing a stable sensory environment and constant reassurance.

Adequate pressure area relief during the acute stages is essential, particularly on hospital gurneys (most preventable pressure sores probably occur in the emergency department).[155] The risks of venous thrombosis are high and can undoubtedly be reduced, although not eliminated, by use of elastic stockings, early mobilization, and subcutaneous heparin. On the other hand, there is very little evidence that symptomatic hemorrhage is significantly worsened by low-dose subcutaneous heparin, although not all orthopaedic surgeons accept this.

Some of the other components of the "orthogeriatric care package" have been evaluated in controlled trials. Malnutrition is a major risk factor both for hip fracture itself and for poor outcome afterward. Nutritional assessment is therefore essential, because trials have shown significant improvements in functional outcome and reduced length of stay in elderly patients given supplementary feeding, either by nasogastric tube[156] or by mouth.[157]

Early mobilization was evaluated as part of an "accelerated rehabilitation package" (which also included access to extra community rehabilitation) in a randomized controlled trial in Australia.[158] There was no significant difference in the proportion of patients returning to their prefracture mobility, but recovery was significantly faster and hospital costs were reduced in the intervention group.

Evidence from trials comparing "traditional" orthopaedic care with collaborative orthogeriatric care remains inconclusive. Of the two older trials, the one from Stirling showed major advantages for orthogeriatric care in terms of length of stay, level of functional ability at discharge, and the proportion returning to their own home,[159,160] whereas that from Glasgow showed no significant difference.[161] A more recent Swedish trial appeared to show the reverse of the results from Stirling, with increased length of stay and institutionalization rates among those randomized to geriatric care.[162] Differences in baseline characteristics between the groups raise doubts about the validity of the randomization, however.

In a randomized trial and cost-benefit analysis of an orthogeriatric unit, set up in an effort to improve slow throughput, patients rehabilitated on the new unit actually stayed in slightly longer than those who remained on the orthopaedic ward, and there was no apparent improvement in outcomes. As well as being new, however, the orthogeriatric unit was hampered by being 3 miles from the main orthopaedic department. Patients waited an average of 18 days before being transferred and nearly one-half of those allocated to receive care on the unit never went there.[163]

The overall message from these trials and from other "before and after" studies seems to be that orthogeriatric care is likely to be most effective when it is started early and when it focuses on older frailer patients.

Other Fractures and Injuries

In comparison with femoral fractures, the amount of tissue damage and systemic upset caused by fractures of the upper limb and other bones is minor, but the disability can still be severe. Despite this, many frail patients with "minor fractures" are not admitted to the hospital at all. The majority of these patients either live alone or with elderly relatives who may be equally frail, so it is most important to assess their ability to cope before they are sent home.[164] This should include an investigation of the causes of the accident or fall and assessment of the usual risk factors, such as poor vision or balance, muscle weakness, or multiple medication.[165] Some system of follow-up, whether by means of an outreach service or by close liaison with community agencies, should be organized.[166]

A survey of elderly people with upper limb fractures in North East England[167] showed that despite many difficulties with activities such as shopping, laundry, and housework, most patients coped well with support. This was provided mainly by relatives and friends, and statutory services made relatively little contribution, although the injury did increase demands on home aids, nursing, and warden services. Demand for chiropodists, bath attendants, and physiotherapists was nearly always unmet. Immobilization of the shoulder was more disabling than of the wrist and it made little difference which side was affected. Those living with a companion reported greater disability than those who were having to cope alone.[167]

These fractures are more often treated by immobilization than by internal fixation and the need to stabilize the fracture must be weighed against the dangers of prolonged immobilization of a joint or limb. Nowadays a lightweight functional brace is generally preferred to a plaster cast as it allows exercises to start earlier.[168] These are necessary to reduce the inevitable rapid muscle wasting, as well as edema formation around the fracture. The modern trend is toward earlier mobilization and exercise of the limb and this appears to produce better results.[169]

Particular attention should always be paid to assessing, maintaining, and restoring hand function[170] and a watch should be kept for late complications.[171] Whether traditional physical treatments such as "electrotherapy" have significant benefits is still uncertain,[172] but the newer technique of patterned neuromuscular stimulation may well improve muscle function after immobilization, and has been used to help restore hand function after neuropathic wasting.[173]

Brain and Spinal Injuries

Although a substantial proportion of patients with disabling spinal and closed head injuries are aged over 65 years,[174] services for these conditions are not dominated by elderly patients. Thus geriatricians rarely play a leading role in organizing rehabilitation, as they do in stroke for instance. They are also rarely involved in acute care, which may be unfortunate as complication rates for elderly patients with severe injuries are often high during the acute phase and outcomes poor.[175,176]

On the other hand, elderly people with less severe trauma (subdural hematoma, central cord syndrome, etc.), usually following a fall,[177] often require rehabilitation in the hospital. Most of these patients will improve with time, as will those with spinal artery strokes, although as always, comorbidity may be the crucial factor and must be carefully assessed. Head injury in elderly people may be a trigger for the development of Alzheimer's disease[178] and the long-term risks of cognitive decline are substantial.

In other respects, management should follow the standard pattern for patients of all ages,[179] paying particular attention to prevention of complications, such as pressure sores, contractures, and respiratory, bowel, and bladder problems. Low-pressure mattresses, such as the large-cell "airwave" system,[180] are almost certainly cost effective in protecting tissue viability in comatose or paraplegic patients, but during the rehabilitation phase, fluidized bead, water, and net beds may seriously hamper recovery of environmental awareness, bed mobility, and postural control.

Bladder catheters are usually needed, at least for a while, to prevent the complications of retention and severe incontinence. Bladder training drill is often useful,[181] and elderly paraplegic patients who are cognitively intact can successfully master the technique of intermittent self-catheterization.[182]

Rehabilitation of Elderly Amputees

Since the World War II, the emphasis of amputee rehabilitation has changed radically, from a service geared to the treatment of young men with war injuries to one designed predominantly for elderly patients with vascular disease. In the last 30 years, progress in vascular surgery has improved the survival of ischemic limbs and general technical improvements mean that those amputations that are performed are far more likely to be below the knee.[183]

Preservation of the knee joint drastically reduces the energy costs of walking[184] as well as the psychological morbidity, and is often crucial to successful rehabilitation. The surgeon is thus always a key member of the rehabilitation team. Good pre- and postoperative medical and nursing care is also essential, to detect and deal with any associated conditions (such as diabetes) or complications that might affect healing of the stump. Factors influencing prognosis include the patient's nutritional state[185] and the hemoglobin level (both high and low levels are bad).[186] Stump bandaging can help to reduce edema but must be done with great care to avoid worsening ischemia. Similar efforts must be made to protect the viability of the remaining foot, so good access to chiropody is important.

Good interdisciplinary team care is also necessary, partly because of the technical expertise required but also to provide essential psychological support at all stages. The importance of psychological factors in successful rehabilitation has long been realized.[187,188] Both patients and relatives need support,[189] and the greatest stress is often around the time of discharge.[190] Amputees often benefit from contact with other amputees and group therapy may help to relieve their fear of the future. There is thus a strong argument for keeping patients in a specialized rehabilitation unit, at least until the feasibility of walking has been established, limb fitting has begun, and longer term goals have been set. Those patients who are anxious to get home as soon as possible are likely to need a lot of help from community services, including occupational therapy.

Today there is great emphasis on early mobilization, using a temporary prosthesis or early walking aid (EWA). Where possible the physiotherapist should assess the patient preoperatively, outline the likely rehabilitation program, and begin taking measures to improve muscle strength and prevent contractures. Ideally, bed exercises should begin on the first postoperative day and the patient should get up to begin balance training within 3 or 4 days, introducing the EWA at the end of the first week. This helps reduce stump edema, allows balance and gait training to begin, and considerably shortens the time to first casting.[191]

Devices such as the pneumatic postamputation mobility aid,[192] which is suitable for transtibial, through-knee, and most transfemoral amputees, allow the patient's future walking potential to be assessed. Those who are unable to stand independently or walk between parallel bars, after a period of training with an EWA, are unlikely to benefit from a definitive prosthesis. On the other hand, patients who manage to use an EWA mostly adapt quickly to walking with a fitted limb, especially transtibial amputees. Elderly patients with transfemoral amputations may still have difficulty in learning to put on and take off a prosthesis, however.

The prosthetist is another essential member of the rehabilitation team, who must liaise closely with the physiotherapist and occupational therapist to design and modify a device that optimizes comfort and gait stability. Sometimes if wound healing is delayed or if the stump is likely to change shape rapidly a temporary inexpensive limb may be used for several months.[193] On the other hand, modern modular prostheses are relatively quick to construct, easy to change, lighter, more comfortable, and look much better. Advanced "energy storing" prosthetic feet, although expensive, can have advantages for elderly patients,[194] and the extra cost may be more than offset by improving the chances that the prosthesis is actually used, and so increasing mobility and independence.[195]

Wheelchairs

A substantial proportion of patients with spinal cord injuries and amputations will become long-term wheelchair users. In Britain, wheelchairs are usually provided via limb-fitting centers on indefinite free loan. Some people prefer to buy their own, mainly to avoid delays, but expert advice should always be sought before doing so. Details of size and design, suitable cushions, straps and other accessories, and whether the chair is attendant propelled, self-propelled (with large rear wheels), or electric, should be discussed with a physio- or occupational therapist.[196]

The therapist will also teach the necessary skills of transferring from bed, toilet, and chair to wheelchair, with or without help and sometimes using a hoist. The home will need to be assessed for ease of wheelchair access and any necessary modifications made as soon as possible to avoid substantial delays in discharge. Good maintenance of wheelchairs is essential, although often neglected.[197]

Arthritis

Arthritis is by far the most common cause of locomotor disability, affecting up to one-half of all people over the age of 75 years to some degree,[33] and at least contributing to immobility in one-half of all patients admitted to elderly care wards.[198] Radiologic changes are even more common, but often bear little relationship to symptoms and disability. For instance, in osteoarthritis of the knee, quadriceps weakness and pain are much better predictors of future function than x-ray appearances.[199]

Management depends on the distribution of arthritis and its effect on functional ability, the degree of inflammation, and the general condition of the patient. Unless joints are acutely inflamed, the relationship between arthritis and disability is rarely straightforward, as it is commonly associated with other chronic and disabling conditions, even in the general elderly population.[200]

The fact that arthritis may be but one of several factors contributing to disability may influence the argument in either direction, when considering joint replacement. Although surgery may be more hazardous in patients with cardiorespiratory disease, and although it may not restore complete health, the absolute benefits of correcting any one condition when their combined effects are multiplicative may be much greater. By the same token, effective treatment of any of the other conditions, together with weight loss where necessary may substantially reduce the problems caused by arthritis. Once again, therefore, close collaboration among physician, surgeon, and therapist is essential to ensure that the right patients (of all ages) are selected for surgery, on and that resources are used in a fairer and more effective way.[201]

Nonsurgical management of chronic arthritis aims to control pain and stiffness, as well as improving function by increasing muscle strength and general fitness. The specific effect of physical treatments such as ultrasonics, short-wave diathermy, or hot wax is still uncertain but there is no doubt that these often have marked general benefits on well-being. Such nonspecific or placebo effects are an essential part of rehabilitation and, far from being denigrated, should be reinforced wherever possible. Progress will come from a better understanding of how these general confidence-building measures work, allowing them to be applied in a more cost-effective way.

Exercises to improve muscle strength are often the mainstay of therapy, particularly in arthritis of the knee. Pain and effusion in the knee joint leads to reflex inhibition of quadriceps, causing muscle wasting and leading in turn to joint instability and further damage.[202] Exercise, sometimes combined with splinting, aspiration of effusions, and corticosteroid injection,[203] aims to break this cycle. Exercise needs to be done frequently (preferably at least daily) and should be supervised, or at least closely monitored, although controlled trials have shown benefit from both hospital-based and home exercise programs.[204–206]

On the other hand, when joints are acutely inflamed the most urgent need is for rest. The beneficial effects of bed rest and joint immobilization on local and general inflammation in acute arthritis have been demonstrated in several studies over many years.[207–211] Other physical treatments may have some additional benefit but the specific method used does not seem to matter.[212] The advantages of immobilization must, however, be weighed against the dangers of rapid muscle wasting[213] and general deconditioning in elderly people, possibly compounded by the use of corticosteroids. Thus regimens that combine rest, splinting and physical treatments with exercise must be devised.[214] Hot or cold packs may be applied to reduce pain before periods of exercise, and the patient must be monitored carefully during and after each session to ensure that inflammatory symptoms are not being worsened.

Isometric exercise is one way of strengthening muscle without increasing joint stress,[215] but there is evidence that dynamic exercise can be done safely and is more effective.[216,217] Mechanical devices can be used to unload weight-bearing joints during exercise, enabling the intensity of aerobic training to be increased.[218] Using water buoyancy to achieve the same effect in hydrotherapy is a more pleasant alternative,[219] and other recreational exercises can be introduced at a later stage.[220]

In a recent randomized trial, a period of inpatient multidisciplinary team care was compared with conventional outpatient treatment in patients with active rheumatoid arthritis.[221] Eleven days of inpatient treatment seemed to produce an early and long-lasting improvement in markers of disease activity, as well as a beneficial effect on emotional well-being, although there was no significant difference in functional ability between the groups.[221] The study may have been too small to detect a worthwhile difference in functional outcome using relatively insensitive measures, but it is also possible that the beneficial effects of rest on inflamed joints were offset by the adverse effects of even a brief period of relative inactivity. Patients who have been assessed in the hospital are more likely to get to know about the wide range of aids and devices available for people with arthritis.[222]

Parkinson's Disease

Medication plays a much bigger role in the rehabilitation of patients with Parkinson's disease than in most other conditions (see also Ch. 38). Physicians should therefore apply the "rehabilitation model" to their use of drugs, assessing which symptoms or functional deficits are causing most distress, setting goals, and taking care to monitor the response to treatment.

Extrapyramidal disturbances with Parkinsonian symptoms are a common feature of many degenerative diseases and are often provoked or exacerbated in frail people by dopamine-blocking medication. Phenothiazines and related drugs, given for confusional states and (often inappropriately) for "dizziness," are the worst offenders. On the other hand, patients with vascular pseudo-parkinsonism rarely show significant response to L-dopa, so it should only be continued after a carefully monitored trial has shown clear benefit.

True idiopathic Parkinson's disease usually presents insidiously and unilaterally in the absence of cognitive impairment. Such patients are often well aware that the disease is likely to progress, so apparently mild problems in the early stages may cause considerable anxiety. Communication difficulties due to dysarthria, exacerbated by lack of facial expression, are a frequent cause of embarrassment and distress. Thus psychological support, relaxation therapy, and counseling are of prime importance.

More serious mental problems such as delirium, depression, pseudodementia, and eventually, in a proportion of cases, true dementia are discussed elsewhere.[223]

As the disease progresses, more serious physical problems occur, including instability and falls, difficulty in initiating movement and "freezing" when walking through doorways, swallowing problems, and difficulty turning over in bed. Performance of everyday activities such as feeding, walking, and dressing may be painfully slow, and there is increasing difficulty getting in and out of chairs and using the toilet.

Regular functional assessment, including measurement of the time taken to perform everyday activities, is important in monitoring the impact of changes in medication or rehabilitation therapy. Many patients show marked diurnal variation in performance, so wherever possible assessments should be made at the same time of day, especially in relation to medication.

Assessment and treatment of associated pathology are important. In addition to the psychological factors already mentioned, other locomotor disorders and cardiorespiratory disease may markedly worsen disability in Parkinsonian patients and should be aggressively treated.[224] Many falls may be due to postural hypotension and simple measures such as review of medication, elastic support stockings, and tilting the head of the bed may help. Acute medical and surgical illness often presents late in patients with Parkinson's disease and can have disastrous effects on physical function.[225] Early mobilization and active rehabilitation are therefore essential during the recovery phase.

The approach to rehabilitation is essentially pragmatic and empirical, dealing with specific problems as they arise. Special tricks may be tried, such as counting or the use of other distracting maneuvers during the initiation of a movement, or looking slightly upward when entering a room to avoid freezing and falling. Walking aids may sometimes be modified to encourage the patient to take longer steps and avoid tripping. Wheeled walking frames are generally preferable to normal Zimmers, which interrupt the gait pattern and tend to encourage backward leaning and falls.

Physiotherapy tends to focus on improving postural awareness, trunk rotation, weight transference, and heel-toe walking. Whether or not detailed analysis of the Parkinsonian gait[226] is helpful in planning therapy is still uncertain, but functional exercises and walking practice almost certainly help to improve confidence. In one small study, exercises done twice a day improved patients' walking speed,[227] and a more intensive physiotherapy regimen has also been shown to improve motor function and self-care in the short term.[228] In both studies, longer term benefits proved difficult to maintain, however.

Certain forms of speech therapy may be useful,[229,230] and simple occupational therapy interventions such as provision of aids can be extremely helpful,[231] although the need for particular aids varies through the course of the illness.[232] Attempts to demonstrate the benefits of structured rehabilitation programs in controlled trials have had little success,[233] but much larger studies with longer follow-up are probably necessary.

Nevertheless there is little doubt that a commonsense approach to providing practical advice and dealing with specific problems can help tremendously, at least in the short term.[234] It is therefore of concern that in a community survey of people with Parkinson's disease in Scotland, 40 percent of respondents said they had no regular medical review.[235] Although two-thirds or more had difficulty with walking or other everyday activities, or were troubled by speech difficulties, only 25 percent said that they had seen an occupational therapist, 7 percent a physiotherapist, and only 4 percent a speech therapist.[235]

Stroke

The reasons why most stroke patients tend to improve if they survive the acute stages are far from clear (see also Ch. 35). Possible mechanisms include improvement in blood flow and restoration of function in the "ischemic penumbra" surrounding the cerebral infarct or hematoma, or gradual resolution of diaschisis ("remote functional depression"), which can affect areas of brain remote from the lesion.

A more promising target for conventional, learning-based rehabilitation therapy is the process by which specific functions are reorganized within the brain after damage, so-called neural plasticity. This has been demonstrated many times in animal experiments, and more recently in patients, using neurophysiologic and functional imaging techniques. The time-scale may be anything from a few days to a few weeks (aging may slow recovery), and the process is very sensitive to environmental and behavioral factors. In laboratory experiments, animals kept in an "enriched environment," where they are interacting with other animals, do consistently better than those kept in isolation without behavioral stimulation.[236]

The overall chemical environment of the brain is likely to have profound effects on all these processes, and experiments have shown that various drugs given at different times can have substantial positive or negative effects on functional recovery.[237] As yet, though, the results are difficult to interpret and certainly not directly applicable to clinical practice.

Other mechanisms of functional recovery are more familiar to clinicians and more readily understood. These include the use of mental tricks (either conscious or unconscious) or physical devices to compensate for various neurologic impairments, such as deficits in attention, concentration, memory, perception, or speech. There is no obvious reason why this process should be time limited, which may explain why significant improvements are often seen in patients given a course of therapy for a specific problem many months after the stroke.[238] Interventions of this kind are usually aimed at reducing disability without altering the underlying impairment.

As yet we do not know how best to promote and direct these processes, either by pharmacologic or by physical means, although the next few years may well see experimental work translated into clinical practice. For the time being clinicians should simply apply the principles of interdisciplinary rehabilitation, learned through experience and validated by properly designed clinical trials, and avoid dogma based on inadequately tested theories.

For all our lack of theoretical understanding, the last few years have clearly shown that interdisciplinary stroke rehabilitation, as provided in well-organized units, works remarkably well. The landmark meta-analysis of randomized trials,[38,239] showing that about 1 patient in 10 will be saved from dying or going into long-term institutional care if treated on a stroke unit rather than on a general ward, has revolutionized attitudes to stroke care. In absolute terms, the benefits of stroke unit care are as great as virtually any other medical treatment, so there can be no doubt that every acute hospital should have an organized stroke service.[240,241]

Although the realization that organized, inpatient stroke care is so effective has given tremendous encouragement to all those working in the specialty, we still do not know which components of the black box produce the benefit. Retrospective analysis of the differences between stroke unit and general ward care in the randomized trials suggest that basic training and a sense of involvement of all staff (especially nurses) in rehabilitation, sharing of expertise, and good communication are the hallmarks of a successful service.[242]

Early, comprehensive rehabilitation assessment and goal setting probably also make a key contribution to the success of stroke units. The patient's neurologic and other impairments, including deficits of concentration, language comprehension, visuospatial perception, sensation, and balance, must be documented, preferably using standardized measures that can detect change. Precise outcome cannot be predicted accurately in individual patients until they are well along the recovery curve, but general statements can be made, which should be encouraging wherever possible. For instance, patients who recover bladder control at any stage tend to do well, regardless of the extent of the motor deficit or other adverse factors.[243]

Another important area that has not received enough attention until recently is swallowing assessment. About one-third of conscious stroke patients have significant swallowing difficulty in the first 24 hours after onset[244,245] and detection and management of this problem is often poor.[246,247] Surveys in several hospitals have shown that only about one-half of the patients with dysphagia, and thus at risk of aspiration and chest infection, had appropriate precautions taken with feeding in the first few days.[247] A multicenter study to evaluate a ward-based dysphagia management policy, whereby all stroke patients are screened on admission by a nurse trained in the use of a simple standardized bedside swallowing assessement and appropriate cases referred for full assessment by a speech therapist, is under way.

Other complications that can be avoided by skilled handling include contractures and painful shoulders.[248] Acute joint pain is quite common in the affected limbs and corticosteroid injections are often helpful.[249] Other associated conditions are extremely common in elderly stroke patients and vigorous treatment can undoubtedly improve overall outcome.

As yet there is much less evidence of the effectiveness of the specific therapies used in stroke rehabilitation than of the package as a whole. Despite years of debate, none of the rival schools of physiotherapy has been convincingly shown to have any advantage over the others.[250] In the treatment of language, cognitive, perceptual, or praxis deficits, therapy has generally relied on repeated practice in specific tasks. This tends to produce a short-term improvement in performance on those tasks, but until recently[251] there has been little sign that it leads to a generalized improvement in function, when compared to "nonspecific stimulation."

This has led to a common misconception, particularly among doctors, that certain treatments, such as speech therapy for aphasia,[252] have been shown to be useless. Although in many trials, patients receiving "active therapy" have done no better than those in the control group, both groups have done surprisingly well, sometimes showing improvement long after the time when spontaneous neurologic recovery can be expected. This suggests that something about the process of taking part in the trial itself might be beneficial, and in fact skilled assessement and monitoring of progress performed by experts constitutes the essence of rehabilitation, whether or not a specific course of therapy is given as well. All therapists have a vital role in giving information and advice to patients and relatives, as well as providing more formal education in basic techniques to other members of the team.

Because recovery depends so much on the patient's own efforts, psychological and emotional reactions are of the utmost importance. Both anxiety and depression are extremely common, although all psychological disturbances are much harder to define operationally because of the presence of neurologic and communication deficits. Depression and emotionalism (frequent crying or laughing, often in "inappropriate" situations) are almost certainly distinct entities,[253] but may yet respond to similar treatments. From the clinician's point of view, the real question is whether the various forms of apathy, anxiety, and misery seen after stroke are likely to respond to treatment. The best way to assess such response is in terms of functional recovery, and now that relatively safe antidepressants are available, a large, pragmatic trial should be done.

Despite its acute onset, stroke has lifelong effects, not just on the patient but on the whole family. The hospital stay often accounts for only a small part of the course of the illness and discharge should therefore be seen not as the end but as the beginning of the main rehabilitation process. The family should already have been involved from an early stage in learning correct methods of lifting and handling and other ways of helping recovery, and it would seem best to reinforce this involvement by continuing formal rehabilitation at home. Two trials comparing domiciliary with hospital-based rehabilitation after discharge from inpatient care have broadly confirmed this impression,[254] although in one of the studies there was a strong suggestion that some frail elderly patients might have benefited from closer supervision in a day hospital.[255]

The overall aim of rehabilitation in the community should be to empower the patient, enabling him or her to adjust to a new physical environment, new family relationships, and new social roles. Unfortunately the structure and philosophy of health and social services in most countries conspire to make hospital discharge a particularly difficult and stressful time for patients facing life with new disabilities, and many opportunities are lost. Numerous studies have shown that discharge arrangements are often chaotic and communication between hospital and community teams poor. Above all there is no sense that coordinated plans are being made for the future or specific, realistic goals set.

The belief that "everything that can be done has already been done" contributes to a sense of hopelessness and abandonment. Where further rehabilitation is provided it usually focuses on physical disabilities, which tend to become less important as time goes by,[256] and little account is taken of any needs beyond basic self-care.[257] Embarrassment in social situations, inability to drive or enjoy leisure activities, fears and misconceptions about the stroke, and altered dynamics within the family all contribute to the "long-term misery" that afflicts even minimally disabled stroke survivors, as well as adding to caregiver strain and ill-health.

In theory, rehabilitation programs or coping strategies can be devised to help with all these things, and different approaches to preventing or alleviating long-term misery are now being evaluated in controlled trials.

Effectiveness of Rehabilitation Services

How Can We Measure Effectiveness?

There is still only limited agreement on the most appropriate measures of rehabilitation outcome, either for individuals or for groups of patients. Roberts and colleagues[258] asked 89 geriatricians and 44 elderly day hospital patients to estimate the relative importance of 12 possible measures for assessing the performance of geriatric medical services. Both groups gave high priority to "reducing disability" and "improving quality of life," and low priority to "reducing mortality." Geriatricians gave greater weight than patients to "effective medical treatment," "consumer satisfaction," "problem resolution," and "efficient use of resources." There was less consensus among patients but they tended to give higher priority to "reducing carer burden," "improving mental health," and "avoiding institutional care."[258]

Most researchers would like to be able to use simple and valid measures of "handicap" or "quality of life" but there are still formidable practical, theoretical, and even philosophical problems to be overcome.[24] Many elderly patients will have difficulty in answering questionnaires, for instance, and although significant progress is being made in combining the different dimensions of handicap into a meaningful scale,[259] any measure based on the concept of the degree to which the subject is able to fulfill his or her usual "social role" is bound to be difficult to interpret when there is so much uncertainty about the proper role of elderly people in society in general.

On the other hand the concept of disability is clearer and more objective (although several studies show that older people tend to accept some degree of disability as "normal"), and relatively simple and effective measurement scales are now coming into widespread use. In practice, however, the amount of valid data from studies that have included such disability measures is quite small, and in drawing general conclusions about the effectiveness of services we mostly have to make use of crude or indirect measures of outcome, such as fatality or long-term institutionalization rates.

Effectiveness of Rehabilitation: What We Know

Given these uncertainties about definitions and difficulties in measuring outcome, it should be clear that it is very hard to draw general conclusions about the effectiveness of rehabilitation. There are many other methodologic difficulties, some of which are described below, in getting unbiased information on effectiveness, so definite answers are difficult to achieve.

Certain principles are accepted by clinicians almost as axioms, however (see the accompanying box). Postacute care cannot be effective in isolation. Full assessment and rehabilitation must begin at least on the acute ward, if not sooner. "Anticipatory care" in the community is being increasingly demanded of primary care teams, although clinical trials of elderly "screening" programs have so far produced somewhat divergent results. The evidence suggests that anticipatory care can sometimes reduce hospital admission and possibly long-term institutionalization and mortality rates, but there is little improvement in functional outcome or perceived quality of life, and the increased clinical activity generated by the results of screening may strain existing resources.

Although the evidence that delay in starting rehabilitative care slows recovery and worsens overall outcome is not based on controlled trials, it has been accepted for many years as an article of faith by British geriatricians.[260] There are a number

Rehabilitation of older people: axioms

- Rehabilitation starts on day one (i.e., on the acute ward)
- Accurate medical diagnosis essential
- Full rehabilitation assessment essential
- Clear plan (specific goals) for every patient
- Teamwork and communication essential
- Stimulating, enabling, confidence-building environment vital
- Must make use of patient's personal qualities and resources
- Families and caregivers need as much support as the patient
- Rehabilitation *really* starts on the day of discharge

Rehabilitation of older people: facts of life

Practice will always vary according to local preference and culture

Resources will never be adequate

Resources will never be matched to needs ("inverse care law")

Outcome depends much more on the patient and family than on the treatment given

Patients and staff usually have different agendas

"Nice" patients will always get more than their fair share of attention

Patients always miss half their therapy sessions

"The best" practice is often the enemy of "the good"

Whether or not an "established" therapy is known to be effective, it is virtually impossible to compare it with "no treatment"

Observing and evaluating clinical practice nearly always alters it

Rehabilitation is never cheap

of other propositions (see the accompanying box) that although not axiomatic, are accepted as facts of life and are unlikely to change or to be rigorously tested in clinical trials.

As we have seen, many trials have been done to evaluate packages of organized interdisciplinary care for specific conditions such as stroke and lower limb fractures, and to assess various components of the rehabilitation black box, including methods of pressure sore prevention, continence promotion and techniques for restoring muscle strength, fitness, balance, and cognitive function. One common feature of the organized, interdisciplinary services evaluated in the "care package" trials is that every patient receives a full assessment of all their medical problems, impairments, and disabilities, instead of just the presenting medical condition.

The first randomized study of comprehensive geriatric assessment (CGA), published in 1984, caused tremendous interest as it appeared to show spectacular benefits in comparison with routine medical care (according to the North American model). Mortality was reduced by half, the costs of hospital care were lower and functional status and morale significantly higher, in those allocated to the Geriatric Assessment Unit.[261]

In a recent statistical overview, 120 published trials were found in which this principle of CGA was compared with conventional medical care.[262] Unfortunately, 84 of these studies had to be rejected because of methodologic defects, but a meta-analysis was done on the remaining studies, in which a total of about 10,000 patients had been randomly allocated to some kind of CGA or to "routine care."[262] The studies evaluated CGA performed in five different settings: the hospital geriatric evaluation and management unit (GEMU), inpatient geriatrics consultation services (IGCS), the home assessment service (HAS), the hospital-home (i.e., postdischarge) assessment service (HHAS), and the outpatient assessment service (OAS). The main results are shown in Table 110-2.

Results from the hospital-based studies (GEMU and IGCS), and those from community-based studies (HAS, HHAS, OAS), have been combined in the form of odds ratios (OR) for the three types of outcome shown. Although very few of the individual studies were large enough to produce a clear result, some definite trends emerged when they were combined. The odds for each outcome (the proportion of patients "achieving" the outcome divided by the proportion not achieving it) in the CGA group are divided by those in the control group to calculate the OR (an OR of 1 indicates equality between the groups, and greater than 1 indicates that more patients in the intervention group achieve the specified outcome).

In terms of producing improvements in physical function, the results were disappointing, but a marked improvement in cognitive function in patients receiving CGA was demonstrated in the hospital-based trials. Reductions in rates of hospital admission and readmission were modest, but still statistically significant, when the hospital and community-based studies were combined.[262]

Table 110-2 Meta-analysis of comprehensive geriatric assessment (CGA) trials[a]

	Odds Ratios: CGA vs Controls		
	Hospital Admissions or Readmissions	**Physical Function Improvement (1 year+)**	**Cognitive Function Improvement (6 months+)**
Institutional (GEMU and IGCS)	(0.9)	(1.2)	1.8
Community (HAS, HHAS, OAS)	(0.9)	(1.0)	(1.0)
All	0.9	(1.1)	1.4

Abbreviations: GEMU, geriatric evaluation and management unit; IGCS, inpatient geriatrics consultation services; HAS, home assessment service; HHAS, hospital-home assessment service; OAS, outpatient assessment service.

[a] *For data in parentheses,* $P > 0.05$.

(From Stuck et al.,[262] with permission.)

Compared to those receiving routine care (i.e., no special assessments), CGA patients were significantly more likely to be living at home (as opposed to being dead or in nursing homes) at follow-up (OR 1.68 for GEMU, 1.49 for HHAS, and 1.20 for HAS). The effectiveness of CGA was largely dependent on the ability of the geriatric assessment teams to implement their own recommendations. This may explain why IGCS and OAS (OR 1.26 and 0.96) showed no significant benefit on this outcome measure.

Effectiveness of Rehabilitation: What We Need to Know

Many more trials have been published in the years since this overview was performed, and more are in progress. On the whole there has been a marked improvement in study design and a general trend toward better results, possibly because the services being evaluated are becoming better organized and better targeted. Thus a clear picture is beginning to emerge of the overall benefits of "comprehensive geriatric care" (of which rehabilitation is always a major part), but there is not yet enough detail to indicate how best to organize services, and still very limited information on the effectiveness of specific therapy techniques.

As in most other fields of medicine, there are wide variations in service organization and in clinical practice, even between neighboring units. Such variations are nearly always due to uncertainties among clinicians about which treatments work and which style of practice is best, and such contentious issues can only be settled by controlled trials. The list of things that we need to know if we are to provide effective and efficient services for elderly patients is almost limitless, but the accompanying box gives a rough indication of the sort of trials that need to be done to answer some of the important questions.

Questions for collaborative trials of elderly rehabilitation

What is the best way of identifying "remediable disability" in elderly people in the community? (GP screening, case finding, nurses, health visitors, volunteers, postal, etc.)

What should we do about it? (Social support, community rehabilitation, community geriatricians, day hospitals, specialist clinics, etc.)

What is the best way to manage the "Geriatric Giants"? (Falls, complications of immobility, cognitive impairment, incontinence, etc.)

Can rehabilitation be done equally well or better at home? (Initial home care or early discharge)

Can groups of patients be identified who will not benefit from rehabilitation?

Can better interdisciplinary collaboration (team notes, goal setting) improve outcome?

What is the optimum (most cost-effective) amount of therapy (per week)?

Is limited physio/occupational/speech therapy time better spent treating the patient or training staff and caregivers?

Can "basic" therapy be provided by rehabilitation nurses rather than specialist therapists?

Can effective rehabilitation be provided in nursing homes?

Day hospital versus "augmented" (Social Services) day center versus domiciliary rehabilitation

Should rehabilitation concentrate less on restoration of function and more on social readjustment?

What is the best way of supporting caregivers? (Daytime respite, night care, domiciliary services, support groups, etc.)

The Future

The next few years will undoubtedly see progress in answering some of these practical questions. Such answers will only ever apply to the situation in which the trials are done, however, and the questions themselves will change as social, political, and economic circumstances evolve and as basic science progresses. Regardless of whether we will ever understand the mechanisms of aging well enough to manipulate them for clinical benefit, the impact of aging on society is already changing profoundly as a result of medical progress.

Better understanding of cardiorespiratory and muscle physiology is already changing rehabilitation practice, and experimental studies are beginning to shed light on the processes of repair and readaptation within the central nervous system. These processes are sensitive both to the chemical and to the behavioural environment, so new drug treatments and techniques of behavioural stimulation are sure to be developed and to have an enormous impact on clinical outcome.

Functional electrical stimulation (FES) will also be increasingly and effectively used in many different situations. Unfortunately, the early development of FES was marred by an excess of clinical zeal and opportunism, which pushed the applications way ahead of the theory, and false hopes were raised. Much harm was done in Britain by the highly publicized case of a policeman, paralyzed after a gunshot injury, who traveled to the United States for FES treatment and killed himself after failing to walk independently. More recent applications of FES have been more modest but more successful, and theoretical knowledge is advancing steadily.

The potential scope of rehabilitation through scientific progress is almost limitless, but however sophisticated the technology, its successful application will always require thorough interdisciplinary assessment of the patient's impairments, disabilities, and handicaps; the setting of specific goals, and careful monitoring of progress.

References

1. Young J: Rehabilitation and older people. BMJ 1996;313: 677–681
2. Warren M: Care of the chronic sick aged. Lancet 1946;1: 841–843
3. Kirkwood TBL, Wolff SP: The biological basis of aging. Age Ageing 1995;24:167–171
4. Olshansky SJ, Carnes BA, Cassel CK: The aging of the human species. Scientific American 1993;268:46–52
5. Young A: There is no such thing as geriatric medicine, and it's here to stay. Lancet 1989;2:263–265
6. World Health Organization: International Classification of Impairments. Disabilities and Handicaps. WHO, Geneva, 1980
7. Baron JC, VonKummer R, DelZoppo GJ: Treatment of acute ischemic stroke—challenging the concept of a rigid and universal time window. Stroke 1995;26:2219–2221
8. Kozlowski DA, Jones TA, Schallert T: Pruning of dendrites and restoration of function after brain- damage—role of the NMDA receptor. Restor Neurol Neurosci 1994;7:119–126
9. Wade DT, Collen FM, Robb GF, Warlow CP: Physiotherapy intervention late after stroke and mobility. BMJ 1992;304: 609–613
10. Barer D: Assessment in rehabilitation. Rev Clin Gerontol 1993; 3:169–186
11. Warner SC, Williams JI: The meaning in life scale: determining the reliability and validity of a measure. J Chron Dis 1987;40: 503–512
12. Velozo CA, Magalhaes LC, Pan AW, Leiter P: Functional scale discrimination at admission and discharge: Rasch analysis of the Level of Rehabilitation Scale-III. Arch Phys Med Rehabil 1995;76:705–712
13. Tallis RC: Measurement and the future of rehabilitation. Marjory Warren Lecture 1988. Geriatric Med 1989;19:31–40
14. Mahoney FJ, Barthel DW: Functional evaluation: the Barthel Index. Md State Med J 1965; 14:61–65
15. Collin C, Wade DT, Davies S, Horne V: The Barthel ADL Index: a reliability study. Int Disabil Stud 1988;10:61–63
16. Hodkinson HM: Evaluation of a mental test score for assessment of mental impairment in the elderly. Age Ageing 1972;1: 233–238
17. Jitapunkul S, Pillay I, Ebrahim SB: The Abbreviated Mental Test: its use and validity. Age Ageing 1991;20:332–336
18. Yesavage JA: Geriatric Depression Scale. Psychopharmacol Bull 1988;24:709–711
19. Royal College of Physicians and British Geriatrics Society Joint Workshops: Standardised Assessment Scales for Elderly People. Royal College of Physicians, London, 1992
20. Rubenstein LZ, Josephson KR, Wieland Gd et al: Effectiveness of a geriatric evaluation unit. A randomized clinical trial. N Engl J Med 1989;311:1664–1670
21. Miller ST, Applegate WB, Elam JT, Graney MJ: Influence of diagnostic classification on outcomes and charges in geriatric assessment and rehabilitation. J Am Geriatr Soc 1994;42: 11–15
22. Epstein AM, Hall JA, Besdine R et al: The emergence of geriatric assessment units. The "new technology of geriatrics". Ann Int Med 1987;106:299–303
23. Mair A: Report of Subcommittee of the Standing Medical Advisory Committee, Scottish Health Service Council on Medical Rehabilitation. HMSO Edinburgh, 1972
24. Ebrahim SB: The goals of rehabilitation for older people. Rev Clin Gerontol 1994;4:93–95
25. Chiou IL, Burnett CN: Values of activities of daily living. A survey of stroke patients and their home therapists. Phys Ther 1985;65:901–906
26. Davis A, Davis S, Moss N et al: First steps towards an interdisciplinary approach to rehabilitation. Clin Rehabil 1992;6: 237–244
27. McGrath JR, Davis AM: Rehabilitation: where are we going and how do we get there? Clin Rehabil 1992;6:225–235
28. Adams GF, Hurwitz LJ: Mental barriers to recovery from stroke. Lancet 1963;2:533–573
29. Garcia CA, Tweedy JR, Blass JP: Underdiagnosis of cognitive impairment in a rehabilitation setting. J Am Geriatr Soc 1984; 32:339–342
30. Brocklehurst JC, Andrews K: Geriatric medicine—the style of practice. Age Ageing 1985;14:1–7
31. Cochrane AL: Effectiveness and efficiency. Nuffield Provincial Hospitals Trust, London, 1972
32. Ostfeld A: Using epidemiological data to plan services for the elderly. Public Health Rep 1988;103: 5202
33. Martin J, Meltzer H, Elliot D: The prevalence of disability among adults. OPCS surveys of disability in Great Britain. Report 1. HMSO, London, 1988
34. Katz S, Branch LG, Branson MH et al: Active life expectancy. N Engl J Med 1983;309:1218–1224
35. Anonymous: Caring for people. Community care in the next decade and beyond HMSO, London, 1989
36. Andrews K: Demographic changes and resources for the elderly. BMJ 1985;290:1023–1024
37. Gloag D: Rehabilitation of the elderly. I: Settings and services. BMJ 1985;290:455–457
38. Dennis M, Langhorne P: So stroke units save lives: where do we go from here?BMJ 1994;309:1273–1277
39. Grundy E: Demography and old age. J Am Geriatr Soc 1983; 31:325–332
40. Jagger C, Spiers NA, Clarke M: Factors associated with decline in function, institutionalization and mortality of elderly people. Age Ageing 1993;22:190–197
41. Isaacs B, Neville Y: The needs of old people. The "interval" as a method of measurement. Br J Prev Soc Med 1976;30: 79–85
42. Jagger C, Clarke M, Cook AJ: Mental and physical health of elderly people: five-year follow-up of a total population. Age Ageing 1989;18:77–82
43. Patrick DL, Peach H: Disablement in the Community. Oxford University Press, Oxford, 1989
44. Anderson R: Living With Chronic Illness. Unwin Hyman, London, 1988
45. Jones D, Vetter NJ: Formal and informal support received by carers of elderly dependants. BMJ 291:643–645

46. Evans LK, Strumpf NE: Tying down the elderly: a review of the literature on physical restraint. J Am Geriatr Soc 1989;36: 65–74
47. Tinker GM: Accidents in a geriatric department. Age Ageing 1979;8:196–198
48. Tinetti M, Liu W-L, Ginter SF: Mechanical restraint use and fall-related injuries among residents of skilled nursing facilities. Ann Intern Med 1992;116:369–374
49. Fulmer TT, O'Malley TA: Inadequate Care of the Elderly. Springer, New York, 1987
50. McCreadie C, Tinker A: Abuse of elderly people in the domestic setting—a U.K. perspective. Age Ageing 1993;22:65–69
51. Vernon M, Bennett G: "Elder abuse": the case for greater involvement of geriatricians. Age Ageing 1995;24:177–179
52. Gray JAM, Bassey EJ, Young A: The risks of inactivity. In pp. 78–94. Gray JAM (ed): Prevention of Diseases in the Elderly. Churchill Livingstone, London, 1985
53. Boyd RV: What is a "Social problem" in geriatrics. pp. 143–157. In Arie T (ed): Health Care of the Elderly. Croom Helm, London, 1981
54. Young A: Exercise physiology in geriatric practice. Acta Med Scand Suppl 1986;711:227–232
55. McMurdo ME, Rennie L: A controlled trial of exercise by residents of old people's homes. Age Ageing 1993;22:11–15
56. McMurdo ME, Rennie LM: Improvements in quadriceps strength with regular seated exercise in the institutionalized elderly. Arch Phys Med Rehabil 1994;75:600–603
57. Sauvage LR Jr, Myklebust BM, CrowPan J et al: A clinical trial of strengthening and aerobic exercise to improve gait and balance in elderly male nursing home residents. Am J Phys Med Rehabil 1992; 71:333–342
58. McMurdo MET, Burnett L: Randomised controlled trial of exercise in the elderly. Gerontology 1992; 38:292–298
59. Elward K, Larson EB: Benefits of exercise for older adults. A review of existing evidence and current recommendations for the general population. Clin Geriatr Med 1992;8:35–50
60. McMurdo MET, Johnstone R: A randomized controlled trial of a home exercise program for elderly people with poor mobility. Age Ageing 1995;24:425–428
61. Cunningham C, Horgan F, Keane N et al: Detection of disability by different members of an interdisciplinary team. Clin Rehabil 1996;10:247–254
62. Stone SP, Ali B, Auberleek I, et al: The Barthel Index in clinical practice: use on a rehabilitation ward for elderly people. J Roy Coll Phys (Lond) 1994;28:419–423
63. Dunn RB, Lewis PA: Compliance with standardised assessment scales for elderly people among consultant geriatricians in Wessex. BMJ 1993;307:606
64. Guthrie S, Harvey A: Motivation and its influence on outcome in rehabilitation. Rev Clin Gerontol 1994;4:235–243
65. Gibbon B, Watkins CL, Waters KR, Barer DH: Multidisciplinary team rehabilitation: reality or myth? Clin Rehabil 1994; 8:90
66. Benbow S, Watkins C, Sangster G et al: The availability and reliability of information on the premorbid functional status of stroke patients in hospital. Clin Rehabil 1994;8:281–285
67. Dyson R: Shortage of therapists. BMJ 300:4
68. Sweeney T, Sheahan N, Rice I, et al: Communication disorders in a hospital elderly population. Clin Rehabil 1993;7:113–117
69. Tolson D, Swan IR, McIntosh J: Auditory rehabilitation: needs and realities on long-stay wards for elderly people. Brit J Clin Practice 1995;49:243–245
70. Ebrahim S, Sainsbury R, Watson S: Foot problems of the elderly: a hospital survey. BMJ 1981;283:949–950
71. White EG, Mulley GP: Footcare for very elderly people: a community survey. Age Ageing 1989;18:275–278
72. Ebrahim S, Barer D, Nouri F: An audit of follow up services for stroke patients after discharge from hospital. Int Disabil Studies 1987;9:103–105
73. Townsend J, Piper M, Frank AO et al: Reduction in hospital readmission stay of elderly patients by a community based hospital discharge scheme: a randomised controlled trial. BMJ 1988;297:544–547
74. Davenport RJ, Dennis MS, Warlow CP: Effect of correcting outcome data for casemix: an example from stroke medicine. BMJ 1996;312:1503–1505
75. Barer D, Ellul J, Watkins C: Correcting outcome data for case mix in stroke medicine. BMJ 1996;313:1005–1006(corr)
76. Stolee P, Rockwood K, Fox RA, Streiner DL: The use of goal attainment scaling in a geriatric care setting. J Am Geriatr Soc 1992;40:574–578
77. Gloag D: Aids and the environment. BMJ 1985;290:220–223
78. George J, Binns VE, Clayden AD, Mulley GP: Aids and adaptations for the elderly at home; underprovided, underused, and undermaintained. BMJ 1988;296:1365–1366
79. Mulley G (ed): More Everyday Aids and Appliances. British Medical Journal Publications, London. London, 1991
80. Chamberlain A, Gallop J: The disabled living centre: what does it do? BMJ 1988;297:1523–1527
81. Wolff H: Tools for living: a personal view of new status for aids for the disabled in society. J Biomed Eng 3:329–330
82. Isaacs B: The Challenge of Geriatric Medicine. Oxford University Press, Oxford, 1992
83. MacKnight C, Rockwood K: Assessing mobility in elderly people. A review of performance-based measures of balance, gait and mobility for bedside use. Rev Clin Gerontol 1995;5: 464–486
84. Mathias S, Nayak USL, Isaacs B: Balance in the elderly patient: the "Get up and Go" test. Arch Phys Med Rehabil 1986;67: 387–389
85. Podsiadlo D, Richardson S: The timed "up and go": a test of basic functional mobility for frail elderly persons. J Am Geriatr Soc 1991;39:142–148
86. Berg KO, Maki BE, Williams JI et al: Clinical and laboratory measures of postural balance in an elderly population. Arch Phys Med Rehabil 1992;73:1073–1080
87. Nutt JG, Marsden CD, Thompson PD: Human walking and higher-level gait disorders, particularly in the elderly. Neurology 1993;43:268–279
88. Prudham D, Evans JG: Factors associated with falls in the elderly: a community study. Age Ageing 1981;10:141–146
89. Campbell AJ, Reinken J, Allan BC, Martinez GS: Falls in old age: a study of frequency and related clinical factors. Age Ageing 1981;10:264–270

90. Blake AJ, Morgan K, Bendall MJ et al: Falls by elderly people at home: prevalence and associated factors. Age Ageing 1988; 17:365–372
91. Downton JH, Andrews K: Postural disturbance and psychological symptoms amongst elderly people living at home. Int J Geriatr Psych 1990;5:93–98
92. Nevitt MC, Cummings SR, Kidd S, Black D: Risk factors for recurrent, non-syncopal falls. A prospective study. JAMA 1989; 261:2663–2668
93. Campbell AJ, Borrie MJ, Spears GF et al: Circumstances and consequences of falls experienced by a community population 70 years and over during a prospective study. Age Ageing 1990; 19:136–141
94. Dove AF, Dave SH: Elderly patients in the accident department and their problems. BMJ 1986;292:807–809
95. Reinsch S, MacRae P, Lachenbruch PA, Tobis JS: Why do healthy older adults fall? Behavioral and environmental risks. Phys Occup Ther Geriatr 1992;11:1–15
96. Lipisitz LA, Jonsson PV, Kelley MM, Koestner JS: Causes and correlates of recurrent falls in ambulatory frail elderly. J Gerontol Med Sci 1991;46:M114–122
97. Sattin RW, Huber DAL, DeVito CA et al: The incidence of fall injury events among the elderly in a defined population. Am J Epidemiol 1990;131:1028–1037
98. Tinetti ME, Speechley M, Ginter SF: Risk factors for falls among elderly persons living in the community. N Engl J Med 1988; 319:1701–1707
99. Lipisitz LA, Jonsson PV, Kelley MM, Koestner JS: Causes and correlates of recurrent falls in ambulatory frail elderly. J Gerontol Med Sci 1991;46:M114–122
100. Lord SR, McLean D, Stathers G: Physiological factors associated with injurious falls in older people living in the community. Gerontology 1992;38:338–346
101. Lord SR, Ward JA, Williams P, Anstey KJ: Physiological factors associated with falls in older community-dwelling women. J Am Geriatr Soc 1994;42:1110–1117
102. Tinetti ME, Baker DI, McAvay G et al: A multifactorial intervention to reduce the risk of falling among elderly people living in the community. N Engl J Med 1994;331:821–827
103. Wagner EH, Lacroix AZ, Grothaus L et al: Preventing disability and falls in older adults—a population-based randomized trial. Am J Public Health 1994;84:1800–1806
104. Tinetti ME, Richman D, Powell L: Falls efficacy as a measure of fear of falling. J Gerontol 1990; 45:P239–243
105. Maki BE, Holliday PJ, Topper AK: Fear of falling and postural performance in the elderly. J Gerontol Med Sci 1991;46: M123–131
106. Ringsberg K, Johnell O, Obrant K: Balance and speed of walking of women with Colles' fractures. Physiotherology 1993;79: 689–692
107. Kolanowski AM: The clinical importance of environmental lighting to the elderly. J Gerontol Nurs 1992;18:10–13
108. Tinetti ME, Ginter SF: Identifying mobility dysfunctions in elderly patients. JAMA 1988;259:1190–1193
109. Colledge NR, Wilson JA, Macintyre CCA, Maclennan WJ: The prevalence and characteristics of dizziness in an elderly community. Age Ageing 1994;23:117–120
110. Prudham D, Evans JG. Factors associated with falls in the elderly: a community study. Age Ageing 1981;10:141–146
111. Brocklehurst JC, Robertson D, James-Groom P: Clinical correlates of sway in old age-sensory modalities. Age Ageing 1982; 11:1–10
112. Downton JH, Andrews K: Postural disturbance and psychological symptoms amongst elderly people living at home. Int J Geriatr Psych 1990;5:93–98
113. Shepard NT, Telian SA, Smith-Wheelock M, Raj A: Vestibular and balance rehabilitation therapy. Ann Otol Rhinol Laryngol 1993;102:198–205
114. Yardley L, Luxon LM: Treating dizziness with vestibular rehabilitation. BMJ 1994;308:1252–1253
115. Dix MR, Hallpike CS: The pathology, symptomatology and diagnosis of certain common disorders of the vestibular system. Ann Otol 1952;61:987–1016
116. Epley JM: The canalith repositioning manoeuvre: for treatment of benign positional vertigo. Otolaryngol Head Neck Surg 1992; 107:399–404
117. Colledge NR, Barr-Hamilton RM, Lewis SJ et al: Evaluation of investigations to diagnose the cause of dizziness in elderly people: a community based controlled study. BMJ 1996; 313: 788–792
118. Crilly RG, Willems DA, Trenholm KJ et al: Effect of exercise on postural sway in the elderly. Gerontology 1989;35:137–143
119. Lichtenstein MJ, Shields SL, Shiavi RG, Burger C: Exercise and balance in aged women: a pilot controlled clinical trial. Arch Phys Med Rehabil 1989;70:138–143
120. Fiatarone MA, Marks EC, Ryan ND et al: High-intensity strength training in nonagenarians—effects on skeletal muscle. JAMA 1990;263:3029–3034
121. Nelson ME, Fiatarone MA, Morganti CM et al: Effects of high-intensity strength training on multiple risk factors for osteoporotic fractures. JAMA 1994;272:1909–1914
122. Judge JO, Whipple RH, Wolfson LI: Effects of resistive and balance exercises on isokinetic strength in older persons. J Am Geriatr Soc 1994;42:937–946
123. Woollacott MH, Shumway-Cook A, Nashner LM: Aging and posture control: changes in sensory organization and muscular coordination. Int J Aging Hum Dev 1986;23:97–114
124. Peterka RJ, Black FO: Age-related changes in human posture control: sensory organization tests. J Vestib Res 1990;1:73–85
125. Hu M-H, Woollacott MH: Multisensory training of standing balance in older adults: I. Postural stability and one-leg stance balance. J Gerontol Med Sci 1994;49:M52–61
126. Hu M-H, Woollacott MH: Multisensory training of standing balance in older adults: II. Kinematic and electromyographic postural responses. J Gerontol Med Sci 1994;49:M62–71
127. Kirsteins AE, Dietz F, Hwang S-M: Evaluating the safety and potential use of a weight-bearing exercise, Tai-Chi Chuan, for rheumatoid arthritis patients. Am J Phys Med Rehabil 1991; 70:136–141
128. Judge JO, Underwood M, Gennosa T: Exercise to improve gait velocity in older persons. Arch Phys Med Rehabil 1993;74: 400–406
129. Wolf SL, Kutner NG, Green RC, McNeely E: The Atlanta FICSIT study: two exercise interventions to reduce frailty in elders. J Am Geriatr Soc 1993;41:329–332

130. Province MA, Hadley EC, Hornbrook MC et al: The effects of exercise on falls in elderly patients. JAMA 1995;273: 1341–1347
131. Prajpati C, Watkins C, Cullen H et al: The "s" test—a preliminary study of an instrument for selecting the most appropriate mobility aid, Clin Rehabil 1996;10:314–318
132. Simpson JM: Elderly people at risk of falling: do they want to be taught how to get up again? Clin Rehabil 1995;9:65–69
133. Robbins S, Gouw GJ, McClaran J: Shoe sole thickness and hardness influence balance in older men. J Am Geriatr Soc 1992;40:1089–1094
134. Robbins S, Waked E, McClaran J: Proprioception and stability: foot position awareness as a function of age and footwear. Age Ageing 1995;24:67–72
135. Rubenstein LZ, Robbins AS, Josephson KR et al: The value of assessing falls in an elderly population: a randomized clinical trial. Ann Intern Med 1990;113:308–316
136. Barer D: Continence after stroke: useful predictor or goal of therapy? Age Ageing 1989;18:183–191
137. Walters MD, Realini JP, Dougherty M: Nonsurgical treatment of urinary incontinence, Review. Curr Opin Obste Gynecol 1992;4:554–558
138. Burns PA, Pranikoff K, Nochajski TH et al: A comparison of effectiveness of biofeedback and pelvic muscle exercise treatment of stress incontinence in older community-dwelling women. J Gerontol 1993;48:M167–174
139. Meyer S, Dhenin T, Schmidt N, De Grandi P: Subjective and objective effects of intravaginal electrical myostimulation and biofeedback in patients with genuine stress urinary incontinence. Br J Urol 1992;69:584–588
140. Flynn L, Cell P, Luisi E: Effectiveness of pelvic muscle exercises in reducing urge incontinence among community residing elders. J Gerontol Nurs 1994;20:23–27
141. O'Brien J, Austin M, Sethi P, O'Boyle P: Urinary incontinence: prevalence, need for treatment, and effectiveness of intervention by nurse. BMJ 1991;303:1308–1312
142. McDowell BJ, Burgio KL, Dombrowski M et al: An interdisciplinary approach to the assessment and behavioral treatment of urinary incontinence in geriatric outpatients. J Am Geriatr Soc 1992;40:370–374
143. Resende TL, Brocklehurst JC, ONeill PA: A pilot study on the effect of exercise and abdominal massage on bowel habit in continuing care patients. Clin Rehabil 1993;7:204–209
144. Ouslander JG, Simmons S, Schnelle J et al: Effects of prompted voiding on fecal continence among nursing-home residents. J Am Geriatr Soc 1996;44:424–428
145. Martin AD, Silverthorn KG, Houston CS et al: The incidence of fracture of the proximal femur in two million Canadians from 1972 to 1984. Clin Orthop 1991;266:111–118
146. Boyce WJ, Vessey MP: Rising incidence of fracture of the proximal femur. Lancet 1985;1:150–151
147. Swanson AJG, Murdoch G: Fractured neck of femur: pattern of incidence and implications. Acta Orthop Scand 1993;54: 348–355
148. Boereboom FT, de-Groot RR, Raymakers JA, Duursma SA: The incidence of hip fractures in The Netherlands. Neth J Med 1991;38:51–58
149. Hansen MA, Overgaard K, Nielson VAH et al: No secular increase in the prevalence of vertebral fractures due to postmenopausal osteoporosis. Osteoporosis Int 1991;2:241–246
150. Speechley M, Tinetti M: Falls and injuries in frail and vigorous community elderly persons. J Amer Geriatr Soc 1991;39:46–52
151. Fitzgerald JF, Moore PS, Dittus RS: The care of elderly patients with hip fracture: changes since implementation of the prospective payment system. N Engl J Med 1988;319:1392–1397
152. Kyle RF: Fractures of the proximal part of the femur. J Bone Jt Surg 1994;76A:924–949
153. Flanagan SR, Ragnarsson KT, Ross MK, Wong DK: Rehabilitation of the geriatric orthopaedic patient. Clin Orthop 1995;316: 80–92
154. Sikorski JM, Davis NJ, Senior J: The rapid transit system for patients with fractures of the proximal femur. BMJ 1985;290: 439–443
155. Versluysen M: Pressure sores in elderly patients: The epidemiology related to hip operations. J Bone Jt Surg 1985;67B: 10–13
156. Bastow MD, Rawlings J, Allison SP: Benefits of supplementary tube feeding after fractured neck of femur: a randomised controlled trial. BMJ 1983;287:1589–192
157. Larsson J, Unosson M, Ek AC et al: Effect of dietary supplements on nutritional status and clinical outcome in 501 geriatric patients—a randomised study. Clin Nutr 1990; 9:179–184
158. Cameron I, Lyle D, Quine S: Accelerated rehabilitation after proximal femoral fracture—a randomized control trial. Disabil Rehab 1993;15:29–34
159. Kennie DC, Reid J, Richardson IR et al: Effectiveness of geriatric rehabilitative care after fractures of the proximal femur in elderly women: a randomized clinical trial. BMJ 1988;297: 1083–1086
160. Reid J, Kennie DC: Geriatric rehabilitative care after fractures of the proximal femur: one year follow up of a randomized clinical trial. BMJ 1989;229:25–26
161. Gilchrist WJ, Raymond JN, Hamblen DL, Williams BO: Prospective randomized study of an orthopaedic geriatric inpatient service. BMJ 1988;297:1116–1118
162. Galvard H, Samuelsson S-M: Orthopaedic or geriatric rehabilitation of hip fracture patients: a prospective, randomized, clinically controlled study in Malmö, Sweden. Aging Clin Exp Res 1995;7:11–16
163. Fordham R, Thompsom R, Holmes J, Hodkinson C: A cost-benefit study of geriatric-orthopaedic management of patients with fractured neck of femur. Discussion Paper 14, 1986; York, Centre for Health Economics, University of York
164. Nankhonya JM, Turnbull CJ, Newton JT: Social and functional impact of minor fractures in elderly people. BMJ 1991;303: 1514–1515
165. Rowland K, Maitra AK, Richardson DA et al: The discharge of elderly patients from an accident and emergency department: functional changes and risk of readmission. Age Ageing 1990; 19:415–418
166. Dove AF, Dave SH, Gerrard E: The accident department and age concern. Health Trends 1986; 16:86–88
167. Madhok R, Bhopal RS: Coping with an upper limb fracture? A study of the elderly. Am J Public Health 1992;106:19–28

168. Latta LL, Sarmiento A, Tarr RR: The rationale of functional bracing of fractures. Clin Orthop 1980; 146:28–36

169. Kristiansen Angermann P, Larsen TK: Functional results following fractures of the proximal humerus: a controlled clinically study comparing two methods of immobilisation. Arch Orthop Trauma Surg 1989; 108:339–341

170. Jarus J, Poremba A: Hand function evaluation: a factor analysis study. Am J Occup Ther 1993;47:439–443

171. Seitz WH: Complications and problems in the management of distal radius fractures. Hand Clin 1994; 10:117–123

172. Livesley PJ, Mugglestone A, Whitton J: Electrotherapy and the management of minimally displaced fracture of the neck of the humerus. Injury 1992;23:323–326

173. Petterson T, Smith GP, Oldham JA et al: The use of patterned neuromuscular stimulation to improve hand function following surgery for ulnar neuropathy. J Hand Surg [Br] 1994;19: 430–433

174. Badley EM, Thompson RP, Wood PHN: The prevalence and severity of major disabling conditions —a reappraisal of the Government Social Survey of the Handicapped and Impaired in Great Britain. Int J Epidemiol 1978;7:145–151

175. Rakier A, Guilburd JN, Soustiel JF et al: Head injuries in the elderly. Brain Injury 1995;9:187–193

176. Schiller WR, Knox R, Chleborad W: A five-year experience with severe injuries in elderly patients. Accid Anal Prev 1995; 27:167–174

177. Johnston RA: Management of old people with neck trauma. BMJ 1989;299:633–634

178. Rasmusson DX, Brandt J, Martin DB, Folstein MF: Head injury as a risk factor in Alzheimer's disease. Brain Injury 1995;9: 213–219

179. Grundy D, Russell J, Swain A: ABC of Spinal Cord Injury. British Medical Journal, London 1986

180. Exton-Smith AN, Overstall PW, Wedgewood J, Wallace G: Use of the airwave system to prevent pressure sores in hospital. Lancet 1982;1:1288–1290

181. Abramson AS: Neurogenic bladder: a guide to evaluation and management. Arch Phys Med Rehabil 1983;64:6–10

182. Oakeshott P, Hunt GM: Intermittent self catheterization for patients with urinary incontinence or difficulty emptying the bladder. BJGen Pract 1992;42:253–255

183. Stewart CPU, Jain AS: Dundee revisited—25 years of total amputee service. Prosthet Orthot Int 1993;1:14–20

184. Waters R, Henry R, Antonelli D, Hyslop H: Energy cost of walking amputees: the influence of the level of amputation. J Bone Joint Surg 1976;58A:42–46

185. Pederson NW, Pederson D: Nutrition as a prognostic indicator in amputation. A populative study of 47 cases. Acta Orthop Scand 1992;63:675–678

186. Enerott M, Persson BM: Risk factors of failed healing in amputation for vascular disease Acta Orthop Scand 1993;64: 369–372

187. Kesler HH: Psychological preparation of the amputee. Indust Med Surg 1951;March:107–108

188. Anderson K, Berg S: The relationship between some psychological factors and the outcome of medical rehabilitation. Scand J Rehab Med 1975;7:166–170

189. Caine D: Psychological consideration affecting rehabilitation after amputation. Med J Aust 1973; 2:818–821

190. MacBride A, Rogers J, Whylie B, Freeman S: Psychological factors in the rehabilitation of the elderly amputee. Psychosomatics 1980;21:258–265

191. Condie ME, Jones D, Treweek SP et al: A one year national survey of patients having lower limb amputation in Scotland. Physiotherapy 1996;82:14–20

192. Redhead RG: The early rehabilitation of the lower limb amputees using an early walking aid. Prosthet Orthot Int 1983;7: 88–90

193. Oxyalcin H, Sesli E: Temporary prosthesis fitting for below knee amputation. Prosthet Orthot Int 1989;13:86–89

194. Muxuno N, Aoyama T, Nakajima H et al: Functional evaluation of gait analysis of various ankle foot assemblies used by the below knee amputee. Prosthet Orthot Int 1992;16:174–182

195. Sapp L, Little CE: Functional outcomes in a lower limb amputee population. Prosthet Orthot Int 1995; 19:92–96

196. Young JB: Everyday aids and appliances: wheelchairs. BMJ 1988;296:625–626

197. Mulley GP: Standards of wheelchairs. BMJ 1989;298: 1198–1199

198. Jenkinson ML, Bliss MR, Brain AT, Scott DL: Peripheral arthritis in the elderly: a hospital study. Ann Rheum Dis 1989;48: 227–231

199. McAlindon T, Cooper C, Kirwan JR, Dieppe PA: Determinants of disability in osteoarthritis of the knee. Ann Rheum Dis 1993; 52:258–262

200. Hochberg MC, Kasper J, Williamson J et al: The contribution of osteoarthritis to disability: preliminary data from the Women's Health and Aging Study. J Rheumatol Suppl 1995; 43:16–18

201. Tennant A, Fear J, Pickering A et al: Prevalence of knee problems in population aged 55 years and over: identifying a need for knee arthroplasty. BMJ 1995;310: 1291–1293

202. Young A, Stokes M, Iles JF: Effects of joint pathology on muscle. Clin Orthop Rel Res 219:21–27

203. Gray RG, Gottlieb NL: Intra-articular corticosteroids. An update assessment. Clin Orthop 1983;177: 1983;177:235–263

204. Chamberlain MA, Care G, Harfield B: Physiotherapy in osteoarthritis of the knees; a controlled trial of hospital versus home exercises. Int Rehabil Med 1982;4:101–106

205. Fisher NM, Gresham G, Pendergast DR: Effects of a quantitative progressive rehabilitation program applied unilaterally to the osteoarthritic knee. Arch Phys Med Rehabil 1993;74: 1319–1326

206. Marks R: Quadriceps strength training for osteoarthritis of the knee: a literature review and analysis. Physiotherapy 1993;79: 13–17

207. Harris R, Copp EP: Immobilization of the knee joint in rheumatoid arthritis. Ann Rheum Dis 1962; 21:353–359

208. Partridge REH, Duthie JJR: Controlled trial of the effect of complete immobilization of joints in rheumatoid arthritis. Ann Rheum Dis 1963;22:91–99

209. Gault SJ, Spyker JM: Beneficial effect of immobilization of joints in rheumatoid arthritides; a splint study using sequential analysis. Arthritis Rheum 1969;12:34–44

210. Mills JA, Pinals RS, Ropes MW et al. Value of bed rest in

patients with rheumatoid arthritis. N Engl J Med 1971;284: 453–458

211. Alexander GJM, Girtas C, Bacon PA: Bed rest, activity and the inflammation of rheumatoid arthritis. Br J Rheumatol 1983;22: 134–140

212. Hawkes J, Care D, Dixon JS et al: Comparison of three physiotherapy regimens for hands with rheumatoid arthritis. BMJ 1985;291:1016

213. Kohke F: The effect of limitation of activity on the human body. JAMA 1966;196:825–830

214. Hicks JE: Exercise and patients with inflammatory arthritis. Rheum Dis Clin North Am 1990;16:845–870

215. Minor MM, Hewitt JE, Webel RR et al: Efficacy of physical conditioning in patients with rheumatoid arthritis and osteoarthritis. Arthritis Rheum 1989;32:1396–1405

216. Ekdahl C, Andersoon SI, Moritz U et al: Dynamic versus static training in patients with rheumatoid arthritis. Scand J Rheumatol 1990;19:17–26

217. Lynberg KK, Ramsing BU, Nawrocki A et al: Safe and effective isokinetic knee extension training in rheumatoid arthritis. Arthritis Rheum 1994;37:623–628

218. Mangione KK, Axen K, Hass F: Mechanical unweighting effects on treadmill exercise and pain in elderly people with osteoarthritis of the knee. Phys Ther 1996;76:387–394

219. McNeal RL: Aquatic therapy for patients with rheumatic disease. Rheum Dis Clin North Am 1990;16:915–929

220. Perlman SG, Connell KJ, Clark A et al: Dance-based aerobic exercise for rheumatoid arthritis. Arthritis Care Res 1990;3: 29–35

221. Vliet-Vlieland TP, Zwinderman AH, Vandenbroucke JP et al: A randomized clinical trial of in-patient multidisciplinary treatment versus routine out-patient care in active rheumatoid arthritis. Br J Rheumatol 1996;35:475–482

222. Mann WC, Hurren D, Tomita M: Assistive devices used by home-based elderly persons with arthritis. Am J Occup Ther 1995;49:810–20

223. Baldwin RC, Byrne EJ: Psychiatric aspects of Parkinson's disease. BMJ 1989;299:3–4

224. Sabate M, Rodriguez M, Mendez E et al: Obstructive and restrictive pulmonary dysfunction increases disability in Parkinson disease. Arch Phys Med Rehabil 1996;77:29–34

225. Simon D, Shapira OM, Mor E, Pfefferman R: Parkinson syndrome: A significantly risk factors for the patient with acute surgical disorder. Int Surg 1992;77:313–316

226. Knuttson E: An analysis of Parkinsonian gait. Brain 1972;95: 475–486

227. Banks M, Caird FI: Physiotherapy benefits patients with Parkinson's disease. Clin Rehabil 1989;3:11–16

228. Comella CL, Stebbins GT, Brown-Toms N, Goetz CG: Physical therapy and Parkinson's disease: a controlled clinical trial. Neurology 1994;44:376–378

229. Scott S, Caird FI: Speech therapy for patients with Parkinson's disease. BMJ 1981;283:1088

230. Scott S, Caird FI: Speech therapy for Parkinson's disease. J Neurol Neurosurg Psychiatry 1983;46: 140–144

231. Anonymous: Parkinson's disease patients and their social needs. BMJ 1982;285:900

232. Beattie A, Caird FI: The occupational therapist and the patient with Parkinson's disease. BMJ 1990;280:1354–1355

233. Gibberd FB, Page NGR, Spencer KM et al: Controlled trial of physiotherapy and occupational therapy for Parkinson's disease. BMJ 1981;282:1196

234. Gibberd FB: Management of Parkinson's Disease. BMJ 1987; 294:1393–1396

235. Mutch WJ, Strudwick A, Roy SK, Downie AW: Parkinson's disease: disability, review, and management. BMJ 1986;293: 675–677

236. Johansson BB: Functional outcome in rats transferred to an enriched environment 15 days after focal brain ischemia. Stroke 1996;27:324–326

237. Feeney DM, Sutton RL: Pharmacotherapy for recovery of function after brain injury. Crit Rev Neurobiol 1987;3:135–197

238. Wade DT, Collen FM, Robb GF, Warlow CP: Physiotherapy intervention late after stroke and mobility. BMJ 1992;304: 609–613

239. Stroke Unit Trialists' Collaboration: A systematic review of specialist multidisciplinary team (stroke unit) care for stroke inpatients. In The Cochrane Database of Systematic Reviews (on disk). British Medical Journal Publications, 1996

240. Sandercock P: Managing stroke—the way forward. BMJ 1993; 307:1297–1298

241. Gladman J, Barer D, Langhorne P: Specialist rehabilitation after stroke. BMJ 1996;312:1623–1624

242. Langhorne P, on behalf of the Stroke Unit Trialists' Collaboration: What is a stroke unit? A survey of the randomised trials. Cerebrovasc Dis 1995;5:228

243. Barer D: Continence after stroke: useful predictor or goal of therapy? Age Ageing 1989;18:183–191

244. Gordon C, Hewer RL, Wade D: Dysphagia in the acute stroke. BMJ 1987;295:411–414

245. Barer D: The natural history and functional consequences of dysphagia after hemispheric stroke. J Neurol Neurosurg Psychiatry 1989;52:236–241

246. Ellul J, Barer D, North West Stroke Dysphagia Study Group: Detection and management of dysphagia in patients with acute stroke. Age Ageing 1993;22(suppl 2):P17

247. Ellul J, Barer D: Detection and management of dysphagia in acute stroke by nonspecialist ward staff. Cerebrovasc Dis 1994; 4:251

248. Mulley GP: Avoidable complications of stroke. J R Coll Phys London 1982;16:94–97

249. Chakravarty K, Durkin CJ, Alhillawi AH et al: The incidence of acute arthritis in stroke patients, and its impact on rehabilitation. Q J Med 1993;86:819–823

250. Partridge CJ, de Weerdt W: Different approaches to physiotherapy in stroke. Rev Clin Gerontol 1995;5:199–209

251. Paolucci S, Antonucci G, Guariglia C et al: Facilitatory effect of neglect rehabilitation on the recovery of left hemiplegic stroke patients—a cross-over study. J Neurol 1996;243:308–314

252. Lincoln NB, Jones AC, McGuirke E et al: Effectiveness of speech therapy for aphasic stroke patients: a randomised controlled trial. Lancet 1984;2:197–200

253. House A, Dennis M, Molyneux A et al: Emotionalism after stroke. BMJ 1989; 298:991–994

254. Gladman J, Forster A, Young J: Hospital-based and home-based rehabilitation after discharge from hospital for stroke patients—analysis of 2 trials. Age Ageing 1995;24:49–53

255. Gladman JRF, Lincoln NB, Barer DH: A randomized controlled trial of domiciliary and hospital-based rehabilitation for stroke patients after discharge from hospital. J Neurol Neurosurg Psychiatry 1993; 56:960–966

256. Forster A, Young J: Specialist nurse support for the patients with stroke in the community—a randomized controlled trial. BMJ 1996;312:1642–1646

257. Forster A, Young J: Stroke rehabilitation: can we do better? BMJ 1992;305:1446–1447

258. Roberts H, Khee TS, Philp I: Setting priorities for measures of performance for geriatric medical services. Age Ageing 1994; 23:154–257

259. Harwood RH, Gompertz P, Ebrahim S: Handicap one year after a stroke: validity of a new scale. J Neurol Neurosurg Psychiatry 1994;57:825–829

260. Hodkinson HM, Jeffreys PM: Making hospital geriatrics work. BMJ 1972;4:536–539

261. Rubenstein LZ, Josephson KR, Wieland GD et al: Effectiveness of a geriatric evaluation unit. A randomized clinical trial. N Engl J Med 1984;311:1664–1670

262. Stuck AE, Siu AL, Wieland GD et al: Comprehensive geriatric assessment: a meta-analysis of controlled trials. Lancet 1994; 342:1032–1036

CHAPTER 111

Long-Term Care—United Kingdom

J. C. BROCKLEHURST

The provision of long-term care in the United Kingdom was virtually a state monopoly for 400 years. Unlike other European countries, in England the church played little part in this after the end of the sixteenth century and the impact of care provided by charities and private agencies was minimal until the 1980s (see Ch. 107). With the advent of the National Health Service (NHS) in 1948 beds providing long-term care for elderly and disabled people became part of the service. These included chronic sick wards in municipal hospitals, workhouse infirmaries, and former infectious diseases hospitals and sanatoria. The specialty of Geriatric Medicine developed to provide an ordered and rational management of the patients in these beds (and of the many hundreds on waiting lists to occupy them).

Through the 1950s and 1960s the management of long-term care became the bedrock of geriatric practice. The aim was to minimize the need for such care by careful clinical and social assessment of those who entered it, by providing rehabilitation and increasing support at home. The number of geriatric beds in England remained virtually the same from 1959 (55,000) until 1985 (55,600).[1] From 1986 to 1994 the number of these beds declined from 55,300 to 37,500. Private and voluntary nursing homes, however, increased from 18,200 beds in England in 1983 to 148,500 in 1994.[1] Similar trends were apparent in the residential home sector with a decline of 49 percent in state-provided residential homes and an increase of 136 percent in private and voluntary homes (Table 111-1). Hospitals for patients with mental illness also provided a good deal of long-term care for elderly people but the psychogeriatric specialty was only recognized in official statistics from 1988. In the 7 years from 1988 to 1994 the number of these NHS beds declined by 33 percent (Table 111-1). This startling growth in the independent sector of both nursing homes and residential homes was due to a regulation that allowed state benefit (called supplementary benefit and later income support) to be used to meet fees in independent nursing and residential homes. The total scale of this expenditure increased from £10,000,000 in England and Wales in 1979 to £190 million in 1983, £439 million in 1986,[2] and £2.5 billion in 1992.

This striking social revolution in provision of long-term care was in keeping with the Conservative Government's privatization policies. However, concern about this uncontrolled expenditure led to consideration of other means of provision. These were published in the report "Caring for People" in 1989.[3] The first objective was to promote the development of domiciliary services to enable people to live in their own homes whenever feasible and sensible. Emphasis on proper assessment of need and good case management was recommended, the promotion of a flourishing independent sector along with good quality public services was acknowledged, and a new funding structure for social care was required. The whole of this was to be achieved by transferring the budget for long-term care to the social service departments of the local municipalities and putting a ceiling on such expenditure. Social service departments then became responsible for the assessment of need, offering various choices including wherever possible domiciliary support as an alternative to residential or nursing home care. These recommendations were enshrined in the National Health Service Community Care Act, 1990.[4] When social services determined that admission to a residential or nursing home was required, a means test was applied and individuals with capital of £5,000 or more (later increased to £8,000 and in 1995 to £16,000) were required to fund themselves until their resources had dwindled to the allowed level. Capital included the value of a house that had to be sold unless it was also occupied by an elderly spouse or other long-term relative. These changes were implemented April 1, 1993. They led to a number of problems.

In the years of expansion of independent homes for long-term care it became easy to discharge patients from hospital into the expanding independent sector and health authorities were thereby able to save money by closing long-stay beds. The scale of closures varied considerably from a total closure of geriatric long-stay beds in some Health Authorities to the retention of a large number in others. One major anomaly was the fact that long-term care within the NHS required no payment from the patient, whereas if, because of local variations in provision, he or she was transferred to a residential or nursing home, payment was required that often involved the gradual liquidation of the patient's assets including the house. Indirectly this disinherited the children of such elderly people, a fact that was particularly unpopular among middle-class voters most of whom were homeowners. Some patients or their caregivers refused to accept long-term care in independent homes on this basis and insisted that it should be supplied free of charge by the Health Authority. Guidance in relation to this thorny problem was issued by the government[5] requiring Health Authorities to provide some continuing NHS inpatient care either in their own geriatric beds or in NHS-contracted

Table 111-1 Changes in the numbers of beds in long-term care by different providers from 1983 to 1994

	1983 (Thousands)	1994 (Thousands)	Change (%)
NHS Geriatrics	56	38	−32
Nursing homes' private and voluntary	18	149	+728
Local Authority (Part 3)	116	69	−49
Residential homes, private and voluntary	89	210	+136
Total	279	466	+67
NHS psychogeriatric	1988: 27	1994: 18	−33

(From House of Commons Health Committee,[1] with permission.)

beds in private nursing homes. This applies to people requiring long-term care in a number of special categories detailed in the guidance.

The guidance also provided for specialist care for people in nursing homes (whether placed by social workers or self-financing) without payment by the patient. These included stoma care, continence advice, diabetic advice, physiotherapy, speech therapy, and chiropody as well as equipment not available on the general practitioner's prescription but excluding incontinence supplies.

Provision was also made for patients or their caregivers to request a review of their entitlement to NHS-provided long-term care if the Health Authority had denied this.

Another problem anticipated to arise from the Care in the Community legislation was that resources available to Social Service Departments would limit the possibilities of placement in nursing homes and the provision of care at home, so that discharge of elderly people from hospital who needed such care would lead to "bed blocking." Early reports indicated that this was not the case. One such study comparing the first 6 months of the Act (from April 1, 1993) to the same 6 months a year later for all patients discharged from the Geriatric Department in Bath showed no significant difference in the length of stay in the hospital and no evidence of discharge being delayed.[6] Another study compared all patients 65 years of age and older in the geriatric service at Charing Cross Hospital who had been inpatients for 28 days or more 1 year before the implementation of the Act with a similar group 1 year after its implementation. It found that delay after being declared medically stable decreased by 29 percent during this time including significant improvements in the waiting time for discharge home and discharge to nursing homes.[7] However, a survey carried out in 1995 (2 years after implementation of the act) by postal questionnaire of one in two consultant geriatricians in the country (310 of whom 35 percent responded) suggested that delays in the discharge of medically fit patients were occurring in 82 percent of cases, lasting an average of 17 days, and that the time from the request for discharge to assessment was over 3 weeks.[8] A survey of hospital bed use one day in March 1995 of all patients aged 75 years and older in the hospital in England and Wales showed that 20 percent were waiting to be discharged and one-third of these were waiting placement in residential or nursing homes.[9] Although delay in discharge may suggest a misuse of hospital beds this is not always the case. A policy statement by the British Geriatrics Society and the Association of Directors of Social Services[10] declared that discharge from the hospital to residential or nursing home care represents a major event in the life of an elderly person and should only follow the most comprehensive functional and medical assessment by a specialist in the medicine of old age and always requires the informed consent of the elderly person or, where appropriate, his or her advocate. It emphasized that the recovery of elderly people from serious illness requires more time than for those who are younger.

Another reported consequence of care in the community was that too many people appeared to be placed in residential homes who would be more appropriately placed in nursing homes, the cost of residential homes being less than that of nursing homes.[11]

The Quality of Long-Term Care

There is no mechanism for the routine inspection of the quality of long-term care within the NHS. The responsibility for maintaining this falls on consultant geriatricians or old age psychiatrists with whom rests the ultimate responsibility for all such patients. A government agency—The Hospital Advisory Service, later renamed The Health Advisory Service—however, was set up in 1969 in response to a series of reports of patients mistreated in psychiatric hospitals.[12] The Hospital (Health) Advisory Service was charged with visiting geriatric and psychiatric departments of hospitals in rotation, the intention being to advise and encourage good practice rather than to admonish. A panel consisting of a consultant geriatrician, manager, nurse, and therapist would spend 1 to 2 weeks in a hospital and a detailed report and recommendations to the Health Authority would follow. For some time these had a limited circulation but later became generally available. There were many criticisms of long-term care.[13] In 1992 The Health Advisory Service was given a wider brief that continued to include visits to geriatric and psychogeriatric hospital departments but now at the request of a Health Authority or a ministerial enquiry where there was thought to be some problem in the service provision.

Nursing and residential homes, on the other hand, are subject by law to inspection—by the Health Authority in the case of nursing homes and Social Service Departments for residential homes. The inspecting agencies are obliged to visit each home twice a year, one of these being unannounced but may also visit as often as they feel necessary. They have the ability to close down any home when this is felt to be in the public interest.[14] The use of precirculated questionnaires is recommended and the visiting panel should include a lay assessor. Generally it includes individuals responsible for inspection of nursing, management, fire risks, health, and safety. A detailed scheme for such use has been produced by the Social Service Inspectorate.[15]

Quality Indicators

Much has been written about indicators of general quality of long-term care. Two of the earliest reviews[16,17] reported findings of two separate working parties. Their proposals have since been developed in two main areas: psychosocial measures and clinical measures. The first of these has been admirably stated in "Homes Are for Living in",[15] which reviews quality in six main domains, namely privacy, dignity, independence, choice, rights, and fulfillment. The second is reviewed in working parties of the Royal College of Physicians of London and the British Geriatrics Society,[18,19] which review mainly clinical domains of care such as promotion of continence, prevention of pressure sores, and prevention of falls and accidents. Guidelines are provided under 12 such domains. A separate audit system—the CARE scheme (continuous assessment, review, and evaluation)[20]—was developed from these guidelines and has since been evaluated as an audit method.[21] This is considered further in Chapter 116, which also reviews other quality assessment systems.

The six psychosocial qualities[15] are those that most people would wish for themselves if they were to live in an institutionalized form of long-term care. They are considered in further detail as follows.

Choice

Defined as "opportunities to select independently from a range of options," choice requires a variety of spaces and facilities within the structure of the home. It includes choice as to form of address, food preferences, who to associate with in the home, the time to go to bed and to get up, and involvement in decisions about oneself and about the facility.

Independence

Defined as "opportunity to act or think without reference to another person, including a willingness to incur a degree of calculated risk," independence includes the provision of personal space over which one has control, control of medication and financial affairs, freedom to move around, and ability to challenge practice.

Dignity

Defined as "recognition of the intrinsic value of people regardless of circumstances; by respecting their uniqueness and their personal needs: treating with respect," dignity involves aspects of toilet provision and dress, knocking on doors, speaking to individuals in wheelchairs before moving them, admission procedures, and dealing with death.

Privacy

Defined as "the right of an individual to be left alone or undisturbed and free from intrusion or public attention into their affairs," privacy includes personal and private space, door locks, a private facility for meeting visitors if desired and for eating in if that is the patient's preference.

Fulfillment

Defined as "the realization of personal aspirations and abilities in all aspects of daily life," fulfillment involves a stimulating environment (buildings and grounds), the availability of activities (recreational, social, and creative), and appropriate aids and adaptations.

Rights

Defined as "the maintenance of all entitlements associated with citizenship—legal, moral, social." These include a clean and well-maintained accommodation, personal safety and security of possessions, confidentiality of information, access to staff including general practitioner and manager, and a clearly understood complaints procedure.

All of these values must be governed by the physical and mental state of the patient, which is ipso facto one of varying degrees of physical and mental handicap. The following elements in the provision of long-term care will assist in achieving these values.

Advocates

In appropriate cases another person may speak for the resident in relation to the staff or the wider world. Legal procedures may be involved—power of attorney, enduring power of attorney, and action by the Court of Protection. Informal advocates, however, may simply be relatives, caregivers or volunteers. The last, voluntary advocates, are especially important for individuals who cannot speak for themselves and have no relation to other caregivers. Such informal advocates should undergo training provided, for example, by the charity Age Concern. Recent reviews of informal advocacy are available.[22,23]

Involvement of relatives

Relatives and informal caregivers often experience a feeling a failure that they can no longer cope and some may even feel guilt that their relative or friend has had to enter a nursing home or other form of long-term care.[24] They may also have real concerns about the care being received and about their own communication with staff members. They may welcome being able to contribute in some way to the care, possibly as a volunteer in the home or hospital,[25] Relatives committees[26] may act as a focus for in-house discussion groups as well as organizing social occasions and fund-raising.

Patients' concerns

The time of admission to long-term care may be viewed with fear: fear of entry into an unknown environment involving close living with strangers, conforming with rules governing daily life, and fear of dependency on staff[27]. Management procedures must therefore be in place concerning introduction to the home and a protocol for the time of admission.

National Health Service Nursing Homes

In the 1980s a number of NHS nursing homes were set up as a reaction to the generally unsuitable long-stay wards of most geriatric units. Two attempts to compare the differences between these two settings by randomizing the allocation of suitable patients to one or the other have been reported. The first was a series of three NHS nursing homes established in different parts of the country, remote from hospitals. Patients requiring long-term care in those three areas were identified by consultant geriatricians in their usual practice.[28–31] The second trial within the City and Hackney Health Authority made similar comparisons between the two NHS nursing homes built on the hospital grounds and geriatric long-stay wards.[32,33] In both studies the nursing homes had the advantage of being "purpose built" or adapted for long-term care and had their own kitchens, although the City and Hackney long-stay wards had an associated recreational club that was the most popular element in the whole comparison. Findings in the two trials were equivocal, with little difference in the matter of choice as to the location and content of meals, going to bed and getting up, or of score on a life satisfaction scale, although in the nursing homes more patients had their own clothes, personal belongings, and privacy. The hospital patients were involved in more activities (partly because of the recreational club). Observational studies on the mood and behavior of the residents, however (as distinct from the processes of care) did show clear advantages in the NHS nursing homes.[34] In reviewing these studies Bond[35] concluded that small, home-like, and community-based units allowing privacy, choice, and more personalized care were preferable to conventional hospital accommodation.

A comparison among five private (for profit) nursing homes and five hospital long-stay wards in Leicestershire selected at random used a dependency score and a specially derived quality-of-care score.[36] The most striking difference between the residents was the greater dependency of patients in hospital continuing care regarding confusion and incontinence; this limited the scope for intersector comparisons on choice, etc. Little difference was shown in most scores, the hospital being higher in general care and activities and the nursing homes in homeliness and buildings.

A major difference between long-term care in the hospital and in nursing homes lies in the medical supervision. In the NHS all long-stay patients are in the nominal charge of a consultant physician in Geriatric Medicine. Two studies of consultant involvement[37,38] show similar results: 66 and 60 percent carrying out ward rounds once weekly or more often, although 15 percent visited the wards only monthly or less frequently. Consultants viewed their main role as providing expert medical advice and supporting nurses' morale.[38] Day-to-day care was carried out by junior hospital doctors or general practitioners. In nursing homes all care is provided by general practitioners, usually on an episodic rather than a routine basis. The feasibility of consultant geriatricians being involved in medical care of nursing home patients would seem to be logistically impossible, although the NHS allows for domiciliary consultation on individual patients in nursing homes at their general practitioner's request. Possible benefits of consultant review of all patients in a nursing home[39] included identifying previously undetected problems in medical management in 20 percent (5 of 25) of patients; more important, it identified a lack of understanding on the part of care staff of the appropriate response to various medical symptoms, due to the lack of guidance policies that might have been produced by general practitioners or Health Authority staff. One effect of audit using the CARE scheme in nursing homes[21] was an increase in written policies and procedures in both nursing homes and long-stay wards. A postal survey among geriatricians carried out by the British Geriatrics Society[40] showed that one-half of respondents were against involvement with patients in nursing homes although one-third were in favor of this.

Daily Life in Long-Term Care

If life for patients in long-term care is to have any meaning, every day should hold something to look forward to. This is not easily achieved. Residents are in the last stage of their lives, probably associated with considerable physical or mental disability and an increasing awareness of approaching death, spent in surroundings that are ordered by necessity rather than choice. It requires an unusually positive philosophy of life as well as a high-quality home for the resident to say "this is the best possible home, I am glad I came here."[41] The most important part of the equation is the attitude and personality of the staff.

Meaningful daily life must fulfill the six qualities of long-term care already discussed (privacy, fulfillment, rights, choice, independence, and dignity) as much as possible. Apart from the physical surroundings and meals this requires some structure to the day, with opportunities for quietness, recreation, religious observance, and, in some cases, intimacy with others. These ideals are more easily provided in a small rather than a large home[42] or by separation of a large home into small independently functioning units. It means some separation of noisy and confused residents from others, in turn requiring a variety of public spaces or separate units.

A recreation program should be developed by a trained activities organizer, ideally with a special activities room or studio.[19,43] The beneficial effects of a recreational program may be thought of as self-evident but there is some research to support it.[44–46]

Pet therapy (e.g., the occasional introduction of dogs to the residents) is becoming popular.[47] The use of massage and aromatherapy—providing sensory stimuli and opportunities for engagement with staff—are well received although a controlled trial showed that the opportunity for one-to-one conversation was the most important part of the treatment session.[48] The desire of some residents for opportunities of intimacy must also be considered.[49] Programs of exercise graded to the abilities of the residents are also important.[50]

One aspect of care that needs careful consideration is dealing with the death of a resident. This bereavement will impinge both on some staff members and on a number of residents, all of whom are likely to derive comfort from some form of recognition of the life of the deceased.

Proper clinical care is essential, including prevention of pressure sores, maintenance of continence, avoiding falls and accidents, identification and treatment of depression, and avoiding over medication. Staff knowledge, skills, and attitudes are all important. Work must be patient centered and not task oriented,[51–53] a situation aided by using key workers, patient biographies, and well thought out training, both inhouse and elsewhere.[54–57]

Respite Care

The idea of intermittent admission to provide respite for caregivers was first described by Delargy[58] in his article "Six Weeks In, Six Weeks Out." Since then there have been numbers of reports of such schemes,[59–62] Rai and colleagues[60] suggested that benefits might be outweighed by associated mortality. However, Howarth and colleagues[61] specifically investigated this claim and showed that among 407 patients studied mortality was no higher while they were in hospital than during an equal period awaiting admission. Homer and Gilleard[62] studied 58 caregivers and their dependents who received inpatient respite care, measuring caregiver stress before admission and changes in the patients' function during admission. The majority of patients showed an improvement in functioning during the period of admission, particularly those who were not demented and those who were being looked after by highly stressed caregivers. Caregivers, on the other hand, showed no observable improvement in their emotional wellbeing but many expressed a wish for more respite than they were currently offered.

Planned intermittent admissions are now widely practiced both in geriatric medicine and in residential and nursing homes. The program in Oxford was reviewed in detail by Robertson and colleagues.[63] They divided intermittent admissions into three types: (1) "The floating bed" for a 3-day, 2-night admission, usually every 2 weeks, (2) "intermittent readmission for longer periods (e.g., 7 days each 3 months), and (3) "holiday admissions" usually for 2 weeks prearranged to coincide with the timing of the caregiver's holiday. They reviewed 50 patients in one or the other of these programs. The major diagnosis and cause of disability was stroke and although their study was uncontrolled and therefore was limited in its usefulness, it was clear that the primary care teams and the patients' caregivers in particular were very satisfied with the arrangements.

Palliative Care

Palliative care is discussed in Chapter 115.

Conclusion

Long-term care for elderly people is becoming more prevalent in keeping with demographic changes. In the United Kingdom the revolutionary change in the last 10 years has been the growth in the independent—particularly the private—sector. This has diminished the role of consultant geriatricians in long-term care, with the major responsibility for planning and provision now falling on managers and nurses. General practitioners provide medical care for individual patients, but play little part in guiding policy.

The need for quality standards is now well recognized, but their implementation requires further development.

References

1. House of Commons Health Committee: Long Term Care: NHS Responsibilities for Meeting Continuing Health Care Needs. Vol. 1. p. VIII. HMSO, London, 1995
2. Care of Elderly People: Market Survey. 8th Ed. Laing and Buisson, London, 1995
3. Secretary of State for Health and Social Services, Wales and Scotland: Caring for People: Community Care in the Next Decade and Beyond. CM89 (White paper) HMSO, London, 1989
4. National Health Service and Community Care Act, 1990: HMSO, London, 1990
5. Department of Health: NHS Responsibilities for Meeting Continuing Health Care Needs. Department of Health, London, 1995
6. Lewis PA, Dunn RB, Vetter NJ: NHS and Community Care Act 1990 and Discharge from Hospital to Private Residential and Nursing Homes. BMJ 1994;309:28–29
7. Ajayi V, Miskeloy FG, Walton IG: The NHS and Community Care Act 1990: is it a success for elderly people? BMJ 1995; 310:439–440
8. Health Policy and Ecomomic Research Unit, British Medical Association: Survey on the Impact of the Implementation of the Community Care Reforms: psychiatrists and geriatricians. British Medical Association, London, 1995

9. Annual Report 1994/1995: National Health Service Executive. HMSO, London, 1995
10. British Geriatrics Society: The Discharge of Elderly Persons From Hospital for Community Care: A Joint Policy Statement by the British Geriatrics Society, the Association of Directors of Social Services and the Royal College of Nursing. British Geriatrics Society Compendium document. Sec 7.1, London, 1995
11. The NHS Health Advisory Service: Making a Mark: The Annual Report of the Director for 1994/1995. HMSO, London, 1995
12. Robb B: Sans Everything—A Case to Answer. Thomas Nelson & Sons Ltd, London, 1967
13. Denham M, Lubel D: Peer review and services for elderly patients. BMJ 1990;300:1635–1636
14. Department of Health: Regulation of Residential Care Homes. LAC 1995 (12): London Department of Health, London, 1995
15. Department of Health Social Services Inspectorate: Homes Are for Living in. HMSO, London, 1989
16. Report of Centre for Policy on Ageing: A Better Home Life. Centre for Policy on Ageing, London, 1996
17. National Institute for Social Work: Residential Care, a Positive Choice. HMSO, London, 1988
18. Report of the Royal College of Physicians and British Geriatrics Society: High Quality Long Term Care for Elderly People: Guidelines and Audit Measures. Royal College of Physicians, London, 1992
19. Report of the Royal College of Physicians: Clinical Guidelines For Enhancing the Health of Older People in Long Term Care. Royal College of Physicians, London, 1997
20. Research Unit of the Royal College of Physicians: The CARE Scheme (Continuous Assessment, Review and Evaluation): Clinical Audit of Long Term Care of Elderly People. 2nd Ed. Royal College of Physicians, London, 1997
21. Brocklehurst J, Dickinson E: Improving the quality of care for older people. Lessons from the CARE scheme. Quality in Health Care (in press) 1997
22. Wertheimer A: Speaking Out—Citizen Advocacy and Older People. Centre for Policy on Ageing, London, 1993
23. Dunning A: Citizen Advocacy With Older People—A Code of Good Practice. Centre for Policy on Ageing, London, 1995
24. White D: Being the Relative of Someone in a Home. The Relatives Association, London, 1994
25. Duncan MT, Morgan DL: Sharing the care: family care givers view of their relationships with nursing home staff. Gerontologist 1994;34:235–244
26. Leeming JT, Luke A: Multidisciplinary meetings with relatives of elderly hospital patients in continuing care wards. Age Ageing 1977;6:1–5
27. Social Service Inspectorate, Department of Health: Implementing Caring for Older People; "the F Factor" Reasons Why Some Older People Choose Residential Care. Department of Health, London, 1994
28. Bond J, Atkinson A, Gregson BA, Newell DJ: Pragmatic and explanatory trials in the evaluation of the experimental National Health Service nursing homes. Age Ageing 1989;18:89–95
29. Bond J, Gregson BA, Atkinson A, Newell DJ: Implementation of a multicentred randomised controlled trial in the evaluation of the experimental National Health Service nursing homes. Age Ageing 1989;18:96–102
30. Bond J, Gregson BA, Atkinson A: Measurement of outcomes within a multicentred randomised controlled trial in the evaluation of the experimental National Health Service nursing homes. Age Ageing 1989;18:292–302
31. Bond J, Bond S, Donaldson C et al: Evaluation of an innovation in the continuing care of very frail elderly people. Ageing Society 1989;9:347–381
32. Bowling A, Formby J, Grant K, Ebrahim S: A randomised controlled trial of nursing home and long stay and geriatric ward care for elderly people. Age Ageing 1991; 20:316–324
33. Bowling A, Formby J: Hospital and nursing home care for the elderly in an inner city health district. Nursing Times 1992;88: 51–54
34. Clarke P, Bowling A: Quality of every day life in long stay institutions for the elderly: an observational study of long term hospital and nursing home care. Social Sci Med, 1990;30:1201–1210
35. Bond J: National Health Service nursing homes again. Age Ageing 1991;20:313–315
36. Wood P, Castleden M: The dependency, quality and staffing of institutions for elderly people. Health Trends 1993;25:97–101
37. Andrews K, Brocklehurst J: British Geriatric Medicine in the 1980s. pp. 46–48. Kings Fund Publishing Office, London, 1987
38. Black JM, Knight PV: Continuing hospital care in Scotland: a survey of consultant geriatricians. Health Bull 1991;49/2: 146–151
39. Pearson J, Challis L, Beaumont CE: Problems of care in a private nursing home. BMJ 1990;301:371–372
40. Newsletter. British Geriatrics Society, London, November 1993
41. White D: Best Possible Home. Relatives Association, London, 1994
42. Kayser-Jones JS: The impact of the environment on the quality of care in nursing homes: a social-psychological perspective. Holistic Nurs Pract 1991;5:29–38
43. Andrews K, Brocklehurst J: British Geriatric Medicine in the 1980s. p. 49. King Edward's Hospital for London, London, 1987
44. McCormack D, Whitehead A: The effect of providing recreational activities on the engagement level of longstay geriatric patients. Age Ageing 1981;10:287–291
45. Davies ADM, Snaith PA: The social behaviour of geriatric patients at mealtimes: an observational and interventional study. Age Ageing 1980;9:93–99
46. Wikström BM, Theorell T, Sandström S: Psychophysiological effects of stimulation with pictures of works of art in old age. Int J Psychosom 1992;39:68–75
47. Frances G, Turner JT, Johnson SB: Domestic animal visitation as a therapy with adult home residents. Int J Nurs Studies 1985; 22:201–206
48. Frazer J, Kerr JR: Psychophysiological effects of back massage on elderly institutionalised patients. J Adv Nurs 1993;18:238–245
49. Bullard-Poe L, Powell C, Mulligan T: The importance of intimacy to men living in nursing homes. Arch Sexual Behav 1994;23: 231–236
50. Fiatarone MA, O'Neill EFF, O'Ryan ND et al: Exercise training and nutritional supplementation for physical frailty in very elderly people. N Engl J Med 1994;330:1769–1775

51. Wells T: Problems in Geriatric Nursing Care. Churchill Livingstone, Edinburgh, 1980
52. Reed J, Bond S: Nurses assessment of elderly patients in hospital. Int J Nurs Studies 1991;13:418–419
53. Waters K: Getting dressed in the morning: styles of staff/patient interaction on rehabilitation hospital wards for elderly people. J Adv Nurs 1994;19:239–248
54. Kihlgren M, Kuremeyr D, Narberg A et al: Nurse-patient interaction after training in integrity-promoting care in a longterm ward: analysis of video recorded morning care sessions. Int J Nurs Studies 1993;30:1–13
55. Gilloran A, Robertson A, McGlew T, McKee K: Improving work satisfaction among nursing staff and quality of care for elderly persons with dementia: some policy implications. Ageing Society 1995;15:375–391
56. Nowlan MR, Grant G, Nowlan J: Busy doing nothing—activity and interaction levels among differing populations of elderly people. J Adv Nurs 1995;22:528–538
57. Nowlan MR, Owens RG, Nowlan J: Continuing professional education: identifying the characteristics of an effective system. J Adv Nurs 1995;21:551–560
58. Delargy J: Six weeks in, six weeks out. A geriatric hospital scheme for rehabilitating the aged and relieving their relatives. Lancet 1957;1:418–419
59. Isaacs B, Thompson J: Holiday admissions to a geriatric unit. Lancet 1960;1:969–971
60. Rai GS, Bielawska C, Murphy PJ, Wright G: Hazards for elderly people admitted for respite ("Holiday admission") and social care ("Social admission"). BMJ 1986;292:240
61. Haworth S, Clarke C, Bayliss R et al: Mortality in elderly patients admitted for respite care. BMJ 1990;300:844–847
62. Homer AC, Gilleard CJ: The effect of inpatient respite care on elderly patients and their carers. Age Ageing 1994;23:274–276
63. Robertson D, Griffiths A, Cosin LZ: A community based continuancy care programme for elderly disabled. J Gerontol 1977;32: 334–339

CHAPTER 112

The American Nursing Home

JOSEPH G. OUSLANDER

The purpose of this chapter is to give non-American readers a brief perspective on the role of the nursing home in the care of the geriatric population in the United States. An American nursing home is an institution that provides health, social, and recreational services to chronically ill people who, for a variety of reasons, cannot be managed in their own home. There are several different types of nursing homes in the United States, and the number of beds in each facility varies considerably. Because of the way that health and social services are funded, and the regulations imposed on nursing homes by the federal and state governments, nursing homes tend to follow a medical rather than a social model. Thus, most American nursing homes look like and are administered in a manner similar to small acute care hospitals, rather than residential homes in which skilled nursing, medical, and other services are available.

At any one time about 5 percent, or 1.8 million, of America's population age 65 years and older is in a nursing home. But this is a deceiving statistic, for several reasons. First, the rate of nursing home use varies considerably with age and sex. Among those 65 to 74 years of age less than 3 percent are in a nursing home; among those 85 years of age and older about 15 percent of men and 25 percent of women are in a nursing home, and close to one-half in this age group die in a nursing home or shortly after discharge from a nursing home to an acute care hospital.[1] Second, a subgroup of nursing home patients stay for only a short period of time. Thus, this lifetime risk of entering a nursing home is underestimated by the prevalence data cited above. It is now estimated that Americans who were 65 years old in the year 1990 have a 43 percent chance of spending some time in a nursing home; the chance is greater for women (about 50 percent) then for men (about 33 percent).[2] Third, for every elderly American in a nursing home, there are two or three with a similar clinical and functional status living at home. The primary factors that determine whether an American enters a nursing home include their medical and functional status, the availability and accessibility of noninstitutional community-based long-term care services, and economic factors.[1,3] Despite the growth of community-based long-term care programs and the increasing number of assisted living facilities, the need for nursing home care is expected to continue to grow. This is in large part due to the decreasing availability of children, especially daughters (who provide the most support to frail older Americans and who are increasingly joining the work force, thus limiting their caregiving abilities) and to economic factors. Economic factors are critical, and are very different in the United States than in countries with a national health program. Thus, in order to understand the American nursing home, one must understand how long-term care is financed in the United States.[1,4,5]

Economic Considerations

Health care for elderly Americans is funded in four basic ways: (1) private health insurance, (2) Medicare, (3) Medicaid, and (4) out-of-pocket expenditures. Although insurance companies are increasingly developing long-term care policies, private insurance plays a very small role in paying for nursing home care in the United States at the present time. Medicare is a federally administered health insurance program for the elderly. The vast majority of elderly Americans qualify for basic Medicare coverage at age 65 by contributions they or a spouse have made during their working years. Although most elderly Americans believe that Medicare will pay for nursing home care, it is not until they or a relative needs nursing home care that reality sets in. Less than 5 percent of Medicare expenditures go to nursing home care, and less than 5 percent of nursing home care is funded by Medicare.[3] Medicare will pay for up to 100 days of nursing home care after an acute illness, but only under specific circumstances. In order to qualify for Medicare reimbursement for nursing home care, nursing home admission must follow a 3-day stay in an acute care hospital, and the patient must require continuous "skilled" nursing care and/or active rehabilitation with carefully documented potential and progress.[6,7] Patients recovering from a hip fracture or stroke with good rehabilitation potential, and patients with unstable medical conditions (such as those requiring intravenous medications) will qualify for some Medicare coverage, usually for a few weeks. Patients with dementia and chronic functional disabilities, on the other hand, are viewed as requiring "custodial" care, and do not qualify for Medicare coverage. Thus, the vast majority of funding for nursing home care comes from Medicaid and out-of-pocket expenditures. Medicaid is a state-administered medical welfare program for the poor; one has to have very limited assets (for example, less than $2,000, excluding a house) to qualify. This has created a phenomenon known as "spend down"; elderly Americans must spend down their assets to pay for nursing home care until they become poor enough to qualify for Medicaid, which will then cover their nursing home care. Because private pay rates for most nursing homes are in the range of $3,000 to $4,000 per month, spend down occurs quickly for most elderly Americans who enter a nursing home.[3]

The growth of managed, capitated systems of care is substantially impacting the nursing home industry in certain areas of the United States with a high penetration of managed care (e.g., California, Oregon, Arizona, Minnesota, Washington, Florida). In a capitated system of care, an insurance company (health maintenance organization) receives a fixed rate per Medicare beneficiary per month. One of the main ways of saving money in this system is to reduce the number of acute hospitals days. As a result, patients in these capitated health plans are being discharged very quickly from acute hospitals into nursing homes while still subacutely ill. In addition, because in capitated systems there is no 3-day acute hospital requirement for Medicare reimbursement of nursing home days, some subacutely ill patients completely bypass the acute hospital. For example, patients with deep vein thrombosis, or mild pneumonia or cellulitis requiring intravenous antibiotics, are commonly directly admitted to nursing homes without an acute hospital stay. These economic incentives are driving the growth of a new level of nursing home care in the United States called "subacute care" (discussed later in this chapter).

Nursing home care in the United States is presently a $60 billion industry, and the costs are expected to rise rapidly over the next several decades.[3,5] There are community-based long-term care services that may delay nursing home admission for some elderly patients, but these services are still evolving, some of them are rare (such as day hospitals), in most areas long-term care services are poorly coordinated and difficult for elderly people and their families to locate, and they are generally not reimbursed by Medicare or private insurance. Thus, it is not surprising that the delivery and costs of long-term care have recently become major societal issues for US citizens as well as the politicians that govern the country.[5,8–10]

Characteristics of Nursing Homes

In the United States there are more nursing home beds than acute care hospital beds. There are between 6,000 and 7,000 acute care hospitals with a total of approximately 1 million beds, and there are over 15,000 nursing homes with over 1.5 million beds. Table 112-1 outlines selected characteristics of nursing homes in the United States. Three-quarters are run for profit, and a large proportion of these are run by organizations that own several or a chain of nursing homes. Most are under 100 beds in size. Thus, the typical American nursing home is a privately owned and operated free-standing facility of between 50 and 200 beds. Some nursing homes are hospital-based, occupying an unused ward in an acute care hospital. Others are located on the campus of a multilevel long-term care community, such as a "life care" or "continuing care retirement" community. The federal and state governments also operate some nursing homes, including over 100 in the Veterans Administration system that serves veterans of US armed forces.

Table 112-1 Selected characteristics of American nursing homes

Total number of nursing homes	15,142
Total number of licensed nursing home beds	1,658,310
For-profit nursing homes	73%
Nonprofit or church-related nursing homes	22%
Government-run nursing homes	4%
Beds licensed as skilled care (as opposed to intermediate custodial care)	45%
Nursing home size (in number of licensed beds)	
50–100	48%
101–150	32%
151–200	13%
201+	7%
Nursing homes Medicare certified	68%
Nursing home revenue from Medicaid	56%

(Data from Ref. 50.)

Nursing Home Staff

The key staff in an American nursing home are the administrator, who is responsible for the day-to-day operation of the facility, and the director of nurses, who supervises the bulk of the facility's employees. Most nursing homes have very few registered and licensed nurses; staff ratios average about one registered nurse for each 50 beds and one licensed vocational nurse for each 25 to 30 beds. Over 90 percent of the hands-on care in American nursing homes is provided by nurse's aides, who are generally poorly educated, frequently do not speak English (especially in some areas of the United States), and are poorly paid (generally under $5.00 per hour). In small and average size facilities, other members of the multidisciplinary team, including the rehabilitation therapists, social workers, activity therapists, and dietitians are part-time and work under contract, rather than as employees of the nursing home. Ancillary services, such as bioclinical laboratory, radiography, dentistry, and podiatry are also provided by outside contracts. Only in very large facilities will one find full-time multidisciplinary staff who provide the types of services mentioned above.

Nursing Home Patients

Patients in American nursing homes are generally characterized as predominantly elderly women with impaired mobility and dementia. It is true that close to three-quarters of nursing home residents are women and older than 75 years of age, over one-half are nonambulatory and need assistance in transfer-

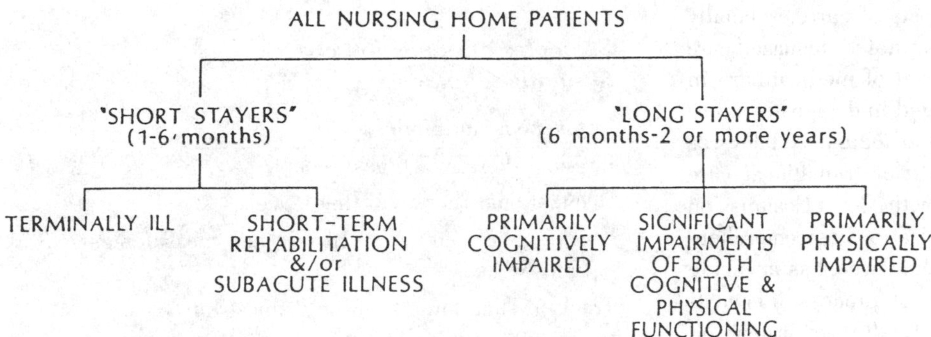

Figure 112-1 Types of patients in American nursing homes. (From Kane et al.,[1] with permission.)

ring, and over one-half have some degree of dementia.[4] But this type of characterization masks the heterogeneity of the nursing home population. Patients in American nursing homes can be broadly characterized based on their length of stay: "short" (i.e., 1 to 6 months) versus "long." Short stayers can be subdivided into two groups: patients who enter the nursing home for short-term rehabilitation after an acute illness (e.g., hip fracture, stroke), and patients who are medically unstable or terminally ill who are either quickly discharged to an acute hospital or die in the nursing home. The proportion of nursing home patients who are short stayers is growing because patients are being rapidly discharged from acute hospitals, and, as mentioned earlier, some acutely ill patients in capitated systems of care are admitted directly to nursing homes in order to avoid costly acute hospital stays. Long stayers can be subdivided into three groups: those with primarily cognitive impairment (e.g., the ambulatory, wandering patient with Alzheimer's disease), those with primarily impairments of physical functioning (e.g., the patient with severe arthritis or end-stage heart or lung disease), and patients with both cognitive and physical impairments. Figure 112-1 illustrates this subgrouping of the nursing home population. Obviously patients may move from one subgroup to another when acute illnesses intervene, chronic illness develops or progresses, or cognitive function declines.

Conceptualizing nursing home patients in this manner has important implications for the goals of nursing home care, for quality assurance, and even for the structure of the nursing home environment. The goals of caring for a previously healthy patient undergoing rehabilitation after a hip fracture are obviously very different than the goals of caring for a patient with advanced dementia and related behavioral disorders, or the goals of caring for a patient with a terminal malignancy. Similarly, from the perspective of quality assurance, processes and outcomes of care relevant for one subgroup of patients may be inappropriate or irrelevant to another subgroup. From a structural standpoint, many American nursing homes attempt to geographically separate different subgroups of patients. This approach offers many potential advantages when it is feasible: The physical environment can be modified for certain types of patients (e.g., wanderers), the staff can be trained and develop expertise in managing specific types of care (e.g., terminal or hospice type care, or rehabilitative care), and patients are often more comfortable when they are around others to whom they can relate. The latter is especially true for cognitively intact patients who are often very distressed by constant interaction, especially at mealtimes, with patients who have dementia and associated behavioral disorders.

Medical Care

The goals of medical care in American nursing homes are listed in the accompanying box. Although these goals appropriately focus on several nonmedical aspects of care, the increasing acuity of medical conditions of patients in nursing homes and the influence these conditions have on function and quality of life, demand that physicians be intimately involved in nursing home care.[4,11]

Goals of care in American nursing homes

- Provide a safe and supportive environment for chronically ill and dependent people
- Restore and maintain the highest possible level of functional independence
- Preserve individual autonomy
- Maximize quality of life, perceived well-being, and life satisfaction
- Provide comfort and dignity for terminally ill patients and their loved ones
- Stabilize and delay progression, whenever possible, of chronic medical conditions
- Prevent acute medical and iatrogenic illnesses, and identify and treat them rapidly when they do occur
- Provide rehabilitation-oriented interdisciplinary care to subacutely ill patients

(Adapted from Ouslander et al.[4])

Financial pressure to reduce the costs of care, especially acute hospital care, and the growth of capitated, managed care has led to the emergence of a new level of medical care in nursing homes: "subacute care." Provided in designated units within free-standing nursing homes and in acute hospital wards that have been designated as subacute or transitional care units, subacute care has been defined by the Joint Commission on Accreditation of Health Care Organizations as comprehensive inpatient care designed for someone who has an acute illness, injury, or exacerbation of a disease process. It is goal-oriented treatment rendered immediately after, or instead of, acute hospitalization to treat one or more specific active complex medical conditions or to administer one or more technically complex treatments, in the context of a person's underlying long-term conditions and overall situation. Generally, the individual's condition is such that the care does not depend heavily on high-technology monitoring or complex diagnostic procedures. Subacute care requires the coordinated services of an interdisciplinary team including physicians, nurses, and other relevant professional disciplines, who are trained and knowledgeable to assess and manage these specific conditions and perform the necessary procedures. Subacute care is given as part of a specifically defined program, regardless of the site. It is generally more intensive than traditional nursing facility care and less than acute care. It requires frequent (daily or weekly) recurrent patient assessment and review of the clinical course and treatment plan for a limited (several days to several months) time period, until the condition is stabilized or a predetermined treatment course is completed.

Examples of admission criteria to subacute units

- Intravenous antibiotics
- Physical therapy 5 times/week
- Occupational therapy 5 times/week
- Weaning oxygen with blood gas measurements 3 times/week
- Tracheal suctioning at least 2 times/shift
- Respiratory therapy treatment 3 times/day or more frequently
- Capillary blood glucose monitoring 2 times/day with insulin coverage
- Injectable medications every 8 hours or 2 times/day
- Wound care (sterile) daily
- Tube feeding
- Laboratory monitoring every 2 to 3 days
- Renal dialysis with monitoring
- Bladder training
- Pain management (parenteral)
- Skilled nursing observation of congestive heart, liver, or renal failure

The accompanying box illustrates examples of conditions typically treated in subacute units. Subacute care poses a number of challenges for the American nursing home. Nursing staff must become trained and experienced in the management of more acutely ill patients. There is a more rapid turnover of patients, which requires more intensive discharge planning. Diagnostic testing (laboratory tests, x-rays, etc.) must be available with a rapid turnover time. More comprehensive and integrated interdisciplinary involvement, especially by rehabilitative staff, is necessary. Structural changes in the nursing home may be required, such as in-room oxygen and larger therapy areas. The nursing home administration must be capable of accurately tracking costs of care, associated revenues, and patient outcomes. Finally, more intense involvement of medical staff than is typical in most American nursing homes is essential.

The vast majority of American nursing homes are too small to have a full-time medical staff or even a full-time medical director, although a small proportion of the larger facilities have both. Most facilities have a loosely organized medical staff supervised by a medical director who works part-time for the nursing home and is paid on an hourly, monthly, or annual basis.[12] Because most American nursing homes are run for profit and have an open medical staff, numerous primary care physicians may be involved in a single nursing home. It is common for dozens of physicians to provide primary care for only a few patients in a small or medium-sized facility. This situation can make it difficult for nursing home nursing staff to develop effective communication and rapport with the medical staff, as well as make it difficult for the medical director to monitor policies, procedures, and standards for medical care.

The role of the primary physician in the American nursing home is to perform a comprehensive medical evaluation at the time of admission, to periodically reassess the patient's progress (visits at 30 to 60-day intervals are required), and to assess acute and subacute changes when they occur.[4,13] Thus, physicians usually visit nursing homes only once or twice a month, depending on the number of patients they have in a given facility. Because physicians are generally not in the nursing home, various regulations and their interpretation result in nursing staff frequently calling physicians to report a variety of problems, such as weight loss, laboratory values, and falls. In addition, acute changes in residents' conditions are generally reported by telephone, often resulting in transfer of the patient to the emergency ward of an acute care hospital for further evaluation.[14–16] The lack of physician presence in the American nursing home therefore results in many unnecessary phone calls and the overuse of acute care hospital emergency wards for patient evaluation. One potential solution to this inefficient way of handling these problems is the involvement of physicians' assistants and/or nurse practitioners.[4,17–20] They are trained in basic patient care assessment techniques, and generally manage acute and subacute conditions using standard protocols under the supervision of a physician. They may be hired by the nursing home and/or by a physician or a group of physicians, and spend a substantial amount of their time in the nursing home.

Quality of Care

Unfortunately, the quality of medical care provided in most American nursing homes is far from optimal.[9,21] Many treatable conditions, such as depression and urinary incontinence, are undiagnosed or misdiagnosed[22–25]; documentation in medical records is poor; many medications, especially psychotropic drugs and antimicrobials, are overused or misused[25,26–29]; and there is little if any input from psychiatrists or psychologists despite the high prevalence of mental morbidity among nursing home patients.[23,24,30]

There are several factors that contribute to this less than optimal quality of care, including educational, attitudinal, and financial. Very few American physicians have had any training in geriatric medicine. Most medical schools have no required geriatric curriculum, and there are less than 2,000 physicians with postgraduate training in geriatric medicine.[31] Even among the latter, the majority do not spend a lot of time in nursing homes. Only a small proportion of practicing physicians visit nursing homes.[32] Many physicians have the same attitude as the American public: the nursing home is the last stop on the way to death, and once in a nursing home there is little that can be done to improve the medical situation. To compound the educational and attitudinal barriers, caring for patients in the nursing home is not a financially rewarding activity. In addition to the financial disincentive, it is a logistical problem for physicians with busy office and hospital practices to go to the nursing home frequently.[31] Thus, there are strong incentives for physicians to not visit nursing homes and to send nursing home patients to acute care hospitals when a patient's condition changes. Admission to an acute care hospital is not only much more expensive than care in the nursing home, the transfer can be physically and emotionally disruptive for nursing home patients and their families, and the acute care hospital is fraught with iatrogenic hazards for this patient population (such as adverse drug reactions, falls, delirium, and pressure sores).[15,33]

New federal rules and regulations, implemented in 1991,[10] should help improve the quality of nursing home care. They contain many provisions pertaining to nursing home patient rights and quality of care, and require an active quality assurance committee in each nursing home. The regulations also mandate a comprehensive, multidisciplinary assessment containing specific data (the Minimum Data Set or MDS). The MDS must be completed on admission, annually, and at the time of every major change in status; selected items on the MDS must be updated quarterly. The MDS is one component of the Resident Assessment Instrument, the other being the Resident Assessment Protocols (RAPs). The RAPs are "triggered" by specific items from the MDS, and basically represent clinical practice guidelines for 18 conditions common in the nursing home patient population.[13]

Ethical Issues

Ethical issues arise on a daily basis in the care of nursing home patients. Ethical considerations play an important role in decisions about the intensity of care provided to very elderly and terminally ill nursing home patients.[34–38] It is beyond the scope of this chapter to discuss these considerations in any detail; however, a few key issues will be briefly mentioned. One of the goals of nursing home care is to preserve individual autonomy (see Box). The high prevalence of dementia among nursing home patients makes this complicated. There are no validated methods of determining when patients with dementia are no longer capable of making health care decisions for themselves, and no well-established standards for surrogate decision makers.[39,40] Advance directives, such as a durable power of attorney for health care, offers a potential solution by enabling a person, while still capable, to designate a surrogate decision maker and state his or her preferences in the event of serious illness.[40] The increased use of advance directives and their incorporation into nursing home medical records will hopefully preserve individual autonomy and at the same time help guide physicians in managing serious illnesses that arise in their nursing home patients.

Future Perspectives

Although many American nursing homes provide excellent care, the overall quality of care in this setting must be improved—especially given the projected enormous need for and costs of nursing home care over the next several decades. At least three approaches will be required: changes in the way that nursing home care is financed, education and training, and research. The potential costs of nursing home care in the United States over the next several decades are staggering. At the present time the federal government is experimenting with a prospective payment system that would base reimbursement for nursing home care on the resources required to care for specific subgroups of nursing home patients, and the prevalence of the different subgroups in a particular facility (so-called RUGS or Resource Utilization Groups).[41] The subgrouping will be based on assessment data that all nursing homes are required to collect as part of the MDS. In theory, RUGS will distribute reimbursement more equitably based on patient's needs. There is one caveat about this reimbursement scheme; it may create an incentive to keep patients sicker and more dependent to achieve higher reimbursement rates. Appropriate adjustments will have to be incorporated for rehabilitative approaches to care. New approaches to quality assurance are also being developed. Increasingly, principles of total quality management and continuous quality improvement are being applied in nursing homes.[41,42] Quality indicators are being developed that are derived from MDS data.[43] These and other quality indicators will be used by regulatory agencies to target more specific quality assurance activities on a state, regional, or national basis.

However, more than financial changes and regulations will be necessary to improve care in American nursing homes. Education in geriatric medicine, gerontology, and long-term care must increase for physicians, nurses, and all other health care professional who care for nursing home patients.[44–46] The United States has made great studies in this regard over the last decade, but much more must be done to meet the tremendous needs for adequately trained health professionals over the next several decades. Very importantly, the nursing home must increasingly become a research laboratory.[47–49] A broad range of research is needed. Basic studies will help determine the causes, treatment, and prevention of conditions that lead to nursing home admission, such as Alzheimer's disease and osteoporosis. Clinical trials will assist in identifying the most effective strategies for managing common conditions among nursing home patients, such as urinary incontinence, depression, and behavioral disorders associated with dementia. Nonbiomedical research is also needed to address issues of quality of life and ethics, which are so important in the nursing home population. Health services research will help identify methods of defining, measuring, and improving quality of care, and in determining the most cost-effective strategies for managing many aspects of nursing home care. Only through this type of multifaceted research will we learn more about caring for the millions of people who will spend some time in an American nursing home over the next several decades.

References

1. Kane RA, Ouslander JG, Abrass IB: Essentials of Clinical Geriatrics. 3rd Ed. McGraw-Hill, New York, 1993
2. Kemper D, Murtaugh C: Lifetime use of nursing home care. N Engl J Med 1991;324:595–600
3. Kane RA, Kane RL: Long-term care: principles, programs and policies. Springer-Verlag New York, 1987
4. Ouslander JG, Osterweil D, Morley J: Medical Care in the Nursing Home. 2nd Ed. McGraw-Hill, New York, 1996
5. Weiner J: Financing long-term care. A proposal by the American College of Physician and the American Geriatrics Society. JAMA 1994;271:1525–1529
6. Loeser WD, Dickstein ES, Schiavone LD: Medicare coverage in nursing homes: a broken promise. N Engl J Med 1981;304: 353–355
7. Smits HL, Feder J, Scanlon W: Medicare's nursing home benefit: variations in interpretation. N Engl J Med 1981;307: 353–356
8. Harrington C, Cassel C, Estes CL et al: A national long-term care program for the United States: a caring vision. JAMA 1991; 266:3023–3029
9. Institute of Medicine: Improving the Quality of Care in Nursing Homes. National Academy Press, Washington, DC, 1986
10. Kane RL: Improving the quality of long-term care. JAMA 1995; 273:1376–1380
11. Department of Health and Human Services, Health Care Financing Administration: Medicare and Medicaid: Conditions of Participation for long-term care facilities; Final rule with requests for comments. Federal Register. February 1989;54: 5317–5373
12. Levenson S (ed): Medical Direction in Long-Term Care. 2nd Ed. Carolina Academic Press, Durham, NC, 1993
13. Levenstein MR, Ouslander JG, Rubenstein LZ, Forsythe SB: Yield of routine annual laboratory tests in a skilled nursing home population. JAMA 1987;258:1909–1915
14. Kayser-Jones JS, Wiener CL, Barbaccia JC: Factors contributing to the hospitalization of nursing home residents. Gerontologist 1989;29:502–510
15. Rubenstein LZ, Ouslander JG, Wieland D: Dynamics and clinical implications of the nursing home: hospital interface. Clin Geriatr Med 1988;4:471–491
16. Weiner JM, Skaggs J: Current Approaches to Integrating Acute and Long-Term Care Financing and Services. American Association of Retired Persons Public Policy Institute, Publication No. 9516, Washington, DC, December 1995
17. Martin SE, Turner CL, Mendelsohn S, Ouslander JG. Assessment and initial management of acute medical problems in a nursing home. In Bosker G (ed): Principles and Practice of Acute Geriatric Medicine. CV Mosby, St. Louis, MO, 1989
18. Kane RA, Kane RL, Arnold S, Garrard J et al: Geriatric nurse practitioners as nursing home employees: implementing the role. Gerontologist 1988;28:469–477
19. Kane RA, Garrard J, Skay L et al: Effects of a geriatric nurse practitioner on process and outcome of nursing home care. Am J Public Health 1989;79:1271–1277
20. Wieland D, Rubenstein LZ, Ouslander JG, Martin SE: Organizing an academic nursing home: impacts on institutionalized elderly. JAMA 1986;255:2622–2627
21. Vladek B: Unloving Care: The Nursing Home Tragedy. Basic Books, New York, 1980
22. Ouslander JG, Kane RL, Abrass IB: Urinary incontinence in elderly nursing home patients. JAMA 1982;248:1194–1198
23. Borson S, Liptzin B, Nininger J et al: Psychiatry in the nursing home. Am J Psychiatry 1987;144:1412–1418
24. Rovner B, German PS, Brant LJ et al: Depression and mortality in the nursing home. JAMA 1991;265:993–996
25. Zimmer JG, Bentley DW, Valenti WM et al: Systemic antibiotic use in nursing homes: a quality assessment. J Am Geriatr Soc 1986;34:703–710
26. Beers M, Avorn J, Soumerai B et al: Psychoactive medication use in intermediate-care facility residents. JAMA 1988;260: 3016–2030
27. Ray WA, Federspeil CF, Schaffner W: A study of antipsychotic drug use in nursing homes: epidemiologic evidence suggesting misuse. Am J Public Health 1980;70:485–491
28. Beers MH, Ouslander JG, Fingold SF et al: Inappropriate medication prescribing in skilled nursing facilities. Ann Intern Med 1992;117:684–689
29. Avorn J, Gurwitz JH: Drug use in the nursing home. Ann Intern Med 1995;123:195–204
30. Zimmer JG, Watson N, Treat A: Behavioral problems among patients in skilled nursing facilities. Am J Public Health 1984; 74:1118–1121
31. Rowe JW, Grossman E, Bond E: The institute of medicine committee on leadership for academic geriatric medicine. Academic

geriatrics for the year 2000. N Engl J Med 1984;316: 1425–1428

32. Mitchell JB, Hewes HT: Why won't physicians make nursing home visits? Gerontologist 1986;26:650–654
33. Tresch DD, Simpson WM, Burton JR: Relationship of long-term and acute-care facilities: the problem of patient transfer and continuity of care. J Am Geriatr Soc 1985;33:819–826
34. Besdine RW: Decisions to withhold treatment from nursing home residents. J Am Geriatr Soc 1983;30:602–606
35. Volicer L, Rheaume Y, Brown J et al: Hospice approach to the treatment of patients with advanced dementia of the Alzheimer's type. JAMA 1986;256:2210–2213
36. Lynn J (ed): No Extraordinary Means—The Choice to Forego Life-Sustaining Food and Water. University Press, Bloomington, IN, 1986
37. Uhlman RF, Clark H, Pearlman RA et al: Medical management decisions in nursing home patients: principles and policy recommendations. Ann Intern Med 1987;106:879–885
38. AGS Ethics Committee: The care of dying patients. A position statement from the American Geriatrics Society. J Am Geriatr Soc 1995;43:577–578
39. Freedman M, Stuss DT, Gordon M: Assessment of competency: the role of neurobehavioral deficits. Ann Intern Med 1991;115: 203–208
40. Emanuel EJ, Emanuel LL: Advance care planning as a process: structuring the discussions in practice. J Am Geriatr Soc 1995; 43:440–446
41. Blumenthal D: Total quality management and physicians' clinical decisions. JAMA 1993;269:2775–2778
42. Schnelle JF, Ouslander JG, Osterweil D, Blumenthal S: Total quality management: administrative and clinical applications in nursing homes. J Am Geriatr Soc 1993;41:1259–1266
43. Zimmerman DR, Karon SL, Arling G et al: Development and testing of nursing home quality indicators. Health Care Financing Review 1995;16:107–127
44. Aiken LH, Mezey MD, Lynaugh JE, Buck CR: Teaching nursing homes: prospects for improving long-term care. J Am Geriatr Soc 1985;33:196–201
45. Riesenberg D: The teaching nursing home: a golden annex to the ivory tower. JAMA 1987;257:3119–3120
46. Libow LS: The teaching nursing home: past, present and future. J Am Geriatr Soc 1984;32:598–603
47. Lipsitz LA, Pluchino FC, Wright SM: Biomedical research in the nursing home: methodological issues and subject recruitment results. J Am Geriatr Soc 1987;35:629–634
48. Rubenstein LZ, Wieland D (eds): Improving Care in the Nursing Home: Comprehensive Reviews of Clinical Research. Sage, London, 1993
49. Ouslander JG, Schnelle JF: Research in nursing homes: practical aspects. J Am Geriatr Soc 1993;41:182–187
50. Marion Merrell Dow Managed Care Digest, Long Term Care Edition, Marion Merrell Dow, Kansas City, MO, 1994

CHAPTER 113

Psychogeriatric Services

TOM ARIE

DAVID JOLLEY

Psychogeriatrics has developed from a number of initiatives in the late 1960s into a new specialty of psychiatry; in 1989 it was formally recognized as such in the United Kingdom. The extent and pace of progress has varied from one country to another, but in many developed countries, and in a few developing countries, there are now psychiatrists and associated workers in the other health professions who specialize in the psychiatry of old age. The U.K. models of services have often guided progress in other countries, but many other countries have much that is new and impressive.[1]

The purpose of psychogeriatric services is to deploy and enhance the skills of the health professions in meeting the needs of mentally ill old people, and in supporting those who care for them. Supporting the caregivers is as important as the more obviously medical function, and recent years have seen a growth of research on how professional inputs can most effectively be matched to the needs and characteristics of caregivers.[2–4]

Origins of Psychogeriatric Services

Until the 1960s the main activity in old age psychiatry was research—epidemiologic, genetic, neuropathologic, and clinical—and even these fields were then cultivated by relatively few workers. In the 1960s, and accelerating during the 1970s, a new preoccupation became evident with planning, delivery, and monitoring of services. This derived from the growing pressure of the aging of populations, and particularly the rapid increase in the numbers of the very aged, which was everywhere pressing upon services.

The development of geriatric medicine, together with progress in epidemiology, evaluation, and organization in health services generally, and particularly in psychiatry, were available for the new "psychogeriatricians", achievements in clinical psychiatry exceeded by far the extent to which the aged were benefiting from them.[5]

Governments also were becoming aware of the need to give priority to these developments, although the direction that they should take, and the degree of differentiation from other services that was appropriate, were still subjects of controversy. These trends in Britain have been described by Arie.[6]

By 1986 some 250 consultants were providing specialized psychiatry services for nearly 70 percent of the elderly population of the United Kingdom[7] and a survey[8] in 1993 identified 405 consultants working with populations ranging from 9,000 to 40,000 older people. At least 24 health districts out of the 199 districts in England and Wales remained unable to name one consultant specializing in this work. Despite these local variations, it is possible to define a "typical" psychogeriatric service, its sphere of responsibility, its facilities, the nature and ratios of the different staff involved, and their patterns of working together. "Style" is an important characteristic of such services: those attributes, over and above types and levels of resources, that determine whether they achieve what is required or not. The organization and style[9] of psychogeriatric services, and educational issues, together with the many relevant policy statements from government, from the Royal Colleges, and from individuals, which have led and reflected these developments, were reviewed in an influential Joint Report from the Royal College of Physicians in London and the Royal College of Psychiatrists in 1989,[10] which will be brought up to date in a further Joint Report to be published in 1997/1998.

A Typical Psychogeriatric Service

A psychogeriatric service normally accepts any psychiatric referrals of persons aged above 65 years ("organic" and "functional" alike) within a defined geographic area. "About" 65 years is important, because here as everywhere flexibility is appropriate. Generally the catchment area is the size of a typical British health district—some 200,000 people—of whom in Britain some 16 percent will be aged over 65 years, making 32,000 people over the age of 65 years of whom some 45 percent will be over 75 years of age. Where amalgamation of health districts has occurred, or where the organization of National Health Service (NHS) Trusts brings administrative responsibility for larger populations together, it is necessary to subdivide activities to this sort of level to facilitate effective working arrangements. How far the service is able to provide for those younger people who have organic mental disorders (presenile dementias, brain trauma, etc.) who may need services similar to those provided for the elderly will depend on the extent of its resources, and on what is available elsewhere locally. In some areas specialist services for patients with presenile dementia have been created and are popular.

Patients who have grown old with enduring or relapsing psychiatric disorders that began earlier in life are often referred to as "graduates." Twenty, and even 10, years ago most graduates lived on back wards of large mental hospitals and were conveniently regarded as the responsibility of the general psychiatry services in whose care they had remained for decades. This was an important consideration, because pioneer psychogeriatricians would have been unable to fulfill their declared responsibility for older people falling ill within the community if they had diverted their energies to the graduates. Matters have changed in the interim: few beds now remain in the large mental hospitals and are most likely to close soon. Original graduates and the next generations who follow them are found in private households, hostels, and other residential establishments, and may have fallen out of touch with the teams that knew them in the acute phases of their illnesses. In addition, their original consultants may have retired or otherwise moved on. Thus whereas it has always been the case that "Old Age" services would take over the care of graduates when they became confused or physically frail, it is increasingly expected that they will accept responsibility for older patients as a 65th birthday gift. Where the Old Age service is reasonably endowed with manpower and other resources, this is a healthy arrangement and may lead to improved patterns of care and mobilization of appropriate responses to the needs of patients. The work is, however, demanding. It is clear that this group of patients has been relatively neglected up to this point and improvement in their care requires more manpower of all sorts and better quality and greater quantity of appropriate facilities.[11]

A few services confine themselves, or are confined by colleagues, to seeing only patients with organic disorders, or patients whose disorders appear to the referrers to be organic. This was one strategy that early services used in their attempts to survive with very limited manpower and reflected a determination to reach those patients to whom no one else would give time. A related strategy restricted responsibilities to those over the age of 75 years. As manpower has improved and the competence of specialist services has been recognized, these restrictive practices have been largely abandoned.

With regard to dementia, the ambulant, severely behaviorally disturbed patient has been a core interest and responsibility of psychogeriatrics, whereas geriatric medicine has provided for physically ill patients who happen to be suffering from dementia, including those patients whose needs for care and nursing include impaired mobility derived from a number of pathologies including dementia. Increased awareness of the potential for better care and support of families, including counseling, when patients are seen early in the course of their illness and followed through its career, has expanded the role and responsibilities of Old Age Psychiatry services in the management of dementia.

Assessment, investigation, and treatment of acute confusional states (delirium) are usually seen as the responsibility of Geriatric Medicine because most such syndromes arise as complications of physical illnesses or medication regimens. Where there are major behavioral problems, the psychiatric team can and should offer other advice and help and some patients will benefit from follow-up by that team.

At least one-third, and sometimes more than one-half, of referrals to a comprehensive service will be suffering from depression or other "functional" psychiatric disorders of late life: They usually account for a majority of patients in the under-75 age group and a minority in the over-75 age group.

Referral rates vary but are likely to run at between 1 and 2 percent of those over 65 years of age per annum (300 to 600 in a population of 30,000 elderly), and a similar number of known patients carried into each year as an established caseload receiving active support and treatment. All services deploy to greater or lesser extent a similar range of facilities and staff, although the extent to which different services rely on particular facilities or types of staff varies greatly. Most services expect to take responsibility for their patients from the first point of referral and to follow them through to death or to a time when they can return to primary care supervision.

The Facilities

Along with the crucial network of extramural staff and facilities, three basic hospital facilities are essential: acute admission or assessment units, longer-stay/respite units, and day patient facilities.

Admission units

Whenever possible admission units should be in a general hospital, because elderly patients even when appropriately referred to psychiatrists often have serious physical disorders, or require access to a wide range of investigative resources. There is a need for 1 to 2 beds per 1,000 old people at risk; 30 to 60 beds will usually be appropriate for a typical health district and these should be distributed in wards of no more than 20 to 24 beds. Whether organic and functional patients are admitted to separate wards, or to subareas of the same ward, must depend on the nature of local facilities, although some segregation is desirable. Plenty of day space is essential, and this also makes it easier to organize time and activities appropriate to groups of differing needs. The pros and cons of mixing patients with contrasting characteristics are often argued with great passion, but there is little objective evaluation of best practice. Well-resourced and well-run units are usually well-liked and successful, whatever their chosen patient mix. This issue is not unique to psychogeriatrics, but arises in other settings in which heterogeneous sick people are looked after.

When this type of ward is in a general hospital, access to other medical, and especially geriatric, facilities should be easy; when admissions are accepted in a psychiatric hospital or a community hospital, with poor investigative resources, then there remains merit in having available an additional facility in a general hospital or in the acute geriatric unit (if that is not in the general hospital) where staff of both services can work together. Such a unit ensures that patients who need joint care and investigation by physicians and psychiatrists can receive it, and it can be a fruitful focus for collaboration between the services, giving the confidence that comes from working side by side. Such joint units may be purpose-planned and built or established by rearrangement of existing facilities.[12,13]

Longer-stay units

The traditional dormitory wards of mental hospitals have been replaced by more appropriate, smaller units serving neighborhoods; these may be public, voluntary, or private. In the 1980s there was a huge expansion in Britain of private residential and nursing care for the aged, stimulated by government policy and funding arrangements. Britain has experienced a period of tension and mistrust between the general population, professionals, and the management of Health Authorities and Social Service Departments wherein the very desirable move from outmoded mental hospital wards to well-sited, well-equipped, local units has been contaminated by a switch of funding from NHS (free at access) funding to means tested funding.[14] This perverse and finance-driven error has now been addressed and Health Authorities have been reminded of their responsibilities to provide long-stay care for the most severely ill and disturbed patients from their population. An exercise of reprovision of NHS-funded facilities and agreement of access criteria is now in progress.[15,16] Norman[17] offers an informed review of different types of long-stay units for people with dementia. Problems of morale of staff and of monitoring of standards loom large; the long-stay sector is the Achilles' heel of services for the elderly. The Health Advisory Service, which is responsible for visiting and reporting on units for the elderly and the mentally ill, as well as for other groups for whom long-term care is needed, has rightly given special emphasis to psychogeriatrics.[18,19] Paramount is the need to provide stimulation and activity, and to maintain the highest level of function of which the resident is capable, together with dignity and choice.[20,21] Such units should also offer respite and holiday admission. It is preferable that they be linked with day hospital units[22] and they should develop a role in supporting nursing homes and other residential units where mentally ill older people are receiving care.[23] Long-stay care is a core activity of psychogeriatric services and the long-stay unit is an active component of a complex interactive system, not a "dead end street."

Day hospitals

Day hospitals are an essential arm of psychogeriatric services.[24] The original target of three places per 1,000 elderly people is rarely attained, but a facility to admit day patients, whether to a separate unit or to the ward areas, is essential. Day care, one of psychiatry's gifts to medicine, is among the few good new ideas in this field. The original hope that day hospitals would be useful chiefly as savers of inpatient beds has been only partly fulfilled, with savings occurring mainly through deferring inpatient care rather than replacing it altogether.[25] In this and other respects there are important differences in the function of a day hospital between psychogeriatric and medical geriatrics.[26]

The main functions of a day hospital in psychogeriatrics are to extend treatment and care to a wider range of patients and to give relief to a wider range of supporters. In psychogeriatrics there are few patients (although there are some) that come only for specific treatments or investigations, in contrast with medical geriatric day hospital; the majority have continuing disabilities, functional or organic. The main groups of attenders are the following:

1. Patients from the inpatient unit, for whom the day hospital acts as a steppingstone to full independence.
2. Patients otherwise coping fairly satisfactorily in the community, for whom attendance perhaps 1 day a week is an "umbilical cord" that, if severed, promptly results in breakdown.
3. Patients who need a short period of observation, investigation, or treatment, ranging occasionally from electroplexy to, more commonly, treatment of some intercurrent derangement that disturbs an otherwise adequate equilibrium.
4. A large group of dependent patients, the great majority of whom suffer from dementias, with behavioral problems with which nonpsychiatric day centers cannot cope, whose families are enabled to continue to care for them at home provided they are able to spend days (sometimes every weekday and, occasionally, when this is feasible, also at the weekend) at a day hospital.

There are also a few patients with dementia who live alone, and who are not too deteriorated, who can be supported through the day hospital. The otherwise unsupported person with dementia living alone at home has a high likelihood of breaking down rapidly to the point of needing institutional care, and the mortality rate is high.[27]

The cause of severance from the day hospital for the majority of dependent attenders is usually deterioration to the point of needing inpatient treatment, or through death. It detracts in no way from the value of the day hospital to emphasize that most organic patients are discharged because they get worse rather than because they improve. Day hospitals function not only as components of the specialist Old Age Psychiatry service but also have a role in collaborating with, and supporting, other forms of day care available to the population at risk. This includes Geriatric Day Hospital care and day care, which may be provided by Social Services, or the voluntary or charitable sectors.[24]

Staffing and Teamwork

Teamwork, an important feature of geriatric services, is central also in psychogeriatrics.[28] This concept has not been clearly defined, but its essence is that people work together across professional boundaries, and that, except where there are legal or knowledge-based constraints, roles overlap and members of the team derive their duties from the assessed needs of the patients, rather than merely from their professional labels or from the prescription of the "leader" of the team.

The team is similar to that in geriatric medicine, although with differences of emphasis. Medical input is from psychiatrists and their trainees, sometimes assisted by family doctors on a sessional basis. The bedrock of staffing is nurses, and senior nurses should generally be doubly qualified in both psychiatric and general nursing if they are to cope properly with the high prevalence of physical disabilities in the mentally ill elderly population.

Community psychiatric nurses, either working outward from the hospital team in the support of patients at home, or based in the community and liaising with the hospital team, are potent agents in facilitating both early referral and continuing care and support of established cases. Of the remedial therapists occupational therapists have the longest history of involvement in psychiatry, but physiotherapists are increasingly necessary and valuable. Access to speech therapy is important too, and a few services now include a speech therapist as an integral part of the core team. In addition, teams grow in potential when they include other therapists: chiropodists, dentists, pharmacists, dieticians, and others.

The practicalities of a district psychogeriatric service mean that it involves a number of teams, including "teams within teams." Thus a large district may have several Community Health Teams for the Elderly, each based within its own locality and interacting with other community teams (Primary Health Care, Social Services, etc.) as well as with each other, and with teams associated with day hospitals, long-stay/respite units, and the assessment/treatment units. Some individuals, including the consultants, are members of a number of teams, whereas others belong to one team only. The skill and success of services depend on achieving healthy functioning of individual teams and their summing and integration into a productive whole. Staff must be enabled to become a team in a real sense; mere "sessions" of multiple individuals whose center of gravity is elsewhere, even if they add up to approximately enough "whole-time equivalents," are unlikely to be capable of forming a real team in which members have confidence in each other.

Social work provision in Britain, which is complicated by its separation from the Health Service, must be negotiated with the local social services; it ranges from excellent in style and quantity to grossly deficient. However, social services departments increasingly are finding it beneficial to invest in supporting psychogeriatric units, which can greatly ease the pressure on overstretched social services.

Clinical psychologists have been slower to move into psychogeriatric work in Britain than in some other countries. The nature and level of their training makes them potentially rich contributors, and their work may embrace psychological treatments such as behavior modification in individuals or groups, for instance by planning token economies, or "reality orientation"; they could conduct groups for staff or for relatives, or more formal psychotherapeutic work.[29] Psychometric testing is a relatively small, although sometimes essential part of their work, but functional assessment is fundamental.[30]

Many services, through lack of resources or recruitment difficulties, depend largely on untrained staff, who for practical purposes are local housewives, sometimes working part-time. In nursing they are nursing auxiliaries, but occupational and physiotherapy helpers, psychologists' assistants, and even untrained speech therapy helpers may play a valuable part. Often the unprofessionalized outlook of such people is an invigorating asset.

Volunteers

Volunteers can fill a multitude of useful roles, although their full potential is unlikely to be achieved unless there exists a Volunteers Organizer to recruit, deploy, support, and encourage them. The quality and availability of volunteers will differ from area to area; in an age likely to see a continuing high level of unemployment, they may become increasingly available.

Staff ratios

Adequate staff ratios are essential. Without them there will either be neglect, or substitutes for staff in the form of restraints and coercion. Staff shortage is the enemy of dignity and choice, and leads to restrictive, regimented care and "playing safe."

There are no firm guidelines on staff levels, although the Royal College of Psychiatrists has issued tentative ones.[31–34] It is unlikely that there will be adequate care on a 20-bed psychogeriatric ward if there are fewer than four or five nurses, at least two of them fully trained, on duty at any time of the day, and there should be two or three at night. Lower levels are seen often, and higher levels occasionally, although rarely in Britain. Similarly day hospitals and Community Mental Health Teams require appropriate staffing levels to perform optimally. Community psychiatric nurses should not each have more than 40 active cases.

At the consultant level the Royal College of Psychiatrists recommends one whole time equivalent for 10,000 people aged 65 years and older, with support from a similar ratio of junior doctors.

Style of Services

The object of psychogeriatric services, as indeed of all services, is that what users of services receive should match their assessed needs, rather than that it should be constrained merely by what is available in that compartment of services into which they happen to have fallen. It follows that assessment must be meticulous and open-minded and collaboration between services must be easy and comfortable. This is easier said that done, but it needs to be said.

The components of "style" have been discussed by Arie and Jolley[9]; suffice it here to say that a service must seek to be available without fuss of defensiveness (and because demand always threatens to outrun resources by far, defensiveness comes all too easily). It must be willing to try new ways of helping; sometimes the users of services themselves come up with the best ideas. It must capitalize on its assets of personality (and should make use of this in selection of staff) rather than merely limiting roles to those defined by professional credentials. It must above all by practical helpfulness and sharing of responsibility, strive to win the confidence of those who use the service, and of potential users. The interests of the various groups of users may point in different directions: families and neighbors may press for relief by admission while the patient clings firmly to a wish to stay at home. Resources are likely to be short, and pressures from the community will compete with those from hospital colleagues for transfer of patients who are "blocking" their acute beds; the staff of one's service may press for protection against a pressure of admissions that exceeds their capacity to cope, or against frank overcrowding. Yet winning the confidence of all three groups—the public, colleagues, and one's own staff—is essential if one is to keep the show successfully on the road.

These principles may sound general, but they are of intense practical importance. Two features of the modus operandi of services need special emphasis: domiciliary assessment, and collaboration between services.

Domiciliary Assessment

In psychogeriatrics all referred patients from the community, however urgent, should first be seen at home. This is not the case in medical geriatrics, where many patients will be acutely ill and have life-threatening illnesses and need to be admitted into the hospital quickly. There is no psychogeriatric crisis so urgent that it will not benefit by the patient's being first assessed (preferably by a senior psychiatrist) in his or her normal setting, but such assessment must be prompt.

The case for universal domiciliary assessment in psychogeriatrics rests on issues such as the following. Psychiatric problems in elderly people comprise derangements of function, and this is best assessed in the normal setting; moves to unfamiliar surroundings may grossly distort it. In the home the characteristics of the setting can be observed: its amenities, warmth, supply of food (and whether it is being eaten), whether the bed is slept in, whether there are accumulations of empty bottles, and so on.

It is often difficult for family doctors, social workers, or even family members to communicate all the information that the specialist needs. The picture, therefore, may look quite different when seen at home from what was described in the referral message. The essential sources of collateral information—relatives, neighbors, visiting friends—may often be brought to the scene only by a crisis that has occurred. They may subsequently "disappear," or be unable to come up to the hospital, yet to have their information available at the time of decision-making following a first contact is invaluable.

The very process of moving an old person may exacerbate the disorder, especially if the patient is already confused. Moreover, hospitalization, the most crucial of all decisions, may pre-empt more appropriate solutions, and above all may undermine the essential aim of maintaining an older person whenever possible in his or her own home. The "hole" in the community left by a person who is removed, even temporarily, has a way of closing rapidly, and it may be very difficult to resettle that person, however good the eventual outcome. Last, the initial visit may establish what the likely resources are, both material and human, that may assist in eventual resettlement.

Collaboration

Collaboration means being ready to support each other, and each other's patients: older people's disorders are commonly mixed. Collaboration with nonmedical professional services, already emphasized, is crucial. At the center of medical collaboration is that with family physicians and that between psychiatrists and geriatric physicians.

Liaison with primary care

The specialized service is interdependent with the teams around the family doctor. The care of elderly mentally ill people is central to good family practice. Identification of those at special risk, case-finding, and surveillance, aimed where possible at prevention and early intervention (where the health visitor has a growing new role) is where psychogeriatrics begins, and that task largely depends on the primary care team.[35]

General practitioners are now required to offer yearly health checks to all patients aged 75 years and older[36] and these checks should include a review of mood and cognitive function. There has not been a flood of extra referrals to Old Age Psychiatry as a result of this exercise and many doubt how useful it can be. General practitioners often know their elderly patients very well, although there are conflicting evaluations of how accurately they estimate mental well-being.[37–39] It is certainly the case that many older people with serious psychiatric disorder are not referred from primary to secondary resources and this may mean that they are denied the most effective treatments.[40] It is a task for the future that specialist services with better resources achieve closer relationships with primary care teams.

Liaison with hospital services

An encouraging feature of the growth of psychogeriatrics in the United Kingdom has been the ease with which professional bodies representing psychiatry and geriatrics have reached agreement on issues that have come to them, and the Standing Joint Committee of the British Geriatrics Society and the Royal College of Psychiatrists has agreed on a series of Guidelines for Collaboration.[41] Their essence is goodwill and good sense and the aim to provide a dependable service in which patients, having made contact with one part of the service, have ready access to all other parts. Emphasized also is the importance of keeping an open mind; patients with a psychiatric history who develop a new illness need to be reassessed de novo rather than merely being automatically labeled "psychiatric," and vice versa with medical illness.

Specialist Old Age Psychiatry services are only beginning to realize the potential of liaison with other specialists. Where there has been only one consultant psychogeriatrician to three or four consultant geriatricians, interaction between even these closely allied colleagues has been superficial. The relationship is changing as Geriatric Medicine consolidates rather than expands its manpower and ratios of 1:1 are becoming possible.

Notwithstanding these advances, the opportunity for effective contribution to other services (Accident and Emergency Department, Orthopedics, Genito urinary Medicine) is there to be explored when manpower allows. A complication of the hospital scene has been the realignment of Geriatric Medicine with General Medicine in many newly created "acute" NHS Trusts. Driven by a desire to make new investigations and modern treatment available to all patients irrespective of age and to bring together the skills of both medical disciplines, this movement has sometimes seemed to be at the expense of commitment to those patients with complex multiple pathology who require long-term rehabilitation and supportive efforts, in conjunction with colleagues (including psychogeriatric services). Many specialist Geriatric Services are spending less time in "community" activities now than they did a decade ago and this is not something with which specialist Old Age Psychiatry feels comfortable. Perhaps a further round of evolution will see Community Mental Health Teams for the Elderly working in tandem with Community Health Teams for the Physically Ill Elderly while encouraging and supporting collaboration with other specialists within the hospitals.

Community Care

The origin of this cosy alliterative phrase is obscure; it would be better if it were restricted to care of people in their own homes,[42] but more commonly it is contrasted with care in hospitals and thus includes many forms of institutional care, such as nursing homes. The ideological issues inherent in such a dichotomy are intricate but, in this context, it suffices to say that a psychogeriatric service should regard itself as belonging to its community, its staff moving freely between the hospital and the nonhospital, the hospital being one of the community's most potent resources for maintaining function and independence. The Community Care Act of 1989[43] gave social services departments a lead role in coordinating and financing community care. Provided resources are adequate, there are obvious advantages in bringing together an often overcompartmentalized system of support, but only time will tell whether social services will be capable of the flexibility that is demanded by the intertwining of health and social needs. Many services are now using the Care Programme Approach much vaunted by government and arising out of the influential studies of David Challis and Bleddyn Davies in Kent.[44] This encourages a systematic application of agreed good practice, allied to a system of recording and review that has a cost in time and mutual tolerance, but should minimize errors and is likely to be useful in arguing the case for additional essential resources.

Education and Training

The main educational function in regard to doctors is the training of psychiatrists, who should rotate through the unit, but cross-training with geriatric physicians and general (internal) physicians, and family doctors, is integral to its role. Arie[45] has described the teaching role of the Nottingham University department for the elderly in which psychiatric and medical services, along with orthopaedic, are combined, facilitating cooperation, teaching, and research. The RCP/RCPsych Report[10] reviewed education and training. In addition all allied professions, including social work, are beginning to see the need to Develop Educational Programms that address, both the theoretical issues and practicalities of care arising from the increasing numbers of elderly people with mental illness that they encounter. There will be advantage in multidisciplinary training and education courses shared by the professions, but these are, as yet, dreams for the future rather than reality.

There is a rising demand for information and education from interested lay people who may be involved with caring for a relative or simply inquisitive for knowledge in this area. It is at least possible that explorations of this nature will strengthen, or even discover, resources and ideas for better management of psychiatric disorders within the older population.

Preventive Approaches

Energies and initiatives during the past 30 years have been devoted to coping with demands arising from established needs. It is now possible to begin to look beyond this reactive mode toward a strategy for limiting the emergence of new psychiatric disorders in late life (perhaps by educational approaches to modify lifestyle and to improve and maintain physical well-being) and to limit the damage arising from illnesses once they occur (by early recognition, effective treatment, and thorough, reactive follow-up).[46] This should prove to be an effective emergent theme in psychogeriatrics over the next few decades.

Conclusion

This chapter is merely an outline, with emphasis on ideas. The reader will find more detail and further numerical data, in the references provided. However, given a basic adequacy of skill and resources, and a rational scheme of organization, it is ideas and style that determine whether or not things work.

References

1. Jolley D, Arie T: Developments in psychogeriatric services. Ch. 11. In Arie T (ed): Recent Advances in Psychogeriatrics 2. Churchill Livingstone, Edinburgh, 1972

2. Gilleard C: Carers: recent research findings. Ch. 12. In Arie T (ed): Recent Advances in Psychogeriatrics 2. Churchill Livingstone, Edinburgh, 1992
3. Levin E, Sinclair I, Gorbach P: Families, Services and Confusion in Old Age. Avebury, Aldershot, 1989
4. Qureshi H, Walker A: The Caring Relationship. Macmillan, London, 1989
5. Jolley D, Arie T: Organisation of psychogeriatric services. Br J Psychiatry 1978;132:1–11
6. Arie T: Martin Roth and the psychogeriatricians. pp. 231–238. In Davison K, Kerr A (eds): Contemporary Themes in Psychiatry. Gaskell, London, 1989
7. Wattis J: Geographical variations in the provision of psychiatric services for old people. Age Ageing 1988;17:171–180
8. Jolley D, Benbow SM: The everyday work of geriatric psychiatrists. Int J Geriatr Psychiatry 1997;12:109–113
9. Arie T, Jolley D: Making services work: organisation and style of psychogeriatric services. In Levy R, Post F (eds): The Psychiatry of Late Life. Blackwell Scientific, London, 1982;222–251
10. RCP/RCPsych: Care of Elderly People With Mental Illness: Specialist Services and Medical Training. Royal College of Physicians of London and Royal College of Psychiatrists, London, 1989
11. Campbell P: Graduates. pp. 779–818. In Jacoby R, Oppenheimer C (eds): Psychiatry in the Elderly. Oxford Medical Publications, Oxford, 1991
12. Arie T, Dunn TB: A do-it-yourself psychiatric-geriatric joint patient clinic. Lancet 1973;2:313–316
13. Pitt B, Silver CP: The combined approach to geriatrics and psychiatry. Age Ageing 1980;9:33–37
14. Jolley D: The future of long-term care as a public health provision. Rev Clin Gerontol 1994;4:1–3
15. Department of Health: NHS Responsibilities for Meeting Continuing Care health care needs. HSG(95)8. HMSO, London, 1995
16. Wattis JP, Fairbairn A: Toward a consensus on continuing care for older adults with psychiatric disorder. Int J Geriatr Psychiatry 1996;11:163–168
17. Norman A: Severe Dementia: The Provision of Long Stay Care. Centre for Policy on Ageing, London, 1987
18. HAS: The Rising Tide. Developing Services for Mental Illness in Old Age. NHS Health Advisory Service, Sutton, Surrey, 1983
19. HAS: Comprehensive Health Services for Elderly People. NHS Health Advisory Services, Sutton, Surrey, 1993
20. Center for Policy on Ageing: A Better Home Life: Good Practice for Residential and Nursing Home Care. Centre for Policy on Ageing, London, 1996
21. Jones K, Fowles AJ: Ideas on Institutions: Analysing the Literature on Long Term Care and Custody. Routledge & Kegan Paul, London, 1984
22. Jolley S, Jolley D: Psychiatric disorders in old age. pp. 268–296. In Bennett D, Freeman H (eds): Community Psychiatry. Churchill Livingstone, Edinburgh, 1991
23. Jolley D: Independent means. Care of the Elderly, October, pp. 376–378, 1994
24. Jolley D: The development of day hospitals and day hospital care. pp. 905–910. In Copeland J, Abou-Saleh M, Blazer D (eds): Principles and Practice of Geriatric Medicine. John Wiley, Chichester, 1994
25. Greene JG, Timbury GC: A geriatric psychiatry day hospital service. Age Ageing 1979;8:49–53
26. Arie T: Day care in geriatric psychiatry. Gerontol Clin 1975;17: 31–39
27. Bergmann K, Foster EM, Justice AW et al: Management of the demented elderly patient in the community. Br J Psychiatry 1978;132:441–447
28. Lindesay J (ed): Working Out: Setting Up and Running Community Psychogeriatric Teams. Research and Development for Psychiatry, London, 1991
29. Hanley I, Hodge J: Psychological Approaches to the Care of the Elderly. Croom Helm, London, 1984
30. Wattis J, Hindmarsh I: Psychological Assessment of the Elderly. Churchill Livingstone, Edinburgh, 1988
31. Royal College of Psychiatrists: Nursing needs for the elderly mentally infirm. Bull R Coll Psychiatr 1978;January:4–5
32. Royal College of Psychiatrists: Guidelines on consultant posts in psychiatry of old age. Bull R Coll Psychiatr 1987;11:240–242
33. Royal College of Psychiatrists: Mental Health of the Nation. Royal College of Psychiatrists, London, 1993
34. Royal College of Psychiatrists: Caring for a Community: The Community Care Policy of the Royal College of Psychiatrists, Royal College of Psychiatrists, London, 1995
35. Williamson J: Screening, surveillance and case-finding. pp. 194–213. In Arie T (ed): Health Care of the Elderly. Croom Helm, London and Johns Hopkins Press, Baltimore
36. Department of Health and the Welsh Office: General Practice in the National Health Service: A New Contract. HMSO, London, 1989
37. Hallewell C, Pettit W: Dementia: assessment and diagnosis in primary health care. Dementia Concern Conference, Regent's College, London, 1993
38. Ilife S, Haines A, Gallivan S et al: Assessment of elderly people in general practice 1: social circumstances and mental state. Br J Gen Pract 1991;41:9–12
39. O'Connor D, Pollitt PA, Hyde JB et al: Do general practitioners miss dementia in their elderly patients? BMJ 1988;297; 1107–1110
40. Cattell H, Jolley D: One hundred cases of suicide in elderly people. Br J Psychiatry 1995;166:451–457
41. Royal College of Psychiatrists: Guidelines for collaboration between geriatric physicians and psychiatrists in the care of the elderly. Bull R Coll Psychiatry 1971; November:168–169. (Reprinted in Arie and Jolley 1982[9] and revised in Psychiatr Bull 1982;16:583–584)
42. Acheson ED: That over-used word 'community'. Health Trends 1985;17:3
43. Department of Health: Caring for People. Community Care in the Next Decade and Beyond. Her Majesty's Stationery Office, London, 1989
44. Challis D, Davies B: Case Management in Community Care. Gower, Aldershot, 1986
45. Arie T: Education in the care of the elderly. Bull NY Acad Med 1985:61:492–500
46. Jolley D: Old age psychiatry. pp. 148–156. In Paykel ES, Jenkins R (eds): Prevention in Psychiatry. Gaskell, London, 1995

CHAPTER 114

The Geriatric Day Hospital

J. C. BROCKLEHURST

The development of day hospitals as adjuvants to inpatient care has been a striking feature of British geriatric practice that has now spread to many parts of the world. The first purpose-built geriatric day hospital was opened at Cowley Road, Oxford, in 1958. It had been preceded by the reception of day patients within hospital geriatric departments. There are now day hospitals in almost all health districts. In 1994 there were over 600 geriatric day hospitals in England.[1] In general, day hospitals follow a medical, paramedical, and nursing model rather than a social one. In Great Britain, social day centers provide a parallel service for elderly people who are not disabled or whose disabilities do not require the assistance of nurses in activities of daily living and who have completed courses of rehabilitation. Day centers are provided by statutory and voluntary agencies and are of considerable variety.[2] Reviews of day hospitals in different countries are available, including Great Britain,[3–7] The United States,[8] Canada,[9] and Israel.[10] Psychogeriatric day hospitals (reviewed by Peace[11]) are discussed in Chapter 113. Day hospitals are also used in terminal care[12] (see Ch. 115).

Day hospitals attempt to dissociate the investigational and therapeutic aspect of hospital treatment from the hotel aspect, which often requires patients to be looked after at night and throughout the weekend when no investigation or treatment is being carried out. The day hospital also allows a close and prolonged supervision of patients suffering from chronic disease who, if isolated completely from hospital care, would almost certainly deteriorate and require readmission.

Variants in day hospital provision include a traveling day hospital[13] in which a group of staff move between different centers on each day in the week for management of psychogeriatric patients. Mobile day centers have also been described[14] but not a mobile day hospital. Nevertheless the development of domiciliary physiotherapy, occupational therapy, speech therapy, and nursing is certainly replacing part of the role of the day hospital.[15]

Effectiveness of Geriatric Day Hospitals

Although geriatric day hospitals are highly regarded both by staff and by patients[16] the evidence for their effectiveness is ambivalent. A number of observational studies[17–19] have indicated improvements during attendance on the Barthel and other scales of activities of daily living and an opportunistic study carried out during a 16-week closure of a geriatric day hospital indicated an increase in deaths and acute admissions of the day hospital attenders resulting from the closure.[20] There have been a few randomized controlled trials comparing day hospital attendance with other forms of treatment and these are discussed below.

The Functions of a Geriatric Day Hospital

Elderly people attend day hospitals for a number of different reasons, and it is important that the staff are aware in each individual case of the main reason for attendance. Principal reasons include functional assessment, rehabilitation, maintenance, social care of disabled people, caregiver's relief, and medical and nursing procedures. Table 114-1 shows the reasons for day hospital attendance among new patients compared with cross-sections of those at various stages of their day hospital attendance. Although rehabilitation and assessment are the most important reasons for initial referral, it is clear that the needs of individual patients change while attending and social care, relatives' relief, and maintenance then become more important. In many cases, assessment is carried out on a single visit.

Social care for mentally confused elderly people is largely a function of psychogeriatric day hospitals.

Assessment

Assessment of function (physical, psychological, social) is an integral and continuing part of geriatric practice. Such assessments may form a periodic component of rehabilitation. However, many patients are referred to day hospitals specifically for functional assessment,[21] usually by an occupational therapist, in relation to their ability to cope in their home environment. Assessment and rehabilitation are closely related.

Rehabilitation

Rehabilitation may be continued from a period of inpatient admission or may be provided from an early stage at the day hospital (for instance, in patients with mild-moderate strokes who may be treated at the day hospital without previous hospital admission).

Table 114-1 Main reasons for acceptance and attendance for geriatric day hospital care[a]

<table>
<tr><th></th><th colspan="3">Acceptance</th><th colspan="2">During Attendance</th></tr>
<tr><th></th><th>U.K. (1982)[b]</th><th>U.K. (1980)[c]</th><th>Israel (1985)[d]</th><th>U.K. (1980)[b]</th><th>Israel (1985)[c]</th></tr>
<tr><td>Assessment</td><td>7</td><td>20</td><td>[e]</td><td>0</td><td>[e]</td></tr>
<tr><td>Rehabilitation</td><td>42</td><td>55</td><td>80</td><td>43</td><td>29</td></tr>
<tr><td>Medical</td><td>17</td><td rowspan="2">8</td><td rowspan="2">6</td><td rowspan="2">19</td><td rowspan="2">12</td></tr>
<tr><td>Nursing</td><td>3</td></tr>
<tr><td>Maintenance</td><td>23</td><td>11</td><td>11</td><td>21</td><td>47</td></tr>
<tr><td>Social/respite care</td><td>7</td><td>5</td><td>1</td><td>17</td><td>8</td></tr>
<tr><td>Other</td><td>1</td><td>3</td><td>3</td><td>0</td><td>4</td></tr>
</table>

[a] *Figures are percent of patients.*
[b] *Data from Royal College of Physicians.*[7]
[c] *Data from Brocklehurst and Tucker.*[5]
[d] *Data from Cohen and Schwertz.*[19]
[e] *Category not recorded.*

Maintenance

Because rehabilitation anticipates improvement there must come a time when patients reach their optimum level of functioning and so rehabilitation is at an end. Some older people will manage to maintain the level of functioning they have achieved by their own efforts aided sometimes by their relatives. Others, however, will deteriorate if all contact with physical therapy is withdrawn, and this may be because they lack confidence at home or because their caregivers are overprotective. Maintenance treatment at the day hospital involves attendance one or more times a week to "top up" with physical therapy and maintain an optimal level of physical functioning.[10,22]

Social Care

Social care usually involves attendances arranged to relieve the caregivers and to maintain the stability of the patient and the caregivers at home. Older people who are not disabled should receive this type of care at a social day center. However, the most demanding patients are those who need assistance with personal care and hygiene and who may have problems with incontinence and balance. For them, the facilities of a day hospital are required.

Medical and Nursing Procedures

Medical and nursing procedures include medical and nursing observations and the management of therapy.[23] Patients should not attend day hospitals primarily for such procedures if they can equally well be carried out at home and if there is no other reason for the patient's attendance. Some medical or social emergencies can be dealt with at the day hospital, obviating the need for inpatient admission.[24]

There is a considerable variation in the reasons for attendance among different day hospitals. Perhaps the most controversial issue is the extent to which the day hospital should be used to provide social support for frail elderly people no longer requiring rehabilitation or even maintenance care. It is argued that the day hospital should have an acute and dynamic function and that the best indicator of its success is its turnover.[25] Most geriatricians accept social care (described also as chronic attendance[22]) as a legitimate function of the day hospital, and Nolan[26] has argued that it ought to be given a great deal more emphasis than is at present the case. From an activity analysis of 18 randomly selected patients attending two day hospitals (a total of 5,383 observations) he found that although approximately 34 percent of the time was spent in therapeutic activity, in fact by far the largest part of this was diversional therapy consisting principally of craft work with the addition of quizzes, films, discussions, etc. By contrast, only 1 percent of the observed time was spent in contact with medical staff. He argued that for older and more disabled individuals, who formed the majority of attenders, the day hospital was a major part of their "coping strategy." It allowed continued existence in the community and had important social and affective dimensions with implications for their "perceived self-esteem." He also indicated that some form of treatment, however minimal, was important because it afforded hope and legitimized their attendance. They valued particularly the opportunity for a bath and also group exercise. The caregivers of such patients were also enthusiastic about the benefits of the day hospital. It gave them a break from the demands of caring and in addition they saw it as a source of advice and a sharing of caring. They, too, appreciated the bathing facility, and their greatest concern was the possibility of discharge.

Number of Places Required

The Department of Health allows two geriatric day hospital places and two psychogeriatric day places for every 1,000 people aged 65 years, and over in the catchment area served by these services.[27] It may be that these figures are overgenerous.[5,25] It is generally agreed that geriatric and psychogeriatric day hospitals should be separate although they may share some services.

Characteristics of Patients Attending Day Hospitals

A number of profiles of patients attending day hospitals have been published.[5,28–31] The main diagnosis of attendees (Table 114-2) reflects the disease basis of geriatric practice except that dementia is underreported, a result of the widespread availability in the United Kingdom of psychogeriatric day hospitals. Many patients continue attending until they are either admitted to the hospital or become ill and die at home. Much larger numbers of stroke patients, on the other hand, are able to be discharged at the completion of a successful course of treatment. The patients are, however, very dependent. In one survey 13 percent were wheelchair patients.[28]

The great majority of geriatric day patients attend 1 or 2 days a week (e.g., 88 percent in Ref. 5 and 93 percent in Ref. 22). A very small proportion attend 4 or 5 days a week, mainly for rehabilitation. The duration of attendance varies considerably among different day hospitals, and many elderly patients have more than one period of attendance. Brocklehurst and Tucker's[5] survey in 1980 showed that 39 percent had attended for up to 3 months, 17 percent between 3 and 6 months, and 43 percent for longer than 6 months. A 1992 survey[7] showed that in 31 percent of day hospitals more than one-quarter of the patients attended longer than 6 months and 10 percent for more than a year.

Martinez and colleagues[22] proposed to classify day hospital patients by the frequency of their attendance: namely, once only, short-term (two to six attendances), medium-term (seven or more attendances), and chronic attenders for whom the intention was that they should continue attending until death or admission to the hospital. This classification would seem to have clear advantages in comparing day hospitals with each other and defining the role of the day hospital.

Table 114-2 Diagnoses of 283 patients attending geriatric day hospitals

	Main Diagnosis (%)	Secondary Diagnoses (%)
Stroke	30	33
Arthritis	18	25
Fractured neck of femur	5	6
Parkinson's disease	5	6
Falls	5	8
Dementia	4	5
Leg ulcer	4	5
Other	26	54

(From Royal College of Physicians,[7] with permission.)

Attenders drop out for various reasons; in one survey 15 percent of attendances were lost because patients felt unwell or did not wish to continue attending.[29] Earlier studies also showed 15 percent who stopped attending because they did not think the day hospital was beneficial or else they found the journey too difficult[28] and 6 percent who refused to continue.[30]

The Evaluation of the Role of a Geriatric Day Hospital

A number of attempts have been made to compare day hospital treatment with inpatient or other alternative forms of care. The results have been equivocal. Eight randomized controlled trials have been reported and these are summarized in Table 114-3. They all have their limitations. Two studies[36–39] include only stroke patients comparing day hospital with domiciliary rehabilitation after discharge from the hospital. In one of these[37–39] day hospital care is provided for the intervention group only if it was judged to be needed following initial assessment. A third study involving only stroke patients[42] randomized them to either a neurologist or a geriatrician on admission and all of the latter were treated at the day hospital following discharge. The study by Cummings and colleagues[34] involved a rehabilitation day hospital treating patients of all ages and the intervention group attended the day hospital following a brief inpatient admission. This was compared with usual inpatient care. The majority of subjects were described as "old and frail." The New Zealand study[33] involved a newly opened day hospital randomizing patients over the age of 55 years referred from the hospital and from general practitioners. The large VA study in America[40,41] included a number of entry criteria, only one of which was required for entry into the trial: residence in a nursing home; dependence in ambulation, dressing, or toileting; bowel incontinence; or significant cognitive impairment. Patients at intake demonstrated major impairment of function and high levels of prior use of health care services although not all of these would necessarily have indicated the appropriateness of day hospital attendance.

The general conclusion to be reached from these trials is that day hospital attendance only occasionally leads to improvement in physical function or mood. More often it prevents hospital admission, and in one case diminished mortality. The cost in most cases was greater for the day hospital group than for the alternative. The main criticism of these trials is that improvement in activities of daily living and in mental function are not the only outcomes to be assessed in day hospital treatment. Also the day hospital attendance did not appear to be tailored to individual needs, generally being on a fixed formula of twice a week for a given period and in one case five times weekly.

Few attempts have been made to evaluate the various functions of day hospital care other than rehabilitation. Zeeli and Isaacs[29] assessed attenders at 3 months on the basis of whether or not they had achieved the objectives set for them at the beginning of attendance. Improvement in mobility was

Table 114-3 Summary of randomized controlled trials in evaluating geriatric day hospital care

Reference	Subjects		Outcome	Intervention Group Compared With Controls
Wan, 1980[31] Weissart, 1980[32] (USA)	Intervention Control	194 190	at 12/12	Mortality ↓ ADLs ↑ (but no change if deaths excluded) Mental function, Morale, Social activity: No difference
Tucker, 1984[33] (New Zealand)	Intervention Control	59 50	at 5/12	Mood ↑ Bed days as in patient ↓ ADLs—no difference
Cummings, 1985[34] (USA)	Intervention Control	48 48	at 3/12	ADLs ↑ Psychological adjustment, Household activity, Medical problems: No difference
Eagle, 1991[35] (Canada)	Intervention Control	55 58	at 12/12	Bed days as in patient ↓ ADLs, Quality of life: No difference
Young, 1992[36] (UK)	Intervention Control	61 63	at 6/12	ADLs—control better
Gladman, 1992[37–39] (UK)	Intervention Control	76 79	at 12/12	"Bad outcome" (death or institutionalization) ↓ ADLs, General health: No difference
Hendrick, 1993[40] Rothman, 1993[41] (USA)	Intervention Control	367 302	at 12/12	Sickness impact profile, General health, Psychological distress, Mental function: No difference
Hui, 1995[42] (Hong Kong)	Intervention Control	60 60	at 6/12	ADLs ↑ Outpatient visits ↓

Abbreviation: ADLs, activities of daily living.

achieved in 68 percent (of 47 patients) and in social, mental, and behavioral state in 33 percent (of 9 patients). In another study[43] 12 percent of 403 attenders were classified as "maintenance" and in all cases this was achieved. The reduced number of "bad outcome" cases in the controlled trial of stroke patients[37–39] referred to above also supports the maintenance role of day hospital care.

One study investigated the effects of a 16-week closure of a geriatric day hospital due to industrial action.[20] Patients who should have attended during that time were matched with a control group the year before and the year following the closure. This indicated significantly more deaths and acute admissions in the day hospital group as a consequence of the closure.

A number of observational (before and after) studies on patients attending day hospitals have been published showing substantial improvements for individual patients in a number of measures.[44–46]

Transportation

Adequate transportation is a *sine qua non* of geriatric day care. Ideally, day hospital patients should come in well-heated vehicles with comfortable individual seats equipped with safety belts, from which they can have a good view of the passing scene. These matters are important because some of the patients are likely to spend an hour or more in the vehicle on each journey, and for most patients this will represent their only excursion from the enclosure of their homes and so the journey itself is likely to be of great interest to them. A vehicle may carry 6 to 10 passengers and must be equipped with a lift that will take both disabled people and patients in wheelchairs. Unfortunately, some vehicles used are "multipurpose," that is, they are equipped with stretchers and the like to cope with emergencies, have frosted windows, and are unsuitable for transporting day patients.[5]

Transportation schedules should be regular so that patients arrive at times when the therapists expect them and so that they leave on time at the end of the day. The driver and other crew members are important people in the day hospital team; their attitude toward the patients will affect the success of the day hospital. They must be tolerant and encouraging and also able to report reasons for nonattendance of individual patients to the day hospital staff. Ambulance crews are divided equally between those who enjoy this work and those who do not.[5]

One problem with a proportion of cases is travel sickness, and 19 percent of attendees have been described as suffering from this at some time (almost one-half of these having a previous history of travel sickness).[47] This was particularly a problem with closed vehicles used also for emergency purposes. Another problem is that many patients spend a long time waiting prepared for their journey (for instance, an average of 60 minutes)[29] partly because of uncertainty of the time when the ambulance will arrive. Curiously, men found the journey less enjoyable than did women.[48]

Medical Supervision

The importance of medical supervision cannot be overemphasized. The day hospital is similar to an inpatient ward and requires the daily attendance of medical staff, together with regular review of all patients by the consultant geriatrician.[22] This is usually best carried out as a case conference in which therapists, nurses, and social workers participate. To maintain a dynamic function the day hospital must discharge patients in the same way as assessment and rehabilitation wards do. This, therefore, requires the closest regular medical surveillance. Discharge is greatly facilitated if adequate social day centers are available in the area to which patients may be transferred. If these are not available then the day hospital should be prepared to continue attendance for social reasons.

Buildings

Many day hospitals are purpose built and others are adapted from existing premises, including hospital wards. All provide a reception area, a dining and general activities area, and a therapy area that may consist of separate occupational therapy and physiotherapy departments or these may be combined. Offices for nursing and medical staff, speech therapists, chiropodists, and social workers are usually provided together with consultation and treatment rooms. The importance of siting the day hospital in association with the geriatric acute or rehabilitation wards has been emphasized.[22,28] Comprehensive reviews of day hospital design have been published in England[49] and Scotland.[50]

Outcome

Efficiency and cost effectiveness of a day hospital will depend, among other things, on the care with which appropriate patients are selected. Zeeli and Isaacs,[29] reviewing 100 patients attending two day hospitals, found that only one-half completed their planned treatment and one-third completed the objectives as set by the referring doctor. A study of 61 patients referred by general practitioners for attendance at a day hospital[51] showed that following home assessment by the consultant, only 54 percent were regarded as appropriate. Alternative management was suggested for most of the others, including referral to a day center, to an outpatient clinic, or a social worker or a domiciliary physiotherapist, and, in a small proportion, hospital admission. It was noted that many general practitioners had a very hazy perception of the purpose of the geriatric day hospital.

As with other forms of medical care, the importance of audit in improving effectiveness of use of day hospitals is becoming recognized. However, standard scales of function such as the Barthel Index and Nottingham ADL Scale are not recommended as useful for day hospital patients.[52]

The Royal College of Physicians of London has published an audit package[53] for geriatric day hospitals based on guidelines derived from the report Geriatric Day Hospitals: Their Role and Guidelines for Good Practice.[7] Two instruments for audit of patient satisfaction with day hospital care have also been published.[54,55]

Cost Effectiveness

A review of National Health Service (NHS) day hospitals for elderly people in England was carried out in 1993 by the National Audit Office.[1] This was based on visits to 22 day hospitals. Recommendations were made as to action required by the NHS Executive as follows:

- Review availability of research on the cost effectiveness of care provided by day hospitals
- Encourage further research if appropriate
- Disseminate relevant information and findings to purchasers and providers

Subsequently, following a report by the Comptroller and Auditor General, the Committee of Public Accounts of the House of Commons examined the services provided by day hospitals, and the management of the service.[56] Among their conclusions were the following:

1. There was a lack of NHS guidelines on the type of day hospital care that could be provided.
2. Health authorities should require the review of all patients' care plans and monitor day hospitals' performance against that requirement.
3. NHS Executive should establish criteria against which effectiveness of the service to patients can be assessed.
4. NHS Executive should encourage day hospitals to develop systems to provide relevant and reliable information about their performance in relation to those criteria.
5. All health authorities should require hospitals to identify where underusage of day hospitals occurs and take steps to secure more efficient use of resources.
6. NHS Executive should encourage day hospitals to develop systems to provide relevant and usable information on their costs.

The National Audit Office[1] estimated the cost of the 16,000 day hospital places each day in England in 1994 as £125 million per annum. The cost is subject to considerable variation depending on the nature and location of the day hospital, the number of staff, and the form of transportation in particular. The subject is reviewed in the report "Geriatric Day Hospitals"[7] and dealt with at length in the Adult Day Care Evaluation Study of the Department of Veteran Affairs in the United States.[57,58].

References

1. National Audit Office: National Health Service Day Hospitals for Elderly People in England. HMSO, London, 1994
2. Carter J: Day Services for Adults: National Institute of Social Services Library No 40. Allen & Unwin, London, 1981
3. Department of Health and Social Security: Adult Training Centres for Mentally Handicapped People and Day Centres for Mentally Ill, Elderly and Younger Physically Handicapped People in England at 31 March 1986. Government Statistical Service, London, 1986
4. Tester S: Caring by Day: A Study of Day Care Services for Older People. Policy Studies in Ageing. No. 8. Centre for Policy on Ageing, London, 1989
5. Brocklehurst JC, Tucker JS: Progress in Geriatric Day Care. King Edward's Hospital Fund for London, London, 1980
6. Vetter NJ, Smith A: Geriatric day hospital. Age Ageing 1989; 18:36–363
7. Royal College of Physicians: Geriatric Day Hospitals: Their Role and Guidelines for Good Practice. Royal College of Physicians, London, 1994
8. Eagle DJ, Guyatt G, Patterson C, Turpie I: Day hospitals cost effectiveness—a summary. Gerontologist 1987;27:735–740
9. Chappell ML, Blandford AA: Adult day care and medical and hospital claims. Gerontologist 1987;27:773–779
10. Cohen MA, Schwartz R: Geriatric Rehabilitation Day Hospitals in Israel: An Evaluation. Brookdale Institute of Gerontology and Adult Human Development, JDC Hill, Jerusalem, 1985
11. Peace SM: Review of day hospital provision in psychogeriatrics. Health Trends 1982;14:92–95
12. Wilkes E, Crowther AGO, Greaves CWKH: A different kind of day hospital—for patients with pre-terminal cancer and chronic disease. In Corr CA, Corr DM (eds): Hospice Care Principles and Practice. Faber & Faber, New York, 1983
13. Evans N, Kendal I, Lovelock R, Powell J: Something to Look Forward to: An Evaluation of a Travelling Day Hospital for Elderly Mentally Ill People. SSRIU Report No. 15. Portsmouth Polytechnic and Hampshire Services Department, Portsmouth, 1986
14. Kaim-Caudle PR: The Sunderland Mobile Day Centre. University of Durham Department of Sociology and Social Administration. Help the Aged, London, 1977
15. Young B, Forster A: Day hospital and home physiotherapy for stroke patients: a comparative cost-effectiveness study. R Coll Physicians 1993;27:252–258
16. Stephenson C, Wilson S, Gladman JR: Patient and carer satisfaction in geriatric day hospitals. Disabil Rehabil 1995;17:252–255
17. MacLennan WJ, Ghosh UK, Richie RT: How does a day hospital work? Health Bull (Edin) 1985;43:105–116
18. Tremblay SD: Day Hospital Evaluation: A Quebec Study. MA Thesis, Montreal Université de Sherbrooke, 1992
19. Cohen MA, Schwartz R: Geriatric Rehabilitation Day Hospitals in Isreal: An Evaluation. Hopedale Institute of Gerontology and Adult Human Development in Israel, Jerusalem, 1985
20. Berry P: Increase of acute admissions and deaths after closing a geriatric day hospital. BMJ 1986;292:176–178
21. Sui AL, Moreshita L, Bloustein B: Comprehensive geriatric assessment in a day hospital. J Am Gerontol Soc 1994;42: 1094–1049
22. Martinez FM, Carpenter AJ, Williamson J: The dynamics of a geriatric day hospital. Age Ageing 1984;13:34–41
23. Bliss MR, Schofield M: A pilot leg ulcer clinic in a geriatric day hospital. Age Ageing 1993;22:279–284
24. Pathy MS: Day hospitals for geriatric patients. Lancet 1969;2: 533–535
25. Martin A, Millard PH: The New Patients Index—a method of measuring the activity of day hospitals. Age Ageing 1975;4: 119–121
26. Nolan MR: The future role of day hospitals for the elderly: the case of nursing initiative. J Adv Nursing 1987;12:683–690
27. Department of Health and Social Services (DHSS): Hospital Geriatric Services 1971. London, DHSS, 1971
28. Brocklehurst JC: The Geriatric Day Hospital. King Edward's Memorial Hospital Fund for London, London, 1970
29. Zeeli D, Isaacs B: The efficiency and effectiveness of geriatric day hospitals. Postgrad Med J 1988;64:683–686
30. Rai GS, Murphy P: Analysis of a geriatric day hospital. Age Ageing 1985;14:139–142
31. Wan TH, Weissart WC, Livierates BB: Geriatric day care and homemaker services: an experimental study. J Gerontol 1980; 35:256–274
32. Weissart WC, Wan TH, Livierates BB, Katz S: The effects and costs of day care services for the chronically ill. Medical Care 1980;18:567–584
33. Tucker MA, Davison JG, Ogle SJ: Day hospital rehabilitation—effectiveness and cost in the elderly: a randomised controlled trial. BMJ 1984;289:1209–1212
34. Cummings V, Kerner JF, Arones S, Steinbock C: Day hospital service in rehabilitation medicine, an evaluation. Arch Phys Med Rehabil 1985;66:86–91
35. Eagle DJ, Guyatt G, Patterson C et al: The effectiveness of a geriatric day hospital. Can Med Assoc J 1991;144:699–704
36. Young JB, Forster A: The Bradford Community Stroke Trial: results of 6 months. BMJ 1992;304:1085–1089
37. Gladman JRF: Day hospital for elderly people. BMJ 1992;305: 55
38. Gladman JRF, Lincoln NB, Barer DH: A randomised controlled trial of a domiciliary rehabilitation service for elderly stroke patients after discharge from hospital. Neurol Neurosurg Psychiatry 1993;56:960–966
39. Gladman JRF, Lincoln NB, for DOMINO Study Group: Follow-up of controlled trial of domiciliary stroke rehabilitation after hospital discharge (Domino Study). Age Ageing 1994;23:9–13
40. Hendrick SC, Rothman ML, Chapko M et al: Overview and patient recruitment in the adult day health care evaluation study. Medical Care 1993;31(Suppl): SS3–14

41. Rothman ML, Hendrick SC, Bulcroft KA et al: Effects of VA adult day health care on health outcomes and satisfaction with care. Medical Care 1993;31(Suppl):SS38–SS49
42. Hui E, Lum CM, Woo J et al: Outcomes of elderly stroke patients. Day hospital versus conventional medical management. Stroke 1995;26:1616–1619
43. Du X, Goodfellow J, Broughton D et al: Routine Outcomes Measurement in Elderly Patients in a Geriatric Day Hospital. University of Newcastle and CASPE Research, 1992
44. MacLennan WJ, Ghosh UK, Ritchie RT: How does a day hospital work? Health Bull 1985;43:109–116
45. Lokk J, Arnetz B: Impact on health care. Consumption of an experimental day care intervention. Scand J Care Sci 1994;8: 95–98
46. Trembay SD: Day Hospital Evaluation: A Quebec Study. MA Thesis, Montreal Université de Sherbrooke, 1992
47. Stokoe D, Zuccollo G: Travel sickness in patients attending a geriatric day hospital. Age Ageing 1985;14:308–311
48. Peach H, Pathy MS: Evaluation of patients' assessment of day hospital care. Br J Prevent Social Med 1977;31:209–210
49. Bacon V, Dubber M: Buildings Used for the Day Care of Elderly People. Buildings Research Team, School of Architecture, Oxford Polytechnic, Oxford, 1987
50. Scottish Hospital Centre: Day Hospitals for Geriatric Patients. Scottish Hospital Centre, Edinburgh, 1983
51. George J, Young JB: General practitioners and the geriatric day hospital. Health Trends 1989;21:24–25
52. Parker SG, Du X, Bardsley MJ et al: Measuring outcomes in care of the elderly. J R Coll Phys 1994;28:428–433
53. Dickinson E, Brocklehurst J: Clinical Audit Scheme for Geriatric Day Hospitals. Royal College of Physicians, London, 1994
54. Montplaisir ML, Tremblay SD: An Evaluation Kit for Day Hospital Development. Montreal Centre Hospitalea Cote-des-Neiges, Montreal, 1986
55. Stephenson C, Wilson S, Gladman JR: Patient and carer satisfaction in geriatric day hospitals. Disabil Rehabil, 1995;17: 252–255
56. Committee of Public Accounts in House of Commons: National Health Service Day Hospitals for Elderly People in England: together with the Proceedings of the Committee Relating to the Report and Minutes of Evidence. HMSO, London, 1995
57. Ehreth J, Chapco M, Hendrick SC, Savarino JE: Cost of VA adult day health care programmes and their effect on utilisation and cost of care. Medical Care 1993;31(suppl):SS50–SS61
58. Ehreth J, Chapco M, Hedrick SC: Comparison of utilisation and cost among contract adult day health care, VA adult day health care and customary care. Medical Care 1993;31(suppl):SS84–93

CHAPTER 115

Palliative Care

JOHN WELSH
MARIE FALLON

> No moral impulse seems more deeply embedded than the need to relieve suffering . . . it has become a foundation-stone for the practice of medicine and it is at the core of the social and welfare programmes of all civilised nations.[1]

Palliative care is defined as "the active total care of patients whose disease is not responsive to curative treatment. Control of pain, of other symptoms and of psychological, social and spiritual problems is paramount. The goal of palliative care is achievement of the best possible quality of life for patients and their families."[2]

Palliative care is not new but its re-emergence to a position of prominence owes much to the efforts of the pioneers of the modern hospice movement. Dame C. Saunders, who founded St. Christophers Hospice, London, in 1967 is the mother figure of this modern focus. The stimulus and motivation for this phenomenon was largely due to a reaction to change in the mainstream medical thrust occurring during the first half of this century. Medicine's traditional emphasis on relief of symptoms was obfuscated by a healthy scientific quest to find the cause of illnesses. This change in emphasis, coinciding with major technological and investigational advances, unconsciously produced a focus on the etiology of disease. The end point became cure and person-centered medicine suffered. By the late 1950s and early 1960s the pioneers of hospice were forced to move out of the National Health Service into the charitable sector to provide for, and to meet, needs that had become subordinated in the quest to understand and conquer all.

The underpinning tenet of the modern hospice movement is the philosophy of the importance of care for the whole person, and features of palliative care philosophy are listed in the accompanying box. Whole person care comprises attention to physical, psychological, social, and spiritual needs, all of which are affected to varying degrees by chronic progressive incurable illness. The needs of the family are also assessed and met by relevant team members. The term *unit of care* was coined by Dame C. Saunders to signify the patient and family who are the focus of care.

The first hospice for dying people is said to have been founded in Lyons, France, by Madamoiselle Garnier in 1842.[3] There has been a rapid growth in the number of hospice services in the United Kingdom and there are now 217 inpatient units providing a total of 3,215 beds,[4] compared with 106 units in 1987.[5]

Palliative medicine became a specialty in the United Kingdom in 1987, recognized by the Royal Colleges of Physicians, and there is now a recognized training pathway for future consultants.

Palliative care is an all-embracing phrase, but in reality is divided into levels of specialism. The following definitions of the different forms or levels of palliative care are adapted from Findlay and Jones.[6]

1. *Basic palliative care:* Care delivery with a palliative approach is a core skill that every health professional in whatever setting dealing with chronic incurable disease should possess.
2. *Specialist palliative care:* Care provided by a multidisciplinary team, led by clinicians with recognized specialist palliative medicine training. The team works collaboratively with those providing a palliative approach and deals with the more complex problems.
3. *Specialist palliative intervention:* This is noncurative treatment aimed specifically at modifying the illness. This treatment is performed by specialists in medicine, clinical and medical oncology, or surgery.

The term *hospice* is tending to be replaced by the term *specialist palliative care service* (SPCS). An SPCS may be based within a specialist palliative care unit (SPCU) sited in a hospital, in the grounds of a hospital, or be free standing, as the traditional hospice.

The traditional hospice provides specialist palliative care and ideally comprises:

1. Inpatient facilities
2. Day hospice/units
3. Home care service
4. Educational service
5. Domiciliary and hospital medical/nursing advisory service
6. Bereavement service
7. 24-hour telephone advisory service.[7]

The above bears remarkable similarities to the geriatric model. The analogy can be taken further as the modern SPCU acts as an assessment and rehabilitation facility with a full multidisciplinary team and liaises closely with the community.

An SPCS responds to referrals from primary health care and from secondary and tertiary centers. The involvement of an SPCS may lead to inpatient care in the SPCU; attendance

Palliative care philosophy

- Affirms life and regards dying as a normal process
- Neither hastens nor postpones death
- Provides relief from pain and other distressing physical symptoms
- Supplies integrative psychosomatic and spiritual care for patients
- Offers a system to help patients live as actively as possible until their death
- Offers a support system for the family to enable them to cope during the patient's illness and subsequently in their bereavement

at the day unit; involvement of the SPCS's home care team; an advisory, liaison, and supportive input to the patient and family; or support and advice to those health professionals already involved.

The three chief categories admitted to inpatient units are patients with the potential for rehabilitation after symptom control, those admitted for respite, which, in effect includes reassessment, and those admitted who are in the terminal stage of their illness and will not live long. The average length of stay in UK hospices is 14 days, and the average discharge rate is 50 percent.[8] Traditionally 94 percent of patients admitted to palliative care programs have cancer,[9] the remainder chiefly comprising motor neuron disease and human immunodeficiency virus or acquired immunodeficiency syndrome.

Most health care professionals feel adept at providing palliative care, but how good are their efforts? There is evidence of poor knowledge of pain control.[10] A survey of 145 physicians, of whom 73 percent were primary care physicians, identified knowledge about 14 fundamental cancer pain principles. It found that there were deficits in 9 out of 14 of these principles. Inappropriate attitudes to managing cancer pain were found in only 2 of 9 cancer pain management concepts.[11] Similarly a Cancer Relief Macmillan Fund survey[12] found that 50 percent of a sample of general practitioners (GP) rated themselves as inadequate or worse in dealing with terminally ill patients. The study demonstrated that the appointment of a GP facilitator in palliative care improved peer knowledge. Complaints about care in the National Health Service are increasing,[13] the majority concerning poor communication between professionals and relatives especially around the time of death.

Education and Training

Education and training is the major area in which substantial improvement in quality of care can be made in a cost-efficient manner. Critical mass experience is often lacking for individual general practitioners. Ongoing interactive problem-based educational programs should therefore be widely available. Postgraduate and basic educational needs must be assessed locally and learning programs established. Curricula exist for medical students, GPs, palliative medicine specialist registrars,[14] and for nurses.[15,16] The General Medical Council[17,18] has recommended that medical graduates should be better equipped to meet the demands of this sensitive area. Major revision of the traditional medical curriculum is under way and one of the innovations in many British medical schools is a more prolonged and intensive period of training in communication skills. Thus it appears that some of the educational deficiencies are being recognized and remedied.

Symptoms

Tolerance to illness in the elderly may be reduced by pre-existing, usually progressive, alterations in normal physiology that occur with aging. Declining physiologic reserves can result in an exaggerated response to illness and associated symptoms. In addition reduced tolerance to treatment and slower recovery may be apparent.[19]

Cancer is predominantly a disease of the elderly with the incidence increasing with age.[20] In Europe 22 percent of all deaths are due to cancer and 150,000 cancer deaths per annum occur in Great Britain.[21] Fifty percent of cancer occurs in only 15 percent of the population (i.e., those over 65 years of age).[20] Likewise, in the United States 50 percent of all cancers occur in those over 65 years of age.[20] Therefore, the geriatrician will see a large number of cancer patients, many of whom will have pain.[22]

There is an increasing tendency to site-specialization in medicine. However, palliative care is an exception as there is a remarkable similarity of symptoms experienced by patients with a wide spectrum of different progressive incurable conditions. Research is lacking on symptoms suffered by those with nonmalignant progressive incurable conditions but studies in this area show considerable distress in noncancer patients. Cartwright and Seale[23] found similarities in symptoms between cancer and noncancer patients. In 639 adults over 75 years of age the incidence of pain was 75 percent in those with cancer, compared with an incidence in noncancer patients of 68 percent. Pain intensity in patients with cancer was more severe but the duration of pain in noncancer cases was longer. In particular chronic pain, in this case defined as pain present for more than 1 year, was particularly common after stroke. Nausea, vomiting, anorexia, and constipation were significantly more common in cancer patients.

In a study of 1,000 patients with different cancer types, the most common symptoms reported were pain, easy fatigue, weakness, anorexia and weight loss, xerostomia, constipation, and dyspnea.[24]

Palliative care focuses on relief of symptoms caused by an illness, not primarily on an attempt to modify the underlying incurable disease. As with any medical problem the approach to symptom control is one of taking a careful history; listening attentively; careful examination; appropriate investigations (avoiding the unnecessary); and analysis and diagnosis of the pathogenesis of the symptom.

Appropriate treatment should be instigated with as much information given as the patient desires. The information should be presented at the patient's pace, free of jargon and given in an understandable and empathic manner. With the patient's consent, the family should be included in this information exchange. Control of cancer-related symptoms is generally achieved by drugs, the average number of medications being six per day.[25] Control of symptoms in patients with preexisting disease will inevitably lead to polypharmacy. Care must be taken to review drug regimens regularly and to be aware of potential interactions. Prescribing principles for the elderly are described in Chapter 11 and will not be considered here. Many of the symptoms and principles of management described below are shared in both malignant and nonmalignant conditions. Symptoms will be illustrated mainly by the use of cancer cases. Various important symptoms are now considered.

Misconceptions about opioids among physicians

- Poor pain assessment
- Reluctance to follow pain guidelines
- Reluctance to prescribe analgesia regularly
- Reluctance to prescribe maximally tolerated analgesia with respect to the severity of pain
- Belief that opioid side effects are unpreventable
- Belief that oral opioids are ineffective
- Belief that use of opioids for analgesia will induce psychological dependence
- Belief that tolerance to opioid analgesia will develop
- Belief that tolerance to certain side effects will not develop
- Belief that complete pain relief in patients with cancer is unattainable

Pain Control

Chronic pain affects the person functionally, physically, and psychosocially.[26] The influence of pain on these components of the whole person must be accurately assessed. The study of pain and pain control in the elderly is a neglected area. Less than 1 percent of approximately 4,000 articles on pain published per annum concern pain in the elderly.[27] Ferrell[28] reviewed eight textbooks of geriatric nursing, finding that of 5,000 pages only 18 pages were devoted to pain and its management.

This is further put in perspective when it is considered that the incidence of pain in the elderly is probably higher than in younger age groups. However there is conflicting evidence. Evidence exists to support the view that there is no difference in incidence of pain in patients below 65 years of age and those above 65 years of age[29,30] Epidemiologic studies in the United Kingdom on this topic are lacking but Bowling and Browne[31] reported a survey of 662 persons over the age of 85 years showing that 70 percent complained of pain. In an American study[32] the prevalence of pain in patients 60 years old and older was found to be 25 percent, being double that of younger patients who had a prevalence of 12 percent. Other studies have estimated the prevalence of pain in elderly patients to vary between 45 and 80 percent.[33–36]

Despite the high incidence of pain in all ages it appears from several hospital studies that, in general, control of this symptom is suboptimal.[37–42] The findings do not appear to have altered over time. Closs et al.[43] showed a similar lack of pain control in the elderly. There is evidence of a number of deficiencies in the knowledge of physicians in relation to cancer pain treatment.[44–46] These deficits relate to both knowledge and attitudes.

Control of pain is underpinned by accurate assessment. Assessment of pain in the elderly may be difficult for several reasons.[47] First, the elderly may report pain differently from younger age groups. This may be because they perceive aging and pain as inevitable. Second, cultural differences and differences in the perception of suffering add to the problem. Third, cognitive impairment, dysphasia, or dementia may make pain assessment difficult.[48,49] Fourth, there may be a reluctance by staff to administer analgesia out of an exaggerated fear of side effects, especially respiratory depression. Finally, there may be a perception that the elderly do not experience the same intensity of pain.[50] It is well known that elderly patients may have painless abdominal catastrophes[51,52] or "silent" myocardial infarction.[53] However, the mechanism of this phenomenon is not known and may not be related to aging as such.

Age-related reduction in pain intensity has not been shown experimentally.[54–57] Clinical experience supports this and a study by Wendy et al.[58] found that 75 percent of 239 cancer patients over 65 years of age had pain on admission to hospice care. This figure correlates well with the incidence of pain in the general hospice population.[30] There was no statistically significant difference between the intensity of pain in the study sample and a younger comparison group with advanced cancer.[58] However, discrepancies exist between patients', caregivers' and professionals' perception of pain intensity. Grossman et al.[59] found that correlation between the physicians' and caregivers' rating of pain and that of the patient were close when the patient reported mild pain, with a concordance of 78 percent. When pain intensity increased to a moderate or severe level, the concordance level fell to 27 percent.

It has recently been shown in a large prospective study[60] of over 2,000 patients with cancer that 88 percent of pain problems can be adequately controlled by adherence to the World Health Organization, (WHO) guidelines[61] for pain control. Other studies have confirmed these results using the WHO guidelines.[62–64] Despite this, the public has a perception that if they develop cancer a painful death is inevitable. In addition to chronic pain, which is defined as a baseline pain present for more than 3 months, breakthrough and incident pain exist.[65]

Breakthrough pain occurs without warning and is perceived above the baseline pain. Incident pain is predictable pain associated with a particular function, for instance, standing, walking, or inspiration. For diagnostic and therapeutic purposes pain types can be divided into the following:

1. Somatic pain
2. Uisceral pain
3. Neuropathic pain
4. Sympathetically mediated pain
5. Mixed etiology
6. Emotional pain or anguish

Pains are commonly of mixed etiology, further complicating their management.

The approach to successful pain management involves obtaining a careful history from which the type and severity of pain and its influence on function and psyche can be ascertained. This must be followed by a thorough examination to establish a diagnosis or differential diagnoses. Relevant investigations should be carried out, providing the patient is fit enough and a positive or negative result is likely to influence treatment. Pain relief should not be withheld until all investigations have been completed.

Depending on the severity of the pain, appropriate analgesia should be prescribed. The WHO analgesic ladder[61] (Fig. 115-1) is the "gold standard." Step one of the ladder is for mild pain and involves the use of basic analgesics such as paracetamol. Step two, for moderate pain, requires the use of weak opioids (e.g., codeine). Step three, for severe pain, employs strong opioids, commonly morphine. At all stages adjuvant analgesics, such as nonsteroidal anti-inflammatory drugs, should be prescribed as appropriate. An adjuvant analgesic is defined as a drug that has a primary indication other than pain, but is analgesic in some painful conditions.[66,67] Table 115-1 lists examples of adjuvant analgesics and their indications. The patient should be introduced to the ladder at whichever level is appropriate to the degree of pain experienced. Before moving up a step the maximum tolerated dose of analgesia together with an adjuvant analgesic should have been tried. There is no gain in moving laterally on the ladder (unless one equipotent analgesic is better tolerated).

Aide-memoire when assessing pain

P = provoking or palliating factors
Q = quality of pain (e.g., dull, burning, stabbing)
R = radiation or referral of pain
S = severity of pain
T = timing of pain (e.g., constant, intermittent)

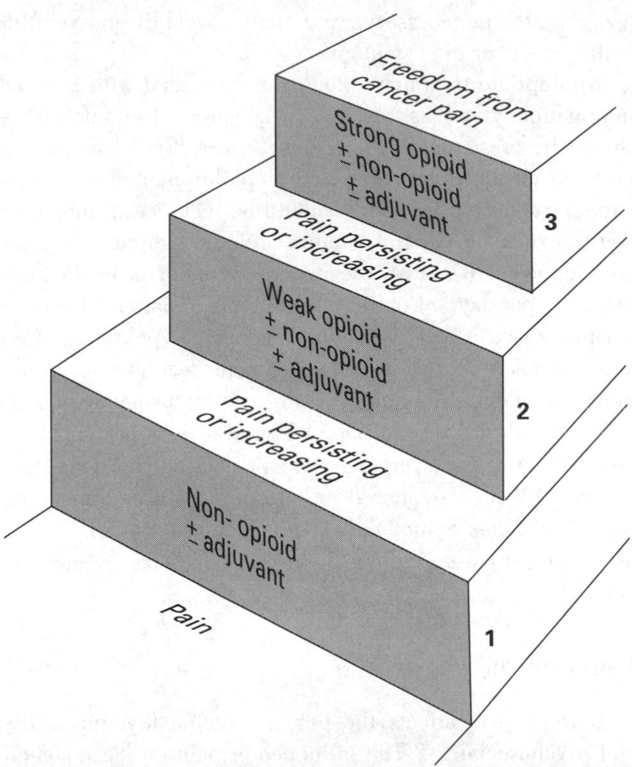

Figure 115-1 The three-step analgesic ladder. (From World Health Organization,[2] with permission.)

The basic guidelines for the use of analgesia in chronic pain are the following:

1. Assess the patient's pain carefully. Remember pain is what the patient says hurts.[68]
2. Use the oral route if possible.
3. Prescribe therapeutic doses of analgesia regularly, the frequency being dependent on the known pharmacokinetics of that drug.
4. Titrate the dose of drug to the individual's analgesic requirements.
5. Provide effective analgesia for breakthrough or incident pain.
6. Reassess pain control regularly.
7. Assess and treat the psychosocial dimension of chronic pain.
8. Pay attention to bowel function; invariably a regular laxative will be required.
9. Prescribe appropriate adjuvant therapy as indicated by the nature of the pain.
10. Keep the patient (and family) informed as fully as they desire.

The strong opioid most commonly used on a worldwide basis is morphine and the reader is referred to two reviews describing morphine's clinical use.[69,70] There are numerous different for-

Table 115-1 Adjuvant analgesics

Drug	Indication	Dose
Dexamethasone	Soft tissue infiltration Hepatic capsular pain Nerve compression pain Nerve infiltration pain Spinal cord compression Raised intracranial pressure	12–16 mg/24 hr
Amitriptyline	Neuropathic pain (especially if altered sensation and constant)	10–150 mg/24 hr
Carbamazepine	Neuropathic pain (especially if lancinating)	200–600 mg/24 hr
Nonsteroidal anti-inflammatory drugs	Bone pain Any inflammatory pain	Depends on choice of drug
Bisphosphonates	Bone pain	

mulations and in uncontrolled severe pain use of an immediate-release morphine gives greater flexibility for dosage change than sustained-release preparations.[71] Morphine has a half-life of about 3 hours,[72,73] and for effective analgesia the immediate-release formulation should be given regularly every 4 hours. Provision for relief of breakthrough pain must be made. The dose of opioid required for breakthrough pain is one-sixth of the total 24-hour oral morphine dose. An immediate-release morphine formulation should be used to determine a patient's morphine requirement. Thereafter a sustained-release morphine preparation can be substituted.

In comparisons of the pharmacokinetic parameters of morphine in young and elderly patients, the elderly study group had a decreased morphine clearance with a trend to a smaller volume of distribution. Also the elderly group had a greater area under the plasma concentration-time curve. The time to reach maximum concentrations was the same in both groups.[74,75] In clinical practice this means that the starting dose will generally be reduced to prevent undue adverse reactions. Successful pain management in the elderly is often complicated because of renal, hepatic, or gastrointestinal impairment. Elderly patients generally require a lower dose of morphine than younger patients,[76] but each patient's morphine dose should be titrated individually to achieve the best therapeutic outcome. Clinical prescribing guidelines are suggested in the the accompanying box.

The oral route should be used if possible. Morphine is a safe drug when used according to accepted guidelines. The only ceiling to morphine dose escalation is the adverse effect profile. If appropriately titrated, doses of several grams have been used safely.[77] If the patient cannot tolerate the oral route, the opioid should be given subcutaneously. Diamorphine is more soluble in water than morphine and is the opioid of choice for injection in the United Kingdom.[78–80] The oral morphine to subcutaneous diamorphine conversion factor is shown in the box. In emaciated patients it is less painful to administer appropriate drugs subcutaneously than intramuscularly.

The accompanying box shows some of the side effects of morphine.[81] Tolerance to some of the adverse effects such as nausea, vomiting, and sedation occurs. Tolerance to constipation, xerostomia,[82] and the analgesic effect does not occur. Nausea and vomiting will occur in approximately 40 percent of opioid naive patients.[83] The antiemetic of choice is haloperidol in a dose of 1.5 mg orally twice a day. Normally this can be discontinued after 3 or 4 days.

Constipation requires a dual-action laxative, such as co-danthramer, with dose titration as indicated. Prescription of laxatives should be proactive, not reactive. Drowsiness will usually resolve after a few days but care should be taken to avoid concurrent sedating medicines. Dry mouth requires regular mouth care and prompt and effective treatment of any infection.

A transdermal therapeutic system (TTS) with fentanyl has recently been introduced in the United Kingdom, but has been available in the United States for some time. Fentanyl is a potent μ-agonist, hence its action can be reversed by naloxone. Fentanyl is a step 3 analgesic used for severe pain. The first

Key points–morphine

Start with immediate release morphine 4-hourly orally.

Generally the starting dose will be 2.5 or 5 mg every 4 hours.

Prescribe morphine at one-sixth of the total 24-hour dose for breakthrough or incident pain.

Titrate the dose against the individual's level of pain and side-effect profile.

Increase the dose by 20 to 50 percent or by the amount of breakthrough morphine used in the previous 24 hours.

When pain is controlled, convert to a sustained-release formulation in an equivalent dosage.

Prescribe a regular laxative, unless a contraindication exists.

Conversion of oral morphine to subcutaneous diamorphine

Total 24-hour dose of oral morphine (mg) divided by 2 or 3. For example, if the oral morphine dose is 60 mg in 24 hours = SC diamorphine 20 or 30 mg in 24 hours.

fentanyl patch applied has a slow onset of action reaching therapeutic plasma levels after 8 to 16 hours.[84] Due to the slow onset of action, TTS fentanyl should be reserved for patients whose pain has been previously stabilized on immediate-release morphine. Breakthrough pain should be treated using immediate-release morphine. Fentanyl has an important role in controlling pain although its use currently requires careful surveillance. Pharmacokinetic parameters after TTS fentanyl are not significantly altered in elderly patients,[85] but when given intravenously in elderly patients fentanyl has a reduced clearance and prolonged half-life.[86]

The rectal route may be chosen for administration of analgesia. Morphine, dextromoramide, and oxycodone suppositories are available. The dose and frequency of administration of morphine rectally is identical to the oral route.[87,88]

Difficult pain

Some pains prove more difficult to control. Generally these pains are classified as "opioid poorly responsive". However, opioids should be titrated to their maximally tolerated dose before arriving at this conclusion. Careful reappraisal of the etiology of the pain and use of appropriate adjuvant agents and nondrug interventions should be considered.

There has been a major interest in pain research in the past 20 years and knowledge of the nociceptive and antinociceptive pathways has increased greatly. The etiology of pains (often neuropathic) that are less opioid responsive is clearer following recognition of the role of AMPA (RS-α-amino-3-hydroxy-5-methylisoxazole-4-proprionic acid) and NMDA (N-methyl-D-aspartate) receptors.[89] If the NMDA receptor pathway is activated, central sensitization develops, frequently accompanied by a clinical triad of signs and symptoms. This triad, comprising allodynia, hyperesthesia, and hyperpathia, is indicative of central sensitization. Morphine acts as an analgesic by its pure agonistic effect on μ-receptors but is inactive at the NMDA receptor. Ketamine, an anesthetic agent, has analgesic properties at low doses and is an NMDA receptor antagonist. Its use as an analgesic in this situation is being evaluated.[90]

Pain due to nerve compression or infiltration may respond to high-dose dexamethasone added to the analgesic regimen.[91]

Side effects of opioids

Common
- Nausea/vomiting
- Xerostomia
- Constipation
- Drowsiness
- Loss of concentration

Less common
- Urinary retention
- Itch (uncommon in adults)
- Hypotension
- Bronchospasm
- Myoclonus
- Respiratory depression
- Gastric stasis
- Sweating

Morphine-induced confusion

Patients who are morphine toxic generally exhibit signs of somnolence, hallucinations, confusion, myoclonus,[92] hypotension, and respiratory depression.[93] However, more subtle signs, such as mild agitation or restlessness, can occur. In this situation the dose of morphine should be reduced. Adjuvant drugs should be prescribed in a morphine-sparing attempt. A careful reappraisal of the patient's drug regimen and level of anxiety should be made. Hallucinations can be controlled by a small dose of haloperidol. Morphine toxicity is usually a result of inappropriate dose escalation, poor pain assesment, deteriorating renal function, and failure to appreciate and treat underlying and associated psychological factors.

Nausea and Vomiting

Nausea and/or vomiting occur in 60 percent of patients with advanced cancer.[94,95] It is distressing and if persistent can rapidly result in symptoms of dehydration and hypovolemia in elderly patients. Vomiting and retching is a complex reflex process. Nausea is mediated via autonomic stimulation of somatic nerves. The vomiting center coordinates the process, receiving input and integrating this from several sources. Figure 115-2 is a diagramatic representation of the mechanisms of vomiting.

It is important to determine the etiology in each patient as the treatment selected depends on the cause. Evaluation will include examination, including fundoscopy and usually rectal examination. Blood analysis is often necessary and may reveal a reversible cause (e.g., hypercalcemia or digoxin toxicity). A review of all drugs is important, especially opioids. Sometimes patients find it difficult to differentiate among expectoration, regurgitation, and vomiting. A specific question about cough may be helpful as cough-induced retching resulting in vomiting requires treatment of the cause of the cough. Causes of nausea and vomiting in advanced cancer are listed in Table 115-2.

Management of nausea and vomiting

Management hinges on correction of the reversible, employing nondrug measures as appropriate and prescribing the correct antiemetic.

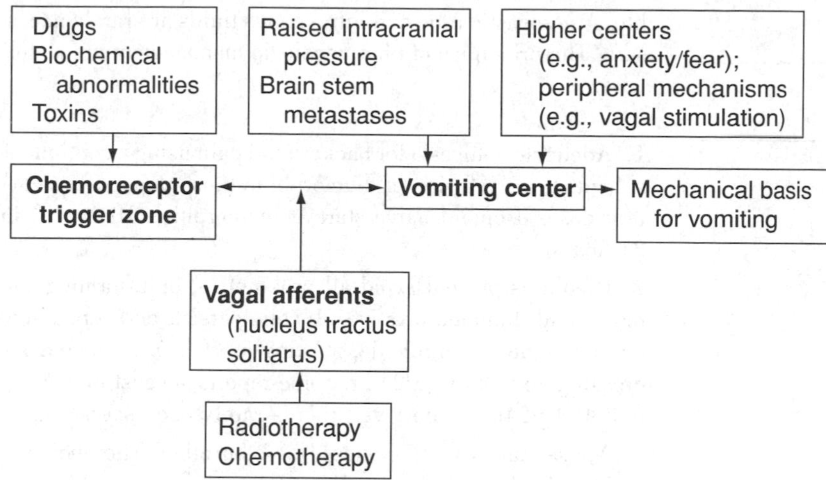

Figure 115-2 Coordination of nausea and vomiting.

Nondrug measures may include avoiding the smell or even the sight of food, avoiding exposure to foods that precipitate nausea, and presenting food in small, attractive quantities.

The choice of antiemetic depends on (1) knowledge of which emetic receptor(s) through which the cause of the vomiting is mediated, and (2) the receptor specificity of the antiemetic. Unless the cause can be removed, drug therapy must be administered regularly. The formulation of the antiemetic will depend on the pervasiveness and severity of the symptom. Oral, rectal, and parenteral preparations are available.

Table 115-2 Causes of nausea and vomiting in advanced cancer

Caused by cancer
Metabolic
Gastroparesis (paraneoplastic visceral neuropathy)
Hepatomegaly
Tense ascites
Bowel obstruction
Partial
Complete
Constipation
Cough
Raised intracranial pressure
Pain
Anxiety
Caused by cancer and/or debility
Cough
Infection
Caused by treatment
Radiotherapy
Chemotherapy
Surgery
Drugs
Concurrent causes
Peptic ulcer
Functional dyspepsia
Hiatal hernia

If a persistent pattern of vomiting is established, parenteral administration may be necessary. In the palliative care setting the subcutaneous route with a continuous infusion using a Graseby or similar lightweight portable pump is frequently used. This pump has the advantage of being small, suitable for use at home, and allowing a mixture of antiemetic and analgesia as indicated.[96] For patients wishing to avoid needles, the per rectal route is an alternative (cyclizine, prochlorperazine, chlorpromazine, and domperidone are available in suppository form). Table 115-3 offers a systematic approach to antiemetic prescribing.

Intestinal Obstruction

Until the advent of the modern palliative care approach to malignant gastrointestinal obstruction, such patients had only two treatment options: palliative surgery, which carried high morbidity and mortality rates,[97] or conservative management with intravenous fluids, nothing by mouth, and a nasogastric tube. The latter has obvious physical and psychological drawbacks. The use of appropriate analgesics and antiemetic drugs by continuous subcutaneous infusion has been shown to control symptoms.[98] Malignant gastrointestinal obstruction is encountered most commonly in patients with advanced abdominal or pelvic cancers. It occurs in 10 to 28 percent of primary bowel cancer, 5 percent of primary ovarian cancer, and in over 40 percent of patients with advanced ovarian cancer.[99]

The following recommendations apply to those patients who have no tumoricidal options open to them or who are awaiting tumoricidal treatment to take effect.

The etiology of bowel obstruction in advanced malignancy can be complicated and should not automatically be assumed to be due to tumor alone. Adhesions, constipation, drugs, unrelated benign conditions, or a combination of factors should be considered. Obstruction may be complete or partial, persistent or transient, high or low, single or at multiple sites.

Table 115-3 Choice of antiemetic

Cause of Nausea and Vomiting	Antiemetic
Drug-induced	Haloperidol 1.5–3 mg nocte Prochlorperazine 5–10 mg
Radiotherapy	Haloperidol 1.5–5 mg bid
Chemotherapy	5-HT_3 receptor antagonist (e.g., ondansetron) Metoclopramide (high dose) Dexamethasone
Metabolic	Haloperidol 5–20 mg/24 hr
Raised intracranial pressure	Cyclicine 50–100 mg tds
Middle ear pressure/irritation	Hyoscine (Kwells) 0.3 mg SL tds–qds
Bowel obstruction[a]	Hyoscine butylbromide 60–120 mg SC/24 hr Octreotide 300–600 μg SC/24 hr
Delayed gastric emptying	Metoclopramide 10–20 mg qds Domperidone 10–20 mg qds Cisapride 10–20 mg bid
Drug-related gastric irritation	Treat gastritis; change medication as necessary

[a] *See section on malignant gastrointestinal obstruction. Haloperidol, cyclicine metoclopramide, hyoscine butylbromide, octreotide, and dexamethasone can all be given by continuous subcutaneous infusion. Mixing dexamethasone with other drugs in a driver syringe is not recommended, but it can be given with diamorphine. Cyclizine is not compatible with octreotide.*

There is almost always an element of continuous abdominal pain from the underlying cancer. Vomiting and intestinal colic occurs in about 80 percent of patients.[100] Distention varies with the level of obstruction and bowel habit may vary from absolute constipation to diarrhea. Bowel sounds may be hyperactive but may also be absent.

Plain abdominal x-rays may confirm constipation. Computed tomography or magnetic resonance imaging can demonstrate obstruction at more than one level and are of use in deciding the technical feasibility of palliative surgery. Surgical intervention is unlikely to be successful in the following situations:

1. Radiologic or previous surgical evidence that technically a surgical procedure will not be successful.
2. Diffuse intra-abdominal carcinomatosis (diffuse palpable intra-abdominal tumors).
3. Massive ascites that reaccumulates rapidly after paracentesis.[101]
4. Poor general physical status.

Medical management of malignant gastrointestinal obstruction hinges on an accurate assessment with attempts to reverse the reversible (e.g., constipation), and to palliate the irreversible. A nasogastic tube and intravenous fluids are rarely necessary. The principles of pharmacologic management are as follows:

1. Adequate analgesia for background pain using a continuous subcutaneous infusion of diamorphine (dose depends on current dose. If opioid naive start at diamorphine 10 mg SC in 24 hours).
2. If colic is present avoid all prokinetics, bulk-forming, osmotic, and stimulant laxatives. If colic persists add subcutaneous hyoscine butylbromide, starting at 60 mg/24 hr and increasing up to 200 mg/24 hr. Some reports suggest increasing to 380 mg/24hr,[102] however, this is rarely necessary.
3. Nausea and vomiting should be controlled. The choice of antiemetic depends on whether the patient is experiencing colic. If the symptoms are suggestive of an incomplete obstruction and colic is not a feature, a trial of the prokinetic, metoclopromide 60 mg SC/24 hr is worthwhile. If the obstruction is more functional than mechanical this may resolve the problem. For other patients with nausea and vomiting haloperidol 5 to 20 mg/24 hr or cyclizine 100 to 150 mg/24 hr are used as first-line treatment. Haloperidol is a dopamine antagonist with its main effect at the chemoreceptor trigger zone, whereas cyclizine acts on histamine and muscarinic cholinergic receptors, its main site of action being the vomiting center.
A general principle in palliative medicine is to use the least number of drugs possible, thus avoiding unnecessary side effects. If control with the first antiemetic is not achieved, the second should be added, and if successful, a trial without the first advocated.
4. Persistent large-volume vomiting despite the above steps may respond to the somatostatin analog, octreotide. This drug is antisecretory and proabsorptive with the resultant net effect of decreasing the volume of fluid in the gut lumen.[103,104] This has the effect of eliminating vomiting completely or reducing volume and frequency of vomiting. Octreotide has also been shown to decrease forward peristalsis and may have direct analgesic activity.[104] Octreotide does not have a direct antiemetic action and if background nausea still exists, it can be combined with haloperidol in a syringe for continuous SC infusion.[105]

A starting dose of 300 μg/24 hr is recommended as this is the mean dose required to control vomiting.[106] Titration beyond 600 μg/24 hr is usually unhelpful. However, this has also to be judged on a clinical basis. Clinical impression and a recent study[107] suggest that the higher the obstruction, the higher the dose of octreotide required.

Octreotide, although expensive, is undoubtedly cost effective in many patients. Some proponents of high-dose hyoscine butylbromide suggest that this is as effective as octreotide in large-volume vomiting due to malignant obstruction. A randomized controlled trial is currently under way to compare the two treatments.

Diamorphine, octreotide, and haloperidol can be mixed in the same syringe and infused using a portable syringe driver.

Octreotide does not appear compatible with cyclizine, methotrimeprazine, or dexamethasone in the same syringe.[106]

Steroids can be useful in some cases of malignant obstruction. The postulated mechanism is a reduction of peritumor inflammatory edema. The dose used is dexamethasone 8 to 16 mg/24 hr by intravenous or subcutaneous route. There are, however, no trials with steroids in this situation.

The role of laxatives in obstruction depends on the analysis of the situation. If a single colonic or rectal obstruction is suspected, then a fecal softening laxative is justified (e.g., docusate). In the more usual situation of small bowel obstruction, laxatives have no role. Where obstruction is due to a combination of tumor compressing the bowel and hard impacted stool in the bowel lumen, both rectal and stoma suppositories and enemas can tip the balance in favor of the bowel opening.

Dietary advice in obstruction depends on the symptoms present. Many patients even with complete obstruction can eat and drink in modest amounts when symptoms are controlled. Diet is often liquid and low residue.

The symptom of dry mouth is usually best dealt with by frequent sips of cool fluids and ice to suck, along with regular mouth care. Administration of intravenous fluid is less helpful in dealing with the symptom of dry mouth per se, largely because this symptom is a complex physical and emotional phenomenon that depends on many factors. It may, however, be entirely appropriate to administer intravenous or subcutaneous fluids to some patients,[108] and this has to be judged on an individual basis. The majority of patients with malignant obstruction who are unsuitable for surgery can be managed by appropriate drug regimens. A few patients, usually with a high obstruction, may require a venting gastrostomy. This procedure needs to be properly evaluated in clinical trials.

Cachexia and Anorexia

Nausea and vomiting may exacerbate anorexia and, if they are controlled, appetite may improve. However, cachexia occurs in 90 percent of patients with advanced cancer and will further reduce mobility and exacerbate weakness due to depletion of muscle mass.[109] Enteral and parenteral feeding does not reverse this syndrome,[110] but in a double-blind placebo-controlled study, Downer[111] showed that the use of megesterol acetate improved appetite and general well-being. There may be a dose response curve to megesterol acetate as shown by Tchekmedyian.[112] Megesterol acetate is generally well tolerated but fluid retention may be problematic.[113] In a double-blind-placebo controlled study of patients attending an oncology clinic, prednisolone 15 mg/day was shown to be statistically superior to placebo in improving appetite.[114]

Constipation

Constipation is one of the most troublesome and persistent symptoms in patients with advanced cancer. Forty-five percent of patients complain of constipation on admission to a hospice.[115] The etiology is usually multifactorial but the common causes are listed in the box. Prevention is the mainstay of management. Good general symptom control, attention to toileting arrangements, mobility, diet, fluid intake, and prescription of an appropriate laxative in a therapeutic dose, are all essential elements in the prevention and management of constipation.

Causes of constipation

Inactivity/poor mobility
Poor diet
Poor fluid intake
Drugs
- Opioids
- Anticholinergics
- Antacids
- Anticonvulsants
- Iron
- Vincristine

Cancer-related
- Tumor in bowel wall
- Tumor causing extrinsic compression of bowel
- Hypercalcemia
- Cord compression

Other illnesses
Unsatisfactory toileting arrangement

The choice of laxative will depend on the bowel history but there frequently needs to be a combination of a stimulant and a softener (e.g., codanthramer or codanthrusate alone, or senna and lactulose given together). The dose should be titrated until the desired effect is achieved. Rectal laxatives are overprescribed, often because an inadequate dose of an oral laxative is used. However, some conditions such as spinal cord compression necessitate the use of regular rectal laxatives. In these situations a careful balance between oral and rectal laxatives gives pseudocontrol of the bowel.

Fecal impaction leading to overflow diarrhea, urinary incontinence, or urinary retention is not uncommon in a patient with cancer who has become bedbound and is taking constipating medication. Diarrhea secondary to impaction is frequently mistreated by antidiarrheal drugs.

The sequence of undiagnosed constipation leading to abdominal pain, which then is treated inappropriately by opioids, is unfortunately common in advanced cancer. This vicious circle causes much distress for patients.

The prevention and management of constipation is multifactorial; however, there is definite evidence that immobility can be a greater causal component in constipation than opioids.[116] Aggressive titration of laxatives in immobile patients is advised.

Terminal Restlessness

It is a fundamental right of humanity that when natural death approaches the passage from life to death should be dignified and peaceful with no undue distress. Moreover, it

Some causes of terminal restlessness

Unrelieved pain
Psychosocial factors: anxiety, fear, unfinished business
Retention of urine
Full rectum, impaction
Dry mouth
Infection: chest, urine, wound
Metabolic (e.g., hypercalcemia, hypoglycemia)
Cerebral metastases
Hiccoughs
Dyspnea
Cough
Drugs
Dehydration

has also been shown that the quality of care, manner of dying, and support given to relatives influences the bereavement outcome of survivors. Pain or restlessness prior to death are unacceptable and distressing for all, not least the dying. The underlying principle of continuing attention to whole person care is vital. The patient may be fearful and anxious about what is happening. As the patient enters the terminal phase the approach to care must continue to be diligent and attention to psychological, spiritual, and physical needs should continue. Careful positioning, ensuring an optimum environment, and attention to the remaining basic needs of the person may alone settle distress.

A study by Wilson et al.[117] showed that 32 percent of elderly patients in a long-stay ward and 41 percent in an assessment ward were distressed in the last week of life. Agitation was the most common manifestation of distress. Restlessness was especially prominent if there were respiratory symptoms or cardiac decompensation. Fifty-six percent of the 150 patients studied were taking opioids. However, the average dose was low at 2.5 to 5 mg immediate-release morphine 4-hourly orally. This dose range, if compared with the average dose in an SPCU is low. The median dose of oral morphine in 955 inpatients at St. Christophers Hospice was 10 mg 4 hourly.[118] In a terminally restless patient there should be an attempt to determine the etiology of the distress (see the accompanying box).

If a cause for terminal restlessness is diagnosed, a decision must be made as to whether to treat the cause or palliate the symptom. If the decision is taken to palliate the cause of the distress, various drugs are available.

Analgesia must be continued and if swallowing becomes difficult an alternative route, usually subcutaneously, should be used. Additional analgesia should be available for breakthrough pain, calculated as described earlier in this chapter.

The level of sedation required and nature of the distress will usually dictate which medication is used. Midazolam, haloperidol, methotrimeprazine, and indirectly hyoscine hydrobromide are commonly used. Midazolam is used subcutaneously in a driver syringe in doses ranging from 5 to 80 mg/24 hr.[119] The dose varies and for anxiety that cannot be alleviated by counseling and personal support a low dose of 5 to 20 mg/24 hr is normally sufficient, especially in elderly patients. If pain is present diamorphine is compatible with midazolam and can be mixed in the same driver syringe. Midazolam also raises the seizure threshold. Dosage increase, if necessary, may be made in increments of 10 to 15 mg in 24 hours. Haloperidol is indicated in cases of agitation with altered sensorium. This drug can be administered via a driver syringe subcutaneously in doses between 2.5 and 25 mg/24 hr.

Methotrimeprazine, a phenothiazine, has antiemetic, antipsychotic, and sedative properties and is claimed to have analgesic properties.[120] It can be administered subcutaneously via a driver syringe and is a potent sedating agent. In the elderly patient haloperidol is safer than methotrimeprazine. Figure 115-3 summarizes the approach.

If oropharyngeal secretions accumulate and produce a "rattle or gurgle," usually the patient is unconscious and unaware. The noise is distressing for relatives and other patients. Excessive secretions may be eased by using hyoscine hydrobromide if sedation is also desired. Hyoscine butylbromide is an alternative if sedation is not required. Diazepam (5 to 10 mg) or chlorpromazine (50 or 100 mg) can be administered rectally.

Dyspnea

Dyspnea is an unpleasant awareness of difficulty in breathing. Dyspnea, like pain, is subjective and involves both the perception of the symptom by the patient and his or her reac-

Figure 115-3 Treatment of terminal restlessness.

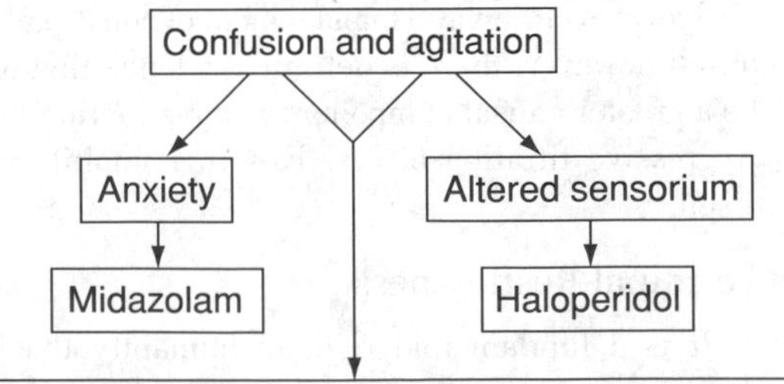

tion to that sensation. The symptom can be very variable even in the same patient not only because its severity is usually directly related to activity, but also because the speed of onset, more than the severity, may influence the patient's perception of breathlessness. In addition, patient's previous experience of a symptom, whether suffered by themselves or witnessed in others, undoubtedly colors their reaction.

There is frequently considerable disparity between doctors' and patients' assessments of symptoms, and indeed patients and their close relatives may well have differing points of view.[121] The tumors most commonly associated with dyspnea are lung, colorectal, breast, and prostate cancers.[122,123] Dyspnea in patients with cancer may be caused by the tumor itself, the treatment of the tumor, pre-existing cardiorespiratory disease, infection, or any combination of these factors. Anemia, pulmonary emboli, or congestive heart failure may arise as a manifestation of debility caused by both the disease and its treatment. Dyspnea has been noted as the most common severe symptom in the last days of life.[124] In a longitudinal survey of 1,700 inpatient hospice patients in the United States, 70 percent of patients with a wide range of malignancies had dyspnea in the last weeks of life.[123] The same rate was reported in patients with lung cancer.[125] In one study neither lung nor heart disease could be identified as the cause of this symptom in one-quarter of patients.[123] The explanation given by the authors in this case was debility of terminal cancer, while an alternative explanation could be functional dyspnea.[126]

The pathogenesis of dyspnea is poorly understood and like pain is likely to be much more complex than previously thought. Factors as diverse as chemical stimulation of the respiratory center in the medulla and the tone of bronchial, diaphragmatic, and intercostal muscles are important. The innervation of the lung is complex and includes excitatory cholinergic parasympathetic and inhibitory adrenergic sympathetic neurons. More recently a nonadrenergic-noncholinergic network has been described. These latter are opioid receptors and together with endogenous opioids, have been demonstrated in the lung.[127–129] There is growing evidence that they have an important role in the pathophysiology of breathlessness.[130,131]

The multiple aspects of the physiology of respiration are summarized in Figure 115-4.

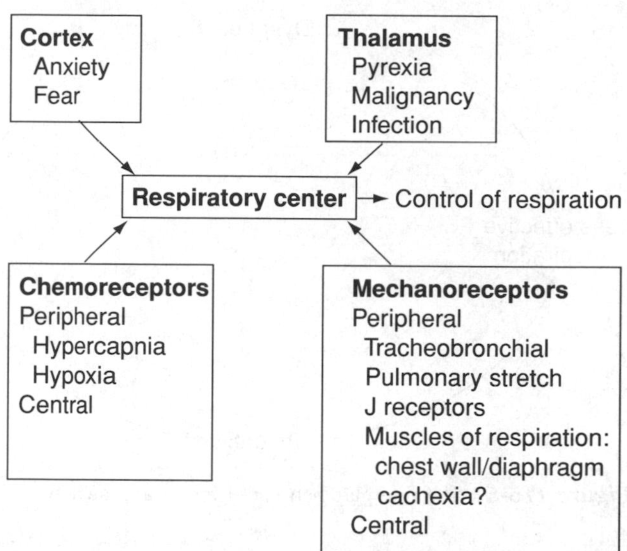

Figure 115-4 The physiology of respiration.

Symptomatic treatment of dyspnea

The fundamental principles are a comprehensive clinical assessment, analysis of symptomatology, and reversal of the reversible and symptomatic relief of the irreversible based on the underlying cause(s). It is important to remember that a dyspneic patient is often an anxious patient (see Fig. 115-5).

In cases where a reversible cause is identified, symptomatic relief should not be witheld while more definitive treatment is being applied, such as aspiration of pleural or ascitic fluid, radiotherapy, chemotherapy, treatment of infection, or laser therapy. The approaches, to symptomatic treatment are, broadly, nonpharmacologic and pharmacologic. The former include the following:

- Explanation and reassurance
- Calm presence
- Comfortable position
- Walking aid
- Bed rest
- Bed downstairs
- Cool air use of a fan
- Wheelchair
- Help with activities of daily living
- Breathing exercises
- Relaxation therapy

Pharmacologic intervention should be integrated with the above as follows. A low-dose systemic opioid, usually morphine, is the treatment of choice of most palliative medicine physicians for dyspnea in malignant disease.[132,133] Although many physicians worry about the respiratory depressant effect of opioids, this is not normally a problem if care is given to the choice of dose and dose titration. There is clinical evidence that patients with chronic obstructive pulmonary disease (COPD) and high arterial carbon dioxide levels tolerate opioids well.[134,135]

Several factors must be considered before choosing the route and dose of opioid. Among these factors are (1) history of exposure to opioids (whether or not opioid naive); (2) current opioid dose and side effect profile; (3) renal function; (4)Co-existing COPD. A typical starting dose for oral morphine would be 5 mg 4-hourly (but see below). For a patient already on morphine, the dose should be gently titrated against dyspnea and adverse effects, using the same principles as in pain control.

Titration is always better achieved by using a 4-hourly immediate-release morphine preparation. This allows specific questions, such as time to onset of action, degree of relief, and duration of action, to be answered more accurately by the

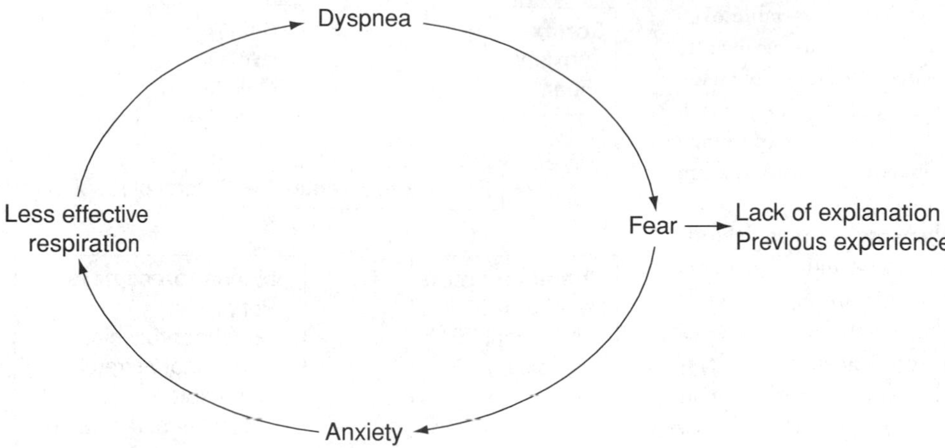

Figure 115-5 The interplay between dyspnea and anxiety.

patient. Subsequently a more efficient titration to reach the desired balance between control of dyspnea and adverse effects is achieved. A dose equal to the individual 4-hourly dose should be prescribed for breakthrough dyspnea at any time.

Often in elderly opioid-naive patients a smaller starting dose of immediate-release morphine such as 2.5 mg 4-hourly may be sufficient. In renal dysfunction as little as 2.5 mg immediate-release morphine 6-hourly or less can reach a better balance between control of dyspnea and adverse effects. There is no evidence that sustained-release morphine compounds are less effective than immediate-release morphine preparations in control of dyspnea. If a stable immediate-release morphine dose is reached this can be converted to sustained-release morphine compound for ease of administration for the patient.

The mechanism of action of opioids in the control of dyspnea is not fully understood and is certainly complex, probably involving several areas. Morphine acts on (1) the cerebral cortex; (2) the respiratory center; (3) stretch (J) receptors in the lungs; (4) peripheral opioid receptors in the lungs; and (5) the cardiovascular system.

Morphine can also be given by nebulizer.[136] Clinical experience suggests nebulized morphine may help to control dyspnea in patients with interstitial lung disease, rather than in patients with encasing lung disease. In a randomized controlled trial in dyspneic patients with cancer no difference in efficacy was found between nebulized morphine and nebulized saline.[137]

There is no evidence that diazepam has any central or peripheral effect on dyspnea per se. However, in the patient who becomes anxious, with resultant worsening of dyspnea, it has an obvious role. The dose of diazepam will vary with the individual patient from 2 mg nocte to 10 mg tds and 20 mg nocte. In patients unable to swallow medication, midazolam is the anxiolytic of choice by continuous subcutaneous infusion. A starting dose of midazolam would be 10 mg over 24 hours.

Nebulized salbutamol has an interesting role in dyspnea due to malignancy. It seems to have much more than a bronchodilator effect and is often of use in the absence of clinical bronchospasm. Salbutamol has been shown to increase voluntary muscle strength.[138]

Nebulized 0.9 percent saline (2 to 5 ml) is also an interesting drug with much more than a mucolytic action. Although clinical research is lacking, the general impression is that it can be an effective treatment for the relief of dyspnea.[139] Nebulized lignocaine is disappointing in both the treatment of intractable cough and of dyspnea, performing poorly against saline in one study.[139]

In patients with cancer-related dyspnea, the benefit of oxygen is not dependent on correction of hypoxia; a trial of oxygen therapy is the only way to determine benefit, not improvement in blood gases. This has only been investigated superficially,[140] and needs to be looked at in more detail.

In summary, dyspnea is a common symptom that needs to be analyzed in the individual patient. All reversible factors should be dealt with and steps taken to give symptomatic relief. A combined approach is necessary to deal with the physical symptomatology and accompanying anxiety. A stepwise approach using simple methods such as nebulized saline and salbutamol, progressing to systemic opioid therapy is advised. A combination of treatments is often required.

Conclusion

Palliative care involves an active, analytical approach to the whole person and his or her problems. It may be introduced at the time of diagnosis of an incurable progressive condition and should not be restricted to the terminal phase of life. It involves reversing the reversible and palliating the irreversible. Care of relatives is important. Although the principles of palliative care are typically applied to the cancer patient, they should also be applied to patients with nonmalignant conditions.

References

1. Callaghan D: The Troubled Dream of Life: In Search of a Peaceful Death. p. 94. Simon & Schuster, New York, 1993
2. World Health Organisation: Cancer Pain Relief and Palliative Care. World Health Organisation, Geneva, 1990

3. Doyle D, Hanks G, MacDonald N (eds): Oxford Textbook of Palliative Medicine. p. 3. Oxford University Press, Oxford, 1993
4. Directory of Hospice and Palliative Care Services in the United Kingdom and Republic of Ireland. p. 1x. St. Christophers Hospice Information Service, London, 1996
5. Lunt B, Hillier R: St. Christophers Hospice Information Service, London, 1987
6. Findlay IG, Jones RVH: Outreach palliative care services: definitions in palliative care. BMJ 1995;311:754
7. National Council for Hospice and Specialist Palliative Care Services: Specialist Palliative Care: A Statement of Definitions. Occasional paper 8, London, 1995
8. Eve A, Smith AM: Palliative care services in Britain and Ireland—update 1991. Palliat Med 1994;8:19–27
9. Directory of Hospice and Palliative Care Services in the United Kingdom and Republic of Ireland. p. X. St. Christophers Hospice Information Service, London, 1996
10. Hamilton J, Edgar L: A survey examining nurses' knowledge of pain control. J Pain Symptom Manage 1992;7:18–26
11. Elliot TE, Murray DM, Elliot BA et al: Physician knowledge and attitudes about cancer pain management: a survey from the Minnesota Cancer Pain Project. J Pain Symptom Manage 1995;10:494–504
12. Cancer Relief Macmillan Fund. p. X. In G.P. Facilitators Project. Section B Project Activities 1992–94
13. Reid W: Just for the Record. The Department of Health. Redhouse Lane Communications, 1995
14. Palliative Medicine Curriculum. Association of Palliative Medicine of Great Britain and Ireland, 1992
15. A Core Curriculum for a Post Basic Course in Palliative Nursing. The International Society for Nurses in Cancer Care approved by the Cancer and Palliative Care Unit. WHO, Geneva, 1991
16. A Core Curriculum for Post-Basic Nursing. The Commission of the European Communities and the European Oncology Nursing Society, Brussels, 1991
17. Recommendations on General Clinical Training. General Medical Council. Kiek & Read, London, 1992
18. Tomorrow's Doctors. Recommendations on undergraduate Medical Education: General Medical Council. Kiek & Read, London 1993
19. Leventhal EA: The dilemma of cancer in the elderly. pp. 1–13. In Veeth JM, Meyer J (eds): Cancer and the Elderly. Karger, Basel, 1986
20. Crawford J, Cohen HJ: Relationship of cancer and aging. Clin Geriatr Med 1987;3:419–431
21. Office of Population Censuses and Surveys (OPCS): Monitor 1992. HMSO, London, 1993
22. Roy R, Thomas MR: Elderly persons with and without pain. A comparative study. Clin J Pain 1987;3:102–106
23. Cartwright A, Seale C: The Year Before Death. pp. 113–116. Aldershot, Ashgate Publishing, Avelbury, 1994
24. Donnelly S, Walsh D: The symptoms of advanced cancer. Semin Oncol 1995;22:67–72
25. Leishman JG, McGovern EM, McKay S et al: An Audit of the Pharmaceutical Care Provided to Terminally Ill Patients in the Hospice and Community. Clinical Resource and Audit Group, Scottish Office Home and Health Department, Edinburgh, 1995
26. Portenoy RK, Miransky J, Thaler HT: Pain in ambulatory patients with lung or colon cancer, prevalence, characteristics and impact. Cancer 1992;70:1616–1624
27. Melding PS: Is there such a thing as geriatric pain? Pain 1991; 46:119–121
28. Ferrell BA: Pain management in elderly people. J Am Geriatr Soc 1991;39:64–73
29. Stein WM, Mieck RP: Cancer pain in the elderly hospice patient. J Pain Symptom Manage 1993;8:474–482
30. Twycross RG: Incidence of pain. Clin Oncol 1984;3:5–15
31. Bowling A, Browne PD: Social networks, health and emotional well-being among the oldest old in London. J Gerontol 1991; 46:20–32
32. Kane RL, Ouslander JG, Abrass IB: Essentials of Clinical Geriatrics. 2nd Ed. McGraw-Hill, New York, 1989
33. Roy R: A psychological perspective on chronic pain and depression in the elderly. Social Work Health Care 1986;12: 27–36
34. Lau-Ting C, Poon WO: Aches and pains among Singapore elderly. Singapore Med J 1988;29:164–167
35. Ferrell BA, Ferrell BR, Osterweil D: Pain in the nursing home. J Am Geriatr Soc 1990;39:64–73
36. Davis MA: Epidemiology of osteoarthritis. Clin Geriatr Med 1988;4:241–255
37. Marks RM, Sachar EJ: Undertreatment of medical inpatients with narcotic analgesics. Ann Intern Med 1973;78:173–181
38. Sriwatanakul K, Weis OF, Alloza JL et al: Analysis of narcotic usage in the treatment of postoperative pain. JAMA 1983;250: 926–929
39. Melzack R, Abbott FV, Zackon W et al: Pain on a surgical ward: a survey of the duration and intensity of pain and the effectiveness of medication. Pain 1987;29:67–72
40. Seers CJ: Pain, Anxiety and Recovery in Patients Undergoing Surgery. Unpublished PhD thesis, Department of Nursing Studies, University of London, London, 1987
41. Carr ECJ: Post operative pain: patient's expectations and experiences. J Adv Nurs 1990;15:89–100
42. Kuhn S, Cook K, Collins M et al: Preception of pain after surgery. BMJ 1990;300:1687–1690
43. Closs SJ, Fairtlough HL, Tierney AJ, Currie CT: Pain in elderly orthopaedic patients. J Clin Nurs 1993;2:41–45
44. Cleeland CS, Cleeland LM, Dar R, Rinchardt LC: Factors influencing physicians' management of cancer pain. Cancer 1986;58:796–800
45. Elliot TE, Elliot BA: Physician attitudes and beliefs about use of morphine for cancer pain. J Pain Symptom Manage 1992; 7:141–148
46. Rife BL, Inik N, Painter JD: A comparative study of the attitudes of physicians and nurses toward the management of cancer pain. J Pain Symptom Manage 1993;8:132–139
47. Closs SJ: Pain in elderly patients: a neglected phenomenon? J Adv Nurs 1994;19:1072–1081
48. Reid W, Stott DJ: Pain relief in elderly patients. Ther Update 1993;Sept:309–316

49. Hayes R: Pain assessment in the elderly. Br J Nurs 1995;4: 1199–1204
50. Fordyce WE: Evaluating and managing chronic pain. Geriatrics 1978;33:59–62
51. Bender JS: Approach to the acute abdomen. Med Clin North Am 1989;73:1413–1422
52. Clinch D: Absence of abdominal pain in elderly patients with peptic ulcer. Age Ageing 1984;13:120–123
53. Bayer AJ, Chada JS, Farag RR, Pathy MS: Changing presentation of myocardial infarctions with increasing old age. J Am Geriatr Soc 1986;34:263–266
54. Collins G, Stone LA: Pain sensitivity, age and activity level in chronic schizophrenics and in normals. Br J Psychiatry 1965;112:33
55. Harkins SW, Chapman CR: Detection and decision factors in pain perception in young and elderly men. Pain 1976;2:253
56. Harkins SW, Chapman CR: The perception of induced dental pain in young and elderly women. J Gerontol 1977;428–435
57. Tucker MA, Andrew MF, Ogle SJ, Davison JG: Age associated change in pain threshold measured by transcutaneous neuronal electrical stimulation. Age Ageing 1989;18:241–246
58. Wendy M, Stein MD, Ralph P, Miech MD: Cancer pain in the elderly hospice patient. J Pain Symptom Manage 1993;8: 474–482
59. Grossman SA, Shiedler VR, Sweden K et al: Correlation of patient and care giver rating of cancer pain. J Pain Symptom Manage 1991;6:53–57
60. Zech DFJ, Grond S, Lynch J et al: Validation of World Health Organisation guidelines for cancer pain relief: a ten year prospective study. Pain 1995;63:65–76
61. World Health Organization: Cancer Pain Relief and Palliative Care. Report of a World Health Organization Expert Committee. Technical Report Series 804. W.H.O, Geneva, 1990
62. Takeda F: Results of field testing in Japan of the W.H.O. draft interim guidelines on relief of cancer pain. Pain Clin 1986; 1:83–89
63. Ventafridda V, Tambburini M, Carceni A et al: A Validation study of the W.H.O. method for cancer pain relief. Cancer 1987;59:851–856
64. Walker VA, Hoskin PJ, Hanks GW, White ID: Evaluation of W.H.O. analgesic guidelines for cancer pain in a hospital-based palliative care unit. J Pain Symptom Manage 1988;3: 145–149
65. Portenoy RK, Hagen NA: Breakthrough pain: definition, prevalence and characteristics. Pain 1990;41:273–281
66. Portenoy RK: Adjuvant analgesics in pain management. pp. 187–203. In Doyle D, Hanks G, MacDonald N (eds): Oxford Textbook of Palliative Medicine. Oxford University Press, Oxford, 1993
67. Russell K, Portenoy MD, Steven D, Waldman MD: Adjuvant analgesics in pain management 2. J Pain Symptom Manage 1994;9:390–391
68. McCaffery M: Nursing Management of the Patient With Pain. Lippincott-Raven, Philadephia, 1972
69. Gorman DJ: Opioid analgesics in the management of pain in patients with cancer: an update. Palliat Med 1991;5:277–294
70. Report of an Expert Working Group of the European Association for Palliative Care: Morphine in cancer pain: modes of administration. BMJ 1996;312:823–826
71. Hanks GW: Controlled release morphine in advanced cancer: the European experience. Cancer 1989;63:2378–2382
72. Sawe J: High dose morphine and methadone in cancer patients. Clinical pharmacokinetics: considerations of oral treatment. Clin Pharmacokinet 1986;11:87–106
73. Portenoy RK, Foley KM, Stulman J et al: Plasma morphine and morphine-6-glucuronide during morphine therapy for cancer pain: plasma profiles, steady state concentrations and the consequences of renal failure. Pain 1991;47:13–19
74. Owen JA, Sitar DS, Barger L et al: Age related morphine kinetics. Clin Pharmacol Ther 1983;34:364–368
75. Baille SP, Bateman ON, Coates PE, Woodhouse KW: Age and the pharmacokinetics of morphine. Age Ageing 1989;18: 258–262
76. Rees WD: Opioid needs of terminal care patients: variations with age and primary site. Clin Oncol 1990;2:79–83
77. Smith KJ, Miller AJ, McKellar J, Court M: Morphine at gramme doses: kinetics, dynamics and clinical need. Postgrad Med 1991;67:55–59
78. Diamorphine hydrochloride. In Dollery C (ed): Therapeutic Drugs. Vol. 1. Churchill Livingstone, London, 1991
79. Martindale: p. 63. In Reynolds J (ed): The Extra Pharmacopoeia: 31st Ed. Royal Pharmaceutical Society, London, 1996
80. The Pharmaceutical Codex. 12th Ed. In Lus W (ed): Morphine. Pharmaceutical Press, London, 1994
81. Portenoy RK: Management of common opioid side effects during long-term therapy of cancer pain. Ann Acad Med Singapore 1994;23:160–170
82. White ID, Hoskin PJ, Hanks GW, Bliss JM: Morphine and dryness of the mouth. BMJ 1989;298:1222–1223
83. Inturrisi CE, Hanks G: Opioid analgesic therapy. pp. 166–181. In Doyle D, Hanks G, MacDonald N (eds): Oxford Textbook of Palliative Medicine. Oxford University Press, Oxford, 1993
84. Plezia PM, Kramer TH, Linford J: Transdermal fentanyl: pharmacokinetics and preliminary clinical evaluation. Pharmacotherapy 1989;9:2–9
85. Data on file Janssen Pharmaceutical, Rowbotham, N91173, 1992
86. Bentley JB, Borel JD, Gillespie TJ et al: Fentanyl pharmacokinetics in obese and non-obese patients. Anesthesiology 1981; 55:A177
87. Pannueti I, Rossi AP, Lafelice G: Control of chronic pain in very advanced cancer patients with morphine hydrochloride administered by oral, rectal and sublingual route. Clinical report and preliminary results on morphine pharmokinetics. Pharmacol Res Commun 1982;14:369–380
88. Raiko RF, Healy N, Pav J et al: The comparative bio-availability of M.S. Contin tablets following rectal and oral administration. pp. 235–241. In Twycross RG (ed): The Edinburgh Symposium on Pain Control and Medical Education. Royal Society of Medicine, London, 1989
89. Woolf CJ, Thompson SWN: The induction and maintenance of central sensitization is dependent on N-methyl-D-aspartic acid receptor activation; implications for the treatment of post-injury pain hypersensitivity states. Pain 1991;44:293–299

90. Fallon MT, Welsh J: What is the role of ketamine in pain control? Eur J Palliat Care 1996;3:143–146

91. Vecht ChJ, Haaxma-Reiche H, van Putten WLJ et al: Initial bolus of conventional versus high dose dexamethasone in metastatic spinal cord compression. Neurology 1989;39:1255–1257

92. Snodgrass SR: Myoclonus: analysis of monoamine, GABA and other systems. FASEB 1990;4:2775–2788

93. Schug SA, Zech D, Grond S et al: A long term survey of morphine in cancer pain patients. J Pain Symptom Manage 1992;7:259–265

94. Curtis EB, Krech R, Walsh TD: Common symptoms in patients with advanced cancer. J Palliat Care 1991;7:25–29

95. Dunlop DM: A study of the relative frequency and importance of gastrointestinal symptoms and weakness in patients with far advanced cancer: student paper. Palliat Med 1989;4:37–43

96. Johnson I, Paterson S: Drugs used in combination in the syringe driver: a survey of hospice practice. Palliat Med 1992;6:125–130

97. Chan A, Woodruff K: Intestinal obstruction in patients with widespread intra-abdominal malignancy. J Pain Symptom Manage 1992;7:339–342

98. Baines MJ, Oliver DJ, Carter RL: Medical management of intestinal obstruction in patients with advanced malignant disease: a clinical and pathological study. Lancet 1985;2:990–993

99. Ripamonti C: Malignant bowel obstruction in advanced and terminal cancer patients. Eur J Palliat Care 1994;1:16–19

100. Twycross R: Symptom management in advanced cancer. p. 175. Radcliffe Medical Press, Oxford, 1995

101. Krebs H, Goplerud DR: Surgical management of bowel obstruction in advanced ovarian cancer. Obstet Gynecol 1983;61:327–330

102. Ventafridda V, Ripamonti C, Catraceni A et al: The management of inoperable gastrointestinal obstruction in terminal cancer patients. Tumori 1990;76:389–393

103. Mercadante S: The role of octreotide in palliative care. J Pain Symptom Manage 1994;9:406–411

104. Fallon MT: Physiology of somatostatin and its synthetic analogue octreotide. Eur J Palliat Care 1994;1:20–22

105. Mercadante S, Spoldi E, Caraceni A et al: Octreotide in relieving gastrointestinal symptoms due to bowel obstruction. Palliat Med 1993;7:42–46

106. Riley J, Fallon MT: The use of octreotide in malignant intestinal obstruction. Eur J Palliat Care 1994;1:23–25

107. Riley J, Khoo D, Waxman J: Randomised and controlled trial of octreotide versus placebo in malignant gastrointestinal obstruction. (in press)—details still awaited

108. Fainsinger RL, MacEachern T, Miller MJ et al: The use of hypodermoclysis for rehydration in terminally ill cancer patients. J Pain Symptom Manage 1994;9:298–302

109. Erick RE: Current concepts in anorexia and cachexia. Am J Hospice Care 1987;4:13–15

110. Bruera E: Clinical management of anorexia and cachexia in patients with advanced cancer. Oncology 1992;2:35–42

111. Downer S: Double blind placebo controlled trial of response to medroxyprogestron in cancer cachexia. Br J Cancer 1993;67:1102–1105

112. Tchekmedyian NS: High dose megesterol acetate—a possible treatment for cachexia. JAMA 1987;257:1195–1198

113. Schmall J: Megesterol acetate in cancer cachexia. Semin Oncol 1991;18:32–34

114. Willox JC, Corr J, Shaw J et al: Prednisolone as an appetite stimulant in patients with advanced cancer. BMJ 1984;288:27

115. St. Christophers Hospice. Annual Statistics. St. Christophers Hospice, London, 1986

116. Fallon MT, Hanks GW: Morphine, constipation and performance status in advanced cancer patients. Palliat Med (accepted for publication)

117. Wilson JA, Lawson PM, Smith RG: The treatment of terminally ill geriatric patients. Palliat Med 1987;1:149–153

118. Twycross R: Pain Relief in Advanced Cancer. p. 313. Churchill Livingstone, Singapore, 1994

119. McNamara P, Minton M, Twycross RG: Use of midazolam in palliative care. Palliat Med 1991;5:244–249

120. Beaver WT, Wallenstein S, Houde RW, Rogers A: A comparison of the analgesic effects of methotrimeprazine and morphine in patients with cancer. Clin Pharmacol Ther 1966;7:436–446

121. Higginson I, Wade A, McCarthy M: Palliative care: views of patients and their families. BMJ 1990;301:277–281

122. Ruben DB, Mor V: Dyspnoea in terminally ill cancer patients. Chest 1986;89:234–236

123. Heyse-Moore LH, Ross V, Mullee MA: How much of a problem is dyspnoea in advanced cancer? Palliat Med 1991;5:20–26

124. Higginson I, McCarthy M: Measuring symptoms in terminal cancer: are pain and dyspnoea controlled? J R Soc Med 1989;82:264–267

125. Krech RL, Davis J, Dedan W, Curtis EB: Symptoms of lung cancer. Palliat Med 1992;6:309–315

126. Davis CL: The therapeutics of dyspnoea. pp. 85–98. In Cancer Surveys Volume 21: Palliative Medicine: Problem Areas in Pain and Symptom Management. Cold Spring Harbor Laboratory Press, New York, 1994

127. Hughes J, Kosterlitz HW, Smith TW: The distribution of methionine-enkephalin and leucine-enkephalin in the brain and peripheral tissues. Br J Pharmacol 1977;61:639–647

128. Miedle A, Manigalt I, Wajda IJ: Distribution of opiate-like substances in rat tissues. Neurochem Res 1979;4:399–410

129. Hedner T, Cassuto J: Opioids and opioid receptors in peripheral tissues. Scand J Gastroenterol 1987;130 (suppl):27–40

130. Frossard M, Barnes PJ: MU opioid receptors modulate noncholinergic constrictor nerves in guinea-pig airways. Eur J Pharmacol 1987;141:519–522

131. Belvisi MG, Rogers DF, Barnes PJ: Neurogenic plasma extravasation: inhibition by morphine in guinea-pig airways in vivo. J Appl Physiol 1989;60:268–272

132. Hoskin PJ, Hanks GW: The management of symptoms in advanced cancer: experience in a hospital-based continuing care unit. J R Soc Med 1988;81:341–344

133. Ahmedzai S: Palliation of respiratory symptoms. pp. 362–365. In Doyle D, Hanks GW, MacDonald N (eds): Oxford Textbook of Palliative Medicine. Oxford University Press, Oxford, 1993

134. Gray JMB, Henry DA, Paice B et al: Acute respiratory failure and CNS-depressing drugs. Postgrad Med J 1981;57:279–282

135. Walsh TD: Opiates and respiratory function in advanced cancer. Recent Results Cancer Res 1984;89:115–117

136. Davis CL: The pharmacokinetics of nebulised morphine. Abstract 995 presented at the 7th World Congress on Pain. IASP Publications, Seattle, 1993

137. Davis CL, Penn K, Daniels J, Slevin M: Single dose randomised controlled trial of nebulised morphine in patients with cancer related breathlessness. Palliat Med 1996;10:64–65

138. Matineau L: Salbutamol, a β-adrenoceptor agonist, increases skeletal muscle strength in young men. Clin Sci 1992;83: 615–621

139. Wilcock A, Corcoran R, Tattersfield AE: Safety and efficacy of nebulised lignocaine in patients with cancer and breathlessness. Palliat Med 1994;8:35–38

140. Bruera E, de Stoutz N, Velasco-Leiva A et al: Effects of oxygen on dyspnoea in hypoxaemic terminal cancer patients. Lancet 1993;342:13–14

CHAPTER 116

Quality Improvement

EDWARD DICKINSON

It is significant that a chapter on quality improvement should appear for the first time in this textbook. This topic may sit uncomfortably for some in a textbook of geriatric medicine and gerontology but will undoubtedly have been encountered by practitioners and is of undisputed importance to the future health care of older people.

Fashion or Fact of Life?

There is no doubt that quality improvement has arrived in health care. Indeed, it is likely to be a prime concern in health systems into the next millennium. Initiatives in quality improvement have the greatest potential to achieve meaningful enhancements in the effectiveness, efficiency, equity, and humanity of health care. Some believe that the focus on quality is merely a management fashion or fad. However, this is a misguided view as will be argued in this chapter from three main standpoints. First, a number of influences have converged to place quality improvement firmly on the agenda, some generic and some specific to different health care systems. Second, the growing theoretical underpinning concerning quality improvement that now exists is beginning to be recognized, understood, and valued. Third, practical experience is accumulating and bringing confidence in more robust approaches to quality improvement than have been previously seen. The approaches of different countries varies but in the UK clinical audit is the prime quality improvement mechanism and is used as a case study of quality improvement.

A Central Consideration in Health Care of Older People

Nowhere is more appropriate than the health care of older people for leading edge quality improvement development. The history, current approaches, nature, and likely future of the care of older people provides ideal ground for such activities. Historically, the systematic application of quality improvement in the health care of older people builds on the firm foundation of the history of struggle for higher quality. The development of geriatric medicine and the care of older people is largely based on persistent striving at a local level for more and better services in the face of policy weakness, professional neglect, and resource starvation, coupled with poor training and a neglected research base. Currently, the team-based approach of the care of older people is ideally suited to modern methods of quality improvement that take a wider view of care than the activities of one professional group. The important aspect of the nature of the care of older people is its complexity. The demands of care involving different disciplines, specialties, and sectors are exacting and amenable to the very best quality improvement techniques. As regards the future, trends toward older populations and more community-based care mean that health systems will be under greater pressure to perform to the highest quality standards.

The purpose of this chapter is to provide the reader with theoretical understanding of and practical insights into quality improvement in health care with a special emphasis on the health care of older people. There is a deliberate inclusion of the clinical, managerial, and strategic perspectives because this continuum reflects the real background against which development is occurring. There are five main sections. The first two provide background material. To understand the wider context of quality improvement, the drivers toward quality and its origins are analyzed. This leads to consideration of the concepts and definitions of quality with an emphasis on how quality links with the other key functions of a health system. The next three sections are essentially practical. There is a description of practical principles of quality improvement, followed by a section on clinical audit. These are intended to contain generalizable messages for other approaches to quality improvement. The last section looks more widely at ways in which international collaboration might contribute to this process.

The Arrival of Quality Improvement

Although quality improvement seems to have advanced rather suddenly, a look at changes inside and outside health systems reveals a curious predictability in this change. For the unconvinced there is ample evidence that quality improvement is maturing rapidly from a marginal to a mainstream activity.

Revolutions in Health Care

Those with very long time horizons will like the idea of sequential revolutions in health care.[1] At first there is rapid expansion in the range and nature of health care activities.

This occurs mainly because of technological advances and the application of these new technologies. Ultimately this change results in concern about the costs of care. This might be expressed by governments or third-party payers who may take a variety of actions to control costs. However, in the third revolution, there is a reaction to the narrow focus on costs and a shift to ideas of accountability and quality. This might occur from a combination of consumer pressure, management influence, and a wider interest in outcomes as well as inputs. Cost containment is not palatable to consumers who grow accustomed to steady service improvement. Cost containment is largely an anathema to professional staff who are often not cost aware and do not wish to see cost control stand in the way of medical advances. Cost containment is also politically uncomfortable. Finally, there is the recognition that enormous amounts of money are wasted because of poor quality care through mistakes, duplication, and rework.[2] This makes third-party payers interested also.[3]

Causes of Change

At a more detailed level, multiple factors are promoting quality improvement with political, economic, social, and technologic perspectives. Health care systems throughout the world are facing the crisis of a mismatch between what is demanded and what is available. The crisis exists for patients, professionals, and policy makers. Political influences rank high among the causes of change, as health is usually high on the political agenda. Within many health care systems there is now a competitive market, either fully fledged or "internal markets" as in the United Kingdom. This brings with it the pressure to secure sustainable competitive advantage; many health managers have learned from colleagues in other sectors that achieving high quality is a most effective pathway to reach this goal. Health care consumes a high level of resources and this has led to questioning of the effectiveness and efficiency of health care. For example, within the United Kingdom the Audit Commission has been active in evaluating value for money in the National Health Service (NHS).[4] Much of this has been interpreted as steps to control the previous autonomy of doctors,[5] particularly in the face of unexplained variations in health care.[6,7] In social terms, there is a clear rise in consumerism as a result of secular changes in society and, in the United Kingdom, under the influence of governmental initiatives such as the Patient's Charter.[8] From the technology perspective, much of the blame for increasing costs is often laid at the door of new medical technologies while paradoxically it may be higher volume, low-cost activities that are responsible. Included in the drivers to change are also the powerful developments of the clinical guidelines "industry," clinical effectiveness, evidence-based medicine, and clinical audit itself.

Diffusion From Industry

These forces for the adoption of quality in health services have collided fortuitously with a diffusion of quality improvement into health care from other sectors of the economy. The story began in the manufacturing industry. After World War II, the rebuilding of Japanese industry provoked serious interest in quality improvement techniques and the success of this approach has been plain to see. Early workers, such as Deming and Juran, have become known as quality gurus. These and other gurus differ on details but have much in common: a focus on process, the need for management commitment, and a preventative perspective.[9] Although Deming was a statistician by profession, his ideas about quality management are strong on human aspects of work and the process (Table 116-1). During the late 1970s the growth of the service industry sector led to the development of interest in service quality improvement, with its special needs such as the unique role of customers in service operations. In the 1980s the interest in quality improvement diffused into the public sector and inevitably into health care.

Reality or Fantasy?

There is now plenty of evidence that quality improvement is becoming firmly established in health care (Table 116-2) and it is clear that this is occurring in many countries.[10] This is shown in many diverse ways. There are new societies and associations for those interested in this area. For example, the International Society for Quality in Health Care has a worldwide membership and permanent secretariat. The European Forum on Quality Management includes a special interest section on public services. There are new types of staff working in health care in quality or clinical audit departments. Physical evidence of quality improvement activities (such as reports, banners, or citations) is becoming more prominent in health care facilities. There are also awards for quality improvement: one of the best known is the Golden Helix Award for Quality Improvement in European Healthcare. To promote and share knowledge, there are new journals such as *Quality in Health Care* and *Evidence Based Medicine*; moreover, general journals are now more likely to contain papers and articles about quality improvement. Go to any professional conference and you will find seminars, talks, or posters on quality issues or projects. Indeed, there are now research and development institutions devoted to this area, such as the Institute for Healthcare Improvement in Boston, Massachusetts. It is clearly evident that quality is consuming much time, interest, and commitment.

The next section builds on this explanation of why quality improvement is firmly on the agenda to develop a deeper understanding of quality improvement.

Quality Improvement

Although quality improvement may have arrived, it is probably not yet a reliable concept in the minds of all health care professionals. The rapid advent of quality improvement has created some confusion as to definition, purpose, and philosophy. Not least, clashing and failed expectations have been generated because of quality improvement failures at an organizational level.

Table 116-1 Deming's Principles

Constancy of purpose	Create constancy of purpose by continual improvements of products and services. Take a long-term view, to stay competitive in business.
The new philosophy	Adopt the new philosophy of continual improvement. The new realities mean that commonly accepted delays and defective workmanship can no longer be tolerated. A transformation of Western management approach is needed.
Cease dependence on inspection	Stop depending on mass inspection. Build quality into the product in the first place. Demand statistical evidence of quality being built into manufacturing and purchasing functions.
End "lowest tender" contracts	End the practice of awarding business on the basis of price alone. Instead require other meaningful measures of quality beyond price. Work to minimize total cost not just initial cost. Move toward a single supplier for any one item on a long-term relationship of loyalty and trust.
Find problems: improve every process	It is management's job to improve the system continually by identifying problems and eliminating them to improve quality, increase productivity, and decrease costs.
Institute training on the job	This includes management, to make better use of all employers.
Institute leadership	Adopt and institute leadership aimed at helping people and machines do a better job. Supervisors should help people forget about the numbers game and concentrate on quality of products, which will automatically improve productivity.
Drive out fear	Drive out fear, so that everyone works effectively for the company, encourage top down and bottom up communication.
Break down barriers	People in different departments must work as a team to deal effectively with problems with products and services.
Eliminate exhortations	Eliminate numeric goals, slogans, exhortations (such as zero defects), and production targets for the work force because most quality problems have to do with processes and systems that are created by managers and are beyond the power of the employees. Such exhortations are simply a source of aggravations.
Eliminate numeric targets	Focus on quality.
Permit pride of workmanship	Remove the barriers that rob hourly paid workers and people in management of their right to pride of workmanship. Abolish performance appraisal and management by objectives.
Encourage education and retraining	Institute a rigorous program of education and encourage self-improvement in everyone.
Top management commitment	Structure top management to empower them to achieve the above 13 preceding points and take action to make the total transformation happen.

Existing Turmoil

This section begins the process of explaining what quality improvement is by looking at definitions and concepts to prepare the reader for the next section, which deals with more practical aspects. But before even trying to clarify the meaning of quality improvement, it is important to state that generally quality in health care is in a confused state at the moment. This is partly because of the speed of development, partly because of disparate interests, and partly because of the failure to use knowledge, understanding, and experience of other areas such as industry. The net effect is that the activities and management of quality are confused.

Table 116-2 Evidence for increasing quality momentum

Prizes	Golden Helix Award, Hospital Doctor Quality Awards, British Geriatrics Society Audit Prize
Associations	International Society for Quality in Health Care, Clinical Audit Association, Deming Association in Health Care, Association for Quality in Health Care
Conferences and seminars	Quality Forum of the Royal Society of Medicine, European Forum on Quality in Healthcare
Journals	*Quality in Health Care, Audit News, Evidence Based Medicine*

For example, the language of quality presents a substantial barrier. A multiplicity of terms are used in relation to quality—quality assurance, total quality management, kaizen, to name a few. A handbook of quality assurance in health care[11] details at least nine quality techniques. The disparate language has been parodied by Shaw who offered three columns of words that can be used to make up titles for 96 different quality activities[12] (Table 116-3). Many of those working in health care are showered with initiatives, activities, jargon, and buzz words. One effect of this is that the focus for quality improvement may be indistinct and the credibility of quality improvement lost. Much of the blame for this must lie with inadequate management. It seems clear that to succeed with quality improvement a clear, sustained, and committed approach is needed. The introduction of clinical audit in the United King-

Table 116-3 Words for quality

Pick one word from each column		
Medical	Care	Evaluation
Health	Standards	Assessment
Clinical	Activity	Assurance
Professional	Quality	Audit
		Review
		Meeting

dom illustrates these types of difficulties. Four features lead to uncertainty among clinicians:

- Confusion with other quality activities (such as those carried out by a quality department)
- No clear commitment of time
- Inadequate information base
- Difficulty implementing change when need for change identified by audit

The failure to harmonize agendas is illustrated by the clear separation of two quality initiatives—the Patients Charter and clinical audit—with resulting doubts and cynicism.

A Definition

A useful working definition of high quality care is "doing the right things well." Although this may seem rather trite, it is a useful working form of the longer definition of Brooks and Kosecoff:[13]

The performance of specific activities in a manner that either increases or at least prevents the deterioration in health status that would have occurred as a function of a disease or condition. Employing this definition, quality of care has two components: 1. The selection of the right activity or task or combination of activities, and 2. The best performance of those activities in a manner that produces the best outcome.

The "right things" are those for which there is agreement that they should be done derived from primary research, meta-analysis, clinical guidelines, contracts for care, and local care pathways. Doing things "well" demands that we understand the dimensions of quality so that we can judge performance in an appropriate fashion. Maxwell[14] has proposed six dimensions of quality and a list of possible dimensions is shown in the accompanying box, shortened by some to the following:

- Effectiveness/efficiency
- Equity
- Humanity

However, these lists of dimensions can be criticized as being rather provider or professionally based. There are alternatives that have been developed through quality models in other service industries and prompt us to consider the perspectives that should be used to specify quality.

Possible dimensions of quality

Relevance
Equity
Accessibility
Continuity and coordination
Ethical
Effectiveness
Efficiency
Social acceptability

Whose Quality?

Perhaps the best known alternative approach is the Gap Service Quality Model (GSQM).[15] Based on research, the way that the quality of services is judged by consumers was characterized. Several dimensions of service quality were identified, as shown in the accompanying box. The currency by which service quality is addressed with the GSQM is satisfaction. However, this is not the narrow view of satisfaction often encountered in health services but satisfaction based on the wide range of attributes shown, including technical effectiveness. Consumer satisfaction depends on the balance between consumer's expectation and the perceived level of service. Thus, a consumer with low expectations will be satisfied with a low level of service but a consumer with high expectations will be difficult to satisfy. The key determinant of perceived quality is the gap between expected and perceived service levels (as illustrated in Fig. 116-1). Quality can be improved by managing this gap and the subgaps that it comprises:

- *Gap 1.* Not knowing what customers expect
- *Gap 2.* Not having adequate service standards

Service quality dimensions

Access
Communication
Courtesy
Credibility
Reliability
Responsiveness
Security
Tangibles
Understanding

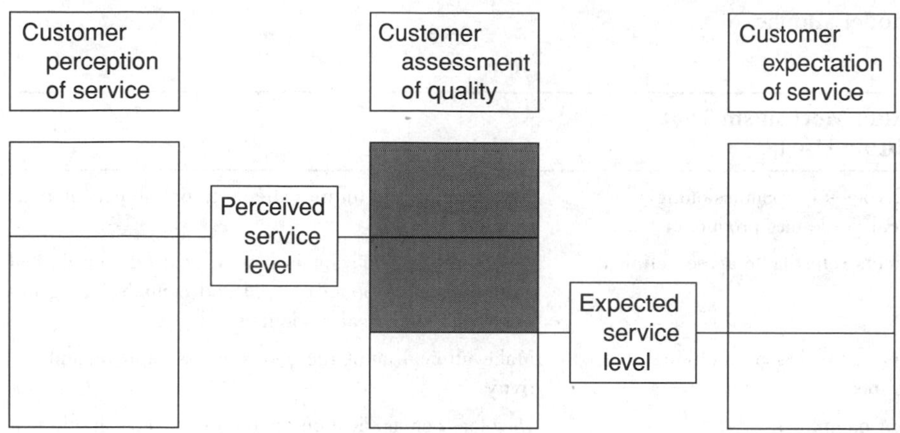

Figure 116-1 The Gap Service Quality Model. A satisfied customer: the perceived level of service (left bar) is higher than the expected level of service (right bar) and thus the customer's assessment of quality is favorable (shaded zone of center bar). (From Dickinson,[16] with permission.)

- *Gap 3.* Not delivering service according to specified standard
- *Gap 4.* Not communicating with customers
- *Gap 5.* Not listening to staff
- *Gap 6.* Not listening to past customers

Although this language and approach may seem alien to health services because it appears to dilute the importance of professionals and reduce judgments about health services to mere satisfaction, this is probably an overemotional and simplistic reaction. In using the services of an accountant, we would expect that the accountancy computations to be absolutely accurate. Indeed, we would be very concerned if they were not. However, we do not judge the quality of our accountant solely on mathematical accuracy. Thus, patients are likely to expect clinical effectiveness, preserving the technical core of interest to the professions, but only as a component of the overall quality of health care. By looking at quality in this way, opportunities appear to exist for melding together professional and consumer views in a complementary way. Defining quality in terms of patient expectations then becomes a broader exercise but not one that diminishes the importance of technical excellence and clinical effectiveness.[16]

Moreover, it is possible to map existing activities in the health service onto the GSQM framework and in this way begin to form a coherent and comprehensive quality improvement approach (Table 116-4). At the core of this is clinical audit for quality improvement, based on assessing implementation of agreed clinical guidelines. This approach matches the proposals of the US Agency for Health Care Policy and Research for measuring performance related to clinical practice guidelines.[17] The introduction of "league tables" in the United Kingdom has been controversial but mirrors the movement in the United States for managed care organizations to distribute "report cards" of their performance for their "customers."[18]

Improvement, Assurance, or Control?

One often hears of quality initiatives referred to as quality assurance. However, this term is now becoming less used as it does not accurately describe the ideal. "Assurance" is widely interpreted as checking the quality of a product or service once it has been manufactured or delivered. There are two problems. First, the process of assurance is too late—the focus needs to be on quality right from the beginning; it also lacks the important dynamic of quality improvement that is described in the next section. Thus, *quality improvement* is the preferred term for effective quality; it is often called continuous quality improvement (CQI) and is closely allied to the concepts of total quality management (TQM).[19]

Quality in Organizations

Finally in this section, there is need to dwell on how quality improvement links with other activities of the organization. Experience in the health service has often been that there are poor links with other functions such as management, finance, and training. Interesting work in the UK NHS suggests very strongly that where clinical audit has worked this has been achieved through its integration into the mainstream of activities.[20] Thus, successful audit programs shared critical factors such as the following:

- Clinical leadership
- Vision, strategy objectives, and planning
- Audit staff and support with basic structure and system
- Training and education
- Understanding and involvement of clinicians
- Supportive organizational environment

Others have described common problems reflecting these findings.[21,22]

Table 116-4 The gap service quality model and the UK National Health Service

Gap	Existing Mechanism That Might Be Used	Activity
Not knowing what customers expect	Local voices in commissioning Clinical guidelines production	Ask patients and future patients to define expectations from service.
Not having adequate service standards	Contracts referring to agreed clinical guidelines	Communicate with commissioners about existing clinical guidelines. Add organizational and commissioning implications to clinical guidelines.
Not delivering service according to specified standard	Clinical audit based on clinical guidelines	Make clinical audit the core quality improvement activity.
Not communicating with customers	Patient pamphlets League tables	Develop communication materials based on clinical guidelines and their implementation.
Not listening to staff		Build managerial mechanisms to respond to clinical audit findings.
Not listening to past customers	Satisfaction surveys	Promote active listening and meaningful communication.

Apart from internal challenges in developing quality improvement such as clinical audit, there may be external influences. For example, in the United Kingdom, commissioners of health care may have quite different expectations.[23] The experience of industry suggests the need to harmonize thinking—successful programs have enjoyed top management commitment and have been placed center stage—often to secure competitive advantage. This need for top management commitment appears to be generic as it has also been experienced in the business re-engineering projects in the NHS.[24]

This section has detailed some of the important underlying ideas of quality improvement at a conceptual and organizational level. The next section discusses how to turn these ideas into reality.

How to Improve Quality: Pathways to Success

Being clear about definitions and dimensions of quality is needed but is not sufficient to achieve success in quality improvement; there are some major steps to take and these are described. Experience suggests that these are most difficult steps to take and so they are considered generically in this section and more specifically in the section on clinical audit.

Choose the Correct Paradigm

The first practical step is to decide which paradigm is being followed. There is a strong temptation to adopt the approach of inspection; that is, there is an individual or team whose job is to check up on quality. Although they may be internal to the organization, they are external to the care delivery team. This approach is based on the precept that people are to be distrusted. Although much easier to adopt and put into action, there is broad agreement that this approach is doomed to failure. A far more powerful and effective approach is an internal approach; service staff are given resources to examine their own work and set objectives for improvement. This empowerment model is based on the idea that people are honest and committed; the latter is a recurrent value that is expressed when considering professional staff in health services. The contrast between these two approaches is shown in Table 116-5. The potential for clinical audit to develop along the empowerment paradigm is strengthened by a survey of UK provider units that described the potential for stimulating organizational change, changing the culture, and developing sensitivity to patients' needs.[25]

Guarantee "Top Management Commitment"

The second practical step is to ensure that the quality activity improvement enjoys top management commitment and in this, that words and deeds match. Too often, senior managers pay lip service to quality initiatives and they fail. Too often senior managers fail to provide adequate resources for quality and they fail. Too often senior managers confuse a variety of

Table 116-5 Inspection or empowerment

	Inspection	Empowerment
Value	Distrust	Trust
Focus	Regulation for safety	Management for quality improvement
Locus	External	Internal
Time frame	Intermittent	Constant
Stance	Reactive	Proactive
Coverage	Regulation oriented	Problem oriented
Style	Mechanistic	Developmental
Results	Punishment	Reward and recognition

Table 116-6 The quality toolbox

Tool	Description	Example
Quality method	Schemes of activities that staff will carry out	Clinical audit
Quality standard	Objectives to assess performances	Clinical guideline
Quality measure	Measures to enable comparisons	Case mix or outcome measure
Quality support system	Infrastructure to support quality improvement	Clinical audit staff, records, and administrative systems

(From Dickinson,[31] with permission.)

quality initiatives and they fail. Staff need to be absolutely confident that they are being led in a committed fashion toward success. This is achievable in real terms at a local level.[26]

Follow the Quality Cycle or Spiral

The third key to practical success is to make activities cyclical so that the quality of care can spiral upward. The purposes of this dynamic are twofold. First, in carrying out each clinical audit, there needs to be purposeful movement toward improvement. Thus, the team needs to consider the results of the audit against agreed standards of care and decide on objectives and a plan for improvement. A re-audit will disclose whether these objectives have been realized and indicate future areas for action. Second, there is a need to revisit the different topics of audit regularly. This highlights one of the difficulties of quality improvement in a complex service—it may be hard to audit everything; this indicates a need to prioritize on the basis of importance and, initially, likelihood of success.

Learning From Others—the Quality Tools

With the right paradigm, commitment, and quality spiral approach, what else could be needed? Two other complementary considerations are recommended. First, many of the basics of quality improvement will have already been developed by others. Thus, it is worth trying to find out if there is some transferrable knowledge. This might be obtainable from a professional organization, college, or quality organization. For example, the British Geriatrics Society publishes a compendium of its policy documents[27] and a catalog of existing guidelines has been produced.[28] Scanning recent journal issues may be fruitful. In the United Kingdom, services of the National Audit Centre, the Eli Lily Primary Care Audit Centre, the National R & D Network in the Health Care of Older People, or the National Clinical Guidelines Register—the two later initiatives are coordinated from the Royal College of Physicians of London—are available. More locally it may be helpful to contact colleagues in neighboring localities to seek out successful clinical audits. There are now published directories of activities.[29,30] Similar approaches will probably work in other countries depending on the local configuration of such resources. Indeed, much of the learning, particularly that in international journals, may be useful. Second, think in terms of the quality toolbox (Table 116-6) to make sense of what others are doing and what you propose. Usually at least two quality tools will need to be used and often all four will be required.

The Case of Clinical Audit

In this chapter clinical audit is used as a case study for learning about quality improvement. Clinical audit was introduced in the United Kingdom at the end of the 1980s and has now become the main quality improvement technique used by clinicians. This development has not been without major pitfalls although levels of involvement are now high and some successes can be claimed.

What Is Clinical Audit?

Clinical audit has been mentioned already in this chapter but there is a need to clarify the topic of discussion. Clinical audit has been defined as the "systematic critical analysis of the quality of medical care, including the procedures used for diagnosis and treatment, the use of resources and the resulting outcome for the patient."[32] The difference foci for audit activities are well established as structure, process, and outcome[33] (Table 116-7). The cyclical nature of audit has been described. From the start audit was promoted as an educational activity, endorsed by professional associations.[34,35] The early stages of debate and discussion clarified the boundaries of audit so that it became clear what clinical audit is not. Clinical audit is not clinical research although they often share the activity of systematic collection of standardized data. Clinical audit is not simply counting. Clinical audit is not necessarily complicated. It can be done just as effectively with a pencil and paper as with a highly powered computerized system.

Practical points include the following:

- *Define the quality activity*
- *Obtain support from the professionals who will be involved*
- *Open up a debate on the meaning of the definition*

Can Clinical Audit Fit in?

Clinical audit is now seen to fit quite well with a number of other important concurrent developments in the health care system that have been grouped under the banner of "clinical effectiveness." A bundle of similar initiatives is concerned

Table 116-7 The foci for clinical audit

Focus: Short Description	Structure: Resources	Process: Activities	Outcome: Results
Example	Buildings	Technical care	Health status
	Vehicles	Communication	Handicap
	Equipment	Coordination	Disability
	Staff and training	Teamwork	Impairment
	Policies and procedures	Timeliness	Mortality
	Intangibles—culture and philosophy		Satisfaction
	Finance		Caregiver's views
	Management systems		Avoidance of complications

with basing practice on existing knowledge. Evidence-based medicine is the new slogan for basing practice on what is known from trials.[37] Such evidence should form the basis for standards used in clinical audit. In some cases, conflicting trials or disparate evidence will need to be synthesized in a systematic manner to enable clear conclusions to be drawn from the research—this is the job of the Cochrane Collaboration (see International section). Clinical Guidelines are a tool for packaging the results of trials and systematic reviews in a format for use. Another approach is that of Getting Research into Practice (GRIP).[38] The second group of initiatives is concerned with systematizing data collection; thus, work on minimum datasets may contribute to clinical audit. Linked with this is the assessment of case mix. Several systems to assess case mix are being developed: ACME,[39] resource utilization groups (RUGs),[40] etc.; they all seek to categorize patients into groups that are homogeneous with respect to some important variable such as disease severity, length of stay, or resource use. Such measures will be useful to make valid comparisons of the results of audit over time or between units, hospitals, regions, or countries. Another form of comparison at an organizational level is accreditation. In the United Kingdom there are two main schemes: the Kings Fund Organisational Audit and South Thames NHS accreditation scheme. An exciting development would be linking accreditation to clinical audit.

Clinical effectiveness

Clinical guidance
- Reports of Royal Colleges and Specialist Societies
- Effective Health Care Bulletins
- Needs assessments
- Clinical guidelines
- Systematic reviews

Health technology assessment
- Population screening
- Cancer services
- Cardiovascular services
- Diagnostic and imaging services
- Other services

(From NHS Executive,[36] with permission.)

This could be achieved by making evidence of a healthy clinical audit program a requirement for accreditation. This would eliminate the "inspection" element of accreditation, strengthen confidence in clinical audit being undertaken as an internal activity, and preserve the empowerment paradigm of clinical audit. Finally, Joss and Kogan[41] demonstrate the potential for audit to respond to different TQM objectives. The closeness of fit is important in the development of new approaches; it has been argued that a lack of "fit" is one of the reasons why management experience often does not transfer well from industry to public health systems.[19]

Practical points include the following:

- *Think about the fit between your quality activity and other developments*
- *Consider developments in "political," research, and information technology spheres*
- *Stick with the empowerment paradigm*

Early Experience

Like any change in an established system, the introduction of clinical audit has not been completely successful. Indeed, concerns about value for money have prompted the attentions of the National Audit Office.[42] Their investigations in Scotland found a reasonably good uptake of clinical audit—60 percent of specialties in Scotland were participants and about 50 percent of primary care physicians—but there were constraints due to shortage of time, shortage of support staff, and the limitations of information technology. These may indicate a lack of top management commitment. At a local level, resources have been deployed in setting up departments of clinical audit and audit staff but it was difficult to obtain a reliable figure for the cost of clinical audit to set against the, albeit anecdotal, benefits seen in every hospital and practice visited. Although the audit cycle seems to be widely understood, a small proportion of reports of audits are of a "full cycle" nature.

Other work has identified fragmentation in audit; for example, misunderstanding of tribal boundaries was described in a study of nursing experience.[43] In relation to the therapy professions, audit has been found to be more often unprofessional.[44] A further issue is the role of purchasers. A regional project found little active involvement of them in clinical audit systems. Yet, the increasing detail of quality specifications in contracts indicates the increasing pressure for monitoring information that could be obtained through clinical audit. Thus, however much clinical audit is considered as a "good thing," significant challenges still exist in its implementation. The myriad evaluative studies have also indicated the major obstacles and areas requiring attention for clinical audit to fulfill its potential.[45–47]

Learning points include the following:

- *Anticipate difficulties in introduction because in general staff dislike change and threats*
- *Consider an incremental approach*
- *Work out the true resource implications and commit to them*
- *Consider the future roles of a range of stakeholders*
- *Make sure activities are cyclical*

Consolidation

Clinical audit appears to have now reached a stage of consolidation with a great deal of activity among the professionals and a restatement of the policy line by central government.[48] There is now a wealth of experience to tap into. An estimated 20,000 projects have taken place[49] with the majority of consultants (83 percent) and general practitioners (86 percent) participating. At the 1995 national meetings of the British Geriatrics Society, about 8 percent of all abstracts were concerned with audit; a wide range of subject matter was represented, ranging from service issues (such as nursing home entry), to geriatric syndromes (such as incontinence), to specific disorders (such as pelvic fracture and hypertension).[50,51]

A particular feature has been the execution of large-scale audit projects at a national level, building on the established tradition of large confidential enquiries. These include Confidential Enquiry into Maternal Deaths, and Confidential Enquiry into Perioperative Deaths.

This has been mirrored in the health care of older people and related areas:

- *Hip fracture*: in two regions (Scotland and East Anglia) there are large-scale ongoing audits of hip fracture care.[52,53]
- *Long-term care*: a large-scale full cycle audit of the quality of this neglected aspect of care has been carried out by the Royal College of Physicians. This used the CARE scheme, which is a ready-made clinical audit scheme based on a set of national clinical guidelines.[54–56]
- *Day hospital care*: a multicenter full cycle audit has been running using a ready-made audit scheme.[57]
- *National chronic wound audit*: this is an ongoing full cycle audit that is unusual in three respects: secondary care, community care, and primary care sectors are participating; the audit looks at processes of care and patient views; and staff from a wide range of backgrounds are taking part.
- *Stroke*: clinical audit in this area has been facilitated by a stroke audit package, complete with data collection and comparison software.[58]
- *Disabled people*: this is an ongoing developmental project concerned with hospital facilities for disabled people.[59]

In addition, further work is coming forward on postacute care, falls, osteoporosis, and confusion.

Practical points include the following:

- *Tap into the many local, regional, national, and international projects*
- *Learn from the experiences of others*
- *Consider using a ready-made audit scheme*

Challenges

The remaining challenges to clinical audit have recently been elucidated by the UK NHS Executive[48] as achieving:

- Multidisciplinary audit
- Multisectoral audit
- Patient-focused audit
- Links between audit and management
- Links between audit and education
- Clarity of purpose between providers and purchasers to avoid the policing conflict

Although the experience of the United Kingdom in the development of clinical audit has been used as an example of an approach to quality improvement, the move toward quality is an international movement. Thus, the next section illustrates some of the possibilities for international development.

International Collaboration

As indicated at the beginning of this chapter, quality improvement is relevant to most health care systems. Not surprisingly therefore is the beginning of international collaboration in activities of relevance to quality improvement.

Assembling Evidence—the Cochrane Collaboration

The major thrust toward assembling the evidence of the effectiveness of interventions is the Cochrane Collaboration.[60] The Cochrane Collaboration is an international network committed to producing and disseminating systematic reviews of health care research (also known as Cochrane Reviews). The Cochrane Collaboration was launched in 1993, based on Archie Cochrane's idea that health services should deliver care that research has shown to be effective.[61] He called for systematic reviews of randomized controlled trials of health care and suggested these should be organized by specialty. Cochrane Reviews are carried out in a very precise way and use the technique of meta-analysis to pool the results of trials.[62] They are designed to assist people in keeping up-to-date in their practice. Cochrane Reviews are quite distinct from traditional overviews, which have fallen into disrepute. Cochrane Reviews are regularly updated and maintained in an electronic database called the Cochrane Library (formerly called the Cochrane Database of Systematic Reviews or CDSR)[63] This is widely available and gives fast and easy access to research information. For each Cochrane Review there is a structured report, full citation of the studies included, and tabulations of the results with a graphic presentation of them (the latter forms the basis of the Cochrane Collaboration logo). The Cochrane Collaboration is guided by six principles: collaboration, building on peoples existing enthusiasm and interest, minimizing duplication of effort, avoidance of bias, keeping up to date, and ensuring access. To manage this massive effort and to preserve the collaborative spirit, the Cochrane Collaboration consists of different entities with different roles: Cochrane Centres, Collaborative Review Groups, Methods Working Groups, a Consumer Network, and the Fields. The interests of older people will be served by the Field known as the Cochrane Collaboration Field in the Health Care of Older People. This involves those concerned with both physical and psychological aspects of health in promoting the perspectives of older people in the work of the Collaboration.[64] There is liaison with a number of Cochrane groups producing systematic reviews because much of their work is of great relevance to the health care of older people.[65]

Setting Standards—Clinical Guidelines

The production of clinical guidelines is quickly becoming an international activity. It is highly likely that the clinical guidelines on the same subject will be similar despite being produced in different countries and the cultural differences in health care. Yet, there has been little serious collaborative work. However, there would be great advantages in joint production if culture-free topics could be identified. The avoidance of drug-induced iatrogenesis is a possible candidate as are the prevention of falls and the prevention of pressure sores.

Clinical Audit

A more recent development has been the advent of international audit projects. For example, there are two European initiatives concerned with hip fracture and stroke. The hip fracture audit originated in Sweden, is being replicated in Scotland, and is developing in other countries. The European Stroke Database (ESDB) is a wide-ranging collaboration involving over 100 centers in 15 European countries that aims to standardize basic data collection in all aspects of stroke care to create a "common clinical language." There is a free flexible "Basic Stroke Register" pack including free database software, data files, and an automated analysis system [D. Barer, personal communication].

Conclusion

This chapter has examined quality improvement in health services for older people in a comprehensive way, describing both theoretical and practical aspects of the subject. Advances have been made but significant challenges remain as illustrated by the case of clinical audit.

Links to research need to be much firmer. Although there are some positive moves in the right direction, much of this effort is hampered by the inadequacy of research. Health care of older people has encountered a triple jeopardy. First, older people have been systematically excluded from trials that would have produced useful information. [66,67] Second, common problems among older people have been under-researched such as incontinence and dementia. Third, gerontology has generally suffered from the relative underinvestment in health services research that is now being addressed.[68]

It is now recognized that one of the most important features of health systems for older people is their complexity and the need for research into systems of care. Funders have an ongoing responsibility to ensure that appropriate research is carried out to meet the practical needs of health services and these may be revealed when writing clinical guidelines or carrying out quality improvement activities.

Consideration of the research issues also demonstrates the paucity of information on the effectiveness of quality improvement activities such as clinical audit itself. Continuation remains largely an act of faith but one that has been grasped in industry and seems highly likely to continue in health services.

References

1. Relman AS: Assessment and accountability: the third revolution. N Engl J Med 1988;319:1220–1228
2. Berwick DM, Enthoven A, Bunker JP: Quality management in the NHS: the doctor's role I. In Smith R (ed): Audit in Action. British Medical Journal, London, 1992
3. Palmer RH: Quality health care. JAMA 1995;275:1851–1852
4. Audit Commission: Lying in Wait: The Use of Medical Beds in Acute Hospitals. HMSO, London, 1992
5. Office of Health Economics: Managing the NHS: Past, Present and Agenda for the Future. OHE, London, 1994
6. McPherson K: How should health policy be modified by the evidence of medical practice variations. In Marinker M (ed): Controversies in Health Care Policies. Challenges to Practice. British Medical Journal, London, 1994
7. Coulter A, Seagrove A, McPherson K: Relation between general practice's outpatient referral rates and rates of elective admission to hospital. BMJ 1990;301:273–277
8. Department of Health: The Patients' Charter: Raising the Standard. Department of Health, London, 1991
9. Speller S: Service Quality—the Missing Link. The Need for a Conceptual Model: A Case Study. Middlesex University Thesis, London, 1991
10. Reerink E: Arcadia revisited: quality assurance in hospitals in the Netherlands. In Smith R (ed): Audit in Action. British Medical Journal, London, 1992

11. Ellis R, Whittington D: Quality Assurance in Health Care. A Handbook. Edward Arnold, London, 1993
12. Shaw CD: The background. In Smith R (ed): Audit in Action. British Medical Journal, London, 1992
13. Brooks RH, Kosekoff JB: Evaluating the quality of medical care. Milbank Memorial Fund Q 1966;44(suppl):166–206
14. Maxwell RJ: Quality assessment in health. BMJ 1984;288: 1470–1472
15. Parasuraman A, Zeithaml VA, Berry LL: A conceptual model of service quality and its implications for future research. J Marketing 1985;49:41–50
16. Dickinson EJ: Developing Health Services for Patients. The Role of a Service Quality Model. Middlesex University Thesis, London, 1995
17. Agency for Health Care Policy and Research: Using Clinical Practice Guidelines to Evaluate Quality of Care, Volume 2: Methods. Department of Health and Human Services, Rockville, MD, 1995
18. US General Accounting Office. Health Care: Employers and Individual Consumers Want Additional Information on Quality. US General Accounting Office, Washington DC, 1995
19. Pollitt C: Business approaches to quality improvement: why they are hard for the NHS to swallow. Quality Health Care 1996; 5:104–110
20. Walshe K: The traits of success in clinical audit. In Walshe K (ed): Evaluating Clinical Audit: Past Errors, Future Directions. Royal Society of Medicine Press, London, 1995
21. Buxton MJ: Achievements of audit in the NHS. Quality Health Care 1994;3(suppl):31–34
22. Kerrison S, Packwood T, Buxton M: Monitoring medical audit. In Robinson R, Le Grand J (eds): Evaluating the NHS Reforms. King's Fund Centre, London, 1985 (Project paper No. 57)
23. Thomson R, Eliot C, Pugh E: Clinical audit and the purchaser-provider interaction: different attitudes and expectations in the United Kingdom. Quality Health Care 1996;65:97–103
24. Brindle D: Back to basics of the bar. Guardian 1996;24 July: 11
25. Buttery Y, Walshe K, Coles J, Bennett J: The Development of Audit. Findings of a National Survey of Health Care Provider Units in England. CASPE Research, London, 1994
26. Essex Rivers Healthcare: Quality Management Strategy. Essex Rivers Healthcare, Cochester, 1994
27. British Geriatrics Society: Guidelines, Policy Statements and Statements of Good Practice. British Geriatrics Society, London, 1995
28. Age Concern and Royal College of Physicians: Gold Standards. Age Concern, London, 1995
29. Smith R (ed): Audit in Action. British Medical Journal, London, 1992
30. NHS Management Executive: A-Z of Quality. A Guide to Quality Initiatives in the NHS. HMSO, London, 1993
31. Dickinson EJ: The quality movement. In Mayer PP, Dickinson EJ, Sandler M (eds): Excellent Care for Elderly People. Chapman & Hall, London, 1997
32. Department of Health: Working for Patients. HMSO, London, 1989
33. Donabedian A: Evaluating the quality of medical care. Milbank Memorial Fund Q 1966;44 (suppl):166–206
34. Royal College of Physicians: Medical Audit. A First Report. What, Why and How? Royal College of Physicians, London, 1989
35. Royal College of Physicians: Medical Audit. A Second Report. Royal College of Physicians, London, 1993
36. NHS Executive: Information on Clinical Effectiveness. Department of Health, London, 1996
37. Sackett DL et al: Evidence based medicine. BMJ 1996;312: 71–72
38. West Midlands Regional GRIP Group: Getting to GRIPs with stroke. GRIPKIT 1996/7. West Midlands NHS Executive Regional Office, Birmingham, 1996
39. Dunstan EJ, Amar K, Watt A et al: First steps in building ACME—an admission case-mix system for the elderly. Age Ageing 1996;25:102–108
40. Carpenter GI, Main A, Turner GF: Casemix for the elderly inpatient: resource utilisation groups (RUGs) validation project. Age Ageing 195;24:5–13
41. Joss R, Kogan M: Advancing Quality. Total Quality Management in the National Health Service. Open University Press, Buckingham, 1995
42. Payne B: Clinical audit: is it value for money? In Walshe K (ed): Evaluating Clinical Audit: Past Errors, Future Directions. Royal Society of Medicine, London, 1995
43. Kitson A, Harvey G, Morrell C: Does clinical audit improve the quality of nursing care? In Walshe K (ed): Evaluating Clinical Audit: Past Lessons, Future Directions. Royal Society of Medicine, London, 1996
44. Packwood T: Clinical audit in four therapy professions: results of an evaluation. In Walshe K (ed): Evaluating Clinical Audit: Past Lessons, Future Directions. Royal Society of Medicine, London, 1996
45. CASPE: Audit Activities of the Medical Royal Colleges and Their Faculties in England. CASPE Research, London, 1995
46. CASPE: Evaluating Audit: Provider Audit in England. A review of Twenty Nine programmes. CASPE Research, London, 1995
47. CASPE: Evaluating Medical Audit: Nursing and Therapy Audit: A Review of the Regions Role. CASPE Research, London, 1995
48. NHS Executive: Clinical Audit in the NHS. Using Clinical Audit in the NHS: A Position Statement. Department of Health, London, 1996
49. National Audit Office: Clinical Audit in England. National Audit Office, London, 1995
50. British Geriatrics Society: Communications to the Spring meeting of the British Geriatrics Society. Age Ageing 1995;24:suppl 2
51. British Geriatrics Society: Communications to the Autumn meeting of the British Geriatrics Society. Age Ageing 1996;25: suppl 2
52. Currie CT, Mountain JA: Mortality after hip fracture: a prospective study of 1214 consecutive admissions. Age Ageing 1996; 25(suppl 1):P24
53. Todd CJ, Freeman CJ, Camilleri-Ferrante C et al: Differences in mortality after fracture of the hip: the East Anglian audit. BMJ 1995;310:904–908

54. Brocklehurst J, Dickinson E: Improving the quality of long term care for older people. Lessons from the CARE scheme. Quality Health Care, 1997
55. Brocklehurst J, Dickinson E: Autonomy for elderly people in long term care. Age Ageing 1996;25:329–332
56. Research Unit of the Royal College of Physicians: The CARE Scheme (Continuous Assessment Review and Evaluation). Clinical Audit of Long Term Care of Elderly People. Royal College of Physicians, London, 1992
57. Research Unit of the Royal College of Physicians: Clinical Audit Scheme for Geriatric Day Hospitals. Royal College of Physicians, London, 1994
58. Royal College of Physicians and UK Stroke Audit Group: Stroke Audit Package. Royal College of Physicians, London, 1994
59. Royal College of Physicians and The Prince of Wales Advisory Group on Disability: A Charter for Disabled People Using Hospitals. Royal College of Physicians, London, 1992
60. Godlee F: The Cochrane Collaboration: deserves the support of doctors and governments. BMJ 1994;309:969–700
61. Cochrane AL: Effectiveness and Efficiency: Random Reflections on Health Services. Nuffield Provincial Hospitals Trust, London, 1972
62. Sackett DL, Oxman AD (eds): Cochrane Collaboration: Cochrane Collaboration Handbook. Cochrane Collaboration, Oxford, 1995
63. Cochrane Library 1996 Issue 2. BMJ Publishing Group and Update Software, Oxford, 1996
64. Dickinson E, Rochon P: Cochrane Collaboration in Health Care of the Elderly. Age Ageing 1995;24:265–266
65. Stroke Unit Trialists' Collaboration: A systematic review of specialist multidisciplinary team (stroke unit) care for stroke inpatients. In Warlow C, van Gijn J, Sandercock P (eds): Stroke Module of the Cochrane Database of Systematic Reviews [updated June 3, 1996]. Available in The Cochrane Library [database on disk and CDROM]. The Cochrane Collaboration; Issue 2. Update Software, Oxford, 1996
66. Gurwitz JH, Col NF, Avorn J: The exclusion of the elderly and women from clinical trials in acute myocardial infarction. JAMA 1992;268:1417–1422
67. Trimble EL, Carter CL, Cain D et al: Representation of older patients in cancer treatment trials. Cancer 1994;74:2208–2214
68. Medical Research Council: The Health of the UK's Elderly People. Research Issues and Opportunities. MRC, London, 1994

CHAPTER 117

Ethical Issues in Geriatric Medicine

JOHN HARRIS

Let's begin with a principle. A good one might be this: *An individual's entitlement to the concern, respect, and protection of the community does not diminish with age*. We might call this the first principle of gerontology. This principle has, I hope, a certain degree of initial plausibility, both as a general moral principle and as an appropriate one for geriatric medicine. Clearly this principle is itself the application of a more general principle. That more general principle is sometimes called the equality principle, which states that *each person is entitled to the same concern, respect, and protection of society as is accorded to any other person in the community*. The equality principle has the advantage of being generally accepted and versions of it are enshrined in many national constitutions throughout the world (the United States and France, for example). The first principle of gerontology simply reminds us that the equality principle applies as much in the face of discrimination on the basis of chronologic age or life expectancy as it does to discrimination on the basis of gender, race, and other arbitrary features.[1] We will soon explore the consequences of accepting such a principle for geriatric medicine and gerontology; this will help to show just how plausible a principle this is and also will allow us to review some of the most important ethical dilemmas that arise within gerontology. But why start with such a principle? Where do such principles come from?

Moral principles are not just plucked from the air, but neither are they derived from unassailable premises or immutable absolutes. They articulate central elements of a shared morality. Like the "Ten Commandments" they remind us of that morality and our commitment to it, and like the famous commandments they require interpretation. Does the proscription on killing include animals and plants? Are some commandments more important than others? Is the prohibition against coveting neighbors' oxen as important as that against coveting neighbors' wives?

However, moral principles also differ from commandments in important ways. Unlike commandments they do not attempt self-justification; they do not purport to explain *why* they ought to be accepted. So, when we articulate a moral principle we are reminding ourselves of what we believe to be an important part of the morality we accept. We should follow the principle *because* we accept the morality, but the principle cannot give us *reasons for* accepting the morality. When we encounter a principle we need first to reflect on our morality to see whether and how the principle fits with it. We then need to explore the consequences of accepting the principle to see whether we can adhere to it consistently with other moral beliefs we share and wish to retain. If the principle can be applied consistently with our general morality well and good, if not, we have to choose whether to abandon the principle or abandon the elements of our morality that are not consistent with it.

Ethics-Based Medicine

Let's now attempt this process with our principle and see what working through this process tells us about ethics-based medicine.

The principle with which we began, that an individual's entitlement to the concern, respect, and protection of the community does not diminish with age, is clearly part of a bigger idea, an idea that deals with entitlements or rights and in particular with entitlements to concern, respect, and protection. This group of entitlements is often termed *respect for persons* and we will need to analyze this idea into its constituent parts. But before doing so we must examine another assumption that has been made.

I'm assuming that medical ethics, or health care ethics as it is now more usually termed, is part of ethics more generally and that what it is ethical to do to and for people within a health care system, or "clinically," is constrained by our general morality. The assumption being made then is that the delivery of health care, both individually and within a health care system, is a dimension of our more general obligations to one another and in particular, that it is entailed by those commitments we have to honor other people's entitlements to concern, respect, and protection. In short, the duties of health care professionals, insofar as they are ethical duties, are derived from general morality and are not part of a particular ethics of health care. The ethical *dilemmas* that arise within a health service may be different from those arising within a prison service, for example, but the principles that inform the *resolution* of those dilemmas are drawn from our general morality.

Resistance to this idea often comes from a confusion about the different sorts of normative systems that operate within any society. Our general morality is just one of the normative systems that operate within society, albeit the one to which all others are answerable. Other general normative systems include the rules governing good manners or etiquette, and, of course, the legal system. Then there are the rules of particular professions, occupations, corporations, or clubs that are often rather misleading, referred to as codes of professional ethics or corporate ethics. All or any of these normative systems may enjoin or forbid things in the name of morality, and the operation of these normative systems may generate ethical dilemmas. But the breach or observance of the requirements of any of these systems is not of itself an ethical issue except insofar as it *also* involves our general morality. For example, although it is always wrong (incorrect) to break the law, it is not always morally wrong. The law requires us to drive on the left in the United Kingdom. There is nothing unethical about driving on the right except insofar as it is dangerous to do so where others are conforming to the law. If it is morally wrong to commit murder it is so not because law forbids it; rather the law forbids it because it is morally wrong.

Medical or health care ethics may then be construed as the ethical code of a particular profession of professions or of the health care system. So construed it has limited force and will appeal, at most, only to members of those professions, or perhaps, more pessimistically, to those who wish to continue to be members of those professions. As we shall construe it, however, it is the application of our general morality to the dilemmas of health care.[2] Thus construed, health care ethics applies as much to patients and their friends and relatives, as it does to doctors and nurses and it is as concerned with the general obligations of society to provide health care as it is with doctors' duties to deliver it.

Respect for Persons

Respect for persons, which is the basis of any ethics of care, and of which our first principle of gerontology is an expression, involves four crucial elements. They are (1) concern for the welfare of others; (2) respect for their wishes; (3) respect for the intrinsic value of their lives; and (4) respect for their interests.

When I suggest that these four elements are crucial to any respectable conception of respect for persons I mean simply that no one could claim to respect persons if their attitude to others failed to take account of these four elements. This, of course, does not take us very far because we need to know both how to *understand* each of these elements, and also, of course, how to *prioritize* them. Obviously people can have self-harming preferences, and where they do we need to decide whether it is more important to respect their wishes or demonstrate concern for their welfare.

However, these four dimensions of what it is to respect persons provide a useful framework for considering the ethics of geriatric medicine and gerontology because they remind us of the particular ethical dilemmas facing all those involved in patient care.

Achieving the right balance between concern for welfare and respect for wishes not only serves to remind us that welfare is not an end in itself but an instrumental good that, at a certain level, frees individuals to create their own lives, but also invites us to consider whether and to what extent individuals are in fact capable of authentic choices. Thinking about the intrinsic value of lives reminds us that many people think that the intrinsic value of lives differs between individuals and that this provides a basis for prioritization not only between individuals but between groups of individuals, young and old, for example. Finally, thinking about just what is involved in respecting people's interests reminds us that it is not always in someone's interests to remain alive or to have their life prolonged and that we may have a legitimate interest both in the manner and the timing of our own death.

The agenda we have set for ourselves can thus be seen to embrace some of the more traditional "headings" of medical ethics in the context of geriatric medicine: euthanasia, informed consent (especially in the mentally incompetent patient), equity and rationing, and limiting treatment (do not resuscitate orders and withholding aggressive treatments). We can now work through this agenda and see where and to what extent the first principle of gerontology can be of use in resolving the dilemmas we will encounter.

Euthanasia

Euthanasia is in a sense the ultimate issue for any ethic of respect for persons, and advocacy of any form of euthanasia is sometimes thought to be inconsistent with such an ethic. I shall be concerned with two types of euthanasia: voluntary, where the individual herself wishes to die and has clearly expressed such a wish, and nonvoluntary, where the individual is no longer competent, but it is believed euthanasia is in the individual's best interests or where it is believed the individual would have wished to die in these circumstances. We will start by trying to clarify the ethics of voluntary euthanasia. Where respect for the intrinsic value of life, and indeed concern for another's welfare, seem to conflict with respect for that person's wishes, what should we do? We must consider these two possible conflicts separately.

Welfare Versus Wishes

To resolve the apparent conflict between concern for welfare and respect for wishes we need to remind ourselves of the point of valuing liberty—freedom of choice. The point of autonomy, the point of choosing and having the freedom to choose between competing conceptions of how, and indeed why, to live is simply that it is only thus that our lives become in any real sense our own. The value of our lives is the value we give to our lives. And we do this, so far as this is possible at all, by shaping our lives for ourselves. Our own choices, decisions, and preferences help to make us what we are, for each helps us to confirm and modify our own character and enables us to develop and to understand ourselves. So autonomy, as the ability and the freedom to make the choices that shape our lives, is quite crucial in giving to each life its own special and peculiar value.

Concern for welfare, and the paternalist control it is so often used to justify, ceases to be legitimate at the point at which, so far from being productive of autonomy, so far from enabling the individual to create her own life, it operates to frustrate the individual's own attempts to create her own life for herself. And of course this also applies in the limiting case of suicide or, of course, to voluntary euthanasia, where the individual's attempts to create her own life involve creating its ending also.

Welfare thus conceived has a point, as does concern for the welfare of others; it is not simply a good in itself. We need welfare, broadly conceived in terms of health, freedom from pain, mobility, shelter, nourishment, and so on, precisely because welfare is *liberating*. It is what we need to be able to pursue our lives to best advantage. So where concern for welfare and respect for wishes are incompatible one with another, concern for welfare must give way to respect for autonomy.

Does Voluntary Euthanasia Conflict With an Ethic of Valuing Life?

This question has been much illuminated by recent debates surrounding the issue of persistent vegetative state (PVS) and we will try to resolve it by considering the issues raised by PVS. This is the condition that was at issue in two crucial cases of highest jurisdiction in the United States and in the United Kingdom, those of Nancy Cruzan and Tony Bland. We will take the Bland case as our exemplar.[3,4] Both Nancy Cruzan and Tony Bland had been left in a PVS following accidents. This is an unconscious state that, after 6 months' to a year's duration, is accepted as permanent and irreversible. People in PVS do not require life support as this is usually understood, although they do require tube feeding and hydration. They are not, nor without assistance will they become, "dead" according to any of the current criteria or accepted definitions of death.

Tony Bland's parents asked the courts to rule that his death could be brought about by withdrawal of feeding and withholding of other life-sustaining measures including antibiotics. After withdrawal of feeding he was expected to succumb to infections from which he would die without antibiotics. In advance of the various hearings, it had been expected that the issue in court would turn on whether it was lawful to withdraw feeding and starve someone to death. There were legal precedents for decisions to withdraw life-sustaining *medical* treatment, but few considered feeding to be a "treatment" and hence something that doctors could withdraw on the basis of their judgments as to whether the measure at issue was in the patient's best interests or could be afforded by the health care system. To their credit the courts did not attempt to stretch the meaning of "medical treatment" to cover feeding, thus attempting to give the doctors clinical discretion in the matter, but squarely faced the issue of whether or not Tony Bland should continue alive.

The three judges of the Court of Appeal and the five judges in the House of Lords were unanimous in concluding, albeit for very different and sometimes inconsistent reasons, that it was lawful to withdraw feeding in order to end Tony Bland's life. Their decision was in effect one permitting nonvoluntary euthanasia. Because Tony Bland was not dead, and would not die unless the Law Lords permitted a definite course of action that would result in his death, their decision to the effect that it was permissible to end his life when it otherwise would have continued indefinitely, effectively brought his life to an end. And indeed, such a decision was sought by Tony Bland's parents for precisely that reason. Because the Law Lords knew that Bland's parents fully intended to halt tube feeding if they permitted it, they knew Tony Bland's life or death hung on their decision.

If we ask what justified the nonvoluntary euthanasia of Tony Bland, I believe none of the reasons given by the various judges is satisfactory. If it is believed that there is a sanctity that attaches to the lives of humans then, as a live human, Tony Bland does not relevantly differ from others whom it is wrong to kill. If, however, it is the lives of *persons* that are sacred in this sense and if the value of their lives is expressed in terms of the respect due to persons in virtue of their personhood, we get a different answer. For although a live human being, Tony Bland, at the time of the courts' deliberations, was no longer a person. Respect for persons no longer applied to him.

It is always helpful in ethics to try to present a clear and positive account, if only to provide those who disagree with all they require for effective refutation. We should, however, note two obvious sorts of objection to the above account. The first would be, and was indeed, presented by the Law Lords who rejected the idea that end-of-life decisions such as those taken in the case of Tony Bland amount to euthanasia. The Lords held that even decisions such as theirs, which effectively brought about the death of an individual, did not in law amount to euthanasia.

Of course, opponents of euthanasia also differ from the position defended above, although they can, and often do, agree with accounts such as this in all its essentials. The point of difference between those who reject euthansia and those who defend it usually turns, as I have indicated, on whether or not the sanctity of existence applies to humans or rather to persons. If to the former, then euthanasia must be rejected; if to the latter a different conclusion follows.[5] To be clearer about why this is so we must look more closely at the idea of personhood.

Personhood

We have so far avoided addressing specifically the question of just what it is that makes individuals persons, but we must now say something about this absolutely crucial idea. Personhood is that set of characteristics that distinguishes persons from other creatures, such as most animals and all plants, and that accounts for the special importance we attach to persons. It is the sense of self, the characteristics that enable us to have a life in which we can take an interest and which enables us to have interests that we wish to see protected. When personhood has permanently disappeared, as in PVS, we are inclined to use language that suggests that the individual we once knew is no longer there although the living human body they once animated is still present. I do not have space here to do justice to the concept of personhood. I have tried to do so elsewhere.[2] However, I do not believe that any sense can be made, for example, of the various legal judgments in the Bland case without resort to such a concept. In the words of Lord Keith of Kinkel in his judgment in that case, "It is, however, perhaps permissible to say that to an individual with no cognitive capacity whatever, and no prospect of ever recovering any such capacity in this world, it must be a matter of complete indifference whether he lives or dies."[4] Lord Keith's, perhaps unconscious, use of the term "individual" rather than that of "person" in this part of his judgment makes the point I am trying to express, namely that not all human beings are persons.

The Idea of Respect for Persons

Respect for persons requires that it is persons who will be respected and hence their interests. Where, however, the person no longer exists, the interests of the former person, although still worthy of our respect, must of necessity give way to the significant interests or preferences of actual people. Thus John's interest, if he can be said to have one, in a further 30 years of life in a PVS would give way to the significant interests or preferences of any actual persons, persons to whom the satisfaction, or not, of their desires can continue to matter. And this would surely accord with our intuitions here. We would not, I imagine, think that someone who could no longer benefit from, or appreciate the life he was leading, should have that life sustained, when to do so would cost the lives of others who could appreciate, and benefit from, their continued existence.[2]

If euthanasia is to be permitted, this will not be because everyone should accept that it is right, nor because to fail to do so violates a defensible conception of the sanctity of life, but simply because to deny a person control of what, on any analysis, must be one of the most important decisions of life, is a form of tyranny, which like all acts of tyranny is an ultimate denial of respect for persons.[6]

We have looked at some of the arguments that would sustain approval of voluntary euthanasia and euthanasia where an individual has permanently ceased to be a person, as in the case of PVS. The most problematic cases of euthanasia, however, are those where consent is itself problematic and before drawing any conclusions about these we must look at the issue of consent more generally.

Consent

The centrality of consent in health care ethics is a function of the importance accorded to autonomy; and autonomy itself, as we have suggested, is part of our concept of the person. It is because we accept that the meaning and purpose of an individual's life are largely acts of self-creation that we are concerned to protect those attempts at self-creation even where we are convinced that they are misguided or even self-harming. However, although the importance of consent derives from our concept of the person, its procedural primacy in health care is owed to the common law tradition that protects individuals from assaults, that is, from unlawful touchings. It is consent that makes laying your hands on someone else lawful—hence the importance of obtaining valid consents to all medical procedures that involve interventions that compromise the bodily integrity of patients.

Just as forcing someone to go on living when they find life intolerable is a terrible form of tyranny and constitutes a denial of the ethic of respect for persons, so also does treating someone who has not consented and who is capable of choosing for herself whether or not she wants treatment. This principle is a cornerstone of medical ethics and is endorsed by the law in most jurisdictions. Both ethics and prudence therefore combine to support it. However, there are many cases where consent is problematic or cannot be obtained prior to treatment and these raise not only special problems of justification, but also special problems of explaining why interventions are justified.

Problematic Consent

Because there are so many cases in health care practice that necessitate touching patients in circumstances where their consent cannot be obtained and where knowledge of their wishes is absent, the law has contrived various fictional consents to protect well-intentioned practitioners from the guilt of unlawful conduct. The moral necessity of obtaining a valid consent where this can be obtained does not require further discussion. To violate the bodily integrity of persons who reject such violation is a form of tyranny and should be accepted and treated as such. We must, however, look more closely at those cases where consent or its refusal is problematic, and at the fictionalized consents that are often manufactured in these circumstances.

There are a number of instances in health care where the patient's consent is appealed to and used, where her actual consent is unobtainable. These are circumstances in which the patient is either unconscious or unable to process the information required to give a valid consent, or is temporarily or permanently lacking the relevant capacity to consent. In such cases terms like *proxy consent*, *substituted judgment*, *presumed consent*, or even *retrospective consent* are used to justify treating a patient. However, not only are these all fictions, but they totally fail to be justifications for treating the patient in particular ways.

Here of course we shall be advancing a thesis that runs counter to much contemporary thinking on consent that seems at home with attributing consent to individuals who are totally unaware that they are supposed to be consenting or are unaware at the time the consent is operative (as in the case of retrospective consent).

The reason why it is right to do what presumed consent or substituted judgment seems to suggest in these cases, is simply because treating the patient in the proposed ways is in his best interests and to fail to treat him would be deliberately to harm him. It is the principle that we should do no harm that justifies treating the patient in particular ways. The justification for treatment is not that the patient consented, nor that he would have, nor that it is safe to presume that he would have, nor that he will when he regains consciousness or competence, but simply that it is the right thing to do, and it is right precisely *because* it is in his best interests. That it is the "best interests"' test that is operative is shown by the fact that we do not presume consent to things that are not in the patient's best interests, even where it is clear that he would have consented. We do not infuse known heavy smokers with cigarette smoke while they are unconscious even where it is reasonable to suppose they would have consented and patients are often denied access to alcoholic beverages or cigarettes, even when they specifically request them.

Of course, we do not give beneficial treatment to patients who have refused them, say by advanced directive, because to do so would constitute an assault and a violation of their will. But it is not a violation of someone's will, nor is it an assault, to give a treatment they have not refused, the withholding of which would constitute an injury. And the reason it is not a violation is not because they have consented in some notional or fictional sense, but because it is the right thing to do. And the reason it is the right thing to do is that to fail or omit to do it would injure the patient. It is the infliction of that injury, by act or omission,[7,8] that would constitute the violation or assault. In short, if someone has not indicated clearly that it would be a violation of his will to refrain from injuring him, then we should not injure him.

It is widely held that not only should we not harm people who do not want to be harmed, we also should not harm even those who do want to be harmed, and that this is sufficient reason not to withhold treatment the absence of which would harm. This raises the question of the right to harm oneself. What of the responsibilities of the shopkeeper who sells cigarettes? Two points need to be made here. The first is that the shopkeeper, as we have here suggested, has sufficient moral reason not to sell cigarettes and would not be wrong to refuse to do so regardless of the preferences of his customers. Second, the delivery of health care is not straightforwardly like the marketplace, despite recent UK government attempts to make it so, and health professionals have often refused to give "treatments," for example, those they regard as mutilating, regardless of the expressed preferences of patients for such treatments.

Not only do we not need the concept of implied or assumed or proxy consent, because it literally does not work; we do not need it because it misleads us as to the character and meaning of our actions. The nineteenth century philosopher Jeremy Benthan was rightly scathing of fictional consents, and he remarked[9]:

In English law, fiction is a syphilis, which runs in every vein, and carries into every part of the system the principle of rottenness. Fiction of use to justice? Exactly as swindling is to trade. It affords presumptive and conclusive evidence of moral turpitude in those by whom it was invented and first employed.

So where, in medical contexts, we act in the best interests of patients who cannot consent, we do so, I suggest, because we rightly believe we should not harm those in our care and not because some irrelevant person or the law has constructed a consent. This does not help with the vexed problem of who is and who is not competent to consent, but it does explain the justification for intervening in the lives of those we are satisfied are not able to give the consents that would otherwise be required.

If the treatment of those whose consent is impaired is problematic, and decisions to discharge them from care equally so, what of research?

Research on Cognitively Impaired Elderly Subjects

There is nothing special about research on cognitively impaired elderly subjects. Cognitive impairment is only significant in this context insofar as it also involves impairment of autonomy and the elderly are not importantly different from other age groups from the point of view of consent.[10]

First we should note the difficulty of distinguishing between research and therapy. Many definitions have been provided and most rely at some point on making the distinction by reference to the intentions of those carrying out the work.[11,12] However, any distinctions based on intent are at best suspect and at worst susceptible to manipulation. The intentions of people are usually mixed and confused. Medical staff may, and doubtless often do, simultaneously intend to do many things when they treat their patients. They may intend to care for patients, offer relief of symptoms, identify and eradicate causes of disease, hone their medical skills, further their careers, satisfy their curiosity, generate research data, carry out instructions, and so on. Identifying *primary* intent is hardly more helpful because it either relies on a degree of self-awareness that few can achieve, or it simply stipulates one of many possible or actual intentions as paramount for the purposes of bringing the activity into an appropriate or permitted category.

This does not mean that there is no distinction to be drawn between research and therapy, but rather that the distinction cannot be drawn sufficiently clearly to sustain claims that therapy is justified whereas research is not. This is perhaps less worrying than might at first appear. The work supposedly done by the distinction between research and therapy might as easily be accomplished by concentrating on the degree of advantage to the patient. We could say that interventions, whether motivated by research or therapeutic imperatives, are permissible if either the patient accepts and consents to the interventions, or, where consent is unobtainable, that the interventions are the best available treatment for the patient, whether or not they also constitute research.

However, it is worth pursuing the distinction between therapeutic and nontherapeutic research a bit further, because, insofar as it is coherent, it relies on a suspiciously narrow view about the definition of "therapeutic" and also about what is, in fact, in every patient's best interests.

The following two claims are often made in this context: (1) The patient's interests are paramount: (2) Research on patients who cannot consent for themselves must be either (i) therapeutic *or* (ii) In the patient's own interests *or* of potential benefit for the patient herself *or* (iii) If not directly for the benefit of the particular patient in question, at least for the benefit of the category of patients to which the subject belongs, so that for example, if the patient has Alzheimer's disease, then research will only be justified if the research will be of benefit if not to the patient herself, at least to other patients with Alzheimer's disease. Neither claim seems sustainable and since the claims are often repeated, it is worth taking a moment to see why this is so.

The patient's interests cannot be paramount for the simple and sufficient reason that being or becoming a patient is not the sort of thing that could conceivably increase either your rights or your moral claims. All people are morally important and with respect to one another each has a claim to equal consideration. No one has a claim to overriding consideration. To say that the patient's interests are paramount, if it means anything, must be seen as a way of reasserting that health professionals are concerned primarily for the patients in their care and may have special contractual duties to them. However, as a general remark about the obligations of the health care system, or of society, it is not sustainable.

The second claim is equally problematic. To assert that research must be therapeutic or in the patient's own interests is not plausible when interpreted as confining research to work that will benefit particular patients directly, in the sense that they will themselves, so to speak, "feel the benefit" or that it will serve their continuing interests.

Let's look at the idea of what is or is not in someone's interests first. We must be wary of being too conservative about what does or does not benefit someone or of defining someone's interests too narrowly. We all benefit from living in a society in which medical research is carried out and which utilizes the benefits of past research. It is both of benefit to patients and it is in their interests to be patients in a society that pursues and actively accepts the benefits of research and where research and its fruits are given a high priority. We all have benefited and continue to benefit from research that was not targeted on us, indeed most of us will have benefited from research undertaken before we were born. We all benefit from vaccines. Some diseases (smallpox) have been eradicated as a result of vaccines, so that vaccination is no longer needed. For current diseases, even if we do not accept vaccination, we benefit substantially from the fact that there are vaccines and from the fact that others, perhaps less selfish or ignorant, do accept vaccination, for this reduces the incidence of diseases to which we, or our children, may be exposed. (Of course those who reject vaccination may be more intelligent if they can count on the rest of us being less intelligent, for then they can "ride free" on the back of our public spiritedness.) Standards of public health are higher and we all benefit. We benefit from research into the causes of diseases that has not only resulted in treatments but has generated screening programs and preventive strategies. Of course, screening programs are arguably a mixed blessing and can cause gratuitous anxiety, particularly where treatment is problematic. We all also benefit from the knowledge that research is ongoing, into diseases or conditions from which we do not currently suffer but to which we may succumb. It makes us feel more secure and gives us hope for the future, for ourselves and our descendants, and others for whom we care. If this is right, then I have a strong general interest that there be research, and in all well founded research; not excluding but not exclusively, research on me and on my condition. All such research is also of clear benefit to me. A narrow interpretation of the requirement that research be of benefit to the subject of the research is, I believe, perverse. If the claim that research on subjects who cannot consent for themselves is justified only if narrowly targeted on conditions from which those subjects currently suffer, and which will likely bear fruit in time to be of direct benefit to them is to be sustained, then it requires separate argument and support. There is no reason, however, to take this narrow interpretation as the standard one.

The third suggestion, that research that is not directly beneficial to the patient be confined to research that will benefit the category of patients to which the subject belongs is also untenable. What arguments sustain the idea that the most appropriate reference group is that of fellow sufferers from a particular disease, Alzheimer's, for example? Surely any moral obligation I have to accept risk or harm for the benefit of others is not plausibly confined to others who are narrowly like me. This is surely close to claiming that research should be confined to others who are "black like me" or "English like me" or "God-fearing like me"? The most appropriate category is surely "human like me."

Justice

Where I benefit from research but refuse to participate in it I am clearly acting unfairly in some sense. I am free-riding on the back of the contribution of others. Although we may conclude that people are ultimately entitled to act unfairly in this way if they choose, that they should not normally be compelled to contribute or participate, there is no reason to presume that those who cannot consent would have wished to be free riders. Indeed, as we have argued, there is no justification for any presumptions about their willingness to consent, in the absence of clear indications about their preferences. What is clear, I believe, is that there is no basis for any presumption that those who cannot consent should be excluded from research, whether that research is targeted on their condition or not. Nor, of course, is there any basis for the presumption that those who cannot consent should be, so to speak, "professional research subjects." They should neither be automatically included in research perhaps because they happen to be readily available in institutions or under continuing care, nor should they be automatically excluded.

We have been talking very generally and assuming a favorable risk/benefit balance for the research subjects: namely that the risks and pain, discomfort, or inconvenience of the research are minimal, and the projected benefits clear. There is clearly a trade-off between risks and benefits and a fairly steep upward curve where we demand that the benefits be clear and urgent before we will accept significant risks or pain inconvenience and so on for ourselves. We should surely apply the same standards to those who cannot consent. I cannot say anything useful or original about this balance. Clearly I will only accept significant risk of death for myself if without accepting such risk there is an almost certainly and substantially worse outcome for myself or those I care about. However, even here the risks are not plausibly undertaken only to benefit oneself. Live kidney donors, for example, clearly accept significant risks for others and we usually applaud their decision to do so.

We should note also that while generally we judge the decision whether or not to participate in research, as one for individuals to make for themselves, whether or not we reserve the right to criticize their decision, we do not accept that there is no obligation to take risks in the public interest nor that compulsion is always ruled out in such cases. There clearly is an obligation (sometimes) to make sacrifices for the community or an entitlement of the community to deny autonomy and violate bodily integrity in the public interest and this obligation is recognized in a number of ways. The following brief list of areas in which this is already recognized and accepted to some extent will serve as a reminder:

- Control of dangerous drugs
- Control of road traffic
- Vaccination
- Screening tests
- Blood donation
- Quarantine for communicable disease
- Compulsory military service
- Detention under mental health acts
- Restriction on sexual and professional activities with the human immunodeficiency virus

An example that seems to illustrate, and to an extent explain, our attitude to the imposition of risk in the public interest involves the following story. Imagine an ocean liner on a cruise. The captain receives a radio message that there is another ship in distress some miles to the north. There are 200 people aboard this other ship and his liner has 1,000 aboard. His is the only ship that can effect the rescue before the stricken ship will founder. He knows that if he diverts into the storm he will impose some risk on his passengers and crew. There will be a small but significant risk of death for all. The storm is a bad one but the modern liner should be able to cope. There is a greater, but still small, risk of death for a few of his passengers and crew in the rough and tumble of the rescue. Finally, because the storm is severe, he will almost certainly be subjecting his many elderly passengers to risk of minor injuries in the rough seas and certainly to discomfort, fear, and inconvenience. Significantly, we don't have to ask what he should do. The captain knows he must attempt the rescue and subject his passengers and crew to the attendant risks and few would disagree. He also knows that he can and must do so without asking for the consent of his passengers and crew, for they would be wrong to withhold their consent and the captain would be wrong to act on it.

The list of areas in which, I believe, similar decisions are made in our society shows that the principles involved are not unfamiliar or indeed unacceptable. Why then should we assume, when considering the ethics of research involving say, congnitively impaired elderly subjects, that different principles should apply?

First, let's just remind ourselves what these principles are, and then go on to see if they are constrained in any way by the situation of patients whose consent is problematic. The principles involved are all dimensions of the principle of equality from which our first principle of gerontology was derived. That principle is, it will be remembered, *that each person is entitled to the same concern, respect, and protection of society as is accorded to any other person in the community*. This principle reminds us that the passengers on the stricken liner have as good a claim to our protection as any other persons (although they may not be fellow citizens), and that although we are not obliged to afford that protection at all costs, we are obliged to act morally when the costs of so doing are reasonable given the importance of what is at stake. I hope it is obvious that if acting morally were only obligatory when doing so was cost free to the agent, morality would not exist. It is not plausible to believe that the costs of acting morally fall only on those competent to consent. So long as we ensure that such costs do not fall *more heavily* on those not competent to consent than on others I can see no sound argument for exempting them from the demands of morality. They may not be *accountable* in law, if they do wrong, but there is no reason to ensure that they do wrong, by exempting them from their moral obligations. The fact that the moral obligations in question are not mandatory, in that competent individuals may not, usually, be coerced into fulfilling them, does not seem to be a reason for exempting those not competent to consent. We do not allow children (or we should not) to do wrong because some adults may freely do so. However we constrain children not only because we are, in part, morally responsible for their actions, but also because this is part of an education process. The right parallel with adults who lack competence might be to include them in research when, although not competent to consent or refuse, they make no overt objection to inclusion or complaint about it. Where they do object or complain, we should perhaps respect that, albeit incompetent, rejection of this particular moral obligation.

Doubtless this defense of the idea that there can be an obligation to participate in research in certain circumstances, whether those who participate are capable of consenting or not, will strike some as controversial. The prohibition of research on those incapable of consent except where the research is in their own therapeutic interest is a principle founded on the highest of motives, that of the need to protect the vulnerable. However, the same motive animates the position defended here. It is not only the incompetent who are vulnerable in the requisite sense. We are all vulnerable unless research is pursued. The issue is one of balance. If research can be pursued without recourse to those whose consent is dubious, then so much the better. This should be our first choice. However, if such a prohibition jeopardizes our capacity to pursue well-founded research then perhaps we should remember that free-riding is not an attractive principle, nor is it a moral principle. We should not, as I have indicated, assume that those incompetent to consent would wish to be free riders, nor that they be excluded from discharging an obligation of good citizenship that we all share.

We must now turn to the vexed question of the application of constraints on resources to the treatment of older people.

Equity and Resources

In discussing the problem of what an equitable distribution of resources for gerontology and geriatric medicine would look like I want to try to do two modest things. The first is to outline what I believe a principled approach to care of the elderly would look like, and the second is to say why at least one, and by implication most, of the alternatives are far from equitable. We must begin by returning to the equality principle, which we identified as the "parent" of the first principle of gerontology.[13]

The Equality Principle Revisited

I shall again assume that it is accepted that no allocation of public resources should discriminate unfairly between rival claimants or groups of claimants and that this happens when each person's claim to the equal concern, respect, and protection of the community, of the society in which they live, is not respected.

The principle of equality involves the idea that people's lives and fundamental interests are of equal importance and that they must in consequence be given equal weight and be equally protected. This principle has powerful intellectual appeal and intuitive force. It is often enough to discredit a proposal or a theory simply to show that it violates this principle. When measures are said to be discriminatory or unfair it is this principle that is in play.

If people's lives and fundamental interests are of equal value then it is unjust to treat people differently in ways that effectively accord different values to their lives or fundamental interests. Deliberately to give one person a better chance of remaining healthy and of having as long a life as possible than another is to value their life and their fundamental interest in health more than the person not so benefited. It is to discriminate in their favor. Where literally all cannot be benefited, equality requires that the method of selecting who will benefit and who will not is fair. This is why scarce resources that bear upon the value of life or the fundamental interests of persons must be allocated justly.

No Dogs in Mangers

One method of allocation of a scarce resource that apparently satisfies the requirements of justice is not to allocate that resource to anyone! All are then treated equally, in the sense that they are all left equally without benefit of the resource in question.

Another superficially distinct but in fact morally similar procedure might be to go on redistributing resources until a distribution was achieved that satisfies the "envy test," that is, one in which no one envies anyone else's life chances as provided by those resources.

This is often thought to be a viable application of the requirements of justice and indeed to constitute a just allocation of resources. The fallacy of such a supposition is easily illustrated. The principle of justice, and indeed the principle of equality, are *moral* principles, that is, they are principles with some moral content, principles that are designed to be more than impartial, that are designed among other things to respect and to do justice to persons. In some sense this must involve some benevolent attitude to persons that is often abbreviated as "respect for person." Such an attitude to others is as different as it is possible to be from simply showing *an equality of lack of respect* or *an equal indifference to the fate of others*.

The failure to allocate resources that would save lives or protect individuals could not then be part of a claim to satisfy the requirements of equality because this principle has at its heart the claim that people's lives and fundamental interests *are of value, that they matter*. Anyone who denied life-saving resources, or resources that would protect life and other fundamental interests, is not valuing the lives of those to whom she denies these protections. Although she is treating them all equally in the sense of treating them all *the same*, she is not treating them *as equals*, as people who matter and hence matter equally.[14] The alternative dog-in-the-manger approach treats all people as *equally unimportant* and hence as equally without value.

It is an integral part of the equality principle that people's moral claims are not diminished by who they are, or how old they are, or by how rich or poor, or powerful or weak they are or by the quality of their lives. The equality principle covers young and old, healthy and sick, weak and strong, regardless of race, creed, color and gender, quality of life, or life expectancy.

Equal Protection

Of the three elements into which the equality principle must be analyzed (concern, respect, and protection) perhaps the most important in the context of resource allocation is that of equal protection.

All governments and would-be governments boast the strongest commitment to national defense. The question that is seldom asked is what is national defense for, what justifies its prominent place in national priorities? The simplistic answer is that without national defense there might be no nation and hence no national priorities. But pressed further, it is reasonable to ask what values and interests national defense subserves.

Arguably protecting citizens against threats to their lives, liberties, and fundamental interests is the first priority for any state. This is the classic argument for the obligation to obey the Sovereign. In 1651 Thomas Hobbes wrote: "The obligation of subjects to the sovereign, is understood to last as long, and no longer, than the power lasteth, by which he is able to protect them."[15] On this view, any citizen's obligation to the State and to obey its laws is conditional upon the State for its part protecting that citizen against threats to her life and liberty.

If we go back to Hobbes and reflect on what citizens want and need in the way of protection I believe we will find that in most contemporary societies the most significant threats to life and liberty come not from the threat of armed aggression from without, but from absence of health care and other social welfare measures within. For most citizens threats to their lives and curtailment of liberty looms not in the form of soldiers with "snow on their boots" but from illness and accident. This is why it is arguable that the obligation to provide health care, and in particular life-saving health care, takes precedence over the obligation to provide defense forces against external (and often mythical) enemies.

There is a very good principle that states that real and present dangers should be met before future and speculative ones. This is why we are often willing to spend limitless amounts on rescue and less on longer term measures that would protect comparable numbers of lives. If a building collapses we do not tell those buried beneath or their relatives that the budget for digging survivors out has been exhausted and further rescue work must wait until the next financial year.

Another feature of the nation state's obligation to defend its citizens that is often overlooked is its egalitarian nature. Just as each citizen owes his or her obligatons to obey the law regardless of such features as race, religion, gender, or age, so the state must discharge its obligation of protection with the same impartiality. This seems unproblematic until we recall that recent developments in the allocation of health care resources are moving increasingly in the direction of valuing the lives of different groups of citizens at less than par.

The Anti-Ageist Argument

Implicit in this discussion has been an argument against ageism in the distribution of resources for health care. This argument can be stated thus[2]:

All of us who wish to go on living have something that each of us values equally although for each it is different in character, for some a much richer prize than for others, and none of us know its true extent. This things is of course "the rest of our lives." So long as we do not know the date of our deaths then for each of us the "rest of our lives" is of indefinite duration. Whether we are 17 or 70, in perfect health or suffering from a terminal disease we each have the rest of our lives to lead. So long as we each wish to live out the rest of our lives, however long that turns out to be, then if we do not deserve to die, we each suffer the same injustice if our wishes are deliberately frustrated and we are cut off prematurely.

An important element of anti-agism expressed in this way is that it links opposition to discrimination on the basis of chronologic age to discrimination on the basis of life expectancy. These are not necessarily linked. Some people have defended what might be termed a "fair innings argument."[2,16] This suggests that people are entitled to every opportunity to live a fair life span—perhaps the traditional three score years and ten. Up to that point they have equal entitlement to health care, beyond the fair innings they are given very low priority. This argument is tempting because it explains the strong intuition people have that there is something wrong with treating the claims of an octogenarian and those of a 20-year-old as equal. However, the fair innings argument has a number of defects. It assumes that the value of a life is to be measured in units of lifetime, the more the better up to a certain point but thereafter extreme discounting begins. The problem is that people value particular events within their life disproportionately to the time required to experience those events. Although the fair innings argument gives great importance to a life having shape and structure, these things are again not necessarily only achieved within a particular time span. On the fair innings argument Nelson Mandela's entitlement to life-saving care from the community was over before he left Victor Verster prison; the long road to freedom would have ended before (personal) freedom was achieved. And it is not only for such as Mandela that the most important part of their life might well begin after a so-called fair innings had been achieved.

Without the vast detail of each person's life and his hopes and aspirations within that detail, we cannot hope to do justice between lives. I believe the only sensible alternative is to count each life for one and none for more than one, whatever the differences in age and in other quality considerations.

It is this outlook that explains why murder is always wrong and wrong to the same degree. When you rob someone of life you take from them not only all they have but all they will ever have; it is a difference in degree so radical that it makes for a difference in the quality of the act. However, the wrongness consists in taking from them something that they want. That is why, as has been suggested, voluntary euthanasia is not wrong and murder is.

Those who believe in discriminating in favor of the young or against the old must believe that insofar as murder is an injustice it is less of an injustice to murder the old than the young and because they also believe that life years are a commodity like any other[17] it is clear that in robbing people of life you take less from them the less life expectancy they have.

Fairness and Quality of Life

The same ideas that underpin discrimination against the old on the grounds of fairness would also entail trying to equalize quality as well as quantity of life. The argument here would be that resources required for survival should be distributed not only so as to favor the young but also so as to favor those whose quality of life has been relatively poor.

Two patients . . . both about 40 years old . . . need a liver transplant but only one suitable liver is available. One of the patients [the first] has had a much worse life than the other. In this case it seems most fair to give the liver to the first person. This supports the life time view.[17]

Again, such a view has some appeal but it has two major problems, one practical and the other theoretical.

The practical problem is that we could never make decisions as to how to allocate life-saving or indeed other scarce resources between people until we had their whole (and very complete and detailed) life history. Without it all sorts of injustices would be compounded. This problem is related to that we noted attendant upon the fair innings approach. Better again to treat each person as counting for one and none for more than one than even to embark on the massively invasive (of privacy) data collection that it would be necessary to hold and have instantly available on each and every citizen and that could never be complete, accurate, or proof against abuse. This incidentally is also the reason why it is wrong to discriminate against smokers, for example in the provision of coronary artery bypass grafts.

The theoretical problem is that if it is right to attempt to even out quality of life as between people then we should do so as a matter of public policy throughout society, not simply in the rare cases where resource allocation decisions in health care arise. This might have to include making sure that no one lived longer than the person who has the shortest life span and no one was happier than the most miserable. This might be dysfunctional in terms of species survival unless a different principle can support leveling up rather than leveling down.

Ultimately we will be comparing different moral priorities. However, there is much to be said for taking individual persons and their wishes and fundamental interests as what matters from the point of view of morality. This means that we must recognize that although their lives will all differ in length, happiness, and success, in short in the degree to which their fundamental interests are satisfied, that people matter morally despite these differences not because of them.

I have defended an argument that shows why we should decline to discriminate against the old. Many think that this is precisely what we *should* do.[17,18] Their arguments either support a fair innings or suggest that an evidence-based medicine requires the maximization of life years to be gained from treatment. If health gain is defined in terms of life years gained then the old will very often lose out. There is no doubt that it is highly attractive to health care providers to measure health gain in terms of life years per treatment and that this accords with our intuitions or our commonsense morality on some occasions. It seems fairer to rescue the 30-year-old rather than the 90-year-old, other things being equal. However, it seems less obvious that we ought always to prefer the 30-year-old to the 32-year-old. If we generalize the ethic of preferring to maximize life years gained from treatment or care then geriatric medicine will always be a low priority and palliative care will not rank at all! Maybe this is the right model of care for out society but I doubt it. I have suggested, on the contrary, that the business of health care is not the maximization of health gain defined in this way, but rather the extension of the obligation to show concern, respect, and protection to all citizens regardless of such things as race, gender, and age. The two approaches not only reflect different interpretation of an ethics of health care delivery but also of different conceptions of morality. I have here defended one such conception, the defense of the alternative must be left to others.[17,18]

Decisions to Limit Treatment

We are now in a position to turn to our final topic, which concerns decisions to limit treatment. When may these legitimately be taken and by whom? Here again it is useful to remind ourselves of the first principle of gerontology and of the purpose of this branch of medicine. If the health care system is rightly seen as a dimension of the community's commitment to the protection of the individual, then so long as the delivery of that care does in fact protect, and no more important values are compromised by the delivery of that protection, then clearly it should continue. We have seen that lack of resources for more important dimensions of protection or for more important candidates for care are often suggested as such more important values. To try to be clear about the ethics of decisions to limit or end treatment we will assume that other claims on the relevant resources are not the principal issue and that we are concerned with the question of when it is appropriate to decide to limit or end particular treatments for individual patients. Let's start with a patient-centered approach to this problem and discuss the patient's own wishes.

A Classic Case

One dilemma in geriatric medicine always seems to be a priority for practitioners. It concerns the dilemmas surrounding the decision to discharge home a frail patient where it is feared that this may involve some risk to his health or life and it is unclear how aware of this risk the patient may be and perhaps where caregivers who may be family members or even neighbors are worried by this risk. Among the questions that arise are the following: (1) How much risk can or should we allow a person to take with his own health? (2) Is it reasonable to think the level of risk varies with the level of competence? (3) What consideration should be given to the wishes of caregivers in view of their very real concerns?

The difficulty of these dilemmas arises not so much from any problems about answering questions such as these but rather from the difficulty of knowing enough about the terms used in the questions. It is clear from the present discussion of issues such as "euthanasia" and "informed consent" that people are permitted to take whatever risks she likes, within the law, with their own health. The wishes of caregivers are important but such wishes cannot be permitted to imprison a competent individual within a context from which he has elected to remove himself. The problem of this classic case is simply that it is often unclear just how competent the patient is to make a decision to leave a protected environment and equally unclear just how competently be will be able to function at home. However, what ethics can contribute here is perhaps the reflection that we are talking of the liberty of the individual. That liberty should not be constrained lightly and the presumption must be that the individual is competent to make decisions unless there is clear evidence to the contrary.

We have seen that to attempt to treat a competent patient against her own wishes is not only unethical but also, in most jurisdictions, a criminal act. Where the patient is not competent and the treatment is in the patient's interests, then again as we have seen, the ethics are simple. We should not injure the patient by withholding beneficial treatment.

Advance Directives or "Living Wills"

Much discussion has arisen about the ethics of advance directives. However they are, I believe, both straightforward and unproblematic. All decisions we take bind us to a certain extent for the future. If I now consent to the administration of an anesthetic, I cannot revoke that consent until I wake up. If I decide to bind myself in the event of my losing competence in the future the principle is the same, even if the loss of competence will be permanent rather than temporary. So long as my instructions are clear, then any treatment of me contrary to those instructions is unethical and probably unlawful.

We should note two features of advance directives. The first is that I can only direct people to forbear. I have no power to command others to do things to me. Although this must be so it does not follow that health professionals or others can disregard my positive wishes. If health professionals would normally act on a patient request for treatment, the fact that the request is expressed in advance should make no difference to the willingness to act. Second the directive, while it may be written or oral, must be clear and unequivocally the patient's own authentic request. Health professionals should be wary of hearsay. To give a concrete example, if an unconscious patient is admitted needing treatment and the person accompanying him, ostensibly his wife, says "he wouldn't have wanted that" or "he always said never to let that happen to him," this of itself is not adequate evidence of the existence of an advance directive. The accompanying person may not be related to the patient, nor if she is, may she be a reliable guide either to his wishes or his best interests. Relatives often have vested interests, inheritance prospects for example. Certainly nothing should be done on the basis of uncorroborated claims about the patient's wishes from unauthenticated sources, which is irrevocable or contrary to the patient's interests. Normally advance directives will be written in due form and the patient's general practitioner should be aware of their existence in advance of their being needed.

Do Not Resuscitate

When might it be legitimate to mark a patient "DNR" or "not for 222" (or "333" or whatever the dial code for the resuscitation team is in a particular institution)? What does such an instruction mean? It means that a relatively simple and inexpensive procedure, albeit one that may be painful and undignified for the patient, that offers a chance of reversing an immediately life-threatening event, will not be attempted. It is an instruction to take the earliest opportunity to ensure that a particular life comes to an end. Such an instruction could only be ethical in two sets of circumstances. The first is where the patient himself has expressly directed that no such treatment be given. The second is where the patient's life has deteriorated to such an extent that continued life as a person is no longer possible. This latter was in essence the nature of the decision taken by the House of Lords in the case of Tony Bland.[4] The Law Lords took their decision with the aim of ending Tony Bland's life and in the knowledge that this would be the effect of their decision. Although the Law Lords insisted that this did not amount to nonvoluntary euthanasia, I see no way of distinguishing their end-of-life decision in the Bland case and cases of nonvoluntary euthanasia. Tony Bland had not and could not have consented and the decision taken by the Law Lords was a classic "end-of-life" decision of the sort contemplated by those who defend euthanasia.

Certainly, wherever a patient can herself be consulted about whether or not she wants to go on living then this should be done, and a DNR decision should only be taken if the patient understands the effects of such a decision and explicitly rejects resuscitation. A DNR decision is not a matter of clinical judgment, because the question of whether a life is worth living, or whether or not it is better that it should end, is not a clinical question. These are moral and mortal questions. Moreover they are questions, the answer to which is a matter of life or death to the patient, and wherever patients have a life as a person in which they continue to be interested, then any decision to end that life when it could continue that is not requested by the patient is a gross and emphatic violation.

This is perhaps a dramatic way of putting the dilemma but I believe it to be justified. To take a decision not to initiate life-saving treatment is in these cases ethically analogous to a decision to withdraw life-sustaining treatment, as in the Bland case. There are differences between decisions not to initiate treatment and decisions to withdraw it, but they are not relevant here. Such differences have to do with the commitment to patients that ongoing treatment represents, its possibly contractual nature, and so on.[7,19]

Against the position I have just articulated it might be claimed that decisions not to resuscitate have traditionally been regarded as clinical matters, and for good reason. Only a clinician is in a position to know when resuscitation will be futile and when the individual concerned is too frail to benefit from attempts at resuscitation. However, both these objections involve a misunderstanding or at least an equivocation over the meaning of the word "futile." If a procedure is genuinely futile, in that nothing that the patient wants or could possibly want can thereby be achieved, then this is a sufficient reason for not attempting it. Or, if the patient is so frail that attempts at resuscitation are simply not possible, then again this is a sufficient reason for not attempting them, and judgments of clinicians in either case are not in dispute. The phrase I used was deliberate and perhaps needs repeating; it was "wherever patients have a life as a person in which they continue to be interested, then any decision to end that life when it could continue which is not requested by the patient is a gross and emphatic violation." The crucial idea here is that of the patient having a life *in which he continues to be interested* and which *could continue*. What must be capable of continuance is the sort of life the patient wants to continue to lead (if such a life is the only alternative) and that might possibly be restored by resuscitation. If resuscitation could not restore such a life then it will indeed be futile. The decision as to whether resuscitation could restore such a life *is* a clinical decision. However, the decision as to whether or not a life is worth living to a particular individual is not a clinical matter. It is and *could only be* a matter for the individual herself.

It is sometimes said that it is unethical to attempt resuscitation when there is only a scant prospect of it proving successful, and therefore, where clinicians judge the chances of success in resuscitation small, they not only need not attempt it, but should not attempt it. Or, if the patient will be hurt or injured by the attempt at resuscitation and the chances of success are so small as to make the infliction of such hurt or injury problematic, then again clinicians often suggest that they are the right people to make the judgment. However, if this were true, it would be unethical to attempt cardiopulmonary resuscitation at the curbside following a traffic accident where the prospects of success were slim. But rescue services usually think it their duty (and surely rightly) to make all attempts to preserve life in such circumstances. This shows that it is not the slim chances of success that are the determining factor in such decisions, but rather that a prior decision has been taken that *this patient is not worth saving*, or would have no prospect of meaningful life if saved, or it would be a cruelty to save them. My argument is that such a prior decision not to resuscitate is only ethical if requested by the patient or if the patient has permanently lost personhood, or is in such irreversible and unendurable pain that euthanasia would be judged justified. The rule of thumb on DNR must surely be: "think of it as euthanasia and, in the absence of a patient clearly refusing resuscitation, only take such a decision where you are satisfied that euthanasia would itself be justified in the circumstances or where resuscitation would be literally and clearly futile."

If this conclusion seems extreme, it is perhaps because we have hitherto drawn too rigid a distinction between acts we have accepted as euthanasia properly so called, and a host of end-of-life decisions, which, while having the same effect as decisions for euthanasia, have for historical or legal reasons escaped being so described. My contention has been that any decision that has the effect of ending or shortening a life that could continue, amounts to euthanasia. That decision can be justified in a number of ways. There are, we have noted, three principal justifications. The first is because the person whose life it is wants to die. This is voluntary euthanasia and should be accepted. The second principal justification is where the individual has permanently lost personhood, as in PVS. And the final justification is where CPR would be literally and clearly futile, either because there is no prospect of its extending life significantly or because the patient is so frail that attempting it in the circumstances would be to inflict pointless injury.

Acknowledgments

I would like to thank Ray Tallis and Sarah Hobson for very helpful comments on an earlier draft of this chapter.

References

1. Harris J: What is the good of health care? Bioethics 1996;10
2. Harris J: The Value of Life. Routledge & Kegan Paul, London, 1985
3. *Cruzan v. Director, Missouri Department of Health*, 497, U.S. 261 (1990)
4. *Airdale NHS Trust V. Bland* [1993] 1 All ER 858 (H.L.)
5. Keown J: (ed): Euthanasia Examined: Ethical Clinical and Legal Perspectives. pp. 6–71. Cambridge University Press, Cambridge, 1995
6. Dworkin R: Life's Dominion. HarperCollins, London, 1993
7. Harris J: Violence & Responsibility. Routledge & Kegan Paul, London, 1980
8. Lord Mustil, judgment in *Airedale NH Trust v Bland* [1993] 1 All England Rep. 821 H.L.
9. Steiner H: A Theory of Rights. p. 258. Blackwell, Oxford, 1994
10. Hirsch S, Harris J (eds): Consent and the Incompetent Patient. The Royal College of Psychiatrists, 1988
11. British Medical Association: Medical Ethics Today: Its Practice and Philosophy. pp 219–229. BMA, London, 1993
12. Ciba Foundation Study Group: Medical research: civil liability and compensation for personal injury—a discussion paper. BMJ 1980;280:1172–1175
13. Harris J: More & Better Justice. pp. 75–97. In Mendus M, Bell M (eds): Philosophy and Medical Welfare. Cambridge, University Press, Cambridge, 1988
14. Dworkin R: Taking Rights Seriously. Duckworth, London, 1977
15. Hobbes T: Leviathan. Oakshott M (ed). Basil Blackwell, Oxford, 1960 (originally published 1651)
16. Callahan C: What Kind of Life: The Limits of Medical Progress. 1990
17. Kappel K, Sandoe P: QALYs, age and fairness. Bioethics, 1992;6
18. Singer P, McKie J, Kuhse H, Richardson J: "Double jeopardy and the use of QALYs in health care allocation." Medical Ethics 1995;21
19. Glover J: Causing Death and Saving Lives. Penguin, Harmondsworth, 1977

Index

Page numbers followed by f indicate figures; those followed by t indicate tables.